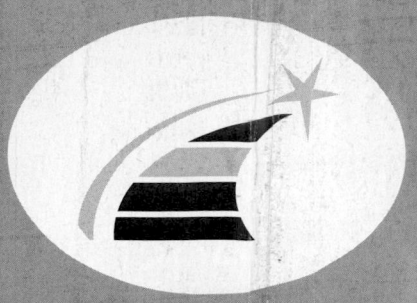

Make the most o[illegible] Physician Coding Exam Review!

1. Assess! Take the Pre-Exam

Use the Pre-Exam located on the companion Evolve site to gauge your strengths and weaknesses, develop a plan for focused study, and gain a better understanding of the testing process.

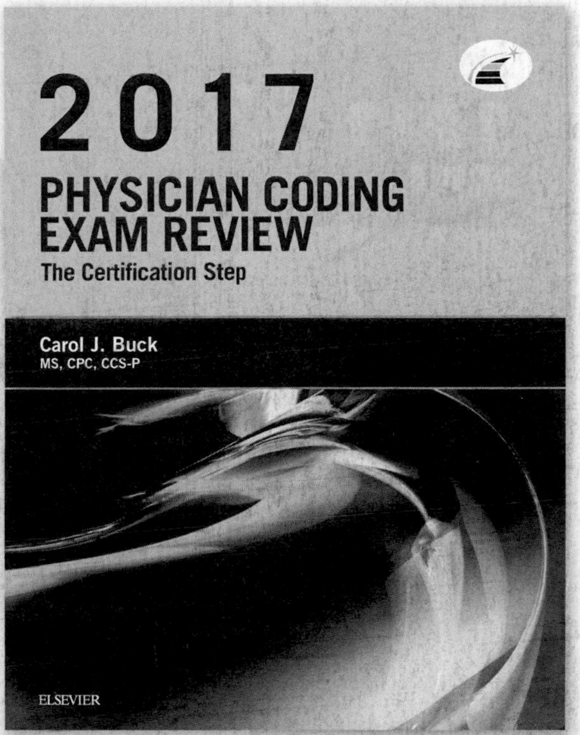

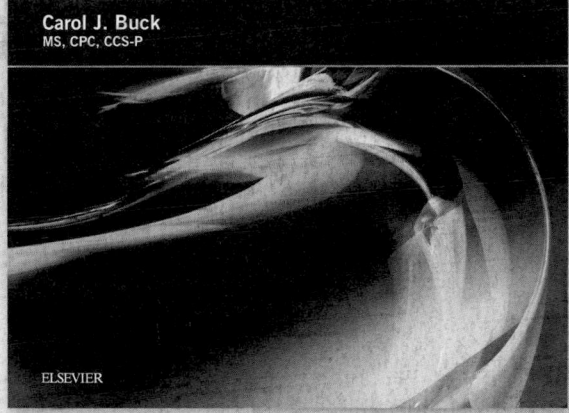

ISBN: 978-0-323-43122-4

2. Study!

Use the quizzes in this book to sharpen your skills and build competency.

3. Apply! Take the Post-Exam

After studying, apply your knowledge to the Post-Exam located on the companion Evolve site. When finished, you'll receive scores for both the Pre- and Post-Exams and a breakdown of incorrect answers to help you identify areas where you need more detailed study and review.

4. Test! Take the Final Exam

Gauge your readiness for the actual physician coding exam with the Final Exam. Boost your test-taking confidence and ensure certification success.

Perfect your understanding and prepare for certification—start your review now!

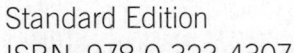

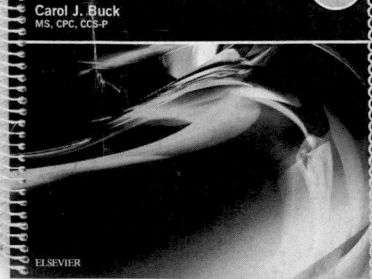

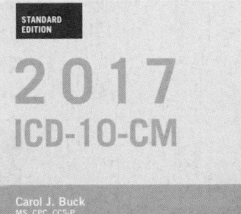

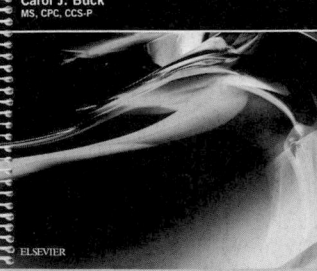

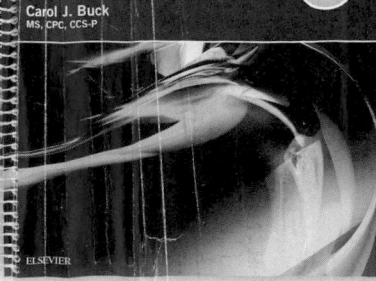

STANDARD EDITION

2017 ICD-10-CM

INCLUDES NETTER'S ANATOMY ART

Carol J. Buck
MS, CPC, CCS-P

Former Program Director
Medical Secretary Programs
Northwest Technical College
East Grand Forks, Minnesota

ELSEVIER

ELSEVIER

3251 Riverport Lane
St. Louis, Missouri 63043

2017 ICD-10-CM STANDARD EDITION

ISBN: 978-0-323-43119-4

Library of Congress Cataloging-in-Publication Data
Names: Buck, Carol J., author.
Title: 2017 ICD-10-CM / Carol J. Buck.
Other titles: ICD-10-CM
Description: Standard edition. | St. Louis, Missouri : Elsevier Inc., [2017] | Includes index. | Preceded by 2016 ICD-10-CM / Carol J. Buck. Standard edition. [2016].
Identifiers: LCCN 2016016064 | ISBN 9780323431194 (pbk.)
Subjects: | MESH: International statistical classification of diseases and related health problems. 10th revision. Clinical modification. | Disease--classification | International Classification of Diseases | Clinical Coding--standards
Classification: LCC RB115 | NLM WB 15 | DDC 616.001/2--dc23 LC record available at https://lccn.loc.gov/2016016064

Director, Private Sector Education & Professional/References: Jeanne R. Olson
Content Development Manager: Luke Held
Associate Content Development Specialist: Anna Miller
Publishing Services Manager: Jeffrey Patterson
Project Manager: Lisa A. P. Bushey
Design Manager: Julia Dummitt

Printed in the United States of America

Last digit is the print number: 9 8 7 6 5 4 3 2 1

DEDICATION

To all the brave medical coders who transitioned the nation into a new coding system.
Decades of waiting finally concluded with the implementation of I-10,
and you have been the pioneers leading the way.

With greatest appreciations for your efforts!

Carol J. Buck, MS, CPC, CCS-P

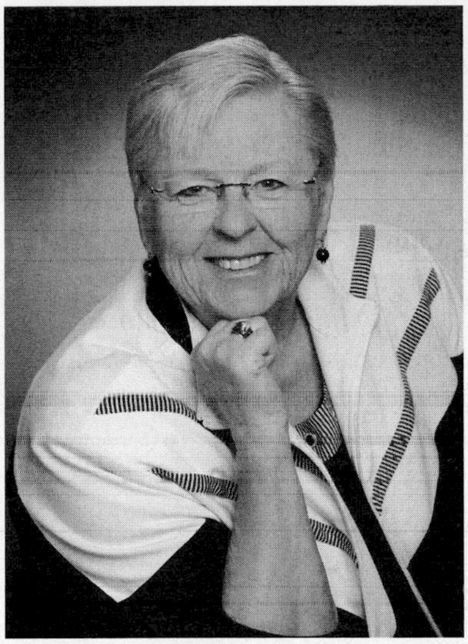

DEVELOPMENT OF THIS EDITION

Query Team

Patricia Cordy Henricksen, MS, CHCA, CPC-I, CPC, CCP-P, ASC-PM
Auditing and Coding Educator
Soterion Medical Services
Lexington, Kentucky

Jackie L. Grass, CPC
Coding and Reimbursement Specialist
Grand Forks, North Dakota

Kathleen Buchda, CPC, CPMA
Revenue Recognition
New Richmond, Wisconsin

Editorial Consultant

Jenna Price, CPC-A
President
Price Editorial Services, LLC
St. Louis, Missouri

Elsevier/MC Strategies Revenue Cycle, Coding and Compliance Staff

"Experts in providing e-learning on revenue cycle, coding and compliance."

Deborah Neville, RHIA, CCS-P
Director

Lynn-Marie D. Wozniak, MS, RHIT
Content Manager

Sandra L. Macica, MS, RHIA, CCS, ROCC
Content Manager

CONTENTS

ICD-10-CM

GUIDE TO USING THE 2017 ICD-10-CM STANDARD

Medical coding has long been a part of the health care profession. Through the years medical coding systems have become more complex and extensive. Today, medical coding is an intricate and immense process that is present in every health care setting. The increased use of electronic submissions for health care services only increases the need for coders who understand the coding process.

2017 ICD-10-CM Standard Edition was developed to help meet the needs of coding professionals at all levels by offering a comprehensive coding text at a reasonable price.

All material strictly adheres to the latest government versions available at the time of printing. Updates from the *Definitions of Medicare Code Edits* (MCE) will be posted to the companion website (www. codingupdates.com) when available.

Illustrations and Items

The ICD-10-CM Tabular List contains illustrations, pictures, and items to assist you in understanding difficult terminology, diseases/conditions, or coding in a specific category. Items are always printed in [redacted] ink so that the added material is not mistaken for official notations or instructions. [redacted] ink is used for other annotations in the text. Your ideas on what other descriptions or illustrations should be in future editions of this text are always appreciated.

Instructional Notations

Includes Notes

Includes

The word 'Includes' appears immediately under certain categories to further define, or give examples of, the content of the category.

Excludes Notes

The ICD-10-CM has two types of excludes notes. Each note has a different definition for use, but they are both similar in that they indicate that codes excluded from each other are independent of each other.

Excludes1

A type 1 Excludes note is a pure excludes. It means "NOT CODED HERE!" An Excludes1 note indicates that the code excluded should never be used at the same time as the code above the Excludes1 note. An Excludes1 is for use when two conditions cannot occur together, such as a congenital form versus an acquired form of the same condition.

Excludes2

A type 2 Excludes note represents "NOT INCLUDED HERE." An Excludes2 note indicates that the condition excluded is not part of the condition it is excluded from but a patient may have both conditions at the same time. When an Excludes2 note appears under a code, it is acceptable to use both the code and the excluded code together.

Code First/Use Additional Code notes (etiology/manifestation paired codes)

Certain conditions have both an underlying etiology and multiple body system manifestations due to the underlying etiology. For such conditions the ICD-10-CM has a coding convention that requires the underlying condition be sequenced first, followed by the manifestation. Wherever such a combination exists, there is a "use additional code" note at the etiology code, and a "code first" note at the manifestation code. These instructional notes indicate the proper sequencing order of the codes, etiology followed by manifestation.

In most cases the manifestation codes will have in the code title, "in diseases classified elsewhere." Codes with this title are a component of the etiology/manifestation convention. The code title indicates that it is a manifestation code. "In diseases classified elsewhere" codes are never permitted to be used as first-listed or principal diagnosis codes. They must be used in conjunction with an underlying condition code, and they must be listed following the underlying condition.

Use additional

The words indicate an instructional note that another code may be needed.

Code first

The words indicate an instructional note that directs the coder to sequence the underlying condition before the manifestation.

Code also

A "code also" note instructs that two codes may be required to fully describe a condition, but the sequencing of the two codes is discretionary, depending on the severity of the conditions and the reason for the encounter.

Unspecified

The highlight indicates that although the code is valid as a principal (first-listed) diagnosis, it is not as specific as other codes without the highlight.

7th characters and placeholder X

For codes less than 6 characters that require a 7th character a placeholder X should be assigned for all characters less than 6. The 7th character must always be the 7th character of a code.

Annotated

Throughout the manual, revisions, additions, and deleted codes or words are indicated by the following symbols:

- ⇐ **Revised:** Revisions within the line or code from the previous edition are indicated by the arrow.
- ◀ **New:** Additions to the previous edition are indicated by the triangle.
- ~~deleted~~ **Deleted:** Deletions from the previous edition are struck through.

ICD-10-CM Tabular List Symbols

- ● **Use Additional Character(s):** The blue stop sign cautions that the code requires additional character(s) to ensure the greatest specificity.
- X For codes less than 6 characters that require a 7th character, a placeholder X should be assigned for all characters less than 6. The 7th character must always be the 7th character of a code.
- **OGCR** The *Official Guidelines for Coding and Reporting* symbol includes the placement of a portion of a guideline as that guideline pertains to the code by which it is located. The complete OGCR are located in Part I.

SYMBOLS AND CONVENTIONS

ICD-10-CM Tabular

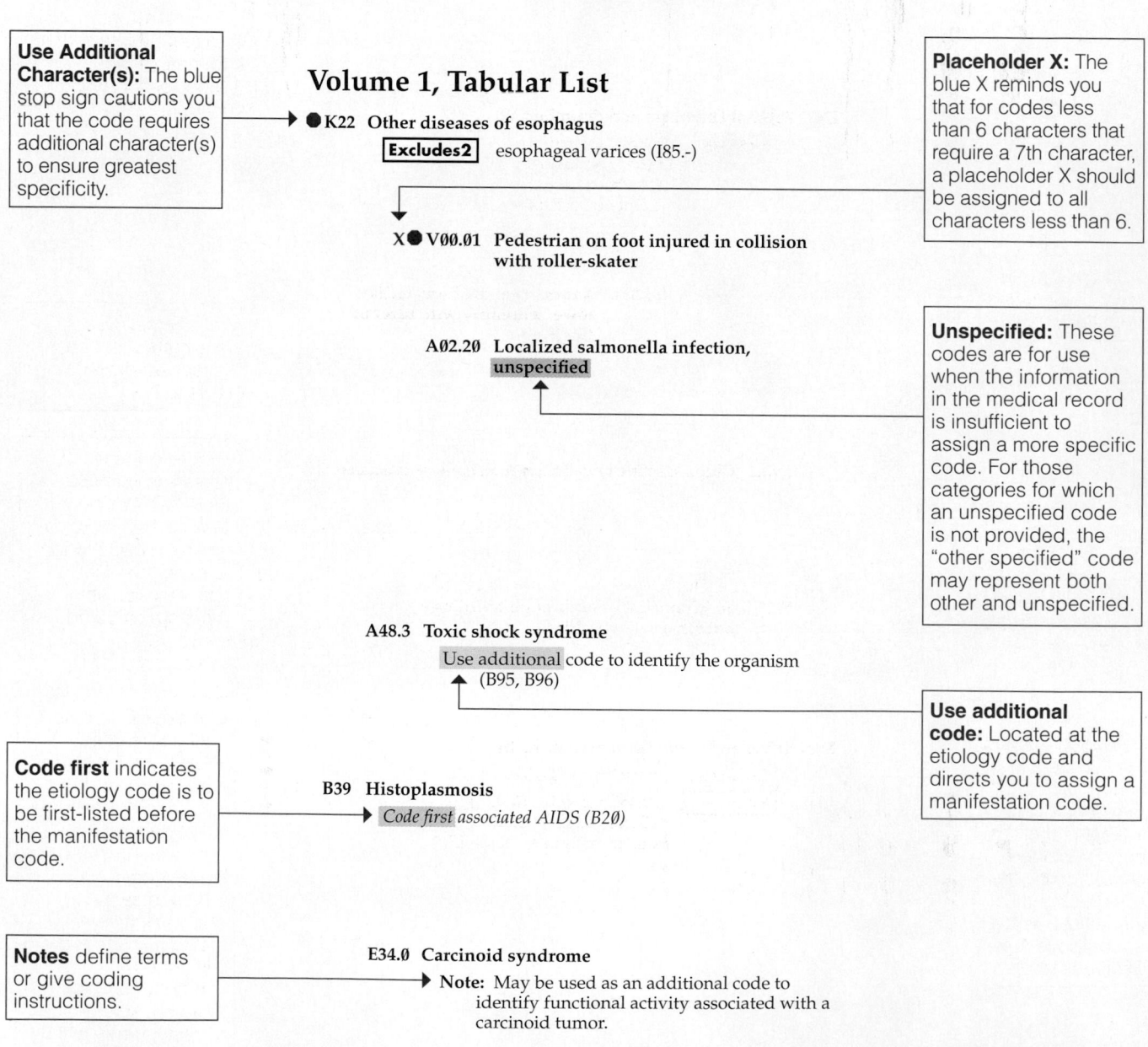

Use Additional Character(s): The blue stop sign cautions you that the code requires additional character(s) to ensure greatest specificity.

Volume 1, Tabular List

● **K22 Other diseases of esophagus**

Excludes2 esophageal varices (I85.-)

Placeholder X: The blue X reminds you that for codes less than 6 characters that require a 7th character, a placeholder X should be assigned to all characters less than 6.

X● **VØØ.Ø1 Pedestrian on foot injured in collision with roller-skater**

AØ2.2Ø Localized salmonella infection, unspecified

Unspecified: These codes are for use when the information in the medical record is insufficient to assign a more specific code. For those categories for which an unspecified code is not provided, the "other specified" code may represent both other and unspecified.

A48.3 Toxic shock syndrome

Use additional code to identify the organism (B95, B96)

Use additional code: Located at the etiology code and directs you to assign a manifestation code.

Code first indicates the etiology code is to be first-listed before the manifestation code.

B39 Histoplasmosis

Code first associated AIDS (B2Ø)

Notes define terms or give coding instructions.

E34.Ø Carcinoid syndrome

Note: May be used as an additional code to identify functional activity associated with a carcinoid tumor.

Codes or index entries are for purposes of illustration only and may not be current.

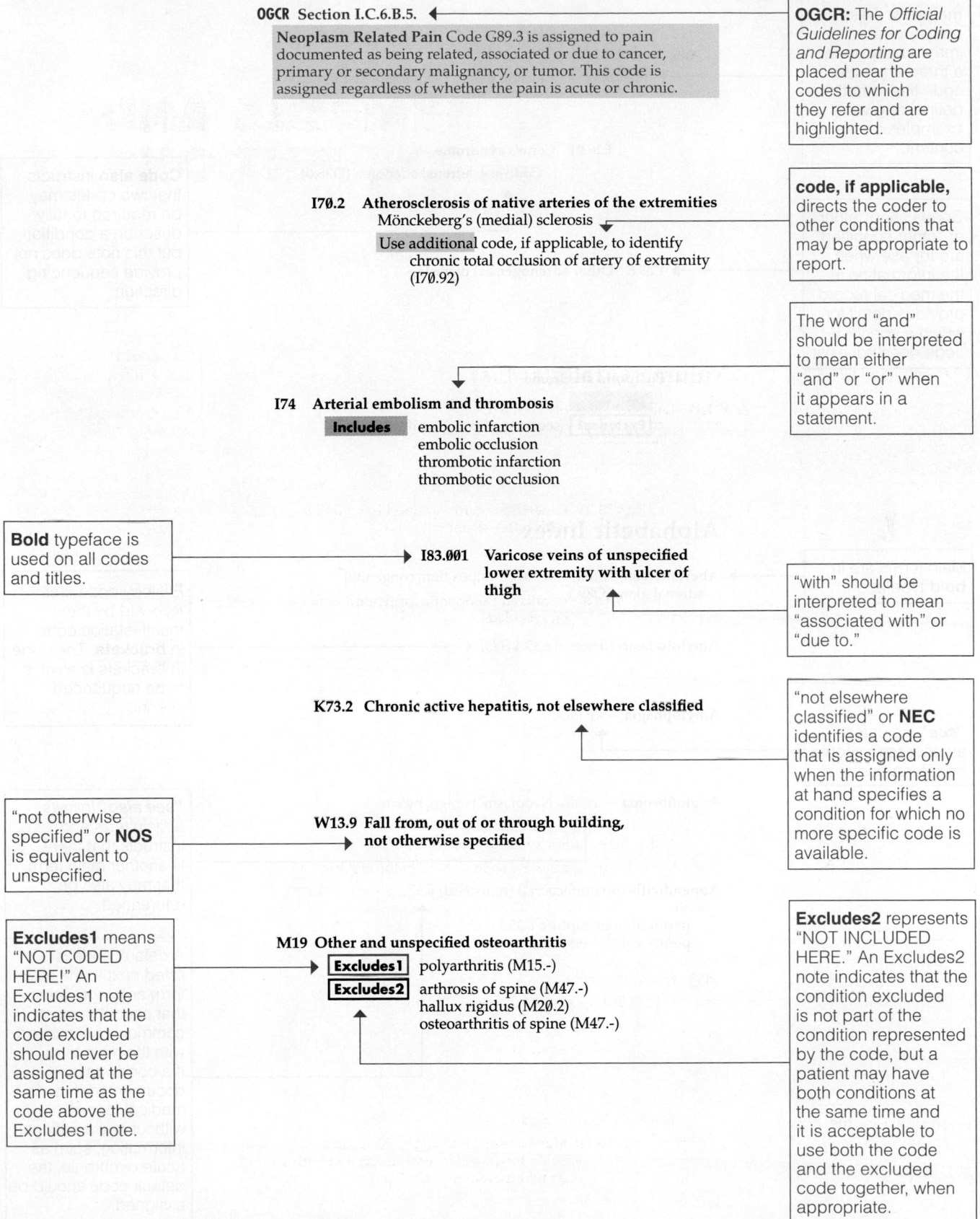

OGCR Section I.C.6.B.5.

Neoplasm Related Pain Code G89.3 is assigned to pain documented as being related, associated or due to cancer, primary or secondary malignancy, or tumor. This code is assigned regardless of whether the pain is acute or chronic.

OGCR: The *Official Guidelines for Coding and Reporting* are placed near the codes to which they refer and are highlighted.

I7Ø.2 Atherosclerosis of native arteries of the extremities
Mönckeberg's (medial) sclerosis
Use additional code, if applicable, to identify chronic total occlusion of artery of extremity (I7Ø.92)

code, if applicable, directs the coder to other conditions that may be appropriate to report.

The word "and" should be interpreted to mean either "and" or "or" when it appears in a statement.

I74 Arterial embolism and thrombosis
Includes embolic infarction
embolic occlusion
thrombotic infarction
thrombotic occlusion

Bold typeface is used on all codes and titles.

I83.ØØ1 Varicose veins of unspecified lower extremity with ulcer of thigh

"with" should be interpreted to mean "associated with" or "due to."

K73.2 Chronic active hepatitis, not elsewhere classified

"not elsewhere classified" or **NEC** identifies a code that is assigned only when the information at hand specifies a condition for which no more specific code is available.

"not otherwise specified" or **NOS** is equivalent to unspecified.

W13.9 Fall from, out of or through building, not otherwise specified

Excludes1 means "NOT CODED HERE!" An Excludes1 note indicates that the code excluded should never be assigned at the same time as the code above the Excludes1 note.

M19 Other and unspecified osteoarthritis
Excludes1 polyarthritis (M15.-)
Excludes2 arthrosis of spine (M47.-)
hallux rigidus (M2Ø.2)
osteoarthritis of spine (M47.-)

Excludes2 represents "NOT INCLUDED HERE." An Excludes2 note indicates that the condition excluded is not part of the condition represented by the code, but a patient may have both conditions at the same time and it is acceptable to use both the code and the excluded code together, when appropriate.

Codes or index entries are for purposes of illustration only and may not be current.

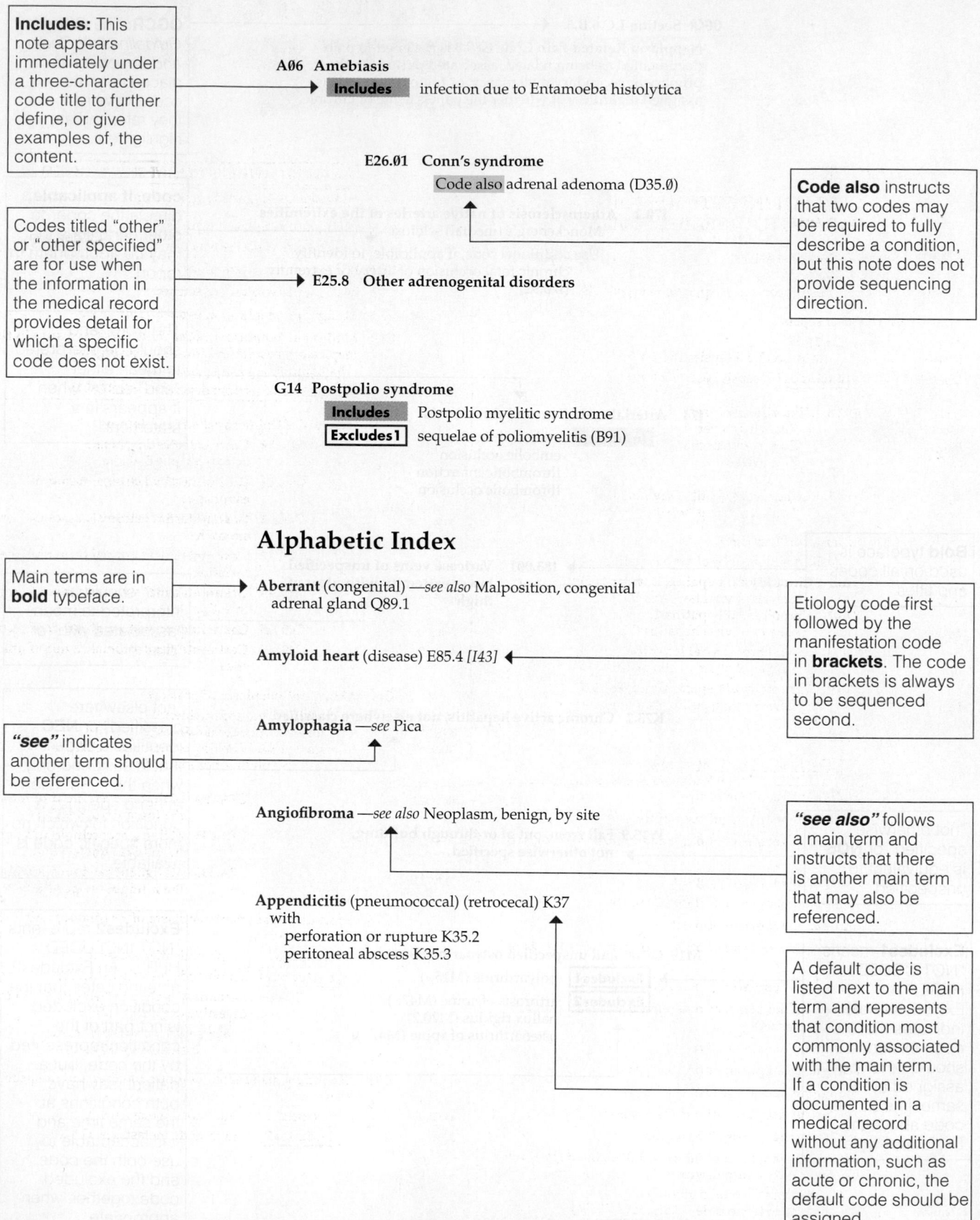

Includes: This note appears immediately under a three-character code title to further define, or give examples of, the content.

AØ6 Amebiasis
Includes infection due to Entamoeba histolytica

E26.Ø1 Conn's syndrome
Code also adrenal adenoma (D35.Ø)

Code also instructs that two codes may be required to fully describe a condition, but this note does not provide sequencing direction.

Codes titled "other" or "other specified" are for use when the information in the medical record provides detail for which a specific code does not exist.

E25.8 Other adrenogenital disorders

G14 Postpolio syndrome
Includes Postpolio myelitic syndrome
Excludes1 sequelae of poliomyelitis (B91)

Alphabetic Index

Main terms are in **bold** typeface.

Aberrant (congenital) —*see also* Malposition, congenital
adrenal gland Q89.1

Amyloid heart (disease) E85.4 *[I43]*

Etiology code first followed by the manifestation code in **brackets**. The code in brackets is always to be sequenced second.

Amylophagia —*see* Pica

"see" indicates another term should be referenced.

Angiofibroma —*see also* Neoplasm, benign, by site

"see also" follows a main term and instructs that there is another main term that may also be referenced.

Appendicitis (pneumococcal) (retrocecal) K37
with
perforation or rupture K35.2
peritoneal abscess K35.3

A default code is listed next to the main term and represents that condition most commonly associated with the main term. If a condition is documented in a medical record without any additional information, such as acute or chronic, the default code should be assigned.

Codes or index entries are for purposes of illustration only and may not be current.

GUIDE TO THE 2017 ICD-10-CM UPDATES

CHAPTER 1

CERTAIN INFECTIOUS AND PARASITIC DISEASES (AØØ-B99)

A4Ø Streptococcal sepsis
Code first
Revised postprocedural streptococcal sepsis (T81.4-)

A41 Other sepsis
Code first
Revised postprocedural sepsis (T81.4-)
Deleted **Excludes1** sepsis NOS (A41.9)

New **A92.5 Zika virus disease**
New Zika virus fever
New Zika virus infection
New Zika NOS

B17.9 Acute viral hepatitis, unspecified
New Acute infectious hepatitis NOS

B18 Chronic viral hepatitis
New **Includes** Carrier of viral hepatitis

B18.1 Chronic viral hepatitis B without delta-agent
New Carrier of viral hepatitis B

B18.2 Chronic viral hepatitis C
New Carrier of viral hepatitis C

B18.8 Other chronic viral hepatitis
New Carrier of other viral hepatitis

B18.9 Chronic viral hepatitis, unspecified
New Carrier of unspecified viral hepatitis

CHAPTER 2

NEOPLASMS (CØØ-D49)

CØØ Malignant neoplasm of lip
CØ1 Malignant neoplasm of base of tongue
CØ2 Malignant neoplasm of other and unspecified parts of tongue
CØ3 Malignant neoplasm of gum
CØ4 Malignant neoplasm of floor of mouth
CØ5 Malignant neoplasm of palate
CØ6 Malignant neoplasm of other and unspecified parts of mouth
CØ7 Malignant neoplasm of parotid gland
CØ8 Malignant neoplasm of other and unspecified major salivary glands
CØ9 Malignant neoplasm of tonsil
C1Ø Malignant neoplasm of oropharynx
C11 Malignant neoplasm of nasopharynx
C12 Malignant neoplasm of pyriform sinus
C13 Malignant neoplasm of hypopharynx
C14 Malignant neoplasm of other and ill-defined sites in the lip, oral cavity and pharynx
Use additional code to identify:
Revised history of tobacco dependence (Z87.891)

MALIGNANT NEOPLASM OF DIGESTIVE ORGANS (C15-C26)
New **Excludes2** gastrointestinal stromal tumors (C49.A-)

C25 Malignant neoplasm of pancreas
New Code also exocrine pancreatic insufficiency (K86.81)

C32 Malignant neoplasm of larynx
C33 Malignant neoplasm of trachea
C34 Malignant neoplasm of bronchus and lung
C39 Malignant neoplasm of other and ill-defined sites in the respiratory system and intrathoracic organs
Use additional code to identify:
Revised history of tobacco dependence (Z87.891)

New **C49.A Gastrointestinal stromal tumor**
New **C49.AØ Gastrointestinal stromal tumor, unspecified site**
New **C49.A1 Gastrointestinal stromal tumor of esophagus**
New **C49.A2 Gastrointestinal stromal tumor of stomach**
New **C49.A3 Gastrointestinal stromal tumor of small intestine**
New **C49.A4 Gastrointestinal stromal tumor of large intestine**
New **C49.A5 Gastrointestinal stromal tumor of rectum**
New **C49.A9 Gastrointestinal stromal tumor of other sites**

C61 Malignant neoplasm of prostate
New Use additional code to identify:
New hormone sensitivity status (Z19.1-Z19.2)
New rising PSA following treatment for malignant neoplasm of prostate (R97.21)

Revised **C7A.Ø94 Malignant carcinoid tumor of the foregut unspecified**
Revised **C7A.Ø95 Malignant carcinoid tumor of the midgut unspecified**
Revised **C7A.Ø96 Malignant carcinoid tumor of the hindgut unspecified**

C78 Secondary malignant neoplasm of respiratory and digestive organs
Deleted **Excludes1** lymph node metastases (C77.0)
New **Excludes2** lymph node metastases (C77.0)

C78.89 Secondary malignant neoplasm of other digestive organs
New Code also exocrine pancreatic insufficiency (K86.81)

C79 Secondary malignant neoplasm of other and unspecified sites
Deleted **Excludes1** lymph node metastases (C77.0)
New **Excludes2** lymph node metastases (C77.0)

Revised C81.1 **Nodular sclerosis Hodgkin lymphoma**
New Nodular sclerosis classical Hodgkin lymphoma
Revised C81.10 **Nodular sclerosis Hodgkin lymphoma, unspecified site**
Revised C81.11 **Nodular sclerosis Hodgkin lymphoma, lymph nodes of head, face, and neck**
Revised C81.12 **Nodular sclerosis Hodgkin lymphoma, intrathoracic lymph nodes**
Revised C81.13 **Nodular sclerosis Hodgkin lymphoma, intra-abdominal lymph nodes**
Revised C81.14 **Nodular sclerosis Hodgkin lymphoma, lymph nodes of axilla and upper limb**
Revised C81.15 **Nodular sclerosis Hodgkin lymphoma, lymph nodes of inguinal region and lower limb**
Revised C81.16 **Nodular sclerosis Hodgkin lymphoma, intrapelvic lymph nodes**
Revised C81.17 **Nodular sclerosis Hodgkin lymphoma, spleen**
Revised C81.18 **Nodular sclerosis Hodgkin lymphoma, lymph nodes of multiple sites**
Revised C81.19 **Nodular sclerosis Hodgkin lymphoma, extranodal and solid organ sites**
Revised C81.2 **Mixed cellularity Hodgkin lymphoma**
New Mixed cellularity classical Hodgkin lymphoma
Revised C81.20 **Mixed cellularity Hodgkin lymphoma, unspecified site**
Revised C81.21 **Mixed cellularity Hodgkin lymphoma, lymph nodes of head, face, and neck**
Revised C81.22 **Mixed cellularity Hodgkin lymphoma, intrathoracic lymph nodes**
Revised C81.23 **Mixed cellularity Hodgkin lymphoma, intra-abdominal lymph nodes**
Revised C81.24 **Mixed cellularity Hodgkin lymphoma, lymph nodes of axilla and upper limb**
Revised C81.25 **Mixed cellularity Hodgkin lymphoma, lymph nodes of inguinal region and lower limb**
Revised C81.26 **Mixed cellularity Hodgkin lymphoma, intrapelvic lymph nodes**
Revised C81.27 **Mixed cellularity Hodgkin lymphoma, spleen**
Revised C81.28 **Mixed cellularity Hodgkin lymphoma, lymph nodes of multiple sites**
Revised C81.29 **Mixed cellularity Hodgkin lymphoma, extranodal and solid organ sites**
Revised C81.3 **Lymphocyte depleted Hodgkin lymphoma**
New Lymphocyte depleted classical Hodgkin lymphoma
Revised C81.30 **Lymphocyte depleted Hodgkin lymphoma, unspecified site**
Revised C81.31 **Lymphocyte depleted Hodgkin lymphoma, lymph nodes of head, face, and neck**
Revised C81.32 **Lymphocyte depleted Hodgkin lymphoma, intrathoracic lymph nodes**
Revised C81.33 **Lymphocyte depleted Hodgkin lymphoma, intra-abdominal lymph nodes**
Revised C81.34 **Lymphocyte depleted Hodgkin lymphoma, lymph nodes of axilla and upper limb**
Revised C81.35 **Lymphocyte depleted Hodgkin lymphoma, lymph nodes of inguinal region and lower limb**
Revised C81.36 **Lymphocyte depleted Hodgkin lymphoma, intrapelvic lymph nodes**
Revised C81.37 **Lymphocyte depleted Hodgkin lymphoma, spleen**
Revised C81.38 **Lymphocyte depleted Hodgkin lymphoma, lymph nodes of multiple sites**
Revised C81.39 **Lymphocyte depleted Hodgkin lymphoma, extranodal and solid organ sites**
Revised C81.4 **Lymphocyte-rich Hodgkin lymphoma**
New Lymphocyte-rich classical Hodgkin lymphoma
Revised C81.40 **Lymphocyte-rich Hodgkin lymphoma, unspecified site**
Revised C81.41 **Lymphocyte-rich Hodgkin lymphoma, lymph nodes of head, face, and neck**
Revised C81.42 **Lymphocyte-rich Hodgkin lymphoma, intrathoracic lymph nodes**
Revised C81.43 **Lymphocyte-rich Hodgkin lymphoma, intra-abdominal lymph nodes**
Revised C81.44 **Lymphocyte-rich Hodgkin lymphoma, lymph nodes of axilla and upper limb**
Revised C81.45 **Lymphocyte-rich Hodgkin lymphoma, lymph nodes of inguinal region and lower limb**
Revised C81.46 **Lymphocyte-rich Hodgkin lymphoma, intrapelvic lymph nodes**
Revised C81.47 **Lymphocyte-rich Hodgkin lymphoma, spleen**
Revised C81.48 **Lymphocyte-rich Hodgkin lymphoma, lymph nodes of multiple sites**
Revised C81.49 **Lymphocyte-rich Hodgkin lymphoma, extranodal and solid organ sites**
Revised C81.7 **Other Hodgkin lymphoma**
New Other classical Hodgkin lymphoma
Revised C81.70 **Other Hodgkin lymphoma, unspecified site**
Revised C81.71 **Other Hodgkin lymphoma, lymph nodes of head, face, and neck**
Revised C81.72 **Other Hodgkin lymphoma, intrathoracic lymph nodes**
Revised C81.73 **Other Hodgkin lymphoma, intra-abdominal lymph nodes**
Revised C81.74 **Other Hodgkin lymphoma, lymph nodes of axilla and upper limb**
Revised C81.75 **Other Hodgkin lymphoma, lymph nodes of inguinal region and lower limb**
Revised C81.76 **Other Hodgkin lymphoma, intrapelvic lymph nodes**
Revised C81.77 **Other Hodgkin lymphoma, spleen**
Revised C81.78 **Other Hodgkin lymphoma, lymph nodes of multiple sites**
Revised C81.79 **Other Hodgkin lymphoma, extranodal and solid organ sites**

C94.20 **Acute megakaryoblastic leukemia not having achieved remission**
Revised Acute megakaryoblastic leukemia with failed remission

D00.0 **Carcinoma in situ of lip, oral cavity and pharynx**
Use additional code to identify:
Revised history of tobacco dependence (Z87.891)

D01.3 **Carcinoma in situ of anus and anal canal**
New Anal intraepithelial neoplasia III [AIN III]
New Severe dysplasia of anus
New **Excludes1** anal intraepithelial neoplasia I and II [AIN I and AIN II] (K62.82)

D02 **Carcinoma in situ of middle ear and respiratory system**
Use additional code to identify:
Revised history of tobacco dependence (Z87.891)

DØ7.5 Carcinoma in situ of prostate

Revised **Excludes1** dysplasia (mild) (moderate) of prostate (N42.3-)

New prostatic intraepithelial neoplasia II [PIN II] (N42.3-)

Revised **D1Ø.3 Benign neoplasm of other and unspecified parts of mouth**

D16.4 Benign neoplasm of bones of skull and face

Deleted **Excludes1** benign neoplasm of lower jaw bone (D16.5)

New **Excludes2** benign neoplasm of lower jaw bone (D16.5)

D27 Benign neoplasm of ovary

Revised **Excludes2** corpus albicans cyst (N83.2-)

Revised corpus luteum cyst (N83.1-)

Revised follicular (atretic) cyst (N83.Ø-)

Revised graafian follicle cyst (N83.Ø-)

Revised ovarian cyst NEC (N83.2-)

Revised ovarian retention cyst (N83.2-)

Revised **D3A.Ø94 Benign carcinoid tumor of the foregut, unspecified**

Revised **D3A.Ø95 Benign carcinoid tumor of the midgut, unspecified**

Revised **D3A.Ø96 Benign carcinoid tumor of the hindgut, unspecified**

Revised **D46.2 Refractory anemia with excess of blasts [RAEB]**

New **D47.Z2 Castleman disease**

New Code also if applicable human herpesvirus 8 infection (B10.89)

New **Excludes2** Kaposi's sarcoma (C46-)

D49.2 Neoplasm of unspecified behavior of bone, soft tissue, and skin

Revised **Excludes1** neoplasm of unspecified behavior of skin of genital organs (D49.59)

New **D49.51 Neoplasm of unspecified behavior of kidney**

New **D49.511 Neoplasm of unspecified behavior of right kidney**

New **D49.512 Neoplasm of unspecified behavior of left kidney**

New **D49.519 Neoplasm of unspecified behavior of unspecified kidney**

New **D49.59 Neoplasm of unspecified behavior of other genitourinary organ**

CHAPTER 3

DISEASES OF THE BLOOD AND BLOOD-FORMING ORGANS AND CERTAIN DISORDERS INVOLVING THE IMMUNE MECHANISM (D5Ø-D89)

D61.81 Pancytopenia

Deleted **Excludes1** pancytopenia (due to) (with) myelodysplastic syndromes (D46.-)

New **Excludes2** pancytopenia (due to) (with) myelodysplastic syndromes (D46.-)

D64.81 Anemia due to antineoplastic chemotherapy

Deleted **Excludes1** anemia in neoplastic disease (D63.Ø)

New **Excludes2** anemia in neoplastic disease (D63.Ø)

D68.62 Lupus anticoagulant syndrome

Revised **Excludes1** lupus anticoagulant (LAC) finding without diagnosis (R76.Ø)

D76 Other specified diseases with participation of lymphoreticular and reticulohistiocytic tissue

New **Excludes1** histiocytic medullary reticulosis (C96.9)

New leukemic reticuloendotheliosis (C91.4-)

New lipomelanotic reticulosis (I89.8)

Deleted leukemic reticuloendotheliosis or reticulosis (C91.4-)

Deleted lipomelanotic reticuloendotheliosis or reticulosis (I89.8)

New malignant reticulosis (C86.Ø)

New nonlipid reticuloendotheliosis (C96.Ø)

Revised **D78.2 Postprocedural hemorrhage of the spleen following a procedure**

Revised **D78.21 Postprocedural hemorrhage of the spleen following a procedure on the spleen**

Revised **D78.22 Postprocedural hemorrhage of the spleen following other procedure**

New **D78.3 Postprocedural hematoma and seroma of the spleen following a procedure**

New **D78.31 Postprocedural hematoma of the spleen following a procedure on the spleen**

New **D78.32 Postprocedural hematoma of the spleen following other procedure**

New **D78.33 Postprocedural seroma of the spleen following a procedure on the spleen**

New **D78.34 Postprocedural seroma of the spleen following other procedure**

New **D89.4 Mast cell activation syndrome and related disorders**

New **Excludes1** aggressive systemic mastocytosis (C96.2)

New cutaneous mastocytosis (Q82.2)

New indolent systemic mastocytosis (D47.Ø)

New malignant mastocytoma (C96.2)

New mast cell leukemia (C94.3-)

New mastocytoma (D47.Ø)

New systemic mastocytosis associated with a clonal hematologic non-mast cell lineage disease (SM-AHNMD) (D47.Ø)

New **D89.4Ø Mast cell activation, unspecified**

New Mast cell activation disorder, unspecified

New Mast cell activation syndrome, NOS

New **D89.41 Monoclonal mast cell activation syndrome**

New **D89.42 Idiopathic mast cell activation syndrome**

New **D89.43 Secondary mast cell activation**

New Secondary mast cell activation syndrome

New Code also underlying etiology, if known

New **D89.49 Other mast cell activation disorder**

New Other mast cell activation syndrome

CHAPTER 4

ENDOCRINE, NUTRITIONAL AND METABOLIC DISEASES (E00-E89)

E08 Diabetes mellitus due to underlying condition

Revised Use additional code to identify control using:
New insulin (Z79.4)
New oral antidiabetic drugs (Z79.84)
New oral hypoglycemic drugs (Z79.84)

E08.32 Diabetes mellitus due to underlying condition with mild nonproliferative diabetic retinopathy

New One of the following 7th characters is to be assigned to codes in subcategory E08.32 to designate laterality of the disease:

New 1 right eye
New 2 left eye
New 3 bilateral
New 9 unspecified eye

E08.33 Diabetes mellitus due to underlying condition with moderate nonproliferative diabetic retinopathy

New One of the following 7th characters is to be assigned to codes in subcategory E08.33 to designate laterality of the disease:

New 1 right eye
New 2 left eye
New 3 bilateral
New 9 unspecified eye

E08.34 Diabetes mellitus due to underlying condition with severe nonproliferative diabetic retinopathy

New One of the following 7th characters is to be assigned to codes in subcategory E08.34 to designate laterality of the disease:

New 1 right eye
New 2 left eye
New 3 bilateral
New 9 unspecified eye

E08.35 Diabetes mellitus due to underlying condition with proliferative diabetic retinopathy

New One of the following 7th characters is to be assigned to codes in subcategory E08.35 to designate laterality of the disease:

New 1 right eye
New 2 left eye
New 3 bilateral
New 9 unspecified eye

New **E08.352 Diabetes mellitus due to underlying condition with proliferative diabetic retinopathy with traction retinal detachment involving the macula**

New **E08.353 Diabetes mellitus due to underlying condition with proliferative diabetic retinopathy with traction retinal detachment not involving the macula**

New **E08.354 Diabetes mellitus due to underlying condition with proliferative diabetic retinopathy with combined traction retinal detachment and rhegmatogenous retinal detachment**

New **E08.355 Diabetes mellitus due to underlying condition with stable proliferative diabetic retinopathy**

New **E08.37 Diabetes mellitus due to underlying condition with diabetic macular edema, resolved following treatment**

New One of the following 7th characters is to be assigned to code E08.37 to designate laterality of the disease:

New 1 right eye
New 2 left eye
New 3 bilateral
New 9 unspecified eye

E09 Drug or chemical induced diabetes mellitus

Revised Use additional code to identify control using:
New insulin (Z79.4)
New oral antidiabetic drugs (Z79.84)
New oral hypoglycemic drugs (Z79.84)

E09.32 Drug or chemical induced diabetes mellitus with mild nonproliferative diabetic retinopathy

New One of the following 7th characters is to be assigned to codes in subcategory E09.32 to designate laterality of the disease:

New 1 right eye
New 2 left eye
New 3 bilateral
New 9 unspecified eye

E09.33 Drug or chemical induced diabetes mellitus with moderate nonproliferative diabetic retinopathy

New One of the following 7th characters is to be assigned to codes in subcategory E09.33 to designate laterality of the disease:

New 1 right eye
New 2 left eye
New 3 bilateral
New 9 unspecified eye

E09.34 Drug or chemical induced diabetes mellitus with severe nonproliferative diabetic retinopathy

New One of the following 7th characters is to be assigned to codes in subcategory E09.34 to designate laterality of the disease:

New 1 right eye
New 2 left eye
New 3 bilateral
New 9 unspecified eye

E09.35 Drug or chemical induced diabetes mellitus with proliferative diabetic retinopathy

New One of the following 7th characters is to be assigned to codes in subcategory E09.35 to designate laterality of the disease:

New	1	right eye
New	2	left eye
New	3	bilateral
New	9	unspecified eye

New **E09.352 Drug or chemical induced diabetes mellitus with proliferative diabetic retinopathy with traction retinal detachment involving the macula**

New **E09.353 Drug or chemical induced diabetes mellitus with proliferative diabetic retinopathy with traction retinal detachment not involving the macula**

New **E09.354 Drug or chemical induced diabetes mellitus with proliferative diabetic retinopathy with combined traction retinal detachment and rhegmatogenous retinal detachment**

New **E09.355 Drug or chemical induced diabetes mellitus with stable proliferative diabetic retinopathy**

New **E09.37 Drug or chemical induced diabetes mellitus with diabetic macular edema, resolved following treatment**

New One of the following 7th characters is to be assigned to code E09.37 to designate laterality of the disease:

New	1	right eye
New	2	left eye
New	3	bilateral
New	9	unspecified eye

E10.32 Type 1 diabetes mellitus with mild nonproliferative diabetic retinopathy

New One of the following 7th characters is to be assigned to codes in subcategory E10.32 to designate laterality of the disease:

New	1	right eye
New	2	left eye
New	3	bilateral
New	9	unspecified eye

E10.33 Type 1 diabetes mellitus with moderate nonproliferative diabetic retinopathy

New One of the following 7th characters is to be assigned to codes in subcategory E10.33 to designate laterality of the disease:

New	1	right eye
New	2	left eye
New	3	bilateral
New	9	unspecified eye

E10.34 Type 1 diabetes mellitus with severe nonproliferative diabetic retinopathy

New One of the following 7th characters is to be assigned to codes in subcategory E10.34 to designate laterality of the disease:

New	1	right eye
New	2	left eye
New	3	bilateral
New	9	unspecified eye

E10.35 Type 1 diabetes mellitus with proliferative diabetic retinopathy

New One of the following 7th characters is to be assigned to codes in subcategory E10.35 to designate laterality of the disease:

New	1	right eye
New	2	left eye
New	3	bilateral
New	9	unspecified eye

New **E10.352 Type 1 diabetes mellitus with proliferative diabetic retinopathy with traction retinal detachment involving the macula**

New **E10.353 Type 1 diabetes mellitus with proliferative diabetic retinopathy with traction retinal detachment not involving the macula**

New **E10.354 Type 1 diabetes mellitus with proliferative diabetic retinopathy with combined traction retinal detachment and rhegmatogenous retinal detachment**

New **E10.355 Type 1 diabetes mellitus with stable proliferative diabetic retinopathy**

New **E10.37 Type 1 diabetes mellitus with diabetic macular edema, resolved following treatment**

One of the following 7th characters is to be assigned to code E10.37 to designate laterality of the disease:

New	1	right eye
New	2	left eye
New	3	bilateral
New	9	unspecified eye

E11 Type 2 diabetes mellitus

Revised Use additional code to identify control using:

New insulin (Z79.4)

New oral antidiabetic drugs (Z79.84)

New oral hypoglycemic drugs (Z79.84)

E11.32 Type 2 diabetes mellitus with mild nonproliferative diabetic retinopathy

New One of the following 7th characters is to be assigned to codes in subcategory E11.32 to designate laterality of the disease:

New	1	right eye
New	2	left eye
New	3	bilateral
New	9	unspecified eye

E11.33 Type 2 diabetes mellitus with moderate nonproliferative diabetic retinopathy

New One of the following 7th characters is to be assigned to codes in subcategory E11.33 to designate laterality of the disease:

New	1	right eye
New	2	left eye
New	3	bilateral
New	9	unspecified eye

E11.34 Type 2 diabetes mellitus with severe nonproliferative diabetic retinopathy

New One of the following 7th characters is to be assigned to codes in subcategory E11.34 to designate laterality of the disease:

New	1	right eye
New	2	left eye
New	3	bilateral
New	9	unspecified eye

E11.35 Type 2 diabetes mellitus with proliferative diabetic retinopathy

New One of the following 7th characters is to be assigned to codes in subcategory E11.35 to designate laterality of the disease:

New	1	right eye
New	2	left eye
New	3	bilateral
New	9	unspecified eye

New **E11.352 Type 2 diabetes mellitus with proliferative diabetic retinopathy with traction retinal detachment involving the macula**

New **E11.353 Type 2 diabetes mellitus with proliferative diabetic retinopathy with traction retinal detachment not involving the macula**

New **E11.354 Type 2 diabetes mellitus with proliferative diabetic retinopathy with combined traction retinal detachment and rhegmatogenous retinal detachment**

New **E11.355 Type 2 diabetes mellitus with stable proliferative diabetic retinopathy**

New **E11.37 Type 2 diabetes mellitus with diabetic macular edema, resolved following treatment**

New One of the following 7th characters is to be assigned to code E11.37 to designate laterality of the disease:

New	1	right eye
New	2	left eye
New	3	bilateral
New	9	unspecified eye

E13 Other specified diabetes mellitus

Revised Use additional code to identify control using:

New insulin (Z79.4)

New oral antidiabetic drugs (Z79.84)

New oral hypoglycemic drugs (Z79.84)

New **Excludes1** type 1 diabetes mellitus (E1Ø.-)

E13.32 Other specified diabetes mellitus with mild nonproliferative diabetic retinopathy

New One of the following 7th characters is to be assigned to codes in subcategory E13.32 to designate laterality of the disease:

New	1	right eye
New	2	left eye
New	3	bilateral
New	9	unspecified eye

E13.33 Other specified diabetes mellitus with moderate nonproliferative diabetic retinopathy

New One of the following 7th characters is to be assigned to codes in subcategory E13.33 to designate laterality of the disease:

New	1	right eye
New	2	left eye
New	3	bilateral
New	9	unspecified eye

E13.34 Other specified diabetes mellitus with severe nonproliferative diabetic retinopathy

New One of the following 7th characters is to be assigned to codes in subcategory E13.34 to designate laterality of the disease:

New	1	right eye
New	2	left eye
New	3	bilateral
New	9	unspecified eye

E13.35 Other specified diabetes mellitus with proliferative diabetic retinopathy

New One of the following 7th characters is to be assigned to codes in subcategory E13.35 to designate laterality of the disease:

New	1	right eye
New	2	left eye
New	3	bilateral
New	9	unspecified eye

New **E13.352 Other specified diabetes mellitus with proliferative diabetic retinopathy with traction retinal detachment involving the macula**

New **E13.353 Other specified diabetes mellitus with proliferative diabetic retinopathy with traction retinal detachment not involving the macula**

New **E13.354 Other specified diabetes mellitus with proliferative diabetic retinopathy with combined traction retinal detachment and rhegmatogenous retinal detachment**

New **E13.355 Other specified diabetes mellitus with stable proliferative diabetic retinopathy**

New **E13.37 Other specified diabetes mellitus with diabetic macular edema, resolved following treatment**

New One of the following 7th characters is to be assigned to code E13.37 to designate laterality of the disease:

New	1	right eye
New	2	left eye
New	3	bilateral
New	9	unspecified eye

E16.Ø Drug-induced hypoglycemia without coma

New **Excludes1** diabetes with hypoglycemia without coma (EØ9.692)

E16.1 Other hypoglycemia

New **Excludes1** diabetes with hypoglycemia (EØ8.649, E1Ø.649, E11.649, E13.649)

E16.2 Hypoglycemia, unspecified

New **Excludes1** diabetes with hypoglycemia (EØ8.649, E1Ø.649, E11.649, E13.649)

E29 Testicular dysfunction

Revised **Excludes1** Klinefelter's syndrome (Q98.Ø-Q98.1, Q98.4)

E66.2 Morbid (severe) obesity with alveolar hypoventilation

New Obesity hypoventilation syndrome (OHS)

E78.Ø Pure hypercholesterolemia

Deleted Familial hypercholesterolemia

Deleted Fredrickson's hyperlipoproteinemia, type IIa

Deleted Hyperbetalipoproteinemia

Deleted Hyperlipidemia, Group A

Deleted Low-density-lipoprotein-type [LDL] hyperlipoproteinemia

New **E78.ØØ Pure hypercholesterolemia, unspecified**

New Fredrickson's hyperlipoproteinemia, type IIa

New Hyperbetalipoproteinemia

New Low-density-lipoprotein-type [LDL] hyperlipoproteinemia

New **E78.01 Familial hypercholesterolemia**

E84 Cystic fibrosis

New Code also exocrine pancreatic insufficiency (K86.81)

E85.Ø Non-neuropathic heredofamilial amyloidosis

Deleted Familial Mediterranean fever

E86 Volume depletion

New Use additional code(s) for any associated disorders of electrolyte and acid-base balance (E87.-)

E88.42 MERRF syndrome

Revised Code also progressive myoclonic epilepsy (G4Ø.3-)

Revised **E89.81 Postprocedural hemorrhage of an endocrine system organ or structure following a procedure**

Revised **E89.81Ø Postprocedural hemorrhage of an endocrine system organ or structure following an endocrine system procedure**

Revised **E89.811 Postprocedural hemorrhage of an endocrine system organ or structure following other procedure**

New **E89.82 Postprocedural hematoma and seroma of an endocrine system organ or structure**

New **E89.82Ø Postprocedural hematoma of an endocrine system organ or structure following an endocrine system procedure**

New **E89.821 Postprocedural hematoma of an endocrine system organ or structure following other procedure**

New **E89.822 Postprocedural seroma of an endocrine system organ or structure following an endocrine system procedure**

New **E89.823 Postprocedural seroma of an endocrine system organ or structure following other procedure**

CHAPTER 5

MENTAL, BEHAVIORAL AND NEURODEVELOPMENTAL DISORDERS (FØ1-F99)

FØ1.5Ø Vascular dementia without behavioral disturbance

New Major neurocognitive disorder without behavioral disturbance

FØ1.51 Vascular dementia with behavioral disturbance

New Major neurocognitive disorder due to vascular disease, with behavioral disturbance

New Major neurocognitive disorder with aggressive behavior

New Major neurocognitive disorder with combative behavior

New Major neurocognitive disorder with violent behavior

FØ2 Dementia in other diseases classified elsewhere

Code first *the underlying physiological condition, such as:*

New dementia with Parkinsonism (G31.83)

New Huntington's disease (G10)

New prion disease (A81.9)

New traumatic brain injury (S06.-)

New **Includes** Major neurocognitive disorder in other diseases classified elsewhere

Deleted **Excludes1** dementia with Parkinsonism (G31.83)

F02.80 Dementia in other diseases classified elsewhere without behavioral disturbance

New Major neurocognitive disorder in other diseases classified elsewhere

F02.81 Dementia in other diseases classified elsewhere with behavioral disturbance

New Major neurocognitive disorder in other diseases classified elsewhere with aggressive behavior

New Major neurocognitive disorder in other diseases classified elsewhere with combative behavior

New Major neurocognitive disorder in other diseases classified elsewhere with violent behavior

F06.1 Catatonic disorder due to known physiological condition

New Catatonia associated with another mental disorder

New Catatonia NOS

F10.10 Alcohol abuse, uncomplicated

New Alcohol use disorder, mild

F10.14 Alcohol abuse with alcohol-induced mood disorder

New Alcohol use disorder, mild, with alcohol-induced bipolar or related disorder

New Alcohol use disorder, mild, with alcohol-induced depressive disorder

F10.20 Alcohol dependence, uncomplicated

New Alcohol use disorder, moderate

New Alcohol use disorder, severe

F10.22 Alcohol dependence with intoxication

Acute drunkenness (in alcoholism)

Deleted **Excludes1** alcohol dependence with withdrawal (F10.23-)

New **Excludes2** alcohol dependence with withdrawal (F10.23-)

F10.23 Alcohol dependence with withdrawal

Deleted **Excludes1** alcohol dependence with intoxication (F10.22-)

New **Excludes2** alcohol dependence with intoxication (F10.22-)

F10.24 Alcohol dependence with alcohol-induced mood disorder

New Alcohol use disorder, moderate, with alcohol-induced bipolar or related disorder

New Alcohol use disorder, moderate, with alcohol-induced depressive disorder

New Alcohol use disorder, severe, with alcohol-induced bipolar or related disorder

New Alcohol use disorder, severe, with alcohol-induced depressive disorder

F10.26 Alcohol dependence with alcohol-induced persisting amnestic disorder

New Alcohol use disorder, moderate, with alcohol-induced major neurocognitive disorder, amnestic-confabulatory type

New Alcohol use disorder, severe, with alcohol-induced major neurocognitive disorder, amnestic-confabulatory type

F10.27 Alcohol dependence with alcohol-induced persisting dementia

New Alcohol use disorder, moderate, with alcohol-induced major neurocognitive disorder, nonamnestic-confabulatory type

New Alcohol use disorder, severe, with alcohol-induced major neurocognitive disorder, nonamnestic-confabulatory type

F10.288 Alcohol dependence with other alcohol-induced disorder

New Alcohol use disorder, moderate, with alcohol-induced mild neurocognitive disorder

New Alcohol use disorder, severe, with alcohol-induced mild neurocognitive disorder

F10.94 Alcohol use, unspecified with alcohol-induced mood disorder

New Alcohol-induced bipolar or related disorder, without use disorder

New Alcohol-induced depressive disorder, without use disorder

F10.959 Alcohol use, unspecified with alcohol-induced psychotic disorder, unspecified

New Alcohol-induced psychotic disorder without use disorder

F10.96 Alcohol use, unspecified with alcohol-induced persisting amnestic disorder

New Alcohol-induced major neurocognitive disorder, amnestic-confabulatory type, without use disorder

F10.97 Alcohol use, unspecified with alcohol-induced persisting dementia

New Alcohol-induced major neurocognitive disorder, nonamnestic-confabulatory type, without use disorder

F10.980 Alcohol use, unspecified with alcohol-induced anxiety disorder

New Alcohol-induced anxiety disorder, without use disorder

F10.981 Alcohol use, unspecified with alcohol-induced sexual dysfunction

New Alcohol-induced sexual dysfunction, without use disorder

F10.982 Alcohol use, unspecified with alcohol-induced sleep disorder

New Alcohol-induced sleep disorder, without use disorder

F10.988 Alcohol use, unspecified with other alcohol-induced disorder

New Alcohol-induced mild neurocognitive disorder, without use disorder

F11.10 Opioid abuse, uncomplicated

New Opioid use disorder, mild

F11.14 Opioid abuse with opioid-induced mood disorder

New Opioid use disorder, mild, with opioid-induced depressive disorder

F11.20 Opioid dependence, uncomplicated
New Opioid use disorder, moderate
New Opioid use disorder, severe

F11.24 Opioid dependence with opioid-induced mood disorder
New Opioid use disorder, moderate, with opioid-induced depressive disorder

F11.921 Opioid use, unspecified with intoxication delirium
New Opioid-induced delirium

F11.94 Opioid use, unspecified with opioid-induced mood disorder
New Opioid-induced depressive disorder, without use disorder

F11.981 Opioid use, unspecified with opioid-induced sexual dysfunction
New Opioid-induced sexual dysfunction, without use disorder

F11.982 Opioid use, unspecified with opioid-induced sleep disorder
New Opioid-induced sleep disorder, without use disorder

F11.988 Opioid use, unspecified with other opioid-induced disorder
New Opioid-induced anxiety disorder, without use disorder

F12.10 Cannabis abuse, uncomplicated
New Cannabis use disorder, mild

F12.188 Cannabis abuse with other cannabis-induced disorder
New Cannabis use disorder, mild, with cannabis-induced sleep disorder

F12.2 Cannabis dependence

F12.20 Cannabis dependence, uncomplicated
New Cannabis use disorder, moderate
New Cannabis use disorder, severe

F12.288 Cannabis dependence with other cannabis-induced disorder
New Cannabis use disorder, moderate, with cannabis-induced sleep disorder
New Cannabis use disorder, severe, with cannabis-induced sleep disorder
New Cannabis withdrawal

F12.959 Cannabis use, unspecified with psychotic disorder, unspecified
New Cannabis-induced psychotic disorder, without use disorder

F12.980 Cannabis use, unspecified with anxiety disorder
New Cannabis-induced anxiety disorder, without use disorder

F12.988 Cannabis use, unspecified with other cannabis-induced disorder
New Cannabis-induced sleep disorder, without use disorder

F13.10 Sedative, hypnotic or anxiolytic abuse, uncomplicated
New Sedative, hypnotic, or anxiolytic use disorder, mild

F13.14 Sedative, hypnotic or anxiolytic abuse with sedative, hypnotic or anxiolytic-induced mood disorder
New Sedative, hypnotic, or anxiolytic use disorder, mild, with sedative, hypnotic, or anxiolytic-induced bipolar or related disorder
New Sedative, hypnotic, or anxiolytic use disorder, mild, with sedative, hypnotic, or anxiolytic-induced depressive disorder

F13.23 Sedative, hypnotic or anxiolytic dependence with withdrawal
New Sedative, hypnotic, or anxiolytic use disorder, moderate
New Sedative, hypnotic, or anxiolytic use disorder, severe

F13.232 Sedative, hypnotic or anxiolytic dependence with withdrawal with perceptual disturbance
New Sedative, hypnotic, or anxiolytic withdrawal with perceptual disturbances

F13.239 Sedative, hypnotic or anxiolytic dependence with withdrawal, unspecified
New Sedative, hypnotic, or anxiolytic withdrawal without perceptual disturbances

F13.24 Sedative, hypnotic or anxiolytic dependence with sedative, hypnotic or anxiolytic-induced mood disorder
New Sedative, hypnotic, or anxiolytic use disorder, moderate, with sedative, hypnotic, or anxiolytic-induced bipolar or related disorder
New Sedative, hypnotic, or anxiolytic use disorder, moderate, with sedative, hypnotic, or anxiolytic-induced depressive disorder
New Sedative, hypnotic, or anxiolytic use disorder, severe, with sedative, hypnotic, or anxiolytic-induced bipolar or related disorder
New Sedative, hypnotic, or anxiolytic use disorder, severe, with sedative, hypnotic, or anxiolytic-induced depressive disorder

F13.27 Sedative, hypnotic or anxiolytic dependence with sedative, hypnotic or anxiolytic-induced persisting dementia
New Sedative, hypnotic, or anxiolytic use disorder, moderate, with sedative, hypnotic, or anxiolytic-induced major neurocognitive disorder
New Sedative, hypnotic, or anxiolytic use disorder, severe, with sedative, hypnotic, or anxiolytic-induced major neurocognitive disorder

F13.288 Sedative, hypnotic or anxiolytic dependence with other sedative, hypnotic or anxiolytic-induced disorder

New Sedative, hypnotic, or anxiolytic use disorder, moderate, with sedative, hypnotic, or anxiolytic-induced mild neurocognitive disorder

New Sedative, hypnotic, or anxiolytic use disorder, severe, with sedative, hypnotic, or anxiolytic-induced mild neurocognitive disorder

F13.921 Sedative, hypnotic or anxiolytic use, unspecified with intoxication delirium

New Sedative, hypnotic, or anxiolytic-induced delirium

F13.94 Sedative, hypnotic or anxiolytic use, unspecified with sedative, hypnotic or anxiolytic-induced mood disorder

New Sedative, hypnotic, or anxiolytic-induced bipolar or related disorder, without use disorder

New Sedative, hypnotic, or anxiolytic-induced depressive disorder, without use disorder

F13.959 Sedative, hypnotic or anxiolytic use, unspecified with sedative, hypnotic or anxiolytic-induced psychotic disorder, unspecified

New Sedative, hypnotic, or anxiolytic-induced psychotic disorder, without use disorder

F13.97 Sedative, hypnotic or anxiolytic use, unspecified with sedative, hypnotic or anxiolytic-induced persisting dementia

New Sedative, hypnotic, or anxiolytic-induced major neurocognitive disorder, without use disorder

F13.980 Sedative, hypnotic or anxiolytic use, unspecified with sedative, hypnotic or anxiolytic-induced anxiety disorder

New Sedative, hypnotic, or anxiolytic-induced anxiety disorder, without use disorder

F13.981 Sedative, hypnotic or anxiolytic use, unspecified with sedative, hypnotic or anxiolytic-induced sexual dysfunction

New Sedative, hypnotic, or anxiolytic-induced sexual dysfunction disorder, without use disorder

F13.982 Sedative, hypnotic or anxiolytic use, unspecified with sedative, hypnotic or anxiolytic-induced sleep disorder

New Sedative, hypnotic, or anxiolytic-induced sleep disorder, without use disorder

F13.988 Sedative, hypnotic or anxiolytic use, unspecified with other sedative, hypnotic or anxiolytic-induced disorder

New Sedative, hypnotic, or anxiolytic-induced mild neurocognitive disorder

F14.10 Cocaine abuse, uncomplicated

New Cocaine use disorder, mild

F14.14 Cocaine abuse with cocaine-induced mood disorder

New Cocaine use disorder, mild, with cocaine-induced bipolar or related disorder

New Cocaine use disorder, mild, with cocaine-induced depressive disorder

F14.188 Cocaine abuse with other cocaine-induced disorder

New Cocaine use disorder, mild, with cocaine-induced obsessive-compulsive or related disorder

F14.20 Cocaine dependence, uncomplicated

New Cocaine use disorder, moderate

New Cocaine use disorder, severe

F14.24 Cocaine dependence with cocaine-induced mood disorder

New Cocaine use disorder, moderate, with cocaine-induced bipolar or related disorder

New Cocaine use disorder, moderate, with cocaine-induced depressive disorder

New Cocaine use disorder, severe, with cocaine-induced bipolar or related disorder

New Cocaine use disorder, severe, with cocaine-induced depressive disorder

F14.288 Cocaine dependence with other cocaine-induced disorder

New Cocaine use disorder, moderate, with cocaine-induced obsessive-compulsive or related disorder

New Cocaine use disorder, severe, with cocaine-induced obsessive-compulsive or related disorder

F14.94 Cocaine use, unspecified with cocaine-induced mood disorder

New Cocaine-induced bipolar or related disorder, without use disorder

New Cocaine-induced depressive disorder, without use disorder

F14.959 Cocaine use, unspecified with cocaine-induced psychotic disorder, unspecified

New Cocaine-induced psychotic disorder, without use disorder

F14.980 Cocaine use, unspecified with cocaine-induced anxiety disorder

New Cocaine-induced anxiety disorder, without use disorder

F14.981 Cocaine use, unspecified with cocaine-induced sexual dysfunction

New Cocaine-induced sexual dysfunction, without use disorder

F14.982 Cocaine use, unspecified with cocaine-induced sleep disorder

New Cocaine-induced sleep disorder, without use disorder

F14.988 Cocaine use, unspecified with other cocaine-induced disorder

New Cocaine-induced obsessive-compulsive or related disorder

F15.10 Other stimulant abuse, uncomplicated

New Amphetamine type substance use disorder, mild

New Other or unspecified stimulant use disorder, mild

F15.122 Other stimulant abuse with intoxication with perceptual disturbance

New Amphetamine or other stimulant use disorder, mild, with amphetamine or other stimulant intoxication, with perceptual disturbances

F15.129 Other stimulant abuse with intoxication, unspecified

New Amphetamine or other stimulant use disorder, mild, with amphetamine or other stimulant intoxication, without perceptual disturbances

F15.14 Other stimulant abuse with stimulant-induced mood disorder

New Amphetamine or other stimulant use disorder, mild, with amphetamine or other stimulant-induced bipolar or related disorder

New Amphetamine or other stimulant use disorder, mild, with amphetamine or other stimulant-induced depressive disorder

F15.188 Other stimulant abuse with other stimulant-induced disorder

New Amphetamine or other stimulant use disorder, mild, with amphetamine or other stimulant-induced obsessive-compulsive or related disorder

F15.20 Other stimulant dependence, uncomplicated

New Amphetamine type substance use disorder, moderate

New Amphetamine type substance use disorder, severe

New Other or unspecified stimulant use disorder, moderate

New Other or unspecified stimulant use disorder, severe

F15.222 Other stimulant dependence with intoxication with perceptual disturbance

New Amphetamine or other stimulant use disorder, moderate, with amphetamine or other stimulant intoxication, with perceptual disturbances

New Amphetamine or other stimulant use disorder, severe, with amphetamine or other stimulant intoxication, with perceptual disturbances

F15.229 Other stimulant dependence with intoxication, unspecified

New Amphetamine or other stimulant use disorder, moderate, with amphetamine or other stimulant intoxication, without perceptual disturbances

New Amphetamine or other stimulant use disorder, severe, with amphetamine or other stimulant intoxication, without perceptual disturbances

F15.23 Other stimulant dependence with withdrawal

New Amphetamine or other stimulant withdrawal

F15.24 Other stimulant dependence with stimulant-induced mood disorder

New Amphetamine or other stimulant use disorder, moderate, with amphetamine or other stimulant-induced bipolar or related disorder

New Amphetamine or other stimulant use disorder, moderate, with amphetamine or other stimulant-induced depressive disorder

New Amphetamine or other stimulant use disorder, severe, with amphetamine or other stimulant-induced bipolar or related disorder

New Amphetamine or other stimulant use disorder, severe, with amphetamine or other stimulant-induced depressive disorder

F15.288 Other stimulant dependence with other stimulant-induced disorder

New Amphetamine or other stimulant use disorder, moderate, with amphetamine or other stimulant-induced obsessive-compulsive or related disorder

New Amphetamine or other stimulant use disorder, severe, with amphetamine or other stimulant-induced obsessive-compulsive or related disorder

F15.921 Other stimulant use, unspecified with intoxication delirium

New Amphetamine or other stimulant-induced delirium

F15.929 Other stimulant use, unspecified with intoxication, unspecified

New Caffeine intoxication

F15.93 Other stimulant use, unspecified with withdrawal

New Caffeine withdrawal

F15.94 Other stimulant use, unspecified with stimulant-induced mood disorder

New Amphetamine or other stimulant-induced bipolar or related disorder, without use disorder

New Amphetamine or other stimulant-induced depressive disorder, without use disorder

F15.959 Other stimulant use, unspecified with stimulant-induced psychotic disorder, unspecified

New Amphetamine or other stimulant-induced psychotic disorder, without use disorder

F15.980 Other stimulant use, unspecified with stimulant-induced anxiety disorder

New Amphetamine or other stimulant-induced anxiety disorder, without use disorder

New Caffeine-induced anxiety disorder, without use disorder

F15.981 Other stimulant use, unspecified with stimulant-induced sexual dysfunction

New Amphetamine or other stimulant-induced sexual dysfunction, without use disorder

F15.982 Other stimulant use, unspecified with stimulant-induced sleep disorder

New Amphetamine or other stimulant-induced sleep disorder, without use disorder

New Caffeine-induced sleep disorder, without use disorder

F15.988 Other stimulant use, unspecified with other stimulant-induced disorder

New Amphetamine or other stimulant-induced obsessive-compulsive or related disorder, without use disorder

F16.10 Hallucinogen abuse, uncomplicated

New Other hallucinogen use disorder, mild

New Phencyclidine use disorder, mild

F16.14 Hallucinogen abuse with hallucinogen-induced mood disorder

New Other hallucinogen use disorder, mild, with other hallucinogen-induced bipolar or related disorder

New Other hallucinogen use disorder, mild, with other hallucinogen-induced depressive disorder

New Phencyclidine use disorder, mild, with phencyclidine-induced bipolar or related disorder

New Phencyclidine use disorder, mild, with phencyclidine-induced depressive disorder

F16.20 Hallucinogen dependence, uncomplicated

New Other hallucinogen use disorder, moderate

New Other hallucinogen use disorder, severe

New Phencyclidine use disorder, moderate

New Phencyclidine use disorder, severe

F16.24 Hallucinogen dependence with hallucinogen-induced mood disorder

New Other hallucinogen use disorder, moderate, with other hallucinogen-induced bipolar or related disorder

New Other hallucinogen use disorder, moderate, with other hallucinogen-induced depressive disorder

New Other hallucinogen use disorder, severe, with other hallucinogen-induced bipolar or related disorder

New Other hallucinogen use disorder, severe, with other hallucinogen-induced depressive disorder

New Phencyclidine use disorder, moderate, with phencyclidine-induced bipolar or related disorder

New Phencyclidine use disorder, moderate, with phencyclidine-induced depressive disorder

New Phencyclidine use disorder, severe, with phencyclidine-induced bipolar or related disorder

New Phencyclidine use disorder, severe, with phencyclidine-induced depressive disorder

F16.921 Hallucinogen use, unspecified with intoxication with delirium

New Other hallucinogen intoxication delirium

F16.94 Hallucinogen use, unspecified with hallucinogen-induced mood disorder

New Other hallucinogen-induced bipolar or related disorder, without use disorder

New Other hallucinogen-induced depressive disorder, without use disorder

New Phencyclidine-induced bipolar or related disorder, without use disorder

New Phencyclidine-induced depressive disorder, without use disorder

F16.959 Hallucinogen use, unspecified with hallucinogen-induced psychotic disorder, unspecified

New Other hallucinogen-induced psychotic disorder, without use disorder

New Phencyclidine-induced psychotic disorder, without use disorder

F16.980 Hallucinogen use, unspecified with hallucinogen-induced anxiety disorder

New Other hallucinogen-induced anxiety disorder, without use disorder

New Phencyclidine-induced anxiety disorder, without use disorder

F17.200 Nicotine dependence, unspecified, uncomplicated

New Tobacco use disorder, mild

New Tobacco use disorder, moderate

New Tobacco use disorder, severe

F17.203 Nicotine dependence unspecified, with withdrawal

New Tobacco withdrawal

F18.10 Inhalant abuse, uncomplicated

New Inhalant use disorder, mild

F18.14 Inhalant abuse with inhalant-induced mood disorder

New Inhalant use disorder, mild, with inhalant-induced depressive disorder

F18.17 Inhalant abuse with inhalant-induced dementia

New Inhalant use disorder, mild, with inhalant-induced major neurocognitive disorder

F18.188 Inhalant abuse with other inhalant-induced disorder

New Inhalant use disorder, mild, with inhalant-induced mild neurocognitive disorder

F18.20 Inhalant dependence, uncomplicated

New Inhalant use disorder, moderate

New Inhalant use disorder, severe

F18.24 Inhalant dependence with inhalant-induced mood disorder

New Inhalant use disorder, moderate, with inhalant-induced depressive disorder

New Inhalant use disorder, severe, with inhalant-induced depressive disorder

F18.27 Inhalant dependence with inhalant-induced dementia

New Inhalant use disorder, moderate, with inhalant-induced major neurocognitive disorder

New Inhalant use disorder, severe, with inhalant-induced major neurocognitive disorder

F18.288 Inhalant dependence with other inhalant-induced disorder

New Inhalant use disorder, moderate, with inhalant-induced mild neurocognitive disorder

New Inhalant use disorder, severe, with inhalant-induced mild neurocognitive disorder

F18.94 Inhalant use, unspecified with inhalant-induced mood disorder

New Inhalant-induced depressive disorder

F18.97 Inhalant use, unspecified with inhalant-induced persisting dementia

New Inhalant-induced major neurocognitive disorder

F18.988 Inhalant use, unspecified with other inhalant-induced disorder

New Inhalant-induced mild neurocognitive disorder

F19.10 Other psychoactive substance abuse, uncomplicated

New Other (or unknown) substance use disorder, mild

F19.14 Other psychoactive substance abuse with psychoactive substance-induced mood disorder

New Other (or unknown) substance use disorder, mild, with other (or unknown) substance-induced bipolar or related disorder

New Other (or unknown) substance use disorder, mild, with other (or unknown) substance-induced depressive disorder

F19.17 Other psychoactive substance abuse with psychoactive substance-induced persisting dementia

New Other (or unknown) substance use disorder, mild, with other (or unknown) substance-induced major neurocognitive disorder

F19.188 Other psychoactive substance abuse with other psychoactive substance-induced disorder

New Other (or unknown) substance use disorder, mild, with other (or unknown) substance-induced mild neurocognitive disorder

New Other (or unknown) substance use disorder, mild, with other (or unknown) substance-induced obsessive-compulsive or related disorder

F19.20 Other psychoactive substance dependence, uncomplicated

New Other (or unknown) substance use disorder, moderate

New Other (or unknown) substance use disorder, severe

F19.24 Other psychoactive substance dependence with psychoactive substance-induced mood disorder

New Other (or unknown) substance use disorder, moderate, with other (or unknown) substance-induced bipolar or related disorder

New Other (or unknown) substance use disorder, moderate, with other (or unknown) substance-induced depressive disorder

New Other (or unknown) substance use disorder, severe, with other (or unknown) substance-induced bipolar or related disorder

New Other (or unknown) substance use disorder, severe, with other (or unknown) substance-induced depressive disorder

F19.27 Other psychoactive substance dependence with psychoactive substance-induced persisting dementia

New Other (or unknown) substance use disorder, moderate, with other (or unknown) substance-induced major neurocognitive disorder

New Other (or unknown) substance use disorder, severe, with other (or unknown) substance-induced major neurocognitive disorder

F19.288 Other psychoactive substance dependence with other psychoactive substance-induced disorder

New Other (or unknown) substance use disorder, moderate, with other (or unknown) substance-induced mild neurocognitive disorder

New Other (or unknown) substance use disorder, severe, with other (or unknown) substance-induced mild neurocognitive disorder

New Other (or unknown) substance use disorder, moderate, with other (or unknown) substance-induced obsessive-compulsive or related disorder

New Other (or unknown) substance use disorder, severe, with other (or unknown) substance-induced obsessive-compulsive or related disorder

F19.921 Other psychoactive substance use, unspecified with intoxication with delirium

New Other (or unknown) substance-induced delirium

F19.94 Other psychoactive substance use, unspecified with psychoactive substance-induced mood disorder

New Other (or unknown) substance-induced bipolar or related disorder, without use disorder

New Other (or unknown) substance-induced depressive disorder, without use disorder

F19.959 Other psychoactive substance use, unspecified with psychoactive substance-induced psychotic disorder, unspecified

New Other or unknown substance-induced psychotic disorder, without use disorder

F19.97 Other psychoactive substance use, unspecified with psychoactive substance-induced persisting dementia

New Other (or unknown) substance-induced major neurocognitive disorder, without use disorder

F19.980 Other psychoactive substance use, unspecified with psychoactive substance-induced anxiety disorder

New Other (or unknown) substance-induced anxiety disorder, without use disorder

F19.981 Other psychoactive substance use, unspecified with psychoactive substance-induced sexual dysfunction

New Other (or unknown) substance-induced sexual dysfunction, without use disorder

F19.982 Other psychoactive substance use, unspecified with psychoactive substance-induced sleep disorder

New Other (or unknown) substance-induced sleep disorder, without use disorder

F19.988 Other psychoactive substance use, unspecified with other psychoactive substance-induced disorder

New Other (or unknown) substance-induced mild neurocognitive disorder, without use disorder

New Other (or unknown) substance-induced obsessive-compulsive or related disorder, without use disorder

F20.3 Undifferentiated schizophrenia

Revised **Excludes2** post-schizophrenic depression (F32.89)

F32.8 Other depressive episodes
Deleted Atypical depression
Deleted Post-schizophrenic depression
Deleted Single episode of 'masked' depression NOS
New **F32.81 Premenstrual dysphoric disorder**
New **Excludes1** premenstrual tension syndrome (N94.3)
New **F32.89 Other specified depressive episodes**
New Atypical depression
New Post-schizophrenic depression
New Single episode of 'masked' depression NOS
F34.1 Dysthymic disorder
New Persistent depressive disorder
F34.8 Other persistent mood [affective] disorders
New **F34.81 Disruptive mood dysregulation disorder**
New **F34.89 Other specified persistent mood disorders**

F42 Obsessive-compulsive disorder
Deleted Anancastic neurosis
Deleted Obsessive-compulsive neurosis
New **F42.2 Mixed obsessional thoughts and acts**
New **F42.3 Hoarding disorder**
New **F42.4 Excoriation (skin-picking) disorder**
New **Excludes1** factitial dermatitis (L98.1)
New other specified behavioral and emotional disorders with onset usually occurring in early childhood and adolescence (F98.8)
New **F42.8 Other obsessive-compulsive disorder**
New Anancastic neurosis
New Obsessive-compulsive neurosis
New **F42.9 Obsessive-compulsive disorder, unspecified**
F43.8 Other reactions to severe stress
New Other specified trauma and stressor-related disorder
F43.9 Reaction to severe stress, unspecified
New Trauma and stressor-related disorder, NOS
F44.0 Dissociative amnesia
New **Excludes1** dissociative amnesia with dissociative fugue (F44.1)
F44.1 Dissociative fugue
Dissociative amnesia with dissociative fugue
F45.1 Undifferentiated somatoform disorder
New Somatic symptom disorder
F45.21 Hypochondriasis
New Illness anxiety disorder
F50.0 Anorexia nervosa
Revised **Excludes1** psychogenic loss of appetite (F50.89)
F50.8 Other eating disorders
Deleted Pica in adults
Deleted Psychogenic loss of appetite
New **F50.81 Binge eating disorder**
New **F50.89 Other specified eating disorder**
New Pica in adults
New Psychogenic loss of appetite
F52.0 Hypoactive sexual desire disorder
Deleted Anhedonia (sexual)
New Sexual anhedonia
F52.22 Female sexual arousal disorder
Deleted Frigidity
F52.32 Male orgasmic disorder
New Delayed ejaculation

F52.6 Dyspareunia not due to a substance or known physiological condition
New Genito-pelvic pain penetration disorder
Revised **Excludes2** dyspareunia (due to a known physiological condition) (N94.1-)
F60.5 Obsessive-compulsive personality disorder
Revised **Excludes2** obsessive-compulsive disorder (F42-)
New **F64.0 Transsexualism**
New Gender identity disorder in adolescence and adulthood
New Gender dysphoria in adolescents and adults
Revised **F64.1 Dual role transvestism**
Deleted Dual role transvestism
Deleted Transvestism
F64.2 Gender identity disorder of childhood
New Gender dysphoria in children
Revised **Excludes1** gender identity disorder in adolescence and adulthood (F64.0)
F80.0 Phonological disorder
New Speech-sound disorder
F80.8 Other developmental disorders of speech or language
New **F80.82 Social pragmatic communication disorder**
New **Excludes1** Asperger's syndrome (F84.5)
New autistic disorder (F84.0)
F84.0 Autistic disorder
New Autism spectrum disorder
F88 Other disorders of psychological development
New Global developmental delay
New Other specified neurodevelopmental disorder
F89 Unspecified disorder of psychological development
New Neurodevelopmental disorder NOS
F91.8 Other conduct disorders
New Other specified conduct disorder
New Other specified disruptive disorder
F91.9 Conduct disorder, unspecified
New Disruptive disorder NOS
F95.0 Transient tic disorder
New Provisional tic disorder
F98 Other behavioral and emotional disorders with onset usually occurring in childhood and adolescence
Revised **Excludes2** obsessive-compulsive disorder (F42-)
F98.4 Stereotyped movement disorders
Revised **Excludes2** compulsions in obsessive-compulsive disorder (F42-)

CHAPTER 6

DISEASES OF THE NERVOUS SYSTEM (G00-G99)

G00.1 Pneumococcal meningitis
New Meningitis due to Streptococcal pneumoniae
G31.84 Mild cognitive impairment, so stated
Revised **Excludes1** cognitive deficits following (sequelae of) cerebral hemorrhage or infarction (I69.01-, I69.11-, I69.21-, I69.31-, I69.81-, I69.91-)

G40 Epilepsy and recurrent seizures

Deleted	**Excludes1**	hippocampal sclerosis (G93.81)
Deleted		mesial temporal sclerosis (G93.81)
Deleted		temporal sclerosis (G93.81)
Deleted		Todd's paralysis (G83.8)
New	**Excludes2**	hippocampal sclerosis (G93.81)
New		mesial temporal sclerosis (G93.81)
New		temporal sclerosis (G93.81)
New		Todd's paralysis (G83.84)

G56.0 Carpal tunnel syndrome

New **G56.03 Carpal tunnel syndrome, bilateral upper limbs**

G56.1 Other lesions of median nerve

New **G56.13 Other lesions of median nerve, bilateral upper limbs**

G56.2 Lesion of ulnar nerve

New **G56.23 Lesion of ulnar nerve, bilateral upper limbs**

G56.3 Lesion of radial nerve

New **G56.33 Lesion of radial nerve, bilateral upper limbs**

G56.4 Causalgia of upper limb

New **G56.43 Causalgia of bilateral upper limbs**

G56.8 Other specified mononeuropathies of upper limb

New **G56.83 Other specified mononeuropathies of bilateral upper limbs**

G56.9 Unspecified mononeuropathy of upper limb

New **G56.93 Unspecified mononeuropathy of bilateral upper limbs**

G57.0 Lesion of sciatic nerve

New **G57.03 Lesion of sciatic nerve, bilateral lower limbs**

G57.1 Meralgia paresthetica

New **G57.13 Meralgia paresthetica, bilateral lower limbs**

G57.2 Lesion of femoral nerve

New **G57.23 Lesion of femoral nerve, bilateral lower limbs**

G57.3 Lesion of lateral popliteal nerve

New **G57.33 Lesion of lateral popliteal nerve, bilateral lower limbs**

G57.4 Lesion of medial popliteal nerve

New **G57.43 Lesion of medial popliteal nerve, bilateral lower limbs**

G57.5 Tarsal tunnel syndrome

New **G57.53 Tarsal tunnel syndrome, bilateral lower limbs**

G57.6 Lesion of plantar nerve

New **G57.63 Lesion of plantar nerve, bilateral lower limbs**

G57.7 Causalgia of lower limb

New **G57.73 Causalgia of bilateral lower limbs**

G57.8 Other specified mononeuropathies of lower limb

New **G57.83 Other specified mononeuropathies of bilateral lower limbs**

G57.9 Unspecified mononeuropathy of lower limb

New **G57.93 Unspecified mononeuropathy of bilateral lower limbs**

G61.8 Other inflammatory polyneuropathies

New **G61.82 Multifocal motor neuropathy**

New MMN

G89 Pain, not elsewhere classified

Revised **Excludes2** pain from prosthetic devices, implants, and grafts (T82.84, T83.84, T84.84, T85.84-)

G97 Intraoperative and postprocedural complications and disorders of nervous system, not elsewhere classified

Revised **G97.5 Postprocedural hemorrhage of a nervous system organ or structure following a procedure**

Revised **G97.51 Postprocedural hemorrhage of a nervous system organ or structure following a nervous system procedure**

Revised **G97.52 Postprocedural hemorrhage of a nervous system organ or structure following other procedure**

New **G97.6 Postprocedural hematoma and seroma of a nervous system organ or structure following a procedure**

New **G97.61 Postprocedural hematoma of a nervous system organ or structure following a nervous system procedure**

New **G97.62 Postprocedural hematoma of a nervous system organ or structure following other procedure**

New **G97.63 Postprocedural seroma of a nervous system organ or structure following a nervous system procedure**

New **G97.64 Postprocedural seroma of a nervous system organ or structure following other procedure**

CHAPTER 7

DISEASES OF THE EYE AND ADNEXA (H00-H59)

H34.81 Central retinal vein occlusion

New One of the following 7th characters is to be assigned to codes in subcategory H34.81 to designate the severity of the occlusion:

New	0	with macular edema
New	1	with retinal neovascularization
New	2	stable
New		Old central retinal vein occlusion

H34.83 Tributary (branch) retinal vein occlusion

New One of the following 7th characters is to be assigned to codes in subcategory H34.83 to designate the severity of the occlusion:

New	0	with macular edema
New	1	with retinal neovascularization
New	2	stable
New		Old tributary (branch) retinal vein occlusion

H35.31 Nonexudative age-related macular degeneration

New Dry age-related macular degeneration

New One of the following 7th characters is to be assigned to codes in subcategory H35.31 to designate the stage of the disease:

New	0	stage unspecified
New	1	early dry stage
New	2	intermediate dry stage
New	3	advanced atrophic without subfoveal involvement
New		advanced dry stage
New	4	advanced atrophic with subfoveal involvement

New **H35.311** Nonexudative age-related macular degeneration, right eye

New **H35.312** Nonexudative age-related macular degeneration, left eye

New **H35.313** Nonexudative age-related macular degeneration, bilateral

New **H35.319** Nonexudative age-related macular degeneration, unspecified eye

H35.32 Exudative age-related macular degeneration

New Wet age-related macular degeneration

New One of the following 7th characters is to be assigned to codes in subcategory H35.32 to designate the stage of the disease:

New	0	stage unspecified
New	1	with active choroidal neovascularization
New	2	with inactive choroidal neovascularization
New		with involuted or regressed neovascularization
New	3	with inactive scar

New **H35.321** Exudative age-related macular degeneration, right eye

New **H35.322** Exudative age-related macular degeneration, left eye

New **H35.323** Exudative age-related macular degeneration, bilateral

New **H35.329** Exudative age-related macular degeneration, unspecified eye

H40.11 Primary open-angle glaucoma

New **H40.111** Primary open-angle glaucoma, right eye

New **H40.112** Primary open-angle glaucoma, left eye

New **H40.113** Primary open-angle glaucoma, bilateral

New **H40.119** Primary open-angle glaucoma, unspecified eye

H42 Glaucoma in diseases classified elsewhere

Revised **Excludes1** glaucoma (in) onchocerciasis (B73.02)

Deleted diabetes mellitus (E08.39, E09.39, E10.39, E11.39, E13.39)

Deleted onchocerciasis (B73.02)

Revised glaucoma (in) syphilis (A52.71)

Revised glaucoma (in) tuberculous (A18.59)

New **Excludes2** glaucoma (in) diabetes mellitus (E08.39, E09.39, E10.39, E11.39, E13.39)

H53.0 Amblyopia ex anopsia

New **H53.04** Amblyopia suspect

New **H53.041** Amblyopia suspect, right eye

New **H53.042** Amblyopia suspect, left eye

New **H53.043** Amblyopia suspect, bilateral

New **H53.049** Amblyopia suspect, unspecified eye

H59 Intraoperative and postprocedural complications and disorders of eye and adnexa, not elsewhere classified

Revised **H59.3** Postprocedural hemorrhage, hematoma, and seroma of eye and adnexa following other procedure

Revised **H59.31** Postprocedural hemorrhage of eye and adnexa following an ophthalmic procedure

Revised **H59.311** Postprocedural hemorrhage of right eye and avdnexa following an ophthalmic procedure

Revised **H59.312** Postprocedural hemorrhage of left eye and adnexa following an ophthalmic procedure

Revised **H59.313** Postprocedural hemorrhage of eye and adnexa following an ophthalmic procedure, bilateral

Revised **H59.319** Postprocedural hemorrhage of unspecified eye and adnexa following an ophthalmic procedure

Revised **H59.32** Postprocedural hemorrhage of eye and adnexa following other procedure

Revised **H59.321** Postprocedural hemorrhage of right eye and adnexa following other procedure

Revised **H59.322** Postprocedural hemorrhage of left eye and adnexa following other procedure

Revised **H59.323** Postprocedural hemorrhage of eye and adnexa following other procedure, bilateral

Revised **H59.329** Postprocedural hemorrhage of unspecified eye and adnexa following other procedure

New **H59.33** Postprocedural hematoma of eye and adnexa following an ophthalmic procedure

New **H59.331** Postprocedural hematoma of right eye and adnexa following an ophthalmic procedure

New **H59.332** Postprocedural hematoma of left eye and adnexa following an ophthalmic procedure

New **H59.333** Postprocedural hematoma of eye and adnexa following an ophthalmic procedure, bilateral

New **H59.339** Postprocedural hematoma of unspecified eye and adnexa following an ophthalmic procedure

New **H59.34** Postprocedural hematoma of eye and adnexa following other procedure

New **H59.341** Postprocedural hematoma of right eye and adnexa following other procedure

New **H59.342** Postprocedural hematoma of left eye and adnexa following other procedure

New **H59.343** Postprocedural hematoma of eye and adnexa following other procedure, bilateral

New **H59.349** Postprocedural hematoma of unspecified eye and adnexa following other procedure

New H59.35 **Postprocedural seroma of eye and adnexa following an ophthalmic procedure**

New H59.351 **Postprocedural seroma of right eye and adnexa following an ophthalmic procedure**

New H59.352 **Postprocedural seroma of left eye and adnexa following an ophthalmic procedure**

New H59.353 **Postprocedural seroma of eye and adnexa following an ophthalmic procedure, bilateral**

New H59.359 **Postprocedural seroma of unspecified eye and adnexa following an ophthalmic procedure**

New H59.36 **Postprocedural seroma of eye and adnexa following other procedure**

New H59.361 **Postprocedural seroma of right eye and adnexa following other procedure**

New H59.362 **Postprocedural seroma of left eye and adnexa following other procedure**

New H59.363 **Postprocedural seroma of eye and adnexa following other procedure, bilateral**

New H59.369 **Postprocedural seroma of unspecified eye and adnexa following other procedure**

CHAPTER 8

DISEASES OF THE EAR AND MASTOID PROCESS (H60-H95)

H65 **Nonsuppurative otitis media**

H66 **Suppurative and unspecified otitis media**

Use additional code to identify:

New history of tobacco dependence (Z87.891)

H90 **Conductive and sensorineural hearing loss**

New H90.A **Conductive and sensorineural hearing loss with restricted hearing on the contralateral side**

New H90.A1 **Conductive hearing loss, unilateral, with restricted hearing on the contralateral side**

New H90.A11 **Conductive hearing loss, unilateral, right ear with restricted hearing on the contralateral side**

New H90.A12 **Conductive hearing loss, unilateral, left ear with restricted hearing on the contralateral side**

New H90.A2 **Sensorineural hearing loss, unilateral, with restricted hearing on the contralateral side**

New H90.A21 **Sensorineural hearing loss, unilateral, right ear, with restricted hearing on the contralateral side**

New H90.A22 **Sensorineural hearing loss, unilateral, left ear, with restricted hearing on the contralateral side**

New H90.A3 **Mixed conductive and sensorineural hearing loss, unilateral with restricted hearing on the contralateral side**

New H90.A31 **Mixed conductive and sensorineural hearing loss, unilateral, right ear with restricted hearing on the contralateral side**

New H90.A32 **Mixed conductive and sensorineural hearing loss, unilateral, left ear with restricted hearing on the contralateral side**

H93 **Other disorders of ear, not elsewhere classified**

New H93.A **Pulsatile tinnitus**

New H93.A1 **Pulsatile tinnitus, right ear**

New H93.A2 **Pulsatile tinnitus, left ear**

New H93.A3 **Pulsatile tinnitus, bilateral**

New H93.A9 **Pulsatile tinnitus, unspecified ear**

H95 **Intraoperative and postprocedural complications and disorders of ear and mastoid process, not elsewhere classified**

Revised H95.4 **Postprocedural hemorrhage of ear and mastoid process following a procedure**

Revised H95.41 **Postprocedural hemorrhage of ear and mastoid process following a procedure on the ear and mastoid process**

Revised H95.42 **Postprocedural hemorrhage of ear and mastoid process following other procedure**

New H95.5 **Postprocedural hematoma and seroma of ear and mastoid process following a procedure**

New H95.51 **Postprocedural hematoma of ear and mastoid process following a procedure on the ear and mastoid process**

New H95.52 **Postprocedural hematoma of ear and mastoid process following other procedure**

New H95.53 **Postprocedural seroma of ear and mastoid process following a procedure on the ear and mastoid process**

New H95.54 **Postprocedural seroma of ear and mastoid process following other procedure**

CHAPTER 9 DISEASES OF THE CIRCULATORY SYSTEM (I00-I99)

This chapter contains the following blocks:

Revised I10-I16 Hypertensive diseases

HYPERTENSIVE DISEASES (I10-I16)

Use additional code to identify:

Revised history of tobacco dependence (Z87.891)

New **Excludes2** hypertensive disease complicating pregnancy, childbirth and the puerperium (O10-O11, O13-O16)

New I16 **Hypertensive crisis**

New Code also any identified hypertensive disease (I10-I15)

New I16.0 **Hypertensive urgency**

New I16.1 **Hypertensive emergency**

New I16.9 **Hypertensive crisis, unspecified**

ISCHEMIC HEART DISEASES (I20-I25)

Revised Use additional code to identify presence of hypertension (I10-I16)

I20 Angina pectoris
Use additional code to identify:
Revised history of tobacco dependence (Z87.891)

I20.8 Other forms of angina pectoris
New Stable angina

I21 ST elevation (STEMI) and non-ST elevation (NSTEMI) myocardial infarction

I22 Subsequent ST elevation (STEMI) and non-ST elevation (NSTEMI) myocardial infarction

I25 Chronic ischemic heart disease
Use additional code to identify:
Revised history of tobacco dependence (Z87.891)

I42 Cardiomyopathy
Deleted **Excludes1** ischemic cardiomyopathy (I25.5)
Deleted peripartum cardiomyopathy (O90.3)
New **Excludes2** ischemic cardiomyopathy (I25.5)
New peripartum cardiomyopathy (O90.3)

I50 Heart failure
Deleted **Excludes1** cardiac arrest (I46.-)
New **Excludes2** cardiac arrest (I46.-)

I50.9 Heart failure, unspecified
Deleted **Excludes1** fluid overload (E87.70)
New **Excludes2** fluid overload (E87.70)

CEREBROVASCULAR DISEASES (I60-I69)

Use additional code to identify presence of:
Revised history of tobacco dependence (Z87.891)

I60 Nontraumatic subarachnoid hemorrhage
Deleted **Excludes1** sequelae of subarachnoid hemorrhage (I69.0-)
New **Excludes2** sequelae of subarachnoid hemorrhage (I69.0-)

I60.2 Nontraumatic subarachnoid hemorrhage from anterior communicating artery
Deleted ~~I60.20 Nontraumatic subarachnoid hemorrhage from unspecified anterior communicating artery~~
Deleted ~~I60.21 Nontraumatic subarachnoid hemorrhage from right anterior communicating artery~~
Deleted ~~I60.22 Nontraumatic subarachnoid hemorrhage from left anterior communicating artery~~

I61 Nontraumatic intracerebral hemorrhage
Deleted **Excludes1** sequelae of intracerebral hemorrhage (I69.1-)
New **Excludes2** sequelae of intracerebral hemorrhage (I69.1-)

I62 Other and unspecified nontraumatic intracranial hemorrhage
Deleted **Excludes1** sequelae of intracerebral hemorrhage (I69.2)
New **Excludes2** sequelae of intracranial hemorrhage (I69.2)

I63 Cerebral infarction
New Use additional code, if known, to indicate National Institutes of Health Stroke Scale (NIHSS) score (R29.7-)
Deleted **Excludes1** sequelae of cerebral infarction (I69.3-)
New **Excludes2** sequelae of cerebral infarction (I69.3-)
New **I63.013 Cerebral infarction due to thrombosis of bilateral vertebral arteries**

I63.03 Cerebral infarction due to thrombosis of carotid artery
New **I63.033 Cerebral infarction due to thrombosis of bilateral carotid arteries**

New **I63.113 Cerebral infarction due to embolism of bilateral vertebral arteries**

New **I63.133 Cerebral infarction due to embolism of bilateral carotid arteries**

New **I63.213 Cerebral infarction due to unspecified occlusion or stenosis of bilateral vertebral arteries**

New **I63.233 Cerebral infarction due to unspecified occlusion or stenosis of bilateral carotid arteries**

New **I63.313 Cerebral infarction due to thrombosis of bilateral middle cerebral arteries**

New **I63.323 Cerebral infarction due to thrombosis of bilateral anterior arteries**

New **I63.333 Cerebral infarction to thrombosis of bilateral posterior arteries**

New **I63.343 Cerebral infarction to thrombosis of bilateral cerebellar arteries**

New **I63.413 Cerebral infarction due to embolism of bilateral middle cerebral arteries**

New **I63.423 Cerebral infarction due to embolism of bilateral anterior cerebral arteries**

New **I63.433 Cerebral infarction due to embolism of bilateral posterior cerebral arteries**

New **I63.443 Cerebral infarction due to embolism of bilateral cerebellar arteries**

New **I63.513 Cerebral infarction due to unspecified occlusion or stenosis of bilateral middle arteries**

New **I63.523** **Cerebral infarction due to unspecified occlusion or stenosis of bilateral anterior arteries**

New **I63.533** **Cerebral infarction due to unspecified occlusion or stenosis of bilateral posterior arteries**

New **I63.543** **Cerebral infarction due to unspecified occlusion or stenosis of bilateral cerebellar arteries**

I67 **Other cerebrovascular diseases**

Deleted **Excludes1** sequelae of the listed conditions (I69.8)

New **Excludes2** sequelae of the listed conditions (I69.8)

New **I69.010** **Attention and concentration deficit following nontraumatic subarachnoid hemorrhage**

New **I69.011** **Memory deficit following nontraumatic subarachnoid hemorrhage**

New **I69.012** **Visuospatial deficit and spatial neglect following nontraumatic subarachnoid hemorrhage**

New **I69.013** **Psychomotor deficit following nontraumatic subarachnoid hemorrhage**

New **I69.014** **Frontal lobe and executive function deficit following nontraumatic subarachnoid hemorrhage**

New **I69.015** **Cognitive social or emotional deficit following nontraumatic subarachnoid hemorrhage**

New **I69.018** **Other symptoms and signs involving cognitive functions following nontraumatic subarachnoid hemorrhage**

New **I69.019** **Unspecified symptoms and signs involving cognitive functions following nontraumatic subarachnoid hemorrhage**

New **I69.110** **Attention and concentration deficit following nontraumatic intracerebral hemorrhage**

New **I69.111** **Memory deficit following nontraumatic intracerebral hemorrhage**

New **I69.112** **Visuospatial deficit and spatial neglect following nontraumatic intracerebral hemorrhage**

New **I69.113** **Psychomotor deficit following nontraumatic intracerebral hemorrhage**

New **I69.114** **Frontal lobe and executive function deficit following nontraumatic intracerebral hemorrhage**

New **I69.115** **Cognitive social or emotional deficit following nontraumatic intracerebral hemorrhage**

New **I69.118** **Other symptoms and signs involving cognitive functions following nontraumatic intracerebral hemorrhage**

New **I69.119** **Unspecified symptoms and signs involving cognitive functions following nontraumatic intracerebral hemorrhage**

I69.123 **Fluency disorder following nontraumatic intracerebral hemorrhage**

Revised Stuttering following nontraumatic intracerebral hemorrhage

I69.21 **Cognitive deficits following other nontraumatic intracranial hemorrhage**

New **I69.210** **Attention and concentration deficit following other nontraumatic intracranial hemorrhage**

New **I69.211** **Memory deficit following other nontraumatic intracranial hemorrhage**

New **I69.212** **Visuospatial deficit and spatial neglect following other nontraumatic intracranial hemorrhage**

New **I69.213** **Psychomotor deficit following other nontraumatic intracranial hemorrhage**

New **I69.214** **Frontal lobe and executive function deficit following other nontraumatic intracranial hemorrhage**

New **I69.215** **Cognitive social or emotional deficit following other nontraumatic intracranial hemorrhage**

New **I69.218** **Other symptoms and signs involving cognitive functions following other nontraumatic intracranial hemorrhage**

New **I69.219** **Unspecified symptoms and signs involving cognitive functions following other nontraumatic intracranial hemorrhage**

I69.223 **Fluency disorder following other nontraumatic intracranial hemorrhage**

Revised Stuttering following other nontraumatic intracranial hemorrhage

New **I69.310** **Attention and concentration deficit following cerebral infarction**

New **I69.311** **Memory deficit following cerebral infarction**

New **I69.312** **Visuospatial deficit and spatial neglect following cerebral infarction**

New **I69.313** **Psychomotor deficit following cerebral infarction**

New **I69.314** **Frontal lobe and executive function deficit following cerebral infarction**

New **I69.315** **Cognitive social or emotional deficit following cerebral infarction**

New **I69.318** **Other symptoms and signs involving cognitive functions following cerebral infarction**

New **I69.319** **Unspecified symptoms and signs involving cognitive functions following cerebral infarction**

I69.323 **Fluency disorder following cerebral infarction**

Revised Stuttering following cerebral infarction

New I69.810 **Attention and concentration deficit following other cerebrovascular disease**

New I69.811 **Memory deficit following other cerebrovascular disease**

New I69.812 **Visuospatial deficit and spatial neglect following other cerebrovascular disease**

New I69.813 **Psychomotor deficit following other cerebrovascular disease**

New I69.814 **Frontal lobe and executive function deficit following other cerebrovascular disease**

New I69.815 **Cognitive social or emotional deficit following other cerebrovascular disease**

New I69.818 **Other symptoms and signs involving cognitive functions following other cerebrovascular disease**

New I69.819 **Unspecified symptoms and signs involving cognitive functions following other cerebrovascular disease**

I69.823 **Fluency disorder following other cerebrovascular disease**

Revised Stuttering following other cerebrovascular disease

New I69.910 **Attention and concentration deficit following unspecified cerebrovascular disease**

New I69.911 **Memory deficit following unspecified cerebrovascular disease**

New I69.912 **Visuospatial deficit and spatial neglect following unspecified cerebrovascular disease**

New I69.913 **Psychomotor deficit following unspecified cerebrovascular disease**

New I69.914 **Frontal lobe and executive function deficit following unspecified cerebrovascular disease**

New I69.915 **Cognitive social or emotional deficit following unspecified cerebrovascular disease**

New I69.918 **Other symptoms and signs involving cognitive functions following unspecified cerebrovascular disease**

New I69.919 **Unspecified symptoms and signs involving cognitive functions following unspecified cerebrovascular disease**

I69.923 **Fluency disorder following unspecified cerebrovascular disease**

Revised Stuttering following unspecified cerebrovascular disease

I70 **Atherosclerosis**

Use additional code to identify:

Revised history of tobacco dependence (Z87.891)

I72 **Other aneurysm**

New **Excludes2** dissection of precerebral artery, congenital (nonruptured) (Q28.1)

New I72.5 **Aneurysm of other precerebral arteries**

New Aneurysm of basilar artery (trunk)

New **Excludes2** aneurysm of carotid artery (I72.0)

New aneurysm of vertebral artery (I72.6)

New dissection of carotid artery (I77.71)

New dissection of other precerebral arteries (I77.75)

New dissection of vertebral artery (I77.74)

New I72.6 **Aneurysm of vertebral artery**

New **Excludes2** dissection of vertebral artery (I77.74)

I74 **Arterial embolism and thrombosis**

Revised **Excludes2** mesenteric embolism and thrombosis (K55.0-)

New I77.70 **Dissection of unspecified artery**

I77.74 **Dissection of vertebral artery**

New **Excludes2** aneurysm of vertebral artery (I72.6)

New I77.75 **Dissection of other precerebral arteries**

New Dissection of basilar artery (trunk)

New **Excludes2** aneurysm of carotid artery (I72.0)

New aneurysm of other precerebral arteries (I72.5)

New aneurysm of vertebral artery (I72.6)

New dissection of carotid artery (I77.71)

New dissection of vertebral artery (I77.74)

New I77.76 **Dissection of artery of upper extremity**

New I77.77 **Dissection of artery of lower extremity**

Revised I77.79 **Dissection of other specified artery**

I82 **Other venous embolism and thrombosis**

Revised **Excludes2** mesenteric (K55.0-)

Deleted I83.1 **Varicose veins of lower extremities with inflammation**

Stasis dermatitis

New I87.2 **Venous insufficiency (chronic) (peripheral)**

Stasis dermatitis

New **Excludes1** stasis dermatitis with varicose veins of lower extremities (I83.1-, I83.2-)

I89 **Other noninfective disorders of lymphatic vessels and lymph nodes**

Revised **Excludes1** chylocele, tunica vaginalis (nonfilarial) NOS (N50.89)

I96 **Gangrene, not elsewhere classified**

Revised **Excludes1** gangrene in diabetes mellitus (E08-E13 with .52)

Revised I97.6 **Postprocedural hemorrhage, hematoma and seroma of a circulatory system organ or structure following a procedure**

Revised I97.61 **Postprocedural hemorrhage of a circulatory system organ or structure following a circulatory system procedure**

Revised I97.610 **Postprocedural hemorrhage of a circulatory system organ or structure following a cardiac catheterization**

Revised I97.611 **Postprocedural hemorrhage of a circulatory system organ or structure following cardiac bypass**

Revised I97.618 **Postprocedural hemorrhage of a circulatory system organ or structure following other circulatory system procedure**

Revised I97.62 **Postprocedural hemorrhage, hematoma and seroma of a circulatory system organ or structure following other procedure**

New I97.620 **Postprocedural hemorrhage of a circulatory system organ or structure following other procedure**

New I97.621 **Postprocedural hematoma of a circulatory system organ or structure following other procedure**

New I97.622 **Postprocedural seroma of a circulatory system organ or structure following other procedure**

New I97.63 **Postprocedural hematoma of a circulatory system organ or structure following a circulatory system procedure**

New I97.630 **Postprocedural hematoma of a circulatory system organ or structure following a cardiac catheterization**

New I97.631 **Postprocedural hematoma of a circulatory system organ or structure following cardiac bypass**

New I97.638 **Postprocedural hematoma of a circulatory system organ or structure following other circulatory system procedure**

New I97.64 **Postprocedural seroma of a circulatory system organ or structure following a circulatory system procedure**

New I97.640 **Postprocedural seroma of a circulatory system organ or structure following a cardiac catheterization**

New I97.641 **Postprocedural seroma of a circulatory system organ or structure following cardiac bypass**

New I97.648 **Postprocedural seroma of a circulatory system organ or structure following other circulatory system procedure**

Revised I97.820 **Postprocedural cerebrovascular infarction following cardiac surgery**

Revised I97.821 **Postprocedural cerebrovascular infarction following other surgery**

CHAPTER 1Ø

DISEASES OF THE RESPIRATORY SYSTEM (JØØ-J99)

J31 **Chronic rhinitis, nasopharyngitis and pharyngitis**
J32 **Chronic sinusitis**
J33 **Nasal polyp**
J35 **Chronic diseases of tonsils and adenoids**
J37 **Chronic laryngitis and laryngotracheitis**
J38 **Diseases of vocal cords and larynx, not elsewhere classified**
J4Ø **Bronchitis, not specified as acute or chronic**
J41 **Simple and mucopurulent chronic bronchitis**
J42 **Unspecified chronic bronchitis**
J43 **Emphysema**
J44 **Other chronic obstructive pulmonary disease**
Use additional code to identify:
Revised history of tobacco dependence (Z87.891)

Deleted **Excludes1** lung diseases due to external agents (J6Ø-J7Ø)

New **Excludes2** lung diseases due to external agents (J60-J70)

J45 **Asthma**
J47 **Bronchiectasis**
Use additional code to identify:
Revised history of tobacco dependence (Z87.891)

J47.Ø **Bronchiectasis with acute lower respiratory infection**
New Use additional code to identify the infection

J81 **Pulmonary edema**
Use additional code to identify:
Revised history of tobacco dependence (Z87.891)

J84.89 **Other specified interstitial pulmonary diseases**
Deleted Organizing pneumonia due to known underlying cause

Revised J95.83 **Postprocedural hemorrhage of a respiratory system organ or structure following a procedure**

Revised J95.83Ø **Postprocedural hemorrhage of a respiratory system organ or structure following a respiratory system procedure**

Revised J95.831 **Postprocedural hemorrhage of a respiratory system organ or structure following other procedure**

New J95.86 **Postprocedural hematoma and seroma of a respiratory system organ or structure following a procedure**

New J95.86Ø **Postprocedural hematoma of a respiratory system organ or structure following a respiratory system procedure**

New J95.861 **Postprocedural hematoma of a respiratory system organ or structure following other procedure**

New J95.862 **Postprocedural seroma of a respiratory system organ or structure following a respiratory system procedure**

New J95.863 **Postprocedural seroma of a respiratory system organ or structure following other procedure**

J98 Other respiratory disorders
Use additional code to identify:
Revised history of tobacco dependence (Z87.891)
J98.5 Diseases of mediastinum, not elsewhere classified
Deleted Fibrosis of mediastinum
Deleted Hernia of mediastinum
Deleted Retraction of mediastinum
Deleted Mediastinitis
New **J98.51 Mediastinitis**
New *Code first underlying condition, if applicable, such as postoperative mediastinitis (T81.-)*
New **J98.59 Other diseases of mediastinum, not elsewhere classified**
New Fibrosis of mediastinum
New Hernia of mediastinum
New Retraction of mediastinum

CHAPTER 11

DISEASES OF THE DIGESTIVE SYSTEM (KØØ-K95)

KØ2 Dental caries
New **Includes** caries of dentine
New dental cavities
New early childhood caries
New pre-eruptive caries
New recurrent caries (dentino enamel junction) (enamel) (to the pulp)

KØ2.52 Dental caries on pit and fissure surface penetrating into dentin
New Primary dental caries, cervical origin

KØ4.Ø Pulpitis
Deleted Reversible pulpitis
Deleted Irreversible pulpitis
New **KØ4.Ø1 Reversible pulpitis**
New **KØ4.Ø2 Irreversible pulpitis**

KØ5 Gingivitis and periodontal diseases
Use additional code to identify:
Revised history of tobacco dependence (Z87.891)

KØ5.ØØ Acute gingivitis, plaque induced
New Plaque induced gingival disease
KØ5.1 Chronic gingivitis
New Pregnancy associated gingivitis
New *Code first, if applicable, diseases of the digestive system complicating pregnancy (O99.61-)*

New **KØ5.211 Aggressive periodontitis, localized, slight**
New **KØ5.212 Aggressive periodontitis, localized, moderate**
New **KØ5.213 Aggressive periodontitis, localized, severe**
New **KØ5.219 Aggressive periodontitis, localized, unspecified severity**
New **KØ5.221 Aggressive periodontitis, generalized, slight**
New **KØ5.222 Aggressive periodontitis, generalized, moderate**
New **KØ5.223 Aggressive periodontitis, generalized, severe**
New **KØ5.229 Aggressive periodontitis, generalized, unspecified severity**

New **KØ5.311 Chronic periodontitis, localized, slight**
New **KØ5.312 Chronic periodontitis, localized, moderate**
New **KØ5.313 Chronic periodontitis, localized, severe**
New **KØ5.319 Chronic periodontitis, localized, unspecified severity**
New **KØ5.321 Chronic periodontitis, generalized, slight**
New **KØ5.322 Chronic periodontitis, generalized, moderate**
New **KØ5.323 Chronic periodontitis, generalized, severe**
New **KØ5.329 Chronic periodontitis, generalized, unspecified severity**
KØ5.5 Other periodontal diseases
New Combined periodontic-endodontic lesion
New Narrow gingival width (of periodontal soft tissue)

New **KØ6.3 Horizontal alveolar bone loss**

KØ6.8 Other specified disorders of gingiva and edentulous alveolar ridge
New Vertical ridge deficiency

KØ8.8 Other specified disorders of teeth and supporting structures
Deleted Enlargement of alveolar ridge NOS
Deleted Irregular alveolar process
Deleted Toothache NOS
New **KØ8.81 Primary occlusal trauma**
New **KØ8.82 Secondary occlusal trauma**
New **KØ8.89 Other specified disorders of teeth and supporting structures**
New Enlargement of alveolar ridge NOS
New Insufficient anatomic crown height
New Insufficient clinical crown length
New Irregular alveolar process
New Toothache NOS

K11 Diseases of salivary glands
K12 Stomatitis and related lesions
K13 Other diseases of lip and oral mucosa
K14 Diseases of tongue
Use additional code to identify:
Revised history of tobacco dependence (Z87.891)

K35.3 Acute appendicitis with localized peritonitis
Revised Acute appendicitis with or without perforation or rupture with peritonitis NOS

NONINFECTIVE ENTERITIS AND COLITIS (K5Ø-K52)
Revised **Excludes1** megacolon (K59.3-)
K52.2 Allergic and dietetic gastroenteritis and colitis
New **Excludes2** allergic eosinophilic colitis (K52.82)
New allergic eosinophilic esophagitis (K2Ø.Ø)
New allergic eosinophilic gastritis (K52.81)
New allergic eosinophilic gastroenteritis (K52.81)
New food protein-induced proctocolitis (K52.82)
New **K52.21 Food protein-induced enterocolitis syndrome**
New Use additional code for hypovolemic shock, if present (R57.1)
New **K52.22 Food protein-induced enteropathy**
K52.29 Other allergic and dietetic gastroenteritis and colitis
New Food hypersensitivity gastroenteritis or colitis
New Immediate gastrointestinal hypersensitivity

New **K52.3 Indeterminate colitis**
New Colonic inflammatory bowel disease unclassified (IBDU)
New **Excludes1** unspecified colitis (K52.9)

K52.81 Eosinophilic gastritis or gastroenteritis
Eosinophilic enteritis
Deleted **Excludes1** eosinophilic esophagitis (K20.0)
New **Excludes2** eosinophilic esophagitis (K20.0)

K52.82 Eosinophilic colitis
New Allergic proctocolitis
New Food-induced eosinophilic proctocolitis
New Food protein-induced proctocolitis
New Milk protein-induced proctocolitis
New **K52.83 Microscopic colitis**
New **K52.831 Collagenous colitis**
New **K52.832 Lymphocytic colitis**
New **K52.838 Other microscopic colitis**
New **K52.839 Microscopic colitis, unspecified**

K52.89 Other specified noninfective gastroenteritis and colitis
Deleted Collagenous colitis
Deleted Lymphocytic colitis
Deleted Microscopic colitis (collagenous or lymphocytic)

K55.0 Acute vascular disorders of intestine
Deleted Acute fulminant ischemic colitis
Deleted Acute intestinal infarction
Deleted Acute small intestine ischemia
Deleted Necrosis of intestine
Deleted Subacute ischemic colitis
New **K55.01 Acute (reversible) ischemia of small intestine**
New **K55.011 Focal (segmental) acute (reversible) ischemia of small intestine**
New **K55.012 Diffuse acute (reversible) ischemia of small intestine**
New **K55.019 Acute (reversible) ischemia of small intestine, extent unspecified**
New **K55.02 Acute infarction of small intestine**
New Gangrene of small intestine
New Necrosis of small intestine
New **K55.021 Focal (segmental) acute infarction of small intestine**
New **K55.022 Diffuse acute infarction of small intestine**
New **K55.029 Acute infarction of small intestine, extent unspecified**
New **K55.03 Acute (reversible) ischemia of large intestine**
New Acute fulminant ischemic colitis
New Subacute ischemic colitis
New **K55.031 Focal (segmental) acute (reversible) ischemia of large intestine**
New **K55.032 Diffuse acute (reversible) ischemia of large intestine**
New **K55.039 Acute (reversible) ischemia of large intestine, extent unspecified**
New **K55.04 Acute infarction of large intestine**
New Gangrene of large intestine
New Necrosis of large intestine
New **K55.041 Focal (segmental) acute infarction of large intestine**
New **K55.042 Diffuse acute infarction of large intestine**
New **K55.049 Acute infarction of large intestine, extent unspecified**
New **K55.05 Acute (reversible) ischemia of intestine, part unspecified**
New **K55.051 Focal (segmental) acute (reversible) ischemia of intestine, part unspecified**
New **K55.052 Diffuse acute (reversible) ischemia of intestine, part unspecified**
New **K55.059 Acute (reversible) ischemia of intestine, part and extent unspecified**
New **K55.06 Acute infarction of intestine, part unspecified**
New Acute intestinal infarction
New Gangrene of intestine
New Necrosis of intestine
New **K55.061 Focal (segmental) acute infarction of intestine, part unspecified**
New **K55.062 Diffuse acute infarction of intestine, part unspecified**
New **K55.069 Acute infarction of intestine, part and extent unspecified**
New **K55.3 Necrotizing enterocolitis**
New **Excludes1** necrotizing enterocolitis of newborn (P77.-)
New **Excludes2** necrotizing enterocolitis due to Clostridium difficile (A04.7)
New **K55.30 Necrotizing enterocolitis, unspecified**
New Necrotizing enterocolitis, NOS
New **K55.31 Stage 1 necrotizing enterocolitis**
New Necrotizing enterocolitis without pneumatosis, without perforation
New **K55.32 Stage 2 necrotizing enterocolitis**
New Necrotizing enterocolitis with pneumatosis, without perforation
New **K55.33 Stage 3 necrotizing enterocolitis**
New Necrotizing enterocolitis with perforation
New Necrotizing enterocolitis with pneumatosis and perforation

New **K58.1 Irritable bowel syndrome with constipation**
New **K58.2 Mixed irritable bowel syndrome**
New **K58.8 Other irritable bowel syndrome**

K59.0 Constipation
New Use additional code for adverse effect, if applicable, to identify drug (T36-T50 with fifth or sixth character 5)
New **K59.03 Drug induced constipation**
New Use additional code for adverse effect, if applicable, to identify drug (T36-T50 with fifth or sixth character 5)
New **K59.04 Chronic idiopathic constipation**
New Functional constipation
New **K59.09 Other constipation**
New Chronic constipation

K59.3 Megacolon, not elsewhere classified
Deleted Toxic colon
New **K59.31 Toxic megacolon**
New **K59.39 Other megacolon**
New Megacolon NOS

K72 Hepatic failure, not elsewhere classified
Deleted Includes acute hepatitis NEC, with hepatic failure
Deleted Excludes1 viral hepatitis with hepatic coma (B15-B19)
New Excludes2 viral hepatitis with hepatic coma (B15-B19)

K72.Ø Acute and subacute hepatic failure
New Acute non-viral hepatitis NOS

K75.Ø Abscess of liver
New Excludes2 acute or subacute hepatitis NOS (B17.9)
New acute or subacute non-viral hepatitis (K72.Ø)
New chronic hepatitis NEC (K73.8)

K76.7 Hepatorenal syndrome
Revised Excludes1 postprocedural hepatorenal syndrome (K91.83)

K85 Acute pancreatitis
Deleted Includes abscess of pancreas
Deleted acute necrosis of pancreas
Deleted gangrene of (gangrenous) pancreas
Deleted hemorrhagic pancreatitis
Deleted infective necrosis of pancreas
Deleted suppurative pancreatitis

New **K85.ØØ Idiopathic acute pancreatitis without necrosis or infection**
New **K85.Ø1 Idiopathic acute pancreatitis with uninfected necrosis**
New **K85.Ø2 Idiopathic acute pancreatitis with infected necrosis**
New **K85.1Ø Biliary acute pancreatitis without necrosis or infection**
New **K85.11 Biliary acute pancreatitis with uninfected necrosis**
New **K85.12 Biliary acute pancreatitis with infected necrosis**
New **K85.2Ø Alcohol induced acute pancreatitis without necrosis or infection**
New **K85.21 Alcohol induced acute pancreatitis with uninfected necrosis**
New **K85.22 Alcohol induced acute pancreatitis with infected necrosis**
New **K85.3Ø Drug induced acute pancreatitis without necrosis or infection**
New **K85.31 Drug induced acute pancreatitis with uninfected necrosis**
New **K85.32 Drug induced acute pancreatitis with infected necrosis**
New **K85.8Ø Other acute pancreatitis without necrosis or infection**
New **K85.81 Other acute pancreatitis with uninfected necrosis**
New **K85.82 Other acute pancreatitis with infected necrosis**
New **K85.9Ø Acute pancreatitis without necrosis or infection, unspecified**
New **K85.91 Acute pancreatitis with uninfected necrosis, unspecified**
New **K85.92 Acute pancreatitis with infected necrosis, unspecified**

K86.Ø Alcohol-induced chronic pancreatitis
New Code also exocrine pancreatic insufficiency (K86.81)
Revised Excludes2 alcohol induced acute pancreatitis (K85.2-)

K86.1 Other chronic pancreatitis
New Code also exocrine pancreatic insufficiency (K86.81)

K86.8 Other specified diseases of pancreas
Deleted Aseptic pancreatic necrosis
Deleted Atrophy of pancreas
Deleted Calculus of pancreas
Deleted Cirrhosis of pancreas
Deleted Fibrosis of pancreas
Deleted Pancreatic fat necrosis
Deleted Pancreatic infantilism
Deleted Pancreatic necrosis NOS
New **K86.81 Exocrine pancreatic insufficiency**
New **K86.89 Other specified diseases of pancreas**
New Aseptic pancreatic necrosis, unrelated to acute pancreatitis
New Atrophy of pancreas
New Calculus of pancreas
New Cirrhosis of pancreas
New Fibrosis of pancreas
New Pancreatic fat necrosis, unrelated to acute pancreatitis
New Pancreatic infantilism
New Pancreatic necrosis NOS, unrelated to acute pancreatitis

K90.Ø Celiac disease
New Celiac disease with steatorrhea
Deleted Idiopathic steatorrhea
New Code also exocrine pancreatic insufficiency (K86.81)

K90.4 Other malabsorption due to intolerance
Deleted Malabsorption due to intolerance to carbohydrate
Deleted Malabsorption due to intolerance to fat
Deleted Malabsorption due to intolerance to protein
Deleted Malabsorption due to intolerance to starch
New **K90.41 Non-celiac gluten sensitivity**
New Gluten sensitivity NOS
New Non-celiac gluten sensitive enteropathy
New **K90.49 Malabsorption due to intolerance, not elsewhere classified**
New Malabsorption due to intolerance to carbohydrate
New Malabsorption due to intolerance to fat
New Malabsorption due to intolerance to protein
New Malabsorption due to intolerance to starch

Revised **K91.61 Intraoperative hemorrhage and hematoma of a digestive system organ or structure complicating a digestive system procedure**
Revised **K91.84 Postprocedural hemorrhage of a digestive system organ or structure following a procedure**
Revised **K91.84Ø Postprocedural hemorrhage of a digestive system organ or structure following a digestive system procedure**
Revised **K91.841 Postprocedural hemorrhage of a digestive system organ or structure following other procedure**

New K91.87 **Postprocedural hematoma and seroma of a digestive system organ or structure following a procedure**

New K91.870 **Postprocedural hematoma of a digestive system organ or structure following a digestive system procedure**

New K91.871 **Postprocedural hematoma of a digestive system organ or structure following other procedure**

New K91.872 **Postprocedural seroma of a digestive system organ or structure following a digestive system procedure**

New K91.873 **Postprocedural seroma of a digestive system organ or structure following other procedure**

CHAPTER 12

DISEASES OF THE SKIN AND SUBCUTANEOUS TISSUE (L00-L99)

L02.2 **Cutaneous abscess, furuncle and carbuncle of trunk**

Revised **Excludes2** abscess of breast (N61.1)

L03.211 **Cellulitis of face**

New **Excludes2** abscess of orbit (H05.01-)

Revised cellulitis of orbit (H05.01-)

New L03.213 **Periorbital cellulitis**

New Preseptal cellulitis

L03.31 **Cellulitis of trunk**

Revised **Excludes2** cellulitis of breast NOS (N61.0)

L05.01 **Pilonidal cyst with abscess**

Deleted Parasacral dimple with abscess

New **Excludes2** congenital sacral dimple (Q82.6)

New parasacral dimple (Q82.6)

L05.91 **Pilonidal cyst without abscess**

Deleted Parasacral dimple

New **Excludes2** congenital sacral dimple (Q82.6)

New parasacral dimple (Q82.6)

DERMATITIS AND ECZEMA (L20-L30)

Revised **Excludes2** stasis dermatitis (I87.2)

L30 **Other and unspecified dermatitis**

Revised **Excludes2** stasis dermatitis (I87.2)

L50.2 **Urticaria due to cold and heat**

New **Excludes2** familial cold urticaria (M04.2)

L70 **Acne**

Revised L70.5 **Acné excoriée**

New Acné excoriée des jeunes filles

Revised L76.2 **Postprocedural hemorrhage of skin and subcutaneous tissue following a procedure**

Revised L76.21 **Postprocedural hemorrhage of skin and subcutaneous tissue following a dermatologic procedure**

Revised L76.22 **Postprocedural hemorrhage of skin and subcutaneous tissue following other procedure**

New L76.3 **Postprocedural hematoma and seroma of skin and subcutaneous tissue following a procedure**

New L76.31 **Postprocedural hematoma of skin and subcutaneous tissue following a dermatologic procedure**

New L76.32 **Postprocedural hematoma of skin and subcutaneous tissue following other procedure**

New L76.33 **Postprocedural seroma of skin and subcutaneous tissue following a dermatologic procedure**

New L76.34 **Postprocedural seroma of skin and subcutaneous tissue following other procedure**

L82 **Seborrheic keratosis**

New **Includes** basal cell papilloma

L89.521 **Pressure ulcer of left ankle, stage 1**

Revised Pressure pre-ulcer skin changes limited to persistent focal edema, left ankle

L98.1 **Factitial dermatitis**

New **Excludes1** Excoriation (skin-picking) disorder (F42.4)

New L98.7 **Excessive and redundant skin and subcutaneous tissue**

New Loose or sagging skin following bariatric surgery weight loss

New Loose or sagging skin following dietary weight loss

New Loose or sagging skin, NOS

New **Excludes2** acquired excess or redundant skin of eyelid (H02.3-)

New congenital excess or redundant skin of eyelid (Q10.3)

New skin changes due to chronic exposure to nonionizing radiation (L57.-)

CHAPTER 13

DISEASES OF THE MUSCULOSKELETAL SYSTEM AND CONNECTIVE TISSUE (M00-M99)

This chapter contains the following blocks:

New	M04	Autoinflammatory syndromes
New	M97	Periprosthetic fracture around internal prosthetic joint

New
AUTOINFLAMMATORY SYNDROMES (M04)

New M04 **Autoinflammatory syndromes**

New **Excludes2** Crohn's disease (K50.-)

New M04.1 **Periodic fever syndromes**

New Familial Mediterranean fever

New Hyperimmunoglobin D syndrome

New Mevalonate kinase deficiency

New Tumor necrosis factor receptor associated periodic syndrome [TRAPS]

New M04.2 **Cryopyrin-associated periodic syndromes**

New Chronic infantile neurological, cutaneous and articular syndrome [CINCA]

New Familial cold autoinflammatory syndrome

New Familial cold urticaria

New Muckle-Wells syndrome

New Neonatal onset multisystemic inflammatory disorder [NOMID]

New **M04.8 Other autoinflammatory syndromes**
New Blau syndrome
New Deficiency of interleukin 1 receptor antagonist [DIRA]
New Majeed syndrome
New Periodic fever, aphthous stomatitis, pharyngitis, and adenopathy syndrome [PFAPA]
New Pyogenic arthritis, pyoderma gangrenosum, and acne syndrome [PAPA]
New **M04.9 Autoinflammatory syndrome, unspecified**

M1A Chronic gout
Deleted **Excludes1** acute gout (M10.-)
New **Excludes2** acute gout (M10.-)

M10 Gout
Deleted Gout NOS
Deleted **Excludes1** chronic gout (M1A.-)
New **Excludes2** chronic gout (M1A.-)

M20.1 Hallux valgus (acquired)
Deleted Bunion
New **Excludes2** bunion (M21.6-)

M21.1 Varus deformity, not elsewhere classified
Revised **Excludes1** metatarsus varus (Q66.22)

M21.6 Other acquired deformities of foot
Revised **Excludes2** deformities of toe (acquired) (M20.1-M20.6-)

New **M21.61 Bunion**
New **M21.611 Bunion of right foot**
New **M21.612 Bunion of left foot**
New **M21.619 Bunion of unspecified foot**
New **M21.62 Bunionette**
New **M21.621 Bunionette of right foot**
New **M21.622 Bunionette of left foot**
New **M21.629 Bunionette of unspecified foot**

New **M25.5 Pain in joint**
New **M25.54 Pain in joints of hand**
New **M25.541 Pain in joints of right hand**
New **M25.542 Pain in joints of left hand**
New **M25.549 Pain in joints of unspecified hand**
New Pain in joints of hand NOS

New **M26.601 Right temporomandibular joint disorder, unspecified**
New **M26.602 Left temporomandibular joint disorder, unspecified**
New **M26.603 Bilateral temporomandibular joint disorder, unspecified**
New **M26.609 Unspecified temporomandibular joint disorder, unspecified side**
New Temporomandibular joint disorder NOS

New **M26.611 Adhesions and ankylosis of right temporomandibular joint**
New **M26.612 Adhesions and ankylosis of left temporomandibular joint**
New **M26.613 Adhesions and ankylosis of bilateral temporomandibular joint**
New **M26.619 Adhesions and ankylosis of temporomandibular joint, unspecified side**

New **M26.621 Arthralgia of right temporomandibular joint**
New **M26.622 Arthralgia of left temporomandibular joint**
New **M26.623 Arthralgia of bilateral temporomandibular joint**
New **M26.629 Arthralgia of temporomandibular joint, unspecified side**

New **M26.631 Articular disc disorder of right temporomandibular joint**
New **M26.632 Articular disc disorder of left temporomandibular joint**
New **M26.633 Articular disc disorder of bilateral temporomandibular joint**
New **M26.639 Articular disc disorder of temporomandibular joint, unspecified side**

M48.5 Collapsed vertebra, not elsewhere classified
New Compression fracture of vertebra NOS

M50.02 Cervical disc disorder with myelopathy, mid-cervical region
Deleted C4-C5 disc disorder with myelopathy
Deleted C5-C6 disc disorder with myelopathy
Deleted C6-C7 disc disorder with myelopathy
New **M50.020 Cervical disc disorder with myelopathy, mid-cervical region, unspecified level**
New **M50.021 Cervical disc disorder at C4-C5 level with myelopathy**
C4-C5 disc disorder with myelopathy
New **M50.022 Cervical disc disorder at C5-C6 level with myelopathy**
C5-C6 disc disorder with myelopathy
New **M50.023 Cervical disc disorder at C6-C7 level with myelopathy**
C6-C7 disc disorder with myelopathy

M50.12 Cervical disc disorder with radiculopathy, mid-cervical region
Deleted C4-C5 disc disorder with radiculopathy
Deleted C5 radiculopathy due to disc disorder
Deleted C5-C6 disc disorder with radiculopathy
Deleted C6 radiculopathy due to disc disorder
Deleted C6-C7 disc disorder with radiculopathy
Deleted C7 radiculopathy due to disc disorder
New **M50.120 Mid-cervical disc disorder, unspecified**
New **M50.121 Cervical disc disorder at C4-C5 level with radiculopathy**
New C4-C5 disc disorder with radiculopathy
New C5 radiculopathy due to disc disorder
New **M50.122 Cervical disc disorder at C5-C6 level with radiculopathy**
New C5-C6 disc disorder with radiculopathy
New C6 radiculopathy due to disc disorder
New **M50.123 Cervical disc disorder at C6-C7 level with radiculopathy**
New C6-C7 disc disorder with radiculopathy
New C7 radiculopathy due to disc disorder

M50.22 Other cervical disc displacement, mid-cervical region
Deleted Other C4-C5 cervical disc displacement
Deleted Other C5-C6 cervical disc displacement
Deleted Other C6-C7 cervical disc displacement
New **M50.220 Other cervical disc displacement, mid-cervical region, unspecified level**
New **M50.221 Other cervical disc displacement at C4-C5 level**
New Other C4-C5 cervical disc displacement
New **M50.222 Other cervical disc displacement at C5-C6 level**
New Other C5-C6 cervical disc displacement
New **M50.223 Other cervical disc displacement at C6-C7 level**
New Other C6-C7 cervical disc displacement

M50.32 Other cervical disc degeneration, mid-cervical region
Deleted Other C4-C5 cervical disc displacement
Deleted Other C5-C6 cervical disc displacement
Deleted Other C6-C7 cervical disc displacement
New **M50.320 Other cervical disc degeneration, mid-cervical region, unspecified level**
New **M50.321 Other cervical disc degeneration at C4-C5 level**
New Other C4-C5 cervical disc degeneration
New **M50.322 Other cervical disc degeneration at C5-C6 level**
New Other C5-C6 cervical disc degeneration
New **M50.323 Other cervical disc degeneration at C6-C7 level**
New Other C6-C7 cervical disc degeneration

M50.82 Other cervical disc disorders, mid-cervical region
Deleted Other C4-C5 cervical disc disorders
Deleted Other C5-C6 cervical disc disorders
Deleted Other C6-C7 cervical disc disorders
New **M50.820 Other cervical disc disorders, mid-cervical region, unspecified level**
New **M50.821 Other cervical disc disorders at C4-C5 level**
New Other C4-C5 cervical disc disorders
New **M50.822 Other cervical disc disorders at C5-C6 level**
New Other C5-C6 cervical disc disorders
New **M50.823 Other cervical disc disorders at C6-C7 level**
New Other C6-C7 cervical disc disorders

M50.92 Cervical disc disorder, unspecified, mid-cervical region
Deleted C4-C5 cervical disc disorder, unspecified
Deleted C5-C6 cervical disc disorder, unspecified
Deleted C6-C7 cervical disc disorder, unspecified
New **M50.920 Unspecified cervical disc disorder, mid-cervical region, unspecified level**
New **M50.921 Unspecified cervical disc disorder at C4-C5 level**
New Unspecified C4-C5 cervical disc disorder
New **M50.922 Unspecified cervical disc disorder at C5-C6 level**
New Unspecified C5-C6 cervical disc disorder
New **M50.923 Unspecified cervical disc disorder at C6-C7 level**
New Unspecified C6-C7 cervical disc disorder

M62.5 Muscle wasting and atrophy, not elsewhere classified
New **Excludes1** sarcopenia (M62.84)

M62.81 Muscle weakness (generalized)
New **Excludes1** muscle weakness in sarcopenia (M62.84)

New **M62.84 Sarcopenia**
New Age-related sarcopenia
New *Code first underlying disease, if applicable, such as:*
New disorders of myoneural junction and muscle disease in diseases classified elsewhere (G73.-)
New other and unspecified myopathies (G72.-)
New primary disorders of muscles (G71.-)

M71.5 Other bursitis, not elsewhere classified
Revised **Excludes2** bursitis of shoulder (M75.5)
bursitis of tibial collateral [Pellegrini-Stieda] (M76.4-)

New **M84.7 Nontraumatic fracture, not elsewhere classified**
New **M84.75 Atypical femoral fracture**
New The appropriate 7th character is to be added to each code from M84.75:

A	initial encounter for fracture
D	subsequent encounter for fracture with routine healing
G	subsequent encounter for fracture with delayed healing
K	subsequent encounter for fracture with nonunion
P	subsequent encounter for fracture with malunion
S	sequela

New **M84.750 Atypical femoral fracture, unspecified**
New **M84.751 Incomplete atypical femoral fracture, right leg**
New **M84.752 Incomplete atypical femoral fracture, left leg**
New **M84.753 Incomplete atypical femoral fracture, unspecified leg**
New **M84.754 Complete transverse atypical femoral fracture, right leg**
New **M84.755 Complete transverse atypical femoral fracture, left leg**
New **M84.756 Complete transverse atypical femoral fracture, unspecified leg**
New **M84.757 Complete oblique atypical femoral fracture, right leg**
New **M84.758 Complete oblique atypical femoral fracture, left leg**
New **M84.759 Complete oblique atypical femoral fracture, unspecified leg**

M90 Osteopathies in diseases classified elsewhere
Revised **Excludes1** diabetes mellitus (E08-E13 with .69-)

M96 Intraoperative and postprocedural complications and disorders of musculoskeletal system, not elsewhere classified

New **Excludes2** periprosthetic fracture around internal prosthetic joint (M97.-)

Revised **M96.83 Postprocedural hemorrhage of a musculoskeletal structure following a procedure**

Revised **M96.830 Postprocedural hemorrhage of a musculoskeletal structure following a musculoskeletal system procedure**

Revised **M96.831 Postprocedural hemorrhage of a musculoskeletal structure following other procedure**

New **M96.84 Postprocedural hematoma and seroma of a musculoskeletal structure following a procedure**

New **M96.840 Postprocedural hematoma of a musculoskeletal structure following a musculoskeletal system procedure**

New **M96.841 Postprocedural hematoma of a musculoskeletal structure following other procedure**

New **M96.842 Postprocedural seroma of a musculoskeletal structure following a musculoskeletal system procedure**

New **M96.843 Postprocedural seroma of a musculoskeletal structure following other procedure**

New **PERIPROSTHETIC FRACTURE AROUND INTERNAL PROSTHETIC JOINT (M97)**

New **M97 Periprosthetic fracture around internal prosthetic joint**

New **Excludes2** fracture of bone following insertion of orthopedic implant, joint prosthesis or bone plate (M96.6-)

New breakage (fracture) of prosthetic joint (T84.01-)

New The appropriate 7th character is to be added to each code from category M97:

New A initial encounter
New D subsequent encounter
New S sequela

New **M97.0 Periprosthetic fracture around internal prosthetic hip joint**

New **M97.01 Periprosthetic fracture around internal prosthetic right hip joint**

New **M97.02 Periprosthetic fracture around internal prosthetic left hip joint**

New **M97.1 Periprosthetic fracture around internal prosthetic knee joint**

New **M97.11 Periprosthetic fracture around internal prosthetic right knee joint**

New **M97.12 Periprosthetic fracture around internal prosthetic left knee joint**

New **M97.2 Periprosthetic fracture around internal prosthetic ankle joint**

New **M97.21 Periprosthetic fracture around internal prosthetic right ankle joint**

New **M97.22 Periprosthetic fracture around internal prosthetic left ankle joint**

New **M97.3 Periprosthetic fracture around internal prosthetic shoulder joint**

New **M97.31 Periprosthetic fracture around internal prosthetic right shoulder joint**

New **M97.32 Periprosthetic fracture around internal prosthetic left shoulder joint**

New **M97.4 Periprosthetic fracture around internal prosthetic elbow joint**

New **M97.41 Periprosthetic fracture around internal prosthetic right elbow joint**

New **M97.42 Periprosthetic fracture around internal prosthetic left elbow joint**

New **M97.8 Periprosthetic fracture around other internal prosthetic joint**

New Periprosthetic fracture around internal prosthetic finger joint

New Periprosthetic fracture around internal prosthetic spinal joint

New Periprosthetic fracture around internal prosthetic toe joint

New Periprosthetic fracture around internal prosthetic wrist joint

New Use additional code to identify the joint (Z96.6-)

New **M97.9 Periprosthetic fracture around unspecified internal prosthetic joint**

CHAPTER 14

DISEASES OF THE GENITOURINARY SYSTEM (N00-N99)

Revised **N10 Acute pyelonephritis**

Revised Acute tubulo-interstitial nephritis

New **N13.0 Hydronephrosis with ureteropelvic junction obstruction**

New Hydronephrosis due to acquired occlusion of ureteropelvic junction

New **Excludes2** Hydronephrosis with ureteropelvic junction obstruction due to calculus (N13.2)

Revised **N13.6 Pyonephrosis**
Conditions in N13.0-N13.5 with infection

N36.0 Urethral fistula

New **Excludes1** urethroscrotal fistula (N50.89)

N36.8 Other specified disorders of urethra

New **Excludes1** congenital urethrocele (Q64.7)

New female urethrocele (N81.0)

N39.42 Incontinence without sensory awareness

New Insensible (urinary) incontinence

N39.49 Other specified urinary incontinence

New **N39.491 Coital incontinence**

New **N39.492 Postural (urinary) incontinence**

N40 Benign prostatic hyperplasia

Deleted **Includes** benign prostatic hyperplasia

New enlarged prostate

Revised **N40.0 Benign prostatic hyperplasia without lower urinary tract symptoms**

Revised **N40.1 Benign prostatic hyperplasia with lower urinary tract symptoms**

N42.3 Dysplasia of prostate

Deleted Prostatic intraepithelial neoplasia I (PIN I)

Deleted Prostatic intraepithelial neoplasia II (PIN II)

Deleted **Excludes1** prostatic intraepithelial neoplasia III (PIN III) (D07.5)

New **N42.30 Unspecified dysplasia of prostate**

New **N42.31 Prostatic intraepithelial neoplasia**

New PIN

New Prostatic intraepithelial neoplasia I (PIN I)

New Prostatic intraepithelial neoplasia II (PIN II)

New **Excludes1** prostatic intraepithelial neoplasia III (PIN III) (D07.5)

New **N42.32 Atypical small acinar proliferation of prostate**

New **N42.39 Other dysplasia of prostate**

N50.8 Other specified disorders of male genital organs

Deleted Atrophy of scrotum, seminal vesicle, spermatic cord, tunica vaginalis and vas deferens

Deleted Edema of scrotum, seminal vesicle, spermatic cord, testis, tunica vaginalis and vas deferens

Deleted Hypertrophy of scrotum, seminal vesicle, spermatic cord, testis, tunica vaginalis and vas deferens

Deleted Ulcer of scrotum, seminal vesicle, spermatic cord, testis, tunica vaginalis and vas deferens

Deleted Chylocele, tunica vaginalis (nonfilarial) NOS

Deleted Urethroscrotal fistula

Deleted Stricture of spermatic cord, tunica vaginalis, and vas deferens

New **N50.81 Testicular pain**

New **N50.811 Right testicular pain**

New **N50.812 Left testicular pain**

New **N50.819 Testicular pain, unspecified**

New **N50.82 Scrotal pain**

New **N50.89 Other specified disorders of the male genital organs**

New Atrophy of scrotum, seminal vesicle, spermatic cord, tunica vaginalis and vas deferens

New Chylocele, tunica vaginalis (nonfilarial) NOS

New Edema of scrotum, seminal vesicle, spermatic cord, tunica vaginalis and vas deferens

New Hypertrophy of scrotum, seminal vesicle, spermatic cord, tunica vaginalis and vas deferens

New Stricture of spermatic cord, tunica vaginalis, and vas deferens

New Ulcer of scrotum, seminal vesicle, spermatic cord, testis, tunica vaginalis and vas deferens

New Urethroscrotal fistula

Revised **N52.3 Postprocedural erectile dysfunction**

New **N52.35 Erectile dysfunction following radiation therapy**

New **N52.36 Erectile dysfunction following interstitial seed therapy**

New **N52.37 Erectile dysfunction following prostate ablative therapy**

New Erectile dysfunction following cryotherapy

New Erectile dysfunction following other prostate ablative therapies

New Erectile dysfunction following ultrasound ablative therapies

Revised **N52.39 Other and unspecified postprocedural erectile dysfunction**

N61 Inflammatory disorders of breast

Deleted Abscess (acute) (chronic) (nonpuerperal) of areola

Deleted Abscess (acute) (chronic) (nonpuerperal) of breast

Deleted Carbuncle of breast

Deleted Infective mastitis (acute) (subacute) (nonpuerperal)

Deleted Mastitis (acute) (subacute) (nonpuerperal) NOS

New **N61.0 Mastitis without abscess**

New Infective mastitis (acute) (nonpuerperal) (subacute)

New Mastitis (acute) (nonpuerperal) (subacute) NOS

New Cellulitis (acute) (nonpuerperal) (subacute) of breast NOS

New Cellulitis (acute) (nonpuerperal) (subacute) of nipple NOS

New **N61.1 Abscess of the breast and nipple**

New Abscess (acute) (chronic) (nonpuerperal) of areola

New Abscess (acute) (chronic) (nonpuerperal) of breast

New Carbuncle of breast

New Mastitis with abscess

N64.1 Fat necrosis of breast

Revised *Code first breast necrosis due to breast graft (T85.898)*

N81 Female genital prolapse

Revised **Excludes1** prolapse and hernia of ovary and fallopian tube (N83.4-)

New **N83.00 Follicular cyst of ovary, unspecified side**

New **N83.01 Follicular cyst of right ovary**

New **N83.02 Follicular cyst of left ovary**

New **N83.10 Corpus luteum cyst of ovary, unspecified side**

New **N83.11 Corpus luteum cyst of right ovary**

New **N83.12 Corpus luteum cyst of left ovary**

N83.20 Unspecified ovarian cysts

New **N83.201 Unspecified ovarian cyst, right side**

New **N83.202 Unspecified ovarian cyst, left side**

New **N83.209 Unspecified ovarian cyst, unspecified side**

New Ovarian cyst, NOS

New **N83.291 Other ovarian cyst, right side**

New **N83.292 Other ovarian cyst, left side**

New **N83.299 Other ovarian cyst, unspecified side**

New **N83.311 Acquired atrophy of right ovary**

New **N83.312 Acquired atrophy of left ovary**

New **N83.319 Acquired atrophy of ovary, unspecified side**

New Acquired atrophy of ovary, NOS

New **N83.321 Acquired atrophy of right fallopian tube**

New **N83.322 Acquired atrophy of left fallopian tube**

New **N83.329 Acquired atrophy of fallopian tube, unspecified side**

New Acquired atrophy of fallopian tube, NOS

New **N83.331 Acquired atrophy of right ovary and fallopian tube**

New **N83.332 Acquired atrophy of left ovary and fallopian tube**

New **N83.339 Acquired atrophy of ovary and fallopian tube, unspecified side**

New Acquired atrophy of ovary and fallopian tube, NOS

New **N83.40 Prolapse and hernia of ovary and fallopian tube, unspecified side**

New Prolapse and hernia of ovary and fallopian tube, NOS

New **N83.41 Prolapse and hernia of right ovary and fallopian tube**

New **N83.42 Prolapse and hernia of left ovary and fallopian tube**

New **N83.511 Torsion of right ovary and ovarian pedicle**

New **N83.512 Torsion of left ovary and ovarian pedicle**

New **N83.519 Torsion of ovary and ovarian pedicle, unspecified side**

New Torsion of ovary and ovarian pedicle, NOS

New **N83.521 Torsion of right fallopian tube**

New **N83.522 Torsion of left fallopian tube**

New **N83.529 Torsion of fallopian tube, unspecified side**

New Torsion of fallopian tube, NOS

N83.6 Hematosalpinx

Revised **Excludes1** tubal pregnancy (O00.1-)

N90.6 Hypertrophy of vulva

Deleted Hypertrophy of labia

New **N90.60 Unspecified hypertrophy of vulva**

New Unspecified hypertrophy of labia

New **N90.61 Childhood asymmetric labium majus enlargement**

New CALME

New **N90.69 Other specified hypertrophy of vulva**

New Other specified hypertrophy of labia

New **N93.1 Pre-pubertal vaginal bleeding**

New **N94.10 Unspecified dyspareunia**

New **N94.11 Superficial (introital) dyspareunia**

New **N94.12 Deep dyspareunia**

New **N94.19 Other specified dyspareunia**

N94.3 Premenstrual tension syndrome

New **Excludes1** Premenstrual dysphoric disorder (F32.81)

Revised **N99.113 Postprocedural anterior bulbous urethral stricture**

New **N99.115 Postprocedural fossa navicularis urethral stricture**

N99.5 Complications of stoma of urinary tract

Revised **Excludes2** mechanical complication of urinary catheter (T83.0-)

Revised **N99.52 Complication of incontinent external stoma of urinary tract**

Revised **N99.520 Hemorrhage of incontinent external stoma of urinary tract**

Revised **N99.521 Infection of incontinent external stoma of urinary tract**

Revised **N99.522 Malfunction of incontinent external stoma of urinary tract**

New **N99.523 Herniation of incontinent stoma of urinary tract**

New **N99.524 Stenosis of incontinent stoma of urinary tract**

Revised **N99.528 Other complication of incontinent external stoma of urinary tract**

Revised **N99.53 Complication of continent stoma of urinary tract**

Revised **N99.530 Hemorrhage of continent stoma of urinary tract**

Revised **N99.531 Infection of continent stoma of urinary tract**

Revised **N99.532 Malfunction of continent stoma of urinary tract**

New **N99.533 Herniation of continent stoma of urinary tract**

New **N99.534 Stenosis of continent stoma of urinary tract**

Revised **N99.538 Other complication of continent stoma of urinary tract**

Revised **N99.82 Postprocedural hemorrhage of a genitourinary system organ or structure following a procedure**

Revised **N99.820 Postprocedural hemorrhage of a genitourinary system organ or structure following a genitourinary system procedure**

Revised **N99.821 Postprocedural hemorrhage of a genitourinary system organ or structure following other procedure**

New **N99.84 Postprocedural hematoma and seroma of a genitourinary system organ or structure following a procedure**

New **N99.840 Postprocedural hematoma of a genitourinary system organ or structure following a genitourinary system procedure**

New **N99.841 Postprocedural hematoma of a genitourinary system organ or structure following other procedure**

New **N99.842 Postprocedural seroma of a genitourinary system organ or structure following a genitourinary system procedure**

New **N99.843 Postprocedural seroma of a genitourinary system organ or structure following other procedure**

CHAPTER 15

PREGNANCY, CHILDBIRTH AND THE PUERPERIUM (O00-O9A)

Revised Use additional code from category Z3A, Weeks of gestation, to identify the specific week of the pregnancy, if known.

O00.0 Abdominal pregnancy

New **O00.00 Abdominal pregnancy without intrauterine pregnancy**

New Abdominal pregnancy NOS

New **O00.01 Abdominal pregnancy with intrauterine pregnancy**

O00.1 Tubal pregnancy

New **O00.10 Tubal pregnancy without intrauterine pregnancy**

New Tubal pregnancy NOS

New **O00.11 Tubal pregnancy with intrauterine pregnancy**

O00.2 Ovarian pregnancy

New **O00.20 Ovarian pregnancy without intrauterine pregnancy**

New Ovarian pregnancy NOS

New **O00.21 Ovarian pregnancy with intrauterine pregnancy**

New **O00.8 Other ectopic pregnancy**

New **O00.80 Other ectopic pregnancy without intrauterine pregnancy**

New Other ectopic pregnancy NOS

New **O00.81 Other ectopic pregnancy with intrauterine pregnancy**

New **O00.9 Ectopic pregnancy, unspecified**

New **O00.90 Unspecified ectopic pregnancy without intrauterine pregnancy**

New Ectopic pregnancy NOS

New **O00.91 Unspecified ectopic pregnancy with intrauterine pregnancy**

Revised **O09.1 Supervision of pregnancy with history of ectopic pregnancy**

Revised **O09.10 Supervision of pregnancy with history of ectopic pregnancy, unspecified trimester**

Revised **O09.11 Supervision of pregnancy with history of ectopic pregnancy, first trimester**

Revised **O09.12 Supervision of pregnancy with history of ectopic pregnancy, second trimester**

Revised **O09.13 Supervision of pregnancy with history of ectopic pregnancy, third trimester**

New **O09.A Supervision of pregnancy with history of molar pregnancy**

New **O09.A0 Supervision of pregnancy with history of molar pregnancy, unspecified trimester**

New **O09.A1 Supervision of pregnancy with history of molar pregnancy, first trimester**

New **O09.A2 Supervision of pregnancy with history of molar pregnancy, second trimester**

New **O09.A3 Supervision of pregnancy with history of molar pregnancy, third trimester**

O09.81 Supervision of pregnancy resulting from assisted reproductive technology

New **Excludes2** gestational carrier status (Z33.3)

New **O11.4 Pre-existing hypertension with pre-eclampsia, complicating childbirth**

New **O11.5 Pre-existing hypertension with pre-eclampsia, complicating the puerperium**

New **O12.04 Gestational edema, complicating childbirth**

New **O12.05 Gestational edema, complicating the puerperium**

New **O12.14 Gestational proteinuria, complicating childbirth**

New **O12.15 Gestational proteinuria, complicating the puerperium**

New **O12.24 Gestational edema with proteinuria, complicating childbirth**

New **O12.25 Gestational edema with proteinuria, complicating the puerperium**

O13 Gestational [pregnancy-induced] hypertension without significant proteinuria

New **Includes** transient hypertension of pregnancy

New **O13.4 Gestational [pregnancy-induced] hypertension without significant proteinuria, complicating childbirth**

New **O13.5 Gestational [pregnancy-induced] hypertension without significant proteinuria, complicating the puerperium**

New **O14.04 Mild to moderate pre-eclampsia, complicating childbirth**

New **O14.05 Mild to moderate pre-eclampsia, complicating the puerperium**

New **O14.14 Severe pre-eclampsia complicating childbirth**

New **O14.15 Severe pre-eclampsia, complicating the puerperium**

New **O14.24 HELLP syndrome, complicating childbirth**

New **O14.25 HELLP syndrome, complicating the puerperium**

New **O14.94 Unspecified pre-eclampsia, complicating childbirth**

New **O14.95 Unspecified pre-eclampsia, complicating the puerperium**

Revised **O15.0 Eclampsia complicating pregnancy**

Revised **O15.00 Eclampsia complicating pregnancy, unspecified trimester**

Revised **O15.02 Eclampsia complicating pregnancy, second trimester**

Revised **O15.03 Eclampsia complicating pregnancy, third trimester**

Revised **O15.1 Eclampsia complicating labor**

Revised **O15.2 Eclampsia complicating the puerperium**

New **O16.4 Unspecified maternal hypertension, complicating childbirth**

New **O16.5 Unspecified maternal hypertension, complicating the puerperium**

Revised **O24.0 Pre-existing type 1 diabetes mellitus, in pregnancy, childbirth and the puerperium**

Revised **O24.01 Pre-existing type 1 diabetes mellitus, in pregnancy**

Revised **O24.011 Pre-existing type 1 diabetes mellitus, in pregnancy, first trimester**

Revised **O24.012 Pre-existing type 1 diabetes mellitus, in pregnancy, second trimester**

Revised **O24.013 Pre-existing type 1 diabetes mellitus, in pregnancy, third trimester**

Revised **O24.019 Pre-existing type 1 diabetes mellitus, in pregnancy, unspecified trimester**

Revised **O24.02 Pre-existing type 1 diabetes mellitus, in childbirth**

Revised **O24.03 Pre-existing type 1 diabetes mellitus, in the puerperium**

Revised **O24.1 Pre-existing type 2 diabetes mellitus, in pregnancy, childbirth and the puerperium**

Revised **O24.11 Pre-existing type 2 diabetes mellitus, in pregnancy**

Revised **O24.111 Pre-existing type 2 diabetes mellitus, in pregnancy, first trimester**

Revised **O24.112 Pre-existing type 2 diabetes mellitus, in pregnancy, second trimester**

Revised **O24.113 Pre-existing type 2 diabetes mellitus, in pregnancy, third trimester**

Revised **O24.119 Pre-existing type 2 diabetes mellitus, in pregnancy, unspecified trimester**

Revised **O24.12 Pre-existing type 2 diabetes mellitus, in childbirth**

Revised **O24.13 Pre-existing type 2 diabetes mellitus, in the puerperium**

New **O24.415 Gestational diabetes mellitus in pregnancy, controlled by oral hypoglycemic drugs**

New Gestational diabetes mellitus in pregnancy, controlled by oral antidiabetic drugs

New **O24.425 Gestational diabetes mellitus in childbirth, controlled by oral hypoglycemic drugs**

New Gestational diabetes mellitus in childbirth, controlled by oral antidiabetic drugs

New **O24.435 Gestational diabetes mellitus in puerperium, controlled by oral hypoglycemic drugs**

New Gestational diabetes mellitus in puerperium, controlled by oral antidiabetic drugs

O33.7 Maternal care for disproportion due to other fetal deformities

New One of the following 7th characters is to be assigned to code O33.7. 7th character 0 is for single gestations and multiple gestations where the fetus is unspecified. 7th characters 1 through 9 are for cases of multiple gestations to identify the fetus for which the code applies. The appropriate code from category O30, Multiple gestation, must also be assigned when assigning code O33.7 with a 7th character of 1 through 9.

New	Ø	not applicable or unspecified
New	1	fetus 1
New	2	fetus 2
New	3	fetus 3
New	4	fetus 4
New	5	fetus 5
New	9	other fetus

O34.Ø Maternal care for congenital malformation of uterus

New Maternal care for double uterus

New Maternal care for uterus bicornis

New **O34.211 Maternal care for low transverse scar from previous cesarean delivery**

New **O34.212 Maternal care for vertical scar from previous cesarean delivery**

New Maternal care for classical scar from previous cesarean delivery

New **O34.219 Maternal care for unspecified type scar from previous cesarean delivery**

New **O34.29 Maternal care due to uterine scar from other previous surgery**

New Maternal care due to uterine scar from other transmural uterine incision

O42.Ø2 Full-term premature rupture of membranes, onset of labor within 24 hours of rupture

Revised Premature rupture of membranes at or after 37 completed weeks of gestation, onset of labor within 24 hours of rupture

O42.12 Full-term premature rupture of membranes, onset of labor more than 24 hours following rupture

Revised Premature rupture of membranes at or after 37 completed weeks of gestation, onset of labor more than 24 hours following rupture

O42.92 Full-term premature rupture of membranes, unspecified as to length of time between rupture and onset of labor

Revised Premature rupture of membranes at or after 37 completed weeks of gestation, unspecified as to length of time between rupture and onset of labor

Revised **O44.Ø Complete placenta previa NOS or without hemorrhage**

Deleted Low implantation of placenta specified as without hemorrhage

New Placenta previa NOS

Revised **O44.ØØ Complete placenta previa NOS or without hemorrhage, unspecified trimester**

Revised **O44.Ø1 Complete placenta previa NOS or without hemorrhage, first trimester**

Revised **O44.Ø2 Complete placenta previa NOS or without hemorrhage, second trimester**

Revised **O44.Ø3 Complete placenta previa NOS or without hemorrhage, third trimester**

Revised **O44.1 Complete placenta previa with hemorrhage**

Deleted Complete placenta previa with hemorrhage

Deleted Low implantation of placenta, NOS or with hemorrhage

Deleted Marginal placenta previa, NOS or with hemorrhage

Deleted Partial placenta previa, NOS or with hemorrhage

Deleted Total placenta previa, NOS or with hemorrhage

Revised **O44.1Ø Complete placenta previa with hemorrhage, unspecified trimester**

Revised **O44.11 Complete placenta previa with hemorrhage, first trimester**

Revised **O44.12 Complete placenta previa with hemorrhage, second trimester**

Revised **O44.13 Complete placenta previa with hemorrhage, third trimester**

New **O44.2 Partial placenta previa without hemorrhage**
Marginal placenta previa, NOS or without hemorrhage

New **O44.20 Partial placenta previa NOS or without hemorrhage, unspecified trimester**

New **O44.21 Partial placenta previa NOS or without hemorrhage, first trimester**

New **O44.22 Partial placenta previa NOS or without hemorrhage, second trimester**

New **O44.23 Partial placenta previa NOS or without hemorrhage, third trimester**

New **O44.3 Partial placenta previa with hemorrhage**

New Marginal placenta previa with hemorrhage

New **O44.30 Partial placenta previa with hemorrhage, unspecified trimester**

New **O44.31 Partial placenta previa with hemorrhage, first trimester**

New **O44.32 Partial placenta previa with hemorrhage, second trimester**

New **O44.33 Partial placenta previa with hemorrhage, third trimester**

New **O44.4 Low lying placenta NOS or without hemorrhage**

New Low implantation of placenta NOS or without hemorrhage

New **O44.40 Low lying placenta NOS or without hemorrhage, unspecified trimester**

New **O44.41 Low lying placenta NOS or without hemorrhage, first trimester**

New **O44.42 Low lying placenta NOS or without hemorrhage, second trimester**

New **O44.43 Low lying placenta NOS or without hemorrhage, third trimester**

New **O44.5 Low lying placenta with hemorrhage**

New Low implantation of placenta with hemorrhage

New **O44.50 Low lying placenta with hemorrhage, unspecified trimester**

New **O44.51 Low lying placenta with hemorrhage, first trimester**

New **O44.52 Low lying placenta with hemorrhage, second trimester**

New **O44.53 Low lying placenta with hemorrhage, third trimester**

New **O70.20 Third degree perineal laceration during delivery, unspecified**

New **O70.21 Third degree perineal laceration during delivery, IIIa**

New Third degree perineal laceration during delivery with less than 50% of external anal sphincter (EAS) thickness torn

New **O70.22 Third degree perineal laceration during delivery, IIIb**

New Third degree perineal laceration during delivery with more than 50% external anal sphincter (EAS) thickness torn

New **O70.23 Third degree perineal laceration during delivery, IIIc**

New Third degree perineal laceration during delivery with both external anal sphincter (EAS) and internal anal sphincter (IAS) torn

Revised **O99.33 Tobacco use disorder complicating pregnancy, childbirth, and the puerperium**

New Smoking complicating pregnancy, childbirth, and the puerperium

New Use additional code from category F17 to identify type of tobacco nicotine dependence

O99.6 Diseases of the digestive system complicating pregnancy, childbirth and the puerperium

New **Excludes2** hemorrhoids in pregnancy (O22.4-)

O99.82 Streptococcus B carrier state complicating pregnancy, childbirth and the puerperium

New **Excludes1** Carrier of streptococcus group B (GBS) in a nonpregnant woman (Z22.330)

CHAPTER 16

CERTAIN CONDITIONS ORIGINATING IN THE PERINATAL PERIOD (P00-P96)

NEWBORN AFFECTED BY MATERNAL FACTORS AND BY COMPLICATIONS OF PREGNANCY, LABOR, AND DELIVERY (P00–P04)

Revised **Note:** These codes are for use when the listed maternal conditions are specified as the cause of confirmed morbidity or potential morbidity which have their origin in the perinatal period (before birth through the first 28 days after birth).

Revised **P00 Newborn affected by maternal conditions that may be unrelated to present pregnancy**

New **Excludes2** encounter for observation of newborn for suspected diseases and conditions ruled out (Z05.-)

New newborn affected by maternal complications of pregnancy (P01.-)

Revised **P00.0 Newborn affected by maternal hypertensive disorders**

Revised Newborn affected by maternal conditions classifiable to O10-O11, O13-O16

Revised **P00.1 Newborn affected by maternal renal and urinary tract diseases**

Revised Newborn affected by maternal conditions classifiable to N00-N39

Revised **P00.2 Newborn affected by maternal infectious and parasitic diseases**

Revised Newborn affected by maternal infectious disease classifiable to A00-B99, J09 and J10

Revised **P00.3 Newborn affected by other maternal circulatory and respiratory diseases**

Revised Newborn affected by maternal conditions classifiable to I00-I99, J00-J99, Q20-Q34 and not included in P00.0, P00.2

Revised **P00.4 Newborn affected by maternal nutritional disorders**

Revised Newborn affected by maternal disorders classifiable to E40-E64

Revised **P00.5 Newborn affected by maternal injury**

Revised Newborn affected by maternal conditions classifiable to O9A.2-

Revised **P00.6 Newborn affected by surgical procedure on mother**

Revised Newborn affected by amniocentesis

Revised **P00.7 Newborn affected by other medical procedures on mother, not elsewhere classified**

Revised Newborn affected by radiation to mother

Revised **P00.8 Newborn affected by other maternal conditions**

Revised **P00.81 Newborn affected by periodontal disease in mother**

Revised **P00.89 Newborn affected by other maternal conditions**

Revised Newborn affected by conditions classifiable to T80-T88

Revised Newborn affected by maternal genital tract or other localized infections

Revised Newborn affected by maternal systemic lupus erythematosus

Revised **P00.9 Newborn affected by unspecified maternal condition**

Revised **P01 Newborn affected by maternal complications of pregnancy**
New **Excludes2** encounter for observation of newborn for suspected diseases and conditions ruled out (Z05.-)
Revised **P01.0 Newborn affected by incompetent cervix**
Revised **P01.1 Newborn affected by premature rupture of membranes**
Revised **P01.2 Newborn affected by oligohydramnios**
Revised **P01.3 Newborn affected by polyhydramnios**
Revised Newborn affected by hydramnios
Revised **P01.4 Newborn affected by ectopic pregnancy**
Revised Newborn affected by abdominal pregnancy
Revised **P01.5 Newborn affected by multiple pregnancy**
Revised Newborn affected by triplet (pregnancy)
Revised Newborn affected by twin (pregnancy)
Revised **P01.6 Newborn affected by maternal death**
Revised **P01.7 Newborn affected by malpresentation before labor**
Revised Newborn affected by breech presentation before labor
Revised Newborn affected by external version before labor
Revised Newborn affected by face presentation before labor
Revised Newborn affected by transverse lie before labor
Revised Newborn affected by unstable lie before labor
Revised **P01.8 Newborn affected by other maternal complications of pregnancy**
Revised **P01.9 Newborn affected by maternal complication of pregnancy, unspecified**
Revised **P02 Newborn affected by complications of placenta, cord and membranes**
New **Excludes2** encounter for observation of newborn for suspected diseases and conditions ruled out (Z05.-)
Revised **P02.0 Newborn affected by placenta previa**
Revised **P02.1 Newborn affected by other forms of placental separation and hemorrhage**
Revised Newborn affected by abruptio placenta
Revised Newborn affected by accidental hemorrhage
Revised Newborn affected by antepartum hemorrhage
Revised Newborn affected by damage to placenta from amniocentesis, cesarean delivery or surgical induction
Revised Newborn affected by maternal blood loss
Revised Newborn affected by premature separation of placenta
Revised **P02.2 Newborn affected by other and unspecified morphological and functional abnormalities of placenta**
Revised **P02.20 Newborn affected by unspecified morphological and functional abnormalities of placenta**
Revised **P02.29 Newborn affected by other morphological and functional abnormalities of placenta**
Revised Newborn affected by placental dysfunction
Revised Newborn affected by placental infarction
Revised Newborn affected by placental insufficiency
Revised **P02.3 Newborn affected by placental transfusion syndromes**
Revised Newborn affected by placental and cord abnormalities resulting in twin-to-twin or other transplacental transfusion
Revised **P02.4 Newborn affected by prolapsed cord**
Revised **P02.5 Newborn affected by other compression of umbilical cord**
Revised Newborn affected by umbilical cord (tightly) around neck
Revised Newborn affected by entanglement of umbilical cord
Revised Newborn affected by knot in umbilical cord
Revised **P02.6 Newborn affected by other and unspecified conditions of umbilical cord**
Revised **P02.60 Newborn affected by unspecified conditions of umbilical cord**
Revised **P02.69 Newborn affected by other conditions of umbilical cord**
Revised Newborn affected by short umbilical cord
Revised Newborn affected by vasa previa
Revised **P02.7 Newborn affected by chorioamnionitis**
Revised Newborn affected by amnionitis
Revised Newborn affected by membranitis
Revised Newborn affected by placentitis
Revised **P02.8 Newborn affected by other abnormalities of membranes**
Revised **P02.9 Newborn affected by abnormality of membranes, unspecified**
Revised **P03 Newborn affected by other complications of labor and delivery**
New **Excludes2** encounter for observation of newborn for suspected diseases and conditions ruled out (Z05.-)
Revised **P03.0 Newborn affected by breech delivery and extraction**
Revised **P03.1 Newborn affected by other malpresentation, malposition and disproportion during labor and delivery**
Revised Newborn affected by contracted pelvis
Revised Newborn affected by conditions classifiable to O64-O66
Revised Newborn affected by persistent occipitoposterior
Revised Newborn affected by transverse lie
Revised **P03.2 Newborn affected by forceps delivery**
Revised **P03.3 Newborn affected by delivery by vacuum extractor [ventouse]**
Revised **P03.4 Newborn affected by Cesarean delivery**
Revised **P03.5 Newborn affected by precipitate delivery**
Revised Newborn affected by rapid second stage
Revised **P03.6 Newborn affected by abnormal uterine contractions**
Revised Newborn affected by conditions classifiable to O62.-, except O62.3
Revised Newborn affected by hypertonic labor
Revised Newborn affected by uterine inertia
Revised **P03.8 Newborn affected by other specified complications of labor and delivery**
Revised **P03.81 Newborn affected by abnormality in fetal (intrauterine) heart rate or rhythm**
Revised **P03.810 Newborn affected by abnormality in fetal (intrauterine) heart rate or rhythm before the onset of labor**
Revised **P03.811 Newborn affected by abnormality in fetal (intrauterine) heart rate or rhythm during labor**
Revised **P03.819 Newborn affected by abnormality in fetal (intrauterine) heart rate or rhythm, unspecified as to time of onset**

Revised **P03.89 Newborn affected by other specified complications of labor and delivery**
Revised Newborn affected by abnormality of maternal soft tissues
Revised Newborn affected by conditions classifiable to O60-O75 and by procedures used in labor and delivery not included in P02.- and P03.0-P03.6
Revised Newborn affected by induction of labor
Revised **P03.9 Newborn affected by complication of labor and delivery, unspecified**

Revised **P04 Newborn affected by noxious substances transmitted via placenta or breast milk**
New **Excludes2** congenital malformations (Q00-Q99)
encounter for observation of newborn for suspected diseases and conditions ruled out (Z05.-)

Revised **P04.0 Newborn affected by maternal anesthesia and analgesia in pregnancy, labor and delivery**
Newborn affected by reactions and intoxications from maternal opiates and tranquilizers administered during labor and delivery
Revised **P04.1 Newborn affected by other maternal medication**
Revised Newborn affected by cancer chemotherapy
Revised Newborn affected by cytotoxic drugs
Revised **P04.2 Newborn affected by maternal use of tobacco**
Newborn affected by exposure in utero to tobacco smoke
Revised **P04.3 Newborn affected by maternal use of alcohol**
P04.4 Newborn affected by maternal use of drugs of
Revised **addiction**
Revised **P04.41 Newborn affected by maternal use of cocaine**
Revised **P04.49 Newborn affected by maternal use of other drugs of addiction**
Revised **Excludes2** newborn affected by maternal anesthesia and analgesia (P04.0)
Revised **P04.5 Newborn affected by maternal use of nutritional chemical substances**
Revised **P04.6 Newborn affected by maternal exposure to environmental chemical substances**
Revised **P04.8 Newborn affected by other maternal noxious substances**
Revised **P04.9 Newborn affected by maternal noxious substance, unspecified**

P05.0 Newborn light for gestational age
New Weight below but length above 10th percentile for gestational age
New **P05.09 Newborn light for gestational age, 2500 grams and over**
New Newborn light for gestational age, other
P05.1 Newborn small for gestational age
New Weight and length below 10th percentile for gestational age
New **P05.19 Newborn small for gestational age, other**
New Newborn small for gestational age, 2500 grams and over

P07 Disorders of newborn related to short gestation and low birth weight, not elsewhere classified
Deleted **Excludes1** low birth weight due to slow fetal growth and fetal malnutrition (P05.-)
P07.0 Extremely low birth weight newborn
New **Excludes1** low birth weight due to slow fetal growth and fetal malnutrition (P05.-)
P07.1 Other low birth weight newborn
New **Excludes1** low birth weight due to slow fetal growth and fetal malnutrition (P05.-)
P96.5 Complication to newborn due to (fetal) intrauterine procedure
Revised **Excludes2** newborn affected by amniocentesis (P00.6)

CHAPTER 17

CONGENITAL MALFORMATIONS, DEFORMATIONS AND CHROMOSOMAL ABNORMALITIES (Q00-Q99)

Q25.1 Coarctation of aorta
New Stenosis of aorta
Q25.2 Atresia of aorta
New **Q25.21 Interruption of aortic arch**
New Atresia of aortic arch
New **Q25.29 Other atresia of aorta**
New Atresia of aorta

Q25.4 Other congenital malformations of aorta
Deleted Absence of aorta
Deleted Aneurysm of sinus of Valsalva (ruptured)
Deleted Aplasia of aorta
Deleted Congenital aneurysm of aorta
Deleted Congenital malformations of aorta
Deleted Congenital dilatation of aorta
Deleted Double aortic arch [vascular ring of aorta]
Deleted Hypoplasia of aorta
Deleted Persistent convolutions of aortic arch
Deleted Persistent right aortic arch
New **Q25.40 Congenital malformation of aorta unspecified**
New **Q25.41 Absence and aplasia of aorta**
New **Q25.42 Hypoplasia of aorta**
New **Q25.43 Congenital aneurysm of aorta**
Congenital aneurysm of aortic root
Congenital aneurysm of aortic sinus
New **Q25.44 Congenital dilation of aorta**
New **Q25.45 Double aortic arch**
Vascular ring of aorta
New **Q25.46 Tortuous aortic arch**
Persistent convolutions of aortic arch
New **Q25.47 Right aortic arch**
Persistent right aortic arch
New **Q25.48 Anomalous origin of subclavian artery**
New **Q25.49 Other congenital malformations of aorta**

Q52.12 Longitudinal vaginal septum
Deleted Longitudinal vaginal septum with or without obstruction
New **Q52.120 Longitudinal vaginal septum, nonobstructing**
New **Q52.121 Longitudinal vaginal septum, obstructing, right side**

New Q52.122 **Longitudinal vaginal septum, obstructing, left side**

New Q52.123 **Longitudinal vaginal septum, microperforate, right side**

New Q52.124 **Longitudinal vaginal septum, microperforate, left side**

New Q52.129 **Other and unspecified longitudinal vaginal septum**

New Q66.21 **Congenital metatarsus primus varus**

New Q66.22 **Congenital metatarsus adductus**

Congenital metatarsus varus

New Q82.6 **Congenital sacral dimple**

New Parasacral dimple

New **Excludes2** pilonidal cyst with abscess (LØ5.Ø1)

New pilonidal cyst without abscess (LØ5.91)

New Q87.82 **Arterial tortuosity syndrome**

CHAPTER 18

SYMPTOMS, SIGNS AND ABNORMAL CLINICAL AND LABORATORY FINDINGS, NOT ELSEWHERE CLASSIFIED (RØØ-R99)

RØØ **Abnormalities of heart beat**

Deleted **Excludes1** specified arrhythmias (I47-I49)

New **Excludes2** specified arrhythmias (I47-I49)

RØ1.1 **Cardiac murmur, unspecified**

New Systolic murmur NOS

SYMPTOMS AND SIGNS INVOLVING THE DIGESTIVE SYSTEM AND ABDOMEN (R1Ø-R19)

Deleted **Excludes1** congenital or infantile pylorospasm (Q4Ø.Ø)

Deleted gastrointestinal hemorrhage (K92.Ø-K92.2)

Deleted intestinal obstruction (K56.-)

Deleted newborn gastrointestinal hemorrhage (P54.Ø-P54.3)

Deleted newborn intestinal obstruction (P76.-)

Deleted pylorospasm (K31.3)

Deleted signs and symptoms involving the urinary system (R3Ø-R39)

Deleted symptoms referable to female genital organs (N94.-)

Deleted symptoms referable to male genital organs (N48-N5Ø)

New **Excludes2** congenital or infantile pylorospasm (Q4Ø.Ø)

New gastrointestinal hemorrhage (K92.Ø-K92.2)

New intestinal obstruction (K56.-)

New newborn gastrointestinal hemorrhage (P54.Ø-P54.3)

New newborn intestinal obstruction (P76.-)

New pylorospasm (K31.3)

New signs and symptoms involving the urinary system (R3Ø-R39)

New symptoms referable to female genital organs (N94.-)

New symptoms referable to male genital organs (N48-N5Ø)

R11 **Nausea and vomiting**

Revised **Excludes1** psychogenic vomiting (F5Ø.89)

New R29.7 **National Institutes of Health Stroke Scale (NIHSS) score**

New *Code first the type of cerebral infarction (I63-)*

New R29.70 **NIHSS score Ø-9**

New R29.7ØØ **NIHSS score Ø**

New R29.7Ø1 **NIHSS score 1**

New R29.7Ø2 **NIHSS score 2**

New R29.7Ø3 **NIHSS score 3**

New R29.7Ø4 **NIHSS score 4**

New R29.7Ø5 **NIHSS score 5**

New R29.7Ø6 **NIHSS score 6**

New R29.7Ø7 **NIHSS score 7**

New R29.7Ø8 **NIHSS score 8**

New R29.7Ø9 **NIHSS score 9**

New R29.71 **NIHSS score 1Ø-19**

New R29.71Ø **NIHSS score 1Ø**

New R29.711 **NIHSS score 11**

New R29.712 **NIHSS score 12**

New R29.713 **NIHSS score 13**

New R29.714 **NIHSS score 14**

New R29.715 **NIHSS score 15**

New R29.716 **NIHSS score 16**

New R29.717 **NIHSS score 17**

New R29.718 **NIHSS score 18**

New R29.719 **NIHSS score 19**

New R29.72 **NIHSS score 2Ø-29**

New R29.72Ø **NIHSS score 2Ø**

New R29.721 **NIHSS score 21**

New R29.722 **NIHSS score 22**

New R29.723 **NIHSS score 23**

New R29.724 **NIHSS score 24**

New R29.725 **NIHSS score 25**

New R29.726 **NIHSS score 26**

New R29.727 **NIHSS score 27**

New R29.728 **NIHSS score 28**

New R29.729 **NIHSS score 29**

New R29.73 **NIHSS score 3Ø-39**

New R29.73Ø **NIHSS score 3Ø**

New R29.731 **NIHSS score 31**

New R29.732 **NIHSS score 32**

New R29.733 **NIHSS score 33**

New R29.734 **NIHSS score 34**

New R29.735 **NIHSS score 35**

New R29.736 **NIHSS score 36**

New R29.737 **NIHSS score 37**

New R29.738 **NIHSS score 38**

New R29.739 **NIHSS score 39**

New R29.74 **NIHSS score 4Ø-42**

New R29.74Ø **NIHSS score 4Ø**

New R29.741 **NIHSS score 41**

New R29.742 **NIHSS score 42**

New R31.21 **Asymptomatic microscopic hematuria**

New AMH

New R31.29 **Other microscopic hematuria**

R39.19 **Other difficulties with micturition**

New R39.191 **Need to immediately re-void**

New R39.192 **Position dependent micturition**

New R39.198 **Other difficulties with micturition**

New R39.82 **Chronic bladder pain**

SYMPTOMS AND SIGNS INVOLVING COGNITION, PERCEPTION, EMOTIONAL STATE AND BEHAVIOR (R4Ø-R46)

Deleted **Excludes1** symptoms and signs constituting part of a pattern of mental disorder (FØ1-F99)

New **Excludes2** symptoms and signs constituting part of a pattern of mental disorder (FØ1-F99)

R4Ø.2 Coma

Revised Note: One code from each subcategory R40.21-R40-23 is required to complete the coma scale

R4Ø.24 Glasgow coma scale, total score

Deleted Use codes R4Ø.21- through R4Ø.23- only when the individual score(s) are documented

New Note: Assign a code from subcategory R4Ø.24, when only the total coma score is documented

New The following appropriate 7th character is to be added to subcategory R40.24-:

New	Ø	unspecified time
New	1	in the field [EMT or ambulance]
New	2	at arrival to emergency department
New	3	at hospital admission
New	4	24 hours or more after hospital admission

R41.84 Other specified cognitive deficit

New **Excludes1** cognitive deficits as sequelae of cerebrovascular disease (I69.Ø1-, I69.11-, I69.21-, I69.31-, I69.81-, I69.91-)

R46.81 Obsessive-compulsive behavior

Revised **Excludes1** obsessive-compulsive disorder (F42-)

R5Ø.82 Postprocedural fever

Revised **Excludes1** postprocedural infection (T81.4-)

R53.1 Weakness

New **Excludes1** sarcopenia (M62.84)

R54 Age-related physical debility

New **Excludes1** sarcopenia (M62.84)

R63.Ø Anorexia

Revised **Excludes1** loss of appetite of nonorganic origin (F5Ø.89)

R65.2 Severe sepsis

Code first underlying infection, such as:

Revised infection following a procedure (T81.4-)

R68.84 Jaw pain

Revised **Excludes1** temporomandibular joint arthralgia (M26.62-)

ABNORMAL FINDINGS ON EXAMINATION OF BLOOD, WITHOUT DIAGNOSIS (R7Ø-R79)

Deleted **Excludes1** abnormalities (of)(on):

Deleted abnormal findings on antenatal screening of mother (O28.-)

Deleted coagulation hemorrhagic disorders (D65-D68)

Deleted lipids (E78.-)

Deleted platelets and thrombocytes (D69.-)

Deleted white blood cells classified elsewhere (D7Ø-D72)

Deleted diagnostic abnormal findings classified elsewhere - see Alphabetical Index

Deleted hemorrhagic and hematological disorders of newborn (P5Ø-P61)

New **Excludes2** abnormal findings on antenatal screening of mother (O28.-)

New abnormalities of lipids (E78.-)

New abnormalities of platelets and thrombocytes (D69.-)

New abnormalities of white blood cells classified elsewhere (D7Ø-D72)

New coagulation hemorrhagic disorders (D65-D68)

New diagnostic abnormal findings classified elsewhere —*see* Alphabetical Index

New hemorrhagic and hematological disorders of newborn (P5Ø-P61)

New **R73.Ø3 Prediabetes**

New Latent diabetes

R73.Ø9 Other abnormal glucose

Deleted Latent diabetes

Deleted Prediabetes

R78.81 Bacteremia

Revised **Excludes1** sepsis-code to specified infection

R82.7 Abnormal findings on microbiological examination of urine

Deleted Positive culture findings of urine

New **R82.71 Bacteriuria**

New **R82.79 Other abnormal findings on microbiological examination of urine**

New Positive culture findings of urine

R93.4 Abnormal findings on diagnostic imaging of urinary organs

Deleted Filling defect of bladder found on diagnostic imaging

Deleted Filling defect of kidney found on diagnostic imaging

Deleted Filling defect of ureter found on diagnostic imaging

Deleted **Excludes1** hypertrophy of kidney (N28.81)

New **Excludes2** hypertrophy of kidney (N28.81)

New **R93.41 Abnormal radiologic findings on diagnostic imaging of renal pelvis, ureter, or bladder**

New Filling defect of bladder found on diagnostic imaging

New Filling defect of renal pelvis found on diagnostic imaging

New Filling defect of ureter found on diagnostic imaging

New	R93.42	Abnormal radiologic findings on diagnostic imaging of kidney
New	R93.421	Abnormal radiologic findings on diagnostic imaging of right kidney
New	R93.422	Abnormal radiologic findings on diagnostic imaging of left kidney
New	R93.429	Abnormal radiologic findings on diagnostic imaging of unspecified kidney
New	R93.49	Abnormal radiologic findings on diagnostic imaging of other urinary organs
New	R97.20	Elevated prostate specific antigen [PSA]
New	R97.21	Rising PSA following treatment for malignant neoplasm of prostate

CHAPTER 19

INJURY, POISONING AND CERTAIN OTHER CONSEQUENCES OF EXTERNAL CAUSES (S00-T88)

	S00.8	Superficial injury of other parts of head
New		Superficial injuries of face [any part]
New	S02.101	Fracture of base of skull, right side
New	S02.102	Fracture of base of skull, left side
New	S02.109	Fracture of base of skull, unspecified side
Revised	S02.110	Type I occipital condyle fracture, unspecified side
Revised	S02.111	Type II occipital condyle fracture, unspecified side
Revised	S02.112	Type III occipital condyle fracture, unspecified side
Revised	S02.118	Other fracture of occiput, unspecified side
New	S02.11A	Type I occipital condyle fracture, right side
New	S02.11B	Type I occipital condyle fracture, left side
New	S02.11C	Type II occipital condyle fracture, right side
New	S02.11D	Type II occipital condyle fracture, left side
New	S02.11E	Type III occipital condyle fracture, right side
New	S02.11F	Type III occipital condyle fracture, left side
New	S02.11G	Other fracture of occiput, right side
New	S02.11H	Other fracture of occiput, left side
New	S02.30	Fracture of orbital floor, unspecified side
New	S02.31	Fracture of orbital floor, right side
New	S02.32	Fracture of orbital floor, left side
Revised	S02.400	Malar fracture, unspecified side
Revised	S02.401	Maxillary fracture, unspecified side
Revised	S02.402	Zygomatic fracture, unspecified side
New	S02.40A	Malar fracture, right side
New	S02.40B	Malar fracture, left side
New	S02.40C	Maxillary fracture, right side
New	S02.40D	Maxillary fracture, left side
New	S02.40E	Zygomatic fracture, right side
New	S02.40F	Zygomatic fracture, left side
Revised	S02.600	Fracture of unspecified part of body of mandible, unspecified side
New	S02.601	Fracture of unspecified part of body of right mandible
New	S02.602	Fracture of unspecified part of body of left mandible
New	S02.610	Fracture of condylar process of mandible, unspecified side
New	S02.611	Fracture of condylar process of right mandible
New	S02.612	Fracture of condylar process of left mandible
New	S02.620	Fracture of subcondylar process of mandible, unspecified side
New	S02.621	Fracture of subcondylar process of right mandible
New	S02.622	Fracture of subcondylar process of left mandible
New	S02.630	Fracture of coronoid process of mandible, unspecified side
New	S02.631	Fracture of coronoid process of right mandible
New	S02.632	Fracture of coronoid process of left mandible
New	S02.640	Fracture of ramus of mandible, unspecified side
New	S02.641	Fracture of ramus of right mandible
New	S02.642	Fracture of ramus of left mandible
New	S02.650	Fracture of angle of mandible, unspecified side
New	S02.651	Fracture of angle of right mandible
New	S02.652	Fracture of angle of left mandible
New	S02.670	Fracture of alveolus of mandible, unspecified side
New	S02.671	Fracture of alveolus of right mandible
New	S02.672	Fracture of alveolus of left mandible
New	S02.80	Fracture of other specified skull and facial bones, unspecified side
New	S02.81	Fracture of other specified skull and facial bones, right side
New	S02.82	Fracture of other specified skull and facial bones, left side
New	S03.00	Dislocation of jaw, unspecified side
New	S03.01	Dislocation of jaw, right side
New	S03.02	Dislocation of jaw, left side
New	S03.03	Dislocation of jaw, bilateral side

New S03.40 **Sprain of jaw, unspecified side**
New S03.41 **Sprain of jaw, right side**
New S03.42 **Sprain of jaw, left side**
New S03.43 **Sprain of jaw, bilateral side**
S06.0 **Concussion**
Revised **Excludes1** concussion with other intracranial injuries classified in subcategories S06.1- to S06.6- , S06.81- and S06.82- code to specified intracranial injury
Deleted ~~S06.0X2 Concussion with loss of consciousness of 31 minutes to 59 minutes~~
Deleted ~~S06.0X3 Concussion with loss of consciousness of 1 hour to 5 hours 59 minutes~~
Deleted ~~S06.0X4 Concussion with loss of consciousness of 6 hours to 24 hours~~
Deleted ~~S06.0X5 Concussion with loss of consciousness greater than 24 hours with return to pre-existing conscious level~~
Deleted ~~S06.0X6 Concussion with loss of consciousness greater than 24 hours without return to pre-existing conscious level with patient surviving~~
Deleted ~~S06.0X7 Concussion with loss of consciousness of any duration with death due to brain injury prior to regaining consciousness~~
Deleted ~~S06.0X8 Concussion with loss of consciousness of any duration with death due to other cause prior to regaining consciousness~~
S06.89 **Other specified intracranial injury**
New **Excludes1** concussion (S06.0X-)
S06.9 **Unspecified intracranial injury**
New Traumatic brain injury NOS
New **Excludes1** conditions classifiable to S06.0- to S06.8-code to specified intracranial injury

S34.101 **Unspecified injury to L_1 level of lumbar spinal cord**
New Unspecified injury to lumbar spinal cord level 1
S34.102 **Unspecified injury to L_2 level of lumbar spinal cord**
New Unspecified injury to lumbar spinal cord level 2
S34.103 **Unspecified injury to L_3 level of lumbar spinal cord**
New Unspecified injury to lumbar spinal cord level 3
S34.104 **Unspecified injury to L_4 level of lumbar spinal cord**
New Unspecified injury to lumbar spinal cord level 4
S34.105 **Unspecified injury to L_5 level of lumbar spinal cord**
New Unspecified injury to lumbar spinal cord level 5

S34.111 **Complete lesion of L_1 level of lumbar spinal cord**
New Complete lesion of lumbar spinal cord level 1
S34.112 **Complete lesion of L_2 level of lumbar spinal cord**
New Complete lesion of lumbar spinal cord level 2
S34.113 **Complete lesion of L_3 level of lumbar spinal cord**
New Complete lesion of lumbar spinal cord level 3
S34.114 **Complete lesion of L_4 level of lumbar spinal cord**
New Complete lesion of lumbar spinal cord level 4
S34.115 **Complete lesion of L_5 level of lumbar spinal cord**
New Complete lesion of lumbar spinal cord level 5
S34.121 **Incomplete lesion of L_1 level of lumbar spinal cord**
New Incomplete lesion of lumbar spinal cord level 1
S34.122 **Incomplete lesion of L_2 level of lumbar spinal cord**
New Incomplete lesion of lumbar spinal cord level 2
S34.123 **Incomplete lesion of L_3 level of lumbar spinal cord**
New Incomplete lesion of lumbar spinal cord level 3
S34.124 **Incomplete lesion of L_4 level of lumbar spinal cord**
New Incomplete lesion of lumbar spinal cord level 4
S34.125 **Incomplete lesion of L_5 level of lumbar spinal cord**
New Incomplete lesion of lumbar spinal cord level 5
Revised S49.031 **Salter-Harris Type III physeal fracture of upper end of humerus, right arm**
Revised S49.032 **Salter-Harris Type III physeal fracture of upper end of humerus, left arm**
Revised S49.039 **Salter-Harris Type III physeal fracture of upper end of humerus, unspecified arm**
Revised S49.13 **Salter-Harris Type III physeal fracture of lower end of humerus**
Revised S49.131 **Salter-Harris Type III physeal fracture of lower end of humerus, right arm**
Revised S49.132 **Salter-Harris Type III physeal fracture of lower end of humerus, left arm**
Revised S49.139 **Salter-Harris Type III physeal fracture of lower end of humerus, unspecified arm**
Revised S54.8X **Injury of other nerves at forearm level**
Revised S54.8X1 **Injury of other nerves at forearm level, right arm**
Revised S54.8X2 **Injury of other nerves at forearm level, left arm**
Revised S54.8X9 **Injury of other nerves at forearm level, unspecified arm**

S92.Ø Fracture of calcaneus

New **Excludes2** Physeal fracture of calcaneus (S99.Ø-)

S92.3 Fracture of metatarsal bone(s)

New **Excludes2** Physeal fracture of metatarsal (S99.1-)

New **S92.4 Fracture of great toe**

Excludes2 Physeal fracture of phalanx of toe (S99.2-)

New **S92.5 Fracture of lesser toe(s)**

Excludes2 Physeal fracture of phalanx of toe (S99.2-)

New **S92.8 Other fracture of foot, except ankle**

New **S92.81 Other fracture of foot**

Sesamoid fracture of foot

New **S92.811 Other fracture of right foot**

New **S92.812 Other fracture of left foot**

New **S92.819 Other fracture of unspecified foot**

S99 Other and unspecified injuries of ankle and foot

Deleted The appropriate 7th character is to be added to each code from subcategories S99

Deleted	A	initial encounter
Deleted	D	subsequent encounter
Deleted	S	sequela

New **S99.Ø Physeal fracture of calcaneus**

New The appropriate 7th character is to be added to each code from subcategories S99.0

New	A	initial encounter for closed fracture
New	B	initial encounter for open fracture
New	D	subsequent encounter for fracture with routine healing
New	G	subsequent encounter for fracture with delayed healing
New	K	subsequent encounter for fracture with nonunion
New	P	subsequent encounter for fracture with malunion
New	S	sequela

New **S99.ØØ Unspecified physeal fracture of calcaneus**

New **S99.ØØ1 Unspecified physeal fracture of right calcaneus**

New **S99.ØØ2 Unspecified physeal fracture of left calcaneus**

New **S99.ØØ9 Unspecified physeal fracture of unspecified calcaneus**

New **S99.Ø1 Salter-Harris Type I physeal fracture of calcaneus**

New **S99.Ø11 Salter-Harris Type I physeal fracture of right calcaneus**

New **S99.Ø12 Salter-Harris Type I physeal fracture of left calcaneus**

New **S99.Ø19 Salter-Harris Type I physeal fracture of unspecified calcaneus**

New **S99.Ø2 Salter-Harris Type II physeal fracture of calcaneus**

New **S99.Ø21 Salter-Harris Type II physeal fracture of right calcaneus**

New **S99.Ø22 Salter-Harris Type II physeal fracture of left calcaneus**

New **S99.Ø29 Salter-Harris Type II physeal fracture of unspecified calcaneus**

New **S99.Ø3 Salter-Harris Type III physeal fracture of calcaneus**

New **S99.Ø31 Salter-Harris Type III physeal fracture of right calcaneus**

New **S99.Ø32 Salter-Harris Type III physeal fracture of left calcaneus**

New **S99.Ø39 Salter-Harris Type III physeal fracture of unspecified calcaneus**

New **S99.Ø4 Salter-Harris Type IV physeal fracture of calcaneus**

New **S99.Ø41 Salter-Harris Type IV physeal fracture of right calcaneus**

New **S99.Ø42 Salter-Harris Type IV physeal fracture of left calcaneus**

New **S99.Ø49 Salter-Harris Type IV physeal fracture of unspecified calcaneus**

New **S99.Ø9 Other physeal fracture of calcaneus**

New **S99.Ø91 Other physeal fracture of right calcaneus**

New **S99.Ø92 Other physeal fracture of left calcaneus**

New **S99.Ø99 Other physeal fracture of unspecified calcaneus**

New **S99.1 Physeal fracture of metatarsal**

New The appropriate 7th character is to be added to each code from subcategories S99.1

New	A	initial encounter for closed fracture
New	B	initial encounter for open fracture
New	D	subsequent encounter for fracture with routine healing
New	G	subsequent encounter for fracture with delayed healing
New	K	subsequent encounter for fracture with nonunion
New	P	subsequent encounter for fracture with malunion
New	S	sequela

New **S99.1Ø Unspecified physeal fracture of metatarsal**

New **S99.1Ø1 Unspecified physeal fracture of right metatarsal**

New **S99.1Ø2 Unspecified physeal fracture of left metatarsal**

New **S99.1Ø9 Unspecified physeal fracture of unspecified metatarsal**

New **S99.11 Salter-Harris Type I physeal fracture of metatarsal**

New **S99.111 Salter-Harris Type I physeal fracture of right metatarsal**

New **S99.112 Salter-Harris Type I physeal fracture of left metatarsal**

New **S99.119 Salter-Harris Type I physeal fracture of unspecified metatarsal**

New **S99.12 Salter-Harris Type II physeal fracture of metatarsal**

New **S99.121 Salter-Harris Type II physeal fracture of right metatarsal**

New **S99.122 Salter-Harris Type II physeal fracture of left metatarsal**

New **S99.129 Salter-Harris Type II physeal fracture of unspecified metatarsal**

New S99.13 **Salter-Harris Type III physeal fracture of metatarsal**
New S99.131 **Salter-Harris Type III physeal fracture of right metatarsal**
New S99.132 **Salter-Harris Type III physeal fracture of left metatarsal**
New S99.139 **Salter-Harris Type III physeal fracture of unspecified metatarsal**
New S99.14 **Salter-Harris Type IV physeal fracture of metatarsal**
New S99.141 **Salter-Harris Type IV physeal fracture of right metatarsal**
New S99.142 **Salter-Harris Type IV physeal fracture of left metatarsal**
New S99.149 **Salter-Harris Type IV physeal fracture of unspecified metatarsal**
New S99.19 **Other physeal fracture of metatarsal**
New S99.191 **Other physeal fracture of right metatarsal**
New S99.192 **Other physeal fracture of left metatarsal**
New S99.199 **Other physeal fracture of unspecified metatarsal**
New S99.2 **Physeal fracture of phalanx of toe**
New The appropriate 7th character is to be added to each code from subcategories S99.2

New A initial encounter for closed fracture
New B initial encounter for open fracture
New D subsequent encounter for fracture with routine healing
New G subsequent encounter for fracture with delayed healing
New K subsequent encounter for fracture with nonunion
New P subsequent encounter for fracture with malunion
New S sequela

New S99.20 **Unspecified physeal fracture of phalanx of toe**
New S99.201 **Unspecified physeal fracture of phalanx of right toe**
New S99.202 **Unspecified physeal fracture of phalanx of right toe**
New S99.209 **Unspecified physeal fracture of phalanx of unspecified toe**
New S99.21 **Salter-Harris Type I physeal fracture of phalanx of toe**
New S99.211 **Salter-Harris Type I physeal fracture of phalanx of right toe**
New S99.212 **Salter-Harris Type I physeal fracture of phalanx of left toe**
New S99.219 **Salter-Harris Type I physeal fracture of phalanx of unspecified toe**
New S99.22 **Salter-Harris Type II physeal fracture of phalanx of toe**
New S99.221 **Salter-Harris Type II physeal fracture of phalanx of right toe**
New S99.222 **Salter-Harris Type II physeal fracture of phalanx of left toe**
New S99.229 **Salter-Harris Type II physeal fracture of phalanx of unspecified toe**
New S99.23 **Salter-Harris Type III physeal fracture of phalanx of toe**
New S99.231 **Salter-Harris Type III physeal fracture of phalanx of right toe**
New S99.232 **Salter-Harris Type III physeal fracture of phalanx of left toe**
New S99.239 **Salter-Harris Type III physeal fracture of phalanx of unspecified toe**
New S99.24 **Salter-Harris Type IV physeal fracture of phalanx of toe**
New S99.241 **Salter-Harris Type IV physeal fracture of phalanx of right toe**
New S99.242 **Salter-Harris Type IV physeal fracture of phalanx of left toe**
New S99.249 **Salter-Harris Type IV physeal fracture of phalanx of unspecified toe**
New S99.29 **Other physeal fracture of phalanx of toe**
New S99.291 **Other physeal fracture of phalanx of right toe**
New S99.292 **Other physeal fracture of phalanx of left toe**
New S99.299 **Other physeal fracture of phalanx of unspecified toe**
S99.8 **Other specified injuries of ankle and foot**
New The appropriate 7th character is to be added to each code from subcategory S99.8

New A initial encounter
New D subsequent encounter
New S sequela

S99.9 **Unspecified injury of ankle and foot**
New The appropriate 7th character is to be added to each code from subcategory S99.9

New A initial encounter
New D subsequent encounter
New S sequela

T17.32 **Food in larynx**
Revised Bones in larynx

T61 **Toxic effect of noxious substances eaten as seafood**
Excludes1 allergic reaction to food, such as:
Deleted gastroenteritis (noninfective) (K52.2)
New food protein-induced enterocolitis syndrome (K52.21)
New food protein-induced enteropathy (K52.22)
New gastroenteritis (noninfective) (K52.29)

T62 **Toxic effect of other noxious substances eaten as food**
Excludes1 allergic reaction to food, such as:
Deleted gastroenteritis (noninfective) (K52.2)
New food protein-induced enterocolitis syndrome (K52.21)
New food protein-induced enteropathy (K52.22)
New gastroenteritis (noninfective) (K52.29)

T78.05 **Anaphylactic reaction due to tree nuts and seeds**
Deleted **Excludes1** anaphylactic reaction due to peanuts (T78.01)
New **Excludes2** anaphylactic reaction due to peanuts (T78.01)

T78.1 Other adverse food reactions, not elsewhere classified

Revised Use additional code to identify the type of reaction, if applicable

Revised **Excludes2** allergic and dietetic gastroenteritis and colitis (K52.29)

New food protein-induced enterocolitis syndrome (K52.21)

New food protein-induced enteropathy (K52.22)

T78.4 Other and unspecified allergy

Excludes1 specified types of allergic reaction such as:

Revised allergic diarrhea (K52.29)

Revised allergic gastroenteritis and colitis (K52.29)

New food protein-induced enterocolitis syndrome (K52.21)

New food protein-induced enteropathy (K52.22)

T80.1 Vascular complications following infusion, transfusion and therapeutic injection

Revised **Excludes2** vascular complications specified as due to prosthetic devices, implants and grafts (T82.8-, T83.8-, T84.8-, T85.8-)

T80.2 Infections following infusion, transfusion and therapeutic injection

Revised **Excludes2** postprocedural infections (T81.4-)

T80.21 Infection due to central venous catheter

New Infection due to pulmonary artery catheter (Swan-Ganz catheter)

T80.211 Bloodstream infection due to central venous catheter

New Bloodstream infection due to pulmonary artery catheter

T80.212 Local infection due to central venous catheter

New Local infection due to pulmonary artery catheter

T80.218 Other infection due to central venous catheter

New Other infection due to pulmonary artery catheter

T80.219 Unspecified infection due to central venous catheter

New Unspecified infection due to pulmonary artery catheter

T80.6 Other serum reactions

Revised **Excludes2** serum hepatitis (B16-B19)

T81.12 Postprocedural septic shock

Revised Postprocedural endotoxic shock resulting from a procedure, not elsewhere classified

Revised Postprocedural gram-negative shock resulting from a procedure, not elsewhere classified

T81.7 Vascular complications following a procedure, not elsewhere classified

Revised **Excludes2** embolism due to prosthetic devices, implants and grafts (T82.8-, T83.81, T84.8-, T85.1-)

Revised **T82.81 Embolism due to cardiac and vascular prosthetic devices, implants and grafts**

Revised **T82.817 Embolism due to cardiac prosthetic devices, implants and grafts**

Revised **T82.818 Embolism due to vascular prosthetic devices, implants and grafts**

Revised **T82.82 Fibrosis due to cardiac and vascular prosthetic devices, implants and grafts**

Revised **T82.827 Fibrosis due to cardiac prosthetic devices, implants and grafts**

Revised **T82.828 Fibrosis due to vascular prosthetic devices, implants and grafts**

Revised **T82.83 Hemorrhage due to cardiac and vascular prosthetic devices, implants and grafts**

Revised **T82.837 Hemorrhage due to cardiac prosthetic devices, implants and grafts**

Revised **T82.838 Hemorrhage due to vascular prosthetic devices, implants and grafts**

Revised **T82.84 Pain due to cardiac and vascular prosthetic devices, implants and grafts**

Revised **T82.847 Pain due to cardiac prosthetic devices, implants and grafts**

Revised **T82.848 Pain due to vascular prosthetic devices, implants and grafts**

Revised **T82.85 Stenosis due to cardiac and vascular prosthetic devices, implants and grafts**

New **T82.855 Stenosis of coronary artery stent**

New In-stent stenosis (restenosis) of coronary artery stent

New Restenosis of coronary artery stent

New **T82.856 Stenosis of peripheral vascular stent**

New In-stent stenosis (restenosis) of peripheral vascular stent

New Restenosis of peripheral vascular stent

Revised **T82.857 Stenosis of other cardiac prosthetic devices, implants and grafts**

Revised **T82.858 Stenosis of other vascular prosthetic devices, implants and grafts**

Revised **T82.86 Thrombosis of cardiac and vascular prosthetic devices, implants and grafts**

Revised **T82.867 Thrombosis due to cardiac prosthetic devices, implants and grafts**

Revised **T82.868 Thrombosis due to vascular prosthetic devices, implants and grafts**

Revised **T83.0 Mechanical complication of urinary catheter**

Revised **T83.01 Breakdown (mechanical) of urinary catheter**

New **T83.011 Breakdown (mechanical) of indwelling urethral catheter**

New **T83.012 Breakdown (mechanical) of nephrostomy catheter**

Revised **T83.018 Breakdown (mechanical) of other urinary catheter**

New Breakdown (mechanical) of Hopkins catheter

New Breakdown (mechanical) of ileostomy catheter

New Breakdown (mechanical) urostomy catheter

Revised	T83.02	**Displacement of urinary catheter**
Revised		Malposition of urinary catheter
New	T83.021	**Displacement of indwelling urethral catheter**
New	T83.022	**Displacement of nephrostomy catheter**
Revised	T83.028	**Displacement of other urinary catheter**
New		Displacement of Hopkins catheter
New		Displacement of ileostomy catheter
New		Displacement of urostomy catheter
Revised	T83.03	**Leakage of urinary catheter**
New	T83.031	**Leakage of indwelling urethral catheter**
New	T83.032	**Leakage of nephrostomy catheter**
Revised	T83.038	**Leakage of other urinary catheter**
New		Leakage of Hopkins catheter
New		Leakage of ileostomy catheter
New		Leakage of urostomy catheter
Revised	T83.09	**Other mechanical complication of urinary catheter**
Revised		Obstruction (mechanical) of urinary catheter
Revised		Perforation of urinary catheter
Revised		Protrusion of urinary catheter
New	T83.091	**Other mechanical complication of indwelling urethral catheter**
New	T83.092	**Other mechanical complication of nephrostomy catheter**
Revised	T83.098	**Other mechanical complication of other urinary catheter**
New		Other mechanical complication of Hopkins catheter
New		Other mechanical complication of ileostomy catheter
New		Other mechanical complication of urostomy catheter
	T83.110	**Breakdown (mechanical) of urinary electronic stimulator device**
New		**Excludes2** Breakdown (mechanical) of electrode (lead) for sacral nerve neuro-stimulator (T85.111)
New		Breakdown (mechanical) of implanted electronic sacral neuro-stimulator, pulse generator or receiver (T85.113)
Revised	T83.111	**Breakdown (mechanical) of implanted urinary sphincter**
Revised	T83.112	**Breakdown (mechanical) of indwelling ureteral stent**
New	T83.113	**Breakdown (mechanical) of other urinary stents**
New		Breakdown (mechanical) of ileal conduit stent
New		Breakdown (mechanical) of nephroureteral stent
	T83.120	**Displacement of urinary electronic stimulator device**
New		**Excludes2** Displacement of electrode (lead) for sacral nerve neuro-stimulator (T85.121)
New		Displacement of implanted electronic sacral neuro-stimulator, pulse generator or receiver (T85.123)
Revised	T83.121	**Displacement of implanted urinary sphincter**
Revised	T83.122	**Displacement of indwelling ureteral stent**
New	T83.123	**Displacement of other urinary stents**
New		Displacement of ileal conduit stent
New		Displacement of nephroureteral stent
	T83.190	**Other mechanical complication of urinary electronic stimulator device**
New		**Excludes2** Other mechanical complication of electrode (lead) for sacral nerve neuro-stimulator (T85.191)
New		Other mechanical complication of implanted electronic sacral neuro-stimulator, pulse generator or receiver (T85.193)
Revised	T83.191	**Other mechanical complication of implanted urinary sphincter**
Revised	T83.192	**Other mechanical complication of indwelling ureteral stent**
New	T83.193	**Other mechanical complication of other urinary stent**
New		Other mechanical complication of ileal conduit stent
New		Other mechanical complication of nephroureteral stent

New T83.24 **Erosion of graft of urinary organ**

New T83.25 **Exposure of graft of urinary organ**

T83.32 **Displacement of intrauterine contraceptive device**

New Missing string of intrauterine contraceptive device

Revised T83.41Ø **Breakdown (mechanical) of implanted penile prosthesis**

New Breakdown (mechanical) of penile prosthesis cylinder

New Breakdown (mechanical) of penile prosthesis pump

New Breakdown (mechanical) of penile prosthesis reservoir

New T83.411 **Breakdown (mechanical) of implanted testicular prosthesis**

Revised T83.42Ø **Displacement of implanted penile prosthesis**

New Displacement of penile prosthesis cylinder

New Displacement of penile prosthesis pump

New Displacement of penile prosthesis reservoir

New T83.421 **Displacement of implanted testicular prosthesis**

Revised T83.49Ø **Other mechanical complication of implanted penile prosthesis**

New Other mechanical complication of penile prosthesis cylinder

New Other mechanical complication of penile prosthesis pump

New Other mechanical complication of penile prosthesis reservoir

New T83.491 **Other mechanical complication of implanted testicular prosthesis**

Revised T83.51 **Infection and inflammatory reaction due to urinary catheter**

New T83.51Ø **Infection and inflammatory reaction due to cystostomy catheter**

New T83.511 **Infection and inflammatory reaction due to indwelling urethral catheter**

New T83.512 **Infection and inflammatory reaction due to nephrostomy catheter**

New T83.518 **Infection and inflammatory reaction due to other urinary catheter**

New Infection and inflammatory reaction due to Hopkins catheter

New Infection and inflammatory reaction due to ileostomy catheter

New Infection and inflammatory reaction due to urostomy catheter

New T83.59Ø **Infection and inflammatory reaction due to implanted urinary neurostimulation device**

New **Excludes2** Infection and inflammatory reaction due to electrode lead of sacral nerve neurostimulator (T85.732)

New Infection and inflammatory reaction due to pulse generator or receiver of sacral nerve neurostimulator (T85.734)

New T83.591 **Infection and inflammatory reaction due to implanted urinary sphincter**

New T83.592 **Infection and inflammatory reaction due to indwelling ureteral stent**

New T83.593 **Infection and inflammatory reaction due to other urinary stents**

New Infection and inflammatory reaction due to ileal conduit stents

New Infection and inflammatory reaction due to nephroureteral stent

New T83.598 **Infection and inflammatory reaction due to other prosthetic device, implant and graft in urinary system**

New T83.61 **Infection and inflammatory reaction due to implanted penile prosthesis**

New Infection and inflammatory reaction due to penile prosthesis cylinder

New Infection and inflammatory reaction due to penile prosthesis pump

New Infection and inflammatory reaction due to penile prosthesis reservoir

New T83.62 **Infection and inflammatory reaction due to implanted testicular prosthesis**

New T83.69 **Infection and inflammatory reaction due to other prosthetic device, implant and graft in genital tract**

Revised T83.711 **Erosion of implanted vaginal mesh to surrounding organ or tissue**

Revised Erosion of implanted vaginal mesh into pelvic floor muscles

New T83.712 **Erosion of implanted urethral mesh to surrounding organ or tissue**

New Erosion of implanted female urethral sling

New Erosion of implanted male urethral sling

New Erosion of implanted urethral mesh into pelvic floor muscles

New T83.713 **Erosion of implanted urethral bulking agent to surrounding organ or tissue**

New T83.714 **Erosion of implanted ureteral bulking agent to surrounding organ or tissue**

Revised T83.718 **Erosion of other implanted mesh to organ or tissue**

New T83.719 **Erosion of other prosthetic materials to surrounding organ or tissue**

T83.72 **Exposure of implanted mesh and other prosthetic materials into surrounding organ or tissue**

New Extrusion of implanted mesh

Revised T83.721 **Exposure of implanted vaginal mesh into vagina**

Revised Exposure of implanted vaginal mesh through vaginal wall

New T83.722 **Exposure of implanted urethral mesh into urethra**

New Exposure of implanted female urethral sling

New Exposure of implanted male urethral sling

New Exposure of implanted urethral mesh through urethral wall

New T83.723 **Exposure of implanted urethral bulking agent into urethra**

New T83.724 **Exposure of implanted ureteral bulking agent into ureter**

Revised T83.728 **Exposure of other implanted mesh into organ or tissue**

New T83.729 **Exposure of other prosthetic materials into organ or tissue**

New T83.79 **Other specified complications due to other genitourinary prosthetic materials**

T83.8 **Other specified complications of genitourinary prosthetic devices, implants and grafts**

Revised T83.81 **Embolism due to genitourinary prosthetic devices, implants and grafts**

Revised T83.82 **Fibrosis due to genitourinary prosthetic devices, implants and grafts**

Revised T83.83 **Hemorrhage due to genitourinary prosthetic devices, implants and grafts**

Revised T83.84 **Pain due to genitourinary prosthetic devices, implants and grafts**

Revised T83.85 **Stenosis due to genitourinary prosthetic devices, implants and grafts**

Revised T83.86 **Thrombosis due to genitourinary prosthetic devices, implants and grafts**

Deleted ~~T84.04 Periprosthetic fracture around internal prosthetic joint~~

Deleted **Excludes2** breakage (fracture) of prosthetic joint (T84.01)

Deleted ~~T84.040 Periprosthetic fracture around internal prosthetic right hip joint~~

Deleted ~~T84.041 Periprosthetic fracture around internal prosthetic left hip joint~~

Deleted ~~T84.042 Periprosthetic fracture around internal prosthetic right knee joint~~

Deleted ~~T84.043 Periprosthetic fracture around internal prosthetic left knee joint~~

Deleted ~~T84.048 Periprosthetic fracture around other internal prosthetic joint~~

Deleted Use additional code to identify the joint (Z96.6-)

Deleted ~~T84.049 Periprosthetic fracture around unspecified internal prosthetic joint~~

Revised T85.110 **Breakdown (mechanical) of implanted electronic neurostimulator of brain electrode (lead)**

Revised T85.111 **Breakdown (mechanical) of implanted electronic neurostimulator of peripheral nerve electrode (lead)**

New Breakdown of electrode (lead) for cranial nerve neurostimulators

New Breakdown of electrode (lead) for gastric neurostimulator

New Breakdown of electrode (lead) for sacral nerve neurostimulator

New Breakdown of electrode (lead) for vagal nerve neurostimulators

Revised T85.112 **Breakdown (mechanical) of implanted electronic neurostimulator of spinal cord electrode (lead)**

New T85.113 **Breakdown (mechanical) of implanted electronic neurostimulator, generator**

New Breakdown (mechanical) of implanted electronic neurostimuator generator, brain, peripheral, gastric, spinal

New Breakdown (mechanical) of implanted electronic sacral neurostimulator, pulse generator or receiver

Revised T85.120 **Displacement of implanted electronic neurostimulator of brain electrode (lead)**

Revised T85.121 **Displacement of implanted electronic neurostimulator of peripheral nerve electrode (lead)**

New Displacement of electrode (lead) for cranial nerve neurostimulators

New Displacement of electrode (lead) for gastric neurostimulator

New Displacement of electrode (lead) for sacral nerve neurostimulator

New Displacement of electrode (lead) for vagal nerve neurostimulators

Revised T85.122 **Displacement of implanted electronic neurostimulator of spinal cord electrode (lead)**

New T85.123 **Displacement of implanted electronic neurostimulator, generator**

New Displacement of implanted electronic neurostimulator generator, brain, peripheral, gastric, spinal

New Displacement of implanted electronic sacral neurostimulator, pulse generator or receiver

Revised T85.190 **Other mechanical complication of implanted electronic neurostimulator of brain electrode (lead)**

Revised T85.191 **Other mechanical complication of implanted electronic neurostimulator of peripheral nerve electrode (lead)**

New Other mechanical complication of electrode (lead) for cranial nerve neurostimulators

New Other mechanical complication of electrode (lead) for gastric neurostimulator

New Other mechanical complication of electrode (lead) for sacral nerve neurostimulator

New Other mechanical complication of electrode (lead) for vagal nerve neurostimulators

Revised T85.192 **Other mechanical complication of implanted electronic neurostimulator of spinal cord electrode (lead)**

New T85.193 **Other mechanical complication of implanted electronic neurostimulator, generator**

New Other mechanical complication of implanted electronic neurostimulator generator, brain, peripheral, gastric, spinal

New Other mechanical complication of implanted electronic sacral neurostimulator, pulse generator or receiver

Revised T85.610 **Breakdown (mechanical) of cranial or spinal infusion catheter**

New Breakdown (mechanical) of epidural infusion catheter

New Breakdown (mechanical) of intrathecal infusion catheter

New Breakdown (mechanical) of subarachnoid infusion catheter

New Breakdown (mechanical) of subdural infusion catheter

New T85.615 **Breakdown (mechanical) of other nervous system device, implant or graft**

New Breakdown (mechanical) of intrathecal infusion pump

Revised T85.620 **Displacement of cranial or spinal infusion catheter**

New Displacement of epidural infusion catheter

New Displacement of intrathecal infusion catheter

New Displacement of subarachnoid infusion catheter

New Displacement of subdural infusion catheter

New T85.625 **Displacement of other nervous system device, implant or graft**

New Displacement of intrathecal infusion pump

Revised T85.630 **Leakage of cranial or spinal infusion catheter**

New Leakage of epidural infusion catheter

New Leakage of intrathecal infusion catheter

New Leakage of subdural infusion catheter

New Leakage of subarachnoid infusion catheter

New T85.635 **Leakage of other nervous system device, implant or graft**

New Leakage of intrathecal infusion pump

Revised T85.690 **Other mechanical complication of cranial or spinal infusion catheter**

New Other mechanical complication of epidural infusion catheter

New Other mechanical complication of intrathecal infusion catheter

New Other mechanical complication of subarachnoid infusion catheter

New Other mechanical complication of subdural infusion catheter

New T85.695 **Other mechanical complication of other nervous system device, implant or graft**

New Other mechanical complication of intrathecal infusion pump

New T85.73 **Infection and inflammatory reaction due to nervous system devices, implants and graft**

New T85.730 **Infection and inflammatory reaction due to ventricular intracranial (communicating) shunt**

New T85.731 **Infection and inflammatory reaction due to implanted electronic neurostimulator of brain, electrode (lead)**

New T85.732 **Infection and inflammatory reaction due to implanted electronic neurostimulator of peripheral nerve, electrode (lead)**

New Infection and inflammatory reaction due to electrode (lead) for cranial nerve neurostimulators

New Infection and inflammatory reaction due to electrode (lead) for gastric neurostimulator

New Infection and inflammatory reaction due to electrode (lead) for sacral nerve neurostimulator

New Infection and inflammatory reaction due to electrode (lead) for vagal nerve neurostimulators

New T85.733 **Infection and inflammatory reaction due to implanted electronic neurostimulator of spinal cord, electrode (lead)**

New T85.734 **Infection and inflammatory reaction due to implanted electronic neurostimulator, generator**

New Generator pocket infection

New T85.735 **Infection and inflammatory reaction due to cranial or spinal infusion catheter**

New Infection and inflammatory reaction due to epidural catheter

New Infection and inflammatory reaction due to intrathecal infusion catheter

New Infection and inflammatory reaction due to subarachnoid catheter

New Infection and inflammatory reaction due to subdural catheter

New T85.738 **Infection and inflammatory reaction due to other nervous system device, implant or graft**

New Infection and inflammatory reaction due to intrathecal infusion pump

New T85.81Ø **Embolism due to nervous system prosthetic devices, implants and grafts**

New T85.818 **Embolism due to other internal prosthetic devices, implants and grafts**

New T85.82Ø **Fibrosis due to nervous system prosthetic devices, implants and grafts**

New T85.828 **Fibrosis due to other internal prosthetic devices, implants and grafts**

New T85.83Ø **Hemorrhage due to nervous system prosthetic devices, implants and grafts**

New T85.838 **Hemorrhage due to other internal prosthetic devices, implants and grafts**

New T85.84Ø **Pain due to nervous system prosthetic devices, implants and grafts**

New T85.848 **Pain due to other internal prosthetic devices, implants and grafts**

New T85.85Ø **Stenosis due to nervous system prosthetic devices, implants and grafts**

New T85.858 **Stenosis due to other internal prosthetic devices, implants and grafts**

New T85.86Ø **Thrombosis due to nervous system prosthetic devices, implants and grafts**

New T85.868 **Thrombosis due to other internal prosthetic devices, implants and grafts**

T85.89 **Other specified complication of internal prosthetic devices, implants and grafts, not elsewhere classified**

New Erosion or breakdown of subcutaneous device pocket

New T85.89Ø **Other specified complication of nervous system prosthetic devices, implants and grafts**

New T85.898 **Other specified complication of other internal prosthetic devices, implants and grafts**

New T88.53 **Unintended awareness under general anesthesia during procedure**

New **Excludes2** personal history of unintended awareness under general anesthesia (Z92.84)

CHAPTER 2Ø

EXTERNAL CAUSES OF MORBIDITY (VØØ-Y99)

This chapter contains the following blocks:

New	X5Ø	Overexertion and strenuous or repetitive movements
Revised	X92-YØ9	Assault

TRANSPORT ACCIDENTS (VØØ-V99)

Deleted **Note:** This section is structured in 12 groups. Those relating to land transport accidents (VØ1-V89) reflect the victim's mode of transport and are subdivided to identify the victim's 'counterpart' or the type of event. The vehicle of which the injured person is an occupant is identified in the first two characters since it is seen as the most important factor to identify for prevention purposes. A transport accident is one in which the vehicle involved must be moving or running or in use for transport purposes at the time of the accident.

New **Note:** This section is structured in 12 groups. Those relating to land transport accidents (VØØ-V89) reflect the victim's mode of transport and are subdivided to identify the victim's 'counterpart' or the type of event. The vehicle of which the injured person is an occupant is identified in the first two characters since it is seen as the most important factor to identify for prevention purposes. A transport accident is one in which the vehicle involved must be moving or running or in use for transport purposes at the time of the accident.

Revised **Note:** Definitions related to transport accidents:

Revised (a) A transport accident (VØØ-V99) is any accident involving a device designed primarily for, or used at the time primarily for, conveying persons or good from one place to another.

Revised (e) A pedestrian is any person involved in an accident who was not at the time of the accident riding in or on a motor vehicle, railway train, streetcar or animal-drawn or other vehicle, or on a pedal cycle or animal. This includes, a person changing a tire, working on a parked car, or a person on foot. It also includes the user of a pedestrian conveyance such as a baby-stroller, ice-skates, skis, sled, roller skates, a skateboard, nonmotorized or motorized wheelchair, motorized mobility scooter, or nonmotorized scooter.

Revised (h) A person on the outside of a vehicle is any person being transported by a vehicle but not occupying the space normally reserved for the driver or passengers, or the space intended for the transport of property. This includes a person travelling on the bodywork, bumper, fender, roof, running board or step of a vehicle, as well as, hanging on the outside of the vehicle.

Revised (k) A motorcycle is a two-wheeled motor vehicle with one or two riding saddles and sometimes with a third wheel for the support of a sidecar. The sidecar is considered part of the motorcycle. This includes a moped, motor scooter, or motorized bicycle.

Revised (n) A car [automobile] is a four-wheeled motor vehicle designed primarily for carrying up to 7 persons. A trailer being towed by the car is considered part of the car. It does not include a van or minivan—see definition (o)

Revised (t) A special vehicle mainly used on industrial premises is a motor vehicle designed primarily for use within the buildings and premises of industrial or commercial establishments. This includes battery-powered airport passenger vehicles or baggage/mail trucks, forklifts, coal-cars in a coal mine, logging cars and trucks used in mines or quarries.

Revised (w) A special all-terrain vehicle is a motor vehicle of special design to enable it to negotiate over rough or soft terrain, snow or sand. Examples of special design are high construction, special wheels and tires, tracks, and support on a cushion of air. This includes snow mobiles, all-terrain vehicles (ATV), and dune buggies. It does not include passenger vehicle designated as sport utility vehicles (SUV).

Deleted ~~V47.01 Driver of sport utility vehicle injured in collision with fixed or stationary object in nontraffic accident~~

Deleted ~~V47.02 Driver of other type car injured in collision with fixed or stationary object in nontraffic accident~~

Deleted ~~V47.11 Passenger of sport utility vehicle injured in collision with fixed or stationary object in nontraffic accident~~

Deleted ~~V47.12 Passenger of other type car injured in collision with fixed or stationary object in nontraffic accident~~

Deleted ~~V47.31 Unspecified occupant of sport utility vehicle injured in collision with fixed or stationary object in nontraffic accident~~

Deleted ~~V47.32 Unspecified occupant of other type car injured in collision with fixed or stationary object in nontraffic accident~~

Deleted ~~V47.51 Driver of sport utility vehicle injured in collision with fixed or stationary object in traffic accident~~

Deleted ~~V47.52 Driver of other type car injured in collision with fixed or stationary object in traffic accident~~

Deleted ~~V47.61 Passenger of sport utility vehicle injured in collision with fixed or stationary object in traffic accident~~

Deleted ~~V47.62 Passenger of other type car injured in collision with fixed or stationary object in traffic accident~~

Deleted ~~V47.91 Unspecified occupant of sport utility vehicle injured in collision with fixed or stationary object in traffic accident~~

Deleted ~~V47.92 Unspecified occupant of other type car injured in collision with fixed or stationary object in traffic accident~~

EXPOSURE TO INANIMATE MECHANICAL FORCES (W2Ø-W49)

Revised **Excludes1** assault (X92-YØ9)

W25 Contact with sharp glass
Excludes2 glass embedded in skin (W45)

Revised **W26 Contact with other sharp objects**
New **Excludes2** sharp object(s) embedded in skin (W45)
New **W26.2 Contact with edge of stiff paper**
New Paper cut
New **W26.8 Contact with other sharp object(s), not elsewhere classified**
New Contact with tin can lid
New **W26.9 Contact with unspecified sharp object(s)**

W45 Foreign body or object entering through skin
New **Includes** foreign body or object embedded in skin
nail embedded in skin
Revised **Excludes2** contact with other sharp object(s) (W26.-)
Deleted ~~W45.1 Paper entering through skin~~
Deleted ~~Paper cut~~
Deleted ~~W45.2 Lid of can entering through skin~~

W89 Exposure to man-made visible and ultraviolet light
Deleted **Excludes2** exposure to sunlight (X32)
New **Excludes1** exposure to sunlight (X32)

X32 Exposure to sunlight
Deleted **Excludes1** radiation-related disorders of the skin and subcutaneous tissue (L55-L59)

X39.Ø Exposure to natural radiation
Revised **Excludes1** contact with and (suspected) exposure to radon and other naturally occuring radiation (Z77.123)

New
OVEREXERTION AND STRENUOUS OR REPETITIVE MOVEMENTS (X5Ø)

New **X5Ø Overexertion and strenuous or repetitive movements**
New The appropriate 7th character is to be added to each code from category X5Ø

New A initial encounter
New D subsequent encounter
New S sequela

New **X5Ø.Ø Overexertion from strenuous movement or load**
New Lifting heavy objects
New Lifting weights
New **X5Ø.1 Overexertion from prolonged static or awkward postures**
New Prolonged bending
New Prolonged kneeling
New Prolonged reaching
New Prolonged sitting
New Prolonged standing
New Prolonged twisting
New Static bending
New Static kneeling
New Static reaching
New Static sitting
New Static standing
New Static twisting

New **X50.3 Overexertion from repetitive movements**
New Use of hand as hammer
New **Excludes2** Overuse from prolonged static or awkward postures (X50.1)

New **X50.9 Other and unspecified overexertion or strenuous movements or postures**
New Contact pressure
New Contact stress

Deleted **ASSAULT (X92-Y08)**

New **ASSAULT (X92-Y09)**

MISADVENTURES TO PATIENTS DURING SURGICAL AND MEDICAL CARE (Y62-Y69)

New **Excludes1** surgical and medical procedures as the cause of abnormal reaction of the patient, without mention of misadventure at the time of the procedure (Y83-Y84)

Deleted **Excludes2** surgical and medical procedures as the cause of abnormal reaction of the patient, without mention of misadventure at the time of the procedure (Y83-Y84)

MEDICAL DEVICES ASSOCIATED WITH ADVERSE INCIDENTS IN DIAGNOSTIC AND THERAPEUTIC USE (Y70-Y82)

Deleted **Excludes1** misadventure to patients during surgical and medical care, classifiable to (Y62-Y69)

Deleted later complications following use of medical devices without breakdown or malfunctioning of device (Y83-Y84)

New **Excludes2** breakdown or malfunctioning of medical device (after implantation) (during procedure) (ongoing use) (Y70-Y82)

New later complications following use of medical devices without breakdown or malfunctioning of device (Y83-Y84)

New misadventure to patients during surgical and medical care, classifiable to (Y62-Y69)

New surgical and other medical procedures as the cause of abnormal reaction of the patient, or of later complication, without mention of misadventure at the time of the procedure (Y83-Y84)

SURGICAL AND OTHER MEDICAL PROCEDURES AS THE CAUSE OF ABNORMAL REACTION OF THE PATIENT, OR OF LATER COMPLICATION, WITHOUT MENTION OF MISADVENTURE AT THE TIME OF THE PROCEDURE (Y83-Y84)

New **Excludes2** breakdown or malfunctioning of medical device (after implantation) (during procedure) (ongoing use) (Y70-Y82)

Revised **Y92.4 Street, highway and other paved roadways as the place of occurrence of the external cause**

New **Y93.85 Activity, choking game**
New Activity, blackout game
New Activity, fainting game
New Activity, pass out game

CHAPTER 21

FACTORS INFLUENCING HEALTH STATUS AND CONTACT WITH HEALTH SERVICES (Z00-Z99)

This chapter contains the following blocks:

Deleted	Z20-Z28	Persons with potential health hazards related to communicable diseases
New	Z19	Hormone sensitivity malignancy status
New	Z20-Z29	Persons with potential health hazards related to communicable diseases

Z01.411 Encounter for gynecological examination (general) (routine) with abnormal findings
New Use additional code to identify any abnormal findings

Z01.419 Encounter for gynecological examination (general) (routine) without abnormal findings
Deleted Use additional code to identify any abnormal findings

New **Z05 Encounter for observation and evaluation of newborn for suspected diseases and conditions ruled out**
New This category is to be used for newborns, within the neonatal period (the first 28 days of life), who are suspected of having an abnormal condition unrelated to exposure from the mother or the birth process, but without signs or symptoms, and which, after examination and observation, is ruled out.

New **Excludes2** newborn observation for suspected condition, related to exposure from the mother or birth process (P00-P04)

New **Z05.0 Observation and evaluation of newborn for suspected cardiac condition ruled out**

New **Z05.1 Observation and evaluation of newborn for suspected infectious condition ruled out**

New **Z05.2 Observation and evaluation of newborn for suspected neurological condition ruled out**

New **Z05.3 Observation and evaluation of newborn for suspected respiratory condition ruled out**

New **Z05.4 Observation and evaluation of newborn for suspected genetic, metabolic or immunologic condition ruled out**

New **Z05.41 Observation and evaluation of newborn for suspected genetic condition ruled out**

New **Z05.42 Observation and evaluation of newborn for suspected metabolic condition ruled out**

New **Z05.43 Observation and evaluation of newborn for suspected immunologic condition ruled out**

New **Z05.5 Observation and evaluation of newborn for suspected gastrointestinal condition ruled out**

New **Z05.6 Observation and evaluation of newborn for suspected genitourinary condition ruled out**

New **Z05.7 Observation and evaluation of newborn for suspected skin, subcutaneous, musculoskeletal and connective tissue condition ruled out**

New **Z05.71 Observation and evaluation of newborn for suspected skin and subcutaneous tissue condition ruled out**

New **Z05.72 Observation and evaluation of newborn for suspected musculoskeletal condition ruled out**

New **Z05.73 Observation and evaluation of newborn for suspected connective tissue condition ruled out**

New **Z05.8 Observation and evaluation of newborn for other specified suspected condition ruled out**

New **Z05.9 Observation and evaluation of newborn for unspecified suspected condition ruled out**

Z12.4 Encounter for screening for malignant neoplasm of cervix

Deleted **Excludes1** encounter for screening for human papillomavirus (Z11.51)

New **Excludes2** encounter for screening for human papillomavirus (Z11.51)

New **HORMONE SENSITIVITY MALIGNANCY STATUS (Z19)**

New **Z19 Hormone sensitivity malignancy status**
New *Code first* malignant neoplasm —*see* Table of Neoplasms, by site, malignant
New **Z19.1 Hormone sensitive malignancy status**
New **Z19.2 Hormone resistant malignancy status**
New Castrate resistant prostate malignancy status

Deleted **PERSONS WITH POTENTIAL HEALTH HAZARDS RELATED TO COMMUNICABLE DISEASES (Z20-Z28)**

New **PERSONS WITH POTENTIAL HEALTH HAZARDS RELATED TO COMMUNICABLE DISEASES (Z20-Z29)**

Z22 Carrier of infectious disease
New **Excludes2** carrier of viral hepatitis (B18.-)
Z22.330 Carrier of Group B streptococcus
New **Excludes1** Carrier of streptococcus group B (GBS) complicating pregnancy, childbirth and the puerperium (O99.82-)
Deleted ~~**Z22.5 Carrier of viral hepatitis**~~
Deleted ~~**Z22.50 Carrier of unspecified viral hepatitis**~~
Deleted ~~**Z22.51 Carrier of viral hepatitis B**~~
Deleted ~~Hepatitis B surface antigen [HBsAg] carrier~~
Deleted ~~**Z22.52 Carrier of viral hepatitis C**~~
Deleted ~~**Z22.59 Carrier of other viral hepatitis**~~
New **Z29 Encounter for other prophylactic measures**
New **Excludes1** desensitization to allergens (Z51.6)
New prophylactic surgery (Z40.-)
New **Z29.1 Encounter for prophylactic immunotherapy**
New Encounter for administration of immunoglobulin
New **Z29.11 Encounter for prophylactic immunotherapy for respiratory syncytial virus (RSV)**
New **Z29.12 Encounter for prophylactic antivenin**
New **Z29.13 Encounter for prophylactic Rho(D) immune globulin**
New **Z29.14 Encounter for prophylactic rabies immune globin**
New **Z29.3 Encounter for prophylactic fluoride administration**
New **Z29.8 Encounter for other specified prophylactic measures**
New **Z29.9 Encounter for prophylactic measures, unspecified**
New **Z30.015 Encounter for initial prescription of vaginal ring hormonal contraceptive**
New **Z30.016 Encounter for initial prescription of transdermal patch hormonal contraceptive device**
New **Z30.017 Encounter for initial prescription of implantable subdermal contraceptive**
New **Z30.018 Encounter for initial prescription of other contraceptives**
New Encounter for initial prescription of barrier contraception
New Encounter for initial prescription of diaphragm
New **Z30.44 Encounter for surveillance of vaginal ring hormonal contraceptive device**
New **Z30.45 Encounter for surveillance of transdermal patch hormonal contraceptive device**
New **Z30.46 Encounter for surveillance of implantable subdermal contraceptive**
New Encounter for checking, reinsertion or removal of implantable subdermal contraceptive
New **Z30.49 Encounter for surveillance of other contraceptives**
New Encounter for surveillance of barrier contraception
New Encounter for surveillance of diaphragm
New **Z31.7 Encounter for procreative management and counseling for gestational carrier**
New **Excludes1** pregnant state, gestational carrier (Z33.3)
Z33.1 Pregnant state, incidental
New **Excludes1** pregnant state, gestational carrier (Z33.3)
New **Z33.3 Pregnant state, gestational carrier**
New **Excludes1** encounter for procreative management and counseling for gestational carrier (Z31.7)

Z3A Weeks of gestation
Revised **Note:** Codes from category Z3A are for use, only on the maternal record, to indicate the weeks of gestation of the pregnancy, if known.

Z45.01 Encounter for adjustment and management of cardiac pacemaker
New Encounter for adjustment and management of cardiac resynchronization therapy pacemaker (CRT-P)
Z45.02 Encounter for adjustment and management of automatic implantable cardiac defibrillator
New Encounter for adjustment and management of cardiac resynchronization therapy defibrillator (CRT-D)
Revised **Z51 Encounter for other aftercare and medical care**
New **Z51.6 Encounter for desensitization to allergens**
New **Z53.3 Procedure converted to open procedure**
New **Z53.31 Laparoscopic surgical procedure converted to open procedure**
New **Z53.32 Thoracoscopic surgical procedure converted to open procedure**
New **Z53.33 Arthroscopic surgical procedure converted to open procedure**
New **Z53.39 Other specified procedure converted to open procedure**

Z77 Other contact with and (suspected) exposures hazardous to health

Revised **Excludes2** newborn affected by noxious substances transmitted via placenta or breast milk (PØ4.-)

Z79 Long term (current) drug therapy

New **Excludes2** long term (current) use of oral antidiabetic drugs (Z79.84)

New long term (current) use of oral hypoglycemic drugs (Z79.84)

New **Z79.84 Long term (current) use of oral hypoglycemic drugs**

New Long term (current) use of oral antidiabetic drugs

New **Excludes2** long term (current) use of insulin (Z79.4)

Z79.891 Long term (current) use of opiate analgesic

Revised **Excludes1** methodone use NOS (F11.9-)

New **Z83.42 Family history of familial hypercholesterolemia**

New **Z84.82 Family history of sudden infant death syndrome**

New Family history of SIDS

Z85 Personal history of malignant neoplasm

Use additional code to identify:

Revised history of tobacco dependence (Z87.891)

Z85.8 Personal history of malignant neoplasms of other organs and systems

Revised Conditions classifiable to CØØ-C14, C4Ø-C49, C69-C75, C7A.Ø98, C76-C79

Z86.ØØ Personal history of in-situ neoplasm

New Conditions classifiable to DØØ-DØ9

Z86.ØØ1 Personal history of in-situ neoplasm of cervix uteri

New Personal history of cervical intraepithelial neoplasia III [CIN III]

Z86.ØØ8 Personal history of in-situ neoplasm of other site

New Personal history of vaginal intraepithelial neoplasia III [VAIN III]

New Personal history of vulvar intraepithelial neoplasia III [VIN III]

Z87.41 Personal history of dysplasia of the female genital tract

New **Excludes1** personal history of intraepithelial neoplasia III of female genital tract (Z87.ØØ1, Z87.ØØ8)

Z9Ø.41 Acquired absence of pancreas

New Code also exocrine pancreatic insufficiency (K86.81)

New **Z92.84 Personal history of unintended awareness under general anesthesia**

New **Excludes2** unintended awareness under general anesthesia during procedure (T88.53)

Z95.Ø Presence of cardiac pacemaker

New Presence of cardiac resynchronization therapy (CRT-P) pacemaker

New **Excludes1** adjustment or management of cardiac device (Z45.Ø-)

Z95.1 Presence of aortocoronary bypass graft

New Presence of coronary artery bypass graft

Z95.81Ø Presence of automatic (implantable) cardiac defibrillator

New Presence of cardiac resynchronization therapy defibrillator (CRT-D)

New Presence of cardioverter-defibrillator (ICD)

Z97.5 Presence of (intrauterine) contraceptive device

Revised **Excludes1** checking, reinsertion or removal of implantable subdermal contraceptive (Z3Ø.46)

New checking, reinsertion or removal of intrauterine contraceptive device (Z3Ø.43-)

Z98.89 Other specified postprocedural states

Deleted Personal history of surgery, not elsewhere classified

New **Z98.89Ø Other specified postprocedural states**

New Personal history of surgery, not elsewhere classified

New **Z98.891 History of uterine scar from previous surgery**

New **Excludes1** Maternal care due to uterine scar from previous surgery (O34.2-)

Z99.2 Dependence on renal dialysis

Deleted **Excludes1** noncompliance with renal dialysis (Z91.15)

New **Excludes2** noncompliance with renal dialysis (Z91.15)

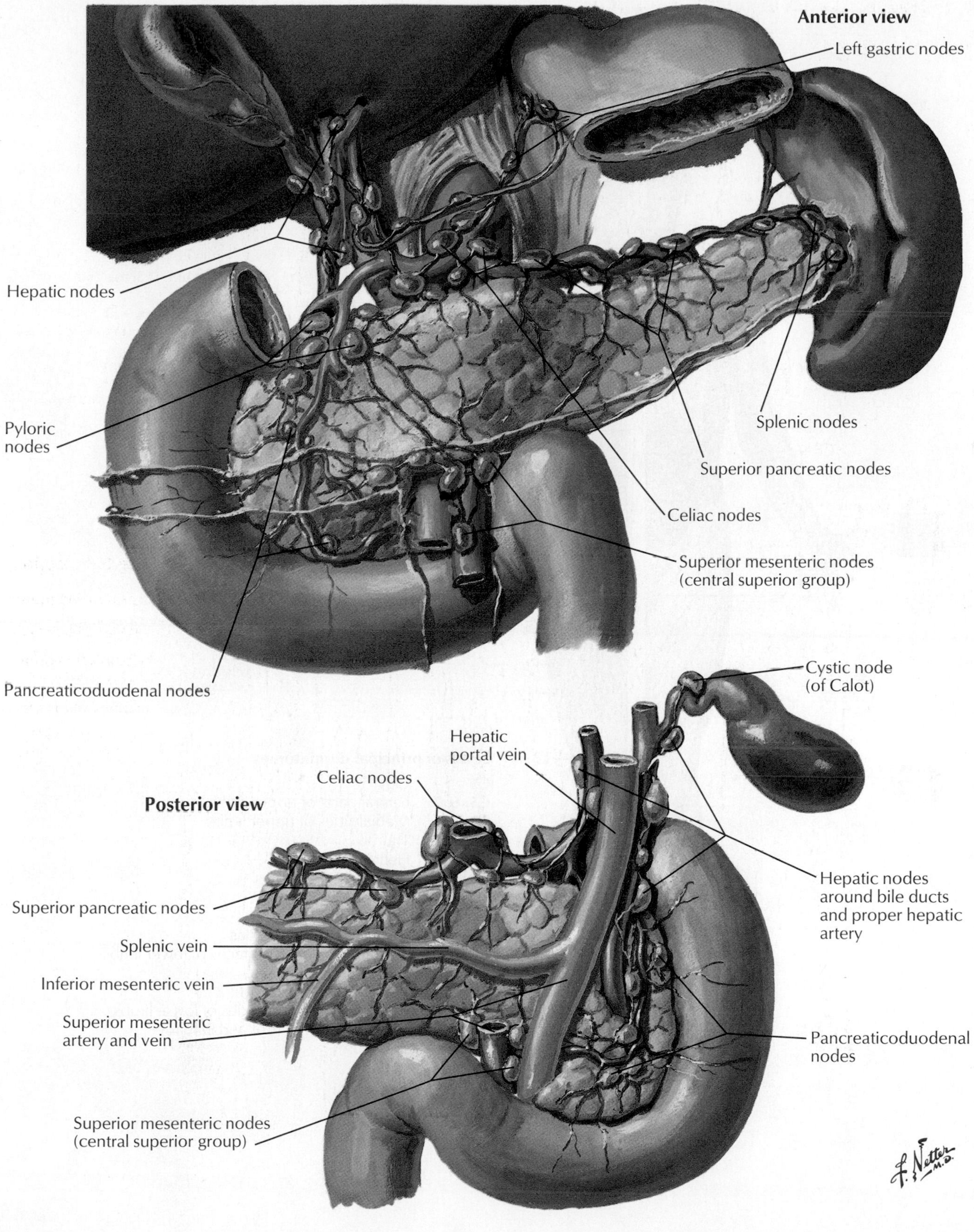

Plate 315 Lymph Vessels and Nodes of Pancreas. (Netter: Atlas of Human Anatomy, 4 ed, 2006, Saunders.)

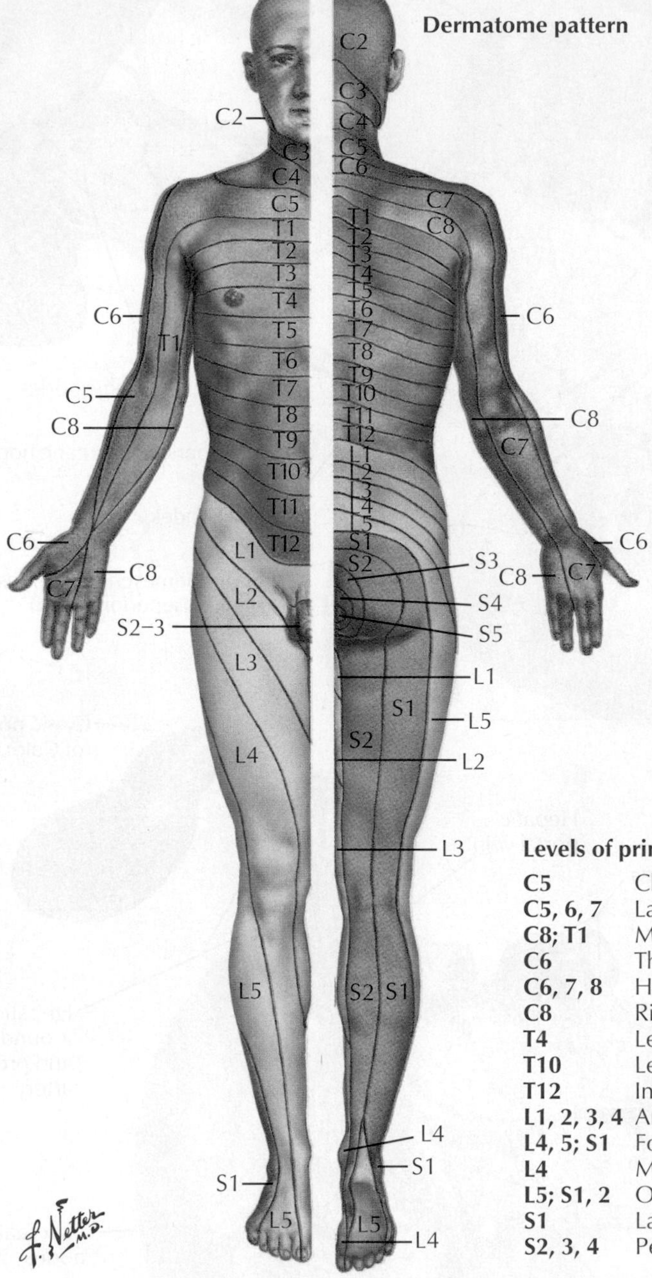

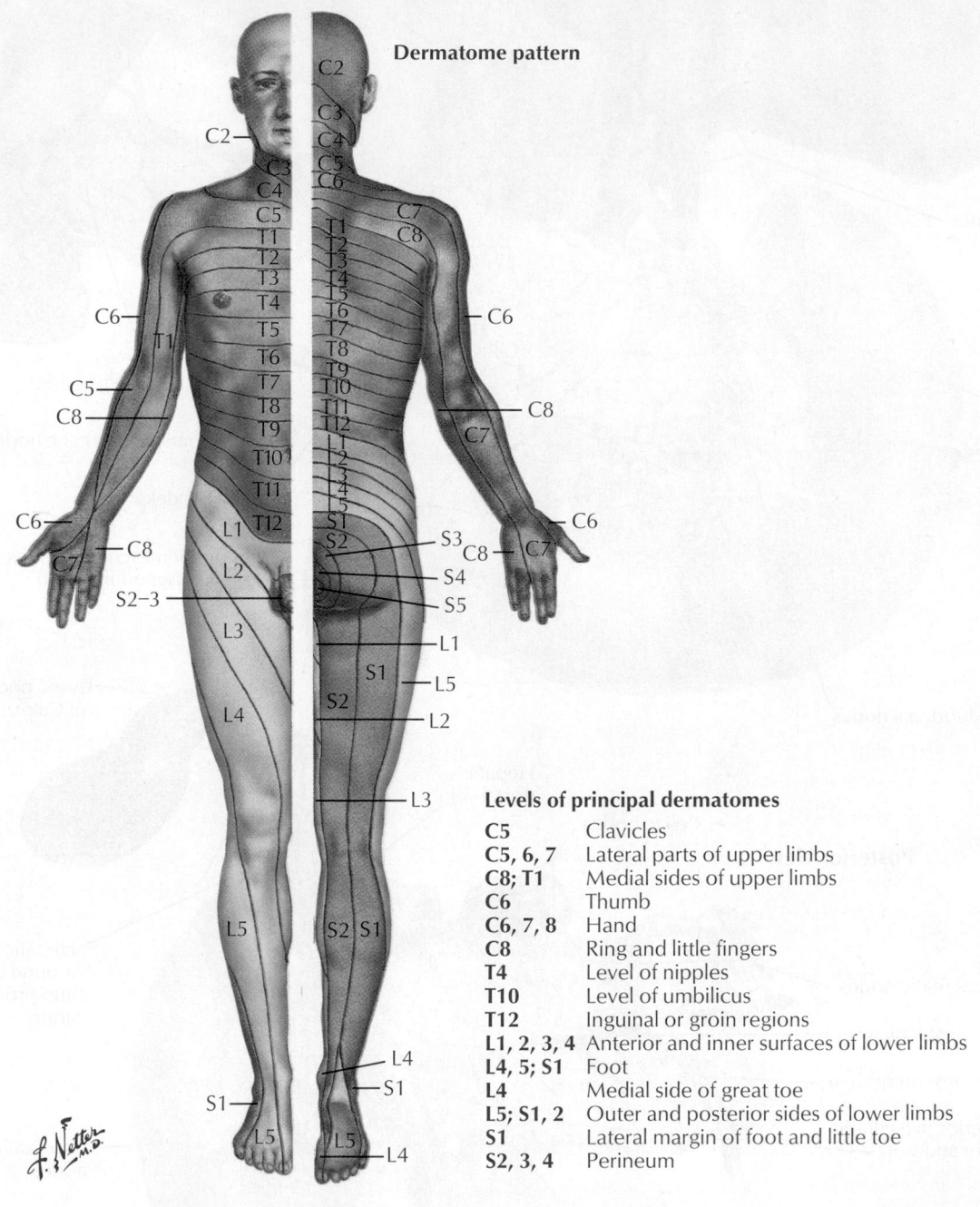

Levels of principal dermatomes

C5	Clavicles
C5, 6, 7	Lateral parts of upper limbs
C8; T1	Medial sides of upper limbs
C6	Thumb
C6, 7, 8	Hand
C8	Ring and little fingers
T4	Level of nipples
T10	Level of umbilicus
T12	Inguinal or groin regions
L1, 2, 3, 4	Anterior and inner surfaces of lower limbs
L4, 5; S1	Foot
L4	Medial side of great toe
L5; S1, 2	Outer and posterior sides of lower limbs
S1	Lateral margin of foot and little toe
S2, 3, 4	Perineum

Plate 164 Dermatomes. (Netter: Atlas of Human Anatomy, 4 ed, 2006, Saunders.)

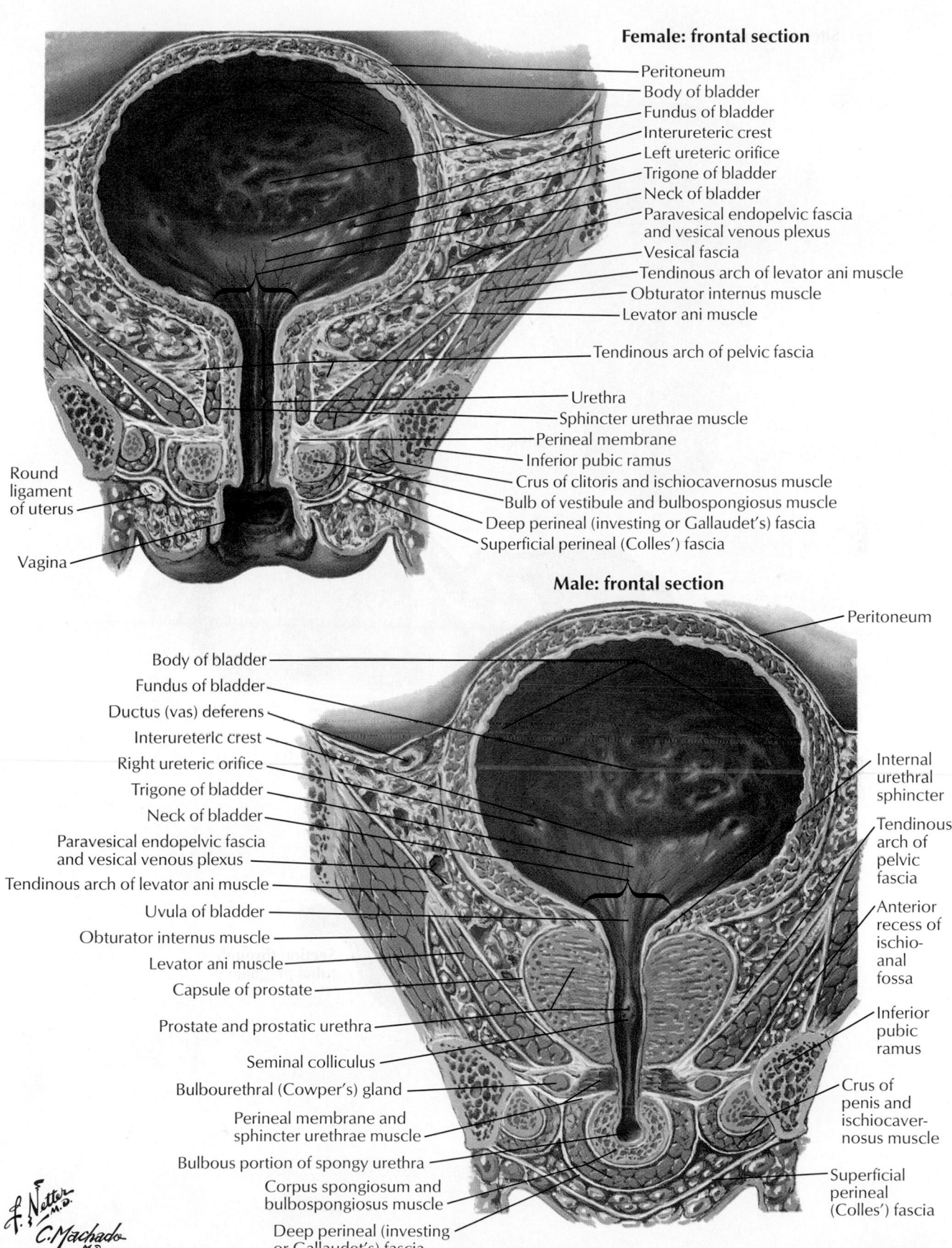

Female: frontal section

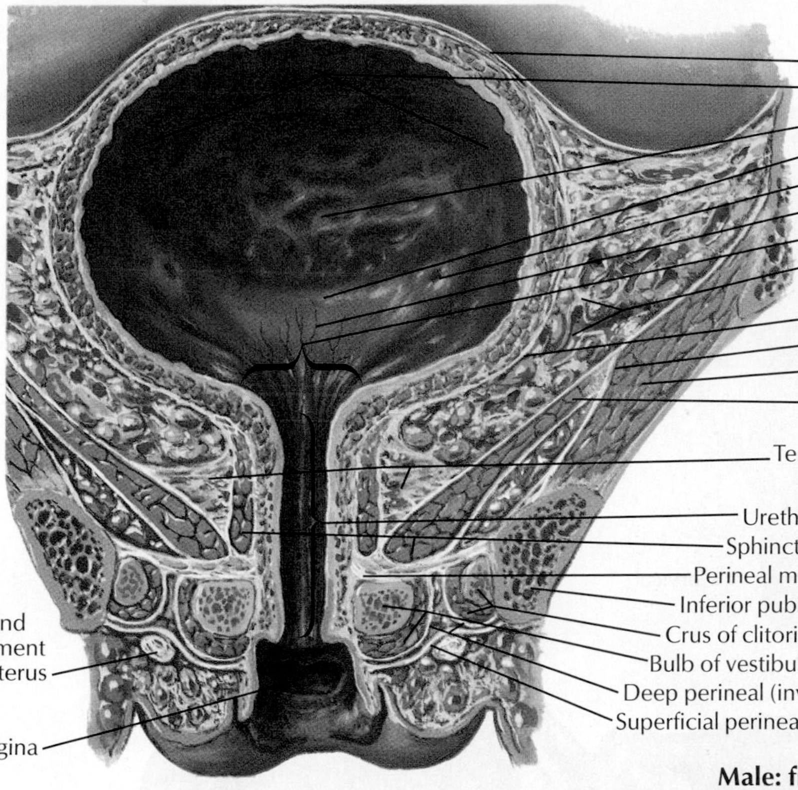
Peritoneum
Body of bladder
Fundus of bladder
Interureteric crest
Left ureteric orifice
Trigone of bladder
Neck of bladder
Paravesical endopelvic fascia and vesical venous plexus
Vesical fascia
Tendinous arch of levator ani muscle
Obturator internus muscle
Levator ani muscle
Tendinous arch of pelvic fascia
Urethra
Sphincter urethrae muscle
Perineal membrane
Inferior pubic ramus
Crus of clitoris and ischiocavernosus muscle
Bulb of vestibule and bulbospongiosus muscle
Deep perineal (investing or Gallaudet's) fascia
Superficial perineal (Colles') fascia
Round ligament of uterus
Vagina

Male: frontal section

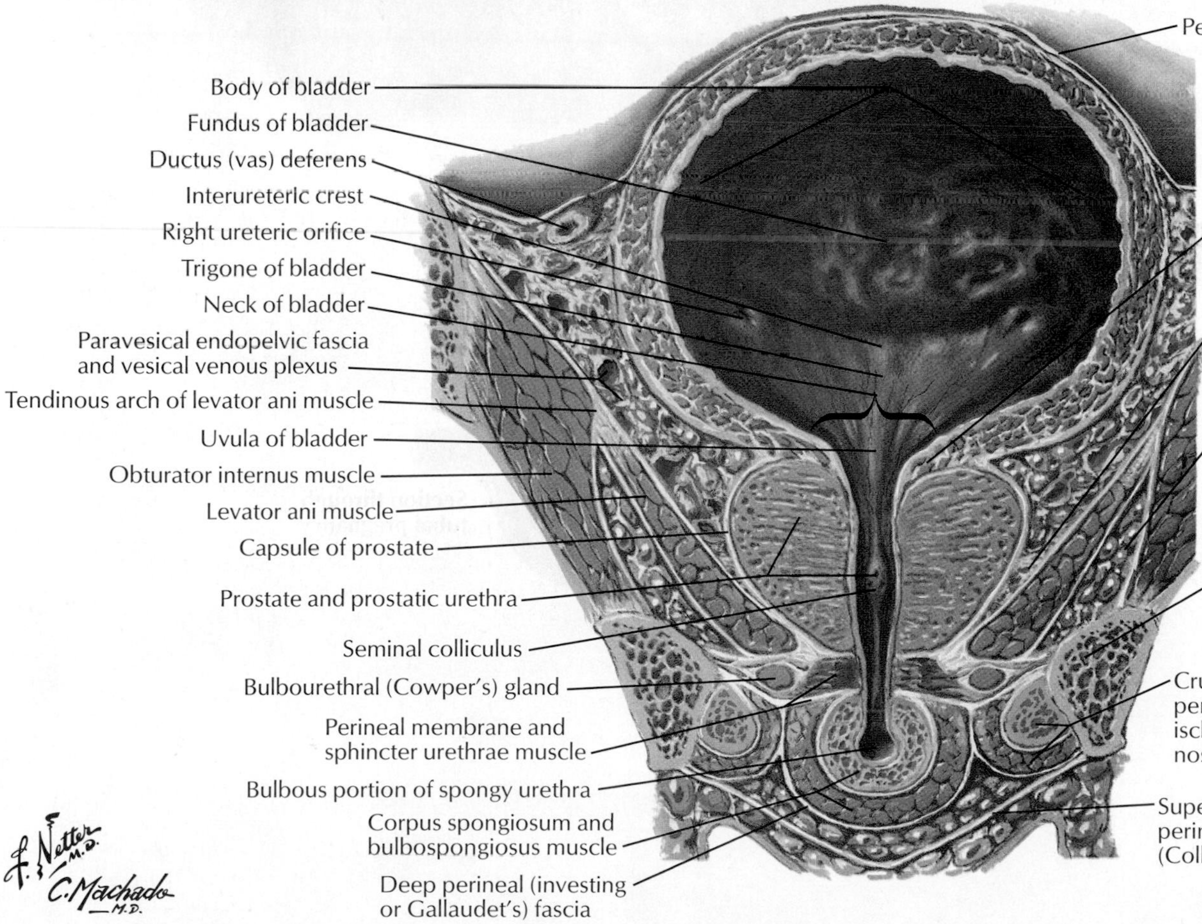
Peritoneum
Body of bladder
Fundus of bladder
Ductus (vas) deferens
Interureteric crest
Right ureteric orifice
Trigone of bladder
Neck of bladder
Paravesical endopelvic fascia and vesical venous plexus
Tendinous arch of levator ani muscle
Uvula of bladder
Obturator internus muscle
Levator ani muscle
Capsule of prostate
Prostate and prostatic urethra
Seminal colliculus
Bulbourethral (Cowper's) gland
Perineal membrane and sphincter urethrae muscle
Bulbous portion of spongy urethra
Corpus spongiosum and bulbospongiosus muscle
Deep perineal (investing or Gallaudet's) fascia
Internal urethral sphincter
Tendinous arch of pelvic fascia
Anterior recess of ischio-anal fossa
Inferior pubic ramus
Crus of penis and ischiocaver-nosus muscle
Superficial perineal (Colles') fascia
F. Netter M.D.
C. Machado M.D.

Plate 366 Urinary Bladder: Female and Male. (Netter: Atlas of Human Anatomy, 4 ed, 2006, Saunders.)

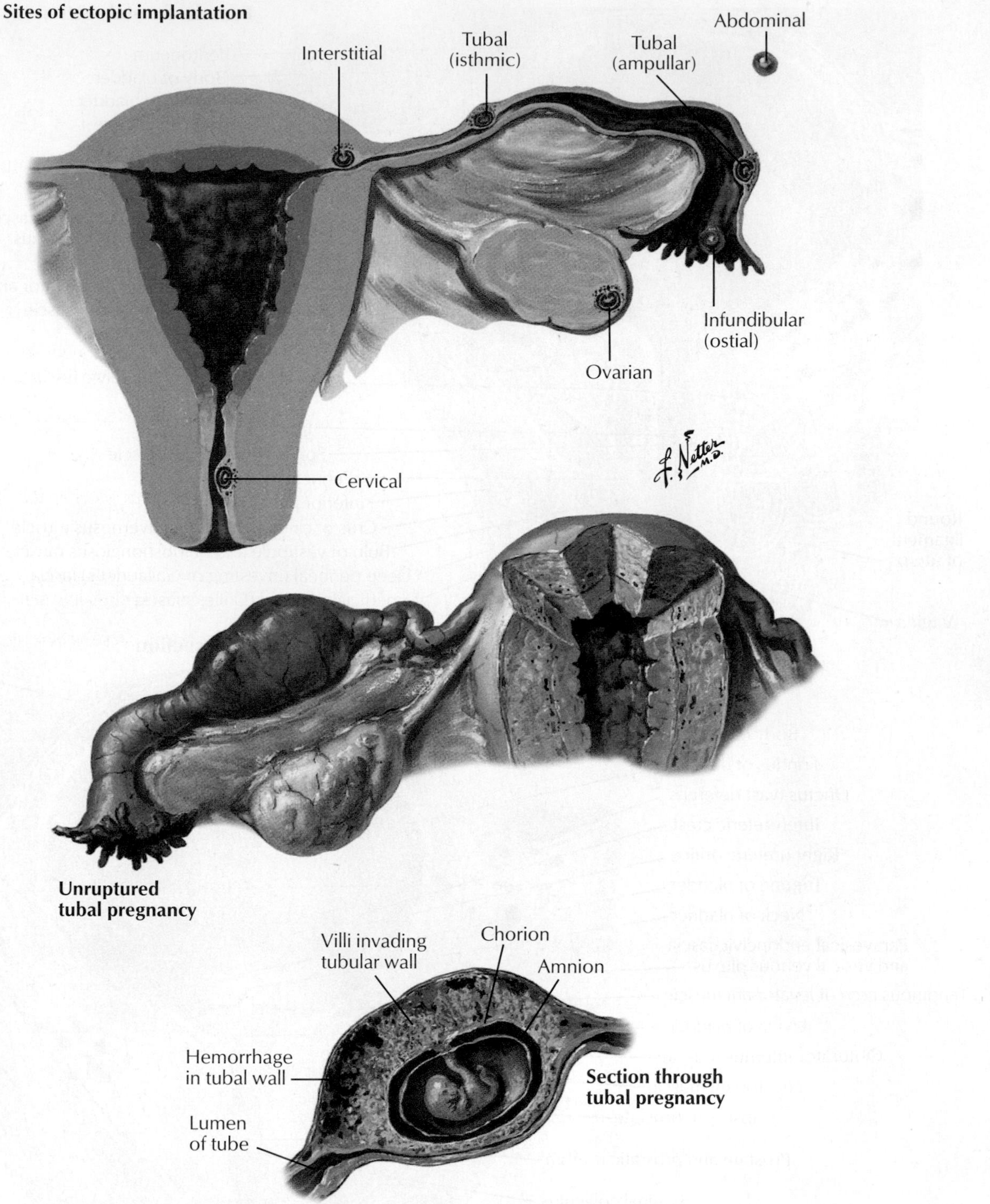

Plate 375 Ectopic Pregnancy. (Netter: Atlas of Human Anatomy, 4 ed, 2006, Saunders.)

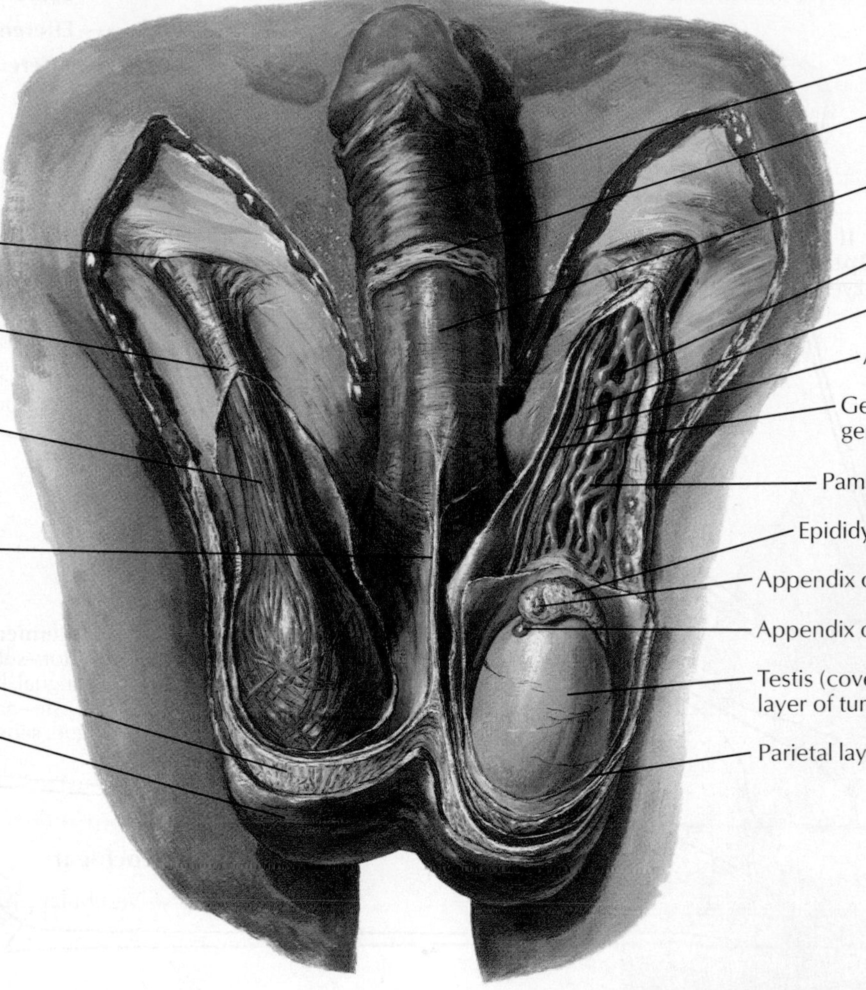

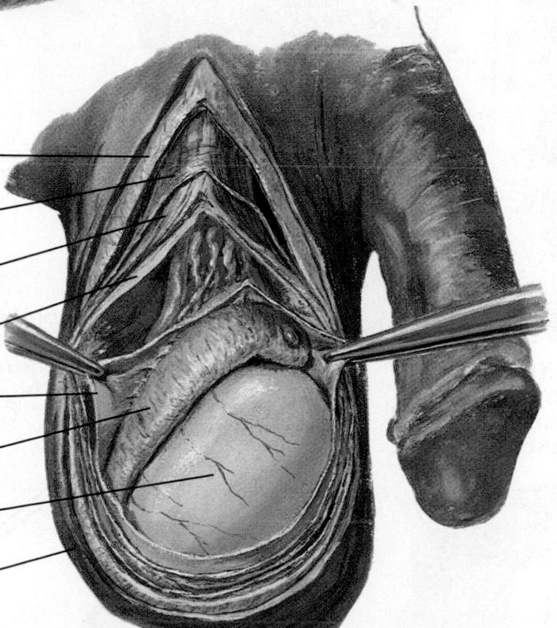

NETTER'S ANATOMY ILLUSTRATIONS

Plate 387 Scrotum and Contents. (Netter: Atlas of Human Anatomy, 4 ed, 2006, Saunders.)

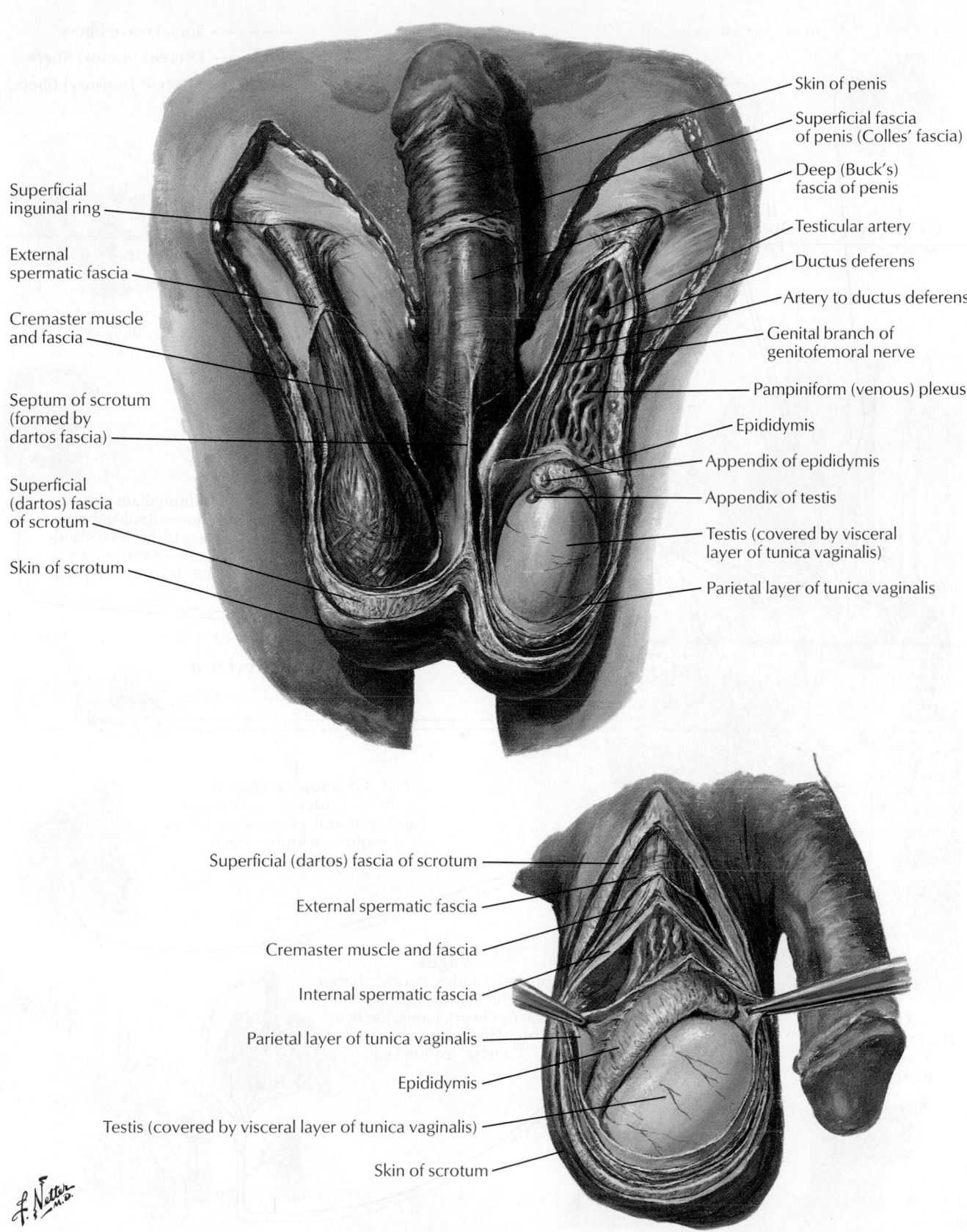

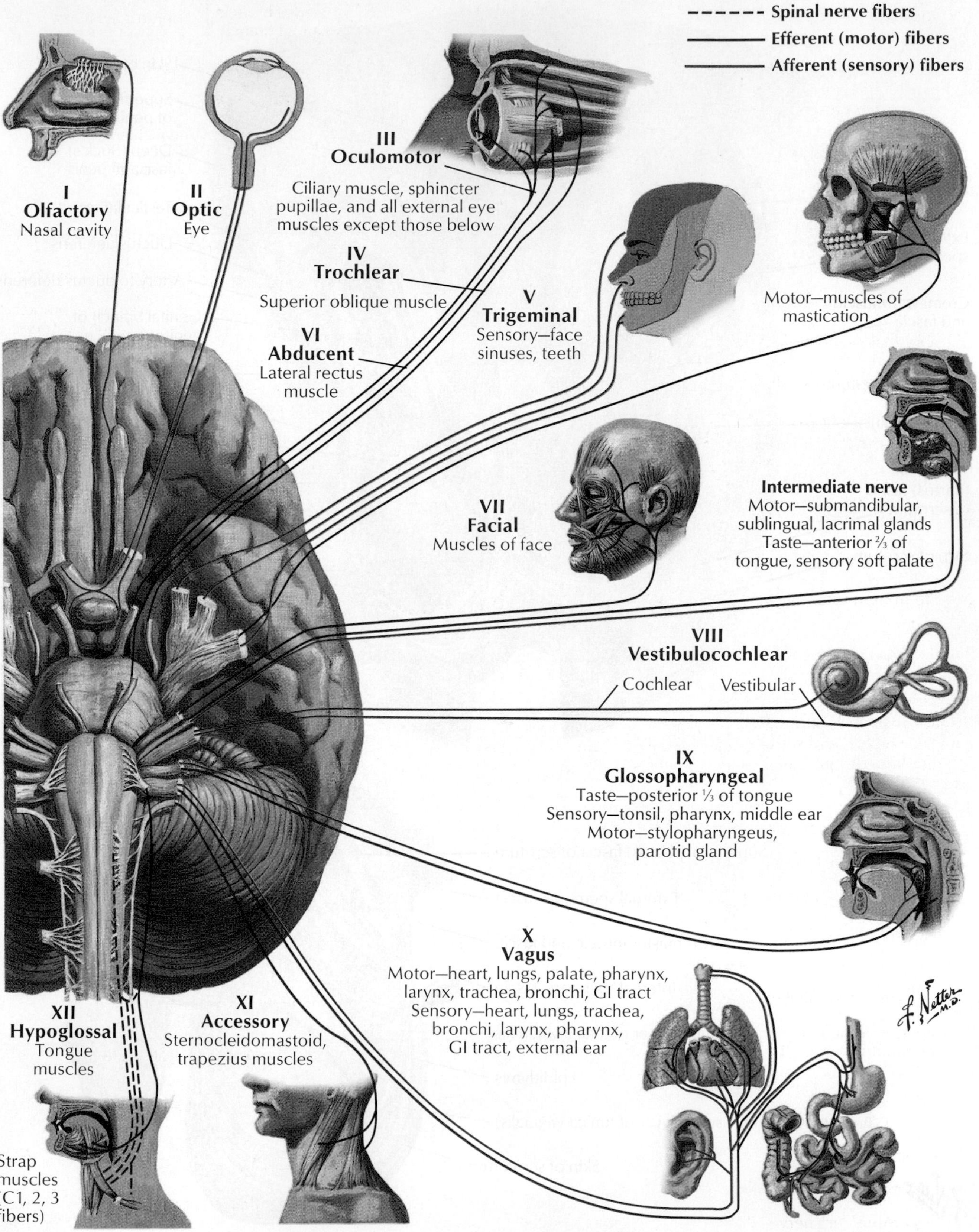

Plate 118 Cranial Nerves (Motor and Sensory Distribution): Schema. (Netter: Atlas of Human Anatomy, 4 ed, 2006, Saunders.)

Superior view

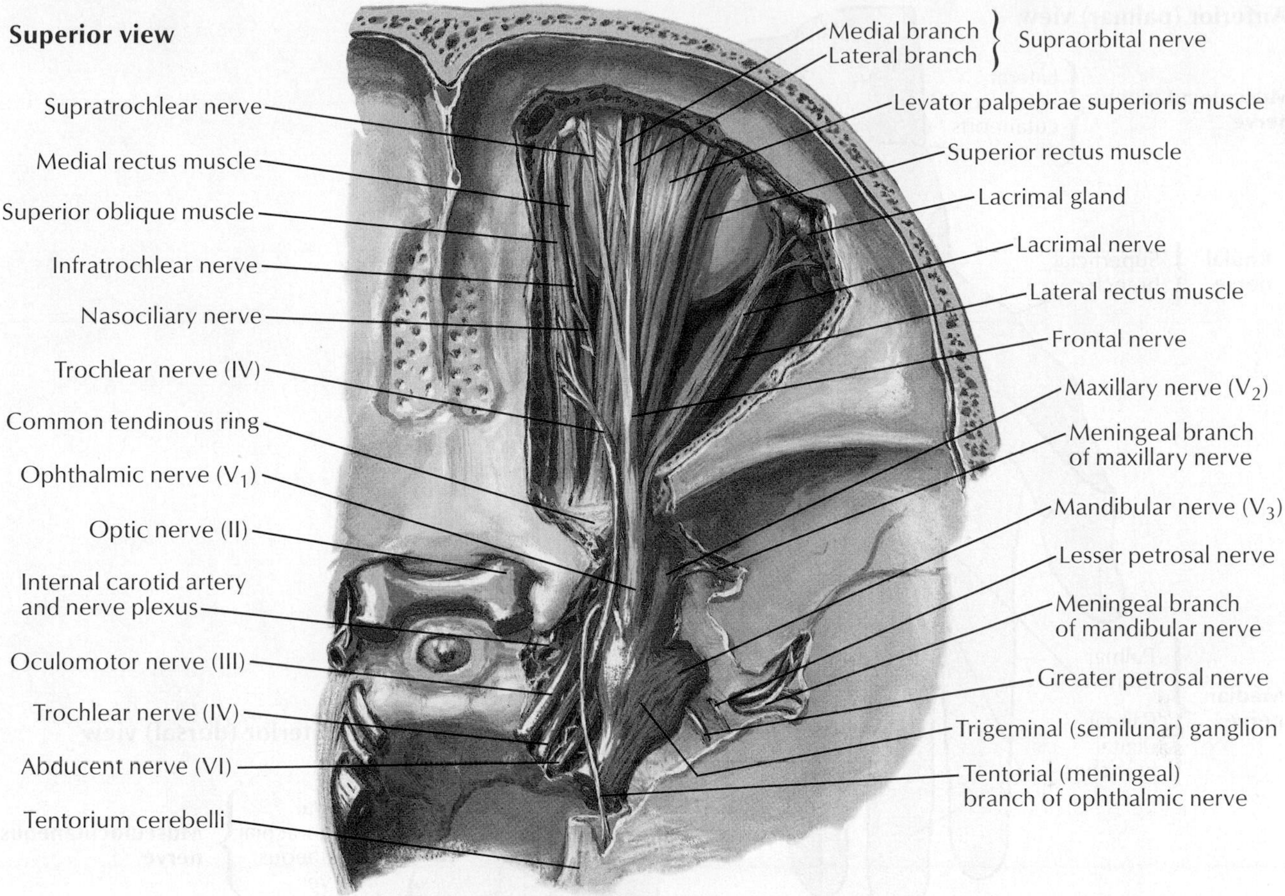

Superior view:
levator palpebrae superioris, superior rectus, and superior oblique muscles partially cut away

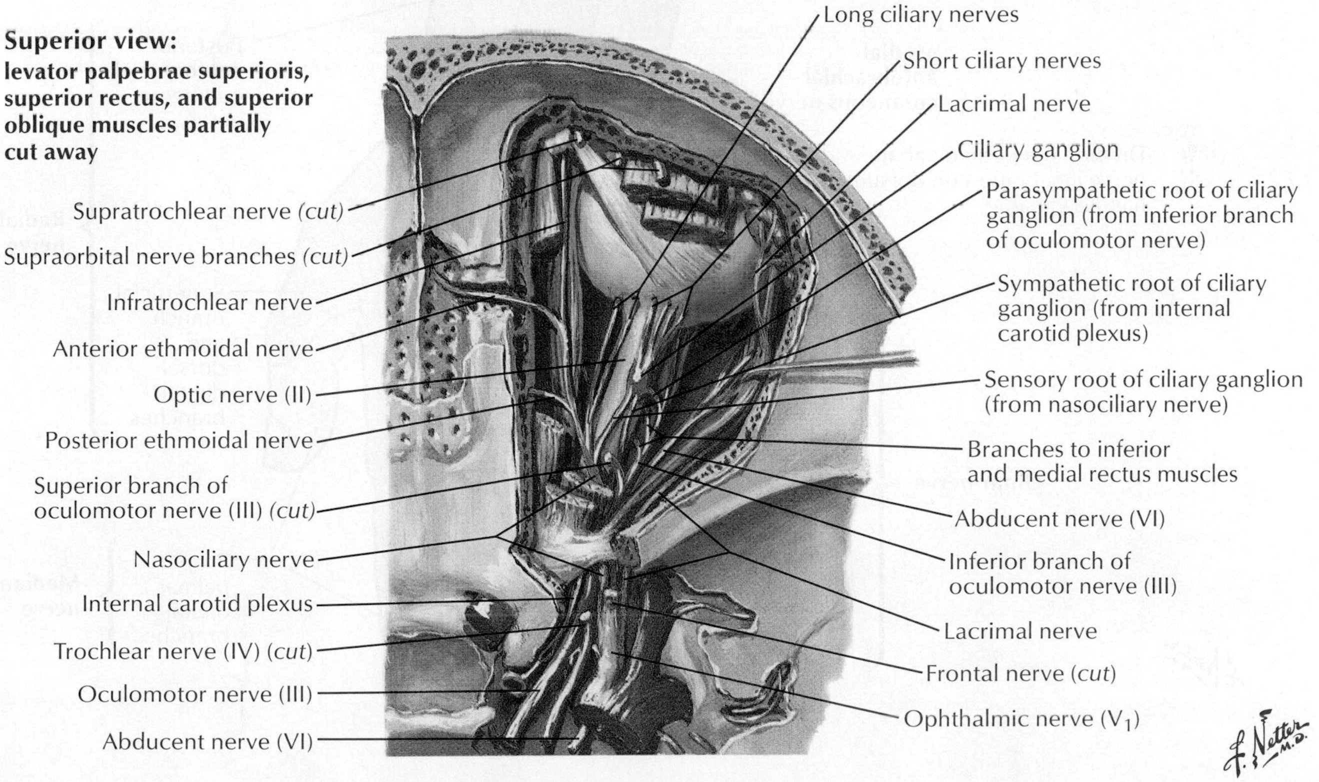

Plate 86 Nerves of Orbit. (Netter: Atlas of Human Anatomy, 4 ed, 2006, Saunders.)

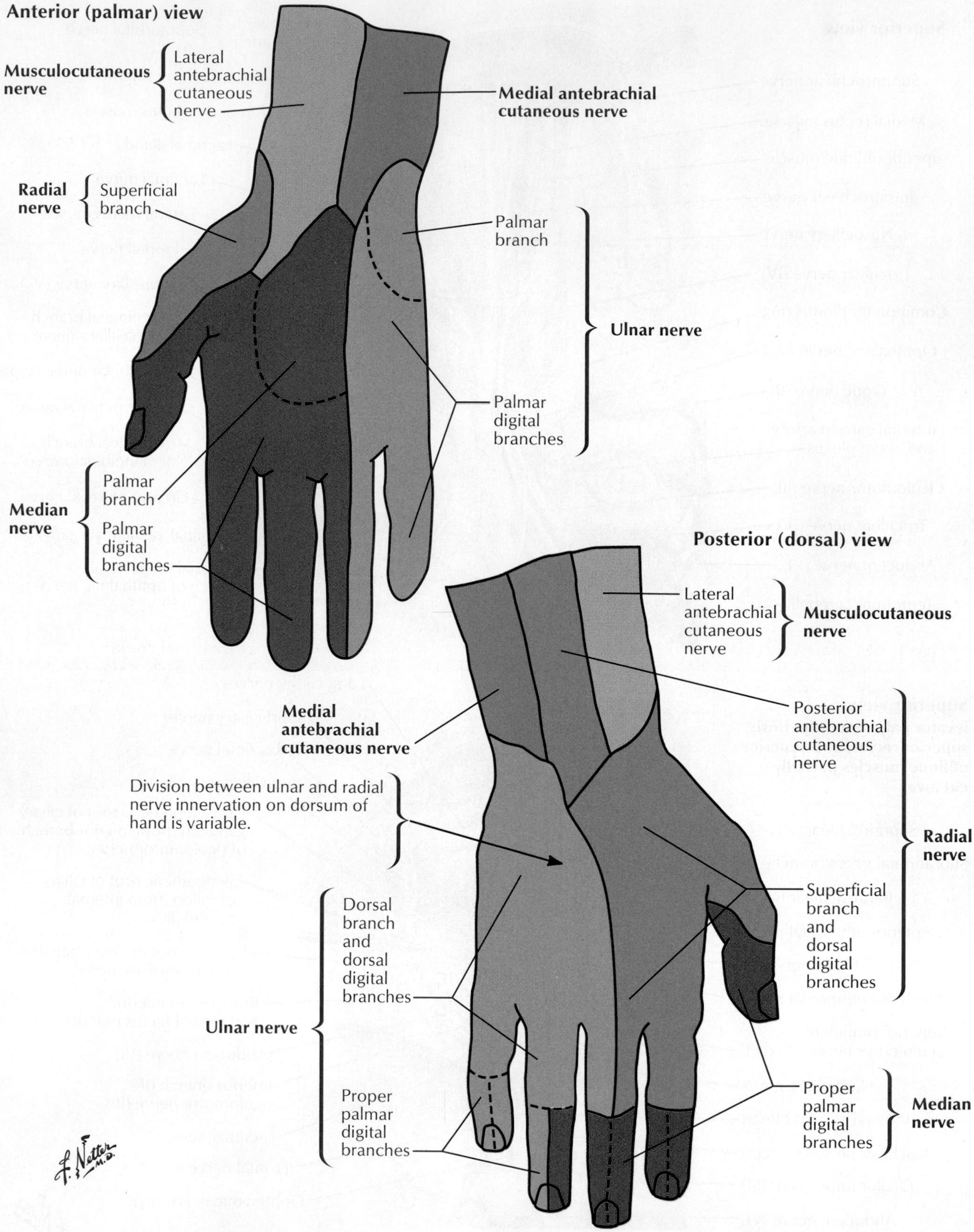

Plate 472 Cutaneous Innervation of Wrist and Hand. (Netter: Atlas of Human Anatomy, 4 ed, 2006, Saunders.)

Anterior view

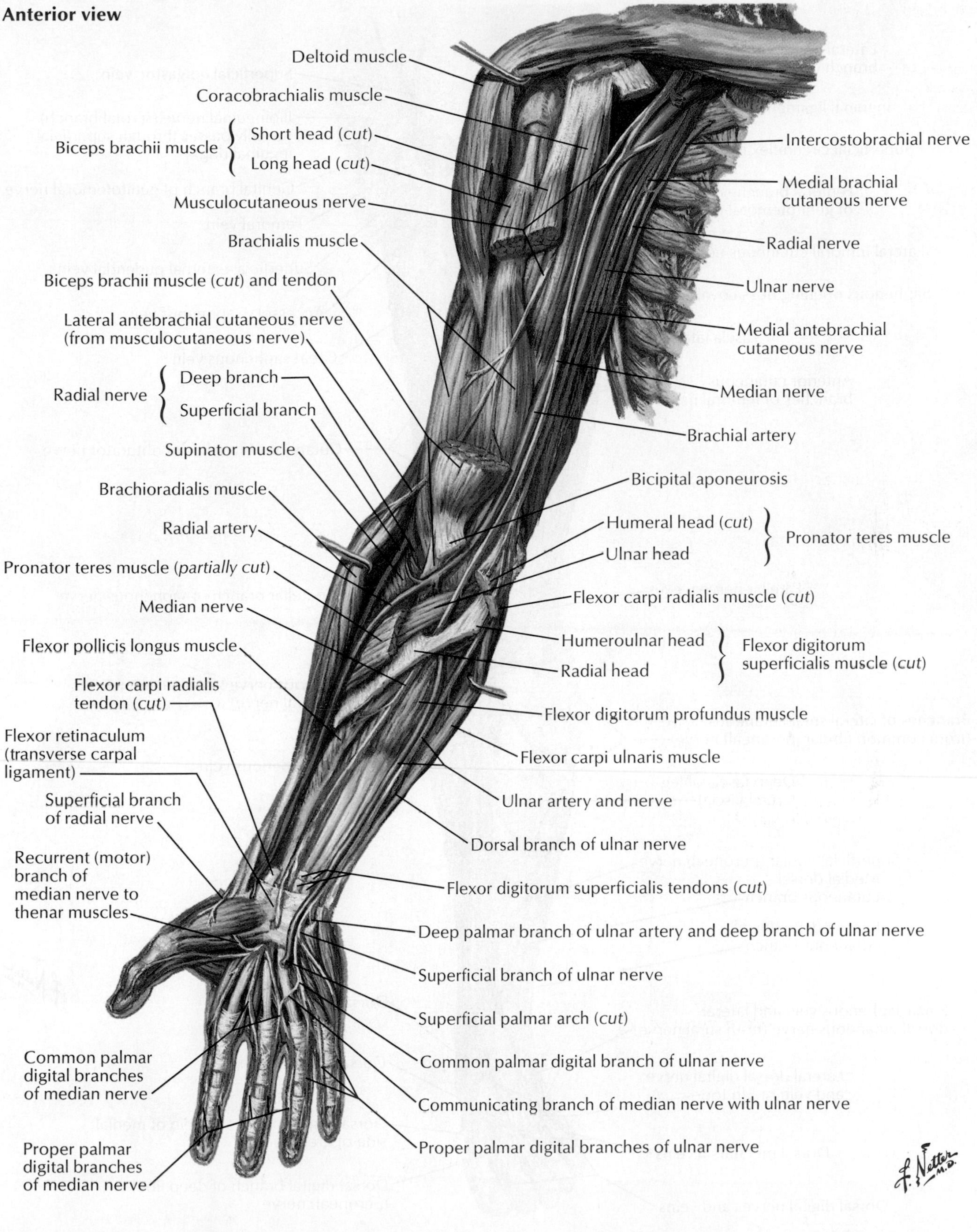

Plate 473 Arteries and Nerves of Upper Limb. (Netter: Atlas of Human Anatomy, 4 ed, 2006, Saunders.)

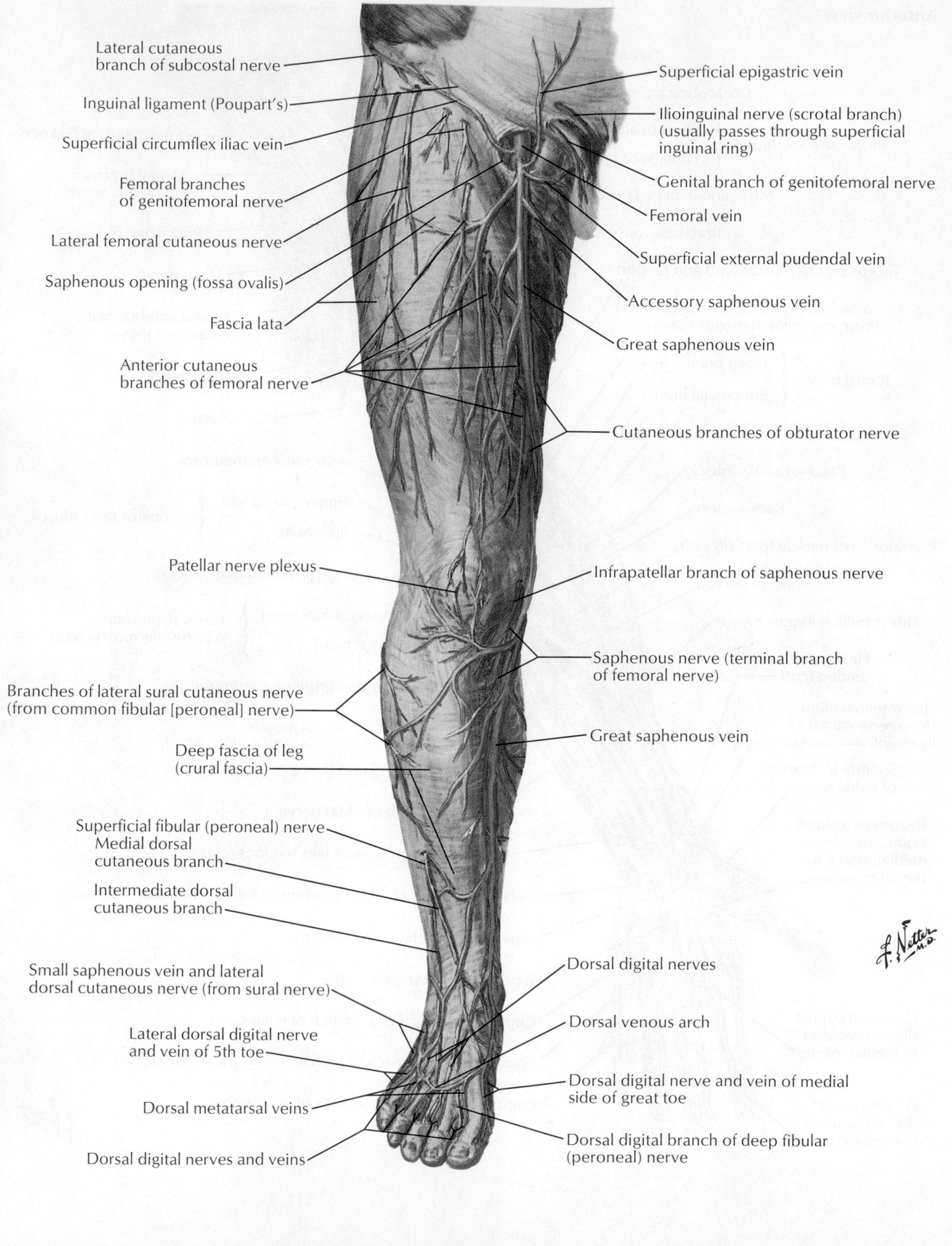
Lateral cutaneous branch of subcostal nerve
Inguinal ligament (Poupart's)
Superficial circumflex iliac vein
Femoral branches of genitofemoral nerve
Lateral femoral cutaneous nerve
Saphenous opening (fossa ovalis)
Fascia lata
Anterior cutaneous branches of femoral nerve
Patellar nerve plexus
Branches of lateral sural cutaneous nerve (from common fibular [peroneal] nerve)
Deep fascia of leg (crural fascia)
Superficial fibular (peroneal) nerve
Medial dorsal cutaneous branch
Intermediate dorsal cutaneous branch
Small saphenous vein and lateral dorsal cutaneous nerve (from sural nerve)
Lateral dorsal digital nerve and vein of 5th toe
Dorsal metatarsal veins
Dorsal digital nerves and veins
Superficial epigastric vein
Ilioinguinal nerve (scrotal branch) (usually passes through superficial inguinal ring)
Genital branch of genitofemoral nerve
Femoral vein
Superficial external pudendal vein
Accessory saphenous vein
Great saphenous vein
Cutaneous branches of obturator nerve
Infrapatellar branch of saphenous nerve
Saphenous nerve (terminal branch of femoral nerve)
Great saphenous vein
Dorsal digital nerves
Dorsal venous arch
Dorsal digital nerve and vein of medial side of great toe
Dorsal digital branch of deep fibular (peroneal) nerve
F. Netter M.D.

Plate 544 Superficial Nerves and Veins of Lower Limb: Anterior View. (Netter: Atlas of Human Anatomy, 4 ed, 2006, Saunders.)

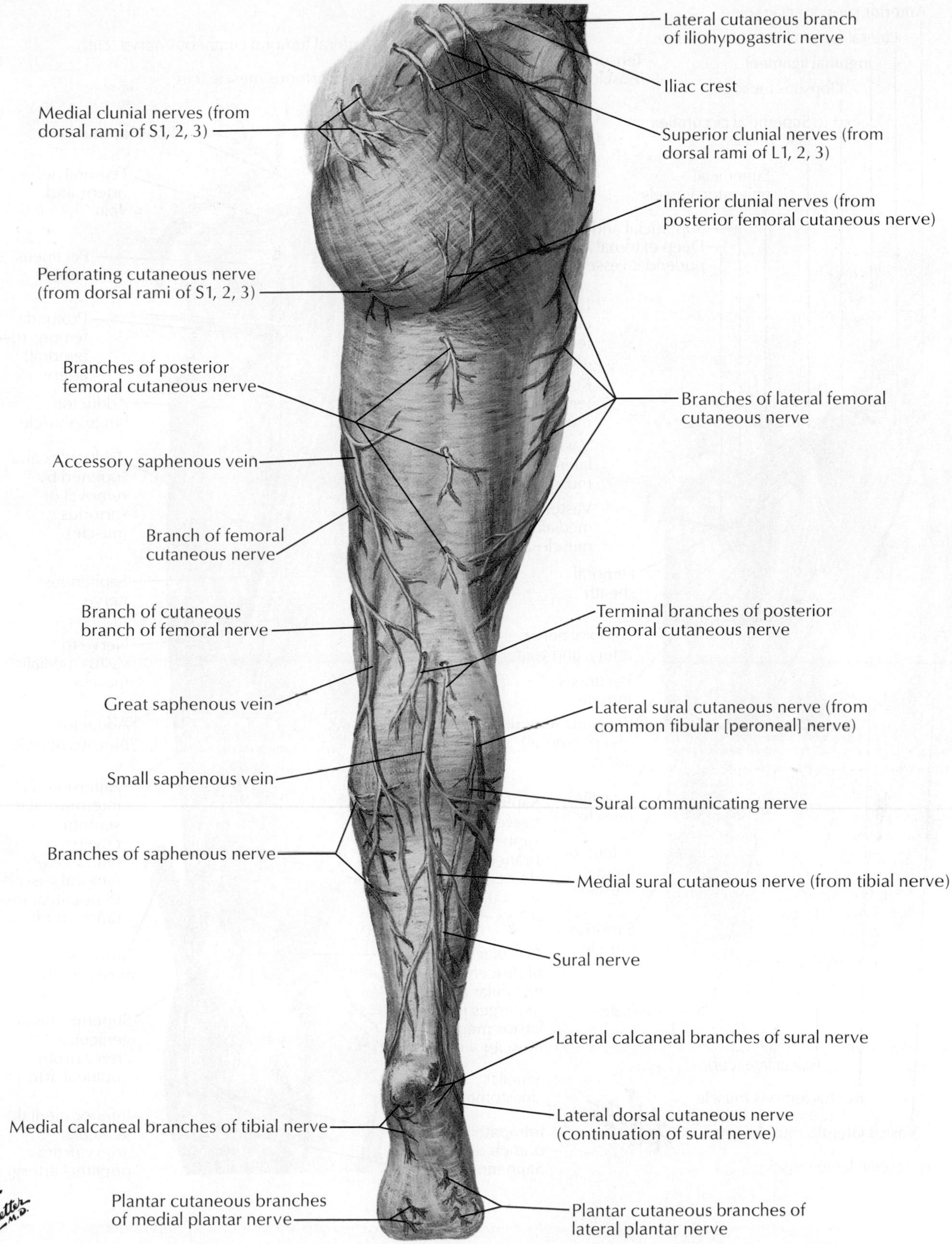

Plate 545 Superficial Nerves and Veins of Lower Limb: Posterior View. (Netter: Atlas of Human Anatomy, 4 ed, 2006, Saunders.)

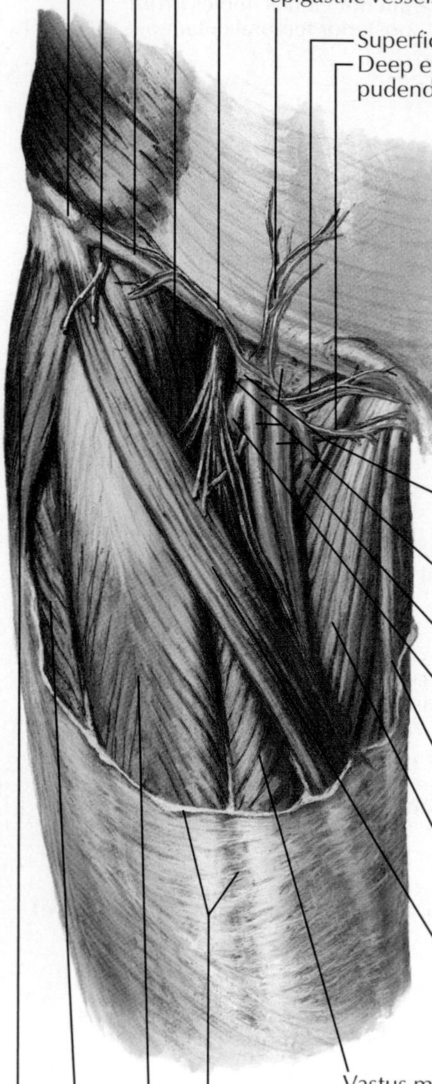
Anterior superior iliac spine
Lateral femoral cutaneous nerve
Inguinal ligament
Iliopsoas muscle
Superficial circumflex iliac vessels
Superficial epigastric vessels
Superficial and Deep external pudendal vessels
Femoral sheath
Femoral nerve, artery, and vein
Pectineus muscle
Profunda femoris (deep femoral) artery
Gracilis muscle
Adductor longus muscle
Sartorius muscle
Vastus medialis muscle
Fascia lata (cut)
Rectus femoris muscle
Vastus lateralis muscle
Tensor fasciae latae muscle
F. Netter M.D.

Superficial dissections

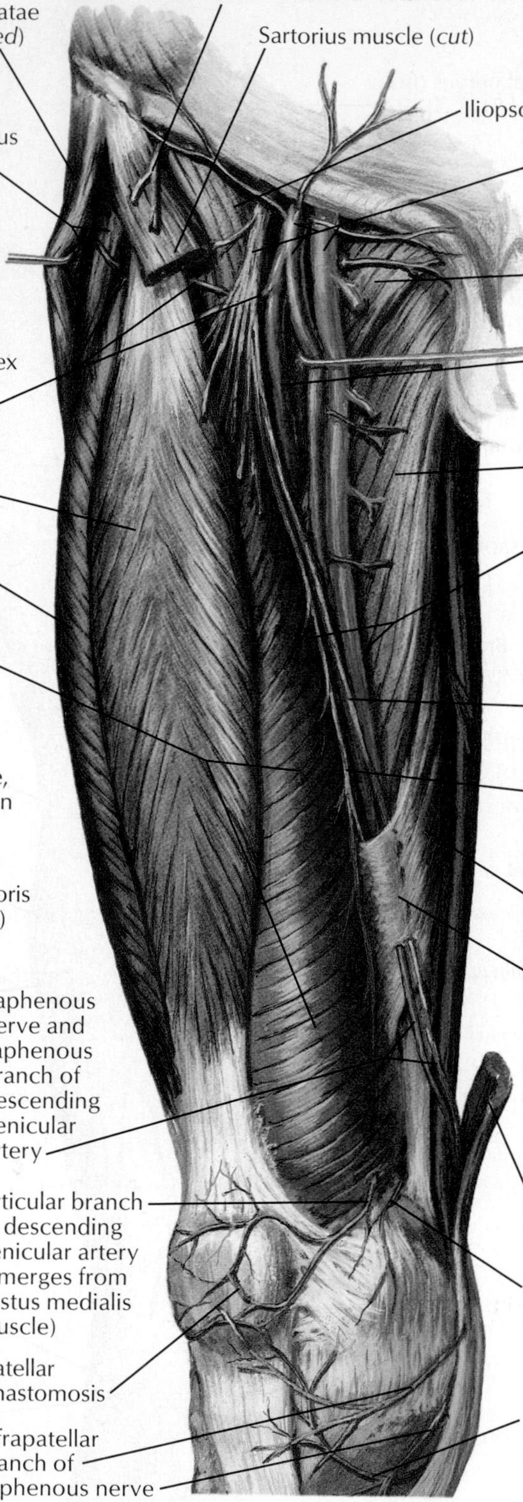
Tensor fasciae latae muscle (retracted)
Gluteus minimus and medius muscles
Lateral femoral cutaneous nerve (cut)
Sartorius muscle (cut)
Iliopsoas muscle
Femoral nerve, artery, and vein
Pectineus muscle
Profunda femoris (deep femoral) artery
Lateral circumflex femoral artery
Rectus femoris muscle
Vastus lateralis muscle
Vastus medialis muscle
Adductor longus muscle
Adductor canal (opened by removal of sartorius muscle)
Saphenous nerve
Nerve to vastus medialis muscle
Adductor magnus muscle
Anteromedial intermuscular septum covers entrance of femoral vessels to popliteal fossa (adductor hiatus)
Saphenous nerve and saphenous branch of descending genicular artery
Sartorius muscle (cut)
Articular branch of descending genicular artery (emerges from vastus medialis muscle)
Superior medial genicular artery (from popliteal artery)
Patellar anastomosis
Infrapatellar branch of Saphenous nerve
Inferior medial genicular artery (from popliteal artery)

Plate 500 Arteries and Nerves of Thigh: Anterior Views. (Netter: Atlas of Human Anatomy, 4 ed, 2006, Saunders.)

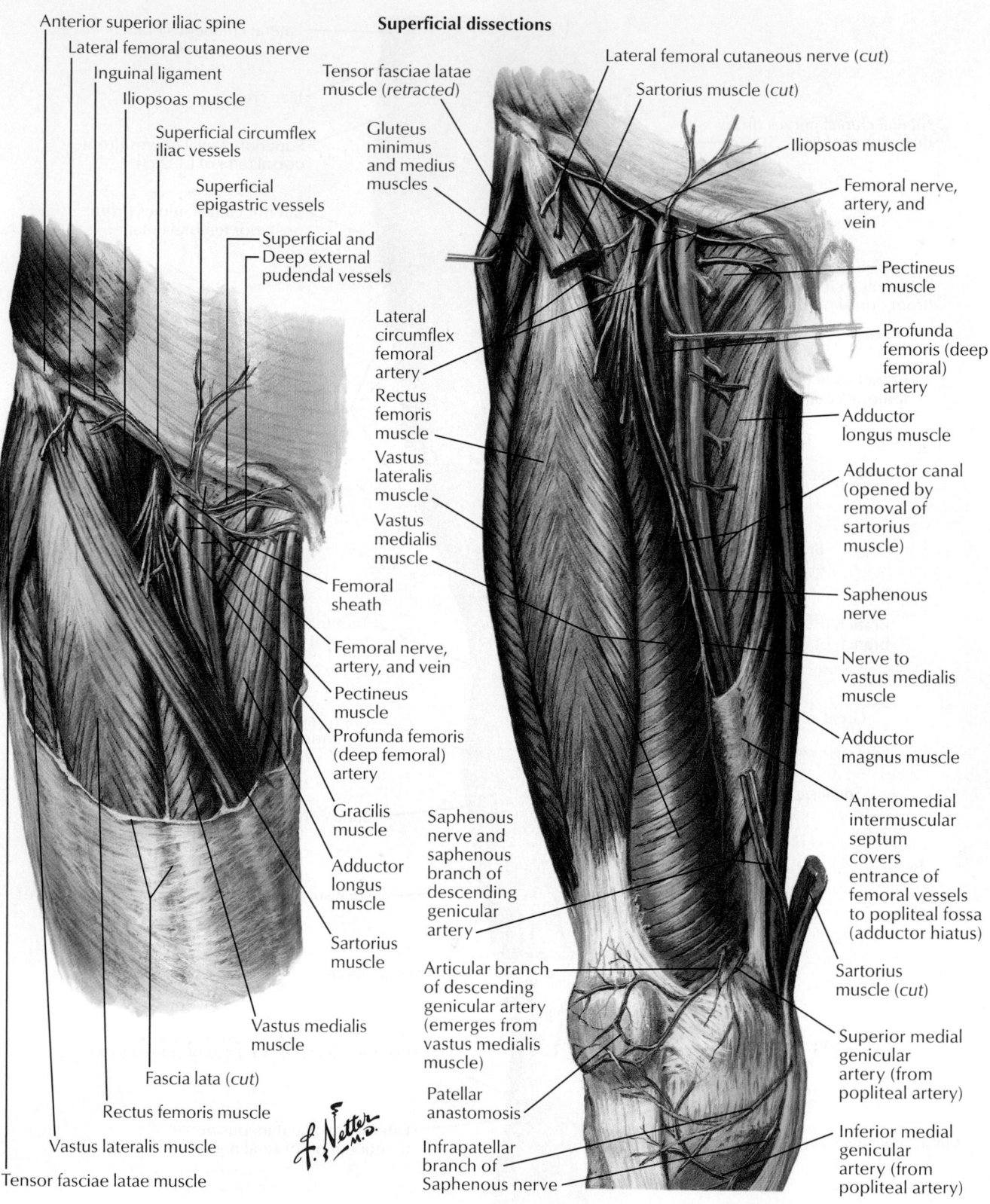

Deep dissection

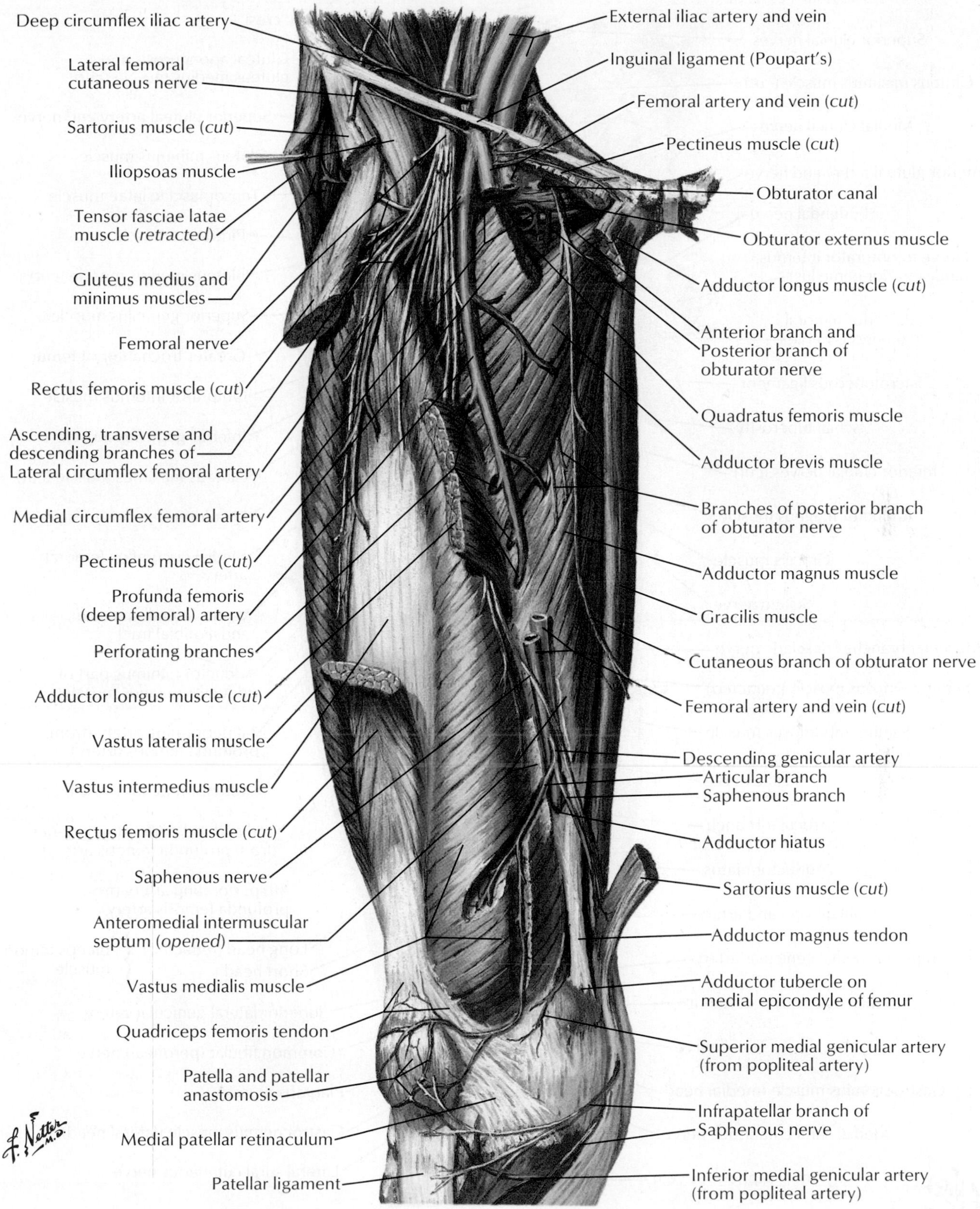

Deep circumflex iliac artery
Lateral femoral cutaneous nerve
Sartorius muscle (*cut*)
Iliopsoas muscle
Tensor fasciae latae muscle (*retracted*)
Gluteus medius and minimus muscles
Femoral nerve
Rectus femoris muscle (*cut*)
Ascending, transverse and descending branches of Lateral circumflex femoral artery
Medial circumflex femoral artery
Pectineus muscle (*cut*)
Profunda femoris (deep femoral) artery
Perforating branches
Adductor longus muscle (*cut*)
Vastus lateralis muscle
Vastus intermedius muscle
Rectus femoris muscle (*cut*)
Saphenous nerve
Anteromedial intermuscular septum (*opened*)
Vastus medialis muscle
Quadriceps femoris tendon
Patella and patellar anastomosis
Medial patellar retinaculum
Patellar ligament
External iliac artery and vein
Inguinal ligament (Poupart's)
Femoral artery and vein (*cut*)
Pectineus muscle (*cut*)
Obturator canal
Obturator externus muscle
Adductor longus muscle (*cut*)
Anterior branch and Posterior branch of obturator nerve
Quadratus femoris muscle
Adductor brevis muscle
Branches of posterior branch of obturator nerve
Adductor magnus muscle
Gracilis muscle
Cutaneous branch of obturator nerve
Femoral artery and vein (*cut*)
Descending genicular artery
Articular branch
Saphenous branch
Adductor hiatus
Sartorius muscle (*cut*)
Adductor magnus tendon
Adductor tubercle on medial epicondyle of femur
Superior medial genicular artery (from popliteal artery)
Infrapatellar branch of Saphenous nerve
Inferior medial genicular artery (from popliteal artery)
F. Netter M.D.

NETTER'S ANATOMY ILLUSTRATIONS

Plate 501 Arteries and Nerves of Thigh: Posterior View. (Netter: Atlas of Human Anatomy, 4 ed, 2006, Saunders.)

Deep dissection

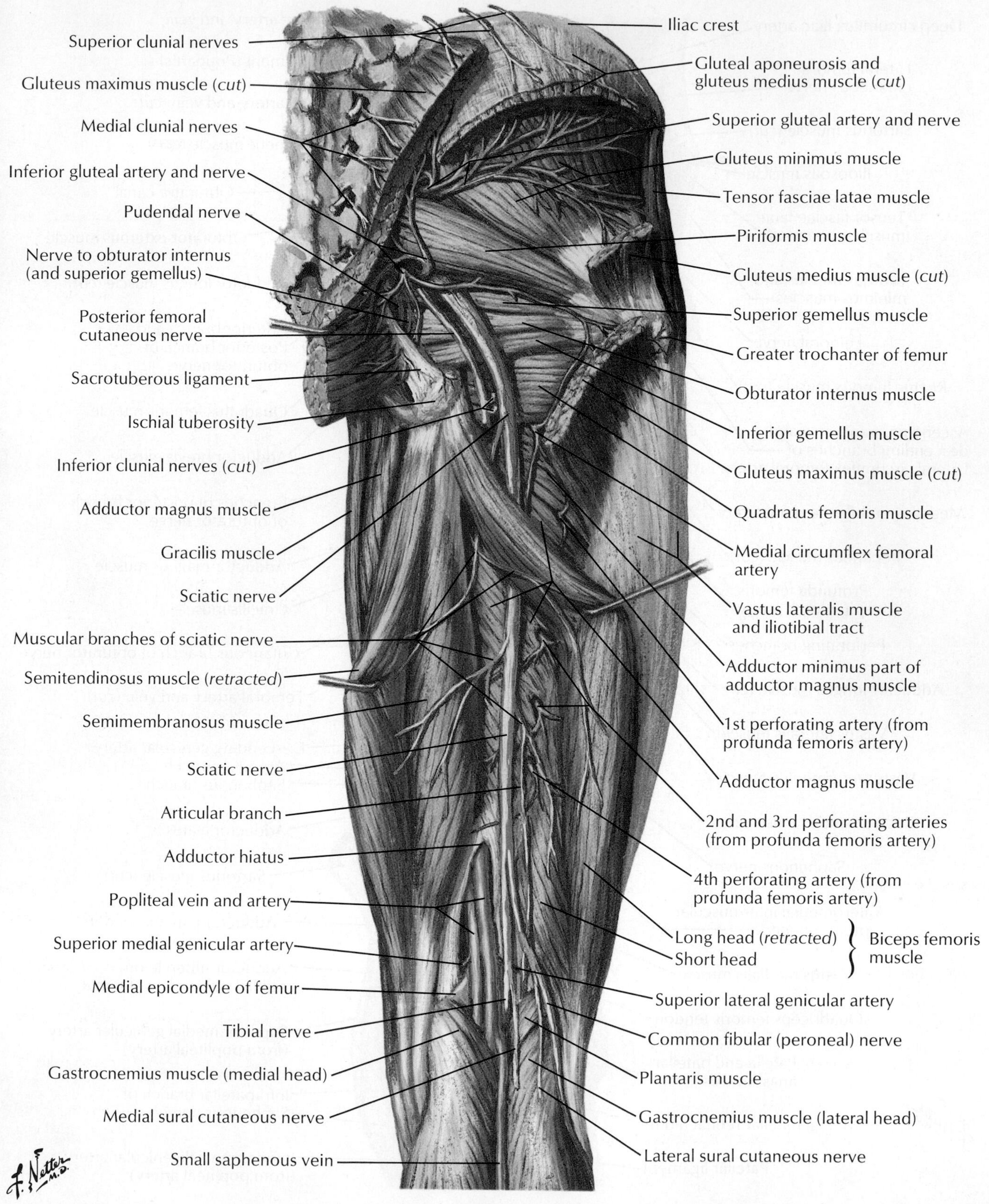

Superior clunial nerves
Gluteus maximus muscle (*cut*)
Medial clunial nerves
Inferior gluteal artery and nerve
Pudendal nerve
Nerve to obturator internus (and superior gemellus)
Posterior femoral cutaneous nerve
Sacrotuberous ligament
Ischial tuberosity
Inferior clunial nerves (*cut*)
Adductor magnus muscle
Gracilis muscle
Sciatic nerve
Muscular branches of sciatic nerve
Semitendinosus muscle (*retracted*)
Semimembranosus muscle
Sciatic nerve
Articular branch
Adductor hiatus
Popliteal vein and artery
Superior medial genicular artery
Medial epicondyle of femur
Tibial nerve
Gastrocnemius muscle (medial head)
Medial sural cutaneous nerve
Small saphenous vein
Iliac crest
Gluteal aponeurosis and gluteus medius muscle (*cut*)
Superior gluteal artery and nerve
Gluteus minimus muscle
Tensor fasciae latae muscle
Piriformis muscle
Gluteus medius muscle (*cut*)
Superior gemellus muscle
Greater trochanter of femur
Obturator internus muscle
Inferior gemellus muscle
Gluteus maximus muscle (*cut*)
Quadratus femoris muscle
Medial circumflex femoral artery
Vastus lateralis muscle and iliotibial tract
Adductor minimus part of adductor magnus muscle
1st perforating artery (from profunda femoris artery)
Adductor magnus muscle
2nd and 3rd perforating arteries (from profunda femoris artery)
4th perforating artery (from profunda femoris artery)
Long head (*retracted*)
Short head
Biceps femoris muscle
Superior lateral genicular artery
Common fibular (peroneal) nerve
Plantaris muscle
Gastrocnemius muscle (lateral head)
Lateral sural cutaneous nerve
F. Netter M.D.

Plate 502 Arteries and Nerves of Thigh: Posterior View. (Netter: Atlas of Human Anatomy, 4 ed, 2006, Saunders.)

Horizontal section

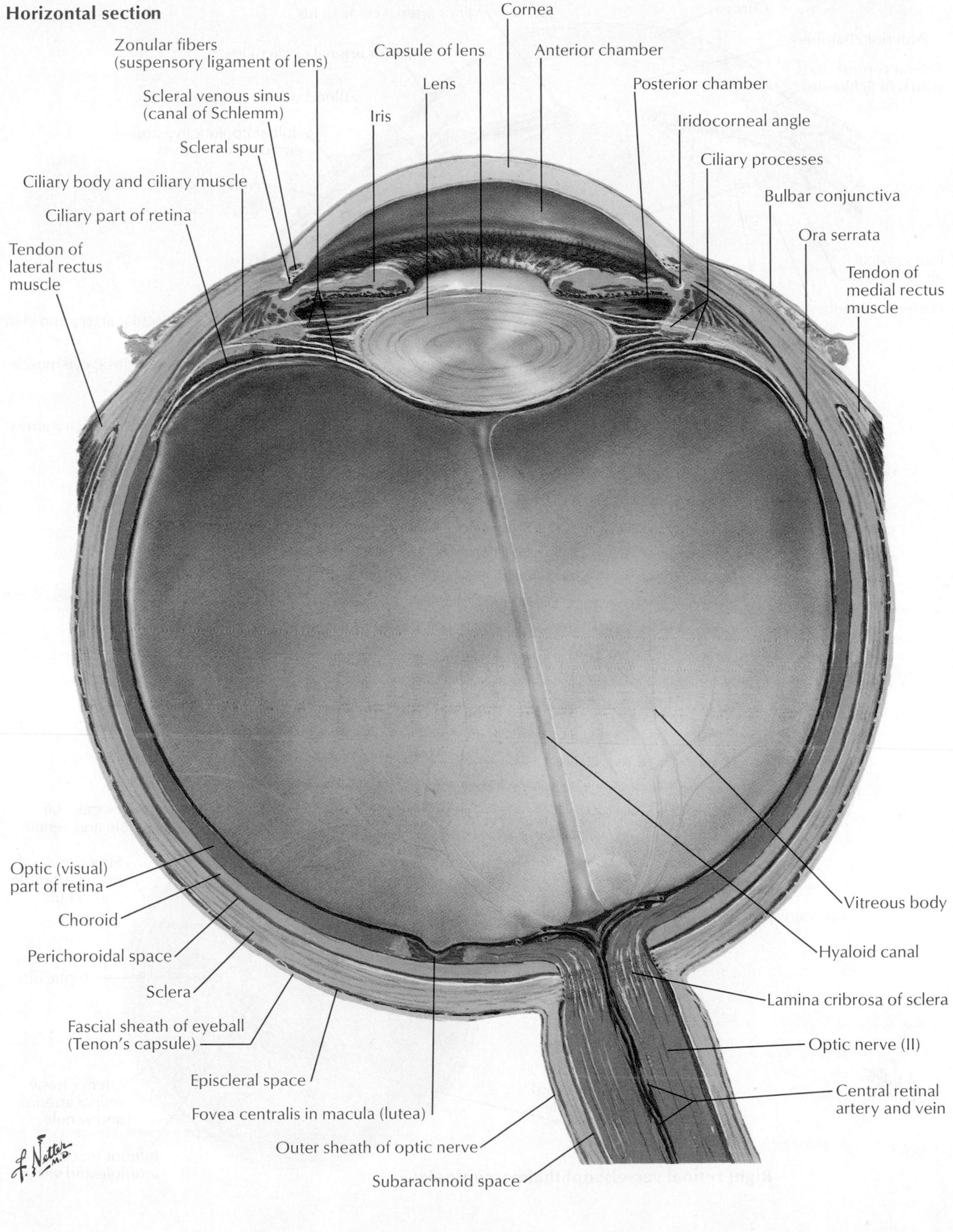

Cornea
Zonular fibers (suspensory ligament of lens)
Capsule of lens
Anterior chamber
Lens
Posterior chamber
Scleral venous sinus (canal of Schlemm)
Iris
Iridocorneal angle
Scleral spur
Ciliary processes
Ciliary body and ciliary muscle
Bulbar conjunctiva
Ciliary part of retina
Ora serrata
Tendon of lateral rectus muscle
Tendon of medial rectus muscle
Optic (visual) part of retina
Vitreous body
Choroid
Perichoroidal space
Hyaloid canal
Sclera
Lamina cribrosa of sclera
Fascial sheath of eyeball (Tenon's capsule)
Optic nerve (II)
Episcleral space
Central retinal artery and vein
Fovea centralis in macula (lutea)
Outer sheath of optic nerve
Subarachnoid space
F. Netter M.D.

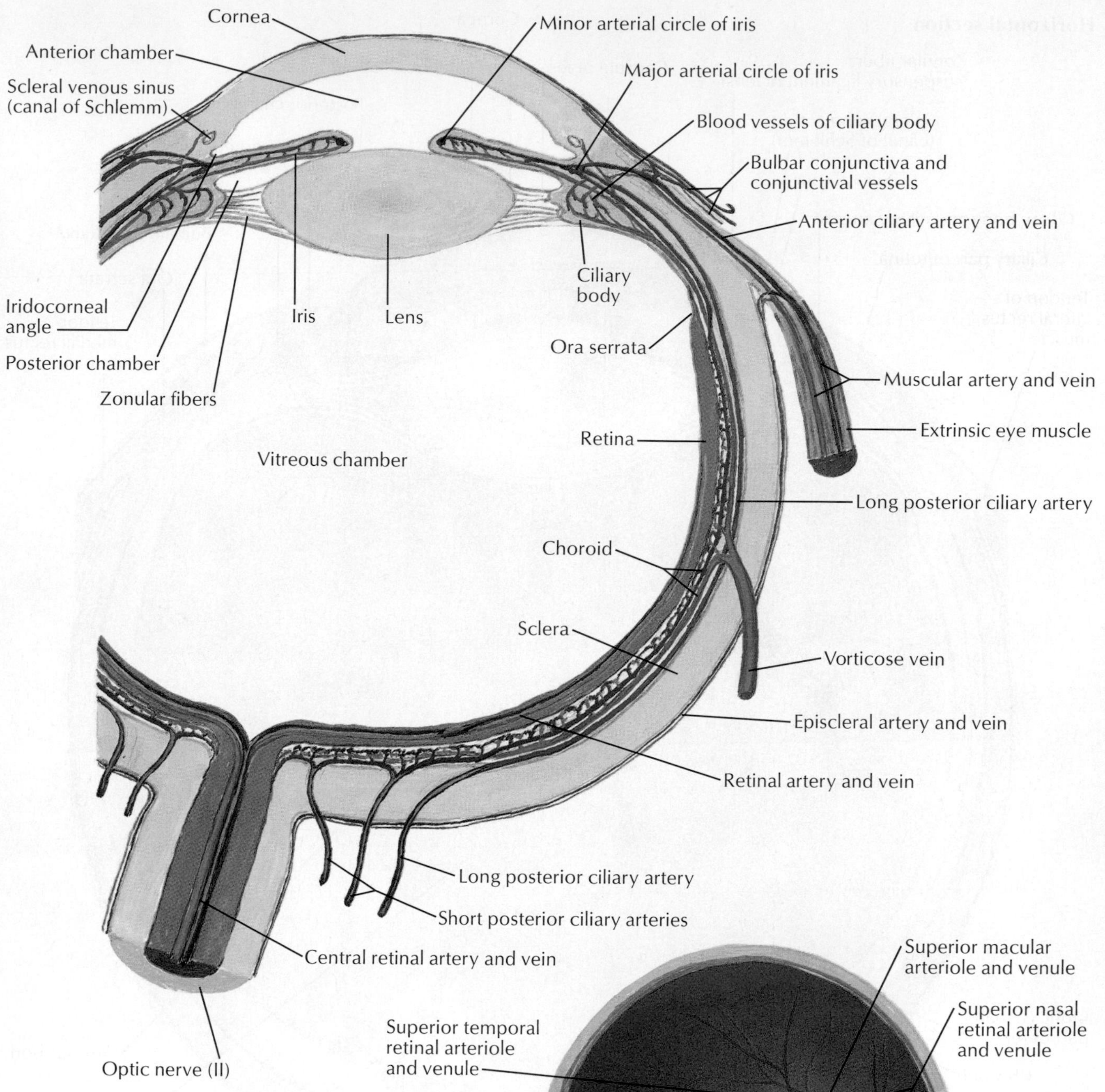

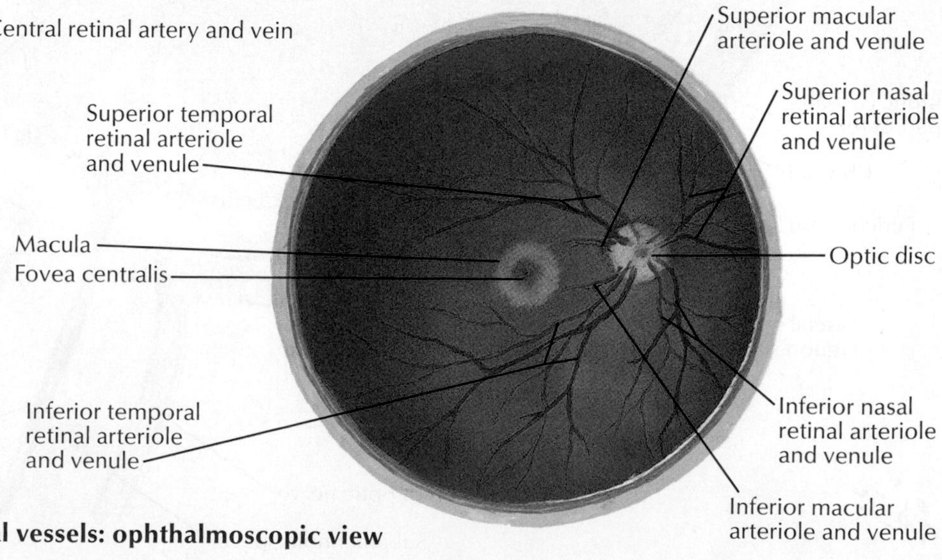

Right retinal vessels: ophthalmoscopic view

Plate 90 Intrinsic Arteries and Veins of Eye. (Netter: Atlas of Human Anatomy, 4 ed, 2006, Saunders.)

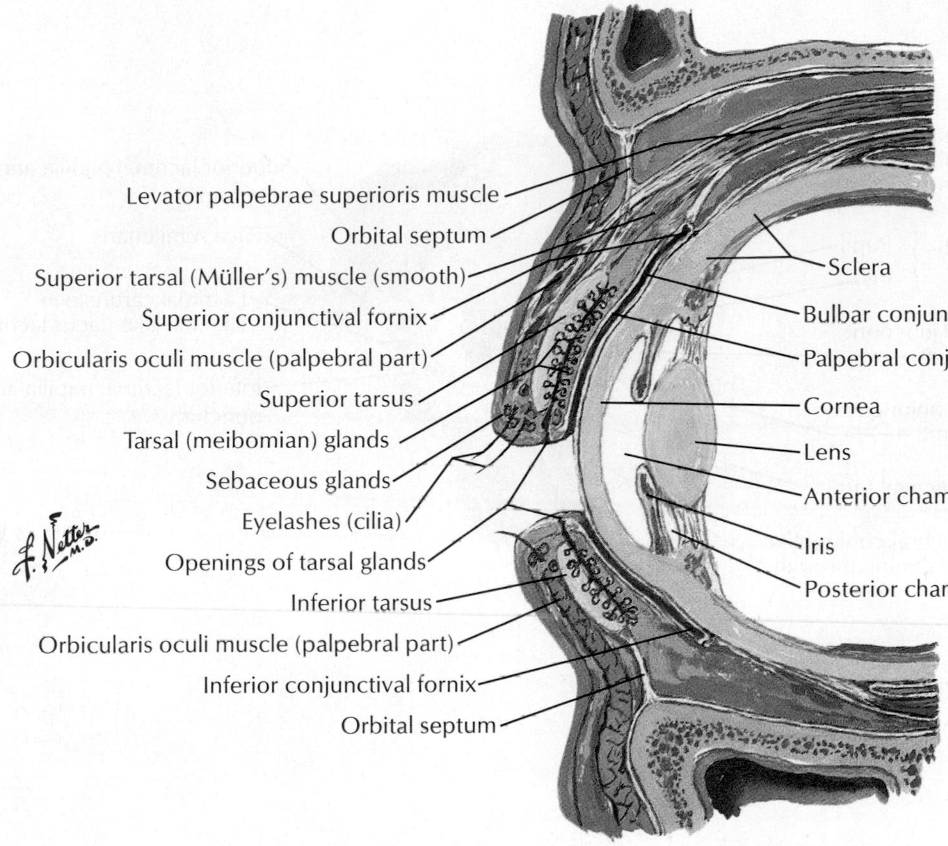

Plate 81, Middle Eyelids. (Netter: Atlas of Human Anatomy, 4 ed, 2006, Saunders.)

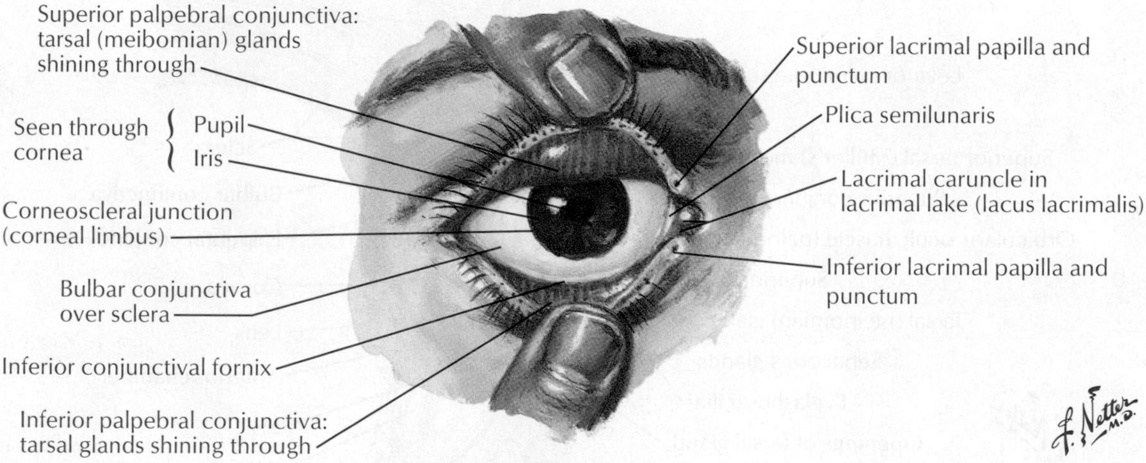

Plate 81, Upper Eyelid. (Netter: Atlas of Human Anatomy, 4 ed, 2006, Saunders.)

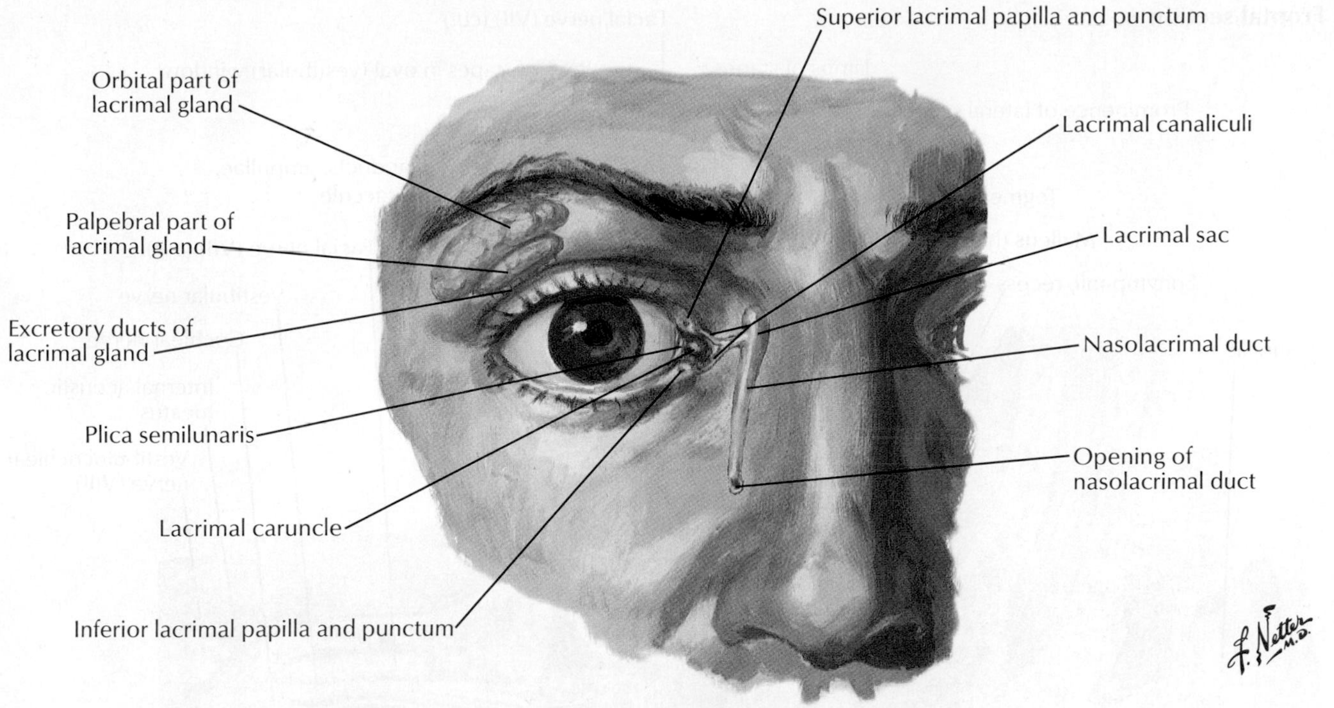

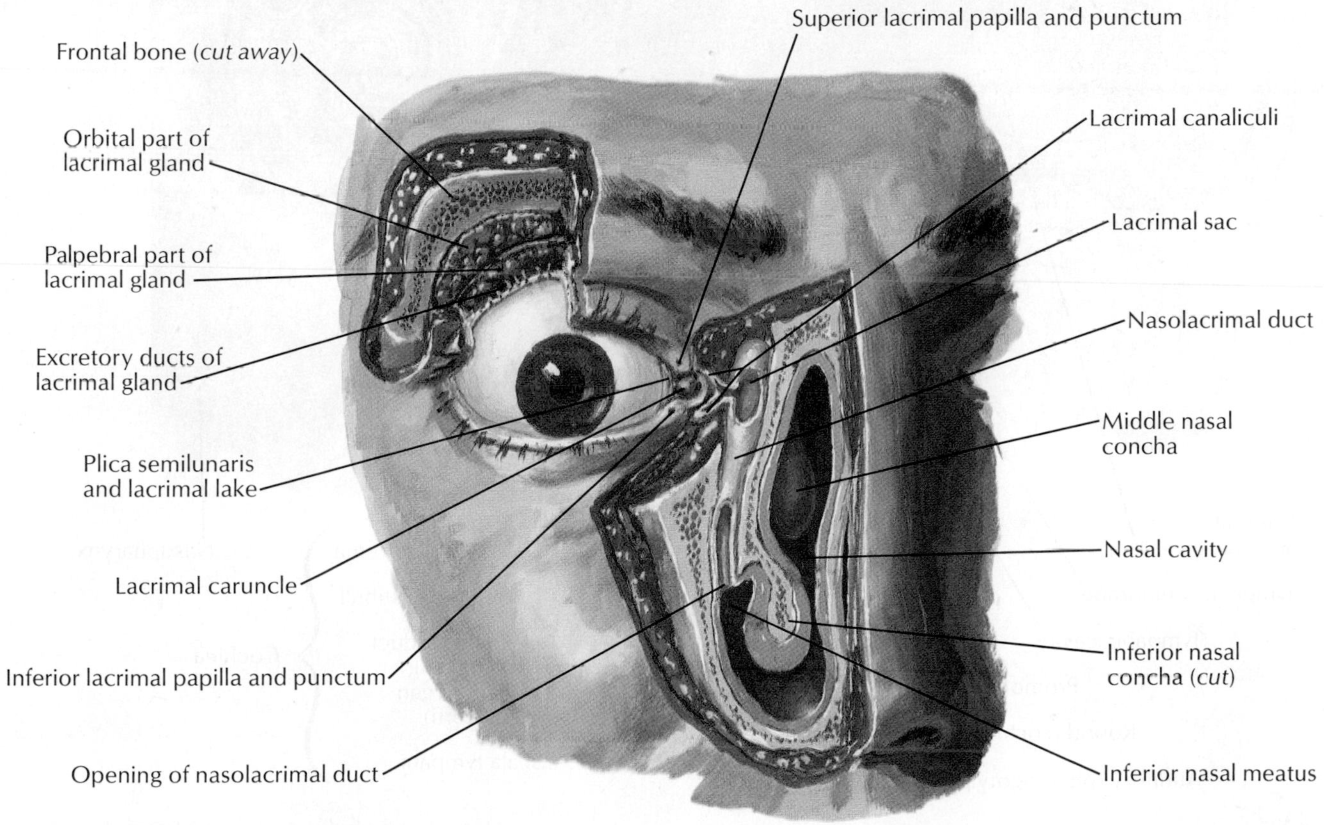

NETTER'S ANATOMY ILLUSTRATIONS

Plate 82 Lacrimal Apparatus. (Netter: Atlas of Human Anatomy, 4 ed, 2006, Saunders.)

Frontal section

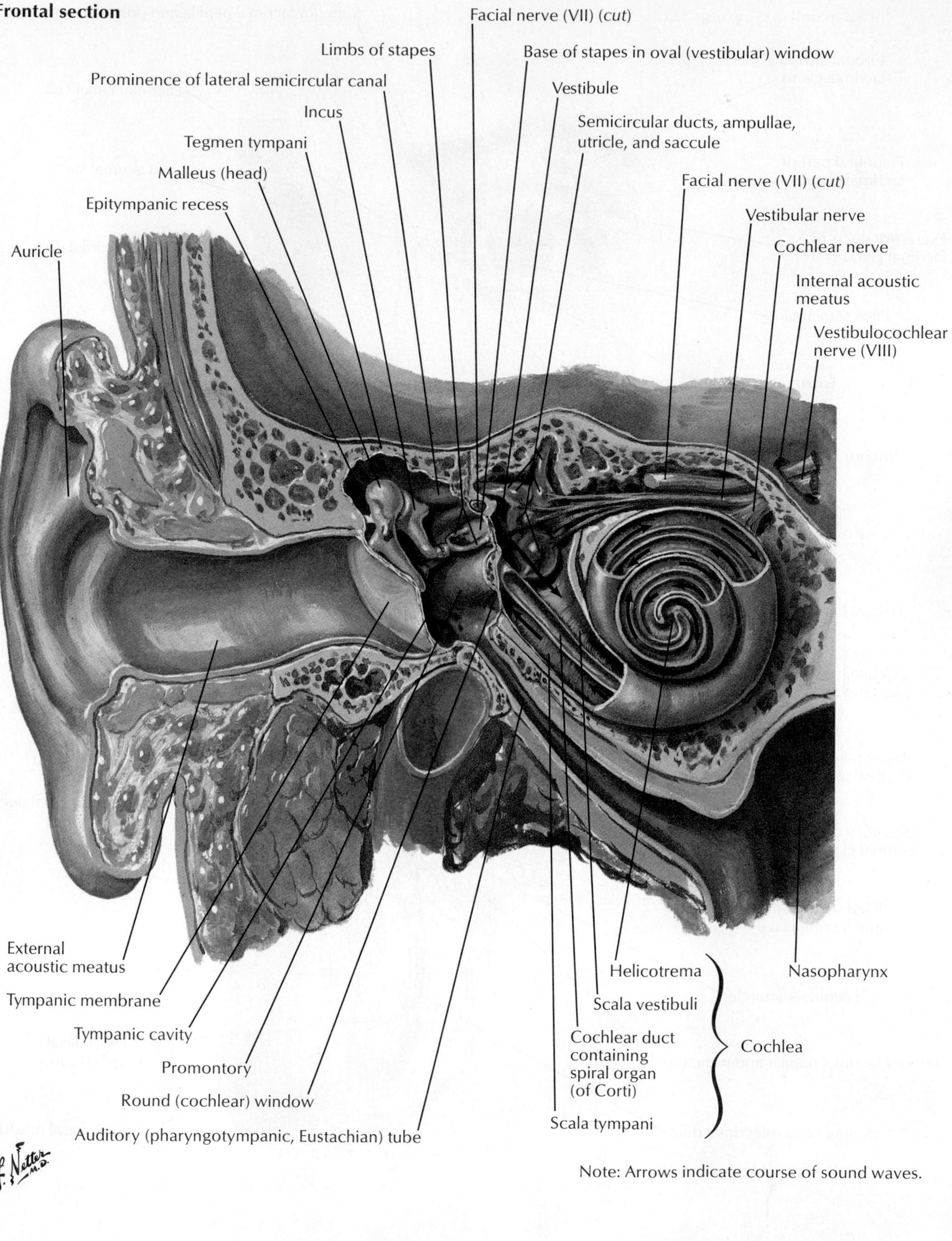

Plate 92 Pathway of Sound Reception. (Netter: Atlas of Human Anatomy, 4 ed, 2006, Saunders.)

Medial wall of tympanic cavity: lateral view

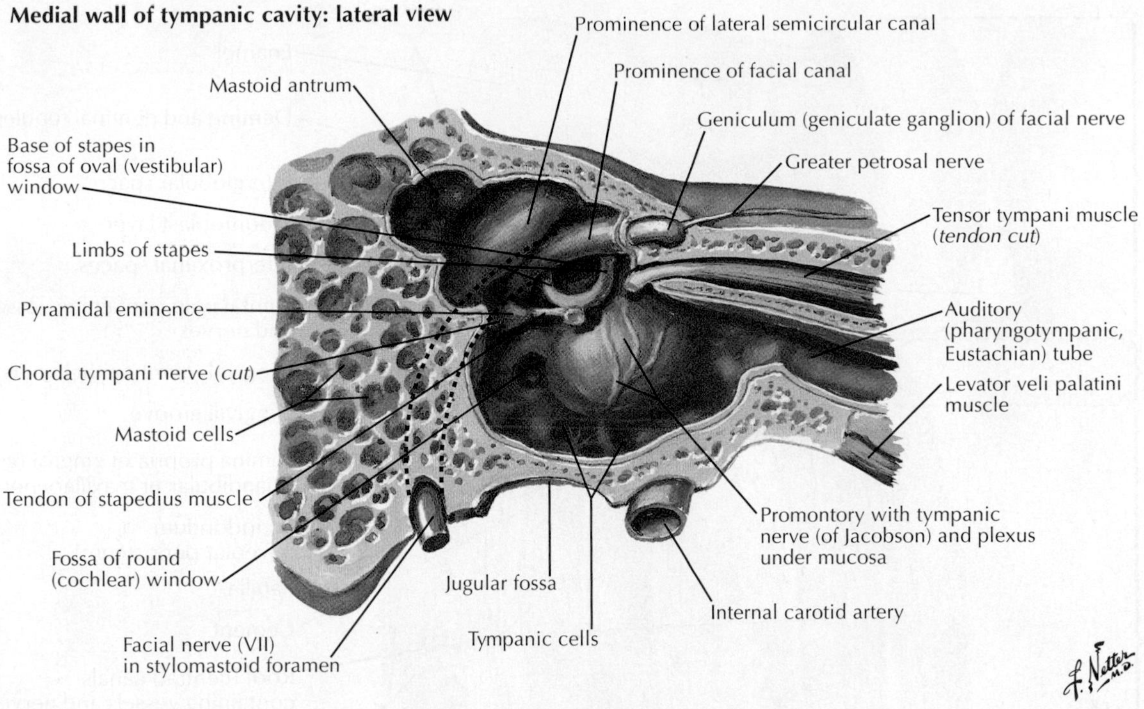

Plate 94 Tympanic Cavity. (Netter: Atlas of Human Anatomy, 4 ed, 2006, Saunders.)

Otoscopic view of right tympanic membrane

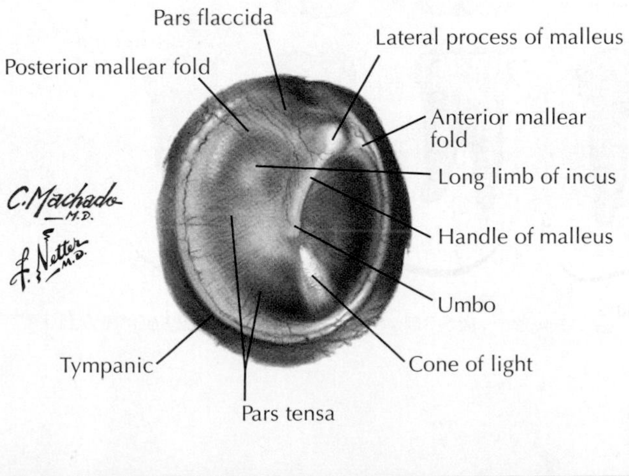

Plate 93 Tympanic Cavity. (Netter: Atlas of Human Anatomy, 4 ed, 2006, Saunders.)

Dissected right bony labyrinth (otic capsule): membranous labyrinth removed

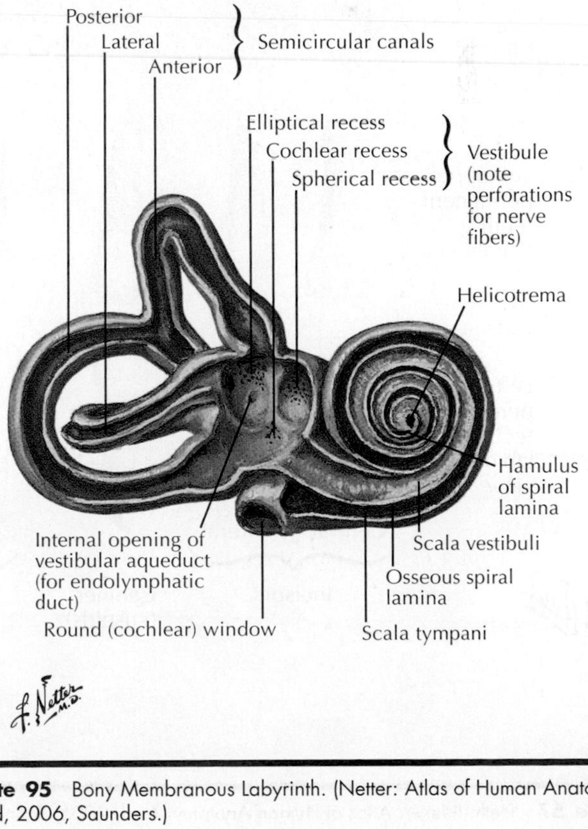

Plate 95 Bony Membranous Labyrinth. (Netter: Atlas of Human Anatomy, 4 ed, 2006, Saunders.)

NETTER'S ANATOMY ILLUSTRATIONS

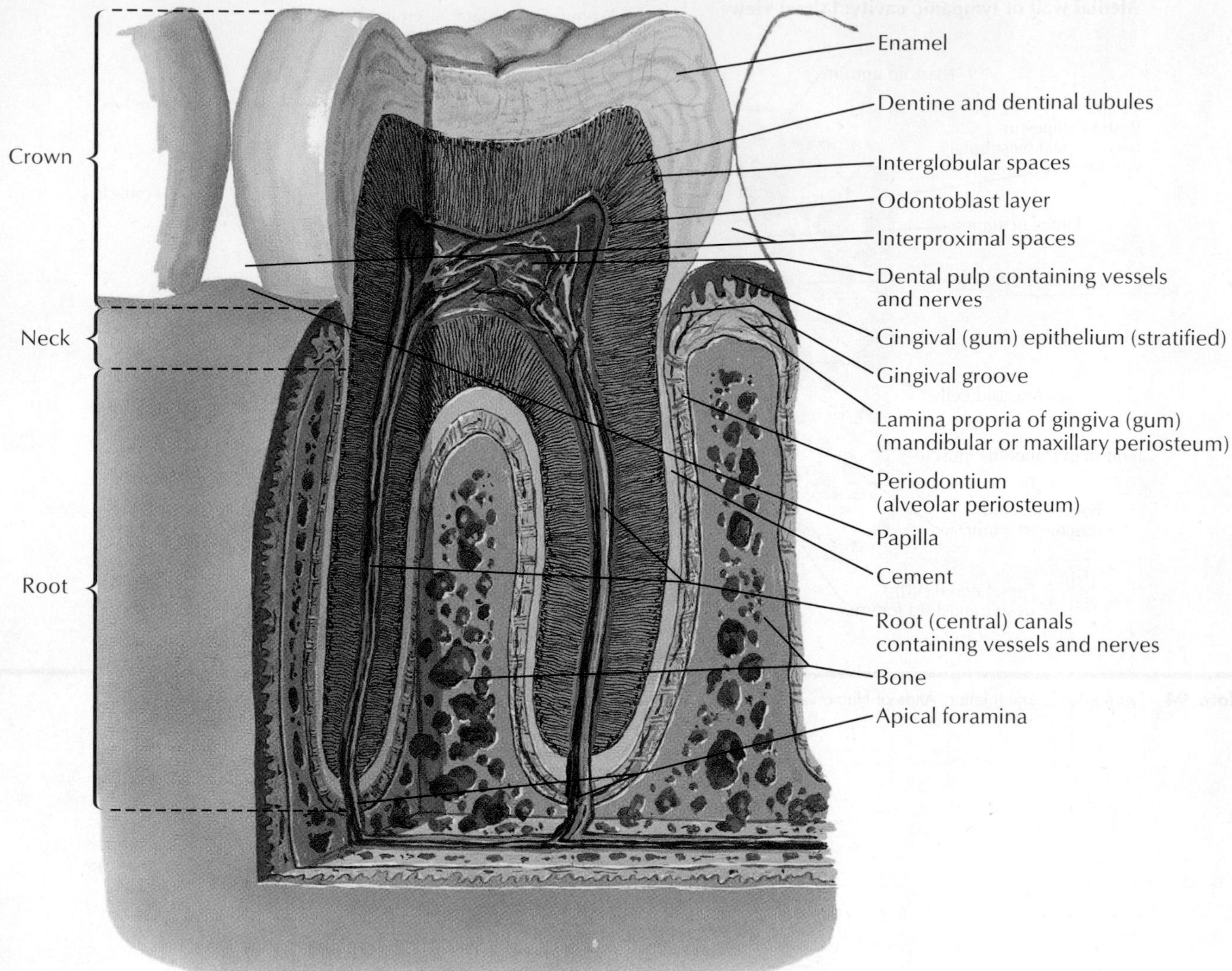
Crown
Neck
Root
Enamel
Dentine and dentinal tubules
Interglobular spaces
Odontoblast layer
Interproximal spaces
Dental pulp containing vessels and nerves
Gingival (gum) epithelium (stratified)
Gingival groove
Lamina propria of gingiva (gum) (mandibular or maxillary periosteum)
Periodontium (alveolar periosteum)
Papilla
Cement
Root (central) canals containing vessels and nerves
Bone
Apical foramina

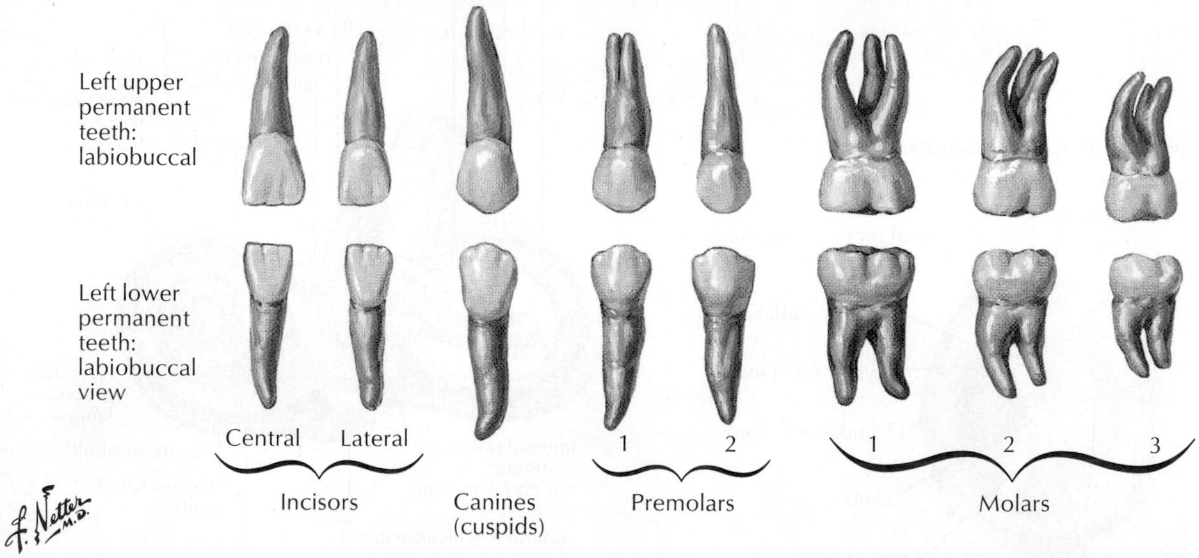
Left upper permanent teeth: labiobuccal
Left lower permanent teeth: labiobuccal view
Central
Lateral
Incisors
Canines (cuspids)
1
2
Premolars
1
2
3
Molars
F. Netter M.D.

Plate 57 Teeth. (Netter: Atlas of Human Anatomy, 4 ed, 2006, Saunders.)

Tongue

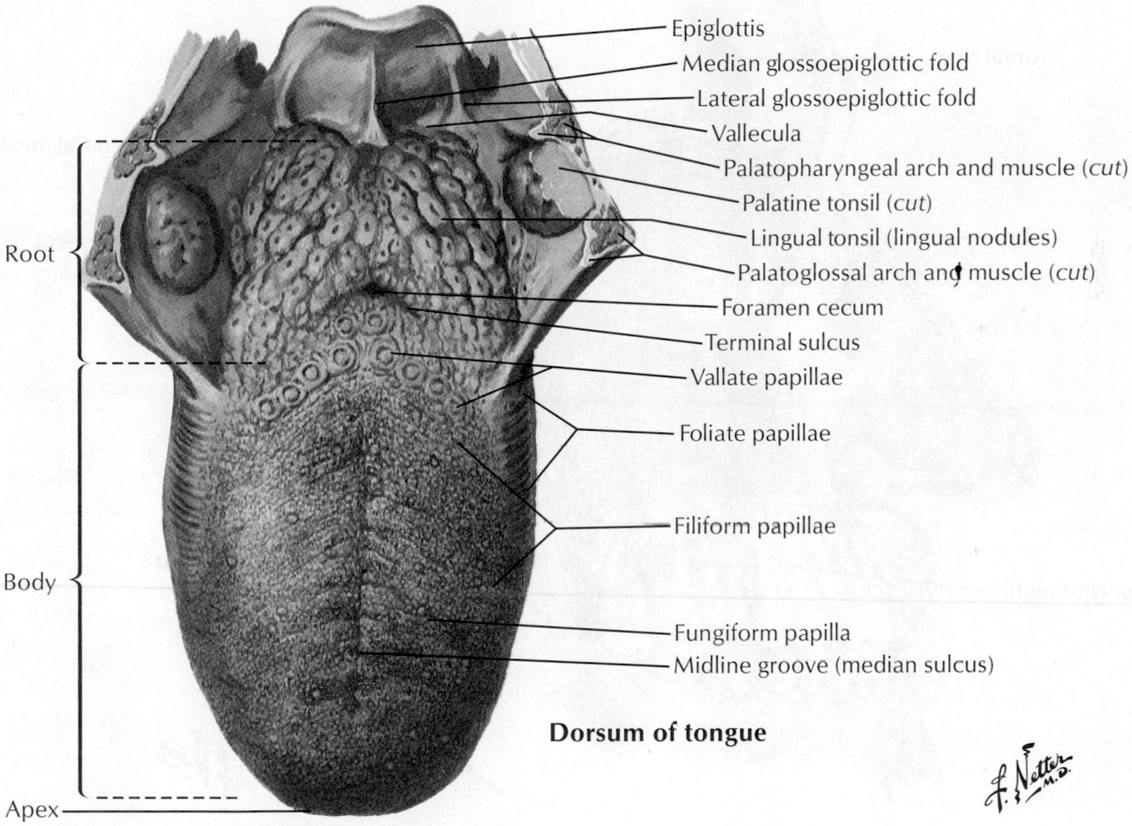

Plate 58 Tongue. (Netter: Atlas of Human Anatomy, 4 ed, 2006, Saunders.)

NETTER'S ANATOMY ILLUSTRATIONS

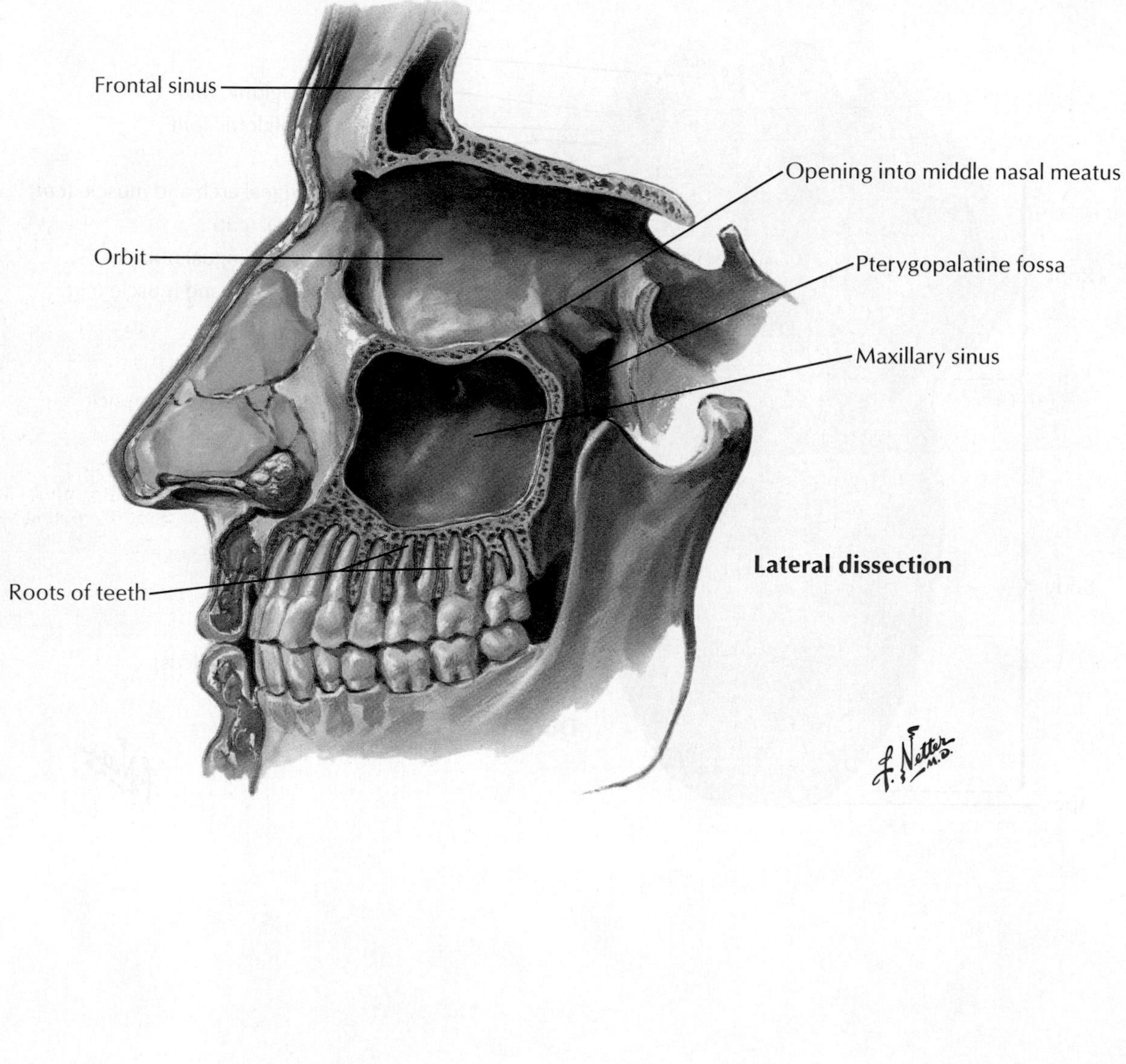

Plate 49 Paranasal Sinuses. (Netter: Atlas of Human Anatomy, 4 ed, 2006, Saunders.)

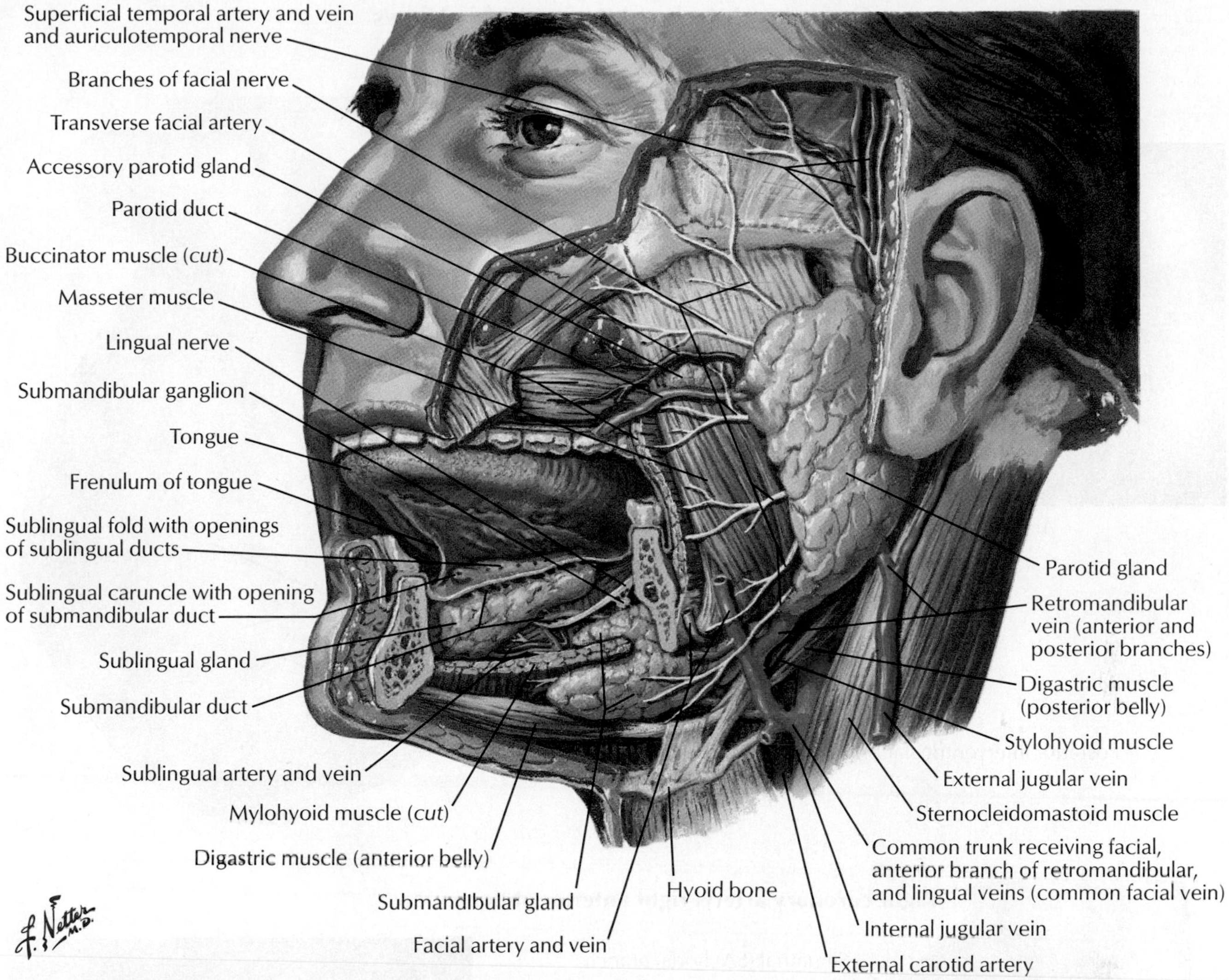

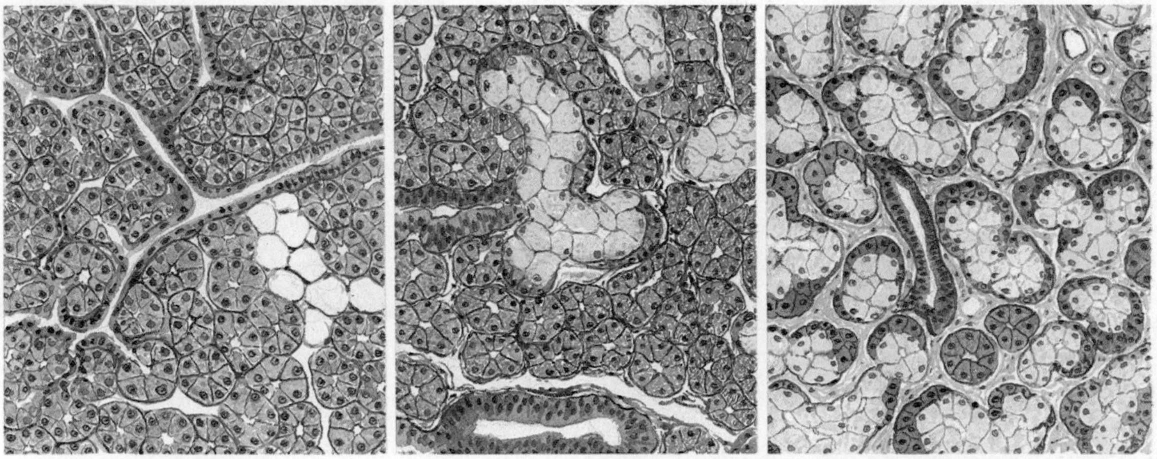

Parotid gland: totally serous

Submandibular gland: mostly serous, partially mucous

Sublingual gland: almost completely mucous

Plate 61 Salivary Glands. (Netter: Atlas of Human Anatomy, 4 ed, 2006, Saunders.)

Coronary Arteries: Arteriographic Views

Right coronary artery: left anterior oblique view

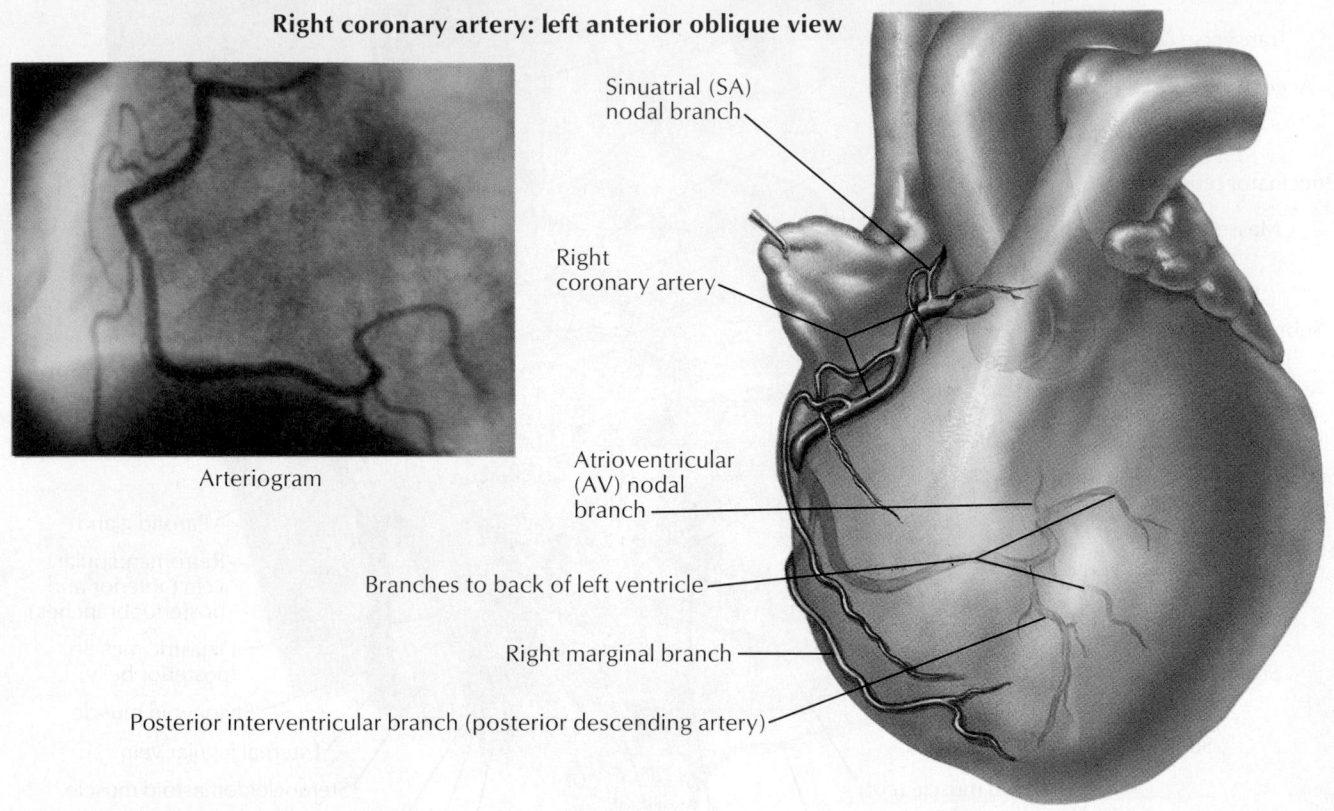

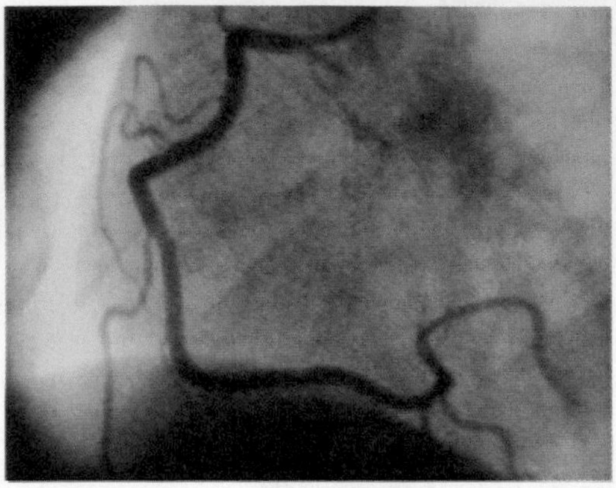

Arteriogram

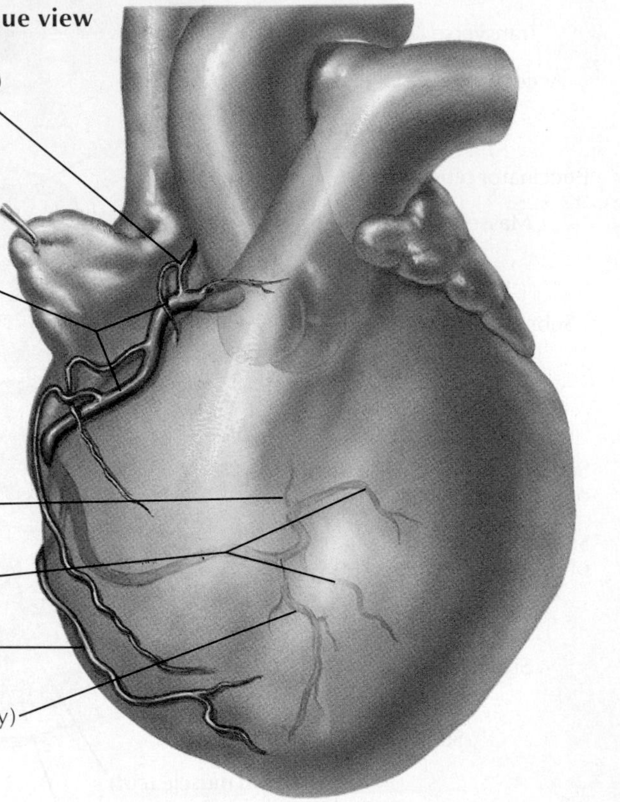

Right coronary artery: right anterior oblique view

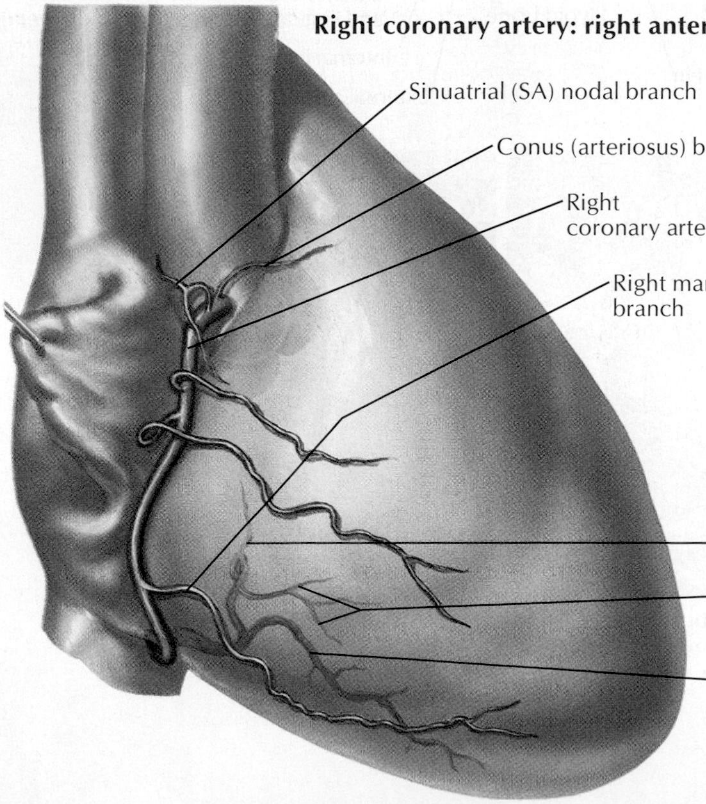

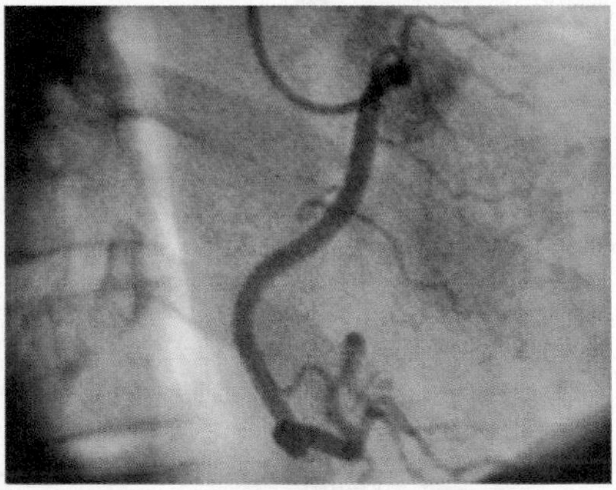

Arteriogram

Left coronary artery: left anterior oblique view

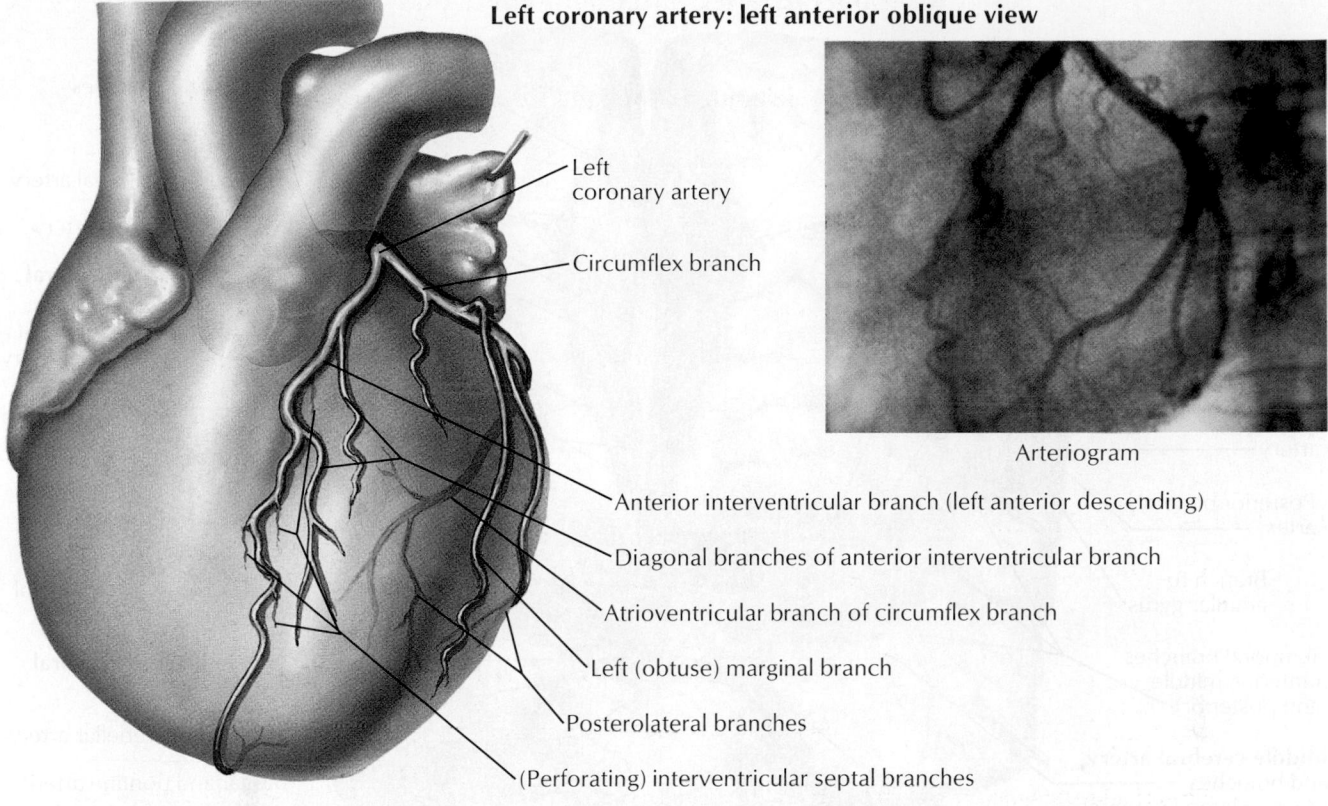

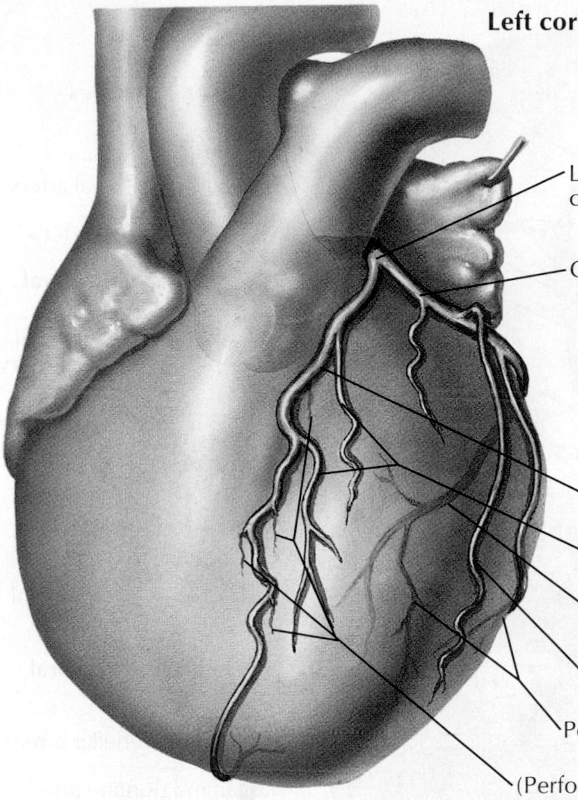

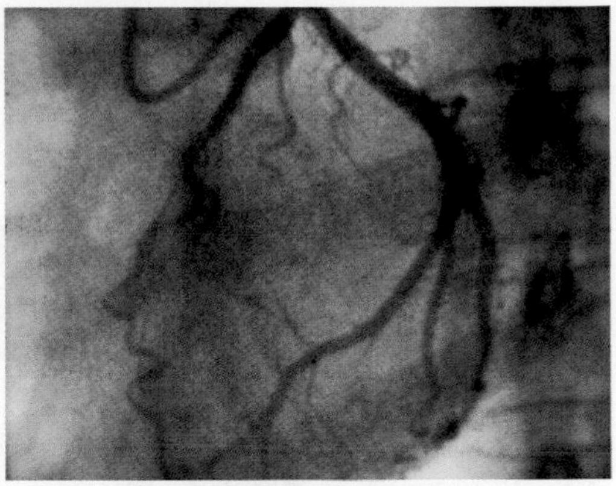

Arteriogram

Left coronary artery: right anterior oblique view

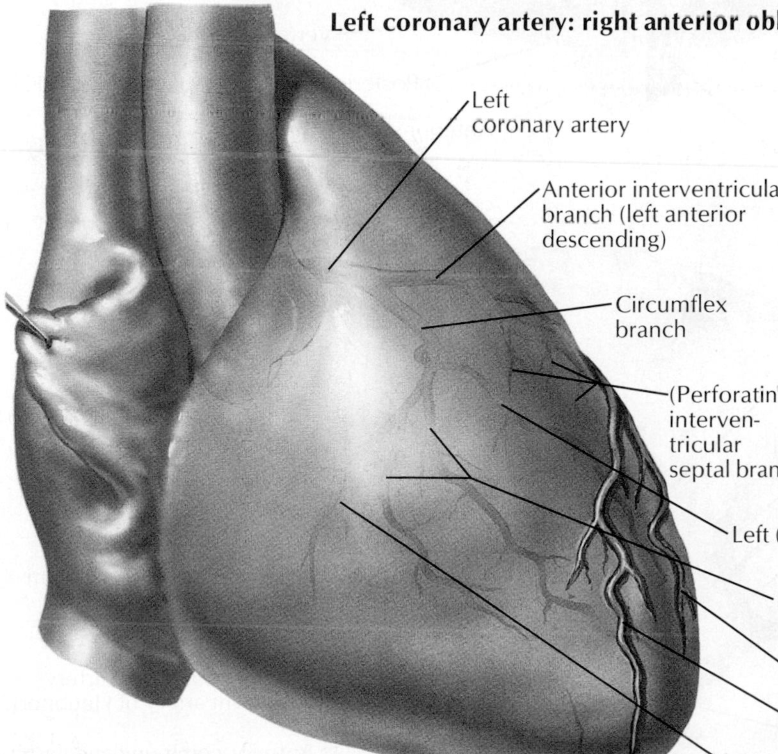

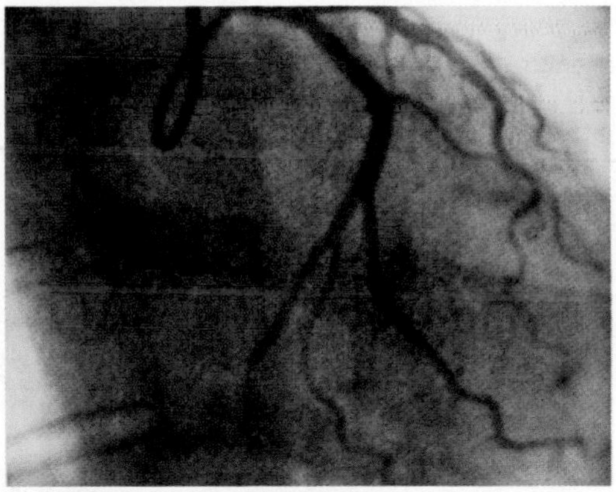

Arteriogram

NETTER'S ANATOMY ILLUSTRATIONS

Plate 219 Coronary Arteries: Arteriographic Views. (Netter: Atlas of Human Anatomy, 4 ed, 2006, Saunders.)

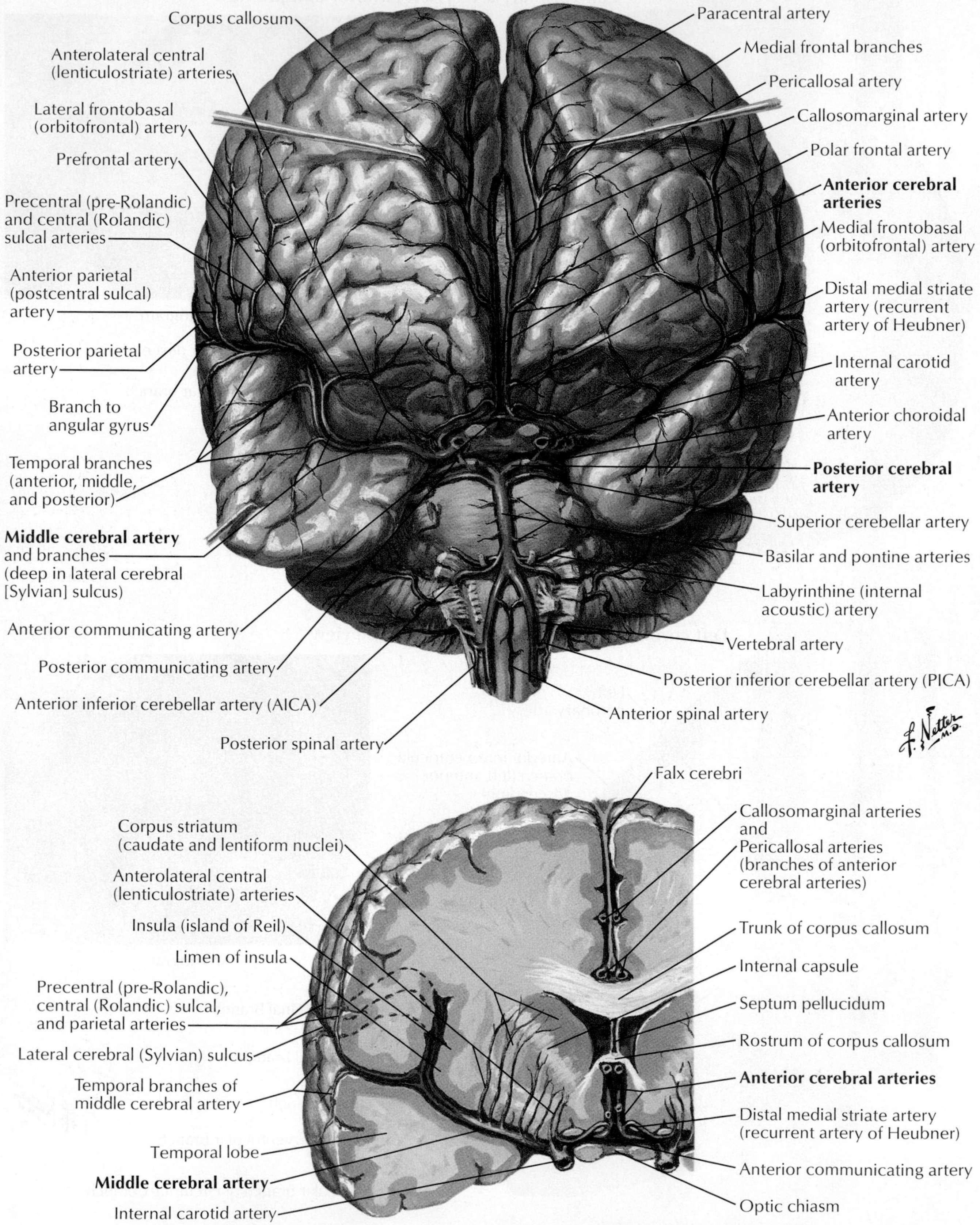
Corpus callosum
Anterolateral central (lenticulostriate) arteries
Lateral frontobasal (orbitofrontal) artery
Prefrontal artery
Precentral (pre-Rolandic) and central (Rolandic) sulcal arteries
Anterior parietal (postcentral sulcal) artery
Posterior parietal artery
Branch to angular gyrus
Temporal branches (anterior, middle, and posterior)
Middle cerebral artery and branches (deep in lateral cerebral [Sylvian] sulcus)
Anterior communicating artery
Posterior communicating artery
Anterior inferior cerebellar artery (AICA)
Posterior spinal artery
Paracentral artery
Medial frontal branches
Pericallosal artery
Callosomarginal artery
Polar frontal artery
Anterior cerebral arteries
Medial frontobasal (orbitofrontal) artery
Distal medial striate artery (recurrent artery of Heubner)
Internal carotid artery
Anterior choroidal artery
Posterior cerebral artery
Superior cerebellar artery
Basilar and pontine arteries
Labyrinthine (internal acoustic) artery
Vertebral artery
Posterior inferior cerebellar artery (PICA)
Anterior spinal artery
F. Netter M.D.
Falx cerebri
Corpus striatum (caudate and lentiform nuclei)
Anterolateral central (lenticulostriate) arteries
Insula (island of Reil)
Limen of insula
Precentral (pre-Rolandic), central (Rolandic) sulcal, and parietal arteries
Lateral cerebral (Sylvian) sulcus
Temporal branches of middle cerebral artery
Temporal lobe
Middle cerebral artery
Internal carotid artery
Callosomarginal arteries and Pericallosal arteries (branches of anterior cerebral arteries)
Trunk of corpus callosum
Internal capsule
Septum pellucidum
Rostrum of corpus callosum
Anterior cerebral arteries
Distal medial striate artery (recurrent artery of Heubner)
Anterior communicating artery
Optic chiasm

Plate 141 Arteries of Brain: Frontal View and Section. (Netter: Atlas of Human Anatomy, 4 ed, 2006, Saunders.)

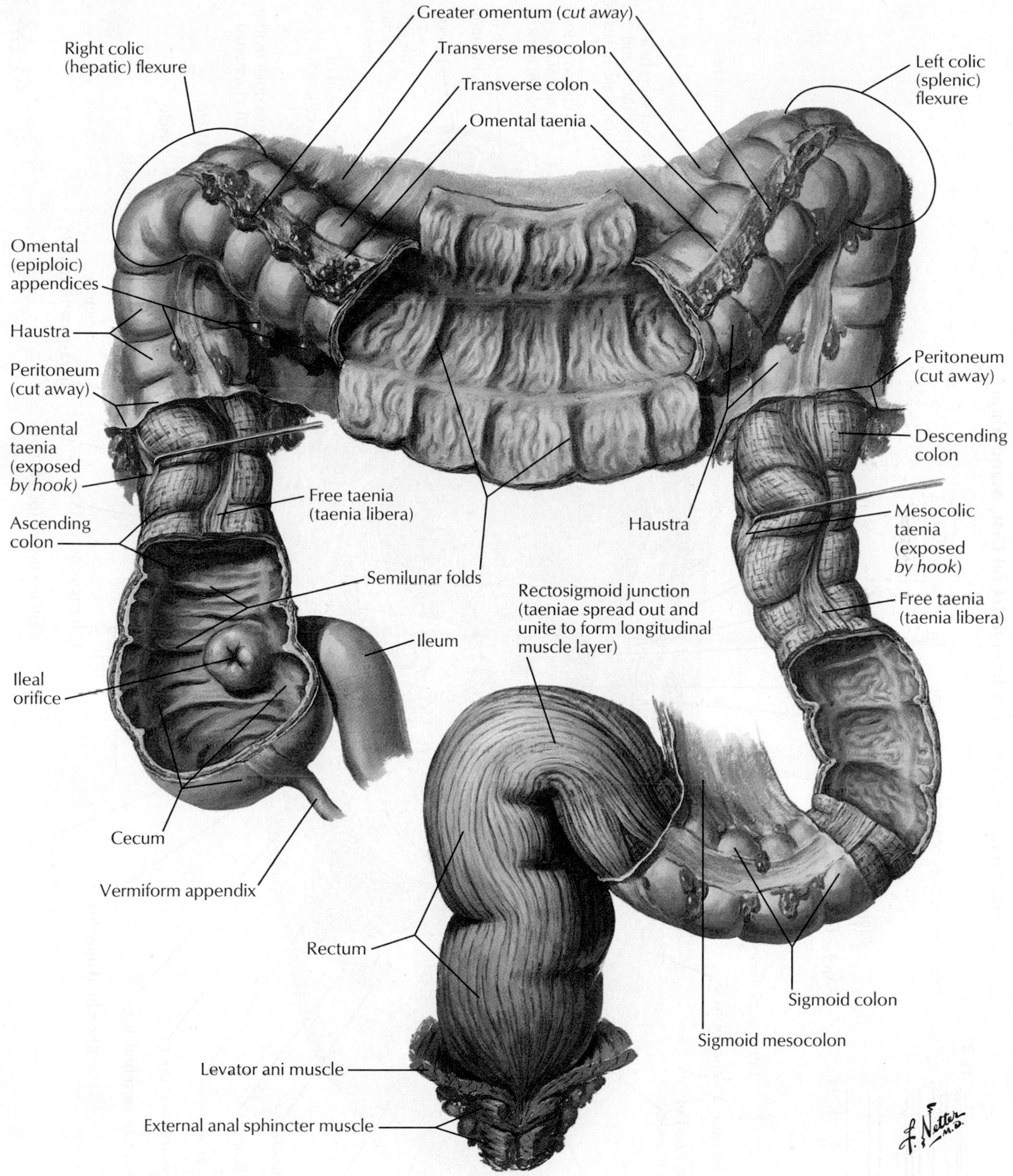

Plate 284 Mucosa and Musculature of Large Intestine. (Netter: Atlas of Human Anatomy, 4 ed, 2006, Saunders.)

Transverse Section: T3–4 Intervertebral Disc, Manubrium

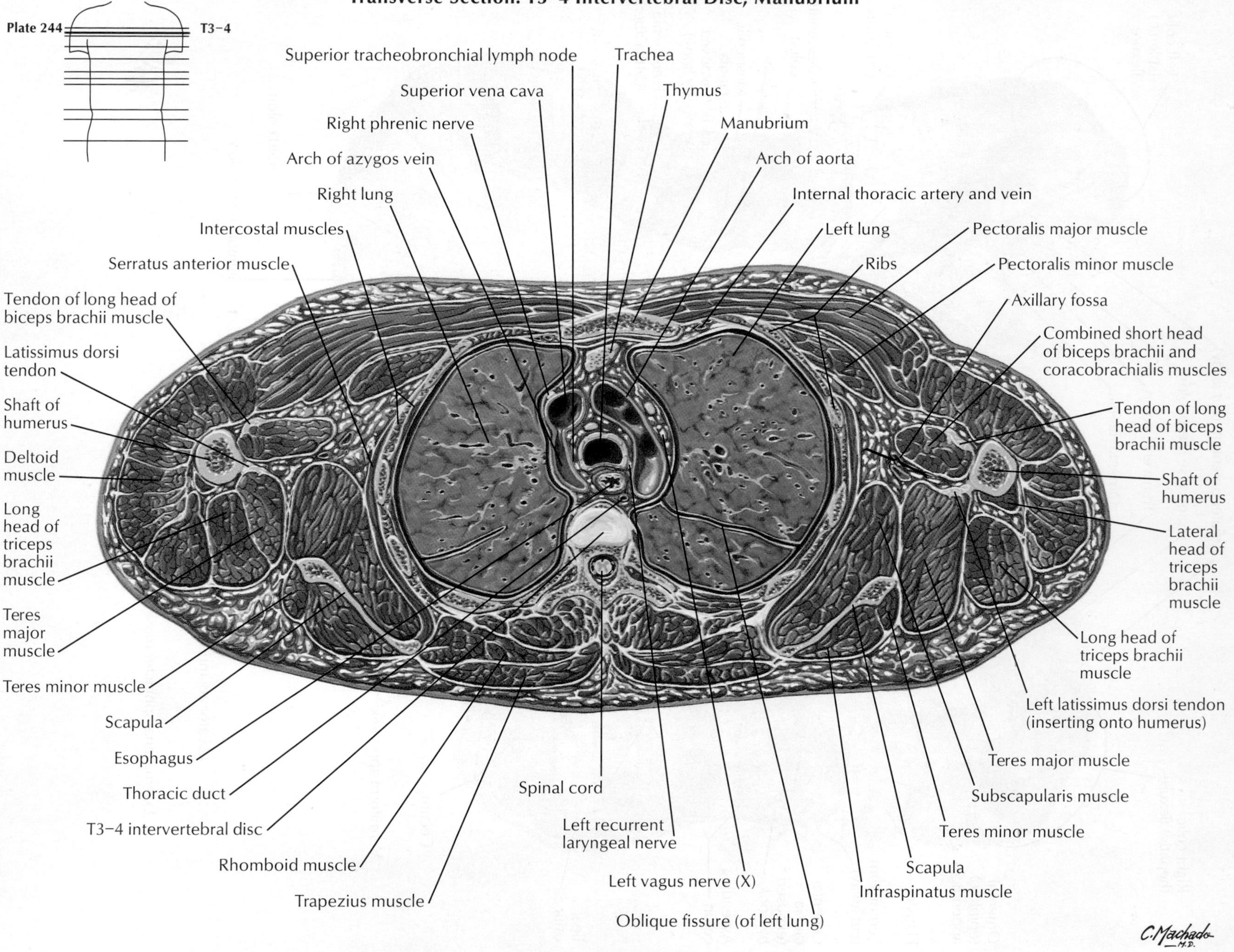

Plate 244 Cross Section of Thorax at T3-4 Disc Level. (Netter: Atlas of Human Anatomy, 4 ed, 2006, Saunders.)

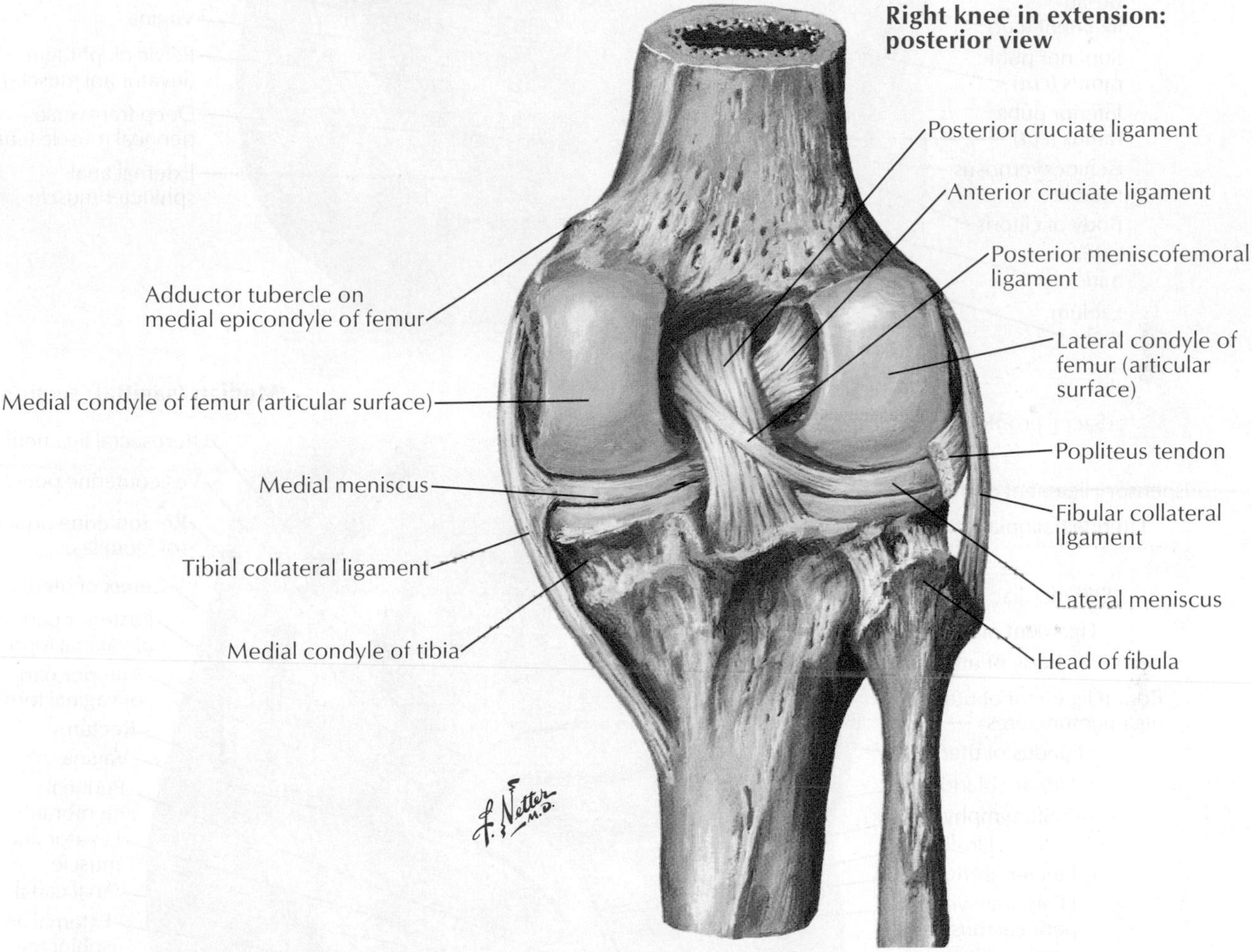

Plate 509 Knee: Cruciate and Collateral Ligaments. (Netter: Atlas of Human Anatomy, 4 ed, 2006, Saunders.)

Paramedian (sagittal) dissection

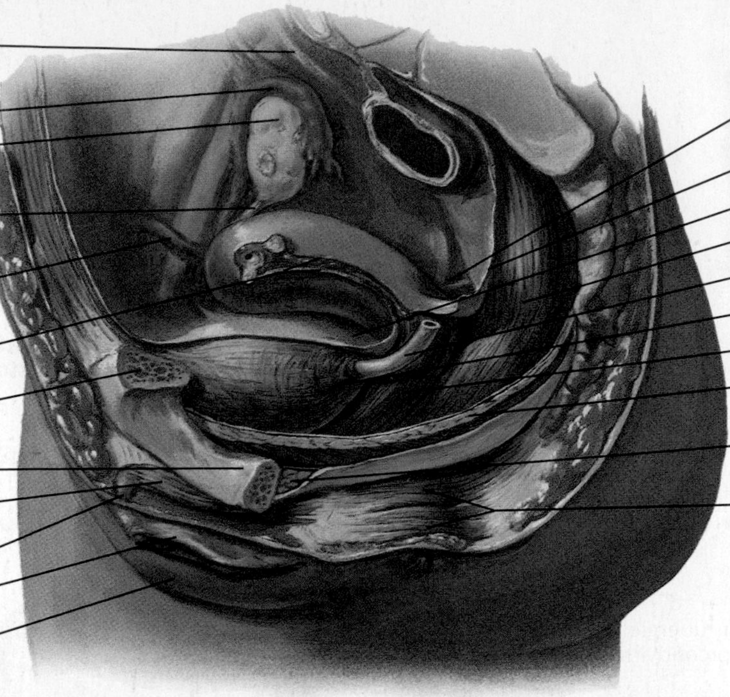

Median (sagittal) section

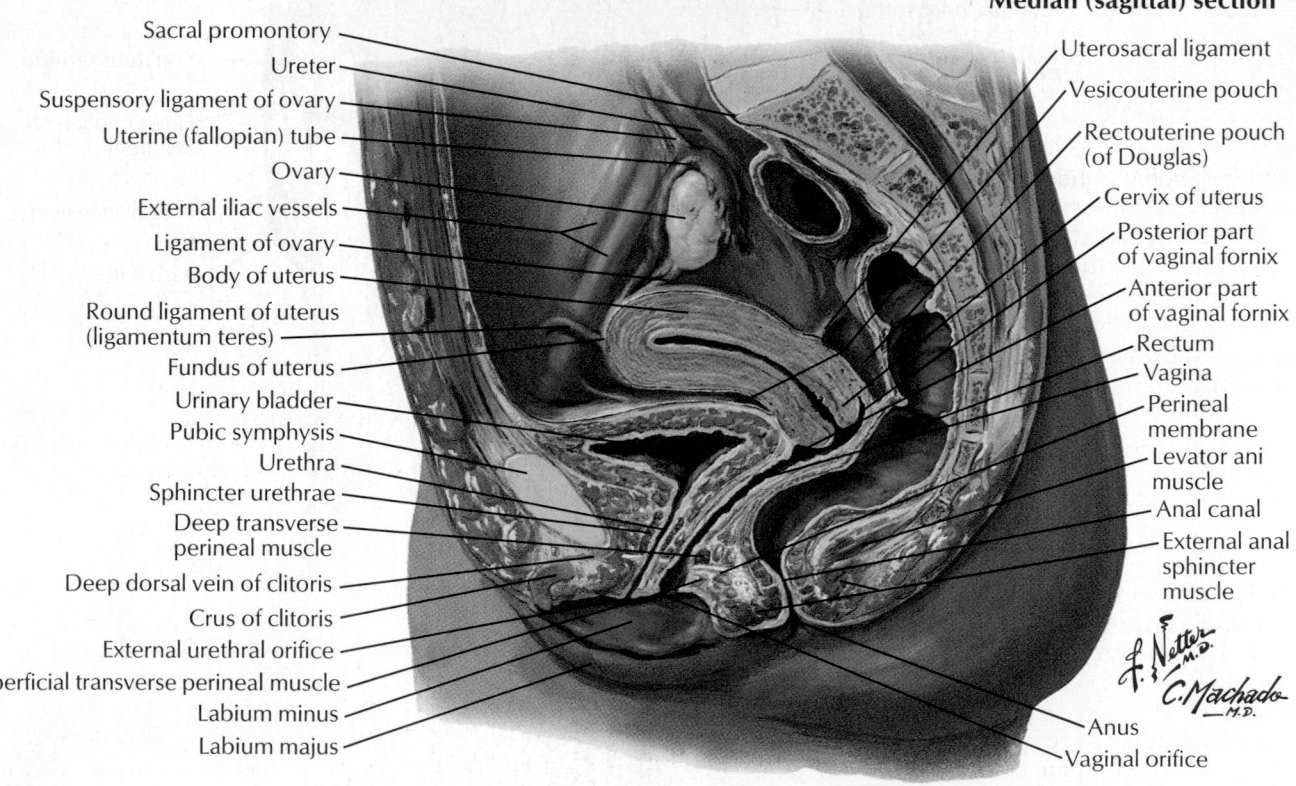

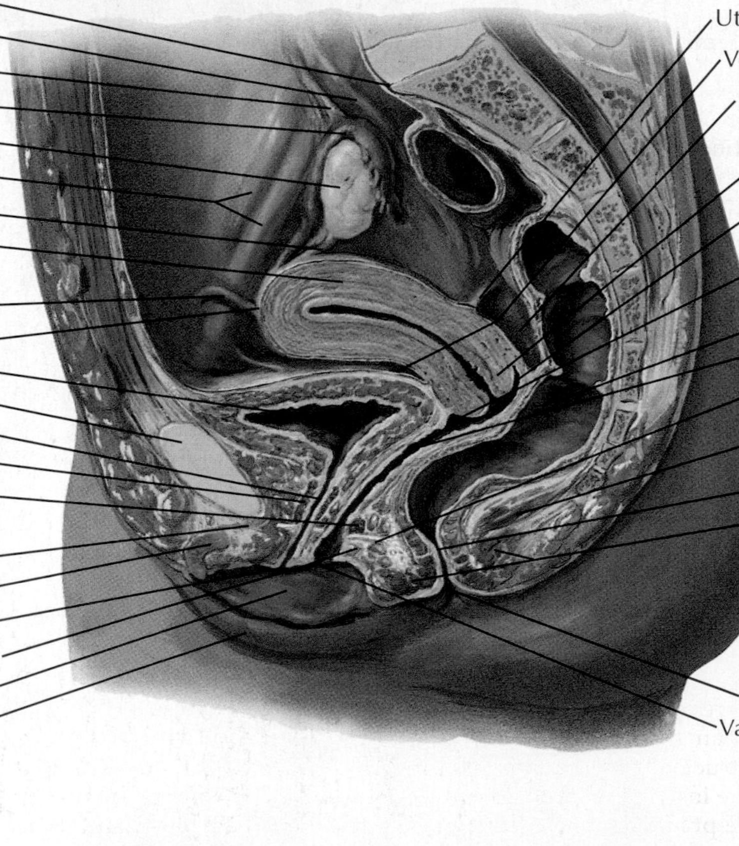

Plate 360 Pelvic Viscera and Perineum: Female. (Netter: Atlas of Human Anatomy, 4 ed, 2006, Saunders.)

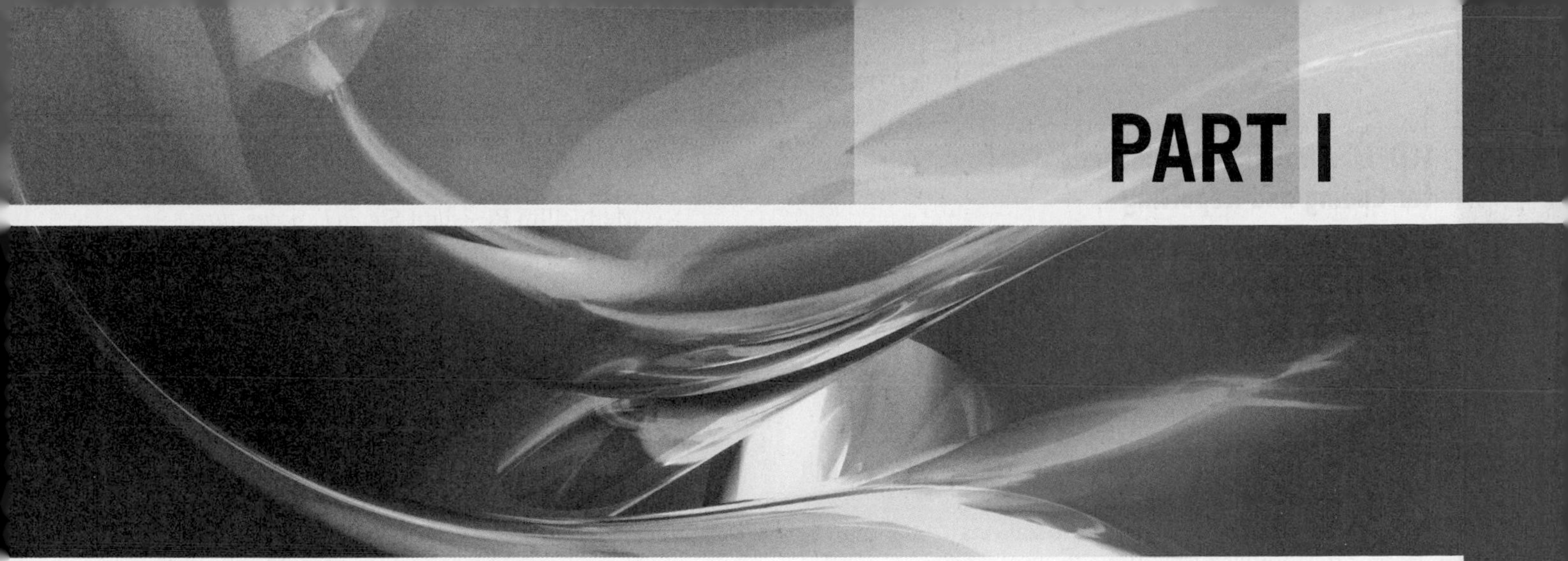

PART I

Introduction

ICD-10-CM Official Guidelines for Coding and Reporting 2017

Narrative changes appear in bold text

Items underlined have been moved within the guidelines since the 2016 version

***Italics* are used to indicate revisions to heading changes**

The Centers for Medicare and Medicaid Services (CMS) and the National Center for Health Statistics (NCHS), two departments within the U.S. Federal Government's Department of Health and Human Services (DHHS) provide the following guidelines for coding and reporting using the International Classification of Diseases, 10th Revision, Clinical Modification (ICD-10-CM). These guidelines should be used as a companion document to the official version of the ICD-10-CM as published on the NCHS website. The ICD-10-CM is a morbidity classification published by the United States for classifying diagnoses and reason for visits in all health care settings. The ICD-10-CM is based on the ICD-10, the statistical classification of disease published by the World Health Organization (WHO).

These guidelines have been approved by the four organizations that make up the Cooperating Parties for the ICD-10-CM: the American Hospital Association (AHA), the American Health Information Management Association (AHIMA), CMS, and NCHS.

These guidelines are a set of rules that have been developed to accompany and complement the official conventions and instructions provided within the ICD-10-CM itself. The instructions and conventions of the classification take precedence over guidelines. These guidelines are based on the coding and sequencing instructions in the Tabular List and Alphabetic Index of ICD-10-CM, but provide additional instruction. Adherence to these guidelines when assigning ICD-10-CM diagnosis codes is required under the Health Insurance Portability and Accountability Act (HIPAA). The diagnosis codes (Tabular List and Alphabetic Index) have been adopted under HIPAA for all healthcare settings. A joint effort between the healthcare provider and the coder is essential to achieve complete and accurate documentation, code assignment, and reporting of diagnoses and procedures. These guidelines have been developed to assist both the healthcare provider and the coder in identifying those diagnoses that are to be reported. The importance of consistent, complete documentation in the medical record cannot be overemphasized. Without such documentation accurate coding cannot be achieved. The entire record should be reviewed to determine the specific reason for the encounter and the conditions treated.

The term encounter is used for all settings, including hospital admissions. In the context of these guidelines, the term provider is used throughout the guidelines to mean physician or any qualified health care practitioner who is legally accountable for establishing the patient's diagnosis. Only this set of guidelines, approved by the Cooperating Parties, is official.

The guidelines are organized into sections. Section I includes the structure and conventions of the classification and general guidelines that apply to the entire classification, and chapter-specific guidelines that correspond to the chapters as they are arranged in the classification. Section II includes guidelines for selection of principal diagnosis for non-outpatient settings. Section III includes guidelines for reporting additional diagnoses in non-outpatient settings. Section IV is for outpatient coding and reporting. It is necessary to review all sections of the guidelines to fully understand all of the rules and instructions needed to code properly.

ICD-10-CM Official Guidelines for Coding and Reporting

Section I. Conventions, general coding guidelines and chapter specific guidelines

A. Conventions for the ICD-10-CM
   1. The Alphabetic Index and Tabular List
   2. Format and Structure:
   3. Use of codes for reporting purposes
   4. Placeholder character
   5. 7th Characters
   6. Abbreviations
      a. Alphabetic Index abbreviations
      b. Tabular List abbreviations
   7. Punctuation
   8. Use of "and"
   9. Other and Unspecified codes
      a. "Other" codes
      b. "Unspecified" codes
   1Ø. Includes Notes
   11. Inclusion terms
   12. Excludes Notes
      a. Excludes1
      b. Excludes2
   13. Etiology/manifestation convention ("code first", "use additional code" and "in diseases classified elsewhere" notes)
   14. "And"
   15. "With"
   16. "See" and "See Also"
   17. "Code also note"
   18. Default codes
   19. Code assignment and Clinical Criteria

B. General Coding Guidelines
   1. Locating a code in the ICD-10-CM
   2. Level of Detail in Coding
   3. Code or codes from AØØ.Ø through T88.9, ZØØ-Z99.8
   4. Signs and symptoms
   5. Conditions that are an integral part of a disease process
   6. Conditions that are not an integral part of a disease process
   7. Multiple coding for a single condition
   8. Acute and Chronic Conditions
   9. Combination Code
   1Ø. Sequela (Late Effects)
   11. Impending or Threatened Condition
   12. Reporting Same Diagnosis Code More than Once
   13. Laterality
   14. Documentation for BMI, *Depth of* Non-pressure ulcers, Pressure Ulcer Stages, Coma Scale, and *NIH Stroke Scale*
   15. Syndromes
   16. Documentation of Complications of Care
   17. Borderline Diagnosis
   18. Use of Sign/Symptom/Unspecified Codes

C. Chapter-Specific Coding Guidelines
   1. Chapter 1: Certain Infectious and Parasitic Diseases (AØØ-B99)
      a. Human Immunodeficiency Virus (HIV) Infections
      b. Infectious agents as the cause of diseases classified to other chapters
      c. Infections resistant to antibiotics
      d. Sepsis, Severe Sepsis, and Septic Shock
      e. Methicillin Resistant *Staphylococcus aureus* (MRSA) Conditions
      f. Zika virus infection
   2. Chapter 2: Neoplasms (CØØ-D49)
      a. Treatment directed at the malignancy
      b. Treatment of secondary site
      c. Coding and sequencing of complications
      d. Primary malignancy previously excised
      e. Admissions/Encounters involving chemotherapy, immunotherapy and radiation therapy
      f. Admission/encounter to determine extent of malignancy
      g. Symptoms, signs, and abnormal findings listed in Chapter 18 associated with neoplasms
      h. Admission/encounter for pain control/management
      i. Malignancy in two or more noncontiguous sites
      j. Disseminated malignant neoplasm, unspecified
      k. Malignant neoplasm without specification of site
      l. Sequencing of neoplasm codes
      m. Current malignancy versus personal history of malignancy
      n. Leukemia, Multiple Myeloma, and Malignant Plasma Cell Neoplasms in remission versus personal history
      o. Aftercare following surgery for neoplasm
      p. Follow-up care for completed treatment of a malignancy
      q. Prophylactic organ removal for prevention of malignancy
      r. Malignant neoplasm associated with transplanted organ
   3. Chapter 3: Disease of the blood and blood-forming organs and certain disorders involving the immune mechanism (D5Ø-D89)
   4. Chapter 4: Endocrine, Nutritional, and Metabolic Diseases (EØØ-E89)
      a. Diabetes mellitus
   5. Chapter 5: Mental, Behavioral and Neurodevelopmental disorders (FØ1 – F99)
      a. Pain disorders related to psychological factors
      b. Mental and behavioral disorders due to psychoactive substance use
   6. Chapter 6: Diseases of the Nervous System (GØØ-G99)
      a. Dominant/nondominant side
      b. Pain - Category G89
   7. Chapter 7: Diseases of the Eye and Adnexa (HØØ-H59)
      a. Glaucoma
   8. Chapter 8: Diseases of the Ear and Mastoid Process (H6Ø-H95)
   9. Chapter 9: Diseases of the Circulatory System (IØØ-I99)
      a. Hypertension
      b. Atherosclerotic Coronary Artery Disease and Angina
      c. Intraoperative and Postprocedural Cerebrovascular Accident
      d. Sequelae of Cerebrovascular Disease
      e. Acute myocardial infarction (AMI)

10. Chapter 10: Diseases of the Respiratory System (J00-J99)
    a. Chronic Obstructive Pulmonary Disease [COPD] and Asthma
    b. Acute Respiratory Failure
    c. Influenza due to certain identified influenza viruses
    d. Ventilator associated Pneumonia
11. Chapter 11: Diseases of the Digestive System (K00-K95)
12. Chapter 12: Diseases of the Skin and Subcutaneous Tissue (L00-L99)
    a. Pressure ulcer stage codes
13. Chapter 13: Diseases of the Musculoskeletal System and Connective Tissue (M00-M99)
    a. Site and laterality
    b. Acute traumatic versus chronic or recurrent musculoskeletal conditions
    c. Coding of Pathologic Fractures
    d. Osteoporosis
14. Chapter 14: Diseases of Genitourinary System (N00-N99)
    a. Chronic kidney disease
15. Chapter 15: Pregnancy, Childbirth, and the Puerperium (O00-O9A)
    a. General Rules for Obstetric Cases
    b. Selection of OB Principal or First-listed Diagnosis
    c. Pre-existing conditions versus conditions due to the pregnancy
    d. Pre-existing hypertension in pregnancy
    e. Fetal Conditions Affecting the Management of the Mother
    f. HIV Infection in Pregnancy, Childbirth and the Puerperium
    g. Diabetes mellitus in pregnancy
    h. Long term use of insulin and oral hypoglycemics
    i. Gestational (pregnancy induced) diabetes
    j. Sepsis and septic shock complicating abortion, pregnancy, childbirth and the puerperium
    k. Puerperal sepsis
    l. Alcohol and tobacco use during pregnancy, childbirth and the puerperium
    m. Poisoning, toxic effects, adverse effects and underdosing in a pregnant patient
    n. Normal Delivery, Code O80
    o. The Peripartum and Postpartum Periods
    p. Code O94, Sequelae of complication of pregnancy, childbirth, and the puerperium
    q. Termination of Pregnancy and Spontaneous abortions
    r. Abuse in a pregnant patient
16. Chapter 16: Certain Conditions Originating in the Perinatal Period (P00-P96)
    a. General Perinatal Rules
    b. Observation and Evaluation of Newborns for Suspected Conditions not Found
    c. Coding Additional Perinatal Diagnoses
    d. Prematurity and Fetal Growth Retardation
    e. Low birth weight and immaturity status
    f. Bacterial Sepsis of Newborn
    g. Stillbirth
17. Chapter 17: Congenital malformations, deformations, and chromosomal abnormalities (Q00-Q99)
18. Chapter 18: Symptoms, signs, and abnormal clinical and laboratory findings, not elsewhere classified (R00-R99)
    a. Use of symptom codes
    b. Use of a symptom code with a definitive diagnosis code
    c. Combination codes that include symptoms
    d. Repeated falls
    e. Coma scale
    f. Functional quadriplegia
    g. SIRS due to Non-Infectious Process
    h. Death NOS
    i. NIHSS Stroke Scale
19. Chapter 19: Injury, poisoning, and certain other consequences of external causes (S00-T88)
    a. Application of 7th Characters in Chapter 19
    b. Coding of Injuries
    c. Coding of Traumatic Fractures
    d. Coding of Burns and Corrosions
    e. Adverse Effects, Poisoning, Underdosing and Toxic Effects
    f. Adult and child abuse, neglect and other maltreatment
    g. Complications of care
20. Chapter 20: External Causes of Morbidity (V00-Y99)
    a. General External Cause Coding Guidelines
    b. Place of Occurrence Guideline
    c. Activity Code
    d. Place of Occurrence, Activity, and Status Codes Used with other External Cause Code
    e. If the Reporting Format Limits the Number of External Cause Codes
    f. Multiple External Cause Coding Guidelines
    g. Child and Adult Abuse Guideline
    h. Unknown or Undetermined Intent Guideline
    i. Sequelae (Late Effects) of External Cause Guidelines
    j. Terrorism Guidelines
    k. External cause status
21. Chapter 21: Factors influencing health status and contact with health services (Z00-Z99)
    a. Use of Z codes in any healthcare setting
    b. Z Codes indicate a reason for an encounter
    c. Categories of Z Codes

Section II. Selection of Principal Diagnosis

A. Codes for symptoms, signs, and ill-defined conditions
B. Two or more interrelated conditions, each potentially meeting the definition for principal diagnosis
C. Two or more diagnoses that equally meet the definition for principal diagnosis
D. Two or more comparative or contrasting conditions
E. A symptom(s) followed by contrasting/comparative diagnoses
F. Original treatment plan not carried out
G. Complications of surgery and other medical care
H. Uncertain Diagnosis

GUIDELINES (ICD-10-CM)

I. Admission from Observation Unit
1. Admission Following Medical Observation
2. Admission Following Post-Operative Observation
J. Admission from Outpatient Surgery
K. Admissions/Encounters for Rehabilitation

Section III. Reporting Additional Diagnoses

A. Previous conditions
B. Abnormal findings
C. Uncertain Diagnosis

Section IV. Diagnostic Coding and Reporting Guidelines for Outpatient Services

A. Selection of first-listed condition
1. Outpatient Surgery
2. Observation Stay
B. Codes from AØØ.Ø through T88.9, ZØØ-Z99
C. Accurate reporting of ICD-10-CM diagnosis codes
D. Codes that describe symptoms and signs
E. Encounters for circumstances other than a disease or injury
F. Level of Detail in Coding
1. ICD-10-CM codes with 3, 4, 5, 6, or 7 characters
2. Use of full number of characters required for a code
G. ICD-10-CM code for the diagnosis, condition, problem, or other reason for encounter/visit
H. Uncertain diagnosis
I. Chronic diseases
J. Code all documented conditions that coexist
K. Patients receiving diagnostic services only
L. Patients receiving therapeutic services only
M. Patients receiving preoperative evaluations only
N. Ambulatory surgery
O. Routine outpatient prenatal visits
P. Encounters for general medical examinations with abnormal findings
Q. Encounters for routine health screenings

Appendix I: Present on Admission Reporting Guidelines

Section I. Conventions, general coding guidelines and chapter specific guidelines

The conventions, general guidelines and chapter-specific guidelines are applicable to all health care settings unless otherwise indicated. The conventions and instructions of the classification take precedence over guidelines.

A. Conventions for the ICD-10-CM

The conventions for the ICD-10-CM are the general rules for use of the classification independent of the guidelines. These conventions are incorporated within the Alphabetic Index and Tabular List of the ICD-10-CM as instructional notes.

1. The Alphabetic Index and Tabular List
The ICD-10-CM is divided into the Alphabetic Index, an alphabetical list of terms and their corresponding code, and the Tabular List, a structured list of codes divided into chapters based on body system or condition. The Alphabetic Index consists of the following parts: the Index of Diseases and Injury, the Index of External Causes of Injury, the Table of Neoplasms and the Table of Drugs and Chemicals.

See Section I.C2. General guidelines
See Section I.C.19. Adverse effects, poisoning, underdosing and toxic effects

2. Format and Structure:
The ICD-10-CM Tabular List contains categories, subcategories and codes. Characters for categories, subcategories and codes may be either a letter or a number. All categories are 3 characters. A three-character category that has no further subdivision is equivalent to a code. Subcategories are either 4 or 5 characters. Codes may be 3, 4, 5, 6 or 7 characters. That is, each level of subdivision after a category is a subcategory. The final level of subdivision is a code. Codes that have applicable 7th characters are still referred to as codes, not subcategories. A code that has an applicable 7th character is considered invalid without the 7th character.

The ICD-10-CM uses an indented format for ease in reference

3. Use of codes for reporting purposes
For reporting purposes only codes are permissible, not categories or subcategories, and any applicable 7th character is required.

4. Placeholder character
The ICD-10-CM utilizes a placeholder character "X". The "X" is used as a placeholder at certain codes to allow for future expansion. An example of this is at the poisoning, adverse effect and underdosing codes, categories T36-T5Ø. Where a placeholder exists, the X must be used in order for the code to be considered a valid code.

5. 7th Characters
Certain ICD-10-CM categories have applicable 7th characters. The applicable 7th character is required for all codes within the category, or as the notes in the Tabular List instruct. The 7th character must always be the 7th character in the data field. If a code that requires a 7th character is not 6 characters, a placeholder X must be used to fill in the empty characters.

6. Abbreviations

a. Alphabetic Index abbreviations

NEC "Not elsewhere classifiable"
This abbreviation in the Alphabetic Index represents "other specified". When a specific code is not available for a condition the Alphabetic Index directs the coder to the "other specified" code in the Tabular List.

NOS "Not otherwise specified"
This abbreviation is the equivalent of unspecified.

b. **Tabular List abbreviations**

NEC "Not elsewhere classifiable"
This abbreviation in the Tabular List represents "other specified". When a specific code is not available for a condition, the Tabular List includes an NEC entry under a code to identify the code as the "other specified" code.

NOS "Not otherwise specified"
This abbreviation is the equivalent of unspecified.

7. **Punctuation**

[ ] Brackets are used in the Tabular List to enclose synonyms, alternative wording or explanatory phrases. Brackets are used in the Alphabetic Index to identify manifestation codes.

( ) Parentheses are used in both the Alphabetic Index and Tabular List to enclose supplementary words that may be present or absent in the statement of a disease or procedure without affecting the code number to which it is assigned. The terms within the parentheses are referred to as nonessential modifiers. The nonessential modifiers in the Alphabetic Index to Diseases apply to subterms following a main term except when a nonessential modifier and a subentry are mutually exclusive, the subentry takes precedence. For example, in the ICD-10-CM Alphabetic Index under the main term Enteritis, "acute" is a nonessential modifier and "chronic" is a subentry. In this case, the nonessential modifier "acute" does not apply to the subentry "chronic".

: Colons are used in the Tabular List after an incomplete term which needs one or more of the modifiers following the colon to make it assignable to a given category.

8. **Use of "and".**
See Section I.A.14. Use of the term "And"

9. **Other and Unspecified codes**

a. **"Other" codes**
Codes titled "other" or "other specified" are for use when the information in the medical record provides detail for which a specific code does not exist. Alphabetic Index entries with NEC in the line designate "other" codes in the Tabular List. These Alphabetic Index entries represent specific disease entities for which no specific code exists so the term is included within an "other" code.

b. **"Unspecified" codes**
Codes titled "unspecified" are for use when the information in the medical record is insufficient to assign a more specific code. For those categories for which an unspecified code is not provided, the "other specified" code may represent both other and unspecified.
See Section I.B.18 Use of Signs/Symptom/Unspecified Codes

10. **Includes Notes**
This note appears immediately under a three-character code title to further define, or give examples of, the content of the category.

11. **Inclusion terms**
List of terms is included under some codes. These terms are the conditions for which that code is to be used. The terms may be synonyms of the code title, or, in the case of "other specified" codes, the terms are a list of the various conditions assigned to that code. The inclusion terms are not necessarily exhaustive. Additional terms found only in the Alphabetic Index may also be assigned to a code.

12. **Excludes Notes**
The ICD-10-CM has two types of excludes notes. Each type of note has a different definition for use but they are all similar in that they indicate that codes excluded from each other are independent of each other.

a. **Excludes1**
A type 1 Excludes note is a pure excludes note. It means "NOT CODED HERE!" An Excludes1 note indicates that the code excluded should never be used at the same time as the code above the Excludes1 note. An Excludes1 is used when two conditions cannot occur together, such as a congenital form versus an acquired form of the same condition.

An exception to the Excludes1 definition is the circumstance when the two conditions are unrelated to each other. If it is not clear whether the two conditions involving an Excludes1 note are related or not, query the provider. For example, code F45.8, Other somatoform disorders, has an Excludes1 note for "sleep related teeth grinding (G47.63)," because "teeth grinding" is an inclusion term under F45.8. Only one of these two codes should be assigned for teeth grinding. However psychogenic dysmenorrhea is also an inclusion term under F45.8, and a patient could have both this condition and sleep related teeth grinding. In this case, the two conditions are clearly unrelated to each other, and so it would be appropriate to report F45.8 and G47.63 together.

b. **Excludes2**
A Type 2 Excludes note represents "Not included here." An excludes2 note indicates that the condition excluded is not part of the condition represented by the code, but a patient may have both conditions at the same time. When an Excludes2 note appears under a code, it is acceptable to use both the code and the excluded code together, when appropriate.

13. **Etiology/manifestation convention ("code first", "use additional code" and "in diseases classified elsewhere" notes)**
Certain conditions have both an underlying etiology and multiple body system manifestations

due to the underlying etiology. For such conditions, the ICD-10-CM has a coding convention that requires the underlying condition be sequenced first, **if applicable,** followed by the manifestation. Wherever such a combination exists, there is a "use additional code" note at the etiology code, and a "code first" note at the manifestation code. These instructional notes indicate the proper sequencing order of the codes, etiology followed by manifestation.

In most cases the manifestation codes will have in the code title, "in diseases classified elsewhere." Codes with this title are a component of the etiology/ manifestation convention. The code title indicates that it is a manifestation code. "In diseases classified elsewhere" codes are never permitted to be used as first-listed or principal diagnosis codes. They must be used in conjunction with an underlying condition code and they must be listed following the underlying condition. See category FØ2, Dementia in other diseases classified elsewhere, for an example of this convention.

There are manifestation codes that do not have "in diseases classified elsewhere" in the title. For such codes, there is a "use additional code" note at the etiology code and a "code first" note at the manifestation code and the rules for sequencing apply.

In addition to the notes in the Tabular List, these conditions also have a specific Alphabetic Index entry structure. In the Alphabetic Index both conditions are listed together with the etiology code first followed by the manifestation codes in brackets. The code in brackets is always to be sequenced second.

An example of the etiology/manifestation convention is dementia in Parkinson's disease. In the Alphabetic Index, code G2Ø is listed first, followed by code FØ2.8Ø or FØ2.81 in brackets. Code G2Ø represents the underlying etiology, Parkinson's disease, and must be sequenced first, whereas codes FØ2.8Ø and FØ2.81 represent the manifestation of dementia in diseases classified elsewhere, with or without behavioral disturbance.

"Code first" and "Use additional code" notes are also used as sequencing rules in the classification for certain codes that are not part of an etiology/manifestation combination.

See Section I.B.7. Multiple coding for a single condition.

14. **"And"**
The word "and" should be interpreted to mean either "and" or "or" when it appears in a title.

For example, cases of "tuberculosis of bones", "tuberculosis of joints" and "tuberculosis of bones and joints" are classified to subcategory A18.Ø, Tuberculosis of bones and joints.

15. **"With"**
The word "with" should be interpreted to mean "associated with" or "due to" when it appears in a code title, the Alphabetic Index, or an instructional note in the Tabular List. **The classification presumes a causal relationship between the two conditions linked by these terms in the Alphabetic Index or Tabular List. These conditions should be coded as related even in the absence of provider documentation explicitly linking them, unless the documentation clearly states the conditions are unrelated. For conditions not specifically linked by these relational terms in the classification, provider documentation must link the conditions in order to code them as related.**

The word "with" in the Alphabetic Index is sequenced immediately following the main term, not in alphabetical order.

16. **"See" and "See Also"**
The "see" instruction following a main term in the Alphabetic Index indicates that another term should be referenced. It is necessary to go to the main term referenced with the "see" note to locate the correct code.

A "see also" instruction following a main term in the Alphabetic Index instructs that there is another main term that may also be referenced that may provide additional Alphabetic Index entries that may be useful. It is not necessary to follow the "see also" note when the original main term provides the necessary code.

17. **"Code also" note**
A "code also" note instructs that two codes may be required to fully describe a condition, but this note does not provide sequencing direction.

18. **Default codes**
A code listed next to a main term in the ICD-10-CM Alphabetic Index is referred to as a default code. The default code represents that condition that is most commonly associated with the main term, or is the unspecified code for the condition. If a condition is documented in a medical record (for example, appendicitis) without any additional information, such as acute or chronic, the default code should be assigned.

19. **Code assignment and Clinical Criteria**
The assignment of a diagnosis code is based on the provider's diagnostic statement that the condition exists. The provider's statement that the patient has a particular condition is sufficient. Code assignment is not based on clinical criteria used by the provider to establish the diagnosis.

B. **General Coding Guidelines**

1. **Locating a code in the ICD-10-CM**
To select a code in the classification that corresponds to a diagnosis or reason for visit documented in a medical record, first locate the term in the Alphabetic Index, and then verify the code in the Tabular List. Read and be guided by instructional notations that appear in both the Alphabetic Index and the Tabular List.

It is essential to use both the Alphabetic Index and Tabular List when locating and assigning a code. The Alphabetic Index does not always provide the full code. Selection of the full code, including laterality and any applicable 7th character can only be done in the Tabular List. A dash (-) at the end of an Alphabetic Index entry indicates that additional characters are required. Even if a dash is not included at the Alphabetic Index entry, it is necessary to refer to the Tabular List to verify that no 7th character is required.

2. **Level of Detail in Coding**
Diagnosis codes are to be used and reported at their highest number of characters available.
ICD-10-CM diagnosis codes are composed of codes with 3, 4, 5, 6 or 7 characters. Codes with three characters are included in ICD-10-CM as the heading of a category of codes that may be further subdivided by the use of fourth and/or fifth characters and/or sixth characters, which provide greater detail.
A three-character code is to be used only if it is not further subdivided. A code is invalid if it has not been coded to the full number of characters required for that code, including the 7th character, if applicable.

3. **Code or codes from A00.0 through T88.9, Z00-Z99.8**
The appropriate code or codes from A00.0 through T88.9, Z00-Z99.8 must be used to identify diagnoses, symptoms, conditions, problems, complaints or other reason(s) for the encounter/visit.

4. **Signs and symptoms**
Codes that describe symptoms and signs, as opposed to diagnoses, are acceptable for reporting purposes when a related definitive diagnosis has not been established (confirmed) by the provider. Chapter 18 of ICD-10-CM, Symptoms, Signs, and Abnormal Clinical and Laboratory Findings, Not Elsewhere Classified (codes R00.0 - R99) contains many, but not all codes for symptoms.
See Section I.B.18 Use of Signs/Symptom/ Unspecified Codes

5. **Conditions that are an integral part of a disease process**
Signs and symptoms that are associated routinely with a disease process should not be assigned as additional codes, unless otherwise instructed by the classification.

6. **Conditions that are not an integral part of a disease process**
Additional signs and symptoms that may not be associated routinely with a disease process should be coded when present.

7. **Multiple coding for a single condition**
In addition to the etiology/manifestation convention that requires two codes to fully describe a single condition that affects multiple body systems, there are other single conditions that also require more than one code. "Use additional code" notes are found in the Tabular List at codes that are not part of an etiology/manifestation pair where a secondary code is useful to fully describe a condition. The sequencing rule is the same as the etiology/manifestation pair, "use additional code" indicates that a secondary code should be added.
For example, for bacterial infections that are not included in chapter 1, a secondary code from category B95, Streptococcus, Staphylococcus, and Enterococcus, as the cause of diseases classified elsewhere, or B96, Other bacterial agents as the cause of diseases classified elsewhere, may be required to identify the bacterial organism causing the infection. A "use additional code" note will normally be found at the infectious disease code, indicating a need for the organism code to be added as a secondary code.
"Code first" notes are also under certain codes that are not specifically manifestation codes but may be due to an underlying cause. When there is a "code first" note and an underlying condition is present, the underlying condition should be sequenced first.
"Code, if applicable, any causal condition first," notes indicate that this code may be assigned as a principal diagnosis when the causal condition is unknown or not applicable. If a causal condition is known, then the code for that condition should be sequenced as the principal or first-listed diagnosis.
Multiple codes may be needed for sequela, complication codes and obstetric codes to more fully describe a condition. See the specific guidelines for these conditions for further instruction.

8. **Acute and Chronic Conditions**
If the same condition is described as both acute (subacute) and chronic, and separate subentries exist in the Alphabetic Index at the same indentation level, code both and sequence the acute (subacute) code first.

9. **Combination Code**
A combination code is a single code used to classify:
Two diagnoses, or
A diagnosis with an associated secondary process (manifestation)
A diagnosis with an associated complication
Combination codes are identified by referring to subterm entries in the Alphabetic Index and by reading the inclusion and exclusion notes in the Tabular List.
Assign only the combination code when that code fully identifies the diagnostic conditions involved or when the Alphabetic Index so directs. Multiple coding should not be used when the classification provides a combination code that clearly identifies all of the elements documented in the diagnosis. When the combination code lacks necessary specificity in describing the manifestation or complication, an additional code should be used as a secondary code.

10. **Sequela (Late Effects)**
A sequela is the residual effect (condition produced) after the acute phase of an illness or injury has terminated. There is no time limit on when a sequela code can be used. The residual may

GUIDELINES (ICD-10-CM)

be apparent early, such as in cerebral infarction, or it may occur months or years later, such as that due to a previous injury. Examples of sequela include: scar formation resulting from a burn, deviated septum due to a nasal fracture, and infertility due to tubal occlusion from old tuberculosis. Coding of sequela generally requires two codes sequenced in the following order: the condition or nature of the sequela is sequenced first. The sequela code is sequenced second.

An exception to the above guidelines are those instances where the code for the sequela is followed by a manifestation code identified in the Tabular List and title, or the sequela code has been expanded (at the fourth, fifth or sixth character levels) to include the manifestation(s). The code for the acute phase of an illness or injury that led to the sequela is never used with a code for the late effect.

See Section I.C.9. Sequelae of cerebrovascular disease

See Section I.C.15. Sequelae of complication of pregnancy, childbirth and the puerperium

See Section I.C.19. Application of 7th characters for Chapter 19

11. **Impending or Threatened Condition**
Code any condition described at the time of discharge as "impending" or "threatened" as follows:

If it did occur, code as confirmed diagnosis.

If it did not occur, reference the Alphabetic Index to determine if the condition has a subentry term for "impending" or "threatened" and also reference main term entries for "Impending" and for "Threatened."

If the subterms are listed, assign the given code.

If the subterms are not listed, code the existing underlying condition(s) and not the condition described as impending or threatened.

12. **Reporting Same Diagnosis Code More than Once**
Each unique ICD-10-CM diagnosis code may be reported only once for an encounter. This applies to bilateral conditions when there are no distinct codes identifying laterality or two different conditions classified to the same ICD-10-CM diagnosis code.

13. **Laterality**
Some ICD-10-CM codes indicate laterality, specifying whether the condition occurs on the left, right or is bilateral. If no bilateral code is provided and the condition is bilateral, assign separate codes for both the left and right side. If the side is not identified in the medical record, assign the code for the unspecified side.

When a patient has a bilateral condition and each side is treated during separate encounters, assign the "bilateral" code (as the condition still exists on both sides), including for the encounter to treat the first side. For the second encounter for treatment after one side has previously been treated and the condition no longer exists on that side, assign the appropriate unilateral code for the side where the condition still exists (e.g., cataract surgery performed on each eye in separate encounters). The bilateral code would not be assigned for the subsequent encounter, as the patient no longer has the condition in the previously-treated site. If the treatment on the first side did not completely resolve the condition, then the bilateral code would still be appropriate.

14. **Documentation for BMI, *Depth of* Non-pressure ulcers, Pressure Ulcer Stages, Coma Scale, *and NIH Stroke Scale***
For the Body Mass Index (BMI), depth of non-pressure chronic ulcers, pressure ulcer stage, **coma scale, and NIH stroke scale (NIHSS) codes,** code assignment may be based on medical record documentation from clinicians who are not the patient's provider (i.e., physician or other qualified healthcare practitioner legally accountable for establishing the patient's diagnosis), since this information is typically documented by other clinicians involved in the care of the patient (e.g., a dietitian often documents the BMI, a nurse often documents the pressure ulcer stages**, and an emergency medical technician often documents the coma scale**). However, the associated diagnosis (such as overweight, obesity, **acute stroke,** or pressure ulcer) must be documented by the patient's provider. If there is conflicting medical record documentation, either from the same clinician or different clinicians, the patient's attending provider should be queried for clarification.

The BMI**, coma scale, and NIHSS** codes should only be reported as secondary diagnoses.

15. **Syndromes**
Follow the Alphabetic Index guidance when coding syndromes. In the absence of Alphabetic Index guidance, assign codes for the documented manifestations of the syndrome. Additional codes for manifestations that are not an integral part of the disease process may also be assigned when the condition does not have a unique code.

16. **Documentation of Complications of Care**
Code assignment is based on the provider's documentation of the relationship between the condition and the care or procedure**, unless otherwise instructed by the classification.** The guideline extends to any complications of care, regardless of the chapter the code is located in. It is important to note that not all conditions that occur during or following medical care or surgery are classified as complications. There must be a cause-and-effect relationship between the care provided and the condition, and an indication in the documentation that it is a complication. Query the provider for clarification, if the complication is not clearly documented.

17. **Borderline Diagnosis**
If the provider documents a "borderline" diagnosis at the time of discharge, the diagnosis is coded as confirmed, unless the classification provides a specific entry (e.g., borderline diabetes). If a borderline condition has a specific index entry in ICD-10-CM, it should be coded as such. Since

borderline conditions are not uncertain diagnoses, no distinction is made between the care setting (inpatient versus outpatient). Whenever the documentation is unclear regarding a borderline condition, coders are encouraged to query for clarification.

18. Use of Sign/Symptom/Unspecified Codes

Sign/symptom and "unspecified" codes have acceptable, even necessary, uses. While specific diagnosis codes should be reported when they are supported by the available medical record documentation and clinical knowledge of the patient's health condition, there are instances when signs/symptoms or unspecified codes are the best choices for accurately reflecting the healthcare encounter. Each healthcare encounter should be coded to the level of certainty known for that encounter.

If a definitive diagnosis has not been established by the end of the encounter, it is appropriate to report codes for sign(s) and/or symptom(s) in lieu of a definitive diagnosis. When sufficient clinical information isn't known or available about a particular health condition to assign a more specific code, it is acceptable to report the appropriate "unspecified" code (e.g., a diagnosis of pneumonia has been determined, but not the specific type). Unspecified codes should be reported when they are the codes that most accurately reflect what is known about the patient's condition at the time of that particular encounter. It would be inappropriate to select a specific code that is not supported by the medical record documentation or conduct medically unnecessary diagnostic testing in order to determine a more specific code.

C. Chapter-Specific Coding Guidelines

In addition to general coding guidelines, there are guidelines for specific diagnoses and/or conditions in the classification. Unless otherwise indicated, these guidelines apply to all health care settings. Please refer to Section II for guidelines on the selection of principal diagnosis.

1. Chapter 1: Certain Infectious and Parasitic Diseases (A00-B99)

a. Human Immunodeficiency Virus (HIV) Infections

1) Code only confirmed cases

Code only confirmed cases of HIV infection/illness. This is an exception to the hospital inpatient guideline Section II, H.

In this context, "confirmation" does not require documentation of positive serology or culture for HIV; the provider's diagnostic statement that the patient is HIV positive, or has an HIV-related illness is sufficient.

2) Selection and sequencing of HIV codes

(a) Patient admitted for HIV-related condition

If a patient is admitted for an HIV-related condition, the principal diagnosis should be B20, Human immunodeficiency virus [HIV] disease followed by additional diagnosis codes for all reported HIV-related conditions.

(b) Patient with HIV disease admitted for unrelated condition

If a patient with HIV disease is admitted for an unrelated condition (such as a traumatic injury), the code for the unrelated condition (e.g., the nature of injury code) should be the principal diagnosis. Other diagnoses would be B20 followed by additional diagnosis codes for all reported HIV-related conditions.

(c) Whether the patient is newly diagnosed

Whether the patient is newly diagnosed or has had previous admissions/encounters for HIV conditions is irrelevant to the sequencing decision.

(d) Asymptomatic human immunodeficiency virus

Z21, Asymptomatic human immunodeficiency virus [HIV] infection status, is to be applied when the patient without any documentation of symptoms is listed as being "HIV positive," "known HIV," "HIV test positive," or similar terminology. Do not use this code if the term "AIDS" is used or if the patient is treated for any HIV-related illness or is described as having any condition(s) resulting from his/her HIV positive status; use B20 in these cases.

(e) Patients with inconclusive HIV serology

Patients with inconclusive HIV serology, but no definitive diagnosis or manifestations of the illness, may be assigned code R75, Inconclusive laboratory evidence of human immunodeficiency virus [HIV].

(f) Previously diagnosed HIV-related illness

Patients with any known prior diagnosis of an HIV-related illness should be coded to B20. Once a patient has developed an HIV-related illness, the patient should always be assigned code B20 on every subsequent admission/encounter. Patients previously diagnosed with any HIV illness (B20) should never be assigned to R75 or Z21, Asymptomatic human immunodeficiency virus [HIV] infection status.

(g) HIV Infection in Pregnancy, Childbirth and the Puerperium

During pregnancy, childbirth or the puerperium, a patient admitted (or presenting for a health care encounter) because of an HIV-related illness should receive a principal diagnosis code of O98.7-, Human immunodeficiency [HIV] disease complicating pregnancy, childbirth and the puerperium, followed by B20 and the code(s) for the HIV-related illness(es). Codes from Chapter 15 always take sequencing priority.

Patients with asymptomatic HIV infection status admitted (or presenting for a health care encounter) during pregnancy, childbirth, or the puerperium should receive codes of O98.7- and Z21.

(h) Encounters for testing for HIV

If a patient is being seen to determine his/her HIV status, use code Z11.4, Encounter for screening for human immunodeficiency virus [HIV]. Use additional codes for any associated high risk behavior.

If a patient with signs or symptoms is being seen for HIV testing, code the signs and symptoms. An additional counseling code Z71.7, Human immunodeficiency virus [HIV] counseling, may be used if counseling is provided during the encounter for the test.

When a patient returns to be informed of his/her HIV test results and the test result is negative, use code Z71.7, Human immunodeficiency virus [HIV] counseling.

If the results are positive, see previous guidelines and assign codes as appropriate.

b. Infectious agents as the cause of diseases classified to other chapters

Certain infections are classified in chapters other than Chapter 1 and no organism is identified as part of the infection code. In these instances, it is necessary to use an additional code from Chapter 1 to identify the organism. A code from category B95, Streptococcus, Staphylococcus, and Enterococcus as the cause of diseases classified to other chapters, B96, Other bacterial agents as the cause of diseases classified to other chapters, or B97, Viral agents as the cause of diseases classified to other chapters, is to be used as an additional code to identify the organism. An instructional note will be found at the infection code advising that an additional organism code is required.

c. Infections resistant to antibiotics

Many bacterial infections are resistant to current antibiotics. It is necessary to identify all infections documented as antibiotic resistant. Assign a code from category Z16, Resistance to antimicrobial drugs, following the infection code only if the infection code does not identify drug resistance.

d. Sepsis, Severe Sepsis, and Septic Shock

1) Coding of Sepsis and Severe Sepsis

(a) Sepsis

For a diagnosis of sepsis, assign the appropriate code for the underlying systemic infection. If the type of infection or causal organism is not further specified, assign code A41.9, Sepsis, unspecified organism.

A code from subcategory R65.2, Severe sepsis, should not be assigned unless severe sepsis or an associated acute organ dysfunction is documented.

(i) Negative or inconclusive blood cultures and sepsis

Negative or inconclusive blood cultures do not preclude a diagnosis of sepsis in patients with clinical evidence of the condition, however, the provider should be queried.

(ii) Urosepsis

The term urosepsis is a nonspecific term. It is not to be considered synonymous with sepsis. It has no default code in the Alphabetic Index. Should a provider use this term, he/she must be queried for clarification.

(iii) Sepsis with organ dysfunction

If a patient has sepsis and associated acute organ dysfunction or multiple organ dysfunction (MOD), follow the instructions for coding severe sepsis.

(iv) Acute organ dysfunction that is not clearly associated with the sepsis

If a patient has sepsis and an acute organ dysfunction, but the medical record documentation indicates that the acute organ dysfunction is related to a medical condition other than the sepsis, do not assign a code from subcategory R65.2, Severe sepsis. An acute organ dysfunction must be associated with the sepsis in order to assign the severe sepsis code. If the documentation is not clear as to whether an acute organ dysfunction is related to the sepsis or another medical condition, query the provider.

(b) Severe sepsis

The coding of severe sepsis requires a minimum of 2 codes: first a code for the underlying systemic infection, followed by a code from subcategory R65.2, Severe sepsis. If the causal organism is not documented, assign code A41.9, Sepsis, unspecified organism, for the infection. Additional code(s) for the associated acute organ dysfunction are also required.

Due to the complex nature of severe sepsis, some cases may require querying the provider prior to assignment of the codes.

2) Septic shock

(a) Septic shock generally refers to circulatory failure associated with severe sepsis, and therefore, it represents a type of acute organ dysfunction.

For all cases of septic shock, the code for the systemic infection should be sequenced first, followed by code R65.21, Severe sepsis with septic shock or code T81.12, Postprocedural septic shock. Any additional codes for the other acute organ dysfunctions should also be assigned. As noted in the sequencing instructions in the Tabular List, the code for septic shock cannot be assigned as a principal diagnosis.

3) Sequencing of severe sepsis

If severe sepsis is present on admission, and meets the definition of principal diagnosis, the underlying systemic infection should be assigned as principal diagnosis followed by the appropriate code from subcategory R65.2 as required by the sequencing rules in the Tabular List. A code from subcategory R65.2 can never be assigned as a principal diagnosis.

When severe sepsis develops during an encounter (it was not present on admission) the underlying systemic infection and the appropriate code from subcategory R65.2 should be assigned as secondary diagnoses.

Severe sepsis may be present on admission but the diagnosis may not be confirmed until sometime after admission. If the documentation is not clear whether severe sepsis was present on admission, the provider should be queried.

4) Sepsis and severe sepsis with a localized infection

If the reason for admission is both sepsis or severe sepsis and a localized infection, such as pneumonia or cellulitis, a code(s) for the underlying systemic infection should be assigned first and the code for the localized infection should be assigned as a secondary diagnosis. If the patient has severe sepsis, a code from subcategory R65.2 should also be assigned as a secondary diagnosis. If the patient is admitted with a localized infection, such as pneumonia, and sepsis/severe sepsis doesn't develop until after admission, the localized infection should be assigned first, followed by the appropriate sepsis/severe sepsis codes.

5) Sepsis due to a postprocedural infection

(a) Documentation of causal relationship

As with all postprocedural complications, code assignment is based on the provider's documentation of the relationship between the infection and the procedure.

(b) Sepsis due to a postprocedural infection

For such cases, the postprocedural infection code, such as, T80.2, Infections following infusion, transfusion, and therapeutic injection, T81.4, Infection following a procedure, T88.0, Infection following immunization, or O86.0, Infection of obstetric surgical wound, should be coded first, followed by the code for the specific infection. If the patient has severe sepsis the appropriate code from subcategory R65.2 should also be assigned with the additional code(s) for any acute organ dysfunction.

(c) Postprocedural infection and postprocedural septic shock

In cases where a postprocedural infection has occurred and has resulted in severe sepsis the code for the precipitating complication such as code T81.4, Infection following a procedure, or O86.0, Infection of obstetrical surgical wound should be coded first followed by code R65.20, Severe sepsis without septic shock. A Code for the systemic infection should also be assigned.

If a postprocedural infection has resulted in postprocedural septic shock, the code for the precipitating complication such as code T81.4, Infection following a procedure, or O86.0, Infection of obstetrical surgical wound should be coded first followed by code T81.12-, Postprocedural septic shock. A code for the systemic infection should also be assigned.

6) Sepsis and severe sepsis associated with a noninfectious process (condition)

In some cases a noninfectious process (condition), such as trauma, may lead to an infection which can result in sepsis or severe sepsis. If sepsis or severe sepsis is documented as associated with a noninfectious condition, such as a burn or serious injury, and this condition meets the definition for principal diagnosis, the code for the noninfectious condition should be sequenced first, followed by the code for the resulting infection. If severe sepsis is present, a code from subcategory R65.2 should also be assigned with any associated organ dysfunction(s) codes. It is not necessary to assign a code from subcategory R65.1, Systemic inflammatory response syndrome (SIRS) of non-infectious origin, for these cases.

If the infection meets the definition of principal diagnosis it should be sequenced before the non-infectious condition. When both the associated non-infectious condition and the infection meet the definition of principal diagnosis either may be assigned as principal diagnosis.

Only one code from category R65, Symptoms and signs specifically associated with systemic inflammation and infection, should be assigned. Therefore, when a non-infectious condition leads to an infection resulting in severe sepsis, assign the appropriate code from subcategory R65.2, Severe sepsis. Do not additionally assign a code from subcategory R65.1, Systemic inflammatory response syndrome (SIRS) of non-infectious origin.

See Section I.C.18. SIRS due to non-infectious process

7) Sepsis and septic shock complicating abortion, pregnancy, childbirth, and the puerperium

See Section I.C.15. Sepsis and septic shock complicating abortion, pregnancy, childbirth and the puerperium

8) Newborn sepsis

See Section I.C.16. f. Bacterial sepsis of Newborn

e. Methicillin Resistant Staphylococcus aureus (MRSA) Conditions

1) Selection and sequencing of MRSA codes

(a) Combination codes for MRSA infection

When a patient is diagnosed with an infection that is due to methicillin resistant *Staphylococcus aureus* (MRSA), and that infection has a combination code that includes the causal organism (e.g., sepsis, pneumonia) assign the appropriate combination code for the condition (e.g., code A41.02, Sepsis

GUIDELINES (ICD-10-CM)

due to Methicillin resistant Staphylococcus aureus or code J15.212, Pneumonia due to Methicillin resistant Staphylococcus aureus). Do not assign code B95.62, Methicillin resistant Staphylococcus aureus infection as the cause of diseases classified elsewhere, as an additional code because the combination code includes the type of infection and the MRSA organism. Do not assign a code from subcategory Z16.11, Resistance to penicillins, as an additional diagnosis.

See Section C.1. for instructions on coding and sequencing of sepsis and severe sepsis.

(b) Other codes for MRSA infection

When there is documentation of a current infection (e.g., wound infection, stitch abscess, urinary tract infection) due to MRSA, and that infection does not have a combination code that includes the causal organism, assign the appropriate code to identify the condition along with code B95.62, Methicillin resistant Staphylococcus aureus infection as the cause of diseases classified elsewhere for the MRSA infection. Do not assign a code from subcategory Z16.11, Resistance to penicillins.

(c) Methicillin susceptible Staphylococcus aureus (MSSA) and MRSA colonization

The condition or state of being colonized or carrying MSSA or MRSA is called colonization or carriage, while an individual person is described as being colonized or being a carrier. Colonization means that MSSA or MSRA is present on or in the body without necessarily causing illness. A positive MRSA colonization test might be documented by the provider as "MRSA screen positive" or "MRSA nasal swab positive".

Assign code Z22.322, Carrier or suspected carrier of Methicillin resistant Staphylococcus aureus, for patients documented as having MRSA colonization. Assign code Z22.321, Carrier or suspected carrier of Methicillin susceptible Staphylococcus aureus, for patient documented as having MSSA colonization. Colonization is not necessarily indicative of a disease process or as the cause of a specific condition the patient may have unless documented as such by the provider.

(d) MRSA colonization and infection

If a patient is documented as having both MRSA colonization and infection during a hospital admission, code Z22.322, Carrier or suspected carrier of Methicillin resistant Staphylococcus aureus, and a code for the MRSA infection may both be assigned.

f. Zika virus infections

1) Code only confirmed cases

Code only a confirmed diagnosis of Zika virus (A92.5, Zika virus disease) as documented by the provider. This is an exception to the hospital inpatient guideline Section II, H.

In this context, "confirmation" does not require documentation of the type of test performed; the physician's diagnostic statement that the condition is confirmed is sufficient. This code should be assigned regardless of the stated mode of transmission.

If the provider documents "suspected", "possible" or "probable" Zika, do not assign code A92.5. Assign a code(s) explaining the reason for encounter (such as fever, rash, or joint pain) or Z20.828, Contact with and (suspected) exposure to other viral communicable diseases.

2. Chapter 2: Neoplasms (C00-D49)

General guidelines

Chapter 2 of the ICD-10-CM contains the codes for most benign and all malignant neoplasms. Certain benign neoplasms, such as prostatic adenomas, may be found in the specific body system chapters. To properly code a neoplasm it is necessary to determine from the record if the neoplasm is benign, in-situ, malignant, or of uncertain histologic behavior. If malignant, any secondary (metastatic) sites should also be determined.

Primary malignant neoplasms overlapping site boundaries

A primary malignant neoplasm that overlaps two or more contiguous (next to each other) sites should be classified to the subcategory/ code .8 ('overlapping lesion'), unless the combination is specifically indexed elsewhere. For multiple neoplasms of the same site that are not contiguous such as tumors in different quadrants of the same breast, codes for each site should be assigned.

Malignant neoplasm of ectopic tissue

Malignant neoplasms of ectopic tissue are to be coded to the site of origin mentioned, e.g., ectopic pancreatic malignant neoplasms involving the stomach are coded to pancreas, unspecified (C25.9).

The neoplasm table in the Alphabetic Index should be referenced first. However, if the histological term is documented, that term should be referenced first, rather than going immediately to the Neoplasm Table, in order to determine which column in the Neoplasm Table is appropriate. For example, if the documentation indicates "adenoma," refer to the term in the Alphabetic Index to review the entries under this term and the instructional note to "see also neoplasm, by site, benign." The table provides the proper code based on the type of neoplasm and the site. It is important to select the proper column in the table that corresponds to the type of neoplasm. The Tabular List should then be referenced to verify that the correct code has been selected from the table and that a more specific site code does not exist.

See Section I.C.21. Factors influencing health status and contact with health services, Status, for information regarding Z15.0, codes for genetic susceptibility to cancer.

a. Treatment directed at the malignancy
If the treatment is directed at the malignancy, designate the malignancy as the principal diagnosis.

The only exception to this guideline is if a patient admission/encounter is solely for the administration of chemotherapy, immunotherapy or radiation therapy, assign the appropriate Z51.— code as the first-listed or principal diagnosis, and the diagnosis or problem for which the service is being performed as a secondary diagnosis.

b. Treatment of secondary site
When a patient is admitted because of a primary neoplasm with metastasis and treatment is directed toward the secondary site only, the secondary neoplasm is designated as the principal diagnosis even though the primary malignancy is still present.

c. Coding and sequencing of complications
Coding and sequencing of complications associated with the malignancies or with the therapy thereof are subject to the following guidelines:

1) Anemia associated with malignancy
When admission/encounter is for management of an anemia associated with the malignancy, and the treatment is only for anemia, the appropriate code for the malignancy is sequenced as the principal or first-listed diagnosis followed by the appropriate code for the anemia (such as code D63.Ø, Anemia in neoplastic disease).

2) Anemia associated with chemotherapy, immunotherapy and radiation therapy
When the admission/encounter is for management of an anemia associated with an adverse effect of the administration of chemotherapy or immunotherapy and the only treatment is for the anemia, the anemia code is sequenced first followed by the appropriate codes for the neoplasm and the adverse effect (T45.1X5, Adverse effect of antineoplastic and immunosuppressive drugs).

When the admission/encounter is for management of an anemia associated with an adverse effect of radiotherapy, the anemia code should be sequenced first, followed by the appropriate neoplasm code and code Y84.2, Radiological procedure and radiotherapy as the cause of abnormal reaction of the patient, or of later complication, without mention of misadventure at the time of the procedure.

3) Management of dehydration due to the malignancy
When the admission/encounter is for management of dehydration due to the malignancy and only the dehydration is being treated (intravenous rehydration), the dehydration is sequenced first, followed by the code(s) for the malignancy.

4) Treatment of a complication resulting from a surgical procedure
When the admission/encounter is for treatment of a complication resulting from a surgical procedure, designate the complication as the principal or first-listed diagnosis if treatment is directed at resolving the complication.

d. Primary malignancy previously excised
When a primary malignancy has been previously excised or eradicated from its site and there is no further treatment directed to that site and there is no evidence of any existing primary malignancy, a code from category Z85, Personal history of malignant neoplasm, should be used to indicate the former site of the malignancy. Any mention of extension, invasion, or metastasis to another site is coded as a secondary malignant neoplasm to that site. The secondary site may be the principal or first-listed with the Z85 code used as a secondary code.

e. Admissions/Encounters involving chemotherapy, immunotherapy and radiation therapy

1) Episode of care involves surgical removal of neoplasm
When an episode of care involves the surgical removal of a neoplasm, primary or secondary site, followed by adjunct chemotherapy or radiation treatment during the same episode of care, the code for the neoplasm should be assigned as principal or first-listed diagnosis.

2) Patient admission/encounter solely for administration of chemotherapy, immunotherapy and radiation therapy
If a patient admission/encounter is solely for the administration of chemotherapy, immunotherapy or radiation therapy assign code Z51.Ø, Encounter for antineoplastic radiation therapy, or Z51.11, Encounter for antineoplastic chemotherapy, or Z51.12, Encounter for antineoplastic immunotherapy as the first-listed or principal diagnosis. If a patient receives more than one of these therapies during the same admission more than one of these codes may be assigned, in any sequence.

The malignancy for which the therapy is being administered should be assigned as a secondary diagnosis.

3) Patient admitted for radiation therapy, chemotherapy or immunotherapy and develops complications
When a patient is admitted for the purpose of radiotherapy, immunotherapy or chemotherapy and develops complications such as uncontrolled nausea and vomiting or dehydration, the principal or first-listed diagnosis is Z51.Ø, Encounter for antineoplastic radiation therapy, or Z51.11, Encounter for antineoplastic chemotherapy, or Z51.12, Encounter for antineoplastic immunotherapy followed by any codes for the complications.

f. Admission/encounter to determine extent of malignancy
When the reason for admission/encounter is to determine the extent of the malignancy, or for a procedure such as paracentesis or thoracentesis, the primary malignancy or appropriate metastatic site is designated as the principal or first-listed diagnosis, even though chemotherapy or radiotherapy is administered.

g. Symptoms, signs, and abnormal findings listed in Chapter 18 associated with neoplasms

Symptoms, signs, and ill-defined conditions listed in Chapter 18 characteristic of, or associated with, an existing primary or secondary site malignancy cannot be used to replace the malignancy as principal or first-listed diagnosis, regardless of the number of admissions or encounters for treatment and care of the neoplasm.

See section I.C.21. Factors influencing health status and contact with health services, Encounter for prophylactic organ removal.

h. Admission/encounter for pain control/ management

See Section I.C.6. for information on coding admission/ encounter for pain control/management.

i. Malignancy in two or more noncontiguous sites

A patient may have more than one malignant tumor in the same organ. These tumors may represent different primaries or metastatic disease, depending on the site. Should the documentation be unclear, the provider should be queried as to the status of each tumor so that the correct codes can be assigned.

j. Disseminated malignant neoplasm, unspecified

Code C8Ø.Ø, Disseminated malignant neoplasm, unspecified, is for use only in those cases where the patient has advanced metastatic disease and no known primary or secondary sites are specified. It should not be used in place of assigning codes for the primary site and all known secondary sites.

k. Malignant neoplasm without specification of site

Code C8Ø.1, Malignant (primary) neoplasm, unspecified, equates to Cancer, unspecified. This code should only be used when no determination can be made as to the primary site of a malignancy. This code should rarely be used in the inpatient setting.

l. Sequencing of neoplasm codes

1) Encounter for treatment of primary malignancy

If the reason for the encounter is for treatment of a primary malignancy, assign the malignancy as the principal/first-listed diagnosis. The primary site is to be sequenced first, followed by any metastatic sites.

2) Encounter for treatment of secondary malignancy

When an encounter is for a primary malignancy with metastasis and treatment is directed toward the metastatic (secondary) site(s) only, the metastatic site(s) is designated as the principal/ first-listed diagnosis. The primary malignancy is coded as an additional code.

3) Malignant neoplasm in a pregnant patient

When a pregnant woman has a malignant neoplasm, a code from subcategory O9A.1-, Malignant neoplasm complicating pregnancy, childbirth, and the puerperium, should be sequenced first, followed by the appropriate code from Chapter 2 to indicate the type of neoplasm.

4) Encounter for complication associated with a neoplasm

When an encounter is for management of a complication associated with a neoplasm, such as dehydration, and the treatment is only for the complication, the complication is coded first, followed by the appropriate code(s) for the neoplasm.

The exception to this guideline is anemia. When the admission/encounter is for management of an anemia associated with the malignancy, and the treatment is only for anemia, the appropriate code for the malignancy is sequenced as the principal or first-listed diagnosis followed by code D63.Ø, Anemia in neoplastic disease.

5) Complication from surgical procedure for treatment of a neoplasm

When an encounter is for treatment of a complication resulting from a surgical procedure performed for the treatment of the neoplasm, designate the complication as the principal/ first-listed diagnosis. See guideline regarding the coding of a current malignancy versus personal history to determine if the code for the neoplasm should also be assigned.

6) Pathologic fracture due to a neoplasm

When an encounter is for a pathological fracture due to a neoplasm, and the focus of treatment is the fracture, a code from subcategory M84.5, Pathological fracture in neoplastic disease, should be sequenced first, followed by the code for the neoplasm.

If the focus of treatment is the neoplasm with an associated pathological fracture, the neoplasm code should be sequenced first, followed by a code from M84.5 for the pathological fracture.

m. Current malignancy versus personal history of malignancy

When a primary malignancy has been excised but further treatment, such as an additional surgery for the malignancy, radiation therapy or chemotherapy is directed to that site, the primary malignancy code should be used until treatment is completed.

When a primary malignancy has been previously excised or eradicated from its site, there is no further treatment (of the malignancy) directed to that site, and there is no evidence of any existing primary malignancy, a code from category Z85, Personal history of malignant neoplasm, should be used to indicate the former site of the malignancy.

See Section I.C.21. Factors influencing health status and contact with health services, History (of)

n. Leukemia, Multiple Myeloma, and Malignant Plasma Cell Neoplasms in remission versus personal history

The categories for leukemia, and category C9Ø, Multiple myeloma and malignant plasma cell neoplasms, have codes indicating whether or not the leukemia has achieved remission. There are also codes Z85.6, Personal history of leukemia, and Z85.79, Personal history of other malignant neoplasms of lymphoid, hematopoietic and related tissues. If the documentation is unclear, as to whether the leukemia has achieved remission, the provider should be queried.

See Section I.C.21. Factors influencing health status and contact with health services, History (of)

o. Aftercare following surgery for neoplasm

See Section I.C.21. Factors influencing health status and contact with health services, Aftercare

p. Follow-up care for completed treatment of a malignancy

See Section I.C.21. Factors influencing health status and contact with health services, Follow-up

q. Prophylactic organ removal for prevention of malignancy

See Section I.C. 21, Factors influencing health status and contact with health services, Prophylactic organ removal

r. Malignant neoplasm associated with transplanted organ

A malignant neoplasm of a transplanted organ should be coded as a transplant complication. Assign first the appropriate code from category T86.-, Complications of transplanted organs and tissue, followed by code C8Ø.2, Malignant neoplasm associated with transplanted organ. Use an additional code for the specific malignancy.

3. Chapter 3: Disease of the blood and blood-forming organs and certain disorders involving the immune mechanism (D5Ø-D89)

Reserved for future guideline expansion

4. Chapter 4: Endocrine, Nutritional, and Metabolic Diseases (EØØ-E89)

a. Diabetes mellitus

The diabetes mellitus codes are combination codes that include the type of diabetes mellitus, the body system affected, and the complications affecting that body system. As many codes within a particular category as are necessary to describe all of the complications of the disease may be used. They should be sequenced based on the reason for a particular encounter. Assign as many codes from categories EØ8 – E13 as needed to identify all of the associated conditions that the patient has.

1) Type of diabetes

The age of a patient is not the sole determining factor, though most type 1 diabetics develop the condition before reaching puberty. For this reason type 1 diabetes mellitus is also referred to as juvenile diabetes.

2) Type of diabetes mellitus not documented

If the type of diabetes mellitus is not documented in the medical record the default is E11.-, Type 2 diabetes mellitus.

3) Diabetes mellitus and the use of insulin oral hypoglycemics

If the documentation in a medical record does not indicate the type of diabetes but does indicate that the patient uses insulin, code E11, Type 2 diabetes mellitus, should be assigned. Code Z79.4, Long-term (current) use of insulin, **or Z79.84, Long term (current) use of oral hypoglycemic drugs,** should also be assigned to indicate that the patient uses insulin **or hypoglycemic drugs**. Code Z79.4 should not be assigned if insulin is given temporarily to bring a type 2 patient's blood sugar under control during an encounter.

4) Diabetes mellitus in pregnancy and gestational diabetes

See Section I.C.15. Diabetes mellitus in pregnancy.

See Section I.C.15. Gestational (pregnancy induced) diabetes

5) Complications due to insulin pump malfunction

(a) Underdose of insulin due to insulin pump failure

An underdose of insulin due to an insulin pump failure should be assigned to a code from subcategory T85.6, Mechanical complication of other specified internal and external prosthetic devices, implants and grafts, that specifies the type of pump malfunction, as the principal or first-listed code, followed by code T38.3X6-, Underdosing of insulin and oral hypoglycemic [antidiabetic] drugs. Additional codes for the type of diabetes mellitus and any associated complications due to the underdosing should also be assigned.

(b) Overdose of insulin due to insulin pump failure

The principal or first-listed code for an encounter due to an insulin pump malfunction resulting in an overdose of insulin, should also be T85.6-, Mechanical complication of other specified internal and external prosthetic devices, implants and grafts, followed by code T38.3X1-, Poisoning by insulin and oral hypoglycemic [antidiabetic] drugs, accidental (unintentional).

6) Secondary diabetes mellitus

Codes under categories EØ8, Diabetes mellitus due to underlying condition, EØ9, Drug or chemical induced diabetes mellitus and E13, Other specified diabetes mellitus, identify complications/manifestations associated with secondary diabetes mellitus. Secondary diabetes is always caused by another condition or event (e.g., cystic fibrosis, malignant neoplasm of pancreas, pancreatectomy, adverse effect of drug, or poisoning).

(a) Secondary diabetes mellitus and the use of insulin or hypoglycemic drugs

For patients who routinely use insulin **or hypoglycemic drugs,** code Z79.4, Long-term (current) use of insulin, **or Z79.84, Long term (current) use of oral hypoglycemic drugs** should also be assigned. Code Z79.4 should not be assigned if insulin is given temporarily to bring a patient's blood sugar under control during an encounter.

(b) Assigning and sequencing secondary diabetes codes and its causes

The sequencing of the secondary diabetes codes in relationship to codes for the cause of the diabetes is based on the Tabular List instructions for categories EØ8, EØ9 and E13.

(i) **Secondary diabetes mellitus due to pancreatectomy** For postpancreatectomy diabetes mellitus (lack of insulin due to the surgical removal of all or part of the pancreas), assign code E89.1, Postprocedural hypoinsulinemia. Assign a code from category E13 and a code from subcategory Z90.41-, Acquired absence of pancreas, as additional codes.

(ii) **Secondary diabetes due to drugs** Secondary diabetes may be caused by an adverse effect of correctly administered medications, poisoning or sequela of poisoning.

See section I.C.19.e for coding of adverse effects and poisoning, and section I.C.20 for external cause code reporting.

5. **Chapter 5: Mental, Behavioral and Neurodevelopmental disorders (F01 – F99)**

a. **Pain disorders related to psychological factors**

Assign code F45.41, for pain that is exclusively related to psychological disorders. As indicated by the Excludes 1 note under category G89, a code from category G89 should not be assigned with code F45.41

Code F45.42, Pain disorders with related psychological factors, should be used with a code from category G89, Pain, not elsewhere classified, if there is documentation of a psychological component for a patient with acute or chronic pain.

See Section I.C.6. Pain

c. **Mental and behavioral disorders due to psychoactive substance use**

1) **In Remission**

Selection of codes for "in remission" for categories F10-F19, Mental and behavioral disorders due to psychoactive substance use (categories F10-F19 with -.21) requires the provider's clinical judgment. The appropriate codes for "in remission" are assigned only on the basis of provider documentation (as defined in the Official Guidelines for Coding and Reporting).

2) **Psychoactive Substance Use, Abuse And Dependence**

When the provider documentation refers to use, abuse and dependence of the same substance (e.g. alcohol, opioid, cannabis, etc.), only one code should be assigned to identify the pattern of use based on the following hierarchy:

- If both use and abuse are documented, assign only the code for abuse
- If both abuse and dependence are documented, assign only the code for dependence
- If use, abuse and dependence are all documented, assign only the code for dependence
- If both use and dependence are documented, assign only the code for dependence.

3) **Psychoactive Substance Use**

As with all other diagnoses, the codes for psychoactive substance use (F10.9-, F11.9-, F12.9-, F13.9-, F14.9-, F15.9-, F16.9-) should only be assigned based on provider documentation and when they meet the definition of a reportable diagnosis (see Section III, Reporting Additional Diagnoses). The codes are to be used only when the psychoactive substance use is associated with a mental or behavioral disorder, and such a relationship is documented by the provider.

6. **Chapter 6: Diseases of the Nervous System (G00-G99)**

a. **Dominant/nondominant side**

Codes from category G81, Hemiplegia and hemiparesis, and subcategories, G83.1, Monoplegia of lower limb, G83.2, Monoplegia of upper limb, and G83.3, Monoplegia, unspecified, identify whether the dominant or nondominant side is affected. Should the affected side be documented, but not specified as dominant or nondominant, and the classification system does not indicate a default, code selection is as follows:

- For ambidextrous patients, the default should be dominant.
- If the left side is affected, the default is non-dominant.
- If the right side is affected, the default is dominant.

b. **Pain - Category G89**

1) **General coding information**

Codes in category G89, Pain, not elsewhere classified, may be used in conjunction with codes from other categories and chapters to provide more detail about acute or chronic pain and neoplasm-related pain, unless otherwise indicated below.

If the pain is not specified as acute or chronic, post-thoracotomy, postprocedural, or neoplasm-related, do not assign codes from category G89.

A code from category G89 should not be assigned if the underlying (definitive) diagnosis is known, unless the reason for the encounter is pain control/management and not management of the underlying condition.

When an admission or encounter is for a procedure aimed at treating the underlying condition (e.g., spinal fusion, kyphoplasty), a code for the underlying condition (e.g., vertebral fracture, spinal stenosis) should be assigned as the principal diagnosis. No code from category G89 should be assigned.

(a) **Category G89 Codes as Principal or First-Listed Diagnosis**

Category G89 codes are acceptable as principal diagnosis or the first-listed code:

- When pain control or pain management is the reason for the admission/encounter (e.g., a patient with displaced intervertebral disc, nerve impingement and severe back pain presents for injection of steroid into the spinal canal). The underlying cause of the pain

GUIDELINES (ICD-10-CM)

should be reported as an additional diagnosis, if known.

- When a patient is admitted for the insertion of a neurostimulator for pain control, assign the appropriate pain code as the principal or first-listed diagnosis. When an admission or encounter is for a procedure aimed at treating the underlying condition and a neurostimulator is inserted for pain control during the same admission/encounter, a code for the underlying condition should be assigned as the principal diagnosis and the appropriate pain code should be assigned as a secondary diagnosis.

(b) Use of Category G89 Codes in Conjunction with Site Specific Pain Codes

(i) Assigning Category G89 and Site-Specific Pain Codes

Codes from category G89 may be used in conjunction with codes that identify the site of pain (including codes from chapter 18) if the category G89 code provides additional information. For example, if the code describes the site of the pain, but does not fully describe whether the pain is acute or chronic, then both codes should be assigned.

(ii) Sequencing of Category G89 Codes with Site-Specific Pain Codes

The sequencing of category G89 codes with site-specific pain codes (including chapter 18 codes), is dependent on the circumstances of the encounter/admission as follows:

- If the encounter is for pain control or pain management, assign the code from category G89 followed by the code identifying the specific site of pain (e.g., encounter for pain management for acute neck pain from trauma is assigned code G89.11, Acute pain due to trauma, followed by code M54.2, Cervicalgia, to identify the site of pain).
- If the encounter is for any other reason except pain control or pain management, and a related definitive diagnosis has not been established (confirmed) by the provider, assign the code for the specific site of pain first, followed by the appropriate code from category G89.

2) Pain due to devices, implants and grafts

See Section I.C.19. Pain due to medical devices

3) Postoperative Pain

The provider's documentation should be used to guide the coding of postoperative pain, as well as *Section III. Reporting Additional Diagnoses* and *Section IV. Diagnostic Coding and Reporting in the Outpatient Setting.*

The default for post-thoracotomy and other postoperative pain not specified as acute or chronic is the code for the acute form.

Routine or expected postoperative pain immediately after surgery should not be coded.

(a) Postoperative pain not associated with specific postoperative complication

Postoperative pain not associated with a specific postoperative complication is assigned to the appropriate postoperative pain code in category G89.

(b) Postoperative pain associated with specific postoperative complication

Postoperative pain associated with a specific postoperative complication (such as painful wire sutures) is assigned to the appropriate code(s) found in Chapter 19, Injury, poisoning, and certain other consequences of external causes. If appropriate, use additional code(s) from category G89 to identify acute or chronic pain (G89.18 or G89.28).

4) Chronic pain

Chronic pain is classified to subcategory G89.2. There is no time frame defining when pain becomes chronic pain. The provider's documentation should be used to guide use of these codes.

5) Neoplasm Related Pain

Code G89.3 is assigned to pain documented as being related, associated or due to cancer, primary or secondary malignancy, or tumor. This code is assigned regardless of whether the pain is acute or chronic.

This code may be assigned as the principal or first-listed code when the stated reason for the admission/encounter is documented as pain control/pain management. The underlying neoplasm should be reported as an additional diagnosis.

When the reason for the admission/encounter is management of the neoplasm and the pain associated with the neoplasm is also documented, code G89.3 may be assigned as an additional diagnosis. It is not necessary to assign an additional code for the site of the pain.

See Section I.C.2 for instructions on the sequencing of neoplasms for all other stated reasons for the admission/encounter (except for pain control/pain management).

6) Chronic pain syndrome

Central pain syndrome (G89.Ø) and chronic pain syndrome (G89.4) are different than the term "chronic pain," and therefore codes should only be used when the provider has specifically documented this condition.

See Section I.C.5. Pain disorders related to psychological factors

7. Chapter 7: Diseases of the Eye and Adnexa (HØØ-H59)

a. Glaucoma

1) Assigning Glaucoma Codes

Assign as many codes from category H4Ø, Glaucoma, as needed to identify the type of glaucoma, the affected eye, and the glaucoma stage.

2) **Bilateral glaucoma with same type and stage**

When a patient has bilateral glaucoma and both eyes are documented as being the same type and stage, and there is a code for bilateral glaucoma, report only the code for the type of glaucoma, bilateral, with the seventh character for the stage.

When a patient has bilateral glaucoma and both eyes are documented as being the same type and stage, and the classification does not provide a code for bilateral glaucoma (i.e. subcategories H40.10, H40.11 and H40.20) report only one code for the type of glaucoma with the appropriate seventh character for the stage.

3) **Bilateral glaucoma stage with different types or stages**

When a patient has bilateral glaucoma and each eye is documented as having a different type or stage, and the classification distinguishes laterality, assign the appropriate code for each eye rather than the code for bilateral glaucoma.

When a patient has bilateral glaucoma and each eye is documented as having a different type, and the classification does not distinguish laterality (i.e. subcategories H40.10, H40.11 and H40.20), assign one code for each type of glaucoma with the appropriate seventh character for the stage.

When a patient has bilateral glaucoma and each eye is documented as having the same type, but different stage, and the classification does not distinguish laterality (i.e. subcategories H40.10, H40.11 and H40.20), assign a code for the type of glaucoma for each eye with the seventh character for the specific glaucoma stage documented for each eye.

4) **Patient admitted with glaucoma and stage evolves during the admission**

If a patient is admitted with glaucoma and the stage progresses during the admission, assign the code for highest stage documented.

5) **Indeterminate stage glaucoma**

Assignment of the seventh character "4" for "indeterminate stage" should be based on the clinical documentation. The seventh character "4" is used for glaucomas whose stage cannot be clinically determined. This seventh character should not be confused with the seventh character "0", unspecified, which should be assigned when there is no documentation regarding the stage of the glaucoma.

8. **Chapter 8: Diseases of the Ear and Mastoid Process (H60-H95)**

Reserved for future guideline expansion

9. **Chapter 9: Diseases of the Circulatory System (I00-I99)**

a. Hypertension

The classification presumes a causal relationship between hypertension and heart involvement and between hypertension and kidney involvement, as the two conditions are linked by the term "with" in the Alphabetic Index. These conditions should be coded as related even in the absence of provider documentation explicitly linking them, unless the documentation clearly states the conditions are unrelated.

For hypertension and conditions not specifically linked by relational terms such as "with," "associated with" or "due to" in the classification, provider documentation must link the conditions in order to code them as related.

1) **Hypertension with Heart Disease**

Hypertension with heart conditions classified to I50.- or I51.4-I51.9, are assigned to, a code from category I11, Hypertensive heart disease. Use an additional code from category I50, Heart failure, to identify the type of heart failure in those patients with heart failure.

The same heart conditions (I50.-, I51.4-I51.9) with hypertension are coded separately **if the provider has specifically documented a different cause**. Sequence according to the circumstances of the admission/encounter.

2) **Hypertensive Chronic Kidney Disease**

Assign codes from category I12, Hypertensive chronic kidney disease, when both hypertension and a condition classifiable to category N18, Chronic kidney disease (CKD), are present. **CKD should not be coded as hypertensive if the physician has specifically documented a different cause.**

The appropriate code from category N18 should be used as a secondary code with a code from category I12 to identify the stage of chronic kidney disease.

See Section I.C.14. Chronic kidney disease.

If a patient has hypertensive chronic kidney disease and acute renal failure, an additional code for the acute renal failure is required.

3) **Hypertensive Heart and Chronic Kidney Disease**

Assign codes from combination category I13, Hypertensive heart and chronic kidney disease, when **there is hypertension with both heart and kidney involvement.** If heart failure is present, assign an additional code from category I50 to identify the type of heart failure.

The appropriate code from category N18, Chronic kidney disease, should be used as a secondary code with a code from category I13 to identify the stage of chronic kidney disease.

See Section I.C.14. Chronic kidney disease.

The codes in category I13, Hypertensive heart and chronic kidney disease, are combination codes that include hypertension, heart disease and chronic kidney disease. The Includes note at I13 specifies that the conditions included at I11 and I12 are included together in I13. If a patient has hypertension, heart disease and chronic kidney disease then a code from I13 should be used, not individual codes for hypertension, heart disease and chronic kidney disease, or codes from I11 or I12.

For patients with both acute renal failure and chronic kidney disease an additional code for acute renal failure is required.

4) Hypertensive Cerebrovascular Disease

For hypertensive cerebrovascular disease, first assign the appropriate code from categories I6Ø-I69, followed by the appropriate hypertension code.

5) Hypertensive Retinopathy

Subcategory H35.Ø, Background retinopathy and retinal vascular changes, should be used with a code from category I1Ø – I15, Hypertensive disease to include the systemic hypertension. The sequencing is based on the reason for the encounter.

6) Hypertension, Secondary

Secondary hypertension is due to an underlying condition. Two codes are required: one to identify the underlying etiology and one from category I15 to identify the hypertension. Sequencing of codes is determined by the reason for admission/encounter.

7) Hypertension, Transient

Assign code RØ3.Ø, Elevated blood pressure reading without diagnosis of hypertension, unless patient has an established diagnosis of hypertension. Assign code O13.-, Gestational [pregnancy-induced] hypertension without significant proteinuria, or O14.-, Pre-eclampsia, for transient hypertension of pregnancy.

8) Hypertension, Controlled

This diagnostic statement usually refers to an existing state of hypertension under control by therapy. Assign the appropriate code from categories I1Ø-I15, Hypertensive diseases.

9) Hypertension, Uncontrolled

Uncontrolled hypertension may refer to untreated hypertension or hypertension not responding to current therapeutic regimen. In either case, assign the appropriate code from categories I1Ø-I15, Hypertensive diseases.

10) Hypertensive Crisis

Assign a code from category I16, Hypertensive crisis, for documented hypertensive urgency, hypertensive emergency or unspecified hypertensive crisis. Code also any identified hypertensive disease (I1Ø-I15). The sequencing is based on the reason for the encounter.

b. Atherosclerotic Coronary Artery Disease and Angina

ICD-10-CM has combination codes for atherosclerotic heart disease with angina pectoris. The subcategories for these codes are I25.11, Atherosclerotic heart disease of native coronary artery with angina pectoris and I25.7, Atherosclerosis of coronary artery bypass graft(s) and coronary artery of transplanted heart with angina pectoris.

When using one of these combination codes it is not necessary to use an additional code for angina pectoris. A causal relationship can be assumed in a patient with both atherosclerosis and angina pectoris, unless the documentation indicates the angina is due to something other than the atherosclerosis.

If a patient with coronary artery disease is admitted due to an acute myocardial infarction (AMI), the AMI should be sequenced before the coronary artery disease.

See Section I.C.9. Acute myocardial infarction (AMI)

c. Intraoperative and Postprocedural Cerebrovascular Accident

Medical record documentation should clearly specify the cause-and-effect relationship between the medical intervention and the cerebrovascular accident in order to assign a code for intraoperative or postprocedural cerebrovascular accident.

Proper code assignment depends on whether it was an infarction or hemorrhage and whether it occurred intraoperatively or postoperatively. If it was a cerebral hemorrhage, code assignment depends on the type of procedure performed.

d. Sequelae of Cerebrovascular Disease

1) Category I69, Sequelae of Cerebrovascular disease

Category I69 is used to indicate conditions classifiable to categories I6Ø-I67 as the causes of sequela (neurologic deficits), themselves classified elsewhere. These "late effects" include neurologic deficits that persist after initial onset of conditions classifiable to categories I6Ø-I67. The neurologic deficits caused by cerebrovascular disease may be present from the onset or may arise at any time after the onset of the condition classifiable to categories I6Ø-I67.

Codes from category I69, Sequelae of cerebrovascular disease, that specify hemiplegia, hemiparesis and monoplegia identify whether the dominant or nondominant side is affected. Should the affected side be documented, but not specified as dominant or nondominant, and the classification system does not indicate a default, code selection is as follows:

- For ambidextrous patients, the default should be dominant.
- If the left side is affected, the default is non-dominant.
- If the right side is affected, the default is dominant.

2) Codes from category I69 with codes from I6Ø-I67

Codes from category I69 may be assigned on a health care record with codes from I6Ø-I67, if the patient has a current cerebrovascular disease and deficits from an old cerebrovascular disease.

3) Codes from category I69 and Personal history of transient ischemic attack (TIA) and cerebral infarction (Z86.73)

Codes from category I69 should not be assigned if the patient does not have neurologic deficits.

See Section I.C.21. 4. History (of) for use of personal history codes

GUIDELINES (ICD-10-CM)

e. **Acute myocardial infarction (AMI)**

1) **ST elevation myocardial infarction (STEMI) and non ST elevation myocardial infarction (NSTEMI)**

The ICD-10-CM codes for acute myocardial infarction (AMI) identify the site, such as anterolateral wall or true posterior wall. Subcategories I21.Ø-I21.2 and code I21.3 are used for ST elevation myocardial infarction (STEMI). Code I21.4, Non-ST elevation (NSTEMI) myocardial infarction, is used for non ST elevation myocardial infarction (NSTEMI) and nontransmural MIs.

If NSTEMI evolves to STEMI, assign the STEMI code. If STEMI converts to NSTEMI due to thrombolytic therapy, it is still coded as STEMI.

For encounters occurring while the myocardial infarction is equal to, or less than, four weeks old, including transfers to another acute setting or a postacute setting, and the myocardial infarction **meets the definition for "other diagnoses" (see Section III, Reporting Additional Diagnoses),** codes from category I21 may continue to be reported. For encounters after the 4 week time frame and the patient is still receiving care related to the myocardial infarction, the appropriate aftercare code should be assigned, rather than a code from category I21. For old or healed myocardial infarctions not requiring further care, code I25.2, Old myocardial infarction, may be assigned.

2) **Acute myocardial infarction, unspecified**

Code I21.3, ST elevation (STEMI) myocardial infarction of unspecified site, is the default for unspecified acute myocardial infarction. If only STEMI or transmural MI without the site is documented, assign code I21.3.

3) **AMI documented as nontransmural or subendocardial but site provided**

If an AMI is documented as nontransmural or subendocardial, but the site is provided, it is still coded as a subendocardial AMI.

See Section I.C.21.3 for information on coding status post administration of tPA in a different facility within the last 24 hours.

4) **Subsequent acute myocardial infarction**

A code from category I22, Subsequent ST elevation (STEMI) and non ST elevation (NSTEMI) myocardial infarction, is to be used when a patient who has suffered an AMI has a new AMI within the 4 week time frame of the initial AMI. A code from category I22 must be used in conjunction with a code from category I21. The sequencing of the I22 and I21 codes depends on the circumstances of the encounter.

1Ø. **Chapter 1Ø: Diseases of the Respiratory System (JØØ-J99)**

a. **Chronic Obstructive Pulmonary Disease [COPD] and Asthma**

1) **Acute exacerbation of chronic obstructive bronchitis and asthma**

The codes in categories J44 and J45 distinguish between uncomplicated cases and those in acute exacerbation. An acute exacerbation is a worsening or a decompensation of a chronic condition. An acute exacerbation is not equivalent to an infection superimposed on a chronic condition, though an exacerbation may be triggered by an infection.

b. **Acute Respiratory Failure**

1) **Acute respiratory failure as principal diagnosis**

A code from subcategory J96.Ø, Acute respiratory failure, or subcategory J96.2, Acute and chronic respiratory failure, may be assigned as a principal diagnosis when it is the condition established after study to be chiefly responsible for occasioning the admission to the hospital, and the selection is supported by the Alphabetic Index and Tabular List. However, chapter-specific coding guidelines (such as obstetrics, poisoning, HIV, newborn) that provide sequencing direction take precedence.

2) **Acute respiratory failure as secondary diagnosis**

Respiratory failure may be listed as a secondary diagnosis if it occurs after admission, or if it is present on admission, but does not meet the definition of principal diagnosis.

3) **Sequencing of acute respiratory failure and another acute condition**

When a patient is admitted with respiratory failure and another acute condition, (e.g., myocardial infarction, cerebrovascular accident, aspiration pneumonia), the principal diagnosis will not be the same in every situation. This applies whether the other acute condition is a respiratory or nonrespiratory condition. Selection of the principal diagnosis will be dependent on the circumstances of admission. If both the respiratory failure and the other acute condition are equally responsible for occasioning the admission to the hospital, and there are no chapter-specific sequencing rules, the guideline regarding two or more diagnoses that equally meet the definition for principal diagnosis *(Section II, C.)* may be applied in these situations.

If the documentation is not clear as to whether acute respiratory failure and another condition are equally responsible for occasioning the admission, query the provider for clarification.

c. **Influenza due to certain identified influenza viruses**

Code only confirmed cases of influenza due to certain identified influenza viruses (category JØ9), and due to other identified influenza virus (category J1Ø). This is an exception to the hospital inpatient guideline Section II, H. (Uncertain Diagnosis).

In this context, "confirmation" does not require documentation of positive laboratory testing specific for avian or other novel influenza A or other identified influenza virus. However, coding should be based on the provider's diagnostic statement that the patient has avian influenza, or other novel influenza A, for category JØ9, or has another particular identified strain of influenza, such as H1N1 or H3N2, but not identified as novel or variant, for category J1Ø.

If the provider records "suspected" or "possible" or "probable" avian influenza, or novel influenza, or other identified influenza, then the appropriate influenza code from category J11, Influenza due to unidentified influenza virus, should be assigned. A code from category JØ9, Influenza due to certain identified influenza viruses, should not be assigned nor should a code from category J1Ø, Influenza due to other identified influenza virus.

d. Ventilator associated Pneumonia

1) Documentation of Ventilator associated Pneumonia

As with all procedural or postprocedural complications, code assignment is based on the provider's documentation of the relationship between the condition and the procedure.

Code J95.851, Ventilator associated pneumonia, should be assigned only when the provider has documented ventilator associated pneumonia (VAP). An additional code to identify the organism (e.g., Pseudomonas aeruginosa, code B96.5) should also be assigned. Do not assign an additional code from categories J12-J18 to identify the type of pneumonia.

Code J95.851 should not be assigned for cases where the patient has pneumonia and is on a mechanical ventilator and the provider has not specifically stated that the pneumonia is ventilator-associated pneumonia. If the documentation is unclear as to whether the patient has a pneumonia that is a complication attributable to the mechanical ventilator, query the provider.

2) Ventilator associated Pneumonia Develops after Admission

A patient may be admitted with one type of pneumonia (e.g., code J13, Pneumonia due to Streptococcus pneumonia) and subsequently develop VAP. In this instance, the principal diagnosis would be the appropriate code from categories J12-J18 for the pneumonia diagnosed at the time of admission. Code J95.851, Ventilator associated pneumonia, would be assigned as an additional diagnosis when the provider has also documented the presence of ventilator associated pneumonia.

11. Chapter 11: Diseases of the Digestive System (KØØ-K95)

Reserved for future guideline expansion

12. Chapter 12: Diseases of the Skin and Subcutaneous Tissue (LØØ-L99)

a. Pressure ulcer stage codes

1) Pressure ulcer stages

Codes from category L89, Pressure ulcer, identify the site of the pressure ulcer as well as the stage of the ulcer.

The ICD-10-CM classifies pressure ulcer stages based on severity, which is designated by stages 1-4, unspecified stage and unstageable.

Assign as many codes from category L89 as needed to identify all the pressure ulcers the patient has, if applicable.

2) Unstageable pressure ulcers

Assignment of the code for unstageable pressure ulcer (L89.--Ø) should be based on the clinical documentation. These codes are used for pressure ulcers whose stage cannot be clinically determined (e.g., the ulcer is covered by eschar or has been treated with a skin or muscle graft) and pressure ulcers that are documented as deep tissue injury but not documented as due to trauma. This code should not be confused with the codes for unspecified stage (L89.--9). When there is no documentation regarding the stage of the pressure ulcer, assign the appropriate code for unspecified stage (L89.--9).

3) Documented pressure ulcer stage

Assignment of the pressure ulcer stage code should be guided by clinical documentation of the stage or documentation of the terms found in the Alphabetic Index. For clinical terms describing the stage that are not found in the Alphabetic Index, and there is no documentation of the stage, the provider should be queried.

4) Patients admitted with pressure ulcers documented as healed

No code is assigned if the documentation states that the pressure ulcer is completely healed.

5) Patients admitted with pressure ulcers documented as healing

Pressure ulcers described as healing should be assigned the appropriate pressure ulcer stage code based on the documentation in the medical record. If the documentation does not provide information about the stage of the healing pressure ulcer, assign the appropriate code for unspecified stage.

If the documentation is unclear as to whether the patient has a current (new) pressure ulcer or if the patient is being treated for a healing pressure ulcer, query the provider.

For ulcers that were present on admission but healed at the time of discharge, assign the code for the site and stage of the pressure ulcer at the time of admission.

6) Patient admitted with pressure ulcer evolving into another stage during the admission

If a patient is admitted with a pressure ulcer at one stage and it progresses to a higher stage, **two separate codes should be assigned: one code for the site and stage of the ulcer on admission and a second code for the same ulcer site and the highest stage reported during the stay.**

13. Chapter 13: Diseases of the Musculoskeletal System and Connective Tissue (MØØ-M99)

a. Site and laterality

Most of the codes within Chapter 13 have site and laterality designations. The site represents the bone, joint or the muscle involved. For some conditions where more than one bone, joint or

GUIDELINES (ICD-10-CM)

muscle is usually involved, such as osteoarthritis, there is a "multiple sites" code available. For categories where no multiple site code is provided and more than one bone, joint or muscle is involved, multiple codes should be used to indicate the different sites involved.

1) Bone versus joint

For certain conditions, the bone may be affected at the upper or lower end, (e.g., avascular necrosis of bone, M87, Osteoporosis, M8Ø, M81). Though the portion of the bone affected may be at the joint, the site designation will be the bone, not the joint.

b. Acute traumatic versus chronic or recurrent musculoskeletal conditions

Many musculoskeletal conditions are a result of previous injury or trauma to a site, or are recurrent conditions. Bone, joint or muscle conditions that are the result of a healed injury are usually found in chapter 13. Recurrent bone, joint or muscle conditions are also usually found in chapter 13. Any current, acute injury should be coded to the appropriate injury code from chapter 19. Chronic or recurrent conditions should generally be coded with a code from chapter 13. If it is difficult to determine from the documentation in the record which code is best to describe a condition, query the provider.

c. Coding of Pathologic Fractures

7th character A is for use as long as the patient is receiving active treatment for the fracture. While the patient may be seen by a new or different provider over the course of treatment for a pathological fracture, assignment of the 7th character is based on whether the patient is undergoing active treatment and not whether the provider is seeing the patient for the first time.

7th character, D is to be used for encounters after the patient has completed active treatment. The other 7th characters, listed under each subcategory in the Tabular List, are to be used for subsequent encounters for **routine care of fractures during the healing and recovery phase as well as** treatment of problems associated with the healing, such as malunions, nonunions, and sequelae.

Care for complications of surgical treatment for fracture repairs during the healing or recovery phase should be coded with the appropriate complication codes.

See Section I.C.19. Coding of traumatic fractures.

d. Osteoporosis

Osteoporosis is a systemic condition, meaning that all bones of the musculoskeletal system are affected. Therefore, site is not a component of the codes under category M81, Osteoporosis without current pathological fracture. The site codes under category M8Ø, Osteoporosis with current pathological fracture, identify the site of the fracture, not the osteoporosis.

1) Osteoporosis without pathological fracture

Category M81, Osteoporosis without current pathological fracture, is for use for patients with osteoporosis who do not currently have a pathologic fracture due to the osteoporosis, even if they have had a fracture in the past. For patients with a history of osteoporosis fractures, status code Z87.31Ø, Personal history of (healed) osteoporosis fracture, should follow the code from M81.

2) Osteoporosis with current pathological fracture

Category M8Ø, Osteoporosis with current pathological fracture, is for patients who have a current pathologic fracture at the time of an encounter. The codes under M8Ø identify the site of the fracture. A code from category M8Ø, not a traumatic fracture code, should be used for any patient with known osteoporosis who suffers a fracture, even if the patient had a minor fall or trauma, if that fall or trauma would not usually break a normal, healthy bone.

14. Chapter 14: Diseases of Genitourinary System (NØØ-N99)

a. Chronic kidney disease

1) Stages of chronic kidney disease (CKD)

The ICD-10-CM classifies CKD based on severity. The severity of CKD is designated by stages 1-5. Stage 2, code N18.2, equates to mild CKD; stage 3, code N18.3, equates to moderate CKD; and stage 4, code N18.4, equates to severe CKD. Code N18.6, End stage renal disease (ESRD), is assigned when the provider has documented end-stage-renal disease (ESRD).

If both a stage of CKD and ESRD are documented, assign code N18.6 only.

2) Chronic kidney disease and kidney transplant status

Patients who have undergone kidney transplant may still have some form of chronic kidney disease CKD because the kidney transplant may not fully restore kidney function. Therefore, the presence of CKD alone does not constitute a transplant complication. Assign the appropriate N18 code for the patient's stage of CKD and code Z94.Ø, Kidney transplant status. If a transplant complication such as failure or rejection or other transplant complication is documented, see section I.C.19.g for information on coding complications of a kidney transplant. If the documentation is unclear as to whether the patient has a complication of the transplant, query the provider.

3) Chronic kidney disease with other conditions

Patients with CKD may also suffer from other serious conditions, most commonly diabetes mellitus and hypertension. The sequencing of the CKD code in relationship to codes for other contributing conditions is based on the conventions in the Tabular List.

See I.C.9. Hypertensive chronic kidney disease.

See I.C.19. Chronic kidney disease and kidney transplant complications.

15. Chapter 15: Pregnancy, Childbirth, and the Puerperium (O00-O9A)

a. General Rules for Obstetric Cases

1) Codes from chapter 15 and sequencing priority

Obstetric cases require codes from chapter 15, codes in the range O00-O9A, Pregnancy, Childbirth, and the Puerperium. Chapter 15 codes have sequencing priority over codes from other chapters. Additional codes from other chapters may be used in conjunction with chapter 15 codes to further specify conditions. Should the provider document that the pregnancy is incidental to the encounter, then code Z33.1, Pregnant state, incidental, should be used in place of any chapter 15 codes. It is the provider's responsibility to state that the condition being treated is not affecting the pregnancy.

2) Chapter 15 codes used only on the maternal record

Chapter 15 codes are to be used only on the maternal record, never on the record of the newborn.

3) Final character for trimester

The majority of codes in Chapter 15 have a final character indicating the trimester of pregnancy. The timeframes for the trimesters are indicated at the beginning of the chapter. If trimester is not a component of a code it is because the condition always occurs in a specific trimester, or the concept of trimester of pregnancy is not applicable. Certain codes have characters for only certain trimesters because the condition does not occur in all trimesters, but it may occur in more than just one.

Assignment of the final character for trimester should be based on the provider's documentation of the trimester (or number of weeks) for the current admission/encounter. This applies to the assignment of trimester for pre-existing conditions as well as those that develop during or are due to the pregnancy. The provider's documentation of the number of weeks may be used to assign the appropriate code identifying the trimester.

Whenever delivery occurs during the current admission, and there is an "in childbirth" option for the obstetric complication being coded, the "in childbirth" code should be assigned.

4) Selection of trimester for inpatient admissions that encompass more than one trimester

In instances when a patient is admitted to a hospital for complications of pregnancy during one trimester and remains in the hospital into a subsequent trimester, the trimester character for the antepartum complication code should be assigned on the basis of the trimester when the complication developed, not the trimester of the discharge. If the condition developed prior to the current admission/encounter or represents a pre-existing condition, the trimester character for the trimester at the time of the admission/encounter should be assigned.

5) Unspecified trimester

Each category that includes codes for trimester has a code for "unspecified trimester." The "unspecified trimester" code should rarely be used, such as when the documentation in the record is insufficient to determine the trimester and it is not possible to obtain clarification.

6) 7th character for Fetus Identification

Where applicable, a 7th character is to be assigned for certain categories (O31, O32, O33.3 - O33.6, O35, O36, O40, O41, O60.1, O60.2, O64, and O69) to identify the fetus for which the complication code applies.

Assign 7th character "0":

- For single gestations
- When the documentation in the record is insufficient to determine the fetus affected and it is not possible to obtain clarification.
- When it is not possible to clinically determine which fetus is affected.

b. Selection of OB Principal or First-listed Diagnosis

1) Routine outpatient prenatal visits

For routine outpatient prenatal visits when no complications are present, a code from category Z34, Encounter for supervision of normal pregnancy, should be used as the first-listed diagnosis. These codes should not be used in conjunction with chapter 15 codes.

2) *Supervision of High-Risk Pregnancy*

Codes from category O09, Supervision of high-risk pregnancy, are intended for use only during the prenatal period. For complications during the labor or delivery episode as a result of a high-risk pregnancy, assign the applicable complication codes from Chapter 15. If there are no complications during the labor or delivery episode, assign code O80, Encounter for full-term uncomplicated delivery.

For routine prenatal outpatient visits for patients with high-risk pregnancies, a code from category O09, Supervision of high-risk pregnancy, should be used as the first-listed diagnosis. Secondary chapter 15 codes may be used in conjunction with these codes if appropriate.

3) Episodes when no delivery occurs

In episodes when no delivery occurs, the principal diagnosis should correspond to the principal complication of the pregnancy which necessitated the encounter. Should more than one complication exist, all of which are treated or monitored, any of the complications codes may be sequenced first.

4) When a delivery occurs

When an obstetric patient is admitted and delivers during that admission, the condition that prompted the admission should be sequenced as the principal diagnosis. If multiple conditions prompted the admission, sequence the one most related to the delivery as the principal

GUIDELINES (ICD-10-CM)

diagnosis. A code for any complication of the delivery should be assigned as an additional diagnosis. In cases of cesarean delivery, if the patient was admitted with a condition that resulted in the performance of a cesarean procedure, that condition should be selected as the principal diagnosis. If the reason for the admission was unrelated to the condition resulting in the cesarean delivery, the condition related to the reason for the admission should be selected as the principal diagnosis.

5) Outcome of delivery

A code from category Z37, Outcome of delivery, should be included on every maternal record when a delivery has occurred. These codes are not to be used on subsequent records or on the newborn record.

c. Pre-existing conditions versus conditions due to the pregnancy

Certain categories in Chapter 15 distinguish between conditions of the mother that existed prior to pregnancy (pre-existing) and those that are a direct result of pregnancy. When assigning codes from Chapter 15, it is important to assess if a condition was pre-existing prior to pregnancy or developed during or due to the pregnancy in order to assign the correct code.

Categories that do not distinguish between pre-existing and pregnancy-related conditions may be used for either. It is acceptable to use codes specifically for the puerperium with codes complicating pregnancy and childbirth if a condition arises postpartum during the delivery encounter.

d. Pre-existing hypertension in pregnancy

Category O1Ø, Pre-existing hypertension complicating pregnancy, childbirth and the puerperium, includes codes for hypertensive heart and hypertensive chronic kidney disease. When assigning one of the O1Ø codes that includes hypertensive heart disease or hypertensive chronic kidney disease, it is necessary to add a secondary code from the appropriate hypertension category to specify the type of heart failure or chronic kidney disease.

See Section I.C.9. Hypertension.

e. Fetal Conditions Affecting the Management of the Mother

1) Codes from categories O35 and O36

Codes from categories O35, Maternal care for known or suspected fetal abnormality and damage, and O36, Maternal care for other fetal problems, are assigned only when the fetal condition is actually responsible for modifying the management of the mother, i.e., by requiring diagnostic studies, additional observation, special care, or termination of pregnancy. The fact that the fetal condition exists does not justify assigning a code from this series to the mother's record.

2) In utero surgery

In cases when surgery is performed on the fetus, a diagnosis code from category O35, Maternal care for known or suspected fetal abnormality and damage, should be assigned identifying the fetal condition. Assign the appropriate procedure code for the procedure performed.

No code from Chapter 16, the perinatal codes, should be used on the mother's record to identify fetal conditions. Surgery performed in utero on a fetus is still to be coded as an obstetric encounter.

f. HIV Infection in Pregnancy, Childbirth and the Puerperium

During pregnancy, childbirth or the puerperium, a patient admitted because of an HIV-related illness should receive a principal diagnosis from subcategory O98.7-, Human immunodeficiency [HIV] disease complicating pregnancy, childbirth and the puerperium, followed by the code(s) for the HIV-related illness(es).

Patients with asymptomatic HIV infection status admitted during pregnancy, childbirth, or the puerperium should receive codes of O98.7- and Z21, Asymptomatic human immunodeficiency virus [HIV] infection status.

g. Diabetes mellitus in pregnancy

Diabetes mellitus is a significant complicating factor in pregnancy. Pregnant women who are diabetic should be assigned a code from category O24, Diabetes mellitus in pregnancy, childbirth, and the puerperium, first, followed by the appropriate diabetes code(s) (EØ8-E13) from Chapter 4.

h. Long term use of insulin and oral hypoglycemics

Code Z79.4, Long-term (current) use of insulin, or **code Z79.84, Long-term (current) use of oral hypoglycemic drugs,** should also be assigned if the diabetes mellitus is being treated with insulin **or oral medications. If the patient is treated with both oral medications and insulin, only the code for insulin-controlled should be assigned.**

i. Gestational (pregnancy induced) diabetes

Gestational (pregnancy induced) diabetes can occur during the second and third trimester of pregnancy in women who were not diabetic prior to pregnancy. Gestational diabetes can cause complications in the pregnancy similar to those of pre-existing diabetes mellitus. It also puts the woman at greater risk of developing diabetes after the pregnancy. Codes for gestational diabetes are in subcategory O24.4, Gestational diabetes mellitus. No other code from category O24, Diabetes mellitus in pregnancy, childbirth, and the puerperium, should be used with a code from O24.4.

The codes under subcategory O24.4 include diet controlled, insulin controlled, **and controlled by oral hypoglycemic drugs.** If a patient with gestational diabetes is treated with both diet and insulin, only the code for insulin-controlled is required. **If a patient with gestational diabetes is treated with both diet and oral hypoglycemic medications, only the code for "controlled by oral hypoglycemic drugs" is required.** Code Z79.4, Long-term (current) use of insulin **or code Z79.84, Long-term (current) use of oral hypoglycemic drugs,** should not be assigned with codes from subcategory O24.4.

An abnormal glucose tolerance in pregnancy is assigned a code from subcategory O99.81, Abnormal glucose complicating pregnancy, childbirth, and the puerperium.

j. Sepsis and septic shock complicating abortion, pregnancy, childbirth and the puerperium

When assigning a chapter 15 code for sepsis complicating abortion, pregnancy, childbirth, and the puerperium, a code for the specific type of infection should be assigned as an additional diagnosis. If severe sepsis is present, a code from subcategory R65.2, Severe sepsis, and code(s) for associated organ dysfunction(s) should also be assigned as additional diagnoses.

k. Puerperal sepsis

Code O85, Puerperal sepsis, should be assigned with a secondary code to identify the causal organism (e.g., for a bacterial infection, assign a code from category B95-B96, Bacterial infections in conditions classified elsewhere). A code from category A4Ø, Streptococcal sepsis, or A41, Other sepsis, should not be used for puerperal sepsis. If applicable, use additional codes to identify severe sepsis (R65.2-) and any associated acute organ dysfunction.

l. Alcohol and tobacco use during pregnancy, childbirth and the puerperium

1) Alcohol use during pregnancy, childbirth and the puerperium

Codes under subcategory O99.31, Alcohol use complicating pregnancy, childbirth, and the puerperium, should be assigned for any pregnancy case when a mother uses alcohol during the pregnancy or postpartum. A secondary code from category F1Ø, Alcohol related disorders, should also be assigned to identify manifestations of the alcohol use.

2) Tobacco use during pregnancy, childbirth and the puerperium

Codes under subcategory O99.33, Smoking (tobacco) complicating pregnancy, childbirth, and the puerperium, should be assigned for any pregnancy case when a mother uses any type of tobacco product during the pregnancy or postpartum. A secondary code from category F17, Nicotine dependence, should also be assigned to identify the type of nicotine dependence.

m. Poisoning, toxic effects, adverse effects and underdosing in a pregnant patient

A code from subcategory O9A.2, Injury, poisoning and certain other consequences of external causes complicating pregnancy, childbirth, and the puerperium, should be sequenced first, followed by the appropriate injury, poisoning, toxic effect, adverse effect or underdosing code, and then the additional code(s) that specifies the condition caused by the poisoning, toxic effect, adverse effect or underdosing.

See Section I.C.19. Adverse effects, poisoning, underdosing and toxic effects.

n. Normal Delivery, Code O8Ø

1) Encounter for full term uncomplicated delivery

Code O8Ø should be assigned when a woman is admitted for a full-term normal delivery and delivers a single, healthy infant without any complications antepartum, during the delivery, or postpartum during the delivery episode. Code O8Ø is always a principal diagnosis. It is not to be used if any other code from chapter 15 is needed to describe a current complication of the antenatal, delivery, or perinatal period. Additional codes from other chapters may be used with code O8Ø if they are not related to or are in any way complicating the pregnancy.

2) Uncomplicated delivery with resolved antepartum complication

Code O8Ø may be used if the patient had a complication at some point during the pregnancy, but the complication is not present at the time of the admission for delivery.

3) Outcome of delivery for O8Ø

Z37.Ø, Single live birth, is the only outcome of delivery code appropriate for use with O8Ø.

o. The Peripartum and Postpartum Periods

1) Peripartum and Postpartum periods

The postpartum period begins immediately after delivery and continues for six weeks following delivery. The peripartum period is defined as the last month of pregnancy to five months postpartum.

2) Peripartum and postpartum complication

A postpartum complication is any complication occurring within the six-week period.

3) Pregnancy-related complications after 6 week period

Chapter 15 codes may also be used to describe pregnancy-related complications after the peripartum or postpartum period if the provider documents that a condition is pregnancy related.

4) Admission for routine postpartum care following delivery outside hospital

When the mother delivers outside the hospital prior to admission and is admitted for routine postpartum care and no complications are noted, code Z39.Ø, Encounter for care and examination of mother immediately after delivery, should be assigned as the principal diagnosis.

5) Pregnancy associated cardiomyopathy

Pregnancy associated cardiomyopathy, code O90.3, is unique in that it may be diagnosed in the third trimester of pregnancy but may continue to progress months after delivery. For this reason, it is referred to as peripartum cardiomyopathy. Code O90.3 is only for use when the cardiomyopathy develops as a result of pregnancy in a woman who did not have pre-existing heart disease.

p. Code O94, Sequelae of complication of pregnancy, childbirth, and the puerperium

1) Code O94

Code O94, Sequelae of complication of pregnancy, childbirth, and the puerperium, is for use in those cases when an initial complication of a pregnancy develops a sequelae requiring care or treatment at a future date.

2) After the initial postpartum period

This code may be used at any time after the initial postpartum period.

3) Sequencing of Code O94

This code, like all sequela codes, is to be sequenced following the code describing the sequelae of the complication.

q. *Termination of Pregnancy and Spontaneous abortions*

1) Abortion with Liveborn Fetus

When an attempted termination of pregnancy results in a liveborn fetus assign code Z33.2, Encounter for elective termination of pregnancy and a code from category Z37, Outcome of Delivery.

2) Retained Products of Conception following an abortion

Subsequent encounters for retained products of conception following a spontaneous abortion or elective termination of pregnancy are assigned the appropriate code from category O03, Spontaneous abortion, or codes O07.4, Failed attempted termination of pregnancy without complication and Z33.2, Encounter for elective termination of pregnancy. This advice is appropriate even when the patient was discharged previously with a discharge diagnosis of complete abortion.

3) Complications leading to abortion

Codes from Chapter 15 may be used as additional codes to identify any documented complications of the pregnancy in conjunction with codes in categories in O07 and O08.

r. Abuse in a pregnant patient

For suspected or confirmed cases of abuse of a pregnant patient, a code(s) from subcategories O9A.3, Physical abuse complicating pregnancy, childbirth, and the puerperium, O9A.4, Sexual abuse complicating pregnancy, childbirth, and the puerperium, and O9A.5, Psychological abuse complicating pregnancy, childbirth, and the puerperium, should be sequenced first, followed by the appropriate codes (if applicable) to identify any associated current injury due to physical abuse, sexual abuse, and the perpetrator of abuse.

See Section I.C.19. Adult and child abuse, neglect and other maltreatment.

16. Chapter 16: Certain Conditions Originating in the Perinatal Period (P00-P96)

For coding and reporting purposes the perinatal period is defined as before birth through the 28th day following birth. The following guidelines are provided for reporting purposes

a. General Perinatal Rules

1) Use of Chapter 16 Codes

Codes in this chapter are <u>never</u> for use on the maternal record. Codes from Chapter 15, the obstetric chapter, are never permitted on the newborn record. Chapter 16 codes may be used throughout the life of the patient if the condition is still present.

2) Principal Diagnosis for Birth Record

When coding the birth episode in a newborn record, assign a code from category Z38, Liveborn infants according to place of birth and type of delivery, as the principal diagnosis. A code from category Z38 is assigned only once, to a newborn at the time of birth. If a newborn is transferred to another institution, a code from category Z38 should not be used at the receiving hospital.

A code from category Z38 is used only on the newborn record, not on the mother's record.

3) Use of Codes from other Chapters with Codes from Chapter 16

Codes from other chapters may be used with codes from chapter 16 if the codes from the other chapters provide more specific detail. Codes for signs and symptoms may be assigned when a definitive diagnosis has not been established. If the reason for the encounter is a perinatal condition, the code from chapter 16 should be sequenced first.

4) Use of Chapter 16 Codes after the Perinatal Period

Should a condition originate in the perinatal period, and continue throughout the life of the patient, the perinatal code should continue to be used regardless of the patient's age.

5) Birth process or community acquired conditions

If a newborn has a condition that may be either due to the birth process or community acquired and the documentation does not indicate which it is, the default is due to the birth process and the code from Chapter 16 should be used. If the condition is community-acquired, a code from Chapter 16 should not be assigned.

6) Code all clinically significant conditions

All clinically significant conditions noted on routine newborn examination should be coded. A condition is clinically significant if it requires:

- clinical evaluation; or
- therapeutic treatment; or
- diagnostic procedures; or

- extended length of hospital stay; or
- increased nursing care and/or monitoring; or
- has implications for future health care needs

Note: The perinatal guidelines listed above are the same as the general coding guidelines for "additional diagnoses", except for the final point regarding implications for future health care needs. Codes should be assigned for conditions that have been specified by the provider as having implications for future health care needs.

b. Observation and Evaluation of Newborns for Suspected Conditions not Found

1) Assign a code from category Z05, Observation and evaluation of newborns and infants for suspected conditions ruled out, to identify those instances when a healthy newborn is evaluated for a suspected condition that is determined after study not to be present. Do not use a code from category Z05 when the patient has identified signs or symptoms of a suspected problem; in such cases code the sign or symptom.

2) A code from category Z05 may also be assigned as a principal or first-listed code for readmissions or encounters when the code from category Z38 code no longer applies. Codes from category Z05 are for use only for healthy newborns and infants for which no condition after study is found to be present.

3) Z05 on a birth record

A code from category Z05 is to be used as a secondary code after the code from category Z38, Liveborn infants according to place of birth and type of delivery.

c. Coding Additional Perinatal Diagnoses

1) Assigning codes for conditions that require treatment

Assign codes for conditions that require treatment or further investigation, prolong the length of stay, or require resource utilization.

2) Codes for conditions specified as having implications for future health care needs

Assign codes for conditions that have been specified by the provider as having implications for future health care needs.

Note: This guideline should not be used for adult patients.

d. Prematurity and Fetal Growth Retardation

Providers utilize different criteria in determining prematurity. A code for prematurity should not be assigned unless it is documented. Assignment of codes in categories PØ5, Disorders of newborn related to slow fetal growth and fetal malnutrition, and PØ7, Disorders of newborn related to short gestation and low birth weight, not elsewhere classified, should be based on the recorded birth weight and estimated gestational age. Codes from category PØ5 should not be assigned with codes from category PØ7.

When both birth weight and gestational age are available, two codes from category PØ7 should be assigned, with the code for birth weight sequenced before the code for gestational age.

e. Low birth weight and immaturity status

Codes from category PØ7, Disorders of newborn related to short gestation and low birth weight, not elsewhere classified, are for use for a child or adult who was premature or had a low birth weight as a newborn and this is affecting the patient's current health status.

See Section I.C.21. Factors influencing health status and contact with health services, Status.

f. Bacterial Sepsis of Newborn

Category P36, Bacterial sepsis of newborn, includes congenital sepsis. If a perinate is documented as having sepsis without documentation of congenital or community acquired, the default is congenital and a code from category P36 should be assigned. If the P36 code includes the causal organism, an additional code from category B95, Streptococcus, Staphylococcus, and Enterococcus as the cause of diseases classified elsewhere, or B96, Other bacterial agents as the cause of diseases classified elsewhere, should not be assigned. If the P36 code does not include the causal organism, assign an additional code from category B96. If applicable, use additional codes to identify severe sepsis (R65.2-) and any associated acute organ dysfunction.

g. Stillbirth

Code P95, Stillbirth, is only for use in institutions that maintain separate records for stillbirths. No other code should be used with P95. Code P95 should not be used on the mother's record.

17. Chapter 17: Congenital malformations, deformations, and chromosomal abnormalities (QØØ-Q99)

Assign an appropriate code(s) from categories QØØ-Q99, Congenital malformations, deformations, and chromosomal abnormalities when a malformation/deformation or chromosomal abnormality is documented. A malformation/deformation/or chromosomal abnormality may be the principal/first-listed diagnosis on a record or a secondary diagnosis.

When a malformation/deformation/or chromosomal abnormality does not have a unique code assignment, assign additional code(s) for any manifestations that may be present.

When the code assignment specifically identifies the malformation/deformation/or chromosomal abnormality, manifestations that are an inherent component of the anomaly should not be coded separately. Additional codes should be assigned for manifestations that are not an inherent component.

Codes from Chapter 17 may be used throughout the life of the patient. If a congenital malformation or deformity has been corrected, a personal history code should be used to identify the history of the malformation or deformity. Although present at birth, malformation/deformation/or chromosomal abnormality may not be identified until later in life. Whenever the condition is diagnosed by the physician, it is appropriate to assign a code from codes Q00-Q99.

For the birth admission, the appropriate code from category Z38, Liveborn infants, according to place of birth and type of delivery, should be sequenced as the principal diagnosis, followed by any congenital anomaly codes, Q00-Q99.

18. Chapter 18: Symptoms, signs, and abnormal clinical and laboratory findings, not elsewhere classified (R00-R99)

Chapter 18 includes symptoms, signs, abnormal results of clinical or other investigative procedures, and ill-defined conditions regarding which no diagnosis classifiable elsewhere is recorded. Signs and symptoms that point to a specific diagnosis have been assigned to a category in other chapters of the classification.

a. Use of symptom codes

Codes that describe symptoms and signs are acceptable for reporting purposes when a related definitive diagnosis has not been established (confirmed) by the provider.

b. Use of a symptom code with a definitive diagnosis code

Codes for signs and symptoms may be reported in addition to a related definitive diagnosis when the sign or symptom is not routinely associated with that diagnosis, such as the various signs and symptoms associated with complex syndromes. The definitive diagnosis code should be sequenced before the symptom code.

Signs or symptoms that are associated routinely with a disease process should not be assigned as additional codes, unless otherwise instructed by the classification.

c. Combination codes that include symptoms

ICD-10-CM contains a number of combination codes that identify both the definitive diagnosis and common symptoms of that diagnosis. When using one of these combination codes, an additional code should not be assigned for the symptom.

d. Repeated falls

Code R29.6, Repeated falls, is for use for encounters when a patient has recently fallen and the reason for the fall is being investigated.

Code Z91.81, History of falling, is for use when a patient has fallen in the past and is at risk for future falls. When appropriate, both codes R29.6 and Z91.81 may be assigned together.

e. Coma scale

The coma scale codes (R40.2-) can be used in conjunction with traumatic brain injury codes, acute cerebrovascular disease or sequelae of cerebrovascular disease codes. These codes are primarily for use by trauma registries, but they may be used in any setting where this information is collected. **The coma scale may also be used to assess the status of the central nervous system for other non-trauma conditions, such as monitoring patients in the intensive care unit regardless of medical condition.** The coma scale codes should be sequenced after the diagnosis code(s).

These codes, one from each subcategory, are needed to complete the scale. The 7th character indicates when the scale was recorded. The 7th character should match for all three codes.

At a minimum, report the initial score documented on presentation at your facility. This may be a score from the emergency medicine technician (EMT) or in the emergency department. If desired, a facility may choose to capture multiple coma scale scores.

Assign code R40.24, Glasgow coma scale, total score, when only the total score is documented in the medical record and not the individual score(s).

f. Functional quadriplegia

Functional quadriplegia (code R53.2) is the lack of ability to use one's limbs or to ambulate due to extreme debility. It is not associated with neurologic deficit or injury, and code R53.2 should not be used for cases of neurologic quadriplegia. It should only be assigned if functional quadriplegia is specifically documented in the medical record.

g. SIRS due to Non-Infectious Process

The systemic inflammatory response syndrome (SIRS) can develop as a result of certain non-infectious disease processes, such as trauma, malignant neoplasm, or pancreatitis. When SIRS is documented with a noninfectious condition, and no subsequent infection is documented, the code for the underlying condition, such as an injury, should be assigned, followed by code R65.10, Systemic inflammatory response syndrome (SIRS) of non-infectious origin without acute organ dysfunction, or code R65.11, Systemic inflammatory response syndrome (SIRS) of non-infectious origin with acute organ dysfunction. If an associated acute organ dysfunction is documented, the appropriate code(s) for the specific type of organ dysfunction(s) should be assigned in addition to code R65.11. If acute organ dysfunction is documented, but it cannot be determined if the acute organ dysfunction is associated with SIRS or due to another condition (e.g., directly due to the trauma), the provider should be queried.

h. Death NOS

Code R99, Ill-defined and unknown cause of mortality, is only for use in the very limited circumstance when a patient who has already died is brought into an emergency department or other healthcare facility and is pronounced dead upon arrival. It does not represent the discharge disposition of death.

i. NIHSS Stroke Scale

The NIH stroke scale (NIHSS) codes (R29.7- -) can be used in conjunction with acute stroke codes (I63) to identify the patient's neurological status and the severity of the stroke. The stroke scale codes should be sequenced after the acute stroke diagnosis code(s).

At a minimum, report the initial score documented. If desired, a facility may choose to capture multiple stroke scale scores.

See Section I.B.14. for information concerning the medical record documentation that may be used for assignment of the NIHSS codes.

19. Chapter 19: Injury, poisoning, and certain other consequences of external causes (S00-T88)

a. Application of 7th Characters in Chapter 19

Most categories in chapter 19 have a 7th character requirement for each applicable code. Most categories in this chapter have three 7th character values (with the exception of fractures): A, initial encounter, D, subsequent encounter and S, sequela. Categories for traumatic fractures have additional 7th character values. While the patient may be seen by a new or different provider over the course of treatment for an injury, assignment of the 7th character is based on whether the patient is undergoing active treatment and not whether the provider is seeing the patient for the first time.

For complication codes, active treatment refers to treatment for the condition described by the code, even though it may be related to an earlier precipitating problem. For example, code T84.50XA, Infection and inflammatory reaction due to unspecified internal joint prosthesis, initial encounter, is used when active treatment is provided for the infection, even though the condition relates to the prosthetic device, implant or graft that was placed at a previous encounter.

7th character "A", initial encounter is used **for each encounter where** the patient is receiving active treatment for the condition.

7th character "D" subsequent encounter is used for encounters after the patient has **completed** active treatment of the condition and is receiving routine care for the condition during the healing or recovery phase.

The aftercare Z codes should not be used for aftercare for conditions such as injuries or poisonings, where 7th characters are provided to identify subsequent care. For example, for aftercare of an injury, assign the acute injury code with the 7th character "D" (subsequent encounter).

7th character "S", sequela, is for use for complications or conditions that arise as a direct result of a condition, such as scar formation after a burn. The scars are sequelae of the burn. When using 7th character "S", it is necessary to use both the injury code that precipitated the sequela and the code for the sequela itself. The "S" is added only to the injury code, not the sequela code. The 7th character "S" identifies the injury responsible for the sequela. The specific type of sequela (e.g. scar) is sequenced first, followed by the injury code.

See Section I.B.10. Sequelae, (Late Effects)

b. Coding of Injuries

When coding injuries, assign separate codes for each injury unless a combination code is provided, in which case the combination code is assigned. Code T07, Unspecified multiple injuries should not be assigned in the inpatient setting unless information for a more specific code is not available. Traumatic injury codes (S00-T14.9) are not to be used for normal, healing surgical wounds or to identify complications of surgical wounds.

The code for the most serious injury, as determined by the provider and the focus of treatment, is sequenced first.

1) Superficial injuries

Superficial injuries such as abrasions or contusions are not coded when associated with more severe injuries of the same site.

2) Primary injury with damage to nerves/ blood vessels

When a primary injury results in minor damage to peripheral nerves or blood vessels, the primary injury is sequenced first with additional code(s) for injuries to nerves and spinal cord (such as category S04), and/or injury to blood vessels (such as category S15). When the primary injury is to the blood vessels or nerves, that injury should be sequenced first.

c. Coding of Traumatic Fractures

The principles of multiple coding of injuries should be followed in coding fractures. Fractures of specified sites are coded individually by site in accordance with both the provisions within categories S02, S12, S22, S32, S42, S49, S52, S59, S62, S72, S79, S82, S89, S92 and the level of detail furnished by medical record content.

A fracture not indicated as open or closed should be coded to closed. A fracture not indicated whether displaced or not displaced should be coded to displaced.

More specific guidelines are as follows:

1) Initial vs. Subsequent Encounter for Fractures

Traumatic fractures are coded using the appropriate 7th character for initial encounter (A, B, C) **for each encounter where** the patient is receiving active treatment for the fracture. The appropriate 7th character for initial encounter should also be assigned for a patient who delayed seeking treatment for the fracture or nonunion.

Fractures are coded using the appropriate 7th character for subsequent care for encounters after the patient has completed active treatment of the fracture and is receiving routine care for the fracture during the healing or recovery phase.

Care for complications of surgical treatment for fracture repairs during the healing or recovery phase should be coded with the appropriate complication codes.

Care of complications of fractures, such as malunion and nonunion, should be reported with the appropriate 7th character for subsequent care with nonunion (K, M, N,) or subsequent care with malunion (P, Q, R).

Malunion/nonunion: The appropriate 7th character for initial encounter should also be assigned for a patient who delayed seeking treatment for the fracture or nonunion.

The open fracture designations in the assignment of the 7th character for fractures of the forearm, femur and lower leg, including ankle are based on the Gustilo open fracture classification. When the Gustilo classification type is not specified for an open fracture, the 7th character for open fracture type I or II should be assigned (B, E, H, M, Q).

A code from category M8Ø, not a traumatic fracture code, should be used for any patient with known osteoporosis who suffers a fracture, even if the patient had a minor fall or trauma, if that fall or trauma would not usually break a normal, healthy bone.

See Section I.C.13. Osteoporosis.

The aftercare Z codes should not be used for aftercare for traumatic fractures. For aftercare of a traumatic fracture, assign the acute fracture code with the appropriate 7th character.

2) Multiple fractures sequencing

Multiple fractures are sequenced in accordance with the severity of the fracture.

d. Coding of Burns and Corrosions

The ICD-10-CM makes a distinction between burns and corrosions. The burn codes are for thermal burns, except sunburns, that come from a heat source, such as a fire or hot appliance. The burn codes are also for burns resulting from electricity and radiation. Corrosions are burns due to chemicals. The guidelines are the same for burns and corrosions.

Current burns (T2Ø-T25) are classified by depth, extent and by agent (X code). Burns are classified by depth as first degree (erythema), second degree (blistering), and third degree (full-thickness involvement). Burns of the eye and internal organs (T26-T28) are classified by site, but not by degree.

1) Sequencing of burn and related condition codes

Sequence first the code that reflects the highest degree of burn when more than one burn is present.

a. When the reason for the admission or encounter is for treatment of external multiple burns, sequence first the code that reflects the burn of the highest degree.

b. When a patient has both internal and external burns, the circumstances of admission govern the selection of the principal diagnosis or first-listed diagnosis.

c. When a patient is admitted for burn injuries and other related conditions such as smoke inhalation and/or respiratory failure, the circumstances of admission govern the selection of the principal or first-listed diagnosis.

2) Burns of the same local site

Classify burns of the same local site (three-character category level, T2Ø-T28) but of different degrees to the subcategory identifying the highest degree recorded in the diagnosis.

3) Non-healing burns

Non-healing burns are coded as acute burns.

Necrosis of burned skin should be coded as a non-healed burn.

4) Infected Burn

For any documented infected burn site, use an additional code for the infection.

5) Assign separate codes for each burn site

When coding burns, assign separate codes for each burn site. Category T3Ø, Burn and corrosion, body region unspecified is extremely vague and should rarely be used.

6) Burns and Corrosions Classified According to Extent of Body Surface Involved

Assign codes from category T31, Burns classified according to extent of body surface involved, or T32, Corrosions classified according to extent of body surface involved, when the site of the burn is not specified or when there is a need for additional data. It is advisable to use category T31 as additional coding when needed to provide data for evaluating burn mortality, such as that needed by burn units. It is also advisable to use category T31 as an additional code for reporting purposes when there is mention of a third-degree burn involving 2Ø percent or more of the body surface.

Categories T31 and T32 are based on the classic "rule of nines" in estimating body surface involved: head and neck are assigned nine percent, each arm nine percent, each leg 18 percent, the anterior trunk 18 percent, posterior trunk 18 percent, and genitalia one percent. Providers may change these percentage assignments where necessary to accommodate infants and children who have proportionately larger heads than adults, and patients who have large buttocks, thighs, or abdomen that involve burns.

7) Encounters for treatment of sequela of burns

Encounters for the treatment of the late effects of burns or corrosions (i.e., scars or joint contractures) should be coded with a burn or corrosion code with the 7th character "S" for sequela.

8) Sequelae with a late effect code and current burn

When appropriate, both a code for a current burn or corrosion with 7th character "A" or "D" and a burn or corrosion code with 7th character "S" may be assigned on the same record (when both a current burn and sequelae of an old burn exist). Burns and corrosions do not heal at the same rate and a current healing wound may still exist with sequela of a healed burn or corrosion.

See Section I.B.1Ø. Sequela, (Late Effects)

9) Use of an external cause code with burns and corrosions

An external cause code should be used with burns and corrosions to identify the source and intent of the burn, as well as the place where it occurred.

GUIDELINES (ICD-10-CM)

e. Adverse Effects, Poisoning , Underdosing and Toxic Effects

Codes in categories T36-T65 are combination codes that include the substance that was taken as well as the intent. No additional external cause code is required for poisonings, toxic effects, adverse effects and underdosing codes.

1) Do not code directly from the Table of Drugs

Do not code directly from the Table of Drugs and Chemicals. Always refer back to the Tabular List.

2) Use as many codes as necessary to describe

Use as many codes as necessary to describe completely all drugs, medicinal or biological substances.

3) If the same code would describe the causative agent

If the same code would describe the causative agent for more than one adverse reaction, poisoning, toxic effect or underdosing, assign the code only once.

4) If two or more drugs, medicinal or biological substances

If two or more drugs, medicinal or biological substances are reported, code each individually unless a combination code is listed in the Table of Drugs and Chemicals.

5) The occurrence of drug toxicity is classified in ICD-10-CM as follows:

(a) Adverse Effect

When coding an adverse effect of a drug that has been correctly prescribed and properly administered, assign the appropriate code for the nature of the adverse effect followed by the appropriate code for the adverse effect of the drug (T36-T5Ø). The code for the drug should have a 5th or 6th character "5" (for example T36.ØX5-) Examples of the nature of an adverse effect are tachycardia, delirium, gastrointestinal hemorrhaging, vomiting, hypokalemia, hepatitis, renal failure, or respiratory failure.

(b) Poisoning

When coding a poisoning or reaction to the improper use of a medication (e.g., overdose, wrong substance given or taken in error, wrong route of administration), first assign the appropriate code from categories T36-T5Ø. The poisoning codes have an associated intent as their 5th or 6th character (accidental, intentional self-harm, assault and undetermined). **If the intent of the poisoning is unknown or unspecified, code the intent as accidental intent. The undetermined intent is only for use if the documentation in the record specifies that the intent cannot be determined.** Use additional code(s) for all manifestations of poisonings.

If there is also a diagnosis of abuse or dependence of the substance, the abuse or dependence is assigned as an additional code.

Examples of poisoning include:

(i) Error was made in drug prescription Errors made in drug prescription or in the administration of the drug by provider, nurse, patient, or other person.

(ii) Overdose of a drug intentionally taken If an overdose of a drug was intentionally taken or administered and resulted in drug toxicity, it would be coded as a poisoning.

(iii) Nonprescribed drug taken with correctly prescribed and properly administered drug.
If a nonprescribed drug or medicinal agent was taken in combination with a correctly prescribed and properly administered drug, any drug toxicity or other reaction resulting from the interaction of the two drugs would be classified as a poisoning.

(iv) Interaction of drug(s) and alcohol. When a reaction results from the interaction of a drug(s) and alcohol, this would be classified as poisoning.

See Section I.C.4. if poisoning is the result of insulin pump malfunctions.

(c) Underdosing

Underdosing refers to taking less of a medication than is prescribed by a provider or a manufacturer's instruction. For underdosing, assign the code from categories T36-T5Ø (fifth or sixth character "6").

Codes for underdosing should never be assigned as principal or first-listed codes. If a patient has a relapse or exacerbation of the medical condition for which the drug is prescribed because of the reduction in dose, then the medical condition itself should be coded.

Noncompliance (Z91.12-, Z91.13-) or complication of care (Y63.6-Y63.9) codes are to be used with an underdosing code to indicate intent, if known.

(d) Toxic Effects

When a harmful substance is ingested or comes in contact with a person, this is classified as a toxic effect. The toxic effect codes are in categories T51-T65.

Toxic effect codes have an associated intent: accidental, intentional self-harm, assault and undetermined.

f. Adult and child abuse, neglect and other maltreatment

Sequence first the appropriate code from categories T74.- (Adult and child abuse, neglect and other maltreatment, confirmed) or T76.- (Adult and child

GUIDELINES (ICD-10-CM)

abuse, neglect and other maltreatment, suspected) for abuse, neglect and other maltreatment, followed by any accompanying mental health or injury code(s).

If the documentation in the medical record states abuse or neglect it is coded as confirmed (T74.-). It is coded as suspected if it is documented as suspected (T76.-).

For cases of confirmed abuse or neglect an external cause code from the assault section (X92-**YØ9**) should be added to identify the cause of any physical injuries. A perpetrator code (YØ7) should be added when the perpetrator of the abuse is known. For suspected cases of abuse or neglect, do not report external cause or perpetrator code.

If a suspected case of abuse, neglect or mistreatment is ruled out during an encounter code ZØ4.71, Encounter for examination and observation following alleged physical adult abuse, ruled out, or code ZØ4.72, Encounter for examination and observation following alleged child physical abuse, ruled out, should be used, not a code from T76.

If a suspected case of alleged rape or sexual abuse is ruled out during an encounter code ZØ4.41, Encounter for examination and observation following alleged **adult rape** or code ZØ4.42, Encounter for examination and observation following alleged **child** rape, should be used, not a code from T76.

See Section I.C.15. Abuse in a pregnant patient.

g. Complications of care

1) General guidelines for complications of care

(a) Documentation of complications of care

See Section I.B.16. for information on documentation of complications of care.

2) Pain due to medical devices

Pain associated with devices, implants or grafts left in a surgical site (for example painful hip prosthesis) is assigned to the appropriate code(s) found in Chapter 19, Injury, poisoning, and certain other consequences of external causes. Specific codes for pain due to medical devices are found in the T code section of the ICD-10-CM. Use additional code(s) from category G89 to identify acute or chronic pain due to presence of the device, implant or graft (G89.18 or G89.28).

3) Transplant complications

(a) Transplant complications other than kidney

Codes under category T86, Complications of transplanted organs and tissues, are for use for both complications and rejection of transplanted organs. A transplant complication code is only assigned if the complication affects the function of the transplanted organ. Two codes are required to fully describe a transplant complication: the appropriate code from category T86 and a secondary code that identifies the complication.

Pre-existing conditions or conditions that develop after the transplant are not coded as complications unless they affect the function of the transplanted organs.

See I.C.21. for transplant organ removal status

See I.C.2. for malignant neoplasm associated with transplanted organ.

(b) Kidney transplant complications

Patients who have undergone kidney transplant may still have some form of chronic kidney disease (CKD) because the kidney transplant may not fully restore kidney function. Code T86.1- should be assigned for documented complications of a kidney transplant, such as transplant failure or rejection or other transplant complication. Code T86.1- should not be assigned for post kidney transplant patients who have chronic kidney (CKD) unless a transplant complication such as transplant failure or rejection is documented. If the documentation is unclear as to whether the patient has a complication of the transplant, query the provider.

Conditions that affect the function of the transplanted kidney, other than CKD, should be assigned a code from subcategory T86.1, Complications of transplanted organ, Kidney, and a secondary code that identifies the complication.

For patients with CKD following a kidney transplant, but who do not have a complication such as failure or rejection, *see section I.C.14. Chronic kidney disease and kidney transplant status.*

4) Complication codes that include the external cause

As with certain other T codes, some of the complications of care codes have the external cause included in the code. The code includes the nature of the complication as well as the type of procedure that caused the complication. No external cause code indicating the type of procedure is necessary for these codes.

5) Complications of care codes within the body system chapters

Intraoperative and postprocedural complication codes are found within the body system chapters with codes specific to the organs and structures of that body system. These codes should be sequenced first, followed by a code(s) for the specific complication, if applicable.

2Ø. Chapter 2Ø: External Causes of Morbidity (VØØ-Y99)

The external causes of morbidity codes should never be sequenced as the first-listed or principal diagnosis.

External cause codes are intended to provide data for injury research and evaluation of injury prevention strategies. These codes capture how the injury or health condition happened (cause), the intent (unintentional or accidental; or intentional, such as suicide or assault), the place where the event occurred the activity of the patient at the time of the event, and the person's status (e.g., civilian, military).

There is no national requirement for mandatory ICD-10-CM external cause code reporting. Unless a provider is subject to a state-based external cause code reporting mandate or these codes are required by a particular payer, reporting of ICD-10-CM codes in Chapter 20, External Causes of Morbidity, is not required. In the absence of a mandatory reporting requirement, providers are encouraged to voluntarily report external cause codes, as they provide valuable data for injury research and evaluation of injury prevention strategies.

a. General External Cause Coding Guidelines

1) Used with any code in the range of A00.0-T88.9, Z00-Z99

An external cause code may be used with any code in the range of A00.0-T88.9, Z00-Z99, classification that is a health condition due to an external cause. Though they are most applicable to injuries, they are also valid for use with such things as infections or diseases due to an external source, and other health conditions, such as a heart attack that occurs during strenuous physical activity.

2) External cause code used for length of treatment

Assign the external cause code, with the appropriate 7th character (initial encounter, subsequent encounter or sequela) for each encounter for which the injury or condition is being treated.

Most categories in chapter 20 have a 7th character requirement for each applicable code. Most categories in this chapter have three 7th character values: A, initial encounter, D, subsequent encounter and S, sequela. While the patient may be seen by a new or different provider over the course of treatment for an injury or condition, assignment of the 7th character for external cause should match the 7th character of the code assigned for the associated injury or condition for the encounter.

3) Use the full range of external cause codes

Use the full range of external cause codes to completely describe the cause, the intent, the place of occurrence and if applicable, the activity of the patient at the time of the event, and the patient's status, for all injuries, and other health conditions due to an external cause.

4) Assign as many external cause codes as necessary

Assign as many external cause codes as necessary to fully explain each cause. If only one external code can be recorded, assign the code most related to the principal diagnosis.

5) The selection of the appropriate external cause code

The selection of the appropriate external cause code is guided by the Alphabetic Index of External Causes and by Inclusion and Exclusion notes in the Tabular List.

6) External cause code can never be a principal diagnosis

An external cause code can never be a principal (first-listed) diagnosis.

7) Combination external cause codes

Certain of the external cause codes are combination codes that identify sequential events that result in an injury, such as a fall which results in striking against an object. The injury may be due to either event or both. The combination external cause code used should correspond to the sequence of events regardless of which caused the most serious injury.

8) No external cause code needed in certain circumstances

No external cause code from Chapter 20 is needed if the external cause and intent are included in a code from another chapter (e.g. T36.0X1- Poisoning by penicillins, accidental (unintentional)).

b. Place of Occurrence Guideline

Codes from category Y92, Place of occurrence of the external cause, are secondary codes for use after other external cause codes to identify the location of the patient at the time of injury or other condition.

Generally, a place of occurrence code is assigned only once, at the initial encounter for treatment. However, in the rare instance that a new injury occurs during hospitalization, an additional place of occurrence code may be assigned. No 7th characters are used for Y92. Only one code from Y92 should be recorded on a medical record.

Do not use place of occurrence code Y92.9 if the place is not stated or is not applicable.

c. Activity Code

Assign a code from category Y93, Activity code, to describe the activity of the patient at the time the injury or other health condition occurred.

An activity code is used only once, at the initial encounter for treatment. Only one code from Y93 should be recorded on a medical record.

The activity codes are not applicable to poisonings, adverse effects, misadventures or sequela.

Do not assign Y93.9, Unspecified activity, if the activity is not stated.

A code from category Y93 is appropriate for use with external cause and intent codes if identifying the activity provides additional information about the event.

d. Place of Occurrence, Activity, and Status Codes Used with other External Cause Code

When applicable, place of occurrence, activity, and external cause status codes are sequenced after the main external cause code(s). Regardless of the number of external cause codes assigned, there should be only one place of occurrence code, one activity code, and one external cause status code assigned to an encounter.

e. If the Reporting Format Limits the Number of External Cause Codes

If the reporting format limits the number of external cause codes that can be used in reporting clinical data, report the code for the cause/intent most related to the principal diagnosis. If the format permits capture of additional external cause codes, the cause/intent, including medical misadventures, of the additional events should be reported rather than the codes for place, activity, or external status.

f. Multiple External Cause Coding Guidelines

More than one external cause code is required to fully describe the external cause of an illness or injury. The assignment of external cause codes should be sequenced in the following priority:

If two or more events cause separate injuries, an external cause code should be assigned for each cause. The first-listed external cause code will be selected in the following order:

External codes for child and adult abuse take priority over all other external cause codes.

See Section I.C.19., Child and Adult abuse guidelines.

External codes for terrorism events take priority over all other external cause codes except child and adult abuse.

External cause codes for cataclysmic events take priority over all other external cause codes except child and adult abuse and terrorism.

External cause codes for transport accidents take priority over all other external cause codes except cataclysmic events, child and adult abuse and terrorism.

Activity and external cause status codes are assigned following all causal (intent) external cause codes.

The first-listed external cause code should correspond to the cause of the most serious diagnosis due to an assault, accident, or self-harm, following the order of hierarchy listed above.

g. Child and Adult Abuse Guideline

Adult and child abuse, neglect and maltreatment are classified as assault. Any of the assault codes may be used to indicate the external cause of any injury resulting from the confirmed abuse.

For confirmed cases of abuse, neglect and maltreatment, when the perpetrator is known, a code from Y07, Perpetrator of maltreatment and neglect, should accompany any other assault codes.

See Section I.C.19. Adult and child abuse, neglect and other maltreatment

h. Unknown or Undetermined Intent Guideline

If the intent (accident, self-harm, assault) of the cause of an injury or other condition is unknown or unspecified, code the intent as accidental intent. All transport accident categories assume accidental intent.

1) Use of undetermined intent

External cause codes for events of undetermined intent are only for use if the documentation in the record specifies that the intent cannot be determined.

i. Sequelae (Late Effects) of External Cause Guidelines

1) Sequelae external cause codes

Sequela are reported using the external cause code with the 7th character "S" for sequela. These codes should be used with any report of a late effect or sequela resulting from a previous injury.

See Section I.B.10. Sequela, (Late Effects)

2) Sequela external cause code with a related current injury

A sequela external cause code should never be used with a related current nature of injury code.

3) Use of sequela external cause codes for subsequent visits

Use a late effect external cause code for subsequent visits when a late effect of the initial injury is being treated. Do not use a late effect external cause code for subsequent visits for follow-up care (e.g., to assess healing, to receive rehabilitative therapy) of the injury when no late effect of the injury has been documented.

j. Terrorism Guidelines

1) Cause of injury identified by the Federal Government (FBI) as terrorism

When the cause of an injury is identified by the Federal Government (FBI) as terrorism, the first-listed external cause code should be a code from category Y38, Terrorism. The definition of terrorism employed by the FBI is found at the inclusion note at the beginning of category Y38. Use additional code for place of occurrence (Y92.-). More than one Y38 code may be assigned if the injury is the result of more than one mechanism of terrorism.

2) Cause of an injury is suspected to be the result of terrorism

When the cause of an injury is suspected to be the result of terrorism a code from category Y38 should not be assigned. Suspected cases should be classified as assault.

3) Code Y38.9, Terrorism, secondary effects

Assign code Y38.9, Terrorism, secondary effects, for conditions occurring subsequent to the terrorist event. This code should not be assigned for conditions that are due to the initial terrorist act.

It is acceptable to assign code Y38.9 with another code from Y38 if there is an injury due to the initial terrorist event and an injury that is a subsequent result of the terrorist event.

k. External cause status

A code from category Y99, External cause status, should be assigned whenever any other external cause code is assigned for an encounter, including an Activity code, except for the events noted below. Assign a code from category Y99, External cause status, to indicate the work status of the person at the time the event occurred. The status code indicates whether the event occurred during military activity, whether a non-military person was at work, whether an individual including a student or volunteer was involved in a non-work activity at the time of the causal event.

A code from Y99, External cause status, should be assigned, when applicable, with other external cause codes, such as transport accidents and falls. The external cause status codes are not applicable to poisonings, adverse effects, misadventures or late effects.

Do not assign a code from category Y99 if no other external cause codes (cause, activity) are applicable for the encounter.

An external cause status code is used only once, at the initial encounter for treatment. Only one code from Y99 should be recorded on a medical record.

Do not assign code Y99.9, Unspecified external cause status, if the status is not stated.

21. Chapter 21: Factors influencing health status and contact with health services (Z00-Z99)

Note: The chapter specific guidelines provide additional information about the use of Z codes for specified encounters.

a. Use of Z codes in any healthcare setting

Z codes are for use in any healthcare setting. Z codes may be used as either a first-listed (principal diagnosis code in the inpatient setting) or secondary code, depending on the circumstances of the encounter. Certain Z codes may only be used as first-listed or principal diagnosis.

b. Z Codes indicate a reason for an encounter

Z codes are not procedure codes. A corresponding procedure code must accompany a Z code to describe any procedure performed.

c. Categories of Z Codes

1) Contact/Exposure

Category Z20 indicates contact with, and suspected exposure to, communicable diseases. These codes are for patients who do not show any sign or symptom of a disease but are suspected to have been exposed to it by close personal contact with an infected individual or are in an area where a disease is epidemic.

Category Z77, Other contact with and (suspected) exposures hazardous to health, indicates contact with and suspected exposures hazardous to health.

Contact/exposure codes may be used as a first-listed code to explain an encounter for testing, or, more commonly, as a secondary code to identify a potential risk.

2) Inoculations and vaccinations

Code Z23 is for encounters for inoculations and vaccinations. It indicates that a patient is being seen to receive a prophylactic inoculation against a disease. Procedure codes are required to identify the actual administration of the injection and the type(s) of immunizations given. Code Z23 may be used as a secondary code if the inoculation is given as a routine part of preventive health care, such as a well-baby visit.

3) Status

Status codes indicate that a patient is either a carrier of a disease or has the sequelae or residual of a past disease or condition. This includes such things as the presence of prosthetic or mechanical devices resulting from past treatment. A status code is informative, because the status may affect the course of treatment and its outcome. A status code is distinct from a history code. The history code indicates that the patient no longer has the condition.

A status code should not be used with a diagnosis code from one of the body system chapters, if the diagnosis code includes the information provided by the status code. For example, code Z94.1, Heart transplant status, should not be used with a code from subcategory T86.2, Complications of heart transplant. The status code does not provide additional information. The complication code indicates that the patient is a heart transplant patient.

For encounters for weaning from a mechanical ventilator, assign a code from subcategory J96.1, Chronic respiratory failure, followed by code Z99.11, Dependence on respirator [ventilator] status.

The status Z codes/categories are:

Z14 Genetic carrier

Genetic carrier status indicates that a person carries a gene, associated with a particular disease, which may be passed to offspring who may develop that disease. The person does not have the disease and is not at risk of developing the disease.

Z15 Genetic susceptibility to disease Genetic susceptibility indicates that a person has a gene that increases the risk of that person developing the disease.

Codes from category Z15 should not be used as principal or first-listed codes. If the patient has the condition to which he/she is susceptible, and that condition is the reason for the encounter, the code for the current condition should be sequenced first. If the patient is being seen for follow-up after completed treatment for this condition, and the condition no longer exists, a follow-up code should be sequenced first, followed by the appropriate personal history and genetic susceptibility codes. If the purpose of the encounter is genetic counseling associated with procreative management, code Z31.5, Encounter for genetic counseling, should be assigned as the first-listed code, followed by a code from category Z15. Additional codes should be assigned for any applicable family or personal history.

Z16 Resistance to antimicrobial drugs

This code indicates that a patient has a condition that is resistant to antimicrobial drug treatment. Sequence the infection code first.

GUIDELINES (ICD-10-CM)

Z17 Estrogen receptor status
Z18 Retained foreign body fragments
Z19 Hormone sensitivity malignancy status
Z21 Asymptomatic HIV infection status This code indicates that a patient has tested positive for HIV but has manifested no signs or symptoms of the disease.
Z22 Carrier of infectious disease Carrier status indicates that a person harbors the specific organisms of a disease without manifest symptoms and is capable of transmitting the infection.
Z28.3 Underimmunization status
Z33.1 Pregnant state, incidental This code is a secondary code only for use when the pregnancy is in no way complicating the reason for visit. Otherwise, a code from the obstetric chapter is required.
Z66 Do not resuscitate

This code may be used when it is documented by the provider that a patient is on do not resuscitate status at any time during the stay.

Z67 Blood type
Z68 Body mass index (BMI)

As with all other secondary diagnosis codes, the BMI codes should only be assigned when they meet the definition of a reportable diagnosis (see Section III, Reporting Additional Diagnoses).

Z74.Ø1 Bed confinement status
Z76.82 Awaiting organ transplant status
Z78 Other specified health status

Code Z78.1, Physical restraint status, may be used when it is documented by the provider that a patient has been put in restraints during the current encounter. Please note that this code should not be reported when it is documented by the provider that a patient is temporarily restrained during a procedure.

Z79 Long-term (current) drug therapy

Codes from this category indicate a patient's continuous use of a prescribed drug (including such things as aspirin therapy) for the long-term treatment of a condition or for prophylactic use. It is not for use for patients who have addictions to drugs. This subcategory is not for use of medications for detoxification or maintenance programs to prevent withdrawal symptoms in patients with drug dependence (e.g., methadone maintenance for opiate dependence). Assign the appropriate code for the drug dependence instead.

Assign a code from Z79 if the patient is receiving a medication for an extended period as a prophylactic measure (such as for the prevention of deep vein thrombosis) or as treatment of a chronic condition (such as arthritis) or a disease requiring a lengthy course of treatment (such as cancer). Do not assign a code from category Z79 for medication being administered for a brief period of time to treat an acute illness or injury (such as a course of antibiotics to treat acute bronchitis).

Z88 Allergy status to drugs, medicaments and biological substances Except: Z88.9, Allergy status to unspecified drugs, medicaments and biological substances status
Z89 Acquired absence of limb
Z9Ø Acquired absence of organs, not elsewhere classified
Z91.Ø- Allergy status, other than to drugs and biological substances
Z92.82 Status post administration of tPA (rtPA) in a different facility within the last 24 hours prior to admission to a current facility Assign code Z92.82, Status post administration of tPA (rtPA) in a different facility within the last 24 hours prior to admission to current facility, as a secondary diagnosis when a patient is received by transfer into a facility and documentation indicates they were administered tissue plasminogen activator (tPA) within the last 24 hours prior to admission to the current facility. This guideline applies even if the patient is still receiving the tPA at the time they are received into the current facility. The appropriate code for the condition for which the tPA was administered (such as cerebrovascular disease or myocardial infarction) should be assigned first. Code Z92.82 is only applicable to the receiving facility record and not to the transferring facility record.
Z93 Artificial opening status
Z94 Transplanted organ and tissue status
Z95 Presence of cardiac and vascular implants and grafts
Z96 Presence of other functional implants
Z97 Presence of other devices
Z98 Other postprocedural states

Assign code Z98.85, Transplanted organ removal status, to indicate that a transplanted organ has been previously removed. This code should not be assigned for the encounter in which the transplanted organ is removed. The complication necessitating removal of the transplant organ should be assigned for that encounter.

See section I.C.19. for information on the coding of organ transplant complications.

Z99 Dependence on enabling machines and devices, not elsewhere classified

Note: Categories Z89-Z9Ø and Z93-Z99 are for use only if there are no complications or malfunctions of the organ or tissue replaced, the amputation site or the equipment on which the patient is dependent.

4) History (of)

There are two types of history Z codes, personal and family. Personal history codes explain a patient's past medical condition that no longer exists and is not receiving any treatment, but that has the potential for recurrence, and therefore may require continued monitoring.

Family history codes are for use when a patient has a family member(s) who has had a particular disease that causes the patient to be at higher risk of also contracting the disease.

Personal history codes may be used in conjunction with follow-up codes and family history codes may be used in conjunction with screening codes to explain the need for a test or procedure. History codes are also acceptable on any medical record regardless of the reason for visit. A history of an illness, even if no longer present, is important information that may alter the type of treatment ordered.

The history Z code categories are:

Z8Ø	Family history of primary malignant neoplasm
Z81	Family history of mental and behavioral disorders
Z82	Family history of certain disabilities and chronic diseases (leading to disablement)
Z83	Family history of other specific disorders
Z84	Family history of other conditions
Z85	Personal history of malignant neoplasm
Z86	Personal history of certain other diseases
Z87	Personal history of other diseases and conditions
Z91.4-	Personal history of psychological trauma, not elsewhere classified
Z91.5	Personal history of self-harm
Z91.8-	Other specified personal risk factors, not elsewhere classified Exception: Z91.83, Wandering in diseases classified elsewhere
Z92	Personal history of medical treatment Except: Z92.Ø, Personal history of contraception Except: Z92.82, Status post administration of tPA (rtPA) in a different facility within the last 24 hours prior to admission to a current facility

5) Screening

Screening is the testing for disease or disease precursors in seemingly well individuals so that early detection and treatment can be provided for those who test positive for the disease (e.g., screening mammogram).

The testing of a person to rule out or confirm a suspected diagnosis because the patient has some sign or symptom is a diagnostic examination, not a screening. In these cases, the sign or symptom is used to explain the reason for the test.

A screening code may be a first-listed code if the reason for the visit is specifically the screening exam. It may also be used as an additional code if the screening is done during an office visit for other health problems. A screening code is not necessary if the screening is inherent to a routine examination, such as a pap smear done during a routine pelvic examination.

Should a condition be discovered during the screening then the code for the condition may be assigned as an additional diagnosis.

The Z code indicates that a screening exam is planned. A procedure code is required to confirm that the screening was performed.

The screening Z codes/categories:

Z11	Encounter for screening for infectious and parasitic diseases
Z12	Encounter for screening for malignant neoplasms
Z13	Encounter for screening for other diseases and disorders Except: Z13.9, Encounter for screening, unspecified
Z36	Encounter for antenatal screening for mother

6) Observation

There are **three** observation Z code categories. They are for use in very limited circumstances when a person is being observed for a suspected condition that is ruled out. The observation codes are not for use if an injury or illness or any signs or symptoms related to the suspected condition are present. In such cases the diagnosis/symptom code is used with the corresponding external cause code.

The observation codes are to be used as principal diagnosis only. **The only exception to this is when the principal diagnosis is required to be a code from category Z38, Liveborn infants according to place of birth and type of delivery. Then a code from category ZØ5, Encounter for observation and evaluation of newborn for suspected diseases and conditions ruled out, is sequenced after the Z38 code.** Additional codes may be used in addition to the observation code, but only if they are unrelated to the suspected condition being observed.

Codes from subcategory ZØ3.7 Encounter for suspected maternal and fetal conditions ruled out, may either be used as a first-listed or as an additional code assignment depending on the case. They are for use in very limited circumstances on a maternal record when an encounter is for a suspected maternal or fetal condition that is ruled out during that encounter (for example, a maternal or fetal condition may be suspected due to an abnormal test result). These codes should not be used when the condition is confirmed. In those cases, the confirmed condition should be coded. In addition, these codes are not for use if an illness or any signs or symptoms related to the suspected condition or problem are present. In such cases the diagnosis/symptom code is used.

GUIDELINES (ICD-10-CM)

Additional codes may be used in addition to the code from subcategory Z03.7, but only if they are unrelated to the suspected condition being evaluated.

Codes from subcategory Z03.7 may not be used for encounters for antenatal screening of mother. *See Section I.C.21. Screening.*

For encounters for suspected fetal condition that are inconclusive following testing and evaluation, assign the appropriate code from category O35, O36, O40 or O41.

The observation Z code categories:

Z03	Encounter for medical observation for suspected diseases and conditions ruled out
Z04	Encounter for examination and observation for other reasons Except: Z04.9, Encounter for examination and observation for unspecified reason
Z05	**Encounter for observation and evaluation of newborn for suspected diseases and conditions ruled out**

7) Aftercare

Aftercare visit codes cover situations when the initial treatment of a disease has been performed and the patient requires continued care during the healing or recovery phase, or for the long-term consequences of the disease. The aftercare Z code should not be used if treatment is directed at a current, acute disease. The diagnosis code is to be used in these cases.

Exceptions to this rule are codes Z51.0, Encounter for antineoplastic radiation therapy, and codes from subcategory Z51.1, Encounter for antineoplastic chemotherapy and immunotherapy. These codes are to be first-listed, followed by the diagnosis code when a patient's encounter is solely to receive radiation therapy, chemotherapy, or immunotherapy for the treatment of a neoplasm. If the reason for the encounter is more than one type of antineoplastic therapy, code Z51.0 and a code from subcategory Z51.1 may be assigned together, in which case one of these codes would be reported as a secondary diagnosis.

The aftercare Z codes should also not be used for aftercare for injuries. For aftercare of an injury, assign the acute injury code with the appropriate 7th character (for subsequent encounter).

The aftercare codes are generally first-listed to explain the specific reason for the encounter. An aftercare code may be used as an additional code when some type of aftercare is provided in addition to the reason for admission and no diagnosis code is applicable. An example of this would be the closure of a colostomy during an encounter for treatment of another condition.

Aftercare codes should be used in conjunction with other aftercare codes or diagnosis codes to provide better detail on the specifics of an aftercare encounter visit, unless otherwise directed by the classification. Should a patient receive multiple types of antineoplastic therapy during the same encounter, code Z51.0, Encounter for antineoplastic radiation therapy, and codes from subcategory Z51.1, Encounter for antineoplastic chemotherapy and immunotherapy, may be used together on a record. The sequencing of multiple aftercare codes depends on the circumstances of the encounter.

Certain aftercare Z code categories need a secondary diagnosis code to describe the resolving condition or sequelae. For others, the condition is included in the code title.

Additional Z code aftercare category terms include fitting and adjustment, and attention to artificial openings.

Status Z codes may be used with aftercare Z codes to indicate the nature of the aftercare. For example code Z95.1, Presence of aortocoronary bypass graft, may be used with code Z48.812, Encounter for surgical aftercare following surgery on the circulatory system, to indicate the surgery for which the aftercare is being performed. A status code should not be used when the aftercare code indicates the type of status, such as using Z43.0, Encounter for attention to tracheostomy, with Z93.0, Tracheostomy status.

The aftercare Z category/codes:

Z42	Encounter for plastic and reconstructive surgery following medical procedure or healed injury
Z43	Encounter for attention to artificial openings
Z44	Encounter for fitting and adjustment of external prosthetic device
Z45	Encounter for adjustment and management of implanted device
Z46	Encounter for fitting and adjustment of other devices
Z47	Orthopedic aftercare
Z48	Encounter for other postprocedural aftercare
Z49	Encounter for care involving renal dialysis
Z51	Encounter for other aftercare **and medical care**

8) Follow-up

The follow-up codes are used to explain continuing surveillance following completed treatment of a disease, condition, or injury. They imply that the condition has been fully treated and no longer exists. They should not be confused with aftercare codes, or injury codes with a 7th character for subsequent encounter, that explain ongoing care of a healing condition or its sequelae. Follow-up codes may be used in conjunction with history codes to provide the full picture of the healed condition and its treatment. The follow-up code is sequenced first, followed by the history code.

A follow-up code may be used to explain multiple visits. Should a condition be found to have recurred on the follow-up visit, then the diagnosis code for the condition should be assigned in place of the follow-up code.

The follow-up Z code categories:

Z08	Encounter for follow-up examination after completed treatment for malignant neoplasm
Z09	Encounter for follow-up examination after completed treatment for conditions other than malignant neoplasm
Z39	Encounter for maternal postpartum care and examination

9) Donor

Codes in category Z52, Donors of organs and tissues, are used for living individuals who are donating blood or other body tissue. These codes are only for individuals donating for others, not for self-donations. They are not used to identify cadaveric donations.

10) Counseling

Counseling Z codes are used when a patient or family member receives assistance in the aftermath of an illness or injury, or when support is required in coping with family or social problems. They are not used in conjunction with a diagnosis code when the counseling component of care is considered integral to standard treatment.

The counseling Z codes/categories:

Z30.0-	Encounter for general counseling and advice on contraception
Z31.5	Encounter for genetic counseling
Z31.6-	Encounter for general counseling and advice on procreation
Z32.2	Encounter for childbirth instruction
Z32.3	Encounter for childcare instruction
Z69	Encounter for mental health services for victim and perpetrator of abuse
Z70	Counseling related to sexual attitude, behavior and orientation
Z71	Persons encountering health services for other counseling and medical advice, not elsewhere classified
Z76.81	Expectant mother prebirth pediatrician visit

11) Encounters for Obstetrical and Reproductive Services

See Section I.C.15. Pregnancy, Childbirth, and the Puerperium, for further instruction on the use of these codes.

Z codes for pregnancy are for use in those circumstances when none of the problems or complications included in the codes from the Obstetrics chapter exist (a routine prenatal visit or postpartum care). Codes in category Z34, Encounter for supervision of normal pregnancy, are always first listed and are not to be used with any other code from the OB chapter.

Codes in category Z3A, Weeks of gestation, may be assigned to provide additional information about the pregnancy. **Category Z3A codes should not be assigned for pregnancies with abortive outcomes (categories O00-O08), elective termination of pregnancy (code Z33.32), nor for postpartum conditions, as category Z3A is not applicable to these conditions.** The date of the admission should be used to determine weeks of gestation for inpatient admissions that encompass more than one gestational week.

The outcome of delivery, category Z37, should be included on all maternal delivery records. It is always a secondary code. Codes in category Z37 should not be used on the newborn record.

Z codes for family planning (contraceptive) or procreative management and counseling should be included on an obstetric record either during the pregnancy or the postpartum stage, if applicable.

Z codes/categories for obstetrical and reproductive services:

Z30	Encounter for contraceptive management
Z31	Encounter for procreative management
Z32.2	Encounter for childbirth instruction
Z32.3	Encounter for childcare instruction
Z33	Pregnant state
Z34	Encounter for supervision of normal pregnancy
Z36	Encounter for antenatal screening of mother
Z3A	Weeks of gestation
Z37	Outcome of delivery
Z39	Encounter for maternal postpartum care and examination
Z76.81	Expectant mother prebirth pediatrician visit

12) Newborns and Infants

See Section I.C.16. Newborn (Perinatal) Guidelines, for further instruction on the use of these codes.

Newborn Z codes/categories:

Z76.1	Encounter for health supervision and care of foundling
Z00.1-	Encounter for routine child health examination
Z38	Liveborn infants according to place of birth and type of delivery

13) Routine and administrative examinations

The Z codes allow for the description of encounters for routine examinations, such as, a general check-up, or, examinations for administrative purposes, such as, a pre-employment physical. The codes are not to be used if the examination is for diagnosis of a suspected condition or for treatment purposes. In such cases the diagnosis code is used. During a routine exam, should a diagnosis or condition be discovered, it should be coded as an additional code. Pre-existing and chronic conditions and history codes may also be included as additional codes as long as the examination is for administrative purposes and not focused on any particular condition.

Some of the codes for routine health examinations distinguish between "with" and "without" abnormal findings. Code assignment depends on the information that is known at the time the encounter is being coded. For example, if no abnormal findings were found during the examination, but the encounter is being coded before test results are back, it is acceptable to assign the code for "without abnormal findings." When assigning a code for "with abnormal findings," additional code(s) should be assigned to identify the specific abnormal finding(s).

Pre-operative examination and pre-procedural laboratory examination Z codes are for use only in those situations when a patient is being cleared for a procedure or surgery and no treatment is given.

The Z codes/categories for routine and administrative examinations:

Z00	Encounter for general examination without complaint, suspected or reported diagnosis
Z01	Encounter for other special examination without complaint, suspected or reported diagnosis
Z02	Encounter for administrative examination Except: Z02.9, Encounter for administrative examinations, unspecified
Z32.0-	Encounter for pregnancy test

14) Miscellaneous Z codes

The miscellaneous Z codes capture a number of other health care encounters that do not fall into one of the other categories. Certain of these codes identify the reason for the encounter; others are for use as additional codes that provide useful information on circumstances that may affect a patient's care and treatment.

Prophylactic Organ Removal

For encounters specifically for prophylactic removal of an organ (such as prophylactic removal of breasts due to a genetic susceptibility to cancer or a family history of cancer), the principal or first-listed code should be a code from category Z40, Encounter for prophylactic surgery, followed by the appropriate codes to identify the associated risk factor (such as genetic susceptibility or family history).

If the patient has a malignancy of one site and is having prophylactic removal at another site to prevent either a new primary malignancy or metastatic disease, a code for the malignancy should also be assigned in addition to a code from subcategory Z40.0, Encounter for prophylactic surgery for risk factors related to malignant neoplasms. A Z40.0 code should not be assigned if the patient is having organ removal for treatment of a malignancy, such as the removal of the testes for the treatment of prostate cancer.

Miscellaneous Z codes/categories:

Z28	Immunization not carried out Except: Z28.3, Underimmunization status
Z29	**Encounter for other prophylactic measures**
Z40	Encounter for prophylactic surgery
Z41	Encounter for procedures for purposes other than remedying health state Except: Z41.9, Encounter for procedure for purposes other than remedying health state, unspecified
Z53	Persons encountering health services for specific procedures and treatment, not carried out
Z55	Problems related to education and literacy
Z56	Problems related to employment and unemployment
Z57	Occupational exposure to risk factors
Z58	Problems related to physical environment
Z59	Problems related to housing and economic circumstances
Z60	Problems related to social environment
Z62	Problems related to upbringing
Z63	Other problems related to primary support group, including family circumstances
Z64	Problems related to certain psychosocial circumstances
Z65	Problems related to other psychosocial circumstances
Z72	Problems related to lifestyle **Note: These codes should be assigned only when the documentation specifies that the patient has an associated problem**
Z73	Problems related to life management difficulty
Z74	Problems related to care provider dependency Except: Z74.01, Bed confinement status
Z75	Problems related to medical facilities and other health care
Z76.0	Encounter for issue of repeat prescription
Z76.3	Healthy person accompanying sick person
Z76.4	Other boarder to healthcare facility
Z76.5	Malingerer [conscious simulation]
Z91.1-	Patient's noncompliance with medical treatment and regimen
Z91.83	Wandering in diseases classified elsewhere
Z91.89	Other specified personal risk factors, not elsewhere classified

15) Nonspecific Z codes

Certain Z codes are so non-specific, or potentially redundant with other codes in the classification, that there can be little justification for their use in the inpatient setting. Their use in the outpatient setting should be limited to those instances when there is no further documentation to permit more precise coding. Otherwise, any sign or symptom or any other reason for visit that is captured in another code should be used.

Nonspecific Z codes/categories:

Z02.9	Encounter for administrative examinations, unspecified
Z04.9	Encounter for examination and observation for unspecified reason
Z13.9	Encounter for screening, unspecified

Z41.9 Encounter for procedure for purposes other than remedying health state, unspecified
Z52.9 Donor of unspecified organ or tissue
Z86.59 Personal history of other mental and behavioral disorders
Z88.9 Allergy status to unspecified drugs, medicaments and biological substances status
Z92.Ø Personal history of contraception

16) Z Codes That May Only be Principal/First-Listed Diagnosis

The following Z codes/categories may only be reported as the principal/first-listed diagnosis, except when there are multiple encounters on the same day and the medical records for the encounters are combined:

ZØØ Encounter for general examination without complaint, suspected or reported diagnosis Except: ZØØ.6
ZØ1 Encounter for other special examination without complaint, suspected or reported diagnosis
ZØ2 Encounter for administrative examination
ZØ3 Encounter for medical observation for suspected diseases and conditions ruled out
ZØ4 Encounter for examination and observation for other reasons
Z33.2 Encounter for elective termination of pregnancy
Z31.81 Encounter for male factor infertility in female patient
Z31.83 Encounter for assisted reproductive fertility procedure cycle
Z31.84 Encounter for fertility preservation procedure
Z34 Encounter for supervision of normal pregnancy
Z39 Encounter for maternal postpartum care and examination
Z38 Liveborn infants according to place of birth and type of delivery
Z42 Encounter for plastic and reconstructive surgery following medical procedure or healed injury
Z51.Ø Encounter for antineoplastic radiation therapy
Z51.1- Encounter for antineoplastic chemotherapy and immunotherapy
Z52 Donors of organs and tissues Except: Z52.9, Donor of unspecified organ or tissue
Z76.1 Encounter for health supervision and care of foundling
Z76.2 Encounter for health supervision and care of other healthy infant and child
Z99.12 Encounter for respirator [ventilator] dependence during power failure

Section II. Selection of Principal Diagnosis

The circumstances of inpatient admission always govern the selection of principal diagnosis. The principal diagnosis is defined in the Uniform Hospital Discharge Data Set (UHDDS) as "that condition established after study to be chiefly responsible for occasioning the admission of the patient to the hospital for care."

The UHDDS definitions are used by hospitals to report inpatient data elements in a standardized manner. These data elements and their definitions can be found in the July 31, 1985, Federal Register (Vol. 5Ø, No, 147), pp. 31Ø38-4Ø.

Since that time the application of the UHDDS definitions has been expanded to include all nonoutpatient settings (acute care, short term, long term care and psychiatric hospitals; home health agencies; rehab facilities; nursing homes, etc). **The UHDDS definitions also apply to hospice services (all levels of care).**

In determining principal diagnosis, coding conventions in the ICD-10-CM, the Tabular List and Alphabetic Index take precedence over these official coding guidelines. *(See Section I.A., Conventions for the ICD-10-CM)*

The importance of consistent, complete documentation in the medical record cannot be overemphasized. Without such documentation the application of all coding guidelines is a difficult, if not impossible, task.

A. Codes for symptoms, signs, and ill-defined conditions

Codes for symptoms, signs, and ill-defined conditions from Chapter 18 are not to be used as principal diagnosis when a related definitive diagnosis has been established.

B. Two or more interrelated conditions, each potentially meeting the definition for principal diagnosis.

When there are two or more interrelated conditions (such as diseases in the same ICD-10-CM chapter or manifestations characteristically associated with a certain disease) potentially meeting the definition of principal diagnosis, either condition may be sequenced first, unless the circumstances of the admission, the therapy provided, the Tabular List, or the Alphabetic Index indicate otherwise.

C. Two or more diagnoses that equally meet the definition for principal diagnosis

In the unusual instance when two or more diagnoses equally meet the criteria for principal diagnosis as determined by the circumstances of admission, diagnostic workup and/or therapy provided, and the Alphabetic Index, Tabular List, or another coding guidelines does not provide sequencing direction, any one of the diagnoses may be sequenced first.

D. Two or more comparative or contrasting conditions.

In those rare instances when two or more contrasting or comparative diagnoses are documented as "either/or" (or similar terminology), they are coded as if the diagnoses were confirmed and the diagnoses are sequenced according to the circumstances of the admission. If no further determination can be made as to which diagnosis should be principal, either diagnosis may be sequenced first.

E. A symptom(s) followed by contrasting/ comparative diagnoses

GUIDELINE HAS BEEN DELETED EFFECTIVE OCTOBER 1, 2014

F. Original treatment plan not carried out

Sequence as the principal diagnosis the condition, which after study occasioned the admission to the hospital, even though treatment may not have been carried out due to unforeseen circumstances.

G. Complications of surgery and other medical care

When the admission is for treatment of a complication resulting from surgery or other medical care, the complication code is sequenced as the principal diagnosis. If the complication is classified to the T80-T88 series and the code lacks the necessary specificity in describing the complication, an additional code for the specific complication should be assigned.

H. Uncertain Diagnosis

If the diagnosis documented at the time of discharge is qualified as "probable", "suspected", "likely", "questionable", "possible", or "still to be ruled out", or other similar terms indicating uncertainty, code the condition as if it existed or was established. The bases for these guidelines are the diagnostic workup, arrangements for further workup or observation, and initial therapeutic approach that correspond most closely with the established diagnosis.

Note: This guideline is applicable only to inpatient admissions to short-term, acute, long-term care and psychiatric hospitals.

I. Admission from Observation Unit

1. Admission Following Medical Observation

When a patient is admitted to an observation unit for a medical condition, which either worsens or does not improve, and is subsequently admitted as an inpatient of the same hospital for this same medical condition, the principal diagnosis would be the medical condition which led to the hospital admission.

2. Admission Following Post-Operative Observation

When a patient is admitted to an observation unit to monitor a condition (or complication) that develops following outpatient surgery, and then is subsequently admitted as an inpatient of the same hospital, hospitals should apply the Uniform Hospital Discharge Data Set (UHDDS) definition of principal diagnosis as "that condition established after study to be chiefly responsible for occasioning the admission of the patient to the hospital for care."

J. Admission from Outpatient Surgery

When a patient receives surgery in the hospital's outpatient surgery department and is subsequently admitted for continuing inpatient care at the same hospital, the following guidelines should be followed in selecting the principal diagnosis for the inpatient admission:

- If the reason for the inpatient admission is a complication, assign the complication as the principal diagnosis.
- If no complication, or other condition, is documented as the reason for the inpatient admission, assign the reason for the outpatient surgery as the principal diagnosis.
- If the reason for the inpatient admission is another condition unrelated to the surgery, assign the unrelated condition as the principal diagnosis.

K. Admissions/Encounters for Rehabilitation

When the purpose for the admission/encounter is rehabilitation, sequence first the code for the condition for which the service is being performed. For example, for an admission/encounter for rehabilitation for right-sided dominant hemiplegia following a cerebrovascular infarction, report code I69.351, Hemiplegia and hemiparesis following cerebral infarction affecting right dominant side, as the first-listed or principal diagnosis.

If the condition for which the rehabilitation service is no longer present, report the appropriate aftercare code as the first-listed or principal diagnosis. For example, if a patient with severe degenerative osteoarthritis of the hip, underwent hip replacement and the current encounter/ admission is for rehabilitation, report code Z47.1, Aftercare following joint replacement surgery, as the first-listed or principal diagnosis.

See Section I.C.21.c.7, Factors influencing health states and contact with health services, Aftercare.

Section III. Reporting Additional Diagnoses

GENERAL RULES FOR OTHER (ADDITIONAL) DIAGNOSES

For reporting purposes the definition for "other diagnoses" is interpreted as additional conditions that affect patient care in terms of requiring:

clinical evaluation; or
therapeutic treatment; or
diagnostic procedures; or
extended length of hospital stay; or
increased nursing care and/or monitoring.

The UHDDS item #11-b defines Other Diagnoses as "all conditions that coexist at the time of admission, that develop subsequently, or that affect the treatment received and/or the length of stay. Diagnoses that relate to an earlier episode which have no bearing on the current hospital stay are to be excluded." UHDDS definitions apply to inpatients in acute care, short-term, long term care and psychiatric hospital setting. The UHDDS definitions are used by acute care short-term hospitals to report inpatient data elements in a standardized manner. These data elements and their definitions can be found in the July 31, 1985, Federal Register (Vol. 5Ø, No, 147), pp. 31Ø38-4Ø.

Since that time the application of the UHDDS definitions has been expanded to include all nonoutpatient settings (acute care, short term, long term care and psychiatric hospitals; home health agencies; rehab facilities; nursing homes, etc). **The UHDDS definitions also apply to hospice services (all levels of care).**

The following guidelines are to be applied in designating "other diagnoses" when neither the Alphabetic Index nor the Tabular List in ICD-10-CM provide direction. The listing of the diagnoses in the patient record is the responsibility of the attending provider.

A. Previous conditions

If the provider has included a diagnosis in the final diagnostic statement, such as the discharge summary or the face sheet, it should ordinarily be coded. Some providers include in the diagnostic statement resolved conditions or diagnoses and status-post procedures from previous admission that have no bearing on the current stay. Such conditions are not to be reported and are coded only if required by hospital policy.

However, history codes (categories Z8Ø-Z87) may be used as secondary codes if the historical condition or family history has an impact on current care or influences treatment.

B. Abnormal findings

Abnormal findings (laboratory, x-ray, pathologic, and other diagnostic results) are not coded and reported unless the provider indicates their clinical significance. If the findings are outside the normal range and the attending provider has ordered other tests to evaluate the condition or prescribed treatment, it is appropriate to ask the provider whether the abnormal finding should be added.

Please note: This differs from the coding practices in the outpatient setting for coding encounters for diagnostic tests that have been interpreted by a provider.

C. Uncertain Diagnosis

If the diagnosis documented at the time of discharge is qualified as "probable", "suspected", "likely", "questionable", "possible", or "still to be ruled out" or other similar terms indicating uncertainty, code the condition as if it existed or was established. The bases for these guidelines are the diagnostic workup, arrangements for further workup or observation, and initial therapeutic approach that correspond most closely with the established diagnosis.

Note: This guideline is applicable only to inpatient admissions to short-term, acute, long-term care and psychiatric hospitals.

Section IV. Diagnostic Coding and Reporting Guidelines for Outpatient Services

These coding guidelines for outpatient diagnoses have been approved for use by hospitals/ providers in coding and reporting hospital-based outpatient services and provider-based office visits. **Guidelines in Section I, Conventions, general coding guidelines and chapter-specific guidelines, should also be applied for outpatient services and office visits.**

Information about the use of certain abbreviations, punctuation, symbols, and other conventions used in the ICD-10-CM Tabular List (code numbers and titles), can be found in Section IA of these guidelines, under "Conventions Used in the Tabular List." Section I.B. contains general guidelines that apply to the entire classification. Section I.C. contains chapter-specific guidelines that correspond to the chapters as they are arranged in the classification. Information about the correct sequence to use in finding a code is also described in Section I.

The terms encounter and visit are often used interchangeably in describing outpatient service contacts and, therefore, appear together in these guidelines without distinguishing one from the other.

Though the conventions and general guidelines apply to all settings, coding guidelines for outpatient and provider reporting of diagnoses will vary in a number of instances from those for inpatient diagnoses, recognizing that:

The Uniform Hospital Discharge Data Set (UHDDS) definition of principal diagnosis **does not apply to hospital-based outpatient services and provider-based office visits.**

Coding guidelines for inconclusive diagnoses (probable, suspected, rule out, etc.) were developed for inpatient reporting and do not apply to outpatients.

A. Selection of first-listed condition

In the outpatient setting, the term first-listed diagnosis is used in lieu of principal diagnosis.

In determining the first-listed diagnosis the coding conventions of ICD-10-CM, as well as the general and disease specific guidelines take precedence over the outpatient guidelines.

Diagnoses often are not established at the time of the initial encounter/visit. It may take two or more visits before the diagnosis is confirmed.

The most critical rule involves beginning the search for the correct code assignment through the Alphabetic Index. Never begin searching initially in the Tabular List as this will lead to coding errors.

1. Outpatient Surgery

When a patient presents for outpatient surgery (same day surgery), code the reason for the surgery as the first-listed diagnosis (reason for the encounter), even if the surgery is not performed due to a contraindication.

2. Observation Stay

When a patient is admitted for observation for a medical condition, assign a code for the medical condition as the first-listed diagnosis.

When a patient presents for outpatient surgery and develops complications requiring admission to observation, code the reason for the surgery as the first reported diagnosis (reason for the encounter), followed by codes for the complications as secondary diagnoses.

B. Codes from A00.0 through T88.9, Z00-Z99
The appropriate code(s) from A00.0 through T88.9, Z00-Z99 must be used to identify diagnoses, symptoms, conditions, problems, complaints, or other reason(s) for the encounter/visit.

C. Accurate reporting of ICD-10-CM diagnosis codes
For accurate reporting of ICD-10-CM diagnosis codes, the documentation should describe the patient's condition, using terminology which includes specific diagnoses as well as symptoms, problems, or reasons for the encounter. There are ICD-10-CM codes to describe all of these.

D. Codes that describe symptoms and signs
Codes that describe symptoms and signs, as opposed to diagnoses, are acceptable for reporting purposes when a diagnosis has not been established (confirmed) by the provider. Chapter 18 of ICD-10-CM, Symptoms, Signs, and Abnormal Clinical and Laboratory Findings Not Elsewhere Classified (codes R00-R99) contain many, but not all codes for symptoms.

E. Encounters for circumstances other than a disease or injury
ICD-10-CM provides codes to deal with encounters for circumstances other than a disease or injury. The Factors Influencing Health Status and Contact with Health Services codes (Z00-Z99) are provided to deal with occasions when circumstances other than a disease or injury are recorded as diagnosis or problems.

See Section I.C.21. Factors influencing health status and contact with health services.

F. Level of Detail in Coding

1. ICD-10-CM codes with 3, 4, 5, 6 or 7 characters
ICD-10-CM is composed of codes with 3, 4, 5, 6 or 7 characters. Codes with three characters are included in ICD-10-CM as the heading of a category of codes that may be further subdivided by the use of fourth, fifth, sixth or seventh characters to provide greater specificity.

2. Use of full number of characters required for a code
A three-character code is to be used only if it is not further subdivided. A code is invalid if it has not been coded to the full number of characters required for that code, including the 7th character, if applicable.

G. ICD-10-CM code for the diagnosis, condition, problem, or other reason for encounter/visit
List first the ICD-10-CM code for the diagnosis, condition, problem, or other reason for encounter/visit shown in the medical record to be chiefly responsible for the services provided. List additional codes that describe any coexisting conditions. In some cases the first-listed diagnosis may be a symptom when a diagnosis has not been established (confirmed) by the physician.

H. Uncertain diagnosis
Do not code diagnoses documented as "probable", "suspected," "questionable," "rule out," or "working diagnosis" or other similar terms indicating uncertainty. Rather, code the condition(s) to the highest degree of certainty for that encounter/visit, such as symptoms, signs, abnormal test results, or other reason for the visit.

Please note: This differs from the coding practices used by short-term, acute care, long-term care and psychiatric hospitals.

I. Chronic diseases
Chronic diseases treated on an ongoing basis may be coded and reported as many times as the patient receives treatment and care for the condition(s)

J. Code all documented conditions that coexist
Code all documented conditions that coexist at the time of the encounter/visit, and require or affect patient care treatment or management. Do not code conditions that were previously treated and no longer exist. However, history codes (categories Z80-Z87) may be used as secondary codes if the historical condition or family history has an impact on current care or influences treatment.

K. Patients receiving diagnostic services only
For patients receiving diagnostic services only during an encounter/visit, sequence first the diagnosis, condition, problem, or other reason for encounter/visit shown in the medical record to be chiefly responsible for the outpatient services provided during the encounter/visit. Codes for other diagnoses (e.g., chronic conditions) may be sequenced as additional diagnoses.

For encounters for routine laboratory/radiology testing in the absence of any signs, symptoms, or associated diagnosis, assign Z01.89, Encounter for other specified special examinations. If routine testing is performed during the same encounter as a test to evaluate a sign, symptom, or diagnosis, it is appropriate to assign both the Z code and the code describing the reason for the non-routine test.

For outpatient encounters for diagnostic tests that have been interpreted by a physician, and the final report is available at the time of coding, code any confirmed or definitive diagnosis(es) documented in the interpretation. Do not code related signs and symptoms as additional diagnoses.

Please note: This differs from the coding practice in the hospital inpatient setting regarding abnormal findings on test results.

L. Patients receiving therapeutic services only
For patients receiving therapeutic services only during an encounter/visit, sequence first the diagnosis, condition, problem, or other reason for encounter/visit shown in the medical record to be chiefly responsible for the outpatient services provided during the encounter/visit. Codes for other diagnoses (e.g., chronic conditions) may be sequenced as additional diagnoses.

The only exception to this rule is that when the primary reason for the admission/encounter is chemotherapy or radiation therapy, the appropriate Z code for the service is listed first, and the diagnosis or problem for which the service is being performed listed second.

M. Patients receiving preoperative evaluations only
For patients receiving preoperative evaluations only, sequence first a code from subcategory Z01.81, Encounter for pre-procedural examinations, to describe the pre-op consultations. Assign a code for the condition to describe the reason for the surgery as an additional diagnosis. Code also any findings related to the pre-op evaluation.

N. Ambulatory surgery
For ambulatory surgery, code the diagnosis for which the surgery was performed. If the postoperative diagnosis is known to be different from the preoperative diagnosis at the time the diagnosis is confirmed, select the postoperative diagnosis for coding, since it is the most definitive.

O. Routine outpatient prenatal visits
See Section I.C.15. Routine outpatient prenatal visits.

P. Encounters for general medical examinations with abnormal findings
The subcategories for encounters for general medical examinations, Z00.0-, provide codes for with and without abnormal findings. Should a general medical examination result in an abnormal finding, the code for general medical examination with abnormal finding should be assigned as the first-listed diagnosis. **An examination with abnormal findings refers to a condition/diagnosis that is newly identified or a change in severity of a chronic condition (such as uncontrolled hypertension, or an acute exacerbation of chronic obstructive pulmonary disease) during a routine physical examination.** A secondary code for the abnormal finding should also be coded.

Q. Encounters for routine health screenings
See Section I.C.21. Factors influencing health status and contact with health services, Screening

GUIDELINES (ICD-10-CM)

Appendix I
Present on Admission Reporting Guidelines

Introduction

These guidelines are to be used as a supplement to the *ICD-10-CM Official Guidelines for Coding and Reporting* to facilitate the assignment of the Present on Admission (POA) indicator for each diagnosis and external cause of injury code reported on claim forms (UB-04 and 837 Institutional).

These guidelines are not intended to replace any guidelines in the main body of the *ICD-10-CM Official Guidelines for Coding and Reporting*. The POA guidelines are not intended to provide guidance on when a condition should be coded, but rather, how to apply the POA indicator to the final set of diagnosis codes that have been assigned in accordance with Sections I, II, and III of the official coding guidelines. Subsequent to the assignment of the ICD-10-CM codes, the POA indicator should then be assigned to those conditions that have been coded.

As stated in the Introduction to the ICD-10-CM Official Guidelines for Coding and Reporting, a joint effort between the healthcare provider and the coder is essential to achieve complete and accurate documentation, code assignment, and reporting of diagnoses and procedures. The importance of consistent, complete documentation in the medical record cannot be overemphasized. Medical record documentation from any provider involved in the care and treatment of the patient may be used to support the determination of whether a condition was present on admission or not. In the context of the official coding guidelines, the term "provider" means a physician or any qualified healthcare practitioner who is legally accountable for establishing the patient's diagnosis.

These guidelines are not a substitute for the provider's clinical judgment as to the determination of whether a condition was/was not present on admission. The provider should be queried regarding issues related to the linking of signs/symptoms, timing of test results, and the timing of findings.

Please see the CDC website for the detailed list of ICD-10-CM codes that do not require the use of a POA indicator (ftp://ftp.cdc.gov/pub/Health_Statistics/NCHS/Publications/ICD10CM/2017/). The conditions on this exempt list represent categories and/or codes for circumstances regarding the healthcare encounter or factors influencing health status that do not represent a current disease or injury or are always present on admission.

General Reporting Requirements

All claims involving inpatient admissions to general acute care hospitals or other facilities that are subject to a law or regulation mandating collection of present on admission information.

Present on admission is defined as present at the time the order for inpatient admission occurs—conditions that develop during an outpatient encounter, including emergency department, observation, or outpatient surgery, are considered as present on admission.

POA indicator is assigned to principal and secondary diagnoses (as defined in Section II of the Official Guidelines for Coding and Reporting) and the external cause of injury codes.

Issues related to inconsistent, missing, conflicting or unclear documentation must still be resolved by the provider.

If a condition would not be coded and reported based on UHDDS definitions and current official coding guidelines, then the POA indicator would not be reported.

Reporting Options

Y - Yes

N - No

U - Unknown

W - Clinically undetermined

Unreported/Not used - (Exempt from POA reporting)

Reporting Definitions

Y = present at the time of inpatient admission

N = not present at the time of inpatient admission

U = documentation is insufficient to determine if condition is present on admission

W = provider is unable to clinically determine whether condition was present on admission or not

Timeframe for POA Identification and Documentation

There is no required timeframe as to when a provider (per the definition of "provider" used in these guidelines) must identify or document a condition to be present on admission. In some clinical situations, it may not be possible for a provider to make a definitive diagnosis (or a condition may not be recognized or reported by the patient) for a period of time after admission. In some cases it may be several days before the provider arrives at a definitive diagnosis. This does not mean that the condition was not present on admission. Determination of whether the condition was present on admission or not will be based on the applicable POA guideline as identified in this document, or on the provider's best clinical judgment.

If at the time of code assignment the documentation is unclear as to whether a condition was present on admission or not, it is appropriate to query the provider for clarification.

Assigning the POA Indicator

Condition is on the "Exempt from Reporting" list

Leave the "present on admission" field blank if the condition is on the list of ICD-10-CM codes for which this field is not applicable. This is the only circumstance in which the field may be left blank.

POA Explicitly Documented

Assign Y for any condition the provider explicitly documents as being present on admission.

Assign N for any condition the provider explicitly documents as not present at the time of admission.

Conditions diagnosed prior to inpatient admission

Assign "Y" for conditions that were diagnosed prior to admission (example: hypertension, diabetes mellitus, asthma)

Conditions diagnosed during the admission but clearly present before admission

Assign "Y" for conditions diagnosed during the admission that were clearly present but not diagnosed until after admission occurred.

Diagnoses subsequently confirmed after admission are considered present on admission if at the time of admission they are documented as suspected, possible, rule out, differential diagnosis, or constitute an underlying cause of a symptom that is present at the time of admission.

Condition develops during outpatient encounter prior to inpatient admission

Assign Y for any condition that develops during an outpatient encounter prior to a written order for inpatient admission.

Documentation does not indicate whether condition was present on admission

Assign "U" when the medical record documentation is unclear as to whether the condition was present on admission. "U" should not be routinely assigned and used only in very limited circumstances. Coders are encouraged to query the providers when the documentation is unclear.

Documentation states that it cannot be determined whether the condition was or was not present on admission

Assign "W" when the medical record documentation indicates that it cannot be clinically determined whether or not the condition was present on admission.

Chronic condition with acute exacerbation during the admission

If a single code identifies both the chronic condition and the acute exacerbation, see POA guidelines pertaining to **codes that contain multiple clinical concepts**.

If a single code only identifies the chronic condition and not the acute exacerbation (e.g., acute exacerbation of chronic leukemia), assign "Y."

Conditions documented as possible, probable, suspected, or rule out at the time of discharge

If the final diagnosis contains a possible, probable, suspected, or rule out diagnosis, and this diagnosis was based on signs, symptoms or clinical findings suspected at the time of inpatient admission, assign "Y."

If the final diagnosis contains a possible, probable, suspected, or rule out diagnosis, and this diagnosis was based on signs, symptoms or clinical findings that were not present on admission, assign "N".

Conditions documented as impending or threatened at the time of discharge

If the final diagnosis contains an impending or threatened diagnosis, and this diagnosis is based on symptoms or clinical findings that were present on admission, assign "Y".

If the final diagnosis contains an impending or threatened diagnosis, and this diagnosis is based on symptoms or clinical findings that were not present on admission, assign "N".

Acute and Chronic Conditions

Assign "Y" for acute conditions that are present at time of admission and N for acute conditions that are not present at time of admission.

Assign "Y" for chronic conditions, even though the condition may not be diagnosed until after admission.

If a single code identifies both an acute and chronic condition, see the POA guidelines for codes **that contain multiple clinical concepts.**

Codes **That Contain Multiple Clinical Concepts**

Assign "N" if at least one of the clinical concepts included in the code was not present on admission (e.g., COPD with acute exacerbation and the exacerbation was not present on admission; gastric ulcer that does not start bleeding until after admission; asthma patient develops status asthmaticus after admission).

Assign "Y" if all of the **clinical concepts included in the code** were present on admission (e.g., **duodenal ulcer that perforates prior to admission**).

For infection codes that include the causal organism, assign "Y" if the infection (or signs of the infection) **were** present on admission, even though the culture results may not be known until after admission (e.g., patient is admitted with pneumonia and the provider documents Pseudomonas as the causal organism a few days later).

Same Diagnosis Code for Two or More Conditions

When the same ICD-10-CM diagnosis code applies to two or more conditions during the same encounter (e.g. two separate conditions classified to the same ICD-10-CM diagnosis code):

Assign "Y" if all conditions represented by the single ICD-10-CM code were present on admission (e.g. bilateral unspecified age-related cataracts).

Assign "N" if any of the conditions represented by the single ICD-10-CM code was not present on admission (e.g. traumatic secondary and recurrent hemorrhage and seroma is assigned to a single code T79.2, but only one of the conditions was present on admission).

Obstetrical conditions

Whether or not the patient delivers during the current hospitalization does not affect assignment of the POA indicator. The determining factor for POA assignment is whether the pregnancy complication or obstetrical condition described by the code was present at the time of admission or not.

If the pregnancy complication or obstetrical condition was present on admission (e.g., patient admitted in preterm labor), assign "Y".

If the pregnancy complication or obstetrical condition was not present on admission (e.g., 2nd degree laceration during delivery, postpartum hemorrhage that occurred during current hospitalization, fetal distress develops after admission), assign "N".

If the obstetrical code includes more than one diagnosis and any of the diagnoses identified by the code were not present on admission assign "N".

(e.g., Category O11, Pre-existing hypertension with pre-eclampsia)

Perinatal conditions

Newborns are not considered to be admitted until after birth. Therefore, any condition present at birth or that developed in utero is considered present at admission and should be assigned "Y". This includes conditions that occur during delivery (e.g., injury during delivery, meconium aspiration, exposure to streptococcus B in the vaginal canal).

Congenital conditions and anomalies

Assign "Y" for congenital conditions and anomalies except for categories Q00-Q99, Congenital anomalies, which are on the exempt list. Congenital conditions are always considered present on admission.

External cause of injury codes

Assign "Y" for any external cause code representing an external cause of morbidity that occurred prior to inpatient admission (e.g., patient fell out of bed at home, patient fell out of bed in emergency room prior to admission).

Assign "N" for any external cause code representing an external cause of morbidity that occurred during inpatient hospitalization (e.g., patient fell out of hospital bed during hospital stay, patient experienced an adverse reaction to a medication administered after inpatient admission).

PART II

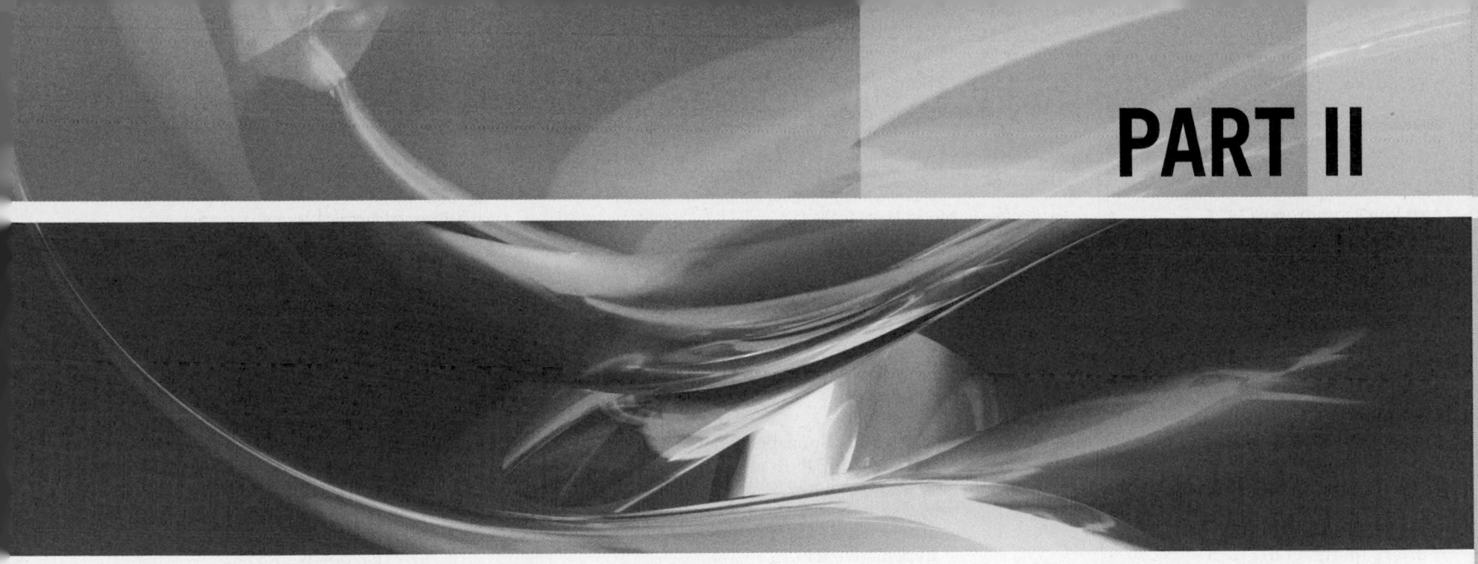

Alphabetic Index

ICD-10-CM INDEX TO DISEASES AND INJURIES

A

- **Aarskog's syndrome** Q87.1
- **Abandonment** —*see* Maltreatment
- **Abasia** (-astasia) (hysterical) F44.4
- **Abderhalden-Kaufmann-Lignac syndrome** (cystinosis) E72.Ø4
- **Abdomen, abdominal** —*see also* condition
  - acute R1Ø.Ø
  - angina K55.1
  - muscle deficiency syndrome Q79.4
- **Abdominalgia** —*see* Pain, abdominal
- **Abduction contracture, hip or other joint** —*see* Contraction, joint
- **Aberrant** (congenital) —*see also* Malposition, congenital
  - adrenal gland Q89.1
  - artery (peripheral) Q27.8
    - basilar NEC Q28.1
    - cerebral Q28.3
    - coronary Q24.5
    - digestive system Q27.8
    - eye Q15.8
    - lower limb Q27.8
    - precerebral Q28.1
    - pulmonary Q25.79
    - renal Q27.2
    - retina Q14.1
    - specified site NEC Q27.8
    - subclavian Q27.8
    - upper limb Q27.8
    - vertebral Q28.1
  - breast Q83.8
  - endocrine gland NEC Q89.2
  - hepatic duct Q44.5
  - pancreas Q45.3
  - parathyroid gland Q89.2
  - pituitary gland Q89.2
  - sebaceous glands, mucous membrane, mouth, congenital Q38.6
  - spleen Q89.Ø9
  - subclavian artery Q27.8
  - thymus (gland) Q89.2
  - thyroid gland Q89.2
  - vein (peripheral) NEC Q27.8
    - cerebral Q28.3
    - digestive system Q27.8
    - lower limb Q27.8
    - precerebral Q28.1
    - specified site NEC Q27.8
    - upper limb Q27.8
- **Aberration**
  - distantial —*see* Disturbance, visual
  - mental F99
- **Abetalipoproteinemia** E78.6
- **Abiotrophy** R68.89
- **Ablatio, ablation**
  - retinae —*see* Detachment, retina
- **Ablepharia, ablepharon** Q1Ø.3
- **Abnormal, abnormality, abnormalities** —*see also* Anomaly
  - acid-base balance (mixed) E87.4
  - albumin R77.Ø
  - alphafetoprotein R77.2
  - alveolar ridge KØ8.9
  - anatomical relationship Q89.9
  - apertures, congenital, diaphragm Q79.1
  - auditory perception H93.29-
    - diplacusis —*see* Diplacusis
    - hyperacusis —*see* Hyperacusis
    - recruitment —*see* Recruitment, auditory
    - threshold shift —*see* Shift, auditory threshold
  - autosomes Q99.9
    - fragile site Q95.5
  - basal metabolic rate R94.8
  - biosynthesis, testicular androgen E29.1
  - bleeding time R79.1

- **Abnormal, abnormality, abnormalities** —*(Continued)*
  - blood level (of)
    - cobalt R79.Ø
    - copper R79.Ø
    - iron R79.Ø
    - lithium R78.89
    - magnesium R79.Ø
    - mineral NEC R79.Ø
    - zinc R79.Ø
  - blood pressure
    - elevated RØ3.Ø
    - low reading (nonspecific) RØ3.1
  - blood sugar R73.Ø9
  - blood-gas level R79.81
  - bowel sounds R19.15
    - absent R19.11
    - hyperactive R19.12
  - brain scan R94.Ø2
  - breathing RØ6.9
  - caloric test R94.138
  - cerebrospinal fluid R83.9
    - cytology R83.6
    - drug level R83.2
    - enzyme level R83.Ø
    - hormones R83.1
    - immunology R83.4
    - microbiology R83.5
    - nonmedicinal level R83.3
    - specified type NEC R83.8
  - chemistry, blood R79.9
    - C-reactive protein R79.82
    - drugs —*see* Findings, abnormal, in blood
    - gas level R79.81
    - minerals R79.Ø
    - pancytopenia D61.818
    - PTT R79.1
    - specified NEC R79.89
    - toxins —*see* Findings, abnormal, in blood
  - chest sounds (friction) (rales) RØ9.89
  - chromosome, chromosomal Q99.9
    - with more than three X chromosomes, female Q97.1
    - analysis result R89.8
      - bronchial washings R84.8
      - cerebrospinal fluid R83.8
      - cervix uteri NEC R87.89
      - nasal secretions R84.8
      - nipple discharge R89.8
      - peritoneal fluid R85.89
      - pleural fluid R84.8
      - prostatic secretions R86.8
      - saliva R85.89
      - seminal fluid R86.8
      - sputum R84.8
      - synovial fluid R89.8
      - throat scrapings R84.8
      - vagina R87.89
      - vulva R87.89
      - wound secretions R89.8
    - dicentric replacement Q93.2
    - ring replacement Q93.2
    - sex Q99.8
      - female phenotype Q97.9
        - specified NEC Q97.8
      - male phenotype Q98.9
        - specified NEC Q98.8
      - structural male Q98.6
    - specified NEC Q99.8
  - clinical findings NEC R68.89
  - coagulation D68.9
    - newborn, transient P61.6
    - profile R79.1
    - time R79.1
  - communication —*see* Fistula
  - conjunctiva, vascular H11.41-
  - coronary artery Q24.5
  - cortisol-binding globulin E27.8
  - course, eustachian tube Q17.8

- **Abnormal, abnormality, abnormalities** —*(Continued)*
  - creatinine clearance R94.4
  - cytology
    - anus R85.619
      - atypical squamous cells cannot exclude high grade squamous intraepithelial lesion (ASC-H) R85.611
      - atypical squamous cells of undetermined significance (ASC-US) R85.61Ø
      - cytologic evidence of malignancy R85.614
      - high grade squamous intraepithelial lesion (HGSIL) R85.613
      - human papillomavirus (HPV) DNA test
        - high risk positive R85.81
        - low risk postive R85.82
      - inadequate smear R85.615
      - low grade squamous intraepithelial lesion (LGSIL) R85.612
      - satisfactory anal smear but lacking transformation zone R85.616
      - specified NEC R85.618
      - unsatisfactory smear R85.615
    - female genital organs —*see* Abnormal, Papanicolaou (smear)
  - dark adaptation curve H53.61
  - dentofacial NEC —*see* Anomaly, dentofacial
  - development, developmental Q89.9
    - central nervous system QØ7.9
  - diagnostic imaging
    - abdomen, abdominal region NEC R93.5
    - biliary tract R93.2
    - bladder R93.41 ◀
    - breast R92.8
    - central nervous system NEC R9Ø.89
    - cerebrovascular NEC R9Ø.89
    - coronary circulation R93.1
    - digestive tract NEC R93.3
    - gastrointestinal (tract) R93.3
    - genitourinary organs R93.8
    - head R93.Ø
    - heart R93.1
    - intrathoracic organ NEC R93.8
    - kidney R93.42- ◀
    - limbs R93.6
    - liver R93.2
    - lung (field) R91.8
    - musculoskeletal system NEC R93.7
    - renal pelvis R93.41 ◀
    - retroperitoneum R93.5
    - site specified NEC R93.8
    - skin and subcutaneous tissue R93.8
    - skull R93.Ø
    - ~~urinary organs R93.4~~
    - urinary organs specified NEC R93.49 ◀
    - ureter R93.41 ◀
  - direction, teeth, fully erupted M26.3Ø
  - ear ossicles, acquired NEC H74.39-
    - ankylosis —*see* Ankylosis, ear ossicles
    - discontinuity —*see* Discontinuity, ossicles, ear
    - partial loss —*see* Loss, ossicles, ear (partial)
  - Ebstein Q22.5
  - echocardiogram R93.1
  - echoencephalogram R9Ø.81
  - echogram —*see* Abnormal, diagnostic imaging
  - electrocardiogram [ECG] [EKG] R94.31
  - electroencephalogram [EEG] R94.Ø1
  - electrolyte —*see* Imbalance, electrolyte
  - electromyogram [EMG] R94.131
  - electro-oculogram [EOG] R94.11Ø
  - electrophysiological intracardiac studies R94.39
  - electroretinogram [ERG] R94.111
  - erythrocytes
    - congenital, with perinatal jaundice D58.9
  - feces (color) (contents) (mucus) R19.5

◀ New ◀ Revised ~~deleted~~ Deleted

A

Abnormal, abnormality, abnormalities — *(Continued)*
specimen
digestive organs (peritoneal fluid) (saliva) R85.9
cytology R85.69
drug level R85.2
enzyme level R85.0
histology R85.7
hormones R85.1
immunology R85.4
microbiology R85.5
nonmedicinal level R85.3
specified type NEC R85.89
female genital organs (secretions) (smears) R87.9
cytology R87.69
cervix R87.619
human papillomavirus (HPV) DNA test
high risk positive R87.810
low risk positive R87.820
inadequate (unsatisfactory) smear R87.615
non-atypical endometrial cells R87.618
specified NEC R87.618
vagina R87.629
human papillomavirus (HPV) DNA test
high risk positive R87.811
low risk positive R87.821
inadequate (unsatisfactory) smear R87.625
vulva R87.69
drug level R87.2
enzyme level R87.0
histological R87.7
hormones R87.1
immunology R87.4
microbiology R87.5
nonmedicinal level R87.3
specified type NEC R87.89
male genital organs (prostatic secretions) (semen) R86.9
cytology R86.6
drug level R86.2
enzyme level R86.0
histological R86.7
hormones R86.1
immunology R86.4
microbiology R86.5
nonmedicinal level R86.3
specified type NEC R86.8
nipple discharge —*see* Abnormal, specimen, specified
respiratory organs (bronchial washings) (nasal secretions) (pleural fluid) (sputum) R84.9
cytology R84.6
drug level R84.2
enzyme level R84.0
histology R84.7
hormones R84.1
immunology R84.4
microbiology R84.5
nonmedicinal level R84.3
specified type NEC R84.8
specified organ, system and tissue NOS R89.9
cytology R89.6
drug level R89.2
enzyme level R89.0
histology R89.7
hormones R89.1
immunology R89.4
microbiology R89.5
nonmedicinal level R89.3
specified type NEC R89.8
synovial fluid —*see* Abnormal, specimen, specified

Abnormal, abnormality, abnormalities — *(Continued)*
specimen *(Continued)*
thorax (bronchial washings) (pleural fluids) —*see* Abnormal, specimen, respiratory organs
vagina (secretion) (smear) R87.629
vulva (secretion) (smear) R87.69
wound secretion —*see* Abnormal, specimen, specified
spermatozoa —*see* Abnormal, specimen, male genital organs
sputum (amount) (color) (odor) R09.3
stool (color) (contents) (mucus) R19.5
bloody K92.1
guaiac positive R19.5
synchondrosis Q78.8
thermography —*see also* Abnormal, diagnostic imaging R93.8
thyroid-binding globulin E07.89
tooth, teeth (form) (size) K00.2
toxicology (findings) R78.9
transport protein E88.09
tumor marker NEC R97.8
ultrasound results —*see* Abnormal, diagnostic imaging
umbilical cord complicating delivery O69.9
urination NEC R39.198 ⟸
urine (constituents) R82.90
bile R82.2
cytological examination R82.8
drugs R82.5
fat R82.0
glucose R81
heavy metals R82.6
hemoglobin R82.3
histological examination R82.8
ketones R82.4
microbiological examination (culture) R82.79 ⟸
myoglobin R82.1
positive culture R82.79 ⟸
protein —*see* Proteinuria
specified substance NEC R82.99
chromoabnormality NEC R82.91
substances nonmedical R82.6
uterine hemorrhage —*see* Hemorrhage, uterus
vectorcardiogram R94.39
visually evoked potential (VEP) R94.112
white blood cells D72.9
specified NEC D72.89
X-ray examination —*see* Abnormal, diagnostic imaging

Abnormity (any organ or part) —*see* Anomaly
Abocclusion M26.29
hemolytic disease (newborn) P55.1
incompatibility reaction ABO —*see* Complication (s), transfusion, incompatibility reaction, ABO
Abolition, language R48.8
Aborter, habitual or recurrent —*see* Loss (of), pregnancy, recurrent
Abortion (complete) (spontaneous) O03.9
with
retained products of conception - see Abortion, incomplete
attempted (elective) (failed) O07.4
complicated by O07.30
afibrinogenemia O07.1
cardiac arrest O07.36
chemical damage of pelvic organ (s) O07.34
circulatory collapse O07.31
cystitis O07.38
defibrination syndrome O07.1
electrolyte imbalance O07.33
embolism (air) (amniotic fluid) (blood clot) (fat) (pulmonary) (septic) (soap) O07.2
endometritis O07.0

Abortion *(Continued)*
attempted *(Continued)*
complicated by *(Continued)*
genital tract and pelvic infection O07.0
hemolysis O07.1
hemorrhage (delayed) (excessive) O07.1
infection
genital tract or pelvic O07.0
urinary tract tract O07.38
intravascular coagulation O07.1
laceration of pelvic organ(s) O07.34
metabolic disorder O07.33
oliguria O07.32
oophoritis O07.0
parametritis O07.0
pelvic peritonitis O07.0
perforation of pelvic organ(s) O07.34
renal failure or shutdown O07.32
salpingitis or salpingo-oophoritis O07.0
sepsis O07.37
shock O07.31
specified condition NEC O07.39
tubular necrosis (renal) O07.32
uremia O07.32
urinary tract infection O07.38
venous complication NEC O07.35
embolism (air) (amniotic fluid) (blood clot) (fat) (pulmonary) (septic) (soap) O07.2
complicated (by) (following) O03.80
afibrinogenemia O03.6
cardiac arrest O03.86
chemical damage of pelvic organ (s) O03.84
circulatory collapse O03.81
cystitis O03.88
defibrination syndrome O03.6
electrolyte imbalance O03.83
embolism (air) (amniotic fluid) (blood clot) (fat) (pulmonary) (septic) (soap) O03.7
endometritis O03.5
genital tract and pelvic infection O03.5
hemolysis O03.6
hemorrhage (delayed) (excessive) O03.6
infection
genital tract or pelvic O03.5
urinary tract O03.88
intravascular coagulation O03.6
laceration of pelvic organ (s) O03.84
metabolic disorder O03.83
oliguria O03.82
oophoritis O03.5
parametritis O03.5
pelvic peritonitis O03.5
perforation of pelvic organ (s) O03.84
renal failure or shutdown O03.82
salpingitis or salpingo-oophoritis O03.5
sepsis O03.87
shock O03.81
specified condition NEC O03.89
tubular necrosis (renal) O03.82
uremia O03.82
urinary tract infection O03.88
venous complication NEC O03.85
embolism (air) (amniotic fluid) (blood clot) (fat) (pulmonary) (septic) (soap) O03.7
failed —*see* Abortion, attempted
habitual or recurrent N96
with current abortion —*see* categories O03-O06
without current pregnancy N96
care in current pregnancy O26.2-
incomplete (spontaneous) O03.4
complicated (by) (following) O03.30
afibrinogenemia O03.1
cardiac arrest O03.36
chemical damage of pelvic organ (s) O03.34
circulatory collapse O03.31
cystitis O03.38

Abortion *(Continued)*
  incomplete *(Continued)*
    complicated *(Continued)*
      defibrination syndrome O03.1
      electrolyte imbalance O03.33
      embolism (air) (amniotic fluid) (blood clot) (fat) (pulmonary) (septic) (soap) O03.2
      endometritis O03.0
      genital tract and pelvic infection O03.0
      hemolysis O03.1
      hemorrhage (delayed) (excessive) O03.1
      infection
        genital tract or pelvic O03.0
        urinary tract O03.38
      intravascular coagulation O03.1
      laceration of pelvic organ (s) O03.34
      metabolic disorder O03.33
      oliguria O03.32
      oophoritis O03.0
      parametritis O03.0
      pelvic peritonitis O03.0
      perforation of pelvic organ (s) O03.34
      renal failure or shutdown O03.32
      salpingitis or salpingo-oophoritis O03.0
      sepsis O03.37
      shock O03.31
      specified condition NEC O03.39
      tubular necrosis (renal) O03.32
      uremia O03.32
      urinary infection O03.38
      venous complication NEC O03.35
        embolism (air) (amniotic fluid) (blood clot) (fat) (pulmonary) (septic) (soap) O03.2
  induced (encounter for) Z33.2
    complicated by O04.80
      afibrinogenemia O04.6
      cardiac arrest O04.86
      chemical damage of pelvic organ (s) O04.84
      circulatory collapse O04.81
      cystitis O04.88
      defibrination syndrome O04.6
      electrolyte imbalance O04.83
      embolism (air) (amniotic fluid) (blood clot) (fat) (pulmonary) (septic) (soap) O04.7
      endometritis O04.5
      genital tract and pelvic infection O04.5
      hemolysis O04.6
      hemorrhage (delayed) (excessive) O04.6
      infection
        genital tract or pelvic O04.5
        urinary tract O04.88
      intravascular coagulation O04.6
      laceration of pelvic organ (s) O04.84
      metabolic disorder O04.83
      oliguria O04.82
      oophoritis O04.5
      parametritis O04.5
      pelvic peritonitis O04.5
      perforation of pelvic organ (s) O04.84
      renal failure or shutdown O04.82
      salpingitis or salpingo-oophoritis O04.5
      sepsis O04.87
      shock O04.81
      specified condition NEC O04.89
      tubular necrosis (renal) O04.82
      uremia O04.82
      urinary tract infection O04.88
      venous complication NEC O04.85
        embolism (air) (amniotic fluid) (blood clot) (fat) (pulmonary) (septic) (soap) O04.7
  missed O02.1
  spontaneous —*see* Abortion (complete) (spontaneous)
    threatened O20.0
  threatened (spontaneous) O20.0

Abortion *(Continued)*
  tubal O00.10 ⬅
    with intrauterine pregnancy O00.11 ◀
Abortus fever A23.1
Aboulomania F60.7
Abrami's disease D59.8
Abramov-Fiedler myocarditis (acute isolated myocarditis) I40.1
Abrasion T14.8
  abdomen, abdominal (wall) S30.811
  alveolar process S00.512
  ankle S90.51-
  antecubital space —*see* Abrasion, elbow
  anus S30.817
  arm (upper) S40.81-
  auditory canal —*see* Abrasion, ear
  auricle —*see* Abrasion, ear
  axilla —*see* Abrasion, arm
  back, lower S30.810
  breast S20.11-
  brow S00.81
  buttock S30.810
  calf —*see* Abrasion, leg
  canthus —*see* Abrasion, eyelid
  cheek S00.81
    internal S00.512
  chest wall —*see* Abrasion, thorax
  chin S00.81
  clitoris S30.814
  cornea S05.0-
  costal region —*see* Abrasion, thorax
  dental K03.1
  digit (s)
    foot —*see* Abrasion, toe
    hand —*see* Abrasion, finger
  ear S00.41-
  elbow S50.31-
  epididymis S30.813
  epigastric region S30.811
  epiglottis S10.11
  esophagus (thoracic) S27.818
    cervical S10.11
  eyebrow —*see* Abrasion, eyelid
  eyelid S00.21-
  face S00.81
  finger (s) S60.41-
    index S60.41-
    little S60.41-
    middle S60.41-
    ring S60.41-
  flank S30.811
  foot (except toe (s) alone) S90.81-
    toe —*see* Abrasion, toe
  forearm S50.81-
    elbow only —*see* Abrasion, elbow
  forehead S00.81
  genital organs, external
    female S30.816
    male S30.815
  groin S30.811
  gum S00.512
  hand S60.51-
  head S00.91
    ear —*see* Abrasion, ear
    eyelid —*see* Abrasion, eyelid
    lip S00.511
    nose S00.31
    oral cavity S00.512
    scalp S00.01
    specified site NEC S00.81
  heel —*see* Abrasion, foot
  hip S70.21-
  inguinal region S30.811
  interscapular region S20.419
  jaw S00.81
  knee S80.21-
  labium (majus) (minus) S30.814
  larynx S10.11
  leg (lower) S80.81-
    knee —*see* Abrasion, knee
    upper —*see* Abrasion, thigh

Abrasion *(Continued)*
  lip S00.511
  lower back S30.810
  lumbar region S30.810
  malar region S00.81
  mammary —*see* Abrasion, breast
  mastoid region S00.81
  mouth S00.512
  nail
    finger —*see* Abrasion, finger
    toe —*see* Abrasion, toe
  nape S10.81
  nasal S00.31
  neck S10.91
    specified site NEC S10.81
    throat S10.11
  nose S00.31
  occipital region S00.01
  oral cavity S00.512
  orbital region —*see* Abrasion, eyelid
  palate S00.512
  palm —*see* Abrasion, hand
  parietal region S00.01
  pelvis S30.810
  penis S30.812
  perineum
    female S30.814
    male S30.810
  periocular area —*see* Abrasion, eyelid
  phalanges
    finger —*see* Abrasion, finger
    toe —*see* Abrasion, toe
  pharynx S10.11
  pinna —*see* Abrasion, ear
  popliteal space —*see* Abrasion, knee
  prepuce S30.812
  pubic region S30.810
  pudendum
    female S30.816
    male S30.815
  sacral region S30.810
  scalp S00.01
  scapular region —*see* Abrasion, shoulder
  scrotum S30.813
  shin —*see* Abrasion, leg
  shoulder S40.21-
  skin NEC T14.8
  sternal region S20.319
  submaxillary region S00.81
  submental region S00.81
  subungual
    finger (s) —*see* Abrasion, finger
    toe (s) —*see* Abrasion, toe
  supraclavicular fossa S10.81
  supraorbital S00.81
  temple S00.81
  temporal region S00.81
  testis S30.813
  thigh S70.31-
  thorax, thoracic (wall) S20.91
    back S20.41-
    front S20.31-
  throat S10.11
  thumb S60.31-
  toe (s) (lesser) S90.416
    great S90.41-
  tongue S00.512
  tooth, teeth (dentifrice) (habitual) (hard tissues) (occupational) (ritual) (traditional) K03.1
  trachea S10.11
  tunica vaginalis S30.813
  tympanum, tympanic membrane —*see* Abrasion, ear
  uvula S00.512
  vagina S30.814
  vocal cords S10.11
  vulva S30.814
  wrist S60.81-
Abrism —*see* Poisoning, food, noxious, plant

A

Abruptio placentae O45.9-
  with
    afibrinogenemia O45.Ø1-
    coagulation defect O45.ØØ-
      specified NEC O45.Ø9-
    disseminated intravascular coagulation O45.Ø2-
    hypofibrinogenemia O45.Ø1-
  specified NEC O45.8-
Abruption, placenta —*see* Abruptio placentae
Abscess (connective tissue) (embolic) (fistulous) (infective) (metastatic) (multiple) (pernicious) (pyogenic) (septic) LØ2.91
  with
    diverticular disease (intestine) K57.8Ø
      with bleeding K57.81
      large intestine K57.2Ø
        with
          bleeding K57.21
          small intestine K57.4Ø
            with bleeding K57.41
      small intestine K57.ØØ
        with
          bleeding K57.Ø1
          large intestine K57.4Ø
            with bleeding K57.41
    lymphangitis - code by site under Abscess
  abdomen, abdominal
    cavity K65.1
    wall LØ2.211
  abdominopelvic K65.1
  accessory sinus —*see* Sinusitis
  adrenal (capsule) (gland) E27.8
  alveolar KØ4.7
    with sinus KØ4.6
  amebic AØ6.4
    brain (and liver or lung abscess) AØ6.6
    genitourinary tract AØ6.82
    liver (without mention of brain or lung abscess) AØ6.4
    lung (and liver) (without mention of brain abscess) AØ6.5
    specified site NEC AØ6.89
    spleen AØ6.89
  anerobic A48.Ø
  ankle —*see* Abscess, lower limb
  anorectal K61.2
  antecubital space —*see* Abscess, upper limb
  antrum (chronic) (Highmore) —*see* Sinusitis, maxillary
  anus K61.Ø
  apical (tooth) KØ4.7
    with sinus (alveolar) KØ4.6
  appendix K35.3
  areola (acute) (chronic) (nonpuerperal) N61.1 ⬅
    puerperal, postpartum or gestational —*see* Infection, nipple
  arm (any part) —*see* Abscess, upper limb
  artery (wall) I77.89
  atheromatous I77.2
  auricle, ear —*see* Abscess, ear, external
  axilla (region) LØ2.41-
    lymph gland or node LØ4.2
  back (any part, except buttock) LØ2.212
  Bartholin's gland N75.1
    with
      abortion —*see* Abortion, by type complicated by, sepsis
      ectopic or molar pregnancy OØ8.Ø
    following ectopic or molar pregnancy OØ8.Ø
  Bezold's —*see* Mastoiditis, acute
  bilharziasis B65.1
  bladder (wall) —*see* Cystitis, specified type NEC
  bone (subperiosteal) —*see also* Osteomyelitis, specified type NEC
    accessory sinus (chronic) —*see* Sinusitis
    chronic or old —*see* Osteomyelitis, chronic
    jaw (lower) (upper) M27.2

Abscess *(Continued)*
  bone *(Continued)*
    mastoid —*see* Mastoiditis, acute, subperiosteal
    petrous —*see* Petrositis
    spinal (tuberculous) A18.Ø1
      nontuberculous —*see* Osteomyelitis, vertebra
  bowel K63.Ø
  brain (any part) (cystic) (otogenic) GØ6.Ø
    amebic (with abscess of any other site) AØ6.6
    gonococcal A54.82
    pheomycotic (chromomycotic) B43.1
    tuberculous A17.81
  breast (acute) (chronic) (nonpuerperal) N61.1 ⬅
    newborn P39.Ø
    puerperal, postpartum, gestational —*see* Mastitis, obstetric, purulent
  broad ligament N73.2
    acute N73.Ø
    chronic N73.1
  Brodie's (localized) (chronic) M86.8X-
  bronchi J98.Ø9
  buccal cavity K12.2
  bulbourethral gland N34.Ø
  bursa M71.ØØ
    ankle M71.Ø7-
    elbow M71.Ø2-
    foot M71.Ø7-
    hand M71.Ø4-
    hip M71.Ø5-
    knee M71.Ø6-
    multiple sites M71.Ø9
    pharyngeal J39.1
    shoulder M71.Ø1-
    specified site NEC M71.Ø8
    wrist M71.Ø3-
  buttock LØ2.31
  canthus —*see* Blepharoconjunctivitis
  cartilage —*see* Disorder, cartilage, specified type NEC
  cecum K35.3
  cerebellum, cerebellar GØ6.Ø
    sequelae GØ9
  cerebral (embolic) GØ6.Ø
    sequelae GØ9
  cervical (meaning neck) LØ2.11
    lymph gland or node LØ4.Ø
  cervix (stump) (uteri) —*see* Cervicitis
  cheek (external) LØ2.Ø1
    inner K12.2
  chest J86.9
    with fistula J86.Ø
    wall LØ2.213
  chin LØ2.Ø1
  choroid —*see* Inflammation, chorioretinal
  circumtonsillar J36
  cold (lung) (tuberculous) —*see also* Tuberculosis, abscess, lung
    articular —*see* Tuberculosis, joint
  colon (wall) K63.Ø
  colostomy K94.Ø2
  conjunctiva —*see* Conjunctivitis, acute
  cornea H16.31-
  corpus
    cavernosum N48.21
    luteum —*see* Oophoritis
  Cowper's gland N34.Ø
  cranium GØ6.Ø
  cul-de-sac (Douglas') (posterior) —*see* Peritonitis, pelvic, female
  cutaneous —*see* Abscess, by site
  dental KØ4.7
    with sinus (alveolar) KØ4.6
  dentoalveolar KØ4.7
    with sinus KØ4.6
  diaphragm, diaphragmatic K65.1
  Douglas' cul-de-sac or pouch —*see* Peritonitis, pelvic, female
  Dubois A5Ø.59

Abscess *(Continued)*
  ear (middle) —*see also* Otitis, media, suppurative
    acute —*see* Otitis, media, suppurative, acute
    external H6Ø.Ø-
  entamebic —*see* Abscess, amebic
  enterostomy K94.12
  epididymis N45.4
  epidural GØ6.2
    brain GØ6.Ø
    spinal cord GØ6.1
  epiglottis J38.7
  epiploon, epiploic K65.1
  erysipelatous —*see* Erysipelas
  esophagus K2Ø.8
  ethmoid (bone) (chronic) (sinus) J32.2
  external auditory canal —*see* Abscess, ear, external
  extradural GØ6.2
    brain GØ6.Ø
      sequelae GØ9
    spinal cord GØ6.1
  extraperitoneal K68.19
  eye —*see* Endophthalmitis, purulent
  eyelid HØØ.Ø3-
  face (any part, except ear, eye and nose) LØ2.Ø1
  fallopian tube —*see* Salpingitis
  fascia M72.8
  fauces J39.1
  fecal K63.Ø
  femoral (region) —*see* Abscess, lower limb
  filaria, filarial —*see* Infestation, filarial
  finger (any) —*see also* Abscess, hand
    nail —*see* Cellulitis, finger
  foot LØ2.61-
  forehead LØ2.Ø1
  frontal sinus (chronic) J32.1
  gallbladder K81.Ø
  genital organ or tract
    female (external) N76.4
    male N49.9
      multiple sites N49.8
      specified NEC N49.8
  gestational mammary O91.11-
  gestational subareolar O91.11-
  gingival —*see* Peridontitis, aggressive, localized ⬅
  gland, glandular (lymph) (acute) —*see* Lymphadenitis, acute
  gluteal (region) LØ2.31
  gonorrheal —*see* Gonococcus
  groin LØ2.214
  gum —*see* Peridontitis, aggressive, localized ⬅
  hand LØ2.51-
  head NEC LØ2.811
    face (any part, except ear, eye and nose) LØ2.Ø1
  heart —*see* Carditis
  heel —*see* Abscess, foot
  helminthic —*see* Infestation, helminth
  hepatic (cholangitic) (hematogenic) (lymphogenic) (pylephlebitic) K75.Ø
    amebic AØ6.4
  hip (region) —*see* Abscess, lower limb
  ileocecal K35.3
  ileostomy (bud) K94.12
  iliac (region) LØ2.214
    fossa K35.3
  infraclavicular (fossa) —*see* Abscess, upper limb
  inguinal (region) LØ2.214
    lymph gland or node LØ4.1
  intestine, intestinal NEC K63.Ø
    rectal K61.1
  intra-abdominal —*see also* Abscess, peritoneum K65.1
    ~~postoperative T81.4~~
      ~~retroperitoneal K68.11~~
    postprocedural T81.43 ◀
      retroperitoneal K68.11 ◀
  intra-muscular, postprocedural T81.42 ◀

Abscess *(Continued)*
intracranial G06.0
intramammary —*see* Abscess, breast
intraorbital —*see* Abscess, orbit
intraperitoneal K65.1
intrasphincteric (anus) K61.4
intraspinal G06.1
intratonsillar J36
ischiorectal (fossa) K61.3
jaw (bone) (lower) (upper) M27.2
joint —*see* Arthritis, pyogenic or pyemic
spine (tuberculous) A18.01
nontuberculous —*see* Spondylopathy, infective
kidney N15.1
with calculus N20.0
with hydronephrosis N13.6
puerperal (postpartum) O86.21
knee —*see also* Abscess, lower limb
joint M00.9
labium (majus) (minus) N76.4
lacrimal
caruncle —*see* Inflammation, lacrimal, passages, acute
gland —*see* Dacryoadenitis
passages (duct) (sac) —*see* Inflammation, lacrimal, passages, acute
lacunar N34.0
larynx J38.7
lateral (alveolar) K04.7
with sinus K04.6
leg (any part) —*see* Abscess, lower limb
lens H27.8
lingual K14.0
tonsil J36
lip K13.0
Littre's gland N34.0
liver (cholangitic) (hematogenic) (lymphogenic) (pylephlebitic) (pyogenic) K75.0
amebic (due to Entamoeba histolytica) (dysenteric) (tropical) A06.4
with
brain abscess (and liver or lung abscess) A06.6
lung abscess A06.5
loin (region) L02.211
lower limb L02.41-
lumbar (tuberculous) A18.01
nontuberculous L02.212
lung (miliary) (putrid) J85.2
with pneumonia J85.1
due to specified organism (*see* Pneumonia, in (due to))
amebic (with liver abscess) A06.5
with
brain abscess A06.6
pneumonia A06.5
lymph, lymphatic, gland or node (acute) —*see also* Lymphadenitis, acute
mesentery I88.0
malar M27.2
mammary gland —*see* Abscess, breast
marginal, anus K61.0
mastoid —*see* Mastoiditis, acute
maxilla, maxillary M27.2
molar (tooth) K04.7
with sinus K04.6
premolar K04.7
sinus (chronic) J32.0
mediastinum J85.3
meibomian gland —*see* Hordeolum
meninges G06.2
mesentery, mesenteric K65.1
mesosalpinx —*see* Salpingitis
mons pubis L02.215
mouth (floor) K12.2
muscle —*see* Myositis, infective
myocardium I40.0
nabothian (follicle) —*see* Cervicitis
nasal J32.9
nasopharyngeal J39.1

Abscess *(Continued)*
navel L02.216
newborn P38.9
with mild hemorrhage P38.1
without hemorrhage P38.9
neck (region) L02.11
lymph gland or node L04.0
nephritic —*see* Abscess, kidney
nipple N61.1 ◄
associated with
lactation —*see* Pregnancy, complicated by ◄
pregnancy —*see* Pregnancy, complicated by
nose (external) (fossa) (septum) J34.0
sinus (chronic) —*see* Sinusitis
omentum K65.1
operative wound T81.40 ◄
orbit, orbital —*see* Cellulitis, orbit
otogenic G06.0
ovary, ovarian (corpus luteum) —*see* Oophoritis
oviduct —*see* Oophoritis
palate (soft) K12.2
hard M27.2
palmar (space) —*see* Abscess, hand
pancreas (duct) —*see* Pancreatitis, acute
parafrenal N48.21
parametric, parametrium N73.2
acute N73.0
chronic N73.1
paranephric N15.1
parapancreatic —*see* Pancreatitis, acute
parapharyngeal J39.0
pararectal K61.1
parasinus —*see* Sinusitis
parauterine (*see also* Disease, pelvis, inflammatory) N73.2
paravaginal —*see* Vaginitis
parietal region (scalp) L02.811
parodontal —*see* Peridontitis, aggressive, localized ◄
parotid (duct) (gland) K11.3
region K12.2
pectoral (region) L02.213
pelvis, pelvic
female —*see* Disease, pelvis, inflammatory
male, peritoneal K65.1
penis N48.21
gonococcal (accessory gland) (periurethral) A54.1
perianal K61.0
periapical K04.7
with sinus (alveolar) K04.6
periappendicular K35.3
pericardial I30.1
pericecal K35.3
pericemental —*see* Peridontitis, aggressive, localized ◄
pericholecystic —*see* Cholecystitis, acute
pericoronal —*see* Peridontitis, aggressive, localized ◄
peridental —*see* Peridontitis, aggressive, localized ◄
perimetric —*see also* Disease, pelvis, inflammatory N73.2
perinephric, perinephritic —*see* Abscess, kidney
perineum, perineal (superficial) L02.215
urethra N34.0
periodontal (parietal) —*see* Peridontitis, aggressive, localized ◄
apical K04.7
periosteum, periosteal —*see also* Osteomyelitis, specified type NEC
with osteomyelitis —*see also* Osteomyelitis, specified type NEC
acute —*see* Osteomyelitis, acute
chronic —*see* Osteomyelitis, chronic
peripharyngeal J39.0
peripleuritic J86.9
with fistula J86.0

Abscess *(Continued)*
periprostatic N41.2
perirectal K61.1
perirenal (tissue) —*see* Abscess, kidney
perisinuous (nose) —*see* Sinusitis
peritoneum, peritoneal (perforated) (ruptured) K65.1
with appendicitis K35.3
pelvic
female —*see* Peritonitis, pelvic, female
male K65.1
postoperative T81.43 ◄
puerperal, postpartum, childbirth O85
tuberculous A18.31
peritonsillar J36
perityphlic K35.3
periureteral N28.89
periurethral N34.0
gonococcal (accessory gland) (periurethral) A54.1
periuterine —*see also* Disease, pelvis, inflammatory N73.2
perivesical —*see* Cystitis, specified type NEC
petrous bone —*see* Petrositis
phagedenic NOS L02.91
chancroid A57
pharynx, pharyngeal (lateral) J39.1
pilonidal L05.01
pituitary (gland) E23.6
pleura J86.9
with fistula J86.0
popliteal —*see* Abscess, lower limb
postcecal K35.3
postlaryngeal J38.7
postnasal J34.0
postoperative (any site) T81.40 ◄
retroperitoneal K68.11
postpharyngeal J39.0
posttonsillar J36
post-typhoid A01.09
pouch of Douglas —*see* Peritonitis, pelvic, female
premammary —*see* Abscess, breast
prepatellar —*see* Abscess, lower limb
prostate N41.2
gonococcal (acute) (chronic) A54.22
psoas muscle K68.12
puerperal - code by site under Puerperal, abscess
pulmonary —*see* Abscess, lung
pulp, pulpal (dental) K04.01 ◄
irreversible K04.02 ◄
reversible K04.01 ◄
rectovaginal septum K63.0
rectovesical —*see* Cystitis, specified type NEC
rectum K61.1
renal —*see* Abscess, kidney
retina —*see* Inflammation, chorioretinal
retrobulbar —*see* Abscess, orbit
retrocecal K65.1
retrolaryngeal J38.7
retromammary —*see* Abscess, breast
retroperitoneal NEC K68.19
postprocedural K68.11
retropharyngeal J39.0
retrouterine —*see* Peritonitis, pelvic, female
retrovesical —*see* Cystitis, specified type NEC
root, tooth K04.7
with sinus (alveolar) K04.6
round ligament —*see also* Disease, pelvis, inflammatory N73.2
rupture (spontaneous) NOS L02.91
sacrum (tuberculous) A18.01
nontuberculous M46.28
salivary (duct) (gland) K11.3
scalp (any part) L02.811
scapular —*see* Osteomyelitis, specified type NEC
sclera —*see* Scleritis
scrofulous (tuberculous) A18.2
scrotum N49.2

A

Abscess *(Continued)*
seminal vesicle N49.Ø
septal, dental KØ4.7
with sinus (alveolar) KØ4.6
serous —*see* Periostitis
shoulder (region) —*see* Abscess, upper limb
sigmoid K63.Ø
sinus (accessory) (chronic) (nasal) —*see also* Sinusitis
intracranial venous (any) GØ6.Ø
Skene's duct or gland N34.Ø
skin —*see* Abscess, by site
specified site NEC LØ2.818
spermatic cord N49.1
sphenoidal (sinus) (chronic) J32.3
spinal cord (any part) (staphylococcal) GØ6.1
tuberculous A17.81
spine (column) (tuberculous) A18.Ø1
epidural GØ6.1
nontuberculous —*see* Osteomyelitis, vertebra
spleen D73.3
amebic AØ6.89
stitch T81.48 (revised)
subarachnoid GØ6.2
brain GØ6.Ø
spinal cord GØ6.1
subareolar —*see* Abscess, breast
subcecal K35.3
subcutaneous —*see also* Abscess, by site
pheomycotic (chromomycotic) B43.2
postprocedural T81.41 (new)
subdiaphragmatic K65.1
subdural GØ6.2
brain GØ6.Ø
sequelae GØ9
spinal cord GØ6.1
subgaleal LØ2.811
subhepatic K65.1
sublingual K12.2
gland K11.3
submammary —*see* Abscess, breast
submandibular (region) (space) (triangle) K12.2
gland K11.3
submaxillary (region) LØ2.Ø1
gland K11.3
submental LØ2.Ø1
gland K11.3
subperiosteal —*see* Osteomyelitis, specified type NEC
subphrenic K65.1
postoperative T81.43 (revised)
suburethral N34.Ø
sudoriparous L75.8
supraclavicular (fossa) —*see* Abscess, upper limb
suprapelvic, acute N73.Ø
suprarenal (capsule) (gland) E27.8
sweat gland L74.8
tear duct —*see* Inflammation, lacrimal, passages, acute
temple LØ2.Ø1
temporal region LØ2.Ø1
temporosphenoidal GØ6.Ø
tendon (sheath) M65.ØØ
ankle M65.Ø7-
foot M65.Ø7-
forearm M65.Ø3-
hand M65.Ø4-
lower leg M65.Ø6-
pelvic region M65.Ø5-
shoulder region M65.Ø1-
specified site NEC M65.Ø8
thigh M65.Ø5-
upper arm M65.Ø2-
testis N45.4
thigh —*see* Abscess, lower limb
thorax J86.9
with fistula J86.Ø
throat J39.1
thumb —*see also* Abscess, hand
nail —*see* Cellulitis, finger

Abscess *(Continued)*
thymus (gland) E32.1
thyroid (gland) EØ6.Ø
toe (any) —*see also* Abscess, foot
nail —*see* Cellulitis, toe
tongue (staphylococcal) K14.Ø
tonsil (s) (lingual) J36
tonsillopharyngeal J36
tooth, teeth (root) KØ4.7
with sinus (alveolar) KØ4.6
supporting structures NEC —*see* Peridontitis, aggressive, localized (revised)
trachea J39.8
trunk LØ2.219
abdominal wall LØ2.211
back LØ2.212
chest wall LØ2.213
groin LØ2.214
perineum LØ2.215
umbilicus LØ2.216
tubal —*see* Salpingitis
tuberculous —*see* Tuberculosis, abscess
tubo-ovarian —*see* Salpingo-oophoritis
tunica vaginalis N49.1
umbilicus LØ2.216
upper
limb LØ2.41-
respiratory J39.8
urethral (gland) N34.Ø
urinary N34.Ø
uterus, uterine (wall) —*see also* Endometritis
ligament —*see also* Disease, pelvis, inflammatory N73.2
neck —*see* Cervicitis
uvula K12.2
vagina (wall) —*see* Vaginitis
vaginorectal —*see* Vaginitis
vas deferens N49.1
vermiform appendix K35.3
vertebra (column) (tuberculous) A18.Ø1
nontuberculous —*see* Osteomyelitis, vertebra
vesical —*see* Cystitis, specified type NEC
vesico-uterine pouch —*see* Peritonitis, pelvic, female
vitreous (humor) —*see* Endophthalmitis, purulent
vocal cord J38.3
von Bezold's —*see* Mastoiditis, acute
vulva N76.4
vulvovaginal gland N75.1
web space —*see* Abscess, hand
wound T81.4Ø (revised)
wrist —*see* Abscess, upper limb

Absence (of) (organ or part) (complete or partial)
adrenal (gland) (congenital) Q89.1
acquired E89.6
albumin in blood E88.Ø9
alimentary tract (congenital) Q45.8
upper Q4Ø.8
alveolar process (acquired) —*see* Anomaly, alveolar
ankle (acquired) Z89.44-
anus (congenital) Q42.3
with fistula Q42.2
aorta (congenital) Q25.41 (revised)
appendix, congenital Q42.8
arm (acquired) Z89.2Ø-
above elbow Z89.22-
congenital (with hand present) —*see* Agenesis, arm, with hand present
and hand —*see* Agenesis, forearm, and hand
below elbow Z89.21-
congenital (with hand present) —*see* Agenesis, arm, with hand present
and hand —*see* Agenesis, forearm, and hand
congenital —*see* Defect, reduction, upper limb

Absence *(Continued)*
arm *(Continued)*
shoulder (following explantation of shoulder joint prosthesis) (joint) (with or without presence of antibiotic-impregnated cement spacer) Z89.23-
congenital (with hand present) —*see* Agenesis, arm, with hand present
artery (congenital) (peripheral) Q27.8
brain Q28.3
coronary Q24.5
pulmonary Q25.79
specified NEC Q27.8
umbilical Q27.Ø
atrial septum (congenital) Q21.1
auditory canal (congenital) (external) Q16.1
auricle (ear), congenital Q16.Ø
bile, biliary duct, congenital Q44.5
bladder (acquired) Z9Ø.6
congenital Q64.5
bowel sounds R19.11
brain QØØ.Ø
part of QØ4.3
breast (s) (and nipple (s)) (acquired) Z9Ø.1-
congenital Q83.8
broad ligament Q5Ø.6
bronchus (congenital) Q32.4
canaliculus lacrimalis, congenital Q1Ø.4
cerebellum (vermis) QØ4.3
cervix (acquired) (with uterus) Z9Ø.71Ø
with remaining uterus Z9Ø.712
congenital Q51.5
chin, congenital Q18.8
cilia (congenital) Q1Ø.3
acquired —*see* Madarosis
clitoris (congenital) Q52.6
coccyx, congenital Q76.49
cold sense R2Ø.8
congenital
lumen —*see* Atresia
organ or site NEC —*see* Agenesis
septum —*see* Imperfect, closure
corpus callosum QØ4.Ø
cricoid cartilage, congenital Q31.8
diaphragm (with hernia), congenital Q79.1
digestive organ (s) or tract, congenital Q45.8
acquired NEC Z9Ø.49
upper Q4Ø.8
ductus arteriosus Q28.8
duodenum (acquired) Z9Ø.49
congenital Q41.Ø
ear, congenital Q16.9
acquired H93.8-
auricle Q16.Ø
external Q16.Ø
inner Q16.5
lobe, lobule Q17.8
middle, except ossicles Q16.4
ossicles Q16.3
ossicles Q16.3
ejaculatory duct (congenital) Q55.4
endocrine gland (congenital) NEC Q89.2
acquired E89.89
epididymis (congenital) Q55.4
acquired Z9Ø.79
epiglottis, congenital Q31.8
esophagus (congenital) Q39.8
acquired (partial) Z9Ø.49
eustachian tube (congenital) Q16.2
extremity (acquired) Z89.9
congenital Q73.Ø
knee (following explantation of knee joint prosthesis) (joint) (with or without presence of antibiotic-impregnated cement spacer) Z89.52-
lower (above knee) Z89.619
below knee Z89.51-
upper —*see* Absence, arm
eye (acquired) Z9Ø.Ø1
congenital Q11.1
muscle (congenital) Q1Ø.3

◄ New ◄ Revised ~~deleted~~ Deleted

Absence *(Continued)*
eyeball (acquired) Z90.01
eyelid (fold) (congenital) Q10.3
acquired Z90.01
face, specified part NEC Q18.8
fallopian tube (s) (acquired) Z90.79
congenital Q50.6
family member (causing problem in home) NEC —*see also* Disruption, family Z63.32
femur, congenital —*see* Defect, reduction, lower limb, longitudinal, femur
fibrinogen (congenital) D68.2
acquired D65
finger (s) (acquired) Z89.02-
congenital —*see* Agenesis, hand
foot (acquired) Z89.43-
congenital —*see* Agenesis, foot
forearm (acquired) —*see* Absence, arm, below elbow
gallbladder (acquired) Z90.49
congenital Q44.0
gamma globulin in blood D80.1
hereditary D80.0
genital organs
acquired (female) (male) Z90.79
female, congenital Q52.8
external Q52.71
internal NEC Q52.8
male, congenital Q55.8
genitourinary organs, congenital NEC
female Q52.8
male Q55.8
globe (acquired) Z90.01
congenital Q11.1
glottis, congenital Q31.8
hand and wrist (acquired) Z89.11-
congenital —*see* Agenesis, hand
head, part (acquired) NEC Z90.09
heat sense R20.8
hip (following explantation of hip joint prosthesis) (joint) (with or without presence of antibiotic-impregnated cement spacer) Z89.62-
hymen (congenital) Q52.4
ileum (acquired) Z90.49
congenital Q41.2
immunoglobulin, isolated NEC D80.3
IgA D80.2
IgG D80.3
IgM D80.4
incus (acquired) —*see* Loss, ossicles, ear
congenital Q16.3
inner ear, congenital Q16.5
intestine (acquired) (small) Z90.49
congenital Q41.9
specified NEC Q41.8
large Z90.49
congenital Q42.9
specified NEC Q42.8
iris, congenital Q13.1
jejunum (acquired) Z90.49
congenital Q41.1
joint
acquired
hip (following explantation of hip joint prosthesis) (with or without presence of antibiotic-impregnated cement spacer) Z89.62-
knee (following explantation of knee joint prosthesis) (with or without presence of antibiotic-impregnated cement spacer) Z89.52-
shoulder (following explantation of shoulder joint prosthesis) (with or without presence of antibiotic-impregnated cement spacer) Z89.23-
congenital NEC Q74.8
kidney (s) (acquired) Z90.5
congenital Q60.2
bilateral Q60.1
unilateral Q60.0

Absence *(Continued)*
knee (following explantation of knee joint prosthesis) (joint) (with or without presence of antibiotic-impregnated cement spacer) Z89.52-
labyrinth, membranous Q16.5
larynx (congenital) Q31.8
acquired Z90.02
leg (acquired) (above knee) Z89.61-
below knee (acquired) Z89.51-
congenital —*see* Defect, reduction, lower limb
lens (acquired) —*see also* Aphakia
congenital Q12.3
post cataract extraction Z98.4-
limb (acquired) —*see* Absence, extremity
lip Q38.6
liver (congenital) Q44.7
lung (fissure) (lobe) (bilateral) (unilateral) (congenital) Q33.3
acquired (any part) Z90.2
menstruation —*see* Amenorrhea
muscle (congenital) (pectoral) Q79.8
ocular Q10.3
neck, part Q18.8
neutrophil —*see* Agranulocytosis
nipple (s) (with breast (s)) (acquired) Z90.1-
congenital Q83.2
nose (congenital) Q30.1
acquired Z90.09
organ
of Corti, congenital Q16.5
or site, congenital NEC Q89.8
acquired NEC Z90.89
osseous meatus (ear) Q16.4
ovary (acquired)
bilateral Z90.722
congenital
bilateral Q50.02
unilateral Q50.01
unilateral Z90.721
oviduct (acquired)
bilateral Z90.722
congenital Q50.6
unilateral Z90.721
pancreas (congenital) Q45.0
acquired Z90.410
complete Z90.410
partial Z90.411
total Z90.410
parathyroid gland (acquired) E89.2
congenital Q89.2
patella, congenital Q74.1
penis (congenital) Q55.5
acquired Z90.79
pericardium (congenital) Q24.8
pituitary gland (congenital) Q89.2
acquired E89.3
prostate (acquired) Z90.79
congenital Q55.4
pulmonary valve Q22.0
punctum lacrimale (congenital) Q10.4
radius, congenital —*see* Defect, reduction, upper limb, longitudinal, radius
rectum (congenital) Q42.1
with fistula Q42.0
acquired Z90.49
respiratory organ NOS Q34.9
rib (acquired) Z90.89
congenital Q76.6
sacrum, congenital Q76.49
salivary gland (s), congenital Q38.4
scrotum, congenital Q55.29
seminal vesicles (congenital) Q55.4
acquired Z90.79
septum
atrial (congenital) Q21.1
between aorta and pulmonary artery Q21.4
ventricular (congenital) Q20.4
sex chromosome
female phenotype Q97.8
male phenotype Q98.8

Absence *(Continued)*
skull bone (congenital) Q75.8
with
anencephaly Q00.0
encephalocele —*see* Encephalocele
hydrocephalus Q03.9
with spina bifida —*see* Spina bifida, by site, with hydrocephalus
microcephaly Q02
spermatic cord, congenital Q55.4
spine, congenital Q76.49
spleen (congenital) Q89.01
acquired Z90.81
sternum, congenital Q76.7
stomach (acquired) (partial) Z90.3
congenital Q40.2
superior vena cava, congenital Q26.8
teeth, tooth (congenital) K00.0
acquired (complete) K08.109
class I K08.101
class II K08.102
class III K08.103
class IV K08.104
due to
caries K08.139
class I K08.131
class II K08.132
class III K08.133
class IV K08.134
periodontal disease K08.129
class I K08.121
class II K08.122
class III K08.123
class IV K08.124
specified NEC K08.199
class I K08.191
class II K08.192
class III K08.193
class IV K08.194
trauma K08.119
class I K08.111
class II K08.112
class III K08.113
class IV K08.114
partial K08.409
class I K08.401
class II K08.402
class III K08.403
class IV K08.404
due to
caries K08.439
class I K08.431
class II K08.432
class III K08.433
class IV K08.434
periodontal disease K08.429
class I K08.421
class II K08.422
class III K08.423
class IV K08.424
specified NEC K08.499
class I K08.491
class II K08.492
class III K08.493
class IV K08.494
trauma K08.419
class I K08.411
class II K08.412
class III K08.413
class IV K08.414
tendon (congenital) Q79.8
testis (congenital) Q55.0
acquired Z90.79
thumb (acquired) Z89.01-
congenital —*see* Agenesis, hand
thymus gland Q89.2
thyroid (gland) (acquired) E89.0
cartilage, congenital Q31.8
congenital E03.1

A

Absence *(Continued)*
  toe (s) (acquired) Z89.42-
    with foot —*see* Absence, foot and ankle
    congenital —*see* Agenesis, foot
    great Z89.41-
  tongue, congenital Q38.3
  trachea (cartilage), congenital Q32.1
  transverse aortic arch, congenital Q25.49 ⬅
  tricuspid valve Q22.4
  umbilical artery, congenital Q27.Ø
  upper arm and forearm with hand present, congenital —*see* Agenesis, arm, with hand present
  ureter (congenital) Q62.4
    acquired Z9Ø.6
  urethra, congenital Q64.5
  uterus (acquired) Z9Ø.71Ø
    with cervix Z9Ø.71Ø
    with remaining cervical stump Z9Ø.711
    congenital Q51.Ø
  uvula, congenital Q38.5
  vagina, congenital Q52.Ø
  vas deferens (congenital) Q55.4
    acquired Z9Ø.79
  vein (peripheral) congenital NEC Q27.8
    cerebral Q28.3
    digestive system Q27.8
    great Q26.8
    lower limb Q27.8
    portal Q26.5
    precerebral Q28.1
    specified site NEC Q27.8
    upper limb Q27.8
  vena cava (inferior) (superior), congenital Q26.8
  ventricular septum Q2Ø.4
  vertebra, congenital Q76.49
  vulva, congenital Q52.71
  wrist (acquired) Z89.12-
Absorbent system disease I87.8
Absorption
  carbohydrate, disturbance K9Ø.49 ⬅
  chemical —*see* Table of Drugs and Chemicals
    through placenta (newborn) PØ4.9
      environmental substance PØ4.6
      nutritional substance PØ4.5
      obstetric anesthetic or analgesic drug PØ4.Ø
  drug NEC —*see* Table of Drugs and Chemicals
    addictive
      through placenta (newborn) PØ4.49
        cocaine PØ4.41
    medicinal
      through placenta (newborn) PØ4.1
    through placenta (newborn) PØ4.1
      obstetric anesthetic or analgesic drug PØ4.Ø
  fat, disturbance K9Ø.49 ⬅
    pancreatic K9Ø.3
  noxious substance —*see* Table of Drugs and Chemicals
  protein, disturbance K9Ø.49 ⬅
  starch, disturbance K9Ø.49 ⬅
  toxic substance —*see* Table of Drugs and Chemicals
  uremic —*see* Uremia
Abstinence symptoms, syndrome
  alcohol F1Ø.239
    with delirium F1Ø.231
  cocaine F14.23
  neonatal P96.1
  nicotine —*see* Dependence, drug, nicotine, with, withdrawal
  opioid F11.93
    with dependence F11.23
Abstinence symptoms, syndrome *(Continued)*
  psychoactive NEC F19.939
    with
      delirium F19.931
      dependence F19.239
        with
          delirium F19.231
          perceptual disturbance F19.232
        uncomplicated F19.23Ø
      perceptual disturbance F19.932
    uncomplicated F19.93Ø
  sedative F13.939
    with
      delirium F13.931
      dependence F13.239
        with
          delirium F13.231
          perceptual disturbance F13.232
        uncomplicated F13.23Ø
      perceptual disturbance F13.932
    uncomplicated F13.93Ø
  stimulant NEC F15.93
    with dependence F15.23
Abulia R68.89
Abulomania F6Ø.7
Abuse
  adult —*see* Maltreatment, adult
    as reason for
      couple seeking advice (including offender) Z63.Ø
  alcohol (non-dependent) F1Ø.1Ø
    with
      anxiety disorder F1Ø.18Ø
      intoxication F1Ø.129
        with delirium F1Ø.121
        uncomplicated F1Ø.12Ø
      mood disorder F1Ø.14
      other specified disorder F1Ø.188
      psychosis F1Ø.159
        delusions F1Ø.15Ø
        hallucinations F1Ø.151
      sexual dysfunction F1Ø.181
      sleep disorder F1Ø.182
      unspecified disorder F1Ø.19
    counseling and surveillance Z71.41
  amphetamine (or related substance) —*see* Abuse, drug, stimulant NEC
  analgesics (non-prescribed) (over the counter) F55.8
  antacids F55.Ø
  antidepressants —*see* Abuse, drug, psychoactive NEC
  anxiolytic —*see* Abuse, drug, sedative
  barbiturates —*see* Abuse, drug, sedative
  caffeine —*see* Abuse, drug, stimulant NEC
  cannabis, cannabinoids —*see* Abuse, drug, cannabis
  child —*see* Maltreatment, child
  cocaine —*see* Abuse, drug, cocaine
  drug NEC (non-dependent) F19.1Ø
    with sleep disorder F19.182
    amphetamine type —*see* Abuse, drug, stimulant NEC
    analgesics (non-prescribed) (over the counter) F55.8
    antacids F55.Ø
    antidepressants —*see* Abuse, drug, psychoactive NEC
    anxiolytics —*see* Abuse, drug, sedative
    barbiturates —*see* Abuse, drug, sedative
    caffeine —*see* Abuse, drug, stimulant NEC
    cannabis F12.1Ø
      with
        anxiety disorder F12.18Ø
        intoxication F12.129
          with
            delirium F12.121
            perceptual disturbance F12.122
          uncomplicated F12.12Ø
        other specified disorder F12.188
Abuse *(Continued)*
  drug NEC *(Continued)*
    cannabis *(Continued)*
      with *(Continued)*
        psychosis F12.159
          delusions F12.15Ø
          hallucinations F12.151
        unspecified disorder F12.19
    cocaine F14.1Ø
      with
        anxiety disorder F14.18Ø
        intoxication F14.129
          with
            delirium F14.121
            perceptual disturbance F14.122
          uncomplicated F14.12Ø
        mood disorder F14.14
        other specified disorder F14.188
        psychosis F14.159
          delusions F14.15Ø
          hallucinations F14.151
        sexual dysfunction F14.181
        sleep disorder F14.182
        unspecified disorder F14.19
    counseling and surveillance Z71.51
    hallucinogen F16.1Ø
      with
        anxiety disorder F16.18Ø
        flashbacks F16.183
        intoxication F16.129
          with
            delirium F16.121
            perceptual disturbance F16.122
          uncomplicated F16.12Ø
        mood disorder F16.14
        other specified disorder F16.188
        perception disorder, persisting F16.183
        psychosis F16.159
          delusions F16.15Ø
          hallucinations F16.151
        unspecified disorder F16.19
    hashish —*see* Abuse, drug, cannabis
    herbal or folk remedies F55.1
    hormones F55.3
    hypnotics —*see* Abuse, drug, sedative
    inhalant F18.1Ø
      with
        anxiety disorder F18.18Ø
        dementia, persisting F18.17
        intoxication F18.129
          with delirium F18.121
          uncomplicated F18.12Ø
        mood disorder F18.14
        other specified disorder F18.188
        psychosis F18.159
          delusions F18.15Ø
          hallucinations F18.151
        unspecified disorder F18.19
    laxatives F55.2
    LSD —*see* Abuse, drug, hallucinogen
    marihuana —*see* Abuse, drug, cannabis
    morphine type (opioids) —*see* Abuse, drug, opioid
    opioid F11.1Ø
      with
        intoxication F11.129
          with
            delirium F11.121
            perceptual disturbance F11.122
          uncomplicated F11.12Ø
        mood disorder F11.14
        other specified disorder F11.188
        psychosis F11.159
          delusions F11.15Ø
          hallucinations F11.151
        sexual dysfunction F11.181
        sleep disorder F11.182
        unspecified disorder F11.19
    PCP (phencyclidine) (or related substance) —*see* Abuse, drug, hallucinogen

Abuse *(Continued)*
drug NEC *(Continued)*
psychoactive NEC F19.10
with
amnestic disorder F19.16
anxiety disorder F19.180
dementia F19.17
intoxication F19.129
with
delirium F19.121
perceptual disturbance F19.122
uncomplicated F19.120
mood disorder F19.14
other specified disorder F19.188
psychosis F19.159
delusions F19.150
hallucinations F19.151
sexual dysfunction F19.181
sleep disorder F19.182
unspecified disorder F19.19
sedative, hypnotic or anxiolytic F13.10
with
anxiety disorder F13.180
intoxication F13.129
with delirium F13.121
uncomplicated F13.120
mood disorder F13.14
other specified disorder F13.188
psychosis F13.159
delusions F13.150
hallucinations F13.151
sexual dysfunction F13.181
sleep disorder F13.182
unspecified disorder F13.19
solvent —*see* Abuse, drug, inhalant
steroids F55.3
stimulant NEC F15.10
with
anxiety disorder F15.180
intoxication F15.129
with
delirium F15.121
perceptual disturbance F15.122
uncomplicated F15.120
mood disorder F15.14
other specified disorder F15.188
psychosis F15.159
delusions F15.150
hallucinations F15.151
sexual dysfunction F15.181
sleep disorder F15.182
unspecified disorder F15.19
tranquilizers —*see* Abuse, drug, sedative
vitamins F55.4
hallucinogens —*see* Abuse, drug, hallucinogen
hashish —*see* Abuse, drug, cannabis
herbal or folk remedies F55.1
hormones F55.3
hypnotic —*see* Abuse, drug, sedative
inhalant —*see* Abuse, drug, inhalant
laxatives F55.2
LSD —*see* Abuse, drug, hallucinogen
marihuana —*see* Abuse, drug, cannabis
morphine type (opioids) —*see* Abuse, drug, opioid
non-psychoactive substance NEC F55.8
antacids F55.0
folk remedies F55.1
herbal remedies F55.1
hormones F55.3
laxatives F55.2
steroids F55.3
vitamins F55.4
opioids —*see* Abuse, drug, opioid
PCP (phencyclidine) (or related substance) —*see* Abuse, drug, hallucinogen
physical (adult) (child) —*see* Maltreatment
psychoactive substance —*see* Abuse, drug, psychoactive NEC

Abuse *(Continued)*
psychological (adult) (child) —*see* Maltreatment
sedative —*see* Abuse, drug, sedative
sexual —*see* Maltreatment
solvent —*see* Abuse, drug, inhalant
steroids F55.3
vitamins F55.4
Acalculia R48.8
developmental F81.2
Acanthamebiasis (with) B60.10
conjunctiva B60.12
keratoconjunctivitis B60.13
meningoencephalitis B60.11
other specified B60.19
Acanthocephaliasis B83.8
Acanthocheilonemiasis B74.4
Acanthocytosis E78.6
Acantholysis L11.9
Acanthosis (acquired) (nigricans) L83
benign Q82.8
congenital Q82.8
seborrheic L82.1
inflamed L82.0
tongue K14.3
Acapnia E87.3
Acarbia E87.2
Acardia, acardius Q89.8
Acardiacus amorphus Q89.8
Acardiotrophia I51.4
Acariasis B88.0
scabies B86
Acarodermatitis (urticarioides) B88.0
Acarophobia F40.218
Acatalasemia, acatalasia E80.3
Acathisia (drug induced) G25.71
Accelerated atrioventricular conduction I45.6
Accentuation of personality traits (type A) Z73.1
Accessory (congenital)
adrenal gland Q89.1
anus Q43.4
appendix Q43.4
atrioventricular conduction I45.6
auditory ossicles Q16.3
auricle (ear) Q17.0
biliary duct or passage Q44.5
bladder Q64.79
blood vessels NEC Q27.9
coronary Q24.5
bone NEC Q79.8
breast tissue, axilla Q83.1
carpal bones Q74.0
cecum Q43.4
chromosome (s) NEC (nonsex) Q92.9
with complex rearrangements NEC Q92.5
seen only at prometaphase Q92.8
13 —*see* Trisomy, 13
18 —*see* Trisomy, 18
21 —*see* Trisomy, 21
partial Q92.9
sex
female phenotype Q97.8
coronary artery Q24.5
cusp (s), heart valve NEC Q24.8
pulmonary Q22.3
cystic duct Q44.5
digit (s) Q69.9
ear (auricle) (lobe) Q17.0
endocrine gland NEC Q89.2
eye muscle Q10.3
eyelid Q10.3
face bone (s) Q75.8
fallopian tube (fimbria) (ostium) Q50.6
finger (s) Q69.0
foreskin N47.8
frontonasal process Q75.8

Accessory *(Continued)*
gallbladder Q44.1
genital organ (s)
female Q52.8
external Q52.79
internal NEC Q52.8
male Q55.8
genitourinary organs NEC Q89.8
female Q52.8
male Q55.8
hallux Q69.2
heart Q24.8
valve NEC Q24.8
pulmonary Q22.3
hepatic ducts Q44.5
hymen Q52.4
intestine (large) (small) Q43.4
kidney Q63.0
lacrimal canal Q10.6
leaflet, heart valve NEC Q24.8
ligament, broad Q50.6
liver Q44.7
duct Q44.5
lobule (ear) Q17.0
lung (lobe) Q33.1
muscle Q79.8
navicular of carpus Q74.0
nervous system, part NEC Q07.8
nipple Q83.3
nose Q30.8
organ or site not listed —*see* Anomaly, by site
ovary Q50.31
oviduct Q50.6
pancreas Q45.3
parathyroid gland Q89.2
parotid gland (and duct) Q38.4
pituitary gland Q89.2
preauricular appendage Q17.0
prepuce N47.8
renal arteries (multiple) Q27.2
rib Q76.6
cervical Q76.5
roots (teeth) K00.2
salivary gland Q38.4
sesamoid bones Q74.8
foot Q74.2
hand Q74.0
skin tags Q82.8
spleen Q89.09
sternum Q76.7
submaxillary gland Q38.4
tarsal bones Q74.2
teeth, tooth K00.1
tendon Q79.8
thumb Q69.1
thymus gland Q89.2
thyroid gland Q89.2
toes Q69.2
tongue Q38.3
tooth, teeth K00.1
tragus Q17.0
ureter Q62.5
urethra Q64.79
urinary organ or tract NEC Q64.8
uterus Q51.2
vagina Q52.10
valve, heart NEC Q24.8
pulmonary Q22.3
vertebra Q76.49
vocal cords Q31.8
vulva Q52.79
Accident
birth —*see* Birth, injury
cardiac —*see* Infarct, myocardium
cerebral I63.9
cerebrovascular (embolic) (ischemic) (thrombotic) I63.9
aborted I63.9
hemorrhagic —*see* Hemorrhage, intracranial, intracerebral

A

Accident *(Continued)*
  cerebrovascular *(Continued)*
    old (without sequelae) Z86.73
      with sequelae (of) —*see* Sequelae, infarction, cerebral
  coronary —*see* Infarct, myocardium
  craniovascular I63.9
  vascular, brain I63.9
Accidental —*see* condition
Accommodation (disorder) —*see also* condition
  hysterical paralysis of F44.89
  insufficiency of H52.4
  paresis —*see* Paresis, of accommodation
  spasm —*see* Spasm, of accommodation
Accouchement —*see* Delivery
Accreta placenta O43.21-
Accretio cordis (nonrheumatic) I31.Ø
Accretions, tooth, teeth KØ3.6
Acculturation difficulty Z6Ø.3
Accumulation secretion, prostate N42.89
Acephalia, acephalism, acephalus, acephaly QØØ.Ø
Acephalobrachia monster Q89.8
Acephalochirus monster Q89.8
Acephalogaster Q89.8
Acephalostomus monster Q89.8
Acephalothorax Q89.8
Acerophobia F4Ø.298
Acetonemia R79.89
  in Type 1 diabetes E1Ø.1Ø
    with coma E1Ø.11
Acetonuria R82.4
Achalasia (cardia) (esophagus) K22.Ø
  congenital Q39.5
  pylorus Q4Ø.Ø
  sphincteral NEC K59.8
Ache (s) —*see* Pain
Acheilia Q38.6
Achillobursitis —*see* Tendinitis, Achilles
Achillodynia —*see* Tendinitis, Achilles
Achlorhydria, achlorhydric (neurogenic) K31.83
  anemia D5Ø.8
  diarrhea K31.83
  psychogenic F45.8
  secondary to vagotomy K91.1
Achluophobia F4Ø.228
Acholia K82.8
Acholuric jaundice (familial) (splenomegalic) —*see also* Spherocytosis
  acquired D59.8
Achondrogenesis Q77.Ø
Achondroplasia (osteosclerosis congenita) Q77.4
Achroma, cutis L8Ø
Achromat (ism), achromatopsia (acquired) (congenital) H53.51
Achromia, congenital —*see* Albinism
Achromia parasitica B36.Ø
Achylia gastrica K31.89
  psychogenic F45.8
Acid
  burn —*see* Corrosion
  deficiency
    amide nicotinic E52
    ascorbic E54
    folic E53.8
    nicotinic E52
    pantothenic E53.8
  intoxication E87.2
  peptic disease K3Ø
  phosphatase deficiency E83.39
  stomach K3Ø
    psychogenic F45.8
Acidemia E87.2
  argininosuccinic E72.22
  isovaleric E71.11Ø
  metabolic (newborn) P19.9
    first noted before onset of labor P19.Ø
    first noted during labor P19.1
    noted at birth P19.2
Acidemia *(Continued)*
  methylmalonic E71.12Ø
  pipecolic E72.3
  propionic E71.121
Acidity, gastric (high) K3Ø
  psychogenic F45.8
Acidocytopenia —*see* Agranulocytosis
Acidocytosis D72.1
Acidopenia —*see* Agranulocytosis
Acidosis (lactic) (respiratory) E87.2
  in Type 1 diabetes E1Ø.1Ø
    with coma E1Ø.11
  kidney, tubular N25.89
  lactic E87.2
  metabolic NEC E87.2
    with respiratory acidosis E87.4
    late, of newborn P74.Ø
  mixed metabolic and respiratory, newborn P84
  newborn P84
  renal (hyperchloremic) (tubular) N25.89
  respiratory E87.2
    complicated by
      metabolic
        acidosis E87.4
        alkalosis E87.4
Aciduria
  argininosuccinic E72.22
  glutaric (type I) E72.3
    type II E71.313
    type III E71.5-
  orotic (congenital) (hereditary) (pyrimidine deficiency) E79.8
    anemia D53.Ø
Acladiosis (skin) B36.Ø
Aclasis, diaphyseal Q78.6
Acleistocardia Q21.1
Aclusion —*see* Anomaly, dentofacial, malocclusion
Acne L7Ø.9
  artificialis L7Ø.8
  atrophica L7Ø.2
  cachecticorum (Hebra) L7Ø.8
  conglobata L7Ø.1
  cystic L7Ø.Ø
  decalvans L66.2
  ~~excoriée des jeunes filles L70.5~~
  excoriée (des jeunes filles) L7Ø.5 ◀
  frontalis L7Ø.2
  indurata L7Ø.Ø
  infantile L7Ø.4
  keloid L73.Ø
  lupoid L7Ø.2
  necrotic, necrotica (miliaris) L7Ø.2
  neonatal L7Ø.4
  nodular L7Ø.Ø
  occupational L7Ø.8
  picker's L7Ø.5
  pustular L7Ø.Ø
  rodens L7Ø.2
  rosacea L71.9
  specified NEC L7Ø.8
  tropica L7Ø.3
  varioliformis L7Ø.2
  vulgaris L7Ø.Ø
Acnitis (primary) A18.4
Acosta's disease T7Ø.29
Acoustic —*see* condition
Acousticophobia F4Ø.298
Acquired —*see also* condition
  immunodeficiency syndrome (AIDS) B2Ø
Acrania QØØ.Ø
Acroangiodermatitis I78.9
Acroasphyxia, chronic I73.89
Acrobystitis N47.7
Acrocephalopolysyndactyly Q87.Ø
Acrocephalosyndactyly Q87.Ø
Acrocephaly Q75.Ø
Acrochondrohyperplasia —*see* Syndrome, Marfan's
Acrocyanosis I73.8
  newborn P28.2
    meaning transient blue hands and feet - omit code
Acrodermatitis L3Ø.8
  atrophicans (chronica) L9Ø.4
  continua (Hallopeau) L4Ø.2
  enteropathica (hereditary) E83.2
  Hallopeau's L4Ø.2
  infantile papular L44.4
  perstans L4Ø.2
  pustulosa continua L4Ø.2
  recalcitrant pustular L4Ø.2
Acrodynia —*see* Poisoning, mercury
Acromegaly, acromegalia E22.Ø
Acromelalgia I73.81
Acromicria, acromikria Q79.8
Acronyx L6Ø.Ø
Acropachy, thyroid —*see* Thyrotoxicosis
Acroparesthesia (simple) (vasomotor) I73.89
Acropathy, thyroid —*see* Thyrotoxicosis
Acrophobia F4Ø.241
Acroposthitis N47.7
Acroscleriasis, acroscleroderma, acrosclerosis —*see* Sclerosis, systemic
Acrosphacelus I96
Acrospiroma, eccrine —*see* Neoplasm, skin, benign
Acrostealgia —*see* Osteochondropathy
Acrotrophodynia —*see* Immersion
ACTH ectopic syndrome E24.3
Actinic —*see* condition
Actinobacillosis, actinobacillus A28.8
  mallei A24.Ø
  muris A25.1
Actinomyces israelii (infection) —*see* Actinomycosis
Actinomycetoma (foot) B47.1
Actinomycosis, actinomycotic A42.9
  with pneumonia A42.Ø
  abdominal A42.1
  cervicofacial A42.2
  cutaneous A42.89
  gastrointestinal A42.1
  pulmonary A42.Ø
  sepsis A42.7
  specified site NEC A42.89
Actinoneuritis G62.82
Action, heart
  disorder I49.9
  irregular I49.9
    psychogenic F45.8
Activated protein C resistance D68.51
Activation ◀
  mast cell (disorder) (syndrome) D89.4Ø ◀
    idiopathic D89.42 ◀
    monoclonal D89.41 ◀
    secondary D89.43 ◀
    specified type NEC D89.49 ◀
Active —*see* condition
Acute —*see also* condition
  abdomen R1Ø.Ø
  gallbladder —*see* Cholecystitis, acute
Acyanotic heart disease (congenital) Q24.9
Acystia Q64.5
Adair-Dighton syndrome (brittle bones and blue sclera, deafness) Q78.Ø
Adamantinoblastoma —*see* Ameloblastoma
Adamantinoma —*see also* Cyst, calcifying odontogenic
  long bones C4Ø.9Ø
    lower limb C4Ø.2-
    upper limb C4Ø.Ø-
  malignant C41.1
    jaw (bone) (lower) C41.1
      upper C41.Ø
  tibial C4Ø.2-
Adamantoblastoma —*see* Ameloblastoma
Adams-Stokes (-Morgagni) disease or syndrome I45.9
Adaption reaction —*see* Disorder, adjustment

◀ New ◀ Revised ~~deleted~~ Deleted

- **Adenocarcinoma** *(Continued)*
  - papillary *(Continued)*
    - intraductal *(Continued)*
      - specified site NEC —*see* Neoplasm, in situ, by site
      - unspecified site DØ5.1-
    - serous
      - specified site —*see* Neoplasm, malignant, by site
      - unspecified site C56.9
  - papillocystic
    - specified site —*see* Neoplasm, malignant, by site
    - unspecified site C56.9
  - pseudomucinous
    - specified site —*see* Neoplasm, malignant, by site
    - unspecified site C56.9
  - renal cell C64-
  - sebaceous —*see* Neoplasm, skin, malignant, by site
  - serous —*see also* Neoplasm, malignant, by site
    - papillary
      - specified site —*see* Neoplasm, malignant, by site
      - unspecified site C56.9
  - sweat gland —*see* Neoplasm, skin, malignant
  - water-clear cell C75.Ø
- **Adenocarcinoma-in-situ** —*see also* Neoplasm, in situ, by site
  - breast DØ5.9-
- **Adenofibroma**
  - clear cell —*see* Neoplasm, benign, by site
  - endometrioid D27.9
    - borderline malignancy D39.1Ø
    - malignant C56-
  - mucinous
    - specified site —*see* Neoplasm, benign, by site
    - unspecified site D27.9
  - papillary
    - specified site —*see* Neoplasm, benign, by site
    - unspecified site D27.9
  - prostate —*see* Enlargement, enlarged, prostate
  - serous
    - specified site —*see* Neoplasm, benign, by site
    - unspecified site D27.9
  - specified site —*see* Neoplasm, benign, by site
  - unspecified site D27.9
- **Adenofibrosis**
  - breast —*see* Fibroadenosis, breast
  - endometrioid N8Ø.Ø
- **Adenoiditis** (chronic) J35.Ø2
  - with tonsillitis J35.Ø3
  - acute JØ3.9Ø
    - recurrent JØ3.91
    - specified organism NEC JØ3.8Ø
      - recurrent JØ3.81
    - staphylococcal JØ3.8Ø
      - recurrent JØ3.81
    - streptococcal JØ3.ØØ
      - recurrent JØ3.Ø1
- **Adenoids** —*see* condition
- **Adenolipoma** —*see* Neoplasm, benign, by site
- **Adenolipomatosis, Launois-Bensaude** E88.89
- **Adenolymphoma**
  - specified site —*see* Neoplasm, benign, by site
  - unspecified site D11.9
- **Adenoma** —*see also* Neoplasm, benign, by site
  - acidophil
    - specified site —*see* Neoplasm, benign, by site
    - unspecified site D35.2
  - acidophil-basophil, mixed
    - specified site —*see* Neoplasm, benign, by site
    - unspecified site D35.2
- **Adenoma** *(Continued)*
  - adrenal (cortical) D35.ØØ
    - clear cell D35.ØØ
    - compact cell D35.ØØ
    - glomerulosa cell D35.ØØ
    - heavily pigmented variant D35.ØØ
    - mixed cell D35.ØØ
  - alpha-cell
    - pancreas D13.7
    - specified site NEC —*see* Neoplasm, benign, by site
    - unspecified site D13.7
  - alveolar D14.3Ø
  - apocrine
    - breast D24-
    - specified site NEC —*see* Neoplasm, skin, benign, by site
    - unspecified site D23.9
  - basal cell D11.9
  - basophil
    - specified site —*see* Neoplasm, benign, by site
    - unspecified site D35.2
  - basophil-acidophil, mixed
    - specified site —*see* Neoplasm, benign, by site
    - unspecified site D35.2
  - beta-cell
    - pancreas D13.7
    - specified site NEC —*see* Neoplasm, benign, by site
    - unspecified site D13.7
  - bile duct D13.4
    - common D13.5
    - extrahepatic D13.5
    - intrahepatic D13.4
    - specified site NEC —*see* Neoplasm, benign, by site
    - unspecified site D13.4
  - black D35.ØØ
  - bronchial D38.1
    - cylindroid type —*see* Neoplasm, lung, malignant
  - ceruminous D23.2-
  - chief cell D35.1
  - chromophobe
    - specified site —*see* Neoplasm, benign, by site
    - unspecified site D35.2
  - colloid
    - specified site —*see* Neoplasm, benign, by site
    - unspecified site D34
  - duct
  - eccrine, papillary —*see* Neoplasm, skin, benign
  - endocrine, multiple
    - single specified site —*see* Neoplasm, uncertain behavior, by site
    - two or more specified sites D44-
    - unspecified site D44.9
  - endometrioid —*see also* Neoplasm, benign
    - borderline malignancy —*see* Neoplasm, uncertain behavior, by site
  - eosinophil
    - specified site —*see* Neoplasm, malignant, by site
    - unspecified site D35.2
  - fetal
    - specified site —*see* Neoplasm, benign, by site
    - unspecified site D34
  - follicular
    - specified site —*see* Neoplasm, benign, by site
    - unspecified site D34
  - hepatocellular D13.4
  - Hurthle cell D34
  - islet cell
    - pancreas D13.7
    - specified site NEC —*see* Neoplasm, benign, by site
    - unspecified site D13.7
- **Adenoma** *(Continued)*
  - liver cell D13.4
  - macrofollicular
    - specified site —*see* Neoplasm, benign, by site
    - unspecified site D34
  - malignant, malignum —*see* Neoplasm, malignant, by site
  - microcystic
    - pancreas D13.6
    - specified site NEC —*see* Neoplasm, benign, by site
    - unspecified site D13.6
  - microfollicular
    - specified site —*see* Neoplasm, benign, by site
    - unspecified site D34
  - mucoid cell
    - specified site —*see* Neoplasm, benign, by site
    - unspecified site D35.2
  - multiple endocrine
    - single specified site —*see* Neoplasm, uncertain behavior, by site
    - two or more specified sites D44-
    - unspecified site D44.9
  - nipple D24-
  - papillary —*see also* Neoplasm, benign, by site
    - eccrine —*see* Neoplasm, skin, benign, by site
  - Pick's tubular
    - specified site —*see* Neoplasm, benign, by site
    - unspecified site
      - female D27.9
      - male D29.2Ø
  - pleomorphic
    - carcinoma in —*see* Neoplasm, salivary gland, malignant
      - specified site —*see* Neoplasm, malignant, by site
      - unspecified site CØ8.9
  - polypoid —*see also* Neoplasm, benign
    - adenocarcinoma in —*see* Neoplasm, malignant, by site
    - adenocarcinoma in situ —*see* Neoplasm, in situ, by site
  - prostate —*see* Neoplasm, benign, prostate
  - rete cell D29.2Ø
  - sebaceous —*see* Neoplasm, skin, benign
  - Sertoli cell
    - specified site —*see* Neoplasm, benign, by site
    - unspecified site
      - female D27.9
      - male D29.2Ø
  - skin appendage —*see* Neoplasm, skin, benign
  - sudoriferous gland —*see* Neoplasm, skin, benign
  - sweat gland —*see* Neoplasm, skin, benign
  - testicular
    - specified site —*see* Neoplasm, benign, by site
    - unspecified site
      - female D27.9
      - male D29.2Ø
  - tubular —*see also* Neoplasm, benign, by site
    - adenocarcinoma in —*see* Neoplasm, malignant, by site
    - adenocarcinoma in situ —*see* Neoplasm, in situ, by site
    - Pick's
      - specified site —*see* Neoplasm, benign
      - unspecified site
        - female D27.9
        - male D29.2Ø
  - tubulovillous —*see also* Neoplasm, benign, by site
    - adenocarcinoma in —*see* Neoplasm, malignant, by site
    - adenocarcinoma in situ —*see* Neoplasm, in situ, by site

Adenoma *(Continued)*
villous —*see* Neoplasm, uncertain behavior, by site
adenocarcinoma in —*see* Neoplasm, malignant, by site
adenocarcinoma in situ —*see* Neoplasm, in situ, by site
water-clear cell D35.1
Adenomatosis
endocrine (multiple) E31.2Ø
single specified site —*see* Neoplasm, uncertain behavior, by site
erosive of nipple D24-
pluriendocrine —*see* Adenomatosis, endocrine
pulmonary D38.1
malignant —*see* Neoplasm, lung, malignant
specified site —*see* Neoplasm, benign, by site
unspecified site D12.6
Adenomatous
goiter (nontoxic) EØ4.9
with hyperthyroidism —*see* Hyperthyroidism, with, goiter, nodular
toxic —*see* Hyperthyroidism, with, goiter, nodular
Adenomyoma —*see also* Neoplasm, benign, by site
prostate —*see* Enlarged, prostate
Adenomyometritis N8Ø.Ø
Adenomyosis N8Ø.Ø
Adenopathy (lymph gland) R59.9
generalized R59.1
inguinal R59.Ø
localized R59.Ø
mediastinal R59.Ø
mesentery R59.Ø
syphilitic (secondary) A51.49
tracheobronchial R59.Ø
tuberculous A15.4
primary (progressive) A15.7
tuberculous —*see also* Tuberculosis, lymph gland
tracheobronchial A15.4
primary (progressive) A15.7
Adenosalpingitis —*see* Salpingitis
Adenosarcoma —*see* Neoplasm, malignant, by site
Adenosclerosis I88.8
Adenosis (sclerosing) **breast** —*see* Fibroadenosis, breast
Adenovirus, as cause of disease classified elsewhere B97.Ø
Adentia (complete) (partial) —*see* Absence, teeth
Adherent —*see also* Adhesions
labia (minora) N9Ø.89
pericardium (nonrheumatic) I31.Ø
rheumatic IØ9.2
placenta (with hemorrhage) O72.Ø
without hemorrhage O73.Ø
prepuce, newborn N47.Ø
scar (skin) L9Ø.5
tendon in scar L9Ø.5
Adhesions, adhesive (postinfective) K66.Ø
with intestinal obstruction K56.5
abdominal (wall) —*see* Adhesions, peritoneum
appendix K38.8
bile duct (common) (hepatic) K83.8
bladder (sphincter) N32.89
bowel —*see* Adhesions, peritoneum
cardiac I31.Ø
rheumatic IØ9.2
cecum —*see* Adhesions, peritoneum
cervicovaginal N88.1
congenital Q52.8
postpartal O9Ø.89
old N88.1
cervix N88.1
ciliary body NEC —*see* Adhesions, iris
Adhesions, adhesive *(Continued)*
clitoris N9Ø.89
colon —*see* Adhesions, peritoneum
common duct K83.8
congenital —*see also* Anomaly, by site
fingers —*see* Syndactylism, complex, fingers
omental, anomalous Q43.3
peritoneal Q43.3
tongue (to gum or roof of mouth) Q38.3
conjunctiva (acquired) H11.21-
congenital Q15.8
cystic duct K82.8
diaphragm —*see* Adhesions, peritoneum
due to foreign body —*see* Foreign body
duodenum —*see* Adhesions, peritoneum
ear
middle H74.1-
epididymis N5Ø.89
epidural —*see* Adhesions, meninges
epiglottis J38.7
eyelid HØ2.59
female pelvis N73.6
gallbladder K82.8
globe H44.89
heart I31.Ø
rheumatic IØ9.2
ileocecal (coil) —*see* Adhesions, peritoneum
ileum —*see* Adhesions, peritoneum
intestine —*see also* Adhesions, peritoneum
with obstruction K56.5
intra-abdominal —*see* Adhesions, peritoneum
iris H21.5Ø-
anterior H21.51-
goniosynechiae H21.52-
posterior H21.54-
to corneal graft T85.898
joint —*see* Ankylosis
knee M23.8X
temporomandibular M26.61-
labium (majus) (minus), congenital Q52.5
liver —*see* Adhesions, peritoneum
lung J98.4
mediastinum J98.59
meninges (cerebral) (spinal) G96.12
congenital QØ7.8
tuberculous (cerebral) (spinal) A17.Ø
mesenteric —*see* Adhesions, peritoneum
nasal (septum) (to turbinates) J34.89
ocular muscle —*see* Strabismus, mechanical
omentum —*see* Adhesions, peritoneum
ovary N73.6
congenital (to cecum, kidney or omentum) Q5Ø.39
paraovarian N73.6
pelvic (peritoneal)
female N73.6
postprocedural N99.4
male —*see* Adhesions, peritoneum
postpartal (old) N73.6
tuberculous A18.17
penis to scrotum (congenital) Q55.8
periappendiceal —*see also* Adhesions, peritoneum
pericardium (nonrheumatic) I31.Ø
focal I31.8
rheumatic IØ9.2
tuberculous A18.84
pericholecystic K82.8
perigastric —*see* Adhesions, peritoneum
periovarian N73.6
periprostatic N42.89
perirectal —*see* Adhesions, peritoneum
perirenal N28.89
peritoneum, peritoneal (postinfective) (postprocedural) K66.Ø
with obstruction (intestinal) K56.5
congenital Q43.3
pelvic, female N73.6
postprocedural N99.4
Adhesions, adhesive *(Continued)*
peritoneum, peritoneal *(Continued)*
postpartal, pelvic N73.6
to uterus N73.6
peritubal N73.6
periureteral N28.89
periuterine N73.6
perivesical N32.89
perivesicular (seminal vesicle) N5Ø.89
pleura, pleuritic J94.8
tuberculous NEC A15.6
pleuropericardial J94.8
postoperative (gastrointestinal tract) K66.Ø
with obstruction K91.3
due to foreign body accidentally left in wound —*see* Foreign body, accidentally left during a procedure
pelvic peritoneal N99.4
urethra —*see* Stricture, urethra, postprocedural
vagina N99.2
postpartal, old (vulva or perineum) N9Ø.89
preputial, prepuce N47.5
pulmonary J98.4
pylorus —*see* Adhesions, peritoneum
sciatic nerve —*see* Lesion, nerve, sciatic
seminal vesicle N5Ø.89
shoulder (joint) —*see* Capsulitis, adhesive
sigmoid flexure —*see* Adhesions, peritoneum
spermatic cord (acquired) N5Ø.89
congenital Q55.4
spinal canal G96.12
stomach —*see* Adhesions, peritoneum
subscapular —*see* Capsulitis, adhesive
temporomandibular M26.61-
tendinitis —*see also* Tenosynovitis, specified type NEC
shoulder —*see* Capsulitis, adhesive
testis N44.8
tongue, congenital (to gum or roof of mouth) Q38.3
acquired K14.8
trachea J39.8
tubo-ovarian N73.6
tunica vaginalis N44.8
uterus N73.6
internal N85.6
to abdominal wall N73.6
vagina (chronic) N89.5
postoperative N99.2
vitreomacular H43.82-
vitreous H43.89
vulva N9Ø.89
Adiaspiromycosis B48.8
Adie (-Holmes) **pupil or syndrome** —*see* Anomaly, pupil, function, tonic pupil
Adiponecrosis neonatorum P83.8
Adiposis —*see also* Obesity
cerebralis E23.6
dolorosa E88.2
Adiposity —*see also* Obesity
heart —*see* Degeneration, myocardial
localized E65
Adiposogenital dystrophy E23.6
Adjustment
disorder —*see* Disorder, adjustment
implanted device —*see* Encounter (for), adjustment (of)
prosthesis, external —*see* Fitting
reaction —*see* Disorder, adjustment
Administration of tPA (rtPA) in a different facility within the last 24 hours prior to admission to current facility Z92.82
Admission (for) —*see also* Encounter (for)
adjustment (of)
artificial
arm Z44.ØØ-
complete Z44.Ø1-
partial Z44.Ø2-
eye Z44.2

A

- **Admission** *(Continued)*
  - adjustment *(Continued)*
    - artificial *(Continued)*
      - leg Z44.1Ø-
        - complete Z44.11-
        - partial Z44.12-
    - brain neuropacemaker Z46.2
      - implanted Z45.42
    - breast
      - implant Z45.81
      - prosthesis (external) Z44.3
    - colostomy belt Z46.89
    - contact lenses Z46.Ø
    - cystostomy device Z46.6
    - dental prosthesis Z46.3
    - device NEC
      - abdominal Z46.89
      - implanted Z45.89
        - cardiac Z45.Ø9
          - defibrillator (with synchronous cardiace pacemaker) Z45.Ø2
          - pacemaker (cardiac resynchronization therapy (CRT-P)) Z45.Ø18 ⬅
            - pulse generator Z45.Ø1Ø
          - resynchronization therapy defibrillator (CRT-D) Z45.Ø2 ◀
        - hearing device Z45.328
          - bone conduction Z45.32Ø
          - cochlear Z45.321
        - infusion pump Z45.1
        - nervous system Z45.49
          - CSF drainage Z45.41
          - hearing device —*see* Admission, adjustment, device, implanted, hearing device
          - neuropacemaker Z45.42
          - visual substitution Z45.31
        - specified NEC Z45.89
        - vascular access Z45.2
        - visual substitution Z45.31
      - nervous system Z46.2
        - implanted —*see* Admission, adjustment, device, implanted, nervous system
      - orthodontic Z46.4
      - prosthetic Z44.9
        - arm —*see* Admission, adjustment, artificial, arm
        - breast Z44.3
        - dental Z46.3
        - eye Z44.2
        - leg —*see* Admission, adjustment, artificial, leg
        - specified type NEC Z44.8
      - substitution
        - auditory Z46.2
          - implanted —*see* Admission, adjustment, device, implanted, hearing device
        - nervous system Z46.2
          - implanted —*see* Admission, adjustment, device, implanted, nervous system
        - visual Z46.2
          - implanted Z45.31
      - urinary Z46.6
    - hearing aid Z46.1
      - implanted —*see* Admission, adjustment, device, implanted, hearing device
    - ileostomy device Z46.89
    - intestinal appliance or device NEC Z46.89
    - neuropacemaker (brain) (peripheral nerve) (spinal cord) Z46.2
      - implanted Z45.42
    - orthodontic device Z46.4
    - orthopedic (brace) (cast) (device) (shoes) Z46.89
    - pacemaker (cardiac resynchronization therapy (CRT-P)) ⬅
      - cardiac Z45.Ø18
        - pulse generator Z45.Ø1Ø
    - pacemaker *(Continued)*
      - nervous system Z46.2
        - implanted Z45.42
    - portacath (port-a-cath) Z45.2
    - prosthesis Z44.9
      - arm —*see* Admission, adjustment, artificial, arm
      - breast Z44.3
      - dental Z46.3
      - eye Z44.2
      - leg —*see* Admission, adjustment, artificial, leg
      - specified NEC Z44.8
    - spectacles Z46.Ø
  - aftercare (*see also* Aftercare) Z51.89
    - postpartum
      - immediately after delivery Z39.Ø
      - routine follow-up Z39.2
    - radiation therapy (antineoplastic) Z51.Ø
  - attention to artificial opening (of) Z43.9
    - artificial vagina Z43.7
    - colostomy Z43.3
    - cystostomy Z43.5
    - enterostomy Z43.4
    - gastrostomy Z43.1
    - ileostomy Z43.2
    - jejunostomy Z43.4
    - nephrostomy Z43.6
    - specified site NEC Z43.8
      - intestinal tract Z43.4
      - urinary tract Z43.6
    - tracheostomy Z43.Ø
    - ureterostomy Z43.6
    - urethrostomy Z43.6
  - breast augmentation or reduction Z41.1
  - breast reconstruction following mastectomy Z42.1
  - change of
    - dressing (nonsurgical) Z48.ØØ
    - neuropacemaker device (brain) (peripheral nerve) (spinal cord) Z46.2
      - implanted Z45.42
    - surgical dressing Z48.Ø1
  - circumcision, ritual or routine (in absence of diagnosis) Z41.2
  - clinical research investigation (control) (normal comparison) (participant) ZØØ.6
  - contraceptive management Z30.9
  - cosmetic surgery NEC Z41.1
  - counseling (*see also* Counseling)
    - dietary Z71.3
    - gestational carrier Z31.7 ◀
    - HIV Z71.7
    - human immunodeficiency virus Z71.7
    - nonattending third party Z71.Ø
    - procreative management NEC Z31.69
  - delivery, full-term, uncomplicated O8Ø
    - cesarean, without indication O82
  - desensitization to allergens Z51.6 ◀
  - dietary surveillance and counseling Z71.3
  - ear piercing Z41.3
  - examination at health care facility (adult) —*see also* Examination ZØØ.ØØ
    - with abnormal findings ZØØ.Ø1
    - clinical research investigation (control) (normal comparison) (participant) ZØØ.6
    - dental ZØ1.2Ø
      - with abnormal findings ZØ1.21
    - donor (potential) ZØØ.5
    - ear ZØ1.1Ø
      - with abnormal findings NEC ZØ1.118
    - eye ZØ1.ØØ
      - with abnormal findings ZØ1.Ø1
    - general, specified reason NEC ZØØ.8
    - hearing ZØ1.1Ø
      - with abnormal findings NEC ZØ1.118
    - postpartum checkup Z39.2
    - psychiatric (general) ZØØ.8
      - requested by authority ZØ4.6
    - vision ZØ1.ØØ
      - with abnormal findings ZØ1.Ø1
  - fitting (of)
    - artificial
      - arm —*see* Admission, adjustment, artificial, arm
      - eye Z44.2
      - leg —*see* Admission, adjustment, artificial, leg
    - brain neuropacemaker Z46.2
      - implanted Z45.42
    - breast prosthesis (external) Z44.3
    - colostomy belt Z46.89
    - contact lenses Z46.Ø
    - cystostomy device Z46.6
    - dental prosthesis Z46.3
    - dentures Z46.3
    - device NEC
      - abdominal Z46.89
      - nervous system Z46.2
        - implanted —*see* Admission, adjustment, device, implanted, nervous system
      - orthodontic Z46.4
      - prosthetic Z44.9
        - breast Z44.3
        - dental Z46.3
        - eye Z44.2
      - substitution
        - auditory Z46.2
          - implanted —*see* Admission, adjustment, device, implanted, hearing device
        - nervous system Z46.2
          - implanted —*see* Admission, adjustment, device, implanted, nervous system
        - visual Z46.2
          - implanted Z45.31
    - hearing aid Z46.1
    - ileostomy device Z46.89
    - intestinal appliance or device NEC Z46.89
    - neuropacemaker (brain) (peripheral nerve) (spinal cord) Z46.2
      - implanted Z45.42
    - orthodontic device Z46.4
    - orthopedic device (brace) (cast) (shoes) Z46.89
    - prosthesis Z44.9
      - arm —*see* Admission, adjustment, artificial, arm
      - breast Z44.3
      - dental Z46.3
      - eye Z44.2
      - leg —*see* Admission, adjustment, artificial, leg
      - specified type NEC Z44.8
    - spectacles Z46.Ø
  - follow-up examination ZØ9
  - intrauterine device management Z3Ø.431
    - initial prescription Z3Ø.Ø14
  - mental health evaluation ZØØ.8
    - requested by authority ZØ4.6
  - observation —*see* Observation
  - Papanicolaou smear, cervix Z12.4
    - for suspected malignant neoplasm Z12.4
  - plastic and reconstructive surgery following medical procedure or healed injury NEC Z42.8
  - plastic surgery, cosmetic NEC Z41.1
  - postpartum observation
    - immediately after delivery Z39.Ø
    - routine follow-up Z39.2
  - poststerilization (for restoration) Z31.Ø
    - aftercare Z31.42
  - procreative management Z31.9
  - prophylactic (measure) —*see also* Encounter, prophylactic measures ⬅
    - organ removal Z4Ø.ØØ
      - breast Z4Ø.Ø1
      - ovary Z4Ø.Ø2

A

Admission *(Continued)*
- prophylactic *(Continued)*
  - organ removal *(Continued)*
    - specified organ NEC Z40.09
    - testes Z40.09
  - vaccination Z23
- psychiatric examination (general) Z00.8
  - requested by authority Z04.6
- radiation therapy (antineoplastic) Z51.0
- reconstructive surgery following medical procedure or healed injury NEC Z42.8
- removal of
  - cystostomy catheter Z43.5
  - drains Z48.03
  - dressing (nonsurgical) Z48.00
  - implantable subdermal contraceptive Z30.46 ◀
  - intrauterine contraceptive device Z30.432
  - neuropacemaker (brain) (peripheral nerve) (spinal cord) Z46.2
    - implanted Z45.42
  - staples Z48.02
  - surgical dressing Z48.01
  - sutures Z48.02
  - ureteral stent Z46.6
- respirator [ventilator] use during power failure Z99.12
- restoration of organ continuity (poststerilization) Z31.0
  - aftercare Z31.42
- sensitivity test —*see also* Test, skin
  - allergy NEC Z01.82
  - Mantoux Z11.1
- tuboplasty following previous sterilization Z31.0
  - aftercare Z31.42
- vasoplasty following previous sterilization Z31.0
  - aftercare Z31.42
- vision examination Z01.00
  - with abnormal findings Z01.01
- waiting period for admission to other facility Z75.1

Adnexitis (suppurative) —*see* Salpingo-oophoritis
Adolescent X-linked adrenoleukodystrophy E71.521
Adrenal (gland) —*see* condition
Adrenalism, tuberculous A18.7
Adrenalitis, adrenitis E27.8
- autoimmune E27.1
- meningococcal, hemorrhagic A39.1

Adrenarche, premature E27.0
Adrenocortical syndrome —*see* Cushing's, syndrome
Adrenogenital syndrome E25.9
- acquired E25.8
- congenital E25.0
- salt loss E25.0

Adrenogenitalism, congenital E25.0
Adrenoleukodystrophy E71.529
- neonatal E71.511
- X-linked E71.529
  - Addison only phenotype E71.528
  - Addison-Schilder E71.528
  - adolescent E71.521
  - adrenomyeloneuropathy E71.522
  - childhood cerebral E71.520
  - other specified E71.528

Adrenomyeloneuropathy E71.522
Adventitious bursa —*see* Bursopathy, specified type NEC
Adverse effect —*see* Table of Drugs and Chemicals, categories T36-T50, with 6th character 5
Advice —*see* Counseling
Adynamia (episodica) (hereditary) (periodic) G72.3
Aeration lung imperfect, newborn —*see* Atelectasis
Aerobullosis T70.3
Aerocele —*see* Embolism, air
Aerodermectasia
- subcutaneous (traumatic) T79.7

Aerodontalgia T70.29
Aeroembolism T70.3
Aerogenes capsulatus infection A48.0
Aero-otitis media T70.0
Aerophagy, aerophagia (psychogenic) F45.8
Aerophobia F40.228
Aerosinusitis T70.1
Aerotitis T70.0
Affection —*see* Disease
Afibrinogenemia —*see also* Defect, coagulation D68.8
- acquired D65
- congenital D68.2
- following ectopic or molar pregnancy O08.1
- in abortion —*see* Abortion, by type, complicated by, afibrinogenemia
- puerperal O72.3

African
- sleeping sickness B56.9
- tick fever A68.1
- trypanosomiasis B56.9
  - gambian B56.0
  - rhodesian B56.1

Aftercare —*see also* Care Z51.89
- following surgery (for) (on)
  - amputation Z47.81
  - attention to
    - drains Z48.03
    - dressings (nonsurgical) Z48.00
      - surgical Z48.01
    - sutures Z48.02
  - circulatory system Z48.812
  - delayed (planned) wound closure Z48.1
  - digestive system Z48.815
  - explantation of joint prosthesis (staged procedure)
    - hip Z47.32
    - knee Z47.33
    - shoulder Z47.31
  - genitourinary system Z48.816
  - joint replacement Z47.1
  - neoplasm Z48.3
  - nervous system Z48.811
  - oral cavity Z48.814
  - organ transplant
    - bone marrow Z48.290
    - heart Z48.21
    - heart-lung Z48.280
    - kidney Z48.22
    - liver Z48.23
    - lung Z48.24
    - multiple organs NEC Z48.288
    - specified NEC Z48.298
  - orthopedic NEC Z47.89
  - planned wound closure Z48.1
  - removal of internal fixation device Z47.2
  - respiratory system Z48.813
  - scoliosis Z47.82
  - sense organs Z48.810
  - skin and subcutaneous tissue Z48.817
  - specified body system
    - circulatory Z48.812
    - digestive Z48.815
    - genitourinary Z48.816
    - nervous Z48.811
    - oral cavity Z48.814
    - respiratory Z48.813
    - sense organs Z48.810
    - skin and subcutaneous tissue Z48.817
    - teeth Z48.814
  - specified NEC Z48.89
  - spinal Z48.89
  - teeth Z48.814
- fracture — code to fracture with seventh character D
- involving
  - removal of
    - drains Z48.03
    - dressings (nonsurgical) Z48.00
    - staples Z48.02
    - surgical dressings Z48.01
    - sutures Z48.02
  - neuropacemaker (brain) (peripheral nerve) (spinal cord) Z46.2
    - implanted Z45.42
  - orthopedic NEC Z47.89
  - postprocedural —*see* Aftercare, following surgery

After-cataract —*see* Cataract, secondary
Agalactia (primary) O92.3
- elective, secondary or therapeutic O92.5

Agammaglobulinemia (acquired (secondary)) (nonfamilial) D80.1
- with
  - immunoglobulin-bearing B-lymphocytes D80.1
  - lymphopenia D81.9
- autosomal recessive (Swiss type) D80.0
- Bruton's X-linked D80.0
- common variable (CVAgamma) D80.1
- congenital sex-linked D80.0
- hereditary D80.0
- lymphopenic D81.9
- Swiss type (autosomal recessive) D80.0
- X-linked (with growth hormone deficiency) (Bruton) D80.0 ⬅

Aganglionosis (bowel) (colon) Q43.1
Age (old) —*see* Senility
Agenesis
- adrenal (gland) Q89.1
- alimentary tract (complete) (partial) NEC Q45.8
  - upper Q40.8
- anus, anal (canal) Q42.3
  - with fistula Q42.2
- aorta Q25.41 ⬅
- appendix Q42.8
- arm (complete) Q71.0-
  - with hand present Q71.1-
- artery (peripheral) Q27.9
  - brain Q28.3
  - coronary Q24.5
  - pulmonary Q25.79
  - specified NEC Q27.8
  - umbilical Q27.0
- auditory (canal) (external) Q16.1
- auricle (ear) Q16.0
- bile duct or passage Q44.5
- bladder Q64.5
- bone Q79.9
- brain Q00.0
  - part of Q04.3
- breast (with nipple present) Q83.8
  - with absent nipple Q83.0
- bronchus Q32.4
- canaliculus lacrimalis Q10.4
- carpus —*see* Agenesis, hand
- cartilage Q79.9
- cecum Q42.8
- cerebellum Q04.3
- cervix Q51.5
- chin Q18.8
- cilia Q10.3
- circulatory system, part NOS Q28.9
- clavicle Q74.0
- clitoris Q52.6
- coccyx Q76.49
- colon Q42.9
  - specified NEC Q42.8
- corpus callosum Q04.0
- cricoid cartilage Q31.8
- diaphragm (with hernia) Q79.1
- digestive organ (s) or tract (complete) (partial) NEC Q45.8
  - upper Q40.8
- ductus arteriosus Q28.8
- duodenum Q41.0

A

Agenesis *(Continued)*
  ear Q16.9
    auricle Q16.Ø
    lobe Q17.8
  ejaculatory duct Q55.4
  endocrine (gland) NEC Q89.2
  epiglottis Q31.8
  esophagus Q39.8
  eustachian tube Q16.2
  eye Q11.1
    adnexa Q15.8
  eyelid (fold) Q1Ø.3
  face
    bones NEC Q75.8
    specified part NEC Q18.8
  fallopian tube Q5Ø.6
  femur —*see* Defect, reduction, lower limb, longitudinal, femur
  fibula —*see* Defect, reduction, lower limb, longitudinal, fibula
  finger (complete) (partial) —*see* Agenesis, hand
  foot (and toes) (complete) (partial) Q72.3-
  forearm (with hand present) —*see* Agenesis, arm, with hand present
    and hand Q71.2-
  gallbladder Q44.Ø
  gastric Q4Ø.2
  genitalia, genital (organ (s))
    female Q52.8
      external Q52.71
      internal NEC Q52.8
    male Q55.8
  glottis Q31.8
  hair Q84.Ø
  hand (and fingers) (complete) (partial) Q71.3-
  heart Q24.8
    valve NEC Q24.8
      pulmonary Q22.Ø
  hepatic Q44.7
  humerus —*see* Defect, reduction, upper limb
  hymen Q52.4
  ileum Q41.2
  incus Q16.3
  intestine (small) Q41.9
    large Q42.9
      specified NEC Q42.8
  iris (dilator fibers) Q13.1
  jaw M26.Ø9
  jejunum Q41.1
  kidney (s) (partial) Q6Ø.2
    bilateral Q6Ø.1
    unilateral Q6Ø.Ø
  labium (majus) (minus) Q52.71
  labyrinth, membranous Q16.5
  lacrimal apparatus Q1Ø.4
  larynx Q31.8
  leg (complete) Q72.Ø-
    with foot present Q72.1-
    lower leg (with foot present) —*see* Agenesis, leg, with foot present
      and foot Q72.2-
  lens Q12.3
  limb (complete) Q73.Ø
    lower —*see* Agenesis, leg
    upper —*see* Agenesis, arm
  lip Q38.Ø
  liver Q44.7
  lung (fissure) (lobe) (bilateral) (unilateral) Q33.3
  mandible, maxilla M26.Ø9
  metacarpus —*see* Agenesis, hand
  metatarsus —*see* Agenesis, foot
  muscle Q79.8
    eyelid Q1Ø.3
    ocular Q15.8
  musculoskeletal system NEC Q79.8
  nail (s) Q84.3
  neck, part Q18.8
  nerve QØ7.8
  nervous system, part NEC QØ7.8

Agenesis *(Continued)*
  nipple Q83.2
  nose Q3Ø.1
  nuclear QØ7.8
  organ
    of Corti Q16.5
    or site not listed —*see* Anomaly, by site
  osseous meatus (ear) Q16.1
  ovary
    bilateral Q5Ø.Ø2
    unilateral Q5Ø.Ø1
  oviduct Q5Ø.6
  pancreas Q45.Ø
  parathyroid (gland) Q89.2
  parotid gland (s) Q38.4
  patella Q74.1
  pelvic girdle (complete) (partial) Q74.2
  penis Q55.5
  pericardium Q24.8
  pituitary (gland) Q89.2
  prostate Q55.4
  punctum lacrimale Q1Ø.4
  radioulnar —*see* Defect, reduction, upper limb
  radius —*see* Defect, reduction, upper limb, longitudinal, radius
  rectum Q42.1
    with fistula Q42.Ø
  renal Q6Ø.2
    bilateral Q6Ø.1
    unilateral Q6Ø.Ø
  respiratory organ NEC Q34.8
  rib Q76.6
  roof of orbit Q75.8
  round ligament Q52.8
  sacrum Q76.49
  salivary gland Q38.4
  scapula Q74.Ø
  scrotum Q55.29
  seminal vesicles Q55.4
  septum
    atrial Q21.1
    between aorta and pulmonary artery Q21.4
    ventricular Q2Ø.4
  shoulder girdle (complete) (partial) Q74.Ø
  skull (bone) Q75.8
    with
      anencephaly QØØ.Ø
      encephalocele —*see* Encephalocele
      hydrocephalus QØ3.9
        with spina bifida —*see* Spina bifida, by site, with hydrocephalus
      microcephaly QØ2
  spermatic cord Q55.4
  spinal cord QØ6.Ø
  spine Q76.49
  spleen Q89.Ø1
  sternum Q76.7
  stomach Q4Ø.2
  submaxillary gland (s) (congenital) Q38.4
  tarsus —*see* Agenesis, foot
  tendon Q79.8
  testicle Q55.Ø
  thymus (gland) Q89.2
  thyroid (gland) EØ3.1
    cartilage Q31.8
  tibia —*see* Defect, reduction, lower limb, longitudinal, tibia
  tibiofibular —*see* Defect, reduction, lower limb, specified type NEC
  toe (and foot) (complete) (partial) —*see* Agenesis, foot
  tongue Q38.3
  trachea (cartilage) Q32.1
  ulna —*see* Defect, reduction, upper limb, longitudinal, ulna
  upper limb —*see* Agenesis, arm
  ureter Q62.4
  urethra Q64.5
  urinary tract NEC Q64.8

Agenesis *(Continued)*
  uterus Q51.Ø
  uvula Q38.5
  vagina Q52.Ø
  vas deferens Q55.4
  vein (s) (peripheral) Q27.9
    brain Q28.3
    great NEC Q26.8
    portal Q26.5
  vena cava (inferior) (superior) Q26.8
  vermis of cerebellum QØ4.3
  vertebra Q76.49
  vulva Q52.71
Ageusia R43.2
Agitated —*see* condition
Agitation R45.1
Aglossia (congenital) Q38.3
Aglossia-adactylia syndrome Q87.Ø
Aglycogenosis E74.ØØ
Agnosia (body image) (other senses) (tactile) R48.1
  developmental F88
  verbal R48.1
    auditory R48.1
      developmental F8Ø.2
    developmental F8Ø.2
  visual (object) R48.3
Agoraphobia F4Ø.ØØ
  with panic disorder F4Ø.Ø1
  without panic disorder F4Ø.Ø2
Agrammatism R48.8
Agranulocytopenia —*see* Agranulocytosis
Agranulocytosis (chronic) (cyclical) (genetic) (infantile) (periodic) (pernicious) (*see also* Neutropenia) D7Ø.9
  congenital D7Ø.Ø
  cytoreductive cancer chemotherapy sequela D7Ø.1
  drug-induced D7Ø.2
    due to cytoreductive cancer chemotherapy D7Ø.1
  due to infection D7Ø.3
  secondary D7Ø.4
    drug-induced D7Ø.2
      due to cytoreductive cancer chemotherapy D7Ø.1
Agraphia (absolute) R48.8
  with alexia R48.Ø
  developmental F81.81
Ague (dumb) —*see* Malaria
Agyria QØ4.3
Ahumada-del Castillo syndrome E23.Ø
Aichomophobia F4Ø.298
AIDS (related complex) B2Ø
Ailment heart —*see* Disease, heart
Ailurophobia F4Ø.218
Ainhum (disease) L94.6
AIN —*see* Neoplasia, intraepithelial, anal ◀
AIPHI (acute idiopathic pulmonary hemorrhage in infants (over 28 days old)) RØ4.81
Air
  anterior mediastinum J98.2
  compressed, disease T7Ø.3
  conditioner lung or pneumonitis J67.7
  embolism (artery) (cerebral) (any site) T79.Ø
    with ectopic or molar pregnancy OØ8.2
    due to implanted device NEC —*see* Complications, by site and type, specified NEC
    following
      abortion —*see* Abortion by type, complicated by, embolism
      ectopic or molar pregnancy OØ8.2
      infusion, therapeutic injection or transfusion T8Ø.Ø
    in pregnancy, childbirth or puerperium —*see* Embolism, obstetric
    traumatic T79.Ø
  hunger, psychogenic F45.8
  rarefied, effects of —*see* Effect, adverse, high altitude
  sickness T75.3

A

- **Airplane sickness** T75.3
- **Akathisia** (drug-induced) (treatment- induced) G25.71
  - neuroleptic induced (acute) G25.71
- **Akinesia** R29.898
- **Akinetic mutism** R41.89
- **Akureyri's disease** G93.3
- **Alactasia, congenital** E73.0
- **Alagille's syndrome** Q44.7
- **Alastrim** B03
- **Albers-Schönberg syndrome** Q78.2
- **Albert's syndrome** —*see* Tendinitis, Achilles
- **Albinism, albino** E70.30
  - with hematologic abnormality E70.339
    - Chédiak-Higashi syndrome E70.330
    - Hermansky-Pudlak syndrome E70.331
    - other specified E70.338
  - I E70.320
  - II E70.321
  - ocular E70.319
    - autosomal recessive E70.311
    - other specified E70.318
    - X-linked E70.310
  - oculocutaneous E70.329
    - other specified E70.328
    - tyrosinase (ty) negative E70.320
    - tyrosinase (ty) positive E70.321
  - other specified E70.39
- **Albinismus** E70.30
- **Albright** (-McCune)(-Sternberg) **syndrome** Q78.1
- **Albuminous** —*see* condition
- **Albuminuria, albuminuric** (acute) (chronic) (subacute) —*see also* Proteinuria R80.9
  - complicating pregnancy —*see* Proteinuria, gestational
    - with
      - gestational hypertension —*see* Pre-eclampsia
      - pre-existing hypertension —*see* Hypertension, complicating pregnancy, pre-existing, with, pre-eclampsia
  - gestational —*see* Proteinuria, gestational
    - with
      - gestational hypertension —*see* Pre-eclampsia
      - pre-existing hypertension —*see* Hypertension, complicating pregnancy, pre-existing, with, pre-eclampsia
  - orthostatic R80.2
  - postural R80.2
  - pre-eclamptic —*see* Pre-eclampsia
  - scarlatinal A38.8
- **Albuminurophobia** F40.298
- **Alcaptonuria** E70.29
- **Alcohol, alcoholic, alcohol-induced**
  - addiction (without remission) F10.20
    - with remission F10.21
  - amnestic disorder, persisting F10.96
    - with dependence F10.26
  - anxiety disorder F10.980 ◀
  - bipolar and related disorder F10.94 ◀
  - brain syndrome, chronic F10.97
    - with dependence F10.27
  - cardiopathy I42.6
  - counseling and surveillance Z71.41
    - family member Z71.42
  - delirium (acute) (tremens) (withdrawal) F10.231
    - with intoxication F10.921
      - in
        - abuse F10.121
        - dependence F10.221
  - dementia F10.97
    - with dependence F10.27
  - depressive disorder F10.94 ◀
  - deterioration F10.97
    - with dependence F10.27

Alcohol, alcoholic, alcohol-induced *(Continued)*
  - hallucinosis (acute) F10.951
    - in
      - abuse F10.151
      - dependence F10.251
  - insanity F10.959
  - intoxication (acute) (without dependence) F10.129
    - with
      - delirium F10.121
      - dependence F10.229
        - with delirium F10.221
        - uncomplicated F10.220
    - uncomplicated F10.120
  - jealousy F10.988
  - Korsakoff's, Korsakov's, Korsakow's F10.26
  - liver K70.9
    - acute —*see* Disease, liver, alcoholic, hepatitis
  - major neurocognitive disorder, amnestic-confabulatory type F10.96 ◀
  - major neurocognitive disorder, nonamnestic-confabulatory type F10.97 ◀
  - mania (acute) (chronic) F10.959
  - mild neurocognitive disorder F10.988 ◀
  - paranoia, paranoid (type) psychosis F10.950
  - pellagra E52
  - poisoning, accidental (acute) NEC —*see* Table of Drugs and Chemicals, alcohol, poisoning
  - psychosis —*see* Psychosis, alcoholic
  - psychotic disorder F10.959 ◀
  - sexual dysfunction F10.981 ◀
  - sleep disorder F10.982 ◀
  - withdrawal (without convulsions) F10.239
    - with delirium F10.231
- **Alcoholism** (chronic) (without remission) F10.20
  - with
    - psychosis —*see* Psychosis, alcoholic
    - remission F10.21
  - Korsakov's F10.96
    - with dependence F10.26
- **Alder (-Reilly) anomaly or syndrome** (leukocyte granulation) D72.0
- **Aldosteronism** E26.9
  - familial (type I) E26.02
  - glucocorticoid-remediable E26.02
  - primary (due to (bilateral) adrenal hyperplasia) E26.09
  - primary NEC E26.09
  - secondary E26.1
  - specified NEC E26.89
- **Aldosteronoma** D44.10
- **Aldrich(-Wiskott) syndrome** (eczema-thrombocytopenia) D82.0
- **Alektorophobia** F40.218
- **Aleppo boil** B55.1
- **Aleukemic** —*see* condition Aleukia
  - congenital D70.0
  - hemorrhagica D61.9
    - congenital D61.09
  - splenica D73.1
- **Alexia** R48.0
  - developmental F81.0
  - secondary to organic lesion R48.0
- **Algoneurodystrophy** M89.00
  - ankle M89.07-
  - foot M89.07-
  - forearm M89.03-
  - hand M89.04-
  - lower leg M89.06-
  - multiple sites M89.0-
  - shoulder M89.01-
  - specified site NEC M89.08
  - thigh M89.05-
  - upper arm M89.02-
- **Algophobia** F40.298
- **Alienation, mental** —*see* Psychosis
- **Alkalemia** E87.3
- **Alkalosis** E87.3
  - metabolic E87.3
    - with respiratory acidosis E87.4
  - respiratory E87.3
- **Alkaptonuria** E70.29
- **Allen-Masters syndrome** N83.8
- **Allergy, allergic** (reaction) (to) T78.40
  - air-borne substance NEC (rhinitis) J30.89
  - alveolitis (extrinsic) J67.9
    - due to
      - Aspergillus clavatus J67.4
      - Cryptostroma corticale J67.6
      - organisms (fungal, thermophilic actinomycete) growing in ventilation (air conditioning) systems J67.7
    - specified type NEC J67.8
  - anaphylactic reaction or shock T78.2
  - angioneurotic edema T78.3
  - animal (dander) (epidermal) (hair) (rhinitis) J30.81
  - bee sting (anaphylactic shock) —*see* Toxicity, venom, arthropod, bee
  - biological —*see* Allergy, drug
  - colitis —*see also* Colitis, allergic K52.29 ⇐
  - dander (animal) (rhinitis) J30.81
  - dandruff (rhinitis) J30.81
  - dental restorative material (existing) K08.55
  - dermatitis —*see* Dermatitis, contact, allergic
  - diathesis —*see* History, allergy
  - drug, medicament & biological (any) (external) (internal) T78.40
    - correct substance properly administered —*see* Table of Drugs and Chemicals, by drug, adverse effect
    - wrong substance given or taken NEC (by accident) —*see* Table of Drugs and Chemicals, by drug, poisoning
  - due to pollen J30.1
  - dust (house) (stock) (rhinitis) J30.89
    - with asthma —*see* Asthma, allergic extrinsic
  - eczema —*see* Dermatitis, contact, allergic
  - epidermal (animal) (rhinitis) J30.81
  - feathers (rhinitis) J30.89
  - food (any) (ingested) NEC T78.1
    - anaphylactic shock —*see* Shock, anaphylactic, due to food
    - dermatitis —*see* Dermatitis, due to, food
    - dietary counseling and surveillance Z71.3
    - in contact with skin L23.6
    - rhinitis J30.5
    - status (without reaction) Z91.018
      - eggs Z91.012
      - milk products Z91.011
      - peanuts Z91.010
      - seafood Z91.013
      - specified NEC Z91.018
  - gastrointestinal —*see also* specific type of allergic reaction ⇐
    - meaning colitis —*see also* Colitis, allergic) K52.29 ◀
    - meaning gastroenteritis —*see also* Gastroenteritis, allergic) K52.29 ◀
    - meaning other adverse food reaction not elsewhere classified T78.1 ◀
  - grain J30.1
  - grass (hay fever) (pollen) J30.1
    - asthma —*see* Asthma, allergic extrinsic
  - hair (animal) (rhinitis) J30.81
  - history (of) —*see* History, allergy
  - horse serum —*see* Allergy, serum
  - inhalant (rhinitis) J30.89
    - pollen J30.1
  - kapok (rhinitis) J30.89
  - medicine —*see* Allergy, drug
  - milk protein —*see also* Allergy, food Z91.011 ⇐
    - anaphylactic reaction T78.07 ◀
    - dermatitis L27.2 ◀
    - enterocolitis syndrome K52.21 ◀
    - enteropathy K52.22 ◀
    - gastroenteritis K52.29 ◀

Allergy, allergic *(Continued)*
milk protein *(Continued)*
gastroesophageal reflux —*see also* Reaction, adverse, food) K21.9 ◀
with esophagitis K21.Ø ◀
proctocolitis K52.82 ◀]
nasal, seasonal due to pollen J3Ø.1
pneumonia J82
pollen (any) (hay fever) J3Ø.1
asthma —*see* Asthma, allergic extrinsic
primrose J3Ø.1
primula J3Ø.1
proctocolitis K52.82 ◀
purpura D69.Ø
ragweed (hay fever) (pollen) J3Ø.1
asthma —*see* Asthma, allergic extrinsic
rose (pollen) J3Ø.1
seasonal NEC J3Ø.2
Senecio jacobae (pollen) J3Ø.1
serum —*see also* Reaction, serum T8Ø.69
anaphylactic shock T8Ø.59
shock (anaphylactic) T78.2
due to
administration of blood and blood products T8Ø.51
adverse effect of correct medicinal substance properly administered T88.6
immunization T8Ø.52
serum NEC T8Ø.59
vaccination T8Ø.52
specific NEC T78.49
tree (any) (hay fever) (pollen) J3Ø.1
asthma —*see* Asthma, allergic extrinsic
upper respiratory J3Ø.9
urticaria L5Ø.Ø
vaccine —*see* Allergy, serum
wheat —*see* Allergy, food
Allescheriasis B48.2
Alligator skin disease Q8Ø.9
Allocheiria, allochiria R2Ø.8
Almeida's disease —*see* Paracoccidioidomycosis
Alopecia (hereditaria) (seborrheica) L65.9
androgenic L64.9
drug-induced L64.Ø
specified NEC L64.8
areata L63.9
ophiasis L63.2
specified NEC L63.8
totalis L63.Ø
universalis L63.1
cicatricial L66.9
specified NEC L66.8
circumscripta L63.9
congenital, congenitalis Q84.Ø
due to cytotoxic drugs NEC L65.8
mucinosa L65.2
postinfective NEC L65.8
postpartum L65.Ø
premature L64.8
specific (syphilitic) A51.32
specified NEC L65.8
syphilitic (secondary) A51.32
totalis (capitis) L63.Ø
universalis (entire body) L63.1
X-ray L58.1
Alpers' disease G31.81
Alpine sickness T7Ø.29
Alport syndrome Q87.81
ALTE (apparent life threatening event) in newborn and infant R68.13
Alteration (of), **Altered**
~~awareness, transient R4Ø.4~~
awareness ◀
transient R4Ø.4 ◀
unintended under general anesthesia, during procedure T88.53 ◀
mental status R41.82
pattern of family relationships affecting child Z62.898

Alteration (of), **Altered** *(Continued)*
sensation
following
cerebrovascular disease I69.998
cerebral infarction I69.398
intracerebral hemorrhage I69.198
nontraumatic intracranial hemorrhage NEC I69.298
specified disease NEC I69.898
subarachnoid hemorrhage I69.Ø98
Alternating —*see* condition
Altitude, high (effects) —*see* Effect, adverse, high altitude
Aluminosis (of lung) J63.Ø
Alveolitis
allergic (extrinsic) —*see* Pneumonitis, hypersensitivity
due to
Aspergillus clavatus J67.4
Cryptostroma corticale J67.6
fibrosing (cryptogenic) (idiopathic) J84.112
jaw M27.3
sicca dolorosa M27.3
Alveolus, alveolar —*see* condition
Alymphocytosis D72.81Ø
thymic (with immunodeficiency) D82.1
Alymphoplasia, thymic D82.1
Alzheimer's disease or sclerosis —*see* Disease, Alzheimer's
Amastia (with nipple present) Q83.8
with absent nipple Q83.Ø
Amathophobia F4Ø.228
Amaurosis (acquired) (congenital) —*see also* Blindness
fugax G45.3
hysterical F44.6
Leber's congenital H35.5Ø
uremic —*see* Uremia
Amaurotic idiocy (infantile) (juvenile) (late) E75.4
Amaxophobia F4Ø.248
Ambiguous genitalia Q56.4
Amblyopia (congenital) (ex anopsia) (partial) (suppression) H53.ØØ-
anisometropic —*see* Amblyopia, refractive
deprivation H53.Ø1-
hysterical F44.6
nocturnal —*see also* Blindness, night
vitamin A deficiency E5Ø.5
refractive H53.Ø2-
strabismic H53.Ø3-
suspect H53.Ø4- ◀
tobacco H53.8
toxic NEC H53.8
uremic —*see* Uremia
Ameba, amebic (histolytica) —*see also* Amebiasis
abscess (liver) AØ6.4
Amebiasis AØ6.9
with abscess —*see* Abscess, amebic
acute AØ6.Ø
chronic (intestine) AØ6.1
with abscess —*see* Abscess, amebic
cutaneous AØ6.7
cutis AØ6.7
cystitis AØ6.81
genitourinary tract NEC AØ6.82
hepatic —*see* Abscess, liver, amebic
intestine AØ6.Ø
nondysenteric colitis AØ6.2
skin AØ6.7
specified site NEC AØ6.89
Ameboma (of intestine) AØ6.3
Amelia Q73.Ø
lower limb —*see* Agenesis, leg
upper limb —*see* Agenesis, arm
Ameloblastoma —*see also* Cyst, calcifying odontogenic
long bones C4Ø.9-
lower limb C4Ø.2-
upper limb C4Ø.Ø-
malignant C41.1
jaw (bone) (lower) C41.1
upper C41.Ø
tibial C4Ø.2-

Amelogenesis imperfecta KØØ.5
nonhereditaria (segmentalis) KØØ.4
Amenorrhea N91.2
hyperhormonal E28.8
primary N91.Ø
secondary N91.1
Amentia —*see* Disability, intellectual
Meynert's (nonalcoholic) FØ4
American
leishmaniasis B55.2
mountain tick fever A93.2
Ametropia —*see* Disorder, refraction
AMH (asymptomatic microscopic hematuria) R31.21 ◀
Amianthosis J61
Amimia R48.8
Amino-acid disorder E72.9
anemia D53.Ø
Aminoacidopathy E72.9
Aminoaciduria E72.9
Amnes (t)ic syndrome (post-traumatic) FØ4
induced by
alcohol F1Ø.96
with dependence F1Ø.26
psychoactive NEC F19.96
with
abuse F19.16
dependence F19.26
sedative F13.96
with dependence F13.26
Amnesia R41.3
anterograde R41.1
auditory R48.8
dissociative F44.Ø
with dissociative fugue F44.1 ◀
hysterical F44.Ø
postictal in epilepsy —*see* Epilepsy
psychogenic F44.Ø
retrograde R41.2
transient global G45.4
Amnion, amniotic —*see* condition
Amnionitis —*see* Pregnancy, complicated by
Amok F68.8
Amoral traits F6Ø.89
Amphetamine (or other stimulant) —induced ◀
anxiety disorder F15.98Ø ◀
bipolar and related disorder F15.94 ◀
delirium F15.921 ◀
depressive disorder F15.94 ◀
obsessive-compulsive and related disorder F15.988 ◀
psychotic disorder F15.959 ◀
sexual dysfunction F15.981 ◀
sleep disorder F15.982 ◀
stimulant withdrawal F15.23 ◀
Ampulla
lower esophagus K22.8
phrenic K22.8
Amputation —*see also* Absence, by site, acquired
neuroma (postoperative) (traumatic) —*see* Complications, amputation stump, neuroma
stump (surgical)
abnormal, painful, or with complication (late) —*see* Complications, amputation stump
healed or old NOS Z89.9
traumatic (complete) (partial)
arm (upper) (complete) S48.91-
at
elbow S58.Ø1-
partial S58.Ø2-
shoulder joint (complete) S48.Ø1-
partial S48.Ø2-
between
elbow and wrist (complete) S58.11-
partial S58.12-
shoulder and elbow (complete) S48.11-
partial S48.12-
partial S48.92-

A

Amputation *(Continued)*
- traumatic *(Continued)*
  - breast (complete) S28.21-
    - partial S28.22-
  - clitoris (complete) S38.211
    - partial S38.212
  - ear (complete) SØ8.11-
    - partial SØ8.12-
  - finger (complete) (metacarpophalangeal) S68.11-
    - index S68.11-
    - little S68.11-
    - middle S68.11-
    - partial S68.12-
      - index S68.12-
      - little S68.12-
      - middle S68.12-
      - ring S68.12-
    - ring S68.11-
    - thumb —*see* Amputation, traumatic, thumb
    - transphalangeal (complete) S68.61-
      - index S68.61-
      - little S68.61-
      - middle S68.61-
      - partial S68.62-
        - index S68.62-
        - little S68.62-
        - middle S68.62-
        - ring S68.62-
      - ring S68.61-
  - foot (complete) S98.91-
    - at ankle level S98.Ø1-
      - partial S98.Ø2-
    - midfoot S98.31-
      - partial S98.32-
    - partial S98.92-
  - forearm (complete) S58.91-
    - at elbow level (complete) S58.Ø1-
      - partial S58.Ø2-
    - between elbow and wrist (complete) S58.11-
      - partial S58.12-
    - partial S58.92-
  - genital organ (s) (external)
    - female (complete) S38.211
      - partial S38.212
    - male
      - penis (complete) S38.221
        - partial S38.222
      - scrotum (complete) S38.231
        - partial S38.232
      - testes (complete) S38.231
        - partial S38.232
  - hand (complete) (wrist level) S68.41-
    - finger (s) alone —*see* Amputation, traumatic, finger
    - partial S68.42-
    - thumb alone —*see* Amputation, traumatic, thumb
    - transmetacarpal (complete) S68.71-
      - partial S68.72-
  - head
    - ear —*see* Amputation, traumatic, ear
    - nose (partial) SØ8.812
      - complete SØ8.811
    - part SØ8.89
      - scalp SØ8.Ø
  - hip (and thigh) (complete) S78.91-
    - at hip joint (complete) S78.Ø1-
      - partial S78.Ø2-
    - between hip and knee (complete) S78.11-
      - partial S78.12-
    - partial S78.92-
  - labium (majus) (minus) (complete) S38.21-
    - partial S38.21-
  - leg (lower) S88.91-
    - at knee level S88.Ø1-
      - partial S88.Ø2-
    - between knee and ankle S88.11-
      - partial S88.12-
    - partial S88.92-

Amputation *(Continued)*
- traumatic *(Continued)*
  - nose (partial) SØ8.812
    - complete SØ8.811
  - penis (complete) S38.221
    - partial S38.222
  - scrotum (complete) S38.231
    - partial S38.232
  - shoulder —*see* Amputation, traumatic, arm
    - at shoulder joint —*see* Amputation, traumatic, arm, at shoulder joint
  - testes (complete) S38.231
    - partial S38.232
  - thigh —*see* Amputation, traumatic, hip
  - thorax, part of S28.1
    - breast —*see* Amputation, traumatic, breast
  - thumb (complete) (metacarpophalangeal) S68.Ø1-
    - partial S68.Ø2-
    - transphalangeal (complete) S68.51-
      - partial S68.52-
  - toe (lesser) S98.13-
    - great S98.11-
      - partial S98.12-
    - more than one S98.21-
      - partial S98.22-
    - partial S98.14-
  - vulva (complete) S38.211
    - partial S38.212

Amputee (bilateral) (old) Z89.9
Amsterdam dwarfism Q87.1
Amusia R48.8
- developmental F8Ø.89

Amyelencephalus, amyelencephaly QØØ.Ø
Amyelia QØ6.Ø
Amygdalitis —*see* Tonsillitis
Amygdalolith J35.8
Amyloid heart (disease) E85.4 *[I43]*
Amyloidosis (generalized) (primary) E85.9
- with lung involvement E85.4 *[J99]*
- familial E85.2
- genetic E85.2
- heart E85.4 *[I43]*
- ~~hemodialysis-associated E85.3~~
- liver E85.4 *[K77]*
- localized E85.4
- neuropathic heredofamilial E85.1
- non-neuropathic heredofamilial E85.Ø
- organ limited E85.4
- Portuguese E85.1
- pulmonary E85.4 *[J99]*
- secondary systemic E85.3
- skin (lichen) (macular) E85.4 *[L99]*
- specified NEC E85.8
- subglottic E85.4 *[J99]*

Amylopectinosis (brancher enzyme deficiency) E74.Ø3
Amylophagia —*see* Pica
Amyoplasia congenita Q79.8
Amyotonia M62.89
- congenita G7Ø.2

Amyotrophia, amyotrophy, amyotrophic G71.8
- congenita Q79.8
- diabetic —*see* Diabetes, amyotrophy
- lateral sclerosis G12.21
- neuralgic G54.5
- spinal progressive G12.21

Anacidity, gastric K31.83
- psychogenic F45.8

Anaerosis of newborn P28.89
Analbuminemia E88.Ø9
Analgesia —*see* Anesthesia
Analphalipoproteinemia E78.6
Anaphylactic
- purpura D69.Ø
- shock or reaction —*see* Shock, anaphylactic

Anaphylactoid shock or reaction —*see* Shock, anaphylactic
Anaphylactoid syndrome of pregnancy O88.Ø1-
Anaphylaxis —*see* Shock, anaphylactic
Anaplasia cervix —*see also* Dysplasia, cervix N87.9
Anaplasmosis, human A77.49
Anarthria R47.1
Anasarca R6Ø.1
- cardiac —*see* Failure, heart, congestive
- lung J18.2
- newborn P83.2
- nutritional E43
- pulmonary J18.2
- renal NØ4.9

Anastomosis
- aneurysmal —*see* Aneurysm
- arteriovenous ruptured brain I6Ø.8
- intestinal K63.89
  - complicated NEC K91.89
    - involving urinary tract N99.89
- retinal and choroidal vessels (congenital) Q14.8

Anatomical narrow angle H4Ø.Ø3-
Ancylostoma, ancylostomiasis (braziliense) (caninum) (ceylanicum) (duodenale) B76.Ø
- Necator americanus B76.1

Andersen's disease (glycogen storage) E74.Ø9
Anderson-Fabry disease E75.21
Andes disease T7Ø.29
Andrews' disease (bacterid) LØ8.89
Androblastoma
- benign
  - specified site —*see* Neoplasm, benign, by site
  - unspecified site
    - female D27.9
    - male D29.2Ø
- malignant
  - specified site —*see* Neoplasm, malignant, by site
  - unspecified site
    - female C56.9
    - male C62.9Ø
- specified site —*see* Neoplasm, uncertain behavior, by site
- tubular
  - with lipid storage
    - specified site —*see* Neoplasm, benign, by site
    - unspecified site
      - female D27.9
      - male D29.2Ø
  - specified site —*see* Neoplasm, benign, by site
  - unspecified site
    - female D27.9
    - male D29.2Ø
- unspecified site
  - female D39.1Ø
  - male D4Ø.1Ø

Androgen insensitivity syndrome —*see also* Syndrome, androgen insensitivity E34.5Ø
Androgen resistance syndrome —*see also* Syndrome, androgen insensitivity E34.5Ø
Android pelvis Q74.2
- with disproportion (fetopelvic) O33.3
  - causing obstructed labor O65.3

Androphobia F4Ø.29Ø
Anectasis, pulmonary (newborn) —*see* Atelectasis
Anemia (essential) (general) (hemoglobin deficiency) (infantile) (primary) (profound) D64.9
- with (due to) (in)
  - disorder of
    - anaerobic glycolysis D55.2
    - pentose phosphate pathway D55.1
  - koilonychia D5Ø.9
- achlorhydric D5Ø.8
- achrestic D53.1
- Addison (-Biermer) (pernicious) D51.Ø
- agranulocytic —*see* Agranulocytosis
- amino-acid-deficiency D53.Ø

- **Anemia** *(Continued)*
  - aplastic D61.9
    - congenital D61.Ø9
    - drug-induced D61.1
    - due to
      - drugs D61.1
      - external agents NEC D61.2
      - infection D61.2
      - radiation D61.2
    - idiopathic D61.3
    - red cell (pure) D6Ø.9
      - chronic D6Ø.Ø
      - congenital D61.Ø1
      - specified type NEC D6Ø.8
      - transient D6Ø.1
    - specified type NEC D61.89
    - toxic D61.2
  - aregenerative
    - congenital D61.Ø9
  - asiderotic D5Ø.9
  - atypical (primary) D64.9
  - Baghdad spring D55.Ø
  - Balantidium coli AØ7.Ø
  - Biermer's (pernicious) D51.Ø
  - blood loss (chronic) D5Ø.Ø
    - acute D62
  - bothriocephalus B7Ø.Ø *[D63.8]*
  - brickmaker's B76.9 *[D63.8]*
  - cerebral I67.89
  - childhood D58.9
  - chlorotic D5Ø.8
  - chronic
    - blood loss D5Ø.Ø
    - hemolytic D58.9
      - idiopathic D59.9
    - simple D53.9
  - chronica congenita aregenerativa D61.Ø9
  - combined system disease NEC D51.Ø *[G32.Ø]*
    - due to dietary vitamin B12 deficiency D51.3 *[G32.Ø]*
  - complicating pregnancy, childbirth or puerperium —*see* Pregnancy, complicated by (management affected by), anemia
  - congenital P61.4
    - aplastic D61.Ø9
    - due to isoimmunization NOS P55.9
    - dyserythropoietic, dyshematopoietic D64.4
    - following fetal blood loss P61.3
    - Heinz body D58.2
    - hereditary hemolytic NOS D58.9
    - pernicious D51.Ø
    - spherocytic D58.Ø
  - Cooley's (erythroblastic) D56.1
  - cytogenic D51.Ø
  - deficiency D53.9
    - 2, 3 diphosphoglycurate mutase D55.2
    - 2, 3 PG D55.2
    - 6 phosphogluconate dehydrogenase D55.1
    - 6-PGD D55.1
    - amino-acid D53.Ø
    - combined B12 and folate D53.1
    - enzyme D55.9
      - drug-induced (hemolytic) D59.2
      - glucose-6-phosphate dehydrogenase (G6PD) D55.Ø
      - glycolytic D55.2
      - nucleotide metabolism D55.3
      - related to hexose monophosphate (HMP) shunt pathway NEC D55.1
      - specified type NEC D55.8
    - erythrocytic glutathione D55.1
    - folate D52.9
      - dietary D52.Ø
      - drug-induced D52.1
    - folic acid D52.9
      - dietary D52.Ø
      - drug-induced D52.1
    - G SH D55.1
    - G6PD D55.Ø
    - GGS-R D55.1

- **Anemia** *(Continued)*
  - deficiency *(Continued)*
    - glucose-6-phosphate dehydrogenase D55.Ø
    - glutathione reductase D55.1
    - glyceraldehyde phosphate dehydrogenase D55.2
    - hexokinase D55.2
    - iron D5Ø.9
      - secondary to blood loss (chronic) D5Ø.Ø
    - nutritional D53.9
      - with
        - poor iron absorption D5Ø.8
        - specified deficiency NEC D53.8
    - phosphofructo-aldolase D55.2
    - phosphoglycerate kinase D55.2
    - PK D55.2
    - protein D53.Ø
    - pyruvate kinase D55.2
    - transcobalamin II D51.2
    - triose-phosphate isomerase D55.2
    - vitamin B12 NOS D51.9
      - dietary D51.3
      - due to
        - intrinsic factor deficiency D51.Ø
        - selective vitamin B12 malabsorption with proteinuria D51.1
      - pernicious D51.Ø
      - specified type NEC D51.8
  - Diamond-Blackfan (congenital hypoplastic) D61.Ø1
  - dibothriocephalus B7Ø.Ø *[D63.8]*
  - dimorphic D53.1
  - diphasic D53.1
  - Diphyllobothrium (Dibothriocephalus) B7Ø.Ø *[D63.8]*
  - due to (in) (with)
    - antineoplastic chemotherapy D64.81
    - blood loss (chronic) D5Ø.Ø
      - acute D62
    - chemotherapy, antineoplastic D64.81
    - chronic disease classified elsewhere NEC D63.8
    - chronic kidney disease D63.1
    - deficiency
      - amino-acid D53.Ø
      - copper D53.8
      - folate (folic acid) D52.9
        - dietary D52.Ø
        - drug-induced D52.1
      - molybdenum D53.8
      - protein D53.Ø
      - zinc D53.8
    - dietary vitamin B12 deficiency D51.3
    - disorder of
      - glutathione metabolism D55.1
      - nucleotide metabolism D55.3
    - drug —*see* Anemia, by type —*see also* Table of Drugs and Chemicals
    - end stage renal disease D63.1
    - enzyme disorder D55.9
    - fetal blood loss P61.3
    - fish tapeworm (D latum) infestation B7Ø.Ø *[D63.8]*
    - hemorrhage (chronic) D5Ø.Ø
      - acute D62
    - impaired absorption D5Ø.9
    - loss of blood (chronic) D5Ø.Ø
      - acute D62
    - myxedema EØ3.9 *[D63.8]*
    - Necator americanus B76.1 *[D63.8]*
    - prematurity P61.2
    - selective vitamin B12 malabsorption with proteinuria D51.1
    - transcobalamin II deficiency D51.2
  - Dyke-Young type (secondary) (symptomatic) D59.1
  - dyserythropoietic (congenital) D64.4
  - dyshematopoietic (congenital) D64.4
  - Egyptian B76.9 *[D63.8]*
  - elliptocytosis —*see* Elliptocytosis
  - enzyme-deficiency, drug-induced D59.2

- **Anemia** *(Continued)*
  - epidemic —*see also* Ancylostomiasis B76.9 *[D63.8]*
  - erythroblastic
    - familial D56.1
    - newborn —*see also* Disease, hemolytic P55.9
    - of childhood D56.1
  - erythrocytic glutathione deficiency D55.1
  - erythropoietin-resistant anemia (EPO resistant anemia) D63.1
  - Faber's (achlorhydric anemia) D5Ø.9
  - factitious (self-induced blood letting) D5Ø.Ø
  - familial erythroblastic D56.1
  - Fanconi's (congenital pancytopenia) D61.Ø9
  - favism D55.Ø
  - fish tapeworm (D. latum) infestation B7Ø.Ø *[D63.8]*
  - folate (folic acid) deficiency D52.9
  - glucose-6-phosphate dehydrogenase (G6PD) deficiency D55.Ø
  - glutathione-reductase deficiency D55.1
  - goat's milk D52.Ø
  - granulocytic —*see* Agranulocytosis
  - Heinz body, congenital D58.2
  - hemolytic D58.9
    - acquired D59.9
      - with hemoglobinuria NEC D59.6
      - autoimmune NEC D59.1
      - infectious D59.4
      - specified type NEC D59.8
      - toxic D59.4
    - acute D59.9
      - due to enzyme deficiency specified type NEC D55.8
      - Lederer's D59.1
    - autoimmune D59.1
      - drug-induced D59.Ø
    - chronic D58.9
      - idiopathic D59.9
    - cold type (secondary) (symptomatic) D59.1
    - congenital (spherocytic) —*see* Spherocytosis
    - due to
      - cardiac conditions D59.4
      - drugs (nonautoimmune) D59.2
        - autoimmune D59.Ø
      - enzyme disorder D55.9
        - drug-induced D59.2
      - presence of shunt or other internal prosthetic device D59.4
    - familial D58.9
    - hereditary D58.9
      - due to enzyme disorder D55.9
        - specified type NEC D55.8
      - specified type NEC D58.8
    - idiopathic (chronic) D59.9
    - mechanical D59.4
    - microangiopathic D59.4
    - nonautoimmune D59.4
      - drug-induced D59.2
    - nonspherocytic
      - congenital or hereditary NEC D55.8
        - glucose-6-phosphate dehydrogenase deficiency D55.Ø
        - pyruvate kinase deficiency D55.2
        - type
          - I D55.1
          - II D55.2
      - type
        - I D55.1
        - II D55.2
    - secondary D59.4
      - autoimmune D59.1
    - specified (hereditary) type NEC D58.8
    - Stransky-Regala type —*see also* Hemoglobinopathy D58.8
    - symptomatic D59.4
      - autoimmune D59.1
    - toxic D59.4
    - warm type (secondary) (symptomatic) D59.1

Anemia *(Continued)*
hemorrhagic (chronic) D5Ø.Ø
acute D62
Herrick's D57.1
hexokinase deficiency D55.2
hookworm B76.9 *[D63.8]*
hypochromic (idiopathic) (microcytic) (normoblastic) D5Ø.9
due to blood loss (chronic) D5Ø.Ø
acute D62
familial sex-linked D64.Ø
pyridoxine-responsive D64.3
sideroblastic, sex-linked D64.Ø
hypoplasia, red blood cells D61.9
congenital or familial D61.Ø1
hypoplastic (idiopathic) D61.9
congenital or familial (of childhood) D61.Ø1
hypoproliferative (refractive) D61.9
idiopathic D64.9
aplastic D61.3
hemolytic, chronic D59.9
in (due to) (with)
chronic kidney disease D63.1
end stage renal disease D63.1
failure, kidney (renal) D63.1
neoplastic disease —*see also* Neoplasm D63.Ø
intertropical —*see also* Ancylostomiasis D63.8
iron deficiency D5Ø.9
secondary to blood loss (chronic) D5Ø.Ø
acute D62
specified type NEC D5Ø.8
Joseph-Diamond-Blackfan (congenital hypoplastic) D61.Ø1
Lederer's (hemolytic) D59.1
leukoerythroblastic D61.82
macrocytic D53.9
nutritional D52.Ø
tropical D52.8
malarial (*see also* Malaria) B54 *[D63.8]*
malignant (progressive) D51.Ø
malnutrition D53.9
marsh (*see also* Malaria) B54 *[D63.8]*
Mediterranean (with other hemoglobinopathy) D56.9
megaloblastic D53.1
combined B12 and folate deficiency D53.1
hereditary D51.1
nutritional D52.Ø
orotic aciduria D53.Ø
refractory D53.1
specified type NEC D53.1
megalocytic D53.1
microcytic (hypochromic) D5Ø.9
due to blood loss (chronic) D5Ø.Ø
acute D62
familial D56.8
microdrepanocytosis D57.4Ø
microelliptopoikilocytic (Rietti-Greppi-Micheli) D56.9
miner's B76.9 *[D63.8]*
myelodysplastic D46.9
myelofibrosis D75.81
myelogenous D64.89
myelopathic D64.89
myelophthisic D61.82
myeloproliferative D47.Z9
newborn P61.4
due to
ABO (antibodies, isoimmunization, maternal/fetal incompatibility) P55.1
Rh (antibodies, isoimmunization, maternal/fetal incompatibility) P55.Ø
following fetal blood loss P61.3
posthemorrhagic (fetal) P61.3
nonspherocytic hemolytic —*see* Anemia, hemolytic, nonspherocytic

Anemia *(Continued)*
normocytic (infectional) D64.9
due to blood loss (chronic) D5Ø.Ø
acute D62
myelophthisic D61.82
nutritional (deficiency) D53.9
with
poor iron absorption D5Ø.8
specified deficiency NEC D53.8
megaloblastic D52.Ø
of prematurity P61.2
orotaciduric (congenital) (hereditary) D53.Ø
osteosclerotic D64.89
ovalocytosis (hereditary) —*see* Elliptocytosis
paludal —*see also* Malaria B54 *[D63.8]*
pernicious (congenital) (malignant) (progressive) D51.Ø
pleochromic D64.89
of sprue D52.8
posthemorrhagic (chronic) D5Ø.Ø
acute D62
newborn P61.3
postoperative (postprocedural)
due to (acute) blood loss D62
chronic blood loss D5Ø.Ø
specified NEC D64.9
postpartum O9Ø.81
pressure D64.89
progressive D64.9
malignant D51.Ø
pernicious D51.Ø
protein-deficiency D53.Ø
pseudoleukemica infantum D64.89
pure red cell D6Ø.9
congenital D61.Ø1
pyridoxine-responsive D64.3
pyruvate kinase deficiency D55.2
refractory D46.4
with
excess of blasts D46.2Ø
1 (RAEB 1) D46.21
2 (RAEB 2) D46.22
in transformation (RAEB T) —*see* Leukemia, acute myeloblastic
hemochromatosis D46.1
sideroblasts (ring) (RARS) D46.1
without ring sideroblasts, so stated D46.Ø
without sideroblasts without excess of blasts D46.Ø
megaloblastic D53.1
sideroblastic D46.1
sideropenic D5Ø.9
Rietti-Greppi-Micheli D56.9
scorbutic D53.2
secondary to
blood loss (chronic) D5Ø.Ø
acute D62
hemorrhage (chronic) D5Ø.Ø
acute D62
semiplastic D61.89
sickle-cell —*see* Disease, sickle-cell
sideroblastic D64.3
hereditary D64.Ø
hypochromic, sex-linked D64.Ø
pyridoxine-responsive NEC D64.3
refractory D46.1
secondary (due to)
disease D64.1
drugs and toxins D64.2
specified type NEC D64.3
sideropenic (refractory) D5Ø.9
due to blood loss (chronic) D5Ø.Ø
acute D62
simple chronic D53.9
specified type NEC D64.89
spherocytic (hereditary) —*see* Spherocytosis
splenic D64.89
splenomegalic D64.89
stomatocytosis D58.8
syphilitic (acquired) (late) A52.79 *[D63.8]*
target cell D64.89

Anemia *(Continued)*
thalassemia D56.9
thrombocytopenic —*see* Thrombocytopenia
toxic D61.2
tropical B76.9 *[D63.8]*
macrocytic D52.8
tuberculous A18.89 *[D63.8]*
vegan D51.3
vitamin
B6-responsive D64.3
B12 deficiency (dietary) pernicious D51.Ø
von Jaksch's D64.89
Witts' (achlorhydric anemia) D5Ø.8
Anemophobia F4Ø.228
Anencephalus, anencephaly QØØ.Ø
Anergasia —*see* Psychosis, organic
Anesthesia, anesthetic R2Ø.Ø
complication or reaction NEC —*see also* Complications, anesthesia T88.59
due to
correct substance properly administered —*see* Table of Drugs and Chemicals, by drug, adverse effect
overdose or wrong substance given —*see* Table of Drugs and Chemicals, by drug, poisoning
unintended awareness under general anesthesia during procedure T88.53 ◀
personal history of Z92.84 ◀
cornea H18.81-
dissociative F44.6
functional (hysterical) F44.6
hyperesthetic, thalamic G89.Ø
hysterical F44.6
local skin lesion R2Ø.Ø
sexual (psychogenic) F52.1
shock (due to) T88.2
skin R2Ø.Ø
testicular N5Ø.9
Anetoderma (maculosum) (of) L9Ø.8
Jadassohn-Pellizzari L9Ø.2
Schweniger-Buzzi L9Ø.1
Aneurin deficiency E51.9
Aneurysm (anastomotic) (artery) (cirsoid) (diffuse) (false) (fusiform) (multiple) (saccular) I72.9
abdominal (aorta) I71.4
ruptured I71.3
syphilitic A52.Ø1
aorta, aortic (nonsyphilitic) I71.9
abdominal I71.4
ruptured I71.3
arch I71.2
ruptured I71.1
arteriosclerotic I71.9
ruptured I71.8
ascending I71.2
ruptured I71.1
congenital Q25.43 ⬅
descending I71.9
abdominal I71.4
ruptured I71.3
ruptured I71.8
thoracic I71.2
ruptured I71.1
root Q25.43 ◀
ruptured I71.8
sinus, congenital Q25.43 ⬅
syphilitic A52.Ø1
thoracic I71.2
ruptured I71.1
thoracoabdominal I71.6
ruptured I71.5
thorax, thoracic (arch) I71.2
ruptured I71.1
transverse I71.2
ruptured I71.1
valve (heart) —*see also* Endocarditis, aortic I35.8

A

Aneurysm *(Continued)*
  arteriosclerotic I72.9
    cerebral I67.1
      ruptured —*see* Hemorrhage, intracranial, subarachnoid
  arteriovenous (congenital) —*see also* Malformation, arteriovenous
    acquired I77.0
      brain I67.1
      coronary I25.41
      pulmonary I28.0
    brain Q28.2
      ruptured I60.8
    peripheral —*see* Malformation, arteriovenous, peripheral
    precerebral vessels Q28.0
    specified site NEC —*see also* Malformation, arteriovenous
      acquired I77.0
  basal —*see* Aneurysm, brain
  basilar (trunk) I72.5 ◀
  berry (congenital) (nonruptured) I67.1
    ruptured I60.7
  brain I67.1
    arteriosclerotic I67.1
      ruptured —*see* Hemorrhage, intracranial, subarachnoid
    arteriovenous (congenital) (nonruptured) Q28.2
      acquired I67.1
        ruptured I60.8
      ruptured I60.8
    berry (congenital) (nonruptured) I67.1
      ruptured —*see also* Hemorrhage, intracranial, subarachnoid I60.7
    congenital Q28.3
      aorta (root) (sinus) Q25.43 ◀
      ruptured I60.7
    meninges I67.1
      ruptured I60.8
    miliary (congenital) (nonruptured) I67.1
      ruptured —*see also* Hemorrhage, intracranial, subarachnoid I60.7
    mycotic I33.0
    ruptured —*see* Hemorrhage, intracranial, subarachnoid
    syphilitic (hemorrhage) A52.05
  cardiac (false) —*see also* Aneurysm, heart I25.3
  carotid artery (common) (external) I72.0
    internal (intracranial) I67.1
      extracranial portion I72.0
    ruptured into brain I60.0-
    syphilitic A52.09
      intracranial A52.05
  cavernous sinus I67.1
    arteriovenous (congenital) (nonruptured) Q28.3
      ruptured I60.8
  celiac I72.8
  central nervous system, syphilitic A52.05
  cerebral —*see* Aneurysm, brain
  chest —*see* Aneurysm, thorax
  circle of Willis I67.1
    congenital Q28.3
      ruptured I60.6
    ruptured I60.6
  common iliac artery I72.3
  congenital (peripheral) Q27.8
    aorta (root) (sinus) Q25.43 ◀
    brain Q28.3
      ruptured I60.7
    coronary Q24.5
    digestive system Q27.8
    lower limb Q27.8
    pulmonary Q25.79
    retina Q14.1
    specified site NEC Q27.8
    upper limb Q27.8
  conjunctiva —*see* Abnormality, conjunctiva, vascular
  conus arteriosus —*see* Aneurysm, heart

Aneurysm *(Continued)*
  coronary (arteriosclerotic) (artery) I25.41
    arteriovenous, congenital Q24.5
    congenital Q24.5
    ruptured —*see* Infarct, myocardium
    syphilitic A52.06
    vein I25.89
  cylindroid (aorta) I71.9
    ruptured I71.8
    syphilitic A52.01
  ductus arteriosus Q25.0
  endocardial, infective (any valve) I33.0
  femoral (artery) (ruptured) I72.4
  gastroduodenal I72.8
  gastroepiploic I72.8
  heart (wall) (chronic or with a stated duration of over 4 weeks) I25.3
    valve —*see* Endocarditis
  hepatic I72.8
  iliac (common) (artery) (ruptured) I72.3
  infective I72.9
    endocardial (any valve) I33.0
  innominate (nonsyphilitic) I72.8
    syphilitic A52.09
  interauricular septum —*see* Aneurysm, heart
  interventricular septum —*see* Aneurysm, heart
  intrathoracic (nonsyphilitic) I71.2
    ruptured I71.1
    syphilitic A52.01
  lower limb I72.4
  lung (pulmonary artery) I28.1
  mediastinal (nonsyphilitic) I72.8
    syphilitic A52.09
  miliary (congenital) I67.1
    ruptured —*see* Hemorrhage, intracerebral, subarachnoid, intracranial
  mitral (heart) (valve) I34.8
  mural —*see* Aneurysm, heart
  mycotic I72.9
    endocardial (any valve) I33.0
    ruptured, brain —*see* Hemorrhage, intracerebral, subarachnoid
  myocardium —*see* Aneurysm, heart
  neck I72.0
  pancreaticoduodenal I72.8
  patent ductus arteriosus Q25.0
  peripheral NEC I72.8
    congenital Q27.8
      digestive system Q27.8
      lower limb Q27.8
      specified site NEC Q27.8
      upper limb Q27.8
  popliteal (artery) (ruptured) I72.4
  ~~precerebral, congenital (nonruptured) Q28.1~~
  precerebral ◀
    congenital (nonruptured) Q28.1 ◀
    specified site, NEC I72.5 ◀
  pulmonary I28.1
    arteriovenous Q25.72
      acquired I28.0
    syphilitic A52.09
    valve (heart) —*see* Endocarditis, pulmonary
  racemose (peripheral) I72.9
    congenital —*see* Aneurysm, congenital
  radial I72.1
  Rasmussen NEC A15.0
  renal (artery) I72.2
  retina —*see also* Disorder, retina, microaneurysms
    congenital Q14.1
    diabetic —*see* Diabetes, microaneurysms, retinal
  sinus of Valsalva Q25.49 ⬅
  specified NEC I72.8
  spinal (cord) I72.8
    syphilitic (hemorrhage) A52.09
  splenic I72.8

Aneurysm *(Continued)*
  subclavian (artery) (ruptured) I72.8
    syphilitic A52.09
  superior mesenteric I72.8
  syphilitic (aorta) A52.01
    central nervous system A52.05
    congenital (late) A50.54 *[I79.0]*
    spine, spinal A52.09
  thoracoabdominal (aorta) I71.6
    ruptured I71.5
    syphilitic A52.01
  thorax, thoracic (aorta) (arch) (nonsyphilitic) I71.2
    ruptured I71.1
    syphilitic A52.01
  traumatic (complication) (early), specified site —*see* Injury, blood vessel
  tricuspid (heart) (valve) I07.8
  ulnar I72.1
  upper limb (ruptured) I72.1
  valve, valvular —*see* Endocarditis
  visceral NEC I72.8
  venous —*see also* Varix I86.8
    congenital Q27.8
      digestive system Q27.8
      lower limb Q27.8
      specified site NEC Q27.8
      upper limb Q27.8
  ventricle —*see* Aneurysm, heart
  vertebral artery I72.6 ◀
  visceral NEC I72.8
Angelman syndrome Q93.5
Anger R45.4
Angiectasis, angiectopia I99.8
Angiitis I77.6
  allergic granulomatous M30.1
  hypersensitivity M31.0
  necrotizing M31.9
    specified NEC M31.8
  nervous system, granulomatous I67.7
Angina (attack) (cardiac) (chest) (heart) (pectoris) (syndrome) (vasomotor) I20.9
  with
    atherosclerotic heart disease —*see* Arteriosclerosis, coronary (artery)
    documented spasm I20.1
  abdominal K55.1
  accelerated —*see* Angina, unstable
  agranulocytic —*see* Agranulocytosis
  angiospastic —*see* Angina, with documented spasm
  aphthous B08.5
  crescendo —*see* Angina, unstable
  croupous J05.0
  cruris I73.9
  de novo effort —*see* Angina, unstable
  diphtheritic, membranous A36.0
  equivalent I20.8
  exudative, chronic J37.0
  following acute myocardial infarction I23.7
  gangrenous diphtheritic A36.0
  intestinal K55.1
  Ludovici K12.2
  Ludwig's K12.2
  malignant diphtheritic A36.0
  membranous J05.0
    diphtheritic A36.0
    Vincent's A69.1
  mesenteric K55.1
  monocytic —*see* Mononucleosis, infectious
  of effort —*see* Angina, specified NEC
  phlegmonous J36
    diphtheritic A36.0
  post-infarctional I23.7
  pre-infarctional —*see* Angina, unstable
  Prinzmetal —*see* Angina, with documented spasm
  progressive —*see* Angina, unstable
  pseudomembranous A69.1
  pultaceous, diphtheritic A36.0

A

◀ New ⬅ Revised ~~deleted~~ Deleted

Angina *(Continued)*
- spasm-induced —*see* Angina, with documented spasm
- specified NEC I20.8
- stable I20.8 ⇐
- stenocardia —*see* Angina, specified NEC
- stridulous, diphtheritic A36.2
- tonsil J36
- trachealis J05.0
- unstable I20.0
- variant —*see* Angina, with documented spasm
- Vincent's A69.1
- worsening effort —*see* Angina, unstable

Angioblastoma —*see* Neoplasm, connective tissue, uncertain behavior
Angiocholecystitis —*see* Cholecystitis, acute
Angiocholitis —*see also* Cholecystitis, acute K83.0
Angiodysgenesis spinalis G95.19
Angiodysplasia (cecum) (colon) K55.20
- with bleeding K55.21
- duodenum (and stomach) K31.819
  - with bleeding K31.811
- stomach (and duodenum) K31.819
  - with bleeding K31.811

Angioedema (allergic) (any site) (with urticaria) T78.3
- hereditary D84.1

Angioendothelioma —*see* Neoplasm, uncertain behavior, by site
- benign D18.00
  - intra-abdominal D18.03
  - intracranial D18.02
  - skin D18.01
  - specified site NEC D18.09
- bone —*see* Neoplasm, bone, malignant
- Ewing's —*see* Neoplasm, bone, malignant

Angioendotheliomatosis C85.8-
Angiofibroma —*see also* Neoplasm, benign, by site
- juvenile
  - specified site —*see* Neoplasm, benign, by site
  - unspecified site D10.6

Angiohemophilia (A) (B) D68.0
Angioid streaks (choroid) (macula) (retina) H35.33
Angiokeratoma —*see* Neoplasm, skin, benign
- corporis diffusum E75.21

Angioleiomyoma —*see* Neoplasm, connective tissue, benign
Angiolipoma —*see also* Lipoma
- infiltrating —*see* Lipoma

Angioma —*see also* Hemangioma, by site
- capillary I78.1
- hemorrhagicum hereditaria I78.0
- intra-abdominal D18.03
- intracranial D18.02
- malignant —*see* Neoplasm, connective tissue, malignant
- plexiform D18.00
  - intra-abdominal D18.03
  - intracranial D18.02
  - skin D18.01
  - specified site NEC D18.09
- senile I78.1
- serpiginosum L81.7
- skin D18.01
- specified site NEC D18.09
- spider I78.1
- stellate I78.1
- venous Q28.3

Angiomatosis Q82.8
- bacillary A79.89
- encephalotrigeminal Q85.8
- hemorrhagic familial I78.0
- hereditary familial I78.0
- liver K76.4

Angiomyolipoma —*see* Lipoma
Angiomyoliposarcoma —*see* Neoplasm, connective tissue, malignant
Angiomyoma —*see* Neoplasm, connective tissue, benign
Angiomyosarcoma —*see* Neoplasm, connective tissue, malignant
Angiomyxoma —*see* Neoplasm, connective tissue, uncertain behavior
Angioneurosis F45.8
Angioneurotic edema (allergic) (any site) (with urticaria) T78.3
- hereditary D84.1

Angiopathia, angiopathy I99.9
- cerebral I67.9
  - amyloid E85.4 *[I68.0]*
- diabetic (peripheral) —*see* Diabetes, angiopathy
- peripheral I73.9
  - diabetic —*see* Diabetes, angiopathy
  - specified type NEC I73.89
- retinae syphilitica A52.05
- retinalis (juvenilis)
  - diabetic —*see* Diabetes, retinopathy
  - proliferative —*see* Retinopathy, proliferative

Angiosarcoma —*see also* Neoplasm, connective tissue, malignant
- liver C22.3

Angiosclerosis —*see* Arteriosclerosis
Angiospasm (peripheral) (traumatic) (vessel) I73.9
- brachial plexus G54.0
- cerebral G45.9
- cervical plexus G54.2
- nerve
  - arm —*see* Mononeuropathy, upper limb
    - axillary G54.0
    - median —*see* Lesion, nerve, median
    - ulnar —*see* Lesion, nerve, ulnar
  - axillary G54.0
  - leg —*see* Mononeuropathy, lower limb
    - median —*see* Lesion, nerve, median
    - plantar —*see* Lesion, nerve, plantar
    - ulnar —*see* Lesion, nerve, ulnar

Angiospastic disease or edema I73.9
Angiostrongyliasis
- due to
  - Parastrongylus
    - cantonensis B83.2
    - costaricensis B81.3
- intestinal B81.3

Anguillulosis —*see* Strongyloidiasis
Angulation
- cecum —*see* Obstruction, intestine
- coccyx (acquired) —*see also* subcategory M43.8
  - congenital NEC Q76.49
- femur (acquired) —*see also* Deformity, limb, specified type NEC, thigh
  - congenital Q74.2
- intestine (large) (small) —*see* Obstruction, intestine
- sacrum (acquired) —*see also* subcategory M43.8
  - congenital NEC Q76.49
- sigmoid (flexure) —*see* Obstruction, intestine
- spine —*see* Dorsopathy, deforming, specified NEC
- tibia (acquired) —*see also* Deformity, limb, specified type NEC, lower leg
  - congenital Q74.2
- ureter N13.5
  - with infection N13.6
- wrist (acquired) —*see also* Deformity, limb, specified type NEC, forearm
  - congenital Q74.0

Angulus infectiosus (lips) K13.0
Anhedonia R45.84
- sexual F52.0 ◀

Anhidrosis L74.4
~~Anhydration, anhydremia E86.0~~
- ~~with~~
  - ~~hypernatremia E87.0~~
  - ~~hyponatremia E87.1~~

Anhydration E86.0 ◀
Anhydremia E86.0
- ~~with~~
  - ~~hypernatremia E87.0~~
  - ~~hyponatremia E87.1~~

Anidrosis L74.4
Aniridia (congenital) Q13.1
Anisakiasis (infection) (infestation) B81.0
Anisakis larvae infestation B81.0
Aniseikonia H52.32
Anisocoria (pupil) H57.02
- congenital Q13.2

Anisocytosis R71.8
Anisometropia (congenital) H52.31
Ankle —*see* condition
Ankyloblepharon (eyelid) (acquired) —*see also* Blepharophimosis
- filiforme (adnatum) (congenital) Q10.3
- total Q10.3

Ankyloglossia Q38.1
Ankylosis (fibrous) (osseous) (joint) M24.60
- ankle M24.67-
- arthrodesis status Z98.1
- cricoarytenoid (cartilage) (joint) (larynx) J38.7
- dental K03.5
- ear ossicles H74.31-
- elbow M24.62-
- foot M24.67-
- hand M24.64-
- hip M24.65-
- incostapedial joint (infectional) —*see* Ankylosis, ear ossicles
- jaw (temporomandibular) M26.61- ⇐
- knee M24.66-
- lumbosacral (joint) M43.27
- postoperative (status) Z98.1
- produced by surgical fusion, status Z98.1
- sacro-iliac (joint) M43.28
- shoulder M24.61-
- spine (joint) —*see also* Fusion, spine
  - spondylitic —*see* Spondylitis, ankylosing
- surgical Z98.1
- temporomandibular M26.61- ⇐
- tooth, teeth (hard tissues) K03.5
- wrist M24.63-

Ankylostoma —*see* Ancylostoma
Ankylostomiasis —*see* Ancylostomiasis
Ankylurethria —*see* Stricture, urethra
Annular —*see also* condition
- detachment, cervix N88.8
- organ or site, congenital NEC —*see* Distortion
- pancreas (congenital) Q45.1

Anodontia (complete) (partial) (vera) K00.0
- acquired K08.10

Anomaly, anomalous (congenital) (unspecified type) Q89.9
- abdominal wall NEC Q79.59
- acoustic nerve Q07.8
- adrenal (gland) Q89.1
- Alder (-Reilly) (leukocyte granulation) D72.0
- alimentary tract Q45.9
  - upper Q40.9
- alveolar M26.70
  - hyperplasia M26.79
    - mandibular M26.72
    - maxillary M26.71
  - hypoplasia M26.79
    - mandibular M26.74
    - maxillary M26.73
  - ridge (process) M26.79
  - specified NEC M26.79
- ankle (joint) Q74.2
- anus Q43.9
- aorta (arch) NEC Q25.40 ⇐
  - coarctation (preductal) (postductal) Q25.1
- aortic cusp or valve Q23.9
- appendix Q43.8
- apple peel syndrome Q41.1
- aqueduct of Sylvius Q03.0
  - with spina bifida —*see* Spina bifida, with hydrocephalus

Anomaly, anomalous *(Continued)*
arm Q74.Ø
arteriovenous NEC
coronary Q24.5
gastrointestinal Q27.33
acquired —*see* Angiodysplasia
artery (peripheral) Q27.9
basilar NEC Q28.1
cerebral Q28.3
coronary Q24.5
digestive system Q27.8
eye Q15.8
great Q25.9
specified NEC Q25.8
lower limb Q27.8
peripheral Q27.9
specified NEC Q27.8
pulmonary NEC Q25.79
renal Q27.2
retina Q14.1
specified site NEC Q27.8
subclavian Q27.8
origin Q25.48 ◀
umbilical Q27.Ø
upper limb Q27.8
vertebral NEC Q28.1
aryteno-epiglottic folds Q31.8
atrial
bands or folds Q2Ø.8
septa Q21.1
atrioventricular
excitation I45.6
septum Q21.Ø
auditory canal Q17.8
auricle
ear Q17.8
causing impairment of hearing Q16.9
heart Q2Ø.8
Axenfeld's Q15.Ø
back Q89.9
band
atrial Q2Ø.8
heart Q24.8
ventricular Q24.8
Bartholin's duct Q38.4
biliary duct or passage Q44.5
bladder Q64.7Ø
absence Q64.5
diverticulum Q64.6
exstrophy Q64.1Ø
cloacal Q64.12
extroversion Q64.19
specified type NEC Q64.19
supravesical fissure Q64.11
neck obstruction Q64.31
specified type NEC Q64.79
bone Q79.9
arm Q74.Ø
face Q75.9
leg Q74.2
pelvic girdle Q74.2
shoulder girdle Q74.Ø
skull Q75.9
with
anencephaly QØØ.Ø
encephalocele —*see* Encephalocele
hydrocephalus QØ3.9
with spina bifida —*see* Spina bifida, by site, with hydrocephalus
microcephaly QØ2
brain (multiple) QØ4.9
vessel Q28.3
breast Q83.9
broad ligament Q5Ø.6
bronchus Q32.4
bulbus cordis Q21.9
bursa Q79.9
canal of Nuck Q52.4
canthus Q1Ø.3
capillary Q27.9

Anomaly, anomalous *(Continued)*
cardiac Q24.9
chambers Q2Ø.9
specified NEC Q2Ø.8
septal closure Q21.9
specified NEC Q21.8
valve NEC Q24.8
pulmonary Q22.3
cardiovascular system Q28.8
carpus Q74.Ø
caruncle, lacrimal Q1Ø.6
cascade stomach Q4Ø.2
cauda equina QØ6.3
cecum Q43.9
cerebral QØ4.9
vessels Q28.3
cervix Q51.9
Chédiak-Higashi(-Steinbrinck) (congenital gigantism of peroxidase granules) E7Ø.33Ø
cheek Q18.9
chest wall Q67.8
bones Q76.9
chin Q18.9
chordae tendineae Q24.8
choroid Q14.3
plexus QØ7.8
chromosomes, chromosomal Q99.9
D (1) —*see* condition, chromosome 13
E (3) —*see* condition, chromosome 18
G —*see* condition, chromosome 21
sex
female phenotype Q97.8
gonadal dysgenesis (pure) Q99.1
Klinefelter's Q98.4
male phenotype Q98.9
Turner's Q96.9
specified NEC Q99.8
cilia Q1Ø.3
circulatory system Q28.9
clavicle Q74.Ø
clitoris Q52.6
coccyx Q76.49
colon Q43.9
common duct Q44.5
communication
coronary artery Q24.5
left ventricle with right atrium Q21.Ø
concha (ear) Q17.3
connection
portal vein Q26.5
pulmonary venous Q26.4
partial Q26.3
total Q26.2
renal artery with kidney Q27.2
cornea (shape) Q13.4
coronary artery or vein Q24.5
cranium —*see* Anomaly, skull
cricoid cartilage Q31.8
cystic duct Q44.5
dental
alveolar —*see* Anomaly, alveolar
arch relationship M26.2Ø
specified NEC M26.29
dentofacial M26.9
alveolar —*see* Anomaly, alveolar
dental arch relationship M26.2Ø
specified NEC M26.29
functional M26.5Ø
specified NEC M26.59
jaw-cranial base relationship M26.1Ø
asymmetry M26.12
maxillary M26.11
specified type NEC M26.19
jaw size M26.ØØ
macrogenia M26.Ø5
mandibular
hyperplasia M26.Ø3
hypoplasia M26.Ø4
maxillary
hyperplasia M26.Ø1
hypoplasia M26.Ø2

Anomaly, anomalous *(Continued)*
dentofacial *(Continued)*
jaw size *(Continued)*
microgenia M26.Ø6
specified type NEC M26.Ø9
malocclusion M26.4
dental arch relationship NEC M26.29
jaw-cranial base relationship —*see* Anomaly, dentofacial, jaw-cranial base relationship
jaw size —*see* Anomaly, dentofacial, jaw size
specified type NEC M26.89
temporomandibular joint M26.6Ø- ⬅
adhesions M26.61- ⬅
ankylosis M26.61- ⬅
arthralgia M26.62- ⬅
articular disc M26.63- ⬅
specified type NEC M26.69
tooth position, fully erupted M26.3Ø
specified NEC M26.39
dermatoglyphic Q82.8
diaphragm (apertures) NEC Q79.1
digestive organ (s) or tract Q45.9
lower Q43.9
upper Q4Ø.9
distance, interarch (excessive) (inadequate) M26.25
distribution, coronary artery Q24.5
ductus
arteriosus Q25.Ø
botalli Q25.Ø
duodenum Q43.9
dura (brain) QØ4.9
spinal cord QØ6.9
ear (external) Q17.9
causing impairment of hearing Q16.9
inner Q16.5
middle (causing impairment of hearing) Q16.4
ossicles Q16.3
Ebstein's (heart) (tricuspid valve) Q22.5
ectodermal Q82.9
Eisenmenger's (ventricular septal defect) Q21.8
ejaculatory duct Q55.4
elbow Q74.Ø
endocrine gland NEC Q89.2
epididymis Q55.4
epiglottis Q31.8
esophagus Q39.9
eustachian tube Q17.8
eye Q15.9
anterior segment Q13.9
specified NEC Q13.89
posterior segment Q14.9
specified NEC Q14.8
ptosis (eyelid) Q1Ø.Ø
specified NEC Q15.8
eyebrow Q18.8
eyelid Q1Ø.3
ptosis Q1Ø.Ø
face Q18.9
bone(s) Q75.9
fallopian tube Q5Ø.6
fascia Q79.9
femur NEC Q74.2
fibula NEC Q74.2
finger Q74.Ø
fixation, intestine Q43.3
flexion (joint) NOS Q74.9
hip or thigh Q65.89
foot NEC Q74.2
varus (congenital) Q66.3
foramen
Botalli Q21.1
ovale Q21.1
forearm Q74.Ø
forehead Q75.8
form, teeth KØØ.2
fovea centralis Q14.1

Anomaly, anomalous *(Continued)*
  frontal bone —*see* Anomaly, skull
  gallbladder (position) (shape) (size) Q44.1
  Gartner's duct Q52.4
  gastrointestinal tract Q45.9
  genitalia, genital organ (s) or system
    female Q52.9
      external Q52.7Ø
      internal NOS Q52.9
    male Q55.9
      hydrocele P83.5
      specified NEC Q55.8
  genitourinary NEC
    female Q52.9
    male Q55.9
  Gerbode Q21.Ø
  glottis Q31.8
  granulation or granulocyte, genetic (constitutional) (leukocyte) D72.Ø
  gum Q38.6
  gyri Q07.9
  hair Q84.2
  hand Q74.Ø
  hard tissue formation in pulp K04.3
  head —*see* Anomaly, skull
  heart Q24.9
    auricle Q2Ø.8
    bands or folds Q24.8
    fibroelastosis cordis I42.4
    obstructive NEC Q22.6
    patent ductus arteriosus (Botalli) Q25.Ø
    septum Q21.9
      auricular Q21.1
      interatrial Q21.1
      interventricular Q21.Ø
        with pulmonary stenosis or atresia, dextraposition of aorta and hypertrophy of right ventricle Q21.3
      specified NEC Q21.8
      ventricular Q21.Ø
        with pulmonary stenosis or atresia, dextraposition of aorta and hypertrophy of right ventricle Q21.3
    tetralogy of Fallot Q21.3
    valve NEC Q24.8
      aortic
        bicuspid valve Q23.1
        insufficiency Q23.1
        stenosis Q23.Ø
          subaortic Q24.4
      mitral
        insufficiency Q23.3
        stenosis Q23.2
      pulmonary Q22.3
        atresia Q22.Ø
        insufficiency Q22.2
        stenosis Q22.1
          infundibular Q24.3
          subvalvular Q24.3
      tricuspid
        atresia Q22.4
        stenosis Q22.4
    ventricle Q2Ø.8
  heel NEC Q74.2
  Hegglin's D72.Ø
  hemianencephaly QØØ.Ø
  hemicephaly QØØ.Ø
  hemicrania QØØ.Ø
  hepatic duct Q44.5
  hip NEC Q74.2
  hourglass stomach Q4Ø.2
  humerus Q74.Ø
  hydatid of Morgagni
    female Q5Ø.5
    male (epididymal) Q55.4
      testicular Q55.29
  hymen Q52.4
  hypersegmentation of neutrophils, hereditary D72.Ø

Anomaly, anomalous *(Continued)*
  hypophyseal Q89.2
  ileocecal (coil) (valve) Q43.9
  ileum Q43.9
  ilium NEC Q74.2
  integument Q84.9
    specified NEC Q84.8
  interarch distance (excessive) (inadequate) M26.25
  intervertebral cartilage or disc Q76.49
  intestine (large) (small) Q43.9
    with anomalous adhesions, fixation or malrotation Q43.3
  iris Q13.2
  ischium NEC Q74.2
  jaw —*see* Anomaly, dentofacial
    alveolar —*see* Anomaly, alveolar
  jaw-cranial base relationship —*see* Anomaly, dentofacial, jaw-cranial base relationship
  jejunum Q43.8
  joint Q74.9
    specified NEC Q74.8
  Jordan's D72.Ø
  kidney(s) (calyx) (pelvis) Q63.9
    artery Q27.2
    specified NEC Q63.8
  Klippel-Feil (brevicollis) Q76.1
  knee Q74.1
  labium (majus) (minus) Q52.7Ø
  labyrinth, membranous Q16.5
  lacrimal apparatus or duct Q1Ø.6
  larynx, laryngeal (muscle) Q31.9
    web (bed) Q31.Ø
  lens Q12.9
  leukocytes, genetic D72.Ø
    granulation (constitutional) D72.Ø
  lid (fold) Q1Ø.3
  ligament Q79.9
    broad Q5Ø.6
    round Q52.8
  limb Q74.9
    lower NEC Q74.2
      reduction deformity —*see* Defect, reduction, lower limb
    upper Q74.Ø
  lip Q38.Ø
  liver Q44.7
    duct Q44.5
  lower limb NEC Q74.2
  lumbosacral (joint) (region) Q76.49
    kyphosis —*see* Kyphosis, congenital
    lordosis —*see* Lordosis, congenital
  lung (fissure) (lobe) Q33.9
  mandible —*see* Anomaly, dentofacial
  maxilla —*see* Anomaly, dentofacial
  May (-Hegglin) D72.Ø
  meatus urinarius NEC Q64.79
  meningeal bands or folds QØ7.9
    constriction of QØ7.8
    spinal QØ6.9
  meninges QØ7.9
    cerebral QØ4.8
    spinal QØ6.9
  meningocele QØ5.9
  mesentery Q45.9
  metacarpus Q74.Ø
  metatarsus NEC Q74.2
  middle ear Q16.4
    ossicles Q16.3
  mitral (leaflets) (valve) Q23.9
    insufficiency Q23.3
    specified NEC Q23.8
    stenosis Q23.2
  mouth Q38.6
  Müllerian —*see also* Anomaly, by site
    uterus NEC Q51.818
  multiple NEC Q89.7
  muscle Q79.9
    eyelid Q1Ø.3
  musculoskeletal system, except limbs Q79.9

Anomaly, anomalous *(Continued)*
  myocardium Q24.8
  nail Q84.6
  narrowness, eyelid Q1Ø.3
  nasal sinus (wall) Q3Ø.8
  neck (any part) Q18.9
  nerve QØ7.9
    acoustic QØ7.8
    optic QØ7.8
  nervous system (central) QØ7.9
  nipple Q83.9
  nose, nasal (bones) (cartilage) (septum) (sinus) Q3Ø.9
    specified NEC Q3Ø.8
  ocular muscle Q15.8
  omphalomesenteric duct Q43.Ø
  opening, pulmonary veins Q26.4
  optic
    disc Q14.2
    nerve QØ7.8
  opticociliary vessels Q13.2
  orbit (eye) Q1Ø.7
  organ Q89.9
    of Corti Q16.5
  origin
    artery
      innominate Q25.8
      pulmonary Q25.79
      renal Q27.2
      subclavian Q25.48 ⬅
  osseous meatus (ear) Q16.1
  ovary Q5Ø.39
  oviduct Q5Ø.6
  palate (hard) (soft) NEC Q38.5
  pancreas or pancreatic duct Q45.3
  papillary muscles Q24.8
  parathyroid gland Q89.2
  paraurethral ducts Q64.79
  parotid (gland) Q38.4
  patella Q74.1
  Pelger-Huët (hereditary hyposegmentation) D72.Ø
  pelvic girdle NEC Q74.2
  pelvis (bony) NEC Q74.2
    rachitic E64.3
  penis (glans) Q55.69
  pericardium Q24.8
  peripheral vascular system Q27.9
  Peter's Q13.4
  pharynx Q38.8
  pigmentation L81.9
    congenital Q82.8
  pituitary (gland) Q89.2
  pleural (folds) Q34.Ø
  portal vein Q26.5
    connection Q26.5
  position, tooth, teeth, fully erupted M26.3Ø
    specified NEC M26.39
  precerebral vessel Q28.1
  prepuce Q55.69
  prostate Q55.4
  pulmonary Q33.9
    artery NEC Q25.79
    valve Q22.3
      atresia Q22.Ø
      insufficiency Q22.2
      specified type NEC Q22.3
      stenosis Q22.1
        infundibular Q24.3
        subvalvular Q24.3
    venous connection Q26.4
      partial Q26.3
      total Q26.2
  pupil Q13.2
    function H57.ØØ
      anisocoria H57.Ø2
      Argyll Robertson pupil H57.Ø1
      miosis H57.Ø3
      mydriasis H57.Ø4
      specified type NEC H57.Ø9
      tonic pupil H57.Ø5-

Anomaly, anomalous *(Continued)*
- pylorus Q4Ø.3
- radius Q74.Ø
- rectum Q43.9
- reduction (extremity) (limb)
  - femur (longitudinal) —*see* Defect, reduction, lower limb, longitudinal, femur
  - fibula (longitudinal) —*see* Defect, reduction, lower limb, longitudinal, fibula
  - lower limb —*see* Defect, reduction, lower limb
  - radius (longitudinal) —*see* Defect, reduction, upper limb, longitudinal, radius
  - tibia (longitudinal) —*see* Defect, reduction, lower limb, longitudinal, tibia
  - ulna (longitudinal) —*see* Defect, reduction, upper limb, longitudinal, ulna
  - upper limb —*see* Defect, reduction, upper limb
- refraction —*see* Disorder, refraction
- renal Q63.9
  - artery Q27.2
  - pelvis Q63.9
    - specified NEC Q63.8
- respiratory system Q34.9
  - specified NEC Q34.8
- retina Q14.1
- rib Q76.6
  - cervical Q76.5
- Rieger's Q13.81
- rotation —*see* Malrotation
  - hip or thigh Q65.89
- round ligament Q52.8
- sacroiliac (joint) NEC Q74.2
- sacrum NEC Q76.49
  - kyphosis —*see* Kyphosis, congenital
  - lordosis —*see* Lordosis, congenital
- saddle nose, syphilitic A5Ø.57
- salivary duct or gland Q38.4
- scapula Q74.Ø
- scrotum —*see* Malformation, testis and scrotum
- sebaceous gland Q82.9
- seminal vesicles Q55.4
- sense organs NEC QØ7.8
- sex chromosomes NEC —*see also* Anomaly, chromosomes
  - female phenotype Q97.8
  - male phenotype Q98.9
- shoulder (girdle) (joint) Q74.Ø
- sigmoid (flexure) Q43.9
- simian crease Q82.8
- sinus of Valsalva Q25.49 ⬅
- skeleton generalized Q78.9
- skin (appendage) Q82.9
- skull Q75.9
  - with
    - anencephaly QØØ.Ø
    - encephalocele —*see* Encephalocele
    - hydrocephalus QØ3.9
      - with spina bifida —*see* Spina bifida, by site, with hydrocephalus
    - microcephaly QØ2
- specified organ or site NEC Q89.8
- spermatic cord Q55.4
- spine, spinal NEC Q76.49
  - column NEC Q76.49
    - kyphosis —*see* Kyphosis, congenital
    - lordosis —*see* Lordosis, congenital
  - cord QØ6.9
  - nerve root QØ7.8
- spleen Q89.Ø9
  - agenesis Q89.Ø1
- stenonian duct Q38.4
- sternum NEC Q76.7
- stomach Q4Ø.3
- submaxillary gland Q38.4
- tarsus NEC Q74.2

Anomaly, anomalous *(Continued)*
- tendon Q79.9
- testis —*see* Malformation, testis and scrotum
- thigh NEC Q74.2
- thorax (wall) Q67.8
  - bony Q76.9
- throat Q38.8
- thumb Q74.Ø
- thymus gland Q89.2
- thyroid (gland) Q89.2
  - cartilage Q31.8
- tibia NEC Q74.2
  - saber A5Ø.56
- toe Q74.2
- tongue Q38.3
- tooth, teeth KØØ.9
  - eruption KØØ.6
  - position, fully erupted M26.3Ø
  - spacing, fully erupted M26.3Ø
- trachea (cartilage) Q32.1
- tragus Q17.9
- tricuspid (leaflet) (valve) Q22.9
  - atresia or stenosis Q22.4
  - Ebstein's Q22.5
- Uhl's (hypoplasia of myocardium, right ventricle) Q24.8
- ulna Q74.Ø
- umbilical artery Q27.Ø
- union
  - cricoid cartilage and thyroid cartilage Q31.8
  - thyroid cartilage and hyoid bone Q31.8
  - trachea with larynx Q31.8
- upper limb Q74.Ø
- urachus Q64.4
- ureter Q62.8
  - obstructive NEC Q62.39
    - cecoureterocele Q62.32
    - orthotopic ureterocele Q62.31
- urethra Q64.7Ø
  - absence Q64.5
  - double Q64.74
  - fistula to rectum Q64.73
  - obstructive Q64.39
    - stricture Q64.32
  - prolapse Q64.71
  - specified type NEC Q64.79
- urinary tract Q64.9
- uterus Q51.9
  - with only one functioning horn Q51.4
- uvula Q38.5
- vagina Q52.4
- valleculae Q31.8
- valve (heart) NEC Q24.8
  - coronary sinus Q24.5
  - inferior vena cava Q24.8
  - pulmonary Q22.3
  - sinus coronario Q24.5
  - venae cavae inferioris Q24.8
- vas deferens Q55.4
- vascular Q27.9
  - brain Q28.3
  - ring Q25.45 ⬅
- vein (s) (peripheral) Q27.9
  - brain Q28.3
  - cerebral Q28.3
  - coronary Q24.5
  - developmental Q28.3
  - great Q26.9
    - specified NEC Q26.8
- vena cava (inferior) (superior) Q26.9
- venous —*see* Anomaly, vein (s)
- venous return Q26.8
- ventricular
  - bands or folds Q24.8
  - septa Q21.Ø
- vertebra Q76.49
  - kyphosis —*see* Kyphosis, congenital
  - lordosis —*see* Lordosis, congenital

Anomaly, anomalous *(Continued)*
- vesicourethral orifice Q64.79
- vessel (s) Q27.9
  - optic papilla Q14.2
  - precerebral Q28.1
- vitelline duct Q43.Ø
- vitreous body or humor Q14.Ø
- vulva Q52.7Ø
- wrist (joint) Q74.Ø

Anomia R48.8

Anonychia (congenital) Q84.3
- acquired L6Ø.8

Anophthalmos, anophthalmus (congenital) (globe) Q11.1
- acquired Z9Ø.Ø1

Anopia, anopsia H53.46-
- quadrant H53.46-

Anorchia, anorchism, anorchidism Q55.Ø

Anorexia R63.Ø
- hysterical F44.89
- nervosa F5Ø.ØØ
  - atypical F5Ø.9
  - binge-eating type F5Ø.2
    - with purging F5Ø.Ø2
  - restricting type F5Ø.Ø1

Anorgasmy, psychogenic (female) F52.31
- male F52.32

Anosmia R43.Ø
- hysterical F44.6
- postinfectional J39.8

Anosognosia R41.89

Anosteoplasia Q78.9

Anovulatory cycle N97.Ø

Anoxemia RØ9.Ø2
- newborn P84

Anoxia (pathological) RØ9.Ø2
- altitude T7Ø.29
- cerebral G93.1
  - complicating
    - anesthesia (general) (local) or other sedation T88.59
      - in labor and delivery O74.3
      - in pregnancy O29.21-
      - postpartum, puerperal O89.2
    - delivery (cesarean) (instrumental) O75.4
  - during a procedure G97.81
  - newborn P84
  - resulting from a procedure G97.82
- due to
  - drowning T75.1
  - high altitude T7Ø.29
- heart —*see* Insufficiency, coronary
- intrauterine P84
- myocardial —*see* Insufficiency, coronary
- newborn P84
- spinal cord G95.11
- systemic (by suffocation) (low content in atmosphere) —*see* Asphyxia, traumatic

Anteflexion —*see* Anteversion

Antenatal
- care (normal pregnancy) Z34.9Ø
- screening (encounter for) of mother Z36

Antepartum —*see* condition

Anterior —*see* condition

Antero-occlusion M26.22Ø

Anteversion
- cervix —*see* Anteversion, uterus
- femur (neck), congenital Q65.89
- uterus, uterine (cervix) (postinfectional) (postpartal, old) N85.4
  - congenital Q51.818
  - in pregnancy or childbirth —*see* Pregnancy, complicated by

Anthophobia F4Ø.228

Anthracosilicosis J6Ø

Anthracosis (lung) (occupational) J6Ø
- lingua K14.3

Anthrax A22.9
with pneumonia A22.1
cerebral A22.8
colitis A22.2
cutaneous A22.Ø
gastrointestinal A22.2
inhalation A22.1
intestinal A22.2
meningitis A22.8
pulmonary A22.1
respiratory A22.1
sepsis A22.7
specified manifestation NEC A22.8
Anthropoid pelvis Q74.2
with disproportion (fetopelvic) O33.Ø
Anthropophobia F4Ø.1Ø
generalized F4Ø.11
Antibodies, maternal (blood group) —*see* Isoimmunization, affecting management of pregnancy
anti-D —*see* Isoimmunization, affecting management of pregnancy, Rh
newborn P55.Ø
Antibody
anticardiolipin R76.Ø
with
hemorrhagic disorder D68.312
hypercoagulable state D68.61
antiphosphatidylglycerol R76.Ø
with
hemorrhagic disorder D68.312
hypercoagulable state D68.61
antiphosphatidylinositol R76.Ø
with
hemorrhagic disorder D68.312
hypercoagulable state D68.61
antiphosphatidylserine R76.Ø
with
hemorrhagic disorder D68.312
hypercoagulable state D68.61
antiphospholipid R76.Ø
with
hemorrhagic disorder D68.312
hypercoagulable state D68.61
Anticardiolipin syndrome D68.61
Anticoagulant, circulating (intrinsic) —*see also* - Disorder, hemorrhagic D68.318
drug-induced (extrinsic) —*see also* - Disorder, hemorrhagic D68.32
iatrogenic D68.32 ◀
Antidiuretic hormone syndrome E22.2
Antimonial cholera —*see* Poisoning, antimony
Antiphospholipid
antibody
with hemorrhagic disorder D68.312
syndrome D68.61
Antisocial personality F6Ø.2
Antithrombinemia —*see* Circulating anticoagulants
Antithromboplastinemia D68.318
Antithromboplastinogenemia D68.318
Antitoxin complication or reaction —*see* Complications, vaccination
Antlophobia F4Ø.228
Antritis J32.Ø
maxilla J32.Ø
acute JØ1.ØØ
recurrent JØ1.Ø1
stomach K29.6Ø
with bleeding K29.61
Antrum, antral —*see* condition
Anuria R34
calculous (impacted) (recurrent) —*see also* Calculus, urinary N2Ø.9
following
abortion —*see* Abortion by type complicated by, renal failure
ectopic or molar pregnancy OØ8.4
newborn P96.Ø
postprocedural N99.Ø

Anuria *(Continued)*
postrenal N13.8
traumatic (following crushing) T79.5
Anus, anal —*see* condition
Anusitis K62.89
Anxiety F41.9
depression F41.8
episodic paroxysmal F41.Ø
generalized F41.1
hysteria F41.8
neurosis F41.1
panic type F41.Ø
reaction F41.1
separation, abnormal (of childhood) F93.Ø
specified NEC F41.8
state F41.1
Aorta, aortic —*see* condition
Aortectasia —*see* Ectasia, aorta
with aneurysm —*see* Aneurysm, aorta
Aortitis (nonsyphilitic) (calcific) I77.6
arteriosclerotic I7Ø.Ø
Doehle-Heller A52.Ø2
luetic A52.Ø2
rheumatic —*see* Endocarditis, acute, rheumatic
specific (syphilitic) A52.Ø2
syphilitic A52.Ø2
congenital A5Ø.54 *[I79.1]*
Apathetic thyroid storm —*see* Thyrotoxicosis
Apathy R45.3
Apeirophobia F4Ø.228
Apepsia K3Ø
psychogenic F45.8
Aperistalsis, esophagus K22.Ø
Apertognathia M26.29
Apert's syndrome Q87.Ø
Aphagia R13.Ø
psychogenic F5Ø.9
Aphakia (acquired) (postoperative) H27.Ø-
congenital Q12.3
Aphasia (amnestic) (global) (nominal) (semantic) (syntactic) R47.Ø1
acquired, with epilepsy (Landau-Kleffner syndrome) —*see* Epilepsy, specified NEC
auditory (developmental) F8Ø.2
developmental (receptive type) F8Ø.2
expressive type F8Ø.1
Wernicke's F8Ø.2
following
cerebrovascular disease I69.92Ø
cerebral infarction I69.32Ø
intracerebral hemorrhage I69.12Ø
nontraumatic intracranial hemorrhage NEC I69.22Ø
specified disease NEC I69.82Ø
subarachnoid hemorrhage I69.Ø2Ø
primary progressive G31.Ø1 *[FØ2.8Ø]*
with behavioral disturbance G31.Ø1 *[FØ2.81]*
progressive isolated G31.Ø1 *[FØ2.8Ø]*
with behavioral disturbance G31.Ø1 *[FØ2.81]*
sensory F8Ø.2
syphilis, tertiary A52.19
Wernicke's (developmental) F8Ø.2
Aphonia (organic) R49.1
hysterical F44.4
psychogenic F44.4
Aphthae, aphthous —*see also* condition
Bednar's K12.Ø
cachectic K14.Ø
epizootic BØ8.8
fever BØ8.8
oral (recurrent) K12.Ø
stomatitis (major) (minor) K12.Ø
thrush B37.Ø
ulcer (oral) (recurrent) K12.Ø
genital organ (s) NEC
female N76.6
male N5Ø.89 ⬅
larynx J38.7

Apical —*see* condition
Apiphobia F4Ø.218
Aplasia —*see also* Agenesis
abdominal muscle syndrome Q79.4
alveolar process (acquired) —*see* Anomaly, alveolar
congenital Q38.6
aorta (congenital) Q25.41 ⬅
axialis extracorticalis (congenita) E75.29
bone marrow (myeloid) D61.9
congenital D61.Ø1
brain QØØ.Ø
part of QØ4.3
bronchus Q32.4
cementum KØØ.4
cerebellum QØ4.3
cervix (congenital) Q51.5
congenital pure red cell D61.Ø1
corpus callosum QØ4.Ø
cutis congenita Q84.8
erythrocyte congenital D61.Ø1
extracortical axial E75.29
eye Q11.1
fovea centralis (congenital) Q14.1
gallbladder, congenital Q44.Ø
iris Q13.1
labyrinth, membranous Q16.5
limb (congenital) Q73.8
lower —*see* Defect, reduction, lower limb
upper —*see* Agenesis, arm
lung, congenital (bilateral) (unilateral) Q33.3
pancreas Q45.Ø
parathyroid-thymic D82.1
Pelizaeus-Merzbacher E75.29
penis Q55.5
prostate Q55.4
red cell (with thymoma) D6Ø.9
acquired D6Ø.9
due to drugs D6Ø.9
adult D6Ø.9
chronic D6Ø.Ø
congenital D61.Ø1
constitutional D61.Ø1
due to drugs D6Ø.9
hereditary D61.Ø1
of infants D61.Ø1
primary D61.Ø1
pure D61.Ø1
due to drugs D6Ø.9
specified type NEC D6Ø.8
transient D6Ø.1
round ligament Q52.8
skin Q84.8
spermatic cord Q55.4
spleen Q89.Ø1
testicle Q55.Ø
thymic, with immunodeficiency D82.1
thyroid (congenital) (with myxedema) EØ3.1
uterus Q51.Ø
ventral horn cell QØ6.1
Apnea, apneic (of) (spells) RØ6.81
newborn NEC P28.4
obstructive P28.4
sleep (central) (obstructive) (primary) P28.3
prematurity P28.4
sleep G47.3Ø
central (primary) G47.31
in conditions classified elsewhere G47.37
obstructive (adult) (pediatric) G47.33
primary central G47.31
specified NEC G47.39
Apneumatosis, newborn P28.Ø
Apocrine metaplasia (breast) —*see* Dysplasia, mammary, specified type NEC
Apophysitis (bone) —*see also* Osteochondropathy
calcaneus M92.8
juvenile M92.9

A

Apoplectiform convulsions (cerebral ischemia) I67.82
Apoplexia, apoplexy, apoplectic
adrenal A39.1
heart (auricle) (ventricle) —*see* Infarct, myocardium
heat T67.Ø
hemorrhagic (stroke) —*see* Hemorrhage, intracranial
meninges, hemorrhagic —*see* Hemorrhage, intracranial, subarachnoid
uremic N18.9 *[I68.8]*
Appearance
bizarre R46.1
specified NEC R46.89
very low level of personal hygiene R46.Ø
Appendage
epididymal (organ of Morgagni) Q55.4
intestine (epiploic) Q43.8
preauricular Q17.Ø
testicular (organ of Morgagni) Q55.29
Appendicitis (pneumococcal) (retrocecal) K37
with
perforation or rupture K35.2
peritoneal abscess K35.3
peritonitis NEC K35.3
generalized (with perforation or rupture) K35.2
localized (with perforation or rupture) K35.3
acute (catarrhal) (fulminating) (gangrenous) (obstructive) (retrocecal) (suppurative) K35.8Ø
with
peritoneal abscess K35.3
peritonitis NEC K35.3
generalized (with perforation or rupture) K35.2
localized (with perforation or rupture) K35.3
specified NEC K35.89
amebic AØ6.89
chronic (recurrent) K36
exacerbation —*see* Appendicitis, acute
gangrenous —*see* Appendicitis, acute
healed (obliterative) K36
interval K36
neurogenic K36
obstructive K36
recurrent K36
relapsing K36
subacute (adhesive) K36
subsiding K36
suppurative —*see* Appendicitis, acute
tuberculous A18.32
Appendicopathia oxyurica B8Ø
Appendix, appendicular —*see also* condition
epididymis Q55.4
Morgagni
female Q5Ø.5
male (epididymal) Q55.4
testicular Q55.29
testis Q55.29
Appetite
depraved —*see* Pica
excessive R63.2
lack or loss —*see also* Anorexia R63.Ø
nonorganic origin F5Ø.89
psychogenic F5Ø.89
perverted (hysterical) —*see* Pica
Apple peel syndrome Q41.1
Apprehension state F41.1
Apprehensiveness, abnormal F41.9
Approximal wear KØ3.Ø
Apraxia (classic) (ideational) (ideokinetic) (ideomotor) (motor) (verbal) R48.2
following
cerebrovascular disease I69.99Ø
cerebral infarction I69.39Ø
intracerebral hemorrhage I69.19Ø
Apraxia *(Continued)*
following *(Continued)*
cerebrovascular disease *(Continued)*
nontraumatic intracranial hemorrhage NEC I69.29Ø
specified disease NEC I69.89Ø
subarachnoid hemorrhage I69.Ø9Ø
oculomotor, congenital H51.8
Aptyalism K11.7
Apudoma —*see* Neoplasm, uncertain behavior, by site
Aqueous misdirection H4Ø.83-
Arabicum elephantiasis —*see* Infestation, filarial
Arachnitis —*see* Meningitis
Arachnodactyly —*see* Syndrome, Marfan's
Arachnoiditis (acute) (adhesive) (basal) (brain) (cerebrospinal) —*see* Meningitis
Arachnophobia F4Ø.21Ø
Arboencephalitis, Australian A83.4
Arborization block (heart) I45.5
ARC (AIDS-related complex) B2Ø
Arches —*see* condition
Arcuate uterus Q51.81Ø
Arcuatus uterus Q51.81Ø
Arcus (cornea) **senilis** —*see* Degeneration, cornea, senile
Arc-welder's lung J63.4
Areflexia R29.2
Areola —*see* condition
Argentaffinoma —*see also* Neoplasm, uncertain behavior, by site
malignant —*see* Neoplasm, malignant, by site
syndrome E34.Ø
Argininemia E72.21
Argininosuccinic aciduria E72.22
Argyll Robertson phenomenon, pupil or syndrome (syphilitic) A52.19
atypical H57.Ø9
nonsyphilitic H57.Ø9
Argyria, argyriasis
conjunctival H11.13-
from drug or medicament —*see* Table of Drugs and Chemicals, by substance
Argyrosis, conjunctival H11.13-
Arhinencephaly QØ4.1
Ariboflavinosis E53.Ø
Arm —*see* condition
Arnold-Chiari disease, obstruction or syndrome (type II) QØ7.ØØ
with
hydrocephalus QØ7.Ø2
with spina bifida QØ7.Ø3
spina bifida QØ7.Ø1
with hydrocephalus QØ7.Ø3
type III —*see* Encephalocele
type IV QØ4.8
Aromatic amino-acid metabolism disorder E7Ø.9
specified NEC E7Ø.8
Arousals, confusional G47.51
Arrest, arrested
cardiac I46.9
complicating
abortion —*see* Abortion, by type, complicated by, cardiac arrest
anesthesia (general) (local) or other sedation —*see* Table of Drugs and Chemicals, by drug
in labor and delivery O74.2
in pregnancy O29.11-
postpartum, puerperal O89.1
delivery (cesarean) (instrumental) O75.4
due to
cardiac condition I46.2
specified condition NEC I46.8
intraoperative I97.71-
newborn P29.81
postprocedural I97.12-
obstetric procedure O75.4
Arrest, arrested *(Continued)*
cardiorespiratory —*see* Arrest, cardiac
circulatory —*see* Arrest, cardiac
deep transverse O64.Ø
development or growth
bone —*see* Disorder, bone, development or growth
child R62.5Ø
tracheal rings Q32.1
epiphyseal
complete
femur M89.15-
humerus M89.12-
tibia M89.16-
ulna M89.13-
forearm M89.13-
specified NEC M89.13-
ulna —*see* Arrest, epiphyseal, by type, ulna
lower leg M89.16-
specified NEC M89.168
tibia —*see* Arrest, epiphyseal, by type, tibia
partial
femur M89.15-
humerus M89.12-
tibia M89.16-
ulna M89.13-
specified NEC M89.18
granulopoiesis —*see* Agranulocytosis
growth plate —*see* Arrest, epiphyseal
heart —*see* Arrest, cardiac
legal, anxiety concerning Z65.3
physeal —*see* Arrest, epiphyseal
respiratory RØ9.2
newborn P28.81
sinus I45.5
spermatogenesis (complete) —*see* Azoospermia
incomplete —*see* Oligospermia
transverse (deep) O64.Ø
Arrhenoblastoma
benign
specified site —*see* Neoplasm, benign, by site
unspecified site
female D27.9
male D29.2Ø
malignant
specified site —*see* Neoplasm, malignant, by site
unspecified site
female C56.9
male C62.9Ø
specified site —*see* Neoplasm, uncertain behavior, by site
unspecified site
female D39.1Ø
male D4Ø.1Ø
Arrhythmia (auricle)(cardiac) (juvenile) (nodal) (reflex)(sinus)(supraventricular) (transitory)(ventricle) I49.9
block I45.9
extrasystolic I49.49
newborn
bradycardia P29.12
occurring before birth PØ3.819
before onset of labor PØ3.81Ø
during labor PØ3.811
tachycardia P29.11
psychogenic F45.8
specified NEC I49.8
vagal R55
ventricular re-entry I47.Ø
Arrillaga-Ayerza syndrome (pulmonary sclerosis with pulmonary hypertension) I27.Ø
Arsenical pigmentation L81.8
from drug or medicament —*see* Table of Drugs and Chemicals
Arsenism —*see* Poisoning, arsenic

A

Arterial —*see* condition
Arteriofibrosis —*see* Arteriosclerosis
Arteriolar sclerosis —*see* Arteriosclerosis
Arteriolith —*see* Arteriosclerosis
Arteriolitis I77.6
necrotizing, kidney I77.5
renal —*see* Hypertension, kidney
Arteriolosclerosis —*see* Arteriosclerosis
Arterionephrosclerosis —*see* Hypertension, kidney
Arteriopathy I77.9
Arteriosclerosis, arteriosclerotic (diffuse) (obliterans) (of) (senile) (with calcification) I70.90
aorta I70.0
arteries of extremities —*see* Arteriosclerosis, extremities
brain I67.2
bypass graft
coronary —*see* Arteriosclerosis, coronary, bypass graft
extremities —*see* Arteriosclerosis, extremities, bypass graft
cardiac —*see* Disease, heart, ischemic, atherosclerotic
cardiopathy —*see* Disease, heart, ischemic, atherosclerotic
cardiorenal —*see* Hypertension, cardiorenal
cardiovascular —*see* Disease, heart, ischemic, atherosclerotic
carotid —*see also* Occlusion, artery, carotid I65.2-
central nervous system I67.2
cerebral I67.2
cerebrovascular I67.2
coronary (artery) I25.10
bypass graft I25.810
with
angina pectoris I25.709
with documented spasm I25.701
specified type NEC I25.708
unstable I25.700
ischemic chest pain I25.709
autologous artery I25.810
with
angina pectoris I25.729
with documented spasm I25.721
specified type I25.728
unstable I25.720
ischemic chest pain I25.729
autologous vein I25.810
with
angina pectoris I25.719
with documented spasm I25.711
specified type I25.718
unstable I25.710
ischemic chest pain I25.719
nonautologous biological I25.810
with
angina pectoris I25.739
with documented spasm I25.731
specified type I25.738
unstable I25.730
ischemic chest pain I25.739
specified type NEC I25.810
with
angina pectoris I25.799
with documented spasm I25.791
specified type I25.798
unstable I25.790
ischemic chest pain I25.799
due to
calcified coronary lesion (severely) I25.84
lipid rich plaque I25.83
native vessel
with
angina pectoris I25.119
with documented spasm I25.111
specified type NEC I25.118
unstable I25.110
ischemic chest pain I25.119

Arteriosclerosis, arteriosclerotic *(Continued)*
coronary *(Continued)*
transplanted heart I25.811
bypass graft I25.812
with
angina pectoris I25.769
with documented spasm I25.761
specified type I25.768
unstable I25.760
ischemic chest pain I25.769
native coronary artery I25.811
with
angina pectoris I25.759
with documented spasm I25.751
specified type I25.758
unstable I25.750
ischemic chest pain I25.759
extremities (native arteries) I70.209
bypass graft I70.309
autologous vein graft I70.409
leg I70.409
with
gangrene (and intermittent claudication, rest pain and ulcer) I70.469
intermittent claudication I70.419
rest pain (and intermittent claudication) I70.429
bilateral I70.403
with
gangrene (and intermittent claudication, rest pain and ulcer) I70.463
intermittent claudication I70.413
rest pain (and intermittent claudication) I70.423
specified type NEC I70.493
left I70.402
with
gangrene (and intermittent claudication, rest pain and ulcer) I70.462
intermittent claudication I70.412
rest pain (and intermittent claudication) I70.422
ulceration (and intermittent claudication and rest pain) I70.449
ankle I70.443
calf I70.442
foot site NEC I70.445
heel I70.444
lower leg NEC I70.448
midfoot I70.444
thigh I70.441
specified type NEC I70.492
right I70.401
with
gangrene (and intermittent claudication, rest pain and ulcer) I70.461
intermittent claudication I70.411
rest pain (and intermittent claudication) I70.421
ulceration (and intermittent claudication and rest pain) I70.439
ankle I70.433
calf I70.432
foot site NEC I70.435
heel I70.434
lower leg NEC I70.438
midfoot I70.434
thigh I70.431
specified type NEC I70.491
specified type NEC I70.499

Arteriosclerosis, arteriosclerotic *(Continued)*
extremities *(Continued)*
bypass graft *(Continued)*
autologous vein graft *(Continued)*
specified NEC I70.408
with
gangrene (and intermittent claudication, rest pain and ulcer) I70.468
intermittent claudication I70.418
rest pain (and intermittent claudication) I70.428
ulceration (and intermittent claudication and rest pain) I70.45
specified type NEC I70.498
leg I70.309
with
gangrene (and intermittent claudication, rest pain and ulcer) I70.369
intermittent claudication I70.319
rest pain (and intermittent claudication) I70.329
bilateral I70.303
with
gangrene (and intermittent claudication, rest pain and ulcer) I70.363
intermittent claudication I70.313
rest pain (and intermittent claudication) I70.323
specified type NEC I70.393
left I70.302
with
gangrene (and intermittent claudication, rest pain and ulcer) I70.362
intermittent claudication I70.312
rest pain (and intermittent claudication) I70.322
ulceration (and intermittent claudication and rest pain) I70.349
ankle I70.343
calf I70.342
foot site NEC I70.345
heel I70.344
lower leg NEC I70.348
midfoot I70.344
thigh I70.341
specified type NEC I70.392
right I70.301
with
gangrene (and intermittent claudication, rest pain and ulcer) I70.361
intermittent claudication I70.311
rest pain (and intermittent claudication) I70.321
ulceration (and intermittent claudication and rest pain) I70.339
ankle I70.333
calf I70.332
foot site NEC I70.335
heel I70.334
lower leg NEC I70.338
midfoot I70.334
thigh I70.331
specified type NEC I70.391
specified type NEC I70.399
nonautologous biological graft I70.509
leg I70.509
with
gangrene (and intermittent claudication, rest pain and ulcer) I70.569
intermittent claudication I70.519
rest pain (and intermittent claudication) I70.529

A

- **Arteriosclerosis, arteriosclerotic** *(Continued)*
  - extremities *(Continued)*
    - leg I70.209
      - with
        - gangrene (and intermittent claudication, rest pain and ulcer) I70.269
        - intermittent claudication I70.219
        - rest pain (and intermittent claudication) I70.229
      - bilateral I70.203
        - with
          - gangrene (and intermittent claudication, rest pain and ulcer) I70.263
          - intermittent claudication I70.213
          - rest pain (and intermittent claudication) I70.223
        - specified type NEC I70.293
      - left I70.202
        - with
          - gangrene (and intermittent claudication, rest pain and ulcer) I70.262
          - intermittent claudication I70.212
          - rest pain (and intermittent claudication) I70.222
          - ulceration (and intermittent claudication and rest pain) I70.249
            - ankle I70.243
            - calf I70.242
            - foot site NEC I70.245
            - heel I70.244
            - lower leg NEC I70.248
            - midfoot I70.244
            - thigh I70.241
        - specified type NEC I70.292
      - right I70.201
        - with
          - gangrene (and intermittent claudication, rest pain and ulcer) I70.261
          - intermittent claudication I70.211
          - rest pain (and intermittent claudication) I70.221
          - ulceration (and intermittent claudication and rest pain) I70.239
            - ankle I70.233
            - calf I70.232
            - foot site NEC I70.235
            - heel I70.234
            - lower leg NEC I70.238
            - midfoot I70.234
            - thigh I70.231
        - specified type NEC I70.291
      - specified type NEC I70.299
    - specified site NEC I70.208
      - with
        - gangrene (and intermittent claudication, rest pain and ulcer) I70.268
        - intermittent claudication I70.218
        - rest pain (and intermittent claudication) I70.228
        - ulceration (and intermittent claudication and rest pain) I70.25
      - specified type NEC I70.298
  - generalized I70.91
  - heart (disease) —*see* Arteriosclerosis, coronary (artery)
  - kidney —*see* Hypertension, kidney
  - medial —*see* Arteriosclerosis, extremities
  - mesenteric (artery) K55.1
  - Mönckeberg's —*see* Arteriosclerosis, extremities
  - myocarditis I51.4
  - peripheral (of extremities) —*see* Arteriosclerosis, extremities
  - pulmonary (idiopathic) I27.0

- **Arteriosclerosis, arteriosclerotic** *(Continued)*
  - renal (arterioles) —*see also* Hypertension, kidney
    - artery I70.1
  - retina (vascular) I70.8 *[H35.0-]*
  - specified artery NEC I70.8
  - spinal (cord) G95.19
  - vertebral (artery) I67.2
- **Arteriospasm** I73.9
- **Arteriovenous** —*see* condition
- **Arteritis** I77.6
  - allergic M31.0
  - aorta (nonsyphilitic) I77.6
    - syphilitic A52.02
  - aortic arch M31.4
  - brachiocephalic M31.4
  - brain I67.7
    - syphilitic A52.04
  - cerebral I67.7
    - in
      - diseases classified elsewhere I68.2
      - systemic lupus erythematosus M32.19
    - listerial A32.89
    - syphilitic A52.04
    - tuberculous A18.89
  - coronary (artery) I25.89
    - rheumatic I01.8
      - chronic I09.89
    - syphilitic A52.06
  - cranial (left) (right), giant cell M31.6
  - deformans —*see* Arteriosclerosis
  - giant cell NEC M31.6
    - with polymyalgia rheumatica M31.5
  - necrosing or necrotizing M31.9
    - specified NEC M31.8
  - nodosa M30.0
  - obliterans —*see* Arteriosclerosis
  - pulmonary I28.8
  - rheumatic —*see* Fever, rheumatic
  - senile —*see* Arteriosclerosis
  - suppurative I77.2
  - syphilitic (general) A52.09
    - brain A52.04
    - coronary A52.06
    - spinal A52.09
  - temporal, giant cell M31.6
  - young female aortic arch syndrome M31.4
- **Artery, arterial** —*see also* condition
  - abscess I77.89
  - single umbilical Q27.0
- **Arthralgia** (allergic) —*see also* Pain, joint
  - in caisson disease T70.3
  - temporomandibular M26.62
- **Arthritis, arthritic** (acute) (chronic) (nonpyogenic) (subacute) M19.90
  - allergic —*see* Arthritis, specified form NEC
  - ankylosing (crippling) (spine) —*see also* Spondylitis, ankylosing
    - sites other than spine —*see* Arthritis, specified form NEC
  - atrophic —*see* Osteoarthritis
    - spine —*see* Spondylitis, ankylosing
  - back —*see* Spondylopathy, inflammatory
  - blennorrhagic (gonococcal) A54.42
  - Charcot's —*see* Arthropathy, neuropathic
    - diabetic —*see* Diabetes, arthropathy, neuropathic
    - syringomyelic G95.0
  - chylous (filarial) —*see also* category M01 B74.9
  - climacteric (any site) NEC —*see* Arthritis, specified form NEC
  - crystal (-induced) —*see* Arthritis, in, crystals
  - deformans —*see* Osteoarthritis
  - degenerative —*see* Osteoarthritis
  - due to or associated with
    - acromegaly E22.0
    - brucellosis —*see* Brucellosis
    - caisson disease T70.3
    - diabetes —*see* Diabetes, arthropathy
    - dracontiasis —*see also* category M01 B72

- **Arthritis, arthritic** *(Continued)*
  - due to or associated with *(Continued)*
    - enteritis NEC
      - regional —*see* Enteritis, regional
    - erysipelas —*see also* category M01 A46
    - erythema
      - epidemic A25.1
      - nodosum L52
    - filariasis NOS B74.9
    - glanders A24.0
    - helminthiasis —*see also* category M01 B83.9
    - hemophilia D66 *[M36.2]*
    - Henoch-(Schönlein) purpura D69.0 *[M36.4]*
    - human parvovirus —*see also* category M01 B97.6
    - infectious disease NEC —*see* category M01
    - leprosy (*see also* category M01) —*see also* Leprosy A30.9
    - Lyme disease A69.23
    - mycobacteria —*see also* category M01 A31.8
    - parasitic disease NEC —*see also* category M01 B89
    - paratyphoid fever (*see also* category M01) —*see also* Fever, paratyphoid A01.4
    - rat bite fever —*see also* category M01 A25.1
    - regional enteritis —*see* Enteritis, regional
    - respiratory disorder NOS J98.9
    - serum sickness —*see also* Reaction, serum T80.69
    - syringomyelia G95.0
    - typhoid fever A01.04
  - epidemic erythema A25.1
  - febrile —*see* Fever, rheumatic
  - gonococcal A54.42
  - gouty (acute) —*see* Gout
  - in (due to)
    - acromegaly —*see also* subcategory M14.8- E22.0
    - amyloidosis —*see also* subcategory M14.8- E85.4
    - bacterial disease —*see also* subcategory M01 A49.9
    - Behçet's syndrome M35.2
    - caisson disease —*see also* subcategory M14.8- T70.3
    - coliform bacilli (Escherichia coli) —*see* Arthritis, in, pyogenic organism NEC
    - crystals M11.9
      - dicalcium phosphate —*see* Arthritis, in, crystals, specified type NEC
      - hydroxyapatite M11.0-
      - pyrophosphate —*see* Arthritis, in, crystals, specified type NEC
      - specified type NEC M11.80
        - ankle M11.87-
        - elbow M11.82-
        - foot joint M11.87-
        - hand joint M11.84-
        - hip M11.85-
        - knee M11.86-
        - multiple sites M11.8-
        - shoulder M11.81-
        - vertebrae M11.88
        - wrist M11.83-
    - dermatoarthritis, lipoid E78.81
    - dracontiasis (dracunculiasis) —*see also* category M01 B72
    - endocrine disorder NEC —*see also* subcategory M14.8- E34.9
    - enteritis, infectious NEC —*see also* category M01 A09
      - specified organism NEC —*see also* category M01 A08.8
    - erythema
      - multiforme —*see also* subcategory M14.8- L51.9
      - nodosum —*see also* subcategory M14.8- L52
    - gout —*see* Gout

A

Arthritis, arthritic *(Continued)*
in *(Continued)*
helminthiasis NEC —*see also* category M01 B83.9
hemochromatosis —*see also* subcategory M14.8- E83.118
hemoglobinopathy NEC D58.2 *[M36.3]*
hemophilia NEC D66 *[M36.2]*
Hemophilus influenzae M00.8- *[B96.3]*
Henoch(-Schönlein) purpura D69.0 *[M36.4]*
hyperparathyroidism NEC —*see also* subcategory M14.8- E21.3
hypersensitivity reaction NEC T78.49 *[M36.4]*
hypogammaglobulinemia —*see also* subcategory M14.8- D80.1
hypothyroidism NEC —*see also* subcategory M14.8- E03.9
infection —*see* Arthritis, pyogenic or pyemic
spine —*see* Spondylopathy, infective
infectious disease NEC —*see* category M01
leprosy —*see also* category M01 A30.9
leukemia NEC C95.9- *[M36.1]*
lipoid dermatoarthritis E78.81
Lyme disease A69.23
Mediterranean fever, familial —*see also* subcategory M14.8- M04.1
Meningococcus A39.83
metabolic disorder NEC —*see also* subcategory M14.8- E88.9
multiple myelomatosis C90.0- *[M36.1]*
mumps B26.85
mycosis NEC —*see also* category M01 B49
myelomatosis (multiple) C90.0- *[M36.1]*
neurological disorder NEC G98.0
ochronosis —*see also* subcategory M14.8- E70.29
O'nyong-nyong —*see also* category M01 A92.1
parasitic disease NEC —*see also* category M01 B89
paratyphoid fever —*see also* category M01 A01.4
Pseudomonas —*see* Arthritis, pyogenic, bacterial NEC
psoriasis L40.50
pyogenic organism NEC —*see* Arthritis, pyogenic, bacterial NEC
Reiter's disease —*see* Reiter's disease
respiratory disorder NEC —*see also* subcategory M14.8- J98.9
reticulosis, malignant —*see also* subcategory M14.8- C86.0
rubella B06.82
Salmonella (arizonae) (cholerae-suis) (enteritidis) (typhimurium) A02.23
sarcoidosis D86.86
specified bacteria NEC —*see* Arthritis, pyogenic, bacterial NEC
sporotrichosis B42.82
syringomyelia G95.0
thalassemia NEC D56.9 *[M36.3]*
tuberculosis —*see* Tuberculosis, arthritis
typhoid fever A01.04
urethritis, Reiter's —*see* Reiter's disease
viral disease NEC —*see also* category M01 B34.9
infectious or infective —*see also* Arthritis, pyogenic or pyemic
spine —*see* Spondylopathy, infective
juvenile M08.90
with systemic onset —*see* Still's disease
ankle M08.97-
elbow M08.92-
foot joint M08.97-
hand joint M08.94-
hip M08.95-
knee M08.96-
multiple site M08.99

Arthritis, arthritic *(Continued)*
juvenile *(Continued)*
pauciarticular M08.40
ankle M08.47-
elbow M08.42-
foot joint M08.47-
hand joint M08.44-
hip M08.45-
knee M08.46-
shoulder M08.41-
vertebrae M08.48
wrist M08.43-
psoriatic L40.54
rheumatoid —*see* Arthritis, rheumatoid, juvenile
shoulder M08.91-
specified type NEC M08.80
ankle M08.87-
elbow M08.82-
foot joint M08.87-
hand joint M08.84-
hip M08.85-
knee M08.86-
multiple site M08.89
shoulder M08.81-
specified joint NEC M08.88
vertebrae M08.88
wrist M08.83-
vertebra M08.98
wrist M08.93-
meaning osteoarthritis —*see* Osteoarthritis
meningococcal A39.83
menopausal (any site) NEC —*see* Arthritis, specified form NEC
mutilans (psoriatic) L40.52
mycotic NEC —*see also* category M01 B49
neuropathic (Charcot) —*see* Arthropathy, neuropathic
diabetic —*see* Diabetes, arthropathy, neuropathic
nonsyphilitic NEC G98.0
syringomyelic G95.0
ochronotic —*see also* subcategory M14.8- E70.29
palindromic (any site) —*see* Rheumatism, palindromic
pneumococcal M00.10
ankle M00.17-
elbow M00.12-
foot joint —*see* Arthritis, pneumococcal, ankle
hand joint M00.14-
hip M00.15-
knee M00.16-
multiple site M00.19
shoulder M00.11-
vertebra M00.18
wrist M00.13-
postdysenteric —*see* Arthropathy, postdysenteric
postmeningococcal A39.84
postrheumatic, chronic —*see* Arthropathy, postrheumatic, chronic
primary progressive —*see also* Arthritis, specified form NEC
spine —*see* Spondylitis, ankylosing
psoriatic L40.50
purulent (any site except spine) —*see* Arthritis, pyogenic or pyemic
spine —*see* Spondylopathy, infective
pyogenic or pyemic (any site except spine) M00.9
bacterial NEC M00.80
ankle M00.87-
elbow M00.82-
foot joint —*see* Arthritis, pyogenic, bacterial NEC, ankle
hand joint M00.84-
hip M00.85-
knee M00.86-
multiple site M00.89

Arthritis, arthritic *(Continued)*
pyogenic or pyemic *(Continued)*
bacterial NEC *(Continued)*
shoulder M00.81-
vertebra M00.88
wrist M00.83-
pneumococcal —*see* Arthritis, pneumococcal
spine —*see* Spondylopathy, infective
staphylococcal —*see* Arthritis, staphylococcal
streptococcal —*see* Arthritis, streptococcal NEC
pneumococcal —*see* Arthritis, pneumococcal
reactive —*see* Reiter's disease
rheumatic —*see also* Arthritis, rheumatoid
acute or subacute —*see* Fever, rheumatic
rheumatoid M06.9
with
carditis —*see* Rheumatoid, carditis
endocarditis —*see* Rheumatoid, carditis
heart involvement NEC —*see* Rheumatoid, carditis
lung involvement —*see* Rheumatoid, lung
myocarditis —*see* Rheumatoid, carditis
myopathy —*see* Rheumatoid, myopathy
pericarditis —*see* Rheumatoid, carditis
polyneuropathy —*see* Rheumatoid, polyneuropathy
rheumatoid factor —*see* Arthritis, rheumatoid, seropositive
splenoadenomegaly and leukopenia —*see* Felty's syndrome
vasculitis —*see* Rheumatoid, vasculitis
visceral involvement NEC —*see* Rheumatoid, arthritis, with involvement of organs NEC
juvenile (with or without rheumatoid factor) M08.00
ankle M08.07-
elbow M08.02-
foot joint M08.07-
hand joint M08.04-
hip M08.05-
knee M08.06-
multiple site M08.09
shoulder M08.01-
vertebra M08.08
wrist M08.03-
seronegative M06.00
ankle M06.07-
elbow M06.02-
foot joint M06.07-
hand joint M06.04-
hip M06.05-
knee M06.06-
multiple sites M06.09
shoulder M06.01-
vertebra M06.08
wrist M06.03-
seropositive M05.9
without organ involvement M05.70
ankle M05.77-
elbow M05.72-
foot joint M05.77-
hand joint M05.74-
hip M05.75-
knee M05.76-
multiple sites M05.79
shoulder M05.71-
vertebra —*see* Spondylitis, ankylosing
wrist M05.73-
specified NEC M05.80
ankle M05.87-
elbow M05.82-
foot joint M05.87-
hand joint M05.84-
hip M05.85-
knee M05.86-

Arthritis, arthritic *(Continued)*
- rheumatoid *(Continued)*
  - specified NEC *(Continued)*
    - multiple sites M05.89
    - shoulder M05.81-
    - vertebra —*see* Spondylitis, ankylosing
    - wrist M05.83-
  - specified type NEC M06.80
    - ankle M06.87-
    - elbow M06.82-
    - foot joint M06.87-
    - hand joint M06.84-
    - hip M06.85-
    - knee M06.86-
    - multiple site M06.89
    - shoulder M06.81-
    - vertebra M06.88
    - wrist M06.83-
  - spine —*see* Spondylitis, ankylosing
- rubella B06.82
- scorbutic —*see also* subcategory M14.8- E54
- senile or senescent —*see* Osteoarthritis
- septic (any site except spine) —*see* Arthritis, pyogenic or pyemic
  - spine —*see* Spondylopathy, infective
- serum (nontherapeutic) (therapeutic) —*see* Arthropathy, postimmunization
- specified form NEC M13.80
  - ankle M13.87-
  - elbow M13.82-
  - foot joint M13.87-
  - hand joint M13.84-
  - hip M13.85-
  - knee M13.86-
  - multiple site M13.89
  - shoulder M13.81-
  - specified joint NEC M13.88
  - wrist M13.83-
- spine —*see also* Spondylopathy, inflammatory
  - infectious or infective NEC —*see* Spondylopathy, infective
  - Marie-Strümpell —*see* Spondylitis, ankylosing
  - pyogenic —*see* Spondylopathy, infective
  - rheumatoid —*see* Spondylitis, ankylosing
  - traumatic (old) —*see* Spondylopathy, traumatic
  - tuberculous A18.01
- staphylococcal M00.00
  - ankle M00.07-
  - elbow M00.02-
  - foot joint —*see* Arthritis, staphylococcal, ankle
  - hand joint M00.04-
  - hip M00.05-
  - knee M00.06-
  - multiple site M00.09
  - shoulder M00.01-
  - vertebra M00.08
  - wrist M00.03-
- streptococcal NEC M00.20
  - ankle M00.27-
  - elbow M00.22-
  - foot joint —*see* Arthritis, streptococcal, ankle
  - hand joint M00.24-
  - hip M00.25-
  - knee M00.26-
  - multiple site M00.29
  - shoulder M00.21-
  - vertebra M00.28
  - wrist M00.23-
- suppurative —*see* Arthritis, pyogenic or pyemic
- syphilitic (late) A52.16
  - congenital A50.55 *[M12.80]*
- syphilitica deformans (Charcot) A52.16
- temporomandibular M26.69
- toxic of menopause (any site) —*see* Arthritis, specified form NEC

Arthritis, arthritic *(Continued)*
- transient —*see* Arthropathy, specified form NEC
- traumatic (chronic) —*see* Arthropathy, traumatic
- tuberculous A18.02
  - spine A18.01
- uratic —*see* Gout ⬅
- urethritica (Reiter's) —*see* Reiter's disease
- vertebral —*see* Spondylopathy, inflammatory
- villous (any site) —*see* Arthropathy, specified form NEC

Arthrocele —*see* Effusion, joint
Arthrodesis status Z98.1
Arthrodynia —*see also* Pain, joint
Arthrodysplasia Q74.9
Arthrofibrosis, joint —*see* Ankylosis
Arthrogryposis (congenital) Q68.8
- multiplex congenita Q74.3

Arthrokatadysis M24.7
Arthropathy (*see also* Arthritis) M12.9
- Charcot's —*see* Arthropathy, neuropathic
  - diabetic —*see* Diabetes, arthropathy, neuropathic
  - syringomyelic G95.0
- cricoarytenoid J38.7
- crystal(-induced) —*see* Arthritis, in, crystals
- diabetic NEC —*see* Diabetes, arthropathy
- distal interphalangeal, psoriatic L40.51
- enteropathic M07.60
  - ankle M07.67-
  - elbow M07.62-
  - foot joint M07.67-
  - hand joint M07.64-
  - hip M07.65-
  - knee M07.66-
  - multiple site M07.69
  - shoulder M07.61-
  - vertebra M07.68
  - wrist M07.63-
- following intestinal bypass M02.00
  - ankle M02.07-
  - elbow M02.02-
  - foot joint M02.07-
  - hand joint M02.04-
  - hip M02.05-
  - knee M02.06-
  - multiple site M02.09
  - shoulder M02.01-
  - vertebra M02.08
  - wrist M02.03-
- gouty —*see also* Gout ⬅
  - in (due to)
    - Lesch-Nyhan syndrome E79.1 *[M14.8-]*
    - sickle-cell disorders D57- *[M14.8-]*
- hemophilic NEC D66 *[M36.2]*
  - in (due to)
    - hyperparathyroidism NEC E21.3 *[M14.8-]*
    - metabolic disease NOS E88.9 *[M14.8-]*
- in (due to)
  - acromegaly E22.0 *[M14.8-]*
  - amyloidosis E85.4 *[M14.8-]*
  - blood disorder NOS D75.9 *[M36.3]*
  - diabetes —*see* Diabetes, arthropathy
  - endocrine disease NOS E34.9 *[M14.8-]*
  - erythema
    - multiforme L51.9 *[M14.8-]*
    - nodosum L52 *[M14.8-]*
- hemochromatosis E83.118 *[M14.8-]*
  - hemoglobinopathy NEC D58.2 *[M36.3]*
  - hemophilia NEC D66 *[M36.2]*
  - Henoch-Schönlein purpura D69.0 *[M36.4]*
  - hyperthyroidism E05.90 *[M14.8-]*
  - hypothyroidism E03.9 *[M14.8-]*
  - infective endocarditis I33.0 *[M12.80]*
  - leukemia NEC C95.9- *[M36.1]*
  - malignant histiocytosis C96.A *[M36.1]*
  - metabolic disease NOS E88.9 *[M14.8-]*
  - multiple myeloma C90.0- *[M36.1]*
  - neoplastic disease NOS (*see also* Neoplasm) D49.9 *[M36.1]*

Arthropathy *(Continued)*
- hemochromatosis *(Continued)*
  - nutritional deficiency —*see also* subcategory M14.8- E63.9
  - psoriasis NOS L40.50
  - sarcoidosis D86.86
  - syphilis (late) A52.77
    - congenital A50.55 *[M12.80]*
  - thyrotoxicosis —*see also* subcategory M14.8- E05.90
  - ulcerative colitis K51.90 *[M07.60]*
  - viral hepatitis (postinfectious) NEC B19.9 *[M12.80]*
  - Whipple's disease —*see also* subcategory M14.8- K90.81
- Jaccoud —*see* Arthropathy, postrheumatic, chronic
- juvenile —*see* Arthritis, juvenile
  - psoriatic L40.54
- mutilans (psoriatic) L40.52
- neuropathic (Charcot) M14.60
  - ankle M14.67-
  - diabetic —*see* Diabetes, arthropathy, neuropathic
  - elbow M14.62-
  - foot joint M14.67-
  - hand joint M14.64-
  - hip M14.65-
  - knee M14.66-
  - multiple site M14.69
  - nonsyphilitic NEC G98.0
  - shoulder M14.61-
  - syringomyelic G95.0
  - vertebra M14.68
  - wrist M14.63-
- osteopulmonary —*see* Osteoarthropathy, hypertrophic, specified NEC
- postdysenteric M02.10
  - ankle M02.17-
  - elbow M02.12-
  - foot joint M02.17-
  - hand joint M02.14-
  - hip M02.15-
  - knee M02.16-
  - multiple site M02.19
  - shoulder M02.11-
  - vertebra M02.18
  - wrist M02.13-
- postimmunization M02.20
  - ankle M02.27-
  - elbow M02.22-
  - foot joint M02.27-
  - hand joint M02.24-
  - hip M02.25-
  - knee M02.26-
  - multiple site M02.29
  - shoulder M02.21-
  - vertebra M02.28
  - wrist M02.23-
- postinfectious NEC B99 *[M12.80]*
  - in (due to)
    - enteritis due to Yersinia enterocolitica A04.6 *[M12.80]*
    - syphilis A52.77
    - viral hepatitis NEC B19.9 *[M12.80]*
- postrheumatic, chronic (Jaccoud) M12.00
  - ankle M12.07-
  - elbow M12.02-
  - foot joint M12.07-
  - hand joint M12.04-
  - hip M12.05-
  - knee M12.06-
  - multiple site M12.09
  - shoulder M12.01-
  - specified joint NEC M12.08
  - vertebrae M12.08
  - wrist M12.03-
- psoriatic NEC L40.59
  - interphalangeal, distal L40.51

A

Arthropathy *(Continued)*
reactive M02.9
in (due to)
infective endocarditis I33.0 *[M02.9]*
specified type NEC M02.80
ankle M02.87-
elbow M02.82-
foot joint M02.87-
hand joint M02.84-
hip M02.85-
knee M02.86-
multiple site M02.89
shoulder M02.81-
vertebra M02.88
wrist M02.83-
specified form NEC M12.80
ankle M12.87-
elbow M12.82-
foot joint M12.87-
hand joint M12.84-
hip M12.85-
knee M12.86-
multiple site M12.89
shoulder M12.81-
specified joint NEC M12.88
vertebrae M12.88
wrist M12.83-
syringomyelic G95.0
tabes dorsalis A52.16
tabetic A52.16
transient —*see* Arthropathy, specified form NEC
traumatic M12.50
ankle M12.57-
elbow M12.52-
foot joint M12.57-
hand joint M12.54-
hip M12.55-
knee M12.56-
multiple site M12.59
shoulder M12.51-
specified joint NEC M12.58
vertebrae M12.58
wrist M12.53-
Arthropyosis —*see* Arthritis, pyogenic or pyemic
Arthrosis (deformans) (degenerative) (localized) —*see also* Osteoarthritis M19.90
spine —*see* Spondylosis
Arthus' phenomenon or reaction T78.41
due to
drug —*see* Table of Drugs and Chemicals, by drug
Articular —*see* condition
Articulation, reverse (teeth) M26.24
Artificial
insemination complication —*see* Complications, artificial, fertilization
opening status (functioning) (without complication) Z93.9
anus (colostomy) Z93.3
colostomy Z93.3
cystostomy Z93.50
appendico-vesicostomy Z93.52
cutaneous Z93.51
specified NEC Z93.59
enterostomy Z93.4
gastrostomy Z93.1
ileostomy Z93.2
intestinal tract NEC Z93.4
jejunostomy Z93.4
nephrostomy Z93.6
specified site NEC Z93.8
tracheostomy Z93.0
ureterostomy Z93.6
urethrostomy Z93.6
urinary tract NEC Z93.6
vagina Z93.8
vagina status Z93.8
Arytenoid —*see* condition
Asbestosis (occupational) J61
ASC-H (atypical squamous cells cannot exclude high grade squamous intraepithelial lesion on cytologic smear)
anus R85.611
cervix R87.611
vagina R87.621
ASC-US (atypical squamous cells of undetermined significance on cytologic smear)
anus R85.610
cervix R87.610
vagina R87.620
Ascariasis B77.9
with
complications NEC B77.89
intestinal complications B77.0
pneumonia, pneumonitis B77.81
Ascaridosis, ascaridiasis —*see* Ascariasis
Ascaris (infection) (infestation) (lumbricoides) —*see* Ascariasis
Ascending —*see* condition
Aschoff's bodies —*see* Myocarditis, rheumatic
Ascites (abdominal) R18.8
cardiac I50.9
chylous (nonfilarial) I89.8
filarial —*see* Infestation, filarial
due to
cirrhosis, alcoholic K70.31
hepatitis
alcoholic K70.11
chronic active K71.51
S. japonicum B65.2
heart I50.9
malignant R18.0
pseudochylous R18.8
syphilitic A52.74
tuberculous A18.31
Aseptic —*see* condition
Asherman's syndrome N85.6
Asialia K11.7
Asiatic cholera —*see* Cholera
Asimultagnosia (simultanagnosia) R48.3
Askin's tumor —*see* Neoplasm, connective tissue, malignant
Asocial personality F60.2
Asomatognosia R41.4
Aspartylglucosaminuria E77.1
Asperger's disease or syndrome F84.5
Aspergilloma —*see* Aspergillosis
Aspergillosis (with pneumonia) B44.9
bronchopulmonary, allergic B44.81
disseminated B44.7
generalized B44.7
pulmonary NEC B44.1
allergic B44.81
invasive B44.0
specified NEC B44.89
tonsillar B44.2
Aspergillus (flavus) (fumigatus) (infection) (terreus) —*see* Aspergillosis
Aspermatogenesis —*see* Azoospermia
Aspermia (testis) —*see* Azoospermia
Asphyxia, asphyxiation (by) R09.01
antenatal P84
birth P84
bunny bag —*see* Asphyxia, due to, mechanical threat to breathing, trapped in bed clothes
crushing S28.0
drowning T75.1
gas, fumes, or vapor —*see* Table of Drugs and Chemicals
inhalation —*see* Inhalation
intrauterine P84
local I73.00
with gangrene I73.01
mucus —*see also* Foreign body, respiratory tract, causing asphyxia
newborn P84
Asphyxia, asphyxiation *(Continued)*
pathological R09.01
postnatal P84
mechanical —*see* Asphyxia, due to, mechanical threat to breathing
prenatal P84
reticularis R23.1
strangulation —*see* Asphyxia, due to, mechanical threat to breathing
submersion T75.1
traumatic T71.9
due to
crushed chest S28.0
foreign body (in) —*see* Foreign body, respiratory tract, causing asphyxia
low oxygen content of ambient air T71.20
due to
being trapped in
low oxygen environment T71.29
in car trunk T71.221
circumstances undetermined T71.224
done with intent to harm by another person T71.223
self T71.222
in refrigerator T71.231
circumstances undetermined T71.234
done with intent to harm by another person T71.233
self T71.232
cave-in T71.21
mechanical threat to breathing (accidental) T71.191
circumstances undetermined T71.194
done with intent to harm by another person T71.193
self T71.192
hanging T71.161
circumstances undetermined T71.164
done with intent to harm by another person T71.163
self T71.162
plastic bag T71.121
circumstances undetermined T71.124
done with intent to harm by another person T71.123
self T71.122
smothering
in furniture T71.151
circumstances undetermined T71.154
done with intent to harm by another person T71.153
self T71.152
under
another person's body T71.141
circumstances undetermined T71.144
done with intent to harm T71.143
pillow T71.111
circumstances undetermined T71.114
done with intent to harm by another person T71.113
self T71.112
trapped in bed clothes T71.131
circumstances undetermined T71.134
done with intent to harm by another person T71.133
self T71.132
vomiting, vomitus —*see* Foreign body, respiratory tract, causing asphyxia
Aspiration
amniotic (clear) fluid (newborn) P24.10
with
pneumonia (pneumonitis) P24.11
respiratory symptoms P24.11

A

Aspiration *(Continued)*
  blood
    newborn (without respiratory symptoms) P24.20
      with
        pneumonia (pneumonitis) P24.21
        respiratory symptoms P24.21
    specified age NEC *—see* Foreign body, respiratory tract
  bronchitis J69.0
  food or foreign body (with asphyxiation) *—see* Asphyxia, food
  liquor (amnii) (newborn) P24.10
    with
      pneumonia (pneumonitis) P24.11
      respiratory symptoms P24.11
  meconium (newborn) (without respiratory symptoms) P24.00
    with
      pneumonitis (pneumonitis) P24.01
      respiratory symptoms P24.01
  milk (newborn) (without respiratory symptoms) P24.30
    with
      pneumonia (pneumonitis) P24.31
      respiratory symptoms P24.31
    specified age NEC *—see* Foreign body, respiratory tract
  mucus *—see also* Foreign body, by site, causing asphyxia
    newborn P24.10
      with
        pneumonia (pneumonitis) P24.11
        respiratory symptoms P24.11
  neonatal P24.9
    specific NEC (without respiratory symptoms) P24.80
      with
        pneumonia (pneumonitis) P24.81
        respiratory symptoms P24.81
  newborn P24.9
    specific NEC (without respiratory symptoms) P24.80
      with
        pneumonia (pneumonitis) P24.81
        respiratory symptoms P24.81
  pneumonia J69.0
  pneumonitis J69.0
  syndrome of newborn *—see* Aspiration, by substance, with pneumonia
  vernix caseosa (newborn) P24.80
    with
      pneumonia (pneumonitis) P24.81
      respiratory symptoms P24.81
  vomitus *—see also* Foreign body, respiratory tract
    newborn (without respiratory symptoms) P24.30
      with
        pneumonia (pneumonitis) P24.31
        respiratory symptoms P24.31
Asplenia (congenital) Q89.01
  postsurgical Z90.81
Assam fever B55.0
Assault, sexual *—see* Maltreatment
Assmann's focus NEC A15.0
Astasia (-abasia) (hysterical) F44.4
Asteatosis cutis L85.3
Astereognosia, astereognosis R48.1
Asterixis R27.8
  in liver disease K71.3
Asteroid hyalitis *—see* Deposit, crystalline
Asthenia, asthenic R53.1
  cardiac *—see also* Failure, heart I50.9
    psychogenic F45.8
  cardiovascular *—see also* Failure, heart I50.9
    psychogenic F45.8
  heart *—see also* Failure, heart I50.9
    psychogenic F45.8
Asthenia, asthenic *(Continued)*
  hysterical F44.4
  myocardial *—see also* Failure, heart I50.9
    psychogenic F45.8
  nervous F48.8
  neurocirculatory F45.8
  neurotic F48.8
  psychogenic F48.8
  psychoneurotic F48.8
  psychophysiologic F48.8
  reaction (psychophysiologic) F48.8
  senile R54
Asthenopia *—see also* Discomfort, visual
  hysterical F44.6
  psychogenic F44.6
Asthenospermia *—see* Abnormal, specimen, male genital organs
Asthma, asthmatic (bronchial) (catarrh) (spasmodic) J45.909
  with
    chronic obstructive bronchitis J44.9
      with
        acute lower respiratory infection J44.0
        exacerbation (acute) J44.1
    chronic obstructive pulmonary disease J44.9
      with
        acute lower respiratory infection J44.0
        exacerbation (acute) J44.1
    exacerbation (acute) J45.901
    hay fever *—see* Asthma, allergic extrinsic
    rhinitis, allergic *—see* Asthma, allergic extrinsic
    status asthmaticus J45.902
  allergic extrinsic J45.909
    with
      exacerbation (acute) J45.901
      status asthmaticus J45.902
  atopic *—see* Asthma, allergic extrinsic
  cardiac *—see* Failure, ventricular, left
  cardiobronchial I50.1
  childhood J45.909
    with
      exacerbation (acute) J45.901
      status asthmaticus J45.902
  chronic obstructive J44.9
    with
      acute lower respiratory infection J44.0
      exacerbation (acute) J44.1
  collier's J60
  cough variant J45.991
  detergent J69.8
  due to
    detergent J69.8
    inhalation of fumes J68.3
  eosinophilic J82
  extrinsic, allergic *—see* Asthma, allergic extrinsic
  grinder's J62.8
  hay *—see* Asthma, allergic extrinsic
  heart I50.1
  idiosyncratic *—see* Asthma, nonallergic
  intermittent (mild) J45.20
    with
      exacerbation (acute) J45.21
      status asthmaticus J45.22
  intrinsic, nonallergic *—see* Asthma, nonallergic
  Kopp's E32.8
  late-onset J45.909
    with
      exacerbation (acute) J45.901
      status asthmaticus J45.902
  mild intermittent J45.20
    with
      exacerbation (acute) J45.21
      status asthmaticus J45.22
Asthma, asthmatic *(Continued)*
  mild persistent J45.30
    with
      exacerbation (acute) J45.31
      status asthmaticus J45.32
  Millar's (laryngismus stridulus) J38.5
  miner's J60
  mixed J45.909
    with
      exacerbation (acute) J45.901
      status asthmaticus J45.902
  moderate persistent J45.40
    with
      exacerbation (acute) J45.41
      status asthmaticus J45.42
  nervous *—see* Asthma, nonallergic
  nonallergic (intrinsic) J45.909
    with
      exacerbation (acute) J45.901
      status asthmaticus J45.902
  persistent
    mild J45.30
      with
        exacerbation (acute) J45.31
        status asthmaticus J45.32
    moderate J45.40
      with
        exacerbation (acute) J45.41
        status asthmaticus J45.42
    severe J45.50
      with
        exacerbation (acute) J45.51
        status asthmaticus J45.52
  platinum J45.998
  pneumoconiotic NEC J64
  potter's J62.8
  predominantly allergic J45.909
  psychogenic F54
  pulmonary eosinophilic J82
  red cedar J67.8
  Rostan's I50.1
  sandblaster's J62.8
  sequoiosis J67.8
  severe persistent J45.50
    with
      exacerbation (acute) J45.51
      status asthmaticus J45.52
  specified NEC J45.998
  stonemason's J62.8
  thymic E32.8
  tuberculous *—see* Tuberculosis, pulmonary
  Wichmann's (laryngismus stridulus) J38.5
  wood J67.8
Astigmatism (compound) (congenital) H52.20-
  irregular H52.21-
  regular H52.22-
Astraphobia F40.220
Astroblastoma
  specified site *—see* Neoplasm, malignant, by site
  unspecified site C71.9
Astrocytoma (cystic)
  anaplastic
    specified site *—see* Neoplasm, malignant, by site
    unspecified site C71.9
  fibrillary
    specified site *—see* Neoplasm, malignant, by site
    unspecified site C71.9
  fibrous
    specified site *—see* Neoplasm, malignant, by site
    unspecified site C71.9
  gemistocytic
    specified site *—see* Neoplasm, malignant, by site
    unspecified site C71.9
  juvenile
    specified site *—see* Neoplasm, malignant, by site
    unspecified site C71.9

A

Astrocytoma *(Continued)*
  pilocytic
    specified site *—see* Neoplasm, malignant, by site
    unspecified site C71.9
  piloid
    specified site *—see* Neoplasm, malignant, by site
    unspecified site C71.9
  protoplasmic
    specified site *—see* Neoplasm, malignant, by site
    unspecified site C71.9
  specified site NEC *—see* Neoplasm, malignant, by site
  subependymal D43.2
    giant cell
      specified site *—see* Neoplasm, uncertain behavior, by site
      unspecified site D43.2
    specified site *—see* Neoplasm, uncertain behavior, by site
    unspecified site D43.2
  unspecified site C71.9
Astroglioma
  specified site *—see* Neoplasm, malignant, by site
  unspecified site C71.9
Asymbolia R48.8
Asymmetry *—see also* Distortion
  between native and reconstructed breast N65.1
  face Q67.Ø
  jaw (lower) *—see* Anomaly, dentofacial, jaw-cranial base relationship, asymmetry
Asynergia, asynergy R27.8
  ventricular I51.89
Asystole (heart) *—see* Arrest, cardiac
At risk
  for falling Z91.81
Ataxia, ataxy, ataxic R27.Ø
  acute R27.8
  brain (hereditary) G11.9
  cerebellar (hereditary) G11.9
    with defective DNA repair G11.3
    alcoholic G31.2
    early-onset G11.1
    in
      alcoholism G31.2
      myxedema EØ3.9 *[G13.2]*
      neoplastic disease *—see also* Neoplasm D49.9 *[G32.81]* (Revised)
      specified disease NEC G32.81
    late-onset (Marie's) G11.2
  cerebral (hereditary) G11.9
  congenital nonprogressive G11.Ø
  family, familial *—see* Ataxia, hereditary
  following
    cerebrovascular disease I69.993
      cerebral infarction I69.393
      intracerebral hemorrhage I69.193
      nontraumatic intracranial hemorrhage NEC I69.293
      specified disease NEC I69.893
      subarachnoid hemorrhage I69.Ø93
  Friedreich's (heredofamilial) (cerebellar) (spinal) G11.1
  gait R26.Ø
    hysterical F44.4
  general R27.8
  gluten M35.9 *[G32.81]*
    with celiac disease K9Ø.Ø *[G32.81]*
  hereditary G11.9
    with neuropathy G6Ø.2
    cerebellar *—see* Ataxia, cerebellar
    spastic G11.4
    specified NEC G11.8
    spinal (Friedreich's) G11.1
  heredofamilial *—see* Ataxia, hereditary
  Hunt's G11.1
  hysterical F44.4

Ataxia, ataxy, ataxic *(Continued)*
  locomotor (progressive) (syphilitic) (partial) (spastic) A52.11
    diabetic *—see* Diabetes, ataxia
  Marie's (cerebellar) (heredofamilial) (late-onset) G11.2
  nonorganic origin F44.4
  nonprogressive, congenital G11.Ø
  psychogenic F44.4
  Roussy-Lévy G6Ø.Ø
  Sanger-Brown's (hereditary) G11.2
  spastic hereditary G11.4
  spinal
    hereditary (Friedreich's) G11.1
    progressive (syphilitic) A52.11
  spinocerebellar, X-linked recessive G11.1
  telangiectasia (Louis-Bar) G11.3
Ataxia-telangiectasia (Louis-Bar) G11.3
Atelectasis (massive) (partial) (pressure) (pulmonary) J98.11
  newborn P28.1Ø
    due to resorption P28.11
    partial P28.19
    primary P28.Ø
    secondary P28.19
  primary (newborn) P28.Ø
  tuberculous *—see* Tuberculosis, pulmonary
Atelocardia Q24.9
Atelomyelia QØ6.1
Atheroembolism
  of
    extremities
      lower I75.Ø2-
      upper I75.Ø1-
    kidney I75.81
    specified NEC I75.89
Atheroma, atheromatous *—see also* Arteriosclerosis I7Ø.9Ø
  aorta, aortic I7Ø.Ø
    valve *—see also* Endocarditis, aortic I35.8
  aorto-iliac I7Ø.Ø
  artery *—see* Arteriosclerosis
  basilar (artery) I67.2
  carotid (artery) (common) (internal) I67.2
  cerebral (arteries) I67.2
  coronary (artery) I25.1Ø
    with angina pectoris *—see* Arteriosclerosis, coronary (artery)
  degeneration *—see* Arteriosclerosis
  heart, cardiac *—see* Disease, heart, ischemic, atherosclerotic
  mitral (valve) I34.8
  myocardium, myocardial *—see* Disease, heart, ischemic, atherosclerotic
  pulmonary valve (heart) *—see also* Endocarditis, pulmonary I37.8
  tricuspid (heart) (valve) I36.8
  valve, valvular *—see* Endocarditis
  vertebral (artery) I67.2
Atheromatosis *—see* Arteriosclerosis
Atherosclerosis *—see also* Arteriosclerosis
  coronary
    artery I25.1Ø
      with angina pectoris *—see* Arteriosclerosis, coronary (artery),
    due to
      calcified coronary lesion (severely) I25.84
      lipid rich plaque I25.83
  transplanted heart I25.811
    bypass graft I25.812
      with angina pectoris *—see* Arteriosclerosis, coronary (artery)
    native coronary artery I25.811
      with angina pectoris *—see* Arteriosclerosis, coronary (artery)
Athetosis (acquired) R25.8
  bilateral (congenital) G8Ø.3
  congenital (bilateral) (double) G8Ø.3
  double (congenital) G8Ø.3
  unilateral R25.8

Athlete's
  foot B35.3
  heart I51.7
Athrepsia E41
Athyrea (acquired) *—see also* Hypothyroidism
  congenital EØ3.1
Atonia, atony, atonic
  bladder (sphincter) (neurogenic) N31.2
  capillary I78.8
  cecum K59.8
    psychogenic F45.8
  colon *—see* Atony, intestine
  congenital P94.2
  esophagus K22.8
  intestine K59.8
    psychogenic F45.8
  stomach K31.89
    neurotic or psychogenic F45.8
  uterus (during labor) O62.2
    with hemorrhage (postpartum) O72.1
    postpartum (with hemorrhage) O72.1
      without hemorrhage O75.89
Atopy *—see* History, allergy
Atransferrinemia, congenital E88.Ø9
Atresia, atretic
  alimentary organ or tract NEC Q45.8
    upper Q4Ø.8
  ani, anus, anal (canal) Q42.3
    with fistula Q42.2
  aorta (ring) Q25.29 (Revised)
  aortic (orifice) (valve) Q23.Ø
    arch Q25.21 (Revised)
    congenital with hypoplasia of ascending aorta and defective development of left ventricle (with mitral stenosis) Q23.4
    in hypoplastic left heart syndrome Q23.4
  aqueduct of Sylvius QØ3.Ø
    with spina bifida *—see* Spina bifida, with hydrocephalus
  artery NEC Q27.8
    cerebral Q28.3
    coronary Q24.5
    digestive system Q27.8
    eye Q15.8
    lower limb Q27.8
    pulmonary Q25.5
    specified site NEC Q27.8
    umbilical Q27.Ø
    upper limb Q27.8
  auditory canal (external) Q16.1
  bile duct (common) (congenital) (hepatic) Q44.2
    acquired *—see* Obstruction, bile duct
  bladder (neck) Q64.39
    obstruction Q64.31
  bronchus Q32.4
  cecum Q42.8
  cervix (acquired) N88.2
    congenital Q51.828
    in pregnancy or childbirth *—see* Anomaly, cervix, in pregnancy or childbirth
      causing obstructed labor O65.5
  choana Q3Ø.Ø
  colon Q42.9
    specified NEC Q42.8
  common duct Q44.2
  cricoid cartilage Q31.8
  cystic duct Q44.2
    acquired K82.8
      with obstruction K82.Ø
  digestive organs NEC Q45.8
  duodenum Q41.Ø
  ear canal Q16.1
  ejaculatory duct Q55.4
  epiglottis Q31.8
  esophagus Q39.Ø
    with tracheoesophageal fistula Q39.1
  eustachian tube Q17.8
  fallopian tube (congenital) Q5Ø.6
    acquired N97.1

Atresia, atretic *(Continued)*
- follicular cyst N83.Ø- ◄
- foramen of
  - Luschka QØ3.1
    - with spina bifida —*see* Spina bifida, with hydrocephalus
  - Magendie QØ3.1
    - with spina bifida —*see* Spina bifida, with hydrocephalus
- gallbladder Q44.1
- genital organ
  - external
    - female Q52.79
    - male Q55.8
  - internal
    - female Q52.8
    - male Q55.8
- glottis Q31.8
- gullet Q39.Ø
  - with tracheoesophageal fistula Q39.1
- heart valve NEC Q24.8
  - pulmonary Q22.Ø
  - tricuspid Q22.4
- hymen Q52.3
  - acquired (postinfective) N89.6
- ileum Q41.2
- intestine (small) Q41.9
  - large Q42.9
    - specified NEC Q42.8
- iris, filtration angle Q15.Ø
- jejunum Q41.1
- lacrimal apparatus Q1Ø.4
- larynx Q31.8
- meatus urinarius Q64.33
- mitral valve Q23.2
  - in hypoplastic left heart syndrome Q23.4
- nares (anterior) (posterior) Q3Ø.Ø
- nasopharynx Q34.8
- nose, nostril Q3Ø.Ø
  - acquired J34.89
- organ or site NEC Q89.8
- osseous meatus (ear) Q16.1
- oviduct (congenital) Q5Ø.6
  - acquired N97.1
- parotid duct Q38.4
  - acquired K11.8
- pulmonary (artery) Q25.5
  - valve Q22.Ø
- pulmonic Q22.Ø
- pupil Q13.2
- rectum Q42.1
  - with fistula Q42.Ø
- salivary duct Q38.4
  - acquired K11.8
- sublingual duct Q38.4
  - acquired K11.8
- submandibular duct Q38.4
  - acquired K11.8
- submaxillary duct Q38.4
  - acquired K11.8
- thyroid cartilage Q31.8
- trachea Q32.1
- tricuspid valve Q22.4
- ureter Q62.1Ø
  - pelvic junction Q62.11
  - vesical orifice Q62.12
- ureteropelvic junction Q62.11
- ureterovesical orifice Q62.12
- urethra (valvular) Q64.39
  - stricture Q64.32
- urinary tract NEC Q64.8
- uterus Q51.818
  - acquired N85.8
- vagina (congenital) Q52.4
  - acquired (postinfectional) (senile) N89.5
- vas deferens Q55.3
- vascular NEC Q27.8
  - cerebral Q28.3
  - digestive system Q27.8

Atresia, atretic *(Continued)*
- vascular NEC *(Continued)*
  - lower limb Q27.8
  - specified site NEC Q27.8
  - upper limb Q27.8
- vein NEC Q27.8
  - digestive system Q27.8
  - great Q26.8
  - lower limb Q27.8
  - portal Q26.5
  - pulmonary Q26.3
  - specified site NEC Q27.8
  - upper limb Q27.8
- vena cava (inferior) (superior) Q26.8
- vesicourethral orifice Q64.31
- vulva Q52.79
  - acquired N9Ø.5

Atrichia, atrichosis —*see* Alopecia

Atrophia —*see also* Atrophy
- cutis senilis L9Ø.8
  - due to radiation L57.8
- gyrata of choroid and retina H31.23
- senilis R54
  - dermatological L9Ø.8
    - due to radiation (nonionizing) (solar) L57.8
- unguium L6Ø.3
  - congenita Q84.6

Atrophie blanche (en plaque) (de Milian) L95.Ø

Atrophoderma, atrophodermia (of) L9Ø.9
- diffusum (idiopathic) L9Ø.4
- maculatum L9Ø.8
  - et striatum L9Ø.8
    - due to syphilis A52.79
  - syphilitic A51.39
- neuriticum L9Ø.8
- Pasini and Pierini L9Ø.3
- ~~pigmentosum Q82.1~~
- reticulatum symmetricum faciei L66.4
- senile L9Ø.8
  - due to radiation (nonionizing) (solar) L57.8
- vermiculata (cheeks) L66.4

Atrophy, atrophic (of)
- adrenal (capsule) (gland) E27.49
  - primary (autoimmune) E27.1
- alveolar process or ridge (edentulous) KØ8.2Ø
- anal sphincter (disuse) N81.84
- appendix K38.8
- arteriosclerotic —*see* Arteriosclerosis
- bile duct (common) (hepatic) K83.8
- bladder N32.89
  - neurogenic N31.8
- blanche (en plaque) (of Milian) L95.Ø
- bone (senile) NEC —*see also* Disorder, bone, specified type NEC
  - due to
    - tabes dorsalis (neurogenic) A52.11
- brain (cortex) (progressive) G31.9
  - frontotemporal circumscribed G31.Ø1 *[FØ2.8Ø]*
    - with behavioral disturbance G31.Ø1 *[FØ2.81]*
  - senile NEC G31.1
- breast N64.2
  - obstetric —*see* Disorder, breast, specified type NEC
- buccal cavity K13.79
- cardiac —*see* Degeneration, myocardial
- cartilage (infectional) (joint) —*see* Disorder, cartilage, specified NEC
- cerebellar —*see* Atrophy, brain
- cerebral —*see* Atrophy, brain
- cervix (mucosa) (senile) (uteri) N88.8
  - menopausal N95.8
- Charcot-Marie-Tooth G6Ø.Ø
- choroid (central) (macular) (myopic) (retina) H31.1Ø-
  - diffuse secondary H31.12-
  - gyrate H31.23
  - senile H31.11-
- ciliary body —*see* Atrophy, iris

Atrophy, atrophic *(Continued)*
- conjunctiva (senile) H11.89
- corpus cavernosum N48.89
- cortical —*see* Atrophy, brain
- cystic duct K82.8
- Déjérine-Thomas G23.8
- disuse NEC —*see* Atrophy, muscle
- Duchenne-Aran G12.21
- ear H93.8-
- edentulous alveolar ridge KØ8.2Ø
- endometrium (senile) N85.8
  - cervix N88.8
- enteric K63.89
- epididymis N5Ø.89 ◄
- eyeball —*see* Disorder, globe, degenerated condition, atrophy
- eyelid (senile) —*see* Disorder, eyelid, degenerative
- facial (skin) L9Ø.9
- fallopian tube (senile) N83.32- ◄
  - with ovary N83.33- ◄
- fascioscapulohumeral (Landouzy- Déjérine) G71.Ø
- fatty, thymus (gland) E32.8
- gallbladder K82.8
- gastric K29.4Ø
  - with bleeding K29.41
- gastrointestinal K63.89
- glandular I89.8
- globe H44.52-
- gum —*see also* Recession, gingival KØ6.Ø ◄
- hair L67.8
- heart (brown) —*see* Degeneration, myocardial
- hemifacial Q67.4
  - Romberg G51.8
- infantile E41
  - paralysis, acute —*see* Poliomyelitis, paralytic
- intestine K63.89
- iris (essential) (progressive) H21.26-
  - specified NEC H21.29
- kidney (senile) (terminal) —*see also* Sclerosis, renal N26.1
  - congenital or infantile Q6Ø.5
    - bilateral Q6Ø.4
    - unilateral Q6Ø.3
  - hydronephrotic —*see* Hydronephrosis
- lacrimal gland (primary) HØ4.14-
  - secondary HØ4.15-
- Landouzy-Déjérine G71.Ø
- laryngitis, infective J37.Ø
- larynx J38.7
- Leber's optic (hereditary) H47.22
- lip K13.Ø
- liver (yellow) K72.9Ø
  - with coma K72.91
  - acute, subacute K72.ØØ
    - with coma K72.Ø1
  - chronic K72.1Ø
    - with coma K72.11
- lung (senile) J98.4
- macular (dermatological) L9Ø.8
  - syphilitic, skin A51.39
    - striated A52.79
- mandible (edentulous) KØ8.2Ø
  - minimal KØ8.21
  - moderate KØ8.22
  - severe KØ8.23
- maxilla KØ8.2Ø
  - minimal KØ8.24
  - moderate KØ8.25
  - severe KØ8.26
- muscle, muscular (diffuse) (general) (idiopathic) (primary) M62.5Ø
  - ankle M62.57-
  - Duchenne-Aran G12.21
  - foot M62.57-
  - forearm M62.53-
  - hand M62.54-
  - infantile spinal G12.Ø
  - lower leg M62.56-

A

- **Atrophy, atrophic** *(Continued)*
  - muscle, muscular *(Continued)*
    - multiple sites M62.59
    - myelopathic —*see* Atrophy, muscle, spinal
    - myotonic G71.11
    - neuritic G58.9
    - neuropathic (peroneal) (progressive) G60.0
    - pelvic (disuse) N81.84
    - peroneal G60.0
    - progressive (bulbar) G12.21
      - adult G12.1
      - infantile (spinal) G12.0
      - spinal G12.9
        - adult G12.1
        - infantile G12.0
    - pseudohypertrophic G71.0
    - shoulder region M62.51-
    - specified site NEC M62.58
    - spinal G12.9
      - adult form G12.1
      - Aran-Duchenne G12.21
      - childhood form, type II G12.1
      - distal G12.1
      - hereditary NEC G12.1
      - infantile, type I (Werdnig- Hoffmann) G12.0
      - juvenile form, type III (Kugelberg-Welander) G12.1
      - progressive G12.21
      - scapuloperoneal form G12.1
      - specified NEC G12.8
    - syphilitic A52.78
    - thigh M62.55-
    - upper arm M62.52-
  - myocardium —*see* Degeneration, myocardial
  - myometrium (senile) N85.8
    - cervix N88.8
  - myopathic NEC —*see* Atrophy, muscle
  - myotonia G71.11
  - nail L60.3
  - nasopharynx J31.1
  - nerve —*see also* Disorder, nerve
    - abducens —*see* Strabismus, paralytic, sixth nerve
    - accessory G52.8
    - acoustic or auditory —*see* subcategory H93.3
    - cranial G52.9
      - eighth (auditory) —*see* subcategory H93.3
      - eleventh (accessory) G52.8
      - fifth (trigeminal) G50.8
      - first (olfactory) G52.0
      - fourth (trochlear) —*see* Strabismus, paralytic, fourth nerve
      - second (optic) H47.20
      - sixth (abducens) —*see* Strabismus, paralytic, sixth nerve
      - tenth (pneumogastric) (vagus) G52.2
      - third (oculomotor) —*see* Strabismus, paralytic, third nerve
      - twelfth (hypoglossal) G52.3
    - hypoglossal G52.3
    - oculomotor —*see* Strabismus, paralytic, third nerve
    - olfactory G52.0
    - optic (papillomacular bundle)
      - syphilitic (late) A52.15
        - congenital A50.44
    - pneumogastric G52.2
    - trigeminal G50.8
    - trochlear —*see* Strabismus, paralytic, fourth nerve
    - vagus (pneumogastric) G52.2
  - neurogenic, bone, tabetic A52.11
  - nutritional E41
  - old age R54
  - olivopontocerebellar G23.8

- **Atrophy, atrophic** *(Continued)*
  - optic (nerve) H47.20
    - glaucomatous H47.23-
    - hereditary H47.22
    - primary H47.21-
    - specified type NEC H47.29-
    - syphilitic (late) A52.15
      - congenital A50.44
  - orbit H05.31-
  - ovary (senile) N83.31-
    - with fallopian tube N83.33-
  - oviduct (senile) —*see* Atrophy, fallopian tube
  - palsy, diffuse (progressive) G12.22
  - pancreas (duct) (senile) K86.89
  - parotid gland K11.0
  - pelvic muscle N81.84
  - penis N48.89
  - pharynx J39.2
  - pluriglandular E31.8
    - autoimmune E31.0
  - polyarthritis M15.9
  - prostate N42.89
  - pseudohypertrophic (muscle) G71.0
  - renal —*see also* Sclerosis, renal N26.1
  - retina, retinal (postinfectional) H35.89
  - rhinitis J31.0
  - salivary gland K11.0
  - scar L90.5
  - sclerosis, lobar (of brain) G31.09 *[F02.80]*
    - with behavioral disturbance G31.09 *[F02.81]*
  - scrotum N50.89
  - seminal vesicle N50.89
  - senile R54
    - due to radiation (nonionizing) (solar) L57.8
  - skin (patches) (spots) L90.9
    - degenerative (senile) L90.8
    - due to radiation (nonionizing) (solar) L57.8
    - senile L90.8
  - spermatic cord N50.89
  - spinal (acute) (cord) G95.89
    - muscular —*see* Atrophy, muscle, spinal
    - paralysis G12.20
      - acute —*see* Poliomyelitis, paralytic
      - meaning progressive muscular atrophy G12.21
  - spine (column) —*see* Spondylopathy, specified NEC
  - spleen (senile) D73.0
  - stomach K29.40
    - with bleeding K29.41
  - striate (skin) L90.6
    - syphilitic A52.79
  - subcutaneous L90.9
  - sublingual gland K11.0
  - submandibular gland K11.0
  - submaxillary gland K11.0
  - Sudeck's —*see* Algoneurodystrophy
  - suprarenal (capsule) (gland) E27.49
    - primary E27.1
  - systemic affecting central nervous system
    - in
      - myxedema E03.9 *[G13.2]*
      - neoplastic disease —*see also* Neoplasm D49.9 *[G13.1]*
      - specified disease NEC G13.8
  - tarso-orbital fascia, congenital Q10.3
  - testis N50.0
  - thenar, partial —*see* Syndrome, carpal tunnel
  - thymus (fatty) E32.8
  - thyroid (gland) (acquired) E03.4
    - with cretinism E03.1
    - congenital (with myxedema) E03.1
  - tongue (senile) K14.8
    - papillae K14.4
  - trachea J39.8
  - tunica vaginalis N50.89
  - turbinate J34.89
  - tympanic membrane (nonflaccid) H73.82-
    - flaccid H73.81-
  - upper respiratory tract J39.8

- **Atrophy, atrophic** *(Continued)*
  - uterus, uterine (senile) N85.8
    - cervix N88.8
    - due to radiation (intended effect) N85.8
      - adverse effect or misadventure N99.89
  - vagina (senile) N95.2
  - vas deferens N50.89
  - vascular I99.8
  - vertebra (senile) —*see* Spondylopathy, specified NEC
  - vulva (senile) N90.5
  - Werdnig-Hoffmann G12.0
  - yellow —*see* Failure, hepatic
- **Attack, attacks**
  - with alteration of consciousness (with automatisms) —*see* Epilepsy, localization-related, symptomatic, with complex partial seizures
  - without alteration of consciousness —*see* Epilepsy, localization-related, symptomatic, with simple partial seizures
  - Adams-Stokes I45.9
  - akinetic —*see* Epilepsy, generalized, specified NEC
  - angina —*see* Angina
  - atonic —*see* Epilepsy, generalized, specified NEC
  - benign shuddering G25.83
  - cataleptic —*see* Catalepsy
  - coronary —*see* Infarct, myocardium
  - cyanotic, newborn P28.2
  - drop NEC R55
  - epileptic —*see* Epilepsy
  - heart —*see* infarct, myocardium
  - hysterical F44.9
  - jacksonian —*see* Epilepsy, localization-related, symptomatic, with simple partial seizures
  - myocardium, myocardial —*see* Infarct, myocardium
  - myoclonic —*see* Epilepsy, generalized, specified NEC
  - panic F41.0
  - psychomotor —*see* Epilepsy, localization-related, symptomatic, with complex partial seizures
  - salaam —*see* Epilepsy, spasms
  - schizophreniform, brief F23
  - shuddering, benign G25.83
  - Stokes-Adams I45.9
  - syncope R55
  - transient ischemic (TIA) G45.9
    - specified NEC G45.8
  - unconsciousness R55
    - hysterical F44.89
  - vasomotor R55
  - vasovagal (paroxysmal) (idiopathic) R55
- **Attention** (to)
  - artificial
    - opening (of) Z43.9
      - digestive tract NEC Z43.4
        - colon Z43.3
        - ilium Z43.2
        - stomach Z43.1
      - specified NEC Z43.8
      - trachea Z43.0
      - urinary tract NEC Z43.6
        - cystostomy Z43.5
        - nephrostomy Z43.6
        - ureterostomy Z43.6
        - urethrostomy Z43.6
      - vagina Z43.7
  - colostomy Z43.3
  - cystostomy Z43.5
  - deficit disorder or syndrome F98.8
    - with hyperactivity —*see* Disorder, attention-deficit hyperactivity
  - gastrostomy Z43.1
  - ileostomy Z43.2

◄ New ◄■■ Revised ~~deleted~~ Deleted

Attention *(Continued)*
jejunostomy Z43.4
nephrostomy Z43.6
surgical dressings Z48.01
sutures Z48.02
tracheostomy Z43.0
ureterostomy Z43.6
urethrostomy Z43.6
Attrition
gum —*see also* Recession, gingival K06.0
tooth, teeth (excessive) (hard tissues) K03.0
Atypical, atypism —*see also* condition
cells (on cytolgocial smear) (endocervical) (endometrial) (glandular)
cervix R87.619
vagina R87.629
cervical N87.9
endometrium N85.9
hyperplasia N85.00
parenting situation Z62.9
Auditory —*see* condition
Aujeszky's disease B33.8
Aurantiasis, cutis E67.1
Auricle, auricular —*see also* condition
cervical Q18.2
Auriculotemporal syndrome G50.8
Austin Flint murmur (aortic insufficiency) I35.1
Australian
Q fever A78
X disease A83.4
Autism, autistic (childhood) (infantile) F84.0
atypical F84.9
spectrum disorder F84.0
Autodigestion R68.89
Autoerythrocyte sensitization (syndrome) D69.2
Autographism L50.3
Autoimmune
disease (systemic) M35.9
inhibitors to clotting factors D68.311
lymphoproliferative syndrome [ALPS] D89.82
thyroiditis E06.3
Autointoxication R68.89
Automatism G93.89
with temporal sclerosis G93.81
epileptic —*see* Epilepsy, localization- related, symptomatic, with complex partial seizures
Automatism *(Continued)*
paroxysmal, idiopathic —*see* Epilepsy, localization-related, symptomatic, with complex partial seizures
Autonomic, autonomous
bladder (neurogenic) N31.2
hysteria seizure F44.5
Autosensitivity, erythrocyte D69.2
Autosensitization, cutaneous L30.2
Autosome —*see* condition by chromosome involved
Autotopagnosia R48.1
Autotoxemia R68.89
Autumn —*see* condition
Avellis' syndrome G46.8
Aversion
oral R63.3
newborn P92.-
nonorganic origin F98.2
sexual F52.1
Aviator's
disease or sickness —*see* Effect, adverse, high altitude
ear T70.0
Avitaminosis (multiple) —*see also* Deficiency, vitamin E56.9
B E53.9
with
beriberi E51.11
pellagra E52
B2 E53.0
B6 E53.1
B12 E53.8
D E55.9
with rickets E55.0
G E53.0
K E56.1
nicotinic acid E52
AVNRT (atrioventricular nodal re-entrant tachycardia) I47.1
AVRT (atrioventricular nodal re-entrant tachycardia) I47.1
Avulsion (traumatic)
blood vessel —*see* Injury, blood vessel
bone —*see* Fracture, by site
cartilage —*see also* Dislocation, by site
symphyseal (inner), complicating delivery O71.6
external site other than limb —*see* Wound, open, by site
Avulsion *(Continued)*
eye S05.7-
head (intracranial)
external site NEC S08.89
scalp S08.0
internal organ or site —*see* Injury, by site
joint —*see also* Dislocation, by site
capsule —*see* Sprain, by site
kidney S37.06-
ligament —*see* Sprain, by site
limb —*see also* Amputation, traumatic, by site
skin and subcutaneous tissue —*see* Wound, open, by site
muscle —*see* Injury, muscle
nerve (root) —*see* Injury, nerve
scalp S08.0
skin and subcutaneous tissue —*see* Wound, open, by site
spleen S36.032
symphyseal cartilage (inner), complicating delivery O71.6
tendon —*see* Injury, muscle
tooth S03.2
Awareness of heart beat R00.2
Axenfeld's
anomaly or syndrome Q15.0
degeneration (calcareous) Q13.4
Axilla, axillary —*see also* condition
breast Q83.1
Axonotmesis —*see* Injury, nerve
Ayerza's disease or syndrome (pulmonary artery sclerosis with pulmonary hypertension) I27.0
Azoospermia (organic) N46.01
due to
drug therapy N46.021
efferent duct obstruction N46.023
infection N46.022
radiation N46.024
specified cause NEC N46.029
systemic disease N46.025
Azotemia R79.89
meaning uremia N19
Aztec ear Q17.3
Azygos
continuation inferior vena cava Q26.8
lobe (lung) Q33.1

A

B

- **Baastrup's disease** —*see* Kissing spine
- **Babesiosis** B60.0
- **Babington's disease** (familial hemorrhagic telangiectasia) I78.0
- **Babinski's syndrome** A52.79
- **Baby**
  - crying constantly R68.11
  - floppy (syndrome) P94.2
- **Bacillary** —*see* condition
- **Bacilluria** R82.71
- **Bacillus** —*see also* Infection, bacillus
  - abortus infection A23.1
  - anthracis infection A22.9
  - coli infection —*see also* Escherichia coli B96.20
  - Flexner's A03.1
  - mallei infection A24.0
  - Shiga's A03.0
  - suipestifer infection —*see* Infection, salmonella
- **Back** —*see* condition
- **Backache** (postural) M54.9
  - sacroiliac M53.3
  - specified NEC M54.89
- **Backflow** —*see* Reflux
- **Backward reading** (dyslexia) F81.0
- **Bacteremia** R78.81
  - with sepsis —*see* Sepsis
- **Bactericholia** —*see* Cholecystitis, acute
- **Bacterid, bacteride** (pustular) L40.3
- **Bacterium, bacteria, bacterial**
  - agent NEC, as cause of disease classified elsewhere B96.89
  - in blood —*see* Bacteremia
  - in urine —*see* Bacteriuria
- **Bacteriuria, bacteruria** R82.71
  - asymptomatic R82.71
- **Bacteroides**
  - fragilis, as cause of disease classified elsewhere B96.6
- **Bad**
  - heart —*see* Disease, heart
  - trip
    - due to drug abuse —*see* Abuse, drug, hallucinogen
    - due to drug dependence —*see* Dependence, drug, hallucinogen
- **Baelz's disease** (cheilitis glandularis apostematosa) K13.0
- **Baerensprung's disease** (eczema marginatum) B35.6
- **Bagasse disease or pneumonitis** J67.1
- **Bagassosis** J67.1
- **Baker's cyst** —*see* Cyst, Baker's
- **Bakwin-Krida syndrome** (metaphyseal dysplasia) Q78.5
- **Balancing side interference** M26.56
- **Balanitis** (circinata) (erosiva) (gangrenosa) (phagedenic) (vulgaris) N48.1
  - amebic A06.82
  - candidal B37.42
  - due to Haemophilus ducreyi A57
  - gonococcal (acute) (chronic) A54.09
  - xerotica obliterans N48.0
- **Balanoposthitis** N47.6
  - gonococcal (acute) (chronic) A54.09
  - ulcerative (specific) A63.8
- **Balanorrhagia** —*see* Balanitis
- **Balantidiasis, balantidiosis** A07.0
- **Bald tongue** K14.4
- **Baldness** —*see also* Alopecia
  - male-pattern —*see* Alopecia, androgenic
- **Balkan grippe** A78
- **Balloon disease** —*see* Effect, adverse, high altitude
- **Balo's disease** (concentric sclerosis) G37.5
- **Bamberger-Marie disease** —*see* Osteoarthropathy, hypertrophic, specified type NEC
- **Bancroft's filariasis** B74.0
- **Band** (s)
  - adhesive —*see* Adhesions, peritoneum
  - anomalous or congenital —*see also* Anomaly, by site
    - heart (atrial) (ventricular) Q24.8
    - intestine Q43.3
    - omentum Q43.3
  - cervix N88.1
  - constricting, congenital Q79.8
  - gallbladder (congenital) Q44.1
  - intestinal (adhesive) —*see* Adhesions, peritoneum
  - obstructive
    - intestine K56.5
    - peritoneum K56.5
  - periappendiceal, congenital Q43.3
  - peritoneal (adhesive) —*see* Adhesions, peritoneum
  - uterus N73.6
    - internal N85.6
  - vagina N89.5
- **Bandemia** D72.825
- **Bandl's ring** (contraction), **complicating delivery** O62.4
- **Bangkok hemorrhagic fever** A91
- **Bang's disease** (brucella abortus) A23.1
- **Bankruptcy, anxiety concerning** Z59.8
- **Bannister's disease** T78.3
  - hereditary D84.1
- **Banti's disease or syndrome** (with cirrhosis) (with portal hypertension) K76.6
- **Bar, median, prostate** —*see* Enlargement, enlarged, prostate
- **Barcoo disease or rot** —*see* Ulcer, skin
- **Barlow's disease** E54
- **Barodontalgia** T70.29
- **Baron Münchausen syndrome** —*see* Disorder, factitious
- **Barosinusitis** T70.1
- **Barotitis** T70.0
- **Barotrauma** T70.29
  - odontalgia T70.29
  - otitic T70.0
  - sinus T70.1
- **Barraquer** (-Simons) **disease or syndrome** (progressive lipodystrophy) E88.1
- **Barré-Guillain disease or syndrome** G61.0
- **Barré-Liéou syndrome** (posterior cervical sympathetic) M53.0
- **Barrel chest** M95.4
- **Barrett's**
  - disease —*see* Barrett's, esophagus
  - esophagus K22.70
    - with dysplasia K22.719
      - high grade K22.711
      - low grade K22.710
    - without dysplasia K22.70
  - syndrome —*see* Barrett's, esophagus
  - ulcer K22.10
    - with bleeding K22.11
    - without bleeding K22.10
- **Barth syndrome** E78.71
- **Bársony** (-Polgár) (-Teschendorf) **syndrome** (corkscrew esophagus) K22.4
- **Bartholinitis** (suppurating) N75.8
  - gonococcal (acute) (chronic) (with abscess) A54.1
- **Bartonellosis** A44.9
  - cutaneous A44.1
  - mucocutaneous A44.1
  - specified NEC A44.8
  - systemic A44.0
- **Barton's fracture** S52.56-
- **Bartter's syndrome** E26.81
- **Basal** —*see* condition
- **Basan's** (hidrotic) **ectodermal dysplasia** Q82.4
- **Baseball finger** —*see* Dislocation, finger
- **Basedow's disease** (exophthalmic goiter) —*see* Hyperthyroidism, with, goiter
- **Basic** —*see* condition
- **Basilar** —*see* condition
- **Bason's** (hidrotic) **ectodermal dysplasia** Q82.4
- **Basopenia** —*see* Agranulocytosis
- **Basophilia** D72.824
- **Basophilism** (cortico-adrenal) (Cushing's) (pituitary) E24.0
- **Bassen-Kornzweig disease or syndrome** E78.6
- **Bat ear** Q17.5
- **Bateman's**
  - disease B08.1
  - purpura (senile) D69.2
- **Bathing cramp** T75.1
- **Bathophobia** F40.248
- **Batten** (-Mayou) **disease** E75.4
  - retina E75.4 *[H36]*
- **Batten-Steinert syndrome** G71.11
- **Battered** —*see* Maltreatment
- **Battey Mycobacterium infection** A31.0
- **Battle exhaustion** F43.0
- **Battledore placenta** O43.19-
- **Baumgarten-Cruveilhier cirrhosis, disease or syndrome** K74.69
- **Bauxite fibrosis** (of lung) J63.1
- **Bayle's disease** (general paresis) A52.17
- **Bazin's disease** (primary) (tuberculous) A18.4
- **Beach ear** —*see* Swimmer's, ear
- **Beaded hair** (congenital) Q84.1
- **Béal conjunctivitis or syndrome** B30.2
- **Beard's disease** (neurasthenia) F48.8
- **Beat** (s)
  - atrial, premature I49.1
  - ectopic I49.49
  - elbow —*see* Bursitis, elbow
  - escaped, heart I49.49
  - hand —*see* Bursitis, hand
  - knee —*see* Bursitis, knee
  - premature I49.40
    - atrial I49.1
    - auricular I49.1
    - supraventricular I49.1
- **Beau's**
  - disease or syndrome —*see* Degeneration, myocardial
  - lines (transverse furrows on fingernails) L60.4
- **Bechterev's syndrome** —*see* Spondylitis, ankylosing
- **Beck's syndrome** (anterior spinal artery occlusion) I65.8
- **Becker's**
  - cardiomyopathy I42.8
  - disease
    - idiopathic mural endomyocardial disease I42.3
    - myotonia congenita, recessive form G71.12
  - dystrophy G71.0
  - pigmented hairy nevus D22.5
- **Beckwith-Wiedemann syndrome** Q87.3
- **Bed confinement status** Z74.01
- **Bed sore** —*see* Ulcer, pressure, by site
- **Bedbug bite** (s) —*see* Bite (s), by site, superficial, insect
- **Bedclothes, asphyxiation or suffocation by** —*see* Asphyxia, traumatic, due to, mechanical, trapped
- **Bednar's**
  - aphthae K12.0
  - tumor —*see* Neoplasm, malignant, by site
- **Bedridden** Z74.01
- **Bedsore** —*see* Ulcer, pressure, by site
- **Bedwetting** —*see* Enuresis
- **Bee sting** (with allergic or anaphylactic shock) —*see* Toxicity, venom, arthropod, bee
- **Beer drinker's heart** (disease) I42.6
- **Begbie's disease** (exophthalmic goiter) —*see* Hyperthyroidism, with, goiter
- **Behavior**
  - antisocial
    - adult Z72.811
    - child or adolescent Z72.810
  - disorder, disturbance —*see* Disorder, conduct
  - disruptive —*see* Disorder, conduct

B

◄ New ◄ Revised ~~deleted~~ Deleted

Behavior *(Continued)*
- drug seeking Z76.5
- inexplicable R46.2
- marked evasiveness R46.5
- obsessive-compulsive R46.81
- overactivity R46.3
- poor responsiveness R46.4
- self-damaging (life-style) Z72.89
- sleep-incompatible Z72.821
- slowness R46.4
- specified NEC R46.89
- strange (and inexplicable) R46.2
- suspiciousness R46.5
- type A pattern Z73.1
- undue concern or preoccupation with stressful events R46.6
- verbosity and circumstantial detail obscuring reason for contact R46.7

Behcet's disease or syndrome M35.2
Behr's disease —*see* Degeneration, macula
Beigel's disease or morbus (white piedra) B36.2
Bejel A65
Bekhterev's syndrome —*see* Spondylitis, ankylosing
Belching —*see* Eructation
Bell's
- mania F30.8
- palsy, paralysis G51.0
  - infant or newborn P11.3
- spasm G51.3

Bence Jones albuminuria or proteinuria NEC R80.3
Bends T70.3
Benedikt's paralysis or syndrome G46.3
Benign (*see also* condition)
- prostatic hyperplasia —*see* Hyperplasia, prostate

Bennett's fracture (displaced) S62.21-
Benson's disease —*see* Deposit, crystalline
Bent
- back (hysterical) F44.4
- nose M95.0
  - congenital Q67.4

Bereavement (uncomplicated) Z63.4
Bergeron's disease (hysterical chorea) F44.4
Berger's disease —*see* Nephropathy, IgA
Beriberi (dry) E51.11
- heart (disease) E51.12
- polyneuropathy E51.11
- wet E51.12
  - involving circulatory system E51.11

Berlin's disease or edema (traumatic) S05.8X-
Berlock (berloque) **dermatitis** L56.2
Bernard-Horner syndrome G90.2
Bernard-Soulier disease or thrombopathia D69.1
Bernhardt (-Roth) **disease** —*see* Mononeuropathy, lower limb, meralgia paresthetica
Bernheim's syndrome —*see* Failure, heart, congestive
Bertielliasis B71.8
Berylliosis (lung) J63.2
Besnier-Boeck (-Schaumann) **disease** —*see* Sarcoidosis
Besnier's
- lupus pernio D86.3
- prurigo L20.0

Bestiality F65.89
Best's disease H35.50
Beta-mercaptolactate-cysteine disulfiduria E72.09
Betalipoproteinemia, broad or floating E78.2
Betting and gambling Z72.6
- pathological (compulsive) F63.0

Bezoar T18.9
- intestine T18.3
- stomach T18.2

Bezold's abscess —*see* Mastoiditis, acute
Bianchi's syndrome R48.8
Bicornate or bicornis uterus Q51.3
- in pregnancy or childbirth O34.0-
  - causing obstructed labor O65.5

Bicuspid aortic valve Q23.1
Biedl-Bardet syndrome Q87.89
Bielschowsky (-Jansky) **disease** E75.4
Biermer's (pernicious) **anemia or disease** D51.0
Biett's disease L93.0
Bifid (congenital)
- apex, heart Q24.8
- clitoris Q52.6
- kidney Q63.8
- nose Q30.2
- patella Q74.1
- scrotum Q55.29
- toe NEC Q74.2
- tongue Q38.3
- ureter Q62.8
- uterus Q51.3
- uvula Q35.7

Biforis uterus (suprasimplex) Q51.3
Bifurcation (congenital)
- gallbladder Q44.1
- kidney pelvis Q63.8
- renal pelvis Q63.8
- rib Q76.6
- tongue, congenital Q38.3
- trachea Q32.1
- ureter Q62.8
- urethra Q64.74
- vertebra Q76.49

Big spleen syndrome D73.1
Bigeminal pulse R00.8
Bilateral —*see* condition
Bile
- duct —*see* condition
- pigments in urine R82.2

Bilharziasis —*see also* Schistosomiasis
- chyluria B65.0
- cutaneous B65.3
- galacturia B65.0
- hematochyluria B65.0
- intestinal B65.1
- lipemia B65.9
- lipuria B65.0
- oriental B65.2
- piarhemia B65.9
- pulmonary NOS B65.9 *[J99]*
  - pneumonia B65.9 *[J17]*
- tropical hematuria B65.0
- vesical B65.0

Biliary —*see* condition
Bilirubin metabolism disorder E80.7
- specified NEC E80.6

Bilirubinemia, familial nonhemolytic E80.4
Bilirubinuria R82.2
Biliuria R82.2
Bilocular stomach K31.2
Binswanger's disease I67.3
Biparta, bipartite
- carpal scaphoid Q74.0
- patella Q74.1
- vagina Q52.10

Bird
- face Q75.8
- fancier's disease or lung J67.2

Birt-Hogg-Dube syndrome Q87.89
Birth
- complications in mother —*see* Delivery, complicated
- compression during NOS P15.9
- defect —*see* Anomaly
- immature (less than 37 completed weeks) —*see* Preterm, newborn
  - extremely (less than 28 completed weeks) —*see* Immaturity, extreme
- inattention, at or after —*see* Maltreatment, child, neglect
- injury NOS P15.9
  - basal ganglia P11.1
  - brachial plexus NEC P14.3

Birth *(Continued)*
- injury NOS *(Continued)*
  - brain (compression) (pressure) P11.2
  - central nervous system NOS P11.9
  - cerebellum P11.1
  - cerebral hemorrhage P10.1
  - external genitalia P15.5
  - eye P15.3
  - face P15.4
  - fracture
    - bone P13.9
      - specified NEC P13.8
    - clavicle P13.4
    - femur P13.2
    - humerus P13.3
    - long bone, except femur P13.3
    - radius and ulna P13.3
    - skull P13.0
    - spine P11.5
    - tibia and fibula P13.3
  - intracranial P11.2
    - laceration or hemorrhage P10.9
      - specified NEC P10.8
  - intraventricular hemorrhage P10.2
  - laceration
    - brain P10.1
    - by scalpel P15.8
    - peripheral nerve P14.9
  - liver P15.0
  - meninges
    - brain P11.1
    - spinal cord P11.5
  - nerve
    - brachial plexus P14.3
    - cranial NEC (except facial) P11.4
    - facial P11.3
    - peripheral P14.9
    - phrenic (paralysis) P14.2
  - paralysis
    - facial nerve P11.3
    - spinal P11.5
  - penis P15.5
  - rupture
    - spinal cord P11.5
  - scalp P12.9
  - scalpel wound P15.8
  - scrotum P15.5
  - skull NEC P13.1
    - fracture P13.0
  - specified type NEC P15.8
  - spinal cord P11.5
  - spine P11.5
  - spleen P15.1
  - sternomastoid (hematoma) P15.2
  - subarachnoid hemorrhage P10.3
  - subcutaneous fat necrosis P15.6
  - subdural hemorrhage P10.0
  - tentorial tear P10.4
  - testes P15.5
  - vulva P15.5
- lack of care, at or after —*see* Maltreatment, child, neglect
- neglect, at or after —*see* Maltreatment, child, neglect
- palsy or paralysis, newborn, NOS (birth injury) P14.9
- premature (infant) —*see* Preterm, newborn
- shock, newborn P96.89
- trauma —*see* Birth, injury
- weight
  - 4000 grams to 4499 grams P08.1
  - 4500 grams or more P08.0
  - low (2499 grams or less) —*see* Low, birthweight
    - extremely (999 grams or less) —*see* Low, birthweight, extreme

Birthmark Q82.5
Bisalbuminemia E88.09
Biskra's button B55.1

B

Bite *(Continued)*
neck *(Continued)*
superficial NEC S10.97
insect S10.96
throat S11.85
superficial NEC S10.17
insect S10.16
nose (septum) (sinus) S01.25
superficial NEC S00.37
insect S00.36
occipital region —*see* Bite, scalp
oral cavity S01.552
superficial NEC S00.572
insect S00.562
orbital region —*see* Bite, eyelid
palate —*see* Bite, oral cavity
palm —*see* Bite, hand
parietal region —*see* Bite, scalp
pelvis S31.050
with penetration into retroperitoneal space S31.051
superficial NEC S30.870
insect S30.860
penis S31.25
superficial NEC S30.872
insect S30.862
perineum
female —*see* Bite, vulva
male —*see* Bite, pelvis
periocular area (with or without lacrimal passages) —*see* Bite, eyelid
phalanges
finger —*see* Bite, finger
toe —*see* Bite, toe
pharynx S11.25
superficial NEC S10.17
insect S10.16
pinna —*see* Bite, ear
poisonous —*see* Venom
popliteal space —*see* Bite, knee
prepuce —*see* Bite, penis
pubic region —*see* Bite, abdomen, wall
rectovaginal septum —*see* Bite, vulva
red bug B88.0
reptile NEC —*see also* Venom, bite, reptile
nonvenomous —*see* Bite, by site
snake —*see* Venom, bite, snake
sacral region —*see* Bite, back, lower
sacroiliac region —*see* Bite, back, lower
salivary gland —*see* Bite, oral cavity
scalp S01.05
superficial NEC S00.07
insect S00.06
scapular region —*see* Bite, shoulder
scrotum S31.35
superficial NEC S30.873
insect S30.863
sea-snake (venomous) —*see* Toxicity, venom, snake, sea snake
shin —*see* Bite, leg
shoulder S41.05-
superficial NEC S40.27-
insect S40.26-
snake —*see also* Venom, bite, snake
nonvenomous —*see* Bite, by site
spermatic cord —*see* Bite, testis
spider (venomous) —*see* Toxicity, venom, spider
nonvenomous —*see* Bite, by site, superficial, insect
sternal region —*see* Bite, thorax, front
submaxillary region —*see* Bite, head, specified site NEC
submental region —*see* Bite, head, specified site NEC
subungual
finger (s) —*see* Bite, finger
toe —*see* Bite, toe
superficial —*see* Bite, by site, superficial
supraclavicular fossa S11.85

Bite *(Continued)*
supraorbital —*see* Bite, head, specified site NEC
temple, temporal region —*see* Bite, head, specified site NEC
temporomandibular area —*see* Bite, cheek
testis S31.35
superficial NEC S30.873
insect S30.863
thigh S71.15-
superficial NEC S70.37-
insect S70.36-
thorax, thoracic (wall) S21.95
back S21.25-
with penetration into thoracic cavity S21.45-
breast —*see* Bite, breast
front S21.15-
with penetration into thoracic cavity S21.35-
superficial NEC S20.97
back S20.47-
front S20.37-
insect S20.96
back S20.46-
front S20.36-
throat —*see* Bite, neck, throat
thumb S61.05-
with
damage to nail S61.15-
superficial NEC S60.37-
insect S60.36-
thyroid S11.15
superficial NEC S10.87
insect S10.86
toe (s) S91.15-
with
damage to nail S91.25-
great S91.15-
with
damage to nail S91.25-
lesser S91.15-
with
damage to nail S91.25-
superficial NEC S90.47-
great S90.47-
insect S90.46-
great S90.46-
tongue S01.552
trachea S11.025
superficial NEC S10.17
insect S10.16
tunica vaginalis —*see* Bite, testis
tympanum, tympanic membrane —*see* Bite, ear
umbilical region S31.155
uvula —*see* Bite, oral cavity
vagina —*see* Bite, vulva
venomous —*see* Venom
vocal cords S11.035
superficial NEC S10.17
insect S10.16
vulva S31.45
superficial NEC S30.874
insect S30.864
wrist S61.55-
superficial NEC S60.87-
insect S60.86-

Biting, cheek or lip K13.1
Biventricular failure (heart) I50.9
Björck (-Thorson) **syndrome** (malignant carcinoid) E34.0
Black
death A20.9
eye S00.1-
hairy tongue K14.3
heel (foot) S90.3-
lung (disease) J60
palm (hand) S60.22-
Blackfan-Diamond anemia or syndrome (congenital hypoplastic anemia) D61.01
Blackhead L70.0
Blackout R55
Bladder —*see* condition
Blast (air) (hydraulic) (immersion) (underwater)
blindness S05.8X-
injury
abdomen or thorax —*see* Injury, by site
ear (acoustic nerve trauma) —*see* Injury, nerve, acoustic, specified type NEC
syndrome NEC T70.8
Blastoma —*see* Neoplasm, malignant, by site
pulmonary —*see* Neoplasm, lung, malignant
Blastomycosis, blastomycotic B40.9
Brazilian —*see* Paracoccidioidomycosis
cutaneous B40.3
disseminated B40.7
European —*see* Cryptococcosis
generalized B40.7
keloidal B48.0
North American B40.9
primary pulmonary B40.0
pulmonary B40.2
acute B40.0
chronic B40.1
skin B40.3
South American —*see* Paracoccidioidomycosis
specified NEC B40.89
Bleb (s) R23.8
emphysematous (lung) (solitary) J43.9
endophthalmitis H59.43
filtering (vitreous), after glaucoma surgery Z98.83
inflammed (infected), postprocedural H59.40
stage 1 H59.41
stage 2 H59.42
stage 3 H59.43
lung (ruptured) J43.9
congenital —*see* Atelectasis
newborn P25.8
subpleural (emphysematous) J43.9
Blebitis, postprocedural H59.40
stage 1 H59.41
stage 2 H59.42
stage 3 H59.43
Bleeder (familial) (hereditary) —*see* Hemophilia
Bleeding —*see also* Hemorrhage
anal K62.5
anovulatory N97.0
atonic, following delivery O72.1
capillary I78.8
puerperal O72.2
contact (postcoital) N93.0
due to uterine subinvolution N85.3
ear —*see* Otorrhagia
excessive, associated with menopausal onset N92.4
familial —*see* Defect, coagulation
following intercourse N93.0
gastrointestinal K92.2
hemorrhoids —*see* Hemorrhoids
intermenstrual (regular) N92.3
irregular N92.1
intraoperative —*see* Complication, intraoperative, hemorrhage
irregular N92.6
menopausal N92.4
newborn, intraventricular —*see* Newborn, affected by, hemorrhage, intraventricular
nipple N64.59
nose R04.0
ovulation N92.3
postclimacteric N95.0
postcoital N93.0
postmenopausal N95.0
postoperative —*see* Complication, postprocedural, hemorrhage
preclimacteric N92.4
pre-pubertal vaginal N93.1 ◀
puberty (excessive, with onset of menstrual periods) N92.2

B

Bleeding *(Continued)*
  rectum, rectal K62.5
    newborn P54.2
  tendencies *—see* Defect, coagulation
  throat R04.1
  tooth socket (post-extraction) K91.840
  umbilical stump P51.9
  uterus, uterine NEC N93.9
    climacteric N92.4
    dysfunctional of functional N93.8
    menopausal N92.4
    preclimacteric or premenopausal N92.4
    unrelated to menstrual cycle N93.9
  vagina, vaginal (abnormal) N93.9
    dysfunctional or functional N93.8
    newborn P54.6
    pre-pubertal N93.1 ◀
  vicarious N94.89
Blennorrhagia, blennorrhagic *—see* Gonorrhea
Blennorrhea (acute) (chronic) *—see also* Gonorrhea
  inclusion (neonatal) (newborn) P39.1
  lower genitourinary tract (gonococcal) A54.00
  neonatorum (gonococcal ophthalmia) A54.31
Blepharelosis *—see* Entropion
Blepharitis (angularis) (ciliaris) (eyelid) (marginal) (nonulcerative) H01.009
  herpes zoster B02.39
  left H01.006
    lower H01.005
    upper H01.004
  right H01.003
    lower H01.002
    upper H01.001
  squamous H01.029
    left H01.026
      lower H01.025
      upper H01.024
    right H01.023
      lower H01.022
      upper H01.021
  ulcerative H01.019
    left H01.016
      lower H01.015
      upper H01.014
    right H01.013
      lower H01.012
      upper H01.011
Blepharochalasis H02.30
  congenital Q10.0
  left H02.36
    lower H02.35
    upper H02.34
  right H02.33
    lower H02.32
    upper H02.31
Blepharoclonus H02.59
Blepharoconjunctivitis H10.50-
  angular H10.52-
  contact H10.53-
  ligneous H10.51-
Blepharophimosis (eyelid) H02.529
  congenital Q10.3
  left H02.526
    lower H02.525
    upper H02.524
  right H02.523
    lower H02.522
    upper H02.521
Blepharoptosis H02.40-
  congenital Q10.0
  mechanical H02.41-
  myogenic H02.42-
  neurogenic H02.43-
  paralytic H02.43-
Blepharopyorrhea, gonococcal A54.39
Blepharospasm G24.5
  drug induced G24.01
Blighted ovum O02.0

Blind *—see also* Blindness
  bronchus (congenital) Q32.4
  loop syndrome K90.2
    congenital Q43.8
  sac, fallopian tube (congenital) Q50.6
  spot, enlarged *—see* Defect, visual field, localized, scotoma, blind spot area
  tract or tube, congenital NEC *—see* Atresia, by site
Blindness (acquired) (congenital) (both eyes) H54.0
  blast S05.8X-
  color *—see* Deficiency, color vision
  concussion S05.8X-
  cortical H47.619
    left brain H47.612
    right brain H47.611
  day H53.11
  due to injury (current episode) S05.9-
    sequelae — code to injury with seventh character S
  eclipse (total) *—see* Retinopathy, solar
  emotional (hysterical) F44.6
  face H53.16
  hysterical F44.6
  legal (both eyes) (USA definition) H54.8
  mind R48.8
  night H53.60
    abnormal dark adaptation curve H53.61
    acquired H53.62
    congenital H53.63
    specified type NEC H53.69
    vitamin A deficiency E50.5
  one eye (other eye normal) H54.40
    left (normal vision on right) H54.42
      low vision on right H54.12
    low vision, other eye H54.10
    right (normal vision on left) H54.41
      low vision on left H54.11
  psychic R48.8
  river B73.01
  snow *—see* Photokeratitis
  sun, solar *—see* Retinopathy, solar
  transient *—see* Disturbance, vision, subjective, loss, transient
  traumatic (current episode) S05.9-
  word (developmental) F81.0
    acquired R48.0
    secondary to organic lesion R48.0
Blister (nonthermal)
  abdominal wall S30.821
  alveolar process S00.522
  ankle S90.52-
  antecubital space *—see* Blister, elbow
  anus S30.827
  arm (upper) S40.82-
  auditory canal *—see* Blister, ear
  auricle *—see* Blister, ear
  axilla *—see* Blister, arm
  back, lower S30.820
  beetle dermatitis L24.89
  breast S20.12-
  brow S00.82
  calf *—see* Blister, leg
  canthus *—see* Blister, eyelid
  cheek S00.82
    internal S00.522
  chest wall *—see* Blister, thorax
  chin S00.82
  costal region *—see* Blister, thorax
  digit (s)
    foot *—see* Blister, toe
    hand *—see* Blister, finger
  due to burn *—see* Burn, by site, second degree
  ear S00.42-
  elbow S50.32-
  epiglottis S10.12
  esophagus, cervical S10.12
  eyebrow *—see* Blister, eyelid
  eyelid S00.22-
  face S00.82

Blister *(Continued)*
  fever B00.1
  finger (s) S60.429
    index S60.42-
    little S60.42-
    middle S60.42-
    ring S60.42-
  foot (except toe (s) alone) S90.82-
    toe *—see* Blister, toe
  forearm S50.82-
    elbow only *—see* Blister, elbow
  forehead S00.82
  fracture - omit code
  genital organ
    female S30.826
    male S30.825
  gum S00.522
  hand S60.52-
  head S00.92
    ear *—see* Blister, ear
    eyelid *—see* Blister, eyelid
    lip S00.521
    nose S00.32
    oral cavity S00.522
    scalp S00.02
    specified site NEC S00.82
  heel *—see* Blister, foot
  hip S70.22-
  interscapular region S20.429
  jaw S00.82
  knee S80.22-
  larynx S10.12
  leg (lower) S80.82-
    knee *—see* Blister, knee
    upper *—see* Blister, thigh
  lip S00.521
  malar region S00.82
  mammary *—see* Blister, breast
  mastoid region S00.82
  mouth S00.522
  multiple, skin, nontraumatic R23.8
  nail
    finger *—see* Blister, finger
    toe *—see* Blister, toe
  nasal S00.32
  neck S10.92
    specified site NEC S10.82
    throat S10.12
  nose S00.32
  occipital region S00.02
  oral cavity S00.522
  orbital region *—see* Blister, eyelid
  palate S00.522
  palm *—see* Blister, hand
  parietal region S00.02
  pelvis S30.820
  penis S30.822
  periocular area *—see* Blister, eyelid
  phalanges
    finger *—see* Blister, finger
    toe *—see* Blister, toe
  pharynx S10.12
  pinna *—see* Blister, ear
  popliteal space *—see* Blister, knee
  scalp S00.02
  scapular region *—see* Blister, shoulder
  scrotum S30.823
  shin *—see* Blister, leg
  shoulder S40.22-
  sternal region S20.329
  submaxillary region S00.82
  submental region S00.82
  subungual
    finger (s) *—see* Blister, finger
    toe (s) *—see* Blister, toe
  supraclavicular fossa S10.82
  supraorbital S00.82
  temple S00.82
  temporal region S00.82
  testis S30.823
  thermal *—see* Burn, second degree, by site

◀ New ⟸ Revised ~~deleted~~ Deleted

Blister *(Continued)*
  thigh S70.32-
  thorax, thoracic (wall) S20.92
    back S20.42-
    front S20.32-
  throat S10.12
  thumb S60.32-
  toe (s) S90.42-
    great S90.42-
  tongue S00.522
  trachea S10.12
  tympanum, tympanic membrane —*see* Blister, ear
  upper arm —*see* Blister, arm (upper)
  uvula S00.522
  vagina S30.824
  vocal cords S10.12
  vulva S30.824
  wrist S60.82-
Bloating R14.0
Bloch-Sulzberger disease or syndrome Q82.3
Block, blocked
  alveolocapillary J84.10
  arborization (heart) I45.5
  arrhythmic I45.9
  atrioventricular (incomplete) (partial) I44.30
    with atrioventricular dissociation I44.2
    complete I44.2
      congenital Q24.6
    congenital Q24.6
    first degree I44.0
    second degree (types I and II) I44.1
    specified NEC I44.39
    third degree I44.2
    types I and II I44.1
  auriculoventricular —*see* Block, atrioventricular
  bifascicular (cardiac) I45.2
  bundle-branch (complete) (false) (incomplete) I45.4
    bilateral I45.2
    left I44.7
      with right bundle branch block I45.2
      hemiblock I44.60
        anterior I44.4
        posterior I44.5
      incomplete I44.7
        with right bundle branch block I45.2
    right I45.10
      with
        left bundle branch block I45.2
        left fascicular block I45.2
      specified NEC I45.19
    Wilson's type I45.19
  cardiac I45.9
  conduction I45.9
    complete I44.2
  fascicular (left) I44.60
    anterior I44.4
    posterior I44.5
    right I45.0
    specified NEC I44.69
  foramen Magendie (acquired) G91.1
    congenital Q03.1
      with spina bifida —*see* Spina bifida, by site, with hydrocephalus
  heart I45.9
    bundle branch I45.4
      bilateral I45.2
    complete (atrioventricular) I44.2
    congenital Q24.6
    first degree (atrioventricular) I44.0
    second degree (atrioventricular) I44.1
    specified type NEC I45.5
    third degree (atrioventricular) I44.2
  hepatic vein I82.0
  intraventricular (nonspecific) I45.4
    bundle branch
      bilateral I45.2
  kidney N28.9
    postcystoscopic or postprocedural N99.0

Block, blocked *(Continued)*
  Mobitz (types I and II) I44.1
  myocardial —*see* Block, heart
  nodal I45.5
  organ or site, congenital NEC —*see* Atresia, by site
  portal (vein) I81
  second degree (types I and II) I44.1
  sinoatrial I45.5
  sinoauricular I45.5
  third degree I44.2
  trifascicular I45.3
  tubal N97.1
  vein NOS I82.90
  Wenckebach (types I and II) I44.1
Blockage —*see* Obstruction
Blocq's disease F44.4
Blood
  constituents, abnormal R78.9
  disease D75.9
  donor —*see* Donor, blood
  dyscrasia D75.9
    with
      abortion —*see* Abortion, by type, complicated by, hemorrhage
      ectopic pregnancy O08.1
      molar pregnancy O08.1
    following ectopic or molar pregnancy O08.1
    newborn P61.9
    puerperal, postpartum O72.3
  flukes NEC —*see* Schistosomiasis
  in
    feces K92.1
      occult R19.5
    urine —*see* Hematuria
  mole O02.0
  occult in feces R19.5
  pressure
    decreased, due to shock following injury T79.4
    examination only Z01.30
    fluctuating I99.8
    high —*see* Hypertension
      borderline R03.0
      incidental reading, without diagnosis of hypertension R03.0
    low —*see also* Hypotension
      incidental reading, without diagnosis of hypotension R03.1
  spitting —*see* Hemoptysis
  staining cornea —*see* Pigmentation, cornea, stromal
  transfusion
    reaction or complication —*see* Complications, transfusion
  type
    A (Rh positive) Z67.10
      Rh negative Z67.11
    AB (Rh positive) Z67.30
      Rh negative Z67.31
    B (Rh positive) Z67.20
      Rh negative Z67.21
    O (Rh positive) Z67.40
      Rh negative Z67.41
    Rh (positive) Z67.90
      negative Z67.91
  vessel rupture —*see* Hemorrhage
  vomiting —*see* Hematemesis
Blood-forming organs, disease D75.9
Bloodgood's disease —*see* Mastopathy, cystic
Bloom (-Machacek)(-Torre) **syndrome** Q82.8
Blount's disease or osteochondrosis —*see* Osteochondrosis, juvenile, tibia
Blue
  baby Q24.9
  diaper syndrome E72.09
  dome cyst (breast) —*see* Cyst, breast
  dot cataract Q12.0

Blue *(Continued)*
  nevus D22.9
  sclera Q13.5
    with fragility of bone and deafness Q78.0
  toe syndrome I75.02-
Blueness —*see* Cyanosis
Blues, postpartal O90.6
  baby O90.6
Blurring, visual H53.8
Blushing (abnormal) (excessive) R23.2
BMI —*see* Body, mass index
Boarder, hospital NEC Z76.4
  accompanying sick person Z76.3
  healthy infant or child Z76.2
    foundling Z76.1
Bockhart's impetigo L01.02
Bodechtel-Guttman disease (subacute sclerosing panencephalitis) A81.1
Boder-Sedgwick syndrome (ataxia-telangiectasia) G11.3
Body, bodies
  Aschoff's —*see* Myocarditis, rheumatic
  asteroid, vitreous —*see* Deposit, crystalline
  cytoid (retina) —*see* Occlusion, artery, retina
  drusen (degenerative) (macula) (retinal) —*see also* Degeneration, macula, drusen
    optic disc —*see* Drusen, optic disc
  foreign —*see* Foreign body
  loose
    joint, except knee —*see* Loose, body, joint
      knee M23.4-
    sheath, tendon —*see* Disorder, tendon, specified type NEC
  mass index (BMI)
    adult
      19 or less Z68.1
      20.0-20.9 Z68.20
      21.0-21.9 Z68.21
      22.0-22.9 Z68.22
      23.0-23.9 Z68.23
      24.0-24.9 Z68.24
      25.0-25.9 Z68.25
      26.0-26.9 Z68.26
      27.0-27.9 Z68.27
      28.0-28.9 Z68.28
      29.0-29.9 Z68.29
      30.0-30.9 Z68.30
      31.0-31.9 Z68.31
      32.0-32.9 Z68.32
      33.0-33.9 Z68.33
      34.0-34.9 Z68.34
      35.0-35.9 Z68.35
      36.0-36.9 Z68.36
      37.0-37.9 Z68.37
      38.0-38.9 Z68.38
      39.0-39.9 Z68.39
      40.0-44.9 Z68.41
      45.0-49.9 Z68.42
      50.0-59.9 Z68.43
      60.0-69.9 Z68.44
      70 and over Z68.45
    pediatric
      5th percentile to less than 85th percentile for age Z68.52
      85th percentile to less than 95th percentile for age Z68.53
      greater than or equal to ninety-fifth percentile for age Z68.54
      less than fifth percentile for age Z68.51
  Mooser's A75.2
  rice —*see also* Loose, body, joint
    knee M23.4-
  rocking F98.4
Boeck's
  disease or sarcoid —*see* Sarcoidosis
  lupoid (miliary) D86.3
Boerhaave's syndrome (spontaneous esophageal rupture) K22.3
Boggy
  cervix N88.8
  uterus N85.8

B

Boil —*see also* Furuncle, by site
- Aleppo B55.1
- Baghdad B55.1
- Delhi B55.1
- lacrimal
  - gland —*see* Dacryoadenitis
  - passages (duct) (sac) —*see* Inflammation, lacrimal, passages, acute
- Natal B55.1
- orbit, orbital —*see* Abscess, orbit
- tropical B55.1

Bold hives —*see* Urticaria

Bombé, iris —*see* Membrane, pupillary

Bone —*see* condition

Bonnevie-Ullrich syndrome —*see also* Turner's syndrome Q87.1 ⇐

Bonnier's syndrome —*see* subcategory H81.8

Bonvale dam fever T73.3

Bony block of joint —*see* Ankylosis

BOOP (bronchiolitis obliterans organized pneumonia) J84.89

Borderline
- diabetes mellitus R73.Ø3 ⇐
- hypertension RØ3.Ø
- osteopenia M85.8-
- pelvis, with obstruction during labor O65.1
- personality F6Ø.3

Borna disease A83.9

Bornholm disease B33.Ø

Boston exanthem A88.Ø

Botalli, ductus (patent) (persistent) Q25.Ø

Bothriocephalus latus infestation B7Ø.Ø

Botulism (foodborne intoxication) AØ5.1
- infant A48.51
- non-foodborne A48.52
- wound A48.52

Bouba —*see* Yaws

Bouchard's nodes (with arthropathy) M15.2

Bouffée délirante F23

Bouillaud's disease or syndrome (rheumatic heart disease) IØ1.9

Bourneville's disease Q85.1

Boutonniere deformity (finger) —*see* Deformity, finger, boutonniere

Bouveret (-Hoffmann) syndrome (paroxysmal tachycardia) I47.9

Bovine heart —*see* Hypertrophy, cardiac

Bowel —*see* condition

Bowen's
- dermatosis (precancerous) —*see* Neoplasm, skin, in situ
- disease —*see* Neoplasm, skin, in situ
- epithelioma —*see* Neoplasm, skin, in situ
- type
  - epidermoid carcinoma-in-situ —*see* Neoplasm, skin, in situ
  - intraepidermal squamous cell carcinoma —*see* Neoplasm, skin, in situ

Bowing
- femur —*see also* Deformity, limb, specified type NEC, thigh
  - congenital Q68.3
- fibula —*see also* Deformity, limb, specified type NEC, lower leg
  - congenital Q68.4
- forearm —*see* Deformity, limb, specified type NEC, forearm
- leg (s), long bones, congenital Q68.5
- radius —*see* Deformity, limb, specified type NEC, forearm
- tibia —*see also* Deformity, limb, specified type NEC, lower leg
  - congenital Q68.4

Bowleg (s) (acquired) M21.16-
- congenital Q68.5
- rachitic E64.3

Boyd's dysentery AØ3.2

Brachial —*see* condition

Brachycardia RØØ.1

Brachycephaly Q75.Ø

Bradley's disease AØ8.19

Bradyarrhythmia, cardiac I49.8

Bradycardia (sinoatrial) (sinus) (vagal) RØØ.1
- neonatal P29.12
- reflex G9Ø.Ø9
- tachycardia syndrome I49.5

Bradykinesia R25.8

Bradypnea RØ6.89

Bradytachycardia I49.5

Brailsford's disease or osteochondrosis —*see* Osteochondrosis, juvenile, radius

Brain —*see also* condition
- death G93.82
- syndrome —*see* Syndrome, brain

Branched-chain amino-acid disorder E71.2

Branchial —*see* condition
- cartilage, congenital Q18.2

Branchiogenic remnant (in neck) Q18.Ø

Brandt's syndrome (acrodermatitis enteropathica) E83.2

Brash (water) R12

Bravais-jacksonian epilepsy —*see* Epilepsy, localization-related, symptomatic, with simple partial seizures

Braxton Hicks contractions —*see* False, labor

Brazilian leishmaniasis B55.2

BRBPR K62.5

Break, retina (without detachment) H33.3Ø-
- with retinal detachment —*see* Detachment, retina
- horseshoe tear H33.31-
- multiple H33.33-
- round hole H33.32-

Breakdown
- device, graft or implant —*see also* Complications, by site and type, mechanical T85.618
  - arterial graft NEC —*see* Complication, cardiovascular device, mechanical, vascular
  - breast (implant) T85.41
  - catheter NEC T85.618
    - cystostomy T83.Ø1Ø
    - dialysis (renal) T82.41
      - intraperitoneal T85.611
    - Hopkins T83.Ø18 ◄
    - ileostomy T83.Ø18 ◄
    - infusion NEC T82.514
      - cranial T85.61Ø ◄
      - epidural T85.61Ø ◄
      - intrathecal T85.61Ø ◄
      - spinal T85.61Ø ⇐
      - subarachnoid T85.61Ø ◄
      - subdural T85.61Ø ◄
    - ~~urinary (indwelling) T83.Ø18~~
    - nephrostomy T83.Ø12 ◄
    - urethral indwelling T83.Ø11 ◄
    - urinary NEC T83.Ø18 ◄
    - urostomy T83.Ø18 ◄
  - electronic (electrode) (pulse generator) (stimulator)
    - bone T84.31Ø
    - cardiac T82.119
      - electrode T82.11Ø
      - pulse generator T82.111
      - specified type NEC T82.118
    - nervous system —*see* Complication, prosthetic device, mechanical, electronic nervous system stimulator
    - urinary —*see* Complication, genitourinary, device, urinary, mechanical
  - fixation, internal (orthopedic) NEC —*see* Complication, fixation device, mechanical
  - gastrointestinal —*see* Complications, prosthetic device, mechanical, gastrointestinal device
  - genital NEC T83.418
    - intrauterine contraceptive device T83.31
    - penile prosthesis (cylinder) (implanted) (pump) (resevoir) T83.41Ø ⇐
    - testicular prosthesis T83.411 ◄

Breakdown *(Continued)*
- device, graft or implant *(Continued)*
  - heart NEC —*see* Complication, cardiovascular device, mechanical
  - intrathecal infusion pump T85.615 ◄
  - joint prosthesis —*see* Complications..., joint prosthesis,internal, mechanical, by site
  - nervous system, specified device NEC T85.615 ◄
  - ocular NEC —*see* Complications, prosthetic device, mechanical, ocular device
  - orthopedic NEC —*see* Complication, orthopedic, device, mechanical
  - specified NEC T85.618
  - subcutaneous device pocket ◄
    - nervous system prosthetic device, implant, or graft T85.89Ø ◄
    - other internal prosthetic device, implant, or graft T85.898 ◄
  - sutures, permanent T85.612
    - used in bone repair —*see* Complications, fixation device, internal (orthopedic), mechanical
  - urinary NEC T83.118 ⇐
    - graft T83.21
    - sphincter, implanted T83.111 ◄
    - stent (ileal conduit) (nephroureteral) T83.113 ◄
    - ureteral indwelling T83.112 ◄
  - vascular NEC —*see* Complication, cardiovascular device, mechanical
  - ventricular intracranial shunt T85.Ø1
- nervous F48.8
- perineum O9Ø.1
- respirator J95.85Ø
  - specified NEC J95.859
- ventilator J95.85Ø
  - specified NEC J95.859

Breast —*see also* condition
- buds E3Ø.1
  - in newborn P96.89
- dense R92.2
- nodule N63

Breath
- foul R19.6
- holder, child RØ6.89
- holding spell RØ6.89
- shortness RØ6.Ø2

Breathing
- labored —*see* Hyperventilation
- mouth RØ6.5
  - causing malocclusion M26.5
- periodic RØ6.3
  - high altitude G47.32

Breathlessness RØ6.81

Breda's disease —*see* Yaws

Breech presentation (mother) O32.1
- causing obstructed labor O64.1
- footling O32.8
  - causing obstructed labor O64.8
- incomplete O32.8
  - causing obstructed labor O64.8

Breisky's disease N9Ø.4

Brennemann's syndrome I88.Ø

Brenner
- tumor (benign) D27.9
  - borderline malignancy D39.1-
  - malignant C56
  - proliferating D39.1

Bretonneau's disease or angina A36.Ø

Breus' mole OØ2.Ø

Brevicollis Q76.49

Brickmakers' anemia B76.9 *[D63.8]*

Bridge, myocardial Q24.5

Bright red blood per rectum (BRBPR) K62.5

Bright's disease —*see also* Nephritis
- arteriosclerotic —*see* Hypertension, kidney

Brill (-Zinsser) disease (recrudescent typhus) A75.1
- flea-borne A75.2
- louse-borne A75.1

B

◄ New ⇐ Revised ~~deleted~~ Deleted

Brill-Symmers' disease C82.90
Brion-Kayser disease —*see* Fever, parathyroid
Briquet's disorder or syndrome F45.0
Brissaud's
  infantilism or dwarfism E23.0
  motor-verbal tic F95.2
Brittle
  bones disease Q78.0
  nails L60.3
    congenital Q84.6
Broad —*see also* condition
  beta disease E78.2
  ligament laceration syndrome N83.8
Broad- or floating-betalipoproteinemia E78.2
Brock's syndrome (atelectasis due to enlarged lymph nodes) J98.19
Brocq-Duhring disease (dermatitis herpetiformis) L13.0
Brodie's abscess or disease M86.8X-
Broken
  arches —*see also* Deformity, limb, flat foot
  arm (meaning upper limb) —*see* Fracture, arm
  back —*see* Fracture, vertebra
  bone —*see* Fracture
  implant or internal device —*see* Complications, by site and type, mechanical
  leg (meaning lower limb) —*see* Fracture, leg
  nose S02.2
  tooth, teeth —*see* Fracture, tooth
Bromhidrosis, bromidrosis L75.0
Bromidism, bromism G92
  chronic (dependence) F13.20
  due to
    correct substance properly administered —*see* Table of Drugs and Chemicals, by drug, adverse effect
    overdose or wrong substance given or taken —*see* Table of Drugs and Chemicals, by drug, poisoning
Bromidrosiphobia F40.298
Bronchi, bronchial —*see* condition
Bronchiectasis (cylindrical) (diffuse) (fusiform) (localized) (saccular) J47.9
  with
    acute
      bronchitis J47.0
      lower respiratory infection J47.0
    exacerbation (acute) J47.1
  congenital Q33.4
  tuberculous NEC —*see* Tuberculosis, pulmonary
Bronchiolectasis —*see* Bronchiectasis
Bronchiolitis (acute) (infective) (subacute) J21.9
  with
    bronchospasm or obstruction J21.9
    influenza, flu or grippe —*see* Influenza, with, respiratory manifestations NEC
  chemical (chronic) J68.4
    acute J68.0
  chronic (fibrosing) (obliterative) J44.9
  due to
    external agent —*see* Bronchitis, acute, due to
    human metapneumovirus J21.1
    respiratory syncytial virus J21.0
    specified organism NEC J21.8
  fibrosa obliterans J44.9
  influenzal —*see* Influenza, with, respiratory manifestations NEC
  obliterans J42
    with organizing pneumonia (BOOP) J84.89
  obliterative (chronic) (subacute) J44.9
    due to chemicals, gases, fumes or vapors (inhalation) J68.4
    due to fumes or vapors J68.4
  respiratory, interstitial lung disease J84.115
Bronchitis (diffuse) (fibrinous) (hypostatic) (infective) (membranous) J40
  with
    influenza, flu or grippe —*see* Influenza, with, respiratory manifestations NEC
Bronchitis *(Continued)*
  with *(Continued)*
    obstruction (airway) (lung) J44.9
    tracheitis (15 years of age and above) J40
      acute or subacute J20.9
      chronic J42
      under 15 years of age J20.9
  acute or subacute (with bronchospasm or obstruction) J20.9
    with
      bronchiectasis J47.0
      chronic obstructive pulmonary disease J44.0
    chemical (due to gases, fumes or vapors) J68.0
    due to
      fumes or vapors J68.0
      Haemophilus influenzae J20.1
      Mycoplasma pneumoniae J20.0
      radiation J70.0
      specified organism NEC J20.8
      Streptococcus J20.2
      virus
        coxsackie J20.3
        echovirus J20.7
        parainfluenzae J20.4
        respiratory syncytial J20.5
        rhinovirus J20.6
    viral NEC J20.8
  allergic (acute) J45.909
    with
      exacerbation (acute) J45.901
      status asthmaticus J45.902
  arachidic T17.528
  aspiration (due to fumes or vapors) J68.0
  asthmatic J45.9
    chronic J44.9
      with
        acute lower respiratory infection J44.0
        exacerbation (acute) J44.1
  capillary —*see* Pneumonia, broncho
  caseous (tuberculous) A15.5
  Castellani's A69.8
  catarrhal (15 years of age and above) J40
    acute —*see* Bronchitis, acute
    chronic J41.0
    under 15 years of age J20.9
  chemical (acute) (subacute) J68.0
    chronic J68.4
    due to fumes or vapors J68.0
      chronic J68.4
  chronic J42
    with
      airways obstruction J44.9
      tracheitis (chronic) J42
    asthmatic (obstructive) J44.9
    catarrhal J41.0
    chemical (due to fumes or vapors) J68.4
    due to
      chemicals, gases, fumes or vapors (inhalation) J68.4
      radiation J70.1
      tobacco smoking J41.0
    emphysematous J44.9
    mucopurulent J41.1
    non-obstructive J41.0
    obliterans J44.9
    obstructive J44.9
    purulent J41.1
    simple J41.0
  croupous —*see* Bronchitis, acute
  due to gases, fumes or vapors (chemical) J68.0
  emphysematous (obstructive) J44.9
  exudative —*see* Bronchitis, acute
  fetid J41.1
  grippal —*see* Influenza, with, respiratory manifestations NEC
  in those under 15 years age —*see* Bronchitis, acute
    chronic —*see* Bronchitis, chronic
Bronchitis *(Continued)*
  influenzal —*see* Influenza, with, respiratory manifestations NEC
  mixed simple and mucopurulent J41.8
  moulder's J62.8
  mucopurulent (chronic) (recurrent) J41.1
    acute or subacute J20.9
    simple (mixed) J41.8
  obliterans (chronic) J44.9
  obstructive (chronic) (diffuse) J44.9
  pituitous J41.1
  pneumococcal, acute or subacute J20.2
  pseudomembranous, acute or subacute —*see* Bronchitis, acute
  purulent (chronic) (recurrent) J41.1
    acute or subacute —*see* Bronchitis, acute
  putrid J41.1
  senile (chronic) J42
  simple and mucopurulent (mixed) J41.8
  smokers' J41.0
  spirochetal NEC A69.8
  subacute —*see* Bronchitis, acute
  suppurative (chronic) J41.1
    acute or subacute —*see* Bronchitis, acute
  tuberculous A15.5
  under 15 years of age —*see* Bronchitis, acute
    chronic —*see* Bronchitis, chronic
  viral NEC, acute or subacute —*see also* Bronchitis, acute J20.8
Bronchoalveolitis J18.0
Bronchoaspergillosis B44.1
Bronchocele meaning goiter E04.0
Broncholithiasis J98.09
  tuberculous NEC A15.5
Bronchomalacia J98.09
  congenital Q32.2
Bronchomycosis NOS B49 *[J99]*
  candidal B37.1
Bronchopleuropneumonia —*see* Pneumonia, broncho
Bronchopneumonia —*see* Pneumonia, broncho
Bronchopneumonitis —*see* Pneumonia, broncho
Bronchopulmonary —*see* condition
Bronchopulmonitis —*see* Pneumonia, broncho
Bronchorrhagia (*see* Hemoptysis)
Bronchorrhea J98.09
  acute J20.9
  chronic (infective) (purulent) J42
Bronchospasm (acute) J98.01
  with
    bronchiolitis, acute J21.9
    bronchitis, acute (conditions in J20) —*see* Bronchitis, acute
  due to external agent —*see* condition, respiratory, acute, due to
  exercise induced J45.990
Bronchospirochetosis A69.8
  Castellani A69.8
Bronchostenosis J98.09
Bronchus —*see* condition
Brontophobia F40.220
Bronze baby syndrome P83.8
Brooke's tumor —*see* Neoplasm, skin, benign
Brown enamel of teeth (hereditary) K00.5
Brown's sheath syndrome H50.61-
Brown-Séquard disease, paralysis or syndrome G83.81
Bruce sepsis A23.0
Brucellosis (infection) A23.9
  abortus A23.1
  canis A23.3
  dermatitis A23.9
  melitensis A23.0
  mixed A23.8
  sepsis A23.9
    melitensis A23.0
    specified NEC A23.8
  suis A23.2
Bruck-de Lange disease Q87.1
Bruck's disease —*see* Deformity, limb

B

Brugsch's syndrome Q82.8
Bruise (skin surface intact) —*see also* Contusion
- with
  - open wound —*see* Wound, open
  - internal organ —*see* Injury, by site
- newborn P54.5
- scalp, due to birth injury, newborn P12.3
- umbilical cord O69.5

Bruit (arterial) R09.89
- cardiac R01.1

Brush burn —*see* Abrasion, by site
Bruton's X-linked agammaglobulinemia D80.0
Bruxism
- psychogenic F45.8
- sleep related G47.63

Bubbly lung syndrome P27.0
Bubo I88.8
- blennorrhagic (gonococcal) A54.89
- chancroidal A57
- climatic A55
- due to Haemophilus ducreyi A57
- gonococcal A54.89
- indolent (nonspecific) I88.8
- inguinal (nonspecific) I88.8
  - chancroidal A57
  - climatic A55
  - due to H. ducreyi A57
  - infective I88.8
- scrofulous (tuberculous) A18.2
- soft chancre A57
- suppurating —*see* Lymphadenitis, acute
- syphilitic (primary) A51.0
  - congenital A50.07
- tropical A55
- virulent (chancroidal) A57

Bubonic plague A20.0
Bubonocele —*see* Hernia, inguinal
Buccal —*see* condition
Buchanan's disease or osteochondrosis M91.0
Buchem's syndrome (hyperostosis corticalis) M85.2
Bucket-handle fracture or tear (semilunar cartilage) —*see* Tear, meniscus
Budd-Chiari syndrome (hepatic vein thrombosis) I82.0
Budgerigar fancier's disease or lung J67.2
Buds
- breast E30.1
  - in newborn P96.89

Buerger's disease (thromboangiitis obliterans) I73.1
Bulbar —*see* condition
Bulbus cordis (left ventricle) (persistent) Q21.8
Bulimia (nervosa) F50.2
- atypical F50.9
- normal weight F50.9

Bulky
- stools R19.5
- uterus N85.2

Bulla (e) R23.8
- lung (emphysematous) (solitary) J43.9
  - newborn P25.8

Bullet wound —*see also* Wound, open
- fracture - code as Fracture, by site
- internal organ —*see* Injury, by site

Bundle
- branch block (complete) (false) (incomplete) —*see* Block, bundle-branch
- of His —*see* condition

Bunion M21.61- ⬅
- tailor's M21.62- ◀

Bunionette M21.62- ◀
Buphthalmia, buphthalmos (congenital) Q15.0
Burdwan fever B55.0
Bürger-Grütz disease or syndrome E78.3
Buried
- penis (congenital) Q55.64
  - acquired N48.83
- roots K08.3

Burke's syndrome K86.89 ⬅
Burkitt
- cell leukemia C91.0-
- lymphoma (malignant) C83.7-
  - small noncleaved, diffuse C83.7-
  - spleen C83.77
  - undifferentiated C83.7-
- tumor C83.7-
- type
  - acute lymphoblastic leukemia C91.0-
  - undifferentiated C83.7-

Burn (electricity) (flame) (hot gas, liquid or hot object) (radiation) (steam) (thermal) T30.0
- abdomen, abdominal (muscle) (wall) T21.02
  - first degree T21.12
  - second degree T21.22
  - third degree T21.32
- above elbow T22.039
  - first degree T22.139
  - left T22.032
    - first degree T22.132
    - second degree T22.232
    - third degree T22.332
  - right T22.031
    - first degree T22.131
    - second degree T22.231
    - third degree T22.331
  - second degree T22.239
  - third degree T22.339
- acid (caustic) (external) (internal) —*see* Corrosion, by site
- alimentary tract NEC T28.2
  - esophagus T28.1
  - mouth T28.0
  - pharynx T28.0
- alkaline (caustic) (external) (internal) —*see* Corrosion, by site
- ankle T25.019
  - first degree T25.119
  - left T25.012
    - first degree T25.112
    - second degree T25.212
    - third degree T25.312
  - multiple with foot —*see* Burn, lower, limb, multiple, ankle and foot
  - right T25.011
    - first degree T25.111
    - second degree T25.211
    - third degree T25.311
  - second degree T25.219
  - third degree T25.319
- anus —*see* Burn, buttock
- arm (lower) (upper) —*see* Burn, upper, limb
- axilla T22.049
  - first degree T22.149
  - left T22.042
    - first degree T22.142
    - second degree T22.242
    - third degree T22.342
  - right T22.041
    - first degree T22.141
    - second degree T22.241
    - third degree T22.341
  - second degree T22.249
  - third degree T22.349
- back (lower) T21.04
  - first degree T21.14
  - second degree T21.24
  - third degree T21.34
  - upper T21.03
    - first degree T21.13
    - second degree T21.23
    - third degree T21.33
- blisters - code as Burn, second degree, by site
- breast (s) —*see* Burn, chest wall
- buttock (s) T21.05
  - first degree T21.15
  - second degree T21.25
  - third degree T21.35

Burn *(Continued)*
- calf T24.039
  - first degree T24.139
  - left T24.032
    - first degree T24.132
    - second degree T24.232
    - third degree T24.332
  - right T24.031
    - first degree T24.131
    - second degree T24.231
    - third degree T24.331
  - second degree T24.239
  - third degree T24.339
- canthus (eye) —*see* Burn, eyelid
- caustic acid or alkaline —*see* Corrosion, by site
- cervix T28.3
- cheek T20.06
  - first degree T20.16
  - second degree T20.26
  - third degree T20.36
- chemical (acids) (alkalines) (caustics) (external) (internal) —*see* Corrosion, by site
- chest wall T21.01
  - first degree T21.11
  - second degree T21.21
  - third degree T21.31
- chin T20.03
  - first degree T20.13
  - second degree T20.23
  - third degree T20.33
- colon T28.2
- conjunctiva (and cornea) —*see* Burn, cornea
- cornea (and conjunctiva) T26.1-
  - chemical —*see* Corrosion, cornea
- corrosion (external) (internal) —*see* Corrosion, by site
- deep necrosis of underlying tissue - code as Burn, third degree, by site
- dorsum of hand T23.069
  - first degree T23.169
  - left T23.062
    - first degree T23.162
    - second degree T23.262
    - third degree T23.362
  - right T23.061
    - first degree T23.161
    - second degree T23.261
    - third degree T23.361
  - second degree T23.269
  - third degree T23.369
- due to ingested chemical agent —*see* Corrosion, by site
- ear (auricle) (external) (canal) T20.01
  - first degree T20.11
  - second degree T20.21
  - third degree T20.31
- elbow T22.029
  - first degree T22.129
  - left T22.022
    - first degree T22.122
    - second degree T22.222
    - third degree T22.322
  - right T22.021
    - first degree T22.121
    - second degree T22.221
    - third degree T22.321
  - second degree T22.229
  - third degree T22.329
- epidermal loss - code as Burn, second degree, by site
- erythema, erythematous - code as Burn, first degree, by site
- esophagus T28.1
- extent (percentage of body surface)
  - less than 10 percent T31.0
  - 10-19 percent T31.10
    - with 0-9 percent third degree burns T31.10
    - with 10-19 percent third degree burns T31.11

- **Burn** *(Continued)*
  - hand *(Continued)*
    - second degree T23.209
    - third degree T23.309
    - thumb —*see* Burn, thumb
  - head (and face) (and neck) T20.00
    - cheek —*see* Burn, cheek
    - chin —*see* Burn, chin
    - ear —*see* Burn, ear
    - eye (s) only —*see* Burn, eye
    - first degree T20.10
    - forehead —*see* Burn, forehead
    - lip —*see* Burn, lip
    - multiple sites T20.09
      - first degree T20.19
      - second degree T20.29
      - third degree T20.39
    - neck —*see* Burn, neck
    - nose —*see* Burn, nose
    - scalp —*see* Burn, scalp
    - second degree T20.20
    - third degree T20.30
  - hip (s) —*see* Burn, thigh ⟸
  - inhalation —*see* Burn, respiratory tract
    - caustic or corrosive substance (fumes) —*see* Corrosion, respiratory tract
  - internal organ (s) T28.40
    - alimentary tract T28.2
      - esophagus T28.1
    - eardrum T28.41
    - esophagus T28.1
    - from caustic or corrosive substance (swallowing) NEC —*see* Corrosion, by site
    - genitourinary T28.3
    - mouth T28.0
    - pharynx T28.0
    - respiratory tract —*see* Burn, respiratory tract
    - specified organ NEC T28.49
  - interscapular region —*see* Burn, back, upper
  - intestine (large) (small) T28.2
  - knee T24.029
    - first degree T24.129
    - left T24.022
      - first degree T24.122
      - second degree T24.222
      - third degree T24.322
    - right T24.021
      - first degree T24.121
      - second degree T24.221
      - third degree T24.321
    - second degree T24.229
    - third degree T24.329
  - labium (majus) (minus) —*see* Burn, genital organs, external, female
  - lacrimal apparatus, duct, gland or sac —*see* Burn, eye, specified site NEC
  - larynx T27.0
    - with lung T27.1
  - leg (s) (lower) (upper) —*see* Burn, lower, limb
  - lightning —*see* Burn, by site
  - limb (s)
    - lower (except ankle or foot alone) —*see* Burn, lower, limb
    - upper —*see* Burn, upper limb
  - lip (s) T20.02
    - first degree T20.12
    - second degree T20.22
    - third degree T20.32
  - lower
    - back —*see* Burn, back
    - limb T24.009
      - ankle —*see* Burn, ankle
      - calf —*see* Burn, calf
      - first degree T24.109
      - foot —*see* Burn, foot
      - hip —*see* Burn, thigh
      - knee —*see* Burn, knee

- **Burn** *(Continued)*
  - lower *(Continued)*
    - limb *(Continued)*
      - left T24.002
        - first degree T24.102
        - second degree T24.202
        - third degree T24.302
      - multiple sites, except ankle and foot T24.099
        - ankle and foot T25.099
          - first degree T25.199
          - left T25.092
            - first degree T25.192
            - second degree T25.292
            - third degree T25.392
          - right T25.091
            - first degree T25.191
            - second degree T25.291
            - third degree T25.391
          - second degree T25.299
          - third degree T25.399
        - first degree T24.199
        - left T24.092
          - first degree T24.192
          - second degree T24.292
          - third degree T24.392
        - right T24.091
          - first degree T24.191
          - second degree T24.291
          - third degree T24.391
        - second degree T24.299
        - third degree T24.399
      - right T24.001
        - first degree T24.101
        - second degree T24.201
        - third degree T24.301
      - second degree T24.209
      - thigh —*see* Burn, thigh
      - third degree T24.309
      - toe —*see* Burn, toe
  - lung (with larynx and trachea) T27.1
  - mouth T28.0
  - neck T20.07
    - first degree T20.17
    - second degree T20.27
    - third degree T20.37
  - nose (septum) T20.04
    - first degree T20.14
    - second degree T20.24
    - third degree T20.34
  - ocular adnexa —*see* Burn, eye
  - orbit region —*see* Burn, eyelid
  - palm T23.059
    - first degree T23.159
    - left T23.052
      - first degree T23.152
      - second degree T23.252
      - third degree T23.352
    - right T23.051
      - first degree T23.151
      - second degree T23.251
      - third degree T23.351
    - second degree T23.259
    - third degree T23.359
  - partial thickness - code as Burn, unspecified degree, by site
  - pelvis —*see* Burn, trunk
  - penis —*see* Burn, genital organs, external, male
  - perineum
    - female —*see* Burn, genital organs, external, female
    - male —*see* Burn, genital organs, external, male
  - periocular area —*see* Burn, eyelid
  - pharynx T28.0
  - rectum T28.2
  - respiratory tract T27.3
    - larynx —*see* Burn, larynx
    - specified part NEC T27.2
    - trachea —*see* Burn, trachea

- **Burn** *(Continued)*
  - sac, lacrimal —*see* Burn, eye, specified site NEC
  - scalp T20.05
    - first degree T20.15
    - second degree T20.25
    - third degree T20.35
  - scapular region T22.069
    - first degree T22.169
    - left T22.062
      - first degree T22.162
      - second degree T22.262
      - third degree T22.362
    - right T22.061
      - first degree T22.161
      - second degree T22.261
      - third degree T22.361
    - second degree T22.269
    - third degree T22.369
  - sclera —*see* Burn, eye, specified site NEC
  - scrotum —*see* Burn, genital organs, external, male
  - shoulder T22.059
    - first degree T22.159
    - left T22.052
      - first degree T22.152
      - second degree T22.252
      - third degree T22.352
    - right T22.051
      - first degree T22.151
      - second degree T22.251
      - third degree T22.351
    - second degree T22.259
    - third degree T22.359
  - stomach T28.2
  - temple —*see* Burn, head
  - testis —*see* Burn, genital organs, external, male
  - thigh T24.019
    - first degree T24.119
    - left T24.012
      - first degree T24.112
      - second degree T24.212
      - third degree T24.312
    - right T24.011
      - first degree T24.111
      - second degree T24.211
      - third degree T24.311
    - second degree T24.219
    - third degree T24.319
  - thorax (external) —*see* Burn, trunk
  - throat (meaning pharynx) T28.0
  - thumb (s) T23.019
    - first degree T23.119
    - left T23.012
      - first degree T23.112
      - second degree T23.212
      - third degree T23.312
    - multiple sites with fingers T23.049
      - first degree T23.149
      - left T23.042
        - first degree T23.142
        - second degree T23.242
        - third degree T23.342
      - right T23.041
        - first degree T23.141
        - second degree T23.241
        - third degree T23.341
      - second degree T23.249
      - third degree T23.349
    - right T23.011
      - first degree T23.111
      - second degree T23.211
      - third degree T23.311
    - second degree T23.219
    - third degree T23.319
  - toe T25.039
    - first degree T25.139
    - left T25.032
      - first degree T25.132
      - second degree T25.232
      - third degree T25.332

B

Burn *(Continued)*
toe *(Continued)*
right T25.Ø31
first degree T25.131
second degree T25.231
third degree T25.331
second degree T25.239
third degree T25.339
tongue T28.Ø
tonsil (s) T28.Ø
trachea T27.Ø
with lung T27.1
trunk T21.ØØ
abdominal wall —*see* Burn, abdominal wall
anus —*see* Burn, buttock
axilla —*see* Burn, upper limb
back —*see* Burn, back
breast —*see* Burn, chest wall
buttock —*see* Burn, buttock
chest wall —*see* Burn, chest wall
first degree T21.1Ø
flank —*see* Burn, abdominal wall
genital
female —*see* Burn, genital organs, external, female
male —*see* Burn, genital organs, external, male
groin —*see* Burn, abdominal wall
interscapular region —*see* Burn, back, upper
labia —*see* Burn, genital organs, external, female
lower back —*see* Burn, back
penis —*see* Burn, genital organs, external, male
perineum
female —*see* Burn, genital organs, external, female
male —*see* Burn, genital organs, external, male
scapula region —*see* Burn, scapular region
scrotum —*see* Burn, genital organs, external, male
second degree T21.2Ø
specified site NEC T21.Ø9
first degree T21.19
second degree T21.29
third degree T21.39
testes —*see* Burn, genital organs, external, male
third degree T21.3Ø
upper back —*see* Burn, back, upper
vulva —*see* Burn, genital organs, external, female
unspecified site with extent of body surface involved specified
less than 1Ø percent T31.Ø
1Ø-19 percent (Ø-9 percent third degree) T31.1Ø
with 1Ø-19 percent third degree T31.11
2Ø-29 percent (Ø-9 percent third degree) T31.2Ø
with
1Ø-19 percent third degree T31.21
2Ø-29 percent third degree T31.22
3Ø-39 percent (Ø-9 percent third degree) T31.3Ø
with
1Ø-19 percent third degree T31.31
2Ø-29 percent third degree T31.32
3Ø-39 percent third degree T31.33
4Ø-49 percent (Ø-9 percent third degree) T31.4Ø
with
1Ø-19 percent third degree T31.41
2Ø-29 percent third degree T31.42
3Ø-39 percent third degree T31.43
4Ø-49 percent third degree T31.44

Burn *(Continued)*
unspecified site with extent of body surface involved specified *(Continued)*
5Ø-59 percent (Ø-9 percent third degree) T31.5Ø
with
1Ø-19 percent third degree T31.51
2Ø-29 percent third degree T31.52
3Ø-39 percent third degree T31.53
4Ø-49 percent third degree T31.54
5Ø-59 percent third degree T31.55
6Ø-69 percent (Ø-9 percent third degree) T31.6Ø
with
1Ø-19 percent third degree T31.61
2Ø-29 percent third degree T31.62
3Ø-39 percent third degree T31.63
4Ø-49 percent third degree T31.64
5Ø-59 percent third degree T31.65
6Ø-69 percent third degree T31.66
7Ø-79 percent (Ø-9 percent third degree) T31.7Ø
with
1Ø-19 percent third degree T31.71
2Ø-29 percent third degree T31.72
3Ø-39 percent third degree T31.73
4Ø-49 percent third degree T31.74
5Ø-59 percent third degree T31.75
6Ø-69 percent third degree T31.76
7Ø-79 percent third degree T31.77
8Ø-89 percent (Ø-9 percent third degree) T31.8Ø
with
1Ø-19 percent third degree T31.81
2Ø-29 percent third degree T31.82
3Ø-39 percent third degree T31.83
4Ø-49 percent third degree T31.84
5Ø-59 percent third degree T31.85
6Ø-69 percent third degree T31.86
7Ø-79 percent third degree T31.87
8Ø-89 percent third degree T31.88
9Ø percent or more (Ø-9 percent third degree) T31.9Ø
with
1Ø-19 percent third degree T31.91
2Ø-29 percent third degree T31.92
3Ø-39 percent third degree T31.93
4Ø-49 percent third degree T31.94
5Ø-59 percent third degree T31.95
6Ø-69 percent third degree T31.96
7Ø-79 percent third degree T31.97
8Ø-89 percent third degree T31.98
9Ø-99 percent third degree T31.99
upper limb T22.ØØ
above elbow —*see* Burn, above elbow
axilla —*see* Burn, axilla
elbow —*see* Burn, elbow
first degree T22.1Ø
forearm —*see* Burn, forearm
hand —*see* Burn, hand
interscapular region —*see* Burn, back, upper
multiple sites T22.Ø99
first degree T22.199
left T22.Ø92
first degree T22.192
second degree T22.292
third degree T22.392
right T22.Ø91
first degree T22.191
second degree T22.291
third degree T22.391
second degree T22.299
third degree T22.399
scapular region —*see* Burn, scapular region
second degree T22.2Ø
shoulder —*see* Burn, shoulder
third degree T22.3Ø
wrist —*see* Burn, wrist
uterus T28.3
vagina T28.3

Burn *(Continued)*
vulva —*see* Burn, genital organs, external, female
wrist T23.Ø79
first degree T23.179
left T23.Ø72
first degree T23.172
second degree T23.272
third degree T23.372
multiple sites with hand T23.Ø99
first degree T23.199
left T23.Ø92
first degree T23.192
second degree T23.292
third degree T23.392
right T23.Ø91
first degree T23.191
second degree T23.291
third degree T23.391
second degree T23.299
third degree T23.399
right T23.Ø71
first degree T23.171
second degree T23.271
third degree T23.371
second degree T23.279
third degree T23.379
Burnett's syndrome E83.52
Burning
feet syndrome E53.9
sensation R2Ø.8
tongue K14.6
Burn-out (state) Z73.Ø
Burns' disease or osteochondrosis —*see* Osteochondrosis, juvenile, ulna
Bursa —*see* condition
Bursitis M71.9
Achilles —*see* Tendinitis, Achilles
adhesive —*see* Bursitis, specified NEC
ankle —*see* Enthesopathy, lower limb, ankle, specified type NEC
calcaneal —*see* Enthesopathy, foot, specified type NEC
collateral ligament, tibial —*see* Bursitis, tibial collateral
due to use, overuse, pressure —*see also* Disorder, soft tissue, due to use, specified type NEC
specified NEC —*see* Disorder, soft tissue, due to use, specified NEC
Duplay's M75.Ø
elbow NEC M7Ø.3-
olecranon M7Ø.2-
finger —*see* Disorder, soft tissue, due to use, specified type NEC, hand
foot —*see* Enthesopathy, foot, specified type NEC
gonococcal A54.49
gouty —*see* Gout ⬅
hand M7Ø.1-
hip NEC M7Ø.7-
trochanteric M7Ø.6-
infective NEC M71.1Ø
abscess —*see* Abscess, bursa
ankle M71.17-
elbow M71.12-
foot M71.17-
hand M71.14-
hip M71.15-
knee M71.16-
multiple sites M71.19
shoulder M71.11-
specified site NEC M71.18
wrist M71.13-
ischial —*see* Bursitis, hip
knee NEC M7Ø.5-
prepatellar M7Ø.4-
occupational NEC —*see also* Disorder, soft tissue, due to, use
olecranon —*see* Bursitis, elbow, olecranon
pharyngeal J39.1

B

Bursitis *(Continued)*
popliteal —*see* Bursitis, knee
prepatellar M70.4-
radiohumeral M77.8
rheumatoid M06.20
ankle M06.27-
elbow M06.22-
foot joint M06.27-
hand joint M06.24-
hip M06.25-
knee M06.26-
multiple site M06.29
shoulder M06.21-
vertebra M06.28
wrist M06.23-
scapulohumeral —*see* Bursitis, shoulder
semimembranous muscle (knee) —*see* Bursitis, knee
shoulder M75.5-
adhesive —*see* Capsulitis, adhesive
specified NEC M71.50
ankle M71.57-
due to use, overuse or pressure —*see* Disorder, soft tissue, due to, use
elbow M71.52-
foot M71.57-
hand M71.54-

Bursitis *(Continued)*
specified NEC *(Continued)*
hip M71.55-
knee M71.56-
shoulder —*see* Bursitis, shoulder
specified site NEC M71.58
tibial collateral M76.4-
wrist M71.53-
subacromial —*see* Bursitis, shoulder
subcoracoid —*see* Bursitis, shoulder
subdeltoid —*see* Bursitis, shoulder
syphilitic A52.78
Thornwaldt, Tornwaldt J39.2
tibial collateral M76.4- (Revised)
toe —*see* Enthesopathy, foot, specified type NEC
trochanteric (area) —*see* Bursitis, hip, trochanteric
wrist —*see* Bursitis, hand
Bursopathy M71.9
specified type NEC M71.80
ankle M71.87-
elbow M71.82-
foot M71.87-
hand M71.84-
hip M71.85-
knee M71.86-

Bursopathy *(Continued)*
specified type NEC *(Continued)*
multiple sites M71.89
shoulder M71.81-
specified site NEC M71.88
wrist M71.83-
Burst stitches or sutures (complication of surgery) T81.31
external operation wound T81.31
internal operation wound T81.32
Buruli ulcer A31.1
Bury's disease L95.1
Buschke's
disease B45.3
scleredema —*see* Sclerosis, systemic
Busse-Buschke disease B45.3
Buttock —*see* condition
Button
Biskra B55.1
Delhi B55.1
oriental B55.1
Buttonhole deformity (finger) —*see* Deformity, finger, boutonniere
Bwamba fever A92.8
Byssinosis J66.0
Bywaters' syndrome T79.5

B

◄ New   ◄■■ Revised   ~~deleted~~ Deleted

C

- **Cachexia** R64
  - cancerous R64
  - cardiac —*see* Disease, heart
  - dehydration E86.Ø
    - ~~with~~
      - ~~hypernatremia E87.Ø~~
      - ~~hyponatremia E87.1~~
  - due to malnutrition R64
  - exophthalmic —*see* Hyperthyroidism
  - heart —*see* Disease, heart
  - hypophyseal E23.Ø
  - hypopituitary E23.Ø
  - lead —*see* Poisoning, lead
  - malignant R64
  - marsh —*see* Malaria
  - nervous F48.8
  - old age R54
  - paludal —*see* Malaria
  - pituitary E23.Ø
  - renal N28.9
  - saturnine —*see* Poisoning, lead
  - senile R54
  - Simmonds' E23.Ø
  - splenica D73.Ø
  - strumipriva EØ3.4
  - tuberculous NEC —*see* Tuberculosis
- **Café au lait spots** L81.3
- **Caffeine-induced** ◀
  - anxiety disorder F15.980 ◀
  - sleep disorder F15.982 ◀
- **Caffey's syndrome** Q78.8
- **Caisson disease** T70.3
- **Cake kidney** Q63.1
- **Caked breast** (puerperal, postpartum) O92.79
- **Calabar swelling** B74.3
- **Calcaneal spur** —*see* Spur, bone, calcaneal
- **Calcaneo-apophysitis** M92.8
- **Calcareous** —*see* condition
- **Calcicosis** J62.8
- **Calciferol** (vitamin D) deficiency E55.9
  - with rickets E55.Ø
- **Calcification**
  - adrenal (capsule) (gland) E27.49
    - tuberculous E35 *[B9Ø.8]*
  - aorta I7Ø.Ø
  - artery (annular) —*see* Arteriosclerosis
  - auricle (ear) —*see* Disorder, pinna, specified type NEC
  - basal ganglia G23.8
  - bladder N32.89
    - due to Schistosoma hematobium B65.Ø
  - brain (cortex) —*see* Calcification, cerebral
  - bronchus J98.Ø9
  - bursa M71.4Ø
    - ankle M71.47-
    - elbow M71.42-
    - foot M71.47-
    - hand M71.44-
    - hip M71.45-
    - knee M71.46-
    - multiple sites M71.49
    - shoulder M75.3-
    - specified site NEC M71.48
    - wrist M71.43-
  - cardiac —*see* Degeneration, myocardial
  - cerebral (cortex) G93.89
    - artery I67.2
  - cervix (uteri) N88.8
  - choroid plexus G93.89
  - conjunctiva —*see* Concretion, conjunctiva
  - corpora cavernosa (penis) N48.89
  - cortex (brain) —*see* Calcification, cerebral
  - dental pulp (nodular) KØ4.2
  - dentinal papilla KØØ.4
  - fallopian tube N83.8
  - falx cerebri G96.19
  - gallbladder K82.8
  - general E83.59
- **Calcification** *(Continued)*
  - heart —*see also* Degeneration, myocardial
    - valve —*see* Endocarditis
  - idiopathic infantile arterial (IIAC) Q28.8
  - intervertebral cartilage or disc (postinfective) —*see* Disorder, disc, specified NEC
  - intracranial —*see* Calcification, cerebral
  - joint —*see* Disorder, joint, specified type NEC
  - kidney N28.89
    - tuberculous N29 *[B9Ø.1]*
  - larynx (senile) J38.7
  - lens —*see* Cataract, specified NEC
  - lung (active) (postinfectional) J98.4
    - tuberculous B9Ø.9
  - lymph gland or node (postinfectional) I89.8
    - tuberculous —*see also* Tuberculosis, lymph gland B9Ø.8
  - mammographic R92.1
  - massive (paraplegic) —*see* Myositis, ossificans, in, quadriplegia
  - medial —*see* Arteriosclerosis, extremities
  - meninges (cerebral) (spinal) G96.19
  - metastatic E83.59
  - Mönckeberg's —*see* Arteriosclerosis, extremities
  - muscle M61.9
    - due to burns —*see* Myositis, ossificans, in, burns
    - paralytic —*see* Myositis, ossificans, in, quadriplegia
    - specified type NEC M61.4Ø
      - ankle M61.47-
      - foot M61.47-
      - forearm M61.43-
      - hand M61.44-
      - lower leg M61.46-
      - multiple sites M61.49
      - pelvic region M61.45-
      - shoulder region M61.41-
      - specified site NEC M61.48
      - thigh M61.45-
      - upper arm M61.42-
  - myocardium, myocardial —*see* Degeneration, myocardial
  - ovary N83.8
  - pancreas K86.89 ⬅
  - penis N48.89
  - periarticular —*see* Disorder, joint, specified type NEC
  - pericardium —*see also* Pericarditis I31.1
  - pineal gland E34.8
  - pleura J94.8
    - postinfectional J94.8
    - tuberculous NEC B9Ø.9
  - pulpal (dental) (nodular) KØ4.2
  - sclera H15.89
  - spleen D73.89
  - subcutaneous L94.2
  - suprarenal (capsule) (gland) E27.49
  - tendon (sheath) —*see also* Tenosynovitis, specified type NEC
    - with bursitis, synovitis or tenosynovitis —*see* Tendinitis, calcific
  - trachea J39.8
  - ureter N28.89
  - vitreous —*see* Deposit, crystalline
- **Calcified** —*see* Calcification
- **Calcinosis** (interstitial) (tumoral) (universalis) E83.59
  - with Raynaud's phenomenon, esophageal dysfunction, sclerodactyly, telangiectasia (CREST syndrome) M34.1
  - circumscripta (skin) L94.2
  - cutis L94.2
- **Calciphylaxis** —*see also* Calcification, by site E83.59
- **Calcium**
  - deposits —*see* Calcification, by site
  - metabolism disorder E83.5Ø
  - salts or soaps in vitreous —*see* Deposit, crystalline
- **Calciuria** R82.99
- **Calculi** —*see* Calculus
- **Calculosis, intrahepatic** —*see* Calculus, bile duct
- **Calculus, calculi, calculous**
  - ampulla of Vater —*see* Calculus, bile duct
  - anuria (impacted) (recurrent) —*see also* Calculus, urinary N2Ø.9
  - appendix K38.1
  - bile duct (common) (hepatic) K8Ø.5Ø
    - with
      - calculus of gallbladder —*see* Calculus, gallbladder and bile duct
      - cholangitis K8Ø.3Ø
        - with
          - cholecystitis —*see* Calculus, bile duct, with cholecystitis
          - obstruction K8Ø.31
        - acute K8Ø.32
          - with
            - chronic cholangitis K8Ø.36
              - with obstruction K8Ø.37
            - obstruction K8Ø.33
        - chronic K8Ø.34
          - with
            - acute cholangitis K8Ø.36
              - with obstruction K8Ø.37
            - obstruction K8Ø.35
      - cholecystitis (with cholangitis) K8Ø.4Ø
        - with obstruction K8Ø.41
        - acute K8Ø.42
          - with
            - chronic cholecystitis K8Ø.46
              - with obstruction K8Ø.47
            - obstruction K8Ø.43
        - chronic K8Ø.44
          - with
            - acute cholecystitis K8Ø.46
              - with obstruction K8Ø.47
            - obstruction K8Ø.45
      - obstruction K8Ø.51
  - biliary —*see also* Calculus, gallbladder
    - specified NEC K8Ø.8Ø
      - with obstruction K8Ø.81
  - bilirubin, multiple —*see* Calculus, gallbladder
  - bladder (encysted) (impacted) (urinary) (diverticulum) N21.Ø
  - bronchus J98.Ø9
  - calyx (kidney) (renal) —*see* Calculus, kidney
  - cholesterol (pure) (solitary) —*see* Calculus, gallbladder
  - common duct (bile) —*see* Calculus, bile duct
  - conjunctiva —*see* Concretion, conjunctiva
  - cystic N21.Ø
    - duct —*see* Calculus, gallbladder
  - dental (subgingival) (supragingival) KØ3.6
  - diverticulum
    - bladder N21.Ø
    - kidney N2Ø.Ø
  - epididymis N5Ø.89 ⬅
  - gallbladder K8Ø.2Ø
    - with
      - bile duct calculus —*see* Calculus, gallbladder and bile duct
      - cholecystitis K8Ø.1Ø
        - with obstruction K8Ø.11
        - acute K8Ø.ØØ
          - with
            - chronic cholecystitis K8Ø.12
              - with obstruction K8Ø.13
            - obstruction K8Ø.Ø1
        - chronic K8Ø.1Ø
          - with
            - acute cholecystitis K8Ø.12
              - with obstruction K8Ø.13
            - obstruction K8Ø.11
        - specified NEC K8Ø.18
          - with obstruction K8Ø.19
      - obstruction K8Ø.21

C

Calculus, calculi, calculous *(Continued)*
- gallbladder and bile duct K80.70
  - with
    - cholecystitis K80.60
      - with obstruction K80.61
      - acute K80.62
        - with
          - chronic cholecystitis K80.66
            - with obstruction K80.67
          - obstruction K80.63
      - chronic K80.64
        - with
          - acute cholecystitis K80.66
            - with obstruction K80.67
          - obstruction K80.65
    - obstruction K80.71
- hepatic (duct) —*see* Calculus, bile duct
- hepatobiliary K80.80
  - with obstruction K80.81
- ileal conduit N21.8
- intestinal (impaction) (obstruction) K56.49
- kidney (impacted) (multiple) (pelvis) (recurrent) (staghorn) N20.0
  - with calculus, ureter N20.2
  - congenital Q63.8
- lacrimal passages —*see* Dacryolith
- liver (impacted) —*see* Calculus, bile duct
- lung J98.4
- mammographic R92.1
- nephritic (impacted) (recurrent) —*see* Calculus, kidney
- nose J34.89
- pancreas (duct) K86.89 ⬅
- parotid duct or gland K11.5
- pelvis, encysted —*see* Calculus, kidney
- prostate N42.0
- pulmonary J98.4
- pyelitis (impacted) (recurrent) N20.0
  - with hydronephrosis N13.2
- pyelonephritis (impacted) (recurrent) —*see* category N20
  - with hydronephrosis N13.2
- renal (impacted) (recurrent) —*see* Calculus, kidney
- salivary (duct) (gland) K11.5
- seminal vesicle N50.89 ⬅
- staghorn —*see* Calculus, kidney
- Stensen's duct K11.5
- stomach K31.89
- sublingual duct or gland K11.5
  - congenital Q38.4
- submandibular duct, gland or region K11.5
- submaxillary duct, gland or region K11.5
- suburethral N21.8
- tonsil J35.8
- tooth, teeth (subgingival) (supragingival) K03.6
- tunica vaginalis N50.89 ⬅
- ureter (impacted) (recurrent) N20.1
  - with calculus, kidney N20.2
    - with hydronephrosis N13.2
      - with infection N13.6
- urethra (impacted) N21.1
- urinary (duct) (impacted) (passage) (tract) N20.9
  - with hydronephrosis N13.2
    - with infection N13.6
  - in (due to)
  - lower N21.9
    - specified NEC N21.8
- vagina N89.8
- vesical (impacted) N21.0
- Wharton's duct K11.5
- xanthine E79.8 *[N22]*

Calicectasis N28.89

Caliectasis N28.89

California
- disease B38.9
- encephalitis A83.5

Caligo cornea —*see* Opacity, cornea, central

Callositas, callosity (infected) L84

Callus (infected) L84
- bone —*see* Osteophyte
  - excessive, following fracture - code as Sequelae of fracture

CALME (childhood asymmetric labium majus enlargement) N90.61 ◀

Calorie deficiency or malnutrition —*see also* Malnutrition E46

Calvé-Perthes disease —*see* Legg-Calve-Perthes disease

Calvé's disease —*see* Osteochondrosis, juvenile, spine

Calvities —*see* Alopecia, androgenic

Cameroon fever —*see* Malaria

Camptocormia (hysterical) F44.4

Camurati-Engelmann syndrome Q78.3

Canal —*see also* condition
- atrioventricular common Q21.2

Canaliculitis (lacrimal) (acute) (subacute) H04.33-
- Actinomyces A42.89
- chronic H04.42-

Canavan's disease E75.29

Canceled procedure (surgical) Z53.9
- because of
  - contraindication Z53.09
    - smoking Z53.01
  - left against medical advice (AMA) Z53.21
  - patient's decision Z53.20
    - for reasons of belief or group pressure Z53.1
    - specified reason NEC Z53.29
  - specified reason NEC Z53.8

Cancer —*see also* Neoplasm, by site, malignant
- bile duct type, liver C22.1
- blood —*see* Leukemia
- breast —*see also* Neoplasm, breast, malignant C50.91-
- hepatocellular C22.0
- lung —*see also* Neoplasm, lung, malignant C34.90-
- ovarian —*see also* Neoplasm, ovary, malignant C56.9-
- unspecified site (primary) C80.1

Cancer (o)**phobia** F45.29

Cancerous —*see* Neoplasm, malignant, by site

Cancrum oris A69.0

Candidiasis, candidal B37.9
- balanitis B37.42
- bronchitis B37.1
- cheilitis B37.83
- congenital P37.5
- cystitis B37.41
- disseminated B37.7
- endocarditis B37.6
- enteritis B37.82
- esophagitis B37.81
- intertrigo B37.2
- lung B37.1
- meningitis B37.5
- mouth B37.0
- nails B37.2
- neonatal P37.5
- onychia B37.2
- oral B37.0
- osteomyelitis B37.89
- otitis externa B37.84
- paronychia B37.2
- perionyxis B37.2
- pneumonia B37.1
- proctitis B37.82
- pulmonary B37.1
- pyelonephritis B37.49
- sepsis B37.7
- skin B37.2
- specified site NEC B37.89
- stomatitis B37.0
- systemic B37.7
- urethritis B37.41
- urogenital site NEC B37.49
- vagina B37.3
- vulva B37.3
- vulvovaginitis B37.3

Candidid L30.2

Candidosis —*see* Candidiasis

Candiru infection or infestation B88.8

Canities (premature) L67.1
- congenital Q84.2

Canker (mouth) (sore) K12.0
- rash A38.9

Cannabinosis J66.2

Cannabis induced ◀
- anxiety disorder F12.980 ◀
- psychotic disorder F12.959 ◀
- sleep disorder F12.988 ◀

Canton fever A75.9

Cantrell's syndrome Q87.89

Capillariasis (intestinal) B81.1
- hepatic B83.8

Capillary —*see* condition

Caplan's syndrome —*see* Rheumatoid, lung

Capsule —*see* condition

Capsulitis (joint) —*see also* Enthesopathy
- adhesive (shoulder) M75.0-
- hepatic K65.8
- labyrinthine —*see* Otosclerosis, specified NEC
- thyroid E06.9

Caput
- crepitus Q75.8
- medusae I86.8
- succedaneum P12.81

Car sickness T75.3

Carapata (disease) A68.0

Carate —*see* Pinta

Carbon lung J60

Carbuncle L02.93
- abdominal wall L02.231
- anus K61.0
- auditory canal, external —*see* Abscess, ear, external
- auricle ear —*see* Abscess, ear, external
- axilla L02.43-
- back (any part) L02.232
- breast N61.1 ⬅
- buttock L02.33
- cheek (external) L02.03
- chest wall L02.233
- chin L02.03
- corpus cavernosum N48.21
- ear (any part) (external) (middle) —*see* Abscess, ear, external
- external auditory canal —*see* Abscess, ear, external
- eyelid —*see* Abscess, eyelid
- face NEC L02.03
- femoral (region) —*see* Carbuncle, lower limb
- finger —*see* Carbuncle, hand
- flank L02.231
- foot L02.63-
- forehead L02.03
- genital —*see* Abscess, genital
- gluteal (region) L02.33
- groin L02.234
- hand L02.53-
- head NEC L02.831
- heel —*see* Carbuncle, foot
- hip —*see* Carbuncle, lower limb
- kidney —*see* Abscess, kidney
- knee —*see* Carbuncle, lower limb
- labium (majus) (minus) N76.4
- lacrimal
  - gland —*see* Dacryoadenitis
  - passages (duct) (sac) —*see* Inflammation, lacrimal, passages, acute
- leg —*see* Carbuncle, lower limb
- lower limb L02.43-
- malignant A22.0
- navel L02.236
- neck L02.13
- nose (external) (septum) J34.0
- orbit, orbital —*see* Abscess, orbit
- palmar (space) —*see* Carbuncle, hand
- partes posteriores L02.33
- pectoral region L02.233
- penis N48.21

Carbuncle *(Continued)*
perineum L02.235
pinna —*see* Abscess, ear, external
popliteal —*see* Carbuncle, lower limb
scalp L02.831
seminal vesicle N49.0
shoulder —*see* Carbuncle, upper limb
specified site NEC L02.838
temple (region) L02.03
thumb —*see* Carbuncle, hand
toe —*see* Carbuncle, foot
trunk L02.239
abdominal wall L02.231
back L02.232
chest wall L02.233
groin L02.234
perineum L02.235
umbilicus L02.236
umbilicus L02.236
upper limb L02.43-
urethra N34.0
vulva N76.4
Carbunculus —*see* Carbuncle
Carcinoid (tumor) —*see* Tumor, carcinoid
Carcinoidosis E34.0
Carcinoma (malignant) —*see also* Neoplasm, by site, malignant
acidophil
specified site —*see* Neoplasm, malignant, by site
unspecified site C75.1
acidophil-basophil, mixed
specified site —*see* Neoplasm, malignant, by site
unspecified site C75.1
adnexal (skin) —*see* Neoplasm, skin, malignant
adrenal cortical C74.0-
alveolar —*see* Neoplasm, lung, malignant
cell —*see* Neoplasm, lung, malignant
ameloblastic C41.1
upper jaw (bone) C41.0
apocrine
breast —*see* Neoplasm, breast, malignant
specified site NEC —*see* Neoplasm, skin, malignant
unspecified site C44.99
basal cell (pigmented) (*see also* Neoplasm, skin, malignant) C44.91
fibro-epithelial —*see* Neoplasm, skin, malignant
morphea —*see* Neoplasm, skin, malignant
multicentric —*see* Neoplasm, skin, malignant
basaloid
basal-squamous cell, mixed —*see* Neoplasm, skin, malignant
basophil
specified site —*see* Neoplasm, malignant, by site
unspecified site C75.1
basophil-acidophil, mixed
specified site —*see* Neoplasm, malignant, by site
unspecified site C75.1
basosquamous —*see* Neoplasm, skin, malignant
bile duct
with hepatocellular, mixed C22.0
liver C22.1
specified site NEC —*see* Neoplasm, malignant, by site
unspecified site C22.1
branchial or branchiogenic C10.4
bronchial or bronchogenic —*see* Neoplasm, lung, malignant
bronchiolar —*see* Neoplasm, lung, malignant
bronchioloalveolar —*see* Neoplasm, lung, malignant
C cell
specified site —*see* Neoplasm, malignant, by site
unspecified site C73
ceruminous C44.29-

Carcinoma *(Continued)*
cervix uteri
in situ D06.9
endocervix D06.0
exocervix D06.1
specified site NEC D06.7
chorionic
specified site —*see* Neoplasm, malignant, by site
unspecified site
female C58
male C62.90
chromophobe
specified site —*see* Neoplasm, malignant, by site
unspecified site C75.1
cloacogenic
specified site —*see* Neoplasm, malignant, by site
unspecified site C21.2
diffuse type
specified site —*see* Neoplasm, malignant, by site
unspecified site C16.9
duct (cell)
with Paget's disease —*see* Neoplasm, breast, malignant
infiltrating
with lobular carcinoma (in situ)
specified site —*see* Neoplasm, malignant, by site
unspecified site (female) C50.91-
male C50.92-
specified site —*see* Neoplasm, malignant, by site
unspecified site (female) C50.91-
male C50.92-
ductal
with lobular
specified site —*see* Neoplasm, malignant, by site
unspecified site (female) C50.91-
male C50.92-
ductular, infiltrating
specified site —*see* Neoplasm, malignant, by site
unspecified site (female) C50.91-
male C50.92-
embryonal
liver C22.7
endometrioid
specified site —*see* Neoplasm, malignant, by site
unspecified site
female C56.9
male C61
eosinophil
specified site —*see* Neoplasm, malignant, by site
unspecified site C75.1
epidermoid —*see also* Neoplasm, skin malignant
in situ, Bowen's type —*see* Neoplasm, skin, in situ
fibroepithelial, basal cell —*see* Neoplasm, skin, malignant
follicular
with papillary (mixed) C73
moderately differentiated C73
pure follicle C73
specified site —*see* Neoplasm, malignant, by site
trabecular C73
unspecified site C73
well differentiated C73
generalized, with unspecified primary site C80.0
glycogen-rich —*see* Neoplasm, breast, malignant
granulosa cell C56-
hepatic cell C22.0

Carcinoma *(Continued)*
hepatocellular C22.0
with bile duct, mixed C22.0
fibrolamellar C22.0
hepatocholangiolitic C22.0
Hurthle cell C73
in
adenomatous
polyposis coli C18.9
pleomorphic adenoma —*see* Neoplasm, salivary glands, malignant
situ —*see* Carcinoma-in-situ
infiltrating
duct
with lobular
specified site —*see* Neoplasm, malignant, by site
unspecified site (female) C50.91-
male C50.92-
with Paget's disease —*see* Neoplasm, breast, malignant
specified site —*see* Neoplasm, malignant
unspecified site (female) C50.91-
male C50.92-
ductular
specified site —*see* Neoplasm, malignant
unspecified site (female) C50.91-
male C50.92-
lobular
specified site —*see* Neoplasm, malignant
unspecified site (female) C50.91-
male C50.92-
inflammatory
specified site —*see* Neoplasm, malignant
unspecified site (female) C50.91-
male C50.92-
intestinal type
specified site —*see* Neoplasm, malignant, by site
unspecified site C16.9
intracystic
noninfiltrating —*see* Neoplasm, in situ, by site
intraductal (noninfiltrating)
with Paget's disease —*see* Neoplasm, breast, malignant
breast D05.1-
papillary
with invasion
specified site —*see* Neoplasm, malignant, by site
unspecified site (female) C50.91-
male C50.92-
breast D05.1-
specified site NEC —*see* Neoplasm, in situ, by site
unspecified site (female) D05.1-
specified site NEC —*see* Neoplasm, in situ, by site
unspecified site (female) D05.1-
intraepidermal —*see* Neoplasm, in situ
squamous cell, Bowen's type —*see* Neoplasm, skin, in situ
intraepithelial —*see* Neoplasm, in situ, by site
squamous cell —*see* Neoplasm, in situ, by site
intraosseous C41.1
upper jaw (bone) C41.0
islet cell
with exocrine, mixed
specified site —*see* Neoplasm, malignant, by site
unspecified site C25.9
pancreas C25.4
specified site NEC —*see* Neoplasm, malignant, by site
unspecified site C25.4

◀ New ⟸ Revised ~~deleted~~ Deleted

Carcinoma *(Continued)*
juvenile, breast —*see* Neoplasm, breast, malignant
large cell
small cell
specified site —*see* Neoplasm, malignant, by site
unspecified site C34.9Ø
Leydig cell (testis)
specified site —*see* Neoplasm, malignant, by site
unspecified site
female C56.9
male C62.9Ø
lipid-rich (female) C5Ø.91-
male C5Ø.92-
liver cell C22.Ø
liver NEC C22.7
lobular (infiltrating)
with intraductal
specified site —*see* Neoplasm, malignant, by site
unspecified site (female) C5Ø.91-
male C5Ø.92-
noninfiltrating
breast DØ5.Ø-
specified site NEC —*see* Neoplasm, in situ, by site
unspecified site DØ5.Ø-
specified site —*see* Neoplasm, malignant, by site
unspecified site (female) C5Ø.91-
male C5Ø.92-
medullary
with
amyloid stroma
specified site —*see* Neoplasm, malignant, by site
unspecified site C73
lymphoid stroma
specified site —*see* Neoplasm, malignant, by site
unspecified site (female) C5Ø.91-
male C5Ø.92-
Merkel cell C4A.9
anal margin C4A.51
anal skin C4A.51
canthus C4A.1-
ear and external auricular canal C4A.2-
external auricular canal C4A.2-
eyelid, including canthus C4A.1-
face C4A.3Ø
specified NEC C4A.39
hip C4A.7-
lip C4A.Ø
lower limb, including hip C4A.7-
neck C4A.4
nodal presentation C7B.1
nose C4A.31
overlapping sites C4A.8
perianal skin C4A.51
scalp C4A.4
secondary C7B.1
shoulder C4A.6-
skin of breast C4A.52
trunk NEC C4A.59
upper limb, including shoulder C4A.6-
visceral metastatic C7B.1
metastatic —*see* Neoplasm, secondary
metatypical —*see* Neoplasm, skin, malignant
morphea, basal cell —*see* Neoplasm, skin, malignant
mucoid
cell
specified site —*see* Neoplasm, malignant, by site
unspecified site C75.1
neuroendocrine —*see also* Tumor, neuroendocrine
high grade, any site C7A.1
poorly differentiated, any site C7A.1

Carcinoma *(Continued)*
nonencapsulated sclerosing C73
noninfiltrating
intracystic —*see* Neoplasm, in situ, by site
intraductal
breast DØ5.1-
papillary
breast DØ5.1-
specified site NEC —*see* Neoplasm, in situ, by site
unspecified site DØ5.1-
specified site —*see* Neoplasm, in situ, by site
unspecified site DØ5.1-
lobular
breast DØ5.Ø-
specified site NEC —*see* Neoplasm, in situ, by site
unspecified site (female) DØ5.Ø-
oat cell
specified site —*see* Neoplasm, malignant, by site
unspecified site C34.9Ø
odontogenic C41.1
upper jaw (bone) C41.Ø
papillary
with follicular (mixed) C73
follicular variant C73
intraductal (noninfiltrating)
with invasion
specified site —*see* Neoplasm, malignant, by site
unspecified site (female) C5Ø.91-
male C5Ø.92-
breast DØ5.1-
specified site NEC —*see* Neoplasm, in situ, by site
unspecified site DØ5.1-
serous
specified site —*see* Neoplasm, malignant, by site
surface
specified site —*see* Neoplasm, malignant, by site
unspecified site C56.9
unspecified site C56.9
papillocystic
specified site —*see* Neoplasm, malignant, by site
unspecified site C56.9
parafollicular cell
specified site —*see* Neoplasm, malignant, by site
unspecified site C73
pilomatrix —*see* Neoplasm, skin, malignant
pseudomucinous
specified site —*see* Neoplasm, malignant, by site
unspecified site C56.9
renal cell C64-
Schmincke —*see* Neoplasm, nasopharynx, malignant
Schneiderian
specified site —*see* Neoplasm, malignant, by site
unspecified site C3Ø.Ø
sebaceous —*see* Neoplasm, skin, malignant
secondary —*see also* Neoplasm, secondary, by site
Merkel cell C7B.1
secretory, breast —*see* Neoplasm, breast, malignant
serous
papillary
specified site —*see* Neoplasm, malignant, by site
unspecified site C56.9
surface, papillary
specified site —*see* Neoplasm, malignant, by site
unspecified site C56.9

Carcinoma *(Continued)*
Sertoli cell
specified site —*see* Neoplasm, malignant, by site
unspecified site C62.9Ø
female C56.9
male C62.9Ø
skin appendage —*see* Neoplasm, skin, malignant
small cell
fusiform cell
specified site —*see* Neoplasm, malignant, by site
unspecified site C34.9Ø
intermediate cell
specified site —*see* Neoplasm, malignant, by site
unspecified site C34.9Ø
large cell
specified site —*see* Neoplasm, malignant, by site
unspecified site C34.9Ø
solid
with amyloid stroma
specified site —*see* Neoplasm, malignant, by site
unspecified site C73
microinvasive
specified site —*see* Neoplasm, malignant, by site
unspecified site C53.9
sweat gland —*see* Neoplasm, skin, malignant
theca cell C56.-
thymic C37
unspecified site (primary) C8Ø.1
water-clear cell C75.Ø
Carcinoma-in-situ —*see also* Neoplasm, in situ, by site
breast NOS DØ5.9-
specified type NEC DØ5.8-
epidermoid —*see also* Neoplasm, in situ, by site
with questionable stromal invasion
cervix DØ6.9
specified site NEC —*see* Neoplasm, in situ, by site
unspecified site DØ6.9
Bowen's type —*see* Neoplasm, skin, in situ
intraductal
breast DØ5.1-
specified site NEC —*see* Neoplasm, in situ, by site
unspecified site DØ5.1-
lobular
with
infiltrating duct
breast (female) C5Ø.91-
male C5Ø.92-
specified site NEC —*see* Neoplasm, malignant
unspecified site (female) C5Ø.91-
male C5Ø.92-
intraductal
breast DØ5.8-
specified site NEC —*see* Neoplasm, in situ, by site
unspecified site (female) DØ5.8-
breast DØ5.Ø-
specified site NEC —*see* Neoplasm, in situ, by site
unspecified site DØ5.Ø-
squamous cell —*see also* Neoplasm, in situ, by site
with questionable stromal invasion
cervix DØ6.9
specified site NEC —*see* Neoplasm, in situ, by site
unspecified site DØ6.9
Carcinomaphobia F45.29

C

Carcinomatosis C80.0
peritonei C78.6
unspecified site (primary) (secondary) C80.0
Carcinosarcoma —*see* Neoplasm, malignant, by site
embryonal —*see* Neoplasm, malignant, by site
Cardia, cardial —*see* condition
Cardiac —*see also* condition
death, sudden —*see* Arrest, cardiac
pacemaker
in situ Z95.0
management or adjustment Z45.018
tamponade I31.4
Cardialgia —*see* Pain, precordial
Cardiectasis —*see* Hypertrophy, cardiac
Cardiochalasia K21.9
Cardiomalacia I51.5
Cardiomegalia glycogenica diffusa E74.02 *[I43]*
Cardiomegaly —*see also* Hypertrophy, cardiac
congenital Q24.8
glycogen E74.02 *[I43]*
idiopathic I51.7
Cardiomyoliposis I51.5
Cardiomyopathy (familial) (idiopathic) I42.9
alcoholic I42.6
amyloid E85.4 *[I43]*
arteriosclerotic —*see* Disease, heart, ischemic, atherosclerotic
beriberi E51.12
cobalt-beer I42.6
congenital I42.4
congestive I42.0
constrictive NOS I42.5
dilated I42.0
due to
alcohol I42.6
beriberi E51.12
cardiac glycogenosis E74.02 *[I43]*
drugs I42.7
external agents NEC I42.7
Friedreich's ataxia G11.1
myotonia atrophica G71.11 *[I43]*
progressive muscular dystrophy G71.0
glycogen storage E74.02 *[I43]*
hypertensive —*see* Hypertension, heart
hypertrophic (nonobstructive) I42.2
obstructive I42.1
congenital Q24.8
in
Chagas' disease (chronic) B57.2
acute B57.0
sarcoidosis D86.85
ischemic I25.5
metabolic E88.9 *[I43]*
thyrotoxic E05.90 *[I43]*
with thyroid storm E05.91 *[I43]*
newborn I42.8
congenital I42.4
nutritional E63.9 *[I43]*
beriberi E51.12
obscure of Africa I42.8
peripartum O90.3
postpartum O90.3
restrictive NEC I42.5
rheumatic I09.0
secondary I42.9
stress induced I51.81
takotsubo I51.81
thyrotoxic E05.90 *[I43]*
with thyroid storm E05.91 *[I43]*
toxic NEC I42.7
tuberculous A18.84
viral B33.24
Cardionephritis —*see* Hypertension, cardiorenal
Cardionephropathy —*see* Hypertension, cardiorenal
Cardionephrosis —*see* Hypertension, cardiorenal
Cardiopathia nigra I27.0
Cardiopathy —*see also* Disease, heart I51.9
idiopathic I42.9
mucopolysaccharidosis E76.3 *[I52]*
Cardiopericarditis —*see* Pericarditis
Cardiophobia F45.29
Cardiorenal —*see* condition
Cardiorrhexis —*see* Infarct, myocardium
Cardiosclerosis —*see* Disease, heart, ischemic, atherosclerotic
Cardiosis —*see* Disease, heart
Cardiospasm (esophagus) (reflex) (stomach) K22.0
congenital Q39.5
with megaesophagus Q39.5
Cardiostenosis —*see* Disease, heart
Cardiosymphysis I31.0
Cardiovascular —*see* condition
Carditis (acute) (bacterial) (chronic) (subacute) I51.89
meningococcal A39.50
rheumatic —*see* Disease, heart, rheumatic
rheumatoid —*see* Rheumatoid, carditis
viral B33.20
Care (of) (for) (following)
child (routine) Z76.2
family member (handicapped) (sick)
creating problem for family Z63.6
provided away from home for holiday relief Z75.5
unavailable, due to
absence (person rendering care) (sufferer) Z74.2
inability (any reason) of person rendering care Z74.2
foundling Z76.1
holiday relief Z75.5
improper —*see* Maltreatment
lack of (at or after birth) (infant) —*see* Maltreatment, child, neglect
lactating mother Z39.1
palliative Z51.5
postpartum
immediately after delivery Z39.0
routine follow-up Z39.2
respite Z75.5
unavailable, due to
absence of person rendering care Z74.2
inability (any reason) of person rendering care Z74.2
well-baby Z76.2
Caries
bone NEC A18.03
dental (dentino enamel junction) (early childhood) (of dentine) (pre-eruptive) (recurrent) (to the pulp) K02.9 ⬅
arrested (coronal) (root) K02.3
chewing surface
limited to enamel K02.51
penetrating into dentin K02.52
penetrating into pulp K02.53
coronal surface
chewing surface
limited to enamel K02.51
penetrating into dentin K02.52
penetrating into pulp K02.53
pit and fissure surface
limited to enamel K02.51
penetrating into dentin K02.52
penetrating into pulp K02.53
smooth surface
limited to enamel K02.61
penetrating into dentin K02.62
penetrating into pulp K02.63
pit and fissure surface
limited to enamel K02.51
penetrating into dentin K02.52
penetrating into pulp K02.53
primary, cervical origin K02.52 ◄
root K02.7
Caries *(Continued)*
dental *(Continued)*
smooth surface
limited to enamel K02.61
penetrating into dentin K02.62
penetrating into pulp K02.63
external meatus —*see* Disorder, ear, external, specified type NEC
hip (tuberculous) A18.02
initial (tooth)
chewing surface K02.51
pit and fissure surface K02.51
smooth surface K02.61
knee (tuberculous) A18.02
labyrinth —*see* subcategory H83.8
limb NEC (tuberculous) A18.03
mastoid process (chronic) —*see* Mastoiditis, chronic
tuberculous A18.03
middle ear —*see* subcategory H74.8
nose (tuberculous) A18.03
orbit (tuberculous) A18.03
ossicles, ear —*see* Abnormal, ear ossicles
petrous bone —*see* Petrositis
root (dental) (tooth) K02.7
sacrum (tuberculous) A18.01
spine, spinal (column) (tuberculous) A18.01
syphilitic A52.77
congenital (early) A50.02 *[M90.80]*
tooth, teeth —*see* Caries, dental
tuberculous A18.03
vertebra (column) (tuberculous) A18.01
Carious teeth —*see* Caries, dental
Carneous mole O02.0
Carnitine insufficiency E71.40
Carotid body or sinus syndrome G90.01
Carotidynia G90.01
Carotinemia (dietary) E67.1
Carotinosis (cutis) (skin) E67.1
Carpal tunnel syndrome —*see* Syndrome, carpal tunnel
Carpenter's syndrome Q87.0
Carpopedal spasm —*see* Tetany
Carr-Barr-Plunkett syndrome Q97.1
Carrier (suspected) of
amebiasis Z22.1
bacterial disease NEC Z22.39
diphtheria Z22.2
intestinal infectious NEC Z22.1
typhoid Z22.0
meningococcal Z22.31
sexually transmitted Z22.4
specified NEC Z22.39
staphylococcal (Methicillin susceptible) Z22.321
Methicillin resistant Z22.322
streptococcal Z22.338
group B Z22.330
complicating pregnancy or delivery O99.82- ◄
typhoid Z22.0
cholera Z22.1
diphtheria Z22.2
gastrointestinal pathogens NEC Z22.1
genetic Z14.8
cystic fibrosis Z14.1
hemophilia A (asymptomatic) Z14.01
symptomatic Z14.02
gestational, pregnant Z33.1 ◄
gonorrhea Z22.4
HAA (hepatitis Australian-antigen) B18.8 ⬅
HB (c)(s)-AG B18.1 ⬅
hepatitis (viral) B18.9 ⬅
Australia-antigen (HAA) B18.8 ⬅
B surface antigen (HBsAg) B18.1 ⬅
with acute delta- (super)infection B17.0
C B18.2 ⬅
specified NEC B18.8 ⬅
human T-cell lymphotropic virus type-1 (HTLV-1) infection Z22.6

Carrier of *(Continued)*
infectious organism Z22.9
specified NEC Z22.8
meningococci Z22.31
Salmonella typhosa Z22.Ø
serum hepatitis —*see* Carrier, hepatitis
staphylococci (Methicillin susceptible) Z22.321
Methicillin resistant Z22.322
streptococci Z22.338
group B Z22.33Ø
complicating pregnancy or delivery O99.82- ◀
syphilis Z22.4
typhoid Z22.Ø
venereal disease NEC Z22.4
Carrion's disease A44.Ø
Carter's relapsing fever (Asiatic) A68.1
Cartilage —*see* condition
Caruncle (inflamed)
conjunctiva (acute) —*see* Conjunctivitis, acute
labium (majus) (minus) N9Ø.89
lacrimal —*see* Inflammation, lacrimal, passages
myrtiform N89.8
urethral (benign) N36.2
Cascade stomach K31.2
Caseation lymphatic gland (tuberculous) A18.2
Cassidy (-Scholte) syndrome (malignant carcinoid) E34.Ø
Castellani's disease A69.8
Castration, traumatic, male S38.231
Casts in urine R82.99
Cat
cry syndrome Q93.4
ear Q17.3
eye syndrome Q92.8
Catabolism, senile R54
Catalepsy (hysterical) F44.2
schizophrenic F2Ø.2
Cataplexy (idiopathic) —*see* - Narcolepsy
Cataract (cortical) (immature) (incipient) H26.9
with
neovascularization —*see* Cataract, complicated
age-related —*see* Cataract, senile
anterior
and posterior axial embryonal Q12.Ø
pyramidal Q12.Ø
associated with
galactosemia E74.21 *[H28]*
myotonic disorders G71.19 *[H28]*
blue Q12.Ø
central Q12.Ø
cerulean Q12.Ø
complicated H26.2Ø
with
neovascularization H26.21-
ocular disorder H26.22-
glaucomatous flecks H26.23-
congenital Q12.Ø
coraliform Q12.Ø
coronary Q12.Ø
crystalline Q12.Ø
diabetic —*see* Diabetes, cataract
drug-induced H26.3-
due to
ocular disorder —*see* Cataract, complicated
radiation H26.8
electric H26.8
extraction status Z98.4-
glass-blower's H26.8
heat ray H26.8
heterochromic —*see* Cataract, complicated
hypermature —*see* Cataract, senile, morgagnian type
in (due to)
chronic iridocyclitis —*see* Cataract, complicated
diabetes —*see* Diabetes, cataract
endocrine disease E34.9 *[H28]*
eye disease —*see* Cataract, complicated

Cataract *(Continued)*
in (due to) *(Continued)*
hypoparathyroidism E2Ø.9 *[H28]*
malnutrition-dehydration E46 *[H28]*
metabolic disease E88.9 *[H28]*
myotonic disorders G71.19 *[H28]*
nutritional disease E63.9 *[H28]*
infantile —*see* Cataract, presenile
irradiational —*see* Cataract, specified NEC
juvenile —*see* Cataract, presenile
malnutrition-dehydration E46 *[H28]*
morgagnian —*see* Cataract, senile, morgagnian type
myotonic G71.19 *[H28]*
myxedema E03.9 *[H28]*
nuclear
embryonal Q12.Ø
sclerosis —*see* Cataract, senile, nuclear
presenile H26.ØØ-
combined forms H26.Ø6-
cortical H26.Ø1-
lamellar —*see* Cataract, presenile, cortical
nuclear H26.Ø3-
specified NEC H26.Ø9
subcapsular polar (anterior) H26.Ø4-
posterior H26.Ø5-
zonular —*see* Cataract, presenile, cortical
secondary H26.4Ø
Soemmering's ring H26.41-
specified NEC H26.49-
to eye disease —*see* Cataract, complicated
senile H25.9
brunescens —*see* Cataract, senile, nuclear
combined forms H25.81-
coronary —*see* Cataract, senile, incipient
cortical H25.Ø1-
hypermature —*see* Cataract, senile, morgagnian type
incipient (mature) (total) H25.Ø9-
cortical —*see* Cataract, senile, cortical
subcapsular —*see* Cataract, senile, subcapsular
morgagnian type (hypermature) H25.2-
nuclear (sclerosis) H25.1-
polar subcapsular (anterior) (posterior) —*see* Cataract, senile, incipient
punctate —*see* Cataract, senile, incipient
specified NEC H25.89
subcapsular polar (anterior) H25.Ø3-
posterior H25.Ø4-
snowflake —*see* Diabetes, cataract
specified NEC H26.8
toxic —*see* Cataract, drug-induced
traumatic H26.1Ø-
localized H26.11-
partially resolved H26.12-
total H26.13-
zonular (perinuclear) Q12.Ø
Cataracta —*see also* Cataract
brunescens —*see* Cataract, senile, nuclear
centralis pulverulenta Q12.Ø
cerulea Q12.Ø
complicata —*see* Cataract, complicated
congenita Q12.Ø
coralliformis Q12.Ø
coronaria Q12.Ø
diabetic —*see* Diabetes, cataract
membranacea
accreta —*see* Cataract, secondary
congenita Q12.Ø
nigra —*see* Cataract, senile, nuclear
sunflower —*see* Cataract, complicated
Catarrh, catarrhal (acute) (febrile) (infectious) (inflammation) (*see also* condition) JØØ
bronchial —*see* Bronchitis
chest —*see* Bronchitis
chronic J31.Ø
due to congenital syphilis A5Ø.Ø3
enteric —*see* Enteritis
eustachian H68.ØØ9
fauces —*see* Pharyngitis

Catarrh, catarrhal *(Continued)*
gastrointestinal —*see* Enteritis
gingivitis KØ5.ØØ
nonplaque induced KØ5.Ø1
plaque induced KØ5.ØØ
hay —*see* Fever, hay
intestinal —*see* Enteritis
larynx, chronic J37.Ø
liver B15.9
with hepatic coma B15.Ø
lung —*see* Bronchitis
middle ear, chronic —*see* Otitis, media, nonsuppurative, chronic, serous
mouth K12.1
nasal (chronic) —*see* Rhinitis
nasobronchial J31.1
nasopharyngeal (chronic) J31.1
acute JØØ
pulmonary —*see* Bronchitis
spring (eye) (vernal) —*see* Conjunctivitis, acute, atopic
summer (hay) —*see* Fever, hay
throat J31.2
tubotympanal —*see also* Otitis, media, nonsuppurative
chronic —*see* Otitis, media, nonsuppurative, chronic, serous
Catatonia (schizophrenic) F2Ø.2
Catatonic
disorder due to known physiologic condition FØ6.1
schizophrenia F2Ø.2
stupor R4Ø.1
Cat-scratch —*see also* Abrasion
disease or fever A28.1
Cauda equina —*see* condition
Cauliflower ear M95.1-
Causalgia (upper limb) G56.4-
lower limb G57.7-
Cause
external, general effects T75.89
Caustic burn —*see* Corrosion, by site
Cavare's disease (familial periodic paralysis) G72.3
Cave-in, injury
crushing (severe) —*see* Crush
suffocation —*see* Asphyxia, traumatic, due to low oxygen, due to cave-in
Cavernitis (penis) N48.29
Cavernositis N48.29
Cavernous —*see* condition
Cavitation of lung —*see also* Tuberculosis, pulmonary
nontuberculous J98.4
Cavities, dental —*see* Caries, dental
Cavity
lung —*see* Cavitation of lung
optic papilla Q14.2
pulmonary —*see* Cavitation of lung
Cavovarus foot, congenital Q66.1
Cavus foot (congenital) Q66.7
acquired —*see* Deformity, limb, foot, specified NEC
Cazenave's disease L1Ø.2
Cecitis K52.9
with perforation, peritonitis, or rupture K65.8
Cecum —*see* condition
Celiac
artery compression syndrome I77.4
disease (with steatorrhea) K9Ø.Ø ⬅
infantilism K9Ø.Ø
Cell (s), cellular —*see also* condition
in urine R82.99
Cellulitis (diffuse) (phlegmonous) (septic) (suppurative) LØ3.9Ø
abdominal wall LØ3.311
anaerobic A48.Ø
ankle —*see* Cellulitis, lower limb
anus K61.Ø
arm —*see* Cellulitis, upper limb
auricle (ear) —*see* Cellulitis, ear

Cellulitis *(Continued)*
  axilla LØ3.11-
  back (any part) LØ3.312
  breast (acute) (nonpuerperal) (subacute) N61.Ø ◀
    nipple N61.Ø ◀
  broad ligament
    acute N73.Ø
  buttock LØ3.317
  cervical (meaning neck) LØ3.221
  cervix (uteri) —*see* Cervicitis
  cheek (external) LØ3.211
    internal K12.2
  chest wall LØ3.313
  chronic LØ3.9Ø
  clostridial A48.Ø
  corpus cavernosum N48.22
  digit
    finger —*see* Cellulitis, finger
    toe —*see* Cellulitis, toe
  Douglas' cul-de-sac or pouch
    acute N73.Ø
  drainage site (following operation) T81.48 ⬅
  ear (external) H6Ø.1-
  eosinophilic (granulomatous) L98.3
  erysipelatous —*see* Erysipelas
  external auditory canal —*see* Cellulitis, ear
  eyelid —*see* Abscess, eyelid
  face NEC LØ3.211
  finger (intrathecal) (periosteal) (subcutaneous) (subcuticular) LØ3.Ø1-
  foot —*see* Cellulitis, lower limb
  gangrenous —*see* Gangrene
  genital organ NEC
    female (external) N76.4
    male N49.9
      multiple sites N49.8
      specified NEC N49.8
  gluteal (region) LØ3.317
  gonococcal A54.89
  groin LØ3.314
  hand —*see* Cellulitis, upper limb
  head NEC LØ3.811
    face (any part, except ear, eye and nose) LØ3.211
  heel —*see* Cellulitis, lower limb
  hip —*see* Cellulitis, lower limb
  jaw (region) LØ3.211
  knee —*see* Cellulitis, lower limb
  labium (majus) (minus) —*see* Vulvitis
  lacrimal passages —*see* Inflammation, lacrimal, passages
  larynx J38.7
  leg —*see* Cellulitis, lower limb
  lip K13.Ø
  lower limb LØ3.11-
    toe —*see* Cellulitis, toe
  mouth (floor) K12.2
  multiple sites, so stated LØ3.9Ø
  nasopharynx J39.1
  navel LØ3.316
    newborn P38.9
      with mild hemorrhage P38.1
      without hemorrhage P38.9
  neck (region) LØ3.221
  nipple (acute) (nonpuerperal) (subacute) N61.Ø ◀
  nose (septum) (external) J34.Ø
  orbit, orbital HØ5.Ø1-
  palate (soft) K12.2
  pectoral (region) LØ3.313
  pelvis, pelvic (chronic)
    female —*see also* Disease, pelvis, inflammatory N73.2
      acute N73.Ø
    following ectopic or molar pregnancy OØ8.Ø
    male K65.Ø
  penis N48.22
  perineal, perineum LØ3.315
  periorbital LØ3.213 ◀

Cellulitis *(Continued)*
  perirectal K61.1
  peritonsillar J36
  periurethral N34.Ø
  periuterine —*see also* Disease, pelvis, inflammatory N73.2
    acute N73.Ø
  pharynx J39.1
  preseptal LØ3.213 ◀
  rectum K61.1
  retroperitoneal K68.9
  round ligament
    acute N73.Ø
  scalp (any part) LØ3.811
  scrotum N49.2
  seminal vesicle N49.Ø
  shoulder —*see* Cellulitis, upper limb
  specified site NEC LØ3.818
  submandibular (region) (space) (triangle) K12.2
    gland K11.3
  submaxillary (region) K12.2
    gland K11.3
  thigh —*see* Cellulitis, lower limb
  thumb (intrathecal) (periosteal) (subcutaneous) (subcuticular) —*see* Cellulitis, finger
  toe (intrathecal) (periosteal) (subcutaneous) (subcuticular) LØ3.Ø3-
  tonsil J36
  trunk LØ3.319
    abdominal wall LØ3.311
    back (any part) LØ3.312
    buttock LØ3.317
    chest wall LØ3.313
    groin LØ3.314
    perineal, perineum LØ3.315
    umbilicus LØ3.316
  tuberculous (primary) A18.4
  umbilicus LØ3.316
  upper limb LØ3.11-
    axilla —*see* Cellulitis, axilla
    finger —*see* Cellulitis, finger
    thumb —*see* Cellulitis, finger
  vaccinal T88.Ø
  vocal cord J38.3
  vulva —*see* Vulvitis
  wrist —*see* Cellulitis, upper limb
Cementoblastoma, benign —*see* Cyst, calcifying odontogenic
Cementoma —*see* Cyst, calcifying odontogenic
Cementoperiostitis —*see* Periodontitis
Cementosis KØ3.4
Central auditory processing disorder H93.25
Central pain syndrome G89.Ø
Cephalematocele, cephal (o)hematocele
  newborn P52.8
    birth injury P1Ø.8
  traumatic —*see* Hematoma, brain
Cephalematoma, cephalhematoma (calcified)
  newborn (birth injury) P12.Ø
  traumatic —*see* Hematoma, brain
Cephalgia, cephalalgia —*see also* Headache
  histamine G44.ØØ9
    intractable G44.ØØ1
    not intractable G44.ØØ9
  trigeminal autonomic (TAC) NEC G44.Ø99
    intractable G44.Ø91
    not intractable G44.Ø99
Cephalic —*see* condition
Cephalitis —*see* Encephalitis
Cephalocele —*see* Encephalocele
Cephalomenia N94.89
Cephalopelvic —*see* condition
Cerclage (with cervical incompetence) **in pregnancy** —*see* Incompetence, cervix, in pregnancy
Cerebellitis —*see* Encephalitis
Cerebellum, cerebellar —*see* condition
Cerebral —*see* condition
Cerebritis —*see* Encephalitis

Cerebro-hepato-renal syndrome Q87.89
Cerebromalacia —*see* Softening, brain
  sequelae of cerebrovascular disease I69.398
Cerebroside lipidosis E75.22
Cerebrospasticity (congenital) G8Ø.1
Cerebrospinal —*see* condition
Cerebrum —*see* condition
Ceroid-lipofuscinosis, neuronal E75.4
Cerumen (accumulation) (impacted) H61.2-
Cervical —*see also* condition
  auricle Q18.2
  dysplasia in pregnancy —*see* Abnormal, cervix, in pregnancy or childbirth
  erosion in pregnancy —*see* Abnormal, cervix, in pregnancy or childbirth
  fibrosis in pregnancy —*see* Abnormal, cervix, in pregnancy or childbirth
  fusion syndrome Q76.1
  rib Q76.5
  shortening (complicating pregnancy) O26.87-
Cervicalgia M54.2
Cervicitis (acute) (chronic) (nonvenereal) (senile (atrophic)) (subacute) (with ulceration) N72
  with
    abortion —*see* Abortion, by type complicated by genital tract and pelvic infection
    ectopic pregnancy OØ8.Ø
    molar pregnancy OØ8.Ø
  chlamydial A56.Ø9
  gonococcal A54.Ø3
  herpesviral A6Ø.Ø3
  puerperal (postpartum) O86.11
  syphilitic A52.76
  trichomonal A59.Ø9
  tuberculous A18.16
Cervicocolpitis (emphysematosa) (*see also* Cervicitis) N72
Cervix —*see* condition
Cesarean delivery, previous, affecting management of pregnancy O34.219 ⬅
  classical (vertical) scar O34.212 ◀
  low transverse scar O34.211 ◀
Céstan (-Chenais) **paralysis or syndrome** G46.3
Céstan-Raymond syndrome I65.8
Cestode infestation B71.9
  specified type NEC B71.8
Cestodiasis B71.9
Chabert's disease A22.9
Chacaleh E53.8
Chafing L3Ø.4
Chagas' (-Mazza) **disease** (chronic) B57.2
  with
    cardiovascular involvement NEC B57.2
    digestive system involvement B57.3Ø
      megacolon B57.32
      megaesophagus B57.31
      other specified B57.39
    megacolon B57.32
    megaesophagus B57.31
    myocarditis B57.2
    nervous system involvement B57.4Ø
      meningitis B57.41
      meningoencephalitis B57.42
      other specified B57.49
    specified organ involvement NEC B57.5
  acute (with) B57.1
    cardiovascular NEC B57.Ø
    myocarditis B57.Ø
Chagres fever B5Ø.9
Chairridden Z74.Ø9
Chalasia (cardiac sphincter) K21.9
Chalazion HØØ.19
  left HØØ.16
    lower HØØ.15
    upper HØØ.14
  right HØØ.13
    lower HØØ.12
    upper HØØ.11

C

- **Chalcosis** —*see also* Disorder, globe, degenerative, chalcosis
  - cornea —*see* Deposit, cornea
  - crystalline lens —*see* Cataract, complicated
  - retina H35.89
- **Chalicosis** (pulmonum) J62.8
- **Chancre** (any genital site) (hard) (hunterian) (mixed) (primary) (seronegative) (seropositive) (syphilitic) A51.Ø
  - congenital A5Ø.Ø7
  - conjunctiva NEC A51.2
  - Ducrey's A57
  - extragenital A51.2
  - eyelid A51.2
  - lip A51.2
  - nipple A51.2
  - Nisbet's A57
  - of
    - carate A67.Ø
    - pinta A67.Ø
    - yaws A66.Ø
  - palate, soft A51.2
  - phagedenic A57
  - simple A57
  - soft A57
    - bubo A57
    - palate A51.2
  - urethra A51.Ø
  - yaws A66.Ø
- **Chancroid** (anus) (genital) (penis) (perineum) (rectum) (urethra) (vulva) A57
- **Chandler's disease** (osteochondritis dissecans, hip) —*see* Osteochondritis, dissecans, hip
- **Change** (s) (in) (of) —*see also* Removal
  - arteriosclerotic —*see* Arteriosclerosis
  - bone —*see also* Disorder, bone
    - diabetic —*see* Diabetes, bone change
  - bowel habit R19.4
  - cardiorenal (vascular) —*see* Hypertension, cardiorenal
  - cardiovascular —*see* Disease, cardiovascular
  - circulatory I99.9
  - cognitive (mild) (organic) R41.89
  - color, tooth, teeth
    - during formation KØØ.8
    - posteruptive KØ3.7
  - contraceptive device Z3Ø.433
  - corneal membrane H18.3Ø
    - Bowman's membrane fold or rupture H18.31-
    - Descemet's membrane
      - fold H18.32-
      - rupture H18.33-
  - coronary —*see* Disease, heart, ischemic
  - degenerative, spine or vertebra —*see* Spondylosis
  - dental pulp, regressive KØ4.2
  - dressing (nonsurgical) Z48.ØØ
    - surgical Z48.Ø1
  - heart —*see* Disease, heart
  - hip joint —*see* Derangement, joint, hip
  - hyperplastic larynx J38.7
  - hypertrophic
    - nasal sinus J34.89
    - turbinate, nasal J34.3
    - upper respiratory tract J39.8
  - indwelling catheter Z46.6
  - inflammatory —*see also* Inflammation
    - sacroiliac M46.1
  - job, anxiety concerning Z56.1
  - joint —*see* Derangement, joint
  - life —*see* Menopause
  - mental status R41.82
  - minimal (glomerular) —*see also* NØØ-NØ7
    - with fourth character .Ø NØ5.Ø
  - myocardium, myocardial —*see* Degeneration, myocardial - of life —*see* Menopause
  - pacemaker Z45.Ø18
    - pulse generator Z45.Ø1Ø

- **Change** *(Continued)*
  - personality (enduring) F68.8
    - due to (secondary to)
      - general medical condition FØ7.Ø
    - secondary (nonspecific) F6Ø.89
  - regressive, dental pulp KØ4.2
  - renal —*see* Disease, renal
  - retina H35.9
    - myopic H44.2-
  - sacroiliac joint M53.3
  - senile —*see also* condition R54
  - sensory R2Ø.8
  - skin R23.9
    - acute, due to ultraviolet radiation L56.9
      - specified NEC L56.8
    - chronic, due to nonionizing radiation L57.9
      - specified NEC L57.8
    - cyanosis R23.Ø
    - flushing R23.2
    - pallor R23.1
    - petechiae R23.3
    - specified change NEC R23.8
    - swelling —*see* Mass, localized
    - texture R23.4
  - trophic
    - arm —*see* Mononeuropathy, upper limb
    - leg —*see* Mononeuropathy, lower limb
  - vascular I99.9
  - vasomotor I73.9
  - voice R49.9
    - psychogenic F44.4
    - specified NEC R49.8
- **Changing sleep-work schedule, affecting sleep** G47.26
- **Changuinola fever** A93.1
- **Chapping skin** T69.8
- **Charcot-Marie-Tooth disease, paralysis or syndrome** G6Ø.Ø
- **Charcot's**
  - arthropathy —*see* Arthropathy, neuropathic
  - cirrhosis K74.3
  - disease (tabetic arthropathy) A52.16
  - joint (disease) (tabetic) A52.16
    - diabetic —*see* Diabetes, with, arthropathy
    - syringomyelic G95.Ø
  - syndrome (intermittent claudication) I73.9
- **CHARGE association** Q89.8
- **Charley-horse** (quadriceps) M62.831
  - traumatic (quadriceps) S76.11-
- **Charlouis' disease** —*see* Yaws
- **Cheadle's disease** E54
- **Checking** (of)
  - cardiac pacemaker (battery) (electrode (s)) Z45.Ø18
    - pulse generator Z45.Ø1Ø
  - implantable subdermal contraceptive Z3Ø.46 ◀
  - intrauterine contraceptive device Z3Ø.431
- **Check-up** —*see* Examination
- **Chédiak-Higashi** (-Steinbrinck) **syndrome** (congenital gigantism of peroxidase granules) E7Ø.33Ø
- **Cheek** —*see* condition
- **Cheese itch** B88.Ø
- **Cheese-washer's lung** J67.8
- **Cheese-worker's lung** J67.8
- **Cheilitis** (acute) (angular) (catarrhal) (chronic) (exfoliative) (gangrenous) (glandular) (infectional) (suppurative) (ulcerative) (vesicular) K13.Ø
  - actinic (due to sun) L56.8
    - other than from sun L59.8
  - candidal B37.83
- **Cheilodynia** K13.Ø
- **Cheiloschisis** —*see* Cleft, lip
- **Cheilosis** (angular) K13.Ø
  - with pellagra E52
  - due to
    - vitamin B2 (riboflavin) deficiency E53.Ø
- **Cheiromegaly** M79.89
- **Cheiropompholyx** L3Ø.1
- **Cheloid** —*see* Keloid

- **Chemical burn** —*see* Corrosion, by site
- **Chemodectoma** —*see* Paraganglioma, nonchromaffin
- **Chemosis, conjunctiva** —*see* Edema, conjunctiva
- **Chemotherapy** (session) (for)
  - cancer Z51.11
  - neoplasm Z51.11
- **Cherubism** M27.8
- **Chest** —*see* condition
- **Cheyne-Stokes breathing** (respiration) RØ6.3
- **Chiari's**
  - disease or syndrome (hepatic vein thrombosis) I82.Ø
  - malformation
    - type I G93.5
    - type II —*see* Spina bifida
  - net Q24.8
- **Chicago disease** B4Ø.9
- **Chickenpox** —*see* Varicella
- **Chiclero ulcer or sore** B55.1
- **Chigger** (infestation) B88.Ø
- **Chignon** (disease) B36.8
  - newborn (from vacuum extraction) (birth injury) P12.1
- **Chilaiditi's syndrome** (subphrenic displacement, colon) Q43.3
- **Chilblain** (s) (lupus) T69.1
- **Child**
  - custody dispute Z65.3
- **Childbirth** —*see* Delivery
- **Childhood**
  - cerebral X-linked adrenoleukodystrophy E71.52Ø
  - period of rapid growth ZØØ.2
- **Chill** (s) R68.83
  - with fever R5Ø.9
  - without fever R68.83
  - congestive in malarial regions B54
- **Chilomastigiasis** AØ7.8
- **Chimera 46,XX/46,XY** Q99.Ø
- **Chin** —*see* condition
- **Chinese dysentery** AØ3.9
- **Chionophobia** F4Ø.228
- **Chitral fever** A93.1
- **Chlamydia, chlamydial** A74.9
  - cervicitis A56.Ø9
  - conjunctivitis A74.Ø
  - cystitis A56.Ø1
  - endometritis A56.11
  - epididymitis A56.19
  - female
    - pelvic inflammatory disease A56.11
    - pelviperitonitis A56.11
  - orchitis A56.19
  - peritonitis A74.81
  - pharyngitis A56.4
  - proctitis A56.3
  - psittaci (infection) A7Ø
  - salpingitis A56.11
  - sexually-transmitted infection NEC A56.8
  - specified NEC A74.89
  - urethritis A56.Ø1
  - vulvovaginitis A56.Ø2
- **Chlamydiosis** —*see* Chlamydia
- **Chloasma** (skin) (idiopathic) (symptomatic) L81.1
  - eyelid HØ2.719
    - hyperthyroid EØ5.9Ø *[HØ2.719]*
      - with thyroid storm EØ5.91 *[HØ2.719]*
    - left HØ2.716
      - lower HØ2.715
      - upper HØ2.714
    - right HØ2.713
      - lower HØ2.712
      - upper HØ2.711
- **Chloroma** C92.3-
- **Chlorosis** D5Ø.9
  - Egyptian B76.9 *[D63.8]*
  - miner's B76.9 *[D63.8]*
- **Chlorotic anemia** D5Ø.8

C

Chocolate cyst (ovary) N8Ø.1
Choked
- disc or disk *—see* Papilledema
- on food, phlegm, or vomitus NOS *—see* Foreign body, by site
- while vomiting NOS *—see* Foreign body, by site

Chokes (resulting from bends) T7Ø.3
Choking sensation RØ9.89
Cholangiectasis K83.8
Cholangiocarcinoma
- with hepatocellular carcinoma, combined C22.Ø
- liver C22.1
- specified site NEC *—see* Neoplasm, malignant, by site
- unspecified site C22.1

Cholangiohepatitis K83.8
- due to fluke infestation B66.1

Cholangiohepatoma C22.Ø
Cholangiolitis (acute) (chronic) (extrahepatic) (gangrenous) (intrahepatic) K83.Ø
- paratyphoidal *—see* Fever, paratyphoid
- typhoidal AØ1.Ø9

Cholangioma D13.4
- malignant *—see* Cholangiocarcinoma

Cholangitis (ascending) (primary) (recurrent) (sclerosing) (secondary) (stenosing) (suppurative) K83.Ø
- with calculus, bile duct *—see* Calculus, bile duct, with cholangitis
- chronic nonsuppurative destructive K74.3

Cholecystectasia K82.8
Cholecystitis K81.9
- with
  - calculus, stones in
    - bile duct (common) (hepatic) *—see* Calculus, bile duct, with cholecystitis
    - cystic duct *—see* Calculus, gallbladder, with cholecystitis
    - gallbladder *—see* Calculus, gallbladder, with cholecystitis
  - choledocholithiasis *—see* Calculus, bile duct, with cholecystitis
  - cholelithiasis *—see* Calculus, gallbladder, with cholecystitis
- acute (emphysematous) (gangrenous) (suppurative) K81.Ø
  - with
    - calculus, stones in
      - cystic duct *—see* Calculus, gallbladder, with cholecystitis, acute
      - gallbladder *—see* Calculus, gallbladder, with cholecystitis, acute
    - choledocholithiasis *—see* Calculus, bile duct, with cholecystitis, acute
    - cholelithiasis *—see* Calculus, gallbladder, with cholecystitis, acute
    - chronic cholecystitis K81.2
      - with gallbladder calculus K8Ø.12
        - with obstruction K8Ø.13
- chronic K81.1
  - with acute cholecystitis K81.2
    - with gallbladder calculus K8Ø.12
      - with obstruction K8Ø.13
- emphysematous (acute) *—see* Cholecystitis, acute
- gangrenous *—see* Cholecystitis, acute
- paratyphoidal, current AØ1.4
- suppurative *—see* Cholecystitis, acute
- typhoidal AØ1.Ø9

Cholecystolithiasis *—see* Calculus, gallbladder
Choledochitis (suppurative) K83.Ø
Choledocholith *—see* Calculus, bile duct
Choledocholithiasis (common duct) (hepatic duct) *—see* Calculus, bile duct
- cystic *—see* Calculus, gallbladder
- typhoidal AØ1.Ø9

Cholelithiasis (cystic duct) (gallbladder) (impacted) (multiple) *—see* Calculus, gallbladder
- bile duct (common) (hepatic) *—see* Calculus, bile duct
- hepatic duct *—see* Calculus, bile duct
- specified NEC K8Ø.8Ø
  - with obstruction K8Ø.81

Cholemia *—see also* Jaundice
- familial (simple) (congenital) E8Ø.4
- Gilbert's E8Ø.4

Choleperitoneum, choleperitonitis K65.3
Cholera (Asiatic) (epidemic) (malignant) AØØ.9
- antimonial *—see* Poisoning, antimony
- classical AØØ.Ø
- due to Vibrio cholerae Ø1 AØØ.9
  - biovar cholerae AØØ.Ø
  - biovar eltor AØØ.1
  - el tor AØØ.1
- el tor AØØ.1

Cholerine *—see* Cholera
Cholestasis NEC K83.1
- with hepatocyte injury K71.Ø
- due to total parenteral nutrition (TPN) K76.89
- pure K71.Ø

Cholesteatoma (ear) (middle) (with reaction) H71.9-
- attic H71.Ø-
- external ear (canal) H6Ø.4-
- mastoid H71.2-
- postmastoidectomy cavity (recurrent) *—see* Complications, postmastoidectomy, recurrent cholesteatoma
- recurrent (postmastoidectomy) *—see* Complications, postmastoidectomy, recurrent cholesteatoma
- tympanum H71.1-

Cholesteatosis, diffuse H71.3-
Cholesteremia E78.ØØ (Revised)
Cholesterin in vitreous *—see* Deposit, crystalline
Cholesterol
- deposit
  - retina H35.89
  - vitreous *—see* Deposit, crystalline
- elevated (high) E78.ØØ (Revised)
  - with elevated (high) triglycerides E78.2
  - screening for Z13.22Ø
- imbibition of gallbladder K82.4

Cholesterolemia (essential) (pure) E78.ØØ (Revised)
- familial E78.Ø1 (New)
- hereditary E78.Ø1 (New)

Cholesterolosis, cholesterosis (gallbladder) K82.4
- cerebrotendinous E75.5

Cholocolic fistula K82.3
Choluria R82.2
Chondritis M94.8X9
- aurical H61.Ø3-
- costal (Tietze's) M94.Ø
- external ear H61.Ø3-
- patella, posttraumatic *—see* Chondromalacia, patella
- pinna H61.Ø3-
- purulent M94.8X-
- tuberculous NEC A18.Ø2
  - intervertebral A18.Ø1

Chondroblastoma *—see also* Neoplasm, bone, benign
- malignant *—see* Neoplasm, bone, malignant

Chondrocalcinosis M11.2Ø
- ankle M11.27-
- elbow M11.22-
- familial M11.1Ø
  - ankle M11.17-
  - elbow M11.12-
  - foot joint M11.17-
  - hand joint M11.14-
  - hip M11.15-
  - knee M11.16-
  - multiple site M11.19
  - shoulder M11.11-
  - vertebrae M11.18
  - wrist M11.13-
- foot joint M11.27-
- hand joint M11.24-
- hip M11.25-
- knee M11.26-
- multiple site M11.29
- shoulder M11.21-
- specified type NEC M11.2Ø
  - ankle M11.27-
  - elbow M11.22-
  - foot joint M11.27-
  - hand joint M11.24-
  - hip M11.25-
  - knee M11.26-
  - multiple site M11.29
  - shoulder M11.21-
  - vertebrae M11.28
  - wrist M11.23-
- vertebrae M11.28
- wrist M11.23-

Chondrodermatitis nodularis helicis or anthelicis *—see* Perichondritis, ear
Chondrodysplasia Q78.9
- with hemangioma Q78.4
- calcificans congenita Q77.3
- fetalis Q77.4
- metaphyseal (Jansen's) (McKusick's) (Schmid's) Q78.8 (Revised)
- punctata Q77.3

Chondrodystrophy, chondrodystrophia (familial) (fetalis) (hypoplastic) Q78.9
- calcificans congenita Q77.3
- myotonic (congenital) G71.13
- punctata Q77.3

Chondroectodermal dysplasia Q77.6
Chondrogenesis imperfecta Q77.4
Chondrolysis M94.35-
Chondroma *—see also* Neoplasm, cartilage, benign
- juxtacortical *—see* Neoplasm, bone, benign
- periosteal *—see* Neoplasm, bone, benign

Chondromalacia (systemic) M94.2Ø
- acromioclavicular joint M94.21-
- ankle M94.27-
- elbow M94.22-
- foot joint M94.27-
- glenohumeral joint M94.21-
- hand joint M94.24-
- hip M94.25-
- knee M94.26-
  - patella M22.4-
- multiple sites M94.29
- patella M22.4-
- rib M94.28
- sacroiliac joint M94.259
- shoulder M94.21-
- sternoclavicular joint M94.21-
- vertebral joint M94.28
- wrist M94.23-

Chondromatosis *—see also* Neoplasm, cartilage, uncertain behavior
- internal Q78.4

Chondromyxosarcoma *—see* Neoplasm, cartilage, malignant
Chondro-osteodysplasia (Morquio-Brailsford type) E76.219
Chondro-osteodystrophy E76.29
Chondro-osteoma *—see* Neoplasm, bone, benign
Chondropathia tuberosa M94.Ø
Chondrosarcoma *—see* Neoplasm, cartilage, malignant
- juxtacortical *—see* Neoplasm, bone, malignant
- mesenchymal *—see* Neoplasm, connective tissue, malignant
- myxoid *—see* Neoplasm, cartilage, malignant

Chordee (nonvenereal) N48.89
- congenital Q54.4
- gonococcal A54.Ø9

C

Chorditis (fibrinous) (nodosa) (tuberosa) J38.2
Chordoma —*see* Neoplasm, vertebral (column), malignant
Chorea (chronic) (gravis) (posthemiplegic) (senile) (spasmodic) G25.5
- with
  - heart involvement I02.0
    - active or acute (conditions in I01-) I02.0
    - rheumatic I02.9
      - with valvular disorder I02.0
  - rheumatic heart disease (chronic) (inactive) (quiescent) — code to rheumatic heart condition involved
- drug-induced G25.4
- habit F95.8
- hereditary G10
- Huntington's G10
- hysterical F44.4
- minor I02.9
  - with heart involvement I02.0
- progressive G25.5
  - hereditary G10
- rheumatic (chronic) I02.9
  - with heart involvement I02.0
- Sydenham's I02.9
  - with heart involvement —*see* Chorea, with rheumatic heart disease
  - nonrheumatic G25.5

Choreoathetosis (paroxysmal) G25.5
Chorioadenoma (destruens) D39.2
Chorioamnionitis O41.12-
Chorioangioma D26.7
Choriocarcinoma —*see* Neoplasm, malignant, by site
- combined with
  - embryonal carcinoma —*see* Neoplasm, malignant, by site
  - other germ cell elements —*see* Neoplasm, malignant, by site
  - teratoma —*see* Neoplasm, malignant, by site
- specified site —*see* Neoplasm, malignant, by site
- unspecified site
  - female C58
  - male C62.90

Chorioencephalitis (acute) (lymphocytic) (serous) A87.2
Chorioepithelioma —*see* Choriocarcinoma
Choriomeningitis (acute) (lymphocytic) (serous) A87.2
Chorionepithelioma —*see* Choriocarcinoma
Chorioretinitis —*see also* Inflammation, chorioretinal
- disseminated —*see also* Inflammation, chorioretinal, disseminated
  - in neurosyphilis A52.19
- Egyptian B76.9 *[D63.8]*
- focal —*see also* Inflammation, chorioretinal, focal
- histoplasmic B39.9 *[H32]*
- in (due to)
  - histoplasmosis B39.9 *[H32]*
  - syphilis (secondary) A51.43
    - late A52.71
  - toxoplasmosis (acquired) B58.01
    - congenital (active) P37.1 *[H32]*
  - tuberculosis A18.53
- juxtapapillary, juxtapapillaris —*see* Inflammation, chorioretinal, focal, juxtapapillary
- leprous A30.9 *[H32]*
- miner's B76.9 *[D63.8]*
- progressive myopia (degeneration) H44.2-
- syphilitic (secondary) A51.43
  - congenital (early) A50.01 *[H32]*
    - late A50.32
  - late A52.71
- tuberculous A18.53

Chorioretinopathy, central serous H35.71-
Choroid —*see* condition
Choroideremia H31.21
Choroiditis —*see* Chorioretinitis
Choroidopathy —*see* Disorder, choroid
Choroidoretinitis —*see* Chorioretinitis
Choroidoretinopathy, central serous —*see* Chorioretinopathy, central serous
Christian-Weber disease M35.6
Christmas disease D67
Chromaffinoma —*see also* Neoplasm, benign, by site
- malignant —*see* Neoplasm, malignant, by site

Chromatopsia —*see* Deficiency, color vision
Chromhidrosis, chromidrosis L75.1
Chromoblastomycosis —*see* Chromomycosis
Chromoconversion R82.91
Chromomycosis B43.9
- brain abscess B43.1
- cerebral B43.1
- cutaneous B43.0
- skin B43.0
- specified NEC B43.8
- subcutaneous abscess or cyst B43.2

Chromophytosis B36.0
Chromosome —*see* condition by chromosome involved
- D (1) —*see* condition, chromosome 13
- E (3) —*see* condition, chromosome 18
- G —*see* condition, chromosome 21

Chromotrichomycosis B36.8
Chronic —*see* condition
- fracture —*see* Fracture, pathological

Churg-Strauss syndrome M30.1
Chyle cyst, mesentery I89.8
Chylocele (nonfilarial) I89.8
- filarial —*see also* Infestation, filarial B74.9 *[N51]*
- tunica vaginalis N50.89 ⬅
  - filarial —*see also* Infestation, filarial B74.9 *[N51]*

Chylomicronemia (fasting) (with hyperprebetalipoproteinemia) E78.3
Chylopericardium I31.3
- acute I30.9

Chylothorax (nonfilarial) I89.8
- filarial —*see also* Infestation, filarial B74.9 *[J91.8]*

Chylous —*see* condition
Chyluria (nonfilarial) R82.0
- due to
  - bilharziasis B65.0
  - Brugia (malayi) B74.1
    - timori B74.2
  - schistosomiasis (bilharziasis) B65.0
  - Wuchereria (bancrofti) B74.0
- filarial —*see* Infestation, filarial

Cicatricial (deformity) —*see* Cicatrix
Cicatrix (adherent) (contracted) (painful) (vicious) —*see also* Scar L90.5
- adenoid (and tonsil) J35.8
- alveolar process M26.79
- anus K62.89
- auricle —*see* Disorder, pinna, specified type NEC
- bile duct (common) (hepatic) K83.8
- bladder N32.89
- bone —*see* Disorder, bone, specified type NEC
- brain G93.89
- cervix (postoperative) (postpartal) N88.1
- common duct K83.8
- cornea H17.9
  - tuberculous A18.59
- duodenum (bulb), obstructive K31.5
- esophagus K22.2
- eyelid —*see* Disorder, eyelid function
- hypopharynx J39.2
- lacrimal passages —*see* Obstruction, lacrimal
- larynx J38.7
- lung J98.4
- middle ear —*see* subcategory H74.8
- mouth K13.79

Cicatrix *(Continued)*
- muscle M62.89
  - with contracture —*see* Contraction, muscle NEC
- nasopharynx J39.2
- palate (soft) K13.79
- penis N48.89
- pharynx J39.2
- prostate N42.89
- rectum K62.89
- retina —*see* Scar, chorioretinal
- semilunar cartilage —*see* Derangement, meniscus
- seminal vesicle N50.89 ⬅
- skin L90.5
  - infected L08.89
  - postinfective L90.5
  - tuberculous B90.8
- specified site NEC L90.5
- throat J39.2
- tongue K14.8
- tonsil (and adenoid) J35.8
- trachea J39.8
- tuberculous NEC B90.9
- urethra N36.8
- uterus N85.8
- vagina N89.8
  - postoperative N99.2
- vocal cord J38.3
- wrist, constricting (annular) L90.5

CIDP (chronic inflammatory demyelinating polyneuropathy) G61.81
CIN —*see* Neoplasia, intraepithelial, cervix
CINCA (chronic infantile neurological, cutaneous and articular syndrome) M04.2 ◀
Cinchonism —*see* Deafness, ototoxic
- correct substance properly administered —*see* Table of Drugs and Chemicals, by drug, adverse effect
- overdose or wrong substance given or taken —*see* Table of Drugs and Chemicals, by drug, poisoning

Circle of Willis —*see* condition
Circular —*see* condition
Circulating anticoagulants —*see also* - Disorder, hemorrhagic D68.318
- due to drugs —*see also* - Disorder, hemorrhagic D68.32
- following childbirth O72.3

Circulation
- collateral, any site I99.8
- defective (lower extremity) I99.8
  - congenital Q28.9
- embryonic Q28.9
- failure (peripheral) R57.9
  - newborn P29.89
- fetal, persistent P29.3
- heart, incomplete Q28.9

Circulatory system —*see* condition
Circulus senilis (cornea) —*see* Degeneration, cornea, senile
Circumcision (in absence of medical indication) (ritual) (routine) Z41.2
Circumscribed —*see* condition
Circumvallate placenta O43.11-
Cirrhosis, cirrhotic (hepatic) (liver) K74.60
- alcoholic K70.30
  - with ascites K70.31
- atrophic —*see* Cirrhosis, liver
- Baumgarten-Cruveilhier K74.69
- biliary (cholangiolitic) (cholangitic) (hypertrophic) (obstructive) (pericholangiolitic) K74.5
  - due to
    - Clonorchiasis B66.1
    - flukes B66.3
  - primary K74.3
  - secondary K74.4
- cardiac (of liver) K76.1
- Charcot's K74.3

C

Cirrhosis, cirrhotic *(Continued)*
cholangiolitic, cholangitic, cholostatic (primary) K74.3
congestive K76.1
Cruveilhier-Baumgarten K74.69
cryptogenic (liver) K74.69
due to
hepatolenticular degeneration E83.01
Wilson's disease E83.01
xanthomatosis E78.2
fatty K76.0
alcoholic K70.0
Hanot's (hypertrophic) K74.3
hepatic —*see* Cirrhosis, liver
hypertrophic K74.3
Indian childhood K74.69
kidney —*see* Sclerosis, renal
Laennec's K70.30
with ascites K70.31
alcoholic K70.30
with ascites K70.31
nonalcoholic K74.69
liver K74.60
alcoholic K70.30
with ascites K70.31
fatty K70.0
congenital P78.81
syphilitic A52.74
lung (chronic) J84.10
macronodular K74.69
alcoholic K70.30
with ascites K70.31
micronodular K74.69
alcoholic K70.30
with ascites K70.31
mixed type K74.69
monolobular K74.3
nephritis —*see* Sclerosis, renal
nutritional K74.69
alcoholic K70.30
with ascites K70.31
obstructive —*see* Cirrhosis, biliary
ovarian N83.8
pancreas (duct) K86.89 ⬅
pigmentary E83.110
portal K74.69
alcoholic K70.30
with ascites K70.31
postnecrotic K74.69
alcoholic K70.30
with ascites K70.31
pulmonary J84.10
renal —*see* Sclerosis, renal
spleen D73.2
stasis K76.1
Todd's K74.3
unilobar K74.3
xanthomatous (biliary) K74.5
due to xanthomatosis (familial) (metabolic) (primary) E78.2
Cistern, subarachnoid R93.0
Citrullinemia E72.23
Citrullinuria E72.23
Civatte's disease or poikiloderma L57.3
Clam digger's itch B65.3
Clammy skin R23.1
Clap —*see* Gonorrhea
Clarke-Hadfield syndrome (pancreatic infantilism) K86.89 ⬅
Clark's paralysis G80.9
Clastothrix L67.8
Claude Bernard-Horner syndrome G90.2
traumatic —*see* Injury, nerve, cervical sympathetic
Claude's disease or syndrome G46.3
Claudicatio venosa intermittens I87.8
~~Claudication, intermittent I73.9~~
~~cerebral (artery) G45.9~~
~~spinal cord (arteriosclerotic) G95.19~~
~~syphilitic A52.09~~
~~venous (axillary) I87.8~~
Claudication (intermittent) I73.9 ◀
cerebral (artery) G45.9 ◀
spinal cord (arteriosclerotic) G95.19 ◀
syphilitic A52.09 ◀
venous (axillary) I87.8 ◀
Claustrophobia F40.240
Clavus (infected) L84
Clawfoot (congenital) Q66.89
acquired —*see* Deformity, limb, clawfoot
Clawhand (acquired) —*see also* Deformity, limb, clawhand
congenital Q68.1
Clawtoe (congenital) Q66.89
acquired —*see* Deformity, toe, specified NEC
Clay eating —*see* Pica
Cleansing of artificial opening —*see* Attention to, artificial, opening
Cleft (congenital) —*see also* Imperfect, closure
alveolar process M26.79
branchial (cyst) (persistent) Q18.2
cricoid cartilage, posterior Q31.8
foot Q72.7 ◀
hand Q71.6 ◀
lip (unilateral) Q36.9
with cleft palate Q37.9
hard Q37.1
with soft Q37.5
soft Q37.3
with hard Q37.5
bilateral Q36.0
with cleft palate Q37.8
hard Q37.0
with soft Q37.4
soft Q37.2
with hard Q37.4
median Q36.1
nose Q30.2
palate Q35.9
with cleft lip (unilateral) Q37.9
bilateral Q37.8
hard Q35.1
with
cleft lip (unilateral) Q37.1
bilateral Q37.0
soft Q35.5
with cleft lip (unilateral) Q37.5
bilateral Q37.4
medial Q35.5
soft Q35.3
with
cleft lip (unilateral) Q37.3
bilateral Q37.2
hard Q35.5
with cleft lip (unilateral) Q37.5
bilateral Q37.4
penis Q55.69
scrotum Q55.29
thyroid cartilage Q31.8
uvula Q35.7
Cleidocranial dysostosis Q74.0
Cleptomania F63.2
Clicking hip (newborn) R29.4
Climacteric (female) —*see also* Menopause
arthritis (any site) NEC —*see* Arthritis, specified form NEC
depression (single episode) F32.89 ⬅
recurrent episode F33.8 ◀
male (symptoms) (syndrome) NEC N50.89 ⬅
melancholia (single episode) F32.89 ◀
recurrent episode F33.8 ◀
paranoid state F22
polyarthritis NEC —*see* Arthritis, specified form NEC
symptoms (female) N95.1
Clinical research investigation (clinical trial) (control subject) (normal comparison) (participant) Z00.6
Clitoris —*see* condition **Cloaca** (persistent) Q43.7
Clonorchiasis, clonorchis infection (liver) B66.1
Clonus R25.8
Closed bite M26.29
Clostridium (C.) **perfringens, as cause of disease classified elsewhere** B96.7
Closure
congenital, nose Q30.0
cranial sutures, premature Q75.0
defective or imperfect NEC —*see* Imperfect, closure
fistula, delayed —*see* Fistula
foramen ovale, imperfect Q21.1
hymen N89.6
interauricular septum, defective Q21.1
interventricular septum, defective Q21.0
lacrimal duct —*see also* Stenosis, lacrimal, duct
congenital Q10.5
nose (congenital) Q30.0
acquired M95.0
of artificial opening —*see* Attention to, artificial, opening
primary angle, without glaucoma damage H40.06-
vagina N89.5
valve —*see* Endocarditis
vulva N90.5
Clot (blood) —*see also* Embolism
artery (obstruction) (occlusion) —*see* Embolism
bladder N32.89
brain (intradural or extradural) —*see* Occlusion, artery, cerebral
circulation I74.9
heart —*see also* Infarct, myocardium
not resulting in infarction I51.3 ⬅
vein —*see* Thrombosis
Clouded state R40.1
epileptic —*see* Epilepsy, specified NEC
paroxysmal —*see* Epilepsy, specified NEC
Cloudy antrum, antra J32.0
Clouston's (hidrotic) **ectodermal dysplasia** Q82.4
Clubbed nail pachydermoperiostosis M89.40 *[L62]*
Clubbing of finger (s) (nails) R68.3
Clubfinger R68.3
congenital Q68.1
Clubfoot (congenital) Q66.89
acquired —*see* Deformity, limb, clubfoot
equinovarus Q66.0
paralytic —*see* Deformity, limb, clubfoot
Clubhand (congenital) (radial) Q71.4-
acquired —*see* Deformity, limb, clubhand
Clubnail R68.3
congenital Q84.6
Clump, kidney Q63.1
Clumsiness, clumsy child syndrome F82
Cluttering F98.81
Clutton's joints A50.51 *[M12.80]*
Coagulation, intravascular (diffuse) (disseminated) —*see also* Defibrination syndrome
complicating abortion —*see* Abortion, by type, complicated by, intravascular coagulation
following ectopic or molar pregnancy O08.1
Coagulopathy —*see also* Defect, coagulation
consumption D65
intravascular D65
newborn P60
Coalition
calcaneo-scaphoid Q66.89
tarsal Q66.89
Coalminer's
elbow —*see* Bursitis, elbow, olecranon
lung or pneumoconiosis J60
Coalworker's lung or pneumoconiosis J60
Coarctation
aorta (preductal) (postductal) Q25.1
pulmonary artery Q25.71
Coated tongue K14.3

◀ New ⬅ Revised ~~deleted~~ Deleted

Coats' disease (exudative retinopathy) *—see* Retinopathy, exudative
Cocaine-induced ◀
  anxiety disorder F14.98Ø ◀
  bipolar and related disorder F14.94 ◀
  depressive disorder F14.94 ◀
  obsessive-compulsive and related disorder F14.988 ◀
  psychotic disorder F14.959 ◀
  sleep disorder F14.982 ◀
  sexual dysfunction F14.981 ◀
Cocainism *—see* Disorder, cocaine use ⬅
Coccidioidomycosis B38.9
  cutaneous B38.3
  disseminated B38.7
  generalized B38.7
  meninges B38.4
  prostate B38.81
  pulmonary B38.2
    acute B38.Ø
    chronic B38.1
  skin B38.3
  specified NEC B38.89
Coccidioidosis *—see* Coccidioidomycosis
Coccidiosis (intestinal) AØ7.3
Coccydynia, coccygodynia M53.3
Coccyx *—see* condition
Cochin-China diarrhea K9Ø.1
Cockayne's syndrome Q87.1
Cocked up toe *—see* Deformity, toe, specified NEC
Cock's peculiar tumor L72.3
Codman's tumor *—see* Neoplasm, bone, benign
Coenurosis B71.8
Coffee-worker's lung J67.8
Cogan's syndrome H16.32-
  oculomotor apraxia H51.8
Coitus, painful (female) N94.1Ø ⬅
  male N53.12
  psychogenic F52.6
Cold JØØ
  with influenza, flu, or grippe *—see* Influenza, with, respiratory manifestations NEC
  agglutinin disease or hemoglobinuria (chronic) D59.1
  bronchial *—see* Bronchitis
  chest *—see* Bronchitis
  common (head) JØØ
  effects of T69.9
    specified effect NEC T69.8
  excessive, effects of T69.9
    specified effect NEC T69.8
  exhaustion from T69.8
  exposure to T69.9
    specified effect NEC T69.8
  head JØØ
  injury syndrome (newborn) P8Ø.Ø
  on lung *—see* Bronchitis
  rose J3Ø.1
  sensitivity, auto-immune D59.1
  virus JØØ
Coldsore BØØ.1
Colibacillosis A49.8
  as the cause of other disease (*see also* Escherichia coli) B96.2Ø
  generalized A41.5Ø
Colic (bilious) (infantile) (intestinal) (recurrent) (spasmodic) R1Ø.83
  abdomen R1Ø.83
    psychogenic F45.8
  appendix, appendicular K38.8
  bile duct *—see* Calculus, bile duct
  biliary *—see* Calculus, bile duct
  common duct *—see* Calculus, bile duct
  cystic duct *—see* Calculus, gallbladder
  Devonshire NEC *—see* Poisoning, lead
  gallbladder *—see* Calculus, gallbladder
  gallstone *—see* Calculus, gallbladder
    gallbladder or cystic duct *—see* Calculus, gallbladder

Colic *(Continued)*
  hepatic (duct) *—see* Calculus, bile duct
  hysterical F45.8
  kidney N23
  lead NEC *—see* Poisoning, lead
  mucous K58.9
    with diarrhea K58.Ø
    psychogenic F54
  nephritic N23
  painter's NEC *—see* Poisoning, lead
  pancreas K86.89 ⬅
  psychogenic F45.8
  renal N23
  saturnine NEC *—see* Poisoning, lead
  ureter N23
  urethral N36.8
    due to calculus N21.1
  uterus NEC N94.89
    menstrual *—see* Dysmenorrhea
  worm NOS B83.9
Colicystitis *—see* Cystitis
Colitis (acute) (catarrhal) (chronic) (noninfective) (hemorrhagic) (*see also* Enteritis) K52.9
  allergic K52.29 ⬅
    with ◀
      food protein-induced enterocolitis syndrome K52.21 ◀
      proctocolitis K52.82 ◀
  amebic (acute) *—see also* Amebiasis AØ6.Ø
    nondysenteric AØ6.2
  anthrax A22.2
  bacillary *—see* Infection, Shigella
  balantidial AØ7.Ø
  Clostridium difficile AØ4.7
  coccidial AØ7.3
  collagenous K52.831 ⬅
  cystica superficialis K52.89
  dietary counseling and surveillance (for) Z71.3
  dietetic *—see also* Colitis, allergic K52.29 ⬅
  drug-induced K52.1
  due to radiation K52.Ø
  eosinophilic K52.82
  food hypersensitivity *—see also* Colitis, allergic K52.29 ⬅
  giardial AØ7.1
  granulomatous *—see* Enteritis, regional, large intestine
  infectious *—see* Enteritis, infectious
  indeterminate, so stated K52.3 ◀
  ischemic K55.9
    acute (subacute) *—see also* Ischemia, intestine, acute K55.Ø39 ⬅
    chronic K55.1
    due to mesenteric artery insufficiency K55.1
    fulminant (acute) *—see also* Ischemia, intestine, acute K55.Ø39 ⬅
  left sided K51.5Ø
    with
      abscess K51.514
      complication K51.519
        specified NEC K51.518
      fistula K51.513
      obstruction K51.512
      rectal bleeding K51.511
  lymphocytic K52.832 ⬅
  membranous
    psychogenic F54
  microscopic K52.839 ⬅
    specified NEC K52.838 ◀
  mucous *—see* Syndrome, irritable, bowel
    psychogenic F54
  noninfective K52.9
    specified NEC K52.89
  polyposa *—see* Polyp, colon, inflammatory
  protozoal AØ7.9
  pseudomembranous AØ4.7
  pseudomucinous *—see* Syndrome, irritable, bowel

Colitis *(Continued)*
  regional *—see* Enteritis, regional, large intestine
  segmental *—see* Enteritis, regional, large intestine
  septic *—see* Enteritis, infectious
  spastic K58.9
    with diarrhea K58.Ø
    psychogenic F54
  staphylococcal AØ4.8
    foodborne AØ5.Ø
  subacute ischemic *—see also* Ischemia, intestine, acute K55.Ø39 ⬅
  thromboulcerative *—see also* Ischemia, intestine, acute K55.Ø39 ⬅
  toxic NEC K52.1
    due to Clostridium difficile AØ4.7
  transmural *—see* Enteritis, regional, large intestine
  trichomonal AØ7.8
  tuberculous (ulcerative) A18.32
  ulcerative (chronic) K51.9Ø
    with
      complication K51.919
        abscess K51.914
        fistula K51.913
        obstruction K51.912
        rectal bleeding K51.911
        specified complication NEC K51.918
    enterocolitis *—see* Enterocolitis, ulcerative
    ileocolitis *—see* Ileocolitis, ulcerative
    mucosal proctocolitis *—see* Proctocolitis, mucosal
    proctitis *—see* Proctitis, ulcerative
    pseudopolyposis *—see* Polyp, colon, inflammatory
    psychogenic F54
    rectosigmoiditis *—see* Rectosigmoiditis, ulcerative
    specified type NEC K51.8Ø
      with
        complication K51.819
          abscess K51.814
          fistula K51.813
          obstruction K51.812
          rectal bleeding K51.811
          specified complication NEC K51.818
Collagenosis, collagen disease (nonvascular) (vascular) M35.9
  cardiovascular I42.8
  reactive perforating L87.1
  specified NEC M35.8
Collapse R55
  adrenal E27.2
  cardiorespiratory R57.Ø
  cardiovascular R57.Ø
    newborn P29.89
  circulatory (peripheral) R57.9
    during or after labor and delivery O75.1
    following ectopic or molar pregnancy OØ8.3
    newborn P29.89
  during or
    after labor and delivery O75.1
    resulting from a procedure, not elsewhere classified T81.1Ø
  external ear canal *—see* Stenosis, external ear canal
  general R55
  heart *—see* Disease, heart
  heat T67.1
  hysterical F44.89
  labyrinth, membranous (congenital) Q16.5
  lung (massive) *—see also* Atelectasis J98.19
    pressure due to anesthesia (general) (local) or other sedation T88.2
      during labor and delivery O74.1
      in pregnancy O29.Ø2-
      postpartum, puerperal O89.Ø9
  myocardial *—see* Disease, heart

Collapse *(Continued)*
- nervous F48.8
- neurocirculatory F45.8
- nose M95.0
- postoperative T81.10
- pulmonary —*see also* Atelectasis J98.19
  - newborn —*see* Atelectasis
- trachea J39.8
- tracheobronchial J98.09
- valvular —*see* Endocarditis
- vascular (peripheral) R57.9
  - during or after labor and delivery O75.1
  - following ectopic or molar pregnancy O08.3
  - newborn P29.89
- vertebra M48.50-
  - cervical region M48.52-
  - cervicothoracic region M48.53-
  - in (due to)
    - metastasis —*see* Collapse, vertebra, in, specified disease NEC
    - osteoporosis —*see also* Osteoporosis M80.88
      - cervical region M80.88
      - cervicothoracic region M80.88
      - lumbar region M80.88
      - lumbosacral region M80.88
      - multiple sites M80.88
      - occipito-atlanto-axial region M80.88
      - sacrococcygeal region M80.88
      - thoracic region M80.88
      - thoracolumbar region M80.88
    - specified disease NEC M48.50-
      - cervical region M48.52-
      - cervicothoracic region M48.53-
      - lumbar region M48.56-
      - lumbosacral region M48.57-
      - occipito-atlanto-axial region M48.51-
      - sacrococcygeal region M48.58-
      - thoracic region M48.54-
      - thoracolumbar region M48.55-
  - lumbar region M48.56-
  - lumbosacral region M48.57-
  - occipito-atlanto-axial region M48.51-
  - sacrococcygeal region M48.58-
  - thoracic region M48.54-
  - thoracolumbar region M48.55-

Collateral —*see also* condition
- circulation (venous) I87.8
- dilation, veins I87.8

Colles' fracture S52.53-
Collet (-Sicard) **syndrome** G52.7
Collier's asthma or lung J60
Collodion baby Q80.2
Colloid nodule (of thyroid) (cystic) E04.1
Coloboma (iris) Q13.0
- eyelid Q10.3
- fundus Q14.8
- lens Q12.2
- optic disc (congenital) Q14.2
  - acquired H47.31-

Coloenteritis —*see* Enteritis
Colon —*see* condition
Colonization
- MRSA (Methicillin resistant Staphylococcus aureus) Z22.322
- MSSA (Methicillin susceptible Staphylococcus aureus) Z22.321
- status —*see* Carrier (suspected) of

Coloptosis K63.4
Color blindness —*see* Deficiency, color vision
Colostomy
- attention to Z43.3
- fitting or adjustment Z46.89
- malfunctioning K94.03
- status Z93.3

Colpitis (acute) —*see* Vaginitis
Colpocele N81.5
Colpocystitis —*see* Vaginitis
Colpospasm N94.2
Column, spinal, vertebral —*see* condition

Coma R40.20
- with
  - motor response (none) R40.231
    - abnormal R40.233
    - extension R40.232
    - flexion withdrawal R40.234
  - motor response (none) *(Continued)*
    - localizes pain R40.235
    - obeys commands R40.236
  - opening of eyes (never) R40.211
    - in response to
      - pain R40.212
      - sound R40.213
    - spontaneous R40.214
  - verbal response (none) R40.221
    - confused conversation R40.224
    - inappropriate words R40.223
    - incomprehensible words R40.222
    - oriented R40.225
- eclamptic —*see* Eclampsia
- epileptic —*see* Epilepsy
- Glasgow, scale score —*see* Glasgow coma scale
- hepatic —*see* Failure, hepatic, by type, with coma
- hyperglycemic (diabetic) —*see* Diabetes, by type, with hyperosmolarity, with coma
- hyperosmolar (diabetic) —*see* Diabetes, by type, with hyperosmolarity, with coma
- hypoglycemic (diabetic) —*see* Diabetes, by type, with hypoglycemia, with coma
  - nondiabetic E15
- in diabetes —*see* Diabetes, coma
- insulin-induced —*see* Coma, hypoglycemic
- myxedematous E03.5
- newborn P91.5
- persistent vegetative state R40.3
- specified NEC, without documented Glasgow coma scale score, or with partial Glasgow coma scale score reported R40.244

Comatose —*see* Coma
Combat fatigue F43.0
Combined —*see* condition
Comedo, comedones (giant) L70.0
Comedocarcinoma —*see also* Neoplasm, breast, malignant
- noninfiltrating
  - breast D05.8-
  - specified site —*see* Neoplasm, in situ, by site
  - unspecified site D05.8-

Comedomastitis —*see* Ectasia, mammary duct
Comminuted fracture - code as Fracture, closed
Common
- arterial trunk Q20.0
- atrioventricular canal Q21.2
- atrium Q21.1
- cold (head) J00
- truncus (arteriosus) Q20.0
- variable immunodeficiency —*see* Immunodeficiency, common variable
- ventricle Q20.4

Commotio, commotion (current)
- brain —*see* Injury, intracranial, concussion
- cerebri —*see* Injury, intracranial, concussion
- retinae S05.8X-
- spinal cord —*see* Injury, spinal cord, by region
- spinalis —*see* Injury, spinal cord, by region

Communication
- between
  - base of aorta and pulmonary artery Q21.4
  - left ventricle and right atrium Q20.5
  - pericardial sac and pleural sac Q34.8
  - pulmonary artery and pulmonary vein, congenital Q25.72
- congenital between uterus and digestive or urinary tract Q51.7

Compartment syndrome (deep) (posterior) (traumatic) T79.A0
- abdomen T79.A3
- lower extremity (hip, buttock, thigh, leg, foot, toes) T79.A2
- nontraumatic
  - abdomen M79.A3
  - lower extremity (hip, buttock, thigh, leg, foot, toes) M79.A2-
  - specified site NEC M79.A9
  - upper extremity (shoulder, arm, forearm, wrist, hand, fingers) M79.A1-
- specified site NEC T79.A9
- upper extremity (shoulder, arm, forearm, wrist, hand, fingers) T79.A1

Compensation
- failure —*see* Disease, heart
- neurosis, psychoneurosis —*see* Disorder, factitious

Complaint —*see also* Disease
- bowel, functional K59.9
  - psychogenic F45.8
- intestine, functional K59.9
  - psychogenic F45.8
- kidney —*see* Disease, renal
- miners' J60

Complete —*see* condition
Complex
- Addison-Schilder E71.528
- cardiorenal —*see* Hypertension, cardiorenal
- Costen's M26.69
- disseminated mycobacterium avium-intracellulare (DMAC) A31.2
- Eisenmenger's (ventricular septal defect) I27.89
- hypersexual F52.8
- jumped process, spine —*see* Dislocation, vertebra
- primary, tuberculous A15.7
- Schilder-Addison E71.528
- subluxation (vertebral) M99.19
  - abdomen M99.19
  - acromioclavicular M99.17
  - cervical region M99.11
  - cervicothoracic M99.11
  - costochondral M99.18
  - costovertebral M99.18
  - head region M99.10
  - hip M99.15
  - lower extremity M99.16
  - lumbar region M99.13
  - lumbosacral M99.13
  - occipitocervical M99.10
  - pelvic region M99.15
  - pubic M99.15
  - rib cage M99.18
  - sacral region M99.14
  - sacrococcygeal M99.14
  - sacroiliac M99.14
  - specified NEC M99.19
  - sternochondral M99.18
  - sternoclavicular M99.17
  - thoracic region M99.12
  - thoracolumbar M99.12
  - upper extremity M99.17
- Taussig-Bing (transposition, aorta and overriding pulmonary artery) Q20.1

Complication (s) (from) (of)
- accidental puncture or laceration during a procedure (of) —*see* Complications, intraoperative (intraprocedural), puncture or laceration
- amputation stump (surgical) (late) NEC T87.9
  - dehiscence T87.81
  - infection or inflammation T87.40
    - lower limb T87.4-
    - upper limb T87.4-
  - necrosis T87.50
    - lower limb T87.5-
    - upper limb T87.5-

◄ New ⟸ Revised ~~deleted~~ Deleted

C

- **Complication** *(Continued)*
  - amputation stump (surgical) (late) (NEC) *(Continued)*
    - neuroma T87.3Ø
      - lower limb T87.3-
      - upper limb T87.3-
    - specified type NEC T87.89
  - anastomosis (and bypass) —*see also* Complications, prosthetic device or implant
    - intestinal (internal) NEC K91.89
      - involving urinary tract N99.89
    - urinary tract (involving intestinal tract) N99.89
    - vascular —*see* Complications, cardiovascular device or implant
  - anesthesia, anesthetic —*see also* Anesthesia, complication T88.59
    - brain, postpartum, puerperal O89.2
    - cardiac
      - in
        - labor and delivery O74.2
        - pregnancy O29.19-
      - postpartum, puerperal O89.1
    - central nervous system
      - in
        - labor and delivery O74.3
        - pregnancy O29.29-
      - postpartum, puerperal O89.2
    - difficult or failed intubation T88.4
      - in pregnancy O29.6-
    - failed sedation (conscious) (moderate) during procedure T88.52
    - general, unintended awareness during procedure T88.53 ◀
    - hyperthermia, malignant T88.3
    - hypothermia T88.51
    - intubation failure T88.4
    - malignant hyperthermia T88.3
    - pulmonary
      - in
        - labor and delivery O74.1
        - pregnancy NEC O29.Ø9-
      - postpartum, puerperal O89.Ø9
    - shock T88.2
    - spinal and epidural
      - in
        - labor and delivery NEC O74.6
          - headache O74.5
        - pregnancy NEC O29.5X-
      - postpartum, puerperal NEC O89.5
        - headache O89.4
    - unintended awareness under general anesthesia during procedure T88.53 ◀
  - anti-reflux device —*see* Complications, esophageal anti-reflux device
  - aortic (bifurcation) graft —*see* Complications, graft, vascular
  - aortocoronary (bypass) graft —*see* Complications, coronary artery (bypass) graft
  - aortofemoral (bypass) graft —*see* Complications, extremity artery (bypass) graft
  - arteriovenous
    - fistula, surgically created T82.9
      - embolism T82.818
      - fibrosis T82.828
      - hemorrhage T82.838
      - infection or inflammation T82.7
      - mechanical
        - breakdown T82.51Ø
        - displacement T82.52Ø
        - leakage T82.53Ø
        - malposition T82.52Ø
        - obstruction T82.59Ø
        - perforation T82.59Ø
        - protrusion T82.59Ø
      - pain T82.848
      - specified type NEC T82.898
      - stenosis T82.858
      - thrombosis T82.868

- **Complication** *(Continued)*
  - arteriovenous *(Continued)*
    - shunt, surgically created T82.9
      - embolism T82.818
      - fibrosis T82.828
      - hemorrhage T82.838
      - infection or inflammation T82.7
      - mechanical
        - breakdown T82.511
        - displacement T82.521
        - leakage T82.531
        - malposition T82.521
        - obstruction T82.591
        - perforation T82.591
        - protrusion T82.591
      - pain T82.848
      - specified type NEC T82.898
      - stenosis T82.858
      - thrombosis T82.868
  - arthroplasty —*see* Complications, joint prosthesis
  - artificial
    - fertilization or insemination N98.9
      - attempted introduction (of)
        - embryo in embryo transfer N98.3
        - ovum following in vitro fertilization N98.2
      - hyperstimulation of ovaries N98.1
      - infection N98.Ø
      - specified NEC N98.8
    - heart T82.9
      - embolism T82.817
      - fibrosis T82.827
      - hemorrhage T82.837
      - infection or inflammation T82.7
      - mechanical
        - breakdown T82.512
        - displacement T82.522
        - leakage T82.532
        - malposition T82.522
        - obstruction T82.592
        - perforation T82.592
        - protrusion T82.592
      - pain T82.847
      - specified type NEC T82.897
      - stenosis T82.857
      - thrombosis T82.867
    - opening
      - cecostomy —*see* Complications, colostomy
      - colostomy —*see* Complications, colostomy
      - cystostomy —*see* Complications, cystostomy
      - enterostomy —*see* Complications, enterostomy
      - gastrostomy —*see* Complications, gastrostomy
      - ileostomy —*see* Complications, enterostomy
      - jejunostomy —*see* Complications, enterostomy
      - nephrostomy —*see* Complications, stoma, urinary tract
      - tracheostomy —*see* Complications, tracheostomy
      - ureterostomy —*see* Complications, stoma, urinary tract
      - urethrostomy —*see* Complications, stoma, urinary tract
  - balloon implant or device
    - gastrointestinal T85.9
      - embolism T85.818 ⬅
      - fibrosis T85.828 ⬅
      - hemorrhage T85.838 ⬅
      - infection and inflammation T85.79
      - pain T85.848 ⬅
      - specified type NEC T85.898 ⬅
      - stenosis T85.858 ⬅
      - thrombosis T85.868 ⬅

- **Complication** *(Continued)*
  - balloon implant or device *(Continued)*
    - vascular (counterpulsation) T82.9
      - embolism T82.818
      - fibrosis T82.828
      - hemorrhage T82.838
      - infection or inflammation T82.7
      - mechanical
        - breakdown T82.513
        - displacement T82.523
        - leakage T82.533
        - malposition T82.523
        - obstruction T82.593
        - perforation T82.593
        - protrusion T82.593
      - pain T82.848
      - specified type NEC T82.898
      - stenosis T82.858
      - thrombosis T82.868
  - bariatric procedure
    - gastric band procedure K95.Ø9
      - infection K95.Ø1
    - specified procedure NEC K95.89
      - infection K95.81
  - bile duct implant (prosthetic) T85.9
    - embolism T85.818 ⬅
    - fibrosis T85.828 ⬅
    - hemorrhage T85.838 ⬅
    - infection and inflammation T85.79
    - mechanical
      - breakdown T85.51Ø
      - displacement T85.52Ø
      - malfunction T85.51Ø
      - malposition T85.52Ø
      - obstruction T85.59Ø
      - perforation T85.59Ø
      - protrusion T85.59Ø
      - specified NEC T85.59Ø
    - pain T85.848 ⬅
    - specified type NEC T85.898 ⬅
    - stenosis T85.858 ⬅
    - thrombosis T85.868 ⬅
  - bladder device (auxiliary) —*see* Complications, genitourinary, device or implant, urinary system
  - bleeding (postoperative) —*see* Complication, postoperative, hemorrhage
    - intraoperative —*see* Complication, intraoperative, hemorrhage
  - blood vessel graft —*see* Complications, graft, vascular
  - bone
    - device NEC T84.9
      - embolism T84.81
      - fibrosis T84.82
      - hemorrhage T84.83
      - infection or inflammation T84.7
      - mechanical
        - breakdown T84.318
        - displacement T84.328
        - malposition T84.328
        - obstruction T84.398
        - perforation T84.398
        - protrusion T84.398
      - pain T84.84
      - specified type NEC T84.89
      - stenosis T84.85
      - thrombosis T84.86
    - graft —*see* Complications, graft, bone
    - growth stimulator (electrode) —*see* Complications, electronic stimulator device, bone
    - marrow transplant —*see* Complications, transplant, bone, marrow
  - brain neurostimulator (electrode) —*see* Complications, electronic stimulator device, brain
  - breast implant (prosthetic) T85.9
    - capsular contracture T85.44
    - embolism T85.818 ⬅
    - fibrosis T85.828 ⬅

- **Complication** *(Continued)*
  - catheter NEC *(Continued)*
    - intraperitoneal dialysis *(Continued)*
      - hemorrhage T85.838 ⟸
      - infection and inflammation T85.71
      - mechanical
        - breakdown T85.611
        - displacement T85.621
        - leakage T85.631
        - malfunction T85.611
        - malposition T85.621
        - obstruction T85.691
        - perforation T85.691
        - protrusion T85.691
        - specified NEC T85.691
      - pain T85.848 ⟸
      - specified type NEC T85.898 ⟸
      - stenosis T85.858 ⟸
      - thrombosis T85.868 ⟸
    - intrathecal infusion ◀
      - infection and inflammation T85.735 ◀
      - mechanical ◀
        - breakdown T85.610 ◀
        - displacement T85.620 ◀
        - leakage T85.630 ◀
        - malfunction T85.690 ◀
        - malposition T85.620 ◀
        - obstruction T85.690 ◀
        - perforation T85.690 ◀
        - protrusion T85.690 ◀
        - specified NEC T85.690 ◀
    - intravenous infusion T82.9
      - embolism T82.818
      - fibrosis T82.828
      - hemorrhage T82.838
      - infection or inflammation T82.7
      - mechanical
        - breakdown T82.514
        - displacement T82.524
        - leakage T82.534
        - malposition T82.524
        - obstruction T82.594
        - perforation T82.594
        - protrusion T82.594
      - pain T82.848
      - specified type NEC T82.898
      - stenosis T82.858
      - thrombosis T82.868
    - spinal infusion ◀
      - infection and inflammation T85.735 ◀
      - mechanical ◀
        - breakdown T85.610 ◀
        - displacement T85.620 ◀
        - leakage T85.630 ◀
        - malfunction T85.690 ◀
        - malposition T85.620 ◀
        - obstruction T85.690 ◀
        - perforation T85.690 ◀
        - protrusion T85.690 ◀
        - specified NEC T85.690 ◀
    - subarachnoid infusion ◀
      - infection and inflammation T85.735 ◀
      - mechanical ◀
        - breakdown T85.610 ◀
        - displacement T85.620 ◀
        - leakage T85.630 ◀
        - malfunction T85.690 ◀
        - malposition T85.620 ◀
        - obstruction T85.690 ◀
        - perforation T85.690 ◀
        - protrusion T85.690 ◀
        - specified NEC T85.690 ◀
    - subdural infusion T85.9
      - embolism T85.810 ⟸
      - fibrosis T85.820 ⟸
      - hemorrhage T85.830 ⟸
      - infection and inflammation T85.735 ⟸
      - mechanical
        - breakdown T85.610
        - displacement T85.620
        - leakage T85.630

- **Complication** *(Continued)*
  - catheter NEC *(Continued)*
    - subdural infusion *(Continued)*
      - mechanical *(Continued)*
        - malfunction T85.610
        - malposition T85.620
        - obstruction T85.690
        - perforation T85.690
        - protrusion T85.690
        - specified NEC T85.690
      - pain T85.840 ⟸
      - specified type NEC T85.890 ⟸
      - stenosis T85.850 ⟸
      - thrombosis T85.860 ⟸
    - ~~urethral, indwelling T83.9~~
      - ~~displacement T83.028~~
      - ~~embolism T83.81~~
      - ~~fibrosis T83.82~~
      - ~~hemorrhage T83.83~~
      - ~~infection and inflammation T83.51~~
      - ~~leakage T83.038~~
      - ~~malposition T83.028~~
      - ~~mechanical~~
        - ~~breakdown T83.018~~
      - ~~obstruction (mechanical) T83.098~~
      - ~~pain T83.84~~
      - ~~perforation T83.098~~
      - ~~protrusion T83.098~~
      - ~~specified type NEC T83.098~~
      - ~~stenosis T83.85~~
      - ~~thrombosis T83.86~~
    - ~~urinary (indwelling) —*see* Complications, catheter, urethral, indwelling~~
    - urethral T83.9 ◀
      - displacement T83.028 ◀
      - embolism T83.81 ◀
      - fibrosis T83.82 ◀
      - hemorrhage T83.83 ◀
      - indwelling ◀
        - breakdown T83.011 ◀
        - displacement T83.021 ◀
        - infection and inflammation T83.511 ◀
        - leakage T83.031 ◀
        - specified complication NEC T83.091 ◀
      - infection and inflammation T83.511 ◀
      - leakage T83.038 ◀
      - malposition T83.028 ◀
      - mechanical ◀
        - breakdown T83.011 ◀
      - obstruction (mechanical) T83.091 ◀
      - pain T83.84 ◀
      - perforation T83.091 ◀
      - protrusion T83.091 ◀
      - specified type NEC T83.091 ◀
      - stenosis T83.85 ◀
      - thrombosis T83.86 ◀
    - urinary NEC ◀
      - breakdown T83.018 ◀
      - displacement T83.028 ◀
      - infection and inflammation T83.518 ◀
      - leakage T83.038 ◀
      - specified complication NEC T83.098 ◀
  - cecostomy (stoma) —*see* Complications, colostomy
  - cesarean delivery wound NEC O90.89
    - disruption O90.0
    - hematoma O90.2
    - infection (following delivery) O86.0
  - chemotherapy (antineoplastic) NEC T88.7
  - chin implant (prosthetic) —*see* Complication, prosthetic device or implant, specified NEC
  - circulatory system I99.8
    - intraoperative I97.88
    - postprocedural I97.89
      - following cardiac surgery I97.19-
        - postcardiotomy syndrome I97.0
      - hypertension I97.3
      - lymphedema after mastectomy I97.2
      - postcardiotomy syndrome I97.0
      - specified NEC I97.89

- **Complication** *(Continued)*
  - colostomy (stoma) K94.00
    - hemorrhage K94.01
    - infection K94.02
    - malfunction K94.03
    - mechanical K94.03
    - specified complication NEC K94.09
  - contraceptive device, intrauterine —*see* Complications, intrauterine, contraceptive device
  - cord (umbilical) —*see* Complications, umbilical cord
  - corneal graft —*see* Complications, graft, cornea
  - coronary artery (bypass) graft T82.9
    - atherosclerosis —*see* Arteriosclerosis, coronary (artery)
    - embolism T82.818
    - fibrosis T82.828
    - hemorrhage T82.838
    - infection and inflammation T82.7
    - mechanical
      - breakdown T82.211
      - displacement T82.212
      - leakage T82.213
      - malposition T82.212
      - obstruction T82.218
      - perforation T82.218
      - protrusion T82.218
      - specified NEC T82.218
    - pain T82.848
    - specified type NEC T82.898 ⟸
    - stenosis T82.858
    - thrombosis T82.868
  - counterpulsation device (balloon), intra-aortic —*see* Complications, balloon implant, vascular
  - cystostomy (stoma) N99.518
    - catheter —*see* Complications, catheter, cystostomy
    - hemorrhage N99.510
    - infection N99.511
    - malfunction N99.512
    - specified type NEC N99.518
  - delivery —*see also* Complications, obstetric O75.9
    - procedure (instrumental) (manual) (surgical) O75.4
    - specified NEC O75.89
  - dialysis (peritoneal) (renal) —*see also* Complications, infusion
    - catheter (vascular) —*see* Complication, catheter, dialysis
      - peritoneal, intraperitoneal —*see* Complications, catheter, intraperitoneal
  - dorsal column (spinal) neurostimulator —*see* Complications, electronic stimulator device, spinal cord
  - drug NEC T88.7
  - ear procedure —*see also* Disorder, ear
    - intraoperative H95.88-
      - hematoma —*see* Complications, intraoperative, hematoma (of), ear ⟸
      - hemorrhage —*see* Complications, intraoperative, hemorrhage (of), ear ⟸
      - laceration —*see* Complications, intraoperative, puncture or laceration..., ear
      - seroma —*see* Complications, postprocedural, seroma (of), mastoid process ◀
      - specified NEC H95.88-
    - postoperative H95.89-
      - external ear canal stenosis H95.81-
      - hematoma —*see* Complications, postprocedural, hemorrhage (hematoma) (of), ear

◀ New ⟸ Revised ~~deleted~~ Deleted

C

New ◄ Revised ◄ ~~deleted~~ Deleted

- **Complication** *(Continued)*
  - genitourinary *(Continued)*
    - device or implant *(Continued)*
      - urinary system *(Continued)*
        - electronic stimulator —*see* Complications, electronic stimulator device, urinary
        - indwelling urethral catheter —*see* Complications, catheter, urethral, indwelling
        - infection or inflammation T83.598 ⬅
          - ~~indwelling urinary catheter T83.51~~
          - indwelling urethral catheter T83.511 ◀
        - kidney transplant —*see* Complication, transplant, kidney
        - organ graft —*see* Complication, graft, urinary organ
        - specified type NEC T83.89
          - embolism T83.81
          - fibrosis T83.82
          - hemorrhage T83.83
          - mechanical T83.198
            - breakdown T83.118
            - displacement T83.128
            - malfunction T83.118
            - malposition T83.128
            - obstruction T83.198
            - perforation T83.198
            - protrusion T83.198
            - specified NEC T83.198
        - sphincter, implanted T83.191 ◀
        - stent (ileal conduit) (nephroureteral) T83.193 ◀
          - ureteral indwelling T83.192 ◀
          - pain T83.84
          - specified complication NEC T83.89
          - stenosis T83.85
          - thrombosis T83.86
        - sphincter implant —*see* Complications, implant, urinary sphincter
    - postprocedural
      - pelvic peritoneal adhesions N99.4
      - renal failure N99.0
      - specified NEC N99.89
      - stoma —*see* Complications, stoma, urinary tract
      - urethral stricture —*see* Stricture, urethra, postprocedural
      - vaginal
        - adhesions N99.2
        - vault prolapse N99.3
  - graft (bypass) (patch) —*see also* Complications, prosthetic device or implant
    - aorta —*see* Complications, graft, vascular
    - arterial —*see* Complication, graft, vascular
    - bone T86.839
      - failure T86.831
      - infection T86.832
      - mechanical T84.318
        - breakdown T84.318
        - displacement T84.328
        - protrusion T84.398
        - specified type NEC T84.398
      - rejection T86.830
      - specified type NEC T86.838
    - carotid artery —*see* Complications, graft, vascular
    - cornea T86.849
      - failure T86.841
      - infection T86.842
      - mechanical T85.398
        - breakdown T85.318
        - displacement T85.328
        - protrusion T85.398
        - specified type NEC T85.398
      - rejection T86.840
      - retroprosthetic membrane T85.398
      - specified type NEC T86.848

- **Complication** *(Continued)*
  - graft *(Continued)*
    - femoral artery (bypass) —*see* Complication, extremity artery (bypass) graft
    - genital organ or tract —*see* Complications, genitourinary, device or implant, genital tract
    - muscle T84.9
      - breakdown T84.410
      - displacement T84.420
      - embolism T84.81
      - fibrosis T84.82
      - hemorrhage T84.83
      - infection and inflammation T84.7
      - mechanical NEC T84.490
      - pain T84.84
      - specified type NEC T84.89
      - stenosis T84.85
      - thrombosis T84.86
    - nerve —*see* Complication, prosthetic device or implant, specified NEC
    - skin —*see* Complications, prosthetic device or implant, skin graft
    - tendon T84.9
      - breakdown T84.410
      - displacement T84.420
      - embolism T84.81
      - fibrosis T84.82
      - hemorrhage T84.83
      - infection and inflammation T84.7
      - mechanical NEC T84.490
      - pain T84.84
      - specified type NEC T84.89
      - stenosis T84.85
      - thrombosis T84.86
    - urinary organ T83.9
      - embolism T83.81
      - fibrosis T83.82
      - hemorrhage T83.83
      - infection and inflammation T83.598 ⬅
        - indwelling urethral catheter T83.511 ⬅
      - mechanical
        - breakdown T83.21
        - displacement T83.22
        - erosion T83.24 ◀
        - exposure T83.25 ◀
        - leakage T83.23
        - malposition T83.22
        - obstruction T83.29
        - perforation T83.29
        - protrusion T83.29
        - specified NEC T83.29
      - pain T83.84
      - specified type NEC T83.89
      - stenosis T83.85
      - thrombosis T83.86
    - vascular T82.9
      - embolism T82.818
      - femoral artery —*see* Complication, extremity artery (bypass) graft
      - fibrosis T82.828
      - hemorrhage T82.838
      - mechanical
        - breakdown T82.319
          - aorta (bifurcation) T82.310
          - carotid artery T82.311
          - specified vessel NEC T82.318
        - displacement T82.329
          - aorta (bifurcation) T82.320
          - carotid artery T82.321
          - specified vessel NEC T82.328
        - leakage T82.339
          - aorta (bifurcation) T82.330
          - carotid artery T82.331
          - specified vessel NEC T82.338
        - malposition T82.329
          - aorta (bifurcation) T82.320
          - carotid artery T82.321
          - specified vessel NEC T82.328

- **Complication** *(Continued)*
  - graft *(Continued)*
    - vascular *(Continued)*
      - mechanical *(Continued)*
        - obstruction T82.399
          - aorta (bifurcation) T82.390
          - carotid artery T82.391
          - specified vessel NEC T82.398
        - perforation T82.399
          - aorta (bifurcation) T82.390
          - carotid artery T82.391
          - specified vessel NEC T82.398
        - protrusion T82.399
          - aorta (bifurcation) T82.390
          - carotid artery T82.391
          - specified vessel NEC T82.398
      - pain T82.848
      - specified complication NEC T82.898
      - stenosis T82.858
      - thrombosis T82.868
  - heart I51.9
    - assist device
      - infection and inflammation T82.7
    - following acute myocardial infarction —*see* Complications, following, acute myocardial infarction
    - postoperative—*see* Complications, circulatory system
    - transplant —*see* Complication, transplant, heart
      - and lung (s) —*see* Complications, transplant, heart, with lung
    - valve
      - graft (biological) T82.9
        - embolism T82.817
        - fibrosis T82.827
        - hemorrhage T82.837
        - infection and inflammation T82.7
        - mechanical T82.228
          - breakdown T82.221
          - displacement T82.222
          - leakage T82.223
          - malposition T82.222
          - obstruction T82.228
          - perforation T82.228
          - protrusion T82.228
        - pain T82.847
        - specified type NEC T82.897
        - stenosis T82.857
        - thrombosis T82.867
      - prosthesis T82.9
        - embolism T82.817
        - fibrosis T82.827
        - hemorrhage T82.837
        - infection or inflammation T82.6
        - mechanical T82.09
          - breakdown T82.01
          - displacement T82.02
          - leakage T82.03
          - malposition T82.02
          - obstruction T82.09
          - perforation T82.09
          - protrusion T82.09
        - pain T82.847
        - specified type NEC T82.897
          - mechanical T82.09
        - stenosis T82.857
        - thrombosis T82.867
  - hematoma
    - intraoperative —*see* Complication, intraoperative, hemorrhage
    - postprocedural —*see* Complication, postprocedural, hematoma ⬅
  - hemodialysis —*see* Complications, dialysis
  - hemorrhage
    - intraoperative —*see* Complication, intraoperative, hemorrhage
    - postprocedural —*see* Complication, postprocedural, hemorrhage

Complication *(Continued)*
- ileostomy (stoma) —*see* Complications, enterostomy
- immunization (procedure) —*see* Complications, vaccination
- implant —*see also* Complications, by site and type
  - urinary sphincter T83.9
    - embolism T83.81
    - fibrosis T83.82
    - hemorrhage T83.83
    - infection and inflammation T83.591 ⬅
    - mechanical
      - breakdown T83.111
      - displacement T83.121
      - leakage T83.191
      - malposition T83.121
      - obstruction T83.191
      - perforation T83.191
      - protrusion T83.191
      - specified NEC T83.191
    - pain T83.84
    - specified type NEC T83.89
    - stenosis T83.85
    - thrombosis T83.86
- infusion (procedure) T8Ø.9Ø
  - air embolism T8Ø.Ø
  - blood —*see* Complications, transfusion
  - catheter —*see* Complications, catheter
  - infection T8Ø.29
  - pump —*see* Complications, cardiovascular, device or implant
  - sepsis T8Ø.29
  - serum reaction —*see also* Reaction, serum T8Ø.69
    - anaphylactic shock —*see also* Shock, anaphylactic T8Ø.59
  - specified type NEC T8Ø.89
- inhalation therapy NEC T81.81
- injection (procedure) T8Ø.9Ø
  - drug reaction —*see* Reaction, drug
  - infection T8Ø.29
  - sepsis T8Ø.29
  - serum (prophylactic) (therapeutic) —*see* Complications, vaccination
  - specified type NEC T8Ø.89
  - vaccine (any) —*see* Complications, vaccination
- inoculation (any) —*see* Complications, vaccination
- insulin pump
  - infection and inflammation T85.72
  - mechanical
    - breakdown T85.614
    - displacement T85.624
    - leakage T85.633
    - malposition T85.624
    - obstruction T85.694
    - perforation T85.694
    - protrusion T85.694
    - specified NEC T85.694
- intestinal pouch NEC K91.858
- intraocular lens (prosthetic) T85.9
  - embolism T85.818 ⬅
  - fibrosis T85.828 ⬅
  - hemorrhage T85.838 ⬅
  - infection and inflammation T85.79
  - mechanical
    - breakdown T85.21
    - displacement T85.22
    - malposition T85.22
    - obstruction T85.29
    - perforation T85.29
    - protrusion T85.29
    - specified NEC T85.29
  - pain T85.848 ⬅
  - specified type NEC T85.898 ⬅
  - stenosis T85.858 ⬅
  - thrombosis T85.868 ⬅

Complication *(Continued)*
- intraoperative (intraprocedural)
  - cardiac arrest
    - during cardiac surgery I97.71Ø
    - during other surgery I97.711
  - cardiac functional disturbance NEC
    - during cardiac surgery I97.79Ø
    - during other surgery I97.791
  - hemorrhage (hematoma) (of)
    - circulatory system organ or structure
      - during cardiac bypass I97.411
      - during cardiac catheterization I97.41Ø
      - during other circulatory system procedure I97.418
      - during other procedure I97.42
    - digestive system organ
      - during procedure on digestive system K91.61
      - during procedure on other organ K91.62
    - ear
      - during procedure on ear and mastoid process H95.21
      - during procedure on other organ H95.22
    - endocrine system organ or structure
      - during procedure on endocrine system organ or structure E36.Ø1
      - during procedure on other organ E36.Ø2
    - eye and adnexa
      - during ophthalmic procedure H59.11-
      - during other procedure H59.12-
    - genitourinary organ or structure
      - during procedure on genitourinary organ or structure N99.61
      - during procedure on other organ N99.62
    - mastoid process
      - during procedure on ear and mastoid process H95.21
      - during procedure on other organ H95.22
    - musculoskeletal structure
      - during musculoskeletal surgery M96.81Ø
      - during non-orthopedic surgery M96.811
      - during orthopedic surgery M96.81Ø
    - nervous system
      - during a nervous system procedure G97.31
      - during other procedure G97.32
    - respiratory system
      - during other procedure J95.62
      - during procedure on respiratory system organ or structure J95.61
    - skin and subcutaneous tissue
      - during a dermatologic procedure L76.Ø1
      - during a procedure on other organ L76.Ø2
    - spleen
      - during a procedure on other organ D78.Ø2
      - during a procedure on the spleen D78.Ø1
  - puncture or laceration (accidental) (unintentional) (of)
    - brain
      - during a nervous system procedure G97.48
      - during other procedure G97.49
    - circulatory system organ or structure
      - during circulatory system procedure I97.51
      - during other procedure I97.52
    - digestive system
      - during procedure on digestive system K91.71
      - during procedure on other organ K91.72

Complication *(Continued)*
- intraoperative *(Continued)*
  - puncture or laceration *(Continued)*
    - ear
      - during procedure on ear and mastoid process H95.31
      - during procedure on other organ H95.32
    - endocrine system organ or structure
      - during procedure on endocrine system organ or structure E36.11
      - during procedure on other organ E36.12
    - eye and adnexa
      - during ophthalmic procedure H59.21-
      - during other procedure H59.22-
    - genitourinary organ or structure
      - during procedure on genitourinary organ or structure N99.71
      - during procedure on other organ N99.72
    - mastoid process
      - during procedure on ear and mastoid process H95.31
      - during procedure on other organ H95.32
    - musculoskeletal structure
      - during musculoskeletal surgery M96.82Ø
      - during non-orthopedic surgery M96.821
      - during orthopedic surgery M96.82Ø
    - nervous system
      - during a nervous system procedure G97.48
      - during other procedure G97.49
    - respiratory system
      - during other procedure J95.72
      - during procedure on respiratory system organ or structure J95.71
    - skin and subcutaneous tissue
      - during a dermatologic procedure L76.11
      - during a procedure on other organ L76.12
    - spleen
      - during a procedure on other organ D78.12
      - during a procedure on the spleen D78.11
  - specified NEC
    - circulatory system I97.88
    - digestive system K91.81
    - ear H95.88
    - endocrine system E36.8
    - eye and adnexa H59.88
    - genitourinary system N99.81
    - mastoid process H95.88
    - musculoskeletal structure M96.89
    - nervous system G97.81
    - respiratory system J95.88
    - skin and subcutaneous tissue L76.81
    - spleen D78.81
- intraperitoneal catheter (dialysis) (infusion) —*see* Complications, catheter, intraperitoneal
- intrathecal infusion pump ◀
  - infection and inflammation T85.738 ◀
  - mechanical ◀
    - breakdown T85.615 ◀
    - displacement T85.625 ◀
    - leakage T85.635 ◀
    - malfunction T85.695 ◀
    - malposition T85.625 ◀
    - obstruction T85.695 ◀
    - perforation T85.695 ◀
    - protrusion T85.695 ◀
    - specified NEC T85.695 ◀
- intrauterine
  - contraceptive device
    - embolism T83.81
    - fibrosis T83.82

C

Complication *(Continued)*
intrauterine *(Continued)*
contraceptive device *(Continued)*
hemorrhage T83.83
infection and inflammation T83.69
mechanical
breakdown T83.31
displacement T83.32
malposition T83.32
obstruction T83.39
perforation T83.39
protrusion T83.39
specified NEC T83.39
pain T83.84
specified type NEC T83.89
stenosis T83.85
thrombosis T83.86
procedure (fetal), to newborn P96.5
jejunostomy (stoma) —*see* Complications, enterostomy
joint prosthesis, internal T84.9
breakage (fracture) T84.01-
dislocation T84.02-
fracture T84.01-
infection or inflammation T84.50
hip T84.5-
knee T84.5-
specified joint NEC T84.59
instability T84.02-
malposition —*see* Complications, joint prosthesis, mechanical, displacement
mechanical
breakage, broken T84.01-
dislocation T84.02-
fracture T84.01-
instability T84.02-
leakage —*see* Complications, joint prosthesis, mechanical, specified NEC
loosening T84.039
hip T84.03-
knee T84.03-
specified joint NEC T84.038
obstruction —*see* Complications, joint prosthesis, mechanical, specified NEC
perforation —*see* Complications, joint prosthesis, mechanical, specified NEC
~~periprosthetic~~
~~fracture T84.049~~
~~hip T84.04-~~
~~knee T84.04-~~
~~other specified joint T84.048~~
osteolysis T84.059 ◄
hip T84.05- ◄
knee T84.05- ◄
other specified joint T84.058 ◄
protrusion —*see* Complications, joint prosthesis, mechanical, specified NEC
specified complication NEC T84.099
hip T84.09-
knee T84.09-
other specified joint T84.098
subluxation T84.02-
wear of articular bearing surface T84.069
hip T84.06-
knee T84.06-
other specified joint T84.068
specified joint NEC T84.89
embolism T84.81
fibrosis T84.82
hemorrhage T84.83
pain T84.84
specified complication NEC T84.89
stenosis T84.85
thrombosis T84.86
subluxation T84.02-
kidney transplant —*see* Complications, transplant, kidney

Complication *(Continued)*
labor O75.9
specified NEC O75.89
liver transplant (immune or nonimmune) —*see* Complications, transplant, liver
lumbar puncture G97.1
cerebrospinal fluid leak G97.0
headache or reaction G97.1
lung transplant —*see* Complications, transplant, lung
and heart —*see* Complications, transplant, lung, with heart
male genital N50.9
device, implant or graft —*see* Complications, genitourinary, device or implant, genital tract
postprocedural or postoperative —*see* Complications, genitourinary, postprocedural
specified NEC N99.89
mastoid (process) procedure
intraoperative H95.88-
hematoma —*see* Complications, intraoperative, hemorrhage (hematoma) (of), mastoid process
hemorrhage —*see* Complications, intraoperative, hemorrhage (hematoma) (of), mastoid process
laceration —*see* Complications, intraoperative, puncture or laceration..., mastoid process
specified NEC H95.88-
postmastoidectomy —*see* Complications, postmastoidectomy
postoperative H95.89-
external ear canal stenosis H95.81-
hematoma —*see* Complications..., postprocedural, hematoma (of), mastoid process
hemorrhage —*see* Complications..., postprocedural, hemorrhage (of), mastoid process
postmastoidectomy —*see* Complications, postmastoidectomy
seroma —*see* Complications, postprocedural, seroma (of), mastoid process ◄
specified NEC H95.89-
mastoidectomy cavity —*see* Complications, postmastoidectomy
mechanical —*see* Complications, by site and type, mechanical
medical procedures (*see also* Complication(s), intraoperative) T88.9
metabolic E88.9
postoperative E89.89
specified NEC E89.89
molar pregnancy NOS O08.9
damage to pelvic organs O08.6
embolism O08.2
genital infection O08.0
hemorrhage (delayed) (excessive) O08.1
metabolic disorder O08.5
renal failure O08.4
shock O08.3
specified type NEC O08.0
venous complication NEC O08.7
musculoskeletal system —*see also* Complication, intraoperative (intraprocedural), by site
device, implant or graft NEC —*see* Complications, orthopedic, device or implant
internal fixation (nail) (plate) (rod) —*see* Complications, fixation device, internal
joint prosthesis —*see* Complications, joint prosthesis

Complication *(Continued)*
musculoskeletal system *(Continued)*
postoperative (postprocedural) M96.89
with osteoporosis —*see* Osteoporosis
fracture following insertion of device —*see* Fracture, following insertion of orthopedic implant, joint prosthesis or bone plate
joint instability after prosthesis removal M96.89
lordosis M96.4
postlaminectomy syndrome NEC M96.1
kyphosis M96.2
pseudarthrosis M96.0
specified complication NEC M96.89
post radiation M96.89
kyphosis M96.3
scoliosis M96.5
specified complication NEC M96.89
nephrostomy (stoma) —*see* Complications, stoma, urinary tract, external NEC
nervous system G98.8
central G96.9
device, implant or graft —*see also* Complication, prosthetic device or implant, specified NEC
electronic stimulator (electrode (s)) —*see* Complications, electronic stimulator device
specified NEC ◄
infection and inflammation T85.738 ◄
mechanical T85.695 ◄
breakdown T85.615 ◄
displacement T85.625 ◄
leakage T85.635 ◄
malfunction T85.695 ◄
malposition T85.625 ◄
obstruction T85.695 ◄
perforation T85.695 ◄
protrusion T85.695 ◄
specified NEC T85.695 ◄
ventricular shunt —*see* Complications, ventricular shunt
electronic stimulator (electrode (s)) —*see* Complications, electronic stimulator device
postprocedural G97.82
intracranial hypotension G97.2
specified NEC G97.82
spinal fluid leak G97.0
newborn, due to intrauterine (fetal) procedure P96.5
nonabsorbable (permanent) sutures —*see* Complication, sutures, permanent
obstetric O75.9
procedure (instrumental) (manual) (surgical) specified NEC O75.4
specified NEC O75.89
surgical wound NEC O90.89
hematoma O90.2
infection O86.0
ocular lens implant —*see* Complications, intraocular lens
ophthalmologic
postprocedural bleb —*see* Blebitis
orbital prosthesis T85.9
embolism T85.818
fibrosis T85.828
hemorrhage T85.838
infection and inflammation T85.79
mechanical
breakdown T85.31-
displacement T85.32-
malposition T85.32-
obstruction T85.39-
perforation T85.39-
protrusion T85.39-
specified NEC T85.39-
pain T85.848
specified type NEC T85.898
stenosis T85.858
thrombosis T85.868

Complication *(Continued)*
- organ or tissue transplant (partial) (total) —*see* Complications, transplant
- orthopedic —*see also* Disorder, soft tissue
  - device or implant T84.9
    - bone
      - device or implant —*see* Complication, bone, device NEC
      - graft —*see* Complication, graft, bone
    - breakdown T84.418
    - displacement T84.428
    - electronic bone stimulator —*see* Complications, electronic stimulator device, bone
    - embolism T84.81
    - fibrosis T84.82
    - fixation device —*see* Complication, fixation device, internal
    - hemorrhage T84.83
    - infection or inflammation T84.7
    - joint prosthesis —*see* Complication, joint prosthesis, internal
    - malfunction T84.418
    - malposition T84.428
    - mechanical NEC T84.498
    - muscle graft —*see* Complications, graft, muscle
    - obstruction T84.498
    - pain T84.84
    - perforation T84.498
    - protrusion T84.498
    - specified complication NEC T84.89
    - stenosis T84.85
    - tendon graft —*see* Complications, graft, tendon
    - thrombosis T84.86
  - fracture (following insertion of device) —*see* Fracture, following insertion of orthopedic implant, joint prosthesis or bone plate
  - postprocedural M96.89
    - fracture —*see* Fracture, following insertion of orthopedic implant, joint prosthesis or bone plate
    - postlaminectomy syndrome NEC M96.1
      - kyphosis M96.3
      - lordosis M96.4
    - postradiation
      - kyphosis M96.2
      - scoliosis M96.5
    - pseudarthrosis post-fusion M96.0
    - specified type NEC M96.89
- pacemaker (cardiac) —*see* Complications, cardiovascular device or implant, electronic
- pancreas transplant —*see* Complications, transplant, pancreas
- penile prosthesis (implant) —*see* Complications, prosthetic device, penile
- perfusion NEC T80.90
- perineal repair (obstetrical) NEC O90.89
  - disruption O90.1
  - hematoma O90.2
  - infection (following delivery) O86.0
- phototherapy T88.9
  - specified NEC T88.8
- postmastoidectomy NEC H95.19-
  - cyst, mucosal H95.13-
  - granulation H95.12-
  - inflammation, chronic H95.11-
  - recurrent cholesteatoma H95.0-
- postoperative —*see* Complications, postprocedural
  - circulatory —*see* Complications, circulatory system
  - ear —*see* Complications, ear
  - endocrine —*see* Complications, endocrine
  - eye —*see* Complications, eye
  - lumbar puncture G97.1
    - cerebrospinal fluid leak G97.0

Complication *(Continued)*
- postoperative *(Continued)*
  - nervous system (central) (peripheral) —*see* Complications, nervous system
  - respiratory system —*see* Complications, respiratory system
- postprocedural —*see also* Complications, surgical procedure
  - cardiac arrest
    - following cardiac surgery I97.120
    - following other surgery I97.121
  - cardiac functional disturbance NEC
    - following cardiac surgery I97.190
    - following other surgery I97.191
  - cardiac insufficiency
    - following cardiac surgery I97.110
    - following other surgery I97.111
  - chorioretinal scars following retinal surgery H59.81-
  - following cataract surgery
    - cataract (lens) fragments H59.02-
    - cystoid macular edema H59.03-
    - specified NEC H59.09-
    - vitreous (touch) syndrome H59.01-
  - heart failure
    - following cardiac surgery I97.130
    - following other surgery I97.131
  - hematoma (of) ◀
    - circulatory system organ or structure ◀
      - following cardiac bypass I97.631 ◀
      - following cardiac catheterization I97.630 ◀
      - following other circulatory system procedure I97.638 ◀
      - following other procedure I97.621 ◀
    - digestive system ◀
      - following procedure on digestive system K91.870 ◀
      - following procedure on other organ K91.871 ◀
    - ear ◀
      - following other procedure H95.52 ◀
      - following procedure on ear and mastoid process H95.51 ◀
    - endocrine system ◀
      - following endocrine system procedure E89.820 ◀
      - following other procedure E89.821 ◀
    - eye and adnexa ◀
      - following ophthalmic procedure H59.33- ◀
      - following other procedure H59.34- ◀
    - genitourinary organ or structure ◀
      - following procedure on genitourinary organ or structure N99.840 ◀
      - following procedure on other organ N99.841 ◀
    - mastoid process ◀
      - following other procedure H95.52 ◀
      - following procedure on ear and mastoid process H95.51 ◀
    - musculoskeletal structure ◀
      - following musculoskeletal surgery M96.840 ◀
      - following non-orthopedic surgery M96.841 ◀
      - following orthopedic surgery M96.840 ◀
    - nervous system ◀
      - following nervous system procedure G97.61 ◀
      - following other procedure G97.62 ◀
    - respiratory system ◀
      - following other procedure J95.861 ◀
      - following procedure on respiratory system organ or structure J95.860 ◀
    - skin and subcutaneous tissue ◀
      - following dermatologic procedure L76.31 ◀
      - following procedure on other organ L76.32 ◀

Complication *(Continued)*
- postprocedural *(Continued)*
  - hematoma *(Continued)*
    - spleen ◀
      - following procedure on other organ D78.32 ◀
      - following procedure on the spleen D78.31 ◀
  - hemorrhage (of) ⬅
    - circulatory system organ or structure
      - ~~following a cardiac bypass I97.611~~
      - ~~following a cardiac catheterization I97.610~~
      - following cardiac bypass I97.611 ◀
      - following cardiac catheterization I97.610 ◀
      - following other circulatory system procedure I97.618
      - following other procedure I97.620 ⬅
    - digestive system
      - following procedure on digestive system K91.840
      - following procedure on other organ K91.841
    - ear
      - following other procedure H95.42
      - following procedure on ear and mastoid process H95.41
    - endocrine system
      - following endocrine system procedure E89.810
      - following other procedure E89.811
    - eye and adnexa
      - following ophthalmic procedure H59.31-
      - following other procedure H59.32-
    - genitourinary organ or structure
      - following procedure on genitourinary organ or structure N99.820
      - following procedure on other organ N99.821
    - mastoid process
      - following other procedure H95.42
      - following procedure on ear and mastoid process H95.41
    - musculoskeletal structure
      - following musculoskeletal surgery M96.830
      - following non-orthopedic surgery M96.831
      - following orthopedic surgery M96.830
    - nervous system
      - ~~following a nervous system procedure G97.51~~
      - following nervous system procedure G97.51
      - following other procedure G97.52
    - respiratory system
      - following other procedure J95.831
      - following procedure on respiratory system organ or structure J95.830
    - skin and subcutaneous tissue
      - ~~following a dermatologic procedure L76.21~~
      - following dermatologic procedure L76.21 ◀
      - following a procedure on other organ L76.22
    - spleen
      - following procedure on other organ D78.22
      - following procedure on the spleen D78.21
  - seroma (of) ◀
    - circulatory system organ or structure ◀
      - following cardiac bypass I97.641 ◀
      - following cardiac catheterization I97.640 ◀
      - following other circulatory system procedure I97.648 ◀
      - following other procedure I97.622 ◀

C

- **Complication** *(Continued)*
  - postprocedural *(Continued)*
    - seroma *(Continued)*
      - digestive system ◀
        - following procedure on digestive system K91.872 ◀
        - following procedure on other organ K91.873 ◀
      - ear ◀
        - following other procedure H95.54 ◀
        - following procedure on ear and mastoid process H95.53 ◀
      - endocrine system ◀
        - following endocrine system procedure E89.822 ◀
        - following other procedure E89.823 ◀
      - eye and adnexa ◀
        - following ophthalmic procedure H59.35- ◀
        - following other procedure H59.36- ◀
      - genitourinary organ or structure ◀
        - following procedure on genitourinary organ or structure N99.842 ◀
        - following procedure on other organ N99.843 ◀
      - mastoid process ◀
        - following other procedure H95.54 ◀
        - following procedure on ear and mastoid process H95.53 ◀
      - musculoskeletal structure ◀
        - following musculoskeletal surgery M96.842 ◀
        - following non-orthopedic surgery M96.843 ◀
        - following orthopedic surgery M96.842 ◀
      - nervous system ◀
        - following nervous system procedure G97.63 ◀
        - following other procedure G97.64 ◀
      - respiratory system ◀
        - following other procedure J95.863 ◀
        - following procedure on respiratory system organ or structure J95.862 ◀
      - skin and subcutaneous tissue ◀
        - following dermatologic procedure L76.33 ◀
        - following procedure on other organ L76.34 ◀
      - spleen ◀
        - following procedure on other organ D78.34 ◀
        - following procedure on the spleen D78.33 ◀
    - specified NEC
      - circulatory system I97.89
      - digestive K91.89
      - ear H95.89
      - endocrine E89.89
      - eye and adnexa H59.89
      - genitourinary N99.89
      - mastoid process H95.89
      - metabolic E89.89
      - musculoskeletal structure M96.89
      - nervous system G97.82
      - respiratory system J95.89
      - skin and subcutaneous tissue L76.82
      - spleen D78.89
  - pregnancy NEC —*see* Pregnancy, complicated by
  - prosthetic device or implant T85.9
    - bile duct —*see* Complications, bile duct implant
    - breast —*see* Complications, breast implant
    - bulking agent ◀
      - ureteral ◀
        - erosion T83.714 ◀
        - exposure T83.724 ◀
      - urethral ◀
        - erosion T83.713 ◀
        - exposure T83.723 ◀
- **Complication** *(Continued)*
  - prosthetic device or implant *(Continued)*
    - cardiac and vascular NEC —*see* Complications, cardiovascular device or implant
    - corneal transplant —*see* Complications, graft, cornea
    - electronic nervous system stimulator —*see* Complications, electronic stimulator device
    - epidural infusion catheter —*see* Complications, catheter, epidural
    - esophageal anti-reflux device —*see* Complications, esophageal anti-reflux device
    - genital organ or tract —*see* Complications, genitourinary, device or implant, genital tract
      - specified NEC T83.79 ◀
    - heart valve —*see* Complications, heart, valve, prosthesis
    - infection or inflammation T85.79
      - intestine transplant T86.892
      - liver transplant T86.43
      - lung transplant T86.812
      - pancreas transplant T86.892
      - skin graft T86.822
    - intraocular lens —*see* Complications, intraocular lens
    - intraperitoneal (dialysis) catheter —*see* Complications, catheter, intraperitoneal
    - joint —*see* Complications, joint prosthesis, internal
    - mechanical NEC T85.698
      - dialysis catheter (vascular) —*see also* Complication, catheter, dialysis, mechanical
        - peritoneal —*see* Complication, catheter, intraperitoneal, mechanical
      - gastrointestinal device T85.598
      - ocular device T85.398
      - subdural (infusion) catheter T85.690
      - suture, permanent T85.692
        - that for bone repair —*see* Complications, fixation device, internal (orthopedic), mechanical
      - ventricular shunt
        - breakdown T85.01
        - displacement T85.02
        - leakage T85.03
        - malposition T85.02
        - obstruction T85.09
        - perforation T85.09
        - protrusion T85.09
        - specified NEC T85.09
    - mesh
      - erosion (to surrounding organ or tissue) T83.717 ⇐
        - urethral (into pelvic floor muscles) T83.712 ◀
        - vaginal (into pelvic floor muscles) T83.711
      - exposure (into surrounding organ or tissue) T83.727 ⇐
        - urethral (through urethral wall) T83.722 ◀
        - vaginal (into vagina) (through vaginal wall) T83.721
    - orbital —*see* Complications, orbital prosthesis
    - penile T83.9
      - embolism T83.81
      - fibrosis T83.82
      - hemorrhage T83.83
      - infection and inflammation T83.61 ⇐
      - mechanical
        - breakdown T83.410
        - displacement T83.420
        - leakage T83.490
        - malposition T83.420
- **Complication** *(Continued)*
  - prosthetic device or implant *(Continued)*
    - penile *(Continued)*
      - mechanical *(Continued)*
        - obstruction T83.490
        - perforation T83.490
        - protrusion T83.490
        - specified NEC T83.490
      - pain T83.84
      - specified type NEC T83.89
      - stenosis T83.85
      - thrombosis T83.86
    - prosthetic materials NEC
      - erosion (to surrounding organ or tissue) T83.718
        - ~~vaginal (into pelvic floor muscles) T83.711~~
      - exposure (into surrounding organ or tissue) T83.728
        - ~~vaginal (into vagina) (through vaginal wall) T83.721~~
    - skin graft T86.829
      - artificial skin or decellularized allodermis
        - embolism T85.818 ⇐
        - fibrosis T85.828 ⇐
        - hemorrhage T85.838 ⇐
        - infection and inflammation T85.79
        - mechanical
          - breakdown T85.613
          - displacement T85.623
          - malfunction T85.613
          - malposition T85.623
          - obstruction T85.693
          - perforation T85.693
          - protrusion T85.693
          - specified NEC T85.693
        - pain T85.848 ⇐
        - specified type NEC T85.898 ⇐
        - stenosis T85.858 ⇐
        - thrombosis T85.868 ⇐
      - failure T86.821
      - infection T86.822
      - rejection T86.820
      - specified NEC T86.828
    - sling ◀
      - urethral (female) (male) ◀
        - erosion T83.712 ◀
        - exposure T83.722 ◀
    - specified NEC T85.9
      - embolism T85.818 ⇐
      - fibrosis T85.828 ⇐
      - hemorrhage T85.838 ⇐
      - infection and inflammation T85.79
      - mechanical
        - breakdown T85.618
        - displacement T85.628
        - leakage T85.638
        - malfunction T85.618
        - malposition T85.628
        - obstruction T85.698
        - perforation T85.698
        - protrusion T85.698
        - specified NEC T85.698
      - pain T85.848 ⇐
      - specified type NEC T85.898 ⇐
      - stenosis T85.858 ⇐
      - thrombosis T85.868 ⇐
    - subdural infusion catheter —*see* Complications, catheter, subdural
    - sutures —*see* Complications, sutures
    - urinary organ or tract NEC —*see* Complications, genitourinary, device or implant, urinary system
    - vascular —*see* Complications, cardiovascular device or implant
    - ventricular shunt —*see* Complications, ventricular shunt (device)
  - puerperium —*see* Puerperal
  - puncture, spinal G97.1
    - cerebrospinal fluid leak G97.0
    - headache or reaction G97.1

C

Complication *(Continued)*
- pyelogram N99.89
- radiation
  - kyphosis M96.2
  - scoliosis M96.5
- reattached
  - extremity (infection) (rejection)
    - lower T87.1X-
    - upper T87.ØX-
  - specified body part NEC T87.2
- reconstructed breast
  - asymmetry between native and reconstructed breast N65.1
  - deformity N65.Ø
  - disproportion between native and reconstructed breast N65.1
  - excess tissue N65.Ø
  - misshappen N65.Ø
- reimplant NEC —*see also* Complications, prosthetic device or implant
  - limb (infection) (rejection) —*see* Complications, reattached, extremity
  - organ (partial) (total) —*see* Complications, transplant
  - prosthetic device NEC —*see* Complications, prosthetic device
- renal N28.9
  - allograft —*see* Complications, transplant, kidney
  - dialysis —*see* Complications, dialysis
- respirator
  - mechancial J95.85Ø
    - specified NEC J95.859
- respiratory system J98.9
  - device, implant or graft —*see* Complication, prosthetic device or implant, specified NEC
  - lung transplant —*see* Complications, prosthetic device or implant, lung transplant
  - postoperative J95.89
    - air leak J95.812
    - Mendelson's syndrome (chemical pneumonitis) J95.4
    - pneumothorax J95.811
    - pulmonary insufficiency (acute) (after nonthoracic surgery) J95.2
      - chronic J95.3
      - following thoracic surgery J95.1
    - respiratory failure (acute) J95.821
      - acute and chronic J95.822
    - specified NEC J95.89
    - subglottic stenosis J95.5
    - tracheostomy complication —*see* Complications, tracheostomy
  - therapy T81.89
- sedation during labor and delivery O74.9
  - cardiac O74.2
  - central nervous system O74.3
  - pulmonary NEC O74.1
- shunt —*see also* Complications, prosthetic device or implant
  - arteriovenous —*see* Complications, arteriovenous, shunt
  - ventricular (communicating) —*see* Complications, ventricular shunt
- skin
  - graft T86.829
    - failure T86.821
    - infection T86.822
    - rejection T86.82Ø
    - specified type NEC T86.828
- spinal
  - anesthesia —*see* Complications, anesthesia, spinal
  - catheter (epidural) (subdural) —*see* Complications, catheter
  - puncture or tap G97.1
    - cerebrospinal fluid leak G97.Ø
    - headache or reaction G97.1

Complication *(Continued)*
- stent
  - bile duct —*see* Complications, bile duct prosthesis
  - ureteral indwelling ◀
    - breakdown T83.112 ◀
    - displacement T83.122 ◀
    - leakage T83.192 ◀
    - malposition T83.122 ◀
    - obstruction T83.192 ◀
    - perforation T83.192 ◀
    - protrusion T83.192 ◀
    - specified NEC T83.192 ◀
  - urinary (ileal conduit) (nephroureteral) T83.193 ◀
    - embolism T83.81 ◀
    - fibrosis T83.82 ◀
    - hemorrhage T83.83 ◀
    - infection and inflammation T83.593 ◀
    - mechanical ◀
      - breakdown T83.113 ◀
      - displacement T83.123 ◀
      - leakage T83.193 ◀
      - malposition T83.123 ◀
      - obstruction T83.193 ◀
      - perforation T83.193 ◀
      - protrusion T83.193 ◀
      - specified NEC T83.193 ◀
    - pain T83.84 ◀
    - specified type NEC T83.89 ◀
    - stenosis T83.85 ◀
    - thrombosis T83.86 ◀
  - vascular ◀
    - end stent stenosis —*see* Restenosis, stent ◀
    - in stent stenosis —*see* Restenosis, stent ◀
- stoma
  - digestive tract
    - colostomy —*see* Complications, colostomy
    - enterostomy —*see* Complications, enterostomy
    - esophagostomy —*see* Complications, esophagostomy
    - gastrostomy —*see* Complications, gastrostomy
  - urinary tract N99.528 ⟵
    - continent N99.538 ◀
      - hemorrhage N99.53Ø ◀
      - herniation N99.533 ◀
      - infection N99.531 ◀
      - malfunction N99.532 ◀
      - specified type NEC N99.538 ◀
      - stenosis N99.534 ◀
    - cystostomy —*see* Complications, cystostomy
    - external NOS N99.528
      - ~~hemorrhage N99.52Ø~~
      - ~~infection N99.521~~
      - ~~malfunction N99.522~~
      - ~~specified type NEC N99.528~~
    - hemorrhage N99.52Ø ⟵
    - herniation N99.523 ◀
    - incontinent N99.528 ◀
      - hemorrhage N99.52Ø ◀
      - herniation N99.523 ◀
      - infection N99.521 ◀
      - malfunction N99.522 ◀
      - specified type NEC N99.528 ◀
      - stenosis N99.524 ◀
    - infection N99.521 ⟵
    - malfunction N99.522 ⟵
    - specified type NEC N99.528 ⟵
    - stenosis N99.524 ◀
- stomach banding —*see* Complication (s), bariatric procedure
- stomach stapling —*see* Complication (s), bariatric procedure
- surgical material, nonabsorbable —*see* Complication, suture, permanent

Complication *(Continued)*
- surgical procedure (on) T81.9
  - amputation stump (late) —*see* Complications, amputation stump
  - cardiac —*see* Complications, circulatory system
  - cholesteatoma, recurrent —*see* Complications, postmastoidectomy, recurrent cholesteatoma
  - circulatory (early) —*see* Complications, circulatory system
  - digestive system —*see* Complications, gastrointestinal
  - dumping syndrome (postgastrectomy) K91.1
  - ear —*see* Complications, ear
  - elephantiasis or lymphedema I97.89
    - postmastectomy I97.2
  - emphysema (surgical) T81.82
  - endocrine —*see* Complications, endocrine
  - eye —*see* Complications, eye
  - fistula (persistent postoperative) T81.83
  - foreign body inadvertently left in wound (sponge) (suture) (swab) —*see* Foreign body, accidentally left during a procedure
  - gastrointestinal —*see* Complications, gastrointestinal
  - genitourinary NEC N99.89
  - hematoma
    - intraoperative —*see* Complication, intraoperative, hemorrhage
    - postprocedural —*see* Complication, postprocedural, hematoma ⟵
  - hemorrhage
    - intraoperative —*see* Complication, intraoperative, hemorrhage
    - postprocedural —*see* Complication, postprocedural, hemorrhage
  - hepatic failure K91.82
  - hyperglycemia (postpancreatectomy) E89.1
  - hypoinsulinemia (postpancreatectomy) E89.1
  - hypoparathyroidism (postparathyroidectomy) E89.2
  - hypopituitarism (posthypophysectomy) E89.3
  - hypothyroidism (post-thyroidectomy) E89.Ø
  - intestinal obstruction K91.3
  - intracranial hypotension following ventricular shunting (ventriculostomy) G97.2
  - lymphedema I97.89
    - postmastectomy I97.2
  - malabsorption (postsurgical) NEC K91.2
    - osteoporosis —*see* Osteoporosis, postsurgical malabsorption
  - mastoidectomy cavity NEC —*see* Complications, postmastoidectomy
  - metabolic E89.89
    - specified NEC E89.89
  - musculoskeletal —*see* Complications, musculoskeletal system
  - nervous system (central) (peripheral) —*see* Complications, nervous system
  - ovarian failure E89.4Ø
    - asymptomatic E89.4Ø
    - symptomatic E89.41
  - peripheral vascular —*see* Complications, surgical procedure, vascular
  - postcardiotomy syndrome I97.Ø
  - postcholecystectomy syndrome K91.5
  - postcommissurotomy syndrome I97.Ø
  - postgastrectomy dumping syndrome K91.1
  - postlaminectomy syndrome NEC M96.1
    - kyphosis M96.3
  - postmastectomy lymphedema syndrome I97.2
  - postmastoidectomy cholesteatoma —*see* Complications, postmastoidectomy, recurrent cholesteatoma

◀ New ⟵ Revised ~~deleted~~ Deleted

Complication *(Continued)*
surgical procedure *(Continued)*
postvagotomy syndrome K91.1
postvalvulotomy syndrome I97.Ø
pulmonary insufficiency (acute) J95.2
chronic J95.3
following thoracic surgery J95.1
reattached body part —*see* Complications, reattached
respiratory —*see* Complications, respiratory system
shock (hypovolemic) T81.19
spleen (postoperative) D78.89
intraoperative D78.81
stitch abscess T81.48
subglottic stenosis (postsurgical) J95.5
testicular hypofunction E89.5
transplant —*see* Complications, organ or tissue transplant
urinary NEC N99.89
vaginal vault prolapse (posthysterectomy) N99.3
vascular (peripheral)
artery T81.719
mesenteric T81.71Ø
renal T81.711
specified NEC T81.718
vein T81.72
wound infection T81.4Ø
suture, permanent (wire) NEC T85.9
with repair of bone —*see* Complications, fixation device, internal
embolism T85.818
fibrosis T85.828
hemorrhage T85.838
infection and inflammation T85.79
mechanical
breakdown T85.612
displacement T85.622
malfunction T85.612
malposition T85.622
obstruction T85.692
perforation T85.692
protrusion T85.692
specified NEC T85.692
pain T85.848
specified type NEC T85.898
stenosis T85.858
thrombosis T85.868
tracheostomy J95.ØØ
granuloma J95.Ø9
hemorrhage J95.Ø1
infection J95.Ø2
malfunction J95.Ø3
mechanical J95.Ø3
obstruction J95.Ø3
specified type NEC J95.Ø9
tracheo-esophageal fistula J95.Ø4
transfusion (blood) (lymphocytes) (plasma) T8Ø.92
air embolism T8Ø.Ø
circulatory overload E87.71
febrile nonhemolytic transfusion reaction R5Ø.84
hemochromatosis E83.111
hemolysis T8Ø.89
hemolytic reaction (antigen unspecified) T8Ø.919
incompatibility reaction (antigen unspecified) T8Ø.919
ABO T8Ø.3Ø
delayed serologic (DSTR) T8Ø.39
hemolytic transfusion reaction (HTR) (unspecified time after transfusion) T8Ø.319
acute (AHTR) (less than 24 hours after transfusion) T8Ø.31Ø
delayed (DHTR) (24 hours or more after transfusion) T8Ø.311
specified NEC T8Ø.39

Complication *(Continued)*
transfusion *(Continued)*
incompatibility reaction *(Continued)*
acute (antigen unspecified) T8Ø.91Ø
delayed (antigen unspecified) T8Ø.911
delayed serologic (DSTR) T8Ø.89
Non-ABO (minor antigens (Duffy) (Kell) (Kidd) (Lewis) (M) (N) (P) (S)) T8Ø.AØ
delayed serologic (DSTR) T8Ø.A9
hemolytic transfusion reaction (HTR) (unspecified time after transfusion) T8Ø.A19
acute (AHTR) (less than 24 hours after transfusion) T8Ø.A1Ø
delayed (DHTR) (24 hours or more after transfusion) T8Ø.A11
specified NEC T8Ø.A9
Rh (antigens (C) (c) (D) (E) (e)) (factor) T8Ø.4Ø
delayed serologic (DSTR) T8Ø.49
hemolytic transfusion reaction (HTR) (unspecified time after transfusion) T8Ø.419
acute (AHTR) (less than 24 hours after transfusion) T8Ø.41Ø
delayed (DHTR) (24 hours or more after transfusion) T8Ø.411
specified NEC T8Ø.49
infection T8Ø.29
acute T8Ø.22
reaction NEC T8Ø.89
sepsis T8Ø.29
shock T8Ø.89
transplant T86.9Ø
bone T86.839
failure T86.831
infection T86.832
rejection T86.83Ø
specified type NEC T86.838
bone marrow T86.ØØ
failure T86.Ø2
infection T86.Ø3
rejection T86.Ø1
specified type NEC T86.Ø9
cornea T86.849
failure T86.841
infection T86.842
rejection T86.84Ø
specified type NEC T86.848
failure T86.92
heart T86.2Ø
with lung T86.3Ø
cardiac allograft vasculopathy T86.29Ø
failure T86.32
infection T86.33
rejection T86.31
specified type NEC T86.39
failure T86.22
infection T86.23
rejection T86.21
specified type NEC T86.298
infection T86.93
intestine T86.859
failure T86.851
infection T86.852
rejection T86.85Ø
specified type NEC T86.858
kidney T86.1Ø
failure T86.12
infection T86.13
rejection T86.11
specified type NEC T86.19
liver T86.4Ø
failure T86.42
infection T86.43
rejection T86.41
specified type NEC T86.49
lung T86.819
with heart T86.3Ø
failure T86.32
infection T86.33

Complication *(Continued)*
transplant *(Continued)*
lung *(Continued)*
with heart *(Continued)*
rejection T86.31
specified type NEC T86.39
failure T86.811
infection T86.812
rejection T86.81Ø
specified type NEC T86.818
malignant neoplasm C8Ø.2
pancreas T86.899
failure T86.891
infection T86.892
rejection T86.89Ø
specified type NEC T86.898
peripheral blood stem cells T86.5
post-transplant lymphoproliferative disorder (PTLD) D47.Z1
rejection T86.91
skin T86.829
failure T86.821
infection T86.822
rejection T86.82Ø
specified type NEC T86.828
specified
tissue T86.899
failure T86.891
infection T86.892
rejection T86.89Ø
specified type NEC T86.898
type NEC T86.99
stem cell (from peripheral blood) (from umbilical cord) T86.5
umbilical cord stem cells T86.5
trauma (early) T79.9
specified NEC T79.8
ultrasound therapy NEC T88.9
umbilical cord NEC
complicating delivery O69.9
specified NEC O69.89
umbrella device, vascular T82.9
embolism T82.818
fibrosis T82.828
hemorrhage T82.838
infection or inflammation T82.7
mechanical
breakdown T82.515
displacement T82.525
leakage T82.535
malposition T82.525
obstruction T82.595
perforation T82.595
protrusion T82.595
pain T82.848
specified type NEC T82.898
stenosis T82.858
thrombosis T82.868
urethral catheter —*see* Complications, catheter, urethral, indwelling
vaccination T88.1
anaphylaxis NEC T8Ø.52
arthropathy —*see* Arthropathy, postimmunization
cellulitis T88.Ø
encephalitis or encephalomyelitis GØ4.Ø2
infection (general) (local) NEC T88.Ø
meningitis GØ3.8
myelitis GØ4.Ø2
protein sickness T8Ø.62
rash T88.1
reaction (allergic) T88.1
serum T8Ø.62
sepsis T88.Ø
serum intoxication, sickness, rash, or other serum reaction NEC T8Ø.62
anaphylactic shock T8Ø.52
shock (allergic) (anaphylactic) T8Ø.52
vaccinia (generalized) (localized) T88.1
vas deferens device or implant —*see* Complications, genitourinary, device or implant, genital tract

Complication *(Continued)*
vascular I99.9
device or implant T82.9
embolism T82.818
fibrosis T82.828
hemorrhage T82.838
infection or inflammation T82.7
mechanical
breakdown T82.519
specified device NEC T82.518
displacement T82.529
specified device NEC T82.528
leakage T82.539
specified device NEC T82.538
malposition T82.529
specified device NEC T82.528
obstruction T82.599
specified device NEC T82.598
perforation T82.599
specified device NEC T82.598
protrusion T82.599
specified device NEC T82.598
pain T82.848
specified type NEC T82.898
stenosis T82.858
thrombosis T82.868
dialysis catheter —*see* Complication, catheter, dialysis
following infusion, therapeutic injection or transfusion T8Ø.1
graft T82.9
embolism T82.818
fibrosis T82.828
hemorrhage T82.838
mechanical
breakdown T82.319
aorta (bifurcation) T82.31Ø
carotid artery T82.311
specified vessel NEC T82.318
displacement T82.329
aorta (bifurcation) T82.32Ø
carotid artery T82.321
specified vessel NEC T82.328
leakage T82.339
aorta (bifurcation) T82.33Ø
carotid artery T82.331
specified vessel NEC T82.338
malposition T82.329
aorta (bifurcation) T82.32Ø
carotid artery T82.321
specified vessel NEC T82.328
obstruction T82.399
aorta (bifurcation) T82.39Ø
carotid artery T82.391
specified vessel NEC T82.398
perforation T82.399
aorta (bifurcation) T82.39Ø
carotid artery T82.391
specified vessel NEC T82.398
protrusion T82.399
aorta (bifurcation) T82.39Ø
carotid artery T82.391
specified vessel NEC T82.398
pain T82.848
specified complication NEC T82.898
stenosis T82.858
thrombosis T82.868
postoperative —*see* Complications, postoperative, circulatory
vena cava device (filter) (sieve) (umbrella) —*see* Complications, umbrella device, vascular
ventilation therapy NEC T81.81
ventilator
mechanical J95.85Ø
specified NEC J95.859
ventricular (communicating) shunt (device) T85.9
embolism T85.81Ø
fibrosis T85.82Ø
hemorrhage T85.83Ø

Complication *(Continued)*
ventricular shunt *(Continued)*
infection and inflammation T85.73Ø
mechanical
breakdown T85.Ø1
displacement T85.Ø2
leakage T85.Ø3
malposition T85.Ø2
obstruction T85.Ø9
perforation T85.Ø9
protrusion T85.Ø9
specified NEC T85.Ø9
pain T85.84Ø
specified type NEC T85.89Ø
stenosis T85.85Ø
thrombosis T85.86Ø
wire suture, permanent (implanted) —*see* Complications, suture, permanent
Compressed air disease T7Ø.3
Compression
with injury - code by Nature of injury
artery I77.1
celiac, syndrome I77.4
brachial plexus G54.Ø
brain (stem) G93.5
due to
contusion (diffuse) —*see* Injury, intracranial, diffuse
focal —*see* Injury, intracranial, focal
injury NEC —*see* Injury, intracranial, diffuse
traumatic —*see* Injury, intracranial, diffuse
bronchus J98.Ø9
cauda equina G83.4
celiac (artery) (axis) I77.4
cerebral —*see* Compression, brain
cervical plexus G54.2
cord
spinal —*see* Compression, spinal
umbilical —*see* Compression, umbilical cord
cranial nerve G52.9
eighth —*see* subcategory H93.3
eleventh G52.8
fifth G5Ø.8
first G52.Ø
fourth —*see* Strabismus, paralytic, fourth nerve
ninth G52.1
second —*see* Disorder, nerve, optic
seventh G52.8
sixth —*see* Strabismus, paralytic, sixth nerve
tenth G52.2
third —*see* Strabismus, paralytic, third nerve
twelfth G52.3
diver's squeeze T7Ø.3
during birth (newborn) P15.9
esophagus K22.2
eustachian tube —*see* Obstruction, eustachian tube, cartilaginous
facies Q67.1
fracture
nontraumatic NOS —*see* Collapse, vertebra
pathological —*see* Fracture, pathological
traumatic —*see* Fracture, traumatic
heart —*see* Disease, heart
intestine —*see* Obstruction, intestine
laryngeal nerve, recurrent G52.2
with paralysis of vocal cords and larynx J38.ØØ
bilateral J38.Ø2
unilateral J38.Ø1
lumbosacral plexus G54.1
lung J98.4
lymphatic vessel I89.Ø
medulla —*see* Compression, brain
nerve —*see also* Disorder, nerve G58.9
arm NEC —*see* Mononeuropathy, upper limb

Compression *(Continued)*
nerve *(Continued)*
axillary G54.Ø
cranial —*see* Compression, cranial nerve
leg NEC —*see* Mononeuropathy, lower limb
median (in carpal tunnel) —*see* Syndrome, carpal tunnel
optic —*see* Disorder, nerve, optic
plantar —*see* Lesion, nerve, plantar
posterior tibial (in tarsal tunnel) —*see* Syndrome, tarsal tunnel
root or plexus NOS (in) G54.9
intervertebral disc disorder NEC —*see* Disorder, disc, with, radiculopathy
with myelopathy —*see* Disorder, disc, with, myelopathy
neoplastic disease —*see also* Neoplasm D49.9 *[G55]*
spondylosis —*see* Spondylosis, with radiculopathy
sciatic (acute) —*see* Lesion, nerve, sciatic
sympathetic G9Ø.8
traumatic —*see* Injury, nerve
ulnar —*see* Lesion, nerve, ulnar
upper extremity NEC —*see* Mononeuropathy, upper limb
spinal (cord) G95.2Ø
by displacement of intervertebral disc NEC —*see also* Disorder, disc, with, myelopathy
nerve root NOS G54.9
due to displacement of intervertebral disc NEC —*see* Disorder, disc, with, radiculopathy
with myelopathy —*see* Disorder, disc, with, myelopathy
specified NEC G95.29
spondylogenic (cervical) (lumbar, lumbosacral) (thoracic) —*see* Spondylosis, with myelopathy NEC
anterior —*see* Syndrome, anterior, spinal artery, compression
traumatic —*see* Injury, spinal cord, by region
subcostal nerve (syndrome) —*see* Mononeuropathy, upper limb, specified NEC
sympathetic nerve NEC G9Ø.8
syndrome T79.5
trachea J39.8
ulnar nerve (by scar tissue) —*see* Lesion, nerve, ulnar
umbilical cord
complicating delivery O69.2
cord around neck O69.1
prolapse O69.Ø
specified NEC O69.2
ureter N13.5
vein I87.1
vena cava (inferior) (superior) I87.1
Compulsion, compulsive
gambling F63.Ø
neurosis F42.8
personality F6Ø.5
states F42.8
swearing F42.8
in Gilles de la Tourette's syndrome F95.2
tics and spasms F95.9
Concato's disease (pericardial polyserositis) A19.9
nontubercular I31.1
pleural —*see* Pleurisy, with effusion
Concavity chest wall M95.4
Concealed penis Q55.69
Concern (normal) **about sick person in family** Z63.6
Concrescence (teeth) KØØ.2
Concretio cordis I31.1
rheumatic IØ9.2

C

◀ New   Revised   ~~deleted~~ Deleted

Concretion —*see also* Calculus
- appendicular K38.1
- canaliculus —*see* Dacryolith
- clitoris N90.89
- conjunctiva H11.12-
- eyelid —*see* Disorder, eyelid, specified type NEC
- lacrimal passages —*see* Dacryolith
- prepuce (male) N47.8
- salivary gland (any) K11.5
- seminal vesicle N50.89 ◀
- tonsil J35.8

Concussion (brain) (cerebral) (current) S06.0X9 ◀
- with ◀
  - loss of consciousness of 30 minutes or less S06.0X1 ◀
  - loss of consciousness of unspecified duration S06.0X9 ◀
- blast (air) (hydraulic) (immersion) (underwater)
  - abdomen or thorax —*see* Injury, blast, by site
  - ear with acoustic nerve injury —*see* Injury, nerve, acoustic, specified type NEC
- cauda equina S34.3
- conus medullaris S34.02
- ocular S05.8X-
- spinal (cord)
  - cervical S14.0
  - lumbar S34.01
  - sacral S34.02
  - thoracic S24.0
- syndrome F07.81
- **Without loss of consciousness** S06.0X0 ◀

Condition —*see* Disease

Conditions arising in the perinatal period —*see* Newborn, affected by

Conduct disorder —*see* Disorder, conduct

Condyloma A63.0
- acuminatum A63.0
- gonorrheal A54.09
- latum A51.31
- syphilitic A51.31
  - congenital A50.07
- venereal, syphilitic A51.31

Conflagration —*see also* Burn
- asphyxia (by inhalation of gases, fumes or vapors) —*see also* Table of Drugs and Chemicals T59.9-

Conflict (with) —*see also* Discord
- family Z73.9
- marital Z63.0
  - involving divorce or estrangement Z63.5
- parent-child Z62.820
  - parent-adopted child Z62.821
  - parent-biological child Z62.820
  - parent-foster child Z62.822
- social role NEC Z73.5

Confluent —*see* condition

Confusion, confused R41.0
- epileptic F05
- mental state (psychogenic) F44.89
- psychogenic F44.89
- reactive (from emotional stress, psychological trauma) F44.89

Confusional arousals G47.51

Congelation T69.9

Congenital —*see also* condition
- aortic septum Q25.49 ◀
- intrinsic factor deficiency D51.0
- malformation —*see* Anomaly

Congestion, congestive
- bladder N32.89
- bowel K63.89
- brain G93.89
- breast N64.59
- bronchial J98.09
- catarrhal J31.0
- chest R09.89
- chill, malarial —*see* Malaria

Congestion, congestive *(Continued)*
- circulatory NEC I99.8
- duodenum K31.89
- eye —*see* Hyperemia, conjunctiva
- facial, due to birth injury P15.4
- general R68.89
- glottis J37.0
- heart —*see* Failure, heart, congestive
- hepatic K76.1
- hypostatic (lung) —*see* Edema, lung
- intestine K63.89
- kidney N28.89
- labyrinth —*see* subcategory H83.8
- larynx J37.0
- liver K76.1
- lung R09.89
  - active or acute —*see* Pneumonia
- malaria, malarial —*see* Malaria
- nasal R09.81
- nose R09.81
- orbit, orbital —*see also* Exophthalmos
  - inflammatory (chronic) —*see* Inflammation, orbit
- ovary N83.8
- pancreas K86.89 ◀
- pelvic, female N94.89
- pleural J94.8
- prostate (active) N42.1
- pulmonary —*see* Congestion, lung
- renal N28.89
- retina H35.81
- seminal vesicle N50.1
- spinal cord G95.19
- spleen (chronic) D73.2
- stomach K31.89
- trachea —*see* Tracheitis
- urethra N36.8
- uterus N85.8
  - with subinvolution N85.3
- venous (passive) I87.8
- viscera R68.89

Congestive —*see* Congestion

Conical
- cervix (hypertrophic elongation) N88.4
- cornea —*see* Keratoconus
- teeth K00.2

Conjoined twins Q89.4

Conjugal maladjustment Z63.0
- involving divorce or estrangement Z63.5

Conjunctiva —*see* condition

Conjunctivitis (staphylococcal) (streptococcal) NOS H10.9
- Acanthamoeba B60.12
- acute H10.3-
  - atopic H10.1-
  - chemical —*see also* Corrosion, cornea H10.21-
  - mucopurulent H10.02-
    - follicular H10.01-
  - pseudomembranous H10.22-
  - serous except viral H10.23-
    - viral —*see* Conjunctivitis, viral
  - toxic H10.21-
- adenoviral (acute) (follicular) B30.1
- allergic (acute) —*see* Conjunctivitis, acute, atopic
  - chronic H10.45
    - vernal H10.44
- anaphylactic —*see* Conjunctivitis, acute, atopic
- Apollo B30.3
- atopic (acute) —*see* Conjunctivitis, acute, atopic
- Béal's B30.2
- blennorrhagic (gonococcal) (neonatorum) A54.31
- chemical (acute) —*see also* Corrosion, cornea H10.21-
- chlamydial A74.0
  - due to trachoma A71.1
  - neonatal P39.1

Conjunctivitis *(Continued)*
- chronic (nodosa) (petrificans) (phlyctenular) H10.40-
  - allergic H10.45
    - vernal H10.44
  - follicular H10.43-
  - giant papillary H10.41-
  - simple H10.42-
  - vernal H10.44
- coxsackievirus 24 B30.3
- diphtheritic A36.86
- due to
  - dust —*see* Conjunctivitis, acute, atopic
  - filariasis B74.9
  - mucocutaneous leishmaniasis B55.2
- enterovirus type 70 (hemorrhagic) B30.3
- epidemic (viral) B30.9
  - hemorrhagic B30.3
- gonococcal (neonatorum) A54.31
- granular (trachomatous) A71.1
  - sequelae (late effect) B94.0
- hemorrhagic (acute) (epidemic) B30.3
- herpes zoster B02.31
- in (due to)
  - Acanthamoeba B60.12
  - adenovirus (acute) (follicular) B30.1
  - Chlamydia A74.0
  - coxsackievirus 24 B30.3
  - diphtheria A36.86
  - enterovirus type 70 (hemorrhagic) B30.3
  - filariasis B74.9
  - gonococci A54.31
  - herpes (simplex) virus B00.53
    - zoster B02.31
  - infectious disease NEC B99
  - meningococci A39.89
  - mucocutaneous leishmaniasis B55.2
  - rosacea L71.9
  - syphilis (late) A52.71
  - zoster B02.31
- inclusion A74.0
- infantile P39.1
  - gonococcal A54.31
- Koch-Weeks' —*see* Conjunctivitis, acute, mucopurulent
- light —*see* Conjunctivitis, acute, atopic
- ligneous —*see* Blepharoconjunctivitis, ligneous
- meningococcal A39.89
- mucopurulent —*see* Conjunctivitis, acute, mucopurulent
- neonatal P39.1
  - gonococcal A54.31
- Newcastle B30.8
- of Béal B30.2
- parasitic
  - filariasis B74.9
  - mucocutaneous leishmaniasis B55.2
- Parinaud's H10.89
- petrificans H10.89
- rosacea L71.9
- specified NEC H10.89
- swimming-pool B30.1
- trachomatous A71.1
  - acute A71.0
  - sequelae (late effect) B94.0
- traumatic NEC H10.89
- tuberculous A18.59
- tularemic A21.1
- tularensis A21.1
- viral B30.9
  - due to
    - adenovirus B30.1
    - enterovirus B30.3
  - specified NEC B30.8

Conjunctivochalasis H11.82-

Connective tissue —*see* condition

Conn's syndrome E26.01

Conradi (-Hunermann) **disease** Q77.3

Consanguinity Z84.3
- counseling Z71.89

- **Conscious simulation** (of illness) Z76.5
- **Consecutive** —*see* condition
- **Consolidation lung** (base) —*see* Pneumonia, lobar
- **Constipation** (atonic) (neurogenic) (simple) (spastic) K59.00
  - chronic K59.09 ◀
    - idiopathic K59.04 ◀
  - drug-induced K59.03 ⬅
  - functional K59.04 ◀
  - outlet dysfunction K59.02
  - psychogenic F45.8
  - slow transit K59.01
  - specified NEC K59.09
- **Constitutional** —*see also* condition
  - substandard F60.7
- **Constitutionally substandard** F60.7
- **Constriction** —*see also* Stricture
  - auditory canal —*see* Stenosis, external ear canal
  - bronchial J98.09
  - duodenum K31.5
  - esophagus K22.2
  - external
    - abdomen, abdominal (wall) S30.841
    - alveolar process S00.542
    - ankle S90.54-
    - antecubital space —*see* Constriction, external, forearm
    - arm (upper) S40.84-
    - auricle —*see* Constriction, external, ear
    - axilla —*see* Constriction, external, arm
    - back, lower S30.840
    - breast S20.14-
    - brow S00.84
    - buttock S30.840
    - calf —*see* Constriction, external, leg
    - canthus —*see* Constriction, external, eyelid
    - cheek S00.84
      - internal S00.542
    - chest wall —*see* Constriction, external, thorax
    - chin S00.84
    - clitoris S30.844
    - costal region —*see* Constriction, external, thorax
    - digit (s)
      - foot —*see* Constriction, external, toe
      - hand —*see* Constriction, external, finger
    - ear S00.44-
    - elbow S50.34-
    - epididymis S30.843
    - epigastric region S30.841
    - esophagus, cervical S10.14
    - eyebrow —*see* Constriction, external, eyelid
    - eyelid S00.24-
    - face S00.84
    - finger (s) S60.44-
      - index S60.44-
      - little S60.44-
      - middle S60.44-
      - ring S60.44-
    - flank S30.841
    - foot (except toe (s) alone) S90.84-
      - toe —*see* Constriction, external, toe
    - forearm S50.84-
      - elbow only —*see* Constriction, external, elbow
    - forehead S00.84
    - genital organs, external
      - female S30.846
      - male S30.845
    - groin S30.841
    - gum S00.542
    - hand S60.54-
    - head S00.94
      - ear —*see* Constriction, external, ear
      - eyelid —*see* Constriction, external, eyelid
      - lip S00.541
      - nose S00.34
      - oral cavity S00.542

Constriction *(Continued)*

- external *(Continued)*
  - head *(Continued)*
    - scalp S00.04
    - specified site NEC S00.84
  - heel —*see* Constriction, external, foot
  - hip S70.24-
  - inguinal region S30.841
  - interscapular region S20.449
  - jaw S00.84
  - knee S80.24-
  - labium (majus) (minus) S30.844
  - larynx S10.14
  - leg (lower) S80.84-
    - knee —*see* Constriction, external, knee
    - upper —*see* Constriction, external, thigh
  - lip S00.541
  - lower back S30.840
  - lumbar region S30.840
  - malar region S00.84
  - mammary —*see* Constriction, external, breast
  - mastoid region S00.84
  - mouth S00.542
  - nail
    - finger —*see* Constriction, external, finger
    - toe —*see* Constriction, external, toe
  - nasal S00.34
  - neck S10.94
    - specified site NEC S10.84
    - throat S10.14
  - nose S00.34
  - occipital region S00.04
  - oral cavity S00.542
  - orbital region —*see* Constriction, external, eyelid
  - palate S00.542
  - palm —*see* Constriction, external, hand
  - parietal region S00.04
  - pelvis S30.840
  - penis S30.842
  - perineum
    - female S30.844
    - male S30.840
  - periocular area —*see* Constriction, external, eyelid
  - phalanges
    - finger —*see* Constriction, external, finger
    - toe —*see* Constriction, external, toe
  - pharynx S10.14
  - pinna —*see* Constriction, external, ear
  - popliteal space —*see* Constriction, external, knee
  - prepuce S30.842
  - pubic region S30.840
  - pudendum
    - female S30.846
    - male S30.845
  - sacral region S30.840
  - scalp S00.04
  - scapular region —*see* Constriction, external, shoulder
  - scrotum S30.843
  - shin —*see* Constriction, external, leg
  - shoulder S40.24-
  - sternal region S20.349
  - submaxillary region S00.84
  - submental region S00.84
  - subungual
    - finger (s) —*see* Constriction, external, finger
    - toe (s) —*see* Constriction, external, toe
  - supraclavicular fossa S10.84
  - supraorbital S00.84
  - temple S00.84
  - temporal region S00.84
  - testis S30.843
  - thigh S70.34-
  - thorax, thoracic (wall) S20.94
    - back S20.44-
    - front S20.34-

Constriction *(Continued)*

- external *(Continued)*
  - throat S10.14
  - thumb S60.34-
  - toe (s) (lesser) S90.44-
    - great S90.44-
  - tongue S00.542
  - trachea S10.14
  - tunica vaginalis S30.843
  - uvula S00.542
  - vagina S30.844
  - vulva S30.844
  - wrist S60.84-
- gallbladder —*see* Obstruction, gallbladder
- intestine —*see* Obstruction, intestine
- larynx J38.6
  - congenital Q31.8
    - specified NEC Q31.8
    - subglottic Q31.1
- organ or site, congenital NEC —*see* Atresia, by site
- prepuce (acquired) (congenital) N47.1
- pylorus (adult hypertrophic) K31.1
  - congenital or infantile Q40.0
  - newborn Q40.0
- ring dystocia (uterus) O62.4
- spastic —*see also* Spasm
  - ureter N13.5
- ureter N13.5
  - with infection N13.6
- urethra —*see* Stricture, urethra
- visual field (peripheral) (functional) —*see* Defect, visual field

- **Constrictive** —*see* condition
- **Consultation**
  - without complaint or sickness Z71.9
    - feared complaint unfounded Z71.1
    - specified reason NEC Z71.89
  - medical —*see* Counseling, medical
  - religious Z71.81
  - specified reason NEC Z71.89
  - spiritual Z71.81
- **Consumption** —*see* Tuberculosis
- **Contact** (with) —*see also* Exposure (to)
  - acariasis Z20.7
  - AIDS virus Z20.6
  - air pollution Z77.110
  - algae and algae toxins Z77.121
  - algae bloom Z77.121
  - anthrax Z20.810
  - aromatic (hazardous) compounds NEC Z77.028
  - aromatic amines Z77.020
  - aromatic dyes NOS Z77.028
  - arsenic Z77.010
  - asbestos Z77.090
  - bacterial disease NEC Z20.818
  - benzene Z77.021
  - blue-green algae bloom Z77.121
  - body fluids (potentially hazardous) Z77.21
  - brown tide Z77.121
  - chemicals (chiefly nonmedicinal) (hazardous) NEC Z77.098
  - cholera Z20.09
  - chromium compounds Z77.018
  - communicable disease Z20.9
    - bacterial NEC Z20.818
    - specified NEC Z20.89
    - viral NEC Z20.828
  - cyanobacteria bloom Z77.121
  - dyes Z77.098
  - Escherichia coli (E. coli) Z20.01
  - fiberglass —*see* Table of Drugs and Chemicals, fiberglass
  - German measles Z20.4
  - gonorrhea Z20.2
  - hazardous metals NEC Z77.018
  - hazardous substances NEC Z77.29
  - hazards in the physical environment NEC Z77.128
  - hazards to health NEC Z77.9

C

Contact *(Continued)*
HIV Z20.6
HTLV-III/LAV Z20.6
human immunodeficiency virus (HIV) Z20.6
infection Z20.9
specified NEC Z20.89
infestation (parasitic) NEC Z20.7
intestinal infectious disease NEC Z20.09
Escherichia coli (E. coli) Z20.01
lead Z77.011
meningococcus Z20.811
mold (toxic) Z77.120
nickel dust Z77.018
noise Z77.122
parasitic disease Z20.7
pediculosis Z20.7
pfiesteria piscicida Z77.121
poliomyelitis Z20.89
pollution
air Z77.110
environmental NEC Z77.118
soil Z77.112
water Z77.111
polycyclic aromatic hydrocarbons Z77.028
rabies Z20.3
radiation, naturally occurring NEC Z77.123
radon Z77.123
red tide (Florida) Z77.121
rubella Z20.4
sexually-transmitted disease Z20.2
smallpox (laboratory) Z20.89
syphilis Z20.2
tuberculosis Z20.1
uranium Z77.012
varicella Z20.820
venereal disease Z20.2
viral disease NEC Z20.828
viral hepatitis Z20.5
water pollution Z77.111
Contamination, food —*see* Intoxication, foodborne
Contraception, contraceptive
advice Z30.09
counseling Z30.09
device (intrauterine) (in situ) Z97.5
causing menorrhagia T83.83
checking Z30.431
complications —*see* Complications, intrauterine, contraceptive device
in place Z97.5
initial prescription Z30.014
reinsertion Z30.433
removal Z30.432
replacement Z30.433
emergency (postcoital) Z30.012
initial prescription Z30.019
barrier Z30.018 ◀
diaphragm Z30.018 ◀
injectable Z30.013
intrauterine device Z30.014
pills Z30.011
postcoital (emergency) Z30.012
specified type NEC Z30.018
subdermal implantable Z30.017 ◀
transdermal patch hormonal Z30.016 ◀
vaginal ring hormonal Z30.015 ◀
maintenance Z30.40
barrier Z30.49 ◀
diaphragm Z30.49 ◀
examination Z30.8
injectable Z30.42
intrauterine device Z30.431
pills Z30.41
specified type NEC Z30.49
subdermal implantable Z30.46 ◀
transdermal patch hormonal Z30.45 ◀
vaginal ring hormonal Z30.44 ◀
management Z30.9
specified NEC Z30.8
postcoital (emergency) Z30.012
prescription Z30.019
repeat Z30.40

Contraception, contraceptive *(Continued)*
sterilization Z30.2
surveillance (drug) —*see* Contraception, maintenance
Contraction (s), contracture, contracted
Achilles tendon —*see also* Short, tendon, Achilles
congenital Q66.89
amputation stump (surgical) (flexion) (late) next proximal joint T87.89
anus K59.8
bile duct (common) (hepatic) K83.8
bladder N32.89
neck or sphincter N32.0
bowel, cecum, colon or intestine, any part —*see* Obstruction, intestine
Braxton Hicks —*see* False, labor
breast implant, capsular T85.44
bronchial J98.09
burn (old) —*see* Cicatrix
cervix —*see* Stricture, cervix
cicatricial —*see* Cicatrix
conjunctiva, trachomatous, active A71.1
sequelae (late effect) B94.0
Dupuytren's M72.0
eyelid —*see* Disorder, eyelid function
fascia (lata) (postural) M72.8
Dupuytren's M72.0
palmar M72.0
plantar M72.2
finger NEC —*see also* Deformity, finger
congenital Q68.1
joint —*see* Contraction, joint, hand
flaccid —*see* Contraction, paralytic
gallbladder K82.0
heart valve —*see* Endocarditis
hip —*see* Contraction, joint, hip
hourglass
bladder N32.89
congenital Q64.79
gallbladder K82.0
congenital Q44.1
stomach K31.89
congenital Q40.2
psychogenic F45.8
uterus (complicating delivery) O62.4
hysterical F44.4
internal os —*see* Stricture, cervix
joint (abduction) (acquired) (adduction) (flexion) (rotation) M24.50
ankle M24.57-
congenital NEC Q68.8
hip Q65.89
elbow M24.52-
foot joint M24.57-
hand joint M24.54-
hip M24.55-
congenital Q65.89
hysterical F44.4
knee M24.56-
shoulder M24.51-
wrist M24.53-
kidney (granular) (secondary) N26.9
congenital Q63.8
hydronephritic —*see* Hydronephrosis
Page N26.2
pyelonephritic —*see* Pyelitis, chronic
tuberculous A18.11
ligament —*see also* Disorder, ligament
congenital Q79.8
muscle (postinfective) (postural) NEC M62.40
with contracture of joint —*see* Contraction, joint
ankle M62.47-
congenital Q79.8
sternocleidomastoid Q68.0
extraocular —*see* Strabismus
eye (extrinsic) —*see* Strabismus
foot M62.47-
forearm M62.43-
hand M62.44-

Contraction, contracture, contracted *(Continued)*
muscle *(Continued)*
hysterical F44.4
ischemic (Volkmann's) T79.6
lower leg M62.46-
multiple sites M62.49
pelvic region M62.45-
posttraumatic —*see* Strabismus, paralytic
psychogenic F45.8
conversion reaction F44.4
shoulder region M62.41-
specified site NEC M62.48
thigh M62.45-
upper arm M62.42-
neck —*see* Torticollis
ocular muscle —*see* Strabismus
organ or site, congenital NEC —*see* Atresia, by site
outlet (pelvis) —*see* Contraction, pelvis
palmar fascia M72.0
paralytic
joint —*see* Contraction, joint
muscle —*see also* Contraction, muscle NEC
ocular —*see* Strabismus, paralytic
pelvis (acquired) (general) M95.5
with disproportion (fetopelvic) O33.1
causing obstructed labor O65.1
inlet O33.2
mid-cavity O33.3
outlet O33.3
plantar fascia M72.2
premature
atrium I49.1
auriculoventricular I49.49
heart I49.49
junctional I49.2
supraventricular I49.1
ventricular I49.3
prostate N42.89
pylorus NEC —*see also* Pylorospasm
psychogenic F45.8
rectum, rectal (sphincter) K59.8
ring (Bandl's) (complicating delivery) O62.4
scar —*see* Cicatrix
spine —*see* Dorsopathy, deforming
sternocleidomastoid (muscle), congenital Q68.0
stomach K31.89
hourglass K31.89
congenital Q40.2
psychogenic F45.8
psychogenic F45.8
tendon (sheath) M62.40
with contracture of joint —*see* Contraction, joint
Achilles —*see* Short, tendon, Achilles
ankle M62.47-
Achilles —*see* Short, tendon, Achilles
foot M62.47-
forearm M62.43-
hand M62.44-
lower leg M62.46-
multiple sites M62.49
neck M62.48
pelvic region M62.45-
shoulder region M62.41-
specified site NEC M62.48
thigh M62.45-
thorax M62.48
trunk M62.48
upper arm M62.42-
toe —*see* Deformity, toe, specified NEC
ureterovesical orifice (postinfectional) N13.5
with infection N13.6
urethra —*see also* Stricture, urethra
orifice N32.0
uterus N85.8
abnormal NEC O62.9
clonic (complicating delivery) O62.4
dyscoordinate (complicating delivery) O62.4

Contraction, contracture, contracted *(Continued)*
uterus *(Continued)*
hourglass (complicating delivery) O62.4
hypertonic O62.4
hypotonic NEC O62.2
inadequate
primary O62.0
secondary O62.1
incoordinate (complicating delivery) O62.4
poor O62.2
tetanic (complicating delivery) O62.4
vagina (outlet) N89.5
vesical N32.89
neck or urethral orifice N32.0
visual field —*see* Defect, visual field, generalized
Volkmann's (ischemic) T79.6
Contusion (skin surface intact) T14.8
abdomen, abdominal (muscle) (wall) S30.1
adnexa, eye NEC S05.8X-
adrenal gland S37.812
alveolar process S00.532
ankle S90.0-
antecubital space —*see* Contusion, forearm
anus S30.3
arm (upper) S40.02-
lower (with elbow) —*see* Contusion, forearm
auditory canal —*see* Contusion, ear
auricle —*see* Contusion, ear
axilla —*see* Contusion, arm, upper
back —*see also* Contusion, thorax, back
lower S30.0
bile duct S36.13
bladder S37.22
bone NEC T14.8
brain (diffuse) —*see* Injury, intracranial, diffuse
focal —*see* Injury, intracranial, focal
brainstem S06.38-
breast S20.0-
broad ligament S37.892
brow S00.83
buttock S30.0
canthus, eye S00.1-
cauda equina S34.3
cerebellar, traumatic S06.37-
cerebral S06.33-
left side S06.32-
right side S06.31-
cheek S00.83
internal S00.532
chest (wall) —*see* Contusion, thorax
chin S00.83
clitoris S30.23
colon —*see* Injury, intestine, large, contusion
common bile duct S36.13
conjunctiva S05.1-
with foreign body (in conjunctival sac) —*see* Foreign body, conjunctival sac
conus medullaris (spine) S34.139
cornea —*see* Contusion, eyeball
with foreign body —*see* Foreign body, cornea
corpus cavernosum S30.21
cortex (brain) (cerebral) —*see* Injury, intracranial, diffuse
focal —*see* Injury, intracranial, focal
costal region —*see* Contusion, thorax
cystic duct S36.13
diaphragm S27.802
duodenum S36.420
ear S00.43-
elbow S50.0-
with forearm —*see* Contusion, forearm
epididymis S30.22
epigastric region S30.1
epiglottis S10.0
esophagus (thoracic) S27.812
cervical S10.0
eyeball S05.1-

C

Contusion *(Continued)*
eyebrow S00.1-
eyelid (and periocular area) S00.1-
face NEC S00.83
fallopian tube S37.529
bilateral S37.522
unilateral S37.521
femoral triangle S30.1
finger (s) S60.00
with damage to nail (matrix) S60.10
index S60.02-
with damage to nail S60.12-
little S60.05-
with damage to nail S60.15-
middle S60.03-
with damage to nail S60.13-
ring S60.04-
with damage to nail S60.14-
thumb —*see* Contusion, thumb
flank S30.1
foot (except toe (s) alone) S90.3-
toe —*see* Contusion, toe
forearm S50.1-
elbow only —*see* Contusion, elbow
forehead S00.83
gallbladder S36.122
genital organs, external
female S30.202
male S30.201
globe (eye) —*see* Contusion, eyeball
groin S30.1
gum S00.532
hand S60.22-
finger (s) —*see* Contusion, finger
wrist —*see* Contusion, wrist
head S00.93
ear —*see* Contusion, ear
eyelid —*see* Contusion, eyelid
lip S00.531
nose S00.33
oral cavity S00.532
scalp S00.03
specified part NEC S00.83
heart —*see also* Injury, heart S26.91 ◀
heel —*see* Contusion, foot
hepatic duct S36.13
hip S70.0-
ileum S36.428
iliac region S30.1
inguinal region S30.1
interscapular region S20.229
intra-abdominal organ S36.92
colon —*see* Injury, intestine, large, contusion
liver S36.112
pancreas —*see* Contusion, pancreas
rectum S36.62
small intestine —*see* Injury, intestine, small, contusion
specified organ NEC S36.892
spleen —*see* Contusion, spleen
stomach S36.32
iris (eye) —*see* Contusion, eyeball
jaw S00.83
jejunum S36.428
kidney S37.01-
major (greater than 2 cm) S37.02-
minor (less than 2 cm) S37.01-
knee S80.0-
labium (majus) (minus) S30.23
lacrimal apparatus, gland or sac S05.8X-
larynx S10.0
leg (lower) S80.1-
knee —*see* Contusion, knee
lens —*see* Contusion, eyeball
lip S00.531
liver S36.112
lower back S30.0
lumbar region S30.0
lung S27.329
bilateral S27.322
unilateral S27.321

Contusion *(Continued)*
malar region S00.83
mastoid region S00.83
membrane, brain —*see* Injury, intracranial, diffuse
focal —*see* Injury, intracranial, focal
mesentery S36.892
mesosalpinx S37.892
mouth S00.532
muscle —*see* Contusion, by site
nail
finger —*see* Contusion, finger, with damage to nail
toe —*see* Contusion, toe, with damage to nail
nasal S00.33
neck S10.93
specified site NEC S10.83
throat S10.0
nerve —*see* Injury, nerve
newborn P54.5
nose S00.33
occipital
lobe (brain) —*see* Injury, intracranial, diffuse
focal —*see* Injury, intracranial, focal
region (scalp) S00.03
orbit (region) (tissues) S05.1-
ovary S37.429
bilateral S37.422
unilateral S37.421
palate S00.532
pancreas S36.229
body S36.221
head S36.220
tail S36.222
parietal
lobe (brain) —*see* Injury, intracranial, diffuse
focal —*see* Injury, intracranial, focal
region (scalp) S00.03
pelvic organ S37.92
adrenal gland S37.812
bladder S37.22
fallopian tube —*see* Contusion, fallopian tube
kidney —*see* Contusion, kidney
ovary —*see* Contusion, ovary
prostate S37.822
specified organ NEC S37.892
ureter S37.12
urethra S37.32
uterus S37.62
pelvis S30.0
penis S30.21
perineum
female S30.23
male S30.0
periocular area S00.1-
peritoneum S36.81
periurethral tissue —*see* Contusion, urethra
pharynx S10.0
pinna —*see* Contusion, ear
popliteal space —*see* Contusion, knee
prepuce S30.21
prostate S37.822
pubic region S30.1
pudendum
female S30.202
male S30.201
quadriceps femoris —*see* Contusion, thigh
rectum S36.62
retroperitoneum S36.892
round ligament S37.892
sacral region S30.0
scalp S00.03
due to birth injury P12.3
scapular region —*see* Contusion, shoulder
sclera —*see* Contusion, eyeball

◀ New ⟸ Revised ~~deleted~~ Deleted

Contusion *(Continued)*
scrotum S30.22
seminal vesicle S37.892
shoulder S40.01-
skin NEC T14.8
small intestine —*see* Injury, intestine, small, contusion
spermatic cord S30.22
spinal cord —*see* Injury, spinal cord, by region
cauda equina S34.3
conus medullaris S34.139
spleen S36.029
major S36.021
minor S36.020
sternal region S20.219
stomach S36.32
subconjunctival S05.1-
subcutaneous NEC T14.8
submaxillary region S00.83
submental region S00.83
subperiosteal NEC T14.8
subungual
finger —*see* Contusion, finger, with damage to nail
toe —*see* Contusion, toe, with damage to nail
supraclavicular fossa S10.83
supraorbital S00.83
suprarenal gland S37.812
temple (region) S00.83
temporal
lobe (brain) —*see* Injury, intracranial, diffuse
focal —*see* Injury, intracranial, focal
region S00.83
testis S30.22
thigh S70.1-
thorax (wall) S20.20
back S20.22-
front S20.21-
throat S10.0
thumb S60.01-
with damage to nail S60.11-
toe (s) (lesser) S90.12-
with damage to nail S90.22-
great S90.11-
with damage to nail S90.21-
specified type NEC S90.221
tongue S00.532
trachea (cervical) S10.0
thoracic S27.52
tunica vaginalis S30.22
tympanum, tympanic membrane —*see* Contusion, ear
ureter S37.12
urethra S37.32
urinary organ NEC S37.892
uterus S37.62
uvula S00.532
vagina S30.23
vas deferens S37.892
vesical S37.22
vocal cord (s) S10.0
vulva S30.23
wrist S60.21-
Conus (congenital) (any type) Q14.8
cornea —*see* Keratoconus
medullaris syndrome G95.81
Conversion hysteria, neurosis or reaction F44.9
Converter, tuberculosis (test reaction) R76.11
Conviction (legal), **anxiety concerning** Z65.0
with imprisonment Z65.1
Convulsions (idiopathic) —*see also* Seizure(s) R56.9
apoplectiform (cerebral ischemia) I67.82
~~benign neonatal (familial) —see Epilepsy, generalized, idiopathic~~
dissociative F44.5
epileptic —*see* Epilepsy
epileptiform, epileptoid —*see* Seizure, epileptiform
Convulsions *(Continued)*
ether (anesthetic) —*see* Table of Drugs and Chemicals, by drug
febrile R56.00
with status epilepticus G40.901
complex R56.01
with status epilepticus G40.901
simple R56.00
hysterical F44.5
infantile P90
epilepsy —*see* Epilepsy
jacksonian —*see* Epilepsy, localization-related, symptomatic, with simple partial seizures
myoclonic G25.3
~~neonatal, benign (familial) —see Epilepsy, generalized, idiopathic~~
newborn P90
obstetrical (nephritic) (uremic) —*see* Eclampsia
paretic A52.17
post traumatic R56.1
psychomotor —*see* Epilepsy, localization-related, symptomatic, with complex partial seizures
recurrent R56.9
reflex R25.8
scarlatinal A38.8
tetanus, tetanic —*see* Tetanus
thymic E32.8
Convulsive —*see also* Convulsions
Cooley's anemia D56.1
Coolie itch B76.9
Cooper's
disease —*see* Mastopathy, cystic
hernia —*see* Hernia, abdomen, specified site NEC
Copra itch B88.0
Coprophagy F50.89 ⇐
Coprophobia F40.298
Coproporphyria, hereditary E80.29
Cor
biloculare Q20.8
bovis, bovinum —*see* Hypertrophy, cardiac
pulmonale (chronic) I27.81
acute I26.09
triatriatum, triatrium Q24.2
triloculare Q20.8
biatrium Q20.4
biventriculare Q21.1
Corbus' disease (gangrenous balanitis) N48.1
Cord —*see also* condition
around neck (tightly) (with compression)
complicating delivery O69.1
bladder G95.89
tabetic A52.19
Cordis ectopia Q24.8
Corditis (spermatic) N49.1
Corectopia Q13.2
Cori's disease (glycogen storage) E74.03
Corkhandler's disease or lung J67.3
Corkscrew esophagus K22.4
Corkworker's disease or lung J67.3
Corn (infected) L84
Cornea —*see also* condition
donor Z52.5
plana Q13.4
Cornelia de Lange syndrome Q87.1
Cornu cutaneum L85.8
Cornual gestation or pregnancy O00.80 ⇐
with intrauterine pregnancy O00.81 ◀
Coronary (artery) —*see* condition
Coronavirus, as cause of disease classified elsewhere B97.29
SARS-associated B97.21
Corpora —*see also* condition
amylacea, prostate N42.89
cavernosa —*see* condition
Corpulence —*see* Obesity
Corpus —*see* condition
Corrected transposition Q20.5
Corrosion (injury) (acid) (caustic) (chemical) (lime) (external) (internal) T30.4
abdomen, abdominal (muscle) (wall) T21.42
first degree T21.52
second degree T21.62
third degree T21.72
above elbow T22.439
first degree T22.539
left T22.432
first degree T22.532
second degree T22.632
third degree T22.732
right T22.431
first degree T22.531
second degree T22.631
third degree T22.731
second degree T22.639
third degree T22.739
alimentary tract NEC T28.7
ankle T25.419
first degree T25.519
left T25.412
first degree T25.512
second degree T25.612
third degree T25.712
multiple with foot —*see* Corrosion, lower, limb, multiple, ankle and foot
right T25.411
first degree T25.511
second degree T25.611
third degree T25.711
second degree T25.619
third degree T25.719
anus —*see* Corrosion, buttock
arm (s) (meaning upper limb (s)) —*see* Corrosion, upper limb
axilla T22.449
first degree T22.549
left T22.442
first degree T22.542
second degree T22.642
third degree T22.742
right T22.441
first degree T22.541
second degree T22.641
third degree T22.741
second degree T22.649
third degree T22.749
back (lower) T21.44
first degree T21.54
second degree T21.64
third degree T21.74
upper T21.43
first degree T21.53
second degree T21.63
third degree T21.73
blisters - code as Corrosion, second degree, by site
breast (s) —*see* Corrosion, chest wall
buttock (s) T21.45
first degree T21.55
second degree T21.65
third degree T21.75
calf T24.439
first degree T24.539
left T24.432
first degree T24.532
second degree T24.632
third degree T24.732
right T24.431
first degree T24.531
second degree T24.631
third degree T24.731
second degree T24.639
third degree T24.739
canthus (eye) —*see* Corrosion, eyelid
cervix T28.8
cheek T20.46
first degree T20.56
second degree T20.66
third degree T20.76

Corrosion (Continued)
chest wall T21.41
first degree T21.51
second degree T21.61
third degree T21.71
chin T20.43
first degree T20.53
second degree T20.63
third degree T20.73
colon T28.7
conjunctiva (and cornea) —see Corrosion, cornea
cornea (and conjunctiva) T26.6-
deep necrosis of underlying tissue - code as Corrosion, third degree, by site
dorsum of hand T23.469
first degree T23.569
left T23.462
first degree T23.562
second degree T23.662
third degree T23.762
right T23.461
first degree T23.561
second degree T23.661
third degree T23.761
second degree T23.669
third degree T23.769
ear (auricle) (external) (canal) T20.41
drum T28.91
first degree T20.51
second degree T20.61
third degree T20.71
elbow T22.429
first degree T22.529
left T22.422
first degree T22.522
second degree T22.622
third degree T22.722
right T22.421
first degree T22.521
second degree T22.621
third degree T22.721
second degree T22.629
third degree T22.729
entire body —see Corrosion, multiple body regions
epidermal loss - code as Corrosion, second degree, by site
epiglottis T27.4
erythema, erythematous - code as Corrosion, first degree, by site
esophagus T28.6
extent (percentage of body surface)
less than 10 percent T32.0
10-19 percent (0-9 percent third degree) T32.10
with 10-19 percent third degree T32.11
20-29 percent (0-9 percent third degree) T32.20
with
10-19 percent third degree T32.21
20-29 percent third degree T32.22
30-39 percent (0-9 percent third degree) T32.30
with
10-19 percent third degree T32.31
20-29 percent third degree T32.32
30-39 percent third degree T32.33
40-49 percent (0-9 percent third degree) T32.40
with
10-19 percent third degree T32.41
20-29 percent third degree T32.42
30-39 percent third degree T32.43
40-49 percent third degree T32.44
50-59 percent (0-9 percent third degree) T32.50
with
10-19 percent third degree T32.51
20-29 percent third degree T32.52

Corrosion (Continued)
extent (Continued)
50-59 percent (Continued)
with (Continued)
30-39 percent third degree T32.53
40-49 percent third degree T32.54
50-59 percent third degree T32.55
60-69 percent (0-9 percent third degree) T32.60
with
10-19 percent third degree T32.61
20-29 percent third degree T32.62
30-39 percent third degree T32.63
40-49 percent third degree T32.64
50-59 percent third degree T32.65
60-69 percent third degree T32.66
70-79 percent (0-9 percent third degree) T32.70
with
10-19 percent third degree T32.71
20-29 percent third degree T32.72
30-39 percent third degree T32.73
40-49 percent third degree T32.74
50-59 percent third degree T32.75
60-69 percent third degree T32.76
70-79 percent third degree T32.77
80-89 percent (0-9 percent third degree) T32.80
with
10-19 percent third degree T32.81
20-29 percent third degree T32.82
30-39 percent third degree T32.83
40-49 percent third degree T32.84
50-59 percent third degree T32.85
60-69 percent third degree T32.86
70-79 percent third degree T32.87
80-89 percent third degree T32.88
90 percent or more (0-9 percent third degree) T32.90
with
10-19 percent third degree T32.91
20-29 percent third degree T32.92
30-39 percent third degree T32.93
40-49 percent third degree T32.94
50-59 percent third degree T32.95
60-69 percent third degree T32.96
70-79 percent third degree T32.97
80-89 percent third degree T32.98
90-99 percent third degree T32.99
extremity —see Corrosion, limb
eye (s) and adnexa T26.9-
with resulting rupture and destruction of eyeball T26.7-
conjunctival sac —see Corrosion, cornea
cornea —see Corrosion, cornea
lid —see Corrosion, eyelid
periocular area —see Corrosion eyelid
specified site NEC T26.8-
eyeball —see Corrosion, eye
eyelid (s) T26.5-
face —see Corrosion, head
finger T23.429
first degree T23.529
left T23.422
first degree T23.522
second degree T23.622
third degree T23.722
multiple sites (without thumb) T23.439
with thumb T23.449
first degree T23.549
left T23.442
first degree T23.542
second degree T23.642
third degree T23.742
right T23.441
first degree T23.541
second degree T23.641
third degree T23.741
second degree T23.649
third degree T23.749

Corrosion (Continued)
finger (Continued)
multiple sites (Continued)
first degree T23.539
left T23.432
first degree T23.532
second degree T23.632
third degree T23.732
right T23.431
first degree T23.531
second degree T23.631
third degree T23.731
second degree T23.639
third degree T23.739
right T23.421
first degree T23.521
second degree T23.621
third degree T23.721
second degree T23.629
third degree T23.729
flank —see Corrosion, abdomen
foot T25.429
first degree T25.529
left T25.422
first degree T25.522
second degree T25.622
third degree T25.722
multiple with ankle —see Corrosion, lower, limb, multiple, ankle and foot
right T25.421
first degree T25.521
second degree T25.621
third degree T25.721
second degree T25.629
third degree T25.729
forearm T22.419
first degree T22.519
left T22.412
first degree T22.512
second degree T22.612
third degree T22.712
right T22.411
first degree T22.511
second degree T22.611
third degree T22.711
second degree T22.619
third degree T22.719
forehead T20.46
first degree T20.56
second degree T20.66
third degree T20.76
fourth degree - code as Corrosion, third degree, by site
full thickness skin loss - code as Corrosion, third degree, by site
gastrointestinal tract NEC T28.7
genital organs
external
female T21.47
first degree T21.57
second degree T21.67
third degree T21.77
male T21.46
first degree T21.56
second degree T21.66
third degree T21.76
internal T28.8
groin —see Corrosion, abdominal wall
hand (s) T23.409
back —see Corrosion, dorsum of hand
finger —see Corrosion, finger
first degree T23.509
left T23.402
first degree T23.502
second degree T23.602
third degree T23.702
multiple sites with wrist T23.499
first degree T23.599
left T23.492
first degree T23.592
second degree T23.692
third degree T23.792

C

◄ New ⟸ Revised ~~deleted~~ Deleted

Corrosion *(Continued)*
hand (s) *(Continued)*
multiple sites *(Continued)*
right T23.491
first degree T23.591
second degree T23.691
third degree T23.791
second degree T23.699
third degree T23.799
palm —*see* Corrosion, palm
right T23.401
first degree T23.501
second degree T23.601
third degree T23.701
second degree T23.609
third degree T23.709
thumb —*see* Corrosion, thumb
head (and face) (and neck) T20.40
cheek —*see* Corrosion, cheek
chin —*see* Corrosion, chin
ear —*see* Corrosion, ear
eye (s) only —*see* Corrosion, eye
first degree T20.50
forehead —*see* Corrosion, forehead
lip —*see* Corrosion, lip
multiple sites T20.49
first degree T20.59
second degree T20.69
third degree T20.79
neck —*see* Corrosion, neck
nose —*see* Corrosion, nose
scalp —*see* Corrosion, scalp
second degree T20.60
third degree T20.70
hip (s) —*see* Corrosion, lower, limb
inhalation —*see* Corrosion, respiratory tract
internal organ (s) (*see also* Corrosion, by site) T28.90
alimentary tract T28.7
esophagus T28.6
esophagus T28.6
genitourinary T28.8
mouth T28.5
pharynx T28.5
specified organ NEC T28.99
interscapular region —*see* Corrosion, back, upper
intestine (large) (small) T28.7
knee T24.429
first degree T24.529
left T24.422
first degree T24.522
second degree T24.622
third degree T24.722
right T24.421
first degree T24.521
second degree T24.621
third degree T24.721
second degree T24.629
third degree T24.729
labium (majus) (minus) —*see* Corrosion, genital organs, external, female
lacrimal apparatus, duct, gland or sac —*see* Corrosion, eye, specified site NEC
larynx T27.4
with lung T27.5
leg (s) (meaning lower limb (s)) —*see* Corrosion, lower limb
limb (s)
lower —*see* Corrosion, lower, limb
upper —*see* Corrosion, upper limb
lip (s) T20.42
first degree T20.52
second degree T20.62
third degree T20.72
lower
back —*see* Corrosion, back
limb T24.409
ankle —*see* Corrosion, ankle
calf —*see* Corrosion, calf

Corrosion *(Continued)*
lower *(Continued)*
limb *(Continued)*
first degree T24.509
foot —*see* Corrosion, foot
hip —*see* Corrosion, thigh
knee —*see* Corrosion, knee
left T24.402
first degree T24.502
second degree T24.602
third degree T24.702
multiple sites, except ankle and foot T24.499
ankle and foot T25.499
first degree T25.599
left T25.492
first degree T25.592
second degree T25.692
third degree T25.792
right T25.491
first degree T25.591
second degree T25.691
third degree T25.791
second degree T25.699
third degree T25.799
first degree T24.599
left T24.492
first degree T24.592
second degree T24.692
third degree T24.792
right T24.491
first degree T24.591
second degree T24.691
third degree T24.791
second degree T24.699
third degree T24.799
right T24.401
first degree T24.501
second degree T24.601
third degree T24.701
second degree T24.609
thigh —*see* Corrosion, thigh
third degree T24.709
lung (with larynx and trachea) T27.5
mouth T28.5
neck T20.47
first degree T20.57
second degree T20.67
third degree T20.77
nose (septum) T20.44
first degree T20.54
second degree T20.64
third degree T20.74
ocular adnexa —*see* Corrosion, eye
orbit region —*see* Corrosion, eyelid
palm T23.459
first degree T23.559
left T23.452
first degree T23.552
second degree T23.652
third degree T23.752
right T23.451
first degree T23.551
second degree T23.651
third degree T23.751
second degree T23.659
third degree T23.759
partial thickness - code as Corrosion, unspecified degree, by site
pelvis —*see* Corrosion, trunk
penis —*see* Corrosion, genital organs, external, male
perineum
female —*see* Corrosion, genital organs, external, female
male —*see* Corrosion, genital organs, external, male
periocular area —*see* Corrosion, eyelid
pharynx T28.5
rectum T28.7

Corrosion *(Continued)*
respiratory tract T27.7
larynx —*see* Corrosion, larynx
specified part NEC T27.6
trachea —*see* Corrosion, larynx
sac, lacrimal —*see* Corrosion, eye, specified site NEC
scalp T20.45
first degree T20.55
second degree T20.65
third degree T20.75
scapular region T22.469
first degree T22.569
left T22.462
first degree T22.562
second degree T22.662
third degree T22.762
right T22.461
first degree T22.561
second degree T22.661
third degree T22.761
second degree T22.669
third degree T22.769
sclera —*see* Corrosion, eye, specified site NEC
scrotum —*see* Corrosion, genital organs, external, male
shoulder T22.459
first degree T22.559
left T22.452
first degree T22.552
second degree T22.652
third degree T22.752
right T22.451
first degree T22.551
second degree T22.651
third degree T22.751
second degree T22.659
third degree T22.759
stomach T28.7
temple —*see* Corrosion, head
testis —*see* Corrosion, genital organs, external, male
thigh T24.419
first degree T24.519
left T24.412
first degree T24.512
second degree T24.612
third degree T24.712
right T24.411
first degree T24.511
second degree T24.611
third degree T24.711
second degree T24.619
third degree T24.719
thorax (external) —*see* Corrosion, trunk
throat (meaning pharynx) T28.5
thumb (s) T23.419
first degree T23.519
left T23.412
first degree T23.512
second degree T23.612
third degree T23.712
multiple sites with fingers T23.449
first degree T23.549
left T23.442
first degree T23.542
second degree T23.642
third degree T23.742
right T23.441
first degree T23.541
second degree T23.641
third degree T23.741
second degree T23.649
third degree T23.749
right T23.411
first degree T23.511
second degree T23.611
third degree T23.711
second degree T23.619
third degree T23.719

Corrosion *(Continued)*
toe T25.439
first degree T25.539
left T25.432
first degree T25.532
second degree T25.632
third degree T25.732
right T25.431
first degree T25.531
second degree T25.631
third degree T25.731
second degree T25.639
third degree T25.739
tongue T28.5
tonsil (s) T28.5
total body —*see* Corrosion, multiple body regions
trachea T27.4
with lung T27.5
trunk T21.40
abdominal wall —*see* Corrosion, abdominal wall
anus —*see* Corrosion, buttock
axilla —*see* Corrosion, upper limb
back —*see* Corrosion, back
breast —*see* Corrosion, chest wall
buttock —*see* Corrosion, buttock
chest wall —*see* Corrosion, chest wall
first degree T21.50
flank —*see* Corrosion, abdominal wall
genital
female —*see* Corrosion, genital organs, external, female
male —*see* Corrosion, genital organs, external, male
groin —*see* Corrosion, abdominal wall
interscapular region —*see* Corrosion, back, upper
labia —*see* Corrosion, genital organs, external, female
lower back —*see* Corrosion, back
penis —*see* Corrosion, genital organs, external, male
perineum
female —*see* Corrosion, genital organs, external, female
male —*see* Corrosion, genital organs, external, male
scapular region —*see* Corrosion, upper limb
scrotum —*see* Corrosion, genital organs, external, male
second degree T21.60
shoulder —*see* Corrosion, upper limb
specified site NEC T21.49
first degree T21.59
second degree T21.69
third degree T21.79
testes —*see* Corrosion, genital organs, external, male
third degree T21.70
upper back —*see* Corrosion, back, upper
vagina T28.8
vulva —*see* Corrosion, genital organs, external, female
unspecified site with extent of body surface involved specified
less than 10 percent T32.0
10-19 percent (0-9 percent third degree) T32.10
with 10-19 percent third degree T32.11
20-29 percent (0-9 percent third degree) T32.20
with
10-19 percent third degree T32.21
20-29 percent third degree T32.22
30-39 percent (0-9 percent third degree) T32.30
with
10-19 percent third degree T32.31
20-29 percent third degree T32.32
30-39 percent third degree T32.33

Corrosion *(Continued)*
unspecified site with extent of body surface involved specified *(Continued)*
40-49 percent (0-9 percent third degree) T32.40
with
10-19 percent third degree T32.41
20-29 percent third degree T32.42
30-39 percent third degree T32.43
40-49 percent third degree T32.44
50-59 percent (0-9 percent third degree) T32.50
with
10-19 percent third degree T32.51
20-29 percent third degree T32.52
30-39 percent third degree T32.53
40-49 percent third degree T32.54
50-59 percent third degree T32.55
60-69 percent (0-9 percent third degree) T32.60
with
10-19 percent third degree T32.61
20-29 percent third degree T32.62
30-39 percent third degree T32.63
40-49 percent third degree T32.64
50-59 percent third degree T32.65
60-69 percent third degree T32.66
70-79 percent (0-9 percent third degree) T32.70
with
10-19 percent third degree T32.71
20-29 percent third degree T32.72
30-39 percent third degree T32.73
40-49 percent third degree T32.74
50-59 percent third degree T32.75
60-69 percent third degree T32.76
70-79 percent third degree T32.77
80-89 percent (0-9 percent third degree) T32.80
with
10-19 percent third degree T32.81
20-29 percent third degree T32.82
30-39 percent third degree T32.83
40-49 percent third degree T32.84
50-59 percent third degree T32.85
60-69 percent third degree T32.86
70-79 percent third degree T32.87
80-89 percent third degree T32.88
90 percent or more (0-9 percent third degree) T32.90
with
10-19 percent third degree T32.91
20-29 percent third degree T32.92
30-39 percent third degree T32.93
40-49 percent third degree T32.94
50-59 percent third degree T32.95
60-69 percent third degree T32.96
70-79 percent third degree T32.97
80-89 percent third degree T32.98
90-99 percent third degree T32.99
upper limb (axilla) (scapular region) T22.40
above elbow —*see* Corrosion, above elbow
axilla —*see* Corrosion, axilla
elbow —*see* Corrosion, elbow
first degree T22.50
forearm —*see* Corrosion, forearm
hand —*see* Corrosion, hand
interscapular region —*see* Corrosion, back, upper
multiple sites T22.499
first degree T22.599
left T22.492
first degree T22.592
second degree T22.692
third degree T22.792
right T22.491
first degree T22.591
second degree T22.691
third degree T22.791
second degree T22.699
third degree T22.799

Corrosion *(Continued)*
upper limb (axilla) (scapular region) *(Continued)*
scapular region —*see* Corrosion, scapular region
second degree T22.60
shoulder —*see* Corrosion, shoulder
third degree T22.70
wrist —*see* Corrosion, hand
uterus T28.8
vagina T28.8
vulva —*see* Corrosion, genital organs, external, female
wrist T23.479
first degree T23.579
left T23.472
first degree T23.572
second degree T23.672
third degree T23.772
multiple sites with hand T23.499
first degree T23.599
left T23.492
first degree T23.592
second degree T23.692
third degree T23.792
right T23.491
first degree T23.591
second degree T23.691
third degree T23.791
second degree T23.699
third degree T23.799
right T23.471
first degree T23.571
second degree T23.671
third degree T23.771
second degree T23.679
third degree T23.779
Corrosive burn —*see* Corrosion
Corsican fever —*see* Malaria
Cortical —*see* condition
Cortico-adrenal —*see* condition
Coryza (acute) J00
with grippe or influenza —*see* Influenza, with, respiratory manifestations NEC
syphilitic
congenital (chronic) A50.05
Costen's syndrome or complex M26.69
Costiveness —*see* Constipation
Costochondritis M94.0
Cot death R99
Cotard's syndrome F22
Cotia virus B08.8
Cotton wool spots (retinal) H35.81
Cotungo's disease —*see* Sciatica
Cough (affected) (chronic) (epidemic) (nervous) R05
with hemorrhage —*see* Hemoptysis
bronchial R05
with grippe or influenza —*see* Influenza, with, respiratory manifestations NEC
functional F45.8
hysterical F45.8
laryngeal, spasmodic R05
psychogenic F45.8
smokers' J41.0
tea taster's B49
Counseling (for) Z71.9
abuse NEC
perpetrator Z69.82
victim Z69.81
alcohol abuser Z71.41
family Z71.42
child abuse
nonparental
perpetrator Z69.021
victim Z69.020
parental
perpetrator Z69.011
victim Z69.010

◄ New ◄ Revised ~~deleted~~ Deleted

Counseling *(Continued)*
consanguinity Z71.89
contraceptive Z3Ø.Ø9
dietary Z71.3
drug abuser Z71.51
family member Z71.52
family Z71.89
fertility preservation (prior to cancer therapy) (prior to removal of gonads) Z31.62
for non-attending third party Z71.Ø
related to sexual behavior or orientation Z7Ø.2
genetic NEC Z31.5
gestational carrier Z31.7 ◀
health (advice) (education) (instruction) —*see* Counseling, medical
human immunodeficiency virus (HIV) Z71.7
impotence Z7Ø.1
insulin pump use Z46.81
medical (for) Z71.9
boarding school resident Z59.3
consanguinity Z71.89
feared complaint and no disease found Z71.1
human immunodeficiency virus (HIV) Z71.7
institutional resident Z59.3
on behalf of another Z71.Ø
related to sexual behavior or orientation Z7Ø.2
person living alone Z6Ø.2
specified reason NEC Z71.89
natural family planning
procreative Z31.61
to avoid pregnancy Z3Ø.Ø2
perpetrator (of)
abuse NEC Z69.82
child abuse
non-parental Z69.Ø21
parental Z69.Ø11
rape NEC Z69.82
spousal abuse Z69.12
procreative NEC Z31.69
fertility preservation (prior to cancer therapy) (prior to removal of gonads) Z31.62
using natural family planning Z31.61
promiscuity Z7Ø.1
rape victim Z69.81
religious Z71.81
sex, sexual (related to) Z7Ø.9
attitude (s) Z7Ø.Ø
behavior or orientation Z7Ø.1
combined concerns Z7Ø.3
non-responsiveness Z7Ø.1
on behalf of third party Z7Ø.2
specified reason NEC Z7Ø.8
specified reason NEC Z71.89
spiritual Z71.81
spousal abuse (perpetrator) Z69.12
victim Z69.11
substance abuse Z71.89
alcohol Z71.41
drug Z71.51
tobacco Z71.6
tobacco use Z71.6
use (of)
insulin pump Z46.81
victim (of)
abuse Z69.81
child abuse
by parent Z69.Ø1Ø
non-parental Z69.Ø2Ø
rape NEC Z69.81
Coupled rhythm RØØ.8
Couvelaire syndrome or uterus (complicating delivery) O45.8X-
Cowperitis —*see* Urethritis
Cowper's gland —*see* condition
Cowpox BØ8.Ø1Ø
due to vaccination T88.1
Coxa
magna M91.4-
plana M91.2-
valga (acquired) —*see also* Deformity, limb, specified type NEC, thigh
congenital Q65.81
sequelae (late effect) of rickets E64.3
vara (acquired) —*see also* Deformity, limb, specified type NEC, thigh
congenital Q65.82
sequelae (late effect) of rickets E64.3
Coxalgia, coxalgic (nontuberculous) —*see also* Pain, joint, hip
tuberculous A18.Ø2
Coxitis —*see* Monoarthritis, hip
Coxsackie (virus) (infection) B34.1
as cause of disease classified elsewhere B97.11
carditis B33.2Ø
central nervous system NEC A88.8
endocarditis B33.21
enteritis AØ8.39
meningitis (aseptic) A87.Ø
myocarditis B33.22
pericarditis B33.23
pharyngitis BØ8.5
pleurodynia B33.Ø
specific disease NEC B33.8
Crabs, meaning pubic lice B85.3
Crack baby PØ4.41
Cracked nipple N64.Ø
associated with
lactation O92.13
pregnancy O92.11-
puerperium O92.12
Cracked tooth KØ3.81
Cradle cap L21.Ø
Craft neurosis F48.8
Cramp (s) R25.2
abdominal —*see* Pain, abdominal
bathing T75.1
colic R1Ø.83
psychogenic F45.8
due to immersion T75.1
fireman T67.2
heat T67.2
immersion T75.1
intestinal —*see* Pain, abdominal
psychogenic F45.8
leg, sleep related G47.62
limb (lower) (upper) NEC R25.2
sleep related G47.62
linotypist's F48.8
organic G25.89
muscle (limb) (general) R25.2
due to immersion T75.1
psychogenic F45.8
occupational (hand) F48.8
organic G25.89
salt-depletion E87.1
sleep related, leg G47.62
stoker's T67.2
swimmer's T75.1
telegrapher's F48.8
organic G25.89
typist's F48.8
organic G25.89
uterus N94.89
menstrual —*see* Dysmenorrhea
writer's F48.8
organic G25.89
Cranial —*see* condition
Craniocleidodysostosis Q74.Ø
Craniofenestria (skull) Q75.8
Craniolacunia (skull) Q75.8
Craniopagus Q89.4
Craniopathy, metabolic M85.2
Craniopharyngeal —*see* condition
Craniopharyngioma D44.4
Craniorachischisis (totalis) QØØ.1
Cranioschisis Q75.8
Craniostenosis Q75.Ø
Craniosynostosis Q75.Ø
Craniotabes (cause unknown) M83.8
neonatal P96.3
rachitic E64.3
syphilitic A5Ø.56
Cranium —*see* condition
Craw-craw —*see* Onchocerciasis
Creaking joint —*see* Derangement, joint, specified type NEC
Creeping
eruption B76.9
palsy or paralysis G12.22
Crenated tongue K14.8
Creotoxism AØ5.9
Crepitus
caput Q75.8
joint —*see* Derangement, joint, specified type NEC
Crescent or conus choroid, congenital Q14.3
CREST syndrome M34.1
Cretin, cretinism (congenital) (endemic) (nongoitrous) (sporadic) EØØ.9
pelvis
with disproportion (fetopelvic) O33.Ø
causing obstructed labor O65.Ø
type
hypothyroid EØØ.1
mixed EØØ.2
myxedematous EØØ.1
neurological EØØ.Ø
Creutzfeldt-Jakob disease or syndrome (with dementia) A81.ØØ
familial A81.Ø9
iatrogenic A81.Ø9
specified NEC A81.Ø9
sporadic A81.Ø9
variant (vCJD) A81.Ø1
Crib death R99
Cribriform hymen Q52.3
Cri-du-chat syndrome Q93.4
Crigler-Najjar disease or syndrome E8Ø.5
Crime, victim of Z65.4
Crimean hemorrhagic fever A98.Ø
Criminalism F6Ø.2
Crisis
abdomen R1Ø.Ø
acute reaction F43.Ø
addisonian E27.2
adrenal (cortical) E27.2
celiac K9Ø.Ø
Dietl's N13.8
emotional —*see also* Disorder, adjustment
acute reaction to stress F43.Ø
specific to childhood and adolescence F93.8
glaucomatocyclitic —*see* Glaucoma, secondary, inflammation
heart —*see* Failure, heart
nitritoid I95.2
correct substance properly administered —*see* Table of Drugs and Chemicals, by drug, adverse effect
overdose or wrong substance given or taken —*see* Table of Drugs and Chemicals, by drug, poisoning
oculogyric H51.8
psychogenic F45.8
Pel's (tabetic) A52.11
psychosexual identity F64.2
renal N28.Ø
sickle-cell D57.ØØ
with
acute chest syndrome D57.Ø1
splenic sequestration D57.Ø2
state (acute reaction) F43.Ø
tabetic A52.11
thyroid —*see* Thyrotoxicosis with thyroid storm
thyrotoxic —*see* Thyrotoxicosis with thyroid storm

C

- **Crocq's disease** (acrocyanosis) I73.89
- **Crohn's disease** *—see* Enteritis, regional
- **Crooked septum, nasal** J34.2
- **Cross syndrome** E7Ø.328
- **Crossbite** (anterior) (posterior) M26.24
- **Cross-eye** *—see* Strabismus, convergent concomitant
- **Croup, croupous** (catarrhal) (infectious) (inflammatory) (nondiphtheritic) JØ5.Ø
  - bronchial J2Ø.9
  - diphtheritic A36.2
  - false J38.5
  - spasmodic J38.5
    - diphtheritic A36.2
  - stridulous J38.5
    - diphtheritic A36.2
- **Crouzon's disease** Q75.1
- **Crowding, tooth, teeth, fully erupted** M26.31
- **CRST syndrome** M34.1
- **Cruchet's disease** A85.8
- **Cruelty in children** *—see also* Disorder, conduct
- **Crural ulcer** *—see* Ulcer, lower limb
- **Crush, crushed, crushing** T14.8
  - abdomen S38.1
  - ankle S97.Ø-
  - arm (upper) (and shoulder) S47.-
  - axilla *—see* Crush, arm
  - back, lower S38.1
  - buttock S38.1
  - cheek SØ7.Ø
  - chest S28.Ø
  - cranium SØ7.1
  - ear SØ7.Ø
  - elbow S57.Ø-
  - extremity
    - lower
      - ankle *—see* Crush, ankle
      - below knee *—see* Crush, leg
      - foot *—see* Crush, foot
      - hip *—see* Crush, hip
      - knee *—see* Crush, knee
      - thigh *—see* Crush, thigh
      - toe *—see* Crush, toe
    - upper
      - below elbow S67.9-
      - elbow *—see* Crush, elbow
      - finger *—see* Crush, finger
      - forearm *—see* Crush, forearm
      - hand *—see* Crush, hand
      - thumb *—see* Crush, thumb
      - upper arm *—see* Crush, arm
      - wrist *—see* Crush, wrist
  - face SØ7.Ø
  - finger (s) S67.1-
    - with hand (and wrist) *—see* Crush, hand, specified site NEC
    - index S67.19-
    - little S67.19-
    - middle S67.19-
    - ring S67.19-
    - thumb *—see* Crush, thumb
  - foot S97.8-
    - toe *—see* Crush, toe
  - forearm S57.8-
  - genitalia, external
    - female S38.ØØ2
      - vagina S38.Ø3
      - vulva S38.Ø3
    - male S38.ØØ1
      - penis S38.Ø1
      - scrotum S38.Ø2
      - testis S38.Ø2
  - hand (except fingers alone) S67.2-
    - with wrist S67.4-
  - head SØ7.9
    - specified NEC SØ7.8
  - heel *—see* Crush, foot
  - hip S77.Ø-
    - with thigh S77.2-
  - internal organ (abdomen, chest, or pelvis) NEC T14.8
- **Crush, crushed, crushing** *(Continued)*
  - knee S87.Ø-
  - labium (majus) (minus) S38.Ø3
  - larynx S17.Ø
  - leg (lower) S87.8-
    - knee *—see* Crush, knee
  - lip SØ7.Ø
  - lower
    - back S38.1
    - leg *—see* Crush, leg
  - neck S17.9
  - nerve *—see* Injury, nerve
  - nose SØ7.Ø
  - pelvis S38.1
  - penis S38.Ø1
  - scalp SØ7.8
  - scapular region *—see* Crush, arm
  - scrotum S38.Ø2
  - severe, unspecified site T14.8
  - shoulder (and upper arm) *—see* Crush, arm
  - skull SØ7.1
  - syndrome (complication of trauma) T79.5
  - testis S38.Ø2
  - thigh S77.1-
    - with hip S77.2-
  - throat S17.8
  - thumb S67.Ø-
    - with hand (and wrist) *—see* Crush, hand, specified site NEC
  - toe (s) S97.1Ø-
    - great S97.11-
    - lesser S97.12-
  - trachea S17.Ø
  - vagina S38.Ø3
  - vulva S38.Ø3
  - wrist S67.3-
    - with hand S67.4-
- **Crusta lactea** L21.Ø
- **Crusts** R23.4
- **Crutch paralysis** *—see* Injury, brachial plexus
- **Cruveilhier-Baumgarten cirrhosis, disease or syndrome** K74.69
- **Cruveilhier's atrophy or disease** G12.8
- **Crying** (constant) (continuous) (excessive)
  - child, adolescent, or adult R45.83
  - infant (baby) (newborn) R68.11
- **Cryofibrinogenemia** D89.2
- **Cryoglobulinemia** (essential) (idiopathic) (mixed) (primary) (purpura) (secondary) (vasculitis) D89.1
  - with lung involvement D89.1 *[J99]*
- **Cryptitis** (anal) (rectal) K62.89
- **Cryptococcosis, cryptococcus** (infection) (neoformans) B45.9
  - bone B45.3
  - cerebral B45.1
  - cutaneous B45.2
  - disseminated B45.7
  - generalized B45.7
  - meningitis B45.1
  - meningocerebralis B45.1
  - osseous B45.3
  - pulmonary B45.Ø
  - skin B45.2
  - specified NEC B45.8
- **Cryptopapillitis** (anus) K62.89
- **Cryptophthalmos** Q11.2
  - syndrome Q87.Ø
- **Cryptorchid, cryptorchism, cryptorchidism** Q53.9
  - bilateral Q53.2Ø
    - abdominal Q53.21
    - perineal Q53.22
  - unilateral Q53.1Ø
    - abdominal Q53.11
    - perineal Q53.12
- **Cryptosporidiosis** AØ7.2
  - hepatobiliary B88.8
  - respiratory B88.8
- **Cryptostromosis** J67.6
- **Crystalluria** R82.99
- **Cubitus**
  - congenital Q68.8
  - valgus (acquired) M21.Ø-
    - congenital Q68.8
    - sequelae (late effect) of rickets E64.3
  - varus (acquired) M21.1-
    - congenital Q68.8
    - sequelae (late effect) of rickets E64.3
- **Cultural deprivation or shock** Z6Ø.3
- **Curling esophagus** K22.4
- **Curling's ulcer** *—see* Ulcer, peptic, acute
- **Curschmann (-Batten) (-Steinert) disease or syndrome** G71.11
- **Curse, Ondine's** *—see* Apnea, sleep
- **Curvature**
  - organ or site, congenital NEC *—see* Distortion
  - penis (lateral) Q55.61
  - Pott's (spinal) A18.Ø1
  - radius, idiopathic, progressive (congenital) Q74.Ø
  - spine (acquired) (angular) (idiopathic) (incorrect) (postural) *—see* Dorsopathy, deforming
    - congenital Q67.5
    - due to or associated with
      - Charcot-Marie-Tooth disease *—see also* subcategory M49.8 G6Ø.Ø
      - osteitis
        - deformans M88.88
        - fibrosa cystica *—see also* subcategory M49.8 E21.Ø
      - tuberculosis (Pott's curvature) A18.Ø1
    - sequelae (late effect) of rickets E64.3
    - tuberculous A18.Ø1
- **Cushingoid due to steroid therapy** E24.2
  - correct substance properly administered *—see* Table of Drugs and Chemicals, by drug, adverse effect
  - overdose or wrong substance given or taken *—see* Table of Drugs and Chemicals, by drug, poisoning
- **Cushing's**
  - syndrome or disease E24.9
    - drug-induced E24.2
    - iatrogenic E24.2
    - pituitary-dependent E24.Ø
    - specified NEC E24.8
  - ulcer *—see* Ulcer, peptic, acute
- **Cusp, Carabelli** - omit code
- **Cut** (external) *—see also* Laceration
  - muscle *—see* Injury, muscle
- **Cutaneous** *—see also* condition
  - hemorrhage R23.3
  - larva migrans B76.9
- **Cutis** *—see also* condition
  - hyperelastica Q82.8
    - acquired L57.4
  - laxa (hyperelastica) *—see* Dermatolysis
  - marmorata R23.8
  - osteosis L94.2
  - pendula *—see* Dermatolysis
  - rhomboidalis nuchae L57.2
  - verticis gyrata Q82.8
    - acquired L91.8
- **Cyanosis** R23.Ø
  - due to
    - patent foramen botalli Q21.1
    - persistent foramen ovale Q21.1
  - enterogenous D74.8
  - paroxysmal digital *—see* Raynaud's disease
    - with gangrene I73.Ø1
  - retina, retinal H35.89
- **Cyanotic heart disease** I24.9
  - congenital Q24.9
- **Cycle**
  - anovulatory N97.Ø
  - menstrual, irregular N92.6
- **Cyclencephaly** QØ4.9
- **Cyclical vomiting** (*see also* Vomiting, cyclical) G43.AØ
  - psychogenic F5Ø.89 ⟸

C

Cyclitis —*see also* Iridocyclitis H20.9
chronic —*see* Iridocyclitis, chronic
Fuchs' heterochromic H20.81-
granulomatous —*see* Iridocyclitis, chronic
lens-induced —*see* Iridocyclitis, lens-induced
posterior H30.2-
Cycloid personality F34.0
Cyclophoria H50.54
Cyclopia, cyclops Q87.0
Cyclopism Q87.0
Cyclosporiasis A07.4
Cyclothymia F34.0
Cyclothymic personality F34.0
Cyclotropia H50.41-
Cylindroma —*see also* Neoplasm, malignant, by site
eccrine dermal —*see* Neoplasm, skin, benign
skin —*see* Neoplasm, skin, benign
Cylindruria R82.99
Cynanche
diphtheritic A36.2
tonsillaris J36
Cynophobia F40.218
Cynorexia R63.2
Cyphosis —*see* Kyphosis
Cyprus fever —*see* Brucellosis
Cyst (colloid) (mucous) (simple) (retention)
adenoid (infected) J35.8
adrenal gland E27.8
congenital Q89.1
air, lung J98.4
allantoic Q64.4
alveolar process (jaw bone) M27.40
amnion, amniotic O41.8X-
aneurysmal M27.49 ◀
anterior
chamber (eye) —*see* Cyst, iris
nasopalatine K09.1
antrum J34.1
anus K62.89
apical (tooth) (periodontal) K04.8
appendix K38.8
arachnoid, brain (acquired) G93.0
congenital Q04.6
arytenoid J38.7
Baker's M71.2-
ruptured M66.0
tuberculous A18.02
Bartholin's gland N75.0
bile duct (common) (hepatic) K83.5
bladder (multiple) (trigone) N32.89
blue dome (breast) —*see* Cyst, breast
bone (local) NEC M85.60
aneurysmal M85.50
ankle M85.57-
foot M85.57-
forearm M85.53-
hand M85.54-
jaw M27.49
lower leg M85.56-
multiple site M85.59
neck M85.58
rib M85.58
shoulder M85.51-
skull M85.58
specified site NEC M85.58
thigh M85.55-
toe M85.57-
upper arm M85.52-
vertebra M85.58
solitary M85.40
ankle M85.47-
fibula M85.46-
foot M85.47-
hand M85.44-
humerus M85.42-
jaw M27.49
neck M85.48
pelvis M85.45-

Cyst *(Continued)*
bone NEC *(Continued)*
solitary *(Continued)*
radius M85.43-
rib M85.48
shoulder M85.41-
skull M85.48
specified site NEC M85.48
tibia M85.46-
toe M85.47-
ulna M85.43-
vertebra M85.48
specified type NEC M85.60
ankle M85.67-
foot M85.67-
forearm M85.63-
hand M85.64-
jaw M27.40
developmental (nonodontogenic) K09.1
odontogenic K09.0
latent M27.0
lower leg M85.66-
multiple site M85.69
neck M85.68
rib M85.68
shoulder M85.61-
skull M85.68
specified site NEC M85.68
thigh M85.65-
toe M85.67-
upper arm M85.62-
vertebra M85.68
brain (acquired) G93.0
congenital Q04.6
hydatid B67.99 *[G94]*
third ventricle (colloid), congenital Q04.6
branchial (cleft) Q18.0
branchiogenic Q18.0
breast (benign) (blue dome) (pedunculated) (solitary) N60.0-
involution —*see* Dysplasia, mammary, specified type NEC
sebaceous —*see* Dysplasia, mammary, specified type NEC
broad ligament (benign) N83.8
bronchogenic (mediastinal) (sequestration) J98.4
congenital Q33.0
buccal K09.8
bulbourethral gland N36.8
bursa, bursal NEC M71.30
with rupture —*see* Rupture, synovium
ankle M71.37-
elbow M71.32-
foot M71.37-
hand M71.34-
hip M71.35-
multiple sites M71.39
pharyngeal J39.2
popliteal space —*see* Cyst, Baker's
shoulder M71.31-
specified site NEC M71.38
wrist M71.33-
calcifying odontogenic D16.5
upper jaw (bone) (maxilla) D16.4
canal of Nuck (female) N94.89
congenital Q52.4
canthus —*see* Cyst, conjunctiva
carcinomatous —*see* Neoplasm, malignant, by site
cauda equina G95.89
cavum septi pellucidi —*see* Cyst, brain
celomic (pericardium) Q24.8
cerebellopontine (angle) —*see* Cyst, brain
cerebellum —*see* Cyst, brain
cerebral —*see* Cyst, brain
cervical lateral Q18.0 ⬅
cervix NEC N88.8
embryonic Q51.6
nabothian N88.8

Cyst *(Continued)*
chiasmal optic NEC —*see* Disorder, optic, chiasm
chocolate (ovary) N80.1
choledochus, congenital Q44.4
chorion O41.8X-
choroid plexus G93.0
ciliary body —*see* Cyst, iris
clitoris N90.7
colon K63.89
common (bile) duct K83.5
congenital NEC Q89.8
adrenal gland Q89.1
epiglottis Q31.8
esophagus Q39.8
fallopian tube Q50.4
kidney Q61.00
more than one (multiple) Q61.02
specified as polycystic Q61.3
adult type Q61.2
infantile type NEC Q61.19
collecting duct dilation Q61.11
solitary Q61.01
larynx Q31.8
liver Q44.6
lung Q33.0
mediastinum Q34.1
ovary Q50.1
oviduct Q50.4
periurethral (tissue) Q64.79
prepuce Q55.69
salivary gland (any) Q38.4
sublingual Q38.6
submaxillary gland Q38.6
thymus (gland) Q89.2
tongue Q38.3
ureterovesical orifice Q62.8
vulva Q52.79
conjunctiva H11.44-
cornea H18.89-
corpora quadrigemina G93.0
corpus
albicans N83.29- ⬅
luteum (hemorrhagic) (ruptured) N83.1- ⬅
Cowper's gland (benign) (infected) N36.8
cranial meninges G93.0
craniobuccal pouch E23.6
craniopharyngeal pouch E23.6
cystic duct K82.8
Cysticercus —*see* Cysticercosis
Dandy-Walker Q03.1
with spina bifida —*see* Spina bifida
dental (root) K04.8
developmental K09.0
eruption K09.0
primordial K09.0
dentigerous (mandible) (maxilla) K09.0
dermoid —*see* Neoplasm, benign, by site
with malignant transformation C56.-
implantation
external area or site (skin) NEC L72.0
iris —*see* Cyst, iris, implantation
vagina N89.8
vulva N90.7
mouth K09.8
oral soft tissue K09.8
sacrococcygeal —*see* Cyst, pilonidal
developmental K09.1
odontogenic K09.0
oral region (nonodontogenic) K09.1
ovary, ovarian Q50.1
dura (cerebral) G93.0
spinal G96.19
ear (external) Q18.1
echinococcal —*see* Echinococcus
embryonic
cervix uteri Q51.6
fallopian tube Q50.4
vagina Q51.6

C

Cyst *(Continued)*
  endometrium, endometrial (uterus) N85.8
    ectopic —*see* Endometriosis
  enterogenous Q43.8
  epidermal, epidermoid (inclusion) (*see also* Cyst, skin) L72.0
    mouth K09.8
    oral soft tissue K09.8
  epididymis N50.3
  epiglottis J38.7
  epiphysis cerebri E34.8
  epithelial (inclusion) L72.0
  epoophoron Q50.5
  eruption K09.0
  esophagus K22.8
  ethmoid sinus J34.1
  external female genital organs NEC N90.7
  eye NEC H57.8
    congenital Q15.8
  eyelid (sebaceous) H02.829
    infected —*see* Hordeolum
    left H02.826
      lower H02.825
      upper H02.824
    right H02.823
      lower H02.822
      upper H02.821
  fallopian tube N83.8
    congenital Q50.4
  fimbrial (twisted) Q50.4
  fissural (oral region) K09.1
  follicle (graafian) (hemorrhagic) N83.0- ⬅
    nabothian N88.8
  follicular (atretic) (hemorrhagic) (ovarian) N83.0- ⬅
    dentigerous K09.0
    odontogenic K09.0
    skin L72.9
      specified NEC L72.8
  frontal sinus J34.1
  gallbladder K82.8
  ganglion —*see* Ganglion
  Gartner's duct Q52.4
  gingiva K09.0
  gland of Moll —*see* Cyst, eyelid
  globulomaxillary K09.1
  graafian follicle (hemorrhagic) N83.0- ⬅
  granulosal lutein (hemorrhagic) N83.1- ⬅
  hemangiomatous D18.00
    intra-abdominal D18.03
    intracranial D18.02
    skin D18.01
    specified site NEC D18.09
  hemorrhagic M27.49 ◄
  hydatid —*see also* Echinococcus B67.90
    brain B67.99 *[G94]*
    liver —*see also* Cyst, liver, hydatid B67.8
    lung NEC B67.99 *[J99]*
    Morgagni
      female Q50.5
      male (epididymal) Q55.4
        testicular Q55.29
    specified site NEC B67.99
  hymen N89.8
    embryonic Q52.4
  hypopharynx J39.2
  hypophysis, hypophyseal (duct) (recurrent) E23.6
    cerebri E23.6
  implantation (dermoid)
    external area or site (skin) NEC L72.0
    iris —*see* Cyst, iris, implantation
    vagina N89.8
    vulva N90.7
  incisive canal K09.1
  inclusion (epidermal) (epithelial) (epidermoid) (squamous) L72.0
    not of skin - code under Cyst, by site
  intestine (large) (small) K63.89
  intracranial —*see* Cyst, brain
  intraligamentous —*see also* Disorder, ligament
    knee —*see* Derangement, knee

Cyst *(Continued)*
  intrasellar E23.6
  iris H21.309
    exudative H21.31-
    idiopathic H21.30-
    implantation H21.32-
    parasitic H21.33-
    pars plana (primary) H21.34-
      exudative H21.35-
  jaw (bone) M27.40
    aneurysmal M27.49
    developmental (odontogenic) K09.0
    fissural K09.1
    hemorrhagic M27.49
    traumatic M27.49
  joint NEC —*see* Disorder, joint, specified type NEC
  kidney (acquired) N28.1
    calyceal —*see* Hydronephrosis
    congenital Q61.00
    more than one (multiple) Q61.02
      specified as polycystic Q61.3
        adult type (autosomal dominant) Q61.2
        infantile type (autosomal recessive) NEC Q61.19
          collecting duct dilation Q61.11
    pyelogenic —*see* Hydronephrosis
    simple N28.1
    solitary (single) Q61.01
      acquired N28.1
  labium (majus) (minus) N90.7
    sebaceous N90.7
  lacrimal —*see also* Disorder, lacrimal system, specified NEC
    gland H04.13-
    passages or sac —*see* Disorder, lacrimal system, specified NEC
  larynx J38.7
  lateral periodontal K09.0
  lens H27.8
    congenital Q12.8
  lip (gland) K13.0
  liver (idiopathic) (simple) K76.89
    congenital Q44.6
    hydatid B67.8
      granulosus B67.0
      multilocularis B67.5
  lung J98.4
    congenital Q33.0
    giant bullous J43.9
  lutein N83.1- ⬅
  lymphangiomatous D18.1
  lymphoepithelial, oral soft tissue K09.8
  macula —*see* Degeneration, macula, hole
  malignant —*see* Neoplasm, malignant, by site
  mammary gland —*see* Cyst, breast
  mandible M27.40
    dentigerous K09.0
    radicular K04.8
  maxilla M27.40
    dentigerous K09.0
    radicular K04.8
  medial, face and neck Q18.8
  median
    anterior maxillary K09.1
    palatal K09.1
  mediastinum, congenital Q34.1
  meibomian (gland) —*see* Chalazion
    infected —*see* Hordeolum
  membrane, brain G93.0
  meninges (cerebral) G93.0
    spinal G96.19
  meniscus, knee —*see* Derangement, knee, meniscus, cystic
  mesentery, mesenteric K66.8
    chyle I89.8
  mesonephric duct
    female Q50.5
    male Q55.4
  milk N64.89

Cyst *(Continued)*
  Morgagni (hydatid)
    female Q50.5
    male (epididymal) Q55.4
      testicular Q55.29
  mouth K09.8
  Müllerian duct Q50.4
    appendix testis Q55.29
    cervix Q51.6
    fallopian tube Q50.4
    female Q50.4
    male Q55.29
    prostatic utricle Q55.4
    vagina (embryonal) Q52.4
  multilocular (ovary) D39.10
    benign —*see* Neoplasm, benign, by site
  myometrium N85.8
  nabothian (follicle) (ruptured) N88.8
  nasoalveolar K09.1
  nasolabial K09.1
  nasopalatine (anterior) (duct) K09.1
  nasopharynx J39.2
  neoplastic —*see* Neoplasm, uncertain behavior, by site
    benign —*see* Neoplasm, benign, by site
  nervous system NEC G96.8
  neuroenteric (congenital) Q06.8
  nipple —*see* Cyst, breast
  nose (turbinates) J34.1
    sinus J34.1
  odontogenic, developmental K09.0
  omentum (lesser) K66.8
    congenital Q45.8
  ora serrata —*see* Cyst, retina, ora serrata
  oral
    region K09.9
      developmental (nonodontogenic) K09.1
      specified NEC K09.8
    soft tissue K09.9
      specified NEC K09.8
  orbit H05.81-
  ovary, ovarian (twisted) N83.20- ⬅
    adherent N83.20- ⬅
    chocolate N80.1
    corpus
      albicans N83.29- ⬅
      luteum (hemorrhagic) N83.1- ⬅
    dermoid D27.9
    developmental Q50.1
    due to failure of involution NEC N83.20- ⬅
    endometrial N80.1
    follicular (graafian) (hemorrhagic) N83.0- ⬅
    hemorrhagic N83.20- ⬅
    in pregnancy or childbirth O34.8-
      with obstructed labor O65.5
    multilocular D39.10
    pseudomucinous D27.9
    retention N83.29- ⬅
    serous N83.20- ⬅
    specified NEC N83.29- ⬅
    theca lutein (hemorrhagic) N83.1- ⬅
    tuberculous A18.18
  oviduct N83.8
  palate (median) (fissural) K09.1
  palatine papilla (jaw) K09.1
  pancreas, pancreatic (hemorrhagic) (true) K86.2
    congenital Q45.2
    false K86.3
  paralabral
    hip M24.85-
    shoulder S43.43-
  paramesonephric duct Q50.4
    female Q50.4
    male Q55.29
  paranephric N28.1
  paraphysis, cerebri, congenital Q04.6
  parasitic B89
  parathyroid (gland) E21.4
  paratubal N83.8
  paraurethral duct N36.8
  paroophoron Q50.5

◄ New ⬅ Revised ~~deleted~~ Deleted

- **Cystadenoma** *(Continued)*
  - mucinous *(Continued)*
    - papillary *(Continued)*
      - specified site —*see* Neoplasm, benign, by site
      - unspecified site D27.9
    - specified site —*see* Neoplasm, benign, by site
    - unspecified site D27.9
  - papillary
    - borderline malignancy
      - ovary C56-
      - specified site NEC —*see* Neoplasm, uncertain behavior, by site
      - unspecified site C56.9
    - lymphomatosum
      - specified site —*see* Neoplasm, benign, by site
      - unspecified site D11.9
    - mucinous
      - borderline malignancy
        - ovary C56.-
        - specified site NEC —*see* Neoplasm, uncertain behavior, by site
        - unspecified site C56.9
      - specified site —*see* Neoplasm, benign, by site
      - unspecified site D27.9
    - pseudomucinous
      - borderline malignancy
        - ovary C56.-
        - specified site NEC —*see* Neoplasm, uncertain behavior, by site
        - unspecified site C56.9
      - specified site —*see* Neoplasm, benign, by site
      - unspecified site D27.9
    - serous
      - borderline malignancy
        - ovary C56.-
        - specified site NEC —*see* Neoplasm, uncertain behavior, by site
        - unspecified site C56.9
      - specified site —*see* Neoplasm, benign, by site
      - unspecified site D27.9
    - specified site —*see* Neoplasm, benign, by site
    - unspecified site D27.9
  - pseudomucinous
    - borderline malignancy
      - ovary C56.-
      - specified site NEC —*see* Neoplasm, uncertain behavior, by site
      - unspecified site C56.9
    - papillary
      - borderline malignancy
        - ovary C56.-
        - specified site NEC —*see* Neoplasm, uncertain behavior, by site
        - unspecified site C56.9
      - specified site —*see* Neoplasm, benign, by site
      - unspecified site D27.9
    - specified site —*see* Neoplasm, benign, by site
    - unspecified site D27.9
  - serous
    - borderline malignancy
      - ovary C56.-
      - specified site NEC —*see* Neoplasm, uncertain behavior, by site
      - unspecified site C56.9
    - papillary
      - borderline malignancy
        - ovary C56.-
        - specified site NEC —*see* Neoplasm, uncertain behavior, by site
        - unspecified site C56.9
      - specified site —*see* Neoplasm, benign, by site
      - unspecified site D27.9
    - specified site —*see* Neoplasm, benign, by site
    - unspecified site D27.9
- **Cystathionine synthase deficiency** E72.11
- **Cystathioninemia** E72.19
- **Cystathioninuria** E72.19
- **Cystic** —*see also* condition
  - breast (chronic) —*see* Mastopathy, cystic
  - corpora lutea (hemorrhagic) N83.1- ⬅
  - duct —*see* condition
  - eyeball (congenital) Q11.Ø
  - fibrosis —*see* Fibrosis, cystic
  - kidney (congenital) Q61.9
    - adult type Q61.2
    - infantile type NEC Q61.19
      - collecting duct dilatation Q61.11
    - medullary Q61.5
  - liver, congenital Q44.6
  - lung disease J98.4
    - congenital Q33.Ø
  - mastitis, chronic —*see* Mastopathy, cystic
  - medullary, kidney Q61.5
  - meniscus —*see* Derangement, knee, meniscus, cystic
  - ovary N83.2Ø- ⬅
- **Cysticercosis, cysticerciasis** B69.9
  - with
    - epileptiform fits B69.Ø
    - myositis B69.81
  - brain B69.Ø
  - central nervous system B69.Ø
  - cerebral B69.Ø
  - ocular B69.1
  - specified NEC B69.89
- **Cysticercus cellulose infestation** —*see* Cysticercosis
- **Cystinosis** (malignant) E72.Ø4
- **Cystinuria** E72.Ø1
- **Cystitis** (exudative) (hemorrhagic) (septic) (suppurative) N3Ø.9Ø
  - with
    - fibrosis —*see* Cystitis, chronic, interstitial
    - hematuria N3Ø.91
    - leukoplakia —*see* Cystitis, chronic, interstitial
    - malakoplakia —*see* Cystitis, chronic, interstitial
    - metaplasia —*see* Cystitis, chronic, interstitial
    - prostatitis N41.3
  - acute N3Ø.ØØ
    - with hematuria N3Ø.Ø1
    - of trigone N3Ø.3Ø
      - with hematuria N3Ø.31
  - allergic —*see* Cystitis, specified type NEC
  - amebic AØ6.81
  - bilharzial B65.9 *[N33]*
  - blennorrhagic (gonococcal) A54.Ø1
  - bullous —*see* Cystitis, specified type NEC
  - calculous N21.Ø
  - chlamydial A56.Ø1
  - chronic N3Ø.2Ø
    - with hematuria N3Ø.21
    - interstitial N3Ø.1Ø
      - with hematuria N3Ø.11
    - of trigone N3Ø.3Ø
      - with hematuria N3Ø.31
    - specified NEC N3Ø.2Ø
      - with hematuria N3Ø.21
  - cystic (a) —*see* Cystitis, specified type NEC
  - diphtheritic A36.85
  - echinococcal
    - granulosus B67.39
    - multilocularis B67.69
  - emphysematous —*see* Cystitis, specified type NEC
  - encysted —*see* Cystitis, specified type NEC
  - eosinophilic —*see* Cystitis, specified type NEC
  - follicular —*see* Cystitis, of trigone
  - gangrenous —*see* Cystitis, specified type NEC
  - glandularis —*see* Cystitis, specified type NEC
  - gonococcal A54.Ø1
  - incrusted —*see* Cystitis, specified type NEC
  - interstitial (chronic) —*see* Cystitis, chronic, interstitial
  - irradiation N3Ø.4Ø
    - with hematuria N3Ø.41
  - irritation —*see* Cystitis, specified type NEC
  - malignant —*see* Cystitis, specified type NEC
  - of trigone N3Ø.3Ø
    - with hematuria N3Ø.31
  - panmural —*see* Cystitis, chronic, interstitial
  - polyposa —*see* Cystitis, specified type NEC
  - prostatic N41.3
  - puerperal (postpartum) O86.22
  - radiation —*see* Cystitis, irradiation
  - specified type NEC N3Ø.8Ø
    - with hematuria N3Ø.81
  - subacute —*see* Cystitis, chronic
  - submucous —*see* Cystitis, chronic, interstitial
  - syphilitic (late) A52.76
  - trichomonal A59.Ø3
  - tuberculous A18.12
  - ulcerative —*see* Cystitis, chronic, interstitial
- **Cystocele** (-urethrocele)
  - female N81.1Ø
    - with prolapse of uterus —*see* Prolapse, uterus
    - lateral N81.12
    - midline N81.11
    - paravaginal N81.12
  - in pregnancy or childbirth O34.8-
    - causing obstructed labor O65.5
  - male N32.89
- **Cystolithiasis** N21.Ø
- **Cystoma** —*see also* Neoplasm, benign, by site
  - endometrial, ovary N8Ø.1
  - mucinous
    - specified site —*see* Neoplasm, benign, by site
    - unspecified site D27.9
  - serous
    - specified site —*see* Neoplasm, benign, by site
    - unspecified site D27.9
  - simple (ovary) N83.29- ⬅
- **Cystoplegia** N31.2
- **Cystoptosis** N32.89
- **Cystopyelitis** —*see* Pyelonephritis
- **Cystorrhagia** N32.89
- **Cystosarcoma phyllodes** D48.6-
  - benign D24-
  - malignant —*see* Neoplasm, breast, malignant
- **Cystostomy**
  - attention to Z43.5
  - complication —*see* Complications, cystostomy
  - status Z93.5Ø
    - appendico-vesicostomy Z93.52
    - cutaneous Z93.51
    - specified NEC Z93.59
- **Cystourethritis** —*see* Urethritis
- **Cystourethrocele** —*see also* Cystocele
  - female N81.1Ø
    - with uterine prolapse —*see* Prolapse, uterus
    - lateral N81.12
    - midline N81.11
    - paravaginal N81.12
  - male N32.89
- **Cytomegalic inclusion disease**
  - congenital P35.1
- **Cytomegalovirus infection** B25.9
- **Cytomycosis** (reticuloendothelial) B39.4
- **Cytopenia** D75.9
  - refractory
    - with multilineage dysplasia D46.A
      - and ring sideroblasts (RCMD RS) D46.B
- **Czerny's disease** (periodic hydrarthrosis of the knee) —*see* Effusion, joint, knee

D

- **Daae** (-Finsen) **disease** (epidemic pleurodynia) B33.0
- **Dabney's grip** B33.0
- **Da Costa's syndrome** F45.8
- **Dacryoadenitis, dacryadenitis** H04.00-
  - acute H04.01-
  - chronic H04.02-
- **Dacryocystitis** H04.30-
  - acute H04.32-
  - chronic H04.41-
  - neonatal P39.1
  - phlegmonous H04.31-
  - syphilitic A52.71
    - congenital (early) A50.01
  - trachomatous, active A71.1
    - sequelae (late effect) B94.0
- **Dacryocystoblenorrhea** —*see* Inflammation, lacrimal, passages, chronic
- **Dacryocystocele** —*see* Disorder, lacrimal system, changes
- **Dacryolith, dacryolithiasis** H04.51-
- **Dacryoma** —*see* Disorder, lacrimal system, changes
- **Dacryopericystitis** —*see* Dacryocystitis
- **Dacryops** H04.11-
- **Dacryostenosis** —*see also* Stenosis, lacrimal
  - congenital Q10.5
- **Dactylitis**
  - bone —*see* Osteomyelitis
  - sickle-cell D57.00
    - Hb C D57.219
    - Hb SS D57.00
    - specified NEC D57.819
  - skin L08.9
  - syphilitic A52.77
  - tuberculous A18.03
- **Dactylolysis spontanea** (ainhum) L94.6
- **Dactylosymphysis** Q70.9
  - fingers —*see* Syndactylism, complex, fingers
  - toes —*see* Syndactylism, complex, toes
- **Damage**
  - arteriosclerotic —*see* Arteriosclerosis
  - brain (nontraumatic) G93.9
    - anoxic, hypoxic G93.1
      - resulting from a procedure G97.82
    - child NEC G80.9
    - due to birth injury P11.2
  - cardiorenal (vascular) —*see* Hypertension, cardiorenal
  - cerebral NEC —*see* Damage, brain
  - coccyx, complicating delivery O71.6
  - coronary —*see* Disease, heart, ischemic
  - eye, birth injury P15.3
  - liver (nontraumatic) K76.9
    - alcoholic K70.9
    - due to drugs —*see* Disease, liver, toxic
    - toxic —*see* Disease, liver, toxic
  - medication T88.7
  - pelvic
    - joint or ligament, during delivery O71.6
    - organ NEC
      - during delivery O71.5
      - following ectopic or molar pregnancy O08.6
  - renal —*see* Disease, renal
  - subendocardium, subendocardial —*see* Degeneration, myocardial
  - vascular I99.9
- **Dana-Putnam syndrome** (subacute combined sclerosis with pernicious anemia) —*see* Degeneration, combined
- **Danbolt** (-Cross) **syndrome** (acrodermatitis enteropathica) E83.2
- **Dandruff** L21.0
- **Dandy-Walker syndrome** Q03.1
  - with spina bifida —*see* Spina bifida
- **Danlos' syndrome** Q79.6
- **Darier** (-White) **disease** (congenital) Q82.8
  - meaning erythema annulare centrifugum L53.1
- **Darier-Roussy sarcoid** D86.3
- **Darling's disease or histoplasmosis** B39.4
- **Darwin's tubercle** Q17.8
- **Dawson's** (inclusion body) **encephalitis** A81.1
- **De Beurmann** (-Gougerot) **disease** B42.1
- **De la Tourette's syndrome** F95.2
- **De Lange's syndrome** Q87.1
- **De Morgan's spots** (senile angiomas) I78.1
- **De Quervain's**
  - disease (tendon sheath) M65.4
  - syndrome E34.51
  - thyroiditis (subacute granulomatous thyroiditis) E06.1
- **De Toni-Fanconi** (-Debré) **syndrome** E72.09
  - with cystinosis E72.04
- **Dead**
  - fetus, retained (mother) O36.4
    - early pregnancy O02.1
  - labyrinth —*see* subcategory H83.2
  - ovum, retained O02.0
- **Deaf nonspeaking NEC** H91.3
- **Deafmutism** (acquired) (congenital) NEC H91.3
  - hysterical F44.6
  - syphilitic, congenital —*see also* subcategory H94.8 A50.09
- **Deafness** (acquired) (complete) (hereditary) (partial) H91.9-
  - with blue sclera and fragility of bone Q78.0
  - auditory fatigue —*see* Deafness, specified type NEC
  - aviation T70.0
    - nerve injury —*see* Injury, nerve, acoustic, specified type NEC
  - boilermaker's —*see* subcategory H83.3
  - central —*see* Deafness, sensorineural
  - conductive H90.2
    - ~~and sensorineural, mixed H90.8~~
      - ~~bilateral H90.6~~
    - and sensorineural ◀
      - mixed H90.8 ◀
        - bilateral H90.6 ◀
    - bilateral H90.0
    - unilateral H90.1-
      - with restricted hearing on the contralateral side H90.A- ◀
  - congenital H90.5
    - with blue sclera and fragility of bone Q78.0
  - due to toxic agents —*see* Deafness, ototoxic
  - emotional (hysterical) F44.6
  - functional (hysterical) F44.6
  - high frequency H91.9-
  - hysterical F44.6
  - low frequency H91.9-
  - mental R48.8
  - mixed conductive and sensorineural H90.8
    - bilateral H90.6
    - unilateral H90.7-
  - nerve —*see* Deafness, sensorineural
  - neural —*see* Deafness, sensorineural
  - noise-induced —*see also* subcategory H83.3
    - nerve injury —*see* Injury, nerve, acoustic, specified type NEC
  - nonspeaking H91.3
  - ototoxic —*see* subcategory H91.0
  - perceptive —*see* Deafness, sensorineural
  - psychogenic (hysterical) F44.6
  - sensorineural H90.5
    - ~~and conductive, mixed H90.8~~
      - ~~bilateral H90.6~~
    - and conductive ◀
      - mixed H90.8 ◀
        - bilateral H90.6 ◀
    - bilateral H90.3
    - unilateral H90.4-
      - with restricted hearing on the contralateral side H90.A- ◀
  - sensory —*see* Deafness, sensorineural
  - specified type NEC —*see* subcategory H91.8
  - sudden (idiopathic) H91.2-
- **Deafness** (*Continued*)
  - syphilitic A52.15
  - transient ischemic H93.01-
  - traumatic —*see* Injury, nerve, acoustic, specified type NEC
  - word (developmental) H93.25
- **Death** (cause unknown) (of) (unexplained) (unspecified cause) R99
  - brain G93.82
  - cardiac (sudden) (with successful resuscitation) — code to underlying disease
    - family history of Z82.41
    - personal history of Z86.74
  - family member (assumed) Z63.4
- **Debility** (chronic) (general) (nervous) R53.81
  - congenital or neonatal NOS P96.9
  - nervous R53.81
  - old age R54
  - senile R54
- **Débove's disease** (splenomegaly) R16.1
- **Decalcification**
  - bone —*see* Osteoporosis
  - teeth K03.89
- **Decapsulation, kidney** N28.89
- **Decay**
  - dental —*see* Caries, dental
  - senile R54
  - tooth, teeth —*see* Caries, dental
- **Deciduitis** (acute)
  - following ectopic or molar pregnancy O08.0
- **Decline** (general) —*see* Debility
  - cognitive, age-associated R41.81
- **Decompensation**
  - cardiac (acute) (chronic) —*see* Disease, heart
  - cardiovascular —*see* Disease, cardiovascular
  - heart —*see* Disease, heart
  - hepatic —*see* Failure, hepatic
  - myocardial (acute) (chronic) —*see* Disease, heart
  - respiratory J98.8
- **Decompression sickness** T70.3
- **Decrease** (d)
  - absolute neutrophile count —*see* Neutropenia
  - blood
    - platelets —*see* Thrombocytopenia
    - pressure R03.1
      - due to shock following
        - injury T79.4
        - operation T81.19
  - estrogen E28.39
    - postablative E89.40
      - asymptomatic E89.40
      - symptomatic E89.41
  - fragility of erythrocytes D58.8
  - function
    - lipase (pancreatic) K90.3
    - ovary in hypopituitarism E23.0
    - parenchyma of pancreas K86.89 ⟸
    - pituitary (gland) (anterior) (lobe) E23.0
      - posterior (lobe) E23.0
  - functional activity R68.89
  - glucose R73.09
  - hematocrit R71.0
  - hemoglobin R71.0
  - leukocytes D72.819
    - specified NEC D72.818
  - libido R68.82
  - lymphocytes D72.810
  - platelets D69.6
  - respiration, due to shock following injury T79.4
  - sexual desire R68.82
  - tear secretion NEC —*see* Syndrome, dry eye
  - tolerance
    - fat K90.49 ⟸
    - glucose R73.09
    - pancreatic K90.3
    - salt and water E87.8
  - vision NEC H54.7
  - white blood cell count D72.819
    - specified NEC D72.818

◀ New ⟸ Revised ~~deleted~~ Deleted

- **Decubitus** (ulcer) —*see* Ulcer, pressure, by site
  - cervix N86
- **Deepening acetabulum** —*see* Derangement, joint, specified type NEC, hip
- **Defect, defective** Q89.9
  - 3-beta-hydroxysteroid dehydrogenase E25.Ø
  - 11-hydroxylase E25.Ø
  - 21-hydroxylase E25.Ø
  - abdominal wall, congenital Q79.59
  - antibody immunodeficiency D8Ø.9
  - aorticopulmonary septum Q21.4
  - atrial septal (ostium secundum type) Q21.1
    - following acute myocardial infarction (current complication) I23.1
    - ostium primum type Q21.2
  - atrioventricular
    - canal Q21.2
    - septum Q21.2
  - auricular septal Q21.1
  - bilirubin excretion NEC E8Ø.6
  - biosynthesis, androgen (testicular) E29.1
  - bulbar septum Q21.Ø
  - catalase E8Ø.3
  - cell membrane receptor complex (CR3) D71
  - circulation I99.9
    - congenital Q28.9
    - newborn Q28.9
  - coagulation (factor) —*see also* Deficiency, factor D68.9
    - with
      - ectopic pregnancy OØ8.1
      - molar pregnancy OØ8.1
    - acquired D68.4
    - antepartum with hemorrhage —*see* Hemorrhage, antepartum, with coagulation defect
    - due to
      - liver disease D68.4
      - vitamin K deficiency D68.4
    - hereditary NEC D68.2
    - intrapartum O67.Ø
    - newborn, transient P61.6
    - postpartum O72.3
    - specified type NEC D68.8
  - complement system D84.1
  - conduction (heart) I45.9
    - bone —*see* Deafness, conductive
  - congenital, organ or site not listed —*see* Anomaly, by site
  - coronary sinus Q21.1
  - cushion, endocardial Q21.2
  - degradation, glycoprotein E77.1
  - dental bridge, crown, fillings —*see* Defect, dental restoration
  - dental restoration KØ8.5Ø
    - specified NEC KØ8.59
  - dentin (hereditary) KØØ.5
  - Descemet's membrane, congenital Q13.89
  - developmental —*see also* Anomaly
    - cauda equina QØ6.3
  - diaphragm
    - with elevation, eventration or hernia —*see* Hernia, diaphragm
    - congenital Q79.1
      - with hernia Q79.Ø
      - gross (with hernia) Q79.Ø
  - ectodermal, congenital Q82.9
  - Eisenmenger's Q21.8
  - enzyme
    - catalase E8Ø.3
    - peroxidase E8Ø.3
  - esophagus, congenital Q39.9
  - extensor retinaculum M62.89
  - fibrin polymerization D68.2
  - filling
    - bladder R93.41 ⬅
    - kidney R93.42- ⬅
    - renal pelvis R93.41 ◀
    - stomach R93.3
    - ureter R93.41 ⬅
    - urinary organs, specified NEC R93.49 ◀

- **Defect, defective** *(Continued)*
  - Gerbode Q21.Ø
  - glycoprotein degradation E77.1
  - Hageman (factor) D68.2
  - hearing —*see* Deafness
  - high grade F7Ø
  - interatrial septal Q21.1
  - interauricular septal Q21.1
  - interventricular septal Q21.Ø
    - with dextroposition of aorta, pulmonary stenosis and hypertrophy of right ventricle Q21.3
    - in tetralogy of Fallot Q21.3
  - learning (specific) —*see* Disorder, learning
  - lymphocyte function antigen-1 (LFA-1) D84.Ø
  - lysosomal enzyme, post-translational modification E77.Ø
  - major osseous M89.7Ø
    - ankle M89.77-
    - carpus M89.74-
    - clavicle M89.71-
    - femur M89.75-
    - fibula M89.76-
    - fingers M89.74-
    - foot M89.77-
    - forearm M89.73-
    - hand M89.74-
    - humerus M89.72-
    - lower leg M89.76-
    - metacarpus M89.74-
    - metatarsus M89.77-
    - multiple sites M89.79
    - pelvic region M89.75-
    - pelvis M89.75-
    - radius M89.73-
    - scapula M89.71-
    - shoulder region M89.71-
    - specified NEC M89.78
    - tarsus M89.77-
    - thigh M89.75-
    - tibia M89.76-
    - toes M89.77-
    - ulna M89.73-
  - mental —*see* Disability, intellectual
  - modification, lysosomal enzymes, post-translational E77.Ø
  - obstructive, congenital
    - renal pelvis Q62.39
    - ureter Q62.39
      - atresia —*see* Atresia, ureter
      - cecoureterocele Q62.32
      - megaureter Q62.2
      - orthotopic ureterocele Q62.31
  - osseous, major M89.7Ø
    - ankle M89.77-
    - carpus M89.74-
    - clavicle M89.71-
    - femur M89.75-
    - fibula M89.76-
    - fingers M89.74-
    - foot M89.77-
    - forearm M89.73-
    - hand M89.74-
    - humerus M89.72-
    - lower leg M89.76-
    - metacarpus M89.74-
    - metatarsus M89.77-
    - multiple sites M89.9
    - pelvic region M89.75-
    - pelvis M89.75-
    - radius M89.73-
    - scapula M89.71-
    - shoulder region M89.71-
    - specified NEC M89.78
    - tarsus M89.77-
    - thigh M89.75-
    - tibia M89.76-
    - toes M89.77-
    - ulna M89.73-
  - osteochondral NEC —*see also* Deformity M95.8-

- **Defect, defective** *(Continued)*
  - ostium
    - primum Q21.2
    - secundum Q21.1
  - peroxidase E8Ø.3
  - placental blood supply —*see* Insufficiency, placental
  - platelets, qualitative D69.1
    - constitutional D68.Ø
  - postural NEC, spine —*see* Dorsopathy, deforming
  - reduction
    - limb Q73.8
      - lower Q72.9-
        - absence —*see* Agenesis, leg
          - foot —*see* Agenesis, foot
        - longitudinal
          - femur Q72.4-
          - fibula Q72.6-
          - tibia Q72.5-
        - specified type NEC Q72.89-
        - split foot Q72.7-
      - specified type NEC Q73.8
      - upper Q71.9-
        - absence —*see* Agenesis, arm
          - forearm —*see* Agenesis, forearm
          - hand —*see* Agenesis, hand
        - lobster-claw hand Q71.6-
        - longitudinal
          - radius Q71.4-
          - ulna Q71.5-
        - specified type NEC Q71.89-
  - renal pelvis Q63.8
    - obstructive Q62.39
  - respiratory system, congenital Q34.9
  - restoration, dental KØ8.5Ø
    - specified NEC KØ8.59
  - retinal nerve bundle fibers H35.89
  - septal (heart) NOS Q21.9
    - acquired (atrial) (auricular) (ventricular) (old) I51.Ø
    - atrial Q21.1
      - concurrent with acute myocardial infarction —*see* Infarct, myocardium
      - following acute myocardial infarction (current complication) I23.1
    - ventricular —*see also* Defect, ventricular septal Q21.Ø
  - sinus venosus Q21.1
  - speech R47.9
    - developmental F8Ø.9
    - specified NEC R47.89
  - Taussig-Bing (aortic transposition and overriding pulmonary artery) Q2Ø.1
  - teeth, wedge KØ3.1
  - vascular (local) I99.9
    - congenital Q27.9
  - ventricular septal Q21.Ø
    - concurrent with acute myocardial infarction —*see* Infarct, myocardium
    - following acute myocardial infarction (current complication) I23.2
    - in tetralogy of Fallot Q21.3
  - vision NEC H54.7
  - visual field H53.4Ø
    - bilateral
      - heteronymous H53.47
      - homonymous H53.46-
    - generalized contraction H53.48-
    - localized
      - arcuate H53.43-
      - scotoma (central area) H53.41-
        - blind spot area H53.42-
      - sector H53.43-
      - specified type NEC H53.45-
  - voice R49.9
    - specified NEC R49.8
  - wedge, tooth, teeth (abrasion) KØ3.1
- **Deferentitis** N49.1
  - gonorrheal (acute) (chronic) A54.23

Defibrination (syndrome) D65
  antepartum —*see* Hemorrhage, antepartum, with coagulation defect, disseminated intravascular coagulation
  following ectopic or molar pregnancy O08.1
  intrapartum O67.0
  newborn P60
  postpartum O72.3
Deficiency, deficient
  3-beta hydroxysteroid dehydrogenase E25.0
  11-hydroxylase E25.0
  21-hydroxylase E25.0
  5-alpha reductase (with male pseudohermaphroditism) E29.1
  abdominal muscle syndrome Q79.4
  AC globulin (congenital) (hereditary) D68.2
    acquired D68.4
  accelerator globulin (Ac G) (blood) D68.2
  acid phosphatase E83.39
  activating factor (blood) D68.2
  adenosine deaminase (ADA) D81.3
  aldolase (hereditary) E74.19
  alpha-1-antitrypsin E88.01
  amino-acids E72.9
  anemia —*see* Anemia
  aneurin E51.9
  antibody with
    hyperimmunoglobulinemia D80.6
    near-normal immunoglobins D80.6
  antidiuretic hormone E23.2
  anti-hemophilic
    factor (A) D66
      B D67
      C D68.1
    globulin (AHG) NEC D66
  antithrombin (antithrombin III) D68.59
  ascorbic acid E54
  attention (disorder) (syndrome) F98.8
    with hyperactivity —*see* Disorder, attention-deficit hyperactivity
  autoprothrombin
    I D68.2
    II D67
    C D68.2
  beta-glucuronidase E76.29
  biotin E53.8
  biotin-dependent carboxylase D81.819
  biotinidase D81.810
  brancher enzyme (amylopectinosis) E74.03
  C1 esterase inhibitor (C1-INH) D84.1
  calciferol E55.9
    with
      adult osteomalacia M83.8
      rickets —*see* Rickets
  calcium (dietary) E58
  calorie, severe E43
    with marasmus E41
      and kwashiorkor E42
  cardiac —*see* Insufficiency, myocardial
  carnitine E71.40
    due to
      hemodialysis E71.43
      inborn errors of metabolism E71.42
      Valproic acid therapy E71.43
    iatrogenic E71.43
    muscle palmityltransferase E71.314
    primary E71.41
    secondary E71.448
  carotene E50.9
  central nervous system G96.8
  ceruloplasmin (Wilson) E83.01
  choline E53.8
  Christmas factor D67
  chromium E61.4
  clotting (blood) —*see also* Deficiency, coagulation factor D68.9
  clotting factor NEC (hereditary) —*see also* Deficiency, factor D68.2
  coagulation NOS D68.9
    with
      ectopic pregnancy O08.1
      molar pregnancy O08.1

Deficiency, deficient *(Continued)*
  coagulation NOS *(Continued)*
    acquired (any) D68.4
    antepartum hemorrhage —*see* Hemorrhage, antepartum, with coagulation defect
    clotting factor NEC —*see also* Deficiency, factor D68.2
    due to
      hyperprothrombinemia D68.4
      liver disease D68.4
      vitamin K deficiency D68.4
    newborn, transient P61.6
    postpartum O72.3
    specified NEC D68.8
  cognitive F09
  color vision H53.50
    achromatopsia H53.51
    acquired H53.52
    deuteranomaly H53.53
    protanomaly H53.54
    specified type NEC H53.59
    tritanomaly H53.55
  combined glucocorticoid and mineralocorticoid E27.49
  contact factor D68.2
  copper (nutritional) E61.0
  corticoadrenal E27.40
    primary E27.1
  craniofacial axis Q75.0
  cyanocobalamin E53.8
  debrancher enzyme (limit dextrinosis) E74.03
  dehydrogenase
    long chain/very long chain acyl CoA E71.310
    medium chain acyl CoA E71.311
    short chain acyl CoA E71.312
  diet E63.9
  dihydropyrimidine dehydrogenase (DPD) E88.89
  disaccharidase E73.9
  edema —*see* Malnutrition, severe
  endocrine E34.9
  energy-supply —*see* Malnutrition
  enzymes, circulating NEC E88.09
  ergosterol E55.9
    with
      adult osteomalacia M83.8
      rickets —*see* Rickets
  essential fatty acid (EFA) E63.0
  factor —*see also* Deficiency, coagulation
    Hageman D68.2
    I (congenital) (hereditary) D68.2
    II (congenital) (hereditary) D68.2
    IX (congenital) (functional) (hereditary) (with functional defect) D67
    multiple (congenital) D68.8
      acquired D68.4
    V (congenital) (hereditary) D68.2
    VII (congenital) (hereditary) D68.2
    VIII (congenital) (functional) (hereditary) (with functional defect) D66
      with vascular defect D68.0
    X (congenital) (hereditary) D68.2
    XI (congenital) (hereditary) D68.1
    XII (congenital) (hereditary) D68.2
    XIII (congenital) (hereditary) D68.2
  femoral, proximal focal (congenital) —*see* Defect, reduction, lower limb, longitudinal, femur
  fibrin-stabilizing factor (congenital) (hereditary) D68.2
    acquired D68.4
  fibrinase D68.2
  fibrinogen (congenital) (hereditary) D68.2
    acquired D65
  folate E53.8
  folic acid E53.8
  foreskin N47.3
  fructokinase E74.11
  fructose 1,6-diphosphatase E74.19

Deficiency, deficient *(Continued)*
  fructose-1-phosphate aldolase E74.19
  galactokinase E74.29
  galactose-1-phosphate uridyl transferase E74.29
  gammaglobulin in blood D80.1
    hereditary D80.0
  glass factor D68.2
  glucocorticoid E27.49
    mineralocorticoid E27.49
  glucose-6-phosphatase E74.01
  glucose-6-phosphate dehydrogenase anemia D55.0
  glucuronyl transferase E80.5
  glycogen synthetase E74.09
  gonadotropin (isolated) E23.0
  growth hormone (idiopathic) (isolated) E23.0
  Hageman factor D68.2
  hemoglobin D64.9
  hepatophosphorylase E74.09
  homogentisate 1,2-dioxygenase E70.29
  hormone
    anterior pituitary (partial) NEC E23.0
      growth E23.0
    growth (isolated) E23.0
    pituitary E23.0
    testicular E29.1
  hypoxanthine-(guanine)-phosphoribosyltransferase (HG-PRT) (total HG-PRT) E79.1
  immunity D84.9
    cell-mediated D84.8
      with thrombocytopenia and eczema D82.0
    combined D81.9
    humoral D80.9
    IgA (secretory) D80.2
    IgG D80.3
    IgM D80.4
  immuno —*see* Immunodeficiency
  immunoglobulin, selective
    A (IgA) D80.2
    G (IgG) (subclasses) D80.3
    M (IgM) D80.4
  inositol (B complex) E53.8
  intrinsic
    factor (congenital) D51.0
    sphincter N36.42
      with urethral hypermobility N36.43
  iodine E61.8
    congenital syndrome —*see* Syndrome, iodine-deficiency, congenital
  iron E61.1
    anemia D50.9
  kalium E87.6
  kappa-light chain D80.8
  labile factor (congenital) (hereditary) D68.2
    acquired D68.4
  lacrimal fluid (acquired) —*see also* Syndrome, dry eye
    congenital Q10.6
  lactase
    congenital E73.0
    secondary E73.1
  Laki-Lorand factor D68.2
  lecithin cholesterol acyltransferase E78.6
  lipocaic K86.89 ⟸
  lipoprotein (familial) (high density) E78.6
  liver phosphorylase E74.09
  lysosomal alpha-1, 4 glucosidase E74.02
  magnesium E61.2
  major histocompatibility complex
    class I D81.6
    class II D81.7
  manganese E61.3
  menadione (vitamin K) E56.1
    newborn P53
  mental (familial) (hereditary) —*see* Disability, intellectual
  methylenetetrahydrofolate reductase (MTHFR) E72.12

D

Deficiency, deficient *(Continued)*
- mevalonate kinase MØ4.1 ◀
- mineral NEC E61.8
- mineralocorticoid E27.49
  - with glucocorticoid E27.49
- molybdenum (nutritional) E61.5
- moral F6Ø.2
- multiple nutrient elements E61.7
- muscle
  - carnitine (palmityltransferase) E71.314
  - phosphofructokinase E74.Ø9
- myoadenylate deaminase E79.2
- myocardial —*see* Insufficiency, myocardial
- myophosphorylase E74.Ø4
- NADH diaphorase or reductase (congenital) D74.Ø
- NADH-methemoglobin reductase (congenital) D74.Ø
- natrium E87.1
- niacin (amide) (-tryptophan) E52
- nicotinamide E52
- nicotinic acid E52
- number of teeth —*see* Anodontia
- nutrient element E61.9
  - multiple E61.7
  - specified NEC E61.8
- nutrition, nutritional E63.9
  - sequelae —*see* Sequelae, nutritional deficiency
  - specified NEC E63.8
- of interleukin 1 receptor antagonist [DIRA] MØ4.8 ◀
- ornithine transcarbamylase E72.4
- ovarian E28.39
- oxygen —*see* Anoxia
- pantothenic acid E53.8
- parathyroid (gland) E2Ø.9
- perineum (female) N81.89
- phenylalanine hydroxylase E7Ø.1
- phosphoenolpyruvate carboxykinase E74.4
- phosphofructokinase E74.19
- phosphomannomutuse E74.8
- phosphomannose isomerase E74.8
- phosphomannosyl mutase E74.8
- phosphorylase kinase, liver E74.Ø9
- pituitary hormone (isolated) E23.Ø
- plasma thromboplastin
  - antecedent (PTA) D68.1
  - component (PTC) D67
- platelet NEC D69.1
  - constitutional D68.Ø
- polyglandular E31.8
  - autoimmune E31.Ø
- potassium (K) E87.6
- prepuce N47.3
- proaccelerin (congenital) (hereditary) D68.2
  - acquired D68.4
- proconvertin factor (congenital) (hereditary) D68.2
  - acquired D68.4
- protein —*see also* Malnutrition E46
  - anemia D53.Ø
  - C D68.59
  - S D68.59
- prothrombin (congenital) (heredItary) D68.2
  - acquired D68.4
- Prower factor D68.2
- pseudocholinesterase E88.Ø9
- PTA (plasma thromboplastin antecedent) D68.1
- PTC (plasma thromboplastin component) D67
- purine nucleoside phosphorylase (PNP) D81.5
- pyracin (alpha) (beta) E53.1
- pyridoxal E53.1
- pyridoxamine E53.1
- pyridoxine (derivatives) E53.1
- pyruvate
  - carboxylase E74.4
  - dehydrogenase E74.4
- riboflavin (vitamin B2) E53.Ø

Deficiency, deficient *(Continued)*
- salt E87.1
- secretion
  - ovary E28.39
  - salivary gland (any) K11.7
  - urine R34
- selenium (dietary) E59
- serum antitrypsin, familial E88.Ø1
- short stature homeobox gene (SHOX)
  - with
    - dyschondrosteosis Q78.8
    - short stature (idiopathic) E34.3
    - Turner's syndrome Q96.9
- sodium (Na) E87.1
- SPCA (factor VII) D68.2
- sphincter, intrinsic N36.42
  - with urethral hypermobility N36.43
- stable factor (congenital) (hereditary) D68.2
  - acquired D68.4
- Stuart-Prower (factor X) D68.2
- sucrase E74.39
- sulfatase E75.29
- sulfite oxidase E72.19
- thiamin, thiaminic (chloride) E51.9
  - beriberi (dry) E51.11
    - wet E51.12
- thrombokinase D68.2
  - newborn P53
- thyroid (gland) —*see* Hypothyroidism
- tocopherol E56.Ø
- tooth bud KØØ.Ø
- transcobalamine II (anemia) D51.2
- vanadium E61.6
- vascular I99.9
- vasopressin E23.2
- vertical ridge KØ6.8 ◀
- viosterol —*see* Deficiency, calciferol
- vitamin (multiple) NOS E56.9
  - A E5Ø.9
    - with
      - Bitot's spot (corneal) E5Ø.1
      - follicular keratosis E5Ø.8
      - keratomalacia E5Ø.4
      - manifestations NEC E5Ø.8
      - night blindness E5Ø.5
      - scar of cornea, xerophthalmic E5Ø.6
      - xeroderma E5Ø.8
      - xerophthalmia E5Ø.7
      - xerosis
        - conjunctival E5Ø.Ø
          - and Bitot's spot E5Ø.1
        - cornea E5Ø.2
          - and ulceration E5Ø.3
    - sequelae E64.1
  - B (complex) NOS E53.9
    - with
      - beriberi (dry) E51.11
        - wet E51.12
      - pellagra E52
  - B1 NOS E51.9
    - beriberi (dry) E51.11
      - with circulatory system manifestations E51.11
      - wet E51.12
  - B12 E53.8
  - B2 (riboflavin) E53.Ø
  - B6 E53.1
  - C E54
    - sequelae E64.2
  - D E55.9
    - with
      - adult osteomalacia M83.8
      - rickets —*see* Rickets
    - 25-hydroxylase E83.32
  - E E56.Ø
  - folic acid E53.8
  - G E53.Ø
  - group B E53.9
    - specified NEC E53.8

Deficiency, deficient *(Continued)*
- vitamin *(Continued)*
  - H (biotin) E53.8
  - K E56.1
    - of newborn P53
  - nicotinic E52
  - P E56.8
  - PP (pellagra-preventing) E52
  - specified NEC E56.8
  - thiamin E51.9
    - beriberi —*see* Beriberi
- zinc, dietary E6Ø

Deficit —*see also* Deficiency
- attention and concentration R41.84Ø
  - following ◀
    - cerebral infarction I69.31Ø ◀
    - cerebrovascular disease I69.91Ø ◀
      - specified disease NEC I69.81Ø ◀
    - nontraumatic ◀
      - intracerebral hemorrhage I69.11Ø ◀
      - specified intracranial hemorrhage NEC I69.21Ø ◀
      - subarachnoid hemorrhage I69.Ø1Ø ◀
  - disorder —*see* Attention, deficit
- ~~cognitive communication R41.841~~
- cognitive ◀
  - communication R41.841 ◀
  - emotional ◀
    - following ◀
      - cerebral infarction I69.315 ◀
      - cerebrovascular disease I69.915 ◀
        - specified disease NEC I69.815 ◀
      - nontraumatic ◀
        - intracerebral hemorrhage I69.115 ◀
        - specified intracranial hemorrhage NEC I69.215 ◀
        - subarachnoid hemorrhage I69.Ø15 ◀
  - following ◀
    - cerebral infarction I69.319 ◀
    - cerebrovascular disease I69.919 ◀
      - specified disease NEC I69.819 ◀
    - nontraumatic ◀
      - intracerebral hemorrhage I69.119 ◀
      - specified intracranial hemorrhage NEC I69.219 ◀
      - subarachnoid hemorrhage I69.Ø19 ◀
  - social ◀
    - following ◀
      - cerebral infarction I69.315 ◀
      - cerebrovascular disease I69.915 ◀
        - specified disease NEC I69.815 ◀
      - nontraumatic ◀
        - intracerebral hemorrhage I69.115 ◀
        - specified intracranial hemorrhage NEC I69.215 ◀
        - subarachnoid hemorrhage I69.Ø15 ◀
- cognitive NEC R41.89
  - following
    - cerebral infarction I69.318 ◀‖‖
    - cerebrovascular disease I69.918 ◀‖‖
      - specified disease NEC I69.818 ◀‖‖
    - ~~intracerebral hemorrhage I69.11~~
    - ~~nontraumatic intracranial hemorrhage NEC I69.21~~
    - nontraumatic ◀
      - intracerebral hemorrhage I69.118 ◀
      - specified intracranial hemorrhage NEC I69.218 ◀
      - subarachnoid hemorrhage I69.Ø18 ◀
    - ~~subarachnoid hemorrhage I69.Ø1~~
- concentration R41.84Ø
- executive function R41.844
  - following ◀
    - cerebral infarction I69.314 ◀
    - cerebrovascular disease I69.914 ◀
      - specified disease NEC I69.814 ◀
    - nontraumatic ◀
      - intracerebral hemorrhage I69.114 ◀
      - specified intracranial hemorrhage NEC I69.214 ◀
      - subarachnoid hemorrhage I69.Ø14 ◀

D

D

- **Deformity** *(Continued)*
  - foot *(Continued)*
    - specified type NEC —*see* Deformity, limb, foot, specified NEC
    - valgus (congenital) Q66.6
      - acquired —*see* Deformity, valgus, ankle
    - varus (congenital) NEC Q66.3
      - acquired —*see* Deformity, varus, ankle
  - forearm (acquired) —*see also* Deformity, limb, forearm
    - congenital Q68.8
  - forehead (acquired) M95.2
    - congenital Q75.8
  - frontal bone (acquired) M95.2
    - congenital Q75.8
  - gallbladder (congenital) Q44.1
    - acquired K82.8
  - gastrointestinal tract (congenital) NOS Q45.9
    - acquired K63.89
  - genitalia, genital organ (s) or system NEC
    - female (congenital) Q52.9
      - acquired N94.89
      - external Q52.70
    - male (congenital) Q55.9
      - acquired N50.89 (Revised)
  - globe (eye) (congenital) Q15.8
    - acquired H44.89
  - gum, acquired NEC K06.8
  - hand (acquired) —*see* Deformity, limb, hand
    - congenital Q68.1
  - head (acquired) M95.2
    - congenital Q75.8
  - heart (congenital) Q24.9
    - septum Q21.9
      - auricular Q21.1
      - ventricular Q21.0
    - valve (congenital) NEC Q24.8
      - acquired —*see* Endocarditis
  - heel (acquired) —*see* Deformity, foot
  - hepatic duct (congenital) Q44.5
    - acquired K83.8
  - hip (joint) (acquired) —*see also* Deformity, limb, thigh
    - congenital Q65.9
    - due to (previous) juvenile osteochondrosis —*see* Coxa, plana
    - flexion —*see* Contraction, joint, hip
  - hourglass —*see* Contraction, hourglass
  - humerus (acquired) M21.82-
    - congenital Q74.0
  - hypophyseal (congenital) Q89.2
  - ileocecal (coil) (valve) (acquired) K63.89
    - congenital Q43.9
  - ileum (congenital) Q43.9
    - acquired K63.89
  - ilium (acquired) M95.5
    - congenital Q74.2
  - integument (congenital) Q84.9
  - intervertebral cartilage or disc (acquired) —*see* Disorder, disc, specified NEC
  - intestine (large) (small) (congenital) NOS Q43.9
    - acquired K63.89
  - intrinsic minus or plus (hand) —*see* Deformity, limb, specified type NEC, forearm
  - iris (acquired) H21.89
    - congenital Q13.2
  - ischium (acquired) M95.5
    - congenital Q74.2
  - jaw (acquired) (congenital) M26.9
  - joint (acquired) NEC M21.90
    - congenital Q68.8
    - elbow M21.92-
    - hand M21.94-
    - hip M21.95-
    - knee M21.96-
    - shoulder M21.92-
    - wrist M21.93-
  - kidney (s) (calyx) (pelvis) (congenital) Q63.9
    - acquired N28.89
    - artery (congenital) Q27.2
      - acquired I77.89
  - Klippel-Feil (brevicollis) Q76.1
  - knee (acquired) NEC —*see also* Deformity, limb, lower leg
    - congenital Q68.2
  - labium (majus) (minus) (congenital) Q52.79
    - acquired N90.89
  - lacrimal passages or duct (congenital) NEC Q10.6
    - acquired —*see* Disorder, lacrimal system, changes
  - larynx (muscle) (congenital) Q31.8
    - acquired J38.7
    - web (glottic) Q31.0
  - leg (upper) (acquired) NEC —*see also* Deformity, limb, thigh
    - congenital Q68.8
    - lower leg —*see* Deformity, limb, lower leg
  - lens (acquired) H27.8
    - congenital Q12.9
  - lid (fold) (acquired) —*see also* Disorder, eyelid, specified type NEC
    - congenital Q10.3
  - ligament (acquired) —*see* Disorder, ligament
    - congenital Q79.9
  - limb (acquired) M21.90
    - clawfoot M21.53-
    - clawhand M21.51-
    - clubfoot M21.54-
    - clubhand M21.52-
    - congenital, except reduction deformity Q74.9
    - flat foot M21.4-
    - flexion M21.20
      - ankle M21.27-
      - elbow M21.22-
      - finger M21.24-
      - hip M21.25-
      - knee M21.26-
      - shoulder M21.21-
      - toe M21.27-
      - wrist M21.23-
    - foot
      - claw —*see* Deformity, limb, clawfoot
      - club —*see* Deformity, limb, clubfoot
      - drop M21.37-
      - flat —*see* Deformity, limb, flat foot
      - specified NEC M21.6X-
    - forearm M21.93-
    - hand M21.94-
    - lower leg M21.96-
    - specified type NEC M21.80
      - forearm M21.83-
      - lower leg M21.86-
      - thigh M21.85-
      - upper arm M21.82-
    - thigh M21.95-
    - unequal length M21.70
      - short site is
        - femur M21.75-
        - fibula M21.76-
        - humerus M21.72-
        - radius M21.73-
        - tibia M21.76-
        - ulna M21.73-
    - upper arm M21.92-
    - valgus —*see* Deformity, valgus
    - varus —*see* Deformity, varus
    - wrist drop M21.33-
  - lip (acquired) NEC K13.0
    - congenital Q38.0
  - liver (congenital) Q44.7
    - acquired K76.89
  - lumbosacral (congenital) (joint) (region) Q76.49
    - acquired —*see* subcategory M43.8
    - kyphosis —*see* Kyphosis, congenital
    - lordosis —*see* Lordosis, congenital
  - lung (congenital) Q33.9
    - acquired J98.4
  - lymphatic system, congenital Q89.9
  - Madelung's (radius) Q74.0
  - mandible (acquired) (congenital) M26.9
  - maxilla (acquired) (congenital) M26.9
  - meninges or membrane (congenital) Q07.9
    - cerebral Q04.8
      - acquired G96.19
    - spinal cord (congenital) G96.19
      - acquired G96.19
  - metacarpus (acquired) —*see* Deformity, limb, forearm
    - congenital Q74.0
  - metatarsus (acquired) —*see* Deformity, foot
    - congenital Q66.9
  - middle ear (congenital) Q16.4
    - ossicles Q16.3
  - mitral (leaflets) (valve) I05.8
    - parachute Q23.2
    - stenosis, congenital Q23.2
  - mouth (acquired) K13.79
    - congenital Q38.6
  - multiple, congenital NEC Q89.7
  - muscle (acquired) M62.89
    - congenital Q79.9
      - sternocleidomastoid Q68.0
  - musculoskeletal system (acquired) M95.9
    - congenital Q79.9
    - specified NEC M95.8
  - nail (acquired) L60.8
    - congenital Q84.6
  - nasal —*see* Deformity, nose
  - neck (acquired) M95.3
    - congenital Q18.9
      - sternocleidomastoid Q68.0
  - nervous system (congenital) Q07.9
  - nipple (congenital) Q83.9
    - acquired N64.89
  - nose (acquired) (cartilage) M95.0
    - bone (turbinate) M95.0
    - congenital Q30.9
      - bent or squashed Q67.4
    - saddle M95.0
      - syphilitic A50.57
    - septum (acquired) J34.2
      - congenital Q30.8
    - sinus (wall) (congenital) Q30.8
      - acquired M95.0
    - syphilitic (congenital) A50.57
      - late A52.73
  - ocular muscle (congenital) Q10.3
    - acquired —*see* Strabismus, mechanical
  - opticociliary vessels (congenital) Q13.2
  - orbit (eye) (acquired) H05.30
    - atrophy —*see* Atrophy, orbit
    - congenital Q10.7
    - due to
      - bone disease NEC H05.32-
      - trauma or surgery H05.33-
    - enlargement —*see* Enlargement, orbit
    - exostosis —*see* Exostosis, orbit
  - organ of Corti (congenital) Q16.5
  - ovary (congenital) Q50.39
    - acquired N83.8
  - oviduct, acquired N83.8
  - palate (congenital) Q38.5
    - acquired M27.8
    - cleft (congenital) —*see* Cleft, palate
  - pancreas (congenital) Q45.3
    - acquired K86.89 (Revised)
  - parathyroid (gland) Q89.2
  - parotid (gland) (congenital) Q38.4
    - acquired K11.8
  - patella (acquired) —*see* Disorder, patella, specified NEC
  - pelvis, pelvic (acquired) (bony) M95.5
    - with disproportion (fetopelvic) O33.0
      - causing obstructed labor O65.0

Deformity *(Continued)*
pelvis, pelvic *(Continued)*
congenital Q74.2
rachitic sequelae (late effect) E64.3
penis (glans) (congenital) Q55.69
acquired N48.89
pericardium (congenital) Q24.8
acquired —*see* Pericarditis
pharynx (congenital) Q38.8
acquired J39.2
pinna, acquired —*see also* Disorder, pinna, deformity
congenital Q17.9
pituitary (congenital) Q89.2
posture —*see* Dorsopathy, deforming
prepuce (congenital) Q55.69
acquired N47.8
prostate (congenital) Q55.4
acquired N42.89
pupil (congenital) Q13.2
acquired —*see* Abnormality, pupillary
pylorus (congenital) Q40.3
acquired K31.89
rachitic (acquired), old or healed E64.3
radius (acquired) —*see also* Deformity, limb, forearm
congenital Q68.8
rectum (congenital) Q43.9
acquired K62.89
reduction (extremity) (limb), congenital (*see also* condition and site) Q73.8
brain Q04.3
lower —*see* Defect, reduction, lower limb
upper —*see* Defect, reduction, upper limb
renal —*see* Deformity, kidney
respiratory system (congenital) Q34.9
rib (acquired) M95.4
congenital Q76.6
cervical Q76.5
rotation (joint) (acquired) —*see* Deformity, limb, specified site NEC
congenital Q74.9
hip —*see* Deformity, limb, specified type NEC, thigh
congenital Q65.89
sacroiliac joint (congenital) Q74.2
acquired —*see* subcategory M43.8
sacrum (acquired) —*see* subcategory M43.8
saddle
back —*see* Lordosis
nose M95.0
syphilitic A50.57
salivary gland or duct (congenital) Q38.4
acquired K11.8
scapula (acquired) M95.8
congenital Q68.8
scrotum (congenital) —*see also* Malformation, testis and scrotum
acquired N50.89 ⬅
seminal vesicles (congenital) Q55.4
acquired N50.89 ⬅
septum, nasal (acquired) J34.2
shoulder (joint) (acquired) —*see* Deformity, limb, upper arm
congenital Q74.0
contraction —*see* Contraction, joint, shoulder
sigmoid (flexure) (congenital) Q43.9
acquired K63.89
skin (congenital) Q82.9
skull (acquired) M95.2
congenital Q75.8
with
anencephaly Q00.0
encephalocele —*see* Encephalocele
hydrocephalus Q03.9
with spina bifida —*see* Spina bifida, by site, with hydrocephalus
microcephaly Q02

Deformity *(Continued)*
soft parts, organs or tissues (of pelvis)
in pregnancy or childbirth NEC O34.8-
causing obstructed labor O65.5
spermatic cord (congenital) Q55.4
acquired N50.89 ⬅
torsion —*see* Torsion, spermatic cord
spinal —*see* Dorsopathy, deforming
column (acquired) —*see* Dorsopathy, deforming
congenital Q67.5
cord (congenital) Q06.9
acquired G95.89
nerve root (congenital) Q07.9
spine (acquired) —*see also* Dorsopathy, deforming
congenital Q67.5
rachitic E64.3
specified NEC —*see* Dorsopathy, deforming, specified NEC
spleen
acquired D73.89
congenital Q89.09
Sprengel's (congenital) Q74.0
sternocleidomastoid (muscle), congenital Q68.0
sternum (acquired) M95.4
congenital NEC Q76.7
stomach (congenital) Q40.3
acquired K31.89
submandibular gland (congenital) Q38.4
submaxillary gland (congenital) Q38.4
acquired K11.8
talipes —*see* Talipes
testis (congenital) —*see also* Malformation, testis and scrotum
acquired N44.8
torsion —*see* Torsion, testis
thigh (acquired) —*see also* Deformity, limb, thigh
congenital NEC Q68.8
thorax (acquired) (wall) M95.4
congenital Q67.8
sequelae of rickets E64.3
thumb (acquired) —*see also* Deformity, finger
congenital NEC Q68.1
thymus (tissue) (congenital) Q89.2
thyroid (gland) (congenital) Q89.2
cartilage Q31.8
acquired J38.7
tibia (acquired) —*see also* Deformity, limb, specified type NEC, lower leg
congenital NEC Q68.8
saber (syphilitic) A50.56
toe (acquired) M20.6-
congenital Q66.9
hallux rigidus M20.2-
hallux valgus M20.1-
hallux varus M20.3-
hammer toe M20.4-
specified NEC M20.5X-
tongue (congenital) Q38.3
acquired K14.8
tooth, teeth K00.2
trachea (rings) (congenital) Q32.1
acquired J39.8
transverse aortic arch (congenital) Q25.49 ⬅
tricuspid (leaflets) (valve) I07.8
atresia or stenosis Q22.4
Ebstein's Q22.5
trunk (acquired) M95.8
congenital Q89.9
ulna (acquired) —*see also* Deformity, limb, forearm
congenital NEC Q68.8
urachus, congenital Q64.4
ureter (opening) (congenital) Q62.8
acquired N28.89
urethra (congenital) Q64.79
acquired N36.8

Deformity *(Continued)*
urinary tract (congenital) Q64.9
urachus Q64.4
uterus (congenital) Q51.9
acquired N85.8
uvula (congenital) Q38.5
vagina (acquired) N89.8
congenital Q52.4
valgus NEC M21.00
ankle M21.07-
elbow M21.02-
hip M21.05-
knee M21.06-
valve, valvular (congenital) (heart) Q24.8
acquired —*see* Endocarditis
varus NEC M21.10
ankle M21.17-
elbow M21.12-
hip M21.15
knee M21.16-
tibia —*see* Osteochondrosis, juvenile, tibia
vas deferens (congenital) Q55.4
acquired N50.89 ⬅
vein (congenital) Q27.9
great Q26.9
vertebra —*see* Dorsopathy, deforming
vertical talus (congenital) Q66.80
left foot Q66.82
right foot Q66.81
vesicourethral orifice (acquired) N32.89
congenital NEC Q64.79
vessels of optic papilla (congenital) Q14.2
visual field (contraction) —*see* Defect, visual field
vitreous body, acquired H43.89
vulva (congenital) Q52.79
acquired N90.89
wrist (joint) (acquired) —*see also* Deformity, limb, forearm
congenital Q68.8
contraction —*see* Contraction, joint, wrist

Degeneration, degenerative
adrenal (capsule) (fatty) (gland) (hyaline) (infectional) E27.8
amyloid —*see also* Amyloidosis E85.9
anterior cornua, spinal cord G12.29
anterior labral S43.49-
aorta, aortic I70.0
fatty I77.89
aortic valve (heart) —*see* Endocarditis, aortic
arteriovascular —*see* Arteriosclerosis
artery, arterial (atheromatous) (calcareous) —*see also* Arteriosclerosis
cerebral, amyloid E85.4 *[I68.0]*
medial —*see* Arteriosclerosis, extremities
articular cartilage NEC —*see* Derangement, joint, articular cartilage, by site
atheromatous —*see* Arteriosclerosis
basal nuclei or ganglia G23.9
specified NEC G23.8
bone NEC —*see* Disorder, bone, specified type NEC
brachial plexus G54.0
brain (cortical) (progressive) G31.9
alcoholic G31.2
arteriosclerotic I67.2
childhood G31.9
specified NEC G31.89
cystic G31.89
congenital Q04.6
in
alcoholism G31.2
beriberi E51.2
cerebrovascular disease I67.9
congenital hydrocephalus Q03.9
with spina bifida —*see also* Spina bifida
Fabry-Anderson disease E75.21
Gaucher's disease E75.22
Hunter's syndrome E76.1

- **Degeneration, degenerative** *(Continued)*
  - brain *(Continued)*
    - in *(Continued)*
      - lipidosis
        - cerebral E75.4
        - generalized E75.6
      - mucopolysaccharidosis —*see* Mucopolysaccharidosis
      - myxedema EØ3.9 *[G32.89]*
      - neoplastic disease —*see also* Neoplasm D49.6 *[G32.89]*
      - Niemann-Pick disease E75.249 *[G32.89]*
      - sphingolipidosis E75.3 *[G32.89]*
      - vitamin B12 deficiency E53.8 *[G32.89]*
    - senile NEC G31.1
  - breast N64.89
  - Bruch's membrane —*see* Degeneration, choroid
  - capillaries (fatty) I78.8
    - amyloid E85.8 *[I79.8]*
  - cardiac —*see also* Degeneration, myocardial
    - valve, valvular —*see* Endocarditis
  - cardiorenal —*see* Hypertension, cardiorenal
  - cardiovascular —*see also* Disease, cardiovascular
    - renal —*see* Hypertension, cardiorenal
  - cerebellar NOS G31.9
    - alcoholic G31.2
    - primary (hereditary) (sporadic) G11.9
  - cerebral —*see* Degeneration, brain
  - cerebrovascular I67.9
    - due to hypertension I67.4
  - cervical plexus G54.2
  - cervix N88.8
    - due to radiation (intended effect) N88.8
      - adverse effect or misadventure N99.89
  - chamber angle H21.21-
  - changes, spine or vertebra —*see* Spondylosis
  - chorioretinal —*see also* Degeneration, choroid
    - hereditary H31.2Ø
  - choroid (colloid) (drusen) H31.1Ø-
    - atrophy —*see* Atrophy, choroidal
    - hereditary —*see* Dystrophy, choroidal, hereditary
  - ciliary body H21.22-
  - cochlear —*see* subcategory H83.8
  - combined (spinal cord) (subacute) E53.8 *[G32.Ø]*
    - with anemia (pernicious) D51.Ø *[G32.Ø]*
      - due to dietary vitamin B12 deficiency D51.3 *[G32.Ø]*
    - in (due to)
      - vitamin B12 deficiency E53.8 *[G32.Ø]*
        - anemia D51.9 *[G32.Ø]*
  - conjunctiva H11.1Ø
    - concretions —*see* Concretion, conjunctiva
    - deposits —*see* Deposit, conjunctiva
    - pigmentations —*see* Pigmentation, conjunctiva
    - pinguecula —*see* Pinguecula
    - xerosis —*see* Xerosis, conjunctiva
  - cornea H18.4Ø
    - calcerous H18.43
      - band keratopathy H18.42-
    - familial, hereditary —*see* Dystrophy, cornea
    - hyaline (of old scars) H18.49
    - keratomalacia —*see* Keratomalacia
    - nodular H18.45-
    - peripheral H18.46-
    - senile H18.41-
    - specified type NEC H18.49
  - cortical (cerebellar) (parenchymatous) G31.89
    - alcoholic G31.2
    - diffuse, due to arteriopathy I67.2
  - corticobasal G31.85
  - cutis L98.8
    - amyloid E85.4 *[L99]*
  - dental pulp KØ4.2
  - disc disease —*see* Degeneration, intervertebral disc NEC

- **Degeneration, degenerative** *(Continued)*
  - dorsolateral (spinal cord) —*see* Degeneration, combined
  - extrapyramidal G25.9
  - eye, macular —*see also* Degeneration, macula
    - congenital or hereditary —*see* Dystrophy, retina
  - facet joints —*see* Spondylosis
  - fatty
    - liver NEC K76.Ø
      - alcoholic K7Ø.Ø
  - grey matter (brain) (Alpers') G31.81
  - heart —*see also* Degeneration, myocardial
    - amyloid E85.4 *[I43]*
    - atheromatous —*see* Disease, heart, ischemic, atherosclerotic
    - ischemic —*see* Disease, heart, ischemic
  - hepatolenticular (Wilson's) E83.Ø1
  - hepatorenal K76.7
  - hyaline (diffuse) (generalized)
    - localized —*see* Degeneration, by site
  - infrapatellar fat pad M79.4
  - intervertebral disc NOS
    - with
      - myelopathy —*see* Disorder, disc, with, myelopathy
      - radiculitis or radiculopathy —*see* Disorder, disc, with, radiculopathy
    - cervical, cervicothoracic —*see* Disorder, disc, cervical, degeneration
      - with
        - myelopathy —*see* Disorder, disc, cervical, with myelopathy
        - neuritis, radiculitis or radiculopathy —*see* Disorder, disc, cervical, with neuritis
    - lumbar region M51.36
      - with
        - myelopathy M51.Ø6
        - neuritis, radiculitis, radiculopathy or sciatica M51.16
    - lumbosacral region M51.37
      - with
        - neuritis, radiculitis, radiculopathy or sciatica M51.17
    - sacrococcygeal region M53.3
    - thoracic region M51.34
      - with
        - myelopathy M51.Ø4
        - neuritis, radiculitis, radiculopathy M51.14
    - thoracolumbar region M51.35
      - with
        - myelopathy M51.Ø5
        - neuritis, radiculitis, radiculopathy M51.15
  - intestine, amyloid E85.4
  - iris (pigmentary) H21.23-
  - ischemic —*see* Ischemia
  - joint disease —*see* Osteoarthritis
  - kidney N28.89
    - amyloid E85.4 *[N29]*
    - cystic, congenital Q61.9
    - fatty N28.89
    - polycystic Q61.3
      - adult type (autosomal dominant) Q61.2
      - infantile type (autosomal recessive) NEC Q61.19
        - collecting duct dilatation Q61.11
  - Kuhnt-Junius —*see also* Degeneration, macula H35.32- ⬅
  - lens —*see* Cataract
  - lenticular (familial) (progressive) (Wilson's) (with cirrhosis of liver) E83.Ø1
  - liver (diffuse) NEC K76.89
    - amyloid E85.4 *[K77]*
    - cystic K76.89
      - congenital Q44.6
    - fatty NEC K76.Ø
      - alcoholic K7Ø.Ø

- **Degeneration, degenerative** *(Continued)*
  - liver *(Continued)*
    - hypertrophic K76.89
    - parenchymatous, acute or subacute K72.ØØ
      - with coma K72.Ø1
    - pigmentary K76.89
    - toxic (acute) K71.9
  - lung J98.4
  - lymph gland I89.8
    - hyaline I89.8
  - macula, macular (acquired) (age-related) (senile) H35.3Ø
    - angioid streaks H35.33
    - atrophic age-related H35.31- ⬅
    - congenital or hereditary —*see* Dystrophy, retina
    - cystoid H35.35-
    - drusen H35.36-
    - dry age-related H35.31- ◀
    - exudative H35.32- ⬅
    - hole H35.34-
    - nonexudative H35.31- ⬅
    - puckering H35.37-
    - toxic H35.38-
    - wet age-related H35.32- ◀
  - membranous labyrinth, congenital (causing impairment of hearing) Q16.5
  - meniscus —*see* Derangement, meniscus
  - mitral —*see* Insufficiency, mitral
  - Mönckeberg's —*see* Arteriosclerosis, extremities
  - motor centers, senile G31.1
  - multi-system G9Ø.3
  - mural —*see* Degeneration, myocardial
  - muscle (fatty) (fibrous) (hyaline) (progressive) M62.89
    - heart —*see* Degeneration, myocardial
  - myelin, central nervous system G37.9
  - myocardial, myocardium (fatty) (hyaline) (senile) I51.5
    - with rheumatic fever (conditions in IØØ) IØ9.Ø
      - active, acute or subacute IØ1.2
        - with chorea IØ2.Ø
      - inactive or quiescent (with chorea) IØ9.Ø
    - hypertensive —*see* Hypertension, heart
    - rheumatic —*see* Degeneration, myocardial, with rheumatic fever
    - syphilitic A52.Ø6
  - nasal sinus (mucosa) J32.9
    - frontal J32.1
    - maxillary J32.Ø
  - nerve —*see* Disorder, nerve
  - nervous system G31.9
    - alcoholic G31.2
    - amyloid E85.4 *[G99.8]*
    - autonomic G9Ø.9
    - fatty G31.89
    - specified NEC G31.89
  - nipple N64.89
  - olivopontocerebellar (hereditary) (familial) G23.8
  - osseous labyrinth —*see* subcategory H83.8
  - ovary N83.8
    - cystic N83.2Ø- ⬅
    - microcystic N83.2Ø- ⬅
  - pallidal pigmentary (progressive) G23.Ø
  - pancreas K86.89 ⬅
    - tuberculous A18.83
  - penis N48.89
  - pigmentary (diffuse) (general)
    - localized —*see* Degeneration, by site
    - pallidal (progressive) G23.Ø
  - pineal gland E34.8
  - pituitary (gland) E23.6
  - popliteal fat pad M79.4
  - posterolateral (spinal cord) —*see* Degeneration, combined
  - pulmonary valve (heart) I37.8
  - pulp (tooth) KØ4.2

D

Degeneration, degenerative *(Continued)*
pupillary margin H21.24-
renal *—see* Degeneration, kidney
retina H35.9
hereditary (cerebroretinal) (congenital) (juvenile) (macula) (peripheral) (pigmentary) *—see* Dystrophy, retina
Kuhnt-Junius *—see also* Degeneration, macula H35.32- (Revised)
macula (cystic) (exudative) (hole) (nonexudative) (pseudohole) (senile) (toxic) *—see* Degeneration, macula
peripheral H35.40
lattice H35.41-
microcystoid H35.42-
paving stone H35.43-
secondary
pigmentary H35.45-
vitreoretinal H35.46-
senile reticular H35.44-
pigmentary (primary) *—see also* Dystrophy, retina
secondary *—see* Degeneration, retina, peripheral, secondary
posterior pole *—see* Degeneration, macula
saccule, congenital (causing impairment of hearing) Q16.5
senile R54
brain G31.1
cardiac, heart or myocardium *—see* Degeneration, myocardial
motor centers G31.1
vascular *—see* Arteriosclerosis
sinus (cystic) *—see also* Sinusitis
polypoid J33.1
skin L98.8
amyloid E85.4 *[L99]*
colloid L98.8
spinal (cord) G31.89
amyloid E85.4 *[G32.89]*
combined (subacute) *—see* Degeneration, combined
dorsolateral *—see* Degeneration, combined
familial NEC G31.89
fatty G31.89
funicular *—see* Degeneration, combined
posterolateral *—see* Degeneration, combined
subacute combined *—see* Degeneration, combined
tuberculous A17.81
spleen D73.0
amyloid E85.4 *[D77]*
stomach K31.89
striatonigral G23.2
suprarenal (capsule) (gland) E27.8
synovial membrane (pulpy) *—see* Disorder, synovium, specified type NEC
tapetoretinal *—see* Dystrophy, retina
thymus (gland) E32.8
fatty E32.8
thyroid (gland) E07.89
tricuspid (heart) (valve) I07.9
tuberculous NEC *—see* Tuberculosis
turbinate J34.89
uterus (cystic) N85.8
vascular (senile) *—see* Arteriosclerosis
hypertensive *—see* Hypertension
vitreoretinal, secondary *—see* Degeneration, retina, peripheral, secondary, vitreoretinal
vitreous (body) H43.81-
Wallerian *—see* Disorder, nerve
Wilson's hepatolenticular E83.01
Deglutition
paralysis R13.0
hysterical F44.4
pneumonia J69.0
Degos' disease I77.89
Dehiscence (of)
amputation stump T87.81
cesarean wound O90.0

Dehiscence *(Continued)*
closure of
cornea T81.31
craniotomy T81.32
fascia (muscular) (superficial) T81.32
internal organ or tissue T81.32
laceration (external) (internal) T81.33
ligament T81.32
mucosa T81.31
muscle or muscle flap T81.32
ribs or rib cage T81.32
skin and subcutaneous tissue (full-thickness) (superficial) T81.31
skull T81.32
sternum (sternotomy) T81.32
tendon T81.32
traumatic laceration (external) (internal) T81.33
episiotomy O90.1
operation wound NEC T81.31
external operation wound (superficial) T81.31
internal operation wound (deep) T81.32
perineal wound (postpartum) O90.1
traumatic injury wound repair T81.33
wound T81.30
traumatic repair T81.33
Dehydration E86.0
~~hypertonic E87.0~~
~~hypotonic E87.1~~
newborn P74.1
Déjérine-Roussy syndrome G93.89
Déjérine-Sottas disease or neuropathy (hypertrophic) G60.0
Déjérine-Thomas atrophy G23.8
Delay, delayed
any plane in pelvis
complicating delivery O66.9
birth or delivery NOS O63.9
closure, ductus arteriosus (Botalli) P29.3
coagulation *—see* Defect, coagulation
conduction (cardiac) (ventricular) I45.9
delivery, second twin, triplet, etc O63.2
development R62.50
global F88
intellectual (specific) F81.9
language F80.9
due to hearing loss F80.4
learning F81.9
pervasive F84.9
physiological R62.50
specified stage NEC R62.0
reading F81.0
sexual E30.0
speech F80.9
due to hearing loss F80.4
spelling F81.81
ejaculation F52.32 ◀
gastric emptying K30
menarche E30.0
menstruation (cause unknown) N91.0
milestone R62.0
passage of meconium (newborn) P76.0
primary respiration P28.9
puberty (constitutional) E30.0
separation of umbilical cord P96.82
sexual maturation, female E30.0
sleep phase syndrome G47.21
union, fracture *—see* Fracture, by site
vaccination Z28.9
Deletion (s)
autosome Q93.9
identified by fluorescence in situ hybridization (FISH) Q93.89
identified by in situ hybridization (ISH) Q93.89
chromosome
with complex rearrangements NEC Q93.7
part of NEC Q93.5
seen only at prometaphase Q93.89

Deletion *(Continued)*
chromosome *(Continued)*
short arm
4 Q93.3
5p Q93.4
22q11.2 Q93.81
specified NEC Q93.89
long arm chromosome 18 or 21 Q93.89
with complex rearrangements NEC Q93.7
microdeletions NEC Q93.88
Delhi boil or button B55.1
Delinquency (juvenile) (neurotic) F91.8
group Z72.810
Delinquent immunization status Z28.3
Delirium, delirious (acute or subacute) (not alcohol or drug-induced) (with dementia) R41.0
alcoholic (acute) (tremens) (withdrawal) F10.921
with intoxication F10.921
in
abuse F10.121
dependence F10.221
due to (secondary to)
alcohol
intoxication F10.921
in
abuse F10.121
dependence F10.221
withdrawal F10.231
amphetamine intoxication F15.921
in
abuse F15.121
dependence F15.221
anxiolytic
intoxication F13.921
in
abuse F13.121
dependence F13.221
withdrawal F13.231
cannabis intoxication (acute) F12.921
in
abuse F12.121
dependence F12.221
cocaine intoxication (acute) F14.921
in
abuse F14.121
dependence F14.221
general medical condition F05
hallucinogen intoxication F16.921
in
abuse F16.121
dependence F16.221
hypnotic
intoxication F13.921
in
abuse F13.121
dependence F13.221
withdrawal F13.231
inhalant intoxication (acute) F18.921
in
abuse F18.121
dependence F18.221
multiple etiologies F05
opioid intoxication (acute) F11.921
in
abuse F11.121
dependence F11.221
other (or unknown) substance F19.921 ◀
phencyclidine intoxication (acute) F16.921
in
abuse F16.121
dependence F16.221
psychoactive substance NEC intoxication (acute) F19.921
in
abuse F19.121
dependence F19.221

D

Delirium, delirious *(Continued)*
due to *(Continued)*
sedative
intoxication F13.921
in
abuse F13.121
dependence F13.221
withdrawal F13.231
unknown etiology FØ5
exhaustion F43.Ø
hysterical F44.89
postprocedural (postoperative) FØ5
puerperal FØ5
thyroid —*see* Thyrotoxicosis with thyroid storm
traumatic —*see* Injury, intracranial
tremens (alcohol-induced) F1Ø.231
sedative-induced F13.231
Delivery (childbirth) (labor)
arrested active phase O62.1
cesarean (for)
without indication O82
abnormal
pelvis (bony) (deformity) (major) NEC
with disproportion (fetopelvic) O33.Ø
with obstructed labor O65.Ø
presentation or position O32.9
abruptio placentae —*see also* Abruptio placentae Ø45.9-
acromion presentation O32.2
atony, uterus O62.2
breech presentation O32.1
incomplete O32.8
brow presentation O32.3
cephalopelvic disproportion O33.9
cerclage O34.3-
chin presentation O32.3
cicatrix of cervix O34.4-
contracted pelvis (general)
inlet O33.2
outlet O33.3
cord presentation or prolapse O69.Ø
cystocele O34.8-
deformity (acquired) (congenital)
pelvic organs or tissues NEC O34.8-
pelvis (bony) NEC O33.Ø
disproportion NOS O33.9
eclampsia —*see* Eclampsia
face presentation O32.3
failed
forceps O66.5
induction of labor O61.9
instrumental O61.1
mechanical O61.1
medical O61.Ø
specified NEC O61.8
surgical O61.1
trial of labor NOS O66.4Ø
following previous cesarean delivery O66.41
vacuum extraction O66.5
ventouse O66.5
fetal-maternal hemorrhage O43.Ø1-
hemorrhage (intrapartum) O67.9
with coagulation defect O67.Ø
specified cause NEC O67.8
high head at term O32.4
hydrocephalic fetus O33.6
incarceration of uterus O34.51-
incoordinate uterine action O62.4
increased size, fetus O33.5
inertia, uterus O62.2
primary O62.Ø
secondary O62.1
lateroversion, uterus O34.59-
mal lie O32.9
malposition
fetus O32.9
pelvic organs or tissues NEC O34.8-
uterus NEC O34.59-

Delivery *(Continued)*
cesarean *(Continued)*
malpresentation NOS O32.9
oblique presentation O32.2
occurring after 37 completed weeks of gestation but before 39 completed weeks gestation due to (spontaneous) onset of labor O75.82
oversize fetus O33.5
pelvic tumor NEC O34.8-
placenta previa O44.Ø- ←
complete O44.Ø- ◄
with hemorrhage O44.1- ◄
~~without hemorrhage O44.Ø-~~
placental insufficiency O36.51-
planned, occurring after 37 completed weeks of gestation but before 39 completed weeks gestation due to (spontaneous) onset of labor O75.82
polyp, cervix O34.4-
causing obstructed labor O65.5
poor dilatation, cervix O62.Ø
pre-eclampsia O14.94 ←
mild O14.Ø4 ←
moderate O14.Ø4 ←
severe O14.14 ←
with hemolysis, elevated liver enzymes and low platelet count (HELLP) O14.24 ←
previous
cesarean delivery O34.219 ←
classical (vertical) scar O34.212 ◄
low transverse scar O34.211 ◄
surgery (to)
cervix O34.4-
gynecological NEC O34.8-
rectum O34.7-
uterus O34.29
vagina O34.6-
prolapse
arm or hand O32.2
uterus O34.52-
prolonged labor NOS O63.9
rectocele O34.8-
retroversion
uterus O34.53-
rigid
cervix O34.4-
pelvic floor O34.8-
perineum O34.7-
vagina O34.6-
vulva O34.7-
sacculation, pregnant uterus O34.59-
scar (s)
cervix O34.4-
cesarean delivery O34.219 ←
classical (vertical) O34.212 ◄
low transverse O34.211 ◄
transmural uterine O34.29 ◄
uterus O34.29
Shirodkar suture in situ O34.3-
shoulder presentation O32.2
stenosis or stricture, cervix O34.4-
~~streptococcus B carrier state O99.824~~
streptococcus group B (GBS) carrier state O99.824 ◄
transmural uterine scar O34.29 ◄
transverse presentation or lie O32.2
tumor, pelvic organs or tissues NEC O34.8-
cervix O34.4-
umbilical cord presentation or prolapse O69.Ø
completely normal case O8Ø
complicated O75.9
by
abnormal, abnormality (of)
forces of labor O62.9
specified type NEC O62.8
glucose O99.814
uterine contractions NOS O62.9
abruptio placentae —*see also* Abruptio placentae O45.9-

Delivery *(Continued)*
complicated *(Continued)*
by *(Continued)*
abuse
physical O9A.32
psychological O9A.52
sexual O9A.42
adherent placenta O72.Ø
without hemorrhage O73.Ø
alcohol use O99.314
anemia (pre-existing) O99.Ø2
anesthetic death O74.8
annular detachment of cervix O71.3
atony, uterus O62.2
attempted vacuum extraction and forceps O66.5
Bandl's ring O62.4
bariatric surgery status O99.844
biliary tract disorder O26.62
bleeding —*see* Delivery, complicated by, hemorrhage
blood disorder NEC O99.12
cervical dystocia (hypotonic) O62.2
primary O62.Ø
secondary O62.1
circulatory system disorder O99.42
compression of cord (umbilical) NEC O69.2
condition NEC O99.89
contraction, contracted ring O62.4
cord (umbilical)
around neck
with compression O69.1
without compression O69.81
bruising O69.5
complication O69.9
specified NEC O69.89
compression NEC O69.2
entanglement O69.2
without compression O69.82
hematoma O69.5
presentation O69.Ø
prolapse O69.Ø
short O69.3
thrombosis (vessels) O69.5
vascular lesion O69.5
Couvelaire uterus O45.8X-
damage to (injury to) NEC
perineum O71.82
periurethral tissue O71.82
vulva O71.82
delay following rupture of membranes (spontaneous) —*see* Pregnancy, complicated by, premature rupture of membranes
depressed fetal heart tones O76
diabetes O24.92
gestational O24.429
diet controlled O24.42Ø
insulin controlled O24.424
oral drug controlled (antidiabetic) (hypoglycemic) O24.425 ◄
pre-existing O24.32
specified NEC O24.82
type 1 O24.Ø2
type 2 O24.12
diastasis recti (abdominis) O71.89
dilatation
bladder O66.8
cervix incomplete, poor or slow O62.Ø
disease NEC O99.89
disruptio uteri —*see* Delivery, complicated by, rupture, uterus
drug use O99.324
dysfunction, uterus NOS O62.9
hypertonic O62.4
hypotonic O62.2
primary O62.Ø
secondary O62.1
incoordinate O62.4
eclampsia O15.1
embolism (pulmonary) —*see* Embolism, obstetric

◄ New ← Revised ~~deleted~~ Deleted

Delivery *(Continued)*
complicated *(Continued)*
by *(Continued)*
endocrine, nutritional or metabolic disease NEC O99.284
failed
attempted vaginal birth after previous cesarean delivery O66.41
induction of labor O61.9
instrumental O61.1
mechanical O61.1
medical O61.Ø
specified NEC O61.8
surgical O61.1
trial of labor O66.4Ø
female genital mutilation O65.5
fetal
abnormal acid-base balance O68
acidemia O68
acidosis O68
alkalosis O68
death, early OØ2.1
deformity O66.3
heart rate or rhythm (abnormal) (non-reassuring) O76
hypoxia O77.8
stress O77.9
due to drug administration O77.1
electrocardiographic evidence of O77.8
specified NEC O77.8
ultrasound evidence of O77.8
fever during labor O75.2
gastric banding status O99.844
gastric bypass status O99.844
gastrointestinal disease NEC O99.62
~~gestational diabetes O24.429~~
~~diet controlled O24.42Ø~~
~~insulin (and diet) controlled O24.424~~
gestational ◀
diabetes O24.429 ◀
diet controlled O24.42Ø ◀
insulin (and diet) controlled O24.424 ◀
oral drug controlled (antidiabetic) (hypoglycemic) O24.425 ◀
edema O12.Ø4 ◀
with proteinuria O12.24 ◀
proteinuria O12.14 ◀
gonorrhea O98.22
hematoma O71.7
ischial spine O71.7
pelvic O71.7
vagina O71.7
vulva or perineum O71.7
hemorrhage (uterine) O67.9
associated with
afibrinogenemia O67.Ø
coagulation defect O67.Ø
hyperfibrinolysis O67.Ø
hypofibrinogenemia O67.Ø
due to
low implantation of placenta O44.5- ◀
low-lying placenta O44.5- ⬅
placenta previa O44.1-
marginal O44.3- ◀
partial O44.3- ◀
premature separation of placenta (normally implanted) (*see also* Abruptio placentae) O45.9-
retained placenta O72.Ø
uterine leiomyoma O67.8
placenta NEC O67.8
postpartum NEC (atonic) (immediate) O72.1
with retained or trapped placenta O72.Ø
delayed O72.2
secondary O72.2
third stage O72.Ø

Delivery *(Continued)*
complicated *(Continued)*
by *(Continued)*
hourglass contraction, uterus O62.4
hypertension, hypertensive (pre-existing) —*see* Hypertension, complicated by, childbirth (labor)
hypotension O26.5-
incomplete dilatation (cervix) O62.Ø
incoordinate uterus contractions O62.4
inertia, uterus O62.2
during latent phase of labor O62.Ø
primary O62.Ø
secondary O62.1
infection (maternal) O98.92
carrier state NEC O99.834
gonorrhea O98.22
human immunodeficiency virus (HIV) O98.72
sexually transmitted NEC O98.32
specified NEC O98.82
syphilis O98.12
tuberculosis O98.Ø2
viral hepatitis O98.42
viral NEC O98.52
injury (to mother) (*see also* Delivery, complicated, by, damage to) O71.9
nonobstetric O9A.22
caused by abuse —*see* Delivery, complicated by, abuse
intrauterine fetal death, early OØ2.1
inversion, uterus O71.2
laceration (perineal) O7Ø.9
anus (sphincter) O7Ø.4
with third degree laceration —*see also* Delivery, complicated, by, laceration, perineum, third degree O7Ø.2Ø ⬅
with mucosa O7Ø.3
without third degree laceration O7Ø.4
bladder (urinary) O71.5
bowel O71.5
cervix (uteri) O71.3
fourchette O7Ø.Ø
hymen O7Ø.Ø
labia O7Ø.Ø
pelvic
floor O7Ø.1
organ NEC O71.5
perineum, perineal O7Ø.9
first degree O7Ø.Ø
fourth degree O7Ø.3
muscles O7Ø.1
second degree O7Ø.1
skin O7Ø.Ø
slight O7Ø.Ø
third degree O7Ø.2Ø ⬅
with ◀
both external anal sphincter (EAS) and internal anal sphincter (IAS) torn (IIIc) O7Ø.23 ◀
less than 5Ø% of external anal sphincter (EAS) thickness torn (IIIa) O7Ø.21 ◀
more than 5Ø% external anal sphincter (EAS) thickness torn (IIIb) O7Ø.22 ◀
IIIa O7Ø.21 ◀
IIIb O7Ø.22 ◀
IIIc O7Ø.23 ◀
peritoneum (pelvic) O71.5
rectovaginal (septum) (without perineal laceration) O71.4
with perineum —*see also* Delivery, complicated, by, laceration, perineum, third degree O7Ø.2Ø ⬅
with anal or rectal mucosa O7Ø.3

Delivery *(Continued)*
complicated *(Continued)*
by *(Continued)*
laceration *(Continued)*
specified NEC O71.89
sphincter ani —*see* Delivery, complicated, by, laceration, anus (sphincter)
urethra O71.5
uterus O71.81
before labor O71.81
vagina, vaginal (deep) (high) (without perineal laceration) O71.4
with perineum O7Ø.Ø
muscles, with perineum O7Ø.1
vulva O7Ø.Ø
liver disorder O26.62
malignancy O9A.12
malnutrition O25.2
malposition, malpresentation
without obstruction O32.9 —*see also* Delivery, complicated by, obstruction
breech O32.1
compound O32.6
face (brow) (chin) O32.3
footling O38.8
high head O32.4
oblique O32.2
specified NEC O32.8
transverse O32.2
unstable lie O32.Ø
placenta O44.Ø- ⬅
~~without hemorrhage O44.Ø-~~
with hemorrhage O44.1- ◀
uterus or cervix O65.5
meconium in amniotic fluid O77.Ø
mental disorder NEC O99.344
metrorrhexis —*see* Delivery, complicated by, rupture, uterus
nervous system disorder O99.354
obesity (pre-existing) O99.214
obesity surgery status O99.844
obstetric trauma O71.9
specified NEC O71.89
obstructed labor
due to
breech (complete) (frank) presentation O64.1
incomplete O64.8
brow presentation O64.3
buttock presentation O64.1
chin presentation O64.2
compound presentation O64.5
contracted pelvis O65.1
deep transverse arrest O64.Ø
deformed pelvis O65.Ø
dystocia (fetal) O66.9
due to
conjoined twins O66.3
fetal
abnormality NEC O66.3
ascites O66.3
hydrops O66.3
meningomyelocele O66.3
sacral teratoma O66.3
tumor O66.3
hydrocephalic fetus O66.3
shoulder O66.Ø
face presentation O64.2
fetopelvic disproportion O65.4
footling presentation O64.8
impacted shoulders O66.Ø
incomplete rotation of fetal head O64.Ø
large fetus O66.2
locked twins O66.1
malposition O64.9
specified NEC O64.8
malpresentation O64.9
specified NEC O64.8

D

Delivery *(Continued)*
complicated *(Continued)*
by *(Continued)*
obstructed labor *(Continued)*
due to *(Continued)*
multiple fetuses NEC O66.6
pelvic
abnormality (maternal) O65.9
organ O65.5
specified NEC O65.8
contraction
inlet O65.2
mid-cavity O65.3
outlet O65.3
persistent (position)
occipitoiliac O64.Ø
occipitoposterior O64.Ø
occipitosacral O64.Ø
occipitotransverse O64.Ø
prolapsed arm O64.4
shoulder presentation O64.4
specified NEC O66.8
pathological retraction ring, uterus O62.4
penetration, pregnant uterus by instrument O71.1
perforation —*see* Delivery, complicated by, laceration
placenta, placental
ablatio —*see also* Abruptio placentae O45.9-
abnormality O43.9-
specified NEC O43.89-
abruptio —*see also* Abruptio placentae O45.9-
accreta O43.21-
adherent (with hemorrhage) O72.Ø
without hemorrhage O73.Ø
detachment (premature) —*see also* Abruptio placentae O45.9-
disorder O43.9-
specified NEC O43.89-
hemorrhage NEC O67.8
increta O43.22-
low (implantation) (lying) O44.4- ⬅
~~without hemorrhage O44.Ø-~~
with hemorrhage O44.5- ◀
malformation O43.1Ø-
malposition O44.Ø- ⬅
without hemorrhage O44.1- ⬅
percreta O43.23-
previa (central) (complete) (lateral) (total) O44.Ø- ⬅
~~without hemorrhage O44.Ø-~~
with hemorrhage O44.1- ◀
marginal O44.2- ◀
with hemorrhage O44.3- ◀
partial O44.2- ◀
with hemorrhage O44.3- ◀
retained (with hemorrhage) O72.Ø
without hemorrhage O73.Ø
separation (premature) O45.9-
specified NEC O45.8X-
vicious insertion O44.1-
precipitate labor O62.3
premature rupture, membranes (*see also* Pregnancy, complicated by, premature rupture of membranes) O42.9Ø
prolapse
arm or hand O32.2
cord (umbilical) O69.Ø
foot or leg O32.8
uterus O34.52-
prolonged labor O63.9
first stage O63.Ø
second stage O63.1
protozoal disease (maternal) O98.62
respiratory disease NEC O99.52
retained membranes or portions of placenta O72.2
without hemorrhage O73.1
retarded birth O63.9

Delivery *(Continued)*
complicated *(Continued)*
by *(Continued)*
retention of secundines (with hemorrhage) O72.Ø
without hemorrhage O73.Ø
partial O72.2
without hemorrhage O73.1
rupture
bladder (urinary) O71.5
cervix O71.3
pelvic organ NEC O71.5
urethra O71.5
uterus (during or after labor) O71.1
before labor O71.Ø-
separation, pubic bone (symphysis pubis) O71.6
shock O75.1
shoulder presentation O64.4
skin disorder NEC O99.72
spasm, cervix O62.4
stenosis or stricture, cervix O65.5
~~streptococcus B carrier state O99.824~~
streptococcus group B (GBS) carrier state O99.824 ◀
subluxation of symphysis (pubis) O26.72
syphilis (maternal) O98.12
tear —*see* Delivery, complicated by, laceration
tetanic uterus O62.4
trauma (obstetrical) —*see also* Delivery, complicated, by, damage to O71.9
non-obstetric O9A.22
periurethral O71.82
specified NEC O71.89
tuberculosis (maternal) O98.Ø2
tumor, pelvic organs or tissues NEC O65.5
umbilical cord around neck
with compression O69.1
without compression O69.81
uterine inertia O62.2
during latent phase of labor O62.Ø
primary O62.Ø
secondary O62.1
vasa previa O69.4
velamentous insertion of cord O43.12-
specified complication NEC O75.89
delayed NOS O63.9
following rupture of membranes
artificial O75.5
second twin, triplet, etc. O63.2
forceps, low following failed vacuum extraction O66.5
missed (at or near term) O36.4
normal O8Ø
obstructed —*see* Delivery, complicated by, obstruction
precipitate O62.3
preterm —*see also* Pregnancy, complicated by, preterm labor O6Ø.1Ø
spontaneous O8Ø
term pregnancy NOS O8Ø
uncomplicated O8Ø
vaginal, following previous cesarean delivery O34.219 ⬅
classical (vertical) scar O34.212 ◀
low transverse scar O34.211 ◀
Delusions (paranoid) —*see* Disorder, delusional
Dementia (degenerative (primary)) (old age) (persisting) FØ3.9Ø
with
aggressive behavior FØ3.91
behavioral disturbance FØ3.91
combative behavior FØ3.91
Lewy bodies G31.83 *[FØ2.8Ø]*
with behavioral disturbance G31.83 *[FØ2.81]*
Parkinson's disease G2Ø *[FØ2.8Ø]*
with behavioral disturbance G2Ø *[FØ2.81]*

Dementia *(Continued)*
with *(Continued)*
Parkinsonism G31.83 *[FØ2.8Ø]*
with behavioral disturbance G31.83 *[FØ2.81]*
violent behavior FØ3.91
alcoholic F1Ø.97
with dependence F1Ø.27
Alzheimer's type —*see* Disease, Alzheimer's
arteriosclerotic —*see* Dementia, vascular
atypical, Alzheimer's type —*see* Disease, Alzheimer's, specified NEC
congenital —*see* Disability, intellectual
frontal (lobe) G31.Ø9 *[FØ2.8Ø]*
with behavioral disturbance G31.Ø9 *[FØ2.81]*
frontotemporal G31.Ø9 *[FØ2.8Ø]*
with behavioral disturbance G31.Ø9 *[FØ2.81]*
specified NEC G31.Ø9 *[FØ2.8Ø]*
with behavioral disturbance G31.Ø9 *[FØ2.81]*
in (due to)
alcohol F1Ø.97
with dependence F1Ø.27
Alzheimer's disease —*see* Disease, Alzheimer's
arteriosclerotic brain disease —*see* Dementia, vascular
cerebral lipidoses E75.- *[FØ2.8Ø]*
with behavioral disturbance E75.- *[FØ2.81]*
Creutzfeldt-Jakob disease —*see also* Creutzfeldt-Jakob disease or syndrome (with dementia) A81.ØØ
epilepsy G4Ø.- *[FØ2.8Ø]*
with behavioral disturbance G4Ø.- *[FØ2.81]*
hepatolenticular degeneration E83.Ø1 *[FØ2.8Ø]*
with behavioral disturbance E83.Ø1 *[FØ2.81]*
human immunodeficiency virus (HIV) disease B2Ø *[FØ2.8Ø]*
with behavioral disturbance B2Ø *[FØ2.81]*
Huntington's disease or chorea G1Ø
hypercalcemia E83.52 *[FØ2.8Ø]*
with behavioral disturbance E83.52 *[FØ2.81]*
hypothyroidism, acquired EØ3.9 *[FØ2.8Ø]*
with behavioral disturbance EØ3.9 *[FØ2.81]*
due to iodine deficiency EØ1.8 *[FØ2.8Ø]*
with behavioral disturbance EØ1.8 *[FØ2.81]*
inhalants F18.97
with dependence F18.27
multiple
etiologies FØ3
sclerosis G35 *[FØ2.8Ø]*
with behavioral disturbance G35 *[FØ2.81]*
neurosyphilis A52.17 *[FØ2.8Ø]*
with behavioral disturbance A52.17 *[FØ2.81]*
juvenile A5Ø.49 *[FØ2.8Ø]*
with behavioral disturbance A5Ø.49 *[FØ2.81]*
niacin deficiency E52 *[FØ2.8Ø]*
with behavioral disturbance E52 *[FØ2.81]*
paralysis agitans G2Ø *[FØ2.8Ø]*
with behavioral disturbance G2Ø *[FØ2.81]*
Parkinson's disease G2Ø *[FØ2.8Ø]*
pellagra E52 *[FØ2.8Ø]*
with behavioral disturbance E52 *[FØ2.81]*
Pick's G31.Ø1 *[FØ2.8Ø]*
with behavioral disturbance G31.Ø1 *[FØ2.81]*
polyarteritis nodosa M3Ø.Ø *[FØ2.8Ø]*
with behavioral disturbance M3Ø.Ø *[FØ2.81]*

D

◀ New ⬅ Revised ~~deleted~~ Deleted

Dementia *(Continued)*
in *(Continued)*
psychoactive drug F19.97
with dependence F19.27
inhalants F18.97
with dependence F18.27
sedatives, hypnotics or anxiolytics F13.97
with dependence F13.27
sedatives, hypnotics or anxiolytics F13.97
with dependence F13.27
systemic lupus erythematosus M32.- *[F02.80]*
with behavioral disturbance M32.- *[F02.81]*
trypanosomiasis
African B56.9 *[F02.80]*
with behavioral disturbance B56.9 *[F02.81]*
unknown etiology F03
vitamin B12 deficiency E53.8 *[F02.80]*
with behavioral disturbance E53.8 *[F02.81]*
volatile solvents F18.97
with dependence F18.27
infantile, infantilis F84.3
Lewy body G31.83 *[F02.80]*
with behavioral disturbance G31.83 *[F02.81]*
multi-infarct —*see* Dementia, vascular
paralytica, paralytic (syphilitic) A52.17 *[F02.80]*
with behavioral disturbance A52.17 *[F02.81]*
juvenilis A50.45
paretic A52.17
praecox —*see* Schizophrenia
presenile F03
Alzheimer's type —*see* Disease, Alzheimer's, early onset
primary degenerative F03
progressive, syphilitic A52.17
senile F03
with acute confusional state F05
Alzheimer's type —*see* Disease, Alzheimer's, late onset
depressed or paranoid type F03
vascular (acute onset) (mixed) (multi-infarct) (subcortical) F01.50
with behavioral disturbance F01.51
Demineralization, bone —*see* Osteoporosis
Demodex folliculorum (infestation) B88.0
Demophobia F40.248
Demoralization R45.3
Demyelination, demyelinization
central nervous system G37.9
specified NEC G37.8
corpus callosum (central) G37.1
disseminated, acute G36.9
specified NEC G36.8
global G35
in optic neuritis G36.0
Dengue (classical) (fever) A90
hemorrhagic A91
sandfly A93.1
Dennie-Marfan syphilitic syndrome A50.45
Dens evaginatus, in dente or invaginatus K00.2
Dense breasts R92.2
Density
increased, bone (disseminated) (generalized) (spotted) —*see* Disorder, bone, density and structure, specified type NEC
lung (nodular) J98.4
Dental —*see also* condition
examination Z01.20
with abnormal findings Z01.21
restoration
aesthetically inadequate or displeasing K08.56
Dental *(Continued)*
restoration *(Continued)*
defective K08.50
specified NEC K08.59
failure of marginal integrity K08.51
failure of periodontal anatomical integrity K08.54
Dentia praecox K00.6
Denticles (pulp) K04.2
Dentigerous cyst K09.0
Dentin
irregular (in pulp) K04.3
opalescent K00.5
secondary (in pulp) K04.3
sensitive K03.89
Dentinogenesis imperfecta K00.5
Dentinoma —*see* Cyst, calcifying odontogenic
Dentition (syndrome) K00.7
delayed K00.6
difficult K00.7
precocious K00.6
premature K00.6
retarded K00.6
Dependence (on) (syndrome) F19.20
with remission F19.21
alcohol (ethyl) (methyl) (without remission) F10.20
with
amnestic disorder, persisting F10.26
anxiety disorder F10.280
dementia, persisting F10.27
intoxication F10.229
with delirium F10.221
uncomplicated F10.220
mood disorder F10.24
psychotic disorder F10.259
with
delusions F10.250
hallucinations F10.251
remission F10.21
sexual dysfunction F10.281
sleep disorder F10.282
specified disorder NEC F10.288
withdrawal F10.239
with
delirium F10.231
perceptual disturbance F10.232
uncomplicated F10.230
counseling and surveillance Z71.41
amobarbital —*see* Dependence, drug, sedative
amphetamine (s) (type) —*see* Dependence, drug, stimulant NEC
amytal (sodium) —*see* Dependence, drug, sedative
analgesic NEC F55.8
anesthetic (agent) (gas) (general) (local) NEC —*see* Dependence, drug, psychoactive NEC
anxiolytic NEC —*see* Dependence, drug, sedative
barbital (s) —*see* Dependence, drug, sedative
barbiturate (s) (compounds) (drugs classifiable to T42) —*see* Dependence, drug, sedative
benzedrine —*see* Dependence, drug, stimulant NEC
bhang —*see* Dependence, drug, cannabis
bromide (s) NEC —*see* Dependence, drug, sedative
caffeine —*see* Dependence, drug, stimulant NEC
cannabis (sativa) (indica) (resin) (derivatives) (type) —*see* Dependence, drug, cannabis
chloral (betaine) (hydrate) —*see* Dependence, drug, sedative
chlordiazepoxide —*see* Dependence, drug, sedative
coca (leaf) (derivatives) —*see* Dependence, drug, cocaine
cocaine —*see* Dependence, drug, cocaine
Dependence *(Continued)*
codeine —*see* Dependence, drug, opioid
combinations of drugs F19.20
dagga —*see* Dependence, drug, cannabis
demerol —*see* Dependence, drug, opioid
dexamphetamine —*see* Dependence, drug, stimulant NEC
dexedrine —*see* Dependence, drug, stimulant NEC
dextromethorphan —*see* Dependence, drug, opioid
dextromoramide —*see* Dependence, drug, opioid
dextro-nor-pseudo-ephedrine —*see* Dependence, drug, stimulant NEC
dextrorphan —*see* Dependence, drug, opioid
diazepam —*see* Dependence, drug, sedative
dilaudid —*see* Dependence, drug, opioid
D-lysergic acid diethylamide —*see* Dependence, drug, hallucinogen
drug NEC F19.20
with sleep disorder F19.282
cannabis F12.20
with
anxiety disorder F12.280
intoxication F12.229
with
delirium F12.221
perceptual disturbance F12.222
uncomplicated F12.220
other specified disorder F12.288
psychosis F12.259
delusions F12.250
hallucinations F12.251
unspecified disorder F12.29
in remission F12.21
cocaine F14.20
with
anxiety disorder F14.280
intoxication F14.229
with
delirium F14.221
perceptual disturbance F14.222
uncomplicated F14.220
mood disorder F14.24
other specified disorder F14.288
psychosis F14.259
delusions F14.250
hallucinations F14.251
sexual dysfunction F14.281
sleep disorder F14.282
unspecified disorder F14.29
withdrawal F14.23
in remission F14.21
withdrawal symptoms in newborn P96.1
counseling and surveillance Z71.51
hallucinogen F16.20
with
anxiety disorder F16.280
flashbacks F16.283
intoxication F16.229
with delirium F16.221
uncomplicated F16.220
mood disorder F16.24
other specified disorder F16.288
perception disorder, persisting F16.283
psychosis F16.259
delusions F16.250
hallucinations F16.251
unspecified disorder F16.29
in remission F16.21
in remission F19.21
inhalant F18.20
with
anxiety disorder F18.280
dementia, persisting F18.27
intoxication F18.229
with delirium F18.221
uncomplicated F18.220
mood disorder F18.24
other specified disorder F18.288

D

Dependence *(Continued)*
drug NEC *(Continued)*
inhalant *(Continued)*
with *(Continued)*
psychosis F18.259
delusions F18.250
hallucinations F18.251
unspecified disorder F18.29
in remission F18.21
nicotine F17.200
with disorder F17.209
remission F17.201
specified disorder NEC F17.208
withdrawal F17.203
chewing tobacco F17.220
with disorder F17.229
remission F17.221
specified disorder NEC F17.228
withdrawal F17.223
cigarettes F17.210
with disorder F17.219
remission F17.211
specified disorder NEC F17.218
withdrawal F17.213
specified product NEC F17.290
with disorder F17.299
remission F17.291
specified disorder NEC F17.298
withdrawal F17.293
opioid F11.20
with
intoxication F11.229
with
delirium F11.221
perceptual disturbance F11.222
uncomplicated F11.220
mood disorder F11.24
other specified disorder F11.288
psychosis F11.259
delusions F11.250
hallucinations F11.251
sexual dysfunction F11.281
sleep disorder F11.282
unspecified disorder F11.29
withdrawal F11.23
in remission F11.21
psychoactive NEC F19.20
with
amnestic disorder F19.26
anxiety disorder F19.280
dementia F19.27
intoxication F19.229
with
delirium F19.221
perceptual disturbance F19.222
uncomplicated F19.220
mood disorder F19.24
other specified disorder F19.288
psychosis F19.259
delusions F19.250
hallucinations F19.251
sexual dysfunction F19.281
sleep disorder F19.282
unspecified disorder F19.29
withdrawal F19.239
with
delirium F19.231
perceptual disturbance F19.232
uncomplicated F19.230
sedative, hypnotic or anxiolytic F13.20
with
amnestic disorder F13.26
anxiety disorder F13.280
dementia, persisting F13.27
intoxication F13.229
with delirium F13.221
uncomplicated F13.220
mood disorder F13.24
other specified disorder F13.288

Dependence *(Continued)*
drug NEC *(Continued)*
sedative, hypnotic or anxiolytic *(Continued)*
with *(Continued)*
psychosis F13.259
delusions F13.250
hallucinations F13.251
sexual dysfunction F13.281
sleep disorder F13.282
unspecified disorder F13.29
withdrawal F13.239
with
delirium F13.231
perceptual disturbance F13.232
uncomplicated F13.230
in remission F13.21
stimulant NEC F15.20
with
anxiety disorder F15.280
intoxication F15.229
with
delirium F15.221
perceptual disturbance F15.222
uncomplicated F15.220
mood disorder F15.24
other specified disorder F15.288
psychosis F15.259
delusions F15.250
hallucinations F15.251
sexual dysfunction F15.281
sleep disorder F15.282
unspecified disorder F15.29
withdrawal F15.23
in remission F15.21
ethyl
alcohol (without remission) F10.20
with remission F10.21
bromide —*see* Dependence, drug, sedative
carbamate F19.20
chloride F19.20
morphine —*see* Dependence, drug, opioid
ganja —*see* Dependence, drug, cannabis
glue (airplane) (sniffing) —*see* Dependence, drug, inhalant
glutethimide —*see* Dependence, drug, sedative
hallucinogenics —*see* Dependence, drug, hallucinogen
hashish —*see* Dependence, drug, cannabis
hemp —*see* Dependence, drug, cannabis
heroin (salt) (any) —*see* Dependence, drug, opioid
hypnotic NEC —*see* Dependence, drug, sedative
Indian hemp —*see* Dependence, drug, cannabis
inhalants —*see* Dependence, drug, inhalant
khat —*see* Dependence, drug, stimulant NEC
laudanum —*see* Dependence, drug, opioid
LSD (-25) (derivatives) —*see* Dependence, drug, hallucinogen
luminal —*see* Dependence, drug, sedative
lysergic acid —*see* Dependence, drug, hallucinogen
maconha —*see* Dependence, drug, cannabis
marihuana —*see* Dependence, drug, cannabis
meprobamate —*see* Dependence, drug, sedative
mescaline —*see* Dependence, drug, hallucinogen
methadone —*see* Dependence, drug, opioid
methamphetamine (s) —*see* Dependence, drug, stimulant NEC
methaqualone —*see* Dependence, drug, sedative
methyl
alcohol (without remission) F10.20
with remission F10.21
bromide —*see* Dependence, drug, sedative
morphine —*see* Dependence, drug, opioid

Dependence *(Continued)*
methyl *(Continued)*
phenidate —*see* Dependence, drug, stimulant NEC
sulfonal —*see* Dependence, drug, sedative
morphine (sulfate) (sulfite) (type) —*see* Dependence, drug, opioid
narcotic (drug) NEC —*see* Dependence, drug, opioid
nembutal —*see* Dependence, drug, sedative
neraval —*see* Dependence, drug, sedative
neravan —*see* Dependence, drug, sedative
neurobarb —*see* Dependence, drug, sedative
nicotine —*see* Dependence, drug, nicotine
nitrous oxide F19.20
nonbarbiturate sedatives and tranquilizers with similar effect —*see* Dependence, drug, sedative
on
artificial heart (fully implantable) (mechanical) Z95.812
aspirator Z99.0
care provider (because of) Z74.9
impaired mobility Z74.09
need for
assistance with personal care Z74.1
continuous supervision Z74.3
no other household member able to render care Z74.2
specified reason NEC Z74.8
machine Z99.89
enabling NEC Z99.89
specified type NEC Z99.89
renal dialysis (hemodialysis) (peritoneal) Z99.2
respirator Z99.11
ventilator Z99.11
wheelchair Z99.3
opiate —*see* Dependence, drug, opioid
opioids —*see* Dependence, drug, opioid
opium (alkaloids) (derivatives) (tincture) —*see* Dependence, drug, opioid
oxygen (long-term) (supplemental) Z99.81
paraldehyde —*see* Dependence, drug, sedative
paregoric —*see* Dependence, drug, opioid
PCP (phencyclidine) (or related substance) —*see* Dependence, drug, hallucinogen ◄
pentobarbital —*see* Dependence, drug, sedative
pentobarbitone (sodium) —*see* Dependence, drug, sedative
pentothal —*see* Dependence, drug, sedative
peyote —*see* Dependence, drug, hallucinogen
phencyclidine (PCP) (or related substance) —*see* Dependence, drug, hallucinogen ◄
phenmetrazine —*see* Dependence, drug, stimulant NEC
phenobarbital —*see* Dependence, drug, sedative
polysubstance F19.20
psilocibin, psilocin, psilocyn, psilocyline —*see* Dependence, drug, hallucinogen
psychostimulant NEC —*see* Dependence, drug, stimulant NEC
secobarbital —*see* Dependence, drug, sedative
seconal —*see* Dependence, drug, sedative
sedative NEC —*see* Dependence, drug, sedative
specified drug NEC —*see* Dependence, drug
stimulant NEC —*see* Dependence, drug, stimulant NEC
substance NEC —*see* Dependence, drug
supplemental oxygen Z99.81
tobacco —*see* Dependence, drug, nicotine
counseling and surveillance Z71.6
tranquilizer NEC —*see* Dependence, drug, sedative
vitamin B6 E53.1
volatile solvents —*see* Dependence, drug, inhalant

D

- **Dependency**
  - care-provider Z74.9
  - passive F6Ø.7
  - reactions (persistent) F6Ø.7
- **Depersonalization** (in neurotic state) (neurotic) (syndrome) F48.1
- **Depletion**
  - extracellular fluid E86.9
  - plasma E86.1
  - potassium E87.6
    - nephropathy N25.89
  - salt or sodium E87.1
    - causing heat exhaustion or prostration T67.4
    - nephropathy N28.9
  - volume NOS E86.9
- **Deployment** (current) (military) status Z56.82
  - in theater or in support of military war, peacekeeping and humanitarian operations Z56.82
  - personal history of Z91.82
    - military war, peacekeeping and humanitarian deployment (current or past conflict) Z91.82
  - returned from Z91.82
- **Depolarization, premature** I49.4Ø
  - atrial I49.1
  - junctional I49.2
  - specified NEC I49.49
  - ventricular I49.3
- **Deposit**
  - bone in Boeck's sarcoid D86.89
  - calcareous, calcium *—see* Calcification
  - cholesterol
    - retina H35.89
    - vitreous (body) (humor) *—see* Deposit, crystalline
  - conjunctiva H11.11-
  - cornea H18.ØØ-
    - argentous H18.Ø2-
    - due to metabolic disorder H18.Ø3-
    - Kayser-Fleischer ring H18.Ø4-
    - pigmentation *—see* Pigmentation, cornea
  - crystalline, vitreous (body) (humor) H43.2-
  - hemosiderin in old scars of cornea *—see* Pigmentation, cornea, stromal
  - metallic in lens *—see* Cataract, specified NEC
  - skin R23.8
  - tooth, teeth (betel) (black) (green) (materia alba) (orange) (tobacco) KØ3.6
  - urate, kidney *—see* Calculus, kidney
- **Depraved appetite** *—see* Pica
- **Depressed**
  - HDL cholesterol E78.6
- **Depression** (acute) (mental) F32.9
  - agitated (single episode) F32.2
  - anaclitic *—see* Disorder, adjustment
  - anxiety F41.8
    - persistent F34.1
  - arches *—see also* Deformity, limb, flat foot
  - atypical (single episode) F32.89 ⬅
    - recurrent episode F33.8 ◀
  - basal metabolic rate R94.8
  - bone marrow D75.89
  - central nervous system RØ9.2
  - cerebral R29.818
    - newborn P91.4
  - cerebrovascular I67.9
  - chest wall M95.4
  - climacteric (single episode) F32.89 ⬅
    - recurrent episode F33.8 ◀
  - endogenous (without psychotic symptoms) F33.2
    - with psychotic symptoms F33.3
  - functional activity R68.89
  - hysterical F44.89
  - involutional (single episode) F32.89 ⬅
    - recurrent episode F33.8 ◀
  - major F32.9
    - with psychotic symptoms F32.3
    - recurrent *—see* Disorder, depressive, recurrent
  - manic-depressive *—see* Disorder, depressive, recurrent
  - masked (single episode) F32.89 ⬅
  - medullary G93.89
  - menopausal (single episode) F32.89 ⬅
    - recurrent episode F33.8 ◀
  - metatarsus *—see* Depression, arches
  - monopolar F33.9
  - nervous F34.1
  - neurotic F34.1
  - nose M95.Ø
  - postnatal F53
  - postpartum F53
  - post-psychotic of schizophrenia F32.89 ⬅
  - post-schizophrenic F32.89 ⬅
  - psychogenic (reactive) (single episode) F32.9
  - psychoneurotic F34.1
  - psychotic (single episode) F32.3
    - recurrent F33.3
  - reactive (psychogenic) (single episode) F32.9
    - psychotic (single episode) F32.3
  - recurrent *—see* Disorder, depressive, recurrent
  - respiratory center G93.89
  - seasonal *—see* Disorder, depressive, recurrent
  - senile FØ3
  - severe, single episode F32.2
  - situational F43.21
  - skull Q67.4
  - specified NEC (single episode) F32.89 ⬅
  - sternum M95.4
  - visual field *—see* Defect, visual field
  - vital (recurrent) (without psychotic symptoms) F33.2
    - with psychotic symptoms F33.3
    - single episode F32.2
- **Deprivation**
  - cultural Z6Ø.3
  - effects NOS T73.9
    - specified NEC T73.8
  - emotional NEC Z65.8
    - affecting infant or child *—see* Maltreatment, child, psychological
  - food T73.Ø
  - protein *—see* Malnutrition
  - sleep Z72.82Ø
  - social Z6Ø.4
    - affecting infant or child *—see* Maltreatment, child, psychological
  - specified NEC T73.8
  - vitamins *—see* Deficiency, vitamin
  - water T73.1
- **Derangement**
  - ankle (internal) *—see* Derangement, joint, ankle
  - cartilage (articular) NEC *—see* Derangement, joint, articular cartilage, by site
    - recurrent *—see* Dislocation, recurrent
  - cruciate ligament, anterior, current injury *—see* Sprain, knee, cruciate, anterior
  - elbow (internal) *—see* Derangement, joint, elbow
  - hip (joint) (internal) (old) *—see* Derangement, joint, hip
  - joint (internal) M24.9
    - ankylosis *—see* Ankylosis
    - articular cartilage M24.1Ø
      - ankle M24.17-
      - elbow M24.12-
      - foot M24.17-
      - hand M24.14-
      - hip M24.15-
      - knee NEC M23.9-
      - loose body *—see* Loose, body
      - shoulder M24.11-
      - wrist M24.13-
    - contracture *—see* Contraction, joint
    - current injury *—see also* Dislocation
      - knee, meniscus or cartilage *—see* Tear, meniscus
    - dislocation
      - pathological *—see* Dislocation, pathological
      - recurrent *—see* Dislocation, recurrent
    - knee *—see* Derangement, knee
    - ligament *—see* Disorder, ligament
    - loose body *—see* Loose, body
    - recurrent *—see* Dislocation, recurrent
    - specified type NEC M24.8Ø
      - ankle M24.87-
      - elbow M24.82-
      - foot joint M24.87-
      - hand joint M24.84-
      - hip M24.85-
      - shoulder M24.81-
      - wrist M24.83-
    - temporomandibular M26.69
  - knee (recurrent) M23.9-
    - ligament disruption, spontaneous M23.6Ø-
      - anterior cruciate M23.61-
      - capsular M23.67-
      - instability, chronic M23.5-
      - lateral collateral M23.64-
      - medial collateral M23.63-
      - posterior cruciate M23.62-
    - loose body M23.4-
    - meniscus M23.3Ø-
      - cystic M23.ØØ-
        - lateral M23.ØØ2
          - anterior horn M23.Ø4-
          - posterior horn M23.Ø5-
          - specified NEC M23.Ø6-
        - medial M23.ØØ5
          - anterior horn M23.Ø1-
          - posterior horn M23.Ø2-
          - specified NEC M23.Ø3-
      - degenerate *—see* Derangement, knee, meniscus, specified NEC
      - detached *—see* Derangement, knee, meniscus, specified NEC
      - due to old tear or injury M23.2Ø-
        - lateral M23.2Ø-
          - anterior horn M23.24-
          - posterior horn M23.25-
          - specified NEC M23.26-
        - medial M23.2Ø-
          - anterior horn M23.21-
          - posterior horn M23.22-
          - specified NEC M23.23-
      - retained *—see* Derangement, knee, meniscus, specified NEC
      - specified NEC M23.3Ø-
        - lateral M23.3Ø-
          - anterior horn M23.34-
          - posterior horn M23.35-
          - specified NEC M23.36-
        - medial M23.3Ø-
          - anterior horn M23.31-
          - posterior horn M23.32-
          - specified NEC M23.33-
    - old M23.8X-
    - specified NEC *—see* subcategory M23.8
  - low back NEC *—see* Dorsopathy, specified NEC
  - meniscus *—see* Derangement, knee, meniscus
  - mental *—see* Psychosis
  - patella, specified NEC *—see* Disorder, patella, derangement NEC
  - semilunar cartilage (knee) *—see* Derangement, knee, meniscus, specified NEC
  - shoulder (internal) *—see* Derangement, joint, shoulder
- **Dercum's disease** E88.2
- **Derealization** (neurotic) F48.1
- **Dermal** *—see* condition
- **Dermaphytid** *—see* Dermatophytosis

D

- **Dermatitis** (eczematous) L3Ø.9
  - ab igne L59.Ø
  - acarine B88.Ø
  - actinic (due to sun) L57.8
    - other than from sun L59.8
  - allergic —*see* Dermatitis, contact, allergic
  - ambustionis, due to burn or scald —*see* Burn
  - amebic AØ6.7
  - ammonia L22
  - arsenical (ingested) L27.8
  - artefacta L98.1
    - psychogenic F54
  - atopic L2Ø.9
    - psychogenic F54
    - specified NEC L2Ø.89
  - autoimmune progesterone L3Ø.8
  - berlock, berloque L56.2
  - blastomycotic B4Ø.3
  - blister beetle L24.89
  - bullous, bullosa L13.9
    - mucosynechial, atrophic L12.1
    - seasonal L3Ø.8
    - specified NEC L13.8
  - calorica L59.Ø
    - due to burn or scald —*see* Burn
  - caterpillar L24.89
  - cercarial B65.3
  - combustionis L59.Ø
    - due to burn or scald —*see* Burn
  - congelationis T69.1
  - contact (occupational) L25.9
    - allergic L23.9
      - due to
        - adhesives L23.1
        - cement L23.5
        - chemical products NEC L23.5
        - chromium L23.Ø
        - cosmetics L23.2
        - dander (cat) (dog) L23.81
        - drugs in contact with skin L23.3
        - dyes L23.4
        - food in contact with skin L23.6
        - hair (cat) (dog) L23.81
        - insecticide L23.5
        - metals L23.Ø
        - nickel L23.Ø
        - plants, non-food L23.7
        - plastic L23.5
        - rubber L23.5
        - specified agent NEC L23.89
    - due to
      - cement L25.3
      - chemical products NEC L25.3
      - cosmetics L25.Ø
      - dander (cat) (dog) L23.81
      - drugs in contact with skin L25.1
      - dyes L25.2
      - food in contact with skin L25.4
      - hair (cat) (dog) L23.81
      - plants, non-food L25.5
      - specified agent NEC L25.8
    - irritant L24.9
      - due to
        - cement L24.5 ⟸
        - chemical products NEC L24.5
        - cosmetics L24.3
        - detergents L24.Ø
        - drugs in contact with skin L24.4
        - food in contact with skin L24.6
        - oils and greases L24.1
        - plants, non-food L24.7
        - solvents L24.2
        - specified agent NEC L24.89
  - contusiformis L52
  - diabetic —*see* EØ8-E13 with .62Ø
  - diaper L22
  - diphtheritica A36.3
  - dry skin L85.3
  - due to
    - acetone (contact) (irritant) L24.2
    - acids (contact) (irritant) L24.5

- **Dermatitis** *(Continued)*
  - due to *(Continued)*
    - adhesive (s) (allergic) (contact) (plaster) L23.1
      - irritant L24.5
    - alcohol (irritant) (skin contact) (substances in category T51) L24.2
      - taken internally L27.8
    - alkalis (contact) (irritant) L24.5
    - arsenic (ingested) L27.8
    - carbon disulfide (contact) (irritant) L24.2
    - caustics (contact) (irritant) L24.5
    - cement (contact) L25.3
    - cereal (ingested) L27.2
    - chemical (s) NEC L25.3
      - taken internally L27.8
    - chlorocompounds L24.2
    - chromium (contact) (irritant) L24.81
    - coffee (ingested) L27.2
    - cold weather L3Ø.8
    - cosmetics (contact) L25.Ø
      - allergic L23.2
      - irritant L24.3
    - cyclohexanes L24.2
    - dander (cat) (dog) L23.81
    - Demodex species B88.Ø
    - Dermanyssus gallinae B88.Ø
    - detergents (contact) (irritant) L24.Ø
    - dichromate L24.81
    - drugs and medicaments (generalized) (internal use) L27.Ø
      - external —*see* Dermatitis, due to, drugs, in contact with skin
      - in contact with skin L25.1
        - allergic L23.3
        - irritant L24.4
      - localized skin eruption L27.1
      - specified substance —*see* Table of Drugs and Chemicals
    - dyes (contact) L25.2
      - allergic L23.4
      - irritant L24.89
    - epidermophytosis —*see* Dermatophytosis
    - esters L24.2
    - external irritant NEC L24.9
    - fish (ingested) L27.2
    - flour (ingested) L27.2
    - food (ingested) L27.2
      - in contact with skin L25.4
    - fruit (ingested) L27.2
    - furs (allergic) (contact) L23.81
    - glues —*see* Dermatitis, due to, adhesives
    - glycols L24.2
    - greases NEC (contact) (irritant) L24.1
    - hair (cat) (dog) L23.81
    - hot
      - objects and materials —*see* Burn
      - weather or places L59.Ø
    - hydrocarbons L24.2
    - infrared rays L59.8
    - ingestion, ingested substance L27.9
      - chemical NEC L27.8
      - drugs and medicaments —*see* Dermatitis, due to, drugs
      - food L27.2
      - specified NEC L27.8
    - insecticide in contact with skin L24.5
    - internal agent L27.9
      - drugs and medicaments (generalized) —*see* Dermatitis, due to, drugs
      - food L27.2
    - irradiation —*see* Dermatitis, due to, radioactive substance
    - ketones L24.2
    - lacquer tree (allergic) (contact) L23.7
    - light (sun) NEC L57.8
      - acute L56.8
      - other L59.8
    - Liponyssoides sanguineus B88.Ø
    - low temperature L3Ø.8
    - meat (ingested) L27.2

- **Dermatitis** *(Continued)*
  - due to *(Continued)*
    - metals, metal salts (contact) (irritant) L24.81
    - milk (ingested) L27.2
    - nickel (contact) (irritant) L24.81
    - nylon (contact) (irritant) L24.5
    - oils NEC (contact) (irritant) L24.1
    - paint solvent (contact) (irritant) L24.2
    - petroleum products (contact) (irritant) (substances in T52) L24.2
    - plants NEC (contact) L25.5
      - allergic L23.7
      - irritant L24.7
    - plasters (adhesive) (any) (allergic) (contact) L23.1
      - irritant L24.5
    - plastic (contact) L25.3
    - preservatives (contact) —*see* Dermatitis, due to, chemical, in contact with skin
    - primrose (allergic) (contact) L23.7
    - primula (allergic) (contact) L23.7
    - radiation L59.8
      - nonionizing (chronic exposure) L57.8
      - sun NEC L57.8
        - acute L56.8
    - radioactive substance L58.9
      - acute L58.Ø
      - chronic L58.1
    - radium L58.9
      - acute L58.Ø
      - chronic L58.1
    - ragweed (allergic) (contact) L23.7
    - Rhus (allergic) (contact) (diversiloba) (radicans) (toxicodendron) (venenata) (verniciflua) L23.7
    - rubber (contact) L24.5
    - Senecio jacobaea (allergic) (contact) L23.7
    - solvents (contact) (irritant) (substances in categories T52) L24.2
    - specified agent NEC (contact) L25.8
      - allergic L23.89
      - irritant L24.89
    - sunshine NEC L57.8
      - acute L56.8
    - tetrachlorethylene (contact) (irritant) L24.2
    - toluene (contact) (irritant) L24.2
    - turpentine (contact) L24.2
    - ultraviolet rays (sun NEC) (chronic exposure) L57.8
      - acute L56.8
    - vaccine or vaccination L27.Ø
      - specified substance —*see* Table of Drugs and Chemicals
    - varicose veins —*see* Varix, leg, with, inflammation
    - X-rays L58.9
      - acute L58.Ø
      - chronic L58.1
  - dyshydrotic L3Ø.1
  - dysmenorrheica N94.6
  - escharotica —*see* Burn
  - exfoliative, exfoliativa (generalized) L26
    - neonatorum LØØ
  - eyelid —*see also* Dermatosis, eyelid
    - allergic HØ1.119
      - left HØ1.116
        - lower HØ1.115
        - upper HØ1.114
      - right HØ1.113
        - lower HØ1.112
        - upper HØ1.111
    - contact —*see* Dermatitis, eyelid, allergic
    - due to
      - Demodex species B88.Ø
      - herpes (zoster) BØ2.39
        - simplex BØØ.59

Dermatitis *(Continued)*
  eyelid *(Continued)*
    eczematous H01.139
      left H01.136
        lower H01.135
        upper H01.134
      right H01.133
        lower H01.132
        upper H01.131
  facta, factitia, factitial L98.1
    psychogenic F54
  flexural NEC L20.82
  friction L30.4
  fungus B36.9
    specified type NEC B36.8
  gangrenosa, gangrenous infantum L08.0
  harvest mite B88.0
  heat L59.0
  herpesviral, vesicular (ear) (lip) B00.1
  herpetiformis (bullous) (erythematous) (pustular) (vesicular) L13.0
    juvenile L12.2
    senile L12.0
  hiemalis L30.8
  hypostatic, hypostatica —*see* Varix, leg, with, inflammation
  infectious eczematoid L30.3
  infective L30.3
  irritant —*see* Dermatitis, contact, irritant
  Jacquet's (diaper dermatitis) L22
  Leptus B88.0
  lichenified NEC L28.0
  medicamentosa (generalized) (internal use) —*see* Dermatitis, due to drugs
  mite B88.0
  multiformis L13.0
    juvenile L12.2
  napkin L22
  neurotica L13.0
  nummular L30.0
  papillaris capillitii L73.0
  pellagrous E52
  perioral L71.0
  photocontact L56.2
  polymorpha dolorosa L13.0
  pruriginosa L13.0
  pruritic NEC L30.8
  psychogenic F54
  purulent L08.0
  pustular
    contagious B08.02
    subcorneal L13.1
  pyococcal L08.0
  pyogenica L08.0
  repens L40.2
  Ritter's (exfoliativa) L00
  Schamberg's L81.7
  schistosome B65.3
  seasonal bullous L30.8
  seborrheic L21.9
    infantile L21.1
    specified NEC L21.8
  sensitization NOS L23.9
  septic L08.0
  solare L57.8
  specified NEC L30.8
  stasis I87.2
    ~~with varicose ulcer —see Varix, leg, with ulcer, with inflammation~~
    with ◀
      varicose ulcer —*see* Varix, leg, with ulcer, with inflammation ◀
      varicose veins —*see* Varix, leg, with, inflammation ◀
    due to postthrombotic syndrome —*see* Syndrome, postthrombotic
  suppurative L08.0
  traumatic NEC L30.4
  trophoneurotica L13.0
  ultraviolet (sun) (chronic exposure) L57.8
    acute L56.8

Dermatitis *(Continued)*
  varicose —*see* Varix, leg, with, inflammation
  vegetans L10.1
  verrucosa B43.0
  vesicular, herpesviral B00.1
Dermatoarthritis, lipoid E78.81
Dermatochalasis, eyelid H02.839
  left H02.836
    lower H02.835
    upper H02.834
  right H02.833
    lower H02.832
    upper H02.831
Dermatofibroma (lenticulare) —*see* Neoplasm, skin, benign
  protuberans —*see* Neoplasm, skin, uncertain behavior
Dermatofibrosarcoma (pigmented) (protuberans) —*see* Neoplasm, skin, malignant
Dermatographia L50.3
Dermatolysis (exfoliativa) (congenital) Q82.8
  acquired L57.4
  eyelids —*see* Blepharochalasis
  palpebrarum —*see* Blepharochalasis
  senile L57.4
Dermatomegaly NEC Q82.8
Dermatomucosomyositis M33.10
  with
    myopathy M33.12
    respiratory involvement M33.11
    specified organ involvement NEC M33.19
Dermatomycosis B36.9
  furfuracea B36.0
  specified type NEC B36.8
Dermatomyositis (acute) (chronic) —*see also* Dermatopolymyositis
  in (due to) neoplastic disease —*see also* Neoplasm D49.9 *[M36.0]*
Dermatoneuritis of children —*see* Poisoning, mercury
Dermatophilosis A48.8
Dermatophytid L30.2
Dermatophytide —*see* Dermatophytosis
Dermatophytosis (epidermophyton) (infection) (Microsporum) (tinea) (Trichophyton) B35.9
  beard B35.0
  body B35.4
  capitis B35.0
  corporis B35.4
  deep-seated B35.8
  disseminated B35.8
  foot B35.3
  granulomatous B35.8
  groin B35.6
  hand B35.2
  nail B35.1
  perianal (area) B35.6
  scalp B35.0
  specified NEC B35.8
Dermatopolymyositis M33.90
  with
    myopathy M33.92
    respiratory involvement M33.91
    specified organ involvement NEC M33.99
  in neoplastic disease (*see also* Neoplasm) D49.9 *[M36.0]*
  juvenile M33.00
    with
      myopathy M33.02
      respiratory involvement M33.01
      specified organ involvement NEC M33.09
  specified NEC M33.10
    myopathy M33.12
    respiratory involvement M33.11
    specified organ involvement NEC M33.19

Dermatopolyneuritis —*see* Poisoning, mercury
Dermatorrhexis Q79.6
  acquired L57.4
Dermatosclerosis —*see also* Scleroderma
  localized L94.0
Dermatosis L98.9
  Andrews' L08.89
  Bowen's —*see* Neoplasm, skin, in situ
  bullous L13.9
    specified NEC L13.8
  exfoliativa L26
  eyelid (noninfectious)
    dermatitis —*see* Dermatitis, eyelid
    discoid lupus erythematosus —*see* Lupus, erythematosus, eyelid
    xeroderma —*see* Xeroderma, acquired, eyelid
  factitial L98.1
  febrile neutrophilic L98.2
  gonococcal A54.89
  herpetiformis L13.0
    juvenile L12.2
  linear IgA L13.8
  menstrual NEC L98.8
  neutrophilic, febrile L98.2
  occupational —*see* Dermatitis, contact
  papulosa nigra L82.1
  pigmentary L81.9
    progressive L81.7
    Schamberg's L81.7
  psychogenic F54
  purpuric, pigmented L81.7
  pustular, subcorneal L13.1
  transient acantholytic L11.1
Dermographia, dermographism L50.3
Dermoid (cyst) —*see also* Neoplasm, benign, by site
  with malignant transformation C56-
  due to radiation (nonionizing) L57.8
Dermopathy
  infiltrative with thyrotoxicosis —*see* Thyrotoxicosis
  nephrogenic fibrosing L90.8
Dermophytosis —*see* Dermatophytosis
Descemetocele H18.73-
Descemet's membrane —*see* condition
Descending —*see* condition
Descensus uteri —*see* Prolapse, uterus
Desert
  rheumatism B38.0
  sore —*see* Ulcer, skin
Desertion (newborn) —*see* Maltreatment
Desmoid (extra-abdominal) (tumor) —*see* Neoplasm, connective tissue, uncertain behavior
  abdominal D48.1
Despondency F32.9
Desquamation, skin R23.4
Destruction, destructive —*see also* Damage
  articular facet —*see also* Derangement, joint, specified type NEC
    knee M23.8X-
    vertebra —*see* Spondylosis
  bone —*see also* Disorder, bone, specified type NEC
    syphilitic A52.77
  joint —*see also* Derangement, joint, specified type NEC
    sacroiliac M53.3
  rectal sphincter K62.89
  septum (nasal) J34.89
  tuberculous NEC —*see* Tuberculosis
  tympanum, tympanic membrane (nontraumatic) —*see* Disorder, tympanic membrane, specified NEC
  vertebral disc —*see* Degeneration, intervertebral disc
Destructiveness —*see also* Disorder, conduct
  adjustment reaction —*see* Disorder, adjustment

D

Desultory labor O62.2
Detachment
- cartilage —*see* Sprain
- cervix, annular N88.8
  - complicating delivery O71.3
- choroid (old) (postinfectional) (simple) (spontaneous) H31.40-
  - hemorrhagic H31.41-
  - serous H31.42-
- ligament —*see* Sprain
- meniscus (knee) —*see also* Derangement, knee, meniscus, specified NEC
  - current injury —*see* Tear, meniscus
  - due to old tear or injury —*see* Derangement, knee, meniscus, due to old tear
- retina (without retinal break) (serous) H33.2-
  - with retinal:
    - break H33.00-
      - giant H33.03-
      - multiple H33.02-
      - single H33.01-
    - dialysis H33.04-
  - pigment epithelium —*see* Degeneration, retina, separation of layers, pigment epithelium detachment
  - rhegmatogenous —*see* Detachment, retina, with retinal, break
  - specified NEC H33.8
  - total H33.05-
  - traction H33.4-
- vitreous (body) H43.81

Detergent asthma J69.8
Deterioration
- epileptic F06.8
- general physical R53.81
- heart, cardiac —*see* Degeneration, myocardial
- mental —*see* Psychosis
- myocardial, myocardium —*see* Degeneration, myocardial
- senile (simple) R54

Deuteranomaly (anomalous trichromat) H53.53
Deuteranopia (complete) (incomplete) H53.53
Development
- abnormal, bone Q79.9
- arrested R62.50
  - bone —*see* Arrest, development or growth, bone
  - child R62.50
  - due to malnutrition E45
- defective, congenital —*see also* Anomaly, by site
  - cauda equina Q06.3
  - left ventricle Q24.8
    - in hypoplastic left heart syndrome Q23.4
  - valve Q24.8
    - pulmonary Q22.3
- delayed (*see also* Delay, development) R62.50
  - arithmetical skills F81.2
  - language (skills) (expressive) F80.1
  - learning skill F81.9
  - mixed skills F88
  - motor coordination F82
  - reading F81.0
  - specified learning skill NEC F81.89
  - speech F80.9
  - spelling F81.81
  - written expression F81.81
- imperfect, congenital —*see also* Anomaly, by site
  - heart Q24.9
  - lungs Q33.6
- incomplete
  - bronchial tree Q32.4
  - organ or site not listed —*see* Hypoplasia, by site
  - respiratory system Q34.9
- sexual, precocious NEC E30.1
- tardy, mental (*see also* Disability, intellectual) F79

Developmental —*see* condition
- ~~testing, child —see Examination, child~~
- testing, infant or child —*see* Examination, child ◀

Devergie's disease (pityriasis rubra pilaris) L44.0
Deviation (in)
- conjugate palsy (eye) (spastic) H51.0
- esophagus (acquired) K22.8
- eye, skew H51.8
- midline (jaw) (teeth) (dental arch) M26.29
  - specified site NEC —*see* Malposition
- nasal septum J34.2
  - congenital Q67.4
- opening and closing of the mandible M26.53
- organ or site, congenital NEC —*see* Malposition, congenital
- septum (nasal) (acquired) J34.2
  - congenital Q67.4
- sexual F65.9
  - bestiality F65.89
  - erotomania F52.8
  - exhibitionism F65.2
  - fetishism, fetishistic F65.0
    - transvestism F65.1
  - frotteurism F65.81
  - masochism F65.51
  - multiple F65.89
  - necrophilia F65.89
  - nymphomania F52.8
  - pederosis F65.4
  - pedophilia F65.4
  - sadism, sadomasochism F65.52
  - satyriasis F52.8
  - specified type NEC F65.89
  - transvestism F64.1
  - voyeurism F65.3
- teeth, midline M26.29
- trachea J39.8
- ureter, congenital Q62.61

Device
- cerebral ventricle (communicating) in situ Z98.2
- contraceptive —*see* Contraceptive, device
- drainage, cerebrospinal fluid, in situ Z98.2

Devic's disease G36.0
Devil's
- grip B33.0
- pinches (purpura simplex) D69.2

Devitalized tooth K04.99
Devonshire colic —*see* Poisoning, lead
Dextraposition, aorta Q20.3
- in tetralogy of Fallot Q21.3

Dextrinosis, limit (debrancher enzyme deficiency) E74.03
Dextrocardia (true) Q24.0
- with
  - complete transposition of viscera Q89.3
  - situs inversus Q89.3

Dextrotransposition, aorta Q20.3
d-glycericacidemia E72.59
Dhat syndrome F48.8
Dhobi itch B35.6
Di George's syndrome D82.1
Di Guglielmo's disease C94.0-
Diabetes, diabetic (mellitus) (sugar) E11.9
- with
  - amyotrophy E11.44
  - arthropathy NEC E11.618
  - autonomic (poly)neuropathy E11.43
  - cataract E11.36
  - Charcot's joints E11.610
  - chronic kidney disease E11.22
  - circulatory complication NEC E11.59
  - complication E11.8
    - specified NEC E11.69
  - dermatitis E11.620
  - foot ulcer E11.621
  - gangrene E11.52
  - gastroparalysis E11.43 ◀
  - gastroparesis E11.43

Diabetes, diabetic *(Continued)*
- with *(Continued)*
  - glomerulonephrosis, intracapillary E11.21
  - glomerulosclerosis, intercapillary E11.21
  - hyperglycemia E11.65
  - hyperosmolarity E11.00
    - with coma E11.01
  - hypoglycemia E11.649
    - with coma E11.641
  - kidney complications NEC E11.29
  - Kimmelsteil-Wilson disease E11.21
  - loss of protective sensation (LOPS) —*see* Diabetes, by type, with neuropathy
  - mononeuropathy E11.41
  - myasthenia E11.44
  - necrobiosis lipoidica E11.620
  - nephropathy E11.21
  - neuralgia E11.42
  - neurologic complication NEC E11.49
  - neuropathic arthropathy E11.610
  - neuropathy E11.40
  - ophthalmic complication NEC E11.39
  - oral complication NEC E11.638
  - osteomyelitis E11.69 ◀
  - periodontal disease E11.630
  - peripheral angiopathy E11.51
    - with gangrene E11.52
  - polyneuropathy E11.42
  - renal complication NEC E11.29
  - renal tubular degeneration E11.29
  - retinopathy E11.319
    - with macular edema E11.311
      - resolved following treatment E11.37 ◀
    - nonproliferative E11.329
      - with macular edema E11.321
      - mild E11.329
        - with macular edema E11.321
      - moderate E11.339
        - with macular edema E11.331
      - severe E11.349
        - with macular edema E11.341
    - proliferative E11.359
      - ~~with macular edema E11.351~~
      - with ◀
        - combined traction retinal detachment and rhegmatogenous retinal detachment E11.354 ◀
        - macular edema E11.351 ◀
        - stable proliferative diabetic retinopathy E11.355 ◀
        - traction retinal detachment involving the macula E11.352 ◀
        - traction retinal detachment not involving the macula E11.353 ◀
  - skin complication NEC E11.628
  - skin ulcer NEC E11.622
- brittle —*see* Diabetes, type 1 ◀
- bronzed E83.110
- complicating pregnancy —*see* Pregnancy, complicated by, diabetes
- dietary counseling and surveillance Z71.3
- due to ◀
  - autoimmune process —*see* Diabetes, type 1 ◀
  - immune mediated pancreatic islet beta-cell destruction —*see* Diabetes, type 1 ◀
- due to drug or chemical E09.9
  - with
    - amyotrophy E09.44
    - arthropathy NEC E09.618
    - autonomic (poly)neuropathy E09.43
    - cataract E09.36
    - Charcot's joints E09.610
    - chronic kidney disease E09.22
    - circulatory complication NEC E09.59
    - complication E09.8
      - specified NEC E09.69

D

Diabetes, diabetic *(Continued)*
  specified type NEC *(Continued)*
    with *(Continued)*
      retinopathy *(Continued)*
        proliferative E13.359
          ~~with macular edema E13.351~~
          with ◀
            combined traction retinal detachment and rhegmatogenous retinal detachment E13.354 ◀
            macular edema E13.351 ◀
            stable proliferative diabetic retinopathy E13.355 ◀
            traction retinal detachment involving the macula E13.352 ◀
            traction retinal detachment not involving the macula E13.353 ◀
      skin complication NEC E13.628
      skin ulcer NEC E13.622
  steroid-induced —*see* Diabetes, due to, drug or chemical
  type 1 E10.9
    with
      amyotrophy E10.44
      arthropathy NEC E10.618
      autonomic (poly)neuropathy E10.43
      cataract E10.36
      Charcot's joints E10.610
      chronic kidney disease E10.22
      circulatory complication NEC E10.59
      complication E10.8
        specified NEC E10.69
      dermatitis E10.620
      foot ulcer E10.621
      gangrene E10.52
      gastroparalysis E10.43 ◀
      gastroparesis E10.43
      glomerulonephrosis, intracapillary E10.21
      glomerulosclerosis, intercapillary E10.21
      hyperglycemia E10.65
      hypoglycemia E10.649
        with coma E10.641
      ketoacidosis E10.10
        with coma E10.11
      kidney complications NEC E10.29
      Kimmelsteil-Wilson disease E10.21
      mononeuropathy E10.41
      myasthenia E10.44
      necrobiosis lipoidica E10.620
      nephropathy E10.21
      neuralgia E10.42
      neurologic complication NEC E10.49
      neuropathic arthropathy E10.610
      neuropathy E10.40
      ophthalmic complication NEC E10.39
      oral complication NEC E10.638
      periodontal disease E10.630
      peripheral angiopathy E10.51
        with gangrene E10.52
      polyneuropathy E10.42
      renal complication NEC E10.29
      renal tubular degeneration E10.29
      retinopathy E10.319
        with macular edema E10.311
          resolved following treatment E10.37 ◀
        nonproliferative E10.329
          with macular edema E10.321
          mild E10.329
            with macular edema E10.321
          moderate E10.339
            with macular edema E10.331
          severe E10.349
            with macular edema E10.341

Diabetes, diabetic *(Continued)*
  type 1 *(Continued)*
    with *(Continued)*
      retinopathy *(Continued)*
        proliferative E10.359
          ~~with macular edema E10.351~~
          with ◀
            combined traction retinal detachment and rhegmatogenous retinal detachment E13.354 ◀
            macular edema E13.351 ◀
            stable proliferative diabetic retinopathy E13.355 ◀
            traction retinal detachment involving the macula E13.352 ◀
            traction retinal detachment not involving the macula E13.353 ◀
      skin complication NEC E10.628
      skin ulcer NEC E10.622
  type 2 E11.9
    with
      amyotrophy E11.44
      arthropathy NEC E11.618
      autonomic (poly)neuropathy E11.43
      cataract E11.36
      Charcot's joints E11.610
      chronic kidney disease E11.22
      circulatory complication NEC E11.59
      complication E11.8
        specified NEC E11.69
      dermatitis E11.620
      foot ulcer E11.621
      gangrene E11.52
      gastroparalysis E11.43 ◀
      gastroparesis E11.43
      glomerulonephrosis, intracapillary E11.21
      glomerulosclerosis, intercapillary E11.21
      hyperglycemia E11.65
      hyperosmolarity E11.00
        with coma E11.01
      hypoglycemia E11.649
        with coma E11.641
      kidney complications NEC E11.29
      Kimmelsteil-Wilson disease E11.21
      mononeuropathy E11.41
      myasthenia E11.44
      necrobiosis lipoidica E11.620
      nephropathy E11.21
      neuralgia E11.42
      neurologic complication NEC E11.49
      neuropathic arthropathy E11.610
      neuropathy E11.40
      ophthalmic complication NEC E11.39
      oral complication NEC E11.638
      periodontal disease E11.630
      peripheral angiopathy E11.51
        with gangrene E11.52
      polyneuropathy E11.42
      renal complication NEC E11.29
      renal tubular degeneration E11.29
      retinopathy E11.319
        with macular edema E11.311
          resolved following treatment E11.37 ◀
        nonproliferative E11.329
          with macular edema E11.321
          mild E11.329
            with macular edema E11.321
          moderate E11.339
            with macular edema E11.331
          severe E11.349
            with macular edema E11.341
        proliferative E11.359
          ~~with macular edema E11.351~~
          with ◀
            combined traction retinal detachment and rhegmatogenous retinal detachment E11.354 ◀

Diabetes, diabetic *(Continued)*
  type 2 *(Continued)*
    with *(Continued)*
      retinopathy *(Continued)*
        proliferative *(Continued)*
          with *(Continued)*
            macular edema E11.351 ◀
            stable proliferative diabetic retinopathy E11.355 ◀
            traction retinal detachment involving the macula E11.352 ◀
            traction retinal detachment not involving the macula E11.353 ◀
      skin complication NEC E11.628
      skin ulcer NEC E11.622
  uncontrolled ◀
    meaning ◀
      hyperglycemia —*see* Diabetes, by type, with, hyperglycemia ◀
      hypoglycemia —*see* Diabetes, by type, with, hypoglycemia ◀
Diacyclothrombopathia D69.1
Diagnosis deferred R69
Dialysis (intermittent) (treatment)
  noncompliance (with) Z91.15
  renal (hemodialysis) (peritoneal), status Z99.2
  retina, retinal —*see* Detachment, retina, with retinal, dialysis
Diamond-Blackfan anemia (congenital hypoplastic) D61.01
Diamond-Gardener syndrome (autoerythrocyte sensitization) D69.2
Diaper rash L22
Diaphoresis (excessive) R61
Diaphragm —*see* condition
Diaphragmalgia R07.1
Diaphragmatitis, diaphragmitis J98.6
Diaphysial aclasis Q78.6
Diaphysitis —*see* Osteomyelitis, specified type NEC
Diarrhea, diarrheal (disease) (infantile) (inflammatory) R19.7
  achlorhydric K31.83
  allergic K52.29 ⟵
    due to ◀
      colitis —*see* Colitis, allergic ◀
      enteritis —*see* Enteritis, allergic ◀
  amebic —*see also* Amebiasis A06.0
    with abscess —*see* Abscess, amebic
    acute A06.0
    chronic A06.1
    nondysenteric A06.2
  bacillary —*see* Dysentery, bacillary
  balantidial A07.0
  cachectic NEC K52.89
  Chilomastix A07.8
  choleriformis A00.1
  chronic (noninfectious) K52.9
  coccidial A07.3
  Cochin-China K90.1
    strongyloidiasis B78.0
  Dientamoeba A07.8
  dietetic —*see also* Diarrhea, allergic K52.29 ⟵
  drug-induced K52.1
  due to
    bacteria A04.9
      specified NEC A04.8
    Campylobacter A04.5
    Capillaria philippinensis B81.1
    Clostridium difficile A04.7
    Clostridium perfringens (C) (F) A04.8
    Cryptosporidium A07.2
    drugs K52.1
    Escherichia coli A04.4
      enteroaggregative A04.4
      enterohemorrhagic A04.3
      enteroinvasive A04.2
      enteropathogenic A04.0

◀ New ⟵ Revised ~~deleted~~ Deleted

- **Diarrhea, diarrheal** *(Continued)*
  - due to *(Continued)*
    - Escherichia coli *(Continued)*
      - enterotoxigenic A04.1
      - specified NEC A04.4
    - food hypersensitivity —*see also* Diarrhea, allergic K52.29 ⬅
    - Necator americanus B76.1
    - S. japonicum B65.2
    - specified organism NEC A08.8
      - bacterial A04.8
      - viral A08.39
    - Staphylococcus A04.8
    - Trichuris trichiuria B79
    - virus —*see* Enteritis, viral
    - Yersinia enterocolitica A04.6
  - dysenteric A09
  - endemic A09
  - epidemic A09
  - flagellate A07.9
  - Flexner's (ulcerative) A03.1
  - functional K59.1
    - following gastrointestinal surgery K91.89
    - psychogenic F45.8
  - Giardia lamblia A07.1
  - giardial A07.1
  - hill K90.1
  - infectious A09
  - malarial —*see* Malaria
  - mite B88.0
  - mycotic NEC B49
  - neonatal (noninfectious) P78.3
  - nervous F45.8
  - neurogenic K59.1
  - noninfectious K52.9
  - postgastrectomy K91.1
  - postvagotomy K91.1
  - protozoal A07.9
    - specified NEC A07.8
  - psychogenic F45.8
  - specified
    - bacterium NEC A04.8
    - virus NEC A08.39
  - strongyloidiasis B78.0
  - toxic K52.1
  - trichomonal A07.8
  - tropical K90.1
  - tuberculous A18.32
  - viral —*see* Enteritis, viral
- **Diastasis**
  - cranial bones M84.88
    - congenital NEC Q75.8
  - joint (traumatic) —*see* Dislocation
  - muscle M62.00
    - ankle M62.07-
    - congenital Q79.8
    - foot M62.07-
    - forearm M62.03-
    - hand M62.04-
    - lower leg M62.06-
    - pelvic region M62.05-
    - shoulder region M62.01-
    - specified site NEC M62.08
    - thigh M62.05-
    - upper arm M62.02-
  - recti (abdomen)
    - complicating delivery O71.89
    - congenital Q79.59
- **Diastema, tooth, teeth, fully erupted** M26.32
- **Diastematomyelia** Q06.2
- **Diataxia, cerebral** G80.4
- **Diathesis**
  - allergic —*see* History, allergy
  - bleeding (familial) D69.9
  - cystine (familial) E72.00
  - gouty —*see* Gout
  - hemorrhagic (familial) D69.9
    - newborn NEC P53
  - spasmophilic R29.0
- **Diaz's disease or osteochondrosis** (juvenile) (talus) —*see* Osteochondrosis, juvenile, tarsus
- **Dibothriocephalus, dibothriocephaliasis** (latus) (infection) (infestation) B70.0
  - larval B70.1
- **Dicephalus, dicephaly** Q89.4
- **Dichotomy, teeth** K00.2
- **Dichromat, dichromatopsia** (congenital) —*see* Deficiency, color vision
- **Dichuchwa** A65
- **Dicroceliasis** B66.2
- **Didelphia, didelphys** —*see* Double uterus
- **Didymytis** N45.1
  - with orchitis N45.3
- **Dietary**
  - inadequacy or deficiency E63.9
  - surveillance and counseling Z71.3
- **Dietl's crisis** N13.8
- **Dieulafoy lesion** (hemorrhagic)
  - duodenum K31.82
  - esophagus K22.8
  - intestine (colon) K63.81
  - stomach K31.82
- **Difficult, difficulty** (in)
  - acculturation Z60.3
  - feeding R63.3
    - newborn P92.9
      - breast P92.5
      - specified NEC P92.8
    - nonorganic (infant or child) F98.29
  - intubation, in anesthesia T88.4
  - mechanical, gastroduodenal stoma K91.89
    - causing obstruction K91.3
  - micturition ◀
    - need to immediately re-void R39.191 ◀
    - position dependent R39.192 ◀
    - specified NEC R39.198 ◀
  - reading (developmental) F81.0
    - secondary to emotional disorders F93.9
  - spelling (specific) F81.81
    - with reading disorder F81.89
    - due to inadequate teaching Z55.8
  - swallowing —*see* Dysphagia
  - walking R26.2
  - work
    - conditions NEC Z56.5
    - schedule Z56.3
- **Diffuse** —*see* condition
- **DiGeorge's syndrome** (thymic hypoplasia) D82.1
- **Digestive** —*see* condition
- **Dihydropyrimidine dehydrogenase disease** (DPD) E88.89
- **Diktyoma** —*see* Neoplasm, malignant, by site
- **Dilaceration, tooth** K00.4
- **Dilatation**
  - anus K59.8
    - venule —*see* Hemorrhoids
  - aorta (focal) (general) —*see* Ectasia, aorta
    - with aneurysm —*see* Aneurysm, aorta
    - congenital Q25.44 ◀
  - artery —*see* Aneurysm
  - bladder (sphincter) N32.89
    - congenital Q64.79
  - blood vessel I99.8
  - bronchial J47.9
    - with
      - exacerbation (acute) J47.1
      - lower respiratory infection J47.0
  - calyx (due to obstruction) —*see* Hydronephrosis
  - capillaries I78.8
  - cardiac (acute) (chronic) —*see also* Hypertrophy, cardiac
    - congenital Q24.8
      - valve NEC Q24.8
        - pulmonary Q22.3
    - valve —*see* Endocarditis
  - cavum septi pellucidi Q06.8
  - cervix (uteri) —*see also* Incompetency, cervix
    - incomplete, poor, slow complicating delivery O62.0
- **Dilatation** *(Continued)*
  - colon K59.39 ⬅
    - congenital Q43.1
    - psychogenic F45.8
    - toxic K59.31 ◀
  - common duct (acquired) K83.8
    - congenital Q44.5
  - cystic duct (acquired) K82.8
    - congenital Q44.5
  - duct, mammary —*see* Ectasia, mammary duct
  - duodenum K59.8
  - esophagus K22.8
    - congenital Q39.5
    - due to achalasia K22.0
  - eustachian tube, congenital Q17.8
  - gallbladder K82.8
  - gastric —*see* Dilatation, stomach
  - heart (acute) (chronic) —*see also* Hypertrophy, cardiac
    - congenital Q24.8
    - valve —*see* Endocarditis
  - ileum K59.8
    - psychogenic F45.8
  - jejunum K59.8
    - psychogenic F45.8
  - kidney (calyx) (collecting structures) (cystic) (parenchyma) (pelvis) (idiopathic) N28.89
  - lacrimal passages or duct —*see* Disorder, lacrimal system, changes
  - lymphatic vessel I89.0
  - mammary duct —*see* Ectasia, mammary duct
  - Meckel's diverticulum (congenital) Q43.0
    - malignant —*see* Table of Neoplasms, small intestine, malignant
  - myocardium (acute) (chronic) —*see* Hypertrophy, cardiac organ or site, congenital NEC —*see* Distortion
  - pancreatic duct K86.89 ⬅
  - pericardium —*see* Pericarditis
  - pharynx J39.2
  - prostate N42.89
  - pulmonary
    - artery (idiopathic) I28.8
    - valve, congenital Q22.3
  - pupil H57.04
  - rectum K59.39 ⬅
  - saccule, congenital Q16.5
  - salivary gland (duct) K11.8
  - sphincter ani K62.89
  - stomach K31.89
    - acute K31.0
    - psychogenic F45.8
  - submaxillary duct K11.8
  - trachea, congenital Q32.1
  - ureter (idiopathic) N28.82
    - congenital Q62.2
    - due to obstruction N13.4
  - urethra (acquired) N36.8
  - vasomotor I73.9
  - vein I86.8
  - ventricular, ventricle (acute) (chronic) —*see also* Hypertrophy, cardiac
    - cerebral, congenital Q04.8
  - venule NEC I86.8
  - vesical orifice N32.89
- **Dilated, dilation** —*see* Dilatation
- **Diminished, diminution**
  - hearing (acuity) —*see* Deafness
  - sense or sensation (cold) (heat) (tactile) (vibratory) R20.8
  - vision NEC H54.7
  - vital capacity R94.2
- **Diminuta taenia** B71.0
- **Dimitri-Sturge-Weber disease** Q85.8
- **Dimple**
  - ~~parasacral, pilonidal or postanal —see Cyst, pilonidal~~
  - congenital sacral Q82.6 ◀
  - parasacral Q82.6 ◀
  - pilonidal or postanal —*see* Cyst, pilonidal ◀

- **Dioctophyme renalis** (infection) (infestation) B83.8
- **Dipetalonemiasis** B74.4
- **Diphallus** Q55.69
- **Diphtheria, diphtheritic** (gangrenous) (hemorrhagic) A36.9
  - carrier (suspected) Z22.2
  - cutaneous A36.3
  - faucial A36.Ø
  - infection of wound A36.3
  - laryngeal A36.2
  - myocarditis A36.81
  - nasal, anterior A36.89
  - nasopharyngeal A36.1
  - neurological complication A36.89
  - pharyngeal A36.Ø
  - specified site NEC A36.89
  - tonsillar A36.Ø
- **Diphyllobothriasis** (intestine) B7Ø.Ø
  - larval B7Ø.1
- **Diplacusis** H93.22-
- **Diplegia** (upper limbs) G83.Ø
  - congenital (cerebral) G8Ø.8
  - facial G51.Ø
  - lower limbs G82.2Ø
  - spastic G8Ø.1
- **Diplococcus, diplococcal** —*see* condition
- **Diplopia** H53.2
- **Dipsomania** F1Ø.2Ø
  - with
    - psychosis —*see* Psychosis, alcoholic
  - remission F1Ø.21
- **Dipylidiasis** B71.1
- **DIRA** (deficiency of interleukin 1 receptor antagonist) MØ4.8 ◀
- **Direction, teeth, abnormal, fully erupted** M26.3Ø
- **Dirofilariasis** B74.8
- **Dirt-eating child** F98.3
- **Disability, disabilities**
  - heart —*see* Disease, heart
  - intellectual F79
    - with
      - autistic features F84.9
    - mild (I.Q. 5Ø-69) F7Ø
    - moderate (I.Q. 35-49) F71
    - profound (I.Q. under 2Ø) F73
    - severe (I.Q. 2Ø-34) F72
    - specified level NEC F78
  - knowledge acquisition F81.9
  - learning F81.9
  - limiting activities Z73.6
  - spelling, specific F81.81
- **Disappearance of family member** Z63.4
- **Disarticulation** —*see* Amputation
  - meaning traumatic amputation —*see* Amputation, traumatic
- **Discharge** (from)
  - abnormal finding in —*see* Abnormal, specimen
  - breast (female) (male) N64.52
  - diencephalic autonomic idiopathic —*see* Epilepsy, specified NEC
  - ear —*see also* Otorrhea
    - blood —*see* Otorrhagia
  - excessive urine R35.8
  - nipple N64.52
  - penile R36.9
  - postnasal RØ9.82
  - prison, anxiety concerning Z65.2
  - urethral R36.9
    - without blood R36.Ø
    - hematospermia R36.1
  - vaginal N89.8
- **Discitis, diskitis** M46.4Ø
  - cervical region M46.42
  - cervicothoracic region M46.43
  - lumbar region M46.46
  - lumbosacral region M46.47
  - multiple sites M46.49
  - occipito-atlanto-axial region M46.41

- **Discitis, diskitis** *(Continued)*
  - pyogenic —*see* Infection, intervertebral disc, pyogenic
  - sacrococcygeal region M46.48
  - thoracic region M46.44
  - thoracolumbar region M46.45
- **Discoid**
  - meniscus (congenital) Q68.6
  - semilunar cartilage (congenital) —*see* Derangement, knee, meniscus, specified NEC
- **Discoloration**
  - nails L6Ø.8
  - teeth (posteruptive) KØ3.7
    - during formation KØØ.8
- **Discomfort**
  - chest RØ7.89
  - visual H53.14-
- **Discontinuity, ossicles, ear** H74.2-
- **Discord** (with)
  - boss Z56.4
  - classmates Z55.4
  - counselor Z64.4
  - employer Z56.4
  - family Z63.8
  - fellow employees Z56.4
  - in-laws Z63.1
  - landlord Z59.2
  - lodgers Z59.2
  - neighbors Z59.2
  - probation officer Z64.4
  - social worker Z64.4
  - teachers Z55.4
  - workmates Z56.4
- **Discordant connection**
  - atrioventricular (congenital) Q2Ø.5
  - ventriculoarterial Q2Ø.3
- **Discrepancy**
  - centric occlusion maximum intercuspation M26.55
  - leg length (acquired) —*see* Deformity, limb, unequal length
    - congenital —*see* Defect, reduction, lower limb
  - uterine size date O26.84-
- **Discrimination**
  - ethnic Z6Ø.5
  - political Z6Ø.5
  - racial Z6Ø.5
  - religious Z6Ø.5
  - sex Z6Ø.5
- **Disease, diseased** —*see also* Syndrome
  - absorbent system I87.8
  - acid-peptic K3Ø
  - Acosta's T7Ø.29
  - Adams-Stokes (-Morgagni) (syncope with heart block) I45.9
  - Addison's anemia (pernicious) D51.Ø
  - adenoids (and tonsils) J35.9
  - adrenal (capsule) (cortex) (gland) (medullary) E27.9
    - hyperfunction E27.Ø
    - specified NEC E27.8
  - ainhum L94.6
  - airway
    - obstructive, chronic J44.9
      - due to
        - cotton dust J66.Ø
        - specific organic dusts NEC J66.8
    - reactive —*see* Asthma
  - akamushi (scrub typhus) A75.3
  - Albers-Schönberg (marble bones) Q78.2
  - Albert's —*see* Tendinitis, Achilles
  - alimentary canal K63.9
  - alligator-skin Q8Ø.9
    - acquired L85.Ø
  - alpha heavy chain C88.3
  - alpine T7Ø.29
  - altitude T7Ø.2Ø

- **Disease, diseased** *(Continued)*
  - alveolar ridge
    - edentulous KØ6.9
      - specified NEC KØ6.8
  - alveoli, teeth KØ8.9
  - Alzheimer's G3Ø.9 *[FØ2.8Ø]*
    - with behavioral disturbance G3Ø.9 *[FØ2.81]*
    - early onset G3Ø.Ø *[FØ2.8Ø]*
      - with behavioral disturbance G3Ø.Ø *[FØ2.81]*
    - late onset G3Ø.1 *[FØ2.8Ø]*
      - with behavioral disturbance G3Ø.1 *[FØ2.81]*
    - specified NEC G3Ø.8 *[FØ2.8Ø]*
      - with behavioral disturbance G3Ø.8 *[FØ2.81]*
  - amyloid —*see* Amyloidosis
  - Andersen's (glycogenosis IV) E74.Ø9
  - Andes T7Ø.29
  - Andrews' (bacterid) LØ8.89
  - angiospastic I73.9
    - cerebral G45.9
    - vein I87.8
  - anterior
    - chamber H21.9
    - horn cell G12.29
  - antiglomerular basement membrane (anti-GBM) antibody M31.Ø
    - tubulo-interstitial nephritis N12
  - antral —*see* Sinusitis, maxillary
  - anus K62.9
    - specified NEC K62.89
  - aorta (nonsyphilitic) I77.9
    - syphilitic NEC A52.Ø2
  - aortic (heart) (valve) I35.9
    - rheumatic IØ6.9
  - Apollo B3Ø.3
  - aponeuroses —*see* Enthesopathy
  - appendix K38.9
    - specified NEC K38.8
  - aqueous (chamber) H21.9
  - Arnold-Chiari —*see* Arnold-Chiari disease
  - arterial I77.9
    - occlusive —*see* Occlusion, by site
      - due to stricture or stenosis I77.1
  - arteriocardiorenal —*see* Hypertension, cardiorenal
  - arteriolar (generalized) (obliterative) I77.9
  - arteriorenal —*see* Hypertension, kidney
  - arteriosclerotic —*see also* Arteriosclerosis
    - cardiovascular —*see* Disease, heart, ischemic, atherosclerotic
    - coronary (artery) —*see* Disease, heart, ischemic, atherosclerotic
    - heart —*see* Disease, heart, ischemic, atherosclerotic
  - artery I77.9
    - cerebral I67.9
    - coronary I25.1Ø
      - with angina pectoris —*see* Arteriosclerosis, coronary (artery),
  - arthropod-borne NOS (viral) A94
    - specified type NEC A93.8
  - atticoantral, chronic H66.2Ø
    - left H66.22
      - with right H66.23
    - right H66.21
      - with left H66.23
  - auditory canal —*see* Disorder, ear, external
  - auricle, ear NEC —*see* Disorder, pinna
  - Australian X A83.4
  - autoimmune (systemic) NOS M35.9
    - hemolytic (cold type) (warm type) D59.1
      - drug-induced D59.Ø
    - thyroid EØ6.3
  - aviator's —*see* Effect, adverse, high altitude
  - ~~Ayala's Q78.5~~
  - Ayerza's (pulmonary artery sclerosis with pulmonary hypertension) I27.Ø

Disease, diseased *(Continued)*
Babington's (familial hemorrhagic telangiectasia) I78.0
bacterial A49.9
specified NEC A48.8
zoonotic A28.9
specified type NEC A28.8
Baelz's (cheilitis glandularis apostematosa) K13.0
bagasse J67.1
balloon —*see* Effect, adverse, high altitude
Bang's (brucella abortus) A23.1
Bannister's T78.3
barometer makers' —*see* Poisoning, mercury
Barraquer (-Simons') (progressive lipodystrophy) E88.1
Barrett's —*see* Barrett's, esophagus
Bartholin's gland N75.9
basal ganglia G25.9
degenerative G23.9
specified NEC G23.8
specified NEC G25.89
Basedow's (exophthalmic goiter) —*see* Hyperthyroidism, with, goiter (diffuse)
Bateman's B08.1
Batten-Steinert G71.11
Battey A31.0
Beard's (neurasthenia) F48.8
Becker
idiopathic mural endomyocardial I42.3
myotonia congenita G71.12
Begbie's (exophthalmic goiter) —*see* Hyperthyroidism, with, goiter (diffuse)
behavioral, organic F07.9
Beigel's (white piedra) B36.2
Benson's —*see* Deposit, crystalline
Bernard-Soulier (thrombopathy) D69.1
Bernhardt (-Roth) —*see* Mononeuropathy, lower limb, meralgia paresthetica
Biermer's (pernicious anemia) D51.0
bile duct (common) (hepatic) K83.9
with calculus, stones —*see* Calculus, bile duct
specified NEC K83.8
biliary (tract) K83.9
specified NEC K83.8
Billroth's —*see* Spina bifida
bird fancier's J67.2
black lung J60
bladder N32.9
in (due to)
schistosomiasis (bilharziasis) B65.0 *[N33]*
specified NEC N32.89
bleeder's D66
blood D75.9
forming organs D75.9
vessel I99.9
Bloodgood's —*see* Mastopathy, cystic
Bodechtel-Guttmann (subacute sclerosing panencephalitis) A81.1
bone —*see also* Disorder, bone
aluminum M83.4
fibrocystic NEC
jaw M27.49
bone-marrow D75.9
Borna A83.9
Bornholm (epidemic pleurodynia) B33.0
Bouchard's (myopathic dilatation of the stomach) K31.0
Bouillaud's (rheumatic heart disease) I01.9
Bourneville (-Brissaud) (tuberous sclerosis) Q85.1
Bouveret (-Hoffmann) (paroxysmal tachycardia) I47.9
bowel K63.9
functional K59.9
psychogenic F45.8
brain G93.9
arterial, artery I67.9
arteriosclerotic I67.2
congenital Q04.9

Disease, diseased *(Continued)*
brain *(Continued)*
degenerative —*see* Degeneration, brain
inflammatory —*see* Encephalitis
organic G93.9
arteriosclerotic I67.2
parasitic NEC B71.9 *[G94]*
senile NEC G31.1
specified NEC G93.89
breast (*see also* Disorder, breast) N64.9
cystic (chronic) —*see* Mastopathy, cystic
fibrocystic —*see* Mastopathy, cystic
Paget's
female, unspecified side C50.91-
male, unspecified side C50.92-
specified NEC N64.89
Breda's —*see* Yaws
Bretonneau's (diphtheritic malignant angina) A36.0
Bright's —*see* Nephritis
arteriosclerotic —*see* Hypertension, kidney
Brill's (recrudescent typhus) A75.1
Brill-Zinsser (recrudescent typhus) A75.1
Brion-Kayser —*see* Fever, paratyphoid
broad
beta E78.2
ligament (noninflammatory) N83.9
inflammatory —*see* Disease, pelvis, inflammatory
specified NEC N83.8
Brocq-Duhring (dermatitis herpetiformis) L13.0
Brocq's
meaning
dermatitis herpetiformis L13.0
prurigo L28.2
bronchopulmonary J98.4
bronchus NEC J98.09
bronze Addison's E27.1
tuberculous A18.7
budgerigar fancier's J67.2
Buerger's (thromboangiitis obliterans) I73.1
bullous L13.9
chronic of childhood L12.2
specified NEC L13.8
Bürger-Grütz (essential familial hyperlipemia) E78.3
bursa —*see* Bursopathy
caisson T70.3
California —*see* Coccidioidomycosis
capillaries I78.9
specified NEC I78.8
Carapata A68.0
cardiac —*see* Disease, heart
cardiopulmonary, chronic I27.9
cardiorenal (hepatic) (hypertensive) (vascular) —*see* Hypertension, cardiorenal
cardiovascular (atherosclerotic) I25.10
with angina pectoris —*see* Arteriosclerosis, coronary (artery),
congenital Q28.9
hypertensive —*see* Hypertension, heart
newborn P29.9
specified NEC P29.89
renal (hypertensive) —*see* Hypertension, cardiorenal
syphilitic (asymptomatic) A52.00
cartilage —*see* Disorder, cartilage
Castellani's A69.8
Castleman (unicentric) (multicentric) D47.Z2 ◀
HHV-8-associated —*see also* Herpesvirus, human, 8 D47.Z2 ◀
cat-scratch A28.1
Cavare's (familial periodic paralysis) G72.3
cecum K63.9
celiac (adult) (infantile) (with steatorrhea) K90.0 ⬅
cellular tissue L98.9

Disease, diseased *(Continued)*
central core G71.2
cerebellar, cerebellum —*see* Disease, brain
cerebral —*see also* Disease, brain
degenerative —*see* Degeneration, brain
cerebrospinal G96.9
cerebrovascular I67.9
acute I67.89
embolic I63.4-
thrombotic I63.3-
arteriosclerotic I67.2
specified NEC I67.89
cervix (uteri) (noninflammatory) N88.9
inflammatory —*see* Cervicitis
specified NEC N88.8
Chabert's A22.9
Chandler's (osteochondritis dissecans, hip) —*see* Osteochondritis, dissecans, hip
Charlouis —*see* Yaws
Chédiak-Steinbrinck (-Higashi) (congenital gigantism of peroxidase granules) E70.330
chest J98.9
Chiari's (hepatic vein thrombosis) I82.0
Chicago B40.9
Chignon B36.8
chigo, chigoe B88.1
childhood granulomatous D71
Chinese liver fluke B66.1
chlamydial A74.9
specified NEC A74.89
cholecystic K82.9
choroid H31.9
specified NEC H31.8
Christmas D67
chronic bullous of childhood L12.2
chylomicron retention E78.3
ciliary body H21.9
specified NEC H21.89
circulatory (system) NEC I99.8
newborn P29.9
syphilitic A52.00
congenital A50.54
coagulation factor deficiency (congenital) —*see* Defect, coagulation
coccidioidal —*see* Coccidioidomycosis
cold
agglutinin or hemoglobinuria D59.1
paroxysmal D59.6
hemagglutinin (chronic) D59.1
collagen NOS (nonvascular) (vascular) M35.9
specified NEC M35.8
colon K63.9
functional K59.9
congenital Q43.2
ischemic —*see also* Ischemia, intestine, acute K55.039 ⬅
colonic inflammatory bowel, unclassified (IBDU) K52.3 ◀
combined system —*see* Degeneration, combined
compressed air T70.3
Concato's (pericardial polyserositis) A19.9
nontubercular I31.1
pleural —*see* Pleurisy, with effusion
conjunctiva H11.9
chlamydial A74.0
specified NEC H11.89
viral B30.9
specified NEC B30.8
connective tissue, systemic (diffuse) M35.9
in (due to)
hypogammaglobulinemia D80.1 *[M36.8]*
ochronosis E70.29 *[M36.8]*
specified NEC M35.8
Conor and Bruch's (boutonneuse fever) A77.1
Cooper's —*see* Mastopathy, cystic
Cori's (glycogenosis III) E74.03
corkhandler's or corkworker's J67.3
cornea H18.9
specified NEC H18.89-

D

Disease, diseased *(Continued)*
- coronary (artery) —*see* Disease, heart, ischemic, atherosclerotic
  - congenital Q24.5
  - ostial, syphilitic (aortic) (mitral) (pulmonary) A52.Ø3
- corpus cavernosum N48.9
  - specified NEC N48.89
- Cotugno's —*see* Sciatica
- coxsackie (virus) NEC B34.1
- cranial nerve NOS G52.9
- Creutzfeldt-Jakob —*see* Creutzfeldt- Jakob disease or syndrome
- Crocq's (acrocyanosis) I73.89
- Crohn's —*see* Enteritis, regional
- Curschmann G71.11
- cystic
  - breast (chronic) —*see* Mastopathy, cystic
  - kidney, congenital Q61.9
  - liver, congenital Q44.6
  - lung J98.4
    - congenital Q33.Ø
- cytomegalic inclusion (generalized) B25.9
  - with pneumonia B25.Ø
  - congenital P35.1
- cytomegaloviral B25.9
  - specified NEC B25.8
- Czerny's (periodic hydrarthrosis of the knee) —*see* Effusion, joint, knee
- Daae (-Finsen) (epidemic pleurodynia) B33.Ø
- Darling's —*see* Histoplasmosis capsulati
- Débove's (splenomegaly) R16.1
- deer fly —*see* Tularemia
- Degos' I77.8
- demyelinating, demyelinizating (nervous system) G37.9
  - multiple sclerosis G35
  - specified NEC G37.8
- dense deposit —*see also* NØØ-NØ7 with fourth character .6 NØ5.6
- deposition, hydroxyapatite —*see* Disease, hydroxyapatite deposition
- de Quervain's (tendon sheath) M65.4
  - thyroid (subacute granulomatous thyroiditis) EØ6.1
- Devergie's (pityriasis rubra pilaris) L44.Ø
- Devic's G36.Ø
- diaphorase deficiency D74.Ø
- diaphragm J98.6
- diarrheal, infectious NEC AØ9
- digestive system K92.9
  - specified NEC K92.89
- disc, degenerative —*see* Degeneration, intervertebral disc
- discogenic —*see also* Displacement, intervertebral disc NEC
  - with myelopathy —*see* Disorder, disc, with, myelopathy
- diverticular —*see* Diverticula
- Dubois (thymus) A5Ø.59 *[E35]*
- Duchenne-Griesinger G71.Ø
- Duchenne's
  - muscular dystrophy G71.Ø
  - pseudohypertrophy, muscles G71.Ø
- ductless glands E34.9
- Duhring's (dermatitis herpetiformis) L13.Ø
- duodenum K31.9
  - specified NEC K31.89
- Dupré's (meningism) R29.1
- Dupuytren's (muscle contracture) M72.Ø
- Durand-Nicholas-Favre (climatic bubo) A55
- Duroziez's (congenital mitral stenosis) Q23.2
- ear —*see* Disorder, ear
- Eberth's —*see* Fever, typhoid
- Ebola (virus) A98.4
- Ebstein's heart Q22.5
- Echinococcus —*see* Echinococcus
- echovirus NEC B34.1
- Eddowes' (brittle bones and blue sclera) Q78.Ø
- edentulous (alveolar) ridge KØ6.9
  - specified NEC KØ6.8

Disease, diseased *(Continued)*
- Edsall's T67.2
- Eichstedt's (pityriasis versicolor) B36.Ø
- Ellis-van Creveld (chondroectodermal dysplasia) Q77.6
- end stage renal (ESRD) N18.6
  - due to hypertension I12.Ø
- endocrine glands or system NEC E34.9
- endomyocardial (eosinophilic) I42.3
- English (rickets) E55.Ø
- enteroviral, enterovirus NEC B34.1
  - central nervous system NEC A88.8
- epidemic B99.9
  - specified NEC B99.8
- epididymis N5Ø.9
- Erb (-Landouzy) G71.Ø
- Erdheim-Chester (ECD) E88.89
- esophagus K22.9
  - functional K22.4
  - psychogenic F45.8
  - specified NEC K22.8
- Eulenburg's (congenital paramyotonia) G71.19
- eustachian tube —*see* Disorder, eustachian tube
- external
  - auditory canal —*see* Disorder, ear, external
  - ear —*see* Disorder, ear, external
- extrapyramidal G25.9
  - specified NEC G25.89
- eye H57.9
  - anterior chamber H21.9
  - inflammatory NEC H57.8
  - muscle (external) —*see* Strabismus
  - specified NEC H57.8
  - syphilitic —*see* Oculopathy, syphilitic
- eyeball H44.9
  - specified NEC H44.89
- eyelid —*see* Disorder, eyelid
  - specified NEC —*see* Disorder, eyelid, specified type NEC
- eyeworm of Africa B74.3
- facial nerve (seventh) G51.9
  - newborn (birth injury) P11.3
- Fahr (of brain) G23.8
- Fahr Volhard (of kidney) I12.-
- fallopian tube (noninflammatory) N83.9
  - inflammatory —*see* Salpingo-oophoritis
  - specified NEC N83.8
- familial periodic paralysis G72.3
- Fanconi's (congenital pancytopenia) D61.Ø9
- fascia NEC —*see also* Disorder, muscle
  - inflammatory —*see* Myositis
  - specified NEC M62.89
- Fauchard's (periodontitis) —*see* Periodontitis
- Favre-Durand-Nicolas (climatic bubo) A55
- Fede's K14.Ø
- Feer's —*see* Poisoning, mercury
- female pelvic inflammatory —*see also* Disease, pelvis, inflammatory N73.9
  - syphilitic (secondary) A51.42
  - tuberculous A18.17
- Fernels' (aortic aneurysm) I71.9
- fibrocaseous of lung —*see* Tuberculosis, pulmonary
- fibrocystic —*see* Fibrocystic disease
- Fiedler's (leptospiral jaundice) A27.Ø
- fifth BØ8.3
- file-cutter's —*see* Poisoning, lead
- fish-skin Q8Ø.9
  - acquired L85.Ø
- Flajani (-Basedow) (exophthalmic goiter) —*see* Hyperthyroidism, with, goiter (diffuse)
- flax-dresser's J66.1
- fluke —*see* Infestation, fluke
- foot and mouth BØ8.8
- foot process NØ4.9
- Forbes' (glycogenosis III) E74.Ø3
- Fordyce-Fox (apocrine miliaria) L75.2
- Fordyce's (ectopic sebaceous glands) (mouth) Q38.6

Disease, diseased *(Continued)*
- Forestier's (rhizomelic pseudopolyarthritis) M35.3
  - meaning ankylosing hyperostosis —*see* Hyperostosis, ankylosing
- Fothergill's
  - neuralgia —*see* Neuralgia, trigeminal
  - scarlatina anginosa A38.9
- Fournier (gangrene) N49.3
  - female N76.89
- fourth BØ8.8
- Fox (-Fordyce) (apocrine miliaria) L75.2
- Francis' —*see* Tularemia
- Franklin C88.2
- Frei's (climatic bubo) A55
- Friedreich's
  - combined systemic or ataxia G11.1
  - myoclonia G25.3
- frontal sinus —*see* Sinusitis, frontal
- fungus NEC B49
- Gaisböck's (polycythemia hypertonica) D75.1
- gallbladder K82.9
  - calculus —*see* Calculus, gallbladder
  - cholecystitis —*see* Cholecystitis
  - cholesterolosis K82.4
  - fistula —*see* Fistula, gallbladder
  - hydrops K82.1
  - obstruction —*see* Obstruction, gallbladder
  - perforation K82.2
  - specified NEC K82.8
- gamma heavy chain C88.2
- Gamna's (siderotic splenomegaly) D73.2
- Gamstorp's (adynamia episodica hereditaria) G72.3
- Gandy-Nanta (siderotic splenomegaly) D73.2
- ganister J62.8
- gastric —*see* Disease, stomach
- gastroesophageal reflux (GERD) K21.9
  - with esophagitis K21.Ø
- gastrointestinal (tract) K92.9
  - amyloid E85.4
  - functional K59.9
    - psychogenic F45.8
  - specified NEC K92.89
- Gee (-Herter) (-Heubner) (-Thaysen) (nontropical sprue) K9Ø.Ø
- genital organs
  - female N94.9
  - male N5Ø.9
- Gerhardt's (erythromelalgia) I73.81
- Gibert's (pityriasis rosea) L42
- Gierke's (glycogenosis I) E74.Ø1
- Gilles de la Tourette's (motor-verbal tic) F95.2
- gingiva KØ6.9
  - plaque induced KØ5.ØØ ◀
  - specified NEC KØ6.8
- gland (lymph) I89.9
- Glanzmann's (hereditary hemorrhagic thrombasthenia) D69.1
- glass-blower's (cataract) —*see* Cataract, specified NEC
  - salivary gland hypertrophy K11.1
- Glisson's —*see* Rickets
- globe H44.9
  - specified NEC H44.89
- glomerular —*see also* Glomerulonephritis
  - with edema —*see* Nephrosis
  - acute —*see* Nephritis, acute
  - chronic —*see* Nephritis, chronic
  - minimal change NØ5.Ø
  - rapidly progressive NØ1.9
- glycogen storage E74.ØØ
  - Andersen's E74.Ø9
  - Cori's E74.Ø3
  - Forbes' E74.Ø3
  - generalized E74.ØØ
  - glucose-6-phosphatase deficiency E74.Ø1
  - heart E74.Ø2 *[I43]*
  - hepatorenal E74.Ø9
  - Hers' E74.Ø9
  - liver and kidney E74.Ø9

D

Disease, diseased *(Continued)*
glycogen storage *(Continued)*
McArdle's E74.Ø4
muscle phosphofructokinase E74.Ø9
myocardium E74.Ø2 *[I43]*
Pompe's E74.Ø2
Tauri's E74.Ø9
type Ø E74.Ø9
type I E74.Ø1
type II E74.Ø2
type III E74.Ø3
type IV E74.Ø9
type V E74.Ø4
type VI-XI E74.Ø9
Von Gierke's E74.Ø1
Goldstein's (familial hemorrhagic telangiectasia) I78.Ø
gonococcal NOS A54.9
graft-versus-host (GVH) D89.813
acute D89.81Ø
acute on chronic D89.812
chronic D89.811
grainhandler's J67.8
granulomatous (childhood) (chronic) D71
Graves' (exophthalmic goiter) —*see* Hyperthyroidism, with, goiter (diffuse)
Griesinger's —*see* Ancylostomiasis
Grisel's M43.6
Gruby's (tinea tonsurans) B35.Ø
Guillain-Barré G61.Ø
Guinon's (motor-verbal tic) F95.2
gum KØ6.9
gynecological N94.9
H (Hartnup's) E72.Ø2
Haff —*see* Poisoning, mercury
Hageman (congenital factor XII deficiency) D68.2
hair (color) (shaft) L67.9
follicles L73.9
specified NEC L73.8
Hamman's (spontaneous mediastinal emphysema) J98.2
hand, foot and mouth BØ8.4
Hansen's —*see* Leprosy
Hantavirus, with pulmonary manifestations B33.4
with renal manifestations A98.5
Harada's H3Ø.81-
Hartnup (pellagra-cerebellar ataxia-renal aminoaciduria) E72.Ø2
Hart's (pellagra-cerebellar ataxia-renal aminoaciduria) E72.Ø2
Hashimoto's (struma lymphomatosa) EØ6.3
Hb —*see* Disease, hemoglobin
heart (organic) I51.9
with
pulmonary edema (acute) —*see also* Failure, ventricular, left I5Ø.1
rheumatic fever (conditions in IØØ)
active IØ1.9
with chorea IØ2.Ø
specified NEC IØ1.8
inactive or quiescent (with chorea) IØ9.9
specified NEC IØ9.89
amyloid E85.4 *[I43]*
aortic (valve) I35.9
arteriosclerotic or sclerotic (senile) —*see* Disease, heart, ischemic, atherosclerotic
artery, arterial —*see* Disease, heart, ischemic, atherosclerotic
beer drinkers' I42.6
beriberi (wet) E51.12
black I27.Ø
congenital Q24.9
cyanotic Q24.9
specified NEC Q24.8
coronary —*see* Disease, heart, ischemic
cryptogenic I51.9

Disease, diseased *(Continued)*
heart *(Continued)*
fibroid —*see* Myocarditis
functional I51.89
psychogenic F45.8
glycogen storage E74.Ø2 *[I43]*
gonococcal A54.83
hypertensive —*see* Hypertension, heart
hyperthyroid —*see also* Hyperthyroidism EØ5.9Ø *[I43]*
with thyroid storm EØ5.91 *[I43]*
ischemic (chronic or with a stated duration of over 4 weeks) I25.9
atherosclerotic (of) I25.1Ø
with angina pectoris —*see* Arteriosclerosis, coronary (artery)
coronary artery bypass graft —*see* Arteriosclerosis, coronary (artery),
cardiomyopathy I25.5
diagnosed on ECG or other special investigation, but currently presenting no symptoms I25.6
silent I25.6
specified form NEC I25.89
kyphoscoliotic I27.1
meningococcal A39.5Ø
endocarditis A39.51
myocarditis A39.52
pericarditis A39.53
mitral IØ5.9
specified NEC IØ5.8
muscular —*see* Degeneration, myocardial
psychogenic (functional) F45.8
pulmonary (chronic) I27.9
in schistosomiasis B65.9 *[I52]*
specified NEC I27.89
rheumatic (chronic) (inactive) (old) (quiescent) (with chorea) IØ9.9
active or acute IØ1.9
with chorea (acute) (rheumatic) (Sydenham's) IØ2.Ø
specified NEC IØ9.89
senile —*see* Myocarditis
syphilitic A52.Ø6
aortic A52.Ø3
aneurysm A52.Ø1
congenital A5Ø.54 *[I52]*
thyrotoxic —*see also* Thyrotoxicosis EØ5.9Ø *[I43]*
with thyroid storm EØ5.91 *[I43]*
valve, valvular (obstructive) (regurgitant) —*see also* Endocarditis
congenital NEC Q24.8
pulmonary Q22.3
vascular —*see* Disease, cardiovascular
heavy chain NEC C88.2
alpha C88.3
gamma C88.2
mu C88.2
Hebra's
pityriasis
maculata et circinata L42
rubra pilaris L44.Ø
prurigo L28.2
hematopoietic organs D75.9
hemoglobin or Hb
abnormal (mixed) NEC D58.2
with thalassemia D56.9
AS genotype D57.3
Bart's D56.Ø
C (Hb-C) D58.2
with other abnormal hemoglobin NEC D58.2
elliptocytosis D58.1
Hb-S D57.2-
sickle-cell D57.2-
thalassemia D56.8
Constant Spring D58.2
D (Hb-D) D58.2

Disease, diseased *(Continued)*
hemoglobin or Hb *(Continued)*
E (Hb-E) D58.2
E-beta thalassemia D56.5
elliptocytosis D58.1
H (Hb-H) (thalassemia) D56.Ø
with other abnormal hemoglobin NEC D56.9
Constant Spring D56.Ø
I thalassemia D56.9
M D74.Ø
S or SS D57.1
SC D57.2-
SD D57.8-
SE D57.8-
spherocytosis D58.Ø
unstable, hemolytic D58.2
hemolytic (newborn) P55.9
autoimmune (cold type) (warm type) D59.1
drug-induced D59.Ø
due to or with
incompatibility
ABO (blood group) P55.1
blood (group) (Duffy) (K(ell)) (Kidd) (Lewis) (M) (S) NEC P55.8
Rh (blood group) (factor) P55.Ø
Rh negative mother P55.Ø
specified type NEC P55.8
unstable hemoglobin D58.2
hemorrhagic D69.9
newborn P53
Henoch (-Schönlein) (purpura nervosa) D69.Ø
hepatic —*see* Disease, liver
hepatobiliary K83.9
toxic K71.9
hepatolenticular E83.Ø1
heredodegenerative NEC
spinal cord G95.89
herpesviral, disseminated BØØ.7
Hers' (glycogenosis VI) E74.Ø9
Herter (-Gee) (-Heubner) (nontropical sprue) K9Ø.Ø
Heubner-Herter (nontropical sprue) K9Ø.Ø
high fetal gene or hemoglobin thalassemia D56.9
Hildenbrand's —*see* Typhus
hip (joint) M25.9
congenital Q65.89
suppurative MØØ.9
tuberculous A18.Ø2
His (-Werner) (trench fever) A79.Ø
Hodgson's I71.2
ruptured I71.1
Holla —*see* Spherocytosis
hookworm B76.9
specified NEC B76.8
host-versus-graft D89.813
acute D89.81Ø
acute on chronic D89.812
chronic D89.811
human immunodeficiency virus (HIV) B2Ø
Huntington's G1Ø
Hutchinson's (cheiropompholyx) —*see* Hutchinson's disease
hyaline (diffuse) (generalized)
membrane (lung) (newborn) P22.Ø
adult J8Ø
hydatid —*see* Echinococcus
hydroxyapatite deposition M11.ØØ
ankle M11.Ø7-
elbow M11.Ø2-
foot joint M11.Ø7-
hand joint M11.Ø4-
hip M11.Ø5-
knee M11.Ø6-
multiple site M11.Ø9
shoulder M11.Ø1-
vertebra M11.Ø8
wrist M11.Ø3-
hyperkinetic —*see* Hyperkinesia
hypertensive —*see* Hypertension

D

- **Disease, diseased** *(Continued)*
  - hypophysis E23.7
  - Iceland G93.3
  - I-cell E77.Ø
  - immune D89.9
  - immunoproliferative (malignant) C88.9
    - small intestinal C88.3
    - specified NEC C88.8
  - inclusion B25.9
    - salivary gland B25.9
  - infectious, infective B99.9
    - congenital P37.9
      - specified NEC P37.8
      - viral P35.9
        - specified type NEC P35.8
    - specified NEC B99.8
  - inflammatory
    - penis N48.29
      - abscess N48.21
      - cellulitis N48.22
    - prepuce N47.7
      - balanoposthitis N47.6
    - tubo-ovarian *—see* Salpingo-oophoritis
  - intervertebral disc *—see also* Disorder, disc
    - with myelopathy *—see* Disorder, disc, with, myelopathy
    - cervical, cervicothoracic *—see* Disorder, disc, cervical
      - with
        - myelopathy *—see* Disorder, disc, cervical, with myelopathy
        - neuritis, radiculitis or radiculopathy *—see* Disorder, disc, cervical, with neuritis
        - specified NEC *—see* Disorder, disc, cervical, specified type NEC
    - lumbar (with)
      - myelopathy M51.Ø6
      - neuritis, radiculitis, radiculopathy or sciatica M51.16
      - specified NEC M51.86
    - lumbosacral (with)
      - neuritis, radiculitis, radiculopathy or sciatica M51.17
      - specified NEC M51.87
    - specified NEC *—see* Disorder, disc, specified NEC
    - thoracic (with)
      - myelopathy M51.Ø4
      - neuritis, radiculitis or radiculopathy M51.14
      - specified NEC M51.84
    - thoracolumbar (with)
      - myelopathy M51.Ø5
      - neuritis, radiculitis or radiculopathy M51.15
      - specified NEC M51.85
  - intestine K63.9
    - functional K59.9
      - psychogenic F45.8
      - specified NEC K59.8
    - organic K63.9
    - protozoal AØ7.9
    - specified NEC K63.89
  - iris H21.9
    - specified NEC H21.89
  - iron metabolism or storage E83.1Ø
  - island (scrub typhus) A75.3
  - itai-itai *—see* Poisoning, cadmium
  - Jakob-Creutzfeldt *—see* Creutzfeldt- Jakob disease or syndrome
  - jaw M27.9
    - fibrocystic M27.49
    - specified NEC M27.8
  - jigger B88.1
  - joint *—see also* Disorder, joint
    - Charcot's *—see* Arthropathy, neuropathic (Charcot)
    - degenerative *—see* Osteoarthritis
      - multiple M15.9
      - spine *—see* Spondylosis

- **Disease, diseased** *(Continued)*
  - joint *(Continued)*
    - hypertrophic *—see* Osteoarthritis
    - sacroiliac M53.3
    - specified NEC *—see* Disorder, joint, specified type NEC
    - spine NEC *—see* Dorsopathy
    - suppurative *—see* Arthritis, pyogenic or pyemic
  - Jourdain's (acute gingivitis) KØ5.ØØ
    - nonplaque induced KØ5.Ø1
    - plaque induced KØ5.ØØ
  - Kaschin-Beck (endemic polyarthritis) M12.1Ø
    - ankle M12.17-
    - elbow M12.12-
    - foot joint M12.17-
    - hand joint M12.14-
    - hip M12.15-
    - knee M12.16-
    - multiple site M12.19
    - shoulder M12.11-
    - vertebra M12.18
    - wrist M12.13-
  - Katayama B65.2
  - Kedani (scrub typhus) A75.3
  - Keshan E59
  - kidney (functional) (pelvis) N28.9
    - chronic N18.9
      - hypertensive *—see* Hypertension, kidney
      - stage 1 N18.1
      - stage 2 (mild) N18.2
      - stage 3 (moderate) N18.3
      - stage 4 (severe) N18.4
      - stage 5 N18.5
    - complicating pregnancy *—see* Pregnancy, complicated by, renal disease
    - cystic (congenital) Q61.9
    - diabetic - see EØ8-E13 with .22
    - fibrocystic (congenital) Q61.8
    - hypertensive *—see* Hypertension, kidney
    - in (due to)
      - schistosomiasis (bilharziasis) B65.9 *[N29]*
    - multicystic Q61.4
    - polycystic Q61.3
      - adult type Q61.2
      - childhood type NEC Q61.19
        - collecting duct dilatation Q61.11
  - Kimmelstiel (-Wilson) (intercapillary polycystic (congenital) glomerulosclerosis) *—see* EØ8-E13 with .21
  - Kimura D21.9
    - specified site (see Neoplasm, connective tissue benign)
  - Kinnier Wilson's (hepatolenticular degeneration) E83.Ø1
  - kissing *—see* Mononucleosis, infectious
  - Klebs' *—see also* Glomerulonephritis NØ5.-
  - Klippel-Feil (brevicollis) Q76.1
  - Köhler-Pellegrini-Stieda (calcification, knee joint) *—see* Bursitis, tibial collateral
  - Kok Q89.8
  - König's (osteochondritis dissecans) *—see* Osteochondritis, dissecans
  - Korsakoff's (nonalcoholic) FØ4
    - alcoholic F1Ø.96
      - with dependence F1Ø.26
  - Kostmann's (infantile genetic agranulocytosis) D7Ø.Ø
  - kuru A81.81
  - Kyasanur Forest A98.2
  - labyrinth, ear *—see* Disorder, ear, inner
  - lacrimal system *—see* Disorder, lacrimal system
  - Lafora's *—see* Epilepsy, generalized, idiopathic
  - Lancereaux-Mathieu (leptospiral jaundice) A27.Ø
  - Landry's G61.Ø
  - Larrey-Weil (leptospiral jaundice) A27.Ø
  - larynx J38.7

- **Disease, diseased** *(Continued)*
  - legionnaires' A48.1
    - nonpneumonic A48.2
  - Lenegre's I44.2
  - lens H27.9
    - specified NEC H27.8
  - Lev's (acquired complete heart block) I44.2
  - Lewy body (dementia) G31.83 *[FØ2.8Ø]*
    - with behavioral disturbance G31.83 *[FØ2.81]*
  - Lichtheim's (subacute combined sclerosis with pernicious anemia) D51.Ø
  - Lightwood's (renal tubular acidosis) N25.89
  - Lignac's (cystinosis) E72.Ø4
  - lip K13.Ø
  - lipid-storage E75.6
    - specified NEC E75.5
  - Lipschütz's N76.6
  - liver (chronic) (organic) K76.9
    - alcoholic (chronic) K7Ø.9
      - acute *—see* Disease, liver, alcoholic, hepatitis
      - cirrhosis K7Ø.3Ø
        - with ascites K7Ø.31
      - failure K7Ø.4Ø
        - with coma K7Ø.41
      - fatty liver K7Ø.Ø
      - fibrosis K7Ø.2
      - hepatitis K7Ø.1Ø
        - with ascites K7Ø.11
      - sclerosis K7Ø.2
    - cystic, congenital Q44.6
    - drug-induced (idiosyncratic) (toxic) (predictable) (unpredictable) *—see* Disease, liver, toxic
    - end stage K72.9Ø
      - due to hepatitis *—see* Hepatitis
    - fatty, nonalcoholic (NAFLD) K76.Ø
      - alcoholic K7Ø.Ø
    - fibrocystic (congenital) Q44.6
    - fluke
      - Chinese B66.1
      - oriental B66.1
      - sheep B66.3
    - glycogen storage E74.Ø9 *[K77]*
    - in (due to)
      - schistosomiasis (bilharziasis) B65.9 *[K77]*
    - inflammatory K75.9
      - alcoholic K7Ø.1
      - specified NEC K75.89
    - polycystic (congenital) Q44.6
    - toxic K71.9
      - with
        - cholestasis K71.Ø
        - cirrhosis (liver) K71.7
        - fibrosis (liver) K71.7
        - focal nodular hyperplasia K71.8
        - hepatic granuloma K71.8
        - hepatic necrosis K71.1Ø
          - with coma K71.11
        - hepatitis NEC K71.6
          - acute K71.2
          - chronic
            - active K71.5Ø
              - with ascites K71.51
            - lobular K71.4
            - persistent K71.3
          - lupoid K71.5Ø
            - with ascites K71.51
        - peliosis hepatis K71.8
        - veno-occlusive disease (VOD) of liver K71.8
    - veno-occlusive K76.5
  - Lobo's (keloid blastomycosis) B48.Ø
  - Lobstein's (brittle bones and blue sclera) Q78.Ø
  - Ludwig's (submaxillary cellulitis) K12.2
  - lumbosacral region M53.87
  - lung J98.4
    - black J6Ø
    - congenital Q33.9
    - cystic J98.4
      - congenital Q33.Ø

Disease, diseased *(Continued)*
- lung *(Continued)*
  - fibroid (chronic) —*see* Fibrosis, lung
  - fluke B66.4
    - oriental B66.4
  - in
    - amyloidosis E85.4 *[J99]*
    - sarcoidosis D86.0
    - Sjögren's syndrome M35.02
    - systemic
      - lupus erythematosus M32.13
      - sclerosis M34.81
  - interstitial J84.9
    - of childhood, specified NEC J84.848
    - respiratory bronchiolitis J84.115
    - specified NEC J84.89
  - obstructive (chronic) J44.9
    - with
      - acute
        - bronchitis J44.0
        - exacerbation NEC J44.1
        - lower respiratory infection J44.0
      - alveolitis, allergic J67.9
      - asthma J44.9
      - bronchiectasis J47.9
        - with
          - exacerbation (acute) J47.1
          - lower respiratory infection J47.0
      - bronchitis J44.9
        - with
          - exacerbation (acute) J44.1
          - lower respiratory infection J44.0
      - emphysema J44.9
      - hypersensitivity pneumonitis J67.9
    - decompensated J44.1
      - with
        - exacerbation (acute) J44.1
  - polycystic J98.4
    - congenital Q33.0
  - rheumatoid (diffuse) (interstitial) —*see* Rheumatoid, lung
- Lutembacher's (atrial septal defect with mitral stenosis) Q21.1
- Lyme A69.20
- lymphatic (gland) (system) (channel) (vessel) I89.9
- lymphoproliferative D47.9
  - specified NEC D47.Z9
  - T-gamma D47.Z9
  - X-linked D82.3
- Magitot's M27.2
- malarial —*see* Malaria
- malignant —*see also* Neoplasm, malignant, by site
- Manson's B65.1
- maple bark J67.6
- maple-syrup-urine E71.0
- Marburg (virus) A98.3
- Marion's (bladder neck obstruction) N32.0
- Marsh's (exophthalmic goiter) —*see* Hyperthyroidism, with, goiter (diffuse)
- mastoid (process) —*see* Disorder, ear, middle
- Mathieu's (leptospiral jaundice) A27.0
- Maxcy's A75.2
- McArdle (-Schmid-Pearson) (glycogenosis V) E74.04
- mediastinum J98.59 ⬅
- medullary center (idiopathic) (respiratory) G93.89
- Meige's (chronic hereditary edema) Q82.0
- meningococcal —*see* Infection, meningococcal
- mental F99
  - organic F09
- mesenchymal M35.9
- mesenteric embolic —*see also* Ischemia, intestine, acute K55.039 ⬅
- metabolic, metabolism E88.9
  - bilirubin E80.7
- metal-polisher's J62.8
- metastatic —*see also* Neoplasm, secondary, by site C79.9

Disease, diseased *(Continued)*
- microvascular — code to condition
- microvillus
  - atrophy Q43.8
  - inclusion (MVD) Q43.8
- middle ear —*see* Disorder, ear, middle
- Mikulicz' (dryness of mouth, absent or decreased lacrimation) K11.8
- Milroy's (chronic hereditary edema) Q82.0
- Minamata —*see* Poisoning, mercury
- minicore G71.2
- Minor's G95.19
- Minot's (hemorrhagic disease, newborn) P53
- Minot-von Willebrand-Jürgens (angiohemophilia) D68.0
- Mitchell's (erythromelalgia) I73.81
- mitral (valve) I05.9
  - nonrheumatic I34.9
- mixed connective tissue M35.1
- moldy hay J67.0
- Monge's T70.29
- Morgagni-Adams-Stokes (syncope with heart block) I45.9
- Morgagni's (syndrome) (hyperostosis frontalis interna) M85.2
- Morton's (with metatarsalgia) —*see* Lesion, nerve, plantar
- Morvan's G60.8
- motor neuron (bulbar) (familial) (mixed type) (spinal) G12.20
  - amyotrophic lateral sclerosis G12.21
  - progressive bulbar palsy G12.22
  - specified NEC G12.29
- moyamoya I67.5
- mu heavy chain disease C88.2
- multicore G71.2
- muscle —*see also* Disorder, muscle
  - inflammatory —*see* Myositis
  - ocular (external) —*see* Strabismus
- musculoskeletal system, soft tissue —*see also* Disorder, soft tissue
  - specified NEC —*see* Disorder, soft tissue, specified type NEC
- mushroom workers' J67.5
- mycotic B49
- myelodysplastic, not classified C94.6
- myeloproliferative, not classified C94.6
  - chronic D47.1
- myocardium, myocardial —*see also* Degeneration, myocardial I51.5
  - primary (idiopathic) I42.9
- myoneural G70.9
- Naegeli's D69.1
- nails L60.9
  - specified NEC L60.8
- Nairobi (sheep virus) A93.8
- nasal J34.9
- nemaline body G71.2
- nerve —*see* Disorder, nerve
- nervous system G98.8
  - autonomic G90.9
  - central G96.9
    - specified NEC G96.8
  - congenital Q07.9
  - parasympathetic G90.9
  - specified NEC G98.8
  - sympathetic G90.9
  - vegetative G90.9
- neuromuscular system G70.9
- Newcastle B30.8
- Nicolas (-Durand)-Favre (climatic bubo) A55
- nipple N64.9
  - Paget's C50.01-
    - female C50.01-
    - male C50.02-
- Nishimoto (-Takeuchi) I67.5
- nonarthropod-borne NOS (viral) B34.9
  - enterovirus NEC B34.1
- nonautoimmune hemolytic D59.4
  - drug-induced D59.2

Disease, diseased *(Continued)*
- Nonne-Milroy-Meige (chronic hereditary edema) Q82.0
- nose J34.9
- nucleus pulposus —*see* Disorder, disc
- nutritional E63.9
- oast-house-urine E72.19
- ocular
  - herpesviral B00.50
  - zoster B02.30
- obliterative vascular I77.1
- Ohara's —*see* Tularemia
- Opitz's (congestive splenomegaly) D73.2
- Oppenheim-Urbach (necrobiosis lipoidica diabeticorum) —*see* E08-E13 with .620
- optic nerve NEC —*see* Disorder, nerve, optic
  - orbit —*see* Disorder, orbit
- Oriental liver fluke B66.1
- Oriental lung fluke B66.4
- Ormond's N13.5
- Oropouche virus A93.0
- Osler-Rendu (familial hemorrhagic telangiectasia) I78.0
- osteofibrocystic E21.0
- Otto's M24.7
- outer ear —*see* Disorder, ear, external
- ovary (noninflammatory) N83.9
  - cystic N83.20- ⬅
  - inflammatory —*see* Salpingo-oophoritis
  - polycystic E28.2
  - specified NEC N83.8
- Owren's (congenital) —*see* Defect, coagulation
- pancreas K86.9
  - cystic K86.2
  - fibrocystic E84.9
  - specified NEC K86.89 ⬅
- panvalvular I08.9
  - specified NEC I08.8
- parametrium (noninflammatory) N83.9
- parasitic B89
  - cerebral NEC B71.9 *[G94]*
  - intestinal NOS B82.9
  - mouth B37.0
  - skin NOS B88.9
  - specified type —*see* Infestation
  - tongue B37.0
- parathyroid (gland) E21.5
  - specified NEC E21.4
- Parkinson's G20
- parodontal K05.6
- Parrot's (syphilitic osteochondritis) A50.02
- Parry's (exophthalmic goiter) —*see* Hyperthyroidism, with, goiter (diffuse)
- Parson's (exophthalmic goiter) —*see* Hyperthyroidism, with, goiter (diffuse)
- Paxton's (white piedra) B36.2
- pearl-worker's —*see* Osteomyelitis, specified type NEC
- Pellegrini-Stieda (calcification, knee joint) —*see* Bursitis, tibial collateral
- pelvis, pelvic
  - female NOS N94.9
    - specified NEC N94.89
  - gonococcal (acute) (chronic) A54.24
  - inflammatory (female) N73.9
    - acute N73.0
    - chlamydial A56.11 ◀
    - chronic N73.1
    - specified NEC N73.8
    - syphilitic (secondary) A51.42
      - late A52.76
    - tuberculous A18.17
  - organ, female N94.9
  - peritoneum, female NEC N94.89
- penis N48.9
  - inflammatory N48.29
    - abscess N48.21
    - cellulitis N48.22
  - specified NEC N48.89

D

Disease, diseased *(Continued)*
periapical tissues NOS K04.90
periodontal K05.6
specified NEC K05.5
periosteum —*see* Disorder, bone, specified type NEC
peripheral
arterial I73.9
autonomic nervous system G90.9
nerves —*see* Polyneuropathy
vascular NOS I73.9
peritoneum K66.9
pelvic, female NEC N94.89
specified NEC K66.8
persistent mucosal (middle ear) H66.20
left H66.22
with right H66.23
right H66.21
with left H66.23
Petit's —*see* Hernia, abdomen, specified site NEC
pharynx J39.2
specified NEC J39.2
Phocas' —*see* Mastopathy, cystic
photochromogenic (acid-fast bacilli) (pulmonary) A31.0
nonpulmonary A31.9
Pick's G31.01 *[F02.80]*
with behavioral disturbance G31.01 *[F02.81]*
brain G31.01 *[F02.80]* ◀
with behavioral disturbance G31.01 *[F02.81]* ◀
of pericardium (pericardial pseudocirrhosis of liver) I31.1 ◀
pigeon fancier's J67.2
pineal gland E34.8
pink —*see* Poisoning, mercury
Pinkus' (lichen nitidus) L44.1
pinworm B80
Piry virus A93.8
pituitary (gland) E23.7
pituitary-snuff-taker's J67.8
pleura (cavity) J94.9
specified NEC J94.8
pneumatic drill (hammer) T75.21
Pollitzer's (hidradenitis suppurativa) L73.2
polycystic
kidney or renal Q61.3
adult type Q61.2
childhood type NEC Q61.19
collecting duct dilatation Q61.11
liver or hepatic Q44.6
lung or pulmonary J98.4
congenital Q33.0
ovary, ovaries E28.2
spleen Q89.09
polyethylene T84.05-
Pompe's (glycogenosis II) E74.02
Posadas-Wernicke B38.9
Potain's (pulmonary edema) —*see* Edema, lung
prepuce N47.8
inflammatory N47.7
balanoposthitis N47.6
Pringle's (tuberous sclerosis) Q85.1
prion, central nervous system A81.9
specified NEC A81.89
prostate N42.9
specified NEC N42.89
protozoal B64
acanthamebiasis —*see* Acanthamebiasis
African trypanosomiasis —*see* African trypanosomiasis
babesiosis B60.0
Chagas disease —*see* Chagas disease
intestine, intestinal A07.9
leishmaniasis —*see* Leishmaniasis
malaria —*see* Malaria
naegleriasis B60.2

Disease, diseased *(Continued)*
protozoal *(Continued)*
pneumocystosis B59
specified organism NEC B60.8
toxoplasmosis —*see* Toxoplasmosis
pseudo-Hurler's E77.0
psychiatric F99
psychotic —*see* Psychosis
Puente's (simple glandular cheilitis) K13.0
puerperal —*see also* Puerperal O90.89
pulmonary —*see also* Disease, lung
artery I28.9
chronic obstructive J44.9
with
acute bronchitis J44.0
exacerbation (acute) J44.1
lower respiratory infection (acute) J44.0
decompensated J44.1
with
exacerbation (acute) J44.1
heart I27.9
specified NEC I27.89
hypertensive (vascular) I27.0
valve I37.9
rheumatic I09.89
pulp (dental) NOS K04.90
pulseless M31.4
Putnam's (subacute combined sclerosis with pernicious anemia) D51.0
Pyle (-Cohn) (metaphyseal dysplasia) Q78.5 ⟸
ragpicker's or ragsorter's A22.1
Raynaud's —*see* Raynaud's disease
reactive airway —*see* Asthma
Reclus' (cystic) —*see* Mastopathy, cystic
rectum K62.9
specified NEC K62.89
Refsum's (heredopathia atactica polyneuritiformis) G60.1
renal (functional) (pelvis) —*see also* Disease, kidney N28.9
with
edema —*see* Nephrosis
glomerular lesion —*see* Glomerulonephritis
with edema —*see* Nephrosis
interstitial nephritis N12
acute N28.9
chronic —*see also* Disease, kidney, chronic N18.9
cystic, congenital Q61.9
diabetic —*see* E08-E13 with .22
end-stage (failure) N18.6
due to hypertension I12.0
fibrocystic (congenital) Q61.8
hypertensive —*see* Hypertension, kidney
lupus M32.14
phosphate-losing (tubular) N25.0
polycystic (congenital) Q61.3
adult type Q61.2
childhood type NEC Q61.19
collecting duct dilatation Q61.11
rapidly progressive N01.9
subacute N01.9
Rendu-Osler-Weber (familial hemorrhagic telangiectasia) I78.0
renovascular (arteriosclerotic) —*see* Hypertension, kidney
respiratory (tract) J98.9
acute or subacute NOS J06.9
due to
chemicals, gases, fumes or vapors (inhalation) J68.3
external agent J70.9
specified NEC J70.8
radiation J70.0
smoke inhalation J70.5
noninfectious J39.8

Disease, diseased *(Continued)*
respiratory *(Continued)*
chronic NOS J98.9
due to
chemicals, gases, fumes or vapors J68.4
external agent J70.9
specified NEC J70.8
radiation J70.1
newborn P27.9
specified NEC P27.8
due to
chemicals, gases, fumes or vapors J68.9
acute or subacute NEC J68.3
chronic J68.4
external agent J70.9
specified NEC J70.8
newborn P28.9
specified type NEC P28.89
upper J39.9
acute or subacute J06.9
noninfectious NEC J39.8
specified NEC J39.8
streptococcal J06.9
retina, retinal H35.9
Batten's or Batten-Mayou E75.4 *[H36]*
specified NEC H35.89
rheumatoid —*see* Arthritis, rheumatoid
rickettsial NOS A79.9
specified type NEC A79.89
Riga (-Fede) (cachectic aphthae) K14.0
Riggs' (compound periodontitis) —*see* Periodontitis
Ritter's L00
Rivalta's (cervicofacial actinomycosis) A42.2
Robles' (onchocerciasis) B73.01
Roger's (congenital interventricular septal defect) Q21.0
Rosenthal's (factor XI deficiency) D68.1
Ross River B33.1
Rossbach's (hyperchlorhydria) K30
Rotes Quérol —*see* Hyperostosis, ankylosing
Roth (-Bernhardt) —*see* Mononeuropathy, lower limb, meralgia paresthetica
Runeberg's (progressive pernicious anemia) D51.0
sacroiliac NEC M53.3
salivary gland or duct K11.9
inclusion B25.9
specified NEC K11.8
virus B25.9
sandworm B76.9
Schimmelbusch's —*see* Mastopathy, cystic
Schmorl's —*see* Schmorl's disease or nodes
Schönlein (-Henoch) (purpura rheumatica) D69.0
Schottmüller's —*see* Fever, paratyphoid
Schultz's (agranulocytosis) —*see* Agranulocytosis
Schwalbe-Ziehen-Oppenheim G24.1
Schwartz-Jampel G71.13
sclera H15.9
specified NEC H15.89
scrofulous (tuberculous) A18.2
scrotum N50.9
sebaceous glands L73.9
semilunar cartilage, cystic —*see also* Derangement, knee, meniscus, cystic
seminal vesicle N50.9
serum NEC —*see also* Reaction, serum T80.69
sexually transmitted A64
anogenital
herpesviral infection —*see* Herpes, anogenital
warts A63.0
chancroid A57
chlamydial infection —*see* Chlamydia
gonorrhea —*see* Gonorrhea
granuloma inguinale A58
specified organism NEC A63.8

D

Disease, diseased *(Continued)*
sexually transmitted *(Continued)*
syphilis —*see* Syphilis
trichomoniasis —*see* Trichomoniasis
Sézary C84.1-
shimamushi (scrub typhus) A75.3
shipyard B30.0
sickle-cell D57.1
with crisis (vasoocclusive pain) D57.00
with
acute chest syndrome D57.01
splenic sequestration D57.02
elliptocytosis D57.8-
Hb-C D57.20
with crisis (vasoocclusive pain) D57.219
with
acute chest syndrome D57.211
splenic sequestration D57.212
without crisis D57.20
Hb-SD D57.80
with crisis D57.819
with
acute chest syndrome D57.811
splenic sequestration D57.812
Hb-SE D57.80
with crisis D57.819
with
acute chest syndrome D57.811
splenic sequestration D57.812
specified NEC D57.80
with crisis D57.819
with
acute chest syndrome D57.811
splenic sequestration D57.812
spherocytosis D57.80
with crisis D57.819
with
acute chest syndrome D57.811
splenic sequestration D57.812
thalassemia D57.40
with crisis (vasoocclusive pain) D57.419
with
acute chest syndrome D57.411
splenic sequestration D57.412
without crisis D57.40
silo-filler's J68.8
bronchitis J68.0
pneumonitis J68.0
pulmonary edema J68.1
simian B B00.4
Simons' (progressive lipodystrophy) E88.1
sin nombre virus B33.4
sinus —*see* Sinusitis
Sirkari's B55.0
sixth B08.20
due to human herpesvirus 6 B08.21
due to human herpesvirus 7 B08.22
skin L98.9
due to metabolic disorder NEC E88.9 *[L99]*
specified NEC L98.8
slim (HIV) B20
small vessel I73.9
Sneddon-Wilkinson (subcorneal pustular dermatosis) L13.1
South African creeping B88.0
spinal (cord) G95.9
congenital Q06.9
specified NEC G95.89
spine —*see also* Spondylopathy
joint —*see* Dorsopathy
tuberculous A18.01
spinocerebellar (hereditary) G11.9
specified NEC G11.8
spleen D73.9
amyloid E85.4 *[D77]*
organic D73.9
polycystic Q89.09
postinfectional D73.89
sponge-diver's —*see* Toxicity, venom, marine animal, sea anemone

Disease, diseased *(Continued)*
Startle Q89.8
Steinert's G71.11
Sticker's (erythema infectiosum) B08.3
Stieda's (calcification, knee joint) —*see* Bursitis, tibial collateral
Stokes' (exophthalmic goiter) —*see* Hyperthyroidism, with, goiter (diffuse)
Stokes-Adams (syncope with heart block) I45.9
stomach K31.9
functional, psychogenic F45.8
specified NEC K31.89
stonemason's J62.8
storage
glycogen —*see* Disease, glycogen storage
mucopolysaccharide —*see* Mucopolysaccharidosis
striatopallidal system NEC G25.89
Stuart-Prower (congenital factor X deficiency) D68.2
Stuart's (congenital factor X deficiency) D68.2
subcutaneous tissue —*see* Disease, skin
supporting structures of teeth K08.9
specified NEC K08.89 (Revised)
suprarenal (capsule) (gland) E27.9
hyperfunction E27.0
specified NEC E27.8
sweat glands L74.9
specified NEC L74.8
Sweeley-Klionsky E75.21
Swift (-Feer) —*see* Poisoning, mercury
swimming-pool granuloma A31.1
Sylvest's (epidemic pleurodynia) B33.0
sympathetic nervous system G90.9
synovium —*see* Disorder, synovium
syphilitic —*see* Syphilis
systemic tissue mast cell C96.2
tanapox (virus) B08.71
Tangier E78.6
Tarral-Besnier (pityriasis rubra pilaris) L44.0
Tauri's E74.09
tear duct —*see* Disorder, lacrimal system
tendon, tendinous —*see also* Disorder, tendon
nodular —*see* Trigger finger
terminal vessel I73.9
testis N50.9
thalassemia Hb-S —*see* Disease, sickle-cell, thalassemia
Thaysen-Gee (nontropical sprue) K90.0
Thomsen G71.12
throat J39.2
septic J02.0
thromboembolic —*see* Embolism
thymus (gland) E32.9
specified NEC E32.8
thyroid (gland) E07.9
heart —*see also* Hyperthyroidism E05.90 *[I43]*
with thyroid storm E05.91 *[I43]*
specified NEC E07.8
Tietze's M94.0
tongue K14.9
specified NEC K14.89
tonsils, tonsillar (and adenoids) J35.9
tooth, teeth K08.9
hard tissues K03.9
specified NEC K03.89
pulp NEC K04.99
specified NEC K08.89 (Revised)
Tourette's F95.2
trachea NEC J39.8
tricuspid I07.9
nonrheumatic I36.9
triglyceride-storage E75.5
trophoblastic —*see* Mole, hydatidiform
tsutsugamushi A75.3
tube (fallopian) (noninflammatory) N83.9
inflammatory —*see* Salpingitis
specified NEC N83.8
tuberculous NEC —*see* Tuberculosis

Disease, diseased *(Continued)*
tubo-ovarian (noninflammatory) N83.9
inflammatory —*see* Salpingo-oophoritis
specified NEC N83.8
tubotympanic, chronic —*see* Otitis, media, suppurative, chronic, tubotympanic
tubulo-interstitial N15.9
specified NEC N15.8
tympanum —*see* Disorder, tympanic membrane
Uhl's Q24.8
Underwood's (sclerema neonatorum) P83.0
Unverricht (-Lundborg) —*see* Epilepsy, generalized, idiopathic
Urbach-Oppenheim (necrobiosis lipoidica diabeticorum) —*see* E08-E13 with .620
ureter N28.9
in (due to)
schistosomiasis (bilharziasis) B65.0 *[N29]*
urethra N36.9
specified NEC N36.8
urinary (tract) N39.9
bladder N32.9
specified NEC N32.89
specified NEC N39.8
uterus (noninflammatory) N85.9
infective —*see* Endometritis
inflammatory —*see* Endometritis
specified NEC N85.8
uveal tract (anterior) H21.9
posterior H31.9
vagabond's B85.1
vagina, vaginal (noninflammatory) N89.9
inflammatory NEC N76.89
specified NEC N89.8
valve, valvular I38
multiple I08.9
specified NEC I08.8
van Creveld-von Gierke (glycogenosis I) E74.01
vas deferens N50.9
vascular I99.9
arteriosclerotic —*see* Arteriosclerosis
ciliary body NEC —*see* Disorder, iris, vascular
hypertensive —*see* Hypertension
iris NEC —*see* Disorder, iris, vascular
obliterative I77.1
peripheral I73.9
occlusive I99.8
peripheral (occlusive) I73.9
in diabetes mellitus —*see* E08-E13 with .51
vasomotor I73.9
vasospastic I73.9
vein I87.9
venereal —*see also* Disease, sexually transmitted A64
chlamydial NEC A56.8
anus A56.3
genitourinary NOS A56.2
pharynx A56.4
rectum A56.3
fifth A55
sixth A55
specified nature or type NEC A63.8
vertebra, vertebral —*see also* Spondylopathy
disc —*see* Disorder, disc
vibration —*see* Vibration, adverse effects
viral, virus —*see also* Disease, by type of virus B34.9
arbovirus NOS A94
arthropod-borne NOS A94
congenital P35.9
specified NEC P35.8
Hanta (with renal manifestations) (Dobrava) (Puumala) (Seoul) A98.5
with pulmonary manifestations (Andes) (Bayou) (Bermejo) (Black Creek Canal) (Choclo) (Juquitiba) (Laguna negra) (Lechiguanas) (New York) (Oran) (Sin nombre) B33.4

Disease, diseased *(Continued)*
viral, virus *(Continued)*
Hantaan (Korean hemorrhagic fever) A98.5
human immunodeficiency (HIV) B20
Kunjin A83.4
nonarthropod-borne NOS B34.9
Powassan A84.8
Rocio (encephalitis) A83.6
Sin nombre (Hantavirus) (cardio)-pulmonary syndrome B33.4
Tahyna B33.8
vesicular stomatitis A93.8
vitreous H43.9
specified NEC H43.89
vocal cord J38.3
Volkmann's, acquired T79.6
von Eulenburg's (congenital paramyotonia) G71.19
von Gierke's (glycogenosis I) E74.01
von Graefe's —*see* Strabismus, paralytic, ophthalmoplegia, progressive
von Willebrand (-Jürgens) (angiohemophilia) D68.0
Vrolik's (osteogenesis imperfecta) Q78.0
vulva (noninflammatory) N90.9
inflammatory NEC N76.89
specified NEC N90.89
Wallgren's (obstruction of splenic vein with collateral circulation) I87.8
Wassilieff's (leptospiral jaundice) A27.0
wasting NEC R64
due to malnutrition E41
Waterhouse-Friderichsen A39.1
Wegner's (syphilitic osteochondritis) A50.02
Weil's (leptospiral jaundice of lung) A27.0
Weir Mitchell's (erythromelalgia) I73.81
Werdnig-Hoffmann G12.0
Wermer's E31.21
Werner-His (trench fever) A79.0
Werner-Schultz (neutropenic splenomegaly) D73.81
Wernicke-Posadas B38.9
whipworm B79
white blood cells D72.9
specified NEC D72.89
white matter R90.82
white-spot, meaning lichen sclerosus et atrophicus L90.0
penis N48.0
vulva N90.4
Wilkie's K55.1
Wilkinson-Sneddon (subcorneal pustular dermatosis) L13.1
Willis' —*see* Diabetes
Wilson's (hepatolenticular degeneration) E83.01
woolsorter's A22.1
yaba monkey tumor B08.72
yaba pox (virus) B08.72
Zika virus A92.5 ◀
zoonotic, bacterial A28.9
specified type NEC A28.8
Disfigurement (due to scar) L90.5
Disgerminoma —*see* Dysgerminoma
DISH (diffuse idiopathic skeletal hyperostosis) —*see* Hyperostosis, ankylosing
Disinsertion, retina —*see* Detachment, retina
Dislocatable hip, congenital Q65.6
Dislocation (articular)
with fracture —*see* Fracture
acromioclavicular (joint) S43.10-
with displacement
100%-200% S43.12-
more than 200% S43.13-
inferior S43.14-
posterior S43.15-
ankle S93.0-
astragalus —*see* Dislocation, ankle
atlantoaxial S13.121
atlantooccipital S13.111

Dislocation *(Continued)*
atloidooccipital S13.111
breast bone S23.29
capsule, joint code by site under Dislocation
carpal (bone) —*see* Dislocation, wrist
carpometacarpal (joint) NEC S63.05-
thumb S63.04-
cartilage (joint) - code by site under Dislocation
cervical spine (vertebra) —*see* Dislocation, vertebra, cervical
chronic —*see* Dislocation, recurrent
clavicle —*see* Dislocation, acromioclavicular joint
coccyx S33.2
congenital NEC Q68.8
coracoid —*see* Dislocation, shoulder
costal cartilage S23.29
costochondral S23.29
cricoarytenoid articulation S13.29
cricothyroid articulation S13.29
dorsal vertebra —*see* Dislocation, vertebra, thoracic
ear ossicle —*see* Discontinuity, ossicles, ear
elbow S53.10-
congenital Q68.8
pathological —*see* Dislocation, pathological NEC, elbow
radial head alone —*see* Dislocation, radial head
recurrent —*see* Dislocation, recurrent, elbow
traumatic S53.10-
anterior S53.11-
lateral S53.14-
medial S53.13-
posterior S53.12-
specified type NEC S53.19-
eye, nontraumatic —*see* Luxation, globe
eyeball, nontraumatic —*see* Luxation, globe
femur
distal end —*see* Dislocation, knee
proximal end —*see* Dislocation, hip
fibula
distal end —*see* Dislocation, ankle
proximal end —*see* Dislocation, knee
finger S63.25-
index S63.25-
interphalangeal S63.27-
distal S63.29-
index S63.29-
little S63.29-
middle S63.29-
ring S63.29-
index S63.27-
little S63.27-
middle S63.27-
proximal S63.28-
index S63.28-
little S63.28-
middle S63.28-
ring S63.28-
ring S63.27-
little S63.25-
metacarpophalangeal S63.26-
index S63.26-
little S63.26-
middle S63.26-
ring S63.26-
middle S63.25-
recurrent —*see* Dislocation, recurrent, finger
ring S63.25-
thumb —*see* Dislocation, thumb
foot S93.30-
recurrent —*see* Dislocation, recurrent, foot
specified site NEC S93.33-
tarsal joint S93.31-
tarsometatarsal joint S93.32-
toe —*see* Dislocation, toe

Dislocation *(Continued)*
fracture —*see* Fracture
glenohumeral (joint) —*see* Dislocation, shoulder
glenoid —*see* Dislocation, shoulder
habitual —*see* Dislocation, recurrent
hip S73.00-
anterior S73.03-
obturator S73.02-
central S73.04-
congenital (total) Q65.2
bilateral Q65.1
partial Q65.5
bilateral Q65.4
unilateral Q65.3-
unilateral Q65.0-
developmental M24.85-
pathological —*see* Dislocation, pathological NEC, hip
posterior S73.01-
recurrent —*see* Dislocation, recurrent, hip
humerus, proximal end —*see* Dislocation, shoulder
incomplete —*see* Subluxation, by site
incus —*see* Discontinuity, ossicles, ear
infracoracoid —*see* Dislocation, shoulder
innominate (pubic junction) (sacral junction) S33.39
acetabulum —*see* Dislocation, hip
interphalangeal (joint (s))
finger S63.279
distal S63.29-
index S63.29-
little S63.29-
middle S63.29-
ring S63.29-
index S63.27-
little S63.27-
middle S63.27-
proximal S63.28-
index S63.28-
little S63.28-
middle S63.28-
ring S63.28-
ring S63.27-
foot or toe —*see* Dislocation, toe
thumb S63.12-
distal joint S63.14-
proximal joint S63.13-
jaw (cartilage) (meniscus) S03.0- ⬅
joint prosthesis —*see* Complications, joint prosthesis, mechanical, displacement, by site
knee S83.106
cap —*see* Dislocation, patella
congenital Q68.2
old M23.8X-
patella —*see* Dislocation, patella
pathological —*see* Dislocation, pathological NEC, knee
proximal tibia
anteriorly S83.11-
laterally S83.14-
medially S83.13-
posteriorly S83.12-
recurrent —*see also* Derangement, knee, specified NEC
specified type NEC S83.19-
lacrimal gland H04.16-
lens (complete) H27.10-
anterior H27.12-
congenital Q12.1
ocular implant —*see* Complications, intraocular lens
partial H27.11-
posterior H27.13-
traumatic S05.8X-
ligament code by site under Dislocation
lumbar (vertebra) —*see* Dislocation, vertebra, lumbar

Dislocation *(Continued)*
- lumbosacral (vertebra) —*see also* Dislocation, vertebra, lumbar
  - congenital Q76.49
- mandible S03.0- ⬅
- meniscus (knee) —*see* Tear, meniscus
  - other sites code by site under Dislocation
- metacarpal (bone)
  - distal end —*see* Dislocation, finger
  - proximal end S63.06-
- metacarpophalangeal (joint)
  - finger S63.26-
    - index S63.26-
    - little S63.26-
    - middle S63.26-
    - ring S63.26-
  - thumb S63.11-
- metatarsal (bone) —*see* Dislocation, foot
- metatarsophalangeal (joint (s)) —*see* Dislocation, toe
- midcarpal (joint) S63.03-
- midtarsal (joint) —*see* Dislocation, foot
- neck S13.20
  - specified site NEC S13.29
  - vertebra —*see* Dislocation, vertebra, cervical
- nose (septal cartilage) S03.1
- occipitoatloid S13.111
- old —*see* Derangement, joint, specified type NEC
- ossicles, ear —*see* Discontinuity, ossicles, ear
- partial —*see* Subluxation, by site
- patella S83.006
  - congenital Q74.1
  - lateral S83.01-
  - recurrent (nontraumatic) M22.0-
    - incomplete M22.1-
  - specified type NEC S83.09-
- pathological NEC M24.30
  - ankle M24.37-
  - elbow M24.32-
  - foot joint M24.37-
  - hand joint M24.34-
  - hip M24.35-
  - knee M24.36-
  - lumbosacral joint —*see* subcategory M53.2
  - pelvic region —*see* Dislocation, pathological, hip
  - sacroiliac —*see* subcategory M53.2
  - shoulder M24.31-
  - wrist M24.33-
- pelvis NEC S33.30
  - specified NEC S33.39
- phalanx
  - finger or hand —*see* Dislocation, finger
  - foot or toe —*see* Dislocation, toe
- prosthesis, internal —*see* Complications, prosthetic device, by site, mechanical
- radial head S53.006
  - anterior S53.01-
  - posterior S53.02-
  - specified type NEC S53.09-
- radiocarpal (joint) S63.02-
- radiohumeral (joint) —*see* Dislocation, radial head
- radioulnar (joint)
  - distal S63.01-
  - proximal —*see* Dislocation, elbow
- radius
  - distal end —*see* Dislocation, wrist
  - proximal end —*see* Dislocation, radial head
- recurrent M24.40
  - ankle M24.47-
  - elbow M24.42-
  - finger M24.44-
  - foot joint M24.47-
  - hand joint M24.44-
  - hip M24.45-
  - knee M24.46-
    - patella —*see* Dislocation, patella, recurrent

Dislocation *(Continued)*
- recurrent *(Continued)*
  - patella —*see* Dislocation, patella, recurrent
  - sacroiliac —*see* subcategory M53.2
  - shoulder M24.41-
  - toe M24.47-
  - vertebra —*see also* subcategory M43.5
    - atlantoaxial M43.4
      - with myelopathy M43.3
  - wrist M24.43-
- rib (cartilage) S23.29
- sacrococcygeal S33.2
- sacroiliac (joint) (ligament) S33.2
  - congenital Q74.2
  - recurrent —*see* subcategory M53.2
- sacrum S33.2
- scaphoid (bone) (hand) (wrist) —*see* Dislocation, wrist
  - foot —*see* Dislocation, foot
- scapula —*see* Dislocation, shoulder, girdle, scapula
- semilunar cartilage, knee —*see* Tear, meniscus
- septal cartilage (nose) S03.1
- septum (nasal) (old) J34.2
- sesamoid bone code by site under Dislocation
- shoulder (blade) (ligament) (joint) (traumatic) S43.006
  - acromioclavicular —*see* Dislocation, acromioclavicular
  - chronic —*see* Dislocation, recurrent, shoulder
  - congenital Q68.8
  - girdle S43.30-
    - scapula S43.31-
    - specified site NEC S43.39-
  - humerus S43.00-
    - anterior S43.01-
    - inferior S43.03-
    - posterior S43.02-
  - pathological —*see* Dislocation, pathological NEC, shoulder
  - recurrent —*see* Dislocation, recurrent, shoulder
  - specified type NEC S43.08-
- spine
  - cervical —*see* Dislocation, vertebra, cervical
  - congenital Q76.49
  - due to birth trauma P11.5
  - lumbar —*see* Dislocation, vertebra, lumbar
  - thoracic —*see* Dislocation, vertebra, thoracic
- spontaneous —*see* Dislocation, pathological
- sternoclavicular (joint) S43.206
  - anterior S43.21-
  - posterior S43.22-
- sternum S23.29
- subglenoid —*see* Dislocation, shoulder
- symphysis pubis S33.4
- talus —*see* Dislocation, ankle
- tarsal (bone (s)) (joint (s)) —*see* Dislocation, foot
- tarsometatarsal (joint (s)) —*see* Dislocation, foot
- temporomandibular (joint) S03.0- ⬅
- thigh, proximal end —*see* Dislocation, hip
- thorax S23.20
  - specified site NEC S23.29
  - vertebra —*see* Dislocation, vertebra
- thumb S63.10-
  - interphalangeal joint —*see* Dislocation, interphalangeal (joint), thumb
  - metacarpophalangeal joint —*see* Dislocation, metacarpophalangeal (joint), thumb
- thyroid cartilage S13.29
- tibia
  - distal end —*see* Dislocation, ankle
  - proximal end —*see* Dislocation, knee
- tibiofibular (joint)
  - distal —*see* Dislocation, ankle
  - superior —*see* Dislocation, knee

Dislocation *(Continued)*
- toe (s) S93.106
  - great S93.10-
    - interphalangeal joint S93.11-
    - metatarsophalangeal joint S93.12-
  - interphalangeal joint S93.119
  - lesser S93.106
    - interphalangeal joint S93.11-
    - metatarsophalangeal joint S93.12-
  - metatarsophalangeal joint S93.12-
- tooth S03.2
- trachea S23.29
- ulna
  - distal end S63.07-
  - proximal end —*see* Dislocation, elbow
- ulnohumeral (joint) —*see* Dislocation, elbow
- vertebra (articular process) (body) (traumatic)
  - cervical S13.101
    - atlantoaxial joint S13.121
    - atlantooccipital joint S13.111
    - atloidooccipital joint S13.111
    - joint between
      - C0 and C1 S13.111
      - C1 and C2 S13.121
      - C2 and C3 S13.131
      - C3 and C4 S13.141
      - C4 and C5 S13.151
      - C5 and C6 S13.161
      - C6 and C7 S13.171
      - C7 and T1 S13.181
    - occipitoatloid joint S13.111
  - congenital Q76.49
  - lumbar S33.101
    - joint between
      - L1 and L2 S33.111
      - L2 and L3 S33.121
      - L3 and L4 S33.131
      - L4 and L5 S33.141
  - nontraumatic —*see* Displacement, intervertebral disc
  - partial —*see* Subluxation, by site
  - recurrent NEC —*see* subcategory M43.5
  - thoracic S23.101
    - joint between
      - T1 and T2 S23.111
      - T2 and T3 S23.121
      - T3 and T4 S23.123
      - T4 and T5 S23.131
      - T5 and T6 S23.133
      - T6 and T7 S23.141
      - T7 and T8 S23.143
      - T8 and T9 S23.151
      - T9 and T10 S23.153
      - T10 and T11 S23.161
      - T11 and T12 S23.163
      - T12 and L1 S23.171
- wrist (carpal bone) S63.006
  - carpometacarpal joint —*see* Dislocation, carpometacarpal (joint)
  - distal radioulnar joint —*see* Dislocation, radioulnar (joint), distal
  - metacarpal bone, proximal —*see* Dislocation, metacarpal (bone), proximal end
  - midcarpal —*see* Dislocation, midcarpal (joint)
  - radiocarpal joint —*see* Dislocation, radiocarpal (joint)
  - recurrent —*see* Dislocation, recurrent, wrist
  - specified site NEC S63.09-
  - ulna —*see* Dislocation, ulna, distal end
- xiphoid cartilage S23.29

Disorder (of) —*see also* Disease
- acantholytic L11.9
  - specified NEC L11.8
- acute
  - psychotic —*see* Psychosis, acute
  - stress F43.0

- Disorder *(Continued)*
  - adjustment (grief) F43.20
    - with
      - anxiety F43.22
        - with depressed mood F43.23
      - conduct disturbance F43.24
        - with emotional disturbance F43.25
      - depressed mood F43.21
        - with anxiety F43.23
      - other specified symptom F43.29
  - adrenal (capsule) (gland) (medullary) E27.9
    - specified NEC E27.8
  - adrenogenital E25.9
    - drug-induced E25.8
    - iatrogenic E25.8
    - idiopathic E25.8
  - adult personality (and behavior) F69
    - specified NEC F68.8
  - affective (mood) —*see* Disorder, mood
  - aggressive, unsocialized F91.1
  - alcohol-related F10.99
    - with
      - amnestic disorder, persisting F10.96
      - anxiety disorder F10.980
      - dementia, persisting F10.97
      - intoxication F10.929
        - with delirium F10.921
        - uncomplicated F10.920
      - mood disorder F10.94
      - other specified F10.988
      - psychotic disorder F10.959
        - with
          - delusions F10.950
          - hallucinations F10.951
      - sexual dysfunction F10.981
      - sleep disorder F10.982
  - alcohol use ◀
    - mild F10.10 ◀
      - with ◀
        - alcohol-induced ◀
          - anxiety disorder F10.180 ◀
          - bipolar and related disorder F10.14 ◀
          - depressive disorder F10.14 ◀
          - psychotic disorder F10.159 ◀
          - sexual dysfunction F10.181 ◀
          - sleep disorder F10.182 ◀
        - alcohol intoxication F10.129 ◀
          - delirium F10.121 ◀
    - moderate or severe F10.20 ◀
      - with ◀
        - alcohol-induced ◀
          - anxiety disorder F10.280 ◀
          - bipolar and related disorder F10.24 ◀
          - depressive disorder F10.24 ◀
          - major neurocognitive disorder, amnestic-confabulatory type F10.26 ◀
          - major neurocognitive disorder, nonamnestic-confabulatory type F10.27 ◀
          - mild neurocognitive disorder F10.288 ◀
          - psychotic disorder F10.259 ◀
          - sexual dysfunction F10.281 ◀
          - sleep disorder F10.282 ◀
        - alcohol intoxication F10.229 ◀
          - delirium F10.221 ◀
  - allergic —*see* Allergy
  - alveolar NEC J84.09
  - amino-acid
    - cystathioninuria E72.19
    - cystinosis E72.04
    - cystinuria E72.01
    - glycinuria E72.09
    - homocystinuria E72.11
    - metabolism —*see* Disturbance, metabolism, amino-acid
      - specified NEC E72.8
    - neonatal, transitory P74.8
- Disorder *(Continued)*
  - amino-acid *(Continued)*
    - renal transport NEC E72.09
    - transport NEC E72.09
  - amnesic, amnestic
    - alcohol-induced F10.96
      - with dependence F10.26
    - due to (secondary to) general medical condition F04
    - psychoactive NEC-induced F19.96
      - with
        - abuse F19.16
        - dependence F19.26
    - sedative, hypnotic or anxiolytic-induced F13.96
      - with dependence F13.26
  - amphetamine-type substance use ◀
    - mild F15.10 ◀
    - moderate F15.20 ◀
    - severe F15.20 ◀
  - amphetamine (or other stimulant) use ◀
    - mild ◀
      - with ◀
        - amphetamine (or other stimulant) -induced ◀
          - anxiety disorder F15.180 ◀
          - bipolar and related disorder F15.14 ◀
          - depressive disorder F15.14 ◀
          - obsessive-compulsive and related disorder F15.188 ◀
          - psychotic disorder F15.159 ◀
          - sexual dysfunction F15.181 ◀
        - amphetamine, cocaine, or other stimulant intoxication ◀
          - with perceptual disturbances F15.122 ◀
          - without perceptual disturbances F15.129 ◀
        - intoxication delirium F15.121 ◀
    - moderate or severe ◀
      - with ◀
        - amphetamine (or other stimulant) -induced ◀
          - anxiety disorder F15.280 ◀
          - obsessive-compulsive and related disorder F15.288 ◀
          - sexual dysfunction F15.281 ◀
          - bipolar and related disorder F15.24 ◀
          - depressive disorder F15.24 ◀
          - psychotic disorder F15.259 ◀
        - amphetamine, cocaine, or other stimulant intoxication ◀
          - with perceptual disturbances F15.222 ◀
          - without perceptual disturbances F15.229 ◀
        - intoxication delirium F15.221 ◀
  - anaerobic glycolysis with anemia D55.2
  - anxiety F41.9
    - due to (secondary to)
      - alcohol F10.980
      - amphetamine F15.980
        - in
          - abuse F15.180
          - dependence F15.280
      - anxiolytic F13.980
        - in
          - abuse F13.180
          - dependence F13.280
      - caffeine F15.980
        - in
          - abuse F15.180
          - dependence F15.280
      - cannabis F12.980
        - in
          - abuse F12.180
          - dependence F12.280
- Disorder *(Continued)*
  - anxiety *(Continued)*
    - due to *(Continued)*
      - cocaine F14.980
        - in
          - abuse F14.180
          - dependence F14.180
      - general medical condition F06.4
      - hallucinogen F16.980
        - in
          - abuse F16.180
          - dependence F16.280
      - hypnotic F13.980
        - in
          - abuse F13.180
          - dependence F13.280
      - inhalant F18.980
        - in
          - abuse F18.180
          - dependence F18.280
      - phencyclidine F16.980
        - in
          - abuse F16.180
          - dependence F16.280
      - psychoactive substance NEC F19.980
        - in
          - abuse F19.180
          - dependence F19.280
      - sedative F13.980
        - in
          - abuse F13.180
          - dependence F13.280
      - volatile solvents F18.980
        - in
          - abuse F18.180
          - dependence F18.280
    - generalized F41.1
    - illness F45.21 ◀
    - mixed
      - with depression (mild) F41.8
      - specified NEC F41.3
    - organic F06.4
    - phobic F40.9
      - of childhood F40.8
    - specified NEC F41.8
  - aortic valve —*see* Endocarditis, aortic
  - aromatic amino-acid metabolism E70.9
    - specified NEC E70.8
  - arteriole NEC I77.89
  - artery NEC I77.89
  - articulation —*see* Disorder, joint
  - attachment (childhood)
    - disinhibited F94.2
    - reactive F94.1
  - attention-deficit hyperactivity (adolescent) (adult) (child) F98.8 ⟸
    - combined type F90.2
    - hyperactive type F90.1
    - inattentive type F90.0
    - specified type NEC F90.8
  - attention-deficit without hyperactivity (adolescent) (adult) (child) F90.0
  - auditory processing (central) H93.25
  - autism spectrum F84.0 ◀
  - autistic F84.0
  - autonomic nervous system G90.9
    - specified NEC G90.8
  - ~~avoidant, child or adolescent F40.10~~
  - avoidant ◀
    - child or adolescent F40.10 ◀
    - restrictive food intake F50.89 ◀
  - balance
    - acid-base E87.8
      - mixed E87.4
    - electrolyte E87.8
    - fluid NEC E87.8
  - behavioral (disruptive) —*see* Disorder, conduct
  - beta-amino-acid metabolism E72.8
  - bile acid and cholesterol metabolism E78.70
    - Barth syndrome E78.71
    - other specified E78.79
    - Smith-Lemli-Opitz syndrome E78.72

◀ New ⟸ Revised ~~deleted~~ Deleted

Disorder *(Continued)*
- bilirubin excretion E80.6
- binge eating F50.81 ◀
- binocular
  - movement H51.9
    - convergence
      - excess H51.12
      - insufficiency H51.11
    - internuclear ophthalmoplegia *—see* Ophthalmoplegia, internuclear
    - palsy of conjugate gaze H51.0
    - specified type NEC H51.8
  - vision NEC *—see* Disorder, vision, binocular
- bipolar (I) F31.9
  - current episode
    - depressed F31.9
      - with psychotic features F31.5
      - without psychotic features F31.30
        - mild F31.31
        - moderate F31.32
        - severe (without psychotic features) F31.4
          - with psychotic features F31.5
    - hypomanic F31.0
    - manic F31.9
      - with psychotic features F31.2
      - without psychotic features F31.10
        - mild F31.11
        - moderate F31.12
        - severe (without psychotic features) F31.13
          - with psychotic features F31.2
    - mixed F31.60
      - mild F31.61
      - moderate F31.62
      - severe (without psychotic features) F31.63
        - with psychotic features F31.64
    - severe depression (without psychotic features) F31.4
      - with psychotic features F31.5
  - II F31.81
  - in remission (currently) F31.70
    - in full remission
      - most recent episode
        - depressed F31.76
        - hypomanic F31.72
        - manic F31.74
        - mixed F31.78
    - in partial remission
      - most recent episode
        - depressed F31.75
        - hypomanic F31.71
        - manic F31.73
        - mixed F31.77
  - organic F06.30
  - single manic episode F30.9
    - mild F30.11
    - moderate F30.12
    - hhsevere (without psychotic symptoms) F30.13
      - with psychotic symptoms F30.2
  - specified NEC F31.89
- bladder N32.9
  - functional NEC N31.9
  - in schistosomiasis B65.0 *[N33]*
  - specified NEC N32.89
- bleeding D68.9
- blood D75.9
  - in congenital early syphilis A50.09 *[D77]*
- body dysmorphic F45.22
- bone M89.9
  - continuity M84.9
    - specified type NEC M84.80
      - ankle M84.87-
      - fibula M84.86-
      - foot M84.87-
      - hand M84.84-

Disorder *(Continued)*
- bone *(Continued)*
  - continuity *(Continued)*
    - specified type *(Continued)*
      - humerus M84.82-
      - neck M84.88
      - pelvis M84.859
      - radius M84.83-
      - rib M84.88
      - shoulder M84.81-
      - skull M84.88
      - thigh M84.85-
      - tibia M84.86-
      - ulna M84.83-
      - vertebra M84.88
  - density and structure M85.9
    - cyst *—see also* Cyst, bone, specified type NEC
      - aneurysmal *—see* Cyst, bone, aneurysmal
      - solitary *—see* Cyst, bone, solitary
    - diffuse idiopathic skeletal hyperostosis *—see* Hyperostosis, ankylosing
    - fibrous dysplasia (monostotic) *—see* Dysplasia, fibrous, bone
    - fluorosis *—see* Fluorosis, skeletal
    - hyperostosis of skull M85.2
    - osteitis condensans *—see* Osteitis, condensans
    - specified type NEC M85.8-
      - ankle M85.87-
      - foot M85.87-
      - forearm M85.83-
      - hand M85.84-
      - lower leg M85.86-
      - multiple sites M85.89
      - neck M85.88
      - rib M85.88
      - shoulder M85.81-
      - skull M85.88
      - thigh M85.85-
      - upper arm M85.82-
      - vertebra M85.88
  - development and growth NEC M89.20
    - carpus M89.24-
    - clavicle M89.21-
    - femur M89.25-
    - fibula M89.26-
    - finger M89.24-
    - humerus M89.22-
    - ilium M89.259
    - ischium M89.259
    - metacarpus M89.24-
    - metatarsus M89.27-
    - multiple sites M89.29
    - neck M89.28
    - radius M89.23-
    - rib M89.28
    - scapula M89.21-
    - skull M89.28
    - tarsus M89.27-
    - tibia M89.26-
    - toe M89.27-
    - ulna M89.23-
    - vertebra M89.28
  - specified type NEC M89.8X-
- brachial plexus G54.0
- branched-chain amino-acid metabolism E71.2
  - specified NEC E71.19
- breast N64.9
  - agalactia *—see* Agalactia
  - associated with
    - lactation O92.70
      - specified NEC O92.79
    - pregnancy O92.20
      - specified NEC O92.29
    - puerperium O92.20
      - specified NEC O92.29

Disorder *(Continued)*
- breast *(Continued)*
  - cracked nipple *—see* Cracked nipple
  - galactorrhea *—see* Galactorrhea
  - hypogalactia O92.4
  - lactation disorder NEC O92.79
  - mastitis *—see* Mastitis
  - nipple infection *—see* Infection, nipple
  - retracted nipple *—see* Retraction, nipple
  - specified type NEC N64.89
- Briquet's F45.0
- bullous, in diseases classified elsewhere L14
- caffeine use ◀
  - mild ◀
    - with ◀
      - caffeine-induced ◀
        - anxiety disorder F15.180 ◀
        - sleep disorder F15.182 ◀
  - moderate or severe ◀
    - with ◀
      - caffeine-induced ◀
        - anxiety disorder F15.280 ◀
        - sleep disorder F15.282 ◀
- cannabis use
  - ~~due to drug abuse —see Abuse, drug, cannabis~~
  - ~~due to drug dependence —see Dependence, drug, cannabis~~
  - mild F12.10 ◀
    - with ◀
      - cannabis-induced ◀
        - anxiety disorder F12.180 ◀
        - psychotic disorder F12.159 ◀
        - sleep disorder F12.188 ◀
      - cannabis intoxication delirium F12.121 ◀
        - with perceptual disturbances F12.122 ◀
        - without perceptual disturbances F12.129 ◀
  - moderate or severe F12.20 ◀
    - with ◀
      - cannabis-induced ◀
        - anxiety disorder F12.280 ◀
        - psychotic disorder F12.259 ◀
        - sleep disorder F12.288 ◀
      - cannabis intoxication ◀
        - with perceptual disturbances F12.222 ◀
        - without perceptual disturbances F12.229 ◀
      - delirium F12.221 ◀
- carbohydrate
  - absorption, intestinal NEC E74.39
  - metabolism (congenital) E74.9
    - specified NEC E74.8
- cardiac, functional I51.89
- carnitine metabolism E71.40
- cartilage M94.9
  - articular NEC *—see* Derangement, joint, articular cartilage
    - chondrocalcinosis *—see* Chondrocalcinosis
  - specified type NEC M94.8X-
    - articular *—see* Derangement, joint, articular cartilage
    - multiple sites M94.8X0
- catatonia (due to known physiological condition) (with another mental disorder) F06.1 ◀
- catatonic
  - due to (secondary to) known physiological condition F06.1
  - organic F06.1
- central auditory processing H93.25
- cervical
  - region NEC M53.82
  - root (nerve) NEC G54.2
- character NOS F60.9
- childhood disintegrative NEC F84.3

D

Disorder *(Continued)*
cholesterol and bile acid metabolism E78.70
Barth syndrome E78.71
other specified E78.79
Smith-Lemli-Opitz syndrome E78.72
choroid H31.9
atrophy —*see* Atrophy, choroid
degeneration —*see* Degeneration, choroid
detachment —*see* Detachment, choroid
dystrophy —*see* Dystrophy, choroid
hemorrhage —*see* Hemorrhage, choroid
rupture —*see* Rupture, choroid
scar —*see* Scar, chorioretinal
solar retinopathy —*see* Retinopathy, solar
specified type NEC H31.8
ciliary body —*see* Disorder, iris
degeneration —*see* Degeneration, ciliary body
coagulation (factor) (*see also* Defect, coagulation) D68.9
newborn, transient P61.6
cocaine use ◀
mild F14.10 ◀
with ◀
amphetamine, cocaine, or other stimulant intoxication ◀
with perceptual disturbances F14.122 ◀
without perceptual disturbances F14.129 ◀
cocaine-induced ◀
anxiety disorder F14.180 ◀
bipolar and related disorder F14.14 ◀
depressive disorder F14.14 ◀
obsessive-compulsive and related disorder F14.188 ◀
psychotic disorder F14.159 ◀
sexual dysfunction F14.181 ◀
sleep disorder F14.182 ◀
cocaine intoxication delirium F14.121 ◀
moderate or severe F14.20 ◀
with ◀
amphetamine, cocaine, or other stimulant intoxication ◀
with perceptual disturbances F14.222 ◀
without perceptual disturbances F14.229 ◀
cocaine-induced ◀
anxiety disorder F14.280 ◀
bipolar and related disorder F14.24 ◀
depressive disorder F14.24 ◀
obsessive-compulsive and related disorder F14.288 ◀
psychotic disorder F14.259 ◀
sexual dysfunction F14.281 ◀
sleep disorder F14.282 ◀
cocaine intoxication delirium F14.221 ◀
coccyx NEC M53.3
cognitive F09
due to (secondary to) general medical condition F09
persisting R41.89
due to
alcohol F10.97
with dependence F10.27
anxiolytics F13.97
with dependence F13.27
hypnotics F13.97
with dependence F13.27
sedatives F13.97
with dependence F13.27
specified substance NEC F19.97
with
abuse F19.17
dependence F19.27

Disorder *(Continued)*
communication F80.9
social pragmatic F80.82 ◀
conduct (childhood) F91.9
adjustment reaction —*see* Disorder, adjustment
adolescent onset type F91.2
childhood onset type F91.1
compulsive F63.9
confined to family context F91.0
depressive F91.8
group type F91.2
hyperkinetic —*see* Disorder, attention-deficit hyperactivity
oppositional defiance F91.3
socialized F91.2
solitary aggressive type F91.1
specified NEC F91.8
unsocialized (aggressive) F91.1
conduction, heart I45.9
congenital glycosylation (CDG) E74.8
conjunctiva H11.9
infection —*see* Conjunctivitis
connective tissue, localized L94.9
specified NEC L94.8
conversion (functional neurological symptom disorder)
with ◀
abnormal movement F44.4 ◀
anesthesia or sensory loss F44.6 ◀
attacks or seizures F44.5 ◀
mixed symptoms F44.7 ◀
special sensory symptoms F44.6 ◀
speech symptoms F44.4 ◀
swallowing symptoms F44.4 ◀
weakness or paralysis F44.4 ◀
convulsive (secondary) —*see* Convulsions
cornea H18.9
deformity —*see* Deformity, cornea
degeneration —*see* Degeneration, cornea
deposits —*see* Deposit, cornea
due to contact lens H18.82-
specified as edema —*see* Edema, cornea
edema —*see* Edema, cornea
keratitis —*see* Keratitis
keratoconjunctivitis —*see* Keratoconjunctivitis
membrane change —*see* Change, corneal membrane
neovascularization —*see* Neovascularization, cornea
scar —*see* Opacity, cornea
specified type NEC H18.89-
ulcer —*see* Ulcer, cornea
corpus cavernosum N48.9
cranial nerve —*see* Disorder, nerve, cranial
cyclothymic F34.0
defiant oppositional F91.3
delusional (persistent) (systematized) F22
induced F24
depersonalization F48.1
depressive F32.9
major F32.9
with psychotic symptoms F32.3
in remission (full) F32.5
partial F32.4
recurrent F33.9
single episode F32.9
mild F32.0
moderate F32.1
severe (without psychotic symptoms) F32.2
with psychotic symptoms F32.3
organic F06.31
persistent F34.1 ◀
recurrent F33.9
current episode
mild F33.0
moderate F33.1

Disorder *(Continued)*
depressive *(Continued)*
recurrent *(Continued)*
current episode *(Continued)*
severe (without psychotic symptoms) F33.2
with psychotic symptoms F33.3
in remission F33.40
full F33.42
partial F33.41
specified NEC F33.8
single episode —*see* Episode, depressive
specified NEC F32.89 ◀
developmental F89
arithmetical skills F81.2
coordination (motor) F82
expressive writing F81.81
language F80.9
expressive F80.1
mixed receptive and expressive F80.2
receptive type F80.2
specified NEC F80.89
learning F81.9
arithmetical F81.2
reading F81.0
mixed F88
motor coordination or function F82
pervasive F84.9
specified NEC F84.8
phonological F80.0
reading F81.0
scholastic skills —*see also* Disorder, learning
mixed F81.89
specified NEC F88
speech F80.9
articulation F80.0
specified NEC F80.89
written expression F81.81
diaphragm J98.6
digestive (system) K92.9
newborn P78.9
specified NEC P78.89
postprocedural —*see* Complication, gastrointestinal
psychogenic F45.8
disc (intervertebral) M51.9
with
myelopathy
cervical region M50.00
cervicothoracic region M50.03
high cervical region M50.01
lumbar region M51.06
mid-cervical region M50.020
sacrococcygeal region M53.3
thoracic region M51.04
thoracolumbar region M51.05
radiculopathy
cervical region M50.10
cervicothoracic region M50.13
high cervical region M50.11
lumbar region M51.16
lumbosacral region M51.17
mid-cervical region M50.120
sacrococcygeal region M53.3
thoracic region M51.14
thoracolumbar region M51.15
cervical M50.90
with
myelopathy M50.00
C2-C3 M50.01
C3-C4 M50.01
C4-C5 M50.021
C5-C6 M50.022
C6-C7 M50.023
C7-T1 M50.03
cervicothoracic region M50.03
high cervical region M50.01
mid-cervical region M50.020

◀ New ⟵ Revised ~~deleted~~ Deleted

Disorder *(Continued)*
disc *(Continued)*
cervical *(Continued)*
with *(Continued)*
neuritis, radiculitis or radiculopathy M50.10
C2-C3 M50.11
C3-C4 M50.11
C4-C5 M50.121 ⬅
C5-C6 M50.122 ⬅
C6-C7 M50.123 ⬅
C7-T1 M50.13
cervicothoracic region M50.13
high cervical region M50.11
mid-cervical region M50.120 ⬅
C2-C3 M50.91
C3-C4 M50.91
C4-C5 M50.921 ⬅
C5-C6 M50.922 ⬅
C6-C7 M50.923 ⬅
C7-T1 M50.93
cervicothoracic region M50.93
degeneration M50.30
C2-C3 M50.31
C3-C4 M50.31
C4-C5 M50.321 ⬅
C5-C6 M50.322 ⬅
C6-C7 M50.323 ⬅
C7-T1 M50.33
cervicothoracic region M50.33
high cervical region M50.31
mid-cervical region M50.320 ⬅
displacement M50.20
C2-C3 M50.21
C3-C4 M50.21
C4-C5 M50.221 ⬅
C5-C6 M50.222 ⬅
C6-C7 M50.223 ⬅
C7-T1 M50.23
cervicothoracic region M50.23
high cervical region M50.21
mid-cervical region M50.220 ⬅
high cervical region M50.91
mid-cervical region M50.920 ⬅
specified type NEC M50.80
C2-C3 M50.81
C3-C4 M50.81
C4-C5 M50.821 ⬅
C5-C6 M50.822 ⬅
C6-C7 M50.823 ⬅
C7-T1 M50.83
cervicothoracic region M50.83
high cervical region M50.81
mid-cervical region M50.820 ⬅
specified NEC
lumbar region M51.86
lumbosacral region M51.87
sacrococcygeal region M53.3
thoracic region M51.84
thoracolumbar region M51.85
disinhibited attachment (childhood) F94.2
disintegrative, childhood NEC F84.3
disruptive F91.9 ◀
mood dysregulation F34.81 ◀
specified NEC F91.8 ◀
disruptive behavior F91.9 ⬅
dissocial personality F60.2
dissociative F44.9
affecting
motor function F44.4
and sensation F44.7
sensation F44.6
and motor function F44.7
brief reactive F43.0
due to (secondary to) general medical condition F06.8
mixed F44.7
organic F06.8
other specified NEC F44.89
double heterozygous sickling —*see* Disease, sickle-cell

Disorder *(Continued)*
dream anxiety F51.5
drug induced hemorrhagic D68.32
drug related F19.99
abuse —*see* Abuse, drug
dependence —*see* Dependence, drug
dysmorphic body F45.22 ⬅
dysthymic F34.1
ear H93.9-
bleeding —*see* Otorrhagia
deafness —*see* Deafness
degenerative H93.09-
discharge —*see* Otorrhea
external H61.9-
auditory canal stenosis —*see* Stenosis, external ear canal
exostosis —*see* Exostosis, external ear canal
impacted cerumen —*see* Impaction, cerumen
otitis —*see* Otitis, externa
perichondritis —*see* Perichondritis, ear
pinna —*see* Disorder, pinna
specified type NEC H61.89-
in diseases classified elsewhere H62.8X-
inner H83.9-
vestibular dysfunction —*see* Disorder, vestibular function
middle H74.9-
adhesive H74.1-
ossicle —*see* Abnormal, ear ossicles
polyp —*see* Polyp, ear (middle)
specified NEC, in diseases classified elsewhere H75.8-
postprocedural —*see* Complications, ear, procedure
specified NEC, in diseases classified elsewhere H94.8-
eating (adult) (psychogenic) F50.9
anorexia —*see* Anorexia
binge F50.81 ◀
bulimia F50.2
child F98.29
pica F98.3
rumination disorder F98.21
pica F50.89 ⬅
childhood F98.3
electrolyte (balance) NEC E87.8
with
abortion —*see* Abortion by type complicated by specified condition NEC
ectopic pregnancy O08.5
molar pregnancy O08.5
acidosis (metabolic) (respiratory) E87.2
alkalosis (metabolic) (respiratory) E87.3
elimination, transepidermal L87.9
specified NEC L87.8
emotional (persistent) F34.9
of childhood F93.9
specified NEC F93.8
endocrine E34.9
postprocedural E89.89
specified NEC E89.89
erectile (male) (organic) —*see also* Dysfunction, sexual, male, erectile N52.9
nonorganic F52.21
erythematous —*see* Erythema
esophagus K22.9
functional K22.4
psychogenic F45.8
eustachian tube H69.9-
infection —*see* Salpingitis, eustachian
obstruction —*see* Obstruction, eustachian tube
patulous —*see* Patulous, eustachian tube
specified NEC H69.8-

Disorder *(Continued)*
extrapyramidal G25.9
in diseases classified elsewhere —*see* category G26
specified type NEC G25.89
eye H57.9
postprocedural —*see* Complication, postprocedural, eye
eyelid H02.9
cyst —*see* Cyst, eyelid
degenerative H02.70
chloasma —*see* Chloasma, eyelid
madarosis —*see* Madarosis
specified type NEC H02.79
vitiligo —*see* Vitiligo, eyelid
xanthelasma —*see* Xanthelasma
dermatochalasis —*see* Dermato-chalasis
edema —*see* Edema, eyelid
elephantiasis —*see* Elephantiasis, eyelid
foreign body, retained —*see* Foreign body, retained, eyelid
function H02.59
abnormal innervation syndrome —*see* Syndrome, abnormal innervation
blepharochalasis —*see* Blepharochalasis
blepharoclonus —*see* Blepharoclonus
blepharophimosis —*see* Blepharophimosis
blepharoptosis —*see* Blepharoptosis
lagophthalmos —*see* Lagophthalmos
lid retraction —*see* Retraction, lid
hypertrichosis —*see* Hypertrichosis, eyelid
specified type NEC H02.89
vascular H02.879
left H02.876
lower H02.875
upper H02.874
right H02.873
lower H02.872
upper H02.871
factitious F68.10
with predominantly
physical symptoms F68.12
with psychological symptoms F68.13
psychological symptoms F68.11
with physical symptoms F68.13
factor, coagulation —*see* Defect, coagulation
fatty acid
metabolism E71.30
specified NEC E71.39
oxidation
LCAD E71.310
MCAD E71.311
SCAD E71.312
specified deficiency NEC E71.318
feeding (infant or child) —*see also* Disorder, eating R63.3-
feigned (with obvious motivation) Z76.5
without obvious motivation —*see* Disorder, factitious
female
hypoactive sexual desire F52.0
orgasmic F52.31
sexual arousal F52.22
fibroblastic M72.9
specified NEC M72.8
fluency
adult onset F98.5
childhood onset F80.81
following
cerebral infarction I69.323
cerebrovascular disease I69.923
specified disease NEC I69.823
intracerebral hemorrhage I69.123
nontraumatic intracranial hemorrhage NEC I69.223
subarachnoid hemorrhage I69.023
in conditions classified elsewhere R47.82
fluid balance E87.8
follicular (skin) L73.9
specified NEC L73.8

D

- **Disorder** *(Continued)*
  - fructose metabolism E74.10
    - essential fructosuria E74.11
    - fructokinase deficiency E74.11
    - fructose-1, 6-diphosphatase deficiency E74.19
    - hereditary fructose intolerance E74.12
    - other specified E74.19
  - functional polymorphonuclear neutrophils D71
  - gallbladder, biliary tract and pancreas in diseases classified elsewhere K87
  - gamma-glutamyl cycle E72.8
  - gastric (functional) K31.9
    - motility K30
    - psychogenic F45.8
    - secretion K30
  - gastrointestinal (functional) NOS K92.9
    - newborn P78.9
    - psychogenic F45.8
  - gender-identity or -role F64.9
    - childhood F64.2
    - effect on relationship F66
    - of adolescence or adulthood F64.0 ⬅
      - nontranssexual F64.8 ◀
    - specified NEC F64.8
    - uncertainty F66
  - genito-pelvic pain penetration F52.6 ◀
  - genitourinary system
    - female N94.9
    - male N50.9
    - psychogenic F45.8
  - globe H44.9
    - degenerated condition H44.50
      - absolute glaucoma H44.51-
      - atrophy H44.52-
      - leucocoria H44.53-
    - degenerative H44.30
      - chalcosis H44.31-
      - myopia H44.2-
      - siderosis H44.32-
      - specified type NEC H44.39-
    - endophthalmitis —*see* Endophthalmitis
    - foreign body, retained —*see* Foreign body, intraocular, old, retained
    - hemophthalmos —*see* Hemophthalmos
    - hypotony H44.40
      - due to
        - ocular fistula H44.42-
        - specified disorder NEC H44.43-
      - flat anterior chamber H44.41-
      - primary H44.44-
    - luxation —*see* Luxation, globe
    - specified type NEC H44.89
  - glomerular (in) N05.9
    - amyloidosis E85.4 *[N08]*
    - cryoglobulinemia D89.1 *[N08]*
    - disseminated intravascular coagulation D65 *[N08]*
    - Fabry's disease E75.21 *[N08]*
    - familial lecithin cholesterol acyltransferase deficiency E78.6 *[N08]*
    - Goodpasture's syndrome M31.0
    - hemolytic-uremic syndrome D59.3
    - Henoch (-Schönlein) purpura D69.0 *[N08]*
    - malariae malaria B52.0
    - microscopic polyangiitis M31.7 *[N08]*
    - multiple myeloma C90.0- *[N08]*
    - mumps B26.83
    - schistosomiasis B65.9 *[N08]*
    - sepsis NEC A41.- *[N08]*
      - streptococcal A40.- *[N08]*
    - sickle-cell disorders D57.- *[N08]*
    - strongyloidiasis B78.9 *[N08]*
    - subacute bacterial endocarditis I33.0 *[N08]*
    - syphilis A52.75
    - systemic lupus erythematosus M32.14
    - thrombotic thrombocytopenic purpura M31.1 *[N08]*
    - Waldenström macroglobulinemia C88.0 *[N08]*
    - Wegener's granulomatosis M31.31
- **Disorder** *(Continued)*
  - gluconeogenesis E74.4
  - glucosaminoglycan metabolism —*see* Disorder, metabolism, glucosaminoglycan
  - glycine metabolism E72.50
    - d-glycericacidemia E72.59
    - hyperhydroxyprolinemia E72.59
    - hyperoxaluria E72.53
    - hyperprolinemia E72.59
    - non-ketotic hyperglycinemia E72.51
    - oxalosis E72.53
    - oxaluria E72.53
    - sarcosinemia E72.59
    - trimethylaminuria E72.52
  - glycoprotein metabolism E77.9
    - specified NEC E77.8
  - habit (and impulse) F63.9
    - involving sexual behavior NEC F65.9
    - specified NEC F63.89
  - hallucinogen use ◀
    - mild F16.10 ◀
      - with ◀
        - hallucinogen-induced ◀
          - anxiety disorder F16.180 ◀
          - bipolar and related disorder F16.14 ◀
          - depressive disorder F16.14 ◀
          - psychotic disorder F16.159 ◀
        - hallucinogen intoxication delirium F16.121 ◀
        - other hallucinogen intoxication F16.129 ◀
    - moderate or severe F16.20 ◀
      - with ◀
        - hallucinogen-induced ◀
          - anxiety disorder F16.280 ◀
          - bipolar and related disorder F16.24 ◀
          - depressive disorder F16.24 ◀
          - psychotic disorder F16.259 ◀
        - hallucinogen intoxication delirium F16.221 ◀
        - other hallucinogen intoxication F16.229 ◀
  - heart action I49.9
  - hematological D75.9
    - newborn (transient) P61.9
      - specified NEC P61.8
  - hematopoietic organs D75.9
  - hemorrhagic NEC D69.9
    - drug-induced D68.32
    - due to
      - extrinsic circulating anticoagulants D68.32
      - increase in
        - anti-IIa D68.32
        - anti-Xa D68.32
      - intrinsic
        - circulating anticoagulants D68.318
        - increase in
          - antithrombin D68.318
          - anti-VIIIa D68.318
          - anti-IXa D68.318
          - anti-XIa D68.318
    - following childbirth O72.3
  - hemostasis —*see* Defect, coagulation
  - histidine metabolism E70.40
    - histidinemia E70.41
    - other specified E70.49
  - hoarding F42.3 ◀
  - hyperkinetic —*see* Disorder, attention-deficit hyperactivity
  - hyperleucine-isoleucinemia E71.19
  - hypervalinemia E71.19
  - hypoactive sexual desire F52.0
  - hypochondriacal F45.20
    - body dysmorphic F45.22
    - neurosis F45.21
    - other specified F45.29
- **Disorder** *(Continued)*
  - identity
    - dissociative F44.81
    - illness anxiety F45.21 ◀
    - of childhood F93.8
  - immune mechanism (immunity) D89.9
    - specified type NEC D89.89
  - impaired renal tubular function N25.9
    - specified NEC N25.89
  - impulse (control) F63.9
  - inflammatory
    - pelvic, in diseases classified elsewhere —*see* category N74
    - penis N48.29
      - abscess N48.21
      - cellulitis N48.22
  - inhalant use ◀
    - mild F18.10 ◀
      - with ◀
        - inhalant-induced ◀
          - anxiety disorder F18.180 ◀
          - depressive disorder F18.14 ◀
          - major neurocognitive disorder F18.17 ◀
          - mild neurocognitive disorder F18.188 ◀
          - psychotic disorder F18.159 ◀
        - inhalant intoxication F18.129 ◀
        - inhalant intoxication delirium F18.121 ◀
    - moderate or severe F18.20 ◀
      - with ◀
        - inhalant-induced ◀
          - anxiety disorder F18.280 ◀
          - depressive disorder F18.24 ◀
          - major neurocognitive disorder F18.27 ◀
          - mild neurocognitive disorder F18.288 ◀
          - psychotic disorder F18.259 ◀
        - inhalant intoxication F18.229 ◀
        - inhalant intoxication delirium F18.221 ◀
  - integument, newborn P83.9
    - specified NEC P83.8
  - intermittent explosive F63.81
  - internal secretion pancreas —*see* Increased, secretion, pancreas, endocrine
  - intestine, intestinal
    - carbohydrate absorption NEC E74.39
      - postoperative K91.2
    - functional NEC K59.9
      - postoperative K91.89
    - psychogenic F45.8
    - vascular K55.9
      - chronic K55.1
      - specified NEC K55.8
  - intraoperative (intraprocedural) —*see* Complications, intraoperative
  - involuntary emotional expression (IEED) F48.2
  - iris H21.9
    - adhesions —*see* Adhesions, iris
    - atrophy —*see* Atrophy, iris
    - chamber angle recession —*see* Recession, chamber angle
    - cyst —*see* Cyst, iris
    - degeneration —*see* Degeneration, iris
    - in diseases classified elsewhere H22
    - iridodialysis —*see* Iridodialysis
    - iridoschisis —*see* Iridoschisis
    - miotic pupillary cyst —*see* Cyst, pupillary
    - pupillary
      - abnormality —*see* Abnormality, pupillary
      - membrane —*see* Membrane, pupillary
    - specified type NEC H21.89
    - vascular NEC H21.1X-
  - iron metabolism E83.10
    - specified NEC E83.19

D

◀ New ⬅ Revised ~~deleted~~ Deleted

Disorder *(Continued)*
isovaleric acidemia E71.11Ø
jaw, developmental M27.Ø
temporomandibular —*see also* Anomaly, dentofacial, temporomandibular joint M26.6Ø- ⬅
joint M25.9
derangement —*see* Derangement, joint
effusion —*see* Effusion, joint
fistula —*see* Fistula, joint
hemarthrosis —*see* Hemarthrosis
instability —*see* Instability, joint
osteophyte —*see* Osteophyte
pain —*see* Pain, joint
psychogenic F45.8
specified type NEC M25.8Ø
ankle M25.87-
elbow M25.82-
foot joint M25.87-
hand joint M25.84-
hip M25.85-
knee M25.86-
shoulder M25.81-
wrist M25.83-
stiffness —*see* Stiffness, joint
ketone metabolism E71.32
kidney N28.9
functional (tubular) N25.9
in
schistosomiasis B65.9 *[N29]*
tubular function N25.9
specified NEC N25.89
lacrimal system HØ4.9
changes HØ4.69
fistula —*see* Fistula, lacrimal
gland HØ4.19
atrophy —*see* Atrophy, lacrimal gland
cyst —*see* Cyst, lacrimal, gland
dacryops —*see* Dacryops
dislocation —*see* Dislocation, lacrimal gland
dry eye syndrome —*see* Syndrome, dry eye
infection —*see* Dacryoadenitis
granuloma —*see* Granuloma, lacrimal
inflammation —*see* Inflammation, lacrimal
obstruction —*see* Obstruction, lacrimal
specified NEC HØ4.89
lactation NEC O92.79
language (developmental) F8Ø.9
expressive F8Ø.1
mixed receptive and expressive F8Ø.2
receptive F8Ø.2
late luteal phase dysphoric N94.89
learning (specific) F81.9
acalculia R48.8
alexia R48.Ø
mathematics F81.2
reading F81.Ø
specified NEC F81.89
spelling F81.81
written expression F81.81
lens H27.9
aphakia —*see* Aphakia
cataract —*see* Cataract
dislocation —*see* Dislocation, lens
specified type NEC H27.8
ligament M24.2Ø
ankle M24.27-
attachment, spine —*see* Enthesopathy, spinal
elbow M24.22-
foot joint M24.27-
hand joint M24.24-
hip M24.25-
knee —*see* Derangement, knee, specified NEC
shoulder M24.21-
vertebra M24.28
wrist M24.23-

Disorder *(Continued)*
ligamentous attachments —*see also* Enthesopathy
spine —*see* Enthesopathy, spinal
lipid
metabolism, congenital E78.9
storage E75.6
specified NEC E75.5
lipoprotein
deficiency (familial) E78.6
metabolism E78.9
specified NEC E78.89
liver K76.9
malarial B54 *[K77]*
low back —*see also* Dorsopathy, specified NEC
lumbosacral
plexus G54.1
root (nerve) NEC G54.4
lung, interstitial, drug-induced J7Ø.4
acute J7Ø.2
chronic J7Ø.3
lymphoproliferative, post-transplant (PTLD) D47.Z1
lysine and hydroxylysine metabolism E72.3
major neurocognitive —*see* Dementia, in (due to) ◀
male
erectile (organic) —*see also* Dysfunction, sexual, male, erectile N52.9
nonorganic F52.21
hypoactive sexual desire F52.Ø
orgasmic F52.32
manic F3Ø.9
organic FØ6.33
mast cell activation —*see* Activation, mast cell ◀
mastoid —*see also* Disorder, ear, middle
postprocedural —*see* Complications, ear, procedure
meniscus —*see* Derangement, knee, meniscus
menopausal N95.9
specified NEC N95.8
menstrual N92.6
psychogenic F45.8
specified NEC N92.5
mental (or behavioral) (nonpsychotic) F99
due to (secondary to)
amphetamine
due to drug abuse —*see* Abuse, drug, stimulant
due to drug dependence —*see* Dependence, drug, stimulant
brain disease, damage and dysfunction FØ9
caffeine use
due to drug abuse —*see* Abuse, drug, stimulant
due to drug dependence —*see* Dependence, drug, stimulant
cannabis use
due to drug abuse —*see* Abuse, drug, cannabis
due to drug dependence —*see* Dependence, drug, cannabis
general medical condition FØ9
sedative or hypnotic use
due to drug abuse —*see* Abuse, drug, sedative
due to drug dependence —*see* Dependence, drug, sedative
tobacco (nicotine) use —*see* Dependence, drug, nicotine
following organic brain damage FØ7.9
frontal lobe syndrome FØ7.Ø
personality change FØ7.Ø
postconcussional syndrome FØ7.81
specified NEC FØ7.89
infancy, childhood or adolescence F98.9
neurotic —*see* Neurosis
organic or symptomatic FØ9

Disorder *(Continued)*
mental *(Continued)*
presenile, psychotic FØ3
problem NEC
psychoneurotic —*see* Neurosis
psychotic —*see* Psychosis
puerperal F53
senile, psychotic NEC FØ3
metabolic, amino acid, transitory, newborn P74.8
metabolism NOS E88.9
amino-acid E72.9
aromatic E7Ø.9
albinism —*see* Albinism
histidine E7Ø.4Ø
histidinemia E7Ø.41
other specified E7Ø.49
hyperphenylalaninemia E7Ø.1
classical phenylketonuria E7Ø.Ø
other specified E7Ø.8
tryptophan E7Ø.5
tyrosine E7Ø.2Ø
hypertyrosinemia E7Ø.21
other specified E7Ø.29
branched chain E71.2
3-methylglutaconic aciduria E71.111
hyperleucine-isoleucinemia E71.19
hypervalinemia E71.19
isovaleric acidemia E71.11Ø
maple syrup urine disease E71.Ø
methylmalonic acidemia E71.12Ø
organic aciduria NEC E71.118
other specified E71.19
proprionate NEC E71.128
proprionic acidemia E71.121
glycine E72.5Ø
d-glycericacidemia E72.59
hyperhydroxyprolinemia E72.59
hyperoxaluria E72.53
hyperprolinemia E72.59
non-ketotic hyperglycinemia E72.51
other specified E72.59
sarcosinemia E72.59
trimethylaminuria E72.52
hydroxylysine E72.3
lysine E72.3
ornithine E72.4
other specified E72.8
beta-amino acid E72.8
gamma-glutamyl cycle E72.8
straight-chain E72.8
sulfur-bearing E72.1Ø
homocystinuria E72.11
methylenetetrahydrofolate reductase deficiency E72.12
other specified E72.19
bile acid and cholesterol metabolism E78.7Ø
bilirubin E8Ø.7
specified NEC E8Ø.6
calcium E83.5Ø
hypercalcemia E83.52
hypocalcemia E83.51
other specified E83.59
carbohydrate E74.9
specified NEC E74.8
cholesterol and bile acid metabolism E78.7Ø
congenital E88.9
copper E83.ØØ
specified type NEC E83.Ø9
Wilson's disease E83.Ø1
cystinuria E72.Ø1
fructose E74.1Ø
galactose E74.2Ø
glucosaminoglycan E76.9
mucopolysaccharidosis —*see* Mucopolysaccharidosis
specified NEC E76.8
glutamine E72.8
glycine E72.5Ø

D

Disorder *(Continued)*
metabolism *(Continued)*
glycogen storage (hepatorenal) E74.09
glycoprotein E77.9
specified NEC E77.8
glycosaminoglycan E76.9
specified NEC E76.8
in labor and delivery O75.89
iron E83.10
isoleucine E71.19
leucine E71.19
lipoid E78.9
lipoprotein E78.9
specified NEC E78.89
magnesium E83.40
hypermagnesemia E83.41
hypomagnesemia E83.42
other specified E83.49
mineral E83.9
specified NEC E83.89
mitochondrial E88.40
MELAS syndrome E88.41
MERRF syndrome (myoclonic epilepsy associated with ragged-red fibers) E88.42
other specified E88.49
ornithine E72.4
phosphatases E83.30
phosphorus E83.30
acid phosphatase deficiency E83.39
hypophosphatasia E83.39
hypophosphatemia E83.39
familial E83.31
other specified E83.39
pseudovitamin D deficiency E83.32
plasma protein NEC E88.09
porphyrin —*see* Porphyria
postprocedural E89.89
specified NEC E89.89
purine E79.9
specified NEC E79.8
pyrimidine E79.9
specified NEC E79.8
pyruvate E74.4
serine E72.8
sodium E87.8
specified NEC E88.89
threonine E72.8
valine E71.19
zinc E83.2
methylmalonic acidemia E71.120
micturition NEC —*see also* Difficulty, micturition R39.198 ⬅
feeling of incomplete emptying R39.14
hesitancy R39.11
poor stream R39.12
psychogenic F45.8
split stream R39.13
straining R39.16
urgency R39.15
mild neurocognitive G31.84 ◀
mitochondrial metabolism E88.40
mitral (valve) —*see* Endocarditis, mitral
mixed
anxiety and depressive F41.8
of scholastic skills (developmental) F81.89
receptive expressive language F80.2
mood F39
bipolar —*see* Disorder, bipolar
depressive —*see* Disorder, depressive
due to (secondary to)
alcohol F10.94
amphetamine F15.94
in
abuse F15.14
dependence F15.24
anxiolytic F13.94
in
abuse F13.14
dependence F13.24

Disorder *(Continued)*
mood *(Continued)*
due to *(Continued)*
cocaine F14.94
in
abuse F14.14
dependence F14.24
general medical condition F06.30
hallucinogen F16.94
in
abuse F16.14
dependence F16.24
hypnotic F13.94
in
abuse F13.14
dependence F13.24
inhalant F18.94
in
abuse F18.14
dependence F18.24
opioid F11.94
in
abuse F11.14
dependence F11.24
phencyclidine (PCP) F16.94
in
abuse F16.14
dependence F16.24
physiological condition F06.30
with
depressive features F06.31
major depressive-like episode F06.32
manic features F06.33
mixed features F06.34
psychoactive substance NEC F19.94
in
abuse F19.14
dependence F19.24
sedative F13.94
in
abuse F13.14
dependence F13.24
volatile solvents F18.94
in
abuse F18.14
dependence F18.24
manic episode F30.9
with psychotic symptoms F30.2
without psychotic symptoms F30.10
mild F30.11
moderate F30.12
severe F30.13
in remission (full) F30.4
partial F30.3
specified type NEC F30.8
organic F06.30
right hemisphere F07.89
persistent F34.9
cyclothymia F34.0
dysthymia F34.1
specified type NEC F34.89 ⬅
recurrent F39
right hemisphere organic F07.89
movement G25.9
drug-induced G25.70
akathisia G25.71
specified NEC G25.79
hysterical F44.4
in diseases classified elsewhere —*see* category G26
periodic limb G47.61
sleep related G47.61
sleep related NEC G47.69
specified NEC G25.89
stereotyped F98.4
treatment-induced G25.9
multiple personality F44.81
muscle M62.9
attachment, spine —*see* Enthesopathy, spinal

Disorder *(Continued)*
muscle *(Continued)*
in trichinellosis —*see* Trichinellosis, with muscle disorder
psychogenic F45.8
specified type NEC M62.89
tone, newborn P94.9
specified NEC P94.8
muscular
attachments —*see also* Enthesopathy
spine —*see* Enthesopathy, spinal
urethra N36.44
musculoskeletal system, soft tissue —*see* Disorder, soft tissue
postprocedural M96.89
psychogenic F45.8
myoneural G70.9
due to lead G70.1
specified NEC G70.89
toxic G70.1
myotonic NEC G71.19
nail, in diseases classified elsewhere L62
neck region NEC —*see* Dorsopathy, specified NEC
neonatal onset multisystemic inflammatory (NOMID) M04.2 ◀
nerve G58.9
abducent NEC —*see* Strabismus, paralytic, sixth nerve
accessory G52.8
acoustic —*see* subcategory H93.3
auditory —*see* subcategory H93.3
auriculotemporal G50.8
axillary G54.0
cerebral —*see* Disorder, nerve, cranial
cranial G52.9
eighth —*see* subcategory H93.3
eleventh G52.8
fifth G50.9
first G52.0
fourth NEC —*see* Strabismus, paralytic, fourth nerve
multiple G52.7
ninth G52.1
second NEC —*see* Disorder, nerve, optic
seventh NEC G51.8
sixth NEC —*see* Strabismus, paralytic, sixth nerve
specified NEC G52.8
tenth G52.2
third NEC —*see* Strabismus, paralytic, third nerve
twelfth G52.3
entrapment —*see* Neuropathy, entrapment
facial G51.9
specified NEC G51.8
femoral —*see* Lesion, nerve, femoral
glossopharyngeal NEC G52.1
hypoglossal G52.3
intercostal G58.0
lateral
cutaneous of thigh —*see* Mononeuropathy, lower limb, meralgia paresthetica
popliteal —*see* Lesion, nerve, popliteal
lower limb —*see* Mononeuropathy, lower limb
medial popliteal —*see* Lesion, nerve, popliteal, medial
median NEC —*see* Lesion, nerve, median
multiple G58.7
oculomotor NEC —*see* Strabismus, paralytic, third nerve
olfactory G52.0
optic NEC H47.09-
hemorrhage into sheath —*see* Hemorrhage, optic nerve
ischemic H47.01-
peroneal —*see* Lesion, nerve, popliteal
phrenic G58.8
plantar —*see* Lesion, nerve, plantar

D

Disorder (Continued)
  nerve (Continued)
    pneumogastric G52.2
    posterior tibial —see Syndrome, tarsal tunnel
    radial —see Lesion, nerve, radial
    recurrent laryngeal G52.2
    root G54.9
      cervical G54.2
      lumbosacral G54.1
      specified NEC G54.8
      thoracic G54.3
    sciatic NEC —see Lesion, nerve, sciatic
    specified NEC G58.8
      lower limb —see Mononeuropathy, lower limb, specified NEC
      upper limb —see Mononeuropathy, upper limb, specified NEC
    sympathetic G90.9
    tibial —see Lesion, nerve, popliteal, medial
    trigeminal G50.9
      specified NEC G50.8
    trochlear NEC —see Strabismus, paralytic, fourth nerve
    ulnar —see Lesion, nerve, ulnar
    upper limb —see Mononeuropathy, upper limb
    vagus G52.2
  nervous system G98.8
    autonomic (peripheral) G90.9
      specified NEC G90.8
    central G96.9
      specified NEC G96.8
    parasympathetic G90.9
    specified NEC G98.8
    sympathetic G90.9
    vegetative G90.9
  neurocognitive ◄
    major ◄
      with ◄
        aggressive behavior F01.51 ◄
        combative behavior F01.51 ◄
        violent behavior F01.51 ◄
      due to vascular disease, with behavioral disturbance F01.51 ◄
      in (due to) (other diseases classified elsewhere) —see also Dementia, in (due to) F02.80 ◄
        with ◄
          aggressive behavior F02.81 ◄
          combative behavior F02.81 ◄
          violent behavior F02.81 ◄
      without behavioral disturbance F01.50 ◄
    mild G31.84 ◄
  neurodevelopmental F89 ◄
    specified NEC F88 ◄
  neurohypophysis NEC E23.3
  neurological NEC R29.818
  neuromuscular G70.9
    hereditary NEC G71.9
    specified NEC G70.89
    toxic G70.1
  neurotic F48.9
    specified NEC F48.8
  neutrophil, polymorphonuclear D71
  nicotine use —see Dependence, drug, nicotine
  nightmare F51.5
  nose J34.9
    specified NEC J34.89
  obsessive-compulsive F42.9 ⬅
  odontogenesis NOS K00.9
  opioid use
    with
      opioid-induced psychotic disorder F11.959
        with
          delusions F11.950
          hallucinations F11.951

Disorder (Continued)
  opioid use (Continued)
    due to drug abuse —see Abuse, drug, opioid
    due to drug dependence —see Dependence, drug, opioid
    mild F11.10 ◄
      with ◄
        opioid-induced ◄
          anxiety disorder F11.188 ◄
          depressive disorder F11.14 ◄
          sexual dysfunction F11.181 ◄
        opioid intoxication ◄
          with perceptual disturbances F11.122 ◄
          delirium F11.121 ◄
          without perceptual disturbances F11.129 ◄
    moderate or severe F11.20 ◄
      with ◄
        opioid-induced ◄
          anxiety disorder F11.288 ◄
          anxiety disorder F11.988 ◄
          depressive disorder F11.24 ◄
          depressive disorder F11.94 ◄
          sexual dysfunction F11.281 ◄
          sexual dysfunction F11.981 ◄
        opioid intoxication ◄
          with perceptual disturbances F11.222 ◄
          delirium F11.221 ◄
          without perceptual disturbances F11.229 ◄
  oppositional defiant F91.3
  optic
    chiasm H47.49
      due to
        inflammatory disorder H47.41
        neoplasm H47.42
        vascular disorder H47.43
    disc H47.39-
      coloboma —see Coloboma, optic disc
      drusen —see Drusen, optic disc
      pseudopapilledema —see Pseudopapilledema
    radiations —see Disorder, visual, pathway
    tracts —see Disorder, visual, pathway
  orbit H05.9
    cyst —see Cyst, orbit
    deformity —see Deformity, orbit
    edema —see Edema, orbit
    enophthalmos —see Enophthalmos
    exophthalmos —see Exophthalmos
    hemorrhage —see Hemorrhage, orbit
    inflammation —see Inflammation, orbit
    myopathy —see Myopathy, extraocular muscles
    retained foreign body —see Foreign body, orbit, old
    specified type NEC H05.89
  organic
    anxiety F06.4
    catatonic F06.1
    delusional F06.2
    dissociative F06.8
    emotionally labile (asthenic) F06.8
    mood (affective) F06.30
    schizophrenia-like F06.2
  orgasmic (female) F52.31
    male F52.32
  ornithine metabolism E72.4
  overanxious F41.1
    of childhood F93.8
  pain
    with related psychological factors F45.42
    exclusively related to psychological factors F45.41
    genito-pelvic penetration disorder F52.6 ◄
  pancreatic internal secretion E16.9
    specified NEC E16.8

Disorder (Continued)
  panic F41.0
    with agoraphobia F40.01
  papulosquamous L44.9
    in diseases classified elsewhere L45
    specified NEC L44.8
  paranoid F22
    induced F24
    shared F24
  parathyroid (gland) E21.5
    specified NEC E21.4
  parietoalveolar NEC J84.09
  paroxysmal, mixed R56.9
  patella M22.9-
    chondromalacia —see Chondromalacia, patella
    derangement NEC M22.3X-
    recurrent
      dislocation —see Dislocation, patella, recurrent
      subluxation —see Dislocation, patella, recurrent, incomplete
    specified NEC M22.8X-
  patellofemoral M22.2X-
  pentose phosphate pathway with anemia D55.1
  perception, due to hallucinogens F16.983
    in
      abuse F16.183
      dependence F16.283
  peripheral nervous system NEC G64
  peroxisomal E71.50
    biogenesis
      neonatal adrenoleukodystrophy E71.511
      specified disorder NEC E71.518
      Zellweger syndrome E71.510
    rhizomelic chondrodysplasia punctata E71.540
    specified form NEC E71.548
      group 1 E71.518
      group 2 E71.53
      group 3 E71.542
    X-linked adrenoleukodystrophy E71.529
      adolescent E71.521
      adrenomyeloneuropathy E71.522
      childhood E71.520
      specified form NEC E71.528
    Zellweger-like syndrome E71.541
  persistent
    (somatoform) pain F45.41
    affective (mood) F34.9
  personality —see also Personality F60.9
    affective F34.0
    aggressive F60.3
    amoral F60.2
    anankastic F60.5
    antisocial F60.2
    anxious F60.6
    asocial F60.2
    asthenic F60.7
    avoidant F60.6
    borderline F60.3
    change (secondary) due to general medical condition F07.0
    compulsive F60.5
    cyclothymic F34.0
    dependent (passive) F60.7
    depressive F34.1
    dissocial F60.2
    emotional instability F60.3
    expansive paranoid F60.0
    explosive F60.3
    following organic brain damage F07.9
    histrionic F60.4
    hyperthymic F34.0
    hypothymic F34.1
    hysterical F60.4
    immature F60.89
    inadequate F60.7

D

Disorder *(Continued)*
personality *(Continued)*
labile F6Ø.3
mixed (nonspecific) F6Ø.89
moral deficiency F6Ø.2
narcissistic F6Ø.81
negativistic F6Ø.89
obsessional F6Ø.5
obsessive (-compulsive) F6Ø.5
organic FØ7.9
overconscientious F6Ø.5
paranoid F6Ø.Ø
passive (-dependent) F6Ø.7
passive-aggressive F6Ø.89
pathological NEC F6Ø.9
pseudosocial F6Ø.2
psychopathic F6Ø.2
schizoid F6Ø.1
schizotypal F21
self-defeating F6Ø.7
specified NEC F6Ø.89
type A F6Ø.5
unstable (emotional) F6Ø.3
pervasive, developmental F84.9
phencyclidine use ◀
mild F16.1Ø ◀
with ◀
phencyclidine-induced ◀
anxiety disorder F16.18Ø ◀
bipolar and related disorder F16.14 ◀
depressive disorder F16.14 ◀
psychotic disorder F16.159 ◀
phencyclidine intoxication F16.129 ◀
phencyclidine intoxication delirium F16.121 ◀
moderate or severe F16.2Ø ◀
with ◀
phencyclidine-induced ◀
anxiety disorder F16.28Ø ◀
bipolar and related disorder F16.24 ◀
depressive disorder F16.24 ◀
psychotic disorder F16.259 ◀
phencyclidine intoxication F16.229 ◀
phencyclidine intoxication delirium F16.221 ◀
phobic anxiety, childhood F4Ø.8
phosphate-losing tubular N25.Ø
pigmentation L81.9
choroid, congenital Q14.3
diminished melanin formation L81.6
iron L81.8
specified NEC L81.8
pinna (noninfective) H61.1Ø-
deformity, acquired H61.11-
hematoma H61.12-
perichondritis —*see* Perichondritis, ear
specified type NEC H61.19-
pituitary gland E23.7
iatrogenic (postprocedural) E89.3
specified NEC E23.6
platelets D69.1
plexus G54.9
specified NEC G54.8
polymorphonuclear neutrophils D71
porphyrin metabolism —*see* Porphyria
postconcussional FØ7.81
posthallucinogen perception F16.983
in
abuse F16.183
dependence F16.283
postmenopausal N95.9
specified NEC N95.8
postprocedural (postoperative) —*see* Complications, postprocedural
post-transplant lymphoproliferative D47.z1
post-traumatic stress (PTSD) F43.1Ø
acute F43.11
chronic F43.12

Disorder *(Continued)*
premenstrual dysphoric (PMDD) F32.81 ◀
prepuce N47.8
propionic acidemia E71.121
prostate N42.9
specified NEC N42.89
psychogenic NOS —*see also* condition F45.9
anxiety F41.8
appetite F5Ø.9
asthenic F48.8
cardiovascular (system) F45.8
compulsive F42.8 ◀
cutaneous F54
depressive F32.9
digestive (system) F45.8
dysmenorrheic F45.8
dyspneic F45.8
endocrine (system) F54
eye NEC F45.8
feeding —*see* Disorder, eating
functional NEC F45.8
gastric F45.8
gastrointestinal (system) F45.8
genitourinary (system) F45.8
heart (function) (rhythm) F45.8
hyperventilatory F45.8
hypochondriacal —*see* Disorder, hypochondriacal
intestinal F45.8
joint F45.8
learning F81.9
limb F45.8
lymphatic (system) F45.8
menstrual F45.8
micturition F45.8
monoplegic NEC F44.4
motor F44.4
muscle F45.8
musculoskeletal F45.8
neurocirculatory F45.8
obsessive F42.8 ◀
occupational F48.8
organ or part of body NEC F45.8
paralytic NEC F44.4
phobic F4Ø.9
physical NEC F45.8
rectal F45.8
respiratory (system) F45.8
rheumatic F45.8
sexual (function) F52.9
skin (allergic) (eczematous) F54
sleep F51.9
specified part of body NEC F45.8
stomach F45.8
psychological F99
associated with
disease classified elsewhere F54
sexual
development F66
relationship F66
uncertainty about gender identity F64.9 ◀
psychomotor NEC F44.4
hysterical F44.4
psychoneurotic —*see also* Neurosis
mixed NEC F48.8
psychophysiologic —*see* Disorder, somatoform
psychosexual F65.9
development F66
identity of childhood F64.2
psychosomatic NOS —*see* Disorder, somatoform
multiple F45.Ø
undifferentiated F45.1
psychotic —*see* Psychosis
transient (acute) F23
puberty E3Ø.9
specified NEC E3Ø.8
pulmonary (valve) —*see* Endocarditis, pulmonary

Disorder *(Continued)*
purine metabolism E79.9
pyrimidine metabolism E79.9
pyruvate metabolism E74.4
reactive attachment (childhood) F94.1
reading R48.Ø
developmental (specific) F81.Ø
receptive language F8Ø.2
receptor, hormonal, peripheral —*see also* Syndrome, androgen insensitivity E34.5Ø
recurrent brief depressive F33.8
reflex R29.2
refraction H52.7
aniseikonia H52.32
anisometropia H52.31
astigmatism —*see* Astigmatism
hypermetropia —*see* Hypermetropia
myopia —*see* Myopia
presbyopia H52.4
specified NEC H52.6
relationship F68.8
due to sexual orientation F66
REM sleep behavior G47.52
renal function, impaired (tubular) N25.9
resonance R49.9
specified NEC R49.8
respiratory function, impaired —*see also* Failure, respiration
postprocedural —*see* Complication, postoperative, respiratory system
psychogenic F45.8
retina H35.9
angioid streaks H35.33
changes in vascular appearance H35.Ø1-
degeneration —*see* Degeneration, retina
dystrophy (hereditary) —*see* Dystrophy, retina
edema H35.81
hemorrhage —*see* Hemorrhage, retina
ischemia H35.82
macular degeneration —*see* Degeneration, macula
microaneurysms H35.Ø4-
microvascular abnormality NEC H35.Ø9
neovascularization —*see* Neovascularization, retina
retinopathy —*see* Retinopathy
separation of layers H35.7Ø
central serous chorioretinopathy H35.71-
pigment epithelium detachment (serous) H35.72-
hemorrhagic H35.73-
specified type NEC H35.89
telangiectasis —*see* Telangiectasis, retina
vasculitis —*see* Vasculitis, retina
retroperitoneal K68.9
right hemisphere organic affective FØ7.89
rumination (infant or child) F98.21
sacrum, sacrococcygeal NEC M53.3
schizoaffective F25.9
bipolar type F25.Ø
depressive type F25.1
manic type F25.Ø
mixed type F25.Ø
specified NEC F25.8
schizoid of childhood F84.5
schizophreniform F2Ø.81
brief F23
schizotypal (personality) F21
secretion, thyrocalcitonin EØ7.Ø
sedative, hypnotic, or anxiolytic use ◀
mild F13.1Ø ◀
with ◀
sedative, hypnotic, or anxiolytic-induced ◀
anxiety disorder F13.18Ø ◀
bipolar and related disorder F13.14 ◀

D

◀ New ◀ Revised ~~deleted~~ Deleted

Disorder *(Continued)*
sedative, hypnotic, or anxiolytic use *(Continued)*
mild *(Continued)*
with *(Continued)*
sedative, hypnotic, or anxiolytic-induced *(Continued)*
depressive disorder F13.14 ◀
psychotic disorder F13.159 ◀
sexual dysfunction F13.181 ◀
sedative, hypnotic, or anxiolytic intoxication F13.129 ◀
sedative, hypnotic, or anxiolytic intoxication delirium F13.121 ◀
moderate or severe F13.2Ø ◀
with ◀
sedative, hypnotic, or anxiolytic-induced ◀
anxiety disorder F13.28Ø ◀
bipolar and related disorder F13.24 ◀
depressive disorder F13.24 ◀
major neurocognitive disorder F13.27 ◀
mild neurocognitive disorder F13.288 ◀
psychotic disorder F13.259 ◀
sexual dysfunction F13.281 ◀
sedative, hypnotic, or anxiolytic intoxication F13.229 ◀
sedative, hypnotic, or anxiolytic intoxication delirium F13.221 ◀
seizure —*see also* Epilepsy G4Ø.9Ø9
intractable G4Ø.919
with status epilepticus G4Ø.911
semantic pragmatic F8Ø.89
with autism F84.Ø
sense of smell R43.1
psychogenic F45.8
separation anxiety, of childhood F93.Ø
sexual
arousal, female F52.22
aversion F52.1
function, psychogenic F52.9
maturation F66
nonorganic F52.9
preference —*see also* Deviation, sexual F65.9
fetishistic transvestism F65.1
relationship F66
shyness, of childhood and adolescence F4Ø.1Ø
sibling rivalry F93.8
sickle-cell (sickling) (homozygous) —*see* Disease, sickle-cell
heterozygous D57.3
specified type NEC D57.8-
trait D57.3
sinus (nasal) J34.9
specified NEC J34.89
skin L98.9
atrophic L9Ø.9
specified NEC L9Ø.8
granulomatous L92.9
specified NEC L92.8
hypertrophic L91.9
specified NEC L91.8
infiltrative NEC L98.6
newborn P83.9
specified NEC P83.8
picking F42.4 ◀
psychogenic (allergic) (eczematous) F54
sleep G47.9
breathing-related —*see* Apnea, sleep
circadian rhythm G47.2Ø
advance sleep phase type G47.22
delayed sleep phase type G47.21
due to
alcohol
abuse F1Ø.182
dependence F1Ø.282
use F1Ø.982

Disorder *(Continued)*
sleep *(Continued)*
circadian rhythm *(Continued)*
due to *(Continued)*
amphetamines
abuse F15.182
dependence F15.282
use F15.982
caffeine
abuse F15.182
dependence F15.282
use F15.982
cocaine
abuse F14.182
dependence F14.282
use F14.982
drug NEC
abuse F19.182
dependence F19.282
use F19.982
opioid
abuse F11.182
dependence F11.282
use F11.982
psychoactive substance NEC
abuse F19.182
dependence F19.282
use F19.982
sedative, hypnotic, or anxiolytic
abuse F13.182
dependence F13.282
use F13.982
stimulant NEC
abuse F15.182
dependence F15.282
use F15.982
free running type G47.24
in conditions classified elsewhere G47.27
irregular sleep wake type G47.23
jet lag type G47.25
shift work type G47.26
specified NEC G47.29
due to
alcohol
abuse F1Ø.182
dependence F1Ø.282
use F1Ø.982
amphetamine
abuse F15.182
dependence F15.282
use F15.982
anxiolytic
abuse F13.182
dependence F13.282
use F13.982
caffeine
abuse F15.182
dependence F15.282
use F15.982
cocaine
abuse F14.182
dependence F14.282
use F14.982
drug NEC
abuse F19.182
dependence F19.282
use F19.982
hypnotic
abuse F13.182
dependence F13.282
use F13.982
opioid
abuse F11.182
dependence F11.282
use F11.982
psychoactive substance NEC
abuse F19.182
dependence F19.282
use F19.982

Disorder *(Continued)*
sleep *(Continued)*
due to *(Continued)*
sedative
abuse F13.182
dependence F13.282
use F13.982
stimulant NEC
abuse F15.182
dependence F15.282
use F15.982
emotional F51.9
excessive somnolence —*see* Hypersomnia
hypersomnia type —*see* Hypersomnia
initiating or maintaining —*see* Insomnia
nightmares F51.5
nonorganic F51.9
specified NEC F51.8
parasomnia type G47.5Ø
specified NEC G47.8
terrors F51.4
walking F51.3
sleep-wake pattern or schedule —*see* Disorder, sleep, circadian rhythm
social
anxiety of childhood F4Ø.1Ø
functioning in childhood F94.9
specified NEC F94.8
pragmatic F8Ø.82 ◀
soft tissue M79.9
ankle M79.9
due to use, overuse and pressure M7Ø.9Ø
ankle M7Ø.97-
bursitis —*see* Bursitis
foot M7Ø.97-
forearm M7Ø.93-
hand M7Ø.94-
lower leg M7Ø.96-
multiple sites M7Ø.99
pelvic region M7Ø.95-
shoulder region M7Ø.91-
specified site NEC M7Ø.98
specified type NEC M7Ø.8Ø
ankle M7Ø.87-
foot M7Ø.87-
forearm M7Ø.83-
hand M7Ø.84-
lower leg M7Ø.86-
multiple sites M7Ø.89
pelvic region M7Ø.85-
shoulder region M7Ø.81-
specified site NEC M7Ø.88
thigh M7Ø.85-
upper arm M7Ø.82-
thigh M7Ø.95-
upper arm M7Ø.92-
foot M79.9
forearm M79.9
hand M79.9
lower leg M79.9
multiple sites M79.9
occupational —*see* Disorder, soft tissue, due to use, overuse and pressure
pelvic region M79.9
shoulder region M79.9
specified type NEC M79.89
thigh M79.9
upper arm M79.9
somatic symptom F45.1 ◀
somatization F45.Ø
somatoform F45.9
pain (persistent) F45.41
somatization (multiple) (long-lasting) F45.Ø
specified NEC F45.8
undifferentiated F45.1
somnolence, excessive —*see* Hypersomnia
specific
arithmetical F81.2
developmental, of motor F82
reading F81.Ø

D

- **Disorder** *(Continued)*
  - specific *(Continued)*
    - speech and language F8Ø.9
    - spelling F81.81
    - written expression F81.81
  - speech R47.9
    - articulation (functional) (specific) F8Ø.Ø
    - developmental F8Ø.9
    - specified NEC R47.89
  - speech-sound F8Ø.Ø ◀
  - spelling (specific) F81.81
  - spine —*see also* Dorsopathy
    - ligamentous or muscular attachments, peripheral —*see* Enthesopathy, spinal
    - specified NEC —*see* Dorsopathy, specified NEC
  - stereotyped, habit or movement F98.4
  - stimulant use (other) (unspecified) ◀
    - mild F15.1Ø ◀
    - moderate or severe F15.2Ø ◀
  - stomach (functional) —*see* Disorder, gastric
  - stress F43.9
    - acute F43.Ø ◀
    - post-traumatic F43.1Ø
      - acute F43.11
      - chronic F43.12
  - substance use (other) (unknown) ◀
    - mild F19.1Ø ◀
      - with substance-induced ◀
        - anxiety disorder F19.18Ø ◀
        - bipolar and related disorder F19.14 ◀
        - depressive disorder F19.14 ◀
        - major neurocognitive disorder F19.17 ◀
        - mild neurocognitive disorder F19.188 ◀
        - obsessive-compulsive and related disorder F19.188 ◀
        - sexual dysfunction F19.181 ◀
      - substance intoxication F19.129 ◀
      - substance intoxication delirium F19.121 ◀
    - moderate or severe F19.2Ø ◀
      - with substance-induced ◀
        - anxiety disorder F19.28Ø ◀
        - bipolar and related disorder F19.24 ◀
        - depressive disorder F19.24 ◀
        - major neurocognitive disorder F19.27 ◀
        - mild neurocognitive disorder F19.288 ◀
        - obsessive-compulsive and related disorder F19.288 ◀
        - sexual dysfunction F19.281 ◀
      - substance intoxication F19.229 ◀
      - substance intoxication delirium F19.221 ◀
  - sulfur-bearing amino-acid metabolism E72.1Ø
  - sweat gland (eccrine) L74.9
    - apocrine L75.9
      - specified NEC L75.8
    - specified NEC L74.8
  - synovium M67.9Ø
    - acromioclavicular M67.91-
    - ankle M67.97-
    - elbow M67.92-
    - foot M67.97-
    - forearm M67.93-
    - hand M67.94-
    - hip M67.95-
    - knee M67.96-
    - multiple sites M67.99
    - rupture —*see* Rupture, synovium
    - shoulder M67.91-
    - specified type NEC M67.8Ø
      - acromioclavicular M67.81-
      - ankle M67.87-
      - elbow M67.82-
      - foot M67.87-
      - hand M67.84-
      - hip M67.85-

- **Disorder** *(Continued)*
  - synovium *(Continued)*
    - specified type *(Continued)*
      - knee M67.86-
      - multiple sites M67.89
      - wrist M67.83-
    - synovitis —*see* Synovitis
    - upper arm M67.92-
    - wrist M67.93-
  - temperature regulation, newborn P81.9
    - specified NEC P81.8
  - temporomandibular joint M26.6Ø- ⬅
  - tendon M67.9Ø
    - acromioclavicular M67.91-
    - ankle M67.97-
    - contracture —*see* Contracture, tendon
    - elbow M67.92-
    - foot M67.97-
    - forearm M67.93-
    - hand M67.94-
    - hip M67.95-
    - knee M67.96-
    - multiple sites M67.99
    - rupture —*see* Rupture, tendon
    - shoulder M67.91-
    - specified type NEC M67.8Ø
      - acromioclavicular M67.81-
      - ankle M67.87-
      - elbow M67.82-
      - foot M67.87-
      - hand M67.84-
      - hip M67.85-
      - knee M67.86-
      - multiple sites M67.89
      - trunk M67.88
      - wrist M67.83-
    - synovitis —*see* Synovitis
    - tendinitis —*see* Tendinitis
    - tenosynovitis —*see* Tenosynovitis
    - trunk M67.98
    - upper arm M67.92-
    - wrist M67.93-
  - thoracic root (nerve) NEC G54.3
  - thyrocalcitonin hypersecretion EØ7.Ø
  - thyroid (gland) EØ7.9
    - function NEC, neonatal, transitory P72.2
    - iodine-deficiency related EØ1.8
    - specified NEC EØ7.89
  - tic —*see* Tic
  - tobacco use ◀
    - mild Z72.Ø ◀
    - moderate F17.2ØØ ◀
    - severe F17.2ØØ ◀
  - tooth KØ8.9
    - development KØØ.9
      - specified NEC KØØ.8
    - eruption KØØ.6
  - Tourette's F95.2
  - trance and possession F44.89
  - trauma and stressor-related F43.9 ◀
    - other specified F43.8 ◀
  - tricuspid (valve) —*see* Endocarditis, tricuspid
  - tryptophan metabolism E7Ø.5
  - tubular, phosphate-losing N25.Ø
  - tubulo-interstitial (in)
    - brucellosis A23.9 *[N16]*
    - cystinosis E72.Ø4
    - diphtheria A36.84
    - glycogen storage disease E74.ØØ *[N16]*
    - leukemia NEC C95.9- *[N16]*
    - lymphoma NEC C85.9- *[N16]*
    - mixed cryoglobulinemia D89.1 *[N16]*
    - multiple myeloma C9Ø.Ø- *[N16]*
    - Salmonella infection AØ2.25
    - sarcoidosis D86.84
    - sepsis A41.9 *[N16]*
      - streptococcal A4Ø.9 *[N16]*
    - systemic lupus erythematosus M32.15
    - toxoplasmosis B58.83
    - transplant rejection T86.91 *[N16]*
    - Wilson's disease E83.Ø1 *[N16]*

- **Disorder** *(Continued)*
  - tubulo-renal function, impaired N25.9
    - specified NEC N25.89
  - tympanic membrane H73.9-
    - atrophy —*see* Atrophy, tympanic membrane
    - infection —*see* Myringitis
    - perforation —*see* Perforation, tympanum
    - specified NEC H73.89-
  - unsocialized aggressive F91.1
  - urea cycle metabolism E72.2Ø
    - argininemia E72.21
    - arginosuccinic aciduria E72.22
    - citrullinemia E72.23
    - ornithine transcarbamylase deficiency E72.4
    - other specified E72.29
  - ureter (in) N28.9
    - schistosomiasis B65.Ø *[N29]*
    - tuberculosis A18.11
  - urethra N36.9
    - specified NEC N36.8
  - urinary system N39.9
    - specified NEC N39.8
  - valve, heart
    - aortic —*see* Endocarditis, aortic
    - mitral —*see* Endocarditis, mitral
    - pulmonary —*see* Endocarditis, pulmonary
    - rheumatic
      - aortic —*see* Endocarditis, aortic, rheumatic
      - mitral —*see* Endocarditis, mitral
      - pulmonary —*see* Endocarditis, pulmonary, rheumatic
      - tricuspid —*see* Endocarditis, tricuspid
    - tricuspid —*see* Endocarditis, tricuspid
  - vestibular function H81.9-
    - specified NEC —*see* subcategory H81.8
      - in diseases classified elsewhere H82.-
    - vertigo —*see* Vertigo
  - vision, binocular H53.3Ø
    - abnormal retinal correspondence H53.31
    - diplopia H53.2
    - fusion with defective stereopsis H53.32
    - simultaneous perception H53.33
    - suppression H53.34
  - visual
    - cortex
      - blindness H47.619
        - left brain H47.612
        - right brain H47.611
      - due to
        - inflammatory disorder H47.629
          - left brain H47.622
          - right brain H47.621
        - neoplasm H47.639
          - left brain H47.632
          - right brain H47.631
        - vascular disorder H47.649
          - left brain H47.642
          - right brain H47.641
    - pathway H47.9
      - due to
        - inflammatory disorder H47.51-
        - neoplasm H47.52-
        - vascular disorder H47.53-
      - optic chiasm —*see* Disorder, optic, chiasm
  - vitreous body H43.9
    - crystalline deposits —*see* Deposit, crystalline
    - degeneration —*see* Degeneration, vitreous
    - hemorrhage —*see* Hemorrhage, vitreous
    - opacities —*see* Opacity, vitreous
    - prolapse —*see* Prolapse, vitreous
    - specified type NEC H43.89
  - voice R49.9
    - specified type NEC R49.8
  - volatile solvent use
    - due to drug abuse —*see* Abuse, drug, inhalant
    - due to drug dependence —*see* Dependence, drug, inhalant

D

- **Disorder** *(Continued)*
  - white blood cells D72.9
    - specified NEC D72.89
  - withdrawing, child or adolescent F40.10
- **Disorientation** R41.0
- **Displacement, displaced**
  - acquired traumatic of bone, cartilage, joint, tendon NEC —*see* Dislocation
  - adrenal gland (congenital) Q89.1
  - appendix, retrocecal (congenital) Q43.8
  - auricle (congenital) Q17.4
  - bladder (acquired) N32.89
    - congenital Q64.19
  - brachial plexus (congenital) Q07.8
  - brain stem, caudal (congenital) Q04.8
  - canaliculus (lacrimalis), congenital Q10.6
  - cardia through esophageal hiatus (congenital) Q40.1
  - cerebellum, caudal (congenital) Q04.8
  - cervix —*see* Malposition, uterus
  - colon (congenital) Q43.3
  - device, implant or graft —*see also* Complications, by site and type, mechanical T85.628
    - arterial graft NEC —*see* Complication, cardiovascular device, mechanical, vascular
    - breast (implant) T85.42
    - catheter NEC T85.628
      - dialysis (renal) T82.42
        - intraperitoneal T85.621
      - infusion NEC T82.524
        - spinal (epidural) (subdural) T85.620
      - urinary ⬅
        - cystostomy T83.020
        - Hopkins T83.028 ◀
        - ileostomy T83.028 ◀
        - indwelling T83.021 ◀
        - nephrostomy T83.022 ◀
        - specified NEC T83.028 ◀
        - urostomy T83.028 ◀
    - electronic (electrode) (pulse generator) (stimulator) —*see* Complication, electronic stimulator
    - fixation, internal (orthopedic) NEC —*see* Complication, fixation device, mechanical
    - gastrointestinal —*see* Complications, prosthetic device, mechanical, gastrointestinal device
    - genital NEC T83.428
      - intrauterine contraceptive device (string) T83.32 ⬅
      - penile prosthesis (cylinder) (implanted) (pump) (resevoir) T83.420 ⬅
      - testicular prosthesis T83.421 ◀
    - heart NEC —*see* Complication, cardiovascular device, mechanical
    - joint prosthesis —*see* Complications, joint prosthesis, mechanical
    - ocular —*see* Complications, prosthetic device, mechanical, ocular device
    - orthopedic NEC —*see* Complication, orthopedic, device or graft, mechanical
    - specified NEC T85.628
    - urinary NEC T83.128 ⬅
      - graft T83.22
      - sphincter, implanted T83.121 ◀
      - stent (ileal conduit) (nephroureteral) T83.123 ◀
      - ureteral indwelling T83.122 ◀
    - vascular NEC —*see* Complication, cardiovascular device, mechanical
    - ventricular intracranial shunt T85.02
  - electronic stimulator
    - bone T84.320
    - cardiac —*see* Complications, cardiac device, electronic

- **Displacement, displaced** *(Continued)*
  - electronic stimulator *(Continued)*
    - nervous system —*see* Complication, prosthetic device, mechanical, electronic nervous system stimulator
    - urinary —*see* Complications, electronic stimulator, urinary
  - esophageal mucosa into cardia of stomach, congenital Q39.8
  - esophagus (acquired) K22.8
    - congenital Q39.8
  - eyeball (acquired) (lateral) (old) —*see* Displacement, globe
    - congenital Q15.8
    - current —*see* Avulsion, eye
  - fallopian tube (acquired) N83.4- ⬅
    - congenital Q50.6
    - opening (congenital) Q50.6
  - gallbladder (congenital) Q44.1
  - gastric mucosa (congenital) Q40.2
  - globe (acquired) (old) (lateral) H05.21-
    - current —*see* Avulsion, eye
  - heart (congenital) Q24.8
    - acquired I51.89
  - hymen (upward) (congenital) Q52.4
  - intervertebral disc NEC
    - with myelopathy —*see* Disorder, disc, with, myelopathy
    - cervical, cervicothoracic (with) M50.20
      - myelopathy —*see* Disorder, disc, cervical, with myelopathy
      - neuritis, radiculitis or radiculopathy —*see* Disorder, disc, cervical, with neuritis
    - due to trauma —*see* Dislocation, vertebra
    - lumbar region M51.26
      - with
        - neuritis, radiculitis, radiculopathy or sciatica M51.16
    - lumbosacral region M51.27
      - with
        - myelopathy M51.07
        - neuritis, radiculitis, radiculopathy or sciatica M51.17
    - sacrococcygeal region M53.3
    - thoracic region M51.24
      - with
        - myelopathy M51.04
        - neuritis, radiculitis, radiculopathy M51.14
    - thoracolumbar region M51.25
      - with
        - myelopathy M51.05
        - neuritis, radiculitis, radiculopathy M51.15
  - intrauterine device (string) T83.32 ⬅
  - kidney (acquired) N28.83
    - congenital Q63.2
  - lachrymal, lacrimal apparatus or duct (congenital) Q10.6
  - lens, congenital Q12.1
  - macula (congenital) Q14.1
  - Meckel's diverticulum Q43.0
    - malignant —*see* Table of Neoplasms, small intestine, malignant
  - nail (congenital) Q84.6
    - acquired L60.8
  - opening of Wharton's duct in mouth Q38.4
  - organ or site, congenital NEC —*see* Malposition, congenital
  - ovary (acquired) N83.4- ⬅
    - congenital Q50.39
    - free in peritoneal cavity (congenital) Q50.39
    - into hernial sac N83.4- ⬅
  - oviduct (acquired) N83.4- ⬅
    - congenital Q50.6
  - parathyroid (gland) E21.4
  - parotid gland (congenital) Q38.4

- **Displacement, displaced** *(Continued)*
  - punctum lacrimale (congenital) Q10.6
  - sacro-iliac (joint) (congenital) Q74.2
    - current injury S33.2
    - old —*see* subcategory M53.2
  - salivary gland (any) (congenital) Q38.4
  - spleen (congenital) Q89.09
  - stomach, congenital Q40.2
  - sublingual duct Q38.4
  - tongue (downward) (congenital) Q38.3
  - tooth, teeth, fully erupted M26.30
    - horizontal M26.33
    - vertical M26.34
  - trachea (congenital) Q32.1
  - ureter or ureteric opening or orifice (congenital) Q62.62
  - uterine opening of oviducts or fallopian tubes Q50.6
  - uterus, uterine —*see* Malposition, uterus
  - ventricular septum Q21.0
    - with rudimentary ventricle Q20.4
- **Disproportion**
  - between native and reconstructed breast N65.1
  - fiber-type G71.2
- **Disruptio uteri** —*see* Rupture, uterus
- **Disruption** (of)
  - ciliary body NEC H21.89
  - closure of
    - cornea T81.31
    - craniotomy T81.32
    - fascia (muscular) (superficial) T81.32
    - internal organ or tissue T81.32
    - laceration (external) (internal) T81.33
    - ligament T81.32
    - mucosa T81.31
    - muscle or muscle flap T81.32
    - ribs or rib cage T81.32
    - skin and subcutaneous tissue (full-thickness) (superficial) T81.31
    - skull T81.32
    - sternum (sternotomy) T81.32
    - tendon T81.32
    - traumatic laceration (external) (internal) T81.33
  - family Z63.8
    - due to
      - absence of family member due to military deployment Z63.31
      - absence of family member NEC Z63.32
      - alcoholism and drug addiction in family Z63.72
      - bereavement Z63.4
      - death (assumed) or disappearance of family member Z63.4
      - divorce or separation Z63.5
      - drug addiction in family Z63.72
      - return of family member from military deployment (current or past conflict) Z63.71
      - stressful life events NEC Z63.79
  - iris NEC H21.89
  - ligament (s) —*see also* Sprain
    - knee
      - current injury —*see* Dislocation, knee
      - old (chronic) —*see* Derangement, knee, ligament, instability, chronic
      - spontaneous NEC —*see* Derangement, knee, disruption ligament
  - ossicular chain —*see* Discontinuity, ossicles, ear
  - pelvic ring (stable) S32.810
    - unstable S32.811
  - traumatic injury wound repair T81.33
  - wound T81.30
    - episiotomy O90.1
    - operation T81.31
      - cesarean O90.0
      - external operation wound (superficial) T81.31
      - internal operation wound (deep) T81.32
    - perineal (obstetric) O90.1
  - traumatic injury repair T81.33

Dissatisfaction with
employment Z56.9
school environment Z55.4
Dissecting —*see* condition
Dissection
aorta I71.ØØ
abdominal I71.Ø2
thoracic I71.Ø1
thoracoabdominal I71.Ø3
artery I77.7Ø ⬅
basilar (trunk) I77.75 ◀
carotid I77.71
cerebral (nonruptured) I67.Ø
ruptured —*see* Hemorrhage, intracranial, subarachnoid
coronary I25.42
extremity ◀
lower I77.77 ◀
upper I77.76 ◀
iliac I77.72
precerebral ◀
congenital (nonruptured) Q28.1 ◀
specified site NEC I77.75 ◀
renal I77.73
specified NEC I77.79
vertebral I77.74
traumatic —*see* Wound, open, by site
vascular I99.8
wound —*see* Wound, open
Disseminated —*see* condition
Dissociation
auriculoventricular or atrioventricular (AV) (any degree) (isorhythmic) I45.89
with heart block I44.2
interference I45.89
Dissociative reaction, state F44.9
Dissolution, vertebra —*see* Osteoporosis
Distension, distention
abdomen R14.Ø
bladder N32.89
cecum K63.89
colon K63.89
gallbladder K82.8
intestine K63.89
kidney N28.89
liver K76.89
seminal vesicle N5Ø.89 ⬅
stomach K31.89
acute K31.Ø
psychogenic F45.8
ureter —*see* Dilatation, ureter
uterus N85.8
Distoma hepaticum infestation B66.3
Distomiasis B66.9
bile passages B66.3
hemic B65.9
hepatic B66.3
due to Clonorchis sinensis B66.1
intestinal B66.5
liver B66.3
due to Clonorchis sinensis B66.1
lung B66.4
pulmonary B66.4
Distomolar (fourth molar) KØØ.1
Disto-occlusion (Division I) (Division II) M26.212
Distortion (s) (congenital)
adrenal (gland) Q89.1
arm NEC Q68.8
bile duct or passage Q44.5
bladder Q64.79
brain QØ4.9
cervix (uteri) Q51.9
chest (wall) Q67.8
bones Q76.8
clavicle Q74.Ø
clitoris Q52.6
coccyx Q76.49
common duct Q44.5
coronary Q24.5
cystic duct Q44.5

Distortion *(Continued)*
ear (auricle) (external) Q17.3
inner Q16.5
middle Q16.4
ossicles Q16.3
endocrine NEC Q89.2
eustachian tube Q17.8
eye (adnexa) Q15.8
face bone (s) NEC Q75.8
fallopian tube Q5Ø.6
femur NEC Q68.8
fibula NEC Q68.8
finger (s) Q68.1
foot Q66.9
genitalia, genital organ (s)
female Q52.8
external Q52.79
internal NEC Q52.8
gyri QØ4.8
hand bone (s) Q68.1
heart (auricle) (ventricle) Q24.8
valve (cusp) Q24.8
hepatic duct Q44.5
humerus NEC Q68.8
hymen Q52.4
intrafamilial communications Z63.8
jaw NEC M26.89
labium (majus) (minus) Q52.79
leg NEC Q68.8
lens Q12.8
liver Q44.7
lumbar spine Q76.49
with disproportion O33.8
causing obstructed labor O65.Ø
lumbosacral (joint) (region) Q76.49
kyphosis —*see* Kyphosis, congenital
lordosis —*see* Lordosis, congenital
nerve QØ7.8
nose Q3Ø.8
organ
of Corti Q16.5
or site not listed —*see* Anomaly, by site
ossicles, ear Q16.3
oviduct Q5Ø.6
pancreas Q45.3
parathyroid (gland) Q89.2
pituitary (gland) Q89.2
radius NEC Q68.8
sacroiliac joint Q74.2
sacrum Q76.49
scapula Q74.Ø
shoulder girdle Q74.Ø
skull bone (s) NEC Q75.8
with
anencephalus QØØ.Ø
encephalocele —*see* Encephalocele
hydrocephalus QØ3.9
with spina bifida —*see* Spina bifida, with hydrocephalus
microcephaly QØ2
spinal cord QØ6.8
spine Q76.49
kyphosis —*see* Kyphosis, congenital
lordosis —*see* Lordosis, congenital
spleen Q89.Ø9
sternum NEC Q76.7
thorax (wall) Q67.8
bony Q76.8
thymus (gland) Q89.2
thyroid (gland) Q89.2
tibia NEC Q68.8
toe (s) Q66.9
tongue Q38.3
trachea (cartilage) Q32.1
ulna NEC Q68.8
ureter Q62.8
urethra Q64.79
causing obstruction Q64.39
uterus Q51.9
vagina Q52.4

Distortion *(Continued)*
vertebra Q76.49
kyphosis —*see* Kyphosis, congenital
lordosis —*see* Lordosis, congenital
visual —*see also* Disturbance, vision
shape and size H53.15
vulva Q52.79
wrist (bones) (joint) Q68.8
Distress
abdomen —*see* Pain, abdominal
acute respiratory RØ6.ØØ ⬅
syndrome (adult) (child) J8Ø ◀
epigastric R1Ø.13
fetal P84
complicating pregnancy —*see* Stress, fetal
gastrointestinal (functional) K3Ø
psychogenic F45.8
intestinal (functional) NOS K59.9
psychogenic F45.8
maternal, during labor and delivery O75.Ø
respiratory (adult) (child) RØ6.ØØ ⬅
~~adult J8Ø~~
~~child J8Ø~~
newborn P22.9
specified NEC P22.8
orthopnea RØ6.Ø1
psychogenic F45.8
shortness of breath RØ6.Ø2
specified type NEC RØ6.Ø9
Distribution vessel, atypical Q27.9
coronary artery Q24.5
precerebral Q28.1
Districhiasis L68.8
Disturbance (s) —*see also* Disease
absorption K9Ø.9
calcium E58
carbohydrate K9Ø.49 ⬅
fat K9Ø.49 ⬅
pancreatic K9Ø.3
protein K9Ø.49 ⬅
starch K9Ø.49 ⬅
vitamin —*see* Deficiency, vitamin
acid-base equilibrium E87.8
mixed E87.4
activity and attention (with hyperkinesis) —*see* Disorder, attention-deficit hyperactivity
amino acid transport E72.ØØ
assimilation, food K9Ø.9
auditory nerve, except deafness —*see* subcategory H93.3
behavior —*see* Disorder, conduct
blood clotting (mechanism) —*see also* Defect, coagulation D68.9
cerebral
nerve —*see* Disorder, nerve, cranial
status, newborn P91.9
specified NEC P91.8
circulatory I99.9
conduct —*see also* Disorder, conduct F91.9
adjustment reaction —*see* Disorder, adjustment
compulsive F63.9
disruptive F91.9
hyperkinetic —*see* Disorder, attention-deficit hyperactivity
socialized F91.2
specified NEC F91.8
unsocialized F91.1
coordination R27.8
cranial nerve —*see* Disorder, nerve, cranial
deep sensibility —*see* Disturbance, sensation
digestive K3Ø
psychogenic F45.8
electrolyte —*see also* Imbalance, electrolyte
newborn, transitory P74.4
hyperammonemia P74.6
potassium balance P74.3
sodium balance P74.2
specified type NEC P74.4

◀ New ⬅ Revised ~~deleted~~ Deleted

Disturbance *(Continued)*
- emotions specific to childhood and adolescence F93.9
  - with
    - anxiety and fearfulness NEC F93.8
    - elective mutism F94.0
    - oppositional disorder F91.3
    - sensitivity (withdrawal) F40.10
    - shyness F40.10
    - social withdrawal F40.10
  - involving relationship problems F93.8
  - mixed F93.8
  - specified NEC F93.8
- endocrine (gland) E34.9
  - neonatal, transitory P72.9
    - specified NEC P72.8
- equilibrium R42
- fructose metabolism E74.10
- gait —*see* Gait
  - hysterical F44.4
  - psychogenic F44.4
- gastrointestinal (functional) K30
  - psychogenic F45.8
- habit, child F98.9
- hearing, except deafness and tinnitus —*see* Abnormal, auditory perception
- heart, functional (conditions in I44-I50)
  - due to presence of (cardiac) prosthesis I97.19-
  - postoperative I97.89
    - cardiac surgery I97.19-
- hormones E34.9
- innervation uterus (parasympathetic) (sympathetic) N85.8
- keratinization NEC
  - gingiva K05.10
    - nonplaque induced K05.11
    - plaque induced K05.10
  - lip K13.0
  - oral (mucosa) (soft tissue) K13.29
  - tongue K13.29
- learning (specific) —*see* Disorder, learning
- memory —*see* Amnesia
  - mild, following organic brain damage F06.8
- mental F99
  - associated with diseases classified elsewhere F54
- metabolism E88.9
  - with
    - abortion —*see* Abortion, by type with other specified complication
    - ectopic pregnancy O08.5
    - molar pregnancy O08.5
  - amino-acid E72.9
    - aromatic E70.9
    - branched-chain E71.2
    - straight-chain E72.8
    - sulfur-bearing E72.10
  - ammonia E72.20
  - arginine E72.21
  - arginosuccinic acid E72.22
  - carbohydrate E74.9
  - cholesterol E78.9
  - citrulline E72.23
  - cystathionine E72.19
  - general E88.9
  - glutamine E72.8
  - histidine E70.40
  - homocystine E72.19
  - hydroxylysine E72.3
  - in labor or delivery O75.89
  - iron E83.10
  - lipoid E78.9
  - lysine E72.3
  - methionine E72.19
  - neonatal, transitory P74.9
    - calcium and magnesium P71.9
      - specified type NEC P71.8

Disturbance *(Continued)*
- metabolism *(Continued)*
  - neonatal, transitory *(Continued)*
    - carbohydrate metabolism P70.9
      - specified type NEC P70.8
    - specified NEC P74.8
  - ornithine E72.4
  - phosphate E83.39
  - sodium NEC E87.8
  - threonine E72.8
  - tryptophan E70.5
  - tyrosine E70.20
  - urea cycle E72.20
- motor R29.2
- nervous, functional R45.0
- neuromuscular mechanism (eye), due to syphilis A52.15
- nutritional E63.9
  - nail L60.3
- ocular motion H51.9
  - psychogenic F45.8
- oculogyric H51.8
  - psychogenic F45.8
- oculomotor H51.9
  - psychogenic F45.8
- olfactory nerve R43.1
- optic nerve NEC —*see* Disorder, nerve, optic
- oral epithelium, including tongue NEC K13.29
- perceptual due to
  - alcohol withdrawal F10.232
  - amphetamine intoxication F15.922
    - in
      - abuse F15.122
      - dependence F15.222
  - anxiolytic withdrawal F13.232
  - cannabis intoxication (acute) F12.922
    - in
      - abuse F12.122
      - dependence F12.222
  - cocaine intoxication (acute) F14.922
    - in
      - abuse F14.122
      - dependence F14.222
  - hypnotic withdrawal F13.232
  - opioid intoxication (acute) F11.922
    - in
      - abuse F11.122
      - dependence F11.222
  - phencyclidine intoxication (acute) F16.122 ◄
    - ~~in~~
      - ~~abuse F19.122~~
      - ~~dependence F19.222~~
  - sedative withdrawal F13.232
- personality (pattern) (trait) —*see also* Disorder, personality F60.9
  - following organic brain damage F07.9
- polyglandular E31.9
  - specified NEC E31.8
- potassium balance, newborn P74.3
- psychogenic F45.9
- psychomotor F44.4
- psychophysical visual H53.16
- pupillary —*see* Anomaly, pupil, function
- reflex R29.2
- rhythm, heart I49.9
- salivary secretion K11.7
- sensation (cold) (heat) (localization) (tactile discrimination) (texture) (vibratory) NEC R20.9
  - hysterical F44.6
  - skin R20.9
    - anesthesia R20.0
    - hyperesthesia R20.3
    - hypoesthesia R20.1
    - paresthesia R20.2
    - specified type NEC R20.8
  - smell R43.9
    - and taste (mixed) R43.8
    - anosmia R43.0

Disturbance *(Continued)*
- sensation *(Continued)*
  - smell *(Continued)*
    - parosmia R43.1
    - specified NEC R43.8
  - taste R43.9
    - and smell (mixed) R43.8
    - parageusia R43.2
    - specified NEC R43.8
- sensory —*see* Disturbance, sensation
- situational (transient) —*see also* Disorder, adjustment
  - acute F43.0
- sleep G47.9
  - nonorganic origin F51.9
- smell —*see* Disturbance, sensation, smell
- sociopathic F60.2
- sodium balance, newborn P74.2
- speech R47.9
  - developmental F80.9
  - specified NEC R47.89
- stomach (functional) K31.9
- sympathetic (nerve) G90.9
- taste —*see* Disturbance, sensation, taste
- temperature
  - regulation, newborn P81.9
    - specified NEC P81.8
  - sense R20.8
    - hysterical F44.6
- tooth
  - eruption K00.6
  - formation K00.4
  - structure, hereditary NEC K00.5
- touch —*see* Disturbance, sensation
- vascular I99.9
  - arteriosclerotic —*see* Arteriosclerosis
- vasomotor I73.9
- vasospastic I73.9
- vision, visual H53.9
  - following
    - cerebral infarction I69.398
    - cerebrovascular disease I69.998
      - specified NEC I69.898
    - intracerebral hemorrhage I69.198
    - nontraumatic intracranial hemorrhage NEC I69.298
    - specified disease NEC I69.898
    - subarachnoid hemorrhage I69.098
  - psychophysical H53.16
  - specified NEC H53.8
  - subjective H53.10
    - day blindness H53.11
    - discomfort H53.14-
    - distortions of shape and size H53.15
    - loss
      - sudden H53.13-
      - transient H53.12-
    - specified type NEC H53.19
- voice R49.9
  - psychogenic F44.4
  - specified NEC R49.8

Diuresis R35.8

Diver's palsy, paralysis or squeeze T70.3

Diverticulitis (acute) K57.92
- bladder —*see* Cystitis
- ileum —*see* Diverticulitis, intestine, small
- intestine K57.92
  - with
    - abscess, perforation or peritonitis K57.80
      - with bleeding K57.81
    - bleeding K57.93
  - congenital Q43.8
  - large K57.32
    - with
      - abscess, perforation or peritonitis K57.20
        - with bleeding K57.21

D

- **Diverticulitis** *(Continued)*
  - intestine *(Continued)*
    - large *(Continued)*
      - with *(Continued)*
        - bleeding K57.33
        - small intestine K57.52
          - with
            - abscess, perforation or peritonitis K57.40
              - with bleeding K57.41
            - bleeding K57.53
    - small K57.12
      - with
        - abscess, perforation or peritonitis K57.00
          - with bleeding K57.01
        - bleeding K57.13
        - large intestine K57.52
          - with
            - abscess, perforation or peritonitis K57.40
              - with bleeding K57.41
            - bleeding K57.53
- **Diverticulosis** K57.90
  - with bleeding K57.91
  - large intestine K57.30
    - with
      - bleeding K57.31
      - small intestine K57.50
        - with bleeding K57.51
  - small intestine K57.10
    - with
      - bleeding K57.11
      - large intestine K57.50
        - with bleeding K57.51
- **Diverticulum, diverticula** (multiple) K57.90
  - appendix (noninflammatory) K38.2
  - bladder (sphincter) N32.3
    - congenital Q64.6
  - bronchus (congenital) Q32.4
    - acquired J98.09
  - calyx, calyceal (kidney) N28.89
  - cardia (stomach) K31.4
  - cecum —*see* Diverticulosis, intestine, large
    - congenital Q43.8
  - colon —*see* Diverticulosis, intestine, large
    - congenital Q43.8
  - duodenum —*see* Diverticulosis, intestine, small
    - congenital Q43.8
  - epiphrenic (esophagus) K22.5
  - esophagus (congenital) Q39.6
    - acquired (epiphrenic) (pulsion) (traction) K22.5
  - eustachian tube —*see* Disorder, eustachian tube, specified NEC
  - fallopian tube N83.8
  - gastric K31.4
  - heart (congenital) Q24.8
  - ileum —*see* Diverticulosis, intestine, small
  - jejunum —*see* Diverticulosis, intestine, small
  - kidney (pelvis) (calyces) N28.89
    - with calculus —*see* Calculus, kidney
  - Meckel's (displaced) (hypertrophic) Q43.0
    - malignant —*see* Table of Neoplasms, small intestine, malignant
  - midthoracic K22.5
  - organ or site, congenital NEC —*see* Distortion
  - pericardium (congenital) (cyst) Q24.8
    - acquired I31.8
  - pharyngoesophageal (congenital) Q39.6
    - acquired K22.5
  - pharynx (congenital) Q38.7
  - rectosigmoid —*see* Diverticulosis, intestine, large
    - congenital Q43.8
  - rectum —*see* Diverticulosis, intestine, large
  - Rokitansky's K22.5
  - seminal vesicle N50.89
  - sigmoid —*see* Diverticulosis, intestine, large
    - congenital Q43.8
- **Diverticulum, diverticula** *(Continued)*
  - stomach (acquired) K31.4
    - congenital Q40.2
  - trachea (acquired) J39.8
  - ureter (acquired) N28.89
    - congenital Q62.8
  - ureterovesical orifice N28.89
  - urethra (acquired) N36.1
    - congenital Q64.79
  - ventricle, left (congenital) Q24.8
  - vesical N32.3
    - congenital Q64.6
  - Zenker's (esophagus) K22.5
- **Division**
  - cervix uteri (acquired) N88.8
  - glans penis Q55.69
  - labia minora (congenital) Q52.79
  - ligament (partial or complete) (current) —*see also* Sprain
    - with open wound —*see* Wound, open
  - muscle (partial or complete) (current) —*see also* Injury, muscle
    - with open wound —*see* Wound, open
  - nerve (traumatic) —*see* Injury, nerve
  - spinal cord —*see* Injury, spinal cord, by region
  - vein I87.8
- **Divorce, causing family disruption** Z63.5
- **Dix-Hallpike neurolabyrinthitis** —*see* Neuronitis, vestibular
- **Dizziness** R42
  - hysterical F44.89
  - psychogenic F45.8
- **DMAC** (disseminated mycobacterium avium-intracellulare complex) A31.2
- **DNR** (do not resuscitate) Z66
- **Doan-Wiseman syndrome** (primary splenic neutropenia) —*see* Agranulocytosis
- **Doehle-Heller aortitis** A52.02
- **Dog bite** —*see* Bite
- **Dohle body panmyelopathic syndrome** D72.0
- **Dolichocephaly** Q67.2
- **Dolichocolon** Q43.8
- **Dolichostenomelia** —*see* Syndrome, Marfan's
- **Donohue's syndrome** E34.8
- **Donor** (organ or tissue) Z52.9
  - blood (whole) Z52.000
    - autologous Z52.010
    - specified component (lymphocytes) (platelets) NEC Z52.008
      - autologous Z52.018
      - specified donor NEC Z52.098
    - specified donor NEC Z52.090
    - stem cells Z52.001
      - autologous Z52.011
      - specified donor NEC Z52.091
  - bone Z52.20
    - autologous Z52.21
    - marrow Z52.3
    - specified type NEC Z52.29
  - cornea Z52.5
  - egg (Oocyte) Z52.819
    - age 35 and over Z52.812
      - anonymous recipient Z52.812
      - designated recipient Z52.813
    - under age 35 Z52.810
      - anonymous recipient Z52.810
      - designated recipient Z52.811
  - kidney Z52.4
  - liver Z52.6
  - lung Z52.89
  - lymphocyte —*see* Donor, blood, specified components NEC
  - Oocyte —*see* Donor, egg
  - platelets Z52.008
  - potential, examination of Z00.5
  - semen Z52.89
  - skin Z52.10
    - autologous Z52.11
    - specified type NEC Z52.19
- **Donor** *(Continued)*
  - specified organ or tissue NEC Z52.89
  - sperm Z52.89
- **Donovanosis** A58
- **Dorsalgia** M54.9
  - psychogenic F45.41
  - specified NEC M54.89
- **Dorsopathy** M53.9
  - deforming M43.9
    - specified NEC —*see* subcategory M43.8
  - specified NEC M53.80
    - cervical region M53.82
    - cervicothoracic region M53.83
    - lumbar region M53.86
    - lumbosacral region M53.87
    - occipito-atlanto-axial region M53.81
    - sacrococcygeal region M53.88
    - thoracic region M53.84
    - thoracolumbar region M53.85
- **Double**
  - albumin E88.09
  - aortic arch Q25.45
  - auditory canal Q17.8
  - auricle (heart) Q20.8
  - bladder Q64.79
  - cervix Q51.820
    - with doubling of uterus (and vagina) Q51.10
      - with obstruction Q51.11
  - inlet ventricle Q20.4
  - kidney with double pelvis (renal) Q63.0
  - meatus urinarius Q64.75
  - monster Q89.4
  - outlet
    - left ventricle Q20.2
    - right ventricle Q20.1
  - pelvis (renal) with double ureter Q62.5
  - tongue Q38.3
  - ureter (one or both sides) Q62.5
    - with double pelvis (renal) Q62.5
  - urethra Q64.74
  - urinary meatus Q64.75
  - uterus Q51.2
    - with
      - doubling of cervix (and vagina) Q51.10
        - with obstruction Q51.11
    - in pregnancy or childbirth O34.59-
      - causing obstructed labor O65.5
  - vagina Q52.10
    - with doubling of uterus (and cervix) Q51.10
      - with obstruction Q51.11
  - vision H53.2
  - vulva Q52.79
- **Douglas' pouch, cul-de-sac** —*see* condition
- **Down syndrome** Q90.9
  - meiotic nondisjunction Q90.0
  - mitotic nondisjunction Q90.1
  - mosaicism Q90.1
  - translocation Q90.2
- **DPD** (dihydropyrimidine dehydrogenase deficiency) E88.89
- **Dracontiasis** B72
- **Dracunculiasis, dracunculosis** B72
- **Dream state, hysterical** F44.89
- **Drepanocytic anemia** —*see* Disease, sickle-cell
- **Dresbach's syndrome** (elliptocytosis) D58.1
- **Dreschlera** (hawaiiensis) (infection) B43.8
- **Dressler's syndrome** I24.1
- **Drift, ulnar** —*see* Deformity, limb, specified type NEC, forearm
- **Drinking** (alcohol)
  - excessive, to excess NEC (without dependence) F10.10
    - habitual (continual) (without remission) F10.20
      - with remission F10.21
- **Drip, postnasal** (chronic) R09.82
  - due to
    - allergic rhinitis —*see* Rhinitis, allergic
    - common cold J00

Drip, postnasal *(Continued)*
due to *(Continued)*
gastroesophageal reflux —*see* Reflux, gastroesophageal
nasopharyngitis —*see* Nasopharyngitis
other known condition — code to condition
sinusitis —*see* Sinusitis
Droop
facial R29.81Ø
cerebrovascular disease I69.992
cerebral infarction I69.392
intracerebral hemorrhage I69.192
nontraumatic intracranial hemorrhage NEC I69.292
specified disease NEC I69.892
subarachnoid hemorrhage I69.Ø92
Drop (in)
attack NEC R55
finger —*see* Deformity, finger
foot —*see* Deformity, limb, foot, drop
hematocrit (precipitous) R71.Ø
hemoglobin R71.Ø
toe —*see* Deformity, toe, specified NEC
wrist —*see* Deformity, limb, wrist drop
Dropped heart beats I45.9
Dropsy, dropsical —*see also* Hydrops
abdomen R18.8
brain —*see* Hydrocephalus
cardiac, heart —*see* Failure, heart, congestive
gangrenous —*see* Gangrene
heart —*see* Failure, heart, congestive
kidney —*see* Nephrosis
lung —*see* Edema, lung
newborn due to isoimmunization P56.Ø
pericardium —*see* Pericarditis
Drowned, drowning (near) T75.1
Drowsiness R4Ø.Ø
Drug
abuse counseling and surveillance Z71.51
addiction —*see* Dependence
dependence —*see* Dependence
habit —*see* Dependence
harmful use —*see* Abuse, drug
induced fever R5Ø.2
overdose —*see* Table of Drugs and Chemicals, by drug, poisoning
poisoning —*see* Table of Drugs and Chemicals, by drug, poisoning
resistant organism infection —*see also* Resistant, organism, to, drug Z16.3Ø
therapy
long term (current) (prophylactic) —*see* Therapy, drug long-term (current) (prophylactic)
short term - omit code
wrong substance given or taken in error —*see* Table of Drugs and Chemicals, by drug, poisoning
Drunkenness (without dependence) F1Ø.129
acute in alcoholism F1Ø.229
chronic (without remission) F1Ø.2Ø
with remission F1Ø.21
pathological (without dependence) F1Ø.129
with dependence F1Ø.229
sleep F51.9
Drusen
macula (degenerative) (retina) —*see* Degeneration, macula, drusen
optic disc H47.32-
Dry, dryness —*see also* condition
larynx J38.7
mouth R68.2
due to dehydration E86.Ø
nose J34.89
socket (teeth) M27.3
throat J39.2
DSAP L56.5
Duane's syndrome H5Ø.81-
Dubin-Johnson disease or syndrome E8Ø.6
Dubois' disease (thymus gland) A5Ø.59 *[E35]*
Dubowitz' syndrome Q87.1
Duchenne-Aran muscular atrophy G12.21
Duchenne-Griesinger disease G71.Ø
Duchenne's
disease or syndrome
motor neuron disease G12.22
muscular dystrophy G71.Ø
locomotor ataxia (syphilitic) A52.11
paralysis
birth injury P14.Ø
due to or associated with
motor neuron disease G12.22
muscular dystrophy G71.Ø
Ducrey's chancre A57
Duct, ductus —*see* condition
Duhring's disease (dermatitis herpetiformis) L13.Ø
Dullness, cardiac (decreased) (increased) RØ1.2
Dumb ague —*see* Malaria
Dumbness —*see* Aphasia
Dumdum fever B55.Ø
Dumping syndrome (postgastrectomy) K91.1
Duodenitis (nonspecific) (peptic) K29.8Ø
with bleeding K29.81
Duodenocholangitis —*see* Cholangitis
Duodenum, duodenal —*see* condition
Duplay's bursitis or periarthritis —*see* Tendinitis, calcific, shoulder
Duplication, duplex —*see also* Accessory
alimentary tract Q45.8
anus Q43.4
appendix (and cecum) Q43.4
biliary duct (any) Q44.5
bladder Q64.79
cecum (and appendix) Q43.4
cervix Q51.82Ø
chromosome NEC
with complex rearrangements NEC Q92.5
seen only at prometaphase Q92.8
cystic duct Q44.5
digestive organs Q45.8
esophagus Q39.8
frontonasal process Q75.8
intestine (large) (small) Q43.4
kidney Q63.Ø
liver Q44.7
pancreas Q45.3
penis Q55.69
respiratory organs NEC Q34.8
salivary duct Q38.4
spinal cord (incomplete) QØ6.2
stomach Q4Ø.2
Dupré's disease (meningism) R29.1
Dupuytren's contraction or disease M72.Ø
Durand-Nicolas-Favre disease A55
Durotomy (inadvertent) (incidental) G97.41
Duroziez's disease (congenital mitral stenosis) Q23.2
Dutton's relapsing fever (West African) A68.1
Dwarfism E34.3
achondroplastic Q77.4
congenital E34.3
constitutional E34.3
hypochondroplastic Q77.4
hypophyseal E23.Ø
infantile E34.3
Laron-type E34.3
Lorain (-Levi) type E23.Ø
metatropic Q77.8
nephrotic-glycosuric (with hypophosphatemic rickets) E72.Ø9
nutritional E45
pancreatic K86.89 ◄
pituitary E23.Ø
renal N25.Ø
thanatophoric Q77.1
Dyke-Young anemia (secondary) (symptomatic) D59.1
Dysacusis —*see* Abnormal, auditory perception
Dysadrenocortism E27.9
hyperfunction E27.Ø
Dysarthria R47.1
following
cerebral infarction I69.322
cerebrovascular disease I69.922
specified disease NEC I69.822
intracerebral hemorrhage I69.122
nontraumatic intracranial hemorrhage NEC I69.222
subarachnoid hemorrhage I69.Ø22
Dysautonomia (familial) G9Ø.1
Dysbarism T7Ø.3
Dysbasia R26.2
angiosclerotica intermittens I73.9
hysterical F44.4
lordotica (progressiva) G24.1
nonorganic origin F44.4
psychogenic F44.4
Dysbetalipoproteinemia (familial) E78.2
Dyscalculia R48.8
developmental F81.2
Dyschezia K59.ØØ
Dyschondroplasia (with hemangiomata) Q78.4
Dyschromia (skin) L81.9
Dyscollagenosis M35.9
Dyscranio-pygo-phalangy Q87.Ø
Dyscrasia
blood (with) D75.9
antepartum hemorrhage —*see* Hemorrhage, antepartum, with coagulation defect
intrapartum hemorrhage O67.Ø
newborn P61.9
specified type NEC P61.8
puerperal, postpartum O72.3
polyglandular, pluriglandular E31.9
Dysendocrinism E34.9
Dysentery, dysenteric (catarrhal) (diarrhea) (epidemic) (hemorrhagic) (infectious) (sporadic) (tropical) AØ9
abscess, liver AØ6.4
amebic —*see also* Amebiasis AØ6.Ø
with abscess —*see* Abscess, amebic
acute AØ6.Ø
chronic AØ6.1
arthritis —*see also* category MØ1 AØ9
bacillary —*see also* category MØ1 AØ3.9
bacillary AØ3.9
arthritis —*see also* category MØ1 AØ3.9
Boyd AØ3.2
Flexner AØ3.1
Schmitz (-Stutzer) AØ3.Ø
Shiga (-Kruse) AØ3.Ø
Shigella AØ3.9
boydii AØ3.2
dysenteriae AØ3.Ø
flexneri AØ3.1
group A AØ3.Ø
group B AØ3.1
group C AØ3.2
group D AØ3.3
sonnei AØ3.3
specified type NEC AØ3.8
Sonne AØ3.3
specified type NEC AØ3.8
balantidial AØ7.Ø
Balantidium coli AØ7.Ø
Boyd's AØ3.2
candidal B37.82
Chilomastix AØ7.8
Chinese AØ3.9
coccidial AØ7.3
Dientamoeba (fragilis) AØ7.8
Embadomonas AØ7.8
Entamoeba, entamebic —*see* Dysentery, amebic
Flexner-Boyd AØ3.2
Flexner's AØ3.1

Dysfunction *(Continued)*
symbolic R48.9
specified type NEC R48.8
temporomandibular (joint) M26.69
joint-pain syndrome M26.62- ←
testicular (endocrine) E29.9
specified NEC E29.8
thymus E32.9
thyroid E07.9
ureterostomy (stoma) *—see* Complications, stoma, urinary tract
urethrostomy (stoma) *—see* Complications, stoma, urinary tract
uterus, complicating delivery O62.9
hypertonic O62.4
hypotonic O62.2
primary O62.0
secondary O62.1
ventricular I51.9
with congestive heart failure I50.9-
left, reversible, following sudden emotional stress I51.81
Dysgenesis
gonadal (due to chromosomal anomaly) Q96.9
pure Q99.1
renal Q60.5
bilateral Q60.4
unilateral Q60.3
reticular D72.0
tidal platelet D69.3
Dysgerminoma
specified site *—see* Neoplasm, malignant, by site
unspecified site
female C56.9
male C62.90
Dysgeusia R43.2
Dysgraphia R27.8
Dyshidrosis, dysidrosis L30.1
Dyskaryotic cervical smear R87.619
Dyskeratosis L85.8
cervix *—see* Dysplasia, cervix
congenital Q82.8
uterus NEC N85.8
Dyskinesia G24.9
biliary (cystic duct or gallbladder) K82.8
drug induced
orofacial G24.01
esophagus K22.4
hysterical F44.4
intestinal K59.8
nonorganic origin F44.4
orofacial (idiopathic) G24.4
drug induced G24.01
psychogenic F44.4
subacute, drug induced G24.01
tardive G24.01
neuroleptic induced G24.01
trachea J39.8
tracheobronchial J98.09
Dyslalia (developmental) F80.0
Dyslexia R48.0
developmental F81.0
Dyslipidemia E78.5
depressed HDL cholesterol E78.6
elevated fasting triglycerides E78.1
Dysmaturity *—see also* Light for dates
pulmonary (newborn) (Wilson-Mikity) P27.0
Dysmenorrhea (essential) (exfoliative) N94.6
congestive (syndrome) N94.6
primary N94.4
psychogenic F45.8
secondary N94.5
Dysmetabolic syndrome X E88.81
Dysmetria R27.8
Dysmorphism (due to)
alcohol Q86.0
exogenous cause NEC Q86.8
hydantoin Q86.1
warfarin Q86.2
Dysmorphophobia (nondelusional) F45.22
delusional F22
Dysnomia R47.01
Dysorexia R63.0
psychogenic F50.89 ←
Dysostosis
cleidocranial, cleidocranialis Q74.0
craniofacial Q75.1
Fairbank's (idiopathic familial generalized osteophytosis) Q78.9
mandibulofacial (incomplete) Q75.4
multiplex E76.01
oculomandibular Q75.5
Dyspareunia (female) N94.10 ←
deep N94.12 ◀
male N53.12
nonorganic F52.6
psychogenic F52.6
secondary N94.19 ←
specified NEC N94.19 ◀
superficial (introital) N94.11 ◀
Dyspepsia R10.13
atonic K30
functional (allergic) (congenital) (gastrointestinal) (occupational) (reflex) K30
intestinal K59.8
nervous F45.8
neurotic F45.8
psychogenic F45.8
Dysphagia R13.10
cervical R13.19
following
cerebral infarction I69.391
cerebrovascular disease I69.991
specified NEC I69.891
intracerebral hemorrhage I69.191
nontraumatic intracranial hemorrhage NEC I69.291
specified disease NEC I69.891
subarachnoid hemorrhage I69.091
functional (hysterical) F45.8
hysterical F45.8
nervous (hysterical) F45.8
neurogenic R13.19
oral phase R13.11
oropharyngeal phase R13.12
pharyngeal phase R13.13
pharyngoesophageal phase R13.14
psychogenic F45.8
sideropenic D50.1
spastica K22.4
specified NEC R13.19
Dysphagocytosis, congenital D71
Dysphasia R47.02
developmental
expressive type F80.1
receptive type F80.2
following
cerebrovascular disease I69.921
cerebral infarction I69.321
intracerebral hemorrhage I69.121
nontraumatic intracranial hemorrhage NEC I69.221
specified disease NEC I69.821
subarachnoid hemorrhage I69.021
Dysphonia R49.0
functional F44.4
hysterical F44.4
psychogenic F44.4
spastica J38.3
~~Dysphoria, postpartal O90.6~~
Dysphoria ◀
gender ◀
in ◀
adolescence and adulthood F64.0 ◀
children F64.2 ◀
postpartal O90.6 ◀
Dyspituitarism E23.3
Dysplasia *—see also* Anomaly
acetabular, congenital Q65.89
alveolar capillary, with vein misalignment J84.843
anus (histologically confirmed) (mild) (moderate) K62.82
severe D01.3
arrhythmogenic right ventricular I42.8
arterial, fibromuscular I77.3
asphyxiating thoracic (congenital) Q77.2
brain Q07.9
bronchopulmonary, perinatal P27.1
cervix (uteri) N87.9
mild N87.0
moderate N87.1
severe D06.9
chondroectodermal Q77.6
colon D12.6
craniometaphyseal Q78.58 ←
dentinal K00.5
diaphyseal, progressive Q78.3
dystrophic Q77.5
ectodermal (anhidrotic) (congenital) (hereditary) Q82.4
hydrotic Q82.8
epithelial, uterine cervix *—see* Dysplasia, cervix
eye (congenital) Q11.2
fibrous
bone NEC (monostotic) M85.00
ankle M85.07-
foot M85.07-
forearm M85.03-
hand M85.04-
lower leg M85.06-
multiple site M85.09
neck M85.08
rib M85.08
shoulder M85.01-
skull M85.08
specified site NEC M85.08
thigh M85.05-
toe M85.07-
upper arm M85.02-
vertebra M85.08
diaphyseal, progressive Q78.3
jaw M27.8
polyostotic Q78.1
florid osseous *—see also* Cyst, calcifying odontogenic
high grade, focal D12.6
hip, congenital Q65.89
joint, congenital Q74.8
kidney Q61.4
multicystic Q61.4
leg Q74.2
lung, congenital (not associated with short gestation) Q33.6
mammary (gland) (benign) N60.9-
cyst (solitary) *—see* Cyst, breast
cystic *—see* Mastopathy, cystic
duct ectasia *—see* Ectasia, mammary duct
fibroadenosis *—see* Fibroadenosis, breast
fibrosclerosis *—see* Fibrosclerosis, breast
specified type NEC N60.8-
metaphyseal Q78.5 ←
muscle Q79.8
oculodentodigital Q87.0
periapical (cemental) (cemento-osseous) *—see* Cyst, calcifying odontogenic
periosteum *—see* Disorder, bone, specified type NEC
polyostotic fibrous Q78.1
prostate *—see also* Neoplasia, intraepithelial, prostate N42.30 ←
severe D07.5
specified NEC N42.39 ◀
renal Q61.4
multicystic Q61.4
retinal, congenital Q14.1

D

Dysplasia *(Continued)*
right ventricular, arrhythmogenic I42.8
septo-optic Q04.4
skin L98.8
spinal cord Q06.1
spondyloepiphyseal Q77.7
thymic, with immunodeficiency D82.1
vagina N89.3
mild N89.0
moderate N89.1
severe NEC D07.2
vulva N90.3
mild N90.0
moderate N90.1
severe NEC D07.1
Dyspnea (nocturnal) (paroxysmal) R06.00
asthmatic (bronchial) J45.909
with
bronchitis J45.909
with
exacerbation (acute) J45.901
status asthmaticus J45.902
chronic J44.9
exacerbation (acute) J45.901
status asthmaticus J45.902
cardiac —*see* Failure, ventricular, left
cardiac —*see* Failure, ventricular, left
functional F45.8
hyperventilation R06.4
hysterical F45.8
newborn P28.89
psychogenic F45.8
shortness of breath R06.02
specified type NEC R06.09
Dyspraxia R27.8
developmental (syndrome) F82
Dysproteinemia E88.09
Dysreflexia, autonomic G90.4
Dysrhythmia
cardiac I49.9
newborn
bradycardia P29.12
occurring before birth P03.819
before onset of labor P03.810
during labor P03.811
tachycardia P29.11
postoperative I97.89
cerebral or cortical —*see* Epilepsy
Dyssomnia —*see* Disorder, sleep
Dyssynergia
biliary K83.8
bladder sphincter N36.44
cerebellaris myoclonica (Hunt's ataxia) G11.1
Dysthymia F34.1
Dysthyroidism E07.9
Dystocia O66.9
affecting newborn P03.1
cervical (hypotonic) O62.2
affecting newborn P03.6
primary O62.0
secondary O62.1
contraction ring O62.4
Dystocia *(Continued)*
fetal O66.9
abnormality NEC O66.3
conjoined twins O66.3
oversize O66.2
maternal O66.9
positional O64.9
shoulder (girdle) O66.0
causing obstructed labor O66.0
uterine NEC O62.4
Dystonia G24.9
deformans progressiva G24.1
drug induced NEC G24.09
acute G24.02
specified NEC G24.09
familial G24.1
idiopathic G24.1
familial G24.1
nonfamilial G24.2
orofacial G24.4
lenticularis G24.8
musculorum deformans G24.1
neuroleptic induced (acute) G24.02
orofacial (idiopathic) G24.4
oromandibular G24.4
due to drug G24.01
specified NEC G24.8
torsion (familial) (idiopathic) G24.1
acquired G24.8
genetic G24.1
symptomatic (nonfamilial) G24.2
Dystonic movements R25.8
Dystrophy, dystrophia
adiposogenital E23.6
Becker's type G71.0
cervical sympathetic G90.2
choroid (hereditary) H31.20
central areolar H31.22
choroideremia H31.21
gyrate atrophy H31.23
specified type NEC H31.29
cornea (hereditary) H18.50
endothelial H18.51
epithelial H18.52
granular H18.53
lattice H18.54
macular H18.55
specified type NEC H18.59
Duchenne's type G71.0
due to malnutrition E45
Erb's G71.0
Fuchs' H18.51
Gower's muscular G71.0
hair L67.8
infantile neuraxonal G31.89
Landouzy-Déjérine G71.0
Leyden-Möbius G71.0
muscular G71.0
benign (Becker type) G71.0
congenital (hereditary) (progressive) (with specific morphological abnormalities of the muscle fiber) G71.0
myotonic G71.11
Dystrophy, dystrophia *(Continued)*
muscular *(Continued)*
distal G71.0
Duchenne type G71.0
Emery-Dreifuss G71.0
Erb type G71.0
facioscapulohumeral G71.0
Gower's G71.0
hereditary (progressive) G71.0
Landouzy-Déjérine type G71.0
limb-girdle G71.0
myotonic G71.11
progressive (hereditary) G71.0
Charcot-Marie (-Tooth) type G60.0
pseudohypertrophic (infantile) G71.0
severe (Duchenne type) G71.0
myocardium, myocardial —*see* Degeneration, myocardial
nail L60.3
congenital Q84.6
nutritional E45
ocular G71.0
oculocerebrorenal E72.03
oculopharyngeal G71.0
ovarian N83.8
polyglandular E31.8
reflex (neuromuscular) (sympathetic) —*see* Syndrome, pain, complex regional I
retinal (hereditary) H35.50
in
lipid storage disorders E75.6 *[H36]*
systemic lipidoses E75.6 *[H36]*
involving
pigment epithelium H35.54
sensory area H35.53
pigmentary H35.52
vitreoretinal H35.51
Salzmann's nodular —*see* Degeneration, cornea, nodular
scapuloperoneal G71.0
skin NEC L98.8
sympathetic (reflex) —*see* Syndrome, pain, complex regional I
cervical G90.2
tapetoretinal H35.54
thoracic, asphyxiating Q77.2
unguium L60.3
congenital Q84.6
vitreoretinal H35.51
vulva N90.4
yellow (liver) —*see* Failure, hepatic
Dysuria R30.0
psychogenic F45.8

D

E

- **Eales' disease** H35.Ø6-
- **Ear** —*see also* condition
  - piercing Z41.3
  - ~~tropical B36.8~~
  - tropical NEC B36.9 *[H62.4Ø]* ◀
  - in ◀
    - aspergillosis B44.89 ◀
    - candidiasis B37.84 ◀
    - moniliasis B37.84 ◀
  - wax (impacted) H61.2Ø
    - left H61.22
      - with right H61.23
    - right H61.21
      - with left H61.23
- **Earache** —*see* subcategory H92.Ø
- **Early satiety** R68.81
- **Eaton-Lambert syndrome**—*see* Syndrome, Lambert-Eaton
- **Eberth's disease** (typhoid fever) AØ1.ØØ
- **Ebola virus disease** A98.4
- **Ebstein's** anomaly or syndrome (heart) Q22.5
- **Eccentro-osteochondrodysplasia** E76.29
- **Ecchondroma** —*see* Neoplasm, bone, benign
- **Ecchondrosis** D48.Ø
- **Ecchymosis** R58
  - conjunctiva —*see* Hemorrhage, conjunctiva
  - eye (traumatic) —*see* Contusion, eyeball
  - eyelid (traumatic) —*see* Contusion, eyelid
  - newborn P54.5
  - spontaneous R23.3
  - traumatic —*see* Contusion
- **Echinococciasis** —*see* Echinococcus
- **Echinococcosis** —*see* Echinococcus
- **Echinococcus** (infection) B67.9Ø
  - granulosus B67.4
    - bone B67.2
    - liver B67.Ø
    - lung B67.1
    - multiple sites B67.32
    - specified site NEC B67.39
    - thyroid B67.31 ⬅
  - liver NOS B67.8
    - granulosus B67.Ø
    - multilocularis B67.5
  - lung NEC B67.99
    - granulosus B67.1
    - multilocularis B67.69
  - multilocularis B67.7
    - liver B67.5
    - multiple sites B67.61
    - specified site NEC B67.69
  - specified site NEC B67.99
    - granulosus B67.39
    - multilocularis B67.69
  - thyroid NEC B67.99
    - granulosus B67.31 ⬅
    - multilocularis B67.69 *[E35]*
- **Echinorhynchiasis** B83.8
- **Echinostomiasis** B66.8
- **Echolalia** R48.8
- **Echovirus**, as cause of disease classified elsewhere B97.12
- **Eclampsia, eclamptic** (coma) (convulsions) (delirium) (with hypertension) NEC O15.9
  - complicating ◀
    - labor and delivery O15.1 ◀
    - postpartum O15.2 ◀
    - pregnancy O15.Ø- ◀
    - puerperium O15.2 ◀
  - ~~during labor and delivery O15.1~~
  - ~~postpartum O15.2~~
  - ~~pregnancy O15.Ø-~~
  - ~~puerperal O15.2~~
- **Economic circumstances affecting care** Z59.9
- **Economo's disease** A85.8
- **Ectasia, ectasis**
  - annuloaortic I35.8
  - aorta I77.819
    - with aneurysm —*see* Aneurysm, aorta
    - abdominal I77.811

- **Ectasia, ectasis** *(Continued)*
  - aorta *(Continued)*
    - thoracic I77.81Ø
    - thoracoabdominal I77.812
  - breast —*see* Ectasia, mammary duct
  - capillary I78.8
  - cornea H18.71-
  - gastric antral vascular (GAVE) K31.819
    - with hemorrhage K31.811
    - without hemorrhage K31.819
  - mammary duct N6Ø.4-
  - salivary gland (duct) K11.8
  - sclera —*see* Sclerectasia
- **Ecthyma** LØ8.Ø
  - contagiosum BØ8.Ø2
  - gangrenosum LØ8.Ø
  - infectiosum BØ8.Ø2
- **Ectocardia** Q24.8
- **Ectodermal dysplasia** (anhidrotic) Q82.4
- **Ectodermosis erosiva pluriorificialis** L51.1
- **Ectopic, ectopia** (congenital)
  - abdominal viscera Q45.8
    - due to defect in anterior abdominal wall Q79.59
  - ACTH syndrome E24.3
  - adrenal gland Q89.1
  - anus Q43.5
  - atrial beats I49.1
  - beats I49.49
    - atrial I49.1
    - ventricular I49.3
  - bladder Q64.1Ø
  - bone and cartilage in lung Q33.5
  - brain QØ4.8
  - breast tissue Q83.8
  - cardiac Q24.8
  - cerebral QØ4.8
  - cordis Q24.8
  - endometrium —*see* Endometriosis
  - gastric mucosa Q4Ø.2
  - gestation —*see* Pregnancy, by site
  - heart Q24.8
  - hormone secretion NEC E34.2
  - kidney (crossed) (pelvis) Q63.2
  - lens, lentis Q12.1
  - mole —*see* Pregnancy, by site
  - organ or site NEC —*see* Malposition, congenital
  - pancreas Q45.3
  - pregnancy —*see* Pregnancy, ectopic
  - pupil —*see* Abnormality, pupillary
  - renal Q63.2
  - sebaceous glands of mouth Q38.6
  - spleen Q89.Ø9
  - testis Q53.ØØ
    - bilateral Q53.Ø2
    - unilateral Q53.Ø1
  - thyroid Q89.2
  - tissue in lung Q33.5
  - ureter Q62.63
  - ventricular beats I49.3
  - vesicae Q64.1Ø
- **Ectromelia** Q73.8
  - lower limb —*see* Defect, reduction, limb, lower, specified type NEC
  - upper limb —*see* Defect, reduction, limb, upper, specified type NEC
- **Ectropion** HØ2.1Ø9
  - cervix N86
    - with cervicitis N72
  - congenital Q1Ø.1
  - eyelid (paralytic) HØ2.1Ø9
    - cicatricial HØ2.119
      - left HØ2.116
        - lower HØ2.115
        - upper HØ2.114
      - right HØ2.113
        - lower HØ2.112
        - upper HØ2.111
    - congenital Q1Ø.1

- **Ectropion** *(Continued)*
  - eyelid *(Continued)*
    - left HØ2.1Ø6
      - lower HØ2.1Ø5
      - upper HØ2.1Ø4
    - mechanical HØ2.129
      - left HØ2.126
        - lower HØ2.125
        - upper HØ2.124
      - right HØ2.123
        - lower HØ2.122
        - upper HØ2.121
    - right HØ2.1Ø3
      - lower HØ2.1Ø2
      - upper HØ2.1Ø1
    - senile HØ2.139
      - left HØ2.136
        - lower HØ2.135
        - upper HØ2.134
      - right HØ2.133
        - lower HØ2.132
        - upper HØ2.131
    - spastic HØ2.149
      - left HØ2.146
        - lower HØ2.145
        - upper HØ2.144
      - right HØ2.143
        - lower HØ2.142
        - upper HØ2.141
  - iris H21.89
  - lip (acquired) K13.Ø
    - congenital Q38.Ø
  - urethra N36.8
  - uvea H21.89
- **Eczema** (acute) (chronic) (erythematous) (fissum) (rubrum) (squamous) (*see also* Dermatitis) L3Ø.9
  - contact —*see* Dermatitis, contact
  - dyshydrotic L3Ø.1
  - external ear —*see* Otitis, externa, acute, eczematoid
  - flexural L2Ø.82
  - herpeticum BØØ.Ø
  - hypertrophicum L28.Ø
  - hypostatic —*see* Varix, leg, with, inflammation
  - impetiginous LØ1.1
  - infantile (due to any substance) L2Ø.83
    - intertriginous L21.1
    - seborrheic L21.1
  - intertriginous NEC L3Ø.4
    - infantile L21.1
  - intrinsic (allergic) L2Ø.84
  - lichenified NEC L28.Ø
  - marginatum (hebrae) B35.6
  - pustular L3Ø.3
  - stasis I87.2 ⬅
    - with varicose veins —*see* Varix, leg, with, inflammation ◀
  - vaccination, vaccinatum T88.1
  - varicose —*see* Varix, leg, with, inflammation
- **Eczematid** L3Ø.2
- **Eddowes** (-Spurway) **syndrome** Q78.Ø
- **Edema, edematous** (infectious) (pitting) (toxic) R6Ø.9
  - with nephritis —*see* Nephrosis
  - allergic T78.3
  - amputation stump (surgical) (sequelae (late effect)) T87.89
  - angioneurotic (allergic) (any site) (with urticaria) T78.3
    - hereditary D84.1
  - angiospastic I73.9
  - Berlin's (traumatic) SØ5.8X-
  - brain (cytotoxic) (vasogenic) G93.6
    - due to birth injury P11.Ø
    - newborn (anoxia or hypoxia) P52.4
      - birth injury P11.Ø
    - traumatic —*see* Injury, intracranial, cerebral edema
  - cardiac —*see* Failure, heart, congestive

Edema, edematous *(Continued)*
cardiovascular —*see* Failure, heart, congestive
cerebral —*see* Edema, brain
cerebrospinal —*see* Edema, brain
cervix (uteri) (acute) N88.8
puerperal, postpartum O9Ø.89
chronic hereditary Q82.Ø
circumscribed, acute T78.3
hereditary D84.1
conjunctiva H11.42-
cornea H18.2-
idiopathic H18.22-
secondary H18.23-
due to contact lens H18.21-
due to
lymphatic obstruction I89.Ø
salt retention E87.Ø
epiglottis —*see* Edema, glottis
essential, acute T78.3
hereditary D84.1
extremities, lower —*see* Edema, legs
eyelid NEC HØ2.849
left HØ2.846
lower HØ2.845
upper HØ2.844
right HØ2.843
lower HØ2.842
upper HØ2.841
familial, hereditary Q82.Ø
famine —*see* Malnutrition, severe
generalized R6Ø.1
glottis, glottic, glottidis (obstructive) (passive) J38.4
allergic T78.3
hereditary D84.1
heart —*see* Failure, heart, congestive
heat T67.7
hereditary Q82.Ø
inanition —*see* Malnutrition, severe
intracranial G93.6
iris H21.89
joint —*see* Effusion, joint
larynx —*see* Edema, glottis
legs R6Ø.Ø
due to venous obstruction I87.1
hereditary Q82.Ø
localized R6Ø.Ø
due to venous obstruction I87.1
lower limbs —*see* Edema, legs
lung J81.1
with heart condition or failure —*see* Failure, ventricular, left
acute J81.Ø
chemical (acute) J68.1
chronic J68.1
chronic J81.1
due to
chemicals, gases, fumes or vapors (inhalation) J68.1
external agent J7Ø.9
specified NEC J7Ø.8
radiation J7Ø.1
due to
chemicals, fumes or vapors (inhalation) J68.1
external agent J7Ø.9
specified NEC J7Ø.8
high altitude T7Ø.29
near drowning T75.1
radiation J7Ø.Ø
meaning failure, left ventricle I5Ø.1
lymphatic I89.Ø
due to mastectomy I97.2
macula H35.81
cystoid, following cataract surgery —*see* Complications, postprocedural, following cataract surgery
diabetic —*see* Diabetes, by type, with, retinopathy, with macular edema
malignant —*see* Gangrene, gas
Milroy's Q82.Ø

Edema, edematous *(Continued)*
nasopharynx J39.2
newborn P83.3Ø
hydrops fetalis —*see* Hydrops, fetalis
specified NEC P83.39
nutritional —*see also* Malnutrition, severe
with dyspigmentation, skin and hair E4Ø
optic disc or nerve —*see* Papilledema
orbit HØ5.22-
pancreas K86.89 ⬅
papilla, optic —*see* Papilledema
penis N48.89
periodic T78.3
hereditary D84.1
pharynx J39.2
pulmonary —*see* Edema, lung
Quincke's T78.3
hereditary D84.1
renal —*see* Nephrosis
retina H35.81
diabetic —*see* Diabetes, by type, with, retinopathy, with macular edema
salt E87.Ø
scrotum N5Ø.89 ⬅
seminal vesicle N5Ø.89 ⬅
spermatic cord N5Ø.89 ⬅
spinal (cord) (vascular) (nontraumatic) G95.19
starvation —*see* Malnutrition, severe
stasis —*see* Hypertension, venous, (chronic)
subglottic —*see* Edema, glottis
supraglottic —*see* Edema, glottis
testis N44.8
tunica vaginalis N5Ø.89 ⬅
vas deferens N5Ø.89 ⬅
vulva (acute) N9Ø.89
Edentulism —*see* Absence, teeth, acquired
Edsall's disease T67.2
Educational handicap Z55.9
specified NEC Z55.8
Edward's syndrome —*see* Trisomy, 18
Effect, adverse
abnormal gravitational (G) forces or states T75.81
abuse —*see* Maltreatment
air pressure T7Ø.9
specified NEC T7Ø.8
altitude (high) —*see* Effect, adverse, high altitude
anesthesia —*see also* Anesthesia T88.59
in labor and delivery O74.9
~~in pregnancy NEC O29.3-~~
local, toxic
in labor and delivery O74.4-
in pregnancy NEC O29.3- ◀
postpartum, puerperal O89.3
postpartum, puerperal O89.9
specified NEC T88.59
in labor and delivery O74.8
postpartum, puerperal O89.8
spinal and epidural T88.59
headache T88.59
in labor and delivery O74.5
postpartum, puerperal O89.4
specified NEC
in labor and delivery O74.6
postpartum, puerperal O89.5
antitoxin —*see* Complications, vaccination
atmospheric pressure T7Ø.9
due to explosion T7Ø.8
high T7Ø.3
low —*see* Effect, adverse, high altitude
specified effect NEC T7Ø.8
biological, correct substance properly administered —*see* Effect, adverse, drug
blood (derivatives) (serum) (transfusion) —*see* Complications, transfusion
chemical substance —*see* Table of Drugs and Chemicals
cold (temperature) (weather) T69.9
chilblains T69.1
frostbite —*see* Frostbite
specified effect NEC T69.8

Effect, adverse *(Continued)*
drugs and medicaments T88.7
specified drug —*see* Table of Drugs and Chemicals, by drug, adverse effect
specified effect — code to condition
electric current, electricity (shock) T75.4
burn —*see* Burn
exertion (excessive) T73.3
exposure —*see* Exposure
external cause NEC T75.89
foodstuffs T78.1
allergic reaction —*see* Allergy, food
causing anaphylaxis —*see* Shock, anaphylactic, due to food
noxious —*see* Poisoning, food, noxious
gases, fumes, or vapors T59.9-
specified agent —*see* Table of Drugs and Chemicals
glue (airplane) sniffing
due to drug abuse —*see* Abuse, drug, inhalant
due to drug dependence —*see* Dependence, drug, inhalant
heat —*see* Heat
high altitude NEC T7Ø.29
anoxia T7Ø.29
on
ears T7Ø.Ø
sinuses T7Ø.1
polycythemia D75.1
high pressure fluids T7Ø.4
hot weather —*see* Heat
hunger T73.Ø
immersion, foot —*see* Immersion
immunization —*see* Complications, vaccination
immunological agents —*see* Complications, vaccination
infrared (radiation) (rays) NOS T66
dermatitis or eczema L59.8
infusion —*see* Complications, infusion
lack of care of infants —*see* Maltreatment, child
lightning —*see* Lightning
medical care T88.9
specified NEC T88.8
medicinal substance, correct, properly administered —*see* Effect, adverse, drug
motion T75.3
noise, on inner ear —*see* subcategory H83.3
overheated places —*see* Heat
psychosocial, of work environment Z56.5
radiation (diagnostic) (infrared) (natural source) (therapeutic) (ultraviolet) (X-ray) NOS T66
dermatitis or eczema —*see* Dermatitis, due to, radiation
fibrosis of lung J7Ø.1
pneumonitis J7Ø.Ø
pulmonary manifestations
acute J7Ø.Ø
chronic J7Ø.1
skin L59.9
radioactive substance NOS
dermatitis or eczema —*see* Radiodermatitis
reduced temperature T69.9
immersion foot or hand —*see* Immersion
specified effect NEC T69.8
serum NEC (*see also* Reaction, serum) T8Ø.69
specified NEC T78.8
external cause NEC T75.89
strangulation —*see* Asphyxia, traumatic
submersion T75.1
thirst T73.1
toxic —*see* Toxicity
transfusion —*see* Complications, transfusion
ultraviolet (radiation) (rays) NOS T66
burn —*see* Burn
dermatitis or eczema —*see* Dermatitis, due to, ultraviolet rays
acute L56.8

Effect, adverse *(Continued)*
- vaccine (any) *—see* Complications, vaccination
- vibration *—see* Vibration, adverse effects
- water pressure NEC T7Ø.9
  - specified NEC T7Ø.8
- weightlessness T75.82
- whole blood *—see* Complications, transfusion
- work environment Z56.5

Effect (s) (of) (from) *—see* Effect, adverse NEC
Effects, late *—see* Sequelae
Effluvium
- anagen L65.1
- telogen L65.Ø

Effort syndrome (psychogenic) F45.8
Effusion
- amniotic fluid *—see* Pregnancy, complicated by, prematue rupture of membranes
- brain (serous) G93.6
- bronchial *—see* Bronchitis
- cerebral G93.6
- cerebrospinal *—see also* Meningitis
  - vessel G93.6
- chest *—see* Effusion, pleura
- chylous, chyliform (pleura) J94.Ø
- intracranial G93.6
- joint M25.4Ø
  - ankle M25.47-
  - elbow M25.42-
  - foot joint M25.47-
  - hand joint M25.44-
  - hip M25.45-
  - knee M25.46-
  - shoulder M25.41-
  - specified joint NEC M25.48
  - wrist M25.43-
- malignant pleural J91.Ø
- meninges *—see* Meningitis
- pericardium, pericardial (noninflammatory) I31.3
  - acute *—see* Pericarditis, acute
- peritoneal (chronic) R18.8
- pleura, pleurisy, pleuritic, pleuropericardial J9Ø
  - chylous, chyliform J94.Ø
  - due to systemic lupus erythematosis M32.13
  - influenzal *—see* Influenza, with, respiratory manifestations NEC
  - malignant J91.Ø
  - newborn P28.89
  - tuberculous NEC A15.6
    - primary (progressive) A15.7
- spinal *—see* Meningitis
- thorax, thoracic *—see* Effusion, pleura

Egg shell nails L6Ø.3
- congenital Q84.6

Egyptian splenomegaly B65.1
Ehlers-Danlos syndrome Q79.6
Ehrlichiosis A77.4Ø
- due to
  - E. chafeensis A77.41
  - E. sennetsu A79.81
  - specified organism NEC A77.49

Eichstedt's disease B36.Ø
Eisenmenger's
- complex or syndrome I27.89
- defect Q21.8

Ejaculation
- delayed F52.32 ◀
- painful N53.12
- premature F52.4
- retarded N53.11
- retrograde N53.14
- semen, painful N53.12
  - psychogenic F52.6

Ekbom's syndrome (restless legs) G25.81
Ekman's syndrome (brittle bones and blue sclera) Q78.Ø
Elastic skin Q82.8
- acquired L57.4

Elastofibroma *—see* Neoplasm, connective tissue, benign
Elastoma (juvenile) Q82.8
- Miescher's L87.2

Elastomyofibrosis I42.4
Elastosis
- actinic, solar L57.8
- atrophicans (senile) L57.4
- perforans serpiginosa L87.2
- senilis L57.4

Elbow *—see* condition
Electric current, electricity, effects (concussion) (fatal) (nonfatal) (shock) T75.4
- burn *—see* Burn

Electric feet syndrome E53.8
Electrocution T75.4
- from electroshock gun (taser) T75.4

Electrolyte imbalance E87.8
- with
  - abortion *—see* Abortion by type, complicated by, electrolyte imbalance
  - ectopic pregnancy OØ8.5
  - molar pregnancy OØ8.5

Elephantiasis (nonfilarial) I89.Ø
- arabicum *—see* Infestation, filarial
- bancroftian B74.Ø
- congenital (any site) (hereditary) Q82.Ø
- due to
  - Brugia (malayi) B74.1
    - timori B74.2
  - mastectomy I97.2
  - Wuchereria (bancrofti) B74.Ø
- eyelid HØ2.859
  - left HØ2.856
    - lower HØ2.855
    - upper HØ2.854
  - right HØ2.853
    - lower HØ2.852
    - upper HØ2.851
- filarial, filariensis *—see* Infestation, filarial
- glandular I89.Ø
- graecorum A3Ø.9
- lymphangiectatic I89.Ø
- lymphatic vessel I89.Ø
  - due to mastectomy I97.2
- scrotum (nonfilarial) I89.Ø
- streptococcal I89.Ø
- surgical I97.89
  - postmastectomy I97.2
- telangiectodes I89.Ø
- vulva (nonfilarial) N9Ø.89

Elevated, elevation
- antibody titer R76.Ø
- basal metabolic rate R94.8
- blood pressure *—see also* Hypertension
  - reading (incidental) (isolated) (nonspecific), no diagnosis of hypertension RØ3.Ø
- blood sugar R73.9
- body temperature (of unknown origin) R5Ø.9
- C-reactive protein (CRP) R79.82
- cancer antigen 125 [CA 125] R97.1
- carcinoembryonic antigen [CEA] R97.Ø
- cholesterol E78.ØØ ⇐
  - with high triglycerides E78.2
- conjugate, eye H51.Ø
- diaphragm, congenital Q79.1
- erythrocyte sedimentation rate R7Ø.Ø
- fasting glucose R73.Ø1
- fasting triglycerides E78.1
- finding on laboratory examination *—see* Findings, abnormal, inconclusive, without diagnosis, by type of exam
- GFR (glomerular filtration rate) *—see* Findings, abnormal, inconclusive, without diagnosis, by type of exam
- glucose tolerance (oral) R73.Ø2
- immunoglobulin level R76.8
- indoleacetic acid R82.5
- lactic acid dehydrogenase (LDH) level R74.Ø
- leukocytes D72.829
- lipoprotein a level E78.8

Elevated, elevation *(Continued)*
- liver function
  - study R94.5
  - test R79.89
    - alkaline phosphatase R74.8
    - aminotransferase R74.Ø
    - bilirubin R17
    - hepatic enzyme R74.8
    - lactate dehydrogenase R74.Ø
- lymphocytes D72.82Ø
- prostate specific antigen [PSA] R97.2Ø ⇐
- Rh titer *—see* Complication (s), transfusion, incompatibility reaction, Rh (factor)
- scapula, congenital Q74.Ø
- sedimentation rate R7Ø.Ø
- SGOT R74.Ø
- SGPT R74.Ø
- transaminase level R74.Ø
- triglycerides E78.1
  - with high cholesterol E78.2
- tumor associated antigens [TAA] NEC R97.8
- tumor specific antigens [TSA] NEC R97.8
- urine level of
  - 17-ketosteroids R82.5
  - catecholamine R82.5
  - indoleacetic acid R82.5
  - steroids R82.5
  - vanillylmandelic acid (VMA) R82.5
- venous pressure I87.8
- white blood cell count D72.829
  - specified NEC D72.828

Elliptocytosis (congenital) (hereditary) D58.1
- Hb C (disease) D58.1
- hemoglobin disease D58.1
- sickle-cell (disease) D57.8-
  - trait D57.3

Ellison-Zollinger syndrome E16.4
Ellis-van Creveld syndrome (chondroectodermal dysplasia) Q77.6
Elongated, elongation (congenital) *—see also* Distortion
- bone Q79.9
- cervix (uteri) Q51.828
  - acquired N88.4
  - hypertrophic N88.4
- colon Q43.8
- common bile duct Q44.5
- cystic duct Q44.5
- frenulum, penis Q55.69
- labia minora (acquired) N9Ø.69 ⇐
- ligamentum patellae Q74.1
- petiolus (epiglottidis) Q31.8
- tooth, teeth KØØ.2
- uvula Q38.6

Eltor cholera AØØ.1
Emaciation (due to malnutrition) E41
Embadomoniasis AØ7.8
Embedded tooth, teeth KØ1.Ø
- root only KØ8.3

Embolic *—see* condition
Embolism (multiple) (paradoxical) I74.9
- air (any site) (traumatic) T79.Ø
  - following
    - abortion *—see* Abortion by type complicated by embolism
    - ectopic pregnancy OØ8.2
    - infusion, therapeutic injection or transfusion T8Ø.Ø
    - molar pregnancy OØ8.2
    - procedure NEC
      - artery T81.719
        - mesenteric T81.71Ø
        - renal T81.711
        - specified NEC T81.718
      - vein T81.72
  - in pregnancy, childbirth or puerperium *—see* Embolism, obstetric
- amniotic fluid (pulmonary) *—see also* Embolism, obstetric
  - following
    - abortion *—see* Abortion by type complicated by embolism

E

E

Embolism *(Continued)*
  vein *(Continued)*
    basilic I82.61-
      chronic I82.71-
    brachial I82.62-
      chronic I82.72-
    brachiocephalic (innominate) I82.29Ø
      chronic I82.291
    cephalic I82.61-
      chronic I82.71-
    chronic I82.91
    deep (DVT) I82.4Ø-
      calf I82.4Z-
        chronic I82.5Z-
      lower leg I82.4Z-
        chronic I82.5Z-
      thigh I82.4Y-
        chronic I82.5Y-
      upper leg I82.4Y
        chronic I82.5y--
    femoral I82.41-
      chronic I82.51-
    iliac (iliofemoral) I82.42-
      chronic I82.52-
    innominate I82.29Ø
      chronic I82.291
    internal jugular I82.C1-
      chronic I82.C2-
    lower extremity
      deep I82.4Ø-
        chronic I82.5Ø-
        specified NEC I82.49-
          chronic NEC I82.59-
      distal
        deep I82.4Z-
      proximal
        deep I82.4Y-
          chronic I82.5Y-
      superficial I82.81-
    popliteal I82.43-
      chronic I82.53-
    radial I82.62-
      chronic I82.72-
    renal I82.3
    saphenous (greater) (lesser) I82.81-
    specified NEC I82.89Ø
      chronic NEC I82.891
    subclavian I82.B1-
      chronic I82.B2-
    thoracic NEC I82.29Ø
      chronic I82.291
    tibial I82.44-
      chronic I82.54-
    ulnar I82.62-
      chronic I82.72-
    upper extremity I82.6Ø-
      chronic I82.7Ø-
      deep I82.62-
        chronic I82.72-
      superficial I82.61-
        chronic I82.71-
  vena cava
    inferior (acute) I82.22Ø
      chronic I82.221
    superior (acute) I82.21Ø
      chronic I82.211
  venous sinus GØ8
  vessels of brain —*see* Occlusion, artery, cerebral
Embolus —*see* Embolism
Embryoma —*see also* Neoplasm, uncertain behavior, by site
  benign —*see* Neoplasm, benign, by site
  kidney C64.-
  liver C22.Ø
  malignant —*see also* Neoplasm, malignant, by site
    kidney C64.-
    liver C22.Ø
    testis C62.9-
      descended (scrotal) C62.1-
      undescended C62.Ø-
Embryoma *(Continued)*
  testis C62.9-
    descended (scrotal) C62.1-
    undescended C62.Ø-
Embryonic
  circulation Q28.9
  heart Q28.9
  vas deferens Q55.4
Embryopathia NOS Q89.9
Embryotoxon Q13.4
Emesis —*see* Vomiting
Emotional lability R45.86
Emotionality, pathological F6Ø.3
Emotogenic disease —*see* Disorder, psychogenic
Emphysema (atrophic) (bullous) (chronic) (interlobular) (lung) (obstructive) (pulmonary) (senile) (vesicular) J43.9
  cellular tissue (traumatic) T79.7
    surgical T81.82
  centrilobular J43.2
  compensatory J98.3
  congenital (interstitial) P25.Ø
  conjunctiva H11.89
  connective tissue (traumatic) T79.7
    surgical T81.82
  due to chemicals, gases, fumes or vapors J68.4
  eyelid (s) —*see* Disorder, eyelid, specified type NEC
    surgical T81.82
    traumatic T79.7
  interstitial J98.2
    congenital P25.Ø
    perinatal period P25.Ø
  laminated tissue T79.7
    surgical T81.82
  mediastinal J98.2
    newborn P25.2
  orbit, orbital —*see* Disorder, orbit, specified type NEC
  panacinar J43.1
  panlobular J43.1
  specified NEC J43.8
  subcutaneous (traumatic) T79.7
    nontraumatic J98.2
    postprocedural T81.82
    surgical T81.82
  surgical T81.82
  thymus (gland) (congenital) E32.8
  traumatic (subcutaneous) T79.7
  unilateral J43.Ø
Empty nest syndrome Z6Ø.Ø
Empyema (acute) (chest) (double) (pleura) (supradiaphragmatic) (thorax) J86.9
  with fistula J86.Ø
  accessory sinus (chronic) —*see* Sinusitis
  antrum (chronic) —*see* Sinusitis, maxillary
  brain (any part) —*see* Abscess, brain
  ethmoidal (chronic) (sinus) —*see* Sinusitis, ethmoidal
  extradural —*see* Abscess, extradural
  frontal (chronic) (sinus) —*see* Sinusitis, frontal
  gallbladder K81.Ø
  mastoid (process) (acute) —*see* Mastoiditis, acute
  maxilla, maxillary M27.2
    sinus (chronic) —*see* Sinusitis, maxillary
  nasal sinus (chronic) —*see* Sinusitis
  sinus (accessory) (chronic) (nasal) —*see* Sinusitis
  sphenoidal (sinus) (chronic) —*see* Sinusitis, sphenoidal
  subarachnoid —*see* Abscess, extradural
  subdural —*see* Abscess, subdural
  tuberculous A15.6
  ureter —*see* Ureteritis
  ventricular —*see* Abscess, brain
En coup de sabre lesion L94.1
Enamel pearls KØØ.2
Enameloma KØØ.2
Enanthema, viral BØ9
Encephalitis (chronic) (hemorrhagic) (idiopathic) (nonepidemic) (spurious) (subacute) GØ4.9Ø
  acute —*see also* Encephalitis, viral A86
    disseminated GØ4.ØØ
      infectious GØ4.Ø1
      noninfectious GØ4.81
      postimmunization (postvaccination) GØ4.Ø2
      postinfectious GØ4.Ø1
    inclusion body A85.8
    necrotizing hemorrhagic GØ4.3Ø
      postimmunization GØ4.32
      postinfectious GØ4.31
      specified NEC GØ4.39
  arboviral, arbovirus NEC A85.2
  arthropod-borne NEC (viral) A85.2
  Australian A83.4
  California (virus) A83.5
  Central European (tick-borne) A84.1
  Czechoslovakian A84.1
  Dawson's (inclusion body) A81.1
  diffuse sclerosing A81.1
  disseminated, acute GØ4.ØØ
  due to
    cat scratch disease A28.1
    human immunodeficiency virus (HIV) disease B2Ø *[GØ5.3]*
    malaria —*see* Malaria
    rickettsiosis —*see* Rickettsiosis
    smallpox inoculation GØ4.Ø2
    typhus —*see* Typhus
  Eastern equine A83.2
  endemic (viral) A86
  epidemic NEC (viral) A86
  equine (acute) (infectious) (viral) A83.9
    Eastern A83.2
    Venezuelan A92.2
    Western A83.1
  Far Eastern (tick-borne) A84.Ø
  following vaccination or other immunization procedure GØ4.Ø2
  herpes zoster BØ2.Ø
  herpesviral BØØ.4
    due to herpesvirus 6 B1Ø.Ø1
    due to herpesvirus 7 B1Ø.Ø9
    specified NEC B1Ø.Ø9
  Ilheus (virus) A83.8
  in (due to)
    actinomycosis A42.82
    adenovirus A85.1
    African trypanosomiasis B56.9 *[GØ5.3]*
    Chagas' disease (chronic) B57.42
    cytomegalovirus B25.8
    enterovirus A85.Ø
    herpes (simplex) virus BØØ.4
      due to herpesvirus 6 B1Ø.Ø1
      due to herpesvirus 7 B1Ø.Ø9
      specified NEC B1Ø.Ø9
    infectious disease NEC B99 *[GØ5.3]*
    influenza —*see* Influenza, with, encephalopathy
    listeriosis A32.12
    measles BØ5.Ø
    mumps B26.2
    naegleriasis B6Ø.2
    parasitic disease NEC B89 *[GØ5.3]*
    poliovirus A8Ø.9 *[GØ5.3]*
    rubella BØ6.Ø1
    syphilis
      congenital A5Ø.42
      late A52.14
    systemic lupus erythematosus M32.19
    toxoplasmosis (acquired) B58.2
      congenital P37.1
    tuberculosis A17.82
    zoster BØ2.Ø

E

Encephalitis *(Continued)*
inclusion body A81.1
infectious (acute) (virus) NEC A86
Japanese (B type) A83.Ø
La Crosse A83.5
lead —*see* Poisoning, lead
lethargica (acute) (infectious) A85.8
louping ill A84.8
lupus erythematosus, systemic M32.19
lymphatica A87.2
Mengo A85.8
meningococcal A39.81
Murray Valley A83.4
otitic NEC H66.4Ø *[GØ5.3]*
parasitic NOS B71.9
periaxial G37.Ø
periaxialis (concentrica) (diffuse) G37.5
postchickenpox BØ1.11
postexanthematous NEC BØ9
postimmunization GØ4.Ø2
postinfectious NEC GØ4.Ø1
postmeasles BØ5.Ø
postvaccinal GØ4.Ø2
postvaricella BØ1.11
postviral NEC A86
Powassan A84.8
Rasmussen GØ4.81
Rio Bravo A85.8
Russian
autumnal A83.Ø
spring-summer (taiga) A84.Ø
saturnine —*see* Poisoning, lead
specified NEC GØ4.81
St. Louis A83.3
subacute sclerosing A81.1
summer A83.Ø
suppurative GØ4.81
tick-borne A84.9
Torula, torular (cryptococcal) B45.1
toxic NEC G92
trichinosis B75 *[GØ5.3]*
type
B A83.Ø
C A83.3
van Bogaert's A81.1
Venezuelan equine A92.2
Vienna A85.8
viral, virus A86
arthropod-borne NEC A85.2
mosquito-borne A83.9
Australian X disease A83.4
California virus A83.5
Eastern equine A83.2
Japanese (B type) A83.Ø
Murray Valley A83.4
specified NEC A83.8
St. Louis A83.3
type B A83.Ø
type C A83.3
Western equine A83.1
tick-borne A84.9
biundulant A84.1
central European A84.1
Czechoslovakian A84.1
diphasic meningoencephalitis A84.1
Far Eastern A84.Ø
Russian spring-summer (taiga) A84.Ø
specified NEC A84.8
specified type NEC A85.8
Western equine A83.1
Encephalocele QØ1.9
frontal QØ1.Ø
nasofrontal QØ1.1
occipital QØ1.2
specified NEC QØ1.8
Encephalocystocele —*see* Encephalocele
Encephaloduroarteriomyosynangiosis (EDAMS) I67.5
Encephalomalacia (brain) (cerebellar) (cerebral) —*see* Softening, brain
Encephalomeningitis —*see* Meningoencephalitis
Encephalomeningocele —*see* Encephalocele
Encephalomeningomyelitis —*see* Meningoencephalitis
Encephalomyelitis —*see also* Encephalitis GØ4.9Ø
acute disseminated GØ4.ØØ
infectious GØ4.Ø1
noninfectious GØ4.81
postimmunization GØ4.Ø2
postinfectious GØ4.Ø1
acute necrotizing hemorrhagic GØ4.3Ø
postimmunization GØ4.32
postinfectious GØ4.31
specified NEC GØ4.39
benign myalgic G93.3
equine A83.9
Eastern A83.2
Venezuelan A92.2
Western A83.1
in diseases classified elsewhere GØ5.3
myalgic, benign G93.3
postchickenpox BØ1.11
postinfectious NEC GØ4.Ø1
postmeasles BØ5.Ø
postvaccinal GØ4.Ø2
postvaricella BØ1.11
rubella BØ6.Ø1
specified NEC GØ4.81
Venezuelan equine A92.2
Encephalomyelocele —*see* Encephalocele
Encephalomyelomeningitis —*see* Meningoencephalitis
Encephalomyelopathy G96.9
Encephalomyeloradiculitis (acute) G61.Ø
Encephalomyeloradiculoneuritis (acute) (Guillain-Barré) G61.Ø
Encephalomyeloradiculopathy G96.9
Encephalopathia hyperbilirubinemica, newborn P57.9
due to isoimmunization (conditions in P55) P57.Ø
Encephalopathy (acute) G93.4Ø
acute necrotizing hemorrhagic GØ4.3Ø
postimmunization GØ4.32
postinfectious GØ4.31
specified NEC GØ4.39
alcoholic G31.2
anoxic —*see* Damage, brain, anoxic
arteriosclerotic I67.2
centrolobar progressive (Schilder) G37.Ø
congenital QØ7.9
degenerative, in specified disease NEC G32.89
due to
drugs (*see also* Table of Drugs and Chemicals) G92
demyelinating callosal G37.1
hepatic —*see* Failure, hepatic
hyperbilirubinemic, newborn P57.9
due to isoimmunization (conditions in P55) P57.Ø
hypertensive I67.4
hypoglycemic E16.2
hypoxic —*see* Damage, brain, anoxic
hypoxic ischemic P91.6Ø
mild P91.61
moderate P91.62
severe P91.63
in (due to) (with)
birth injury P11.1
hyperinsulinism E16.1 *[G94]*
influenza —*see* Influenza, with, encephalopathy
lack of vitamin (*see also* Deficiency, vitamin) E56.9 *[G32.89]*
neoplastic disease (*see also* Neoplasm) D49.9 *[G13.1]*
serum (*see also* Reaction, serum) T8Ø.69
syphilis A52.17
Encephalopathy *(Continued)*
in *(Continued)*
trauma (postconcussional) FØ7.81
current injury —*see* Injury, intracranial
vaccination GØ4.Ø2
lead —*see* Poisoning, lead
metabolic G93.41
drug induced G92
toxic G92
myoclonic, early, symptomatic —*see* Epilepsy, generalized, specified NEC
necrotizing, subacute (Leigh) G31.82
pellagrous E52 *[G32.89]*
portosystemic —*see* Failure, hepatic
postcontusional FØ7.81
current injury —*see* Injury, intracranial, diffuse
posthypoglycemic (coma) E16.1 *[G94]*
postradiation G93.89
saturnine —*see* Poisoning, lead
septic G93.41
specified NEC G93.49
spongioform, subacute (viral) A81.Ø9
toxic G92
metabolic G92
traumatic (postconcussional) FØ7.81
current injury —*see* Injury, intracranial
vitamin B deficiency NEC E53.9 *[G32.89]*
vitamin B1 E51.2
Wernicke's E51.2
Encephalorrhagia —*see* Hemorrhage, intracranial, intracerebral
Encephalosis, posttraumatic FØ7.81
Enchondroma —*see also* Neoplasm, bone, benign
Enchondromatosis (cartilaginous) (multiple) Q78.4
Encopresis R15.9
functional F98.1
nonorganic origin F98.1
psychogenic F98.1
Encounter (with health service) (for) Z76.89
adjustment and management (of)
breast implant Z45.81
implanted device NEC Z45.89
myringotomy device (stent) (tube) Z45.82
administrative purpose only ZØ2.9
examination for
adoption ZØ2.82
armed forces ZØ2.3
disability determination ZØ2.71
driving license ZØ2.4
employment ZØ2.1
insurance ZØ2.6
medical certificate NEC ZØ2.79
paternity testing ZØ2.81
residential institution admission ZØ2.2
school admission ZØ2.Ø
sports ZØ2.5
specified reason NEC ZØ2.89
aftercare —*see* Aftercare
antenatal screening Z36
assisted reproductive fertility procedure cycle Z31.83
blood typing ZØ1.83
Rh typing ZØ1.83
breast augmentation or reduction Z41.1
breast implant exchange (different material) (different size) Z45.81
breast reconstruction following mastectomy Z42.1
check-up —*see* Examination
chemotherapy for neoplasm Z51.11
colonoscopy, screening Z12.11
counseling —*see* Counseling
delivery, full-term, uncomplicated O8Ø
cesarean, without indication O82
desensitization to allergens Z51.6 ◀
ear piercing Z41.3
examination —*see* Examination

E

Endocarditis *(Continued)*
mitral *(Continued)*
arteriosclerotic I34.8
nonrheumatic I34.8
acute or subacute I33.9
specified NEC I05.8
monilial B37.6
multiple valves I08.9
specified disorders I08.8
mycotic (acute) (any valve) (subacute) I33.0
pneumococcal (acute) (any valve) (subacute) I33.0
pulmonary (chronic) (heart) (valve) I37.8
with rheumatic fever (conditions in I00)
active —*see* Endocarditis, acute, rheumatic
inactive or quiescent (with chorea) I09.89
with aortic, mitral or tricuspid disease I08.8
acute or subacute I33.9
rheumatic I01.1
with chorea (acute) (rheumatic) (Sydenham's) I02.0
arteriosclerotic I37.8
congenital Q22.2
rheumatic (chronic) (inactive) (with chorea) I09.89
active or acute I01.1
with chorea (acute) (rheumatic) (Sydenham's) I02.0
syphilitic A52.03
purulent (acute) (any valve) (subacute) I33.0
Q fever A78 *[I39]*
rheumatic (chronic) (inactive) (with chorea) I09.1
active or acute (aortic) (mitral) (pulmonary) (tricuspid) I01.1
with chorea (acute) (rheumatic) (Sydenham's) I02.0
rheumatoid —*see* Rheumatoid, carditis
septic (acute) (any valve) (subacute) I33.0
streptococcal (acute) (any valve) (subacute) I33.0
subacute —*see* Endocarditis, acute
suppurative (acute) (any valve) (subacute) I33.0
syphilitic A52.03
toxic I33.9
tricuspid (chronic) (heart) (inactive) (rheumatic) (valve) (with chorea) I07.9
with
aortic (valve) disease I08.2
mitral (valve) disease I08.3
mitral (valve) disease I08.1
aortic (valve) disease I08.3
rheumatic fever (conditions in I00)
active —*see* Endocarditis, acute, rheumatic
inactive or quiescent (with chorea) I07.8
active or acute I01.1
with chorea (acute) (rheumatic) (Sydenham's) I02.0
arteriosclerotic I36.8
nonrheumatic I36.8
acute or subacute I33.9
specified cause, except rheumatic I36.8
tuberculous —*see* Tuberculosis, endocarditis
typhoid A01.02
ulcerative (acute) (any valve) (subacute) I33.0
vegetative (acute) (any valve) (subacute) I33.0
verrucous (atypical) (nonbacterial) (nonrheumatic) M32.11
Endocardium, endocardial —*see also* condition
cushion defect Q21.2
Endocervicitis —*see also* Cervicitis
due to intrauterine (contraceptive) device T83.69 ⬅
hyperplastic N72
Endocrine —*see* condition
Endocrinopathy, pluriglandular E31.9
Endodontic
overfill M27.52
underfill M27.53
Endodontitis K04.01 ⬅
irreversible K04.02 ◀
reversible K04.01 ◀
Endomastoiditis —*see* Mastoiditis
Endometrioma N80.9
Endometriosis N80.9
appendix N80.5
bladder N80.8
bowel N80.5
broad ligament N80.3
cervix N80.0
colon N80.5
cul-de-sac (Douglas') N80.3
exocervix N80.0
fallopian tube N80.2
female genital organ NEC N80.8
gallbladder N80.8
in scar of skin N80.6
internal N80.0
intestine N80.5
lung N80.8
myometrium N80.0
ovary N80.1
parametrium N80.3
pelvic peritoneum N80.3
peritoneal (pelvic) N80.3
rectovaginal septum N80.4
rectum N80.5
round ligament N80.3
skin (scar) N80.6
specified site NEC N80.8
stromal D39.0
umbilicus N80.8
uterus (internal) N80.0
vagina N80.4
vulva N80.8
Endometritis (decidual) (nonspecific) (purulent) (senile (atrophic) (suppurative) N71.9
with ectopic pregnancy O08.0
acute N71.0
blenorrhagic (gonococcal) (acute) (chronic) A54.24
cervix, cervical (with erosion or ectropion) —*see also* Cervicitis
hyperplastic N72
chlamydial A56.11
chronic N71.1
following
abortion —*see* Abortion by type complicated by genital infection
ectopic or molar pregnancy O08.0
gonococcal, gonorrheal (acute) (chronic) A54.24
hyperplastic —*see also* Hyperplasia, endometrial N85.00-
cervix N72
puerperal, postpartum, childbirth O86.12
subacute N71.0
tuberculous A18.17
Endometrium —*see* condition
Endomyocardiopathy, South African I42.3
Endomyocarditis —*see* Endocarditis
Endomyofibrosis I42.3
Endomyometritis —*see* Endometritis
Endopericarditis —*see* Endocarditis
Endoperineuritis —*see* Disorder, nerve
Endophlebitis —*see* Phlebitis
Endophthalmia —*see* Endophthalmitis, purulent
Endophthalmitis (acute) (infective) (metastatic) (subacute) H44.009
bleb associated H59.4 —*see also* Bleb, inflammed (infected), postprocedural
gonorrheal A54.39
in (due to)
cysticercosis B69.1
onchocerciasis B73.01
toxocariasis B83.0
Endophthalmitis *(Continued)*
panuveitis —*see* Panuveitis
parasitic H44.12-
purulent H44.00-
panophthalmitis —*see* Panophthalmitis
vitreous abscess H44.02-
specified NEC H44.19
sympathetic —*see* Uveitis, sympathetic
Endosalpingioma D28.2
Endosalpingiosis N94.89
Endosteitis —*see* Osteomyelitis
Endothelioma, bone —*see* Neoplasm, bone, malignant
Endotheliosis (hemorrhagic infectional) D69.8
Endotoxemia — code to condition
Endotrachelitis —*see* Cervicitis
Engelmann (-Camurati) **syndrome** Q78.3
English disease —*see* Rickets
Engman's disease L30.3
Engorgement
breast N64.59
newborn P83.4
puerperal, postpartum O92.79
lung (passive) —*see* Edema, lung
pulmonary (passive) —*see* Edema, lung
stomach K31.89
venous, retina —*see* Occlusion, retina, vein, engorgement
Enlargement, enlarged —*see also* Hypertrophy
adenoids J35.2
with tonsils J35.3
alveolar ridge K08.89 ⬅
congenital —*see* Anomaly, alveolar
apertures of diaphragm (congenital) Q79.1
gingival K06.1
heart, cardiac —*see* Hypertrophy, cardiac
labium majus, childhood asymmetric (CALME) N90.61 ◀
lacrimal gland, chronic H04.03-
liver —*see* Hypertrophy, liver
lymph gland or node R59.9
generalized R59.1
localized R59.0
orbit H05.34-
organ or site, congenital NEC —*see* Anomaly, by site
parathyroid (gland) E21.0
pituitary fossa R93.0
prostate N40.0
with lower urinary tract symptoms (LUTS) N40.1
without lower urinary tract symptoms (LUTS) N40.0
sella turcica R93.0
spleen —*see* Splenomegaly
thymus (gland) (congenital) E32.0
thyroid (gland) —*see* Goiter
tongue K14.8
tonsils J35.1
with adenoids J35.3
uterus N85.2
Enophthalmos H05.40-
due to
orbital tissue atrophy H05.41-
trauma or surgery H05.42-
Enostosis M27.8
Entamebic, entamebiasis —*see* Amebiasis
Entanglement
umbilical cord (s) O69.2
with compression O69.2
without compression O69.82
around neck (with compression) O69.1
without compression O69.81
of twins in monoamniotic sac O69.2
Enteralgia —*see* Pain, abdominal
Enteric —*see* condition
Enteritis (acute) (diarrheal) (hemorrhagic) (noninfective) K52.9 ⬅
adenovirus A08.2
aertrycke infection A02.0

E

- **Enteritis** *(Continued)*
  - allergic K52.29 ⬅
    - with ◄
      - eosinophilic gastritis or gastroenteritis K52.81 ◄
      - food protein-induced enterocolitis syndrome K52.21 ◄
      - food protein-induced enteropathy K52.22 ◄
  - amebic (acute) AØ6.Ø
    - with abscess —*see* Abscess, amebic
    - chronic AØ6.1
      - with abscess —*see* Abscess, amebic
      - nondysenteric AØ6.2
    - nondysenteric AØ6.2
  - astrovirus AØ8.32
  - bacillary NOS AØ3.9
  - bacterial AØ4.9
    - specified NEC AØ4.8
  - calicivirus AØ8.31
  - candidal B37.82
  - Chilomastix AØ7.8
  - choleriformis AØØ.1
  - chronic (noninfectious) K52.9
    - ulcerative —*see* Colitis, ulcerative
  - cicatrizing (chronic) —*see* Enteritis, regional, small intestine
  - Clostridium
    - botulinum (food poisoning) AØ5.1
    - difficile AØ4.7
  - coccidial AØ7.3
  - coxsackie virus AØ8.39
  - dietetic —*see also* Enteritis, allergic K52.29 ⬅
  - drug-induced K52.1
  - due to
    - astrovirus AØ8.32
    - calicivirus AØ8.31
    - coxsackie virus AØ8.39
    - drugs K52.1
    - echovirus AØ8.39
    - enterovirus NEC AØ8.39
    - food hypersensitivity —*see also* Enteritis, allergic K52.29 ⬅
    - infectious organism (bacterial) (viral) —*see* Enteritis, infectious
    - torovirus AØ8.39
    - Yersinia enterocolitica AØ4.6
  - echovirus AØ8.39
  - eltor AØØ.1
  - enterovirus NEC AØ8.39
  - eosinophilic K52.81
  - epidemic (infectious) AØ9
  - fulminant —*see also* Ischemia, intestine, acute K55.Ø19 ⬅
  - gangrenous —*see* Enteritis, infectious
  - giardial AØ7.1
  - infectious NOS AØ9
    - due to
      - adenovirus AØ8.2
      - Aerobacter aerogenes AØ4.8
      - Arizona (bacillus) AØ2.Ø
      - bacteria NOS AØ4.9
        - specified NEC AØ4.8
      - Campylobacter AØ4.5
      - Clostridium difficile AØ4.7
      - Clostridium perfringens AØ4.8
      - Enterobacter aerogenes AØ4.8
      - enterovirus AØ8.39
      - Escherichia coli AØ4.4
        - enteroaggregative AØ4.4
        - enterohemorrhagic AØ4.3
        - enteroinvasive AØ4.2
        - enteropathogenic AØ4.Ø
        - enterotoxigenic AØ4.1
        - specified NEC AØ4.4
      - specified
        - bacteria NEC AØ4.8
        - virus NEC AØ8.39
      - Staphylococcus AØ4.8
- **Enteritis** *(Continued)*
  - infectious NOS *(Continued)*
    - due to *(Continued)*
      - virus NEC AØ8.4
        - specified type NEC AØ8.39
      - Yersinia enterocolitica AØ4.6
    - specified organism NEC AØ8.8
  - influenzal —*see* Influenza, with, digestive manifestations
  - ischemic K55.9
    - acute —*see also* Ischemia, intestine, acute K55.Ø19 ⬅
    - chronic K55.1
  - microsporidial AØ7.8
  - mucomembranous, myxomembranous —*see* Syndrome, irritable bowel
  - mucous —*see* Syndrome, irritable bowel
  - necroticans AØ5.2
  - necrotizing of newborn —*see* Enterocolitis, necrotizing, in newborn
  - neurogenic —*see* Syndrome, irritable bowel
  - newborn necrotizing —*see* Enterocolitis, necrotizing, in newborn
  - noninfectious K52.9
  - norovirus AØ8.11
  - parasitic NEC B82.9
  - paratyphoid (fever) —*see* Fever, paratyphoid
  - protozoal AØ7.9
    - specified NEC AØ7.8
  - radiation K52.Ø
  - regional (of) K5Ø.9Ø
    - with
      - complication K5Ø.919
        - abscess K5Ø.914
        - fistula K5Ø.913
        - intestinal obstruction K5Ø.912
        - rectal bleeding K5Ø.911
        - specified complication NEC K5Ø.918
    - colon —*see* Enteritis, regional, large intestine
    - duodenum —*see* Enteritis, regional, small intestine
    - ileum —*see* Enteritis, regional, small intestine
    - jejunum —*see* Enteritis, regional, small intestine
    - large bowel —*see* Enteritis, regional, large intestine
    - large intestine (colon) (rectum) K5Ø.1Ø
      - with
        - complication K5Ø.119
          - abscess K5Ø.114
          - fistula K5Ø.113
          - intestinal obstruction K5Ø.112
          - rectal bleeding K5Ø.111
          - small intestine (duodenum) (ileum) (jejunum) involvement K5Ø.8Ø
            - with
              - complication K5Ø.819
                - abscess K5Ø.814
                - fistula K5Ø.813
                - intestinal obstruction K5Ø.812
                - rectal bleeding K5Ø.811
                - specified complication NEC K5Ø.818
          - specified complication NEC K5Ø.118
    - rectum —*see* Enteritis, regional, large intestine
    - small intestine (duodenum) (ileum) (jejunum) K5Ø.ØØ
      - with
        - complication K5Ø.Ø19
          - abscess K5Ø.Ø14
          - fistula K5Ø.Ø13
          - intestinal obstruction K5Ø.Ø12
- **Enteritis** *(Continued)*
  - regional *(Continued)*
    - small intestine *(Continued)*
      - with *(Continued)*
        - complication *(Continued)*
          - large intestine (colon) (rectum) involvement K5Ø.8Ø
            - with
              - complication K5Ø.819
                - abscess K5Ø.814
                - fistula K5Ø.813
                - intestinal obstruction K5Ø.812
                - rectal bleeding K5Ø.811
                - specified complication NEC K5Ø.818
          - rectal bleeding K5Ø.Ø11
          - specified complication NEC K5Ø.Ø18
  - rotaviral AØ8.Ø
  - Salmonella, salmonellosis (arizonae) (cholerae-suis) (enteritidis) (typhimurium) AØ2.Ø
  - segmental —*see* Enteritis, regional
  - septic AØ9
  - Shigella —*see* Infection, Shigella
  - small round structured NEC AØ8.19
  - spasmodic, spastic —*see* Syndrome, irritable bowel
  - staphylococcal AØ4.8
    - due to food AØ5.Ø
  - torovirus AØ8.39
  - toxic NEC K52.1
    - due to Clostridium difficile AØ4.7
  - trichomonal AØ7.8
  - tuberculous A18.32
  - typhosa AØ1.ØØ
  - ulcerative (chronic) —*see* Colitis, ulcerative
  - viral AØ8.4
    - adenovirus AØ8.2
    - enterovirus AØ8.39
    - Rotavirus AØ8.Ø
    - small round structured NEC AØ8.19
    - specified NEC AØ8.39
    - virus specified NEC AØ8.39
- **Enterobiasis** B8Ø
- **Enterobius vermicularis** (infection) (infestation) B8Ø
- **Enterocele** —*see also* Hernia, abdomen
  - pelvic, pelvis (acquired) (congenital) N81.5
  - vagina, vaginal (acquired) (congenital) NEC N81.5
- **Enterocolitis** —*see also* Enteritis K52.9
  - due to Clostridium difficile AØ4.7
  - fulminant ischemic —*see also* Ischemia, intestine, acute K55.Ø59 ⬅
  - granulomatous —*see* Enteritis, regional
  - hemorrhagic (acute) —*see also* Ischemia, intestine, acute K55.Ø59 ⬅
    - chronic K55.1
  - infectious NEC AØ9
  - ischemic K55.9
  - necrotizing K55.3Ø ⬅
    - with ◄
      - perforation K55.33 ◄
      - pneumatosis K55.32 ◄
        - and perforation K55.33 ◄
    - due to Clostridium difficile AØ4.7
    - in non-newborn K55.3Ø ◄
      - stage 1 (without pneumatosis, without perforation) K55.31 ◄
      - stage 2 (with pneumatosis, without perforation) K55.32 ◄
      - stage 3 (with pneumatosis, with perforation) K55.33 ◄
    - in newborn P77.9
      - stage 1 (without pneumatosis, without perforation) P77.1
      - stage 2 (with pneumatosis, without perforation) P77.2
      - stage 3 (with pneumatosis, with perforation) P77.3
    - without pneumatosis or perforation K55.31 ◄

E

- **Enterocolitis** *(Continued)*
  - noninfectious K52.9
    - newborn —*see* Enterocolitis, necrotizing, in newborn
  - pseudomembranous (newborn) A04.7
  - radiation K52.0
    - newborn —*see* Enterocolitis, necrotizing, in newborn
  - ulcerative (chronic) —*see* Pancolitis, ulcerative (chronic)
- **Enterogastritis** —*see* Enteritis
- **Enteropathy** K63.9
  - food protein-induced enterocolitis K52.22 ◀
  - gluten-sensitive K90.0
    - non-celiac K90.41 ◀
  - hemorrhagic, terminal —*see also* Ischemia, intestine, acute K55.059 ◀━
  - protein-losing K90.49 ◀━
- **Enteroperitonitis** —*see* Peritonitis
- **Enteroptosis** K63.4
- **Enterorrhagia** K92.2
- **Enterospasm** —*see also* Syndrome, irritable, bowel
  - psychogenic F45.8
- **Enterostenosis** —*see also* Obstruction, intestine K56.69
- **Enterostomy**
  - complication —*see* Complication, enterostomy
  - status Z93.4
- **Enterovirus, as cause of disease classified elsewhere** B97.10
  - coxsackievirus B97.11
  - echovirus B97.12
  - other specified B97.19
- **Enthesopathy** (peripheral) M77.9
  - Achilles tendinitis —*see* Tendinitis, Achilles
  - ankle and tarsus M77.9
    - specified type NEC —*see* Enthesopathy, foot, specified type NEC
  - anterior tibial syndrome M76.81-
  - calcaneal spur —*see* Spur, bone, calcaneal
  - elbow region M77.8
    - lateral epicondylitis —*see* Epicondylitis, lateral
    - medial epicondylitis —*see* Epicondylitis, medial
  - foot NEC M77.9
    - metatarsalgia —*see* Metatarsalgia
    - specified type NEC M77.5-
  - forearm M77.9
  - gluteal tendinitis —*see* Tendinitis, gluteal
  - hand M77.9
  - hip —*see* Enthesopathy, lower limb, specified type NEC
  - iliac crest spur —*see* Spur, bone, iliac crest
  - iliotibial band syndrome —*see* Syndrome, iliotibial band
  - knee —*see* Enthesopathy, lower limb, lower leg, specified type NEC
  - lateral epicondylitis —*see* Epicondylitis, lateral
  - lower limb (excluding foot) M76.9
    - Achilles tendinitis —*see* Tendinitis, Achilles
    - anterior tibial syndrome M76.81-
    - gluteal tendinitis —*see* Tendinitis, gluteal
    - iliac crest spur —*see* Spur, bone, iliac crest
    - iliotibial band syndrome —*see* Syndrome, iliotibial band
    - patellar tendinitis —*see* Tendinitis, patellar
    - pelvic region —*see* Enthesopathy, lower limb, specified type NEC
    - peroneal tendinitis —*see* Tendinitis, peroneal
    - posterior tibial syndrome M76.82-
    - psoas tendinitis —*see* Tendinitis, psoas
    - shoulder M77.9
    - specified type NEC M76.89-
    - tibial collateral bursitis —*see* Bursitis, tibial collateral
- **Enthesopathy** *(Continued)*
  - medial epicondylitis —*see* Epicondylitis, medial
  - multiple sites M77.9
  - patellar tendinitis —*see* Tendinitis, patellar
  - pelvis M77.9
  - periarthritis of wrist —*see* Periarthritis, wrist
  - peroneal tendinitis —*see* Tendinitis, peroneal
  - posterior tibial syndrome M76.82-
  - psoas tendinitis —*see* Tendinitis, psoas
  - shoulder region —*see* Lesion, shoulder
  - specified site NEC M77.9
  - specified type NEC M77.8
  - spinal M46.00
    - cervical region M46.02
    - cervicothoracic region M46.03
    - lumbar region M46.06
    - lumbosacral region M46.07
    - multiple sites M46.09
    - occipito-atlanto-axial region M46.01
    - sacrococcygeal region M46.08
    - thoracic region M46.04
    - thoracolumbar region M46.05
  - tibial collateral bursitis —*see* Bursitis, tibial collateral
  - upper arm M77.9
  - wrist and carpus NEC M77.8
    - calcaneal spur —*see* Spur, bone, calcaneal
    - periarthritis of wrist —*see* Periarthritis, wrist
- **Entomophobia** F40.218
- **Entomophthoromycosis** B46.8
- **Entrance, air into vein** —*see* Embolism, air
- **Entrapment, nerve** —*see* Neuropathy, entrapment
- **Entropion** (eyelid) (paralytic) H02.009
  - cicatricial H02.019
    - left H02.016
      - lower H02.015
      - upper H02.014
    - right H02.013
      - lower H02.012
      - upper H02.011
  - congenital Q10.2
  - left H02.006
    - lower H02.005
    - upper H02.004
  - mechanical H02.029
    - left H02.026
      - lower H02.025
      - upper H02.024
    - right H02.023
      - lower H02.022
      - upper H02.021
  - right H02.003
    - lower H02.002
    - upper H02.001
  - senile H02.039
    - left H02.036
      - lower H02.035
      - upper H02.034
    - right H02.033
      - lower H02.032
      - upper H02.031
  - spastic H02.049
    - left H02.046
      - lower H02.045
      - upper H02.044
    - right H02.043
      - lower H02.042
      - upper H02.041
- **Enucleated eye** (traumatic, current) S05.7-
- **Enuresis** R32
  - functional F98.0
  - habit disturbance F98.0
  - nocturnal N39.44
    - psychogenic F98.0
  - nonorganic origin F98.0
  - psychogenic F98.0
- **Eosinopenia** —*see* Agranulocytosis
- **Eosinophilia** (allergic) (hereditary) (idiopathic) (secondary) D72.1
  - with
    - angiolymphoid hyperplasia (ALHE) D18.01
  - infiltrative J82
  - Löffler's J82
  - peritoneal —*see* Peritonitis, eosinophilic
  - pulmonary NEC J82
  - tropical (pulmonary) J82
- **Eosinophilia-myalgia syndrome** M35.8
- **Ependymitis** (acute) (cerebral) (chronic) (granular) —*see* Encephalomyelitis
- **Ependymoblastoma**
  - specified site —*see* Neoplasm, malignant, by site
  - unspecified site C71.9
- **Ependymoma** (epithelial) (malignant)
  - anaplastic
    - specified site —*see* Neoplasm, malignant, by site
    - unspecified site C71.9
  - benign
    - specified site —*see* Neoplasm, benign, by site
    - unspecified site D33.2
  - myxopapillary D43.2
    - specified site —*see* Neoplasm, uncertain behavior, by site
    - unspecified site D43.2
  - papillary D43.2
    - specified site —*see* Neoplasm, uncertain behavior, by site
    - unspecified site D43.2
  - specified site —*see* Neoplasm, malignant, by site
  - unspecified site C71.9
- **Ependymopathy** G93.89
- **Ephelis, ephelides** L81.2
- **Epiblepharon** (congenital) Q10.3
- **Epicanthus, epicanthic fold** (eyelid) (congenital) Q10.3
- **Epicondylitis** (elbow)
  - lateral M77.1-
  - medial M77.0-
- **Epicystitis** —*see* Cystitis
- **Epidemic** —*see* condition
- **Epidermidalization, cervix** —*see* Dysplasia, cervix
- **Epidermis, epidermal** —*see* condition
- **Epidermodysplasia verruciformis** B07.8
- **Epidermolysis**
  - bullosa (congenital) Q81.9
    - acquired L12.30
      - drug-induced L12.31
      - specified cause NEC L12.35
    - dystrophica Q81.2
    - letalis Q81.1
    - simplex Q81.0
    - specified NEC Q81.8
  - necroticans combustiformis L51.2
    - due to drug —*see* Table of Drugs and Chemicals, by drug
- **Epidermophytid** —*see* Dermatophytosis
- **Epidermophytosis** (infected) —*see* Dermatophytosis
- **Epididymis** —*see* condition
- **Epididymitis** (acute) (nonvenereal) (recurrent) (residual) N45.1
  - with orchitis N45.3
  - blennorrhagic (gonococcal) A54.23
  - caseous (tuberculous) A18.15
  - chlamydial A56.19
  - filarial —*see also* Infestation, filarial B74.9 *[N51]*
  - gonococcal A54.23
  - syphilitic A52.76
  - tuberculous A18.15
- **Epididymo-orchitis** —*see also* Epididymitis N45.3
- **Epidural** —*see* condition

◀ New ◀━ Revised ~~deleted~~ Deleted

Epigastrium, epigastric —*see* condition
Epigastrocele —*see* Hernia, ventral
Epiglottis —*see* condition
Epiglottitis, epiglottiditis (acute) J05.10
  with obstruction J05.11
  chronic J37.0
Epignathus Q89.4
Epilepsia partialis continua —*see also* Kozhevnikof's epilepsy G40.1-
Epilepsy, epileptic, epilepsia (attack) (cerebral) (convulsion) (fit) (seizure) G40.909

Note: the following terms are to be considered equivalent to intractable: pharmacoresistant (pharmacologically resistant), treatment resistant, refractory (medically) and poorly controlled

  with
    complex partial seizures —*see* Epilepsy, localization-related, symptomatic, with complex partial seizures
    grand mal seizures on awakening —*see* Epilepsy, generalized, specified NEC
    myoclonic absences —*see* Epilepsy, generalized, specified NEC
    myoclonic-astatic seizures —*see* Epilepsy, generalized, specified NEC
    simple partial seizures —*see* Epilepsy, localization-related, symptomatic, with simple partial seizures
  akinetic —*see* Epilepsy, generalized, specified NEC
  benign childhood with centrotemporal EEG spikes —*see* Epilepsy, localization-related, idiopathic
  benign myoclonic in infancy G40.80-
  Bravais-jacksonian —*see* Epilepsy, localization-related, symptomatic, with simple partial seizures
  childhood
    with occipital EEG paroxysms —*see* Epilepsy, localization-related, idiopathic
    absence G40.A09
      intractable G40.A19
        with status epilepticus G40.A11
        without status epilepticus G40.A19
      not intractable G40.A09
        with status epilepticus G40.A01
        without status epilepticus G40.A09
  climacteric —*see* Epilepsy, specified NEC
  cysticercosis B69.0
  deterioration (mental) F06.8
  due to syphilis A52.19
  focal —*see* Epilepsy, localization-related, symptomatic, with simple partial seizures
  generalized
    idiopathic G40.309
      intractable G40.319
        with status epilepticus G40.311
        without status epilepticus G40.319
      not intractable G40.309
        with status epilepticus G40.301
        without status epilepticus G40.309
    specified NEC G40.409
      intractable G40.419
        with status epilepticus G40.411
        without status epilepticus G40.419
      not intractable G40.409
        with status epilepticus G40.401
        without status epilepticus G40.409
  impulsive petit mal —*see* Epilepsy, juvenile myoclonic
  intractable G40.919
    with status epilepticus G40.911
    without status epilepticus G40.919

Epilepsy, epileptic, epilepsia *(Continued)*
  juvenile absence G40.A09
    intractable G40.A19
      with status epilepticus G40.A11
      without status epilepticus G40.A19
    not intractable G40.A09
      with status epilepticus G40.A01
      without status epilepticus G40.A09
  juvenile myoclonic G40.B11
    intractable G40.B19
      with status epilepticus G40.B11
      without status epilepticus G40.B19
    not intractable G40.B09
      with status epilepticus G40.B01
      without status epilepticus G40.B09
  localization-related (focal) (partial)
    idiopathic G40.009
      with seizures of localized onset G40.009
        intractable G40.019
          with status epilepticus G40.011
          without status epilepticus G40.019
        not intractable G40.009
          with status epilepticus G40.001
          without status epilepticus G40.009
    symptomatic
      with complex partial seizures G40.209
        intractable G40.219
          with status epilepticus G40.211
          without status epilepticus G40.219
        not intractable G40.209
          with status epilepticus G40.201
          without status epilepticus G40.209
      with simple partial seizures G40.109
        intractable G40.119
          with status epilepticus G40.111
          without status epilepticus G40.119
        not intractable G40.109
          with status epilepticus G40.101
          without status epilepticus G40.109
  myoclonus, myoclonic —*see* Epilepsy, generalized, specified NEC
    progressive —*see* Epilepsy, generalized, idiopathic
  not intractable G40.909
    with status epilepticus G40.901
    without status epilepticus G40.909
  on awakening —*see* Epilepsy, generalized, specified NEC
  parasitic NOS B71.9 *[G94]*
  partialis continua —*see also* Kozhevnikof's epilepsy G40.1-
  peripheral —*see* Epilepsy, specified NEC
  procursiva —*see* Epilepsy, localization-related, symptomatic, with simple partial seizures
  progressive (familial) myoclonic —*see* Epilepsy, generalized, idiopathic
  reflex —*see* Epilepsy, specified NEC
  related to
    alcohol G40.509
      not intractable G40.509
        with status epilepticus G40.501
        without status epliepticus G40.509
    drugs G40.509
      not intractable G40.509
        with status epilepticus G40.501
        without status epliepticus G40.509
    external causes G40.509
      not intractable G40.509
        with status epilepticus G40.501
        without status epliepticus G40.509
    hormonal changes G40.509
      not intractable G40.509
        with status epilepticus G40.501
        without status epliepticus G40.509
    sleep deprivation G40.509
      not intractable G40.509
        with status epilepticus G40.501
        without status epliepticus G40.509

Epilepsy, epileptic, epilepsia *(Continued)*
  related to *(Continued)*
    stress G40.509
      not intractable G40.509
        with status epilepticus G40.501
        without status epliepticus G40.509
  somatomotor —*see* Epilepsy, localization-related, symptomatic, with simple partial seizures
  somatosensory —*see* Epilepsy, localization-related, symptomatic, with simple partial seizures
  spasms G40.822
    intractable G40.824
      with status epilepticus G40.823
      without status epilepticus G40.824
    not intractable G40.822
      with status epilepticus G40.821
      without status epilepticus G40.822
  specified NEC G40.802
    intractable G40.804
      with status epilepticus G40.803
      without status epilepticus G40.804
    not intractable G40.802
      with status epilepticus G40.801
      without status epilepticus G40.802
  syndromes
    generalized
      idiopathic G40.309
        intractable G40.319
          with status epilepticus G40.311
          without status epilepticus G40.319
        not intractable G40.309
          with status epilepticus G40.301
          without status epilepticus G40.309
      specified NEC G40.409
        intractable G40.419
          with status epilepticus G40.411
          without status epilepticus G40.419
        not intractable G40.409
          with status epilepticus G40.401
          without status epilepticus G40.409
    localization-related (focal) (partial)
      idiopathic G40.009
        with seizures of localized onset G40.009
          intractable G40.019
            with status epilepticus G40.011
            without status epilepticus G40.019
          not intractable G40.009
            with status epilepticus G40.001
            without status epilepticus G40.009
      symptomatic
        with complex partial seizures G40.209
          intractable G40.219
            with status epilepticus G40.211
            without status epilepticus G40.219
          not intractable G40.209
            with status epilepticus G40.201
            without status epilepticus G40.209
        with simple partial seizures G40.109
          intractable G40.119
            with status epilepticus G40.111
            without status epilepticus G40.119
          not intractable G40.109
            with status epilepticus G40.101
            without status epilepticus G40.109
    specified NEC G40.802
      intractable G40.804
        with status epilepticus G40.803
        without status epilepticus G40.804
      not intractable G40.802
        with status epilepticus G40.801
        without status epilepticus G40.802
  tonic (-clonic) —*see* Epilepsy, generalized, specified NEC
  twilight F05

E

Epilepsy, epileptic, epilepsia *(Continued)*
uncinate (gyrus) —*see* Epilepsy, localization-related, symptomatic, with complex partial seizures
Unverricht (-Lundborg) (familial myoclonic) —*see* Epilepsy, generalized, idiopathic
visceral —*see* Epilepsy, specified NEC
visual —*see* Epilepsy, specified NEC
Epiloia Q85.1
Epimenorrhea N92.Ø
Epipharyngitis —*see* Nasopharyngitis
Epiphora HØ4.2Ø-
due to
excess lacrimation HØ4.21-
insufficient drainage HØ4.22-
Epiphyseal arrest —*see* Arrest, epiphyseal
Epiphyseolysis, epiphysiolysis —*see* Osteochondropathy
Epiphysitis —*see also* Osteochondropathy
juvenile M92.9
syphilitic (congenital) A5Ø.Ø2
Epiplocele —*see* Hernia, abdomen
Epiploitis —*see* Peritonitis
Epiplosarcomphalocele —*see* Hernia, umbilicus
Episcleritis (suppurative) H15.1Ø-
in (due to)
syphilis A52.71
tuberculosis A18.51
nodular H15.12-
periodica fugax H15.11-
angioneurotic —*see* Edema, angioneurotic
syphilitic (late) A52.71
tuberculous A18.51
Episode
affective, mixed F39
depersonalization (in neurotic state) F48.1
depressive F32.9
major F32.9
mild F32.Ø
moderate F32.1
severe (without psychotic symptoms) F32.2
with psychotic symptoms F32.3
recurrent F33.9
brief F33.8
specified NEC F32.89 ◀
hypomanic F3Ø.8
manic F3Ø.9
with
psychotic symptoms F3Ø.2
remission (full) F3Ø.4
partial F3Ø.3
without psychotic symptoms F3Ø.1Ø
mild F3Ø.11
moderate F3Ø.12
severe (without psychotic symptoms) F3Ø.13
with psychotic symptoms F3Ø.2
other specified F3Ø.8
recurrent F31.89
psychotic F23
organic FØ6.8
schizophrenic (acute) NEC, brief F23
Epispadias (female) (male) Q64.Ø
Episplenitis D73.89
Epistaxis (multiple) RØ4.Ø
hereditary I78.Ø
vicarious menstruation N94.89
Epithelioma (malignant) —*see also* Neoplasm, malignant, by site
adenoides cysticum —*see* Neoplasm, skin, benign
basal cell —*see* Neoplasm, skin, malignant
benign —*see* Neoplasm, benign, by site
Bowen's —*see* Neoplasm, skin, in situ
calcifying, of Malherbe —*see* Neoplasm, skin, benign
external site —*see* Neoplasm, skin, malignant
intraepidermal, Jadassohn —*see* Neoplasm, skin, benign
squamous cell —*see* Neoplasm, malignant, by site
Epitheliomatosis pigmented Q82.1
Epitheliopathy, multifocal placoid pigment H3Ø.14-
Epithelium, epithelial —*see* condition
Epituberculosis (with atelectasis) (allergic) A15.7
Eponychia Q84.6
Epstein's
nephrosis or syndrome —*see* Nephrosis
pearl KØ9.8
Epulis (gingiva) (fibrous) (giant cell) KØ6.8
Equinia A24.Ø
Equinovarus (congenital) (talipes) Q66.Ø
acquired —*see* Deformity, limb, clubfoot
Equivalent
convulsive (abdominal) —*see* Epilepsy, specified NEC
epileptic (psychic) —*see* Epilepsy, localization-related, symptomatic, with complex partial seizures
Erb (-Duchenne) **paralysis** (birth injury) (newborn) P14.Ø
Erb's
disease G71.Ø
palsy, paralysis (brachial) (birth) (newborn) P14.Ø
spinal (spastic) syphilitic A52.17
pseudohypertrophic muscular dystrophy G71.Ø
Erb-Goldflam disease or syndrome G7Ø.ØØ
with exacerbation (acute) G7Ø.Ø1
in crisis G7Ø.Ø1
Erdheim's syndrome (acromegalic macrospondylitis) E22.Ø
Erection, painful (persistent) —*see* Priapism
Ergosterol deficiency (vitamin D) E55.9
with
adult osteomalacia M83.8
rickets —*see* Rickets
Ergotism —*see also* Poisoning, food, noxious, plant
from ergot used as drug (migraine therapy) —*see* Table of Drugs and Chemicals
Erosio interdigitalis blastomycetica B37.2
Erosion
artery I77.2
without rupture I77.89
bone —*see* Disorder, bone, density and structure, specified NEC
bronchus J98.Ø9
cartilage (joint) —*see* Disorder, cartilage, specified type NEC
cervix (uteri) (acquired) (chronic) (congenital) N86
with cervicitis N72
cornea (nontraumatic) —*see* Ulcer, cornea
recurrent H18.83-
traumatic —*see* Abrasion, cornea
dental (idiopathic) (occupational) (due to diet, drugs or vomiting) KØ3.2
duodenum, postpyloric —*see* Ulcer, duodenum
esophagus K22.1Ø
with bleeding K22.11
gastric —*see* Ulcer, stomach
gastrojejunal —*see* Ulcer, gastrojejunal
implanted mesh —*see* Complications, mesh
intestine K63.3
lymphatic vessel I89.8
pylorus, pyloric (ulcer) —*see* Ulcer, stomach
spine, aneurysmal A52.Ø9
stomach —*see* Ulcer, stomach
subcutaneous device pocket ◀
nervous system prosthetic device, implant, or graft T85.89Ø ◀
other internal prosthetic device, implant, or graft T85.898 ◀
teeth (idiopathic) (occupational) (due to diet, drugs or vomiting) KØ3.2
urethra N36.8
uterus N85.8
Erotomania F52.8
Error
metabolism, inborn —*see* Disorder, metabolism
refractive —*see* Disorder, refraction
Eructation R14.2
nervous or psychogenic F45.8
Eruption
creeping B76.9
drug (generalized) (taken internally) L27.Ø
fixed L27.1
in contact with skin —*see* Dermatitis, due to drugs
localized L27.1
Hutchinson, summer L56.4
Kaposi's varicelliform BØØ.Ø
napkin L22
polymorphous light (sun) L56.4
recalcitrant pustular L13.8
ringed R23.8
skin (nonspecific) R21
creeping (meaning hookworm) B76.9
due to inoculation/vaccination (generalized) —*see also* Dermatitis, due to, vaccine L27.Ø
localized L27.1
erysipeloid A26.Ø
feigned L98.1
Kaposi's varicelliform BØØ.Ø
lichenoid L28.Ø
meaning dermatitis —*see* Dermatitis
toxic NEC L53.Ø
tooth, teeth, abnormal (incomplete) (late) (premature) (sequence) KØØ.6
vesicular R23.8
Erysipelas (gangrenous) (infantile) (newborn) (phlegmonous) (suppurative) A46
external ear A46 *[H62.4Ø]*
puerperal, postpartum O86.89
Erysipeloid A26.9
cutaneous (Rosenbach's) A26.Ø
disseminated A26.8
sepsis A26.7
specified NEC A26.8
Erythema, erythematous (infectional) (inflammation) L53.9
ab igne L59.Ø
annulare (centrifugum) (rheumaticum) L53.1
arthriticum epidemicum A25.1
brucellum —*see* Brucellosis
chronic figurate NEC L53.3
chronicum migrans (Borrelia burgdorferi) A69.2Ø
diaper L22
due to
chemical NEC L53.Ø
in contact with skin L24.5
drug (internal use) —*see* Dermatitis, due to, drugs
elevatum diutinum L95.1
endemic E52
epidemic, arthritic A25.1
figuratum perstans L53.3
gluteal L22
heat - code by site under Burn, first degree
ichthyosiforme congenitum bullous Q8Ø.3
in diseases classified elsewhere L54
induratum (nontuberculous) L52
tuberculous A18.4
infectiosum BØ8.3
intertrigo L3Ø.4
iris L51.9
marginatum L53.2
in (due to) acute rheumatic fever IØØ
medicamentosum —*see* Dermatitis, due to, drugs
migrans A26.Ø
chronicum A69.2Ø
tongue K14.1

E

Erythema, erythematous *(Continued)*
multiforme (major) (minor) L51.9
bullous, bullosum L51.1
conjunctiva L51.1
nonbullous L51.0
pemphigoides L12.0
specified NEC L51.8
napkin L22
neonatorum P83.8
toxic P83.1
nodosum L52
tuberculous A18.4
palmar L53.8
pernio T69.1
rash, newborn P83.8
scarlatiniform (recurrent) (exfoliative) L53.8
solare L55.0
specified NEC L53.8
toxic, toxicum NEC L53.0
newborn P83.1
tuberculous (primary) A18.4
Erythematous, erythematosus —*see* condition
Erythermalgia (primary) I73.81
Erythralgia I73.81
Erythrasma L08.1
Erythredema (polyneuropathy) —*see* Poisoning, mercury
Erythremia (acute) C94.0-
chronic D45
secondary D75.1
Erythroblastopenia —*see also* Aplasia, red cell D60.9
congenital D61.01
Erythroblastophthisis D61.09
Erythroblastosis (fetalis) (newborn) P55.9
due to
ABO (antibodies) (incompatibility) (isoimmunization) P55.1
Rh (antibodies) (incompatibility) (isoimmunization) P55.0
Erythrocyanosis (crurum) I73.89
Erythrocythemia —*see* Erythremia
Erythrocytosis (megalosplenic) (secondary) D75.1
familial D75.0
oval, hereditary —*see* Elliptocytosis
secondary D75.1
stress D75.1
Erythroderma (secondary) —*see also* Erythema L53.9
bullous ichthyosiform, congenital Q80.3
desquamativum L21.1
ichthyosiform, congenital (bullous) Q80.3
neonatorum P83.8
psoriaticum L40.8
Erythrodysesthesia, palmar plantar (PPE) L27.1
Erythrogenesis imperfecta D61.09
Erythroleukemia C94.0-
Erythromelalgia I73.81
Erythrophagocytosis D75.89
Erythrophobia F40.298
Erythroplakia, oral epithelium, and tongue K13.29
Erythroplasia (Queyrat) D07.4
specified site —*see* Neoplasm, skin, in situ
unspecified site D07.4
Escherichia coli (E. coli), as cause of disease classified elsewhere B96.20
non-O157 Shiga toxin-producing (with known O group) B96.22
non-Shiga toxin-producing B96.29
O157 with confirmation of Shiga toxin when H antigen is unknown, or is not H7 B96.21
O157:H- (nonmotile) with confirmation of Shiga toxin B96.21
O157:H7 with or without confirmation of Shiga toxin-production B96.21
Shiga toxin-producing (with unspecified O group) (STEC) B96.23

Escherichia coli *(Continued)*
O157 B96.21
O157:H7 with or without confirmation of Shiga toxin-production B96.21
specified NEC B96.22
specified NEC B96.29
Esophagismus K22.4
Esophagitis (acute) (alkaline) (chemical) (chronic) (infectional) (necrotic) (peptic) (postoperative) K20.9
candidal B37.81
due to gastrointestinal reflux disease K21.0
eosinophilic K20.0
reflux K21.0
specified NEC K20.8
tuberculous A18.83
ulcerative K22.10
with bleeding K22.11
Esophagocele K22.5
Esophagomalacia K22.8
Esophagospasm K22.4
Esophagostenosis K22.2
Esophagostomiasis B81.8
Esophagotracheal —*see* condition
Esophagus —*see* condition
Esophoria H50.51
convergence, excess H51.12
divergence, insufficiency H51.8
Esotropia —*see* Strabismus, convergent concomitant
Espundia B55.2
Essential —*see* condition
Esthesioneuroblastoma C30.0
Esthesioneurocytoma C30.0
Esthesioneuroepithelioma C30.0
Esthiomene A55
Estivo-autumnal malaria (fever) B50.9
Estrangement (marital) Z63.5
parent-child NEC Z62.890
Estriasis —*see* Myiasis
Ethanolism —*see* Alcoholism
Etherism —*see* Dependence, drug, inhalant
Ethmoid, ethmoidal —*see* condition
Ethmoiditis (chronic) (nonpurulent) (purulent) —*see also* Sinusitis, ethmoidal
influenzal —*see* Influenza, with, respiratory manifestations NEC
Woakes' J33.1
Ethylism —*see* Alcoholism
Eulenburg's disease (congenital paramyotonia) G71.19
Eumycetoma B47.0
Eunuchoidism E29.1
hypogonadotropic E23.0
European blastomycosis —*see* Cryptococcosis
Eustachian —*see* condition
Evaluation (for) (of)
development state
adolescent Z00.3
period of
delayed growth in childhood Z00.70
with abnormal findings Z00.71
rapid growth in childhood Z00.2
puberty Z00.3
growth and developmental state (period of rapid growth) Z00.2
delayed growth Z00.70
with abnormal findings Z00.71
mental health (status) Z00.8
requested by authority Z04.6
period of
delayed growth in childhood Z00.70
with abnormal findings Z00.71
rapid growth in childhood Z00.2
suspected condition —*see* Observation
Evans syndrome D69.41
Event, apparent life threatening in newborn and infant (ALTE) R68.13
Eventration —*see also* Hernia, ventral
colon into chest —*see* Hernia, diaphragm
diaphragm (congenital) Q79.1

Eversion
bladder N32.89
cervix (uteri) N86
with cervicitis N72
foot NEC —*see also* Deformity, valgus, ankle
congenital Q66.6
punctum lacrimale (postinfectional) (senile) H04.52-
ureter (meatus) N28.89
urethra (meatus) N36.8
uterus N81.4
Evidence
cytologic
of malignancy on anal smear R85.614
of malignancy on cervical smear R87.614
of malignancy on vaginal smear R87.624
Evisceration
birth injury P15.8
traumatic NEC
eye —*see* Enucleated eye
Evulsion —*see* Avulsion
Ewing's sarcoma or tumor —*see* Neoplasm, bone, malignant
Examination (for) (following) (general) (of) (routine) Z00.00
with abnormal findings Z00.01
abuse, physical (alleged), ruled out
adult Z04.71
child Z04.72
adolescent (development state) Z00.3
alleged rape or sexual assault (victim), ruled out
adult Z04.41
child Z04.42
allergy Z01.82
annual (adult) (periodic) (physical) Z00.00
with abnormal findings Z00.01
gynecological Z01.419
with abnormal findings Z01.411
antibody response Z01.84
blood —*see* Examination, laboratory
blood pressure Z01.30
with abnormal findings Z01.31
cancer staging —*see* Neoplasm, malignant, by site
cervical Papanicolaou smear Z12.4
as part of routine gynecological examination Z01.419
with abnormal findings Z01.411
child (over 28 days old) Z00.129
with abnormal findings Z00.121
under 28 days old —*see* Newborn, examination
clinical research control or normal comparison (control) (participant) Z00.6
contraceptive (drug) maintenance (routine) Z30.8
device (intrauterine) Z30.431
dental Z01.20
with abnormal findings Z01.21
developmental —*see* Examination, child
donor (potential) Z00.5
ear Z01.10
with abnormal findings NEC Z01.118
eye Z01.00
with abnormal findings Z01.01
following
accident NEC Z04.3
transport Z04.1
work Z04.2
assault, alleged, ruled out
adult Z04.71
child Z04.72
motor vehicle accident Z04.1
treatment (for) Z09
combined NEC Z09
fracture Z09
malignant neoplasm Z08
malignant neoplasm Z08
mental disorder Z09
specified condition NEC Z09

Examination *(Continued)*
follow-up (routine) (following) Z09
chemotherapy NEC Z09
malignant neoplasm Z08
fracture Z09
malignant neoplasm Z08
postpartum Z39.2
psychotherapy Z09
radiotherapy NEC Z09
malignant neoplasm Z08
surgery NEC Z09
malignant neoplasm Z08
gynecological Z01.419
with abnormal findings Z01.411
for contraceptive maintenance Z30.8
health *—see* Examination, medical
hearing Z01.10
with abnormal findings NEC Z01.118
following failed hearing screening Z01.110
immunity status testing Z01.84
laboratory (as part of a general medical examination) Z00.00
with abnormal findings Z00.01
preprocedural Z01.812
lactating mother Z39.1
medical (adult) (for) (of) Z00.00
with abnormal findings Z00.01
administrative purpose only Z02.9
specified NEC Z02.89
admission to
armed forces Z02.3
old age home Z02.2
prison Z02.89
residential institution Z02.2
school Z02.0
following illness or medical treatment Z02.0
summer camp Z02.89
adoption Z02.82
blood alcohol or drug level Z02.83
camp (summer) Z02.89
clinical research, normal subject (control) (participant) Z00.6
control subject in clinical research (normal comparison) (participant) Z00.6
donor (potential) Z00.5
driving license Z02.4
general (adult) Z00.00
with abnormal findings Z00.01
immigration Z02.89
insurance purposes Z02.6
marriage Z02.89
medicolegal reasons NEC Z04.8
naturalization Z02.89
participation in sport Z02.5
paternity testing Z02.81
population survey Z00.8
pre-employment Z02.1
pre-operative *—see* Examination, pre-procedural
pre-procedural
cardiovascular Z01.810
respiratory Z01.811
specified NEC Z01.818
preschool children
for admission to school Z02.0
prisoners
for entrance into prison Z02.89
recruitment for armed forces Z02.3
specified NEC Z00.8
sport competition Z02.5
medicolegal reason NEC Z04.8
newborn *—see* Newborn, examination
pelvic (annual) (periodic) Z01.419
with abnormal findings Z01.411
period of rapid growth in childhood Z00.2
periodic (adult) (annual) (routine) Z00.00
with abnormal findings Z00.01
physical (adult) *—see also* Examination, medical Z00.00
sports Z02.5

Examination *(Continued)*
postpartum
immediately after delivery Z39.0
routine follow-up Z39.2
pre-chemotherapy (antineoplastic) Z01.818
prenatal (normal pregnancy) *—see also* Pregnancy, normal Z34.9-
pre-procedural (pre-operative)
cardiovascular Z01.810
laboratory Z01.812
respiratory Z01.811
specified NEC Z01.818
prior to chemotherapy (antineoplastic) Z01.818
psychiatric NEC Z00.8
follow-up not needing further care Z09
requested by authority Z04.6
radiological (as part of a general medical examination) Z00.00
with abnormal findings Z00.01
repeat cervical smear to confirm findings of recent normal smear following initial abnormal smear Z01.42
skin (hypersensitivity) Z01.82
special *—see also* Examination, by type Z01.89
specified type NEC Z01.89
specified type or reason NEC Z04.8
teeth Z01.20
with abnormal findings Z01.21
urine *—see* Examination, laboratory
vision Z01.00
with abnormal findings Z01.01
Exanthem, exanthema *—see also* Rash
with enteroviral vesicular stomatitis B08.4
Boston A88.0
epidemic with meningitis A88.0 *[G02]*
subitum B08.20
due to human herpesvirus 6 B08.21
due to human herpesvirus 7 B08.22
viral, virus B09
specified type NEC B08.8
Excess, excessive, excessively
alcohol level in blood R78.0
androgen (ovarian) E28.1
attrition, tooth, teeth K03.0
carotene, carotin (dietary) E67.1
cold, effects of T69.9
specified effect NEC T69.8
convergence H51.12
crying
in child, adolescent, or adult R45.83
in infant R68.11
development, breast N62
divergence H51.8
drinking (alcohol) NEC (without dependence) F10.10
habitual (continual) (without remission) F10.20
eating R63.2
estrogen E28.0
fat *—see also* Obesity
in heart *—see* Degeneration, myocardial
localized E65
foreskin N47.8
gas R14.0
glucagon E16.3
heat *—see* Heat
intermaxillary vertical dimension of fully erupted teeth M26.37
interocclusal distance of fully erupted teeth M26.37
kalium E87.5
large
colon K59.39 ⬅
congenital Q43.8
infant P08.0
organ or site, congenital NEC *—see* Anomaly, by site
long
organ or site, congenital NEC *—see* Anomaly, by site

Excess, excessive, excessively *(Continued)*
menstruation (with regular cycle) N92.0
with irregular cycle N92.1
napping Z72.821
natrium E87.0
number of teeth K00.1
nutrient (dietary) NEC R63.2
potassium (K) E87.5
salivation K11.7
secretion *—see also* Hypersecretion
milk O92.6
sputum R09.3
sweat R61
sexual drive F52.8
short
organ or site, congenital NEC *—see* Anomaly, by site
umbilical cord in labor or delivery O69.3
~~skin, eyelid (acquired) —see Blepharochalasis~~
~~congenital Q10.3~~
skin L98.7 ◀
and subcutaneous tissue L98.7 ◀
eyelid (acquired) *—see* Blepharochalasis ◀
congenital Q10.3 ◀
sodium (Na) E87.0
spacing of fully erupted teeth M26.32
sputum R09.3
sweating R61
thirst R63.1
due to deprivation of water T73.1
tuberosity of jaw M26.07
vitamin
A (dietary) E67.0
administered as drug (prolonged intake) *—see* Table of Drugs and Chemicals, vitamins, adverse effect
overdose or wrong substance given or taken *—see* Table of Drugs and Chemicals, vitamins, poisoning
D (dietary) E67.3
administered as drug (prolonged intake) *—see* Table of Drugs and Chemicals, vitamins, adverse effect
overdose or wrong substance given or taken *—see* Table of Drugs and Chemicals, vitamins, poisoning
weight
gain R63.5
loss R63.4
Excitability, abnormal, under minor stress (personality disorder) F60.3
Excitation
anomalous atrioventricular I45.6
psychogenic F30.8
reactive (from emotional stress, psychological trauma) F30.8
Excitement
hypomanic F30.8
manic F30.9
mental, reactive (from emotional stress, psychological trauma) F30.8
state, reactive (from emotional stress, psychological trauma) F30.8
Excoriation (traumatic) *—see also* Abrasion
neurotic L98.1
skin picking disorder F42.4 ◀
Exfoliation
due to erythematous conditions according to extent of body surface involved L49.0
10-19 percent of body surface L49.1
20-29 percent of body surface L49.2
30-39 percent of body surface L49.3
40-49 percent of body surface L49.4
50-59 percent of body surface L49.5
60-69 percent of body surface L49.6
70-79 percent of body surface L49.7
80-89 percent of body surface L49.8
90-99 percent of body surface L49.9
less than 10 percent of body surface L49.0
teeth, due to systemic causes K08.0

E

Exfoliative *—see* condition

Exhaustion, exhaustive (physical NEC) R53.83
- battle F43.0
- cardiac *—see* Failure, heart
- delirium F43.0
- due to
  - cold T69.8
  - excessive exertion T73.3
  - exposure T73.2
  - neurasthenia F48.8
- heart *—see* Failure, heart
- heat *—see also* Heat, exhaustion T67.5
  - due to
    - salt depletion T67.4
    - water depletion T67.3
- maternal, complicating delivery O75.81
- mental F48.8
- myocardium, myocardial *—see* Failure, heart
- nervous F48.8
- old age R54
- psychogenic F48.8
- psychosis F43.0
- senile R54
- vital NEC Z73.0

Exhibitionism F65.2

Exocervicitis *—see* Cervicitis

Exomphalos Q79.2
- meaning hernia *—see* Hernia, umbilicus

Exophoria H50.52
- convergence, insufficiency H51.11
- divergence, excess H51.8

Exophthalmos H05.2-
- congenital Q15.8
- constant NEC H05.24-
- displacement, globe *—see* Displacement, globe
- due to thyrotoxicosis (hyperthyroidism) *—see* Hyperthyroidism, with, goiter (diffuse)
- dysthyroid *—see* Hyperthyroidism, with, goiter (diffuse)
- goiter *—see* Hyperthyroidism, with, goiter (diffuse)
- intermittent NEC H05.25-
- malignant *—see* Hyperthyroidism, with, goiter (diffuse)
- orbital
  - edema *—see* Edema, orbit
  - hemorrhage *—see* Hemorrhage, orbit
- pulsating NEC H05.26-
- thyrotoxic, thyrotropic *—see* Hyperthyroidism, with, goiter (diffuse)

Exostosis *—see also* Disorder, bone
- cartilaginous *—see* Neoplasm, bone, benign
- congenital (multiple) Q78.6
- external ear canal H61.81-
- gonococcal A54.49
- jaw (bone) M27.8
- multiple, congenital Q78.6
- orbit H05.35-
- osteocartilaginous *—see* Neoplasm, bone, benign
- syphilitic A52.77

Exotropia *—see* Strabismus, divergent concomitant

Explanation of
- investigation finding Z71.2
- medication Z71.89

Exposure (to) *—see also* Contact, with T75.89
- acariasis Z20.7
- AIDS virus Z20.6
- air pollution Z77.110
- algae and algae toxins Z77.121
- algae bloom Z77.121
- anthrax Z20.810
- aromatic amines Z77.020
- aromatic (hazardous) compounds NEC Z77.028
- aromatic dyes NOS Z77.028

Exposure *(Continued)*
- arsenic Z77.010
- asbestos Z77.090
- bacterial disease NEC Z20.818
- benzene Z77.021
- blue-green algae bloom Z77.121
- body fluids (potentially hazardous) Z77.21
- brown tide Z77.121
- chemicals (chiefly nonmedicinal) (hazardous) NEC Z77.098
- cholera Z20.09
- chromium compounds Z77.018
- cold, effects of T69.9
  - specified effect NEC T69.8
- communicable disease Z20.9
  - bacterial NEC Z20.818
  - specified NEC Z20.89
  - viral NEC Z20.828
- cyanobacteria bloom Z77.121
- disaster Z65.5
- discrimination Z60.5
- dyes Z77.098
- effects of T73.9
- environmental tobacco smoke (acute) (chronic) Z77.22
- Escherichia coli (E. coli) Z20.01
- exhaustion due to T73.2
- fiberglass *—see* Table of Drugs and Chemicals, fiberglass
- German measles Z20.4
- gonorrhea Z20.2
- hazardous metals NEC Z77.018
- hazardous substances NEC Z77.29
- hazards in the physical environment NEC Z77.128
- hazards to health NEC Z77.9
- human immunodeficiency virus (HIV) Z20.6
- human T-lymphotropic virus type-1 (HTLV-1) Z20.89
- implanted
  - mesh *—see* Complications, mesh
  - prosthetic materials NEC *—see* Complications, prosthetic materials NEC
- infestation (parasitic) NEC Z20.7
- intestinal infectious disease NEC Z20.09
  - Escherichia coli (E. coli) Z20.01
- lead Z77.011
- meningococcus Z20.811
- mold (toxic) Z77.120
- nickel dust Z77.018
- noise Z77.122
- occupational
  - air contaminants NEC Z57.39
  - dust Z57.2
  - environmental tobacco smoke Z57.31
  - extreme temperature Z57.6
  - noise Z57.0
  - radiation Z57.1
  - risk factors Z57.9
    - specified NEC Z57.8
  - toxic agents (gases) (liquids) (solids) (vapors) in agriculture Z57.4
  - toxic agents (gases) (liquids) (solids) (vapors) in industry NEC Z57.5
  - vibration Z57.7
- parasitic disease NEC Z20.7
- pediculosis Z20.7
- persecution Z60.5
- pfiesteria piscicida Z77.121
- poliomyelitis Z20.89
- pollution
  - air Z77.110
  - environmental NEC Z77.118
  - soil Z77.112
  - water Z77.111
- polycyclic aromatic hydrocarbons Z77.028

Exposure *(Continued)*
- prenatal (drugs) (toxic chemicals) *—see* Newborn, affected by, noxious substances transmitted via placenta or breast milk (Revised)
- rabies Z20.3
- radiation, naturally occurring NEC Z77.123
- radon Z77.123
- red tide (Florida) Z77.121
- rubella Z20.4
- second hand tobacco smoke (acute) (chronic) Z77.22
  - in the perinatal period P96.81
- sexually-transmitted disease Z20.2
- smallpox (laboratory) Z20.89
- syphilis Z20.2
- terrorism Z65.4
- torture Z65.4
- tuberculosis Z20.1
- uranium Z77.012
- varicella Z20.820
- venereal disease Z20.2
- viral disease NEC Z20.828
- war Z65.5
- water pollution Z77.111

Exsanguination *—see* Hemorrhage

Exstrophy
- abdominal contents Q45.8
- bladder Q64.10
  - cloacal Q64.12
  - specified type NEC Q64.19
  - supravesical fissure Q64.11

Extensive *—see* condition

Extra *—see also* Accessory
- marker chromosomes (normal individual) Q92.61
  - in abnormal individual Q92.62
- rib Q76.6
  - cervical Q76.5

Extrasystoles (supraventricular) I49.49
- atrial I49.1
- auricular I49.1
- junctional I49.2
- ventricular I49.3

Extrauterine gestation or pregnancy *—see* Pregnancy, by site

Extravasation
- blood R58
- chyle into mesentery I89.8
- pelvicalyceal N13.8
- pyelosinus N13.8
- urine (from ureter) R39.0
- vesicant agent
  - antineoplastic chemotherapy T80.810
  - other agent NEC T80.818

Extremity *—see* condition, limb

Extrophy *—see* Exstrophy

Extroversion
- bladder Q64.19
- uterus N81.4
  - complicating delivery O71.2
  - postpartal (old) N81.4

Extruded tooth (teeth) M26.34

Extrusion
- breast implant (prosthetic) T85.42
- eye implant (globe) (ball) T85.328
- intervertebral disc *—see* Displacement, intervertebral disc
- ocular lens implant (prosthetic) *—see* Complications, intraocular lens
- vitreous *—see* Prolapse, vitreous

Exudate
- pleural *—see* Effusion, pleura
- retina H35.89

Exudative *—see* condition

Eye, eyeball, eyelid *—see* condition

Eyestrain *—see* Disturbance, vision, subjective

Eyeworm disease of Africa B74.3

E

F

Faber's syndrome (achlorhydric anemia) D50.9
Fabry (-Anderson) **disease** E75.21
Faciocephalalgia, autonomic —*see also* Neuropathy, peripheral, autonomic G90.09
Factor (s)
psychic, associated with diseases classified elsewhere F54
psychological
affecting physical conditions F54
or behavioral
affecting general medical condition F54
associated with disorders or diseases classified elsewhere F54
Fahr disease (of brain) G23.8
Fahr Volhard disease (of kidney) I12.-
Failure, failed
abortion —*see* Abortion, attempted
aortic (valve) I35.8
rheumatic I06.8
attempted abortion —*see* Abortion, attempted
biventricular I50.9
bone marrow —*see* Anemia, aplastic
cardiac —*see* Failure, heart
cardiorenal (chronic) I50.9
hypertensive I13.2
cardiorespiratory (*see also* Failure, heart) R09.2
cardiovascular (chronic) —*see* Failure, heart
cerebrovascular I67.9
cervical dilatation in labor O62.0
circulation, circulatory (peripheral) R57.9
newborn P29.89
compensation —*see* Disease, heart
compliance with medical treatment or regimen —*see* Noncompliance
congestive —*see* Failure, heart, congestive
dental implant (endosseous) M27.69
due to
failure of dental prosthesis M27.63
lack of attached gingiva M27.62
occlusal trauma (poor prosthetic design) M27.62
parafunctional habits M27.62
periodontal infection (peri-implantitis) M27.62
poor oral hygiene M27.62
osseointegration M27.61
due to
complications of systemic disease M27.61
poor bone quality M27.61
iatrogenic M27.61
post-osseointegration
biological M27.62
due to complications of systemic disease M27.62
iatrogenic M27.62
mechanical M27.63
pre-integration M27.61
pre-osseointegration M27.61
specified NEC M27.69
descent of head (at term) of pregnancy (mother) O32.4
endosseous dental implant —*see* Failure, dental implant
engagement of head (term of pregnancy) (mother) O32.4
erection (penile) —*see also* Dysfunction, sexual, male, erectile N52.9
~~nonorgqanic F52.21~~
nonorganic F52.21 ◀
examination (s), anxiety concerning Z55.2
expansion terminal respiratory units (newborn) (primary) P28.0
forceps NOS (with subsequent cesarean delivery) O66.5
gain weight (child over 28 days old) R62.51
adult R62.7
newborn P92.6

Failure, failed *(Continued)*
genital response (male) F52.21
female F52.22
heart (acute) (senile) (sudden) I50.9
with
acute pulmonary edema —*see* Failure, ventricular, left
decompensation —*see* Failure, heart, congestive
dilatation —*see* Disease, heart
arteriosclerotic I70.90
biventricular I50.9
combined left-right sided I50.9
compensated I50.9
complicating
anesthesia (general) (local) or other sedation
in labor and delivery O74.2
in pregnancy O29.12-
postpartum, puerperal O89.1
delivery (cesarean) (instrumental) O75.4
congestive (compensated) (decompensated) I50.9
with rheumatic fever (conditions in I00)
active I01.8
inactive or quiescent (with chorea) I09.81
newborn P29.0
rheumatic (chronic) (inactive) (with chorea) I09.81
active or acute I01.8
with chorea I02.0
decompensated I50.9
degenerative —*see* Degeneration, myocardial
diastolic (congestive) I50.30
acute (congestive) I50.31
and (on) chronic (congestive) I50.33
chronic (congestive) I50.32
and (on) acute (congestive) I50.33
combined with systolic (congestive) I50.40
acute (congestive) I50.41
and (on) chronic (congestive) I50.43
chronic (congestive) I50.42
and (on) acute (congestive) I50.43
due to presence of cardiac prosthesis I97.13-
following cardiac surgery I97.13-
high output NOS I50.9
hypertensive —*see* Hypertension, heart
left (ventricular) —*see* Failure, ventricular, left
low output (syndrome) NOS I50.9
newborn P29.0
organic —*see* Disease, heart
peripartum O90.3
postprocedural I97.13-
rheumatic (chronic) (inactive) I09.9
right (ventricular) (secondary to left heart failure) —*see* Failure, heart, congestive
systolic (congestive) I50.20
acute (congestive) I50.21
and (on) chronic (congestive) I50.23
chronic (congestive) I50.22
and (on) acute (congestive) I50.23
combined with diastolic (congestive) I50.40
acute (congestive) I50.41
and (on) chronic (congestive) I50.43
chronic (congestive) I50.42
and (on) acute (congestive) I50.43
thyrotoxic —*see also* Thyrotoxicosis E05.90 *[I43]*
with thyroid storm E05.91 *[I43]*
valvular —*see* Endocarditis

Failure, failed *(Continued)*
hepatic K72.90
with coma K72.91
acute or subacute K72.00
with coma K72.01
due to drugs K71.10
with coma K71.11
alcoholic (acute) (chronic) (subacute) K70.40
with coma K70.41
chronic K72.10
with coma K72.11
due to drugs (acute) (subacute) (chronic) K71.10
with coma K71.11
due to drugs (acute) (subacute) (chronic) K71.10
with coma K71.11
postprocedural K91.82
hepatorenal K76.7
induction (of labor) O61.9
abortion —*see* Abortion, attempted
by
oxytocic drugs O61.0
prostaglandins O61.0
instrumental O61.1
mechanical O61.1
medical O61.0
specified NEC O61.8
surgical O61.1
intubation during anesthesia T88.4
in pregnancy O29.6-
labor and delivery O74.7
postpartum, puerperal O89.6
involution, thymus (gland) E32.0
kidney —*see also* Disease, kidney, chronic N19
acute —*see also* Failure, renal, acute N17.9-
diabetic —*see* E08-E13 with .22
lactation (complete) O92.3
partial O92.4
Leydig's cell, adult E29.1
liver —*see* Failure, hepatic
menstruation at puberty N91.0
mitral I05.8
myocardial, myocardium —*see also* Failure, heart I50.9
chronic —*see also* Failure, heart, congestive I50.9
congestive —*see also* Failure, heart, congestive I50.9
orgasm (female) (psychogenic) F52.31
male F52.32
ovarian (primary) E28.39
iatrogenic E89.40
asymptomatic E89.40
symptomatic E89.41
postprocedural (postablative) (postirradiation) (postsurgical) E89.40
asymptomatic E89.40
symptomatic E89.41
ovulation causing infertility N97.0
polyglandular, autoimmune E31.0
prosthetic joint implant —*see* Complications, joint prosthesis, mechanical, breakdown, by site
renal N19
with
tubular necrosis (acute) N17.0
acute N17.9
with
cortical necrosis N17.1
medullary necrosis N17.2
tubular necrosis N17.0
specified NEC N17.8
chronic N18.9
hypertensive —*see* Hypertension, kidney
congenital P96.0
end stage (chronic) N18.6
due to hypertension I12.0

Failure, failed *(Continued)*
- renal *(Continued)*
  - following
    - abortion —*see* Abortion by type complicated by specified condition NEC
    - crushing T79.5
    - ectopic or molar pregnancy O08.4
    - labor and delivery (acute) O90.4
  - hypertensive —*see* Hypertension, kidney
  - postprocedural N99.Ø
- respiration, respiratory J96.9
  - with
    - hypercapnia J96.92
    - hypoxia J96.91
  - acute J96.ØØ
    - with
      - hypercapnia J96.Ø2
      - hypoxia J96.Ø1
  - acute and (on) chronic J96.2Ø
    - with
      - hypercapnia J96.22
      - hypoxia J96.21
  - center G93.89
  - chronic J96.1Ø
    - with
      - hypercapnia J96.12
      - hypoxia J96.11
  - newborn P28.5
  - postprocedural (acute) J95.821
    - acute and chronic J95.822
- rotation
  - cecum Q43.3
  - colon Q43.3
  - intestine Q43.3
  - kidney Q63.2
- sedation (conscious) (moderate) during procedure T88.52
  - history of Z92.83
- segmentation —*see also* Fusion
  - fingers —*see* Syndactylism, complex, fingers
  - vertebra Q76.49
    - with scoliosis Q76.3
- seminiferous tubule, adult E29.1
- senile (general) R54
- sexual arousal (male) F52.21
  - female F52.22
- testicular endocrine function E29.1
- to thrive (child over 28 days old) R62.51
  - adult R62.7
  - newborn P92.6
- transplant T86.92
  - bone T86.831
    - marrow T86.Ø2
  - cornea T86.841
  - heart T86.22
    - with lung (s) T86.32
  - intestine T86.851
  - kidney T86.12
  - liver T86.42
  - lung (s) T86.811
    - with heart T86.32
  - pancreas T86.891
  - skin (allograft) (autograft) T86.821
  - specified organ or tissue NEC T86.891
  - stem cell (peripheral blood) (umbilical cord) T86.5
- trial of labor (with subsequent cesarean delivery) O66.4Ø
  - following previous cesarean delivery O66.41
- tubal ligation N99.89
- urinary —*see* Disease, kidney, chronic
- vacuum extraction NOS (with subsequent cesarean delivery) O66.5
- vasectomy N99.89
- ventouse NOS (with subsequent cesarean delivery) O66.5

Failure, failed *(Continued)*
- ventricular —*see also* Failure, heart I5Ø.9
  - left I5Ø.1
    - with rheumatic fever (conditions in IØØ)
      - active IØ1.8
        - with chorea IØ2.Ø
      - inactive or quiescent (with chorea) IØ9.81
    - rheumatic (chronic) (inactive) (with chorea) IØ9.81
      - active or acute IØ1.8
        - with chorea IØ2.Ø
  - right —*see also* Failure, heart, congestive I5Ø.9
- vital centers, newborn P91.8

Fainting (fit) R55

Fallen arches —*see* Deformity, limb, flat foot

Falling, falls (repeated) R29.6
- any organ or part —*see* Prolapse

Fallopian
- insufflation Z31.41
- tube —*see* condition

Fallot's
- pentalogy Q21.8
- tetrad or tetralogy Q21.3
- triad or trilogy Q22.3

False —*see also* condition
- croup J38.5
- joint —*see* Nonunion, fracture
- labor (pains) O47.9
  - at or after 37 completed weeks of gestation O47.1
  - before 37 completed weeks of gestation O47.Ø-
- passage, urethra (prostatic) N36.5
- pregnancy F45.8

Family, familial —*see also* condition
- disruption Z63.8
  - involving divorce or separation Z63.5
- Li-Fraumeni (syndrome) Z15.Ø1
- planning advice Z3Ø.Ø9
- problem Z63.9
  - specified NEC Z63.8
- retinoblastoma C69.2-

Famine (effects of) T73.Ø
- edema —*see* Malnutrition, severe

Fanconi (-de Toni)(-Debré) syndrome E72.Ø9
- with cystinosis E72.Ø4

Fanconi's anemia (congenital pancytopenia) D61.Ø9

Farber's disease or syndrome E75.29

Farcy A24.Ø

Farmer's
- lung J67.Ø
- skin L57.8

Farsightedness —*see* Hypermetropia

Fascia —*see* condition

Fasciculation R25.3

Fasciitis M72.9
- diffuse (eosinophilic) M35.4
- infective M72.8
  - necrotizing M72.6
- necrotizing M72.6
- nodular M72.4
- perirenal (with ureteral obstruction) N13.5
  - with infection N13.6
- plantar M72.2
- specified NEC M72.8
- traumatic (old) M72.8
  - current - code by site under Sprain

Fascioliasis B66.3

Fasciolopsis, fasciolopsiasis (intestinal) B66.5

Fascioscapulohumeral myopathy G71.Ø

Fast pulse RØØ.Ø

Fat
- embolism —*see* Embolism, fat
- excessive —*see also* Obesity
  - in heart —*see* Degeneration, myocardial
- in stool R19.5

Fat *(Continued)*
- localized (pad) E65
  - heart —*see* Degeneration, myocardial
  - knee M79.4
  - retropatellar M79.4
- necrosis
  - breast N64.1
  - mesentery K65.4
  - omentum K65.4
- pad E65
  - knee M79.4

Fatigue R53.83
- auditory deafness —*see* Deafness
- chronic R53.82
- combat F43.Ø
- general R53.83
  - psychogenic F48.8
- heat (transient) T67.6
- muscle M62.89
- myocardium —*see* Failure, heart
- neoplasm-related R53.Ø
- nervous, neurosis F48.8
- operational F48.8
- psychogenic (general) F48.8
- senile R54
- voice R49.8

Fatness —*see* Obesity

Fatty —*see also* condition
- apron E65
- degeneration —*see* Degeneration, fatty
- heart (enlarged) —*see* Degeneration, myocardial
- liver NEC K76.Ø
  - alcoholic K7Ø.Ø
  - nonalcoholic K76.Ø
- necrosis —*see* Degeneration, fatty

Fauces —*see* condition

Fauchard's disease (periodontitis) —*see* Periodontitis

Faucitis JØ2.9

Favism (anemia) D55.Ø

Favus —*see* Dermatophytosis

Fazio-Londe disease or syndrome G12.1

Fear complex or reaction F4Ø.9

Fear of —*see* Phobia

Feared complaint unfounded Z71.1

Febris, febrile —*see also* Fever
- flava —*see also* Fever, yellow A95.9
- melitensis A23.Ø
- pestis —*see* Plague
- recurrens —*see* Fever, relapsing
- rubra A38.9

Fecal
- incontinence R15.9
- smearing R15.1
- soiling R15.1
- urgency R15.2

Fecalith (impaction) K56.41
- appendix K38.1
- congenital P76.8

Fede's disease K14.Ø

Feeble rapid pulse due to shock following injury T79.4

Feeble-minded F7Ø

Feeding
- difficulties R63.3
- problem R63.3
  - newborn P92.9
    - specified NEC P92.8
  - nonorganic (adult) —*see* Disorder, eating

Feeling (of)
- foreign body in throat RØ9.89

Feer's disease —*see* Poisoning, mercury

Feet —*see* condition

Feigned illness Z76.5

Feil-Klippel syndrome (brevicollis) Q76.1

Feinmesser's (hidrotic) **ectodermal dysplasia** Q82.4

Felinophobia F4Ø.218

- **Felon** —*see also* Cellulitis, digit
  - with lymphangitis —*see* Lymphangitis, acute, digit
- **Felty's syndrome** MØ5.ØØ
  - ankle MØ5.Ø7-
  - elbow MØ5.Ø2-
  - foot joint MØ5.Ø7-
  - hand joint MØ5.Ø4-
  - hip MØ5.Ø5-
  - knee MØ5.Ø6-
  - multiple site MØ5.Ø9
  - shoulder MØ5.Ø1-
  - vertebra —*see* Spondylitis, ankylosing
  - wrist MØ5.Ø3-
- **Female genital cutting status** —*see* Female genital mutilation status (FGM)
- **Female genital mutilation status** (FGM) N9Ø.81Ø
  - specified NEC N9Ø.818
  - type I (clitorectomy status) N9Ø.811
  - type II (clitorectomy with excision of labia minora status) N9Ø.812
  - type III (infibulation status) N9Ø.813
  - type IV N9Ø.818
- **Femur, femoral** —*see* condition
- **Fenestration, fenestrated** —*see also* Imperfect, closure
  - aortico-pulmonary Q21.4
  - cusps, heart valve NEC Q24.8
    - pulmonary Q22.3
  - pulmonic cusps Q22.3
- **Fernell's disease** (aortic aneurysm) I71.9
- **Fertile eunuch syndrome** E23.Ø
- **Fetid**
  - breath R19.6
  - sweat L75.Ø
- **Fetishism** F65.Ø
  - transvestic F65.1
- **Fetus, fetal** —*see also* condition
  - alcohol syndrome (dysmorphic) Q86.Ø
  - compressus O31.Ø-
  - hydantoin syndrome Q86.1
  - lung tissue P28.Ø
  - papyraceous O31.Ø-
- **Fever** (inanition) (of unknown origin) (persistent) (with chills) (with rigor) R5Ø.9
  - abortus A23.1
  - Aden (dengue) A9Ø
  - African tick-borne A68.1
  - American
    - mountain (tick) A93.2
    - spotted A77.Ø
  - aphthous BØ8.8
  - arbovirus, arboviral A94
    - hemorrhagic A94
    - specified NEC A93.8
  - Argentinian hemorrhagic A96.Ø
  - Assam B55.Ø
  - Australian Q A78
  - Bangkok hemorrhagic A91
  - Barmah forest A92.8
  - Bartonella A44.Ø
  - bilious, hemoglobinuric B5Ø.8
  - blackwater B5Ø.8
  - blister BØØ.1
  - Bolivian hemorrhagic A96.1
  - Bonvale dam T73.3
  - boutonneuse A77.1
  - brain —*see* Encephalitis
  - Brazilian purpuric A48.4
  - breakbone A9Ø
  - Bullis A77.Ø
  - Bunyamwera A92.8
  - Burdwan B55.Ø
  - Bwamba A92.8
  - Cameroon —*see* Malaria
  - Canton A75.9
  - catarrhal (acute) JØØ
    - chronic J31.Ø
  - cat-scratch A28.1
  - Central Asian hemorrhagic A98.Ø
  - cerebral —*see* Encephalitis

Fever *(Continued)*

  - cerebrospinal meningococcal A39.Ø
  - Chagres B5Ø.9
  - Chandipura A92.8
  - Changuinola A93.1
  - Charcot's (biliary) (hepatic) (intermittent) —*see* Calculus, bile duct
  - Chikungunya (viral) (hemorrhagic) A92.Ø
  - Chitral A93.1
  - Colombo —*see* Fever, paratyphoid
  - Colorado tick (virus) A93.2
  - congestive (remittent) —*see* Malaria
  - Congo virus A98.Ø
  - continued malarial B5Ø.9
  - Corsican —*see* Malaria
  - Crimean-Congo hemorrhagic A98.Ø
  - Cyprus —*see* Brucellosis
  - dandy A9Ø
  - deer fly —*see* Tularemia
  - dengue (virus) A9Ø
    - hemorrhagic A91
    - sandfly A93.1
  - desert B38.Ø
  - drug induced R5Ø.2
  - due to
    - conditions classified elsewhere R5Ø.81
    - heat T67.Ø
  - enteric AØ1.ØØ
  - enteroviral exanthematous (Boston exanthem) A88.Ø
  - ephemeral (of unknown origin) R5Ø.9
  - epidemic hemorrhagic A98.5
  - erysipelatous —*see* Erysipelas
  - estivo-autumnal (malarial) B5Ø.9
  - famine A75.Ø
  - five day A79.Ø
  - following delivery O86.4
  - Fort Bragg A27.89
  - gastroenteric AØ1.ØØ
  - gastromalarial —*see* Malaria
  - Gibraltar —*see* Brucellosis
  - glandular —*see* Mononucleosis, infectious
  - Guama (viral) A92.8
  - Haverhill A25.1
  - hay (allergic) J3Ø.1
    - with asthma (bronchial) J45.9Ø9
      - with
        - exacerbation (acute) J45.9Ø1
        - status asthmaticus J45.9Ø2
    - due to
      - allergen other than pollen J3Ø.89
      - pollen, any plant or tree J3Ø.1
  - heat (effects) T67.Ø
  - hematuric, bilious B5Ø.8
  - hemoglobinuric (malarial) (bilious) B5Ø.8
  - hemorrhagic (arthropod-borne) NOS A94
    - with renal syndrome A98.5
    - arenaviral A96.9
      - specified NEC A96.8
    - Argentinian A96.Ø
    - Bangkok A91
    - Bolivian A96.1
    - Central Asian A98.Ø
    - Chikungunya A92.Ø
    - Crimean-Congo A98.Ø
    - dengue (virus) A91
    - epidemic A98.5
    - Junin (virus) A96.Ø
    - Korean A98.5
    - Kyasanur forest A98.2
    - Machupo (virus) A96.1
    - mite-borne A93.8
    - mosquito-borne A92.8
    - Omsk A98.1
    - Philippine A91
    - Russian A98.5
    - Singapore A91
    - Southeast Asia A91
    - Thailand A91

Fever *(Continued)*

  - hemorrhagic NOS *(Continued)*
    - tick-borne NEC A93.8
    - viral A99
      - specified NEC A98.8
  - hepatic —*see* Cholecystitis
  - herpetic —*see* Herpes
  - icterohemorrhagic A27.Ø
  - Indiana A93.8
  - infective B99.9
    - specified NEC B99.8
  - intermittent (bilious) —*see also* Malaria
    - of unknown origin R5Ø.9
    - pernicious B5Ø.9
  - iodide R5Ø.2
  - Japanese river A75.3
  - jungle —*see also* Malaria
    - yellow A95.Ø
  - Junin (virus) hemorrhagic A96.Ø
  - Katayama B65.2
  - kedani A75.3
  - Kenya (tick) A77.1
  - Kew Garden A79.1
  - Korean hemorrhagic A98.5
  - Lassa A96.2
  - Lone Star A77.Ø
  - Machupo (virus) hemorrhagic A96.1
  - malaria, malarial —*see* Malaria
  - Malta A23.9
  - Marseilles A77.1
  - marsh —*see* Malaria
  - Mayaro (viral) A92.8
  - Mediterranean —*see also* Brucellosis A23.9
    - familial MØ4.1 ⟸
    - tick A77.1
  - meningeal —*see* Meningitis
  - Meuse A79.Ø
  - Mexican A75.2
  - mianeh A68.1
  - miasmatic —*see* Malaria
  - mosquito-borne (viral) A92.9
    - hemorrhagic A92.8
  - mountain —*see also* Brucellosis
    - meaning Rocky Mountain spotted fever A77.Ø
    - tick (American) (Colorado) (viral) A93.2
  - Mucambo (viral) A92.8
  - mud A27.9
  - Neapolitan —*see* Brucellosis
  - neutropenic D7Ø.9
  - newborn P81.9
    - environmental P81.Ø
  - Nine-Mile A78
  - non-exanthematous tick A93.2
  - North Asian tick-borne A77.2
  - Omsk hemorrhagic A98.1
  - O'nyong-nyong (viral) A92.1
  - Oropouche (viral) A93.Ø
  - Oroya A44.Ø
  - paludal —*see* Malaria
  - Panama (malarial) B5Ø.9
  - Pappataci A93.1
  - paratyphoid AØ1.4
    - A AØ1.1
    - B AØ1.2
    - C AØ1.3
  - parrot A7Ø
  - periodic (Mediterranean) MØ4.1 ⟸
  - persistent (of unknown origin) R5Ø.9
  - petechial A39.Ø
  - pharyngoconjunctival B3Ø.2
  - Philippine hemorrhagic A91
  - phlebotomus A93.1
  - Piry (virus) A93.8
  - Pixuna (viral) A92.8
  - Plasmodium ovale B53.Ø
  - polioviral (nonparalytic) A8Ø.4
  - Pontiac A48.2
  - postimmunization R5Ø.83
  - postoperative R5Ø.82
    - due to infection T81.4Ø ⟸

Fever *(Continued)*
- posttransfusion R5Ø.84
- postvaccination R5Ø.83
- presenting with conditions classified elsewhere R5Ø.81
- pretibial A27.89
- puerperal O86.4
- Q A78
- quadrilateral A78
- quartan (malaria) B52.9
- Queensland (coastal) (tick) A77.3
- quintan A79.Ø
- rabbit —*see* Tularemia
- rat-bite A25.9
  - due to
    - Spirillum A25.Ø
    - Streptobacillus moniliformis A25.1
- recurrent —*see* Fever, relapsing
- relapsing (Borrelia) A68.9
  - Carter's (Asiatic) A68.1
  - Dutton's (West African) A68.1
  - Koch's A68.9
  - louse-borne A68.Ø
  - Novy's
    - louse-borne A68.Ø
    - tick-borne A68.1
  - Obermeyer's (European) A68.Ø
  - tick-borne A68.1
- remittent (bilious) (congestive) (gastric) —*see* Malaria
- rheumatic (active) (acute) (chronic) (subacute) IØØ
  - with central nervous system involvement IØ2.9
  - active with heart involvement —*see* category IØ1
  - inactive or quiescent with
    - cardiac hypertrophy IØ9.89
    - carditis IØ9.9
    - endocarditis IØ9.1
      - aortic (valve) IØ6.9
        - with mitral (valve) disease IØ8.Ø
      - mitral (valve) IØ5.9
        - with aortic (valve) disease IØ8.Ø
      - pulmonary (valve) IØ9.89
      - tricuspid (valve) IØ7.8
    - heart disease NEC IØ9.89
    - heart failure (congestive) (conditions in I5Ø.9) IØ9.81
    - left ventricular failure (conditions in I5Ø.1) IØ9.81
    - myocarditis, myocardial degeneration (conditions in I51.4) IØ9.Ø
    - pancarditis IØ9.9
    - pericarditis IØ9.2
- Rift Valley (viral) A92.4
- Rocky Mountain spotted A77.Ø
- rose J3Ø.1
- Ross River B33.1
- Russian hemorrhagic A98.5
- San Joaquin (Valley) B38.Ø
- sandfly A93.1
- Sao Paulo A77.Ø
- scarlet A38.9
- seven day (leptospirosis) (autumnal) (Japanese) A27.89
  - dengue A9Ø
- shin-bone A79.Ø
- Singapore hemorrhagic A91
- solar A9Ø
- Songo A98.5
- sore BØØ.1
- South African tick-bite A68.1
- Southeast Asia hemorrhagic A91
- spinal —*see* Meningitis
- spirillary A25.Ø
- splenic —*see* Anthrax
- spotted A77.9
  - American A77.Ø
  - Brazilian A77.Ø
  - cerebrospinal meningitis A39.Ø

Fever *(Continued)*
- spotted *(Continued)*
  - Colombian A77.Ø
  - due to Rickettsia
    - australis A77.3
    - conorii A77.1
    - rickettsii A77.Ø
    - sibirica A77.2
    - specified type NEC A77.8
  - Ehrlichiosis A77.4Ø
    - due to
      - E. chafeensis A77.41
      - specified organism NEC A77.49
  - Rocky Mountain A77.Ø
- steroid R5Ø.2
- streptobacillary A25.1
- subtertian B5Ø.9
- Sumatran mite A75.3
- sun A9Ø
- swamp A27.9
- swine AØ2.8
- sylvatic, yellow A95.Ø
- Tahyna B33.8
- tertian —*see* Malaria, tertian
- Thailand hemorrhagic A91
- thermic T67.Ø
- three-day A93.1
- tick
  - American mountain A93.2
  - Colorado A93.2
  - Kemerovo A93.8
  - Mediterranean A77.1
  - mountain A93.2
  - nonexanthematous A93.2
  - Quaranfil A93.8
- tick-bite NEC A93.8
- tick-borne (hemorrhagic) NEC A93.8
- trench A79.Ø
- tsutsugamushi A75.3
- typhogastric AØ1.ØØ
- typhoid (abortive) (hemorrhagic) (intermittent) (malignant) AØ1.ØØ
  - complicated by
    - arthritis AØ1.Ø4
    - heart involvement AØ1.Ø2
    - meningitis AØ1.Ø1
    - osteomyelitis AØ1.Ø5
    - pneumonia AØ1.Ø3
    - specified NEC AØ1.Ø9
- typhomalarial —*see* Malaria
- typhus —*see* Typhus (fever)
- undulant —*see* Brucellosis
- unknown origin R5Ø.9
- uveoparotid D86.89
- valley B38.Ø
- Venezuelan equine A92.2
- vesicular stomatitis A93.8
- viral hemorrhagic —*see* Fever, hemorrhagic, by type of virus
- Volhynian A79.Ø
- Wesselsbron (viral) A92.8
- West
  - African B5Ø.8
  - Nile (viral) A92.3Ø
    - with
      - complications NEC A92.39
      - cranial nerve disorders A92.32
      - encephalitis A92.31
      - encephalomyelitis A92.31
      - neurologic manifestation NEC A92.32
      - optic neuritis A92.32
      - polyradiculitis A92.32
- Whitmore's —*see* Melioidosis
- Wolhynian A79.Ø
- worm B83.9
- yellow A95.9
  - jungle A95.Ø
  - sylvatic A95.Ø
  - urban A95.1
- Zika virus A92.5 ◀

Fibrillation
- atrial or auricular (established) I48.91
  - chronic I48.2
  - paroxysmal I48.Ø
  - permanent I48.2
  - persistent I48.1
- cardiac I49.8
- heart I49.8
- muscular M62.89
- ventricular I49.Ø1

Fibrin
- ball or bodies, pleural (sac) J94.1
- chamber, anterior (eye) (gelatinous exudate) —*see* Iridocyclitis, acute

Fibrinogenolysis —*see* Fibrinolysis

Fibrinogenopenia D68.8
- acquired D65
- congenital D68.2

Fibrinolysis (hemorrhagic) (acquired) D65
- antepartum hemorrhage —*see* Hemorrhage, antepartum, with coagulation defect
- following
  - abortion —*see* Abortion by type complicated by hemorrhage
  - ectopic or molar pregnancy OØ8.1
- intrapartum O67.Ø
- newborn, transient P6Ø
- postpartum O72.3

Fibrinopenia (hereditary) D68.2
- acquired D68.4

Fibrinopurulent —*see* condition

Fibrinous —*see* condition

Fibroadenoma
- cellular intracanalicular D24-
- giant D24-
- intracanalicular
  - cellular D24-
  - giant D24-
  - specified site —*see* Neoplasm, benign, by site
  - unspecified site D24-
- juvenile D24-
- pericanalicular
  - specified site —*see* Neoplasm, benign, by site
  - unspecified site D24-
- phyllodes D24-
- prostate D29.1
- specified site NEC —*see* Neoplasm, benign, by site
- unspecified site D24-

Fibroadenosis, breast (chronic) (cystic) (diffuse) (periodic) (segmental) N6Ø.2-

Fibroangioma —*see also* Neoplasm, benign, by site
- juvenile
  - specified site —*see* Neoplasm, benign, by site
  - unspecified site D1Ø.6

Fibrochondrosarcoma —*see* Neoplasm, cartilage, malignant

Fibrocystic
- disease —*see also* Fibrosis, cystic
  - breast —*see* Mastopathy, cystic
  - jaw M27.49
  - kidney (congenital) Q61.8
  - liver Q44.6
  - pancreas E84.9
- kidney (congenital) Q61.8

Fibrodysplasia ossificans progressiva —*see* Myositis, ossificans, progressiva

Fibroelastosis (cordis) (endocardial) (endomyocardial) I42.4

Fibroid (tumor) —*see also* Neoplasm, connective tissue, benign
- disease, lung (chronic) —*see* Fibrosis, lung
- heart (disease) —*see* Myocarditis
- in pregnancy or childbirth O34.1-
  - causing obstructed labor O65.5
- induration, lung (chronic) —*see* Fibrosis, lung
- lung —*see* Fibrosis, lung

Fibroid *(Continued)*
pneumonia (chronic) —*see* Fibrosis, lung
uterus D25.9
Fibrolipoma —*see* Lipoma
Fibroliposarcoma —*see* Neoplasm, connective tissue, malignant
Fibroma —*see also* Neoplasm, connective tissue, benign
ameloblastic —*see* Cyst, calcifying odontogenic
bone (nonossifying) —*see* Disorder, bone, specified type NEC
ossifying —*see* Neoplasm, bone, benign
cementifying —*see* Neoplasm, bone, benign
chondromyxoid —*see* Neoplasm, bone, benign
desmoplastic —*see* Neoplasm, connective tissue, uncertain behavior
durum —*see* Neoplasm, connective tissue, benign
fascial —*see* Neoplasm, connective tissue, benign
invasive —*see* Neoplasm, connective tissue, uncertain behavior
molle —*see* Lipoma
myxoid —*see* Neoplasm, connective tissue, benign
nasopharynx, nasopharyngeal (juvenile) D10.6
nonosteogenic (nonossifying) —*see* Dysplasia, fibrous
odontogenic (central) —*see* Cyst, calcifying odontogenic
ossifying —*see* Neoplasm, bone, benign
periosteal —*see* Neoplasm, bone, benign
soft —*see* Lipoma
Fibromatosis M72.9
abdominal —*see* Neoplasm, connective tissue, uncertain behavior
aggressive —*see* Neoplasm, connective tissue, uncertain behavior
congenital generalized —*see* Neoplasm, connective tissue, uncertain behavior
Dupuytren's M72.0
gingival K06.1
palmar (fascial) M72.0
plantar (fascial) M72.2
pseudosarcomatous (proliferative) (subcutaneous) M72.4
retroperitoneal D48.3
specified NEC M72.8
Fibromyalgia M79.7
Fibromyoma —*see also* Neoplasm, connective tissue, benign
uterus (corpus) —*see also* Leiomyoma, uterus
in pregnancy or childbirth —*see* Fibroid, in pregnancy or childbirth
causing obstructed labor O65.5
Fibromyositis M79.7
Fibromyxolipoma D17.9
Fibromyxoma —*see* Neoplasm, connective tissue, benign
Fibromyxosarcoma —*see* Neoplasm, connective tissue, malignant
Fibro-odontoma, ameloblastic —*see* Cyst, calcifying odontogenic
Fibro-osteoma —*see* Neoplasm, bone, benign
Fibroplasia, retrolental H35.17
Fibropurulent —*see* condition
Fibrosarcoma —*see also* Neoplasm, connective tissue, malignant
ameloblastic C41.1
upper jaw (bone) C41.0
congenital —*see* Neoplasm, connective tissue, malignant
fascial —*see* Neoplasm, connective tissue, malignant
infantile —*see* Neoplasm, connective tissue, malignant

Fibrosarcoma *(Continued)*
odontogenic C41.1
upper jaw (bone) C41.0
periosteal —*see* Neoplasm, bone, malignant
Fibrosclerosis
breast N60.3-
multifocal M35.5
penis (corpora cavernosa) N48.6
Fibrosis, fibrotic
adrenal (gland) E27.8
amnion O41.8X-
anal papillae K62.89
arteriocapillary —*see* Arteriosclerosis
bladder N32.89
interstitial —*see* Cystitis, chronic, interstitial
localized submucosal —*see* Cystitis, chronic, interstitial
panmural —*see* Cystitis, chronic, interstitial
breast —*see* Fibrosclerosis, breast
capillary —*see also* Arteriosclerosis I70.90
lung (chronic) —*see* Fibrosis, lung
cardiac —*see* Myocarditis
cervix N88.8
chorion O41.8X-
corpus cavernosum (sclerosing) N48.6
cystic (of pancreas) E84.9
with
distal intestinal obstruction syndrome E84.19
fecal impaction E84.19
intestinal manifestations NEC E84.19
pulmonary manifestations E84.0
specified manifestations NEC E84.8
due to device, implant or graft —*see also* Complications, by site and type, specified NEC T85.828 ◄═
arterial graft NEC T82.828
breast (implant) T85.828 ◄═
catheter NEC T85.828 ◄═
dialysis (renal) T82.828
intraperitoneal T85.828 ◄═
infusion NEC T82.828
spinal (epidural) (subdural) T85.820 ◄═
urinary (indwelling) T83.82
electronic (electrode) (pulse generator) (stimulator)
bone T84.82
cardiac T82.827
nervous system (brain) (peripheral nerve) (spinal) T85.820 ◄═
urinary T83.82
fixation, internal (orthopedic) NEC T84.82
gastrointestinal (bile duct) (esophagus) T85.828 ◄═
genital NEC T83.82
heart NEC T82.827
joint prosthesis T84.82
ocular (corneal graft) (orbital implant) NEC T85.828 ◄═
orthopedic NEC T84.82
specified NEC T85.828 ◄═
urinary NEC T83.82
vascular NEC T82.828
ventricular intracranial shunt T85.820 ◄═
ejaculatory duct N50.89 ◄═
endocardium —*see* Endocarditis
endomyocardial (tropical) I42.3
epididymis N50.89 ◄═
eye muscle —*see* Strabismus, mechanical
heart —*see* Myocarditis
hepatic —*see* Fibrosis, liver
hepatolienal (portal hypertension) K76.6
hepatosplenic (portal hypertension) K76.6
infrapatellar fat pad M79.4
intrascrotal N50.89 ◄═
kidney N26.9
liver K74.0
with sclerosis K74.2
alcoholic K70.2

Fibrosis, fibrotic *(Continued)*
lung (atrophic) (chronic) (confluent) (massive) (perialveolar) (peribronchial) J84.10
with
anthracosilicosis J60
anthracosis J60
asbestosis J61
bagassosis J67.1
bauxite J63.1
berylliosis J63.2
byssinosis J66.0
calcicosis J62.8
chalicosis J62.8
dust reticulation J64
farmer's lung J67.0
ganister disease J62.8
graphite J63.3
pneumoconiosis NOS J64
siderosis J63.4
silicosis J62.8
capillary J84.10
congenital P27.8
diffuse (idiopathic) J84.10
chemicals, gases, fumes or vapors (inhalation) J68.4
interstitial J84.10
acute J84.114
talc J62.0
following radiation J70.1
idiopathic J84.112
postinflammatory J84.10
silicotic J62.8
tuberculous —*see* Tuberculosis, pulmonary
lymphatic gland I89.8
median bar —*see* Hyperplasia, prostate
mediastinum (idiopathic) J98.59 ◄═
meninges G96.19
myocardium, myocardial —*see* Myocarditis
ovary N83.8
oviduct N83.8
pancreas K86.89 ◄═
penis NEC N48.6
pericardium I31.0
perineum, in pregnancy or childbirth O34.7-
causing obstructed labor O65.5
pleura J94.1
popliteal fat pad M79.4
prostate (chronic) —*see* Hyperplasia, prostate
pulmonary —*see also* Fibrosis, lung J84.10
congenital P27.8
idiopathic J84.112
rectal sphincter K62.89
retroperitoneal, idiopathic (with ureteral obstruction) N13.5
with infection N13.6
sclerosing mesenteric (idiopathic) K65.4
scrotum N50.89 ◄═
seminal vesicle N50.89 ◄═
senile R54
skin L90.5
spermatic cord N50.89 ◄═
spleen D73.89
in schistosomiasis (bilharziasis) B65.9 *[D77]*
subepidermal nodular —*see* Neoplasm, skin, benign
submucous (oral) (tongue) K13.5
testis N44.8
chronic, due to syphilis A52.76
thymus (gland) E32.8
tongue, submucous K13.5
tunica vaginalis N50.89 ◄═
uterus (non-neoplastic) N85.8
vagina N89.8
valve, heart —*see* Endocarditis
vas deferens N50.89 ◄═
vein I87.8
Fibrositis (periarticular) M79.7
nodular, chronic (Jaccoud's) (rheumatoid) —*see* Arthropathy, postrheumatic, chronic

◄ New ◄═ Revised ~~deleted~~ Deleted

Fibrothorax J94.1
Fibrotic —*see* Fibrosis
Fibrous —*see* condition
Fibroxanthoma —*see also* Neoplasm, connective tissue, benign
  atypical —*see* Neoplasm, connective tissue, uncertain behavior
  malignant —*see* Neoplasm, connective tissue, malignant
Fibroxanthosarcoma —*see* Neoplasm, connective tissue, malignant
Fiedler's
  disease (icterohemorrhagic leptospirosis) A27.0
  myocarditis (acute) I40.1
Fifth disease B08.3
  venereal A55
Filaria, filarial, filariasis —*see* Infestation, filarial
Filatov's disease —*see* Mononucleosis, infectious
File-cutter's disease —*see* Poisoning, lead
Filling defect
  biliary tract R93.2
  bladder R93.41 ⬅
  duodenum R93.3
  gallbladder R93.2
  gastrointestinal tract R93.3
  intestine R93.3
  kidney R93.42- ⬅
  stomach R93.3
  ureter R93.41 ⬅
  urinary organs, specified NEC R93.49 ◀
Fimbrial cyst Q50.4
Financial problem affecting care NOS Z59.9
  bankruptcy Z59.8
  foreclosure on loan Z59.8
Findings, abnormal, inconclusive, without diagnosis —*see also* Abnormal
  17-ketosteroids, elevated R82.5
  acetonuria R82.4
  alcohol in blood R78.0
  anisocytosis R71.8
  antenatal screening of mother O28.9
    biochemical O28.1
    chromosomal O28.5
    cytological O28.2
    genetic O28.5
    hematological O28.0
    radiological O28.4
    specified NEC O28.8
    ultrasonic O28.3
  antibody titer, elevated R76.0
  anticardiolipin antibody R76.0
  antiphosphatidylglycerol antibody R76.0
  antiphosphatidylinositol antibody R76.0
  antiphosphatidylserine antibody R76.0
  antiphospholipid antibody R76.0
  bacteriuria R82.71 ⬅
  bicarbonate E87.8
  bile in urine R82.2
  blood sugar R73.09
    high R73.9
    low (transient) E16.2
  body fluid or substance, specified NEC R88.8
  casts, urine R82.99
  catecholamines R82.5
  cells, urine R82.99
  chloride E87.8
  cholesterol E78.9
    high E78.00 ⬅
      with high triglycerides E78.2
  chyluria R82.0
  cloudy
    dialysis effluent R88.0
    urine R82.90
  creatinine clearance R94.4
  crystals, urine R82.99
  culture
    blood R78.81
    positive —*see* Positive, culture
  echocardiogram R93.1

Findings, abnormal, inconclusive, without diagnosis *(Continued)*
  electrolyte level, urinary R82.99
  function study NEC R94.8
    bladder R94.8
    endocrine NEC R94.7
      thyroid R94.6
    kidney R94.4
    liver R94.5
    pancreas R94.8
    placenta R94.8
    pulmonary R94.2
    spleen R94.8
  gallbladder, nonvisualization R93.2
  glucose (tolerance test) (non-fasting) R73.09
  glycosuria R81
  heart
    shadow R93.1
    sounds R01.2
  hematinuria R82.3
  hematocrit drop (precipitous) R71.0
  hemoglobinuria R82.3
  human papillomavirus (HPV) DNA test positive
    cervix
      high risk R87.810
      low risk R87.820
    vagina
      high risk R87.811
      low risk R87.821
  in blood (of substance not normally found in blood) R78.9
    addictive drug NEC R78.4
    alcohol (excessive level) R78.0
    cocaine R78.2
    hallucinogen R78.3
    heavy metals (abnormal level) R78.79
    lead R78.71
    lithium (abnormal level) R78.89
    opiate drug R78.1
    psychotropic drug R78.5
    specified substance NEC R78.89
    steroid agent R78.6
  indoleacetic acid, elevated R82.5
  ketonuria R82.4
  lactic acid dehydrogenase (LDH) R74.0
  liver function test R79.89
  mammogram NEC R92.8
    calcification (calculus) R92.1
    inconclusive result (due to dense breasts) R92.2
    microcalcification R92.0
  mediastinal shift R93.8
  melanin, urine R82.99
  myoglobinuria R82.1
  neonatal screening P09
  nonvisualization of gallbladder R93.2
  odor of urine NOS R82.90
  Papanicolaou cervix R87.619
    non-atypical endometrial cells R87.618
  pneumoencephalogram R93.0
  poikilocytosis R71.8
  potassium (deficiency) E87.6
    excess E87.5
  PPD R76.11
  radiologic (X-ray) R93.8
    abdomen R93.5
    biliary tract R93.2
    breast R92.8
    gastrointestinal tract R93.3
    genitourinary organs R93.8
    head R93.0
    inconclusive due to excess body fat of patient R93.9
    intrathoracic organs NEC R93.1
    placenta R93.8
    retroperitoneum R93.5
    skin R93.8
    skull R93.0
    subcutaneous tissue R93.8

Findings, abnormal, inconclusive, without diagnosis *(Continued)*
  red blood cell (count) (morphology) (sickling) (volume) R71.8
  scan NEC R94.8
    bladder R94.8
    bone R94.8
    kidney R94.4
    liver R93.2
    lung R94.2
    pancreas R94.8
    placental R94.8
    spleen R94.8
    thyroid R94.6
  sedimentation rate, elevated R70.0
  SGOT R74.0
  SGPT R74.0
  sodium (deficiency) E87.1
    excess E87.0
  specified body fluid NEC R88.8
  stress test R94.39
  thyroid (function) (metabolic rate) (scan) (uptake) R94.6
  transaminase (level) R74.0
  triglycerides E78.9
    high E78.1
      with high cholesterol E78.2
  tuberculin skin test (without active tuberculosis) R76.11
  urine R82.90
    acetone R82.4
    bacteria R82.71 ⬅
    bile R82.2
    casts or cells R82.99
    chyle R82.0
    culture positive R82.79 ⬅
    glucose R81
    hemoglobin R82.3
    ketone R82.4
    sugar R81
  vanillylmandelic acid (VMA), elevated R82.5
  vectorcardiogram (VCG) R94.39
  ventriculogram R93.0
  white blood cell (count) (differential) (morphology) D72.9
  xerography R92.8
Finger —*see* condition
Fire, Saint Anthony's —*see* Erysipelas
Fire-setting
  pathological (compulsive) F63.1
Fish hook stomach K31.89
Fishmeal-worker's lung J67.8
Fissure, fissured
  anus, anal K60.2
    acute K60.0
    chronic K60.1
    congenital Q43.8
  ear, lobule, congenital Q17.8
  epiglottis (congenital) Q31.8
  larynx J38.7
    congenital Q31.8
  lip K13.0
    congenital —*see* Cleft, lip
  nipple N64.0
    associated with
      lactation O92.13
      pregnancy O92.11-
      puerperium O92.12
  nose Q30.2
  palate (congenital) —*see* Cleft, palate
  skin R23.4
  spine (congenital) —*see also* Spina bifida
    with hydrocephalus —*see* Spina bifida, by site, with hydrocephalus
  tongue (acquired) K14.5
    congenital Q38.3
Fistula (cutaneous) L98.8
  abdomen (wall) K63.2
    bladder N32.2
    intestine NEC K63.2

◀ New ⬅ Revised ~~deleted~~ Deleted

Fistula *(Continued)*
abdomen *(Continued)*
ureter N28.89
uterus N82.5
abdominorectal K63.2
abdominosigmoidal K63.2
abdominothoracic J86.Ø
abdominouterine N82.5
congenital Q51.7
abdominovesical N32.2
accessory sinuses —*see* Sinusitis
actinomycotic —*see* Actinomycosis
alveolar antrum —*see* Sinusitis, maxillary
alveolar process KØ4.6
anorectal K6Ø.5
antrobuccal —*see* Sinusitis, maxillary
antrum —*see* Sinusitis, maxillary
anus, anal (recurrent) (infectional) K6Ø.3
congenital Q43.6
with absence, atresia and stenosis Q42.2
tuberculous A18.32
aorta-duodenal I77.2
appendix, appendicular K38.3
arteriovenous (acquired) (nonruptured) I77.Ø
brain I67.1
congenital Q28.2
ruptured I6Ø.8
ruptured I6Ø.8
cerebral —*see* Fistula, arteriovenous, brain
congenital (peripheral) —*see also* Malformation, arteriovenous
brain Q28.2
ruptured I6Ø.8
coronary Q24.5
pulmonary Q25.72
coronary I25.41
congenital Q24.5
pulmonary I28.Ø
congenital Q25.72
surgically created (for dialysis) Z99.2
complication —*see* Complication, arteriovenous, fistula, surgically created
traumatic —*see* Injury, blood vessel
artery I77.2
aural (mastoid) —*see* Mastoiditis, chronic
auricle —*see also* Disorder, pinna, specified type NEC
congenital Q18.1
Bartholin's gland N82.8
bile duct (common) (hepatic) K83.3
with calculus, stones —*see* Calculus, bile duct
biliary (tract) —*see* Fistula, bile duct
bladder (sphincter) NEC —*see also* Fistula, vesico- N32.2
into seminal vesicle N32.2
bone —*see also* Disorder, bone, specified type NEC
with osteomyelitis, chronic —*see* Osteomyelitis, chronic, with draining sinus
brain G93.89
arteriovenous (acquired) I67.1
congenital Q28.2
branchial (cleft) Q18.Ø
branchiogenous Q18.Ø
breast N61.Ø
puerperal, postpartum or gestational, due to mastitis (purulent) —*see* Mastitis, obstetric, purulent
bronchial J86.Ø
bronchocutaneous, bronchomediastinal, bronchopleural, bronchopleuromediastinal (infective) J86.Ø
tuberculous NEC A15.5
bronchoesophageal J86.Ø
congenital Q39.2
with atresia of esophagus Q39.1
bronchovisceral J86.Ø

Fistula *(Continued)*
buccal cavity (infective) K12.2
cecosigmoidal K63.2
cecum K63.2
cerebrospinal (fluid) G96.Ø
cervical, lateral Q18.1
cervicoaural Q18.1
cervicosigmoidal N82.4
cervicovesical N82.1
cervix N82.8
chest (wall) J86.Ø
cholecystenteric —*see* Fistula, gallbladder
cholecystocolic —*see* Fistula, gallbladder
cholecystocolonic —*see* Fistula, gallbladder
cholecystoduodenal —*see* Fistula, gallbladder
cholecystogastric —*see* Fistula, gallbladder
cholecystointestinal —*see* Fistula, gallbladder
choledochoduodenal —*see* Fistula, bile duct
cholocolic K82.3
coccyx —*see* Sinus, pilonidal
colon K63.2
colostomy K94.Ø9
common duct —*see* Fistula, bile duct
congenital, site not listed —*see* Anomaly, by site
coronary, arteriovenous I25.41
congenital Q24.5
costal region J86.Ø
cul-de-sac, Douglas' N82.8
cystic duct —*see also* Fistula, gallbladder
congenital Q44.5
dental KØ4.6
diaphragm J86.Ø
duodenum K31.6
ear (external) (canal) —*see* Disorder, ear, external, specified type NEC
enterocolic K63.2
enterocutaneous K63.2
enterouterine N82.4
congenital Q51.7
enterovaginal N82.4
congenital Q52.2
large intestine N82.3
small intestine N82.2
enterovesical N32.1
epididymis N5Ø.89
tuberculous A18.15
esophagobronchial J86.Ø
congenital Q39.2
with atresia of esophagus Q39.1
esophagocutaneous K22.8
esophagopleural-cutaneous J86.Ø
esophagotracheal J86.Ø
congenital Q39.2
with atresia of esophagus Q39.1
esophagus K22.8
congenital Q39.2
with atresia of esophagus Q39.1
ethmoid —*see* Sinusitis, ethmoidal
eyeball (cornea) (sclera) —*see* Disorder, globe, hypotony
eyelid HØ1.8
fallopian tube, external N82.5
fecal K63.2
congenital Q43.6
from periapical abscess KØ4.6
frontal sinus —*see* Sinusitis, frontal
gallbladder K82.3
with calculus, cholelithiasis, stones —*see* Calculus, gallbladder
gastric K31.6
gastrocolic K31.6
congenital Q4Ø.2
tuberculous A18.32
gastroenterocolic K31.6
gastroesophageal K31.6
gastrojejunal K31.6
gastrojejunocolic K31.6

Fistula *(Continued)*
genital tract (female) N82.9
specified NEC N82.8
to intestine NEC N82.4
to skin N82.5
hepatic artery-portal vein, congenital Q26.6
hepatopleural J86.Ø
hepatopulmonary J86.Ø
ileorectal or ileosigmoidal K63.2
ileovaginal N82.2
ileovesical N32.1
ileum K63.2
in ano K6Ø.3
tuberculous A18.32
inner ear (labyrinth) —*see* subcategory H83.1
intestine NEC K63.2
intestinocolonic (abdominal) K63.2
intestinoureteral N28.89
intestinouterine N82.4
intestinovaginal N82.4
large intestine N82.3
small intestine N82.2
intestinovesical N32.1
ischiorectal (fossa) K61.3
jejunum K63.2
joint M25.1Ø
ankle M25.17-
elbow M25.12-
foot joint M25.17-
hand joint M25.14-
hip M25.15-
knee M25.16-
shoulder M25.11-
specified joint NEC M25.18
tuberculous —*see* Tuberculosis, joint
vertebrae M25.18
wrist M25.13-
kidney N28.89
labium (majus) (minus) N82.8
labyrinth —*see* subcategory H83.1
lacrimal (gland) (sac) HØ4.61-
lacrimonasal duct —*see* Fistula, lacrimal
laryngotracheal, congenital Q34.8
larynx J38.7
lip K13.Ø
congenital Q38.Ø
lumbar, tuberculous A18.Ø1
lung J86.Ø
lymphatic I89.8
mammary (gland) N61.Ø
mastoid (process) (region) —*see* Mastoiditis, chronic
maxillary J32.Ø
medial, face and neck Q18.8
mediastinal J86.Ø
mediastinobronchial J86.Ø
mediastinocutaneous J86.Ø
middle ear —*see* subcategory H74.8
mouth K12.2
nasal J34.89
sinus —*see* Sinusitis
nasopharynx J39.2
nipple N64.Ø
nose J34.89
oral (cutaneous) K12.2
maxillary J32.Ø
nasal (with cleft palate) —*see* Cleft, palate
orbit, orbital —*see* Disorder, orbit, specified type NEC
oroantral J32.Ø
oviduct, external N82.5
palate (hard) M27.8
pancreatic K86.89
pancreaticoduodenal K86.89
parotid (gland) K11.4
region K12.2
penis N48.89
perianal K6Ø.3
pericardium (pleura) (sac) —*see* Pericarditis
pericecal K63.2
perineorectal K6Ø.4
perineosigmoidal K63.2

F

Fistula *(Continued)*
perineum, perineal (with urethral involvement) NEC N36.0
tuberculous A18.13
ureter N28.89
perirectal K60.4
tuberculous A18.32
peritoneum K65.9
pharyngoesophageal J39.2
pharynx J39.2
branchial cleft (congenital) Q18.0
pilonidal (infected) (rectum) —*see* Sinus, pilonidal
pleura, pleural, pleurocutaneous, pleuroperitoneal J86.0
tuberculous NEC A15.6
pleuropericardial I31.8
portal vein-hepatic artery, congenital Q26.6
postauricular H70.81-
postoperative, persistent T81.83
specified site —*see* Fistula, by site
preauricular (congenital) Q18.1
prostate N42.89
pulmonary J86.0
arteriovenous I28.0
congenital Q25.72
tuberculous —*see* Tuberculosis, pulmonary
pulmonoperitoneal J86.0
rectolabial N82.4
rectosigmoid (intercommunicating) K63.2
rectoureteral N28.89
rectourethral N36.0
congenital Q64.73
rectouterine N82.4
congenital Q51.7
rectovaginal N82.3
congenital Q52.2
tuberculous A18.18
rectovesical N32.1
congenital Q64.79
rectovesicovaginal N82.3
rectovulval N82.4
congenital Q52.79
rectum (to skin) K60.4
congenital Q43.6
with absence, atresia and stenosis Q42.0
tuberculous A18.32
renal N28.89
retroauricular —*see* Fistula, postauricular
salivary duct or gland (any) K11.4
congenital Q38.4
scrotum (urinary) N50.89 (Revised)
tuberculous A18.15
semicircular canals —*see* subcategory H83.1
sigmoid K63.2
to bladder N32.1
sinus —*see* Sinusitis
skin L98.8
to genital tract (female) N82.5
splenocolic D73.89
stercoral K63.2
stomach K31.6
sublingual gland K11.4
submandibular gland K11.4
submaxillary (gland) K11.4
region K12.2
thoracic J86.0
duct I89.8
thoracoabdominal J86.0
thoracogastric J86.0
thoracointestinal J86.0
thorax J86.0
thyroglossal duct Q89.2
thyroid E07.89
trachea, congenital (external) (internal) Q32.1
tracheoesophageal J86.0
congenital Q39.2
with atresia of esophagus Q39.1
following tracheostomy J95.04
traumatic arteriovenous —*see* Injury, blood vessel, by site

Fistula *(Continued)*
tuberculous - code by site under Tuberculosis
typhoid A01.09
umbilicourinary Q64.8
urachus, congenital Q64.4
ureter (persistent) N28.89
ureteroabdominal N28.89
ureterorectal N28.89
ureterosigmoido-abdominal N28.89
ureterovaginal N82.1
ureterovesical N32.2
urethra N36.0
congenital Q64.79
tuberculous A18.13
urethroperineal N36.0
urethroperineovesical N32.2
urethrorectal N36.0
congenital Q64.73
urethroscrotal N50.89 (Revised)
urethrovaginal N82.1
urethrovesical N32.2
urinary (tract) (persistent) (recurrent) N36.0
uteroabdominal N82.5
congenital Q51.7
uteroenteric, uterointestinal N82.4
congenital Q51.7
uterorectal N82.4
congenital Q51.7
uteroureteric N82.1
uterourethral Q51.7
uterovaginal N82.8
uterovesical N82.1
congenital Q51.7
uterus N82.8
vagina (postpartal) (wall) N82.8
vaginocutaneous (postpartal) N82.5
vaginointestinal NEC N82.4
large intestine N82.3
small intestine N82.2
vaginoperineal N82.5
vasocutaneous, congenital Q55.7
vesical NEC N32.2
vesicoabdominal N32.2
vesicocervicovaginal N82.1
vesicocolic N32.1
vesicocutaneous N32.2
vesicoenteric N32.1
vesicointestinal N32.1
vesicometrorectal N82.4
vesicoperineal N32.2
vesicorectal N32.1
congenital Q64.79
vesicosigmoidal N32.1
vesicosigmoidovaginal N82.3
vesicoureteral N32.2
vesicoureterovaginal N82.1
vesicourethral N32.2
vesicourethrorectal N32.1
vesicouterine N82.1
congenital Q51.7
vesicovaginal N82.0
vulvorectal N82.4
congenital Q52.79

Fit R56.9
epileptic —*see* Epilepsy
fainting R55
hysterical F44.5
newborn P90

Fitting (and adjustment) (of)
artificial
arm —*see* Admission, adjustment, artificial, arm
breast Z44.3
eye Z44.2
leg —*see* Admission, adjustment, artificial, leg
automatic implantable cardiac defibrillator (with synchronous cardiac pacemaker) Z45.02

Fitting *(Continued)*
brain neuropacemaker Z46.2
implanted Z45.42
cardiac defibrillator —*see* Fitting (and adjustment) (of), automatic implantable cardiac defibrillator
catheter, non-vascular Z46.82
colostomy belt Z46.89
contact lenses Z46.0
CRT-D (resynchronization therapy defibrillator) Z45.02 (New)
CRT-P (cardiac resynchronization therapy pacemaker) Z45.018 (New)
pulse generator Z45.010 (New)
cystostomy device Z46.6
defibrillator, cardiac —*see* Fitting (and adjustment) (of), automatic implantable cardiac defibrillator
dentures Z46.3
device NOS Z46.9
abdominal Z46.89
gastrointestinal NEC Z46.59
implanted NEC Z45.89
nervous system Z46.2
implanted —*see* Admission, adjustment, device, implanted, nervous system
orthodontic Z46.4
orthoptic Z46.0
orthotic Z46.89
prosthetic (external) Z44.9
breast Z44.3
dental Z46.3
eye Z44.2
specified NEC Z44.8
specified NEC Z46.89
substitution
auditory Z46.2
implanted —*see* Admission, adjustment, device, implanted, hearing device
nervous system Z46.2
implanted —*see* Admission, adjustment, device, implanted, nervous system
visual Z46.2
implanted Z45.31
urinary Z46.6
gastric lap band Z46.51
gastrointestinal appliance NEC Z46.59
glasses (reading) Z46.0
hearing aid Z46.1
ileostomy device Z46.89
insulin pump Z46.81
intestinal appliance NEC Z46.89
myringotomy device (stent) (tube) Z45.82
neuropacemaker Z46.2
implanted Z45.42
non-vascular catheter Z46.82
orthodontic device Z46.4
orthopedic device (brace) (cast) (corset) (shoes) Z46.89
pacemaker (cardiac) (cardiac resynchronization therapy (CRT-P)) Z45.018 (Revised)
nervous system (brain) (peripheral nerve) (spinal cord) Z46.2
implanted Z45.42
pulse generator Z45.010
portacath (port-a-cath) Z45.2
prosthesis (external) Z44.9
arm —*see* Admission, adjustment, artificial, arm
breast Z44.3
dental Z46.3
eye Z44.2
leg —*see* Admission, adjustment, artificial, leg
specified NEC Z44.8
spectacles Z46.0
wheelchair Z46.89

F

- **Fitzhugh-Curtis syndrome**
  - due to
    - Chlamydia trachomatis A74.81
    - Neisseria gonorrhorea (gonococcal peritonitis) A54.85
- **Fitz's syndrome** (acute hemorrhagic pancreatitis) —*see also* Pancreatitis, acute K85.80
- **Fixation**
  - joint —*see* Ankylosis
  - larynx J38.7
  - stapes —*see* Ankylosis, ear ossicles
    - deafness —*see* Deafness, conductive
  - uterus (acquired) —*see* Malposition, uterus
  - vocal cord J38.3
- **Flabby ridge** K06.8
- **Flaccid** —*see also* condition
  - palate, congenital Q38.5
- **Flail**
  - chest S22.5-
    - newborn (birth injury) P13.8
  - joint (paralytic) M25.20
    - ankle M25.27-
    - elbow M25.22-
    - foot joint M25.27-
    - hand joint M25.24-
    - hip M25.25-
    - knee M25.26-
    - shoulder M25.21-
    - specified joint NEC M25.28
    - wrist M25.23-
- **Flajani's disease** —*see* Hyperthyroidism, with, goiter (diffuse)
- **Flap, liver** K71.3
- **Flashbacks** (residual to hallucinogen use) F16.283
- **Flat**
  - chamber (eye) —*see* Disorder, globe, hypotony, flat anterior chamber
  - chest, congenital Q67.8
  - foot (acquired) (fixed type) (painful) (postural) —*see also* Deformity, limb, flat foot
    - congenital (rigid) (spastic (everted)) Q66.5-
    - rachitic sequelae (late effect) E64.3
  - organ or site, congenital NEC —*see* Anomaly, by site
  - pelvis M95.5
    - with disproportion (fetopelvic) O33.0
      - causing obstructed labor O65.0
    - congenital Q74.2
- **Flatau-Schilder disease** G37.0
- **Flatback syndrome** M40.30
  - lumbar region M40.36
  - lumbosacral region M40.37
  - thoracolumbar region M40.35
- **Flattening**
  - head, femur M89.8X5
  - hip —*see* Coxa, plana
  - lip (congenital) Q18.8
  - nose (congenital) Q67.4
    - acquired M95.0
- **Flatulence** R14.3
  - psychogenic F45.8
- **Flatus** R14.3
  - vaginalis N89.8
- **Flax-dresser's disease** J66.1
- **Flea bite** —*see* Injury, bite, by site, superficial, insect
- **Flecks, glaucomatous** (subcapsular) —*see* Cataract, complicated
- **Fleischer** (-Kayser) **ring** (cornea) H18.04-
- **Fleshy mole** O02.0
- **Flexibilitas cerea** —*see* Catalepsy
- **Flexion**
  - amputation stump (surgical) T87.89
  - cervix —*see* Malposition, uterus
  - contracture, joint —*see* Contraction, joint
  - deformity, joint —*see also* Deformity, limb, flexion M21.20
    - hip, congenital Q65.89
  - uterus —*see also* Malposition, uterus
    - lateral —*see* Lateroversion, uterus
- **Flexner-Boyd dysentery** A03.2
- **Flexner's dysentery** A03.1
- **Flexure** —*see* Flexion
- **Flint murmur** (aortic insufficiency) I35.1
- **Floater, vitreous** —*see* Opacity, vitreous
- **Floating**
  - cartilage (joint) —*see also* Loose, body, joint
    - knee —*see* Derangement, knee, loose body
  - gallbladder, congenital Q44.1
  - kidney N28.89
    - congenital Q63.8
  - spleen D73.89
- **Flooding** N92.0
- **Floor** —*see* condition
- **Floppy**
  - baby syndrome (nonspecific) P94.2
  - iris syndrome (intraoperative) (IFIS) H21.81
  - nonrheumatic mitral valve syndrome I34.1
- **Flu** —*see also* Influenza
  - avian —*see also* Influenza, due to, identified novel influenza A virus J09.X2
  - bird —*see also* Influenza, due to, identified novel influenza A virus J09.X2
  - intestinal NEC A08.4
  - swine (viruses that normally cause infections in pigs) —*see also* Influenza, due to, identified novel influenza A virus J09.X2
- **Fluctuating blood pressure** I99.8
- **Fluid**
  - abdomen R18.8
  - chest J94.8
  - heart —*see* Failure, heart, congestive
  - joint —*see* Effusion, joint
  - loss (acute) E86.9
    - ~~with~~
      - ~~hypernatremia E87.0~~
      - ~~hyponatremia E87.1~~
  - lung —*see* Edema, lung
  - overload E87.70
    - specified NEC E87.79
  - peritoneal cavity R18.8
  - pleural cavity J94.8
  - retention R60.9
- **Flukes NEC** —*see also* Infestation, fluke
  - blood NEC —*see* Schistosomiasis
  - liver B66.3
- **Fluor** (vaginalis) N89.8
  - trichomonal or due to Trichomonas (vaginalis) A59.00
- **Fluorosis**
  - dental K00.3
  - skeletal M85.10
    - ankle M85.17-
    - foot M85.17-
    - forearm M85.13-
    - hand M85.14-
    - lower leg M85.16-
    - multiple site M85.19
    - neck M85.18
    - rib M85.18
    - shoulder M85.11-
    - skull M85.18
    - specified site NEC M85.18
    - thigh M85.15-
    - toe M85.17-
    - upper arm M85.12-
    - vertebra M85.18
- **Flush syndrome** E34.0
- **Flushing** R23.2
  - menopausal N95.1
- **Flutter**
  - atrial or auricular I48.92
    - atypical I48.4
    - type I I48.3
    - type II I48.4
    - typical I48.3
  - heart I49.8
    - atrial or auricular I48.92
      - atypical I48.4
      - type I I48.3
      - type II I48.4
      - typical I48.3
    - ventricular I49.02
  - ventricular I49.02
- **FNHTR** (febrile nonhemolytic transfusion reaction) R50.84
- **Fochier's abscess** - code by site under Abscess
- **Focus, Assmann's** —*see* Tuberculosis, pulmonary
- **Fogo selvagem** L10.3
- **Foix-Alajouanine syndrome** G95.19
- **Fold, folds** (anomalous) —*see also* Anomaly, by site
  - Descemet's membrane —*see* Change, corneal membrane, Descemet's, fold
  - epicanthic Q10.3
  - heart Q24.8
- **Folie à deux** F24
- **Follicle**
  - cervix (nabothian) (ruptured) N88.8
  - graafian, ruptured, with hemorrhage N83.0-
  - nabothian N88.8
- **Follicular** —*see* condition
- **Folliculitis** (superficial) L73.9
  - abscedens et suffodiens L66.3
  - cyst N83.0-
  - decalvans L66.2
  - deep —*see* Furuncle, by site
  - gonococcal (acute) (chronic) A54.01
  - keloid, keloidalis L73.0
  - pustular L01.02
  - ulerythematosa reticulata L66.4
- **Folliculome lipidique**
  - specified site —*see* Neoplasm, benign, by site
  - unspecified site
    - female D27.9
    - male D29.20
- **Følling's disease** E70.0
- **Follow-up** —*see* Examination, follow-up
- **Fong's syndrome** (hereditary osteo-onychodysplasia) Q87.2
- **Food**
  - allergy L27.2
  - asphyxia (from aspiration or inhalation) —*see* Foreign body, by site
  - choked on —*see* Foreign body, by site
  - deprivation T73.0
    - specified kind of food NEC E63.8
  - intoxication —*see* Poisoning, food
  - lack of T73.0
  - poisoning —*see* Poisoning, food
  - rejection NEC —*see* Disorder, eating
  - strangulation or suffocation —*see* Foreign body, by site
  - toxemia —*see* Poisoning, food
- **Foot** —*see* condition
- **Foramen ovale** (nonclosure) (patent) (persistent) Q21.1
- **Forbes' glycogen storage disease** E74.03
- **Fordyce-Fox disease** L75.2
- **Fordyce's disease** (mouth) Q38.6
- **Forearm** —*see* condition
- **Foreign body**
  - with
    - laceration —*see* Laceration, by site, with foreign body
    - puncture wound —*see* Puncture, by site, with foreign body
  - accidentally left following a procedure T81.509
    - aspiration T81.506
      - resulting in
        - adhesions T81.516
        - obstruction T81.526
        - perforation T81.536
        - specified complication NEC T81.596

Foreign body *(Continued)*
accidentally left following a procedure *(Continued)*
cardiac catheterization T81.505
resulting in
acute reaction T81.60
aseptic peritonitis T81.61
specified NEC T81.69
adhesions T81.515
obstruction T81.525
perforation T81.535
specified complication NEC T81.595
causing
acute reaction T81.60
aseptic peritonitis T81.61
specified complication NEC T81.69
adhesions T81.519
aseptic peritonitis T81.61
obstruction T81.529
perforation T81.539
specified complication NEC T81.599
endoscopy T81.504
resulting in
adhesions T81.514
obstruction T81.524
perforation T81.534
specified complication NEC T81.594
immunization T81.503
resulting in
adhesions T81.513
obstruction T81.523
perforation T81.533
specified complication NEC T81.593
infusion T81.501
resulting in
adhesions T81.511
obstruction T81.521
perforation T81.531
specified complication NEC T81.591
injection T81.503
resulting in
adhesions T81.513
obstruction T81.523
perforation T81.533
specified complication NEC T81.593
kidney dialysis T81.502
resulting in
adhesions T81.512
obstruction T81.522
perforation T81.532
specified complication NEC T81.592
packing removal T81.507
resulting in
acute reaction T81.60
aseptic peritonitis T81.61
specified NEC T81.69
adhesions T81.517
obstruction T81.527
perforation T81.537
specified complication NEC T81.597
puncture T81.506
resulting in
adhesions T81.516
obstruction T81.526
perforation T81.536
specified complication NEC T81.596
specified procedure NEC T81.508
resulting in
acute reaction T81.60
aseptic peritonitis T81.61
specified NEC T81.69
adhesions T81.518
obstruction T81.528
perforation T81.538
specified complication NEC T81.598
surgical operation T81.500
resulting in
acute reaction T81.60
aseptic peritonitis T81.61
specified NEC T81.69

Foreign body *(Continued)*
accidentally left following a procedure *(Continued)*
surgical operation *(Continued)*
resulting in *(Continued)*
adhesions T81.510
obstruction T81.520
perforation T81.530
specified complication NEC T81.590
transfusion T81.501
resulting in
adhesions T81.511
obstruction T81.521
perforation T81.531
specified complication NEC T81.591
alimentary tract T18.9
anus T18.5
colon T18.4
esophagus —*see* Foreign body, esophagus
mouth T18.0
multiple sites T18.8
rectosigmoid (junction) T18.5
rectum T18.5
small intestine T18.3
specified site NEC T18.8
stomach T18.2
anterior chamber (eye) S05.5-
auditory canal —*see* Foreign body, entering through orifice, ear
bronchus T17.508
causing
asphyxiation T17.500
food (bone) (seed) T17.520
gastric contents (vomitus) T17.510
specified type NEC T17.590
injury NEC T17.508
food (bone) (seed) T17.528
gastric contents (vomitus) T17.518
specified type NEC T17.598
canthus —*see* Foreign body, conjunctival sac
ciliary body (eye) S05.5-
conjunctival sac T15.1-
cornea T15.0-
entering through orifice
accessory sinus T17.0
alimentary canal T18.9
multiple parts T18.8
specified part NEC T18.8
alveolar process T18.0
antrum (Highmore's) T17.0
anus T18.5
appendix T18.4
auditory canal —*see* Foreign body, entering through orifice, ear
auricle —*see* Foreign body, entering through orifice, ear
bladder T19.1
bronchioles —*see* Foreign body, respiratory tract, specified site NEC
bronchus (main) —*see* Foreign body, bronchus
buccal cavity T18.0
canthus (inner) —*see* Foreign body, conjunctival sac
cecum T18.4
cervix (canal) (uteri) T19.3
colon T18.4
conjunctival sac —*see* Foreign body, conjunctival sac
cornea —*see* Foreign body, cornea
digestive organ or tract NOS T18.9
multiple parts T18.8
specified part NEC T18.8
duodenum T18.3
ear (external) T16.-
esophagus —*see* Foreign body, esophagus
eye (external) NOS T15.9-
conjunctival sac —*see* Foreign body, conjunctival sac
cornea —*see* Foreign body, cornea
specified part NEC T15.8-

Foreign body *(Continued)*
entering through orifice *(Continued)*
eyeball —*see also* Foreign body, entering through orifice, eye, specified part NEC
with penetrating wound —*see* Puncture, eyeball
eyelid —*see also* Foreign body, conjunctival sac
with
laceration —*see* Laceration, eyelid, with foreign body
puncture —*see* Puncture, eyelid, with foreign body
superficial injury —*see* Foreign body, superficial, eyelid
gastrointestinal tract T18.9
multiple parts T18.8
specified part NEC T18.8
genitourinary tract T19.9
multiple parts T19.8
specified part NEC T19.8
globe —*see* Foreign body, entering through orifice, eyeball
gum T18.0
Highmore's antrum T17.0
hypopharynx —*see* Foreign body, pharynx
ileum T18.3
intestine (small) T18.3
large T18.4
lacrimal apparatus (punctum) —*see* Foreign body, entering through orifice, eye, specified part NEC
large intestine T18.4
larynx —*see* Foreign body, larynx
lung —*see* Foreign body, respiratory tract, specified site NEC
maxillary sinus T17.0
mouth T18.0
nasal sinus T17.0
nasopharynx —*see* Foreign body, pharynx
nose (passage) T17.1
nostril T17.1
oral cavity T18.0
palate T18.0
penis T19.4
pharynx —*see* Foreign body, pharynx
piriform sinus —*see* Foreign body, pharynx
rectosigmoid (junction) T18.5
rectum T18.5
respiratory tract —*see* Foreign body, respiratory tract
sinus (accessory) (frontal) (maxillary) (nasal) T17.0
piriform —*see* Foreign body, pharynx
small intestine T18.3
stomach T18.2
suffocation by —*see* Foreign body, by site
tear ducts or glands —*see* Foreign body, entering through orifice, eye, specified part NEC
throat —*see* Foreign body, pharynx
tongue T18.0
tonsil, tonsillar (fossa) —*see* Foreign body, pharynx
trachea —*see* Foreign body, trachea
ureter T19.8
urethra T19.0
uterus (any part) T19.3
vagina T19.2
vulva T19.2
esophagus T18.108
causing
injury NEC T18.108
food (bone) (seed) T18.128
gastric contents (vomitus) T18.118
specified type NEC T18.198
tracheal compression T18.100
food (bone) (seed) T18.120
gastric contents (vomitus) T18.110
specified type NEC T18.190

F

Foreign body *(Continued)*
felling of, in throat R09.89
fragment —*see* Retained, foreign body fragments (type of)
genitourinary tract T19.9
bladder T19.1
multiple parts T19.8
penis T19.4
specified site NEC T19.8
urethra T19.0
uterus T19.3
IUD Z97.5
vagina T19.2
contraceptive device Z97.5
vulva T19.2
granuloma (old) (soft tissue) —*see also* Granuloma, foreign body
skin L92.3
in
laceration —*see* Laceration, by site, with foreign body
puncture wound —*see* Puncture, by site, with foreign body
soft tissue (residual) M79.5
inadvertently left in operation wound —*see* Foreign body, accidentally left during a procedure
ingestion, ingested NOS T18.9
inhalation or inspiration —*see* Foreign body, by site
internal organ, not entering through a natural orifice - code as specific injury with foreign body
intraocular S05.5-
old, retained (nonmagnetic) H44.70-
anterior chamber H44.71-
ciliary body H44.72-
iris H44.72-
lens H44.73-
magnetic H44.60-
anterior chamber H44.61-
ciliary body H44.62-
iris H44.62-
lens H44.63-
posterior wall H44.64-
specified site NEC H44.69-
vitreous body H44.65-
posterior wall H44.74-
specified site NEC H44.79-
vitreous body H44.75-
iris —*see* Foreign body, intraocular
lacrimal punctum —*see* Foreign body, entering through orifice, eye, specified part NEC
larynx T17.308
causing
asphyxiation T17.300
food (bone) (seed) T17.320
gastric contents (vomitus) T17.310
specified type NEC T17.390
injury NEC T17.308
food (bone) (seed) T17.328
gastric contents (vomitus) T17.318
specified type NEC T17.398
lens —*see* Foreign body, intraocular
ocular muscle S05.4-
old, retained —*see* Foreign body, orbit, old
old or residual
soft tissue (residual) M79.5
operation wound, left accidentally —*see* Foreign body, accidentally left during a procedure
orbit S05.4-
old, retained H05.5-
pharynx T17.208
causing
asphyxiation T17.200
food (bone) (seed) T17.220
gastric contents (vomitus) T17.210
specified type NEC T17.290

Foreign body *(Continued)*
pharynx *(Continued)*
causing *(Continued)*
injury NEC T17.208
food (bone) (seed) T17.228
gastric contents (vomitus) T17.218
specified type NEC T17.298
respiratory tract T17.908
bronchioles —*see* Foreign body, respiratory tract, specified site NEC
bronchus —*see* Foreign body, bronchus
causing
asphyxiation T17.900
food (bone) (seed) T17.920
gastric contents (vomitus) T17.910
specified type NEC T17.990
injury NEC T17.908
food (bone) (seed) T17.928
gastric contents (vomitus) T17.918
specified type NEC T17.998
larynx —*see* Foreign body, larynx
lung —*see* Foreign body, respiratory tract, specified site NEC
multiple parts —*see* Foreign body, respiratory tract, specified site NEC
nasal sinus T17.0
nasopharynx —*see* Foreign body, pharynx
nose T17.1
nostril T17.1
pharynx —*see* Foreign body, pharynx
specified site NEC T17.808
causing
asphyxiation T17.800
food (bone) (seed) T17.820
gastric contents (vomitus) T17.810
specified type NEC T17.890
injury NEC T17.808
food (bone) (seed) T17.828
gastric contents (vomitus) T17.818
specified type NEC T17.898
throat —*see* Foreign body, pharynx
trachea —*see* Foreign body, trachea
retained (old) (nonmagnetic) (in)
anterior chamber (eye) —*see* Foreign body, intraocular, old, retained, anterior chamber
magnetic —*see* Foreign body, intraocular, old, retained, magnetic, anterior chamber
ciliary body —*see* Foreign body, intraocular, old, retained, ciliary body
magnetic —*see* Foreign body, intraocular, old, retained, magnetic, ciliary body
eyelid H02.819
left H02.816
lower H02.815
upper H02.814
right H02.813
lower H02.812
upper H02.811
fragments —*see* Retained, foreign body fragments (type of)
globe —*see* Foreign body, intraocular, old, retained
magnetic —*see* Foreign body, intraocular, old, retained, magnetic
intraocular —*see* Foreign body, intraocular, old, retained
magnetic —*see* Foreign body, intraocular, old, retained, magnetic
iris —*see* Foreign body, intraocular, old, retained, iris
magnetic —*see* Foreign body, intraocular, old, retained, magnetic, iris
lens —*see* Foreign body, intraocular, old, retained, lens
magnetic —*see* Foreign body, intraocular, old, retained, magnetic, lens
muscle —*see* Foreign body, retained, soft tissue

Foreign body *(Continued)*
retained *(Continued)*
orbit —*see* Foreign body, orbit, old
posterior wall of globe —*see* Foreign body, intraocular, old, retained, posterior wall
magnetic —*see* Foreign body, intraocular, old, retained, magnetic, posterior wall
retrobulbar —*see* Foreign body, orbit, old, retrobulbar
soft tissue M79.5
vitreous —*see* Foreign body, intraocular, old, retained, vitreous body
magnetic —*see* Foreign body, intraocular, old, retained, magnetic, vitreous body
retina S05.5-
superficial, without open wound
abdomen, abdominal (wall) S30.851
alveolar process S00.552
ankle S90.55-
antecubital space —*see* Foreign body, superficial, forearm
anus S30.857
arm (upper) S40.85-
auditory canal —*see* Foreign body, superficial, ear
auricle —*see* Foreign body, superficial, ear
axilla —*see* Foreign body, superficial, arm
back, lower S30.850
breast S20.15-
brow S00.85
buttock S30.850
calf —*see* Foreign body, superficial, leg
canthus —*see* Foreign body, superficial, eyelid
cheek S00.85
internal S00.552
chest wall —*see* Foreign body, superficial, thorax
chin S00.85
clitoris S30.854
costal region —*see* Foreign body, superficial, thorax
digit (s)
foot —*see* Foreign body, superficial, toe
hand —*see* Foreign body, superficial, finger
ear S00.45-
elbow S50.35-
epididymis S30.853
epigastric region S30.851
epiglottis S10.15
esophagus, cervical S10.15
eyebrow —*see* Foreign body, superficial, eyelid
eyelid S00.25-
face S00.85
finger (s) S60.459
index S60.45-
little S60.45-
middle S60.45-
ring S60.45-
flank S30.851
foot (except toe (s) alone) S90.85-
toe —*see* Foreign body, superficial, toe
forearm S50.85-
elbow only —*see* Foreign body, superficial, elbow
forehead S00.85
genital organs, external
female S30.856
male S30.855
groin S30.851
gum S00.552
hand S60.55-
head S00.95
ear —*see* Foreign body, superficial, ear
eyelid —*see* Foreign body, superficial, eyelid

Foreign body *(Continued)*
superficial, without open wound *(Continued)*
head *(Continued)*
lip S00.551
nose S00.35
oral cavity S00.552
scalp S00.05
specified site NEC S00.85
heel —*see* Foreign body, superficial, foot
hip S70.25-
inguinal region S30.851
interscapular region S20.459
jaw S00.85
knee S80.25-
labium (majus) (minus) S30.854
larynx S10.15
leg (lower) S80.85-
knee —*see* Foreign body, superficial, knee
upper —*see* Foreign body, superficial, thigh
lip S00.551
lower back S30.850
lumbar region S30.850
malar region S00.85
mammary —*see* Foreign body, superficial, breast
mastoid region S00.85
mouth S00.552
nail
finger —*see* Foreign body, superficial, finger
toe —*see* Foreign body, superficial, toe
nape S10.85
nasal S00.35
neck S10.95
specified site NEC S10.85
throat S10.15
nose S00.35
occipital region S00.05
oral cavity S00.552
orbital region —*see* Foreign body, superficial, eyelid
palate S00.552
palm —*see* Foreign body, superficial, hand
parietal region S00.05
pelvis S30.850
penis S30.852
perineum
female S30.854
male S30.850
periocular area —*see* Foreign body, superficial, eyelid
phalanges
finger —*see* Foreign body, superficial, finger
toe —*see* Foreign body, superficial, toe
pharynx S10.15
pinna —*see* Foreign body, superficial, ear
popliteal space —*see* Foreign body, superficial, knee
prepuce S30.852
pubic region S30.850
pudendum
female S30.856
male S30.855
sacral region S30.850
scalp S00.05
scapular region —*see* Foreign body, superficial, shoulder
scrotum S30.853
shin —*see* Foreign body, superficial, leg
shoulder S40.25-
sternal region S20.359
submaxillary region S00.85
submental region S00.85
subungual
finger (s) —*see* Foreign body, superficial, finger
toe (s) —*see* Foreign body, superficial, toe

Foreign body *(Continued)*
superficial, without open wound *(Continued)*
supraclavicular fossa S10.85
supraorbital S00.85
temple S00.85
temporal region S00.85
testis S30.853
thigh S70.35-
thorax, thoracic (wall) S20.95
back S20.45-
front S20.35-
throat S10.15
thumb S60.35-
toe (s) (lesser) S90.456
great S90.45-
tongue S00.552
trachea S10.15
tunica vaginalis S30.853
tympanum, tympanic membrane —*see* Foreign body, superficial, ear
uvula S00.552
vagina S30.854
vocal cords S10.15
vulva S30.854
wrist S60.85-
swallowed T18.9
trachea T17.408
causing
asphyxiation T17.400
food (bone) (seed) T17.420
gastric contents (vomitus) T17.410
specified type NEC T17.490
injury NEC T17.408
food (bone) (seed) T17.428
gastric contents (vomitus) T17.418
specified type NEC T17.498
type of fragment —*see* Retained, foreign body fragments (type of)
vitreous (humor) S05.5-
Forestier's disease (rhizomelic pseudopolyarthritis) M35.3-
meaning ankylosing hyperostosis —*see* Hyperostosis, ankylosing
Formation
hyalin in cornea —*see* Degeneration, cornea
sequestrum in bone (due to infection) —*see* Osteomyelitis, chronic
valve
colon, congenital Q43.8
ureter (congenital) Q62.39
Formication R20.2
Fort Bragg fever A27.89
Fossa —*see also* condition
pyriform —*see* condition
Foster-Kennedy syndrome H47.14-
Fothergill's
disease (trigeminal neuralgia) —*see also* Neuralgia, trigeminal
scarlatina anginosa A38.9
Foul breath R19.6
Foundling Z76.1
Fournier disease or gangrene N49.3
female N76.89
Fourth
cranial nerve —*see* condition
molar K00.1
Foville's (peduncular) **disease or syndrome** G46.3
Fox (-Fordyce) disease (apocrine miliaria) L75.2
Fracture, burst —*see* Fracture, traumatic, by site
Fracture, chronic —*see* Fracture, pathological
Fracture, insufficiency —*see* Fracture, pathologic, by site
Fracture, nontraumatic, NEC ◀
atypical ◀
femur M84.750- ◀
complete ◀
oblique M84.759 ◀
left side M84.758 ◀
right side M84.757 ◀

Fracture, nontraumatic *(Continued)*
atypical *(Continued)*
femur *(Continued)*
complete *(Continued)*
transverse M84.756 ◀
left side M84.755 ◀
right side M84.754 ◀
incomplete M84.753 ◀
left side M84.752 ◀
right side M84.751 ◀
Fracture, pathological (pathologic) —*see also* Fracture, traumatic M84.40
ankle M84.47-
carpus M84.44-
clavicle M84.41-
compression (not due to trauma) —*see also* Collapse, vertebra M48.50- ◀
dental implant M27.63
dental restorative material K08.539
with loss of material K08.531
without loss of material K08.530
due to
neoplastic disease NEC —*see also* Neoplasm M84.50
ankle M84.57-
carpus M84.54-
clavicle M84.51-
femur M84.55-
fibula M84.56-
finger M84.54-
hip M84.559
humerus M84.52-
ilium M84.550
ischium M84.550
metacarpus M84.54-
metatarsus M84.57-
neck M84.58
pelvis M84.550
radius M84.53-
rib M84.58
scapula M84.51-
skull M84.58
specified site NEC M84.58
tarsus M84.57-
tibia M84.56-
toe M84.57-
ulna M84.53-
vertebra M84.58
osteoporosis M80.00 ⟸
disuse —*see* Osteoporosis, specified type NEC, with pathological fracture
drug-induced —*see* Osteoporosis, drug induced, with pathological fracture
idiopathic —*see* Osteoporosis, specified type NEC, with pathological fracture
postmenopausal —*see* Osteoporosis, postmenopausal, with pathological fracture
postoophorectomy —*see* Osteoporosis, postoophorectomy, with pathological fracture
postsurgical malabsorption —*see* Osteoporosis, specified type NEC, with pathological fracture
specified cause NEC —*see* Osteoporosis, specified type NEC, with pathological fracture
specified disease NEC M84.60
ankle M84.67-
carpus M84.64-
clavicle M84.61-
femur M84.65-
fibula M84.66-
finger M84.64-
hip M84.65-
humerus M84.62-
ilium M84.650
ischium M84.650
metacarpus M84.64-
metatarsus M84.67-

◀ New ⟸ Revised ~~deleted~~ Deleted

- **Fracture, pathological** *(Continued)*
  - due to *(Continued)*
    - specified disease NEC *(Continued)*
      - neck M84.68
      - radius M84.63-
      - rib M84.68
      - scapula M84.61-
      - skull M84.68
      - tarsus M84.67-
      - tibia M84.66-
      - toe M84.67-
      - ulna M84.63-
      - vertebra M84.68
  - femur M84.45-
  - fibula M84.46-
  - finger M84.44-
  - hip M84.459
  - humerus M84.42-
  - ilium M84.454
  - ischium M84.454
  - joint prosthesis —*see* Complications, joint prosthesis, mechanical, breakdown, by site
    - periprosthetic —*see* Fracture, pathological, periprosthetic ⬅
  - metacarpus M84.44-
  - metatarsus M84.47-
  - neck M84.48
  - pelvis M84.454
  - periprosthetic M97.9 ◀
    - ankle M97.2- ◀
    - elbow M97.4- ◀
    - finger M97.8 ◀
    - hip M97.Ø- ◀
    - knee M97.1- ◀
    - other specified joint M97.8 ◀
    - shoulder M97.3- ◀
    - spinal joint M97.8 ◀
    - toe joint M97.8 ◀
    - wrist joint M97.8 ◀
  - radius M84.43-
  - restorative material (dental) KØ8.539
    - with loss of material KØ8.531
    - without loss of material KØ8.53Ø
  - rib M84.48
  - scapula M84.41-
  - skull M84.48
  - tarsus M84.47-
  - tibia M84.46-
  - toe M84.47-
  - ulna M84.43-
  - vertebra M84.48
- **Fracture, traumatic** (abduction) (adduction) (separation) —*see also* Fracture, pathological T14.8
  - acetabulum S32.4Ø-
    - column
      - anterior (displaced) (iliopubic) S32.43-
        - nondisplaced S32.436
      - posterior (displaced) (ilioischial) S32.443
        - nondisplaced S32.44-
    - dome (displaced) S32.48-
      - nondisplaced S32.48
    - specified NEC S32.49-
    - transverse (displaced) S32.45-
      - with associated posterior wall fracture (displaced) S32.46-
        - nondisplaced S32.46-
      - nondisplaced S32.45-
    - wall
      - anterior (displaced) S32.41-
        - nondisplaced S32.41-
      - medial (displaced) S32.47-
        - nondisplaced S32.47-
      - posterior (displaced) S32.42-
        - with associated transverse fracture (displaced) S32.46-
          - nondisplaced S32.46-
        - nondisplaced S32.42-

- **Fracture, traumatic** *(Continued)*
  - acromion —*see* Fracture, scapula, acromial process
  - ankle S82.899
    - bimalleolar (displaced) S82.84-
      - nondisplaced S82.84-
    - lateral malleolus only (displaced) S82.6-
      - nondisplaced S82.6-
    - medial malleolus (displaced) S82.5-
      - associated with Maisonneuve's fracture —*see* Fracture, Maisonneuve's
      - nondisplaced S82.5-
    - talus —*see* Fracture, tarsal, talus
    - trimalleolar (displaced) S82.85-
      - nondisplaced S82.85-
  - arm (upper) —*see also* Fracture, humerus, shaft
    - humerus —*see* Fracture, humerus
    - radius —*see* Fracture, radius
    - ulna —*see* Fracture, ulna
  - astragalus —*see* Fracture, tarsal, talus
  - atlas —*see* Fracture, neck, cervical vertebra, first
  - axis —*see* Fracture, neck, cervical vertebra, second
  - back —*see* Fracture, vertebra
  - Barton's —*see* Barton's fracture
  - base of skull —*see* Fracture, skull, base
  - basicervical (basal) (femoral) S72.Ø
  - Bennett's —*see* Bennett's fracture
  - bimalleolar —*see* Fracture, ankle, bimalleolar
  - blow-out SØ2.3- ⬅
  - bone NEC T14.8
    - birth injury P13.9
    - following insertion of orthopedic implant, joint prosthesis or bone plate —*see* Fracture, following insertion of orthopedic implant, joint prosthesis or bone plate
    - in (due to) neoplastic disease NEC —*see* Fracture, pathological, due to, neoplastic disease
    - pathological (cause unknown) —*see* Fracture, pathological
  - breast bone —*see* Fracture, sternum
  - bucket handle (semilunar cartilage) —*see* Tear, meniscus
  - burst —*see* Fracture, traumatic, by site
  - calcaneus —*see* Fracture, tarsal, calcaneus
  - carpal bone (s) S62.1Ø-
    - capitate (displaced) S62.13-
      - nondisplaced S62.13-
    - cuneiform —*see* Fracture, carpal bone, triquetrum
    - hamate (body) (displaced) S62.143
      - hook process (displaced) S62.15-
        - nondisplaced S62.15-
      - nondisplaced S62.14-
    - larger multangular —*see* Fracture, carpal bones, trapezium
    - lunate (displaced) S62.12-
      - nondisplaced S62.12-
    - navicular S62.ØØ-
      - distal pole (displaced) S62.Ø1-
        - nondisplaced S62.Ø1-
      - middle third (displaced) S62.Ø2-
        - nondisplaced S62.Ø2-
      - proximal third (displaced) S62.Ø3-
        - nondisplaced S62.Ø3-
      - volar tuberosity —*see* Fracture, carpal bones, navicular, distal pole
    - os magnum —*see* Fracture, carpal bones, capitate
    - pisiform (displaced) S62.16-
      - nondisplaced S62.16-
    - semilunar —*see* Fracture, carpal bones, lunate
    - smaller multangular —*see* Fracture, carpal bones, trapezoid

- **Fracture, traumatic** *(Continued)*
  - carpal bone (s) *(Continued)*
    - trapezium (displaced) S62.17-
      - nondisplaced S62.17-
    - trapezoid (displaced) S62.18-
      - nondisplaced S62.18-
    - triquetrum (displaced) S62.11-
      - nondisplaced S62.11-
    - unciform —*see* Fracture, carpal bones, hamate
  - cervical —*see* Fracture, vertebra, cervical
  - clavicle S42.ØØ-
    - acromial end (displaced) S42.Ø3-
      - nondisplaced S42.Ø3-
    - birth injury P13.4
    - lateral end —*see* Fracture, clavicle, acromial end
    - shaft (displaced) S42.Ø2-
      - nondisplaced S42.Ø2-
    - sternal end (anterior) (displaced) S42.Ø1-
      - nondisplaced S42.Ø1-
      - posterior S42.Ø1-
  - coccyx S32.2
  - collapsed —*see* Collapse, vertebra
  - collar bone —*see* Fracture, clavicle
  - Colles' —*see* Colles' fracture
  - ~~compression, not due to trauma —see Collapse, vertebra~~
  - coronoid process —*see* Fracture, ulna, upper end, coronoid process
  - corpus cavernosum penis S39.84Ø
  - costochondral cartilage S23.41
  - costochondral, costosternal junction —*see* Fracture, rib
  - cranium —*see* Fracture, skull
  - cricoid cartilage S12.8
  - cuboid (ankle) —*see* Fracture, tarsal, cuboid
  - cuneiform
    - foot —*see* Fracture, tarsal, cuneiform
    - wrist —*see* Fracture, carpal, triquetrum
  - delayed union —*see* Delay, union, fracture
  - dental restorative material KØ8.539
    - with loss of material KØ8.531
    - without loss of material KØ8.53Ø
  - due to
    - birth injury —*see* Birth, injury, fracture
    - osteoporosis —*see* Osteoporosis, with fracture
  - Dupuytren's —*see* Fracture, ankle, lateral malleolus
  - elbow S42.4Ø-
  - ethmoid (bone) (sinus) —*see* Fracture, skull, base
  - face bone SØ2.92
  - fatigue —*see also* Fracture, stress
    - vertebra M48.4Ø
      - cervical region M48.42
      - cervicothoracic region M48.43
      - lumbar region M48.46
      - lumbosacral region M48.47
      - occipito-atlanto-axial region M48.41
      - sacrococcygeal region M48.48
      - thoracic region M48.44
      - thoracolumbar region M48.45
  - femur, femoral S72.9-
    - basicervical (basal) S72.Ø
    - birth injury P13.2
    - capital epiphyseal S79.Ø1-
    - condyles, epicondyles —*see* Fracture, femur, lower end
    - distal end —*see* Fracture, femur, lower end
    - epiphysis
      - head —*see* Fracture, femur, upper end, epiphysis
      - lower —*see* Fracture, femur, lower end, epiphysis
      - upper —*see* Fracture, femur, upper end, epiphysis
    - following insertion of implant, prosthesis or plate M96.66-

Fracture, traumatic *(Continued)*
femur, femoral *(Continued)*
head —*see* Fracture, femur, upper end, head
intertrochanteric —*see* Fracture, femur, trochanteric
intratrochanteric —*see* Fracture, femur, trochanteric
lower end S72.4Ø-
condyle (displaced) S72.41-
lateral (displaced) S72.42-
nondisplaced S72.42-
medial (displaced) S72.43-
nondisplaced S72.43-
nondisplaced S72.41-
epiphysis (displaced) S72.44-
nondisplaced S72.44-
physeal S79.1Ø-
Salter-Harris
Type I S79.11-
Type II S79.12-
Type III S79.13-
Type IV S79.14-
specified NEC S79.19-
specified NEC S72.49-
supracondylar (displaced) S72.45-
with intracondylar extension (displaced) S72.46-
nondisplaced S72.46-
nondisplaced S72.45-
torus S72.47-
neck —*see* Fracture, femur, upper end, neck
pertrochanteric —*see* Fracture, femur, trochanteric
shaft (lower third) (middle third) (upper third) S72.3Ø-
comminuted (displaced) S72.35-
nondisplaced S72.35-
oblique (displaced) S72.33-
nondisplaced S72.33-
segmental (displaced) S72.36-
nondisplaced S72.36-
specified NEC S72.39-
spiral (displaced) S72.34-
nondisplaced S72.34-
transverse (displaced) S72.32-
nondisplaced S72.32-
specified site NEC —*see* subcategory S72.8
subcapital (displaced) S72.Ø1-
subtrochanteric (region) (section) (displaced) S72.2-
nondisplaced S72.2-
transcervical —*see* Fracture, femur, upper end, neck
transtrochanteric —*see* Fracture, femur, trochanteric
trochanteric S72.1Ø-
apophyseal (displaced) S72.13-
nondisplaced S72.13-
greater trochanter (displaced) S72.11-
nondisplaced S72.11-
intertrochanteric (displaced) S72.14-
nondisplaced S72.14-
lesser trochanter (displaced) S72.12-
nondisplaced S72.12-
upper end S72.ØØ-
apophyseal (displaced) S72.13-
nondisplaced S72.13-
cervicotrochanteric —*see* Fracture, femur, upper end, neck, base
epiphysis (displaced) S72.Ø2-
nondisplaced S72.Ø2-
head S72.Ø5-
articular (displaced) S72.Ø6-
nondisplaced S72.Ø6-
specified NEC S72.Ø9-
intertrochanteric (displaced) S72.14-
nondisplaced S72.14-
intracapsular S72.Ø1-
midcervical (displaced) S72.Ø3-
nondisplaced S72.Ø3-

Fracture, traumatic *(Continued)*
femur, femoral *(Continued)*
upper end *(Continued)*
neck S72.ØØ-
base (displaced) S72.Ø4-
nondisplaced S72.Ø4-
specified NEC S72.Ø9-
pertrochanteric —*see* Fracture, femur, upper end, trochanteric
physeal S79.ØØ-
Salter-Harris type I S79.Ø1-
specified NEC S79.Ø9-
subcapital (displaced) S72.Ø1-
subtrochanteric (displaced) S72.2-
nondisplaced S72.2-
transcervical —*see* Fracture, femur, upper end, midcervical
trochanteric S72.1Ø-
greater (displaced) S72.11-
nondisplaced S72.11-
lesser (displaced) S72.12-
nondisplaced S72.12-
fibula (shaft) (styloid) S82.4Ø-
comminuted (displaced) S82.45-
nondisplaced S82.45-
following insertion of implant, prosthesis or plate M96.67-
involving ankle or malleolus —*see* Fracture, fibula, lateral malleolus
lateral malleolus (displaced) S82.6-
nondisplaced S82.6-
lower end
physeal S89.3Ø-
Salter-Harris
Type I S89.31-
Type II S89.32-
specified NEC S89.39-
specified NEC S82.83-
torus S82.82-
oblique (displaced) S82.43-
nondisplaced S82.43-
segmental (displaced) S82.46-
nondisplaced S82.46-
specified NEC S82.49-
spiral (displaced) S82.44-
nondisplaced S82.44-
transverse (displaced) S82.42-
nondisplaced S82.42-
upper end
physeal S89.2Ø-
Salter-Harris
Type I S89.21-
Type II S89.22-
specified NEC S89.29-
specified NEC S82.83-
torus S82.81-
finger (except thumb) S62.6Ø-
distal phalanx (displaced) S62.63-
nondisplaced S62.66-
index S62.6Ø-
distal phalanx (displaced) S62.63-
nondisplaced S62.66-
medial phalanx (displaced) S62.62-
nondisplaced S62.65-
proximal phalanx (displaced) S62.61-
nondisplaced S62.64-
little S62.6Ø-
distal phalanx (displaced) S62.63-
nondisplaced S62.66-
medial phalanx (displaced) S62.62-
nondisplaced S62.65-
proximal phalanx (displaced) S62.61-
nondisplaced S62.64-
medial phalanx (displaced) S62.62-
nondisplaced S62.65-
middle S62.6Ø-
distal phalanx (displaced) S62.63-
nondisplaced S62.66-
medial phalanx (displaced) S62.62-
nondisplaced S62.65-

Fracture, traumatic *(Continued)*
finger *(Continued)*
middle *(Continued)*
proximal phalanx (displaced) S62.61-
nondisplaced S62.64-
proximal phalanx (displaced) S62.61-
nondisplaced S62.64-
ring S62.6Ø-
distal phalanx (displaced) S62.63-
nondisplaced S62.66-
medial phalanx (displaced) S62.62-
nondisplaced S62.65-
proximal phalanx (displaced) S62.61-
nondisplaced S62.64-
thumb —*see* Fracture, thumb
following insertion (intraoperative) (postoperative) of orthopedic implant, joint prosthesis or bone plate M96.69
femur M96.66-
fibula M96.67-
humerus M96.62-
pelvis M96.65
radius M96.63-
specified bone NEC M96.69
tibia M96.67-
ulna M96.63-
foot S92.9Ø-
astragalus —*see* Fracture, tarsal, talus
calcaneus —*see* Fracture, tarsal, calcaneus
cuboid —*see* Fracture, tarsal, cuboid
cuneiform —*see* Fracture, tarsal, cuneiform
metatarsal —*see* Fracture, metatarsal
navicular —*see* Fracture, tarsal, navicular
sesamoid S92.81- ◀
specified NEC S92.81- ◀
talus —*see* Fracture, tarsal, talus
tarsal —*see* Fracture, tarsal
toe —*see* Fracture, toe
forearm S52.9-
radius —*see* Fracture, radius
ulna —*see* Fracture, ulna
fossa (anterior) (middle) (posterior) SØ2.19
frontal (bone) (skull) SØ2.Ø
sinus SØ2.19
glenoid (cavity) (scapula) —*see* Fracture, scapula, glenoid cavity
greenstick —*see* Fracture, by site
hallux —*see* Fracture, toe, great
hand S62.9-
carpal —*see* Fracture, carpal bone
finger (except thumb) —*see* Fracture, finger
metacarpal —*see* Fracture, metacarpal
navicular (scaphoid) (hand) —*see* Fracture, carpal bone, navicular
thumb —*see* Fracture, thumb
healed or old
with complications - code by Nature of the complication
heel bone —*see* Fracture, tarsal, calcaneus
Hill-Sachs S42.29-
hip —*see* Fracture, femur, neck
humerus S42.3Ø-
anatomical neck —*see* Fracture, humerus, upper end
articular process —*see* Fracture, humerus, lower end
capitellum —*see* Fracture, humerus, lower end, condyle, lateral
distal end —*see* Fracture, humerus, lower end
epiphysis
lower —*see* Fracture, humerus, lower end, physeal
upper —*see* Fracture, humerus, upper end, physeal
external condyle —*see* Fracture, humerus, lower end, condyle, lateral
following insertion of implant, prosthesis or plate M96.62-
great tuberosity —*see* Fracture, humerus, upper end, greater tuberosity

F

- **Fracture, traumatic** *(Continued)*
  - humerus *(Continued)*
    - intercondylar —*see* Fracture, humerus, lower end
    - internal epicondyle —*see* Fracture, humerus, lower end, epicondyle, medial
    - lesser tuberosity —*see* Fracture, humerus, upper end, lesser tuberosity
    - lower end S42.40-
      - condyle
        - lateral (displaced) S42.45-
          - nondisplaced S42.45-
        - medial (displaced) S42.46-
          - nondisplaced S42.46-
      - epicondyle
        - lateral (displaced) S42.43-
          - nondisplaced S42.43-
        - medial (displaced) S42.44-
          - incarcerated S42.44-
          - nondisplaced S42.44-
      - physeal S49.10-
        - Salter-Harris
          - Type I S49.11-
          - Type II S49.12-
          - Type III S49.13-
          - Type IV S49.14-
        - specified NEC S49.19-
      - specified NEC (displaced) S42.49-
        - nondisplaced S42.49-
      - supracondylar (simple) (displaced) S42.41-
        - with intercondylar fracture —*see* Fracture, humerus, lower end ◀
        - comminuted (displaced) S42.42-
          - nondisplaced S42.42-
        - nondisplaced S42.41-
      - torus S42.48-
      - transcondylar (displaced) S42.47-
        - nondisplaced S42.47-
    - proximal end —*see* Fracture, humerus, upper end
    - shaft S42.30-
      - comminuted (displaced) S42.35-
        - nondisplaced S42.35-
      - greenstick S42.31-
      - oblique (displaced) S42.33-
        - nondisplaced S42.33-
      - segmental (displaced) S42.36-
        - nondisplaced S42.36-
      - specified NEC S42.39-
      - spiral (displaced) S42.34-
        - nondisplaced S42.34-
      - transverse (displaced) S42.32-
        - nondisplaced S42.32-
    - supracondylar —*see* Fracture, humerus, lower end
    - surgical neck —*see* Fracture, humerus, upper end, surgical neck
    - trochlea —*see* Fracture, humerus, lower end, condyle, medial
    - tuberosity —*see* Fracture, humerus, upper end
    - upper end S42.20-
      - anatomical neck —*see* Fracture, humerus, upper end, specified NEC
      - articular head —*see* Fracture, humerus, upper end, specified NEC
      - epiphysis —*see* Fracture, humerus, upper end, physeal
      - greater tuberosity (displaced) S42.25-
        - nondisplaced S42.25-
      - lesser tuberosity (displaced) S42.26-
        - nondisplaced S42.26-
      - physeal S49.00-
        - Salter-Harris
          - Type I S49.01-
          - Type II S49.02-
          - Type III S49.03-
          - Type IV S49.04-
        - specified NEC S49.09-

- **Fracture, traumatic** *(Continued)*
  - humerus *(Continued)*
    - upper end *(Continued)*
      - specified NEC (displaced) S42.29-
        - nondisplaced S42.29-
      - surgical neck (displaced) S42.21-
        - four-part S42.24-
        - nondisplaced S42.21-
        - three-part S42.23-
        - two-part (displaced) S42.22-
          - nondisplaced S42.22-
      - torus S42.27-
      - transepiphyseal —*see* Fracture, humerus, upper end, physeal
  - hyoid bone S12.8
  - ilium S32.30-
    - with disruption of pelvic ring —*see* Disruption, pelvic ring
    - avulsion (displaced) S32.31-
      - nondisplaced S32.31-
    - specified NEC S32.39-
  - impaction, impacted - code as Fracture, by site
  - innominate bone —*see* Fracture, ilium
  - instep —*see* Fracture, foot
  - ischium S32.60-
    - with disruption of pelvic ring —*see* Disruption, pelvic ring
    - avulsion (displaced) S32.61-
      - nondisplaced S32.61-
    - specified NEC S32.69-
  - jaw (bone) (lower) —*see* Fracture, mandible
    - upper —*see* Fracture, maxilla
  - joint prosthesis —*see* Complications, joint prosthesis, mechanical, breakdown, by site
    - periprosthetic —*see* Fracture, traumatic, periprosthetic ⟸
  - knee cap —*see* Fracture, patella
  - larynx S12.8
  - late effects —*see* Sequelae, fracture
  - leg (lower) S82.9-
    - ankle —*see* Fracture, ankle
    - femur —*see* Fracture, femur
    - fibula —*see* Fracture, fibula
    - malleolus —*see* Fracture, ankle
    - patella —*see* Fracture, patella
    - specified site NEC S82.89-
    - tibia —*see* Fracture, tibia
  - lumbar spine —*see* Fracture, vertebra, lumbar
  - lumbosacral spine S32.9
  - Maisonneuve's (displaced) S82.86-
    - nondisplaced S82.86-
  - malar bone —*see also* Fracture, maxilla S02.400
    - left side S02.40B ◀
    - right side S02.40A ◀
  - malleolus —*see* Fracture, ankle
  - malunion —*see* Fracture, by site
  - mandible (lower jawbone) S02.609
    - alveolus S02.67- ⟸
    - angle (of jaw) S02.65- ⟸
    - body, unspecified S02.600-
      - left side S02.602 ◀
      - right side S02.601 ◀
    - condylar process S02.61- ⟸
    - coronoid process S02.63- ⟸
    - ramus, unspecified S02.64- ⟸
    - specified site NEC S02.69
    - subcondylar process S02.62- ⟸
    - symphysis S02.66
  - manubrium (sterni) S22.21
    - dissociation from sternum S22.23
  - march —*see* Fracture, traumatic, stress, by site
  - maxilla, maxillary (bone) (sinus) (superior) (upper jaw) S02.401
    - alveolus S02.42
    - inferior —*see* Fracture, mandible
    - LeFort I S02.411
    - LeFort II S02.412
    - LeFort III S02.413

- **Fracture, traumatic** *(Continued)*
  - maxilla, maxillary *(Continued)*
    - left side S02.40D ◀
    - right side S02.40C ◀
  - metacarpal S62.309
    - base (displaced) S62.319
      - nondisplaced S62.349
    - fifth S62.30-
      - base (displaced) S62.31-
        - nondisplaced S62.34-
      - neck (displaced) S62.33-
        - nondisplaced S62.36-
      - shaft (displaced) S62.32-
        - nondisplaced S62.35-
      - specified NEC S62.398
    - first S62.20-
      - base NEC (displaced) S62.23-
        - nondisplaced S62.23-
      - Bennett's —*see* Bennett's fracture
      - neck (displaced) S62.25-
        - nondisplaced S62.25-
      - shaft (displaced) S62.24-
        - nondisplaced S62.24-
      - specified NEC S62.29-
    - fourth S62.30-
      - base (displaced) S62.31-
        - nondisplaced S62.34-
      - neck (displaced) S62.33-
        - nondisplaced S62.36-
      - shaft (displaced) S62.32-
        - nondisplaced S62.35-
      - specified NEC S62.39-
    - neck (displaced) S62.33-
      - nondisplaced S62.36-
    - Rolando's —*see* Rolando's fracture
    - second S62.30-
      - base (displaced) S62.31-
        - nondisplaced S62.34-
      - neck (displaced) S62.33-
        - nondisplaced S62.36-
      - shaft (displaced) S62.32-
        - nondisplaced S62.35-
      - specified NEC S62.39-
    - shaft (displaced) S62.32-
      - nondisplaced S62.35-
    - specified NEC S62.399
    - third S62.30-
      - base (displaced) S62.31-
        - nondisplaced S62.34-
      - neck (displaced) S62.33-
        - nondisplaced S62.36-
      - shaft (displaced) S62.32-
        - nondisplaced S62.35-
      - specified NEC S62.39-
  - metastatic —*see* Fracture, pathological, due to, neoplastic disease —*see also* Neoplasm
  - metatarsal bone S92.30-
    - fifth (displaced) S92.35-
      - nondisplaced S92.35-
    - first (displaced) S92.31-
      - nondisplaced S92.31-
    - fourth (displaced) S92.34-
      - nondisplaced S92.34-
    - physeal S99.10- ◀
      - Salter-Harris ◀
        - Type I S99.11- ◀
        - Type II S99.12- ◀
        - Type III S99.13- ◀
        - Type IV S99.14- ◀
      - specified NEC S99.19- ◀
    - second (displaced) S92.32-
      - nondisplaced S92.32-
    - third (displaced) S92.33-
      - nondisplaced S92.33-
  - Monteggia's —*see* Monteggia's fracture
  - multiple
    - hand (and wrist) NEC —*see* Fracture, by site
    - ribs —*see* Fracture, rib, multiple

F

◀ New ⟸ Revised ~~deleted~~ Deleted

F

Fracture, traumatic *(Continued)*
  sesamoid bone
    foot S92.81- ◀
    hand —*see* Fracture, carpal
    other —*see* Fracture, traumatic, by site ◀
    ~~other - code by site under Fracture~~
  shepherd's —*see* Fracture, tarsal, talus
  shoulder (girdle) S42.9-
    blade —*see* Fracture, scapula
  sinus (ethmoid) (frontal) S02.19
  skull S02.91
    base S02.10- ◀━
      occiput S02.119
        condyle S02.113
          type I S02.110
            left side S02.11B ◀
            right side S02.11A ◀
          type II S02.111
            left side S02.11D ◀
            right side S02.11C ◀
          type III S02.112
            left side S02.11F ◀
            right side S02.11E ◀
          specified NEC S02.118 ◀
            left side S02.11H ◀
            right side S02.11G ◀
        ~~specified NEC S02.118~~
      specified NEC S02.19- ◀━
    birth injury P13.0
    frontal bone S02.0
    parietal bone S02.0
    specified site NEC S02.8
    temporal bone S02.19
    vault S02.0
  Smith's —*see* Smith's fracture
  sphenoid (bone) (sinus) S02.19
  spine —*see* Fracture, vertebra
  spinous process —*see* Fracture, vertebra
  spontaneous (cause unknown) —*see* Fracture, pathological
  stave (of thumb) —*see* Fracture, metacarpal, first
  sternum S22.20
    with flail chest —*see* Flail, chest
    body S22.22
    manubrium S22.21
    xiphoid (process) S22.24
  stress M84.30
    ankle M84.37-
    carpus M84.34-
    clavicle M84.31-
    femoral neck M84.359
    femur M84.35-
    fibula M84.36-
    finger M84.34-
    hip M84.359
    humerus M84.32-
    ilium M84.350
    ischium M84.350
    metacarpus M84.34-
    metatarsus M84.37-
    neck —*see* Fracture, fatigue, vertebra
    pelvis M84.350
    radius M84.33-
    rib M84.38
    scapula M84.31-
    skull M84.38
    tarsus M84.37-
    tibia M84.36-
    toe M84.37-
    ulna M84.33-
    vertebra —*see* Fracture, fatigue, vertebra
  supracondylar, elbow —*see* Fracture, humerus, lower end, supracondylar
  symphysis pubis —*see* Fracture, pubis
  talus (ankle bone) —*see* Fracture, tarsal, talus
  tarsal bone (s) S92.20-
    astragalus —*see* Fracture, tarsal, talus
    calcaneus S92.00-
      anterior process (displaced) S92.02-
        nondisplaced S92.02-

Fracture, traumatic *(Continued)*
  tarsal bone *(Continued)*
    calcaneus *(Continued)*
      body (displaced) S92.01-
        nondisplaced S92.01-
      extraarticular NEC (displaced) S92.05-
        nondisplaced S92.05-
      intraarticular (displaced) S92.06-
        nondisplaced S92.06-
      physeal S99.00- ◀
        Salter-Harris ◀
          Type I S99.01- ◀
          Type II S99.02- ◀
          Type III S99.03- ◀
          Type IV S99.04- ◀
        specified NEC S99.09- ◀
      tuberosity (displaced) S92.04-
        avulsion (displaced) S92.03-
          nondisplaced S92.03-
        nondisplaced S92.04-
    cuboid (displaced) S92.21-
      nondisplaced S92.21-
    cuneiform
      intermediate (displaced) S92.23-
        nondisplaced S92.23-
      lateral (displaced) S92.22-
        nondisplaced S92.22-
      medial (displaced) S92.24-
        nondisplaced S92.24-
    navicular (displaced) S92.25-
      nondisplaced S92.25-
    scaphoid —*see* Fracture, tarsal, navicular
    talus S92.10-
      avulsion (displaced) S92.15-
        nondisplaced S92.15-
      body (displaced) S92.12-
        nondisplaced S92.12-
      dome (displaced) S92.14-
        nondisplaced S92.14-
      head (displaced) S92.12-
        nondisplaced S92.12-
      lateral process (displaced) S92.14-
        nondisplaced S92.14-
      neck (displaced) S92.11-
        nondisplaced S92.11-
      posterior process (displaced) S92.13-
        nondisplaced S92.13-
      specified NEC S92.19-
  temporal bone (styloid) S02.19
  thorax (bony) S22.9
    with flail chest —*see* Flail, chest
    rib S22.3-
      multiple S22.4-
        with flail chest —*see* Flail, chest
    sternum S22.20
      body S22.22
      manubrium S22.21
      xiphoid process S22.24
    vertebra (displaced) S22.009
      burst (stable) S22.001
        unstable S22.002
      eighth S22.069
        burst (stable) S22.061
          unstable S22.062
        specified type NEC S22.068
        wedge compression S22.060
      eleventh S22.089
        burst (stable) S22.081
          unstable S22.082
        specified type NEC S22.088
        wedge compression S22.080
      fifth S22.059
        burst (stable) S22.051
          unstable S22.052
        specified type NEC S22.058
        wedge compression S22.050
      first S22.019
        burst (stable) S22.011
          unstable S22.012
        specified type NEC S22.018
        wedge compression S22.010

Fracture, traumatic *(Continued)*
  thorax *(Continued)*
    vertebra *(Continued)*
      fourth S22.049
        burst (stable) S22.041
          unstable S22.042
        specified type NEC S22.048
        wedge compression S22.040
      ninth S22.079
        burst (stable) S22.071
          unstable S22.072
        specified type NEC S22.078
        wedge compression S22.070
      nondisplaced S22.001
      second S22.029
        burst (stable) S22.021
          unstable S22.022
        specified type NEC S22.028
        wedge compression S22.020
      seventh S22.069
        burst (stable) S22.061
          unstable S22.062
        specified type NEC S22.068
        wedge compression S22.060
      sixth S22.059
        burst (stable) S22.051
          unstable S22.052
        specified type NEC S22.058
        wedge compression S22.050
      specified type NEC S22.008
      tenth S22.079
        burst (stable) S22.071
          unstable S22.072
        specified type NEC S22.078
        wedge compression S22.070
      third S22.039
        burst (stable) S22.031
          unstable S22.032
        specified type NEC S22.038
        wedge compression S22.030
      twelfth S22.089
        burst (stable) S22.081
          unstable S22.082
        specified type NEC S22.088
        wedge compression S22.080
      wedge compression S22.000
  thumb S62.50-
    distal phalanx (displaced) S62.52-
      nondisplaced S62.52-
    proximal phalanx (displaced) S62.51-
      nondisplaced S62.51-
  thyroid cartilage S12.8
  tibia (shaft) S82.20-
    comminuted (displaced) S82.25-
      nondisplaced S82.25-
    condyles —*see* Fracture, tibia, upper end
    distal end —*see* Fracture, tibia, lower end
    epiphysis
      lower —*see* Fracture, tibia, lower end
      upper —*see* Fracture, tibia, upper end
    following insertion of implant, prosthesis or plate M96.67-
    head (involving knee joint) —*see* Fracture, tibia, upper end
    intercondyloid eminence —*see* Fracture, tibia, upper end
    involving ankle or malleolus —*see* Fracture, ankle, medial malleolus
    lower end S82.30-
      physeal S89.10-
        Salter-Harris
          Type I S89.11-
          Type II S89.12-
          Type III S89.13-
          Type IV S89.14-
        specified NEC S89.19-
      pilon (displaced) S82.87-
        nondisplaced S82.87-
      specified NEC S82.39-
      torus S82.31-

◀ New ◀━ Revised ~~deleted~~ Deleted

Fracture, traumatic *(Continued)*
- tibia *(Continued)*
  - malleolus —*see* Fracture, ankle, medial malleolus
  - oblique (displaced) S82.23-
    - nondisplaced S82.23-
  - pilon —*see* Fracture, tibia, lower end, pilon
  - proximal end —*see* Fracture, tibia, upper end
  - segmental (displaced) S82.26-
    - nondisplaced S82.26-
  - specified NEC S82.29-
  - spine —*see* Fracture, upper end, spine
  - spiral (displaced) S82.24-
    - nondisplaced S82.24-
  - transverse (displaced) S82.22-
    - nondisplaced S82.22-
  - tuberosity —*see* Fracture, tibia, upper end, tuberosity
  - upper end S82.10-
    - bicondylar (displaced) S82.14-
      - nondisplaced S82.14-
    - lateral condyle (displaced) S82.12-
      - nondisplaced S82.12-
    - medial condyle (displaced) S82.13-
      - nondisplaced S82.13-
    - physeal S89.00-
      - Salter-Harris
        - Type I S89.01-
        - Type II S89.02-
        - Type III S89.03-
        - Type IV S89.04-
      - specified NEC S89.09-
    - plateau —*see* Fracture, tibia, upper end, bicondylar
    - specified NEC S82.19-
    - spine (displaced) S82.11-
      - nondisplaced S82.11-
    - torus S82.16-
    - tuberosity (displaced) S82.15-
      - nondisplaced S82.15-
- toe S92.91-
  - great (displaced) S92.40-
    - distal phalanx (displaced) S92.42-
      - nondisplaced S92.42-
    - nondisplaced S92.40-
    - proximal phalanx (displaced) S92.41-
      - nondisplaced S92.41-
    - specified NEC S92.49-
  - lesser (displaced) S92.50-
    - distal phalanx (displaced) S92.53-
      - nondisplaced S92.53-
    - medial phalanx (displaced) S92.52-
      - nondisplaced S92.52-
    - nondisplaced S92.50-
    - proximal phalanx (displaced) S92.51-
      - nondisplaced S92.51-
    - specified NEC S92.59-
  - physeal ◀
    - phalanx S99.20- ◀
      - Salter-Harris ◀
        - Type I S99.21- ◀
        - Type II S99.22- ◀
        - Type III S99.23- ◀
        - Type IV S99.24- ◀
      - specified NEC S99.29- ◀
- tooth (root) S02.5
- trachea (cartilage) S12.8
- transverse process —*see* Fracture, vertebra
- trapezium or trapezoid bone —*see* Fracture, carpal
- trimalleolar —*see* Fracture, ankle, trimalleolar
- triquetrum (cuneiform of carpus) —*see* Fracture, carpal, triquetrum
- trochanter —*see* Fracture, femur, trochanteric
- tuberosity (external) —*see* Fracture, traumatic, by site ⬅
- ulna (shaft) S52.20-
  - bent bone S52.28-
  - coronoid process —*see* Fracture, ulna, upper end, coronoid process
  - distal end —*see* Fracture, ulna, lower end
  - following insertion of implant, prosthesis or plate M96.63-
  - head S52.00-
  - lower end S52.60-
    - physeal S59.00-
      - Salter-Harris
        - Type I S59.01-
        - Type II S59.02-
        - Type III S59.03-
        - Type IV S59.04-
      - specified NEC S59.09-
    - specified NEC S52.69-
    - styloid process (displaced) S52.61-
      - nondisplaced S52.61-
    - torus S52.62-
  - proximal end —*see* Fracture, ulna, upper end
  - shaft S52.20-
    - comminuted (displaced) S52.25-
      - nondisplaced S52.25-
    - greenstick S52.21-
    - Monteggia's —*see* Monteggia's fracture
    - oblique (displaced) S52.23-
      - nondisplaced S52.23-
    - segmental (displaced) S52.26-
      - nondisplaced S52.26-
    - specified NEC S52.29-
    - spiral (displaced) S52.24-
      - nondisplaced S52.24-
    - transverse (displaced) S52.22-
      - nondisplaced S52.22-
  - upper end S52.00-
    - coronoid process (displaced) S52.04-
      - nondisplaced S52.04-
    - olecranon process (displaced) S52.02-
      - with intraarticular extension S52.03-
      - nondisplaced S52.02-
        - with intraarticular extension S52.03-
    - specified NEC S52.09-
    - torus S52.01-
- unciform —*see* Fracture, carpal, hamate
- vault of skull S02.0
- vertebra, vertebral (arch) (body) (column) (neural arch) (pedicle) (spinous process) (transverse process)
  - atlas —*see* Fracture, neck, cervical vertebra, first
  - axis —*see* Fracture, neck, cervical vertebra, second
  - cervical (teardrop) S12.9
    - axis —*see* Fracture, neck, cervical vertebra, second
    - first (atlas) —*see* Fracture, neck, cervical vertebra, first
    - second (axis) —*see* Fracture, neck, cervical vertebra, second
  - chronic M84.48
  - coccyx S32.2
  - dorsal —*see* Fracture, thorax, vertebra
  - lumbar S32.009
    - burst (stable) S32.001
      - unstable S32.002
    - fifth S32.059
      - burst (stable) S32.051
        - unstable S32.052
      - specified type NEC S32.058
      - wedge compression S32.050
    - first S32.019
      - burst (stable) S32.011
        - unstable S32.012
      - specified type NEC S32.018
      - wedge compression S32.010
    - fourth S32.049
      - burst (stable) S32.041
        - unstable S32.042
      - specified type NEC S32.048
      - wedge compression S32.040
    - second S32.029
      - burst (stable) S32.021
        - unstable S32.022
      - specified type NEC S32.028
      - wedge compression S32.020
    - specified type NEC S32.008
    - third S32.039
      - burst (stable) S32.031
        - unstable S32.032
      - specified type NEC S32.038
      - wedge compression S32.030
    - wedge compression S32.000
  - metastatic —*see* Collapse, vertebra, in, specified disease NEC —*see also* Neoplasm
  - newborn (birth injury) P11.5
  - sacrum S32.10
    - specified NEC S32.19
    - Type
      - 1 S32.14
      - 2 S32.15
      - 3 S32.16
      - 4 S32.17
    - Zone
      - I S32.119
        - displaced (minimally) S32.111
          - severely S32.112
        - nondisplaced S32.110
      - II S32.129
        - displaced (minimally) S32.121
          - severely S32.122
        - nondisplaced S32.120
      - III S32.139
        - displaced (minimally) S32.131
          - severely S32.132
        - nondisplaced S32.130
  - thoracic —*see* Fracture, thorax, vertebra
- vertex S02.0
- vomer (bone) S02.2
- wrist S62.10-
  - carpal —*see* Fracture, carpal bone
  - navicular (scaphoid) (hand) —*see* Fracture, carpal, navicular
- xiphisternum, xiphoid (process) S22.24
- zygoma S02.442
  - left side S02.40F ◀
  - right side S02.40E ◀

Fragile, fragility
- autosomal site Q95.5
- bone, congenital (with blue sclera) Q78.0
- capillary (hereditary) D69.8
- hair L67.8
- nails L60.3
- non-sex chromosome site Q95.5
- X chromosome Q99.2

Fragilitas
- crinium L67.8
- ossium (with blue sclerae) (hereditary) Q78.0
- unguium L60.3
  - congenital Q84.6

Fragments, cataract (lens)**, following cataract surgery** H59.02-
- retained foreign body —*see* Retained, foreign body fragments (type of)

Frailty (frail) R54
- mental R41.81

Frambesia, frambesial (tropica) —*see also* Yaws
- initial lesion or ulcer A66.0
- primary A66.0

Frambeside
- gummatous A66.4
- of early yaws A66.2

Frambesioma A66.1
Franceschetti-Klein (-Wildervanck) **disease or syndrome** Q75.4
Francis' disease —*see* Tularemia
Franklin disease C88.2
Frank's essential thrombocytopenia D69.3
Fraser's syndrome Q87.Ø
Freckle (s) L81.2
  malignant melanoma in —*see* Melanoma
  melanotic (Hutchinson's) —*see* Melanoma, in situ
  retinal D49.81
Frederickson's hyperlipoproteinemia, type
  I and V E78.3
  IIA E78.ØØ
  IIB and III E78.2
  IV E78.1
Freeman Sheldon syndrome Q87.Ø
Freezing —*see also* Effect, adverse, cold T69.9
Freiberg's disease (infraction of metatarsal head or osteochondrosis) —*see* Osteochondrosis, juvenile, metatarsus
Frei's disease A55
Fremitus, friction, cardiac RØ1.2
Frenum, frenulum
  external os Q51.828
  tongue (shortening) (congenital) Q38.1
Frequency micturition (nocturnal) R35.Ø
  psychogenic F45.8
Frey's syndrome
  auriculotemporal G5Ø.8
  hyperhidrosis L74.52
Friction
  burn —*see* Burn, by site
  fremitus, cardiac RØ1.2
  precordial RØ1.2
  sounds, chest RØ9.89
Friderichsen-Waterhouse syndrome or disease A39.1
Friedländer's B (bacillus) **NEC** —*see also* condition A49.8
Friedreich's
  ataxia G11.1
  combined systemic disease G11.1
  facial hemihypertrophy Q67.4
  sclerosis (cerebellum) (spinal cord) G11.1
Frigidity F52.22
Fröhlich's syndrome E23.6
Frontal —*see also* condition
  lobe syndrome FØ7.Ø
Frostbite (superficial) T33.9Ø
  with
    partial thickness skin loss —*see* Frostbite (superficial), by site
    tissue necrosis T34.9Ø
  abdominal wall T33.3
    with tissue necrosis T34.3
  ankle T33.81-
    with tissue necrosis T34.81-
  arm T33.4-
  with tissue necrosis T34.4-
    finger (s) —*see* Frostbite, finger
    hand —*see* Frostbite, hand
    wrist —*see* Frostbite, wrist
  ear T33.Ø1-
    with tissue necrosis T34.Ø1-
  face T33.Ø9
    with tissue necrosis T34.Ø9
  finger T33.53-
    with tissue necrosis T34.53-
  foot T33.82-
    with tissue necrosis T34.82-
  hand T33.52-
    with tissue necrosis T34.52-
  head T33.Ø9
    with tissue necrosis T34.Ø9
    ear —*see* Frostbite, ear
    nose —*see* Frostbite, nose
  hip (and thigh) T33.6-
    with tissue necrosis T34.6-

Frostbite *(Continued)*
  knee T33.7-
    with tissue necrosis T34.7-
  leg T33.9-
    with tissue necrosis T34.9-
    ankle —*see* Frostbite, ankle
    foot —*see* Frostbite, foot
    knee —*see* Frostbite, knee
    lower T33.7-
      with tissue necrosis T34.7-
    thigh —*see* Frostbite, hip
    toe —*see* Frostbite, toe
  limb
    lower T33.99
      with tissue necrosis T34.99
    upper —*see* Frostbite, arm
  neck T33.1
    with tissue necrosis T34.1
  nose T33.Ø2
    with tissue necrosis T34.Ø2
  pelvis T33.3
    with tissue necrosis T34.3
  specified site NEC T33.99
    with tissue necrosis T34.99
  thigh —*see* Frostbite, hip
  thorax T33.2
    with tissue necrosis T34.2
  toes T33.83-
    with tissue necrosis T34.83-
  trunk T33.99
    with tissue necrosis T34.99
  wrist T33.51-
    with tissue necrosis T34.51-
Frotteurism F65.81
Frozen —*see also* Effect, adverse, cold T69.9
  pelvis (female) N94.89
    male K66.8
  shoulder —*see* Capsulitis, adhesive
Fructokinase deficiency E74.11
Fructose 1,6 diphosphatase deficiency E74.19
Fructosemia (benign) (essential) E74.12
Fructosuria (benign) (essential) E74.11
Fuchs'
  black spot (myopic) H44.2-
  dystrophy (corneal endothelium) H18.51
  heterochromic cyclitis —*see* Cyclitis, Fuchs' heterochromic
Fucosidosis E77.1
Fugue R68.89
  dissociative F44.1
  hysterical (dissociative) F44.1
  postictal in epilepsy —*see* Epilepsy
  reaction to exceptional stress (transient) F43.Ø
Fulminant, fulminating —*see* condition
Functional —*see also* condition
  bleeding (uterus) N93.8
Functioning, intellectual, borderline R41.83
Fundus —*see* condition
Fungemia NOS B49
Fungus, fungous
  cerebral G93.89
  disease NOS B49
  infection —*see* Infection, fungus
Funiculitis (acute) (chronic) (endemic) N49.1
  gonococcal (acute) (chronic) A54.23
  tuberculous A18.15
Funnel
  breast (acquired) M95.4
    congenital Q67.6
    sequelae (late effect) of rickets E64.3
  chest (acquired) M95.4
    congenital Q67.6
    sequelae (late effect) of rickets E64.3
  pelvis (acquired) M95.5
    with disproportion (fetopelvic) O33.3
      causing obstructed labor O65.3
    congenital Q74.2
FUO (fever of unknown origin) R5Ø.9
Furfur L21.Ø
  microsporon B36.Ø

Furrier's lung J67.8
Furrowed K14.5
  nail (s) (transverse) L6Ø.4
    congenital Q84.6
  tongue K14.5
    congenital Q38.3
Furuncle LØ2.92
  abdominal wall LØ2.221
  ankle —*see* Furuncle, lower limb
  antecubital space —*see* Furuncle, upper limb
  anus K61.Ø
  arm —*see* Furuncle, upper limb
  auditory canal, external —*see* Abscess, ear, external
  auricle (ear) —*see* Abscess, ear, external
  axilla (region) LØ2.42-
  back (any part) LØ2.222
  breast N61.1
  buttock LØ2.32
  cheek (external) LØ2.Ø2
  chest wall LØ2.223
  chin LØ2.Ø2
  corpus cavernosum N48.21
  ear, external —*see* Abscess, ear, external
  external auditory canal —*see* Abscess, ear, external
  eyelid —*see* Abscess, eyelid
  face LØ2.Ø2
  femoral (region) —*see* Furuncle, lower limb
  finger —*see* Furuncle, hand
  flank LØ2.221
  foot LØ2.62-
  forehead LØ2.Ø2
  gluteal (region) LØ2.32
  groin LØ2.224
  hand LØ2.52-
  head LØ2.821
    face LØ2.Ø2
  hip —*see* Furuncle, lower limb
  kidney —*see* Abscess, kidney
  knee —*see* Furuncle, lower limb
  labium (majus) (minus) N76.4
  lacrimal
    gland —*see* Dacryoadenitis
    passages (duct) (sac) —*see* Inflammation, lacrimal, passages, acute
  leg (any part) —*see* Furuncle, lower limb
  lower limb LØ2.42-
  malignant A22.Ø
  mouth K12.2
  navel LØ2.226
  neck LØ2.12
  nose J34.Ø
  orbit, orbital —*see* Abscess, orbit
  palmar (space) —*see* Furuncle, hand
  partes posteriores LØ2.32
  pectoral region LØ2.223
  penis N48.21
  perineum LØ2.225
  pinna —*see* Abscess, ear, external
  popliteal —*see* Furuncle, lower limb
  prepatellar —*see* Furuncle, lower limb
  scalp LØ2.821
  seminal vesicle N49.Ø
  shoulder —*see* Furuncle, upper limb
  specified site NEC LØ2.828
  submandibular K12.2
  temple (region) LØ2.Ø2
  thumb —*see* Furuncle, hand
  toe —*see* Furuncle, foot
  trunk LØ2.229
    abdominal wall LØ2.221
    back LØ2.222
    chest wall LØ2.223
    groin LØ2.224
    perineum LØ2.225
    umbilicus LØ2.226
  umbilicus LØ2.226
  upper limb LØ2.42-
  vulva N76.4

F

Furunculosis —*see* Furuncle
Fused —*see* Fusion, fused
Fusion, fused (congenital)
  astragaloscaphoid Q74.2
  atria Q21.1
  auditory canal Q16.1
  auricles, heart Q21.1
  binocular with defective stereopsis H53.32
  bone Q79.8
  cervical spine M43.22
  choanal Q30.0
  commissure, mitral valve Q23.2
  cusps, heart valve NEC Q24.8
    mitral Q23.2
    pulmonary Q22.1
    tricuspid Q22.4
  ear ossicles Q16.3
  fingers Q70.0-
  hymen Q52.3
  joint (acquired) —*see also* Ankylosis
    congenital Q74.8
  kidneys (incomplete) Q63.1
  labium (majus) (minus) Q52.5
  larynx and trachea Q34.8
Fusion, fused *(Continued)*
  limb, congenital Q74.8
    lower Q74.2
    upper Q74.0
  lobes, lung Q33.8
  lumbosacral (acquired) M43.27
    arthrodesis status Z98.1
    congenital Q76.49
    postprocedural status Z98.1
  nares, nose, nasal, nostril (s) Q30.0
  organ or site not listed —*see* Anomaly, by site
  ossicles Q79.9
    auditory Q16.3
  pulmonic cusps Q22.1
  ribs Q76.6
  sacroiliac (joint) (acquired) M43.28
    arthrodesis status Z98.1
    congenital Q74.2
    postprocedural status Z98.1
  spine (acquired) NEC M43.20
    arthrodesis status Z98.1
    cervical region M43.22
    cervicothoracic region M43.23
    congenital Q76.49
Fusion, fused *(Continued)*
  spine *(Continued)*
    lumbar M43.26
    lumbosacral region M43.27
    occipito-atlanto-axial region M43.21
    postoperative status Z98.1
    sacrococcygeal region M43.28
    thoracic region M43.24
    thoracolumbar region M43.25
  sublingual duct with submaxillary duct at opening in mouth Q38.4
  testes Q55.1
  toes Q70.2
  tooth, teeth K00.2
  trachea and esophagus Q39.8
  twins Q89.4
  vagina Q52.4
  ventricles, heart Q21.0
  vertebra (arch) —*see* Fusion, spine
  vulva Q52.5
Fusospirillosis (mouth) (tongue) (tonsil) A69.1
Fussy baby R68.12

F

G

- **Gain in weight** (abnormal) (excessive) —*see also* Weight, gain
- **Gaisböck's disease** (polycythemia hypertonica) D75.1
- **Gait abnormality** R26.9
  - ataxic R26.Ø
  - falling R29.6
  - hysterical (ataxic) (staggering) F44.4
  - paralytic R26.1
  - spastic R26.1
  - specified type NEC R26.89
  - staggering R26.Ø
  - unsteadiness R26.81
  - walking difficulty NEC R26.2
- **Galactocele** (breast) N64.89
  - puerperal, postpartum O92.79
- **Galactokinase deficiency** E74.29
- **Galactophoritis** N61.Ø
  - gestational, puerperal, postpartum O91.2-
- **Galactorrhea** O92.6
  - not associated with childbirth N64.3
- **Galactosemia** (classic) (congenital) E74.21
- **Galactosuria** E74.29
- **Galacturia** R82.Ø
  - schistosomiasis (bilharziasis) B65.Ø
- **Galeazzi's fracture** S52.37-
- **Galen's vein** —*see* condition
- **Galeophobia** F4Ø.218
- **Gall duct** —*see* condition
- **Gallbladder** —*see also* condition
  - acute K81.Ø
- **Gallop rhythm** RØØ.8
- **Gallstone** (colic) (cystic duct) (gallbladder) (impacted) (multiple) —*see also* Calculus, gallbladder
  - with
    - cholecystitis —*see* Calculus, gallbladder, with cholecystitis
  - bile duct (common) (hepatic) —*see* Calculus, bile duct
  - causing intestinal obstruction K56.3
  - specified NEC K8Ø.8Ø
    - with obstruction K8Ø.81
- **Gambling** Z72.6
  - pathological (compulsive) F63.Ø
- **Gammopathy** (of undetermined significance [MGUS]) D47.2
  - associated with lymphoplasmacytic dyscrasia D47.2
  - monoclonal D47.2
  - polyclonal D89.Ø
- **Gamna's disease** (siderotic splenomegaly) D73.1
- **Gamophobia** F4Ø.298
- **Gampsodactylia** (congenital) Q66.7
- **Gamstorp's disease** (adynamia episodica hereditaria) G72.3
- **Gandy-Nanta disease** (siderotic splenomegaly) D73.1
- **Gang**
  - membership offenses Z72.81Ø
- **Gangliocytoma** D36.1Ø
- **Ganglioglioma** —*see* Neoplasm, uncertain behavior, by site
- **Ganglion** (compound) (diffuse) (joint) (tendon (sheath)) M67.4Ø
  - ankle M67.47-
  - foot M67.47-
  - forearm M67.43-
  - hand M67.44-
  - lower leg M67.46-
  - multiple sites M67.49
  - of yaws (early) (late) A66.6
  - pelvic region M67.45-
  - periosteal —*see* Periostitis
  - shoulder region M67.41-
  - specified site NEC M67.48
  - thigh region M67.45-
  - tuberculous A18.Ø9
  - upper arm M67.42-
  - wrist M67.43-
- **Ganglioneuroblastoma** —*see* Neoplasm, nerve, malignant
- **Ganglioneuroma** D36.1Ø
  - malignant —*see* Neoplasm, nerve, malignant
- **Ganglioneuromatosis** D36.1Ø
- **Ganglionitis**
  - fifth nerve —*see* Neuralgia, trigeminal
  - gasserian (postherpetic) (postzoster) BØ2.21
  - geniculate G51.1
    - newborn (birth injury) P11.3
    - postherpetic, postzoster BØ2.21
  - herpes zoster BØ2.21
  - postherpetic geniculate BØ2.21
- **Gangliosidosis** E75.1Ø
  - GM1 E75.19
  - GM2 E75.ØØ
    - other specified E75.Ø9
    - Sandhoff disease E75.Ø1
    - Tay-Sachs disease E75.Ø2
  - GM3 E75.19
  - mucolipidosis IV E75.11
- **Gangosa** A66.5
- **Gangrene, gangrenous** (connective tissue) (dropsical) (dry) (moist) (skin) (ulcer) —*see also* Necrosis I96
  - with diabetes (mellitus) —*see* Diabetes, gangrene
  - abdomen (wall) I96
  - alveolar M27.3
  - appendix K35.8Ø
    - with
      - perforation or rupture K35.2
      - peritoneal abscess K35.3
      - peritonitis NEC K35.3
        - generalized (with perforation or rupture) K35.2
        - localized (with perforation or rupture) K35.3
  - arteriosclerotic (general) (senile) —*see* Arteriosclerosis, extremities, with, gangrene
  - auricle I96
  - Bacillus welchii A48.Ø
  - bladder (infectious) —*see* Cystitis, specified type NEC
  - bowel, cecum, or colon —*see* Gangrene, intestine
  - Clostridium perfringens or welchii A48.Ø
  - cornea H18.89-
  - corpora cavernosa N48.29
    - noninfective N48.89
  - cutaneous, spreading I96
  - decubital —*see* Ulcer, pressure, by site
  - diabetic (any site) —*see* Diabetes, gangrene
  - emphysematous —*see* Gangrene, gas
  - epidemic —*see* Poisoning, food, noxious, plant
  - epididymis (infectional) N45.1
  - erysipelas —*see* Erysipelas
  - extremity (lower) (upper) I96
  - Fournier N49.3
    - female N76.89
  - fusospirochetal A69.Ø
  - gallbladder —*see* Cholecystitis, acute
  - gas (bacillus) A48.Ø
    - following
      - abortion —*see* Abortion by type complicated by infection
      - ectopic or molar pregnancy OØ8.Ø
  - glossitis K14.Ø
  - hernia —*see* Hernia, by site, with gangrene
  - intestine, intestinal (hemorrhagic) (massive) —*see also* Infarct, intestine K55.Ø69
    - with
      - mesenteric embolism —*see also* Infarct, intestine K55.Ø69
      - obstruction —*see* Obstruction, intestine
  - laryngitis JØ4.Ø
  - limb (lower) (upper) I96

Gangrene, gangrenous *(Continued)*

  - lung J85.Ø
    - spirochetal A69.8
  - lymphangitis I89.1
  - Meleney's (synergistic) —*see* Ulcer, skin
  - mesentery —*see also* Infarct, intestine K55.Ø69
    - with
      - embolism —*see also* Infarct, intestine K55.Ø69
      - intestinal obstruction —*see* Obstruction, intestine
  - mouth A69.Ø
  - ovary —*see* Oophoritis
  - pancreas —*see* Pancreatitis, acute
  - penis N48.29
    - noninfective N48.89
  - perineum I96
  - pharynx —*see also* Pharyngitis
    - Vincent's A69.1
  - presenile I73.1
  - progressive synergistic —*see* Ulcer, skin
  - pulmonary J85.Ø
  - pulpal (dental) KØ4.1
  - quinsy J36
  - Raynaud's (symmetric gangrene) I73.Ø1
  - retropharyngeal J39.2
  - scrotum N49.3
    - noninfective N5Ø.89
  - senile (atherosclerotic) —*see* Arteriosclerosis, extremities, with, gangrene
  - spermatic cord N49.1
    - noninfective N5Ø.89
  - spine I96
  - spirochetal NEC A69.8
  - spreading cutaneous I96
  - stomatitis A69.Ø
  - symmetrical I73.Ø1
  - testis (infectional) N45.2
    - noninfective N44.8
  - throat —*see also* Pharyngitis
    - diphtheritic A36.Ø
    - Vincent's A69.1
  - thyroid (gland) EØ7.89
  - tooth (pulp) KØ4.1
  - tuberculous NEC —*see* Tuberculosis
  - tunica vaginalis N49.1
    - noninfective N5Ø.89
  - umbilicus I96
  - uterus —*see* Endometritis
  - uvulitis K12.2
  - vas deferens N49.1
    - noninfective N5Ø.89
  - vulva N76.89
- **Ganister disease** J62.8
- **Ganser's syndrome** (hysterical) F44.89
- **Gardner-Diamond syndrome** (autoerythrocyte sensitization) D69.2
- **Gargoylism** E76.Ø1
- **Garré's disease, osteitis** (sclerosing), **osteomyelitis** —*see* Osteomyelitis, specified type NEC
- **Garrod's pad, knuckle** M72.1
- **Gartner's duct**
  - cyst Q52.4
  - persistent Q5Ø.6
- **Gas** R14.3
  - asphyxiation, inhalation, poisoning, suffocation NEC —*see* Table of Drugs and Chemicals
  - excessive R14.Ø
  - gangrene A48.Ø
    - following
      - abortion —*see* Abortion by type complicated by infection
      - ectopic or molar pregnancy OØ8.Ø
  - on stomach R14.Ø
  - pains R14.1
- **Gastralgia** —*see also* Pain, abdominal
- **Gastrectasis** K31.Ø
  - psychogenic F45.8
- **Gastric** —*see* condition

Gastrinoma
- malignant
  - pancreas C25.4
  - specified site NEC —*see* Neoplasm, malignant, by site
  - unspecified site C25.4
- specified site —*see* Neoplasm, uncertain behavior
- unspecified site D37.9

Gastritis (simple) K29.7Ø
- with bleeding K29.71
- acute (erosive) K29.ØØ
  - with bleeding K29.Ø1
- alcoholic K29.2Ø
  - with bleeding K29.21
- allergic K29.6Ø
  - with bleeding K29.61
- atrophic (chronic) K29.4Ø
  - with bleeding K29.41
- chronic (antral) (fundal) K29.5Ø
  - with bleeding K29.51
  - atrophic K29.4Ø
    - with bleeding K29.41
  - superficial K29.3Ø
    - with bleeding K29.31
- dietary counseling and surveillance Z71.3
- due to diet deficiency E63.9
- eosinophilic K52.81
- giant hypertrophic K29.6Ø
  - with bleeding K29.61
- granulomatous K29.6Ø
  - with bleeding K29.61
- hypertrophic (mucosa) K29.6Ø
  - with bleeding K29.61
- nervous F54
- spastic K29.6Ø
  - with bleeding K29.61
- specified NEC K29.6Ø
  - with bleeding K29.61
- superficial chronic K29.3Ø
  - with bleeding K29.31
- tuberculous A18.83
- viral NEC AØ8.4

Gastrocarcinoma —*see* Neoplasm, malignant, stomach

Gastrocolic —*see* condition

Gastrodisciasis, gastrodiscoidiasis B66.8

Gastroduodenitis K29.9Ø
- with bleeding K29.91
- virus, viral AØ8.4
  - specified type NEC AØ8.39

Gastrodynia —*see* Pain, abdominal

Gastroenteritis (acute) (chronic) (noninfectious) (*see also* Enteritis) K52.9
- allergic K52.29 ⬅
  - with ◀
    - eosinophilic gastritis or gastroenteritis K52.81 ◀
    - food protein-induced enterocolitis syndrome K52.21 ◀
    - food protein-induced enteropathy K52.22 ◀
- dietetic —*see also* Gastroenteritis, allergic K52.29 ⬅
- drug-induced K52.1
- due to
  - Cryptosporidium AØ7.2
  - drugs K52.1
  - food poisoning —*see* Intoxication, foodborne
  - radiation K52.Ø
- eosinophilic K52.81
- epidemic (infectious) AØ9
- food hypersensitivity —*see also* Gastroenteritis, allergic K52.29 ⬅
- infectious —*see* Enteritis, infectious
- influenzal —*see* Influenza, with gastroenteritis
- noninfectious K52.9
  - specified NEC K52.89
- rotaviral AØ8.Ø

Gastroenteritis *(Continued)*
- Salmonella AØ2.Ø
- toxic K52.1
- viral NEC AØ8.4
  - acute infectious AØ8.39
    - type Norwalk AØ8.11
  - infantile (acute) AØ8.39
  - Norwalk agent AØ8.11
  - rotaviral AØ8.Ø
  - severe of infants AØ8.39
  - specified type NEC AØ8.39

Gastroenteropathy —*see also* Gastroenteritis K52.9
- acute, due to Norovirus AØ8.11
- acute, due to Norwalk agent AØ8.11
- infectious AØ9

Gastroenteroptosis K63.4

Gastroesophageal laceration-hemorrhage syndrome K22.6

Gastrointestinal —*see* condition

Gastrojejunal —*see* condition

Gastrojejunitis —*see also* Enteritis K52.9

Gastrojejunocolic —*see* condition

Gastroliths K31.89

Gastromalacia K31.89

Gastroparalysis K31.84
- diabetic —*see* Diabetes, gastroparalysis

Gastroparesis K31.84
- diabetic —*see* Diabetes, by type, with gastroparesis

Gastropathy K31.9
- congestive portal K31.89
- erythematous K29.7Ø
- exudative K9Ø.89
- portal hypertensive K31.89

Gastroptosis K31.89

Gastrorrhagia K92.2
- psychogenic F45.8

Gastroschisis (congenital) Q79.3

Gastrospasm (neurogenic) (reflex) K31.89
- neurotic F45.8
- psychogenic F45.8

Gastrostaxis —*see* Gastritis, with bleeding

Gastrostenosis K31.89

Gastrostomy
- attention to Z43.1
- status Z93.1

Gastrosuccorrhea (continuous) (intermittent) K31.89
- neurotic F45.8
- psychogenic F45.8

Gatophobia F4Ø.218

Gaucher's disease or splenomegaly (adult) (infantile) E75.22

Gee (-Herter)(-Thaysen) disease (nontropical sprue) K9Ø.Ø

Gélineau's syndrome G47.419
- with cataplexy G47.411

Gemination, tooth, teeth KØØ.2

Gemistocytoma
- specified site —*see* Neoplasm, malignant, by site
- unspecified site C71.9

General, generalized —*see* condition

Genetic
- carrier (status)
  - cystic fibrosis Z14.1
  - hemophilia A (asymptomatic) Z14.Ø1
    - symptomatic Z14.Ø2
  - specified NEC Z14.8
- susceptibility to disease NEC Z15.89
  - malignant neoplasm Z15.Ø9
    - breast Z15.Ø1
    - endometrium Z15.Ø4
    - ovary Z15.Ø2
    - prostate Z15.Ø3
    - specified NEC Z15.Ø9
  - multiple endocrine neoplasia Z15.81

Genital —*see* condition

Genito-anorectal syndrome A55

Genitourinary system —*see* condition

Genu
- congenital Q74.1
- extrorsum (acquired) —*see also* Deformity, varus, knee
  - congenital Q74.1
  - sequelae (late effect) of rickets E64.3
- introrsum (acquired) —*see also* Deformity, valgus, knee
  - congenital Q74.1
  - sequelae (late effect) of rickets E64.3
- rachitic (old) E64.3
- recurvatum (acquired) —*see also* Deformity, limb, specified type NEC, lower leg
  - congenital Q68.2
  - sequelae (late effect) of rickets E64.3
- valgum (acquired) (knock-knee) M21.Ø6-
  - congenital Q74.1
  - sequelae (late effect) of rickets E64.3
- varum (acquired) (bowleg) M21.16-
  - congenital Q74.1
  - sequelae (late effect) of rickets E64.3

Geographic tongue K14.1

Geophagia —*see* Pica

Geotrichosis B48.3
- stomatitis B48.3

Gephyrophobia F4Ø.242

Gerbode defect Q21.Ø

GERD (gastroesophageal reflux disease) K21.9

Gerhardt's
- disease (erythromelalgia) I73.81
- syndrome (vocal cord paralysis) J38.ØØ
  - bilateral J38.Ø2
  - unilateral J38.Ø1

German measles —*see also* Rubella
- exposure to Z2Ø.4

Germinoblastoma (diffuse) C85.9-
- follicular C82.9-

Germinoma —*see* Neoplasm, malignant, by site

Gerontoxon —*see* Degeneration, cornea, senile

Gerstmann-Sträussler-Scheinker syndrome (GSS) A81.82

Gerstmann's syndrome R48.8
- developmental F81.2

Gestation (period) —*see also* Pregnancy
- ectopic —*see* Pregnancy, by site
- multiple O3Ø.9-
  - greater than quadruplets —*see* Pregnancy, multiple (gestation), specified NEC
  - specified NEC —*see* Pregnancy, multiple (gestation), specified NEC

Gestational
- mammary abscess O91.11-
- purulent mastitis O91.11-
- subareolar abscess O91.11-

Ghon tubercle, primary infection A15.7

Ghost
- teeth KØØ.4
- vessels (cornea) H16.41-

Ghoul hand A66.3

Gianotti-Crosti disease L44.4

Giant
- cell
  - epulis KØ6.8
  - peripheral granuloma KØ6.8
- esophagus, congenital Q39.5
- kidney, congenital Q63.3
- urticaria T78.3
  - hereditary D84.1

Giardiasis AØ7.1

Gibert's disease or pityriasis L42

Giddiness R42
- hysterical F44.89
- psychogenic F45.8

Gierke's disease (glycogenosis I) E74.Ø1

Gigantism (cerebral) (hypophyseal) (pituitary) E22.Ø
- constitutional E34.4

Gilbert's disease or syndrome E8Ø.4

Gilchrist's disease B4Ø.9

Gilford-Hutchinson disease E34.8

G

◀ New ⬅ Revised ~~deleted~~ Deleted

- **Gilles de la Tourette's disease or syndrome** (motor-verbal tic) F95.2
- **Gingivitis** K05.10
  - acute (catarrhal) K05.00
    - necrotizing A69.1
    - nonplaque induced K05.01
    - plaque induced K05.00
  - chronic (desquamative) (hyperplastic) (simple marginal) (pregnancy associated) (ulcerative) K05.10
    - nonplaque induced K05.11
    - plaque induced K05.10
  - expulsiva —*see* Periodontitis
  - necrotizing ulcerative (acute) A69.1
  - pellagrous E52
    - acute necrotizing A69.1
  - Vincent's A69.1
- **Gingivoglossitis** K14.0
- **Gingivopericementitis** —*see* Periodontitis
- **Gingivosis** —*see* Gingivitis, chronic
- **Gingivostomatitis** K05.10
  - herpesviral B00.2
  - necrotizing ulcerative (acute) A69.1
- **Gland, glandular** —*see* condition
- **Glanders** A24.0
- **Glanzmann (-Naegeli) disease or thrombasthenia** D69.1
- **Glasgow coma scale**
  - total score
    - 3-8 R40.243
    - 9-12 R40.242
    - 13-15 R40.241
- **Glass-blower's disease** (cataract) —*see* Cataract, specified NEC
- **Glaucoma** H40.9
  - with
    - increased episcleral venous pressure H40.81-
    - pseudoexfoliation of lens —*see* Glaucoma, open angle, primary, capsular
  - absolute H44.51-
  - angle-closure (primary) H40.20-
    - acute (attack) (crisis) H40.21-
    - chronic H40.22-
    - intermittent H40.23-
    - residual stage H40.24-
  - borderline H40.00-
  - capsular (with pseudoexfoliation of lens) —*see* Glaucoma, open angle, primary, capsular
  - childhood Q15.0
  - closed angle —*see* Glaucoma, angle-closure
  - congenital Q15.0
  - corticosteroid-induced —*see* Glaucoma, secondary, drugs
  - hypersecretion H40.82-
  - in (due to)
    - amyloidosis E85.4 *[H42]*
    - aniridia Q13.1 *[H42]*
    - concussion of globe —*see* Glaucoma, secondary, trauma
    - dislocation of lens —*see* Glaucoma, secondary
    - disorder of lens NEC —*see* Glaucoma, secondary
    - drugs —*see* Glaucoma, secondary, drugs
    - endocrine disease NOS E34.9 *[H42]*
    - eye
      - inflammation —*see* Glaucoma, secondary, inflammation
      - trauma —*see* Glaucoma, secondary, trauma
    - hypermature cataract —*see* Glaucoma, secondary
    - iridocyclitis —*see* Glaucoma, secondary, inflammation
    - lens disorder —*see* Glaucoma, secondary,
    - Lowe's syndrome E72.03 *[H42]*
    - metabolic disease NOS E88.9 *[H42]*
    - ocular disorders NEC —*see* Glaucoma, secondary
- **Glaucoma** *(Continued)*
  - in (due to) *(Continued)*
    - onchocerciasis B73.02
    - pupillary block —*see* Glaucoma, secondary
    - retinal vein occlusion —*see* Glaucoma, secondary
    - Rieger's anomaly Q13.81 *[H42]*
    - rubeosis of iris —*see* Glaucoma, secondary
    - tumor of globe —*see* Glaucoma, secondary
  - infantile Q15.0
  - low tension —*see* Glaucoma, open angle, primary, low-tension
  - malignant H40.83-
  - narrow angle —*see* Glaucoma, angle-closure
  - newborn Q15.0
  - noncongestive (chronic) —*see* Glaucoma, open angle
  - nonobstructive —*see* Glaucoma, open angle
  - obstructive —*see also* Glaucoma, angle-closure
    - due to lens changes —*see* Glaucoma, secondary
  - open angle H40.10-
    - primary H40.11-
      - capsular (with pseudoexfoliation of lens) H40.14-
      - low-tension H40.12-
      - pigmentary H40.13-
      - residual stage H40.15-
  - phacolytic —*see* Glaucoma, secondary
  - pigmentary —*see* Glaucoma, open angle, primary, pigmentary
  - postinfectious —*see* Glaucoma, secondary, inflammation
  - secondary (to) H40.5-
    - drugs H40.6-
    - inflammation H40.4-
    - trauma H40.3-
  - simple (chronic) H40.11-
  - simplex H40.11-
  - specified type NEC H40.89
  - suspect H40.00-
  - syphilitic A52.71
  - traumatic —*see also* Glaucoma, secondary, trauma
    - newborn (birth injury) P15.3
  - tuberculous A18.59
- **Glaucomatous flecks** (subcapsular) —*see* Cataract, complicated
- **Glazed tongue** K14.4
- **Gleet** (gonococcal) A54.01
- **Glénard's disease** K63.4
- **Glioblastoma** (multiforme)
  - with sarcomatous component
    - specified site —*see* Neoplasm, malignant, by site
    - unspecified site C71.9
  - giant cell
    - specified site —*see* Neoplasm, malignant, by site
    - unspecified site C71.9
  - specified site —*see* Neoplasm, malignant, by site
  - unspecified site C71.9
- **Glioma** (malignant)
  - astrocytic
    - specified site —*see* Neoplasm, malignant, by site
    - unspecified site C71.9
  - mixed
    - specified site —*see* Neoplasm, malignant, by site
    - unspecified site C71.9
  - nose Q30.8
  - specified site NEC —*see* Neoplasm, malignant, by site
  - subependymal D43.2
    - specified site —*see* Neoplasm, uncertain behavior, by site
    - unspecified site D43.2
  - unspecified site C71.9
- **Gliomatosis cerebri** C71.0
- **Glioneuroma** —*see* Neoplasm, uncertain behavior, by site
- **Gliosarcoma**
  - specified site —*see* Neoplasm, malignant, by site
  - unspecified site C71.9
- **Gliosis** (cerebral) G93.89
  - spinal G95.89
- **Glisson's disease** —*see* Rickets
- **Globinuria** R82.3
- **Globus** (hystericus) F45.8
- **Glomangioma** D18.00
  - intra-abdominal D18.03
  - intracranial D18.02
  - skin D18.01
  - specified site NEC D18.09
- **Glomangiomyoma** D18.00
  - intra-abdominal D18.03
  - intracranial D18.02
  - skin D18.01
  - specified site NEC D18.09
- **Glomangiosarcoma** —*see* Neoplasm, connective tissue, malignant
- **Glomerular**
  - disease in syphilis A52.75
  - nephritis —*see* Glomerulonephritis
- **Glomerulitis** —*see* Glomerulonephritis
- **Glomerulonephritis** —*see also* Nephritis N05.9
  - with
    - edema —*see* Nephrosis
    - minimal change N05.0
    - minor glomerular abnormality N05.0
  - acute N00.9
  - chronic N03.9
  - crescentic (diffuse) NEC —*see also* N00-N07 with fourth character .7 N05.7
  - dense deposit —*see also* N00-N07 with fourth character .6 N05.6
  - diffuse
    - crescentic —*see also* N00-N07 with fourth character .7 N05.7
    - endocapillary proliferative —*see also* N00N07 with fourth character .4 N05.4
    - membranous —*see also* N00-N07 with fourth character .2 N05.2
    - mesangial proliferative —*see also* N00-N07 with fourth character .3 N05.3
    - mesangiocapillary —*see also* N00-N07 with fourth character .5 N05.5
    - sclerosing N05.8
  - endocapillary proliferative (diffuse) NEC —*see also* N00-N07 with fourth character .4 N05.4
  - extracapillary NEC —*see also* N00-N07 with fourth character .7 N05.7
  - focal (and segmental) —*see also* N00-N07 with fourth character .1 N05.1
  - hypocomplementemic —*see* Glomerulonephritis, membranoproliferative
  - IgA —*see* Nephropathy, IgA
  - immune complex (circulating) NEC N05.8
  - in (due to)
    - amyloidosis E85.4 *[N08]*
    - bilharziasis B65.9 *[N08]*
    - cryoglobulinemia D89.1 *[N08]*
    - defibrination syndrome D65 *[N08]*
    - diabetes mellitus —*see* Diabetes, glomerulosclerosis
    - disseminated intravascular coagulation D65 *[N08]*
    - Fabry (-Anderson) disease E75.21 *[N08]*
    - Goodpasture's syndrome M31.0
    - hemolytic-uremic syndrome D59.3
    - Henoch (-Schönlein) purpura D69.0 *[N08]*
    - lecithin cholesterol acyltransferase deficiency E78.6 *[N08]*

◄ New ⬅ Revised ~~deleted~~ Deleted

Glomerulonephritis *(Continued)*
in *(Continued)*
microscopic polyangiitis M31.7 *[N08]*
multiple myeloma C90.0- *[N08]*
Plasmodium malariae B52.0
schistosomiasis B65.9 *[N08]*
sepsis A41.9- *[N08]*
streptococcal A40- *[N08]*
sickle-cell disorders D57.- *[N08]*
strongyloidiasis B78.9 *[N08]*
subacute bacterial endocarditis I33.0 *[N08]*
syphilis (late) congenital A50.59 *[N08]*
systemic lupus erythematosus M32.14
thrombotic thrombocytopenic purpura M31.1 *[N08]*
typhoid fever A01.09
Waldenström macroglobulinemia C88.0 *[N08]*
Wegener's granulomatosis M31.31
latent or quiescent N03.9
lobular, lobulonodular —*see* Glomerulonephritis, membranoproliferative
membranoproliferative (diffuse) (type 1 or 3) —*see also* N00-N07 with fourth character .5 N05.5
dense deposit (type 2) NEC —*see also* N00-N07 with fourth character .6 N05.6
membranous (diffuse) NEC —*see also* N00-N07 with fourth character .2 N05.2
mesangial
IgA/IgG —*see* Nephropathy, IgA
proliferative (diffuse) NEC —*see also* N00-N07 with fourth character .3 N05.3
mesangiocapillary (diffuse) NEC —*see also* N00-N07 with fourth character .5 N05.5
necrotic, necrotizing NEC —*see also* N00-N07 with fourth character .8 N05.8
nodular —*see* Glomerulonephritis, membranoproliferative
poststreptococcal NEC N05.9
acute N00.9
chronic N03.9
rapidly progressive N01.9
proliferative NEC —*see also* N00-N07 with fourth character .8 N05.8
diffuse (lupus) M32.14
rapidly progressive N01.9
sclerosing, diffuse N05.8
specified pathology NEC —*see also* N00-N07 with fourth character .8 N05.8
subacute N01.9
Glomerulopathy —*see* Glomerulonephritis
Glomerulosclerosis —*see also* Sclerosis, renal
intercapillary (nodular) (with diabetes) —*see* Diabetes, glomerulosclerosis
intracapillary —*see* Diabetes, glomerulosclerosis
Glossagra K14.6
Glossalgia K14.6
Glossitis (chronic superficial) (gangrenous) (Moeller's) K14.0
areata exfoliativa K14.1
atrophic K14.4
benign migratory K14.1
cortical superficial, sclerotic K14.0
Hunter's D51.0
interstitial, sclerous K14.0
median rhomboid K14.2
pellagrous E52
superficial, chronic K14.0
Glossocele K14.8
Glossodynia K14.6
exfoliativa K14.4
Glossoncus K14.8
Glossopathy K14.9
Glossophytia K14.3
Glossoplegia K14.8
Glossoptosis K14.8
Glossopyrosis K14.6
Glossotrichia K14.3
Glossy skin L90.8
Glottis —*see* condition
Glottitis —*see also* Laryngitis J04.0
Glucagonoma
pancreas
benign D13.7
malignant C25.4
uncertain behavior D37.8
specified site NEC
benign —*see* Neoplasm, benign, by site
malignant —*see* Neoplasm, malignant, by site
uncertain behavior —*see* Neoplasm, uncertain behavior, by site
unspecified site
benign D13.7
malignant C25.4
uncertain behavior D37.8
Glucoglycinuria E72.51
Glucose-galactose malabsorption E74.39
Glue
ear —*see* Otitis, media, nonsuppurative, chronic, mucoid
sniffing (airplane) —*see* Abuse, drug, inhalant
dependence —*see* Dependence, drug, inhalant
Glutaric aciduria E72.3
Glycinemia E72.51
Glycinuria (renal) (with ketosis) E72.09
Glycogen
infiltration —*see* Disease, glycogen storage
storage disease —*see* Disease, glycogen storage
Glycogenosis (diffuse) (generalized) —*see also* Disease, glycogen storage
cardiac E74.02 *[I43]*
diabetic, secondary —*see* Diabetes, glycogenosis, secondary
pulmonary interstitial J84.842
Glycopenia E16.2
Glycosuria R81
renal E74.8
Gnathostoma spinigerum (infection) (infestation), **gnathostomiasis** (wandering swelling) B83.1
Goiter (plunging) (substernal) E04.9
with
hyperthyroidism (recurrent) —*see* Hyperthyroidism, with, goiter
thyrotoxicosis —*see* Hyperthyroidism, with, goiter
adenomatous —*see* Goiter, nodular
cancerous C73
congenital (nontoxic) E03.0
diffuse E03.0
parenchymatous E03.0
transitory, with normal functioning P72.0
cystic E04.2
due to iodine-deficiency E01.1
due to
enzyme defect in synthesis of thyroid hormone E07.1
iodine-deficiency (endemic) E01.2
dyshormonogenetic (familial) E07.1
endemic (iodine-deficiency) E01.2
diffuse E01.0
multinodular E01.1
exophthalmic —*see* Hyperthyroidism, with, goiter
iodine-deficiency (endemic) E01.2
diffuse E01.0
multinodular E01.1
nodular E01.1
lingual Q89.2
lymphadenoid E06.3
malignant C73
Goiter *(Continued)*
multinodular (cystic) (nontoxic) E04.2
toxic or with hyperthyroidism E05.20
with thyroid storm E05.21
neonatal NEC P72.0
nodular (nontoxic) (due to) E04.9
with
hyperthyroidism E05.20
with thyroid storm E05.21
thyrotoxicosis E05.20
with thyroid storm E05.21
endemic E01.1
iodine-deficiency E01.1
sporadic E04.9
toxic E05.20
with thyroid storm E05.21
nontoxic E04.9
diffuse (colloid) E04.0
multinodular E04.2
simple E04.0
specified NEC E04.8
uninodular E04.1
simple E04.0
toxic —*see* Hyperthyroidism, with, goiter
uninodular (nontoxic) E04.1
toxic or with hyperthyroidism E05.10
with thyroid storm E05.11
Goiter-deafness syndrome E07.1
Goldberg syndrome Q89.8
Goldberg-Maxwell syndrome E34.51
Goldblatt's hypertension or kidney I70.1
Goldenhar (-Gorlin) **syndrome** Q87.0
Goldflam-Erb disease or syndrome G70.00
with exacerbation (acute) G70.01
in crisis G70.01
Goldscheider's disease Q81.8
Goldstein's disease (familial hemorrhagic telangiectasia) I78.0
Golfer's elbow —*see* Epicondylitis, medial
Gonadoblastoma
specified site —*see* Neoplasm, uncertain behavior, by site
unspecified site
female D39.10
male D40.10
Gonecystitis —*see* Vesiculitis
Gongylonemiasis B83.8
Goniosynechiae —*see* Adhesions, iris, goniosynechiae
Gonococcemia A54.86
Gonococcus, gonococcal (disease) (infection) —*see also* condition A54.9
anus A54.6
bursa, bursitis A54.49
conjunctiva, conjunctivitis (neonatorum) A54.31
endocardium A54.83
eye A54.30
conjunctivitis A54.31
iridocyclitis A54.32
keratitis A54.33
newborn A54.31
other specified A54.39
fallopian tubes (acute) (chronic) A54.24
genitourinary (organ) (system) (tract) (acute)
lower A54.00
with abscess (accessory gland) (periurethral) A54.1
upper —*see also* condition A54.29
heart A54.83
iridocyclitis A54.32
joint A54.42
lymphatic (gland) (node) A54.89
meninges, meningitis A54.81
musculoskeletal A54.40
arthritis A54.42
osteomyelitis A54.43
other specified A54.49
spondylopathy A54.41
pelviperitonitis A54.24
pelvis (acute) (chronic) A54.24

- **Gonococcus, gonococcal** *(Continued)*
  - pharynx A54.5
  - proctitis A54.6
  - pyosalpinx (acute) (chronic) A54.24
  - rectum A54.6
  - skin A54.89
  - specified site NEC A54.89
  - tendon sheath A54.49
  - throat A54.5
  - urethra (acute) (chronic) A54.Ø1
    - with abscess (accessory gland) (periurethral) A54.1
  - vulva (acute) (chronic) A54.Ø2
- **Gonocytoma**
  - specified site —*see* Neoplasm, uncertain behavior, by site
  - unspecified site
    - female D39.1Ø
    - male D4Ø.1Ø
- **Gonorrhea** (acute) (chronic) A54.9
  - Bartholin's gland (acute) (chronic) (purulent) A54.Ø2
    - with abscess (accessory gland) (periurethral) A54.1
  - bladder A54.Ø1
  - cervix A54.Ø3
  - conjunctiva, conjunctivitis (neonatorum) A54.31
  - contact Z2Ø.2
  - Cowper's gland (with abscess) A54.1
  - exposure to Z2Ø.2
  - fallopian tube (acute) (chronic) A54.24
  - kidney (acute) (chronic) A54.21
  - lower genitourinary tract A54.ØØ
    - with abscess (accessory gland) (periurethral) A54.1
  - ovary (acute) (chronic) A54.24
  - pelvis (acute) (chronic) A54.24
    - female pelvic inflammatory disease A54.24
  - penis A54.Ø9
  - prostate (acute) (chronic) A54.22
  - seminal vesicle (acute) (chronic) A54.23
  - specified site not listed —*see also* Gonococcus A54.89
  - spermatic cord (acute) (chronic) A54.23
  - urethra A54.Ø1
    - with abscess (accessory gland) (periurethral) A54.1
  - vagina A54.Ø2
  - vas deferens (acute) (chronic) A54.23
  - vulva A54.Ø2
- **Goodall's disease** AØ8.19
- **Goodpasture's syndrome** M31.Ø
- **Gopalan's syndrome** (burning feet) E53.Ø
- **Gorlin-Chaudry-Moss syndrome** Q87.Ø
- **Gottron's papules** L94.4
- **Gougerot's syndrome** (trisymptomatic) L81.7
- **Gougerot-Blum syndrome** (pigmented purpuric lichenoid dermatitis) L81.7
- **Gougerot-Carteaud disease or syndrome** (confluent reticulate papillomatosis) L83
- **Gouley's syndrome** (constrictive pericarditis) I31.1
- **Goundou** A66.6
- **Gout, chronic** (*see also* Gout, gouty) M1A.9-
  - drug-induced M1A.2Ø
    - ankle M1A.27-
    - elbow M1A.22-
    - foot joint M1A.27-
    - hand joint M1A.24-
    - hip M1A.25-
    - knee M1A.26-
    - multiple site M1A.29-
    - shoulder M1A.21-
    - vertebrae M1A.28
    - wrist M1A.23-
  - idiopathic M1A.ØØ
    - ankle M1A.Ø7-
    - elbow M1A.Ø2-
    - foot joint M1A.Ø7-
    - hand joint M1A.Ø4-
- **Gout, chronic** *(Continued)*
  - idiopathic *(Continued)*
    - hip M1A.Ø5-
    - knee M1A.Ø6-
    - multiple site M1A.Ø9
    - shoulder M1A.Ø1-
    - vertebrae M1A.Ø8
    - wrist M1A.Ø3-
  - in (due to) renal impairment M1A.3Ø
    - ankle M1A.37-
    - elbow M1A.32-
    - foot joint M1A.37-
    - hand joint M1A.34-
    - hip M1A.35-
    - knee M1A.36-
    - multiple site M1A.39
    - shoulder M1A.31-
    - vertebrae M1A.38
    - wrist M1A.33-
  - lead-induced M1A.1Ø
    - ankle M1A.17-
    - elbow M1A.12-
    - foot joint M1A.17-
    - hand joint M1A.14-
    - hip M1A.15-
    - knee M1A.16-
    - multiple site M1A.19
    - shoulder M1A.11-
    - vertebrae M1A.18
    - wrist M1A.13-
  - primary —*see* Gout, chronic, idiopathic
  - saturnine —*see* Gout, chronic, lead-induced
  - secondary NEC M1A.4Ø
    - ankle M1A.47-
    - elbow M1A.42-
    - foot joint M1A.47-
    - hand joint M1A.44-
    - hip M1A.45-
    - knee M1A.46-
    - multiple site M1A.49
    - shoulder M1A.41-
    - vertebrae M1A.48
    - wrist M1A.43-
  - syphilitic —*see also* subcategory M14.8- A52.77
  - tophi M1A.9
- **Gout, gouty** (acute) (attack) (flare) —*see also* Gout, chronic M1Ø.9-
  - drug-induced M1Ø.2Ø
    - ankle M1Ø.27-
    - elbow M1Ø.22-
    - foot joint M1Ø.27-
    - hand joint M1Ø.24-
    - hip M1Ø.25-
    - knee M1Ø.26-
    - multiple site M1Ø.29
    - shoulder M1Ø.21-
    - vertebrae M1Ø.28
    - wrist M1Ø.23-
  - idiopathic M1Ø.ØØ
    - ankle M1Ø.Ø7-
    - elbow M1Ø.Ø2-
    - foot joint M1Ø.Ø7-
    - hand joint M1Ø.Ø4-
    - hip M1Ø.Ø5-
    - knee M1Ø.Ø6-
    - multiple site M1Ø.Ø9
    - shoulder M1Ø.Ø1-
    - vertebrae M1Ø.Ø8
    - wrist M1Ø.Ø3-
  - in (due to) renal impairment M1Ø.3Ø
    - ankle M1Ø.37-
    - elbow M1Ø.32-
    - foot joint M1Ø.37-
    - hand joint M1Ø.34-
    - hip M1Ø.35-
    - knee M1Ø.36-
    - multiple site M1Ø.39
    - shoulder M1Ø.31-
    - vertebrae M1Ø.38
    - wrist M1Ø.33-
- **Gout, gouty** *(Continued)*
  - lead-induced M1Ø.1Ø
    - ankle M1Ø.17-
    - elbow M1Ø.12-
    - foot joint M1Ø.17-
    - hand joint M1Ø.14-
    - hip M1Ø.15-
    - knee M1Ø.16-
    - multiple site M1Ø.19
    - shoulder M1Ø.11-
    - vertebrae M1Ø.18
    - wrist M1Ø.13-
  - primary —*see* Gout, idiopathic
  - saturnine —*see* Gout, lead-induced
  - secondary NEC M1Ø.4Ø
    - ankle M1Ø.47-
    - elbow M1Ø.42-
    - foot joint M1Ø.47-
    - hand joint M1Ø.44-
    - hip M1Ø.45-
    - knee M1Ø.46-
    - multiple site M1Ø.49
    - shoulder M1Ø.41-
    - vertebrae M1Ø.48
    - wrist M1Ø.43-
  - syphilitic —*see also* subcategory M14.8- A52.77
  - tophi NEC —*see* Gout, chronic
- **Gower's**
  - muscular dystrophy G71.Ø
  - syndrome (vasovagal attack) R55
- **Gradenigo's syndrome** —*see* Otitis, media, suppurative, acute
- **Graefe's disease** —*see* Strabismus, paralytic, ophthalmoplegia, progressive
- **Graft-versus-host disease** D89.813
  - acute D89.81Ø
  - acute on chronic D89.812
  - chronic D89.811
- **Grain mite** (itch) B88.Ø
- **Grainhandler's disease or lung** J67.8
- **Grand mal** —*see* Epilepsy, generalized, specified NEC
- **Grand multipara status only** (not pregnant) Z64.1
  - pregnant —*see* Pregnancy, complicated by, grand multiparity
- **Granite worker's lung** J62.8
- **Granular** —*see also* condition
  - inflammation, pharynx J31.2
  - kidney (contracting) —*see* Sclerosis, renal
  - liver K74.69
- **Granulation tissue** (abnormal) (excessive) L92.9
  - postmastoidectomy cavity —*see* Complications, postmastoidectomy, granulation
- **Granulocytopenia** (primary) (malignant) —*see* Agranulocytosis
- **Granuloma** L92.9
  - abdomen K66.8
    - from residual foreign body L92.3
    - pyogenicum L98.Ø
  - actinic L57.5
  - annulare (perforating) L92.Ø
  - apical KØ4.5
  - aural —*see* Otitis, externa, specified NEC
  - beryllium (skin) L92.3
  - bone
    - eosinophilic C96.6
    - from residual foreign body —*see* Osteomyelitis, specified type NEC
    - lung C96.6
  - brain (any site) GØ6.Ø
    - schistosomiasis B65.9 *[GØ7]*
  - canaliculus lacrimalis —*see* Granuloma, lacrimal
  - candidal (cutaneous) B37.2
  - cerebral (any site) GØ6.Ø
  - coccidioidal (primary) (progressive) B38.7
    - lung B38.1
    - meninges B38.4

◀ New ◀━ Revised ~~deleted~~ Deleted

Granuloma *(Continued)*
- colon K63.89
- conjunctiva H11.22-
- dental KØ4.5
- ear, middle —*see* Cholesteatoma
- eosinophilic C96.6
  - bone C96.6
  - lung C96.6
  - oral mucosa K13.4
  - skin L92.2
- eyelid HØ1.8
- facial (e) L92.2
- foreign body (in soft tissue) NEC M6Ø.2Ø
  - ankle M6Ø.27-
  - foot M6Ø.27-
  - forearm M6Ø.23-
  - hand M6Ø.24-
  - in operation wound —*see* Foreign body, accidentally left during a procedure
  - lower leg M6Ø.26-
  - pelvic region M6Ø.25-
  - shoulder region M6Ø.21-
  - skin L92.3
  - specified site NEC M6Ø.28
  - subcutaneous tissue L92.3
  - thigh M6Ø.25-
  - upper arm M6Ø.22-
- gangraenescens M31.2
- genito-inguinale A58
- giant cell (central) (reparative) (jaw) M27.1
  - gingiva (peripheral) KØ6.8
- gland (lymph) I88.8
- hepatic NEC K75.3
  - in (due to)
    - berylliosis J63.2 *[K77]*
    - sarcoidosis D86.89
- Hodgkin C81.9
- ileum K63.89
- infectious B99.9
  - specified NEC B99.8
- inguinale (Donovan) (venereal) A58
- intestine NEC K63.89
- intracranial (any site) GØ6.Ø
- intraspinal (any part) GØ6.1
- iridocyclitis —*see* Iridocyclitis, chronic
- jaw (bone) (central) M27.1
  - reparative giant cell M27.1
- kidney —*see also* Infection, kidney N15.8
- lacrimal HØ4.81-
- larynx J38.7
- lethal midline (faciale (e)) M31.2
- liver NEC —*see* Granuloma, hepatic
- lung (infectious) —*see also* Fibrosis, lung
  - coccidioidal B38.1
  - eosinophilic C96.6
- Majocchi's B35.8
- malignant (facial (e)) M31.2
- mandible (central) M27.1
- midline (lethal) M31.2
- monilial (cutaneous) B37.2
- nasal sinus —*see* Sinusitis
- operation wound T81.89
  - foreign body —*see* Foreign body, accidentally left during a procedure
  - stitch T81.89
  - talc —*see* Foreign body, accidentally left during a procedure
- oral mucosa K13.4
- orbit, orbital HØ5.11-
- paracoccidioidal B41.8
- penis, venereal A58
- periapical KØ4.5
- peritoneum K66.8
  - due to ova of helminths NOS —*see also* Helminthiasis B83.9 *[K67]*
- postmastoidectomy cavity —*see* Complications, postmastoidectomy, recurrent cholesteatoma
- prostate N42.89
- pudendi (ulcerating) A58
- pulp, internal (tooth) KØ3.3

Granuloma *(Continued)*
- pyogenic, pyogenicum (of) (skin) L98.Ø
  - gingiva KØ6.8
  - maxillary alveolar ridge KØ4.5
  - oral mucosa K13.4
- rectum K62.89
- reticulohistiocytic D76.3
- rubrum nasi L74.8
- Schistosoma —*see* Schistosomiasis
- septic (skin) L98.Ø
- silica (skin) L92.3
- sinus (accessory) (infective) (nasal) —*see* Sinusitis
- skin L92.9
  - from residual foreign body L92.3
  - pyogenicum L98.Ø
- spine
  - syphilitic (epidural) A52.19
  - tuberculous A18.Ø1
- stitch (postoperative) T81.89
- suppurative (skin) L98.Ø
- swimming pool A31.1
- talc —*see also* Granuloma, foreign body
  - in operation wound —*see* Foreign body, accidentally left during a procedure
- telangiectaticum (skin) L98.Ø
- tracheostomy J95.Ø9
- trichophyticum B35.8
- tropicum A66.4
- umbilicus L92.9
- urethra N36.8
- uveitis —*see* Iridocyclitis, chronic
- vagina A58
- venereum A58
- vocal cord J38.3

Granulomatosis L92.9
- lymphoid C83.8-
- miliary (listerial) A32.89
- necrotizing, respiratory M31.3Ø
- progressive septic D71
- specified NEC L92.8
- Wegener's M31.3Ø
  - with renal involvement M31.31

Granulomatous tissue (abnormal) (excessive) L92.9
Granulosis rubra nasi L74.8
Graphite fibrosis (of lung) J63.3
Graphospasm F48.8
- organic G25.89

Grating scapula M89.8X1
Gravel (urinary) —*see* Calculus, urinary
Graves' disease —*see* Hyperthyroidism, with, goiter
Gravis —*see* condition
Grawitz tumor C64.-
Gray syndrome (newborn) P93.Ø
Grayness, hair (premature) L67.1
- congenital Q84.2

Green sickness D5Ø.8
Greenfield's disease
- meaning
  - concentric sclerosis (encephalitis periaxialis concentrica) G37.5
  - metachromatic leukodystrophy E75.25

Greenstick fracture - code as Fracture, by site
Grey syndrome (newborn) P93.Ø
Grief F43.21
- prolonged F43.29
- reaction —*see also* Disorder, adjustment F43.2Ø

Griesinger's disease B76.9
Grinder's lung or pneumoconiosis J62.8
Grinding, teeth
- psychogenic F45.8
- sleep related G47.63

Grip
- Dabney's B33.Ø
- devil's B33.Ø

Grippe, grippal —*see also* Influenza
- Balkan A78
- summer, of Italy A93.1

Grisel's disease M43.6
Groin —*see* condition
Grooved tongue K14.5
Ground itch B76.9
Grover's disease or syndrome L11.1
Growing pains, children R29.898
Growth (fungoid) (neoplastic) (new) —*see also* Neoplasm
- adenoid (vegetative) J35.8
- benign —*see* Neoplasm, benign, by site
- malignant —*see* Neoplasm, malignant, by site
- rapid, childhood ZØØ.2
- secondary —*see* Neoplasm, secondary, by site

Gruby's disease B35.Ø
Gubler-Millard paralysis or syndrome G46.3
Guerin-Stern syndrome Q74.3
Guidance, insufficient anterior (occlusal) M26.54
Guillain-Barré disease or syndrome G61.Ø
- sequelae G65.Ø

Guinea worms (infection) (infestation) B72
Guinon's disease (motor-verbal tic) F95.2
Gull's disease EØ3.4
Gum —*see* condition
Gumboil KØ4.7
- with sinus KØ4.6

Gumma (syphilitic) A52.79
- artery A52.Ø9
  - cerebral A52.Ø4
- bone A52.77
  - of yaws (late) A66.6
- brain A52.19
- cauda equina A52.19
- central nervous system A52.3
- ciliary body A52.71
- congenital A5Ø.59
- eyelid A52.71
- heart A52.Ø6
- intracranial A52.19
- iris A52.71
- kidney A52.75
- larynx A52.73
- leptomeninges A52.19
- liver A52.74
- meninges A52.19
- myocardium A52.Ø6
- nasopharynx A52.73
- neurosyphilitic A52.3
- nose A52.73
- orbit A52.71
- palate (soft) A52.79
- penis A52.76
- pericardium A52.Ø6
- pharynx A52.73
- pituitary A52.79
- scrofulous (tuberculous) A18.4
- skin A52.79
- specified site NEC A52.79
- spinal cord A52.19
- tongue A52.79
- tonsil A52.73
- trachea A52.73
- tuberculous A18.4
- ulcerative due to yaws A66.4
- ureter A52.75
- yaws A66.4
  - bone A66.6

Gunn's syndrome QØ7.8
Gunshot wound —*see also* Wound, open
- fracture - code as Fracture, by site
- internal organs —*see* Injury, by site

Gynandrism Q56.Ø
Gynandroblastoma
- specified site —*see* Neoplasm, uncertain behavior, by site
- unspecified site
  - female D39.1Ø
  - male D4Ø.1Ø

Gynecological examination (periodic) (routine) ZØ1.419
- with abnormal findings ZØ1.411

Gynecomastia N62
Gynephobia F4Ø.291
Gyrate scalp Q82.8

H

H (Hartnup's) disease E72.Ø2
Haas' disease or osteochondrosis (juvenile) (head of humerus) —*see* Osteochondrosis, juvenile, humerus
Habit, habituation
  bad sleep Z72.821
  chorea F95.8
  disturbance, child F98.9
  drug —*see* Dependence, drug
  irregular sleep Z72.821
  laxative F55.2
  spasm —*see* Tic
  tic —*see* Tic
Haemophilus (H.) influenzae, as cause of disease classified elsewhere B96.3
Haff disease —*see* Poisoning, mercury
Hageman's factor defect, deficiency or disease D68.2
Haglund's disease or osteochondrosis (juvenile) (os tibiale externum) —*see* Osteochondrosis, juvenile, tarsus
Hailey-Hailey disease Q82.8
Hair —*see also* condition
  plucking F63.3
    in stereotyped movement disorder F98.4
  tourniquet syndrome —*see also* Constriction, external, by site
    finger S6Ø.44-
    penis S3Ø.842
    thumb S6Ø.34-
    toe S9Ø.44-
Hairball in stomach T18.2
Hair-pulling, pathological (compulsive) F63.3
Hairy black tongue K14.3
Half vertebra Q76.49
Halitosis R19.6
Hallerman-Streiff syndrome Q87.Ø
Hallervorden-Spatz disease G23.Ø
Hallopeau's acrodermatitis or disease L4Ø.2
Hallucination R44.3
  auditory R44.Ø
  gustatory R44.2
  olfactory R44.2
  specified NEC R44.2
  tactile R44.2
  visual R44.1
Hallucinosis (chronic) F28
  alcoholic (acute) F1Ø.951
    in
      abuse F1Ø.151
      dependence F1Ø.251
  drug-induced F19.951
    cannabis F12.951
    cocaine F14.951
    hallucinogen F16.151
    in
      abuse F19.151
        cannabis F12.151
        cocaine F14.151
        hallucinogen F16.151
        inhalant F18.151
        opioid F11.151
        sedative, anxiolytic or hypnotic F13.151
        stimulant NEC F15.151
      dependence F19.251
        cannabis F12.251
        cocaine F14.251
        hallucinogen F16.251
        inhalant F18.251
        opioid F11.251
        sedative, anxiolytic or hypnotic F13.251
        stimulant NEC F15.251
    inhalant F18.951
    opioid F11.951
    sedative, anxiolytic or hypnotic F13.951
    stimulant NEC F15.951
  organic FØ6.Ø
Hallux
  deformity (acquired) NEC M2Ø.5X-
  limitus M2Ø.5X-
  malleus (acquired) NEC M2Ø.3-
  rigidus (acquired) M2Ø.2-
    congenital Q74.2
    sequelae (late effect) of rickets E64.3
  valgus (acquired) M2Ø.1-
    congenital Q66.6
  varus (acquired) M2Ø.3-
    congenital Q66.3
Halo, visual H53.19
Hamartoma, hamartoblastoma Q85.9
  epithelial (gingival), odontogenic, central or peripheral —*see* Cyst, calcifying odontogenic
Hamartosis Q85.9
Hamman-Rich syndrome J84.114
Hammer toe (acquired) **NEC** —*see also* Deformity, toe, hammer toe
  congenital Q66.89
  sequelae (late effect) of rickets E64.3
Hand —*see* condition
Hand-foot syndrome L27.1
Handicap, handicapped
  educational Z55.9
    specified NEC Z55.8
Hand-Schüller-Christian disease or syndrome C96.5
Hanging (asphyxia) (strangulation) (suffocation) —*see* Asphyxia, traumatic, due to mechanical threat
Hangnail —*see also* Cellulitis, digit
  with lymphangitis —*see* Lymphangitis, acute, digit
Hangover (alcohol) F1Ø.129
Hanhart's syndrome Q87.Ø
Hanot-Chauffard (-Troisier) **syndrome** E83.19
Hanot's cirrhosis or disease K74.3
Hansen's disease —*see* Leprosy
Hantaan virus disease (Korean hemorrhagic fever) A98.5
Hantavirus disease (with renal manifestations) (Dobrava) (Puumala) (Seoul) A98.5
  with pulmonary manifestations (Andes) (Bayou) (Bermejo) (Black Creek Canal) (Choclo) (Juquitiba) (Laguna negra) (Lechiguanas) (New York) (Oran) (Sin nombre) B33.4
Happy puppet syndrome Q93.5
Harada's disease or syndrome H3Ø.81-
Hardening
  artery —*see* Arteriosclerosis
  brain G93.89
Harelip (complete) (incomplete) —*see* Cleft, lip
Harlequin (newborn) Q8Ø.4
Harley's disease D59.6
Harmful use (of)
  alcohol F1Ø.1Ø
  anxiolytics —*see* Abuse, drug, sedative
  cannabinoids —*see* Abuse, drug, cannabis
  cocaine —*see* Abuse, drug, cocaine
  drug —*see* Abuse, drug
  hallucinogens —*see* Abuse, drug, hallucinogen
  hypnotics —*see* Abuse, drug, sedative -
    opioids —*see* Abuse, drug, opioid
  PCP (phencyclidine) —*see* Abuse, drug, hallucinogen
  sedatives —*see* Abuse, drug, sedative
  stimulants NEC —*see* Abuse, drug, stimulant
Harris' lines —*see* Arrest, epiphyseal
Hartnup's disease E72.Ø2
Harvester's lung J67.Ø
Harvesting ovum for in vitro fertilization Z31.83
Hashimoto's disease or thyroiditis EØ6.3
Hashitoxicosis (transient) EØ6.3
Hassal-Henle bodies or warts (cornea) H18.49
Haut mal —*see* Epilepsy, generalized, specified NEC
Haverhill fever A25.1
Hay fever —*see also* Fever, hay J3Ø.1
Hayem-Widal syndrome D59.8
Haygarth's nodes M15.8
Haymaker's lung J67.Ø
Hb (abnormal)
  Bart's disease D56.Ø
  disease —*see* Disease, hemoglobin
  trait —*see* Trait
Head —*see* condition
Headache R51
  allergic NEC G44.89
  associated with sexual activity G44.82
  chronic daily R51
  cluster G44.ØØ9
    chronic G44.Ø29
      intractable G44.Ø21
      not intractable G44.Ø29
    episodic G44.Ø19
      intractable G44.Ø11
      not intractable G44.Ø19
    intractable G44.ØØ1
    not intractable G44.ØØ9
  cough (primary) G44.83
  daily chronic R51
  drug-induced NEC G44.4Ø
    intractable G44.41
    not intractable G44.4Ø
  exertional (primary) G44.84
  histamine G44.ØØ9
    intractable G44.ØØ1
    not intractable G44.ØØ9
  hypnic G44.81
  lumbar puncture G97.1
  medication overuse G44.4Ø
    intractable G44.41
    not intractable G44.4Ø
  menstrual —*see* Migraine, menstrual
  migraine (type) —*see also* Migraine G43.9Ø9
  nasal septum R51
  neuralgiform, short lasting unilateral, with conjunctival injection and tearing (SUNCT) G44.Ø59
    intractable G44.Ø51
    not intractable G44.Ø59
  new daily persistent (NDPH) G44.52
  orgasmic G44.82
  periodic syndromes in adults and children G43.CØ
    with refractory migraine G43.C1
    intractable G43.C1
    not intractable G43.CØ
    without refractory migraine G43.CØ
  postspinal puncture G97.1
  post-traumatic G44.3Ø9
    acute G44.319
      intractable G44.311
      not intractable G44.319
    chronic G44.329
      intractable G44.321
      not intractable G44.329
    intractable G44.3Ø1
    not intractable G44.3Ø9
  pre-menstrual —*see* Migraine, menstrual
  preorgasmic G44.82
  primary
    cough G44.83
    exertional G44.84
    stabbing G44.85
    thunderclap G44.53
  rebound G44.4Ø
    intractable G44.41
    not intractable G44.4Ø
  short lasting unilateral neuralgiform, with conjunctival injection and tearing (SUNCT) G44.Ø59
    intractable G44.Ø51
    not intractable G44.Ø59
  specified syndrome NEC G44.89

- **Headache** *(Continued)*
  - spinal and epidural anesthesia - induced T88.59
    - in labor and delivery O74.5
    - in pregnancy O29.4-
    - postpartum, puerperal O89.4
  - spinal fluid loss (from puncture) G97.1
  - stabbing (primary) G44.85
  - tension (-type) G44.2Ø9
    - chronic G44.229
      - intractable G44.221
      - not intractable G44.229
    - episodic G44.219
      - intractable G44.211
      - not intractable G44.219
    - intractable G44.2Ø1
    - not intractable G44.2Ø9
  - thunderclap (primary) G44.53
  - vascular NEC G44.1
- **Healthy**
  - infant
    - accompanying sick mother Z76.3
    - receiving care Z76.2
  - person accompanying sick person Z76.3
- **Hearing examination** ZØ1.1Ø
  - with abnormal findings NEC ZØ1.118
  - following failed hearing screening ZØ1.11Ø
  - for hearing conservation and treatment ZØ1.12
- **Heart** —*see* condition
- **Heart beat**
  - abnormality RØØ.9
    - specified NEC RØØ.8
  - awareness RØØ.2
  - rapid RØØ.Ø
  - slow RØØ.1
- **Heartburn** R12
  - psychogenic F45.8
- **Heat** (effects) T67.9
  - apoplexy T67.Ø
  - burn —*see also* Burn L55.9
  - collapse T67.1
  - cramps T67.2
  - dermatitis or eczema L59.Ø
  - edema T67.7
  - erythema - code by site under Burn, first degree
  - excessive T67.9
    - specified effect NEC T67.8
  - exhaustion T67.5
    - anhydrotic T67.3
    - due to
      - salt (and water) depletion T67.4
      - water depletion T67.3
        - with salt depletion T67.4
  - fatigue (transient) T67.6
  - fever T67.Ø
  - hyperpyrexia T67.Ø
  - prickly L74.Ø
  - prostration —*see* Heat, exhaustion
  - pyrexia T67.Ø
  - rash L74.Ø
  - specified effect NEC T67.8
  - stroke T67.Ø
  - sunburn —*see* Sunburn
  - syncope T67.1
- **Heavy-for-dates NEC** (infant) (4ØØØg to 4499g) PØ8.1
  - exceptionally (45ØØg or more) PØ8.Ø
- **Hebephrenia, hebephrenic** (schizophrenia) F2Ø.1
- **Heberden's disease or nodes** (with arthropathy) M15.1
- **Hebra's**
  - pityriasis L26
  - prurigo L28.2
- **Heel** —*see* condition
- **Heerfordt's disease** D86.89
- **Hegglin's anomaly or syndrome** D72.Ø
- **Heilmeyer-Schoner disease** D45
- **Heine-Medin disease** A8Ø.9
- **Heinz body anemia, congenital** D58.2
- **Heliophobia** F4Ø.228
- **Heller's disease or syndrome** F84.3
- **HELLP syndrome** (hemolysis, elevated liver enzymes and low platelet count) O14.2-
  - complicating ◀
    - childbirth O14.24 ◀
    - puerperium O14.25 ◀
- **Helminthiasis** —*see also* Infestation, helminth
  - Ancylostoma B76.Ø
  - intestinal B82.Ø
    - mixed types (types classifiable to more than one of the titles B65.Ø-B81.3 and B81.8) B81.4
    - specified type NEC B81.8
  - mixed types (intestinal) (types classifiable to more than one of the titles B65.Ø-B81.3 and B81.8) B81.4
  - Necator (americanus) B76.1
  - specified type NEC B83.8
- **Heloma** L84
- **Hemangioblastoma** —*see* Neoplasm, connective tissue, uncertain behavior
  - malignant —*see* Neoplasm, connective tissue, malignant
- **Hemangioendothelioma** —*see also* Neoplasm, uncertain behavior, by site
  - benign D18.ØØ
    - intra-abdominal D18.Ø3
    - intracranial D18.Ø2
    - skin D18.Ø1
    - specified site NEC D18.Ø9
  - bone (diffuse) —*see* Neoplasm, bone, malignant
  - epithelioid —*see also* Neoplasm, uncertain behavior, by site
    - malignant —*see* Neoplasm, malignant, by site
  - malignant —*see* Neoplasm, connective tissue, malignant
- **Hemangiofibroma** —*see* Neoplasm, benign, by site
- **Hemangiolipoma** —*see* Lipoma
- **Hemangioma** D18.ØØ
  - arteriovenous D18.ØØ
    - intra-abdominal D18.Ø3
    - intracranial D18.Ø2
    - skin D18.Ø1
    - specified site NEC D18.Ø9
  - capillary D18.ØØ
    - intra-abdominal D18.Ø3
    - intracranial D18.Ø2
    - skin D18.Ø1
    - specified site NEC D18.Ø9
  - cavernous D18.ØØ
    - intra-abdominal D18.Ø3
    - intracranial D18.Ø2
    - skin D18.Ø1
    - specified site NEC D18.Ø9
  - epithelioid D18.ØØ
    - intra-abdominal D18.Ø3
    - intracranial D18.Ø2
    - skin D18.Ø1
    - specified site NEC D18.Ø9
  - histiocytoid D18.ØØ
    - intra-abdominal D18.Ø3
    - intracranial D18.Ø2
    - skin D18.Ø1
    - specified site NEC D18.Ø9
  - infantile D18.ØØ
    - intra-abdominal D18.Ø3
    - intracranial D18.Ø2
    - skin D18.Ø1
    - specified site NEC D18.Ø9
  - intra-abdominal D18.Ø3
  - intracranial D18.Ø2
  - intramuscular D18.ØØ
    - intra-abdominal D18.Ø3
    - intracranial D18.Ø2
    - skin D18.Ø1
    - specified site NEC D18.Ø9
- **Hemangioma** *(Continued)*
  - intrathoracic structures D18.Ø9 ◀
  - juvenile D18.ØØ
  - malignant —*see* Neoplasm, connective tissue, malignant
  - plexiform D18.ØØ
    - intra-abdominal D18.Ø3
    - intracranial D18.Ø2
    - skin D18.Ø1
    - specified site NEC D18.Ø9
  - racemose D18.ØØ
    - intra-abdominal D18.Ø3
    - intracranial D18.Ø2
    - skin D18.Ø1
    - specified site NEC D18.Ø9
  - sclerosing —*see* Neoplasm, skin, benign
  - simplex D18.ØØ
    - intra-abdominal D18.Ø3
    - intracranial D18.Ø2
    - skin D18.Ø1
    - specified site NEC D18.Ø9
  - skin D18.Ø1
  - specified site NEC D18.Ø9
  - venous D18.ØØ
    - intra-abdominal D18.Ø3
    - intracranial D18.Ø2
    - skin D18.Ø1
    - specified site NEC D18.Ø9
  - verrucous keratotic D18.ØØ
    - intra-abdominal D18.Ø3
    - intracranial D18.Ø2
    - skin D18.Ø1
    - specified site NEC D18.Ø9
- **Hemangiomatosis** (systemic) I78.8
  - involving single site —*see* Hemangioma
- **Hemangiopericytoma** —*see also* Neoplasm, connective tissue, uncertain behavior
  - benign —*see* Neoplasm, connective tissue, benign
  - malignant —*see* Neoplasm, connective tissue, malignant
- **Hemangiosarcoma** —*see* Neoplasm, connective tissue, malignant
- **Hemarthrosis** (nontraumatic) M25.ØØ
  - ankle M25.Ø7-
  - elbow M25.Ø2-
  - foot joint M25.Ø7-
  - hand joint M25.Ø4-
  - hip M25.Ø5-
  - in hemophilic arthropathy —*see* Arthropathy, hemophilic
  - knee M25.Ø6-
  - shoulder M25.Ø1-
  - specified joint NEC M25.Ø8
  - traumatic —*see* Sprain, by site
  - vertebrae M25.Ø8
  - wrist M25.Ø3-
- **Hematemesis** K92.Ø
  - with ulcer - code by site under Ulcer, with hemorrhage K27.4
  - newborn, neonatal P54.Ø
    - due to swallowed maternal blood P78.2
- **Hematidrosis** L74.8
- **Hematinuria** —*see also* Hemoglobinuria
  - malarial B5Ø.8
- **Hematobilia** K83.8
- **Hematocele**
  - female NEC N94.89
    - with ectopic pregnancy OØØ.9Ø ⇐
      - with intrauterine pregnancy OØØ.91 ◀
    - ovary N83.8
  - male N5Ø.1
- **Hematochezia** —*see also* Melena K92.1
- **Hematochyluria** —*see also* Infestation, filarial
  - schistosomiasis (bilharziasis) B65.Ø
- **Hematocolpos** (with hematometra or hematosalpinx) N89.7
- **Hematocornea** —*see* Pigmentation, cornea, stromal
- **Hematogenous** —*see* condition

Hematoma (traumatic) (skin surface intact) — *see also* Contusion
  with
    injury of internal organs —*see* Injury, by site
    open wound —*see* Wound, open
  amputation stump (surgical) (late) T87.89
  aorta, dissecting I71.ØØ
    abdominal I71.Ø2
    thoracic I71.Ø1
    thoracoabdominal I71.Ø3
  aortic intramural —*see* Dissection, aorta
  arterial (complicating trauma) —*see* Injury, blood vessel, by site
  auricle —*see* Contusion, ear
    nontraumatic —*see* Disorder, pinna, hematoma
  birth injury NEC P15.8
  brain (traumatic)
    with
      cerebral laceration or contusion (diffuse) —*see* Injury, intracranial, diffuse
        focal —*see* Injury, intracranial, focal
    cerebellar, traumatic SØ6.37-
    intracerebral, traumatic —*see* Injury, intracranial, intracerebral hemorrhage
    newborn NEC P52.4
      birth injury P1Ø.1
    nontraumatic —*see* Hemorrhage, intracranial
    subarachnoid, arachnoid, traumatic —*see* Injury, intracranial, subarachnoid hemorrhage
    subdural, traumatic —*see* Injury, intracranial, subdural hemorrhage
  breast (nontraumatic) N64.89
  broad ligament (nontraumatic) N83.7
    traumatic S37.892
  cerebellar, traumatic SØ6.37-
  cerebral —*see* Hematoma, brain
  cerebrum SØ6.36-
    left SØ6.35-
    right SØ6.34-
  cesarean delivery wound O9Ø.2
  complicating delivery (perineal) (pelvic) (vagina) (vulva) O71.7
  corpus cavernosum (nontraumatic) N48.89
  epididymis (nontraumatic) N5Ø.1
  epidural (traumatic) —*see* Injury, intracranial, epidural hemorrhage
    spinal —*see* Injury, spinal cord, by region
  episiotomy O9Ø.2
  face, birth injury P15.4
  genital organ NEC (nontraumatic)
    female (nonobstetric) N94.89
      traumatic S3Ø.2Ø2
    male N5Ø.1
      traumatic S3Ø.2Ø1
  internal organs —*see* Injury, by site
  intracerebral, traumatic —*see* Injury, intracranial, intracerebral hemorrhage
  intraoperative —*see* Complications, intraoperative, hemorrhage
  labia (nontraumatic) (nonobstetric) N9Ø.8
  liver (subcapsular) (nontraumatic) K76.89
    birth injury P15.Ø
  mediastinum —*see* Injury, intrathoracic
  mesosalpinx (nontraumatic) N83.7
    traumatic S37.898
  muscle - code by site under Contusion
  nontraumatic
    muscle M79.81
    soft tissue M79.81
  obstetrical surgical wound O9Ø.2
  orbit, orbital (nontraumatic) —*see also* Hemorrhage, orbit
    traumatic —*see* Contusion, orbit
  pelvis (female) (nontraumatic) (nonobstetric) N94.89
    obstetric O71.7
    traumatic —*see* Injury, by site

Hematoma *(Continued)*
  penis (nontraumatic) N48.89
    birth injury P15.5
  perianal (nontraumatic) K64.5
  perineal S3Ø.23
    complicating delivery O71.7
  perirenal —*see* Injury, kidney
  pinna —*see* Contusion, ear
    nontraumatic —*see* Disorder, pinna, hematoma
  placenta O43.89-
  postoperative (postprocedural) —*see* Complication, postprocedural, hematoma ⬅ (Revised)
  retroperitoneal (nontraumatic) K66.1
    traumatic S36.892
  scrotum, superficial S3Ø.22
    birth injury P15.5
  seminal vesicle (nontraumatic) N5Ø.1
    traumatic S37.892
  spermatic cord (traumatic) S37.892
    nontraumatic N5Ø.1
  spinal (cord) (meninges) —*see also* Injury, spinal cord, by region
    newborn (birth injury) P11.5
  spleen D73.5
    intraoperative —*see* Complications, intraoperative, hemorrhage, spleen
    postprocedural (postoperative) —*see* Complications, postprocedural, hemorrhage, spleen
  sternocleidomastoid, birth injury P15.2
  sternomastoid, birth injury P15.2
  subarachnoid (traumatic) —*see* Injury, intracranial, subarachnoid hemorrhage
    newborn (nontraumatic) P52.5
      due to birth injury P1Ø.3
    nontraumatic —*see* Hemorrhage, intracranial, subarachnoid
  subdural (traumatic) —*see* Injury, intracranial, subdural hemorrhage
    newborn (localized) P52.8
      birth injury P1Ø.Ø
    nontraumatic —*see* Hemorrhage, intracranial, subdural
  superficial, newborn P54.5
  testis (nontraumatic) N5Ø.1
    birth injury P15.5
  tunica vaginalis (nontraumatic) N5Ø.1
  umbilical cord, complicating delivery O69.5
  uterine ligament (broad) (nontraumatic) N83.7
    traumatic S37.892
  vagina (ruptured) (nontraumatic) N89.8
    complicating delivery O71.7
  vas deferens (nontraumatic) N5Ø.1
    traumatic S37.892
  vitreous —*see* Hemorrhage, vitreous
  vulva (nontraumatic) (nonobstetric) N9Ø.89
    complicating delivery O71.7
    newborn (birth injury) P15.5
Hematometra N85.7
  with hematocolpos N89.7
Hematomyelia (central) G95.19
  newborn (birth injury) P11.5
  traumatic T14.8
Hematomyelitis GØ4.9Ø
Hematoperitoneum —*see* Hemoperitoneum
Hematophobia F4Ø.23Ø
Hematopneumothorax (*see* Hemothorax)
Hematopoiesis, cyclic D7Ø.4
Hematoporphyria —*see* Porphyria
Hematorachis, hematorrhachis G95.19
  newborn (birth injury) P11.5
Hematosalpinx N83.6
  with
    hematocolpos N89.7
    hematometra N85.7
      with hematocolpos N89.7
  infectional —*see* Salpingitis

Hematospermia R36.1
Hematothorax (*see* Hemothorax)
Hematuria R31.9
  benign (familial) (of childhood) —*see also* Hematuria, idiopathic
    essential microscopic R31.1
  due to sulphonamide, sulfonamide —*see* Table of Drugs and Chemicals, by drug
  endemic —*see also* Schistosomiasis B65.Ø
  gross R31.Ø
  idiopathic NØ2.9
    with glomerular lesion
      crescentic (diffuse) glomerulonephritis NØ2.7
      dense deposit disease NØ2.6
      endocapillary proliferative glomerulonephritis NØ2.4
      focal and segmental hyalinosis or sclerosis NØ2.1
      membranoproliferative (diffuse) NØ2.5
      membranous (diffuse) NØ2.2
      mesangial proliferative (diffuse) NØ2.3
      mesangiocapillary (diffuse) NØ2.5
      minor abnormality NØ2.Ø
      proliferative NEC NØ2.8
      specified pathology NEC NØ2.8
  intermittent —*see* Hematuria, idiopathic
  malarial B5Ø.8
  microscopic NEC (with symptoms) R31.29 ⬅ (Revised)
    asymptomatic R31.21 ◀ (New)
    benign essential R31.1
  paroxysmal —*see also* Hematuria, idiopathic
    nocturnal D59.5
  persistent —*see* Hematuria, idiopathic
  recurrent —*see* Hematuria, idiopathic
  tropical —*see also* Schistosomiasis B65.Ø
  tuberculous A18.13
Hemeralopia (day blindness) H53.11
  vitamin A deficiency E5Ø.5
Hemi-akinesia R41.4
Hemianalgesia R2Ø.Ø
Hemianencephaly QØØ.Ø
Hemianesthesia R2Ø.Ø
Hemianopia, hemianopsia (heteronymous) H53.47
  homonymous H53.46-
  syphilitic A52.71
Hemiathetosis R25.8
Hemiatrophy R68.89
  cerebellar G31.9
  face, facial, progressive (Romberg) G51.8
  tongue K14.8
Hemiballism (us) G25.5
Hemicardia Q24.8
Hemicephalus, hemicephaly QØØ.Ø
Hemichorea G25.5
Hemicolitis, left —*see* Colitis, left sided
Hemicrania
  congenital malformation QØØ.Ø
  continua G44.51
  meaning migraine —*see also* Migraine G43.9Ø9
  paroxysmal G44.Ø39
    chronic G44.Ø49
      intractable G44.Ø41
      not intractable G44.Ø49
    episodic G44.Ø39
      intractable G44.Ø31
      not intractable G44.Ø39
    intractable G44.Ø31
    not intractable G44.Ø39
Hemidystrophy —*see* Hemiatrophy
Hemiectromelia Q73.8
Hemihypalgesia R2Ø.8
Hemihypesthesia R2Ø.1
Hemi-inattention R41.4
Hemimelia Q73.8
  lower limb —*see* Defect, reduction, lower limb, specified type NEC
  upper limb —*see* Defect, reduction, upper limb, specified type NEC
Hemiparalysis —*see* Hemiplegia
Hemiparesis —*see* Hemiplegia

H

Hemiparesthesia R2Ø.2
Hemiparkinsonism G2Ø
Hemiplegia G81.9-
alternans facialis G83.89
ascending NEC G81.9Ø
spinal G95.89
congenital (cerebral) G8Ø.8
spastic G8Ø.2
embolic (current episode) I63.4-
flaccid G81.Ø-
following
cerebrovascular disease I69.959
cerebral infarction I69.35-
intracerebral hemorrhage I69.15-
nontraumatic intracranial hemorrhage NEC I69.25-
specified disease NEC I69.85-
stroke NOS I69.35-
subarachnoid hemorrhage I69.Ø5-
hysterical F44.4
newborn NEC P91.8
birth injury P11.9
spastic G81.1-
congenital G8Ø.2
thrombotic (current episode) I63.3-
Hemisection, spinal cord —*see* Injury, spinal cord, by region
Hemispasm (facial) R25.2
Hemisporosis B48.8
Hemitremor R25.1
Hemivertebra Q76.49
failure of segmentation with scoliosis Q76.3
fusion with scoliosis Q76.3
Hemochromatosis E83.119
with refractory anemia D46.1
due to repeated red blood cell transfusion E83.111
hereditary (primary) E83.11Ø
primary E83.11Ø
specified NEC E83.118
Hemoglobin —*see also* condition
abnormal (disease) —*see* Disease, hemoglobin
AS genotype D57.3
Constant Spring D58.2
E-beta thalassemia D56.5
fetal, hereditary persistence (HPFH) D56.4
H Constant Spring D56.Ø
low NOS D64.9
S (Hb S), heterozygous D57.3
Hemoglobinemia D59.9
due to blood transfusion T8Ø.89
paroxysmal D59.6
nocturnal D59.5
Hemoglobinopathy (mixed) D58.2
with thalassemia D56.8
sickle-cell D57.1
with thalassemia D57.4Ø
with crisis (vasoocclusive pain) D57.419
with
acute chest syndrome D57.411
splenic sequestration D57.412
without crisis D57.4Ø
Hemoglobinuria R82.3
with anemia, hemolytic, acquired (chronic) NEC D59.6
cold (agglutinin) (paroxysmal) (with Raynaud's syndrome) D59.6
due to exertion or hemolysis NEC D59.6
intermittent D59.6
malarial B5Ø.8
march D59.6
nocturnal (paroxysmal) D59.5
paroxysmal (cold) D59.6
nocturnal D59.5
Hemolymphangioma D18.1
Hemolysis
intravascular
with
abortion —*see* Abortion, by type, complicated by, hemorrhage
ectopic or molar pregnancy OØ8.1

Hemolysis *(Continued)*
intravascular *(Continued)*
with *(Continued)*
hemorrhage
antepartum —*see* Hemorrhage, antepartum, with coagulation defect
intrapartum —*see also* Hemorrhage, complicating, delivery O67.Ø
postpartum O72.3
neonatal (excessive) P58.9
specified NEC P58.8
Hemolytic —*see* condition
Hemopericardium I31.2
following acute myocardial infarction (current complication) I23.Ø
newborn P54.8
traumatic —*see* Injury, heart, with hemopericardium
Hemoperitoneum K66.1
infectional K65.9
traumatic S36.899
with open wound —*see* Wound, open, with penetration into peritoneal cavity
Hemophilia (classical) (familial) (hereditary) D66
A D66
B D67
C D68.1
acquired D68.311
autoimmune D68.311
calcipriva —*see also* Defect, coagulation D68.4
nonfamilial —*see also* Defect, coagulation D68.4
secondary D68.311
vascular D68.Ø
Hemophthalmos H44.81-
Hemopneumothorax —*see also* Hemothorax
traumatic S27.2
Hemoptysis RØ4.2
newborn P26.9
tuberculous —*see* Tuberculosis, pulmonary
Hemorrhage, hemorrhagic (concealed) R58
abdomen R58
accidental antepartum —*see* Hemorrhage, antepartum
acute idiopathic pulmonary, in infants RØ4.81
adenoid J35.8
adrenal (capsule) (gland) E27.49
medulla E27.8
newborn P54.4
after delivery —*see* Hemorrhage, postpartum
alveolar
lung, newborn P26.8
process KØ8.89
alveolus KØ8.89
amputation stump (surgical) T87.89
anemia (chronic) D5Ø.Ø
acute D62
antepartum (with) O46.9Ø
with coagulation defect O46.ØØ-
afibrinogenemia O46.Ø1-
disseminated intravascular coagulation O46.Ø2-
hypofibrinogenemia O46.Ø1-
specified defect NEC O46.Ø9-
before 2Ø weeks gestation O2Ø.9
specified type NEC O2Ø.8
threatened abortion O2Ø.Ø
due to
abruptio placenta —*see also* Abruptio placentae O45.9-
leiomyoma, uterus —*see* Hemorrhage, antepartum, specified cause NEC
placenta previa O44.1-
specified cause NEC —*see* subcategory O46.8X-
anus (sphincter) K62.5
apoplexy (stroke) —*see* Hemorrhage, intracranial, intracerebral

Hemorrhage, hemorrhagic *(Continued)*
arachnoid —*see* Hemorrhage, intracranial, subarachnoid
artery R58
brain —*see* Hemorrhage, intracranial, intracerebral
basilar (ganglion) I61.Ø
bladder N32.89
bowel K92.2
newborn P54.3
brain (miliary) (nontraumatic) —*see* Hemorrhage, intracranial, intracerebral
due to
birth injury P1Ø.1
syphilis A52.Ø5
epidural or extradural (traumatic) —*see* Injury, intracranial, epidural hemorrhage
newborn P52.4
birth injury P1Ø.1
subarachnoid —*see* Hemorrhage, intracranial, subarachnoid
subdural —*see* Hemorrhage, intracranial, subdural
brainstem (nontraumatic) I61.3
traumatic SØ6.38-
breast N64.59
bronchial tube —*see* Hemorrhage, lung
bronchopulmonary —*see* Hemorrhage, lung
bronchus —*see* Hemorrhage, lung
bulbar I61.5
capillary I78.8
primary D69.8
cecum K92.2
cerebellar, cerebellum (nontraumatic) I61.4
newborn P52.6
traumatic SØ6.37-
cerebral, cerebrum —*see also* Hemorrhage, intracranial, intracerebral
lobe I61.1
newborn (anoxic) P52.4
birth injury P1Ø.1
cerebromeningeal I61.8
cerebrospinal —*see* Hemorrhage, intracranial, intracerebral
cervix (uteri) (stump) NEC N88.8
chamber, anterior (eye) —*see* Hyphema
childbirth —*see* Hemorrhage, complicating, delivery
choroid H31.3Ø-
expulsive H31.31-
ciliary body —*see* Hyphema
cochlea —*see* subcategory H83.8
colon K92.2
complicating
abortion —*see* Abortion, by type, complicated by, hemorrhage
delivery O67.9
associated with coagulation defect (afibrinogenemia) (DIC) (hyperfibrinolysis) O67.Ø
specified cause NEC O67.8
surgical procedure —*see* Hemorrhage, intraoperative
conjunctiva H11.3-
newborn P54.8
cord, newborn (stump) P51.9
corpus luteum (ruptured) cyst N83.1-
cortical (brain) I61.1
cranial —*see* Hemorrhage, intracranial
cutaneous R23.3
due to autosensitivity, erythrocyte D69.2
newborn P54.5
delayed
following ectopic or molar pregnancy OØ8.1
postpartum O72.2
diathesis (familial) D69.9
disease D69.9
newborn P53
specified type NEC D69.8

Hemorrhage, hemorrhagic *(Continued)*
- due to or associated with
  - afibrinogenemia or other coagulation defect (conditions in categories D65-D69)
    - antepartum —*see* Hemorrhage, antepartum, with coagulation defect
    - intrapartum O67.Ø
  - dental implant M27.61
  - device, implant or graft —*see also* Complications, by site and type, specified NEC T85.838
    - arterial graft NEC T82.838
    - breast T85.838
    - catheter NEC T85.838
      - dialysis (renal) T82.838
        - intraperitoneal T85.838
      - infusion NEC T82.838
        - spinal (epidural) (subdural) T85.83Ø
      - urinary (indwelling) T83.83
    - electronic (electrode) (pulse generator) (stimulator)
      - bone T84.83
      - cardiac T82.837
      - nervous system (brain) (peripheral nerve) (spinal) T85.83Ø
      - urinary T83.83
    - fixation, internal (orthopedic) NEC T84.83
    - gastrointestinal (bile duct) (esophagus) T85.838
    - genital NEC T83.83
    - heart NEC T82.837
    - joint prosthesis T84.83
    - ocular (corneal graft) (orbital implant) NEC T85.838
    - orthopedic NEC T84.83
      - bone graft T86.838
    - specified NEC T85.838
    - urinary NEC T83.83
    - vascular NEC T82.838
    - ventricular intracranial shunt T85.838
- duodenum, duodenal K92.2
  - ulcer —*see* Ulcer, duodenum, with hemorrhage
- dura mater —*see* Hemorrhage, intracranial, subdural
- endotracheal —*see* Hemorrhage, lung
- epicranial subaponeurotic (massive), birth injury P12.2
- epidural (traumatic) —*see also* Injury, intracranial, epidural hemorrhage
  - nontraumatic I62.1
- esophagus K22.8
  - varix I85.Ø1
    - secondary I85.11
- excessive, following ectopic gestation (subsequent episode) OØ8.1
- extradural (traumatic) —*see* Injury, intracranial, epidural hemorrhage
  - birth injury P1Ø.8
  - newborn (anoxic) (nontraumatic) P52.8
  - nontraumatic I62.1
- eye NEC H57.8
  - fundus —*see* Hemorrhage, retina
  - lid —*see* Disorder, eyelid, specified type NEC
- fallopian tube N83.6
- fibrinogenolysis —*see* Fibrinolysis
- fibrinolytic (acquired) —*see* Fibrinolysis
- from
  - ear (nontraumatic) —*see* Otorrhagia
  - tracheostomy stoma J95.Ø1
- fundus, eye —*see* Hemorrhage, retina
- funis —*see* Hemorrhage, umbilicus, cord
- gastric —*see* Hemorrhage, stomach
- gastroenteric K92.2
  - newborn P54.3
- gastrointestinal (tract) K92.2
  - newborn P54.3
- genital organ, male N5Ø.1

Hemorrhage, hemorrhagic *(Continued)*
- genitourinary (tract) NOS R31.9
- gingiva KØ6.8
- globe (eye) —*see* Hemophthalmos
- graafian follicle cyst (ruptured) N83.Ø-
- gum KØ6.8
- heart I51.89
- hypopharyngeal (throat) RØ4.1
- intermenstrual (regular) N92.3
  - irregular N92.1
- internal (organs) NEC R58
  - capsule I61.Ø
  - ear —*see* subcategory H83.8
  - newborn P54.8
- intestine K92.2
  - newborn P54.3
- intra-abdominal R58
- intra-alveolar (lung), newborn P26.8
- intracerebral (nontraumatic) —*see* Hemorrhage, intracranial, intracerebral
- intracranial (nontraumatic) I62.9
  - birth injury P1Ø.9
  - epidural, nontraumatic I62.1
  - extradural, nontraumatic I62.1
  - intracerebral (nontraumatic) (in) I61.9
    - brain stem I61.3
    - cerebellum I61.4
    - hemisphere I61.2
      - cortical (superficial) I61.1
      - subcortical (deep) I61.Ø
    - intraoperative
      - during a nervous system procedure G97.31
      - during other procedure G97.32
    - intraventricular I61.5
    - multiple localized I61.6
    - newborn P52.4
      - birth injury P1Ø.1
    - postprocedural
      - following a nervous system procedure G97.51
      - following other procedure G97.52
    - specified NEC I61.8
    - superficial I61.1
    - traumatic (diffuse) —*see* Injury, intracranial, diffuse
      - focal —*see* Injury, intracranial, focal
  - newborn P52.9
    - specified NEC P52.8
  - subarachnoid (nontraumatic) (from) I6Ø.9
    - intracranial (cerebral) artery I6Ø.7
      - anterior communicating I6Ø.2
      - basilar I6Ø.4
      - carotid siphon and bifurcation I6Ø.Ø-
      - communicating I6Ø.7
        - anterior I6Ø.2
        - posterior I6Ø.3-
      - middle cerebral I6Ø.1-
      - posterior communicating I6Ø.3-
      - specified artery NEC I6Ø.6
      - vertebral I6Ø.5-
    - newborn P52.5
      - birth injury P1Ø.3
    - specified NEC I6Ø.8
    - traumatic SØ6.6X-
  - subdural (nontraumatic) I62.ØØ
    - acute I62.Ø1
    - birth injury P1Ø.Ø
    - chronic I62.Ø3
    - newborn (anoxic) (hypoxic) P52.8
      - birth injury P1Ø.Ø
    - spinal G95.19
    - subacute I62.Ø2
    - traumatic —*see* Injury, intracranial, subdural hemorrhage
  - traumatic —*see* Injury, intracranial, focal brain injury

Hemorrhage, hemorrhagic *(Continued)*
- intramedullary NEC G95.19
- intraocular —*see* Hemophthalmos
- intraoperative, intraprocedural —*see* Complication, hemorrhage (hematoma), intraoperative (intraprocedural), by site
- intrapartum —*see* Hemorrhage, complicating, delivery
- intrapelvic
  - female N94.89
  - male K66.1
- intraperitoneal K66.1
- intrapontine I61.3
- intraprocedural —*see* Complication, hemorrhage (hematoma), intraoperative (intraprocedural), by site
- intrauterine N85.7
  - complicating delivery —*see also* Hemorrhage, complicating, delivery O67.9
  - postpartum —*see* Hemorrhage, postpartum
- intraventricular I61.5
  - newborn (nontraumatic) —*see also* Newborn, affected by, hemorrhage P52.3
    - due to birth injury P1Ø.2
    - grade
      - 1 P52.Ø
      - 2 P52.1
      - 3 P52.21
      - 4 P52.22
- intravesical N32.89
- iris (postinfectional) (postinflammatory) (toxic) —*see* Hyphema
- joint (nontraumatic) —*see* Hemarthrosis
- kidney N28.89
- knee (joint) (nontraumatic) —*see* Hemarthrosis, knee
- labyrinth —*see* subcategory H83.8
- lenticular striate artery I61.Ø
- ligature, vessel —*see* Hemorrhage, postoperative
- liver K76.89
- lung RØ4.89
  - newborn P26.9
    - massive P26.1
    - specified NEC P26.8
  - tuberculous —*see* Tuberculosis, pulmonary
- massive umbilical, newborn P51.Ø
- mediastinum —*see* Hemorrhage, lung
- medulla I61.3
- membrane (brain) I6Ø.8
  - spinal cord —*see* Hemorrhage, spinal cord
- meninges, meningeal (brain) (middle) I6Ø.8
  - spinal cord —*see* Hemorrhage, spinal cord
- mesentery K66.1
- metritis —*see* Endometritis
- mouth K13.79
- mucous membrane NEC R58
  - newborn P54.8
- muscle M62.89
- nail (subungual) L6Ø.8
- nasal turbinate RØ4.Ø
  - newborn P54.8
- navel, newborn P51.9
- newborn P54.9
  - specified NEC P54.8
- nipple N64.59
- nose RØ4.Ø
  - newborn P54.8
- omentum K66.1
- optic nerve (sheath) H47.Ø2-
- orbit, orbital HØ5.23-
- ovary NEC N83.8
- oviduct N83.6
- pancreas K86.89
- parathyroid (gland) (spontaneous) E21.4
- parturition —*see* Hemorrhage, complicating, delivery
- penis N48.89
- pericardium, pericarditis I31.2
- peritoneum, peritoneal K66.1
- peritonsillar tissue J35.8
  - due to infection J36

Hemorrhage, hemorrhagic *(Continued)*
petechial R23.3
due to autosensitivity, erythrocyte D69.2
pituitary (gland) E23.6
pleura —*see* Hemorrhage, lung
polioencephalitis, superior E51.2
polymyositis —*see* Polymyositis
pons, pontine I61.3
posterior fossa (nontraumatic) I61.8
newborn P52.6
postmenopausal N95.Ø
postnasal RØ4.Ø
postoperative —*see* Complications, postprocedural, hemorrhage, by site
postpartum NEC (following delivery of placenta) O72.1
delayed or secondary O72.2
retained placenta O72.Ø
third stage O72.Ø
pregnancy —*see* Hemorrhage, antepartum
preretinal —*see* Hemorrhage, retina
prostate N42.1
puerperal —*see* Hemorrhage, postpartum
delayed or secondary O72.2
pulmonary RØ4.89
newborn P26.9
massive P26.1
specified NEC P26.8
tuberculous —*see* Tuberculosis, pulmonary
purpura (primary) D69.3
rectum (sphincter) K62.5
newborn P54.2
recurring, following initial hemorrhage at time of injury T79.2
renal N28.89
respiratory passage or tract RØ4.9
specified NEC RØ4.89
retina, retinal (vessels) H35.6-
diabetic —*see* Diabetes, retinal, hemorrhage
retroperitoneal R58
scalp R58
scrotum N5Ø.1
secondary (nontraumatic) R58
following initial hemorrhage at time of injury T79.2
seminal vesicle N5Ø.1
skin R23.3
newborn P54.5
slipped umbilical ligature P51.8
spermatic cord N5Ø.1
spinal (cord) G95.19
newborn (birth injury) P11.5
spleen D73.5
intraoperative —*see* Complications, intraoperative, hemorrhage, spleen
postprocedural —*see* Complications, postprocedural, hemorrhage, spleen
stomach K92.2
newborn P54.3
ulcer —*see* Ulcer, stomach, with hemorrhage
subarachnoid (nontraumatic) —*see* Hemorrhage, intracranial, subarachnoid
subconjunctival —*see also* Hemorrhage, conjunctiva
birth injury P15.3
subcortical (brain) I61.Ø
subcutaneous R23.3
subdiaphragmatic R58
subdural (acute) (nontraumatic) —*see* Hemorrhage, intracranial, subdural
subependymal
newborn P52.Ø
with intraventricular extension P52.1
and intracerebral extension P52.22
subgaleal P12.2
subhyaloid —*see* Hemorrhage, retina
subperiosteal —*see* Disorder, bone, specified type NEC
subretinal —*see* Hemorrhage, retina
subtentorial —*see* Hemorrhage, intracranial, subdural

Hemorrhage, hemorrhagic *(Continued)*
subungual L6Ø.8
suprarenal (capsule) (gland) E27.49
newborn P54.4
tentorium (traumatic) NEC —*see* Hemorrhage, brain
newborn (birth injury) P1Ø.4
testis N5Ø.1
third stage (postpartum) O72.Ø
thorax —*see* Hemorrhage, lung
throat RØ4.1
thymus (gland) E32.8
thyroid (cyst) (gland) EØ7.89
tongue K14.8
tonsil J35.8
trachea —*see* Hemorrhage, lung
tracheobronchial RØ4.89
newborn P26.Ø
traumatic — code to specific injury
cerebellar —*see* Hemorrhage, brain
intracranial —*see* Hemorrhage, brain
recurring or secondary (following initial hemorrhage at time of injury) T79.2
tuberculous NEC —*see also* Tuberculosis, pulmonary A15.Ø
tunica vaginalis N5Ø.1
ulcer - code by site under Ulcer, with hemorrhage K27.4
umbilicus, umbilical
cord
after birth, newborn P51.9
complicating delivery O69.5
newborn P51.9
massive P51.Ø
slipped ligature P51.8
stump P51.9
urethra (idiopathic) N36.8
uterus, uterine (abnormal) N93.9
climacteric N92.4
complicating delivery —*see* Hemorrhage, complicating, delivery
dysfunctional or functional N93.8
intermenstrual (regular) N92.3
irregular N92.1
postmenopausal N95.Ø
postpartum —*see* Hemorrhage, postpartum
preclimacteric or premenopausal N92.4
prepubertal N93.8
pubertal N92.2
vagina (abnormal) N93.9
newborn P54.6
vas deferens N5Ø.1
vasa previa O69.4
ventricular I61.5
vesical N32.89
viscera NEC R58
newborn P54.8
vitreous (humor) (intraocular) H43.1-
vulva N9Ø.89

Hemorrhoids (bleeding) (without mention of degree) K64.9
1st degree (grade/stage I) (without prolapse outside of anal canal) K64.Ø
2nd degree (grade/stage II) (that prolapse with straining but retract spontaneously) K64.1
3rd degree (grade/stage III) (that prolapse with straining and require manual replacement back inside anal canal) K64.2
4th degree (grade/stage IV) (with prolapsed tissue that cannot be manually replaced) K64.3
complicating
pregnancy O22.4
puerperium O87.2
external K64.4
with
thrombosis K64.5

Hemorrhoids *(Continued)*
internal (without mention of degree) K64.8
prolapsed K64.8
skin tags
anus K64.4
residual K64.4
specified NEC K64.8
strangulated —*see also* Hemorrhoids, by degree K64.8
thrombosed —*see also* Hemorrhoids, by degree K64.5
ulcerated —*see also* Hemorrhoids, by degree K64.8

Hemosalpinx N83.6
with
hematocolpos N89.7
hematometra N85.7
with hematocolpos N89.7

Hemosiderosis (dietary) E83.19
pulmonary, idiopathic E83.1 *[J84.Ø3]*
transfusion T8Ø.89

Hemothorax (bacterial) (nontuberculous) J94.2
newborn P54.8
traumatic S27.1
with pneumothorax S27.2
tuberculous NEC A15.6

Henoch (-Schönlein) **disease or syndrome** (purpura) D69.Ø

Henpue, henpuye A66.6

Hepar lobatum (syphilitic) A52.74

Hepatalgia K76.89

Hepatitis K75.9
acute B17.9
with coma K72.Ø1
with hepatic failure —*see* Failure, hepatic
alcoholic —*see* Hepatitis, alcoholic
infectious B15.9
~~with hepatic coma B15.Ø~~
non-viral K72.Ø
viral B17.9
alcoholic (acute) (chronic) K7Ø.1Ø
with ascites K7Ø.11
amebic —*see* Abscess, liver, amebic
anicteric (viral) —*see* Hepatitis, viral
antigen-associated (HAA) —*see* Hepatitis, B
Australia-antigen (positive) —*see* Hepatitis, B
autoimmune K75.4
B B19.1Ø
with hepatic coma B19.11
acute B16.9
with
delta-agent (coinfection) (without hepatic coma) B16.1
with hepatic coma B16.Ø
hepatic coma (without delta-agent coinfection) B16.2
chronic B18.1
with delta-agent B18.Ø
bacterial NEC K75.89
C (viral) B19.2Ø
with hepatic coma B19.21
acute B17.1Ø
with hepatic coma B17.11
chronic B18.2
catarrhal (acute) B15.9
with hepatic coma B15.Ø
cholangiolitic K75.89
cholestatic K75.89
chronic K73.9
active NEC K73.2
lobular NEC K73.1
persistent NEC K73.Ø
specified NEC K73.8
cytomegaloviral B25.1
due to ethanol (acute) (chronic) —*see* Hepatitis, alcoholic
epidemic B15.9
with hepatic coma B15.Ø
fulminant NEC (viral) —*see* Hepatitis, viral
granulomatous NEC K75.3
herpesviral BØØ.81

H

Hepatitis *(Continued)*
- history of
  - B Z86.19
  - C Z86.19
- homologous serum —*see* Hepatitis, viral, type B
- in (due to)
  - mumps B26.81
  - toxoplasmosis (acquired) B58.1
    - congenital (active) P37.1 *[K77]*
- infectious, infective B15.9
  - ~~with hepatic coma B15.0~~
  - acute (subacute) B17.9
  - chronic B18.9
- inoculation —*see* Hepatitis, viral, type B
- interstitial (chronic) K74.69
- lupoid NEC K75.2
- malignant NEC (with hepatic failure) K72.90
  - with coma K72.91
- neonatal giant cell P59.29
- neonatal (idiopathic) (toxic) P59.29
- newborn P59.29
- postimmunization —*see* Hepatitis, viral, type B
- post-transfusion —*see* Hepatitis, viral, type B
- reactive, nonspecific K75.2
- serum —*see* Hepatitis, viral, type B
- specified type NEC
  - with hepatic failure —*see* Failure, hepatic
- syphilitic (late) A52.74
  - congenital (early) A50.08 *[K77]*
    - late A50.59 *[K77]*
  - secondary A51.45
- toxic —*see also* Disease, liver, toxic K71.6
- tuberculous A18.83
- viral, virus B19.9
  - with hepatic coma B19.0
  - acute B17.9
  - chronic B18.9
    - specified NEC B18.8
    - type
      - B B18.1
        - with delta-agent B18.0
      - C B18.2
  - congenital P35.3
  - coxsackie B33.8 *[K77]*
  - cytomegalic inclusion B25.1
  - in remission, any type — code to Hepatitis, chronic, by type
  - non-A, non-B B17.8
  - specified type NEC (with or without coma) B17.8
  - type
    - A B15.9
      - with hepatic coma B15.0
    - B B19.10
      - with hepatic coma B19.11
      - acute B16.9
        - with
          - delta-agent (coinfection) (without hepatic coma) B16.1
            - with hepatic coma B16.0
          - hepatic coma (without delta-agent coinfection) B16.2
      - chronic B18.1
        - with delta-agent B18.0
    - C B19.20
      - with hepatic coma B19.21
      - acute B17.10
        - with hepatic coma B17.11
      - chronic B18.2
    - E B17.2
    - non-A, non-B B17.8

Hepatization lung (acute) —*see* Pneumonia, lobar
Hepatoblastoma C22.2
Hepatocarcinoma C22.0
Hepatocholangiocarcinoma C22.0
Hepatocholangioma, benign D13.4
Hepatocholangitis K75.89
Hepatolenticular degeneration E83.01
Hepatoma (malignant) C22.0
- benign D13.4
- embryonal C22.0

Hepatomegaly —*see also* Hypertrophy, liver
- with splenomegaly R16.2
- congenital Q44.7
- in mononucleosis
  - gammaherpesviral B27.09
  - infectious specified NEC B27.89

Hepatoptosis K76.89
Hepatorenal syndrome following labor and delivery O90.4
Hepatosis K76.89
Hepatosplenomegaly R16.2
- hyperlipemic (Bürger-Grütz type) E78.3 *[K77]*

Hereditary —*see* condition
Heredodegeneration, macular —*see* Dystrophy, retina
Heredopathia atactica polyneuritiformis G60.1
Heredosyphilis —*see* Syphilis, congenital
Herlitz' syndrome Q81.1
Hermansky-Pudlak syndrome E70.331
Hermaphrodite, hermaphroditism (true) Q56.0
- 46,XX with streak gonads Q99.1
- 46,XX/46,XY Q99.0
- 46,XY with streak gonads Q99.1
- chimera 46,XX/46,XY Q99.0

Hernia, hernial (acquired) (recurrent) K46.9
- with
  - gangrene —*see* Hernia, by site, with, gangrene
  - incarceration —*see* Hernia, by site, with, obstruction
  - irreducible —*see* Hernia, by site, with, obstruction
  - obstruction —*see* Hernia, by site, with, obstruction
  - strangulation —*see* Hernia, by site, with, obstruction
- abdomen, abdominal K46.9
  - with
    - gangrene (and obstruction) K46.1
    - obstruction K46.0
  - femoral —*see* Hernia, femoral
  - incisional —*see* Hernia, incisional
  - inguinal —*see* Hernia, inguinal
  - specified site NEC K45.8
    - with
      - gangrene (and obstruction) K45.1
      - obstruction K45.0
  - umbilical —*see* Hernia, umbilical
  - wall —*see* Hernia, ventral
- appendix —*see* Hernia, abdomen
- bladder (mucosa) (sphincter)
  - congenital (female) (male) Q79.51
  - female —*see* Cystocele
  - male N32.89
- brain, congenital —*see* Encephalocele
- cartilage, vertebra —*see* Displacement, intervertebral disc
- cerebral, congenital —*see also* Encephalocele
  - endaural Q01.8
- ciliary body (traumatic) S05.2-
- colon —*see* Hernia, abdomen
- Cooper's —*see* Hernia, abdomen, specified site NEC
- crural —*see* Hernia, femoral
- diaphragm, diaphragmatic K44.9
  - with
    - gangrene (and obstruction) K44.1
    - obstruction K44.0
  - congenital Q79.0
- direct (inguinal) —*see* Hernia, inguinal
- diverticulum, intestine —*see* Hernia, abdomen
- double (inguinal) —*see* Hernia, inguinal, bilateral
- due to adhesions (with obstruction) K56.5
- epigastric —*see also* Hernia, ventral K43.9
- esophageal hiatus —*see* Hernia, hiatal

Hernia, hernial *(Continued)*
- external (inguinal) —*see* Hernia, inguinal
- fallopian tube N83.4-
- fascia M62.89
- femoral K41.90
  - with
    - gangrene (and obstruction) K41.40
      - not specified as recurrent K41.40
      - recurrent K41.41
    - obstruction K41.30
      - not specified as recurrent K41.30
      - recurrent K41.31
  - bilateral K41.20
    - with
      - gangrene (and obstruction) K41.10
        - not specified as recurrent K41.10
        - recurrent K41.11
      - obstruction K41.00
        - not specified as recurrent K41.00
        - recurrent K41.01
    - not specified as recurrent K41.20
    - recurrent K41.21
  - not specified as recurrent K41.90
  - recurrent K41.91
  - unilateral K41.90
    - with
      - gangrene (and obstruction) K41.40
        - not specified as recurrent K41.40
        - recurrent K41.41
      - obstruction K41.30
        - not specified as recurrent K41.30
        - recurrent K41.31
    - not specified as recurrent K41.90
    - recurrent K41.91
- foramen magnum G93.5
  - congenital Q01.8
- funicular (umbilical) —*see also* Hernia, umbilicus
  - spermatic (cord) —*see* Hernia, inguinal
- gastrointestinal tract —*see* Hernia, abdomen
- Hesselbach's —*see* Hernia, femoral, specified site NEC
- hiatal (esophageal) (sliding) K44.9
  - with
    - gangrene (and obstruction) K44.1
    - obstruction K44.0
  - congenital Q40.1
- hypogastric —*see* Hernia, ventral
- incarcerated —*see also* Hernia, by site, with obstruction
  - with gangrene —*see* Hernia, by site, with gangrene
- incisional K43.92
  - with
    - gangrene (and obstruction) K43.1
    - obstruction K43.0
- indirect (inguinal) —*see* Hernia, inguinal
- inguinal (direct) (external) (funicular) (indirect) (internal) (oblique) (scrotal) (sliding) K40.90
  - with
    - gangrene (and obstruction) K40.40
      - not specified as recurrent K40.40
      - recurrent K40.41
    - obstruction K40.30
      - not specified as recurrent K40.30
      - recurrent K40.31
  - bilateral K40.20
    - with
      - gangrene (and obstruction) K40.10
        - not specified as recurrent K40.10
        - recurrent K40.11
      - obstruction K40.00
        - not specified as recurrent K40.00
        - recurrent K40.01
    - not specified as recurrent K40.20
    - recurrent K40.21
  - not specified as recurrent K40.90
  - recurrent K40.91

H

History (Continued)
family (Continued)
osteoporosis Z82.62
polycystic kidney Z82.71
polyps (colon) Z83.71
psychiatric disorder Z81.8
psychoactive substance abuse NEC Z81.3
respiratory condition NEC Z83.6
asthma and other lower respiratory conditions Z82.5
self-harmful behavior Z81.8
SIDS (sudden infant death syndrome) Z84.82 ◀
skin condition Z84.0
specified condition NEC Z84.89
stroke (cerebrovascular) Z82.3
substance abuse NEC Z81.4
alcohol Z81.1
drug NEC Z81.3
psychoactive NEC Z81.3
tobacco Z81.2
~~sudden cardiac death Z82.41~~
sudden ◀
cardiac death Z82.41 ◀
infant death syndrome (SIDS) Z84.82 ◀
tobacco abuse Z81.2
violence, violent behavior Z81.8
visual loss Z82.1
personal (of) —*see also* History, family (of)
abuse
adult Z91.419
physical and sexual Z91.410
psychological Z91.411
childhood Z62.819
physical Z62.810
psychological Z62.811
sexual Z62.810
alcohol dependence F10.21
allergy (to) Z88.9
analgesic agent NEC Z88.6
anesthetic Z88.4
antibiotic agent NEC Z88.1
anti-infective agent NEC Z88.3
contrast media Z91.041
drugs, medicaments and biological substances Z88.9
specified NEC Z88.8
food Z91.018
additives Z91.02
eggs Z91.012
milk products Z91.011
peanuts Z91.010
seafood Z91.013
specified food NEC Z91.018
insect Z91.038
bee Z91.030
latex Z91.040
medicinal agents Z88.9
specified NEC Z88.8
narcotic agent NEC Z88.5
nonmedicinal agents Z91.048
penicillin Z88.0
serum Z88.7
specified NEC Z91.09
sulfonamides Z88.2
vaccine Z88.7
anaphylactic shock Z87.892
anaphylaxis Z87.892
behavioral disorders Z86.59
benign carcinoid tumor Z86.012
benign neoplasm Z86.018
brain Z86.011
carcinoid Z86.012
colonic polyps Z86.010
brain injury (traumatic) Z87.820
breast implant removal Z98.86
calculi, renal Z87.442
cancer —*see* History, personal (of), malignant neoplasm (of)
cardiac arrest (death), successfully resuscitated Z86.74

History (Continued)
personal (Continued)
cerebral infarction without residual deficit Z86.73
cervical dysplasia Z87.410
chemotherapy for neoplastic condition Z92.21
childhood abuse —*see* History, personal (of), abuse
cleft lip (corrected) Z87.730
cleft palate (corrected) Z87.730
collapsed vertebra (healed) Z87.311
due to osteoporosis Z87.310
combat and operational stress reaction Z86.51
congenital malformation (corrected) Z87.798
circulatory system (corrected) Z87.74
digestive system (corrected) NEC Z87.738
ear (corrected) Z87.720
eye (corrected) Z87.721
face and neck (corrected) Z87.790
genitourinary system (corrected) NEC Z87.718
heart (corrected) Z87.74
integument (corrected) Z87.76
limb (s) (corrected) Z87.76
musculoskeletal system (corrected) Z87.76
neck (corrected) Z87.790
nervous system (corrected) NEC Z87.728
respiratory system (corrected) Z87.75
sense organs (corrected) NEC Z87.728
specified NEC Z87.798
contraception Z92.0
deployment (military) Z91.82
diabetic foot ulcer Z86.31
disease or disorder (of) Z87.898
blood and blood-forming organs Z86.2
circulatory system Z86.79
specified condition NEC Z86.79
connective tissue NEC Z87.39
digestive system Z87.19
colonic polyp Z86.010
peptic ulcer disease Z87.11
specified condition NEC Z87.19
ear Z86.69
endocrine Z86.39
diabetic foot ulcer Z86.31
gestational diabetes Z86.32
specified type NEC Z86.39
eye Z86.69
genital (track) system NEC
female Z87.42
male Z87.438
hematological Z86.2
Hodgkin Z85.71
immune mechanism Z86.2
infectious Z86.19
malaria Z86.13
Methicillin resistant Staphylococcus aureus (MRSA) Z86.14
poliomyelitis Z86.12
specified NEC Z86.19
tuberculosis Z86.11
mental NEC Z86.59
metabolic Z86.39
diabetic foot ulcer Z86.31
gestational diabetes Z86.32
specified type NEC Z86.39
musculoskeletal NEC Z87.39
nervous system Z86.69
nutritional Z86.39
parasitic Z86.19
respiratory system NEC Z87.09
sense organs Z86.69
skin Z87.2
specified site or type NEC Z87.898
subcutaneous tissue Z87.2

History (Continued)
personal (Continued)
disease or disorder (of) (Continued)
trophoblastic Z87.59
urinary system NEC Z87.448
drug dependence —*see* Dependence, drug, by type, in remission
drug therapy
antineoplastic chemotherapy Z92.21
estrogen Z92.23
immunosupression Z92.25
inhaled steroids Z92.240
monoclonal drug Z92.22
specified NEC Z92.29
steroid Z92.241
systemic steroids Z92.241
dysplasia
cervical (mild) (moderate) Z87.410 ⬅
severe (grade III) Z86.001 ◀
prostatic Z87.430
vaginal Z87.411
vulvar (mild) (moderate) Z87.412 ⬅
severe (grade III) Z86.008 ◀
embolism (venous) Z86.718
pulmonary Z86.711
encephalitis Z86.61
estrogen therapy Z92.23
extracorporeal membrane oxygenation (ECMO) Z92.81
failed conscious sedation Z92.83
failed moderate sedation Z92.83
fall, falling Z91.81
fracture (healed)
fatigue Z87.312
fragility Z87.310
osteoporosis Z87.310
pathological NEC Z87.311
stress Z87.312
traumatic Z87.81
gestational diabetes Z86.32
hepatitis
B Z86.19
C Z86.19
Hodgkin disease Z85.71
hyperthermia, malignant Z88.4
hypospadias (corrected) Z87.710
hysterectomy Z90.710
immunosupression therapy Z92.25
in situ neoplasm
breast Z86.000
cervix uteri Z86.001
specified NEC Z86.008
infection NEC Z86.19
central nervous system Z86.61
Methicillin resistant Staphylococcus aureus (MRSA) Z86.14
urinary (tract) Z87.41
injury NEC Z87.828
in utero procedure during pregnancy Z98.870
in utero procedure while a fetus Z98.871
irradiation Z92.3
kidney stones Z87.442
leukemia Z85.6
lymphoma (non-Hodgkin) Z85.72
malignant melanoma (skin) Z85.820
malignant neoplasm (of) Z85.9
accessory sinuses Z85.22
anus NEC Z85.048
carcinoid Z85.040
bladder Z85.51
bone Z85.830
brain Z85.841
breast Z85.3
bronchus NEC Z85.118
carcinoid Z85.110
carcinoid —*see* History, personal (of), malignant neoplasm, by site, carcinoid
cervix Z85.41
colon NEC Z85.038
carcinoid Z85.030

H

History *(Continued)*
- personal *(Continued)*
  - malignant neoplasm *(Continued)*
    - digestive organ Z85.ØØ
      - specified NEC Z85.Ø9
    - endocrine gland NEC Z85.858
    - epididymis Z85.48
    - esophagus Z85.Ø1
    - eye Z85.84Ø
    - gastrointestinal tract —*see* History, malignant neoplasm, digestive organ
    - genital organ
      - female Z85.4Ø
        - specified NEC Z85.44
      - male Z85.45
        - specified NEC Z85.49
    - hematopoietic NEC Z85.79
    - intrathoracic organ Z85.2Ø-
    - kidney NEC Z85.528
      - carcinoid Z85.52Ø
    - large intestine NEC Z85.Ø38
      - carcinoid Z85.Ø3Ø
    - larynx Z85.21
    - liver Z85.Ø5
    - lung NEC Z85.118
      - carcinoid Z85.11Ø
    - mediastinum Z85.29
    - Merkel cell Z85.821
    - middle ear Z85.22
    - nasal cavities Z85.22
    - nervous system NEC Z85.848
    - oral cavity Z85.819
      - specified site NEC Z85.818
    - ovary Z85.43
    - pancreas Z85.Ø7
    - pelvis Z85.53
    - pharynx Z85.819
      - specified site NEC Z85.818
    - pleura Z85.29
    - prostate Z85.46
    - rectosigmoid junction NEC Z85.Ø48
      - carcinoid Z85.Ø4Ø
    - rectum NEC Z85.Ø48
      - carcinoid Z85.Ø4Ø
    - respiratory organ Z85.2Ø
    - sinuses, accessory Z85.22
    - skin NEC Z85.828
      - melanoma Z85.82Ø
      - Merkel cell Z85.821
    - small intestine NEC Z85.Ø68
      - carcinoid Z85.Ø6Ø
    - soft tissue Z85.831
    - specified site NEC Z85.89
    - stomach NEC Z85.Ø28
      - carcinoid Z85.Ø2Ø
    - testis Z85.47
    - thymus NEC Z85.238
      - carcinoid Z85.23Ø
    - thyroid Z85.85Ø
    - tongue Z85.81Ø
    - trachea Z85.12
    - ureter Z85.54
    - urinary organ or tract Z85.5Ø
      - specified NEC Z85.59
    - uterus Z85.42
  - maltreatment Z91.89
  - medical treatment NEC Z92.89
  - melanoma (malignant) (skin) Z85.82Ø
  - meningitis Z86.61
  - mental disorder Z86.59
  - Merkel cell carcinoma (skin) Z85.821
  - Methicillin resistant Staphylococcus aureus (MRSA) Z86.14
  - military deployment Z91.82
  - military war, peacekeeping and humanitarian deployment (current or past conflict) Z91.82
  - myocardial infarction (old) I25.2
  - neglect (in)
    - adult Z91.412
    - childhood Z62.812

History *(Continued)*
- personal *(Continued)*
  - neoplasm
    - benign Z86.Ø18
      - brain Z86.Ø11
      - colon polyp Z86.Ø1Ø
    - in situ
      - breast Z86.ØØØ
      - cervix uteri Z86.ØØ1
      - specified NEC Z86.ØØ8
    - malignant —*see* History of, malignant neoplasm
    - uncertain behavior Z86.Ø3
  - nephrotic syndrome Z87.441
  - nicotine dependence Z87.891
  - noncompliance with medical treatment or regimen —*see* Noncompliance
  - nutritional deficiency Z86.39
  - obstetric complications Z87.59
    - childbirth Z87.59
    - pregnancy Z87.59
    - pre-term labor Z87.51
    - puerperium Z87.59
  - osteoporosis fractures Z87.31
  - parasuicide (attempt) Z91.5
  - physical trauma NEC Z87.828
    - self-harm or suicide attempt Z91.5
  - pneumonia (recurrent) Z87.Ø1
  - poisoning NEC Z91.89
    - self-harm or suicide attempt Z91.5
  - poor personal hygiene Z91.89
  - preterm labor Z87.51
  - procedure during pregnancy Z98.87Ø
  - procedure while a fetus Z98.871
  - prolonged reversible ischemic neurologic deficit (PRINO) Z86.73
  - prostatic dysplasia Z87.43Ø
  - psychiatric disorder NEC Z87.89
  - psychological
    - abuse
      - adult Z91.411
      - child Z62.811
    - trauma, specified NEC Z91.49
  - radiation therapy Z92.3
  - removal
    - implant
      - breast Z98.86
  - renal calculi Z87.442
  - respiratory condition NEC Z87.Ø9
  - retained foreign body fully removed Z87.821
  - risk factors NEC Z91.89
  - self-harm Z91.5
  - self-poisoning attempt Z91.5
  - sex reassignment Z87.89Ø
  - sleep-wake cycle problem Z72.821
  - specified NEC Z87.898
  - steroid therapy (systemic) Z92.241
    - inhaled Z92.24Ø
  - stroke without residual deficits Z86.73
  - substance abuse NEC F1Ø-F19 with fifth character 1
  - sudden cardiac arrest Z86.74
  - sudden cardiac death successfully resuscitated Z86.74
  - suicide attempt Z91.5
  - surgery NEC Z98.89Ø ⬅
    - with uterine scar Z98.891 ◀
    - sex reassignment Z87.89Ø
    - transplant —*see* Transplant
  - thrombophlebitis Z86.72
  - thrombosis (venous) Z86.718
    - pulmonary Z86.711
  - tobacco dependence Z87.891
  - transient ischemic attack (TIA) without residual deficits Z86.73
  - trauma (physical) NEC Z87.828
    - psychological NEC Z91.49
    - self-harm Z91.5
  - traumatic brain injury Z87.82Ø
  - unhealthy sleep-wake cycle Z72.821

History *(Continued)*
- personal *(Continued)*
  - unintended awareness under general anesthesia Z92.84 ◀
  - urinary (recurrent) (tract) infection (s) Z87.44Ø
  - urinary calculi Z87.42
  - uterine scar from previous surgery Z98.891 ◀
  - vaginal dysplasia Z87.411
  - venous thrombosis or embolism Z86.718
    - pulmonary Z86.711
  - vulvar dysplasia Z87.412

His-Werner disease A79.Ø

HIV —*see also* Human, immunodeficiency virus B2Ø
- laboratory evidence (nonconclusive) R75
- nonconclusive test (in infants) R75
- positive, seropositive Z21

Hives (bold) —*see* Urticaria

Hoarseness R49.Ø

Hobo Z59.Ø

Hodgkin disease —*see* Lymphoma, Hodgkin

Hodgson's disease I71.2
- ruptured I71.1

Hoffa-Kastert disease E88.89

Hoffa's disease E88.89

Hoffmann-Bouveret syndrome I47.9

Hoffmann's syndrome EØ3.9 *[G73.7]*

Hole (round)
- macula H35.34-
- retina (without detachment) —*see* Break, retina, round hole
  - with detachment —*see* Detachment, retina, with retinal, break

Holiday relief care Z75.5

Hollenhorst's plaque —*see* Occlusion, artery, retina

Hollow foot (congenital) Q66.7
- acquired —*see* Deformity, limb, foot, specified NEC

Holoprosencephaly QØ4.2

Holt-Oram syndrome Q87.2

Homelessness Z59.Ø

Homesickness —*see* Disorder, adjustment

Homocystinemia, homocystinuria E72.11

Homogentisate 1,2-dioxygenase deficiency E7Ø.29

Homologous serum hepatitis (prophylactic) (therapeutic) —*see* Hepatitis, viral, type B

Honeycomb lung J98.4
- congenital Q33.Ø

Hooded
- clitoris Q52.6
- penis Q55.69

Hookworm (anemia) (disease) (infection) (infestation) B76.9
- specified NEC B76.8

Hordeolum (eyelid) (externum) (recurrent) HØØ.Ø19
- internum HØØ.Ø29
  - left HØØ.Ø26
    - lower HØØ.Ø25
    - upper HØØ.Ø24
  - right HØØ.Ø23
    - lower HØØ.Ø22
    - upper HØØ.Ø21
- left HØØ.Ø16
  - lower HØØ.Ø15
  - upper HØØ.Ø14
- right HØØ.Ø13
  - lower HØØ.Ø12
  - upper HØØ.Ø11

Horn
- cutaneous L85.8
- nail L6Ø.2
  - congenital Q84.6

Horner (-Claude Bernard) **syndrome** G9Ø.2
- traumatic —*see* Injury, nerve, cervical sympathetic

H

- **Horseshoe kidney** (congenital) Q63.1
- **Horton's headache or neuralgia** G44.099
  - intractable G44.091
  - not intractable G44.099
- **Hospital hopper syndrome** —*see* Disorder, factitious
- **Hospitalism in children** —*see* Disorder, adjustment
- **Hostility** R45.5
  - towards child Z62.3
- **Hot flashes**
  - menopausal N95.1
- **Hourglass** (contracture) —*see also* Contraction, hourglass
  - stomach K31.89
    - congenital Q40.2
    - stricture K31.2
- **Household, housing circumstance affecting care** Z59.9
  - specified NEC Z59.8
- **Housemaid's knee** —*see* Bursitis, prepatellar
- **Hudson (-Stähli) line** (cornea) —*see* Pigmentation, cornea, anterior
- **Human**
  - bite (open wound) —*see also* Bite
    - intact skin surface —*see* Bite, superficial
  - herpesvirus —*see* Herpes
  - immunodeficiency virus (HIV) disease (infection) B20
    - asymptomatic status Z21
    - contact Z20.6
    - counseling Z71.7
    - dementia B20 *[F02.80]*
      - with behavioral disturbance B20 *[F02.81]*
    - exposure to Z20.6
    - laboratory evidence R75
    - type-2 (HIV 2) as cause of disease classified elsewhere B97.35
  - papillomavirus (HPV)
    - DNA test positive
      - high risk
        - cervix R87.810
        - vagina R87.811
      - low risk
        - cervix R87.820
        - vagina R87.821
    - screening for Z11.51
  - T-cell lymphotropic virus
    - type-1 (HTLV-I) infection B33.3
      - as cause of disease classified elsewhere B97.33
      - carrier Z22.6
    - type-2 (HTLV-II) as cause of disease classified elsewhere B97.34
- **Humidifier lung or pneumonitis** J67.7
- **Humiliation** (experience) **in childhood** Z62.898
- **Humpback** (acquired) —*see* Kyphosis
- **Hunchback** (acquired) —*see* Kyphosis
- **Hunger** T73.0
  - air, psychogenic F45.8
- **Hungry bone syndrome** E83.81
- **Hunner's ulcer** —*see* Cystitis, chronic, interstitial
- **Hunter's**
  - glossitis D51.0
  - syndrome E76.1
- **Huntington's disease or chorea** G10
  - with dementia G10 *[F02.80]*
    - with behavioral disturbance G10 *[F02.81]*
- **Hunt's**
  - disease or syndrome (herpetic geniculate ganglionitis) B02.21
    - dyssynergia cerebellaris myoclonica G11.1
  - neuralgia B02.21
- **Hurler (-Scheie) disease or syndrome** E76.02
- **Hurst's disease** G36.1
- **Hurthle cell**
  - adenocarcinoma C73
  - adenoma D34
  - carcinoma C73
  - tumor D34
- **Hutchinson-Boeck disease or syndrome** —*see* Sarcoidosis
- **Hutchinson-Gilford disease or syndrome** E34.8
- **Hutchinson's**
  - disease, meaning
    - angioma serpiginosum L81.7
    - pompholyx (cheiropompholyx) L30.1
    - prurigo estivalis L56.4
    - summer eruption or summer prurigo L56.4
  - melanotic freckle —*see* Melanoma, in situ
    - malignant melanoma in —*see* Melanoma
  - teeth or incisors (congenital syphilis) A50.52
  - triad (congenital syphilis) A50.53
- **Hyalin plaque, sclera, senile** H15.89
- **Hyaline membrane** (disease) (lung) (pulmonary) (newborn) P22.0
- **Hyalinosis**
  - cutis (et mucosae) E78.89
  - focal and segmental (glomerular) —*see also* N00-N07 with fourth character .1 N05.1
- **Hyalitis, hyalosis, asteroid** —*see also* Deposit, crystalline
  - syphilitic (late) A52.71
- **Hydatid**
  - cyst or tumor —*see* Echinococcus
  - mole —*see* Hydatidiform mole
  - Morgagni
    - female Q50.5
    - male (epididymal) Q55.4
      - testicular Q55.29
- **Hydatidiform mole** (benign) (complicating pregnancy) (delivered) (undelivered) O01.9
  - classical O01.0
  - complete O01.0
  - incomplete O01.1
  - invasive D39.2
  - malignant D39.2
  - partial O01.1
- **Hydatidosis** —*see* Echinococcus
- **Hydradenitis** (axillaris) (suppurative) L73.2
- **Hydradenoma** —*see* Hidradenoma
- **Hydramnios** O40.-
- **Hydrancephaly, hydranencephaly** Q04.3
  - with spina bifida —*see* Spina bifida, with hydrocephalus
- **Hydrargyrism NEC** —*see* Poisoning, mercury
- **Hydrarthrosis** —*see also* Effusion, joint
  - gonococcal A54.42
  - intermittent M12.40
    - ankle M12.47-
    - elbow M12.42-
    - foot joint M12.47-
    - hand joint M12.44-
    - hip M12.45-
    - knee M12.46-
    - multiple site M12.49
    - shoulder M12.41-
    - specified joint NEC M12.48
    - wrist M12.43-
  - of yaws (early) (late) —*see also* subcategory M14.8- A66.6
  - syphilitic (late) A52.77
    - congenital A50.55 *[M12.80]*
- **Hydremia** D64.89
- **Hydrencephalocele** (congenital) —*see* Encephalocele
- **Hydrencephalomeningocele** (congenital) —*see* Encephalocele
- **Hydroa** R23.8
  - aestivale L56.4
  - vacciniforme L56.4
- **Hydroadenitis** (axillaris) (suppurative) L73.2
- **Hydrocalycosis** —*see* Hydronephrosis
- **Hydrocele** (spermatic cord) (testis) (tunica vaginalis) N43.3
  - canal of Nuck N94.89
  - communicating N43.2
    - congenital P83.5
  - congenital P83.5
  - encysted N43.0
- **Hydrocele** *(Continued)*
  - female NEC N94.89
  - infected N43.1
  - newborn P83.5
  - round ligament N94.89
  - specified NEC N43.2
  - spinalis —*see* Spina bifida
  - vulva N90.89
- **Hydrocephalus** (acquired) (external) (internal) (malignant) (recurrent) G91.9
  - aqueduct Sylvius stricture Q03.0
  - causing disproportion O33.6
    - with obstructed labor O66.3
  - communicating G91.0
  - congenital (external) (internal) Q03.9
    - with spina bifida Q05.4
      - cervical Q05.0
      - dorsal Q05.1
      - lumbar Q05.2
      - lumbosacral Q05.2
      - sacral Q05.3
      - thoracic Q05.1
      - thoracolumbar Q05.1
    - specified NEC Q03.8
  - due to toxoplasmosis (congenital) P37.1
  - foramen Magendie block (acquired) G91.1
    - congenital —*see also* Hydrocephalus, congenital Q03.1
  - in (due to)
    - infectious disease NEC B89 *[G91.4]*
    - neoplastic disease NEC (*see also* Neoplasm) G91.4
    - parasitic disease B89 *[G91.4]*
  - newborn Q03.9
    - with spina bifida —*see* Spina bifida, with hydrocephalus
  - noncommunicating G91.1
  - normal pressure G91.2
    - secondary G91.0
  - obstructive G91.1
  - otitic G93.2
  - post-traumatic NEC G91.3
  - secondary G91.4
    - post-traumatic G91.3
  - specified NEC G91.8
  - syphilitic, congenital A50.49
- **Hydrocolpos** (congenital) N89.8
- **Hydrocystoma** —*see* Neoplasm, skin, benign
- **Hydroencephalocele** (congenital) —*see* Encephalocele
- **Hydroencephalomeningocele** (congenital) —*see* Encephalocele
- **Hydrohematopneumothorax** —*see* Hemothorax
- **Hydromeningitis** —*see* Meningitis
- **Hydromeningocele** (spinal) —*see also* Spina bifida
  - cranial —*see* Encephalocele
- **Hydrometra** N85.8
- **Hydrometrocolpos** N89.8
- **Hydromicrocephaly** Q02
- **Hydromphalos** (since birth) Q45.8
- **Hydromyelia** Q06.4
- **Hydromyelocele** —*see* Spina bifida
- **Hydronephrosis** (atrophic) (early) (functionless) (intermittent) (primary) (secondary) **NEC** N13.30
  - with
    - infection N13.6
    - obstruction (by) (of)
      - renal calculus N13.2
        - with infection N13.6
      - ureteral NEC N13.1
        - with infection N13.6
        - calculus N13.2
          - with infection N13.6
      - ureteropelvic junction (congenital) Q62.0
        - ~~with infection N13.6~~
        - acquired N13.0 ◄
          - with infection N13.6 ◄
    - ureteral stricture NEC N13.1
      - with infection N13.6

Hydronephrosis NEC *(Continued)*
  congenital Q62.Ø
    due to acquired occlusion of ureteropelvic junction N13.Ø ◀
  specified type NEC N13.39
  tuberculous A18.11
Hydropericarditis —*see* Pericarditis
Hydropericardium —*see* Pericarditis
Hydroperitoneum R18.8
Hydrophobia —*see* Rabies
Hydrophthalmos Q15.Ø
Hydropneumohemothorax —*see* Hemothorax
Hydropneumopericarditis —*see* Pericarditis
Hydropneumopericardium —*see* Pericarditis
Hydropneumothorax J94.8
  traumatic —*see* Injury, intrathoracic, lung
  tuberculous NEC A15.6
Hydrops R6Ø.9
  abdominis R18.8
  articulorum intermittens —*see* Hydrarthrosis, intermittent
  cardiac —*see* Failure, heart, congestive
  causing obstructed labor (mother) O66.3
  endolymphatic H81.Ø-
  fetal —*see* Pregnancy, complicated by, hydrops, fetalis
  fetalis P83.2
    due to
      ABO isoimmunization P56.Ø
      alpha thalassemia D56.Ø
      hemolytic disease P56.9Ø
        specified NEC P56.99
      isoimmunization (ABO) (Rh) P56.Ø
      other specified nonhemolytic disease NEC P83.2
      Rh incompatibility P56.Ø
    during pregnancy —*see* Pregnancy, complicated by, hydrops, fetalis
  gallbladder K82.1
  joint —*see* Effusion, joint
  labyrinth H81.Ø
  newborn (idiopathic) P83.2
    due to
      ABO isoimmunization P56.Ø
      alpha thalassemia D56.Ø
      hemolytic disease P56.9Ø
        specified NEC P56.99
      isoimmunization (ABO) (Rh) P56.Ø
      Rh incompatibility P56.Ø
  nutritional —*see* Malnutrition, severe
  pericardium —*see* Pericarditis
  pleura —*see* Hydrothorax
  spermatic cord —*see* Hydrocele
Hydropyonephrosis N13.6
Hydrorachis QØ6.4
Hydrorrhea (nasal) J34.89
  pregnancy —*see* Rupture, membranes, premature
Hydrosadenitis (axillaris) (suppurative) L73.2
Hydrosalpinx (fallopian tube) (follicularis) N7Ø.11
Hydrothorax (double) (pleura) J94.8
  chylous (nonfilarial) I89.8
    filarial —*see also* Infestation, filarial B74.9 *[J91.8]*
  traumatic —*see* Injury, intrathoracic
  tuberculous NEC (non primary) A15.6
Hydroureter —*see also* Hydronephrosis N13.4
  with infection N13.6
  congenital Q62.39
Hydroureteronephrosis —*see* Hydronephrosis
Hydrourethra N36.8
Hydroxykynureninuria E7Ø.8
Hydroxylysinemia E72.3
Hydroxyprolinemia E72.59
Hygiene, sleep
  abuse Z72.821
  inadequate Z72.821
  poor Z72.821
Hygroma (congenital) (cystic) D18.1
  praepatellare, prepatellar —*see* Bursitis, prepatellar

Hymen —*see* condition
Hymenolepis, hymenolepiasis (diminuta) (infection) (infestation) (nana) B71.Ø
Hypalgesia R2Ø.8
Hyperacidity (gastric) K31.89
  psychogenic F45.8
Hyperactive, hyperactivity F9Ø.9
  basal cell, uterine cervix —*see* Dysplasia, cervix
  bowel sounds R19.12
  cervix epithelial (basal) —*see* Dysplasia, cervix
  child F9Ø.9
    attention deficit —*see* Disorder, attention-deficit hyperactivity
  detrusor muscle N32.81
  gastrointestinal K31.89
    psychogenic F45.8
  nasal mucous membrane J34.3
  stomach K31.89
  thyroid (gland) —*see* Hyperthyroidism
Hyperacusis H93.23-
Hyperadrenalism E27.5
Hyperadrenocorticism E24.9
  congenital E25.Ø
  iatrogenic E24.2
    correct substance properly administered —*see* Table of Drugs and Chemicals, by drug, adverse effect
    overdose or wrong substance given or taken —*see* Table of Drugs and Chemicals, by drug, poisoning
  not associated with Cushing's syndrome E27.Ø
  pituitary-dependent E24.Ø
Hyperaldosteronism E26.9
  familial (type I) E26.Ø2
  glucocorticoid-remediable E26.Ø2
  primary (due to (bilateral) adrenal hyperplasia) E26.Ø9
  primary NEC E26.Ø9
  secondary E26.1
  specified NEC E26.89
Hyperalgesia R2Ø.8
Hyperalimentation R63.2
  carotene, carotin E67.1
  specified NEC E67.8
  vitamin
    A E67.Ø
    D E67.3
Hyperaminoaciduria
  arginine E72.21
  cystine E72.Ø1
  lysine E72.3
  ornithine E72.4
Hyperammonemia (congenital) E72.2Ø
Hyperazotemia —*see* Uremia
Hyperbetalipoproteinemia (familial) E78.ØØ ⬅
  with prebetalipoproteinemia E78.2
Hyperbilirubinemia
  constitutional E8Ø.6
  familial conjugated E8Ø.6
  neonatal (transient) —*see* Jaundice, newborn
Hypercalcemia, hypocalciuric, familial E83.52
Hypercalciuria, idiopathic E83.52
Hypercapnia RØ6.89
  newborn P84
Hypercarotenemia, hypercarotinemia (dietary) E67.1
Hypercementosis KØ3.4
Hyperchloremia E87.8
Hyperchlorhydria K31.89
  neurotic F45.8
  psychogenic F45.8
Hypercholesterinemia —*see* Hypercholesterolemia
Hypercholesterolemia (essential) (primary) (pure) E78.ØØ ⬅
  with hyperglyceridemia, endogenous E78.2
  dietary counseling and surveillance Z71.3
  familial E78.Ø1 ◀
  hereditary E78.Ø1 ◀

Hyperchylia gastrica, psychogenic F45.8
Hyperchylomicronemia (familial) (primary) E78.3
  with hyperbetalipoproteinemia E78.3
Hypercoagulable (state) D68.59
  activated protein C resistance D68.51
  antithrombin (III) deficiency D68.59
  factor V Leiden mutation D68.51
  primary NEC D68.59
  protein C deficiency D68.59
  protein S deficiency D68.59
  prothrombin gene mutation D68.52
  secondary D68.69
  specified NEC D68.69
Hypercoagulation (state) D68.59
Hypercorticalism, pituitary-dependent E24.Ø
Hypercorticosolism —*see* Cushing's, syndrome
Hypercorticosteronism E24.2
  correct substance properly administered —*see* Table of Drugs and Chemicals, by drug, adverse effect
  overdose or wrong substance given or taken —*see* Table of Drugs and Chemicals, by drug, poisoning
Hypercortisonism E24.2
  correct substance properly administered —*see* Table of Drugs and Chemicals, by drug, adverse effect
  overdose or wrong substance given or taken —*see* Table of Drugs and Chemicals, by drug, poisoning
Hyperekplexia Q89.8
Hyperelectrolytemia E87.8
Hyperemesis R11.1Ø
  with nausea R11.2
  gravidarum (mild) O21.Ø
    with
      carbohydrate depletion O21.1
      dehydration O21.1
      electrolyte imbalance O21.1
      metabolic disturbance O21.1
    severe (with metabolic disturbance) O21.1
  projectile R11.12
  psychogenic F45.8
Hyperemia (acute) (passive) R68.89
  anal mucosa K62.89
  bladder N32.89
  cerebral I67.89
  conjunctiva H11.43-
  ear internal, acute —*see* subcategory H83.Ø
  enteric K59.8
  eye —*see* Hyperemia, conjunctiva
  eyelid (active) (passive) —*see* Disorder, eyelid, specified type NEC
  intestine K59.8
  iris —*see* Disorder, iris, vascular
  kidney N28.89
  labyrinth —*see* subcategory H83.Ø
  liver (active) K76.89
  lung (passive) —*see* Edema, lung
  pulmonary (passive) —*see* Edema, lung
  renal N28.89
  retina H35.89
  stomach K31.89
Hyperesthesia (body surface) R2Ø.3
  larynx (reflex) J38.7
    hysterical F44.89
  pharynx (reflex) J39.2
    hysterical F44.89
Hyperestrogenism (drug-induced) (iatrogenic) E28.Ø
Hyperexplexia Q89.8
Hyperfibrinolysis —*see* Fibrinolysis
Hyperfructosemia E74.19
Hyperfunction
  adrenal cortex, not associated with Cushing's syndrome E27.Ø
    medulla E27.5
      adrenomedullary E27.5
    virilism E25.9
      congenital E25.Ø

H

Hyperfunction *(Continued)*
  ovarian E28.8
  pancreas K86.89
  parathyroid (gland) E21.3
  pituitary (gland) (anterior) E22.9
    specified NEC E22.8
  polyglandular E31.1
  testicular E29.Ø
Hypergammaglobulinemia D89.2
  polyclonal D89.Ø
  Waldenström D89.Ø
Hypergastrinemia E16.4
Hyperglobulinemia R77.1
Hyperglycemia, hyperglycemic (transient) R73.9
  coma —*see* Diabetes, by type, with coma
  postpancreatectomy E89.1
Hyperglyceridemia (endogenous) (essential) (familial) (hereditary) (pure) E78.1
  mixed E78.3
Hyperglycinemia (non-ketotic) E72.51
Hypergonadism
  ovarian E28.8
  testicular (primary) (infantile) E29.Ø
Hyperheparinemia D68.32
Hyperhidrosis, hyperidrosis R61
  focal
    primary L74.519
      axilla L74.51Ø
      face L74.511
      palms L74.512
      soles L74.513
    secondary L74.52
  generalized R61
  localized
    primary L74.519
      axilla L74.51Ø
      face L74.511
      palms L74.512
      soles L74.513
    secondary L74.52
  psychogenic F45.8
  secondary R61
    focal L74.52
Hyperhistidinemia E7Ø.41
Hyperhomocysteinemia E72.11
Hyperhydroxyprolinemia E72.59
Hyperinsulinism (functional) E16.1
  with
    coma (hypoglycemic) E15
    encephalopathy E16.1 *[G94]*
  ectopic E16.1
  therapeutic misadventure (from administration of insulin) —*see* subcategory T38.3
Hyperkalemia E87.5
Hyperkeratosis —*see also* Keratosis L85.9
  cervix N88.Ø
  due to yaws (early) (late) (palmar or plantar) A66.3
  follicularis Q82.8
    penetrans (in cutem) L87.Ø
  palmoplantaris climacterica L85.1
  pinta A67.1
  senile (with pruritus) L57.Ø
  universalis congenita Q8Ø.8
  vocal cord J38.3
  vulva N9Ø.4
Hyperkinesia, hyperkinetic (disease) (reaction) (syndrome) (childhood) (adolescence) —*see also* Disorder, attention-deficit hyperactivity
  heart I51.89
Hyperleucine-isoleucinemia E71.19
Hyperlipemia, hyperlipidemia E78.5
  combined E78.2
    familial E78.4
  group
    A E78.ØØ
    B E78.1
    C E78.2
    D E78.3
  mixed E78.2
  specified NEC E78.4
Hyperlipidosis E75.6
  hereditary NEC E75.5
Hyperlipoproteinemia E78.5
  Fredrickson's type
    I E78.3
    IIa E78.ØØ
    IIb E78.2
    III E78.2
    IV E78.1
    V E78.3
  low-density-lipoprotein-type (LDL) E78.ØØ
  very-low-density-lipoprotein-type (VLDL) E78.1
Hyperlucent lung, unilateral J43.Ø
Hyperlysinemia E72.3
Hypermagnesemia E83.41
  neonatal P71.8
Hypermenorrhea N92.Ø
Hypermethioninemia E72.19
Hypermetropia (congenital) H52.Ø-
Hypermobility, hypermotility
  cecum —*see* Syndrome, irritable bowel
  coccyx —*see* subcategory M53.2
  colon —*see* Syndrome, irritable bowel
    psychogenic F45.8
  ileum K58.9
  intestine —*see also* Syndrome, irritable bowel K58.9
    psychogenic F45.8
  meniscus (knee) —*see* Derangement, knee, meniscus
  scapula —*see* Instability, joint, shoulder
  stomach K31.89
    psychogenic F45.8
  syndrome M35.7
  urethra N36.41
    with intrinsic sphincter deficiency N36.43
Hypernasality R49.21
Hypernatremia E87.Ø
Hypernephroma C64.-
Hyperopia —*see* Hypermetropia
Hyperorexia nervosa F5Ø.2
Hyperornithinemia E72.4
Hyperosmia R43.1
Hyperosmolality E87.Ø
Hyperostosis (monomelic) —*see also* Disorder, bone, density and structure, specified NEC
  ankylosing (spine) M48.1Ø
    cervical region M48.12
    cervicothoracic region M48.13
    lumbar region M48.16
    lumbosacral region M48.17
    multiple sites M48.19
    occipito-atlanto-axial region M48.11
    sacrococcygeal region M48.18
    thoracic region M48.14
    thoracolumbar region M48.15
  cortical (skull) M85.2
    infantile M89.8X-
  frontal, internal of skull M85.2
  interna frontalis M85.2
  skeletal, diffuse idiopathic —*see* Hyperostosis, ankylosing
  skull M85.2
    congenital Q75.8
  vertebral, ankylosing —*see* Hyperostosis, ankylosing
Hyperovarism E28.8
Hyperoxaluria (primary) E72.53
Hyperparathyroidism E21.3
  primary E21.Ø
  secondary (renal) N25.81
    non-renal E21.1
  specified NEC E21.2
  tertiary E21.2
Hyperpathia R2Ø.8
Hyperperistalsis R19.2
  psychogenic F45.8
Hyperpermeability, capillary I78.8
Hyperphagia R63.2
Hyperphenylalaninemia NEC E7Ø.1
Hyperphoria (alternating) H5Ø.53
Hyperphosphatemia E83.39
Hyperpiesis, hyperpiesia —*see* Hypertension
Hyperpigmentation —*see also* Pigmentation
  melanin NEC L81.4
  postinflammatory L81.Ø
Hyperpinealism E34.8
Hyperpituitarism E22.9
Hyperplasia, hyperplastic
  adenoids J35.2
  adrenal (capsule) (cortex) (gland) E27.8
    with
      sexual precocity (male) E25.9
        congenital E25.Ø
      virilism, adrenal E25.9
        congenital E25.Ø
      virilization (female) E25.9
        congenital E25.Ø
    congenital E25.Ø
      salt-losing E25.Ø
  adrenomedullary E27.5
  angiolymphoid, eosinophilia (ALHE) D18.Ø1
  appendix (lymphoid) K38.Ø
  artery, fibromuscular I77.3
  bone —*see also* Hypertrophy, bone
    marrow D75.89
  breast —*see also* Hypertrophy, breast
    ductal (atypical) N6Ø.9-
  C-cell, thyroid EØ7.Ø
  cementation (tooth) (teeth) KØ3.4
  cervical gland R59.Ø
  cervix (uteri) (basal cell) (endometrium) (polypoid) —*see also* Dysplasia, cervix
    congenital Q51.828
  clitoris, congenital Q52.6
  denture KØ6.2
  endocervicitis N72
  endometrium, endometrial (adenomatous) (benign) (cystic) (glandular) (glandular-cystic) (polypoid) N85.ØØ
    with atypia N85.Ø2
    cervix —*see* Dysplasia, cervix
    complex (without atypia) N85.Ø1
    simple (without atypia) N85.Ø1
  epithelial L85.9
    focal, oral, including tongue K13.29
    nipple N62
    skin L85.9
    tongue K13.29
    vaginal wall N89.3
  erythroid D75.89
  fibromuscular of artery (carotid) (renal) I77.3
  genital
    female NEC N94.89
    male N5Ø.89
  gingiva KØ6.1
  glandularis cystica uteri (interstitialis) —*see also* Hyperplasia, endometrial N85.ØØ-
  gum KØ6.1
  hymen, congenital Q52.4
  irritative, edentulous (alveolar) KØ6.2
  jaw M26.Ø9
    alveolar M26.79
    lower M26.Ø3
      alveolar M26.72
    upper M26.Ø1
      alveolar M26.71
  kidney (congenital) Q63.3
  labia N9Ø.69
    epithelial N9Ø.3
  liver (congenital) Q44.7
    nodular, focal K76.89
  lymph gland or node R59.9
  mandible, mandibular M26.Ø3
    alveolar M26.72
    unilateral condylar M27.8
  maxilla, maxillary M26.Ø1
    alveolar M26.71
  myometrium, myometrial N85.2
  neuroendocrine cell, of infancy J84.841

Hyperplasia, hyperplastic *(Continued)*
nose
lymphoid J34.89
polypoid J33.9
oral mucosa (irritative) K13.6
organ or site, congenital NEC —*see* Anomaly, by site
ovary N83.8
palate, papillary (irritative) K13.6
pancreatic islet cells E16.9
alpha E16.8
with excess
gastrin E16.4
glucagon E16.3
beta E16.1
parathyroid (gland) E21.0
pharynx (lymphoid) J39.2
prostate (adenofibromatous) (nodular) N40.0
with lower urinary tract symptoms (LUTS) N40.1
without lower urinary tract symptoms (LUTS) N40.0
renal artery I77.89
reticulo-endothelial (cell) D75.89
salivary gland (any) K11.1
Schimmelbusch's —*see* Mastopathy, cystic
suprarenal capsule (gland) E27.8
thymus (gland) (persistent) E32.0
thyroid (gland) —*see* Goiter
tonsils (faucial) (infective) (lingual) (lymphoid) J35.1
with adenoids J35.3
unilateral condylar M27.8
uterus, uterine N85.2
endometrium (glandular) —*see also* Hyperplasia, endometrial N85.00-
vulva N90.69 ⬅
epithelial N90.3
Hyperpnea —*see* Hyperventilation
Hyperpotassemia E87.5
Hyperprebetalipoproteinemia (familial) E78.1
Hyperprolactinemia E22.1
Hyperprolinemia (type I) (type II) E72.59
Hyperproteinemia E88.09
Hyperprothrombinemia, causing coagulation factor deficiency D68.4
Hyperpyrexia R50.9
heat (effects) T67.0
malignant, due to anesthetic T88.3
rheumatic —*see* Fever, rheumatic
unknown origin R50.9
Hyper-reflexia R29.2
Hypersalivation K11.7
Hypersecretion
ACTH (not associated with Cushing's syndrome) E27.0
pituitary E24.0
adrenaline E27.5
adrenomedullary E27.5
androgen (testicular) E29.0
ovarian (drug-induced) (iatrogenic) E28.1
calcitonin E07.0
catecholamine E27.5
corticoadrenal E24.9
cortisol E24.9
epinephrine E27.5
estrogen E28.0
gastric K31.89
psychogenic F45.8
gastrin E16.4
glucagon E16.3
hormone (s)
ACTH (not associated with Cushing's syndrome) E27.0
pituitary E24.0
antidiuretic E22.2
growth E22.0

Hypersecretion *(Continued)*
hormone *(Continued)*
intestinal NEC E34.1
ovarian androgen E28.1
pituitary E22.9
testicular E29.0
thyroid stimulating E05.80
with thyroid storm E05.81
insulin —*see* Hyperinsulinism
lacrimal glands —*see* Epiphora
medulloadrenal E27.5
milk O92.6
ovarian androgens E28.1
salivary gland (any) K11.7
thyrocalcitonin E07.0
upper respiratory J39.8
Hypersegmentation, leukocytic, hereditary D72.0
Hypersensitive, hypersensitiveness, hypersensitivity —*see also* Allergy
carotid sinus G90.01
colon —*see* Irritable, colon
drug T88.7
gastrointestinal K52.29 ⬅
immediate K52.29 ◀
psychogenic F45.8
labyrinth —*see* subcategory H83.2
pain R20.8
pneumonitis —*see* Pneumonitis, allergic
reaction T78.40
upper respiratory tract NEC J39.3
Hypersomnia (organic) G47.10
due to
alcohol
abuse F10.182
dependence F10.282
use F10.982
amphetamines
abuse F15.182
dependence F15.282
use F15.982
caffeine
abuse F15.182
dependence F15.282
use F15.982
cocaine
abuse F14.182
dependence F14.282
use F14.982
drug NEC
abuse F19.182
dependence F19.282
use F19.982
medical condition G47.14
mental disorder F51.13
opioid
abuse F11.182
dependence F11.282
use F11.982
psychoactive substance NEC
abuse F19.182
dependence F19.282
use F19.982
sedative, hypnotic, or anxiolytic
abuse F13.182
dependence F13.282
use F13.982
stimulant NEC
abuse F15.182
dependence F15.282
use F15.982
idiopathic G47.11
with long sleep time G47.11
without long sleep time G47.12
menstrual related G47.13
nonorganic origin F51.11
specified NEC F51.19
not due to a substance or known physiological condition F51.11
specified NEC F51.19

Hypersomnia *(Continued)*
primary F51.11
recurrent G47.13
specified NEC G47.19
Hypersplenia, hypersplenism D73.1
Hyperstimulation, ovaries (associated with induced ovulation) N98.1
Hypersusceptibility —*see* Allergy
Hypertelorism (ocular) (orbital) Q75.2
Hypertension, hypertensive (accelerated) (benign) (essential) (idiopathic) (malignant) (systemic) I10
with
heart involvement (conditions in I51.4-I51.9 due to hypertension) —*see* Hypertension, heart
kidney involvement —*see* Hypertension, kidney
benign, intracranial G93.2
borderline R03.0
cardiorenal (disease) I13.10
with heart failure I13.0
with stage 1 through stage 4 chronic kidney disease I13.0
with stage 5 or end stage renal disease I13.2
without heart failure I13.10
with stage 1 through stage 4 chronic kidney disease I13.10
with stage 5 or end stage renal disease I13.11
cardiovascular
disease (arteriosclerotic) (sclerotic) —*see* Hypertension, heart
renal (disease) —*see* Hypertension, cardiorenal
chronic venous —*see* Hypertension, venous (chronic)
complicating
childbirth (labor) O16.4 ⬅
~~with~~
~~heart disease O10.12~~
~~with renal disease O10.32~~
~~renal disease O10.22~~
~~with heart disease O10.32~~
~~essential O10.02~~
pre-existing O10.92 ◀
with ◀
heart disease O10.12 ◀
with renal disease O10.32 ◀
pre-eclampsia O11.4 ◀
renal disease O10.22 ◀
with heart disease O10.32 ◀
essential O10.02 ◀
secondary O10.42
pregnancy O16.-
with edema —*see also* Pre-eclampsia O14.9-
gestational (pregnancy induced) (without proteinuria) O13.- ⬅
with proteinuria O14.9-
mild pre-eclampsia O14.0-
moderate pre-eclampsia O14.0-
severe pre-eclampsia O14.1-
with hemolysis, elevated liver enzymes and low platelet count (HELLP) O14.2-
pre-existing O10.91-
with
heart disease O10.11-
with renal disease O10.31-
pre-eclampsia —*see* category O11 ⬅
renal disease O10.21-
with heart disease O10.31-
essential O10.01-
secondary O10.41-
transient O13.- ◀

H

Hypertension, hypertensive *(Continued)*
complicating *(Continued)*
puerperium pre-existing O16.5 ⬅
~~with~~
~~heart disease O1Ø.13~~
~~with renal disease O1Ø.33~~
~~renal disease O1Ø.23~~
~~with heart disease O1Ø.33~~
~~essential O1Ø.Ø3~~
pre-existing ◀
with ◀
heart disease O1Ø.13 ◀
with renal disease O1Ø.33 ◀
pre-eclampsia O11.5 ◀
renal disease O1Ø.23 ◀
with heart disease O1Ø.33 ◀
essential O1Ø.Ø3 ◀
pregnancy-induced O13.9
secondary O1Ø.43
crisis I16.9 ◀
due to
endocrine disorders I15.2
pheochromocytoma I15.2
renal disorders NEC I15.1
arterial I15.Ø
renovascular disorders I15.Ø
specified disease NEC I15.8
emergency I16.2 ◀
encephalopathy I67.4
gestational (without significant proteinuria) (pregnancy-induced) (transient) O13.-
with significant proteinuria —*see* Pre-eclampsia
complicating ◀
delivery O13.4 ◀
puerperium O13.5 ◀
Goldblatt's I7Ø.1
heart (disease) (conditions in I51.4-I51.9 due to hypertension) I11.9
with
heart failure (congestive) I11.Ø
kidney disease (chronic) —*see* Hypertension, cardiorenal
intracranial (benign) G93.2
kidney I12.9
with
heart disease —*see* Hypertension, cardiorenal
stage 1 through stage 4 chronic kidney disease I12.9
stage 5 chronic kidney disease (CKD) or end stage renal disease (ESRD) I12.Ø
lesser circulation I27.Ø
maternal O16.- ◀
newborn P29.2
pulmonary (persistent) P29.3
ocular H4Ø.Ø5-
pancreatic duct — code to underlying condition
with chronic pancreatitis K86.1
portal (due to chronic liver disease) (idiopathic) K76.6
gastropathy K31.89
in (due to) schistosomiasis (bilharziasis) B65.9 *[K77]*
postoperative I97.3
psychogenic F45.8
pulmonary (artery) (secondary) NEC I27.2
with
cor pulmonale (chronic) I27.2
acute I26.Ø9
right heart ventricular strain/failure I27.2
acute I26.Ø9
of newborn (persistent) P29.3
primary (idiopathic) I27.Ø
renal —*see* Hypertension, kidney
renovascular I15.Ø

Hypertension, hypertensive *(Continued)*
secondary NEC I15.9
due to
endocrine disorders I15.2
pheochromocytoma I15.2
renal disorders NEC I15.1
arterial I15.Ø
renovascular disorders I15.Ø
specified NEC I15.8
transient, of pregnancy O13.- ◀
urgency I16.Ø ◀
venous (chronic)
due to
deep vein thrombosis —*see* Syndrome, postthrombotic
idiopathic I87.3Ø9
with
inflammation I87.32-
with ulcer I87.33-
specified complication NEC I87.39-
ulcer I87.31-
with inflammation I87.33-
asymptomatic I87.3Ø-
Hypertensive urgency —*see* Hypertension
Hyperthecosis ovary E28.8
Hyperthermia (of unknown origin) —*see also* Hyperpyrexia
malignant, due to anesthesia T88.3
newborn P81.9
environmental P81.Ø
Hyperthyroid (recurrent) —*see* Hyperthyroidism
Hyperthyroidism (latent) (pre-adult) (recurrent) EØ5.9Ø
with
goiter (diffuse) EØ5.ØØ
with thyroid storm EØ5.Ø1
nodular (multinodular) EØ5.2Ø
with thyroid storm EØ5.21
uninodular EØ5.1Ø
with thyroid storm EØ5.11
storm EØ5.91
due to ectopic thyroid tissue EØ5.3Ø
with thyroid storm EØ5.31
neonatal, transitory P72.1
specified NEC EØ5.8Ø
with thyroid storm EØ5.81
Hypertony, hypertonia, hypertonicity
bladder N31.8
congenital P94.1
stomach K31.89
psychogenic F45.8
uterus, uterine (contractions) (complicating delivery) O62.4
Hypertrichosis L68.9
congenital Q84.2
eyelid HØ2.869
left HØ2.866
lower HØ2.865
upper HØ2.864
right HØ2.863
lower HØ2.862
upper HØ2.861
lanuginosa Q84.2
acquired L68.1
localized L68.2
specified NEC L68.8
Hypertriglyceridemia, essential E78.1
Hypertrophy, hypertrophic
adenofibromatous, prostate —*see* Enlargement, enlarged, prostate
adenoids (infective) J35.2
with tonsils J35.3
adrenal cortex E27.8
alveolar process or ridge —*see* Anomaly, alveolar
anal papillae K62.89
artery I77.89
congenital NEC Q27.8
digestive system Q27.8
lower limb Q27.8

Hypertrophy, hypertrophic *(Continued)*
artery *(Continued)*
congenital NEC *(Continued)*
specified site NEC Q27.8
upper limb Q27.8
auricular —*see* Hypertrophy, cardiac
Bartholin's gland N75.8
bile duct (common) (hepatic) K83.8
bladder (sphincter) (trigone) N32.89
bone M89.3Ø
carpus M89.34-
clavicle M89.31-
femur M89.35-
fibula M89.36-
finger M89.34-
humerus M89.32-
ilium M89.359
ischium M89.359
metacarpus M89.34-
metatarsus M89.37-
multiple sites M89.39
neck M89.38
radius M89.33-
rib M89.38
scapula M89.31-
skull M89.38
tarsus M89.37-
tibia M89.36-
toe M89.37-
ulna M89.33-
vertebra M89.38
brain G93.89
breast N62
cystic —*see* Mastopathy, cystic
newborn P83.4
pubertal, massive N62
puerperal, postpartum —*see* Disorder, breast, specified type NEC
senile (parenchymatous) N62
cardiac (chronic) (idiopathic) I51.7
with rheumatic fever (conditions in IØØ)
active IØ1.8
inactive or quiescent (with chorea) IØ9.89
congenital NEC Q24.8
fatty —*see* Degeneration, myocardial
hypertensive —*see* Hypertension, heart
rheumatic (with chorea) IØ9.89
active or acute IØ1.8
with chorea IØ2.Ø
valve —*see* Endocarditis
cartilage —*see* Disorder, cartilage, specified type NEC
cecum —*see* Megacolon
cervix (uteri) N88.8
congenital Q51.828
elongation N88.4
clitoris (cirrhotic) N9Ø.89
congenital Q52.6
colon —*see also* Megacolon
congenital Q43.2
conjunctiva, lymphoid H11.89
corpora cavernosa N48.89
cystic duct K82.8
duodenum K31.89
endometrium (glandular) —*see also* Hyperplasia, endometrial N85.ØØ-
cervix N88.8
epididymis N5Ø.89 ⬅
esophageal hiatus (congenital) Q79.1
with hernia —*see* Hernia, hiatal
eyelid —*see* Disorder, eyelid, specified type NEC
fat pad E65
knee (infrapatellar) (popliteal) (prepatellar) (retropatellar) M79.4
foot (congenital) Q74.2
frenulum, frenum (tongue) K14.8
lip K13.Ø
gallbladder K82.8
gastric mucosa K29.6Ø
with bleeding K29.61

Hypertrophy, hypertrophic *(Continued)*
- gland, glandular R59.9
  - generalized R59.1
  - localized R59.Ø
- gum (mucous membrane) KØ6.1
- heart (idiopathic) —*see also* Hypertrophy, cardiac
  - valve —*see also* Endocarditis I38
- hemifacial Q67.4
- hepatic —*see* Hypertrophy, liver
- hiatus (esophageal) Q79.1
- hilus gland R59.Ø
- hymen, congenital Q52.4
- ileum K63.89
- intestine NEC K63.89
- jejunum K63.89
- kidney (compensatory) N28.81
  - congenital Q63.3
- labium (majus) (minus) N9Ø.6Ø ◄
- ligament —*see* Disorder, ligament
- lingual tonsil (infective) J35.1
  - with adenoids J35.3
- lip K13.Ø
  - congenital Q18.6
- liver R16.Ø
  - acute K76.89
  - cirrhotic —*see* Cirrhosis, liver
  - congenital Q44.7
  - fatty —*see* Fatty, liver
- lymph, lymphatic gland R59.9
  - generalized R59.1
  - localized R59.Ø
  - tuberculous —*see* Tuberculosis, lymph gland
- mammary gland —*see* Hypertrophy, breast
- Meckel's diverticulum (congenital) Q43.Ø
  - malignant —*see* Table of Neoplasms, small intestine, malignant
- median bar —*see* Hyperplasia, prostate
- meibomian gland —*see* Chalazion
- meniscus, knee, congenital Q74.1
- metatarsal head —*see* Hypertrophy, bone, metatarsus
- metatarsus —*see* Hypertrophy, bone, metatarsus
- mucous membrane
  - alveolar ridge KØ6.2
  - gum KØ6.1
  - nose (turbinate) J34.3
- muscle M62.89
- muscular coat, artery I77.89
- myocardium —*see also* Hypertrophy, cardiac
  - idiopathic I42.2
- myometrium N85.2
- nail L6Ø.2
  - congenital Q84.5
- nasal J34.89
  - alae J34.89
  - bone J34.89
  - cartilage J34.89
  - mucous membrane (septum) J34.3
  - sinus J34.89
  - turbinate J34.3
- nasopharynx, lymphoid (infectional) (tissue) (wall) J35.2
- nipple N62
- organ or site, congenital NEC —*see* Anomaly, by site - ovary N83.8
- palate (hard) M27.8
  - soft K13.79
- pancreas, congenital Q45.3
- parathyroid (gland) E21.Ø
- parotid gland K11.1
- penis N48.89
- pharyngeal tonsil J35.2
- pharynx J39.2
  - lymphoid (infectional) (tissue) (wall) J35.2
- pituitary (anterior) (fossa) (gland) E23.6
- prepuce (congenital) N47.8
  - female N9Ø.89

Hypertrophy, hypertrophic *(Continued)*
- prostate —*see* Enlargement, enlarged, prostate
  - congenital Q55.4
- pseudomuscular G71.Ø
- pylorus (adult) (muscle) (sphincter) K31.1
  - congenital or infantile Q4Ø.Ø
- rectal, rectum (sphincter) K62.89
- rhinitis (turbinate) J31.Ø
- salivary gland (any) K11.1
  - congenital Q38.4
- scaphoid (tarsal) —*see* Hypertrophy, bone, tarsus
- scar L91.Ø
- scrotum N5Ø.89 ◄
- seminal vesicle N5Ø.89 ◄
- sigmoid —*see* Megacolon
- skin L91.9
  - specified NEC L91.8
- spermatic cord N5Ø.89 ◄
- spleen —*see* Splenomegaly
- spondylitis —*see* Spondylosis
- stomach K31.89
- sublingual gland K11.1
- submandibular gland K11.1
- suprarenal cortex (gland) E27.8
- synovial NEC M67.2Ø
  - acromioclavicular M67.21-
  - ankle M67.27-
  - elbow M67.22-
  - foot M67.27-
  - hand M67.24-
  - hip M67.25-
  - knee M67.26-
  - multiple sites M67.29
  - specified site NEC M67.28
  - wrist M67.23-
- tendon —*see* Disorder, tendon, specified type NEC
- testis N44.8
  - congenital Q55.29
- thymic, thymus (gland) (congenital) E32.Ø
- thyroid (gland) —*see* Goiter
- toe (congenital) Q74.2
  - acquired —*see also* Deformity, toe, specified NEC
- tongue K14.8
  - congenital Q38.2
  - papillae (foliate) K14.3
- tonsils (faucial) (infective) (lingual) (lymphoid) J35.1
  - with adenoids J35.3
- tunica vaginalis N5Ø.89 ◄
- ureter N28.89
- urethra N36.8
- uterus N85.2
  - neck (with elongation) N88.4
  - puerperal O9Ø.89
- uvula K13.79
- vagina N89.8
- vas deferens N5Ø.89 ◄
- vein I87.8
- ventricle, ventricular (heart) —*see also* Hypertrophy, cardiac
  - congenital Q24.8
  - in tetralogy of Fallot Q21.3
- verumontanum N36.8
- vocal cord J38.3
- vulva N9Ø.6Ø ◄
  - stasis (nonfilarial) N9Ø.69 ◄

Hypertropia H5Ø.2-

Hypertyrosinemia E7Ø.21

Hyperuricemia (asymptomatic) E79.Ø

Hypervalinemia E71.19

Hyperventilation (tetany) RØ6.4
- hysterical F45.8
- psychogenic F45.8
- syndrome F45.8

Hypervitaminosis (dietary) NEC E67.8
- A E67.Ø
  - administered as drug (prolonged intake) —*see* Table of Drugs and Chemicals, vitamins, adverse effect
  - overdose or wrong substance given or taken —*see* Table of Drugs and Chemicals, vitamins, poisoning
- B6 E67.2
- D E67.3
  - administered as drug (prolonged intake) —*see* Table of Drugs and Chemicals, vitamins, adverse effect
  - overdose or wrong substance given or taken —*see* Table of Drugs and Chemicals, vitamins, poisoning
- K E67.8
  - administered as drug (prolonged intake) —*see* Table of Drugs and Chemicals, vitamins, adverse effect
  - overdose or wrong substance given or taken —*see* Table of Drugs and Chemicals, vitamins, poisoning

Hypervolemia E87.7Ø
- specified NEC E87.79

Hypesthesia R2Ø.1
- cornea —*see* Anesthesia, cornea

Hyphema H21.Ø
- traumatic SØ5.1-

Hypoacidity, gastric K31.89
- psychogenic F45.8

Hypoadrenalism, hypoadrenia E27.4Ø
- primary E27.1
- tuberculous A18.7

Hypoadrenocorticism E27.4Ø
- pituitary E23.Ø
- primary E27.1

Hypoalbuminemia E88.Ø9

Hypoaldosteronism E27.4Ø

Hypoalphalipoproteinemia E78.6

Hypobarism T7Ø.29

Hypobaropathy T7Ø.29

Hypobetalipoproteinemia (familial) E78.6

Hypocalcemia E83.51
- dietary E58
- neonatal P71.1
  - due to cow's milk P71.Ø
- phosphate-loading (newborn) P71.1

Hypochloremia E87.8

Hypochlorhydria K31.89
- neurotic F45.8
- psychogenic F45.8

Hypochondria, hypochondriac, hypochondriasis (reaction) F45.21
- sleep F51.Ø3

Hypochondrogenesis Q77.Ø

Hypochondroplasia Q77.4

Hypochromasia, blood cells D5Ø.8

Hypodontia —*see* Anodontia

Hypoeosinophilia D72.89

Hypoesthesia R2Ø.1

Hypofibrinogenemia D68.8
- acquired D65
- congenital (hereditary) D68.2

Hypofunction
- adrenocortical E27.4Ø
  - drug-induced E27.3
  - postprocedural E89.6
  - primary E27.1
- adrenomedullary, postprocedural E89.6
- cerebral R29.818
- corticoadrenal NEC E27.4Ø
- intestinal K59.8
- labyrinth —*see* subcategory H83.2
- ovary E28.39
- pituitary (gland) (anterior) E23.Ø
- testicular E29.1
  - postprocedural (postsurgical) (postirradiation) (iatrogenic) E89.5

Hypogalactia O92.4

H

Hypogammaglobulinemia —*see also* Agammaglobulinemia D8Ø.1
hereditary D8Ø.Ø
nonfamilial D8Ø.1
transient, of infancy D8Ø.7
Hypogenitalism (congenital) —*see* Hypogonadism
Hypoglossia Q38.3
Hypoglycemia (spontaneous) E16.2
coma E15
diabetic —*see* Diabetes, coma
diabetic —*see* Diabetes, hypoglycemia
dietary counseling and surveillance Z71.3
drug-induced E16.Ø
with coma (nondiabetic) E15
due to insulin E16.Ø
with coma (nondiabetic) E15
therapeutic misadventure —*see* subcategory T38.3
functional, nonhyperinsulinemic E16.1
iatrogenic E16.Ø
with coma (nondiabetic) E15
in infant of diabetic mother P7Ø.1
gestational diabetes P7Ø.Ø
infantile E16.1
leucine-induced E71.19
neonatal (transitory) P7Ø.4
iatrogenic P7Ø.3
reactive (not drug-induced) E16.1
transitory neonatal P7Ø.4
Hypogonadism
female E28.39
hypogonadotropic E23.Ø
male E29.1
ovarian (primary) E28.39
pituitary E23.Ø
testicular (primary) E29.1
Hypohidrosis, hypoidrosis L74.4
Hypoinsulinemia, postprocedural E89.1
Hypokalemia E87.6
Hypoleukocytosis —*see* Agranulocytosis
Hypolipoproteinemia (alpha) (beta) E78.6
Hypomagnesemia E83.42
neonatal P71.2
Hypomania, hypomanic reaction F3Ø.8
Hypomenorrhea —*see* Oligomenorrhea
Hypometabolism R63.8
Hypomotility
gastrointestinal (tract) K31.89
psychogenic F45.8
intestine K59.8
psychogenic F45.8
stomach K31.89
psychogenic F45.8
Hyponasality R49.22
Hyponatremia E87.1
Hypo-osmolality E87.1
Hypo-ovarianism, hypo-ovarism E28.39
Hypoparathyroidism E2Ø.9
familial E2Ø.8
idiopathic E2Ø.Ø
neonatal, transitory P71.4
postprocedural E89.2
specified NEC E2Ø.8
Hypoperfusion (in)
newborn P96.89
Hypopharyngitis —*see* Laryngopharyngitis
Hypophoria H5Ø.53
Hypophosphatemia, hypophosphatasia (acquired) (congenital) (renal) E83.39
familial E83.31
Hypophyseal, hypophysis —*see also* condition
dwarfism E23.Ø
gigantism E22.Ø
Hypopiesis —*see* Hypotension
Hypopinealism E34.8
Hypopituitarism (juvenile) E23.Ø
drug-induced E23.1
due to
hypophysectomy E89.3
radiotherapy E89.3
Hypopituitarism *(Continued)*
iatrogenic NEC E23.1
postirradiation E89.3
postpartum O99.285
postprocedural E89.3
Hypoplasia, hypoplastic
adrenal (gland), congenital Q89.1
alimentary tract, congenital Q45.8
upper Q4Ø.8
anus, anal (canal) Q42.3
with fistula Q42.2
aorta, aortic Q25.42
ascending, in hypoplastic left heart syndrome Q23.4
valve Q23.1
in hypoplastic left heart syndrome Q23.4
areola, congenital Q83.8
arm (congenital) —*see* Defect, reduction, upper limb
artery (peripheral) Q27.8
brain (congenital) Q28.3
coronary Q24.5
digestive system Q27.8
lower limb Q27.8
pulmonary Q25.79
functional, unilateral J43.Ø
retinal (congenital) Q14.1
specified site NEC Q27.8
umbilical Q27.Ø
upper limb Q27.8
auditory canal Q17.8
causing impairment of hearing Q16.9
biliary duct or passage Q44.5
bone NOS Q79.9
face Q75.8
marrow D61.9
megakaryocytic D69.49
skull —*see* Hypoplasia, skull
brain QØ2
gyri QØ4.3
part of QØ4.3
breast (areola) N64.82
bronchus Q32.4
cardiac Q24.8
carpus —*see* Defect, reduction, upper limb, specified type NEC
cartilage hair Q78.8
cecum Q42.8
cementum KØØ.4
cephalic QØ2
cerebellum QØ4.3
cervix (uteri), congenital Q51.821
clavicle (congenital) Q74.Ø
coccyx Q76.49
colon Q42.9
specified NEC Q42.8
corpus callosum QØ4.Ø
cricoid cartilage Q31.2
digestive organ (s) or tract NEC Q45.8
upper (congenital) Q4Ø.8
ear (auricle) (lobe) Q17.2
middle Q16.4
enamel of teeth (neonatal) (postnatal) (prenatal) KØØ.4
endocrine (gland) NEC Q89.2
endometrium N85.8
epididymis (congenital) Q55.4
epiglottis Q31.2
erythroid, congenital D61.Ø1
esophagus (congenital) Q39.8
eustachian tube Q17.8
eye Q11.2
eyelid (congenital) Q1Ø.3
face Q18.8
bone (s) Q75.8
femur (congenital) —*see* Defect, reduction, lower limb, specified type NEC
fibula (congenital) —*see* Defect, reduction, lower limb, specified type NEC
Hypoplasia, hypoplastic *(Continued)*
finger (congenital) —*see* Defect, reduction, upper limb, specified type NEC
focal dermal Q82.8
foot —*see* Defect, reduction, lower limb, specified type NEC
gallbladder Q44.Ø
genitalia, genital organ (s)
female, congenital Q52.8
external Q52.79
internal NEC Q52.8
in adiposogenital dystrophy E23.6
glottis Q31.2
hair Q84.2
hand (congenital) —*see* Defect, reduction, upper limb, specified type NEC
heart Q24.8
humerus (congenital) —*see* Defect, reduction, upper limb, specified type NEC
intestine (small) Q41.9
large Q42.9
specified NEC Q42.8
jaw M26.Ø9
alveolar M26.79
lower M26.Ø4
alveolar M26.74
upper M26.Ø2
alveolar M26.73
kidney (s) Q6Ø.5
bilateral Q6Ø.4
unilateral Q6Ø.3
labium (majus) (minus), congenital Q52.79
larynx Q31.2
left heart syndrome Q23.4
leg (congenital) —*see* Defect, reduction, lower limb
limb Q73.8
lower (congenital) —*see* Defect, reduction, lower limb
upper (congenital) —*see* Defect, reduction, upper limb
liver Q44.7
lung (lobe) (not associated with short gestation) Q33.6
associated with immaturity, low birth weight, prematurity, or short gestation P28.Ø
mammary (areola), congenital Q83.8
mandible, mandibular M26.Ø4
alveolar M26.74
unilateral condylar M27.8
maxillary M26.Ø2
alveolar M26.73
medullary D61.9
megakaryocytic D69.49
metacarpus —*see* Defect, reduction, upper limb, specified type NEC
metatarsus —*see* Defect, reduction, lower limb, specified type NEC
muscle Q79.8
nail (s) Q84.6
nose, nasal Q3Ø.1
optic nerve H47.Ø3-
osseous meatus (ear) Q17.8
ovary, congenital Q5Ø.39
pancreas Q45.Ø
parathyroid (gland) Q89.2
parotid gland Q38.4
patella Q74.1
pelvis, pelvic girdle Q74.2
penis (congenital) Q55.62
peripheral vascular system Q27.8
digestive system Q27.8
lower limb Q27.8
specified site NEC Q27.8
upper limb Q27.8
pituitary (gland) (congenital) Q89.2
pulmonary (not associated with short gestation) Q33.6
artery, functional J43.Ø
associated with short gestation P28.Ø

Hypoplasia, hypoplastic *(Continued)*
- radioulnar —*see* Defect, reduction, upper limb, specified type NEC
- radius —*see* Defect, reduction, upper limb
- rectum Q42.1
  - with fistula Q42.Ø
- respiratory system NEC Q34.8
- rib Q76.6
- right heart syndrome Q22.6
- sacrum Q76.49
- scapula Q74.Ø
- scrotum Q55.1
- shoulder girdle Q74.Ø
- skin Q82.8
- skull (bone) Q75.8
  - with
    - anencephaly QØØ.Ø
    - encephalocele —*see* Encephalocele
    - hydrocephalus QØ3.9
      - with spina bifida —*see* Spina bifida, by site, with hydrocephalus
    - microcephaly QØ2
- spinal (cord) (ventral horn cell) QØ6.1
- spine Q76.49
- sternum Q76.7
- tarsus —*see* Defect, reduction, lower limb, specified type NEC
- testis Q55.1
- thymic, with immunodeficiency D82.1
- thymus (gland) Q89.2
  - with immunodeficiency D82.1
- thyroid (gland) EØ3.1
  - cartilage Q31.2
- tibiofibular (congenital) —*see* Defect, reduction, lower limb, specified type NEC
- toe —*see* Defect, reduction, lower limb, specified type NEC
- tongue Q38.3
- Turner's KØØ.4
- ulna (congenital) —*see* Defect, reduction, upper limb
- umbilical artery Q27.Ø
- unilateral condylar M27.8
- ureter Q62.8
- uterus, congenital Q51.811
- vagina Q52.4
- vascular NEC peripheral Q27.8
  - brain Q28.3
  - digestive system Q27.8
  - lower limb Q27.8
  - specified site NEC Q27.8
  - upper limb Q27.8
- vein (s) (peripheral) Q27.8
  - brain Q28.3
  - digestive system Q27.8
  - great Q26.8
  - lower limb Q27.8
  - specified site NEC Q27.8
  - upper limb Q27.8
- vena cava (inferior) (superior) Q26.8
- vertebra Q76.49
- vulva, congenital Q52.79
- zonule (ciliary) Q12.8

Hypopotassemia E87.6

Hypoproconvertinemia, congenital (hereditary) D68.2

Hypoproteinemia E77.8

Hypoprothrombinemia (congenital) (hereditary) (idiopathic) D68.2
- acquired D68.4
- newborn, transient P61.6

Hypoptyalism K11.7

Hypopyon (eye) (anterior chamber) —*see* Iridocyclitis, acute, hypopyon

Hypopyrexia R68.Ø

Hyporeflexia R29.2

Hyposecretion
- ACTH E23.Ø
- antidiuretic hormone E23.2
- ovary E28.39
- salivary gland (any) K11.7
- vasopressin E23.2

Hyposegmentation, leukocytic, hereditary D72.Ø

Hyposiderinemia D5Ø.9

Hypospadias Q54.9
- balanic Q54.Ø
- coronal Q54.Ø
- glandular Q54.Ø
- penile Q54.1
- penoscrotal Q54.2
- perineal Q54.3
- specified NEC Q54.8

Hypospermatogenesis —*see* Oligospermia

Hyposplenism D73.Ø

Hypostasis pulmonary, passive —*see* Edema, lung

Hypostatic —*see* condition

Hyposthenuria N28.89

Hypotension (arterial) (constitutional) I95.9
- chronic I95.89
- drug-induced I95.2
- due to (of) hemodialysis I95.3
- iatrogenic I95.89
- idiopathic (permanent) I95.Ø
- intracranial, following ventricular shunting (ventriculostomy) G97.2
- intra-dialytic I95.3
- maternal, syndrome (following labor and delivery) O26.5-
- neurogenic, orthostatic G9Ø.3
- orthostatic (chronic) I95.1
  - due to drugs I95.2
  - neurogenic G9Ø.3
- postoperative I95.81
- postural I95.1
- specified NEC I95.89

Hypothermia (accidental) T68
- due to anesthesia, anesthetic T88.51
- low environmental temperature T68
- neonatal P8Ø.9
  - environmental (mild) NEC P8Ø.8
  - mild P8Ø.8
  - severe (chronic) (cold injury syndrome) P8Ø.Ø
  - specified NEC P8Ø.8
- not associated with low environmental temperature R68.Ø

Hypothyroidism (acquired) EØ3.9
- congenital (without goiter) EØ3.1
  - with goiter (diffuse) EØ3.Ø
- due to
  - exogenous substance NEC EØ3.2
  - iodine-deficiency, acquired EØ1.8
    - subclinical EØ2
  - irradiation therapy E89.Ø
  - medicament NEC EØ3.2
  - P-aminosalicylic acid (PAS) EØ3.2
  - phenylbutazone EØ3.2
  - resorcinol EØ3.2
  - sulfonamide EØ3.2
  - surgery E89.Ø
  - thiourea group drugs EØ3.2
- iatrogenic NEC EØ3.2
- iodine-deficiency (acquired) EØ1.8
  - congenital —*see* Syndrome, iodine-deficiency, congenital
  - subclinical EØ2
- neonatal, transitory P72.2
- postinfectious EØ3.3
- postirradiation E89.Ø
- postprocedural E89.Ø
- postsurgical E89.Ø
- specified NEC EØ3.8
- subclinical, iodine-deficiency related EØ2

Hypotonia, hypotonicity, hypotony
- bladder N31.2
- congenital (benign) P94.2
- eye —*see* Disorder, globe, hypotony

Hypotrichosis —*see* Alopecia

Hypotropia H5Ø.2-

Hypoventilation RØ6.89
- congenital central alveolar G47.35
- sleep related
  - idiopathic nonobstructive alveolar G47.34
  - in conditions classified elsewhere G47.36

Hypovitaminosis —*see* Deficiency, vitamin

Hypovolemia E86.1
- surgical shock T81.19
- traumatic (shock) T79.4

Hypoxemia RØ9.Ø2
- newborn P84
- sleep related, in conditions classified elsewhere G47.36

Hypoxia —*see also* Anoxia RØ9.Ø2
- cerebral, during a procedure NEC G97.81
  - postprocedural NEC G97.82
- intrauterine P84
- myocardial —*see* Insufficiency, coronary
- newborn P84
- sleep-related G47.34

Hypsarhythmia —*see* Epilepsy, generalized, specified NEC

Hysteralgia, pregnant uterus O26.89-

Hysteria, hysterical (conversion) (dissociative state) F44.9
- anxiety F41.8
- convulsions F44.5
- psychosis, acute F44.9

Hysteroepilepsy F44.5

I

IBDU (colonic inflammatory bowel dissease unclassified) K52.3 ◀
Ichthyoparasitism due to Vandellia cirrhosa B88.8
Ichthyosis (congenital) Q8Ø.9
  acquired L85.Ø
  fetalis Q8Ø.4
  hystrix Q8Ø.8
  lamellar Q8Ø.2
  lingual K13.29
  palmaris and plantaris Q82.8
  simplex Q8Ø.Ø
  vera Q8Ø.8
  vulgaris Q8Ø.Ø
  X-linked Q8Ø.1
Ichthyotoxism *—see* Poisoning, fish
  bacterial *—see* Intoxication, foodborne
Icteroanemia, hemolytic (acquired) D59.9
  congenital *—see* Spherocytosis
Icterus *—see also* Jaundice
  conjunctiva R17
  gravis, newborn P55.Ø
  hematogenous (acquired) D59.9
  hemolytic (acquired) D59.9
    congenital *—see* Spherocytosis
  hemorrhagic (acute) (leptospiral) (spirochetal) A27.Ø
    newborn P53
  infectious B15.9
    with hepatic coma B15.Ø
    leptospiral A27.Ø
    spirochetal A27.Ø
  neonatorum *—see* Jaundice, newborn
  newborn P59.9
  spirochetal A27.Ø
Ictus solaris, solis T67.Ø
Ideation
  homicidal R45.85Ø
  suicidal R45.851
Identity disorder (child) F64.9
  gender role F64.2
  psychosexual F64.2
Idioglossia F8Ø.Ø
Idiopathic *—see* condition
Idiot, idiocy (congenital) F73
  amaurotic (Bielschowsky(-Jansky)) (family) (infantile (late)) (juvenile (late)) (Vogt-Spielmeyer) E75.4
  microcephalic QØ2
Id reaction (due to bacteria) L3Ø.2
IgE asthma J45.9Ø9
IIAC (idiopathic infantile arterial calcification) Q28.8
Ileitis (chronic) (noninfectious) *—see also* Enteritis K52.9
  backwash *—see* Pancolitis, ulcerative (chronic)
  infectious AØ9
  regional (ulcerative) *—see* Enteritis, regional, small intestine
  segmental *—see* Enteritis, regional
  terminal (ulcerative) *—see* Enteritis, regional, small intestine
Ileocolitis *—see also* Enteritis K52.9
  infectious AØ9
  regional *—see* Enteritis, regional
Ileostomy
  attention to Z43.2
  malfunctioning K94.13
  status Z93.2
    with complication *—see* Complications, enterostomy
Ileotyphus *—see* Typhoid
Ileum *—see* condition
Ileus (bowel) (colon) (inhibitory) (intestine) K56.7
  adynamic K56.Ø
  due to gallstone (in intestine) K56.3
  duodenal (chronic) K31.5

Ileus *(Continued)*
  gallstone K56.3
  mechanical NEC K56.69
  meconium P76.Ø
    in cystic fibrosis E84.11
    meaning meconium plug (without cystic fibrosis) P76.Ø
  myxedema K59.8
  neurogenic K56.Ø
    Hirschsprung's disease or megacolon Q43.1
  newborn
    due to meconium P76.Ø
      in cystic fibrosis E84.11
      meaning meconium plug (without cystic fibrosis) P76.Ø
    transitory P76.1
  obstructive K56.69
  paralytic K56.Ø
Iliac *—see* condition
Iliotibial band syndrome M76.3-
Illiteracy Z55.Ø
Illness—*see also* Disease R69
  manic-depressive *—see* Disorder, bipolar
Imbalance R26.89
  autonomic G9Ø.8
  constituents of food intake E63.1
  electrolyte E87.8
    with
      abortion *—see* Abortion by type, complicated by, electrolyte imbalance
      molar pregnancy OØ8.5
    due to hyperemesis gravidarum O21.1
    following ectopic or molar pregnancy OØ8.5
    neonatal, transitory NEC P74.4
      potassium P74.3
      sodium P74.2
  endocrine E34.9
  eye muscle NOS H5Ø.9
  hormone E34.9
  hysterical F44.4
  labyrinth *—see* subcategory H83.2
  posture R29.3
  protein-energy *—see* Malnutrition
  sympathetic G9Ø.8
Imbecile, imbecility (I.Q. 35-49) F71
Imbedding, intrauterine device T83.39
Imbibition, cholesterol (gallbladder) K82.4
Imbrication, teeth, fully erupted M26.3Ø
Imerslund (-Gräsbeck) **syndrome** D51.1
Immature *—see also* Immaturity
  birth (less than 37 completed weeks) *—see* Preterm, newborn
    extremely (less than 28 completed weeks) *—see* Immaturity, extreme
  personality F6Ø.89
Immaturity (less than 37 completed weeks) *—see also* Preterm, newborn
  extreme of newborn (less than 28 completed weeks of gestation) (less than 196 completed days of gestation) (unspecified weeks of gestation) PØ7.2Ø
    gestational age
      23 completed weeks (23 weeks, Ø days through 23 weeks, 6 days) PØ7.22
      24 completed weeks (24 weeks, Ø days through 24 weeks, 6 days) PØ7.23
      25 completed weeks (25 weeks, Ø days through 25 weeks, 6 days) PØ7.24
      26 completed weeks (26 weeks, Ø days through 26 weeks, 6 days) PØ7.25
      27 completed weeks (27 weeks, Ø days through 27 weeks, 6 days) PØ7.26
      less than 23 completed weeks PØ7.21
  fetus or infant light-for-dates *—see* Light-for-dates
  lung, newborn P28.Ø
  organ or site NEC *—see* Hypoplasia
  pulmonary, newborn P28.Ø
  reaction F6Ø.89
  sexual (female) (male), after puberty E3Ø.Ø

Immersion T75.1
  foot T69.Ø2-
  hand T69.Ø1-
Immobile, immobility
  complete, due to severe physical disability or frailty R53.2
  intestine K59.8
  syndrome (paraplegic) M62.3
Immune reconstitution (inflammatory) **syndrome [IRIS]** D89.3
Immunization *—see also* Vaccination
  ABO *—see* Incompatibility, ABO
    in newborn P55.1
  complication *—see* Complications, vaccination
  encounter for Z23
  not done (not carried out) Z28.9
    because (of)
      acute illness of patient Z28.Ø1
      allergy to vaccine (or component) Z28.Ø4
      caregiver refusal Z28.82
      chronic illness of patient Z28.Ø2
      contraindication NEC Z28.Ø9
      group pressure Z28.1
      guardian refusal Z28.82
      immune compromised state of patient Z28.Ø3
      parent refusal Z28.82
      patient's belief Z28.1
      patient had disease being vaccinated against Z28.81
      patient refusal Z28.21
      religious beliefs of patient Z28.1
      specified reason NEC Z28.89
        of patient Z28.29
      unspecified patient reason Z28.2Ø
  Rh factor
    affecting management of pregnancy NEC O36.Ø9-
      anti-D antibody O36.Ø1-
    from transfusion *—see* Complication (s), transfusion, incompatibility reaction, Rh (factor)
Immunocytoma C83.Ø-
Immunodeficiency D84.9
  with
    adenosine-deaminase deficiency D81.3
    antibody defects D8Ø.9
      specified type NEC D8Ø.8
    hyperimmunoglobulinemia D8Ø.6
    increased immunoglobulin M (IgM) D8Ø.5
    major defect D82.9
      specified type NEC D82.8
    partial albinism D82.8
    short-limbed stature D82.2
    thrombocytopenia and eczema D82.Ø
  antibody with
    hyperimmunoglobulinemia D8Ø.6
    near-normal immunoglobulins D8Ø.6
  autosomal recessive, Swiss type D8Ø.Ø
  combined D81.9
    biotin-dependent carboxylase D81.819
      biotinidase D81.81Ø
      holocarboxylase synthetase D81.818
      specified type NEC D81.818
    severe (SCID) D81.9
      with
        low or normal B-cell numbers D81.2
        low T- and B-cell numbers D81.1
        reticular dysgenesis D81.Ø
    specified type NEC D81.89
  common variable D83.9
    with
      abnormalities of B-cell numbers and function D83.Ø
      autoantibodies to B- or T-cells D83.2
      immunoregulatory T-cell disorders D83.1
    specified type NEC D83.8
  following hereditary defective response to Epstein-Barr virus (EBV) D82.3

Immunodeficiency *(Continued)*
selective, immunoglobulin
A (IgA) D8Ø.2
G (IgG) (subclasses) D8Ø.3
M (IgM) D8Ø.4
severe combined (SCID) D81.9
specified type NEC D84.8
X-linked, with increased IgM D8Ø.5
Immunotherapy (encounter for)
antineoplastic Z51.12
Impaction, impacted
bowel, colon, rectum —*see also* Impaction, fecal K56.49
by gallstone K56.3
calculus —*see* Calculus
cerumen (ear) (external) H61.2-
cuspid —*see* Impaction, tooth
dental (same or adjacent tooth) KØ1.1
fecal, feces K56.41
fracture —*see* Fracture, by site
gallbladder —*see* Calculus, gallbladder
gallstone (s) —*see* Calculus, gallbladder
bile duct (common) (hepatic) —*see* Calculus, bile duct
cystic duct —*see* Calculus, gallbladder
in intestine, with obstruction (any part) K56.3
intestine (calculous) NEC —*see also* Impaction, fecal K56.49
gallstone, with ileus K56.3
intrauterine device (IUD) T83.39
molar —*see* Impaction, tooth
shoulder, causing obstructed labor O66.Ø
tooth, teeth KØ1.1
turbinate J34.89
Impaired, impairment (function)
auditory discrimination —*see* Abnormal, auditory perception
cognitive, mild, so stated G31.84
dual sensory Z73.82
fasting glucose R73.Ø1
glucose tolerance (oral) R73.Ø2
hearing —*see* Deafness
heart —*see* Disease, heart
kidney N28.9
disorder resulting from N25.9
specified NEC N25.89
liver K72.9Ø
with coma K72.91
mastication KØ8.89 ⟸
mild cognitive, so stated G31.84
mobility
ear ossicles —*see* Ankylosis, ear ossicles
requiring care provider Z74.Ø9
myocardium, myocardial —*see* Insufficiency, myocardial
rectal sphincter R19.8
renal (acute) (chronic) N28.9
disorder resulting from N25.9
specified NEC N25.89
vision NEC H54.7
both eyes H54.3
Impediment, speech R47.9
psychogenic (childhood) F98.8
slurring R47.81
specified NEC R47.89
Impending
coronary syndrome I2Ø.Ø
delirium tremens F1Ø.239
myocardial infarction I2Ø.Ø
Imperception auditory (acquired) —*see also* Deafness
congenital H93.25
Imperfect
aeration, lung (newborn) NEC —*see* Atelectasis
closure (congenital)
alimentary tract NEC Q45.8
lower Q43.8
upper Q4Ø.8
atrioventricular ostium Q21.2

Imperfect *(Continued)*
closure *(Continued)*
atrium (secundum) Q21.1
branchial cleft or sinus Q18.Ø
choroid Q14.3
cricoid cartilage Q31.8
cusps, heart valve NEC Q24.8
pulmonary Q22.3
ductus
arteriosus Q25.Ø
Botalli Q25.Ø
ear drum (causing impairment of hearing) Q16.4
esophagus with communication to bronchus or trachea Q39.1
eyelid Q1Ø.3
foramen
botalli Q21.1
ovale Q21.1
genitalia, genital organ (s) or system
female Q52.8
external Q52.79
internal NEC Q52.8
male Q55.8
glottis Q31.8
interatrial ostium or septum Q21.1
interauricular ostium or septum Q21.1
interventricular ostium or septum Q21.Ø
larynx Q31.8
lip —*see* Cleft, lip
nasal septum Q3Ø.3
nose Q3Ø.2
omphalomesenteric duct Q43.Ø
optic nerve entry Q14.2
organ or site not listed —*see* Anomaly, by site
ostium
interatrial Q21.1
interauricular Q21.1
interventricular Q21.Ø
palate —*see* Cleft, palate
preauricular sinus Q18.1
retina Q14.1
roof of orbit Q75.8
sclera Q13.5
septum
aorticopulmonary Q21.4
atrial (secundum) Q21.1
between aorta and pulmonary artery Q21.4
heart Q21.9
interatrial (secundum) Q21.1
interauricular (secundum) Q21.1
interventricular Q21.Ø
in tetralogy of Fallot Q21.3
nasal Q3Ø.3
ventricular Q21.Ø
with pulmonary stenosis or atresia, dextraposition of aorta, and hypertrophy of right ventricle Q21.3
in tetralogy of Fallot Q21.3
skull Q75.Ø
with
anencephaly QØØ.Ø
encephalocele —*see* Encephalocele
hydrocephalus QØ3.9
with spina bifida —*see* Spina bifida, by site, with hydrocephalus
microcephaly QØ2
spine (with meningocele) —*see* Spina bifida
trachea Q32.1
tympanic membrane (causing impairment of hearing) Q16.4
uterus Q51.818
vitelline duct Q43.Ø
erection —*see* Dysfunction, sexual, male, erectile
fusion —*see* Imperfect, closure
inflation, lung (newborn) —*see* Atelectasis

Imperfect *(Continued)*
posture R29.3
rotation, intestine Q43.3
septum, ventricular Q21.Ø
Imperfectly descended testis —*see* Cryptorchid
Imperforate (congenital) —*see also* Atresia
anus Q42.3
with fistula Q42.2
cervix (uteri) Q51.828
esophagus Q39.Ø
with tracheoesophageal fistula Q39.1
hymen Q52.3
jejunum Q41.1
pharynx Q38.8
rectum Q42.1
with fistula Q42.Ø
urethra Q64.39
vagina Q52.4
Impervious (congenital) —*see also* Atresia
anus Q42.3
with fistula Q42.2
bile duct Q44.2
esophagus Q39.Ø
with tracheoesophageal fistula Q39.1
intestine (small) Q41.9
large Q42.9
specified NEC Q42.8
rectum Q42.1
with fistula Q42.Ø
ureter —*see* Atresia, ureter
urethra Q64.39
Impetiginization of dermatoses LØ1.1
Impetigo (any organism) (any site) (circinate) (contagiosa) (simplex) (vulgaris) LØ1.ØØ
Bockhart's LØ1.Ø2
bullous, bullosa LØ1.Ø3
external ear LØ1.ØØ *[H62.4Ø]*
follicularis LØ1.Ø2
furfuracea L3Ø.5
herpetiformis L4Ø.1
nonobstetrical L4Ø.1
neonatorum LØ1.Ø3
nonbullous LØ1.Ø1
specified type NEC LØ1.Ø9
ulcerative LØ1.Ø9
Impingement (on teeth)
soft tissue
anterior M26.81
posterior M26.82
Implant, endometrial N8Ø.9
Implantation
anomalous —*see* Anomaly, by site
ureter Q62.63
cyst
external area or site (skin) NEC L72.Ø
iris —*see* Cyst, iris, implantation
vagina N89.8
vulva N9Ø.7
dermoid (cyst) —*see* Implantation, cyst
Impotence (sexual) N52.9
counseling Z7Ø.1
organic origin —*see also* Dysfunction, sexual, male, erectile N52.9
psychogenic F52.21
Impression, basilar Q75.8
Imprisonment, anxiety concerning Z65.1
Improper care (child) (newborn) —*see* Maltreatment
Improperly tied umbilical cord (causing hemorrhage) P51.8
Impulsiveness (impulsive) R45.87
Inability to swallow —*see* Aphagia
Inaccessible, inaccessibility
health care NEC Z75.3
due to
waiting period Z75.2
for admission to facility elsewhere Z75.1
other helping agencies Z75.4
Inactive —*see* condition

Inadequate, inadequacy
  aesthetics of dental restoration K08.56
  biologic, constitutional, functional, or social F60.7
  development
    child R62.50
    genitalia
      after puberty NEC E30.0
      congenital
        female Q52.8
          external Q52.79
          internal Q52.8
        male Q55.8
    lungs Q33.6
      associated with short gestation P28.0
    organ or site not listed —*see* Anomaly, by site
  diet (causing nutritional deficiency) E63.9
  eating habits Z72.4
  environment, household Z59.1
  family support Z63.8
  food (supply) NEC Z59.4
    hunger effects T73.0
  functional F60.7
  household care, due to
    family member
      handicapped or ill Z74.2
      on vacation Z75.5
      temporarily away from home Z74.2
    technical defects in home Z59.1
    temporary absence from home of person rendering care Z74.2
  housing (heating) (space) Z59.1
  income (financial) Z59.6
  intrafamilial communication Z63.8
  material resources Z59.9
  mental —*see* Disability, intellectual
  parental supervision or control of child Z62.0
  personality F60.7
  pulmonary
    function R06.89
      newborn P28.5
    ventilation, newborn P28.5
  sample of cytologic smear
    anus R85.615
    cervix R87.615
    vagina R87.625
  social F60.7
    insurance Z59.7
    skills NEC Z73.4
  supervision of child by parent Z62.0
  teaching affecting education Z55.8
  welfare support Z59.7
Inanition R64
  with edema —*see* Malnutrition, severe
  due to
    deprivation of food T73.0
    malnutrition —*see* Malnutrition
  fever R50.9
Inappropriate
  change in quantitative human chorionic gonadotropin (hCG) in early pregnancy O02.81
  diet or eating habits Z72.4
  level of quantitative human chorionic gonadotropin (hCG) for gestational age in early pregnancy O02.81
  secretion
    antidiuretic hormone (ADH) (excessive) E22.2
      deficiency E23.2
    pituitary (posterior) E22.2
Inattention at or after birth —*see* Neglect
Incarceration, incarcerated
  enterocele K46.0
    gangrenous K46.1
  epiplocele K46.0
    gangrenous K46.1
  exomphalos K42.0 ◀
    gangrenous K42.1 ◀
  ~~exophthalmos K42.0~~
    ~~gangrenous K42.1~~

Incarceration, incarcerated *(Continued)*
  hernia —*see also* Hernia, by site, with obstruction
    with gangrene —*see* Hernia, by site, with gangrene
  iris, in wound —*see* Injury, eye, laceration, with prolapse
  lens, in wound —*see* Injury, eye, laceration, with prolapse
  omphalocele K42.0
  prison, anxiety concerning Z65.1
  rupture —*see* Hernia, by site
  sarcoepiplocele K46.0
    gangrenous K46.1
  sarcoepiplomphalocele K42.0
    with gangrene K42.1
  uterus N85.8
    gravid O34.51-
      causing obstructed labor O65.5
Incised wound
  external —*see* Laceration
  internal organs —*see* Injury, by site
Incision, incisional
  hernia K43.2
    with
      gangrene (and obstruction) K43.1
      obstruction K43.0
  surgical, complication —*see* Complications, surgical procedure
  traumatic
    external —*see* Laceration
    internal organs —*see* Injury, by site
Inclusion
  azurophilic leukocytic D72.0
  blennorrhea (neonatal) (newborn) P39.1
  gallbladder in liver (congenital) Q44.1
Incompatibility
  ABO
    affecting management of pregnancy O36.11-
      anti-A sensitization O36.11-
      anti-B sensitization O36.19-
      specified NEC O36.19-
    infusion or transfusion reaction —*see* Complication (s), transfusion, incompatibility reaction, ABO
    newborn P55.1
  blood (group) (Duffy) (K(ell)) (Kidd) (Lewis) (M) (S) NEC
    affecting management of pregnancy O36.11-
      anti-A sensitization O36.11-
      anti-B sensitization O36.19-
    infusion or transfusion reaction T80.89
    newborn P55.8
  divorce or estrangement Z63.5
  Rh (blood group) (factor) Z31.82
    affecting management of pregnancy NEC O36.09-
      anti-D antibody O36.01-
    infusion or transfusion reaction —*see* Complication (s), transfusion, incompatibility reaction, Rh (factor)
    newborn P55.0
  rhesus —*see* Incompatibility, Rh
Incompetency, incompetent, incompetence
  annular
    aortic (valve) —*see* Insufficiency, aortic
    mitral (valve) I34.0
    pulmonary valve (heart) I37.1
  aortic (valve) —*see* Insufficiency, aortic
  cardiac valve —*see* Endocarditis
  cervix, cervical (os) N88.3
    in pregnancy O34.3-
  chronotropic I45.89
    with
      autonomic dysfunction G90.8
      ischemic heart disease I25.89
      left ventricular dysfunction I51.89
      sinus node dysfunction I49.8
  esophagogastric (junction) (sphincter) K22.0

Incompetency, incompetent, incompetence *(Continued)*
  mitral (valve) —*see* Insufficiency, mitral
  pelvic fundus N81.89
  pubocervical tissue N81.82
  pulmonary valve (heart) I37.1
    congenital Q22.3
  rectovaginal tissue N81.83
  tricuspid (annular) (valve) —*see* Insufficiency, tricuspid
  valvular —*see* Endocarditis
    congenital Q24.8
  vein, venous (saphenous) (varicose) —*see* Varix, leg
Incomplete —*see also* condition
  bladder, emptying R33.9
  defecation R15.0
  expansion lungs (newborn) NEC —*see* Atelectasis
  rotation, intestine Q43.3
Inconclusive
  diagnostic imaging due to excess body fat of patient R93.9
  findings on diagnostic imaging of breast NEC R92.8
  mammogram (due to dense breasts) R92.2
Incontinence R32
  anal sphincter R15.9
  coital N39.491 ◀
  feces R15.9
    nonorganic origin F98.1
  insensible (urinary) N39.42 ◀
  overflow N39.490
  postural (urinary) N39.492 ◀
  psychogenic F45.8
  rectal R15.9
  reflex N39.498
  stress (female) (male) N39.3
    and urge N39.46
  urethral sphincter R32
  urge N39.41
    and stress (female) (male) N39.46
  urine (urinary) R32
    continuous N39.45
    due to cognitive impairment, or severe physical disability or immobility R39.81
    functional R39.81
    insensible N39.42 ◀
    mixed (stress and urge) N39.46
    nocturnal N39.44
    nonorganic origin F98.0
    overflow N39.490
    post dribbling N39.43
    postural N39.492 ◀
    reflex N39.498
    specified NEC N39.498
    stress (female) (male) N39.3
      and urge N39.46
    total N39.498
    unaware N39.42
    urge N39.41
      and stress (female) (male) N39.46
Incontinentia pigmenti Q82.3
Incoordinate, incoordination
  esophageal-pharyngeal (newborn) —*see* Dysphagia
  muscular R27.8
  uterus (action) (contractions) (complicating delivery) O62.4
Increase, increased
  abnormal, in development R63.8
  androgens (ovarian) E28.1
  anticoagulants (antithrombin) (anti-VIIIa) (anti-IXa) (anti-Xa) (anti-XIa) —*see* Circulating anticoagulants
  cold sense R20.8
  estrogen E28.0
  function
    adrenal
      cortex —*see* Cushing's, syndrome
      medulla E27.5

◀ New   ◀ Revised   ~~deleted~~ Deleted

Increase, increased *(Continued)*
function *(Continued)*
pituitary (gland) (anterior) (lobe) E22.9
posterior E22.2
heat sense R20.8
intracranial pressure (benign) G93.2
permeability, capillaries I78.8
pressure, intracranial G93.2
secretion
gastrin E16.4
glucagon E16.3
pancreas, endocrine E16.9
growth hormone-releasing hormone E16.8
pancreatic polypeptide E16.8
somatostatin E16.8
vasoactive-intestinal polypeptide E16.8
sphericity, lens Q12.4
splenic activity D73.1
venous pressure I87.8
portal K76.6
Increta placenta O43.22-
Incrustation, cornea, foreign body (lead) (zinc) —*see* Foreign body, cornea
Incyclophoria H50.54
Incyclotropia —*see* Cyclotropia
Indeterminate sex Q56.4
India rubber skin Q82.8
Indigestion (acid) (bilious) (functional) K30
catarrhal K31.89
due to decomposed food NOS A05.9
nervous F45.8
psychogenic F45.8
Indirect —*see* condition
Induratio penis plastica N48.6
Induration, indurated
brain G93.89
breast (fibrous) N64.51
puerperal, postpartum O92.29
broad ligament N83.8
chancre
anus A51.1
congenital A50.07
extragenital NEC A51.2
corpora cavernosa (penis) (plastic) N48.6
liver (chronic) K76.89
lung (black) (chronic) (fibroid) —*see also* Fibrosis, lung J84.10
essential brown J84.03
penile (plastic) N48.6
phlebitic —*see* Phlebitis
skin R23.4
Inebriety (without dependence) —*see* Alcohol, intoxication
Inefficiency, kidney N28.9
Inelasticity, skin R23.4
Inequality, leg (length) (acquired) —*see also* Deformity, limb, unequal length
congenital —*see* Defect, reduction, lower limb
lower leg —*see* Deformity, limb, unequal length
Inertia
bladder (neurogenic) N31.2
stomach K31.89
psychogenic F45.8
uterus, uterine during labor O62.2
during latent phase of labor O62.0
primary O62.0
secondary O62.1
vesical (neurogenic) N31.2
Infancy, infantile, infantilism —*see also* condition
celiac K90.0
genitalia, genitals (after puberty) E30.0
Herter's (nontropical sprue) K90.0
intestinal K90.0
Lorain E23.0
pancreatic K86.89 (Revised)
pelvis M95.5
with disproportion (fetopelvic) O33.1
causing obstructed labor O65.1
Infancy, infantile, infantilism *(Continued)*
pituitary E23.0
renal N25.0
uterus —*see* Infantile, genitalia
Infant (s) —*see also* Infancy
excessive crying R68.11
irritable child R68.12
lack of care —*see* Neglect
liveborn (singleton) Z38.2
born in hospital Z38.00
by cesarean Z38.01
born outside hospital Z38.1
multiple NEC Z38.8
born in hospital Z38.68
by cesarean Z38.69
born outside hospital Z38.7
quadruplet Z38.8
born in hospital Z38.63
by cesarean Z38.64
born outside hospital Z38.7
quintuplet Z38.8
born in hospital Z38.65
by cesarean Z38.66
born outside hospital Z38.7
triplet Z38.8
born in hospital Z38.61
by cesarean Z38.62
born outside hospital Z38.7
twin Z38.5
born in hospital Z38.30
by cesarean Z38.31
born outside hospital Z38.4
of diabetic mother (syndrome of) P70.1
gestational diabetes P70.0
Infantile —*see also* condition
genitalia, genitals E30.0
os, uterine E30.0
penis E30.0
testis E29.1
uterus E30.0
Infantilism —*see* Infancy
Infarct, infarction
adrenal (capsule) (gland) E27.49
appendices epiploicae —*see also* Infarct, intestine K55.069 (Revised)
bowel —*see also* Infarct, intestine K55.069 (Revised)
brain (stem) —*see* Infarct, cerebral
breast N64.89
brewer's (kidney) N28.0
cardiac —*see* Infarct, myocardium
cerebellar —*see* Infarct, cerebral
cerebral —*see also* Occlusion, artery cerebral or precerebral, with infarction I63.9-
aborted I63.9
cortical I63.9
due to
cerebral venous thrombosis, nonpyogenic I63.6
embolism
cerebral arteries I63.4-
precerebral arteries I63.1-
occlusion NEC
cerebral arteries I63.5-
precerebral arteries I63.2-
stenosis NEC
cerebral arteries I63.5-
precerebral arteries I63.2-
thrombosis
cerebral artery I63.3-
precerebral artery I63.0-
intraoperative
during cardiac surgery I97.810
during other surgery I97.811
postprocedural
following cardiac surgery I97.820
following other surgery I97.821
specified NEC I63.8
colon (acute) (agnogenic) (embolic) (hemorrhagic) (nonocclusive) (nonthrombotic) (occlusive) (segmental) (thrombotic) (with gangrene) —*see also* Infarct, intestine K55.049 (Revised)
Infarct, infarction *(Continued)*
coronary artery —*see* Infarct, myocardium
embolic —*see* Embolism
fallopian tube N83.8
gallbladder K82.8
heart —*see* Infarct, myocardium
hepatic K76.3
hypophysis (anterior lobe) E23.6
impending (myocardium) I20.0
intestine (acute) (agnogenic) (embolic) (hemorrhagic) (nonocclusive) (nonthrombotic) (occlusive) (thrombotic) (with gangrene) K55.069 (Revised)
diffuse K55.062 (New)
focal K55.061 (New)
large K55.049 (New)
diffuse K55.042 (New)
focal K55.041 (New)
small K55.029 (New)
diffuse K55.022 (New)
focal K55.021 (New)
kidney N28.0
liver K76.3
lung (embolic) (thrombotic) —*see* Embolism, pulmonary
lymph node I89.8
mesentery, mesenteric (embolic) (thrombotic) (with gangrene) —*see also* Infarct, intestine K55.069 (Revised)
muscle (ischemic) M62.20
ankle M62.27-
foot M62.27-
forearm M62.23-
hand M62.24-
lower leg M62.26-
pelvic region M62.25-
shoulder region M62.21-
specified site NEC M62.28
thigh M62.25-
upper arm M62.22-
myocardium, myocardial (acute) (with stated duration of 4 weeks or less) I21.3
diagnosed on ECG, but presenting no symptoms I25.2
healed or old I25.2
intraoperative
during cardiac surgery I97.790
during other surgery I97.791
non-Q wave I21.4
non-ST elevation (NSTEMI) I21.4
subsequent I22.2
nontransmural I21.4
past (diagnosed on ECG or other investigation, but currently presenting no symptoms) I25.2
postprocedural
following cardiac surgery I97.190
following other surgery I97.191
Q wave (*see also*, Infarct, myocardium, by site) I21.3
ST elevation (STEMI) I21.3
anterior (anteroapical) (anterolateral) (anteroseptal) (Q wave) (wall) I21.09
subsequent I22.0
inferior (diaphragmatic) (inferolateral) (inferoposterior) (wall) NEC I21.19
subsequent I22.1
inferoposterior transmural (Q wave) I21.11
involving
coronary artery of anterior wall NEC I21.09
coronary artery of inferior wall NEC I21.19
diagonal coronary artery I21.02
left anterior descending coronary artery I21.02
left circumflex coronary artery I21.21
left main coronary artery I21.01

(New) New (Revised) Revised ~~deleted~~ Deleted

Infarct, infarction *(Continued)*
myocardium, myocardial *(Continued)*
ST elevation (STEMI) *(Continued)*
involving *(Continued)*
oblique marginal coronary artery I21.21
right coronary artery I21.11
lateral (apical-lateral) (basal-lateral) (high) I21.29
subsequent I22.8
posterior (posterobasal) (posterolateral) (posteroseptal) (true) I21.29
subsequent I22.8
septal I21.29
subsequent I22.8
specified NEC I21.29
subsequent I22.8
subsequent I22.9
subsequent (recurrent) (reinfarction) I22.9
anterior (anteroapical) (anterolateral) (anteroseptal) (wall) I22.Ø
diaphragmatic (wall) I22.1
inferior (diaphragmatic) (inferolateral) (inferoposterior) (wall) I22.1
lateral (apical-lateral) (basal-lateral) (high) I22.8
non-ST elevation (NSTEMI) I22.2
posterior (posterobasal) (posterolateral) (posteroseptal) (true) I22.8
septal I22.8
specified NEC I22.8
ST elevation I22.9
anterior (anteroapical) (anterolateral) (anteroseptal) (wall) I22.Ø
inferior (diaphragmatic) (inferolateral) (inferoposterior) (wall) I22.1
specified NEC I22.8
subendocardial I22.2
transmural I22.9
anterior (anteroapical) (anterolateral) (anteroseptal) (wall) I22.Ø
diaphragmatic (wall) I22.1
inferior (diaphragmatic) (inferolateral) (inferoposterior) (wall) I22.1
lateral (apical-lateral) (basal-lateral) (high) I22.8
posterior (posterobasal) (posterolateral) (posteroseptal) (true) I22.8
specified NEC I22.8
syphilitic A52.Ø6
transmural I21.3
anterior (anteroapical) (anterolateral) (anteroseptal) (Q wave) (wall) NEC I21.Ø9
inferior (diaphragmatic) (inferolateral) (inferoposterior) (Q wave) (wall) NEC I21.19
inferoposterior (Q wave) I21.11
lateral (apical-lateral) (basal-lateral) (high) NEC I21.29
posterior (posterobasal) (posterolateral) (posteroseptal) (true) NEC I21.29
septal NEC I21.29
specified NEC I21.29
nontransmural I21.4
omentum —*see also* Infarct, intestine K55.Ø69
ovary N83.8
pancreas K86.89
papillary muscle —*see* Infarct, myocardium
parathyroid gland E21.4
pituitary (gland) E23.6
placenta O43.81-
prostate N42.89
pulmonary (artery) (vein) (hemorrhagic) —*see* Embolism, pulmonary
renal (embolic) (thrombotic) N28.Ø
retina, retinal (artery) —*see* Occlusion, artery, retina
spinal (cord) (acute) (embolic) (nonembolic) G95.11

Infarct, infarction *(Continued)*
spleen D73.5
embolic or thrombotic I74.8
subendocardial (acute) (nontransmural) I21.4
suprarenal (capsule) (gland) E27.49
testis N5Ø.1
thrombotic —*see also* Thrombosis
artery, arterial —*see* Embolism
thyroid (gland) EØ7.89
ventricle (heart) —*see* Infarct, myocardium
Infecting —*see* condition
Infection, infected, infective (opportunistic) B99.9
with
drug resistant organism —*see* Resistance (to), drug —*see also* specific organism
lymphangitis —*see* Lymphangitis
organ dysfunction (acute) R65.2Ø
with septic shock R65.21
abscess (skin) - code by site under Abscess
Absidia —*see* Mucormycosis
Acanthamoeba —*see* Acanthamebiasis
Acanthocheilonema (perstans) (streptocerca) B74.4
accessory sinus (chronic) —*see* Sinusitis
achorion —*see* Dermatophytosis
Acremonium falciforme B47.Ø
acromioclavicular MØØ.9
Actinobacillus (actinomycetem-comitans) A28.8
mallei A24.Ø
muris A25.1
Actinomadura B47.1
Actinomyces (israelii) —*see also* Actinomycosis A42.9
Actinomycetales —*see* Actinomycosis
actinomycotic NOS —*see* Actinomycosis
adenoid (and tonsil) JØ3.9Ø
chronic J35.Ø2
adenovirus NEC
as cause of disease classified elsewhere B97.Ø
unspecified nature or site B34.Ø
aerogenes capsulatus A48.Ø
aertrycke —*see* Infection, salmonella
alimentary canal NOS —*see* Enteritis, infectious
Allescheria boydii B48.2
Alternaria B48.8
alveolus, alveolar (process) KØ4.7
Ameba, amebic (histolytica) —*see* Amebiasis
amniotic fluid, sac or cavity O41.1Ø-
chorioamnionitis O41.12-
placentitis O41.14-
amputation stump (surgical) —*see* Complication, amputation stump, infection
Ancylostoma (duodenalis) B76.Ø
Anisakiasis, Anisakis larvae B81.Ø
anthrax —*see* Anthrax
antrum (chronic) —*see* Sinusitis, maxillary
anus, anal (papillae) (sphincter) K62.89
arbovirus (arbor virus) A94
specified type NEC A93.8
artificial insemination N98.Ø
Ascaris lumbricoides —*see* Ascariasis
Ascomycetes B47.Ø
Aspergillus (flavus) (fumigatus) (terreus) —*see* Aspergillosis
atypical
acid-fast (bacilli) —*see* Mycobacterium, atypical
mycobacteria —*see* Mycobacterium, atypical
virus A81.9
specified type NEC A81.89
auditory meatus (external) —*see* Otitis, externa, infective
auricle (ear) —*see* Otitis, externa, infective
axillary gland (lymph) LØ4.2

Infection, infected, infective *(Continued)*
Bacillus A49.9
abortus A23.1
anthracis —*see* Anthrax
Ducrey's (any location) A57
Flexner's AØ3.1
Friedländer's NEC A49.8
gas (gangrene) A48.Ø
mallei A24.Ø
melitensis A23.Ø
paratyphoid, paratyphosus AØ1.4
A AØ1.1
B AØ1.2
C AØ1.3
Shiga (-Kruse) AØ3.Ø
suipestifer —*see* Infection, salmonella
swimming pool A31.1
typhosa AØ1.ØØ
welchii —*see* Gangrene, gas
bacterial NOS A49.9
as cause of disease classified elsewhere B96.89
Bacteroides fragilis [B. fragilis] B96.6
Clostridium perfringens [C. perfringens] B96.7
Enterobacter sakazakii B96.89
Enterococcus B95.2
Escherichia coli [E. coli] (*see also* Escherichia coli) B96.2Ø
Helicobacter pylori [H.pylori] B96.81
Hemophilus influenzae [H. influenzae] B96.3
Klebsiella pneumoniae [K. pneumoniae] B96.1
Mycoplasma pneumoniae [M. pneumoniae] B96.Ø
Proteus (mirabilis) (morganii) B96.4
Pseudomonas (aeruginosa) (mallei) (pseudomallei) B96.5
Staphylococcus B95.8
aureus (methicillin susceptible) (MSSA) B95.61
methicillin resistant (MRSA) B95.62
specified NEC B95.7
Streptococcus B95.5
group A B95.Ø
group B B95.1
pneumoniae B95.3
specified NEC B95.4
Vibrio vulnificus B96.82
specified NEC A48.8
Bacterium
paratyphosum AØ1.4
A AØ1.1
B AØ1.2
C AØ1.3
typhosum AØ1.ØØ
Bacteroides NEC A49.8
fragilis, as cause of disease classified elsewhere B96.6
Balantidium coli AØ7.Ø
Bartholin's gland N75.8
Basidiobolus B46.8
bile duct (common) (hepatic) —*see* Cholangitis
bladder —*see* Cystitis
Blastomyces, blastomycotic —*see also* Blastomycosis
brasiliensis —*see* Paracoccidioidomycosis
dermatitidis —*see* Blastomycosis
European —*see* Cryptococcosis
Loboi B48.Ø
North American B4Ø.9
South American —*see* Paracoccidioidomycosis
bleb, postprocedure —*see* Blebitis
bone —*see* Osteomyelitis
Bordetella —*see* Whooping cough
Borrelia bergdorfi A69.2Ø

◀ New ⇐ Revised ~~deleted~~ Deleted

Infection, infected, infective *(Continued)*
lancet fluke B66.2
larynx NEC J38.7
leg (skin) NOS L08.9
Legionella pneumophila A48.1
nonpneumonic A48.2
Leishmania —*see also* Leishmaniasis
aethiopica B55.1
braziliensis B55.2
chagasi B55.0
donovani B55.0
infantum B55.0
major B55.1
mexicana B55.1
tropica B55.1
lentivirus, as cause of disease classified elsewhere B97.31
Leptosphaeria senegalensis B47.0
Leptospira interrogans A27.9
autumnalis A27.89
canicola A27.89
hebdomadis A27.89
icterohaemorrhagiae A27.0
pomona A27.89
specified type NEC A27.89
leptospirochetal NEC —*see* Leptospirosis
Listeria monocytogenes —*see also* Listeriosis
congenital P37.2
Loa loa B74.3
with conjunctival infestation B74.3
eyelid B74.3
Loboa loboi B48.0
local, skin (staphylococcal) (streptococcal) L08.9
abscess - code by site under Abscess
cellulitis - code by site under Cellulitis
specified NEC L08.89
ulcer —*see* Ulcer, skin
Loefflerella mallei A24.0
lung —*see also* Pneumonia J18.9
atypical Mycobacterium A31.0
spirochetal A69.8
tuberculous —*see* Tuberculosis, pulmonary
virus —*see* Pneumonia, viral
lymph gland —*see also* Lymphadenitis, acute
mesenteric I88.0
lymphoid tissue, base of tongue or posterior pharynx, NEC (chronic) J35.03
Madurella (grisea) (mycetomii) B47.0
major
following ectopic or molar pregnancy O08.0
puerperal, postpartum, childbirth O85
Malassezia furfur B36.0
Malleomyces
mallei A24.0
pseudomallei (whitmori) —*see* Melioidosis
mammary gland N61.0
Mansonella (ozzardi) (perstans) (streptocerca) B74.4
mastoid —*see* Mastoiditis
maxilla, maxillary M27.2
sinus (chronic) —*see* Sinusitis, maxillary
mediastinum J98.51
Medina (worm) B72
meibomian cyst or gland —*see* Hordeolum
meninges —*see* Meningitis, bacterial
meningococcal —*see also* condition A39.9
adrenals A39.1
brain A39.81
cerebrospinal A39.0
conjunctiva A39.89
endocardium A39.51
heart A39.50
endocardium A39.51
myocardium A39.52
pericardium A39.53

Infection, infected, infective *(Continued)*
meningococcal *(Continued)*
joint A39.83
meninges A39.0
meningococcemia A39.4
acute A39.2
chronic A39.3
myocardium A39.52
pericardium A39.53
retrobulbar neuritis A39.82
specified site NEC A39.89
mesenteric lymph nodes or glands NEC I88.0
Metagonimus B66.8
metatarsophalangeal M00.9
methicillin
resistant Staphylococcus aureus (MRSA) A49.02
susceptible Staphylococcus aureus (MSSA) A49.01
Microsporum, microsporic —*see* Dermatophytosis
mixed flora (bacterial) NEC A49.8
Monilia —*see* Candidiasis
Monosporium apiospermum B48.2
mouth, parasitic B37.0
Mucor —*see* Mucormycosis
muscle NEC —*see* Myositis, infective
mycelium NOS B49
mycetoma B47.9
actinomycotic NEC B47.1
mycotic NEC B47.0
Mycobacterium, mycobacterial —*see* Mycobacterium
Mycoplasma NEC A49.3
pneumoniae, as cause of disease classified elsewhere B96.0
mycotic NOS B49
pathogenic to compromised host only B48.8
skin NOS B36.9
myocardium NEC I40.0
nail (chronic)
with lymphangitis —*see* Lymphangitis, acute, digit
finger L03.01-
fungus B35.1
ingrowing L60.0
toe L03.03-
fungus B35.1
nasal sinus (chronic) —*see* Sinusitis
nasopharynx —*see* Nasopharyngitis
navel L08.82
Necator americanus B76.1
Neisseria —*see* Gonococcus
Neotestudina rosatii B47.0
newborn P39.9
intra-amniotic NEC P39.2
skin P39.4
specified type NEC P39.8
nipple N61.0
associated with
lactation O91.03
pregnancy O91.01-
puerperium O91.02
Nocardia —*see* Nocardiosis
obstetrical surgical wound (puerperal) O86.0
Oesophagostomum (apiostomum) B81.8
Oestrus ovis —*see* Myiasis
Oidium albicans B37.9
Onchocerca (volvulus) —*see* Onchocerciasis - oncovirus, as cause of disease classified elsewhere B97.32
operation wound T81.40
Opisthorchis (felineus) (viverrini) B66.0
orbit, orbital —*see* Inflammation, orbit
orthopoxvirus NEC B08.09
ovary —*see* Salpingo-oophoritis
Oxyuris vermicularis B80

Infection, infected, infective *(Continued)*
pancreas (acute) —*see* Pancreatitis, acute
abscess —*see* Pancreatitis, acute
specified NEC —*see also* Pancreatitis, acute K85.80
papillomavirus, as cause of disease classified elsewhere B97.7
papovavirus NEC B34.4
Paracoccidioides brasiliensis —*see* Paracoccidioidomycosis
Paragonimus (westermani) B66.4
parainfluenza virus B34.8
parameningococcus NOS A39.9
parapoxvirus B08.60
specified NEC B08.69
parasitic B89
Parastrongylus
cantonensis B83.2
costaricensis B81.3
paratyphoid A01.4
Type A A01.1
Type B A01.2
Type C A01.3
paraurethral ducts N34.2
parotid gland —*see* Sialoadenitis
parvovirus NEC B34.3
as cause of disease classified elsewhere B97.6
Pasteurella NEC A28.0
multocida A28.0
pestis —*see* Plague
pseudotuberculosis A28.0
septica (cat bite) (dog bite) A28.0
tularensis —*see* Tularemia
pelvic, female —*see* Disease, pelvis, inflammatory
Penicillium (marneffei) B48.4
penis (glans) (retention) NEC N48.29
periapical K04.5
peridental, periodontal K05.20
generalized —*see* Peridontitis, aggressive, generalized
localized —*see* Peridontitis, aggressive, localized
perinatal period P39.9
specified type NEC P39.8
perineal repair (puerperal) O86.0
periorbital —*see* Inflammation, orbit
perirectal K62.89
perirenal —*see* Infection, kidney
peritoneal —*see* Peritonitis
periureteral N28.89
Petriellidium boydii B48.2
pharynx —*see also* Pharyngitis
coxsackievirus B08.5
posterior, lymphoid (chronic) J35.03
Phialophora
gougerotii (subcutaneous abscess or cyst) B43.2
jeanselmei (subcutaneous abscess or cyst) B43.2
verrucosa (skin) B43.0
Piedraia hortae B36.3
pinta A67.9
intermediate A67.1
late A67.2
mixed A67.3
primary A67.0
pinworm B80
pityrosporum furfur B36.0
pleuro-pneumonia-like organism (PPLO) NEC A49.3
as cause of disease classified elsewhere B96.0
pneumococcus, pneumococcal NEC A49.1
as cause of disease classified elsewhere B95.3
generalized (purulent) A40.3
with pneumonia J13
Pneumocystis carinii (pneumonia) B59
Pneumocystis jiroveci (pneumonia) B59

◄ New ⬅ Revised ~~deleted~~ Deleted

Infestation *(Continued)*
Acariasis B88.0
demodex folliculorum B88.0
sarcoptes scabiei B86
trombiculae B88.0
Agamofilaria streptocerca B74.4
Ancylostoma, ankylostoma (braziliense) (caninum) (ceylanicum) (duodenale) B76.0
americanum B76.1
new world B76.1
Anisakis larvae, anisakiasis B81.0
arthropod NEC B88.2
Ascaris lumbricoides —*see* Ascariasis
Balantidium coli A07.0
beef tapeworm B68.1
Bothriocephalus (latus) B70.0
larval B70.1
broad tapeworm B70.0
larval B70.1
Brugia (malayi) B74.1
timori B74.2
candiru B88.8
Capillaria
hepatica B83.8
philippinensis B81.1
cat liver fluke B66.0
cestodes B71.9
diphyllobothrium —*see* Infestation, diphyllobothrium
dipylidiasis B71.1
hymenolepiasis B71.0
specified type NEC B71.8
chigger B88.0
chigo, chigoe B88.1
Clonorchis (sinensis) (liver) B66.1
coccidial A07.3
crab-lice B85.3
Cysticercus cellulosae —*see* Cysticercosis
Demodex (folliculorum) B88.0
Dermanyssus gallinae B88.0
Dermatobia (hominis) —*see* Myiasis
Dibothriocephalus (latus) B70.0
larval B70.1
Dicrocoelium dendriticum B66.2
Diphyllobothrium (adult) (latum) (intestinal) (pacificum) B70.0
larval B70.1
Diplogonoporus (grandis) B71.8
Dipylidium caninum B67.4
Distoma hepaticum B66.3
dog tapeworm B67.4
Dracunculus medinensis B72
dragon worm B72
dwarf tapeworm B71.0
Echinococcus —*see* Echinococcus
Echinostomum ilocanum B66.8
Entamoeba (histolytica) —*see* Infection, Ameba
Enterobius vermicularis B80
eyelid
in (due to)
leishmaniasis B55.1
loiasis B74.3
onchocerciasis B73.09
phthiriasis B85.3
parasitic NOS B89
eyeworm B74.3
Fasciola (gigantica) (hepatica) (indica) B66.3
Fasciolopsis (buski) (intestine) B66.5
filarial B74.9
bancroftian B74.0
conjunctiva B74.9
due to
Acanthocheilonema (perstans) (streptocerca) B74.4
Brugia (malayi) B74.1
timori B74.2
Dracunculus medinensis B72
guinea worm B72
loa loa B74.3

Infestation *(Continued)*
filarial *(Continued)*
due to *(Continued)*
Mansonella (ozzardi) (perstans) (streptocerca) B74.4
Onchocerca volvulus B73.00
eye B73.00
eyelid B73.09
Wuchereria (bancrofti) B74.0
Malayan B74.1
ozzardi B74.4
specified type NEC B74.8
fish tapeworm B70.0
larval B70.1
fluke B66.9
blood NOS —*see* Schistosomiasis
cat liver B66.0
intestinal B66.5
lancet B66.2
liver (sheep) B66.3
cat B66.0
Chinese B66.1
due to clonorchiasis B66.1
oriental B66.1
lung (oriental) B66.4
sheep liver B66.3
specified type NEC B66.8
fly larvae —*see* Myiasis
Gasterophilus (intestinalis) —*see* Myiasis
Gastrodiscoides hominis B66.8
Giardia lamblia A07.1
Gnathostoma (spinigerum) B83.1
Gongylonema B83.8
guinea worm B72
helminth B83.9
angiostrongyliasis B83.2
intestinal B81.3
gnathostomiasis B83.1
hirudiniasis, internal B83.4
intestinal B82.0
angiostrongyliasis B81.3
anisakiasis B81.0
ascariasis —*see* Ascariasis
capillariasis B81.1
cysticercosis —*see* Cysticercosis
diphyllobothriasis —*see* Infestation, diphyllobothriasis
dracunculiasis B72
echinococcus —*see* Echinococcosis
enterobiasis B80
filariasis —*see* Infestation, filarial
fluke —*see* Infestation, fluke
hookworm —*see* Infestation, hookworm
mixed (types classifiable to more than one of the titles B65.0-B81.3 and B81.8) B81.4
onchocerciasis —*see* Onchocerciasis
schistosomiasis —*see* Infestation, schistosoma
specified
cestode NEC —*see* Infestation, cestode
type NEC B81.8
strongyloidiasis —*see* Strongyloidiasis
taenia —*see* Infestation, taenia
trichinellosis B75
trichostrongyliasis B81.2
trichuriasis B79
specified type NEC B83.8
syngamiasis B83.3
visceral larva migrans B83.0
Heterophyes (heterophyes) B66.8
hookworm B76.9
ancylostomiasis B76.0
necatoriasis B76.1
specified type NEC B76.8
Hymenolepis (diminuta) (nana) B71.0
intestinal NEC B82.9
leeches (aquatic) (land) —*see* Hirudiniasis
Leishmania —*see* Leishmaniasis
lice, louse —*see* Infestation, Pediculus
Linguatula B88.8

Infestation *(Continued)*
Liponyssoides sanguineus B88.0
Loa loa B74.3
conjunctival B74.3
eyelid B74.3
louse —*see* Infestation, Pediculus
maggots —*see* Myiasis
Mansonella (ozzardi) (perstans) (streptocerca) B74.4
Medina (worm) B72
Metagonimus (yokogawai) B66.8
microfilaria streptocerca —*see* Onchocerciasis
eye B73.00
eyelid B73.09
mites B88.9
scabic B86
Monilia (albicans) —*see* Candidiasis
mouth B37.0
Necator americanus B76.1
nematode NEC (intestinal) B82.0
Ancylostoma B76.0
conjunctiva NEC B83.9
Enterobius vermicularis B80
Gnathostoma spinigerum B83.1
physaloptera B80
specified NEC B81.8
trichostrongylus B81.2
trichuris (trichuria) B79
Oesophagostomum (apiostomum) B81.8
Oestrus ovis —*see also* Myiasis B87.9
Onchocerca (volvulus) —*see* Onchocerciasis
Opisthorchis (felineus) (viverrini) B66.0
orbit, parasitic NOS B89
Oxyuris vermicularis B80
Paragonimus (westermani) B66.4
parasite, parasitic B89
eyelid B89
intestinal NOS B82.9
mouth B37.0
skin B88.9
tongue B37.0
Parastrongylus
cantonensis B83.2
costaricensis B81.3
Pediculus B85.2
body B85.1
capitis (humanus) (any site) B85.0
corporis (humanus) (any site) B85.1
head B85.0
mixed (classifiable to more than one of the titles B85.0-B85.3) B85.4
pubis (any site) B85.3
Pentastoma B88.8
Phthirus (pubis) (any site) B85.3
with any infestation classifiable to B85.0-B85.2 B85.4
pinworm B80
pork tapeworm (adult) B68.0
protozoal NEC B64
intestinal A07.9
specified NEC A07.8
specified NEC B60.8
pubic, louse B85.3
rat tapeworm B71.0
red bug B88.0
roundworm (large) NEC B82.0
Ascariasis —*see also* Ascariasis B77.9
sandflea B88.1
Sarcoptes scabiei B86
scabies B86
Schistosoma B65.9
bovis B65.8
cercariae B65.3
haematobium B65.0
intercalatum B65.8
japonicum B65.2
mansoni B65.1
mattheei B65.8
mekongi B65.8
specified type NEC B65.8
spindale B65.8

- **Infestation** *(Continued)*
  - screw worms —*see* Myiasis
  - skin NOS B88.9
  - Sparganum (mansoni) (proliferum) (baxteri) B7Ø.1
    - larval B7Ø.1
  - specified type NEC B88.8
  - Spirometra larvae B7Ø.1
  - Stellantchasmus falcatus B66.8
  - Strongyloides stercoralis —*see* Strongyloidiasis
  - Taenia B68.9
    - diminuta B71.Ø
    - echinococcus —*see* Echinococcus
    - mediocanellata B68.1
    - nana B71.Ø
    - saginata B68.1
    - solium (intestinal form) B68.Ø
      - larval form —*see* Cysticercosis
  - Taeniarhynchus saginatus B68.1
  - tapeworm B71.9
    - beef B68.1
    - broad B7Ø.Ø
      - larval B7Ø.1
    - dog B67.4
    - dwarf B71.Ø
    - fish B7Ø.Ø
      - larval B7Ø.1
    - pork B68.Ø
    - rat B71.Ø
  - Ternidens diminutus B81.8
  - Tetranychus molestissimus B88.Ø
  - threadworm B8Ø
  - tongue B37.Ø
  - Toxocara (canis) (cati) (felis) B83.Ø
  - trematode (s) NEC —*see* Infestation, fluke
  - Trichinella (spiralis) B75
  - Trichocephalus B79
  - Trichomonas —*see* Trichomoniasis
  - Trichostrongylus B81.2
  - Trichuris (trichiura) B79
  - Trombicula (irritans) B88.Ø
  - Tunga penetrans B88.1
  - Uncinaria americana B76.1
  - Vandellia cirrhosa B88.8
  - whipworm B79
  - worms B83.9
    - intestinal B82.Ø
  - Wuchereria (bancrofti) B74.Ø
- **Infiltrate, infiltration**
  - amyloid (generalized) (localized) —*see* Amyloidosis
  - calcareous NEC R89.7
    - localized —*see* Degeneration, by site
  - calcium salt R89.7
  - cardiac
    - fatty —*see* Degeneration, myocardial
    - glycogenic E74.Ø2 *[I43]*
  - corneal —*see* Edema, cornea
  - eyelid —*see* Inflammation, eyelid
  - glycogen, glycogenic —*see* Disease, glycogen storage
  - heart, cardiac
    - fatty —*see* Degeneration, myocardial
    - glycogenic E74.Ø2 *[I43]*
  - inflammatory in vitreous H43.89
  - kidney N28.89
  - leukemic —*see* Leukemia
  - liver K76.89
    - fatty —*see* Fatty, liver NEC
    - glycogen —*see also* Disease, glycogen storage E74.Ø3 *[K77]*
  - lung R91.8
    - eosinophilic J82
  - lymphatic —*see also* Leukemia, lymphatic C91.9-
    - gland I88.9
  - muscle, fatty M62.89
  - myocardium, myocardial
    - fatty —*see* Degeneration, myocardial
    - glycogenic E74.Ø2 *[I43]*
- **Infiltrate, infiltration** *(Continued)*
  - on chest x-ray R91.8
  - pulmonary R91.8
    - with eosinophilia J82
  - skin (lymphocytic) L98.6
  - thymus (gland) (fatty) E32.8
  - urine R39.Ø
  - vesicant agent
    - antineoplastic chemotherapy T8Ø.81Ø
    - other agent NEC T8Ø.818
  - vitreous body H43.89
- **Infirmity** R68.89
  - senile R54
- **Inflammation, inflamed, inflammatory** (with exudation)
  - abducent (nerve) —*see* Strabismus, paralytic, sixth nerve
  - accessory sinus (chronic) —*see* Sinusitis
  - adrenal (gland) E27.8
  - alveoli, teeth M27.3
    - scorbutic E54
  - anal canal, anus K62.89
  - antrum (chronic) —*see* Sinusitis, maxillary
  - appendix —*see* Appendicitis
  - arachnoid —*see* Meningitis
  - areola N61.Ø ⬅
    - puerperal, postpartum or gestational —*see* Infection, nipple
  - areolar tissue NOS LØ8.9
  - artery —*see* Arteritis
  - auditory meatus (external) —*see* Otitis, externa
  - Bartholin's gland N75.8
  - bile duct (common) (hepatic) or passage —*see* Cholangitis
  - bladder —*see* Cystitis
  - bone —*see* Osteomyelitis
  - brain —*see also* Encephalitis
    - membrane —*see* Meningitis
  - breast N61.Ø ⬅
    - puerperal, postpartum, gestational —*see* Mastitis, obstetric
  - broad ligament —*see* Disease, pelvis, inflammatory
  - bronchi —*see* Bronchitis
  - catarrhal JØØ
  - cecum —*see* Appendicitis
  - cerebral —*see also* Encephalitis
    - membrane —*see* Meningitis
  - cerebrospinal
    - meningococcal A39.Ø
  - cervix (uteri) —*see* Cervicitis
  - chest J98.8
  - chorioretinal H3Ø.9-
    - cyclitis —*see* Cyclitis
    - disseminated H3Ø.1Ø-
      - generalized H3Ø.13-
      - peripheral H3Ø.12-
      - posterior pole H3Ø.11-
    - epitheliopathy —*see* Epitheliopathy
    - focal H3Ø.ØØ-
      - juxtapapillary H3Ø.Ø1-
      - macular H3Ø.Ø4-
      - paramacular —*see* Inflammation, chorioretinal, focal, macular
      - peripheral H3Ø.Ø3-
      - posterior pole H3Ø.Ø2-
    - specified type NEC H3Ø.89-
  - choroid —*see* Inflammation, chorioretinal
  - chronic, postmastoidectomy cavity —*see* Complications, postmastoidectomy, inflammation
  - colon —*see* Enteritis
  - connective tissue (diffuse) NEC —*see* Disorder, soft tissue, specified type NEC
  - cornea —*see* Keratitis
  - corpora cavernosa N48.29
  - cranial nerve —*see* Disorder, nerve, cranial
  - Douglas' cul-de-sac or pouch (chronic) N73.Ø
- **Inflammation, inflamed, inflammatory** *(Continued)*
  - due to device, implant or graft —*see also* Complications, by site and type, infection or inflammation
    - arterial graft T82.7
    - breast (implant) T85.79
    - catheter T85.79
      - dialysis (renal) T82.7
        - intraperitoneal T85.71
      - infusion T82.7
        - cranial T85.735 ◀
        - intrathecal T85.735 ◀
        - spinal (epidural) (subdural) T85.735 ⬅
        - subarachnoid T85.735 ◀
      - urinary T83.518 ⬅
        - cystostomy T83.51Ø ◀
        - Hopkins T83.518 ◀
        - ileostomy T83.518 ◀
        - nephrostomy T83.512 ◀
        - specified NEC T83.518 ◀
        - urethral indwelling T83.511 ◀
        - urostomy T83.518 ◀
    - electronic (electrode) (pulse generator) (stimulator)
      - bone T84.7
      - cardiac T82.7
      - nervous system T85.738 ⬅
        - brain T85.731 ◀
        - cranial nerve T85.732 ◀
        - gastric nerve T85.732 ◀
        - neurostimulator generator T85.734 ◀
        - peripheral nerve T85.732 ◀
        - sacral nerve T85.732 ◀
        - spinal cord T85.733 ◀
        - vagal nerve T85.732 ◀
      - urinary T83.59Ø ⬅
    - fixation, internal (orthopedic) NEC —*see* Complication, fixation device, infection
    - gastrointestinal (bile duct) (esophagus) T85.79
      - neurostimulator electrode (lead) T85.732 ◀
    - genital NEC T83.69 ⬅
    - heart NEC T82.7
      - valve (prosthesis) T82.6
        - graft T82.7
    - joint prosthesis —*see* Complication, joint prosthesis, infection
    - ocular (corneal graft) (orbital implant) NEC T85.79
    - orthopedic NEC T84.7
    - penile (cylinder) (pump) (resevoir) T83.61 ◀
    - specified NEC T85.79
    - testicular T83.62 ◀
    - urinary NEC T83.598 ⬅
      - ileal conduit stent T83.593 ◀
      - implanted neurostimulation T83.59Ø ◀
      - implanted sphincter T83.591 ◀
      - indwelling ureteral stent T83.592 ◀
      - nephroureteral stent T83.593 ◀
      - specified stent NEC T83.593 ◀
    - vascular NEC T82.7
    - ~~ventricular intracranial shunt T85.79~~
    - ventricular intracranial (communicating) shunt T85.73Ø ◀
  - duodenum K29.8Ø
    - with bleeding K29.81
  - dura mater —*see* Meningitis
  - ear (middle) —*see also* Otitis, media
    - external —*see* Otitis, externa
    - inner —*see* subcategory H83.Ø
  - epididymis —*see* Epididymitis
  - esophagus K2Ø.9
  - ethmoidal (sinus) (chronic) —*see* Sinusitis, ethmoidal
  - eustachian tube (catarrhal) —*see* Salpingitis, eustachian

Inflammation, inflamed, inflammatory (*Continued*)
eyelid H01.9
abscess —*see* Abscess, eyelid
blepharitis —*see* Blepharitis
chalazion —*see* Chalazion
dermatosis (noninfectious) —*see* Dermatosis, eyelid
hordeolum —*see* Hordeolum
specified NEC H01.8
fallopian tube —*see* Salpingo-oophoritis
fascia —*see* Myositis
follicular, pharynx J31.2
frontal (sinus) (chronic) —*see* Sinusitis, frontal
gallbladder —*see* Cholecystitis
gastric —*see* Gastritis
gastrointestinal —*see* Enteritis
genital organ (internal) (diffuse)
female —*see* Disease, pelvis, inflammatory
male N49.9
multiple sites N49.8
specified NEC N49.8
gland (lymph) —*see* Lymphadenitis
glottis —*see* Laryngitis
granular, pharynx J31.2
gum K05.10
nonplaque induced K05.11
plaque induced K05.10
heart —*see* Carditis
hepatic duct —*see* Cholangitis
ileoanal (internal) pouch K91.850
ileum —*see also* Enteritis
regional or terminal —*see* Enteritis, regional
intestinal pouch K91.850
intestine (any part) —*see* Enteritis
jaw (acute) (bone) (chronic) (lower) (suppurative) (upper) M27.2
joint NEC —*see* Arthritis
sacroiliac M46.1
kidney —*see* Nephritis
knee (joint) M13.169
tuberculous A18.02
labium (majus) (minus) —*see* Vulvitis
lacrimal
gland —*see* Dacryoadenitis
passages (duct) (sac) —*see also* Dacryocystitis
canaliculitis —*see* Canaliculitis, lacrimal
larynx —*see* Laryngitis
leg NOS L08.9
lip K13.0
liver (capsule) —*see also* Hepatitis
chronic K73.9
suppurative K75.0
lung (acute) —*see also* Pneumonia
chronic J98.4
lymphatic vessel —*see* Lymphangitis
lymph gland or node —*see* Lymphadenitis
maxilla, maxillary M27.2
sinus (chronic) —*see* Sinusitis, maxillary
membranes of brain or spinal cord —*see* Meningitis
meninges —*see* Meningitis
mouth K12.1
muscle —*see* Myositis
myocardium —*see* Myocarditis
nasal sinus (chronic) —*see* Sinusitis
nasopharynx —*see* Nasopharyngitis
navel L08.82
nerve NEC —*see* Neuralgia
nipple N61.0 ◄ (Revised)
puerperal, postpartum or gestational —*see* Infection, nipple
nose —*see* Rhinitis
oculomotor (nerve) —*see* Strabismus, paralytic, third nerve
optic nerve —*see* Neuritis, optic
orbit (chronic) H05.10
acute H05.00
abscess —*see* Abscess, orbit
cellulitis —*see* Cellulitis, orbit

Inflammation, inflamed, inflammatory (*Continued*)
orbit (chronic) (*Continued*)
acute (*Continued*)
osteomyelitis —*see* Osteomyelitis, orbit
periostitis —*see* Periostitis, orbital
tenonitis —*see* Tenonitis, eye
granuloma —*see* Granuloma, orbit
myositis —*see* Myositis, orbital
ovary —*see* Salpingo-oophoritis
oviduct —*see* Salpingo-oophoritis
pancreas (acute) —*see* Pancreatitis
parametrium N73.0
parotid region L08.9
pelvis, female —*see* Disease, pelvis, inflammatory
penis (corpora cavernosa) N48.29
perianal K62.89
pericardium —*see* Pericarditis
perineum (female) (male) L08.9
perirectal K62.89
peritoneum —*see* Peritonitis
periuterine —*see* Disease, pelvis, inflammatory
perivesical —*see* Cystitis
petrous bone (acute) (chronic) —*see* Petrositis
pharynx (acute) —*see* Pharyngitis
pia mater —*see* Meningitis
pleura —*see* Pleurisy
polyp, colon —*see also* Polyp, colon, inflammatory K51.40
prostate —*see also* Prostatitis
specified type NEC N41.8
rectosigmoid —*see* Rectosigmoiditis
rectum —*see also* Proctitis K62.89
respiratory, upper —*see also* Infection, respiratory, upper J06.9
acute, due to radiation J70.0
chronic, due to external agent —*see* condition, respiratory, chronic, due to
due to
chemicals, gases, fumes or vapors (inhalation) J68.2
radiation J70.1
retina —*see* Chorioretinitis
retrocecal —*see* Appendicitis
retroperitoneal —*see* Peritonitis
salivary duct or gland (any) (suppurative) —*see* Sialoadenitis
scorbutic, alveoli, teeth E54
scrotum N49.2
seminal vesicle —*see* Vesiculitis
sigmoid —*see* Enteritis
sinus —*see* Sinusitis
Skene's duct or gland —*see* Urethritis
skin L08.9
spermatic cord N49.1
sphenoidal (sinus) —*see* Sinusitis, sphenoidal
spinal
cord —*see* Encephalitis
membrane —*see* Meningitis
nerve —*see* Disorder, nerve
spine —*see* Spondylopathy, inflammatory
spleen (capsule) D73.89
stomach —*see* Gastritis
subcutaneous tissue L08.9
suprarenal (gland) E27.8
synovial —*see* Tenosynovitis
tendon (sheath) NEC —*see* Tenosynovitis
testis —*see* Orchitis
throat (acute) —*see* Pharyngitis
thymus (gland) E32.8
thyroid (gland) —*see* Thyroiditis
tongue K14.0
tonsil —*see* Tonsillitis
trachea —*see* Tracheitis
trochlear (nerve) —*see* Strabismus, paralytic, fourth nerve
tubal —*see* Salpingo-oophoritis
tuberculous NEC —*see* Tuberculosis

Inflammation, inflamed, inflammatory (*Continued*)
tubo-ovarian —*see* Salpingo-oophoritis
tunica vaginalis N49.1
tympanic membrane —*see* Tympanitis
umbilicus, umbilical L08.82
uterine ligament —*see* Disease, pelvis, inflammatory
uterus (catarrhal) —*see* Endometritis
uveal tract (anterior) NOS —*see also* Iridocyclitis
posterior —*see* Chorioretinitis
vagina —*see* Vaginitis
vas deferens N49.1
vein —*see also* Phlebitis
intracranial or intraspinal (septic) G08
thrombotic I80.9
leg —*see* Phlebitis, leg
lower extremity —*see* Phlebitis, leg
vocal cord J38.3
vulva —*see* Vulvitis
Wharton's duct (suppurative) —*see* Sialoadenitis
Inflation, lung, imperfect (newborn) —*see* Atelectasis
Influenza (bronchial) (epidemic) (respiratory (upper)) (unidentified influenza virus) J11.1
with
digestive manifestations J11.2
encephalopathy J11.81
enteritis J11.2
gastroenteritis J11.2
gastrointestinal manifestations J11.2
laryngitis J11.1
myocarditis J11.82
otitis media J11.83
pharyngitis J11.1
pneumonia J11.00
specified type J11.08
respiratory manifestations NEC J11.1
specified manifestation NEC J11.89
A/H5N1 —*see also* Influenza, due to, identified novel influenza A virus J09.X2
avian —*see also* Influenza, due to, identified novel influenza A virus J09.X2
bird —*see also* Influenza, due to, identified novel influenza A virus J09.X2
novel (2009) H1N1 influenza —*see also* Influenza, due to, identified influenza virus NEC J10.1
novel influenza A/H1N1 —*see also* Influenza, due to, identified influenza virus NEC J10.1
due to
avian (*see also* Influenza, due to, identified novel influenza A virus) J09.X2
identified influenza virus NEC J10.1
with
digestive manifestations J10.2
encephalopathy J10.81
enteritis J10.2
gastroenteritis J10.2
gastrointestinal manifestations J10.2
laryngitis J10.1
myocarditis J10.82
otitis media J10.83
pharyngitis J10.1
pneumonia (unspecified type) J10.00
with same identified influenza virus J10.01
specified type NEC J10.08
respiratory manifestations NEC J10.1
specified manifestation NEC J10.89
identified novel influenza A virus J09.X2
with
digestive manifestations J09.X3
encephalopathy J09.X9
enteritis J09.X3
gastroenteritis J09.X3
gastrointestinal manifestations J09.X3

Influenza *(Continued)*
due to *(Continued)*
identified novel influenza A virus *(Continued)*
with *(Continued)*
laryngitis J09.X2
myocarditis J09.X9
otitis media J09.X9
pharyngitis J09.X2
pneumonia J09.X1
respiratory manifestations NEC J09.X2
specified manifestation NEC J09.X9
upper respiratory symptoms J09.X2
of other animal origin, not bird or swine (*see also* Influenza, due to, identified novel influenza A virus) J09.X2
swine (viruses that normally cause infections in pigs) —*see also* Influenza, due to, identified novel influenza A virus J09.X2
Influenza-like disease —*see* Influenza
Influenzal —*see* Influenza
Infraction, Freiberg's (metatarsal head) —*see* Osteochondrosis, juvenile, metatarsus
Infraeruption of tooth (teeth) M26.34
Infusion complication, misadventure, or reaction —*see* Complications, infusion
Ingestion
chemical —*see* Table of Drugs and Chemicals, by substance, poisoning
drug or medicament
correct substance properly administered —*see* Table of Drugs and Chemicals, by drug, adverse effect
overdose or wrong substance given or taken —*see* Table of Drugs and Chemicals, by drug, poisoning
foreign body —*see* Foreign body, alimentary tract
tularemia A21.3
Ingrowing
hair (beard) L73.1
nail (finger) (toe) L60.0
Inguinal —*see also* condition
testicle Q53.9
bilateral Q53.21
unilateral Q53.11
Inhalant-induced ◀
anxiety disorder F18.980 ◀
depressive disorder F18.94 ◀
major neurocognitive disorder F18.97 ◀
mild neurocognitive disorder F18.988 ◀
psychotic disorder F18.959 ◀
Inhalation
anthrax A22.1
flame T27.3
food or foreign body —*see* Foreign body, by site
gases, fumes, or vapors NEC T59.9-
specified agent —*see* Table of Drugs and Chemicals, by substance
liquid or vomitus —*see* Asphyxia
meconium (newborn) P24.00
with
with respiratory symptoms P24.01
pneumonia (pneumonitis) P24.01
mucus —*see* Asphyxia, mucus
oil or gasoline (causing suffocation) —*see* Foreign body, by site
smoke J70.5
due to chemicals, gases, fumes and vapors J68.9
steam —*see* Toxicity, vapors
stomach contents or secretions —*see* Foreign body, by site
due to anesthesia (general) (local) or other sedation T88.59
in labor and delivery O74.0
in pregnancy O29.01-
postpartum, puerperal O89.01
Inhibition, orgasm
female F52.31
male F52.32
Inhibitor, systemic lupus erythematosus (presence of) D68.62
Iniencephalus, iniencephaly Q00.2
Injection, traumatic jet (air) (industrial) (water) (paint or dye) T70.4
Injury —*see also* specified injury type T14.90
abdomen, abdominal S39.91
blood vessel —*see* Injury, blood vessel, abdomen
cavity —*see* Injury, intra-abdominal
contusion S30.1
internal —*see* Injury, intra-abdominal
intra-abdominal organ —*see* Injury, intra-abdominal
nerve —*see* Injury, nerve, abdomen
open —*see* Wound, open, abdomen
specified NEC S39.81
superficial —*see* Injury, superficial, abdomen
Achilles tendon S86.00-
laceration S86.02-
specified type NEC S86.09-
strain S86.01-
acoustic, resulting in deafness —*see* Injury, nerve, acoustic
adrenal (gland) S37.819
contusion S37.812
laceration S37.813
specified type NEC S37.818
alveolar (process) S09.93
ankle S99.91-
contusion —*see* Contusion, ankle
dislocation —*see* Dislocation, ankle
fracture —*see* Fracture, ankle
nerve —*see* Injury, nerve, ankle
open —*see* Wound, open, ankle
specified type NEC S99.81-
sprain —*see* Sprain, ankle
superficial —*see* Injury, superficial, ankle
anterior chamber, eye —*see* Injury, eye, specified site NEC
anus —*see* Injury, abdomen
aorta (thoracic) S25.00
abdominal S35.00
laceration (minor) (superficial) S35.01
major S35.02
specified type NEC S35.09
laceration (minor) (superficial) S25.01
major S25.02
specified type NEC S25.09
arm (upper) S49.9-
blood vessel —*see* Injury, blood vessel, arm
contusion —*see* Contusion, arm, upper
fracture —*see* Fracture, humerus
lower —*see* Injury, forearm
muscle —*see* Injury, muscle, shoulder
nerve —*see* Injury, nerve, arm
open —*see* Wound, open, arm
specified type NEC S49.8-
superficial —*see* Injury, superficial, arm
artery (complicating trauma) —*see also* Injury, blood vessel, by site
cerebral or meningeal —*see* Injury, intracranial
auditory canal (external) (meatus) S09.91
auricle, auris, ear S09.91
axilla —*see* Injury, shoulder
back —*see* Injury, back, lower
bile duct S36.13
birth —*see also* Birth, injury P15.9
bladder (sphincter) S37.20
at delivery O71.5
contusion S37.22
laceration S37.23
obstetrical trauma O71.5
specified type NEC S37.29
Injury *(Continued)*
blast (air) (hydraulic) (immersion) (underwater) NEC T14.8
acoustic nerve trauma —*see* Injury, nerve, acoustic
bladder —*see* Injury, bladder
brain —*see* Concussion
colon —*see* Injury, intestine, large, blast injury
ear (primary) S09.31-
secondary S09.39-
generalized T70.8
lung —*see* Injury, intrathoracic, lung, blast injury
multiple body organs T70.8
peritoneum S36.81
rectum S36.61
retroperitoneum S36.898
small intestine S36.419
duodenum S36.410
specified site NEC S36.418
specified
intra-abdominal organ NEC S36.898
pelvic organ NEC S37.899
blood vessel NEC T14.8
abdomen S35.9-
aorta —*see* Injury, aorta, abdominal
celiac artery —*see* Injury, blood vessel, celiac artery
iliac vessel —*see* Injury, blood vessel, iliac
laceration S35.91
mesenteric vessel —*see* Injury, mesenteric
portal vein —*see* Injury, blood vessel, portal vein
renal vessel —*see* Injury, blood vessel, renal
specified vessel NEC S35.8X-
splenic vessel —*see* Injury, blood vessel, splenic
vena cava —*see* Injury, vena cava, inferior
ankle —*see* Injury, blood vessel, foot
aorta (abdominal) (thoracic) —*see* Injury, aorta
arm (upper) NEC S45.90-
forearm —*see* Injury, blood vessel, forearm
laceration S45.91-
specified
site NEC S45.80-
laceration S45.81-
specified type NEC S45.89-
type NEC S45.99-
superficial vein S45.30-
laceration S45.31-
specified type NEC S45.39-
axillary
artery S45.00-
laceration S45.01-
specified type NEC S45.09-
vein S45.20-
laceration S45.21-
specified type NEC S45.29-
azygos vein —*see* Injury, blood vessel, thoracic, specified site NEC
brachial
artery S45.10-
laceration S45.11-
specified type NEC S45.19-
vein S45.20-
laceration S45.219
specified type NEC S45.29-
carotid artery (common) (external) (internal, extracranial) S15.00-
internal, intracranial S06.8-
laceration (minor) (superficial) S15.01-
major S15.02-
specified type NEC S15.09-

◀ New ⟵ Revised ~~deleted~~ Deleted

Injury *(Continued)*
blood vessel NEC *(Continued)*
celiac artery S35.219
branch S35.299
laceration (minor) (superficial) S35.291
major S35.292
specified NEC S35.298
laceration (minor) (superficial) S35.211
major S35.212
specified type NEC S35.218
cerebral —*see* Injury, intracranial
deep plantar —*see* Injury, blood vessel, plantar artery
digital (hand) —*see* Injury, blood vessel, finger
dorsal
artery (foot) S95.ØØ-
laceration S95.Ø1-
specified type NEC S95.Ø9-
vein (foot) S95.2Ø-
laceration S95.21-
specified type NEC S95.29-
due to accidental laceration during procedure —*see* Laceration, accidental complicating surgery
extremity —*see* Injury, blood vessel, limb
femoral
artery (common) (superficial) S75.ØØ-
laceration (minor) (superficial) S75.Ø1-
major S75.Ø2-
specified type NEC S75.Ø9-
vein (hip level) (thigh level) S75.1Ø-
laceration (minor) (superficial) S75.11-
major S75.12-
specified type NEC S75.19-
finger S65.5Ø-
index S65.5Ø-
laceration S65.51-
specified type NEC S65.59-
laceration S65.51-
little S65.5Ø-
laceration S65.51-
specified type NEC S65.59-
middle S65.5Ø-
laceration S65.51-
specified type NEC S65.59-
specified type NEC S65.59-
thumb —*see* Injury, blood vessel, thumb
foot S95.9Ø-
dorsal
artery —*see* Injury, blood vessel, dorsal, artery
vein —*see* Injury, blood vessel, dorsal, vein
laceration S95.91-
plantar artery —*see* Injury, blood vessel, plantar artery
specified
site NEC S95.8Ø-
laceration S95.81-
specified type NEC S95.89-
specified type NEC S95.99-
forearm S55.9Ø-
laceration S55.91-
radial artery —*see* Injury, blood vessel, radial artery
specified
site NEC S55.8Ø-
laceration S55.81-
specified type NEC S55.89-
type NEC S55.99-
ulnar artery —*see* Injury, blood vessel, ulnar artery
vein S55.2Ø-
laceration S55.21-
specified type NEC S55.29-
gastric
artery —*see* Injury, mesenteric, artery, branch
vein —*see* Injury, blood vessel, abdomen

Injury *(Continued)*
blood vessel NEC *(Continued)*
gastroduodenal artery —*see* Injury, mesenteric, artery, branch
greater saphenous vein (lower leg level) S85.3Ø-
hip (and thigh) level S75.2Ø-
laceration (minor) (superficial) S75.21-
major S75.22-
specified type NEC S75.29-
laceration S85.31-
specified type NEC S85.39-
hand (level) S65.9Ø-
finger —*see* Injury, blood vessel, finger
laceration S65.91-
palmar arch —*see* Injury, blood vessel, palmar arch
radial artery —*see* Injury, blood vessel, radial artery, hand
specified
site NEC S65.8Ø-
laceration S65.81-
specified type NEC S65.89-
type NEC S65.99-
thumb —*see* Injury, blood vessel, thumb
ulnar artery —*see* Injury, blood vessel, ulnar artery, hand
head S09.Ø
intracranial —*see* Injury, intracranial
multiple S09.Ø
hepatic
artery —*see* Injury, mesenteric, artery
vein —*see* Injury, vena cava, inferior
hip S75.9Ø-
femoral artery —*see* Injury, blood vessel, femoral, artery
femoral vein —*see* Injury, blood vessel, femoral, vein
greater saphenous vein —*see* Injury, blood vessel, greater saphenous, hip level
laceration S75.91-
specified
site NEC S75.8Ø-
laceration S75.81-
specified type NEC S75.89-
type NEC S75.99-
hypogastric (artery) (vein) —*see* Injury, blood vessel, iliac
iliac S35.5-
artery S35.51-
specified vessel NEC S35.5-
uterine vessel —*see* Injury, blood vessel, uterine
vein S35.51-
innominate —*see* Injury, blood vessel, thoracic, innominate
intercostal (artery) (vein) —*see* Injury, blood vessel, thoracic, intercostal
jugular vein (external) S15.2Ø-
internal S15.3Ø-
laceration (minor) (superficial) S15.31-
major S15.32-
specified type NEC S15.39-
laceration (minor) (superficial) S15.21-
major S15.22-
specified type NEC S15.29-
leg (level) (lower) S85.9Ø-
greater saphenous —*see* Injury, blood vessel, greater saphenous
laceration S85.91-
lesser saphenous —*see* Injury, blood vessel, lesser saphenous
peroneal artery —*see* Injury, blood vessel, peroneal artery
popliteal
artery —*see* Injury, blood vessel, popliteal, artery
vein —*see* Injury, blood vessel, popliteal, vein

Injury *(Continued)*
blood vessel NEC *(Continued)*
leg (level) (lower) *(Continued)*
specified
site NEC S85.8Ø-
laceration S85.81-
specified type NEC S85.89-
type NEC S85.99-
thigh —*see* Injury, blood vessel, hip
tibial artery —*see* Injury, blood vessel, tibial artery
lesser saphenous vein (lower leg level) S85.4Ø-
laceration S85.41-
specified type NEC S85.49-
limb
lower —*see* Injury, blood vessel, leg
upper —*see* Injury, blood vessel, arm
lower back —*see* Injury, blood vessel, abdomen
specified NEC —*see* Injury, blood vessel, abdomen, specified, site NEC
mammary (artery) (vein) —*see* Injury, blood vessel, thoracic, specified site NEC
mesenteric (inferior) (superior)
artery —*see* Injury, mesenteric, artery
vein —*see* Injury, mesenteric, vein
neck S15.9
specified site NEC S15.8
ovarian (artery) (vein) —*see* subcategory S35.8
palmar arch (superficial) S65.2Ø-
deep S65.3Ø-
laceration S65.31-
specified type NEC S65.39-
laceration S65.21-
specified type NEC S65.29-
pelvis —*see* Injury, blood vessel, abdomen
specified NEC —*see* Injury, blood vessel, abdomen, specified, site NEC
peroneal artery S85.2Ø-
laceration S85.21-
specified type NEC S85.29-
plantar artery (deep) (foot) S95.1Ø-
laceration S95.11-
specified type NEC S95.19-
popliteal
artery S85.ØØ-
laceration S85.Ø1-
specified type NEC S85.Ø9-
vein S85.5Ø-
laceration S85.51-
specified type NEC S85.59-
portal vein S35.319
laceration S35.311
specified type NEC S35.318
precerebral —*see* Injury, blood vessel, neck
pulmonary (artery) (vein) —*see* Injury, blood vessel, thoracic, pulmonary
radial artery (forearm level) S55.1Ø-
hand and wrist (level) S65.1Ø-
laceration S65.11-
specified type NEC S65.19-
laceration S55.11-
specified type NEC S55.19-
renal
artery S35.4Ø-
laceration S35.41-
specified NEC S35.49-
vein S35.4Ø-
laceration S35.41-
specified NEC S35.49-
saphenous vein (greater) (lower leg level) —*see* Injury, blood vessel, greater saphenous
hip and thigh level —*see* Injury, blood vessel, greater saphenous, hip level
lesser —*see* Injury, blood vessel, lesser saphenous

Injury *(Continued)*
blood vessel NEC *(Continued)*
shoulder
specified NEC —*see* Injury, blood vessel, arm, specified site NEC
superficial vein —*see* Injury, blood vessel, arm, superficial vein
specified NEC T14.8
splenic
artery —*see* Injury, blood vessel, celiac artery, branch
vein S35.329
laceration S35.321
specified NEC S35.328
subclavian —*see* Injury, blood vessel, thoracic, innominate
thigh —*see* Injury, blood vessel, hip
thoracic S25.9Ø
aorta S25.ØØ
laceration (minor) (superficial) S25.Ø1
major S25.Ø2
specified type NEC S25.Ø9
azygos vein —*see* Injury, blood vessel, thoracic, specified, site NEC
innominate
artery S25.1Ø-
laceration (minor) (superficial) S25.11-
major S25.12-
specified type NEC S25.19-
vein S25.3Ø-
laceration (minor) (superficial) S25.31-
major S25.32-
specified type NEC S25.39-
intercostal S25.5Ø-
laceration S25.51-
specified type NEC S25.59-
laceration S25.91
mammary vessel —*see* Injury, blood vessel, thoracic, specified, site NEC
pulmonary S25.4Ø-
laceration (minor) (superficial) S25.41-
major S25.42-
specified type NEC S25.49-
specified
site NEC S25.8Ø-
laceration S25.81-
specified type NEC S25.89-
type NEC S25.99
subclavian —*see* Injury, blood vessel, thoracic, innominate
vena cava (superior) S25.2Ø
laceration (minor) (superficial) S25.21
major S25.22
specified type NEC S25.29
thumb S65.4Ø-
laceration S65.41-
specified type NEC S65.49-
tibial artery S85.1Ø-
anterior S85.13-
laceration S85.14-
specified injury NEC S85.15-
laceration S85.11-
posterior S85.16-
laceration S85.17-
specified injury NEC S85.18-
specified injury NEC S85.12-
ulnar artery (forearm level) S55.ØØ-
hand and wrist (level) S65.ØØ-
laceration S65.Ø1-
specified type NEC S65.Ø9-
laceration S55.Ø1-
specified type NEC S55.Ø9-
upper arm (level) —*see* Injury, blood vessel, arm
superficial vein —*see* Injury, blood vessel, arm, superficial vein
uterine S35.5-
artery S35.53-
vein S35.53-

Injury *(Continued)*
blood vessel NEC *(Continued)*
vena cava —*see* Injury, vena cava
vertebral artery S15.1Ø-
laceration (minor) (superficial) S15.11-
major S15.12-
specified type NEC S15.19-
wrist (level) —*see* Injury, blood vessel, hand
brachial plexus S14.3
newborn P14.3
brain (traumatic) SØ6.9-
diffuse (axonal) SØ6.2X-
focal SØ6.3Ø-
~~traumatic —see category SØ6~~
brainstem SØ6.38-
breast NOS S29.9
broad ligament —*see* Injury, pelvic organ, specified site NEC
bronchus, bronchi —*see* Injury, intrathoracic, bronchus
brow SØ9.9Ø
buttock S39.92
canthus, eye SØ5.9Ø
cardiac plexus —*see* Injury, nerve, thorax, sympathetic
cauda equina S34.3
cavernous sinus —*see* Injury, intracranial
cecum —*see* Injury, colon
celiac ganglion or plexus —*see* Injury, nerve, lumbosacral, sympathetic
cerebellum —*see* Injury, intracranial
cerebral —*see* Injury, intracranial
cervix (uteri) —*see* Injury, uterus
cheek (wall) SØ9.93
chest —*see* Injury, thorax
childbirth (newborn) —*see also* Birth, injury
maternal NEC O71.9
chin SØ9.93
choroid (eye) —*see* Injury, eye, specified site NEC
clitoris S39.94
coccyx —*see also* Injury, back, lower
complicating delivery O71.6
colon —*see* Injury, intestine, large
common bile duct —*see* Injury, liver
conjunctiva (superficial) —*see* Injury, eye, conjunctiva
conus medullaris —*see* Injury, spinal, sacral
cord
spermatic (pelvic region) S37.898
scrotal region S39.848
spinal —*see* Injury, spinal cord, by region
cornea —*see* Injury, eye, specified site NEC
abrasion —*see* Injury, eye, cornea, abrasion
cortex (cerebral) —*see also* Injury, intracranial
visual —*see* Injury, nerve, optic
costal region NEC S29.9
costochondral NEC S29.9
cranial
cavity —*see* Injury, intracranial
nerve —*see* Injury, nerve, cranial
crushing —*see* Crush
cutaneous sensory nerve
cystic duct —*see* Injury, liver
deep tissue —*see* Contusion, by site
meaning pressure ulcer —*see* Ulcer, pressure, unstageable, by site
delivery (newborn) P15.9
maternal NEC O71.9
Descemet's membrane —*see* Injury, eyeball, penetrating
diaphragm —*see* Injury, intrathoracic, diaphragm
duodenum —*see* Injury, intestine, small, duodenum
ear (auricle) (external) (canal) SØ9.91
abrasion —*see* Abrasion, ear
bite —*see* Bite, ear
blister —*see* Blister, ear
bruise —*see* Contusion, ear

Injury *(Continued)*
ear *(Continued)*
contusion —*see* Contusion, ear
external constriction —*see* Constriction, external, ear
hematoma —*see* Hematoma, ear
inner —*see* Injury, ear, middle
laceration —*see* Laceration, ear
middle SØ9.3Ø-
blast —*see* Injury, blast, ear
specified NEC SØ9.39-
puncture —*see* Puncture, ear
superficial —*see* Injury, superficial, ear
eighth cranial nerve (acoustic or auditory) —*see* Injury, nerve, acoustic
elbow S59.9Ø-
contusion —*see* Contusion, elbow
dislocation —*see* Dislocation, elbow
fracture —*see* Fracture, ulna, upper end
open —*see* Wound, open, elbow
specified NEC S59.8Ø-
sprain —*see* Sprain, elbow
superficial —*see* Injury, superficial, elbow
eleventh cranial nerve (accessory) —*see* Injury, nerve, accessory
epididymis S39.94
epigastric region S39.91
epiglottis NEC S19.89
esophageal plexus —*see* Injury, nerve, thorax, sympathetic
esophagus (thoracic part) —*see also* Injury, intrathoracic, esophagus
cervical NEC S19.85
eustachian tube SØ9.3Ø-
eye SØ5.9-
avulsion SØ5.7-
ball —*see* Injury, eyeball
conjunctiva SØ5.Ø-
cornea
abrasion SØ5.Ø-
laceration SØ5.3-
with prolapse SØ5.2-
lacrimal apparatus SØ5.8X-
orbit penetration SØ5.4-
specified site NEC SØ5.8X-
eyeball SØ5.8X-
contusion SØ5.1-
penetrating SØ5.6-
with
foreign body SØ5.5-
prolapse or loss of intraocular tissue SØ5.2-
without prolapse or loss of intraocular tissue SØ5.3-
specified type NEC SØ5.8-
eyebrow SØ9.93
eyelid SØ9.93
abrasion —*see* Abrasion, eyelid
contusion —*see* Contusion, eyelid
open —*see* Wound, open, eyelid
face SØ9.93
fallopian tube S37.5Ø9
bilateral S37.5Ø2
blast injury S37.512
contusion S37.522
laceration S37.532
specified type NEC S37.592
blast injury (primary) S37.519
bilateral S37.512
secondary —*see* Injury, fallopian tube, specified type NEC
unilateral S37.511
contusion S37.529
bilateral S37.522
unilateral S37.521
laceration S37.539
bilateral S37.532
unilateral S37.531
specified type NEC S37.599
bilateral S37.592
unilateral S37.591

Injury *(Continued)*
fallopian tube *(Continued)*
unilateral S37.501
blast injury S37.511
contusion S37.521
laceration S37.531
specified type NEC S37.591
fascia —*see* Injury, muscle
fifth cranial nerve (trigeminal) —*see* Injury, nerve, trigeminal
finger (nail) S69.9-
blood vessel —*see* Injury, blood vessel, finger
contusion —*see* Contusion, finger
dislocation —*see* Dislocation, finger
fracture —*see* Fracture, finger
muscle —*see* Injury, muscle, finger
nerve —*see* Injury, nerve, digital, finger
open —*see* Wound, open, finger
specified NEC S69.8-
sprain —*see* Sprain, finger
superficial —*see* Injury, superficial, finger
first cranial nerve (olfactory) —*see* Injury, nerve, olfactory
flank —*see* Injury, abdomen
foot S99.92-
blood vessel —*see* Injury, blood vessel, foot
contusion —*see* Contusion, foot
dislocation —*see* Dislocation, foot
fracture —*see* Fracture, foot
muscle —*see* Injury, muscle, foot
open —*see* Wound, open, foot
specified type NEC S99.82-
sprain —*see* Sprain, foot
superficial —*see* Injury, superficial, foot
forceps NOS P15.9
forearm S59.91-
blood vessel —*see* Injury, blood vessel, forearm
contusion —*see* Contusion, forearm
fracture —*see* Fracture, forearm
muscle —*see* Injury, muscle, forearm
nerve —*see* Injury, nerve, forearm
open —*see* Wound, open, forearm
specified NEC S59.81-
superficial —*see* Injury, superficial, forearm
forehead S09.90
fourth cranial nerve (trochlear) —*see* Injury, nerve, trochlear
gallbladder S36.129
contusion S36.122
laceration S36.123
specified NEC S36.128
ganglion
celiac, coeliac —*see* Injury, nerve, lumbosacral, sympathetic
gasserian —*see* Injury, nerve, trigeminal
stellate —*see* Injury, nerve, thorax, sympathetic
thoracic sympathetic —*see* Injury, nerve, thorax, sympathetic
gasserian ganglion —*see* Injury, nerve, trigeminal
gastric artery —*see* Injury, blood vessel, celiac artery, branch
gastroduodenal artery —*see* Injury, blood vessel, celiac artery, branch
gastrointestinal tract —*see* Injury, intra-abdominal
with open wound into abdominal cavity —*see* Wound, open, with penetration into peritoneal cavity
colon —*see* Injury, intestine, large
rectum —*see* Injury, intestine, large, rectum
with open wound into abdominal cavity S36.61
small intestine —*see* Injury, intestine, small
specified site NEC —*see* Injury, intra-abdominal, specified, site NEC
stomach —*see* Injury, stomach

Injury *(Continued)*
genital organ (s)
external S39.94
specified NEC S39.848
internal S37.90
fallopian tube —*see* Injury, fallopian tube
ovary —*see* Injury, ovary
prostate —*see* Injury, prostate
seminal vesicle —*see* Injury, pelvis, organ, specified site NEC
uterus —*see* Injury, uterus
vas deferens —*see* Injury, pelvis, organ, specified site NEC
obstetrical trauma O71.9
gland
lacrimal laceration —*see* Injury, eye, specified site NEC
salivary S09.93 ⟸
thyroid NEC S19.84
globe (eye) S05.90
specified NEC S05.8X-
groin —*see* Injury, abdomen
gum S09.90
hand S69.9-
blood vessel —*see* Injury, blood vessel, hand
contusion —*see* Contusion, hand
fracture —*see* Fracture, hand
muscle —*see* Injury, muscle, hand
nerve —*see* Injury, nerve, hand
open —*see* Wound, open, hand
specified NEC S69.8-
sprain —*see* Sprain, hand
superficial —*see* Injury, superficial, hand
head S09.90
with loss of consciousness S06.9-
specified NEC S09.8-
heart S26.90
with hemopericardium S26.00
contusion S26.01
laceration (mild) S26.020
major S26.022
moderate S26.021
specified type NEC S26.09
without hemopericardium S26.10
contusion S26.11
laceration S26.12
specified type NEC S26.19
contusion S26.91
laceration S26.92
specified type NEC S26.99
heel —*see* Injury, foot
hepatic
artery —*see* Injury, blood vessel, celiac artery, branch
duct —*see* Injury, liver
vein —*see* Injury, vena cava, inferior
hip S79.91-
blood vessel —*see* Injury, blood vessel, hip
contusion —*see* Contusion, hip
dislocation —*see* Dislocation, hip
fracture —*see* Fracture, femur, neck
muscle —*see* Injury, muscle, hip
nerve —*see* Injury, nerve, hip
open —*see* Wound, open, hip
specified NEC S79.81-
sprain —*see* Sprain, hip
superficial —*see* Injury, superficial, hip
hymen S39.94
hypogastric
blood vessel —*see* Injury, blood vessel, iliac
plexus —*see* Injury, nerve, lumbosacral, sympathetic
ileum —*see* Injury, intestine, small
iliac region S39.91
instrumental (during surgery) —*see* Laceration, accidental complicating surgery
birth injury —*see* Birth, injury
nonsurgical —*see* Injury, by site

Injury *(Continued)*
instrumental *(Continued)*
obstetrical O71.9
bladder O71.5
cervix O71.3
high vaginal O71.4
perineal NOS O70.9
urethra O71.5
uterus O71.5
with rupture or perforation O71.1
internal T14.8
aorta —*see* Injury, aorta
bladder (sphincter) —*see* Injury, bladder
with
ectopic or molar pregnancy O08.6
following ectopic or molar pregnancy O08.6
obstetrical trauma O71.5
bronchus, bronchi —*see* Injury, intrathoracic, bronchus
cecum —*see* Injury, intestine, large
cervix (uteri) —*see also* Injury, uterus
with ectopic or molar pregnancy O08.6
following ectopic or molar pregnancy O08.6
obstetrical trauma O71.3
chest —*see* Injury, intrathoracic
gastrointestinal tract —*see* Injury, intra-abdominal
heart —*see* Injury, heart
intestine NEC —*see* Injury, intestine
intrauterine —*see* Injury, uterus
mesentery —*see* Injury, intra-abdominal, specified, site NEC
pelvis, pelvic (organ) S37.90
following ectopic or molar pregnancy (subsequent episode) O08.6
obstetrical trauma NEC O71.5
rupture or perforation O71.1
specified NEC S39.83
rectum —*see* Injury, intestine, large, rectum
stomach —*see* Injury, stomach
ureter —*see* Injury, ureter
urethra (sphincter) following ectopic or molar pregnancy O08.6
uterus —*see* Injury, uterus
interscapular area —*see* Injury, thorax
intestine
large S36.509
ascending (right) S36.500
blast injury (primary) S36.510
secondary S36.590
contusion S36.520
laceration S36.530
specified type NEC S36.590
blast injury (primary) S36.519
ascending (right) S36.510
descending (left) S36.512
rectum S36.61
sigmoid S36.513
specified site NEC S36.518
transverse S36.511
contusion S36.529
ascending (right) S36.520
descending (left) S36.522
rectum S36.62
sigmoid S36.523
specified site NEC S36.528
transverse S36.521
descending (left) S36.502
blast injury (primary) S36.512
secondary S36.592
contusion S36.522
laceration S36.532
specified type NEC S36.592
laceration S36.539
ascending (right) S36.530
descending (left) S36.532
rectum S36.63
sigmoid S36.533

Injury *(Continued)*
lumbar, lumbosacral (region) S39.92
plexus —*see* Injury, lumbosacral plexus
lumbosacral plexus S34.4
lung —*see also* Injury, intrathoracic, lung
aspiration J69.Ø
transfusion-related (TRALI) J95.84
lymphatic thoracic duct —*see* Injury, intrathoracic, specified organ NEC
malar region SØ9.93
mastoid region SØ9.9Ø
maxilla SØ9.93
mediastinum —*see* Injury, intrathoracic, specified organ NEC
membrane, brain —*see* Injury, intracranial
meningeal artery —*see* Injury, intracranial, subdural hemorrhage
meninges (cerebral) —*see* Injury, intracranial
mesenteric
artery
branch S35.299
laceration (minor) (superficial) S35.291
major S35.292
specified NEC S35.298
inferior S35.239
laceration (minor) (superficial) S35.231
major S35.232
specified NEC S35.238
superior S35.229
laceration (minor) (superficial) S35.221
major S35.222
specified NEC S35.228
plexus (inferior) (superior) —*see* Injury, nerve, lumbosacral, sympathetic
vein
inferior S35.349
laceration S35.341
specified NEC S35.348
superior S35.339
laceration S35.331
specified NEC S35.338
mesentery —*see* Injury, intra-abdominal, specified site NEC
mesosalpinx —*see* Injury, pelvic organ, specified site NEC
middle ear SØ9.3Ø-
midthoracic region NOS S29.9
mouth SØ9.93
multiple NOS TØ7
muscle (and fascia) (and tendon)
abdomen S39.ØØ1
laceration S39.Ø21
specified type NEC S39.Ø91
strain S39.Ø11
abductor
thumb, forearm level —*see* Injury, muscle, thumb, abductor
adductor
thigh S76.2Ø-
laceration S76.22-
specified type NEC S76.29-
strain S76.21-
ankle —*see* Injury, muscle, foot
anterior muscle group, at leg level (lower) S86.2Ø-
laceration S86.22-
specified type NEC S86.29-
strain S86.21-
arm (upper) —*see* Injury, muscle, shoulder
biceps (parts NEC) S46.2Ø-
laceration S46.22-
long head S46.1Ø-
laceration S46.12-
specified type NEC S46.19-
strain S46.11-
specified type NEC S46.29-
strain S46.21-
extensor
finger (s) (other than thumb) —*see* Injury, muscle, finger by site, extensor

Injury *(Continued)*
muscle *(Continued)*
extensor *(Continued)*
forearm level, specified NEC —*see* Injury, muscle, forearm, extensor
thumb —*see* Injury, muscle, thumb, extensor
toe (large) (ankle level) (foot level) —*see* Injury, muscle, toe, extensor
finger
extensor (forearm level) S56.4Ø-
hand level S66.3Ø9
laceration S66.329
specified type NEC S66.399
strain S66.319
laceration S56.429
specified type NEC S56.499
strain S56.419
flexor (forearm level) S56.1Ø-
hand level S66.1Ø9
laceration S66.129
specified type NEC S66.199
strain S66.119
laceration S56.129
specified type NEC S56.199
strain S56.119
index
extensor (forearm level)
hand level S66.3Ø8
laceration S66.32-
specified type NEC S66.39-
strain S66.31-
specified type NEC S56.492-
flexor (forearm level)
hand level S66.1Ø8
laceration S66.12-
specified type NEC S66.19-
strain S66.11-
specified type NEC S56.19-
strain S56.11-
intrinsic S66.5Ø-
laceration S66.52-
specified type NEC S66.59-
strain S66.51-
intrinsic S66.5Ø9
laceration S66.529
specified type NEC S66.599
strain S66.519
little
extensor (forearm level)
hand level S66.3Ø-
laceration S66.32-
specified type NEC S66.39-
strain S66.31-
laceration S56.42-
specified type NEC S56.49-
strain S56.41-
flexor (forearm level)
hand level S66.1Ø-
laceration S66.12-
specified type NEC S66.19-
strain S66.11-
laceration S56.12-
specified type NEC S56.19-
strain S56.11-
intrinsic S66.5Ø-
laceration S66.52-
specified type NEC S66.59-
strain S66.51-
middle
extensor (forearm level)
hand level S66.3Ø-
laceration S66.32-
specified type NEC S66.39-
strain S66.31-
laceration S56.42-
specified type NEC S56.49-
strain S56.41-

Injury *(Continued)*
muscle *(Continued)*
finger *(Continued)*
middle *(Continued)*
flexor (forearm level)
hand level S66.1Ø-
laceration S66.12-
specified type NEC S66.19-
strain S66.11-
laceration S56.12-
specified type NEC S56.19-
strain S56.11-
intrinsic S66.5Ø-
laceration S66.52-
specified type NEC S66.59-
strain S66.51-
ring
extensor (forearm level)
hand level S66.3Ø-
laceration S66.32-
specified type NEC S66.39-
strain S66.31-
laceration S56.42-
specified type NEC S56.49-
strain S56.41-
flexor (forearm level)
hand level S66.1Ø-
laceration S66.12-
specified type NEC S66.19-
strain S66.11-
laceration S56.12-
specified type NEC S56.19-
strain S56.11-
intrinsic S66.5Ø-
laceration S66.52-
specified type NEC S66.59-
strain S66.51-
flexor
finger(s) (other than thumb) — *see* Injury, muscle, finger
forearm level, specified NEC — *see* Injury, muscle, forearm, flexor
thumb —*see* Injury, muscle, thumb, flexor
toe (long) (ankle level) (foot level) —*see* Injury, muscle, toe, flexor
foot S96.9Ø-
intrinsic S96.2Ø-
laceration S96.22-
specified type NEC S96.29-
strain S96.21-
laceration S96.92-
long extensor, toe —*see* Injury, muscle, toe, extensor
long flexor, toe —*see* Injury, muscle, toe, flexor
specified
site NEC S96.8Ø-
laceration S96.82-
specified type NEC S96.89-
strain S96.81-
type NEC S96.99-
strain S96.91-
forearm (level) S56.9Ø-
extensor S56.5Ø-
laceration S56.52-
specified type NEC S56.59-
strain S56.51-
flexor S56.2Ø-
laceration S56.22-
specified type NEC S56.29-
strain S56.21-
laceration S56.92-
specified S56.99-
site NEC S56.8Ø-
laceration S56.82-
strain S56.81-
type NEC S56.89-
strain S56.91-

Injury (Continued)
muscle (Continued)
hand (level) S66.9Ø-
laceration S66.92-
specified
site NEC S66.8Ø-
laceration S66.82-
specified type NEC S66.89-
strain S66.81-
type NEC S66.99-
strain S66.91-
head SØ9.1Ø
laceration SØ9.12
specified type NEC SØ9.19
strain SØ9.11
hip NEC S76.ØØ-
laceration S76.Ø2-
specified type NEC S76.Ø9-
strain S76.Ø1-
intrinsic
ankle and foot level —*see* Injury, muscle, foot, intrinsic
finger (other than thumb) —*see* Injury, muscle, finger by site, intrinsic
foot (level) —*see* Injury, muscle, foot, intrinsic
thumb —*see* Injury, muscle, thumb, intrinsic
leg (level) (lower) S86.9Ø-
Achilles tendon —*see* Injury, Achilles tendon
anterior muscle group —*see* Injury, muscle, anterior muscle group
laceration S86.92-
peroneal muscle group —*see* Injury, muscle, peroneal muscle group
posterior muscle group —*see* Injury, muscle, posterior muscle group, leg level
specified
site NEC S86.8Ø-
laceration S86.82-
specified type NEC S86.89-
strain S86.81-
type NEC S86.99-
strain S86.91-
long
extensor toe, at ankle and foot level —*see* Injury, muscle, toe, extensor
flexor, toe, at ankle and foot level —*see* Injury, muscle, toe, flexor
head, biceps —*see* Injury, muscle, biceps, long head
lower back S39.ØØ2
laceration S39.Ø22
specified type NEC S39.Ø92
strain S39.Ø12
neck (level) S16.9
laceration S16.2
specified type NEC S16.8
strain S16.1
pelvis S39.ØØ3
laceration S39.Ø23
specified type NEC S39.Ø93
strain S39.Ø13
peroneal muscle group, at leg level (lower) S86.3Ø-
laceration S86.32-
specified type NEC S86.39-
strain S86.31-
posterior muscle (group)
leg level (lower) S86.1Ø-
laceration S86.12-
specified type NEC S86.19-
strain S86.11-
thigh level S76.3Ø-
laceration S76.32-
specified type NEC S76.39-
strain S76.31-

Injury (Continued)
muscle (Continued)
quadriceps (thigh) S76.1Ø-
laceration S76.12-
specified type NEC S76.19-
strain S76.11-
shoulder S46.9Ø-
laceration S46.92-
rotator cuff —*see* Injury, rotator cuff
specified site NEC S46.8Ø-
laceration S46.82-
specified type NEC S46.89-
strain S46.81-
specified type NEC S46.99-
strain S46.91-
thigh NEC (level) S76.9Ø-
adductor —*see* Injury, muscle, adductor, thigh
laceration S76.92-
posterior muscle (group) —*see* Injury, muscle, posterior muscle, thigh level
quadriceps —*see* Injury, muscle, quadriceps
specified
site NEC S76.8Ø-
laceration S76.82-
specified type NEC S76.89-
strain S76.81-
type NEC S76.99-
strain S76.91-
thorax (level) S29.ØØ9
back wall S29.ØØ2
front wall S29.ØØ1
laceration S29.Ø29
back wall S29.Ø22
front wall S29.Ø21
specified type NEC S29.Ø99
back wall S29.Ø92
front wall S29.Ø91
strain S29.Ø19
back wall S29.Ø12
front wall S29.Ø11
thumb
abductor (forearm level) S56.3Ø-
laceration S56.32-
specified type NEC S56.39-
strain S56.31-
extensor (forearm level) S56.3Ø-
hand level S66.2Ø-
laceration S66.22-
specified type NEC S66.29-
strain S66.21-
laceration S56.32-
specified type NEC S56.39-
strain S56.31-
flexor (forearm level) S56.ØØ-
hand level S66.ØØ-
laceration S66.Ø2-
specified type NEC S66.Ø9-
strain S66.Ø1-
laceration S56.Ø2-
specified type NEC S56.Ø9-
strain S56.Ø1-
wrist level —*see* Injury, muscle, thumb, flexor, hand level
intrinsic S66.4Ø-
laceration S66.42-
specified type NEC S66.49-
strain S66.41-
toe —*see also* Injury, muscle, foot
extensor, long S96.1Ø-
laceration S96.12-
specified type NEC S96.19-
strain S96.11-
flexor, long S96.ØØ-
laceration S96.Ø2-
specified type NEC S96.Ø9-
strain S96.Ø1-

Injury (Continued)
muscle (Continued)
triceps S46.3Ø-
laceration S46.32-
specified type NEC S46.39-
strain S46.31-
wrist (and hand) level —*see* Injury, muscle, hand
musculocutaneous nerve —*see* Injury, nerve, musculocutaneous
myocardium —*see* Injury, heart
nape —*see* Injury, neck
nasal (septum) (sinus) SØ9.92
nasopharynx SØ9.92
neck S19.9
specified NEC S19.8Ø
specified site NEC S19.89
nerve NEC T14.8
abdomen S34.9
peripheral S34.6
specified site NEC S34.8
abducens SØ4.4-
contusion SØ4.4-
laceration SØ4.4-
specified type NEC SØ4.4-
abducent —*see* Injury, nerve, abducens
accessory SØ4.7-
contusion SØ4.7-
laceration SØ4.7-
specified type NEC SØ4.7-
acoustic SØ4.6-
contusion SØ4.6-
laceration SØ4.6-
specified type NEC SØ4.6-
ankle S94.9-
cutaneous sensory S94.3-
specified site NEC —*see* subcategory S94.8
anterior crural, femoral —*see* Injury, nerve, femoral
arm (upper) S44.9-
axillary —*see* Injury, nerve, axillary
cutaneous —*see* Injury, nerve, cutaneous, arm
median —*see* Injury, nerve, median, upper arm
musculocutaneous —*see* Injury, nerve, musculocutaneous
radial —*see* Injury, nerve, radial, upper arm
specified site NEC —*see* subcategory S44.8
ulnar —*see* Injury, nerve, ulnar, arm
auditory —*see* Injury, nerve, acoustic
axillary S44.3-
brachial plexus —*see* Injury, brachial plexus
cervical sympathetic S14.5
cranial SØ4.9
contusion SØ4.9
eighth (acoustic or auditory) —*see* Injury, nerve, acoustic
eleventh (accessory) —*see* Injury, nerve, accessory
fifth (trigeminal) —*see* Injury, nerve, trigeminal
first (olfactory) —*see* Injury, nerve, olfactory
fourth (trochlear) —*see* Injury, nerve, trochlear
laceration SØ4.9
ninth (glossopharyngeal) —*see* Injury, nerve, glossopharyngeal
second (optic) —*see* Injury, nerve, optic
seventh (facial) —*see* Injury, nerve, facial
sixth (abducent) —*see* Injury, nerve, abducens
specified
nerve NEC SØ4.89-
contusion SØ4.89-
laceration SØ4.89-
specified type NEC SØ4.89-
type NEC SØ4.9

◀ New ⬅ Revised ~~deleted~~ Deleted

Injury *(Continued)*
nerve NEC *(Continued)*
cranial *(Continued)*
tenth (pneumogastric or vagus) —*see* Injury, nerve, vagus
third (oculomotor) —*see* Injury, nerve, oculomotor
twelfth (hypoglossal) —*see* Injury, nerve, hypoglossal
cutaneous sensory
ankle (level) S94.3-
arm (upper) (level) S44.5-
foot (level) —*see* Injury, nerve, cutaneous sensory, ankle
forearm (level) S54.3-
hip (level) S74.2-
leg (lower level) S84.2-
shoulder (level) —*see* Injury, nerve, cutaneous sensory, arm
thigh (level) —*see* Injury, nerve, cutaneous sensory, hip
deep peroneal —*see* Injury, nerve, peroneal, foot
digital
finger S64.4-
index S64.49-
little S64.49-
middle S64.49-
ring S64.49-
thumb S64.3-
toe —*see* Injury, nerve, ankle, specified site NEC
eighth cranial (acoustic or auditory) —*see* Injury, nerve, acoustic
eleventh cranial (accessory) —*see* Injury, nerve, accessory
facial S04.5-
contusion S04.5-
laceration S04.5-
newborn P11.3
specified type NEC S04.5-
femoral (hip level) (thigh level) S74.1-
fifth cranial (trigeminal) —*see* Injury, nerve, trigeminal
finger (digital) —*see* Injury, nerve, digital, finger
first cranial (olfactory) —*see* Injury, nerve, olfactory
foot S94.9-
cutaneous sensory S94.3-
deep peroneal S94.2-
lateral plantar S94.0-
medial plantar S94.1-
specified site NEC —*see* subcategory S94.8
forearm (level) S54.9-
cutaneous sensory —*see* Injury, nerve, cutaneous sensory, forearm
median —*see* Injury, nerve, median
radial —*see* Injury, nerve, radial
specified site NEC —*see* subcategory S54.8
ulnar —*see* Injury, nerve, ulnar
fourth cranial (trochlear) —*see* Injury, nerve, trochlear
glossopharyngeal S04.89-
specified type NEC S04.89-
hand S64.9-
median —*see* Injury, nerve, median, hand
radial —*see* Injury, nerve, radial, hand
specified NEC —*see* subcategory S64.8
ulnar —*see* Injury, nerve, ulnar, hand
hip (level) S74.9-
cutaneous sensory —*see* Injury, nerve, cutaneous sensory, hip
femoral —*see* Injury, nerve, femoral
sciatic —*see* Injury, nerve, sciatic
specified site NEC —*see* subcategory S74.8

Injury *(Continued)*
nerve NEC *(Continued)*
hypoglossal S04.89-
specified type NEC S04.89-
lateral plantar S94.0-
leg (lower) S84.9-
cutaneous sensory —*see* Injury, nerve, cutaneous sensory, leg
peroneal —*see* Injury, nerve, peroneal
specified site NEC —*see* subcategory S84.8
tibial —*see* Injury, nerve, tibial
upper —*see* Injury, nerve, thigh
lower
back —*see* Injury, nerve, abdomen, specified site NEC
peripheral —*see* Injury, nerve, abdomen, peripheral
limb —*see* Injury, nerve, leg
lumbar plexus —*see* Injury, nerve, lumbosacral, sympathetic
lumbar spinal —*see* Injury, nerve, spinal, lumbar
lumbosacral
plexus —*see* Injury, nerve, lumbosacral, sympathetic
sympathetic S34.5
medial plantar S94.1-
median (forearm level) S54.1-
hand (level) S64.1-
upper arm (level) S44.1-
wrist (level) —*see* Injury, nerve, median, hand
musculocutaneous S44.4-
musculospiral (upper arm level) —*see* Injury, nerve, radial, upper arm
neck S14.9
peripheral S14.4
specified site NEC S14.8
sympathetic S14.5
ninth cranial (glossopharyngeal) —*see* Injury, nerve, glossopharyngeal
oculomotor S04.1-
contusion S04.1-
laceration S04.1-
specified type NEC S04.1-
olfactory S04.81-
specified type NEC S04.81-
optic S04.01-
contusion S04.01-
laceration S04.01-
specified type NEC S04.01-
pelvic girdle —*see* Injury, nerve, hip
pelvis —*see* Injury, nerve, abdomen, specified site NEC
peripheral —*see* Injury, nerve, abdomen, peripheral
peripheral NEC T14.8
abdomen —*see* Injury, nerve, abdomen, peripheral
lower back —*see* Injury, nerve, abdomen, peripheral
neck —*see* Injury, nerve, neck, peripheral
pelvis —*see* Injury, nerve, abdomen, peripheral
specified NEC T14.8
peroneal (lower leg level) S84.1-
foot S94.2-
plexus
brachial —*see* Injury, brachial plexus
celiac, coeliac —*see* Injury, nerve, lumbosacral, sympathetic
mesenteric, inferior —*see* Injury, nerve, lumbosacral, sympathetic
sacral —*see* Injury, lumbosacral plexus
spinal
brachial —*see* Injury, brachial plexus
lumbosacral —*see* Injury, lumbosacral plexus

Injury *(Continued)*
nerve NEC *(Continued)*
pneumogastric —*see* Injury, nerve, vagus
radial (forearm level) S54.2-
hand (level) S64.2-
upper arm (level) S44.2-
wrist (level) —*see* Injury, nerve, radial, hand
root —*see* Injury, nerve, spinal, root
sacral plexus —*see* Injury, lumbosacral plexus
sacral spinal —*see* Injury, nerve, spinal, sacral
sciatic (hip level) (thigh level) S74.0-
second cranial (optic) —*see* Injury, nerve, optic
seventh cranial (facial) —*see* Injury, nerve, facial
shoulder —*see* Injury, nerve, arm
sixth cranial (abducent) —*see* Injury, nerve, abducens
spinal
plexus —*see* Injury, nerve, plexus, spinal
root
cervical S14.2
dorsal S24.2
lumbar S34.21
sacral S34.22
thoracic —*see* Injury, nerve, spinal, root, dorsal
splanchnic —*see* Injury, nerve, lumbosacral, sympathetic
sympathetic NEC —*see* Injury, nerve, lumbosacral, sympathetic
cervical —*see* Injury, nerve, cervical sympathetic
tenth cranial (pneumogastric or vagus) —*see* Injury, nerve, vagus
thigh (level) —*see* Injury, nerve, hip
cutaneous sensory —*see* Injury, nerve, cutaneous sensory, hip
femoral —*see* Injury, nerve, femoral
sciatic —*see* Injury, nerve, sciatic
specified NEC —*see* Injury, nerve, hip
third cranial (oculomotor) —*see* Injury, nerve, oculomotor
thorax S24.9
peripheral S24.3
specified site NEC S24.8
sympathetic S24.4
thumb, digital —*see* Injury, nerve, digital, thumb
tibial (lower leg level) (posterior) S84.0-
toe —*see* Injury, nerve, ankle
trigeminal S04.3-
contusion S04.3-
laceration S04.3-
specified type NEC S04.3-
trochlear S04.2-
contusion S04.2-
laceration S04.2-
specified type NEC S04.2-
twelfth cranial (hypoglossal) —*see* Injury, nerve, hypoglossal
ulnar (forearm level) S54.0-
arm (upper) (level) S44.0-
hand (level) S64.0-
wrist (level) —*see* Injury, nerve, ulnar, hand
vagus S04.89-
specified type NEC S04.89-
wrist (level) —*see* Injury, nerve, hand
ninth cranial nerve (glossopharyngeal) —*see* Injury, nerve, glossopharyngeal
nose (septum) S09.92
obstetrical O71.9
specified NEC O71.89
occipital (region) (scalp) S09.90
lobe —*see* Injury, intracranial
optic chiasm S04.02
optic radiation S04.03-

Injury *(Continued)*
optic tract and pathways S04.03-
orbit, orbital (region) —*see* Injury, eye
penetrating (with foreign body) —*see* Injury, eye, orbit, penetrating
specified NEC —*see* Injury, eye, specified site NEC
ovary, ovarian S37.4Ø9
bilateral S37.4Ø2
contusion S37.422
laceration S37.432
specified type NEC S37.492
blood vessel —*see* Injury, blood vessel, ovarian
contusion S37.429
bilateral S37.422
unilateral S37.421
laceration S37.439
bilateral S37.432
unilateral S37.431
specified type NEC S37.499
bilateral S37.492
unilateral S37.491
unilateral S37.4Ø1
contusion S37.421
laceration S37.431
specified type NEC S37.491
palate (hard) (soft) SØ9.93
pancreas S36.2Ø9
body S36.2Ø1
contusion S36.221
laceration S36.231
major S36.261
minor S36.241
moderate S36.251
specified type NEC S36.291
contusion S36.229
head S36.2ØØ
contusion S36.22Ø
laceration S36.23Ø
major S36.26Ø
minor S36.24Ø
moderate S36.25Ø
specified type NEC S36.29Ø
laceration S36.239
major S36.269
minor S36.249
moderate S36.259
specified type NEC S36.299
tail S36.2Ø2
contusion S36.222
laceration S36.232
major S36.262
minor S36.242
moderate S36.252
specified type NEC S36.292
parietal (region) (scalp) SØ9.9Ø
lobe —*see* Injury, intracranial
patellar ligament (tendon) S76.1Ø-
laceration S76.12-
specified NEC S76.19-
strain S76.11-
pelvis, pelvic (floor) S39.93
complicating delivery O7Ø.1
joint or ligament, complicating delivery O71.6
organ S37.9Ø
with ectopic or molar pregnancy OØ8.6
complication of abortion —*see* Abortion
contusion S37.92
following ectopic or molar pregnancy OØ8.6
laceration S37.93
obstetrical trauma NEC O71.5
specified
site NEC S37.899
contusion S37.892
laceration S37.893
specified type NEC S37.898
type NEC S37.99
specified NEC S39.83

Injury *(Continued)*
penis S39.94
perineum S39.94
peritoneum S36.81
laceration S36.893
periurethral tissue —*see* Injury, urethra
complicating delivery O71.82
phalanges
foot —*see* Injury, foot
hand —*see* Injury, hand
pharynx NEC S19.85
pleura —*see* Injury, intrathoracic, pleura
plexus
brachial —*see* Injury, brachial plexus
cardiac —*see* Injury, nerve, thorax, sympathetic
celiac, coeliac —*see* Injury, nerve, lumbosacral, sympathetic
esophageal —*see* Injury, nerve, thorax, sympathetic
hypogastric —*see* Injury, nerve, lumbosacral, sympathetic
lumbar, lumbosacral —*see* Injury, lumbosacral plexus
mesenteric —*see* Injury, nerve, lumbosacral, sympathetic
pulmonary —*see* Injury, nerve, thorax, sympathetic
postcardiac surgery (syndrome) I97.Ø
prepuce S39.94
prostate S37.829
contusion S37.822
laceration S37.823
specified type NEC S37.828
pubic region S39.94
pudendum S39.94
pulmonary plexus —*see* Injury, nerve, thorax, sympathetic
rectovaginal septum NEC S39.83
rectum —*see* Injury, intestine, large, rectum
retina —*see* Injury, eye, specified site NEC
penetrating —*see* Injury, eyeball, penetrating
retroperitoneal —*see* Injury, intra-abdominal, specified site NEC
rotator cuff (muscle (s)) (tendon (s)) S46.ØØ-
laceration S46.Ø2-
specified type NEC S46.Ø9-
strain S46.Ø1-
round ligament —*see* Injury, pelvic organ, specified site NEC
sacral plexus —*see* Injury, lumbosacral plexus
salivary duct or gland SØ9.93
scalp SØ9.9Ø
newborn (birth injury) P12.9
due to monitoring (electrode) (sampling incision) P12.4
specified NEC P12.89
caput succedaneum P12.81
scapular region —*see* Injury, shoulder
sclera —*see* Injury, eye, specified site NEC
penetrating —*see* Injury, eyeball, penetrating
scrotum S39.94
second cranial nerve (optic) —*see* Injury, nerve, optic
seminal vesicle —*see* Injury, pelvic organ, specified site NEC
seventh cranial nerve (facial) —*see* Injury, nerve, facial
shoulder S49.9-
blood vessel —*see* Injury, blood vessel, arm
contusion —*see* Contusion, shoulder
dislocation —*see* Dislocation, shoulder
fracture —*see* Fracture, shoulder
muscle —*see* Injury, muscle, shoulder
nerve —*see* Injury, nerve, shoulder
open —*see* Wound, open, shoulder
specified type NEC S49.8-

Injury *(Continued)*
shoulder *(Continued)*
sprain —*see* Sprain, shoulder girdle
superficial —*see* Injury, superficial, shoulder
sinus
cavernous —*see* Injury, intracranial
nasal SØ9.92
sixth cranial nerve (abducent) —*see* Injury, nerve, abducens
skeleton, birth injury P13.9
specified part NEC P13.8
skin NEC T14.8
surface intact —*see* Injury, superficial
skull NEC SØ9.9Ø
specified NEC T14.8
spermatic cord (pelvic region) S37.898
scrotal region S39.848
spinal (cord)
cervical (neck) S14.1Ø9
anterior cord syndrome S14.139
C1 level S14.131
C2 level S14.132
C3 level S14.133
C4 level S14.134
C5 level S14.135
C6 level S14.136
C7 level S14.137
C8 level S14.138
Brown-Séquard syndrome S14.149
C1 level S14.141
C2 level S14.142
C3 level S14.143
C4 level S14.144
C5 level S14.145
C6 level S14.146
C7 level S14.147
C8 level S14.148
C1 level S14.1Ø1
C2 level S14.1Ø2
C3 level S14.1Ø3
C4 level S14.1Ø4
C5 level S14.1Ø5
C6 level S14.1Ø6
C7 level S14.1Ø7
C8 level S14.1Ø8
central cord syndrome S14.129
C1 level S14.121
C2 level S14.122
C3 level S14.123
C4 level S14.124
C5 level S14.125
C6 level S14.126
C7 level S14.127
C8 level S14.128
complete lesion S14.119
C1 level S14.111
C2 level S14.112
C3 level S14.113
C4 level S14.114
C5 level S14.115
C6 level S14.116
C7 level S14.117
C8 level S14.118
concussion S14.Ø
edema S14.Ø
incomplete lesion specified NEC S14.159
C1 level S14.151
C2 level S14.152
C3 level S14.153
C4 level S14.154
C5 level S14.155
C6 level S14.156
C7 level S14.157
C8 level S14.158
posterior cord syndrome S14.159
C1 level S14.151
C2 level S14.152
C3 level S14.153
C4 level S14.154
C5 level S14.155

Injury *(Continued)*
spinal *(Continued)*
cervical *(Continued)*
posterior cord syndrome *(Continued)*
C6 level S14.156
C7 level S14.157
C8 level S14.158
dorsal —*see* Injury, spinal, thoracic
lumbar S34.109
complete lesion S34.119
L1 level S34.111
L2 level S34.112
L3 level S34.113
L4 level S34.114
L5 level S34.115
concussion S34.01
edema S34.01
incomplete lesion S34.129
L1 level S34.121
L2 level S34.122
L3 level S34.123
L4 level S34.124
L5 level S34.125
L1 level S34.101
L2 level S34.102
L3 level S34.103
L4 level S34.104
L5 level S34.105
nerve root NEC
cervical —*see* Injury, nerve, spinal, root, cervical
dorsal —*see* Injury, nerve, spinal, root, dorsal
lumbar S34.21
sacral S34.22
thoracic —*see* Injury, nerve, spinal, root, dorsal
plexus
brachial —*see* Injury, brachial plexus
lumbosacral —*see* Injury, lumbosacral plexus
sacral S34.139
complete lesion S34.131
incomplete lesion S34.132
thoracic S24.109
anterior cord syndrome S24.139
T1 level S24.131
T2-T6 level S24.132
T7-T10 level S24.133
T11-T12 level S24.134
Brown-Séquard syndrome S24.149
T1 level S24.141
T2-T6 level S24.142
T7-T10 level S24.143
T11-T12 level S24.144
complete lesion S24.119
T1 level S24.111
T2-T6 level S24.112
T7-T10 level S24.113
T11-T12 level S24.114
concussion S24.0
edema S24.0
incomplete lesion specified NEC S24.159
T1 level S24.151
T2-T6 level S24.152
T7-T10 level S24.153
T11-T12 level S24.154
posterior cord syndrome S24.159
T1 level S24.151
T2-T6 level S24.152
T7-T10 level S24.153
T11-T12 level S24.154
T1 level S24.101
T2-T6 level S24.102
T7-T10 level S24.103
T11-T12 level S24.104
splanchnic nerve —*see* Injury, nerve, lumbosacral, sympathetic

Injury *(Continued)*
spleen S36.00
contusion S36.029
major S36.021
minor S36.020
laceration S36.039
major (massive) (stellate) S36.032
moderate S36.031
superficial (capsular) (minor) S36.030
specified type NEC S36.09
splenic artery —*see* Injury, blood vessel, celiac artery, branch
stellate ganglion —*see* Injury, nerve, thorax, sympathetic
sternal region S29.9
stomach S36.30
contusion S36.32
laceration S36.33
specified type NEC S36.39
subconjunctival —*see* Injury, eye, conjunctiva
subcutaneous NEC T14.8
submaxillary region S09.93
submental region S09.93
subungual
fingers —*see* Injury, hand
toes —*see* Injury, foot
superficial NEC T14.8
abdomen, abdominal (wall) S30.92
abrasion S30.811
bite S30.871
insect S30.861
contusion S30.1
external constriction S30.841
foreign body S30.851
abrasion —*see* Abrasion, by site
adnexa, eye NEC —*see* Injury, eye, specified site NEC
alveolar process —*see* Injury, superficial, oral cavity
ankle S90.91-
abrasion —*see* Abrasion, ankle
bite —*see* Bite, ankle
blister —*see* Blister, ankle
contusion —*see* Contusion, ankle
external constriction —*see* Constriction, external, ankle
foreign body —*see* Foreign body, superficial, ankle
anus S30.98
arm (upper) S40.92-
abrasion —*see* Abrasion, arm
bite —*see* Bite, superficial, arm
blister —*see* Blister, arm (upper)
contusion —*see* Contusion, arm
external constriction —*see* Constriction, external, arm
foreign body —*see* Foreign body, superficial, arm
auditory canal (external) (meatus) —*see* Injury, superficial, ear
auricle —*see* Injury, superficial, ear
axilla —*see* Injury, superficial, arm
back —*see also* Injury, superficial, thorax, back
lower S30.91
abrasion S30.810
contusion S30.0
external constriction S30.840
superficial
bite NEC S30.870
insect S30.860
foreign body S30.850
bite NEC —*see* Bite, superficial NEC, by site
blister —*see* Blister, by site
breast S20.10-
abrasion —*see* Abrasion, breast
bite —*see* Bite, superficial, breast
contusion —*see* Contusion, breast
external constriction —*see* Constriction, external, breast
foreign body —*see* Foreign body, superficial, breast

Injury *(Continued)*
superficial NEC *(Continued)*
brow —*see* Injury, superficial, head, specified NEC
buttock S30.91
calf —*see* Injury, superficial, leg
canthus, eye —*see* Injury, superficial, periocular area
cheek (external) —*see* Injury, superficial, head, specified NEC
internal —*see* Injury, superficial, oral cavity
chest wall —*see* Injury, superficial, thorax
chin —*see* Injury, superficial, head NEC
clitoris S30.95
conjunctiva —*see* Injury, eye, conjunctiva
with foreign body (in conjunctival sac) —*see* Foreign body, conjunctival sac
contusion —*see* Contusion, by site
costal region —*see* Injury, superficial, thorax
digit (s)
hand —*see* Injury, superficial, finger
ear (auricle) (canal) (external) S00.40-
abrasion —*see* Abrasion, ear
bite —*see* Bite, superficial, ear
contusion —*see* Contusion, ear
external constriction —*see* Constriction, external, ear
foreign body —*see* Foreign body, superficial, ear
elbow S50.90-
abrasion —*see* Abrasion, elbow
bite —*see* Bite, superficial, elbow
blister —*see* Blister, elbow
contusion —*see* Contusion, elbow
external constriction —*see* Constriction, external, elbow
foreign body —*see* Foreign body, superficial, elbow
epididymis S30.94
epigastric region S30.92
epiglottis —*see* Injury, superficial, throat
esophagus
cervical —*see* Injury, superficial, throat
external constriction —*see* Constriction, external, by site
extremity NEC T14.8
eyeball NEC —*see* Injury, eye, specified site NEC
eyebrow —*see* Injury, superficial, periocular area
eyelid S00.20-
abrasion —*see* Abrasion, eyelid
bite —*see* Bite, superficial, eyelid
contusion —*see* Contusion, eyelid
external constriction —*see* Constriction, external, eyelid
foreign body —*see* Foreign body, superficial, eyelid
face NEC —*see* Injury, superficial, head, specified NEC
finger (s) S60.949
abrasion —*see* Abrasion, finger
bite —*see* Bite, superficial, finger
blister —*see* Blister, finger
contusion —*see* Contusion, finger
external constriction —*see* Constriction, external, finger
foreign body —*see* Foreign body, superficial, finger
index S60.94-
insect bite —*see* Bite, by site, superficial, insect
little S60.94-
middle S60.94-
ring S60.94-
flank S30.92
foot S90.92-
abrasion —*see* Abrasion, foot
bite —*see* Bite, foot

Injury *(Continued)*
superficial NEC *(Continued)*
foot *(Continued)*
blister —*see* Blister, foot
contusion —*see* Contusion, foot
external constriction —*see* Constriction, external, foot
foreign body —*see* Foreign body, superficial, foot
forearm S50.91-
abrasion —*see* Abrasion, forearm
bite —*see* Bite, forearm, superficial
blister —*see* Blister, forearm
contusion —*see* Contusion, forearm
elbow only —*see* Injury, superficial, elbow
external constriction —*see* Constriction, external, forearm
foreign body —*see* Foreign body, superficial, forearm
forehead —*see* Injury, superficial, head NEC
foreign body —*see* Foreign body, superficial
genital organs, external
female S30.97
male S30.96
globe (eye) —*see* Injury, eye, specified site NEC
groin S30.92
gum —*see* Injury, superficial, oral cavity
hand S60.92-
abrasion —*see* Abrasion, hand
bite —*see* Bite, superficial, hand
contusion —*see* Contusion, hand
external constriction —*see* Constriction, external, hand
foreign body —*see* Foreign body, superficial, hand
head S00.90
ear —*see* Injury, superficial, ear
eyelid —*see* Injury, superficial, eyelid
nose S00.30
oral cavity S00.502
scalp S00.00
specified site NEC S00.80
heel —*see* Injury, superficial, foot
hip S70.91-
abrasion —*see* Abrasion, hip
bite —*see* Bite, superficial, hip
blister —*see* Blister, hip
contusion —*see* Contusion, hip
external constriction —*see* Constriction, external, hip
foreign body —*see* Foreign body, superficial, hip
iliac region —*see* Injury, superficial, abdomen
inguinal region —*see* Injury, superficial, abdomen
insect bite —*see* Bite, by site, superficial, insect
interscapular region —*see* Injury, superficial, thorax, back
jaw —*see* Injury, superficial, head, specified NEC
knee S80.91-
abrasion —*see* Abrasion, knee
bite —*see* Bite, superficial, knee
blister —*see* Blister, knee
contusion —*see* Contusion, knee
external constriction —*see* Constriction, external, knee
foreign body —*see* Foreign body, superficial, knee
labium (majus) (minus) S30.95
lacrimal (apparatus) (gland) (sac) —*see* Injury, eye, specified site NEC
larynx —*see* Injury, superficial, throat
leg (lower) S80.92-
abrasion —*see* Abrasion, leg
bite —*see* Bite, superficial, leg

Injury *(Continued)*
superficial NEC *(Continued)*
leg *(Continued)*
contusion —*see* Contusion, leg
external constriction —*see* Constriction, external, leg
foreign body —*see* Foreign body, superficial, leg
knee —*see* Injury, superficial, knee
limb NEC T14.8
lip S00.501
lower back S30.91
lumbar region S30.91
malar region —*see* Injury, superficial, head, specified NEC
mammary —*see* Injury, superficial, breast
mastoid region —*see* Injury, superficial, head, specified NEC
mouth —*see* Injury, superficial, oral cavity
muscle NEC T14.8
nail NEC T14.8
finger —*see* Injury, superficial, finger
toe —*see* Injury, superficial, toe
nasal (septum) —*see* Injury, superficial, nose
neck S10.90
specified site NEC S10.80
nose (septum) S00.30
occipital region —*see* Injury, superficial, scalp
oral cavity S00.502
orbital region —*see* Injury, superficial, periocular area
palate —*see* Injury, superficial, oral cavity
palm —*see* Injury, superficial, hand
parietal region —*see* Injury, superficial, scalp
pelvis S30.91
girdle —*see* Injury, superficial, hip
penis S30.93
perineum
female S30.95
male S30.91
periocular area S00.20-
abrasion —*see* Abrasion, eyelid
bite —*see* Bite, superficial, eyelid
contusion —*see* Contusion, eyelid
external constriction —*see* Constriction, external, eyelid
foreign body —*see* Foreign body, superficial, eyelid
phalanges
finger —*see* Injury, superficial, finger
toe —*see* Injury, superficial, toe
pharynx —*see* Injury, superficial, throat
pinna —*see* Injury, superficial, ear
popliteal space —*see* Injury, superficial, knee
prepuce S30.93
pubic region S30.91
pudendum
female S30.97
male S30.96
sacral region S30.91
scalp S00.00
scapular region —*see* Injury, superficial, shoulder
sclera —*see* Injury, eye, specified site NEC
scrotum S30.94
shin —*see* Injury, superficial, leg
shoulder S40.91-
abrasion —*see* Abrasion, shoulder
bite —*see* Bite, superficial, shoulder
blister —*see* Blister, shoulder
contusion —*see* Contusion, shoulder
external constriction —*see* Constriction, external, shoulder
foreign body —*see* Foreign body, superficial, shoulder

Injury *(Continued)*
superficial NEC *(Continued)*
skin NEC T14.8
sternal region —*see* Injury, superficial, thorax, front
subconjunctival —*see* Injury, eye, specified site NEC
subcutaneous NEC T14.8
submaxillary region —*see* Injury, superficial, head, specified NEC
submental region —*see* Injury, superficial, head, specified NEC
subungual
finger (s) —*see* Injury, superficial, finger
toe (s) —*see* Injury, superficial, toe
supraclavicular fossa —*see* Injury, superficial, neck
supraorbital —*see* Injury, superficial, head, specified NEC
temple —*see* Injury, superficial, head, specified NEC
temporal region —*see* Injury, superficial, head, specified NEC
testis S30.94
thigh S70.92-
abrasion —*see* Abrasion, thigh
bite —*see* Bite, superficial, thigh
blister —*see* Blister, thigh
contusion —*see* Contusion, thigh
external constriction —*see* Constriction, external, thigh
foreign body —*see* Foreign body, superficial, thigh
thorax, thoracic (wall) S20.90
abrasion —*see* Abrasion, thorax
back S20.40-
bite —*see* Bite, thorax, superficial
blister —*see* Blister, thorax
contusion —*see* Contusion, thorax
external constriction —*see* Constriction, external, thorax
foreign body —*see* Foreign body, superficial, thorax
front S20.30-
throat S10.10
abrasion S10.11
bite S10.17
insect S10.16
blister S10.12
contusion S10.0
external constriction S10.14
foreign body S10.15
thumb S60.93-
abrasion —*see* Abrasion, thumb
bite —*see* Bite, superficial, thumb
blister —*see* Blister, thumb
contusion —*see* Contusion, thumb
external constriction —*see* Constriction, external, thumb
foreign body —*see* Foreign body, superficial, thumb
insect bite —*see* Bite, by site, superficial, insect
specified type NEC S60.39-
toe (s) S90.93-
abrasion —*see* Abrasion, toe
bite —*see* Bite, toe
blister —*see* Blister, toe
contusion —*see* Contusion, toe
external constriction —*see* Constriction, external, toe
foreign body —*see* Foreign body, superficial, toe
great S90.93-
tongue —*see* Injury, superficial, oral cavity
tooth, teeth —*see* Injury, superficial, oral cavity
trachea S10.10
tunica vaginalis S30.94
tympanum, tympanic membrane —*see* Injury, superficial, ear

Injury *(Continued)*
superficial NEC *(Continued)*
uvula —*see* Injury, superficial, oral cavity
vagina S30.95
vocal cords —*see* Injury, superficial, throat
vulva S30.95
wrist S60.91-
supraclavicular region —*see* Injury, neck
supraorbital S09.93
suprarenal gland (multiple) —*see* Injury, adrenal
surgical complication (external or internal site) —*see* Laceration, accidental complicating surgery
temple S09.90
temporal region S09.90
tendon —*see also* Injury, muscle, by site
abdomen —*see* Injury, muscle, abdomen
Achilles —*see* Injury, Achilles tendon
lower back —*see* Injury, muscle, lower back
pelvic organs —*see* Injury, muscle, pelvis
tenth cranial nerve (pneumogastric or vagus) —*see* Injury, nerve, vagus
testis S39.94
thigh S79.92-
blood vessel —*see* Injury, blood vessel, hip
contusion —*see* Contusion, thigh
fracture —*see* Fracture, femur
muscle —*see* Injury, muscle, thigh
nerve —*see* Injury, nerve, thigh
open —*see* Wound, open, thigh
specified NEC S79.82-
superficial —*see* Injury, superficial, thigh
third cranial nerve (oculomotor) —*see* Injury, nerve, oculomotor
thorax, thoracic S29.9
blood vessel —*see* Injury, blood vessel, thorax
cavity —*see* Injury, intrathoracic
dislocation —*see* Dislocation, thorax
external (wall) S29.9
contusion —*see* Contusion, thorax
nerve —*see* Injury, nerve, thorax
open —*see* Wound, open, thorax
specified NEC S29.8
sprain —*see* Sprain, thorax
superficial —*see* Injury, superficial, thorax
fracture —*see* Fracture, thorax
internal —*see* Injury, intrathoracic
intrathoracic organ —*see* Injury, intrathoracic
sympathetic ganglion —*see* Injury, nerve, thorax, sympathetic
throat —*see also* Injury, neck S19.9
thumb S69.9-
blood vessel —*see* Injury, blood vessel, thumb
contusion —*see* Contusion, thumb
dislocation —*see* Dislocation, thumb
fracture —*see* Fracture, thumb
muscle —*see* Injury, muscle, thumb
nerve —*see* Injury, nerve, digital, thumb
open —*see* Wound, open, thumb
specified NEC S69.8-
sprain —*see* Sprain, thumb
superficial —*see* Injury, superficial, thumb
thymus (gland) —*see* Injury, intrathoracic, specified organ NEC
thyroid (gland) NEC S19.84
toe S99.92-
contusion —*see* Contusion, toe
dislocation —*see* Dislocation, toe
fracture —*see* Fracture, toe
muscle —*see* Injury, muscle, toe
open —*see* Wound, open, toe
specified type NEC S99.82-
sprain —*see* Sprain, toe
superficial —*see* Injury, superficial, toe
tongue S09.93
tonsil S09.93

Injury *(Continued)*
tooth S09.93
trachea (cervical) NEC S19.82
thoracic —*see* Injury, intrathoracic, trachea, thoracic
transfusion-related acute lung (TRALI) J95.84
tunica vaginalis S39.94
twelfth cranial nerve (hypoglossal) —*see* Injury, nerve, hypoglossal
ureter S37.10
contusion S37.12
laceration S37.13
specified type NEC S37.19
urethra (sphincter) S37.30
at delivery O71.5
contusion S37.32
laceration S37.33
specified type NEC S37.38
urinary organ S37.899
contusion S37.92
laceration S37.93
specified
site NEC S37.899
contusion S37.892
laceration S37.893
specified type NEC S37.898
type NEC S37.99
uterus, uterine S37.60
with ectopic or molar pregnancy O08.6
blood vessel —*see* Injury, blood vessel, iliac
contusion S37.62
laceration S37.63
cervix at delivery O71.3
rupture associated with obstetrics —*see* Rupture, uterus
specified type NEC S37.69
uvula S09.93
vagina S39.93
abrasion S30.814
bite S31.45
insect S30.864
superficial NEC S30.874
contusion S30.23
crush S38.03
during delivery —*see* Laceration, vagina, during delivery
external constriction S30.844
insect bite S30.864
laceration S31.41
with foreign body S31.42
open wound S31.40
puncture S31.43
with foreign body S31.44
superficial S30.95
foreign body S30.854
vas deferens —*see* Injury, pelvic organ, specified site NEC
vascular NEC T14.8
vein —*see* Injury, blood vessel
vena cava (superior) S25.20
inferior S35.10
laceration (minor) (superficial) S35.11
major S35.12
specified type NEC S35.19
laceration (minor) (superficial) S25.21
major S25.22
specified type NEC S25.29
vesical (sphincter) —*see* Injury, bladder
visual cortex S04.04-
vitreous (humor) S05.90
specified NEC S05.8X-
vocal cord NEC S19.83
vulva S39.94
abrasion S30.814
bite S31.45
insect S30.864
superficial NEC S30.874
contusion S30.23
crush S38.03
during delivery —*see* Laceration, perineum, female, during delivery

Injury *(Continued)*
vulva *(Continued)*
external constriction S30.844
insect bite S30.864
laceration S31.41
with foreign body S31.42
open wound S31.40
puncture S31.43
with foreign body S31.44
superficial S30.95
foreign body S30.854
whiplash (cervical spine) S13.4
wrist S69.9-
blood vessel —*see* Injury, blood vessel, hand
contusion —*see* Contusion, wrist
dislocation —*see* Dislocation, wrist
fracture —*see* Fracture, wrist
muscle —*see* Injury, muscle, hand
nerve —*see* Injury, nerve, hand
open —*see* Wound, open, wrist
specified NEC S69.8-
sprain —*see* Sprain, wrist
superficial —*see* Injury, superficial, wrist
Inoculation —*see also* Vaccination
complication or reaction —*see* Complications, vaccination
Insanity, insane —*see also* Psychosis
adolescent —*see* Schizophrenia
confusional F28
acute or subacute F05
delusional F22
senile F03
Insect
bite —*see* Bite, by site, superficial, insect
venomous, poisoning NEC (by) —*see* Venom, arthropod
Insensitivity
adrenocorticotropin hormone (ACTH) E27.49
androgen E34.50
complete E34.51
partial E34.52
Insertion
cord (umbilical) lateral or velamentous O43.12-
intrauterine contraceptive device (encounter for) —*see* Intrauterine contraceptive device
Insolation (sunstroke) T67.0
Insomnia (organic) G47.00
without objective findings F51.02
adjustment F51.02
adjustment disorder F51.02
behavioral, of childhood Z73.819
combined type Z73.812
limit setting type Z73.811
sleep-onset association type Z73.810
childhood Z73.819
chronic F51.04
somatized tension F51.04
conditioned F51.04
due to
alcohol
abuse F10.182
dependence F10.282
use F10.982
amphetamines
abuse F15.182
dependence F15.282
use F15.982
anxiety disorder F51.05
caffeine
abuse F15.182
dependence F15.282
use F15.982
cocaine
abuse F14.182
dependence F14.282
use F14.982
depression F51.05

- **Insomnia** *(Continued)*
  - due to *(Continued)*
    - drug NEC
      - abuse F19.182
      - dependence F19.282
      - use F19.982
    - medical condition G47.Ø1
    - mental disorder NEC F51.Ø5
    - opioid
      - abuse F11.182
      - dependence F11.282
      - use F11.982
    - psychoactive substance NEC
      - abuse F19.182
      - dependence F19.282
      - use F19.982
    - sedative, hypnotic, or anxiolytic
      - abuse F13.182
      - dependence F13.282
      - use F13.982
    - stimulant NEC
      - abuse F15.182
      - dependence F15.282
      - use F15.982
  - fatal familial (FFI) A81.83
  - idiopathic F51.Ø1
  - learned F51.3
  - nonorganic origin F51.Ø1
  - not due to a substance or known physiological condition F51.Ø1
    - specified NEC F51.Ø9
  - paradoxical F51.Ø3
  - primary F51.Ø1
  - psychiatric F51.Ø5
  - psychophysiologic F51.Ø4
  - related to psychopathology F51.Ø5
  - short-term F51.Ø2
  - specified NEC G47.Ø9
  - stress-related F51.Ø2
  - transient F51.Ø2
- **Inspiration**
  - food or foreign body —*see* Foreign body, by site
  - mucus —*see* Asphyxia, mucus
- **Inspissated bile syndrome** (newborn) P59.1
- **Instability**
  - emotional (excessive) F6Ø.3
  - joint (post-traumatic) M25.3Ø
    - ankle M25.37-
    - due to old ligament injury —*see* Disorder, ligament
    - elbow M25.32-
    - flail —*see* Flail, joint
    - foot M25.37-
    - hand M25.34-
    - hip M25.35-
    - knee M25.36-
    - lumbosacral —*see* subcategory M53.2
    - prosthesis —*see* Complications, joint prosthesis, mechanical, displacement, by site
    - sacroiliac —*see* subcategory M53.2
    - secondary to
      - old ligament injury —*see* Disorder, ligament
      - removal of joint prosthesis M96.89
    - shoulder (region) M25.31-
    - spine —*see* subcategory M53.2
    - wrist M25.33-
  - knee (chronic) M23.5-
  - lumbosacral —*see* subcategory M53.2
  - nervous F48.8
  - personality (emotional) F6Ø.3
  - spine —*see* Instability, joint, spine
  - vasomotor R55
- **Institutional syndrome** (childhood) F94.2
- **Institutionalization, affecting child** Z62.22
  - disinhibited attachment F94.2
- **Insufficiency, insufficient**
  - accommodation, old age H52.4
  - adrenal (gland) E27.4Ø
    - primary E27.1
  - adrenocortical E27.4Ø
    - drug-induced E27.3
    - iatrogenic E27.3
    - primary E27.1
  - anatomic crown height KØ8.89 ◄
  - anterior (occlusal) guidance M26.54
  - anus K62.89
  - aortic (valve) I35.1
    - with
      - mitral (valve) disease IØ8.Ø
        - with tricuspid (valve) disease IØ8.3
      - stenosis I35.2
      - tricuspid (valve) disease IØ8.2
        - with mitral (valve) disease IØ8.3
    - congenital Q23.1
    - rheumatic IØ6.1
      - with
        - mitral (valve) disease IØ8.Ø
          - with tricuspid (valve) disease IØ8.3
        - stenosis IØ6.2
          - with mitral (valve) disease IØ8.Ø
            - with tricuspid (valve) disease IØ8.3
        - tricuspid (valve) disease IØ8.2
          - with mitral (valve) disease IØ8.3
    - specified cause NEC I35.1
    - syphilitic A52.Ø3
  - arterial I77.1
    - basilar G45.Ø
    - carotid (hemispheric) G45.1
    - cerebral I67.81
    - coronary (acute or subacute) I24.8
    - mesenteric K55.1
    - peripheral I73.9
    - precerebral (multiple) (bilateral) G45.2
    - vertebral G45.Ø
  - arteriovenous I99.8
  - biliary K83.8
  - cardiac —*see also* Insufficiency, myocardial
    - due to presence of (cardiac) prosthesis I97.11-
    - postprocedural I97.11-
  - cardiorenal, hypertensive I13.2
  - cardiovascular —*see* Disease, cardiovascular
  - cerebrovascular (acute) I67.81
    - with transient focal neurological signs and symptoms G45.8
  - circulatory NEC I99.8
    - newborn P29.89
  - clinical crown length KØ8.89 ◄
  - convergence H51.11
  - coronary (acute or subacute) I24.8
    - chronic or with a stated duration of over 4 weeks I25.89
  - corticoadrenal E27.4Ø
    - primary E27.1
  - dietary E63.9
  - divergence H51.8
  - food T73.Ø
  - gastroesophageal K22.8
  - gonadal
    - ovary E28.39
    - testis E29.1
  - heart —*see also* Insufficiency, myocardial
    - newborn P29.Ø
    - valve —*see* Endocarditis
  - hepatic —*see* Failure, hepatic
  - idiopathic autonomic G9Ø.Ø9
  - interocclusal distance of fully erupted teeth (ridge) M26.36
  - kidney N28.9
    - acute N28.9
    - chronic N18.9
  - lacrimal (secretion) HØ4.12-
    - passages —*see* Stenosis, lacrimal
  - liver —*see* Failure, hepatic
- **Insufficiency, insufficient** *(Continued)*
  - lung —*see* Insufficiency, pulmonary
  - mental (congenital) —*see* Disability, intellectual
  - mesenteric K55.1
  - mitral (valve) I34.Ø
    - with
      - aortic valve disease IØ8.Ø
        - with tricuspid (valve) disease IØ8.3
      - obstruction or stenosis IØ5.2
        - with aortic valve disease IØ8.Ø
      - tricuspid (valve) disease IØ8.1
        - with aortic (valve) disease IØ8.3
    - congenital Q23.3
    - rheumatic IØ5.1
      - with
        - aortic valve disease IØ8.Ø
          - with tricuspid (valve) disease IØ8.3
        - obstruction or stenosis IØ5.2
          - with aortic valve disease IØ8.Ø
            - with tricuspid (valve) disease IØ8.3
        - tricuspid (valve) disease IØ8.1
          - with aortic (valve) disease IØ8.3
      - active or acute IØ1.1
        - with chorea, rheumatic (Sydenham's) IØ2.Ø
    - specified cause, except rheumatic I34.Ø
  - muscle —*see also* Disease, muscle
    - heart —*see* Insufficiency, myocardial
    - ocular NEC H5Ø.9
  - myocardial, myocardium (with arteriosclerosis) I5Ø.9
    - with
      - rheumatic fever (conditions in IØØ) IØ9.Ø
        - active, acute or subacute IØ1.2
          - with chorea IØ2.Ø
        - inactive or quiescent (with chorea) IØ9.Ø
    - congenital Q24.8
    - hypertensive —*see* Hypertension, heart
    - newborn P29.Ø
    - rheumatic IØ9.Ø
      - active, acute, or subacute IØ1.2
    - syphilitic A52.Ø6
  - nourishment T73.Ø
  - pancreatic K86.89 ⇐
    - exocrine K86.81 ◄
  - parathyroid (gland) E2Ø.9
  - peripheral vascular (arterial) I73.9
  - pituitary E23.Ø
  - placental (mother) O36.51-
  - platelets D69.6
  - prenatal care affecting management of pregnancy OØ9.3-
  - progressive pluriglandular E31.Ø
  - pulmonary J98.4
    - acute, following surgery (nonthoracic) J95.2
      - thoracic J95.1
    - chronic, following surgery J95.3
    - following
      - shock J98.4
      - trauma J98.4
    - newborn P28.5
    - valve I37.1
      - with stenosis I37.2
      - congenital Q22.2
      - rheumatic IØ9.89
        - with aortic, mitral or tricuspid (valve) disease IØ8.8
  - pyloric K31.89
  - renal (acute) N28.9
    - chronic N18.9
  - respiratory RØ6.89
    - newborn P28.5
  - rotation —*see* Malrotation
  - sleep syndrome F51.12

- **Insufficiency, insufficient** *(Continued)*
  - social insurance Z59.7
  - suprarenal E27.40
    - primary E27.1
  - tarso-orbital fascia, congenital Q10.3
  - testis E29.1
  - thyroid (gland) (acquired) E03.9
    - congenital E03.1
  - tricuspid (valve) (rheumatic) I07.1
    - with
      - aortic (valve) disease I08.2
        - with mitral (valve) disease I08.3
      - mitral (valve) disease I08.1
        - with aortic (valve) disease I08.3
      - obstruction or stenosis I07.2
        - with aortic (valve) disease I08.2
          - with mitral (valve) disease I08.3
    - congenital Q22.8
    - nonrheumatic I36.1
      - with stenosis I36.2
  - urethral sphincter R32
  - valve, valvular (heart) —*see* Endocarditis
    - congenital Q24.8
  - vascular I99.8
    - intestine K55.9
      - acute —*see also* Ischemia, intestine, acute K55.059
    - mesenteric K55.1
    - peripheral I73.9
    - renal —*see* Hypertension, kidney
  - velopharyngeal
    - acquired K13.79
    - congenital Q38.8
  - venous (chronic) (peripheral) I87.2
  - ventricular —*see* Insufficiency, myocardial
  - welfare support Z59.7
- **Insufflation, fallopian** Z31.41
- **Insular** —*see* condition
- **Insulinoma**
  - pancreas
    - benign D13.7
    - malignant C25.4
    - uncertain behavior D37.8
  - specified site
    - benign —*see* Neoplasm, by site, benign
    - malignant —*see* Neoplasm, by site, malignant
    - uncertain behavior —*see* Neoplasm, by site, uncertain behavior
  - unspecified site
    - benign D13.7
    - malignant C25.4
    - uncertain behavior D37.8
- **Insuloma** —*see* Insulinoma
- **Interference**
  - balancing side M26.56
  - non-working side M26.56
- **Intermenstrual** —*see* condition
- **Intermittent** —*see* condition
- **Internal** —*see* condition
- **Interrogation**
  - cardiac defibrillator (automatic) (implantable) Z45.02
  - cardiac pacemaker Z45.018
  - cardiac (event) (loop) recorder Z45.09
  - infusion pump (implanted) (intrathecal) Z45.1
  - neurostimulator Z46.2
- **Interruption**
  - aortic arch Q25.21 ◀
  - phase-shift, sleep cycle —*see* Disorder, sleep, circadian rhythm
  - sleep phase-shift, or 24 hour sleep-wake cycle —*see* Disorder, sleep, circadian rhythm
- **Interstitial** —*see* condition
- **Intertrigo** L30.4
  - labialis K13.0
- **Intervertebral disc** —*see* condition
- **Intestine, intestinal** —*see* condition
- **Intolerance**
  - carbohydrate K90.49
  - disaccharide, hereditary E73.0
  - fat NEC K90.49
    - pancreatic K90.3
  - food K90.49
    - dietary counseling and surveillance Z71.3
  - fructose E74.10
    - hereditary E74.12
  - glucose(-galactose) E74.39
  - gluten K90.01
  - lactose E73.9
    - specified NEC E73.8
  - lysine E72.3
  - milk NEC K90.49
    - lactose E73.9
  - protein K90.49
  - starch NEC K90.49
  - sucrose (-isomaltose) E74.31
- **Intoxicated NEC** (without dependence) —*see* Alcohol, intoxication
- **Intoxication**
  - acid E87.2
  - alcoholic (acute) (without dependence) —*see* Alcohol, intoxication
  - alimentary canal K52.1
  - amphetamine (without dependence) —*see* Abuse, drug, stimulant, with intoxication
    - with dependence —*see* Dependence, drug, stimulant, with intoxication
  - anxiolytic (acute) (without dependence) —*see* Abuse, drug, sedative, with intoxication
    - with dependence —*see* Dependence, drug, sedative, with intoxication
  - caffeine F15.929
    - with dependence —*see* Dependence, drug, stimulant, with intoxication
  - cannabinoids (acute) (without dependence) —*see* Use, cannabis, with intoxication
    - ~~with dependence —see Dependence, drug, cannabis, with intoxication~~
    - with ◀
      - abuse —*see* Abuse, drug, cannabis, with intoxication ◀
      - dependence —*see* Dependence, drug, cannabis, with intoxication ◀
  - chemical —*see* Table of Drugs and Chemicals
    - via placenta or breast milk —*see* - Absorption, chemical, through placenta
  - cocaine (acute) (without dependence) —*see* Abuse, drug, cocaine, with intoxication
    - with dependence —*see* Dependence, drug, cocaine, with intoxication
  - drug
    - acute (without dependence) —*see* Abuse, drug, by type with intoxication
      - with dependence —*see* Dependence, drug, by type with intoxication
    - addictive
      - via placenta or breast milk —*see* Absorption, drug, addictive, through placenta
    - newborn P93.8
      - gray baby syndrome P93.0
    - overdose or wrong substance given or taken —*see* Table of Drugs and Chemicals, by drug, poisoning
  - enteric K52.1
  - foodborne A05.9
    - bacterial A05.9
    - classical (Clostridium botulinum) A05.1
    - due to
      - Bacillus cereus A05.4
      - bacterium A05.9
        - specified NEC A05.8
      - Clostridium
        - botulinum A05.1
        - perfringens A05.2
        - welchii A05.2
      - Salmonella A02.9
        - with
          - (gastro) enteritis A02.0
          - localized infection (s) A02.20
            - arthritis A02.23
            - meningitis A02.21
            - osteomyelitis A02.24
            - pneumonia A02.22
            - pyelonephritis A02.25
            - specified NEC A02.29
          - sepsis A02.1
          - specified manifestation NEC A02.8
      - Staphylococcus A05.0
      - Vibrio
        - parahaemolyticus A05.3
        - vulnificus A05.5
    - enterotoxin, staphylococcal A05.0
    - noxious —*see* Poisoning, food, noxious
  - gastrointestinal K52.1
  - hallucinogenic (without dependence) —*see* Abuse, drug, hallucinogen, with intoxication
    - with dependence —*see* Dependence, drug, hallucinogen, with intoxication
  - hypnotic (acute) (without dependence) —*see* Abuse, drug, sedative, with intoxication
    - with dependence —*see* Dependence, drug, sedative, with intoxication
  - inhalant (acute) (without dependence) —*see* Abuse, drug, inhalant, with intoxication
    - with dependence —*see* Dependence, drug, inhalant, with intoxication
  - meaning
    - inebriation —*see* category F10
    - poisoning —*see* Table of Drugs and Chemicals
  - methyl alcohol (acute) (without dependence) —*see* Alcohol, intoxication
  - opioid (acute) (without dependence) —*see* Abuse, drug, opioid, with intoxication
    - with dependence —*see* Dependence, drug, opioid, with intoxication
  - pathologic NEC (without dependence) —*see* Alcohol, intoxication
  - phencyclidine (without dependence) —*see* Abuse, drug, hallucinogen, with intoxication
    - with dependence —*see* Dependence, drug, hallucinogen, with intoxication
  - potassium (K) E87.5
  - psychoactive substance NEC (without dependence) —*see* Abuse, drug, psychoactive NEC, with intoxication
    - with dependence —*see* Dependence, drug, psychoactive NEC, with intoxication
  - sedative (acute) (without dependence) —*see* Abuse, drug, sedative, with intoxication
    - with dependence —*see* Dependence, drug, sedative, with intoxication
  - serum —*see also* Reaction, serum T80.69
  - uremic —*see* Uremia
  - volatile solvents (acute) (without dependence) —*see* Abuse, drug, inhalant, with intoxication
    - with dependence —*see* Dependence, drug, inhalant, with intoxication
  - water E87.79
- **Intracranial** —*see* condition
- **Intrahepatic gallbladder** Q44.1
- **Intraligamentous** —*see* condition
- **Intrathoracic** —*see also* condition
  - kidney Q63.2
- **Intrauterine contraceptive device**
  - checking Z30.431
  - in situ Z97.5
  - insertion Z30.430
    - immediately following removal Z30.433

Intrauterine contraceptive device *(Continued)*
management Z30.431
reinsertion Z30.433
removal Z30.432
replacement Z30.433
retention in pregnancy O26.3-
Intraventricular —*see* condition
Intrinsic deformity —*see* Deformity
Intubation, difficult or failed T88.4
Intumescence, lens (eye) (cataract) —*see* Cataract
Intussusception (bowel) (colon) (enteric) (ileocecal) (ileocolic) (intestine) (rectum) K56.1
appendix K38.8
congenital Q43.8
ureter (with obstruction) N13.5
Invagination (bowel, colon, intestine or rectum) K56.1
Inversion
albumin-globulin (A-G) ratio E88.09
bladder N32.89
cecum —*see* Intussusception
cervix N88.8
chromosome in normal individual Q95.1
circadian rhythm —*see* Disorder, sleep, circadian rhythm
nipple N64.59
congenital Q83.8
gestational —*see* Retraction, nipple
puerperal, postpartum —*see* Retraction, nipple
nyctohemeral rhythm —*see* Disorder, sleep, circadian rhythm
optic papilla Q14.2
organ or site, congenital NEC —*see* Anomaly, by site
sleep rhythm —*see* Disorder, sleep, circadian rhythm
testis (congenital) Q55.29
uterus (chronic) (postinfectional) (postpartal, old) N85.5
postpartum O71.2
vagina (posthysterectomy) N99.3
ventricular Q20.5
Investigation —*see also* Examination Z04.9
clinical research subject (control) (normal comparison) (participant) Z00.6
Involuntary movement, abnormal R25.9
Involution, involutional —*see also* condition
breast, cystic —*see* Dysplasia, mammary, specified type NEC
depression (single episode) F32.89 ⬅
recurrent episode F33.9
melancholia (single episode) F32.89 ⬅
recurrent episode F33.8 ◀
ovary, senile —*see* Atrophy, ovary
thymus failure E32.8
I.Q.
under 20 F73
20-34 F72
35-49 F71
50-69 F70
IRDS (type I) P22.0
type II P22.1
Irideremia Q13.1
Iridis rubeosis —*see* Disorder, iris, vascular
Iridochoroiditis (panuveitis) —*see* Panuveitis
Iridocyclitis H20.9-
acute H20.0-
hypopyon H20.05-
primary H20.01-
recurrent H20.02-
secondary (noninfectious) H20.04-
infectious H20.03-
chronic H20.1-
due to allergy —*see* Iridocyclitis, acute, secondary
endogenous —*see* Iridocyclitis, acute, primary
Fuchs' —*see* Cyclitis, Fuchs' heterochromic
gonococcal A54.32
granulomatous —*see* Iridocyclitis, chronic
herpes, herpetic (simplex) B00.51
zoster B02.32

Iridocyclitis *(Continued)*
hypopyon —*see* Iridocyclitis, acute, hypopyon
in (due to)
ankylosing spondylitis M45.9
gonococcal infection A54.32
herpes (simplex) virus B00.51
zoster B02.32
infectious disease NOS B99
parasitic disease NOS B89 *[H22]*
sarcoidosis D86.83
syphilis A51.43
tuberculosis A18.54
zoster B02.32
lens-induced H20.2-
nongranulomatous —*see* Iridocyclitis, acute
recurrent —*see* Iridocyclitis, acute, recurrent
rheumatic —*see* Iridocyclitis, chronic
subacute —*see* Iridocyclitis, acute
sympathetic —*see* Uveitis, sympathetic
syphilitic (secondary) A51.43
tuberculous (chronic) A18.54
Vogt-Koyanagi H20.82-
Iridocyclochoroiditis (panuveitis) —*see* Panuveitis
Iridodialysis H21.53-
Iridodonesis H21.89
Iridoplegia (complete) (partial) (reflex) H57.09
Iridoschisis H21.25-
Iris —*see also* condition
bombé —*see* Membrane, pupillary
Iritis —*see also* Iridocyclitis
chronic —*see* Iridocyclitis, chronic
diabetic —*see* E08-E13 with .39
due to
herpes simplex B00.51
leprosy A30.9 *[H22]*
gonococcal A54.32
gouty —*see also* Gout, by type M10.9 *[H22]* ⬅
granulomatous —*see* Iridocyclitis, chronic
lens induced —*see* Iridocyclitis, lens-induced
papulosa (syphilitic) A52.71
rheumatic —*see* Iridocyclitis, chronic
syphilitic (secondary) A51.43
congenital (early) A50.01
late A52.71
tuberculous A18.54
Iron —*see* condition
Iron-miner's lung J63.4
Irradiated enamel (tooth, teeth) K03.89
Irradiation effects, adverse T66
Irreducible, irreducibility —*see* condition
Irregular, irregularity
action, heart I49.9
alveolar process K08.89 ⬅
bleeding N92.6
breathing R06.89
contour of cornea (acquired) —*see* Deformity, cornea
congenital Q13.4
contour, reconstructed breast N65.0
dentin (in pulp) K04.3
eye movements H55.89
nystagmus —*see* Nystagmus
saccadic H55.81
labor O62.2
menstruation (cause unknown) N92.6
periods N92.6
prostate N42.9
pupil —*see* Abnormality, pupillary
reconstructed breast N65.0
respiratory R06.89
septum (nasal) J34.2
shape, organ or site, congenital NEC —*see* Distortion
sleep-wake pattern (rhythm) G47.23
Irritable, irritability R45.4
bladder N32.89
bowel (syndrome) K58.9
~~with diarrhea K58.0~~
with ◀
constipation K58.1 ◀
diarrhea K58.0 ◀

Irritable, irritability *(Continued)*
bowel (syndrome) *(Continued)*
mixed K58.2 ◀
psychogenic F45.8
specified NEC K58.8 ◀
bronchial —*see* Bronchitis
cerebral, in newborn P91.3
colon —*see also* Irritable, bowel K58.9 ⬅
with diarrhea K58.0
psychogenic F45.8
duodenum K59.8
heart (psychogenic) F45.8
hip —*see* Derangement, joint, specified type NEC, hip
ileum K59.8
infant R68.12
jejunum K59.8
rectum K59.8
stomach K31.89
psychogenic F45.8
sympathetic G90.8
urethra N36.8
Irritation
anus K62.89
axillary nerve G54.0
bladder N32.89
brachial plexus G54.0
bronchial —*see* Bronchitis
cervical plexus G54.2
cervix —*see* Cervicitis
choroid, sympathetic —*see* Endophthalmitis
cranial nerve —*see* Disorder, nerve, cranial
gastric K31.89
psychogenic F45.8
globe, sympathetic —*see* Uveitis, sympathetic
labyrinth —*see* subcategory H83.2
lumbosacral plexus G54.1
meninges (traumatic) —*see* Injury, intracranial
nontraumatic —*see* Meningismus
nerve —*see* Disorder, nerve
nervous R45.0
penis N48.89
perineum NEC L29.3
peripheral autonomic nervous system G90.8
peritoneum —*see* Peritonitis
pharynx J39.2
plantar nerve —*see* Lesion, nerve, plantar
spinal (cord) (traumatic) —*see also* Injury, spinal cord, by region
nerve G58.9
root NEC —*see* Radiculopathy
nontraumatic —*see* Myelopathy
stomach K31.89
psychogenic F45.8
sympathetic nerve NEC G90.8
ulnar nerve —*see* Lesion, nerve, ulnar
vagina N89.8
Ischemia, ischemic I99.8
bowel (transient)
acute —*see also* Ischemia, intestine, acute K55.059 ⬅
chronic K55.1
due to mesenteric artery insufficiency K55.1
brain —*see* Ischemia, cerebral
cardiac (*see* Disease, heart, ischemic)
cardiomyopathy I25.5
cerebral (chronic) (generalized) I67.82
arteriosclerotic I67.2
intermittent G45.9
newborn P91.0
recurrent focal G45.8
transient G45.9
colon chronic (due to mesenteric artery insufficiency) K55.1
coronary —*see* Disease, heart, ischemic
demand (coronary) —*see also* Angina I24.8
heart (chronic or with a stated duration of over 4 weeks) I25.9
acute or with a stated duration of 4 weeks or less I24.9
subacute I24.9

◀ New ⬅ Revised ~~deleted~~ Deleted

Ischemia, ischemic *(Continued)*
infarction, muscle —*see* Infarct, muscle
intestine (large) (small) (transient) K55.9
acute K55.Ø59 ⬅
diffuse K55.Ø52 ◀
focal K55.Ø51 ◀
large K55.Ø39 ◀
diffuse K55.Ø32 ◀
focal K55.Ø31 ◀
small K55.Ø19 ◀
diffuse K55.Ø12 ◀
focal K55.Ø11 ◀
chronic K55.1
due to mesenteric artery insufficiency K55.1
kidney N28.Ø
mesenteric, acute —*see also* Ischemia, intestine, acute K55.Ø59 ⬅
muscle, traumatic T79.6
myocardium, myocardial (chronic or with a stated duration of over 4 weeks) I25.9
acute, without myocardial infarction I51.3 ⬅
silent (asymptomatic) I25.6
transient of newborn P29.4
renal N28.Ø
retina, retinal —*see* Occlusion, artery, retina
small bowel
acute K55.Ø19 ⬅
diffuse K55.Ø12 ◀
focal K55.Ø11 ◀
chronic K55.1
due to mesenteric artery insufficiency K55.1
spinal cord G95.11
subendocardial —*see* Insufficiency, coronary
supply (coronary) —*see also* Angina I25.9
due to vasospasm I2Ø.1
Ischial spine —*see* condition
Ischialgia —*see* Sciatica
Ischiopagus Q89.4
Ischium, ischial —*see* condition
Ischuria R34
Iselin's disease or osteochondrosis —*see* Osteochondrosis, juvenile, metatarsus
Islands of
parotid tissue in
lymph nodes Q38.6
neck structures Q38.6
submaxillary glands in
fascia Q38.6
lymph nodes Q38.6
neck muscles Q38.6
Islet cell tumor, pancreas D13.7
Isoimmunization NEC —*see also* Incompatibility
affecting management of pregnancy (ABO) (with hydrops fetalis) O36.11-
anti-A sensitization O36.11-
anti-B sensitization O36.19-
anti-c sensitization O36.Ø9-
anti-C sensitization O36.Ø9-
anti-e sensitization O36.Ø9-
anti-E sensitization O36.Ø9-
Rh NEC O36.Ø9-
anti-D antibody O36.Ø1-
specified NEC O36.19-
newborn P55.9
with
hydrops fetalis P56.Ø
kernicterus P57.Ø
ABO (blood groups) P55.1
Rhesus (Rh) factor P55.Ø
specified type NEC P55.8
Isolation, isolated
dwelling Z59.8
family Z63.79
social Z6Ø.4
Isoleucinosis E71.19
Isomerism atrial appendages (with asplenia or polysplenia) Q2Ø.6
Isosporiasis, isosporosis AØ7.3
Isovaleric acidemia E71.11Ø
Issue of
medical certificate ZØ2.79
for disability determination ZØ2.71
Issue of *(Continued)*
repeat prescription (appliance) (glasses) (medicinal substance, medicament, medicine) Z76.Ø
contraception —*see* Contraception
Itch, itching —*see also* Pruritus
baker's L23.6
barber's B35.Ø
bricklayer's L24.5
cheese B88.Ø
clam digger's B65.3
coolie B76.9
copra B88.Ø
dew B76.9
dhobi B35.6
filarial —*see* Infestation, filarial
grain B88.Ø
grocer's B88.Ø
ground B76.9
harvest B88.Ø
jock B35.6
Malabar B35.5
beard B35.Ø
foot B35.3
scalp B35.Ø
meaning scabies B86
Norwegian B86
perianal L29.Ø
poultrymen's B88.Ø
sarcoptic B86
scabies B86
scrub B88.Ø
straw B88.Ø
swimmer's B65.3
water B76.9
winter L29.8
Ivemark's syndrome (asplenia with congenital heart disease) Q89.Ø1
Ivory bones Q78.2
Ixodiasis NEC B88.8

J

Jaccoud's syndrome —*see* Arthropathy, postrheumatic, chronic
Jackson's
membrane Q43.3
paralysis or syndrome G83.89
veil Q43.3
Jacquet's dermatitis (diaper dermatitis) L22
Jadassohn-Pellizari's disease or anetoderma L90.2
Jadassohn's
blue nevus —*see* Nevus
intraepidermal epithelioma —*see* Neoplasm, skin, benign
Jaffe-Lichtenstein (-Uehlinger) **syndrome** —*see* Dysplasia, fibrous, bone NEC
Jakob-Creutzfeldt disease or syndrome —*see* Creutzfeldt-Jakob disease or syndrome
Jaksch-Luzet disease D64.89
Jamaican
neuropathy G92
paraplegic tropical ataxic-spastic syndrome G92
Janet's disease F48.8
Janiceps Q89.4
Jansky-Bielschowsky amaurotic idiocy E75.4
Japanese
B-type encephalitis A83.0
river fever A75.3
Jaundice (yellow) R17
acholuric (familial) (splenomegalic) —*see also* Spherocytosis
acquired D59.8
breast-milk (inhibitor) P59.3
catarrhal (acute) B15.9
with hepatic coma B15.0
cholestatic (benign) R17
due to or associated with
delayed conjugation P59.8
associated with (due to) preterm delivery P59.0
preterm delivery P59.0
epidemic (catarrhal) B15.9
with hepatic coma B15.0
leptospiral A27.0
spirochetal A27.0
familial nonhemolytic (congenital) (Gilbert) E80.4
Crigler-Najjar E80.5
febrile (acute) B15.9
with hepatic coma B15.0
leptospiral A27.0
spirochetal A27.0
hematogenous D59.9
hemolytic (acquired) D59.9
congenital —*see* Spherocytosis

Jaundice *(Continued)*
hemorrhagic (acute) (leptospiral) (spirochetal) A27.0
infectious (acute) (subacute) B15.9
with hepatic coma B15.0
leptospiral A27.0
spirochetal A27.0
leptospiral (hemorrhagic) A27.0
malignant (without coma) K72.90
with coma K72.91
neonatal —*see* Jaundice, newborn
newborn P59.9
due to or associated with
ABO
antibodies P55.1
incompatibility, maternal/fetal P55.1
isoimmunization P55.1
absence or deficiency of enzyme system for bilirubin conjugation (congenital) P59.8
bleeding P58.1
breast milk inhibitors to conjugation P59.3
associated with preterm delivery P59.0
bruising P58.0
Crigler-Najjar syndrome E80.5
delayed conjugation P59.8
associated with preterm delivery P59.0
drugs or toxins
given to newborn P58.42
transmitted from mother P58.41
excessive hemolysis P58.9
due to
bleeding P58.1
bruising P58.0
drugs or toxins
given to newborn P58.42
transmitted from mother P58.41
infection P58.2
polycythemia P58.3
swallowed maternal blood P58.5
specified type NEC P58.8
galactosemia E74.21
Gilbert syndrome E80.4
hemolytic disease P55.9
ABO isoimmunization P55.1
Rh isoimmunization P55.0
specified NEC P55.8
hepatocellular damage P59.20
specified NEC P59.29
hereditary hemolytic anemia P58.8
hypothyroidism, congenital E03.1
incompatibility, maternal/fetal NOS P55.9
infection P58.2

Jaundice *(Continued)*
newborn *(Continued)*
due to or associated with *(Continued)*
inspissated bile syndrome P59.1
isoimmunization NOS P55.9
mucoviscidosis E84.9
polycythemia P58.3
preterm delivery P59.0
Rh
antibodies P55.0
incompatibility, maternal/fetal P55.0
isoimmunization P55.0
specified cause NEC P59.8
swallowed maternal blood P58.5
spherocytosis (congenital) D58.0
nonhemolytic congenital familial (Gilbert) E80.4
nuclear, newborn —*see also* Kernicterus of newborn P57.9
obstructive —*see also* Obstruction, bile duct K83.1
post-immunization —*see* Hepatitis, viral, type, B
post-transfusion —*see* Hepatitis, viral, type, B
regurgitation —*see also* Obstruction, bile duct K83.1
serum (homologous) (prophylactic) (therapeutic) —*see* Hepatitis, viral, type, B
spirochetal (hemorrhagic) A27.0
symptomatic R17
newborn P59.9
Jaw —*see* condition
Jaw-winking phenomenon or syndrome Q07.8
Jealousy
alcoholic F10.988
childhood F93.8
sibling F93.8
Jejunitis —*see* Enteritis
Jejunostomy status Z93.4
Jejunum, jejunal —*see* condition
Jensen's disease —*see* Inflammation, chorioretinal, focal, juxtapapillary
Jerks, myoclonic G25.3
Jervell-Lange-Nielsen syndrome I45.81
Jeune's disease Q77.2
Jigger disease B88.1
Job's syndrome (chronic granulomatous disease) D71
Joint —*see also* condition
mice —*see* Loose, body, joint
knee M23.4-
Jordan's anomaly or syndrome D72.0
Joseph-Diamond-Blackfan anemia (congenital hypoplastic) D61.01
Jungle yellow fever A95.0
Jüngling's disease —*see* Sarcoidosis
Juvenile —*see* condition

◄ New ⟸ Revised ~~deleted~~ Deleted

K

Ketosis NEC E88.89
- diabetic —*see* Diabetes, by type, with ketoacidosis

Kew Garden fever A79.1
Kidney —*see* condition
Kienböck's disease —*see also* Osteochondrosis, juvenile, hand, carpal lunate
- adult M93.1

Kimmelstiel (-Wilson) **disease** —*see* Diabetes, Kimmelstiel (-Wilson) disease
Kimura disease D21.9
- specified site (see Neoplasm, connective tissue benign)

Kink, kinking
- artery I77.1
- hair (acquired) L67.8
- ileum or intestine —*see* Obstruction, intestine
- Lane's —*see* Obstruction, intestine
- organ or site, congenital NEC —*see* Anomaly, by site
- ureter (pelvic junction) N13.5
  - with
    - hydronephrosis N13.1
      - with infection N13.6
    - pyelonephritis (chronic) N11.1
  - congenital Q62.39
- vein (s) I87.8
  - caval I87.1
  - peripheral I87.1

Kinnier Wilson's disease (hepatolenticular degeneration) E83.Ø1
Kissing spine M48.2Ø
- cervical region M48.22
- cervicothoracic region M48.23
- lumbar region M48.26
- lumbosacral region M48.27
- occipito-atlanto-axial region M48.21
- thoracic region M48.24
- thoracolumbar region M48.25

K

Klatskin's tumor C24.Ø
Klauder's disease A26.8
Klebs' disease —*see also* Glomerulonephritis NØ5.-
Klebsiella (K.) **pneumoniae, as cause of disease classified elsewhere** B96.1
Klein (e)**-Levin syndrome** G47.13
Kleptomania F63.2
Klinefelter's syndrome Q98.4
- karyotype 47,XXY Q98.Ø
- male with more than two X chromosomes Q98.1

Klippel-Feil deficiency, disease, or syndrome (brevicollis) Q76.1
Klippel's disease I67.2
Klippel-Trenaunay (-Weber) **syndrome** Q87.2
Klumpke (-Déjerine) **palsy, paralysis** (birth) (newborn) P14.1
Knee —*see* condition
Knock knee (acquired) M21.Ø6-
- congenital Q74.1

Knot (s)
- intestinal, syndrome (volvulus) K56.2
- surfer S89.8-
- umbilical cord (true) O69.2

Knotting (of)
- hair L67.8
- intestine K56.2

Knuckle pad (Garrod's) **M72.1**
Koch's
- infection —*see* Tuberculosis
- relapsing fever A68.9

Koch-Weeks' conjunctivitis —*see* Conjunctivitis, acute, mucopurulent
Köebner's syndrome Q81.8
Köenig's disease (osteochondritis dissecans) —*see* Osteochondritis, dissecans
Köhler-Pellegrini-Steida disease or syndrome (calcification, knee joint) —*see* Bursitis, tibial collateral
Köhler's disease
- patellar —*see* Osteochondrosis, juvenile, patella
- tarsal navicular —*see* Osteochondrosis, juvenile, tarsus

Koilonychia L6Ø.3
- congenital Q84.6

Kojevnikov's, epilepsy —*see* Kozhevnikof's epilepsy
Koplik's spots BØ5.9
Kopp's asthma E32.8
Korsakoff's (Wernicke) **disease, psychosis or syndrome** (alcoholic) F1Ø.96
- with dependence F1Ø.26
- drug-induced
  - due to drug abuse —*see* Abuse, drug, by type, with amnestic disorder
  - due to drug dependence —*see* Dependence, drug, by type, with amnestic disorder
- nonalcoholic FØ4

Korsakov's disease, psychosis or syndrome —*see* Korsakoff's disease
Korsakow's disease, psychosis or syndrome —*see* Korsakoff's disease
Kostmann's disease or syndrome (infantile genetic agranulocytosis) —*see* Agranulocytosis
Kozhevnikof's epilepsy G4Ø.1Ø9
- intractable G4Ø.119
  - with status epilepticus G4Ø.111
  - without status epilepticus G4Ø.119
- not intractable G4Ø.1Ø9
  - with status epilepticus G4Ø.1Ø1
  - without status epilepticus G4Ø.1Ø9

Krabbe's
- disease E75.23
- syndrome, congenital muscle hypoplasia Q79.8

Kraepelin-Morel disease —*see* Schizophrenia
Kraft-Weber-Dimitri disease Q85.8
Kraurosis
- ani K62.89
- penis N48.Ø

Kraurosis *(Continued)*
- vagina N89.8
- vulva N9Ø.4

Kreotoxism AØ5.9
Krukenberg's
- spindle —*see* Pigmentation, cornea, posterior
- tumor C79.6-

Kufs' disease E75.4
Kugelberg-Welander disease G12.1
Kuhnt-Junius degeneration —*see also* Degeneration, macula H35.32- ⬅
Kümmell's disease or spondylitis —*see* Spondylopathy, traumatic
Kupffer cell sarcoma C22.3
Kuru A81.81
Kussmaul's
- disease M3Ø.Ø
- respiration E87.2
  - in diabetic acidosis —*see* Diabetes, by type, with ketoacidosis

Kwashiorkor E4Ø
- marasmic, marasmus type E42

Kyasanur Forest disease A98.2
Kyphoscoliosis, kyphoscoliotic (acquired) —*see also* Scoliosis M41.9
- congenital Q67.5
- heart (disease) I27.1
- sequelae of rickets E64.3
- tuberculous A18.Ø1

Kyphosis, kyphotic (acquired) M4Ø.2Ø9
- cervical region M4Ø.2Ø2
- cervicothoracic region M4Ø.2Ø3
- congenital Q76.419
  - cervical region Q76.412
  - cervicothoracic region Q76.413
  - occipito-atlanto-axial region Q76.411
  - thoracic region Q76.414
  - thoracolumbar region Q76.415
- Morquio-Brailsford type (spinal) —*see also* subcategory M49.8 E76.219
- postlaminectomy M96.3
- postradiation therapy M96.2
- postural (adolescent) M4Ø.ØØ
  - cervicothoracic region M4Ø.Ø3
  - thoracic region M4Ø.Ø4
  - thoracolumbar region M4Ø.Ø5
- secondary NEC M4Ø.1Ø
  - cervical region M4Ø.12
  - cervicothoracic region M4Ø.13
  - thoracic region M4Ø.14
  - thoracolumbar region M4Ø.15
- sequelae of rickets E64.3
- specified type NEC M4Ø.299
  - cervical region M4Ø.292
  - cervicothoracic region M4Ø.293
  - thoracic region M4Ø.294
  - thoracolumbar region M4Ø.295
- syphilitic, congenital A5Ø.56
- thoracic region M4Ø.2Ø4
- thoracolumbar region M4Ø.2Ø5
- tuberculous A18.Ø1

Kyrle disease L87.Ø

L

- **Labia, labium** —*see* condition
- **Labile**
  - blood pressure RØ9.89
  - vasomotor system I73.9
- **Labioglossal paralysis** G12.29
- **Labium leporinum** —*see* Cleft, lip
- **Labor** —*see* Delivery
- **Labored breathing** —*see* Hyperventilation
- **Labyrinthitis** (circumscribed) (destructive) (diffuse) (inner ear) (latent) (purulent) (suppurative) (*see also* subcategory) H83.Ø
  - syphilitic A52.79
- **Laceration**
  - with abortion —*see* Abortion, by type, complicated by laceration of pelvic organs
  - abdomen, abdominal
    - wall S31.119
      - with
        - foreign body S31.129
        - penetration into peritoneal cavity S31.619
          - with foreign body S31.629
      - epigastric region S31.112
        - with
          - foreign body S31.122
          - penetration into peritoneal cavity S31.612
            - with foreign body S31.622
      - left
        - lower quadrant S31.114
          - with
            - foreign body S31.124
            - penetration into peritoneal cavity S31.614
              - with foreign body S31.624
        - upper quadrant S31.111
          - with
            - foreign body S31.121
            - penetration into peritoneal cavity S31.611
              - with foreign body S31.621
      - periumbilic region S31.115
        - with
          - foreign body S31.125
          - penetration into peritoneal cavity S31.615
            - with foreign body S31.625
      - right
        - lower quadrant S31.113
          - with
            - foreign body S31.123
            - penetration into peritoneal cavity S31.613
              - with foreign body S31.623
        - upper quadrant S31.11Ø
          - with
            - foreign body S31.12Ø
            - penetration into peritoneal cavity S31.61Ø
              - with foreign body S31.62Ø
  - accidental, complicating surgery —*see* Complications, surgical, accidental puncture or laceration
  - Achilles tendon S86.Ø2-
  - adrenal gland S37.813
  - alveolar (process) —*see* Laceration, oral cavity
  - ankle S91.Ø1-
    - with
      - foreign body S91.Ø2-
  - antecubital space —*see* Laceration, elbow
  - anus (sphincter) S31.831
    - with
      - ectopic or molar pregnancy OØ8.6
      - foreign body S31.832
    - complicating delivery —*see* Delivery, complicated, by, laceration, anus (sphincter)

Laceration *(Continued)*

  - anus *(Continued)*
    - following ectopic or molar pregnancy OØ8.6
    - nontraumatic, nonpuerperal —*see* Fissure, anus
  - arm (upper) S41.11-
    - with foreign body S41.12-
    - lower —*see* Laceration, forearm
  - auditory canal (external) (meatus) —*see* Laceration, ear
  - auricle, ear —*see* Laceration, ear
  - axilla —*see* Laceration, arm
  - back —*see also* Laceration, thorax, back
    - lower S31.Ø1Ø
      - with
        - foreign body S31.Ø2Ø
          - with penetration into retroperitoneal space S31.Ø21
        - penetration into retroperitoneal space S31.Ø11
  - bile duct S36.13
  - bladder S37.23
    - with ectopic or molar pregnancy OØ8.6
    - following ectopic or molar pregnancy OØ8.6
    - obstetrical trauma O71.5
  - blood vessel —*see* Injury, blood vessel
  - bowel —*see also* Laceration, intestine
    - with ectopic or molar pregnancy OØ8.6
    - complicating abortion —*see* Abortion, by type, complicated by, specified condition NEC
    - following ectopic or molar pregnancy OØ8.6
    - obstetrical trauma O71.5
  - brain (any part) (cortex) (diffuse) (membrane) —*see also* Injury, intracranial, diffuse
    - during birth P1Ø.8
      - with hemorrhage P1Ø.1
    - focal —*see* Injury, intracranial, focal brain injury
  - brainstem SØ6.38-
  - breast S21.Ø1-
    - with foreign body S21.Ø2-
  - broad ligament S37.893
    - with ectopic or molar pregnancy OØ8.6
    - following ectopic or molar pregnancy OØ8.6
    - laceration syndrome N83.8
    - obstetrical trauma O71.6
    - syndrome (laceration) N83.8
  - buttock S31.8Ø1
    - with foreign body S31.8Ø2
    - left S31.821
      - with foreign body S31.822
    - right S31.811
      - with foreign body S31.812
  - calf —*see* Laceration, leg
  - canaliculus lacrimalis —*see* Laceration, eyelid
  - canthus, eye —*see* Laceration, eyelid
  - capsule, joint —*see* Sprain
  - causing eversion of cervix uteri (old) N86
  - central (perineal), complicating delivery O7Ø.9
  - cerebellum, traumatic SØ6.37-
  - cerebral SØ6.33-
    - during birth P1Ø.8
      - with hemorrhage P1Ø.1
    - left side SØ6.32-
    - right side SØ6.31-
  - cervix (uteri)
    - with ectopic or molar pregnancy OØ8.6
    - following ectopic or molar pregnancy OØ8.6
    - nonpuerperal, nontraumatic N88.1
    - obstetrical trauma (current) O71.3
    - old (postpartal) N88.1
    - traumatic S37.63

Laceration *(Continued)*

  - cheek (external) SØ1.41-
    - with foreign body SØ1.42-
    - internal —*see* Laceration, oral cavity
  - chest wall —*see* Laceration, thorax
  - chin —*see* Laceration, head, specified site NEC
  - chordae tendinae NEC I51.1
    - concurrent with acute myocardial infarction —*see* Infarct, myocardium
    - following acute myocardial infarction (current complication) I23.4
  - clitoris —*see* Laceration, vulva
  - colon —*see* Laceration, intestine, large, colon
  - common bile duct S36.13
  - cortex (cerebral) —*see* Injury, intracranial, diffuse
  - costal region —*see* Laceration, thorax
  - cystic duct S36.13
  - diaphragm S27.8Ø3
  - digit (s)
    - foot —*see* Laceration, toe
    - hand —*see* Laceration, finger
  - duodenum S36.43Ø
  - ear (canal) (external) SØ1.31-
    - with foreign body SØ1.32-
    - drum SØ9.2-
  - elbow S51.Ø1-
    - with
      - foreign body S51.Ø2-
  - epididymis —*see* Laceration, testis
  - epigastric region —*see* Laceration, abdomen, wall, epigastric region
  - esophagus K22.8
    - traumatic
      - cervical S11.21
        - with foreign body S11.22
      - thoracic S27.813
  - eye (ball) SØ5.3-
    - with prolapse or loss of intraocular tissue SØ5.2-
    - penetrating SØ5.6-
  - eyebrow —*see* Laceration, eyelid
  - eyelid SØ1.11-
    - with foreign body SØ1.12-
  - face NEC —*see* Laceration, head, specified site NEC
  - fallopian tube S37.539
    - bilateral S37.532
    - unilateral S37.531
  - finger (s) S61.219
    - with
      - damage to nail S61.319
        - with
          - foreign body S61.329
      - foreign body S61.229
    - index S61.218
      - with
        - damage to nail S61.318
          - with
            - foreign body S61.328
        - foreign body S61.228
      - left S61.211
        - with
          - damage to nail S61.311
            - with
              - foreign body S61.321
          - foreign body S61.221
      - right S61.21Ø
        - with
          - damage to nail S61.31Ø
            - with
              - foreign body S61.32Ø
          - foreign body S61.22Ø
    - little S61.218
      - with
        - damage to nail S61.318
          - with
            - foreign body S61.328
        - foreign body S61.228

Laceration *(Continued)*
  finger *(Continued)*
    little *(Continued)*
      left S61.217
        with
          damage to nail S61.317
            with
              foreign body S61.327
          foreign body S61.227
      right S61.216
        with
          damage to nail S61.316
            with
              foreign body S61.326
          foreign body S61.226
    middle S61.218
      with
        damage to nail S61.318
          with
            foreign body S61.328
        foreign body S61.228
      left S61.213
        with
          damage to nail S61.313
            with
              foreign body S61.323
          foreign body S61.223
      right S61.212
        with
          damage to nail S61.312
            with
              foreign body S61.322
          foreign body S61.222
    ring S61.218
      with
        damage to nail S61.318
          with
            foreign body S61.328
        foreign body S61.228
      left S61.215
        with
          damage to nail S61.315
            with
              foreign body S61.325
          foreign body S61.225
      right S61.214
        with
          damage to nail S61.314
            with
              foreign body S61.324
          foreign body S61.224
  flank S31.119
    with foreign body S31.129
  foot (except toe (s) alone) S91.319
    with foreign body S91.329
    left S91.312
      with foreign body S91.322
    right S91.311
      with foreign body S91.321
    toe —*see* Laceration, toe
  forearm S51.819
    with
      foreign body S51.829
    elbow only —*see* Laceration, elbow
    left S51.812
      with
        foreign body S51.822
    right S51.811
      with
        foreign body S51.821
  forehead S01.81
    with foreign body S01.82
  fourchette O70.0
    with ectopic or molar pregnancy O08.6
    complicating delivery O70.0
    following ectopic or molar pregnancy O08.6
  gallbladder S36.123

Laceration *(Continued)*
  genital organs, external
    female S31.512
      with foreign body S31.522
      vagina —*see* Laceration, vagina
      vulva —*see* Laceration, vulva
    male S31.511
      with foreign body S31.521
      penis —*see* Laceration, penis
      scrotum —*see* Laceration, scrotum
      testis —*see* Laceration, testis
  groin —*see* Laceration, abdomen, wall
  gum —*see* Laceration, oral cavity
  hand S61.419
    with
      foreign body S61.429
    finger —*see* Laceration, finger
    left S61.412
      with
        foreign body S61.422
    right S61.411
      with
        foreign body S61.421
    thumb —*see* Laceration, thumb
  head S01.91
    with foreign body S01.92
    cheek —*see* Laceration, cheek
    ear —*see* Laceration, ear
    eyelid —*see* Laceration, eyelid
    lip —*see* Laceration, lip
    nose —*see* Laceration, nose
    oral cavity —*see* Laceration, oral cavity
    scalp S01.01
      with foreign body S01.02
    specified site NEC S01.81
      with foreign body S01.82
    temporomandibular area —*see* Laceration, cheek
  heart —*see* Injury, heart, laceration
  heel —*see* Laceration, foot
  hepatic duct S36.13
  hip S71.019
    with foreign body S71.029
    left S71.012
      with foreign body S71.022
    right S71.011
      with foreign body S71.021
  hymen —*see* Laceration, vagina
  hypochondrium —*see* Laceration, abdomen, wall
  hypogastric region —*see* Laceration, abdomen, wall
  ileum S36.438
  inguinal region —*see* Laceration, abdomen, wall
  instep —*see* Laceration, foot
  internal organ —*see* Injury, by site
  interscapular region —*see* Laceration, thorax, back
  intestine
    large
      colon S36.539
        ascending S36.530
        descending S36.532
        sigmoid S36.533
        specified site NEC S36.538
      rectum S36.63
        transverse S36.531
    small S36.439
      duodenum S36.430
      specified site NEC S36.438
  intra-abdominal organ S36.93
    intestine —*see* Laceration, intestine
    liver —*see* Laceration, liver
    pancreas —*see* Laceration, pancreas
    peritoneum S36.81
    specified site NEC S36.893
    spleen —*see* Laceration, spleen
    stomach —*see* Laceration, stomach

Laceration *(Continued)*
  intracranial NEC —*see also* Injury, intracranial, diffuse
    birth injury P10.9
  jaw —*see* Laceration, head, specified site NEC
  jejunum S36.438
  joint capsule —*see* Sprain, by site
  kidney S37.03-
    major (greater than 3 cm) (massive) (stellate) S37.06-
    minor (less than 1 cm) S37.04-
    moderate (1 to 3 cm) S37.05-
      multiple S37.06-
  knee S81.01-
    with foreign body S81.02-
  labium (majus) (minus) —*see* Laceration, vulva
  lacrimal duct —*see* Laceration, eyelid
  large intestine —*see* Laceration, intestine, large
  larynx S11.011
    with foreign body S11.012
  leg (lower) S81.819
    with foreign body S81.829
    foot —*see* Laceration, foot
    knee —*see* Laceration, knee
    left S81.812
      with foreign body S81.822
    right S81.811
      with foreign body S81.821
    upper —*see* Laceration, thigh
  ligament —*see* Sprain
  lip S01.511
    with foreign body S01.521
  liver S36.113
    major (stellate) S36.116
    minor S36.114
    moderate S36.115
  loin —*see* Laceration, abdomen, wall
  lower back —*see* Laceration, back, lower
  lumbar region —*see* Laceration, back, lower
  lung S27.339
    bilateral S27.332
    unilateral S27.331
  malar region —*see* Laceration, head, specified site NEC
  mammary —*see* Laceration, breast
  mastoid region —*see* Laceration, head, specified site NEC
  meninges —*see* Injury, intracranial, diffuse
  meniscus —*see* Tear, meniscus
  mesentery S36.893
  mesosalpinx S37.893
  mouth —*see* Laceration, oral cavity
  muscle —*see* Injury, muscle, by site, laceration
  nail
    finger —*see* Laceration, finger, with damage to nail
    toe —*see* Laceration, toe, with damage to nail
  nasal (septum) (sinus) —*see* Laceration, nose
  nasopharynx —*see* Laceration, head, specified site NEC
  neck S11.91
    with foreign body S11.92
    involving
      cervical esophagus S11.21
        with foreign body S11.22
      larynx —*see* Laceration, larynx
      pharynx —*see* Laceration, pharynx
      thyroid gland —*see* Laceration, thyroid gland
      trachea —*see* Laceration, trachea
    specified site NEC S11.81
      with foreign body S11.82
  nerve —*see* Injury, nerve
  nose (septum) (sinus) S01.21
    with foreign body S01.22
  ocular NOS S05.3-
    adnexa NOS S01.11-

L

Laceration *(Continued)*
oral cavity S01.512
with foreign body S01.522
orbit (eye) —*see* Wound, open, ocular, orbit
ovary S37.439
bilateral S37.432
unilateral S37.431
palate —*see* Laceration, oral cavity
palm —*see* Laceration, hand
pancreas S36.239
body S36.231
major S36.261
minor S36.241
moderate S36.251
head S36.230
major S36.260
minor S36.240
moderate S36.250
major S36.269
minor S36.249
moderate S36.259
tail S36.232
major S36.262
minor S36.242
moderate S36.252
pelvic S31.010
with
foreign body S31.020
penetration into retroperitoneal cavity S31.021
penetration into retroperitoneal cavity S31.011
floor —*see also* Laceration, back, lower
with ectopic or molar pregnancy O08.6
complicating delivery O70.1
following ectopic or molar pregnancy O08.6
old (postpartal) N81.89
organ S37.93
with ectopic or molar pregnancy O08.6
adrenal gland S37.813
bladder S37.23
fallopian tube —*see* Laceration, fallopian tube
following ectopic or molar pregnancy O08.6
kidney —*see* Laceration, kidney
obstetrical trauma O71.5
ovary —*see* Laceration, ovary
prostate S37.823
specified site NEC S37.893
ureter S37.13
urethra S37.33
uterus S37.63
penis S31.21
with foreign body S31.22
perineum
female S31.41
with
ectopic or molar pregnancy O08.6
foreign body S31.42
during delivery O70.9
first degree O70.0
fourth degree O70.3
second degree O70.1
third degree —*see also* Delivery, complicated, by, laceration, perineum, third degree O70.20 (Revised)
old (postpartal) N81.89
postpartal N81.89
secondary (postpartal) O90.1
male S31.119
with foreign body S31.129
periocular area (with or without lacrimal passages) —*see* Laceration, eyelid
peritoneum S36.893
periumbilic region —*see* Laceration, abdomen, wall, periumbilic

Laceration *(Continued)*
periurethral tissue —*see* Laceration, urethra
phalanges
finger —*see* Laceration, finger
toe —*see* Laceration, toe
pharynx S11.21
with foreign body S11.22
pinna —*see* Laceration, ear
popliteal space —*see* Laceration, knee
prepuce —*see* Laceration, penis
prostate S37.823
pubic region S31.119
with foreign body S31.129
pudendum —*see* Laceration, genital organs, external
rectovaginal septum —*see* Laceration, vagina
rectum S36.63
retroperitoneum S36.893
round ligament S37.893
sacral region —*see* Laceration, back, lower
sacroiliac region —*see* Laceration, back, lower
salivary gland —*see* Laceration, oral cavity
scalp S01.01
with foreign body S01.02
scapular region —*see* Laceration, shoulder
scrotum S31.31
with foreign body S31.32
seminal vesicle S37.893
shin —*see* Laceration, leg
shoulder S41.019
with foreign body S41.029
left S41.012
with foreign body S41.022
right S41.011
with foreign body S41.021
small intestine —*see* Laceration, intestine, small
spermatic cord —*see* Laceration, testis
spinal cord (meninges) —*see also* Injury, spinal cord, by region
due to injury at birth P11.5
newborn (birth injury) P11.5
spleen S36.039
major (massive) (stellate) S36.032
moderate S36.031
superficial (minor) S36.030
sternal region —*see* Laceration, thorax, front
stomach S36.33
submaxillary region —*see* Laceration, head, specified site NEC
submental region —*see* Laceration, head, specified site NEC
subungual
finger (s) —*see* Laceration, finger, with damage to nail
toe (s) —*see* Laceration, toe, with damage to nail
suprarenal gland —*see* Laceration, adrenal gland
temple, temporal region —*see* Laceration, head, specified site NEC
temporomandibular area —*see* Laceration, cheek
tendon —*see* Injury, muscle, by site, laceration
Achilles S86.02-
tentorium cerebelli —*see* Injury, intracranial, diffuse
testis S31.31
with foreign body S31.32
thigh S71.11-
with foreign body S71.12-
thorax, thoracic (wall) S21.91
with foreign body S21.92
back S21.22-
with penetration into thoracic cavity S21.42-
front S21.12-
with penetration into thoracic cavity S21.32-

Laceration *(Continued)*
thorax, thoracic *(Continued)*
back S21.21-
with
foreign body S21.22-
with penetration into thoracic cavity S21.42-
penetration into thoracic cavity S21.41-
breast —*see* Laceration, breast
front S21.11-
with
foreign body S21.12-
with penetration into thoracic cavity S21.32-
penetration into thoracic cavity S21.31-
thumb S61.019
with
damage to nail S61.119
with
foreign body S61.129
foreign body S61.029
left S61.012
with
damage to nail S61.112
with
foreign body S61.122
foreign body S61.022
right S61.011
with
damage to nail S61.111
with
foreign body S61.121
foreign body S61.021
thyroid gland S11.11
with foreign body S11.12
toe (s) S91.119
with
damage to nail S91.219
with
foreign body S91.229
foreign body S91.129
great S91.113
with
damage to nail S91.213
with
foreign body S91.223
foreign body S91.123
left S91.112
with
damage to nail S91.212
with
foreign body S91.222
foreign body S91.122
right S91.111
with
damage to nail S91.211
with
foreign body S91.221
foreign body S91.121
lesser S91.116
with
damage to nail S91.216
with
foreign body S91.226
foreign body S91.126
left S91.115
with
damage to nail S91.215
with
foreign body S91.225
foreign body S91.125
right S91.114
with
damage to nail S91.214
with
foreign body S91.224
foreign body S91.124
tongue —*see* Laceration, oral cavity

Laceration *(Continued)*
trachea S11.Ø21
with foreign body S11.Ø22
tunica vaginalis —*see* Laceration, testis
tympanum, tympanic membrane —*see* Laceration, ear, drum
umbilical region S31.115
with foreign body S31.125
ureter S37.13
urethra S37.33
with or following ectopic or molar pregnancy OØ8.6
obstetrical trauma O71.5
urinary organ NEC S37.893
uterus S37.63
with ectopic or molar pregnancy OØ8.6
following ectopic or molar pregnancy OØ8.6
nonpuerperal, nontraumatic N85.8
obstetrical trauma NEC O71.81
old (postpartal) N85.8
uvula —*see* Laceration, oral cavity
vagina S31.41
with
ectopic or molar pregnancy OØ8.6
foreign body S31.42
during delivery O71.4
with perineal laceration —*see* Laceration, perineum, female, during delivery
following ectopic or molar pregnancy OØ8.6
nonpuerperal, nontraumatic N89.8
old (postpartal) N89.8
vas deferens S37.893
vesical —*see* Laceration, bladder
vocal cords S11.Ø31
with foreign body S11.Ø32
vulva S31.41
with
ectopic or molar pregnancy OØ8.6
foreign body S31.42
complicating delivery O7Ø.Ø
following ectopic or molar pregnancy OØ8.6
nonpuerperal, nontraumatic N9Ø.89
old (postpartal) N9Ø.89
wrist S61.519
with
foreign body S61.529
left S61.512
with
foreign body S61.522
right S61.511
with
foreign body S61.521

Lack of
achievement in school Z55.3
adequate
food Z59.4
intermaxillary vertical dimension of fully erupted teeth M26.36
sleep Z72.82Ø
appetite (*see* Anorexia) R63.Ø
awareness R41.9
care
in home Z74.2
of infant (at or after birth) T76.Ø2
confirmed T74.Ø2
cognitive functions R41.9
coordination R27.9
ataxia R27.Ø
specified type NEC R27.8
development (physiological) R62.5Ø
failure to thrive (child over 28 days old) R62.51
adult R62.7
newborn P92.6
short stature R62.52
specified type NEC R62.59
energy R53.83
financial resources Z59.6

L

Lack of *(Continued)*
food T73.Ø
growth R62.52
heating Z59.1
housing (permanent) (temporary) Z59.Ø
adequate Z59.1
learning experiences in childhood Z62.898
leisure time (affecting life-style) Z73.2
material resources Z59.9
memory —*see also* Amnesia
mild, following organic brain damage FØ6.8
ovulation N97.Ø
parental supervision or control of child Z62.Ø
person able to render necessary care Z74.2
physical exercise Z72.3
play experience in childhood Z62.898
posterior occlusal support M26.57
relaxation (affecting life-style) Z73.2
sexual
desire F52.Ø
enjoyment F52.1
shelter Z59.Ø
sleep (adequate) Z72.82Ø
supervision of child by parent Z62.Ø
support, posterior occlusal M26.57
water T73.1
Lacrimal —*see* condition
Lacrimation, abnormal —*see* Epiphora
Lacrimonasal duct —*see* condition
Lactation, lactating (breast) (puerperal, postpartum)
associated
cracked nipple O92.13
retracted nipple O92.Ø3
defective O92.4
disorder NEC O92.79
excessive O92.6
failed (complete) O92.3
partial O92.4
mastitis NEC —*see* Mastitis, obstetric
mother (care and/or examination) Z39.1
nonpuerperal N64.3
Lacticemia, excessive E87.2
Lacunar skull Q75.8
Laennec's cirrhosis K7Ø.3Ø ⬅
~~alcoholic K7Ø.3Ø~~
~~with ascites K7Ø.31~~
with ascites K7Ø.31 ◀
nonalcoholic K74.69 ◀
Lafora's disease —*see* Epilepsy, generalized, idiopathic
Lag, lid (nervous) —*see* Retraction, lid
Lagophthalmos (eyelid) (nervous) HØ2.2Ø9
cicatricial HØ2.219
left HØ2.216
lower HØ2.215
upper HØ2.214
right HØ2.213
lower HØ2.212
upper HØ2.211
keratoconjunctivitis —*see* Keratoconjunctivitis
left HØ2.2Ø6
lower HØ2.2Ø5
upper HØ2.2Ø4
mechanical HØ2.229
left HØ2.226
lower HØ2.225
upper HØ2.224
right HØ2.223
lower HØ2.222
upper HØ2.221
paralytic HØ2.239
left HØ2.236
lower HØ2.235
upper HØ2.234
right HØ2.233
lower HØ2.232
upper HØ2.231
right HØ2.2Ø3
lower HØ2.2Ø2
upper HØ2.2Ø1

Laki-Lorand factor deficiency —*see* Defect, coagulation, specified type NEC
Lalling F8Ø.Ø
Lambert-Eaton syndrome —*see* Syndrome, Lambert-Eaton
Lambliasis, lambliosis AØ7.1
Landau-Kleffner syndrome —*see* Epilepsy, specified NEC
Landouzy-Déjérine dystrophy or facioscapulohumeral atrophy G71.Ø
Landouzy's disease (icterohemorrhagic leptospirosis) A27.Ø
Landry-Guillain-Barré, syndrome or paralysis G61.Ø
Landry's disease or paralysis G61.Ø
Lane's
band Q43.3
kink —*see* Obstruction, intestine
syndrome K9Ø.2
Langdon Down's syndrome —*see* Trisomy, 21
Lapsed immunization schedule status Z28.3
Large
baby (regardless of gestational age) (4ØØØg to 4499g) PØ8.1
ear, congenital Q17.1
physiological cup Q14.2
stature R68.89
Large-for-dates NEC (infant) (4ØØØg to 4499g) PØ8.1
affecting management of pregnancy O36.6-
exceptionally (45ØØg or more) PØ8.Ø
Larsen-Johansson disease osteochondrosis —*see* Osteochondrosis, juvenile, patella
Larsen's syndrome (flattened facies and multiple congenital dislocations) Q74.8
Larva migrans
cutaneous B76.9
Ancylostoma B76.Ø
visceral B83.Ø
Laryngeal —*see* condition
Laryngismus (stridulus) J38.5
congenital P28.89
diphtheritic A36.2
Laryngitis (acute) (edematous) (fibrinous) (infective) (infiltrative) (malignant) (membranous) (phlegmonous) (pneumococcal) (pseudomembranous) (septic) (subglottic) (suppurative) (ulcerative) JØ4.Ø
with
influenza, flu, or grippe —*see* Influenza, with, laryngitis
tracheitis (acute) —*see* Laryngotracheitis
atrophic J37.Ø
catarrhal J37.Ø
chronic J37.Ø
with tracheitis (chronic) J37.1
diphtheritic A36.2
due to external agent —*see* Inflammation, respiratory, upper, due to
Hemophilus influenzae JØ4.Ø
H. influenzae JØ4.Ø
hypertrophic J37.Ø
influenzal —*see* Influenza, with, respiratory manifestations NEC
obstructive JØ5.Ø
sicca J37.Ø
spasmodic JØ5.Ø
acute JØ4.Ø
streptococcal JØ4.Ø
stridulous JØ5.Ø
syphilitic (late) A52.73
congenital A5Ø.59 *[J99]*
early A5Ø.Ø3 *[J99]*
tuberculous A15.5
Vincent's A69.1
Laryngocele (congenital) (ventricular) Q31.3
Laryngofissure J38.7
congenital Q31.8
Laryngomalacia (congenital) Q31.5

◀ New ⬅ Revised ~~deleted~~ Deleted

◀ New ⟸ Revised ~~deleted~~ Deleted

L

◀ New ⟸ Revised ~~deleted~~ Deleted

Lesion *(Continued)*
- ulcerated or ulcerative —*see* Ulcer, skin
- uterus N85.9
- vagus nerve G52.2
- valvular —*see* Endocarditis
- vascular I99.9
  - affecting central nervous system I67.9
  - following trauma NEC T14.8
  - umbilical cord, complicating delivery O69.5
- warty —*see* Verruca
- white spot (tooth)
  - chewing surface KØ2.51
  - pit and fissure surface KØ2.51
  - smooth surface KØ2.61

Lethargic —*see* condition
Lethargy R53.83
Letterer-Siwe's disease C96.Ø
Leukemia, leukemic C95.9-
- acute basophilic C94.8-
- acute bilineal C95.Ø-
- acute erythroid C94.Ø-
- acute lymphoblastic C91.Ø-
- acute megakaryoblastic C94.2-
- acute megakaryocytic C94.2-
- acute mixed lineage C95.Ø-
- acute monoblastic (monoblastic/monocytic) C93.Ø-
- acute monocytic (monoblastic/monocytic) C93.Ø-
- acute myeloblastic (minimal differentiation) (with maturation) C92.Ø-
- acute myeloid
  - with
    - 11q23-abnormality C92.6-
    - dysplasia of remaining hematopoesis and/or myelodysplastic disease in its history C92.A-
    - multilineage dysplasia C92.A-
    - variation of MLL-gene C92.6-
  - M6 (a)(b) C94.Ø-
  - M7 C94.2-
- acute myelomonocytic C92.5-
- acute promyelocytic C92.4-
- adult T-cell (HTLV-1-associated) (acute variant) (chronic variant) (lymphomatoid variant) (smouldering variant) C91.5-
- aggressive NK-cell C94.8-
- AML (1/ETO) (MØ) (M1) (M2) (without a FAB classification) C92.Ø-
- AML M3 C92.4-
- AML M4 (Eo with inv(16) or t(16;16)) C92.5-
- AML M5 C93.Ø-
- AML M5a C93.Ø-
- AML M5b C93.Ø-
- AML Me with t (15;17) and variants C92.4-
- atypical chronic myeloid, BCR/ABL-negative C92.2-
- biphenotypic acute C95.Ø-
- blast cell C95.Ø-
- Burkitt-type, mature B-cell C91.A-
- chronic lymphocytic, of B-cell type C91.1-
- chronic monocytic C93.1-
- chronic myelogenous (Philadelphia chromosome (Ph1) positive) (t(9;22)) (q34;q11) (with crisis of blast cells) C92.1-
- chronic myeloid, BCR/ABL-positive C92.1-
  - atypical, BCR/ABL-negative C92.2-
- chronic myelomonocytic C93.1-
- chronic neutrophilic D47.1
- CMML (-1) (-2) (with eosinophilia) C93.1-
- granulocytic —*see also* Category C92 C92.9-
- hairy-cell C91.4-
- juvenile myelomonocytic C93.3-
- lymphoid C91.9-
  - specified NEC C91.Z-
- mast cell C94.3-
- mature B-cell, Burkitt-type C91.A-

Leukemia, leukemic *(Continued)*
- monocytic (subacute) C93.9-
  - specified NEC C93.Z-
- myelogenous —*see also* Category C92 C92.9-
- myeloid C92.9-
  - specified NEC C92.Z-
- plasma cell C9Ø.1-
- plasmacytic C9Ø.1-
- prolymphocytic
  - of B-cell type C91.3-
  - of T-cell type C91.6-
- specified NEC C94.8-
- stem cell, of unclear lineage C95.Ø-
- subacute lymphocytic C91.9-
- T-cell large granular lymphocytic C91.Z-
- unspecified cell type C95.9-
  - acute C95.Ø-
  - chronic C95.1-

Leukemoid reaction —*see also* Reaction, leukemoid D72.823-
Leukoaraiosis (hypertensive) I67.81
Leukoariosis —*see* Leukoaraiosis
Leukocoria —*see* Disorder, globe, degenerated condition, leucocoria
Leukocytopenia D72.819
Leukocytosis D72.829
- eosinophilic D72.1

Leukoderma, leukodermia NEC L81.5
- syphilitic A51.39
  - late A52.79

Leukodystrophy E75.29
Leukoedema, oral epithelium K13.29
Leukoencephalitis GØ4.81
- acute (subacute) hemorrhagic G36.1
  - postimmunization or postvaccinal GØ4.Ø2
- postinfectious GØ4.Ø1
- subacute sclerosing A81.1
- van Bogaert's (sclerosing) A81.1

Leukoencephalopathy —*see also* Encephalopathy G93.49
- Binswanger's I67.3
- heroin vapor G92
- metachromatic E75.25
- multifocal (progressive) A81.2
- postimmunization and postvaccinal GØ4.Ø2
- progressive multifocal A81.2
- reversible, posterior G93.6
- van Bogaert's (sclerosing) A81.1
- vascular, progressive I67.3

Leukoerythroblastosis D75.9
Leukokeratosis —*see also* Leukoplakia
- mouth K13.21
- nicotina palati K13.24
- oral mucosa K13.21
- tongue K13.21
- vocal cord J38.3

Leukokraurosis vulva (e) N9Ø.4
Leukoma (cornea) —*see also* Opacity, cornea
- adherent H17.Ø-
- interfering with central vision —*see* Opacity, cornea, central

Leukomalacia, cerebral, newborn P91.2
- periventricular P91.2

Leukomelanopathy, hereditary D72.Ø
Leukonychia (punctata) (striata) L6Ø.8
- congenital Q84.4

Leukopathia unguium L6Ø.8
- congenital Q84.4

Leukopenia D72.819
- basophilic D72.818
- chemotherapy (cancer) induced D7Ø.1
- congenital D7Ø.Ø
- cyclic D7Ø.Ø
- drug induced NEC D7Ø.2
  - due to cytoreductive cancer chemotherapy D7Ø.1
- eosinophilic D72.818
- familial D7Ø.Ø
- infantile genetic D7Ø.Ø
- malignant D7Ø.9
- periodic D7Ø.Ø
- transitory neonatal P61.5

Leukopenic —*see* condition
Leukoplakia
- anus K62.89
- bladder (postinfectional) N32.89
- buccal K13.21
- cervix (uteri) N88.Ø
- esophagus K22.8
- gingiva K13.21
- hairy (oral mucosa) (tongue) K13.3
- kidney (pelvis) N28.89
- larynx J38.7
- lip K13.21
- mouth K13.21
- oral epithelium, including tongue (mucosa) K13.21
- palate K13.21
- pelvis (kidney) N28.89
- penis (infectional) N48.Ø
- rectum K62.89
- syphilitic (late) A52.79
- tongue K13.21
- ureter (postinfectional) N28.89
- urethra (postinfectional) N36.8
- uterus N85.8
- vagina N89.4
- vocal cord J38.3
- vulva N9Ø.4

Leukorrhea N89.8
- due to Trichomonas (vaginalis) A59.ØØ
- trichomonal A59.ØØ

Leukosarcoma C85.9
Levocardia (isolated) Q24.1
- with situs inversus Q89.3

Levotransposition Q2Ø.5
Lev's disease or syndrome (acquired complete heart block) I44.2
Levulosuria —*see* Fructosuria
Levurid L3Ø.2
Lewy body (ies) (dementia) (disease) G31.83
Leyden-Moebius dystrophy G71.Ø
Leydig cell
- carcinoma
  - specified site —*see* Neoplasm, malignant, by site
  - unspecified site
    - female C56.9-
    - male C62.9-
- tumor
  - benign
    - specified site —*see* Neoplasm, benign, by site
    - unspecified site
      - female D27.-
      - male D29.2-
  - malignant
    - specified site —*see* Neoplasm, malignant, by site
    - unspecified site
      - female C56.-
      - male C62.9-
  - specified site —*see* Neoplasm, uncertain behavior, by site
  - unspecified site
    - female D39.1-
    - male D4Ø.1-

Leydig-Sertoli cell tumor
- specified site —*see* Neoplasm, benign, by site
- unspecified site
  - female D27.-
  - male D29.2-

LGSIL (Low grade squamous intraepithelial lesion on cytologic smear of)
- anus R85.612
- cervix R87.612
- vagina R87.622

Liar, pathologic F6Ø.2
Libido
- decreased R68.82

Libman-Sacks disease M32.11
Lice (infestation) B85.2
  body (Pediculus corporis) B85.1
  crab B85.3
  head (Pediculus capitis) B85.0
  mixed (classifiable to more than one of the titles B85.0-B85.3) B85.4
  pubic (Phthirus pubis) B85.3
Lichen L28.0
  albus L90.0
    penis N48.0
    vulva N90.4
  amyloidosis E85.4 *[L99]*
  atrophicus L90.0
    penis N48.0
    vulva N90.4
  congenital Q82.8
  myxedematosus L98.5
  nitidus L44.1
  pilaris Q82.8
    acquired L85.8
  planopilaris L66.1
  planus (chronicus) L43.9
    annularis L43.8
    bullous L43.1
    follicular L66.1
    hypertrophic L43.0
    moniliformis L44.3
    of Wilson L43.9
    specified NEC L43.8
    subacute (active) L43.3
    tropicus L43.3
  ruber
    acuminatus L44.0
    moniliformis L44.3
    planus L43.9
  sclerosus (et atrophicus) L90.0
    penis N48.0
    vulva N90.4
  scrofulosus (primary) (tuberculous) A18.4
  simplex (chronicus) (circumscriptus) L28.0
  striatus L44.2
  urticatus L28.2
Lichenification L28.0
Lichenoides tuberculosis (primary) A18.4
Lichtheim's disease or syndrome —*see* Degeneration, combined
Lien migrans D73.89
Ligament —*see* condition
Light
  for gestational age —*see* Light for dates
  headedness R42
Light-for-dates (infant) P05.00
  with weight of
    499 grams or less P05.01
    500-749 grams P05.02
    750-999 grams P05.03
    1000-1249 grams P05.04
    1250-1499 grams P05.05
    1500-1749 grams P05.06
    1750-1999 grams P05.07
    2000-2499 grams P05.08
    2500 grams and over P05.09 ◀
  affecting management of pregnancy O36.59-
  and small-for-dates —*see* Small for dates
  specified NEC P05.09 ◀
Lightning (effects) (stroke) (struck by) T75.00
  burn —*see* Burn
  foot E53.8
  shock T75.01
  specified effect NEC T75.09
Lightwood-Albright syndrome N25.89
Lightwood's disease or syndrome (renal tubular acidosis) N25.89
Lignac (-de Toni) (-Fanconi) (-Debré) **disease or syndrome** E72.09
  with cystinosis E72.04
Ligneous thyroiditis E06.5
Likoff's syndrome I20.8
Limb —*see* condition
Limbic epilepsy personality syndrome F07.0
Limitation, limited
  activities due to disability Z73.6
  cardiac reserve —*see* Disease, heart
  eye muscle duction, traumatic —*see* Strabismus, mechanical
  mandibular range of motion M26.52
Lindau (-von Hippel) **disease** Q85.8
Line (s)
  Beau's L60.4
  Harris' —*see* Arrest, epiphyseal
  Hudson's (cornea) —*see* Pigmentation, cornea, anterior
  Stähli's (cornea) —*see* Pigmentation, cornea, anterior
Linea corneae senilis —*see* Change, cornea, senile
Lingua
  geographica K14.1
  nigra (villosa) K14.3
  plicata K14.5
  tylosis K13.29
Lingual —*see* condition
Linguatulosis B88.8
Linitis (gastric) **plastica** C16.9
Lip —*see* condition
Lipedema —*see* Edema
Lipemia —*see also* Hyperlipidemia
  retina, retinalis E78.3
Lipidosis E75.6
  cerebral (infantile) (juvenile) (late) E75.4
  cerebroretinal E75.4
  cerebroside E75.22
  cholesterol (cerebral) E75.5
  glycolipid E75.21
  hepatosplenomegalic E78.3
  sphingomyelin —*see* Niemann-Pick disease or syndrome
  sulfatide E75.29
Lipoadenoma —*see* Neoplasm, benign, by site
Lipoblastoma —*see* Lipoma
Lipoblastomatosis —*see* Lipoma
Lipochondrodystrophy E76.01
Lipochrome histiocytosis (familial) D71
Lipodermatosclerosis —*see* Varix, leg, with, inflammation
  ulcerated —*see* Varix, leg, with, ulcer, with inflammation by site
Lipodystrophia progressiva E88.1
Lipodystrophy (progressive) E88.1
  insulin E88.1
  intestinal K90.81
  mesenteric K65.4
Lipofibroma —*see* Lipoma
Lipofuscinosis, neuronal (with ceroidosis) E75.4
Lipogranuloma, sclerosing L92.8
Lipogranulomatosis E78.89
Lipoid —*see also* condition
  histiocytosis D76.3
    essential E75.29
  nephrosis N04.9
  proteinosis of Urbach E78.89
Lipoidemia —*see* Hyperlipidemia
Lipoidosis —*see* Lipidosis
Lipoma D17.9
  fetal D17.9
    fat cell D17.9
  infiltrating D17.9
  intramuscular D17.9
  pleomorphic D17.9
  site classification
    arms (skin) (subcutaneous) D17.2-
    connective tissue D17.30
      intra-abdominal D17.5
      intrathoracic D17.4
      peritoneum D17.79
      retroperitoneum D17.79
      specified site NEC D17.39
      spermatic cord D17.6
    face (skin) (subcutaneous) D17.0
    genitourinary organ NEC D17.72
Lipoma *(Continued)*
  site classification *(Continued)*
    head (skin) (subcutaneous) D17.0
    intra-abdominal D17.5
    intrathoracic D17.4
    kidney D17.71
    legs (skin) (subcutaneous) D17.2-
    neck (skin) (subcutaneous) D17.0
    peritoneum D17.79
    retroperitoneum D17.79
    skin D17.30
      specified site NEC D17.39
    specified site NEC D17.79
    spermatic cord D17.6
    subcutaneous D17.30
      specified site NEC D17.39
    trunk (skin) (subcutaneous) D17.1
    unspecified D17.9
  spindle cell D17.9
Lipomatosis E88.2
  dolorosa (Dercum) E88.2
  fetal —*see* Lipoma
  Launois-Bensaude E88.89
Lipomyoma —*see* Lipoma
Lipomyxoma —*see* Lipoma
Lipomyxosarcoma —*see* Neoplasm, connective tissue, malignant
Lipoprotein metabolism disorder E78.9
Lipoproteinemia E78.5
  broad-beta E78.2
  floating-beta E78.2
  hyper-pre-beta E78.1
Liposarcoma —*see also* Neoplasm, connective tissue, malignant
  dedifferentiated —*see* Neoplasm, connective tissue, malignant
  differentiated type —*see* Neoplasm, connective tissue, malignant
  embryonal —*see* Neoplasm, connective tissue, malignant
  mixed type —*see* Neoplasm, connective tissue, malignant
  myxoid —*see* Neoplasm, connective tissue, malignant
  pleomorphic —*see* Neoplasm, connective tissue, malignant
  round cell —*see* Neoplasm, connective tissue, malignant
  well differentiated type —*see* Neoplasm, connective tissue, malignant
Liposynovitis prepatellaris E88.89
Lipping, cervix N86
Lipschütz disease or ulcer N76.6
Lipuria R82.0
  schistosomiasis (bilharziasis) B65.0
Lisping F80.0
Lissauer's paralysis A52.17
Lissencephalia, lissencephaly Q04.3
Listeriosis, listerellosis A32.9
  congenital (disseminated) P37.2
  cutaneous A32.0
  neonatal, newborn (disseminated) P37.2
  oculoglandular A32.81
  specified NEC A32.89
Lithemia E79.0
Lithiasis —*see* Calculus
Lithosis J62.8
Lithuria R82.99
Litigation, anxiety concerning Z65.3
Little leaguer's elbow —*see* Epicondylitis, medial
Little's disease G80.9
Littre's
  gland —*see* condition
  hernia —*see* Hernia, abdomen
Littritis —*see* Urethritis
Livedo (annularis) (racemosa) (reticularis) R23.1
Liver —*see* condition
Living alone (problems with) Z60.2
  with handicapped person Z74.2

L

◀ New ◀ Revised ~~deleted~~ Deleted

Lloyd's syndrome —*see* Adenomatosis, endocrine
Loa loa, loaiasis, loasis B74.3
Lobar —*see* condition
Lobomycosis B48.Ø
Lobo's disease B48.Ø
Lobotomy syndrome FØ7.Ø
Lobstein (-Ekman) **disease or syndrome** Q78.Ø
Lobster-claw hand Q71.6-
Lobulation (congenital) —*see also* Anomaly, by site
  kidney, Q63.1
  liver, abnormal Q44.7
  spleen Q89.Ø9
Lobule, lobular —*see* condition
Local, localized —*see* condition
Locked twins causing obstructed labor O66.1
Locked-in state G83.5
Locking
  joint —*see* Derangement, joint, specified type NEC
    knee —*see* Derangement, knee
Lockjaw —*see* Tetanus
Löffler's
  endocarditis I42.3
  eosinophilia J82
  pneumonia J82
  syndrome (eosinophilic pneumonitis) J82
Loiasis (with conjunctival infestation) (eyelid) B74.3
Lone Star fever A77.Ø
Long
  labor O63.9
    first stage O63.Ø
    second stage O63.1
  QT syndrome I45.81
Long-term (current) (prophylactic) **drug therapy (use of)**
  agents affecting estrogen receptors and estrogen levels NEC Z79.818
  anastrozole (Arimidex) Z79.811
  antibiotics Z79.2
    short-term use - omit code
  anticoagulants Z79.Ø1
  anti-inflammatory, non-steroidal (NSAID) Z79.1
  antiplatelet Z79.Ø2
  antithrombotics Z79.Ø2
  aromatase inhibitors Z79.811
  aspirin Z79.82
  birth control pill or patch Z79.3
  bisphosphonates Z79.83
  contraceptive, oral Z79.3
  drug, specified NEC Z79.899
  estrogen receptor downregulators Z79.818
  Evista Z79.81Ø
  exemestane (Aromasin) Z79.811
  Fareston Z79.81Ø
  fulvestrant (Faslodex) Z79.818
  gonadotropin-releasing hormone (GnRH) agonist Z79.818
  goserelin acetate (Zoladex) Z79.818
  hormone replacement (postmenopausal) Z79.89Ø
  insulin Z79.4
  letrozole (Femara) Z79.811
  leuprolide acetate (leuprorelin) (Lupron) Z79.818
  megestrol acetate (Megace) Z79.818
  methadone for pain management Z79.891
  Nolvadex Z79.81Ø
  non-steroidal anti-inflammatories (NSAID) Z79.1
  opiate analgesic Z79.891
  ~~oral contraceptive Z79.3~~
  oral ◀
    antidiabetic Z79.84 ◀
    contraceptive Z79.3 ◀
    hypoglycemic Z79.84 ◀
  raloxifene (Evista) Z79.81Ø

Long-term *(Continued)*
  selective estrogen receptor modulators (SERMs) Z79.81Ø
  steroids
    inhaled Z79.51
    systemic Z79.52
  tamoxifen (Nolvadex) Z79.81Ø
  toremifene (Fareston) Z79.81Ø
Longitudinal stripes or grooves, nails L6Ø.8
  congenital Q84.6
Loop
  intestine —*see* Volvulus
  vascular on papilla (optic) Q14.2
Loose —*see also* condition
  body
    joint M24.ØØ
      ankle M24.Ø7-
      elbow M24.Ø2-
      hand M24.Ø4-
      hip M24.Ø5-
      knee M23.4-
      shoulder (region) M24.Ø1-
      specified site NEC M24.Ø8
      toe M24.Ø7-
      vertebra M24.Ø8
      wrist M24.Ø3-
    knee M23.4-
    sheath, tendon —*see* Disorder, tendon, specified type NEC
  cartilage —*see* Loose, body, joint
  skin and subcutaneous tissue (following bariatric surgery weight loss) (following dietary weight loss) L98.7 ◀
  tooth, teeth KØ8.89 ⬅
Loosening
  aseptic
    joint prosthesis —*see* Complications, joint prosthesis, mechanical, loosening, by site
  epiphysis —*see* Osteochondropathy
  mechanical
    joint prosthesis —*see* Complications, joint prosthesis, mechanical, loosening, by site
Looser-Milkman (-Debray) **syndrome** M83.8
Lop ear (deformity) Q17.3
Lorain (-Levi) **short stature syndrome** E23.Ø
Lordosis M4Ø.5Ø
  acquired —*see* Lordosis, specified type NEC
  congenital Q76.429
    lumbar region Q76.426
    lumbosacral region Q76.427
    sacral region Q76.428
    sacrococcygeal region Q76.428
    thoracolumbar region Q76.425
  lumbar region M4Ø.56
  lumbosacral region M4Ø.57
  postsurgical M96.4
  postural —*see* Lordosis, specified type NEC
  rachitic (late effect) (sequelae) E64.3
  sequelae of rickets E64.3
  specified type NEC M4Ø.4Ø
    lumbar region M4Ø.46
    lumbosacral region M4Ø.47
    thoracolumbar region M4Ø.45
  thoracolumbar region M4Ø.55
  tuberculous A18.Ø1
Loss (of)
  appetite (*see* Anorexia) R63.Ø
    hysterical F5Ø.89 ⬅
    nonorganic origin F5Ø.89 ⬅
    psychogenic F5Ø.89 ⬅
  blood —*see* Hemorrhage
  bone —*see* Loss, substance of, bone ◀
  consciousness, transient R55
    traumatic —*see* Injury, intracranial
  control, sphincter, rectum R15.9
    nonorganic origin F98.1
  elasticity, skin R23.4

Loss *(Continued)*
  family (member) in childhood Z62.898
  fluid (acute) E86.9
    ~~with~~
      ~~hypernatremia E87.Ø~~
      ~~hyponatremia E87.1~~
  function of labyrinth —*see* subcategory H83.2
  hair, nonscarring —*see* Alopecia
  hearing —*see also* Deafness
    central NOS H9Ø.5
    conductive H9Ø.2 ◀
      bilateral H9Ø.Ø ◀
      unilateral ◀
        with ◀
          restricted hearing on the contralateral side H9Ø.A1- ◀
          unrestricted hearing on the contralateral side H9Ø.1- ◀
    mixed conductive and sensorineural hearing loss H9Ø.8 ◀
      bilateral H9Ø.6 ◀
      unilateral ◀
        with ◀
          restricted hearing on the contralateral side H9Ø.A3- ◀
          unrestricted hearing on the contralateral side H9Ø.7- ◀
    neural NOS H9Ø.5
    perceptive NOS H9Ø.5
    sensorineural NOS H9Ø.5
      bilateral H9Ø.3 ◀
      unilateral ◀
        with ◀
          restricted hearing on the contralateral side H9Ø.A2- ◀
          unrestricted hearing on the contralateral side H9Ø.4- ◀
    sensory NOS H9Ø.5
  height R29.89Ø
  limb or member, traumatic, current —*see* Amputation, traumatic
  love relationship in childhood Z62.898
  memory —*see also* Amnesia
    mild, following organic brain damage FØ6.8
  mind —*see* Psychosis
  occlusal vertical dimension of fully erupted teeth M26.37
  organ or part —*see* Absence, by site, acquired
  ossicles, ear (partial) H74.32-
  parent in childhood Z63.4
  pregnancy, recurrent N96
    without current pregnancy N96
    care in current pregnancy O26.2-
  recurrent pregnancy —*see* Loss, pregnancy, recurrent
  self-esteem, in childhood Z62.898
  sense of
    smell —*see* Disturbance, sensation, smell
    taste —*see* Disturbance, sensation, taste
    touch R2Ø.8
  sensory R44.9
    dissociative F44.6
  sexual desire F52.Ø
  sight (acquired) (complete) (congenital) —*see* Blindness
  substance of
    bone —*see* Disorder, bone, density and structure, specified NEC
      horizontal alveolar KØ6.3 ◀
    cartilage —*see* Disorder, cartilage, specified type NEC
      auricle (ear) —*see* Disorder, pinna, specified type NEC
    vitreous (humor) H15.89
  tooth, teeth —*see* Absence, teeth, acquired
  vision, visual H54.7
    both eyes H54.3
    one eye H54.6Ø
      left (normal vision on right) H54.62
      right (normal vision on left) H54.61

- **Loss** *(Continued)*
  - vision, visual *(Continued)*
    - specified as blindness —*see* Blindness
    - subjective
      - sudden H53.13-
      - transient H53.12-
  - vitreous —*see* Prolapse, vitreous
  - voice —*see* Aphonia
  - weight (abnormal) (cause unknown) R63.4
- **Louis-Bar syndrome** (ataxia-telangiectasia) G11.3
- **Louping ill** (encephalitis) A84.8
- **Louse, lousiness** —*see* Lice
- **Low**
  - achiever, school Z55.3
  - back syndrome M54.5
  - basal metabolic rate R94.8
  - birthweight (2499 grams or less) P07.10
    - with weight of
      - 1000-1249 grams P07.14
      - 1250-1499 grams P07.15
      - 1500-1749 grams P07.16
      - 1750-1999 grams P07.17
      - 2000-2499 grams P07.18
    - extreme (999 grams or less) P07.00
      - with weight of
        - 499 grams or less P07.01
        - 500-749 grams P07.02
        - 750-999 grams P07.03
    - for gestational age —*see* Light for dates
  - blood pressure —*see also* Hypotension
    - reading (incidental) (isolated) (nonspecific) R03.1
  - cardiac reserve —*see* Disease, heart
  - function —*see also* Hypofunction
    - kidney N28.9
  - hematocrit D64.9
  - hemoglobin D64.9
  - income Z59.6
  - level of literacy Z55.0
  - lying
    - kidney N28.89
    - organ or site, congenital —*see* Malposition, congenital
  - output syndrome (cardiac) —*see* Failure, heart
  - platelets (blood) —*see* Thrombocytopenia
  - reserve, kidney N28.89
  - salt syndrome E87.1
  - self esteem R45.81
  - set ears Q17.4
  - vision H54.2
    - one eye (other eye normal) H54.50
      - left (normal vision on right) H54.52
      - other eye blind —*see* Blindness
      - right (normal vision on left) H54.51
- **Low-density-lipoprotein-type** (LDL) **hyperlipoproteinemia** E78.00 ⬅
- **Lowe's syndrome** E72.03
- **Lown-Ganong-Levine syndrome** I45.6
- **LSD reaction** (acute) (without dependence) F16.90
  - with dependence F16.20
- **L-shaped kidney** Q63.8
- **Ludwig's angina or disease** K12.2
- **Lues** (venerea), **luetic** —*see* Syphilis
- **Luetscher's syndrome** (dehydration) E86.0
- **Lumbago, lumbalgia** M54.5
  - with sciatica M54.4-
    - due to intervertebral disc disorder M51.17
  - due to displacement, intervertebral disc M51.27
    - with sciatica M51.17
- **Lumbar** —*see* condition
- **Lumbarization, vertebra, congenital** Q76.49
- **Lumbermen's itch** B88.0
- **Lump** —*see* Mass
- **Lunacy** —*see* Psychosis
- **Lung** —*see* condition
- **Lupoid** (miliary) **of Boeck** D86.3
- **Lupus**
  - anticoagulant D68.62
    - with
      - hemorrhagic disorder D68.312
      - hypercoagulable state D68.62
    - finding without diagnosis R76.0
  - discoid (local) L93.0
  - erythematosus (discoid) (local) L93.0
    - disseminated —*see* Lupus, erythematosus, systemic
    - eyelid H01.129
      - left H01.126
        - lower H01.125
        - upper H01.124
      - right H01.123
        - lower H01.122
        - upper H01.121
    - profundus L93.2
    - specified NEC L93.2
    - subacute cutaneous L93.1
    - systemic M32.9
      - with organ or system involvement M32.10
        - endocarditis M32.11
        - lung M32.13
        - pericarditis M32.12
        - renal (glomerular) M32.14
          - tubulo-interstitial M32.15
        - specified organ or system NEC M32.19
      - drug-induced M32.0
      - inhibitor (presence of) D68.62
        - with
          - hemorrhagic disorder D68.312
          - hypercoagulable state D68.62
        - finding without diagnosis R76.0
      - specified NEC M32.8
  - exedens A18.4
  - hydralazine M32.0
    - correct substance properly administered —*see* Table of Drugs and Chemicals, by drug, adverse effect
    - overdose or wrong substance given or taken —*see* Table of Drugs and Chemicals, by drug, poisoning
  - nephritis (chronic) M32.14
  - nontuberculous, not disseminated L93.0
  - panniculitis L93.2
  - pernio (Besnier) D86.3
  - systemic —*see* Lupus, erythematosus, systemic
  - tuberculous A18.4
    - eyelid A18.4
  - vulgaris A18.4
    - eyelid A18.4
- **Luteinoma** D27.-
- **Lutembacher's disease or syndrome** (atrial septal defect with mitral stenosis) Q21.1
- **Luteoma** D27.-
- **Lutz** (-Splendore-de Almeida) **disease** —*see* Paracoccidioidomycosis
- **Luxation** —*see also* Dislocation
  - eyeball (nontraumatic) —*see* Luxation, globe
    - birth injury P15.3
  - globe, nontraumatic H44.82-
  - lacrimal gland —*see* Dislocation, lacrimal gland
  - lens (old) (partial) (spontaneous)
    - congenital Q12.1
      - syphilitic A50.39
- **Lycanthropy** F22
- **Lyell's syndrome** L51.2
  - due to drug L51.2
    - correct substance properly administered —*see* Table of Drugs and Chemicals, by drug, adverse effect
    - overdose or wrong substance given or taken —*see* Table of Drugs and Chemicals, by drug, poisoning
- **Lyme disease** A69.20
- **Lymph**
  - gland or node —*see* condition
  - scrotum —*see* Infestation, filarial
- **Lymphadenitis** I88.9
  - with ectopic or molar pregnancy O08.0
  - acute L04.9
    - axilla L04.2
    - face L04.0
    - head L04.0
    - hip L04.3
    - limb
      - lower L04.3
      - upper L04.2
    - neck L04.0
    - shoulder L04.2
    - specified site NEC L04.8
    - trunk L04.1
  - anthracosis (occupational) J60
  - any site, except mesenteric I88.9
    - chronic I88.1
    - subacute I88.1
  - breast
    - gestational —*see* Mastitis, obstetric
    - puerperal, postpartum (nonpurulent) O91.22
  - chancroidal (congenital) A57
  - chronic I88.1
    - mesenteric I88.0
  - due to
    - Brugia (malayi) B74.1
      - timori B74.2
    - chlamydial lymphogranuloma A55
    - diphtheria (toxin) A36.89
    - lymphogranuloma venereum A55
    - Wuchereria bancrofti B74.0
  - following ectopic or molar pregnancy O08.0
  - gonorrheal A54.89
  - infective —*see* Lymphadenitis, acute
  - mesenteric (acute) (chronic) (nonspecific) (subacute) I88.0
    - due to Salmonella typhi A01.09
    - tuberculous A18.39
  - mycobacterial A31.8
  - purulent —*see* Lymphadenitis, acute
  - pyogenic —*see* Lymphadenitis, acute
  - regional, nonbacterial I88.8
  - septic —*see* Lymphadenitis, acute
  - subacute, unspecified site I88.1
  - suppurative —*see* Lymphadenitis, acute
  - syphilitic (early) (secondary) A51.49
    - late A52.79
  - tuberculous —*see* Tuberculosis, lymph gland
  - venereal (chlamydial) A55
- **Lymphadenoid goiter** E06.3
- **Lymphadenopathy** (generalized) R59.1
  - angioimmunoblastic, with dysproteinemia (AILD) C86.5
  - due to toxoplasmosis (acquired) B58.89
    - congenital (acute) (subacute) (chronic) P37.1
  - localized R59.0
  - syphilitic (early) (secondary) A51.49
- **Lymphadenosis** R59.1
- **Lymphangiectasis** I89.0
  - conjunctiva H11.89
  - postinfectional I89.0
  - scrotum I89.0
- **Lymphangiectatic elephantiasis, nonfilarial** I89.0
- **Lymphangioendothelioma** D18.1
  - malignant —*see* Neoplasm, connective tissue, malignant
- **Lymphangioleiomyomatosis** J84.81
- **Lymphangioma** D18.1
  - capillary D18.1
  - cavernous D18.1
  - cystic D18.1
  - malignant —*see* Neoplasm, connective tissue, malignant
- **Lymphangiomyoma** D18.1
- **Lymphangiomyomatosis** J84.81

L

- **Lymphangiosarcoma** —*see* Neoplasm, connective tissue, malignant
- **Lymphangitis** I89.1
  - with
    - abscess - code by site under Abscess
    - cellulitis - code by site under Cellulitis
    - ectopic or molar pregnancy OØ8.Ø
  - acute LØ3.91
    - abdominal wall LØ3.321
    - ankle —*see* Lymphangitis, acute, lower limb
    - arm —*see* Lymphangitis, acute, upper limb
    - auricle (ear) —*see* Lymphangitis, acute, ear
    - axilla LØ3.12-
    - back (any part) LØ3.322
    - buttock LØ3.327
    - cervical (meaning neck) LØ3.222
    - cheek (external) LØ3.212
    - chest wall LØ3.323
    - digit
      - finger —*see* Lymphangitis, acute, finger
      - toe —*see* Lymphangitis, acute, toe
    - ear (external) H6Ø.1-
    - external auditory canal —*see* Lymphangitis, acute, ear
    - eyelid —*see* Abscess, eyelid
    - face NEC LØ3.212
    - finger (intrathecal) (periosteal) (subcutaneous) (subcuticular) LØ3.Ø2-
    - foot —*see* Lymphangitis, acute, lower limb
    - gluteal (region) LØ3.327
    - groin LØ3.324
    - hand —*see* Lymphangitis, acute, upper limb
    - head NEC LØ3.891
      - face (any part, except ear, eye and nose) LØ3.212
    - heel —*see* Lymphangitis, acute, lower limb
    - hip —*see* Lymphangitis, acute, lower limb
    - jaw (region) LØ3.212
    - knee —*see* Lymphangitis, acute, lower limb
    - leg —*see* Lymphangitis, acute, lower limb
    - lower limb LØ3.12-
      - toe —*see* Lymphangitis, acute, toe
    - navel LØ3.326
    - neck (region) LØ3.222
    - orbit, orbital —*see* Cellulitis, orbit
    - pectoral (region) LØ3.323
    - perineal, perineum LØ3.325
    - scalp (any part) LØ3.891
    - shoulder —*see* Lymphangitis, acute, upper limb
    - specified site NEC LØ3.898
    - thigh —*see* Lymphangitis, acute, lower limb
    - thumb (intrathecal) (periosteal) (subcutaneous) (subcuticular) —*see* Lymphangitis, acute, finger
    - toe (intrathecal) (periosteal) (subcutaneous) (subcuticular) LØ3.Ø4-
    - trunk LØ3.329
      - abdominal wall LØ3.321
      - back (any part) LØ3.322
      - buttock LØ3.327
      - chest wall LØ3.323
      - groin LØ3.324
      - perineal, perineum LØ3.325
      - umbilicus LØ3.326
    - umbilicus LØ3.326
    - upper limb LØ3.12-
      - axilla —*see* Lymphangitis, acute, axilla
      - finger —*see* Lymphangitis, acute, finger
      - thumb —*see* Lymphangitis, acute, finger
    - wrist —*see* Lymphangitis, acute, upper limb
  - breast
    - gestational —*see* Mastitis, obstetric
  - chancroidal A57
  - chronic (any site) I89.1

- **Lymphangitis** *(Continued)*
  - due to
    - Brugia (malayi) B74.1
      - timori B74.2
    - Wuchereria bancrofti B74.Ø
  - following ectopic or molar pregnancy OØ8.89
  - penis
    - acute N48.29
    - gonococcal (acute) (chronic) A54.Ø9
  - puerperal, postpartum, childbirth O86.89
  - strumous, tuberculous A18.2
  - subacute (any site) I89.1
  - tuberculous —*see* Tuberculosis, lymph gland
- **Lymphatic** (vessel) —*see* condition
- **Lymphatism** E32.8
- **Lymphectasia** I89.Ø
- **Lymphedema** (acquired) —*see also* Elephantiasis
  - congenital Q82.Ø
  - hereditary (chronic) (idiopathic) Q82.Ø
  - postmastectomy I97.2
  - praecox I89.Ø
  - secondary I89.Ø
  - surgical NEC I97.89
    - postmastectomy (syndrome) I97.2
- **Lymphoblastic** —*see* condition
- **Lymphoblastoma** (diffuse) —*see* Lymphoma, lymphoblastic (diffuse)
  - giant follicular —*see* Lymphoma, lymphoblastic (diffuse)
  - macrofollicular —*see* Lymphoma, lymphoblastic (diffuse)
- **Lymphocele** I89.8
- **Lymphocytic**
  - chorioencephalitis (acute) (serous) A87.2
  - choriomeningitis (acute) (serous) A87.2
  - meningoencephalitis A87.2
- **Lymphocytoma, benign cutis** L98.8
- **Lymphocytopenia** D72.81Ø
- **Lymphocytosis** (symptomatic) D72.82Ø
  - infectious (acute) B33.8
- **Lymphoepithelioma** —*see* Neoplasm, malignant, by site
- **Lymphogranuloma** (malignant) —*see also* Lymphoma, Hodgkin
  - chlamydial A55
  - inguinale A55
  - venereum (any site) (chlamydial) (with stricture of rectum) A55
- **Lymphogranulomatosis** (malignant) —*see also* Lymphoma, Hodgkin
  - benign (Boeck's sarcoid) (Schaumann's) D86.1
- **Lymphohistiocytosis, hemophagocytic** (familial) D76.1
- **Lymphoid** —*see* condition
- **Lymphoma** (of) (malignant) C85.9Ø
  - adult T-cell (HTLV-1-associated) (acute variant) (chronic variant) (lymphomatoid variant) (smouldering variant) C91.5-
  - anaplastic large cell
    - ALK-negative C84.7-
    - ALK-positive C84.6-
    - CD3Ø-positive C84.6-
    - primary cutaneous C86.6
  - angioimmunoblastic T-cell C86.5
  - BALT C88.4
  - B-cell C85.1-
  - B-precursor C83.5-
  - blastic NK-cell C86.4
  - bronchial-associated lymphoid tissue [BALT-lymphoma] C88.4
  - Burkitt (atypical) C83.7-
  - Burkitt-like C83.7-
  - centrocytic C83.1-
  - cutaneous follicle center C82.6-
  - cutaneous T-cell C84.A-
  - diffuse follicle center C82.5-
  - diffuse large cell C83.3-
    - anaplastic C83.3-
    - B-cell C83.3-

- **Lymphoma** *(Continued)*
  - diffuse large cell *(Continued)*
    - CD3Ø-positive C83.3-
    - centroblastic C83.3-
    - immunoblastic C83.3-
    - plasmablastic C83.3-
    - subtype not specified C83.3-
    - T-cell rich C83.3-
  - enteropathy-type (associated) (intestinal) T-cell C86.2
  - extranodal marginal zone B-cell lymphoma of mucosa-associated lymphoid tissue [MALT-lymphoma] C88.4
  - extranodal NK/T-cell, nasal type C86.Ø
  - follicular C82.9-
    - grade
      - I C82.Ø-
      - II C82.1-
      - III C82.2-
      - IIIa C82.3-
      - IIIb C82.4-
    - specified NEC C82.8-
  - hepatosplenic T-cell (alpha-beta) (gamma-delta) C86.1
  - histiocytic C85.9-
    - true C96.A
  - Hodgkin C81.9
    - ~~classical C81.7-~~
      - ~~lymphocyte-rich C81.4-~~
      - ~~lymphocytic depletion C81.3-~~
      - ~~mixed cellularity C81.2-~~
      - ~~nodular sclerosis C81.1-~~
      - ~~specified NEC C81.7-~~
    - lymphocyte-rich (classical) C81.4- ◀
    - lymphocyte depleted (classical) C81.3- ◀
    - mixed cellularity (classical) C81.2- ◀
    - nodular sclerosis (classical) C81.1- ◀
    - specified NEC (classical) C81.7- ◀
    - lymphocyte-rich classical C81.4-
    - lymphocyte depleted classical C81.3-
    - mixed cellularity classical C81.2-
    - nodular
      - lymphocyte predominant C81.Ø-
      - ~~sclerosis classical C81.1-~~
      - sclerosis (classical) C81.1- ◀
  - intravascular large B-cell C83.8-
  - Lennert's C84.4-
  - lymphoblastic (diffuse) C83.5-
  - lymphoblastic B-cell C83.5-
  - lymphoblastic T-cell C83.5-
  - lymphoepithelioid C84.4-
  - lymphoplasmacytic C83.Ø-
    - with IgM-production C88.Ø
  - MALT C88.4
  - mantle cell C83.1-
  - mature T-cell NEC C84.4-
  - mature T/NK-cell C84.9-
    - specified NEC C84.Z-
  - mediastinal (thymic) large B-cell C85.2-
  - Mediterranean C88.3
  - mucosa-associated lymphoid tissue [MALT-lymphoma] C88.4
  - NK/T cell C84.9-
  - nodal marginal zone C83.Ø-
  - non-follicular (diffuse) C83.9-
    - specified NEC C83.8-
  - non-Hodgkin —*see also* Lymphoma, by type C85.9-
    - specified NEC C85.8-
  - non-leukemic variant of B-CLL C83.Ø-
  - peripheral T-cell, not classified C84.4-
  - primary cutaneous
    - anaplastic large cell C86.6
    - CD3Ø-positive large T-cell C86.6
  - primary effusion B-cell C83.8-
  - SALT C88.4
  - skin-associated lymphoid tissue [SALT-lymphoma] C88.4

Lymphoma *(Continued)*
small cell B-cell C83.Ø-
splenic marginal zone C83.Ø-
subcutaneous panniculitis-like T-cell C86.3
T-precursor C83.5-
true histiocytic C96.A
Lymphomatosis —*see* Lymphoma
Lymphopathia venereum, veneris A55
Lymphopenia D72.810
Lymphoplasmacytic leukemia —*see* Leukemia, chronic lymphocytic, B-cell type
Lymphoproliferation, X-linked disease D82.3
Lymphoreticulosis, benign (of inoculation) A28.1
Lymphorrhea I89.8
Lymphosarcoma (diffuse) —*see also* Lymphoma C85.9-
Lymphostasis I89.8
Lypemania —*see* Melancholia
Lysine and hydroxylysine metabolism disorder E72.3
Lyssa —*see* Rabies

◀ New ⟵ Revised ~~deleted~~ Deleted

M

Macacus ear Q17.3
Maceration, wet feet, tropical (syndrome) T69.Ø2-
MacLeod's syndrome J43.Ø
Macrocephalia, macrocephaly Q75.3
Macrocheilia, macrochilia (congenital)Q18.6
Macrocolon —*see also* Megacolon Q43.1
Macrocornea Q15.8
  with glaucoma Q15.Ø
Macrocytic —*see* condition
Macrocytosis D75.89
Macrodactylia, macrodactylism (fingers) (thumbs) Q74.Ø
  toes Q74.2
Macrodontia KØØ.2
Macrogenia M26.Ø5
Macrogenitosomia (adrenal) (male) (praecox) E25.9
  congenital E25.Ø
Macroglobulinemia (idiopathic) (primary) C88.Ø
  monoclonal (essential) D47.2
  Waldenström C88.Ø
Macroglossia (congenital) Q38.2
  acquired K14.8
Macrognathia, macrognathism (congenital) (mandibular) (maxillary) M26.Ø9
Macrogyria (congenital) QØ4.8
Macrohydrocephalus —*see* Hydrocephalus
Macromastia —*see* Hypertrophy, breast
Macrophthalmos Q11.3
  in congenital glaucoma Q15.Ø
Macropsia H53.15
Macrosigmoid K59.39
  congenital Q43.2
Macrospondylitis, acromegalic E22.Ø
Macrostomia (congenital) Q18.4
Macrotia (external ear) (congenital) Q17.1
Macula
  cornea, corneal —*see* Opacity, cornea
  degeneration (atrophic) (exudative) (senile) —*see also* Degeneration, macula
    hereditary —*see* Dystrophy, retina
Maculae ceruleae — B85.1
Maculopathy, toxic —*see* Degeneration, macula, toxic
Madarosis (eyelid) HØ2.729
  left HØ2.726
    lower HØ2.725
    upper HØ2.724
  right HØ2.723
    lower HØ2.722
    upper HØ2.721
Madelung's
  deformity (radius) Q74.Ø
  disease
    radial deformity Q74.Ø
    symmetrical lipomas, neck E88.89
Madness —*see* Psychosis
Madura
  foot B47.9
    actinomycotic B47.1
    mycotic B47.Ø
Maduromycosis B47.Ø
Maffucci's syndrome Q78.4
Magnesium metabolism disorder —*see* Disorder, metabolism, magnesium
Main en griffe (acquired) —*see also* Deformity, limb, clawhand
  congenital Q74.Ø
Maintenance (encounter for)
  antineoplastic chemotherapy Z51.11
  antineoplastic radiation therapy Z51.Ø
  methadone F11.2Ø
Majocchi's
  disease L81.7
  granuloma B35.8
Major —*see* condition
Malabar itch (any site) B35.5
Malabsorption K9Ø.9
  calcium K9Ø.89
  carbohydrate K9Ø.49
  disaccharide E73.9
  fat K9Ø.49
  galactose E74.2Ø
  glucose(-galactose) E74.39
  intestinal K9Ø.9
    specified NEC K9Ø.89
  isomaltose E74.31
  lactose E73.9
  methionine E72.19
  monosaccharide E74.39
  postgastrectomy K91.2
  postsurgical K91.2
  protein K9Ø.49
  starch K9Ø.49
  sucrose E74.39
  syndrome K9Ø.9
    postsurgical K91.2
Malacia, bone (adult) M83.9
  juvenile —*see* Rickets
Malacoplakia
  bladder N32.89
  pelvis (kidney) N28.89
  ureter N28.89
  urethra N36.8
Malacosteon, juvenile —*see* Rickets
Maladaptation —*see* Maladjustment
Maladie de Roger Q21.Ø
Maladjustment
  conjugal Z63.Ø
    involving divorce or estrangement Z63.5
  educational Z55.4
  family Z63.9
  marital Z63.Ø
    involving divorce or estrangement Z63.5
  occupational NEC Z56.89
  simple, adult —*see* Disorder, adjustment
  situational —*see* Disorder, adjustment
  social Z6Ø.9
    due to
      acculturation difficulty Z6Ø.3
      discrimination and persecution (perceived) Z6Ø.5
      exclusion and isolation Z6Ø.4
      life-cycle (phase of life) transition Z6Ø.Ø
      rejection Z6Ø.4
      specified reason NEC Z6Ø.8
Malaise R53.81
Malakoplakia —*see* Malacoplakia
Malaria, malarial (fever) B54
  with
    blackwater fever B5Ø.8
      hemoglobinuric (bilious) B5Ø.8
    hemoglobinuria B5Ø.8
  accidentally induced (therapeutically) - code by type under Malaria
  algid B5Ø.9
  cerebral B5Ø.Ø *[G94]*
  clinically diagnosed (without parasitological confirmation) B54
  congenital NEC P37.4
    falciparum P37.3
  congestion, congestive B54
  continued (fever) B5Ø.9
  estivo-autumnal B5Ø.9
  falciparum B5Ø.9
    with complications NEC B5Ø.8
      cerebral B5Ø.Ø *[G94]*
    severe B5Ø.8
  hemorrhagic B54
  malariae B52.9
    with
      complications NEC B52.8
      glomerular disorder B52.Ø
  malignant (tertian) —*see* Malaria, falciparum
  mixed infections — code to first listed type in B5Ø-B53
  ovale B53.Ø
  parasitologically confirmed NEC B53.8
Malaria, malarial *(Continued)*
  pernicious, acute —*see* Malaria, falciparum
  Plasmodium (P.)
    falciparum NEC —*see* Malaria, falciparum
    malariae NEC B52.9
      with Plasmodium
        falciparum (and or vivax) —*see* Malaria, falciparum
        vivax —*see also* Malaria, vivax
          and falciparum —*see* Malaria, falciparum
    ovale B53.Ø
      with Plasmodium malariae —*see also* Malaria, malariae
        and vivax —*see also* Malaria, vivax
          and falciparum —*see* Malaria, falciparum
    simian B53.1
      with Plasmodium malariae —*see also* Malaria, malariae
        and vivax —*see also* Malaria, vivax
          and falciparum —*see* Malaria, falciparum
    vivax NEC B51.9
      with Plasmodium falciparum —*see* Malaria, falciparum
  quartan —*see* Malaria, malariae
  quotidian —*see* Malaria, falciparum
  recurrent B54
  remittent B54
  specified type NEC (parasitologically confirmed) B53.8
  spleen B54
  subtertian (fever) —*see* Malaria, falciparum
  tertian (benign) —*see also* Malaria, vivax
    malignant B5Ø.9
  tropical B5Ø.9
  typhoid B54
  vivax B51.9
    with
      complications NEC B51.8
      ruptured spleen B51.Ø
Malassez's disease (cystic) N5Ø.89
Malassimilation K9Ø.9
Mal de los pintos —*see* Pinta
Mal de mer T75.3
Maldescent, testis Q53.9
  bilateral Q53.2Ø
    abdominal Q53.21
    perineal Q53.22
  unilateral Q53.1Ø
    abdominal Q53.11
    perineal Q53.12
Maldevelopment —*see also* Anomaly
  brain QØ7.9
  colon Q43.9
  hip Q74.2
    congenital dislocation Q65.2
      bilateral Q65.1
      unilateral Q65.Ø-
  mastoid process Q75.8
  middle ear Q16.4
    except ossicles Q16.4
    ossicles Q16.3
  ossicles Q16.3
  spine Q76.49
  toe Q74.2
Male type pelvis Q74.2
  with disproportion (fetopelvic) O33.3
    causing obstructed labor O65.3
Malformation (congenital) —*see also* Anomaly
  adrenal gland Q89.1
  affecting multiple systems with skeletal changes NEC Q87.5
  alimentary tract Q45.9
    specified type NEC Q45.8
    upper Q4Ø.9
      specified type NEC Q4Ø.8
  aorta Q25.4Ø
    absence Q25.41 ◀
    aneurysm, congenital Q25.43 ◀

Malformation *(Continued)*
aorta *(Continued)*
aplasia Q25.41 ◀
atresia Q25.29 ⬅
aortic arch Q25.21 ◀
coarctation (preductal) (postductal) Q25.1
dilatation, congenital Q25.44 ◀
hypoplasia Q25.42 ◀
patent ductus arteriosus Q25.0
specified type NEC Q25.49 ⬅
stenosis Q25.1 ⬅
supravalvular Q25.3 ◀
aortic valve Q23.9
specified NEC Q23.8
arteriovenous, aneurysmatic (congenital) Q27.30
brain Q28.2
cerebral Q28.2
peripheral Q27.30
digestive system Q27.33
lower limb Q27.32
other specified site Q27.39
renal vessel Q27.34
upper limb Q27.31
precerebral vessels (nonruptured) Q28.0
auricle
ear (congenital) Q17.3
acquired H61.119
left H61.112
with right H61.113
right H61.111
with left H61.113
bile duct Q44.5
bladder Q64.79
aplasia Q64.5
diverticulum Q64.6
exstrophy —*see* Exstrophy, bladder
neck obstruction Q64.31
bone Q79.9
face Q75.9
specified type NEC Q75.8
skull Q75.9
specified type NEC Q75.8
brain (multiple) Q04.9
arteriovenous Q28.2
specified type NEC Q04.8
branchial cleft Q18.2
breast Q83.9
specified type NEC Q83.8
broad ligament Q50.6
bronchus Q32.4
bursa Q79.9
cardiac
chambers Q20.9
specified type NEC Q20.8
septum Q21.9
specified type NEC Q21.8
cerebral Q04.9
vessels Q28.3
cervix uteri Q51.9
specified type NEC Q51.828
Chiari
Type I G93.5
Type II Q07.01
choroid (congenital) Q14.3
plexus Q07.8
circulatory system Q28.9
cochlea Q16.5
cornea Q13.4
coronary vessels Q24.5
corpus callosum (congenital) Q04.0
diaphragm Q79.1
digestive system NEC, specified type NEC Q45.8
dura Q07.9
brain Q04.9
spinal Q06.9
ear Q17.9
causing impairment of hearing Q16.9

Malformation *(Continued)*
ear *(Continued)*
external Q17.9
accessory auricle Q17.0
causing impairment of hearing Q16.9
absence of
auditory canal Q16.1
auricle Q16.0
macrotia Q17.1
microtia Q17.2
misplacement Q17.4
misshapen NEC Q17.3
prominence Q17.5
specified type NEC Q17.8
inner Q16.5
middle Q16.4
absence of eustachian tube Q16.2
ossicles (fusion) Q16.3
ossicles Q16.3
specified type NEC Q17.8
epididymis Q55.4
esophagus Q39.9
specified type NEC Q39.8
eye Q15.9
lid Q10.3
specified NEC Q15.8
fallopian tube Q50.6
genital organ —*see* Anomaly, genitalia
great
artery Q25.9
aorta —*see* Malformation, aorta
pulmonary artery —*see* Malformation, pulmonary, artery
specified type NEC Q25.8
vein Q26.9
anomalous
portal venous connection Q26.5
pulmonary venous connection Q26.4
partial Q26.3
total Q26.2
persistent left superior vena cava Q26.1
portal vein-hepatic artery fistula Q26.6
specified type NEC Q26.8
vena cava stenosis, congenital Q26.0
gum Q38.6
hair Q84.2
heart Q24.9
specified type NEC Q24.8
integument Q84.9
specified type NEC Q84.8
internal ear Q16.5
intestine Q43.9
specified type NEC Q43.8
iris Q13.2
joint Q74.9
ankle Q74.2
lumbosacral Q76.49
sacroiliac Q74.2
specified type NEC Q74.8
kidney Q63.9
accessory Q63.0
giant Q63.3
horseshoe Q63.1
hydronephrosis Q62.0
malposition Q63.2
specified type NEC Q63.8
lacrimal apparatus Q10.6
lingual Q38.3
lip Q38.0
liver Q44.7
lung Q33.9
meninges or membrane (congenital) Q07.9
cerebral Q04.8
spinal (cord) Q06.9
middle ear Q16.4
ossicles Q16.3
mitral valve Q23.9
specified NEC Q23.8
Mondini's (congenital) (malformation, cochlea) Q16.5

Malformation *(Continued)*
mouth (congenital) Q38.6
multiple types NEC Q89.7
musculoskeletal system Q79.9
myocardium Q24.8
nail Q84.6
nervous system (central) Q07.9
nose Q30.9
specified type NEC Q30.8
optic disc Q14.2
orbit Q10.7
ovary Q50.39
palate Q38.5
parathyroid gland Q89.2
pelvic organs or tissues NEC
in pregnancy or childbirth O34.8-
causing obstructed labor O65.5
penis Q55.69
aplasia Q55.5
curvature (lateral) Q55.61
hypoplasia Q55.62
pericardium Q24.8
peripheral vascular system Q27.9
specified type NEC Q27.8
pharynx Q38.8
precerebral vessels Q28.1
prostate Q55.4
pulmonary
arteriovenous Q25.72
artery Q25.9
atresia Q25.5
specified type NEC Q25.79
stenosis Q25.6
valve Q22.3
renal artery Q27.2
respiratory system Q34.9
retina Q14.1
scrotum —*see* Malformation, testis and scrotum
seminal vesicles Q55.4
sense organs NEC Q07.9
skin Q82.9
specified NEC Q89.8
spinal
cord Q06.9
nerve root Q07.8
spine Q76.49
kyphosis —*see* Kyphosis, congenital
lordosis —*see* Lordosis, congenital
spleen Q89.09
stomach Q40.3
specified type NEC Q40.2
teeth, tooth K00.9
tendon Q79.9
testis and scrotum Q55.20
aplasia Q55.0
hypoplasia Q55.1
polyorchism Q55.21
retractile testis Q55.22
scrotal transposition Q55.23
specified NEC Q55.29
thorax, bony Q76.9
throat Q38.8
thyroid gland Q89.2
tongue (congenital) Q38.3
hypertrophy Q38.2
tie Q38.1
trachea Q32.1
tricuspid valve Q22.9
specified type NEC Q22.8
umbilical cord NEC (complicating delivery) O69.89
umbilicus Q89.9
ureter Q62.8
agenesis Q62.4
duplication Q62.5
malposition —*see* Malposition, congenital, ureter
obstructive defect —*see* Defect, obstructive, ureter
vesico-uretero-renal reflux Q62.7

M

- **Malformation** *(Continued)*
  - urethra Q64.79
    - aplasia Q64.5
    - duplication Q64.74
    - posterior valves Q64.2
    - prolapse Q64.71
    - stricture Q64.32
  - urinary system Q64.9
  - uterus Q51.9
    - specified type NEC Q51.818
  - vagina Q52.4
  - vascular system, peripheral Q27.9
  - vas deferens Q55.4
    - atresia Q55.3
  - venous —*see* Anomaly, vein (s)
  - vulva Q52.7Ø
- **Malfunction** —*see also* Dysfunction
  - cardiac electronic device T82.119
    - electrode T82.11Ø
    - pulse generator T82.111
    - specified type NEC T82.118
  - catheter device NEC T85.618
    - cystostomy T83.Ø1Ø
    - dialysis (renal) (vascular) T82.41
      - intraperitoneal T85.611
    - infusion NEC T82.514
      - cranial T85.61Ø ◀
      - epidural T85.61Ø ◀
      - intrathecal T85.61Ø ◀
      - spinal T85.61Ø ⬅
      - subarachnoid T85.61Ø ◀
      - subdural T85.61Ø ◀
    - ~~urinary, indwelling T83.Ø18~~
    - urinary —*see also* Breakdown, device, catheter T83.Ø18 ◀
  - colostomy K94.Ø3
    - valve K94.Ø3
  - cystostomy (stoma) N99.512
    - catheter T83.Ø1Ø
  - enteric stoma K94.13
  - enterostomy K94.13
  - esophagostomy K94.33
  - gastroenteric K31.89
  - gastrostomy K94.23
  - ileostomy K94.13
    - valve K94.13
  - intrathecal infusion pump T85.615 ◀
  - jejunostomy K94.13
  - nervous system device, implant or graft, specified NEC T85.615 ◀
  - pacemaker —*see* Malfunction, cardiac electronic device
  - prosthetic device, internal —*see* Complications, prosthetic device, by site, mechanical
  - tracheostomy J95.Ø3
  - urinary device NEC —*see* Complication, genitourinary, device, urinary, mechanical
  - valve
    - colostomy K94.Ø3
    - heart T82.Ø9
    - ileostomy K94.13
  - vascular graft or shunt NEC —*see* Complication, cardiovascular device, mechanical, vascular
  - ventricular (communicating shunt) T85.Ø1
- **Malherbe's tumor** —*see* Neoplasm, skin, benign
- **Malibu disease** L98.8-
- **Malignancy** —*see also* Neoplasm, malignant, by site
  - unspecified site (primary) C8Ø.1
- **Malignant** —*see* condition
- **Malingerer, malingering** Z76.5
- **Mallet finger** (acquired) —*see* Deformity, finger, mallet finger
  - congenital Q74.Ø
  - sequelae of rickets E64.3
- **Malleus** A24.Ø
- **Mallory's bodies** R89.7
- **Mallory-Weiss syndrome** K22.6
- **Malnutrition** E46
  - degree
    - first E44.1
    - mild (protein) E44.1
    - moderate (protein) E44.Ø
    - second E44.Ø
    - severe (protein-energy) E43
      - intermediate form E42
        - with
          - kwashiorkor (and marasmus) E42
          - marasmus E41
    - third E43
  - following gastrointestinal surgery K91.2
  - intrauterine
    - light-for-dates —*see* Light for dates
    - small-for-dates —*see* Small for dates
  - lack of care, or neglect (child) (infant) T76.Ø2
    - confirmed T74.Ø2
  - malignant E4Ø
  - protein E46
    - calorie E46
      - mild E44.1
      - moderate E44.Ø
      - severe E43
        - intermediate form E42
          - with
            - kwashiorkor (and marasmus) E42
            - marasmus E41
    - energy E46
      - mild E44.1
      - moderate E44.Ø
      - severe E43
        - intermediate form E42
          - with
            - kwashiorkor (and marasmus) E42
            - marasmus E41
  - severe (protein-energy) E43
    - with
      - kwashiorkor (and marasmus) E42
      - marasmus E41
- **Malocclusion** (teeth) M26.4
  - Angle's M26.219
    - class I M26.211
    - class II M26.212
    - class III M26.213
  - due to
    - abnormal swallowing M26.59
    - mouth breathing M26.59
    - tongue, lip or finger habits M26.59
  - temporomandibular (joint) M26.69
- **Malposition**
  - cervix —*see* Malposition, uterus
  - congenital
    - adrenal (gland) Q89.1
    - alimentary tract Q45.8
      - lower Q43.8
      - upper Q4Ø.8
    - aorta Q25.49 ⬅
    - appendix Q43.8
    - arterial trunk Q2Ø.Ø
    - artery (peripheral) Q27.8
      - coronary Q24.5
      - digestive system Q27.8
      - lower limb Q27.8
      - pulmonary Q25.79
      - specified site NEC Q27.8
      - upper limb Q27.8
    - auditory canal Q17.8
      - causing impairment of hearing Q16.9
    - auricle (ear) Q17.4
      - causing impairment of hearing Q16.9
      - cervical Q18.2
    - biliary duct or passage Q44.5
    - bladder (mucosa) —*see* Exstrophy, bladder
    - brachial plexus QØ7.8
    - brain tissue QØ4.8
    - breast Q83.8
    - bronchus Q32.4
- **Malposition** *(Continued)*
  - congenital *(Continued)*
    - cecum Q43.8
    - clavicle Q74.Ø
    - colon Q43.8
    - digestive organ or tract NEC Q45.8
      - lower Q43.8
      - upper Q4Ø.8
    - ear (auricle) (external) Q17.4
      - ossicles Q16.3
    - endocrine (gland) NEC Q89.2
    - epiglottis Q31.8
    - eustachian tube Q17.8
    - eye Q15.8
    - facial features Q18.8
    - fallopian tube Q5Ø.6
    - finger (s) Q68.1
      - supernumerary Q69.Ø
    - foot Q66.9
    - gallbladder Q44.1
    - gastrointestinal tract Q45.8
    - genitalia, genital organ (s) or tract
      - female Q52.8
        - external Q52.79
        - internal NEC Q52.8
      - male Q55.8
    - glottis Q31.8
    - hand Q68.1
    - heart Q24.8
      - dextrocardia Q24.Ø
        - with complete transposition of viscera Q89.3
    - hepatic duct Q44.5
    - hip (joint) Q65.89
    - intestine (large) (small) Q43.8
      - with anomalous adhesions, fixation or malrotation Q43.3
    - joint NEC Q68.8
    - kidney Q63.2
    - larynx Q31.8
    - limb Q68.8
      - lower Q68.8
      - upper Q68.8
    - liver Q44.7
    - lung (lobe) Q33.8
    - nail (s) Q84.6
    - nerve QØ7.8
    - nervous system NEC QØ7.8
    - nose, nasal (septum) Q3Ø.8
    - organ or site not listed —*see* Anomaly, by site
    - ovary Q5Ø.39
    - pancreas Q45.3
    - parathyroid (gland) Q89.2
    - patella Q74.1
    - peripheral vascular system Q27.8
    - pituitary (gland) Q89.2
    - respiratory organ or system NEC Q34.8
    - rib (cage) Q76.6
      - supernumerary in cervical region Q76.5
    - scapula Q74.Ø
    - shoulder Q74.Ø
    - spinal cord QØ6.8
    - spleen Q89.Ø9
    - sternum NEC Q76.7
    - stomach Q4Ø.2
    - symphysis pubis Q74.2
    - thymus (gland) Q89.2
    - thyroid (gland) (tissue) Q89.2
      - cartilage Q31.8
    - toe (s) Q66.9
      - supernumerary Q69.2
    - tongue Q38.3
    - trachea Q32.1
    - ureter Q62.6Ø
      - deviation Q62.61
      - displacement Q62.62
      - ectopia Q62.63
      - specified type NEC Q62.69

M

M

Maroteaux-Lamy syndrome (mild) (severe) E76.29
Marrow (bone)
  arrest D61.9
  poor function D75.89
Marseilles fever A77.1
Marsh fever —*see* Malaria
Marshall's (hidrotic) **ectodermal dysplasia** Q82.4
Marsh's disease (exophthalmic goiter) EØ5.ØØ
  with storm EØ5.Ø1
Masculinization (female) **with adrenal hyperplasia** E25.9
  congenital E25.Ø
Masculinovoblastoma D27.-
Masochism (sexual) F65.51
Mason's lung J62.8
Mass
  abdominal R19.ØØ
    epigastric R19.Ø6
    generalized R19.Ø7
    left lower quadrant R19.Ø4
    left upper quadrant R19.Ø2
    periumbilic R19.Ø5
    right lower quadrant R19.Ø3
    right upper quadrant R19.Ø1
    specified site NEC R19.Ø9
  breast N63
  chest R22.2
  cystic —*see* Cyst
  ear H93.8-
  head R22.Ø
  intra-abdominal (diffuse) (generalized) —*see* Mass, abdominal
  kidney N28.89
  liver R16.Ø
  localized (skin) R22.9
    chest R22.2
    head R22.Ø
    limb
      lower R22.4-
      upper R22.3-
    neck R22.1
    trunk R22.2
  lung R91.8
  malignant —*see* Neoplasm, malignant, by site
  neck R22.1
  pelvic (diffuse) (generalized) —*see* Mass, abdominal
  specified organ NEC —*see* Disease, by site
  splenic R16.1
  substernal thyroid —*see* Goiter
  superficial (localized) R22.9
  umbilical (diffuse) (generalized) R19.Ø9
Massive —*see* condition
Mast cell
  disease, systemic tissue D47.Ø
  leukemia C94.3-
  sarcoma C96.2
  tumor D47.Ø
    malignant C96.2
Mastalgia N64.4
Masters-Allen syndrome N83.8
Mastitis (acute) (diffuse) (nonpuerperal) (subacute) N61.Ø ⬅
  with abscess N61.1 ◀
  chronic (cystic) —*see* Mastopathy, cystic
  cystic (Schimmelbusch's type) —*see* Mastopathy, cystic
  fibrocystic —*see* Mastopathy, cystic
  infective N61.Ø ⬅
    newborn P39.Ø
  interstitial, gestational or puerperal —*see* Mastitis, obstetric
  neonatal (noninfective) P83.4
    infective P39.Ø
  obstetric (interstitial) (nonpurulent)
    associated with
      lactation O91.23
      pregnancy O91.21-
      puerperium O91.22
Mastitis *(Continued)*
  obstetric *(Continued)*
    purulent
      associated with
        lactation O91.13
        pregnancy O91.11-
        puerperium O91.12
  periductal —*see* Ectasia, mammary duct
  phlegmonous —*see* Mastopathy, cystic
  plasma cell —*see* Ectasia, mammary duct
  without abscess N61.Ø ◀
Mastocytoma D47.Ø
  malignant C96.2
Mastocytosis Q82.2
  aggressive systemic C96.2
  indolent systemic D47.Ø
  malignant C96.2
  systemic, associated with clonal hematopoetic non-mast-cell disease (SM-AHNMD) D47.Ø
Mastodynia N64.4
Mastoid —*see* condition
Mastoidalgia —*see* subcategory H92.Ø
Mastoiditis (coalescent) (hemorrhagic) (suppurative) H7Ø.9-
  acute, subacute H7Ø.ØØ-
    complicated NEC H7Ø.Ø9-
    subperiosteal H7Ø.Ø1-
  chronic (necrotic) (recurrent) H7Ø.1-
  in (due to)
    infectious disease NEC B99 *[H75.Ø-]*
    parasitic disease NEC B89 *[H75.Ø-]*
    tuberculosis A18.Ø3
  petrositis —*see* Petrositis
  postauricular fistula —*see* Fistula, postauricular
  specified NEC H7Ø.89-
  tuberculous A18.Ø3
Mastopathy, mastopathia N64.9
  chronica cystica —*see* Mastopathy, cystic
  cystic (chronic) (diffuse) N6Ø.1
    with epithelial proliferation N6Ø.3-
  diffuse cystic —*see* Mastopathy, cystic
  estrogenic, oestrogenica N64.89
  ovarian origin N64.89
Mastoplasia, mastoplastia N62
Masturbation (excessive) F98.8
Maternal care (for) —*see* Pregnancy (complicated by) (management affected by)
Matheiu's disease (leptospiral jaundice) A27.Ø
Mauclaire's disease or osteochondrosis —*see* Osteochondrosis, juvenile, hand, metacarpal
Maxcy's disease A75.2
Maxilla, maxillary —*see* condition
May (-Hegglin) **anomaly or syndrome** D72.Ø
McArdle (-Schmid)(-Pearson) **disease** (glycogen storage) E74.Ø4
McCune-Albright syndrome Q78.1
McQuarrie's syndrome (idiopathic familial hypoglycemia) E16.2
Meadow's syndrome Q86.1
Measles (black) (hemorrhagic) (suppressed) BØ5.9
  with
    complications NEC BØ5.89
    encephalitis BØ5.Ø
    intestinal complications BØ5.4
    keratitis (keratoconjunctivitis) BØ5.81
    meningitis BØ5.1
    otitis media BØ5.3
    pneumonia BØ5.2
  French —*see* Rubella
  German —*see* Rubella
  Liberty —*see* Rubella
Meatitis, urethral —*see* Urethritis
Meatus, meatal —*see* condition
Meat-wrappers' asthma J68.9
Meckel-Gruber syndrome Q61.9
Meckel's diverticulitis, diverticulum (displaced) (hypertrophic) Q43.Ø
Meconium
  ileus, newborn P76.Ø
    in cystic fibrosis E84.11
    meaning meconium plug (without cystic fibrosis) P76.Ø
  obstruction, newborn P76.Ø
    due to fecaliths P76.Ø
    in mucoviscidosis E84.11
  peritonitis P78.Ø
  plug syndrome (newborn) NEC P76.Ø
Median —*see also* condition
  arcuate ligament syndrome I77.4
  bar (prostate) (vesical orifice) —*see* Hyperplasia, prostate
  rhomboid glossitis K14.2
Mediastinal shift R93.8
Mediastinitis (acute) (chronic) J98.51 ⬅
  syphilitic A52.73
  tuberculous A15.8
Mediastinopericarditis —*see also* Pericarditis
  acute I3Ø.9
  adhesive I31.Ø
  chronic I31.8
    rheumatic IØ9.2
Mediastinum, mediastinal —*see* condition
Medicine poisoning —*see* Table of Drugs and Chemicals, by drug, poisoning
Mediterranean
  fever —*see* Brucellosis
    familial MØ4.1 ⬅
    tick A77.1
  kala-azar B55.Ø
  leishmaniasis B55.Ø
  tick fever A77.1
Medulla —*see* condition
Medullary cystic kidney Q61.5
Medullated fibers
  optic (nerve) Q14.8
  retina Q14.1
Medulloblastoma
  desmoplastic C71.6
  specified site —*see* Neoplasm, malignant, by site
  unspecified site C71.6
Medulloepithelioma —*see also* Neoplasm, malignant, by site
  teratoid —*see* Neoplasm, malignant, by site
Medullomyoblastoma
  specified site —*see* Neoplasm, malignant, by site
  unspecified site C71.6
Meekeren-Ehlers-Danlos syndrome Q79.6
Megacolon (acquired) (functional) (not Hirschsprung's disease) (in) K59.39 ⬅
  Chagas' disease B57.32
  congenital, congenitum (aganglionic) Q43.1
  Hirschsprung's (disease) Q43.1
  toxic NEC K59.31 ⬅
    due to Clostridium difficile AØ4.7
Megaesophagus (functional) K22.Ø
  congenital Q39.5
  in (due to) Chagas' disease B57.31
Megalencephaly QØ4.5
Megalerythema (epidemic) BØ8.3
Megaloappendix Q43.8
Megalocephalus, megalocephaly NEC Q75.3
Megalocornea Q15.8
  with glaucoma Q15.Ø
Megalocytic anemia D53.1
Megalodactylia (fingers) (thumbs) (congenital) Q74.Ø
  toes Q74.2
Megaloduodenum Q43.8
Megaloesophagus (functional) K22.Ø
  congenital Q39.5

◀ New ⬅ Revised ~~deleted~~ Deleted

Megalogastria (acquired) K31.89
  congenital Q4Ø.2
Megalophthalmos Q11.3
Megalopsia H53.15
Megalosplenia —*see* Splenomegaly
Megaloureter N28.82
  congenital Q62.2
Megarectum K62.89
Megasigmoid K59.39
  congenital Q43.2
Megaureter N28.82
  congenital Q62.2
Megavitamin-B6 syndrome E67.2
Megrim —*see* Migraine
Meibomian
  cyst, infected —*see* Hordeolum
  gland —*see* condition
  sty, stye —*see* Hordeolum
Meibomitis —*see* Hordeolum
Meige-Milroy disease (chronic hereditary edema) Q82.Ø
Meige's syndrome Q82.Ø
Melalgia, nutritional E53.8
Melancholia F32.9
  climacteric (single episode) F32.89
    recurrent episode F33.8
  hypochondriac F45.29
  intermittent (single episode) F32.89
    recurrent episode F33.8
  involutional (single episode) F32.89
    recurrent episode F33.8
  menopausal (single episode) F32.89
    recurrent episode F33.8
  puerperal F32.89
  reactive (emotional stress or trauma) F32.3
  recurrent F33.9
  senile FØ3
  stuporous (single episode) F32.89
    recurrent episode F33.8
Melanemia R79.89
Melanoameloblastoma —*see* Neoplasm, bone, benign
Melanoblastoma —*see* Melanoma
Melanocarcinoma —*see* Melanoma
Melanocytoma, eyeball D31.9-
Melanocytosis, neurocutaneous Q82.8
Melanoderma, melanodermia L81.4
Melanodontia, infantile KØ3.89
Melanodontoclasia KØ3.89
Melanoepithelioma —*see* Melanoma
Melanoma (malignant) C43.9
  acral lentiginous, malignant —*see* Melanoma, skin, by site
  amelanotic —*see* Melanoma, skin, by site
  balloon cell —*see* Melanoma, skin, by site
  benign —*see* Nevus
  desmoplastic, malignant —*see* Melanoma, skin, by site
  epithelioid cell —*see* Melanoma, skin, by site
    with spindle cell, mixed —*see* Melanoma, skin, by site
  in
    giant pigmented nevus —*see* Melanoma, skin, by site
    Hutchinson's melanotic freckle —*see* Melanoma, skin, by site
    junctional nevus —*see* Melanoma, skin, by site
    precancerous melanosis —*see* Melanoma, skin, by site
  in situ DØ3.9
    abdominal wall DØ3.59
    ala nasi DØ3.39
    ankle DØ3.7-
    anus, anal (margin) (skin) DØ3.51
    arm DØ3.6-
    auditory canal DØ3.2-
    auricle (ear) DØ3.2-
    auricular canal (external) DØ3.2-
    axilla, axillary fold DØ3.59
    back DØ3.59

Melanoma *(Continued)*
  in situ *(Continued)*
    breast DØ3.52
    brow DØ3.39
    buttock DØ3.59
    canthus (eye) DØ3.1-
    cheek (external) DØ3.39
    chest wall DØ3.59
    chin DØ3.39
    choroid DØ3.8
    conjunctiva DØ3.8
    ear (external) DØ3.2-
    external meatus (ear) DØ3.2-
    eye DØ3.8
    eyebrow DØ3.39
    eyelid (lower) (upper) DØ3.1-
    face DØ3.3Ø
      specified NEC DØ3.39
    female genital organ (external) NEC DØ3.8
    finger DØ3.6-
    flank DØ3.59
    foot DØ3.7-
    forearm DØ3.6-
    forehead DØ3.39
    foreskin DØ3.8
    gluteal region DØ3.59
    groin DØ3.59
    hand DØ3.6-
    heel DØ3.7-
    helix DØ3.2-
    hip DØ3.7-
    interscapular region DØ3.59
    iris DØ3.8
    jaw DØ3.39
    knee DØ3.7-
    labium (majus) (minus) DØ3.8
    lacrimal gland DØ3.8
    leg DØ3.7-
    lip (lower) (upper) DØ3.Ø
    lower limb NEC DØ3.7-
    male genital organ (external) NEC DØ3.8
    nail DØ3.9
      finger DØ3.6-
      toe DØ3.7-
    neck DØ3.4
    nose (external) DØ3.39
    orbit DØ3.8
    penis DØ3.8
    perianal skin DØ3.51
    perineum DØ3.51
    pinna DØ3.2-
    popliteal fossa or space DØ3.7-
    prepuce DØ3.8
    pudendum DØ3.8
    retina DØ3.8
    retrobulbar DØ3.8
    scalp DØ3.4
    scrotum DØ3.8
    shoulder DØ3.6-
    specified site NEC DØ3.8
    submammary fold DØ3.52
    temple DØ3.39
    thigh DØ3.7-
    toe DØ3.7-
    trunk NEC DØ3.59
    umbilicus DØ3.59
    upper limb NEC DØ3.6-
    vulva DØ3.8
  juvenile —*see* Nevus
  malignant, of soft parts except skin —*see* Neoplasm, connective tissue, malignant
  metastatic
    breast C79.81
    genital organ C79.82
    specified site NEC C79.89
  neurotropic, malignant —*see* Melanoma, skin, by site
  nodular —*see* Melanoma, skin, by site
  regressing, malignant —*see* Melanoma, skin, by site

Melanoma *(Continued)*
  skin C43.9
    abdominal wall C43.59
    ala nasi C43.31
    ankle C43.7-
    anus, anal (skin) C43.51
    arm C43.6-
    auditory canal (external) C43.2-
    auricle (ear) C43.2-
    auricular canal (external) C43.2-
    axilla, axillary fold C43.59
    back C43.59
    breast (female) (male) C43.52
    brow C43.39
    buttock C43.59
    canthus (eye) C43.1-
    cheek (external) C43.39
    chest wall C43.59
    chin C43.39
    ear (external) C43.2-
    elbow C43.6-
    external meatus (ear) C43.2-
    eyebrow C43.39
    eyelid (lower) (upper) C43.1-
    face C43.3Ø
      specified NEC C43.39
    female genital organ (external) NEC C51.9
    finger C43.6-
    flank C43.59
    foot C43.7-
    forearm C43.6-
    forehead C43.39
    foreskin C6Ø.Ø
    glabella C43.39
    gluteal region C43.59
    groin C43.59
    hand C43.6-
    heel C43.7-
    helix C43.2-
    hip C43.7-
    interscapular region C43.59
    jaw (external) C43.39
    knee C43.7-
    labium C51.9
      majus C51.Ø
      minus C51.1
    leg C43.7-
    lip (lower) (upper) C43.Ø
    lower limb NEC C43.7-
    male genital organ (external) NEC C63.9
    nail
      finger C43.6-
      toe C43.7-
    nasolabial groove C43.39
    nates C43.59
    neck C43.4
    nose (external) C43.31
    overlapping site C43.8
    palpebra C43.1-
    penis C6Ø.9
    perianal skin C43.51
    perineum C43.51
    pinna C43.2-
    popliteal fossa or space C43.7-
    prepuce C6Ø.Ø
    pudendum C51.9
    scalp C43.4
    scrotum C63.2
    shoulder C43.6-
    skin NEC C43.9
    submammary fold C43.52
    temple C43.39
    thigh C43.7-
    toe C43.7-
    trunk NEC C43.59
    umbilicus C43.59
    upper limb NEC C43.6-
    vulva C51.9
      overlapping sites C51.8

M

◀ New ⬅ Revised ~~deleted~~ Deleted

Melanoma *(Continued)*
spindle cell
with epithelioid, mixed —*see* Melanoma, skin, by site
type A C69.4-
type B C69.4-
superficial spreading —*see* Melanoma, skin, by site
Melanosarcoma —*see also* Melanoma
epithelioid cell —*see* Melanoma
Melanosis L81.4
addisonian E27.1
tuberculous A18.7
adrenal E27.1
colon K63.89
conjunctiva —*see* Pigmentation, conjunctiva
congenital Q13.89
cornea (presenile) (senile) —*see also* Pigmentation, cornea
congenital Q13.4
eye NEC H57.8
congenital Q15.8
lenticularis progressiva Q82.1
liver K76.89
precancerous —*see also* Melanoma, in situ
malignant melanoma in —*see* Melanoma
Riehl's L81.4
sclera H15.89
congenital Q13.89
suprarenal E27.1
tar L81.4
toxic L81.4
Melanuria R82.99
MELAS syndrome E88.41
Melasma L81.1
adrenal (gland) E27.1
suprarenal (gland) E27.1
Melena K92.1
with ulcer - code by site under Ulcer, with hemorrhage K27.4
due to swallowed maternal blood P78.2
newborn, neonatal P54.1
due to swallowed maternal blood P78.2
Meleney's
gangrene (cutaneous) —*see* Ulcer, skin
ulcer (chronic undermining) —*see* Ulcer, skin
Melioidosis A24.9
acute A24.1
chronic A24.2
fulminating A24.1
pneumonia A24.1
pulmonary (chronic) A24.2
acute A24.1
subacute A24.2
sepsis A24.1
specified NEC A24.3
subacute A24.2
Melitensis, febris A23.Ø
Melkersson (-Rosenthal) **syndrome** G51.2
Mellitus, diabetes —*see* Diabetes
Melorheostosis (bone) —*see* Disorder, bone, density and structure, specified NEC
Meloschisis Q18.4
Melotia Q17.4
Membrana
capsularis lentis posterior Q13.89
epipapillaris Q14.2
Membranacea placenta O43.19-
Membranaceous uterus N85.8
Membrane (s), membranous —*see also* condition
cyclitic —*see* Membrane, pupillary
folds, congenital —*see* Web
Jackson's Q43.3
over face of newborn P28.9
premature rupture —*see* Rupture, membranes, premature
pupillary H21.4-
persistent Q13.89
retained (with hemorrhage) (complicating delivery) O72.2
without hemorrhage O73.1

Membrane (s), membranous *(Continued)*
secondary cataract —*see* Cataract, secondary
unruptured (causing asphyxia) —*see* Asphyxia, newborn
vitreous —*see* Opacity, vitreous, membranes and strands
Membranitis —*see* Chorioamnionitis
Memory disturbance, lack or loss —*see also* Amnesia
mild, following organic brain damage F06.8
Menadione deficiency E56.1
Menarche
delayed E30.Ø
precocious E30.1
Mendacity, pathologic F60.2
Mendelson's syndrome (due to anesthesia) J95.4
in labor and delivery O74.Ø
in pregnancy O29.Ø1-
obstetric O74.Ø
postpartum, puerperal O89.Ø1
Ménétrier's disease or syndrome K29.6Ø
with bleeding K29.61
Ménière's disease, syndrome or vertigo H81.Ø-
Meninges, meningeal —*see* condition
Meningioma —*see also* Neoplasm, meninges, benign
angioblastic —*see* Neoplasm, meninges, benign
angiomatous —*see* Neoplasm, meninges, benign
endotheliomatous —*see* Neoplasm, meninges, benign
fibroblastic —*see* Neoplasm, meninges, benign
fibrous —*see* Neoplasm, meninges, benign
hemangioblastic —*see* Neoplasm, meninges, benign
hemangiopericytic —*see* Neoplasm, meninges, benign
malignant —*see* Neoplasm, meninges, malignant
meningiothelial —*see* Neoplasm, meninges, benign
meningotheliomatous —*see* Neoplasm, meninges, benign
mixed —*see* Neoplasm, meninges, benign
multiple —*see* Neoplasm, meninges, uncertain behavior
papillary —*see* Neoplasm, meninges, uncertain behavior
psammomatous —*see* Neoplasm, meninges, benign
syncytial —*see* Neoplasm, meninges, benign
transitional —*see* Neoplasm, meninges, benign
Meningiomatosis (diffuse) —*see* Neoplasm, meninges, uncertain behavior
Meningism —*see* Meningismus
Meningismus (infectional) (pneumococcal) R29.1
due to serum or vaccine R29.1
influenzal —*see* Influenza, with, manifestations NEC
Meningitis (basal) (basic) (brain) (cerebral) (cervical) (congestive) (diffuse) (hemorrhagic) infantile) (membranous) (metastatic) (nonspecific) (pontine) (progressive) (simple) (spinal) (subacute) (sympathetic) (toxic) G03.9
abacterial G03.Ø
actinomycotic A42.81
adenoviral A87.1
arbovirus A87.8
aseptic (acute) G03.Ø
bacterial G00.9
Escherichia coli (E. coli) G00.8
Friedländer (bacillus) G00.8
gram-negative G00.9
H. influenzae G00.Ø
Klebsiella G00.8

Meningitis *(Continued)*
bacterial *(Continued)*
pneumococcal G00.1
specified organism NEC G00.8
staphylococcal G00.3
streptococcal (acute) G00.2
benign recurrent (Mollaret) G03.2
candidal B37.5
caseous (tuberculous) A17.Ø
cerebrospinal A39.Ø
chronic NEC G03.1
clear cerebrospinal fluid NEC G03.Ø
coxsackievirus A87.Ø
cryptococcal B45.1
diplococcal (gram positive) A39.Ø
echovirus A87.Ø
enteroviral A87.Ø
eosinophilic B83.2
epidemic NEC A39.Ø
Escherichia coli (E. coli) G00.8
fibrinopurulent G00.9
specified organism NEC G00.8
Friedländer (bacillus) G00.8
gonococcal A54.81
gram-negative cocci G00.9
gram-positive cocci G00.9
Haemophilus (influenzae) G00.Ø
H. influenzae G00.Ø
in (due to)
adenovirus A87.1
African trypanosomiasis B56.9 *[G02]*
anthrax A22.8
bacterial disease NEC A48.8 *[G01]*
Chagas' disease (chronic) B57.41
chickenpox B01.Ø
coccidioidomycosis B38.4
Diplococcus pneumoniae G00.1
enterovirus A87.Ø
herpes (simplex) virus B00.3
zoster B02.1
infectious mononucleosis B27.92
leptospirosis A27.81
Listeria monocytogenes A32.11
Lyme disease A69.21
measles B05.1
mumps (virus) B26.1
neurosyphilis (late) A52.13
parasitic disease NEC B89 *[G02]*
poliovirus A80.9 *[G02]*
preventive immunization, inoculation or vaccination G03.8
rubella B06.02
Salmonella infection A02.21
specified cause NEC G03.8
Streptococcal pneumoniae G00.1 ◀
typhoid fever A01.01
varicella B01.Ø
viral disease NEC A87.8
whooping cough A37.90
zoster B02.1
infectious G00.9
influenzal (H. influenzae) G00.Ø
Klebsiella G00.8
leptospiral (aseptic) A27.81
lymphocytic (acute) (benign) (serous) A87.2
meningococcal A39.Ø
Mima polymorpha G00.8
Mollaret (benign recurrent) G03.2
monilial B37.5
mycotic NEC B49 *[G02]*
Neisseria A39.Ø
nonbacterial G03.Ø
nonpyogenic NEC G03.Ø
ossificans G96.19
~~pneumococcal G00.1~~
pneumococcal streptococcus pneumoniae G00.1 ◀
poliovirus A80.9 *[G02]*
postmeasles B05.1
purulent G00.9
specified organism NEC G00.8

M

Meningitis *(Continued)*
- pyogenic GØØ.9
  - specified organism NEC GØØ.8
- Salmonella (arizonae) (Cholerae-Suis) (enteritidis) (typhimurium) AØ2.21
- septic GØØ.9
  - specified organism NEC GØØ.8
- serosa circumscripta NEC GØ3.Ø
- serous NEC G93.2
- specified organism NEC GØØ.8
- sporotrichosis B42.81
- staphylococcal GØØ.3
- sterile GØ3.Ø
- Streptococcal (acute) GØØ.2 ⬅
  - pneumoniae GØØ.1 ◀
- suppurative GØØ.9
  - specified organism NEC GØØ.8
- syphilitic (late) (tertiary) A52.13
  - acute A51.41
  - congenital A5Ø.41
  - secondary A51.41
- Torula histolytica (cryptococcal) B45.1
- traumatic (complication of injury) T79.8
- tuberculous A17.Ø
- typhoid AØ1.Ø1
- viral NEC A87.9
- Yersinia pestis A2Ø.3

Meningocele (spinal) —*see also* Spina bifida
- with hydrocephalus —*see* Spina bifida, by site, with hydrocephalus
- acquired (traumatic) G96.19
- cerebral —*see* Encephalocele

Meningocerebritis —*see* Meningoencephalitis

Meningococcemia A39.4
- acute A39.2
- chronic A39.3

Meningococcus, meningococcal —*see also* condition A39.9
- adrenalitis, hemorrhagic A39.1
- carrier (suspected) of Z22.31
- meningitis (cerebrospinal) A39.Ø

Meningoencephalitis —*see also* Encephalitis GØ4.9Ø
- acute NEC —*see also* Encephalitis, viral A86
- bacterial NEC GØ4.2
- California A83.5
- diphasic A84.1
- eosinophilic B83.2
- epidemic A39.81
- herpesviral, herpetic BØØ.4
  - due to herpesvirus 6 B1Ø.Ø1
  - due to herpesvirus 7 B1Ø.Ø9
  - specified NEC B1Ø.Ø9
- in (due to)
  - blastomycosis NEC B4Ø.81
  - diseases classified elsewhere GØ5.3
  - free-living amebae B6Ø.2
  - Hemophilus influenzae (H. influenzae) GØØ.Ø ⬅
  - herpes BØØ.4
    - due to herpesvirus 6 B1Ø.Ø1
    - due to herpesvirus 7 B1Ø.Ø9
    - specified NEC B1Ø.Ø9
  - H. influenzae GØØ.Ø
  - Lyme disease A69.22
  - mercury —*see* subcategory T56.1
  - mumps B26.2
  - Naegleria (amebae) (organisms) (fowleri) B6Ø.2
  - Parastrongylus cantonensis B83.2
  - toxoplasmosis (acquired) B58.2
    - congenital P37.1
- infectious (acute) (viral) A86
- influenzal (H. influenzae) GØØ.Ø ⬅
- Listeria monocytogenes A32.12
- lymphocytic (serous) A87.2
- mumps B26.2
- parasitic NEC B89 *[GØ5.3]*
- pneumococcal GØ4.2 ⬅
- primary amebic B6Ø.2

Meningoencephalitis *(Continued)*
- specific (syphilitic) A52.14
- specified organism NEC GØ4.81
- staphylococcal GØ4.2
- streptococcal GØ4.2
- syphilitic A52.14
- toxic NEC G92
  - due to mercury —*see* subcategory T56.1
- tuberculous A17.82
- virus NEC A86

Meningoencephalocele —*see also* Encephalocele
- syphilitic A52.19
  - congenital A5Ø.49

Meningoencephalomyelitis —*see also* Meningoencephalitis
- acute NEC (viral) A86
  - disseminated GØ4.ØØ
    - postimmunization or postvaccination GØ4.Ø2
  - postinfectious GØ4.Ø1
- due to
  - actinomycosis A42.82
  - Torula B45.1
  - Toxoplasma or toxoplasmosis (acquired) B58.2
    - congenital P37.1
- postimmunization or postvaccination GØ4.Ø2

Meningoencephalomyelopathy G96.9

Meningoencephalopathy G96.9

Meningomyelitis —*see also* Meningoencephalitis
- bacterial NEC GØ4.2
- blastomycotic NEC B4Ø.81
- cryptococcal B45.1
- in diseases classified elsewhere GØ5.4
- meningococcal A39.81
- syphilitic A52.14
- tuberculous A17.82

Meningomyelocele —*see also* Spina bifida
- syphilitic A52.19

Meningomyeloneuritis —*see* Meningoencephalitis

Meningoradiculitis —*see* Meningitis

Meningovascular —*see* condition

Menkes' disease or syndrome E83.Ø9
- meaning maple-syrup-urine disease E71.Ø

Menometrorrhagia N92.1

Menopause, menopausal (asymptomatic) (state) Z78.Ø
- arthritis (any site) NEC —*see* Arthritis, specified form NEC
- bleeding N92.4
- depression (single episode) F32.89 ⬅
  - agitated (single episode) F32.2
    - recurrent episode F33.9
  - psychotic (single episode) F32.89 ⬅
    - recurrent episode F33.8 ⬅
  - recurrent episode F33.9
- melancholia (single episode) F32.89 ⬅
  - recurrent episode F33.8 ⬅
- paranoid state F22
- premature E28.319
  - asymptomatic E28.319
    - postirradiation E89.4Ø
    - postsurgical E89.4Ø
  - symptomatic E28.31Ø
    - postirradiation E89.41
    - postsurgical E89.41
- psychosis NEC F28
- symptomatic N95.1
- toxic polyarthritis NEC —*see* Arthritis, specified form NEC

Menorrhagia (primary) N92.Ø
- climacteric N92.4
  - menopausal N92.4
- menopausal N92.4
- postclimacteric N95.Ø
- postmenopausal N95.Ø
- preclimacteric or premenopausal N92.4
- pubertal (menses retained) N92.2

Menostaxis N92.Ø

Menses, retention N94.89

Menstrual —*see* Menstruation

Menstruation
- absent —*see* Amenorrhea
- anovulatory N97.Ø
- cycle, irregular N92.6
- delayed N91.Ø
- disorder N93.9
  - psychogenic F45.8
- during pregnancy O2Ø.8
- excessive (with regular cycle) N92.Ø
  - with irregular cycle N92.1
  - at puberty N92.2
- frequent N92.Ø
- infrequent —*see* Oligomenorrhea
- irregular N92.6
  - specified NEC N92.5
- latent N92.5
- membranous N92.5
- painful —*see also* Dysmenorrhea N94.6
  - primary N94.4
  - psychogenic F45.8
  - secondary N94.5
- passage of clots N92.Ø
- precocious E3Ø.1
- protracted N92.5
- rare —*see* Oligomenorrhea
- retained N94.89
- retrograde N92.5
- scanty —*see* Oligomenorrhea
- suppression N94.89
- vicarious (nasal) N94.89

Mental —*see also* condition
- deficiency —*see* Disability, intellectual
- deterioration —*see* Psychosis
- disorder —*see* Disorder, mental
- exhaustion F48.8
- insufficiency (congenital) —*see* Disability, intellectual
- observation without need for further medical care ZØ3.89
- retardation —*see* Disability, intellectual
- subnormality —*see* Disability, intellectual
- upset —*see* Disorder, mental

Meralgia paresthetica G57.1-

Mercurial —*see* condition

Mercurialism —*see* subcategory T56.1

MERRF syndrome (myoclonic epilepsy associated with ragged-red fiber) E88.42

Merkel cell tumor —*see* Carcinoma, Merkel cell

Merocele —*see* Hernia, femoral

Meromelia
- lower limb —*see* Defect, reduction, lower limb
  - intercalary
    - femur —*see* Defect, reduction, lower limb, specified type NEC
    - tibiofibular (complete) (incomplete) —*see* Defect, reduction, lower limb
- upper limb —*see* Defect, reduction, upper limb
  - intercalary, humeral, radioulnar —*see* Agenesis, arm, with hand present

Merzbacher-Pelizaeus disease E75.29

Mesaortitis —*see* Aortitis

Mesarteritis —*see* Arteritis

Mesencephalitis —*see* Encephalitis

Mesenchymoma —*see also* Neoplasm, connective tissue, uncertain behavior
- benign —*see* Neoplasm, connective tissue, benign
- malignant —*see* Neoplasm, connective tissue, malignant

Mesenteritis
- retractile K65.4
- sclerosing K65.4

Mesentery, mesenteric —*see* condition

M

◀ New ⬅ Revised ~~deleted~~ Deleted

M

M

◄ New ⬅ Revised ~~deleted~~ Deleted

- **Mobile, mobility** *(Continued)*
  - kidney N28.89
  - organ or site, congenital NEC *—see* Malposition, congenital
- **Mobitz heart block** (atrioventricular) I44.1
- **Moebius, Möbius**
  - disease (ophthalmoplegic migraine) *—see* Migraine, ophthalmoplegic
  - syndrome Q87.Ø
    - congenital oculofacial paralysis (with other anomalies) Q87.Ø
    - ophthalmoplegic migraine *—see* Migraine, ophthalmoplegic
- **Moeller's glossitis** K14.Ø
- **Mohr's syndrome** (Types I and II) Q87.Ø
- **Mola destruens** D39.2
- **Molar pregnancy** OØ2.Ø
- **Molarization of premolars** KØØ.2
- **Molding, head** (during birth) - omit code
- **Mole** (pigmented) *—see also* Nevus
  - blood OØ2.Ø
  - Breus' OØ2.Ø
  - cancerous *—see* Melanoma
  - carneous OØ2.Ø
  - destructive D39.2
  - fleshy OØ2.Ø
  - hydatid, hydatidiform (benign) (complicating pregnancy) (delivered) (undelivered) OØ1.9
    - classical OØ1.Ø
    - complete OØ1.Ø
    - incomplete OØ1.1
    - invasive D39.2
    - malignant D39.2
    - partial OØ1.1
  - intrauterine OØ2.Ø
  - invasive (hydatidiform) D39.2
  - malignant
    - meaning
      - malignant hydatidiform mole D39.2
      - melanoma *—see* Melanoma
  - nonhydatidiform OØ2.Ø
  - nonpigmented *—see* Nevus
  - pregnancy NEC OØ2.Ø
  - skin *—see* Nevus
  - tubal OØØ.1Ø ⇐
    - with intrauterine pregnancy OØØ.11 ◀
  - vesicular *—see* Mole, hydatidiform
- **Molimen, molimina** (menstrual) N94.3
- **Molluscum contagiosum** (epitheliale) BØ8.1
- **Mönckeberg's arteriosclerosis, disease, or sclerosis** *—see* Arteriosclerosis, extremities
- **Mondini's malformation** (cochlea) Q16.5
- **Mondor's disease** I8Ø.8
- **Monge's disease** T7Ø.29
- **Monilethrix** (congenital) Q84.1
- **Moniliasis** *—see also* Candidiasis B37.9
  - neonatal P37.5
- **Monitoring** (encounter for)
  - therapeutic drug level Z51.81
- **Monkey malaria** B53.1
- **Monkeypox** BØ4
- **Monoarthritis** M13.1Ø
  - ankle M13.17-
  - elbow M13.12-
  - foot joint M13.17-
  - hand joint M13.14-
  - hip M13.15-
  - knee M13.16-
  - shoulder M13.11-
  - wrist M13.13-
- **Monoblastic** *—see* condition
- **Monochromat** (ism), **monochromatopsia** (acquired) (congenital) H53.51
- **Monocytic** *—see* condition
- **Monocytopenia** D72.818
- **Monocytosis** (symptomatic) D72.821
- **Monomania** *—see* Psychosis
- **Mononeuritis** G58.9
  - cranial nerve *—see* Disorder, nerve, cranial
- **Mononeuritis** *(Continued)*
  - femoral nerve G57.2-
  - lateral
    - cutaneous nerve of thigh G57.1-
    - popliteal nerve G57.3-
  - lower limb G57.9-
    - specified nerve NEC G57.8-
  - medial popliteal nerve G57.4-
  - median nerve G56.1-
  - multiplex G58.7
  - plantar nerve G57.6-
  - posterior tibial nerve G57.5-
  - radial nerve G56.3-
  - sciatic nerve G57.Ø-
  - specified NEC G58.8
  - tibial nerve G57.4-
  - ulnar nerve G56.2-
  - upper limb G56.9-
    - specified nerve NEC G56.8-
  - vestibular *—see* subcategory H93.3
- **Mononeuropathy** G58.9
  - carpal tunnel syndrome *—see* Syndrome, carpal tunnel
  - diabetic NEC *—see* EØ8-E13 with .41
  - femoral nerve *—see* Lesion, nerve, femoral
  - ilioinguinal nerve G57.8-
  - in diseases classified elsewhere *—see* category G59
  - intercostal G58.Ø
  - lower limb G57.9-
    - causalgia *—see* Causalgia, lower limb
    - femoral nerve *—see* Lesion, nerve, femoral
    - meralgia paresthetica G57.1-
    - plantar nerve *—see* Lesion, nerve, plantar
    - popliteal nerve *—see* Lesion, nerve, popliteal
    - sciatic nerve *—see* Lesion, nerve, sciatic
    - specified NEC G57.8-
    - tarsal tunnel syndrome *—see* Syndrome, tarsal tunnel
  - median nerve *—see* Lesion, nerve, median
  - multiplex G58.7
  - obturator nerve G57.8-
  - popliteal nerve *—see* Lesion, nerve, popliteal
  - radial nerve *—see* Lesion, nerve, radial
  - saphenous nerve G57.8-
  - specified NEC G58.8
  - tarsal tunnel syndrome *—see* Syndrome, tarsal tunnel
  - tuberculous A17.83
  - ulnar nerve *—see* Lesion, nerve, ulnar
  - upper limb G56.9-
    - carpal tunnel syndrome *—see* Syndrome, carpal tunnel
    - causalgia *—see* Causalgia
    - median nerve *—see* Lesion, nerve, median
    - radial nerve *—see* Lesion, nerve, radial
    - specified site NEC G56.8-
    - ulnar nerve *—see* Lesion, nerve, ulnar
- **Mononucleosis, infectious** B27.9Ø
  - with
    - complication NEC B27.99
    - meningitis B27.92
    - polyneuropathy B27.91
  - cytomegaloviral B27.1Ø
    - with
      - complication NEC B27.19
      - meningitis B27.12
      - polyneuropathy B27.11
  - Epstein-Barr (virus) B27.ØØ
    - with
      - complication NEC B27.Ø9
      - meningitis B27.Ø2
      - polyneuropathy B27.Ø1
  - gammaherpesviral B27.ØØ
    - with
      - complication NEC B27.Ø9
      - meningitis B27.Ø2
      - polyneuropathy B27.Ø1
- **Mononucleosis, infectious** *(Continued)*
  - specified NEC B27.8Ø
    - with
      - complication NEC B27.89
      - meningitis B27.82
      - polyneuropathy B27.81
- **Monoplegia** G83.3-
  - congenital (cerebral) G8Ø.8
    - spastic G8Ø.1
  - embolic (current episode) I63.4- ⇐
  - following
    - cerebrovascular disease
      - cerebral infarction
        - lower limb I69.34-
        - upper limb I69.33-
      - intracerebral hemorrhage
        - lower limb I69.14-
        - upper limb I69.13-
      - lower limb I69.94-
      - nontraumatic intracranial hemorrhage NEC
        - lower limb I69.24-
        - upper limb I69.23-
      - specified disease NEC
        - lower limb I69.84-
        - upper limb I69.83-
      - stroke NOS
        - lower limb I69.34-
        - upper limb I69.33-
      - subarachnoid hemorrhage
        - lower limb I69.Ø4-
        - upper limb I69.Ø3-
      - upper limb I69.93-
  - hysterical (transient) F44.4
  - lower limb G83.1-
  - psychogenic (conversion reaction) F44.4
  - thrombotic (current episode) I63.3- ⇐
  - transient R29.818
  - upper limb G83.2-
- **Monorchism, monorchidism** Q55.Ø
- **Monosomy** *—see also* Deletion, chromosome Q93.9
  - specified NEC Q93.89
  - whole chromosome
    - meiotic nondisjunction Q93.Ø
    - mitotic nondisjunction Q93.1
    - mosaicism Q93.1
  - X Q96.9
- **Monster, monstrosity** (single) Q89.7
  - acephalic QØØ.Ø
  - twin Q89.4
- **Monteggia's fracture** (-dislocation) S52.27-
- **Mooren's ulcer** (cornea) *—see* Ulcer, cornea, Mooren's
- **Moore's syndrome** *—see* Epilepsy, specified NEC
- **Mooser-Neill reaction** A75.2
- **Mooser's bodies** A75.2
- **Morbidity not stated or unknown** R69
- **Morbilli** *—see* Measles
- **Morbus** *—see also* Disease
  - angelicus, anglorum E55.Ø
  - Beigel B36.2
  - caducus *—see* Epilepsy
  - celiacus K9Ø.Ø
  - comitialis *—see* Epilepsy
  - cordis *—see also* Disease, heart I51.9
    - valvulorum *—see* Endocarditis
  - coxae senilis M16.9
    - tuberculous A18.Ø2
  - hemorrhagicus neonatorum P53
  - maculosus neonatorum P54.5
- **Morel** (-Stewart)(-Morgagni) **syndrome** M85.2
- **Morel-Kraepelin disease** *—see* Schizophrenia
- **Morel-Moore syndrome** M85.2
- **Morgagni's**
  - cyst, organ, hydatid, or appendage
    - female Q5Ø.5
    - male (epididymal) Q55.4
      - testicular Q55.29
  - syndrome M85.2

Morgagni-Stewart-Morel syndrome M85.2
Morgagni-Stokes-Adams syndrome I45.9
Morgagni-Turner (-Albright) **syndrome** Q96.9
Moria FØ7.Ø
Moron (I.Q. 5Ø-69) F7Ø
Morphea L94.Ø
Morphinism (without remission) F11.2Ø
  with remission F11.21
Morphinomania (without remission) F11.2Ø
  with remission F11.21
Morquio (-Ullrich)(-Brailsford) **disease or syndrome** —*see* Mucopolysaccharidosis
Mortification (dry) (moist) —*see* Gangrene
Morton's metatarsalgia (neuralgia)(neuroma) (syndrome) G57.6
Morvan's disease or syndrome G6Ø.8
Mosaicism, mosaic (autosomal) (chromosomal)
  45,X/46,XX Q96.3
  45,X/other cell lines NEC with abnormal sex chromosome Q96.4
  sex chromosome
    female Q97.8
    lines with various numbers of X chromosomes Q97.2
    male Q98.7
  XY Q96.3
Moschowitz' disease M31.1
Mother yaw A66.Ø
Motion sickness (from travel, any vehicle) (from roundabouts or swings) T75.3
Mottled, mottling, teeth (enamel) (endemic) (nonendemic) KØØ.3
Mounier-Kuhn syndrome Q32.4
  with bronchiectasis J47.9
    exacerbation (acute) J47.1
    lower respiratory infection J47.Ø
  acquired J98.Ø9
    with bronchiectasis J47.9
      with
        exacerbation (acute) J47.1
        lower respiratory infection J47.Ø
Mountain
  sickness T7Ø.29
    with polycythemia , acquired (acute) D75.1
  tick fever A93.2
Mouse, joint —*see* Loose, body, joint
  knee M23.4-
Mouth —*see* condition
Movable
  coccyx —*see* subcategory M53.2
  kidney N28.89
    congenital Q63.8
  spleen D73.89
Movements, dystonic R25.8
Moyamoya disease I67.5
MRSA (Methicillin resistant Staphylococcus aureus)
  infection A49.Ø2
    as the cause of diseases classified elsewhere B95.62
  sepsis A41.Ø2
MSSA (Methicillin susceptible Staphylococcus aureus)
  infection A49.Ø1
    as the cause of diseases classified elsewhere B95.61
  sepsis A41.Ø1
Mucha-Habermann disease L41.Ø
Mucinosis (cutaneous) (focal) (papular) (reticular erythematous) (skin) L98.5
  oral K13.79
Mucocele
  appendix K38.8
  buccal cavity K13.79
  gallbladder K82.1
  lacrimal sac, chronic HØ4.43-
  nasal sinus J34.1
  nose J34.1
  salivary gland (any) K11.6
  sinus (accessory) (nasal) J34.1
  turbinate (bone) (middle) (nasal) J34.1
  uterus N85.8
Mucolipidosis
  I E77.1
  II, III E77.Ø
  IV E75.11
Mucopolysaccharidosis E76.3
  beta-gluduronidase deficiency E76.29
  cardiopathy E76.3 *[I52]*
  Hunter's syndrome E76.1
  Hurler's syndrome E76.Ø1
  Hurler-Scheie syndrome E76.Ø2
  Maroteaux-Lamy syndrome E76.29
  Morquio syndrome E76.219
    A E76.21Ø
    B E76.211
    classic E76.21Ø
  Sanfilippo syndrome E76.22
  Scheie's syndrome E76.Ø3
  specified NEC E76.29
  type
    I
      Hurler's syndrome E76.Ø1
      Hurler-Scheie syndrome E76.Ø2
      Scheie's syndrome E76.Ø3
    II E76.1
    III E76.22
    IV E76.219
    IVA E76.21Ø
    IVB E76.211
    VI E76.29
    VII E76.29
Mucormycosis B46.5
  cutaneous B46.3
  disseminated B46.4
  gastrointestinal B46.2
  generalized B46.4
  pulmonary B46.Ø
  rhinocerebral B46.1
  skin B46.3
  subcutaneous B46.3
Mucositis (ulcerative) K12.3Ø
  due to drugs NEC K12.32
  gastrointestinal K92.81
  mouth (oral) (oropharyngeal) K12.3Ø
    due to antineoplastic therapy K12.31
    due to drugs NEC K12.32
    due to radiation K12.33
    specified NEC K12.39
    viral K12.39
  nasal J34.81
  oral cavity —*see* Mucositis, mouth
  oral soft tissues —*see* Mucositis, mouth
  vagina and vulva N76.81
Mucositis necroticans agranulocytica —*see* Agranulocytosis
Mucous —*see also* condition
  patches (syphilitic) A51.39
    congenital A5Ø.Ø7
Mucoviscidosis E84.9
  with meconium obstruction E84.11
Mucus
  asphyxia or suffocation —*see* Asphyxia, mucus
  in stool R19.5
  plug —*see* Asphyxia, mucus
Muguet B37.Ø
Mulberry molars (congenital syphilis) A5Ø.52
Müllerian mixed tumor
  specified site —*see* Neoplasm, malignant, by site
  unspecified site C54.9
Multicystic kidney (development) Q61.4
Multiparity (grand) Z64.1
  affecting management of pregnancy, labor and delivery (supervision only) OØ9.4-
  requiring contraceptive management —*see* Contraception
Multipartita placenta O43.19-
Multiple, multiplex —*see also* condition
  digits (congenital) Q69.9
Multiple, multiplex *(Continued)*
  endocrine neoplasia —*see* Neoplasia, endocrine, multiple [MEN]
  personality F44.81
Mumps B26.9
  arthritis B26.85
  complication NEC B26.89
  encephalitis B26.2
  hepatitis B26.81
  meningitis (aseptic) B26.1
  meningoencephalitis B26.2
  myocarditis B26.82
  oophoritis B26.89
  orchitis B26.Ø
  pancreatitis B26.3
  polyneuropathy B26.84
Mumu —*see also* Infestation, filarial B74.9 *[N51]*
Münchhausen's syndrome —*see* Disorder, factitious
Münchmeyer's syndrome —*see* Myositis, ossificans, progressiva
Mural —*see* condition
Murmur (cardiac) (heart) (organic) RØ1.1
  abdominal R19.15
  aortic (valve) —*see* Endocarditis, aortic
  benign RØ1.Ø
  diastolic —*see* Endocarditis
  Flint I35.1
  functional RØ1.Ø
  Graham Steell I37.1
  innocent RØ1.Ø
  mitral (valve) —*see* Insufficiency, mitral
  nonorganic RØ1.Ø
  presystolic, mitral —*see* Insufficiency, mitral
  pulmonic (valve) I37.8
  systolic RØ1.1 ⟸
  tricuspid (valve) IØ7.9
  valvular —*see* Endocarditis
Murri's disease (intermittent hemoglobinuria) D59.6
Muscle, muscular —*see also* condition
  carnitine (palmityltransferase) deficiency E71.314
Musculoneuralgia —*see* Neuralgia
Mushroom-workers' (pickers') **disease or lung** J67.5
Mushrooming hip —*see* Derangement, joint, specified NEC, hip
Mutation (s)
  factor V Leiden D68.51
  surfactant, of lung J84.83
  prothrombin gene D68.52
Mutism —*see also* Aphasia
  deaf (acquired) (congenital) NEC H91.3
  elective (adjustment reaction) (childhood) F94.Ø
  hysterical F44.4
  selective (childhood) F94.Ø
MVD (microvillus inclusion disease) Q43.8
MVID (microvillus inclusion disease) Q43.8
Myalgia M79.1
  epidemic (cervical) B33.Ø
  traumatic NEC T14.8
Myasthenia G7Ø.9
  congenital G7Ø.2
  cordis —*see* Failure, heart
  developmental G7Ø.2
  gravis G7Ø.ØØ
    with exacerbation (acute) G7Ø.Ø1
    in crisis G7Ø.Ø1
    neonatal, transient P94.Ø
    pseudoparalytica G7Ø.ØØ
      with exacerbation (acute) G7Ø.Ø1
      in crisis G7Ø.Ø1
  stomach, psychogenic F45.8
  syndrome
    in
      diabetes mellitus —*see* EØ8-E13 with .44
      neoplastic disease —*see also* Neoplasm D49.9 *[G73.3]*

Myasthenia *(Continued)*
- syndrome *(Continued)*
  - in *(Continued)*
    - pernicious anemia D51.Ø *[G73.3]*
    - thyrotoxicosis EØ5.9Ø *[G73.3]*
      - with thyroid storm EØ5.91 *[G73.3]*

Myasthenic M62.81
Mycelium infection B49
Mycetismus —*see* Poisoning, food, noxious, mushroom
Mycetoma B47.9
- actinomycotic B47.1
- bone (mycotic) B47.9 *[M9Ø.8Ø]*
- eumycotic B47.Ø
- foot B47.9
  - actinomycotic B47.1
  - mycotic B47.Ø
- madurae NEC B47.9
  - mycotic B47.Ø
- maduromycotic B47.Ø
- mycotic B47.Ø
- nocardial B47.1

Mycobacteriosis —*see* Mycobacterium
Mycobacterium, mycobacterial (infection) A31.9
- anonymous A31.9
- atypical A31.9
  - cutaneous A31.1
  - pulmonary A31.Ø
    - tuberculous —*see* Tuberculosis, pulmonary
  - specified site NEC A31.8
- avium (intracellulare complex) A31.Ø
- balnei A31.1
- Battey A31.Ø
- chelonei A31.8
- cutaneous A31.1
- extrapulmonary systemic A31.8
- fortuitum A31.8
- intracellulare (Battey bacillus) A31.Ø
- kakaferifu A31.8
- kansasii (yellow bacillus) A31.Ø
- kasongo A31.8
- leprae —*see also* Leprosy A3Ø.9
- luciflavum A31.1
- marinum (M. balnei) A31.1
- nonspecific —*see* Mycobacterium, atypical
- pulmonary (atypical) A31.Ø
  - tuberculous —*see* Tuberculosis, pulmonary
- scrofulaceum A31.8
- simiae A31.8
- systemic, extrapulmonary A31.8
- szulgai A31.8
- terrae A31.8
- triviale A31.8
- tuberculosis (human, bovine) —*see* Tuberculosis
- ulcerans A31.1
- xenopi A31.8

Mycoplasma (M.) **pneumoniae, as cause of disease classified elsewhere** B96.Ø
Mycosis, mycotic B49
- cutaneous NEC B36.9
- ear B36.9 ⬅
  - in ◀
    - aspergillosis B44.89 ◀
    - candidiasis B37.84 ◀
    - moniliasis B37.84 ◀
- fungoides (extranodal) (solid organ) C84.Ø-
- mouth B37.Ø
- nails B35.1
- opportunistic B48.8
- skin NEC B36.9
- specified NEC B48.8
- stomatitis B37.Ø
- vagina, vaginitis (candidal) B37.3

Mydriasis (pupil) H57.Ø4
Myelatelia QØ6.1
Myelinolysis, pontine, central G37.2
Myelitis (acute) (ascending) (childhood) (chronic) (descending) (diffuse) (disseminated) (idiopathic) (pressure) (progressive) (spinal cord) (subacute) —*see also* Encephalitis GØ4.91
- herpes simplex BØØ.82
- herpes zoster BØ2.24
- in diseases classified elsewhere GØ5.4
- necrotizing, subacute G37.4
- optic neuritis in G36.Ø
- postchickenpox BØ1.12
- postherpetic BØ2.24
- postimmunization GØ4.Ø2
- postinfectious NEC GØ4.89
- postvaccinal GØ4.Ø2
- specified NEC GØ4.89
- syphilitic (transverse) A52.14
- toxic G92
- transverse (in demyelinating diseases of central nervous system) G37.3
- tuberculous A17.82
- varicella BØ1.12

Myeloblastic —*see* condition
Myeloblastoma
- granular cell —*see also* Neoplasm, connective tissue
  - malignant —*see* Neoplasm, connective tissue, malignant
- tongue D1Ø.1

Myelocele —*see* Spina bifida
Myelocystocele —*see* Spina bifida
Myelocytic —*see* condition
Myelodysplasia D46.9
- specified NEC D46.Z
- spinal cord (congenital) QØ6.1

Myelodysplastic syndrome D46.9
- with
  - 5q deletion D46.C
  - isolated del (5q) chromosomal abnormality C46.C
- specified NEC D46.Z

Myeloencephalitis —*see* Encephalitis
Myelofibrosis D75.81
- with myeloid metaplasia D47.4
- acute C94.4-
- idiopathic (chronic) D47.4
- primary D47.1
- secondary D75.81
  - in myeloproliferative disease D47.4

Myelogenous —*see* condition
Myeloid —*see* condition
Myelokathexis D7Ø.9
Myeloleukodystrophy E75.29
Myelolipoma —*see* Lipoma
Myeloma (multiple) C9Ø.Ø-
- monostotic C9Ø.3
  - plasma cell C9Ø.Ø-
- plasma cell C9Ø.Ø-
- solitary —*see also* Plasmacytoma, solitary C9Ø.3-

Myelomalacia G95.89
Myelomatosis C9Ø.Ø-
Myelomeningitis —*see* Meningoencephalitis
Myelomeningocele (spinal cord) —*see* Spina bifida
Myelo-osteo-musculodysplasia hereditaria Q79.8
Myelopathic
- anemia D64.89
- muscle atrophy —*see* Atrophy, muscle, spinal
- pain syndrome G89.Ø

Myelopathy (spinal cord) G95.9
- drug-induced G95.89
- in (due to)
  - degeneration or displacement, intervertebral disc NEC —*see* Disorder, disc, with, myelopathy
  - infection —*see* Encephalitis
  - intervertebral disc disorder —*see also* Disorder, disc, with, myelopathy
  - mercury —*see* subcategory T56.1
  - neoplastic disease —*see also* Neoplasm D49.9 *[G99.2]*
  - pernicious anemia D51.Ø *[G99.2]*
  - spondylosis —*see* Spondylosis, with myelopathy NEC
- necrotic (subacute) (vascular) G95.19
- radiation-induced G95.89
- spondylogenic NEC —*see* Spondylosis, with myelopathy NEC
- toxic G95.89
- transverse, acute G37.3
- vascular G95.19
- vitamin B12 E53.8 *[G32.Ø]*

Myelophthisis D61.82
Myeloradiculitis GØ4.91
Myeloradiculodysplasia (spinal) QØ6.1
Myelosarcoma C92.3-
Myelosclerosis D75.89
- with myeloid metaplasia D47.4
- disseminated, of nervous system G35
- megakaryocytic D47.4
  - with myeloid metaplasia D47.4

Myelosis
- acute C92.Ø-
- aleukemic C92.9-
- chronic D47.1
- erythremic (acute) C94.Ø-
- megakaryocytic C94.2-
- nonleukemic D72.828
- subacute C92.9-

Myiasis (cavernous) B87.9
- aural B87.4
- creeping B87.Ø
- cutaneous B87.Ø
- dermal B87.Ø
- ear (external) (middle) B87.4
- eye B87.2
- genitourinary B87.81
- intestinal B87.82
- laryngeal B87.3
- nasopharyngeal B87.3
- ocular B87.2
- orbit B87.2
- skin B87.Ø
- specified site NEC B87.89
- traumatic B87.1
- wound B87.1

Myoadenoma, prostate —*see* Hyperplasia, prostate
Myoblastoma
- granular cell —*see also* Neoplasm, connective tissue, benign
  - malignant —*see* Neoplasm, connective tissue, malignant
- tongue D1Ø.1

Myocardial —*see* condition
Myocardiopathy (congestive) (constrictive) (familial) (hypertrophic nonobstructive) (idiopathic) (infiltrative) (obstructive) (primary) (restrictive) (sporadic) —*see also* Cardiomyopathy I42.9
- alcoholic I42.6
- cobalt-beer I42.6
- glycogen storage E74.Ø2 *[I43]*
- hypertrophic obstructive I42.1
- in (due to)
  - beriberi E51.12
  - cardiac glycogenosis E74.Ø2 *[I43]*
  - Friedreich's ataxia G11.1 *[I43]*
  - myotonia atrophica G71.11 *[I43]*
  - progressive muscular dystrophy G71.Ø *[I43]*
- obscure (African) I42.8
- secondary I42.9
- thyrotoxic EØ5.9Ø *[I43]*
  - with storm EØ5.91 *[I43]*
- toxic NEC I42.7

M

- **Myocarditis** (with arteriosclerosis) (chronic) (fibroid) (interstitial) (old) (progressive) (senile) I51.4
  - with
    - rheumatic fever (conditions in I00) I09.0
      - active —*see* Myocarditis, acute, rheumatic
      - inactive or quiescent (with chorea) I09.0
  - active I40.9
    - rheumatic I01.2
      - with chorea (acute) (rheumatic) (Sydenham's) I02.0
  - acute or subacute (interstitial) I40.9
    - due to
      - streptococcus (beta-hemolytic) I01.2
    - idiopathic I40.1
    - rheumatic I01.2
      - with chorea (acute) (rheumatic) (Sydenham's) I02.0
    - specified NEC I40.8
  - aseptic of newborn B33.22
  - bacterial (acute) I40.0
  - Coxsackie (virus) B33.22
  - diphtheritic A36.81
  - eosinophilic I40.1
  - epidemic of newborn (Coxsackie) B33.22
  - Fiedler's (acute) (isolated) I40.1
  - giant cell (acute) (subacute) I40.1
  - gonococcal A54.83
  - granulomatous (idiopathic) (isolated) (nonspecific) I40.1
  - hypertensive —*see* Hypertension, heart
  - idiopathic (granulomatous) I40.1
  - in (due to)
    - diphtheria A36.81
    - epidemic louse-borne typhus A75.0 *[I41]*
    - Lyme disease A69.29
    - sarcoidosis D86.85
    - scarlet fever A38.1
    - toxoplasmosis (acquired) B58.81
    - typhoid A01.02
    - typhus NEC A75.9 *[I41]*
  - infective I40.0
  - influenzal —*see* Influenza, with, myocarditis
  - isolated (acute) I40.1
  - meningococcal A39.52
  - mumps B26.82
  - nonrheumatic, active I40.9
  - parenchymatous I40.9
  - pneumococcal I40.0
  - rheumatic (chronic) (inactive) (with chorea) I09.0
    - active or acute I01.2
      - with chorea (acute) (rheumatic) (Sydenham's) I02.0
  - rheumatoid —*see* Rheumatoid, carditis
  - septic I40.0
  - staphylococcal I40.0
  - suppurative I40.0
  - syphilitic (chronic) A52.06
  - toxic I40.8
    - rheumatic —*see* Myocarditis, acute, rheumatic
  - tuberculous A18.84
  - typhoid A01.02
  - valvular —*see* Endocarditis
  - virus, viral I40.0
    - of newborn (Coxsackie) B33.22
- **Myocardium, myocardial** —*see* condition
- **Myocardosis** —*see* Cardiomyopathy
- **Myoclonus, myoclonic, myoclonia** (familial) (essential) (multifocal) (simplex) G25.3
  - drug-induced G25.3
  - epilepsy —*see also* Epilepsy, generalized, specified NEC G40.4-
    - familial (progressive) G25.3
  - epileptica G40.409
    - with status epilepticus G40.401
  - facial G51.3
  - familial progressive G25.3
  - Friedreich's G25.3
  - jerks G25.3
  - massive G25.3
  - palatal G25.3
  - pharyngeal G25.3
- **Myocytolysis** I51.5
- **Myodiastasis** —*see* Diastasis, muscle
- **Myoendocarditis** —*see* Endocarditis
- **Myoepithelioma** —*see* Neoplasm, benign, by site
- **Myofasciitis** (acute) —*see* Myositis
- **Myofibroma** —*see also* Neoplasm, connective tissue, benign
  - uterus (cervix) (corpus) —*see* Leiomyoma
- **Myofibromatosis** D48.1
  - infantile Q89.8
- **Myofibrosis** M62.89
  - heart —*see* Myocarditis
  - scapulohumeral —*see* Lesion, shoulder, specified NEC
- **Myofibrositis** M79.7
  - scapulohumeral —*see* Lesion, shoulder, specified NEC
- **Myoglobulinuria, myoglobinuria** (primary) R82.1
- **Myokymia, facial** G51.4
- **Myolipoma** —*see* Lipoma
- **Myoma** —*see also* Neoplasm, connective tissue, benign
  - malignant —*see* Neoplasm, connective tissue, malignant
  - prostate D29.1
  - uterus (cervix) (corpus) —*see* Leiomyoma
- **Myomalacia** M62.89
- **Myometritis** —*see* Endometritis
- **Myometrium** —*see* condition
- **Myonecrosis, clostridial** A48.0
- **Myopathy** G72.9
  - acute
    - necrotizing G72.81
    - quadriplegic G72.81
  - alcoholic G72.1
  - benign congenital G71.2
  - central core G71.2
  - centronuclear G71.2
  - congenital (benign) G71.2
  - critical illness G72.81
  - distal G71.0
  - drug-induced G72.0
  - endocrine NEC E34.9 *[G73.7]*
  - extraocular muscles H05.82-
  - facioscapulohumeral G71.0
  - hereditary G71.9
    - specified NEC G71.8
  - immune NEC G72.49
  - in (due to)
    - Addison's disease E27.1 *[G73.7]*
    - alcohol G72.1
    - amyloidosis E85.0 *[G73.7]*
    - cretinism E00.9 *[G73.7]*
    - Cushing's syndrome E24.9 *[G73.7]*
    - drugs G72.0
    - endocrine disease NEC E34.9 *[G73.7]*
    - giant cell arteritis M31.6 *[G73.7]*
    - glycogen storage disease E74.00 *[G73.7]*
    - hyperadrenocorticism E24.9 *[G73.7]*
    - hyperparathyroidism NEC E21.3 *[G73.7]*
    - hypoparathyroidism E20.9 *[G73.7]*
    - hypopituitarism E23.0 *[G73.7]*
    - hypothyroidism E03.9 *[G73.7]*
    - infectious disease NEC B99 *[G73.7]*
    - lipid storage disease E75.6 *[G73.7]*
    - metabolic disease NEC E88.9 *[G73.7]*
    - myxedema E03.9 *[G73.7]*
    - parasitic disease NEC B89 *[G73.7]*
    - polyarteritis nodosa M30.0 *[G73.7]*
    - rheumatoid arthritis —*see* Rheumatoid, myopathy
    - sarcoidosis D86.87
    - scleroderma M34.82
    - sicca syndrome M35.03
    - Sjögren's syndrome M35.03
    - systemic lupus erythematosus M32.19
    - thyrotoxicosis (hyperthyroidism) E05.90 *[G73.7]*
      - with thyroid storm E05.91 *[G73.7]*
    - toxic agent NEC G72.2
  - inflammatory NEC G72.49
  - intensive care (ICU) G72.81
  - limb-girdle G71.0
  - mitochondrial NEC G71.3
  - myotubular G71.2
  - mytonic, proximal (PROMM) G71.11
  - nemaline G71.2
  - ocular G71.0
  - oculopharyngeal G71.0
  - of critical illness G72.81
  - primary G71.9
    - specified NEC G71.8
  - progressive NEC G72.89
  - proximal myotonic (PROMM) G71.11
  - rod G71.2
  - scapulohumeral G71.0
  - specified NEC G72.89
  - toxic G72.2
- **Myopericarditis** —*see also* Pericarditis
  - chronic rheumatic I09.2
- **Myopia** (axial) (congenital) H52.1-
  - degenerative (malignant) H44.2-
  - malignant H44.2-
  - pernicious H44.2-
  - progressive high (degenerative) H44.2-
- **Myosarcoma** —*see* Neoplasm, connective tissue, malignant
- **Myosis** (pupil) H57.03
  - stromal (endolymphatic) D39.0
- **Myositis** M60.9
  - clostridial A48.0
  - due to posture —*see* Myositis, specified type NEC
  - epidemic B33.0
  - fibrosa or fibrous (chronic), Volkmann's T79.6
  - foreign body granuloma —*see* Granuloma, foreign body
  - in (due to)
    - bilharziasis B65.9 *[M63.8-]*
    - cysticercosis B69.81
    - leprosy A30.9 *[M63.8-]*
    - mycosis B49 *[M63.8-]*
    - sarcoidosis D86.87
    - schistosomiasis B65.9 *[M63.8-]*
    - syphilis
      - late A52.78
      - secondary A51.49
    - toxoplasmosis (acquired) B58.82
    - trichinellosis B75 *[M63.8-]*
    - tuberculosis A18.09
  - inclusion body [IBM] G72.41
  - infective M60.009
    - arm M60.002
      - left M60.001
      - right M60.000
    - leg M60.005
      - left M60.004
      - right M60.003
    - lower limb M60.005
      - ankle M60.07-
      - foot M60.07-
      - lower leg M60.06-
      - thigh M60.05-
      - toe M60.07-
    - multiple sites M60.09
    - specified site NEC M60.08
    - upper limb M60.002
      - finger M60.04-
      - forearm M60.03-
      - hand M60.04-
      - shoulder region M60.01-
      - upper arm M60.02-

Myositis *(Continued)*
interstitial M60.10
ankle M60.17-
foot M60.17-
forearm M60.13-
hand M60.14-
lower leg M60.16-
multiple sites M60.19
shoulder region M60.11-
specified site NEC M60.18
thigh M60.15-
upper arm M60.12-
mycotic B49 *[M63.8-]*
ossificans or ossifying (circumscripta) —*see also* Ossification, muscle, specified NEC
in (due to)
burns M61.30
ankle M61.37-
foot M61.37-
forearm M61.33-
hand M61.34-
lower leg M61.36-
multiple sites M61.39
pelvic region M61.35-
shoulder region M61.31-
specified site NEC M61.38
thigh M61.35-
upper arm M61.32-
quadriplegia or paraplegia M61.20
ankle M61.27-
foot M61.27-
forearm M61.23-
hand M61.24-
lower leg M61.26-
multiple sites M61.29
pelvic region M61.25-
shoulder region M61.21-
specified site NEC M61.28
thigh M61.25-
upper arm M61.22-
progressiva M61.10
ankle M61.17-
finger M61.14-
foot M61.17-
forearm M61.13-
hand M61.14-
lower leg M61.16-

Myositis *(Continued)*
ossificans or ossifying *(Continued)*
progressiva *(Continued)*
multiple sites M61.19
pelvic region M61.15-
shoulder region M61.11-
specified site NEC M61.18
thigh M61.15-
toe M61.17-
upper arm M61.12-
traumatica M61.00
ankle M61.07-
foot M61.07-
forearm M61.03-
hand M61.04-
lower leg M61.06-
multiple sites M61.09
pelvic region M61.05-
shoulder region M61.01-
specified site NEC M61.08
thigh M61.05-
upper arm M61.02-
purulent —*see* Myositis, infective
specified type NEC M60.80
ankle M60.87-
foot M60.87-
forearm M60.83-
hand M60.84-
lower leg M60.86-
multiple sites M60.89
pelvic region M60.85-
shoulder region M60.81-
specified site NEC M60.88
thigh M60.85-
upper arm M60.82-
suppurative —*see* Myositis, infective
traumatic (old) —*see* Myositis, specified type NEC
Myospasia impulsiva F95.2
Myotonia (acquisita) (intermittens) M62.89
atrophica G71.11
chondrodystrophic G71.13
congenita (acetazolamide responsive) (dominant) (recessive) G71.12
drug-induced G71.14
dystrophica G71.11
fluctuans G71.19

Myotonia *(Continued)*
levior G71.12
permanens G71.19
symptomatic G71.19
Myotonic pupil —*see* Anomaly, pupil, function, tonic pupil
Myriapodiasis B88.2
Myringitis H73.2-
with otitis media —*see* Otitis, media
acute H73.00-
bullous H73.01-
specified NEC H73.09-
bullous —*see* Myringitis, acute, bullous
chronic H73.1-
Mysophobia F40.228
Mytilotoxism —*see* Poisoning, fish
Myxadenitis labialis K13.0
Myxedema (adult) (idiocy) (infantile) (juvenile) —*see also* Hypothyroidism E03.9
circumscribed E05.90
with storm E05.91
coma E03.5
congenital E00.1
cutis L98.5
localized (pretibial) E05.90
with storm E05.91
papular L98.5
Myxochondrosarcoma —*see* Neoplasm, cartilage, malignant
Myxofibroma —*see* Neoplasm, connective tissue, benign
odontogenic —*see* Cyst, calcifying odontogenic
Myxofibrosarcoma —*see* Neoplasm, connective tissue, malignant
Myxolipoma D17.9
Myxoliposarcoma —*see* Neoplasm, connective tissue, malignant
Myxoma —*see also* Neoplasm, connective tissue, benign
nerve sheath —*see* Neoplasm, nerve, benign
odontogenic —*see* Cyst, calcifying odontogenic
Myxosarcoma —*see* Neoplasm, connective tissue, malignant

M

N

Naegeli's
disease Q82.8
leukemia, monocytic C93.1-
Naegleriasis (with meningoencephalitis) B6Ø.2
Naffziger's syndrome G54.Ø
Naga sore —*see* Ulcer, skin
Nägele's pelvis M95.5
with disproportion (fetopelvic) O33.Ø
causing obstructed labor O65.Ø
Nail —*see also* condition
biting F98.8
patella syndrome Q87.2
Nanism, nanosomia —*see* Dwarfism
Nanophyetiasis B66.8
Nanukayami A27.89
Napkin rash L22
Narcolepsy G47.419
with cataplexy G47.411
in conditions classified elsewhere G47.429
with cataplexy G47.421
Narcosis RØ6.89
Narcotism —*see* Dependence
NARP (Neuropathy, Ataxia and Retinitis pigmentosa) syndrome E88.49
Narrow
anterior chamber angle H4Ø.Ø3-
gingival width (of periodontal soft tissue) KØ5.5 ◀
pelvis —*see* Contraction, pelvis
Narrowing —*see also* Stenosis
artery I77.1
auditory, internal I65.8
basilar —*see* Occlusion, artery, basilar
carotid —*see* Occlusion, artery, carotid
cerebellar —*see* Occlusion, artery, cerebellar
cerebral —*see* Occlusion artery, cerebral
choroidal —*see* Occlusion, artery, cerebral, specified NEC
communicating posterior —*see* Occlusion, artery, cerebral, specified NEC
coronary —*see also* Disease, heart, ischemic, atherosclerotic
congenital Q24.5
syphilitic A5Ø.54 *[I52]*
due to syphilis NEC A52.Ø6
hypophyseal —*see* Occlusion, artery, cerebral, specified NEC
pontine —*see* Occlusion, artery, cerebral, specified NEC
precerebral —*see* Occlusion, artery, precerebral
vertebral —*see* Occlusion, artery, vertebral
auditory canal (external) —*see* Stenosis, external ear canal
eustachian tube —*see* Obstruction, eustachian tube
eyelid —*see* Disorder, eyelid function
larynx J38.6
mesenteric artery —*see also* Ischemia, intestine, acute K55.Ø59 ⬅
palate M26.89
palpebral fissure —*see* Disorder, eyelid function
ureter N13.5
with infection N13.6
urethra —*see* Stricture, urethra
Narrowness, abnormal, eyelid Q1Ø.3
Nasal —*see* condition
Nasolachrymal, nasolacrimal —*see* condition
Nasopharyngeal —*see also* condition
pituitary gland Q89.2
torticollis M43.6
Nasopharyngitis (acute) (infective) (streptococcal) (subacute) JØØ
chronic (suppurative) (ulcerative) J31.1
Nasopharynx, nasopharyngeal —*see* condition
Natal tooth, teeth KØØ.6
Nausea (without vomiting) R11.Ø
with vomiting R11.2
gravidarum —*see* Hyperemesis, gravidarum
marina T75.3
navalis T75.3
Navel —*see* condition
Neapolitan fever —*see* Brucellosis
Near drowning T75.1
Nearsightedness —*see* Myopia
Near-syncope R55
Nebula, cornea —*see* Opacity, cornea
Necator americanus infestation B76.1
Necatoriasis B76.1
Neck —*see* condition
Necrobiosis R68.89
lipoidica NEC L92.1
with diabetes —*see* EØ8-E13 with .62Ø
Necrolysis, toxic epidermal L51.2
due to drug
correct substance properly administered —*see* Table of Drugs and Chemicals, by drug, adverse effect
overdose or wrong substance given or taken —*see* Table of Drugs and Chemicals, by drug, poisoning
Necrophilia F65.89
Necrosis, necrotic (ischemic) —*see also* Gangrene
adrenal (capsule) (gland) E27.49
amputation stump (surgical) (late) T87.5Ø
arm T87.5-
leg T87.5-
antrum J32.Ø
aorta (hyaline) —*see also* Aneurysm, aorta
cystic medial —*see* Dissection, aorta
artery I77.5
bladder (aseptic) (sphincter) N32.89
bone —*see also* Osteonecrosis M87.9
aseptic or avascular —*see* Osteonecrosis
idiopathic M87.ØØ
ethmoid J32.2
jaw M27.2
tuberculous —*see* Tuberculosis, bone
brain I67.89
breast (aseptic) (fat) (segmental) N64.1
bronchus J98.Ø9
central nervous system NEC I67.89
cerebellar I67.89
cerebral I67.89
colon —*see also* Infarct, intestine K55.Ø49 ⬅
cornea H18.89- ⬅
cortical (acute) (renal) N17.1
cystic medial (aorta) —*see* Dissection, aorta
dental pulp KØ4.1
esophagus K22.8
ethmoid (bone) J32.2
eyelid —*see* Disorder, eyelid, degenerative
fat, fatty (generalized) —*see also* Disorder, soft tissue, specified type NEC
abdominal wall K65.4
breast (aseptic) (segmental) N64.1
localized —*see* Degeneration, by site, fatty
mesentery K65.4
omentum K65.4
pancreas K86.89 ⬅
peritoneum K65.4
skin (subcutaneous), newborn P83.Ø
subcutaneous, due to birth injury P15.6
gallbladder —*see* Cholecystitis, acute
heart —*see* Infarct, myocardium
hip, aseptic or avascular —*see* Osteonecrosis, by type, femur
intestine (acute) (hemorrhagic) (massive) —*see also* Infarct, intestine K55.Ø69 ⬅
jaw M27.2
kidney (bilateral) N28.Ø
acute N17.9
cortical (acute) (bilateral) N17.1
with ectopic or molar pregnancy OØ8.4
medullary (bilateral) (in acute renal failure) (papillary) N17.2
Necrosis, necrotic *(Continued)*
kidney *(Continued)*
papillary (bilateral) (in acute renal failure) N17.2
tubular N17.Ø
with ectopic or molar pregnancy OØ8.4
complicating
abortion —*see* Abortion, by type, complicated by, tubular necrosis
ectopic or molar pregnancy OØ8.4
pregnancy —*see* Pregnancy, complicated by, diseases of, specified type or system NEC
following ectopic or molar pregnancy OØ8.4
traumatic T79.5
larynx J38.7
liver (with hepatic failure) (cell) —*see* Failure, hepatic
hemorrhagic, central K76.2
lung J85.Ø
lymphatic gland —*see* Lymphadenitis, acute
mammary gland (fat) (segmental) N64.1
mastoid (chronic) —*see* Mastoiditis, chronic
medullary (acute) (renal) N17.2
mesentery —*see also* Infarct, intestine K55.Ø69 ⬅
fat K65.4
mitral valve —*see* Insufficiency, mitral
myocardium, myocardial —*see* Infarct, myocardium
nose J34.Ø
omentum (with mesenteric infarction) —*see also* Infarct, intestine K55.Ø69 ⬅
fat K65.4
orbit, orbital —*see* Osteomyelitis, orbit
ossicles, ear —*see* Abnormal, ear ossicles
ovary N7Ø.92
pancreas (aseptic) (duct) (fat) K86.89 ⬅
acute (infective) —*see* Pancreatitis, acute
infective —*see* Pancreatitis, acute
papillary (acute) (renal) N17.2
perineum N9Ø.89
peritoneum (with mesenteric infarction) —*see also* Infarct, intestine K55.Ø69 ⬅
fat K65.4
pharynx JØ2.9
in granulocytopenia —*see* Neutropenia
Vincent's A69.1
phosphorus —*see* subcategory T54.2
pituitary (gland) E23.Ø ⬅
postpartum O99.285 ◀
Sheehan O99.285 ◀
pressure —*see* Ulcer, pressure, by site
pulmonary J85.Ø
pulp (dental) KØ4.1
radiation —*see* Necrosis, by site
radium —*see* Necrosis, by site
renal —*see* Necrosis, kidney
sclera H15.89
scrotum N5Ø.89 ⬅
skin or subcutaneous tissue NEC I96
spine, spinal (column) —*see also* Osteonecrosis, by type, vertebra
cord G95.19
spleen D73.5
stomach K31.89
stomatitis (ulcerative) A69.Ø
subcutaneous fat, newborn P83.8
subendocardial (acute) I21.4
chronic I25.89
suprarenal (capsule) (gland) E27.49
testis N5Ø.89 ⬅
thymus (gland) E32.8
tonsil J35.8
trachea J39.8
tuberculous NEC —*see* Tuberculosis
tubular (acute) (anoxic) (renal) (toxic) N17.Ø
postprocedural N99.Ø
vagina N89.8

◀ New ⬅ Revised ~~deleted~~ Deleted

Necrosis, necrotic *(Continued)*
- vertebra *—see also* Osteonecrosis, by type, vertebra
  - tuberculous A18.01
- vulva N90.89
- X-ray *—see* Necrosis, by site

Necrospermia *—see* Infertility, male

Need (for)
- care provider because (of)
  - assistance with personal care Z74.1
  - continuous supervision required Z74.3
  - impaired mobility Z74.09
  - no other household member able to render care Z74.2
  - specified reason NEC Z74.8
- immunization *—see* Vaccination
- vaccination *—see* Vaccination

Neglect
- adult
  - confirmed T74.01
  - history of Z91.412
  - suspected T76.01
- child (childhood)
  - confirmed T74.02
  - history of Z62.812
  - suspected T76.02
- emotional, in childhood Z62.898
- hemispatial R41.4
- left-sided R41.4
- sensory R41.4
- visuospatial R41.4

Neisserian infection NEC *—see* Gonococcus

Nelaton's syndrome G60.8

Nelson's syndrome E24.1

Nematodiasis (intestinal) B82.0
- Ancylostoma B76.0

Neonatal *—see also* Newborn
- acne L70.4
- bradycardia P29.12
- screening, abnormal findings on P09
- tachycardia P29.11
- tooth, teeth K00.6

Neonatorum *—see* condition

Neoplasia
- endocrine, multiple (MEN) E31.20
  - type I E31.21
  - type IIA E31.22
  - type IIB E31.23
- intraepithelial (histologically confirmed)
  - anal (AIN) (histologically confirmed) K62.82
    - grade I K62.82
    - grade II K62.82
    - severe D01.3
  - cervical glandular (histologically confirmed) D06.9
  - cervix (uteri) (CIN) (histologically confirmed) N87.9
    - glandular D06.9
    - grade I N87.0
    - grade II N87.1
    - grade III (severe dysplasia) *—see also* Carcinoma, cervix uteri, in situ D06.9
  - prostate (histologically confirmed) (PIN) N42.31 ⬅
    - grade I N42.31 ⬅
    - grade II N42.31 ⬅
    - grade III (severe dysplasia) D07.5 ◀
    - ~~severe D07.5~~
  - vagina (histologically confirmed) (VAIN) N89.3
    - grade I N89.0
    - grade II N89.1
    - grade III (severe dysplasia) D07.2
  - vulva (histologically confirmed) (VIN) N90.3
    - grade I N90.0
    - grade II N90.1
    - grade III (severe dysplasia) D07.1

Neoplasm, neoplastic *—see also* Table of Neoplasms
- lipomatous, benign *—see* Lipoma

Neovascularization
- ciliary body *—see* Disorder, iris, vascular
- cornea H16.40-
  - deep H16.44-
  - ghost vessels *—see* Ghost, vessels
  - localized H16.43-
  - pannus *—see* Pannus
- iris *—see* Disorder, iris, vascular
- retina H35.05-

Nephralgia N23

Nephritis, nephritic (albuminuric) (azotemic) (congenital) (disseminated) (epithelial) (familial) (focal) (granulomatous) (hemorrhagic) (infantile) (nonsuppurative, excretory) (uremic) N05.9
- with
  - dense deposit disease N05.6
  - diffuse
    - crescentic glomerulonephritis N05.7
    - endocapillary proliferative glomerulonephritis N05.4
    - membranous glomerulonephritis N05.2
    - mesangial proliferative glomerulonephritis N05.3
    - mesangiocapillary glomerulonephritis N05.5
  - edema *—see* Nephrosis
  - focal and segmental glomerular lesions N05.1
  - foot process disease N04.9
  - glomerular lesion
    - diffuse sclerosing N05.8
    - hypocomplementemic *—see* Nephritis, membranoproliferative
    - IgA *—see* Nephropathy, IgA
    - lobular, lobulonodular *—see* Nephritis, membranoproliferative
    - nodular *—see* Nephritis, membranoproliferative
  - lesion of
    - glomerulonephritis, proliferative N05.8
    - renal necrosis N05.9
  - minor glomerular abnormality N05.0
  - specified morphological changes NEC N05.8
- acute N00.9
  - with
    - dense deposit disease N00.6
    - diffuse
      - crescentic glomerulonephritis N00.7
      - endocapillary proliferative glomerulonephritis N00.4
      - membranous glomerulonephritis N00.2
      - mesangial proliferative glomerulonephritis N00.3
      - mesangiocapillary glomerulonephritis N00.5
    - focal and segmental glomerular lesions N00.1
    - minor glomerular abnormality N00.0
    - specified morphological changes NEC N00.8
- amyloid E85.4 *[N08]*
- antiglomerular basement membrane (anti-GBM) antibody NEC
  - in Goodpasture's syndrome M31.0
- antitubular basement membrane (tubulo-interstitial) NEC N12
  - toxic *—see* Nephropathy, toxic
- arteriolar *—see* Hypertension, kidney
- arteriosclerotic *—see* Hypertension, kidney
- ascending *—see* Nephritis, tubulo-interstitial
- atrophic N03.9

Nephritis, nephritic *(Continued)*
- Balkan (endemic) N15.0
- calculous, calculus *—see* Calculus, kidney
- cardiac *—see* Hypertension, kidney
- cardiovascular *—see* Hypertension, kidney
- chronic N03.9
  - with
    - dense deposit disease N03.6
    - diffuse
      - crescentic glomerulonephritis N03.7
      - endocapillary proliferative glomerulonephritis N03.4
      - membranous glomerulonephritis N03.2
      - mesangial proliferative glomerulonephritis N03.3
      - mesangiocapillary glomerulonephritis N03.5
    - focal and segmental glomerular lesions N03.1
    - minor glomerular abnormality N03.0
    - specified morphological changes NEC N03.8
  - arteriosclerotic *—see* Hypertension, kidney
- cirrhotic N26.9
- complicating pregnancy O26.83-
- croupous N00.9
- degenerative *—see* Nephrosis
- diffuse sclerosing N05.8
- due to
  - diabetes mellitus *—see* E08-E13 with .21
  - subacute bacterial endocarditis I33.0
  - systemic lupus erythematosus (chronic) M32.14
  - typhoid fever A01.09
- gonococcal (acute) (chronic) A54.21
- hypocomplementemic *—see* Nephritis, membranoproliferative
- IgA *—see* Nephropathy, IgA
- immune complex (circulating) NEC N05.8
- infective *—see* Nephritis, tubulo-interstitial
- interstitial *—see* Nephritis, tubulo-interstitial
- lead N14.3
- membranoproliferative (diffuse) (type 1 or 3) *—see also* N00-N07 with fourth character .5 N05.5
  - type 2 *—see also* N00-N07 with fourth character .6 N05.6
- minimal change N05.0
- necrotic, necrotizing NEC *—see also* N00-N07 with fourth character .8 N05.8
- nephrotic *—see* Nephrosis
- nodular *—see* Nephritis, membranoproliferative
- polycystic Q61.3
  - adult type Q61.2
  - autosomal
    - dominant Q61.2
    - recessive NEC Q61.19
  - childhood type NEC Q61.19
  - infantile type NEC Q61.19
- poststreptococcal N05.9
  - acute N00.9
  - chronic N03.9
  - rapidly progressive N01.9
- proliferative NEC *—see also* N00-N07 with fourth character .8 N05.8
- purulent *—see* Nephritis, tubulo-interstitial
- rapidly progressive N01.9
  - with
    - dense deposit disease N01.6
    - diffuse
      - crescentic glomerulonephritis N01.7
      - endocapillary proliferative glomerulonephritis N01.4

Nephritis, nephritic *(Continued)*
rapidly progressive *(Continued)*
with *(Continued)*
diffuse *(Continued)*
membranous glomerulonephritis N01.2
mesangial proliferative glomerulonephritis N01.3
mesangiocapillary glomerulonephritis N01.5
focal and segmental glomerular lesions N01.1
minor glomerular abnormality N01.0
specified morphological changes NEC N01.8
salt losing or wasting NEC N28.89
saturnine N14.3
sclerosing, diffuse N05.8
septic —*see* Nephritis, tubulo-interstitial
specified pathology NEC —*see also* N00-N07 with fourth character .8 N05.8
subacute N01.9
suppurative —*see* Nephritis, tubulo-interstitial
syphilitic (late) A52.75
congenital A50.59 *[N08]*
early (secondary) A51.44
toxic —*see* Nephropathy, toxic
tubal, tubular —*see* Nephritis, tubulo-interstitial
tuberculous A18.11
tubulo-interstitial (in) N12
acute (infectious) N10
chronic (infectious) N11.9
nonobstructive N11.8
reflux-associated N11.0
obstructive N11.1
specified NEC N11.8
due to
brucellosis A23.9 *[N16]*
cryoglobulinemia D89.1 *[N16]*
glycogen storage disease E74.00 *[N16]*
Sjögren's syndrome M35.04
vascular —*see* Hypertension, kidney
war N00.9
Nephroblastoma (epithelial) (mesenchymal) C64-
Nephrocalcinosis E83.59 *[N29]*
Nephrocystitis, pustular —*see* Nephritis, tubulo-interstitial
Nephrolithiasis (congenital) (pelvis) (recurrent) —*see also* Calculus, kidney
Nephroma C64-
mesoblastic D41.0-
Nephronephritis —*see* Nephrosis
Nephronophthisis Q61.5
Nephropathia epidemica A98.5
Nephropathy —*see also* Nephritis N28.9
with
edema —*see* Nephrosis
glomerular lesion —*see* Glomerulonephritis
amyloid, hereditary E85.0
analgesic N14.0
with medullary necrosis, acute N17.2
Balkan (endemic) N15.0
chemical —*see* Nephropathy, toxic
diabetic —*see* E08-E13 with .21
drug-induced N14.2
specified NEC N14.1
focal and segmental hyalinosis or sclerosis N02.1
heavy metal-induced N14.3
hereditary NEC N07.9
with
dense deposit disease N07.6
diffuse
crescentic glomerulonephritis N07.7
endocapillary proliferative glomerulonephritis N07.4

Nephropathy *(Continued)*
hereditary NEC *(Continued)*
with *(Continued)*
diffuse *(Continued)*
membranous glomerulonephritis N07.2
mesangial proliferative glomerulonephritis N07.3
mesangiocapillary glomerulonephritis N07.5
focal and segmental glomerular lesions N07.1
minor glomerular abnormality N07.0
specified morphological changes NEC N07.8
hypercalcemic N25.89
hypertensive —*see* Hypertension, kidney
hypokalemic (vacuolar) N25.89
IgA N02.8
with glomerular lesion N02.9
focal and segmental hyalinosis or sclerosis N02.1
membranoproliferative (diffuse) N02.5
membranous (diffuse) N02.2
mesangial proliferative (diffuse) N02.3
mesangiocapillary (diffuse) N02.5
proliferative NEC N02.8
specified pathology NEC N02.8
lead N14.3
membranoproliferative (diffuse) N02.5
membranous (diffuse) N02.2
mesangial (IgA/IgG) —*see* Nephropathy, IgA
proliferative (diffuse) N02.3
mesangiocapillary (diffuse) N02.5
obstructive N13.8
phenacetin N17.2
phosphate-losing N25.0
potassium depletion N25.89
pregnancy-related O26.83-
proliferative NEC (*see also* N00-N07 with fourth character .8) N05.8
protein-losing N25.89
saturnine N14.3
sickle-cell D57.- *[N08]*
toxic NEC N14.4
due to
drugs N14.2
analgesic N14.0
specified NEC N14.1
heavy metals N14.3
vasomotor N17.0
water-losing N25.89
Nephroptosis N28.83
Nephropyosis —*see* Abscess, kidney
Nephrorrhagia N28.89
Nephrosclerosis (arteriolar) (arteriosclerotic) (chronic) (hyaline) —*see also* Hypertension, kidney
hyperplastic —*see* Hypertension, kidney
senile N26.9
Nephrosis, nephrotic (Epstein's) (syndrome) (congenital) N04.9
with
foot process disease N04.9
glomerular lesion N04.1
hypocomplementemic N04.5
acute N04.9
anoxic —*see* Nephrosis, tubular
chemical —*see* Nephrosis, tubular
cholemic K76.7
diabetic —*see* E08-E13 with .21
Finnish type (congenital) Q89.8
hemoglobin N10
hemoglobinuric —*see* Nephrosis, tubular
in
amyloidosis E85.4 *[N08]*
diabetes mellitus —*see* E08-E13 with .21
epidemic hemorrhagic fever A98.5
malaria (malariae) B52.0
ischemic —*see* Nephrosis, tubular
lipoid N04.9

Nephrosis, nephrotic *(Continued)*
lower nephron —*see* Nephrosis, tubular
malarial (malariae) B52.0
minimal change N04.0
myoglobin N10
necrotizing —*see* Nephrosis, tubular
osmotic (sucrose) N25.89
radiation N04.9
syphilitic (late) A52.75
toxic —*see* Nephrosis, tubular
tubular (acute) N17.0
postprocedural N99.0
radiation N04.9
Nephrosonephritis, hemorrhagic (endemic) A98.5
Nephrostomy
attention to Z43.6
status Z93.6
Nerve —*see also* condition
injury —*see* Injury, nerve, by body site
Nerves R45.0
Nervous —*see also* condition R45.0
heart F45.8
stomach F45.8
tension R45.0
Nervousness R45.0
Nesidioblastoma
pancreas D13.7
specified site NEC —*see* Neoplasm, benign, by site
unspecified site D13.7
Nettleship's syndrome Q82.2
Neumann's disease or syndrome L10.1
Neuralgia, neuralgic (acute) M79.2
accessory (nerve) G52.8
acoustic (nerve) —*see* subcategory H93.3
auditory (nerve) —*see* subcategory H93.3
ciliary G44.009
intractable G44.001
not intractable G44.009
cranial
nerve —*see also* Disorder, nerve, cranial
fifth or trigeminal —*see* Neuralgia, trigeminal
postherpetic, postzoster B02.29
ear —*see* subcategory H92.0
facialis vera G51.1
Fothergill's —*see* Neuralgia, trigeminal
glossopharyngeal (nerve) G52.1
Horton's G44.099
intractable G44.091
not intractable G44.099
Hunt's B02.21
hypoglossal (nerve) G52.3
infraorbital —*see* Neuralgia, trigeminal
malarial —*see* Malaria
migrainous G44.009
intractable G44.001
not intractable G44.009
Morton's G57.6-
nerve, cranial —*see* Disorder, nerve, cranial
nose G52.0
occipital M54.81
olfactory G52.0
penis N48.9
perineum R10.2
postherpetic NEC B02.29
trigeminal B02.22
pubic region R10.2
scrotum R10.2
Sluder's G44.89
specified nerve NEC G58.8
spermatic cord R10.2
sphenopalatine (ganglion) G90.09
trifacial —*see* Neuralgia, trigeminal
trigeminal G50.0
postherpetic, postzoster B02.22
vagus (nerve) G52.2
writer's F48.8
organic G25.89

Neurapraxia —*see* Injury, nerve
Neurasthenia F48.8
cardiac F45.8
gastric F45.8
heart F45.8
Neurilemmoma —*see also* Neoplasm, nerve, benign
acoustic (nerve) D33.3
malignant —*see also* Neoplasm, nerve, malignant
acoustic (nerve) C72.4
Neurilemmosarcoma —*see* Neoplasm, nerve, malignant
Neurinoma —*see* Neoplasm, nerve, benign
Neurinomatosis —*see* Neoplasm, nerve, uncertain behavior
Neuritis (rheumatoid) M79.2
abducens (nerve) —*see* Strabismus, paralytic, sixth nerve
accessory (nerve) G52.8
acoustic (nerve) —*see also* subcategory H93.3
in (due to)
infectious disease NEC B99 *[H94.Ø-]*
parasitic disease NEC B89 *[H94.Ø-]*
syphilitic A52.15
alcoholic G62.1
with psychosis —*see* Psychosis, alcoholic
amyloid, any site E85.4 *[G63]*
auditory (nerve) —*see* subcategory H93.3
brachial —*see* Radiculopathy
due to displacement, intervertebral disc —*see* Disorder, disc, cervical, with neuritis
cranial nerve
due to Lyme disease A69.22
eighth or acoustic or auditory —*see* subcategory H93.3
eleventh or accessory G52.8
fifth or trigeminal G51.Ø
first or olfactory G52.Ø
fourth or trochlear —*see* Strabismus, paralytic, fourth nerve
second or optic —*see* Neuritis, optic
seventh or facial G51.8
newborn (birth injury) P11.3
sixth or abducent —*see* Strabismus, paralytic, sixth nerve
tenth or vagus G52.2
third or oculomotor —*see* Strabismus, paralytic, third nerve
twelfth or hypoglossal G52.3
Déjérine-Sottas G6Ø.Ø
diabetic (mononeuropathy) —*see* EØ8-E13 with .41
polyneuropathy —*see* EØ8-E13 with .42
due to
beriberi E51.11
displacement, prolapse or rupture, intervertebral disc —*see* Disorder, disc, with, radiculopathy
herniation, nucleus pulposus M51.9 *[G55]*
endemic E51.11
facial G51.8
newborn (birth injury) P11.3
general —*see* Polyneuropathy
geniculate ganglion G51.1
due to herpes (zoster) BØ2.21
gouty —*see also* Gout, by type M1Ø.9 *[G63]* (Revised)
hypoglossal (nerve) G52.3
ilioinguinal (nerve) G57.9-
infectious (multiple) NEC G61.Ø
interstitial hypertrophic progressive G6Ø.Ø
lumbar M54.16
lumbosacral M54.17
multiple —*see also* Polyneuropathy
endemic E51.11
infective, acute G61.Ø
multiplex endemica E51.11
nerve root —*see* Radiculopathy
oculomotor (nerve) —*see* Strabismus, paralytic, third nerve
Neuritis *(Continued)*
olfactory nerve G52.Ø
optic (nerve) (hereditary) (sympathetic) H46.9
with demyelination G36.Ø
in myelitis G36.Ø
nutritional H46.2
papillitis —*see* Papillitis, optic
retrobulbar H46.1-
specified type NEC H46.8
toxic H46.3
peripheral (nerve) G62.9
multiple —*see* Polyneuropathy
single —*see* Mononeuritis
pneumogastric (nerve) G52.2
postherpetic, postzoster BØ2.29
progressive hypertrophic interstitial G6Ø.Ø
retrobulbar —*see also* Neuritis, optic, retrobulbar
in (due to)
late syphilis A52.15
meningococcal infection A39.82
meningococcal A39.82
syphilitic A52.15
sciatic (nerve) —*see also* Sciatica
due to displacement of intervertebral disc —*see* Disorder, disc, with, radiculopathy
serum —*see also* Reaction, serum T8Ø.69
shoulder-girdle G54.5
specified nerve NEC G58.8
spinal (nerve) root —*see* Radiculopathy
syphilitic A52.15
thenar (median) G56.1-
thoracic M54.14
toxic NEC G62.2
trochlear (nerve) —*see* Strabismus, paralytic, fourth nerve
vagus (nerve) G52.2
Neuroastrocytoma —*see* Neoplasm, uncertain behavior, by site
Neuroavitaminosis E56.9 *[G99.8]*
Neuroblastoma
olfactory C3Ø.Ø
specified site —*see* Neoplasm, malignant, by site
unspecified site C74.9Ø
Neurochorioretinitis —*see* Chorioretinitis
Neurocirculatory asthenia F45.8
Neurocysticercosis B69.Ø
Neurocytoma —*see* Neoplasm, benign, by site
Neurodermatitis (circumscribed) (circumscripta) (local) L28.Ø
atopic L2Ø.81
diffuse (Brocq) L2Ø.81
disseminated L2Ø.81
Neuroencephalomyelopathy, optic G36.Ø
Neuroepithelioma —*see also* Neoplasm, malignant, by site
olfactory C3Ø.Ø
Neurofibroma —*see also* Neoplasm, nerve, benign
melanotic —*see* Neoplasm, nerve, benign
multiple —*see* Neurofibromatosis
plexiform —*see* Neoplasm, nerve, benign
Neurofibromatosis (multiple) (nonmalignant) Q85.ØØ
acoustic Q85.Ø2
malignant —*see* Neoplasm, nerve, malignant
specified NEC Q85.Ø9
type 1 (von Recklinghausen) Q85.Ø1
type 2 Q85.Ø2
Neurofibrosarcoma —*see* Neoplasm, nerve, malignant
Neurogenic —*see also* condition
bladder (*see also* Dysfunction, bladder, neuromuscular) N31.9
cauda equina syndrome G83.4
bowel NEC K59.2
heart F45.8
Neuroglioma —*see* Neoplasm, uncertain behavior, by site
Neurolabyrinthitis (of Dix and Hallpike) —*see* Neuronitis, vestibular
Neurolathyrism —*see* Poisoning, food, noxious, plant
Neuroleprosy A3Ø.9
Neuroma —*see also* Neoplasm, nerve, benign
acoustic (nerve) D33.3
amputation (stump) (traumatic) (surgical complication) (late) T87.3-
arm T87.3-
leg T87.3-
digital (toe) G57.6-
interdigital G58.8 (Revised)
lower limb toe G57.8- (Revised)
upper limb G56.8-
intermetatarsal G57.8-
Morton's G57.6-
nonneoplastic
arm G56.9-
leg G57.9-
lower extremity G57.9-
upper extremity G56.9-
optic (nerve) D33.3
plantar G57.6-
plexiform —*see* Neoplasm, nerve, benign
surgical (nonneoplastic)
arm G56.9-
leg G57.9-
lower extremity G57.9-
upper extremity G56.9-
Neuromyalgia —*see* Neuralgia
Neuromyasthenia (epidemic) (postinfectious) G93.3
Neuromyelitis G36.9
ascending G61.Ø
optica G36.Ø
Neuromyopathy G7Ø.9
paraneoplastic D49.9 *[G13.Ø]*
Neuromyotonia (Isaacs) G71.19
Neuronevus —*see* Nevus
Neuronitis G58.9
ascending (acute) G57.2-
vestibular H81.2-
Neuroparalytic —*see* condition
Neuropathy, neuropathic G62.9
acute motor G62.81
alcoholic G62.1
with psychosis —*see* Psychosis, alcoholic
arm G56.9-
autonomic, peripheral —*see* Neuropathy, peripheral, autonomic
axillary G56.9-
bladder N31.9
atonic (motor) (sensory) N31.2
autonomous N31.2
flaccid N31.2
nonreflex N31.2
reflex N31.1
uninhibited N31.Ø
brachial plexus G54.Ø
cervical plexus G54.2
chronic
progressive segmentally demyelinating G62.89
relapsing demyelinating G62.89
Déjérine-Sottas G6Ø.Ø
diabetic —*see* EØ8-E13 with .4Ø
mononeuropathy —*see* EØ8-E13 with .41
polyneuropathy —*see* EØ8-E13 with .42
entrapment G58.9
iliohypogastric nerve G57.8-
ilioinguinal nerve G57.8-
lateral cutaneous nerve of thigh G57.1-
median nerve G56.Ø-
obturator nerve G57.8-
peroneal nerve G57.3-
posterior tibial nerve G57.5-
saphenous nerve G57.8-
ulnar nerve G56.2-

N

Neuropathy, neuropathic *(Continued)*
  facial nerve G51.9
  hereditary G6Ø.9
    motor and sensory (types I-IV) G6Ø.Ø
    sensory G6Ø.8
    specified NEC G6Ø.8
  hypertrophic G6Ø.Ø
    Charcot-Marie-Tooth G6Ø.Ø
    Déjérine-Sottas G6Ø.Ø
    interstitial progressive G6Ø.Ø
    of infancy G6Ø.Ø
    Refsum G6Ø.1
  idiopathic G6Ø.9
    progressive G6Ø.3
    specified NEC G6Ø.8
  in association with hereditary ataxia G6Ø.2
  intercostal G58.Ø
  ischemic —*see* Disorder, nerve
  Jamaica (ginger) G62.2
  leg NEC G57.9-
  lower extremity G57.9-
  lumbar plexus G54.1
  median nerve G56.1-
  motor and sensory —*see also* Polyneuropathy
    hereditary (types I-IV) G6Ø.Ø
  multifocal motor (MMN) G61.82 ◀
  multiple (acute) (chronic) —*see* Polyneuropathy
  optic (nerve) —*see also* Neuritis, optic
    ischemic H47.Ø1-
  paraneoplastic (sensorial) (Denny Brown) D49.9 *[G13.Ø]*
  peripheral (nerve) —*see also* Polyneuropathy G62.9
    autonomic G9Ø.9
      idiopathic G9Ø.Ø9
      in (due to)
        amyloidosis E85.4 *[G99.Ø]*
        diabetes mellitus —*see* EØ8-E13 with .43
        endocrine disease NEC E34.9 *[G99.Ø]*
        gout M1Ø.ØØ *[G99.Ø]*
        hyperthyroidism EØ5.9Ø *[G99.Ø]*
          with thyroid storm EØ5.91 *[G99.Ø]*
        metabolic disease NEC E88.9 *[G99.Ø]*
    idiopathic G6Ø.9
      progressive G6Ø.3
    in (due to)
      antitetanus serum G62.Ø
      arsenic G62.2
      drugs NEC G62.Ø
      lead G62.2
      organophosphate compounds G62.2
      toxic agent NEC G62.2
  plantar nerves G57.6-
  progressive
    hypertrophic interstitial G6Ø.Ø
    inflammatory G62.81
  radicular NEC —*see* Radiculopathy
  sacral plexus G54.1
  sciatic G57.Ø-
  serum G61.1
  toxic NEC G62.2
  trigeminal sensory G5Ø.8
  ulnar nerve G56.2-
  uremic N18.9 *[G63]*
  vitamin B12 E53.8 *[G63]*
    with anemia (pernicious) D51.Ø *[G63]*
      due to dietary deficiency D51.3 *[G63]*
Neurophthisis —*see also* Disorder, nerve
  peripheral, diabetic —*see* EØ8-E13 with .42
Neuroretinitis —*see* Chorioretinitis
Neuroretinopathy, hereditary optic H47.22
Neurosarcoma —*see* Neoplasm, nerve, malignant
Neurosclerosis —*see* Disorder, nerve
Neurosis, neurotic F48.9
  anankastic F42.8 ⬅
  anxiety (state) F41.1
    panic type F41.Ø
  asthenic F48.8
  bladder F45.8

Neurosis, neurotic *(Continued)*
  cardiac (reflex) F45.8
  cardiovascular F45.8
  character F6Ø.9
  colon F45.8
  compensation F68.1
  compulsive, compulsion F42.8 ⬅
  conversion F44.9
  craft F48.8
  cutaneous F45.8
  depersonalization F48.1
  depressive (reaction) (type) F34.1
  environmental F48.8
  excoriation L98.1
  fatigue F48.8
  functional —*see* Disorder, somatoform
  gastric F45.8
  gastrointestinal F45.8
  heart F45.8
  hypochondriacal F45.21
  hysterical F44.9
  incoordination F45.8
    larynx F45.8
    vocal cord F45.8
  intestine F45.8
  larynx (sensory) F45.8
    hysterical F44.4
  mixed NEC F48.8
  musculoskeletal F45.8
  obsessional F42.8 ⬅
  obsessive-compulsive F42.8 ⬅
  occupational F48.8
  ocular NEC F45.8
  organ —*see* Disorder, somatoform
  pharynx F45.8
  phobic F4Ø.9
  posttraumatic (situational) F43.1Ø
    acute F43.11
    chronic F43.12
  psychasthenic (type) F48.8
  railroad F48.8
  rectum F45.8
  respiratory F45.8
  rumination F45.8
  sexual F65.9
  situational F48.8
  social F4Ø.1Ø
    generalized F4Ø.11
  specified type NEC F48.8
  state F48.9
    with depersonalization episode F48.1
  stomach F45.8
  traumatic F43.1Ø
    acute F43.11
    chronic F43.12
  vasomotor F45.8
  visceral F45.8
  war F48.8
Neurospongioblastosis diffusa Q85.1
Neurosyphilis (arrested) (early) (gumma) (late) (latent) (recurrent) (relapse) A52.3
  with ataxia (cerebellar) (locomotor) (spastic) (spinal) A52.19
  aneurysm (cerebral) A52.Ø5
  arachnoid (adhesive) A52.13
  arteritis (any artery) (cerebral) A52.Ø4
  asymptomatic A52.2
  congenital A5Ø.4Ø
  dura (mater) A52.13
  general paresis A52.17
  hemorrhagic A52.Ø5
  juvenile (asymptomatic) (meningeal) A5Ø.4Ø
  leptomeninges (aseptic) A52.13
  meningeal, meninges (adhesive) A52.13
  meningitis A52.13
  meningovascular (diffuse) A52.13
  optic atrophy A52.15
  parenchymatous (degenerative) A52.19
  paresis, paretic A52.17
    juvenile A5Ø.45

Neurosyphilis *(Continued)*
  remission in (sustained) A52.3
  serological (without symptoms) A52.2
  specified nature or site NEC A52.19
  tabes, tabetic (dorsalis) A52.11
    juvenile A5Ø.45
  taboparesis A52.17
    juvenile A5Ø.45
  thrombosis (cerebral) A52.Ø5
  vascular (cerebral) NEC A52.Ø5
Neurothekeoma —*see* Neoplasm, nerve, benign
Neurotic —*see* Neurosis
Neurotoxemia —*see* Toxemia
Neutroclusion M26.211
Neutropenia, neutropenic (chronic) (genetic) (idiopathic) (immune) (infantile) (malignant) (pernicious) (splenic) D7Ø.9
  congenital (primary) D7Ø.Ø
  cyclic D7Ø.4
  cytoreductive cancer chemotherapy sequela D7Ø.1
  drug-induced D7Ø.2
    due to cytoreductive cancer chemotherapy D7Ø.1
  due to infection D7Ø.3
  fever D7Ø.9
  neonatal, transitory (isoimmune) (maternal transfer) P61.5
  periodic D7Ø.4
  secondary (cyclic) (periodic) (splenic) D7Ø.4
    drug-induced D7Ø.2
      due to cytoreductive cancer chemotherapy D7Ø.1
  toxic D7Ø.8
Neutrophilia, hereditary giant D72.Ø
Nevocarcinoma —*see* Melanoma
Nevus D22.9
  achromic —*see* Neoplasm, skin, benign
  amelanotic —*see* Neoplasm, skin, benign
  angiomatous D18.ØØ
    intra-abdominal D18.Ø3
    intracranial D18.Ø2
    skin D18.Ø1
    specified site NEC D18.Ø9
  araneus I78.1
  balloon cell —*see* Neoplasm, skin, benign
  bathing trunk D48.5
  blue —*see* Neoplasm, skin, benign
    cellular —*see* Neoplasm, skin, benign
    giant —*see* Neoplasm, skin, benign
    Jadassohn's —*see* Neoplasm, skin, benign
    malignant —*see* Melanoma
  capillary D18.ØØ
    intra-abdominal D18.Ø3
    intracranial D18.Ø2
    skin D18.Ø1
    specified site NEC D18.Ø9
  cavernous D18.ØØ
    intra-abdominal D18.Ø3
    intracranial D18.Ø2
    skin D18.Ø1
    specified site NEC D18.Ø9
  cellular —*see* Neoplasm, skin, benign
    blue —*see* Neoplasm, skin, benign
  choroid D31.3-
  comedonicus Q82.5
  conjunctiva D31.Ø-
  dermal —*see* Neoplasm, skin, benign
    with epidermal nevus —*see* Neoplasm, skin, benign
  dysplastic —*see* Neoplasm, skin, benign
  eye D31.9-
  flammeus Q82.5
  hemangiomatous D18.ØØ
    intra-abdominal D18.Ø3
    intracranial D18.Ø2
    skin D18.Ø1
    specified site NEC D18.Ø9
  iris D31.4-
  lacrimal gland D31.5-
  lymphatic D18.1

- **Nevus** *(Continued)*
  - magnocellular
    - specified site —*see* Neoplasm, benign, by site
    - unspecified site D31.40
  - malignant —*see* Melanoma
  - meaning hemangioma D18.00
    - intra-abdominal D18.03
    - intracranial D18.02
    - skin D18.01
    - specified site NEC D18.09
  - mouth (mucosa) D10.30
    - specified site NEC D10.39
    - white sponge Q38.6
  - multiplex Q85.1
  - non-neoplastic I78.1
  - oral mucosa D10.30
    - specified site NEC D10.39
    - white sponge Q38.6
  - orbit D31.6-
  - pigmented
    - giant —*see also* Neoplasm, skin, uncertain behavior D48.5
      - malignant melanoma in —*see* Melanoma
  - portwine Q82.5
  - retina D31.2-
  - retrobulbar D31.6-
  - sanguineous Q82.5
  - senile I78.1
  - skin D22.9
    - abdominal wall D22.5
    - ala nasi D22.39
    - ankle D22.7-
    - anus, anal D22.5
    - arm D22.6-
    - auditory canal (external) D22.2-
    - auricle (ear) D22.2-
    - auricular canal (external) D22.2-
    - axilla, axillary fold D22.5
    - back D22.5
    - breast D22.5
    - brow D22.39
    - buttock D22.5
    - canthus (eye) D22.1-
    - cheek (external) D22.39
    - chest wall D22.5
    - chin D22.39
    - ear (external) D22.2-
    - external meatus (ear) D22.2-
    - eyebrow D22.39
    - eyelid (lower) (upper) D22.1-
    - face D22.30
      - specified NEC D22.39
    - female genital organ (external) NEC D28.0
    - finger D22.6-
    - flank D22.5
    - foot D22.7-
    - forearm D22.6-
    - forehead D22.39
    - foreskin D29.0
    - genital organ (external) NEC
      - female D28.0
      - male D29.9
    - gluteal region D22.5
    - groin D22.5
    - hand D22.6-
    - heel D22.7-
    - helix D22.2-
    - hip D22.7-
    - interscapular region D22.5
    - jaw D22.39
    - knee D22.7-
    - labium (majus) (minus) D28.0
    - leg D22.7-
    - lip (lower) (upper) D22.0
    - lower limb D22.7-
    - male genital organ (external) D29.9
    - nail D22.9
      - finger D22.6-
      - toe D22.7-
    - nasolabial groove D22.39
    - nates D22.5

- **Nevus** *(Continued)*
  - skin *(Continued)*
    - neck D22.4
    - nose (external) D22.39
    - palpebra D22.1-
    - penis D29.0
    - perianal skin D22.5
    - perineum D22.5
    - pinna D22.2-
    - popliteal fossa or space D22.7-
    - prepuce D29.0
    - pudendum D28.0
    - scalp D22.4
    - scrotum D29.4
    - shoulder D22.6-
    - submammary fold D22.5
    - temple D22.39
    - thigh D22.7-
    - toe D22.7-
    - trunk NEC D22.5
    - umbilicus D22.5
    - upper limb D22.6-
    - vulva D28.0
  - specified site NEC —*see* Neoplasm, benign, by site
  - spider I78.1
  - stellar I78.1
  - strawberry Q82.5
  - Sutton's —*see* Neoplasm, skin, benign
  - unius lateris Q82.5
  - Unna's Q82.5
  - vascular Q82.5
  - verrucous Q82.5
- **Newborn** (infant) (liveborn) (singleton) Z38.2
  - abstinence syndrome P96.1
  - acne L70.4
  - affected by ⟸
    - abnormalities of membranes P02.9
      - specified NEC P02.8
    - abruptio placenta P02.1
    - amino-acid metabolic disorder, transitory P74.8
    - amniocentesis (while in utero) P00.6
    - amnionitis P02.7
    - apparent life threatening event (ALTE) R68.13
    - bleeding (into)
      - cerebral cortex P52.22
      - germinal matrix P52.0
      - ventricles P52.1
    - breech delivery P03.0
    - cardiac arrest P29.81
    - cardiomyopathy I42.8
      - congenital I42.4
    - cerebral ischemia P91.0
    - Cesarean delivery P03.4
    - chemotherapy agents P04.1
    - chorioamnionitis P02.7
    - cocaine (crack) P04.41
    - complications of labor and delivery P03.9
      - specified NEC P03.89
    - compression of umbilical cord NEC P02.5
    - contracted pelvis P03.1
    - delivery P03.9
      - Cesarean P03.4
      - forceps P03.2
      - vacuum extractor P03.3
    - entanglement (knot) in umbilical cord P02.5
    - environmental chemicals P04.6
    - fetal (intrauterine)
      - growth retardation P05.9
      - malnutrition not light or small for gestational age P05.2
    - forceps delivery P03.2
    - heart rate abnormalities
      - bradycardia P29.12
      - intrauterine P03.819
        - before onset of labor P03.810
        - during labor P03.811
      - tachycardia P29.11

- **Newborn** *(Continued)*
  - affected by *(Continued)*
    - hemorrhage (antepartum) P02.1
      - cerebellar (nontraumatic) P52.6
      - intracerebral (nontraumatic) P52.4
      - intracranial (nontraumatic) P52.9
        - specified NEC P52.8
      - intraventricular (nontraumatic) P52.3
        - grade 1 P52.0
        - grade 2 P52.1
        - grade 3 P52.21
        - grade 4 P52.22
      - posterior fossa (nontraumatic) P52.6
      - subarachnoid (nontraumatic) P52.5
      - subependymal P52.0
        - with intracerebral extension P52.22
        - with intraventricular extension P52.1
          - with enlargment of ventricles P52.21
        - without intraventricular extension P52.0
    - hypoxic ischemic encephalopathy [HIE] P91.60
      - mild P91.61
      - moderate P91.62
      - severe P91.63
    - induction of labor P03.89
    - intestinal perforation P78.0
    - intrauterine (fetal) blood loss P50.9
      - due to (from)
        - cut end of co-twin cord P50.5
        - hemorrhage into
          - co-twin P50.3
          - maternal circulation P50.4
        - placenta P50.2
        - ruptured cord blood P50.1
        - vasa previa P50.0
      - specified NEC P50.8
    - intrauterine (fetal) hemorrhage P50.9
    - intrauterine (in utero) procedure P96.5
    - malpresentation (malposition) NEC P03.1
    - maternal (complication of) (use of)
      - alcohol P04.3
      - analgesia (maternal) P04.0
      - anesthesia (maternal) P04.0
      - blood loss P02.1
      - circulatory disease P00.3
      - condition P00.9
        - specified NEC P00.89
      - delivery P03.9
        - Cesarean P03.4
        - forceps P03.2
        - vacuum extractor P03.3
      - diabetes mellitus (pre-existing) P70.1
      - disorder P00.9
        - specified NEC P00.89
      - drugs (addictive) (illegal) NEC P04.49
      - ectopic pregnancy P01.4
      - gestational diabetes P70.0
      - hemorrhage P02.1
      - hypertensive disorder P00.0
      - incompetent cervix P01.0
      - infectious disease P00.2
      - injury P00.5
      - labor and delivery P03.9
      - malpresentation before labor P01.7
      - maternal death P01.6
      - medical procedure P00.7
      - medication P04.1
      - multiple pregnancy P01.5
      - nutritional disorder P00.4
      - oligohydramnios P01.2
      - parasitic disease P00.2
      - periodontal disease P00.81
      - placenta previa P02.0
      - polyhydramnios P01.3
      - precipitate delivery P03.5
      - pregnancy P01.9
        - specified P01.8
      - premature rupture of membranes P01.1
      - renal disease P00.1

N

Newborn *(Continued)*
affected by *(Continued)*
maternal *(Continued)*
respiratory disease PØØ.3
surgical procedure PØØ.6
urinary tract disease PØØ.1
uterine contraction (abnormal) PØ3.6
meconium peritonitis P78.Ø
medication (legal) (maternal use) (prescribed) PØ4.1
membrane abnormalities PØ2.9
specified NEC PØ2.8
membranitis PØ2.7
methamphetamine (s) PØ4.49
mixed metabolic and respiratory acidosis P84
neonatal abstinence syndrome P96.1
noxious substances transmitted via placenta or breast milk PØ4.9
specified NEC PØ4.8
nutritional supplements PØ4.5
placenta previa PØ2.Ø
placental
abnormality (functional) (morphological) PØ2.2Ø
specified NEC PØ2.29
dysfunction PØ2.29
infarction PØ2.29
insufficiency PØ2.29
separation NEC PØ2.1
transfusion syndromes PØ2.3
placentitis PØ2.7
precipitate delivery PØ3.5
prolapsed cord PØ2.4
respiratory arrest P28.81
slow intrauterine growth PØ5.9
tobacco PØ4.2
twin to twin transplacental transfusion PØ2.3
umbilical cord (tightly) around neck PØ2.5
umbilical cord condition PØ2.6Ø
short cord PØ2.69
specified NEC PØ2.69
uterine contractions (abnormal) PØ3.6
vasa previa PØ2.69
from intrauterine blood loss P5Ø.Ø
apnea P28.4 ⇐
obstructive P28.4
primary P28.3
~~specified P28.4~~
sleep (central) (obstructive) (primary) P28.3 ◀
born in hospital Z38.ØØ
by cesarean Z38.Ø1
born outside hospital Z38.1
breast buds P96.89
breast engorgement P83.4
check-up —*see* Newborn, examination
convulsion P9Ø
dehydration P74.1
examination
8 to 28 days old ZØØ.111
under 8 days old ZØØ.11Ø
fever P81.9
environmentally-induced P81.Ø
hyperbilirubinemia P59.9
of prematurity P59.Ø
hypernatremia P74.2
hyponatremia P74.2
infection P39.9
candidal P37.5
specified NEC P39.8
urinary tract P39.3
jaundice P59.9 ⇐
due to
breast milk inhibitor P59.3
hepatocellular damage P59.2Ø
specified NEC P59.29
preterm delivery P59.Ø
of prematurity P59.Ø
specified NEC P59.8

Newborn *(Continued)*
late metabolic acidosis P74.Ø
mastitis P39.Ø
infective P39.Ø
noninfective P83.4
multiple born NEC Z38.8
born in hospital Z38.68
by cesarean Z38.69
born outside hospital Z38.7
omphalitis P38.9
with mild hemorrhage P38.1
without hemorrhage P38.9
post-term PØ8.21
prolonged gestation (over 42 completed weeks) PØ8.22
quadruplet Z38.8
born in hospital Z38.63
by cesarean Z38.64
born outside hospital Z38.7
quintuplet Z38.8
born in hospital Z38.65
by cesarean Z38.66
born outside hospital Z38.7
seizure P9Ø
sepsis (congenital) P36.9
due to
anaerobes NEC P36.5
Escherichia coli P36.4
Staphylococcus P36.3Ø
aureus P36.2
specified NEC P36.39
Streptococcus P36.1Ø
group B P36.Ø
specified NEC P36.19
specified NEC P36.8
triplet Z38.8
born in hospital Z38.61
by cesarean Z38.62
born outside hospital Z38.7
twin Z38.5
born in hospital Z38.3Ø
by cesarean Z38.31
born outside hospital Z38.4
vomiting P92.Ø9
bilious P92.Ø1
weight check ZØØ.111
Newcastle conjunctivitis or disease B3Ø.8
Nezelof's syndrome (pure alymphocytosis) D81.4
Niacin (amide) **deficiency** E52
Nicolas (-Durand)-**Favre disease** A55
Nicotine —*see* Tobacco
Nicotinic acid deficiency E52
Niemann-Pick disease or syndrome E75.249
specified NEC E75.248
type
A E75.24Ø
B E75.241
C E75.242
D E75.243
Night
blindness —*see* Blindness, night
sweats R61
terrors (child) F51.4
Nightmares (REM sleep type) F51.5
NIHSS (National Institutes of Health Stroke Scale) **score** R29.7- ◀
Nipple —*see* condition
Nisbet's chancre A57
Nishimoto (-Takeuchi) disease I67.5
Nitritoid crisis or reaction —*see* Crisis, nitritoid
Nitrosohemoglobinemia D74.8
Njovera A65
Nocardiosis, nocardiasis A43.9
cutaneous A43.1
lung A43.Ø
pneumonia A43.Ø
pulmonary A43.Ø
specified site NEC A43.8
Nocturia R35.1
psychogenic F45.8

Nocturnal —*see* condition
Nodal rhythm I49.8
Node (s) —*see also* Nodule
Bouchard's (with arthropathy) M15.2
Haygarth's M15.8
Heberden's (with arthropathy) M15.1
larynx J38.7
lymph —*see* condition
milker's BØ8.Ø3
Osler's I33.Ø
Schmorl's —*see* Schmorl's disease
singer's J38.2
teacher's J38.2
tuberculous —*see* Tuberculosis, lymph gland
vocal cord J38.2
Nodule (s), nodular
actinomycotic —*see* Actinomycosis
breast NEC N63
colloid (cystic), thyroid EØ4.1
cutaneous —*see* Swelling, localized
endometrial (stromal) D26.1
Haygarth's M15.8
inflammatory —*see* Inflammation
juxta-articular
syphilitic A52.77
yaws A66.7
larynx J38.7
lung, solitary (subsegmental branch of the bronchial tree) R91.1
multiple R91.8
milker's BØ8.Ø3
prostate N4Ø.2
with lower urinary tract symptoms (LUTS) N4Ø.3
without lower urinary tract symptoms (LUTS) N4Ø.2
pulmonary, solitary (subsegmental branch of the bronchial tree) R91.1
retrocardiac RØ9.89
rheumatoid MØ6.3Ø
ankle MØ6.37-
elbow MØ6.32-
foot joint MØ6.37-
hand joint MØ6.34-
hip MØ6.35-
knee MØ6.36-
multiple site MØ6.39
shoulder MØ6.31-
vertebra MØ6.38
wrist MØ6.33-
scrotum (inflammatory) N49.2
singer's J38.2
solitary, lung (subsegmental branch of the bronchial tree) R91.1
multiple R91.8
subcutaneous —*see* Swelling, localized
teacher's J38.2
thyroid (cold) (gland) (nontoxic) EØ4.1
with thyrotoxicosis EØ5.2Ø
with thyroid storm EØ5.21
toxic or with hyperthyroidism EØ5.2Ø
with thyroid storm EØ5.21
vocal cord J38.2
Noma (gangrenous) (hospital) (infective) A69.Ø
auricle I96
mouth A69.Ø
pudendi N76.89
vulvae N76.89
Nomad, nomadism Z59.Ø
NOMID (neonatal onset multisystemic inflammatory disorder) MØ4.2 ◀
Nonautoimmune hemolytic anemia D59.4
drug-induced D59.2
Nonclosure —*see also* Imperfect, closure
ductus arteriosus (Botallo's) Q25.Ø
foramen
botalli Q21.1
ovale Q21.1

◀ New ⇐ Revised ~~deleted~~ Deleted

Noncompliance Z91.19
with
dialysis Z91.15
dietary regimen Z91.11
medical treatment Z91.19
medication regimen NEC Z91.14
underdosing —*see also* Table of Drugs and Chemicals, categories T36-T5Ø, with final character 6 Z91.14
intentional NEC Z91.128
due to financial hardship of patient Z91.12Ø
unintentional NEC Z91.138
due to patient's age related debility Z91.13Ø
renal dialysis Z91.15
Nondescent (congenital) —*see also* Malposition, congenital
cecum Q43.3
colon Q43.3
testicle Q53.9
bilateral Q53.2Ø
abdominal Q53.21
perineal Q53.22
unilateral Q53.1Ø
abdominal Q53.11
perineal Q53.12
Nondevelopment
brain QØ2
part of QØ4.3
heart Q24.8
organ or site, congenital NEC —*see* Hypoplasia
Nonengagement
head NEC O32.4
in labor, causing obstructed labor O64.8
Nonexanthematous tick fever A93.2
Nonexpansion, lung (newborn) P28.Ø
Nonfunctioning
cystic duct —*see also* Disease, gallbladder K82.8
gallbladder —*see also* Disease, gallbladder K82.8
kidney N28.9
labyrinth —*see* subcategory H83.2
Non-Hodgkin lymphoma NEC —*see* Lymphoma, non-Hodgkin
Nonimplantation, ovum N97.2
Noninsufflation, fallopian tube N97.1
Non-ketotic hyperglycinemia E72.51
Nonne-Milroy syndrome Q82.Ø
Nonovulation N97.Ø
Nonpatent fallopian tube N97.1
Nonpneumatization, lung NEC P28.Ø
Nonrotation —*see* Malrotation
Nonsecretion, urine —*see* Anuria
Nonunion
fracture —*see* Fracture, by site
joint, following fusion or arthrodesis M96.Ø ◀
organ or site, congenital NEC —*see* Imperfect, closure
symphysis pubis, congenital Q74.2
Nonvisualization, gallbladder R93.2
Nonvital, nonvitalized tooth KØ4.99
Non-working side interference M26.56
Noonan's syndrome Q87.1
Normocytic anemia (infectional) due to blood loss (chronic) D5Ø.Ø
acute D62
Norrie's disease (congenital) Q15.8
North American blastomycosis B4Ø.9
Norwegian itch B86
Nose, nasal —*see* condition
Nosebleed RØ4.Ø
Nose-picking F98.8
Nosomania F45.21
Nosophobia F45.22
Nostalgia F43.2Ø
Notch of iris Q13.2
Notching nose, congenital (tip) Q3Ø.2
Nothnagel's
syndrome —*see* Strabismus, paralytic, third nerve
vasomotor acroparesthesia I73.89
Novy's relapsing fever A68.9
louse-borne A68.Ø
tick-borne A68.1
Noxious
foodstuffs, poisoning by —*see* Poisoning, food, noxious, plant
substances transmitted through placenta or breast milk PØ4.9
Nucleus pulposus —*see* condition
Numbness R2Ø.Ø
Nuns' knee —*see* Bursitis, prepatellar
Nursemaid's elbow S53.Ø3-
Nutcracker esophagus K22.4
Nutmeg liver K76.1
Nutrient element deficiency E61.9
specified NEC E61.8
Nutrition deficient or insufficient —*see also* Malnutrition E46
due to
insufficient food T73.Ø
lack of
care (child) T76.Ø2
adult T76.Ø1
food T73.Ø
Nutritional stunting E45
Nyctalopia (night blindness) —*see* Blindness, night
Nycturia R35.1
psychogenic F45.8
Nymphomania F52.8
Nystagmus H55.ØØ
benign paroxysmal —*see* Vertigo, benign paroxysmal
central positional H81.4-
congenital H55.Ø1
dissociated H55.Ø4
latent H55.Ø2
miners' H55.Ø9
positional
benign paroxysmal H81.4-
central H81.4-
specified form NEC H55.Ø9
visual deprivation H55.Ø3

N

O

Obermeyer's relapsing fever (European) A68.0
Obesity E66.9
~~with alveolar hyperventilation E66.2~~
with alveolar hypoventilation E66.2 ◀
adrenal E27.8
complicating
childbirth O99.214
pregnancy O99.21-
puerperium O99.215
constitutional E66.8
dietary counseling and surveillance Z71.3
drug-induced E66.1
due to
drug E66.1
excess calories E66.09
morbid E66.01
severe E66.01
endocrine E66.8
endogenous E66.8
exogenous E66.09 ◀
familial E66.8
glandular E66.8
hypothyroid —*see* Hypothyroidism
hypoventilation syndrome (OHS) E66.2 ◀
morbid E66.01
~~with alveolar hypoventilation E66.2~~
with ◀
alveolar hypoventilation E66.2 ◀
obesity hypoventilation syndrome (OHS) E66.2 ◀
due to excess calories E66.01
nutritional E66.09
pituitary E23.6
severe E66.01
specified type NEC E66.8
Oblique —*see* condition
Obliteration
appendix (lumen) K38.8
artery I77.1
bile duct (noncalculous) K83.1
common duct (noncalculous) K83.1
cystic duct —*see* Obstruction, gallbladder
disease, arteriolar I77.1
endometrium N85.8
eye, anterior chamber —*see* Disorder, globe, hypotony
fallopian tube N97.1
lymphatic vessel I89.0
due to mastectomy I97.2
organ or site, congenital NEC —*see* Atresia, by site
ureter N13.5
with infection N13.6
urethra —*see* Stricture, urethra
vein I87.8
vestibule (oral) K08.89 ⬅
Observation (following) (for) (without need for further medical care) Z04.9
accident NEC Z04.3
at work Z04.2
transport Z04.1
adverse effect of drug Z03.6
alleged rape or sexual assault (victim), ruled out
adult Z04.41
child Z04.42
criminal assault Z04.8
development state
adolescent Z00.3
period of rapid growth in childhood Z00.2
puberty Z00.3
disease, specified NEC Z03.89
following work accident Z04.2
growth and development state —*see* Observation, development state
injuries (accidental) NEC —*see also* Observation, accident
Observation *(Continued)*
newborn (for) ⬅
suspected condition, related to exposure from the mother or birth process —*see* Newborn, affected by, maternal ◀
ruled out Z05.9 ◀
cardiac Z05.0 ◀
connective tissue Z05.73 ◀
gastrointestinal Z05.5 ◀
genetic Z05.41 ◀
genitourinary Z05.6 ◀
immunologic Z05.43 ◀
infectious Z05.1 ◀
metabolic Z05.42 ◀
musculoskeletal Z05.72 ◀
neurological Z05.2 ◀
respiratory Z05.3 ◀
skin and subcutaneous tissue Z05.71 ◀
specified condition NEC Z05.8 ◀
postpartum
immediately after delivery Z39.0
routine follow-up Z39.2
pregnancy (normal) (without complication) Z34.9-
high risk O09.9-
suicide attempt, alleged NEC Z03.89
self-poisoning Z03.6
suspected, ruled out —*see also* Suspected condition, ruled out
abuse, physical
adult Z04.71
child Z04.72
accident at work Z04.2
adult battering victim Z04.71
child battering victim Z04.72
condition NEC Z03.89
newborn —*see also* Observation, newborn (for), suspected condition, ruled out Z05.9 ⬅
drug poisoning or adverse effect Z03.6
exposure (to)
anthrax Z03.810
biological agent NEC Z03.818
inflicted injury NEC Z04.8
suicide attempt, alleged Z03.89
self-poisoning Z03.6
toxic effects from ingested substance (drug) (poison) Z03.6
toxic effects from ingested substance (drug) (poison) Z03.6
Obsession, obsessional state F42.8 ⬅
mixed thoughts and acts F42.2 ◀
Obsessive-compulsive neurosis or reaction F42.8 ⬅
Obstetric embolism, septic —*see* Embolism, obstetric, septic
Obstetrical trauma (complicating delivery) O71.9
with or following ectopic or molar pregnancy O08.6
specified type NEC O71.89
Obstipation —*see* Constipation
Obstruction, obstructed, obstructive
airway J98.8
with
allergic alveolitis J67.9
asthma J45.909
with
exacerbation (acute) J45.901
status asthmaticus J45.902
bronchiectasis J47.9
with
exacerbation (acute) J47.1
lower respiratory infection J47.0
bronchitis (chronic) J44.9
emphysema J43.9
Obstruction, obstructed, obstructive *(Continued)*
airway *(Continued)*
chronic J44.9
with
allergic alveolitis —*see* Pneumonitis, hypersensitivity
bronchiectasis J47.9
with
exacerbation (acute) J47.1
lower respiratory infection J47.0
due to
foreign body —*see* Foreign body, by site, causing asphyxia
inhalation of fumes or vapors J68.9
laryngospasm J38.5
ampulla of Vater K83.1
aortic (heart) (valve) —*see* Stenosis, aortic
aortoiliac I74.09
aqueduct of Sylvius G91.1
congenital Q03.0
with spina bifida —*see* Spina bifida, by site, with hydrocephalus
Arnold-Chiari —*see* Arnold-Chiari disease
artery (*see also* Embolism, artery) I74.9
basilar (complete) (partial) —*see* Occlusion, artery, basilar
carotid (complete) (partial) —*see* Occlusion, artery, carotid
cerebellar —*see* Occlusion, artery, cerebellar
cerebral (anterior) (middle) (posterior) —*see* Occlusion, artery, cerebral
precerebral —*see* Occlusion, artery, precerebral
renal N28.0
retinal NEC —*see* Occlusion, artery, retina
stent —*see* Restenosis, stent ◀
vertebral (complete) (partial) —*see* Occlusion, artery, vertebral
band (intestinal) K56.69
bile duct or passage (common) (hepatic) (noncalculous) K83.1
with calculus K80.51
congenital (causing jaundice) Q44.3
biliary (duct) (tract) K83.1
gallbladder K82.0
bladder-neck (acquired) N32.0
congenital Q64.31
due to hyperplasia (hypertrophy) of prostate —*see* Hyperplasia, prostate
bowel —*see* Obstruction, intestine
bronchus J98.09
canal, ear —*see* Stenosis, external ear canal
cardia K22.2
caval veins (inferior) (superior) I87.1
cecum —*see* Obstruction, intestine
circulatory I99.8
colon —*see* Obstruction, intestine
common duct (noncalculous) K83.1
coronary (artery) —*see* Occlusion, coronary
cystic duct —*see also* Obstruction, gallbladder
with calculus K80.21
device, implant or graft —*see also* Complications, by site and type, mechanical T85.698
arterial graft NEC —*see* Complication, cardiovascular device, mechanical, vascular
catheter NEC T85.628
cystostomy T83.090
dialysis (renal) T82.49
intraperitoneal T85.691
Hopkins T83.098 ◀
ileostomy T83.098 ◀
infusion NEC T82.594
spinal (epidural) (subdural) T85.690
nephrostomy T83.092 ◀
urethral indwelling T83.091 ◀
urinary T83.098 ◀
~~urinary, indwelling T83.098~~
urostomy T83.098 ◀

◀ New ⬅ Revised ~~deleted~~ Deleted

Obstruction, obstructed, obstructive *(Continued)*
- device, implant or graft *(Continued)*
  - due to infection T85.79
  - gastrointestinal —*see* Complications, prosthetic device, mechanical, gastrointestinal device
  - genital NEC T83.498
    - intrauterine contraceptive device T83.39
    - penile prosthesis (cylinder) (implanted) (pump) (resevoir) T83.490 ⬅
    - testicular prosthesis T83.491 ◀
  - heart NEC —*see* Complication, cardiovascular device, mechanical
  - joint prosthesis —*see* Complications, joint prosthesis, mechanical, specified NEC, by site
  - orthopedic NEC —*see* Complication, orthopedic, device, mechanical
  - specified NEC T85.628
  - urinary NEC —*see also* Complication, genitourinary, device, urinary, mechanical
    - graft T83.29
  - vascular NEC —*see* Complication, cardiovascular device, mechanical
  - ventricular intracranial shunt T85.09
- due to foreign body accidentally left in operative wound T81.529
- duodenum K31.5
- ejaculatory duct N50.89 ⬅
- esophagus K22.2
- eustachian tube (complete) (partial) H68.10-
  - cartilagenous (extrinsic) H68.13-
    - intrinsic H68.12-
  - osseous H68.11-
- fallopian tube (bilateral) N97.1
- fecal K56.41
  - with hernia —*see* Hernia, by site, with obstruction
- foramen of Monro (congenital) Q03.8
  - with spina bifida —*see* Spina bifida, by site, with hydrocephalus
- foreign body —*see* Foreign body
- gallbladder K82.0
  - with calculus, stones K80.21
  - congenital Q44.1
- gastric outlet K31.1
- gastrointestinal —*see* Obstruction, intestine
- hepatic K76.89
  - duct (noncalculous) K83.1
- hepatobiliary K83.1
- ileum —*see* Obstruction, intestine
- iliofemoral (artery) I74.5
- intestine K56.60
  - with
    - adhesions (intestinal) (peritoneal) K56.5
  - adynamic K56.0
  - by gallstone K56.3
  - congenital (small) Q41.9
    - large Q42.9
      - specified part NEC Q42.8
  - neurogenic K56.0
    - Hirschsprung's disease or megacolon Q43.1
  - newborn P76.9
    - due to
      - fecaliths P76.8
      - inspissated milk P76.2
      - meconium (plug) P76.0
        - in mucoviscidosis E84.11
    - specified NEC P76.8
  - postoperative K91.3
  - reflex K56.0
  - specified NEC K56.69
  - volvulus K56.2
- intracardiac ball valve prosthesis T82.09
- jejunum —*see* Obstruction, intestine
- joint prosthesis —*see* Complications, joint prosthesis, mechanical, specified NEC, by site

Obstruction, obstructed, obstructive *(Continued)*
- kidney (calices) N28.89
- labor —*see* Delivery
- lacrimal (passages) (duct)
  - by
    - dacryolith —*see* Dacryolith
    - stenosis —*see* Stenosis, lacrimal
  - congenital Q10.5
  - neonatal H04.53-
- lacrimonasal duct —*see* Obstruction, lacrimal
- lacteal, with steatorrhea K90.2
- laryngitis —*see* Laryngitis
- larynx NEC J38.6
  - congenital Q31.8
- lung J98.4
  - disease, chronic J44.9
- lymphatic I89.0
- meconium (plug)
  - newborn P76.0
    - due to fecaliths P76.0
    - in mucoviscidosis E84.11
- mitral —*see* Stenosis, mitral
- nasal J34.89
- nasolacrimal duct —*see also* Obstruction, lacrimal
  - congenital Q10.5
- nasopharynx J39.2
- nose J34.89
- organ or site, congenital NEC —*see* Atresia, by site
- pancreatic duct K86.89 ⬅
- parotid duct or gland K11.8
- pelviureteral junction N13.5
  - with hydronephrosis N13.0 ◀
  - congenital Q62.39
- pharynx J39.2
- portal (circulation) (vein) I81
- prostate —*see also* Hyperplasia, prostate
  - valve (urinary) N32.0
- pulmonary valve (heart) I37.0
- pyelonephritis (chronic) N11.1
- pylorus
  - adult K31.1
  - congenital or infantile Q40.0
- rectosigmoid —*see* Obstruction, intestine
- rectum K62.4
- renal N28.89
  - outflow N13.8
  - pelvis, congenital Q62.39
- respiratory J98.8
  - chronic J44.9
- retinal (vessels) H34.9
- salivary duct (any) K11.8
  - with calculus K11.5
- sigmoid —*see* Obstruction, intestine
- sinus (accessory) (nasal) J34.89
- Stensen's duct K11.8
- stomach NEC K31.89
  - acute K31.0
  - congenital Q40.2
  - due to pylorospasm K31.3
- submandibular duct K11.8
- submaxillary gland K11.8
  - with calculus K11.5
- thoracic duct I89.0
- thrombotic —*see* Thrombosis
- trachea J39.8
- tracheostomy airway J95.03
- tricuspid (valve) —*see* Stenosis, tricuspid
- upper respiratory, congenital Q34.8
- ureter (functional) (pelvic junction) NEC N13.5
  - with
    - hydronephrosis N13.1
      - with infection N13.6
    - pyelonephritis (chronic) N11.1
  - congenital Q62.39
  - due to calculus —*see* Calculus, ureter

Obstruction, obstructed, obstructive *(Continued)*
- urethra NEC N36.8
  - congenital Q64.39
- urinary (moderate) N13.9
  - due to hyperplasia (hypertrophy) of prostate —*see* Hyperplasia, prostate
  - organ or tract (lower) N13.9
  - prostatic valve N32.0
  - specified NEC N13.8
- uropathy N13.9
- uterus N85.8
- vagina N89.5
- valvular —*see* Endocarditis
- vein, venous I87.1
  - caval (inferior) (superior) I87.1
  - thrombotic —*see* Thrombosis
- vena cava (inferior) (superior) I87.1
- vesical NEC N32.0
- vesicourethral orifice N32.0
  - congenital Q64.31
- vessel NEC I99.8
  - stent —*see* Restenosis, stent ◀

Obturator —*see* condition

Occlusal wear, teeth K03.0

Occlusio pupillae —*see* Membrane, pupillary

Occlusion, occluded
- anus K62.4
  - congenital Q42.3
    - with fistula Q42.2
- aortoiliac (chronic) I74.09
- aqueduct of Sylvius G91.1
  - congenital Q03.0
    - with spina bifida —*see* Spina bifida, by site, with hydrocephalus
- artery —*see also* Embolism, artery I74.9
  - auditory, internal I65.8
  - basilar I65.1
    - with
      - infarction I63.22
        - due to
          - embolism I63.12
          - thrombosis I63.02
  - brain or cerebral I66.9
    - with infarction (due to) I63.5- ⬅
      - embolism I63.4- ⬅
      - thrombosis I63.3- ⬅
  - carotid I65.2-
    - with
      - infarction I63.23-
        - due to
          - embolism I63.13-
          - thrombosis I63.03-
  - cerebellar (anterior inferior) (posterior inferior) (superior) I66.3
    - with infarction I63.54-
      - due to
        - embolism I63.44-
        - thrombosis I63.34-
  - cerebral I66.9
    - with infarction I63.50
      - due to
        - embolism I63.40
          - specified NEC I63.49
        - thrombosis I63.30
          - specified NEC I63.39
    - anterior I66.1-
      - with infarction I63.52-
        - due to
          - embolism I63.42-
          - thrombosis I63.32-
    - middle I66.0-
      - with infarction I63.51-
        - due to
          - embolism I63.41-
          - thrombosis I63.31-
    - posterior I66.2-
      - with infarction I63.53-
        - due to
          - embolism I63.43-
          - thrombosis I63.33-

- **Occlusion, occluded** *(Continued)*
  - artery *(Continued)*
    - cerebral *(Continued)*
      - specified NEC I66.8
        - with infarction I63.59
          - due to
            - embolism I63.4- ⬅
            - thrombosis I63.3- ⬅
    - choroidal (anterior) —*see* Occlusion, artery, cerebral, specified NEC
    - communicating posterior —*see* Occlusion, artery, precerebral, specified NEC
    - complete
      - coronary I25.82
      - extremities I7Ø.92
    - coronary (acute) (thrombotic) (without myocardial infarction) I24.Ø
      - with myocardial infarction —*see* Infarction, myocardium
      - chronic total I25.82
      - complete I25.82
      - healed or old I25.2
      - total (chronic) I25.82
    - hypophyseal —*see* Occlusion, artery, precerebral, specified NEC
    - iliac I74.5
    - lower extremities due to stenosis or stricture I77.1
    - mesenteric (embolic) (thrombotic) —*see also* Infarct, intestine K55.Ø69 ⬅
    - perforating —*see* Occlusion, artery, cerebral, specified NEC
    - peripheral I77.9
      - thrombotic or embolic I74.4
    - pontine —*see* Occlusion, artery, cerebral, specified NEC
    - precerebral I65.9
      - with infarction I63.2Ø
        - due to
          - embolism I63.1Ø
            - specified NEC I63.19
          - thrombosis I63.ØØ
            - specified NEC I63.Ø9
        - specified NEC I63.29
      - basilar —*see* Occlusion, artery, basilar
      - carotid —*see* Occlusion, artery, carotid
      - puerperal O88.23
      - specified NEC I65.8
        - with infarction I63.29
          - due to
            - embolism I63.19
            - thrombosis I63.ØØ
      - vertebral —*see* Occlusion, artery, vertebral
    - renal N28.Ø
    - retinal
      - branch H34.23-
      - central H34.1-
      - partial H34.21-
      - transient H34.Ø-
    - spinal —*see* Occlusion, artery, precerebral, vertebral
    - total (chronic)
      - coronary I25.82
      - extremities I7Ø.92
    - vertebral I65.Ø-
      - with
        - infarction I63.21-
          - due to
            - embolism I63.11-
            - thrombosis I63.Ø1-
  - basilar artery —*see* Occlusion, artery, basilar
  - bile duct (common) (hepatic) (noncalculous) K83.1
  - bowel —*see* Obstruction, intestine
  - carotid (artery) (common) (internal) —*see* Occlusion, artery, carotid
  - centric (of teeth) M26.59
    - maximum intercuspation discrepancy M26.55
  - cerebellar (artery) —*see* Occlusion, artery, cerebellar
  - cerebral (artery) —*see* Occlusion, artery, cerebral
  - cerebrovascular —*see also* Occlusion, artery, cerebral
    - with infarction I63.5- ⬅
  - cervical canal —*see* Stricture, cervix
  - cervix (uteri) —*see* Stricture, cervix
  - choanal Q3Ø.Ø
  - choroidal (artery) —*see* Occlusion, artery, precerebral, specified NEC
  - colon —*see* Obstruction, intestine
  - communicating posterior artery —*see* Occlusion, artery, precerebral, specified NEC
  - coronary (artery) (vein) (thrombotic) —*see also* Infarct, myocardium
    - chronic total I25.82
    - healed or old I25.2
    - not resulting in infarction I24.Ø
    - total (chronic) I25.82
  - cystic duct —*see* Obstruction, gallbladder
  - embolic —*see* Embolism
  - fallopian tube N97.1
    - congenital Q5Ø.6
  - gallbladder —*see also* Obstruction, gallbladder
    - congenital (causing jaundice) Q44.1
  - gingiva, traumatic KØ6.2
  - hymen N89.6
    - congenital Q52.3
  - hypophyseal (artery) —*see* Occlusion, artery, precerebral, specified NEC
  - iliac artery I74.5
  - intestine —*see* Obstruction, intestine
  - lacrimal passages —*see* Obstruction, lacrimal
  - lung J98.4
  - lymph or lymphatic channel I89.Ø
  - mammary duct N64.89
  - mesenteric artery (embolic) (thrombotic) —*see also* Infarct, intestine K55.Ø69 ⬅
  - nose J34.89
    - congenital Q3Ø.Ø
  - organ or site, congenital NEC —*see* Atresia, by site
  - oviduct N97.1
    - congenital Q5Ø.6
  - peripheral arteries
    - due to stricture or stenosis I77.1
    - upper extremity I74.2
  - pontine (artery) —*see* Occlusion, artery, precerebral, specified NEC
  - posterior lingual, of mandibular teeth M26.29
  - precerebral artery —*see* Occlusion, artery, precerebral
  - punctum lacrimale —*see* Obstruction, lacrimal
  - pupil —*see* Membrane, pupillary
  - pylorus, adult —*see also* Stricture, pylorus K31.1
  - renal artery N28.Ø
  - retina, retinal
    - artery —*see* Occlusion, artery, retinal
    - vein (central) H34.81-
      - engorgement H34.82-
      - tributary H34.83-
    - vessels H34.9
  - spinal artery —*see* Occlusion, artery, precerebral, vertebral
  - teeth (mandibular) (posterior lingual) M26.29
  - thoracic duct I89.Ø
  - thrombotic —*see* Thrombosis, artery
  - traumatic
    - edentulous (alveolar) ridge KØ6.2
    - gingiva KØ6.2
    - periodontal KØ5.5
  - tubal N97.1
  - ureter (complete) (partial) N13.5
    - congenital Q62.1Ø
  - ureteropelvic junction N13.5
    - congenital Q62.11
  - ureterovesical orifice N13.5
    - congenital Q62.12
  - urethra —*see* Stricture, urethra
  - uterus N85.8
  - vagina N89.5
  - vascular NEC I99.8
  - vein —*see* Thrombosis
    - retinal —*see* Occlusion, retinal, vein
  - vena cava (inferior) (superior) —*see* Embolism, vena cava
  - ventricle (brain) NEC G91.1
  - vertebral (artery) —*see* Occlusion, artery, vertebral
  - vessel (blood) I99.8
  - vulva N9Ø.5
- **Occult**
  - blood in feces (stools) R19.5
- **Occupational**
  - problems NEC Z56.89
- **Ochlophobia** —*see* Agoraphobia
- **Ochronosis** (endogenous) E7Ø.29
- **Ocular muscle** —*see* condition
- **Oculogyric crisis or disturbance** H51.8
  - psychogenic F45.8
- **Oculomotor syndrome** H51.9
- **Oculopathy**
  - syphilitic NEC A52.71
    - congenital
      - early A5Ø.Ø1
      - late A5Ø.3Ø
    - early (secondary) A51.43
    - late A52.71
- **Oddi's sphincter spasm** K83.4
- **Odontalgia** KØ8.89 ⬅
- **Odontoameloblastoma** —*see* Cyst, calcifying odontogenic
- **Odontoclasia** KØ3.89
- **Odontodysplasia, regional** KØØ.4
- **Odontogenesis imperfecta** KØØ.5
- **Odontoma** (ameloblastic) (complex) (compound) (fibroameloblastic) —*see* Cyst, calcifying odontogenic
- **Odontomyelitis** (closed) (open) KØ4.Ø1 ⬅
  - irreversible KØ4.Ø2 ◀
  - reversible KØ4.Ø1 ◀
- **Odontorrhagia** KØ8.89 ⬅
- **Odontosarcoma, ameloblastic** C41.1
  - upper jaw (bone) C41.Ø
- **Oestriasis** —*see* Myiasis
- **Oguchi's disease** H53.63
- **Ohara's disease** —*see* Tularemia
- **OHS** (obesity hypoventilation syndrome) E66.2 ◀
- **Oidiomycosis** —*see* Candidiasis
- **Oidium albicans infection** —*see* Candidiasis
- **Old** (previous) **myocardial infarction** I25.2
- **Old age** (without mention of debility) R54-
  - dementia FØ3
- **Olfactory** —*see* condition
- **Oligemia** —*see* Anemia
- **Oligoastrocytoma**
  - specified site —*see* Neoplasm, malignant, by site
  - unspecified site C71.9
- **Oligocythemia** D64.9
- **Oligodendroblastoma**
  - specified site —*see* Neoplasm, malignant
  - unspecified site C71.9
- **Oligodendroglioma**
  - anaplastic type
    - specified site —*see* Neoplasm, malignant, by site
    - unspecified site C71.9
  - specified site —*see* Neoplasm, malignant, by site
  - unspecified site C71.9
- **Oligodontia** —*see* Anodontia

Oligoencephalon QØ2
Oligohidrosis L74.4
Oligohydramnios O41.Ø-
Oligohydrosis L74.4
Oligomenorrhea N91.5
primary N91.3
secondary N91.4
Oligophrenia —*see also* Disability, intellectual
phenylpyruvic E7Ø.Ø
Oligospermia N46.11
due to
drug therapy N46.121
efferent duct obstruction N46.123
infection N46.122
radiation N46.124
specified cause NEC N46.129
systemic disease N46.125
Oligotrichia —*see* Alopecia
Oliguria R34
with, complicating or following ectopic or molar pregnancy OØ8.4
postprocedural N99.Ø
Ollier's disease Q78.4
Omenotocele —*see* Hernia, abdomen, specified site NEC
Omentitis —*see* Peritonitis
Omentum, omental —*see* condition
Omphalitis (congenital) (newborn) P38.9
with mild hemorrhage P38.1
without hemorrhage P38.9
not of newborn LØ8.82
tetanus A33
Omphalocele Q79.2
Omphalomesenteric duct, persistent Q43.Ø
Omphalorrhagia, newborn P51.9
Omsk hemorrhagic fever A98.1
Onanism (excessive) F98.8
Onchocerciasis, onchocercosis B73.1
with
eye disease B73.ØØ
endophthalmitis B73.Ø1
eyelid B73.Ø9
glaucoma B73.Ø2
specified NEC B73.Ø9
eye NEC B73.ØØ
eyelid B73.Ø9
Oncocytoma —*see* Neoplasm, benign, by site
Oncovirus, as cause of disease classified elsewhere B97.32
Ondine's curse —*see* Apnea, sleep
Oneirophrenia F23
Onychauxis L6Ø.2
congenital Q84.5
Onychia —*see also* Cellulitis, digit
with lymphangitis —*see* Lymphangitis, acute, digit
candidal B37.2
dermatophytic B35.1
Onychitis —*see also* Cellulitis, digit
with lymphangitis —*see* Lymphangitis, acute, digit
Onychocryptosis L6Ø.Ø
Onychodystrophy L6Ø.3
congenital Q84.6
Onychogryphosis, onychogryposis L6Ø.2
Onycholysis L6Ø.1
Onychomadesis L6Ø.8
Onychomalacia L6Ø.3
Onychomycosis (finger) (toe) B35.1
Onycho-osteodysplasia Q87.2 ⬅
Onychophagia F98.8
Onychophosis L6Ø.8
Onychoptosis L6Ø.8
Onychorrhexis L6Ø.3
congenital Q84.6
Onychoschizia L6Ø.3
Onyxis (finger) (toe) L6Ø.Ø
Onyxitis —*see also* Cellulitis, digit
with lymphangitis —*see* Lymphangitis, acute, digit
Oophoritis (cystic) (infectional) (interstitial) N7Ø.92
with salpingitis N7Ø.93
acute N7Ø.Ø2
with salpingitis N7Ø.Ø3
chronic N7Ø.12
with salpingitis N7Ø.13
complicating abortion —*see* Abortion, by type, complicated by, oophoritis
Oophorocele N83.4- ⬅
Opacity, opacities
cornea H17.-
central H17.1-
congenital Q13.3
degenerative —*see* Degeneration, cornea
hereditary —*see* Dystrophy, cornea
inflammatory —*see* Keratitis
minor H17.81-
peripheral H17.82-
sequelae of trachoma (healed) B94.Ø
specified NEC H17.89
enamel (teeth) (fluoride) (nonfluoride) KØØ.3
lens —*see* Cataract
snowball —*see* Deposit, crystalline
vitreous (humor) NEC H43.39-
congenital Q14.Ø
membranes and strands H43.31-
Opalescent dentin (hereditary) KØØ.5
Open, opening
abnormal, organ or site, congenital —*see* Imperfect, closure
angle with
borderline
findings
high risk H4Ø.Ø2-
low risk H4Ø.Ø1-
intraocular pressure H4Ø.ØØ-
cupping of discs H4Ø.Ø1-
glaucoma (primary) —*see* Glaucoma, open angle
bite
anterior M26.22Ø
posterior M26.221
false —*see* Imperfect, closure
margin on tooth restoration KØ8.51
restoration margins of tooth KØ8.51
wound —*see* Wound, open
Operational fatigue F48.8
Operative —*see* condition
Operculitis —*see* Periodontitis
Operculum —*see* Break, retina
Ophiasis L63.2
Ophthalmia —*see also* Conjunctivitis H1Ø.9
actinic rays —*see* Photokeratitis
allergic (acute) —*see* Conjunctivitis, acute, atopic
blennorrhagic (gonococcal) (neonatorum) A54.31
diphtheritic A36.86
Egyptian A71.1
electrica —*see* Photokeratitis
gonococcal (neonatorum) A54.31
metastatic —*see* Endophthalmitis, purulent
migraine —*see* Migraine, ophthalmoplegic
neonatorum, newborn P39.1
gonococcal A54.31
nodosa H16.24-
purulent —*see* Conjunctivitis, acute, mucopurulent
spring —*see* Conjunctivitis, acute, atopic
sympathetic —*see* Uveitis, sympathetic
Ophthalmitis —*see* Ophthalmia
Ophthalmocele (congenital) Q15.8
Ophthalmoneuromyelitis G36.Ø
Ophthalmoplegia —*see also* Strabismus, paralytic
anterior internuclear —*see* Ophthalmoplegia, internuclear
ataxia-areflexia G61.Ø
diabetic —*see* EØ8-E13 with .39
Ophthalmoplegia *(Continued)*
exophthalmic EØ5.ØØ
with thyroid storm EØ5.Ø1
external H49.88-
progressive H49.4-
with pigmentary retinopathy —*see* Kearns-Sayre syndrome
total H49.3-
internal (complete) (total) H52.51-
internuclear H51.2-
migraine —*see* Migraine, ophthalmoplegic
Parinaud's H49.88-
progressive external —*see* Ophthalmoplegia, external, progressive
supranuclear, progressive G23.1
total (external) —*see* Ophthalmoplegia, external, total
Opioid (s)
abuse —*see* Abuse, drug, opioids
dependence —*see* Dependence, drug, opioids
induced, without use disorder ◀
anxiety disorder F11.988 ◀
delirium F11.921 ◀
depressive disorder F11.94 ◀
sexual dysfunction F11.981 ◀
sleep disorder F11.982 ◀
Opisthognathism M26.Ø9
Opisthorchiasis (felineus) (viverrini) B66.Ø
Opitz' disease D73.2
Opiumism —*see* Dependence, drug, opioid
Oppenheim's disease G7Ø.2
Oppenheim-Urbach disease (necrobiosis lipoidica diabeticorum) —*see* EØ8-E13 with .62Ø
Optic nerve —*see* condition
Orbit —*see* condition
Orchioblastoma C62.9-
Orchitis (gangrenous) (nonspecific) (septic) (suppurative) N45.2
blennorrhagic (gonococcal) (acute) (chronic) A54.23
chlamydial A56.19
filarial —*see also* Infestation, filarial B74.9 *[N51]*
gonococcal (acute) (chronic) A54.23
mumps B26.Ø
syphilitic A52.76
tuberculous A18.15
Orf (virus disease) BØ8.Ø2
Organic —*see also* condition
brain syndrome FØ9
heart —*see* Disease, heart
mental disorder FØ9
psychosis FØ9
Orgasm
anejaculatory N53.13
Oriental
bilharziasis B65.2
schistosomiasis B65.2
Orifice —*see* condition
Origin of both great vessels from right ventricle Q2Ø.1
Ormond's disease (with ureteral obstruction) N13.5
with infection N13.6
Ornithine metabolism disorder E72.4
Ornithinemia (Type I) (Type II) E72.4
Ornithosis A7Ø
Orotaciduria, oroticaciduria (congenital) (hereditary) (pyrimidine deficiency) E79.8
anemia D53.Ø
Orthodontics
adjustment Z46.4
fitting Z46.4
Orthopnea RØ6.Ø1
Orthopoxvirus BØ8.Ø9
specified NEC BØ8.Ø9
Os, uterus —*see* condition
Osgood-Schlatter disease or osteochondrosis —*see* Osteochondrosis, juvenile, tibia

Osler (-Weber)-**Rendu disease** I78.Ø
Osler's nodes I33.Ø
Osmidrosis L75.Ø
Osseous —*see* condition
Ossification
artery —*see* Arteriosclerosis
auricle (ear) —*see* Disorder, pinna, specified type NEC
bronchial J98.Ø9
cardiac —*see* Degeneration, myocardial
cartilage (senile) —*see* Disorder, cartilage, specified type NEC
coronary (artery) —*see* Disease, heart, ischemic, atherosclerotic
diaphragm J98.6
ear, middle —*see* Otosclerosis
falx cerebri G96.19
fontanel, premature Q75.Ø
heart —*see also* Degeneration, myocardial
valve —*see* Endocarditis
larynx J38.7
ligament —*see* Disorder, tendon, specified type NEC
posterior longitudinal —*see* Spondylopathy, specified NEC
meninges (cerebral) (spinal) G96.19
multiple, eccentric centers —*see* Disorder, bone, development or growth
muscle —*see also* Calcification, muscle
due to burns —*see* Myositis, ossificans, in, burns
paralytic —*see* Myositis, ossificans, in, quadriplegia
progressive —*see* Myositis, ossificans, progressiva
specified NEC M61.5Ø
ankle M61.57-
foot M61.57-
forearm M61.53-
hand M61.54-
lower leg M61.56-
multiple sites M61.59
pelvic region M61.55-
shoulder region M61.51-
specified site NEC M61.58
thigh M61.55-
upper arm M61.52-
traumatic —*see* Myositis, ossificans, traumatica
myocardium, myocardial —*see* Degeneration, myocardial
penis N48.89
periarticular —*see* Disorder, joint, specified type NEC
pinna —*see* Disorder, pinna, specified type NEC
rider's bone —*see* Ossification, muscle, specified NEC
sclera H15.89
subperiosteal, post-traumatic M89.8X-
tendon —*see* Disorder, tendon, specified type NEC
trachea J39.8
tympanic membrane —*see* Disorder, tympanic membrane, specified NEC
vitreous (humor) —*see* Deposit, crystalline
Osteitis —*see also* Osteomyelitis
alveolar M27.3
condensans M85.3Ø
ankle M85.37-
foot M85.37-
forearm M85.33-
hand M85.34-
lower leg M85.36-
multiple site M85.39
neck M85.38
rib M85.38
shoulder M85.31-
skull M85.38
Osteitis *(Continued)*
condensans *(Continued)*
specified site NEC M85.38
thigh M85.35-
toe M85.37-
upper arm M85.32-
vertebra M85.38
deformans M88.9
in (due to)
malignant neoplasm of bone C41.9 *[M9Ø.6Ø]*
neoplastic disease —*see also* Neoplasm D49.9 *[M9Ø.6Ø]*
carpus D49.9 *[M9Ø.64-]*
clavicle D49.9 *[M9Ø.61-]*
femur D49.9 *[M9Ø.65-]*
fibula D49.9 *[M9Ø.66-]*
finger D49.9 *[M9Ø.64-]*
humerus D49.9 *[M9Ø.62-]*
ilium D49.9 *[M9Ø.65-]*
ischium D49.9 *[M9Ø.65-]*
metacarpus D49.9 *[M9Ø.64-]*
metatarsus D49.9 *[M9Ø.67-]*
multiple sites D49.9 *[M9Ø.69]*
neck D49.9 *[M9Ø.68]*
radius D49.9 *[M9Ø.63-]*
rib D49.9 *[M9Ø.68]*
scapula D49.9 *[M9Ø.61-]*
skull D49.9 *[M9Ø.68]*
tarsus D49.9 *[M9Ø.67-]*
tibia D49.9 *[M9Ø.66-]*
toe D49.9 *[M9Ø.67-]*
ulna D49.9 *[M9Ø.63-]*
vertebra D49.9 *[M9Ø.68]*
skull M88.Ø
specified NEC —*see* Paget's disease, bone, by site
vertebra M88.1
due to yaws A66.6
fibrosa NEC —*see* Cyst, bone, by site
circumscripta —*see* Dysplasia, fibrous, bone NEC
cystica (generalisata) E21.Ø
disseminata Q78.1
osteoplastica E21.Ø
fragilitans Q78.Ø
Garr's (sclerosing) —*see* Osteomyelitis, specified type NEC
jaw (acute) (chronic) (lower) (suppurative) (upper) M27.2
parathyroid E21.Ø
petrous bone (acute) (chronic) —*see* Petrositis
sclerotic, nonsuppurative —*see* Osteomyelitis, specified type NEC
tuberculosa A18.Ø9
cystica D86.89
multiplex cystoides D86.89
Osteoarthritis M19.9Ø
ankle M19.Ø7-
elbow M19.Ø2-
foot joint M19.Ø7-
generalized M15.9
erosive M15.4
primary M15.Ø
specified NEC M15.8
hand joint M19.Ø4-
first carpometacarpal joint M18.9-
hip M16.1-
bilateral M16.Ø
due to hip dysplasia (unilateral) M16.3-
bilateral M16.2
interphalangeal
distal (Heberden) M15.1
proximal (Bouchard) M15.2
knee M17.9-
bilateral M17.Ø
post-traumatic NEC M19.92
ankle M19.17-
elbow M19.12-
foot joint M19.17-
Osteoarthritis *(Continued)*
post-traumatic NEC *(Continued)*
hand joint M19.14-
first carpometacarpal joint M18.3-
bilateral M18.2
hip M16.5-
bilateral M16.4
knee M17.3-
bilateral M17.2
shoulder M19.11-
wrist M19.13-
primary M19.91
ankle M19.Ø7-
elbow M19.Ø2-
foot joint M19.Ø7-
hand joint M19.Ø4-
first carpometacarpal joint M18.1-
bilateral M18.Ø
hip M16.1-
bilateral M16.Ø
knee M17.1-
bilateral M17.Ø
shoulder M19.Ø1-
spine —*see* Spondylosis
wrist M19.Ø3-
secondary M19.93
ankle M19.27-
elbow M19.22-
foot joint M19.27-
hand joint M19.24-
first carpometacarpal joint M18.5-
bilateral M18.4
hip M16.7
bilateral M16.6
knee M17.5
bilateral M17.4
multiple M15.3
shoulder M19.21-
spine —*see* Spondylosis
wrist M19.23-
shoulder M19.Ø1-
spine —*see* Spondylosis
wrist M19.Ø3-
Osteoarthropathy (hypertrophic) M19.9Ø
ankle —*see* Osteoarthritis, primary, ankle
elbow —*see* Osteoarthritis, primary, elbow
foot joint —*see* Osteoarthritis, primary, foot
hand joint —*see* Osteoarthritis, primary, hand joint
knee joint —*see* Osteoarthritis, primary, knee
multiple site —*see* Osteoarthritis, primary, multiple joint
pulmonary —*see also* Osteoarthropathy, specified type NEC
hypertrophic —*see* Osteoarthropathy, hypertrophic, specified type NEC
secondary —*see* Osteoarthropathy, specified type NEC
secondary hypertrophic —*see* Osteoarthropathy, specified type NEC
shoulder —*see* Osteoarthritis, primary, shoulder
specified joint NEC —*see* Osteoarthritis, primary, specified joint NEC
specified type NEC M89.4Ø
carpus M89.44-
clavicle M89.41-
femur M89.45-
fibula M89.46-
finger M89.44-
humerus M89.42-
ilium M89.459
ischium M89.459
metacarpus M89.44-
metatarsus M89.47-
multiple sites M89.49
neck M89.48
radius M89.43-
rib M89.48
scapula M89.41-
skull M89.48

- **Osteochondrosis** *(Continued)*
  - patellar center (juvenile) (primary) (secondary) —*see* Osteochondrosis, juvenile, patella
  - pelvis (juvenile) M91.0
  - Pierson's M91.0
  - radius (head) (juvenile) —*see* Osteochondrosis, juvenile, radius
  - Scheuermann's —*see* Osteochondrosis, juvenile, spine
  - Sever's —*see* Osteochondrosis, juvenile, tarsus
  - Sinding-Larsen —*see* Osteochondrosis, juvenile, patella
  - spine M42.9
    - adult M42.10
      - cervical region M42.12
      - cervicothoracic region M42.13
      - lumbar region M42.16
      - lumbosacral region M42.17
      - multiple sites M42.19
      - occipito-atlanto-axial region M42.11
      - sacrococcygeal region M42.18
      - thoracic region M42.14
      - thoracolumbar region M42.15
    - juvenile —*see* Osteochondrosis, juvenile, spine
  - symphysis pubis (juvenile) M91.0
  - syphilitic (congenital) A50.02
  - talus (juvenile) —*see* Osteochondrosis, juvenile, tarsus
  - tarsus (navicular) (juvenile) —*see* Osteochondrosis, juvenile, tarsus
  - tibia (proximal) (tubercle) (juvenile) —*see* Osteochondrosis, juvenile, tibia
  - tuberculous —*see* Tuberculosis, bone
  - ulna (lower) (juvenile) —*see* Osteochondrosis, juvenile, ulna
  - van Neck's M91.0
  - vertebral —*see* Osteochondrosis, spine
- **Osteoclastoma** D48.0
  - malignant —*see* Neoplasm, bone, malignant
- **Osteodynia** —*see* Disorder, bone, specified type NEC
- **Osteodystrophy** Q78.9
  - azotemic N25.0
  - congenital Q78.9
  - parathyroid, secondary E21.1
  - renal N25.0
- **Osteofibroma** —*see* Neoplasm, bone, benign
- **Osteofibrosarcoma** —*see* Neoplasm, bone, malignant
- **Osteogenesis imperfecta** Q78.0
- **Osteogenic** —*see* condition
- **Osteolysis** M89.50
  - carpus M89.54-
  - clavicle M89.51-
  - femur M89.55-
  - fibula M89.56-
  - finger M89.54-
  - humerus M89.52-
  - ilium M89.559
  - ischium M89.559
  - joint prosthesis (periprosthetic) —*see* Complications, joint prosthesis, mechanical, periprosthetic, osteolysis, by site
  - metacarpus M89.54-
  - metatarsus M89.57-
  - multiple sites M89.59
  - neck M89.58
  - periprosthetic —*see* Complications, joint prosthesis, mechanical, periprosthetic, osteolysis, by site
  - radius M89.53-
  - rib M89.58
  - scapula M89.51-
  - skull M89.58
- **Osteolysis** *(Continued)*
  - tarsus M89.57-
  - tibia M89.56-
  - toe M89.57-
  - ulna M89.53-
  - vertebra M89.58
- **Osteoma** —*see also* Neoplasm, bone, benign
  - osteoid —*see also* Neoplasm, bone, benign
    - giant —*see* Neoplasm, bone, benign
- **Osteomalacia** M83.9
  - adult M83.9
    - drug-induced NEC M83.5
    - due to
      - malabsorption (postsurgical) M83.2
      - malnutrition M83.3
    - specified NEC M83.8
  - aluminium-induced M83.4
  - infantile —*see* Rickets
  - juvenile —*see* Rickets
  - oncogenic E83.89
  - pelvis M83.8
  - puerperal M83.0
  - senile M83.1
  - vitamin-D-resistant in adults E83.31 *[M90.8-]*
    - carpus E83.31 *[M90.84-]*
    - clavicle E83.31 *[M90.81-]*
    - femur E83.31 *[M90.85-]*
    - fibula E83.31 *[M90.86-]*
    - finger E83.31 *[M90.84-]*
    - humerus E83.31 *[M90.82-]*
    - ilium E83.31 *[M90.859]*
    - ischium E83.31 *[M90.859]*
    - metacarpus E83.31 *[M90.84-]*
    - metatarsus E83.31 *[M90.87-]*
    - multiple sites E83.31 *[M90.89]*
    - neck E83.31 *[M90.88]*
    - radius E83.31 *[M90.83-]*
    - rib E83.31 *[M90.88]*
    - scapula E83.31 *[M90.819]*
    - skull E83.31 *[M90.88]*
    - tarsus E83.31 *[M90.879]*
    - tibia E83.31 *[M90.869]*
    - toe E83.31 *[M90.879]*
    - ulna E83.31 *[M90.839]*
    - vertebra E83.31 *[M90.88]*
- **Osteomyelitis** (general) (infective) (localized) (neonatal) (purulent) (septic) (staphylococcal) (streptococcal) (suppurative) (with periostitis) M86.9
  - acute M86.10
    - carpus M86.14-
    - clavicle M86.11-
    - femur M86.15-
    - fibula M86.16-
    - finger M86.14-
    - hematogenous M86.00
      - carpus M86.04-
      - clavicle M86.01-
      - femur M86.05-
      - fibula M86.06-
      - finger M86.04-
      - humerus M86.02-
      - ilium M86.059
      - ischium M86.059
      - mandible M27.2
      - metacarpus M86.04-
      - metatarsus M86.07-
      - multiple sites M86.09
      - neck M86.08
      - orbit H05.02-
      - petrous bone —*see* Petrositis
      - radius M86.03-
      - rib M86.08
      - scapula M86.01-
      - skull M86.08
      - tarsus M86.07-
      - tibia M86.06-
      - toe M86.07-
      - ulna M86.03-
      - vertebra —*see* Osteomyelitis, vertebra
- **Osteomyelitis** *(Continued)*
  - acute *(Continued)*
    - humerus M86.12-
    - ilium M86.159
    - ischium M86.159
    - mandible M27.2
    - metacarpus M86.14-
    - metatarsus M86.17-
    - multiple sites M86.19
    - neck M86.18
    - orbit H05.02-
    - petrous bone —*see* Petrositis
    - radius M86.13-
    - rib M86.18
    - scapula M86.11-
    - skull M86.18
    - tarsus M86.17-
    - tibia M86.16-
    - toe M86.17-
    - ulna M86.13-
    - vertebra —*see* Osteomyelitis, vertebra
  - chronic (or old) M86.60
    - with draining sinus M86.40
      - carpus M86.44-
      - clavicle M86.41-
      - femur M86.45-
      - fibula M86.46-
      - finger M86.44-
      - humerus M86.42-
      - ilium M86.459
      - ischium M86.459
      - mandible M27.2
      - metacarpus M86.44-
      - metatarsus M86.47-
      - multiple sites M86.49
      - neck M86.48
      - orbit H05.02-
      - petrous bone —*see* Petrositis
      - radius M86.43-
      - rib M86.48
      - scapula M86.41-
      - skull M86.48
      - tarsus M86.47-
      - tibia M86.46-
      - toe M86.47-
      - ulna M86.43-
      - vertebra —*see* Osteomyelitis, vertebra
    - carpus M86.64-
    - clavicle M86.61-
    - femur M86.65-
    - fibula M86.66-
    - finger M86.64-
    - hematogenous NEC M86.50
      - carpus M86.54-
      - clavicle M86.51-
      - femur M86.55-
      - fibula M86.56-
      - finger M86.54-
      - humerus M86.52-
      - ilium M86.559
      - ischium M86.559
      - mandible M27.2
      - metacarpus M86.54-
      - metatarsus M86.57-
      - multifocal M86.30
        - carpus M86.34-
        - clavicle M86.31-
        - femur M86.35-
        - fibula M86.36-
        - finger M86.34-
        - humerus M86.32-
        - ilium M86.359
        - ischium M86.359
        - metacarpus M86.34-
        - metatarsus M86.37-
        - multiple sites M86.39
        - neck M86.38
        - radius M86.33-
        - rib M86.38
        - scapula M86.31-

Osteonecrosis *(Continued)*
  secondary NEC *(Continued)*
    radius M87.33-
    rib M87.38
    scapula M87.319
    skull M87.38
    tarsus M87.379
    tibia M87.366
    toe M87.379
    ulna M87.33-
    vertebra M87.38
  specified type NEC M87.8Ø
    carpus M87.83-
    clavicle M87.81-
    femur M87.85-
    fibula M87.86-
    finger M87.84-
    humerus M87.82-
    ilium M87.85-
    ischium M87.85-
    metacarpus M87.84-
    metatarsus M87.87-
    multiple sites M87.89
    neck M87.88
    radius M87.83-
    rib M87.88-
    scapula M87.81-
    skull M87.88
    tarsus M87.87-
    tibia M87.86-
    toe M87.87-
    ulna M87.83-
    vertebra M87.88
Osteo-onycho-arthro-dysplasia Q87.2 ⬅
Osteo-onychodysplasia, hereditary Q87.2 ⬅
Osteopathia condensans disseminata Q78.8
Osteopathy —*see also* Osteomyelitis, Osteonecrosis, Osteoporosis
  after poliomyelitis M89.6Ø
    carpus M89.64-
    clavicle M89.61-
    femur M89.65-
    fibula M89.66-
    finger M89.64-
    humerus M89.62-
    ilium M89.659
    ischium M89.659
    metacarpus M89.64-
    metatarsus M89.67-
    multiple sites M89.69
    neck M89.68
    radius M89.63-
    rib M89.68
    scapula M89.61-
    skull M89.68
    tarsus M89.67-
    tibia M89.66-
    toe M89.67-
    ulna M89.63-
    vertebra M89.68
  in (due to)
    renal osteodystrophy N25.Ø
    specified diseases classified elsewhere —*see* subcategory M9Ø.8
Osteopenia M85.8-
  borderline M85.8-
Osteoperiostitis —*see* Osteomyelitis, specified type NEC
Osteopetrosis (familial) Q78.2
Osteophyte M25.7Ø
  ankle M25.77-
  elbow M25.72-
  foot joint M25.77-
  hand joint M25.74-
  hip M25.75-
  knee M25.76-
  shoulder M25.71-
  spine M25.78
  vertebrae M25.78
  wrist M25.73-
Osteopoikilosis Q78.8
Osteoporosis (female) (male) M81.Ø
  with current pathological fracture M8Ø.ØØ
  age-related M81.Ø
    with current pathologic fracture M8Ø.ØØ
      carpus M8Ø.Ø4-
      clavicle M8Ø.Ø1-
      fibula M8Ø.Ø6-
      finger M8Ø.Ø4-
      humerus M8Ø.Ø2-
      ilium M8Ø.Ø5-
      ischium M8Ø.Ø5-
      metacarpus M8Ø.Ø4-
      metatarsus M8Ø.Ø7-
      pelvis M8Ø.Ø5-
      radius M8Ø.Ø3-
      scapula M8Ø.Ø1-
      tarsus M8Ø.Ø7-
      tibia M8Ø.Ø6-
      toe M8Ø.Ø7-
      ulna M8Ø.Ø3-
      vertebra M8Ø.Ø8
  disuse M81.8
    with current pathological fracture M8Ø.8Ø
      carpus M8Ø.84-
      clavicle M8Ø.81-
      fibula M8Ø.86-
      finger M8Ø.84-
      humerus M8Ø.82-
      ilium M8Ø.85-
      ischium M8Ø.85-
      metacarpus M8Ø.84-
      metatarsus M8Ø.87-
      pelvis M8Ø.85-
      radius M8Ø.83-
      scapula M8Ø.81-
      tarsus M8Ø.87-
      tibia M8Ø.86-
      toe M8Ø.87-
      ulna M8Ø.83-
      vertebra M8Ø.88
  drug-induced —*see* Osteoporosis, specified type NEC
  idiopathic —*see* Osteoporosis, specified type NEC
  involutional —*see* Osteoporosis, age-related
  Lequesne M81.6
  localized M81.6
  postmenopausal M81.Ø
    with pathological fracture M8Ø.ØØ
      carpus M8Ø.Ø4-
      clavicle M8Ø.Ø1-
      fibula M8Ø.Ø6-
      finger M8Ø.Ø4-
      humerus M8Ø.Ø2-
      ilium M8Ø.Ø5-
      ischium M8Ø.Ø5-
      metacarpus M8Ø.Ø4-
      metatarsus M8Ø.Ø7-
      pelvis M8Ø.Ø5-
      radius M8Ø.Ø3-
      scapula M8Ø.Ø1-
      tarsus M8Ø.Ø7-
      tibia M8Ø.Ø6-
      toe M8Ø.Ø7-
      ulna M8Ø.Ø3-
      vertebra M8Ø.Ø8
  postoophorectomy —*see* Osteoporosis, specified type NEC
  postsurgical malabsorption —*see* Osteoporosis, specified type NEC
  post-traumatic —*see* Osteoporosis, specified type NEC
  senile —*see* Osteoporosis, age-related
  specified type NEC M81.8
    with pathological fracture M8Ø.8Ø
      carpus M8Ø.84-
      clavicle M8Ø.81-
      fibula M8Ø.86-
      finger M8Ø.84-
      humerus M8Ø.82-
      ilium M8Ø.85-
Osteoporosis *(Continued)*
  specified type NEC *(Continued)*
    with pathological fracture *(Continued)*
      ischium M8Ø.85-
      metacarpus M8Ø.84-
      metatarsus M8Ø.87-
      pelvis M8Ø.85-
      radius M8Ø.83-
      scapula M8Ø.81-
      tarsus M8Ø.87-
      tibia M8Ø.86-
      toe M8Ø.87-
      ulna M8Ø.83-
      vertebra M8Ø.88
Osteopsathyrosis (idiopathica) Q78.Ø
Osteoradionecrosis, jaw (acute) (chronic) (lower) (suppurative) (upper) M27.2
Osteosarcoma (any form) —*see* Neoplasm, bone, malignant
Osteosclerosis Q78.2
  acquired M85.8-
  congenita Q77.4
  fragilitas (generalisata) Q78.2
  myelofibrosis D75.81
Osteosclerotic anemia D64.89
Osteosis
  cutis L94.2
  renal fibrocystic N25.Ø
Österreicher-Turner syndrome Q87.2
Ostium
  atrioventriculare commune Q21.2
  primum (arteriosum) (defect) (persistent) Q21.2
  secundum (arteriosum) (defect) (patent) (persistent) Q21.1
Ostrum-Furst syndrome Q75.8
Otalgia —*see* subcategory H92.Ø
Otitis (acute) H66.9Ø
  with effusion —*see also* Otitis, media, nonsuppurative
    purulent —*see* Otitis, media, suppurative
  adhesive —*see* subcategory H74.1
  chronic —*see also* Otitis, media, chronic
    with effusion —*see also* Otitis, media, nonsuppurative, chronic
  externa H6Ø.9-
    abscess —*see* Abscess, ear, external
    acute (noninfective) H6Ø.5Ø-
      actinic H6Ø.51-
      chemical H6Ø.52-
      contact H6Ø.53-
      eczematoid H6Ø.54-
      infective —*see* Otitis, externa, infective
      reactive H6Ø.55-
      specified NEC H6Ø.59-
    cellulitis —*see* Cellulitis, ear
    chronic H6Ø.6-
    diffuse —*see* Otitis, externa, infective, diffuse
    hemorrhagic —*see* Otitis, externa, infective, hemorrhagic
    in (due to)
      aspergillosis B44.89
      candidiasis B37.84
      erysipelas A46 *[H62.4Ø]*
      herpes (simplex) virus infection BØØ.1
        zoster BØ2.8
      impetigo LØ1.ØØ *[H62.4Ø]*
      infectious disease NEC B99 *[H62.4-]*
      mycosis NEC B36.9 *[H62.4Ø]*
      parasitic disease NEC B89 *[H62.4Ø]*
      viral disease NEC B34.9 *[H62.4Ø]*
      zoster BØ2.8
    infective NEC H6Ø.39-
      abscess —*see* Abscess, ear, external
      cellulitis —*see* Cellulitis, ear
      diffuse H6Ø.31-
      hemorrhagic H6Ø.32-
      swimmer's ear —*see* Swimmer's, ear
    malignant H6Ø.2-
    ~~mycotic B36.9 [H62.4Ø]~~

◀ New ⬅ Revised ~~deleted~~ Deleted

Otitis *(Continued)*
externa *(Continued)*
mycotic NEC B36.9 *[H62.4Ø]* ◀
in ◀
aspergillosis B44.89 ◀
candidiasis B37.84 ◀
moniliasis B37.84 ◀
necrotizing —*see* Otitis, externa, malignant
Pseudomonas aeruginosa —*see* Otitis, externa, malignant
reactive —*see* Otitis, externa, acute, reactive
specified NEC —*see* subcategory H6Ø.8
~~tropical B36.8~~
tropical NEC B36.9 *[H62.4Ø]* ◀
in ◀
aspergillosis B44.89 ◀
candidiasis B37.84 ◀
moniliasis B37.84 ◀
insidiosa —*see* Otosclerosis
interna —*see* subcategory H83.Ø
media (hemorrhagic) (staphylococcal) (streptococcal) H66.9-
with effusion (nonpurulent) —*see* Otitis, media, nonsuppurative
acute, subacute H66.9Ø
allergic —*see* Otitis, media, nonsuppurative, acute, allergic
exudative —*see* Otitis, media, suppurative, acute ⬅
mucoid —*see* Otitis, media, nonsuppurative, acute
necrotizing —*see also* Otitis, media, suppurative, acute
in
measles BØ5.3
scarlet fever A38.Ø
nonsuppurative NEC —*see* Otitis, media, nonsuppurative, acute
purulent —*see* Otitis, media, suppurative, acute
sanguinous —*see* Otitis, media, nonsuppurative, acute
secretory —*see* Otitis, media, nonsuppurative, acute, serous
seromucinous —*see* Otitis, media, nonsuppurative, acute
serous —*see* Otitis, media, nonsuppurative, acute, serous
suppurative —*see* Otitis, media, suppurative, acute
allergic —*see* Otitis, media, nonsuppurative
catarrhal —*see* Otitis, media, nonsuppurative
chronic H66.9Ø
with effusion (nonpurulent) —*see* Otitis, media, nonsuppurative, chronic
allergic —*see* Otitis, media, nonsuppurative, chronic, allergic
benign suppurative —*see* Otitis, media, suppurative, chronic, tubotympanic
catarrhal —*see* Otitis, media, nonsuppurative, chronic, serous
exudative —*see* Otitis, media, suppurative, chronic ⬅
mucinous —*see* Otitis, media, nonsuppurative, chronic, mucoid
mucoid —*see* Otitis, media, nonsuppurative, chronic, mucoid
nonsuppurative NEC —*see* Otitis, media, nonsuppurative, chronic
purulent —*see* Otitis, media, suppurative, chronic
secretory —*see* Otitis, media, nonsuppurative, chronic, mucoid
seromucinous —*see* Otitis, media, nonsuppurative, chronic
serous —*see* Otitis, media, nonsuppurative, chronic, serous
suppurative —*see* Otitis, media, suppurative, chronic

Otitis *(Continued)*
media *(Continued)*
chronic *(Continued)*
transudative —*see* Otitis, media, nonsuppurative, chronic, mucoid
exudative —*see* Otitis, media, nonsuppurative
in (due to) (with)
influenza —*see* Influenza, with, otitis media
measles BØ5.3
scarlet fever A38.Ø
tuberculosis A18.6
viral disease NEC B34.- *[H67.-]*
mucoid —*see* Otitis, media, nonsuppurative
nonsuppurative H65.9-
acute or subacute NEC H65.19-
allergic H65.11-
recurrent H65.11-
recurrent H65.19-
secretory —*see* Otitis, media, nonsuppurative, serous
serous H65.Ø-
recurrent H65.Ø-
chronic H65.49-
allergic H65.41-
mucoid H65.3-
serous H65.2-
postmeasles BØ5.3
purulent —*see* Otitis, media, suppurative
secretory —*see* Otitis, media, nonsuppurative
seromucinous —*see* Otitis, media, nonsuppurative
serous —*see* Otitis, media, nonsuppurative
suppurative H66.4-
acute H66.ØØ-
with rupture of ear drum H66.Ø1-
recurrent H66.ØØ-
with rupture of ear drum H66.Ø1-
chronic —*see also* subcategory H66.3
atticoantral H66.2-
benign —*see* Otitis, media, suppurative, chronic, tubotympanic
tubotympanic H66.1-
transudative —*see* Otitis, media, nonsuppurative
tuberculous A18.6
Otocephaly Q18.2
Otolith syndrome —*see* subcategory H81.8
Otomycosis (diffuse) NEC B36.9 *[H62.4Ø]*
in
aspergillosis B44.89
candidiasis B37.84
moniliasis B37.84
Otoporosis —*see* Otosclerosis
Otorrhagia (nontraumatic) H92.2-
traumatic - code by Type of injury
Otorrhea H92.1-
cerebrospinal G96.Ø
Otosclerosis (general) H8Ø.9-
cochlear (endosteal) H8Ø.2-
involving
otic capsule —*see* Otosclerosis, cochlear
oval window
nonobliterative H8Ø.Ø-
obliterative H8Ø.1-
round window —*see* Otosclerosis, cochlear
nonobliterative —*see* Otosclerosis, involving, oval window, nonobliterative
obliterative —*see* Otosclerosis, involving, oval window, obliterative
specified NEC H8Ø.8-
Otospongiosis —*see* Otosclerosis
Otto's disease or pelvis M24.7
Outcome of delivery Z37.9
multiple births Z37.9
all liveborn Z37.5Ø
quadruplets Z37.52
quintuplets Z37.53

Outcome of delivery *(Continued)*
multiple births *(Continued)*
all liveborn *(Continued)*
sextuplets Z37.54
specified number NEC Z37.59
triplets Z37.51
all stillborn Z37.7
some liveborn Z37.6Ø
quadruplets Z37.62
quintuplets Z37.63
sextuplets Z37.64
specified number NEC Z37.69
triplets Z37.61
single NEC Z37.9
liveborn Z37.Ø
stillborn Z37.1
twins NEC Z37.9
both liveborn Z37.2
both stillborn Z37.4
one liveborn, one stillborn Z37.3
Outlet —*see* condition
Ovalocytosis (congenital) (hereditary) —*see* Elliptocytosis
Ovarian —*see* Condition
Ovariocele N83.4- ⬅
Ovaritis (cystic) —*see* Oophoritis
Ovary, ovarian —*see also* condition
resistant syndrome E28.39
vein syndrome N13.8
Overactive —*see also* Hyperfunction
adrenal cortex NEC E27.Ø
bladder N32.81
hypothalamus E23.3
thyroid —*see* Hyperthyroidism
Overactivity R46.3
child —*see* Disorder, attention-deficit hyperactivity
Overbite (deep) (excessive) (horizontal) (vertical) M26.29
Overbreathing —*see* Hyperventilation
Overconscientious personality F6Ø.5
Overdevelopment —*see* Hypertrophy
Overdistension —*see* Distension
Overdose, overdosage (drug) —*see* Table of Drugs and Chemicals, by drug, poisoning
Overeating R63.2
nonorganic origin F5Ø.89 ⬅
psychogenic F5Ø.89 ⬅
Overexertion (effects) (exhaustion) T73.3
Overexposure (effects) T73.9
exhaustion T73.2
Overfeeding —*see* Overeating
newborn P92.4
Overfill, endodontic M27.52
Overgrowth, bone —*see* Hypertrophy, bone
Overhanging of dental restorative material (unrepairable) KØ8.52
Overheated (places) (effects) —*see* Heat
Overjet (excessive horizontal) M26.23
Overlaid, overlying (suffocation) —*see* Asphyxia, traumatic, due to mechanical threat
Overlap, excessive horizontal (teeth) M26.23
Overl apping toe (acquired) —*see also* Deformity, toe, specified NEC
congenital (fifth toe) Q66.89
Overload
circulatory, due to transfusion (blood) (blood components) (TACO) E87.71
fluid E87.7Ø
due to transfusion (blood) (blood components) E87.71
specified NEC E87.79
iron, due to repeated red blood cell transfusions E83.111
potassium (K) E87.5
sodium (Na) E87.Ø
Overnutrition —*see* Hyperalimentation
Overproduction —*see also* Hypersecretion
ACTH E27.Ø
catecholamine E27.5
growth hormone E22.Ø

Overprotection, child by parent Z62.1
Overriding
aorta Q25.49 ⬅
finger (acquired) —*see* Deformity, finger
congenital Q68.1
toe (acquired) —*see also* Deformity, toe, specified NEC
congenital Q66.89
Overstrained R53.83
heart —*see* Hypertrophy, cardiac
Overuse, muscle NEC M7Ø.8-
Overweight E66.3
Overworked R53.83
Oviduct —*see* condition
Ovotestis Q56.Ø
Ovulation (cycle)
failure or lack of N97.Ø
pain N94.Ø
Ovum —*see* condition
Owren's disease or syndrome (parahemophilia) D68.2
Ox heart —*see* Hypertrophy, cardiac
Oxalosis E72.53
Oxaluria E72.53
Oxycephaly, oxycephalic Q75.Ø
syphilitic, congenital A5Ø.Ø2
Oxyuriasis B8Ø
Oxyuris vermicularis (infestation) B8Ø
Ozena J31.Ø

O

P

Pachyderma, pachydermia L85.9
  larynx (verrucosa) J38.7
Pachydermatocele (congenital) Q82.8
Pachydermoperiostosis —*see also* Osteoarthropathy, hypertrophic, specified type NEC
  clubbed nail M89.4Ø *[L62]*
Pachygyria QØ4.3
Pachymeningitis (adhesive) (basal) (brain) (cervical) (chronic) (circumscribed) (external) (fibrous) (hemorrhagic) (hypertrophic) (internal) (purulent) (spinal) (suppurative) —*see* Meningitis
Pachyonychia (congenital) Q84.5
Pacinian tumor —*see* Neoplasm, skin, benign
Pad, knuckle or Garrod's M72.1
Paget-Schroetter syndrome I82.89Ø
Paget's disease
  with infiltrating duct carcinoma —*see* Neoplasm, breast, malignant
  bone M88.9
    carpus M88.84-
    clavicle M88.81-
    femur M88.85-
    fibula M88.86-
    finger M88.84-
    humerus M88.82-
    ilium M88.85-
    in neoplastic disease —*see* Osteitis, deformans, in neoplastic disease
    ischium M88.85-
    metacarpus M88.84-
    metatarsus M88.87-
    multiple sites M88.89
    neck M88.88
    radius M88.83-
    rib M88.88
    scapula M88.81-
    skull M88.Ø
    tarsus M88.87-
    tibia M88.86-
    toe M88.87-
    ulna M88.83-
    vertebra M88.88
  breast (female) C5Ø.Ø1-
    male C5Ø.Ø2-
  extramammary —*see also* Neoplasm, skin, malignant
    anus C21.Ø
      margin C44.59Ø
      skin C44.59Ø
  intraductal carcinoma —*see* Neoplasm, breast, malignant
  malignant —*see* Neoplasm, skin, malignant
    breast (female) C5Ø.Ø1-
      male C5Ø.Ø2-
    unspecified site (female) C5Ø.Ø1-
      male C5Ø.Ø2-
  mammary —*see* Paget's disease, breast
  nipple —*see* Paget's disease, breast
  osteitis deformans —*see* Paget's disease, bone
Pain(s) —*see also* Painful R52
  abdominal R1Ø.9
    colic R1Ø.83
    generalized R1Ø.84
      with acute abdomen R1Ø.Ø
    lower R1Ø.3Ø
      left quadrant R1Ø.32
      pelvic or perineal R1Ø.2
      periumbilical R1Ø.33
      right quadrant R1Ø.31
    rebound —*see* Tenderness, abdominal, rebound
    severe with abdominal rigidity R1Ø.Ø
    tenderness —*see* Tenderness, abdominal
    upper R1Ø.1Ø
      epigastric R1Ø.13
      left quadrant R1Ø.12
      right quadrant R1Ø.11

Pain *(Continued)*
  acute R52
    due to trauma G89.11
    neoplasm related G89.3
    postprocedural NEC G89.18
    post-thoracotomy G89.12
    specified by site — code to Pain, by site
  adnexa (uteri) R1Ø.2
  anginoid —*see* Pain, precordial
  anus K62.89
  arm —*see* Pain, limb, upper
  axillary (axilla) M79.62-
  back (postural) M54.9
  bladder R39.89
    associated with micturition —*see* Micturition, painful
    chronic R39.82 ◀
  bone —*see* Disorder, bone, specified type NEC
  breast N64.4
  broad ligament R1Ø.2
  cancer associated (acute) (chronic) G89.3
  cecum —*see* Pain, abdominal
  cervicobrachial M53.1
  chest (central) RØ7.9
    anterior wall RØ7.89
    atypical RØ7.89
    ischemic I2Ø.9
    musculoskeletal RØ7.89
    non-cardiac RØ7.89
    on breathing RØ7.1
    pleurodynia RØ7.81
    precordial RØ7.2
    wall (anterior) RØ7.89
  chronic G89.29
    associated with significant psychosocial dysfunction G89.4
    due to trauma G89.21
    neoplasm related G89.3
    postoperative NEC G89.28
    postprocedural NEC G89.28
    post-thoracotomy G89.22
    specified NEC G89.29
  coccyx M53.3
  colon —*see* Pain, abdominal
  coronary —*see* Angina
  costochondral RØ7.1
  diaphragm RØ7.1
  due to cancer G89.3
  due to device, implant or graft —*see also* Complications, by site and type, specified NEC T85.848 ⬅
    arterial graft NEC T82.848
    breast (implant) T85.848 ⬅
    catheter NEC T85.848 ⬅
      dialysis (renal) T82.848
        intraperitoneal T85.848 ⬅
      infusion NEC T82.848
        spinal (epidural) (subdural) T85.84Ø ⬅
      urinary (indwelling) T83.84
    electronic (electrode) (pulse generator) (stimulator)
      bone T84.84
      cardiac T82.847
      nervous system (brain) (peripheral nerve) (spinal) T85.84Ø ⬅
      urinary T83.84
    fixation, internal (orthopedic) NEC T84.84
    gastrointestinal (bile duct) (esophagus) T85.848 ⬅
    genital NEC T83.84
    heart NEC T82.847
    infusion NEC T85.848 ⬅
    joint prosthesis T84.84
    ocular (corneal graft) (orbital implant) NEC T85.848 ⬅
    orthopedic NEC T84.84
    specified NEC T85.848 ⬅
    urinary NEC T83.84
    vascular NEC T82.848
    ventricular intracranial shunt T85.84Ø ⬅

Pain *(Continued)*
  due to malignancy (primary) (secondary) G89.3
  ear —*see* subcategory H92.Ø
  epigastric, epigastrium R1Ø.13
  eye —*see* Pain, ocular
  face, facial R51
    atypical G5Ø.1
  female genital organs NEC N94.89
  finger —*see* Pain, limb, upper
  flank —*see* Pain, abdominal
  foot —*see* Pain, limb, lower
  gallbladder K82.9
  gas (intestinal) R14.1
  gastric —*see* Pain, abdominal
  generalized NOS R52
  genital organ
    female N94.89
    male N5Ø.89 ⬅
  groin —*see* Pain, abdominal, lower
  hand —*see* Pain, limb, upper
  head —*see* Headache
  heart —*see* Pain, precordial
  infra-orbital —*see* Neuralgia, trigeminal
  intercostal RØ7.82
  intermenstrual N94.Ø
  jaw R68.84
  joint M25.5Ø
    ankle M25.57-
    elbow M25.52-
    finger M25.54- ⬅
    foot M25.57-
    hand M25.54- ⬅
    hip M25.55-
    knee M25.56-
    shoulder M25.51-
    toe M25.57-
    wrist M25.53-
  kidney N23
  laryngeal RØ7.Ø
  leg —*see* Pain, limb, lower
  limb M79.6Ø9
    lower M79.6Ø-
      foot M79.67-
      lower leg M79.66-
      thigh M79.65-
      toe M79.67-
    upper M79.6Ø-
      axilla M79.62-
      finger M79.64-
      forearm M79.63-
      hand M79.64-
      upper arm M79.62-
  loin M54.5
  low back M54.5
  lumbar region M54.5
  mandibular R68.84
  mastoid —*see* subcategory H92.Ø
  maxilla R68.84
  menstrual —*see also* Dysmenorrhea N94.6
  metacarpophalangeal (joint) —*see* Pain, joint, hand
  metatarsophalangeal (joint) —*see* Pain, joint, foot
  mouth K13.79
  muscle —*see* Myalgia
  musculoskeletal —*see also* Pain, by site M79.1
  myofascial M79.1
  nasal J34.89
  nasopharynx J39.2
  neck NEC M54.2
  nerve NEC —*see* Neuralgia
  neuromuscular —*see* Neuralgia
  nose J34.89
  ocular H57.1-
  ophthalmic —*see* Pain, ocular
  orbital region —*see* Pain, ocular
  ovary N94.89
  over heart —*see* Pain, precordial
  ovulation N94.Ø
  pelvic (female) R1Ø.2

Pain *(Continued)*
  penis N48.89
  pericardial —*see* Pain, precordial
  perineal, perineum R10.2
  pharynx J39.2
  pleura, pleural, pleuritic R07.81
  postoperative NOS G89.18
  postprocedural NOS G89.18
  post-thoracotomy G89.12
  precordial (region) R07.2
  premenstrual N94.3
  psychogenic (persistent) (any site) F45.41
  radicular (spinal) —*see* Radiculopathy
  rectum K62.89
  respiration R07.1
  retrosternal R07.2
  rheumatoid, muscular —*see* Myalgia
  rib R07.81
  root (spinal) —*see* Radiculopathy
  round ligament (stretch) R10.2
  sacroiliac M53.3
  sciatic —*see* Sciatica
  scrotum N50.82 ⬅
  seminal vesicle N50.89 ⬅
  shoulder M25.51-
  spermatic cord N50.89 ⬅
  spinal root —*see* Radiculopathy
  spine M54.9
    cervical M54.2
    low back M54.5
      with sciatica M54.4-
    thoracic M54.6
  stomach —*see* Pain, abdominal
  substernal R07.2
  temporomandibular (joint) M26.62- ⬅
  testis N50.81- ⬅
  thoracic spine M54.6
    with radicular and visceral pain M54.14
  throat R07.0
  tibia —*see* Pain, limb, lower
  toe —*see* Pain, limb, lower
  tongue K14.6
  tooth K08.89 ⬅
  trigeminal —*see* Neuralgia, trigeminal
  tumor associated G89.3
  ureter N23
  urinary (organ) (system) N23
  uterus NEC N94.89
  vagina R10.2
  vertebrogenic (syndrome) M54.89
  vesical R39.89
    associated with micturition —*see* Micturition, painful
  vulva R10.2
Painful —*see also* Pain
  coitus
    female N94.10 ⬅
    male N53.12
    psychogenic F52.6
  ejaculation (semen) N53.12
    psychogenic F52.6
  erection —*see* Priapism
  feet syndrome E53.8
  joint replacement (hip) (knee) T84.84
  menstruation —*see* Dysmenorrhea
    psychogenic F45.8
  micturition —*see* Micturition, painful
  respiration R07.1
  scar NEC L90.5
  wire sutures T81.89
Painter's colic —*see* subcategory T56.0
Palate —*see* condition
Palatoplegia K13.79
Palatoschisis —*see* Cleft, palate
Palilalia R48.8
Palliative care Z51.5
Pallor R23.1
  optic disc, temporal —*see* Atrophy, optic
Palmar —*see also* condition
  fascia —*see* condition

Palpable
  cecum K63.89
  kidney N28.89
  ovary N83.8
  prostate N42.9
  spleen —*see* Splenomegaly
Palpitations (heart) R00.2
  psychogenic F45.8
Palsy —*see also* Paralysis G83.9
  atrophic diffuse (progressive) G12.22
  Bell's —*see also* Palsy, facial
    newborn P11.3
  brachial plexus NEC G54.0
    newborn (birth injury) P14.3
  brain —*see* Palsy, cerebral
  bulbar (progressive) (chronic) G12.22
    of childhood (Fazio-Londe) G12.1
    pseudo NEC G12.29
    supranuclear (progressive) G23.1
  cerebral (congenital) G80.9
    ataxic G80.4
    athetoid G80.3
    choreathetoid G80.3
    diplegic G80.8
      spastic G80.1
    dyskinetic G80.3
      athetoid G80.3
      choreathetoid G80.3
      distonic G80.3
    dystonic G80.3
    hemiplegic G80.8
      spastic G80.2
    mixed G80.8
    monoplegic G80.8
      spastic G80.1
    paraplegic G80.8
      spastic G80.1
    quadriplegic G80.8
      spastic G80.0
    spastic G80.1
      diplegic G80.1
      hemiplegic G80.2
      monoplegic G80.1
      quadriplegic G80.0
      specified NEC G80.1
      tetrapelgic G80.0
    specified NEC G80.8
    syphilitic A52.12
      congenital A50.49
    tetraplegic G80.8
      spastic G80.0
  cranial nerve —*see also* Disorder, nerve, cranial
    multiple G52.7
      in
        infectious disease B99 *[G53]*
        neoplastic disease —*see also* Neoplasm D49.9 *[G53]*
        parasitic disease B89 *[G53]*
        sarcoidosis D86.82
  creeping G12.22
  diver's T70.3
  Erb's P14.0
  facial G51.0
    newborn (birth injury) P11.3
  glossopharyngeal G52.1
  Klumpke (-Déjérine) P14.1
  lead —*see* subcategory T56.0
  median nerve (tardy) G56.1-
  nerve G58.9
    specified NEC G58.8
  peroneal nerve (acute) (tardy) G57.3-
  progressive supranuclear G23.1
  pseudobulbar NEC G12.29
  radial nerve (acute) G56.3-
  seventh nerve —*see also* Palsy, facial
    newborn P11.3
  shaking —*see* Parkinsonism
  spastic (cerebral) (spinal) G80.1
  ulnar nerve (tardy) G56.2-
  wasting G12.29

Paludism —*see* Malaria
Panangiitis M30.0
Panaris, panaritium —*see also* Cellulitis, digit
  with lymphangitis —*see* Lymphangitis, acute, digit
Panarteritis nodosa M30.0
  brain or cerebral I67.7
Pancake heart R93.1
  with cor pulmonale (chronic) I27.81
Pancarditis (acute) (chronic) I51.89
  rheumatic I09.89
    active or acute I01.8
Pancoast's syndrome or tumor C34.1-
Pancolitis, ulcerative (chronic) K51.00
  with
    abscess K51.014
    complication K51.019
    fistula K51.013
    obstruction K51.012
    rectal bleeding K51.011
    specified complication NEC K51.018
Pancreas, pancreatic —*see* condition
Pancreatitis (annular) (apoplectic) (calcareous) (edematous) (hemorrhagic) (malignant) (recurrent) (subacute) (suppurative) K85.90 ⬅
  with necrosis (uninfected) K85.91 ◀
    infected K85.92 ◀
  acute (without necrosis or infection) K85.90 ⬅
    with necrosis (uninfected) K85.91 ◀
      infected K85.92 ◀
    alcohol induced (without necrosis or infection) K85.20 ⬅
      with necrosis (uninfected) K85.21 ◀
        infected K85.22 ◀
    biliary (without necrosis or infection) K85.10 ⬅
      with necrosis (uninfected) K85.11 ◀
        infected K85.12 ◀
    drug induced (without necrosis or infection) K85.30 ⬅
      with necrosis (uninfected) K85.31 ◀
        infected K85.32 ◀
    gallstone (without necrosis or infection) K85.10 ⬅
      with necrosis (uninfected) K85.11 ◀
        infected K85.12 ◀
    idiopathic (without necrosis or infection) K85.00 ⬅
      with necrosis (uninfected) K85.01 ◀
        infected K85.02 ◀
    specified NEC (without necrosis or infection) K85.80 ⬅
      with necrosis (uninfected) K85.81 ◀
        infected K85.82 ◀
  chronic (infectious) K86.1
    alcohol-induced K86.0
    recurrent K86.1
    relapsing K86.1
  cystic (chronic) K86.1
  cytomegaloviral B25.2
  fibrous (chronic) K86.1
  gallstone (without necrosis or infection) K85.10 ⬅
    with necrosis (uninfected) K85.11 ◀
      infected K85.12 ◀
  gangrenous —*see* Pancreatitis, acute ⬅
  interstitial (chronic) K86.1
    acute —*see also* Pancreatitis, acute K85.80 ⬅
  mumps B26.3
  recurrent (chronic) K86.1
  relapsing, chronic K86.1
  syphilitic A52.74
Pancreatoblastoma —*see* Neoplasm, pancreas, malignant
Pancreolithiasis K86.89 ⬅
Pancytolysis D75.89

◀ New ⬅ Revised ~~deleted~~ Deleted

Pancytopenia (acquired) D61.818
- with
  - malformations D61.Ø9
  - myelodysplastic syndrome —*see* Syndrome, myelodysplastic
- antineoplastic chemotherapy induced D61.81Ø
- congenital D61.Ø9
- drug-induced NEC D61.811

Panencephalitis, subacute, sclerosing A81.1
Panhematopenia D61.9
- congenital D61.Ø9
- constitutional D61.Ø9
- splenic, primary D73.1

Panhemocytopenia D61.9
- congenital D61.Ø9
- constitutional D61.Ø9

Panhypogonadism E29.1
Panhypopituitarism E23.Ø
- prepubertal E23.Ø

Panic (attack) (state) F41.Ø
- reaction to exceptional stress (transient) F43.Ø

Panmyelopathy, familial, constitutional D61.Ø9
Panmyelophthisis D61.82
- congenital D61.Ø9

Panmyelosis (acute) (with myelofibrosis) C94.4-
Panner's disease —*see* Osteochondrosis, juvenile, humerus
Panneuritis endemica E51.11
Panniculitis (nodular) (nonsuppurative) M79.3
- back M54.ØØ
  - cervical region M54.Ø2
  - cervicothoracic region M54.Ø3
  - lumbar region M54.Ø6
  - lumbosacral region M54.Ø7
  - multiple sites M54.Ø9
  - occipito-atlanto-axial region M54.Ø1
  - sacrococcygeal region M54.Ø8
  - thoracic region M54.Ø4
  - thoracolumbar region M54.Ø5
- lupus L93.2
- mesenteric K65.4
- neck M54.Ø2
  - cervicothoracic region M54.Ø3
  - occipito-atlanto-axial region M54.Ø1
- relapsing M35.6

Panniculus adiposus (abdominal) E65
Pannus (allergic) (cornea) (degenerativus) (keratic) H16.42-
- abdominal (symptomatic) E65
- trachomatosus, trachomatous (active) A71.1

Panophthalmitis H44.Ø1-
Pansinusitis (chronic) (hyperplastic) (nonpurulent) (purulent) J32.4
- acute JØ1.4Ø
  - recurrent JØ1.41
- tuberculous A15.8

Panuveitis (sympathetic) H44.11-
Panvalvular disease IØ8.9
- specified NEC IØ8.8

PAPA (pyogenic arthritis, pyoderma gangrenosum, and acne syndrome) MØ4.8 ◀
Papanicolaou smear, cervix Z12.4
- as part of routine gynecological examination ZØ1.419
  - with abnormal findings ZØ1.411
- for suspected neoplasm Z12.4
- nonspecific abnormal finding R87.619
- routine ZØ1.419
  - with abnormal findings ZØ1.411

Papilledema (choked disc) H47.1Ø
- associated with
  - decreased ocular pressure H47.12
  - increased intracranial pressure H47.11
  - retinal disorder H47.13
- Foster-Kennedy syndrome H47.14-

Papillitis H46.ØØ
- anus K62.89
- chronic lingual K14.4
- necrotizing, kidney N17.2
- optic H46.Ø-
- rectum K62.89
- renal, necrotizing N17.2
- tongue K14.Ø

Papilloma —*see also* Neoplasm, benign, by site
- acuminatum (female) (male) (anogenital) A63.Ø
- basal cell L82.1 ◀
  - inflamed L82.Ø ◀
- benign pinta (primary) A67.Ø
- bladder (urinary) (transitional cell) D41.4
- choroid plexus (lateral ventricle) (third ventricle) D33.Ø
  - anaplastic C71.5
  - fourth ventricle D33.1
  - malignant C71.5
- renal pelvis (transitional cell) D41.1-
  - benign D3Ø.1-
- Schneiderian
  - specified site —*see* Neoplasm, benign, by site
  - unspecified site D14.Ø
- serous surface
  - borderline malignancy
    - specified site —*see* Neoplasm, uncertain behavior, by site
    - unspecified site D39.1Ø
  - specified site —*see* Neoplasm, benign, by site
  - unspecified site D27.9
- transitional (cell)
  - bladder (urinary) D41.4
  - inverted type —*see* Neoplasm, uncertain behavior, by site
  - renal pelvis D41.1-
  - ureter D41.2-
- ureter (transitional cell) D41.2-
  - benign D3Ø.2-
- urothelial —*see* Neoplasm, uncertain behavior, by site
- villous —*see* Neoplasm, uncertain behavior, by site
  - adenocarcinoma in —*see* Neoplasm, malignant, by site
  - in situ —*see* Neoplasm, in situ
- yaws, plantar or palmar A66.1

Papillomata, multiple, of yaws A66.1
Papillomatosis —*see also* Neoplasm, benign, by site
- confluent and reticulated L83
- cystic, breast —*see* Mastopathy, cystic
- ductal, breast —*see* Mastopathy, cystic
- intraductal (diffuse) —*see* Neoplasm, benign, by site
- subareolar duct D24-

Papillomavirus, as cause of disease classified elsewhere B97.7
Papillon-Léage and Psaume syndrome Q87.Ø
Papule (s) R23.8
- carate (primary) A67.Ø
- fibrous, of nose D22.39
- Gottron's L94.4
- pinta (primary) A67.Ø

Papulosis
- lymphomatoid C86.6
- malignant I77.89

Papyraceous fetus O31.Ø-
Para-albuminemia E88.Ø9
Paracephalus Q89.7
Parachute mitral valve Q23.2
Paracoccidioidomycosis B41.9
- disseminated B41.7
- generalized B41.7
- mucocutaneous-lymphangitic B41.8
- pulmonary B41.Ø
- specified NEC B41.8
- visceral B41.8

Paradentosis KØ5.4
Paraffinoma T88.8
Paraganglioma D44.7
- adrenal D35.Ø-
  - malignant C74.1-
- aortic body D44.7
  - malignant C75.5
- carotid body D44.6
  - malignant C75.4
- chromaffin —*see also* Neoplasm, benign, by site
  - malignant —*see* Neoplasm, malignant, by site
- extra-adrenal D44.7
  - malignant C75.5
    - specified site —*see* Neoplasm, malignant, by site
    - unspecified site C75.5
  - specified site —*see* Neoplasm, uncertain behavior, by site
  - unspecified site D44.7
- gangliocytic D13.2
  - specified site —*see* Neoplasm, benign, by site
  - unspecified site D13.2
- glomus jugulare D44.7
  - malignant C75.5
- jugular D44.7
- malignant C75.5
  - specified site —*see* Neoplasm, malignant, by site
  - unspecified site C75.5
- nonchromaffin D44.7
  - malignant C75.5
    - specified site —*see* Neoplasm, malignant, by site
    - unspecified site C75.5
  - specified site —*see* Neoplasm, uncertain behavior, by site
  - unspecified site D44.7
- parasympathetic D44.7
  - specified site —*see* Neoplasm, uncertain behavior, by site
  - unspecified site D44.7
- specified site —*see* Neoplasm, uncertain behavior, by site
- sympathetic D44.7
  - specified site —*see* Neoplasm, uncertain behavior, by site
  - unspecified site D44.7
- unspecified site D44.7

Parageusia R43.2
- psychogenic F45.8

Paragonimiasis B66.4
Paragranuloma, Hodgkin —*see* Lymphoma, Hodgkin, classical, specified NEC
Parahemophilia —*see also* Defect, coagulation D68.2
Parakeratosis R23.4
- variegata L41.Ø

Paralysis, paralytic (complete) (incomplete) G83.9
- with
  - syphilis A52.17
- abducens, abducent (nerve) —*see* Strabismus, paralytic, sixth nerve
- abductor, lower extremity G57.9-
- accessory nerve G52.8
- accommodation —*see also* Paresis, of accommodation
  - hysterical F44.89
- acoustic nerve (except Deafness) —*see* subcategory H93.3
- agitans —*see also* Parkinsonism G2Ø
  - arteriosclerotic G21.4
- alternating (oculomotor) G83.89
- amyotrophic G12.21

Paralysis, paralytic *(Continued)*
ankle G57.9-
anus (sphincter) K62.89
arm —*see* Monoplegia, upper limb
ascending (spinal), acute G61.0
association G12.29
asthenic bulbar G70.00
with exacerbation (acute) G70.01
in crisis G70.01
ataxic (hereditary) G11.9
general (syphilitic) A52.17
atrophic G58.9
infantile, acute —*see* Poliomyelitis, paralytic
progressive G12.22
spinal (acute) —*see* Poliomyelitis, paralytic
axillary G54.0
Babinski-Nageotte's G83.89
Bell's G51.0
newborn P11.3
Benedikt's G46.3
birth injury P14.9
spinal cord P11.5
bladder (neurogenic) (sphincter) N31.2
bowel, colon or intestine K56.0
brachial plexus G54.0
birth injury P14.3
newborn (birth injury) P14.3
brain G83.9
diplegia G83.0
triplegia G83.89
bronchial J98.09
Brown-Séquard G83.81
bulbar (chronic) (progressive) G12.22
infantile —*see* Poliomyelitis, paralytic
poliomyelitic —*see* Poliomyelitis, paralytic
pseudo G12.29
bulbospinal G70.00
with exacerbation (acute) G70.01
in crisis G70.01
cardiac —*see also* Failure, heart I50.9
cerebrocerebellar, diplegic G80.1
cervical
plexus G54.2
sympathetic G90.09
Céstan-Chenais G46.3
Charcot-Marie-Tooth type G60.0
Clark's G80.9
colon K56.0
compressed air T70.3
compression
arm G56.9-
leg G57.9-
lower extremity G57.9-
upper extremity G56.9-
congenital (cerebral) —*see* Palsy, cerebral
conjugate movement (gaze) (of eye) H51.0
cortical (nuclear) (supranuclear) H51.0
cordis —*see* Failure, heart
cranial or cerebral nerve G52.9
creeping G12.22
crossed leg G83.89
crutch —*see* Injury, brachial plexus
deglutition R13.0
hysterical F44.4
dementia A52.17
descending (spinal) NEC G12.29
diaphragm (flaccid) J98.6
due to accidental dissection of phrenic nerve during procedure —*see* Puncture, accidental complicating surgery
digestive organs NEC K59.8
diplegic —*see* Diplegia
divergence (nuclear) H51.8
diver's T70.3
Duchenne's
birth injury P14.0
due to or associated with
motor neuron disease G12.22
muscular dystrophy G71.0

Paralysis, paralytic *(Continued)*
due to intracranial or spinal birth injury —*see* Palsy, cerebral
embolic (current episode) I63.4- (Revised)
Erb (-Duchenne) (birth) (newborn) P14.0
Erb's syphilitic spastic spinal A52.17
esophagus K22.8
eye muscle (extrinsic) H49.9
intrinsic —*see also* Paresis, of accommodation
facial (nerve) G51.0
birth injury P11.3
congenital P11.3
following operation NEC —*see* Puncture, accidental complicating surgery
newborn (birth injury) P11.3
familial (recurrent) (periodic) G72.3
spastic G11.4
fauces J39.2
finger G56.9-
gait R26.1
gastric nerve (nondiabetic) G52.2
gaze, conjugate H51.0
general (progressive) (syphilitic) A52.17
juvenile A50.45
glottis J38.00
bilateral J38.02
unilateral J38.01
gluteal G54.1
Gubler (-Millard) G46.3
hand —*see* Monoplegia, upper limb
heart —*see* Arrest, cardiac
hemiplegic —*see* Hemiplegia
hyperkalemic periodic (familial) G72.3
hypoglossal (nerve) G52.3
hypokalemic periodic G72.3
hysterical F44.4
ileus K56.0
infantile —*see also* Poliomyelitis, paralytic A80.30
bulbar —*see* Poliomyelitis, paralytic
cerebral —*see* Palsy, cerebral
spastic —*see* Palsy, cerebral, spastic
infective —*see* Poliomyelitis, paralytic
inferior nuclear G83.9
internuclear —*see* Ophthalmoplegia, internuclear
intestine K56.0
iris H57.09
due to diphtheria (toxin) A36.89
ischemic, Volkmann's (complicating trauma) T79.6
Jackson's G83.89
jake —*see* Poisoning, food, noxious, plant
Jamaica ginger (jake) G62.2
juvenile general A50.45
Klumpke (-Déjérine) (birth) (newborn) P14.1
labioglossal (laryngeal) (pharyngeal) G12.29
Landry's G61.0
laryngeal nerve (recurrent) (superior) (unilateral) J38.00
bilateral J38.02
unilateral J38.01
larynx J38.00
bilateral J38.02
due to diphtheria (toxin) A36.2
unilateral J38.01
lateral G12.21
lead —*see* subcategory T56.0
left side —*see* Hemiplegia
leg G83.1-
both —*see* Paraplegia
crossed G83.89
hysterical F44.4
psychogenic F44.4
transient or transitory R29.818
traumatic NEC —*see* Injury, nerve, leg
levator palpebrae superioris —*see* Blepharoptosis, paralytic
limb —*see* Monoplegia
lip K13.0

Paralysis, paralytic *(Continued)*
Lissauer's A52.17
lower limb —*see* Monoplegia, lower limb
both —*see* Paraplegia
lung J98.4
median nerve G56.1-
medullary (tegmental) G83.89
mesencephalic NEC G83.89
tegmental G83.89
middle alternating G83.89
Millard-Gubler-Foville G46.3
monoplegic —*see* Monoplegia
motor G83.9
muscle, muscular NEC G72.89
due to nerve lesion G58.9
eye (extrinsic) H49.9
intrinsic —*see* Paresis, of accommodation
oblique —*see* Strabismus, paralytic, fourth nerve
iris sphincter H21.9
ischemic (Volkmann's) (complicating trauma) T79.6
progressive G12.21
pseudohypertrophic G71.0
musculocutaneous nerve G56.9-
musculospiral G56.9-
nerve —*see also* Disorder, nerve
abducent —*see* Strabismus, paralytic, sixth nerve
accessory G52.8
auditory (except Deafness) —*see* subcategory H93.3
birth injury P14.9
cranial or cerebral G52.9
facial G51.0
birth injury P11.3
congenital P11.3
newborn (birth injury) P11.3
fourth or trochlear —*see* Strabismus, paralytic, fourth nerve
newborn (birth injury) P14.9
oculomotor —*see* Strabismus, paralytic, third nerve
phrenic (birth injury) P14.2
radial G56.3-
seventh or facial G51.0
newborn (birth injury) P11.3
sixth or abducent —*see* Strabismus, paralytic, sixth nerve
syphilitic A52.15
third or oculomotor —*see* Strabismus, paralytic, third nerve
trigeminal G50.9
trochlear —*see* Strabismus, paralytic, fourth nerve
ulnar G56.2-
normokalemic periodic G72.3
ocular H49.9
alternating G83.89
oculofacial, congenital (Moebius) Q87.0
oculomotor (external bilateral) (nerve) —*see* Strabismus, paralytic, third nerve
palate (soft) K13.79
paratrigeminal G50.9
periodic (familial) (hyperkalemic) (hypokalemic) (myotonic) (normokalemic) (potassium sensitive) (secondary) G72.3
peripheral autonomic nervous system —*see* Neuropathy, peripheral, autonomic
peroneal (nerve) G57.3-
pharynx J39.2
phrenic nerve G56.8-
plantar nerve (s) G57.6-
pneumogastric nerve G52.2
poliomyelitis (current) —*see* Poliomyelitis, paralytic
popliteal nerve G57.3-
postepileptic transitory G83.84

Paralysis, paralytic *(Continued)*
progressive (atrophic) (bulbar) (spinal) G12.22
general A52.17
infantile acute —*see* Poliomyelitis, paralytic
supranuclear G23.1
pseudobulbar G12.29
pseudohypertrophic (muscle) G71.Ø
psychogenic F44.4
quadriceps G57.9-
quadriplegic —*see* Tetraplegia
radial nerve G56.3-
rectus muscle (eye) H49.9
recurrent isolated sleep G47.53
respiratory (muscle) (system) (tract) RØ6.81
center NEC G93.89
congenital P28.89
newborn P28.89
right side —*see* Hemiplegia
saturnine —*see* subcategory T56.Ø
sciatic nerve G57.Ø-
senile G83.9
shaking —*see* Parkinsonism
shoulder G56.9-
sleep, recurrent isolated G47.53
spastic G83.9
cerebral —*see* Palsy, cerebral, spastic
congenital (cerebral) —*see* Palsy, cerebral, spastic
familial G11.4
hereditary G11.4
quadriplegic G8Ø.Ø
syphilitic (spinal) A52.17
sphincter, bladder —*see* Paralysis, bladder
spinal (cord) G83.9
accessory nerve G52.8
acute —*see* Poliomyelitis, paralytic
ascending acute G61.Ø
atrophic (acute) —*see also* Poliomyelitis, paralytic
spastic, syphilitic A52.17
congenital NEC —*see* Palsy, cerebral
hereditary G95.89
infantile —*see* Poliomyelitis, paralytic
progressive G12.21
sequelae NEC G83.89
sternomastoid G52.8
stomach K31.84
diabetic —*see* Diabetes, by type, with gastroparesis
nerve G52.2
diabetic —*see* Diabetes, by type, with gastroparesis
stroke —*see* Infarct, brain
subcapsularis G56.8-
supranuclear (progressive) G23.1
sympathetic G9Ø.8
cervical G9Ø.Ø9
nervous system —*see* Neuropathy, peripheral, autonomic
syndrome G83.9
specified NEC G83.89
syphilitic spastic spinal (Erb's) A52.17
thigh G57.9-
throat J39.2
diphtheritic A36.Ø
muscle J39.2
thrombotic (current episode) I63.3- ◄
thumb G56.9-
tick —*see* Toxicity, venom, arthropod, specified NEC
Todd's (postepileptic transitory paralysis) G83.84
toe G57.6-
tongue K14.8
transient R29.5
arm or leg NEC R29.818
traumatic NEC —*see* Injury, nerve
trapezius G52.8
traumatic, transient NEC —*see* Injury, nerve

Paralysis, paralytic *(Continued)*
trembling —*see* Parkinsonism
triceps brachii G56.9-
trigeminal nerve G5Ø.9
trochlear (nerve) —*see* Strabismus, paralytic, fourth nerve
ulnar nerve G56.2-
upper limb —*see* Monoplegia, upper limb
uremic N18.9 *[G99.8]*
uveoparotitic D86.89
uvula K13.79
postdiphtheritic A36.Ø
vagus nerve G52.2
vasomotor NEC G9Ø.8
velum palati K13.79
vesical —*see* Paralysis, bladder
vestibular nerve (except Vertigo) —*see* subcategory H93.3
vocal cords J38.ØØ
bilateral J38.Ø2
unilateral J38.Ø1
Volkmann's (complicating trauma) T79.6
wasting G12.29
Weber's G46.3
wrist G56.9-
Paramedial urethrovesical orifice Q64.79
Paramenia N92.6
Parametritis —*see also* Disease, pelvis, inflammatory N73.2
acute N73.Ø
complicating abortion —*see* Abortion, by type, complicated by, parametritis
Parametrium, parametric —*see* condition
Paramnesia —*see* Amnesia
Paramolar KØØ.1
Paramyloidosis E85.8
Paramyoclonus multiplex G25.3
Paramyotonia (congenita) G71.19
Parangi —*see* Yaws
Paranoia (querulans) F22
senile FØ3
Paranoid
dementia (senile) FØ3
praecox —*see* Schizophrenia
personality F6Ø.Ø
psychosis (climacteric) (involutional) (menopausal) F22
psychogenic (acute) F23
senile FØ3
reaction (acute) F23
chronic F22
schizophrenia F2Ø.Ø
state (climacteric) (involutional) (menopausal) (simple) F22
senile FØ3
tendencies F6Ø.Ø
traits F6Ø.Ø
trends F6Ø.Ø
type, psychopathic personality F6Ø.Ø
Paraparesis —*see* Paraplegia
Paraphasia R47.Ø2
Paraphilia F65.9
Paraphimosis (congenital) N47.2
chancroidal A57
Paraphrenia, paraphrenic (late) F22
schizophrenia F2Ø.Ø
Paraplegia (lower) G82.2Ø
ataxic —*see* Degeneration, combined, spinal cord
complete G82.21
congenital (cerebral) G8Ø.8
spastic G8Ø.1
familial spastic G11.4
functional (hysterical) F44.4
hereditary, spastic G11.4
hysterical F44.4
incomplete G82.22
Pott's A18.Ø1
psychogenic F44.4

Paraplegia *(Continued)*
spastic
Erb's spinal, syphilitic A52.17
hereditary G11.4
tropical GØ4.1
syphilitic (spastic) A52.17
tropical spastic GØ4.1
Parapoxvirus BØ8.6Ø
specified NEC BØ8.69
Paraproteinemia D89.2
benign (familial) D89.2
monoclonal D47.2
secondary to malignant disease D47.2
Parapsoriasis L41.9
en plaques L41.4
guttata L41.1
large plaque L41.4
retiform, retiformis L41.5
small plaque L41.3
specified NEC L41.8
varioliformis (acuta) L41.Ø
Parasitic —*see also* condition
disease NEC B89
stomatitis B37.Ø
sycosis (beard) (scalp) B35.Ø
twin Q89.4
Parasitism B89
intestinal B82.9
skin B88.9
specified —*see* Infestation
Parasitophobia F4Ø.218
Parasomnia G47.5Ø
due to
alcohol
abuse F1Ø.182
dependence F1Ø.282
use F1Ø.982
amphetamines
abuse F15.182
dependence F15.282
use F15.982
caffeine
abuse F15.182
dependence F15.282
use F15.982
cocaine
abuse F14.182
dependence F14.282
use F14.982
drug NEC
abuse F19.182
dependence F19.282
use F19.982
opioid
abuse F11.182
dependence F11.282
use F11.982
psychoactive substance NEC
abuse F19.182
dependence F19.282
use F19.982
sedative, hypnotic, or anxiolytic
abuse F13.182
dependence F13.282
use F13.982
stimulant NEC
abuse F15.182
dependence F15.282
use F15.982
in conditions classified elsewhere G47.54
nonorganic origin F51.8
organic G47.5Ø
specified NEC G47.59
Paraspadias Q54.9
Paraspasmus facialis G51.8
Parasuicide (attempt)
history of (personal) Z91.5
in family Z81.8
Parathyroid gland —*see* condition
Parathyroid tetany E2Ø.9
Paratrachoma A74.Ø

P

Paratyphilitis —*see* Appendicitis
Paratyphoid (fever) —*see* Fever, paratyphoid
Paratyphus —*see* Fever, paratyphoid
Paraurethral duct Q64.79
nonorganic origin F51.5
Paraurethritis —*see also* Urethritis
gonococcal (acute) (chronic) (with abscess) A54.1
Paravaccinia NEC BØ8.Ø4
Paravaginitis —*see* Vaginitis
Parencephalitis —*see also* Encephalitis
sequelae GØ9
Parent-child conflict —*see* Conflict, parent-child
estrangement NEC Z62.89Ø
Paresis —*see also* Paralysis
accommodation —*see* Paresis, of accommodation
Bernhardt's G57.1-
bladder (sphincter) —*see also* Paralysis, bladder
tabetic A52.17
bowel, colon or intestine K56.Ø
extrinsic muscle, eye H49.9
general (progressive) (syphilitic) A52.17
juvenile A5Ø.45
heart —*see* Failure, heart
insane (syphilitic) A52.17
juvenile (general) A5Ø.45
of accommodation H52.52-
peripheral progressive (idiopathic) G6Ø.3
pseudohypertrophic G71.Ø
senile G83.9
syphilitic (general) A52.17
congenital A5Ø.45
vesical NEC N31.2
Paresthesia —*see also* Disturbance, sensation
Bernhardt G57.1-
Paretic —*see* condition
Parinaud's
conjunctivitis H1Ø.89
oculoglandular syndrome H1Ø.89
ophthalmoplegia H49.88
Parkinsonism (idiopathic) (primary) G2Ø
with neurogenic orthostatic hypotension (symptomatic) G9Ø.3
arteriosclerotic G21.4
dementia G31.83 *[FØ2.8Ø]*
with behavioral disturbance G31.83 *[FØ2.81]*
due to
drugs NEC G21.19
neuroleptic G21.11
neuroleptic induced G21.11
postencephalitic G21.3
secondary G21.9
due to
arteriosclerosis G21.4
drugs NEC G21.19
neuroleptic G21.11
encephalitis G21.3
external agents NEC G21.2
syphilis A52.19
specified NEC G21.8
syphilitic A52.19
treatment-induced NEC G21.19
vascular G21.4
Parkinson's disease, syndrome or tremor —*see* Parkinsonism
Parodontitis —*see* Periodontitis
Parodontosis KØ5.4
Paronychia —*see also* Cellulitis, digit
with lymphangitis —*see* Lymphangitis, acute, digit
candidal (chronic) B37.2
tuberculous (primary) A18.4
Parorexia (psychogenic) F5Ø.89
Parosmia R43.1
psychogenic F45.8
Parotid gland —*see* condition
Parotitis, parotiditis (allergic) (nonspecific toxic) (purulent) (septic) (suppurative) —*see also* Sialoadenitis
Parotitis, parotiditis *(Continued)*
epidemic —*see* Mumps
infectious —*see* Mumps
postoperative K91.89
surgical K91.89
Parrot fever A7Ø
Parrot's disease (early congenital syphilitic pseudoparalysis) A5Ø.Ø2
Parry-Romberg syndrome G51.8
Parry's disease or syndrome EØ5.ØØ
with thyroid storm EØ5.Ø1
Pars planitis —*see* Cyclitis
Parsonage (-Aldren)-**Turner syndrome** G54.5
Parson's disease (exophthalmic goiter) EØ5.ØØ
with thyroid storm EØ5.Ø1
Particolored infant Q82.8
Parturition —*see* Delivery
Parulis KØ4.7
with sinus KØ4.6
Parvovirus, as cause of disease classified elsewhere B97.6
Pasini and Pierini's atrophoderma L9Ø.3
Passage
false, urethra N36.5
meconium (newborn) during delivery PØ3.82
of sounds or bougies —*see* Attention to, artificial, opening
Passive —*see* condition
smoking Z77.22
Pasteurella septica A28.Ø
Pasteurellosis —*see* Infection, Pasteurella
PAT (paroxysmal atrial tachycardia) I47.1
Patau's syndrome —*see* Trisomy, 13
Patches
mucous (syphilitic) A51.39
congenital A5Ø.Ø7
smokers' (mouth) K13.24
Patellar —*see* condition
Patent —*see also* Imperfect, closure
canal of Nuck Q52.4
cervix N88.3
ductus arteriosus or Botallo's Q25.Ø
foramen
botalli Q21.1
ovale Q21.1
interauricular septum Q21.1
interventricular septum Q21.Ø
omphalomesenteric duct Q43.Ø
os (uteri) —*see* Patent, cervix
ostium secundum Q21.1
urachus Q64.4
vitelline duct Q43.Ø
Paterson (-Brown)(-Kelly) **syndrome or web** D5Ø.1
Pathologic, pathological —*see also* condition
asphyxia RØ9.Ø1
fire-setting F63.1
gambling F63.Ø
ovum OØ2.Ø
resorption, tooth KØ3.3
stealing F63.2
Pathology (of) —*see* Disease
periradicular, associated with previous endodontic treatment NEC M27.59
Pattern, sleep-wake, irregular G47.23
Patulous —*see also* Imperfect, closure (congenital)
alimentary tract Q45.8
lower Q43.8
upper Q4Ø.8
eustachian tube H69.Ø-
Pause, sinoatrial I49.5
Paxton's disease B36.2
Pearl (s)
enamel KØØ.2
Epstein's KØ9.8
Pearl-worker's disease —*see* Osteomyelitis, specified type NEC
Pectenosis K62.4
Pectoral —*see* condition
Pectus
carinatum (congenital) Q67.7
acquired M95.4
rachitic sequelae (late effect) E64.3
excavatum (congenital) Q67.6
acquired M95.4
rachitic sequelae (late effect) E64.3
recurvatum (congenital) Q67.6
Pedatrophia E41
Pederosis F65.4
Pediculosis (infestation) B85.2
capitis (head-louse) (any site) B85.Ø
corporis (body-louse) (any site) B85.1
eyelid B85.Ø
mixed (classifiable to more than one of the titles B85.Ø-B85.3) B85.4
pubis (pubic louse) (any site) B85.3
vestimenti B85.1
vulvae B85.3
Pediculus (infestation) —*see* Pediculosis
Pedophilia F65.4
Peg-shaped teeth KØØ.2
Pelade —*see* Alopecia, areata
Pelger-Huët anomaly or syndrome D72.Ø
Peliosis (rheumatica) D69.Ø
hepatis K76.4
with toxic liver disease K71.8
Pelizaeus-Merzbacher disease E75.29
Pellagra (alcoholic) (with polyneuropathy) E52
Pellagra-cerebellar-ataxia-renal aminoaciduria syndrome E72.Ø2
Pellegrini (-Stieda) **disease or syndrome** —*see* Bursitis, tibial collateral
Pellizzi's syndrome E34.8
Pel's crisis A52.11
Pelvic —*see also* condition
examination (periodic) (routine) ZØ1.419
with abnormal findings ZØ1.411
kidney, congenital Q63.2
Pelviolithiasis —*see* Calculus, kidney
Pelviperitonitis —*see also* Peritonitis, pelvic
gonococcal A54.24
puerperal O85
Pelvis —*see* condition or type
Pemphigoid L12.9
benign, mucous membrane L12.1
bullous L12.Ø
cicatricial L12.1
juvenile L12.2
ocular L12.1
specified NEC L12.8
Pemphigus L1Ø.9
benign familial (chronic) Q82.8
Brazilian L1Ø.3
circinatus L13.Ø
conjunctiva L12.1
drug-induced L1Ø.5
erythematosus L1Ø.4
foliaceous L1Ø.2
gangrenous —*see* Gangrene
neonatorum LØ1.Ø3
ocular L12.1
paraneoplastic L1Ø.81
specified NEC L1Ø.89
syphilitic (congenital) A5Ø.Ø6
vegetans L1Ø.1
vulgaris L1Ø.Ø
wildfire L1Ø.3
Pendred's syndrome EØ7.1
Pendulous
abdomen, in pregnancy —*see* Pregnancy, complicated by, abnormal, pelvic organs or tissues NEC
breast N64.89
Penetrating wound —*see also* Puncture
with internal injury —*see* Injury, by site
eyeball —*see* Puncture, eyeball
orbit (with or without foreign body) —*see* Puncture, orbit
uterus by instrument with or following ectopic or molar pregnancy OØ8.6

P

Penicillosis B48.4
Penis —*see* condition
Penitis N48.29
Pentalogy of Fallot Q21.8
Pentasomy X syndrome Q97.1
Pentosuria (essential) E74.8
Percreta placenta O43.23-
Peregrinating patient —*see* Disorder, factitious
Perforation, perforated (nontraumatic) (of)
accidental during procedure (blood vessel) (nerve) (organ) —*see* Complication, accidental puncture or laceration
antrum —*see* Sinusitis, maxillary
appendix K35.2
with localized peritonitis K35.3 ◀
atrial septum, multiple Q21.1
attic, ear —*see* Perforation, tympanum, attic
bile duct (common) (hepatic) K83.2
cystic K82.2
bladder (urinary)
with or following ectopic or molar pregnancy O08.6
obstetrical trauma O71.5
traumatic S37.29
at delivery O71.5
bowel K63.1
with or following ectopic or molar pregnancy O08.6
newborn P78.0
obstetrical trauma O71.5
traumatic —*see* Laceration, intestine
broad ligament N83.8
with or following ectopic or molar pregnancy O08.6
obstetrical trauma O71.6
by
device, implant or graft —*see also* Complications, by site and type, mechanical T85.628
arterial graft NEC —*see* Complication, cardiovascular device, mechanical, vascular
breast (implant) T85.49
catheter NEC T85.698
cystostomy T83.090
dialysis (renal) T82.49
intraperitoneal T85.691
infusion NEC T82.594
spinal (epidural) (subdural) T85.690
urinary —*see also* Complications, catheter, urinary T83.098 ◀
electronic (electrode) (pulse generator) (stimulator)
bone T84.390
cardiac T82.199
electrode T82.190
pulse generator T82.191
specified type NEC T82.198
nervous system —*see* Complication, prosthetic device, mechanical, electronic nervous system stimulator
urinary —*see* Complication, genitourinary, device, urinary, mechanical
fixation, internal (orthopedic) NEC —*see* Complication, fixation device, mechanical
gastrointestinal —*see* Complications, prosthetic device, mechanical, gastrointestinal device
genital NEC T83.498
intrauterine contraceptive device T83.39
penile prosthesis T83.490
heart NEC —*see* Complication, cardiovascular device, mechanical
joint prosthesis —*see* Complications, joint prosthesis, mechanical, specified NEC, by site

Perforation, perforated *(Continued)*
by *(Continued)*
urinary *(Continued)*
ocular NEC —*see* Complications, prosthetic device, mechanical, ocular device
orthopedic NEC —*see* Complication, orthopedic, device, mechanical
specified NEC T85.628
urinary NEC —*see also* Complication, genitourinary, device, urinary, mechanical
graft T83.29
~~urinary, indwelling T83.098~~
vascular NEC —*see* Complication, cardiovascular device, mechanical
ventricular intracranial shunt T85.09
foreign body left accidentally in operative wound T81.539
instrument (any) during a procedure, accidental —*see* Puncture, accidental complicating surgery
cecum K35.2
with localized peritonitis K35.3 ◀
cervix (uteri) N88.8
with or following ectopic or molar pregnancy O08.6
obstetrical trauma O71.3
colon K63.1
newborn P78.0
obstetrical trauma O71.5
traumatic —*see* Laceration, intestine, large
common duct (bile) K83.2
cornea (due to ulceration) —*see* Ulcer, cornea, perforated
cystic duct K82.2
diverticulum (intestine) K57.80
with bleeding K57.81
large intestine K57.20
with
bleeding K57.21
small intestine K57.40
with bleeding K57.41
small intestine K57.00
with
bleeding K57.01
large intestine K57.40
with bleeding K57.41
ear drum —*see* Perforation, tympanum
esophagus K22.3
ethmoidal sinus —*see* Sinusitis, ethmoidal
frontal sinus —*see* Sinusitis, frontal
gallbladder K82.2
heart valve —*see* Endocarditis
ileum K63.1
newborn P78.0
obstetrical trauma O71.5
traumatic —*see* Laceration, intestine, small
instrumental, surgical (accidental) (blood vessel) (nerve) (organ) —*see* Puncture, accidental complicating surgery
intestine NEC K63.1
with ectopic or molar pregnancy O08.6
newborn P78.0
obstetrical trauma O71.5
traumatic —*see* Laceration, intestine
ulcerative NEC K63.1
newborn P78.0
jejunum, jejunal K63.1
obstetrical trauma O71.5
traumatic —*see* Laceration, intestine, small
ulcer —*see* Ulcer, gastrojejunal, with perforation
joint prosthesis —*see* Complications, joint prosthesis, mechanical, specified NEC, by site
mastoid (antrum) (cell) —*see* Disorder, mastoid, specified NEC
maxillary sinus —*see* Sinusitis, maxillary
membrana tympani —*see* Perforation, tympanum

Perforation, perforated *(Continued)*
nasal
septum J34.89
congenital Q30.3
syphilitic A52.73
sinus J34.89
congenital Q30.8
due to sinusitis —*see* Sinusitis
palate —*see also* Cleft, palate Q35.9
syphilitic A52.79
palatine vault —*see also* Cleft, palate, hard Q35.1
syphilitic A52.79
congenital A50.59
pars flaccida (ear drum) —*see* Perforation, tympanum, attic
pelvic
floor S31.030
with
ectopic or molar pregnancy O08.6
penetration into retroperitoneal space S31.031
retained foreign body S31.040
with penetration into retroperitoneal space S31.041
following ectopic or molar pregnancy O08.6
obstetrical trauma O70.1
organ S37.99
adrenal gland S37.818
bladder —*see* Perforation, bladder
fallopian tube S37.599
bilateral S37.592
unilateral S37.591
kidney S37.09-
obstetrical trauma O71.5
ovary S37.499
bilateral S37.492
unilateral S37.491
prostate S37.828
specified organ NEC S37.898
ureter —*see* Perforation, ureter
urethra —*see* Perforation, urethra
uterus —*see* Perforation, uterus
perineum —*see* Laceration, perineum
pharynx J39.2
rectum K63.1
newborn P78.0
obstetrical trauma O71.5
traumatic S36.63
root canal space due to endodontic treatment M27.51
sigmoid K63.1
newborn P78.0
obstetrical trauma O71.5
traumatic S36.533
sinus (accessory) (chronic) (nasal) J34.89
sphenoidal sinus —*see* Sinusitis, sphenoidal
surgical (accidental) (by instrument) (blood vessel) (nerve) (organ) —*see* Puncture, accidental complicating surgery
traumatic
external —*see* Puncture
eye —*see* Puncture, eyeball
internal organ —*see* Injury, by site
tympanum, tympanic (membrane) (persistent post-traumatic) (postinflammatory) H72.9-
attic H72.1-
multiple —*see* Perforation, tympanum, multiple
total —*see* Perforation, tympanum, total
central H72.0-
multiple —*see* Perforation, tympanum, multiple
total —*see* Perforation, tympanum, total
marginal NEC —*see* subcategory H72.2
multiple H72.81-
pars flaccida —*see* Perforation, tympanum, attic
total H72.82-
traumatic, current episode S09.2-

Perforation, perforated *(Continued)*
typhoid, gastrointestinal —*see* Typhoid
ulcer —*see* Ulcer, by site, with perforation
ureter N28.89
traumatic S37.19
urethra N36.8
with ectopic or molar pregnancy OØ8.6
following ectopic or molar pregnancy OØ8.6
obstetrical trauma O71.5
traumatic S37.39
at delivery O71.5
uterus
with ectopic or molar pregnancy OØ8.6
by intrauterine contraceptive device T83.39
following ectopic or molar pregnancy OØ8.6
obstetrical trauma O71.1
traumatic S37.69
obstetric O71.1
uvula K13.79
syphilitic A52.79
vagina
obstetrical trauma O71.4
other trauma - see Puncture, vagina
Periadenitis mucosa necrotica recurrens K12.Ø
Periappendicitis (acute) —*see* Appendicitis
Periarteritis nodosa (disseminated) (infectious) (necrotizing) M3Ø.Ø
Periarthritis (joint) —*see also* Enthesopathy
Duplay's M75.Ø-
gonococcal A54.42
humeroscapularis —*see* Capsulitis, adhesive
scapulohumeral —*see* Capsulitis, adhesive
shoulder —*see* Capsulitis, adhesive
wrist M77.2-
Periarthrosis (angioneural) —*see* Enthesopathy
Pericapsulitis, adhesive (shoulder) —*see* Capsulitis, adhesive
Pericarditis (with decompensation) (with effusion) I31.9
with rheumatic fever (conditions in IØØ)
active —*see* Pericarditis, rheumatic
inactive or quiescent IØ9.2
acute (hemorrhagic) (nonrheumatic) (Sicca) I3Ø.9
with chorea (acute) (rheumatic) (Sydenham's) IØ2.Ø
benign I3Ø.8
nonspecific I3Ø.Ø
rheumatic IØ1.Ø
with chorea (acute) (Sydenham's) IØ2.Ø
adhesive or adherent (chronic) (external) (internal) I31.Ø
acute —*see* Pericarditis, acute
rheumatic IØ9.2
bacterial (acute) (subacute) (with serous or seropurulent effusion) I3Ø.1
calcareous I31.1
cholesterol (chronic) I31.8
acute I3Ø.9
chronic (nonrheumatic) I31.9
rheumatic IØ9.2
constrictive (chronic) I31.1
coxsackie B33.23
fibrinocaseous (tuberculous) A18.84
fibrinopurulent I3Ø.1
fibrinous I3Ø.8
fibrous I31.Ø
gonococcal A54.83
idiopathic I3Ø.Ø
in systemic lupus erythematosus M32.12
infective I3Ø.1
meningococcal A39.53
neoplastic (chronic) I31.8
acute I3Ø.9
obliterans, obliterating I31.Ø
plastic I31.Ø
pneumococcal I3Ø.1

Pericarditis *(Continued)*
postinfarction I24.1
purulent I3Ø.1
rheumatic (active) (acute) (with effusion) (with pneumonia) IØ1.Ø
with chorea (acute) (rheumatic) (Sydenham's) IØ2.Ø
chronic or inactive (with chorea) IØ9.2
rheumatoid —*see* Rheumatoid, carditis
septic I3Ø.1
serofibrinous I3Ø.8
staphylococcal I3Ø.1
streptococcal I3Ø.1
suppurative I3Ø.1
syphilitic A52.Ø6
tuberculous A18.84
uremic N18.9 *[I32]*
viral I3Ø.1
Pericardium, pericardial —*see* condition
Pericellulitis —*see* Cellulitis
Pericementitis (chronic) (suppurative) —*see also* Periodontitis
acute KØ5.2Ø
generalized —*see* Peridontitis, aggressive, generalized ⇐
localized —*see* Peridontitis, aggressive, localized ⇐
Perichondritis
auricle —*see* Perichondritis, ear
bronchus J98.Ø9
ear (external) H61.ØØ-
acute H61.Ø1-
chronic H61.Ø2-
external auditory canal —*see* Perichondritis, ear
larynx J38.7
syphilitic A52.73
typhoid AØ1.Ø9
nose J34.89
pinna —*see* Perichondritis, ear
trachea J39.8
Periclasia KØ5.4
Pericoronitis —*see* Periodontitis
Pericystitis N3Ø.9Ø
with hematuria N3Ø.91
Peridiverticulitis (intestine) K57.92
cecum —*see* Diverticulitis, intestine, large
colon —*see* Diverticulitis, intestine, large
duodenum —*see* Diverticulitis, intestine, small
intestine —*see* Diverticulitis, intestine
jejunum —*see* Diverticulitis, intestine, small
rectosigmoid —*see* Diverticulitis, intestine, large
rectum —*see* Diverticulitis, intestine, large
sigmoid —*see* Diverticulitis, intestine, large
Periendocarditis —*see* Endocarditis
Periepididymitis N45.1
Perifolliculitis LØ1.Ø2
abscedens, caput, scalp L66.3
capitis, abscedens (et suffodiens) L66.3
superficial pustular LØ1.Ø2
Perihepatitis K65.8
Perilabyrinthitis (acute) —*see* subcategory H83.Ø
Perimeningitis —*see* Meningitis
Perimetritis —*see* Endometritis
Perimetrosalpingitis —*see* Salpingo-oophoritis
Perineocele N81.81
Perinephric, perinephritic —*see* condition
Perinephritis —*see also* Infection, kidney
purulent —*see* Abscess, kidney
Perineum, perineal —*see* condition
Perineuritis NEC —*see* Neuralgia
Periodic —*see* condition
Periodontitis (chronic) (complex) (compound) (local) (simplex) KØ5.3Ø
acute KØ5.2Ø
generalized KØ5.229 ⇐
moderate KØ5.222 ◄
severe KØ5.223 ◄
slight KØ5.221 ◄

Periodontitis *(Continued)*
acute *(Continued)*
localized KØ5.219 ⇐
moderate KØ5.212 ◄
severe KØ5.213 ◄
slight KØ5.211 ◄
apical KØ4.5
acute (pulpal origin) KØ4.4
generalized KØ5.329 ⇐
moderate KØ5.322 ◄
severe KØ5.323 ◄
slight KØ5.321 ◄
localized KØ5.319 ⇐
moderate KØ5.312 ◄
severe KØ5.313 ◄
slight KØ5.311 ◄
Periodontoclasia KØ5.4
Periodontosis (juvenile) KØ5.4
Periods —*see also* Menstruation
heavy N92.Ø
irregular N92.6
shortened intervals (irregular) N92.1
Perionychia —*see also* Cellulitis, digit
with lymphangitis —*see* Lymphangitis, acute, digit
Perioophoritis —*see* Salpingo-oophoritis
Periorchitis N45.2
Periosteum, periosteal —*see* condition
Periostitis (albuminosa) (circumscribed) (diffuse) (infective) (monomelic) —*see also* Osteomyelitis
alveolar M27.3
alveolodental M27.3
dental M27.3
gonorrheal A54.43
jaw (lower) (upper) M27.2
orbit HØ5.Ø3-
syphilitic A52.77
congenital (early) A5Ø.Ø2 *[M9Ø.8Ø]*
secondary A51.46
tuberculous —*see* Tuberculosis, bone
yaws (hypertrophic) (early) (late) A66.6 *[M9Ø.8Ø]*
Periostosis (hyperplastic) —*see also* Disorder, bone, specified type NEC
with osteomyelitis —*see* Osteomyelitis, specified type NEC
Peripartum
cardiomyopathy O9Ø.3
Periphlebitis —*see* Phlebitis
Periproctitis K62.89
Periprostatitis —*see* Prostatitis
Perirectal —*see* condition
Perirenal —*see* condition
Perisalpingitis —*see* Salpingo-oophoritis
Perisplenitis (infectional) D73.89
Peristalsis, visible or reversed R19.2
Peritendinitis —*see* Enthesopathy
Peritoneum, peritoneal —*see* condition
Peritonitis (adhesive) (bacterial) (fibrinous) (hemorrhagic) (idiopathic) (localized) (perforative) (primary) (with adhesions) (with effusion) K65.9
with or following
abscess K65.1
appendicitis K35.3 ⇐
with perforation or rupture K35.2
generalized K35.2
localized K35.3
diverticular disease (intestine) K57.8Ø
with bleeding K57.81
ectopic or molar pregnancy OØ8.Ø
large intestine K57.2Ø
with
bleeding K57.21
small intestine K57.4Ø
with bleeding K57.41
small intestine K57.ØØ
with
bleeding K57.Ø1
large intestine K57.4Ø
with bleeding K57.41

◄ New ⇐ Revised ~~deleted~~ Deleted

Peritonitis *(Continued)*
  acute (generalized) K65.Ø
  aseptic T81.61
  bile, biliary K65.3
  chemical T81.61
  chlamydial A74.81
  chronic proliferative K65.8
  complicating abortion —*see* Abortion, by type, complicated by, pelvic peritonitis
  congenital P78.1
  diaphragmatic K65.Ø
  diffuse K65.Ø
  diphtheritic A36.89
  disseminated K65.Ø
  due to
    bile K65.3
    foreign
      body or object accidentally left during a procedure (instrument) (sponge) (swab) T81.599
      substance accidentally left during a procedure (chemical) (powder) (talc) T81.61
    talc T81.61
    urine K65.8
  eosinophilic K65.8
    acute K65.Ø
  fibrocaseous (tuberculous) A18.31
  fibropurulent K65.Ø
  following ectopic or molar pregnancy O08.Ø
  general (ized) K65.Ø
  gonococcal A54.85
  meconium (newborn) P78.Ø
  neonatal P78.1
    meconium P78.Ø
  pancreatic K65.Ø
  paroxysmal, familial E85.Ø
    benign E85.Ø
  pelvic
    female N73.5
      acute N73.3
      chronic N73.4
        with adhesions N73.6
    male K65.Ø
  periodic, familial E85.Ø
  proliferative, chronic K65.8
  puerperal, postpartum, childbirth O85
  purulent K65.Ø
  septic K65.Ø
  specified NEC K65.8
  spontaneous bacterial K65.2
  subdiaphragmatic K65.Ø
  subphrenic K65.Ø
  suppurative K65.Ø
  syphilitic A52.74
    congenital (early) A5Ø.Ø8 *[K67]*
  talc T81.61
  tuberculous A18.31
  urine K65.8
Peritonsillar —*see* condition
Peritonsillitis J36
Perityphlitis K37
Periureteritis N28.89
Periurethral —*see* condition
Periurethritis (gangrenous) —*see* Urethritis
Periuterine —*see* condition
Perivaginitis —*see* Vaginitis
Perivasculitis, retinal H35.Ø6-
Perivasitis (chronic) N49.1
Perivesiculitis (seminal) —*see* Vesiculitis
Perlèche NEC K13.Ø
  due to
    candidiasis B37.83
    moniliasis B37.83
    riboflavin deficiency E53.Ø
    vitamin B2 (riboflavin) deficiency E53.Ø
Pernicious —*see* condition
Pernio, perniosis T69.1
Perpetrator (of abuse) —*see* Index to External Causes of Injury, Perpetrator
Persecution
  delusion F22
  social Z6Ø.5
Perseveration (tonic) R48.8
Persistence, persistent (congenital)
  anal membrane Q42.3
    with fistula Q42.2
  arteria stapedia Q16.3
  atrioventricular canal Q21.2
  branchial cleft Q18.Ø
  bulbus cordis in left ventricle Q21.8
  canal of Cloquet Q14.Ø
  capsule (opaque) Q12.8
  cilioretinal artery or vein Q14.8
  cloaca Q43.7
  communication —*see* Fistula, congenital
  convolutions
    aortic arch Q25.46 ⟸
    fallopian tube Q5Ø.6
    oviduct Q5Ø.6
    uterine tube Q5Ø.6
  double aortic arch Q25.45 ⟸
  ductus arteriosus (Botalli) Q25.Ø
  fetal
    circulation P29.3
    form of cervix (uteri) Q51.828
    hemoglobin, hereditary (HPFH) D56.4
  foramen
    Botalli Q21.1
    ovale Q21.1
  Gartner's duct Q52.4
  hemoglobin, fetal (hereditary) (HPFH) D56.4
  hyaloid
    artery (generally incomplete) Q14.Ø
    system Q14.8
  hymen, in pregnancy or childbirth —*see* Pregnancy, complicated by, abnormal, vulva
  lanugo Q84.2
  left
    posterior cardinal vein Q26.8
    root with right arch of aorta Q25.49 ⟸
    superior vena cava Q26.1
  Meckel's diverticulum Q43.Ø
    malignant —*see* Table of Neoplasms, small intestine, malignant
  mucosal disease (middle ear) —*see* Otitis, media, suppurative, chronic, tubotympanic
  nail (s), anomalous Q84.6
  omphalomesenteric duct Q43.Ø
  organ or site not listed —*see* Anomaly, by site
  ostium
    atrioventriculare commune Q21.2
    primum Q21.2
    secundum Q21.1
  ovarian rests in fallopian tube Q5Ø.6
  pancreatic tissue in intestinal tract Q43.8
  primary (deciduous)
    teeth KØØ.6
    vitreous hyperplasia Q14.Ø
  pupillary membrane Q13.89
  rhesus (Rh)titer —*see* Complication (s), transfusion, incompatibility reaction, Rh (factor)
  right aortic arch Q25.47 ⟸
  sinus
    urogenitalis
      female Q52.8
      male Q55.8
    venosus with imperfect incorporation in right auricle Q26.8
  thymus (gland) (hyperplasia) E32.Ø
  thyroglossal duct Q89.2
  thyrolingual duct Q89.2
  truncus arteriosus or communis Q2Ø.Ø
  tunica vasculosa lentis Q12.2
  umbilical sinus Q64.4
  urachus Q64.4
  vitelline duct Q43.Ø
Person (with)
  admitted for clinical research, as a control subject (normal comparison) (participant) ZØØ.6
  awaiting admission to adequate facility elsewhere Z75.1
  concern (normal) about sick person in family Z63.6
  consulting on behalf of another Z71.Ø
  feigning illness Z76.5
  living (in)
    without
      adequate housing (heating) (space) Z59.1
      housing (permanent) (temporary) Z59.Ø
      person able to render necessary care Z74.2
      shelter Z59.Ø
    alone Z6Ø.2
    boarding school Z59.3
    residential institution Z59.3
  on waiting list Z75.1
  sick or handicapped in family Z63.6
Personality (disorder) F6Ø.9
  accentuation of traits (type A pattern) Z73.1
  affective F34.Ø
  aggressive F6Ø.3
  amoral F6Ø.2
  anacastic, anankastic F6Ø.5
  antisocial F6Ø.2
  anxious F6Ø.6
  asocial F6Ø.2
  asthenic F6Ø.7
  avoidant F6Ø.6
  borderline F6Ø.3
  change due to organic condition (enduring) FØ7.Ø
  compulsive F6Ø.5
  cycloid F34.Ø
  cyclothymic F34.Ø
  dependent F6Ø.7
  depressive F34.1
  dissocial F6Ø.2
  dual F44.81
  eccentric F6Ø.89
  emotionally unstable F6Ø.3
  expansive paranoid F6Ø.Ø
  explosive F6Ø.3
  fanatic F6Ø.Ø
  haltlose type F6Ø.89
  histrionic F6Ø.4
  hyperthymic F34.Ø
  hypothymic F34.1
  hysterical F6Ø.4
  immature F6Ø.89
  inadequate F6Ø.7
  labile (emotional) F6Ø.3
  mixed (nonspecific) F6Ø.89 ⟸
  morally defective F6Ø.2
  multiple F44.81
  narcissistic F6Ø.81
  obsessional F6Ø.5
  obsessive (-compulsive) F6Ø.5
  organic FØ7.Ø
  overconscientious F6Ø.5
  paranoid F6Ø.Ø
  passive (-dependent) F6Ø.7
  passive-aggressive F6Ø.89
  pathologic F6Ø.9
  pattern defect or disturbance F6Ø.9
  pseudopsychopathic (organic) FØ7.Ø
  pseudoretarded (organic) FØ7.Ø
  psychoinfantile F6Ø.4
  psychoneurotic NEC F6Ø.89
  psychopathic F6Ø.2
  querulant F6Ø.Ø
  sadistic F6Ø.89
  schizoid F6Ø.1
  self-defeating F6Ø.7
  sensitive paranoid F6Ø.Ø

Personality *(Continued)*
sociopathic (amoral) (antisocial) (asocial) (dissocial) F60.2
specified NEC F60.89
type A Z73.1
unstable (emotional) F60.3
Perthes' disease —*see* Legg-Calvé-Perthes disease
Pertussis (*see also* Whooping cough) A37.90
Perversion, perverted
appetite F50.89
psychogenic F50.89
function
pituitary gland E23.2
posterior lobe E22.2
sense of smell and taste R43.8
psychogenic F45.8
sexual —*see* Deviation, sexual
Pervious, congenital —*see also* Imperfect, closure
ductus arteriosus Q25.0
Pes (congenital) —*see also* Talipes
acquired —*see also* Deformity, limb, foot, specified NEC
planus —*see* Deformity, limb, flat foot
adductus Q66.89
cavus Q66.7
deformity NEC, acquired —*see* Deformity, limb, foot, specified NEC
planus (acquired) (any degree) —*see also* Deformity, limb, flat foot
rachitic sequelae (late effect) E64.3
valgus Q66.6
Pest, pestis —*see* Plague
Petechia, petechiae R23.3
newborn P54.5
Petechial typhus A75.9
Peter's anomaly Q13.4
Petit mal seizure —*see* Epilepsy, generalized, specified NEC
Petit's hernia —*see* Hernia, abdomen, specified site NEC
Petrellidosis B48.2
Petrositis H70.20-
acute H70.21-
chronic H70.22-
Peutz-Jeghers disease or syndrome Q85.8
Peyronie's disease N48.6
PFAPA (periodic fever, aphthous stomatitis, pharyngitis, and adenopathy syndrome) M04.8
Pfeiffer's disease —*see* Mononucleosis, infectious
Phagedena (dry) (moist) (sloughing) —*see also* Gangrene
geometric L88
penis N48.29
tropical —*see* Ulcer, skin
vulva N76.6
Phagedenic —*see* condition
Phakoma H35.89
Phakomatosis —*see also* specific eponymous syndromes Q85.9
Bourneville's Q85.1
specified NEC Q85.8
Phantom limb syndrome (without pain) G54.7
with pain G54.6
Pharyngeal pouch syndrome D82.1
Pharyngitis (acute) (catarrhal) (gangrenous) (infective) (malignant) (membranous) (phlegmonous) (pseudomembranous) (simple) (subacute) (suppurative) (ulcerative) (viral) J02.9
with influenza, flu, or grippe —*see* Influenza, with, pharyngitis
aphthous B08.5
atrophic J31.2
chlamydial A56.4
chronic (atrophic) (granular) (hypertrophic) J31.2
Pharyngitis *(Continued)*
coxsackievirus B08.5
diphtheritic A36.0
enteroviral vesicular B08.5
follicular (chronic) J31.2
fusospirochetal A69.1
gonococcal A54.5
granular (chronic) J31.2
herpesviral B00.2
hypertrophic J31.2
infectional, chronic J31.2
influenzal —*see* Influenza, with, respiratory manifestations NEC
lymphonodular, acute (enteroviral) B08.8
pneumococcal J02.8
purulent J02.9
putrid J02.9
septic J02.0
sicca J31.2
specified organism NEC J02.8
staphylococcal J02.8
streptococcal J02.0
syphilitic, congenital (early) A50.03
tuberculous A15.8
vesicular, enteroviral B08.5
viral NEC J02.8
Pharyngoconjunctivitis, viral B30.2
Pharyngolaryngitis (acute) J06.0
chronic J37.0
Pharyngoplegia J39.2
Pharyngotonsillitis, herpesviral B00.2
Pharyngotracheitis, chronic J42
Pharynx, pharyngeal —*see* condition
Phencyclidine-induced
anxiety disorder F16.980
bipolar and related disorder F16.94
depressive disorder F16.94
psychotic disorder F16.959
Phenomenon
Arthus' —*see* Arthus' phenomenon
jaw-winking Q07.8
lupus erythematosus (LE) cell M32.9
Raynaud's (secondary) I73.00
with gangrene I73.01
vasomotor R55
vasospastic I73.9
vasovagal R55
Wenckebach's I44.1
Phenylketonuria E70.1
classical E70.0
maternal E70.1
Pheochromoblastoma
specified site —*see* Neoplasm, malignant, by site
unspecified site C74.10
Pheochromocytoma
malignant
specified site —*see* Neoplasm, malignant, by site
unspecified site C74.10
specified site —*see* Neoplasm, benign, by site
unspecified site D35.00
Pheohyphomycosis —*see* Chromomycosis
Pheomycosis —*see* Chromomycosis
Phimosis (congenital) (due to infection) N47.1
chancroidal A57
Phlebectasia —*see also* Varix
congenital Q27.4
Phlebitis (infective) (pyemic) (septic) (suppurative) I80.9
antepartum —*see* Thrombophlebitis, antepartum
blue —*see* Phlebitis, leg, deep
breast, superficial I80.8
cavernous (venous) sinus —*see* Phlebitis, intracranial (venous) sinus
cerebral (venous) sinus —*see* Phlebitis, intracranial (venous) sinus
chest wall, superficial I80.8
cranial (venous) sinus —*see* Phlebitis, intracranial (venous) sinus
Phlebitis *(Continued)*
deep (vessels) —*see* Phlebitis, leg, deep
due to implanted device —*see* Complications, by site and type, specified NEC
during or resulting from a procedure T81.72
femoral vein (superficial) I80.1-
femoropopliteal vein I80.0-
gestational —*see* Phlebopathy, gestational
hepatic veins I80.8
iliofemoral —*see* Phlebitis, femoral vein
intracranial (venous) sinus (any) G08
nonpyogenic I67.6
intraspinal venous sinuses and veins G08
nonpyogenic G95.19
lateral (venous) sinus —*see* Phlebitis, intracranial (venous) sinus
leg I80.3
antepartum —*see* Thrombophlebitis, antepartum
deep (vessels) NEC I80.20-
iliac I80.21-
popliteal vein I80.22-
specified vessel NEC I80.29-
tibial vein I80.23-
femoral vein (superficial) I80.1-
superficial (vessels) I80.0-
longitudinal sinus —*see* Phlebitis, intracranial (venous) sinus
lower limb —*see* Phlebitis, leg
migrans, migrating (superficial) I82.1
pelvic
with ectopic or molar pregnancy O08.0
following ectopic or molar pregnancy O08.0
puerperal, postpartum O87.1
popliteal vein —*see* Phlebitis, leg, deep, popliteal
portal (vein) K75.1
postoperative T81.72
pregnancy —*see* Thrombophlebitis, antepartum
puerperal, postpartum, childbirth O87.0
deep O87.1
pelvic O87.1
superficial O87.0
retina —*see* Vasculitis, retina
saphenous (accessory) (great) (long) (small) —*see* Phlebitis, leg, superficial
sinus (meninges) —*see* Phlebitis, intracranial (venous) sinus
specified site NEC I80.8
syphilitic A52.09
tibial vein —*see* Phlebitis, leg, deep, tibial
ulcerative I80.9
leg —*see* Phlebitis, leg
umbilicus I80.8
uterus (septic) —*see* Endometritis
varicose (leg) (lower limb) —*see* Varix, leg, with, inflammation
Phlebofibrosis I87.8
Phleboliths I87.8
Phlebopathy
gestational O22.9-
puerperal O87.9
Phlebosclerosis I87.8
Phlebothrombosis —*see also* Thrombosis
antepartum —*see* Thrombophlebitis, antepartum
pregnancy —*see* Thrombophlebitis, antepartum
puerperal —*see* Thrombophlebitis, puerperal
Phlebotomus fever A93.1
Phlegmasia
alba dolens O87.1
nonpuerperal —*see* Phlebitis, femoral vein
cerulea dolens —*see* Phlebitis, leg, deep
Phlegmon —*see* Abscess
Phlegmonous —*see* condition

◀ New ⟵ Revised ~~deleted~~ Deleted

- **Phlyctenulosis** (allergic) (keratoconjunctivitis) (nontuberculous) *—see also* Keratoconjunctivitis
  - cornea *—see* Keratoconjunctivitis
  - tuberculous A18.52
- **Phobia, phobic** F40.9
  - animal F40.218
    - spiders F40.210
  - examination F40.298
  - reaction F40.9
  - simple F40.298
  - social F40.10
    - generalized F40.11
  - specific (isolated) F40.298
    - animal F40.218
      - spiders F40.210
    - blood F40.230
    - injection F40.231
    - injury F40.233
    - men F40.290
    - natural environment F40.228
      - thunderstorms F40.220
    - situational F40.248
      - bridges F40.242
      - closed in spaces F40.240
      - flying F40.243
      - heights F40.241
    - specified focus NEC F40.298
    - transfusion F40.231
    - women F40.291
  - specified NEC F40.8
    - medical care NEC F40.232
  - state F40.9
- **Phocas' disease** *—see* Mastopathy, cystic
- **Phocomelia** Q73.1
  - lower limb *—see* Agenesis, leg, with foot present
  - upper limb *—see* Agenesis, arm, with hand present
- **Phoria** H50.50
- **Phosphate-losing tubular disorder** N25.0
- **Phosphatemia** E83.39
- **Phosphaturia** E83.39
- **Photodermatitis** (sun) L56.8
  - chronic L57.8
  - due to drug L56.8
  - light other than sun L59.8
- **Photokeratitis** H16.13-
- **Photophobia** H53.14-
- **Photophthalmia** *—see* Photokeratitis
- **Photopsia** H53.19
- **Photoretinitis** *—see* Retinopathy, solar
- **Photosensitivity, photosensitization** (sun) **skin** L56.8
  - light other than sun L59.8
- **Phrenitis** *—see* Encephalitis
- **Phrynoderma** (vitamin A deficiency) E50.8
- **Phthiriasis** (pubis) B85.3
  - with any infestation classifiable to B85.0-B85.2 B85.4
- **Phthirus infestation** *—see* Phthiriasis
- **Phthisis** *—see also* Tuberculosis
  - bulbi (infectional) *—see* Disorder, globe, degenerated condition, atrophy
  - eyeball (due to infection) *—see* Disorder, globe, degenerated condition, atrophy
- **Phycomycosis** *—see* Zygomycosis
- **Physalopteriasis** B81.8
- **Physical restraint status** Z78.1
- **Phytobezoar** T18.9
  - intestine T18.3
  - stomach T18.2
- **Pian** *—see* Yaws
- **Pianoma** A66.1
- **Pica** F50.89 ⬅
  - in adults F50.89 ⬅
  - infant or child F98.3
- **Picking, nose** F98.8
- **Pick-Niemann disease** *—see* Niemann-Pick disease or syndrome
- **Pick's**
  - cerebral atrophy G31.01 *[F02.80]*
    - with behavioral disturbance G31.01 *[F02.81]*
  - disease or syndrome (brain) G31.01 *[F02.80]*
    - with behavioral disturbance G31.01 *[F02.81]*
    - brain G31.01 *[F02.80]* ◀
      - with behavioral disturbance G31.01 *[F02.81]* ◀
    - pericardium (pericardial pseudocirrhosis of liver) I31.1 ◀
  - syndrome ◀
    - brain G31.01 *[F02.80]* ◀
      - with behavioral disturbance G31.01 *[F02.81]* ◀
    - of heart (pericardial pseudocirrhosis of liver) I31.1 ◀
- **Pickwickian syndrome** E66.2
- **Piebaldism** E70.39
- **Piedra** (beard) (scalp) B36.8
  - black B36.3
  - white B36.2
- **Pierre Robin deformity or syndrome** Q87.0
- **Pierson's disease or osteochondrosis** M91.0
- **Pig-bel** A05.2
- **Pigeon**
  - breast or chest (acquired) M95.4
    - congenital Q67.7
    - rachitic sequelae (late effect) E64.3
  - breeder's disease or lung J67.2
  - fancier's disease or lung J67.2
  - toe *—see* Deformity, toe, specified NEC
- **Pigmentation** (abnormal) (anomaly) L81.9
  - conjunctiva H11.13-
  - cornea (anterior) H18.01-
    - posterior H18.05-
    - stromal H18.06-
  - diminished melanin formation NEC L81.6
  - iron L81.8
  - lids, congenital Q82.8
  - limbus corneae *—see* Pigmentation, cornea
  - metals L81.8
  - optic papilla, congenital Q14.2
  - retina, congenital (grouped) (nevoid) Q14.1
  - scrotum, congenital Q82.8
  - tattoo L81.8
- **Piles** *—see also* Hemorrhoids K64.9
- **Pili**
  - annulati or torti (congenital) Q84.1
  - incarnati L73.1
- **Pill roller hand** (intrinsic) *—see* Parkinsonism
- **Pilomatrixoma** *—see* Neoplasm, skin, benign
  - malignant *—see* Neoplasm, skin, malignant
- **Pilonidal** *—see* condition
- **Pimple** R23.8
- **PIN** *—see* Neoplasia, intraepithelial, prostate ◀
- **Pinched nerve** *—see* Neuropathy, entrapment
- **Pindborg tumor** *—see* Cyst, calcifying odontogenic
- **Pineal body or gland** *—see* condition
- **Pinealoblastoma** C75.3
- **Pinealoma** D44.5
  - malignant C75.3
- **Pineoblastoma** C75.3
- **Pineocytoma** D44.5
- **Pinguecula** H11.15-
- **Pingueculitis** H10.81-
- **Pinhole meatus** *—see also* Stricture, urethra N35.9
- **Pink**
  - disease *—see* subcategory T56.1
  - eye *—see* Conjunctivitis, acute, mucopurulent
- **Pinkus' disease** (lichen nitidus) L44.1
- **Pinpoint**
  - meatus *—see* Stricture, urethra
  - os (uteri) *—see* Stricture, cervix
- **Pins and needles** R20.2
- **Pinta** A67.9
  - cardiovascular lesions A67.2
  - chancre (primary) A67.0
- **Pinta** *(Continued)*
  - erythematous plaques A67.1
  - hyperchromic lesions A67.1
  - hyperkeratosis A67.1
  - lesions A67.9
    - cardiovascular A67.2
    - hyperchromic A67.1
    - intermediate A67.1
    - late A67.2
    - mixed A67.3
    - primary A67.0
    - skin (achromic) (cicatricial) (dyschromic) A67.2
      - hyperchromic A67.1
      - mixed (achromic and hyperchromic) A67.3
  - papule (primary) A67.0
  - skin lesions (achromic) (cicatricial) (dyschromic) A67.2
    - hyperchromic A67.1
    - mixed (achromic and hyperchromic) A67.3
  - vitiligo A67.2
- **Pintids** A67.1
- **Pinworm** (disease) (infection) (infestation) B80
- **Piroplasmosis** B60.0
- **Pistol wound** *—see* Gunshot wound
- **Pitchers' elbow** *—see* Derangement, joint, specified type NEC, elbow
- **Pithecoid pelvis** Q74.2
  - with disproportion (fetopelvic) O33.0
    - causing obstructed labor O65.0
- **Pithiatism** F48.8
- **Pitted** *—see* Pitting
- **Pitting** *—see also* Edema R60.9
  - lip R60.0
  - nail L60.8
  - teeth K00.4
- **Pituitary gland** *—see* condition
- **Pituitary-snuff-taker's disease** J67.8
- **Pityriasis** (capitis) L21.0
  - alba L30.5
  - circinata (et maculata) L42
  - furfuracea L21.0
  - Hebra's L26
  - lichenoides L41.0
    - chronica L41.1
    - et varioliformis (acuta) L41.0
  - maculata (et circinata) L30.5
  - nigra B36.1
  - pilaris, Hebra's L44.0
  - rosea L42
  - rotunda L44.8
  - rubra (Hebra) pilaris L44.0
  - simplex L30.5
  - specified type NEC L30.5
  - streptogenes L30.5
  - versicolor (scrotal) B36.0
- **Placenta, placental** *—see* Pregnancy, complicated by (care of) (management affected by), specified condition
- **Placentitis** O41.14-
- **Plagiocephaly** Q67.3
- **Plague** A20.9
  - abortive A20.8
  - ambulatory A20.8
  - asymptomatic A20.8
  - bubonic A20.0
  - cellulocutaneous A20.1
  - cutaneobubonic A20.1
  - lymphatic gland A20.0
  - meningitis A20.3
  - pharyngeal A20.8
  - pneumonic (primary) (secondary) A20.2
  - pulmonary, pulmonic A20.2
  - septicemic A20.7
  - tonsillar A20.8
    - septicemic A20.7
- **Planning, family**
  - contraception Z30.9
  - procreation Z31.69

P

- **Plaque** (s)
  - artery, arterial —*see* Arteriosclerosis
  - calcareous —*see* Calcification
  - coronary, lipid rich I25.83
  - epicardial I31.8
  - erythematous, of pinta A67.1
  - Hollenhorst's —*see* Occlusion, artery, retina
  - lipid rich, coronary I25.83
  - pleural (without asbestos) J92.9
    - with asbestos J92.Ø
  - tongue K13.29
- **Plasmacytoma** C9Ø.3-
  - extramedullary C9Ø.2-
  - medullary C9Ø.Ø-
  - solitary C9Ø.3-
- **Plasmacytopenia** D72.818
- **Plasmacytosis** D72.822
- **Plaster ulcer** —*see* Ulcer, pressure, by site
- **Plateau iris syndrome** (post-iridectomy) (postprocedural) (without glaucoma) H21.82
  - with glaucoma H4Ø.22-
- **Platybasia** Q75.8
- **Platyonychia** (congenital) Q84.6
  - acquired L6Ø.8
- **Platypelloid pelvis** M95.5
  - with disproportion (fetopelvic) O33.Ø
    - causing obstructed labor O65.Ø
  - congenital Q74.2
- **Platyspondylisis** Q76.49
- **Plaut** (-Vincent) **disease** —*see also* Vincent's A69.1
- **Plethora** R23.2
  - newborn P61.1
- **Pleura, pleural** —*see* condition
- **Pleuralgia** RØ7.81
- **Pleurisy** (acute) (adhesive) (chronic) (costal) (diaphragmatic) (double) (dry) (fibrinous) (fibrous) (interlobar) (latent) (plastic) (primary) (residual) (sicca) (sterile) (subacute) (unresolved) RØ9.1
  - with
    - adherent pleura J86.Ø
    - effusion J9Ø
      - chylous, chyliform J94.Ø
      - tuberculous (non primary) A15.6
        - primary (progressive) A15.7
    - tuberculosis —*see* Pleurisy, tuberculous (non primary)
  - encysted —*see* Pleurisy, with effusion
  - exudative —*see* Pleurisy, with effusion
  - fibrinopurulent, fibropurulent —*see* Pyothorax
  - hemorrhagic —*see* Hemothorax
  - pneumococcal J9Ø
  - purulent —*see* Pyothorax
  - septic —*see* Pyothorax
  - serofibrinous —*see* Pleurisy, with effusion
  - seropurulent —*see* Pyothorax
  - serous —*see* Pleurisy, with effusion
  - staphylococcal J86.9
  - streptococcal J9Ø
  - suppurative —*see* Pyothorax
  - traumatic (post) (current) —*see* Injury, intrathoracic, pleura
  - tuberculous (with effusion) (non primary) A15.6
    - primary (progressive) A15.7
- **Pleuritis sicca** —*see* Pleurisy
- **Pleurobronchopneumonia** —*see* Pneumonia, broncho
- **Pleurodynia** RØ7.81
  - epidemic B33.Ø
  - viral B33.Ø
- **Pleuropericarditis** —*see also* Pericarditis
  - acute I3Ø.9
- **Pleuropneumonia** (acute) (bilateral) (double) (septic) —*see also* Pneumonia J18.8
  - chronic —*see* Fibrosis, lung
- **Pleuro-pneumonia-like-organism** (PPLO), **as cause of disease classified elsewhere** B96.Ø
- **Pleurorrhea** —*see* Pleurisy, with effusion
- **Plexitis, brachial** G54.Ø
- **Plica**
  - polonica B85.Ø
  - syndrome, knee M67.5
  - tonsil J35.8
- **Plicated tongue** K14.5
- **Plug**
  - bronchus NEC J98.Ø9
  - meconium (newborn) NEC syndrome P76.Ø
  - mucus —*see* Asphyxia, mucus
- **Plumbism** —*see* subcategory T56.Ø
- **Plummer's disease** EØ5.2Ø
  - with thyroid storm EØ5.21
- **Plummer-Vinson syndrome** D5Ø.1
- **Pluricarential syndrome of infancy** E4Ø
- **Plus** (and minus) **hand** (intrinsic) —*see* Deformity, limb, specified type NEC, forearm
- **Pneumathemia** —*see* Air, embolism
- **Pneumatic hammer** (drill) **syndrome** T75.21
- **Pneumatocele** (lung) J98.4
  - intracranial G93.89
  - tension J44.9
- **Pneumatosis**
  - cystoides intestinalis K63.89
  - intestinalis K63.89
  - peritonei K66.8
- **Pneumaturia** R39.89
- **Pneumoblastoma** —*see* Neoplasm, lung, malignant
- **Pneumocephalus** G93.89
- **Pneumococcemia** A4Ø.3
- **Pneumococcus, pneumococcal** —*see* condition
- **Pneumoconiosis** (due to) (inhalation of) J64
  - with tuberculosis (any type in A15) J65
  - aluminum J63.Ø
  - asbestos J61
  - bagasse, bagassosis J67.1
  - bauxite J63.1
  - beryllium J63.2
  - coal miners' (simple) J6Ø
  - coalworkers' (simple) J6Ø
  - collier's J6Ø
  - cotton dust J66.Ø
  - diatomite (diatomaceous earth) J62.8
  - dust
    - inorganic NEC J63.6
    - lime J62.8
    - marble J62.8
    - organic NEC J66.8
  - fumes or vapors (from silo) J68.9
  - graphite J63.3
  - grinder's J62.8
  - kaolin J62.8
  - mica J62.8
  - millstone maker's J62.8
  - mineral fibers NEC J61
  - miner's J6Ø
  - moldy hay J67.Ø
  - potter's J62.8
  - rheumatoid —*see* Rheumatoid, lung
  - sandblaster's J62.8
  - silica, silicate NEC J62.8
    - with carbon J6Ø
  - stonemason's J62.8
  - talc (dust) J62.Ø
- **Pneumocystis carinii pneumonia** B59
- **Pneumocystis jiroveci** (pneumonia) B59
- **Pneumocystosis** (with pneumonia) B59
- **Pneumohemopericardium** I31.2
- **Pneumohemothorax** J94.2
  - traumatic S27.2
- **Pneumohydropericardium** —*see* Pericarditis
- **Pneumohydrothorax** —*see* Hydrothorax
- **Pneumomediastinum** J98.2
  - congenital or perinatal P25.2
- **Pneumomycosis** B49 *[J99]*
- **Pneumonia** (acute) (double) (migratory) (purulent) (septic) (unresolved) J18.9
  - with
    - influenza —*see* Influenza, with, pneumonia
    - lung abscess J85.1
      - due to specified organism —*see* Pneumonia, in (due to)
  - adenoviral J12.Ø
  - adynamic J18.2
  - alba A5Ø.Ø4
  - allergic (eosinophilic) J82
  - alveolar —*see* Pneumonia, lobar
  - anaerobes J15.8
  - anthrax A22.1
  - apex, apical —*see* Pneumonia, lobar
  - Ascaris B77.81
  - aspiration J69.Ø
    - due to
      - aspiration of microorganisms
        - bacterial J15.9
        - viral J12.9
      - food (regurgitated) J69.Ø
      - gastric secretions J69.Ø
      - milk (regurgitated) J69.Ø
      - oils, essences J69.1
      - solids, liquids NEC J69.8
      - vomitus J69.Ø
    - newborn P24.81
      - amniotic fluid (clear) P24.11
      - blood P24.21
      - food (regurgitated) P24.31
      - liquor (amnii) P24.11
      - meconium P24.Ø1
      - milk P24.31
      - mucus P24.11
      - specified NEC P24.81
      - stomach contents P24.31
    - postprocedural J95.4
  - atypical NEC J18.9
  - bacillus J15.9
    - specified NEC J15.8
  - bacterial J15.9
    - specified NEC J15.8
  - Bacteroides (fragilis) (oralis) (melaninogenicus) J15.8
  - basal, basic, basilar —*see* Pneumonia, by type
  - bronchiolitis obliterans organized (BOOP) J84.89
  - broncho-, bronchial (confluent) (croupous) (diffuse) (disseminated) (hemorrhagic) (involving lobes) (lobar) (terminal) J18.Ø
    - allergic (eosinophilic) J82
    - aspiration —*see* Pneumonia, aspiration
    - bacterial J15.9
      - specified NEC J15.8
    - chronic —*see* Fibrosis, lung
    - diplococcal J13
    - Eaton's agent J15.7
    - Escherichia coli (E. coli) J15.5
    - Friedländer's bacillus J15.Ø
    - Hemophilus influenzae J14
    - hypostatic J18.2
    - inhalation (*see also* Pneumonia, aspiration
      - due to fumes or vapors (chemical) J68.Ø
      - of oils or essences J69.1
    - Klebsiella (pneumoniae) J15.Ø
    - lipid, lipoid J69.1
      - endogenous J84.89
    - Mycoplasma (pneumoniae) J15.7
    - pleuro-pneumonia-like-organisms (PPLO) J15.7
    - pneumococcal J13
    - Proteus J15.6
    - Pseudomonas J15.1
    - Serratia marcescens J15.6
    - specified organism NEC J16.8
    - staphylococcal —*see* Pneumonia, staphylococcal
    - streptococcal NEC J15.4
      - group B J15.3
      - pneumoniae J13
    - viral, virus —*see* Pneumonia, viral

◀ New ⟵ Revised ~~deleted~~ Deleted

Pneumonia *(Continued)*
- Butyrivibrio (fibriosolvens) J15.8
- Candida B37.1
- caseous —*see* Tuberculosis, pulmonary
- catarrhal —*see* Pneumonia, broncho
- chlamydial J16.Ø
  - congenital P23.1
- cholesterol J84.89
- cirrhotic (chronic) —*see* Fibrosis, lung
- Clostridium (haemolyticum) (novyi) J15.8
- confluent —*see* Pneumonia, broncho
- congenital (infective) P23.9
  - due to
    - bacterium NEC P23.6
    - Chlamydia P23.1
    - Escherichia coli P23.4
    - Haemophilus influenzae P23.6
    - infective organism NEC P23.8
    - Klebsiella pneumoniae P23.6
    - Mycoplasma P23.6
    - Pseudomonas P23.5
    - Staphylococcus P23.2
    - Streptococcus (except group B) P23.6
      - group B P23.3
    - viral agent P23.Ø
  - specified NEC P23.8
- croupous —*see* Pneumonia, lobar
- cryptogenic organizing J84.116
- cytomegalic inclusion B25.Ø
- cytomegaloviral B25.Ø
- deglutition —*see* Pneumonia, aspiration
- desquamative interstitial J84.117
- diffuse —*see* Pneumonia, broncho
- diplococcal, diplococcus (broncho-) (lobar) J13
- disseminated (focal) —*see* Pneumonia, broncho
- Eaton's agent J15.7
- embolic, embolism —*see* Embolism, pulmonary
- Enterobacter J15.6
- eosinophilic J82
- Escherichia coli (E. coli) J15.5
- Eubacterium J15.8
- fibrinous —*see* Pneumonia, lobar
- fibroid, fibrous (chronic) —*see* Fibrosis, lung
- Friedländer's bacillus J15.Ø
- Fusobacterium (nucleatum) J15.8
- gangrenous J85.Ø
- giant cell (measles) BØ5.2
- gonococcal A54.84
- gram-negative bacteria NEC J15.6
  - anaerobic J15.8
- Hemophilus influenzae (broncho) (lobar) J14
- human metapneumovirus J12.3
- hypostatic (broncho) (lobar) J18.2
- in (due to)
  - actinomycosis A42.Ø
  - adenovirus J12.Ø
  - anthrax A22.1
  - ascariasis B77.81
  - aspergillosis B44.9
  - Bacillus anthracis A22.1
  - Bacterium anitratum J15.6
  - candidiasis B37.1
  - chickenpox BØ1.2
  - Chlamydia J16.Ø
    - neonatal P23.1
  - coccidioidomycosis B38.2
    - acute B38.Ø
    - chronic B38.1
  - cytomegalovirus disease B25.Ø
  - Diplococcus (pneumoniae) J13
  - Eaton's agent J15.7
  - Enterobacter J15.6
  - Escherichia coli (E. coli) J15.5
  - Friedländer's bacillus J15.Ø
  - fumes and vapors (chemical) (inhalation) J68.Ø
  - gonorrhea A54.84
  - Hemophilus influenzae (H. influenzae) J14

Pneumonia *(Continued)*
- in *(Continued)*
  - Herellea J15.6
  - histoplasmosis B39.2
    - acute B39.Ø
    - chronic B39.1
  - human metapneumovirus J12.3
  - Klebsiella (pneumoniae) J15.Ø
  - measles BØ5.2
  - Mycoplasma (pneumoniae) J15.7
  - nocardiosis, nocardiasis A43.Ø
  - ornithosis A7Ø
  - parainfluenza virus J12.2
  - pleuro-pneumonia-like-organism (PPLO) J15.7
  - pneumococcus J13
  - pneumocystosis (Pneumocystis carinii) (Pneumocystis jiroveci) B59
  - Proteus J15.6
  - Pseudomonas NEC J15.1
    - pseudomallei A24.1
  - psittacosis A7Ø
  - Q fever A78
  - respiratory syncytial virus J12.1
  - rheumatic fever IØØ *[J17]*
  - rubella BØ6.81
  - Salmonella (infection) AØ2.22
    - typhi AØ1.Ø3
  - schistosomiasis B65.9 *[J17]*
  - Serratia marcescens J15.6
  - specified
    - bacterium NEC J15.8
    - organism NEC J16.8
  - spirochetal NEC A69.8
  - Staphylococcus J15.2Ø
    - aureus (methicillin susceptible) (MSSA) J15.211
      - methicillin resistant (MRSA) J15.212
    - specified NEC J15.29
  - Streptococcus J15.4
    - group B J15.3
    - pneumoniae J13
    - specified NEC J15.4
  - toxoplasmosis B58.3
  - tularemia A21.2
  - typhoid (fever) AØ1.Ø3
  - varicella BØ1.2
  - virus —*see* Pneumonia, viral
  - whooping cough A37.91
    - due to
      - Bordetella parapertussis A37.11
      - Bordetella pertussis A37.Ø1
      - specified NEC A37.81
  - Yersinia pestis A2Ø.2
- inhalation of food or vomit —*see* Pneumonia, aspiration
- interstitial J84.9
  - chronic J84.111
  - desquamative J84.117
  - due to
    - collagen vascular disease J84.17
    - known underlying cause J84.17
  - idiopathic NOS J84.111
  - in disease classified elsewhere J84.17
  - lymphocytic (due to collagen vascular disease) (in diseases classified elsewhere) J84.17
  - lymphoid J84.2
  - non-specific J84.89
    - due to
      - collagen vascular disease J84.17
      - known underlying cause J84.17
    - idiopathic J84.113
    - in diseases classified elsewhere J84.17
  - plasma cell B59
  - pseudomonas J15.1
  - usual J84.112
    - due to collagen vascular disease J84.17
    - idiopathic J84.112
    - in diseases classified elsewhere J84.17

Pneumonia *(Continued)*
- Klebsiella (pneumoniae) J15.Ø
- lipid, lipoid (exogenous) J69.1
  - endogenous J84.89
- lobar (disseminated) (double) (interstitial) J18.1
  - bacterial J15.9
    - specified NEC J15.8
  - chronic —*see* Fibrosis, lung
  - Escherichia coli (E. coli) J15.5
  - Friedländer's bacillus J15.Ø
  - Hemophilus influenzae J14
  - hypostatic J18.2
  - Klebsiella (pneumoniae) J15.Ø
  - pneumococcal J13
  - Proteus J15.6
  - Pseudomonas J15.1
  - specified organism NEC J16.8
  - staphylococcal —*see* Pneumonia, staphylococcal
  - streptococcal NEC J15.4
  - Streptococcus pneumoniae J13
  - viral, virus —*see* Pneumonia, viral
- lobular —*see* Pneumonia, broncho
- Löffler's J82
- lymphoid interstitial J84.2
- massive —*see* Pneumonia, lobar
- meconium P24.Ø1
- MRSA (Methicillin resistant Staphylococcus aureus) J15.212 ◀
- MSSA (methicillin susceptible Staphylococcus aureus) J15.211
- multilobar —*see* Pneumonia, by type
- Mycoplasma (pneumoniae) J15.7
- necrotic J85.Ø
- neonatal P23.9
  - aspiration —*see* Aspiration, by substance, with pneumonia
- nitrogen dioxide J68.Ø ⬅
- organizing J84.89
  - due to
    - collagen vascular disease J84.17
    - known underlying cause J84.17
  - in diseases classified elsewhere J84.17
- orthostatic J18.2
- parainfluenza virus J12.2
- parenchymatous —*see* Fibrosis, lung
- passive J18.2
- patchy —*see* Pneumonia, broncho
- Peptococcus J15.8
- Peptostreptococcus J15.8
- plasma cell (of infants) B59
- pleurolobar —*see* Pneumonia, lobar
- pleuro-pneumonia-like organism (PPLO) J15.7
- pneumococcal (broncho) (lobar) J13
- Pneumocystis (carinii) (jiroveci) B59
- postinfectional NEC B99 *[J17]*
- postmeasles BØ5.2
- Proteus J15.6
- Pseudomonas J15.1
- psittacosis A7Ø
- radiation J7Ø.Ø
- respiratory syncytial virus J12.1
- resulting from a procedure J95.89
- rheumatic IØØ *[J17]*
- Salmonella (arizonae) (cholerae-suis) (enteritidis) (typhimurium) AØ2.22
  - typhi AØ1.Ø3
  - typhoid fever AØ1.Ø3
- SARS-associated coronavirus J12.81
- segmented, segmental —*see* Pneumonia, broncho-
- Serratia marcescens J15.6
- specified NEC J18.8
  - bacterium NEC J15.8
  - organism NEC J16.8
  - virus NEC J12.89
- spirochetal NEC A69.8

- **Pneumonia** *(Continued)*
  - staphylococcal (broncho) (lobar) J15.20
    - aureus (methicillin susceptible) (MSSA) J15.211
      - methicillin resistant (MRSA) J15.212
    - specified NEC J15.29
  - static, stasis J18.2
  - streptococcal NEC (broncho) (lobar) J15.4
    - group
      - A J15.4
      - B J15.3
      - specified NEC J15.4
  - Streptococcus pneumoniae J13
  - syphilitic, congenital (early) A50.04
  - traumatic (complication) (early) (secondary) T79.8
  - tuberculous (any) —*see* Tuberculosis, pulmonary
  - tularemic A21.2
  - varicella B01.2
  - Veillonella J15.8
  - ventilator associated J95.851
  - viral, virus (broncho) (interstitial) (lobar) J12.9
    - adenoviral J12.0
    - congenital P23.0
    - human metapneumovirus J12.3
    - parainfluenza J12.2
    - respiratory syncytial J12.1
    - SARS-associated coronavirus J12.81
    - specified NEC J12.89
  - white (congenital) A50.04
- **Pneumonic** —*see* condition
- **Pneumonitis** (acute) (primary) —*see also* Pneumonia
  - air-conditioner J67.7
  - allergic (due to) J67.9
    - organic dust NEC J67.8
    - red cedar dust J67.8
    - sequoiosis J67.8
    - wood dust J67.8
  - aspiration J69.0
    - due to
      - anesthesia J95.4
        - during
          - labor and delivery O74.0
          - pregnancy O29.01-
          - puerperium O89.01
      - fumes or gases J68.0
    - obstetric O74.0
  - chemical (due to gases, fumes or vapors) (inhalation) J68.0
    - due to anesthesia J95.4
  - cholesterol J84.89
  - chronic —*see* Fibrosis, lung
  - congenital rubella P35.0
  - crack (cocaine) J68.0
  - due to
    - beryllium J68.0
    - cadmium J68.0
    - crack (cocaine) J68.0
    - detergent J69.8
    - fluorocarbon-polymer J68.0
    - food, vomit (aspiration) J69.0
    - fumes or vapors J68.0
    - gases, fumes or vapors (inhalation) J68.0
    - inhalation
      - blood J69.8
      - essences J69.1
      - food (regurgitated), milk, vomit J69.0
      - oils, essences J69.1
      - saliva J69.0
      - solids, liquids NEC J69.8
    - manganese J68.0
    - nitrogen dioxide J68.0
    - oils, essences J69.1
    - solids, liquids NEC J69.8
    - toxoplasmosis (acquired) B58.3
      - congenital P37.1
    - vanadium J68.0
    - ventilator J95.851
- **Pneumonitis** *(Continued)*
  - eosinophilic J82
  - hypersensitivity J67.9
    - air conditioner lung J67.7
    - bagassosis J67.1
    - bird fancier's lung J67.2
    - farmer's lung J67.0
    - maltworker's lung J67.4
    - maple bark-stripper's lung J67.6
    - mushroom worker's lung J67.5
    - specified organic dust NEC J67.8
    - suberosis J67.3
  - interstitial (chronic) J84.89
    - acute J84.114
    - lymphoid J84.2
    - non-specific J84.89
      - idiopathic J84.113
  - lymphoid, interstitial J84.2
  - meconium P24.01
  - postanesthetic J95.4
    - correct substance properly administered —*see* Table of Drugs and Chemcials, by drug, adverse effect
    - in labor and delivery O74.0
    - in pregnancy O29.01-
    - obstetric O74.0
    - overdose or wrong substance given or taken (by accident) —*see* Table of Drugs and Chemicals, by drug, poisoning
    - postpartum, puerperal O89.01
  - postoperative J95.4
    - obstetric O74.0
  - radiation J70.0
  - rubella, congenital P35.0
  - ventilation (air-conditioning) J67.7
  - ventilator associated J95.851
  - wood-dust J67.8
- **Pneumonoconiosis** —*see* Pneumoconiosis
- **Pneumoparotid** K11.8
- **Pneumopathy NEC** J98.4
  - alveolar J84.09
  - due to organic dust NEC J66.8
  - parietoalveolar J84.09
- **Pneumopericarditis** —*see also* Pericarditis
  - acute I30.9
- **Pneumopericardium** —*see also* Pericarditis
  - congenital P25.3
  - newborn P25.3
  - traumatic (post) —*see* Injury, heart
- **Pneumophagia** (psychogenic) F45.8
- **Pneumopleurisy, pneumopleuritis** —*see also* Pneumonia J18.8
- **Pneumopyopericardium** I30.1
- **Pneumopyothorax** —*see* Pyopneumothorax
  - with fistula J86.0
- **Pneumorrhagia** —*see also* Hemorrhage, lung
  - tuberculous —*see* Tuberculosis, pulmonary
- **Pneumothorax NOS** J93.9
  - acute J93.83
  - chronic J93.81
  - congenital P25.1
  - perinatal period P25.1
  - postprocedural J95.811
  - specified NEC J93.83
  - spontaneous NOS J93.83
    - newborn P25.1
    - primary J93.11
    - secondary J93.12
    - tension J93.0
  - tense valvular, infectional J93.0
  - tension (spontaneous) J93.0
  - traumatic S27.0
    - with hemothorax S27.2
  - tuberculous —*see* Tuberculosis, pulmonary
- **Podagra** —*see also* Gout M10.9
- **Podencephalus** Q01.9
- **Poikilocytosis** R71.8
- **Poikiloderma** L81.6
  - Civatte's L57.3
  - congenital Q82.8
  - vasculare atrophicans L94.5
- **Poikilodermatomyositis** M33.10
  - with
    - myopathy M33.12
    - respiratory involvement M33.11
    - specified organ involvement NEC M33.19
- **Pointed ear** (congenital) Q17.3
- **Poison ivy, oak, sumac or other plant dermatitis** (allergic) (contact) L23.7
- **Poisoning** (acute) —*see also* Table of Drugs and Chemicals
  - algae and toxins T65.82-
  - Bacillus B (aertrycke) (cholerae (suis)) (paratyphosus) (suipestifer) A02.9
    - botulinus A05.1
  - bacterial toxins A05.9
  - berries, noxious —*see* Poisoning, food, noxious, berries
  - botulism A05.1
  - ciguatera fish T61.0-
  - Clostridium botulinum A05.1
  - death-cap (Amanita phalloides) (Amanita verna) —*see* Poisoning, food, noxious, mushrooms
  - drug —*see* Table of Drugs and Chemicals, by drug, poisoning
  - epidemic, fish (noxious) —*see* Poisoning, seafood
    - bacterial A05.9
  - fava bean D55.0
  - fish (noxious) T61.9-
    - bacterial —*see* Intoxication, foodborne, by agent
    - ciguatera fish —*see* Poisoning, ciguatera fish
    - scombroid fish —*see* Poisoning, scombroid fish
    - specified type NEC T61.77-
  - food (acute) (diseased) (infected) (noxious) NEC T62.9-
    - bacterial —*see* Intoxication, foodborne, by agent
    - due to
      - Bacillus (aertrycke) (choleraesuis) (paratyphosus) (suipestifer) A02.9
        - botulinus A05.1
      - Clostridium (perfringens) (Welchii) A05.2
      - salmonella (aertrycke) (callinarum) (choleraesuis) (enteritidis) (paratyphi) (suipestifer) A02.9
        - with
          - gastroenteritis A02.0
          - sepsis A02.1
      - staphylococcus A05.0
      - Vibrio
        - parahaemolyticus A05.3
        - vulnificus A05.5
    - noxious or naturally toxic T62.9-
      - berries —*see* subcategory T62.1-
      - fish —*see* Poisoning, seafood
      - mushrooms —*see* subcategory T62.0X-
      - plants NEC —*see* subcategory T62.2X-
      - seafood —*see* Poisoning, seafood
      - specified NEC —*see* subcategory T62.8X-
  - ichthyotoxism —*see* Poisoning, seafood
  - kreotoxism, food A05.9
  - latex T65.81-
  - lead T56.0-
  - mushroom —*see* Poisoning, food, noxious, mushroom
  - mussels —*see also* Poisoning, shellfish
    - bacterial —*see* Intoxication, foodborne, by agent
  - nicotine (tobacco) T65.2-
  - noxious foodstuffs —*see* Poisoning, food, noxious
  - plants, noxious —*see* Poisoning, food, noxious, plants NEC
  - ptomaine —*see* Poisoning, food
  - radiation J70.0

Poisoning *(Continued)*
Salmonella (arizonae) (cholerae-suis) (enteritidis) (typhimurium) A02.9
scombroid fish T61.1-
seafood (noxious) T61.9-
bacterial —*see* Intoxication, foodborne, by agent
fish —*see* Poisoning, fish
shellfish —*see* Poisoning, shellfish
specified NEC —*see* subcategory T61.8X-
shellfish (amnesic) (azaspiracid) (diarrheic) (neurotoxic) (noxious) (paralytic) T61.78-
bacterial —*see* Intoxication, foodborne, by agent
ciguatera mollusk —*see* Poisoning, ciguatera fish
specified substance NEC T65.891
Staphylococcus, food A05.0
tobacco (nicotine) T65.2-
water E87.79
Poker spine —*see* Spondylitis, ankylosing
Poland syndrome Q79.8
Polioencephalitis (acute) (bulbar) A80.9
inferior G12.22
influenzal —*see* Influenza, with, encephalopathy
superior hemorrhagic (acute) (Wernicke's) E51.2
Wernicke's E51.2
Polioencephalomyelitis (acute) (anterior) A80.9
with beriberi E51.2
Polioencephalopathy, superior hemorrhagic E51.2
with
beriberi E51.11
pellagra E52
Poliomeningoencephalitis —*see* Meningoencephalitis
Poliomyelitis (acute) (anterior) (epidemic) A80.9
with paralysis (bulbar) —*see* Poliomyelitis, paralytic
abortive A80.4
ascending (progressive) —*see* Poliomyelitis, paralytic
bulbar (paralytic) —*see* Poliomyelitis, paralytic
congenital P35.8
nonepidemic A80.9
nonparalytic A80.4
paralytic A80.30
specified NEC A80.39
vaccine-associated A80.0
wild virus
imported A80.1
indigenous A80.2
spinal, acute A80.9
Poliosis (eyebrow) (eyelashes) L67.1
circumscripta, acquired L67.1
Pollakiuria R35.0
psychogenic F45.8
Pollinosis J30.1
Pollitzer's disease L73.2
Polyadenitis —*see also* Lymphadenitis
malignant A20.0
Polyalgia M79.89
Polyangiitis M30.0
microscopic M31.7
overlap syndrome M30.8
Polyarteritis
microscopic M31.7
nodosa M30.0
with lung involvement M30.1
juvenile M30.2
related condition NEC M30.8
Polyarthralgia —*see* Pain, joint
Polyarthritis, polyarthropathy —*see also* Arthritis M13.0
due to or associated with other specified conditions —*see* Arthritis
Polyarthritis, polyarthropathy *(Continued)*
epidemic (Australian) (with exanthema) B33.1
infective —*see* Arthritis, pyogenic or pyemic
inflammatory M06.4
juvenile (chronic) (seronegative) M08.3
migratory —*see* Fever, rheumatic
rheumatic, acute —*see* Fever, rheumatic
Polyarthrosis M15.9
post-traumatic M15.3
primary M15.0
specified NEC M15.8
Polycarential syndrome of infancy E40
Polychondritis (atrophic) (chronic) —*see also* Disorder, cartilage, specified type NEC
relapsing M94.1
Polycoria Q13.2
Polycystic (disease)
degeneration, kidney Q61.3
autosomal dominant (adult type) Q61.2
autosomal recessive (infantile type) NEC Q61.19
kidney Q61.3
autosomal
dominant Q61.2
recessive NEC Q61.19
autosomal dominant (adult type) Q61.2
autosomal recessive (childhood type) NEC Q61.19
infantile type NEC Q61.19
liver Q44.6
lung J98.4
congenital Q33.0
ovary, ovaries E28.2
spleen Q89.09
Polycythemia (secondary) D75.1
acquired D75.1
benign (familial) D75.0
due to
donor twin P61.1
erythropoietin D75.1
fall in plasma volume D75.1
high altitude D75.1
maternal-fetal transfusion P61.1
stress D75.1
emotional D75.1
erythropoietin D75.1
familial (benign) D75.0
Gaisböck's (hypertonica) D75.1
high altitude D75.1
hypertonica D75.1
hypoxemic D75.1
neonatorum P61.1
nephrogenous D75.1
relative D75.1
secondary D75.1
spurious D75.1
stress D75.1
vera D45
Polycytosis cryptogenica D75.1
Polydactylism, polydactyly Q69.9
toes Q69.2
Polydipsia R63.1
Polydystrophy, pseudo-Hurler E77.0
Polyembryoma —*see* Neoplasm, malignant, by site
Polyglandular
deficiency E31.0
dyscrasia E31.9
dysfunction E31.9
syndrome E31.8
Polyhydramnios O40.-
Polymastia Q83.1
Polymenorrhea N92.0
Polymyalgia M35.3
arteritica, giant cell M31.5
rheumatica M35.3
with giant cell arteritis M31.5
Polymyositis (acute) (chronic) (hemorrhagic) M33.20
with
myopathy M33.22
respiratory involvement M33.21
skin involvement —*see* Dermatopolymyositis
specified organ involvement NEC M33.29
ossificans (generalisata) (progressiva) —*see* Myositis, ossificans, progressiva
Polyneuritis, polyneuritic —*see also* Polyneuropathy
acute (post-)infective G61.0
alcoholic G62.1
cranialis G52.7
demyelinating, chronic inflammatory (CIDP) G61.81
diabetic —*see* Diabetes, polyneuropathy
diphtheritic A36.83
due to lack of vitamin NEC E56.9 *[G63]*
endemic E51.11
erythredema —*see* subcategory T56.1
febrile, acute G61.0
hereditary ataxic G60.1
idiopathic, acute G61.0
infective (acute) G61.0
inflammatory, chronic demyelinating (CIDP) G61.81
nutritional E63.9 *[G63]*
postinfective (acute) G61.0
specified NEC G62.89
Polyneuropathy (peripheral) G62.9
alcoholic G62.1
amyloid (Portuguese) E85.1 *[G63]*
arsenical G62.2
critical illness G62.81
demyelinating, chronic inflammatory (CIDP) G61.81
diabetic —*see* Diabetes, polyneuropathy
drug-induced G62.0
hereditary G60.9
specified NEC G60.8
idiopathic G60.9
progressive G60.3
in (due to)
alcohol G62.1
sequelae G65.2
amyloidosis, familial (Portuguese) E85.1 *[G63]*
antitetanus serum G61.1
arsenic G62.2
sequelae G65.2
avitaminosis NEC E56.9 *[G63]*
beriberi E51.11
collagen vascular disease NEC M35.9 *[G63]*
deficiency (of)
B (-complex) vitamins E53.9 *[G63]*
vitamin B6 E53.1 *[G63]*
diabetes —*see* Diabetes, polyneuropathy
diphtheria A36.83
drug or medicament G62.0
correct substance properly administered —*see* Table of Drugs and Chemicals, by drug, adverse effect
overdose or wrong substance given or taken —*see* Table of Drugs and Chemicals, by drug, poisoning
endocrine disease NEC E34.9 *[G63]*
herpes zoster B02.23
hypoglycemia E16.2 *[G63]*
infectious
disease NEC B99 *[G63]*
mononucleosis B27.91
lack of vitamin NEC E56.9 *[G63]*
lead G62.2
sequelae G65.2
leprosy A30.9 *[G63]*
Lyme disease A69.22
metabolic disease NEC E88.9 *[G63]*
microscopic polyangiitis M31.7 *[G63]*

P

◄ New ◄ Revised ~~deleted~~ Deleted

- **Polyneuropathy** *(Continued)*
  - in *(Continued)*
    - mumps B26.84
    - neoplastic disease —*see also* Neoplasm D49.9 *[G63]*
    - nutritional deficiency NEC E63.9 *[G63]*
    - organophosphate compounds G62.2
      - sequelae G65.2
    - parasitic disease NEC B89 *[G63]*
    - pellagra E52 *[G63]*
    - polyarteritis nodosa M30.0
    - porphyria E80.20 *[G63]*
    - radiation G62.82
    - rheumatoid arthritis —*see* Rheumatoid, polyneuropathy
    - sarcoidosis D86.89
    - serum G61.1
    - syphilis (late) A52.15
      - congenital A50.43
    - systemic
      - connective tissue disorder M35.9 *[G63]*
      - lupus erythematosus M32.19
    - toxic agent NEC G62.2
      - sequelae G65.2
    - triorthocresyl phosphate G62.2
      - sequelae G65.2
    - tuberculosis A17.89
    - uremia N18.9 *[G63]*
    - vitamin B12 deficiency E53.8 *[G63]*
      - with anemia (pernicious) D51.0 *[G63]*
        - due to dietary deficiency D51.3 *[G63]*
    - zoster B02.23
  - inflammatory G61.9
    - chronic demyelinating (CIDP) G61.81
    - sequelae G65.1
    - specified NEC G61.89
  - lead G62.2
    - sequelae G65.2
  - nutritional NEC E63.9 *[G63]*
  - postherpetic (zoster) B02.23
  - progressive G60.3
  - radiation-induced G62.82
  - sensory (hereditary) (idiopathic) G60.8
  - specified NEC G62.89
  - syphilitic (late) A52.15
    - congenital A50.43
- **Polyopia** H53.8
- **Polyorchism, polyorchidism** Q55.21
- **Polyosteoarthritis** —*see also* Osteoarthritis, generalized M15.9-
  - post-traumatic M15.3
  - specified NEC M15.8
- **Polyostotic fibrous dysplasia** Q78.1
- **Polyotia** Q17.0
- **Polyp, polypus**
  - accessory sinus J33.8
  - adenocarcinoma in —*see* Neoplasm, malignant, by site
  - adenocarcinoma in situ in —*see* Neoplasm, in situ, by site
  - adenoid tissue J33.0
  - adenomatous —*see also* Neoplasm, benign, by site
    - adenocarcinoma in —*see* Neoplasm, malignant, by site
    - adenocarcinoma in situ in —*see* Neoplasm, in situ, by site
    - carcinoma in —*see* Neoplasm, malignant, by site
    - carcinoma in situ in —*see* Neoplasm, in situ, by site
    - multiple —*see* Neoplasm, benign
      - adenocarcinoma in —*see* Neoplasm, malignant, by site
      - adenocarcinoma in situ in —*see* Neoplasm, in situ, by site
  - antrum J33.8
  - anus, anal (canal) K62.0

- **Polyp, polypus** *(Continued)*
  - Bartholin's gland N84.3
  - bladder D41.4
  - carcinoma in —*see* Neoplasm, malignant, by site
  - carcinoma in situ in —*see* Neoplasm, in situ, by site
  - cecum D12.0
  - cervix (uteri) N84.1
    - in pregnancy or childbirth —*see* Pregnancy, complicated by, abnormal, cervix
    - mucous N84.1
    - nonneoplastic N84.1
  - choanal J33.0
  - cholesterol K82.4
  - clitoris N84.3
  - colon K63.5
    - adenomatous D12.6
    - ascending D12.2
    - cecum D12.0
    - descending D12.4
    - inflammatory K51.40
      - with
        - abscess K51.414
        - complication K51.419
          - specified NEC K51.418
        - fistula K51.413
        - intestinal obstruction K51.412
        - rectal bleeding K51.411
    - sigmoid D12.5
    - transverse D12.3
  - corpus uteri N84.0
  - dental K04.01 ⬅
    - irreversible K04.02 ◀
    - reversible K04.01 ◀
  - duodenum K31.7
  - ear (middle) H74.4-
  - endometrium N84.0
  - ethmoidal (sinus) J33.8
  - fallopian tube N84.8
  - female genital tract N84.9
    - specified NEC N84.8
  - frontal (sinus) J33.8
  - gallbladder K82.4
  - gingiva, gum K06.8
  - labia, labium (majus) (minus) N84.3
  - larynx (mucous) J38.1
    - adenomatous D14.1
  - malignant —*see* Neoplasm, malignant, by site
  - maxillary (sinus) J33.8
  - middle ear —*see* Polyp, ear (middle)
  - myometrium N84.0
  - nares
    - anterior J33.9
    - posterior J33.0
  - nasal (mucous) J33.9
    - cavity J33.0
    - septum J33.0
  - nasopharyngeal J33.0
  - nose (mucous) J33.9
  - oviduct N84.8
  - pharynx J39.2
  - placenta O90.89
  - prostate —*see* Enlargement, enlarged, prostate
  - pudenda, pudendum N84.3
  - pulpal (dental) K04.01 ⬅
    - irreversible K04.02 ◀
    - reversible K04.01 ◀
  - rectum (nonadenomatous) K62.1
    - adenomatous —*see* Polyp, adenomatous
  - septum (nasal) J33.0
  - sinus (accessory) (ethmoidal) (frontal) (maxillary) (sphenoidal) J33.8
  - sphenoidal (sinus) J33.8
  - stomach K31.7
    - adenomatous D13.1
  - tube, fallopian N84.8
  - turbinate, mucous membrane J33.8
  - umbilical, newborn P83.6
  - ureter N28.89

- **Polyp, polypus** *(Continued)*
  - urethra N36.2
  - uterus (body) (corpus) (mucous) N84.0
    - cervix N84.1
    - in pregnancy or childbirth —*see* Pregnancy, complicated by, tumor, uterus
  - vagina N84.2
  - vocal cord (mucous) J38.1
  - vulva N84.3
- **Polyphagia** R63.2
- **Polyploidy** Q92.7
- **Polypoid** —*see* condition
- **Polyposis** —*see also* Polyp
  - coli (adenomatous) D12.6
    - adenocarcinoma in C18.9
    - adenocarcinoma in situ in —*see* Neoplasm, in situ, by site
    - carcinoma in C18.9
  - colon (adenomatous) D12.6
  - familial D12.6
    - adenocarcinoma in situ in —*see* Neoplasm, in situ, by site
  - intestinal (adenomatous) D12.6
  - malignant lymphomatous C83.1
  - multiple, adenomatous —*see also* Neoplasm, benign D36.9
- **Polyradiculitis** —*see* Polyneuropathy
- **Polyradiculoneuropathy** (acute) (postinfective) (segmentally demyelinating) G61.0
- **Polyserositis**
  - due to pericarditis I31.1
  - pericardial I31.1
  - periodic, familial E85.0
  - tuberculous A19.9
    - acute A19.1
    - chronic A19.8
- **Polysplenia syndrome** Q89.09
- **Polysyndactyly** —*see also* Syndactylism, syndactyly Q70.4
- **Polytrichia** L68.3
- **Polyunguia** Q84.6
- **Polyuria** R35.8
  - nocturnal R35.1
  - psychogenic F45.8
- **Pompe's disease** (glycogen storage) E74.02
- **Pompholyx** L30.1
- **Poncet's disease** (tuberculous rheumatism) A18.09
- **Pond fracture** —*see* Fracture, skull
- **Ponos** B55.0
- **Pons, pontine** —*see* condition
- **Poor**
  - aesthetic of existing restoration of tooth K08.56
  - contractions, labor O62.2
  - gingival margin to tooth restoration K08.51
  - personal hygiene R46.0
  - prenatal care, affecting management of pregnancy —*see* Pregnancy, complicated by, insufficient, prenatal care
  - sucking reflex (newborn) R29.2
  - urinary stream R39.12
  - vision NEC H54.7
- **Poradenitis, nostras inguinalis or venerea** A55
- **Porencephaly** (congenital) (developmental) (true) Q04.6
  - acquired G93.0
  - nondevelopmental G93.0
  - traumatic (post) F07.89
- **Porocephaliasis** B88.8
- **Porokeratosis** Q82.8
- **Poroma, eccrine** —*see* Neoplasm, skin, benign
- **Porphyria** (South African) E80.20
  - acquired E80.20
  - acute intermittent (hepatic) (Swedish) E80.21
  - cutanea tarda (hereditary) (symptomatic) E80.1
  - due to drugs E80.20
    - correct substance properly administered —*see* Table of Drugs and Chemicals, by drug, adverse effect

P

Porphyria *(Continued)*
- due to drugs *(Continued)*
  - overdose or wrong substance given or taken *—see* Table of Drugs and Chemicals, by drug, poisoning
- erythropoietic (congenital) (hereditary) E80.0
- hepatocutaneous type E80.1
- secondary E80.20
- toxic NEC E80.20
- variegata E80.20

Porphyrinuria *—see* Porphyria
Porphyruria *—see* Porphyria
Portal *—see* condition
Port wine nevus, mark, or stain Q82.5
Posadas-Wernicke disease B38.9
Positive
- culture (nonspecific)
  - blood R78.81
  - bronchial washings R84.5
  - cerebrospinal fluid R83.5
  - cervix uteri R87.5
  - nasal secretions R84.5
  - nipple discharge R89.5
  - nose R84.5
    - staphylococcus (Methicillin susceptible) Z22.321
      - Methicillin resistant Z22.322
  - peritoneal fluid R85.5
  - pleural fluid R84.5
  - prostatic secretions R86.5
  - saliva R85.5
  - seminal fluid R86.5
  - sputum R84.5
  - synovial fluid R89.5
  - throat scrapings R84.5
  - urine R82.79 ⬅
  - vagina R87.5
  - vulva R87.5
  - wound secretions R89.5
- PPD (skin test) R76.11
- serology for syphilis A53.0
  - with signs or symptoms - code as Syphilis, by site and stage
  - false R76.8
- skin test, tuberculin (without active tuberculosis) R76.11
- test, human immunodeficiency virus (HIV) R75
- VDRL A53.0
  - with signs or symptoms - code by site and stage under Syphilis A53.9
- Wassermann reaction A53.0

Postcardiotomy syndrome I97.0
Postcaval ureter Q62.62
Postcholecystectomy syndrome K91.5
Postclimacteric bleeding N95.0
Postcommissurotomy syndrome I97.0
Postconcussional syndrome F07.81
Postcontusional syndrome F07.81
Postcricoid region *—see* condition
Post-dates (40-42 weeks) (pregnancy) (mother) O48.0
- more than 42 weeks gestation O48.1

Postencephalitic syndrome F07.89
Posterior *—see* condition
Posterolateral sclerosis (spinal cord) *—see* Degeneration, combined
Postexanthematous *—see* condition
Postfebrile *—see* condition
Postgastrectomy dumping syndrome K91.1
Posthemiplegic chorea *—see* Monoplegia
Posthemorrhagic anemia (chronic) D50.0
- acute D62
- newborn P61.3

Postherpetic neuralgia (zoster) B02.29
- trigeminal B02.22

Posthitis N47.7
Postimmunization complication or reaction — *see* Complications, vaccination
Postinfectious *—see* condition
Postlaminectomy syndrome NEC M96.1
Postleukotomy syndrome F07.0
Postmastectomy lymphedema (syndrome) I97.2
Postmaturity, postmature (over 42 weeks)
- maternal (over 42 weeks gestation) O48.1
- newborn P08.22

Postmeasles complication NEC *—see also* condition B05.89
Postmenopausal
- endometrium (atrophic) N95.8
  - suppurative *—see also* Endometritis N71.9
- osteoporosis *—see* Osteoporosis, postmenopausal

Postnasal drip R09.82
- due to
  - allergic rhinitis *—see* Rhinitis, allergic
  - common cold J00
  - gastroesophageal reflux *—see* Reflux, gastroesophageal
  - nasopharyngitis *—see* Nasopharyngitis
  - other know condition — code to condition
  - sinusitis *—see* Sinusitis

Postnatal *—see* condition
Postoperative (postprocedural) *—see* Complication, postoperative
- pneumothorax, therapeutic Z98.3
- state NEC Z98.890 ⬅

Postpancreatectomy hyperglycemia E89.1
Postpartum *—see* Puerperal
Postphlebitic syndrome *—see* Syndrome, postthrombotic
Postpolio (myelitic) **syndrome** G14
Postpoliomyelitic *—see also* condition
- osteopathy *—see* Osteopathy, after poliomyelitis

Postprocedural *—see also* Postoperative
- hypoinsulinemia E89.1

Postschizophrenic depression F32.89 ⬅
Postsurgery status *—see also* Status (post)
- pneumothorax, therapeutic Z98.3

Post-term (40-42 weeks) (pregnancy) (mother) O48.0
- infant P08.21
- more than 42 weeks gestation (mother) O48.1

Post-traumatic brain syndrome, nonpsychotic F07.81
Post-typhoid abscess A01.09
Postures, hysterical F44.2
Postvaccinal reaction or complication *—see* Complications, vaccination
Postvalvulotomy syndrome I97.0
Potain's
- disease (pulmonary edema) *—see* Edema, lung
- syndrome (gastrectasis with dyspepsia) K31.0

Potter's
- asthma J62.8
- facies Q60.6
- lung J62.8
- syndrome (with renal agenesis) Q60.6

Pott's
- curvature (spinal) A18.01
- disease or paraplegia A18.01
- spinal curvature A18.01
- tumor, puffy *—see* Osteomyelitis, specified type NEC

Pouch
- bronchus Q32.4
- Douglas' *—see* condition
- esophagus, esophageal, congenital Q39.6
  - acquired K22.5
- gastric K31.4
- Hartmann's K82.8
- pharynx, pharyngeal (congenital) Q38.7

Pouchitis K91.850
Poultrymen's itch B88.0
Poverty NEC Z59.6
- extreme Z59.5

Poxvirus NEC B08.8
Prader-Willi syndrome Q87.1
Preauricular appendage or tag Q17.0
Prebetalipoproteinemia (acquired) (essential) (familial) (hereditary) (primary) (secondary) E78.1
- with chylomicronemia E78.3

Precipitate labor or delivery O62.3
Preclimacteric bleeding (menorrhagia) N92.4
Precocious
- adrenarche E30.1
- menarche E30.1
- menstruation E30.1
- pubarche E30.1
- puberty E30.1
  - central E22.8
- sexual development NEC E30.1
- thelarche E30.8

Precocity, sexual (constitutional) (cryptogenic) (female) (idiopathic) (male) E30.1
- with adrenal hyperplasia E25.9
  - congenital E25.0

Precordial pain R07.2
Predeciduous teeth K00.2
Prediabetes, prediabetic R73.03 ⬅
- complicating
  - pregnancy *—see* Pregnancy, complicated by, diseases of, specified type or system NEC
  - puerperium O99.89

Predislocation status of hip at birth Q65.6
Pre-eclampsia O14.9-
- with pre-existing hypertension *—see* Hypertension, complicating pregnancy, pre-existing, with, pre-eclampsia
- complicating ◀
  - childbirth O14.94 ◀
  - puerperium O14.95 ◀
- mild O14.0-
  - complicating ◀
    - childbirth O14.04 ◀
    - puerperium O14.05 ◀
- moderate O14.0-
  - complicating ◀
    - childbirth O14.04 ◀
    - puerperium O14.05 ◀
- severe O14.1-
  - with hemolysis, elevated liver enzymes and low platelet count (HELLP) O14.2-
    - complicating ◀
      - childbirth O14.24 ◀
      - puerperium O14.25 ◀
  - complicating ◀
    - childbirth O14.14 ◀
    - puerperium O14.15 ◀

Pre-eruptive color change, teeth, tooth K00.8
Pre-excitation atrioventricular conduction I45.6
Preglaucoma H40.00-
Pregnancy (single) (uterine) *—see also* Delivery and Puerperal

> Note: The Tabular must be reviewed for assignment of the appropriate character indicating the trimester of the pregnancy
>
> Note: The Tabular must be reviewed for assignment of appropriate seventh character for multiple gestation codes in Chapter 15

- abdominal (ectopic) O00.00 ⬅
  - with intrauterine pregnancy O00.01 ◀
  - with viable fetus O36.7-
- ampullar O00.10 ⬅
  - with intrauterine pregnancy O00.11 ◀
- biochemical O02.81
- broad ligament O00.80 ⬅
  - with intrauterine pregnancy O00.81 ◀
- cervical O00.80 ⬅
  - with intrauterine pregnancy O00.81 ◀
- chemical O02.81
- complicated NOS O26.9-

P

◀ New ⬅ Revised ~~deleted~~ Deleted

- **Pregnancy** *(Continued)*
  - complicated by *(Continued)*
    - fetal *(Continued)*
      - heart rate irregularity (bradycardia) (decelerations) (tachycardia) O76
      - hereditary disease O35.2
      - hydrocephalus O35.Ø
      - intrauterine death O36.4
      - poor growth O36.59-
        - light for dates O36.59-
        - small for dates O36.59-
      - problem O36.9-
        - specified NEC O36.89-
      - reduction (elective) O31.3-
      - selective termination O31.3-
      - spina bifida O35.Ø
      - thrombocytopenia O36.82-
    - fibroid (tumor) (uterus) O34.1-
    - fissure of nipple O92.11-
    - gallstones O99.61-
    - gastric banding status O99.84-
    - gastric bypass status O99.84-
    - genital herpes (asymptomatic) (history of) (inactive) O98.51-
    - genital tract infection O23.9-
    - glomerular diseases (conditions in NØØ-NØ7) O26.83-
      - with hypertension, pre-existing —*see* Hypertension, complicating, pregnancy, pre-existing, with, renal disease
    - gonorrhea O98.21-
    - grand multiparity OØ9.4
    - habitual aborter —*see* Pregnancy, complicated by, recurrent pregnancy loss
    - HELLP syndrome (hemolysis, elevated liver enzymes and low platelet count) O14.2-
    - hemorrhage
      - antepartum —*see* Hemorrhage, antepartum
      - before 2Ø completed weeks gestation O2Ø.9
        - specified NEC O2Ø.8
      - due to premature separation, placenta —*see also* Abruptio placentae O45.9-
      - early O2Ø.9
        - specified NEC O2Ø.8
      - threatened abortion O2Ø.Ø
    - hemorrhoids O22.4-
    - hepatitis (viral) O98.41-
    - herniation of uterus O34.59-
    - high
      - head at term O32.4
      - risk —*see* Supervision (of) (for), high-risk
    - history of in utero procedure during previous pregnancy OØ9.82-
    - HIV O98.71-
    - human immunodeficiency virus (HIV) disease O98.71-
    - hydatidiform mole —*see also* Mole, hydatidiform OØ1.9-
    - hydramnios O4Ø.-
    - hydrocephalic fetus (disproportion) O33.6
    - hydrops
      - amnii O4Ø.-
      - fetalis O36.2-
        - associated with isoimmunization —*see also* Pregnancy, complicated by, isoimmunization O36.11-
    - hydrorrhea O42.9Ø
    - hyperemesis (gravidarum) (mild) —*see also* Hyperemesis, gravidarum O21.Ø-
    - hypertension —*see* Hypertension, complicating pregnancy
    - hypertensive
      - heart and renal disease, pre-existing —*see* Hypertension, complicating, pregnancy, pre-existing, with, heart disease, with renal disease
- **Pregnancy** *(Continued)*
  - complicated by *(Continued)*
    - hypertensive *(Continued)*
      - heart disease, pre-existing —*see* Hypertension, complicating, pregnancy, pre-existing, with, heart disease
      - renal disease, pre-existing —*see* Hypertension, complicating, pregnancy, pre-existing, with, renal disease
    - hypotension O26.5-
    - immune disorders NEC (conditions in D8Ø-D89) O99.11-
    - incarceration, uterus O34.51-
    - incompetent cervix O34.3-
    - inconclusive fetal viability O36.8Ø
    - infection (s) O98.91-
      - amniotic fluid or sac O41.1Ø-
      - bladder O23.1-
      - carrier state NEC O99.83Ø
        - streptococcus B O99.82Ø
      - genital organ or tract O23.9-
        - specified NEC O23.59-
      - genitourinary tract O23.9-
      - gonorrhea O98.21-
      - hepatitis (viral) O98.41-
      - HIV O98.71-
      - human immunodeficiency virus (HIV) O98.71-
      - kidney O23.Ø-
      - nipple O91.Ø1-
      - parasitic disease O98.91-
        - specified NEC O98.81-
      - protozoal disease O98.61-
      - sexually transmitted NEC O98.31-
      - specified type NEC O98.81-
      - syphilis O98.11-
      - tuberculosis O98.Ø1-
      - urethra O23.2-
      - urinary (tract) O23.4-
        - specified NEC O23.3-
      - viral disease O98.51-
    - injury or poisoning (conditions in SØØ-T88) O9A.21-
      - due to abuse
        - physical O9A.31-
        - psychological O9A.51-
        - sexual O9A.41-
    - insufficient
      - prenatal care OØ9.3-
      - weight gain O26.1-
    - insulin resistance O26.89
    - intrauterine fetal death (near term) O36.4
      - early pregnancy OØ2.1
      - multiple gestation (one fetus or more) O31.2-
    - isoimmunization O36.11-
      - anti-A sensitization O36.11-
      - anti-B sensitization O36.19-
      - Rh O36.Ø9-
        - anti-D antibody O36.Ø1-
      - specified NEC O36.19-
    - laceration of uterus NEC O71.81
    - malformation
      - placenta, placental (vessel) O43.1Ø-
        - specified NEC O43.19-
      - uterus (congenital) O34.Ø-
    - malnutrition (conditions in E4Ø-E46) O25.1-
    - maternal hypotension syndrome O26.5-
    - mental disorders (conditions in FØ1-FØ9, F2Ø-F99) O99.34-
      - alcohol use O99.31-
      - drug use O99.32-
      - smoking O99.33-
    - mentum presentation O32.3
    - metabolic disorders O99.28-
    - missed
      - abortion OØ2.1
      - delivery O36.4
- **Pregnancy** *(Continued)*
  - complicated by *(Continued)*
    - multiple gestations O3Ø.9-
      - conjoined twins O3Ø.Ø2-
      - quadruplet —*see* Pregnancy, quadruplet
      - specified complication NEC O31.8X-
      - specified number of multiples NEC —*see* Pregnancy, multiple (gestation), specified NEC
      - triplet —*see* Pregnancy, triplet
      - twin —*see* Pregnancy, twin
    - musculoskeletal condition (conditions is MØØ-M99) O99.89
    - necrosis, liver (conditions in K72) O26.61-
    - neoplasm
      - benign
        - cervix O34.4-
        - corpus uteri O34.1-
        - uterus O34.1-
      - malignant O9A.11-
    - nephropathy NEC O26.83-
    - nervous system condition (conditions in GØØ-G99) O99.35-
    - nutritional diseases NEC O99.28-
    - obesity (pre-existing) O99.21-
    - obesity surgery status O99.84-
    - oblique lie or presentation O32.2
    - older mother —*see* Pregnancy, complicated by, elderly
    - oligohydramnios O41.Ø-
      - with premature rupture of membranes —*see also* Pregnancy, complicated by, premature rupture of membranes O42-
    - onset (spontaneous) of labor after 37 completed weeks of gestation but before 39 completed weeks gestation, with delivery by (planned) cesarean section O75.82
    - oophoritis O23.52-
    - overdose, drug —*see also* Table of Drugs and Chemicals, by drug, poisoning O9A.21-
    - oversize fetus O33.5
    - papyraceous fetus O31.Ø-
    - pelvic inflammatory disease O99.89
    - periodontal disease O99.61-
    - peripheral neuritis O26.82-
    - peritoneal (pelvic) adhesions O99.89
    - phlebitis O22.9-
    - phlebopathy O22.9-
    - phlebothrombosis (superficial) O22.2-
      - deep O22.3-
    - placenta accreta O43.21-
    - placenta increta O43.22-
    - placenta percreta O43.23-
    - placenta previa O44.Ø- ⟸
      - complete O44.Ø- ◀
        - with hemorrhage O44.1- ◀
      - marginal O44.2- ◀
        - with hemorrhage O44.3- ◀
      - partial O44.2- ◀
        - with hemorrhage O44.3- ◀
      - ~~without hemorrhage O44.Ø-~~
    - placental disorder O43.9-
      - specified NEC O43.89-
    - placental dysfunction O43.89-
    - placental infarction O43.81-
    - placental insufficiency O36.51-
    - placental transfusion syndromes
      - fetomaternal O43.Ø1-
      - fetus to fetus O43.Ø2-
      - maternofetal O43.Ø1-
    - placentitis O41.14-
    - pneumonia O99.51-
    - poisoning —*see also* Table of Drugs and Chemicals O9A.21-
    - polyhydramnios O4Ø-
    - polymorphic eruption of pregnancy O26.86
    - poor obstetric history NEC OØ9.29-

P

Pregnancy *(Continued)*
complicated by *(Continued)*
postmaturity (post-term) (4Ø to 42 weeks) O48.Ø
more than 42 completed weeks gestation (prolonged) O48.1
pre-eclampsia O14.9-
mild O14.Ø-
moderate O14.Ø-
severe O14.1-
with hemolysis, elevated liver enzymes and low platelet count (HELLP) O14.2-
premature labor —*see* Pregnancy, complicated by, preterm labor
premature rupture of membranes O42.9Ø
full-term, unspecified as to length of time between rupture and onset of labor O42.92 ◀
with onset of labor
within 24 hours O42.ØØ
~~after 37 weeks gestation O42.02~~
at or after 37 weeks gestation, onset of labor within 24 hours of rupture O42.Ø2 ◀
pre-term (before 37 completed weeks of gestation) O42.Ø1-
after 24 hours O42.1Ø
~~after 37 weeks gestation O42.12~~
at or after 37 weeks gestation, onset of labor more than 24 hours following rupture O42.12 ◀
pre-term (before 37 completed weeks of gestation) O42.11-
~~after 37 weeks gestation O42.92~~
at or after 37 weeks gestation, unspecified as to length of time between rupture and onset of labor O42.92 ◀
~~full-term O42.92~~
pre-term (before 37 completed weeks of gestation) O42.91-
premature separation of placenta —*see also* Abruptio placentae O45.9-
presentation, fetal —*see* Delivery, complicated by, malposition
preterm delivery O6Ø.1Ø
preterm labor
with delivery O6Ø.1Ø
preterm O6Ø.1Ø
term O6Ø.2Ø
second trimester
with preterm delivery
second trimester O6Ø.12
third trimester O6Ø.13
with term delivery O6Ø.22
without delivery O6Ø.Ø2
third trimester
with term delivery O6Ø.23
with third trimester preterm delivery O6Ø.14
without delivery O6Ø.Ø3
without delivery O6Ø.ØØ
second trimester O6Ø.Ø2
third trimester O6Ø.Ø3
previous history of —*see* Pregnancy, supervision of, high-risk
prolapse, uterus O34.52-
proteinuria (gestational) —*see also* Proteinuria, gestational O12.1- ⬅
with edema O12.2-
pruritic urticarial papules and plaques of pregnancy (PUPPP) O26.86
pruritus (neurogenic) O26.89-
psychosis or psychoneurosis (puerperal) F53
ptyalism O26.89-
PUPPP (pruritic urticarial papules and plaques of pregnancy) O26.86
pyelitis O23.Ø-
recurrent pregnancy loss O26.2-

Pregnancy *(Continued)*
complicated by *(Continued)*
renal disease or failure NEC O26.83-
with secondary hypertension, pre-existing —*see* Hypertension, complicating, pregnancy, pre-existing, secondary
hypertensive, pre-existing —*see* Hypertension, complicating, pregnancy, pre-existing, with, renal disease
respiratory condition (conditions in JØØ-J99) O99.51-
retained, retention
dead ovum OØ2.Ø
intrauterine contraceptive device O26.3-
retroversion, uterus O34.53-
Rh immunization, incompatibility or sensitization NEC O36.Ø9-
anti-D antibody O36.Ø1-
rupture
amnion (premature) —*see also* Pregnancy, complicated by, premature rupture of membranes O42-
membranes (premature) —*see also* Pregnancy, complicated by, premature rupture of membranes O42-
uterus (during labor) O71.1
before onset of labor O71.Ø-
salivation (excessive) O26.89-
salpingitis O23.52-
salpingo-oophoritis O23.52-
sepsis (conditions in A4Ø, A41) O98.81-
size date discrepancy (uterine) O26.84-
skin condition (conditions in LØØ-L99) O99.71-
smoking (tobacco) O99.33-
social problem OØ9.7-
specified condition NEC O26.89-
spotting O26.85-
~~streptococcus B carrier state O99.820~~
streptococcus group B (GBS) carrier state O99.82Ø ◀
subluxation of symphysis (pubis) O26.71-
syphilis (conditions in A5Ø-A53) O98.11-
threatened
abortion O2Ø.Ø
labor O47.9
at or after 37 completed weeks of gestation O47.1
before 37 completed weeks of gestation O47.Ø-
thrombophlebitis (superficial) O22.2-
thrombosis O22.9-
cerebral venous O22.5-
cerebrovenous sinus O22.5-
deep O22.3-
tobacco use disorder (smoking) O99.33- ◀
torsion of uterus O34.59-
toxemia O14.9-
transverse lie or presentation O32.2
tuberculosis (conditions in A15-A19) O98.Ø1-
tumor (benign)
cervix O34.4-
malignant O9A.11-
uterus O34.1-
unstable lie O32.Ø
upper respiratory infection O99.51-
urethritis O23.2-
uterine size date discrepancy O26.84-
vaginitis or vulvitis O23.59-
varicose veins (lower extremities) O22.Ø-
genitals O22.1-
legs O22.Ø-
perineal O22.1-
vaginal or vulval O22.1-
venereal disease NEC (conditions in A63.8) O98.31-

Pregnancy *(Continued)*
complicated by *(Continued)*
venous disorders O22.9-
specified NEC O22.8X-
very young mother —*see* Pregnancy, complicated by, young mother
viral diseases (conditions in A8Ø-BØ9, B25-B34) O98.51-
vomiting O21.9
due to diseases classified elsewhere O21.8
hyperemesis gravidarum (mild) —*see also* Hyperemesis, gravidarum O21.Ø-
late (occurring after 2Ø weeks of gestation) O21.2
young mother
multigravida OØ9.62-
primigravida OØ9.61-
concealed OØ9.3-
continuing following
elective fetal reduction of one or more fetus O31.3-
intrauterine death of one or more fetus O31.2-
spontaneous abortion of one or more fetus O31.1-
cornual OØØ.8Ø ⬅
with intrauterine pregnancy OØØ.81 ◀
ectopic (ruptured) OØØ.9Ø ⬅
with intrauterine pregnancy OØØ.91 ◀
abdominal OØØ.ØØ ⬅
~~with viable fetus O36.7-~~
with ◀
intrauterine pregnancy OØØ.Ø1 ◀
viable fetus O36.7- ◀
cervical OØØ.8Ø ⬅
with intrauterine pregnancy OØØ.81 ◀
complicated (by) OØ8.9
afibrinogenemia OØ8.1
cardiac arrest OØ8.81
chemical damage of pelvic organ (s) OØ8.6
circulatory collapse OØ8.3
defibrination syndrome OØ8.1
electrolyte imbalance OØ8.5
embolism (amniotic fluid) (blood clot) (pulmonary) (septic) OØ8.2
endometritis OØ8.Ø
genital tract and pelvic infection OØ8.Ø
hemorrhage (delayed) (excessive) OØ8.1
infection
genital tract or pelvic OØ8.Ø
kidney ØØ8.83
urinary tract OØ8.83
intravascular coagulation OØ8.1
laceration of pelvic organ (s) OØ8.6
metabolic disorder OØ8.5
oliguria OØ8.4
oophoritis OØ8.Ø
parametritis OØ8.Ø
pelvic peritonitis OØ8.Ø
perforation of pelvic organ (s) OØ8.6
renal failure or shutdown OØ8.4
salpingitis or salpingo-oophoritis OØ8.Ø
sepsis OØ8.82
shock OØ8.83
septic OØ8.82
specified condition NEC OØ8.89
tubular necrosis (renal) OØ8.4
uremia OØ8.4
urinary infection OØ8.83
venous complication NEC OØ8.7
embolism OØ8.2
cornual OØØ.8Ø ⬅
with intrauterine pregnancy OØØ.81 ◀
intraligamentous OØØ.8Ø ⬅
with intrauterine pregnancy OØØ.81 ◀

P

P

Pregnancy *(Continued)*
weeks of gestation *(Continued)*
greater than 42 weeks Z3A.49
less than 8 weeks Z3A.01
not specified Z3A.00
Preiser's disease —*see* Osteonecrosis, secondary, due to, trauma, metacarpus
Pre-kwashiorkor —*see* Malnutrition, severe
Preleukemia (syndrome) D46.9
Preluxation, hip, congenital Q65.6
Premature —*see also* condition
adrenarche E27.0
aging E34.8
beats I49.40
atrial I49.1
auricular I49.1
supraventricular I49.1
birth NEC —*see* Preterm, newborn
closure, foramen ovale Q21.8
contraction
atrial I49.1
atrioventricular I49.49
auricular I49.1
auriculoventricular I49.2
heart (extrasystole) I49.49
junctional I49.2
ventricular I49.3
delivery —*see also* Pregnancy, complicated by, preterm labor O60.10
ejaculation F52.4
infant NEC —*see* Preterm, newborn
light-for-dates —*see* Light for dates
labor —*see* Pregnancy, complicated by, preterm labor
lungs P28.0
menopause E28.319
asymptomatic E28.319
symptomatic E28.310
newborn
extreme (less than 28 completed weeks) —*see* Immaturity, extreme
less than 37 completed weeks —*see* Preterm, newborn
puberty E30.1
rupture membranes or amnion —*see* Pregnancy, complicated by, premature rupture of membranes
senility E34.8
thelarche E30.8
ventricular systole I49.3
Prematurity NEC (less than 37 completed weeks) —*see* Preterm, newborn
extreme (less than 28 completed weeks) —*see* Immaturity, extreme
Premenstrual
dysphoric disorder (PMDD) F32.81 ⬅
tension (syndrome) N94.3
Premolarization, cuspids K00.2
Prenatal
care, normal pregnancy —*see* Pregnancy, normal
screening of mother Z36
teeth K00.6
Preparatory care for subsequent treatment NEC
for dialysis Z49.01
peritoneal Z49.02
Prepartum —*see* condition
Preponderance, left or right ventricular I51.7
Prepuce —*see* condition
PRES (posterior reversible encephalopathy syndrome) I67.83
Presbycardia R54
Presbycusis, presbyacusia H91.1-
Presbyesophagus K22.8
Presbyophrenia F03
Presbyopia H52.4
Prescription of contraceptives (initial) Z30.019
barrier Z30.018 ◀
diaphragm Z30.018 ◀
emergency (postcoital) Z30.012

Prescription of contraceptives *(Continued)*
implantable subdermal Z30.017 ⬅
injectable Z30.013
intrauterine contraceptive device Z30.014
pills Z30.011
postcoital (emergency) Z30.012
repeat Z30.40
barrier Z30.49 ◀
diaphragm Z30.49 ◀
implantable subdermal Z30.46 ⬅
injectable Z30.42
pills Z30.41
specified type NEC Z30.49
transdermal patch hormonal Z30.45 ◀
vaginal ring hormonal Z30.44 ◀
specified type NEC Z30.018
transdermal patch hormonal Z30.016 ◀
vaginal ring hormonal Z30.015 ◀
Presence (of)
ankle-joint implant (functional) (prosthesis) Z96.66-
aortocoronary (bypass) graft Z95.1
arterial-venous shunt (dialysis) Z99.2
artificial
eye (globe) Z97.0
heart (fully implantable) (mechanical) Z95.812
valve Z95.2
larynx Z96.3
lens (intraocular) Z96.1
limb (complete) (partial) Z97.1-
arm Z97.1-
bilateral Z97.15
leg Z97.1-
bilateral Z97.16
audiological implant (functional) Z96.29
bladder implant (functional) Z96.0
bone
conduction hearing device Z96.29
implant (functional) NEC Z96.7
joint (prosthesis) —*see* Presence, joint implant
cardiac
defibrillator (functional) (with synchronous cardiac pacemaker)Z95.810
implant or graft Z95.9
specified type NEC Z95.818
pacemaker Z95.0
resynchronization therapy ◀
defibrillator Z95.810 ◀
pacemaker Z95.0 ◀
cerebrospinal fluid drainage device Z98.2
cochlear implant (functional) Z96.21
contact lens (es) Z97.3
coronary artery graft or prosthesis Z95.5
CRT-D (cardiac resynchronization therapy defibrillator) Z95.810 ◀
CRT-P (cardiac resynchronization therapy pacemaker) Z95.0 ◀
cardioverter-defribrillator (ICD) Z95.810 ◀
CSF shunt Z98.2
dental prosthesis device Z97.2
dentures Z97.2
device (external) NEC Z97.8
cardiac NEC Z95.818
heart assist Z95.811
implanted (functional) Z96.9
specified NEC Z96.89
prosthetic Z97.8
ear implant Z96.20
cochlear implant Z96.21
myringotomy tube Z96.22
specified type NEC Z96.29
elbow-joint implant (functional) (prosthesis) Z96.62-
endocrine implant (functional) NEC Z96.49
eustachian tube stent or device (functional) Z96.29
external hearing-aid or device Z97.4
finger-joint implant (functional) (prosthetic) Z96.69-

Presence *(Continued)*
functional implant Z96.9
specified NEC Z96.89
graft
cardiac NEC Z95.818
vascular NEC Z95.828
hearing-aid or device (external) Z97.4
implant (bone) (cochlear) (functional) Z96.21
heart assist device Z95.811
heart valve implant (functional) Z95.2
prosthetic Z95.2
specified type NEC Z95.4
xenogenic Z95.3
hip-joint implant (functional) (prosthesis) Z96.64-
ICD (cardioverter-defribrillator) Z95.810 ◀
implanted device (artificial) (functional) (prosthetic) Z96.9
automatic cardiac defibrillator (with synchronous cardiac pacemaker) Z95.810
cardiac pacemaker Z95.0
cochlear Z96.21
dental Z96.5
heart Z95.812
heart valve Z95.2
prosthetic Z95.2
specified NEC Z95.4
xenogenic Z95.3
insulin pump Z96.41
intraocular lens Z96.1
joint Z96.60
ankle Z96.66-
elbow Z96.62-
finger Z96.69-
hip Z96.64-
knee Z96.65-
shoulder Z96.61-
specified NEC Z96.698
wrist Z96.63-
larynx Z96.3
myringotomy tube Z96.22
otological Z96.20
cochlear Z96.21
eustachian stent Z96.29
myringotomy Z96.22
specified NEC Z96.29
stapes Z96.29
skin Z96.81
skull plate Z96.7
specified NEC Z96.89
urogenital Z96.0
insulin pump (functional) Z96.41
intestinal bypass or anastomosis Z98.0
intraocular lens (functional) Z96.1
intrauterine contraceptive device (IUD) Z97.5
intravascular implant (functional) (prosthetic) NEC Z95.9
coronary artery Z95.5
defibrillator (with synchronous cardiac pacemaker) Z95.810
peripheral vessel (with angioplasty) Z95.820
joint implant (prosthetic) (any) Z96.60
ankle —*see* Presence, ankle joint implant
elbow —*see* Presence, elbow joint implant
finger —*see* Presence, finger joint implant
hip —*see* Presence, hip joint implant
knee —*see* Presence, knee joint implant
shoulder —*see* Presence, shoulder joint implant
specified joint NEC Z96.698
wrist —*see* Presence, wrist joint implant
knee-joint implant (functional) (prosthesis) Z96.65-
laryngeal implant (functional) Z96.3
mandibular implant (dental) Z96.5
myringotomy tube (s) Z96.22
orthopedic-joint implant (prosthetic) (any) —*see* Presence, joint implant

Presence *(Continued)*
otological implant (functional) Z96.29
shoulder-joint implant (functional) (prosthesis) Z96.61-
skull-plate implant Z96.7
spectacles Z97.3
stapes implant (functional) Z96.29
systemic lupus erythematosus [SLE] inhibitor D68.62
tendon implant (functional) (graft) Z96.7
tooth root (s) implant Z96.5
ureteral stent Z96.Ø
urethral stent Z96.Ø
urogenital implant (functional) Z96.Ø
vascular implant or device Z95.9
access port device Z95.828
specified type NEC Z95.828
wrist-joint implant (functional) (prosthesis) Z96.63-
Presenile —*see also* condition
dementia FØ3
premature aging E34.8
Presentation, fetal —*see* Delivery, complicated by, malposition
Prespondylolisthesis (congenital) Q76.2
Pressure
area, skin —*see* Ulcer, pressure, by site
brachial plexus G54.Ø
brain G93.5
injury at birth NEC P11.1
cerebral —*see* Pressure, brain
chest RØ7.89
cone, tentorial G93.5
hyposystolic —*see also* Hypotension
incidental reading, without diagnosis of hypotension RØ3.1
increased
intracranial (benign) G93.2
injury at birth P11.Ø
intraocular H4Ø.Ø5-
lumbosacral plexus G54.1
mediastinum J98.59 ⟸
necrosis (chronic) —*see* Ulcer, pressure, by site
parental, inappropriate (excessive) Z62.6
sore (chronic) —*see* Ulcer, pressure, by site
spinal cord G95.2Ø
ulcer (chronic) —*see* Ulcer, pressure, by site
venous, increased I87.8
Pre-syncope R55
Preterm
delivery (*see also* Pregnancy, complicated by, preterm labor) O6Ø.1Ø
labor —*see* Pregnancy, complicated by, preterm labor
newborn (infant) PØ7.3Ø
gestational age
28 completed weeks (28 weeks, Ø days through 28 weeks, 6 days) PØ7.31
29 completed weeks (29 weeks, Ø days through 29 weeks, 6 days) PØ7.32
3Ø completed weeks (3Ø weeks, Ø days through 3Ø weeks, 6 days) PØ7.33
31 completed weeks (31 weeks, Ø days through 31 weeks, 6 days) PØ7.34
32 completed weeks (32 weeks, Ø days through 32 weeks, 6 days) PØ7.35
33 completed weeks (33 weeks, Ø days through 33 weeks, 6 days) PØ7.36
34 completed weeks (34 weeks, Ø days through 34 weeks, 6 days) PØ7.37
35 completed weeks (35 weeks, Ø days through 35 weeks, 6 days) PØ7.38
36 completed weeks (36 weeks, Ø days through 36 weeks, 6 days) PØ7.39
Previa
placenta (total) (without hemorrhage) O44.Ø- ⟸
~~without hemorrhage O44.Ø-~~
Previa *(Continued)*
placenta *(Continued)*
with hemorrhage O44.1- ◀
complete O44.Ø- ◀
with hemorrhage O44.1- ◀
low —*see also* Delivery, complicated, by, placenta, low O44.4- ◀
with hemorrhage O44.5- ◀
marginal O44.2- ◀
with hemorrhage O44.3- ◀
partial O44.2- ◀
with hemorrhage O44.3- ◀
vasa O69.4
Priapism N48.3Ø
due to
disease classified elsewhere N48.32
drug N48.33
specified cause NEC N48.39
trauma N48.31
Prickling sensation (skin) R2Ø.2
Prickly heat L74.Ø
Primary —*see* condition
Primigravida
elderly, affecting management of pregnancy, labor and delivery (supervision only) —*see* Pregnancy, complicated by, elderly, primigravida
older, affecting management of pregnancy, labor and delivery (supervision only) —*see* Pregnancy, complicated by, elderly, primigravida
very young, affecting management of pregnancy, labor and delivery (supervision only) —*see* Pregnancy, complicated by, young mother, primigravida
Primipara
elderly, affecting management of pregnancy, labor and delivery (supervision only) —*see* Pregnancy, complicated by, elderly, primigravida
older, affecting management of pregnancy, labor and delivery (supervision only) —*see* Pregnancy, complicated by, elderly, primigravida
very young, affecting management of pregnancy, labor and delivery (supervision only) —*see* Pregnancy, complicated by, young mother, primigravida
Primus varus (bilateral) Q66.2
PRIND (Prolonged reversible ischemic neurologic deficit) I63.9
Pringle's disease (tuberous sclerosis)Q85.1
Prinzmetal angina I2Ø.1
Prizefighter ear —*see* Cauliflower ear
Problem (with) (related to)
academic Z55.8
acculturation Z6Ø.3
adjustment (to)
change of job Z56.1
life-cycle transition Z6Ø.Ø
pension Z6Ø.Ø
retirement Z6Ø.Ø
adopted child Z62.821
alcoholism in family Z63.72
atypical parenting situation Z62.9
bankruptcy Z59.8
behavioral (adult) F69
drug seeking Z76.5 ⟸
birth of sibling affecting child Z62.898
care (of)
provider dependency Z74.9
specified NEC Z74.8
sick or handicapped person in family or household Z63.6
child
abuse (affecting the child) —*see* Maltreatment, child
custody or support proceedings Z65.3
in care of non-parental family member Z62.21
Problem *(Continued)*
child *(Continued)*
in foster care Z62.21
in welfare custody Z62.21
living in orphanage or group home Z62.22
child-rearing Z62.9
specified NEC Z62.898
communication (developmental) F8Ø.9
conflict or discord (with)
boss Z56.4
classmates Z55.4
counselor Z64.4
employer Z56.4
family Z63.9
specified NEC Z63.8
probation officer Z64.4
social worker Z64.4
teachers Z55.4
workmates Z56.4
conviction in legal proceedings Z65.Ø
with imprisonment Z65.1
counselor Z64.4
creditors Z59.8
digestive K92.9
drug addict in family Z63.72
ear —*see* Disorder, ear
economic Z59.9
affecting care Z59.9
specified NEC Z59.8
education Z55.9
specified NEC Z55.8
employment Z56.9
change of job Z56.1
discord Z56.4
environment Z56.5
sexual harassment Z56.81
specified NEC Z56.89
stress NEC Z56.6
stressful schedule Z56.3
threat of job loss Z56.2
unemployment Z56.Ø
enuresis, child F98.Ø
eye H57.9
failed examinations (school) Z55.2
falling Z91.81
family —*see also* Disruption, family Z63.9-
specified NEC Z63.8
feeding (elderly) (infant) R63.3
newborn P92.9
breast P92.5
overfeeding P92.4
slow P92.2
specified NEC P92.8
underfeeding P92.3
nonorganic F5Ø.89 ⟸
finance Z59.9
specified NEC Z59.8
foreclosure on loan Z59.8
foster child Z62.822
frightening experience (s) in childhood Z62.898
genital NEC
female N94.9
male N5Ø.9
health care Z75.9
specified NEC Z75.8
hearing —*see* Deafness
homelessness Z59.Ø
housing Z59.9
inadequate Z59.1
isolated Z59.8
specified NEC Z59.8
identity (of childhood) F93.8
illegitimate pregnancy (unwanted) Z64.Ø
illiteracy Z55.Ø
impaired mobility Z74.Ø9
imprisonment or incarceration Z65.1
inadequate teaching affecting education Z55.8
inappropriate (excessive) parental pressure Z62.6

P

- **Problem** *(Continued)*
  - influencing health status NEC Z78.9
  - in-law Z63.1
  - institutionalization, affecting child Z62.22
  - intrafamilial communication Z63.8
  - jealousy, child F93.8
  - landlord Z59.2
  - language (developmental) F80.9
  - learning (developmental) F81.9
  - legal Z65.3
    - conviction without imprisonment Z65.0
    - imprisonment Z65.1
    - release from prison Z65.2
  - life-management Z73.9
    - specified NEC Z73.89
  - life-style Z72.9
    - gambling Z72.6
    - high-risk sexual behavior (heterosexual) Z72.51
      - bisexual Z72.53
      - homosexual Z72.52
    - inappropriate eating habits Z72.4
    - self-damaging behavior NEC Z72.89
    - specified NEC Z72.89
    - tobacco use Z72.0
  - literacy Z55.9
    - low level Z55.0
    - specified NEC Z55.8
  - living alone Z60.2
  - lodgers Z59.2
  - loss of love relationship in childhood Z62.898
  - marital Z63.0
    - involving
      - divorce Z63.5
      - estrangement Z63.5
      - gender identity F66
  - mastication K08.89 ⬅
  - medical
    - care, within family Z63.6
    - facilities Z75.9
      - specified NEC Z75.8
  - mental F48.9
  - multiparity Z64.1
  - negative life events in childhood Z62.9
    - altered pattern of family relationships Z62.898
    - frightening experience Z62.898
    - loss of
      - love relationship Z62.898
      - self-esteem Z62.898
    - physical abuse (alleged) —*see* Maltreatment, child
    - removal from home Z62.29
    - specified event NEC Z62.898
  - neighbor Z59.2
  - neurological NEC R29.818
  - new step-parent affecting child Z62.898
  - none (feared complaint unfounded) Z71.1
  - occupational NEC Z56.89
  - parent-child —*see* Conflict, parent-child
  - personal hygiene Z91.89
  - personality F69
  - phase-of-life transition, adjustment Z60.0
  - presence of sick or disabled person in family or household Z63.79
    - needing care Z63.6
  - primary support group (family) Z63.9
    - specified NEC Z63.8
  - probation officer Z64.4
  - psychiatric F99
  - psychosexual (development) F66
  - psychosocial Z65.9
    - specified NEC Z65.8
  - relationship Z63.9
    - childhood F93.8
  - release from prison Z65.2
  - removal from home affecting child Z62.29
- **Problem** *(Continued)*
  - seeking and accepting known hazardous and harmful
    - behavioral or psychological interventions Z65.8
    - chemical, nutritional or physical interventions Z65.8
  - sexual function (nonorganic) F52.9
  - sight H54.7
  - sleep disorder, child F51.9
  - smell —*see* Disturbance, sensation, smell
  - social
    - environment Z60.9
      - specified NEC Z60.8
    - exclusion and rejection Z60.4
    - worker Z64.4
  - speech R47.9
    - developmental F80.9
    - specified NEC R47.89
  - swallowing —*see* Dysphagia
  - taste —*see* Disturbance, sensation, taste
  - tic, child F95.0
  - underachievement in school Z55.3
  - unemployment Z56.0
    - threatened Z56.2
  - unwanted pregnancy Z64.0
  - upbringing Z62.9
    - specified NEC Z62.898
  - urinary N39.9
  - voice production R47.89
  - work schedule (stressful) Z56.3
- **Procedure** (surgical)
  - converted ◀
    - arthroscopic to open Z53.33 ◀
    - laparoscopic to open Z53.31 ◀
    - specified procedure NEC to open Z53.39 ◀
    - thoracoscopic to open Z53.32 ◀
  - for purpose other than remedying health state Z41.9
    - specified NEC Z41.8
  - not done Z53.9
    - because of
      - administrative reasons Z53.8
      - contraindication Z53.09
        - smoking Z53.01
      - patient's decision Z53.20
        - for reasons of belief or group pressure Z53.1
        - left against medical advice (AMA) Z53.21
        - specified reason NEC Z53.29
      - specified reason NEC Z53.8
- **Procidentia** (uteri) N81.3
- **Proctalgia** K62.89
  - fugax K59.4
  - spasmodic K59.4
- **Proctitis** K62.89
  - amebic (acute) A06.0
  - chlamydial A56.3
  - gonococcal A54.6
  - granulomatous —*see* Enteritis, regional, large intestine
  - herpetic A60.1
  - radiation K62.7
  - tuberculous A18.32
  - ulcerative (chronic) K51.20
    - with
      - complication K51.219
        - abscess K51.214
        - fistula K51.213
        - obstruction K51.212
        - rectal bleeding K51.211
        - specified NEC K51.218
- **Proctocele**
  - female (without uterine prolapse) N81.6
    - with uterine prolapse N81.2
      - complete N81.3
  - male K62.3
- ~~Proctocolitis, mucosal —see Rectosigmoiditis, ulcerative~~
- **Proctocolitis** ◀
  - food-induced eosinophilic K52.82 ◀
  - food protein-induced K52.82 ◀
  - milk protein-induced K52.82 ◀
  - mucosal —*see* Rectosigmoiditis, ulcerative ◀
- **Proctoptosis** K62.3
- **Proctorrhagia** K62.5
- **Proctosigmoiditis** K63.89
  - ulcerative (chronic) —*see* Rectosigmoiditis, ulcerative
- **Proctospasm** K59.4
  - psychogenic F45.8
- **Profichet's disease** —*see* Disorder, soft tissue, specified type NEC
- **Progeria** E34.8
- **Prognathism** (mandibular) (maxillary) M26.19
- **Progonoma** (melanotic) —*see* Neoplasm, benign, by site
- **Progressive** —*see* condition
- **Prolactinoma**
  - specified site —*see* Neoplasm, benign, by site
  - unspecified site D35.2
- **Prolapse, prolapsed**
  - anus, anal (canal) (sphincter) K62.2
  - arm or hand O32.2
    - causing obstructed labor O64.4
  - bladder (mucosa) (sphincter) (acquired)
    - congenital Q79.4
    - female —*see* Cystocele
    - male N32.89
  - breast implant (prosthetic) T85.49
  - cecostomy K94.09
  - cecum K63.4
  - cervix, cervical (hypertrophied) N81.2
    - anterior lip, obstructing labor O65.5
    - congenital Q51.828
    - postpartal, old N81.2
    - stump N81.85
  - ciliary body (traumatic) —*see* Laceration, eye(ball), with prolapse or loss of interocular tissue
  - colon (pedunculated) K63.4
  - colostomy K94.09
  - disc (intervertebral) —*see* Displacement, intervertebral disc
  - eye implant (orbital) T85.398
    - lens (ocular) —*see* Complications, intraocular lens
  - fallopian tube N83.4- ⬅
  - gastric (mucosa) K31.89
  - genital, female N81.9
    - specified NEC N81.89
  - globe, nontraumatic —*see* Luxation, globe
  - ileostomy bud K94.19
  - intervertebral disc —*see* Displacement, intervertebral disc
  - intestine (small) K63.4
  - iris (traumatic) —*see* Laceration, eye(ball), with prolapse or loss of interocular tissue
    - nontraumatic H21.89
  - kidney N28.83
    - congenital Q63.2
  - laryngeal muscles or ventricle J38.7
  - liver K76.89
  - meatus urinarius N36.8
  - mitral (valve) I34.1
  - ocular lens implant —*see* Complications, intraocular lens
  - organ or site, congenital NEC —*see* Malposition, congenital
  - ovary N83.4- ⬅
  - pelvic floor, female N81.89
  - perineum, female N81.89
  - rectum (mucosa) (sphincter) K62.3
    - due to trichuris trichuria B79
  - spleen D73.89
  - stomach K31.89
  - umbilical cord
    - complicating delivery O69.0

P

Prolapse, prolapsed *(Continued)*
- urachus, congenital Q64.4
- ureter N28.89
  - with obstruction N13.5
    - with infection N13.6
- ureterovesical orifice N28.89
- urethra (acquired) (infected) (mucosa) N36.8
  - congenital Q64.71
- urinary meatus N36.8
  - congenital Q64.72
- uterovaginal N81.4
  - complete N81.3
  - incomplete N81.2
- uterus (with prolapse of vagina) N81.4
  - complete N81.3
  - congenital Q51.818
  - first degree N81.2
  - in pregnancy or childbirth —*see* Pregnancy, complicated by, abnormal, uterus
  - incomplete N81.2
  - postpartal (old) N81.4
  - second degree N81.2
  - third degree N81.3
- uveal (traumatic) —*see* Laceration, eye(ball), with prolapse or loss of interocular tissue
- vagina (anterior) (wall) —*see* Cystocele
  - with prolapse of uterus N81.4
    - complete N81.3
    - incomplete N81.2
  - posterior wall N81.6
  - posthysterectomy N99.3
- vitreous (humor) H43.0-
  - in wound —*see* Laceration, eye(ball), with prolapse or loss of interocular tissue
- womb —*see* Prolapse, uterus

Prolapsus, female N81.9
- specified NEC N81.89

Proliferation (s)
- primary cutaneous CD30-positive large T-cell C86.6
- prostate, atypical small acinar N42.32 ◀

Proliferative —*see* condition

Prolonged, prolongation (of)
- bleeding (time) (idiopathic) R79.1
- coagulation (time) R79.1
- gestation (over 42 completed weeks)
  - mother O48.1
  - newborn P08.22
- interval I44.0
- labor O63.9
  - first stage O63.0
  - second stage O63.1
- partial thromboplastin time (PTT) R79.1
- pregnancy (more than 42 weeks gestation) O48.1
- prothrombin time R79.1
- QT interval I45.81
- uterine contractions in labor O62.4

Prominence, prominent
- with disproportion (fetopelvic) O33.0
  - causing obstructed labor O65.0
- auricle (congenital) (ear) Q17.5
- ischial spine or sacral promontory
- nose (congenital) acquired M95.0

Promiscuity —*see* High, risk, sexual behavior

Pronation
- ankle —*see* Deformity, limb, foot, specified NEC
- foot —*see also* Deformity, limb, foot, specified NEC
  - congenital Q74.2

Prophylactic
- administration of
  - antibiotics, long-term Z79.2
    - short-term use - omit code
  - drug —*see also* Long-term (current) drug therapy (use of) Z79.899-
- medication Z79.899

Prophylactic *(Continued)*
- organ removal (for neoplasia management) Z40.00
  - breast Z40.01
  - ovary Z40.02
  - specified site NEC Z40.09
- surgery Z40.9
  - for risk factors related to malignant neoplasm —*see* Prophylactic, organ removal
  - specified NEC Z40.8
- vaccination Z23

Propionic acidemia E71.121

Proptosis (ocular) —*see also* Exophthalmos
- thyroid —*see* Hyperthyroidism, with goiter

Prosecution, anxiety concerning Z65.3

Prosopagnosia R48.3

Prostadynia N42.81

Prostate, prostatic —*see* condition

Prostatism —*see* Hyperplasia, prostate

Prostatitis (congestive) (suppurative) (with cystitis) N41.9
- acute N41.0
- cavitary N41.8
- chronic N41.1
- diverticular N41.8
- due to Trichomonas (vaginalis) A59.02
- fibrous N41.1
- gonococcal (acute) (chronic) A54.22
- granulomatous N41.4
- hypertrophic N41.1
- subacute N41.1
- trichomonal A59.02
- tuberculous A18.14

Prostatocystitis N41.3

Prostatorrhea N42.89

Prostatosis N42.82

Prostration R53.83
- heat —*see also* Heat, exhaustion
  - anhydrotic T67.3
  - due to
    - salt (and water) depletion T67.4
    - water depletion T67.3
- nervous F48.8
- senile R54

Protanomaly (anomalous trichromat) H53.54

Protanopia (complete) (incomplete) H53.54

Protection (against) (from) —*see* Prophylactic

Protein
- deficiency NEC —*see* Malnutrition
- malnutrition —*see* Malnutrition
- sickness —*see also* Reaction, serum T80.69

Proteinemia R77.9

Proteinosis
- alveolar (pulmonary) J84.01
- lipid or lipoid (of Urbach) E78.89

Proteinuria R80.9
- Bence Jones R80.3
- complicating pregnancy —*see* Proteinuria, gestational
- gestational ⇐
  - ~~with edema O12.2-~~
  - complicating ◀
    - childbirth O12.14 ◀
    - pregnancy O12.1- ◀
      - with edema O12.2- ◀
    - puerperium O12.15 ◀
- idiopathic R80.0
- isolated R80.0
  - with glomerular lesion N06.9
    - dense deposit disease N06.6
    - diffuse
      - crescentic glomerulonephritis N06.7
      - endocapillary proliferative glomerulonephritis N06.4
      - mesangiocapillary glomerulonephritis N06.5
    - focal and segmental hyalinosis or sclerosis N06.1
    - membranous (diffuse) N06.2

Proteinuria *(Continued)*
- isolated *(Continued)*
  - with glomerular lesion *(Continued)*
    - mesangial proliferative (diffuse) N06.3
    - minimal change N06.0
    - specified pathology NEC N06.8
- orthostatic R80.2
  - with glomerular lesion —*see* Proteinuria, isolated, with glomerular lesion
- persistent R80.1
  - with glomerular lesion —*see* Proteinuria, isolated, with glomerular lesion
- postural R80.2
  - with glomerular lesion —*see* Proteinuria, isolated, with glomerular lesion
- pre-eclamptic —*see* Pre-eclampsia
- puerperal O12.15 ◀
- specified type NEC R80.8

Proteolysis, pathologic D65

Proteus (mirabilis) (morganii), as cause of disease classified elsewhere B96.4

Prothrombin gene mutation D68.52

Protoporphyria, erythropoietic E80.0

Protozoal —*see also* condition
- disease B64
  - specified NEC B60.8

Protrusion, protrusio
- acetabuli M24.7
- acetabulum (into pelvis) M24.7
- device, implant or graft —*see also* Complications, by site and type, mechanical T85.698
  - arterial graft NEC —*see* Complication, cardiovascular device, mechanical, vascular
  - breast (implant) T85.49
  - catheter NEC T85.698
    - cystostomy T83.090
    - dialysis (renal) T82.49
      - intraperitoneal T85.691
    - infusion NEC T82.594
      - spinal (epidural) (subdural) T85.690
    - ~~urinary, indwelling T83.098~~
    - urinary —*see also* Complications, catheter, urinary T83.098 ◀
  - electronic (electrode) (pulse generator) (stimulator)
    - bone T84.390
    - nervous system —*see* Complication, prosthetic device, mechanical, electronic nervous system stimulator
  - fixation, internal (orthopedic) NEC —*see* Complication, fixation device, mechanical
  - gastrointestinal —*see* Complications, prosthetic device, mechanical, gastrointestinal device
  - genital NEC T83.498
    - intrauterine contraceptive device T83.39
    - penile prosthesis (cylinder) (implanted) (pump) (resevoir) T83.490 ⇐
    - testicular prosthesis T83.491 ◀
  - heart NEC —*see* Complication, cardiovascular device, mechanical
  - joint prosthesis —*see* Complications, joint prosthesis, mechanical, specified NEC, by site
  - ocular NEC —*see* Complications, prosthetic device, mechanical, ocular device
  - orthopedic NEC —*see* Complication, orthopedic, device, mechanical
  - specified NEC T85.628
  - urinary NEC —*see also* Complication, genitourinary, device, urinary, mechanical
    - graft T83.29
  - vascular NEC —*see* Complication, cardiovascular device, mechanical

P

Protrusion, protrusio *(Continued)*
device, implant or graft *(Continued)*
ventricular intracranial shunt T85.Ø9
intervertebral disc —*see* Displacement, intervertebral disc
joint prosthesis —*see* Complications, joint prosthesis, mechanical, specified NEC, by site
nucleus pulposus —*see* Displacement, intervertebral disc
Prune belly (syndrome) Q79.4
Prurigo (ferox) (gravis) (Hebrae) (Hebra's) (mitis) (simplex) L28.2
Besnier's L2Ø.Ø
estivalis L56.4
nodularis L28.1
psychogenic F45.8
Pruritus, pruritic (essential) L29.9
ani, anus L29.Ø
psychogenic F45.8
anogenital L29.3
psychogenic F45.8
due to onchocerca volvulus B73.1
gravidarum —*see* Pregnancy, complicated by, specified pregnancy-related condition NEC
hiemalis L29.8
neurogenic (any site) F45.8
perianal L29.Ø
psychogenic (any site) F45.8
scroti, scrotum L29.1
psychogenic F45.8
senile, senilis L29.8
specified NEC L29.8
psychogenic F45.8
Trichomonas A59.9
vulva, vulvae L29.2
psychogenic F45.8
Pseudarthrosis, pseudoarthrosis (bone) —*see* Nonunion, fracture
clavicle, congenital Q74.Ø
joint, following fusion or arthrodesis M96.Ø
Pseudoaneurysm —*see* Aneurysm
Pseudoangina (pectoris) —*see* Angina
Pseudoangioma I81
Pseudoarteriosus Q28.8
Pseudoarthrosis —*see* Pseudarthrosis
Pseudobulbar affect (PBA) F48.2
Pseudochromhidrosis L67.8
Pseudocirrhosis, liver, pericardial I31.1
Pseudocowpox BØ8.Ø3
Pseudocoxalgia M91.3-
Pseudocroup J38.5
Pseudo-Cushing's syndrome, alcohol-induced E24.4
Pseudocyesis F45.8
Pseudocyst
lung J98.4
pancreas K86.3
retina —*see* Cyst, retina
Pseudoelephantiasis neuroarthritica Q82.Ø
Pseudoexfoliation, capsule (lens) —*see* Cataract, specified NEC
Pseudofolliculitis barbae L73.1
Pseudoglioma H44.89
Pseudohemophilia (Bernuth's) (hereditary) (type B) D68.Ø
Type A D69.8
vascular D69.8
Pseudohermaphroditism Q56.3
adrenal E25.8
female Q56.2
with adrenocortical disorder E25.8
without adrenocortical disorder Q56.2
~~adrenal, congenital E25.Ø~~
adrenal (congenital) E25.Ø ◄
male Q56.1
with
adrenocortical disorder E25.8
androgen resistance E34.51
Pseudohermaphroditism *(Continued)*
male *(Continued)*
with *(Continued)*
cleft scrotum Q56.1
feminizing testis E34.51
5-alpha-reductase deficiency E29.1
without gonadal disorder Q56.1
adrenal E25.8
Pseudo-Hurler's polydystrophy E77.Ø
Pseudohydrocephalus G93.2
Pseudohypertrophic muscular dystrophy (Erb's) G71.Ø
Pseudohypertrophy, muscle G71.Ø
Pseudohypoparathyroidism E2Ø.1
Pseudoinsomnia F51.Ø3
Pseudoleukemia, infantile D64.89
Pseudomembranous —*see* condition
Pseudomeningocele (cerebral) (infective) (post-traumatic) G96.19
postprocedural (spinal) G97.82
Pseudomenses (newborn) P54.6
Pseudomenstruation (newborn) P54.6
Pseudomonas
aeruginosa, as cause of disease classified elsewhere B96.5
mallei infection A24.Ø
as cause of disease classified elsewhere B96.5
pseudomallei, as cause of disease classified elsewhere B96.5
Pseudomyotonia G71.19
Pseudomyxoma peritonei C78.6
Pseudoneuritis, optic (nerve) (disc) (papilla), **congenital** Q14.2
Pseudo-obstruction intestine (acute) (chronic) (idiopathic) (intermittent secondary) (primary) K59.8
Pseudopapilledema H47.33-
congenital Q14.2
Pseudoparalysis
arm or leg R29.818
atonic, congenital P94.2
Pseudopelade L66.Ø
Pseudophakia Z96.1
Pseudopolyarthritis, rhizomelic M35.3
Pseudopolycythemia D75.1
Pseudopseudohypoparathyroidism E2Ø.1
Pseudopterygium H11.81-
Pseudoptosis (eyelid) —*see* Blepharochalasis
Pseudopuberty, precocious
female heterosexual E25.8
male isosexual E25.8
Pseudorickets (renal) N25.Ø
Pseudorubella BØ8.2Ø
Pseudosclerema, newborn P83.8
Pseudosclerosis (brain)
Jakob's —*see* Creutzfeldt-Jakob disease or syndrome
of Westphal (Strüümpell) E83.Ø1
spastic —*see* Creutzfeldt-Jakob disease or syndrome
Pseudotetanus —*see* Convulsions
Pseudotetany R29.Ø
hysterical F44.5
Pseudotruncus arteriosus Q25.49 ⬅
Pseudotuberculosis A28.2
enterocolitis AØ4.8
pasteurella (infection) A28.Ø
Pseudotumor
cerebri G93.2
orbital HØ5.11-
Pseudoxanthoma elasticum Q82.8
Psilosis (sprue) (tropical) K9Ø.1
nontropical K9Ø.Ø
Psittacosis A7Ø
Psoitis M6Ø.88
Psoriasis L4Ø.9
arthropathic L4Ø.5Ø
arthritis mutilans L4Ø.52
distal interphalangeal L4Ø.51
Psoriasis *(Continued)*
arthropathic *(Continued)*
juvenile L4Ø.54
other specified L4Ø.59
spondylitis L4Ø.53
buccal K13.29
flexural L4Ø.8
guttate L4Ø.4
mouth K13.29
nummular L4Ø.Ø
plaque L4Ø.Ø
psychogenic F54
pustular (generalized) L4Ø.1
palmaris et plantaris L4Ø.3
specified NEC L4Ø.8
vulgaris L4Ø.Ø
Psychasthenia F48.8
Psychiatric disorder or problem F99
Psychogenic —*see also* condition
factors associated with physical conditions F54
Psychological and behavioral factors affecting medical condition F59
Psychoneurosis, psychoneurotic —*see also* Neurosis
anxiety (state) F41.1
depersonalization F48.1
hypochondriacal F45.21
hysteria F44.9
neurasthenic F48.8
personality NEC F6Ø.89
Psychopathy, psychopathic
affectionless F94.2
autistic F84.5
constitution, post-traumatic FØ7.81
personality —*see* Disorder, personality
sexual —*see* Deviation, sexual
state F6Ø.2
Psychosexual identity disorder of childhood F64.2
Psychosis, psychotic F29
acute (transient) F23
hysterical F44.9
affective —*see* Disorder, mood
alcoholic F1Ø.959
with
abuse F1Ø.159
anxiety disorder F1Ø.98Ø
with
abuse F1Ø.18Ø
dependence F1Ø.28Ø
delirium tremens F1Ø.231
delusions F1Ø.95Ø
with
abuse F1Ø.15Ø
dependence F1Ø.25Ø
dementia F1Ø.97
with dependence F1Ø.27
dependence F1Ø.259
hallucinosis F1Ø.951
with
abuse F1Ø.151
dependence F1Ø.251
mood disorder F1Ø.94
with
abuse F1Ø.14
dependence F1Ø.24
paranoia F1Ø.95Ø
with
abuse F1Ø.15Ø
dependence F1Ø.25Ø
persisting amnesia F1Ø.96
with dependence F1Ø.26
amnestic confabulatory F1Ø.96
with dependence F1Ø.26
delirium tremens F1Ø.231
Korsakoff's, Korsakov's, Korsakow's F1Ø.26
paranoid type F1Ø.95Ø
with
abuse F1Ø.15Ø
dependence F1Ø.25Ø

P

Psychosis, psychotic *(Continued)*
anergastic *—see* Psychosis, organic
arteriosclerotic (simple type) (uncomplicated) F01.50
with behavioral disturbance F01.51
childhood F84.0
atypical F84.8
climacteric *—see* Psychosis, involutional
confusional F29
acute or subacute F05
reactive F23
cycloid F23
depressive *—see* Disorder, depressive
disintegrative (childhood) F84.3
drug-induced *—see* F11-F19 with .x59
paranoid and hallucinatory states *—see* F11-F19 with .x50 or .x51
due to or associated with
addiction, drug *—see* F11-F19 with .X59
dependence
alcohol F10.259
drug *—see* F11-F19 with .x59
epilepsy F06.8
Huntington's chorea F06.8
ischemia, cerebrovascular (generalized) F06.8
multiple sclerosis F06.8
physical disease F06.8
presenile dementia F03
senile dementia F03
vascular disease (arteriosclerotic) (cerebral) F01.50
with behavioral disturbance F01.51
epileptic F06.8
episode F23
due to or associated with physical condition F06.8
exhaustive F43.0
hallucinatory, chronic F28
hypomanic F30.8
hysterical (acute) F44.9
induced F24
infantile F84.0
atypical F84.8
infective (acute) (subacute) F05
involutional F28
depressive *—see* Disorder, depressive
melancholic *—see* Disorder, depressive
paranoid (state) F22
Korsakoff's, Korsakov's, Korsakow's (nonalcoholic) F04
alcoholic F10.96
in dependence F10.26
induced by other psychoactive substance *—see* categories F11-F19 with .x5x
mania, manic (single episode) F30.2
recurrent type F31.89
manic-depressive *—see* Disorder, bipolar ⬅
menopausal *—see* Psychosis, involutional
mixed schizophrenic and affective F25.8
multi-infarct (cerebrovascular) F01.50
with behavioral disturbance F01.51
nonorganic F29
specified NEC F28
organic F09
due to or associated with
arteriosclerosis (cerebral) *—see* Psychosis, arteriosclerotic
cerebrovascular disease, arteriosclerotic *—see* Psychosis, arteriosclerotic
childbirth *—see* Psychosis, puerperal
Creutzfeldt-Jakob disease or syndrome *—see* Creutzfeldt-Jakob disease or syndrome
dependence, alcohol F10.259
disease
alcoholic liver F10.259
brain, arteriosclerotic *—see* Psychosis, arteriosclerotic

Psychosis, psychotic *(Continued)*
organic *(Continued)*
due to or associated with *(Continued)*
disease *(Continued)*
cerebrovascular F01.50
with behavioral disturbance F01.51
Creutzfeldt-Jakob *—see* Creutzfeldt-Jakob disease or syndrome
endocrine or metabolic F06.8
acute or subacute F05
liver, alcoholic F10.259
epilepsy transient (acute) F05
infection
brain (intracranial) F06.8
acute or subacute F05
intoxication
alcoholic (acute) F10.259
drug F19 with .X59 F11-
ischemia, cerebrovascular (generalized) *—see* Psychosis, arteriosclerotic
puerperium *—see* Psychosis, puerperal
trauma, brain (birth) (from electric current) (surgical) F06.8
acute or subacute F05
infective F06.8
acute or subacute F05
post-traumatic F06.8
acute or subacute F05
paranoiac F22
paranoid (climacteric) (involutional) (menopausal) F22
psychogenic (acute) F23
schizophrenic F20.0
senile F03
postpartum F53
presbyophrenic (type) F03
presenile F03
psychogenic (paranoid) F23
depressive F32.3
puerperal F53
specified type *—see* Psychosis, by type
reactive (brief) (transient) (emotional stress) (psychological trauma) F23
depressive F32.3
recurrent F33.3
excitative type F30.8
schizoaffective F25.9
depressive type F25.1
manic type F25.0
schizophrenia, schizophrenic *—see* Schizophrenia
schizophrenia-like, in epilepsy F06.2
schizophreniform F20.81
affective type F25.9
brief F23
confusional type F23
depressive type F25.1
manic type F25.0
mixed type F25.0
senile NEC F03
depressed or paranoid type F03
simple deterioration F03
specified type — code to condition
shared F24
situational (reactive) F23
symbiotic (childhood) F84.3
symptomatic F09
Psychosomatic *—see* Disorder, psychosomatic
Psychosyndrome, organic F07.9
Psychotic episode due to or associated with physical condition F06.8
Pterygium (eye) H11.00-
amyloid H11.01-
central H11.02-
colli Q18.3
double H11.03-
peripheral
progressive H11.05-
stationary H11.04-
recurrent H11.06-

Ptilosis (eyelid) *—see* Madarosis
Ptomaine (poisoning) *—see* Poisoning, food
Ptosis *—see also* Blepharoptosis
adiposa (false) *—see* Blepharoptosis
breast N64.81
cecum K63.4
colon K63.4
congenital (eyelid) Q10.0
specified site NEC *—see* Anomaly, by site
eyelid *—see* Blepharoptosis
congenital Q10.0
gastric K31.89
intestine K63.4
kidney N28.83
liver K76.89
renal N28.83
splanchnic K63.4
spleen D73.89
stomach K31.89
viscera K63.4
PTP D69.51
Ptyalism (periodic) K11.7
hysterical F45.8
pregnancy *—see* Pregnancy, complicated by, specified pregnancy-related condition NEC
psychogenic F45.8
Ptyalolithiasis K11.5
Pubarche, precocious E30.1
Pubertas praecox E30.1
Puberty (development state) Z00.3
bleeding (excessive) N92.2
delayed E30.0
precocious (constitutional) (cryptogenic) (idiopathic) E30.1
central E22.8
due to
ovarian hyperfunction E28.1
estrogen E28.0
testicular hyperfunction E29.0
premature E30.1
due to
adrenal cortical hyperfunction E25.8
pineal tumor E34.8
pituitary (anterior) hyperfunction E22.8
Puckering, macula *—see* Degeneration, macula, puckering
Pudenda, pudendum *—see* condition
Puente's disease (simple glandular cheilitis) K13.0
Puerperal, puerperium (complicated by, complications)
abnormal glucose (tolerance test) O99.815
abscess
areola O91.02
associated with lactation O91.03
Bartholin's gland O86.19
breast O91.12
associated with lactation O91.13
cervix (uteri) O86.11
genital organ NEC O86.19
kidney O86.21
mammary O91.12
associated with lactation O91.13
nipple O91.02
associated with lactation O91.03
peritoneum O85
subareolar O91.12
associated with lactation O91.13
urinary tract *—see* Puerperal, infection, urinary
uterus O86.12
vagina (wall) O86.13
vaginorectal O86.13
vulvovaginal gland O86.13
adnexitis O86.19
afibrinogenemia, or other coagulation defect O72.3
albuminuria (acute) (subacute) *—see* Proteinuria, gestational
alcohol use O99.315

Puerperal, puerperium *(Continued)*
  anemia O90.81
    pre-existing (pre-pregnancy) O99.03
  anesthetic death O89.8
  apoplexy O99.43
  bariatric surgery status O99.845
  blood disorder NEC O99.13
  blood dyscrasia O72.3
  cardiomyopathy O90.3
  cerebrovascular disorder (conditions in I60-I69) O99.43
  cervicitis O86.11
  circulatory system disorder O99.43
  coagulopathy (any) O72.3
  complications O90.9
    specified NEC O90.89
  convulsions —*see* Eclampsia
  cystitis O86.22
  cystopyelitis O86.29
  delirium NEC F05
  diabetes O24.93
    gestational —*see* Puerperal, gestational diabetes
    pre-existing O24.33
      specified NEC O24.83
      type 1 O24.03
      type 2 O24.13
  digestive system disorder O99.63
  disease O90.9
    breast NEC O92.29
    cerebrovascular (acute) O99.43
    nonobstetric NEC O99.89
    tubo-ovarian O86.19
    Valsuani's O99.03
  disorder O90.9
    biliary tract O26.63
    lactation O92.70
    liver O26.63
    nonobstetric NEC O99.89
  disruption
    cesarean wound O90.0
    episiotomy wound O90.1
    perineal laceration wound O90.1
  drug use O99.325
  eclampsia (with pre-existing hypertension) O15.2
  embolism (pulmonary) (blood clot) —*see* Embolism, obstetric, puerperal
  endocrine, nutritional or metabolic disease NEC O99.285
  endophlebitis —*see* Puerperal, phlebitis
  endotrachelitis O86.11
  failure
    lactation (complete) O92.3
      partial O92.4
    renal, acute O90.4
  fever (of unknown origin) O86.4
    septic O85
  fissure, nipple O92.12
    associated with lactation O92.13
  fistula
    breast (due to mastitis) O91.12
      associated with lactation O91.13
    nipple O91.02
      associated with lactation O91.03
  galactophoritis O91.22
    associated with lactation O91.23
  galactorrhea O92.6
  gastric banding status O99.845
  gastric bypass status O99.845
  gastrointestinal disease NEC O99.63
  ~~gestational diabetes O24.439~~
    ~~diet controlled O24.430~~
    ~~insulin (and diet) controlled O24.434~~
  gestational ◀
    diabetes O24.439 ◀
      diet controlled O24.430 ◀
      insulin (and diet) controlled O24.434 ◀
      oral drug controlled (antidiabetic) (hypoglycemic) O24.435 ◀

Puerperal, puerperium *(Continued)*
  gestational *(Continued)*
    edema O12.05 ◀
      with proteinuria O12.25 ◀
    proteinuria O12.15 ◀
  gonorrhea O98.23
  hematoma, subdural O99.43
  hemiplegia, cerebral O99.355-
    due to cerebrovascular disorder O99.43
  hemorrhage O72.1
    brain O99.43
    bulbar O99.43
    cerebellar O99.43
    cerebral O99.43
    cortical O99.43
    delayed or secondary O72.2
    extradural O99.43
    internal capsule O99.43
    intracranial O99.43
    intrapontine O99.43
    meningeal O99.43
    pontine O99.43
    retained placenta O72.0
    subarachnoid O99.43
    subcortical O99.43
    subdural O99.43
    third stage O72.0
    uterine, delayed O72.2
    ventricular O99.43
  hemorrhoids O87.2
  hepatorenal syndrome O90.4
  hypertension —*see* Hypertension, complicating, puerperium
  hypertrophy, breast O92.29
  induration breast (fibrous) O92.29
  infection O86.4
    cervix O86.11
    generalized O85
    genital tract NEC O86.19
      obstetric surgical wound O86.0
    kidney (bacillus coli) O86.21
    maternal O98.93
      carrier state NEC O99.835
      gonorrhea O98.23
      human immunodeficiency virus (HIV) O98.73
      protozoal O98.63
      sexually transmitted NEC O98.33
      specified NEC O98.83
      ~~streptococcus B carrier state O99.825~~
      streptococcus group B (GBS) carrier state O99.825 ◀
      syphilis O98.13
      tuberculosis O98.03
      viral hepatitis O98.43
      viral NEC O98.53
    nipple O91.02
      associated with lactation O91.03
    peritoneum O85
    renal O86.21
    specified NEC O86.89
    urinary (asymptomatic) (tract) NEC O86.20
      bladder O86.22
      kidney O86.21
      specified site NEC O86.29
      urethra O86.22
    vagina O86.13
    vein —*see* Puerperal, phlebitis
  ischemia, cerebral O99.43
  lymphangitis O86.89
    breast O91.22
      associated with lactation O91.23
  malignancy O9A.13
  malnutrition O25.3
  mammillitis O91.02
    associated with lactation O91.03
  mammitis O91.22
    associated with lactation O91.23
  mania F30.8

Puerperal, puerperium *(Continued)*
  mastitis O91.22
    associated with lactation O91.23
    purulent O91.12
      associated with lactation O91.13
  melancholia —*see* Disorder, depressive
  mental disorder NEC O99.345
  metroperitonitis O85
  metrorrhagia —*see* Hemorrhage, postpartum
  metrosalpingitis O86.19
  metrovaginitis O86.13
  milk leg O87.1
  monoplegia, cerebral O99.43
  mood disturbance O90.6
  necrosis, liver (acute) (subacute) (conditions in subcategory K72.0) O26.63 ◀
    with renal failure O90.4
  nervous system disorder O99.355
  neuritis O90.89
  obesity (pre-existing prior to pregnancy) O99.215
  obesity surgery status O99.845
  occlusion, precerebral artery O99.43
  paralysis
    bladder (sphincter) O90.89
    cerebral O99.43
  paralytic stroke O99.43
  parametritis O85
  paravaginitis O86.13
  pelviperitonitis O85
  perimetritis O86.12
  perimetrosalpingitis O86.19
  perinephritis O86.21
  periphlebitis —*see* Puerperal phlebitis
  peritoneal infection O85
  peritonitis (pelvic) O85
  perivaginitis O86.13
  phlebitis O87.0
    deep O87.1
    pelvic O87.1
    superficial O87.0
  phlebothrombosis, deep O87.1
  phlegmasia alba dolens O87.1
  placental polyp O90.89
  pneumonia, embolic —*see* Embolism, obstetric, puerperal
  pre-eclampsia —*see* Pre-eclampsia
  psychosis F53
  pyelitis O86.21
  pyelocystitis O86.29
  pyelonephritis O86.21
  pyelonephrosis O86.21
  pyemia O85
  pyocystitis O86.29
  pyohemia O85
  pyometra O86.12
  pyonephritis O86.21
  pyosalpingitis O86.19
  pyrexia (of unknown origin) O86.4
  renal
    disease NEC O90.89
    failure O90.4
  respiratory disease NEC O99.53
  retention
    decidua —*see* Retention, decidua
    placenta O72.0
    secundines —*see* Retention, secundines
  retrated nipple O92.02
  salpingo-ovaritis O86.19
  salpingoperitonitis O85
  secondary perineal tear O90.1
  sepsis O85
  sepsis (pelvic) O85
  septic thrombophlebitis O86.81
  skin disorder NEC O99.73
  specified condition NEC O99.89
  stroke O99.43
  subinvolution (uterus) O90.89
  subluxation of symphysis (pubis) O26.73

P

Puerperal, puerperium *(Continued)*
suppuration —*see* Puerperal, abscess
tetanus A34
thelitis O91.02
associated with lactation O91.03
thrombocytopenia O72.3
thrombophlebitis (superficial) O87.0
deep O87.1
pelvic O87.1
septic O86.81
thrombosis (venous) —*see* Thrombosis, puerperal
thyroiditis O90.5
toxemia (eclamptic) (pre-eclamptic) (with convulsions) O15.2
trauma, non-obstetric O9A.23
caused by abuse (physical) (suspected) O9A.33
confirmed O9A.33
psychological (suspected) O9A.53
confirmed O9A.53
sexual (suspected) O9A.43
confirmed O9A.43
uremia (due to renal failure) O90.4
urethritis O86.22
vaginitis O86.13
varicose veins (legs) O87.4
vulva or perineum O87.8
venous O87.9
vulvitis O86.19
vulvovaginitis O86.13
white leg O87.1
Puerperium —*see* Puerperal
Pulmolithiasis J98.4
Pulmonary —*see* condition
Pulpitis (acute) (anachoretic) (chronic) (hyperplastic) (putrescent) (suppurative) (ulcerative) K04.01 ⬅
irreversible K04.02 ⬅
reversible K04.01 ⬅
Pulpless tooth K04.99
Pulse
alternating R00.8
bigeminal R00.8
fast R00.0
feeble, rapid due to shock following injury T79.4
rapid R00.0
weak R09.89
Pulsus alternans or trigeminus R00.8
Punch drunk F07.81
Punctum lacrimale occlusion —*see* Obstruction, lacrimal
Puncture
abdomen, abdominal
wall S31.139
with
foreign body S31.149
penetration into peritoneal cavity S31.639
with foreign body S31.649
epigastric region S31.132
with
foreign body S31.142
penetration into peritoneal cavity S31.632
with foreign body S31.642
left
lower quadrant S31.134
with
foreign body S31.144
penetration into peritoneal cavity S31.634
with foreign body S31.644
upper quadrant S31.131
with
foreign body S31.141
penetration into peritoneal cavity S31.631
with foreign body S31.641

Puncture *(Continued)*
abdomen, abdominal *(Continued)*
wall *(Continued)*
periumbilic region S31.135
with
foreign body S31.145
penetration into peritoneal cavity S31.635
with foreign body S31.645
right
lower quadrant S31.133
with
foreign body S31.143
penetration into peritoneal cavity S31.633
with foreign body S31.643
upper quadrant S31.130
with
foreign body S31.140
penetration into peritoneal cavity S31.630
with foreign body S31.640
accidental, complicating surgery —*see* Complication, accidental puncture or laceration
alveolar (process) —*see* Puncture, oral cavity
ankle S91.039
with
foreign body S91.049
left S91.032
with
foreign body S91.042
right S91.031
with
foreign body S91.041
anus S31.833
with foreign body S31.834
arm (upper) S41.139
with foreign body S41.149
left S41.132
with foreign body S41.142
lower —*see* Puncture, forearm
right S41.131
with foreign body S41.141
auditory canal (external) (meatus) —*see* Puncture, ear
auricle, ear —*see* Puncture, ear
axilla —*see* Puncture, arm
back —*see also* Puncture, thorax, back
lower S31.030
with
foreign body S31.040
with penetration into retroperitoneal space S31.041
penetration into retroperitoneal space S31.031
bladder (traumatic) S37.29
nontraumatic N32.89
breast S21.039
with foreign body S21.049
left S21.032
with foreign body S21.042
right S21.031
with foreign body S21.041
buttock S31.803
with foreign body S31.804
left S31.823
with foreign body S31.824
right S31.813
with foreign body S31.814
by
device, implant or graft —*see* Complications, by site and type, mechanical
foreign body left accidentally in operative wound T81.539
instrument (any) during a procedure, accidental —*see* Puncture, accidental complicating surgery
calf —*see* Puncture, leg
canaliculus lacrimalis —*see* Puncture, eyelid

Puncture *(Continued)*
canthus, eye —*see* Puncture, eyelid
cervical esophagus S11.23
with foreign body S11.24
cheek (external) S01.439
with foreign body S01.449
internal —*see* Puncture, oral cavity
left S01.432
with foreign body S01.442
right S01.431
with foreign body S01.441
chest wall —*see* Puncture, thorax
chin —*see* Puncture, head, specified site NEC
clitoris —*see* Puncture, vulva
costal region —*see* Puncture, thorax
digit (s)
foot —*see* Puncture, toe
hand —*see* Puncture, finger
ear (canal) (external) S01.339
with foreign body S01.349
drum S09.2-
left S01.332
with foreign body S01.342
right S01.331
with foreign body S01.341
elbow S51.039
with
foreign body S51.049
left S51.032
with
foreign body S51.042
right S51.031
with
foreign body S51.041
epididymis —*see* Puncture, testis
epigastric region —*see* Puncture, abdomen, wall, epigastric
epiglottis S11.83
with foreign body S11.84
esophagus
cervical S11.23
with foreign body S11.24
thoracic S27.818
eyeball S05.6-
with foreign body S05.5-
eyebrow —*see* Puncture, eyelid
eyelid S01.13-
with foreign body S01.14-
left S01.132
with foreign body S01.142
right S01.131
with foreign body S01.141
face NEC —*see* Puncture, head, specified site NEC
finger (s) S61.239
with
damage to nail S61.339
with
foreign body S61.349
foreign body S61.249
index S61.238
with
damage to nail S61.338
with
foreign body S61.348
foreign body S61.248
left S61.231
with
damage to nail S61.331
with
foreign body S61.341
foreign body S61.241
right S61.230
with
damage to nail S61.330
with
foreign body S61.340
foreign body S61.240
little S61.238
with
damage to nail S61.338

Puncture *(Continued)*
- pudendum *—see* Puncture, genital organs, external
- rectovaginal septum *—see* Puncture, vagina
- sacral region *—see* Puncture, back, lower
- sacroiliac region *—see* Puncture, back, lower
- salivary gland *—see* Puncture, oral cavity
- scalp S01.Ø3
  - with foreign body SØ1.Ø4
- scapular region *—see* Puncture, shoulder
- scrotum S31.33
  - with foreign body S31.34
- shin *—see* Puncture, leg
- shoulder S41.Ø39
  - with foreign body S41.Ø49
  - left S41.Ø32
    - with foreign body S41.Ø42
  - right S41.Ø31
    - with foreign body S41.Ø41
- spermatic cord *—see* Puncture, testis
- sternal region *—see* Puncture, thorax, front
- submaxillary region *—see* Puncture, head, specified site NEC
- submental region *—see* Puncture, head, specified site NEC
- subungual
  - finger (s) *—see* Puncture, finger, with damage to nail
  - toe *—see* Puncture, toe, with damage to nail
- supraclavicular fossa *—see* Puncture, neck, specified site NEC
- temple, temporal region *—see* Puncture, head, specified site NEC
- temporomandibular area *—see* Puncture, cheek
- testis S31.33
  - with foreign body S31.34
- thigh S71.139
  - with foreign body S71.149
  - left S71.132
    - with foreign body S71.142
  - right S71.131
    - with foreign body S71.141
- thorax, thoracic (wall) S21.93
  - with foreign body S21.94
  - back S21.23-
    - with
      - foreign body S21.24-
        - with penetration S21.44
      - penetration S21.43
  - breast *—see* Puncture, breast
  - front S21.13-
    - with
      - foreign body S21.14-
        - with penetration S21.34
      - penetration S21.33
- throat *—see* Puncture, neck
- thumb S61.Ø39
  - with
    - damage to nail S61.139
      - with
        - foreign body S61.149
    - foreign body S61.Ø49
  - left S61.Ø32
    - with
      - damage to nail S61.132
        - with
          - foreign body S61.142
      - foreign body S61.Ø42
  - right S61.Ø31
    - with
      - damage to nail S61.131
        - with
          - foreign body S61.141
      - foreign body S61.Ø41

Puncture *(Continued)*
- thyroid gland S11.13
  - with foreign body S11.14
- toe (s) S91.139
  - with
    - damage to nail S91.239
      - with
        - foreign body S91.249
    - foreign body S91.149
  - great S91.133
    - with
      - damage to nail S91.233
        - with
          - foreign body S91.243
      - foreign body S91.143
    - left S91.132
      - with
        - damage to nail S91.232
          - with
            - foreign body S91.242
        - foreign body S91.142
    - right S91.131
      - with
        - damage to nail S91.231
          - with
            - foreign body S91.241
        - foreign body S91.141
  - lesser S91.136
    - with
      - damage to nail S91.236
        - with
          - foreign body S91.246
      - foreign body S91.146
    - left S91.135
      - with
        - damage to nail S91.235
          - with
            - foreign body S91.245
        - foreign body S91.145
    - right S91.134
      - with
        - damage to nail S91.234
          - with
            - foreign body S91.244
        - foreign body S91.144
- tongue *—see* Puncture, oral cavity
- trachea S11.Ø23
  - with foreign body S11.Ø24
- tunica vaginalis *—see* Puncture, testis
- tympanum, tympanic membrane S09.2-
- umbilical region S31.135
  - with foreign body S31.145
- uvula *—see* Puncture, oral cavity
- vagina S31.43
  - with foreign body S31.44
- vocal cords S11.Ø33
  - with foreign body S11.Ø34
- vulva S31.43
  - with foreign body S31.44
- wrist S61.539
  - with
    - foreign body S61.549
  - left S61.532
    - with
      - foreign body S61.542
  - right S61.531
    - with
      - foreign body S61.541

PUO (pyrexia of unknown origin) R5Ø.9

Pupillary membrane (persistent) Q13.89

Pupillotonia *—see* Anomaly, pupil, function, tonic pupil

Purpura D69.2
- abdominal D69.Ø
- allergic D69.Ø
- anaphylactoid D69.Ø
- annularis telangiectodes L81.7
- arthritic D69.Ø
- autoerythrocyte sensitization D69.2
- autoimmune D69.Ø

Purpura *(Continued)*
- bacterial D69.Ø
- Bateman's (senile) D69.2
- capillary fragility (hereditary) (idiopathic) D69.8
- cryoglobulinemic D89.1
- Devil's pinches D69.2
- fibrinolytic *—see* Fibrinolysis
- fulminans, fulminous D65
- gangrenous D65
- hemorrhagic, hemorrhagica D69.3
  - not due to thrombocytopenia D69.Ø
- Henoch (-Schönlein) (allergic) D69.Ø
- hypergammaglobulinemic (benign) (Waldenström's) D89.Ø
- idiopathic (thrombocytopenic) D69.3
  - nonthrombocytopenic D69.Ø
- immune thrombocytopenic D69.3
- infectious D69.Ø
- malignant D69.Ø
- neonatorum P54.5
- nervosa D69.Ø
- newborn P54.5
- nonthrombocytopenic D69.2
  - hemorrhagic D69.Ø
  - idiopathic D69.Ø
- nonthrombopenic D69.2
- peliosis rheumatica D69.Ø
- posttransfusion (post-transfusion) (from (fresh) whole blood or blood products) D69.51
- primary D69.49
- red cell membrane sensitivity D69.2
- rheumatica D69.Ø
- Schönlein (-Henoch) (allergic) D69.Ø
- scorbutic E54 *[D77]*
- senile D69.2
- simplex D69.2
- symptomatica D69.Ø
- telangiectasia annularis L81.7
- thrombocytopenic D69.49
  - congenital D69.42
  - hemorrhagic D69.3
  - hereditary D69.42
  - idiopathic D69.3
  - immune D69.3
  - neonatal, transitory P61.Ø
  - thrombotic M31.1
- thrombohemolytic *—see* Fibrinolysis
- thrombolytic *—see* Fibrinolysis
- thrombopenic D69.49
- thrombotic, thrombocytopenic M31.1
- toxic D69.Ø
- vascular D69.Ø
- visceral symptoms D69.Ø

Purpuric spots R23.3

Purulent *—see* condition

Pus
- in
  - stool R19.5
  - urine N39.Ø
- tube (rupture) *—see* Salpingo-oophoritis

Pustular rash LØ8.Ø

Pustule (nonmalignant) LØ8.9
- malignant A22.Ø

Pustulosis palmaris et plantaris L4Ø.3

Putnam (-Dana) **disease or syndrome** *—see* Degeneration, combined

Putrescent pulp (dental) KØ4.1

Pyarthritis, pyarthrosis *—see* Arthritis, pyogenic or pyemic
- tuberculous *—see* Tuberculosis, joint

Pyelectasis *—see* Hydronephrosis

Pyelitis (congenital) (uremic) *—see also* Pyelonephritis
- with
  - calculus *—see* category N2Ø
    - with hydronephrosis N13.2
  - contracted kidney N11.9

P

Pyelitis *(Continued)*
acute N10
chronic N11.9
with calculus —*see* category N20
with hydronephrosis N13.2
cystica N28.84
puerperal (postpartum) O86.21
tuberculous A18.11
Pyelocystitis —*see* Pyelonephritis
Pyelonephritis —*see also* Nephritis, tubulo-interstitial
with
calculus —*see* category N20
with hydronephrosis N13.2
contracted kidney N11.9
acute N10
calculous —*see* category N20
with hydronephrosis N13.2
chronic N11.9
with calculus —*see* category N20
with hydronephrosis N13.2
associated with ureteral obstruction or stricture N11.1
nonobstructive N11.8
with reflux (vesicoureteral) N11.0
obstructive N11.1
specified NEC N11.8
in (due to)
brucellosis A23.9 *[N16]*
cryoglobulinemia (mixed) D89.1 *[N16]*
cystinosis E72.04
diphtheria A36.84
glycogen storage disease E74.09 *[N16]*
leukemia NEC C95.9- *[N16]*
lymphoma NEC C85.90 *[N16]*
multiple myeloma C90.0- *[N16]*
obstruction N11.1
Salmonella infection A02.25
sarcoidosis D86.84
sepsis A41.9 *[N16]*
Sjögren's disease M35.04
toxoplasmosis B58.83
transplant rejection T86.91 *[N16]*
Wilson's disease E83.01 *[N16]*
nonobstructive N12
with reflux (vesicoureteral) N11.0
chronic N11.8
syphilitic A52.75
Pyelonephrosis (obstructive) N11.1
chronic N11.9
Pyelophlebitis I80.8
Pyeloureteritis cystica N28.85
Pyemia, pyemic (fever) (infection) (purulent) —*see also* Sepsis
joint —*see* Arthritis, pyogenic or pyemic
liver K75.1
pneumococcal A40.3
portal K75.1
postvaccinal T88.0
puerperal, postpartum, childbirth O85
specified organism NEC A41.89
tuberculous —*see* Tuberculosis, miliary
Pygopagus Q89.4
Pyknoepilepsy (idiopathic) —*see* Pyknolepsy
Pyknolepsy G40.A09
intractable G40.A19
with status epilepticus G40.A11
without status epilepticus G40.A19
not intractable G40.A09
with status epilepticus G40.A01
without status epilepticus G40.A09
Pylephlebitis K75.1
Pyle's syndrome Q78.5
Pylethrombophlebitis K75.1
Pylethrombosis K75.1
Pyloritis K29.90
with bleeding K29.91
Pylorospasm (reflex) NEC K31.3
congenital or infantile Q40.0
neurotic F45.8
newborn Q40.0
psychogenic F45.8
Pylorus, pyloric —*see* condition
Pyoarthrosis —*see* Arthritis, pyogenic or pyemic
Pyocele
mastoid —*see* Mastoiditis, acute
sinus (accessory) —*see* Sinusitis
turbinate (bone) J32.9
urethra —*see also* Urethritis N34.0
Pyocolpos —*see* Vaginitis
Pyocystitis N30.80
with hematuria N30.81
Pyoderma, pyodermia L08.0
gangrenosum L88
newborn P39.4
Pyoderma, pyodermia *(Continued)*
phagedenic L88
vegetans L08.81
Pyodermatitis L08.0
vegetans L08.81
Pyogenic —*see* condition
Pyohydronephrosis N13.6
Pyometra, pyometrium, pyometritis —*see* Endometritis
Pyomyositis (tropical) —*see* Myositis, infective
Pyonephritis N12
Pyonephrosis N13.6
tuberculous A18.11
Pyo-oophoritis —*see* Salpingo-oophoritis
Pyo-ovarium —*see* Salpingo-oophoritis
Pyopericarditis, pyopericardium I30.1
Pyophlebitis —*see* Phlebitis
Pyopneumopericardium I30.1
Pyopneumothorax (infective) J86.9
with fistula J86.0
tuberculous NEC A15.6
Pyosalpinx, pyosalpingitis —*see also* Salpingo-oophoritis
Pyothorax J86.9
with fistula J86.0
tuberculous NEC A15.6
Pyoureter N28.89
tuberculous A18.11
Pyramidopallidonigral syndrome G20
Pyrexia (of unknown origin) R50.9
atmospheric T67.0
during labor NEC O75.2
heat T67.0
newborn P81.9
environmentally-induced P81.0
persistent R50.9
puerperal O86.4
Pyroglobulinemia NEC E88.09
Pyromania F63.1
Pyrosis R12
Pyuria (bacterial) N39.0

◄ New ⟸ Revised ~~deleted~~ Deleted

Q

Q fever A78
  with pneumonia A78
Quadricuspid aortic valve Q23.8
Quadrilateral fever A78
Quadriparesis —*see* Quadriplegia
  meaning muscle weakness M62.81
Quadriplegia G82.5Ø-
  complete
    C1-C4 level G82.51
    C5-C7 level G82.53
  congenital (cerebral) (spinal) G8Ø.8
    spastic G8Ø.Ø
Quadriplegia *(Continued)*
  embolic (current episode) I63.4- (Revised)
  functional R53.2
  incomplete
    C1-C4 level G82.52
    C5-C7 level G82.54
  thrombotic (current episode) I63.3- (Revised)
  traumatic — code to injury with seventh character S
    current episode —*see* Injury, spinal (cord), cervical
Quadruplet, pregnancy —*see* Pregnancy, quadruplet
Quarrelsomeness F6Ø.3
Queensland fever A77.3
Quervain's disease M65.4
  thyroid EØ6.1
Queyrat's erythroplasia DØ7.4
  penis DØ7.4
  specified site —*see* Neoplasm, skin, in situ
  unspecified site DØ7.4
Quincke's disease or edema T78.3
  hereditary D84.1
Quinsy (gangrenous) J36
Quintan fever A79.Ø
Quintuplet, pregnancy —*see* Pregnancy, quintuplet

R

Rabbit fever —*see* Tularemia
Rabies A82.9
contact Z2Ø.3
exposure to Z2Ø.3
inoculation reaction —*see* Complications, vaccination
sylvatic A82.Ø
urban A82.1
Rachischisis —*see* Spina bifida
Rachitic —*see also* condition
deformities of spine (late effect) (sequelae) E64.3
pelvis (late effect) (sequelae) E64.3
with disproportion (fetopelvic) O33.Ø
causing obstructed labor O65.Ø
Rachitis, rachitism (acute) (tarda) —*see also* Rickets
renalis N25.Ø
sequelae E64.3
Radial nerve —*see* condition
Radiation
burn —*see* Burn
effects NOS T66
sickness NOS T66
therapy, encounter for Z51.Ø
Radiculitis (pressure) (vertebrogenic) —*see* Radiculopathy
Radiculomyelitis —*see also* Encephalitis
toxic, due to
Clostridium tetani A35
Corynebacterium diphtheriae A36.82
Radiculopathy M54.10
cervical region M54.12
cervicothoracic region M54.13
due to
disc disorder
C3 M5Ø.11
C4 M5Ø.11
C5 M5Ø.121 ◄
C6 M5Ø.122 ◄
C7 M5Ø.123 ◄
C8 M5Ø.13
displacement of intervertebral disc —*see* Disorder, disc, with, radiculopathy
leg M54.1-
lumbar region M54.16
lumbosacral region M54.17
occipito-atlanto-axial region M54.11
postherpetic BØ2.29
sacrococcygeal region M54.18
syphilitic A52.11
thoracic region (with visceral pain) M54.14
thoracolumbar region M54.15
Radiodermal burns (acute, chronic, or occupational) —*see* Burn
Radiodermatitis L58.9
acute L58.Ø
chronic L58.1
Radiotherapy session Z51.Ø
RAEB (refractory anemia with excess blasts) D46.2- ◄
Rage, meaning rabies —*see* Rabies
Ragpicker's disease A22.1
Ragsorter's disease A22.1
Raillietiniasis B71.8
Railroad neurosis F48.8
Railway spine F48.8
Raised —*see also* Elevated
antibody titer R76.Ø
Rake teeth, tooth M26.39
Rales RØ9.89
Ramifying renal pelvis Q63.8
Ramsay-Hunt disease or syndrome —*see also* Hunt's disease BØ2.21
meaning dyssynergia cerebellaris myoclonica G11.1
Ranula K11.6
congenital Q38.4
Rape
adult
confirmed T74.21
suspected T76.21
alleged, observation or examination, ruled out
adult ZØ4.41
child ZØ4.42
child
confirmed T74.22
suspected T76.22
Rapid
feeble pulse, due to shock, following injury T79.4
heart (beat) RØØ.Ø
psychogenic F45.8
second stage (delivery) O62.3
time-zone change syndrome —*see* Disorder, sleep, circadian rhythm, psychogenic
Rarefaction, bone —*see* Disorder, bone, density and structure, specified NEC
Rash (toxic) R21
canker A38.9
diaper L22
drug (internal use) L27.Ø
contact —*see also* Dermatitis, due to, drugs, external L25.1
following immunization T88.1
food —*see* Dermatitis, due to, food
heat L74.Ø
napkin (psoriasiform) L22
nettle —*see* Urticaria
pustular LØ8.Ø
rose R21
epidemic BØ6.9
scarlet A38.9
serum —*see also* Reaction, serum T8Ø.69
wandering tongue K14.1
Rasmussen aneurysm —*see* Tuberculosis, pulmonary
Rasmussen encephalitis GØ4.81
Rat-bite fever A25.9
due to Streptobacillus moniliformis A25.1
spirochetal (morsus muris) A25.Ø
Rathke's pouch tumor D44.3
Raymond (-Céstan) **syndrome** I65.8
Raynaud's disease, phenomenon or syndrome (secondary) I73.ØØ
with gangrene (symmetric) I73.Ø1
RDS (newborn) (type I) P22.Ø
type II P22.1
Reaction —*see also* Disorder
adaptation —*see* Disorder, adjustment
adjustment (anxiety) (conduct disorder) (depressiveness) (distress) —*see* Disorder, adjustment
with
mutism, elective (child) (adolescent) F94.Ø
adverse
food (any) (ingested) NEC T78.1
anaphylactic —*see* Shock, anaphylactic, due to food
anaphylactoid —*see* Shock, anaphylactic
affective —*see* Disorder, mood
allergic —*see* Allergy
anaphylactic —*see* Shock, anaphylactic
anesthesia —*see* Anesthesia, complication
antitoxin (prophylactic) (therapeutic) —*see* Complications, vaccination
anxiety F41.1
Arthus —*see* Arthus' phenomenon
asthenic F48.8
combat and operational stress F43.Ø
compulsive F42.8 ⬅
conversion F44.9
crisis, acute F43.Ø
deoxyribonuclease (DNA) (DNase) hypersensitivity D69.2
depressive (single episode) F32.9
affective (single episode) F31.4
recurrent episode F33.9
neurotic F34.1
psychoneurotic F34.1
Reaction *(Continued)*
depressive *(Continued)*
psychotic F32.3
recurrent —*see* Disorder, depressive, recurrent
dissociative F44.9
drug NEC T88.7
addictive —*see* Dependence, drug
transmitted via placenta or breast milk —*see* Absorption, drug, addictive, through placenta
allergic —*see* Allergy, drug
lichenoid L43.2
newborn P93.8
gray baby syndrome P93.Ø
overdose or poisoning (by accident) —*see* Table of Drugs and Chemicals, by drug, poisoning
photoallergic L56.1
phototoxic L56.Ø
withdrawal —*see* Dependence, by drug, with, withdrawal
infant of dependent mother P96.1
newborn P96.1
wrong substance given or taken (by accident) —*see* Table of Drugs and Chemicals, by drug, poisoning
fear F4Ø.9
child (abnormal) F93.8
febrile nonhemolytic transfusion (FNHTR) R5Ø.84
fluid loss, cerebrospinal G97.1
foreign
body NEC —*see* Granuloma, foreign body
in operative wound (inadvertently left) —*see* Foreign body, accidentally left during a procedure
substance accidentally left during a procedure (chemical) (powder) (talc) T81.6Ø
aseptic peritonitis T81.61
body or object (instrument) (sponge) (swab) —*see* Foreign body, accidentally left during a procedure
specified reaction NEC T81.69
grief —*see* Disorder, adjustment
Herxheimer's R68.89
hyperkinetic —*see* Hyperkinesia
hypochondriacal F45.2Ø
hypoglycemic, due to insulin E16.Ø
with coma (diabetic) —*see* Diabetes, coma
nondiabetic E15
therapeutic misadventure —*see* subcategory T38.3
hypomanic F3Ø.8
hysterical F44.9
immunization —*see* Complications, vaccination
incompatibility
ABO blood group (infusion) (transfusion) —*see* Complication (s), transfusion, incompatibility reaction, ABO
delayed serologic T8Ø.39
minor blood group (Duffy) (E) (K(ell)) (Kidd) (Lewis) (M) (N) (P) (S) T8Ø.89
Rh (factor) (infusion) (transfusion) —*see* Complication (s), transfusion, incompatibility reaction, Rh (factor)
inflammatory —*see* Infection
infusion —*see* Complications, infusion
inoculation (immune serum) —*see* Complications, vaccination
insulin T38.3-
involutional psychotic —*see* Disorder, depressive
leukemoid D72.823
basophilic D72.823
lymphocytic D72.823
monocytic D72.823
myelocytic D72.823
neutrophilic D72.823

Reaction *(Continued)*
LSD (acute)
due to drug abuse —*see* Abuse, drug, hallucinogen
due to drug dependence —*see* Dependence, drug, hallucinogen
lumbar puncture G97.1
manic-depressive —*see* Disorder, bipolar
neurasthenic F48.8
neurogenic —*see* Neurosis
neurotic F48.9
neurotic-depressive F34.1
nitritoid —*see* Crisis, nitritoid - obsessive-compulsive F42
nonspecific
to
cell mediated immunity measurement of gamma interferon antigen response without active tuberculosis R76.12
QuantiFERON-TB test (QFT) without active tuberculosis R76.12
tuberculin test —*see also* Reaction, tuberculin skin test R76.11
obsessive-compulsive F42.8 ⇐
organic, acute or subacute —*see* Delirium
paranoid (acute) F23
chronic F22
senile FØ3
passive dependency F6Ø.7
phobic F4Ø.9
post-traumatic stress, uncomplicated Z73.3
psychogenic F99
psychoneurotic —*see also* Neurosis
compulsive F42.8 ⇐
depersonalization F48.1
depressive F34.1
hypochondriacal F45.2Ø
neurasthenic F48.8
obsessive F42.8 ⇐
psychophysiologic —*see* Disorder, somatoform
psychosomatic —*see* Disorder, somatoform
psychotic —*see* Psychosis
scarlet fever toxin —*see* Complications, vaccination
schizophrenic F23
acute (brief) (undifferentiated) F23
latent F21
undifferentiated (acute) (brief) F23
serological for syphilis —*see* Serology for syphilis
serum T8Ø.69
anaphylactic (immediate) —*see also* Shock, anaphylactic T8Ø.59
specified reaction NEC
due to
administration of blood and blood products T8Ø.61
immunization T8Ø.62
serum specified NEC T8Ø.69
vaccination T8Ø.62
situational —*see* Disorder, adjustment
somatization —*see* Disorder, somatoform
spinal puncture G97.1
stress (severe) F43.9
acute (agitation) ("daze") (disorientation) (disturbance of consciousness) (flight reaction) (fugue) F43.Ø
specified NEC F43.8
surgical procedure —*see* Complications, surgical procedure
tetanus antitoxin —*see* Complications, vaccination
toxic, to local anesthesia T81.59 ⇐
in labor and delivery O74.4
in pregnancy O29.3X-
postpartum, puerperal O89.3
toxin-antitoxin —*see* Complications, vaccination

Reaction *(Continued)*
transfusion (blood) (bone marrow) (lymphocytes) (allergic) —*see* Complications, transfusion
tuberculin skin test, abnormal R76.11
vaccination (any) —*see* Complications, vaccination
withdrawing, child or adolescent F93.8
Reactive airway disease —*see* Asthma
Reactive depression —*see* Reaction, depressive
Rearrangement
chromosomal
balanced (in) Q95.9
abnormal individual (autosomal) Q95.2
non-sex (autosomal) chromosomes Q95.2
sex/non-sex chromosomes Q95.3
specified NEC Q95.8
Recalcitrant patient —*see* Noncompliance
Recanalization, thrombus —*see* Thrombosis
Recession, receding
chamber angle (eye) H21.55-
chin M26.Ø9
gingival (generalized) (localized) (postinfective) (postoperative) KØ6.ØØ ⇐
Miller Class I KØ6.Ø1 ◀
Miller Class II KØ6.Ø2 ◀
Miller Class III KØ6.Ø3 ◀
Miller Class IV KØ6.Ø4 ◀
Recklinghausen's disease Q85.Ø1
bones E21.Ø
Reclus' disease (cystic) —*see* Mastopathy, cystic
Recrudescent typhus (fever) A75.1
Recruitment, auditory H93.21-
Rectalgia K62.89
Rectitis K62.89
Rectocele
female (without uterine prolapse) N81.6
with uterine prolapse N81.4
incomplete N81.2
in pregnancy —*see* Pregnancy, complicated by, abnormal, pelvic organs or tissues NEC
male K62.3
Rectosigmoid junction —*see* condition
Rectosigmoiditis K63.89
ulcerative (chronic) K51.3Ø
with
complication K51.319
abscess K51.314
fistula K51.313
obstruction K51.312
rectal bleeding K51.311
specified NEC K51.318
Rectourethral —*see* condition
Rectovaginal —*see* condition
Rectovesical —*see* condition
Rectum, rectal —*see* condition
Recurrent —*see* condition
pregnancy loss —*see* Loss (of), pregnancy, recurrent
Red bugs B88.Ø
Red-cedar lung or pneumonitis J67.8
Red tide —*see also* Table of Drugs and Chemicals T65.82-
Reduced
mobility Z74.Ø9
ventilatory or vital capacity R94.2
Redundant, redundancy
anus (congenital) Q43.8
clitoris N9Ø.89
colon (congenital) Q43.8
foreskin (congenital) N47.8
intestine (congenital) Q43.8
labia N9Ø.69 ⇐
organ or site, congenital NEC —*see* Accessory
panniculus (abdominal) E65
prepuce (congenital) N47.8
pylorus K31.89
rectum (congenital) Q43.8
scrotum N5Ø.89 ⇐

Redundant, redundancy *(Continued)*
sigmoid (congenital) Q43.8
skin L98.7 ⇐
~~eyelids —see Blepharochalasis~~
and subcutaneous tissue L98.7 ◀
of face L57.4 ◀
eyelids —*see* Blepharochalasis ◀
stomach K31.89
Reduplication —*see* Duplication
Reflex R29.2
hyperactive gag J39.2
pupillary, abnormal —*see* Anomaly, pupil, function
vasoconstriction I73.9
vasovagal R55
Reflux K21.9
acid K21.9
esophageal K21.9
with esophagitis K21.Ø
newborn P78.83
gastroesophageal K21.9
with esophagitis K21.Ø
mitral —*see* Insufficiency, mitral
ureteral —*see* Reflux, vesicoureteral
vesicoureteral (with scarring) N13.7Ø
with
nephropathy N13.729
with hydroureter N13.739
bilateral N13.732
unilateral N13.731
without hydroureter N13.729
bilateral N13.722
unilateral N13.721
bilateral N13.722
unilateral N13.721
pyelonephritis (chronic) N11.Ø
without nephropathy N13.71
congenital Q62.7
Reforming, artificial openings —*see* Attention to, artificial, opening
Refractive error —*see* Disorder, refraction
Refsum's disease or syndrome G6Ø.1
Refusal of
food, psychogenic F5Ø.89 ⇐
treatment (because of) Z53.2Ø
left against medical advice (AMA) Z53.21
patient's decision NEC Z53.29
reasons of belief or group pressure Z53.1
Regional —*see* condition
Regurgitation R11.1Ø
aortic (valve) —*see* Insufficiency, aortic
food —*see also* Vomiting
with reswallowing —*see* Rumination
newborn P92.1
gastric contents —*see* Vomiting
heart —*see* Endocarditis
mitral (valve) —*see* Insufficiency, mitral
congenital Q23.3
myocardial —*see* Endocarditis
pulmonary (valve) (heart) I37.1
congenital Q22.2
syphilitic A52.Ø3
tricuspid —*see* Insufficiency, tricuspid
valve, valvular —*see* Endocarditis
congenital Q24.8
vesicoureteral —*see* Reflux, vesicoureteral
Reichmann's disease or syndrome K31.89
Reifenstein syndrome E34.52
~~Reinsertion, contraceptive device Z30.433~~
Reinsertion ◀
implantable subdermal contraceptive Z3Ø.46 ◀
intrauterine contraceptive device Z3Ø.433 ◀
Reiter's disease, syndrome, or urethritis MØ2.3Ø
ankle MØ2.37-
elbow MØ2.32-
foot joint MØ2.37-
hand joint MØ2.34-
hip MØ2.35-
knee MØ2.36-
multiple site MØ2.39

◀ New ⇐ Revised ~~deleted~~ Deleted

R

Reiter's disease, syndrome, or urethritis *(Continued)*
- shoulder M02.31-
- vertebra M02.38
- wrist M02.33-

Rejection
- food, psychogenic F50.89 ⬅
- transplant T86.91
  - bone T86.830
    - marrow T86.01
  - cornea T86.840
  - heart T86.21
    - with lung (s) T86.31
  - intestine T86.850
  - kidney T86.11
  - liver T86.41
  - lung (s) T86.810
    - with heart T86.31
  - organ (immune or nonimmune cause) T86.91
  - pancreas T86.890
  - skin (allograft) (autograft) T86.820
  - specified NEC T86.890
  - stem cell (peripheral blood) (umbilical cord) T86.5

Relapsing fever A68.9
- Carter's (Asiatic) A68.1
- Dutton's (West African) A68.1
- Koch's A68.9
- louse-borne (epidemic) A68.0
- Novy's (American) A68.1
- Obermeyers's (European) A68.0
- Spirillum A68.9
- tick-borne (endemic) A68.1

Relationship
- occlusal
  - open anterior M26.220
  - open posterior M26.221

Relaxation
- anus (sphincter) K62.89
  - psychogenic F45.8
- arch (foot) —*see also* Deformity, limb, flat foot
- back ligaments —*see* Instability, joint, spine
- bladder (sphincter) N31.2
- cardioesophageal K21.9
- cervix —*see* Incompetency, cervix
- diaphragm J98.6
- joint (capsule) (ligament) (paralytic) —*see* Flail, joint
  - congenital NEC Q74.8
- lumbosacral (joint) —*see* subcategory M53.2
- pelvic floor N81.89
- perineum N81.89
- posture R29.3
- rectum (sphincter) K62.89
- sacroiliac (joint) —*see* subcategory M53.2
- scrotum N50.89 ⬅
- urethra (sphincter) N36.44
- vesical N31.2

Release from prison, anxiety concerning Z65.2

Remains
- canal of Cloquet Q14.0
- capsule (opaque) Q14.8

Remittent fever (malarial) B54

Remnant
- canal of Cloquet Q14.0
- capsule (opaque) Q14.8
- cervix, cervical stump (acquired) (postoperative) N88.8
- cystic duct, postcholecystectomy K91.5
- fingernail L60.8
  - congenital Q84.6
- meniscus, knee —*see* Derangement, knee, meniscus, specified NEC
- thyroglossal duct Q89.2
- tonsil J35.8
  - infected (chronic) J35.01
- urachus Q64.4

Removal (from) (of)
- artificial
  - arm Z44.00-
    - complete Z44.01-
    - partial Z44.02-
  - eye Z44.2-
  - leg Z44.10-
    - complete Z44.11-
    - partial Z44.12-
- breast implant Z45.81
- cardiac pulse generator (battery) (end-of-life) Z45.010
- catheter (urinary) (indwelling) Z46.6
  - from artificial opening —*see* Attention to, artificial, opening
  - non-vascular Z46.82
  - vascular NEC Z45.2
- device Z46.9
  - contraceptive Z30.432
    - implantable subdermal Z30.46 ◀
  - implanted NEC Z45.89
  - specified NEC Z46.89
- drains Z48.03
- dressing (nonsurgical) Z48.00
  - surgical Z48.01
- external
  - fixation device — code to fracture with seventh character D
  - prosthesis, prosthetic device Z44.9
    - breast Z44.3-
    - specified NEC Z44.8
- home in childhood (to foster home or institution) Z62.29
- ileostomy Z43.2
- insulin pump Z46.81
- myringotomy device (stent) (tube) Z45.82
- nervous system device NEC Z46.2
  - brain neuropacemaker Z46.2
  - visual substitution device Z46.2
    - implanted Z45.31
- non-vascular catheter Z46.82
- organ, prophylactic (for neoplasia management) —*see* Prophylactic, organ removal
- orthodontic device Z46.4
- staples Z48.02
- stent
  - ureteral Z46.6
- suture Z48.02
- urinary device Z46.6
- vascular access device or catheter Z45.2

Ren
- arcuatus Q63.1
- mobile, mobilis N28.89
  - congenital Q63.8
- unguliformis Q63.1

Renal —*see* condition

Rendu-Osler-Weber disease or syndrome I78.0

Reninoma D41.0-

Renon-Delille syndrome E23.3

Reovirus, as cause of disease classified elsewhere B97.5

Repeated falls NEC R29.6

Replaced chromosome by dicentric ring Q93.2

Replacement by artificial or mechanical device or prosthesis of
- bladder Z96.0
- blood vessel NEC Z95.828
- bone NEC Z96.7
- cochlea Z96.21
- coronary artery Z95.5
- eustachian tube Z96.29
- eye globe Z97.0
- heart Z95.812
  - valve Z95.2
    - prosthetic Z95.2
    - specified NEC Z95.4
    - xenogenic Z95.3
- intestine Z96.89

Replacement by artificial or mechanical device or prosthesis of *(Continued)*
- joint Z96.60
  - hip —*see* Presence, hip joint implant
  - knee —*see* Presence, knee joint implant
  - specified site NEC Z96.698
- larynx Z96.3
- lens Z96.1
- limb (s) —*see* Presence, artificial, limb
- mandible NEC (for tooth root implant (s)) Z96.5
- organ NEC Z96.89
- peripheral vessel NEC Z95.828
- stapes Z96.29
- teeth Z97.2
- tendon Z96.7
- tissue NEC Z96.89
- tooth root (s) Z96.5
- vessel NEC Z95.828
  - coronary (artery) Z95.5

Request for expert evidence Z04.8

Reserve, decreased or low
- cardiac —*see* Disease, heart
- kidney N28.89

Residual —*see also* condition
- ovary syndrome N99.83
- state, schizophrenic F20.5
- urine R39.198 ⬅

Resistance, resistant (to)
- activated protein C D68.51
- complicating pregnancy O26.89
- insulin E88.81
- organism (s)
  - to
    - drug Z16.30 ⬅
      - aminoglycosides Z16.29
      - amoxicillin Z16.11
      - ampicillin Z16.11
      - antibiotic (s) Z16.20
        - multiple Z16.24
        - specified NEC Z16.29
      - antifungal Z16.32
      - antimicrobial (single) Z16.30
        - multiple Z16.35
        - specified NEC Z16.39
      - ~~antimycobacterial (single) Z16.341~~
        - ~~multiple Z16.342~~
      - antimycobacterial (single) Z16.341 ◀
        - multiple Z16.342 ◀
      - antiparasitic Z16.31
      - antiviral Z16.33
      - beta lactam antibiotics Z16.10
        - specified NEC Z16.19
      - cephalosporins Z16.19
      - extended beta lactamase (ESBL) Z16.12
      - fluoroquinolones Z16.23
      - macrolides Z16.29
      - methicillin —*see* MRSA
      - multiple drugs (MDRO)
        - antibiotics Z16.24
        - antimicrobial Z16.35 ◀
        - antimycobacterials Z16.342 ◀
      - penicillins Z16.11
      - quinine (and related compounds) Z16.31
      - quinolones Z16.23
      - sulfonamides Z16.29
      - tetracyclines Z16.29
      - tuberculostatics (single) Z16.341
        - multiple Z16.342
      - vancomycin Z16.21
        - related antibiotics Z16.22
- thyroid hormone E07.89

Resorption
- dental (roots) K03.3
  - alveoli M26.79
- teeth (external) (internal) (pathological) (roots) K03.3

R

◀ New ⬅ Revised ~~deleted~~ Deleted

R

Retinoblastoma C69.2-
  differentiated C69.2-
  undifferentiated C69.2-
Retinochoroiditis —*see also* Inflammation, chorioretinal
  disseminated —*see* Inflammation, chorioretinal, disseminated
    syphilitic A52.71
  focal —*see* Inflammation, chorioretinal
  juxtapapillaris —*see* Inflammation, chorioretinal, focal, juxtapapillary
Retinopathy (background) H35.ØØ
  arteriosclerotic I7Ø.8 *[H35.Ø-]*
  atherosclerotic I7Ø.8 *[H35.Ø-]*
  central serous —*see* Chorioretinopathy, central serous
  Coats H35.Ø2-
  diabetic —*see* Diabetes, retinopathy
  exudative H35.Ø2-
  hypertensive H35.Ø3-
  in (due to)
    diabetes —*see* Diabetes, retinopathy
  sickle-cell disorders D57.- *[H36]*
  of prematurity H35.1Ø-
    stage Ø H35.11-
    stage 1 H35.12-
    stage 2 H35.13-
    stage 3 H35.14-
    stage 4 H35.15-
    stage 5 H35.16-
  pigmentary, congenital —*see* Dystrophy, retina
  proliferative NEC H35.2-
    diabetic —*see* Diabetes, retinopathy, proliferative
    sickle-cell D57.- *[H36]*
  solar H31.Ø2-
Retinoschisis H33.1Ø-
  congenital Q14.1
  specified type NEC H33.19-
Retortamoniasis AØ7.8
Retractile testis Q55.22
Retraction
  cervix —*see* Retroversion, uterus
  drum (membrane) —*see* Disorder, tympanic membrane, specified NEC
  finger —*see* Deformity, finger
  lid HØ2.539
    left HØ2.536
      lower HØ2.535
      upper HØ2.534
    right HØ2.533
      lower HØ2.532
      upper HØ2.531
  lung J98.4
  mediastinum J98.59 ◄
  nipple N64.53
    associated with
      lactation O92.Ø3
      pregnancy O92.Ø1-
      puerperium O92.Ø2
    congenital Q83.8
  palmar fascia M72.Ø
  pleura —*see* Pleurisy
  ring, uterus (Bandl's) (pathological) O62.4
  sternum (congenital) Q76.7
    acquired M95.4
  uterus —*see* Retroversion, uterus
  valve (heart) —*see* Endocarditis
Retrobulbar —*see* condition
Retrocecal —*see* condition
Retrocession —*see* Retroversion
Retrodisplacement —*see* Retroversion
Retroflection, retroflexion —*see* Retroversion
Retrognathia, retrognathism (mandibular) (maxillary) M26.19
Retrograde menstruation N92.5
Retroperineal —*see* condition
Retroperitoneal —*see* condition
Retroperitonitis K68.9
Retropharyngeal —*see* condition
Retroplacental —*see* condition
Retroposition —*see* Retroversion
Retroprosthetic membrane T85.398
Retrosternal thyroid (congenital) Q89.2
Retroversion, retroverted
  cervix —*see* Retroversion, uterus
  female NEC —*see* Retroversion, uterus
  iris H21.89
  testis (congenital) Q55.29
  uterus (acquired) (acute) (any degree) (asymptomatic) (cervix) (postinfectional) (postpartal, old) N85.4
    congenital Q51.818
    in pregnancy O34.53-
Retrovirus, as cause of disease classified elsewhere B97.3Ø
  human
    immunodeficiency, type 2 (HIV 2) B97.35
    T-cell lymphotropic
      type I (HTLV-I) B97.33
      type II (HTLV-II) B97.34
  lentivirus B97.31
  oncovirus B97.32
  specified NEC B97.39
Retrusion, premaxilla (developmental) M26.Ø9
Rett's disease or syndrome F84.2
Reverse peristalsis R19.2
Reye's syndrome G93.7
Rh (factor)
  hemolytic disease (newborn) P55.Ø
  incompatibility, immunization or sensitization
    affecting management of pregnancy NEC O36.Ø9-
      anti-D antibody O36.Ø1-
    newborn P55.Ø
    transfusion reaction —*see* Complication (s), transfusion, incompatibility reaction, Rh (factor)
  negative mother affecting newborn P55.Ø
  titer elevated —*see* Complication (s), transfusion, incompatibility reaction, Rh (factor)
  transfusion reaction —*see* Complication (s), transfusion, incompatibility reaction, Rh (factor)
Rhabdomyolysis (idiopathic) **NEC** M62.82
  traumatic T79.6
Rhabdomyoma —*see also* Neoplasm, connective tissue, benign
  adult —*see* Neoplasm, connective tissue, benign
  fetal —*see* Neoplasm, connective tissue, benign
  glycogenic —*see* Neoplasm, connective tissue, benign
Rhabdomyosarcoma (any type) —*see* Neoplasm, connective tissue, malignant
Rhabdosarcoma —*see* Rhabdomyosarcoma
Rhesus (factor) **incompatibility** —*see* Rh, incompatibility
Rheumatic (acute) (subacute) (chronic)
  adherent pericardium IØ9.2
  coronary arteritis IØ1.9
  degeneration, myocardium IØ9.Ø
  fever (acute) —*see* Fever, rheumatic
  heart —*see* Disease, heart, rheumatic
  myocardial degeneration —*see* Degeneration, myocardium
  myocarditis (chronic) (inactive) (with chorea) IØ9.Ø
    with chorea (acute) (rheumatic) (Sydenham's) IØ2.Ø
    active or acute IØ1.2
  pancarditis, acute IØ1.8
    with chorea (acute (rheumatic) Sydenham's) IØ2.Ø
  pericarditis (active) (acute) (with effusion) (with pneumonia) IØ1.Ø
    with chorea (acute) (rheumatic) (Sydenham's) IØ2.Ø
    chronic or inactive IØ9.2
Rheumatic *(Continued)*
  pneumonia IØØ *[J17]*
  torticollis M43.6
  typhoid fever AØ1.Ø9
Rheumatism (articular) (neuralgic) (nonarticular) M79.Ø
  gout —*see* Arthritis, rheumatoid
  intercostal, meaning Tietze's disease M94.Ø
  palindromic (any site) M12.3Ø
    ankle M12.37-
    elbow M12.32-
    foot joint M12.37-
    hand joint M12.34-
    hip M12.35-
    knee M12.36-
    multiple site M12.39
    shoulder M12.31-
    specified joint NEC M12.38
    vertebrae M12.38
    wrist M12.33-
  sciatic M54.4-
Rheumatoid —*see also* condition
  arthritis —*see also* Arthritis, rheumatoid
    with involvement of organs NEC MØ5.6Ø
      ankle MØ5.67-
      elbow MØ5.62-
      foot joint MØ5.67-
      hand joint MØ5.64-
      hip MØ5.65-
      knee MØ5.66-
      multiple site MØ5.69
      shoulder MØ5.61-
      vertebra —*see* Spondylitis, ankylosing
      wrist MØ5.63-
    seronegative —*see* Arthritis, rheumatoid, seronegative
    seropositive —*see* Arthritis, rheumatoid, seropositive
  carditis MØ5.3Ø
    ankle MØ5.37-
    elbow MØ5.32-
    foot joint MØ5.37-
    hand joint MØ5.34-
    hip MØ5.35-
    knee MØ5.36-
    multiple site MØ5.39
    shoulder MØ5.31-
    vertebra —*see* Spondylitis, ankylosing
    wrist MØ5.33-
  endocarditis —*see* Rheumatoid, carditis
  lung (disease) MØ5.1Ø
    ankle MØ5.17-
    elbow MØ5.12-
    foot joint MØ5.17-
    hand joint MØ5.14-
    hip MØ5.15-
    knee MØ5.16-
    multiple site MØ5.19
    shoulder MØ5.11-
    vertebra —*see* Spondylitis, ankylosing
    wrist MØ5.13-
  myocarditis —*see* Rheumatoid, carditis
  myopathy MØ5.4Ø
    ankle MØ5.47-
    elbow MØ5.42-
    foot joint MØ5.47-
    hand joint MØ5.44-
    hip MØ5.45-
    knee MØ5.46-
    multiple site MØ5.49
    shoulder MØ5.41-
    vertebra —*see* Spondylitis, ankylosing
    wrist MØ5.43-
  pericarditis —*see* Rheumatoid, carditis
  polyarthritis —*see* Arthritis, rheumatoid
  polyneuropathy MØ5.5Ø
    ankle MØ5.57-
    elbow MØ5.52-
    foot joint MØ5.57-
    hand joint MØ5.54-
    hip MØ5.55-

- **Rheumatoid** *(Continued)*
  - polyneuropathy *(Continued)*
    - knee MØ5.56-
    - multiple site MØ5.59
    - shoulder MØ5.51-
    - vertebra —*see* Spondylitis, ankylosing
    - wrist MØ5.53-
  - vasculitis MØ5.2Ø
    - ankle MØ5.27-
    - elbow MØ5.22-
    - foot joint MØ5.27-
    - hand joint MØ5.24-
    - hip MØ5.25-
    - knee MØ5.26-
    - multiple site MØ5.29
    - shoulder MØ5.21-
    - vertebra —*see* Spondylitis, ankylosing
    - wrist MØ5.23-
- **Rhinitis** (atrophic) (catarrhal) (chronic) (croupous) (fibrinous) (granulomatous) (hyperplastic) (hypertrophic) (membranous) (obstructive) (purulent) (suppurative) (ulcerative) J31.Ø
  - with
    - sore throat —*see* Nasopharyngitis
  - acute JØØ
  - allergic J3Ø.9
    - with asthma J45.9Ø9
      - with
        - exacerbation (acute) J45.9Ø1
        - status asthmaticus J45.9Ø2
    - due to
      - food J3Ø.5
      - pollen J3Ø.1
    - nonseasonal J3Ø.89
    - perennial J3Ø.89
    - seasonal NEC J3Ø.2
    - specified NEC J3Ø.89
  - infective JØØ
  - pneumococcal JØØ
  - syphilitic A52.73
    - congenital A5Ø.Ø5 *[J99]*
  - tuberculous A15.8
  - vasomotor J3Ø.Ø
- **Rhinoantritis** (chronic) —*see* Sinusitis, maxillary
- **Rhinodacryolith** —*see* Dacryolith
- **Rhinolith** (nasal sinus) J34.89
- **Rhinomegaly** J34.89
- **Rhinopharyngitis** (acute) (subacute) —*see also* Nasopharyngitis
  - chronic J31.1
  - destructive ulcerating A66.5
  - mutilans A66.5
- **Rhinophyma** L71.1
- **Rhinorrhea** J34.89
  - cerebrospinal (fluid) G96.Ø
  - paroxysmal —*see* Rhinitis, allergic
  - spasmodic —*see* Rhinitis, allergic
- **Rhinosalpingitis** —*see* Salpingitis, eustachian
- **Rhinoscleroma** A48.8
- **Rhinosporidiosis** B48.1
- **Rhinovirus infection NEC** B34.8
- **Rhizomelic chondrodysplasia punctata** E71.54Ø
- **Rhythm**
  - atrioventricular nodal I49.8
  - disorder I49.9
    - coronary sinus I49.8
    - ectopic I49.8
    - nodal I49.8
  - escape I49.9
  - heart, abnormal I49.9
  - idioventricular I44.2
  - nodal I49.8
  - sleep, inversion G47.2-
    - nonorganic origin —*see* Disorder, sleep, circadian rhythm, psychogenic
- **Rhytidosis facialis** L98.8
- **Rib** —*see also* condition
  - cervical Q76.5
- **Riboflavin deficiency** E53.Ø
- **Rice bodies** —*see also* Loose, body, joint
  - knee M23.4-
- **Richter syndrome** —*see* Leukemia, chronic lymphocytic, B-cell type
- **Richter's hernia** —*see* Hernia, abdomen, with obstruction
- **Ricinism** —*see* Poisoning, food, noxious, plant
- **Rickets** (active) (acute) (adolescent) (chest wall) (congenital) (current) (infantile) (intestinal) E55.Ø
  - adult —*see* Osteomalacia
  - celiac K9Ø.Ø
  - hypophosphatemic with nephrotic-glycosuric dwarfism E72.Ø9
  - inactive E64.3
  - kidney N25.Ø
  - renal N25.Ø
  - sequelae, any E64.3
  - vitamin-D-resistant E83.31 *[M9Ø.8Ø]*
- **Rickettsial disease** A79.9
  - specified type NEC A79.89
- **Rickettsialpox** (Rickettsia akari) A79.1
- **Rickettsiosis** A79.9
  - due to
    - Ehrlichia sennetsu A79.81
    - Rickettsia akari (rickettsialpox) A79.1
  - specified type NEC A79.89
  - tick-borne A77.9
  - vesicular A79.1
- **Rider's bone** —*see* Ossification, muscle, specified NEC
- **Ridge, alveolus** —*see also* condition
  - flabby KØ6.8
- **Ridged ear, congenital** Q17.3
- **Riedel's**
  - lobe, liver Q44.7
  - struma, thyroiditis or disease EØ6.5
- **Rieger's anomaly or syndrome** Q13.81
- **Riehl's melanosis** L81.4
- **Rietti-Greppi-Micheli anemia** D56.9
- **Rieux's hernia** —*see* Hernia, abdomen, specified site NEC
- **Riga** (-Fede) **disease** K14.Ø
- **Riggs' disease** —*see* Periodontitis
- **Right aortic arch** Q25.47 ◄
- **Right middle lobe syndrome** J98.11
- **Rigid, rigidity** —*see also* condition
  - abdominal R19.3Ø
    - with severe abdominal pain R1Ø.Ø
    - epigastric R19.36
    - generalized R19.37
    - left lower quadrant R19.34
    - left upper quadrant R19.32
    - periumbilic R19.35
    - right lower quadrant R19.33
    - right upper quadrant R19.31
  - articular, multiple, congenital Q68.8
  - cervix (uteri) in pregnancy —*see* Pregnancy, complicated by, abnormal, cervix
  - hymen (acquired) (congenital) N89.6
  - nuchal R29.1
  - pelvic floor in pregnancy —*see* Pregnancy, complicated by, abnormal, pelvic organs or tissues NEC
  - perineum or vulva in pregnancy —*see* Pregnancy, complicated by, abnormal, vulva
  - spine —*see* Dorsopathy, specified NEC
  - vagina in pregnancy —*see* Pregnancy, complicated by, abnormal, vagina
- **Rigors** R68.89
  - with fever R5Ø.9
- **Riley-Day syndrome** G9Ø.1
- **RIND** (reversible ischemic neurologic deficit) I63.9
- **Ring** (s)
  - aorta (vascular) Q25.45 ⟸
  - Bandl's O62.4
  - contraction, complicating delivery O62.4
- **Ring** (s) *(Continued)*
  - esophageal, lower (muscular) K22.2
  - Fleischer's (cornea) H18.Ø4-
  - hymenal, tight (acquired) (congenital) N89.6
  - Kayser-Fleischer (cornea) H18.Ø4-
  - retraction, uterus, pathological O62.4
  - Schatzki's (esophagus) (lower) K22.2
    - congenital Q39.3
  - Soemmerring's —*see* Cataract, secondary
  - vascular (congenital) Q25.8
    - aorta Q25.45 ⟸
- **Ringed hair** (congenital) Q84.1
- **Ringworm** B35.9
  - beard B35.Ø
  - black dot B35.Ø
  - body B35.4
  - Burmese B35.5
  - corporeal B35.4
  - foot B35.3
  - groin B35.6
  - hand B35.2
  - honeycomb B35.Ø
  - nails B35.1
  - perianal (area) B35.6
  - scalp B35.Ø
  - specified NEC B35.8
  - Tokelau B35.5
- **Rise, venous pressure** I87.8
- **Rising, PSA following treatment for malignant neoplasm of prostate** R97.21 ◄
- **Risk, suicidal**
  - meaning personal history of attempted suicide Z91.5
  - meaning suicidal ideation —*see* Ideation, suicidal
- **Ritter's disease** LØØ
- **Rivalry, sibling** Z62.891
- **Rivalta's disease** A42.2
- **River blindness** B73.Ø1
- **Robert's pelvis** Q74.2
  - with disproportion (fetopelvic) O33.Ø
    - causing obstructed labor O65.Ø
- **Robin** (-Pierre) **syndrome** Q87.Ø
- **Robinow-Silvermann-Smith syndrome** Q87.1
- **Robinson's** (hidrotic) **ectodermal dysplasia or syndrome** Q82.4
- **Robles' disease** B73.Ø1
- **Rocky Mountain** (spotted) **fever** A77.Ø
- **Roetheln** —*see* Rubella
- **Roger's disease** Q21.Ø
- **Rokitansky-Aschoff sinuses** (gallbladder) K82.8
- **Rolando's fracture** (displaced) S62.22-
  - nondisplaced S62.22-
- **Romano-Ward** (prolonged QT interval) **syndrome** I45.81
- **Romberg's disease or syndrome** G51.8
- **Roof, mouth** —*see* condition
- **Rosacea** L71.9
  - acne L71.9
  - keratitis L71.8
  - specified NEC L71.8
- **Rosary, rachitic** E55.Ø
- **Rose**
  - cold J3Ø.1
  - fever J3Ø.1
  - rash R21
    - epidemic BØ6.9
- **Rosenbach's erysipeloid** A26.Ø
- **Rosenthal's disease or syndrome** D68.1
- **Roseola** BØ9
  - infantum BØ8.2Ø
    - due to human herpesvirus 6 BØ8.21
    - due to human herpesvirus 7 BØ8.22
- **Ross River disease or fever** B33.1
- **Rossbach's disease** K31.89
  - psychogenic F45.8
- **Rostan's asthma** (cardiac) —*see* Failure, ventricular, left
- **Rotation**
  - anomalous, incomplete or insufficient, intestine Q43.3

- **Rotation** *(Continued)*
  - cecum (congenital) Q43.3
  - colon (congenital) Q43.3
  - spine, incomplete or insufficient —*see* Dorsopathy, deforming, specified NEC
  - tooth, teeth, fully erupted M26.35
  - vertebra, incomplete or insufficient —*see* Dorsopathy, deforming, specified NEC
- **Rotes Quérol disease or syndrome** —*see* Hyperostosis, ankylosing
- **Roth** (-Bernhardt) **disease or syndrome** —*see* Meralgia paraesthetica
- **Rothmund** (-Thomson) **syndrome** Q82.8
- **Rotor's disease or syndrome** E80.6
- **Round**
  - back (with wedging of vertebrae) —*see* Kyphosis
    - sequelae (late effect) of rickets E64.3
  - worms (large) (infestation) NEC B82.Ø
    - Ascariasis —*see also* Ascariasis B77.9
- **Roussy-Lévy syndrome** G6Ø.Ø
- **Rubella** (German measles) BØ6.9
  - complication NEC BØ6.Ø9
    - neurological BØ6.ØØ
  - congenital P35.Ø
  - contact Z2Ø.4
  - exposure to Z2Ø.4
  - maternal
    - care for (suspected) damage to fetus O35.3
    - manifest rubella in infant P35.Ø
    - suspected damage to fetus affecting management of pregnancy O35.3
  - specified complications NEC BØ6.89
- **Rubeola** (meaning measles) —*see* Measles
  - meaning rubella —*see* Rubella
- **Rubeosis, iris** —*see* Disorder, iris, vascular
- **Rubinstein-Taybi syndrome** Q87.2
- **Rudimentary** (congenital) —*see also* Agenesis
  - arm —*see* Defect, reduction, upper limb
  - bone Q79.9
  - cervix uteri Q51.828
  - eye Q11.2
  - lobule of ear Q17.3
  - patella Q74.1
  - respiratory organs in thoracopagus Q89.4
  - tracheal bronchus Q32.4
  - uterus Q51.818
    - in male Q56.1
  - vagina Q52.Ø
- **Ruled out condition** —*see* Observation, suspected
- **Rumination** R11.1Ø
  - with nausea R11.2
  - disorder of infancy F98.21
  - neurotic F42.8 ⬅
  - newborn P92.1
  - obsessional F42.8 ⬅
  - psychogenic F42.8 ⬅
- **Runeberg's disease** D51.Ø
- **Runny nose** RØ9.89
- **Rupia** (syphilitic) A51.39
  - congenital A5Ø.Ø6
  - tertiary A52.79
- **Rupture, ruptured**
  - abscess (spontaneous) - code by site under Abscess
  - aneurysm —*see* Aneurysm
  - anus (sphincter) —*see* Laceration, anus
  - aorta, aortic I71.8
    - abdominal I71.3
    - arch I71.1
    - ascending I71.1
    - descending I71.8
      - abdominal I71.3
      - thoracic I71.1
    - syphilitic A52.Ø1
    - thoracoabdominal I71.5
    - thorax, thoracic I71.1
    - transverse I71.1
    - traumatic —*see* Injury, aorta, laceration, major

- **Rupture, ruptured** *(Continued)*
  - aorta, aortic *(Continued)*
    - valve or cusp —*see also* Endocarditis, aortic I35.8
  - appendix (with peritonitis) K35.2
    - with localized peritonitis K35.3 ◀
  - arteriovenous fistula, brain I6Ø.8
  - artery I77.2
    - brain —*see* Hemorrhage, intracranial, intracerebral
    - coronary —*see* Infarct, myocardium
    - heart —*see* Infarct, myocardium
    - pulmonary I28.8
    - traumatic (complication) —*see* Injury, blood vessel
  - bile duct (common) (hepatic) K83.2
    - cystic K82.2
  - bladder (sphincter) (nontraumatic) (spontaneous) N32.89
    - following ectopic or molar pregnancy OØ8.6
    - obstetrical trauma O71.5
    - traumatic S37.29
  - blood vessel —*see also* Hemorrhage
    - brain —*see* Hemorrhage, intracranial, intracerebral
    - heart —*see* Infarct, myocardium
    - traumatic (complication) —*see* Injury, blood vessel, laceration, major, by site
  - bone —*see* Fracture
  - bowel (nontraumatic) K63.1
  - brain
    - aneurysm (congenital) —*see also* Hemorrhage, intracranial, subarachnoid
      - syphilitic A52.Ø5
    - hemorrhagic —*see* Hemorrhage, intracranial, intracerebral
  - capillaries I78.8
  - cardiac (auricle) (ventricle) (wall) I23.3
    - with hemopericardium I23.Ø
    - infectional I4Ø.9
    - traumatic —*see* Injury, heart
  - cartilage (articular) (current) —*see also* Sprain
    - knee S83.3-
    - semilunar —*see* Tear, meniscus
  - cecum (with peritonitis) K65.Ø
    - with peritoneal abscess K35.3
    - traumatic S36.598
  - celiac artery, traumatic —*see* Injury, blood vessel, celiac artery, laceration, major
  - cerebral aneurysm (congenital) (*see* Hemorrhage, intracranial, subarachnoid)
  - cervix (uteri)
    - with ectopic or molar pregnancy OØ8.6
    - following ectopic or molar pregnancy OØ8.6
    - obstetrical trauma O71.3
    - traumatic S37.69
  - chordae tendineae NEC I51.1
    - concurrent with acute myocardial infarction —*see* Infarct, myocardium
    - following acute myocardial infarction (current complication) I23.4
  - choroid (direct) (indirect) (traumatic) H31.32-
  - circle of Willis I6Ø.6
  - colon (nontraumatic) K63.1
    - traumatic —*see* Injury, intestine, large
  - cornea (traumatic) —*see* Injury, eye, laceration
  - coronary (artery) (thrombotic) —*see* Infarct, myocardium
  - corpus luteum (infected) (ovary) N83.1- ⬅
  - cyst —*see* Cyst
  - cystic duct K82.2
  - Descemet's membrane —*see* Change, corneal membrane, Descemet's, rupture
    - traumatic —*see* Injury, eye, laceration
  - diaphragm, traumatic —*see* Injury, intrathoracic, diaphragm
  - disc —*see* Rupture, intervertebral disc

- **Rupture, ruptured** *(Continued)*
  - diverticulum (intestine) K57.8Ø
    - with bleeding K57.81
    - bladder N32.3
    - large intestine K57.2Ø
      - with
        - bleeding K57.21
        - small intestine K57.4Ø
          - with bleeding K57.41
    - small intestine K57.ØØ
      - with
        - bleeding K57.Ø1
        - large intestine K57.4Ø
          - with bleeding K57.41
  - duodenal stump K31.89
  - ear drum (nontraumatic) —*see also* Perforation, tympanum
    - traumatic SØ9.2-
      - due to blast injury —*see* Injury, blast, ear
  - esophagus K22.3
  - eye (without prolapse or loss of intraocular tissue) —*see* Injury, eye, laceration
  - fallopian tube NEC (nonobstetric) (nontraumatic) N83.8
    - due to pregnancy OØØ.1Ø ⬅
      - with intrauterine pregnancy OØØ.11 ◀
  - fontanel P13.1
  - gallbladder K82.2
    - traumatic S36.128
  - gastric —*see also* Rupture, stomach
    - vessel K92.2
  - globe (eye) (traumatic) —*see* Injury, eye, laceration
  - graafian follicle (hematoma) N83.Ø- ⬅
  - heart —*see* Rupture, cardiac
  - hymen (nontraumatic) (nonintentional) N89.8
  - internal organ, traumatic —*see* Injury, by site
  - intervertebral disc —*see* Displacement, intervertebral disc
    - traumatic —*see* Rupture, traumatic, intervertebral disc
  - intestine NEC (nontraumatic) K63.1
    - traumatic —*see* Injury, intestine
  - iris —*see also* Abnormality, pupillary
    - traumatic —*see* Injury, eye, laceration
  - joint capsule, traumatic —*see* Sprain
  - kidney (traumatic) S37.Ø6-
    - birth injury P15.8
    - nontraumatic N28.89
  - lacrimal duct (traumatic) —*see* Injury, eye, specified site NEC
  - lens (cataract) (traumatic) —*see* Cataract, traumatic
  - ligament, traumatic —*see* Rupture, traumatic, ligament, by site
  - liver S36.116
    - birth injury P15.Ø
  - lymphatic vessel I89.8
  - marginal sinus (placental) (with hemorrhage) —*see* Hemorrhage, antepartum, specified cause NEC
  - membrana tympani (nontraumatic) —*see* Perforation, tympanum
  - membranes (spontaneous)
    - artificial
      - delayed delivery following O75.5
    - delayed delivery following —*see* Pregnancy, complicated by, premature rupture of membranes
  - meningeal artery I6Ø.8
  - meniscus (knee) —*see also* Tear, meniscus
    - old —*see* Derangement, meniscus
    - site other than knee - code as Sprain
  - mesenteric artery, traumatic —*see* Injury, mesenteric, artery, laceration, major
  - mesentery (nontraumatic) K66.8
    - traumatic —*see* Injury, intra-abdominal, specified, site NEC
  - mitral (valve) I34.8

Rupture, ruptured *(Continued)*
muscle (traumatic) —*see also* Strain
diastasis —*see* Diastasis, muscle
nontraumatic M62.10
ankle M62.17-
foot M62.17-
forearm M62.13-
hand M62.14-
lower leg M62.16-
pelvic region M62.15-
shoulder region M62.11-
specified site NEC M62.18
thigh M62.15-
upper arm M62.12-
traumatic —*see* Strain, by site
musculotendinous junction NEC, nontraumatic —*see* Rupture, tendon, spontaneous
mycotic aneurysm causing cerebral hemorrhage —*see* Hemorrhage, intracranial, subarachnoid
myocardium, myocardial —*see* Rupture, cardiac
traumatic —*see* Injury, heart
nontraumatic, meaning hernia —*see* Hernia
obstructed —*see* Hernia, by site, obstructed
operation wound —*see* Disruption, wound, operation
ovary, ovarian N83.8
corpus luteum cyst N83.1- ◀▮
follicle (graafian) N83.0- ◀▮
oviduct (nonobstetric) (nontraumatic) N83.8
due to pregnancy O00.10 ◀▮
with intrauterine pregnancy O00.11 ◀
pancreas (nontraumatic) K86.89 ◀▮
traumatic S36.299
papillary muscle NEC I51.2
following acute myocardial infarction (current complication) I23.5
pelvic
floor, complicating delivery O70.1
organ NEC, obstetrical trauma O71.5
perineum (nonobstetric) (nontraumatic) N90.89
complicating delivery —*see* Delivery, complicated, by, laceration, anus (sphincter)
postoperative wound —*see* Disruption, wound, operation
prostate (traumatic) S37.828
pulmonary
artery I28.8
valve (heart) I37.8
vein I28.8
vessel I28.8
pus tube —*see* Salpingitis
pyosalpinx —*see* Salpingitis
rectum (nontraumatic) K63.1
traumatic S36.69
retina, retinal (traumatic) (without detachment) —*see also* Break, retina
with detachment —*see* Detachment, retina, with retinal, break
rotator cuff (nontraumatic) M75.10-
complete M75.12-
incomplete M75.11-
sclera —*see* Injury, eye, laceration
sigmoid (nontraumatic) K63.1
traumatic S36.593
spinal cord —*see also* Injury, spinal cord, by region
due to injury at birth P11.5
newborn (birth injury) P11.5
spleen (traumatic) S36.09
birth injury P15.1
congenital (birth injury) P15.1
due to P. vivax malaria B51.0
nontraumatic D73.5
spontaneous D73.5

Rupture, ruptured *(Continued)*
splenic vein R58
traumatic —*see* Injury, blood vessel, splenic vein
stomach (nontraumatic) (spontaneous) K31.89
traumatic S36.39
supraspinatus (complete) (incomplete) (nontraumatic) —*see* Tear, rotator cuff
symphysis pubis
obstetric O71.6
traumatic S33.4
synovium (cyst) M66.10
ankle M66.17-
elbow M66.12-
finger M66.14-
foot M66.17-
forearm M66.13-
hand M66.14-
pelvic region M66.15-
shoulder region M66.11-
specified site NEC M66.18
thigh M66.15-
toe M66.17-
upper arm M66.12-
wrist M66.13-
tendon (traumatic) —*see* Strain
nontraumatic (spontaneous) M66.9
ankle M66.87-
extensor M66.20
ankle M66.27-
foot M66.27-
forearm M66.23-
hand M66.24-
lower leg M66.26-
multiple sites M66.29
pelvic region M66.25-
shoulder region M66.21-
specified site NEC M66.28
thigh M66.25-
upper arm M66.22-
flexor M66.30
ankle M66.37-
foot M66.37-
forearm M66.33-
hand M66.34-
lower leg M66.36-
multiple sites M66.39
pelvic region M66.35-
shoulder region M66.31-
specified site NEC M66.38
thigh M66.35-
upper arm M66.32-
foot M66.87-
forearm M66.83-
hand M66.84-
lower leg M66.86-
multiple sites M66.89
pelvic region M66.85-
shoulder region M66.81-
specified
site NEC M66.88
tendon M66.80
thigh M66.85-
upper arm M66.82-
thoracic duct I89.8
tonsil J35.8
traumatic
aorta —*see* Injury, aorta, laceration, major
diaphragm —*see* Injury, intrathoracic, diaphragm
external site —*see* Wound, open, by site
eye —*see* Injury, eye, laceration
internal organ —*see* Injury, by site
intervertebral disc
cervical S13.0
lumbar S33.0
thoracic S23.0

Rupture, ruptured *(Continued)*
traumatic *(Continued)*
kidney S37.06-
ligament —*see also* Sprain
ankle —*see* Sprain, ankle
carpus —*see* Rupture, traumatic, ligament, wrist
collateral (hand) —*see* Rupture, traumatic, ligament, finger, collateral
finger (metacarpophalangeal) (interphalangeal) S63.40-
collateral S63.41-
index S63.41-
little S63.41-
middle S63.41-
ring S63.41-
index S63.40-
little S63.40-
middle S63.40-
palmar S63.42-
index S63.42-
little S63.42-
middle S63.42-
ring S63.42-
ring S63.40-
specified site NEC S63.499
index S63.49-
little S63.49-
middle S63.49-
ring S63.49-
volar plate S63.43-
index S63.43-
little S63.43-
middle S63.43-
ring S63.43-
foot —*see* Sprain, foot
radial collateral S53.2-
radiocarpal —*see* Rupture, traumatic, ligament, wrist, radiocarpal
ulnar collateral S53.3-
ulnocarpal —*see* Rupture, traumatic, ligament, wrist, ulnocarpal
wrist S63.30-
collateral S63.31-
radiocarpal S63.32-
specified site NEC S63.39-
ulnocarpal (palmar) S63.33-
liver S36.116
membrana tympani —*see* Rupture, ear drum, traumatic
muscle or tendon —*see* Strain
myocardium —*see* Injury, heart
pancreas S36.299
rectum S36.69
sigmoid S36.593
spleen S36.09
stomach S36.39
symphysis pubis S33.4
tympanum, tympanic (membrane) —*see* Rupture, ear drum, traumatic
ureter S37.19
uterus S37.69
vagina —*see* Injury, vagina
vena cava —*see* Injury, vena cava, laceration, major
tricuspid (heart) (valve) I07.8
tube, tubal (nonobstetric) (nontraumatic) N83.8
abscess —*see* Salpingitis
due to pregnancy O00.10 ◀▮
with intrauterine pregnancy O00.11 ◀
tympanum, tympanic (membrane) (nontraumatic) —*see also* Perforation, tympanic membrane H72.9-
traumatic —*see* Rupture, ear drum, traumatic
umbilical cord, complicating delivery O69.89
ureter (traumatic) S37.19
nontraumatic N28.89

R

Rupture, ruptured *(Continued)*
urethra (nontraumatic) N36.8
with ectopic or molar pregnancy O08.6
following ectopic or molar pregnancy O08.6
obstetrical trauma O71.5
traumatic S37.39
uterosacral ligament (nonobstetric) (nontraumatic) N83.8
uterus (traumatic) S37.69
before labor O71.0-
during or after labor O71.1

Rupture, ruptured *(Continued)*
uterus *(Continued)*
nonpuerperal, nontraumatic N85.8
pregnant (during labor) O71.1
before labor O71.0-
vagina —*see* Injury, vagina
valve, valvular (heart) —*see* Endocarditis
varicose vein —*see* Varix
varix —*see* Varix
vena cava R58
traumatic —*see* Injury, vena cava, laceration, major
vesical (urinary) N32.89

Rupture, ruptured *(Continued)*
vessel (blood) R58
pulmonary I28.8
traumatic —*see* Injury, blood vessel
viscus R19.8
vulva complicating delivery O70.0
Russell-Silver syndrome Q87.1
Russian spring-summer type encephalitis A84.0
Rust's disease (tuberculous cervical spondylitis) A18.01
Ruvalcaba-Myhre-Smith syndrome E71.440
Rytand-Lipsitch syndrome I44.2

R

◄ New ⟸ Revised ~~deleted~~ Deleted

S

Saber, sabre shin or tibia (syphilitic) A50.56 *[M90.8-]*
Sac lacrimal —*see* condition
Saccharomyces infection B37.9
Saccharopinuria E72.3
Saccular —*see* condition
Sacculation
aorta (nonsyphilitic) —*see* Aneurysm, aorta
bladder N32.3
intralaryngeal (congenital) (ventricular) Q31.3
larynx (congenital) (ventricular) Q31.3
organ or site, congenital —*see* Distortion
pregnant uterus —*see* Pregnancy, complicated by, abnormal, uterus
ureter N28.89
urethra N36.1
vesical N32.3
Sachs' amaurotic familial idiocy or disease E75.02
Sachs-Tay disease E75.02
Sacks-Libman disease M32.11
Sacralgia M53.3
Sacralization Q76.49
Sacrodynia M53.3
Sacroiliac joint —*see* condition
Sacroiliitis NEC M46.1
Sacrum —*see* condition
Saddle
back —*see* Lordosis
embolus
abdominal aorta I74.01
pulmonary artery I26.92
with acute cor pulmonale I26.02
injury — code to condition
nose M95.0
due to syphilis A50.57
Sadism (sexual) F65.52
Sadness, postpartal O90.6
Sadomasochism F65.50
Saemisch's ulcer (cornea) —*see* Ulcer, cornea, central
Sagging ◀
skin and subcutaneous tissue (following bariatric surgery weight loss) (following dietary weight loss) L98.7 ◀
Sahib disease B55.0
Sailors' skin L57.8
Saint
Anthony's fire —*see* Erysipelas
triad —*see* Hernia, diaphragm
Vitus' dance —*see* Chorea, Sydenham's
Salaam
attack (s) —*see* Epilepsy, spasms
tic R25.8
Salicylism
abuse F55.8
overdose or wrong substance given —*see* Table of Drugs and Chemicals, by drug, poisoning
Salivary duct or gland —*see* condition
Salivation, excessive K11.7
Salmonella —*see* Infection, Salmonella
Salmonellosis A02.0
Salpingitis (catarrhal) (fallopian tube) (nodular) (pseudofollicular) (purulent) (septic) N70.91
with oophoritis N70.93
acute N70.01
with oophoritis N70.03
chlamydial A56.11
chronic N70.11
with oophoritis N70.13
complicating abortion —*see* Abortion, by type, complicated by, salpingitis
ear —*see* Salpingitis, eustachian
eustachian (tube) H68.00-
acute H68.01-
chronic H68.02-
Salpingitis *(Continued)*
follicularis N70.11
with oophoritis N70.13
gonococcal (acute) (chronic) A54.24
interstitial, chronic N70.11
with oophoritis N70.13
isthmica nodosa N70.11
with oophoritis N70.13
specific (gonococcal) (acute) (chronic) A54.24
tuberculous (acute) (chronic) A18.17
venereal (gonococcal) (acute) (chronic) A54.24
Salpingocele N83.4- ⬅
Salpingo-oophoritis (catarrhal) (purulent) (ruptured) (septic) (suppurative) N70.93
acute N70.03
with ectopic or molar pregnancy O08.0
following ectopic or molar pregnancy O08.0
gonococcal A54.24
chronic N70.13
following ectopic or molar pregnancy O08.0
gonococcal (acute) (chronic) A54.24
puerperal O86.19
specific (gonococcal) (acute) (chronic) A54.24
subacute N70.03
tuberculous (acute) (chronic) A18.17
venereal (gonococcal) (acute) (chronic) A54.24
Salpingo-ovaritis —*see* Salpingo-oophoritis
Salpingoperitonitis —*see* Salpingo-oophoritis
Salzmann's nodular dystrophy —*see* Degeneration, cornea, nodular
Sampson's cyst or tumor N80.1
San Joaquin (Valley) **fever** B38.0
Sandblaster's asthma, lung or pneumoconiosis J62.8
Sander's disease (paranoia) F22
Sandfly fever A93.1
Sandhoff's disease E75.01
Sanfilippo (Type B) (Type C) (Type D) **syndrome** E76.22
Sanger-Brown ataxia G11.2
Sao Paulo fever or typhus A77.0
Saponification, mesenteric K65.8
Sarcocele (benign)
syphilitic A52.76
congenital A50.59
Sarcocystosis A07.8
Sarcoepiplocele —*see* Hernia
Sarcoepiplomphalocele Q79.2
Sarcoid —*see also* Sarcoidosis
arthropathy D86.86
Boeck's D86.9
Darier-Roussy D86.3
iridocyclitis D86.83
meningitis D86.81
myocarditis D86.85
myositis D86.87
pyelonephritis D86.84
Spiegler-Fendt L08.89
Sarcoidosis D86.9
with
cranial nerve palsies D86.82
hepatic granuloma D86.89
polyarthritis D86.86
tubulo-interstitial nephropathy D86.84
combined sites NEC D86.89
lung D86.0
and lymph nodes D86.2
lymph nodes D86.1
and lung D86.2
meninges D86.81
skin D86.3
specified type NEC D86.89
Sarcoma (of) —*see also* Neoplasm, connective tissue, malignant
alveolar soft part —*see* Neoplasm, connective tissue, malignant
ameloblastic C41.1
upper jaw (bone) C41.0
botryoid —*see* Neoplasm, connective tissue, malignant
Sarcoma *(Continued)*
botryoides —*see* Neoplasm, connective tissue, malignant
cerebellar C71.6
circumscribed (arachnoidal) C71.6
circumscribed (arachnoidal) cerebellar C71.6
clear cell —*see also* Neoplasm, connective tissue, malignant
kidney C64.-
dendritic cells (accessory cells) C96.4
embryonal —*see* Neoplasm, connective tissue, malignant
endometrial (stromal) C54.1
isthmus C54.0
epithelioid (cell) —*see* Neoplasm, connective tissue, malignant
Ewing's —*see* Neoplasm, bone, malignant
follicular dendritic cell C96.4
germinoblastic (diffuse) —*see* Lymphoma, diffuse, large cell
follicular —*see* Lymphoma, follicular, specified NEC
giant cell (except of bone) —*see also* Neoplasm, connective tissue, malignant
bone —*see* Neoplasm, bone, malignant
glomoid —*see* Neoplasm, connective tissue, malignant
granulocytic C92.3-
hemangioendothelial —*see* Neoplasm, connective tissue, malignant
hemorrhagic, multiple —*see* Sarcoma, Kaposi's
histiocytic C96.A
Hodgkin —*see* Lymphoma, Hodgkin
immunoblastic (diffuse) —*see* Lymphoma, diffuse large cell
interdigitating dendritic cell C96.4
Kaposi's
colon C46.4
connective tissue C46.1
gastrointestinal organ C46.4
lung C46.5-
lymph node (s) C46.3
palate (hard) (soft) C46.2
rectum C46.4
skin C46.0
specified site NEC C46.7
stomach C46.4
unspecified site C46.9
Kupffer cell C22.3
Langerhans cell C96.4
leptomeningeal —*see* Neoplasm, meninges, malignant
liver NEC C22.4
lymphangioendothelial —*see* Neoplasm, connective tissue, malignant
lymphoblastic —*see* Lymphoma, lymphoblastic (diffuse)
lymphocytic —*see* Lymphoma, small cell B-cell
mast cell C96.2
melanotic —*see* Melanoma
meningeal —*see* Neoplasm, meninges, malignant
meningothelial —*see* Neoplasm, meninges, malignant
mesenchymal —*see also* Neoplasm, connective tissue, malignant
mixed —*see* Neoplasm, connective tissue, malignant
mesothelial —*see* Mesothelioma
monstrocellular
specified site —*see* Neoplasm, malignant, by site
unspecified site C71.9
myeloid C92.3-
neurogenic —*see* Neoplasm, nerve, malignant
odontogenic C41.1
upper jaw (bone) C41.0

S

Sarcoma *(Continued)*
- osteoblastic —*see* Neoplasm, bone, malignant
- osteogenic —*see also* Neoplasm, bone, malignant
  - juxtacortical —*see* Neoplasm, bone, malignant
  - periosteal —*see* Neoplasm, bone, malignant
- periosteal —*see also* Neoplasm, bone, malignant
  - osteogenic —*see* Neoplasm, bone, malignant
- pleomorphic cell —*see* Neoplasm, connective tissue, malignant
- reticulum cell (diffuse) —*see* Lymphoma, diffuse large cell
  - nodular —*see* Lymphoma, follicular
  - pleomorphic cell type —*see* Lymphoma, diffuse large cell
- rhabdoid —*see* Neoplasm, malignant, by site
- round cell —*see* Neoplasm, connective tissue, malignant
- small cell —*see* Neoplasm, connective tissue, malignant
- soft tissue —*see* Neoplasm, connective tissue, malignant
- spindle cell —*see* Neoplasm, connective tissue, malignant
- stromal (endometrial) C54.1
  - isthmus C54.Ø
- synovial —*see also* Neoplasm, connective tissue, malignant
  - biphasic —*see* Neoplasm, connective tissue, malignant
  - epithelioid cell —*see* Neoplasm, connective tissue, malignant
  - spindle cell —*see* Neoplasm, connective tissue, malignant

Sarcomatosis
- meningeal —*see* Neoplasm, meninges, malignant
- specified site NEC —*see* Neoplasm, connective tissue, malignant
- unspecified site C8Ø.1

Sarcopenia (age-related) M62.84 ◀
Sarcosinemia E72.59
Sarcosporidiosis (intestinal) AØ7.8
Satiety, early R68.81
Saturnine —*see* condition
Saturnism
- overdose or wrong substance given or taken —*see* Table of Drugs and Chemicals, by drug, poisoning

Satyriasis F52.8
Sauriasis —*see* Ichthyosis
SBE (subacute bacterial endocarditis) I33.Ø
Scabies (any site) B86
Scabs R23.4
Scaglietti-Dagnini syndrome E22.Ø
Scald —*see* Burn
Scalenus anticus (anterior) **syndrome** G54.Ø
Scales R23.4
Scaling, skin R23.4
Scalp —*see* condition
Scapegoating affecting child Z62.3
Scaphocephaly Q75.Ø
Scapulalgia M89.8X1
Scapulohumeral myopathy G71.Ø
Scar, scarring —*see also* Cicatrix L9Ø.5
- adherent L9Ø.5
- atrophic L9Ø.5
- cervix
  - in pregnancy or childbirth —*see* Pregnancy, complicated by, abnormal cervix
- cheloid L91.Ø
- chorioretinal H31.ØØ-
  - posterior pole macula H31.Ø1-
  - postsurgical H59.81-
  - solar retinopathy H31.Ø2-
  - specified type NEC H31.Ø9-

Scar, scarring *(Continued)*
- choroid —*see* Scar, chorioretinal
- conjunctiva H11.24-
- cornea H17.9
  - xerophthalmic —*see also* Opacity, cornea
    - vitamin A deficiency E5Ø.6
- duodenum, obstructive K31.5
- hypertrophic L91.Ø
- keloid L91.Ø
- labia N9Ø.89
- lung (base) J98.4
- macula —*see* Scar, chorioretinal, posterior pole
- muscle M62.89
- myocardium, myocardial I25.2
- painful L9Ø.5
- posterior pole (eye) —*see* Scar, chorioretinal, posterior pole
- retina —*see* Scar, chorioretinal
- trachea J39.8
- transmural uterine, in pregnancy O34.29 ◀
- uterus N85.8
  - in pregnancy O34.29
- vagina N89.8
  - postoperative N99.2
- vulva N9Ø.89

Scarabiasis B88.2
Scarlatina (anginosa) (maligna) (ulcerosa) A38.9
- myocarditis (acute) A38.1
  - old —*see* Myocarditis
- otitis media A38.Ø

Scarlet fever (albuminuria) (angina) A38.9
Schamberg's disease (progressive pigmentary dermatosis) L81.7
Schatzki's ring (acquired) (esophagus) (lower) K22.2
- congenital Q39.3

Schaufenster krankheit I2Ø.8
Schaumann's
- benign lymphogranulomatosis D86.1
- disease or syndrome —*see* Sarcoidosis

Scheie's syndrome E76.Ø3
Schenck's disease B42.1
Scheuermann's disease or osteochondrosis —*see* Osteochondrosis, juvenile, spine
Schilder (-Flatau) **disease** G37.Ø
Schilling-type monocytic leukemia C93.Ø-
Schimmelbusch's disease, cystic mastitis, or hyperplasia —*see* Mastopathy, cystic
Schistosoma infestation —*see* Infestation, Schistosoma
Schistosomiasis B65.9
- with muscle disorder B65.9 *[M63.8Ø]*
  - ankle B65.9 *[M63.87-]*
  - foot B65.9 *[M63.87-]*
  - forearm B65.9 *[M63.83-]*
  - hand B65.9 *[M63.84-]*
  - lower leg B65.9 *[M63.86-]*
  - multiple sites B65.9 *[M63.89]*
  - pelvic region B65.9 *[M63.85-]*
  - shoulder region B65.9 *[M63.81-]*
  - specified site NEC B65.9 *[M63.88]*
  - thigh B65.9 *[M63.85-]*
  - upper arm B65.9 *[M63.82-]*
- Asiatic B65.2
- bladder B65.Ø
- chestermani B65.8
- colon B65.1
- cutaneous B65.3
- due to
  - S. haematobium B65.Ø
  - S. japonicum B65.2
  - S. mansoni B65.1
  - S. mattheii B65.8
- Eastern B65.2
- genitourinary tract B65.Ø
- intestinal B65.1
- lung NEC B65.9 *[J99]*
  - pneumonia B65.9 *[J17]*
- Manson's (intestinal) B65.1

Schistosomiasis *(Continued)*
- oriental B65.2
- pulmonary NEC B65.9 *[J99]*
  - pneumonia B65.9
- Schistosoma
  - haematobium B65.Ø
  - japonicum B65.2
  - mansoni B65.1
- specified type NEC B65.8
- urinary B65.Ø
- vesical B65.Ø

Schizencephaly QØ4.6
Schizoaffective psychosis F25.9
Schizodontia KØØ.2
Schizoid personality F6Ø.1
Schizophrenia, schizophrenic F2Ø.9
- acute (brief) (undifferentiated) F23
- atypical (form) F2Ø.3
- borderline F21
- catalepsy F2Ø.2
- catatonic (type) (excited) (withdrawn) F2Ø.2
- cenesthopathic, cenesthesiopathic F2Ø.89
- childhood type F84.5
- chronic undifferentiated F2Ø.5
- cyclic F25.Ø
- disorganized (type) F2Ø.1
- flexibilitas cerea F2Ø.2
- hebephrenic (type) F2Ø.1
- incipient F21
- latent F21
- negative type F2Ø.5
- paranoid (type) F2Ø.Ø
- paraphrenic F2Ø.Ø
- post-psychotic depression F32.89 ⬅
- prepsychotic F21
- prodromal F21
- pseudoneurotic F21
- pseudopsychopathic F21
- reaction F23
- residual (state) (type) F2Ø.5
- restzustand F2Ø.5
- schizoaffective (type) —*see* Psychosis, schizoaffective
- simple (type) F2Ø.89
- simplex F2Ø.89
- specified type NEC F2Ø.89
- stupor F2Ø.2
- syndrome of childhood F84.5
- undifferentiated (type) F2Ø.3
  - chronic F2Ø.5

Schizothymia (persistent) F6Ø.1
Schlatter-Osgood disease or osteochondrosis —*see* Osteochondrosis, juvenile, tibia
Schlatter's tibia —*see* Osteochondrosis, juvenile, tibia
Schmidt's syndrome (polyglandular, autoimmune) E31.Ø
Schmincke's carcinoma or tumor —*see* Neoplasm, nasopharynx, malignant
Schmitz (-Stutzer) **dysentery** AØ3.Ø
Schmorl's disease or nodes
- lumbar region M51.46
- lumbosacral region M51.47
- sacrococcygeal region M53.3
- thoracic region M51.44
- thoracolumbar region M51.45

Schneiderian
- papilloma —*see* Neoplasm, nasopharynx benign
  - specified site —*see* Neoplasm, benign, by site
  - unspecified site D14.Ø
- specified site —*see* Neoplasm, malignant, by site
- unspecified site C3Ø.Ø

Scholte's syndrome (malignant carcinoid) E34.Ø
Scholz (-Bielchowsky-Henneberg) **disease or syndrome** E75.25
Schönlein (-Henoch) **disease or purpura** (primary) (rheumatic) D69.Ø

Schottmuller's disease A01.4
Schroeder's syndrome (endocrine hypertensive) E27.0
Schüller-Christian disease or syndrome C96.5
Schultze's type acroparesthesia, simple I73.89
Schultz's disease or syndrome —*see* Agranulocytosis
Schwalbe-Ziehen-Oppenheim disease G24.1
Schwannoma —*see also* Neoplasm, nerve, benign
  malignant —*see also* Neoplasm, nerve, malignant
    with rhabdomyoblastic differentiation —*see* Neoplasm, nerve, malignant
  melanocytic —*see* Neoplasm, nerve, benign
  pigmented —*see* Neoplasm, nerve, benign
Schwannomatosis Q85.03
Schwartz (-Jampel) syndrome G71.13
Schwartz-Bartter syndrome E22.2
Schweniger-Buzzi anetoderma L90.1
Sciatic —*see* condition
Sciatica (infective)
  with lumbago M54.4-
    due to intervertebral disc disorder —*see* Disorder, disc, with, radiculopathy
  due to displacement of intervertebral disc (with lumbago) —*see* Disorder, disc, with, radiculopathy
  wallet M54.3-
Scimitar syndrome Q26.8
Sclera —*see* condition
Sclerectasia H15.84-
Scleredema
  adultorum —*see* Sclerosis, systemic
  Buschke's —*see* Sclerosis, systemic
  newborn P83.0
Sclerema (adiposum) (edematosum) (neonatorum) (newborn) P83.0
  adultorum —*see* Sclerosis, systemic
Scleriasis —*see* Scleroderma
Scleritis H15.00-
  with corneal involvement H15.04-
  anterior H15.01-
  brawny H15.02-
  in (due to) zoster B02.34
  posterior H15.03-
  specified type NEC H15.09-
  syphilitic A52.71
  tuberculous (nodular) A18.51
Sclerochoroiditis H31.8
Scleroconjunctivitis —*see* Scleritis
Sclerocystic ovary syndrome E28.2
Sclerodactyly, sclerodactylia L94.3
Scleroderma, sclerodermia (acrosclerotic) (diffuse) (generalized) (progressive) (pulmonary) —*see also* Sclerosis, systemic M34.9-
  circumscribed L94.0
  linear L94.1
  localized L94.0
  newborn P83.8
  systemic M34.9
Sclerokeratitis H16.8
  tuberculous A18.52
Scleroma nasi A48.8
Scleromalacia (perforans) H15.05-
Scleromyxedema L98.5
Sclérose en plaques G35
Sclerosis, sclerotic
  adrenal (gland) E27.8
  Alzheimer's —*see* Disease, Alzheimer's
  amyotrophic (lateral) G12.21
  aorta, aortic I70.0
    valve —*see* Endocarditis, aortic
  artery, arterial, arteriolar, arteriovascular —*see* Arteriosclerosis
  ascending multiple G35
  brain (generalized) (lobular) G37.9
    artery, arterial I67.2
    diffuse G37.0
    disseminated G35

Sclerosis, sclerotic *(Continued)*
  brain *(Continued)*
    insular G35
    Krabbe's E75.23
    miliary G35
    multiple G35
    presenile (Alzheimer's) —*see* Disease, Alzheimer's, early onset
    senile (arteriosclerotic) I67.2
    stem, multiple G35
    tuberous Q85.1
  bulbar, multiple G35
  bundle of His I44.39
  cardiac —*see* Disease, heart, ischemic, atherosclerotic
  cardiorenal —*see* Hypertension, cardiorenal
  cardiovascular —*see also* Disease, cardiovascular
    renal —*see* Hypertension, cardiorenal
  cerebellar —*see* Sclerosis, brain
  cerebral —*see* Sclerosis, brain
  cerebrospinal (disseminated) (multiple) G35
  cerebrovascular I67.2
  choroid —*see* Degeneration, choroid
  combined (spinal cord) —*see also* Degeneration, combined
    multiple G35
  concentric (Balo) G37.5
  cornea —*see* Opacity, cornea
  coronary (artery) I25.10
    with angina pectoris —*see* Arteriosclerosis, coronary (artery),
  corpus cavernosum
    female N90.89
    male N48.6
  diffuse (brain) (spinal cord) G37.0
  disseminated G35
  dorsal G35
  dorsolateral (spinal cord) —*see* Degeneration, combined
  endometrium N85.5
  extrapyramidal G25.9
  eye, nuclear (senile) —*see* Cataract, senile, nuclear
  focal and segmental (glomerular) —*see also* N00-N07 with fourth character .1 N05.1
  Friedreich's (spinal cord) G11.1
  funicular (spermatic cord) N50.89 (Revised)
  general (vascular) —*see* Arteriosclerosis
  gland (lymphatic) I89.8
  hepatic K74.1
    alcoholic K70.2
  hereditary
    cerebellar G11.9
    spinal (Friedreich's ataxia) G11.1
  hippocampal G93.81
  insular G35
  kidney —*see* Sclerosis, renal
  larynx J38.7
  lateral (amyotrophic) (descending) (primary) (spinal) G12.21
  lens, senile nuclear —*see* Cataract, senile, nuclear
  liver K74.1
    with fibrosis K74.2
      alcoholic K70.2
    alcoholic K70.2
    cardiac K76.1
  lung —*see* Fibrosis, lung
  mastoid —*see* Mastoiditis, chronic
  mesial temporal G93.81
  mitral I05.8
  Mönckeberg's (medial) —*see* Arteriosclerosis, extremities
  multiple (brain stem) (cerebral) (generalized) (spinal cord) G35
  myocardium, myocardial —*see* Disease, heart, ischemic, atherosclerotic
  nuclear (senile), eye —*see* Cataract, senile, nuclear

Sclerosis, sclerotic *(Continued)*
  ovary N83.8
  pancreas K86.89 (Revised)
  penis N48.6
  peripheral arteries —*see* Arteriosclerosis, extremities
  plaques G35
  pluriglandular E31.8
  polyglandular E31.8
  posterolateral (spinal cord) —*see* Degeneration, combined
  presenile (Alzheimer's) —*see* Disease, Alzheimer's, early onset
  primary, lateral G12.29
  progressive, systemic M34.0
  pulmonary —*see* Fibrosis, lung
    artery I27.0
    valve (heart) —*see* Endocarditis, pulmonary
  renal N26.9
    with
      cystine storage disease E72.09
      hypertensive heart disease (conditions in I11) —*see* Hypertension, cardiorenal
    arteriolar (hyaline) (hyperplastic) —*see* Hypertension, kidney
  retina (senile) (vascular) H35.00
  senile (vascular) —*see* Arteriosclerosis
  spinal (cord) (progressive) G95.89
    ascending G61.0
    combined —*see also* Degeneration, combined
      multiple G35
      syphilitic A52.11
    disseminated G35
    dorsolateral —*see* Degeneration, combined
    hereditary (Friedreich's) (mixed form) G11.1
    lateral (amyotrophic) G12.21
    multiple G35
    posterior (syphilitic) A52.11
  stomach K31.89
  subendocardial, congenital I42.4
  systemic M34.9
    with
      lung involvement M34.81
      myopathy M34.82
      polyneuropathy M34.83
    drug-induced M34.2
    due to chemicals NEC M34.2
    progressive M34.0
    specified NEC M34.89
  temporal (mesial) G93.81
  tricuspid (heart) (valve) I07.8
  tuberous (brain) Q85.1
  tympanic membrane —*see* Disorder, tympanic membrane, specified NEC
  valve, valvular (heart) —*see* Endocarditis
  vascular —*see* Arteriosclerosis
  vein I87.8
Scoliosis (acquired) (postural) M41.9
  adolescent (idiopathic) —*see* Scoliosis, idiopathic, adolescent (Revised)
  congenital Q67.5
    due to bony malformation Q76.3
    failure of segmentation (hemivertebra) Q76.3
    hemivertebra fusion Q76.3
    postural Q67.5
  idiopathic M41.20
    adolescent M41.129
      cervical region M41.122
      cervicothoracic region M41.123
      lumbar region M41.126
      lumbosacral region M41.127
      thoracic region M41.124
      thoracolumbar region M41.125
    cervical region M41.22
    cervicothoracic region M41.23

S

Scoliosis *(Continued)*
idiopathic *(Continued)*
infantile M41.ØØ
cervical region M41.Ø2
cervicothoracic region M41.Ø3
lumbar region M41.Ø6
lumbosacral region M41.Ø7
sacrococcygeal region M41.Ø8
thoracic region M41.Ø4
thoracolumbar region M41.Ø5
juvenile M41.119
cervical region M41.112
cervicothoracic region M41.113
lumbar region M41.116
lumbosacral region M41.117
thoracic region M41.114
thoracolumbar region M41.115
lumbar region M41.26
lumbosacral region M41.27
thoracic region M41.24
thoracolumbar region M41.25
infantile *—see* Scoliosis, idiopathic, infantile ◀
neuromuscular M41.4Ø
cervical region M41.42
cervicothoracic region M41.43
lumbar region M41.46
lumbosacral region M41.47
occipito-atlanto-axial region M41.41
thoracic region M41.44
thoracolumbar region M41.45
paralytic *—see* Scoliosis, neuromuscular
postradiation therapy M96.5
rachitic (late effect or sequelae) E64.3 *[M49.8Ø]*
cervical region E64.3 *[M49.82]*
cervicothoracic region E64.3 *[M49.83]*
lumbar region E64.3 *[M49.86]*
lumbosacral region E64.3 *[M49.87]*
multiple sites E64.3 *[M49.89]*
occipito-atlanto-axial region E64.3 *[M49.81]*
sacrococcygeal region E64.3 *[M49.88]*
thoracic region E64.3 *[M49.84]*
thoracolumbar region E64.3 *[M49.85]*
sciatic M54.4-
secondary (to) NEC M41.5Ø
cerebral palsy, Friedreich's ataxia, poliomyelitis, neuromuscular disorders *—see* Scoliosis, neuromuscular
cervical region M41.52
cervicothoracic region M41.53
lumbar region M41.56
lumbosacral region M41.57
thoracic region M41.54
thoracolumbar region M41.55
specified form NEC M41.8Ø
cervical region M41.82
cervicothoracic region M41.83
lumbar region M41.86
lumbosacral region M41.87
thoracic region M41.84
thoracolumbar region M41.85
thoracogenic M41.3Ø
thoracic region M41.34
thoracolumbar region M41.35
tuberculous A18.Ø1
Scoliotic pelvis
with disproportion (fetopelvic) O33.Ø
causing obstructed labor O65.Ø
Scorbutus, scorbutic *—see also* Scurvy
anemia D53.2
Score, NIHSS (National Institutes of Health Stroke Scale) R29.7- ◀
Scotoma (arcuate) (Bjerrum) (central) (ring) *—see also* Defect, visual field, localized, scotoma
scintillating H53.19
Scratch *—see* Abrasion
Scratchy throat RØ9.89
Screening (for) Z13.9
alcoholism Z13.89
anemia Z13.Ø
anomaly, congenital Z13.89
antenatal, of mother Z36
arterial hypertension Z13.6
arthropod-borne viral disease NEC Z11.59
bacteriuria, asymptomatic Z13.89
behavioral disorder Z13.89
brain injury, traumatic Z13.85Ø
bronchitis, chronic Z13.83
brucellosis Z11.2
cardiovascular disorder Z13.6
cataract Z13.5
chlamydial diseases Z11.8
cholera Z11.Ø
chromosomal abnormalities (nonprocreative) NEC Z13.79
colonoscopy Z12.11
congenital
dislocation of hip Z13.89
eye disorder Z13.5
malformation or deformation Z13.89
contamination NEC Z13.88
cystic fibrosis Z13.228
dengue fever Z11.59
dental disorder Z13.84
depression Z13.89
developmental handicap Z13.42 ⇐
in early childhood Z13.42 ⇐
infant Z13.41 ◀
diabetes mellitus Z13.1
diphtheria Z11.2
disability, intellectual Z13.42 ⇐
infant Z13.41 ◀
disease or disorder Z13.9
bacterial NEC Z11.2
intestinal infectious Z11.Ø
respiratory tuberculosis Z11.1
blood or blood-forming organ Z13.Ø
cardiovascular Z13.6
Chagas' Z11.6
chlamydial Z11.8
dental Z13.89
developmental Z13.42 ⇐
in child Z13.42 ◀
infant Z13.41 ◀
digestive tract NEC Z13.818
lower GI Z13.811
upper GI Z13.81Ø
ear Z13.5
endocrine Z13.29
eye Z13.5
genitourinary Z13.89
heart Z13.6
human immunodeficiency virus (HIV) infection Z11.4
immunity Z13.Ø
infection
intestinal Z11.Ø
specified NEC Z11.6
infectious Z11.9
mental Z13.89
metabolic Z13.228
neurological Z13.89
nutritional Z13.21
metabolic Z13.228
lipoid disorders Z13.22Ø
protozoal Z11.6
intestinal Z11.Ø
respiratory Z13.83
rheumatic Z13.828
rickettsial Z11.8
sexually-transmitted NEC Z11.3
human immunodeficiency virus (HIV) Z11.4
sickle-cell (trait) Z13.Ø
skin Z13.89
specified NEC Z13.89
spirochetal Z11.8
thyroid Z13.29
Screening *(Continued)*
disease or disorder *(Continued)*
vascular Z13.6
venereal Z11.3
viral NEC Z11.59
human immunodeficiency virus (HIV) Z11.4
intestinal Z11.Ø
elevated titer Z13.89
emphysema Z13.83
encephalitis, viral (mosquito- or tick-borne) Z11.59
exposure to contaminants (toxic) Z13.88
fever
dengue Z11.59
hemorrhagic Z11.59
yellow Z11.59
filariasis Z11.6
galactosemia Z13.228
gastrointestinal condition Z13.818
genetic (nonprocreative)- for procreative management *—see* Testing, genetic, for procreative management
disease carrier status (nonprocreative) Z13.71
specified NEC (nonprocreative) Z13.79
genitourinary condition Z13.89
glaucoma Z13.5
gonorrhea Z11.3
gout Z13.89
helminthiasis (intestinal) Z11.6
hematopoietic malignancy Z12.89
hemoglobinopathies NEC Z13.Ø
hemorrhagic fever Z11.59
Hodgkin disease Z12.89
human immunodeficiency virus (HIV) Z11.4
human papillomavirus Z11.51
hypertension Z13.6
immunity disorders Z13.Ø
infection
mycotic Z11.8
parasitic Z11.8
ingestion of radioactive substance Z13.88
intellectual disability Z13.42 ⇐
infant Z13.41 ◀
intestinal
helminthiasis Z11.6
infectious disease Z11.Ø
leishmaniasis Z11.6
leprosy Z11.2
leptospirosis Z11.8
leukemia Z12.89
lymphoma Z12.89
malaria Z11.6
malnutrition Z13.29
metabolic Z13.228
nutritional Z13.21
measles Z11.59
mental disorder Z13.89
metabolic errors, inborn Z13.228
multiphasic Z13.89
musculoskeletal disorder Z13.828
osteoporosis Z13.82Ø
mycoses Z11.8
myocardial infarction (acute) Z13.6
neoplasm (malignant) (of) Z12.9
bladder Z12.6
blood Z12.89
breast Z12.39
routine mammogram Z12.31
cervix Z12.4
colon Z12.11
genitourinary organs NEC Z12.79
bladder Z12.6
cervix Z12.4
ovary Z12.73
prostate Z12.5
testis Z12.71
vagina Z12.72
hematopoietic system Z12.89

Screening *(Continued)*
neoplasm *(Continued)*
intestinal tract Z12.10
colon Z12.11
rectum Z12.12
small intestine Z12.13
lung Z12.2
lymph (glands) Z12.89
nervous system Z12.82
oral cavity Z12.81
prostate Z12.5
rectum Z12.12
respiratory organs Z12.2
skin Z12.83
small intestine Z12.13
specified site NEC Z12.89
stomach Z12.0
nephropathy Z13.89
nervous system disorders NEC Z13.858
neurological condition Z13.89
osteoporosis Z13.820
parasitic infestation Z11.9
specified NEC Z11.8
phenylketonuria Z13.228
plague Z11.2
poisoning (chemical) (heavy metal) Z13.88
poliomyelitis Z11.59
postnatal, chromosomal abnormalities Z13.89
prenatal, of mother Z36
protozoal disease Z11.6
intestinal Z11.0
pulmonary tuberculosis Z11.1
radiation exposure Z13.88
respiratory condition Z13.83
respiratory tuberculosis Z11.1
rheumatoid arthritis Z13.828
rubella Z11.59
schistosomiasis Z11.6
sexually-transmitted disease NEC Z11.3
human immunodeficiency virus (HIV) Z11.4
sickle-cell disease or trait Z13.0
skin condition Z13.89
sleeping sickness Z11.6
special Z13.9
specified NEC Z13.89
syphilis Z11.3
tetanus Z11.2
trachoma Z11.8
traumatic brain injury Z13.850
trypanosomiasis Z11.6
tuberculosis, respiratory Z11.1
venereal disease Z11.3
viral encephalitis (mosquito- or tick-borne) Z11.59
whooping cough Z11.2
worms, intestinal Z11.6
yaws Z11.8
yellow fever Z11.59
Scrofula, scrofulosis (tuberculosis of cervical lymph glands) A18.2
Scrofulide (primary) (tuberculous) A18.4
Scrofuloderma, scrofulodermia (any site) (primary) A18.4
Scrofulosus lichen (primary) (tuberculous) A18.4
Scrofulous —*see* condition
Scrotal tongue K14.5
Scrotum —*see* condition
Scurvy, scorbutic E54
anemia D53.2
gum E54
infantile E54
rickets E55.0 *[M90.80]*
Sealpox B08.62
Seasickness T75.3
Seatworm (infection) (infestation) B80
Sebaceous —*see also* condition
cyst —*see* Cyst, sebaceous
Seborrhea, seborrheic L21.9
capillitii R23.8
capitis L21.0
dermatitis L21.9
infantile L21.1
eczema L21.9
infantile L21.1
sicca L21.0
Seckel's syndrome Q87.1
Seclusion, pupil —*see* Membrane, pupillary
Second hand tobacco smoke exposure (acute) (chronic) Z77.22
in the perinatal period P96.81
Secondary
dentin (in pulp) K04.3
neoplasm, secondaries —*see* Table of Neoplasms, secondary
Secretion
antidiuretic hormone, inappropriate E22.2
catecholamine, by pheochromocytoma E27.5
hormone
antidiuretic, inappropriate (syndrome) E22.2
by
carcinoid tumor E34.0
pheochromocytoma E27.5
ectopic NEC E34.2
urinary
excessive R35.8
suppression R34
Section
nerve, traumatic —*see* Injury, nerve
Sedative, hypnotic, or anxiolytic-induced ◀
anxiety disorder F13.980 ◀
bipolar and related disorder F13.94 ◀
delirium F13.921 ◀
depressive disorder F13.94 ◀
major neurocognitive disorder F13.97 ◀
mild neurocognitive disorder F13.988 ◀
psychotic disorder F13.959 ◀
sexual dysfunction F13.981 ◀
sleep disorder F13.982 ◀
Segmentation, incomplete (congenital) —*see also* Fusion
bone NEC Q78.8
lumbosacral (joint) (vertebra) Q76.49
Seitelberger's syndrome (infantile neuraxonal dystrophy) G31.89
Seizure(s) —*see also* Convulsions R56.9
akinetic —*see* Epilepsy, generalized, specified NEC
atonic —*see* Epilepsy, generalized, specified NEC
autonomic (hysterical) F44.5
convulsive —*see* Convulsions
cortical (focal) (motor) —*see* Epilepsy, localization-related, symptomatic, with simple partial seizures
disorder —*see also* Epilepsy G40.909
due to stroke —*see* Sequelae (of), disease, cerebrovascular, by type, specified NEC
epileptic —*see* Epilepsy
febrile (simple) R56.00
with status epilepticus G40.901
complex (atypical) (complicated) R56.01
with status epilepticus G40.901
grand mal G40.409
intractable G40.419
with status epilepticus G40.411
without status epilepticus G40.419
not intractable G40.409
with status epilepticus G40.401
without status epilepticus G40.409
heart —*see* Disease, heart
hysterical F44.5
intractable G40.919
with status epilepticus G40.911
Jacksonian (focal) (motor type) (sensory type) —*see* Epilepsy, localization-related, symptomatic, with simple partial seizures
Seizure *(Continued)*
newborn P90
nonspecific epileptic
atonic —*see* Epilepsy, generalized, specified NEC
clonic —*see* Epilepsy, generalized, specified NEC
myoclonic —*see* Epilepsy, generalized, specified NEC
tonic —*see* Epilepsy, generalized, specified NEC
tonic-clonic —*see* Epilepsy, generalized, specified NEC
partial, developing into secondarily generalized seizures
complex —*see* Epilepsy, localization-related, symptomatic, with complex partial seizures
simple —*see* Epilepsy, localization-related, symptomatic, with simple partial seizures
petit mal G40.409
intractable G40.419
with status epilepticus G40.411
without status epilepticus G40.419
not intractable G40.409
with status epilepticus G40.401
without status epilepticus G40.409
post traumatic R56.1
recurrent G40.909
specified NEC G40.89
uncinate —*see* Epilepsy, localization-related, symptomatic, with complex partial seizures
Selenium deficiency, dietary E59
Self-damaging behavior (life-style) Z72.89
Self-harm (attempted)
history (personal) Z91.5
in family Z81.8
Self-mutilation (attempted)
history (personal) Z91.5
in family Z81.8
Self-poisoning
history (personal) Z91.5
in family Z81.8
observation following (alleged) attempt Z03.6
Semicoma R40.1
Seminal vesiculitis N49.0
Seminoma C62.9-
specified site —*see* Neoplasm, malignant, by site
Senear-Usher disease or syndrome L10.4
Senectus R54
Senescence (without mention of psychosis) R54
Senile, senility —*see also* condition R41.81
with
acute confusional state F05
mental changes NOS F03
psychosis NEC —*see* Psychosis, senile
asthenia R54
cervix (atrophic) N88.8
debility R54
endometrium (atrophic) N85.8
fallopian tube (atrophic) —*see* Atrophy, fallopian tube
heart (failure) R54
ovary (atrophic) —*see* Atrophy, ovary
premature E34.8
vagina, vaginitis (atrophic) N95.2
wart L82.1
Sensation
burning (skin) R20.8
tongue K14.6
loss of R20.8
prickling (skin) R20.2
tingling (skin) R20.2
Sense loss
smell —*see* Disturbance, sensation, smell
taste —*see* Disturbance, sensation, taste
touch R20.8

S

- **Sensibility disturbance** (cortical) (deep) (vibratory) R20.9
- **Sensitive, sensitivity** —*see also* Allergy
  - carotid sinus G90.01
  - child (excessive) F93.8
  - cold, autoimmune D59.1
  - dentin K03.89
  - gluten (non-celiac) K90.41 ◀
  - latex Z91.040
  - methemoglobin D74.8
  - tuberculin, without clinical or radiological symptoms R76.11
  - visual
    - glare H53.71
    - impaired contrast H53.72
- **Sensitiver Beziehungswahn** F22
- **Sensitization, auto-erythrocytic** D69.2
- **Separation**
  - anxiety, abnormal (of childhood) F93.0
  - apophysis, traumatic - code as Fracture, by site
  - choroid —*see* Detachment, choroid
  - epiphysis, epiphyseal
    - nontraumatic —*see also* Osteochondropathy, specified type NEC
      - upper femoral —*see* Slipped, epiphysis, upper femoral
    - traumatic - code as Fracture, by site
  - fracture —*see* Fracture
  - infundibulum cardiac from right ventricle by a partition Q24.3
  - joint (traumatic) (current) - code by site under Dislocation
  - pubic bone, obstetrical trauma O71.6
  - retina, retinal —*see* Detachment, retina
  - symphysis pubis, obstetrical trauma O71.6
  - tracheal ring, incomplete, congenital Q32.1
- **Sepsis** (generalized) (unspecified organism) A41.9
  - with
    - organ dysfunction (acute) (multiple) R65.20
      - with septic shock R65.21
  - actinomycotic A42.7
  - adrenal hemorrhage syndrome (meningococcal) A39.1
  - anaerobic A41.4
  - Bacillus anthracis A22.7
  - Brucella —*see also* Brucellosis A23.9
  - candidal B37.7
  - cryptogenic A41.9
  - due to device, implant or graft T85.79
    - arterial graft NEC T82.7
    - breast (implant) T85.79
    - catheter NEC T85.79
      - dialysis (renal) T82.7
        - intraperitoneal T85.71
      - infusion NEC T82.7
        - spinal (cranial) (epidural) (intrathecal) (spinal) (subarachnoid) (subdural) T85.735 ⬅
      - urethral indwelling T83.511 ◀
      - urinary T83.518 ⬅
    - ectopic or molar pregnancy O08.82
    - electronic (electrode) (pulse generator) (stimulator)
      - bone T84.7
      - cardiac T82.7
      - nervous system T85.738 ⬅
        - brain T85.731 ◀
        - neurostimulator generator T85.734 ◀
        - peripheral nerve T85.732 ◀
        - spinal cord T85.733 ◀
      - urinary T83.590 ⬅
    - fixation, internal (orthopedic) —*see* Complication, fixation device, infection
    - gastrointestinal (bile duct) (esophagus) T85.79
      - neurostimulator electrode (lead) T85.732 ◀

Sepsis *(Continued)*
  - due to device, implant or graft *(Continued)*
    - genital T83.69 ⬅
    - heart NEC T82.7
      - valve (prosthesis) T82.6
        - graft T82.7
    - joint prosthesis —*see* Complication, joint prosthesis, infection
    - ocular (corneal graft) (orbital implant) T85.79
    - orthopedic NEC T84.7
      - fixation device, internal —*see* Complication, fixation device, infection
    - specified NEC T85.79
    - vascular T82.7
    - ~~ventricular intracranial shunt T85.79~~
    - ventricular intracranial (communicating) shunt T85.730 ◀
  - during labor O75.3
  - Enterococcus A41.81
  - Erysipelothrix (rhusiopathiae) (erysipeloid) A26.7
  - Escherichia coli (E. coli) A41.5
  - extraintestinal yersiniosis A28.2
  - following
    - abortion (subsequent episode) O08.0
      - current episode —*see* Abortion
    - ectopic or molar pregnancy O08.82
    - immunization T88.0
    - infusion, therapeutic injection or transfusion NEC T80.29
  - gangrenous A41.9
  - gonococcal A54.86
  - Gram-negative (organism) A41.5
    - anaerobic A41.4
  - Haemophilus influenzae A41.3
  - herpesviral B00.7
  - intra-abdominal K65.1
  - intraocular —*see* Endophthalmitis, purulent
  - Listeria monocytogenes A32.7
  - localized — code to specific localized infection
    - in operation wound T81.49 ⬅
    - skin —*see* Abscess
  - malleus A24.0
  - melioidosis A24.1
  - meningeal —*see* Meningitis
  - meningococcal A39.4
    - acute A39.2
    - chronic A39.3
  - MSSA (Methicillin susceptible Staphylococcus aureus) A41.01
  - newborn P36.9
    - due to
      - anaerobes NEC P36.5
      - Escherichia coli P36.4
      - Staphylococcus P36.30
        - aureus P36.2
        - specified NEC P36.39
      - Streptococcus P36.10
        - group B P36.0
        - specified NEC P36.19
    - specified NEC P36.8
  - Pasteurella multocida A28.0
  - pelvic, puerperal, postpartum, childbirth O85
  - pneumococcal A40.3
  - postprocedural T81.49 ⬅
  - puerperal, postpartum, childbirth (pelvic) O85
  - Salmonella (arizonae) (cholerae-suis) (enteritidis) (typhimurium) A02.1
  - severe R65.20
    - with septic shock R65.21
  - Shigella (*see also* Dysentery, bacillary) A03.9
  - skin, localized —*see* Abscess
  - specified organism NEC A41.89
  - Staphylococcus, staphylococcal A41.2
    - aureus (methicillin susceptible) (MSSA) A41.01
      - methicillin resistant (MRSA) A41.02

Sepsis *(Continued)*
  - Staphylococcus, staphylococcal *(Continued)*
    - coagulase-negative A41.1
    - specified NEC A41.1
  - Streptococcus, streptococcal A40.9
    - agalactiae A40.1
    - group
      - A A40.0
      - B A40.1
      - D A41.81
    - neonatal P36.10
      - group B P36.0
      - specified NEC P36.19
    - pneumoniae A40.3
    - pyogenes A40.0
    - specified NEC A40.8
  - tracheostomy stoma J95.02
  - tularemic A21.7
  - umbilical, umbilical cord (newborn) —*see* Sepsis, newborn
  - Yersinia pestis A20.7
- **Septate** —*see* Septum
- **Septic** —*see* condition
  - arm —*see* Cellulitis, upper limb
    - with lymphangitis —*see* Lymphangitis, acute, upper limb
  - embolus —*see* Embolism
  - finger —*see* Cellulitis, digit
    - with lymphangitis —*see* Lymphangitis, acute, digit
  - foot —*see* Cellulitis, lower limb
    - with lymphangitis —*see* Lymphangitis, acute, lower limb
  - gallbladder (acute) K81.0
  - hand —*see* Cellulitis, upper limb
    - with lymphangitis —*see* Lymphangitis, acute, upper limb
  - joint —*see* Arthritis, pyogenic or pyemic
  - leg —*see* Cellulitis, lower limb
    - with lymphangitis —*see* Lymphangitis, acute, lower limb
  - nail —*see also* Cellulitis, digit
    - with lymphangitis —*see* Lymphangitis, acute, digit
  - sore —*see also* Abscess
    - throat J02.0
      - streptococcal J02.0
  - spleen (acute) D73.89
  - teeth, tooth (pulpal origin) K04.4
  - throat —*see* Pharyngitis
  - thrombus —*see* Thrombosis
  - toe —*see* Cellulitis, digit
    - with lymphangitis —*see* Lymphangitis, acute, digit
  - tonsils, chronic J35.01
    - with adenoiditis J35.03
  - uterus —*see* Endometritis
- **Septicemia** A41.9
  - meaning sepsis —*see* Sepsis
- **Septum, septate** (congenital) —*see also* Anomaly, by site
  - anal Q42.3
    - with fistula Q42.2
  - aqueduct of Sylvius Q03.0
    - with spina bifida —*see* Spina bifida, by site, with hydrocephalus
  - uterus (complete) (partial) Q51.2
  - vagina Q52.10
    - in pregnancy —*see* Pregnancy, complicated by, abnormal vagina
      - causing obstructed labor O65.5
    - longitudinal Q52.129 ⬅
      - microperforate ◀
        - left side Q52.124 ◀
        - right side Q52.123 ◀
      - nonobstruction Q52.120 ◀
      - obstructing Q52.129 ◀
        - left side Q52.122 ◀
        - right side Q52.121 ◀
    - transverse Q52.11

S

◀ New ⬅ Revised ~~deleted~~ Deleted

Sequelae (of) —*see also* condition
abscess, intracranial or intraspinal (conditions in G06) G09
amputation — code to injury with seventh character S
burn and corrosion — code to injury with seventh character S
calcium deficiency E64.8
cerebrovascular disease —*see* Sequelae, disease, cerebrovascular
childbirth O94
contusion — code to injury with seventh character S
corrosion —*see* Sequelae, burn and corrosion
crushing injury — code to injury with seventh character S
disease
cerebrovascular I69.90
alteration of sensation I69.998
aphasia I69.920
apraxia I69.990
ataxia I69.993
cognitive deficits I69.91
disturbance of vision I69.998
dysarthria I69.922
dysphagia I69.991
dysphasia I69.921
facial droop I69.992
facial weakness I69.992
fluency disorder I69.923
hemiplegia I69.95-
hemorrhage
intracerebral —*see* Sequelae, hemorrhage, intracerebral
intracranial, nontraumatic NEC —*see* Sequelae, hemorrhage, intracranial, nontraumatic
subarachnoid —*see* Sequelae, hemorrhage, subarachnoid
language deficit I69.928
monoplegia
lower limb I69.84-
upper limb I69.93-
paralytic syndrome I69.96-
specified effect NEC I69.998
specified type NEC I69.80
alteration of sensation I69.898
aphasia I69.820
apraxia I69.890
ataxia I69.893
cognitive deficits I69.81
disturbance of vision I69.898
dysarthria I69.822
dysphagia I69.891
dysphasia I69.821
facial droop I69.892
facial weakness I69.892
fluency disorder I69.823
hemiplegia I69.85-
language deficit I69.828
monoplegia
lower limb I69.84-
upper limb I69.83-
paralytic syndrome I69.86-
specified effect NEC I69.898
speech deficit I69.928
speech deficit I69.828
stroke NOS —*see* Sequelae, stroke NOS
dislocation — code to injury with seventh character S
encephalitis or encephalomyelitis (conditions in G04) G09
in infectious disease NEC B94.8
viral B94.1
external cause — code to injury with seventh character S
foreign body entering natural orifice — code to injury with seventh character S
fracture — code to injury with seventh character S

Sequelae *(Continued)*
frostbite — code to injury with seventh character S
Hansen's disease B92
hemorrhage
intracerebral I69.10
alteration of sensation I69.198
aphasia I69.120
apraxia I69.190
ataxia I69.193
cognitive deficits I69.11
disturbance of vision I69.198
dysarthria I69.122
dysphagia I69.191
dysphasia I69.121
facial droop I69.192
facial weakness I69.192
fluency disorder I69.123
hemiplegia I69.15-
language deficit NEC I69.128
monoplegia
lower limb I69.14-
upper limb I69.13-
paralytic syndrome I69.16-
specified effect NEC I69.198
speech deficit NEC I69.128
intracranial, nontraumatic NEC I69.20
alteration of sensation I69.298
aphasia I69.220
apraxia I69.290
ataxia I69.293
cognitive deficits I69.21
disturbance of vision I69.298
dysarthria I69.222
dysphagia I69.291
dysphasia I69.221
facial droop I69.292
facial weakness I69.292
fluency disorder I69.223
hemiplegia I69.25-
language deficit NEC I69.228
monoplegia
lower limb I69.24-
upper limb I69.23-
paralytic syndrome I69.26-
specified effect NEC I69.298
speech deficit NEC I69.228
subarachnoid I69.00
alteration of sensation I69.098
aphasia I69.020
apraxia I69.090
ataxia I69.093
cognitive deficits —*see* subcategory I69.01- ⬅
disturbance of vision I69.098
dysarthria I69.022
dysphagia I69.091
dysphasia I69.021
facial droop I69.092
facial weakness I69.092
fluency disorder I69.023
hemiplegia I69.05-
language deficit NEC I69.028
monoplegia
lower limb I69.04-
upper limb I69.03-
paralytic syndrome I69.06-
specified effect NEC I69.098
speech deficit NEC I69.028
hepatitis, viral B94.2
hyperalimentation E68
infarction
cerebral I69.30
alteration of sensation I69.398
aphasia I69.320
apraxia I69.390
ataxia I69.393
cognitive deficits I69.31
disturbance of vision I69.398
dysarthria I69.322
dysphagia I69.391

Sequelae *(Continued)*
infarction *(Continued)*
cerebral *(Continued)*
dysphasia I69.321
facial droop I69.392
facial weakness I69.392
fluency disorder I69.323
hemiplegia I69.35-
language deficit NEC I69.328
monoplegia
lower limb I69.34-
upper limb I69.33-
paralytic syndrome I69.36-
specified effect NEC I69.398
speech deficit NEC I69.328
infection, pyogenic, intracranial or intraspinal G09
infectious disease B94.9
specified NEC B94.8
injury — code to injury with seventh character S
leprosy B92
meningitis
bacterial (conditions in G00) G09
other or unspecified cause (conditions in G03) G09
muscle (and tendon) injury — code to injury with seventh character S
myelitis —*see* Sequelae, encephalitis
niacin deficiency E64.8
nutritional deficiency E64.9
specified NEC E64.8
obstetrical condition O94
parasitic disease B94.9
phlebitis or thrombophlebitis of intracranial or intraspinal venous sinuses and veins (conditions in G08) G09
poisoning — code to poisoning with seventh character S
nonmedicinal substance —*see* Sequelae, toxic effect, nonmedicinal substance
poliomyelitis (acute) B91
pregnancy O94
protein-energy malnutrition E64.0
puerperium O94
rickets E64.3
selenium deficiency E64.8
sprain and strain — code to injury with seventh character S
stroke NOS I69.30
alteration in sensation I69.398
aphasia I69.320
apraxia I69.390
ataxia I69.393
cognitive deficits I69.31
disturbance of vision I69.398
dysarthria I69.322
dysphagia I69.391
dysphasia I69.321
facial droop I69.392
facial weakness I69.392
hemiplegia I69.35-
language deficit NEC I69.328
monoplegia
lower limb I69.34-
upper limb I69.33-
paralytic syndrome I69.36-
specified effect NEC I69.398
speech deficit NEC I69.328
tendon and muscle injury — code to injury with seventh character S
thiamine deficiency E64.8
trachoma B94.0
tuberculosis B90.9
bones and joints B90.2
central nervous system B90.0
genitourinary B90.1
pulmonary (respiratory) B90.9
specified organs NEC B90.8

S

Sequelae *(Continued)*
viral
encephalitis B94.1
hepatitis B94.2
vitamin deficiency NEC E64.8
A E64.1
B E64.8
C E64.2
wound, open — code to injury with seventh character S
Sequestration —*see also* Sequestrum
disk —*see* Displacement, intervertebral disk ◀
lung, congenital Q33.2
Sequestrum
bone —*see* Osteomyelitis, chronic
dental M27.2
jaw bone M27.2
orbit —*see* Osteomyelitis, orbit
sinus (accessory) (nasal) —*see* Sinusitis
Sequoiosis lung or pneumonitis J67.8
Serology for syphilis
doubtful
with signs or symptoms - code by site and stage under Syphilis
follow-up of latent syphilis —*see* Syphilis, latent
negative, with signs or symptoms — code by site and stage under Syphilis
positive A53.Ø
with signs or symptoms - code by site and stage under Syphilis
reactivated A53.Ø
Seroma —*see also* Hematoma
postprocedural —*see* Complication, postprocedural, seroma ◀
traumatic, secondary and recurrent T79.2
Seropurulent —*see* condition
Serositis, multiple K65.8
pericardial I31.1
peritoneal K65.8
Serous —*see* condition
Sertoli cell
adenoma
specified site —*see* Neoplasm, benign, by site
unspecified site
female D27.9
male D29.2Ø
carcinoma
specified site —*see* Neoplasm, malignant, by site
unspecified site (male) C62.9-
female C56.9
tumor
with lipid storage
specified site —*see* Neoplasm, benign, by site
unspecified site
female D27.9
male D29.2Ø
specified site —*see* Neoplasm, benign, by site
unspecified site
female D27.9
male D29.2Ø
Sertoli-Leydig cell tumor —*see* Neoplasm, benign, by site
specified site —*see* Neoplasm, benign, by site
unspecified site
female D27.9
male D29.2Ø
Serum
allergy, allergic reaction —*see also* Reaction, serum T8Ø.69
shock —*see also* Shock, anaphylactic T8Ø.59
arthritis —*see also* Reaction, serum T8Ø.69
complication or reaction NEC —*see also* Reaction, serum T8Ø.69

Serum *(Continued)*
disease NEC —*see also* Reaction, serum T8Ø.69
hepatitis —*see also* Hepatitis, viral, type B carrier (suspected) of B18.1 ◀▪
intoxication —*see also* Reaction, serum T8Ø.69
neuritis —*see also* Reaction, serum T8Ø.69
neuropathy G61.1
poisoning NEC —*see also* Reaction, serum T8Ø.69
rash NEC —*see also* Reaction, serum T8Ø.69
reaction NEC —*see also* Reaction, serum T8Ø.69
sickness NEC —*see also* Reaction, serum T8Ø.69
urticaria —*see also* Reaction, serum T8Ø.69
Sesamoiditis M25.8-
Sever's disease or osteochondrosis —*see* Osteochondrosis, juvenile, tarsus
Severe sepsis R65.2Ø
with septic shock R65.21
Sex
chromosome mosaics Q97.8
lines with various numbers of X chromosomes Q97.2
education Z7Ø.8
reassignment surgery status Z87.89Ø
Sextuplet pregnancy —*see* Pregnancy, sextuplet
Sexual
function, disorder of (psychogenic) F52.9
immaturity (female) (male) E3Ø.Ø
impotence (psychogenic) organic origin NEC —*see* Dysfunction, sexual, male
precocity (constitutional) (cryptogenic) (female) (idiopathic) (male) E3Ø.1
Sexuality, pathologic —*see* Deviation, sexual
Sézary disease C84.1-
Shadow, lung R91.8
Shaking palsy or paralysis —*see* Parkinsonism
Shallowness, acetabulum —*see* Derangement, joint, specified type NEC, hip
Shaver's disease J63.1
Sheath (tendon) —*see* condition
Sheathing, retinal vessels H35.Ø1-
Shedding
nail L6Ø.8
premature, primary (deciduous) teeth KØØ.6
Sheehan's disease or syndrome E23.Ø
Shelf, rectal K62.89
Shell teeth KØØ.5
Shellshock (current) F43.Ø
lasting state —*see* Disorder, post-traumatic stress
Shield kidney Q63.1
Shift
auditory threshold (temporary) H93.24-
mediastinal R93.8
Shifting sleep-work schedule (affecting sleep) G47.26
Shiga (-Kruse) dysentery AØ3.Ø
Shiga's bacillus AØ3.Ø
Shigella (dysentery) —*see* Dysentery, bacillary
Shigellosis AØ3.9
Group A AØ3.Ø
Group B AØ3.1
Group C AØ3.2
Group D AØ3.3
Shin splints S86.89
Shingles —*see* Herpes, zoster
Shipyard disease or eye B3Ø.Ø
Shirodkar suture, in pregnancy —*see* Pregnancy, complicated by, incompetent cervix
Shock R57.9
with ectopic or molar pregnancy OØ8.3
adrenal (cortical) (Addisonian) E27.2
adverse food reaction (anaphylactic) —*see* Shock, anaphylactic, due to food
allergic —*see* Shock, anaphylactic

Shock *(Continued)*
anaphylactic T78.2
chemical —*see* Table of Drugs and Chemicals
due to drug or medicinal substance
correct substance properly administered T88.6
overdose or wrong substance given or taken (by accident) —*see* Table of Drugs and Chemicals, by drug, poisoning
due to food (nonpoisonous) T78.ØØ
additives T78.Ø6
dairy products T78.Ø7
eggs T78.Ø8
fish T78.Ø3
shellfish T78.Ø2
fruit T78.Ø4
milk T78.Ø7
nuts T78.Ø5
multiple types T78.Ø5 ◀
peanuts T78.Ø1
peanuts T78.Ø1
seeds T78.Ø5
specified type NEC T78.Ø9
vegetable T78.Ø4
following sting (s) —*see* Venom
immunization T8Ø.52
serum T8Ø.59
blood and blood products T8Ø.51
immunization T8Ø.52
specified NEC T8Ø.59
vaccination T8Ø.52
anaphylactoid —*see* Shock, anaphylactic
anesthetic
correct substance properly administered T88.2
overdose or wrong substance given or taken —*see* Table of Drugs and Chemicals, by drug, poisoning
specified anesthetic —*see* Table of Drugs and Chemicals, by drug, poisoning
cardiogenic R57.Ø
chemical substance —*see* Table of Drugs and Chemicals
complicating ectopic or molar pregnancy OØ8.3
culture —*see* Disorder, adjustment
drug
due to correct substance properly administered T88.6
overdose or wrong substance given or taken (by accident) —*see* Table of Drugs and Chemicals, by drug, poisoning
during or after labor and delivery O75.1
electric T75.4
(taser) T75.4
endotoxic R65.21
postprocedural (resulting from a procedure, not elsewhere classified) T81.12 ◀▪
following
ectopic or molar pregnancy OØ8.3
injury (immediate) (delayed) T79.4
labor and delivery O75.1
food (anaphylactic) —*see* Shock, anaphylactic, due to food
from electroshock gun (taser) T75.4
gram-negative R65.21
postprocedural (resulting from a procedure, not elsewhere classified) T81.12 ◀▪
hematologic R57.8
hemorrhagic
surgery (intraoperative) (postoperative) T81.19
trauma T79.4
hypovolemic R57.1
surgical T81.19
traumatic T79.4

◀ New ◀▪ Revised ~~deleted~~ Deleted

Shock *(Continued)*
insulin E15
therapeutic misadventure —*see* subcategory T38.3
kidney N17.Ø
traumatic (following crushing) T79.5
lightning T75.Ø1
liver K72.ØØ ◀
lung J8Ø
obstetric O75.1
with ectopic or molar pregnancy OØ8.3
following ectopic or molar pregnancy OØ8.3
pleural (surgical) T81.19
due to trauma T79.4
postprocedural (postoperative) T81.1Ø
with ectopic or molar pregnancy OØ8.3
cardiogenic T81.11
endotoxic T81.12
following ectopic or molar pregnancy OØ8.3
gram-negative T81.12
hypovolemic T81.19
septic T81.12
specified type NEC T81.19
psychic F43.Ø
septic (due to severe sepsis) R65.21
specified NEC R57.8
surgical T81.1Ø
taser gun (taser) T75.4
therapeutic misadventure NEC T81.1Ø
thyroxin
overdose or wrong substance given or taken —*see* Table of Drugs and Chemicals, by drug, poisoning
toxic, syndrome A48.3
transfusion —*see* Complications, transfusion
traumatic (immediate) (delayed) T79.4
Shoemaker's chest M95.4
Short, shortening, shortness
arm (acquired) —*see also* Deformity, limb, unequal length
congenital Q71.81-
forearm —*see* Deformity, limb, unequal length
bowel syndrome K91.2
breath RØ6.Ø2
cervical (complicating pregnancy) O26.87-
non-gravid uterus N88.3
common bile duct, congenital Q44.5
cord (umbilical), complicating delivery O69.3
cystic duct, congenital Q44.5
esophagus (congenital) Q39.8
femur (acquired) —*see* Deformity, limb, unequal length, femur
congenital —*see* Defect, reduction, lower limb, longitudinal, femur
frenum, frenulum, linguae (congenital) Q38.1
hip (acquired) —*see also* Deformity, limb, unequal length
congenital Q65.89
leg (acquired) —*see also* Deformity, limb, unequal length
congenital Q72.81-
lower leg —*see also* Deformity, limb, unequal length
limbed stature, with immunodeficiency D82.2
lower limb (acquired) —*see also* Deformity, limb, unequal length
congenital Q72.81-
organ or site, congenital NEC —*see* Distortion
palate, congenital Q38.5
radius (acquired) —*see also* Deformity, limb, unequal length
congenital —*see* Defect, reduction, upper limb, longitudinal, radius
rib syndrome Q77.2
stature (child) (hereditary) (idiopathic) NEC R62.52
constitutional E34.3
due to endocrine disorder E34.3
Laron-type E34.3

Short, shortening, shortness *(Continued)*
tendon —*see also* Contraction, tendon
with contracture of joint —*see* Contraction, joint
Achilles (acquired) M67.Ø-
congenital Q66.89
congenital Q79.8
thigh (acquired) —*see also* Deformity, limb, unequal length, femur
congenital —*see* Defect, reduction, lower limb, longitudinal, femur
tibialis anterior (tendon) —*see* Contraction, tendon
umbilical cord
complicating delivery O69.3
upper limb, congenital —*see* Defect, reduction, upper limb, specified type NEC
urethra N36.8
uvula, congenital Q38.5
vagina (congenital) Q52.4
Shortsightedness —*see* Myopia
Shoshin (acute fulminating beriberi) E51.11
Shoulder —*see* condition
Shovel-shaped incisors KØØ.2
Shower, thromboembolic —*see* Embolism
Shunt
arterial-venous (dialysis) Z99.2
arteriovenous, pulmonary (acquired) I28.Ø
congenital Q25.72
cerebral ventricle (communicating) in situ Z98.2
surgical, prosthetic, with complications —*see* Complications, cardiovascular, device or implant Shutdown, renal N28.9
Shutdown, renal N28.9
Shy-Drager syndrome G9Ø.3
Sialadenitis, sialadenosis (any gland) (chronic) (periodic) (suppurative) —*see* Sialoadenitis
Sialectasia K11.8
Sialidosis E77.1
Sialitis, silitis (any gland) (chronic) (suppurative) —*see* Sialoadenitis
Sialoadenitis (any gland) (periodic) (suppurative) K11.2Ø
acute K11.21
recurrent K11.22
chronic K11.23
Sialoadenopathy K11.9
Sialoangitis —*see* Sialoadenitis
Sialodochitis (fibrinosa) —*see* Sialoadenitis
Sialodocholithiasis K11.5
Sialolithiasis K11.5
Sialometaplasia, necrotizing K11.8
Sialorrhea —*see also* Ptyalism
periodic —*see* Sialoadenitis
Sialosis K11.7
Siamese twin Q89.4
Sibling rivalry Z62.891
Sicard's syndrome G52.7
Sicca syndrome M35.ØØ
with
keratoconjunctivitis M35.Ø1
lung involvement M35.Ø2
myopathy M35.Ø3
renal tubulo-interstitial disorders M35.Ø4
specified organ involvement NEC M35.Ø9
Sick R69
or handicapped person in family Z63.79
needing care at home Z63.6
sinus (syndrome) I49.5
Sick-euthyroid syndrome EØ7.81
Sickle-cell
anemia —*see* Disease, sickle-cell
trait D57.3
Sicklemia —*see also* Disease, sickle-cell
trait D57.3
Sickness
air (travel) T75.3
airplane T75.3
alpine T7Ø.29

Sickness *(Continued)*
altitude T7Ø.2Ø
Andes T7Ø.29
aviator's T7Ø.29
balloon T7Ø.29
car T75.3
compressed air T7Ø.3
decompression T7Ø.3
green D5Ø.8
milk —*see* Poisoning, food, noxious
motion T75.3
mountain T7Ø.29
acute D75.1
protein —*see also* Reaction, serum T8Ø.69
radiation T66
roundabout (motion) T75.3
sea T75.3
serum NEC —*see also* Reaction, serum T8Ø.69
sleeping (African) B56.9
by Trypanosoma B56.9
brucei
gambiense B56.Ø
rhodesiense B56.1
East African B56.1
Gambian B56.Ø
Rhodesian B56.1
West African B56.Ø
swing (motion) T75.3
train (railway) (travel) T75.3
travel (any vehicle) T75.3
Sideropenia —*see* Anemia, iron deficiency
Siderosilicosis J62.8
Siderosis (lung) J63.4
eye (globe) —*see* Disorder, globe, degenerative, siderosis
Siemens' syndrome (ectodermal dysplasia) Q82.8
Sighing RØ6.89
psychogenic F45.8
Sigmoid —*see also* condition
flexure —*see* condition
kidney Q63.1
Sigmoiditis —*see also* Enteritis K52.9
infectious AØ9
noninfectious K52.9
Silfverskjöld's syndrome Q78.9
Silicosiderosis J62.8
Silicosis, silicotic (simple) (complicated) J62.8
with tuberculosis J65
Silicotuberculosis J65
Silo-fillers' disease J68.8
bronchitis J68.Ø
pneumonitis J68.Ø
pulmonary edema J68.1
Silver's syndrome Q87.1
Simian malaria B53.1
Simmonds' cachexia or disease E23.Ø
Simons' disease or syndrome (progressive lipodystrophy) E88.1
Simple, simplex —*see* condition
Simulation, conscious (of illness) Z76.5
Simultanagnosia (asimultagnosia) R48.3
Sin Nombre virus disease (Hantavirus) (cardio)-pulmonary syndrome) B33.4
Sinding-Larsen disease or osteochondrosis —*see* Osteochondrosis, juvenile, patella
Singapore hemorrhagic fever A91
Singer's node or nodule J38.2
Single
atrium Q21.2
coronary artery Q24.5
umbilical artery Q27.Ø
ventricle Q2Ø.4
Singultus RØ6.6
epidemicus B33.Ø
Sinus —*see also* Fistula
abdominal K63.89
arrest I45.5
arrhythmia I49.8
bradycardia RØØ.1
branchial cleft (internal) (external) Q18.Ø
coccygeal —*see* Sinus, pilonidal

S

Sinus *(Continued)*
  dental KØ4.6
  dermal (congenital) QØ6.8
    with abscess QØ6.8
    coccygeal, pilonidal —*see* Sinus, coccygeal
  infected, skin NEC LØ8.89
  marginal, ruptured or bleeding —*see* Hemorrhage, antepartum, specified cause NEC
  medial, face and neck Q18.8
  pause I45.5
  pericranii QØ1.9
  pilonidal (infected) (rectum) LØ5.92
    with abscess LØ5.Ø2
  preauricular Q18.1
  rectovaginal N82.3
  Rokitansky-Aschoff (gallbladder) K82.8
  sacrococcygeal (dermoid) (infected) —*see* Sinus, pilonidal
  tachycardia RØØ.Ø
    paroxysmal I47.1
  tarsi syndrome M25.57- ⬅
  testis N5Ø.89 ⬅
  tract (postinfective) —*see* Fistula
  urachus Q64.4
Sinusitis (accessory) (chronic) (hyperplastic) (nasal) (nonpurulent) (purulent) J32.9
  acute JØ1.9Ø
    ethmoidal JØ1.2Ø
      recurrent JØ1.21
    frontal JØ1.1Ø
      recurrent JØ1.11
    involving more than one sinus, other than pansinusitis JØ1.8Ø
      recurrent JØ1.81
    maxillary JØ1.ØØ
      recurrent JØ1.Ø1
    pansinusitis JØ1.4Ø
      recurrent JØ1.41
    recurrent JØ1.91
    specified NEC JØ1.8Ø
      recurrent JØ1.81
    sphenoidal JØ1.3Ø
      recurrent JØ1.31
  allergic —*see* Rhinitis, allergic
  due to high altitude T7Ø.1
  ethmoidal J32.2
    acute JØ1.2Ø
      recurrent JØ1.21
  frontal J32.1
    acute JØ1.1Ø
      recurrent JØ1.11
  influenzal —*see* Influenza, with, respiratory manifestations NEC
  involving more than one sinus but not pansinusitis J32.8
    acute JØ1.8Ø
      recurrent JØ1.81
  maxillary J32.Ø
    acute JØ1.ØØ
      recurrent JØ1.Ø1
  sphenoidal J32.3
    acute JØ1.3Ø
      recurrent JØ1.31
  tuberculous, any sinus A15.8
Sinusitis-bronchiectasis-situs inversus (syndrome) (triad) Q89.3
Sipple's syndrome E31.22
Sirenomelia (syndrome) Q87.2
Siriasis T67.Ø
Sirkari's disease B55.Ø
Siti A65
Situation, psychiatric F99
Situational
  disturbance (transient) —*see* Disorder, adjustment
    acute F43.Ø
  maladjustment —*see* Disorder, adjustment
  reaction —*see* Disorder, adjustment
    acute F43.Ø

Situs inversus or transversus (abdominalis) (thoracis) Q89.3
Sixth disease BØ8.2Ø
  due to human herpesvirus 6 BØ8.21
  due to human herpesvirus 7 BØ8.22
Sjögren-Larsson syndrome Q87.1
Sjögren's syndrome or disease —*see* Sicca syndrome
Skeletal —*see* condition
Skene's gland —*see* condition
Skenitis —*see* Urethritis
Skerljevo A65
Skevas-Zerfus disease —*see* Toxicity, venom, marine animal, sea anemone
Skin —*see also* condition
  clammy R23.1
  donor —*see* Donor, skin
  hidebound M35.9
Slate-dressers' or slate-miners' lung J62.8
Sleep
  apnea —*see* Apnea, sleep
  deprivation Z72.82Ø
  disorder or disturbance G47.9
    child F51.9
    nonorganic origin F51.9
    specified NEC G47.8
  disturbance G47.9
    nonorganic origin F51.9
  drunkenness F51.9
  rhythm inversion G47.2-
  terrors F51.4
  walking F51.3
    hysterical F44.89
Sleep hygiene
  abuse Z72.821
  inadequate Z72.821
  poor Z72.821
Sleeping sickness —*see* Sickness, sleeping
Sleeplessness —*see* Insomnia
  menopausal N95.11
Sleep-wake schedule disorder G47.2Ø
Slim disease (in HIV infection) B2Ø
Slipped, slipping
  epiphysis (traumatic) —*see also* Osteochondropathy, specified type NEC
    capital femoral (traumatic)
      acute (on chronic) S79.Ø1-
    current traumatic - code as Fracture, by site
    upper femoral (nontraumatic) M93.ØØ-
      acute M93.Ø1-
        on chronic M93.Ø3-
      chronic M93.Ø2-
  intervertebral disc —*see* Displacement, intervertebral disc
  ligature, umbilical P51.8
  patella —*see* Disorder, patella, derangement NEC
  rib M89.8X8
  sacroiliac joint —*see* subcategory M53.2
  tendon —*see* Disorder, tendon
  ulnar nerve, nontraumatic —*see* Lesion, nerve, ulnar
  vertebra NEC —*see* Spondylolisthesis
Slocumb's syndrome E27.Ø
Sloughing (multiple) (phagedena) (skin) —*see also* Gangrene
  abscess —*see* Abscess
  appendix K38.8
  fascia —*see* Disorder, soft tissue, specified type NEC
  scrotum N5Ø.89 ⬅
  tendon —*see* Disorder, tendon
  transplanted organ —*see* Rejection, transplant
  ulcer —*see* Ulcer, skin
Slow
  feeding, newborn P92.2
  flow syndrome, coronary I2Ø.8
  heart(beat) RØØ.1
Slowing, urinary stream R39.198 ⬅
Sluder's neuralgia (syndrome) G44.89

Slurred, slurring speech R47.81
Small (ness)
  for gestational age —*see* Small for dates
  introitus, vagina N89.6
  kidney (unknown cause) N27.9
    bilateral N27.1
    unilateral N27.Ø
  ovary (congenital) Q5Ø.39
  pelvis
    with disproportion (fetopelvic) O33.1
      causing obstructed labor O65.1
  uterus N85.8
  white kidney NØ3.9
Small-and-light-for-dates —*see* Small for dates
Small-for-dates (infant) PØ5.1Ø
  with weight of
    499 grams or less PØ5.11
    5ØØ-749 grams PØ5.12
    75Ø-999 grams PØ5.13
    1ØØØ-1249 grams PØ5.14
    125Ø-1499 grams PØ5.15
    15ØØ-1749 grams PØ5.16
    175Ø-1999 grams PØ5.17
    2ØØØ-2499 grams PØ5.18
    25ØØ grams and over PØ5.19 ◀
  specified NEC PØ5.19 ◀
Smallpox BØ3
Smearing, fecal R15.1
Smith-Lemli-Opitz syndrome E78.72
Smith's fracture S52.54-
Smoker —*see* Dependence, drug, nicotine
Smoker's
  bronchitis J41.Ø
  cough J41.Ø
  palate K13.24
  throat J31.2
  tongue K13.24
Smoking
  passive Z77.22
Smothering spells RØ6.81
Snaggle teeth, tooth M26.39
Snapping
  finger —*see* Trigger finger
  hip —*see* Derangement, joint, specified type NEC, hip
    involving the iliotiblial band M76.3-
  knee —*see* Derangement, knee
    involving the iliotiblial band M76.3-
Sneddon-Wilkinson disease or syndrome (subcorneal pustular dermatosis) L13.1
Sneezing (intractable) RØ6.7
Sniffing
  cocaine
    abuse —*see* Abuse, drug, cocaine
    dependence —*see* Dependence, drug, cocaine
  gasoline
    abuse —*see* Abuse, drug, inhalant
    dependence —*see* Dependence, drug, inhalant
  glue (airplane)
    abuse —*see* Abuse, drug, inhalant
    drug dependence —*see* Dependence, drug, inhalant
Sniffles
  newborn P28.89
Snoring RØ6.83
Snow blindness —*see* Photokeratitis
Snuffles (non-syphilitic) RØ6.5
  newborn P28.89
  syphilitic (infant) A5Ø.Ø5 *[J99]*
Social
  exclusion Z6Ø.4
    due to discrimination or persecution (perceived) Z6Ø.5
  migrant Z59.Ø
    acculturation difficulty Z6Ø.3
  rejection Z6Ø.4
    due to discrimination or persecution Z6Ø.5

S

Social *(Continued)*
role conflict NEC Z73.5
skills inadequacy NEC Z73.4
transplantation Z60.3
Sodoku A25.0
Soemmerring's ring —*see* Cataract, secondary
Soft —*see also* condition
nails L60.3
Softening
bone —*see* Osteomalacia
brain (necrotic) (progressive) G93.89
congenital Q04.8
embolic I63.4-
hemorrhagic —*see* Hemorrhage, intracranial, intracerebral
occlusive I63.5-
thrombotic I63.3-
cartilage M94.2-
patella M22.4-
cerebellar —*see* Softening, brain
cerebral —*see* Softening, brain
cerebrospinal —*see* Softening, brain
myocardial, heart —*see* Degeneration, myocardial
spinal cord G95.89
stomach K31.89
Soldier's
heart F45.8
patches I31.0
Solitary
cyst, kidney N28.1
kidney, congenital Q60.0
Solvent abuse —*see* Abuse, drug, inhalant
dependence —*see* Dependence, drug, inhalant
Somatization reaction, somatic reaction —*see* Disorder, somatoform
Somnambulism F51.3
hysterical F44.89
Somnolence R40.0
nonorganic origin F51.11
Sonne dysentery A03.3
Soor B37.0
Sore
bed —*see* Ulcer, pressure, by site
chiclero B55.1
Delhi B55.1
desert —*see* Ulcer, skin
eye H57.1-
Lahore B55.1
mouth K13.79
canker K12.0
muscle M79.1
Naga —*see* Ulcer, skin
of skin —*see* Ulcer, skin - oriental B55.1
pressure —*see* Ulcer, pressure, by site
skin L98.9
soft A57
throat (acute) —*see also* Pharyngitis
with influenza, flu, or grippe —*see* Influenza, with, respiratory manifestations NEC
chronic J31.2
coxsackie (virus) B08.5
diphtheritic A36.0
herpesviral B00.2
influenzal —*see* Influenza, with, respiratory manifestations NEC
septic J02.0
streptococcal (ulcerative) J02.0
viral NEC J02.8
coxsackie B08.5
tropical —*see* Ulcer, skin
veldt —*see* Ulcer, skin
Soto's syndrome (cerebral gigantism) Q87.3
South African cardiomyopathy syndrome I42.8
Southeast Asian hemorrhagic fever A91
Spacing
abnormal, tooth, teeth, fully erupted M26.30
excessive, tooth, fully erupted M26.32
Spade-like hand (congenital) Q68.1
Spading nail L60.8
congenital Q84.6
Spanish collar N47.1
Sparganosis B70.1
Spasm (s), **spastic, spasticity** —*see also* condition R25.2
accommodation —*see* Spasm, of accommodation
ampulla of Vater K83.4
anus, ani (sphincter) (reflex) K59.4
psychogenic F45.8
artery I73.9
cerebral G45.9
Bell's G51.3
bladder (sphincter, external or internal) N32.89
psychogenic F45.8
bronchus, bronchiole J98.01
cardia K22.0
cardiac I20.1
carpopedal —*see* Tetany
cerebral (arteries) (vascular) G45.9
cervix, complicating delivery O62.4
ciliary body (of accommodation) —*see* Spasm, of accommodation
colon —*see also* Irritable, bowel K58.9
with diarrhea K58.0
psychogenic F45.8
common duct K83.8
compulsive —*see* Tic
conjugate H51.8
coronary (artery) I20.1
diaphragm (reflex) R06.6
epidemic B33.0
psychogenic F45.8
duodenum K59.8
epidemic diaphragmatic (transient) B33.0
esophagus (diffuse) K22.4
psychogenic F45.8
facial G51.3
fallopian tube N83.8
gastrointestinal (tract) K31.89
psychogenic F45.8
glottis J38.5
hysterical F44.4
psychogenic F45.8
conversion reaction F44.4
reflex through recurrent laryngeal nerve J38.5
habit —*see* Tic
heart I20.1
hemifacial (clonic) G51.3
hourglass —*see* Contraction, hourglass
hysterical F44.4
infantile —*see* Epilepsy, spasms
inferior oblique, eye H51.8
intestinal —*see also* Syndrome, irritable bowel K58.9
psychogenic F45.8
larynx, laryngeal J38.5
hysterical F44.4
psychogenic F45.8
conversion reaction F44.4
levator palpebrae superioris —*see* Disorder, eyelid function
muscle NEC M62.838
back M62.830
nerve, trigeminal G51.0
nervous F45.8
nodding F98.4
occupational F48.8
oculogyric H51.8
psychogenic F45.8
of accommodation H52.53-
ophthalmic artery —*see* Occlusion, artery, retina
perineal, female N94.89
peroneo-extensor —*see also* Deformity, limb, flat foot
pharynx (reflex) J39.2
hysterical F45.8
psychogenic F45.8
Spasm (s), **spastic, spasticity** *(Continued)*
psychogenic F45.8
pylorus NEC K31.3
adult hypertrophic K31.89
congenital or infantile Q40.0
psychogenic F45.8
rectum (sphincter) K59.4
psychogenic F45.8
retinal (artery) —*see* Occlusion, artery, retina
sigmoid —*see also* Syndrome, irritable bowel K58.9
psychogenic F45.8
sphincter of Oddi K83.4
stomach K31.89
neurotic F45.8
throat J39.2
hysterical F45.8
psychogenic F45.8
tic F95.9
chronic F95.1
transient of childhood F95.0
tongue K14.8
torsion (progressive) G24.1
trigeminal nerve —*see* Neuralgia, trigeminal
ureter N13.5
urethra (sphincter) N35.9
uterus N85.8
complicating labor O62.4
vagina N94.2
psychogenic F52.5
vascular I73.9
vasomotor I73.9
vein NEC I87.8
viscera —*see* Pain, abdominal
Spasmodic —*see* condition
Spasmophilia —*see* Tetany
Spasmus nutans F98.4
Spastic, spasticity —*see also* Spasm
child (cerebral) (congenital) (paralysis) G80.1
Speaker's throat R49.8
Specific, specified —*see* condition
Speech
defect, disorder, disturbance, impediment R47.9
psychogenic, in childhood and adolescence F98.8
slurring R47.81
specified NEC R47.89
Spencer's disease A08.19
Spens' syndrome (syncope with heart block) I45.9
Sperm counts (fertility testing) Z31.41
postvasectomy Z30.8
reversal Z31.42
Spermatic cord —*see* condition
Spermatocele N43.40
congenital Q55.4
multiple N43.42
single N43.41
Spermatocystitis N49.0
Spermatocytoma C62.9-
specified site —*see* Neoplasm, malignant, by site
Spermatorrhea N50.89
Sphacelus —*see* Gangrene
Sphenoidal —*see* condition
Sphenoiditis (chronic) —*see* Sinusitis, sphenoidal
Sphenopalatine ganglion neuralgia G90.09
Sphericity, increased, lens (congenital) Q12.4
Spherocytosis (congenital) (familial) (hereditary) D58.0
hemoglobin disease D58.0
sickle-cell (disease) D57.8-
Spherophakia Q12.4
Sphincter —*see* condition
Sphincteritis, sphincter of Oddi —*see* Cholangitis
Sphingolipidosis E75.3
specified NEC E75.29

Sphingomyelinosis E75.3
Spicule tooth K00.2
Spider
bite —*see* Toxicity, venom, spider
fingers —*see* Syndrome, Marfan's
nevus I78.1
toes —*see* Syndrome, Marfan's
vascular I78.1
Spiegler-Fendt
benign lymphocytoma L98.8
sarcoid L08.89
Spielmeyer-Vogt disease E75.4
Spina bifida (aperta) Q05.9
with hydrocephalus NEC Q05.4
cervical Q05.5
with hydrocephalus Q05.0
dorsal Q05.6
with hydrocephalus Q05.1
lumbar Q05.7
with hydrocephalus Q05.2
lumbosacral Q05.7
with hydrocephalus Q05.2
occulta Q76.0
sacral Q05.8
with hydrocephalus Q05.3
thoracic Q05.6
with hydrocephalus Q05.1
thoracolumbar Q05.6
with hydrocephalus Q05.1
Spindle, Krukenberg's —*see* Pigmentation, cornea, posterior
Spine, spinal —*see* condition
Spiradenoma (eccrine) —*see* Neoplasm, skin, benign
Spirillosis A25.0
Spirillum
minus A25.0
obermeieri infection A68.0
Spirochetal —*see* condition
Spirochetosis A69.9
arthritic, arthritica A69.9
bronchopulmonary A69.8
icterohemorrhagic A27.0
lung A69.8
Spirometrosis B70.1
Spitting blood —*see* Hemoptysis
Splanchnoptosis K63.4
Spleen, splenic —*see* condition
Splenectasis —*see* Splenomegaly
Splenitis (interstitial) (malignant) (nonspecific) D73.89
malarial —*see also* Malaria B54 *[D77]*
tuberculous A18.85
Splenocele D73.89
Splenomegaly, splenomegalia (Bengal) (cryptogenic) (idiopathic) (tropical) R16.1
with hepatomegaly R16.2
cirrhotic D73.2
congenital Q89.09
congestive, chronic D73.2
Egyptian B65.1
Gaucher's E75.22
malarial —*see also* Malaria B54 *[D77]*
neutropenic D73.81
Niemann-Pick —*see* Niemann-Pick disease or syndrome
siderotic D73.2
syphilitic A52.79
congenital (early) A50.08 *[D77]*
Splenopathy D73.9
Splenoptosis D73.89
Splenosis D73.89
Splinter —*see* Foreign body, superficial, by site
Split, splitting
foot Q72.7-
hand Q71.6 ◀
heart sounds R01.2
lip, congenital —*see* Cleft, lip
nails L60.3
urinary stream R39.13
Spondylarthrosis —*see* Spondylosis
Spondylitis (chronic) —*see also* Spondylopathy, inflammatory
ankylopoietica —*see* Spondylitis, ankylosing
ankylosing (chronic) M45.9
with lung involvement M45.9 *[J99]*
cervical region M45.2
cervicothoracic region M45.3
juvenile M08.1
lumbar region M45.6
lumbosacral region M45.7
multiple sites M45.0
occipito-atlanto-axial region M45.1
sacrococcygeal region M45.8
thoracic region M45.4
thoracolumbar region M45.5
atrophic (ligamentous) —*see* Spondylitis, ankylosing
deformans (chronic) —*see* Spondylosis
gonococcal A54.41
gouty —*see also* Gout, by type, vertebrae M10.08 ⬅
in (due to)
brucellosis A23.9 *[M49.80]*
cervical region A23.9 *[M49.82]*
cervicothoracic region A23.9 *[M49.83]*
lumbar region A23.9 *[M49.86]*
lumbosacral region A23.9 *[M49.87]*
multiple sites A23.9 *[M49.89]*
occipito-atlanto-axial region A23.9 *[M49.81]*
sacrococcygeal region A23.9 *[M49.88]*
thoracic region A23.9 *[M49.84]*
thoracolumbar region A23.9 *[M49.85]*
enterobacteria —*see also* subcategory M49.8 A04.9
tuberculosis A18.01
infectious NEC —*see* Spondylopathy, infective
juvenile ankylosing (chronic) M08.1
Kümmell's —*see* Spondylopathy, traumatic
Marie-Strümpell —*see* Spondylitis, ankylosing
muscularis —*see* Spondylopathy, specified NEC
psoriatic L40.53
rheumatoid —*see* Spondylitis, ankylosing
rhizomelica —*see* Spondylitis, ankylosing
sacroiliac NEC M46.1
senescent, senile —*see* Spondylosis
traumatic (chronic) or post-traumatic —*see* Spondylopathy, traumatic
tuberculous A18.01
typhosa A01.05
Spondylolisthesis (acquired) (degenerative) M43.10
with disproportion (fetopelvic) O33.0
causing obstructed labor O65.0
cervical region M43.12
cervicothoracic region M43.13
congenital Q76.2
lumbar region M43.16
lumbosacral region M43.17
multiple sites M43.19
occipito-atlanto-axial region M43.11
sacrococcygeal region M43.18
thoracic region M43.14
thoracolumbar region M43.15
traumatic (old) M43.10
acute
fifth cervical (displaced) S12.430
nondisplaced S12.431
specified type NEC (displaced) S12.450
nondisplaced S12.451
type III S12.44
fourth cervical (displaced) S12.330
nondisplaced S12.331
specified type NEC (displaced) S12.350
nondisplaced S12.351
type III S12.34
Spondylolisthesis *(Continued)*
traumatic *(Continued)*
acute *(Continued)*
second cervical (displaced) S12.130
nondisplaced S12.131
specified type NEC (displaced) S12.150
nondisplaced S12.151
type III S12.14
seventh cervical (displaced) S12.630
nondisplaced S12.631
specified type NEC (displaced) S12.650
nondisplaced S12.651
type III S12.64
sixth cervical (displaced) S12.530
nondisplaced S12.531
specified type NEC (displaced) S12.550
nondisplaced S12.551
type III S12.54
third cervical (displaced) S12.230
nondisplaced S12.231
specified type NEC (displaced) S12.250
nondisplaced S12.251
type III S12.24
Spondylolysis (acquired) M43.00
cervical region M43.02
cervicothoracic region M43.03
congenital Q76.2
lumbar region M43.06
lumbosacral region M43.07
with disproportion (fetopelvic) O33.0
causing obstructed labor O65.8
multiple sites M43.09
occipito-atlanto-axial region M43.01
sacrococcygeal region M43.08
thoracic region M43.04
thoracolumbar region M43.05
Spondylopathy M48.9
infective NEC M46.50
cervical region M46.52
cervicothoracic region M46.53
lumbar region M46.56
lumbosacral region M46.57
multiple sites M46.59
occipito-atlanto-axial region M46.51
sacrococcygeal region M46.58
thoracic region M46.54
thoracolumbar region M46.55
inflammatory M46.90
cervical region M46.92
cervicothoracic region M46.93
lumbar region M46.96
lumbosacral region M46.97
multiple sites M46.99
occipito-atlanto-axial region M46.91
sacrococcygeal region M46.98
specified type NEC M46.80
cervical region M46.82
cervicothoracic region M46.83
lumbar region M46.86
lumbosacral region M46.87
multiple sites M46.89
occipito-atlanto-axial region M46.81
sacrococcygeal region M46.88
thoracic region M46.84
thoracolumbar region M46.85
thoracic region M46.94
thoracolumbar region M46.95
neuropathic, in
syringomyelia and syringobulbia G95.0
tabes dorsalis A52.11
specified NEC —*see* subcategory M48.8
traumatic M48.30
cervical region M48.32
cervicothoracic region M48.33
lumbar region M48.36
lumbosacral region M48.37
occipito-atlanto-axial region M48.31

S

Spondylopathy *(Continued)*
traumatic *(Continued)*
sacrococcygeal region M48.38
thoracic region M48.34
thoracolumbar region M48.35
Spondylosis M47.9
with
disproportion (fetopelvic) O33.Ø
causing obstructed labor O65.Ø
myelopathy NEC M47.1Ø
cervical region M47.12
cervicothoracic region M47.13
lumbar region M47.16
occipito-atlanto-axial region M47.11
thoracic region M47.14
thoracolumbar region M47.15
radiculopathy M47.2Ø
cervical region M47.22
cervicothoracic region M47.23
lumbar region M47.26
lumbosacral region M47.27
occipito-atlanto-axial region M47.21
sacrococcygeal region M47.28
thoracic region M47.24
thoracolumbar region M47.25
without myelopathy or radiculopathy M47.819
cervical region M47.812
cervicothoracic region M47.813
lumbar region M47.816
lumbosacral region M47.817
occipito-atlanto-axial region M47.811
sacrococcygeal region M47.818
thoracic region M47.814
thoracolumbar region M47.815
specified NEC M47.899
cervical region M47.892
cervicothoracic region M47.893
lumbar region M47.896
lumbosacral region M47.897
occipito-atlanto-axial region M47.891
sacrococcygeal region M47.898
thoracic region M47.894
thoracolumbar region M47.895
traumatic —*see* Spondylopathy, traumatic
Sponge
inadvertently left in operation wound —*see* Foreign body, accidentally left during a procedure
kidney (medullary) Q61.5
Sponge-diver's disease —*see* Toxicity, venom, marine animal, sea anemone
Spongioblastoma (any type) —*see* Neoplasm, malignant, by site
specified site —*see* Neoplasm, malignant, by site
unspecified site C71.9
Spongioneuroblastoma —*see* Neoplasm, malignant, by site
Spontaneous —*see also* condition
fracture (cause unknown) —*see* Fracture, pathological
Spoon nail L6Ø.3
congenital Q84.6
Sporadic —*see* condition
Sporothrix schenckii infection —*see* Sporotrichosis
Sporotrichosis B42.9
arthritis B42.82
disseminated B42.7
generalized B42.7
lymphocutaneous (fixed) (progressive) B42.1
pulmonary B42.Ø
specified NEC B42.89
Spots, spotting (in) (of)
Bitot's —*see also* Pigmentation, conjunctiva
in the young child E5Ø.1
vitamin A deficiency E5Ø.1
Spots, spotting *(Continued)*
café, au lait L81.3
Cayenne pepper I78.1
cotton wool, retina —*see* Occlusion, artery, retina
de Morgan's (senile angiomas) I78.1
Fuchs' black (myopic) H44.2-
intermenstrual (regular) N92.Ø
irregular N92.1
Koplik's BØ5.9
liver L81.4
pregnancy O26.85-
purpuric R23.3
ruby I78.1
Spotted fever —*see* Fever, spotted N92.3
Sprain (joint) (ligament)
acromioclavicular joint or ligament S43.5-
ankle S93.4Ø-
calcaneofibular ligament S93.41-
deltoid ligament S93.42-
internal collateral ligament —*see* Sprain, ankle, specified ligament NEC
specified ligament NEC S93.49-
talofibular ligament —*see* Sprain, ankle, specified ligament NEC
tibiofibular ligament S93.43-
anterior longitudinal, cervical S13.4
atlas, atlanto-axial, atlanto-occipital S13.4
breast bone —*see* Sprain, sternum
calcaneofibular —*see* Sprain, ankle
carpal —*see* Sprain, wrist
carpometacarpal —*see* Sprain, hand, specified site NEC
cartilage
costal S23.41
semilunar (knee) —*see* Sprain, knee, specified site NEC
with current tear —*see* Tear, meniscus
thyroid region S13.5
xiphoid —*see* Sprain, sternum
cervical, cervicodorsal, cervicothoracic S13.4
chondrosternal S23.421
coracoclavicular S43.8-
coracohumeral S43.41-
coronary, knee —*see* Sprain, knee, specified site NEC
costal cartilage S23.41
cricoarytenoid articulation or ligament S13.5
cricothyroid articulation S13.5
cruciate, knee —*see* Sprain, knee, cruciate
deltoid, ankle —*see* Sprain, ankle
dorsal (spine) S23.3
elbow S53.4Ø-
radial collateral ligament S53.43-
radiohumeral S53.41-
rupture
radial collateral ligament —*see* Rupture, traumatic, ligament, radial collateral
ulnar collateral ligament —*see* Rupture, traumatic, ligament, ulnar collateral
specified type NEC S53.49-
ulnar collateral ligament S53.44-
ulnohumeral S53.42-
femur, head —*see* Sprain, hip
fibular collateral, knee —*see* Sprain, knee, collateral
fibulocalcaneal —*see* Sprain, ankle
finger (s) S63.61-
index S63.61-
interphalangeal (joint) S63.63-
index S63.63-
little S63.63-
middle S63.63-
ring S63.63-
little S63.61-
metacarpophalangeal (joint) S63.65-
middle S63.61-
ring S63.61-
Sprain *(Continued)*
finger (s) *(Continued)*
specified site NEC S63.69-
index S63.69-
little S63.69-
middle S63.69-
ring S63.69-
foot S93.6Ø-
specified ligament NEC S93.69-
tarsal ligament S93.61-
tarsometatarsal ligament S93.62-
toe —*see* Sprain, toe
hand S63.9-
finger —*see* Sprain, finger
specified site NEC —*see* subcategory S63.8
thumb —*see* Sprain, thumb
head SØ3.9
hip S73.1Ø-
iliofemoral ligament S73.11-
ischiocapsular (ligament) S73.12-
specified NEC S73.19-
iliofemoral —*see* Sprain, hip
innominate
acetabulum —*see* Sprain, hip
sacral junction S33.6
internal
collateral, ankle —*see* Sprain, ankle
semilunar cartilage —*see* Sprain, knee, specified site NEC
interphalangeal
finger —*see* Sprain, finger, interphalangeal (joint)
toe —*see* Sprain, toe, interphalangeal joint
ischiocapsular —*see* Sprain, hip
ischiofemoral —*see* Sprain, hip
jaw (articular disc) (cartilage) (meniscus) SØ3.4- ⬅
old M26.69
knee S83.9-
collateral ligament S83.4Ø-
lateral (fibular) S83.42-
medial (tibial) S83.41-
cruciate ligament S83.5Ø-
anterior S83.51-
posterior S83.52-
lateral (fibular) collateral ligament S83.42-
medial (tibial) collateral ligament S83.41-
patellar ligament S76.11-
specified site NEC S83.8X-
superior tibiofibular joint (ligament) S83.6-
lateral collateral, knee —*see* Sprain, knee, collateral
lumbar (spine) S33.5
lumbosacral S33.9
mandible (articular disc) SØ3.4- ⬅
old M26.69
medial collateral, knee —*see* Sprain, knee, collateral
meniscus
jaw SØ3.4- ⬅
old M26.69
knee —*see* Sprain, knee, specified site NEC
with current tear —*see* Tear, meniscus
old —*see* Derangement, knee, meniscus, due to old tear
mandible SØ3.4- ⬅
old M26.69
metacarpal (distal) (proximal) —*see* Sprain, hand, specified site NEC
metacarpophalangeal —*see* Sprain, finger, metacarpophalangeal (joint)
metatarsophalangeal —*see* Sprain, toe, metatarsophalangeal joint
midcarpal —*see* Sprain, hand, specified site NEC
midtarsal —*see* Sprain, foot, specified site NEC
neck S13.9
anterior longitudinal cervical ligament S13.4
atlanto-axial joint S13.4

S

Sprain *(Continued)*
neck *(Continued)*
atlanto-occipital joint S13.4
cervical spine S13.4
cricoarytenoid ligament S13.5
cricothyroid ligament S13.5
specified site NEC S13.8
thyroid region (cartilage) S13.5
nose SØ3.8
orbicular, hip —*see* Sprain, hip
patella —*see* Sprain, knee, specified site NEC
patellar ligament S76.11-
pelvis NEC S33.8
phalanx
finger —*see* Sprain, finger
toe —*see* Sprain, toe
pubofemoral —*see* Sprain, hip
radiocarpal —*see* Sprain, wrist
radiohumeral —*see* Sprain, elbow
radius, collateral —*see* Rupture, traumatic, ligament, radial collateral
rib (cage) S23.41
rotator cuff (capsule) S43.42-
sacroiliac (region)
chronic or old —*see* subcategory M53.2
joint S33.6
scaphoid (hand) —*see* Sprain, hand, specified site NEC
scapula (r) —*see* Sprain, shoulder girdle, specified site NEC
semilunar cartilage (knee) —*see* Sprain, knee, specified site NEC
with current tear —*see* Tear, meniscus
old —*see* Derangement, knee, meniscus, due to old tear
shoulder joint S43.4Ø-
acromioclavicular joint (ligament) —*see* Sprain, acromioclavicular joint
blade —*see* Sprain, shoulder, girdle, specified site NEC
coracoclavicular joint (ligament) —*see* Sprain, coracoclavicular joint
coracohumeral ligament —*see* Sprain, coracohumeral joint
girdle S43.9-
specified site NEC S43.8-
rotator cuff —*see* Sprain, rotator cuff
specified site NEC S43.49-
sternoclavicular joint (ligament) —*see* Sprain, sternoclavicular joint
spine
cervical S13.4
lumbar S33.5
thoracic S23.3
sternoclavicular joint S43.6-
sternum S23.429
chondrosternal joint S23.421
specified site NEC S23.428
sternoclavicular (joint) (ligament) S23.42Ø
symphysis
jaw SØ3.4- ⬅
old M26.69
mandibular SØ3.4- ⬅
old M26.69
talofibular —*see* Sprain, ankle
tarsal —*see* Sprain, foot, specified site NEC
tarsometatarsal —*see* Sprain, foot, specified site NEC
temporomandibular SØ3.4- ⬅
old M26.69
thorax S23.9
ribs S23.41
specified site NEC S23.8
spine S23.3
sternum —*see* Sprain, sternum
thumb S63.6Ø-
interphalangeal (joint) S63.62-
metacarpophalangeal (joint) S63.64-
specified site NEC S63.68-
thyroid cartilage or region S13.5

Sprain *(Continued)*
tibia (proximal end) —*see* Sprain, knee, specified site NEC
tibial collateral, knee —*see* Sprain, knee, collateral
tibiofibular
distal —*see* Sprain, ankle
superior —*see* Sprain, knee, specified site NEC
toe (s) S93.5Ø-
great S93.5Ø-
interphalangeal joint S93.51-
great S93.51-
lesser S93.51-
lesser S93.5Ø-
metatarsophalangeal joint S93.52-
great S93.52-
lesser S93.52-
ulna, collateral —*see* Rupture, traumatic, ligament, ulnar collateral
ulnohumeral —*see* Sprain, elbow
wrist S63.5Ø-
carpal S63.51-
radiocarpal S63.52-
specified site NEC S63.59-
xiphoid cartilage —*see* Sprain, sternum
Sprengel's deformity (congenital) Q74.Ø
Sprue (tropical) K9Ø.1
celiac K9Ø.Ø
idiopathic K9Ø.49 ⬅
meaning thrush B37.Ø
nontropical K9Ø.Ø
Spur, bone —*see also* Enthesopathy
calcaneal M77.3-
iliac crest M76.2-
nose (septum) J34.89
Spurway's syndrome Q78.Ø
Sputum
abnormal (amount) (color) (odor) (purulent) RØ9.3
blood-stained RØ4.2
excessive (cause unknown) RØ9.3
Squamous —*see also* condition
epithelium in
cervical canal (congenital) Q51.828
uterine mucosa (congenital) Q51.818
Squashed nose M95.Ø
congenital Q67.4
Squeeze, diver's T7Ø.3
Squint —*see also* Strabismus
accommodative —*see* Strabismus, convergent concomitant
St. Hubert's disease A82.9
Stab —*see also* Laceration
internal organs —*see* Injury, by site
Stafne's cyst or cavity M27.Ø
Staggering gait R26.Ø
hysterical F44.4
Staghorn calculus —*see* Calculus, kidney
Stähli's line (cornea) (pigment) —*see* Pigmentation, cornea, anterior
Stain, staining
meconium (newborn) P96.83
port wine Q82.5
tooth, teeth (hard tissues) (extrinsic) KØ3.6
due to
accretions KØ3.6
deposits (betel) (black) (green) (materia alba) (orange) (soft) (tobacco) KØ3.6
metals (copper) (silver) KØ3.7
nicotine KØ3.6
pulpal bleeding KØ3.7
tobacco KØ3.6
intrinsic KØØ.8
Stammering —*see also* Disorder, fluency F8Ø.81
Standstill
auricular I45.5
cardiac —*see* Arrest, cardiac
sinoatrial I45.5
ventricular —*see* Arrest, cardiac
Stannosis J63.5

Stanton's disease —*see* Melioidosis
Staphylitis (acute) (catarrhal) (chronic) (gangrenous) (membranous) (suppurative) (ulcerative) K12.2
Staphylococcal scalded skin syndrome LØØ
Staphylococcemia A41.2
Staphylococcus, staphylococcal —*see also* condition
as cause of disease classified elsewhere B95.8
aureus (methicillin susceptible) (MSSA) B95.61
methicillin resistant (MRSA) B95.62
specified NEC, as cause of disease classified elsewhere B95.7
Staphyloma (sclera)
cornea H18.72-
equatorial H15.81-
localized (anterior) H15.82-
posticum H15.83-
ring H15.85-
Stargardt's disease —*see* Dystrophy, retina
Starvation (inanition) (due to lack of food) T73.Ø
edema —*see* Malnutrition, severe
Stasis
bile (noncalculous) K83.1
bronchus J98.Ø9
with infection —*see* Bronchitis
cardiac —*see* Failure, heart, congestive
cecum K59.8
colon K59.8
dermatitis I87.2 ⬅
with ◀
varicose ulcer —*see* Varix, leg, with ulcer, with inflammation ◀
varicose veins —*see* Varix, leg, with, inflammation ◀
due to postthrombotic syndrome —*see* Syndrome, postthrombotic ◀
duodenal K31.5
eczema —*see* Varix, leg, with, inflammation
edema —*see* Hypertension, venous (chronic), idiopathic
foot T69.Ø-
ileocecal coil K59.8
ileum K59.8
intestinal K59.8
jejunum K59.8
kidney N19
liver (cirrhotic) K76.1
lymphatic I89.8
pneumonia J18.2
pulmonary —*see* Edema, lung
rectal K59.8
renal N19
tubular N17.Ø
ulcer —*see* Varix, leg, with, ulcer
without varicose veins I87.2
urine —*see* Retention, urine
venous I87.8
State (of)
affective and paranoid, mixed, organic psychotic FØ6.8
agitated R45.1
acute reaction to stress F43.Ø
anxiety (neurotic) F41.1
apprehension F41.1
burn-out Z73.Ø
climacteric, female Z78.Ø
symptomatic N95.1
compulsive F42.8 ⬅
mixed with obsessional thoughts F42.2 ⬅
confusional (psychogenic) F44.89
acute —*see also* Delirium
with
arteriosclerotic dementia FØ1.5Ø
with behavioral disturbance FØ1.51
senility or dementia FØ5
alcoholic F1Ø.231

◀ New ⬅ Revised ~~deleted~~ Deleted

State *(Continued)*
  confusional (psychogenic) *(Continued)*
    epileptic F05
    reactive (from emotional stress, psychological trauma) F44.89
    subacute —*see* Delirium
  convulsive —*see* Convulsions
  crisis F43.Ø
  depressive F32.9
    neurotic F34.1
  dissociative F44.9
  emotional shock (stress) R45.7
  hypercoagulation —*see* Hypercoagulable
  locked-in G83.5
  menopausal Z78.Ø
    symptomatic N95.1
  neurotic F48.9
    with depersonalization F48.1
  obsessional F42.8 ⬅
  oneiroid (schizophrenia-like) F23
  organic
    hallucinatory (nonalcoholic) F06.Ø
    paranoid (-hallucinatory) F06.2
  panic F41.Ø
  paranoid F22
    climacteric F22
    involutional F22
    menopausal F22
    organic F06.2
    senile F03
    simple F22
  persistent vegetative R40.3
  phobic F40.9
  postleukotomy F07.Ø
  ~~pregnant, incidental Z33.1~~
  pregnant ◀
    gestational carrier Z33.3 ◀
    incidental Z33.1 ◀
  psychogenic, twilight F44.89
  psychopathic (constitutional) F60.2
  psychotic, organic —*see also* Psychosis, organic
    mixed paranoid and affective F06.8
    senile or presenile F03
    transient NEC F06.8
      with
        depression F06.31
        hallucinations F06.Ø
  residual schizophrenic F2Ø.5
  restlessness R45.1
  stress (emotional) R45.7
  tension (mental) F48.9
    specified NEC F48.8
  transient organic psychotic NEC F06.8
    depressive type F06.31
    hallucinatory type F06.Ø ⬅
  twilight
    epileptic F05
    psychogenic F44.89
  vegetative, persistent R40.3
  vital exhaustion Z73.Ø
  withdrawal —*see* Withdrawal, state
Status (post) —*see also* Presence (of)
  absence, epileptic —*see* Epilepsy, by type, with status epilepticus
  administration of tPA (rtPA) in a different facility within the last 24 hours prior to admission to the current facility Z92.82
  adrenalectomy (unilateral) (bilateral) E89.6
  anastomosis Z98.Ø
  anginosus I2Ø.9
  angioplasty (peripheral) Z98.62
    with implant Z95.82Ø
    coronary artery Z98.61
      with implant Z95.5
  aortocoronary bypass Z95.1
  arthrodesis Z98.1
  artificial opening (of) Z93.9
    gastrointestinal tract Z93.4
    specified NEC Z93.8

Status *(Continued)*
  artificial opening (of) *(Continued)*
    urinary tract Z93.6
    vagina Z93.8
  asthmaticus —*see* Asthma, by type, with status asthmaticus
  awaiting organ transplant Z76.82
  bariatric surgery Z98.84
  bed confinement Z74.Ø1
  bleb, filtering (vitreous), after glaucoma surgery Z98.83
  breast implant Z98.82
    removal Z98.86
  cataract extraction Z98.4-
  cholecystectomy Z9Ø.49
  clitorectomy N9Ø.811
    with excision of labia minora N9Ø.812
  colectomy (complete) (partial) Z9Ø.49
  colonization —*see* Carrier (suspected) of
  colostomy Z93.3
  convulsivus idiopathicus —*see* Epilepsy, by type, with status epilepticus
  coronary artery angioplasty —*see* Status, angioplasty, coronary artery
  cystectomy (urinary bladder) Z9Ø.6
  cystostomy Z93.5Ø
    appendico-vesicostomy Z93.52
    cutaneous Z93.51
    specified NEC Z93.59
  delinquent immunization Z28.3
  dental Z98.818
    crown Z98.811
    fillings Z98.811
    restoration Z98.811
    sealant Z98.81Ø
    specified NEC Z98.818
  deployment (current) (military) Z56.82
  dialysis (hemodialysis) (peritoneal) Z99.2
  do not resuscitate (DNR) Z66
  donor —*see* Donor
  embedded fragments —*see* Retained, foreign body fragments (type of)
  embedded splinter —*see* Retained, foreign body fragments (type of)
  enterostomy Z93.4
  epileptic, epilepticus —*see also* Epilepsy, by type, with status epilepticus G4Ø.9Ø1
  estrogen receptor
    negative Z17.1
    positive Z17.Ø
  female genital cutting —*see* Female genital mutilation status
  female genital mutilation —*see* Female genital mutilation status
  filtering (vitreous) bleb after glaucoma surgery Z98.83
  gastrectomy (complete) (partial) Z9Ø.3
  gastric banding Z98.84
  gastric bypass for obesity Z98.84
  gastrostomy Z93.1
  human immunodeficiency virus (HIV) infection, asymptomatic Z21
  hysterectomy (complete) (total) Z9Ø.71Ø
    partial (with remaining cervial stump) Z9Ø.711
  ileostomy Z93.2
  implant
    breast Z98.82
  infibulation N9Ø.813
  intestinal bypass Z98.Ø
  jejunostomy Z93.4
  lapsed immunization schedule Z28.3
  laryngectomy Z9Ø.Ø2
  lymphaticus E32.8
  malignancy ◀
    castrate resistant prostate Z19.2 ◀
    hormone resistant Z19.2 ◀
    hormone sensitive Z19.1 ◀
  marmoratus G8Ø.3
  mastectomy (unilateral) (bilateral) Z9Ø.1-

Status *(Continued)*
  military deployment status (current) Z56.82
    in theater or in support of military war, peacekeeping and humanitarian operations Z56.82
  nephrectomy (unilateral) (bilateral) Z9Ø.5
  nephrostomy Z93.6
  obesity surgery Z98.84
  oophorectomy
    bilateral Z9Ø.722
    unilateral Z9Ø.721
  organ replacement
    by artificial or mechanical device or prosthesis of
      artery Z95.828
      bladder Z96.Ø
      blood vessel Z95.828
      breast Z97.8
      eye globe Z97.Ø
      heart Z95.812
        valve Z95.2
      intestine Z97.8
      joint Z96.6Ø
        hip —*see* Presence, hip joint implant
        knee —*see* Presence, knee joint implant
        specified site NEC Z96.698
      kidney Z97.8
      larynx Z96.3
      lens Z96.1
      limbs —*see* Presence, artificial, limb
      liver Z97.8
      lung Z97.8
      pancreas Z97.8
    by organ transplant (heterologous) (homologous) —*see* Transplant
  pacemaker
    brain Z96.89
    cardiac Z95.Ø
    specified NEC Z96.89
  pancreatectomy Z9Ø.41Ø
    complete Z9Ø.41Ø
    partial Z9Ø.411
    total Z9Ø.41Ø
  pneumonectomy (complete) (partial) Z9Ø.2
  pneumothorax, therapeutic Z98.3
  postcommotio cerebri F07.81
  postoperative (postprocedural) NEC Z98.89Ø ⬅
    breast implant Z98.82
    dental Z98.818
      crown Z98.811
      fillings Z98.811
      restoration Z98.811
      sealant Z98.81Ø
      specified NEC Z98.818
    pneumothorax, therapeutic Z98.3
    uterine scar Z98.891 ◀
  postpartum (routine follow-up) Z39.2
    care immediately after delivery Z39.Ø
  postsurgical (postprocedural) NEC Z98.89Ø ⬅
    pneumothorax, therapeutic Z98.3
  pregnancy, incidental Z33.1
  prosthesis coronary angioplasty Z95.5
  pseudophakia Z96.1
  renal dialysis (hemodialysis) (peritoneal) Z99.2
  retained foreign body —*see* Retained, foreign body fragments (type of)
  reversed jejunal transposition (for bypass Z98.Ø
  salpingo-oophorectomy
    bilateral Z9Ø.722
    unilateral Z9Ø.721
  sex reassignment surgery status Z87.89Ø
  shunt
    arteriovenous (for dialysis) Z99.2
    cerebrospinal fluid Z98.2
    ventricular (communicating) (for drainage) Z98.2

Status *(Continued)*
splenectomy Z9Ø.81
thymicolymphaticus E32.8
thymicus E32.8
thymolymphaticus E32.8
thyroidectomy (hypothyroidism) E89.Ø
tooth (teeth) extraction —*see also* Absence, teeth, acquired KØ8.4Ø9
tPA (rtPA) administration in a different facility within the last 24 hours prior to admission to current facility Z92.82
tracheostomy Z93.Ø
transplant —*see* Transplant
organ removed Z98.85
tubal ligation Z98.51
underimmunization Z28.3
ureterostomy Z93.6
urethrostomy Z93.6
vagina, artificial Z93.8
vasectomy Z98.52
wheelchair confinement Z99.3
Stealing
child problem F91.8
in company with others Z72.81Ø
pathological (compulsive) F63.2
Steam burn —*see* Burn
Steatocystoma multiplex L72.2
Steatohepatitis (nonalcoholic) (NASH) K75.81
Steatoma L72.3
eyelid (cystic) —*see* Dermatosis, eyelid
infected —*see* Hordeolum
Steatorrhea (chronic) K9Ø.9
with lacteal obstruction K9Ø.2
idiopathic (adult) (infantile) K9Ø.9
pancreatic K9Ø.3
primary K9Ø.Ø
tropical K9Ø.1
Steatosis E88.89
heart —*see* Degeneration, myocardial
kidney N28.89
liver NEC K76.Ø
Steele-Richardson-Olszewski disease or syndrome G23.1
Steinbrocker's syndrome G9Ø.8
Steinert's disease G71.11
Stein-Leventhal syndrome E28.2
Stein's syndrome E28.2
STEMI —*see also* - Infarct, myocardium, ST elevation I21.3
Stenocardia I2Ø.8
Stenocephaly Q75.8
Stenosis, stenotic (cicatricial) —*see also* Stricture
ampulla of Vater K83.1
anus, anal (canal) (sphincter) K62.4
and rectum K62.4
congenital Q42.3
with fistula Q42.2
aorta (ascending) (supraventricular) (congenital) Q25.1
arteriosclerotic I7Ø.Ø
calcified I7Ø.Ø
supravalvular Q25.3
aortic (valve) I35.Ø
with insufficiency I35.2
congenital Q23.Ø
rheumatic IØ6.Ø
with
incompetency, insufficiency or regurgitation IØ6.2
with mitral (valve) disease IØ8.Ø
with tricuspid (valve) disease IØ8.3
mitral (valve) disease IØ8.Ø
with tricuspid (valve) disease IØ8.3
tricuspid (valve) disease IØ8.2
with mitral (valve) disease IØ8.3
specified cause NEC I35.Ø
syphilitic A52.Ø3

Stenosis, stenotic *(Continued)*
aqueduct of Sylvius (congenital) QØ3.Ø
with spina bifida —*see* Spina bifida, by site, with hydrocephalus
acquired G91.1
artery NEC —*see also* Arteriosclerosis I77.1
celiac I77.4
cerebral —*see* Occlusion, artery, cerebral
extremities —*see* Arteriosclerosis, extremities
precerebral —*see* Occlusion, artery, precerebral
pulmonary (congenital) Q25.6
acquired I28.8
renal I7Ø.1
stent
coronary T82.855
peripheral T82.856
bile duct (common) (hepatic) K83.1
congenital Q44.3
bladder-neck (acquired) N32.Ø
congenital Q64.31
brain G93.89
bronchus J98.Ø9
congenital Q32.3
syphilitic A52.72
cardia (stomach) K22.2
congenital Q39.3
cardiovascular —*see* Disease, cardiovascular
caudal M48.Ø8
cervix, cervical (canal) N88.2
congenital Q51.828
in pregnancy or childbirth —*see* Pregnancy, complicated by, abnormal cervix
colon —*see also* Obstruction, intestine
congenital Q42.9
specified NEC Q42.8
colostomy K94.Ø3
common (bile) duct K83.1
congenital Q44.3
coronary (artery) —*see* Disease, heart, ischemic, atherosclerotic
cystic duct —*see* Obstruction, gallbladder
due to presence of device, implant or graft —*see also* Complications, by site and type, specified NEC T85.858
arterial graft NEC T82.858
breast (implant) T85.858
catheter T85.858
dialysis (renal) T82.858
intraperitoneal T85.858
infusion NEC T82.858
spinal (epidural) (subdural) T85.85Ø
urinary (indwelling) T83.85
fixation, internal (orthopedic) NEC T84.85
gastrointestinal (bile duct) (esophagus) T85.858
genital NEC T83.85
heart NEC T82.857
joint prosthesis T84.85
ocular (corneal graft) (orbital implant) NEC T85.858
orthopedic NEC T84.85
specified NEC T85.858
urinary NEC T83.85
vascular NEC T82.858
ventricular intracranial shunt T85.85Ø
duodenum K31.5
congenital Q41.Ø
ejaculatory duct NEC N5Ø.89
endocervical os —*see* Stenosis, cervix
enterostomy K94.13
esophagus K22.2
congenital Q39.3
syphilitic A52.79
congenital A5Ø.59 *[K23]*
eustachian tube —*see* Obstruction, eustachian tube

Stenosis, stenotic *(Continued)*
external ear canal (acquired) H61.3Ø-
congenital Q16.1
due to
inflammation H61.32-
trauma H61.31-
postprocedural H95.81-
specified cause NEC H61.39-
gallbladder —*see* Obstruction, gallbladder
glottis J38.6
heart valve (congenital) Q24.8
aortic Q23.Ø
mitral Q23.2
pulmonary Q22.1
tricuspid Q22.4
hepatic duct K83.1
hymen N89.6
hypertrophic subaortic (idiopathic) I42.1
ileum K56.69
congenital Q41.2
infundibulum cardia Q24.3
intervertebral foramina —*see also* Lesion, biomechanical, specified NEC
connective tissue M99.79
abdomen M99.79
cervical region M99.71
cervicothoracic M99.71
head region M99.7Ø
lumbar region M99.73
lumbosacral M99.73
occipitocervical M99.7Ø
sacral region M99.74
sacrococcygeal M99.74
sacroiliac M99.74
specified NEC M99.79
thoracic region M99.72
thoracolumbar M99.72
disc M99.79
abdomen M99.79
cervical region M99.71
cervicothoracic M99.71
head region M99.7Ø
lower extremity M99.76
lumbar region M99.73
lumbosacral M99.73
occipitocervical M99.7Ø
pelvic M99.75
rib cage M99.78
sacral region M99.74
sacrococcygeal M99.74
sacroiliac M99.74
specified NEC M99.79
thoracic region M99.72
thoracolumbar M99.72
upper extremity M99.77
osseous M99.69
abdomen M99.69
cervical region M99.61
cervicothoracic M99.61
head region M99.6Ø
lower extremity M99.66
lumbar region M99.63
lumbosacral M99.63
occipitocervical M99.6Ø
pelvic M99.65
rib cage M99.68
sacral region M99.64
sacrococcygeal M99.64
sacroiliac M99.64
specified NEC M99.69
thoracic region M99.62
thoracolumbar M99.62
upper extremity M99.67
subluxation —*see* Stenosis, intervertebral foramina, osseous
intestine —*see also* Obstruction, intestine
congenital (small) Q41.9
large Q42.9
specified NEC Q42.8
specified NEC Q41.8

Stenosis, stenotic *(Continued)*
jejunum K56.69
congenital Q41.1
lacrimal (passage)
canaliculi H04.54-
congenital Q1Ø.5
duct HØ4.55-
punctum HØ4.56-
sac HØ4.57-
lacrimonasal duct —*see* Stenosis, lacrimal, duct
congenital Q1Ø.5
larynx J38.6
congenital NEC Q31.8
subglottic Q31.1
syphilitic A52.73
congenital A5Ø.59 *[J99]*
mitral (chronic) (inactive) (valve) IØ5.Ø
with
aortic valve disease IØ8.Ø
incompetency, insufficiency or regurgitation IØ5.2
active or acute IØ1.1
with rheumatic or Sydenham's chorea IØ2.Ø
congenital Q23.2
specified cause, except rheumatic I34.2
syphilitic A52.Ø3
myocardium, myocardial —*see also* Degeneration, myocardial
hypertrophic subaortic (idiopathic) I42.1
nares (anterior) (posterior) J34.89
congenital Q3Ø.Ø
nasal duct —*see also* Stenosis, lacrimal, duct
congenital Q1Ø.5
nasolacrimal duct —*see also* Stenosis, lacrimal, duct
congenital Q1Ø.5
neural canal —*see also* Lesion, biomechanical, specified NEC
connective tissue M99.49
abdomen M99.49
cervical region M99.41
cervicothoracic M99.41
head region M99.4Ø
lower extremity M99.46
lumbar region M99.43
lumbosacral M99.43
occipitocervical M99.4Ø
pelvic M99.45
rib cage M99.48
sacral region M99.44
sacrococcygeal M99.44
sacroiliac M99.44
specified NEC M99.49
thoracic region M99.42
thoracolumbar M99.42
upper extremity M99.47
intervertebral disc M99.59
abdomen M99.59
cervical region M99.51
cervicothoracic M99.51
head region M99.5Ø
lower extremity M99.56
lumbar region M99.53
lumbosacral M99.53
occipitocervical M99.5Ø
pelvic M99.55
rib cage M99.58
sacral region M99.54
sacrococcygeal M99.54
sacroiliac M99.54
specified NEC M99.59
thoracic region M99.52
thoracolumbar M99.52
upper extremity M99.57
osseous M99.39
abdomen M99.39
cervical region M99.31
cervicothoracic M99.31
head region M99.3Ø

Stenosis, stenotic *(Continued)*
neural canal *(Continued)*
osseous *(Continued)*
lower extremity M99.36
lumbar region M99.33
lumbosacral M99.33
occipitocervical M99.3Ø
pelvic M99.35
rib cage M99.38
sacral region M99.34
sacrococcygeal M99.34
sacroiliac M99.34
specified NEC M99.39
thoracic region M99.32
thoracolumbar M99.32
upper extremity M99.37
subluxation M99.29
cervical region M99.21
cervicothoracic M99.21
head region M99.2Ø
lower extremity M99.26
lumbar region M99.23
lumbosacral M99.23
occipitocervical M99.2Ø
pelvic M99.25
rib cage M99.28
sacral region M99.24
sacrococcygeal M99.24
sacroiliac M99.24
specified NEC M99.29
thoracic region M99.22
thoracolumbar M99.22
upper extremity M99.27
organ or site, congenital NEC —*see* Atresia, by site
papilla of Vater K83.1
pulmonary (artery) (congenital) Q25.6
with ventricular septal defect, transposition of aorta, and hypertrophy of right ventricle Q21.3
acquired I28.8
in tetralogy of Fallot Q21.3
infundibular Q24.3
subvalvular Q24.3
supravalvular Q25.6
valve I37.Ø
with insufficiency I37.2
congenital Q22.1
rheumatic IØ9.89
with aortic, mitral or tricuspid (valve) disease IØ8.8
vein, acquired I28.8
vessel NEC I28.8
pulmonic (congenital) Q22.1
infundibular Q24.3
subvalvular Q24.3
pylorus (hypertrophic) (acquired) K31.1
adult K31.1
congenital Q4Ø.Ø
infantile Q4Ø.Ø
rectum (sphincter) —*see* Stricture, rectum
renal artery I7Ø.1
congenital Q27.1
salivary duct (any) K11.8
sphincter of Oddi K83.1
spinal M48.ØØ
cervical region M48.Ø2
cervicothoracic region M48.Ø3
lumbar region M48.Ø6
lumbosacral region M48.Ø7
occipito-atlanto-axial region M48.Ø1
sacrococcygeal region M48.Ø8
thoracic region M48.Ø4
thoracolumbar region M48.Ø5
stent ◀
vascular ◀
end stent ◀
adjacent to stent —*see* Arteriosclerosis ◀

Stenosis, stenotic *(Continued)*
stent *(Continued)*
vascular *(Continued)*
end stent *(Continued)*
within the stent ◀
coronary T82.855 ◀
peripheral T82.856 ◀
in stent ◀
coronary vessel T82.855 ◀
peripheral vessel T82.856 ◀
stomach, hourglass K31.2
subaortic (congenital) Q24.4
hypertrophic (idiopathic) I42.1
subglottic J38.6
congenital Q31.1
postprocedural J95.5
trachea J39.8
congenital Q32.1
syphilitic A52.73
tuberculous NEC A15.5
tracheostomy J95.Ø3
tricuspid (valve) IØ7.Ø
with
aortic (valve) disease IØ8.2
incompetency, insufficiency or regurgitation IØ7.2
with aortic (valve) disease IØ8.2
with mitral (valve) disease IØ8.3
mitral (valve) disease IØ8.1
with aortic (valve) disease IØ8.3
congenital Q22.4
nonrheumatic I36.Ø
with insufficiency I36.2
tubal N97.1
ureter —*see* Atresia, ureter
ureteropelvic junction, congenital Q62.11
ureterovesical orifice, congenital Q62.12
urethra (valve) —*see also* Stricture, urethra
congenital Q64.32
urinary meatus, congenital Q64.33
vagina N89.5
congenital Q52.4
in pregnancy —*see* Pregnancy, complicated by, abnormal vagina
causing obstructed labor O65.5
valve (cardiac) (heart) —*see also* Endocarditis I38
congenital Q24.8
aortic Q23.Ø
mitral Q23.2
pulmonary Q22.1
tricuspid Q22.4
vena cava (inferior) (superior) I87.1
congenital Q26.Ø
vesicourethral orifice Q64.31
vulva N9Ø.5
Stent jail T82.897
Stercolith (impaction) K56.41
appendix K38.1
Stercoraceous, stercoral ulcer K63.3
anus or rectum K62.6
Stereotypies NEC F98.4
Sterility —*see* Infertility
Sterilization —*see* Encounter (for), sterilization
Sternalgia —*see* Angina
Sternopagus Q89.4
Sternum bifidum Q76.7
Steroid
effects (adverse) (adrenocortical) (iatrogenic)
cushingoid E24.2
correct substance properly administered —*see* Table of Drugs and Chemicals, by drug, adverse effect
overdose or wrong substance given or taken —*see* Table of Drugs and Chemicals, by drug, poisoning

Steroid *(Continued)*
effects *(Continued)*
diabetes —*see* category E09
correct substance properly administered —*see* Table of Drugs and Chemicals, by drug, adverse effect
overdose or wrong substance given or taken —*see* Table of Drugs and Chemicals, by drug, poisoning
fever R50.2
insufficiency E27.3
correct substance properly administered —*see* Table of Drugs and Chemicals, by drug, adverse effect
overdose or wrong substance given or taken —*see* Table of Drugs and Chemicals, by drug, poisoning
responder H40.04-
Stevens-Johnson disease or syndrome L51.1
toxic epidermal necrolysis overlap L51.3
Stewart-Morel syndrome M85.2
Sticker's disease B08.3
Sticky eye —*see* Conjunctivitis, acute, mucopurulent
Stieda's disease —*see* Bursitis, tibial collateral
Stiff neck —*see* Torticollis
Stiff-man syndrome G25.82
Stiffness, joint NEC M25.60-
ankle M25.67-
ankylosis —*see* Ankylosis, joint
contracture —*see* Contraction, joint
elbow M25.62-
foot M25.67-
hand M25.64-
hip M25.65-
knee M25.66-
shoulder M25.61-
wrist M25.63-
Stigmata congenital syphilis A50.59
Stillbirth P95
Still-Felty syndrome —*see* Felty's syndrome
Still's disease or syndrome (juvenile) M08.20
adult-onset M06.1
ankle M08.27-
elbow M08.22-
foot joint M08.27-
hand joint M08.24-
hip M08.25-
knee M08.26-
multiple site M08.29
shoulder M08.21-
vertebra M08.28
wrist M08.23-
Stimulation, ovary E28.1
Sting (venomous) (with allergic or anaphylactic shock) —*see* Table of Drugs and Chemicals, by animal or substance, poisoning
Stippled epiphyses Q78.8
Stitch
abscess T81.48 ◄
burst (in operation wound) —*see* Disruption, wound, operation
Stokes-Adams disease or syndrome I45.9
Stokes' disease E05.00
with thyroid storm E05.01
Stokvis (-Talma) disease D74.8
Stoma malfunction
colostomy K94.03
enterostomy K94.13
gastrostomy K94.23
ileostomy K94.13
tracheostomy J95.03
Stomach —*see* condition
Stomatitis (denture) (ulcerative) K12.1
angular K13.0
due to dietary or vitamin deficiency E53.0
aphthous K12.0
bovine B08.61

Stomatitis *(Continued)*
candidal B37.0
catarrhal K12.1
diphtheritic A36.89
due to
dietary deficiency E53.0
thrush B37.0
vitamin deficiency
B group NEC E53.9
B2 (riboflavin) E53.0
epidemic B08.8
epizootic B08.8
follicular K12.1
gangrenous A69.0
Geotrichum B48.3
herpesviral, herpetic B00.2
herpetiformis K12.0
malignant K12.1
membranous acute K12.1
monilial B37.0
mycotic B37.0
necrotizing ulcerative A69.0
parasitic B37.0
septic K12.1
spirochetal A69.1
suppurative (acute) K12.2
ulceromembranous A69.1
vesicular K12.1
with exanthem (enteroviral) B08.4
virus disease A93.8
Vincent's A69.1
Stomatocytosis D58.8
Stomatomycosis B37.0
Stomatorrhagia K13.79
Stone (s) —*see also* Calculus
bladder (diverticulum) N21.0
cystine E72.09
heart syndrome I50.1
kidney N20.0
prostate N42.0
pulpal (dental) K04.2
renal N20.0
salivary gland or duct (any) K11.5
urethra (impacted) N21.1
urinary (duct) (impacted) (passage) N20.9
bladder (diverticulum) N21.0
lower tract N21.9
specified NEC N21.8
xanthine E79.8 *[N22]*
Stonecutter's lung J62.8
Stonemason's asthma, disease, lung or pneumoconiosis J62.8
Stoppage
heart —*see* Arrest, cardiac
urine —*see* Retention, urine
Storm, thyroid —*see* Thyrotoxicosis
Strabismus (congenital) (nonparalytic) H50.9
concomitant H50.40
convergent —*see* Strabismus, convergent concomitant
divergent —*see* Strabismus, divergent concomitant
convergent concomitant H50.00
accommodative component H50.43
alternating H50.05
with
A pattern H50.06
specified nonconcomitances NEC H50.08
V pattern H50.07
monocular H50.01-
with
A pattern H50.02-
specified noncomitances NEC H50.04-
V pattern H50.03-
intermittent H50.31-
alternating H50.32

Strabismus *(Continued)*
cyclotropia H50.41 ◄
divergent concomitant H50.10
alternating H50.15
with
A pattern H50.16
specified noncomitances NEC H50.18
V pattern H50.17
monocular H50.11-
with
A pattern H50.12-
specified noncomitances NEC H50.14-
V pattern H50.13-
intermittent H50.33-
alternating H50.34
Duane's syndrome H50.81-
due to adhesions, scars H50.69
heterophoria H50.50
alternating H50.55
cyclophoria H50.54
esophoria H50.51
exophoria H50.52
vertical H50.53
heterotropia H50.40
intermittent H50.30
hypertropia H50.2-
hypotropia —*see* Hypertropia
latent H50.50
mechanical H50.60
Brown's sheath syndrome H50.61-
specified type NEC H50.69
monofixation syndrome H50.42
paralytic H49.9
abducens nerve H49.2-
fourth nerve H49.1-
Kearns-Sayre syndrome H49.81-
ophthalmoplegia (external)
progressive H49.4-
with pigmentary retinopathy H49.81-
total H49.3-
sixth nerve H49.2-
specified type NEC H49.88-
third nerve H49.0-
trochlear nerve H49.1-
specified type NEC H50.89
vertical H50.2-
Strain
back S39.012
cervical S16.1
eye NEC —*see* Disturbance, vision, subjective
heart —*see* Disease, heart
low back S39.012
mental NOS Z73.3
work-related Z56.6
muscle (tendon) —*see* Injury, muscle, by site, strain
neck S16.1
physical NOS Z73.3
work-related Z56.6
postural —*see also* Disorder, soft tissue, due to use
psychological NEC Z73.3
tendon —*see* Injury, muscle, by site, strain
Straining, on urination R39.16
Strand, vitreous —*see* Opacity, vitreous, membranes and strands
Strangulation, strangulated —*see also* Asphyxia, traumatic
appendix K38.8
bladder-neck N32.0
bowel or colon K56.2
food or foreign body —*see* Foreign body, by site
hemorrhoids —*see* Hemorrhoids, with complication
hernia —*see also* Hernia, by site, with obstruction
with gangrene —*see* Hernia, by site, with gangrene

Strangulation, strangulated *(Continued)*
intestine (large) (small) K56.2
with hernia —*see also* Hernia, by site, with obstruction
with gangrene —*see* Hernia, by site, with gangrene
mesentery K56.2
mucus —*see* Asphyxia, mucus
omentum K56.2
organ or site, congenital NEC —*see* Atresia, by site
ovary —*see* Torsion, ovary
penis N48.89
foreign body T19.4
rupture —*see* Hernia, by site, with obstruction
stomach due to hernia —*see also* Hernia, by site, with obstruction
with gangrene —*see* Hernia, by site, with gangrene
vesicourethral orifice N32.Ø
Strangury R3Ø.Ø
Straw itch B88.Ø
Strawberry
gallbladder K82.4
mark Q82.5
tongue (red) (white) K14.3
Streak (s)
macula, angioid H35.33
ovarian Q5Ø.32
Strephosymbolia F81.Ø
secondary to organic lesion R48.8
Streptobacillary fever A25.1
Streptobacillosis A25.1
Streptobacillus moniliformis A25.1
Streptococcus, streptococcal —*see also* condition
as cause of disease classified elsewhere B95.5
group
A, as cause of disease classified elsewhere B95.Ø
B, as cause of disease classified elsewhere B95.1
D, as cause of disease classified elsewhere B95.2
pneumoniae, as cause of disease classified elsewhere B95.3
specified NEC, as cause of disease classified elsewhere B95.4
Streptomycosis B47.1
Streptotrichosis A48.8
Stress F43.9
family —*see* Disruption, family
fetal P84
complicating pregnancy O77.9
due to drug administration O77.1
mental NEC Z73.3
work-related Z56.6
physical NEC Z73.3
work-related Z56.6
polycythemia D75.1
reaction —*see also* Reaction, stress F43.9
work schedule Z56.3
Stretching, nerve —*see* Injury, nerve
Striae albicantes, atrophicae or distensae (cutis) L9Ø.6
Stricture —*see also* Stenosis
ampulla of Vater K83.1
anus (sphincter) K62.4
congenital Q42.3
with fistula Q42.2
infantile Q42.3
with fistula Q42.2
aorta (ascending) (congenital) Q25.1 ⬅
arteriosclerotic I7Ø.Ø
calcified I7Ø.Ø
supravalvular, congenital Q25.3
aortic (valve) —*see* Stenosis, aortic
aqueduct of Sylvius (congenital) QØ3.Ø
with spina bifida —*see* Spina bifida, by site, with hydrocephalus
acquired G91.1

Stricture *(Continued)*
artery I77.1
basilar —*see* Occlusion, artery, basilar
carotid —*see* Occlusion, artery, carotid
celiac I77.4
congenital (peripheral) Q27.8
cerebral Q28.3
coronary Q24.5
digestive system Q27.8
lower limb Q27.8
retinal Q14.1
specified site NEC Q27.8
umbilical Q27.Ø
upper limb Q27.8
coronary —*see* Disease, heart, ischemic, atherosclerotic
congenital Q24.5
precerebral —*see* Occlusion, artery, precerebral
pulmonary (congenital) Q25.6
acquired I28.8
renal I7Ø.1
vertebral —*see* Occlusion, artery, vertebral
auditory canal (external) (congenital)
acquired —*see* Stenosis, external ear canal
bile duct (common) (hepatic) K83.1
congenital Q44.3
postoperative K91.89
bladder N32.89
neck N32.Ø
bowel —*see* Obstruction, intestine
brain G93.89
bronchus J98.Ø9
congenital Q32.3
syphilitic A52.72
cardia (stomach) K22.2
congenital Q39.3
cardiac —*see also* Disease, heart
orifice (stomach) K22.2
cecum —*see* Obstruction, intestine
cervix, cervical (canal) N88.2
congenital Q51.828
in pregnancy —*see* Pregnancy, complicated by, abnormal cervix
causing obstructed labor O65.5
colon —*see also* Obstruction, intestine
congenital Q42.9
specified NEC Q42.8
colostomy K94.Ø3
common (bile) duct K83.1
coronary (artery) —*see* Disease, heart, ischemic, atherosclerotic
cystic duct —*see* Obstruction, gallbladder
digestive organs NEC, congenital Q45.8
duodenum K31.5
congenital Q41.Ø
ear canal (external) (congenital) Q16.1
acquired —*see* Stricture, auditory canal, acquired
ejaculatory duct N5Ø.89 ⬅
enterostomy K94.13
esophagus K22.2
congenital Q39.3
syphilitic A52.79
congenital A5Ø.59 *[K23]*
eustachian tube —*see also* Obstruction, eustachian tube
congenital Q17.8
fallopian tube N97.1
gonococcal A54.24
tuberculous A18.17
gallbladder —*see* Obstruction, gallbladder
glottis J38.6
heart —*see also* Disease, heart
valve (*see also* Endocarditis) I38
aortic Q23.Ø
mitral Q23.4
pulmonary Q22.1
tricuspid Q22.4
hepatic duct K83.1
hourglass, of stomach K31.2

Stricture *(Continued)*
hymen N89.6
hypopharynx J39.2
ileum K56.69
congenital Q41.2
intestine —*see also* Obstruction, intestine
congenital (small) Q41.9
large Q42.9
specified NEC Q42.8
specified NEC Q41.8
ischemic K55.1
jejunum K56.69
congenital Q41.1
lacrimal passages —*see also* Stenosis, lacrimal
congenital Q1Ø.5
larynx J38.6
congenital NEC Q31.8
subglottic Q31.1
syphilitic A52.73
congenital A5Ø.59 *[J99]*
meatus
ear (congenital) Q16.1
acquired —*see* Stricture, auditory canal, acquired
osseous (ear) (congenital) Q16.1
acquired —*see* Stricture, auditory canal, acquired
urinarius —*see also* Stricture, urethra
congenital Q64.33
mitral (valve) —*see* Stenosis, mitral
myocardium, myocardial I51.5
hypertrophic subaortic (idiopathic) I42.1
nares (anterior) (posterior) J34.89
congenital Q3Ø.Ø
nasal duct —*see also* Stenosis, lacrimal, duct
congenital Q1Ø.5
nasolacrimal duct —*see also* Stenosis, lacrimal, duct
congenital Q1Ø.5
nasopharynx J39.2
syphilitic A52.73
nose J34.89
congenital Q3Ø.Ø
nostril (anterior) (posterior) J34.89
congenital Q3Ø.Ø
syphilitic A52.73
congenital A5Ø.59 *[J99]*
organ or site, congenital NEC —*see* Atresia, by site
os uteri —*see* Stricture, cervix
osseous meatus (ear) (congenital) Q16.1
acquired —*see* Stricture, auditory canal, acquired
oviduct —*see* Stricture, fallopian tube
pelviureteric junction (congenital) Q62.11
acquired, with hydronephrosis N13.Ø ◀
penis, by foreign body T19.4
pharynx J39.2
prostate N42.89
pulmonary, pulmonic
artery (congenital) Q25.6
acquired I28.8
noncongenital I28.8
infundibulum (congenital) Q24.3
valve I37.Ø
congenital Q22.1
vein, acquired I28.8
vessel NEC I28.8
punctum lacrimale —*see also* Stenosis, lacrimal, punctum
congenital Q1Ø.5
pylorus (hypertrophic) K31.1
adult K31.1
congenital Q4Ø.Ø
infantile Q4Ø.Ø
rectosigmoid K56.69
rectum (sphincter) K62.4
congenital Q42.1
with fistula Q42.Ø

◀ New ⬅ Revised ~~deleted~~ Deleted

- **Stricture** *(Continued)*
  - rectum (sphincter) *(Continued)*
    - due to
      - chlamydial lymphogranuloma A55
      - irradiation K91.89
      - lymphogranuloma venereum A55
    - gonococcal A54.6
    - inflammatory (chlamydial) A55
    - syphilitic A52.74
    - tuberculous A18.32
  - renal artery I7Ø.1
    - congenital Q27.1
  - salivary duct or gland (any) K11.8
  - sigmoid (flexure) —*see* Obstruction, intestine
  - spermatic cord N5Ø.89 ⇐
  - stoma (following) (of)
    - colostomy K94.Ø3
    - enterostomy K94.13
    - gastrostomy K94.23
    - ileostomy K94.13
    - tracheostomy J95.Ø3
  - stomach K31.89
    - congenital Q4Ø.2
    - hourglass K31.2
  - subaortic Q24.4
    - hypertrophic (acquired) (idiopathic) I42.1
  - subglottic J38.6
  - syphilitic NEC A52.79
  - trachea J39.8
    - congenital Q32.1
    - syphilitic A52.73
    - tuberculous NEC A15.5
  - tracheostomy J95.Ø3
  - tricuspid (valve) —*see* Stenosis, tricuspid
  - tunica vaginalis N5Ø.89 ⇐
  - ureter (postoperative) N13.5
    - with
      - hydronephrosis N13.1
        - with infection N13.6
      - pyelonephritis (chronic) N11.1
    - congenital —*see* Atresia, ureter
    - tuberculous A18.11
  - ureteropelvic junction (congenital) Q62.11
    - acquired, with hydronephrosis N13.Ø ◄
  - ureterovesical orifice N13.5
    - with infection N13.6
  - urethra (organic) (spasmodic) N35.9
    - associated with schistosomiasis B65.Ø *[N37]*
    - congenital Q64.39
      - valvular (posterior) Q64.2
    - due to
      - infection —*see* Stricture, urethra, postinfective
      - trauma —*see* Stricture, urethra, post-traumatic
    - gonococcal, gonorrheal A54.Ø1
    - infective NEC —*see* Stricture, urethra, postinfective
    - late effect (sequelae) of injury —*see* Stricture, urethra, post-traumatic
    - postcatheterization —*see* Stricture, urethra, postprocedural
    - postinfective NEC
      - female N35.12
      - male N35.119
        - anterior urethra N35.114
        - bulbous urethra N35.112
        - meatal N35.111
        - membranous urethra N35.113
    - postobstetric N35.Ø21
    - postoperative —*see* Stricture, urethra, postprocedural
    - postprocedural
      - female N99.12
      - male N99.114
        - ~~anterior urethra N99.113~~
        - anterior bulbous urethra N99.113 ◄
        - bulbous urethra N99.111
        - fossa navicularis N99.115 ◄
        - meatal N99.11Ø
        - membranous urethra N99.112
- **Stricture** *(Continued)*
  - urethra (organic) (spasmodic) *(Continued)*
    - post-traumatic
      - female N35.Ø28
        - due to childbirth N35.Ø21
      - male N35.Ø14
        - anterior urethra N35.Ø13
        - bulbous urethra N35.Ø11
        - meatal N35.Ø1Ø
        - membranous urethra N35.Ø12
    - sequela (late effect) of
      - childbirth N35.Ø21
      - injury —*see* Stricture, urethra, post-traumatic
    - specified cause NEC N35.8
    - syphilitic A52.76
    - traumatic —*see* Stricture, urethra, post-traumatic
    - valvular (posterior), congenital Q64.2
  - urinary meatus —*see* Stricture, urethra
  - uterus, uterine (synechiae) N85.6
    - os (external) (internal) —*see* Stricture, cervix
  - vagina (outlet) —*see* Stenosis, vagina
  - valve (cardiac) (heart) —*see also* Endocarditis
    - congenital
      - aortic Q23.Ø
      - mitral Q23.2
      - pulmonary Q22.1
      - tricuspid Q22.4
  - vas deferens N5Ø.89 ⇐
    - congenital Q55.4
  - vein I87.1
  - vena cava (inferior) (superior) NEC I87.1
    - congenital Q26.Ø
  - vesicourethral orifice N32.Ø
    - congenital Q64.31
  - vulva (acquired) N9Ø.5
- **Stridor** RØ6.1
  - congenital (larynx) P28.89
- **Stridulous** —*see* condition
- **Stroke** (apoplectic) (brain) (embolic) (ischemic) (paralytic) (thrombotic) I63.9
  - epileptic —*see* Epilepsy
  - heat T67.Ø
  - in evolution I63.9
  - intraoperative
    - during cardiac surgery I97.81Ø
    - during other surgery I97.811
  - lightning —*see* Lightning
  - meaning
    - cerebral hemorrhage — code to Hemorrhage, intracranial
    - cerebral infarction — code to Infarction, cerebral
  - postprocedural
    - following cardiac surgery I97.82Ø
    - following other surgery I97.821
  - unspecified (NOS) I63.9
- **Stromatosis, endometrial** D39.Ø
- **Strongyloidiasis, strongyloidosis** B78.9
  - cutaneous B78.1
  - disseminated B78.7
  - intestinal B78.Ø
- **Strophulus pruriginosus** L28.2
- **Struck by lightning** —*see* Lightning
- **Struma** —*see also* Goiter
  - Hashimoto EØ6.3
  - lymphomatosa EØ6.3
  - nodosa (simplex) EØ4.9
    - endemic EØ1.2
      - multinodular EØ1.1
    - multinodular EØ4.2
      - iodine-deficiency related EØ1.1
    - toxic or with hyperthyroidism EØ5.2Ø
      - with thyroid storm EØ5.21
      - multinodular EØ5.2Ø
        - with thyroid storm EØ5.21
      - uninodular EØ5.1Ø
        - with thyroid storm EØ5.11
- **Struma** *(Continued)*
  - nodosa (simplex) *(Continued)*
    - toxicosa EØ5.2Ø
      - with thyroid storm EØ5.21
      - multinodular EØ5.2Ø
        - with thyroid storm EØ5.21
      - uninodular EØ5.1Ø
        - with thyroid storm EØ5.11
    - uninodular EØ4.1
  - ovarii D27.-
  - Riedel's EØ6.5
- **Strumipriva cachexia** EØ3.4
- **Strümpell-Marie spine** —*see* Spondylitis, ankylosing
- **Strümpell-Westphal pseudosclerosis** E83.Ø1
- **Stuart deficiency disease** (factor X) D68.2
- **Stuart-Prower factor deficiency** (factor X) D68.2
- **Student's elbow** —*see* Bursitis, elbow, olecranon
- **Stump** —*see* Amputation
- **Stunting, nutritional** E45
- **Stupor** (catatonic) R4Ø.1
  - depressive (single episode) F32.89 ⇐
    - recurrent episode F33.8 ◄
  - dissociative F44.2
  - manic F3Ø.2
  - manic-depressive F31.89
  - psychogenic (anergic) F44.2
  - reaction to exceptional stress (transient) F43.Ø
- **Sturge** (-Weber) (-Dimitri) (-Kalischer) **disease or syndrome** Q85.8
- **Stuttering** F8Ø.81
  - adult onset F98.5
  - childhood onset F8Ø.81
  - following cerebrovascular disease —*see* Disorder, fluency, following cerebrovascular disease
  - in conditions classified elsewhere R47.82
- **Sty, stye** (external) (internal) (meibomian) (zeisian) —*see* Hordeolum
- **Subacidity, gastric** K31.89
  - psychogenic F45.8
- **Subacute** —*see* condition
- **Subarachnoid** —*see* condition
- **Subcortical** —*see* condition
- **Subcostal syndrome, nerve compression** —*see* Mononeuropathy, upper limb, specified site NEC
- **Subcutaneous, subcuticular** —*see* condition
- **Subdural** —*see* condition
- **Subendocardium** —*see* condition
- **Subependymoma**
  - specified site —*see* Neoplasm, uncertain behavior, by site
  - unspecified site D43.2
- **Suberosis** J67.3
- **Subglossitis** —*see* Glossitis
- **Subhemophilia** D66
- **Subinvolution**
  - breast (postlactational) (postpuerperal) N64.89
  - puerperal O9Ø.89
  - uterus (chronic) (nonpuerperal) N85.3
    - puerperal O9Ø.89
- **Sublingual** —*see* condition
- **Sublinguitis** —*see* Sialoadenitis
- **Subluxatable hip** Q65.6
- **Subluxation** —*see also* Dislocation
  - acromioclavicular S43.11-
  - ankle S93.Ø-
  - atlantoaxial, recurrent M43.4
    - with myelopathy M43.3
  - carpometacarpal (joint) NEC S63.Ø5-
    - thumb S63.Ø4-
  - complex, vertebral —*see* Complex, subluxation
  - congenital —*see also* Malposition, congenital
    - hip —*see* Dislocation, hip, congenital, partial

S

◄ New ⇐ Revised ~~deleted~~ Deleted

Sugar
blood
high (transient) R73.9
low (transient) E16.2
in urine R81
Suicide, suicidal (attempted) T14.91
by poisoning —*see* Table of Drugs and Chemicals
history of (personal) Z91.5
in family Z81.8
ideation —*see* Ideation, suicidal
risk
meaning personal history of attempted suicide Z91.5
meaning suicidal ideation —*see* Ideation, suicidal
tendencies
meaning personal history of attempted suicide Z91.5
meaning suicidal ideation —*see* Ideation, suicidal
trauma —*see* nature of injury by site
Suipestifer infection —*see* Infection, salmonella
Sulfhemoglobinemia, sulphemoglobinemia (acquired) (with methemoglobinemia) D74.8
Sumatran mite fever A75.3
Summer —*see* condition
Sunburn L55.9
due to ◀
tanning bed (acute) L56.8 ◀
chronic L57.8 ◀
ultraviolet radiation (acute) L56.8 ◀
chronic L57.8 ◀
first degree L55.Ø
second degree L55.1
third degree L55.2
SUNCT (short lasting unilateral neuralgiform headache with conjunctival injection and tearing) G44.Ø59
intractable G44.Ø51
not intractable G44.Ø59
Sunken acetabulum —*see* Derangement, joint, specified type NEC, hip
Sunstroke T67.Ø
Superfecundation —*see* Pregnancy, multiple
Superfetation —*see* Pregnancy, multiple
Superinvolution (uterus) N85.8
Supernumerary (congenital)
aortic cusps Q23.8
auditory ossicles Q16.3
bone Q79.8
breast Q83.1
carpal bones Q74.Ø
cusps, heart valve NEC Q24.8
aortic Q23.8
mitral Q23.2
pulmonary Q22.3
digit (s) Q69.9
ear (lobule) Q17.Ø
fallopian tube Q5Ø.6
finger Q69.Ø
hymen Q52.4
kidney Q63.Ø
lacrimonasal duct Q1Ø.6
lobule (ear) Q17.Ø
mitral cusps Q23.2
muscle Q79.8
nipple (s) Q83.3
organ or site not listed —*see* Accessory
ossicles, auditory Q16.3
ovary Q5Ø.31
oviduct Q5Ø.6
pulmonary, pulmonic cusps Q22.3
rib Q76.6
cervical or first (syndrome) Q76.5
roots (of teeth) KØØ.2
spleen Q89.Ø9
tarsal bones Q74.2
teeth KØØ.1
Supernumerary *(Continued)*
testis Q55.29
thumb Q69.1
toe Q69.2
uterus Q51.2
vagina Q52.1
vertebra Q76.49
Supervision (of)
contraceptive —*see* Prescription, contraceptives
dietary (for) Z71.3
allergy (food) Z71.3
colitis Z71.3
diabetes mellitus Z71.3
food allergy or intolerance Z71.3
gastritis Z71.3
hypercholesterolemia Z71.3
hypoglycemia Z71.3
intolerance (food) Z71.3
obesity Z71.3
specified NEC Z71.3
healthy infant or child Z76.2
foundling Z76.1
high-risk pregnancy —*see* Pregnancy, complicated by, high, risk
lactation Z39.1
pregnancy —*see* Pregnancy, supervision of
Supplemental teeth KØØ.1
Suppression
binocular vision H53.34
lactation O92.5
menstruation N94.89
ovarian secretion E28.39
renal N28.9
urine, urinary secretion R34
Suppuration, suppurative —*see also* condition
accessory sinus (chronic) —*see* Sinusitis
adrenal gland
antrum (chronic) —*see* Sinusitis, maxillary
bladder —*see* Cystitis
brain GØ6.Ø
sequelae GØ9
breast N61.1 ⬅
puerperal, postpartum or gestational —*see* Mastitis, obstetric, purulent
dental periosteum M27.3
ear (middle) —*see also* Otitis, media
external NEC —*see* Otitis, externa, infective
internal —*see* subcategory H83.Ø
ethmoidal (chronic) (sinus) —*see* Sinusitis, ethmoidal
fallopian tube —*see* Salpingo-oophoritis
frontal (chronic) (sinus) —*see* Sinusitis, frontal
gallbladder (acute) K81.Ø
gum KØ5.2Ø
generalized —*see* Peridontitis, aggressive, generalized ⬅
localized —*see* Peridontitis, aggressive, localized ⬅
intracranial GØ6.Ø
joint —*see* Arthritis, pyogenic or pyemic
labyrinthine —*see* subcategory H83.Ø
lung —*see* Abscess, lung
mammary gland N61.1 ⬅
puerperal, postpartum O91.12
associated with lactation O91.13
maxilla, maxillary M27.2
sinus (chronic) —*see* Sinusitis, maxillary
muscle —*see* Myositis, infective
nasal sinus (chronic) —*see* Sinusitis
pancreas, acute —*see also* Pancreatitis, acute K85.8Ø ⬅
parotid gland —*see* Sialoadenitis
pelvis, pelvic
female —*see* Disease, pelvis, inflammatory
male K65.Ø
pericranial —*see* Osteomyelitis
salivary duct or gland (any) —*see* Sialoadenitis
Suppuration, suppurative *(Continued)*
sinus (accessory) (chronic) (nasal) —*see* Sinusitis
sphenoidal sinus (chronic) —*see* Sinusitis, sphenoidal
thymus (gland) E32.1
thyroid (gland) EØ6.Ø
tonsil —*see* Tonsillitis
uterus —*see* Endometritis
Supraeruption of tooth (teeth) M26.34
Supraglottitis JØ4.3Ø
with obstruction JØ4.31
Suprarenal (gland) —*see* condition
Suprascapular nerve —*see* condition
Suprasellar —*see* condition
Surfer's knots or nodules S89.8-
Surgical
emphysema T81.82
procedures, complication or misadventure —*see* Complications, surgical procedures
shock T81.1Ø
Surveillance (of) (for) —*see also* Observation
alcohol abuse Z71.41
contraceptive —*see* Prescription, contraceptives
dietary Z71.3
drug abuse Z71.51
Susceptibility to disease, genetic Z15.89
malignant neoplasm Z15.Ø9
breast Z15.Ø1
endometrium Z15.Ø4
ovary Z15.Ø2
prostate Z15.Ø3
specified NEC Z15.Ø9
multiple endocrine neoplasia Z15.81
Suspected condition, ruled out —*see also* Observation, suspected
amniotic cavity and membrane ZØ3.71
cervical shortening ZØ3.75
fetal anomaly ZØ3.73
fetal growth ZØ3.74
maternal and fetal conditions NEC ZØ3.79
newborn —*see also* Observation, newborn, suspected condition ruled out ZØ5.9 ◀
oligohydramnios ZØ3.71
placental problem ZØ3.72
polyhydramnios ZØ3.71
Suspended uterus
in pregnancy or childbirth —*see* Pregnancy, complicated by, abnormal uterus
Sutton's nevus D22.9
Suture
burst (in operation wound) T81.31
external operation wound T81.31
internal operation wound T81.32
inadvertently left in operation wound —*see* Foreign body, accidentally left during a procedure
removal Z48.Ø2
Swab inadvertently left in operation wound —*see* Foreign body, accidentally left during a procedure
Swallowed, swallowing
difficulty —*see* Dysphagia
foreign body —*see* Foreign body, alimentary tract
Swan-neck deformity (finger) —*see* Deformity, finger, swan-neck
Swearing, compulsive F42.8 ⬅
in Gilles de la Tourette's syndrome F95.2
Sweat, sweats
fetid L75.Ø
night R61
Sweating, excessive R61
Sweeley-Klionsky disease E75.21
Sweet's disease or dermatosis L98.2
Swelling (of) R6Ø.9
abdomen, abdominal (not referable to any particular organ) —*see* Mass, abdominal
ankle —*see* Effusion, joint, ankle

S

◀ New ⬅ Revised ~~deleted~~ Deleted

Swelling *(Continued)*
arm M79.89
forearm M79.89
breast N63
Calabar B74.3
cervical gland R59.Ø
chest, localized R22.2
ear H93.8-
extremity (lower) (upper) —*see* Disorder, soft tissue, specified type NEC
finger M79.89
foot M79.89
glands R59.9
generalized R59.1
localized R59.Ø
hand M79.89
head (localized) R22.Ø
inflammatory —*see* Inflammation
intra-abdominal —*see* Mass, abdominal
joint —*see* Effusion, joint
leg M79.89
lower M79.89
limb —*see* Disorder, soft tissue, specified type NEC
localized (skin) R22.9
chest R22.2
head R22.Ø
limb
lower —*see* Mass, localized, limb, lower
upper —*see* Mass, localized, limb, upper
neck R22.1
trunk R22.2
neck (localized) R22.1
pelvic —*see* Mass, abdominal
scrotum N5Ø.89
splenic —*see* Splenomegaly
testis N5Ø.89
toe M79.89
umbilical R19.Ø9
wandering, due to Gnathostoma (spinigerum) B83.1
white —*see* Tuberculosis, arthritis
Swift (-Feer) disease
overdose or wrong substance given or taken —*see* Table of Drugs and Chemicals, by drug, poisoning
Swimmer's
cramp T75.1
ear H6Ø.33-
itch B65.3
Swimming in the head R42
Swollen —*see* Swelling
Swyer syndrome Q99.1
Sycosis L73.8
barbae (not parasitic) L73.8
contagiosa (mycotic) B35.Ø
lupoides L73.8
mycotic B35.Ø
parasitic B35.Ø
vulgaris L73.8
Sydenham's chorea —*see* Chorea, Sydenham's
Sylvatic yellow fever A95.Ø
Sylvest's disease B33.Ø
Symblepharon H11.23-
congenital Q1Ø.3
Symond's syndrome G93.2
Sympathetic —*see* condition
Sympatheticotonia G9Ø.8
Sympathicoblastoma
specified site —*see* Neoplasm, malignant, by site
unspecified site C74.9Ø
Sympathogonioma —*see* Sympathicoblastoma
Symphalangy (fingers) (toes) Q7Ø.9
Symptoms NEC R68.89
breast NEC N64.59
development NEC R63.8
factitious, self-induced —*see* Disorder, factitious
Symptoms NEC *(Continued)*
genital organs, female R1Ø.2
involving
abdomen NEC R19.8
appearance NEC R46.89
awareness R41.9
altered mental status R41.82
amnesia —*see* Amnesia
borderline intellectual functioning R41.83
coma —*see* Coma
disorientation R41.Ø
neurologic neglect syndrome R41.4
senile cognitive decline R41.81
specified symptom NEC R41.89
behavior NEC R46.89
cardiovascular system NEC RØ9.89
chest NEC RØ9.89
circulatory system NEC RØ9.89
cognitive functions R41.9
altered mental status R41.82
amnesia —*see* Amnesia
borderline intellectual functioning R41.83
coma —*see* Coma
disorientation R41.Ø
neurologic neglect syndrome R41.4
senile cognitive decline R41.81
specified symptom NEC R41.89
development NEC R62.5Ø
digestive system NEC R19.8
emotional state NEC R45.89
emotional lability R45.86
food and fluid intake R63.8
general perceptions and sensations R44.9
specified NEC R44.8
musculoskeletal system R29.91
specified NEC R29.898
nervous system R29.9Ø
specified NEC R29.818
pelvis NEC R19.8
respiratory system NEC RØ9.89
skin and integument R23.9
urinary system R39.9
menopausal N95.1
metabolism NEC R63.8
neurotic F48.8
of infancy R68.19
pelvis NEC, female R1Ø.2
skin and integument NEC R23.9
subcutaneous tissue NEC R23.9
Sympus Q74.2
Syncephalus Q89.4
Synchondrosis
abnormal (congenital) Q78.8
ischiopubic M91.Ø
Synchysis (scintillans) (senile) (vitreous body) H43.89
Syncope (near) (pre-) R55
anginosa I2Ø.8
bradycardia RØØ.1
cardiac R55
carotid sinus G9Ø.Ø1
due to spinal (lumbar) puncture G97.1
heart R55
heat T67.1
laryngeal RØ5
psychogenic F48.8
tussive RØ5
vasoconstriction R55
vasodepressor R55
vasomotor R55
vasovagal R55
Syndactylism, syndactyly Q7Ø.9
complex (with synostosis)
fingers Q7Ø.Ø-
toes Q7Ø.2-
simple (without synostosis)
fingers Q7Ø.1-
toes Q7Ø.3-
Syndrome —*see also* Disease
5q minus NOS D46.C
48,XXXX Q97.1
49,XXXXX Q97.1
abdominal
acute R1Ø.Ø
muscle deficiency Q79.4
abnormal innervation HØ2.519
left HØ2.516
lower HØ2.515
upper HØ2.514
right HØ2.513
lower HØ2.512
upper HØ2.511
abstinence, neonatal P96.1
acid pulmonary aspiration, obstetric O74.Ø
acquired immunodeficiency —*see* Human, immunodeficiency virus (HIV) disease
acute abdominal R1Ø.Ø
acute respiratory distress (adult) (child) J8Ø
idiopathic J84.114
Adair-Dighton Q78.Ø
Adams-Stokes (-Morgagni) I45.9
adiposogenital E23.6
adrenal
hemorrhage (meningococcal) A39.1
meningococcic A39.1
adrenocortical —*see* Cushing's, syndrome
adrenogenital E25.9
congenital, associated with enzyme deficiency E25.Ø
afferent loop NEC K91.89
Alagille's Q44.7
alcohol withdrawal (without convulsions) —*see* Dependence, alcohol, with, withdrawal
Alder's D72.Ø
Aldrich (-Wiskott) D82.Ø
alien hand R41.4
Alport Q87.81
alveolar hypoventilation E66.2
alveolocapillary block J84.1Ø
amnesic, amnestic (confabulatory) (due to) —*see* Disorder, amnesic
amyostatic (Wilson's disease) E83.Ø1
androgen insensitivity E34.5Ø
complete E34.51
partial E34.52
androgen resistance (*see also* Syndrome, androgen insensitivity) E34.5Ø
Angelman Q93.5
anginal —*see* Angina
ankyloglossia superior Q38.1
anterior
chest wall RØ7.89
cord G83.82
spinal artery G95.19
compression M47.Ø19
cervical region M47.Ø12
cervicothoracic region M47.Ø13
lumbar region M47.Ø16
occipito-atlanto-axial region M47.Ø11
thoracic region M47.Ø14
thoracolumbar region M47.Ø15
tibial M76.81-
antibody deficiency D8Ø.9
agammaglobulinemic D8Ø.1
hereditary D8Ø.Ø
congenital D8Ø.Ø
hypogammaglobulinemic D8Ø.1
hereditary D8Ø.Ø
anticardiolipin (-antibody) D68.61
antiphospholipid (-antibody) D68.61
aortic
arch M31.4
bifurcation I74.Ø9
aortomesenteric duodenum occlusion K31.5
apical ballooning (transient left ventricular) I51.81
arcuate ligament I77.4

S

- **Syndrome** *(Continued)*
  - argentaffin, argintaffinoma E34.0
  - Arnold-Chiari —*see* Arnold-Chiari disease
  - Arrillaga-Ayerza I27.0
  - arterial tortuosity Q87.82 ◀
  - arteriovenous steal T82.898- ◀
  - Asherman's N85.6
  - aspiration, of newborn —*see* Aspiration, by substance, with pneumonia
    - meconium P24.01
  - ataxia-telangiectasia G11.3
  - auriculotemporal G50.8
  - autoerythrocyte sensitization (Gardner-Diamond) D69.2
  - autoimmune lymphoproliferative [ALPS] D89.82
  - autoimmune polyglandular E31.0
  - autoinflammatory M04.9 ◀
    - specified type NEC M04.8 ◀
  - autosomal —*see* Abnormal, autosomes
  - Avellis' G46.8
  - Ayerza (-Arrillaga) I27.0
  - Babinski-Nageotte G83.89
  - Bakwin-Krida Q78.5 ⬅
  - bare lymphocyte D81.6
  - Barré-Guillain G61.0
  - Barré-Liéou M53.0
  - Barrett's —*see* Barrett's, esophagus
  - Barsony-Polgar K22.4
  - Barsony-Teschendorf K22.4
  - Barth E78.71
  - Bartter's E26.81
  - basal cell nevus Q87.89
  - Basedow's E05.00
    - with thyroid storm E05.01
  - basilar artery G45.0
  - Batten-Steinert G71.11
  - battered
    - baby or child —*see* Maltreatment, child, physical abuse
    - spouse —*see* Maltreatment, adult, physical abuse
  - Beals Q87.40
  - Beau's I51.5
  - Beck's I65.8
  - Benedikt's G46.3
  - Béquez César (-Steinbrinck-Chédiak-Higashi) D70.330
  - Bernhardt-Roth —*see* Meralgia paresthetica
  - Bernheim's I50.9
  - big spleen D73.1
  - bilateral polycystic ovarian E28.2
  - Bing-Horton's —*see* Horton's headache
  - Birt-Hogg-Dube syndrome Q87.89
  - Björck (-Thorsen) E34.0
  - black
    - lung J60
    - widow spider bite —*see* Toxicity, venom, spider, black widow
  - Blackfan-Diamond D61.01
  - Blau M04.8 ◀
  - blind loop K90.2
    - congenital Q43.8
    - postsurgical K91.2
  - blue sclera Q78.0
  - blue toe I75.02-
  - Boder-Sedgewick G11.3
  - Boerhaave's K22.3
  - Borjeson Forssman Lehmann Q89.8
  - Bouillaud's I01.9
  - Bourneville (-Pringle) Q85.1
  - Bouveret (-Hoffman) I47.9
  - brachial plexus G54.0
  - bradycardia-tachycardia I49.5
  - brain (nonpsychotic) F09
    - with psychosis, psychotic reaction F09
    - acute or subacute —*see* Delirium
    - congenital —*see* Disability, intellectual
    - organic F09
      - post-traumatic (nonpsychotic) F07.81
      - psychotic F09

- **Syndrome** *(Continued)*
  - brain (nonpsychotic) *(Continued)*
    - personality change F07.0
    - postcontusional F07.81
    - post-traumatic, nonpsychotic F07.81
    - psycho-organic F09
    - psychotic F06.8
  - brain stem stroke G46.3
  - Brandt's (acrodermatitis enteropathica) E83.2
  - broad ligament laceration N83.8
  - Brock's J98.11
  - bronze baby P83.8
  - Brown-Sequard G83.81
  - bubbly lung P27.0
  - Buchem's M85.2
  - Budd-Chiari I82.0
  - bulbar (progressive) G12.22
  - Bürger-Grütz E78.3
  - Burke's K86.89 ⬅
  - Burnett's (milk-alkali) E83.52
  - burning feet E53.9
  - Bywaters' T79.5
  - Call-Fleming I67.841
  - carbohydrate-deficient glycoprotein (CDGS) E77.8
  - carcinogenic thrombophlebitis I82.1
  - carcinoid E34.0
  - cardiac asthma I50.1
  - cardiacos negros I27.0
  - cardiofaciocutaneous Q87.89
  - cardiopulmonary-obesity E66.2
  - cardiorenal —*see* Hypertension, cardiorenal
  - cardiorespiratory distress (idiopathic), newborn P22.0
  - cardiovascular renal —*see* Hypertension, cardiorenal
  - carotid
    - artery (hemispheric) (internal) G45.1
    - body G90.01
    - sinus G90.01
  - carpal tunnel G56.0-
  - Cassidy (-Scholte) E34.0
  - cat-cry Q93.4
  - cat eye Q92.8
  - cauda equina G83.4
  - causalgia —*see* Causalgia
  - celiac K90.0
    - artery compression I77.4
    - axis I77.4
  - central pain G89.0
  - cerebellar
    - hereditary G11.9
    - stroke G46.4
  - cerebellomedullary malformation —*see* Spina bifida
  - cerebral
    - artery
      - anterior G46.1
      - middle G46.0
      - posterior G46.2
    - gigantism E22.0
  - cervical (root) M53.1
    - disc —*see* Disorder, disc, cervical, with neuritis
    - fusion Q76.1
    - posterior, sympathicus M53.0
    - rib Q76.5
    - sympathetic paralysis G90.2
  - cervicobrachial (diffuse) M53.1
  - cervicocranial M53.0
  - cervicodorsal outlet G54.2
  - cervicothoracic outlet G54.0
  - Céstan (-Raymond) I65.8
  - Charcot's (angina cruris) (intermittent claudication) I73.9
  - Charcot-Weiss-Baker G90.09
  - CHARGE Q89.8
  - Chédiak-Higashi (-Steinbrinck) E70.330
  - chest wall R07.1
  - Chiari's (hepatic vein thrombosis) I82.0
  - Chilaiditi's Q43.3

- **Syndrome** *(Continued)*
  - child maltreatment —*see* Maltreatment, child
  - chondrocostal junction M94.0
  - chondroectodermal dysplasia Q77.6
  - chromosome 4 short arm deletion Q93.3
  - chromosome 5 short arm deletion Q93.4
  - chronic
    - infantile neurological, cutaneous and articular (CINCA) M04.2 ◀
    - pain G89.4
      - personality F68.8
  - Clarke-Hadfield K86.89 ⬅
  - Clerambault's automatism G93.89
  - Clouston's (hidrotic ectodermal dysplasia) Q82.4
  - clumsiness, clumsy child F82
  - cluster headache G44.009
    - intractable G44.001
    - not intractable G44.009
  - Coffin-Lowry Q89.8
  - cold injury (newborn) P80.0
  - combined immunity deficiency D81.9
  - compartment (deep) (posterior) (traumatic) T79.A0
    - abdomen T79.A3
    - lower extremity (hip, buttock, thigh, leg, foot, toes) T79.A2
    - nontraumatic
      - abdomen M79.A3
      - lower extremity (hip, buttock, thigh, leg, foot, toes) M79.A2-
      - specified site NEC M79.A9
      - upper extremity (shoulder, arm, forearm, wrist, hand, fingers) M79.A1-
    - postprocedural —*see* Syndrome compartment, nontraumatic
    - specified site NEC T79.A9
    - upper extremity (shoulder, arm, forearm, wrist, hand, fingers) T79.A1
  - complex regional pain —*see* Syndrome, pain, complex regional
  - compression T79.5
    - anterior spinal —*see* Syndrome, anterior, spinal artery, compression
    - cauda equina G83.4
    - celiac artery I77.4
    - vertebral artery M47.029
      - cervical region M47.022
      - occipito-atlanto-axial region M47.021
  - concussion F07.81
  - congenital
    - affecting multiple systems NEC Q87.89
    - central alveolar hypoventilation G47.35
    - facial diplegia Q87.0
    - muscular hypertrophy-cerebral Q87.89
    - oculo-auriculovertebral Q87.0
    - oculofacial diplegia (Moebius) Q87.0
    - rubella (manifest) P35.0
  - congestion-fibrosis (pelvic), female N94.89
  - congestive dysmenorrhea N94.6
  - Conn's E26.01
  - connective tissue M35.9
    - overlap NEC M35.1
  - conus medullaris G95.81
  - cord
    - anterior G83.82
    - posterior G83.83
  - coronary
    - acute NEC I24.9
    - insufficiency or intermediate I20.0
    - slow flow I20.8
  - Costen's (complex) M26.69
  - costochondral junction M94.0
  - costoclavicular G54.0
  - costovertebral E22.0
  - Cowden Q85.8
  - craniovertebral M53.0
  - Creutzfeldt-Jakob —*see* Creutzfeldt-Jakob disease or syndrome
  - cri-du-chat Q93.4

- **Syndrome** *(Continued)*
  - crib death R99
  - cricopharyngeal —*see* Dysphagia
  - croup J05.0
  - CRPS I —*see* Syndrome, pain, complex regional I
  - crush T79.5
  - cubital tunnel —*see* Lesion, nerve, ulnar
  - Curschmann (-Batten) (-Steinert) G71.11
  - Cushing's E24.9
    - alcohol-induced E24.4
    - drug-induced E24.2
    - due to
      - alcohol
      - drugs E24.2
      - ectopic ACTH E24.3
      - overproduction of pituitary ACTH E24.0
    - overdose or wrong substance given or taken —*see* Table of Drugs and Chemicals, by drug, poisoning
    - pituitary-dependent E24.0
    - specified type NEC E24.8
  - cryopyrin-associated periodic M04.2 ◀
  - cryptophthalmos Q87.0
  - cystic duct stump K91.5
  - Dana-Putnam D51.0
  - Danbolt (-Cross) (acrodermatitis enteropathica) E83.2
  - Dandy-Walker Q03.1
    - with spina bifida Q07.01
  - Danlos' Q79.6 ⬅
  - defibrination —*see also* Fibrinolysis
    - with
      - antepartum hemorrhage —*see* Hemorrhage, antepartum, with coagulation defect
      - intrapartum hemorrhage —*see* Hemorrhage, complicating, delivery
    - newborn P60
    - postpartum O72.3
  - Degos' I77.8
  - Déjérine-Roussy G89.0
  - delayed sleep phase G47.21
  - demyelinating G37.9
  - dependence —*see* F10-F19 with fourth character .2
  - depersonalization (-derealization) F48.1
  - De Quervain E34.51
  - de Toni-Fanconi (-Debré) E72.09
    - with cystinosis E72.04
  - diabetes mellitus-hypertension-nephrosis —*see* Diabetes, nephrosis
  - diabetes mellitus in newborn infant P70.2
  - diabetes-nephrosis —*see* Diabetes, nephrosis
  - diabetic amyotrophy —*see* Diabetes, amyotrophy
  - dialysis associated steal T82.898- ◀
  - Diamond-Blackfan D61.01
  - Diamond-Gardener D69.2
  - DIC (diffuse or disseminated intravascular coagulopathy) D65
  - di George's D82.1
  - Dighton's Q78.0
  - disequilibrium E87.8
  - Döhle body-panmyelopathic D72.0
  - dorsolateral medullary G46.4
  - double athetosis G80.3
  - Down (*see also* Down syndrome) Q90.9
  - Dresbach's (elliptocytosis) D58.1
  - Dressler's (postmyocardial infarction) I24.1
    - postcardiotomy I97.0
  - drug withdrawal, infant of dependent mother P96.1
  - dry eye H04.12-
  - due to abnormality
    - chromosomal Q99.9
      - sex
        - female phenotype Q97.9
        - male phenotype Q98.9
      - specified NEC Q99.8

- **Syndrome** *(Continued)*
  - dumping (postgastrectomy) K91.1
    - nonsurgical K31.89
  - Dupré's (meningism) R29.1
  - dysmetabolic X E88.81
  - dyspraxia, developmental F82
  - Eagle-Barrett Q79.4
  - Eaton-Lambert —*see* Syndrome, Lambert-Eaton
  - Ebstein's Q22.5
  - ectopic ACTH E24.3
  - eczema-thrombocytopenia D82.0
  - Eddowes' Q78.0
  - effort (psychogenic) F45.8
  - Ehlers-Danlos Q79.6
  - Eisenmenger's I27.89
  - Ekman's Q78.0
  - electric feet E53.8
  - Ellis-van Creveld Q77.6
  - empty nest Z60.0
  - endocrine-hypertensive E27.0
  - entrapment —*see* Neuropathy, entrapment
  - eosinophilia-myalgia M35.8
  - epileptic —*see also* Epilepsy, by type
    - absence G40.A09
      - intractable G40.A19
        - with status epilepticus G40.A11
        - without status epilepticus G40.A19
      - not intractable G40.A09
        - with status epilepticus G40.A01
        - without status epilepticus G40.A09
  - Erdheim-Chester (ECD) E88.89
  - Erdheim's E22.0
  - erythrocyte fragmentation D59.4
  - Evans D69.41
  - exhaustion F48.8
  - extrapyramidal G25.9
    - specified NEC G25.89
  - eye retraction —*see* Strabismus
  - eyelid-malar-mandible Q87.0
  - Faber's D50.9
  - facial pain, paroxysmal G50.0
  - Fallot's Q21.3
  - familial cold autoinflammatory M04.2 ◀
  - familial eczema-thrombocytopenia (Wiskott-Aldrich) D82.0
  - Fanconi (-de Toni) (-Debré) E72.09
    - with cystinosis E72.04
  - Fanconi's (anemia) (congenital pancytopenia) D61.09
  - fatigue
    - chronic R53.82
    - psychogenic F48.8
  - faulty bowel habit K59.39 ⬅
  - Feil-Klippel (brevicollis) Q76.1
  - Felty's —*see* Felty's syndrome
  - fertile eunuch E23.0
  - fetal
    - alcohol (dysmorphic) Q86.0
    - hydantoin Q86.1
  - Fiedler's I40.1
  - first arch Q87.0
  - fish odor E72.8
  - Fisher's G61.0
  - Fitzhugh-Curtis
    - due to
      - Chlamydia trachomatis A74.81
      - Neisseria gonorrhorea (gonococcal peritonitis) A54.85
  - Fitz's —*see also* Pancreatitis, acute K85.80 ⬅
  - Flajani (-Basedow) E05.00
    - with thyroid storm E05.01
  - flatback —*see* Flatback syndrome
  - floppy
    - baby P94.2
    - iris (intraoeprative) (IFIS) H21.81
    - mitral valve I34.1
  - flush E34.0
  - Foix-Alajouanine G95.19
  - Fong's Q87.2 ⬅

- **Syndrome** *(Continued)*
  - food protein-induced enterocolitis K52.21 ◀
  - foramen magnum G93.5
  - Foster-Kennedy H47.14-
  - Foville's (peduncular) G46.3
  - fragile X Q99.2
  - Franceschetti Q75.4
  - Frey's
    - auriculotemporal G50.8
    - hyperhidrosis L74.52
  - Friderichsen-Waterhouse A39.1
  - Froin's G95.89
  - frontal lobe F07.0
  - Fukuhara E88.49
  - functional
    - bowel K59.9
    - prepubertal castrate E29.1
  - Gaisböck's D75.1
  - ganglion (basal ganglia brain) G25.9
    - geniculi G51.1
  - Gardner-Diamond D69.2
  - gastroesophageal
    - junction K22.0
    - laceration-hemorrhage K22.6
  - gastrojejunal loop obstruction K91.89
  - Gee-Herter-Heubner K90.0
  - Gelineau's G47.419
    - with cataplexy G47.411
  - genito-anorectal A55
  - Gerstmann-Sträussler-Scheinker (GSS) A81.82
  - Gianotti-Crosti L44.4
  - giant platelet (Bernard-Soulier) D69.1
  - Gilles de la Tourette's F95.2
  - goiter-deafness E07.1
  - Goldberg Q89.8
  - Goldberg-Maxwell E34.51
  - Good's D83.8
  - Gopalan' (burning feet) E53.8
  - Gorlin's Q87.89
  - Gougerot-Blum L81.7
  - Gouley's I31.1
  - Gower's R55
  - gray or grey (newborn) P93.0
    - platelet D69.1
  - Gubler-Millard G46.3
  - Guillain-Barré (-Strohl) G61.0
  - gustatory sweating G50.8
  - Hadfield-Clarke K86.89 ⬅
  - hair tourniquet —*see* Constriction, external, by site
  - Hamman's J98.19
  - hand-foot L27.1
  - hand-shoulder G90.8
  - hantavirus (cardio)-pulmonary (HPS) (HCPS) B33.4
  - happy puppet Q93.5
  - Harada's H30.81-
  - Hayem-Faber D50.9
  - headache NEC G44.89
    - complicated NEC G44.59
  - Heberden's I20.8
  - Hedinger's E34.0
  - Hegglin's D72.0
  - HELLP (hemolysis, elevated liver enzymes and low platelet count) O14.2-
    - complicating ◀
      - childbirth O14.24 ◀
      - puerperium O14.25 ◀
  - hemolytic-uremic D59.3
  - hemophagocytic, infection-associated D76.2
  - Henoch-Schönlein D69.0
  - hepatic flexure K59.8
  - hepatopulmonary K76.81
  - hepatorenal K76.7
    - following delivery O90.4
    - postoperative or postprocedural K91.83
    - postpartum, puerperal O90.4
  - hepatourologic K76.7
  - Herter (-Gee) (nontropical sprue) K90.0

◀ New ◀▪▪▪ Revised ~~deleted~~ Deleted

Syndrome *(Continued)*
Miller-Dieker Q93.88
Miller-Fisher G61.0
Minkowski-Chauffard D58.0
Mirizzi's K83.1
MNGIE (Mitochondrial Neurogastrointestinal Encephalopathy) E88.49
Möbius, ophthalmoplegic migraine —*see* Migraine, ophthalmoplegic
monofixation H50.42
Morel-Moore M85.2
Morel-Morgagni M85.2
Morgagni (-Morel) (-Stewart) M85.2
Morgagni-Adams-Stokes I45.9
Mounier-Kuhn Q32.4
with bronchiectasis J47.9
with
exacerbation (acute) J47.1
lower respiratory infection J47.0
acquired J98.09
with bronchiectasis J47.9
with
exacerbation (acute) J47.1
lower respiratory infection J47.0
Muckle-Wells M04.2 ◀
mucocutaneous lymph node (acute febrile) (MCLS) M30.3
multiple endocrine neoplasia (MEN) —*see* Neoplasia, endocrine, multiple (MEN)
multiple operations —*see* Disorder, factitious
myasthenic G70.9
in
diabetes mellitus —*see* Diabetes, amyotrophy
endocrine disease NEC E34.9 *[G73.3]*
neoplastic disease —*see also* Neoplasm D49.9 *[G73.3]*
thyrotoxicosis (hyperthyroidism) E05.90 *[G73.3]*
with thyroid storm E05.91 *[G73.3]*
myelodysplastic D46.9
with
5q deletion D46.C
isolated del (5q) chromosomal abnormality D46.C
lesions, low grade D46.20
specified NEC D46.Z
myelopathic pain G89.0
myeloproliferative (chronic) D47.1
myofascial pain M79.1
Naffziger's G54.0
nail patella Q87.2
NARP (Neuropathy, Ataxia and Retinitis pigmentosa) E88.49
neonatal abstinence P96.1
nephritic —*see also* Nephritis
with edema —*see* Nephrosis
acute N00.9
chronic N03.9
rapidly progressive N01.9
nephrotic (congenital) —*see also* Nephrosis N04.9
with
dense deposit disease N04.6
diffuse
crescentic glomerulonephritis N04.7
endocapillary proliferative glomerulonephritis N04.4
membranous glomerulonephritis N04.2
mesangial proliferative glomerulonephritis N04.3
mesangiocapillary glomerulonephritis N04.5
focal and segmental glomerular lesions N04.1
minor glomerular abnormality N04.0
specified morphological changes NEC N04.8
diabetic —*see* Diabetes, nephrosis

Syndrome *(Continued)*
neurologic neglect R41.4
Nezelof's D81.4
Nonne-Milroy-Meige Q82.0
Nothnagel's vasomotor acroparesthesia I73.89
obesity hypoventilation (OHS) E66.2 ◀
oculomotor H51.9
ophthalmoplegia-cerebellar ataxia —*see* Strabismus, paralytic, third nerve
oral allergy T78.1 ◀
oral-facial-digital Q87.0
organic
affective F06.30
amnesic (not alcohol- or drug-induced) F04
brain F09
depressive F06.31
hallucinosis F06.0
personality F07.0
Ormond's N13.5
oro-facial-digital Q87.0
os trigonum Q68.8
Osler-Weber-Rendu I78.0
osteoporosis-osteomalacia M83.8
Osterreicher-Turner Q87.2 ⟸
otolith —*see* subcategory H81.8
oto-palatal-digital Q87.0
outlet (thoracic) G54.0
ovary
polycystic E28.2
resistant E28.39
sclerocystic E28.2
Owren's D68.2
Paget-Schroetter I82.890
pain —*see also* Pain
complex regional I G90.50
lower limb G90.52-
specified site NEC G90.59
upper limb G90.51-
complex regional II —*see* Causalgia
painful
bruising D69.2
feet E53.8
prostate N42.81
paralysis agitans —*see* Parkinsonism
paralytic G83.9
specified NEC G83.89
Parinaud's H51.0
parkinsonian —*see* Parkinsonism
Parkinson's —*see* Parkinsonism
paroxysmal facial pain G50.0
Parry's E05.00
with thyroid storm E05.01
Parsonage (-Aldren)-Turner G54.5
patella clunk M25.86-
Paterson (-Brown) (-Kelly) D50.1
pectoral girdle I77.89
pectoralis minor I77.89
Pelger-Huet D72.0
pellagra-cerebellar ataxia-renal aminoaciduria E72.02
pellagroid E52
Pellegrini-Stieda —*see* Bursitis, tibial collateral
pelvic congestion-fibrosis, female N94.89
penta X Q97.1
peptic ulcer —*see* Ulcer, peptic
perabduction I77.89
periodic fever M04.1 ◀
periodic fever, aphthous stomatitis, pharyngitis, and adenopathy [PFAPA] M04.8 ◀
periodic headache, in adults and children —*see* Headache, periodic syndromes in adults and children
periurethral fibrosis N13.5
phantom limb (without pain) G54.7
with pain G54.6
pharyngeal pouch D82.1
Pick's —*see* Disease, Pick's ⟸
Pickwickian E66.2

Syndrome *(Continued)*
PIE (pulmonary infiltration with eosinophilia) J82
pigmentary pallidal degeneration (progressive) G23.0
pineal E34.8
pituitary E22.0
placental transfusion —*see* Pregnancy, complicated by, placental transfusion syndromes
plantar fascia M72.2
plateau iris (post-iridectomy) (postprocedural) H21.82
Plummer-Vinson D50.1
pluricarential of infancy E40
plurideficiency E40
pluriglandular (compensatory) E31.8
autoimmune E31.0
pneumatic hammer T75.21
polyangiitis overlap M30.8
polycarential of infancy E40
polyglandular E31.8
autoimmune E31.0
polysplenia Q89.09
pontine NEC G93.89
popliteal
artery entrapment I77.89
web Q87.89
postcardiac injury
postcardiotomy I97.0
postmyocardial infarction I24.1
postcardiotomy I97.0
post chemoembolization — code to associated conditions
postcholecystectomy K91.5
postcommissurotomy I97.0
postconcussional F07.81
postcontusional F07.81
postencephalitic F07.89
posterior
cervical sympathetic M53.0
cord G83.83
fossa compression G93.5
reversible encephalopathy (PRES) I67.83
postgastrectomy (dumping) K91.1
postgastric surgery K91.1
postinfarction I24.1
postlaminectomy NEC M96.1
postleukotomy F07.0
postmastectomy lymphedema I97.2
postmyocardial infarction I24.1
postoperative NEC T81.9
blind loop K90.2
postpartum panhypopituitary (Sheehan) E23.0
postpolio (myelitic) G14
postthrombotic I87.009
with
inflammation I87.02-
with ulcer I87.03-
specified complication NEC I87.09-
ulcer I87.01-
with inflammation I87.03-
asymptomatic I87.00-
postvagotomy K91.1
postvalvulotomy I97.0
postviral NEC G93.3
fatigue G93.3
Potain's K31.0
potassium intoxication E87.5
precerebral artery (multiple) (bilateral) G45.2
preinfarction I20.0
preleukemic D46.9
premature senility E34.8
premenstrual dysphoric F32.89 ⟸
premenstrual tension N94.3
Prinzmetal-Massumi R07.1
prune belly Q79.4
pseudocarpal tunnel (sublimis) —*see* Syndrome, carpal tunnel

S

S

◀ New ⬅ Revised ~~deleted~~ Deleted

Syndrome *(Continued)*
  tumor lysis (following antineoplastic chemotherapy) (spontaneous) NEC E88.3
  tumor necrosis factor receptor associated periodic (TRAPS) MØ4.1 ◀
  Twiddler's (due to)
    automatic implantable defibrillator T82.198
    cardiac pacemaker T82.198
  Unverricht (-Lundborg) *—see* Epilepsy, generalized, idiopathic
  upward gaze H51.8
  uremia, chronic *—see also* Disease, kidney, chronic N18.9
  urethral N34.3
  urethro-oculo-articular *—see* Reiter's disease
  urohepatic K76.7
  vago-hypoglossal G52.7
  van Buchem's M85.2
  van der Hoeve's Q78.Ø
  vascular NEC in cerebrovascular disease G46.8
  vasoconstriction, reversible cerebrovascular I67.841
  vasomotor I73.9
  vasospastic (traumatic) T75.22
  vasovagal R55
  VATER Q87.2
  velo-cardio-facial Q93.81
  vena cava (inferior) (superior) (obstruction) I87.1
  vertebral
    artery G45.Ø
      compression *—see* Syndrome, anterior, spinal artery, compression
    steal G45.Ø
  vertebro-basilar artery G45.Ø
  vertebrogenic (pain) M54.89
  vertiginous *—see* Disorder, vestibular function
  Vinson-Plummer D5Ø.1
  virus B34.9
  visceral larva migrans B83.Ø
  visual disorientation H53.8
  vitamin B6 deficiency E53.1
  vitreal corneal H59.Ø1-
  vitreous (touch) H59.Ø1-
  Vogt-Koyanagi H2Ø.82-
  Volkmann's T79.6
  von Schroetter's I82.89Ø
  von Willebrand (-Jürgen) D68.Ø
  Waldenström-Kjellberg D5Ø.1
  Wallenberg's G46.3
  water retention E87.79
  Waterhouse (-Friderichsen) A39.1
  Weber-Gubler G46.3
  Weber-Leyden G46.3
  Weber's G46.3
  Wegener's M31.3Ø
    with
      kidney involvement M31.31
      lung involvement M31.3Ø
        with kidney involvement M31.31
  Weingarten's (tropical eosinophilia) J82
  Weiss-Baker G9Ø.Ø9
  Werdnig-Hoffman G12.Ø
  Wermer's E31.21
  Werner's E34.8
  Wernicke-Korsakoff (nonalcoholic) FØ4
    alcoholic F1Ø.26
  West's *—see* Epilepsy, spasms
  Westphal-Strümpell E83.Ø1
  wet
    feet (maceration) (tropical) T69.Ø-
    lung, newborn P22.1
  whiplash S13.4
  whistling face Q87.Ø
  Wilkie's K55.1
  Wilkinson-Sneddon L13.1
  Willebrand (-Jürgens) D68.Ø

Syndrome *(Continued)*
  Wilson's (hepatolenticular degeneration) E83.Ø1
  Wiskott-Aldrich D82.Ø
  withdrawal *—see* Withdrawal, state
    drug
      infant of dependent mother P96.1
      therapeutic use, newborn P96.2
  Woakes' (ethmoiditis) J33.1
  Wright's (hyperabduction) I77.89
  X I2Ø.9
  XXXX Q97.1
  XXXXX Q97.1
  XXXXY Q98.1
  XXY Q98.Ø
  yellow nail L6Ø.5
  Zahorsky's BØ8.5
  Zellweger syndrome E71.51Ø
  Zellweger-like syndrome E71.541
Synechia (anterior) (iris) (posterior) (pupil) *—see also* Adhesions, iris
  intra-uterine (traumatic) N85.6
Synesthesia R2Ø.8
Syngamiasis, syngamosis B83.3
Synodontia KØØ.2
Synorchidism, synorchism Q55.1
Synostosis (congenital) Q78.8
  astragalo-scaphoid Q74.2
  radioulnar Q74.Ø
Synovial sarcoma *—see* Neoplasm, connective tissue, malignant
Synovioma (malignant) *—see also* Neoplasm, connective tissue, malignant
  benign *—see* Neoplasm, connective tissue, benign
Synoviosarcoma *—see* Neoplasm, connective tissue, malignant
Synovitis *—see also* Tenosynovitis M65.9 ⟸
  crepitant
    hand M7Ø.Ø-
    wrist M7Ø.Ø3-
  gonococcal A54.49
  gouty *—see* Gout ⟸
  in (due to)
    crystals M65.8-
    gonorrhea A54.49
    syphilis (late) A52.78
    use, overuse, pressure *—see* Disorder, soft tissue, due to use
  infective NEC *—see* Tenosynovitis, infective NEC
  specified NEC *—see* Tenosynovitis, specified type NEC
  syphilitic A52.78
    congenital (early) A5Ø.Ø2
  toxic *—see* Synovitis, transient
  transient M67.3-
    ankle M67.37-
    elbow M67.32-
    foot joint M67.37-
    hand joint M67.34-
    hip M67.35-
    knee M67.36-
    multiple site M67.39
    pelvic region M67.35-
    shoulder M67.31-
    specified joint NEC M67.38
    wrist M67.33-
  traumatic, current *—see* Sprain
  tuberculous *—see* Tuberculosis, synovitis
  villonodular (pigmented) M12.2-
    ankle M12.27-
    elbow M12.22-
    foot joint M12.27-
    hand joint M12.24-
    hip M12.25-
    knee M12.26-
    multiple site M12.29
    pelvic region M12.25-
    shoulder M12.21-
    specified joint NEC M12.28

Synovitis *(Continued)*
  villonodular (pigmented) *(Continued)*
    vertebrae M12.28
    wrist M12.23-
Syphilid A51.39
  congenital A5Ø.Ø6
  newborn A5Ø.Ø6
  tubercular (late) A52.79
Syphilis, syphilitic (acquired) A53.9
  abdomen (late) A52.79
  acoustic nerve A52.15
  adenopathy (secondary) A51.49
  adrenal (gland) (with cortical hypofunction) A52.79
  age under 2 years NOS *—see also* Syphilis, congenital, early
    acquired A51.9
  alopecia (secondary) A51.32
  anemia (late) A52.79 *[D63.8]*
  aneurysm (aorta) (ruptured) A52.Ø1
    central nervous system A52.Ø5
    congenital A5Ø.54 *[I79.Ø]*
  anus (late) A52.74
    primary A51.1
    secondary A51.39
  aorta (arch) (abdominal) (thoracic) A52.Ø2
    aneurysm A52.Ø1
  aortic (insufficiency) (regurgitation) (stenosis)A52.Ø3
    aneurysm A52.Ø1
  arachnoid (adhesive) (cerebral) (spinal) A52.13
  asymptomatic *—see* Syphilis, latent
  ataxia (locomotor) A52.11
  atrophoderma maculatum A51.39
  auricular fibrillation A52.Ø6
  bladder (late) A52.76
  bone A52.77
    secondary A51.46
  brain A52.17
  breast (late) A52.79
  bronchus (late) A52.72
  bubo (primary) A51.Ø
  bulbar palsy A52.19
  bursa (late) A52.78
  cardiac decompensation A52.Ø6
  cardiovascular A52.ØØ
  central nervous system (late) (recurrent) (relapse) (tertiary) A52.3
    with
      ataxia A52.11
      general paralysis A52.17
        juvenile A5Ø.45
      paresis (general) A52.17
        juvenile A5Ø.45
      tabes (dorsalis) A52.11
        juvenile A5Ø.45
      taboparesis A52.17
        juvenile A5Ø.45
    aneurysm A52.Ø5
    congenital A5Ø.4Ø
    juvenile A5Ø.4Ø
    remission in (sustained) A52.3
    serology doubtful, negative, or positive A52.3
    specified nature or site NEC A52.19
    vascular A52.Ø5
  cerebral A52.17
    meningovascular A52.13
    nerves (multiple palsies) A52.15
    sclerosis A52.17
    thrombosis A52.Ø5
  cerebrospinal (tabetic type) A52.12
  cerebrovascular A52.Ø5
  cervix (late) A52.76
  chancre (multiple) A51.Ø
    extragenital A51.2
    Rollet's A51.Ø
  Charcot's joint A52.16
  chorioretinitis A51.43
    congenital A5Ø.Ø1
    late A52.71
    prenatal A5Ø.Ø1

S

Syphilis, syphilitic *(Continued)*
orbit (late) A52.71
organic A53.9
osseous (late) A52.77
osteochondritis (congenital) (early) A50.02 *[M90.80]*
osteoporosis A52.77
ovary (late) A52.76
oviduct (late) A52.76
palate (late) A52.79
pancreas (late) A52.74
paralysis A52.17
general A52.17
juvenile A50.45
paresis (general) A52.17
juvenile A50.45
paresthesia A52.19
Parkinson's disease or syndrome A52.19
paroxysmal tachycardia A52.06
pemphigus (congenital) A50.06
penis (chancre) A51.0
late A52.76
pericardium A52.06
perichondritis, larynx (late) A52.73
periosteum (late) A52.77
congenital (early) A50.02 *[M90.80]*
early (secondary) A51.46
peripheral nerve A52.79
petrous bone (late) A52.77
pharynx (late) A52.73
secondary A51.39
pituitary (gland) A52.79
pleura (late) A52.73
pneumonia, white A50.04
pontine lesion A52.17
portal vein A52.09
primary A51.0
anal A51.1
and secondary —*see* Syphilis, secondary
central nervous system A52.3
extragenital chancre NEC A51.2
fingers A51.2
genital A51.0
lip A51.2
specified site NEC A51.2
tonsils A51.2
prostate (late) A52.76
ptosis (eyelid) A52.71
pulmonary (late) A52.72
artery A52.09
pyelonephritis (late) A52.75
recently acquired, symptomatic A51.9
rectum (late) A52.74
respiratory tract (late) A52.73
retina, late A52.71
retrobulbar neuritis A52.15
salpingitis A52.76
sclera (late) A52.71
sclerosis
cerebral A52.17
coronary A52.06
multiple A52.11
scotoma (central) A52.71
scrotum (late) A52.76

Syphilis, syphilitic *(Continued)*
secondary (and primary) A51.49
adenopathy A51.49
anus A51.39
bone A51.46
chorioretinitis, choroiditis A51.43
hepatitis A51.45
liver A51.45
lymphadenitis A51.49
meningitis (acute) A51.41
mouth A51.39
mucous membranes A51.39
periosteum, periostitis A51.46
pharynx A51.39
relapse (treated, untreated) A51.49
skin A51.39
specified form NEC A51.49
tonsil A51.39
ulcer A51.39
viscera NEC A51.49
vulva A51.39
seminal vesicle (late) A52.76
seronegative with signs or symptoms - code by site and stage under Syphilis
seropositive
with signs or symptoms - code by site and stage under Syphilis
follow-up of latent syphilis —*see* Syphilis, latent
only finding —*see* Syphilis, latent
seventh nerve (paralysis) A52.15
sinus, sinusitis (late) A52.73
skeletal system A52.77
skin (with ulceration) (early) (secondary) A51.39
late or tertiary A52.79
small intestine A52.74
spastic spinal paralysis A52.17
spermatic cord (late) A52.76
spinal (cord) A52.12
spleen A52.79
splenomegaly A52.79
spondylitis A52.77
staphyloma A52.71
stigmata (congenital) A50.59
stomach A52.74
synovium A52.78
tabes dorsalis (late) A52.11
juvenile A50.45
tabetic type A52.11
juvenile A50.45
taboparesis A52.17
juvenile A50.45
tachycardia A52.06
tendon (late) A52.78
tertiary A52.9
with symptoms NEC A52.79
cardiovascular A52.00
central nervous system A52.3
multiple NEC A52.79
specified site NEC A52.79
testis A52.76
thorax A52.73
throat A52.73

Syphilis, syphilitic *(Continued)*
thymus (gland) (late) A52.79
thyroid (late) A52.79
tongue (late) A52.79
tonsil (lingual) (late) A52.73
primary A51.2
secondary A51.39
trachea (late) A52.73
tunica vaginalis (late) A52.76
ulcer (any site) (early) (secondary) A51.39
late A52.79
perforating A52.79
foot A52.11
urethra (late) A52.76
urogenital (late) A52.76
uterus (late) A52.76
uveal tract (secondary) A51.43
late A52.71
uveitis (secondary) A51.43
late A52.71
uvula (late) (perforated) A52.79
vagina A51.0
late A52.76
valvulitis NEC A52.03
vascular A52.00
brain (cerebral) A52.05
ventriculi A52.74
vesicae urinariae (late) A52.76
viscera (abdominal) (late) A52.74
secondary A51.49
vitreous (opacities) (late) A52.71
hemorrhage A52.71
vulva A51.0
late A52.76
secondary A51.39
Syphiloma A52.79
cardiovascular system A52.00
central nervous system A52.3
circulatory system A52.00
congenital A50.59
Syphilophobia F45.29
Syringadenoma —*see also* Neoplasm, skin, benign
papillary —*see* Neoplasm, skin, benign
Syringobulbia G95.0
Syringocystadenoma —*see* Neoplasm, skin, benign
papillary —*see* Neoplasm, skin, benign
Syringoma —*see also* Neoplasm, skin, benign
chondroid —*see* Neoplasm, skin, benign
Syringomyelia G95.0
Syringomyelitis —*see* Encephalitis
Syringomyelocele —*see* Spina bifida
Syringopontia G95.0
System, systemic —*see also* condition
disease, combined —*see* Degeneration, combined
inflammatory response syndrome (SIRS) of non-infectious origin (without organ dysfunction) R65.10
with acute organ dysfunction R65.11
lupus erythematosus M32.9
inhibitor present D68.62

S

◄ New ◄ Revised ~~deleted~~ Deleted

T

Tabacism, tabacosis, tabagism —*see also* Poisoning, tobacco
meaning dependence (without remission) F17.200
with
disorder F17.299
remission F17.211
specified disorder NEC F17.298
withdrawal F17.203
Tabardillo A75.9
flea-borne A75.2
louse-borne A75.0
Tabes, tabetic A52.10
with
central nervous system syphilis A52.10
Charcot's joint A52.16
cord bladder A52.19
crisis, viscera (any) A52.19
paralysis, general A52.17
paresis (general) A52.17
perforating ulcer (foot) A52.19
arthropathy (Charcot) A52.16
bladder A52.19
bone A52.11
cerebrospinal A52.12
congenital A50.45
conjugal A52.10
dorsalis A52.11
juvenile A50.49
juvenile A50.49
latent A52.19
mesenterica A18.39
paralysis, insane, general A52.17
spasmodic A52.17
syphilis (cerebrospinal) A52.12
Taboparalysis A52.17
Taboparesis (remission) A52.17
juvenile A50.45
TAC (trigeminal autonomic cephalgia) NEC G44.099
intractable G44.091
not intractable G44.099
Tache noir S60.22-
Tachyalimentation K91.2
Tachyarrhythmia, tachyrhythmia —*see* Tachycardia
Tachycardia R00.0
atrial (paroxysmal) I47.1
auricular I47.1
AV nodal re-entry (re-entrant) I47.1
junctional (paroxysmal) I47.1
newborn P29.11
nodal (paroxysmal) I47.1
non-paroxysmal AV nodal I45.89
paroxysmal (sustained) (nonsustained) I47.9
with sinus bradycardia I49.5
atrial (PAT) I47.1
atrioventricular (AV) (re-entrant) I47.1
psychogenic F54
junctional I47.1
ectopic I47.1
nodal I47.1
psychogenic (atrial) (supraventricular) (ventricular) F54
supraventricular (sustained) I47.1
psychogenic F54
ventricular I47.2
psychogenic F54
psychogenic F45.8
sick sinus I49.5
sinoauricular NOS R00.0
paroxysmal I47.1
sinus [sinusal] NOS R00.0
paroxysmal I47.1
supraventricular I47.1
ventricular (paroxysmal) (sustained) I47.2
psychogenic F54
Tachygastria K31.89
Tachypnea R06.82
hysterical F45.8
newborn (idiopathic) (transitory) P22.1
psychogenic F45.8
transitory, of newborn P22.1
TACO (transfusion associated circulatory overload) E87.71
Taenia (infection) (infestation) B68.9
diminuta B71.0
echinococcal infestation B67.90
mediocanellata B68.1
nana B71.0
saginata B68.1
solium (intestinal form) B68.0
larval form —*see* Cysticercosis
Taeniasis (intestine) —*see* Taenia
Tag (hypertrophied skin) (infected) L91.8
adenoid J35.8
anus K64.4
hemorrhoidal K64.4
hymen N89.8
perineal N90.89
preauricular Q17.0
sentinel K64.4
skin L91.8
accessory (congenital) Q82.8
anus K64.4
congenital Q82.8
preauricular Q17.0
tonsil J35.8
urethra, urethral N36.8
vulva N90.89
Tahyna fever B33.8
Takahara's disease E80.3
Takayasu's disease or syndrome M31.4
Talcosis (pulmonary) J62.0
Talipes (congenital) Q66.89
acquired, planus —*see* Deformity, limb, flat foot
asymmetric Q66.89
calcaneovalgus Q66.4
calcaneovarus Q66.1
calcaneus Q66.89
cavus Q66.7
equinovalgus Q66.6
equinovarus Q66.0
equinus Q66.89
percavus Q66.7
planovalgus Q66.6
planus (acquired) (any degree) —*see also* Deformity, limb, flat foot
congenital Q66.5-
due to rickets (sequelae) E64.3
valgus Q66.6
varus Q66.3
Tall stature, constitutional E34.4
Talma's disease M62.89
Talon noir S90.3-
hand S60.22-
heel S90.3-
toe S90.1-
Tamponade, heart I31.4
Tanapox (virus disease) B08.71
Tangier disease E78.6
Tantrum, child problem F91.8
Tapeworm (infection) (infestation) —*see* Infestation, tapeworm
Tapia's syndrome G52.7
TAR (thrombocytopenia with absent radius) **syndrome** Q87.2
Tarral-Besnier disease L44.0
Tarsal tunnel syndrome —*see* Syndrome, tarsal tunnel
Tarsalgia —*see* Pain, limb, lower
Tarsitis (eyelid) H01.8
syphilitic A52.71
tuberculous A18.4
Tartar (teeth) (dental calculus) K03.6
Tattoo (mark) L81.8
Tauri's disease E74.09
Taurodontism K00.2
Taussig-Bing syndrome Q20.1
Taybi's syndrome Q87.2
Tay-Sachs amaurotic familial idiocy or disease E75.02
TBI (traumatic brain injury) S06.9 ◄
Teacher's node or nodule J38.2
Tear, torn (traumatic) —*see also* Laceration
with abortion —*see* Abortion
annular fibrosis M51.35
anus, anal (sphincter) S31.831
complicating delivery
with third degree perineal laceration —*see also* Delivery, complicated, by, laceration, perineum, third degree O70.20 ◄
with mucosa O70.3
without third degree perineal laceration O70.4
nontraumatic (healed) (old) K62.81
articular cartilage, old —*see* Derangement, joint, articular cartilage, by site
bladder
with ectopic or molar pregnancy O08.6
following ectopic or molar pregnancy O08.6
obstetrical O71.5
traumatic —*see* Injury, bladder
bowel
with ectopic or molar pregnancy O08.6
following ectopic or molar pregnancy O08.6
obstetrical trauma O71.5
broad ligament
with ectopic or molar pregnancy O08.6
following ectopic or molar pregnancy O08.6
obstetrical trauma O71.6
bucket handle (knee) (meniscus) —*see* Tear, meniscus
capsule, joint —*see* Sprain
cartilage —*see also* Sprain
articular, old —*see* Derangement, joint, articular cartilage, by site
cervix
with ectopic or molar pregnancy O08.6
following ectopic or molar pregnancy O08.6
obstetrical trauma (current) O71.3
old N88.1
traumatic —*see* Injury, uterus
dural G97.41
nontraumatic G96.11
internal organ —*see* Injury, by site
knee cartilage
articular (current) S83.3-
old —*see* Derangement, knee, meniscus, due to old tear
ligament —*see* Sprain
meniscus (knee) (current injury) S83.209
bucket-handle S83.20-
lateral
bucket-handle S83.25-
complex S83.27-
peripheral S83.26-
specified type NEC S83.28-
medial
bucket-handle S83.21-
complex S83.23-
peripheral S83.22-
specified type NEC S83.24-
old —*see* Derangement, knee, meniscus, due to old tear
site other than knee - code as Sprain
specified type NEC S83.20-
muscle —*see* Strain
pelvic
floor, complicating delivery O70.1
organ NEC, obstetrical trauma O71.5
with ectopic or molar pregnancy O08.6
following ectopic or molar pregnancy O08.6
perineal, secondary O90.1

Tear, torn *(Continued)*
periurethral tissue, obstetrical trauma O71.82
with ectopic or molar pregnancy OØ8.6
following ectopic or molar pregnancy OØ8.6
rectovaginal septum —*see* Laceration, vagina
retina, retinal (without detachment) (horseshoe) —*see also* Break, retina, horseshoe
with detachment —*see* Detachment, retina, with retinal, break
rotator cuff (nontraumatic) M75.1Ø-
complete M75.12-
incomplete M75.11-
traumatic S46.Ø1-
capsule S43.42-
semilunar cartilage, knee —*see* Tear, meniscus
supraspinatus (complete) (incomplete) (nontraumatic) —*see also* Tear, rotator cuff M75.1Ø-
tendon —*see* Strain
tentorial, at birth P1Ø.4
umbilical cord
complicating delivery O69.89
urethra
with ectopic or molar pregnancy OØ8.6
following ectopic or molar pregnancy OØ8.6
obstetrical trauma O71.5
uterus —*see* Injury, uterus
vagina —*see* Laceration, vagina
vessel, from catheter —*see* Puncture, accidental complicating surgery
vulva, complicating delivery O7Ø.Ø
Tear-stone —*see* Dacryolith
Teeth —*see also* condition
grinding
psychogenic F45.8
sleep related G47.63
Teething (syndrome) KØØ.7
Telangiectasia, telangiectasis (verrucous) I78.1
ataxic (cerebellar) (Louis-Bar) G11.3
familial I78.Ø
hemorrhagic, hereditary (congenital) (senile) I78.Ø
hereditary, hemorrhagic (congenital) (senile) I78.Ø
juxtafoveal H35.Ø7-
macular H35.Ø7-
parafoveal H35.Ø7-
retinal (idiopathic) (juxtafoveal) (macular) (parafoveal) H35.Ø7-
spider I78.1
Telephone scatologia F65.89
Telescoped bowel or intestine K56.1
congenital Q43.8
Temperature
body, high (of unknown origin) R5Ø.9
cold, trauma from T69.9
newborn P8Ø.Ø
specified effect NEC T69.8
Temple —*see* condition
Temporal —*see* condition
Temporomandibular joint pain-dysfunction syndrome M26.62- ◄
Temporosphenoidal —*see* condition
Tendency
bleeding —*see* Defect, coagulation
suicide
meaning personal history of attempted suicide Z91.5
meaning suicidal ideation —*see* Ideation, suicidal
to fall R29.6
Tenderness, abdominal R1Ø.819
epigastric R1Ø.816
generalized R1Ø.817
left lower quadrant R1Ø.814
left upper quadrant R1Ø.812
periumbilic R1Ø.815
Tenderness, abdominal *(Continued)*
rebound R1Ø.829
epigastric R1Ø.826
generalized R1Ø.827
left lower quadrant R1Ø.824
left upper quadrant R1Ø.822
periumbilic R1Ø.825
right lower quadrant R1Ø.823
right upper quadrant R1Ø.821
right lower quadrant R1Ø.813
right upper quadrant R1Ø.811
Tendinitis, tendonitis —*see also* Enthesopathy
Achilles M76.6-
adhesive —*see* Tenosynovitis, specified type NEC
shoulder —*see* Capsulitis, adhesive
bicipital M75.2-
calcific M65.2-
ankle M65.27-
foot M65.27-
forearm M65.23-
hand M65.24-
lower leg M65.26-
multiple sites M65.29
pelvic region M65.25-
shoulder M75.3-
specified site NEC M65.28
thigh M65.25-
upper arm M65.22-
due to use, overuse, pressure —*see also* Disorder, soft tissue, due to use
specified NEC —*see* Disorder, soft tissue, due to use, specified NEC
gluteal M76.Ø-
patellar M76.5-
peroneal M76.7-
psoas M76.1-
tibial (posterior) M76.82-
anterior M76.81-
trochanteric —*see* Bursitis, hip, trochanteric
Tendon —*see* condition
Tendosynovitis —*see* Tenosynovitis
Tenesmus (rectal) R19.8
vesical R3Ø.1
Tennis elbow —*see* Epicondylitis, lateral
Tenonitis —*see also* Tenosynovitis
eye (capsule) HØ5.Ø4-
Tenontosynovitis —*see* Tenosynovitis
Tenontothecitis —*see* Tenosynovitis
Tenophyte —*see* Disorder, synovium, specified type NEC
Tenosynovitis —*see also* Synovitis M65.9
adhesive —*see* Tenosynovitis, specified type NEC
shoulder —*see* Capsulitis, adhesive
bicipital (calcifying) —*see* Tendinitis, bicipital
gonococcal A54.49
in (due to)
crystals M65.8-
gonorrhea A54.49
syphilis (late) A52.78
use, overuse, pressure —*see also* Disorder, soft tissue, due to use
specified NEC —*see* Disorder, soft tissue, due to use, specified NEC
infective NEC M65.1-
ankle M65.17-
foot M65.17-
forearm M65.13-
hand M65.14-
lower leg M65.16-
multiple sites M65.19
pelvic region M65.15-
shoulder region M65.11-
specified site NEC M65.18
thigh M65.15-
upper arm M65.12-
radial styloid M65.4
shoulder region M65.81-
adhesive —*see* Capsulitis, adhesive
Tenosynovitis *(Continued)*
specified type NEC M65.88-
ankle M65.87-
foot M65.87-
forearm M65.83-
hand M65.84-
lower leg M65.86-
multiple sites M65.89
pelvic region M65.85-
shoulder region M65.81-
specified site NEC M65.88
thigh M65.85-
upper arm M65.82-
tuberculous —*see* Tuberculosis, tenosynovitis
Tenovaginitis —*see* Tenosynovitis
Tension
arterial, high —*see also* Hypertension
without diagnosis of hypertension RØ3.Ø
headache G44.2Ø9
intractable G44.2Ø1
not intractable G44.2Ø9
nervous R45.Ø
pneumothorax J93.Ø
premenstrual N94.3
state (mental) F48.9
Tentorium —*see* condition
Teratencephalus Q89.8
Teratism Q89.7
Teratoblastoma (malignant) —*see* Neoplasm, malignant, by site
Teratocarcinoma —*see also* Neoplasm, malignant, by site
liver C22.7
Teratoma (solid) —*see also* Neoplasm, uncertain behavior, by site
with embryonal carcinoma, mixed —*see* Neoplasm, malignant, by site
with malignant transformation —*see* Neoplasm, malignant, by site
adult (cystic) —*see* Neoplasm, benign, by site
benign —*see* Neoplasm, benign, by site
combined with choriocarcinoma —*see* Neoplasm, malignant, by site
cystic (adult) —*see* Neoplasm, benign, by site
differentiated —*see* Neoplasm, benign, by site
embryonal —*see also* Neoplasm, malignant, by site
liver C22.7
immature —*see* Neoplasm, malignant, by site
liver C22.7
adult, benign, cystic, differentiated type or mature D13.4
malignant —*see also* Neoplasm, malignant, by site
anaplastic —*see* Neoplasm, malignant, by site
intermediate —*see* Neoplasm, malignant, by site
specified site —*see* Neoplasm, malignant, by site
unspecified site C62.9Ø
undifferentiated —*see* Neoplasm, malignant, by site
mature —*see* Neoplasm, uncertain behavior, by site
malignant —*see* Neoplasm, by site, malignant, by site
ovary D27.-
embryonal, immature or malignant C56-
solid —*see* Neoplasm, uncertain behavior, by site
testis C62.9-
adult, benign, cystic, differentiated type or mature D29.2-
scrotal C62.1-
undescended C62.Ø-
Termination
anomalous —*see also* Malposition, congenital
right pulmonary vein Q26.3
pregnancy, elective Z33.2

T

Ternidens diminutus infestation B81.8
Ternidensiasis B81.8
Terror (s) **night** (child) F51.4
Terrorism, victim of Z65.4
Terry's syndrome H44.2-
Tertiary —*see* condition
Test, tests, testing (for)
adequacy (for dialysis)
hemodialysis Z49.31
peritoneal Z49.32
blood pressure Z01.30
abnormal reading —*see* Blood, pressure
blood typing Z01.83
Rh typing Z01.83
blood-alcohol Z04.8
positive —*see* Findings, abnormal, in blood
blood-drug Z04.8
positive —*see* Findings, abnormal, in blood
cardiac pulse generator (battery) Z45.010
fertility Z31.41
genetic
disease carrier status for procreative management
female Z31.430
male Z31.440
male partner of patient with recurrent pregnancy loss Z31.441
procreative management NEC
female Z31.438
male Z31.448
hearing Z01.10
with abnormal findings NEC Z01.118
HIV (human immunodeficiency virus)
nonconclusive (in infants) R75
positive Z21
seropositive Z21
immunity status Z01.84
intelligence NEC Z01.89
laboratory (as part of a general medical examination) Z00.00
with abnormal finding Z00.01
for medicolegal reason NEC Z04.8
male partner of patient with recurrent pregnancy loss Z31.441
Mantoux (for tuberculosis) Z11.1
abnormal result R76.11
pregnancy, positive first pregnancy —*see* Pregnancy, normal, first
procreative Z31.49
fertility Z31.41
skin, diagnostic
allergy Z01.82
special screening examination —*see* Screening, by name of disease
Mantoux Z11.1
tuberculin Z11.1
specified NEC Z01.89
tuberculin Z11.1
abnormal result R76.11
vision Z01.00
with abnormal findings Z01.01
Wassermann Z11.3
positive —*see* Serology for syphilis, positive
Testicle, testicular, testis —*see also* condition
feminization syndrome —*see also* Syndrome, androgen insensitivity E34.51
migrans Q55.29
Tetanus, tetanic (cephalic) (convulsions) A35
with
abortion A34
ectopic or molar pregnancy O08.0
following ectopic or molar pregnancy O08.0
inoculation reaction (due to serum) —*see* Complications, vaccination
neonatorum A33
obstetrical A34
puerperal, postpartum, childbirth A34
Tetany (due to) R29.0
alkalosis E87.3
associated with rickets E55.0
convulsions R29.0
hysterical F44.5
functional (hysterical) F44.5
hyperkinetic R29.0
hysterical F44.5
hyperpnea R06.4
hysterical F44.5
psychogenic F45.8
hyperventilation —*see also* Hyperventilation R06.4
hysterical F44.5
neonatal (without calcium or magnesium deficiency) P71.3
parathyroid (gland) E20.9
parathyroprival E89.2
post- (para)thyroidectomy E89.2
postoperative E89.2
pseudotetany R29.0
psychogenic (conversion reaction) F44.5
Tetralogy of Fallot Q21.3
Tetraplegia (chronic) —*see also* Quadriplegia G82.50-
Thailand hemorrhagic fever A91
Thalassanemia —*see* Thalassemia
Thalassemia (anemia) (disease) D56.9
with other hemoglobinopathy D56.8
alpha (major) (severe) (triple gene defect) D56.0
minor D56.3
silent carrier D56.3
trait D56.3
beta (severe) D56.1
homozygous D56.1
major D56.1
minor D56.3
trait D56.3
delta-beta (homozygous) D56.2
minor D56.3
trait D56.3
dominant D56.8
hemoglobin
C D56.8
E-beta D56.5
intermedia D56.1
major D56.1
minor D56.3
mixed D56.8
sickle-cell —*see* Disease, sickle-cell, thalassemia
specified type NEC D56.8
trait D56.3
variants D56.8
Thanatophoric dwarfism or short stature Q77.1
Thaysen-Gee disease (nontropical sprue) K90.0
Thaysen's disease K90.0
Thecoma D27-
luteinized D27-
malignant C56-
Thelarche, premature E30.8
Thelaziasis B83.8
Thelitis N61.0 ◄
puerperal, postpartum or gestational —*see* Infection, nipple
Therapeutic —*see* condition
Therapy
drug, long-term (current) (prophylactic)
agents affecting estrogen receptors and estrogen levels NEC Z79.818
anastrozole (Arimidex) Z79.811
antibiotics Z79.2
short-term use - omit code
anticoagulants Z79.01
anti-inflammatory Z79.1
antiplatelet Z79.02
antithrombotics Z79.02
aromatase inhibitors Z79.811
aspirin Z79.82
birth control pill or patch Z79.3
Therapy *(Continued)*
drug, long-term *(Continued)*
bisphosphonates Z79.83
contraceptive, oral Z79.3
drug, specified NEC Z79.899
estrogen receptor downregulators Z79.818
Evista Z79.810
exemestane (Aromasin) Z79.811
Fareston Z79.810
fulvestrant (Faslodex) Z79.818
gonadotropin-releasing hormone (GnRH) agonist Z79.818
goserelin acetate (Zoladex) Z79.818
hormone replacement (postmenopausal) Z79.890
insulin Z79.4
letrozole (Femara) Z79.811
leuprolide acetate (leuprorelin) (Lupron) Z79.818
megestrol acetate (Megace) Z79.818
methadone
for pain management Z79.891
maintenance therapy F11.20
Nolvadex Z79.810
opiate analgesic Z79.891
oral contraceptive Z79.3
raloxifene (Evista) Z79.810
selective estrogen receptor modulators (SERMs) Z79.810
short term - omit code
steroids
inhaled Z79.51
systemic Z79.52
tamoxifen (Nolvadex) Z79.810
toremifene (Fareston) Z79.810
Thermic —*see* condition
Thermography (abnormal) —*see also* Abnormal, diagnostic imaging R93.8
breast R92.8
Thermoplegia T67.0
Thesaurismosis, glycogen —*see* Disease, glycogen storage
Thiamin deficiency E51.9
specified NEC E51.8
Thiaminic deficiency with beriberi E51.11
Thibierge-Weissenbach syndrome —*see* Sclerosis, systemic
Thickening
bone —*see* Hypertrophy, bone
breast N64.59
endometrium R93.8
epidermal L85.9
specified NEC L85.8
hymen N89.6
larynx J38.7
nail L60.2
congenital Q84.5
periosteal —*see* Hypertrophy, bone
pleura J92.9
with asbestos J92.0
skin R23.4
subepiglottic J38.7
tongue K14.8
valve, heart —*see* Endocarditis
Thigh —*see* condition
Thinning vertebra —*see* Spondylopathy, specified NEC
Thirst, excessive R63.1
due to deprivation of water T73.1
Thomsen disease G71.12
Thoracic —*see also* condition
kidney Q63.2
outlet syndrome G54.0
Thoracogastroschisis (congenital) Q79.8
Thoracopagus Q89.4
Thorax —*see* condition
Thorn's syndrome N28.89
Thorson-Björck syndrome E34.0
Threadworm (infection) (infestation) B80

◄ New ◄ Revised ~~deleted~~ Deleted

Threatened
  abortion O20.0
    with subsequent abortion O03.9
  job loss, anxiety concerning Z56.2
  labor (without delivery) O47.9
    ~~after 37 completed weeks of gestation O47.1~~
    at or after 37 completed weeks of gestation O47.1 ◄
    before 37 completed weeks of gestation O47.0-
  loss of job, anxiety concerning Z56.2
  miscarriage O20.0
  unemployment, anxiety concerning Z56.2
Three-day fever A93.1
Threshers' lung J67.0
Thrix annulata (congenital) Q84.1
Throat —*see* condition
Thrombasthenia (Glanzmann) (hemorrhagic) (hereditary) D69.1
Thromboangiitis I73.1
  obliterans (general) I73.1
    cerebral I67.89
    vessels
      brain I67.89
      spinal cord I67.89
Thromboarteritis —*see* Arteritis
Thromboasthenia (Glanzmann) (hemorrhagic) (hereditary) D69.1
Thrombocytasthenia (Glanzmann) D69.1
Thrombocythemia (essential) (hemorrhagic) (idiopathic) (primary) D47.3
Thrombocytopathy (dystrophic) (granulopenic) D69.1
Thrombocytopenia, thrombocytopenic D69.6
  with absent radius (TAR) Q87.2
  congenital D69.42
  dilutional D69.59
  due to
    drugs D69.59
    extracorporeal circulation of blood D69.59
    (massive)blood transfusion D69.59
    platelet alloimmunization D69.59
  essential D69.3
  heparin induced (HIT) D75.82
  hereditary D69.42
  idiopathic D69.3
  neonatal, transitory P61.0
    due to
      exchange transfusion P61.0
      idiopathic maternal thrombocytopenia P61.0
      isoimmunization P61.0
  primary NEC D69.49
    idiopathic D69.3
  puerperal, postpartum O72.3
  secondary D69.59
  transient neonatal P61.0
Thrombocytosis, essential D47.3
  primary D47.3
Thromboembolism —*see* Embolism
Thrombopathy (Bernard-Soulier) D69.1
  constitutional D68.0
  Willebrand-Jurgens D68.0
Thrombopenia —*see* Thrombocytopenia
Thrombophilia D68.59
  primary NEC D68.59
  secondary NEC D68.69
  specified NEC D68.69
Thrombophlebitis I80.9
  antepartum O22.2-
    deep O22.3-
    superficial O22.2-
  cavernous (venous) sinus G08
    complicating pregnancy O22.5-
    nonpyogenic I67.6
  cerebral (sinus) (vein) G08
    nonpyogenic I67.6
    sequelae G09
  due to implanted device —*see* Complications, by site and type, specified NEC

Thrombophlebitis *(Continued)*
  during or resulting from a procedure NEC T81.72
  femoral vein (superficial) I80.1-
  femoropopliteal vein I80.0-
  hepatic (vein) I80.8
  idiopathic, recurrent I82.1
  iliofemoral I80.1-
  intracranial venous sinus (any) G08
    nonpyogenic I67.6
    sequelae G09
  intraspinal venous sinuses and veins G08
    nonpyogenic G95.19
  lateral (venous) sinus G08
    nonpyogenic I67.6
  leg I80.299
    superficial I80.0-
  longitudinal (venous) sinus G08
    nonpyogenic I67.6
  lower extremity I80.299
  migrans, migrating I82.1
  pelvic
    with ectopic or molar pregnancy O08.0
    following ectopic or molar pregnancy O08.0
    puerperal O87.1
  popliteal vein —*see* Phlebitis, leg, deep, popliteal
  portal (vein) K75.1
  postoperative T81.72
  pregnancy —*see* Thrombophlebitis, antepartum
  puerperal, postpartum, childbirth O87.0
    deep O87.1
    pelvic O87.1
    septic O86.81
    superficial O87.0
  saphenous (greater) (lesser) I80.0-
  sinus (intracranial) G08
    nonpyogenic I67.6
  specified site NEC I80.8
  tibial vein I80.23-
Thrombosis, thrombotic (bland) (multiple) (progressive) (silent) (vessel) I82.90
  anal K64.5
  antepartum —*see* Thrombophlebitis, antepartum
  aorta, aortic I74.10
    abdominal I74.09
      saddle I74.01
    bifurcation I74.09
    saddle I74.01
    specified site NEC I74.19
    terminal I74.09
    thoracic I74.11
    valve —*see* Endocarditis, aortic
  apoplexy I63.3- ⬅
  artery, arteries (postinfectional) I74.9
    auditory, internal —*see* Occlusion, artery, precerebral, specified NEC
    basilar —*see* Occlusion, artery, basilar
    carotid (common) (internal) —*see* Occlusion, artery, carotid
    cerebellar (anterior inferior) (posterior inferior) (superior) —*see* Occlusion, artery, cerebellar
    cerebral —*see* Occlusion, artery, cerebral
    choroidal (anterior) —*see* Occlusion, artery, cerebral, specified NEC
    communicating, posterior —*see* Occlusion, artery, cerebral, specified NEC
    coronary —*see also* Infarct, myocardium
      not resulting in infarction I24.0
    hepatic I74.8
    hypophyseal —*see* Occlusion, artery, cerebral, specified NEC
    iliac I74.5
    limb I74.4
      lower I74.3
      upper I74.2

Thrombosis, thrombotic *(Continued)*
  artery, arteries *(Continued)*
    meningeal, anterior or posterior —*see* Occlusion, artery, cerebral, specified NEC
    mesenteric (with gangrene) —*see also* Infarct, intestine K55.069 ⬅
    ophthalmic —*see* Occlusion, artery, retina
    pontine —*see* Occlusion, artery, cerebral, specified NEC
    precerebral —*see* Occlusion, artery, precerebral
    pulmonary (iatrogenic) —*see* Embolism, pulmonary
    renal N28.0
    retinal —*see* Occlusion, artery, retina
    spinal, anterior or posterior G95.11
    traumatic NEC T14.8
    vertebral —*see* Occlusion, artery, vertebral
  atrium, auricular —*see also* Infarct, myocardium
    following acute myocardial infarction (current complication) I23.6
    not resulting in infarction I51.3 ⬅
  basilar (artery) —*see* Occlusion, artery, basilar
  brain (artery) (stem) —*see also* Occlusion, artery, cerebral
    due to syphilis A52.05
    puerperal O99.43
    sinus —*see* Thrombosis, intracranial venous sinus
  capillary I78.8
  cardiac —*see also* Infarct, myocardium
    not resulting in infarction I51.3 ⬅
    valve —*see* Endocarditis
  carotid (artery) (common) (internal) —*see* Occlusion, artery, carotid
  cavernous (venous) sinus —*see* Thrombosis, intracranial venous sinus
  cerebellar artery (anterior inferior) (posterior inferior) (superior) I66.3
  cerebral (artery) —*see* Occlusion, artery, cerebral
  cerebrovenous sinus —*see also* Thrombosis, intracranial venous sinus
    puerperium O87.3
  chronic I82.91
  coronary (artery) (vein) —*see also* Infarct, myocardium
    not resulting in infarction I24.0
  corpus cavernosum N48.89
  cortical I66.9
  deep —*see* Embolism, vein, lower extremity
  due to device, implant or graft —*see also* Complications, by site and type, specified NEC T85.868 ⬅
    arterial graft NEC T82.868
    breast (implant) T85.868 ⬅
    catheter NEC T85.868 ⬅
      dialysis (renal) T82.868
        intraperitoneal T85.868 ⬅
      infusion NEC T82.868
        spinal (epidural) (subdural) T85.860 ⬅
      urinary (indwelling) T83.86
    electronic (electrode) (pulse generator) (stimulator)
      bone T84.86
      cardiac T82.867
      nervous system (brain) (peripheral nerve) (spinal) T85.860 ⬅
      urinary T83.86
    fixation, internal (orthopedic) NEC T84.86
    gastrointestinal (bile duct) (esophagus) T85.868 ⬅
    genital NEC T83.86
    heart T82.867
    joint prosthesis T84.86
    ocular (corneal graft) (orbital implant) NEC T85.868 ⬅
    orthopedic NEC T84.86

Thrombosis, thrombotic *(Continued)*
  due to device, implant or graft *(Continued)*
    specified NEC T85.868
    urinary NEC T83.86
    vascular NEC T82.868
    ventricular intracranial shunt T85.86Ø
  during the puerperium —*see* Thrombosis, puerperal
  endocardial —*see also* Infarct, myocardium
    not resulting in infarction I51.3
  eye —*see* Occlusion, retina
  genital organ
    female NEC N94.89
      pregnancy —*see* Thrombophlebitis, antepartum
    male N5Ø.1
  gestational —*see* Phlebopathy, gestational
  heart (chamber) —*see also* Infarct, myocardium
    not resulting in infarction I51.3
  hepatic (vein) I82.Ø
    artery I74.8
  history (of) Z86.718
  intestine (with gangrene) —*see also* Infarct, intestine K55.Ø69
  intracardiac NEC (apical) (atrial) (auricular) (ventricular) (old) I51.3
  intracranial (arterial) I66.9
    venous sinus (any) GØ8
      nonpyogenic origin I67.6
      puerperium O87.3
  intramural —*see also* Infarct, myocardium
    not resulting in infarction I51.3
  intraspinal venous sinuses and veins GØ8
    nonpyogenic G95.19
  kidney (artery) N28.Ø
  lateral (venous) sinus —*see* Thrombosis, intracranial venous sinus
  leg —*see* Thrombosis, vein, lower extremity
    arterial I74.3
  liver (venous) I82.Ø
    artery I74.8
    portal vein I81
  longitudinal (venous) sinus —*see* Thrombosis, intracranial venous sinus
  lower limb —*see* Thrombosis, vein, lower extremity
  lung (iatrogenic) (postoperative) —*see* Embolism, pulmonary
  meninges (brain) (arterial) I66.8
  mesenteric (artery) (with gangrene) —*see also* Infarct, intestine K55.Ø69
    vein (inferior) (superior) I81
  mitral I34.8
  mural —*see also* Infarct, myocardium
    due to syphilis A52.Ø6
    not resulting in infarction I51.3
  omentum (with gangrene) —*see also* Infarct, intestine K55.Ø69
  ophthalmic —*see* Occlusion, retina
  pampiniform plexus (male) N5Ø.1
  parietal —*see also* Infarct, myocardium
    not resulting in infarction I24.Ø
  penis, superficial vein N48.81
  perianal venous K64.5
  peripheral arteries I74.4
    upper I74.2
  personal history (of) Z86.718
  portal I81
    due to syphilis A52.Ø9
  precerebral artery —*see* Occlusion, artery, precerebral
  puerperal, postpartum O87.Ø
    brain (artery) O99.43
      venous (sinus) O87.3
    cardiac O99.43
    cerebral (artery) O99.43
      venous (sinus) O87.3
    superficial O87.Ø

Thrombosis, thrombotic *(Continued)*
  pulmonary (artery) (iatrogenic) (postoperative) (vein) —*see* Embolism, pulmonary
  renal (artery) N28.Ø
    vein I82.3
  resulting from presence of device, implant or graft —*see* Complications, by site and type, specified NEC
  retina, retinal —*see* Occlusion, retina
  scrotum N5Ø.1
  seminal vesicle N5Ø.1
  sigmoid (venous) sinus —*see* Thrombosis, intracranial venous sinus
  sinus, intracranial (any) —*see* Thrombosis, intracranial venous sinus
  specified site NEC I82.89Ø
    chronic I82.891
  spermatic cord N5Ø.1
  spinal cord (arterial) G95.11
    due to syphilis A52.Ø9
    pyogenic origin GØ6.1
  spleen, splenic D73.5
    artery I74.8
  testis N5Ø.1
  traumatic NEC T14.8
  tricuspid IØ7.8
  tumor —*see* Neoplasm, by site
  tunica vaginalis N5Ø.1
  umbilical cord (vessels), complicating delivery O69.5
  vas deferens N5Ø.1
  vein (acute) I82.9Ø
    antecubital I82.61-
      chronic I82.71-
    axillary I82.A1-
      chronic I82.A2-
    basilic I82.61-
      chronic I82.71-
    brachial I82.62-
      chronic I82.72-
    brachiocephalic (innominate) I82.29Ø
      chronic I82.291
    cerebral, nonpyogenic I67.6
    cephalic I82.61-
      chronic I82.71-
    chronic I82.91
    deep (DVT) I82.4Ø-
      calf I82.4Z-
        chronic I82.5Z-
      lower leg I82.4Z-
        chronic I82.5Z-
      thigh I82.4Y-
        chronic I82.5Y-
      upper leg I82.4Y
        chronic I82.5y-
    femoral I82.41-
      chronic I82.51-
    iliac (iliofemoral) I82.42-
      chronic I82.52-
    innominate I82.29Ø
      chronic I82.291
    internal jugular I82.C1-
      chronic I82.C2-
    lower extremity
      deep I82.4Ø-
        chronic I82.5Ø-
        specified NEC I82.49-
          chronic NEC I82.59-
      distal
        deep I82.4Z-
      proximal
        deep I82.4Y-
          chronic I82.5Y-
      superficial I82.81-
    perianal K64.5
    popliteal I82.43-
      chronic I82.53-
    radial I82.62-
      chronic I82.72-
    renal I82.3

Thrombosis, thrombotic *(Continued)*
  vein *(Continued)*
    saphenous (greater) (lesser) I82.81-
    specified NEC I82.89Ø
      chronic NEC I82.891
    subclavian I82.B1-
      chronic I82.B2-
    thoracic NEC I82.29Ø
      chronic I82.291
    tibial I82.44-
      chronic I82.54-
    ulnar I82.62-
      chronic I82.72-
    upper extremity I82.6Ø-
      chronic I82.7Ø-
      deep I82.62-
        chronic I82.72-
      superficial I82.61-
        chronic I82.71-
  vena cava
    inferior I82.22Ø
      chronic I82.221
    superior I82.21Ø
      chronic I82.211
  venous, perianal K64.5
  ventricle —*see also* Infarct, myocardium
    following acute myocardial infarction (current complication) I23.6
    not resulting in infarction I24.Ø
Thrombus —*see* Thrombosis
Thrush —*see also* Candidiasis
  newborn P37.5
  oral B37.Ø
  vaginal B37.3
Thumb —*see also* condition
  sucking (child problem) F98.8
Thymitis E32.8
Thymoma (benign) D15.Ø
  malignant C37
Thymus, thymic (gland) —*see* condition
Thyrocele —*see* Goiter
Thyroglossal —*see also* condition
  cyst Q89.2
  duct, persistent Q89.2
Thyroid (gland) (body) —*see also* condition
  hormone resistance EØ7.89
  lingual Q89.2
  nodule (cystic) (nontoxic) (single) EØ4.1
Thyroiditis EØ6.9
  acute (nonsuppurative) (pyogenic) (suppurative) EØ6.Ø
  autoimmune EØ6.3
  chronic (nonspecific) (sclerosing) EØ6.5
    with thyrotoxicosis, transient EØ6.2
    fibrous EØ6.5
    lymphadenoid EØ6.3
    lymphocytic EØ6.3
    lymphoid EØ6.3
  de Quervain's EØ6.1
  drug-induced EØ6.4
  fibrous (chronic) EØ6.5
  giant-cell (follicular) EØ6.1
  granulomatous (de Quervain) (subacute) EØ6.1
  Hashimoto's (struma lymphomatosa) EØ6.3
  iatrogenic EØ6.4
  ligneous EØ6.5
  lymphocytic (chronic) EØ6.3
  lymphoid EØ6.3
  lymphomatous EØ6.3
  nonsuppurative EØ6.1
  postpartum, puerperal O9Ø.5
  pseudotuberculous EØ6.1
  pyogenic EØ6.Ø
  radiation EØ6.4
  Riedel's EØ6.5
  subacute (granulomatous) EØ6.1
  suppurative EØ6.Ø
  tuberculous A18.81
  viral EØ6.1
  woody EØ6.5

T

Thyrolingual duct, persistent Q89.2
Thyromegaly E01.0
Thyrotoxic
  crisis —*see* Thyrotoxicosis
  heart disease or failure —*see also* Thyrotoxicosis E05.90 *[I43]*
    with thyroid storm E05.91 *[I43]*
  storm —*see* Thyrotoxicosis
Thyrotoxicosis (recurrent) E05.90
  with
    goiter (diffuse) E05.00
      with thyroid storm E05.01
      adenomatous uninodular E05.10
        with thyroid storm E05.11
      multinodular E05.20
        with thyroid storm E05.21
      nodular E05.20
        with thyroid storm E05.21
      uninodular E05.10
        with thyroid storm E05.11
    infiltrative
      dermopathy E05.00
        with thyroid storm E05.01
      ophthalmopathy E05.00
        with thyroid storm E05.01
    single thyroid nodule E05.10
      with thyroid storm E05.11
    thyroid storm E05.91
  due to
    ectopic thyroid nodule or tissue E05.30
      with thyroid storm E05.31
    ingestion of (excessive) thyroid material E05.40
      with thyroid storm E05.41
    overproduction of thyroid-stimulating hormone E05.80
      with thyroid storm E05.81
    specified cause NEC E05.80
      with thyroid storm E05.81
  factitia E05.40
    with thyroid storm E05.41
  heart E05.90 *[I43]*
    with thyroid storm E05.91 *[I43]*
    failure E05.90 *[I43]*
  neonatal (transient) P72.1
  transient with chronic thyroiditis E06.2
Tibia vara —*see* Osteochondrosis, juvenile, tibia
Tic (disorder) F95.9
  breathing F95.8
  child problem F95.0
  compulsive F95.1
  de la Tourette F95.2
  degenerative (generalized) (localized) G25.69
    facial G25.69
  disorder
    chronic
      motor F95.1
      vocal F95.1
    combined vocal and multiple motor F95.2
    transient F95.0
  douloureux G50.0
    atypical G50.1
    postherpetic, postzoster B02.22
  drug-induced G25.61
  eyelid F95.8
  habit F95.9
    chronic F95.1
    transient of childhood F95.0
  lid, transient of childhood F95.0
  motor-verbal F95.2
  occupational F48.8
  orbicularis F95.8
    transient of childhood F95.0
  organic origin G25.69
  postchoreic G25.69
  provisional F95.0 ◀
  psychogenic, compulsive F95.1
  salaam R25.8
  spasm (motor or vocal) F95.9
    chronic F95.1
    transient of childhood F95.0
  specified NEC F95.8
Tick-borne —*see* condition
Tietze's disease or syndrome M94.0
Tight, tightness
  anus K62.89
  chest R07.89
  fascia (lata) M62.89
  foreskin (congenital) N47.1
  hymen, hymenal ring N89.6
  introitus (acquired) (congenital) N89.6
  rectal sphincter K62.89
  tendon —*see* Short, tendon
  urethral sphincter N35.9
Tilting vertebra —*see* Dorsopathy, deforming, specified NEC
Timidity, child F93.8
Tin-miner's lung J63.5
Tinea (intersecta) (tarsi) B35.9
  amiantacea L44.8
  asbestina B35.0
  barbae B35.0
  beard B35.0
  black dot B35.0
  blanca B36.2
  capitis B35.0
  corporis B35.4
  cruris B35.6
  flava B36.0
  foot B35.3
  furfuracea B36.0
  imbricata (Tokelau) B35.5
  kerion B35.0
  manuum B35.2
  microsporic —*see* Dermatophytosis
  nigra B36.1
  nodosa —*see* Piedra
  pedis B35.3
  scalp B35.0
  specified site NEC B35.8
  sycosis B35.0
  tonsurans B35.0
  trichophytic —*see* Dermatophytosis
  unguium B35.1
  versicolor B36.0
Tingling sensation (skin) R20.2
~~Tinnitus (audible) (aurium) (subjective) —see subcategory H93.1~~
Tinnitus NOS H93.1- ◀
  audible H93.1- ◀
  aurium H93.1- ◀
  pulsatile H93.A- ◀
  subjective H93.1- ◀
Tipped tooth (teeth) M26.33
Tipping
  pelvis M95.5
    with disproportion (fetopelvic) O33.0
      causing obstructed labor O65.0
  tooth (teeth), fully erupted M26.33
Tiredness R53.83
Tissue —*see* condition
Tobacco (nicotine)
  abuse —*see* Tobacco, use ◀
  dependence —*see* Dependence, drug, nicotine
  harmful use Z72.0
  heart —*see* Tobacco, toxic effect
  maternal use, affecting newborn P04.2
  toxic effect —*see* Table of Drugs and Chemicals, by substance, poisoning
    chewing tobacco —*see* Table of Drugs and Chemicals, by substance, poisoning
    cigarettes —*see* Table of Drugs and Chemicals, by substance, poisoning
  use Z72.0
    complicating
      childbirth O99.334
      pregnancy O99.33-
      puerperium O99.335
    counseling and surveillance Z71.6
    history Z87.891 ◀
  withdrawal state —*see also* Dependence, drug, nicotine F17.203 ⟸
Tocopherol deficiency E56.0
Todd's
  cirrhosis K74.3
  paralysis (postepileptic) (transitory) G83.84
Toe —*see* condition
Toilet, artificial opening —*see* Attention to, artificial, opening
Tokelau (ringworm) B35.5
Tollwut —*see* Rabies
Tommaselli's disease R31.9
  correct substance properly administered —*see* Table of Drugs and Chemicals, by drug, adverse effect
  overdose or wrong substance given or taken —*see* Table of Drugs and Chemicals, by drug, poisoning
Tongue —*see also* condition
  tie Q38.1
Tonic pupil —*see* Anomaly, pupil, function, tonic pupil
Toni-Fanconi syndrome (cystinosis) E72.09
  with cystinosis E72.04
Tonsil —*see* condition
Tonsillitis (acute) (catarrhal) (croupous) (follicular) (gangrenous) (infective) (lacunar) (lingual) (malignant) (membranous) (parenchymatous) (phlegmonous) (pseudomembranous) (purulent) (septic) (subacute) (suppurative) (toxic) (ulcerative) (vesicular) (viral) J03.90
  chronic J35.01
    with adenoiditis J35.03
  diphtheritic A36.0
  hypertrophic J35.01
    with adenoiditis J35.03
  recurrent J03.91
  specified organism NEC J03.80
    recurrent J03.81
  staphylococcal J03.80
    recurrent J03.81
  streptococcal J03.00
    recurrent J03.01
  tuberculous A15.8
  Vincent's A69.1
Tooth, teeth —*see* condition
Toothache K08.89 ⟸
Topagnosis R20.8
Tophi —*see* Gout, chronic
TORCH infection —*see* Infection, congenital
  without active infection P00.2
Torn —*see* Tear
Tornwaldt's cyst or disease J39.2
Torsion
  accessory tube —*see* Torsion, fallopian tube
  adnexa (female) —*see* Torsion, fallopian tube
  aorta, acquired I77.1
  appendix epididymis N44.04
  appendix testis N44.03
  bile duct (common) (hepatic) K83.8
    congenital Q44.5
  bowel, colon or intestine K56.2
  cervix —*see* Malposition, uterus
  cystic duct K82.8
  dystonia —*see* Dystonia, torsion
  epididymis (appendix) N44.04
  fallopian tube N83.52- ⟸
    with ovary N83.53
  gallbladder K82.8
    congenital Q44.1
  hydatid of Morgagni
    female N83.52- ⟸
    male N44.03
  kidney (pedicle) (leading to infarction) N28.0
  Meckel's diverticulum (congenital) Q43.0
    malignant —*see* Table of Neoplasms, small intestine, malignant
  mesentery K56.2
  omentum K56.2
  organ or site, congenital NEC —*see* Anomaly, by site

T

Torsion *(Continued)*
ovary (pedicle) N83.51- ◀
with fallopian tube N83.53
congenital Q5Ø.2
oviduct —*see* Torsion, fallopian tube
penis (acquired) N48.82
congenital Q55.63
spasm —*see* Dystonia, torsion
spermatic cord N44.Ø2
extravaginal N44.Ø1
intravaginal N44.Ø2
spleen D73.5
testis, testicle N44.ØØ
appendix N44.Ø3
tibia —*see* Deformity, limb, specified type NEC, lower leg
uterus —*see* Malposition, uterus
Torticollis (intermittent) (spastic) M43.6
congenital (sternomastoid) Q68.Ø
due to birth injury P15.8
hysterical F44.4
ocular R29.891
psychogenic F45.8
conversion reaction F44.4
rheumatic M43.6
rheumatoid MØ6.88
spasmodic G24.3
traumatic, current S13.4
Tortipelvis G24.1
Tortuous
aortic arch Q25.46 ◀
artery I77.1
organ or site, congenital NEC —*see* Distortion
retinal vessel, congenital Q14.1
ureter N13.8
urethra N36.8
vein —*see* Varix
Torture, victim of Z65.4
Torula, torular (histolytica) (infection) —*see* Cryptococcosis
Torulosis —*see* Cryptococcosis
Torus (mandibularis) (palatinus) M27.Ø
fracture —*see* Fracture, by site, torus
Touraine's syndrome Q79.8
Tourette's syndrome F95.2
Tourniquet syndrome —*see* Constriction, external, by site
Tower skull Q75.Ø
with exophthalmos Q87.Ø
Toxemia R68.89
bacterial —*see* Sepsis
burn —*see* Burn
eclamptic (with pre-existing hypertension) —*see* Eclampsia
erysipelatous —*see* Erysipelas
fatigue R68.89
food —*see* Poisoning, food
gastrointestinal K52.1
intestinal K52.1
kidney —*see* Uremia
malarial —*see* Malaria
myocardial —*see* Myocarditis, toxic
of pregnancy —*see* Pre-eclampsia
pre-eclamptic —*see* Pre-eclampsia
small intestine K52.1
staphylococcal, due to food AØ5.Ø
stasis R68.89
uremic —*see* Uremia
urinary —*see* Uremia
Toxemica cerebropathia psychica (nonalcoholic) FØ4
alcoholic —*see* Alcohol, amnestic disorder
Toxic (poisoning) —*see also* condition T65.91
effect —*see* Table of Drugs and Chemicals, by substance, poisoning
shock syndrome A48.3
thyroid (gland) —*see* Thyrotoxicosis
Toxicemia —*see* Toxemia
Toxicity —*see* Table of Drugs and Chemicals, by substance, poisoning
fava bean D55.Ø
Toxic *(Continued)*
food, noxious —*see* Poisoning, food
from drug or nonmedicinal substance —*see* Table of Drugs and Chemicals, by drug
Toxicosis —*see also* Toxemia
capillary, hemorrhagic D69.Ø
Toxinfection, gastrointestinal K52.1
Toxocariasis B83.Ø
Toxoplasma, toxoplasmosis (acquired) B58.9
with
hepatitis B58.1
meningoencephalitis B58.2
ocular involvement B58.ØØ
other organ involvement B58.89
pneumonia, pneumonitis B58.3
congenital (acute) (subacute) (chronic) P37.1
maternal, manifest toxoplasmosis in infant (acute) (subacute) (chronic) P37.1
tPA (rtPA) administation in a different facility within the last 24 hours prior to admission to current facility Z92.82
Trabeculation, bladder N32.89
Trachea —*see* condition
Tracheitis (catarrhal) (infantile) (membranous) (plastic) (septal) (suppurative) (viral) JØ4.1Ø
with
bronchitis (15 years of age and above) J4Ø
acute or subacute —*see* Bronchitis, acute
chronic J42
tuberculous NEC A15.5
under 15 years of age J2Ø.9
laryngitis (acute) JØ4.2
chronic J37.1
tuberculous NEC A15.5
acute JØ4.1Ø
with obstruction JØ4.11
chronic J42
with
bronchitis (chronic) J42
laryngitis (chronic) J37.1
diphtheritic (membranous) A36.89
due to external agent —*see* Inflammation, respiratory, upper, due to
syphilitic A52.73
tuberculous A15.5
Trachelitis (nonvenereal) —*see* Cervicitis
Tracheobronchial —*see* condition
Tracheobronchitis (15 years of age and above) —*see also* Bronchitis
due to
Bordetella bronchiseptica A37.8Ø
with pneumonia A37.81
Francisella tularensis A21.8
Tracheobronchomegaly Q32.4
with bronchiectasis J47.9
with
exacerbation (acute) J47.1
lower respiratory infection J47.Ø
acquired J98.Ø9
with bronchiectasis J47.9
with
exacerbation (acute) J47.1
lower respiratory infection J47.Ø
Tracheobronchopneumonitis —*see* Pneumonia, broncho-
Tracheocele (external) (internal) J39.8
congenital Q32.1
Tracheomalacia J39.8
congenital Q32.Ø
Tracheopharyngitis (acute) JØ6.9
chronic J42
due to external agent —*see* Inflammation, respiratory, upper, due to
Tracheostenosis J39.8
Tracheostomy
complication —*see* Complication, tracheostomy
status Z93.Ø
attention to Z43.Ø
malfunctioning J95.Ø3
Trachoma, trachomatous A71.9
active (stage) A71.1
contraction of conjunctiva A71.1
dubium A71.Ø
healed or sequelae B94.Ø
initial (stage) A71.Ø
pannus A71.1
Türck's J37.Ø
Traction, vitreomacular H43.82-
Train sickness T75.3
Trait (s)
Hb-S D57.3
hemoglobin
abnormal NEC D58.2
with thalassemia D56.3
C —*see* Disease, hemoglobin C
S (Hb-S) D57.3
Lepore D56.3
personality, accentuated Z73.1
sickle-cell D57.3
with elliptocytosis or spherocytosis D57.3
type A personality Z73.1
Tramp Z59.Ø
Trance R41.89
hysterical F44.89
Transaminasemia R74.Ø
Transection
abdomen (partial) S38.3
aorta (incomplete) —*see also* Injury, aorta
complete —*see* Injury, aorta, laceration, major
carotid artery (incomplete) —*see also* Injury, blood vessel, carotid, laceration
complete —*see* Injury, blood vessel, carotid, laceration, major
celiac artery (incomplete) S35.211
branch (incomplete) S35.291
complete S35.292
complete S35.212
innominate
artery (incomplete) —*see also* Injury, blood vessel, thoracic, innominate, artery, laceration
complete —*see* Injury, blood vessel, thoracic, innominate, artery, laceration, major
vein (incomplete) —*see also* Injury, blood vessel, thoracic, innominate, vein, laceration
complete —*see* Injury, blood vessel, thoracic, innominate, vein, laceration, major
jugular vein (external) (incomplete) —*see also* Injury, blood vessel, jugular vein, laceration
complete —*see* Injury, blood vessel, jugular vein, laceration, major
internal (incomplete) —*see also* Injury, blood vessel, jugular vein, internal, laceration
complete —*see* Injury, blood vessel, jugular vein, internal, laceration, major
mesenteric artery (incomplete) —*see also* Injury, mesenteric, artery, laceration
complete —*see* Injury, mesenteric artery, laceration, major
pulmonary vessel (incomplete) —*see also* Injury, blood vessel, thoracic, pulmonary, laceration
complete —*see* Injury, blood vessel, thoracic, pulmonary, laceration, major
subclavian —*see* Transection, innominate
vena cava (incomplete) —*see also* Injury, vena cava
complete —*see* Injury, vena cava, laceration, major
vertebral artery (incomplete) —*see also* Injury, blood vessel, vertebral, laceration
complete —*see* Injury, blood vessel, vertebral, laceration, major

T

Transfusion
associated (red blood cell) hemochromatosis E83.111
blood
ABO incompatible —*see* Complication (s), transfusion, incompatibility reaction, ABO
minor blood group (Duffy) (E) (K(ell)) (Kidd) (Lewis) (M) (N) (P) (S) T80.89
reaction or complication —*see* Complications, transfusion
fetomaternal (mother) —*see* Pregnancy, complicated by, placenta, transfusion syndrome
maternofetal (mother) —*see* Pregnancy, complicated by, placenta, transfusion syndrome
placental (syndrome) (mother) —*see* Pregnancy, complicated by, placenta, transfusion syndrome
reaction (adverse) —*see* Complications, transfusion
related acute lung injury (TRALI) J95.84
twin-to-twin —*see* Pregnancy, complicated by, placenta, transfusion syndrome, fetus to fetus
Transient (meaning homeless) —*see also* condition Z59.0
Translocation
balanced autosomal Q95.9
in normal individual Q95.0
chromosomes NEC Q99.8
balanced and insertion in normal individual Q95.0
Down's syndrome Q90.2
trisomy
13 Q91.6
18 Q91.2
21 Q90.2
Translucency, iris —*see* Degeneration, iris
Transmission of chemical substances through the placenta —*see* Absorption, chemical, through placenta
Transparency, lung, unilateral J43.0
Transplant (ed) (status) Z94.9
awaiting organ Z76.82
bone Z94.6
marrow Z94.81
candidate Z76.82
complication —*see* Complication, transplant
cornea Z94.7
heart Z94.1
and lung (s) Z94.3
valve Z95.2
prosthetic Z95.2
specified NEC Z95.4
xenogenic Z95.3
intestine Z94.82
kidney Z94.0
liver Z94.4
lung (s) Z94.2
and heart Z94.3
organ (failure) (infection) (rejection)Z94.9
removal status Z98.85
pancreas Z94.83
skin Z94.5
social Z60.3
specified organ or tissue NEC Z94.89
stem cells Z94.84
tissue Z94.9
Transplants, ovarian, endometrial N80.1
Transposed —*see* Transposition
Transposition (congenital) —*see also* Malposition, congenital
abdominal viscera Q89.3
aorta (dextra) Q20.3
appendix Q43.8
colon Q43.8
corrected Q20.5
great vessels (complete) (partial) Q20.3
Transposition *(Continued)*
heart Q24.0
with complete transposition of viscera Q89.3
intestine (large) (small) Q43.8
reversed jejunal (for bypass) (status) Z98.0
scrotum Q55.23
stomach Q40.2
with general transposition of viscera Q89.3
tooth, teeth, fully erupted M26.30
vessels, great (complete) (partial) Q20.3
viscera (abdominal) (thoracic) Q89.3
Transsexualism F64.0 ⬅
Transverse —*see also* condition
arrest (deep), in labor O64.0
lie (mother) O32.2
causing obstructed labor O64.8
Transvestism, transvestitism (dual-role) F64.1
fetishistic F65.1
Trapped placenta (with hemorrhage) O72.0
without hemorrhage O73.0
TRAPS (tumor necrosis factor receptor associated periodic syndrome) M04.1 ◀
Trauma, traumatism —*see also* Injury
acoustic —*see* subcategory H83.3
birth —*see* Birth, injury
complicating ectopic or molar pregnancy O08.6
during delivery O71.9
following ectopic or molar pregnancy O08.6
obstetric O71.9
specified NEC O71.89
occlusal ◀
primary K08.81 ◀
secondary K08.82 ◀
Traumatic —*see also* condition
brain injury S06.9 ⬅
Treacher Collins syndrome Q75.4
Treitz's hernia —*see* Hernia, abdomen, specified site NEC
Trematode infestation —*see* Infestation, fluke
Trematodiasis —*see* Infestation, fluke
Trembling paralysis —*see* Parkinsonism
Tremor (s) R25.1
drug induced G25.1
essential (benign) G25.0
familial G25.0
hereditary G25.0
hysterical F44.4
intention G25.2
medication induced postural G25.1
mercurial —*see* subcategory T56.1
Parkinson's —*see* Parkinsonism
psychogenic (conversion reaction) F44.4
senilis R54
specified type NEC G25.2
Trench
fever A79.0
foot —*see* Immersion, foot
mouth A69.1
Treponema pallidum infection —*see* Syphilis
Treponematosis
due to
T. pallidum —*see* Syphilis
T. pertenue —*see* Yaws
Triad
Hutchinson's (congenital syphilis) A50.53
Kartagener's Q89.3
Saint's —*see* Hernia, diaphragm
Trichiasis (eyelid) H02.059
with entropion —*see* Entropion
left H02.056
lower H02.055
upper H02.054
right H02.053
lower H02.052
upper H02.051
Trichinella spiralis (infection) (infestation) B75
Trichinellosis, trichiniasis, trichinelliasis, trichinosis B75
with muscle disorder B75 *[M63.80]*
ankle B75 *[M63.87-]*
foot B75 *[M63.87-]*
forearm B75 *[M63.83-]*
hand B75 *[M63.84-]*
lower leg B75 *[M63.86-]*
multiple sites B75 *[M63.89]*
pelvic region B75 *[M63.85-]*
shoulder region B75 *[M63.81-]*
specified site NEC B75 *[M63.88]*
thigh B75 *[M63.85-]*
upper arm B75 *[M63.82-]*
Trichobezoar T18.9
intestine T18.3
stomach T18.2
Trichocephaliasis, trichocephalosis B79
Trichocephalus infestation B79
Trichoclasis L67.8
Trichoepithelioma —*see also* Neoplasm, skin, benign
malignant —*see* Neoplasm, skin, malignant
Trichofolliculoma —*see* Neoplasm, skin, benign
Tricholemmoma —*see* Neoplasm, skin, benign
Trichomoniasis A59.9
bladder A59.03
cervix A59.09
intestinal A07.8
prostate A59.02
seminal vesicles A59.09
specified site NEC A59.8
urethra A59.03
urogenitalis A59.00
vagina A59.01
vulva A59.01
Trichomycosis
axillaris A48.8
nodosa, nodularis B36.8
Trichonodosis L67.8
Trichophytid, trichophyton infection —*see* Dermatophytosis
Trichophytobezoar T18.9
intestine T18.3
stomach T18.2
Trichophytosis —*see* Dermatophytosis
Trichoptilosis L67.8
Trichorrhexis (nodosa) (invaginata) L67.0
Trichosis axillaris A48.8
Trichosporosis nodosa B36.2
Trichostasis spinulosa (congenital) Q84.1
Trichostrongyliasis, trichostrongylosis (small intestine) B81.2
Trichostrongylus infection B81.2
Trichotillomania F63.3
Trichromat, trichromatopsia, anomalous (congenital) H53.55
Trichuriasis B79
Trichuris trichiura (infection) (infestation) (any site) B79
Tricuspid (valve) —*see* condition
Trifid —*see also* Accessory
kidney (pelvis) Q63.8
tongue Q38.3
Trigeminal neuralgia —*see* Neuralgia, trigeminal
Trigeminy R00.8
Trigger finger (acquired) M65.30
congenital Q74.0
index finger M65.32-
little finger M65.35-
middle finger M65.33-
ring finger M65.34-
thumb M65.31-
Trigonitis (bladder) (chronic) (pseudomembranous) N30.30
with hematuria N30.31
Trigonocephaly Q75.0
Trilocular heart —*see* Cor triloculare

Trimethylaminuria E72.52
Tripartite placenta O43.19-
Triphalangeal thumb Q74.Ø
Triple —*see also* Accessory
  kidneys Q63.Ø
  uteri Q51.818
  X, female Q97.Ø
Triplegia G83.89
  congenital G8Ø.8
Triplet (newborn) —*see also* Newborn, triplet
  complicating pregnancy —*see* Pregnancy, triplet
Triplication —*see* Accessory
Triploidy Q92.7
Trismus R25.2
  neonatorum A33
  newborn A33
Trisomy (syndrome) Q92.9
  13 (partial) Q91.7
    meiotic nondisjunction Q91.4
    mitotic nondisjunction Q91.5
    mosaicism Q91.5
    translocation Q91.6
  18 (partial) Q91.3
    meiotic nondisjunction Q91.Ø
    mitotic nondisjunction Q91.1
    mosaicism Q91.1
    translocation Q91.2
  2Ø Q92.8
  21 (partial) Q9Ø.9
    meiotic nondisjunction Q9Ø.Ø
    mitotic nondisjunction Q9Ø.1
    mosaicism Q9Ø.1
    translocation Q9Ø.2
  22 Q92.8
  autosomes Q92.9
  chromosome specified NEC Q92.8
    partial Q92.2
      due to unbalanced translocation Q92.5
    specified NEC Q92.8
    whole (nonsex chromosome)
      meiotic nondisjunction Q92.Ø
      mitotic nondisjunction Q92.1
      mosaicism Q92.1
  due to
    dicentrics —*see* Extra, marker chromosomes
    extra rings —*see* Extra, marker chromosomes
    isochromosomes —*see* Extra, marker chromosomes
  specified NEC Q92.8
  whole chromosome Q92.9
    meiotic nondisjunction Q92.Ø
    mitotic nondisjunction Q92.1
    mosaicism Q92.1
    partial Q92.9
    specified NEC Q92.8
Tritanomaly, tritanopia H53.55
Trombiculosis, trombiculiasis, trombidiosis B88.Ø
Trophedema (congenital) (hereditary) Q82.Ø
Trophoblastic disease —*see also* Mole, hydatidiform OØ1.9
Tropholymphedema Q82.Ø
Trophoneurosis NEC G96.8
  disseminated M34.9
Tropical —*see* condition
Trouble —*see also* Disease
  heart —*see* Disease, heart
  kidney —*see* Disease, renal
  nervous R45.Ø
  sinus —*see* Sinusitis
Trousseau's syndrome (thrombophlebitis migrans) I82.1
Truancy, childhood
  from school Z72.81Ø
Truncus
  arteriosus (persistent) Q2Ø.Ø
  communis Q2Ø.Ø
Trunk —*see* condition
Trypanosomiasis
  African B56.9
    by Trypanosoma brucei
      gambiense B56.Ø
      rhodesiense B56.1
  American —*see* Chagas' disease
  Brazilian —*see* Chagas' disease
  by Trypanosoma
    brucei gambiense B56.Ø
    brucei rhodesiense B56.1
    cruzi —*see* Chagas' disease
  gambiensis, Gambian B56.Ø
  rhodesiensis, Rhodesian B56.1
  South American —*see* Chagas' disease
  where
    African trypanosomiasis is prevalent B56.9
    Chagas' disease is prevalent B57.2
T-shaped incisors KØØ.2
Tsutsugamushi (disease) (fever) A75.3
Tube, tubal, tubular —*see* condition
Tubercle —*see also* Tuberculosis
  brain, solitary A17.81
  Darwin's Q17.8
  Ghon, primary infection A15.7
Tuberculid, tuberculide (indurating, subcutaneous) (lichenoid) (miliary) (papulonecrotic) (primary) (skin) A18.4
Tuberculoma —*see also* Tuberculosis
  brain A17.81
  meninges (cerebral) (spinal) A17.1
  spinal cord A17.81
Tuberculosis, tubercular, tuberculous (calcification) (calcified) (caseous) (chromogenic acid-fast bacilli) (degeneration) (fibrocaseous) (fistula) (interstitial) (isolated circumscribed lesions) (necrosis) (parenchymatous) (ulcerative) A15.9
  with pneumoconiosis (any condition in J6Ø-J64) J65
  abdomen (lymph gland) A18.39
  abscess (respiratory) A15.9
    bone A18.Ø3
      hip A18.Ø2
      knee A18.Ø2
      sacrum A18.Ø1
      specified site NEC A18.Ø3
      spinal A18.Ø1
      vertebra A18.Ø1
    brain A17.81
    breast A18.89
    Cowper's gland A18.15
    dura (mater) (cerebral) (spinal) A17.81
    epidural (cerebral) (spinal) A17.81
    female pelvis A18.17
    frontal sinus A15.8
    genital organs NEC A18.1Ø
    genitourinary A18.1Ø
    gland (lymphatic) —*see* Tuberculosis, lymph gland
    hip A18.Ø2
    intestine A18.32
    ischiorectal A18.32
    joint NEC A18.Ø2
      hip A18.Ø2
      knee A18.Ø2
      specified NEC A18.Ø2
      vertebral A18.Ø1
    kidney A18.11
    knee A18.Ø2
    latent R76.11
    lumbar (spine) A18.Ø1
    lung —*see* Tuberculosis, pulmonary
    meninges (cerebral) (spinal) A17.Ø
    muscle A18.Ø9
    perianal (fistula) A18.32
    perinephritic A18.11
    perirectal A18.32
    rectum A18.32
    retropharyngeal A15.8
    sacrum A18.Ø1
Tuberculosis, tubercular, tuberculous *(Continued)*
  abscess *(Continued)*
    scrofulous A18.2
    scrotum A18.15
    skin (primary) A18.4
    spinal cord A17.81
    spine or vertebra (column) A18.Ø1
    subdiaphragmatic A18.31
    testis A18.15
    urinary A18.13
    uterus A18.17
  accessory sinus —*see* Tuberculosis, sinus
  Addison's disease A18.7
  adenitis —*see* Tuberculosis, lymph gland
  adenoids A15.8
  adenopathy —*see* Tuberculosis, lymph gland
  adherent pericardium A18.84
  adnexa (uteri) A18.17
  adrenal (capsule) (gland) A18.7
  alimentary canal A18.32
  anemia A18.89
  ankle (joint) (bone) A18.Ø2
  anus A18.32
  apex, apical —*see* Tuberculosis, pulmonary
  appendicitis, appendix A18.32
  arachnoid A17.Ø
  artery, arteritis A18.89
    cerebral A18.89
  arthritis (chronic) (synovial) A18.Ø2
    spine or vertebra (column) A18.Ø1
  articular —*see* Tuberculosis, joint
  ascites A18.31
  asthma —*see* Tuberculosis, pulmonary
  axilla, axillary (gland) A18.2
  bladder A18.12
  bone A18.Ø3
    hip A18.Ø2
    knee A18.Ø2
    limb NEC A18.Ø3
    sacrum A18.Ø1
    spine or vertebral column A18.Ø1
  bowel (miliary) A18.32
  brain A17.81
  breast A18.89
  broad ligament A18.17
  bronchi, bronchial, bronchus A15.5
    ectasia, ectasis (bronchiectasis) —*see* Tuberculosis, pulmonary
    fistula A15.5
      primary (progressive) A15.7
    gland or node A15.4
      primary (progressive) A15.7
    lymph gland or node A15.4
      primary (progressive) A15.7
  bronchiectasis —*see* Tuberculosis, pulmonary
  bronchitis A15.5
  bronchopleural A15.6
  bronchopneumonia, bronchopneumonic —*see* Tuberculosis, pulmonary
  bronchorrhagia A15.5
  bronchotracheal A15.5
  bronze disease A18.7
  buccal cavity A18.83
  bulbourethral gland A18.15
  bursa A18.Ø9
  cachexia A15.9
  cardiomyopathy A18.84
  caries —*see* Tuberculosis, bone
  cartilage A18.Ø2
    intervertebral A18.Ø1
  catarrhal —*see* Tuberculosis, respiratory
  cecum A18.32
  cellulitis (primary) A18.4
  cerebellum A17.81
  cerebral, cerebrum A17.81
  cerebrospinal A17.81
    meninges A17.Ø
  cervical (lymph gland or node) A18.2
  cervicitis, cervix (uteri) A18.16
  chest —*see* Tuberculosis, respiratory

◄ New ◄▮▮▮ Revised ~~deleted~~ Deleted

Tuberculosis, tubercular, tuberculous
(Continued)
chorioretinitis A18.53
choroid, choroiditis A18.53
ciliary body A18.54
colitis A18.32
collier's J65
colliquativa (primary) A18.4
colon A18.32
complex, primary A15.7
congenital P37.0
conjunctiva A18.59
connective tissue (systemic) A18.89
contact Z20.1
cornea (ulcer) A18.52
Cowper's gland A18.15
coxae A18.02
coxalgia A18.02
cul-de-sac of Douglas A18.17
curvature, spine A18.01
cutis (colliquativa) (primary) A18.4
cyst, ovary A18.18
cystitis A18.12
dactylitis A18.03
diarrhea A18.32
diffuse —*see* Tuberculosis, miliary
digestive tract A18.32
disseminated —*see* Tuberculosis, miliary
duodenum A18.32
dura (mater) (cerebral) (spinal) A17.0
abscess (cerebral) (spinal) A17.81
dysentery A18.32
ear (inner) (middle) A18.6
bone A18.03
external (primary) A18.4
skin (primary) A18.4
elbow A18.02
emphysema —*see* Tuberculosis, pulmonary
empyema A15.6
encephalitis A17.82
endarteritis A18.89
endocarditis A18.84
aortic A18.84
mitral A18.84
pulmonary A18.84
tricuspid A18.84
endocrine glands NEC A18.82
endometrium A18.17
enteric, enterica, enteritis A18.32
enterocolitis A18.32
epididymis, epididymitis A18.15
epidural abscess (cerebral) (spinal) A17.81
epiglottis A15.5
episcleritis A18.51
erythema (induratum) (nodosum) (primary) A18.4
esophagus A18.83
eustachian tube A18.6
exposure (to) Z20.1
exudative —*see* Tuberculosis, pulmonary
eye A18.50
eyelid (primary) (lupus) A18.4
fallopian tube (acute) (chronic) A18.17
fascia A18.09
fauces A15.8
female pelvic inflammatory disease A18.17
finger A18.03
first infection A15.7
gallbladder A18.83
ganglion A18.09
gastritis A18.83
gastrocolic fistula A18.32
gastroenteritis A18.32
gastrointestinal tract A18.32
general, generalized —*see* Tuberculosis, miliary
genital organs A18.10
genitourinary A18.10
genu A18.02
glandula suprarenalis A18.7
glandular, general A18.2

Tuberculosis, tubercular, tuberculous
(Continued)
glottis A15.5
grinder's J65
gum A18.83
hand A18.03
heart A18.84
hematogenous —*see* Tuberculosis, miliary
hemoptysis —*see* Tuberculosis, pulmonary
hemorrhage NEC —*see* Tuberculosis, pulmonary
hemothorax A15.6
hepatitis A18.83
hilar lymph nodes A15.4
primary (progressive) A15.7
hip (joint) (disease) (bone) A18.02
hydropneumothorax A15.6
hydrothorax A15.6
hypoadrenalism A18.7
hypopharynx A15.8
ileocecal (hyperplastic) A18.32
ileocolitis A18.32
ileum A18.32
iliac spine (superior) A18.03
immunological findings only A15.7
indurativa (primary) A18.4
infantile A15.7
infection A15.9
without clinical manifestations A15.7
infraclavicular gland A18.2
inguinal gland A18.2
inguinalis A18.2
intestine (any part) A18.32
iridocyclitis A18.54
iris, iritis A18.54
ischiorectal A18.32
jaw A18.03
jejunum A18.32
joint A18.02
vertebral A18.01
keratitis (interstitial) A18.52
keratoconjunctivitis A18.52
kidney A18.11
knee (joint) A18.02
kyphosis, kyphoscoliosis A18.01
laryngitis A15.5
larynx A15.5
latent R76.11
leptomeninges, leptomeningitis (cerebral) (spinal) A17.0
lichenoides (primary) A18.4
linguae A18.83
lip A18.83
liver A18.83
lordosis A18.01
lung —*see* Tuberculosis, pulmonary
lupus vulgaris A18.4
lymph gland or node (peripheral) A18.2
abdomen A18.39
bronchial A15.4
primary (progressive) A15.7
cervical A18.2
hilar A15.4
primary (progressive) A15.7
intrathoracic A15.4
primary (progressive) A15.7
mediastinal A15.4
primary (progressive) A15.7
mesenteric A18.39
retroperitoneal A18.39
tracheobronchial A15.4
primary (progressive) A15.7
lymphadenitis —*see* Tuberculosis, lymph gland
lymphangitis —*see* Tuberculosis, lymph gland
lymphatic (gland) (vessel) —*see* Tuberculosis, lymph gland
mammary gland A18.89
marasmus A15.9
mastoiditis A18.03

Tuberculosis, tubercular, tuberculous
(Continued)
mediastinal lymph gland or node A15.4
primary (progressive) A15.7
mediastinitis A15.8
primary (progressive) A15.7
mediastinum A15.8
primary (progressive) A15.7
medulla A17.81
melanosis, Addisonian A18.7
meninges, meningitis (basilar) (cerebral) (cerebrospinal) (spinal) A17.0
meningoencephalitis A17.82
mesentery, mesenteric (gland or node) A18.39
miliary A19.9
acute A19.2
multiple sites A19.1
single specified site A19.0
chronic A19.8
specified NEC A19.8
millstone makers' J65
miner's J65
molder's J65
mouth A18.83
multiple A19.9
acute A19.1
chronic A19.8
muscle A18.09
myelitis A17.82
myocardium, myocarditis A18.84
nasal (passage) (sinus) A15.8
nasopharynx A15.8
neck gland A18.2
nephritis A18.11
nerve (mononeuropathy) A17.83
nervous system A17.9
nose (septum) A15.8
ocular A18.50
omentum A18.31
oophoritis (acute) (chronic) A18.17
optic (nerve trunk) (papilla) A18.59
orbit A18.59
orchitis A18.15
organ, specified NEC A18.89
osseous —*see* Tuberculosis, bone
osteitis —*see* Tuberculosis, bone
osteomyelitis —*see* Tuberculosis, bone
otitis media A18.6
ovary, ovaritis (acute) (chronic) A18.17
oviduct (acute) (chronic) A18.17
pachymeningitis A17.0
palate (soft) A18.83
pancreas A18.83
papulonecrotic (a) (primary) A18.4
parathyroid glands A18.82
paronychia (primary) A18.4
parotid gland or region A18.83
pelvis (bony) A18.03
penis A18.15
peribronchitis A15.5
pericardium, pericarditis A18.84
perichondritis, larynx A15.5
periostitis —*see* Tuberculosis, bone
perirectal fistula A18.32
peritoneum NEC A18.31
peritonitis A18.31
pharynx, pharyngitis A15.8
phlyctenulosis (keratoconjunctivitis) A18.52
phthisis NEC —*see* Tuberculosis, pulmonary
pituitary gland A18.82
pleura, pleural, pleurisy, pleuritis (fibrinous) (obliterative) (purulent) (simple plastic) (with effusion) A15.6
primary (progressive) A15.7
pneumonia, pneumonic —*see* Tuberculosis, pulmonary
pneumothorax (spontaneous) (tense valvular) —*see* Tuberculosis, pulmonary
polyneuropathy A17.89

Tuberculosis, tubercular, tuberculous *(Continued)*
polyserositis A19.9
acute A19.1
chronic A19.8
potter's J65
prepuce A18.15
primary (complex) A15.7
proctitis A18.32
prostate, prostatitis A18.14
pulmonalis —*see* Tuberculosis, pulmonary
pulmonary (cavitated) (fibrotic) (infiltrative) (nodular) A15.Ø
childhood type or first infection A15.7
primary (complex) A15.7
pyelitis A18.11
pyelonephritis A18.11
pyemia —*see* Tuberculosis, miliary
pyonephrosis A18.11
pyopneumothorax A15.6
pyothorax A15.6
rectum (fistula) (with abscess) A18.32
reinfection stage —*see* Tuberculosis, pulmonary
renal A18.11
renis A18.11
respiratory A15.9
primary A15.7
specified site NEC A15.8
retina, retinitis A18.53
retroperitoneal (lymph gland or node) A18.39
rheumatism NEC A18.Ø9
rhinitis A15.8
sacroiliac (joint) A18.Ø1
sacrum A18.Ø1
salivary gland A18.83
salpingitis (acute) (chronic) A18.17
sandblaster's J65
sclera A18.51
scoliosis A18.Ø1
scrofulous A18.2
scrotum A18.15
seminal tract or vesicle A18.15
senile A15.9
septic —*see* Tuberculosis, miliary
shoulder (joint) A18.Ø2
blade A18.Ø3
sigmoid A18.32
sinus (any nasal) A15.8
bone A18.Ø3
epididymis A18.15
skeletal NEC A18.Ø3
skin (any site) (primary) A18.4
small intestine A18.32
soft palate A18.83
spermatic cord A18.15
spine, spinal (column) A18.Ø1
cord A17.81
medulla A17.81
membrane A17.Ø
meninges A17.Ø
spleen, splenitis A18.85
spondylitis A18.Ø1
sternoclavicular joint A18.Ø2
stomach A18.83
stonemason's J65
subcutaneous tissue (cellular) (primary) A18.4
subcutis (primary) A18.4
subdeltoid bursa A18.83
submaxillary (region) A18.83
supraclavicular gland A18.2
suprarenal (capsule) (gland) A18.7
swelling, joint —*see also* category MØ1 (*see also* Tuberculosis, joint) A18.Ø2
symphysis pubis A18.Ø2
synovitis A18.Ø9
articular A18.Ø2
spine or vertebra A18.Ø1
systemic —*see* Tuberculosis, miliary

Tuberculosis, tubercular, tuberculous *(Continued)*
tarsitis A18.4
tendon (sheath) —*see* Tuberculosis, tenosynovitis
tenosynovitis A18.Ø9
spine or vertebra A18.Ø1
testis A18.15
throat A15.8
thymus gland A18.82
thyroid gland A18.81
tongue A18.83
tonsil, tonsillitis A15.8
trachea, tracheal A15.5
lymph gland or node A15.4
primary (progressive) A15.7
tracheobronchial A15.5
lymph gland or node A15.4
primary (progressive) A15.7
tubal (acute) (chronic) A18.17
tunica vaginalis A18.15
ulcer (skin) (primary) A18.4
bowel or intestine A18.32
specified NEC - code under Tuberculosis, by site
unspecified site A15.9
ureter A18.11
urethra, urethral (gland) A18.13
urinary organ or tract A18.13
uterus A18.17
uveal tract A18.54
uvula A18.83
vagina A18.18
vas deferens A18.15
verruca, verrucosa (cutis) (primary) A18.4
vertebra (column) A18.Ø1
vesiculitis A18.15
vulva A18.18
wrist (joint) A18.Ø2

Tuberculum
Carabelli —*see* Note at KØØ.2
occlusal —*see* Note at KØØ.2
paramolare KØØ.2

Tuberosity, enitre maxillary M26.Ø7
Tuberous sclerosis (brain) Q85.1
Tubo-ovarian —*see* condition
Tuboplasty, after previous sterilization Z31.Ø
aftercare Z31.42
Tubotympanitis, catarrhal (chronic) —*see* Otitis, media, nonsuppurative, chronic, serous
Tularemia A21.9
with
conjunctivitis A21.1
pneumonia A21.2
abdominal A21.3
bronchopneumonic A21.2
conjunctivitis A21.1
cryptogenic A21.3
enteric A21.3
gastrointestinal A21.3
generalized A21.7
ingestion A21.3
intestinal A21.3
oculoglandular A21.1
ophthalmic A21.1
pneumonia (any), pneumonic A21.2
pulmonary A21.2
sepsis A21.7
specified NEC A21.8
typhoidal A21.7
ulceroglandular A21.Ø
Tularensis conjunctivitis A21.1
Tumefaction —*see also* Swelling
liver —*see* Hypertrophy, liver
Tumor —*see also* Neoplasm, unspecified behavior, by site
acinar cell —*see* Neoplasm, uncertain behavior, by site
acinic cell —*see* Neoplasm, uncertain behavior, by site

Tumor *(Continued)*
adenocarcinoid —*see* Neoplasm, malignant, by site
adenomatoid —*see also* Neoplasm, benign, by site
odontogenic —*see* Cyst, calcifying odontogenic
adnexal (skin) —*see* Neoplasm, skin, benign, by site
adrenal
cortical (benign) D35.Ø-
malignant C74.Ø-
rest —*see* Neoplasm, benign, by site
alpha-cell
malignant
pancreas C25.4
specified site NEC —*see* Neoplasm, malignant, by site
unspecified site C25.4
pancreas D13.7
specified site NEC —*see* Neoplasm, benign, by site
unspecified site D13.7
aneurysmal —*see* Aneurysm
aortic body D44.7
malignant C75.5
Askin's —*see* Neoplasm, connective tissue, malignant
basal cell —*see also* Neoplasm, skin, uncertain behavior D48.5
Bednar —*see* Neoplasm, skin, malignant
benign (unclassified) —*see* Neoplasm, benign, by site
beta-cell
malignant
pancreas C25.4
specified site NEC —*see* Neoplasm, malignant, by site
unspecified site C25.4
pancreas D13.7
specified site NEC —*see* Neoplasm, benign, by site
unspecified site D13.7
Brenner D27.9
borderline malignancy D39.1-
malignant C56-
proliferating D39.1
bronchial alveolar, intravascular D38.1
Brooke's —*see* Neoplasm, skin, benign
brown fat —*see* Lipoma
Burkitt —*see* Lymphoma, Burkitt
calcifying epithelial odontogenic —*see* Cyst, calcifying odontogenic
carcinoid
benign D3A.ØØ
appendix D3A.Ø2Ø
ascending colon D3A.Ø22
bronchus (lung) D3A.Ø9Ø
cecum D3A.Ø21
colon D3A.Ø29
descending colon D3A.Ø24
duodenum D3A.Ø1Ø
foregut NOS D3A.Ø94
hindgut NOS D3A.Ø96
ileum D3A.Ø12
jejunum D3A.Ø11
kidney D3A.Ø93
large intestine D3A.Ø29
lung (bronchus) D3A.Ø9Ø
midgut NOS D3A.Ø95
rectum D3A.Ø26
sigmoid colon D3A.Ø25
small intestine D3A.Ø19
specified NEC D3A.Ø98
stomach D3A.Ø92
thymus D3A.Ø91
transverse colon D3A.Ø23
malignant C7A.ØØ
appendix C7A.Ø2Ø
ascending colon C7A.Ø22
bronchus (lung) C7A.Ø9Ø

Tumor *(Continued)*
  neuroendocrine D3A.8
    malignant poorly differentiated C7A.1
    secondary NEC C7B.8
    specified NEC C7A.8
  neurogenic olfactory C30.Ø
  nonencapsulated sclerosing C73
  odontogenic (adenomatoid) (benign) (calcifying epithelial) (keratocystic) (squamous) —*see* Cyst, calcifying odontogenic
    malignant C41.1
      upper jaw (bone) C41.Ø
  ovarian stromal D39.1-
  ovary, in pregnancy —*see* Pregnancy, complicated by
  pacinian —*see* Neoplasm, skin, benign
  Pancoast's —*see* Pancoast's syndrome
  papillary —*see also* Papilloma
    cystic D37.9
    mucinous of low malignant potential C56-
      specified site —*see* Neoplasm, malignant, by site
      unspecified site C56.9
    serous of low malignant potential
      specified site —*see* Neoplasm, malignant, by site
      unspecified site C56.9
  pelvic, in pregnancy or childbirth —*see* Pregnancy, complicated by
  phantom F45.8
  phyllodes D48.6-
    benign D24-
    malignant —*see* Neoplasm, breast, malignant
  Pindborg —*see* Cyst, calcifying odontogenic
  placental site trophoblastic D39.2
  plasma cell (malignant) (localized) —*see* Plasmacytoma, solitary
  polyvesicular vitelline
    specified site —*see* Neoplasm, malignant, by site
    unspecified site
      female C56.9
      male C62.9Ø
  Pott's puffy —*see* Osteomyelitis, specified NEC
  Rathke's pouch D44.3
  retinal anlage —*see* Neoplasm, benign, by site
  salivary gland type, mixed —*see* Neoplasm, salivary gland, benign
    malignant —*see* Neoplasm, salivary gland, malignant
  Sampson's N8Ø.1
  Schmincke's —*see* Neoplasm, nasopharynx, malignant
  sclerosing stromal D27-
  sebaceous —*see* Cyst, sebaceous
  secondary —*see* Neoplasm, secondary, by site
    carcinoid C7B.ØØ
      bone C7B.Ø3
      distant lymph nodes C7B.Ø1
      liver C7B.Ø2
      peritoneum C7B.Ø4
      specified NEC C7B.Ø9
    neuroendocrine NEC C7B.8
  serous of low malignant potential
    specified site —*see* Neoplasm, malignant, by site
    unspecified site C56.9
  Sertoli cell —*see* Neoplasm, benign, by site
    with lipid storage
      specified site —*see* Neoplasm, benign, by site
      unspecified site
        female D27.9
        male D29.2Ø
    specified site —*see* Neoplasm, benign, by site
    unspecified site
      female D27.9
      male D29.2Ø

Tumor *(Continued)*
  Sertoli-Leydig cell —*see* Neoplasm, benign, by site
    specified site —*see* Neoplasm, benign, by site
    unspecified site
      female D27.9
      male D29.2Ø
  sex cord(-stromal) —*see* Neoplasm, uncertain behavior, by site
    with annular tubules D39.1-
  skin appendage —*see* Neoplasm, skin, benign
  smooth muscle —*see* Neoplasm, connective tissue, uncertain behavior
  soft tissue
    benign —*see* Neoplasm, connective tissue, benign
    malignant —*see* Neoplasm, connective tissue, malignant
  sternomastoid (congenital) Q68.Ø
  stromal
    endometrial D39.Ø
    gastric D48.1
      benign D21.4
      malignant C16.9
      uncertain behavior D48.1
    gastrointestinal C49.A- ⟸
      benign D21.4
      esophagus C49.A1 ◀
      large intestine C49.A4 ◀
      malignant C49.AØ ⟸
        colon C49.A4 ◀
        duodenum C49.A3 ◀
        esophagus C49.A1 ◀
        ileum C49.A3 ◀
        jejunum C49.A3 ◀
        Meckel diverticulum C49.A3 ◀
        large intestine C49.A4 ◀
        omentum C49.A9 ◀
        peritoneum C49.A9 ◀
        rectum C49.A5 ◀
        small intestine C49.A3 ◀
        specified site NEC C49.A9 ◀
        stomach C49.A2 ◀
      large intestine C49.A4 ◀
      rectum C49.A5 ◀
      small intestine C49.A3 ◀
      specified site NEC C49.A9 ◀
      stomach C49.A2 ◀
      uncertain behavior D48.1
    intestine
      benign D21.4
      malignant ⟸
        large C49.A4 ◀
        small C49.A3 ◀
      uncertain behavior D48.1
    ovarian D39.1-
    stomach C49.A2 ⟸
      benign D21.4
      malignant C49.A2 ⟸
      uncertain behavior D48.1
  sweat gland —*see also* Neoplasm, skin, uncertain behavior
    benign —*see* Neoplasm, skin, benign
    malignant —*see* Neoplasm, skin, malignant
  syphilitic, brain A52.17
  testicular D4Ø.1Ø
  testicular stromal D4Ø.1-
  theca cell D27.-
  theca cell-granulosa cell D39.1-
  Triton, malignant —*see* Neoplasm, nerve, malignant
  trophoblastic, placental site D39.2
  turban D23.4
  uterus (body), in pregnancy or childbirth —*see* Pregnancy, complicated by, tumor, uterus
  vagina, in pregnancy or childbirth —*see* Pregnancy, complicated by
  varicose —*see* Varix

Tumor *(Continued)*
  von Recklinghausen's —*see* Neurofibromatosis
  vulva or perineum, in pregnancy or childbirth —*see* Pregnancy, complicated by
    causing obstructed labor O65.5
  Warthin's —*see* Neoplasm, salivary gland, benign
  Wilms' C64-
  yolk sac —*see* Neoplasm, malignant, by site
    specified site —*see* Neoplasm, malignant, by site
    unspecified site
      female C56.9
      male C62.9Ø
Tumor lysis syndrome (following antineoplastic chemotherapy) (spontaneous) NEC E88.3
Tumorlet —*see* Neoplasm, uncertain behavior, by site
Tungiasis B88.1
Tunica vasculosa lentis Q12.2
Turban tumor D23.4
Türck's trachoma J37.Ø
Turner-Kieser syndrome Q87.2 ⟸
Turner-like syndrome Q87.1
Turner's
  hypoplasia (tooth) KØØ.4
  syndrome Q96.9
    specified NEC Q96.8
  tooth KØØ.4
Turner-Ullrich syndrome Q96.9
Tussis convulsiva —*see* Whooping cough
Twiddler's syndrome (due to)
  automatic implantable defibrillator T82.198
  cardiac pacemaker T82.198
Twilight state
  epileptic FØ5
  psychogenic F44.89
Twin (newborn) —*see also* Newborn, twin
  conjoined Q89.4
  pregnancy —*see* Pregnancy, twin, conjoined
Twinning, teeth KØØ.2
Twist, twisted
  bowel, colon or intestine K56.2
  hair (congenital) Q84.1
  mesentery K56.2
  omentum K56.2
  organ or site, congenital NEC —*see* Anomaly, by site
  ovarian pedicle —*see* Torsion, ovary
Twitching R25.3
Tylosis (acquired) L84
  buccalis K13.29
  linguae K13.29
  palmaris et plantaris (congenital) (inherited) Q82.8
    acquired L85.1
Tympanism R14.Ø
Tympanites (abdominal) (intestinal) R14.Ø
Tympanitis —*see* Myringitis
Tympanosclerosis —*see* subcategory H74.Ø
Tympanum —*see* condition
Tympany
  abdomen R14.Ø
  chest RØ9.89
Type A behavior pattern Z73.1
Typhlitis —*see* Appendicitis
Typhoenteritis —*see* Typhoid
Typhoid (abortive) (ambulant) (any site) (clinical) (fever) (hemorrhagic) (infection) (intermittent) (malignant) (rheumatic) (Widal negative) AØ1.ØØ
  with pneumonia AØ1.Ø3
  abdominal AØ1.Ø9
  arthritis AØ1.Ø4
  carrier (suspected) of Z22.Ø
  cholecystitis (current) AØ1.Ø9
  endocarditis AØ1.Ø2
  heart involvement AØ1.Ø2

T

◀ New ⟸ Revised ~~deleted~~ Deleted

Typhoid *(Continued)*
inoculation reaction —*see* Complications, vaccination
meningitis A01.01
mesenteric lymph nodes A01.09
myocarditis A01.02
osteomyelitis A01.05
perichondritis, larynx A01.09
pneumonia A01.03
specified NEC A01.09
spine A01.05
ulcer (perforating) A01.09
Typhomalaria (fever) —*see* Malaria
Typhomania A01.00
Typhoperitonitis A01.09
Typhus (fever) A75.9
abdominal, abdominalis —*see* Typhoid
African tick A77.1
amarillic A95.9
brain A75.9 *[G94]*

Typhus *(Continued)*
cerebral A75.9 *[G94]*
classical A75.0
due to Rickettsia
prowazekii A75.0
recrudescent A75.1
tsutsugamushi A75.3
typhi A75.2
endemic (flea-borne) A75.2
epidemic (louse-borne) A75.0
exanthematic NEC A75.0
exanthematicus SAI A75.0
brillii SAI A75.1
mexicanus SAI A75.2
typhus murinus A75.2
flea-borne A75.2
India tick A77.1
Kenya (tick) A77.1
louse-borne A75.0
Mexican A75.2

Typhus *(Continued)*
mite-borne A75.3
murine A75.2
North Asian tick-borne A77.2
petechial A75.9
Queensland tick A77.3
rat A75.2
recrudescent A75.1
recurrens —*see* Fever, relapsing
Sao Paulo A77.0
scrub (China) (India) (Malaysia) (New Guinea) A75.3
shop (of Malaysia) A75.2
Siberian tick A77.2
tick-borne A77.9
tropical (mite-borne) A75.3
Tyrosinemia E70.21
newborn, transitory P74.5
Tyrosinosis E70.21
Tyrosinuria E70.29

U

Uhl's anomaly or disease Q24.8
Ulcer, ulcerated, ulcerating, ulceration, ulcerative
alveolar process M27.3
amebic (intestine) AØ6.1
skin AØ6.7
anastomotic —*see* Ulcer, gastrojejunal
anorectal K62.6
antral —*see* Ulcer, stomach
anus (sphincter) (solitary) K62.6
aorta —*see* Aneurysm
aphthous (oral) (recurrent) K12.Ø
genital organ (s)
female N76.6
male N5Ø.89
artery I77.2
atrophic —*see* Ulcer, skin
decubitus —*see* Ulcer, pressure, by site
back L98.429
with
bone necrosis L98.424
exposed fat layer L98.422
muscle necrosis L98.423
skin breakdown only L98.421
Barrett's (esophagus) K22.1Ø
with bleeding K22.11
bile duct (common) (hepatic) K83.8
bladder (solitary) (sphincter) NEC N32.89
bilharzial B65.9 *[N33]*
in schistosomiasis (bilharzial) B65.9 *[N33]*
submucosal —*see* Cystitis, interstitial
tuberculous A18.12
bleeding K27.4
bone —*see* Osteomyelitis, specified type NEC
bowel —*see* Ulcer, intestine
breast N61.1
bronchus J98.Ø9
buccal (cavity) (traumatic) K12.1
Buruli A31.1
buttock L98.419
with
bone necrosis L98.414
exposed fat layer L98.412
muscle necrosis L98.413
skin breakdown only L98.411
cancerous —*see* Neoplasm, malignant, by site
cardia K22.1Ø
with bleeding K22.11
cardioesophageal (peptic) K22.1Ø
with bleeding K22.11
cecum —*see* Ulcer, intestine
cervix (uteri) (decubitus) (trophic) N86
with cervicitis N72
chancroidal A57
chiclero B55.1
chronic (cause unknown) —*see* Ulcer, skin
Cochin-China B55.1
colon —*see* Ulcer, intestine
conjunctiva H1Ø.89
cornea H16.ØØ-
with hypopyon H16.Ø3-
central H16.Ø1-
dendritic (herpes simplex) BØØ.52
marginal H16.Ø4-
Mooren's H16.Ø5-
mycotic H16.Ø6-
perforated H16.Ø7-
ring H16.Ø2-
tuberculous (phlyctenular) A18.52
corpus cavernosum (chronic) N48.5
crural —*see* Ulcer, lower limb
Curling's —*see* Ulcer, peptic, acute
Cushing's —*see* Ulcer, peptic, acute
cystic duct K82.8
cystitis (interstitial) —*see* Cystitis, interstitial
decubitus —*see* Ulcer, pressure, by site
dendritic, cornea (herpes simplex) BØØ.52
diabetes, diabetic —*see* Diabetes, ulcer
Dieulafoy's K25.Ø

Ulcer, ulcerated, ulcerating, ulceration, ulcerative *(Continued)*
due to
infection NEC —*see* Ulcer, skin
radiation NEC L59.8
trophic disturbance (any region) —*see* Ulcer, skin
X-ray L58.1
duodenum, duodenal (eroded) (peptic) K26.9
with
hemorrhage K26.4
and perforation K26.6
perforation K26.5
acute K26.3
with
hemorrhage K26.Ø
and perforation K26.2
perforation K26.1
chronic K26.7
with
hemorrhage K26.4
and perforation K26.6
perforation K26.5
dysenteric AØ9
elusive —*see* Cystitis, interstitial
endocarditis (acute) (chronic) (subacute) I28.8
epiglottis J38.7
esophagus (peptic) K22.1Ø
with bleeding K22.11
due to
aspirin K22.1Ø
with bleeding K22.11
gastrointestinal reflux disease K21.Ø
ingestion of chemical or medicament K22.1Ø
with bleeding K22.11
fungal K22.1Ø
with bleeding K22.11
infective K22.1Ø
with bleeding K22.11
varicose —*see* Varix, esophagus
eyelid (region) HØ1.8
fauces J39.2
Fenwick (-Hunner) (solitary) —*see* Cystitis, interstitial
fistulous —*see* Ulcer, skin
foot (indolent) (trophic) —*see* Ulcer, lower limb
frambesial, initial A66.Ø
frenum (tongue) K14.Ø
gallbladder or duct K82.8
gangrenous —*see* Gangrene
gastric —*see* Ulcer, stomach
gastrocolic —*see* Ulcer, gastrojejunal
gastroduodenal —*see* Ulcer, peptic
gastroesophageal —*see* Ulcer, stomach
gastrointestinal —*see* Ulcer, gastrojejunal
gastrojejunal (peptic) K28.9
with
hemorrhage K28.4
and perforation K28.6
perforation K28.5
acute K28.3
with
hemorrhage K28.Ø
and perforation K28.2
perforation K28.1
chronic K28.7
with
hemorrhage K28.4
and perforation K28.6
perforation K28.5
gastrojejunocolic —*see* Ulcer, gastrojejunal
gingiva KØ6.8
gingivitis KØ5.1Ø
nonplaque induced KØ5.11
plaque induced KØ5.1Ø
glottis J38.7
granuloma of pudenda A58
gum KØ6.8
gumma, due to yaws A66.4

Ulcer, ulcerated, ulcerating, ulceration, ulcerative *(Continued)*
heel —*see* Ulcer, lower limb
hemorrhoid —*see also* Hemorrhoids, by degree K64.8
Hunner's —*see* Cystitis, interstitial
hypopharynx J39.2
hypopyon (chronic) (subacute) —*see* Ulcer, cornea, with hypopyon
hypostaticum —*see* Ulcer, varicose
ileum —*see* Ulcer, intestine
intestine, intestinal K63.3
with perforation K63.1
amebic AØ6.1
duodenal —*see* Ulcer, duodenum
granulocytopenic (with hemorrhage) —*see* Neutropenia
marginal —*see* Ulcer, gastrojejunal
perforating K63.1
newborn P78.Ø
primary, small intestine K63.3
rectum K62.6
stercoraceous, stercoral K63.3
tuberculous A18.32
typhoid (fever) —*see* Typhoid
varicose I86.8
jejunum, jejunal —*see* Ulcer, gastrojejunal
keratitis —*see* Ulcer, cornea
knee —*see* Ulcer, lower limb
labium (majus) (minus) N76.6
laryngitis —*see* Laryngitis
larynx (aphthous) (contact) J38.7
diphtheritic A36.2
leg —*see* Ulcer, lower limb
lip K13.Ø
Lipschütz's N76.6
lower limb (atrophic) (chronic) (neurogenic) (perforating) (pyogenic) (trophic) (tropical) L97.9Ø9
with
bone necrosis L97.9Ø4
exposed fat layer L97.9Ø2
muscle necrosis L97.9Ø3
skin breakdown only L97.9Ø1
ankle L97.3Ø9
with
bone necrosis L97.3Ø4
exposed fat layer L97.3Ø2
muscle necrosis L97.3Ø3
skin breakdown only L97.3Ø1
left L97.329
with
bone necrosis L97.324
exposed fat layer L97.322
muscle necrosis L97.323
skin breakdown only L97.321
right L97.319
with
bone necrosis L97.314
exposed fat layer L97.312
muscle necrosis L97.313
skin breakdown only L97.311
calf L97.2Ø9
with
bone necrosis L97.2Ø4
exposed fat layer L97.2Ø2
muscle necrosis L97.2Ø3
skin breakdown only L97.2Ø1
left L97.229
with
bone necrosis L97.224
exposed fat layer L97.222
muscle necrosis L97.223
skin breakdown only L97.221
right L97.219
with
bone necrosis L97.214
exposed fat layer L97.212
muscle necrosis L97.213
skin breakdown only L97.211
decubitus —*see* Ulcer, pressure, by site

Ulcer, ulcerated, ulcerating, ulceration, ulcerative *(Continued)*
lower limb *(Continued)*
foot specified NEC L97.509
with
bone necrosis L97.504
exposed fat layer L97.502
muscle necrosis L97.503
skin breakdown only L97.501
left L97.529
with
bone necrosis L97.524
exposed fat layer L97.522
muscle necrosis L97.523
skin breakdown only L97.521
right L97.519
with
bone necrosis L97.514
exposed fat layer L97.512
muscle necrosis L97.513
skin breakdown only L97.511
heel L97.409
with
bone necrosis L97.404
exposed fat layer L97.402
muscle necrosis L97.403
skin breakdown only L97.401
left L97.429
with
bone necrosis L97.424
exposed fat layer L97.422
muscle necrosis L97.423
skin breakdown only L97.421
right L97.419
with
bone necrosis L97.414
exposed fat layer L97.412
muscle necrosis L97.413
skin breakdown only L97.411
left L97.929
with
bone necrosis L97.924
exposed fat layer L97.922
muscle necrosis L97.923
skin breakdown only L97.921
lower leg NOS L97.909
with
bone necrosis L97.904
exposed fat layer L97.902
muscle necrosis L97.903
skin breakdown only L97.901
left L97.929
with
bone necrosis L97.924
exposed fat layer L97.922
muscle necrosis L97.923
skin breakdown only L97.921
right L97.919
with
bone necrosis L97.914
exposed fat layer L97.912
muscle necrosis L97.913
skin breakdown only L97.911
specified site NEC L97.809
with
bone necrosis L97.804
exposed fat layer L97.802
muscle necrosis L97.803
skin breakdown only L97.801
left L97.829
with
bone necrosis L97.824
exposed fat layer L97.822
muscle necrosis L97.823
skin breakdown only L97.821
right L97.819
with
bone necrosis L97.814
exposed fat layer L97.812
muscle necrosis L97.813
skin breakdown only L97.811

Ulcer, ulcerated, ulcerating, ulceration, ulcerative *(Continued)*
lower limb *(Continued)*
midfoot L97.409
with
bone necrosis L97.404
exposed fat layer L97.402
muscle necrosis L97.403
skin breakdown only L97.401
left L97.429
with
bone necrosis L97.424
exposed fat layer L97.422
muscle necrosis L97.423
skin breakdown only L97.421
right L97.419
with
bone necrosis L97.414
exposed fat layer L97.412
muscle necrosis L97.413
skin breakdown only L97.411
right L97.919
with
bone necrosis L97.914
exposed fat layer L97.912
muscle necrosis L97.913
skin breakdown only L97.911
thigh L97.109
with
bone necrosis L97.104
exposed fat layer L97.102
muscle necrosis L97.103
skin breakdown only L97.101
left L97.129
with
bone necrosis L97.124
exposed fat layer L97.122
muscle necrosis L97.123
skin breakdown only L97.121
right L97.119
with
bone necrosis L97.114
exposed fat layer L97.112
muscle necrosis L97.113
skin breakdown only L97.111
toe L97.509
with
bone necrosis L97.504
exposed fat layer L97.502
muscle necrosis L97.503
skin breakdown only L97.501
left L97.529
with
bone necrosis L97.524
exposed fat layer L97.522
muscle necrosis L97.523
skin breakdown only L97.521
right L97.519
with
bone necrosis L97.514
exposed fat layer L97.512
muscle necrosis L97.513
skin breakdown only L97.511
leprous A30.1
syphilitic A52.19
varicose —*see* Varix, leg, with, ulcer
luetic —*see* Ulcer, syphilitic
lung J98.4
tuberculous —*see* Tuberculosis, pulmonary
malignant —*see* Neoplasm, malignant, by site
marginal NEC —*see* Ulcer, gastrojejunal
meatus (urinarius) N34.2
Meckel's diverticulum Q43.0
malignant —*see* Table of Neoplasms, small intestine, malignant
Meleney's (chronic undermining) —*see* Ulcer, skin
Mooren's (cornea) —*see* Ulcer, cornea, Mooren's
mycobacterial (skin) A31.1
nasopharynx J39.2

Ulcer, ulcerated, ulcerating, ulceration, ulcerative *(Continued)*
neck, uterus N86
neurogenic NEC —*see* Ulcer, skin
nose, nasal (passage) (infective) (septum) J34.0
skin —*see* Ulcer, skin
spirochetal A69.8
varicose (bleeding) I86.8
oral mucosa (traumatic) K12.1
palate (soft) K12.1
penis (chronic) N48.5
peptic (site unspecified) K27.9
with
hemorrhage K27.4
and perforation K27.6
perforation K27.5
acute K27.3
with
hemorrhage K27.0
and perforation K27.2
perforation K27.1
chronic K27.7
with
hemorrhage K27.4
and perforation K27.6
perforation K27.5
esophagus K22.10
with bleeding K22.11
newborn P78.82
perforating K27.5
skin —*see* Ulcer, skin
peritonsillar J35.8
phagedenic (tropical) —*see* Ulcer, skin
pharynx J39.2
phlebitis —*see* Phlebitis
plaster —*see* Ulcer, pressure, by site
popliteal space —*see* Ulcer, lower limb
postpyloric —*see* Ulcer, duodenum
prepuce N47.7
prepyloric —*see* Ulcer, stomach
pressure (pressure area) L89.9-
ankle L89.5-
back L89.1-
buttock L89.3-
coccyx L89.15-
contiguous site of back, buttock, hip L89.4-
elbow L89.0-
face L89.81-
head L89.81-
heel L89.6-
hip L89.2-
sacral region (tailbone) L89.15-
specified site NEC L89.89-
stage 1 (healing) (pre-ulcer skin changes limited to persistent focal edema)
ankle L89.5-
back L89.1-
buttock L89.3-
coccyx L89.15-
contiguous site of back, buttock, hip L89.4-
elbow L89.0-
face L89.81-
head L89.81-
heel L89.6-
hip L89.2-
sacral region (tailbone) L89.15-
specified site NEC L89.89-
stage 2 (healing) (abrasion, blister, partial thickness skin loss involving epidermis and/or dermis)
ankle L89.5-
back L89.1-
buttock L89.3-
coccyx L89.15-
contiguous site of back, buttock, hip L89.4-
elbow L89.0-
face L89.81-
head L89.81-

Ulcer, ulcerated, ulcerating, ulceration, ulcerative *(Continued)*
pressure *(Continued)*
stage 2 *(Continued)*
heel L89.6-
hip L89.2-
sacral region (tailbone) L89.15-
specified site NEC L89.89-
stage 3 (healing) (full thickness skin loss involving damage or necrosis of subcutaneous tissue)
ankle L89.5-
back L89.1-
buttock L89.3-
coccyx L89.15-
contiguous site of back, buttock, hip L89.4-
elbow L89.Ø-
face L89.81-
head L89.81-
heel L89.6-
hip L89.2-
sacral region (tailbone) L89.15-
specified site NEC L89.89-
stage 4 (healing) (necrosis of soft tissues through to underlying muscle, tendon, or bone)
ankle L89.5-
back L89.1-
buttock L89.3-
coccyx L89.15-
contiguous site of back, buttock, hip L89.4-
elbow L89.Ø-
face L89.81-
head L89.81-
heel L89.6-
hip L89.2-
sacral region (tailbone) L89.15-
specified site NEC L89.89-
unspecified stage
ankle L89.5-
back L89.1-
buttock L89.3-
coccyx L89.15-
contiguous site of back, buttock, hip L89.4-
elbow L89.Ø-
face L89.81-
head L89.81-
heel L89.6-
hip L89.2-
sacral region (tailbone) L89.15-
specified site NEC L89.89-
unstageable
ankle L89.5-
back L89.1-
buttock L89.3-
coccyx L89.15-
contiguous site of back, buttock, hip L89.4-
elbow L89.Ø-
face L89.81-
head L89.81-
heel L89.6-
hip L89.2-
sacral region (tailbone) L89.15-
specified site NEC L89.89-
primary of intestine K63.3
with perforation K63.1
prostate N41.9
pyloric —*see* Ulcer, stomach
rectosigmoid K63.3
with perforation K63.1
rectum (sphincter) (solitary) K62.6
stercoraceous, stercoral K62.6
retina —*see* Inflammation, chorioretinal
rodent —*see also* Neoplasm, skin, malignant
sclera —*see* Scleritis
scrofulous (tuberculous) A18.2

Ulcer, ulcerated, ulcerating, ulceration, ulcerative *(Continued)*
scrotum N5Ø.89
tuberculous A18.15
varicose I86.1
seminal vesicle N5Ø.89
sigmoid —*see* Ulcer, intestine
skin (atrophic) (chronic) (neurogenic) (non-healing) (perforating) (pyogenic) (trophic) (tropical) L98.499
with gangrene —*see* Gangrene
amebic AØ6.7
back —*see* Ulcer, back
buttock —*see* Ulcer, buttock
decubitus —*see* Ulcer, pressure
lower limb —*see* Ulcer, lower limb
mycobacterial A31.1
specified site NEC L98.499
with
bone necrosis L98.494
exposed fat layer L98.492
muscle necrosis L98.493
skin breakdown only L98.491
tuberculous (primary) A18.4
varicose —*see* Ulcer, varicose
sloughing —*see* Ulcer, skin
solitary, anus or rectum (sphincter) K62.6
sore throat JØ2.9
streptococcal JØ2.Ø
spermatic cord N5Ø.89
spine (tuberculous) A18.Ø1
stasis (venous) —*see* Varix, leg, with, ulcer
without varicose veins I87.2
stercoraceous, stercoral K63.3
with perforation K63.1
anus or rectum K62.6
stoma, stomal —*see* Ulcer, gastrojejunal
stomach (eroded) (peptic) (round) K25.9
with
hemorrhage K25.4
and perforation K25.6
perforation K25.5
acute K25.3
with
hemorrhage K25.Ø
and perforation K25.2
perforation K25.1
chronic K25.7
with
hemorrhage K25.4
and perforation K25.6
perforation K25.5
stomal —*see* Ulcer, gastrojejunal
stomatitis K12.1
stress —*see* Ulcer, peptic
strumous (tuberculous) A18.2
submucosal, bladder —*see* Cystitis, interstitial
syphilitic (any site) (early) (secondary) A51.39
late A52.79
perforating A52.79
foot A52.11
testis N5Ø.89
thigh —*see* Ulcer, lower limb
throat J39.2
diphtheritic A36.Ø
toe —*see* Ulcer, lower limb
tongue (traumatic) K14.Ø
tonsil J35.8
diphtheritic A36.Ø
trachea J39.8
trophic —*see* Ulcer, skin
tropical —*see* Ulcer, skin
tuberculous —*see* Tuberculosis, ulcer
tunica vaginalis N5Ø.89
turbinate J34.89
typhoid (perforating) —*see* Typhoid

Ulcer, ulcerated, ulcerating, ulceration, ulcerative *(Continued)*
unspecified site —*see* Ulcer, skin
urethra (meatus) —*see* Urethritis
uterus N85.8
cervix N86
with cervicitis N72
neck N86
with cervicitis N72
vagina N76.5
in Behçet's disease M35.2 *[N77.Ø]*
pessary N89.8
valve, heart I33.Ø
varicose (lower limb, any part) —*see also* Varix, leg, with, ulcer
broad ligament I86.2
esophagus —*see* Varix, esophagus
inflamed or infected —*see* Varix, leg, with ulcer, with inflammation
nasal septum I86.8
perineum I86.3
scrotum I86.1
specified site NEC I86.8
sublingual I86.Ø
vulva I86.3
vas deferens N5Ø.89
vulva (acute) (infectional) N76.6
in (due to)
Behçet's disease M35.2 *[N77.Ø]*
herpesviral (herpes simplex) infection A6Ø.Ø4
tuberculosis A18.18
vulvobuccal, recurring N76.6
X-ray L58.1
yaws A66.4
Ulcerosa scarlatina A38.8
Ulcus —*see also* Ulcer
cutis tuberculosum A18.4
duodeni —*see* Ulcer, duodenum
durum (syphilitic) A51.Ø
extragenital A51.2
gastrojejunale —*see* Ulcer, gastrojejunal
hypostaticum —*see* Ulcer, varicose
molle (cutis) (skin) A57
serpens corneae —*see* Ulcer, cornea, central
ventriculi —*see* Ulcer, stomach
Ulegyria QØ4.8
Ulerythema
ophryogenes, congenital Q84.2
sycosiforme L73.8
Ullrich(-Bonnevie)(-Turner) syndrome —*see also* Turner's syndrome Q87.1
Ullrich-Feichtiger syndrome Q87.Ø
Ulnar —*see* condition
Ulorrhagia, ulorrhea KØ6.8
Umbilicus, umbilical —*see* condition
Unacceptable
contours of tooth KØ8.54
morphology of tooth KØ8.54
Unavailability (of)
bed at medical facility Z75.1
health service-related agencies Z75.4
medical facilities (at) Z75.3
due to
investigation by social service agency Z75.2
lack of services at home Z75.Ø
remoteness from facility Z75.3
waiting list Z75.1
home Z75.Ø
outpatient clinic Z75.3
schooling Z55.1
social service agencies Z75.4
Uncinaria americana infestation B76.1
Uncinariasis B76.9
Uncongenial work Z56.5
Unconscious (ness) —*see* Coma
Underachievement in school Z55.3
Underdevelopment —*see also* Undeveloped
nose Q3Ø.1
sexual E3Ø.Ø

◀ New ⬅ Revised ~~deleted~~ Deleted

- **Underdosing** —*see also* Table of Drugs and Chemicals, categories T36-T50, with final character 6 Z91.14
  - intentional NEC Z91.128
    - due to financial hardship of patient Z91.120
  - unintentional NEC Z91.138
    - due to patient's age related debility Z91.130
- **Underfeeding, newborn** P92.3
- **Underfill, endodontic** M27.53
- **Underimmunization status** Z28.3
- **Undernourishment** —*see* Malnutrition
- **Undernutrition** —*see* Malnutrition
- **Under observation** —*see* Observation
- **Underweight** R63.6
  - for gestational age —*see* Light for dates
- **Underwood's disease** P83.0
- **Undescended** —*see also* Malposition, congenital
  - cecum Q43.3
  - colon Q43.3
  - testicle —*see* Cryptorchid
- **Undeveloped, undevelopment** —*see also* Hypoplasia
  - brain (congenital) Q02
  - cerebral (congenital) Q02
  - heart Q24.8
  - lung Q33.6
  - testis E29.1
  - uterus E30.0
- **Undiagnosed** (disease) R69
- **Undulant fever** —*see* Brucellosis
- **Unemployment, anxiety concerning** Z56.0
  - threatened Z56.2
- **Unequal length** (acquired) (limb) —*see also* Deformity, limb, unequal length
  - leg —*see also* Deformity, limb, unequal length
    - congenital Q72.9-
- **Unextracted dental root** K08.3
- **Unguis incarnatus** L60.0
- **Unhappiness** R45.2
- **Unicornate uterus** Q51.4
- **Unilateral** —*see also* condition
  - development, breast N64.89
  - organ or site, congenital NEC —*see* Agenesis, by site
- **Unilocular heart** Q20.8
- **Union, abnormal** —*see also* Fusion
  - larynx and trachea Q34.8
- **Universal mesentery** Q43.3
- **Unrepairable overhanging of dental restorative materials** K08.52
- **Unsatisfactory**
  - restoration of tooth K08.50
    - specified NEC K08.59
  - sample of cytologic smear
    - anus R85.615
    - cervix R87.615
    - vagina R87.625
  - surroundings Z59.1
    - work Z56.5
- **Unsoundness of mind** —*see* Psychosis
- **Unstable**
  - back NEC —*see* Instability, joint, spine
  - hip (congenital) Q65.6
    - acquired —*see* Derangement, joint, specified type NEC, hip
  - joint —*see* Instability, joint
    - secondary to removal of joint prosthesis M96.89
  - lie (mother) O32.0
  - lumbosacral joint (congenital)
    - acquired —*see* subcategory M53.2
  - sacroiliac —*see* subcategory M53.2
  - spine NEC —*see* Instability, joint, spine
- **Unsteadiness on feet** R26.81
- **Untruthfulness, child problem** F91.8
- **Unverricht(-Lundborg) disease or epilepsy** —*see* Epilepsy, generalized, idiopathic
- **Unwanted pregnancy** Z64.0
- **Upbringing, institutional** Z62.22
  - away from parents NEC Z62.29
  - in care of non-parental family member Z62.21
  - in foster care Z62.21
  - in orphanage or group home Z62.22
  - in welfare custody Z62.21
- **Upper respiratory** —*see* condition
- **Upset**
  - gastric K30
  - gastrointestinal K30
    - psychogenic F45.8
  - intestinal (large) (small) K59.9
    - psychogenic F45.8
  - menstruation N93.9
  - mental F48.9
  - stomach K30
    - psychogenic F45.8
- **Urachus** —*see also* condition
  - patent or persistent Q64.4
- **Urbach-Oppenheim disease** (necrobiosis lipoidica diabeticorum) —*see* E08-E13 with .620
- **Urbach's lipoid proteinosis** E78.89
- **Urbach-Wiethe disease** E78.89
- **Urban yellow fever** A95.1
- **Urea**
  - blood, high —*see* Uremia
  - cycle metabolism disorder —*see* Disorder, urea cycle metabolism
- **Uremia, uremic** N19
  - with
    - ectopic or molar pregnancy O08.4
    - polyneuropathy N18.9 *[G63]*
  - chronic —*see also* Disease, kidney, chronic N18.9
    - due to hypertension —*see* Hypertensive, kidney
  - complicating
    - ectopic or molar pregnancy O08.4
  - congenital P96.0
  - extrarenal R39.2
  - following ectopic or molar pregnancy O08.4
  - newborn P96.0
  - prerenal R39.2
- **Ureter, ureteral** —*see* condition
- **Ureteralgia** N23
- **Ureterectasis** —*see* Hydroureter
- **Ureteritis** N28.89
  - cystica N28.86
  - due to calculus N20.1
    - with calculus, kidney N20.2
      - with hydronephrosis N13.2
  - gonococcal (acute) (chronic) A54.21
  - nonspecific N28.89
- **Ureterocele** N28.89
  - congenital (orthotopic) Q62.31
    - ectopic Q62.32
- **Ureterolith, ureterolithiasis** —*see* Calculus, ureter
- **Ureterostomy**
  - attention to Z43.6
  - status Z93.6
- **Urethra, urethral** —*see* condition
- **Urethralgia** R39.89
- **Urethritis** (anterior) (posterior) N34.2
  - calculous N21.1
  - candidal B37.41
  - chlamydial A56.01
  - diplococcal (gonococcal) A54.01
    - with abscess (accessory gland) (periurethral) A54.1
  - gonococcal A54.01
    - with abscess (accessory gland) (periurethral) A54.1
  - nongonococcal N34.1
    - Reiter's —*see* Reiter's disease
  - nonspecific N34.1
  - nonvenereal N34.1
  - postmenopausal N34.2
  - puerperal O86.22
  - Reiter's —*see* Reiter's disease
- **Urethritis** *(Continued)*
  - specified NEC N34.2
  - trichomonal or due to Trichomonas (vaginalis) A59.03
- **Urethrocele** N81.0
  - with
    - cystocele —*see* Cystocele
    - prolapse of uterus —*see* Prolapse, uterus
- **Urethrolithiasis** (with colic or infection) N21.1
- **Urethrorectal** —*see* condition
- **Urethrorrhagia** N36.8
- **Urethrorrhea** R36.9
- **Urethrostomy**
  - attention to Z43.6
  - status Z93.6
- **Urethrotrigonitis** —*see* Trigonitis
- **Urethrovaginal** —*see* condition
- **Urgency**
  - fecal R15.2
  - hypertensive —*see* Hypertension
  - urinary N39.15 ◄
- **Urhidrosis, uridrosis** L74.8
- **Uric acid in blood** (increased) E79.0
- **Uricacidemia** (asymptomatic) E79.0
- **Uricemia** (asymptomatic) E79.0
- **Uricosuria** R82.99
- **Urinary** —*see* condition
- **Urination**
  - frequent R35.0
  - painful R30.9
- **Urine**
  - blood in —*see* Hematuria
  - discharge, excessive R35.8
  - enuresis, nonorganic origin F98.0
  - extravasation R39.0
  - frequency R35.0
  - incontinence R32
    - nonorganic origin F98.0
  - intermittent stream R39.198 ◄
  - pus in N39.0
  - retention or stasis R33.9
    - organic R33.8
      - drug-induced R33.0
    - psychogenic F45.8
  - secretion
    - deficient R34
    - excessive R35.8
    - frequency R35.0
  - stream
    - intermittent R39.198 ◄
    - slowing R39.198 ◄
    - splitting R39.13
    - weak R39.12
- **Urinemia** —*see* Uremia
- **Urinoma, urethra** N36.8
- **Uroarthritis, infectious** (Reiter's) —*see* Reiter's disease
- **Urodialysis** R34
- **Urolithiasis** —*see* Calculus, urinary
- **Uronephrosis** —*see* Hydronephrosis
- **Uropathy** N39.9
  - obstructive N13.9
    - specified NEC N13.8
  - reflux N13.9
    - specified NEC N13.8
  - vesicoureteral reflux-associated —*see* Reflux, vesicoureteral
- **Urosepsis** — code to condition
- **Urticaria** L50.9
  - with angioneurotic edema T78.3
    - hereditary D84.1
  - allergic L50.0
  - cholinergic L50.5
  - chronic L50.8
  - cold, familial L50.2
  - contact L50.6
  - dermatographic L50.3
  - due to
    - cold or heat L50.2
    - drugs L50.0
    - food L50.0

Urticaria *(Continued)*
  due to *(Continued)*
    inhalants L5Ø.Ø
    plants L5Ø.6
    serum —*see also* Reaction, serum T8Ø.69
  factitial L5Ø.3
  familial cold MØ4.2 ◄
  giant T78.3
    hereditary D84.1
  gigantea T78.3
  idiopathic L5Ø.1
  larynx T78.3
    hereditary D84.1
  neonatorum P83.8
  nonallergic L5Ø.1
  papulosa (Hebra) L28.2
  pigmentosa Q82.2
  recurrent periodic L5Ø.8
  serum —*see also* Reaction, serum T8Ø.69
  solar L56.3
  specified type NEC L5Ø.8
  thermal (cold) (heat) L5Ø.2
  vibratory L5Ø.4
  xanthelasmoidea Q82.2
Use (of)
  alcohol Z72.89 ⟸
    ~~with sleep disorder F1Ø.982~~
    with ◄
      intoxication F1Ø.929 ◄
      sleep disorder F1Ø.982 ◄
    harmful —*see* Abuse, alcohol
  amphetamines —*see* Use, stimulant NEC
  caffeine —*see* Use, stimulant NEC
  cannabis F12.9Ø
    with
      anxiety disorder F12.98Ø
      intoxication F12.929
        with
          delirium F12.921
          perceptual disturbance F12.922
        uncomplicated F12.92Ø
      other specified disorder F12.988
      psychosis F12.959
        delusions F12.95Ø
        hallucinations F12.951
      unspecified disorder F12.99
  cocaine F14.9Ø
    with
      anxiety disorder F14.98Ø
      intoxication F14.929
        with
          delirium F14.921
          perceptual disturbance F14.922
        uncomplicated F14.92Ø
      other specified disorder F14.988
      psychosis F14.959
        delusions F14.95Ø
        hallucinations F14.951
      sexual dysfunction F14.981
      sleep disorder F14.982
      unspecified disorder F14.99
    harmful —*see* Abuse, drug, cocaine
  drug (s) NEC F19.9Ø
    with sleep disorder F19.982
    harmful —*see* Abuse, drug, by type
  hallucinogen NEC F16.9Ø
    with
      anxiety disorder F16.98Ø
      intoxication F16.929
        with
          delirium F16.921
        uncomplicated F16.92Ø
      mood disorder F16.94
      other specified disorder F16.988

Use *(Continued)*
  hallucinogen NEC *(Continued)*
    with *(Continued)*
      perception disorder (flashbacks) F16.983
      psychosis F16.959
        delusions F16.95Ø
        hallucinations F16.951
      unspecified disorder F16.99
    harmful —*see* Abuse, drug, hallucinogen NEC
  inhalants F18.9Ø
    with
      anxiety disorder F18.98Ø
      intoxication F18.929
        with delirium F18.921
        uncomplicated F18.92Ø
      mood disorder F18.94
      other specified disorder F18.988
      persisting dementia F18.97
      psychosis F18.959
        delusions F18.95Ø
        hallucinations F18.951
      unspecified disorder F18.99
    harmful —*see* Abuse, drug, inhalant
  methadone —*see* Use, opioid ⟸
  nonprescribed drugs F19.9Ø
    harmful —*see* Abuse, non-psychoactive substance
  opioid F11.9Ø
    with
      disorder F11.99
        mood F11.94
        sleep F11.982
        specified type NEC F11.988
      intoxication F11.929
        with
          delirium F11.921
          perceptual disturbance F11.922
        uncomplicated F11.92Ø
      withdrawal F11.93
    harmful —*see* Abuse, drug, opioid
  patent medicines F19.9Ø
    harmful —*see* Abuse, non-psychoactive substance
  psychoactive drug NEC F19.9Ø
    with
      anxiety disorder F19.98Ø
      intoxication F19.929
        with
          delirium F19.921
          perceptual disturbance F19.922
        uncomplicated F19.92Ø
      mood disorder F19.94
      other specified disorder F19.988
      persisting
        amnestic disorder F19.96
        dementia F19.97
      psychosis F19.959
        delusions F19.95Ø
        hallucinations F19.951
      sexual dysfunction F19.981
      sleep disorder F19.982
      unspecified disorder F19.99
      withdrawal F19.939
        with
          delirium F19.931
          perceptual disturbance F19.932
        uncomplicated F19.93Ø
    harmful —*see* Abuse, drug NEC, psychoactive NEC

Use *(Continued)*
  sedative, hypnotic, or anxiolytic F13.9Ø
    with
      anxiety disorder F13.98Ø
      intoxication F13.929
        with
          delirium F13.921
        uncomplicated F13.92Ø
      other specified disorder F13.988
      persisting
        amnestic disorder F13.96
        dementia F13.97
      psychosis F13.959
        delusions F13.95Ø
        hallucinations F13.951
      sexual dysfunction F13.981
      sleep disorder F13.982
      unspecified disorder F13.99
    harmful —*see* Abuse, drug, sedative, hypnotic, or anxiolytic
  stimulant NEC F15.9Ø
    with
      anxiety disorder F15.98Ø
      intoxication F15.929
        with
          delirium F15.921
          perceptual disturbance F15.922
        uncomplicated F15.92Ø
      mood disorder F15.94
      other specified disorder F15.988
      psychosis F15.959
        delusions F15.95Ø
        hallucinations F15.951
      sexual dysfunction F15.981
      sleep disorder F15.982
      unspecified disorder F15.99
      withdrawal F15.93
    harmful —*see* Abuse, drug, stimulant NEC
  tobacco Z72.Ø
    with dependence —*see* Dependence, drug, nicotine
  volatile solvents —*see also* Use, inhalant F18.9Ø
    harmful —*see* Abuse, drug, inhalant
Usher-Senear disease or syndrome L1Ø.4
Uta B55.1
Uteromegaly N85.2
Uterovaginal —*see* condition
Uterovesical —*see* condition
Uveal —*see* condition
Uveitis (anterior) —*see also* Iridocyclitis
  acute —*see* Iridocyclitis, acute
  chronic —*see* Iridocyclitis, chronic
  due to toxoplasmosis (acquired) B58.Ø9
    congenital P37.1
  granulomatous —*see* Iridocyclitis, chronic
  heterochromic —*see* Cyclitis, Fuchs' heterochromic
  lens-induced —*see* Iridocyclitis, lens-induced
  posterior —*see* Chorioretinitis
  sympathetic H44.13-
  syphilitic (secondary) A51.43
    congenital (early) A5Ø.Ø1
    late A52.71
  tuberculous A18.54
Uveoencephalitis —*see* Inflammation, chorioretinal
Uveokeratitis —*see* Iridocyclitis
Uveoparotitis D86.89
Uvula —*see* condition
Uvulitis (acute) (catarrhal) (chronic) (membranous) (suppurative) (ulcerative) K12.2

U

◄ New ⟸ Revised ~~deleted~~ Deleted

V

Vaccination (prophylactic)
complication or reaction —*see* Complications, vaccination
delayed Z28.9
encounter for Z23
not done —*see* Immunization, not done, because (of)
Vaccinia (generalized) (localized) T88.1
without vaccination B08.011
congenital P35.8
Vacuum, in sinus (accessory) (nasal) J34.89
Vagabond, vagabondage Z59.0
Vagabond's disease B85.1
Vagina, vaginal —*see* condition
Vaginalitis (tunica) (testis) N49.1
Vaginismus (reflex) N94.2
functional F52.5
nonorganic F52.5
psychogenic F52.5
secondary N94.2
Vaginitis (acute) (circumscribed) (diffuse) (emphysematous) (nonvenereal) (ulcerative) N76.0
with ectopic or molar pregnancy O08.0
amebic A06.82
atrophic, postmenopausal N95.2
bacterial N76.0
blennorrhagic (gonococcal) A54.02
candidal B37.3
chlamydial A56.02
chronic N76.1
due to Trichomonas (vaginalis) A59.01
following ectopic or molar pregnancy O08.0
gonococcal A54.02
with abscess (accessory gland) (periurethral) A54.1
granuloma A58
in (due to)
candidiasis B37.3
herpesviral (herpes simplex) infection A60.04
pinworm infection B80 *[N77.1]*
monilial B37.3
mycotic (candidal) B37.3
postmenopausal atrophic N95.2
puerperal (postpartum) O86.13
senile (atrophic) N95.2
subacute or chronic N76.1
syphilitic (early) A51.0
late A52.76
trichomonal A59.01
tuberculous A18.18
Vaginosis —*see* Vaginitis
Vagotonia G52.2
Vagrancy Z59.0
VAIN —*see* Neoplasia, intraepithelial, vagina
Vallecula —*see* condition
Valley fever B38.0
Valsuani's disease —*see* Anemia, obstetric
Valve, valvular (formation) —*see also* condition
cerebral ventricle (communicating) in situ Z98.2
cervix, internal os Q51.828
congenital NEC —*see* Atresia, by site
ureter (pelvic junction) (vesical orifice) Q62.39
urethra (congenital) (posterior) Q64.2
Valvulitis (chronic) —*see* Endocarditis
Valvulopathy —*see* Endocarditis
Van Bogaert's leukoencephalopathy (sclerosing) (subacute) A81.1
Van Bogaert-Scherer-Epstein disease or syndrome E75.5
Van Buchem's syndrome M85.2
Van Creveld-von Gierke disease E74.01
Van der Hoeve (-de Kleyn) **syndrome** Q78.0
Van der Woude's syndrome Q38.0
Van Neck's disease or osteochondrosis M91.0
Vanishing lung J44.9
Vapor asphyxia or suffocation T59.9
specified agent —*see* Table of Drugs and Chemicals
Variance, lethal ball, prosthetic heart valve T82.09
Variants, thalassemic D56.8
Variations in hair color L67.1
Varicella B01.9
with
complications NEC B01.89
encephalitis B01.11
encephalomyelitis B01.11
meningitis B01.0
myelitis B01.12
pneumonia B01.2
congenital P35.8
Varices —*see* Varix
Varicocele (scrotum) (thrombosed) I86.1
ovary I86.2
perineum I86.3
spermatic cord (ulcerated) I86.1
Varicose
aneurysm (ruptured) I77.0
dermatitis —*see* Varix, leg, with, inflammation
eczema —*see* Varix, leg, with, inflammation
phlebitis —*see* Varix, with, inflammation
tumor —*see* Varix
ulcer (lower limb, any part) —*see also* Varix, leg, with, ulcer
anus —*see also* Hemorrhoids K64.8
esophagus —*see* Varix, esophagus
inflamed or infected —*see* Varix, leg, with ulcer, with inflammation
nasal septum I86.8
perineum I86.3
scrotum I86.1
specified site NEC I86.8
vein —*see* Varix
vessel —*see* Varix, leg
Varicosis, varicosities, varicosity —*see* Varix
Variola (major) (minor) B03
Varioloid B03
Varix (lower limb) (ruptured) I83.90
with
edema I83.899
inflammation I83.10
with ulcer (venous) I83.209
pain I83.819
specified complication NEC I83.899
stasis dermatitis I83.10
with ulcer (venous) I83.209
swelling I83.899
ulcer I83.009
with inflammation I83.209
aneurysmal I77.0
asymptomatic I83.9-
bladder I86.2
broad ligament I86.2
complicating
childbirth (lower extremity) O87.4
anus or rectum O87.2
genital (vagina, vulva or perineum) O87.8
pregnancy (lower extremity) O22.0-
anus or rectum O22.4-
genital (vagina, vulva or perineum) O22.1-
puerperium (lower extremity) O87.4
anus or rectum O87.2
genital (vagina, vulva, perineum) O87.8
congenital (any site) Q27.8
esophagus (idiopathic) (primary) (ulcerated) I85.00
bleeding I85.01
congenital Q27.8
in (due to)
alcoholic liver disease I85.10
bleeding I85.11
cirrhosis of liver I85.10
bleeding I85.11
Varix *(Continued)*
esophagus *(Continued)*
in *(Continued)*
portal hypertension I85.10
bleeding I85.11
schistosomiasis I85.10
bleeding I85.11
toxic liver disease I85.10
bleeding I85.11
secondary I85.10
bleeding I85.11
gastric I86.4
inflamed or infected I83.10
ulcerated I83.209
labia (majora) I86.3
leg (asymptomatic) I83.90
with
edema I83.899
inflammation I83.10
with ulcer —*see* Varix, leg, with, ulcer, with inflammation by site
pain I83.819
specified complication NEC I83.899
swelling I83.899
ulcer I83.009
with inflammation I83.209
ankle I83.003
with inflammation I83.203
calf I83.002
with inflammation I83.202
foot NEC I83.005
with inflammation I83.205
heel I83.004
with inflammation I83.204
lower leg NEC I83.008
with inflammation I83.208
midfoot I83.004
with inflammation I83.204
thigh I83.001
with inflammation I83.201
bilateral (asymptomatic) I83.93
with
edema I83.893
pain I83.813
specified complication NEC I83.893
swelling I83.893
ulcer I83.009
with inflammation I83.209
left (asymptomatic) I83.92
with
edema I83.892
inflammation I83.12
with ulcer —*see* Varix, leg, with, ulcer, with inflammation by site
pain I83.812
specified complication NEC I83.892
swelling I83.892
ulcer I83.029
with inflammation I83.229
ankle I83.023
with inflammation I83.223
calf I83.022
with inflammation I83.222
foot NEC I83.025
with inflammation I83.225
heel I83.024
with inflammation I83.224
lower leg NEC I83.028
with inflammation I83.228
midfoot I83.024
with inflammation I83.224
thigh I83.021
with inflammation I83.221
right (asymptomatic) I83.91
with
edema I83.891
inflammation I83.11
with ulcer —*see* Varix, leg, with, ulcer, with inflammation by site

V

- **Varix** *(Continued)*
  - leg *(Continued)*
    - right *(Continued)*
      - with *(Continued)*
        - pain I83.811
        - specified complication NEC I83.891
        - swelling I83.891
        - ulcer I83.Ø19
          - with inflammation I83.219
          - ankle I83.Ø13
            - with inflammation I83.213
          - calf I83.Ø12
            - with inflammation I83.212
          - foot NEC I83.Ø15
            - with inflammation I83.215
          - heel I83.Ø14
            - with inflammation I83.214
          - lower leg NEC I83.Ø18
            - with inflammation I83.218
          - midfoot I83.Ø14
            - with inflammation I83.214
          - thigh I83.Ø11
            - with inflammation I83.211
  - nasal septum I86.8
  - orbit I86.8
    - congenital Q27.8
  - ovary I86.2
  - papillary I78.1
  - pelvis I86.2
  - perineum I86.3
  - pharynx I86.8
  - placenta O43.89-
  - renal papilla I86.8
  - retina H35.Ø9
  - scrotum (ulcerated) I86.1
  - sigmoid colon I86.8
  - specified site NEC I86.8
  - spinal (cord) (vessels) I86.8
  - spleen, splenic (vein) (with phlebolith) I86.8
  - stomach I86.4
  - sublingual I86.Ø
  - ulcerated I83.ØØ9
    - inflamed or infected I83.2Ø9
  - uterine ligament I86.2
  - vagina I86.8
  - vocal cord I86.8
  - vulva I86.3
- **Vas deferens** —*see* condition
- **Vas deferentitis** N49.1
- **Vasa previa** O69.4
  - hemorrhage from, affecting newborn P5Ø.Ø
- **Vascular** —*see also* condition
  - loop on optic papilla Q14.2
  - spasm I73.9
  - spider I78.1
- **Vascularization, cornea** —*see* Neovascularization, cornea
- **Vasculitis** I77.6
  - allergic D69.Ø
  - cryoglobulinemic D89.1
  - disseminated I77.6
  - hypocomplementemic M31.8
  - kidney I77.89
  - livedoid L95.Ø
  - nodular L95.8
  - retina H35.Ø6-
  - rheumatic —*see* Fever, rheumatic
  - rheumatoid —*see* Rheumatoid, vasculitis
  - skin (limited to) L95.9
    - specified NEC L95.8
- **Vasculopathy, necrotizing** M31.9
  - cardiac allograft T86.29Ø
  - specified NEC M31.8
- **Vasitis** (nodosa) N49.1
  - tuberculous A18.15
- **Vasodilation** I73.9
- **Vasomotor** —*see* condition
- **Vasoplasty, after previous sterilization** Z31.Ø
  - aftercare Z31.42
- **Vasospasm** (vasoconstriction) I73.9
  - cerebral (cerebrovascular) (artery) I67.848
    - reversible I67.841
  - coronary I2Ø.1
  - nerve
    - arm —*see* Mononeuropathy, upper limb
    - brachial plexus G54.Ø
    - cervical plexus G54.2
    - leg —*see* Mononeuropathy, lower limb
  - peripheral NOS I73.9
  - retina (artery) —*see* Occlusion, artery, retina
- **Vasospastic** —*see* condition
- **Vasovagal attack** (paroxysmal) R55
  - psychogenic F45.8
- **VATER syndrome** Q87.2
- **Vater's ampulla** —*see* condition
- **Vegetation, vegetative**
  - adenoid (nasal fossa) J35.8
  - endocarditis (acute) (any valve) (subacute) I33.Ø
  - heart (mycotic) (valve) I33.Ø
- **Veil**
  - Jackson's Q43.3
- **Vein, venous** —*see* condition
- **Veldt sore** —*see* Ulcer, skin
- **Velpeau's hernia** —*see* Hernia, femoral
- **Venereal**
  - bubo A55
  - disease A64
  - granuloma inguinale A58
  - lymphogranuloma (Durand-Nicolas-Favre) A55
- **Venofibrosis** I87.8
- **Venom, venomous** —*see* Table of Drugs and Chemicals, by animal or substance, poisoning
- **Venous** —*see* condition
- **Ventilator lung, newborn** P27.8
- **Ventral** —*see* condition
- **Ventricle, ventricular** —*see also* condition
  - escape I49.3
  - inversion Q2Ø.5
- **Ventriculitis** (cerebral) —*see also* Encephalitis G04.90
- **Ventriculostomy status** Z98.2
- **Vernet's syndrome** G52.7
- **Verneuil's disease** (syphilitic bursitis) A52.78
- **Verruca** (due to HPV) (filiformis) (simplex) (viral) (vulgaris) BØ7.9
  - acuminata A63.Ø
  - necrogenica (primary) (tuberculosa) A18.4
  - plana BØ7.8
  - plantaris BØ7.Ø
  - seborrheica L82.1
    - inflamed L82.Ø
  - senile (seborrheic) L82.1
    - inflamed L82.Ø
  - tuberculosa (primary) A18.4
  - venereal A63.Ø
- **Verrucosities** —*see* Verruca
- **Verruga peruana, peruviana** A44.1
- **Version**
  - with extraction
  - cervix —*see* Malposition, uterus
  - uterus (postinfectional) (postpartal, old) —*see* Malposition, uterus
- **Vertebra, vertebral** —*see* condition
- **Vertical talus** (congenital) Q66.8Ø
  - left foot Q66.82
  - right foot Q66.81
- **Vertigo** R42
  - auditory —*see* Vertigo, aural
  - aural H81.31-
  - benign paroxysmal (positional) H81.1-
  - central (origin) H81.4-
  - cerebral H81.4-
  - Dix and Hallpike (epidemic) —*see* Neuronitis, vestibular
  - due to infrasound T75.23
- **Vertigo** *(Continued)*
  - epidemic A88.1
    - Dix and Hallpike —*see* Neuronitis, vestibular
    - Pedersen's —*see* Neuronitis, vestibular
    - vestibular neuronitis —*see* Neuronitis, vestibular
  - hysterical F44.89
  - infrasound T75.23
  - labyrinthine —*see* subcategory H81.Ø
  - laryngeal RØ5
  - malignant positional H81.4-
  - Ménière's —*see* subcategory H81.4Ø
  - menopausal N95.11
  - otogenic —*see* Vertigo, aural
  - paroxysmal positional, benign —*see* Vertigo, benign paroxysmal
  - Pedersen's (epidemic) —*see* Neuronitis, vestibular
  - peripheral NEC H81.39-
  - positional
    - benign paroxysmal —*see* Vertigo, benign paroxysmal
    - malignant H81.4-
- **Very-low-density-lipoprotein-type** (VLDL) **hyperlipoproteinemia** E78.1
- **Vesania** —*see* Psychosis
- **Vesical** —*see* condition
- **Vesicle**
  - cutaneous R23.8
  - seminal —*see* condition
  - skin R23.8
- **Vesicocolic** —*see* condition
- **Vesicoperineal** —*see* condition
- **Vesicorectal** —*see* condition
- **Vesicourethrorectal** —*see* condition
- **Vesicovaginal** —*see* condition
- **Vesicular** —*see* condition
- **Vesiculitis** (seminal) N49.Ø
  - amebic AØ6.82
  - gonorrheal (acute) (chronic) A54.23
  - trichomonal A59.Ø9
  - tuberculous A18.15
- **Vestibulitis** (ear) —*see also* subcategory H83.Ø
  - nose (external) J34.89
  - vulvar N94.81Ø
- **Vestibulopathy, acute peripheral** (recurrent) —*see* Neuronitis, vestibular
- **Vestige, vestigial** —*see also* Persistence
  - branchial Q18.Ø
  - structures in vitreous Q14.Ø
- **Vibration**
  - adverse effects T75.2Ø
    - pneumatic hammer syndrome T75.21
    - specified effect NEC T75.29
    - vasospastic syndrome T75.22
    - vertigo from infrasound T75.23
  - exposure (occupational) Z57.7
  - vertigo T75.23
- **Vibriosis** A28.9
- **Victim** (of)
  - crime Z65.4
  - disaster Z65.5
  - terrorism Z65.4
  - torture Z65.4
  - war Z65.5
- **Vidal's disease** L28.Ø
- **Villaret's syndrome** G52.7
- **Villous** —*see* condition
- **VIN** —*see* Neoplasia, intraepithelial, vulva
- **Vincent's infection** (angina) (gingivitis) A69.1
  - stomatitis NEC A69.1
- **Vinson-Plummer syndrome** D5Ø.1
- **Violence, physical** R45.6
- **Viosterol deficiency** —*see* Deficiency, calciferol
- **Vipoma** —*see* Neoplasm, malignant, by site
- **Viremia** B34.9
- **Virilism** (adrenal) E25.9
  - congenital E25.Ø
- **Virilization** (female) (suprarenal) E25.9
  - congenital E25.Ø
  - isosexual E28.2

- **Virulent bubo** A57
- **Virus, viral** —*see also* condition
  - as cause of disease classified elsewhere B97.89
  - cytomegalovirus B25.9
  - human immunodeficiency (HIV) —*see* Human, immunodeficiency virus (HIV) disease
  - infection —*see* Infection, virus
  - specified NEC B34.8
  - ~~swine influenza (viruses that normally cause infections in pigs) (see also Influenza, due to, identified novel influenza A virus) J09.X2~~
  - swine influenza (viruses that normally cause infections in pigs) —*see also* Influenza, due to, identified novel influenza A virus J09.X2 ◀
  - West Nile (fever) A92.30
    - with
      - complications NEC A92.39
      - cranial nerve disorders A92.32
      - encephalitis A92.31
      - encephalomyelitis A92.31
      - neurologic manifestation NEC A92.32
      - optic neuritis A92.32
      - polyradiculitis A92.32
- **Viscera, visceral** —*see* condition
- **Visceroptosis** K63.4
- **Visible peristalsis** R19.2
- **Vision, visual**
  - binocular, suppression H53.34
  - blurred, blurring H53.8
    - hysterical F44.6
  - defect, defective NEC H54.7
  - disorientation (syndrome) H53.8
  - disturbance H53.9
    - hysterical F44.6
  - double H53.2
  - examination Z01.00
    - with abnormal findings Z01.01
  - field, limitation (defect) —*see* Defect, visual field
  - hallucinations R44.1
  - halos H53.19
  - loss —*see* Loss, vision
    - sudden —*see* Disturbance, vision, subjective, loss, sudden
  - low (both eyes) —*see* Low, vision
  - perception, simultaneous without fusion H53.33
- **Vitality, lack or want of** R53.83
  - newborn P96.89
- **Vitamin deficiency** —*see* Deficiency, vitamin
- **Vitelline duct, persistent** Q43.0
- **Vitiligo** L80
  - eyelid H02.739
    - left H02.736
      - lower H02.735
      - upper H02.734

- **Vitiligo** *(Continued)*
  - eyelid *(Continued)*
    - right H02.733
      - lower H02.732
      - upper H02.731
  - pinta A67.2
  - vulva N90.89
- **Vitreal corneal syndrome** H59.01-
- **Vitreoretinopathy, proliferative** —*see also* Retinopathy, proliferative
  - with retinal detachment —*see* Detachment, retina, traction
- **Vitreous** —*see also* condition
  - touch syndrome —*see* Complication, postprocedural, following cataract surgery
- **Vocal cord** —*see* condition
- **Vogt-Koyanagi syndrome** H20.82-
- **Vogt's disease or syndrome** G80.3
- **Vogt-Spielmeyer amaurotic idiocy or disease** E75.4
- **Voice**
  - change R49.9
    - specified NEC R49.8
  - loss —*see* Aphonia
- **Volhynian fever** A79.0
- **Volkmann's ischemic contracture or paralysis** (complicating trauma) T79.6
- **Volvulus** (bowel) (colon) (intestine) K56.2 ⬅
  - with perforation K56.2
  - congenital Q43.8
  - duodenum K31.5 ◀
  - fallopian tube —*see* Torsion, fallopian tube
  - oviduct —*see* Torsion, fallopian tube
  - stomach (due to absence of gastrocolic ligament) K31.89
- **Vomiting** R11.10
  - with nausea R11.2
  - without nausea R11.11
  - asphyxia —*see* Foreign body, by site, causing asphyxia, gastric contents
  - bilious (cause unknown) R11.14
    - following gastro-intestinal surgery K91.0
    - in newborn P92.01
  - blood —*see* Hematemesis
  - causing asphyxia, choking, or suffocation —*see* Foreign body, by site
  - cyclical G43.A0
    - with refractory migraine G43.A1
    - intractable G43.A1
    - not intractable G43.A0
    - psychogenic F50.89 ⬅
    - without refractory migraine G43.A0
  - fecal mater R11.13
  - following gastrointestinal surgery K91.0
    - psychogenic F50.89 ⬅

- **Vomiting** *(Continued)*
  - functional K31.89
  - hysterical F50.89 ⬅
  - nervous F50.89 ⬅
  - neurotic F50.89 ⬅
  - newborn NEC P92.09
    - bilious P92.01
  - periodic R11.10
    - psychogenic F50.89 ⬅
  - projectile R11.12
  - psychogenic F50.89 ⬅
  - uremic —*see* Uremia
- **Vomito negro** —*see* Fever, yellow
- **Von Bezold's abscess** —*see* Mastoiditis, acute
- **Von Economo-Cruchet disease** A85.8
- **Von Eulenburg's disease** G71.19
- **Von Gierke's disease** E74.01
- **Von Hippel** (-Lindau) **disease or syndrome** Q85.8
- **Von Jaksch's anemia or disease** D64.89
- **Von Recklinghausen**
  - disease (neurofibromatosis) Q85.01
    - bones E21.0
- **Von Schroetter's syndrome** I82.890
- **Von Willebrand** (-Jurgens)(-Minot) **disease or syndrome** D68.0
- **Von Zumbusch's disease** L40.1
- **Voyeurism** F65.3
- **Vrolik's disease** Q78.0
- **Vulva** —*see* condition
- **Vulvismus** N94.2
- **Vulvitis** (acute) (allergic) (atrophic) (hypertrophic) (intertriginous) (senile) N76.2
  - with ectopic or molar pregnancy O08.0
  - adhesive, congenital Q52.79
  - blennorrhagic (gonococcal) A54.02
  - candidal B37.3
  - chlamydial A56.02
  - due to Haemophilus ducreyi A57
  - following ectopic or molar pregnancy O08.0
  - gonococcal A54.02
    - with abscess (accessory gland) (periurethral) A54.1
  - herpesviral A60.04
  - leukoplakic N90.4
  - monilial B37.3
  - puerperal (postpartum) O86.19
  - subacute or chronic N76.3
  - syphilitic (early) A51.0
    - late A52.76
  - trichomonal A59.01
  - tuberculous A18.18
- **Vulvodynia** N94.819
  - specified NEC N94.818
- **Vulvorectal** —*see* condition
- **Vulvovaginitis** (acute) —*see* Vaginitis

V

W

Waiting list, person on Z75.1
  for organ transplant Z76.82
  undergoing social agency investigation Z75.2
Waldenström
  hypergammaglobulinemia D89.0
  syndrome or macroglobulinemia C88.0
Waldenström-Kjellberg syndrome D50.1
Walking
  difficulty R26.2
    psychogenic F44.4
  sleep F51.3
    hysterical F44.89
Wall, abdominal —*see* condition
Wallenberg's disease or syndrome G46.3
Wallgren's disease I87.8
Wandering
  gallbladder, congenital Q44.1
  in diseases classified elsewhere Z91.83
  kidney, congenital Q63.8
  organ or site, congenital NEC —*see* Malposition, congenital, by site
  pacemaker (heart) I49.8
  spleen D73.89
War neurosis F48.8
Wart (due to HPV) (filiform) (infectious) (viral) B07.9
  anogenital region (venereal) A63.0
  common B07.8
  external genital organs (venereal) A63.0
  flat B07.8
  Hassal-Henle's (of cornea) H18.49
  Peruvian A44.1
  plantar B07.0
  prosector (tuberculous) A18.4
  seborrheic L82.1
    inflamed L82.0
  senile (seborrheic) L82.1
    inflamed L82.0
  tuberculous A18.4
  venereal A63.0
Warthin's tumor —*see* Neoplasm, salivary gland, benign
Wassilieff's disease A27.0
Wasting
  disease R64
    due to malnutrition E41
  extreme (due to malnutrition) E41
  muscle NEC —*see* Atrophy, muscle
Water
  clefts (senile cataract) —*see* Cataract, senile, incipient
  deprivation of T73.1
  intoxication E87.79
  itch B76.9
  lack of T73.1
  loading E87.70
  on
    brain —*see* Hydrocephalus
    chest J94.8
  poisoning E87.79
Waterbrash R12
Waterhouse(-Friderichsen) **syndrome or disease** (meningococcal) A39.1
Water-losing nephritis N25.89
Watermelon stomach K31.819
  with hemorrhage K31.811
  without hemorrhage K31.819
Watsoniasis B66.8
Wax in ear —*see* Impaction, cerumen
Weak, weakening, weakness (generalized) R53.1
  arches (acquired) —*see also* Deformity, limb, flat foot
  bladder (sphincter) R32
  facial R29.810
    following
      cerebrovascular disease I69.992
        cerebral infarction I69.392
        intracerebral hemorrhage I69.192
Weak, weakening, weakness *(Continued)*
  facial *(Continued)*
    following *(Continued)*
      cerebrovascular disease *(Continued)*
        nontraumatic intracranial hemorrhage NEC I69.292
        specified disease NEC I69.892
        stroke I69.392
        subarachnoid hemorrhage I69.092
  foot (double) —*see* Weak, arches
  heart, cardiac —*see* Failure, heart
  mind F70
  muscle M62.81
  myocardium —*see* Failure, heart
  newborn P96.89
  pelvic fundus N81.89
  pubocervical tissue N81.82
  rectovaginal tissue N81.83
  senile R54
  urinary stream R39.12
  valvular —*see* Endocarditis
Wear, worn (with normal or routine use)
  articular bearing surface of internal joint prosthesis —*see* Complications, joint prosthesis, mechanical, wear of articular bearing surfaces, by site
  device, implant or graft —*see* Complications, by site, mechanical complication
  tooth, teeth (approximal) (hard tissues) (interproximal) (occlusal) K03.0
Weather, weathered
  effects of
    cold T69.9
      specified effect NEC T69.8
    hot —*see* Heat
  skin L57.8
Weaver's syndrome Q87.3
Web, webbed (congenital)
  duodenal Q43.8
  esophagus Q39.4
  fingers Q70.1
  larynx (glottic) (subglottic) Q31.0
  neck (pterygium colli) Q18.3
  Paterson-Kelly D50.1
  popliteal syndrome Q87.89
  toes Q70.3
Weber-Christian disease M35.6
Weber-Cockayne syndrome (epidermolysis bullosa) Q81.8
Weber-Gubler syndrome G46.3
Weber-Leyden syndrome G46.3
Weber-Osler syndrome I78.0
Weber's paralysis or syndrome G46.3
Wedge-shaped or wedging vertebra —*see* Collapse, vertebra NEC
Wegener's granulomatosis or syndrome M31.30
  with
    kidney involvement M31.31
    lung involvement M31.30
      with kidney involvement M31.31
Wegner's disease A50.02
Weight
  1000-2499 grams at birth (low) —*see* Low, birthweight
  999 grams or less at birth (extremely low) —*see* Low, birthweight, extreme
  and length below 10th percentile for gestational age P05.1- ◀
  below but length above 10th percentile for gestational age P05.0- ◀
  gain (abnormal) (excessive) R63.5
    in pregnancy —*see* Pregnancy, complicated by, excessive weight gain
      low —*see* Pregnancy, complicated by, insufficient, weight gain
  loss (abnormal) (cause unknown) R63.4
Weightlessness (effect of) T75.82
Weil (l)-Marchesani syndrome Q87.1
Weil's disease A27.0
Weingarten's syndrome J82
Weir Mitchell's disease I73.81
Weiss-Baker syndrome G90.09
Wells' disease L98.3
Wen —*see* Cyst, sebaceous
Wenckebach's block or phenomenon I44.1
Werdnig-Hoffmann syndrome (muscular atrophy) G12.0
Werlhof's disease D69.3
Werner-His disease A79.0
Wermer's disease or syndrome E31.21
Werner's disease or syndrome E34.8
Wernicke-Korsakoff's syndrome or psychosis (alcoholic) F10.96
  with dependence F10.26
  drug-induced
    due to drug abuse —*see* Abuse, drug, by type, with amnestic disorder
    due to drug dependence —*see* Dependence, drug, by type, with amnestic disorder
  nonalcoholic F04
Wernicke-Posadas disease B38.9
Wernicke's
  developmental aphasia F80.2
  disease or syndrome E51.2
  encephalopathy E51.2
  polioencephalitis, superior E51.2
West African fever B50.8
Westphal-Strümpell syndrome E83.01
West's syndrome —*see* Epilepsy, spasms
Wet
  feet, tropical (maceration) (syndrome) —*see* Immersion, foot
  lung (syndrome), newborn P22.1
Wharton's duct —*see* condition
Wheal —*see* Urticaria
Wheezing R06.2
Whiplash injury S13.4
Whipple's disease —*see also* subcategory M14.8- K90.81
Whipworm (disease) (infection) (infestation) B79
Whistling face Q87.0
White —*see also* condition
  kidney, small N03.9
  leg, puerperal, postpartum, childbirth O87.1
  mouth B37.0
  patches of mouth K13.29
  spot lesions, teeth
    chewing surface K02.51
    pit and fissure surface K02.51
    smooth surface K02.61
Whitehead L70.0
Whitlow —*see also* Cellulitis, digit
  with lymphangitis —*see* Lymphangitis, acute, digit
  herpesviral B00.89
Whitmore's disease or fever —*see* Melioidosis
Whooping cough A37.90
  with pneumonia A37.91
    due to Bordetella
      bronchiseptica A37.81
      parapertussis A37.11
      pertussis A37.01
    specified organism NEC A37.81
  due to
    Bordetella
      bronchiseptica A37.80
        with pneumonia A37.81
      parapertussis A37.10
        with pneumonia A37.11
      pertussis A37.00
        with pneumonia A37.01
      specified NEC A37.80
        with pneumonia A37.81
Wichman's asthma J38.5
Wide cranial sutures, newborn P96.3
Widening aorta —*see* Ectasia, aorta
  with aneurysm —*see* Aneurysm, aorta
Wilkie's disease or syndrome K55.1
Wilkinson-Sneddon disease or syndrome L13.1

W

Willebrand (-Jürgens) thrombopathy D68.Ø
Willige-Hunt disease or syndrome G23.1
Wilms' tumor C64-
Wilson-Mikity syndrome P27.Ø
Wilson's
  disease or syndrome E83.Ø1
  hepatolenticular degeneration E83.Ø1
  lichen ruber L43.9
Window —*see also* Imperfect, closure
  aorticopulmonary Q21.4
Winter —*see* condition
Wiskott-Aldrich syndrome D82.Ø
Withdrawal state —*see also* Dependence, drug by type, with withdrawal
  alcohol ◄
    with perceptual disturbances F1Ø.232 ◄
    without perceptual disturbances F1Ø.239 ◄
  caffeine F15.93 ◄
  cannabis F12.288 ◄
  newborn
    correct therapeutic substance properly administered P96.2
    infant of dependent mother P96.1
  therapeutic substance, neonatal P96.2
Witts' anemia D5Ø.8
Witzelsucht FØ7.Ø
Woakes' ethmoiditis or syndrome J33.1
Wolff-Hirschorn syndrome Q93.3
Wolff-Parkinson-White syndrome I45.6
Wolhynian fever A79.Ø
Wolman's disease E75.5
Wood lung or pneumonitis J67.8
Woolly, wooly hair (congenital) (nevus) Q84.1
Woolsorter's disease A22.1
Word
  blindness (congenital) (developmental) F81.Ø
  deafness (congenital) (developmental) H93.25
Worm (s) (infection) (infestation) —*see also* Infestation, helminth
  guinea B72
  in intestine NEC B82.Ø
Worm-eaten soles A66.3
Worn out —*see* Exhaustion
  cardiac
    defibrillator (with synchronous cardiac pacemaker) Z45.Ø2
    pacemaker
      battery Z45.Ø1Ø
      lead Z45.Ø18
  device, implant or graft —*see* Complications, by site, mechanical
Worried well Z71.1
Worries R45.82
Wound, open
  abdomen, abdominal
    wall S31.1Ø9
      with penetration into peritoneal cavity S31.6Ø9
      bite —*see* Bite, abdomen, wall
      epigastric region S31.1Ø2
        with penetration into peritoneal cavity S31.6Ø2
        bite —*see* Bite, abdomen, wall, epigastric region
        laceration —*see* Laceration, abdomen, wall, epigastric region
        puncture —*see* Puncture, abdomen, wall, epigastric region
      laceration —*see* Laceration, abdomen, wall
      left
        lower quadrant S31.1Ø4
          with penetration into peritoneal cavity S31.6Ø4
          bite —*see* Bite, abdomen, wall, left, lower quadrant
          laceration —*see* Laceration, abdomen, wall, left, lower quadrant
          puncture —*see* Puncture, abdomen, wall, left, lower quadrant

Wound, open *(Continued)*
  abdomen, abdominal *(Continued)*
    wall *(Continued)*
      left *(Continued)*
        upper quadrant S31.1Ø1
          with penetration into peritoneal cavity S31.6Ø1
          bite —*see* Bite, abdomen, wall, left, upper quadrant
          laceration —*see* Laceration, abdomen, wall, left, upper quadrant
          puncture —*see* Puncture, abdomen, wall, left, upper quadrant
      periumbilic region S31.1Ø5
        with penetration into peritoneal cavity S31.6Ø5
        bite —*see* Bite, abdomen, wall, periumbilic region
        laceration —*see* Laceration, abdomen, wall, periumbilic region
        puncture —*see* Puncture, abdomen, wall, periumbilic region
      puncture —*see* Puncture, abdomen, wall
      right
        lower quadrant S31.1Ø3
          with penetration into peritoneal cavity S31.6Ø3
          bite —*see* Bite, abdomen, wall, right, lower quadrant
          laceration —*see* Laceration, abdomen, wall, right, lower quadrant
          puncture —*see* Puncture, abdomen, wall, right, lower quadrant
        upper quadrant S31.1ØØ
          with penetration into peritoneal cavity S31.6ØØ
          bite —*see* Bite, abdomen, wall, right, upper quadrant
          laceration —*see* Laceration, abdomen, wall, right, upper quadrant
          puncture —*see* Puncture, abdomen, wall, right, upper quadrant
  alveolar (process) —*see* Wound, open, oral cavity
  ankle S91.ØØ-
    bite —*see* Bite, ankle
    laceration —*see* Laceration, ankle
    puncture —*see* Puncture, ankle
  antecubital space —*see* Wound, open, elbow
  anterior chamber, eye —*see* Wound, open, ocular
  anus S31.839
    bite S31.835
    laceration —*see* Laceration, anus
    puncture —*see* Puncture, anus
  arm (upper) S41.1Ø-
    with amputation —*see* Amputation, traumatic, arm
    bite —*see* Bite, arm
    forearm —*see* Wound, open, forearm
    laceration —*see* Laceration, arm
    puncture —*see* Puncture, arm
  auditory canal (external) (meatus) —*see* Wound, open, ear
  auricle, ear —*see* Wound, open, ear
  axilla —*see* Wound, open, arm
  back —*see also* Wound, open, thorax, back
    lower S31.ØØØ
      with penetration into retroperitoneal space S31.ØØ1
      bite —*see* Bite, back, lower
      laceration —*see* Laceration, back, lower
      puncture —*see* Puncture, back, lower
  bite —*see* Bite
  blood vessel —*see* Injury, blood vessel
  breast S21.ØØ-
    with amputation —*see* Amputation, traumatic, breast

Wound, open *(Continued)*
  breast *(Continued)*
    bite —*see* Bite, breast
    laceration —*see* Laceration, breast
    puncture —*see* Puncture, breast
  buttock S31.8Ø9
    bite —*see* Bite, buttock
    laceration —*see* Laceration, buttock
    left S31.829
    puncture —*see* Puncture, buttock
    right S31.819
  calf —*see* Wound, open, leg
  canaliculus lacrimalis —*see* Wound, open, eyelid
  canthus, eye —*see* Wound, open, eyelid
  cervical esophagus S11.2Ø
    bite S11.25
    laceration —*see* Laceration, esophagus, traumatic, cervical
    puncture —*see* Puncture, cervical esophagus
  cheek (external) SØ1.4Ø-
    bite —*see* Bite, cheek
    internal —*see* Wound, open, oral cavity
    laceration —*see* Laceration, cheek
    puncture —*see* Puncture, cheek
  chest wall —*see* Wound, open, thorax
  chin —*see* Wound, open, head, specified site NEC
  choroid —*see* Wound, open, ocular
  ciliary body (eye) —*see* Wound, open, ocular
  clitoris S31.4Ø
    with amputation —*see* Amputation, traumatic, clitoris
    bite S31.45
    laceration —*see* Laceration, vulva
    puncture —*see* Puncture, vulva
  conjunctiva —*see* Wound, open, ocular
  cornea —*see* Wound, open, ocular
  costal region —*see* Wound, open, thorax
  Descemet's membrane —*see* Wound, open, ocular
  digit (s)
    foot —*see* Wound, open, toe
    hand —*see* Wound, open, finger
  ear (canal) (external) SØ1.3Ø-
    with amputation —*see* Amputation, traumatic, ear
    bite —*see* Bite, ear
    drum SØ9.2-
    laceration —*see* Laceration, ear
    puncture —*see* Puncture, ear
  elbow S51.ØØ-
    bite —*see* Bite, elbow
    laceration —*see* Laceration, elbow
    puncture —*see* Puncture, elbow
  epididymis —*see* Wound, open, testis
  epigastric region S31.1Ø2
    with penetration into peritoneal cavity S31.6Ø2
    bite —*see* Bite, abdomen, wall, epigastric region
    laceration —*see* Laceration, abdomen, wall, epigastric region
    puncture —*see* Puncture, abdomen, wall, epigastric region
  epiglottis —*see* Wound, open, neck, specified site NEC
  esophagus (thoracic) S27.819
    cervical —*see* Wound, open, cervical esophagus
    laceration S27.813
    specified type NEC S27.818
  eye —*see* Wound, open, ocular
  eyeball —*see* Wound, open, ocular
  eyebrow —*see* Wound, open, eyelid
  eyelid SØ1.1Ø-
    bite —*see* Bite, eyelid
    laceration —*see* Laceration, eyelid
    puncture —*see* Puncture, eyelid
  face NEC —*see* Wound, open, head, specified site NEC

W

Wound, open *(Continued)*
  finger (s) S61.209
    with
      amputation —*see* Amputation, traumatic, finger
      damage to nail S61.309
    bite —*see* Bite, finger
    index S61.208
      with
        damage to nail S61.308
      left S61.201
        with
          damage to nail S61.301
      right S61.200
        with
          damage to nail S61.300
    laceration —*see* Laceration, finger
    little S61.208
      with
        damage to nail S61.308
      left S61.207
        with damage to nail S61.307
      right S61.206
        with damage to nail S61.306
    middle S61.208
      with
        damage to nail S61.308
      left S61.203
        with damage to nail S61.303
      right S61.202
        with damage to nail S61.302
    puncture —*see* Puncture, finger
    ring S61.208
      with
        damage to nail S61.308
      left S61.205
        with damage to nail S61.305
      right S61.204
        with damage to nail S61.304
  flank —*see* Wound, open, abdomen, wall
  foot (except toe (s) alone) S91.30-
    with amputation —*see* Amputation, traumatic, foot
    bite —*see* Bite, foot
    laceration —*see* Laceration, foot
    puncture —*see* Puncture, foot
    toe —*see* Wound, open, toe
  forearm S51.80-
    with
      amputation —*see* Amputation, traumatic, forearm
    bite —*see* Bite, forearm
    elbow only —*see* Wound, open, elbow
    laceration —*see* Laceration, forearm
    puncture —*see* Puncture, forearm
  forehead —*see* Wound, open, head, specified site NEC
  genital organs, external
    with amputation —*see* Amputation, traumatic, genital organs
    bite —*see* Bite, genital organ
    female S31.502
      vagina S31.40
      vulva S31.40
    laceration —*see* Laceration, genital organ
    male S31.501
      penis S31.20
      scrotum S31.30
      testes S31.30
    puncture —*see* Puncture, genital organ
  globe (eye) —*see* Wound, open, ocular
  groin —*see* Wound, open, abdomen, wall
  gum —*see* Wound, open, oral cavity
  hand S61.40-
    with
      amputation —*see* Amputation, traumatic, hand
    bite —*see* Bite, hand
    finger (s) —*see* Wound, open, finger
    laceration —*see* Laceration, hand

Wound, open *(Continued)*
  hand *(Continued)*
    puncture —*see* Puncture, hand
    thumb —*see* Wound, open, thumb
  head S01.90
    bite —*see* Bite, head
    cheek —*see* Wound, open, cheek
    ear —*see* Wound, open, ear
    eyelid —*see* Wound, open, eyelid
    laceration —*see* Laceration, head
    lip —*see* Wound, open, lip
    nose S01.20
    oral cavity —*see* Wound, open, oral cavity
    puncture —*see* Puncture, head
    scalp —*see* Wound, open, scalp
    specified site NEC S01.80
    temporomandibular area —*see* Wound, open, cheek
  heel —*see* Wound, open, foot
  hip S71.00-
    with amputation —*see* Amputation, traumatic, hip
    bite —*see* Bite, hip
    laceration —*see* Laceration, hip
    puncture —*see* Puncture, hip
  hymen S31.40
    bite —*see* Bite, vulva
    laceration —*see* Laceration, vagina
    puncture —*see* Puncture, vagina
  hypochondrium S31.109
    bite —*see* Bite, hypochondrium
    laceration —*see* Laceration, hypochondrium
    puncture —*see* Puncture, hypochondrium
  hypogastric region S31.109
    bite —*see* Bite, hypogastric region
    laceration —*see* Laceration, hypogastric region
    puncture —*see* Puncture, hypogastric region
  iliac (region) —*see* Wound, open, inguinal region
  inguinal region S31.109
    bite —*see* Bite, abdomen, wall, lower quadrant
    laceration —*see* Laceration, inguinal region
    puncture —*see* Puncture, inguinal region
  instep —*see* Wound, open, foot
  interscapular region —*see* Wound, open, thorax, back
  intraocular —*see* Wound, open, ocular
  iris —*see* Wound, open, ocular
  jaw —*see* Wound, open, head, specified site NEC
  knee S81.00-
    bite —*see* Bite, knee
    laceration —*see* Laceration, knee
    puncture —*see* Puncture, knee
  labium (majus) (minus) —*see* Wound, open, vulva
  laceration —*see* Laceration, by site
  lacrimal duct —*see* Wound, open, eyelid
  larynx S11.019
    bite —*see* Bite, larynx
    laceration —*see* Laceration, larynx
    puncture —*see* Puncture, larynx
  left
    lower quadrant S31.104
      with penetration into peritoneal cavity S31.604
      bite —*see* Bite, abdomen, wall, left, lower quadrant
      laceration —*see* Laceration, abdomen, wall, left, lower quadrant
      puncture —*see* Puncture, abdomen, wall, left, lower quadrant
    upper quadrant S31.101
      with penetration into peritoneal cavity S31.601
      bite —*see* Bite, abdomen, wall, left, upper quadrant

Wound, open *(Continued)*
  left *(Continued)*
    upper quadrant *(Continued)*
      laceration —*see* Laceration, abdomen, wall, left, upper quadrant
      puncture —*see* Puncture, abdomen, wall, left, upper quadrant
  leg (lower) S81.80-
    with amputation —*see* Amputation, traumatic, leg
    ankle —*see* Wound, open, ankle
    bite —*see* Bite, leg
    foot —*see* Wound, open, foot
    knee —*see* Wound, open, knee
    laceration —*see* Laceration, leg
    puncture —*see* Puncture, leg
    toe —*see* Wound, open, toe
    upper —*see* Wound, open, thigh
  lip S01.501
    bite —*see* Bite, lip
    laceration —*see* Laceration, lip
    puncture —*see* Puncture, lip
  loin S31.109
    bite —*see* Bite, abdomen, wall
    laceration —*see* Laceration, loin
    puncture —*see* Puncture, loin
  lower back —*see* Wound, open, back, lower
  lumbar region —*see* Wound, open, back, lower
  malar region —*see* Wound, open, head, specified site NEC
  mammary —*see* Wound, open, breast
  mastoid region —*see* Wound, open, head, specified site NEC
  mouth —*see* Wound, open, oral cavity
  nail
    finger —*see* Wound, open, finger, with damage to nail
    toe —*see* Wound, open, toe, with damage to nail
  nape (neck) —*see* Wound, open, neck
  nasal (septum) (sinus) —*see* Wound, open, nose
  nasopharynx —*see* Wound, open, head, specified site NEC
  neck S11.90
    bite —*see* Bite, neck
    involving
      cervical esophagus S11.20
      larynx —*see* Wound, open, larynx
      pharynx S11.20
      thyroid S11.10
      trachea (cervical) S11.029
        bite —*see* Bite, trachea
        laceration S11.021
          with foreign body S11.022
        puncture S11.023
          with foreign body S11.024
    laceration —*see* Laceration, neck
    puncture —*see* Puncture, neck
    specified site NEC S11.80
      specified type NEC S11.89
  nose (septum) (sinus) S01.20
    with amputation —*see* Amputation, traumatic, nose
    bite —*see* Bite, nose
    laceration —*see* Laceration, nose
    puncture —*see* Puncture, nose
  ocular S05.90
    avulsion (traumatic enucleation) S05.7-
    eyeball S05.6-
      with foreign body S05.5-
    eyelid —*see* Wound, open, eyelid
    laceration and rupture S05.3-
      with prolapse or loss of intraocular tissue S05.2-
    orbit (penetrating) (with or without foreign body) S05.4-
    periocular area —*see* Wound, open, eyelid
    specified NEC S05.8X-

W

X

Xanthelasma (eyelid) (palpebrarum) H02.60
- left H02.66
  - lower H02.65
  - upper H02.64
- right H02.63
  - lower H02.62
  - upper H02.61

Xanthelasmatosis (essential) E78.2
Xanthinuria, hereditary E79.8
Xanthoastrocytoma
- specified site —*see* Neoplasm, malignant, by site
- unspecified site C71.9

Xanthofibroma —*see* Neoplasm, connective tissue, benign
Xanthogranuloma D76.3
Xanthoma (s), **xanthomatosis** (primary) (familial) (hereditary) E75.5
- with
  - hyperlipoproteinemia
    - Type I E78.3
    - Type III E78.2
    - Type IV E78.1
    - Type V E78.3
- bone (generalisata) C96.5
- cerebrotendinous E75.5
- cutaneotendinous E75.5

Xanthoma (s), **xanthomatosis** *(Continued)*
- disseminatum (skin) E78.2
- eruptive E78.2
- hypercholesterinemic E78.00 ⬅
- hypercholesterolemic E78.00 ⬅
- hyperlipidemic E78.5
- joint E75.5
- multiple (skin) E78.2
- tendon (sheath) E75.5
- tuberosum E78.2
- tuberous E78.2
- tubo-eruptive E78.2
- verrucous, oral mucosa K13.4

Xanthosis R23.8
Xenophobia F40.10
Xeroderma —*see also* Ichthyosis
- acquired L85.0
  - eyelid H01.149
    - left H01.146
      - lower H01.145
      - upper H01.144
    - right H01.143
      - lower H01.142
      - upper H01.141
- pigmentosum Q82.1
- vitamin A deficiency E50.8

Xerophthalmia (vitamin A deficiency) E50.7
- unrelated to vitamin A deficiency —*see* Keratoconjunctivitis

Xerosis
- conjunctiva H11.14-
  - with Bitot's spots —*see also* Pigmentation, conjunctiva
    - vitamin A deficiency E50.1
  - vitamin A deficiency E50.0
- cornea H18.89-
  - with ulceration —*see* Ulcer, cornea
    - vitamin A deficiency E50.3
  - vitamin A deficiency E50.2
- cutis L85.3
- skin L85.3

Xerostomia K11.7
Xiphopagus Q89.4
XO syndrome Q96.9
X-ray (of)
- abnormal findings —*see* Abnormal, diagnostic imaging
- breast (mammogram) (routine) Z12.31
- chest
  - routine (as part of a general medical examination) Z00.00
    - with abnormal findings Z00.01
- routine (as part of a general medical examination) Z00.00
  - with abnormal findings Z00.01

XXXXY syndrome Q98.1
XXY syndrome Q98.0

Y

Yaba pox virus disease B08.72
Yatapoxvirus B08.70
  specified NEC B08.79
Yawning R06.89
  psychogenic F45.8
Yaws A66.9
  bone lesions A66.6
  butter A66.1
  chancre A66.0
  cutaneous, less than five years after infection A66.2
  early (cutaneous) (macular) (maculopapular) (micropapular) (papular) A66.2
    frambeside A66.2
    skin lesions NEC A66.2
  eyelid A66.2
  ganglion A66.6
  gangosis, gangosa A66.5
  gumma, gummata A66.4
    bone A66.6
  gummatous
    frambeside A66.4
    osteitis A66.6
    periostitis A66.6
  hydrarthrosis —*see also* subcategory M14.8- A66.6
  hyperkeratosis (early) (late) A66.3

Yaws *(Continued)*
  initial lesions A66.0
  joint lesions —*see also* subcategory M14.8- A66.6
  juxta-articular nodules A66.7
  late nodular (ulcerated) A66.4
  latent (without clinical manifestations) (with positive serology) A66.8
  mother A66.0
  mucosal A66.7
  multiple papillomata A66.1
  nodular, late (ulcerated) A66.4
  osteitis A66.6
  papilloma, plantar or palmar A66.1
  periostitis (hypertrophic) A66.6
  specified NEC A66.7
  ulcers A66.4
  wet crab A66.1
Yeast infection —*see also* Candidiasis B37.9
Yellow
  atrophy (liver) —*see* Failure, hepatic
  fever —*see* Fever, yellow
  jack —*see* Fever, yellow
  jaundice —*see* Jaundice
  nail syndrome L60.5
Yersiniosis —*see also* Infection, Yersinia
  extraintestinal A28.2
  intestinal A04.6

Z

Zahorsky's syndrome (herpangina) B08.5
Zellweger's syndrome Q87.89
Zenker's diverticulum (esophagus) K22.5
Ziehen-Oppenheim disease G24.1
Zieve's syndrome K70.0
Zika NOS A92.5 ◀
Zinc
  deficiency, dietary E60
  metabolism disorder E83.2
Zollinger-Ellison syndrome E16.4
Zona —*see* Herpes, zoster
Zoophobia F40.218
Zoster (herpes) —*see* Herpes, zoster
Zygomycosis B46.9
  specified NEC B46.8
Zymotic —*see* condition

Z

ICD-10-CM Table of Neoplasms

	Malignant Primary	Malignant Secondary	Ca in situ	Benign	Uncertain Behavior	Unspecified Behavior

The list below gives the code numbers for neoplasms by anatomical site. For each site there are six possible code numbers according to whether the neoplasm in question is malignant, benign, in situ, of uncertain behavior, or of unspecified nature. The description of the neoplasm will often indicate which of the six columns is appropriate; e.g., malignant melanoma of skin, benign fibroadenoma of breast, carcinoma in situ of cervix uteri.

Where such descriptors are not present, the remainder of the Index should be consulted where guidance is given to the appropriate column for each morphological (histological) variety listed; e.g., Mesonephroma—*see Neoplasm, malignant;* Embryoma—*see also Neoplasm, uncertain behavior;* Disease, Bowen's—*see Neoplasm, skin, in situ.* However, the guidance in the Index can be overridden if one of the descriptors mentioned above is present; e.g., malignant adenoma of colon is coded to C18.9 and not to D12.6 as the adjective "Malignant" overrides the Index entry 'Adenoma—*see also Neoplasm, benign.*'

Codes listed with a dash -, following the code have a required additional character for laterality. The Tablular must be reviewed for the complete code.

	Malignant Primary	Malignant Secondary	Ca in situ	Benign	Uncertain Behavior	Unspecified Behavior
Neoplasm, neoplastic	C80.1	C79.9	D09.9	D36.9	D48.9	D49.9
abdomen, abdominal	C76.2	C79.8-	D09.8	D36.7	D48.7	D49.89
cavity	C76.2	C79.8-	D09.8	D36.7	D48.7	D49.89
organ	C76.2	C79.8-	D09.8	D36.7	D48.7	D49.89
viscera	C76.2	C79.8-	D09.8	D36.7	D48.7	D49.89
wall—*see also Neoplasm, abdomen, wall, skin*	C44.509	C79.2-	D04.5	D23.5	D48.5	D49.2
connective tissue	C49.4	C79.8-	—	D21.4	D48.1	D49.2
skin	C44.509					
basal cell carcinoma	C44.519	—	—	—	—	—
specified type NEC	C44.599	—	—	—	—	—
squamous cell carcinoma	C44.529	—	—	—	—	—
abdominopelvic	C76.8	C79.8-	—	D36.7	D48.7	D49.89
accessory sinus—*see Neoplasm, sinus*						
acoustic nerve	C72.4-	C79.49	—	D33.3	D43.3	D49.7
adenoid (pharynx) (tissue)	C11.1	C79.89	D00.08	D10.6	D37.05	D49.0
adipose tissue—*see also Neoplasm, connective tissue*	C49.4	C79.89	—	D21.9	D48.1	D49.2
adnexa (uterine)	C57.4	C79.89	D07.39	D28.7	D39.8	D49.59 ◄
adrenal	C74.9-	C79.7-	D09.3	D35.0-	D44.1-	D49.7
capsule	C74.9-	C79.7-	D09.3	D35.0-	D44.1-	D49.7
cortex	C74.0-	C79.7-	D09.3	D35.0-	D44.1-	D49.7
gland	C74.9-	C79.7-	D09.3	D35.0-	D44.1-	D49.7
medulla	C74.1-	C79.7-	D09.3	D35.0-	D44.1-	D49.7
ala nasi (external)—*see also Neoplasm, skin, nose*	C44.301	C79.2	D04.39	D23.39	D48.5	D49.2
alimentary canal or tract NEC	C26.9	C78.80	D01.9	D13.9	D37.9	D49.0
alveolar	C03.9	C79.89	D00.03	D10.39	D37.09	D49.0
mucosa	C03.9	C79.89	D00.03	D10.39	D37.09	D49.0
lower	C03.1	C79.89	D00.03	D10.39	D37.09	D49.0
upper	C03.0	C79.89	D00.03	D10.39	D37.09	D49.0
ridge or process	C41.1	C79.51	—	D16.5-	D48.0	D49.2
carcinoma	C03.9	C79.8-	—	—	—	—
lower	C03.1	C79.8-	—	—	—	—
upper	C03.0	C79.8-	—	—	—	—
lower	C41.1	C79.51	—	D16.5-	D48.0	D49.2
mucosa	C03.9	C79.89	D00.03	D10.39	D37.09	D49.0
lower	C03.1	C79.89	D00.03	D10.39	D37.09	D49.0
upper	C03.0	C79.89	D00.03	D10.39	D37.09	D49.0
upper	C41.0	C79.51	—	D16.4-	D48.0	D49.2
sulcus	C06.1	C79.89	D00.02	D10.39	D37.09	D49.0
alveolus	C03.9	C79.89	D00.03	D10.39	D37.09	D49.0
lower	C03.1	C79.89	D00.03	D10.39	D37.09	D49.0
upper	C03.0	C79.89	D00.03	D10.39	D37.09	D49.0
ampulla of Vater	C24.1	C78.89	D01.5	D13.5	D37.6	D49.0
ankle NEC	C76.5-	C79.89	D04.7-	D36.7	D48.7	D49.89
anorectum, anorectal (junction)	C21.8	C78.5	D01.3	D12.9	D37.8	D49.0
antecubital fossa or space	C76.4-	C79.89	D04.6-	D36.7	D48.7	D49.89
antrum (Highmore) (maxillary)	C31.0	C78.39	D02.3	D14.0	D38.5	D49.1
pyloric	C16.3	C78.89	D00.2	D13.1	D37.1	D49.0
tympanicum	C30.1	C78.39	D02.3	D14.0	D38.5	D49.1
anus, anal	C21.0	C78.5	D01.3	D12.9	D37.8	D49.0
canal	C21.1	C78.5	D01.3	D12.9	D37.8	D49.0
cloacogenic zone	C21.2	C78.5	D01.3	D12.9	D37.8	D49.0
margin—*see also Neoplasm, anus, skin*	C44.500	C79.2	D04.5	D23.5	D48.5	D49.2
overlapping lesion with rectosigmoid junction or rectum	C21.8	—	—	—	—	—
skin	C44.500	C79.2	D04.5	D23.5	D48.5	D49.2
basal cell carcinoma	C44.510	—	—	—	—	—
specified type NEC	C44.590	—	—	—	—	—
squamous cell carcinoma	C44.520	—	—	—	—	—
sphincter	C21.1	C78.5	D01.3	D12.9	D37.8	D49.0
aorta (thoracic)	C49.3	C79.89	—	D21.3	D48.1	D49.2
abdominal	C49.4	C79.89	—	D21.4	D48.1	D49.2
aortic body	C75.5	C79.89	—	D35.6	D44.7	D49.7
aponeurosis	C49.9	C79.89	—	D21.9	D48.1	D49.2
palmar	C49.1-	C79.89	—	D21.1-	D48.1	D49.2
plantar	C49.2-	C79.89	—	D21.2-	D48.1	D49.2

	Malignant Primary	Malignant Secondary	Ca in situ	Benign	Uncertain Behavior	Unspecified Behavior
appendix	C18.1	C78.5	DØ1.Ø	D12.1	D37.3	D49.Ø
arachnoid	C7Ø.9	C79.49	—	D32.9	D42.9	D49.7
cerebral	C7Ø.Ø	C79.32	—	D32.Ø	D42.Ø	D49.7
spinal	C7Ø.1	C79.49	—	D32.1	D42.1	D49.7
areola	C5Ø.Ø-	C79.81	DØ5.-	D24.-	D48.6-	D49.3
arm NEC	C76.4-	C79.89	DØ4.6-	D36.7	D48.7	D49.89
artery — *see Neoplasm, connective tissue*						
aryepiglottic fold	C13.1	C79.89	DØØ.Ø8	D1Ø.7	D37.Ø5	D49.Ø
hypopharyngeal aspect	C13.1	C79.89	DØØ.Ø8	D1Ø.7	D37.Ø5	D49.Ø
laryngeal aspect	C32.1	C78.39	DØ2.Ø	D14.1	D38.Ø	D49.1
marginal zone	C13.1	C79.89	DØØ.Ø8	D1Ø.7	D37.Ø5	D49.Ø
arytenoid (cartilage)	C32.3	C78.39	DØ2.Ø	D14.1	D38.Ø	D49.1
fold — *see Neoplasm, aryepiglottic*						
associated with transplanted organ	C8Ø.2	—	—	—	—	—
atlas	C41.2	C79.51	—	D16.6	D48.Ø	D49.2
atrium, cardiac	C38.Ø	C79.89	—	D15.1	D48.7	D49.89
auditory						
canal (external) (skin)	C44.2Ø-	C79.2	DØ4.2-	D23.2-	D48.5	D49.2
internal	C3Ø.1	C78.39	DØ2.3	D14.Ø	D38.5	D49.1
nerve	C72.4-	C79.49	—	D33.3	D43.3	D49.7
tube	C3Ø.1	C78.39	DØ2.3	D14.Ø	D38.5	D49.1
opening	C11.2	C79.89	DØØ.Ø8	D1Ø.6	D37.Ø5	D49.Ø
auricle, ear — *see also Neoplasm, skin, ear*	C44.2Ø-	C79.2	DØ4.2-	D23.2-	D48.5	D49.2
auricular canal (external) — *see also Neoplasm, skin, ear*	C44.2Ø-	C79.2	DØ4.2-	D23.2-	D48.5	D49.2
internal	C3Ø.1	C78.39	DØ2.3	D14.Ø	D38.5	D49.2
autonomic nerve or nervous system NEC *(see Neoplasm, nerve, peripheral)*						
axilla, axillary	C76.1	C79.89	DØ9.8	D36.7	D48.7	D49.89
fold — *see also Neoplasm, skin, trunk*	C44.5Ø9	C79.2	DØ4.5	D23.5	D48.5	D49.2
back NEC	C76.8	C79.89	DØ4.5	D36.7	D48.7	D49.89
Bartholin's gland	C51.Ø	C79.82	DØ7.1	D28.Ø	D39.8	D49.59
basal ganglia	C71.Ø	C79.31	—	D33.Ø	D43.Ø	D49.6
basis pedunculi	C71.7	C79.31	—	D33.1	D43.1	D49.6
bile or biliary (tract)	C24.9	C78.89	DØ1.5	D13.5	D37.6	D49.Ø
canaliculi (biliferi) (intrahepatic)	C22.1	C78.7	DØ1.5	D13.4	D37.6	D49.Ø
canals, interlobular	C22.1	C78.89	DØ1.5	D13.4	D37.6	D49.Ø

	Malignant Primary	Malignant Secondary	Ca in situ	Benign	Uncertain Behavior	Unspecified Behavior
bile or biliary *(Continued)*						
duct or passage (common) (cystic) (extrahepatic)	C24.Ø	C78.89	DØ1.5	D13.5	D37.6	D49.Ø
interlobular	C22.1	C78.89	DØ1.5	D13.4	D37.6	D49.Ø
intrahepatic	C22.1	C78.7	DØ1.5	D13.4	D37.6	D49.Ø
and extrahepatic	C24.8	C78.89	DØ1.5	D13.5	D37.6	D49.Ø
bladder (urinary)	C67.9	C79.11	DØ9.Ø	D3Ø.3	D41.4	D49.4
dome	C67.1	C79.11	DØ9.Ø	D3Ø.3	D41.4	D49.4
neck	C67.5	C79.11	DØ9.Ø	D3Ø.3	D41.4	D49.4
orifice	C67.9	C79.11	DØ9.Ø	D3Ø.3	D41.4	D49.4
ureteric	C67.6	C79.11	DØ9.Ø	D3Ø.3	D41.4	D49.4
urethral	C67.5	C79.11	DØ9.Ø	D3Ø.3	D41.4	D49.4
overlapping lesion	C67.8	—	—	—	—	—
sphincter	C67.8	C79.11	DØ9.Ø	D3Ø.3	D41.4	D49.4
trigone	C67.Ø	C79.11	DØ9.Ø	D3Ø.3	D41.4	D49.4
urachus	C67.7	C79.11	DØ9.Ø	D3Ø.3	D41.4	D49.4
wall	C67.9	C79.11	DØ9.Ø	D3Ø.3	D41.4	D49.4
anterior	C67.3	C79.11	DØ9.Ø	D3Ø.3	D41.4	D49.4
lateral	C67.2	C79.11	DØ9.Ø	D3Ø.3	D41.4	D49.4
posterior	C67.4	C79.11	DØ9.Ø	D3Ø.3	D41.4	D49.4
blood vessel — *see Neoplasm, connective tissue*						
bone (periosteum)	C41.9	C79.51	—	D16.9-	D48.Ø	D49.2
acetabulum	C41.4	C79.51	—	D16.8-	D48.Ø	D49.2
ankle	C4Ø.3-	C79.51	—	D16.3-	—	—
arm NEC	C4Ø.Ø-	C79.51	—	D16.Ø-	—	—
astragalus	C4Ø.3-	C79.51	—	D16.3-	—	—
atlas	C41.2	C79.51	—	D16.6-	D48.Ø	D49.2
axis	C41.2	C79.51	—	D16.6-	D48.Ø	D49.2
back NEC	C41.2	C79.51	—	D16.6-	D48.Ø	D49.2
calcaneus	C4Ø.3-	C79.51	—	D16.3-	—	—
calvarium	C41.Ø	C79.51	—	D16.4-	D48.Ø	D49.2
carpus (any)	C4Ø.1-	C79.51	—	D16.1-	—	—
cartilage NEC	C41.9	C79.51	—	D16.9-	D48.Ø	D49.2
clavicle	C41.3	C79.51	—	D16.7-	D48.Ø	D49.2
clivus	C41.Ø	C79.51	—	D16.4-	D48.Ø	D49.2
coccygeal vertebra	C41.4	C79.51	—	D16.8-	D48.Ø	D49.2
coccyx	C41.4	C79.51	—	D16.8-	D48.Ø	D49.2
costal cartilage	C41.3	C79.51	—	D16.7-	D48.Ø	D49.2
costovertebral joint	C41.3	C79.51	—	D16.7-	D48.Ø	D49.2
cranial	C41.Ø	C79.51	—	D16.4-	D48.Ø	D49.2
cuboid	C4Ø.3-	C79.51	—	D16.3-	—	—
cuneiform	C41.9	C79.51	—	D16.9-	D48.Ø	D49.2
elbow	C4Ø.Ø-	C79.51	—	D16.Ø-	—	—

TABLE OF NEOPLASMS

◀ New ⬅ Revised ~~deleted~~ Deleted

	Malignant Primary	Malignant Secondary	Ca in situ	Benign	Uncertain Behavior	Unspecified Behavior
bone *(Continued)*						
ethmoid (labyrinth)	C41.Ø	C79.51	—	D16.4-	D48.Ø	D49.2
face	C41.Ø	C79.51	—	D16.4-	D48.Ø	D49.2
femur (any part)	C4Ø.2-	C79.51	—	D16.2-	—	—
fibula (any part)	C4Ø.2-	C79.51	—	D16.2-	—	—
finger (any)	C4Ø.1-	C79.51	—	D16.1-	—	—
foot	C4Ø.3-	C79.51	—	D16.3-	—	—
forearm	C4Ø.Ø-	C79.51	—	D16.Ø-	—	—
frontal	C41.Ø	C79.51	—	D16.4-	D48.Ø	D49.2
hand	C4Ø.1-	C79.51	—	D16.1-	—	—
heel	C4Ø.3-	C79.51	—	D16.3-	—	—
hip	C41.4	C79.51	—	D16.8-	D48.Ø	D49.2
humerus (any part)	C4Ø.Ø-	C79.51	—	D16.Ø-	—	—
hyoid	C41.Ø	C79.51	—	D16.4-	D48.Ø	D49.2
ilium	C41.4	C79.51	—	D16.8-	D48.Ø	D49.2
innominate	C41.4	C79.51	—	D16.8-	D48.Ø	D49.2
intervertebral cartilage or disc	C41.2	C79.51	—	D16.6-	D48.Ø	D49.2
ischium	C41.4	C79.51	—	D16.8-	D48.Ø	D49.2
jaw (lower)	C41.1	C79.51	—	D16.5-	D48.Ø	D49.2
knee	C4Ø.2-	C79.51	—	D16.2-	—	—
leg NEC	C4Ø.2-	C79.51	—	D16.2-	—	—
limb NEC	C4Ø.9-	C79.51	—	D16.9-	—	—
lower (long bones)	C4Ø.2-	C79.51	—	D16.2-	—	—
short bones	C4Ø.3-	C79.51	—	D16.3-	—	—
upper (long bones)	C4Ø.Ø-	C79.51	—	D16.Ø-	—	—
short bones	C4Ø.1-	C79.51	—	D16.1-	—	—
malar	C41.Ø	C79.51	—	D16.4-	D48.Ø	D49.2
mandible	C41.1	C79.51	—	D16.5-	D48.Ø	D49.2
marrow NEC (any bone)	C96.9	C79.52	—	—	D47.9	D49.89
mastoid	C41.Ø	C79.51	—	D16.4-	D48.Ø	D49.2
maxilla, maxillary (superior)	C41.Ø	C79.51	—	D16.4-	D48.Ø	D49.2
inferior	C41.1	C79.51	—	D16.5-	D48.Ø	D49.2
metacarpus (any)	C4Ø.1-	C79.51	—	D16.1-	—	—
metatarsus (any)	C4Ø.3-	C79.51	—	D16.3-	—	—
overlapping sites	C4Ø.8-	—	—	—	—	—
navicular						
ankle	C4Ø.3-	C79.51	—	—	—	—
hand	C4Ø.1-	C79.51	—	—	—	—
nose, nasal	C41.Ø	C79.51	—	D16.4-	D48.Ø	D49.2
occipital	C41.Ø	C79.51	—	D16.4-	D48.Ø	D49.2
orbit	C41.Ø	C79.51	—	D16.4-	D48.Ø	D49.2
parietal	C41.Ø	C79.51	—	D16.4-	D48.Ø	D49.2
patella	C4Ø.2-	C79.51	—	—	—	—
pelvic	C41.4	C79.51	—	D16.8	D48.Ø	D49.2
bone *(Continued)*						
phalanges						
foot	C4Ø.3-	C79.51	—	—	—	—
hand	C4Ø.1-	C79.51	—	—	—	—
pubic	C41.4	C79.51	—	D16.8	D48.Ø	D49.2
radius (any part)	C4Ø.Ø-	C79.51	—	D16.Ø-	—	—
rib	C41.3	C79.51	—	D16.7	D48.Ø	D49.2
sacral vertebra	C41.4	C79.51	—	D16.8	D48.Ø	D49.2
sacrum	C41.4	C79.51	—	D16.8	D48.Ø	D49.2
scaphoid						
of ankle	C4Ø.3-	C79.51	—	—	—	—
of hand	C4Ø.1-	C79.51	—	—	—	—
scapula (any part)	C4Ø.Ø-	C79.51	—	D16.Ø-	—	—
sella turcica	C41.Ø	C79.51	—	D16.4-	D48.Ø	D49.2
shoulder	C4Ø.Ø-	C79.51	—	D16.Ø-	—	—
skull	C41.Ø	C79.51	—	D16.4-	D48.Ø	D49.2
sphenoid	C41.Ø	C79.51	—	D16.4-	D48.Ø	D49.2
spine, spinal (column)	C41.2	C79.51	—	D16.6	D48.Ø	D49.2
coccyx	C41.4	C79.51	—	D16.8	D48.Ø	D49.2
sacrum	C41.4	C79.51	—	D16.8	D48.Ø	D49.2
sternum	C41.3	C79.51	—	D16.7	D48.Ø	D49.2
tarsus (any)	C4Ø.3-	C79.51	—	—	—	—
temporal	C41.Ø	C79.51	—	D16.4-	D48.Ø	D49.2
thumb	C4Ø.1-	C79.51	—	—	—	—
tibia (any part)	C4Ø.2-	C79.51	—	—	—	—
toe (any)	C4Ø.3-	C79.51	—	—	—	—
trapezium	C4Ø.1-	C79.51	—	—	—	—
trapezoid	C4Ø.1-	C79.51	—	—	—	—
turbinate	C41.Ø	C79.51	—	D16.4-	D48.Ø	D49.2
ulna (any part)	C4Ø.Ø-	C79.51	—	D16.Ø-	—	—
unciform	C4Ø.1-	C79.51	—	—	—	—
vertebra (column)	C41.2	C79.51	—	D16.6	D48.Ø	D49.2
coccyx	C41.4	C79.51	—	D16.8	D48.Ø	D49.2
sacrum	C41.4	C79.51	—	D16.8	D48.Ø	D49.2
vomer	C41.Ø	C79.51	—	D16.4-	D48.Ø	D49.2
wrist	C4Ø.1-	C79.51	—	—	—	—
xiphoid process	C41.3	C79.51	—	D16.7	D48.Ø	D49.2
zygomatic	C41.Ø	C79.51	—	D16.4-	D48.Ø	D49.2
book-leaf (mouth)	CØ6.89	C79.89	DØØ.ØØ	D1Ø.39	D37.Ø9	D49.Ø
bowel — *see Neoplasm, intestine*						
brachial plexus	C47.1-	C79.89	—	D36.12	D48.2	D49.2
brain NEC	C71.9	C79.31	—	D33.2	D43.2	D49.6
basal ganglia	C71.Ø	C79.31	—	D33.Ø	D43.Ø	D49.6
cerebellopontine angle	C71.6	C79.31	—	D33.1	D43.1	D49.6

	Malignant Primary	Malignant Secondary	Ca in situ	Benign	Uncertain Behavior	Unspecified Behavior
brain NEC *(Continued)*						
cerebellum NOS	C71.6	C79.31	—	D33.1	D43.1	D49.6
cerebrum	C71.Ø	C79.31	—	D33.Ø	D43.Ø	D49.6
choroid plexus	C71.7	C79.31	—	D33.1	D43.1	D49.6
corpus callosum	C71.8	C79.31	—	D33.2	D43.2	D49.6
corpus striatum	C71.Ø	C79.31	—	D33.Ø	D43.Ø	D49.6
cortex (cerebral)	C71.Ø	C79.31	—	D33.Ø	D43.Ø	D49.6
frontal lobe	C71.1	C79.31	—	D33.Ø	D43.Ø	D49.6
globus pallidus	C71.Ø	C79.31	—	D33.Ø	D43.Ø	D49.6
hippocampus	C71.2	C79.31	—	D33.Ø	D43.Ø	D49.6
hypothalamus	C71.Ø	C79.31	—	D33.Ø	D43.Ø	D49.6
internal capsule	C71.Ø	C79.31	—	D33.Ø	D43.Ø	D49.6
medulla oblongata	C71.7	C79.31	—	D33.1	D43.1	D49.6
meninges	C7Ø.Ø	C79.32	—	D32.Ø	D42.Ø	D49.7
midbrain	C71.7	C79.31	—	D33.1	D43.1	D49.6
occipital lobe	C71.4	C79.31	—	D33.Ø	D43.Ø	D49.6
overlapping lesion	C71.8	C79.31	—	—	—	—
parietal lobe	C71.3	C79.31	—	D33.Ø	D43.Ø	D49.6
peduncle	C71.7	C79.31	—	D33.1	D43.1	D49.6
pons	C71.7	C79.31	—	D33.1	D43.1	D49.6
stem	C71.7	C79.31	—	D33.1	D43.1	D49.6
tapetum	C71.8	C79.31	—	D33.2	D43.2	D49.6
temporal lobe	C71.2	C79.31	—	D33.Ø	D43.Ø	D49.6
thalamus	C71.Ø	C79.31	—	D33.Ø	D43.Ø	D49.6
uncus	C71.2	C79.31	—	D33.Ø	D43.Ø	D49.6
ventricle (floor)	C71.5	C79.31	—	D33.Ø	D43.Ø	D49.6
fourth	C71.7	C79.31	—	D33.1	D43.1	D49.6
branchial (cleft) (cyst) (vestiges)	C1Ø.4	C79.89	DØØ.Ø8	D1Ø.5	D37.Ø5	D49.Ø
breast (connective tissue) (glandular tissue) (soft parts)	C5Ø.9-	C79.81	DØ5.-	D24.-	D48.6-	D49.3
areola	C5Ø.Ø-	C79.81	DØ5.-	D24.-	D48.6-	D49.3
axillary tail	C5Ø.6-	C79.81	DØ5.-	D24.-	D48.6-	D49.3
central portion	C5Ø.1-	C79.81	DØ5.-	D24.-	D48.6-	D49.3
inner	C5Ø.8-	C79.81	DØ5.-	D24.-	D48.6-	D49.3
lower	C5Ø.8-	C79.81	DØ5.-	D24.-	D48.6-	D49.3
lower-inner quadrant	C5Ø.3-	C79.81	DØ5.-	D24.-	D48.6-	D49.3
lower-outer quadrant	C5Ø.5-	C79.81	DØ5.-	D24.-	D48.6-	D49.3
mastectomy site (skin) — *see also Neoplasm, breast, skin*	C44.5Ø1	C79.2	—	—	—	—
specified as breast tissue	C5Ø.8-	C79.81	—	—	—	—
midline	C5Ø.8-	C79.81	DØ5.-	D24.-	D48.6-	D49.3
nipple	C5Ø.Ø-	C79.81	DØ5.-	D24.-	D48.6-	D49.3
outer	C5Ø.8-	C79.81	DØ5.-	D24.-	D48.6-	D49.3
overlapping lesion	C5Ø.8-	—	—	—	—	—

	Malignant Primary	Malignant Secondary	Ca in situ	Benign	Uncertain Behavior	Unspecified Behavior
breast *(Continued)*						
skin	C44.5Ø1	C79.2	DØ4.5	D23.5	D48.5	D49.2
basal cell carcinoma	C44.511	—	—	—	—	—
specified type NEC	C44.591	—	—	—	—	—
squamous cell carcinoma	C44.521	—	—	—	—	—
tail (axillary)	C5Ø.6-	C79.81	DØ5.-	D24.-	D48.6-	D49.3
upper	C5Ø.8-	C79.81	DØ5.-	D24.-	D48.6-	D49.3
upper-inner quadrant	C5Ø.2-	C79.81	DØ5.-	D24.-	D48.6-	D49.3
upper-outer quadrant	C5Ø.4-	C79.81	DØ5.-	D24.-	D48.6-	D49.3
broad ligament	C57.1	C79.82	DØ7.39	D28.2	D39.8	D49.59
bronchiogenic, bronchogenic (lung)	C34.9-	C78.Ø-	DØ2.2-	D14.3-	D38.1	D49.1
bronchiole	C34.9-	C78.Ø-	DØ2.2-	D14.3-	D38.1	D49.1
bronchus	C34.9-	C78.Ø-	DØ2.2-	D14.3-	D38.1	D49.1
carina	C34.Ø-	C78.Ø-	DØ2.2-	D14.3-	D38.1	D49.1
lower lobe of lung	C34.3-	C78.Ø-	DØ2.2-	D14.3-	D38.1	D49.1
main	C34.Ø-	C78.Ø-	DØ2.2-	D14.3-	D38.1	D49.1
middle lobe of lung	C34.2	C78.Ø-	DØ2.21	D14.31	D38.1	D49.1
overlapping lesion	C34.8-	—	—	—	—	—
upper lobe of lung	C34.1-	C78.Ø-	DØ2.2-	D14.3-	D38.1	D49.1
brow	C44.3Ø9	C79.2	DØ4.39	D23.39	D48.5	D49.2
basal cell carcinoma	C44.319	—	—	—	—	—
specified type NEC	C44.399	—	—	—	—	—
squamous cell carcinoma	C44.329	—	—	—	—	—
buccal (cavity)	CØ6.9	C79.89	DØØ.ØØ	D1Ø.39	D37.Ø9	D49.Ø
commissure	CØ6.Ø	C79.89	DØØ.Ø2	D1Ø.39	D37.Ø9	D49.Ø
groove (lower) (upper)	CØ6.1	C79.89	DØØ.Ø2	D1Ø.39	D37.Ø9	D49.Ø
mucosa	CØ6.Ø	C79.89	DØØ.Ø2	D1Ø.39	D37.Ø9	D49.Ø
sulcus (lower) (upper)	CØ6.1	C79.89	DØØ.Ø2	D1Ø.39	D37.Ø9	D49.Ø
bulbourethral gland	C68.Ø	C79.19	DØ9.19	D3Ø.4	D41.3	D49.59
bursa — *see Neoplasm, connective tissue*						
buttock NEC	C76.3	C79.89	DØ4.5	D36.7	D48.7	D49.89
calf	C76.5-	C79.89	DØ4.7-	D36.7	D48.7	D49.89
calvarium	C41.Ø	C79.51	—	D16.4-	D48.Ø	D49.2
calyx, renal	C65.-	C79.Ø-	DØ9.19	D3Ø.1-	D41.1-	D49.51-
canal						
anal	C21.1	C78.5	DØ1.3	D12.9	D37.8	D49.Ø
auditory (external) — *see also Neoplasm, skin, ear*	C44.2Ø-	C79.2	DØ4.2-	D23.2-	D48.5	D49.2
auricular (external) — *see also Neoplasm, skin, ear*	C44.2Ø-	C79.2	DØ4.2-	D23.2-	D48.5	D49.2
canaliculi, biliary (biliferi) (intrahepatic)	C22.1	C78.7	DØ1.5	D13.4	D37.6	D49.Ø

◀ New ⬅ Revised ~~deleted~~ Deleted

	Malignant Primary	Malignant Secondary	Ca in situ	Benign	Uncertain Behavior	Unspecified Behavior
canthus (eye) (inner) (outer)	C44.1Ø-	C79.2	DØ4.1-	D23.1-	D48.5	D49.2
basal cell carcinoma	C44.11-	—	—	—	—	—
specified type NEC	C44.19-	—	—	—	—	—
squamous cell carcinoma	C44.12-	—	—	—	—	—
capillary — *see Neoplasm, connective tissue*						
caput coli	C18.Ø	C78.5	DØ1.Ø	D12.Ø	D37.4	D49.Ø
carcinoid — *see Tumor, carcinoid*						
cardia (gastric)	C16.Ø	C78.89	DØØ.2	D13.1	D37.1	D49.Ø
cardiac orifice (stomach)	C16.Ø	C78.89	DØØ.2	D13.1	D37.1	D49.Ø
cardio-esophageal junction	C16.Ø	C78.89	DØØ.2	D13.1	D37.1	D49.Ø
cardio-esophagus	C16.Ø	C78.89	DØØ.2	D13.1	D37.1	D49.Ø
carina (bronchus)	C34.Ø-	C78.Ø-	DØ2.2-	D14.3-	D38.1	D49.1
carotid (artery)	C49.Ø	C79.89	—	D21.Ø	D48.1	D49.2
body	C75.4	C79.89	—	D35.5	D44.6	D49.7
carpus (any bone)	C4Ø.1-	C79.51	—	D16.1-	—	—
cartilage (articular) (joint) NEC — *see also Neoplasm, bone*	C41.9	C79.51	—	D16.9-	D48.Ø	D49.2
arytenoid	C32.3	C78.39	DØ2.Ø	D14.1	D38.Ø	D49.1
auricular	C49.Ø	C79.89	—	D21.Ø	D48.1	D49.2
bronchi	C34.Ø-	C78.39	—	D14.3-	D38.1	D49.1
costal	C41.3	C79.51	—	D16.7	D48.Ø	D49.2
cricoid	C32.3	C78.39	DØ2.Ø	D14.1	D38.Ø	D49.1
cuneiform	C32.3	C78.39	DØ2.Ø	D14.1	D38.Ø	D49.1
ear (external)	C49.Ø	C79.89	—	D21.Ø	D48.1	D49.2
ensiform	C41.3	C79.51	—	D16.7	D48.Ø	D49.2
epiglottis	C32.1	C78.39	DØ2.Ø	D14.1	D38.Ø	D49.1
anterior surface	C1Ø.1	C79.89	DØØ.Ø8	D1Ø.5	D37.Ø5	D49.Ø
eyelid	C49.Ø	C79.89	—	D21.Ø	D48.1	D49.2
intervertebral	C41.2	C79.51	—	D16.6	D48.Ø	D49.2
larynx, laryngeal	C32.3	C78.39	DØ2.Ø	D14.1	D38.Ø	D49.1
nose, nasal	C3Ø.Ø	C78.39	DØ2.3	D14.Ø	D38.5	D49.1
pinna	C49.Ø	C79.89	—	D21.Ø	D48.1	D49.2
rib	C41.3	C79.51	—	D16.7	D48.Ø	D49.2
semilunar (knee)	C4Ø.2-	C79.51	—	D16.2-	D48.Ø	D49.2
thyroid	C32.3	C78.39	DØ2.Ø	D14.1	D38.Ø	D49.1
trachea	C33	C78.39	DØ2.1	D14.2	D38.1	D49.1
cauda equina	C72.1	C79.49	—	D33.4	D43.4	D49.7
cavity						
buccal	CØ6.9	C79.89	DØØ.ØØ	D1Ø.3Ø	D37.Ø9	D49.Ø
nasal	C3Ø.Ø	C78.39	DØ2.3	D14.Ø	D38.5	D49.1
oral	CØ6.9	C79.89	DØØ.ØØ	D1Ø.3Ø	D37.Ø9	D49.Ø
peritoneal	C48.2	C78.6	—	D2Ø.1	D48.4	D49.Ø
tympanic	C3Ø.1	C78.39	DØ2.3	D14.Ø	D38.5	D49.1

	Malignant Primary	Malignant Secondary	Ca in situ	Benign	Uncertain Behavior	Unspecified Behavior
cecum	C18.Ø	C78.5	DØ1.Ø	D12.Ø	D37.4	D49.Ø
central nervous system	C72.9	C79.4Ø	—	—	—	—
cerebellopontine (angle)	C71.6	C79.31	—	D33.1	D43.1	D49.6
cerebellum, cerebellar	C71.6	C79.31	—	D33.1	D43.1	D49.6
cerebrum, cerebral (cortex) (hemisphere) (white matter)	C71.Ø	C79.31	—	D33.Ø	D43.Ø	D49.6
meninges	C7Ø.Ø	C79.32	—	D32.Ø	D42.Ø	D49.7
peduncle	C71.7	C79.31	—	D33.1	D43.1	D49.6
ventricle	C71.5	C79.31	—	D33.Ø	D43.Ø	D49.6
fourth	C71.7	C79.31	—	D33.1	D43.1	D49.6
cervical region	C76.Ø	C79.89	DØ9.8	D36.7	D48.7	D49.89
cervix (cervical) (uteri) (uterus)	C53.9	C79.82	DØ6.9	D26.Ø	D39.Ø	D49.59
canal	C53.Ø	C79.82	DØ6.Ø	D26.Ø	D39.Ø	D49.59
endocervix (canal) (gland)	C53.Ø	C79.82	DØ6.Ø	D26.Ø	D39.Ø	D49.59
exocervix	C53.1	C79.82	DØ6.1	D26.Ø	D39.Ø	D49.59
external os	C53.1	C79.82	DØ6.1	D26.Ø	D39.Ø	D49.59
internal os	C53.Ø	C79.82	DØ6.Ø	D26.Ø	D39.Ø	D49.59
nabothian gland	C53.Ø	C79.82	DØ6.Ø	D26.Ø	D39.Ø	D49.59
overlapping lesion	C53.8	—	—	—	—	—
squamocolumnar junction	C53.8	C79.82	DØ6.7	D26.Ø	D39.Ø	D49.59
stump	C53.8	C79.82	DØ6.7	D26.Ø	D39.Ø	D49.59
cheek	C76.Ø	C79.89	DØ9.8	D36.7	D48.7	D49.89
external	C44.3Ø9	C79.2	DØ4.39	D23.39	D48.5	D49.2
basal cell carcinoma	C44.319	—	—	—	—	—
specified type NEC	C44.399	—	—	—	—	—
squamous cell carcinoma	C44.329	—	—	—	—	—
inner aspect	CØ6.Ø	C79.89	DØØ.Ø2	D1Ø.39	D37.Ø9	D49.Ø
internal	CØ6.Ø	C79.89	DØØ.Ø2	D1Ø.39	D37.Ø9	D49.Ø
mucosa	CØ6.Ø	C79.89	DØØ.Ø2	D1Ø.39	D37.Ø9	D49.Ø
chest (wall) NEC	C76.1	C79.89	DØ9.8	D36.7	D48.7	D49.89
chiasma opticum	C72.3-	C79.49	—	D33.3	D43.3	D49.7
chin	C44.3Ø9	C79.2	DØ4.39	D23.39	D48.5	D49.2
basal cell carcinoma	C44.319	—	—	—	—	—
specified type NEC	C44.399	—	—	—	—	—
squamous cell carcinoma	C44.329	—	—	—	—	—
choana	C11.3	C79.89	DØØ.Ø8	D1Ø.6	D37.Ø5	D49.Ø
cholangiole	C22.1	C78.89	DØ1.5	D13.4	D37.6	D49.Ø
choledochal duct	C24.Ø	C78.89	DØ1.5	D13.5	D37.6	D49.Ø
choroid	C69.3-	C79.49	DØ9.2-	D31.3-	D48.7	D49.81
plexus	C71.5	C79.31	—	D33.Ø	D43.Ø	D49.6
ciliary body	C69.4-	C79.49	DØ9.2-	D31.4-	D48.7	D49.89
clavicle	C41.3	C79.51	—	D16.7	D48.Ø	D49.2
clitoris	C51.2	C79.82	DØ7.1	D28.Ø	D39.8	D49.59
clivus	C41.Ø	C79.51	—	D16.4-	D48.Ø	D49.2

	Malignant Primary	Malignant Secondary	Ca in situ	Benign	Uncertain Behavior	Unspecified Behavior
cloacogenic zone	C21.2	C78.5	DØ1.3	D12.9	D37.8	D49.Ø
coccygeal						
body or glomus	C49.5	C79.89	—	D21.5	D48.1	D49.2
vertebra	C41.4	C79.51	—	D16.8	D48.Ø	D49.2
coccyx	C41.4	C79.51	—	D16.8	D48.Ø	D49.2
colon — *see also Neoplasm, intestine, large*	C18.9	C78.5	—	—	—	—
with rectum	C19	C78.5	DØ1.1	D12.7	D37.5	D49.Ø
column, spinal — *see Neoplasm, spine*						
columnella — *see also Neoplasm, skin, face*	C44.39Ø	C79.2	DØ4.39	D23.39	D48.5	D49.2
commissure						
labial, lip	CØØ.6	C79.89	DØØ.Ø1	D1Ø.39	D37.Ø1	D49.Ø
laryngeal	C32.Ø	C78.39	DØ2.Ø	D14.1	D38.Ø	D49.1
common (bile) duct	C24.Ø	C78.89	DØ1.5	D13.5	D37.6	D49.Ø
concha — *see also Neoplasm, skin, ear*	C44.2Ø-	C79.2	DØ4.2-	D23.2-	D48.5	D49.2
nose	C3Ø.Ø	C78.39	DØ2.3	D14.Ø	D38.5	D49.1
conjunctiva	C69.Ø-	C79.49	DØ9.2-	D31.Ø-	D48.7	D49.89
connective tissue NEC	C49.9	C79.89	—	D21.9	D48.1	D49.2

Note: For neoplasms of connective tissue (blood vessel, bursa, fascia, ligament, muscle, peripheral nerves, sympathetic and parasympathetic nerves and ganglia, synovia, tendon, etc.) or of morphological types that indicate connective tissue, code according to the list under "Neoplasm, connective tissue". For sites that do not appear in this list, code to neoplasm of that site; e.g., fibrosarcoma, pancreas (C25.9)

Note: Morphological types that indicate connective tissue appear in their proper place in the alphabetic index with the instruction "*see Neoplasm, connective tissue ....*"

	Malignant Primary	Malignant Secondary	Ca in situ	Benign	Uncertain Behavior	Unspecified Behavior
abdomen	C49.4	C79.89	—	D21.4	D48.1	D49.2
abdominal wall	C49.4	C79.89	—	D21.4	D48.1	D49.2
ankle	C49.2-	C79.89	—	D21.2-	D48.1	D49.2
antecubital fossa or space	C49.1-	C79.89	—	D21.1-	D48.1	D49.2
arm	C49.1-	C79.89	—	D21.1-	D48.1	D49.2
auricle (ear)	C49.Ø	C79.89	—	D21.Ø	D48.1	D49.2
axilla	C49.3	C79.89	—	D21.3	D48.1	D49.2
back	C49.6	C79.89	—	D21.6	D48.1	D49.2
breast — *see Neoplasm, breast*						
buttock	C49.5	C79.89	—	D21.5	D48.1	D49.2
calf	C49.2-	C79.89	—	D21.2-	D48.1	D49.2
cervical region	C49.Ø	C79.89	—	D21.Ø	D48.1	D49.2
cheek	C49.Ø	C79.89	—	D21.Ø	D48.1	D49.2
chest (wall)	C49.3	C79.89	—	D21.3	D48.1	D49.2
chin	C49.Ø	C79.89	—	D21.Ø	D48.1	D49.2
connective tissue NEC *(Continued)*						
diaphragm	C49.3	C79.89	—	D21.3	D48.1	D49.2
ear (external)	C49.Ø	C79.89	—	D21.Ø	D48.1	D49.2
elbow	C49.1-	C79.89	—	D21.1-	D48.1	D49.2
extrarectal	C49.5	C79.89	—	D21.5	D48.1	D49.2
extremity	C49.9	C79.89	—	D21.9	D48.1	D49.2
lower	C49.2-	C79.89	—	D21.2-	D48.1	D49.2
upper	C49.1-	C79.89	—	D21.1-	D48.1	D49.2
eyelid	C49.Ø	C79.89	—	D21.Ø	D48.1	D49.2
face	C49.Ø	C79.89	—	D21.Ø	D48.1	D49.2
finger	C49.1-	C79.89	—	D21.1-	D48.1	D49.2
flank	C49.6	C79.89	—	D21.6	D48.1	D49.2
foot	C49.2-	C79.89	—	D21.2-	D48.1	D49.2
forearm	C49.1-	C79.89	—	D21.1-	D48.1	D49.2
forehead	C49.Ø	C79.89	—	D21.Ø	D48.1	D49.2
gastric	C49.4	C79.89	—	D21.4	D48.1	D49.2
gastrointestinal	C49.4	C79.89	—	D21.4	D48.1	D49.2
gluteal region	C49.5	C79.89	—	D21.5	D48.1	D49.2
great vessels NEC	C49.3	C79.89	—	D21.3	D48.1	D49.2
groin	C49.5	C79.89	—	D21.5	D48.1	D49.2
hand	C49.1-	C79.89	—	D21.1-	D48.1	D49.2
head	C49.Ø	C79.89	—	D21.Ø	D48.1	D49.2
heel	C49.2-	C79.89	—	D21.2-	D48.1	D49.2
hip	C49.2-	C79.89	—	D21.2-	D48.1	D49.2
hypochondrium	C49.4	C79.89	—	D21.4	D48.1	D49.2
iliopsoas muscle	C49.5	C79.89	—	D21.5	D48.1	D49.2
infraclavicular region	C49.3	C79.89	—	D21.3	D48.1	D49.2
inguinal (canal) (region)	C49.5	C79.89	—	D21.5	D48.1	D49.2
intestinal	C49.4	C79.89	—	D21.4	D48.1	D49.2
intrathoracic	C49.3	C79.89	—	D21.3	D48.1	D49.2
ischiorectal fossa	C49.5	C79.89	—	D21.5	D48.1	D49.2
jaw	CØ3.9	C79.89	DØØ.Ø3	D1Ø.39	D48.1	D49.Ø
knee	C49.2-	C79.89	—	D21.2-	D48.1	D49.2
leg	C49.2-	C79.89	—	D21.2-	D48.1	D49.2
limb NEC	C49.9	C79.89	—	D21.9	D48.1	D49.2
lower	C49.2-	C79.89	—	D21.2-	D48.1	D49.2
upper	C49.1-	C79.89	—	D21.1-	D48.1	D49.2
nates	C49.5	C79.89	—	D21.5	D48.1	D49.2
neck	C49.Ø	C79.89	—	D21.Ø	D48.1	D49.2
orbit	C69.6-	C79.49	DØ9.2-	D31.6-	D48.1	D49.89
overlapping lesion	C49.8	—	—	—	—	—
pararectal	C49.5	C79.89	—	D21.5	D48.1	D49.2
para-urethral	C49.5	C79.89	—	D21.5	D48.1	D49.2
paravaginal	C49.5	C79.89	—	D21.5	D48.1	D49.2

◀ New ◀ Revised ~~deleted~~ Deleted

TABLE OF NEOPLASMS

	Malignant Primary	Malignant Secondary	Ca in situ	Benign	Uncertain Behavior	Unspecified Behavior
connective tissue NEC *(Continued)*						
pelvis (floor)	C49.5	C79.89	—	D21.5	D48.1	D49.2
pelvo-abdominal	C49.8	C79.89	—	D21.6	D48.1	D49.2
perineum	C49.5	C79.89	—	D21.5	D48.1	D49.2
perirectal (tissue)	C49.5	C79.89	—	D21.5	D48.1	D49.2
periurethral (tissue)	C49.5	C79.89	—	D21.5	D48.1	D49.2
popliteal fossa or space	C49.2-	C79.89	—	D21.2-	D48.1	D49.2
presacral	C49.5	C79.89	—	D21.5	D48.1	D49.2
psoas muscle	C49.4	C79.89	—	D21.4	D48.1	D49.2
pterygoid fossa	C49.Ø	C79.89	—	D21.Ø	D48.1	D49.2
rectovaginal septum or wall	C49.5	C79.89	—	D21.5	D48.1	D49.2
rectovesical	C49.5	C79.89	—	D21.5	D48.1	D49.2
retroperitoneum	C48.Ø	C78.6	—	D2Ø.Ø	D48.3	D49.Ø
sacrococcygeal region	C49.5	C79.89	—	D21.5	D48.1	D49.2
scalp	C49.Ø	C79.89	—	D21.Ø	D48.1	D49.2
scapular region	C49.3	C79.89	—	D21.3	D48.1	D49.2
shoulder	C49.1-	C79.89	—	D21.1-	D48.1	D49.2
skin (dermis) NEC—*see also Neoplasm, skin, by site*	C44.90	C79.2	DØ4.9	D23.9	D48.5	D49.2
stomach	C49.4	C79.89	—	D21.4	D48.1	D49.2
submental	C49.Ø	C79.89	—	D21.Ø	D48.1	D49.2
supraclavicular region	C49.Ø	C79.89	—	D21.Ø	D48.1	D49.2
temple	C49.Ø	C79.89	—	D21.Ø	D48.1	D49.2
temporal region	C49.Ø	C79.89	—	D21.Ø	D48.1	D49.2
thigh	C49.2-	C79.89	—	D21.2-	D48.1	D49.2
thoracic (duct) (wall)	C49.3	C79.89	—	D21.3	D48.1	D49.2
thorax	C49.3	C79.89	—	D21.3	D48.1	D49.2
thumb	C49.1-	C79.89	—	D21.1-	D48.1	D49.2
toe	C49.2-	C79.89	—	D21.2-	D48.1	D49.2
trunk	C49.6	C79.89	—	D21.6	D48.1	D49.2
umbilicus	C49.4	C79.89	—	D21.4	D48.1	D49.2
vesicorectal	C49.5	C79.89	—	D21.5	D48.1	D49.2
wrist	C49.1-	C79.89	—	D21.1-	D48.1	D49.2
conus medullaris	C72.Ø	C79.49	—	D33.4	D43.4	D49.7
cord (true) (vocal)	C32.Ø	C78.39	DØ2.Ø	D14.1	D38.Ø	D49.1
false	C32.1	C78.39	DØ2.Ø	D14.1	D38.Ø	D49.1
spermatic	C63.1-	C79.82	DØ7.69	D29.8	D4Ø.8	D49.59
spinal (cervical) (lumbar) (thoracic)	C72.Ø	C79.49	—	D33.4	D43.4	D49.7
cornea (limbus)	C69.1-	C79.49	DØ9.2-	D31.1-	D48.7	D49.89
corpus						
albicans	C56.-	C79.6-	DØ7.39	D27.-	D39.1-	D49.59
callosum, brain	C71.Ø	C79.31	—	D33.2	D43.2	D49.6
cavernosum	C6Ø.2	C79.82	DØ7.4	D29.Ø	D4Ø.8	D49.59

	Malignant Primary	Malignant Secondary	Ca in situ	Benign	Uncertain Behavior	Unspecified Behavior
corpus *(Continued)*						
gastric	C16.2	C78.89	DØØ.2	D13.1	D37.1	D49.Ø
overlapping sites	C54.8	—	—	—	—	—
penis	C6Ø.2	C79.82	DØ7.4	D29.Ø	D4Ø.8	D49.59
striatum, cerebrum	C71.Ø	C79.31	—	D33.Ø	D43.Ø	D49.6
uteri	C54.9	C79.82	DØ7.Ø	D26.1	D39.Ø	D49.59
isthmus	C54.Ø	C79.82	DØ7.Ø	D26.1	D39.Ø	D49.59
cortex						
adrenal	C74.Ø-	C79.7-	DØ9.3	D35.Ø-	D44.1-	D49.7
cerebral	C71.Ø	C79.31	—	D33.Ø	D43.Ø	D49.6
costal cartilage	C41.3	C79.51	—	D16.7	D48.Ø	D49.2
costovertebral joint	C41.3	C79.51	—	D16.7	D48.Ø	D49.2
Cowper's gland	C68.Ø	C79.19	DØ9.19	D3Ø.4	D41.3	D49.59
cranial (fossa, any)	C71.9	C79.31	—	D33.2	D43.2	D49.6
meninges	C7Ø.Ø	C79.32	—	D32.Ø	D42.Ø	D49.7
nerve	C72.5Ø	C79.49	—	D33.3	D43.3	D49.7
specified NEC	C72.59	C79.49	—	D33.3	D43.3	D49.7
craniobuccal pouch	C75.2	C79.89	DØ9.3	D35.2	D44.3	D49.7
craniopharyngeal (duct) (pouch)	C75.2	C79.89	DØ9.3	D35.3	D44.4	D49.7
cricoid	C13.Ø	C79.89	DØØ.Ø8	D1Ø.7	D37.Ø5	D49.Ø
cartilage	C32.3	C78.39	DØ2.Ø	D14.1	D38.Ø	D49.1
cricopharynx	C13.Ø	C79.89	DØØ.Ø8	D1Ø.7	D37.Ø5	D49.Ø
crypt of Morgagni	C21.8	C78.5	DØ1.3	D12.9	D37.8	D49.Ø
crystalline lens	C69.4-	C79.49	DØ9.2-	D31.4-	D48.7	D49.89
cul-de-sac (Douglas')	C48.1	C78.6	—	D2Ø.1	D48.4	D49.Ø
cuneiform cartilage	C32.3	C78.39	DØ2.Ø	D14.1	D38.Ø	D49.1
cutaneous—*see Neoplasm, skin*						
cutis—*see Neoplasm, skin*						
cystic (bile) duct (common)	C24.Ø	C78.89	DØ1.5	D13.5	D37.6	D49.Ø
dermis—*see Neoplasm, skin*						
diaphragm	C49.3	C79.89	—	D21.3	D48.1	D49.2
digestive organs, system, tube, or tract NEC	C26.9	C78.89	DØ1.9	D13.9	D37.9	D49.Ø
disc, intervertebral	C41.2	C79.51	—	D16.6	D48.Ø	D49.2
disease, generalized	C8Ø.Ø	—	—	—	—	—
disseminated	C8Ø.Ø	—	—	—	—	—
Douglas' cul-de-sac or pouch	C48.1	C78.6	—	D2Ø.1	D48.4	D49.Ø
duodenojejunal junction	C17.8	C78.4	DØ1.49	D13.39	D37.2	D49.Ø
duodenum	C17.Ø	C78.4	DØ1.49	D13.2	D37.2	D49.Ø
dura (cranial) (mater)	C7Ø.9	C79.49	—	D32.9	D42.9	D49.7
cerebral	C7Ø.Ø	C79.32	—	D32.Ø	D42.Ø	D49.7
spinal	C7Ø.1	C79.49	—	D32.1	D42.1	D49.7

TABLE OF NEOPLASMS

	Malignant Primary	Malignant Secondary	Ca in situ	Benign	Uncertain Behavior	Unspecified Behavior
ear (external) — *see also Neoplasm, skin, ear*	C44.2Ø-	C79.2	DØ4.2-	D23.2-	D48.5	D49.2
auricle or auris — *see also Neoplasm, skin, ear*	C44.2Ø-	C79.2	DØ4.2-	D23.2-	D48.5	D49.2
canal, external — *see also Neoplasm, skin, ear*	C44.2Ø-	C79.2	DØ4.2-	D23.2-	D48.5	D49.2
cartilage	C49.Ø	C79.89	—	D21.Ø	D48.1	D49.2
external meatus — *see also Neoplasm, skin, ear*	C44.2Ø-	C79.2	DØ4.2-	D23.2-	D48.5	D49.2
inner	C3Ø.1	C78.39	DØ2.3	D14.Ø	D38.5	D49.1
lobule — *see also Neoplasm, skin, ear*	C44.2Ø-	C79.2	DØ4.2-	D23.2-	D48.5	D49.2
middle	C3Ø.1	C78.39	DØ2.3	D14.Ø	D38.5	D49.1
overlapping lesion with accessory sinuses	C31.8	—	—	—	—	—
skin	C44.2Ø-	C79.2	DØ4.2-	D23.2-	D48.5	D49.2
basal cell carcinoma	C44.21-	—	—	—	—	—
specified type NEC	C44.29-	—	—	—	—	—
squamous cell carcinoma	C44.22-	—	—	—	—	—
earlobe	C44.2Ø-	C79.2	DØ4.2-	D23.2-	D48.5	D49.2
basal cell carcinoma	C44.21-	—	—	—	—	—
specified type NEC	C44.29-	—	—	—	—	—
squamous cell carcinoma	C44.22-	—	—	—	—	—
ejaculatory duct	C63.7	C79.82	DØ7.69	D29.8	D4Ø.8	D49.59
elbow NEC	C76.4-	C79.89	DØ4.6-	D36.7	D48.7	D49.89
endocardium	C38.Ø	C79.89	—	D15.1	D48.7	D49.89
endocervix (canal) (gland)	C53.Ø	C79.82	DØ6.Ø	D26.Ø	D39.Ø	D49.59
endocrine gland NEC	C75.9	C79.89	DØ9.3	D35.9	D44.9	D49.7
pluriglandular	C75.8	C79.89	DØ9.3	D35.7	D44.9	D49.7
endometrium (gland) (stroma)	C54.1	C79.82	DØ7.Ø	D26.1	D39.Ø	D49.59
ensiform cartilage	C41.3	C79.51	—	D16.7	D48.Ø	D49.2
enteric — *see Neoplasm, intestine*						
ependyma (brain)	C71.5	C79.31	—	D33.Ø	D43.Ø	D49.6
fourth ventricle	C71.7	C79.31	—	D33.1	D43.1	D49.6
epicardium	C38.Ø	C79.89	—	D15.1	D48.7	D49.89
epididymis	C63.Ø-	C79.82	DØ7.69	D29.3-	D4Ø.8	D49.59
epidural	C72.9	C79.49	—	D33.9	D43.9	D49.7
epiglottis	C32.1	C78.39	DØ2.Ø	D14.1	D38.Ø	D49.1
anterior aspect or surface	C1Ø.1	C79.89	DØØ.Ø8	D1Ø.5	D37.Ø5	D49.Ø
cartilage	C32.3	C78.39	DØ2.Ø	D14.1	D38.Ø	D49.1
free border (margin)	C1Ø.1	C79.89	DØØ.Ø8	D1Ø.5	D37.Ø5	D49.Ø
junctional region	C1Ø.8	C79.89	DØØ.Ø8	D1Ø.5	D37.Ø5	D49.Ø
posterior (laryngeal) surface	C32.1	C78.39	DØ2.Ø	D14.1	D38.Ø	D49.1
suprahyoid portion	C32.1	C78.39	DØ2.Ø	D14.1	D38.Ø	D49.1

	Malignant Primary	Malignant Secondary	Ca in situ	Benign	Uncertain Behavior	Unspecified Behavior
esophagogastric junction	C16.Ø	C78.89	DØØ.2	D13.1	D37.1	D49.Ø
esophagus	C15.9	C78.89	DØØ.1	D13.Ø	D37.8	D49.Ø
abdominal	C15.5	C78.89	DØØ.1	D13.Ø	D37.8	D49.Ø
cervical	C15.3	C78.89	DØØ.1	D13.Ø	D37.8	D49.Ø
distal (third)	C15.5	C78.89	DØØ.1	D13.Ø	D37.8	D49.Ø
lower (third)	C15.5	C78.89	DØØ.1	D13.Ø	D37.8	D49.Ø
middle (third)	C15.4	C78.89	DØØ.1	D13.Ø	D37.8	D49.Ø
overlapping lesion	C15.8	—	—	—	—	—
proximal (third)	C15.3	C78.89	DØØ.1	D13.Ø	D37.8	D49.Ø
thoracic	C15.4	C78.89	DØØ.1	D13.Ø	D37.8	D49.Ø
upper (third)	C15.3	C78.89	DØØ.1	D13.Ø	D37.8	D49.Ø
ethmoid (sinus)	C31.1	C78.39	DØ2.3	D14.Ø	D38.5	D49.1
bone or labyrinth	C41.Ø	C79.51	—	D16.4-	D48.Ø	D49.2
eustachian tube	C3Ø.1	C78.39	DØ2.3	D14.Ø	D38.5	D49.1
exocervix	C53.1	C79.82	DØ6.1	D26.Ø	D39.Ø	D49.59
external						
meatus (ear) — *see also Neoplasm, skin, ear*	C44.2Ø-	C79.2	DØ4.2-	D23.2-	D48.5	D49.2
os, cervix uteri	C53.1	C79.82	DØ6.1	D26.Ø	D39.Ø	D49.59
extradural	C72.9	C79.49	—	D33.9	D43.9	D49.7
extrahepatic (bile) duct	C24.Ø	C78.89	DØ1.5	D13.5	D37.6	D49.Ø
overlapping lesion with gallbladder	C24.8	—	—	—	—	—
extraocular muscle	C69.6-	C79.49	DØ9.2-	D31.6-	D48.7	D49.89
extrarectal	C76.3	C79.89	DØ9.8	D36.7	D48.7	D49.89
extremity	C76.8	C79.89	DØ4.8	D36.7	D48.7	D49.89
lower	C76.5-	C79.89	DØ4.7-	D36.7	D48.7	D49.89
upper	C76.4-	C79.89	DØ4.6-	D36.7	D48.7	D49.89
eye NEC	C69.9-	C79.49	DØ9.2	D31.9	D48.7	D49.89
overlapping sites	C69.8	—	—	—	—	—
eyeball	C69.9-	C79.49	DØ9.2-	D31.9-	D48.7	D49.89
eyebrow	C44.3Ø9	C79.2	DØ4.39	D23.39	D48.5	D49.2
basal cell carcinoma	C44.319	—	—	—	—	—
specified type NEC	C44.399	—	—	—	—	—
squamous cell carcinoma	C44.329	—	—	—	—	—
eyelid (lower) (skin) (upper)	C44.1Ø-	—	—	—	—	—
basal cell carcinoma	C44.11-	—	—	—	—	—
cartilage	C49.Ø	C79.89	—	D21.Ø	D48.1	D49.2
specified type NEC	C44.19-	—	—	—	—	—
squamous cell carcinoma	C44.12-	—	—	—	—	—
face NEC	C76.Ø	C79.89	DØ4.39	D36.7	D48.7	D49.89
fallopian tube (accessory)	C57.Ø-	C79.82	DØ7.39	D28.2	D39.8	D49.59
falx (cerebella) (cerebri)	C7Ø.Ø	C79.32	—	D32.Ø	D42.Ø	D49.7

◄ New ⇐ Revised ~~deleted~~ Deleted

	Malignant Primary	Malignant Secondary	Ca in situ	Benign	Uncertain Behavior	Unspecified Behavior
fascia — *see also Neoplasm, connective tissue*						
palmar	C49.1-	C79.89	—	D21.1-	D48.1	D49.2
plantar	C49.2-	C79.89	—	D21.2-	D48.1	D49.2
fatty tissue — *see Neoplasm, connective tissue*						
fauces, faucial NEC	C1Ø.9	C79.89	DØØ.Ø8	D1Ø.5	D37.Ø5	D49.Ø
pillars	CØ9.1	C79.89	DØØ.Ø8	D1Ø.5	D37.Ø5	D49.Ø
tonsil	CØ9.9	C79.89	DØØ.Ø8	D1Ø.4	D37.Ø5	D49.Ø
femur (any part)	C4Ø.2-	—	—	D16.2-	—	—
fetal membrane	C58	C79.82	DØ7.Ø	D26.7	D39.2	D49.59
fibrous tissue — *see Neoplasm, connective tissue*						
fibula (any part)	C4Ø.2-	C79.51	—	D16.2-	—	—
filum terminale	C72.Ø	C79.49	—	D33.4	D43.4	D49.7
finger NEC	C76.4-	C79.89	DØ4.6-	D36.7	D48.7	D49.89
flank NEC	C76.8	C79.89	DØ4.5	D36.7	D48.7	D49.89
follicle, nabothian	C53.Ø	C79.82	DØ6.Ø	D26.Ø	D39.Ø	D49.59
foot NEC	C76.5-	C79.89	DØ4.7-	D36.7	D48.7	D49.89
forearm NEC	C76.4-	C79.89	DØ4.6-	D36.7	D48.7	D49.89
forehead (skin)	C44.3Ø9	C79.2	DØ4.39	D23.39	D48.5	D49.2
basal cell carcinoma	C44.319	—	—	—	—	—
specified type NEC	C44.399	—	—	—	—	—
squamous cell carcinoma	C44.329	—	—	—	—	—
foreskin	C6Ø.Ø	C79.82	DØ7.4	D29.Ø	D4Ø.8	D49.59
fornix						
pharyngeal	C11.3	C79.89	DØØ.Ø8	D1Ø.6	D37.Ø5	D49.Ø
vagina	C52	C79.82	DØ7.2	D28.1	D39.8	D49.59
fossa (of)						
anterior (cranial)	C71.9	C79.31	—	D33.2	D43.2	D49.6
cranial	C71.9	C79.31	—	D33.2	D43.2	D49.6
ischiorectal	C76.3	C79.89	DØ9.8	D36.7	D48.7	D49.89
middle (cranial)	C71.9	C79.31	—	D33.2	D43.2	D49.6
piriform	C12	C79.89	DØØ.Ø8	D1Ø.7	D37.Ø5	D49.Ø
pituitary	C75.1	C79.89	DØ9.3	D35.2	D44.3	D49.7
posterior (cranial)	C71.9	C79.31	—	D33.2	D43.2	D49.6
pterygoid	C49.Ø	C79.89	—	D21.Ø	D48.1	D49.2
pyriform	C12	C79.89	DØØ.Ø8	D1Ø.7	D37.Ø5	D49.Ø
Rosenmuller	C11.2	C79.89	DØØ.Ø8	D1Ø.6	D37.Ø5	D49.Ø
tonsillar	CØ9.Ø	C79.89	DØØ.Ø8	D1Ø.5	D37.Ø5	D49.Ø
fourchette	C51.9	C79.82	DØ7.1	D28.Ø	D39.8	D49.59
frenulum						
labii — *see Neoplasm, lip, internal*						
linguae	CØ2.2	C79.89	DØØ.Ø7	D1Ø.1	D37.Ø2	D49.Ø

	Malignant Primary	Malignant Secondary	Ca in situ	Benign	Uncertain Behavior	Unspecified Behavior
frontal						
bone	C41.Ø	C79.51	—	D16.4-	D48.Ø	D49.2
lobe, brain	C71.1	C79.31	—	D33.Ø	D43.Ø	D49.6
pole	C71.1	C79.31	—	D33.Ø	D43.Ø	D49.6
sinus	C31.2	C78.39	DØ2.3	D14.Ø	D38.5	D49.1
fundus						
stomach	C16.1	C78.89	DØØ.2	D13.1	D37.1	D49.Ø
uterus	C54.3	C79.82	DØ7.Ø	D26.1	D39.Ø	D49.59
gall duct (extrahepatic)	C24.Ø	C78.89	DØ1.5	D13.5	D37.6	D49.Ø
intrahepatic	C22.1	C78.7	DØ1.5	D13.4	D37.6	D49.Ø
gallbladder	C23	C78.89	DØ1.5	D13.5	D37.6	D49.Ø
overlapping lesion with extrahepatic bile ducts	C24.8	—	—	—	—	—
ganglia — *see also Neoplasm, nerve, peripheral*	C47.9	C79.89	—	D36.1Ø	D48.2	D49.2
basal	C71.Ø	C79.31	—	D33.Ø	D43.Ø	D49.6
cranial nerve	C72.5Ø	C79.49	—	D33.3	D43.3	D49.7
Gartner's duct	C52	C79.82	DØ7.2	D28.1	D39.8	D49.59
gastric — *see Neoplasm, stomach*						
gastrocolic	C26.9	C78.89	DØ1.9	D13.9	D37.9	D49.Ø
gastroesophageal junction	C16.Ø	C78.89	DØØ.2	D13.1	D37.1	D49.Ø
gastrointestinal (tract) NEC	C26.9	C78.89	DØ1.9	D13.9	D37.9	D49.Ø
generalized	C8Ø.Ø	—	—	—	—	—
genital organ or tract						
female NEC	C57.9	C79.82	DØ7.3Ø	D28.9	D39.9	D49.59
overlapping lesion	C57.8	—	—	—	—	—
specified site NEC	C57.7	C79.82	DØ7.39	D28.7	D39.8	D49.59
male NEC	C63.9	C79.82	DØ7.6Ø	D29.9	D4Ø.9	D49.59
overlapping lesion	C63.8	—	—	—	—	—
specified site NEC	C63.7	C79.82	DØ7.69	D29.8	D4Ø.8	D49.59
genitourinary tract						
female	C57.9	C79.82	DØ7.3Ø	D28.9	D39.9	D49.59
male	C63.9	C79.82	DØ7.6Ø	D29.9	D4Ø.9	D49.59
gingiva (alveolar) (marginal)	CØ3.9	C79.89	DØØ.Ø3	D1Ø.39	D37.Ø9	D49.Ø
lower	CØ3.1	C79.89	DØØ.Ø3	D1Ø.39	D37.Ø9	D49.Ø
mandibular	CØ3.1	C79.89	DØØ.Ø3	D1Ø.39	D37.Ø9	D49.Ø
maxillary	CØ3.Ø	C79.89	DØØ.Ø3	D1Ø.39	D37.Ø9	D49.Ø
upper	CØ3.Ø	C79.89	DØØ.Ø3	D1Ø.39	D37.Ø9	D49.Ø
gland, glandular (lymphatic) (system) — *see also Neoplasm, lymph gland*						
endocrine NEC	C75.9	C79.89	DØ9.3	D35.9	D44.9	D49.7
salivary — *see Neoplasm, salivary gland*						

TABLE OF NEOPLASMS

	Malignant Primary	Malignant Secondary	Ca in situ	Benign	Uncertain Behavior	Unspecified Behavior
glans penis	C6Ø.1	C79.82	DØ7.4	D29.Ø	D4Ø.8	D49.59
globus pallidus	C71.Ø	C79.31	—	D33.Ø	D43.Ø	D49.6
glomus						
coccygeal	C49.5	C79.89	—	D21.5	D48.1	D49.2
jugularis	C75.5	C79.89	—	D35.6	D44.7	D49.7
glosso-epiglottic fold(s)	C1Ø.1	C79.89	DØØ.Ø8	D1Ø.5	D37.Ø5	D49.Ø
glossopalatine fold	CØ9.1	C79.89	DØØ.Ø8	D1Ø.5	D37.Ø5	D49.Ø
glossopharyngeal sulcus	CØ9.Ø	C79.89	DØØ.Ø8	D1Ø.5	D37.Ø5	D49.Ø
glottis	C32.Ø	C78.39	DØ2.Ø	D14.1	D38.Ø	D49.1
gluteal region	C76.3	C79.89	DØ4.5	D36.7	D48.7	D49.89
great vessels NEC	C49.3	C79.89	—	D21.3	D48.1	D49.2
groin NEC	C76.3	C79.89	DØ4.5	D36.7	D48.7	D49.89
gum	CØ3.9	C79.89	DØØ.Ø3	D1Ø.39	D37.Ø9	D49.Ø
lower	CØ3.1	C79.89	DØØ.Ø3	D1Ø.39	D37.Ø9	D49.Ø
upper	CØ3.Ø	C79.89	DØØ.Ø3	D1Ø.39	D37.Ø9	D49.Ø
hand NEC	C76.4-	C79.89	DØ4.6-	D36.7	D48.7	D49.89
head NEC	C76.Ø	C79.89	DØ4.4	D36.7	D48.7	D49.89
heart	C38.Ø	C79.89	—	D15.1	D48.7	D49.89
heel NEC	C76.5-	C79.89	DØ4.7-	D36.7	D48.7	D49.89
helix — *see also Neoplasm, skin, ear*	C44.2Ø-	C79.2	DØ4.2-	D23.2-	D48.5	D49.2
hematopoietic, hemopoietic tissue NEC	C96.9	—	—	—	—	—
specified NEC	C96.Z	—	—	—	—	—
hemisphere, cerebral	C71.Ø	C79.31	—	D33.Ø	D43.Ø	D49.6
hemorrhoidal zone	C21.1	C78.5	DØ1.3	D12.9	D37.8	D49.Ø
hepatic — *see also Index to disease, by histology*	C22.9	C78.7	DØ1.5	D13.4	D37.6	D49.Ø
duct (bile)	C24.Ø	C78.89	DØ1.5	D13.5	D37.6	D49.Ø
flexure (colon)	C18.3	C78.5	DØ1.Ø	D12.3	D37.4	D49.Ø
primary	C22.8	C78.7	DØ1.5	D13.4	D37.6	D49.Ø
hepatobiliary	C24.9	C79.89	DØ1.5	D13.5	D37.6	D49.Ø
hepatoblastoma	C22.2	C78.7	DØ1.5	D13.4	D37.6	D49.Ø
hepatoma	C22.Ø	C78.7	DØ1.5	D13.4	D37.6	D49.Ø
hilus of lung	C34.Ø-	C78.Ø-	DØ2.2-	D14.3-	D38.1	D49.1
hip NEC	C76.5-	C79.89	DØ4.7-	D36.7	D48.7	D49.89
hippocampus, brain	C71.2	C79.31	—	D33.Ø	D43.Ø	D49.6
humerus (any part)	C4Ø.Ø-	C79.51	—	D16.Ø-	—	—
hymen	C52	C79.82	DØ7.2	D28.1	D39.8	D49.59
hypopharynx, hypopharyngeal NEC	C13.9	C79.89	DØØ.Ø8	D1Ø.7	D37.Ø5	D49.Ø
overlapping lesion	C13.8	—	—	—	—	—
postcricoid region	C13.Ø	C79.89	DØØ.Ø8	D1Ø.7	D37.Ø5	D49.Ø
posterior wall	C13.2	C79.89	DØØ.Ø8	D1Ø.7	D37.Ø5	D49.Ø
pyriform fossa (sinus)	C12	C79.89	DØØ.Ø8	D1Ø.7	D37.Ø5	D49.Ø
hypophysis	C75.1	C79.89	DØ9.3	D35.2	D44.3	D49.7
hypothalamus	C71.Ø	C79.31	—	D33.Ø	D43.Ø	D49.6
ileocecum, ileocecal (coil) (junction) (valve)	C18.Ø	C78.5	DØ1.Ø	D12.Ø	D37.4	D49.Ø
ileum	C17.2	C78.4	DØ1.49	D13.39	D37.2	D49.Ø
ilium	C41.4	C79.51	—	D16.8	D48.Ø	D49.2
immunoproliferative NEC	C88.9	—	—	—	—	—
infraclavicular (region)	C76.1	C79.89	DØ4.5	D36.7	D48.7	D49.89
inguinal (region)	C76.3	C79.89	DØ4.5	D36.7	D48.7	D49.89
insula	C71.Ø	C79.31	—	D33.Ø	D43.Ø	D49.6
insular tissue (pancreas)	C25.4	C78.89	DØ1.7	D13.7	D37.8	D49.Ø
brain	C71.Ø	C79.31	—	D33.Ø	D43.Ø	D49.6
interarytenoid fold	C13.1	C79.89	DØØ.Ø8	D1Ø.7	D37.Ø5	D49.Ø
hypopharyngeal aspect	C13.1	C79.89	DØØ.Ø8	D1Ø.7	D37.Ø5	D49.Ø
laryngeal aspect	C32.1	C78.39	DØ2.Ø	D14.1	D38.Ø	D49.1
marginal zone	C13.1	C79.89	DØØ.Ø8	D1Ø.7	D37.Ø5	D49.Ø
interdental papillae	CØ3.9	C79.89	DØØ.Ø3	D1Ø.39	D37.Ø9	D49.Ø
lower	CØ3.1	C79.89	DØØ.Ø3	D1Ø.39	D37.Ø9	D49.Ø
upper	CØ3.Ø	C79.89	DØØ.Ø3	D1Ø.39	D37.Ø9	D49.Ø
internal						
capsule	C71.Ø	C79.31	—	D33.Ø	D43.Ø	D49.6
os (cervix)	C53.Ø	C79.82	DØ6.Ø	D26.Ø	D39.Ø	D49.59
intervertebral cartilage or disc	C41.2	C79.51	—	D16.6	D48.Ø	D49.2
intestine, intestinal	C26.Ø	C78.8Ø	DØ1.4Ø	D13.9	D37.8	D49.Ø
large	C18.9	C78.5	DØ1.Ø	D12.6	D37.4	D49.Ø
appendix	C18.1	C78.5	DØ1.Ø	D12.1	D37.3	D49.Ø
caput coli	C18.Ø	C78.5	DØ1.Ø	D12.Ø	D37.4	D49.Ø
cecum	C18.Ø	C78.5	DØ1.Ø	D12.Ø	D37.4	D49.Ø
colon	C18.9	C78.5	DØ1.Ø	D12.6	D37.4	D49.Ø
and rectum	C19	C78.5	DØ1.1	D12.7	D37.5	D49.Ø
ascending	C18.2	C78.5	DØ1.Ø	D12.2	D37.4	D49.Ø
caput	C18.Ø	C78.5	DØ1.Ø	D12.Ø	D37.4	D49.Ø
descending	C18.6	C78.5	DØ1.Ø	D12.4	D37.4	D49.Ø
distal	C18.6	C78.5	DØ1.Ø	D12.4	D37.4	D49.Ø
left	C18.6	C78.5	DØ1.Ø	D12.4	D37.4	D49.Ø
overlapping lesion	C18.8	—	—	—	—	—
pelvic	C18.7	C78.5	DØ1.Ø	D12.5	D37.4	D49.Ø
right	C18.2	C78.5	DØ1.Ø	D12.2	D37.4	D49.Ø
sigmoid (flexure)	C18.7	C78.5	DØ1.Ø	D12.5	D37.4	D49.Ø
transverse	C18.4	C78.5	DØ1.Ø	D12.3	D37.4	D49.Ø
hepatic flexure	C18.3	C78.5	DØ1.Ø	D12.3	D37.4	D49.Ø
ileocecum, ileocecal (coil) (valve)	C18.Ø	C78.5	DØ1.Ø	D12.Ø	D37.4	D49.Ø
overlapping lesion	C18.8	—	—	—	—	—

TABLE OF NEOPLASMS

◀ New ◀ Revised ~~deleted~~ Deleted

	Malignant Primary	Malignant Secondary	Ca in situ	Benign	Uncertain Behavior	Unspecified Behavior
intestine, intestinal *(Continued)*						
large *(Continued)*						
sigmoid flexure (lower) (upper)	C18.7	C78.5	DØ1.Ø	D12.5	D37.4	D49.Ø
splenic flexure	C18.5	C78.5	DØ1.Ø	D12.3	D37.4	D49.Ø
small	C17.9	C78.4	DØ1.4Ø	D13.3Ø	D37.2	D49.Ø
duodenum	C17.Ø	C78.4	DØ1.49	D13.2	D37.2	D49.Ø
ileum	C17.2	C78.4	DØ1.49	D13.39	D37.2	D49.Ø
jejunum	C17.1	C78.4	DØ1.49	D13.39	D37.2	D49.Ø
overlapping lesion	C17.8	—	—	—	—	—
tract NEC	C26.Ø	C78.89	DØ1.4Ø	D13.9	D37.8	D49.Ø
intra-abdominal	C76.2	C79.89	DØ9.8	D36.7	D48.7	D49.89
intracranial NEC	C71.9	C79.31	—	D33.2	D43.2	D49.6
intrahepatic (bile) duct	C22.1	C78.7	DØ1.5	D13.4	D37.6	D49.Ø
intraocular	C69.9-	C79.49	DØ9.2-	D31.9-	D48.7	D49.89
intraorbital	C69.6-	C79.49	DØ9.2-	D31.6-	D48.7	D49.89
intrasellar	C75.1	C79.89	DØ9.3	D35.2	D44.3	D49.7
intrathoracic (cavity) (organs)	C76.1	C79.89	DØ9.8	D15.9	D48.7	D49.89
specified NEC	C76.1	C79.89	DØ9.8	D15.7	—	—
iris	C69.4-	C79.49	DØ9.2-	D31.4-	D48.7	D49.89
ischiorectal (fossa)	C76.3	C79.89	DØ9.8	D36.7	D48.7	D49.89
ischium	C41.4	C79.51	—	D16.8	D48.Ø	D49.2
island of Reil	C71.Ø	C79.31	—	D33.Ø	D43.Ø	D49.6
islands or islets of Langerhans	C25.4	C78.89	DØ1.7	D13.7	D37.8	D49.Ø
isthmus uteri	C54.Ø	C79.82	DØ7.Ø	D26.1	D39.Ø	D49.59
jaw	C76.Ø	C79.89	DØ9.8	D36.7	D48.7	D49.89
bone	C41.1	C79.51	—	D16.5-	D48.Ø	D49.2
lower	C41.1	C79.51	—	D16.5-	—	—
upper	C41.Ø	C79.51	—	D16.4-	—	—
carcinoma (any type) (lower) (upper)	C76.Ø	C79.89	—	—	—	—
skin—*see also Neoplasm, skin, face*	C44.3Ø9	C79.2	DØ4.39	D23.39	D48.5	D49.2
soft tissues	CØ3.9	C79.89	DØØ.Ø3	D1Ø.39	D37.Ø9	D49.Ø
lower	CØ3.1	C79.89	DØØ.Ø3	D1Ø.39	D37.Ø9	D49.Ø
upper	CØ3.Ø	C79.89	DØØ.Ø3	D1Ø.39	D37.Ø9	D49.Ø
jejunum	C17.1	C78.4	DØ1.49	D13.39	D37.2	D49.Ø
joint NEC—*see also Neoplasm, bone*	C41.9	C79.51	—	D16.9-	D48.Ø	D49.2
acromioclavicular	C4Ø.Ø-	C79.51	—	D16.Ø-	—	—
bursa or synovial membrane—*see Neoplasm, connective tissue*						
costovertebral	C41.3	C79.51	—	D16.7	D48.Ø	D49.2
sternocostal	C41.3	C79.51	—	D16.7	D48.Ø	D49.2
temporomandibular	C41.1	C79.51	—	D16.5-	D48.Ø	D49.2

	Malignant Primary	Malignant Secondary	Ca in situ	Benign	Uncertain Behavior	Unspecified Behavior
junction						
anorectal	C21.8	C78.5	DØ1.3	D12.9	D37.8	D49.Ø
cardioesophageal	C16.Ø	C78.89	DØØ.2	D13.1	D37.1	D49.Ø
esophagogastric	C16.Ø	C78.89	DØØ.2	D13.1	D37.1	D49.Ø
gastroesophageal	C16.Ø	C78.89	DØØ.2	D13.1	D37.1	D49.Ø
hard and soft palate	CØ5.9	C79.89	DØØ.ØØ	D1Ø.39	D37.Ø9	D49.Ø
ileocecal	C18.Ø	C78.5	DØ1.Ø	D12.Ø	D37.4	D49.Ø
pelvirectal	C19	C78.5	DØ1.1	D12.7	D37.5	D49.Ø
pelviureteric	C65.-	C79.Ø-	DØ9.19	D3Ø.1-	D41.1-	D49.59
rectosigmoid	C19	C78.5	DØ1.1	D12.7	D37.5	D49.Ø
squamocolumnar, of cervix	C53.8	C79.82	DØ6.7	D26.Ø	D39.Ø	D49.59
Kaposi's sarcoma—*see Kaposi's, sarcoma*						
kidney (parenchymal)	C64.-	C79.Ø-	DØ9.19	D3Ø.Ø-	D41.Ø-	D49.51-
calyx	C65.-	C79.Ø-	DØ9.19	D3Ø.1-	D41.1-	D49.51-
hilus	C65.-	C79.Ø-	DØ9.19	D3Ø.1-	D41.1-	D49.51-
pelvis	C65.-	C79.Ø-	DØ9.19	D3Ø.1-	D41.1-	D49.51-
knee NEC	C76.5-	C79.89	DØ4.7-	D36.7	D48.7	D49.89
labia (skin)	C51.9	C79.82	DØ7.1	D28.Ø	D39.8	D49.59
majora	C51.Ø	C79.82	DØ7.1	D28.Ø	D39.8	D49.59
minora	C51.1	C79.82	DØ7.1	D28.Ø	D39.8	D49.59
labial—*see also Neoplasm, lip*	CØØ.9	C79.89	DØØ.Ø1	D1Ø.Ø	D37.Ø1	D49.Ø
sulcus (lower) (upper)	CØ6.1	C79.89	DØØ.Ø2	D1Ø.39	D37.Ø9	D49.Ø
labium (skin)	C51.9	C79.82	DØ7.1	D28.Ø	D39.8	D49.59
majus	C51.Ø	C79.82	DØ7.1	D28.Ø	D39.8	D49.59
minus	C51.1	C79.82	DØ7.1	D28.Ø	D39.8	D49.59
lacrimal						
canaliculi	C69.5-	C79.49	DØ9.2-	D31.5-	D48.7	D49.89
duct (nasal)	C69.5-	C79.49	DØ9.2-	D31.5-	D48.7	D49.89
gland	C69.5-	C79.49	DØ9.2-	D31.5-	D48.7	D49.89
punctum	C69.5-	C79.49	DØ9.2-	D31.5-	D48.7	D49.89
sac	C69.5-	C79.49	DØ9.2-	D31.5-	D48.7	D49.89
Langerhans, islands or islets	C25.4	C78.89	DØ1.7	D13.7	D37.8	D49.Ø
laryngopharynx	C13.9	C79.89	DØØ.Ø8	D1Ø.7	D37.Ø5	D49.Ø
larynx, laryngeal NEC	C32.9	C78.39	DØ2.Ø	D14.1	D38.Ø	D49.1
aryepiglottic fold	C32.1	C78.39	DØ2.Ø	D14.1	D38.Ø	D49.1
cartilage (arytenoid) (cricoid) (cuneiform) (thyroid)	C32.3	C78.39	DØ2.Ø	D14.1	D38.Ø	D49.1
commissure (anterior) (posterior)	C32.Ø	C78.39	DØ2.Ø	D14.1	D38.Ø	D49.1
extrinsic NEC	C32.1	C78.39	DØ2.Ø	D14.1	D38.Ø	D49.1
meaning hypopharynx	C13.9	C79.89	DØØ.Ø8	D1Ø.7	D37.Ø5	D49.Ø
interarytenoid fold	C32.1	C78.39	DØ2.Ø	D14.1	D38.Ø	D49.1
intrinsic	C32.Ø	C78.39	DØ2.Ø	D14.1	D38.Ø	D49.1

TABLE OF NEOPLASMS

◄ New ⬅ Revised ~~deleted~~ Deleted

TABLE OF NEOPLASMS

	Malignant Primary	Malignant Secondary	Ca in situ	Benign	Uncertain Behavior	Unspecified Behavior
larynx, laryngeal NEC *(Continued)*						
overlapping lesion	C32.8	—	—	—	—	—
ventricular band	C32.1	C78.39	D02.0	D14.1	D38.0	D49.1
leg NEC	C76.5-	C79.89	D04.7-	D36.7	D48.7	D49.89
lens, crystalline	C69.4-	C79.49	D09.2-	D31.4-	D48.7	D49.89
lid (lower) (upper)	C44.10-	C79.2	D04.1-	D23.1-	D48.5	D49.2
basal cell carcinoma	C44.11-	—	—	—	—	—
specified type NEC	C44.19-	—	—	—	—	—
squamous cell carcinoma	C44.12-	—	—	—	—	—
ligament — *see also Neoplasm, connective tissue*						
broad	C57.1	C79.82	D07.39	D28.2	D39.8	D49.59
Mackenrodt's	C57.7	C79.82	D07.39	D28.7	D39.8	D49.59
non-uterine — *see Neoplasm, connective tissue*						
round	C57.2	C79.82	—	D28.2	D39.8	D49.59
sacro-uterine	C57.3	C79.82	—	D28.2	D39.8	D49.59
uterine	C57.3	C79.82	—	D28.2	D39.8	D49.59
utero-ovarian	C57.7	C79.82	D07.39	D28.2	D39.8	D49.59
uterosacral	C57.3	C79.82	—	D28.2	D39.8	D49.59
limb	C76.8	C79.89	D04.8	D36.7	D48.7	D49.89
lower	C76.5-	C79.89	D04.7-	D36.7	D48.7	D49.89
upper	C76.4-	C79.89	D04.6-	D36.7	D48.7	D49.89
limbus of cornea	C69.1-	C79.49	D09.2-	D31.1-	D48.7	D49.89
lingual NEC — *see also Neoplasm, tongue*	C02.9	C79.89	D00.07	D10.1	D37.02	D49.0
lingula, lung	C34.1-	C78.0-	D02.2-	D14.3-	D38.1	D49.1
lip	C00.9	C79.89	D00.01	D10.0	D37.01	D49.0
buccal aspect — *see Neoplasm, lip, internal*						
commissure	C00.6	C79.89	D00.01	D10.0	D37.01	D49.0
external	C00.2	C79.89	D00.01	D10.0	D37.01	D49.0
lower	C00.1	C79.89	D00.01	D10.0	D37.01	D49.0
upper	C00.0	C79.89	D00.01	D10.0	D37.01	D49.0
frenulum — *see Neoplasm, lip, internal*						
inner aspect — *see Neoplasm, lip, internal*						
internal	C00.5	C79.89	D00.01	D10.0	D37.01	D49.0
lower	C00.4	C79.89	D00.01	D10.0	D37.01	D49.0
upper	C00.3	C79.89	D00.01	D10.0	D37.01	D49.0
lipstick area	C00.2	C79.89	D00.01	D10.0	D37.01	D49.0
lower	C00.1	C79.89	D00.01	D10.0	D37.01	D49.0
upper	C00.0	C79.89	D00.01	D10.0	D37.01	D49.0

	Malignant Primary	Malignant Secondary	Ca in situ	Benign	Uncertain Behavior	Unspecified Behavior
lip *(Continued)*						
lower	C00.1	C79.89	D00.01	D10.0	D37.01	D49.0
internal	C00.4	C79.89	D00.01	D10.0	D37.01	D49.0
mucosa — *see Neoplasm, lip, internal*						
oral aspect — *see Neoplasm, lip, internal*						
overlapping lesion	C00.8	—	—	—	—	—
with oral cavity or pharynx	C14.8	—	—	—	—	—
skin (commissure) (lower) (upper)	C44.00	C79.2	D04.0	D23.0	D48.5	D49.2
basal cell carcinoma	C44.01	—	—	—	—	—
specified type NEC	C44.09	—	—	—	—	—
squamous cell carcinoma	C44.02	—	—	—	—	—
upper	C00.0	C79.89	D00.01	D10.0	D37.01	D49.0
internal	C00.3	C79.89	D00.01	D10.0	D37.01	D49.0
vermilion border	C00.2	C79.89	D00.01	D10.0	D37.01	D49.0
lower	C00.1	C79.89	D00.01	D10.0	D37.01	D49.0
upper	C00.0	C79.89	D00.01	D10.0	D37.01	D49.0
lipomatous — *see Lipoma, by site*						
liver — *see also Index to disease, by histology*	C22.9	C78.7	D01.5	D13.4	D37.6	D49.0
primary	C22.8	C78.7	D01.5	D13.4	D37.6	D49.0
lumbosacral plexus	C47.5	C79.89	—	D36.16	D48.2	D49.2
lung	C34.9-	C78.0-	D02.2-	D14.3-	D38.1	D49.1
azygos lobe	C34.1-	C78.0-	D02.2-	D14.3-	D38.1	D49.1
carina	C34.0-	C78.0-	D02.2-	D14.3-	D38.1	D49.1
hilus	C34.0-	C78.0-	D02.2-	D14.3-	D38.1	D49.1
lingula	C34.1-	C78.0-	D02.2-	D14.3-	D38.1	D49.1
lobe NEC	C34.9-	C78.0-	D02.2-	D14.3-	D38.1	D49.1
lower lobe	C34.3-	C78.0-	D02.2-	D14.3-	D38.1	D49.1
main bronchus	C34.0-	C78.0-	D02.2-	D14.3-	D38.1	D49.1
mesothelioma — *see Mesothelioma*						
middle lobe	C34.2	C78.0-	D02.21	D14.31	D38.1	D49.1
overlapping lesion	C34.8-	—	—	—	—	—
upper lobe	C34.1-	C78.0-	D02.2-	D14.3-	D38.1	D49.1
lymph, lymphatic channel NEC	C49.9	C79.89	—	D21.9	D48.1	D49.2
gland (secondary)	—	C77.9	—	D36.0	D48.7	D49.89
abdominal	—	C77.2	—	D36.0	D48.7	D49.89
aortic	—	C77.2	—	D36.0	D48.7	D49.89
arm	—	C77.3	—	D36.0	D48.7	D49.89
auricular (anterior) (posterior)	—	C77.0	—	D36.0	D48.7	D49.89

	Malignant Primary	Malignant Secondary	Ca in situ	Benign	Uncertain Behavior	Unspecified Behavior
lymph, lymphatic channel NEC *(Continued)*						
gland *(Continued)*						
axilla, axillary	—	C77.3	—	D36.Ø	D48.7	D49.89
brachial	—	C77.3	—	D36.Ø	D48.7	D49.89
bronchial	—	C77.1	—	D36.Ø	D48.7	D49.89
bronchopulmonary	—	C77.1	—	D36.Ø	D48.7	D49.89
celiac	—	C77.2	—	D36.Ø	D48.7	D49.89
cervical	—	C77.Ø	—	D36.Ø	D48.7	D49.89
cervicofacial	—	C77.Ø	—	D36.Ø	D48.7	D49.89
Cloquet	—	C77.4	—	D36.Ø	D48.7	D49.89
colic	—	C77.2	—	D36.Ø	D48.7	D49.89
common duct	—	C77.2	—	D36.Ø	D48.7	D49.89
cubital	—	C77.3	—	D36.Ø	D48.7	D49.89
diaphragmatic	—	C77.1	—	D36.Ø	D48.7	D49.89
epigastric, inferior	—	C77.1	—	D36.Ø	D48.7	D49.89
epitrochlear	—	C77.3	—	D36.Ø	D48.7	D49.89
esophageal	—	C77.1	—	D36.Ø	D48.7	D49.89
face	—	C77.Ø	—	D36.Ø	D48.7	D49.89
femoral	—	C77.4	—	D36.Ø	D48.7	D49.89
gastric	—	C77.2	—	D36.Ø	D48.7	D49.89
groin	—	C77.4	—	D36.Ø	D48.7	D49.89
head	—	C77.Ø	—	D36.Ø	D48.7	D49.89
hepatic	—	C77.2	—	D36.Ø	D48.7	D49.89
hilar (pulmonary)	—	C77.1	—	D36.Ø	D48.7	D49.89
splenic	—	C77.2	—	D36.Ø	D48.7	D49.89
hypogastric	—	C77.5	—	D36.Ø	D48.7	D49.89
ileocolic	—	C77.2	—	D36.Ø	D48.7	D49.89
iliac	—	C77.5	—	D36.Ø	D48.7	D49.89
infraclavicular	—	C77.3	—	D36.Ø	D48.7	D49.89
inguina, inguinal	—	C77.4	—	D36.Ø	D48.7	D49.89
innominate	—	C77.1	—	D36.Ø	D48.7	D49.89
intercostal	—	C77.1	—	D36.Ø	D48.7	D49.89
intestinal	—	C77.2	—	D36.Ø	D48.7	D49.89
intrabdominal	—	C77.2	—	D36.Ø	D48.7	D49.89
intrapelvic	—	C77.5	—	D36.Ø	D48.7	D49.89
intrathoracic	—	C77.1	—	D36.Ø	D48.7	D49.89
jugular	—	C77.Ø	—	D36.Ø	D48.7	D49.89
leg	—	C77.4	—	D36.Ø	D48.7	D49.89
limb						
lower	—	C77.4	—	D36.Ø	D48.7	D49.89
upper	—	C77.3	—	D36.Ø	D48.7	D49.89
lower limb	—	C77.4	—	D36.Ø	D48.7	D49.89
lumbar	—	C77.2	—	D36.Ø	D48.7	D49.89

	Malignant Primary	Malignant Secondary	Ca in situ	Benign	Uncertain Behavior	Unspecified Behavior
lymph, lymphatic channel NEC *(Continued)*						
gland *(Continued)*						
mandibular	—	C77.Ø	—	D36.Ø	D48.7	D49.89
mediastinal	—	C77.1	—	D36.Ø	D48.7	D49.89
mesenteric (inferior) (superior)	—	C77.2	—	D36.Ø	D48.7	D49.89
midcolic	—	C77.2	—	D36.Ø	D48.7	D49.89
multiple sites in categories C77.Ø - C77.5	—	C77.8	—	D36.Ø	D48.7	D49.89
neck	—	C77.Ø	—	D36.Ø	D48.7	D49.89
obturator	—	C77.5	—	D36.Ø	D48.7	D49.89
occipital	—	C77.Ø	—	D36.Ø	D48.7	D49.89
pancreatic	—	C77.2	—	D36.Ø	D48.7	D49.89
para-aortic	—	C77.2	—	D36.Ø	D48.7	D49.89
paracervical	—	C77.5	—	D36.Ø	D48.7	D49.89
parametrial	—	C77.5	—	D36.Ø	D48.7	D49.89
parasternal	—	C77.1	—	D36.Ø	D48.7	D49.89
parotid	—	C77.Ø	—	D36.Ø	D48.7	D49.89
pectoral	—	C77.3	—	D36.Ø	D48.7	D49.89
pelvic	—	C77.5	—	D36.Ø	D48.7	D49.89
peri-aortic	—	C77.2	—	D36.Ø	D48.7	D49.89
peripancreatic	—	C77.2	—	D36.Ø	D48.7	D49.89
popliteal	—	C77.4	—	D36.Ø	D48.7	D49.89
porta hepatis	—	C77.2	—	D36.Ø	D48.7	D49.89
portal	—	C77.2	—	D36.Ø	D48.7	D49.89
preauricular	—	C77.Ø	—	D36.Ø	D48.7	D49.89
prelaryngeal	—	C77.Ø	—	D36.Ø	D48.7	D49.89
presymphysial	—	C77.5	—	D36.Ø	D48.7	D49.89
pretracheal	—	C77.Ø	—	D36.Ø	D48.7	D49.89
primary (any site) NEC	C96.9	—	—	—	—	—
pulmonary (hiler)	—	C77.1	—	D36.Ø	D48.7	D49.89
pyloric	—	C77.2	—	D36.Ø	D48.7	D49.89
retroperitoneal	—	C77.2	—	D36.Ø	D48.7	D49.89
retropharyngeal	—	C77.Ø	—	D36.Ø	D48.7	D49.89
Rosenmuller's	—	C77.4	—	D36.Ø	D48.7	D49.89
sacral	—	C77.5	—	D36.Ø	D48.7	D49.89
scalene	—	C77.Ø	—	D36.Ø	D48.7	D49.89
site NEC	—	C77.9	—	D36.Ø	D48.7	D49.89
splenic (hilar)	—	C77.2	—	D36.Ø	D48.7	D49.89
subclavicular	—	C77.3	—	D36.Ø	D48.7	D49.89
subinguinal	—	C77.4	—	D36.Ø	D48.7	D49.89
sublingual	—	C77.Ø	—	D36.Ø	D48.7	D49.89
submandibular	—	C77.Ø	—	D36.Ø	D48.7	D49.89

TABLE OF NEOPLASMS

	Malignant Primary	Malignant Secondary	Ca in situ	Benign	Uncertain Behavior	Unspecified Behavior
lymph, lymphatic channel NEC *(Continued)*						
gland *(Continued)*						
submaxillary	—	C77.Ø	—	D36.Ø	D48.7	D49.89
submental	—	C77.Ø	—	D36.Ø	D48.7	D49.89
subscapular	—	C77.3	—	D36.Ø	D48.7	D49.89
supraclavicular	—	C77.Ø	—	D36.Ø	D48.7	D49.89
thoracic	—	C77.1	—	D36.Ø	D48.7	D49.89
tibial	—	C77.4	—	D36.Ø	D48.7	D49.89
tracheal	—	C77.1	—	D36.Ø	D48.7	D49.89
tracheobronchial	—	C77.1	—	D36.Ø	D48.7	D49.89
upper limb	—	C77.3	—	D36.Ø	D48.7	D49.89
Virchow's	—	C77.Ø	—	D36.Ø	D48.7	D49.89
node—*see also Neoplasm, lymph gland*						
primary NEC	C96.9	—	—	—	—	—
vessel—*see also Neoplasm, connective tissue*	C49.9	C79.89	—	D21.9	D48.1	D49.2
Mackenrodt's ligament	C57.7	C79.82	DØ7.39	D28.7	D39.8	D49.59
malar	C41.Ø	C79.51	—	D16.4-	D48.Ø	D49.2
region—*see Neoplasm, cheek*						
mammary gland—*see Neoplasm, breast*						
mandible	C41.1	C79.51	—	D16.5-	D48.Ø	D49.2
alveolar						
mucosa (carcinoma)	CØ3.1	C79.89	DØØ.Ø3	D1Ø.39	D37.Ø9	D49.Ø
ridge or process	C41.1	C79.51	—	D16.5-	D48.Ø	D49.2
marrow (bone) NEC	C96.9	C79.52	—	—	D47.9	D49.89
mastectomy site (skin)—*see also Neoplasm, breast, skin*	C44.5Ø1	C79.2	—	—	—	—
specified as breast tissue	C5Ø.8-	C79.81	—	—	—	—
mastoid (air cells) (antrum) (cavity)	C3Ø.1	C78.39	DØ2.3	D14.Ø	D38.5	D49.1
bone or process	C41.Ø	C79.51	—	D16.4-	D48.Ø	D49.2
maxilla, maxillary (superior)	C41.Ø	C79.51	—	D16.4-	D48.Ø	D49.2
alveolar						
mucosa	CØ3.Ø	C79.89	DØØ.Ø3	D1Ø.39	D37.Ø9	D49.Ø
ridge or process (carcinoma)	C41.Ø	C79.51	—	D16.4-	D48.Ø	D49.2
antrum	C31.Ø	C78.39	DØ2.3	D14.Ø	D38.5	D49.1
carcinoma	CØ3.Ø	C79.51	—	—	—	—
inferior—*see Neoplasm, mandible*						
sinus	C31.Ø	C78.39	DØ2.3	D14.Ø	D38.5	D49.1
meatus external (ear)—*see also Neoplasm, skin, ear*	C44.2Ø-	C79.2	DØ4.2-	D23.2-	D48.5	D49.2
Meckel diverticulum, malignant	C17.3	C78.4	DØ1.49	D13.39	D37.2	D49.Ø

	Malignant Primary	Malignant Secondary	Ca in situ	Benign	Uncertain Behavior	Unspecified Behavior
mediastinum, mediastinal	C38.3	C78.1	—	D15.2	D38.3	D49.89
anterior	C38.1	C78.1	—	D15.2	D38.3	D49.89
posterior	C38.2	C78.1	—	D15.2	D38.3	D49.89
medulla						
adrenal	C74.1-	C79.7-	DØ9.3	D35.Ø-	D44.1-	D49.7
oblongata	C71.7	C79.31	—	D33.1	D43.1	D49.6
meibomian gland	C44.1Ø-	C79.2	DØ4.1-	D23.1-	D48.5	D49.2
basal cell carcinoma	C44.11-	—	—	—	—	—
specified type NEC	C44.19-	—	—	—	—	—
squamous cell carcinoma	C44.12-	—	—	—	—	—
melanoma—*see Melanoma*						
meninges	C7Ø.9	C79.49	—	D32.9	D42.9	D49.7
brain	C7Ø.Ø	C79.32	—	D32.Ø	D42.Ø	D49.7
cerebral	C7Ø.Ø	C79.32	—	D32.Ø	D42.Ø	D49.7
crainial	C7Ø.Ø	C79.32	—	D32.Ø	D42.Ø	D49.7
intracranial	C7Ø.Ø	C79.32	—	D32.Ø	D42.Ø	D49.7
spinal (cord)	C7Ø.1	C79.49	—	D32.1	D42.1	D49.7
meniscus, knee joint (lateral) (medial)	C4Ø.2-	C79.51	—	D16.2-	D48.Ø	D49.2
Merkel cell—*see Carcinoma, Merkel cell*						
mesentery, mesenteric	C48.1	C78.6	—	D2Ø.1	D48.4	D49.Ø
mesoappendix	C48.1	C78.6	—	D2Ø.1	D48.4	D49.Ø
mesocolon	C48.1	C78.6	—	D2Ø.1	D48.4	D49.Ø
mesopharynx—*see Neoplasm, oropharynx*						
mesosalpinx	C57.1	C79.82	DØ7.39	D28.2	D39.8	D49.59
mesothelial tissue—*see Mesothelioma*						
mesothelioma—*see Mesothelioma*						
mesovarium	C57.1	C79.82	DØ7.39	D28.2	D39.8	D49.59
metacarpus (any bone)	C4Ø.1-	C79.51	—	D16.1-	—	—
metastatic NEC—*see also Neoplasm, by site, secondary*	—	C79.9	—	—	—	—
metatarsus (any bone)	C4Ø.3-	C79.51	—	D16.3-	—	—
midbrain	C71.7	C79.31	—	D33.1	D43.1	D49.6
milk duct—*see Neoplasm, breast*						
mons						
pubis	C51.9	C79.82	DØ7.1	D28.Ø	D39.8	D49.59
veneris	C51.9	C79.82	DØ7.1	D28.Ø	D39.8	D49.59
motor tract	C72.9	C79.49	—	D33.9	D43.9	D49.7
brain	C71.9	C79.31	—	D33.2	D43.2	D49.6
cauda equina	C72.1	C79.49	—	D33.4	D43.4	D49.7
spinal	C72.Ø	C79.49	—	D33.4	D43.4	D49.7

◄ New ⟵ Revised ~~deleted~~ Deleted

	Malignant Primary	Malignant Secondary	Ca in situ	Benign	Uncertain Behavior	Unspecified Behavior
mouth	C06.9	C79.89	D00.00	D10.30	D37.09	D49.0
book-leaf	C06.89	C79.89	—	—	—	—
floor	C04.9	C79.89	D00.06	D10.2	D37.09	D49.0
anterior portion	C04.0	C79.89	D00.06	D10.2	D37.09	D49.0
lateral portion	C04.1	C79.89	D00.06	D10.2	D37.09	D49.0
overlapping lesion	C04.8	—	—	—	—	—
overlapping NEC	C06.80	—	—	—	—	—
roof	C05.9	C79.89	D00.00	D10.39	D37.09	D49.0
specified part NEC	C06.89	C79.89	D00.00	D10.39	D37.09	D49.0
vestibule	C06.1	C79.89	D00.00	D10.39	D37.09	D49.0
mucosa						
alveolar (ridge or process)	C03.9	C79.89	D00.03	D10.39	D37.09	D49.0
lower	C03.1	C79.89	D00.03	D10.39	D37.09	D49.0
upper	C03.0	C79.89	D00.03	D10.39	D37.09	D49.0
buccal	C06.0	C79.89	D00.02	D10.39	D37.09	D49.0
cheek	C06.0	C79.89	D00.02	D10.39	D37.09	D49.0
lip — *see Neoplasm, lip, internal*						
nasal	C30.0	C78.39	D02.3	D14.0	D38.5	D49.1
oral	C06.0	C79.89	D00.02	D10.39	D37.09	D49.0
Mullerian duct						
female	C57.7	C79.82	D07.39	D28.7	D39.8	D49.59
male	C63.7	C79.82	D07.69	D29.8	D40.8	D49.59
muscle — *see also Neoplasm, connective tissue*						
extraocular	C69.6-	C79.49	D09.2-	D31.6-	D48.7	D49.89
myocardium	C38.0	C79.89	—	D15.1	D48.7	D49.89
myometrium	C54.2	C79.82	D07.0	D26.1	D39.0	D49.59
myopericardium	C38.0	C79.89	—	D15.1	D48.7	D49.89
nabothian gland (follicle)	C53.0	C79.82	D06.0	D26.0	D39.0	D49.59
nail — *see also Neoplasm, skin, limb*	C44.90	C79.2	D04.9	D23.9	D48.5	D49.2
finger — *see also Neoplasm, skin, limb, upper*	C44.60-	C79.2	D04.6-	D23.6-	D48.5	D49.2
toe — *see also Neoplasm, skin, limb, lower*	C44.70-	C79.2	D04.7-	D23.7-	D48.5	D49.2
nares, naris (anterior) (posterior)	C30.0	C78.39	D02.3	D14.0	D38.5	D49.1
nasal — *see Neoplasm, nose*						
nasolabial groove — *see also Neoplasm, skin, face*	C44.309	C79.2	D04.39	D23.39	D48.5	D49.2
nasolacrimal duct	C69.5-	C79.49	D09.2-	D31.5-	D48.7	D49.89
nasopharynx, nasopharyngeal	C11.9	C79.89	D00.08	D10.6	D37.05	D49.0
floor	C11.3	C79.89	D00.08	D10.6	D37.05	D49.0
overlapping lesion	C11.8	—	—	—	—	—
roof	C11.0	C79.89	D00.08	D10.6	D37.05	D49.0

	Malignant Primary	Malignant Secondary	Ca in situ	Benign	Uncertain Behavior	Unspecified Behavior
nasopharynx, nasopharyngeal *(Continued)*						
wall	C11.9	C79.89	D00.08	D10.6	D37.05	D49.0
anterior	C11.3	C79.89	D00.08	D10.6	D37.05	D49.0
lateral	C11.2	C79.89	D00.08	D10.6	D37.05	D49.0
posterior	C11.1	C79.89	D00.08	D10.6	D37.05	D49.0
superior	C11.0	C79.89	D00.08	D10.6	D37.05	D49.0
nates — *see also Neoplasm, skin, trunk*	C44.509	C79.2	D04.5	D23.5	D48.5	D49.2
neck NEC	C76.0	C79.89	D09.8	D36.7	D48.7	D49.89
skin	C44.40	—	—	—	—	—
basal cell carcinoma	C44.41	—	—	—	—	—
specified type NEC	C44.49	—	—	—	—	—
squamous cell carcinoma	C44.42	—	—	—	—	—
nerve (ganglion)	C47.9	C79.89	—	D36.10	D48.2	D49.2
abducens	C72.59	C79.49	—	D33.3	D43.3	D49.7
accessory (spinal)	C72.59	C79.49	—	D33.3	D43.3	D49.7
acoustic	C72.4-	C79.49	—	D33.3	D43.3	D49.7
auditory	C72.4-	C79.49	—	D33.3	D43.3	D49.7
autonomic NEC — *see also Neoplasm, nerve, peripheral*	C47.9	C79.89	—	D36.10	D48.2	D49.2
brachial	C47.1-	C79.89	—	D36.12	D48.2	D49.2
cranial	C72.50	C79.49	—	D33.3	D43.3	D49.7
specified NEC	C72.59	C79.49	—	D33.3	D43.3	D49.7
facial	C72.59	C79.49	—	D33.3	D43.3	D49.7
femoral	C47.2-	C79.89	—	D36.13	D48.2	D49.2
ganglion NEC — *see also Neoplasm, nerve, peripheral*	C47.9	C79.89	—	D36.10	D48.2	D49.2
glossopharyngeal	C72.59	C79.49	—	D33.3	D43.3	D49.7
hypoglossal	C72.59	C79.49	—	D33.3	D43.3	D49.7
intercostal	C47.3	C79.89	—	D36.14	D48.2	D49.2
lumbar	C47.6	C79.89	—	D36.17	D48.2	D49.2
median	C47.1-	C79.89	—	D36.12	D48.2	D49.2
obturator	C47.2-	C79.89	—	D36.13	D48.2	D49.2
oculomotor	C72.59	C79.49	—	D33.3	D43.3	D49.7
olfactory	C47.2-	C79.49	—	D33.3	D43.3	D49.7
optic	C72.3-	C79.49	—	D33.3	D43.3	D49.7
parasympathetic NEC	C47.9	C79.89	—	D36.10	D48.2	D49.2
peripheral NEC	C47.9	C79.89	—	D36.10	D48.2	D49.2
abdomen	C47.4	C79.89	—	D36.15	D48.2	D49.2
abdominal wall	C47.4	C79.89	—	D36.15	D48.2	D49.2
ankle	C47.2-	C79.89	—	D36.13	D48.2	D49.2

TABLE OF NEOPLASMS

◀ New ⬅ Revised ~~deleted~~ Deleted

	Malignant Primary	Malignant Secondary	Ca in situ	Benign	Uncertain Behavior	Unspecified Behavior
nerve *(Continued)*						
peripheral NEC *(Continued)*						
antecubital fossa or space	C47.1-	C79.89	—	D36.12	D48.2	D49.2
arm	C47.1-	C79.89	—	D36.12	D48.2	D49.2
auricle (ear)	C47.Ø	C79.89	—	D36.11	D48.2	D49.2
axilla	C47.3	C79.89	—	D36.12	D48.2	D49.2
back	C47.6	C79.89	—	D36.17	D48.2	D49.2
buttock	C47.5	C79.89	—	D36.16	D48.2	D49.2
calf	C47.2-	C79.89	—	D36.13	D48.2	D49.2
cervical region	C47.Ø	C79.89	—	D36.11	D48.2	D49.2
cheek	C47.Ø	C79.89	—	D36.11	D48.2	D49.2
chest (wall)	C47.3	C79.89	—	D36.14	D48.2	D49.2
chin	C47.Ø	C79.89	—	D36.11	D48.2	D49.2
ear (external)	C47.Ø	C79.89	—	D36.11	D48.2	D49.2
elbow	C47.1-	C79.89	—	D36.12	D48.2	D49.2
extrarectal	C47.5	C79.89	—	D36.16	D48.2	D49.2
extremity	C47.9	C79.89	—	D36.1Ø	D48.2	D49.2
lower	C47.2-	C79.89	—	D36.13	D48.2	D49.2
upper	C47.1-	C79.89	—	D36.12	D48.2	D49.2
eyelid	C47.Ø	C79.89	—	D36.11	D48.2	D49.2
face	C47.Ø	C79.89	—	D36.11	D48.2	D49.2
finger	C47.1-	C79.89	—	D36.12	D48.2	D49.2
flank	C47.6	C79.89	—	D36.17	D48.2	D49.2
foot	C47.2-	C79.89	—	D36.13	D48.2	D49.2
forearm	C47.1-	C79.89	—	D36.12	D48.2	D49.2
forehead	C47.Ø	C79.89	—	D36.11	D48.2	D49.2
gluteal region	C47.5	C79.89	—	D36.16	D48.2	D49.2
groin	C47.5	C79.89	—	D36.16	D48.2	D49.2
hand	C47.1-	C79.89	—	D36.12	D48.2	D49.2
head	C47.Ø	C79.89	—	D36.11	D48.2	D49.2
heel	C47.2-	C79.89	—	D36.13	D48.2	D49.2
hip	C47.2-	C79.89	—	D36.13	D48.2	D49.2
infraclavicular region	C47.3	C79.89	—	D36.14	D48.2	D49.2
inguinal (canal) (region)	C47.5	C79.89	—	D36.16	D48.2	D49.2
intrathoracic	C47.3	C79.89	—	D36.14	D48.2	D49.2
ischiorectal fossa	C47.5	C79.89	—	D36.16	D48.2	D49.2
knee	C47.2-	C79.89	—	D36.13	D48.2	D49.2
leg	C47.2-	C79.89	—	D36.13	D48.2	D49.2
limb NEC	C47.9	C79.89	—	D36.1Ø	D48.2	D49.2
lower	C47.2-	C79.89	—	D36.13	D48.2	D49.2
upper	C47.1-	C79.89	—	D36.12	D48.2	D49.2
nates	C47.5	C79.89	—	D36.16	D48.2	D49.2
neck	C47.Ø	C79.89	—	D36.11	D48.2	D49.2
orbit	C69.6-	C79.49	—	D31.6-	D48.7	D49.2
nerve *(Continued)*						
peripheral NEC *(Continued)*						
pararectal	C47.5	C79.89	—	D36.16	D48.2	D49.2
paraurethral	C47.5	C79.89	—	D36.16	D48.2	D49.2
paravaginal	C47.5	C79.89	—	D36.16	D48.2	D49.2
pelvis (floor)	C47.5	C79.89	—	D36.16	D48.2	D49.2
pelvoabdominal	C47.8	C79.89	—	D36.17	D48.2	D49.2
perineum	C47.5	C79.89	—	D36.16	D48.2	D49.2
perirectal (tissue)	C47.5	C79.89	—	D36.16	D48.2	D49.2
periurethral (tissue)	C47.5	C79.89	—	D36.16	D48.2	D49.2
popliteal fossa or space	C47.2-	C79.89	—	D36.13	D48.2	D49.2
presacral	C47.5	C79.89	—	D36.16	D48.2	D49.2
pterygoid fossa	C47.Ø	C79.89	—	D36.11	D48.2	D49.2
rectovaginal septum or wall	C47.5	C79.89	—	D36.16	D48.2	D49.2
rectovesical	C47.5	C79.89	—	D36.16	D48.2	D49.2
sacrococcygeal region	C47.5	C79.89	—	D36.16	D48.2	D49.2
scalp	C47.Ø	C79.89	—	D36.11	D48.2	D49.2
scapular region	C47.3	C79.89	—	D36.14	D48.2	D49.2
shoulder	C47.1-	C79.89	—	D36.12	D48.2	D49.2
submental	C47.Ø	C79.89	—	D36.11	D48.2	D49.2
supraclavicular region	C47.Ø	C79.89	—	D36.11	D48.2	D49.2
temple	C47.Ø	C79.89	—	D36.11	D48.2	D49.2
temporal region	C47.Ø	C79.89	—	D36.11	D48.2	D49.2
thigh	C47.2-	C79.89	—	D36.13	D48.2	D49.2
thoracic (duct) (wall)	C47.3	C79.89	—	D36.14	D48.2	D49.2
thorax	C47.3	C79.89	—	D36.14	D48.2	D49.2
thumb	C47.1-	C79.89	—	D36.12	D48.2	D49.2
toe	C47.2-	C79.89	—	D36.13	D48.2	D49.2
trunk	C47.6	C79.89	—	D36.17	D48.2	D49.2
umbilicus	C47.4	C79.89	—	D36.15	D48.2	D49.2
vesicorectal	C47.5	C79.89	—	D36.16	D48.2	D49.2
wrist	C47.1-	C79.89	—	D36.12	D48.2	D49.2
radial	C47.1-	C79.89	—	D36.12	D48.2	D49.2
sacral	C47.5	C79.89	—	D36.16	D48.2	D49.2
sciatic	C47.2-	C79.89	—	D36.13	D48.2	D49.2
spinal NEC	C47.9	C79.89	—	D36.1Ø	D48.2	D49.2
accessory	C72.59	C79.49	—	D33.3	D43.3	D49.7
sympathetic NEC—*see also Neoplasm, nerve, peripheral*	C47.9	C79.89	—	D36.1Ø	D48.2	D49.2
trigeminal	C72.59	C79.49	—	D33.3	D43.3	D49.7
trochlear	C72.59	C79.49	—	D33.3	D43.3	D49.7
ulnar	C47.1-	C79.89	—	D36.12	D48.2	D49.2
vagus	C72.59	C79.49	—	D33.3	D43.3	D49.7

◀ New ⟸ Revised ~~deleted~~ Deleted

	Malignant Primary	Malignant Secondary	Ca in situ	Benign	Uncertain Behavior	Unspecified Behavior
nervous system (central)	C72.9	C79.4Ø	—	D33.9	D43.9	D49.7
autonomic—*see Neoplasm, nerve, peripheral*						
parasympathetic—*see Neoplasm, nerve, peripheral*						
specified site NEC	—	C79.49	—	D33.7	D43.8	—
sympathetic—*see Neoplasm, nerve, peripheral*						
nevus—*see Nevus*						
nipple	C5Ø.Ø-	C79.81	DØ5.-	D24.-	—	—
nose, nasal	C76.Ø	C79.89	DØ9.8	D36.7	D48.7	D49.89
ala (external) (nasi)—*see also Neoplasm, nose, skin*	C44.3Ø1	C79.2	DØ4.39	D23.39	D48.5	D49.2
bone	C41.Ø	C79.51	—	D16.4-	D48.Ø	D49.2
cartilage	C3Ø.Ø	C78.39	DØ2.3	D14.Ø	D38.5	D49.1
cavity	C3Ø.Ø	C78.39	DØ2.3	D14.Ø	D38.5	D49.1
choana	C11.3	C79.89	DØØ.Ø8	D1Ø.6	D37.Ø5	D49.Ø
external (skin)—*see also Neoplasm, nose, skin*	C44.3Ø1	C79.2	DØ4.39	D23.39	D48.5	D49.2
fossa	C3Ø.Ø	C78.39	DØ2.3	D14.Ø	D38.5	D49.1
internal	C3Ø.Ø	C78.39	DØ2.3	D14.Ø	D38.5	D49.1
mucosa	C3Ø.Ø	C78.39	DØ2.3	D14.Ø	D38.5	D49.1
septum	C3Ø.Ø	C78.39	DØ2.3	D14.Ø	D38.5	D49.1
posterior margin	C11.3	C79.89	DØØ.Ø8	D1Ø.6	D37.Ø5	D49.Ø
sinus—*see Neoplasm, sinus*						
skin	C44.3Ø1	C79.2	DØ4.39	D23.39	D48.5	D49.2
basal cell carcinoma	C44.311	—	—	—	—	—
specified type NEC	C44.391	—	—	—	—	—
squamous cell carcinoma	C44.321	—	—	—	—	—
turbinate (mucosa)	C3Ø.Ø	C78.39	DØ2.3	D14.Ø	D38.5	D49.1
bone	C41.Ø	C79.51	—	D16.4-	D48.Ø	D49.2
vestibule	C3Ø.Ø	C78.39	DØ2.3	D14.Ø	D38.5	D49.1
nostril	C3Ø.Ø	C78.39	DØ2.3	D14.Ø	D38.5	D49.1
nucleus pulposus	C41.2	C79.51	—	D16.6	D48.Ø	D49.2
occipital						
bone	C41.Ø	C79.51	—	D16.4-	D48.Ø	D49.2
lobe or pole, brain	C71.4	C79.31	—	D33.Ø	D43.Ø	D49.6
odontogenic—*see Neoplasm, jaw bone*						
olfactory nerve or bulb	C72.2-	C79.49	—	D33.3	D43.3	D49.7
olive (brain)	C71.7	C79.31	—	D33.1	D43.1	D49.6
omentum	C48.1	C78.6	—	D2Ø.1	D48.4	D49.Ø
operculum (brain)	C71.Ø	C79.31	—	D33.Ø	D43.Ø	D49.6

	Malignant Primary	Malignant Secondary	Ca in situ	Benign	Uncertain Behavior	Unspecified Behavior	
optic nerve, chiasm, or tract	C72.3-	C79.49	—	D33.3	D43.3	D49.7	
oral (cavity)	CØ6.9	C79.89	DØØ.ØØ	D1Ø.3Ø	D37.Ø9	D49.Ø	
ill-defined	C14.8	C79.89	DØØ.ØØ	D1Ø.3Ø	D37.Ø9	D49.Ø	
mucosa	CØ6.Ø	C79.89	DØØ.Ø2	D1Ø.39	D37.Ø9	D49.Ø	
orbit	C69.6-	C79.49	DØ9.2-	D31.6-	D48.7	D49.89	
autonomic nerve	C69.6-	C79.49	—	D31.6-	D48.7	D49.2	
bone	C41.Ø	C79.51	—	D16.4-	D48.Ø	D49.2	
eye	C69.6-	C79.49	DØ9.2-	D31.6-	D48.7	D49.89	
peripheral nerves	C69.6-	C79.49	—	D31.6-	D48.7	D49.2	
soft parts	C69.6-	C79.49	DØ9.2-	D31.6-	D48.7	D49.89	
organ of Zuckerkandl	C75.5	C79.89	—	D35.6	D44.7	D49.7	
oropharynx	C1Ø.9	C79.89	DØØ.Ø8	D1Ø.5	D37.Ø5	D49.Ø	
branchial cleft (vestige)	C1Ø.4	C79.89	DØØ.Ø8	D1Ø.5	D37.Ø5	D49.Ø	
junctional region	C1Ø.8	C79.89	DØØ.Ø8	D1Ø.5	D37.Ø5	D49.Ø	
lateral wall	C1Ø.2	C79.89	DØØ.Ø8	D1Ø.5	D37.Ø5	D49.Ø	
overlapping lesion	C1Ø.8	—	—	—	—	—	
pillars or fauces	CØ9.1	C79.89	DØØ.Ø8	D1Ø.5	D37.Ø5	D49.Ø	
posterior wall	C1Ø.3	C79.89	DØØ.Ø8	D1Ø.5	D37.Ø5	D49.Ø	
vallecula	C1Ø.Ø	C79.89	DØØ.Ø8	D1Ø.5	D37.Ø5	D49.Ø	
os							
external	C53.1	C79.82	DØ6.1	D26.Ø	D39.Ø	D49.59	⇐
internal	C53.Ø	C79.82	DØ6.Ø	D26.Ø	D39.Ø	D49.59	⇐
ovary	C56.-	C79.6-	DØ7.39	D27.-	D39.1-	D49.59	⇐
oviduct	C57.Ø-	C79.82	DØ7.39	D28.2	D39.8	D49.59	⇐
palate	CØ5.9	C79.89	DØØ.ØØ	D1Ø.39	D37.Ø9	D49.Ø	
hard	CØ5.Ø	C79.89	DØØ.Ø5	D1Ø.39	D37.Ø9	D49.Ø	
junction of hard and soft palate	CØ5.9	C79.89	DØØ.ØØ	D1Ø.39	D37.Ø9	D49.Ø	
overlapping lesions	CØ5.8	—	—	—	—	—	
soft	CØ5.1	C79.89	DØØ.Ø4	D1Ø.39	D37.Ø9	D49.Ø	
nasopharyngeal surface	C11.3	C79.89	DØØ.Ø8	D1Ø.6	D37.Ø5	D49.Ø	
posterior surface	C11.3	C79.89	DØØ.Ø8	D1Ø.6	D37.Ø5	D49.Ø	
superior surface	C11.3	C79.89	DØØ.Ø8	D1Ø.6	D37.Ø5	D49.Ø	
palatoglossal arch	CØ9.1	C79.89	DØØ.ØØ	D1Ø.5	D37.Ø9	D49.Ø	
palatopharyngeal arch	CØ9.1	C79.89	DØØ.ØØ	D1Ø.5	D37.Ø9	D49.Ø	
pallium	C71.Ø	C79.31	—	D33.Ø	D43.Ø	D49.6	
palpebra	C44.1Ø-	C79.2	DØ4.1-	D23.1-	D48.5	D49.2	
basal cell carcinoma	C44.11-	—	—	—	—	—	
specified type NEC	C44.19-	—	—	—	—	—	
squamous cell carcinoma	C44.12-	—	—	—	—	—	
pancreas	C25.9	C78.89	DØ1.7	D13.6	D37.8	D49.Ø	
body	C25.1	C78.89	DØ1.7	D13.6	D37.8	D49.Ø	
duct (of Santorini) (of Wirsung)	C25.3	C78.89	DØ1.7	D13.6	D37.8	D49.Ø	
ectopic tissue	C25.7	C78.89	—	D13.6	D37.8	D49.Ø	
head	C25.Ø	C78.89	DØ1.7	D13.6	D37.8	D49.Ø	

	Malignant Primary	Malignant Secondary	Ca in situ	Benign	Uncertain Behavior	Unspecified Behavior
pancreas *(Continued)*						
islet cells	C25.4	C78.89	D01.7	D13.7	D37.8	D49.0
neck	C25.7	C78.89	D01.7	D13.6	D37.8	D49.0
overlapping lesion	C25.8	—	—	—	—	—
tail	C25.2	C78.89	D01.7	D13.6	D37.8	D49.0
para-aortic body	C75.5	C79.89	—	D35.6	D44.7	D49.7
paraganglion NEC	C75.5	C79.89	—	D35.6	D44.7	D49.7
parametrium	C57.3	C79.82	—	D28.2	D39.8	D49.59
paranephric	C48.0	C78.6	—	D20.0	D48.3	D49.0
pararectal	C76.3	C79.89	—	D36.7	D48.7	D49.89
parasagittal (region)	C76.0	C79.89	D09.8	D36.7	D48.7	D49.89
parasellar	C72.9	C79.49	—	D33.9	D43.8	D49.7
parathyroid (gland)	C75.0	C79.89	D09.3	D35.1	D44.2	D49.7
paraurethral	C76.3	C79.89	—	D36.7	D48.7	D49.89
gland	C68.1	C79.19	D09.19	D30.8	D41.8	D49.59
paravaginal	C76.3	C79.89	—	D36.7	D48.7	D49.89
parenchyma, kidney	C64.-	C79.0-	D09.19	D30.0-	D41.0-	D49.51-
parietal						
bone	C41.0	C79.51	—	D16.4-	D48.0	D49.2
lobe, brain	C71.3	C79.31	—	D33.0	D43.0	D49.6
paroophoron	C57.1	C79.82	D07.39	D28.2	D39.8	D49.59
parotid (duct) (gland)	C07	C79.89	D00.00	D11.0	D37.030	D49.0
parovarium	C57.1	C79.82	D07.39	D28.2	D39.8	D49.59
patella	C40.20	C79.51	—	—	—	—
peduncle, cerebral	C71.7	C79.31	—	D33.1	D43.1	D49.6
pelvirectal junction	C19	C78.5	D01.1	D12.7	D37.5	D49.0
pelvis, pelvic	C76.3	C79.89	D09.8	D36.7	D48.7	D49.89
bone	C41.4	C79.51	—	D16.8	D48.0	D49.2
floor	C76.3	C79.89	D09.8	D36.7	D48.7	D49.89
renal	C65.-	C79.0-	D09.19	D30.1-	D41.1-	D49.51-
viscera	C76.3	C79.89	D09.8	D36.7	D48.7	D49.89
wall	C76.3	C79.89	D09.8	D36.7	D48.7	D49.89
pelvo-abdominal	C76.8	C79.89	D09.8	D36.7	D48.7	D49.89
penis	C60.9	C79.82	D07.4	D29.0	D40.8	D49.59
body	C60.2	C79.82	D07.4	D29.0	D40.8	D49.59
corpus (cavernosum)	C60.2	C79.82	D07.4	D29.0	D40.8	D49.59
glans	C60.1	C79.82	D07.4	D29.0	D40.8	D49.59
overlapping sites	C60.8	—	—	—	—	—
skin NEC	C60.9	C79.82	D07.4	D29.0	D40.8	D49.59
periadrenal (tissue)	C48.0	C78.6	—	D20.0	D48.3	D49.0
perianal (skin) — *see also Neoplasm, anus, skin*	C44.500	C79.2	D04.5	D23.5	D48.5	D49.2
pericardium	C38.0	C79.89	—	D15.1	D48.7	D49.89
perinephric	C48.0	C78.6	—	D20.0	D48.3	D49.0

	Malignant Primary	Malignant Secondary	Ca in situ	Benign	Uncertain Behavior	Unspecified Behavior
perineum	C76.3	C79.89	D09.8	D36.7	D48.7	D49.89
periodontal tissue NEC	C03.9	C79.89	D00.03	D10.39	D37.09	D49.0
periosteum — *see Neoplasm, bone*						
peripancreatic	C48.0	C78.6	—	D20.0	D48.3	D49.0
peripheral nerve NEC	C47.9	C79.89	—	D36.10	D48.2	D49.2
perirectal (tissue)	C76.3	C79.89	—	D36.7	D48.7	D49.89
perirenal (tissue)	C48.0	C78.6	—	D20.0	D48.3	D49.0
peritoneum, peritoneal (cavity)	C48.2	C78.6	—	D20.1	D48.4	D49.0
benign mesothelial tissue — *see Mesothelioma, benign*						
overlapping lesion	C48.8	—	—	—	—	—
with digestive organs	C26.9	—	—	—	—	—
parietal	C48.1	C78.6	—	D20.1	D48.4	D49.0
pelvic	C48.1	C78.6	—	D20.1	D48.4	D49.0
specified part NEC	C48.1	C78.6	—	D20.1	D48.4	D49.0
peritonsillar (tissue)	C76.0	C79.89	D09.8	D36.7	D48.7	D49.89
periurethral tissue	C76.3	C79.89	—	D36.7	D48.7	D49.89
phalanges						
foot	C40.3-	C79.51	—	D16.3-	—	—
hand	C40.1-	C79.51	—	D16.1-	—	—
pharynx, pharyngeal	C14.0	C79.89	D00.08	D10.9	D37.05	D49.0
bursa	C11.1	C79.89	D00.08	D10.6	D37.05	D49.0
fornix	C11.3	C79.89	D00.08	D10.6	D37.05	D49.0
recess	C11.2	C79.89	D00.08	D10.6	D37.05	D49.0
region	C14.0	C79.89	D00.08	D10.9	D37.05	D49.0
tonsil	C11.1	C79.89	D00.08	D10.6	D37.05	D49.0
wall (lateral) (posterior)	C14.0	C79.89	D00.08	D10.9	D37.05	D49.0
pia mater	C70.9	C79.40	—	D32.9	D42.9	D49.7
cerebral	C70.0	C79.32	—	D32.0	D42.0	D49.7
cranial	C70.0	C79.32	—	D32.0	D42.0	D49.7
spinal	C70.1	C79.49	—	D32.1	D42.1	D49.7
pillars of fauces	C09.1	C79.89	D00.08	D10.5	D37.05	D49.0
pineal (body) (gland)	C75.3	C79.89	D09.3	D35.4	D44.5	D49.7
pinna (ear) NEC — *see also Neoplasm, skin, ear*	C44.20-	C79.2	D04.2-	D23.2-	D48.5	D49.2
piriform fossa or sinus	C12	C79.89	D00.08	D10.7	D37.05	D49.0
pituitary (body) (fossa) (gland) (lobe)	C75.1	C79.89	D09.3	D35.2	D44.3	D49.7
placenta	C58	C79.82	D07.0	D26.7	D39.2	D49.59
pleura, pleural (cavity)	C38.4	C78.2	—	D19.0	D38.2	D49.1
overlapping lesion with heart or mediastinum	C38.8	—	—	—	—	—
parietal	C38.4	C78.2	—	D19.0	D38.2	D49.1
visceral	C38.4	C78.2	—	D19.0	D38.2	D49.1

New   Revised   ~~deleted~~ Deleted

	Malignant Primary	Malignant Secondary	Ca in situ	Benign	Uncertain Behavior	Unspecified Behavior
plexus						
brachial	C47.1-	C79.89	—	D36.12	D48.2	D49.2
cervical	C47.0	C79.89	—	D36.11	D48.2	D49.2
choroid	C71.5	C79.31	—	D33.0	D43.0	D49.6
lumbosacral	C47.5	C79.89	—	D36.16	D48.2	D49.2
sacral	C47.5	C79.89	—	D36.16	D48.2	D49.2
pluriendocrine	C75.8	C79.89	D09.3	D35.7	D44.9	D49.7
pole						
frontal	C71.1	C79.31	—	D33.0	D43.0	D49.6
occipital	C71.4	C79.31	—	D33.0	D43.0	D49.6
pons (varolii)	C71.7	C79.31	—	D33.1	D43.1	D49.6
popliteal fossa or space	C76.5-	C79.89	D04.7-	D36.7	D48.7	D49.89
postcricoid (region)	C13.0	C79.89	D00.08	D10.7	D37.05	D49.0
posterior fossa (cranial)	C71.9	C79.31	—	D33.2	D43.2	D49.6
postnasal space	C11.9	C79.89	D00.08	D10.6	D37.05	D49.0
prepuce	C60.0	C79.82	D07.4	D29.0	D40.8	D49.59
prepylorus	C16.4	C78.89	D00.2	D13.1	D37.1	D49.0
presacral (region)	C76.3	C79.89	—	D36.7	D48.7	D49.89
prostate (gland)	C61	C79.82	D07.5	D29.1	D40.0	D49.59
utricle	C68.0	C79.19	D09.19	D30.4	D41.3	D49.59
pterygoid fossa	C49.0	C79.89	—	D21.0	D48.1	D49.2
pubic bone	C41.4	C79.51	—	D16.8	D48.0	D49.2
pudenda, pudendum (female)	C51.9	C79.82	D07.1	D28.0	D39.8	D49.59
pulmonary — *see also Neoplasm, lung*	C34.9-	C78.0-	D02.2-	D14.3-	D38.1	D49.1
putamen	C71.0	C79.31	—	D33.0	D43.0	D49.6
pyloric						
antrum	C16.3	C78.89	D00.2	D13.1	D37.1	D49.0
canal	C16.4	C78.89	D00.2	D13.1	D37.1	D49.0
pylorus	C16.4	C78.89	D00.2	D13.1	D37.1	D49.0
pyramid (brain)	C71.7	C79.31	—	D33.1	D43.1	D49.6
pyriform fossa or sinus	C12	C79.89	D00.08	D10.7	D37.05	D49.0
radius (any part)	C40.0-	C79.51	—	D16.0-	—	—
Rathke's pouch	C75.1	C79.89	D09.3	D35.2	D44.3	D49.7
rectosigmoid (junction)	C19	C78.5	D01.1	D12.7	D37.5	D49.0
overlapping lesion with anus or rectum	C21.8	—	—	—	—	—
rectouterine pouch	C48.1	C78.6	—	D20.1	D48.4	D49.0
rectovaginal septum or wall	C76.3	C79.89	D09.8	D36.7	D48.7	D49.89
rectovesical septum	C76.3	C79.89	D09.8	D36.7	D48.7	D49.89
rectum (ampulla)	C20	C78.5	D01.2	D12.8	D37.5	D49.0
and colon	C19	C78.5	D01.1	D12.7	D37.5	D49.0
overlapping lesion with anus or rectosigmoid junction	C21.8	—	—	—	—	—

	Malignant Primary	Malignant Secondary	Ca in situ	Benign	Uncertain Behavior	Unspecified Behavior
renal	C64.-	C79.0-	D09.19	D30.0-	D41.0-	D49.51-
calyx	C65.-	C79.0-	D09.19	D30.1-	D41.1-	D49.51-
hilus	C65.-	C79.0-	D09.19	D30.1-	D41.1-	D49.51-
parenchyma	C64.-	C79.0-	D09.19	D30.0-	D41.0-	D49.51-
pelvis	C65.-	C79.0-	D09.19	D30.1-	D41.1-	D49.51-
respiratory						
organs or system NEC	C39.9	C78.30	D02.4	D14.4	D38.6	D49.1
tract NEC	C39.9	C78.30	D02.4	D14.4	D38.5	D49.1
upper	C39.0	C78.30	D02.4	D14.4	D38.5	D49.1
retina	C69.2-	C79.49	D09.2-	D31.2-	D48.7	D49.81
retrobulbar	C69.6-	C79.49	—	D31.6-	D48.7	D49.89
retrocecal	C48.0	C78.6	—	D20.0	D48.3	D49.0
retromolar (area) (triangle) (trigone)	C06.2	C79.89	D00.00	D10.39	D37.09	D49.0
retro-orbital	C76.0	C79.89	D09.8	D36.7	D48.7	D49.89
retroperitoneal (space) (tissue)	C48.0	C78.6	—	D20.0	D48.3	D49.0
retroperitoneum	C48.0	C78.6	—	D20.0	D48.3	D49.0
retropharyngeal	C14.0	C79.89	D00.08	D10.9	D37.05	D49.0
retrovesical (septum)	C76.3	C79.89	D09.8	D36.7	D48.7	D49.89
rhinencephalon	C71.0	C79.31	—	D33.0	D43.0	D49.6
rib	C41.3	C79.51	—	D16.7	D48.0	D49.2
Rosenmuller's fossa	C11.2	C79.89	D00.08	D10.6	D37.05	D49.0
round ligament	C57.2	C79.82	—	D28.2	D39.8	D49.59
sacrococcyx, sacrococcygeal	C41.4	C79.51	—	D16.8	D48.0	D49.2
region	C76.3	C79.89	D09.8	D36.7	D48.7	D49.89
sacrouterine ligament	C57.3	C79.82	—	D28.2	D39.8	D49.59
sacrum, sacral (vertebra)	C41.4	C79.51	—	D16.8	D48.0	D49.2
salivary gland or duct (major)	C08.9	C79.89	D00.00	D11.9	D37.039	D49.0
minor NEC	C06.9	C79.89	D00.00	D10.39	D37.04	D49.0
overlapping lesion	C08.9	—	—	—	—	—
parotid	C07	C79.89	D00.00	D11.0	D37.030	D49.0
pluriglandular	C08.9	C79.89	D00.00	D11.9	D37.039	D49.0
sublingual	C08.1	C79.89	D00.00	D11.7	D37.031	D49.0
submandibular	C08.0	C79.89	D00.00	D11.7	D37.032	D49.0
submaxillary	C08.0	C79.89	D00.00	D11.7	D37.032	D49.0
salpinx (uterine)	C57.0-	C79.82	D07.39	D28.2	D39.8	D49.59
Santorini's duct	C25.3	C78.89	D01.7	D13.6	D37.8	D49.0
scalp	C44.40	C79.2	D04.4	D23.4	D48.5	D49.2
basal cell carcinoma	C44.41	—	—	—	—	—
specified type NEC	C44.49	—	—	—	—	—
squamous cell carcinoma	C44.42	—	—	—	—	—
scapula (any part)	C40.0-	C79.51	—	D16.0-	—	—
scapular region	C76.1	C79.89	D09.8	D36.7	D48.7	D49.89

	Malignant Primary	Malignant Secondary	Ca in situ	Benign	Uncertain Behavior	Unspecified Behavior
scar NEC — *see also Neoplasm, skin, by site*	C44.90	C79.2	D04.9	D23.9	D48.5	D49.2
sciatic nerve	C47.2-	C79.89	—	D36.13	D48.2	D49.2
sclera	C69.4-	C79.49	D09.2-	D31.4-	D48.7	D49.89
scrotum (skin)	C63.2	C79.82	D07.61	D29.4	D40.8	D49.59
sebaceous gland — *see Neoplasm, skin*						
sella turcica	C75.1	C79.89	D09.3	D35.2	D44.3	D49.7
bone	C41.0	C79.51	—	D16.4-	D48.0	D49.2
semilunar cartilage (knee)	C40.2-	C79.51	—	D16.2-	D48.0	D49.2
seminal vesicle	C63.7	C79.82	D07.69	D29.8	D40.8	D49.59
septum						
nasal	C30.0	C78.39	D02.3	D14.0	D38.5	D49.1
posterior margin	C11.3	C79.89	D00.08	D10.6	D37.05	D49.0
rectovaginal	C76.3	C79.89	D09.8	D36.7	D48.7	D49.89
rectovesical	C76.3	C79.89	D09.8	D36.7	D48.7	D49.89
urethrovaginal	C57.9	C79.82	D07.30	D28.9	D39.9	D49.59
vesicovaginal	C57.9	C79.82	D07.30	D28.9	D39.9	D49.59
shoulder NEC	C76.4-	C79.89	D04.6-	D36.7	D48.7	D49.89
sigmoid flexure (lower) (upper)	C18.7	C78.5	D01.0	D12.5	D37.4	D49.0
sinus (accessory)	C31.9	C78.39	D02.3	D14.0	D38.5	D49.1
bone (any)	C41.0	C79.51	—	D16.4-	D48.0	D49.2
ethmoidal	C31.1	C78.39	D02.3	D14.0	D38.5	D49.1
frontal	C31.2	C78.39	D02.3	D14.0	D38.5	D49.1
maxillary	C31.0	C78.39	D02.3	D14.0	D38.5	D49.1
nasal, paranasal NEC	C31.9	C78.39	D02.3	D14.0	D38.5	D49.1
overlapping lesion	C31.8	—	—	—	—	—
pyriform	C12	C79.89	D00.08	D10.7	D37.05	D49.0
sphenoid	C31.3	C78.39	D02.3	D14.0	D38.5	D49.1
skeleton, skeletal NEC	C41.9	C79.51	—	D16.9-	D48.0	D49.2
Skene's gland	C68.1	C79.19	D09.19	D30.8	D41.8	D49.59
skin NOS	C44.90	C79.2	D04.9	D23.9	D48.5	D49.2
abdominal wall	C44.509	C79.2	D04.5	D23.5	D48.5	D49.2
basal cell carcinoma	C44.519	—	—	—	—	—
specified type NEC	C44.599	—	—	—	—	—
squamous cell carcinoma	C44.529	—	—	—	—	—
ala nasi — *see also Neoplasm, nose, skin*	C44.301	C79.2	D04.39	D23.39	D48.5	D49.2
ankle — *see also Neoplasm, skin, limb, lower*	C44.70-	C79.2	D04.7-	D23.7-	D48.5	D49.2
antecubital space — *see also Neoplasm, skin, limb, upper*	C44.60-	C79.2	D04.6-	D23.6-	D48.5	D49.2
skin NOS *(Continued)*						
anus	C44.500	C79.2	D04.5	D23.5	D48.5	D49.2
basal cell carcinoma	C44.510	—	—	—	—	—
specified type NEC	C44.590	—	—	—	—	—
squamous cell carcinoma	C44.520	—	—	—	—	—
arm — *see also Neoplasm, skin, limb, upper*	C44.60-	C79.2	D04.6-	D23.6-	D48.5	D49.2
auditory canal (external) — *see also Neoplasm, skin, ear*	C44.20-	C79.2	D04.2-	D23.2-	D48.5	D49.2
auricle (ear) — *see also Neoplasm, skin, ear*	C44.20-	C79.2	D04.2-	D23.2-	D48.5	D49.2
auricular canal (external) — *see also Neoplasm, skin, ear*	C44.20-	C79.2	D04.2-	D23.2-	D48.5	D49.2
axilla, axillary fold — *see also Neoplasm, skin, trunk*	C44.509	C79.2	D04.5	D23.5	D48.5	D49.2
back — *see also Neoplasm, skin, trunk*	C44.509	C79.2	D04.5	D23.5	D48.5	D49.2
basal cell carcinoma	C44.91					
breast	C44.501	C79.2	D04.5	D23.5	D48.5	D49.2
basal cell carcinoma	C44.511	—	—	—	—	—
specified type NEC	C44.591	—	—	—	—	—
squamous cell carcinoma	C44.521	—	—	—	—	—
brow — *see also Neoplasm, skin, face*	C44.309	C79.2	D04.39	D23.39	D48.5	D49.2
buttock — *see also Neoplasm, skin, trunk*	C44.509	C79.2	D04.5	D23.5	D48.5	D49.2
calf — *see also Neoplasm, skin, limb, lower*	C44.70-	C79.2	D04.7-	D23.7-	D48.5	D49.2
canthus (eye) (inner) (outer)	C44.10-	C79.2	D04.1-	D23.1-	D48.5	D49.2
basal cell carcinoma	C44.11-	—	—	—	—	—
specified type NEC	C44.19-	—	—	—	—	—
squamous cell carcinoma	C44.12-	—	—	—	—	—
cervical region — *see also Neoplasm, skin, neck*	C44.40	C79.2	D04.4	D23.4	D48.5	D49.2
cheek (external) — *see also Neoplasm, skin, face*	C44.309	C79.2	D04.39	D23.39	D48.5	D49.2
chest (wall) — *see also Neoplasm, skin, trunk*	C44.509	C79.2	D04.5	D23.5	D48.5	D49.2
chin — *see also Neoplasm, skin, face*	C44.309	C79.2	D04.39	D23.39	D48.5	D49.2
clavicular area — *see also Neoplasm, skin, trunk*	C44.509	C79.2	D04.5	D23.5	D48.5	D49.2
clitoris	C51.2	C79.82	D07.1	D28.0	D39.8	D49.59
columnella — *see also Neoplasm, skin, face*	C44.309	C79.2	D04.39	D23.39	D48.5	D49.2

◄ New ◄ Revised deleted Deleted

	Malignant Primary	Malignant Secondary	Ca in situ	Benign	Uncertain Behavior	Unspecified Behavior
skin NOS *(Continued)*						
concha — *see also Neoplasm, skin, ear*	C44.2Ø-	C79.2	DØ4.2-	D23.2-	D48.5	D49.2
ear (external)	C44.2Ø-	C79.2	DØ4.2-	D23.2-	D48.5	D49.2
basal cell carcinoma	C44.21-	—	—	—	—	—
specified type NEC	C44.29-	—	—	—	—	—
squamous cell carcinoma	C44.22-	—	—	—	—	—
elbow — *see also Neoplasm, skin, limb, upper*	C44.6Ø-	C79.2	DØ4.6-	D23.6-	D48.5	D49.2
eyebrow — *see also Neoplasm, skin, face*	C44.3Ø9	C79.2	DØ4.39	D23.39	D48.5	D49.2
eyelid	C44.1Ø-	C79.2	DØ4.1-	D23.1-	D48.5	D49.2
basal cell carcinoma	C44.11-	—	—	—	—	—
specified type NEC	C44.19-	—	—	—	—	—
squamous cell carcinoma	C44.12-	—	—	—	—	—
face NOS	C44.3ØØ	C79.2	DØ4.3Ø	D23.3Ø	D48.5	D49.2
basal cell carcinoma	C44.31Ø	—	—	—	—	—
specified type NEC	C44.39Ø	—	—	—	—	—
squamous cell carcinoma	C44.32Ø	—	—	—	—	—
female genital organs (external)	C51.9	C79.82	DØ7.1	D28.Ø	D39.8	D49.59
clitoris	C51.2	C79.82	DØ7.1	D28.Ø	D39.8	D49.59
labium NEC	C51.9	C79.82	DØ7.1	D28.Ø	D39.8	D49.59
majus	C51.Ø	C79.82	DØ7.1	D28.Ø	D39.8	D49.59
minus	C51.1	C79.82	DØ7.1	D28.Ø	D39.8	D49.59
pudendum	C51.9	C79.82	DØ7.1	D28.Ø	D39.8	D49.59
vulva	C51.9	C79.82	DØ7.1	D28.Ø	D39.8	D49.59
finger — *see also Neoplasm, skin, limb, upper*	C44.6Ø-	C79.2	DØ4.6-	D23.6-	D48.5	D49.2
flank — *see also Neoplasm, skin, trunk*	C44.5Ø9	C79.2	DØ4.5	D23.5	D48.5	D49.2
foot — *see also Neoplasm, skin, limb, lower*	C44.7Ø-	C79.2	DØ4.7-	D23.7-	D48.5	D49.2
forearm — *see also Neoplasm, skin, limb, upper*	C44.6Ø-	C79.2	DØ4.6-	D23.6-	D48.5	D49.2
forehead — *see also Neoplasm, skin, face*	C44.3Ø9	C79.2	DØ4.39	D23.39	D48.5	D49.2
glabella — *see also Neoplasm, skin, face*	C44.3Ø9	C79.2	DØ4.39	D23.39	D48.5	D49.2
gluteal region — *see also Neoplasm, skin, trunk*	C44.5Ø9	C79.2	DØ4.5	D23.5	D48.5	D49.2
groin — *see also Neoplasm, skin, trunk*	C44.5Ø9	C79.2	DØ4.5	D23.5	D48.5	D49.2
hand — *see also Neoplasm, skin, limb, upper*	C44.6Ø-	C79.2	DØ4.6-	D23.6-	D48.5	D49.2

	Malignant Primary	Malignant Secondary	Ca in situ	Benign	Uncertain Behavior	Unspecified Behavior
skin NOS *(Continued)*						
head NEC — *see also Neoplasm, skin, scalp*	C44.4Ø	C79.2	DØ4.4	D23.4	D48.5	D49.2
heel — *see also Neoplasm, skin, limb, lower*	C44.7Ø-	C79.2	DØ4.7-	D23.7-	D48.5	D49.2
helix — *see also Neoplasm, skin, ear*	C44.2Ø-	C79.2	DØ4.2-	D23.2-	D48.5	D49.2
hip — *see also Neoplasm, skin, limb, lower*	C44.7Ø-	C79.2	DØ4.7-	D23.7-	D48.5	D49.2
infraclavicular region — *see also Neoplasm, skin, trunk*	C44.5Ø9	C79.2	DØ4.5	D23.5	D48.5	D49.2
inguinal region — *see also Neoplasm, skin, trunk*	C44.5Ø9	C79.2	DØ4.5	D23.5	D48.5	D49.2
jaw — *see also Neoplasm, skin, face*	C44.3Ø9	C79.2	DØ4.39	D23.39	D48.5	D49.2
Kaposi's sarcoma — *see Kaposi's, sarcoma, skin*						
knee — *see also Neoplasm, skin, limb, lower*	C44.7Ø-	C79.2	DØ4.7-	D23.7-	D48.5	D49.2
labia						
majora	C51.Ø	C79.82	DØ7.1	D28.Ø	D39.8	D49.59
minora	C51.1	C79.82	DØ7.1	D28.Ø	D39.8	D49.59
leg — *see also Neoplasm, skin, limb, lower*	C44.7Ø-	C79.2	DØ4.7-	D23.7-	D48.5	D49.2
lid (lower) (upper)	C44.1Ø-	C79.2	DØ4.1-	D23.1-	D48.5	D49.2
basal cell carcinoma	C44.11-	—	—	—	—	—
specified type NEC	C44.19-	—	—	—	—	—
squamous cell carcinoma	C44.12-	—	—	—	—	—
limb NEC	C44.9Ø	C79.2	DØ4.9	D23.9	D48.5	D49.2
basal cell carcinoma	C44.91					
lower	C44.7Ø-	C79.2	DØ4.7-	D23.7-	D48.5	D49.2
basal cell carcinoma	C44.71-	—	—	—	—	—
specified type NEC	C44.79-	—	—	—	—	—
squamous cell carcinoma	C44.72-	—	—	—	—	—
upper	C44.6Ø-	C79.2	DØ4.6-	D23.6-	D48.5	D49.2
basal cell carcinoma	C44.61-	—	—	—	—	—
specified type NEC	C44.69-	—	—	—	—	—
squamous cell carcinoma	C44.62-	—	—	—	—	—
lip (lower) (upper)	C44.ØØ	C79.2	DØ4.Ø	D23.Ø	D48.5	D49.2
basal cell carcinoma	C44.Ø1	—	—	—	—	—
specified type NEC	C44.Ø9	—	—	—	—	—
squamous cell carcinoma	C44.Ø2	—	—	—	—	—

	Malignant Primary	Malignant Secondary	Ca in situ	Benign	Uncertain Behavior	Unspecified Behavior
skin NOS *(Continued)*						
male genital organs	C63.9	C79.82	D07.60	D29.9	D40.8	D49.59
penis	C60.9	C79.82	D07.4	D29.0	D40.8	D49.59
prepuce	C60.0	C79.82	D07.4	D29.0	D40.8	D49.59
scrotum	C63.2	C79.82	D07.61	D29.4	D40.8	D49.59
mastectomy site (skin) — *see also Neoplasm, skin, breast*	C44.501	C79.2	—	—	—	—
specified as breast tissue	C50.8-	C79.81	—	—	—	—
meatus, acoustic (external) — *see also Neoplasm, skin, ear*	C44.20-	C79.2	D04.2-	D23.2-	D48.5	D49.2
melanotic — *see Melanoma*						
Merkel cell — *see Carcinoma, Merkel cell*						
nates — *see also Neoplasm, skin, trunk*	C44.509	C79.2	D04.5	D23.5	D48.5	D49.2
neck	C44.40	C79.2	D04.4	D23.4	D48.5	D49.2
basal cell carcinoma	C44.41	—	—	—	—	—
specified type NEC	C44.49	—	—	—	—	—
squamous cell carcinoma	C44.42	—	—	—	—	—
nevus — *see Nevus, skin*						
nose (external) — *see also Neoplasm, nose, skin*	C44.301	C79.2	D04.39	D23.39	D48.5	D49.2
overlapping lesion	C44.80	—	—	—	—	—
basal cell carcinoma	C44.81	—	—	—	—	—
specified type NEC	C44.89	—	—	—	—	—
squamous cell carcinoma	C44.82	—	—	—	—	—
palm — *see also Neoplasm, skin, limb, upper*	C44.60-	C79.2	D04.6-	D23.6-	D48.5	D49.2
palpebra	C44.10-	C79.2	D04.1-	D23.1-	D48.5	D49.2
basal cell carcinoma	C44.11-	—	—	—	—	—
specified type NEC	C44.19-	—	—	—	—	—
squamous cell carcinoma	C44.12-	—	—	—	—	—
penis NEC	C60.9	C79.82	D07.4	D29.0	D40.8	D49.59
perianal — *see also Neoplasm, skin, anus*	C44.500	C79.2	D04.5	D23.5	D48.5	D49.2
perineum — *see also Neoplasm, skin, anus*	C44.500	C79.2	D04.5	D23.5	D48.5	D49.2
pinna — *see also Neoplasm, skin, ear*	C44.20-	C79.2	D04.2-	D23.2-	D48.5	D49.2
plantar — *see also Neoplasm, skin, limb, lower*	C44.70-	C79.2	D04.7-	D23.7-	D48.5	D49.2
popliteal fossa or space — *see also Neoplasm, skin, limb, lower*	C44.70-	C79.2	D04.7-	D23.7-	D48.5	D49.2
prepuce	C60.0	C79.82	D07.4	D29.0	D40.8	D49.59
skin NOS *(Continued)*						
pubes — *see also Neoplasm, skin, trunk*	C44.509	C79.2	D04.5	D23.5	D48.5	D49.2
sacrococcygeal region — *see also Neoplasm, skin, trunk*	C44.509	C79.2	D04.5	D23.5	D48.5	D49.2
scalp	C44.40	C79.2	D04.4	D23.4	D48.5	D49.2
basal cell carcinoma	C44.41	—	—	—	—	—
specified type NEC	C44.49	—	—	—	—	—
squamous cell carcinoma	C44.42	—	—	—	—	—
scapular region — *see also Neoplasm, skin, trunk*	C44.509	C79.2	D04.5	D23.5	D48.5	D49.2
scrotum	C63.2	C79.82	D07.61	D29.4	D40.8	D49.59
shoulder — *see also Neoplasm, skin, limb, upper*	C44.60-	C79.2	D04.6-	D23.6-	D48.5	D49.2
sole (foot) — *see also Neoplasm, skin, limb, lower*	C44.70-	C79.2	D04.7-	D23.7-	D48.5	D49.2
specified sites NEC	C44.80	C79.2	D04.8	D23.9	D48.5	D49.2
basal cell carcinoma	C44.81	—	—	—	—	—
specified type NEC	C44.89	—	—	—	—	—
squamous cell carcinoma	C44.82	—	—	—	—	—
specified type NEC	C44.99	—	—	—	—	—
squamous cell carcinoma	C44.92	—	—	—	—	—
submammary fold — *see also Neoplasm, skin, trunk*	C44.509	C79.2	D04.5	D23.5	D48.5	D49.2
supraclavicular region — *see also Neoplasm, skin, neck*	C44.40	C79.2	D04.4	D23.4	D48.5	D49.2
temple — *see also Neoplasm, skin, face*	C44.309	C79.2	D04.39	D23.39	D48.5	D49.2
thigh — *see also Neoplasm, skin, limb, lower*	C44.70-	C79.2	D04.7-	D23.7-	D48.5	D49.2
thoracic wall — *see also Neoplasm, skin, trunk*	C44.509	C79.2	D04.5	D23.5	D48.5	D49.2
thumb — *see also Neoplasm, skin, limb, upper*	C44.60-	C79.2	D04.6-	D23.6-	D48.5	D49.2
toe — *see also Neoplasm, skin, limb, lower*	C44.70-	C79.2	D04.7-	D23.7-	D48.5	D49.2
tragus — *see also Neoplasm, skin, ear*	C44.20-	C79.2	D04.2-	D23.2-	D48.5	D49.2
trunk	C44.509	C79.2	D04.5	D23.5	D48.5	D49.2
basal cell carcinoma	C44.519	—	—	—	—	—
specified type NEC	C44.599	—	—	—	—	—
squamous cell carcinoma	C44.529	—	—	—	—	—
umbilicus — *see also Neoplasm, skin, trunk*	C44.509	C79.2	D04.5	D23.5	D48.5	D49.2

◄ New ⇐ Revised ~~deleted~~ Deleted

	Malignant Primary	Malignant Secondary	Ca in situ	Benign	Uncertain Behavior	Unspecified Behavior
skin NOS *(Continued)*						
vulva	C51.9	C79.82	DØ7.1	D28.Ø	D39.8	D49.59
overlapping lesion	C51.8	—	—	—	—	—
wrist — *see also Neoplasm, skin, limb, upper*	C44.6Ø-	C79.2	DØ4.6-	D23.6-	D48.5	D49.2
skull	C41.Ø	C79.51	—	D16.4-	D48.Ø	D49.2
soft parts or tissues — *see Neoplasm, connective tissue*						
specified site NEC	C76.8	C79.89	DØ9.8	D36.7	D48.7	D49.89
spermatic cord	C63.1-	C79.82	DØ7.69	D29.8	D4Ø.8	D49.59
sphenoid	C31.3	C78.39	DØ2.3	D14.Ø	D38.5	D49.1
bone	C41.Ø	C79.51	—	D16.4-	D48.Ø	D49.2
sinus	C31.3	C78.39	DØ2.3	D14.Ø	D38.5	D49.1
sphincter						
anal	C21.1	C78.5	DØ1.3	D12.9	D37.8	D49.Ø
of Oddi	C24.Ø	C78.89	DØ1.5	D13.5	D37.6	D49.Ø
spine, spinal (column)	C41.2	C79.51	—	D16.6	D48.Ø	D49.2
bulb	C71.7	C79.31	—	D33.1	D43.1	D49.6
coccyx	C41.4	C79.51	—	D16.8	D48.Ø	D49.2
cord (cervical) (lumbar) (sacral) (thoracic)	C72.Ø	C79.49	—	D33.4	D43.4	D49.7
dura mater	C7Ø.1	C79.49	—	D32.1	D42.1	D49.7
lumbosacral	C41.2	C79.51	—	D16.6	D48.Ø	D49.2
marrow NEC	C96.9	C79.52	—	—	D47.9	D49.89
membrane	C7Ø.1	C79.49	—	D32.1	D42.1	D49.7
meninges	C7Ø.1	C79.49	—	D32.1	D42.1	D49.7
nerve (root)	C47.9	C79.89	—	D36.1Ø	D48.2	D49.2
pia mater	C7Ø.1	C79.49	—	D32.1	D42.1	D49.7
root	C47.9	C79.89	—	D36.1Ø	D48.2	D49.2
sacrum	C41.4	C79.51	—	D16.8	D48.Ø	D49.2
spleen, splenic NEC	C26.1	C78.89	DØ1.7	D13.9	D37.8	D49.Ø
flexure (colon)	C18.5	C78.5	DØ1.Ø	D12.3	D37.4	D49.Ø
stem, brain	C71.7	C79.31	—	D33.1	D43.1	D49.6
Stensen's duct	CØ7	C79.89	DØØ.ØØ	D11.Ø	D37.Ø3Ø	D49.Ø
sternum	C41.3	C79.51	—	D16.7	D48.Ø	D49.2
stomach	C16.9	C78.89	DØØ.2	D13.1	D37.1	D49.Ø
antrum (pyloric)	C16.3	C78.89	DØØ.2	D13.1	D37.1	D49.Ø
body	C16.2	C78.89	DØØ.2	D13.1	D37.1	D49.Ø
cardia	C16.Ø	C78.89	DØØ.2	D13.1	D37.1	D49.Ø
cardiac orifice	C16.Ø	C78.89	DØØ.2	D13.1	D37.1	D49.Ø
corpus	C16.2	C78.89	DØØ.2	D13.1	D37.1	D49.Ø
fundus	C16.1	C78.89	DØØ.2	D13.1	D37.1	D49.Ø
greater curvature NEC	C16.6	C78.89	DØØ.2	D13.1	D37.1	D49.Ø
lesser curvature NEC	C16.5	C78.89	DØØ.2	D13.1	D37.1	D49.Ø
stomach *(Continued)*						
overlapping lesion	C16.8	—	—	—	—	—
prepylorus	C16.4	C78.89	DØØ.2	D13.1	D37.1	D49.Ø
pylorus	C16.4	C78.89	DØØ.2	D13.1	D37.1	D49.Ø
wall NEC	C16.9	C78.89	DØØ.2	D13.1	D37.1	D49.Ø
anterior NEC	C16.8	C78.89	DØØ.2	D13.1	D37.1	D49.Ø
posterior NEC	C16.8	C78.89	DØØ.2	D13.1	D37.1	D49.Ø
stroma, endometrial	C54.1	C79.82	DØ7.Ø	D26.1	D39.Ø	D49.59
stump, cervical	C53.8	C79.82	DØ6.7	D26.Ø	D39.Ø	D49.59
subcutaneous (nodule) (tissue) NEC — *see Neoplasm, connective tissue*						
subdural	C7Ø.9	C79.32	—	D32.9	D42.9	D49.7
subglottis, subglottic	C32.2	C78.39	DØ2.Ø	D14.1	D38.Ø	D49.1
sublingual	CØ4.9	C79.89	DØØ.Ø6	D1Ø.2	D37.Ø9	D49.Ø
gland or duct	CØ8.1	C79.89	DØØ.ØØ	D11.7	D37.Ø31	D49.Ø
submandibular gland	CØ8.Ø	C79.89	DØØ.ØØ	D11.7	D37.Ø32	D49.Ø
submaxillary gland or duct	CØ8.Ø	C79.89	DØØ.ØØ	D11.7	D37.Ø32	D49.Ø
submental	C76.Ø	C79.89	DØ9.8	D36.7	D48.7	D49.89
subpleural	C34.9-	C78.Ø-	DØ2.2-	D14.3-	D38.1	D49.1
substernal	C38.1	C78.1	—	D15.2	D38.3	D49.89
sudoriferous, sudoriparous gland, site unspecified	C44.9Ø	C79.2	DØ4.9	D23.9	D48.5	D49.2
specified site — *see Neoplasm, skin*						
supraclavicular region	C76.Ø	C79.89	DØ9.8	D36.7	D48.7	D49.89
supraglottis	C32.1	C78.39	DØ2.Ø	D14.1	D38.Ø	D49.1
suprarenal	C74.9-	C79.7-	DØ9.3	D35.Ø-	D44.1-	D49.7
capsule	C74.9-	C79.7-	DØ9.3	D35.Ø-	D44.1-	D49.7
cortex	C74.Ø-	C79.7-	DØ9.3	D35.Ø-	D44.1-	D49.7
gland	C74.9-	C79.7-	DØ9.3	D35.Ø-	D44.1-	D49.7
medulla	C74.1-	C79.7-	DØ9.3	D35.Ø-	D44.1-	D49.7
suprasellar (region)	C71.9	C79.31	—	D33.2	D43.2	D49.6
supratentorial (brain) NEC	C71.Ø	C79.31	—	D33.Ø	D43.Ø	D49.6
sweat gland (apocrine) (eccrine), site unspecified	C44.9Ø	C79.2	DØ4.9	D23.9	D48.5	D49.2
specified site — *see Neoplasm, skin*						
sympathetic nerve or nervous system NEC	C47.9	C79.89	—	D36.1Ø	D48.2	D49.2
symphysis pubis	C41.4	C79.51	—	D16.8	D48.Ø	D49.2
synovial membrane — *see Neoplasm, connective tissue*						
tapetum, brain	C71.8	C79.31	—	D33.2	D43.2	D49.6

	Malignant Primary	Malignant Secondary	Ca in situ	Benign	Uncertain Behavior	Unspecified Behavior
tarsus (any bone)	C4Ø.3-	C79.51	—	D16.3-	—	—
temple (skin) — *see also Neoplasm, skin, face*	C44.3Ø9	C79.2	DØ4.39	D23.39	D48.5	D49.2
temporal						
bone	C41.Ø	C79.51	—	D16.4-	D48.Ø	D49.2
lobe or pole	C71.2	C79.31	—	D33.Ø	D43.Ø	D49.6
region	C76.Ø	C79.89	DØ9.8	D36.7	D48.7	D49.89
skin — *see also Neoplasm, skin, face*	C44.3Ø9	C79.2	DØ4.39	D23.39	D48.5	D49.2
tendon (sheath) — *see Neoplasm, connective tissue*						
tentorium (cerebelli)	C7Ø.Ø	C79.32	—	D32.Ø	D42.Ø	D49.7
testis, testes	C62.9-	C79.82	DØ7.69	D29.2-	D4Ø.1-	D49.59
descended	C62.1-	C79.82	DØ7.69	D29.2-	D4Ø.1-	D49.59
ectopic	C62.Ø-	C79.82	DØ7.69	D29.2-	D4Ø.1-	D49.59
retained	C62.Ø-	C79.82	DØ7.69	D29.2-	D4Ø.1-	D49.59
scrotal	C62.1-	C79.82	DØ7.69	D29.2-	D4Ø.1-	D49.59
undescended	C62.Ø-	C79.82	DØ7.69	D29.2-	D4Ø.1-	D49.59
unspecified whether descended or undescended	C62.9-	C79.82	DØ7.69	D29.2-	D4Ø.1-	D49.59
thalamus	C71.Ø	C79.31	—	D33.Ø	D43.Ø	D49.6
thigh NEC	C76.5-	C79.89	DØ4.7-	D36.7	D48.7	D49.89
thorax, thoracic (cavity) (organs NEC)	C76.1	C79.89	DØ9.8	D36.7	D48.7	D49.89
duct	C49.3	C79.89	—	D21.3	D48.1	D49.2
wall NEC	C76.1	C79.89	DØ9.8	D36.7	D48.7	D49.89
throat	C14.Ø	C79.89	DØØ.Ø8	D1Ø.9	D37.Ø5	D49.Ø
thumb NEC	C76.4-	C79.89	DØ4.6-	D36.7	D48.7	D49.89
thymus (gland)	C37	C79.89	DØ9.3	D15.Ø	D38.4	D49.89
thyroglossal duct	C73	C79.89	DØ9.3	D34	D44.Ø	D49.7
thyroid (gland)	C73	C79.89	DØ9.3	D34	D44.Ø	D49.7
cartilage	C32.3	C78.39	DØ2.Ø	D14.1	D38.Ø	D49.1
tibia (any part)	C4Ø.2-	C79.51	—	D16.2-	—	—
toe NEC	C76.5-	C79.89	DØ4.7-	D36.7	D48.7	D49.89
tongue	CØ2.9	C79.89	DØØ.Ø7	D1Ø.1	D37.Ø2	D49.Ø
anterior (two-thirds) NEC	CØ2.3	C79.89	DØØ.Ø7	D1Ø.1	D37.Ø2	D49.Ø
dorsal surface	CØ2.Ø	C79.89	DØØ.Ø7	D1Ø.1	D37.Ø2	D49.Ø
ventral surface	CØ2.2	C79.89	DØØ.Ø7	D1Ø.1	D37.Ø2	D49.Ø
base (dorsal surface)	CØ1	C79.89	DØØ.Ø7	D1Ø.1	D37.Ø2	D49.Ø
border (lateral)	CØ2.1	C79.89	DØØ.Ø7	D1Ø.1	D37.Ø2	D49.Ø
dorsal surface NEC	CØ2.Ø	C79.89	DØØ.Ø7	D1Ø.1	D37.Ø2	D49.Ø
fixed part NEC	CØ1	C79.89	DØØ.Ø7	D1Ø.1	D37.Ø2	D49.Ø
foreamen cecum	CØ2.Ø	C79.89	DØØ.Ø7	D1Ø.1	D37.Ø2	D49.Ø
frenulum linguae	CØ2.2	C79.89	DØØ.Ø7	D1Ø.1	D37.Ø2	D49.Ø
tongue *(Continued)*						
junctional zone	CØ2.8	C79.89	DØØ.Ø7	D1Ø.1	D37.Ø2	D49.Ø
margin (lateral)	CØ2.1	C79.89	DØØ.Ø7	D1Ø.1	D37.Ø2	D49.Ø
midline NEC	CØ2.Ø	C79.89	DØØ.Ø7	D1Ø.1	D37.Ø2	D49.Ø
mobile part NEC	CØ2.3	C79.89	DØØ.Ø7	D1Ø.1	D37.Ø2	D49.Ø
overlapping lesion	CØ2.8	—	—	—	—	—
posterior (third)	CØ1	C79.89	DØØ.Ø7	D1Ø.1	D37.Ø2	D49.Ø
root	CØ1	C79.89	DØØ.Ø7	D1Ø.1	D37.Ø2	D49.Ø
surface (dorsal)	CØ2.Ø	C79.89	DØØ.Ø7	D1Ø.1	D37.Ø2	D49.Ø
base	CØ1	C79.89	DØØ.Ø7	D1Ø.1	D37.Ø2	D49.Ø
ventral	CØ2.2	C79.89	DØØ.Ø7	D1Ø.1	D37.Ø2	D49.Ø
tip	CØ2.1	C79.89	DØØ.Ø7	D1Ø.1	D37.Ø2	D49.Ø
tonsil	CØ2.4	C79.89	DØØ.Ø7	D1Ø.1	D37.Ø2	D49.Ø
tonsil	CØ9.9	C79.89	DØØ.Ø8	D1Ø.4	D37.Ø5	D49.Ø
fauces, faucial	CØ9.9	C79.89	DØØ.Ø8	D1Ø.4	D37.Ø5	D49.Ø
lingual	CØ2.4	C79.89	DØØ.Ø7	D1Ø.1	D37.Ø2	D49.Ø
overlapping sites	CØ9.8	—	—	—	—	—
palatine	CØ9.9	C79.89	DØØ.Ø8	D1Ø.4	D37.Ø5	D49.Ø
pharyngeal	C11.1	C79.89	DØØ.Ø8	D1Ø.6	D37.Ø5	D49.Ø
pillar (anterior) (posterior)	CØ9.1	C79.89	DØØ.Ø8	D1Ø.5	D37.Ø5	D49.Ø
tonsillar fossa	CØ9.Ø	C79.89	DØØ.Ø8	D1Ø.5	D37.Ø5	D49.Ø
tooth socket NEC	CØ3.9	C79.89	DØØ.Ø3	D1Ø.39	D37.Ø9	D49.Ø
trachea (cartilage) (mucosa)	C33	C78.39	DØ2.1	D14.2	D38.1	D49.1
overlapping lesion with bronchus or lung	C34.8-	—	—	—	—	—
tracheobronchial	C34.8-	C78.39	DØ2.1	D14.2	D38.1	D49.1
overlapping lesion with lung	C34.8-	—	—	—	—	—
tragus — *see also Neoplasm, skin, ear*	C44.2Ø-	C79.2	DØ4.2-	D23.2-	D48.5	D49.2
trunk NEC	C76.8	C79.89	DØ4.5	D36.7	D48.7	D49.89
tubo-ovarian	C57.8	C79.82	DØ7.39	D28.7	D39.8	D49.59
tunica vaginalis	C63.7	C79.82	DØ7.69	D29.8	D4Ø.8	D49.59
turbinate (bone)	C41.Ø	C79.51	—	D16.4-	D48.Ø	D49.2
nasal	C3Ø.Ø	C78.39	DØ2.3	D14.Ø	D38.5	D49.1
tympanic cavity	C3Ø.1	C78.39	DØ2.3	D14.Ø	D38.5	D49.1
ulna (any part)	C4Ø.Ø-	C79.51	—	D16.Ø-	—	—
umbilicus, umbilical — *see also Neoplasm, skin, trunk*	C44.5Ø9	C79.2	DØ4.5	D23.5	D48.5	D49.2
uncus, brain	C71.2	C79.31	—	D33.Ø	D43.Ø	D49.6
unknown site or unspecified	C8Ø.1	C79.9	DØ9.9	D36.9	D48.9	D49.9
urachus	C67.7	C79.11	DØ9.Ø	D3Ø.3	D41.4	D49.4
ureter, ureteral	C66.-	C79.19	DØ9.19	D3Ø.2-	D41.2-	D49.59
orifice (bladder)	C67.6	C79.11	DØ9.Ø	D3Ø.3	D41.4	D49.4
ureter-bladder (junction)	C67.6	C79.11	DØ9.Ø	D3Ø.3	D41.4	D49.4

TABLE OF NEOPLASMS

◄ New ⇐ Revised ~~deleted~~ Deleted

	Malignant Primary	Malignant Secondary	Ca in situ	Benign	Uncertain Behavior	Unspecified Behavior
urethra, urethral (gland)	C68.Ø	C79.19	DØ9.19	D3Ø.4	D41.3	D49.59
orifice, internal	C67.5	C79.11	DØ9.Ø	D3Ø.3	D41.4	D49.4
urethrovaginal (septum)	C57.9	C79.82	DØ7.3Ø	D28.9	D39.8	D49.59
urinary organ or system	C68.9	C79.1Ø	DØ9.1Ø	D3Ø.9	D41.9	D49.59
bladder — *see Neoplasm, bladder*						
overlapping lesion	C68.8	—	—	—	—	—
specified sites NEC	C68.8	C79.19	DØ9.19	D3Ø.8	D41.8	D49.59
utero-ovarian	C57.8	C79.82	DØ7.39	D28.7	D39.8	D49.59
ligament	C57.1	C79.82	DØ7.39	D28.2	D39.8	D49.59
uterosacral ligament	C57.3	C79.82	—	D28.2	D39.8	D49.59
uterus, uteri, uterine	C55	C79.82	DØ7.Ø	D26.9	D39.Ø	D49.59
adnexa NEC	C57.4	C79.82	DØ7.39	D28.7	D39.8	D49.59
body	C54.9	C79.82	DØ7.Ø	D26.1	D39.Ø	D49.59
cervix	C53.9	C79.82	DØ6.9	D26.Ø	D39.Ø	D49.59
cornu	C54.9	C79.82	DØ7.Ø	D26.1	D39.Ø	D49.59
corpus	C54.9	C79.82	DØ7.Ø	D26.1	D39.Ø	D49.59
endocervix (canal) (gland)	C53.Ø	C79.82	DØ6.Ø	D26.Ø	D39.Ø	D49.59
endometrium	C54.1	C79.82	DØ7.Ø	D26.1	D39.Ø	D49.59
exocervix	C53.1	C79.82	DØ6.1	D26.Ø	D39.Ø	D49.59
external os	C53.1	C79.82	DØ6.1	D26.Ø	D39.Ø	D49.59
fundus	C54.3	C79.82	DØ7.Ø	D26.1	D39.Ø	D49.59
internal os	C53.Ø	C79.82	DØ6.Ø	D26.Ø	D39.Ø	D49.59
isthmus	C54.Ø	C79.82	DØ7.Ø	D26.1	D39.Ø	D49.59
ligament	C57.3	C79.82	—	D28.2	D39.8	D49.59
broad	C57.1	C79.82	DØ7.39	D28.2	D39.8	D49.59
round	C57.2	C79.82	—	D28.2	D39.8	D49.59
lower segment	C54.Ø	C79.82	DØ7.Ø	D26.1	D39.Ø	D49.59
myometrium	C54.2	C79.82	DØ7.Ø	D26.1	D39.Ø	D49.59
overlapping sites	C54.8	—	—	—	—	—
squamocolumnar junction	C53.8	C79.82	DØ6.7	D26.Ø	D39.Ø	D49.59
tube	C57.Ø-	C79.82	DØ7.39	D28.2	D39.8	D49.59
utricle, prostatic	C68.Ø	C79.19	DØ9.19	D3Ø.4	D41.3	D49.59
uveal tract	C69.4-	C79.49	DØ9.2-	D31.4-	D48.7	D49.89
uvula	CØ5.2	C79.89	DØØ.Ø4	D1Ø.39	D37.Ø9	D49.Ø
vagina, vaginal (fornix) (vault) (wall)	C52	C79.82	DØ7.2	D28.1	D39.8	D49.59
vaginovesical	C57.9	C79.82	DØ7.3Ø	D28.9	D39.9	D49.59
septum	C57.9	C79.82	DØ7.3Ø	D28.9	D39.9	D49.59
vallecula (epiglottis)	C1Ø.Ø	C79.89	DØØ.Ø8	D1Ø.5	D37.Ø5	D49.Ø
vas deferens	C63.1-	C79.82	DØ7.69	D29.8	D4Ø.8	D49.59
vascular — *see Neoplasm, connective tissue*						
Vater's ampulla	C24.1	C78.89	DØ1.5	D13.5	D37.6	D49.Ø
vein, venous — *see Neoplasm, connective tissue*						
vena cava (abdominal) (inferior)	C49.4	C79.89	—	D21.4	D48.1	D49.2
superior	C49.3	C79.89	—	D21.3	D48.1	D49.2
ventricle (cerebral) (floor) (lateral) (third)	C71.5	C79.31	—	D33.Ø	D43.Ø	D49.6
cardiac (left) (right)	C38.Ø	C79.89	—	D15.1	D48.7	D49.89
fourth	C71.7	C79.31	—	D33.1	D43.1	D49.6
ventricular band of larynx	C32.1	C78.39	DØ2.Ø	D14.1	D38.Ø	D49.1
ventriculus — *see Neoplasm, stomach*						
vermillion border — *see Neoplasm, lip*						
vermis, cerebellum	C71.6	C79.31	—	D33.1	D43.1	D49.6
vertebra (column)	C41.2	C79.51	—	D16.6	D48.Ø	D49.2
coccyx	C41.4	C79.51	—	D16.8-	D48.Ø	D49.2
marrow NEC	C96.9	C79.52	—	—	D47.9	D49.89
sacrum	C41.4	C79.51	—	D16.8-	D48.Ø	D49.2
vesical — *see Neoplasm, bladder*						
vesicle, seminal	C63.7	C79.82	DØ7.69	D29.8	D4Ø.8	D49.59
vesicocervical tissue	C57.9	C79.82	DØ7.3Ø	D28.9	D39.9	D49.59
vesicorectal	C76.3	C79.82	DØ9.8	D36.7	D48.7	D49.89
vesicovaginal	C57.9	C79.82	DØ7.3Ø	D28.9	D39.9	D49.59
septum	C57.9	C79.82	DØ7.3Ø	D28.9	D39.8	D49.59
vessel (blood) — *see Neoplasm, connective tissue*						
vestibular gland, greater	C51.Ø	C79.82	DØ7.1	D28.Ø	D39.8	D49.59
vestibule						
mouth	CØ6.1	C79.89	DØØ.ØØ	D1Ø.39	D37.Ø9	D49.Ø
nose	C3Ø.Ø	C78.39	DØ2.3	D14.Ø	D38.5	D49.1
Virchow's gland	C77.Ø	C77.Ø	—	D36.Ø	D48.7	D49.89
viscera NEC	C76.8	C79.89	DØ9.8	D36.7	D48.7	D49.89
vocal cords (true)	C32.Ø	C78.39	DØ2.Ø	D14.1	D38.Ø	D49.1
false	C32.1	C78.39	DØ2.Ø	D14.1	D38.Ø	D49.1
vomer	C41.Ø	C79.51	—	D16.4-	D48.Ø	D49.2
vulva	C51.9	C79.82	DØ7.1	D28.Ø	D39.8	D49.59
vulvovaginal gland	C51.Ø	C79.82	DØ7.1	D28.Ø	D39.8	D49.59
Waldeyer's ring	C14.2	C79.89	DØØ.Ø8	D1Ø.9	D37.Ø5	D49.Ø
Wharton's duct	CØ8.Ø	C79.89	DØØ.ØØ	D11.7	D37.Ø32	D49.Ø
white matter (central) (cerebral)	C71.Ø	C79.31	—	D33.Ø	D43.Ø	D49.6
windpipe	C33	C78.39	DØ2.1	D14.2	D38.1	D49.1

	Malignant Primary	Malignant Secondary	Ca in situ	Benign	Uncertain Behavior	Unspecified Behavior
Wirsung's duct	C25.3	C78.89	D01.7	D13.6	D37.8	D49.0
wolffian (body) (duct)						
female	C57.7	C79.82	D07.39	D28.7	D39.8	D49.59
male	C63.7	C79.82	D07.69	D29.8	D40.8	D49.59
womb — *see Neoplasm, uterus*						
wrist NEC	C76.4-	C79.89	D04.6-	D36.7	D48.7	D49.89
xiphoid process	C41.3	C79.51	—	D16.7	D48.0	D49.2
Zuckerkandl organ	C75.5	C79.89	—	D35.6	D44.7	D49.7

TABLE OF NEOPLASMS

New Revised ~~deleted~~ Deleted

ICD-10-CM Table of Drugs and Chemicals

Substance	Poisoning, Accidental (Unintentional)	Poisoning, Intentional Self-Harm	Poisoning, Assault	Poisoning, Undetermined	Adverse Effect	Underdosing
#						
1-propanol	T51.3X1	T51.3X2	T51.3X3	T51.3X4	—	—
2-propanol	T51.2X1	T51.2X2	T51.2X3	T51.2X4	—	—
2,4-D (dichlorophen-oxyacetic acid)	T60.3X1	T60.3X2	T60.3X3	T60.3X4	—	—
2,4-toluene diisocyanate	T65.0X1	T65.0X2	T65.0X3	T65.0X4	—	—
2,4,5-T (trichloro-phenoxyacetic acid)	T60.1X1	T60.1X2	T60.1X3	T60.1X4	—	—
14-hydroxydihydro-morphinone	T40.2X1	T40.2X2	T40.2X3	T40.2X4	T40.2X5	T40.2X6
A						
ABOB	T37.5X1	T37.5X2	T37.5X3	T37.5X4	T37.5X5	T37.5X6
Abrine	T62.2X1	T62.2X2	T62.2X3	T62.2X4	—	—
Abrus (seed)	T62.2X1	T62.2X2	T62.2X3	T62.2X4	—	—
Absinthe	T51.0X1	T51.0X2	T51.0X3	T51.0X4	—	—
beverage	T51.0X1	T51.0X2	T51.0X3	T51.0X4	—	—
Acaricide	T60.8X1	T60.8X2	T60.8X3	T60.8X4	—	—
Acebutolol	T44.7X1	T44.7X2	T44.7X3	T44.7X4	T44.7X5	T44.7X6
Acecarbromal	T42.6X1	T42.6X2	T42.6X3	T42.6X4	T42.6X5	T42.6X6
Aceclidine	T44.1X1	T44.1X2	T44.1X3	T44.1X4	T44.1X5	T44.1X6
Acedapsone	T37.0X1	T37.0X2	T37.0X3	T37.0X4	T37.0X5	T37.0X6
Acefylline piperazine	T48.6X1	T48.6X2	T48.6X3	T48.6X4	T48.6X5	T48.6X6
Acemorphan	T40.2X1	T40.2X2	T40.2X3	T40.2X4	T40.2X5	T40.2X6
Acenocoumarin	T45.511	T45.512	T45.513	T45.514	T45.515	T45.516
Acenocoumarol	T45.511	T45.512	T45.513	T45.514	T45.515	T45.516
Acepifylline	T48.6X1	T48.6X2	T48.6X3	T48.6X4	T48.6X5	T48.6X6
Acepromazine	T43.3X1	T43.3X2	T43.3X3	T43.3X4	T43.3X5	T43.3X6
Acesulfamethoxypyridazine	T37.0X1	T37.0X2	T37.0X3	T37.0X4	T37.0X5	T37.0X6
Acetal	T52.8X1	T52.8X2	T52.8X3	T52.8X4	—	—
Acetaldehyde (vapor)	T52.8X1	T52.8X2	T52.8X3	T52.8X4	—	—
liquid	T65.891	T65.892	T65.893	T65.894	—	—
P-Acetamidophenol	T39.1X1	T39.1X2	T39.1X3	T39.1X4	T39.1X5	T39.1X6
Acetaminophen	T39.1X1	T39.1X2	T39.1X3	T39.1X4	T39.1X5	T39.1X6
Acetaminosalol	T39.1X1	T39.1X2	T39.1X3	T39.1X4	T39.1X5	T39.1X6
Acetanilide	T39.1X1	T39.1X2	T39.1X3	T39.1X4	T39.1X5	T39.1X6
Acetarsol	T37.3X1	T37.3X2	T37.3X3	T37.3X4	T37.3X5	T37.3X6
Acetazolamide	T50.2X1	T50.2X2	T50.2X3	T50.2X4	T50.2X5	T50.2X6
Acetiamine	T45.2X1	T45.2X2	T45.2X3	T45.2X4	T45.2X5	T45.2X6
Acetic						
acid	T54.2X1	T54.2X2	T54.2X3	T54.2X4	—	—
with sodium acetate (ointment)	T49.3X1	T49.3X2	T49.3X3	T49.3X4	T49.3X5	T49.3X6
Acetic *(Continued)*						
acid *(Continued)*						
ester (solvent) (vapor)	T52.8X1	T52.8X2	T52.8X3	T52.8X4	—	—
irrigating solution	T50.3X1	T50.3X2	T50.3X3	T50.3X4	T50.3X5	T50.3X6
medicinal (lotion)	T49.2X1	T49.2X2	T49.2X3	T49.2X4	T49.2X5	T49.2X6
anhydride	T65.891	T65.892	T65.893	T65.894	—	—
ether (vapor)	T52.8X1	T52.8X2	T52.8X3	T52.8X4	—	—
Acetohexamide	T38.3X1	T38.3X2	T38.3X3	T38.3X4	T38.3X5	T38.3X6
Acetohydroxamic acid	T50.991	T50.992	T50.993	T50.994	T50.995	T50.996
Acetomenaphthone	T45.7X1	T45.7X2	T45.7X3	T45.7X4	T45.7X5	T45.7X6
Acetomorphine	T40.1X1	T40.1X2	T40.1X3	T40.1X4	—	—
Acetone (oils)	T52.4X1	T52.4X2	T52.4X3	T52.4X4	—	—
chlorinated	T52.4X1	T52.4X2	T52.4X3	T52.4X4	—	—
vapor	T52.4X1	T52.4X2	T52.4X3	T52.4X4	—	—
Acetonitrile	T52.8X1	T52.8X2	T52.8X3	T52.8X4	—	—
Acetophenazine	T43.3X1	T43.3X2	T43.3X3	T43.3X4	T43.3X5	T43.3X6
Acetophenetedin	T39.1X1	T39.1X2	T39.1X3	T39.1X4	T39.1X5	T39.1X6
Acetophenone	T52.4X1	T52.4X2	T52.4X3	T52.4X4	—	—
Acetorphine	T40.2X1	T40.2X2	T40.2X3	T40.2X4	—	—
Acetosulfone (sodium)	T37.1X1	T37.1X2	T37.1X3	T37.1X4	T37.1X5	T37.1X6
Acetrizoate (sodium)	T50.8X1	T50.8X2	T50.8X3	T50.8X4	T50.8X5	T50.8X6
Acetylcarbromal	T42.6X1	T42.6X2	T42.6X3	T42.6X4	T42.6X5	T42.6X6
Acetrizoic acid	T50.8X1	T50.8X2	T50.8X3	T50.8X4	T50.8X5	T50.8X6
Acetyl						
bromide	T53.6X1	T53.6X2	T53.6X3	T53.6X4	—	—
chloride	T53.6X1	T53.6X2	T53.6X3	T53.6X4	—	—
Acetylcholine						
chloride	T44.1X1	T44.1X2	T44.1X3	T44.1X4	T44.1X5	T44.1X6
derivative	T44.1X1	T44.1X2	T44.1X3	T44.1X4	T44.1X5	T44.1X6
Acetylcysteine	T48.4X1	T48.4X2	T48.4X3	T48.4X4	T48.4X5	T48.4X6
Acetyldigitoxin	T46.0X1	T46.0X2	T46.0X3	T46.0X4	T46.0X5	T46.0X6
Acetyldigoxin	T46.0X1	T46.0X2	T46.0X3	T46.0X4	T46.0X5	T46.0X6
Acetyldihydrocodeine	T40.2X1	T40.2X2	T40.2X3	T40.2X4	—	—
Acetyldihydrocodeinone	T40.2X1	T40.2X2	T40.2X3	T40.2X4	—	—
Acetylene (gas)	T59.891	T59.892	T59.893	T59.894	—	—
dichloride	T53.6X1	T53.6X2	T53.6X3	T53.6X4	—	—
incomplete combustion of	T58.11	T58.12	T58.13	T58.14	—	—
industrial	T59.891	T59.892	T59.893	T59.894	—	—
tetrachloride	T53.6X1	T53.6X2	T53.6X3	T53.6X4	—	—
vapor	T53.6X1	T53.6X2	T53.6X3	T53.6X4	—	—
Acetylphenylhydrazine	T39.8X1	T39.8X2	T39.8X3	T39.8X4	T39.8X5	T39.8X6
Acetylpheneturide	T42.6X1	T42.6X2	T42.6X3	T42.6X4	T42.6X5	T42.6X6

Substance	Poisoning, Accidental (Unintentional)	Poisoning, Intentional Self-Harm	Poisoning, Assault	Poisoning, Undetermined	Adverse Effect	Underdosing
Acetylsalicylic acid (salts)	T39.Ø11	T39.Ø12	T39.Ø13	T39.Ø14	T39.Ø15	T39.Ø16
enteric coated	T39.Ø11	T39.Ø12	T39.Ø13	T39.Ø14	T39.Ø15	T39.Ø16
Acetylsulfamethoxypyridazine	T37.ØX1	T37.ØX2	T37.ØX3	T37.ØX4	T37.ØX5	T37.ØX6
Achromycin	T36.4X1	T36.4X2	T36.4X3	T36.4X4	T36.4X5	T36.4X6
ophthalmic preparation	T49.5X1	T49.5X2	T49.5X3	T49.5X4	T49.5X5	T49.5X6
topical NEC	T49.ØX1	T49.ØX2	T49.ØX3	T49.ØX4	T49.ØX5	T49.ØX6
Aciclovir	T37.5X1	T37.5X2	T37.5X3	T37.5X4	T37.5X5	T37.5X6
Acid (corrosive) NEC	T54.2X1	T54.2X2	T54.2X3	T54.2X4	—	—
Acidifying agent NEC	T5Ø.9Ø1	T5Ø.9Ø2	T5Ø.9Ø3	T5Ø.9Ø4	T5Ø.9Ø5	T5Ø.9Ø6
Acipimox	T46.6X1	T46.6X2	T46.6X3	T46.6X4	T46.6X5	T46.6X6
Acitretin	T5Ø.991	T5Ø.992	T5Ø.993	T5Ø.994	T5Ø.995	T5Ø.996
Aclarubicin	T45.1X1	T45.1X2	T45.1X3	T45.1X4	T45.1X5	T45.1X6
Aclatonium napadisilate	T48.1X1	T48.1X2	T48.1X3	T48.1X4	T48.1X5	T48.1X6
Aconite (wild)	T46.991	T46.992	T46.993	T46.994	T46.995	T46.996
Aconitine	T46.991	T46.992	T46.993	T46.994	T46.995	T46.996
Aconitum ferox	T46.991	T46.992	T46.993	T46.994	T46.995	T46.996
Acridine	T65.6X1	T65.6X2	T65.6X3	T65.6X4	—	—
vapor	T59.891	T59.892	T59.893	T59.894	—	—
Acriflavine	T37.91	T37.92	T37.93	T37.94	T37.95	T37.96
Acriflavinium chloride	T49.ØX1	T49.ØX2	T49.ØX3	T49.ØX4	T49.ØX5	T49.ØX6
Acrinol	T49.ØX1	T49.ØX2	T49.ØX3	T49.ØX4	T49.ØX5	T49.ØX6
Acrisorcin	T49.ØX1	T49.ØX2	T49.ØX3	T49.ØX4	T49.ØX5	T49.ØX6
Acrivastine	T45.ØX1	T45.ØX2	T45.ØX3	T45.ØX4	T45.ØX5	T45.ØX6
Acrolein (gas)	T59.891	T59.892	T59.893	T59.894	—	—
liquid	T54.1X1	T54.1X2	T54.1X3	T54.1X4	—	—
Acrylamide	T65.891	T65.892	T65.893	T65.894	—	—
Acrylic resin	T49.3X1	T49.3X2	T49.3X3	T49.3X4	T49.3X5	T49.3X6
Acrylonitrile	T65.891	T65.892	T65.893	T65.894	—	—
Actaea spicata	T62.2X1	T62.2X2	T62.2X3	T62.2X4	—	—
berry	T62.1X1	T62.1X2	T62.1X3	T62.1X4	—	—
Acterol	T37.3X1	T37.3X2	T37.3X3	T37.3X4	T37.3X5	T37.3X6
ACTH	T38.811	T38.812	T38.813	T38.814	T38.815	T38.816
Actinomycin C	T45.1X1	T45.1X2	T45.1X3	T45.1X4	T45.1X5	T45.1X6
Actinomycin D	T45.1X1	T45.1X2	T45.1X3	T45.1X4	T45.1X5	T45.1X6
Activated charcoal — *see also Charcoal, medicinal*	T47.6X1	T47.6X2	T47.6X3	T47.6X4	T47.6X5	T47.6X6
Acyclovir	T37.5X1	T37.5X2	T37.5X3	T37.5X4	T37.5X5	T37.5X6
Adenine	T45.2X1	T45.2X2	T45.2X3	T45.2X4	T45.2X5	T45.2X6
arabinoside	T37.5X1	T37.5X2	T37.5X3	T37.5X4	T37.5X5	T37.5X6
Adenosine (phosphate)	T46.2X1	T46.2X2	T46.2X3	T46.2X4	T46.2X5	T46.2X6
ADH	T38.891	T38.892	T38.893	T38.894	T38.895	T38.896
Adhesive NEC	T65.891	T65.892	T65.893	T65.894	—	—
Adicillin	T36.ØX1	T36.ØX2	T36.ØX3	T36.ØX4	T36.ØX5	T36.ØX6
Adiphenine	T44.3X1	T44.3X2	T44.3X3	T44.3X4	T44.3X5	T44.3X6
Adipiodone	T5Ø.8X1	T5Ø.8X2	T5Ø.8X3	T5Ø.8X4	T5Ø.8X5	T5Ø.8X6
Adjunct, pharmaceutical	T5Ø.9Ø1	T5Ø.9Ø2	T5Ø.9Ø3	T5Ø.9Ø4	T5Ø.9Ø5	T5Ø.9Ø6
Adrenal (extract, cortex or medulla) (glucocorticoids) (hormones) (mineralo corticoids)	T38.ØX1	T38.ØX2	T38.ØX3	T38.ØX4	T38.ØX5	T38.ØX6
ENT agent	T49.6X1	T49.6X2	T49.6X3	T49.6X4	T49.6X5	T49.6X6
ophthalmic preparation	T49.5X1	T49.5X2	T49.5X3	T49.5X4	T49.5X5	T49.5X6
topical NEC	T49.ØX1	T49.ØX2	T49.ØX3	T49.ØX4	T49.ØX5	T49.ØX6
Adrenaline	T44.5X1	T44.5X2	T44.5X3	T44.5X4	T44.5X5	T44.5X6
Adrenalin — *see Adrenaline*						
Adrenergic NEC	T44.9Ø1	T44.9Ø2	T44.9Ø3	T44.9Ø4	T44.9Ø5	T44.9Ø6
blocking agent NEC	T44.8X1	T44.8X2	T44.8X3	T44.8X4	T44.8X5	T44.8X6
beta, heart	T44.7X1	T44.7X2	T44.7X3	T44.7X4	T44.7X5	T44.7X6
specified NEC	T44.991	T44.992	T44.993	T44.994	T44.995	T44.996
Adrenochrome						
(mono) semicarbazone	T46.991	T46.992	T46.993	T46.994	T46.995	T46.996
derivative	T46.991	T46.992	T46.993	T46.994	T46.995	T46.996
Adrenocorticotrophic hormone	T38.811	T38.812	T38.813	T38.814	T38.815	T38.816
Adrenocorticotrophin	T38.811	T38.812	T38.813	T38.814	T38.815	T38.816
Adriamycin	T45.1X1	T45.1X2	T45.1X3	T45.1X4	T45.1X5	T45.1X6
Aerosol spray NEC	T65.91	T65.92	T65.93	T65.94	—	—
Aerosporin	T36.8X1	T36.8X2	T36.8X3	T36.8X4	T36.8X5	T36.8X6
ENT agent	T49.6X1	T49.6X2	T49.6X3	T49.6X4	T49.6X5	T49.6X6
ophthalmic preparation	T49.5X1	T49.5X2	T49.5X3	T49.5X4	T49.5X5	T49.5X6
topical NEC	T49.ØX1	T49.ØX2	T49.ØX3	T49.ØX4	T49.ØX5	T49.ØX6
Aethusa cynapium	T62.2X1	T62.2X2	T62.2X3	T62.2X4	—	—
Afghanistan black	T4Ø.7X1	T4Ø.7X2	T4Ø.7X3	T4Ø.7X4	T4Ø.7X5	T4Ø.7X6
Aflatoxin	T64.Ø1	T64.Ø2	T64.Ø3	T64.Ø4	—	—
Afloqualone	T42.8X1	T42.8X2	T42.8X3	T42.8X4	T42.8X5	T42.8X6
African boxwood	T62.2X1	T62.2X2	T62.2X3	T62.2X4	—	—
Agar	T47.4X1	T47.4X2	T47.4X3	T47.4X4	T47.4X5	T47.4X6
Agonist						
predominantly						
alpha-adrenoreceptor	T44.4X1	T44.4X2	T44.4X3	T44.4X4	T44.4X5	T44.4X6
beta-adrenoreceptor	T44.5X1	T44.5X2	T44.5X3	T44.5X4	T44.5X5	T44.5X6
Agricultural agent NEC	T65.91	T65.92	T65.93	T65.94	—	—
Agrypnal	T42.3X1	T42.3X2	T42.3X3	T42.3X4	T42.3X5	T42.3X6
AHLG	T5Ø.Z11	T5Ø.Z12	T5Ø.Z13	T5Ø.Z14	T5Ø.Z15	T5Ø.Z16
Air contaminant(s), source/type NOS	T65.91	T65.92	T65.93	T65.94	—	—

Substance	Poisoning, Accidental (Unintentional)	Poisoning, Intentional Self-Harm	Poisoning, Assault	Poisoning, Undetermined	Adverse Effect	Underdosing
Ajmaline	T46.2X1	T46.2X2	T46.2X3	T46.2X4	T46.2X5	T46.2X6
Akritoin	T37.8X1	T37.8X2	T37.8X3	T37.8X4	T37.8X5	T37.8X6
Akee	T62.1X1	T62.1X2	T62.1X3	T62.1X4	—	—
Akrinol	T49.ØX1	T49.ØX2	T49.ØX3	T49.ØX4	T49.ØX5	T49.ØX6
Alacepril	T46.4X1	T46.4X2	T46.4X3	T46.4X4	T46.4X5	T46.4X6
Alantolactone	T37.4X1	T37.4X2	T37.4X3	T37.4X4	T37.4X5	T37.4X6
Albamycin	T36.8X1	T36.8X2	T36.8X3	T36.8X4	T36.8X5	T36.8X6
Albendazole	T37.4X1	T37.4X2	T37.4X3	T37.4X4	T37.4X5	T37.4X6
Albumin						
bovine	T45.8X1	T45.8X2	T45.8X3	T45.8X4	T45.8X5	T45.8X6
human serum	T45.8X1	T45.8X2	T45.8X3	T45.8X4	T45.8X5	T45.8X6
salt-poor	T45.8X1	T45.8X2	T45.8X3	T45.8X4	T45.8X5	T45.8X6
normal human serum	T45.8X1	T45.8X2	T45.8X3	T45.8X4	T45.8X5	T45.8X6
Albuterol	T48.6X1	T48.6X2	T48.6X3	T48.6X4	T48.6X5	T48.6X6
Albutoin	T42.ØX1	T42.ØX2	T42.ØX3	T42.ØX4	T42.ØX5	T42.ØX6
Alclometasone	T49.ØX1	T49.ØX2	T49.ØX3	T49.ØX4	T49.ØX5	T49.ØX6
Alcohol	T51.91	T51.92	T51.93	T51.94	—	—
absolute	T51.ØX1	T51.ØX2	T51.ØX3	T51.ØX4	—	—
beverage	T51.ØX1	T51.ØX2	T51.ØX3	T51.ØX4	—	—
allyl	T51.8X1	T51.8X2	T51.8X3	T51.8X4	—	—
amyl	T51.3X1	T51.3X2	T51.3X3	T51.3X4	—	—
antifreeze	T51.1X1	T51.1X2	T51.1X3	T51.1X4	—	—
beverage	T51.ØX1	T51.ØX2	T51.ØX3	T51.ØX4	—	—
butyl	T51.3X1	T51.3X2	T51.3X3	T51.3X4	—	—
dehydrated	T51.ØX1	T51.ØX2	T51.ØX3	T51.ØX4	—	—
beverage	T51.ØX1	T51.ØX2	T51.ØX3	T51.ØX4	—	—
denatured	T51.ØX1	T51.ØX2	T51.ØX3	T51.ØX4	—	—
deterrent NEC	T5Ø.6X1	T5Ø.6X2	T5Ø.6X3	T5Ø.6X4	T5Ø.6X5	T5Ø.6X6
diagnostic (gastric function)	T5Ø.8X1	T5Ø.8X2	T5Ø.8X3	T5Ø.8X4	T5Ø.8X5	T5Ø.8X6
ethyl	T51.ØX1	T51.ØX2	T51.ØX3	T51.ØX4	—	—
beverage	T51.ØX1	T51.ØX2	T51.ØX3	T51.ØX4	—	—
grain	T51.ØX1	T51.ØX2	T51.ØX3	T51.ØX4	—	—
beverage	T51.ØX1	T51.ØX2	T51.ØX3	T51.ØX4	—	—
industrial	T51.ØX1	T51.ØX2	T51.ØX3	T51.ØX4	—	—
isopropyl	T51.2X1	T51.2X2	T51.2X3	T51.2X4	—	—
methyl	T51.1X1	T51.1X2	T51.1X3	T51.1X4	—	—
preparation for consumption	T51.ØX1	T51.ØX2	T51.ØX3	T51.ØX4	—	—
propyl	T51.3X1	T51.3X2	T51.3X3	T51.3X4	—	—
secondary	T51.2X1	T51.2X2	T51.2X3	T51.2X4	—	—
radiator	T51.1X1	T51.1X2	T51.1X3	T51.1X4	—	—
rubbing	T51.2X1	T51.2X2	T51.2X3	T51.2X4	—	—
specified type NEC	T51.8X1	T51.8X2	T51.8X3	T51.8X4	—	—
Alcohol *(Continued)*						
surgical	T51.ØX1	T51.ØX2	T51.ØX3	T51.ØX4	—	—
vapor (from any type of Alcohol)	T59.891	T59.892	T59.893	T59.894	—	—
wood	T51.1X1	T51.1X2	T51.1X3	T51.1X4	—	—
Alcuronium (chloride)	T48.1X1	T48.1X2	T48.1X3	T48.1X4	T48.1X5	T48.1X6
Aldactone	T5Ø.ØX1	T5Ø.ØX2	T5Ø.ØX3	T5Ø.ØX4	T5Ø.ØX5	T5Ø.ØX6
Aldesulfone sodium	T37.1X1	T37.1X2	T37.1X3	T37.1X4	T37.1X5	T37.1X6
Aldicarb	T6Ø.ØX1	T6Ø.ØX2	T6Ø.ØX3	T6Ø.ØX4	—	—
Aldomet	T46.5X1	T46.5X2	T46.5X3	T46.5X4	T46.5X5	T46.5X6
Aldosterone	T5Ø.ØX1	T5Ø.ØX2	T5Ø.ØX3	T5Ø.ØX4	T5Ø.ØX5	T5Ø.ØX6
Aldrin (dust)	T6Ø.1X1	T6Ø.1X2	T6Ø.1X3	T6Ø.1X4	—	—
Aleve — *see Naproxen*						
Alexitol sodium	T47.1X1	T47.1X2	T47.1X3	T47.1X4	T47.1X5	T47.1X6
Alfacalcidol	T45.2X1	T45.2X2	T45.2X3	T45.2X4	T45.2X5	T45.2X6
Alfadolone	T41.1X1	T41.1X2	T41.1X3	T41.1X4	T41.1X5	T41.1X6
Alfaxalone	T41.1X1	T41.1X2	T41.1X3	T41.1X4	T41.1X5	T41.1X6
Alfentanil	T4Ø.4X1	T4Ø.4X2	T4Ø.4X3	T4Ø.4X4	T4Ø.4X5	T4Ø.4X6
Alfuzosin (hydrochloride)	T44.8X1	T44.8X2	T44.8X3	T44.8X4	T44.8X5	T44.8X6
Algae (harmful) (toxin)	T65.821	T65.822	T65.823	T65.824	—	—
Algeldrate	T47.1X1	T47.1X2	T47.1X3	T47.1X4	T47.1X5	T47.1X6
Algin	T47.8X1	T47.8X2	T47.8X3	T47.8X4	T47.8X5	T47.8X6
Alglucerase	T45.3X1	T45.3X2	T45.3X3	T45.3X4	T45.3X5	T45.3X6
Alidase	T45.3X1	T45.3X2	T45.3X3	T45.3X4	T45.3X5	T45.3X6
Alimemazine	T43.3X1	T43.3X2	T43.3X3	T43.3X4	T43.3X5	T43.3X6
Aliphatic thiocyanates	T65.ØX1	T65.ØX2	T65.ØX3	T65.ØX4	—	—
Alizapride	T45.ØX1	T45.ØX2	T45.ØX3	T45.ØX4	T45.ØX5	T45.ØX6
Alkali (caustic)	T54.3X1	T54.3X2	T54.3X3	T54.3X4	—	—
Alkalizing agent NEC	T5Ø.9Ø1	T5Ø.9Ø2	T5Ø.9Ø3	T5Ø.9Ø4	T5Ø.9Ø5	T5Ø.9Ø6
Alkaline antiseptic solution (aromatic)	T49.6X1	T49.6X2	T49.6X3	T49.6X4	T49.6X5	T49.6X6
Alkalinizing agents (medicinal)	T5Ø.9Ø1	T5Ø.9Ø2	T5Ø.9Ø3	T5Ø.9Ø4	T5Ø.9Ø5	T5Ø.9Ø6
Alka-seltzer	T39.Ø11	T39.Ø12	T39.Ø13	T39.Ø14	T39.Ø15	T39.Ø16
Alkavervir	T46.5X1	T46.5X2	T46.5X3	T46.5X4	T46.5X5	T46.5X6
Alkonium (bromide)	T49.ØX1	T49.ØX2	T49.ØX3	T49.ØX4	T49.ØX5	T49.ØX6
Alkylating drug NEC	T45.1X1	T45.1X2	T45.1X3	T45.1X4	T45.1X5	T45.1X6
antimyeloproliferative	T45.1X1	T45.1X2	T45.1X3	T45.1X4	T45.1X5	T45.1X6
lymphatic	T45.1X1	T45.1X2	T45.1X3	T45.1X4	T45.1X5	T45.1X6
Alkylisocyanate	T65.ØX1	T65.ØX2	T65.ØX3	T65.ØX4	—	—
Allantoin	T49.411	T49.412	T49.413	T49.414	T49.415	T49.416
Allegron	T43.ØX1	T43.ØX2	T43.ØX3	T43.ØX4	T43.ØX5	T43.ØX6
Allethrin	T49.ØX1	T49.ØX2	T49.ØX3	T49.ØX4	T49.ØX5	T49.ØX6
Allobarbital	T42.3X1	T42.3X2	T42.3X3	T42.3X4	T42.3X5	T42.3X6

Substance	Poisoning, Accidental (Unintentional)	Poisoning, Intentional Self-Harm	Poisoning, Assault	Poisoning, Undetermined	Adverse Effect	Underdosing
Allopurinol	T50.4X1	T50.4X2	T50.4X3	T50.4X4	T50.4X5	T50.4X6
Allyl						
alcohol	T51.8X1	T51.8X2	T51.8X3	T51.8X4	—	—
disulfide	T46.6X1	T46.6X2	T46.6X3	T46.6X4	T46.6X5	T46.6X6
Allylestrenol	T38.5X1	T38.5X2	T38.5X3	T38.5X4	T38.5X5	T38.5X6
Allylisopropylacetylurea	T42.6X1	T42.6X2	T42.6X3	T42.6X4	T42.6X5	T42.6X6
Allylisopropylmalonylurea	T42.3X1	T42.3X2	T42.3X3	T42.3X4	T42.3X5	T42.3X6
Allylthiourea	T49.3X1	T49.3X2	T49.3X3	T49.3X4	T49.3X5	T49.3X6
Allyltribromide	T42.6X1	T42.6X2	T42.6X3	T42.6X4	T42.6X5	T42.6X6
Allypropymal	T42.3X1	T42.3X2	T42.3X3	T42.3X4	T42.3X5	T42.3X6
Almagate	T47.1X1	T47.1X2	T47.1X3	T47.1X4	T47.1X5	T47.1X6
Almasilate	T47.1X1	T47.1X2	T47.1X3	T47.1X4	T47.1X5	T47.1X6
Almitrine	T50.7X1	T50.7X2	T50.7X3	T50.7X4	T50.7X5	T50.7X6
Aloes	T47.2X1	T47.2X2	T47.2X3	T47.2X4	T47.2X5	T47.2X6
Aloglutamol	T47.1X1	T47.1X2	T47.1X3	T47.1X4	T47.1X5	T47.1X6
Aloin	T47.2X1	T47.2X2	T47.2X3	T47.2X4	T47.2X5	T47.2X6
Aloxidone	T42.2X1	T42.2X2	T42.2X3	T42.2X4	T42.2X5	T42.2X6
Alpha						
acetyldigoxin	T46.0X1	T46.0X2	T46.0X3	T46.0X4	T46.0X5	T46.0X6
adrenergic blocking drug	T44.6X1	T44.6X2	T44.6X3	T44.6X4	T44.6X5	T44.6X6
amylase	T45.3X1	T45.3X2	T45.3X3	T45.3X4	T45.3X5	T45.3X6
tocoferol (acetate)	T45.2X1	T45.2X2	T45.2X3	T45.2X4	T45.2X5	T45.2X6
tocopherol	T45.2X1	T45.2X2	T45.2X3	T45.2X4	T45.2X5	T45.2X6
Alphadolone	T41.1X1	T41.1X2	T41.1X3	T41.1X4	T41.1X5	T41.1X6
Alphaprodine	T40.4X1	T40.4X2	T40.4X3	T40.4X4	T40.4X5	T40.4X6
Alphaxalone	T41.1X1	T41.1X2	T41.1X3	T41.1X4	T41.1X5	T41.1X6
Alprazolam	T42.4X1	T42.4X2	T42.4X3	T42.4X4	T42.4X5	T42.4X6
Alprenolol	T44.7X1	T44.7X2	T44.7X3	T44.7X4	T44.7X5	T44.7X6
Alprostadil	T46.7X1	T46.7X2	T46.7X3	T46.7X4	T46.7X5	T46.7X6
Alsactide	T38.811	T38.812	T38.813	T38.814	T38.815	T38.816
Alseroxylon	T46.5X1	T46.5X2	T46.5X3	T46.5X4	T46.5X5	T46.5X6
Alteplase	T45.611	T45.612	T45.613	T45.614	T45.615	T45.616
Altizide	T50.2X1	T50.2X2	T50.2X3	T50.2X4	T50.2X5	T50.2X6
Altretamine	T45.1X1	T45.1X2	T45.1X3	T45.1X4	T45.1X5	T45.1X6
Alum (medicinal)	T49.4X1	T49.4X2	T49.4X3	T49.4X4	T49.4X5	T49.4X6
nonmedicinal (ammonium) (potassium)	T56.891	T56.892	T56.893	T56.894	—	—
Aluminium, aluminum						
acetate	T49.2X1	T49.2X2	T49.2X3	T49.2X4	T49.2X5	T49.2X6
solution	T49.0X1	T49.0X2	T49.0X3	T49.0X4	T49.0X5	T49.0X6
aspirin	T39.011	T39.012	T39.013	T39.014	T39.015	T39.016
bis (acetylsalicylate)	T39.011	T39.012	T39.013	T39.014	T39.015	T39.016

Substance	Poisoning, Accidental (Unintentional)	Poisoning, Intentional Self-Harm	Poisoning, Assault	Poisoning, Undetermined	Adverse Effect	Underdosing
Aluminium, aluminum *(Continued)*						
carbonate (gel, basic)	T47.1X1	T47.1X2	T47.1X3	T47.1X4	T47.1X5	T47.1X6
chlorhydroxide-complex	T47.1X1	T47.1X2	T47.1X3	T47.1X4	T47.1X5	T47.1X6
chloride	T49.2X1	T49.2X2	T49.2X3	T49.2X4	T49.2X5	T49.2X6
clofibrate	T46.6X1	T46.6X2	T46.6X3	T46.6X4	T46.6X5	T46.6X6
diacetate	T49.2X1	T49.2X2	T49.2X3	T49.2X4	T49.2X5	T49.2X6
glycinate	T47.1X1	T47.1X2	T47.1X3	T47.1X4	T47.1X5	T47.1X6
hydroxide (gel)	T47.1X1	T47.1X2	T47.1X3	T47.1X4	T47.1X5	T47.1X6
hydroxide-magnesium carb. gel	T47.1X1	T47.1X2	T47.1X3	T47.1X4	T47.1X5	T47.1X6
magnesium silicate	T47.1X1	T47.1X2	T47.1X3	T47.1X4	T47.1X5	T47.1X6
nicotinate	T46.7X1	T46.7X2	T46.7X3	T46.7X4	T46.7X5	T46.7X6
ointment (surgical) (topical)	T49.3X1	T49.3X2	T49.3X3	T49.3X4	T49.3X5	T49.3X6
phosphate	T47.1X1	T47.1X2	T47.1X3	T47.1X4	T47.1X5	T47.1X6
salicylate	T39.091	T39.092	T39.093	T39.094	T39.095	T39.096
silicate	T47.1X1	T47.1X2	T47.1X3	T47.1X4	T47.1X5	T47.1X6
sodium silicate	T47.1X1	T47.1X2	T47.1X3	T47.1X4	T47.1X5	T47.1X6
subacetate	T49.2X1	T49.2X2	T49.2X3	T49.2X4	T49.2X5	T49.2X6
sulfate	T49.0X1	T49.0X2	T49.0X3	T49.0X4	T49.0X5	T49.0X6
tannate	T47.6X1	T47.6X2	T47.6X3	T47.6X4	T47.6X5	T47.6X6
topical NEC	T49.3X1	T49.3X2	T49.3X3	T49.3X4	T49.3X5	T49.3X6
Alurate	T42.3X1	T42.3X2	T42.3X3	T42.3X4	T42.3X5	T42.3X6
Alverine	T44.3X1	T44.3X2	T44.3X3	T44.3X4	T44.3X5	T44.3X6
Alvodine	T40.2X1	T40.2X2	T40.2X3	T40.2X4	T40.2X5	T40.2X6
Amanita phalloides	T62.0X1	T62.0X2	T62.0X3	T62.0X4	—	—
Amanitine	T62.0X1	T62.0X2	T62.0X3	T62.0X4	—	—
Amantadine	T42.8X1	T42.8X2	T42.8X3	T42.8X4	T42.8X5	T42.8X6
Ambazone	T49.6X1	T49.6X2	T49.6X3	T49.6X4	T49.6X5	T49.6X6
Ambenonium (chloride)	T44.0X1	T44.0X2	T44.0X3	T44.0X4	T44.0X5	T44.0X6
Ambroxol	T48.4X1	T48.4X2	T48.4X3	T48.4X4	T48.4X5	T48.4X6
Ambuphylline	T48.6X1	T48.6X2	T48.6X3	T48.6X4	T48.6X5	T48.6X6
Ambutonium bromide	T44.3X1	T44.3X2	T44.3X3	T44.3X4	T44.3X5	T44.3X6
Amcinonide	T49.0X1	T49.0X2	T49.0X3	T49.0X4	T49.0X5	T49.0X6
Amdinocilline	T36.0X1	T36.0X2	T36.0X3	T36.0X4	T36.0X5	T36.0X6
Ametazole	T50.8X1	T50.8X2	T50.8X3	T50.8X4	T50.8X5	T50.8X6
Amethocaine	T41.3X1	T41.3X2	T41.3X3	T41.3X4	T41.3X5	T41.3X6
regional	T41.3X1	T41.3X2	T41.3X3	T41.3X4	T41.3X5	T41.3X6
spinal	T41.3X1	T41.3X2	T41.3X3	T41.3X4	T41.3X5	T41.3X6
Amethopterin	T45.1X1	T45.1X2	T45.1X3	T45.1X4	T45.1X5	T45.1X6
Amezinium metilsulfate	T44.991	T44.992	T44.993	T44.994	T44.995	T44.996
Amfebutamone	T43.291	T43.292	T43.293	T43.294	T43.295	T43.296
Amfepramone	T50.5X1	T50.5X2	T50.5X3	T50.5X4	T50.5X5	T50.5X6

◀ New ⬅ Revised ~~deleted~~ Deleted

Substance	Poisoning, Accidental (Unintentional)	Poisoning, Intentional Self-Harm	Poisoning, Assault	Poisoning, Undetermined	Adverse Effect	Underdosing
Amfetamine	T43.621	T43.622	T43.623	T43.624	T43.625	T43.626
Amfetaminil	T43.621	T43.622	T43.623	T43.624	T43.625	T43.626
Amfomycin	T36.8X1	T36.8X2	T36.8X3	T36.8X4	T36.8X5	T36.8X6
Amidefrine mesilate	T48.5X1	T48.5X2	T48.5X3	T48.5X4	T48.5X5	T48.5X6
Amidone	T40.3X1	T40.3X2	T40.3X3	T40.3X4	T40.3X5	T40.3X6
Amidopyrine	T39.2X1	T39.2X2	T39.2X3	T39.2X4	T39.2X5	T39.2X6
Amidotrizoate	T50.8X1	T50.8X2	T50.8X3	T50.8X4	T50.8X5	T50.8X6
Amiflamine	T43.1X1	T43.1X2	T43.1X3	T43.1X4	T43.1X5	T43.1X6
Amikacin	T36.5X1	T36.5X2	T36.5X3	T36.5X4	T36.5X5	T36.5X6
Amikhelline	T46.3X1	T46.3X2	T46.3X3	T46.3X4	T46.3X5	T46.3X6
Amiloride	T50.2X1	T50.2X2	T50.2X3	T50.2X4	T50.2X5	T50.2X6
Aminacrine	T49.0X1	T49.0X2	T49.0X3	T49.0X4	T49.0X5	T49.0X6
Amineptine	T43.011	T43.012	T43.013	T43.014	T43.015	T43.016
Aminitrozole	T37.3X1	T37.3X2	T37.3X3	T37.3X4	T37.3X5	T37.3X6
Aminoacetic acid (derivatives)	T50.3X1	T50.3X2	T50.3X3	T50.3X4	T50.3X5	T50.3X6
Amino acids	T50.3X1	T50.3X2	T50.3X3	T50.3X4	T50.3X5	T50.3X6
Aminoacridine	T49.0X1	T49.0X2	T49.0X3	T49.0X4	T49.0X5	T49.0X6
Aminobenzoic acid (-p)	T49.3X1	T49.3X2	T49.3X3	T49.3X4	T49.3X5	T49.3X6
4-Aminobutyric acid	T43.8X1	T43.8X2	T43.8X3	T43.8X4	T43.8X5	T43.8X6
Aminocaproic acid	T45.621	T45.622	T45.623	T45.624	T45.625	T45.626
Aminofenazone	T39.2X1	T39.2X2	T39.2X3	T39.2X4	T39.2X5	T39.2X6
Aminoethylisothiourium	T45.8X1	T45.8X2	T45.8X3	T45.8X4	T45.8X5	T45.8X6
Aminoglutethimide	T45.1X1	T45.1X2	T45.1X3	T45.1X4	T45.1X5	T45.1X6
Aminohippuric acid	T50.8X1	T50.8X2	T50.8X3	T50.8X4	T50.8X5	T50.8X6
Aminomethylbenzoic acid	T45.691	T45.692	T45.693	T45.694	T45.695	T45.696
Aminometradine	T50.2X1	T50.2X2	T50.2X3	T50.2X4	T50.2X5	T50.2X6
Aminopentamide	T44.3X1	T44.3X2	T44.3X3	T44.3X4	T44.3X5	T44.3X6
Aminophenazone	T39.2X1	T39.2X2	T39.2X3	T39.2X4	T39.2X5	T39.2X6
Aminophenol	T54.0X1	T54.0X2	T54.0X3	T54.0X4	—	—
4-Aminophenol derivatives	T39.1X1	T39.1X2	T39.1X3	T39.1X4	T39.1X5	T39.1X6
Aminophenylpyridone	T43.591	T43.592	T43.593	T43.594	T43.595	T43.596
Aminophylline	T48.6X1	T48.6X2	T48.6X3	T48.6X4	T48.6X5	T48.6X6
Aminopterin sodium	T45.1X1	T45.1X2	T45.1X3	T45.1X4	T45.1X5	T45.1X6
Aminopyrine	T39.2X1	T39.2X2	T39.2X3	T39.2X4	T39.2X5	T39.2X6
8-Aminoquinoline drugs	T37.2X1	T37.2X2	T37.2X3	T37.2X4	T37.2X5	T37.2X6
Aminorex	T50.5X1	T50.5X2	T50.5X3	T50.5X4	T50.5X5	T50.5X6
Aminosalicylic acid	T37.1X1	T37.1X2	T37.1X3	T37.1X4	T37.1X5	T37.1X6
Aminosalylum	T37.1X1	T37.1X2	T37.1X3	T37.1X4	T37.1X5	T37.1X6
Amiodarone	T46.2X1	T46.2X2	T46.2X3	T46.2X4	T46.2X5	T46.2X6
Amiphenazole	T50.7X1	T50.7X2	T50.7X3	T50.7X4	T50.7X5	T50.7X6
Amiquinsin	T46.5X1	T46.5X2	T46.5X3	T46.5X4	T46.5X5	T46.5X6
Amisometradine	T50.2X1	T50.2X2	T50.2X3	T50.2X4	T50.2X5	T50.2X6

Substance	Poisoning, Accidental (Unintentional)	Poisoning, Intentional Self-Harm	Poisoning, Assault	Poisoning, Undetermined	Adverse Effect	Underdosing
Amisulpride	T43.591	T43.592	T43.593	T43.594	T43.595	T43.596
Amitriptyline	T43.021	T43.022	T43.023	T43.024	T43.025	T43.026
Amitriptylinoxide	T43.021	T43.022	T43.023	T43.024	T43.025	T43.026
Amlexanox	T48.6X1	T48.6X2	T48.6X3	T48.6X4	T48.6X5	T48.6X6
Ammonia (fumes) (gas) (vapor)	T59.891	T59.892	T59.893	T59.894	—	—
aromatic spirit	T48.991	T48.992	T48.993	T48.994	T48.995	T48.996
liquid (household)	T54.3X1	T54.3X2	T54.3X3	T54.3X4	—	—
Ammoniated mercury	T49.0X1	T49.0X2	T49.0X3	T49.0X4	T49.0X5	T49.0X6
Ammonium						
acid tartrate	T49.5X1	T49.5X2	T49.5X3	T49.5X4	T49.5X5	T49.5X6
bromide	T42.6X1	T42.6X2	T42.6X3	T42.6X4	T42.6X5	T42.6X6
carbonate	T54.3X1	T54.3X2	T54.3X3	T54.3X4	—	—
chloride	T50.991	T50.992	T50.993	T50.994	T50.995	T50.996
expectorant	T48.4X1	T48.4X2	T48.4X3	T48.4X4	T48.4X5	T48.4X6
compounds (household) NEC	T54.3X1	T54.3X2	T54.3X3	T54.3X4	—	—
fumes (any usage)	T59.891	T59.892	T59.893	T59.894	—	—
industrial	T54.3X1	T54.3X2	T54.3X3	T54.3X4	—	—
ichthyosulronate	T49.4X1	T49.4X2	T49.4X3	T49.4X4	T49.4X5	T49.4X6
mandelate	T37.91	T37.92	T37.93	T37.94	T37.95	T37.96
sulfamate	T60.3X1	T60.3X2	T60.3X3	T60.3X4	—	—
sulfonate resin	T47.8X1	T47.8X2	T47.8X3	T47.8X4	T47.8X5	T47.8X6
Amobarbital (sodium)	T42.3X1	T42.3X2	T42.3X3	T42.3X4	T42.3X5	T42.3X6
Amodiaquine	T37.2X1	T37.2X2	T37.2X3	T37.2X4	T37.2X5	T37.2X6
Amopyroquin(e)	T37.2X1	T37.2X2	T37.2X3	T37.2X4	T37.2X5	T37.2X6
Amoxapine	T43.011	T43.012	T43.013	T43.014	T43.015	T43.016
Amoxicillin	T36.0X1	T36.0X2	T36.0X3	T36.0X4	T36.0X5	T36.0X6
Amperozide	T43.591	T43.592	T43.593	T43.594	T43.595	T43.596
Amphenidone	T43.591	T43.592	T43.593	T43.594	T43.595	T43.596
Amphetamine NEC	T43.621	T43.622	T43.623	T43.624	T43.625	T43.626
Amphomycin	T36.8X1	T36.8X2	T36.8X3	T36.8X4	T36.8X5	T36.8X6
Amphotalide	T37.4X1	T37.4X2	T37.4X3	T37.4X4	T37.4X5	T37.4X6
Amphotericin B	T36.7X1	T36.7X2	T36.7X3	T36.7X4	T36.7X5	T36.7X6
topical	T49.0X1	T49.0X2	T49.0X3	T49.0X4	T49.0X5	T49.0X6
Ampicillin	T36.0X1	T36.0X2	T36.0X3	T36.0X4	T36.0X5	T36.0X6
Amprotropine	T44.3X1	T44.3X2	T44.3X3	T44.3X4	T44.3X5	T44.3X6
Amsacrine	T45.1X1	T45.1X2	T45.1X3	T45.1X4	T45.1X5	T45.1X6
Amygdaline	T62.2X1	T62.2X2	T62.2X3	T62.2X4	—	—
Amyl						
acetate	T52.8X1	T52.8X2	T52.8X3	T52.8X4	—	—
vapor	T59.891	T59.892	T59.893	T59.894	—	—
alcohol	T51.3X1	T51.3X2	T51.3X3	T51.3X4	—	—
chloride	T53.6X1	T53.6X2	T53.6X3	T53.6X4	—	—

Substance	Poisoning, Accidental (Unintentional)	Poisoning, Intentional Self-Harm	Poisoning, Assault	Poisoning, Undetermined	Adverse Effect	Underdosing
Amyl *(Continued)*						
formate	T52.8X1	T52.8X2	T52.8X3	T52.8X4	—	—
nitrite	T46.3X1	T46.3X2	T46.3X3	T46.3X4	T46.3X5	T46.3X6
propionate	T65.891	T65.892	T65.893	T65.894	—	—
Amylase	T47.5X1	T47.5X2	T47.5X3	T47.5X4	T47.5X5	T47.5X6
Amyleine, regional	T41.3X1	T41.3X2	T41.3X3	T41.3X4	T41.3X5	T41.3X6
Amylene						
dichloride	T53.6X1	T53.6X2	T53.6X3	T53.6X4	—	—
hydrate	T51.3X1	T51.3X2	T51.3X3	T51.3X4	—	—
Amylmetacresol	T49.6X1	T49.6X2	T49.6X3	T49.6X4	T49.6X5	T49.6X6
Amylobarbitone	T42.3X1	T42.3X2	T42.3X3	T42.3X4	T42.3X5	T42.3X6
Amylocaine, regional	T41.3X1	T41.3X2	T41.3X3	T41.3X4	T41.3X5	T41.3X6
infiltration (subcutaneous)	T41.3X1	T41.3X2	T41.3X3	T41.3X4	T41.3X5	T41.3X6
nerve block (peripheral) (plexus)	T41.3X1	T41.3X2	T41.3X3	T41.3X4	T41.3X5	T41.3X6
spinal	T41.3X1	T41.3X2	T41.3X3	T41.3X4	T41.3X5	T41.3X6
topical (surface)	T41.3X1	T41.3X2	T41.3X3	T41.3X4	T41.3X5	T41.3X6
Amylopectin	T47.6X1	T47.6X2	T47.6X3	T47.6X4	T47.6X5	T47.6X6
Amytal (sodium)	T42.3X1	T42.3X2	T42.3X3	T42.3X4	T42.3X5	T42.3X6
Anabolic steroid	T38.7X1	T38.7X2	T38.7X3	T38.7X4	T38.7X5	T38.7X6
Analeptic NEC	T50.7X1	T50.7X2	T50.7X3	T50.7X4	T50.7X5	T50.7X6
Analgesic	T39.91	T39.92	T39.93	T39.94	T39.95	T39.96
anti-inflammatory NEC	T39.91	T39.92	T39.93	T39.94	T39.95	T39.96
propionic acid derivative	T39.311	T39.312	T39.313	T39.314	T39.315	T39.316
antirheumatic NEC	T39.4X1	T39.4X2	T39.4X3	T39.4X4	T39.4X5	T39.4X6
aromatic NEC	T39.1X1	T39.1X2	T39.1X3	T39.1X4	T39.1X5	T39.1X6
narcotic NEC	T40.601	T40.602	T40.603	T40.604	T40.605	T40.606
combination	T40.601	T40.602	T40.603	T40.604	T40.605	T40.606
obstetric	T40.601	T40.602	T40.603	T40.604	T40.605	T40.606
non-narcotic NEC	T39.91	T39.92	T39.93	T39.94	T39.95	T39.96
combination	T39.91	T39.92	T39.93	T39.94	T39.95	T39.96
pyrazole	T39.2X1	T39.2X2	T39.2X3	T39.2X4	T39.2X5	T39.2X6
specified NEC	T39.8X1	T39.8X2	T39.8X3	T39.8X4	T39.8X5	T39.8X6
Analgin	T39.2X1	T39.2X2	T39.2X3	T39.2X4	T39.2X5	T39.2X6
Anamirta cocculus	T62.1X1	T62.1X2	T62.1X3	T62.1X4	—	—
Ancillin	T36.0X1	T36.0X2	T36.0X3	T36.0X4	T36.0X5	T36.0X6
Ancrod	T45.691	T45.692	T45.693	T45.694	T45.695	T45.696
Androgen	T38.7X1	T38.7X2	T38.7X3	T38.7X4	T38.7X5	T38.7X6
Androgen-estrogen mixture	T38.7X1	T38.7X2	T38.7X3	T38.7X4	T38.7X5	T38.7X6
Androstalone	T38.7X1	T38.7X2	T38.7X3	T38.7X4	T38.7X5	T38.7X6
Androstanolone	T38.7X1	T38.7X2	T38.7X3	T38.7X4	T38.7X5	T38.7X6
Androsterone	T38.7X1	T38.7X2	T38.7X3	T38.7X4	T38.7X5	T38.7X6
Anemone pulsatilla	T62.2X1	T62.2X2	T62.2X3	T62.2X4	—	—
Anesthesia						
caudal	T41.3X1	T41.3X2	T41.3X3	T41.3X4	T41.3X5	T41.3X6
endotracheal	T41.0X1	T41.0X2	T41.0X3	T41.0X4	T41.0X5	T41.0X6
epidural	T41.3X1	T41.3X2	T41.3X3	T41.3X4	T41.3X5	T41.3X6
inhalation	T41.0X1	T41.0X2	T41.0X3	T41.0X4	T41.0X5	T41.0X6
local	T41.3X1	T41.3X2	T41.3X3	T41.3X4	T41.3X5	T41.3X6
mucosal	T41.3X1	T41.3X2	T41.3X3	T41.3X4	T41.3X5	T41.3X6
muscle relaxation	T48.1X1	T48.1X2	T48.1X3	T48.1X4	T48.1X5	T48.1X6
nerve blocking	T41.3X1	T41.3X2	T41.3X3	T41.3X4	T41.3X5	T41.3X6
plexus blocking	T41.3X1	T41.3X2	T41.3X3	T41.3X4	T41.3X5	T41.3X6
potentiated	T41.201	T41.202	T41.203	T41.204	T41.205	T41.206
rectal	T41.201	T41.202	T41.203	T41.204	T41.205	T41.206
general	T41.201	T41.202	T41.203	T41.204	T41.205	T41.206
local	T41.3X1	T41.3X2	T41.3X3	T41.3X4	T41.3X5	T41.3X6
regional	T41.3X1	T41.3X2	T41.3X3	T41.3X4	T41.3X5	T41.3X6
surface	T41.3X1	T41.3X2	T41.3X3	T41.3X4	T41.3X5	T41.3X6
Anesthetic NEC—*see also Anesthesia*	T41.41	T41.42	T41.43	T41.44	T41.45	T41.46
with muscle relaxant	T41.201	T41.202	T41.203	T41.204	T41.205	T41.206
general	T41.201	T41.202	T41.203	T41.204	T41.205	T41.206
local	T41.3X1	T41.3X2	T41.3X3	T41.3X4	T41.3X5	T41.3X6
gaseous NEC	T41.0X1	T41.0X2	T41.0X3	T41.0X4	T41.0X5	T41.0X6
general NEC	T41.201	T41.202	T41.203	T41.204	T41.205	T41.206
halogenated hydrocarbon derivatives NEC	T41.0X1	T41.0X2	T41.0X3	T41.0X4	T41.0X5	T41.0X6
infiltration NEC	T41.3X1	T41.3X2	T41.3X3	T41.3X4	T41.3X5	T41.3X6
intravenous NEC	T41.1X1	T41.1X2	T41.1X3	T41.1X4	T41.1X5	T41.1X6
local NEC	T41.3X1	T41.3X2	T41.3X3	T41.3X4	T41.3X5	T41.3X6
rectal	T41.201	T41.202	T41.203	T41.204	T41.205	T41.206
general	T41.201	T41.202	T41.203	T41.204	T41.205	T41.206
local	T41.3X1	T41.3X2	T41.3X3	T41.3X4	T41.3X5	T41.3X6
regional NEC	T41.3X1	T41.3X2	T41.3X3	T41.3X4	T41.3X5	T41.3X6
spinal NEC	T41.3X1	T41.3X2	T41.3X3	T41.3X4	T41.3X5	T41.3X6
thiobarbiturate	T41.1X1	T41.1X2	T41.1X3	T41.1X4	T41.1X5	T41.1X6
topical	T41.3X1	T41.3X2	T41.3X3	T41.3X4	T41.3X5	T41.3X6
Aneurine	T45.2X1	T45.2X2	T45.2X3	T45.2X4	T45.2X5	T45.2X6
Angio-Conray	T50.8X1	T50.8X2	T50.8X3	T50.8X4	T50.8X5	T50.8X6
Angiotensin	T44.5X1	T44.5X2	T44.5X3	T44.5X4	T44.5X5	T44.5X6
Angiotensinamide	T44.991	T44.992	T44.993	T44.994	T44.995	T44.996
Anhydrohydroxy-progesterone	T38.5X1	T38.5X2	T38.5X3	T38.5X4	T38.5X5	T38.5X6
Anhydron	T50.2X1	T50.2X2	T50.2X3	T50.2X4	T50.2X5	T50.2X6
Anileridine	T40.4X1	T40.4X2	T40.4X3	T40.4X4	T40.4X5	T40.4X6

◀ New ⬅ Revised ~~deleted~~ Deleted

Substance	Poisoning, Accidental (Unintentional)	Poisoning, Intentional Self-Harm	Poisoning, Assault	Poisoning, Undetermined	Adverse Effect	Underdosing
Aniline (dye) (liquid)	T65.3X1	T65.3X2	T65.3X3	T65.3X4	—	—
analgesic	T39.1X1	T39.1X2	T39.1X3	T39.1X4	T39.1X5	T39.1X6
derivatives, therapeutic NEC	T39.1X1	T39.1X2	T39.1X3	T39.1X4	T39.1X5	T39.1X6
vapor	T65.3X1	T65.3X2	T65.3X3	T65.3X4	—	—
Anise oil	T47.5X1	T47.5X2	T47.5X3	T47.5X4	T47.5X5	T47.5X6
Aniscoropine	T44.3X1	T44.3X2	T44.3X3	T44.3X4	T44.3X5	T44.3X6
Anisidine	T65.3X1	T65.3X2	T65.3X3	T65.3X4	—	—
Anisindione	T45.511	T45.512	T45.513	T45.514	T45.515	T45.516
Anisotropine methyl-bromide	T44.3X1	T44.3X2	T44.3X3	T44.3X4	T44.3X5	T44.3X6
Anistreplase	T45.611	T45.612	T45.613	T45.614	T45.615	T45.616
Anorexiant (central)	T50.5X1	T50.5X2	T50.5X3	T50.5X4	T50.5X5	T50.5X6
Anorexic agents	T50.5X1	T50.5X2	T50.5X3	T50.5X4	T50.5X5	T50.5X6
Ansamycin	T36.6X1	T36.6X2	T36.6X3	T36.6X4	T36.6X5	T36.6X6
Ant (bite) (sting)	T63.421	T63.422	T63.423	T63.424	—	—
Antabuse	T50.6X1	T50.6X2	T50.6X3	T50.6X4	T50.6X5	T50.6X6
Ant poison — *see Insecticide*						
Antacid NEC	T47.1X1	T47.1X2	T47.1X3	T47.1X4	T47.1X5	T47.1X6
Antagonist						
Aldosterone	T50.0X1	T50.0X2	T50.0X3	T50.0X4	T50.0X5	T50.0X6
alpha-adrenoreceptor	T44.6X1	T44.6X2	T44.6X3	T44.6X4	T44.6X5	T44.6X6
anticoagulant	T45.7X1	T45.7X2	T45.7X3	T45.7X4	T45.7X5	T45.7X6
beta-adrenoreceptor	T44.7X1	T44.7X2	T44.7X3	T44.7X4	T44.7X5	T44.7X6
extrapyramidal NEC	T44.3X1	T44.3X2	T44.3X3	T44.3X4	T44.3X5	T44.3X6
folic acid	T45.1X1	T45.1X2	T45.1X3	T45.1X4	T45.1X5	T45.1X6
H2 receptor	T47.0X1	T47.0X2	T47.0X3	T47.0X4	T47.0X5	T47.0X6
heavy metal	T45.8X1	T45.8X2	T45.8X3	T45.8X4	T45.8X5	T45.8X6
narcotic analgesic	T50.7X1	T50.7X2	T50.7X3	T50.7X4	T50.7X5	T50.7X6
opiate	T50.7X1	T50.7X2	T50.7X3	T50.7X4	T50.7X5	T50.7X6
pyrimidine	T45.1X1	T45.1X2	T45.1X3	T45.1X4	T45.1X5	T45.1X6
serotonin	T46.5X1	T46.5X2	T46.5X3	T46.5X4	T46.5X5	T46.5X6
Antazolin(e)	T45.0X1	T45.0X2	T45.0X3	T45.0X4	T45.0X5	T45.0X6
Anterior pituitary hormone NEC	T38.811	T38.812	T38.813	T38.814	T38.815	T38.816
Anthelmintic NEC	T37.4X1	T37.4X2	T37.4X3	T37.4X4	T37.4X5	T37.4X6
Anthiolimine	T37.4X1	T37.4X2	T37.4X3	T37.4X4	T37.4X5	T37.4X6
Anthralin	T49.4X1	T49.4X2	T49.4X3	T49.4X4	T49.4X5	T49.4X6
Anthramycin	T45.1X1	T45.1X2	T45.1X3	T45.1X4	T45.1X5	T45.1X6
Antiadrenergic NEC	T44.8X1	T44.8X2	T44.8X3	T44.8X4	T44.8X5	T44.8X6
Antiallergic NEC	T45.0X1	T45.0X2	T45.0X3	T45.0X4	T45.0X5	T45.0X6
Anti-anemic (drug) (preparation)	T45.8X1	T45.8X2	T45.8X3	T45.8X4	T45.8X5	T45.8X6
Antiandrogen NEC	T38.6X1	T38.6X2	T38.6X3	T38.6X4	T38.6X5	T38.6X6
Antianxiety drug NEC	T43.501	T43.502	T43.503	T43.504	T43.505	T43.506
Antiaris toxicaria	T65.891	T65.892	T65.893	T65.894	—	—

Substance	Poisoning, Accidental (Unintentional)	Poisoning, Intentional Self-Harm	Poisoning, Assault	Poisoning, Undetermined	Adverse Effect	Underdosing
Antiarteriosclerotic drug	T46.6X1	T46.6X2	T46.6X3	T46.6X4	T46.6X5	T46.6X6
Antiasthmatic drug NEC	T48.6X1	T48.6X2	T48.6X3	T48.6X4	T48.6X5	T48.6X6
Antibiotic NEC	T36.91	T36.92	T36.93	T36.94	T36.95	T36.96
aminoglycoside	T36.5X1	T36.5X2	T36.5X3	T36.5X4	T36.5X5	T36.5X6
anticancer	T45.1X1	T45.1X2	T45.1X3	T45.1X4	T45.1X5	T45.1X6
antifungal	T36.7X1	T36.7X2	T36.7X3	T36.7X4	T36.7X5	T36.7X6
antimycobacterial	T36.5X1	T36.5X2	T36.5X3	T36.5X4	T36.5X5	T36.5X6
antineoplastic	T45.1X1	T45.1X2	T45.1X3	T45.1X4	T45.1X5	T45.1X6
cephalosporin (group)	T36.1X1	T36.1X2	T36.1X3	T36.1X4	T36.1X5	T36.1X6
chloramphenicol (group)	T36.2X1	T36.2X2	T36.2X3	T36.2X4	T36.2X5	T36.2X6
ENT	T49.6X1	T49.6X2	T49.6X3	T49.6X4	T49.6X5	T49.6X6
eye	T49.5X1	T49.5X2	T49.5X3	T49.5X4	T49.5X5	T49.5X6
fungicidal (local)	T49.0X1	T49.0X2	T49.0X3	T49.0X4	T49.0X5	T49.0X6
intestinal	T36.8X1	T36.8X2	T36.8X3	T36.8X4	T36.8X5	T36.8X6
b-lactam NEC	T36.1X1	T36.1X2	T36.1X3	T36.1X4	T36.1X5	T36.1X6
local	T49.0X1	T49.0X2	T49.0X3	T49.0X4	T49.0X5	T49.0X6
macrolides	T36.3X1	T36.3X2	T36.3X3	T36.3X4	T36.3X5	T36.3X6
polypeptide	T36.8X1	T36.8X2	T36.8X3	T36.8X4	T36.8X5	T36.8X6
specified NEC	T36.8X1	T36.8X2	T36.8X3	T36.8X4	T36.8X5	T36.8X6
tetracycline (group)	T36.4X1	T36.4X2	T36.4X3	T36.4X4	T36.4X5	T36.4X6
throat	T49.6X1	T49.6X2	T49.6X3	T49.6X4	T49.6X5	T49.6X6
Anticancer agents NEC	T45.1X1	T45.1X2	T45.1X3	T45.1X4	T45.1X5	T45.1X6
Anticholesterolemic drug NEC	T46.6X1	T46.6X2	T46.6X3	T46.6X4	T46.6X5	T46.6X6
Anticholinergic NEC	T44.3X1	T44.3X2	T44.3X3	T44.3X4	T44.3X5	T44.3X6
Anticholinesterase	T44.0X1	T44.0X2	T44.0X3	T44.0X4	T44.0X5	T44.0X6
organophosphorus	T44.0X1	T44.0X2	T44.0X3	T44.0X4	T44.0X5	T44.0X6
insecticide	T60.0X1	T60.0X2	T60.0X3	T60.0X4	—	—
nerve gas	T59.891	T59.892	T59.893	T59.894	—	—
reversible	T44.0X1	T44.0X2	T44.0X3	T44.0X4	T44.0X5	T44.0X6
ophthalmological	T49.5X1	T49.5X2	T49.5X3	T49.5X4	T49.5X5	T49.5X6
Anticoagulant NEC	T45.511	T45.512	T45.513	T45.514	T45.515	T45.516
Antagonist	T45.7X1	T45.7X2	T45.7X3	T45.7X4	T45.7X5	T45.7X6
Anti-common-cold drug NEC	T48.5X1	T48.5X2	T48.5X3	T48.5X4	T48.5X5	T48.5X6
Anticonvulsant	T42.71	T42.72	T42.73	T42.74	T42.75	T42.76
barbiturate	T42.3X1	T42.3X2	T42.3X3	T42.3X4	T42.3X5	T42.3X6
combination (with barbiturate)	T42.3X1	T42.3X2	T42.3X3	T42.3X4	T42.3X5	T42.3X6
hydantoin	T42.0X1	T42.0X2	T42.0X3	T42.0X4	T42.0X5	T42.0X6
hypnotic NEC	T42.6X1	T42.6X2	T42.6X3	T42.6X4	T42.6X5	T42.6X6
oxazolidinedione	T42.2X1	T42.2X2	T42.2X3	T42.2X4	T42.2X5	T42.2X6
pyrimidinedione	T42.6X1	T42.6X2	T42.6X3	T42.6X4	T42.6X5	T42.6X6
specified NEC	T42.6X1	T42.6X2	T42.6X3	T42.6X4	T42.6X5	T42.6X6
succinimide	T42.2X1	T42.2X2	T42.2X3	T42.2X4	T42.2X5	T42.2X6

Substance	Poisoning, Accidental (Unintentional)	Poisoning, Intentional Self-Harm	Poisoning, Assault	Poisoning, Undetermined	Adverse Effect	Underdosing
Anti-D immunoglobulin (human)	T5Ø.Z11	T5Ø.Z12	T5Ø.Z13	T5Ø.Z14	T5Ø.Z15	T5Ø.Z16
Antidepressant NEC	T43.2Ø1	T43.2Ø2	T43.2Ø3	T43.2Ø4	T43.2Ø5	T43.2Ø6
monoamine oxidase inhibitor	T43.1X1	T43.1X2	T43.1X3	T43.1X4	T43.1X5	T43.1X6
selective serotonin norepinephrine reuptake inhibitor	T43.211	T43.212	T43.213	T43.214	T43.215	T43.216
selective serotonin reuptake inhibitor	T43.221	T43.222	T43.223	T43.224	T43.225	T43.226
specified NEC	T43.291	T43.292	T43.293	T43.294	T43.295	T43.296
tetracyclic	T43.Ø21	T43.Ø22	T43.Ø23	T43.Ø24	T43.Ø25	T43.Ø26
triazolopyridine	T43.221	T43.222	T43.223	T43.224	T43.225	T43.226
tricyclic	T43.Ø11	T43.Ø12	T43.Ø13	T43.Ø14	T43.Ø15	T43.Ø16
Antidiabetic NEC	T38.3X1	T38.3X2	T38.3X3	T38.3X4	T38.3X5	T38.3X6
biguanide	T38.3X1	T38.3X2	T38.3X3	T38.3X4	T38.3X5	T38.3X6
and sulfonyl combined	T38.3X1	T38.3X2	T38.3X3	T38.3X4	T38.3X5	T38.3X6
combined	T38.3X1	T38.3X2	T38.3X3	T38.3X4	T38.3X5	T38.3X6
sulfonylurea	T38.3X1	T38.3X2	T38.3X3	T38.3X4	T38.3X5	T38.3X6
Antidiarrheal drug NEC	T47.6X1	T47.6X2	T47.6X3	T47.6X4	T47.6X5	T47.6X6
absorbent	T47.6X1	T47.6X2	T47.6X3	T47.6X4	T47.6X5	T47.6X6
Antidiphtheria serum	T5Ø.Z11	T5Ø.Z12	T5Ø.Z13	T5Ø.Z14	T5Ø.Z15	T5Ø.Z16
Antidiuretic hormone	T38.891	T38.892	T38.893	T38.894	T38.895	T38.896
Antidote NEC	T5Ø.6X1	T5Ø.6X2	T5Ø.6X3	T5Ø.6X4	T5Ø.6X5	T5Ø.6X6
heavy metal	T45.8X1	T45.8X2	T45.8X3	T45.8X4	T45.8X5	T45.8X6
Antidysrhythmic NEC	T46.2X1	T46.2X2	T46.2X3	T46.2X4	T46.2X5	T46.2X6
Antiemetic drug	T45.ØX1	T45.ØX2	T45.ØX3	T45.ØX4	T45.ØX5	T45.ØX6
Antiepilepsy agent	T42.71	T42.72	T42.73	T42.74	T42.75	T42.76
combination	T42.5X1	T42.5X2	T42.5X3	T42.5X4	T42.5X5	T42.5X6
mixed	T42.5X1	T42.5X2	T42.5X3	T42.5X4	T42.5X5	T42.5X6
specified, NEC	T42.6X1	T42.6X2	T42.6X3	T42.6X4	T42.6X5	T42.6X6
Antiestrogen NEC	T38.6X1	T38.6X2	T38.6X3	T38.6X4	T38.6X5	T38.6X6
Antifertility pill	T38.4X1	T38.4X2	T38.4X3	T38.4X4	T38.4X5	T38.4X6
Antifibrinolytic drug	T45.621	T45.622	T45.623	T45.624	T45.625	T45.626
Antifilarial drug	T37.4X1	T37.4X2	T37.4X3	T37.4X4	T37.4X5	T37.4X6
Antiflatulent	T47.5X1	T47.5X2	T47.5X3	T47.5X4	T47.5X5	T47.5X6
Antifreeze	T65.91	T65.92	T65.93	T65.94	—	—
alcohol	T51.1X1	T51.1X2	T51.1X3	T51.1X4	—	—
ethylene glycol	T51.8X1	T51.8X2	T51.8X3	T51.8X4	—	—
Antifungal						
antibiotic (systemic)	T36.7X1	T36.7X2	T36.7X3	T36.7X4	T36.7X5	T36.7X6
anti-infective NEC	T37.91	T37.92	T37.93	T37.94	T37.95	T37.96
disinfectant, local	T49.ØX1	T49.ØX2	T49.ØX3	T49.ØX4	T49.ØX5	T49.ØX6
nonmedicinal (spray)	T6Ø.3X1	T6Ø.3X2	T6Ø.3X3	T6Ø.3X4	—	—
topical	T49.ØX1	T49.ØX2	T49.ØX3	T49.ØX4	T49.ØX5	T49.ØX6
Anti-gastric-secretion drug NEC	T47.1X1	T47.1X2	T47.1X3	T47.1X4	T47.1X5	T47.1X6
Antigonadotrophin NEC	T38.6X1	T38.6X2	T38.6X3	T38.6X4	T38.6X5	T38.6X6
Antihallucinogen	T43.5Ø1	T43.5Ø2	T43.5Ø3	T43.5Ø4	T43.5Ø5	T43.5Ø6
Antihelmintics	T37.4X1	T37.4X2	T37.4X3	T37.4X4	T37.4X5	T37.4X6
Antihemophilic						
factor	T45.8X1	T45.8X2	T45.8X3	T45.8X4	T45.8X5	T45.8X6
fraction	T45.8X1	T45.8X2	T45.8X3	T45.8X4	T45.8X5	T45.8X6
globulin concentrate	T45.7X1	T45.7X2	T45.7X3	T45.7X4	T45.7X5	T45.7X6
human plasma	T45.8X1	T45.8X2	T45.8X3	T45.8X4	T45.8X5	T45.8X6
plasma, dried	T45.7X1	T45.7X2	T45.7X3	T45.7X4	T45.7X5	T45.7X6
Antihemorrhoidal preparation	T49.2X1	T49.2X2	T49.2X3	T49.2X4	T49.2X5	T49.2X6
Antiheparin drug	T45.7X1	T45.7X2	T45.7X3	T45.7X4	T45.7X5	T45.7X6
Antihistamine	T45.ØX1	T45.ØX2	T45.ØX3	T45.ØX4	T45.ØX5	T45.ØX6
Antihookworm drug	T37.4X1	T37.4X2	T37.4X3	T37.4X4	T37.4X5	T37.4X6
Anti-human lymphocytic globulin	T5Ø.Z11	T5Ø.Z12	T5Ø.Z13	T5Ø.Z14	T5Ø.Z15	T5Ø.Z16
Antihyperlipidemic drug	T46.6X1	T46.6X2	T46.6X3	T46.6X4	T46.6X5	T46.6X6
Antihypertensive drug NEC	T46.5X1	T46.5X2	T46.5X3	T46.5X4	T46.5X5	T46.5X6
Anti-infective NEC	T37.91	T37.92	T37.93	T37.94	T37.95	T37.96
anthelmintic	T37.4X1	T37.4X2	T37.4X3	T37.4X4	T37.4X5	T37.4X6
antibiotics	T36.91	T36.92	T36.93	T36.94	T36.95	T36.96
specified NEC	T36.8X1	T36.8X2	T36.8X3	T36.8X4	T36.8X5	T36.8X6
antimalarial	T37.2X1	T37.2X2	T37.2X3	T37.2X4	T37.2X5	T37.2X6
antimycobacterial NEC	T37.1X1	T37.1X2	T37.1X3	T37.1X4	T37.1X5	T37.1X6
antibiotics	T36.5X1	T36.5X2	T36.5X3	T36.5X4	T36.5X5	T36.5X6
antiprotozoal NEC	T37.3X1	T37.3X2	T37.3X3	T37.3X4	T37.3X5	T37.3X6
blood	T37.2X1	T37.2X2	T37.2X3	T37.2X4	T37.2X5	T37.2X6
antiviral	T37.5X1	T37.5X2	T37.5X3	T37.5X4	T37.5X5	T37.5X6
arsenical	T37.8X1	T37.8X2	T37.8X3	T37.8X4	T37.8X5	T37.8X6
bismuth, local	T49.ØX1	T49.ØX2	T49.ØX3	T49.ØX4	T49.ØX5	T49.ØX6
ENT	T49.6X1	T49.6X2	T49.6X3	T49.6X4	T49.6X5	T49.6X6
eye NEC	T49.5X1	T49.5X2	T49.5X3	T49.5X4	T49.5X5	T49.5X6
heavy metals NEC	T37.8X1	T37.8X2	T37.8X3	T37.8X4	T37.8X5	T37.8X6
local NEC	T49.ØX1	T49.ØX2	T49.ØX3	T49.ØX4	T49.ØX5	T49.ØX6
specified NEC	T49.ØX1	T49.ØX2	T49.ØX3	T49.ØX4	T49.ØX5	T49.ØX6
mixed	T37.91	T37.92	T37.93	T37.94	T37.95	T37.96
ophthalmic preparation	T49.5X1	T49.5X2	T49.5X3	T49.5X4	T49.5X5	T49.5X6
topical NEC	T49.ØX1	T49.ØX2	T49.ØX3	T49.ØX4	T49.ØX5	T49.ØX6
Anti-inflammatory drug NEC	T49.ØX1	T49.ØX2	T49.ØX3	T49.ØX4	T49.ØX5	T49.ØX6
local	T49.ØX1	T49.ØX2	T49.ØX3	T49.ØX4	T49.ØX5	T49.ØX6
nonsteroidal NEC	T39.391	T39.392	T39.393	T39.394	T39.395	T39.396
propionic acid derivative	T39.311	T39.312	T39.313	T39.314	T39.315	T39.316
specified NEC	T39.391	T39.392	T39.393	T39.394	T39.395	T39.396

Substance	Poisoning, Accidental (Unintentional)	Poisoning, Intentional Self-Harm	Poisoning, Assault	Poisoning, Undetermined	Adverse Effect	Underdosing
Antikaluretic	T50.3X1	T50.3X2	T50.3X3	T50.3X4	T50.3X5	T50.3X6
Antiknock (tetraethyl lead)	T56.0X1	T56.0X2	T56.0X3	T56.0X4	—	—
Antilipemic drug NEC	T46.6X1	T46.6X2	T46.6X3	T46.6X4	T46.6X5	T46.6X6
Antimalarial	T37.2X1	T37.2X2	T37.2X3	T37.2X4	T37.2X5	T37.2X6
prophylactic NEC	T37.2X1	T37.2X2	T37.2X3	T37.2X4	T37.2X5	T37.2X6
pyrimidine derivative	T37.2X1	T37.2X2	T37.2X3	T37.2X4	T37.2X5	T37.2X6
Antimetabolite	T45.1X1	T45.1X2	T45.1X3	T45.1X4	T45.1X5	T45.1X6
Antimitotic agent	T45.1X1	T45.1X2	T45.1X3	T45.1X4	T45.1X5	T45.1X6
Antimony (compounds) (vapor) NEC	T56.891	T56.892	T56.893	T56.894	—	—
anti-infectives	T37.8X1	T37.8X2	T37.8X3	T37.8X4	T37.8X5	T37.8X6
dimercaptosuccinate	T37.3X1	T37.3X2	T37.3X3	T37.3X4	T37.3X5	T37.3X6
hydride	T56.891	T56.892	T56.893	T56.894	—	—
pesticide (vapor)	T60.8X1	T60.8X2	T60.8X3	T60.8X4	—	—
potassium (sodium) tartrate	T37.8X1	T37.8X2	T37.8X3	T37.8X4	T37.8X5	T37.8X6
sodium dimercaptosuccinate	T37.3X1	T37.3X2	T37.3X3	T37.3X4	T37.3X5	T37.3X6
tartrated	T37.8X1	T37.8X2	T37.8X3	T37.8X4	T37.8X5	T37.8X6
Antimuscarinic NEC	T44.3X1	T44.3X2	T44.3X3	T44.3X4	T44.3X5	T44.3X6
Antimycobacterial drug NEC	T37.1X1	T37.1X2	T37.1X3	T37.1X4	T37.1X5	T37.1X6
antibiotics	T36.5X1	T36.5X2	T36.5X3	T36.5X4	T36.5X5	T36.5X6
combination	T37.1X1	T37.1X2	T37.1X3	T37.1X4	T37.1X5	T37.1X6
Antinausea drug	T45.0X1	T45.0X2	T45.0X3	T45.0X4	T45.0X5	T45.0X6
Antinematode drug	T37.4X1	T37.4X2	T37.4X3	T37.4X4	T37.4X5	T37.4X6
Antineoplastic NEC	T45.1X1	T45.1X2	T45.1X3	T45.1X4	T45.1X5	T45.1X6
alkaloidal	T45.1X1	T45.1X2	T45.1X3	T45.1X4	T45.1X5	T45.1X6
antibiotics	T45.1X1	T45.1X2	T45.1X3	T45.1X4	T45.1X5	T45.1X6
combination	T45.1X1	T45.1X2	T45.1X3	T45.1X4	T45.1X5	T45.1X6
estrogen	T38.5X1	T38.5X2	T38.5X3	T38.5X4	T38.5X5	T38.5X6
steroid	T38.7X1	T38.7X2	T38.7X3	T38.7X4	T38.7X5	T38.7X6
Antiparasitic drug (systemic)	T37.91	T37.92	T37.93	T37.94	T37.95	T37.96
local	T49.0X1	T49.0X2	T49.0X3	T49.0X4	T49.0X5	T49.0X6
specified NEC	T37.8X1	T37.8X2	T37.8X3	T37.8X4	T37.8X5	T37.8X6
Antiparkinsonism drug NEC	T42.8X1	T42.8X2	T42.8X3	T42.8X4	T42.8X5	T42.8X6
Antiperspirant NEC	T49.2X1	T49.2X2	T49.2X3	T49.2X4	T49.2X5	T49.2X6
Antiphlogistic NEC	T39.4X1	T39.4X2	T39.4X3	T39.4X4	T39.4X5	T39.4X6
Antiplatyhelmintic drug	T37.4X1	T37.4X2	T37.4X3	T37.4X4	T37.4X5	T37.4X6
Antiprotozoal drug NEC	T37.3X1	T37.3X2	T37.3X3	T37.3X4	T37.3X5	T37.3X6
blood	T37.2X1	T37.2X2	T37.2X3	T37.2X4	T37.2X5	T37.2X6
local	T49.0X1	T49.0X2	T49.0X3	T49.0X4	T49.0X5	T49.0X6
Antipruritic drug NEC	T49.1X1	T49.1X2	T49.1X3	T49.1X4	T49.1X5	T49.1X6
Antipsychotic drug	T43.501	T43.502	T43.503	T43.504	T43.505	T43.506
specified NEC	T43.591	T43.592	T43.593	T43.594	T43.595	T43.596

Substance	Poisoning, Accidental (Unintentional)	Poisoning, Intentional Self-Harm	Poisoning, Assault	Poisoning, Undetermined	Adverse Effect	Underdosing
Antipyretic	T39.91	T39.92	T39.93	T39.94	T39.95	T39.96
specified NEC	T39.8X1	T39.8X2	T39.8X3	T39.8X4	T39.8X5	T39.8X6
Antipyrine	T39.2X1	T39.2X2	T39.2X3	T39.2X4	T39.2X5	T39.2X6
Antirabies hyperimmune serum	T50.Z11	T50.Z12	T50.Z13	T50.Z14	T50.Z15	T50.Z16
Antirheumatic NEC	T39.4X1	T39.4X2	T39.4X3	T39.4X4	T39.4X5	T39.4X6
Antirigidity drug NEC	T42.8X1	T42.8X2	T42.8X3	T42.8X4	T42.8X5	T42.8X6
Antischistosomal drug	T37.4X1	T37.4X2	T37.4X3	T37.4X4	T37.4X5	T37.4X6
Antiscorpion sera	T50.Z11	T50.Z12	T50.Z13	T50.Z14	T50.Z15	T50.Z16
Antiseborrheics	T49.4X1	T49.4X2	T49.4X3	T49.4X4	T49.4X5	T49.4X6
Antiseptics (external) (medicinal)	T49.0X1	T49.0X2	T49.0X3	T49.0X4	T49.0X5	T49.0X6
Antistine	T45.0X1	T45.0X2	T45.0X3	T45.0X4	T45.0X5	T45.0X6
Antitapeworm drug	T37.4X1	T37.4X2	T37.4X3	T37.4X4	T37.4X5	T37.4X6
Antitetanus immunoglobulin	T50.Z11	T50.Z12	T50.Z13	T50.Z14	T50.Z15	T50.Z16
Antithyroid drug NEC	T38.2X1	T38.2X2	T38.2X3	T38.2X4	T38.2X5	T38.2X6
Antitoxin	T50.Z11	T50.Z12	T50.Z13	T50.Z14	T50.Z15	T50.Z16
diphtheria	T50.Z11	T50.Z12	T50.Z13	T50.Z14	T50.Z15	T50.Z16
gas gangrene	T50.Z11	T50.Z12	T50.Z13	T50.Z14	T50.Z15	T50.Z16
tetanus	T50.Z11	T50.Z12	T50.Z13	T50.Z14	T50.Z15	T50.Z16
Antitoxin, any	T50.901	T50.902	T50.903	T50.904	T50.905	T50.906
Antitrichomonal drug	T37.3X1	T37.3X2	T37.3X3	T37.3X4	T37.3X5	T37.3X6
Antituberculars	T37.1X1	T37.1X2	T37.1X3	T37.1X4	T37.1X5	T37.1X6
antibiotics	T36.5X1	T36.5X2	T36.5X3	T36.5X4	T36.5X5	T36.5X6
Antitussive NEC	T48.3X1	T48.3X2	T48.3X3	T48.3X4	T48.3X5	T48.3X6
codeine mixture	T40.2X1	T40.2X2	T40.2X3	T40.2X4	T40.2X5	T40.2X6
opiate	T40.2X1	T40.2X2	T40.2X3	T40.2X4	T40.2X5	T40.2X6
Antivaricose drug	T46.8X1	T46.8X2	T46.8X3	T46.8X4	T46.8X5	T46.8X6
Antivenin, antivenom (sera)	T50.Z11	T50.Z12	T50.Z13	T50.Z14	T50.Z15	T50.Z16
crotaline	T50.Z11	T50.Z12	T50.Z13	T50.Z14	T50.Z15	T50.Z16
spider bite	T50.Z11	T50.Z12	T50.Z13	T50.Z14	T50.Z15	T50.Z16
Antivertigo drug	T45.0X1	T45.0X2	T45.0X3	T45.0X4	T45.0X5	T45.0X6
Antiviral drug NEC	T37.5X1	T37.5X2	T37.5X3	T37.5X4	T37.5X5	T37.5X6
eye	T49.5X1	T49.5X2	T49.5X3	T49.5X4	T49.5X5	T49.5X6
Antiwhipworm drug	T37.4X1	T37.4X2	T37.4X3	T37.4X4	T37.4X5	T37.4X6
Ant poisons — *see Pesticides*						
Antrol — *see also by specific chemical substance*	T60.91	T60.92	T60.93	T60.94	—	—
fungicide	T60.91	T60.92	T60.93	T60.94	—	—
ANTU (alpha naphthylthiourea)	T60.4X1	T60.4X2	T60.4X3	T60.4X4	—	—
Apalcillin	T36.0X1	T36.0X2	T36.0X3	T36.0X4	T36.0X5	T36.0X6
APC	T48.5X1	T48.5X2	T48.5X3	T48.5X4	T48.5X5	T48.5X6
Aplonidine	T44.4X1	T44.4X2	T44.4X3	T44.4X4	T44.4X5	T44.4X6
Apomorphine	T47.7X1	T47.7X2	T47.7X3	T47.7X4	T47.7X5	T47.7X6

Substance	Poisoning, Accidental (Unintentional)	Poisoning, Intentional Self-Harm	Poisoning, Assault	Poisoning, Undetermined	Adverse Effect	Underdosing
Appetite depressants, central	T50.5X1	T50.5X2	T50.5X3	T50.5X4	T50.5X5	T50.5X6
Apraclonidine (hydrochloride)	T44.4X1	T44.4X2	T44.4X3	T44.4X4	T44.4X5	T44.4X6
Apresoline	T46.5X1	T46.5X2	T46.5X3	T46.5X4	T46.5X5	T46.5X6
Aprindine	T46.2X1	T46.2X2	T46.2X3	T46.2X4	T46.2X5	T46.2X6
Aprobarbital	T42.3X1	T42.3X2	T42.3X3	T42.3X4	T42.3X5	T42.3X6
Apronalide	T42.6X1	T42.6X2	T42.6X3	T42.6X4	T42.6X5	T42.6X6
Aprotinin	T45.621	T45.622	T45.623	T45.624	T45.625	T45.626
Aptocaine	T41.3X1	T41.3X2	T41.3X3	T41.3X4	T41.3X5	T41.3X6
Aqua fortis	T54.2X1	T54.2X2	T54.2X3	T54.2X4	—	—
Ara-A	T37.5X1	T37.5X2	T37.5X3	T37.5X4	T37.5X5	T37.5X6
Ara-C	T45.1X1	T45.1X2	T45.1X3	T45.1X4	T45.1X5	T45.1X6
Arachis oil	T49.3X1	T49.3X2	T49.3X3	T49.3X4	T49.3X5	T49.3X6
cathartic	T47.4X1	T47.4X2	T47.4X3	T47.4X4	T47.4X5	T47.4X6
Aralen	T37.2X1	T37.2X2	T37.2X3	T37.2X4	T37.2X5	T37.2X6
Arecoline	T44.1X1	T44.1X2	T44.1X3	T44.1X4	T44.1X5	T44.1X6
Arginine	T50.991	T50.992	T50.993	T50.994	T50.995	T50.996
glutamate	T50.991	T50.992	T50.993	T50.994	T50.995	T50.996
Argyrol	T49.0X1	T49.0X2	T49.0X3	T49.0X4	T49.0X5	T49.0X6
ENT agent	T49.6X1	T49.6X2	T49.6X3	T49.6X4	T49.6X5	T49.6X6
ophthalmic preparation	T49.5X1	T49.5X2	T49.5X3	T49.5X4	T49.5X5	T49.5X6
Aristocort	T38.0X1	T38.0X2	T38.0X3	T38.0X4	T38.0X5	T38.0X6
ENT agent	T49.6X1	T49.6X2	T49.6X3	T49.6X4	T49.6X5	T49.6X6
ophthalmic preparation	T49.5X1	T49.5X2	T49.5X3	T49.5X4	T49.5X5	T49.5X6
topical NEC	T49.0X1	T49.0X2	T49.0X3	T49.0X4	T49.0X5	T49.0X6
Aromatics, corrosive	T54.1X1	T54.1X2	T54.1X3	T54.1X4	—	—
disinfectants	T54.1X1	T54.1X2	T54.1X3	T54.1X4	—	—
Arsenate of lead	T57.0X1	T57.0X2	T57.0X3	T57.0X4	—	—
herbicide	T57.0X1	T57.0X2	T57.0X3	T57.0X4	—	—
Arsenic, arsenicals (compounds) (dust) (vapor) NEC	T57.0X1	T57.0X2	T57.0X3	T57.0X4	—	—
anti-infectives	T37.8X1	T37.8X2	T37.8X3	T37.8X4	T37.8X5	T37.8X6
pesticide (dust) (fumes)	T57.0X1	T57.0X2	T57.0X3	T57.0X4	—	—
Arsine (gas)	T57.0X1	T57.0X2	T57.0X3	T57.0X4	—	—
Arsphenamine (silver)	T37.8X1	T37.8X2	T37.8X3	T37.8X4	T37.8X5	T37.8X6
Arsthinol	T37.3X1	T37.3X2	T37.3X3	T37.3X4	T37.3X5	T37.3X6
Artane	T44.3X1	T44.3X2	T44.3X3	T44.3X4	T44.3X5	T44.3X6
Arthropod (venomous) NEC	T63.481	T63.482	T63.483	T63.484	—	—
Articaine	T41.3X1	T41.3X2	T41.3X3	T41.3X4	T41.3X5	T41.3X6
Asbestos	T57.8X1	T57.8X2	T57.8X3	T57.8X4	—	—
Ascaridole	T37.4X1	T37.4X2	T37.4X3	T37.4X4	T37.4X5	T37.4X6
Ascorbic acid	T45.2X1	T45.2X2	T45.2X3	T45.2X4	T45.2X5	T45.2X6
Asiaticoside	T49.0X1	T49.0X2	T49.0X3	T49.0X4	T49.0X5	T49.0X6
Asparaginase	T45.1X1	T45.1X2	T45.1X3	T45.1X4	T45.1X5	T45.1X6
Aspidium (oleoresin)	T37.4X1	T37.4X2	T37.4X3	T37.4X4	T37.4X5	T37.4X6
Aspirin (aluminum) (soluble)	T39.011	T39.012	T39.013	T39.014	T39.015	T39.016
Aspoxicillin	T36.0X1	T36.0X2	T36.0X3	T36.0X4	T36.0X5	T36.0X6
Astemizole	T45.0X1	T45.0X2	T45.0X3	T45.0X4	T45.0X5	T45.0X6
Astringent (local)	T49.2X1	T49.2X2	T49.2X3	T49.2X4	T49.2X5	T49.2X6
specified NEC	T49.2X1	T49.2X2	T49.2X3	T49.2X4	T49.2X5	T49.2X6
Astromicin	T36.5X1	T36.5X2	T36.5X3	T36.5X4	T36.5X5	T36.5X6
Ataractic drug NEC	T43.501	T43.502	T43.503	T43.504	T43.505	T43.506
Atenolol	T44.7X1	T44.7X2	T44.7X3	T44.7X4	T44.7X5	T44.7X6
Atonia drug, intestinal	T47.4X1	T47.4X2	T47.4X3	T47.4X4	T47.4X5	T47.4X6
Atophan	T50.4X1	T50.4X2	T50.4X3	T50.4X4	T50.4X5	T50.4X6
Atracurium besilate	T48.1X1	T48.1X2	T48.1X3	T48.1X4	T48.1X5	T48.1X6
Atropine	T44.3X1	T44.3X2	T44.3X3	T44.3X4	T44.3X5	T44.3X6
derivative	T44.3X1	T44.3X2	T44.3X3	T44.3X4	T44.3X5	T44.3X6
methonitrate	T44.3X1	T44.3X2	T44.3X3	T44.3X4	T44.3X5	T44.3X6
Attapulgite	T47.6X1	T47.6X2	T47.6X3	T47.6X4	T47.6X5	T47.6X6
Attenuvax	T50.991	T50.992	T50.993	T50.994	T50.995	T50.996
Auramine	T65.891	T65.892	T65.893	T65.894	—	—
dye	T65.6X1	T65.6X2	T65.6X3	T65.6X4	—	—
fungicide	T60.3X1	T60.3X2	T60.3X3	T60.3X4	—	—
Auranofin	T39.4X1	T39.4X2	T39.4X3	T39.4X4	T39.4X5	T39.4X6
Aurantiin	T46.991	T46.992	T46.993	T46.994	T46.995	T46.996
Aureomycin	T36.4X1	T36.4X2	T36.4X3	T36.4X4	T36.4X5	T36.4X6
ophthalmic preparation	T49.5X1	T49.5X2	T49.5X3	T49.5X4	T49.5X5	T49.5X6
topical NEC	T49.0X1	T49.0X2	T49.0X3	T49.0X4	T49.0X5	T49.0X6
Aurothioglucose	T39.4X1	T39.4X2	T39.4X3	T39.4X4	T39.4X5	T39.4X6
Aurothioglycanide	T39.4X1	T39.4X2	T39.4X3	T39.4X4	T39.4X5	T39.4X6
Aurothiomalate sodium	T39.4X1	T39.4X2	T39.4X3	T39.4X4	T39.4X5	T39.4X6
Aurotioprol	T39.4X1	T39.4X2	T39.4X3	T39.4X4	T39.4X5	T39.4X6
Automobile fuel	T52.0X1	T52.0X2	T52.0X3	T52.0X4	—	—
Autonomic nervous system agent NEC	T44.901	T44.902	T44.903	T44.904	T44.905	T44.906
Avlosulfon	T37.1X1	T37.1X2	T37.1X3	T37.1X4	T37.1X5	T37.1X6
Avomine	T42.6X1	T42.6X2	T42.6X3	T42.6X4	T42.6X5	T42.6X6
Axerophthol	T45.2X1	T45.2X2	T45.2X3	T45.2X4	T45.2X5	T45.2X6
Azacitidine	T45.1X1	T45.1X2	T45.1X3	T45.1X4	T45.1X5	T45.1X6
Azacyclonol	T43.591	T43.592	T43.593	T43.594	T43.595	T43.596
Azadirachta	T60.2X1	T60.2X2	T60.2X3	T60.2X4	—	—
Azanidazole	T37.3X1	T37.3X2	T37.3X3	T37.3X4	T37.3X5	T37.3X6
Azapetine	T46.7X1	T46.7X2	T46.7X3	T46.7X4	T46.7X5	T46.7X6
Azapropazone	T39.2X1	T39.2X2	T39.2X3	T39.2X4	T39.2X5	T39.2X6

Substance	Poisoning, Accidental (Unintentional)	Poisoning, Intentional Self-Harm	Poisoning, Assault	Poisoning, Undetermined	Adverse Effect	Underdosing
Azaribine	T45.1X1	T45.1X2	T45.1X3	T45.1X4	T45.1X5	T45.1X6
Azaserine	T45.1X1	T45.1X2	T45.1X3	T45.1X4	T45.1X5	T45.1X6
Azatadine	T45.0X1	T45.0X2	T45.0X3	T45.0X4	T45.0X5	T45.0X6
Azatepa	T45.1X1	T45.1X2	T45.1X3	T45.1X4	T45.1X5	T45.1X6
Azathioprine	T45.1X1	T45.1X2	T45.1X3	T45.1X4	T45.1X5	T45.1X6
Azelaic acid	T49.0X1	T49.0X2	T49.0X3	T49.0X4	T49.0X5	T49.0X6
Azelastine	T45.0X1	T45.0X2	T45.0X3	T45.0X4	T45.0X5	T45.0X6
Azidocillin	T36.0X1	T36.0X2	T36.0X3	T36.0X4	T36.0X5	T36.0X6
Azidothymidine	T37.5X1	T37.5X2	T37.5X3	T37.5X4	T37.5X5	T37.5X6
Azinphos (ethyl) (methyl)	T60.0X1	T60.0X2	T60.0X3	T60.0X4	—	—
Aziridine (chelating)	T54.1X1	T54.1X2	T54.1X3	T54.1X4	—	—
Azithromycin	T36.3X1	T36.3X2	T36.3X3	T36.3X4	T36.3X5	T36.3X6
Azlocillin	T36.01	T36.02	T36.03	T36.04	T36.05	T36.06
Azobenzene smoke	T65.3X1	T65.3X2	T65.3X3	T65.3X4	—	—
acaricide	T60.8X1	T60.8X2	T60.8X3	T60.8X4	—	—
Azosulfamide	T37.0X1	T37.0X2	T37.0X3	T37.0X4	T37.0X5	T37.0X6
AZT	T37.5X1	T37.5X2	T37.5X3	T37.5X4	T37.5X5	T37.5X6
Aztreonam	T36.1X1	T36.1X2	T36.1X3	T36.1X4	T36.1X5	T36.1X6
Azulfidine	T37.0X1	T37.0X2	T37.0X3	T37.0X4	T37.0X5	T37.0X6
Azuresin	T50.8X1	T50.8X2	T50.8X3	T50.8X4	T50.8X5	T50.8X6
B						
Bacampicillin	T36.0X1	T36.0X2	T36.0X3	T36.0X4	T36.0X5	T36.0X6
Bacillus						
lactobacillus	T47.8X1	T47.8X2	T47.8X3	T47.8X4	T47.8X5	T47.8X6
subtilis	T47.6X1	T47.6X2	T47.6X3	T47.6X4	T47.6X5	T47.6X6
Bacimycin	T49.0X1	T49.0X2	T49.0X3	T49.0X4	T49.0X5	T49.0X6
ophthalmic preparation	T49.5X1	T49.5X2	T49.5X3	T49.5X4	T49.5X5	T49.5X6
Bacitracin zinc	T49.0X1	T49.0X2	T49.0X3	T49.0X4	T49.0X5	T49.0X6
with neomycin	T49.0X1	T49.0X2	T49.0X3	T49.0X4	T49.0X5	T49.0X6
ENT agent	T49.6X1	T49.6X2	T49.6X3	T49.6X4	T49.6X5	T49.6X6
ophthalmic preparation	T49.5X1	T49.5X2	T49.5X3	T49.5X4	T49.5X5	T49.5X6
topical NEC	T49.0X1	T49.0X2	T49.0X3	T49.0X4	T49.0X5	T49.0X6
Baclofen	T42.8X1	T42.8X2	T42.8X3	T42.8X4	T42.8X5	T42.8X6
Baking soda	T50.991	T50.992	T50.993	T50.994	T50.995	T50.996
BAL	T45.8X1	T45.8X2	T45.8X3	T45.8X4	T45.8X5	T45.8X6
Bambuterol	T48.6X1	T48.6X2	T48.6X3	T48.6X4	T48.6X5	T48.6X6
Bamethan (sulfate)	T46.7X1	T46.7X2	T46.7X3	T46.7X4	T46.7X5	T46.7X6
Bamifylline	T48.6X1	T48.6X2	T48.6X3	T48.6X4	T48.6X5	T48.6X6
Bamipine	T45.0X1	T45.0X2	T45.0X3	T45.0X4	T45.0X5	T45.0X6
Baneberry — *see Actaea spicata*						
Banewort — *see Belladonna*						

Substance	Poisoning, Accidental (Unintentional)	Poisoning, Intentional Self-Harm	Poisoning, Assault	Poisoning, Undetermined	Adverse Effect	Underdosing
Barbenyl	T42.3X1	T42.3X2	T42.3X3	T42.3X4	T42.3X5	T42.3X6
Barbexaclone	T42.6X1	T42.6X2	T42.6X3	T42.6X4	T42.6X5	T42.6X6
Barbital	T42.3X1	T42.3X2	T42.3X3	T42.3X4	T42.3X5	T42.3X6
sodium	T42.3X1	T42.3X2	T42.3X3	T42.3X4	T42.3X5	T42.3X6
Barbitone	T42.3X1	T42.3X2	T42.3X3	T42.3X4	T42.3X5	T42.3X6
Barbiturate NEC	T42.3X1	T42.3X2	T42.3X3	T42.3X4	T42.3X5	T42.3X6
with tranquilizer	T42.3X1	T42.3X2	T42.3X3	T42.3X4	T42.3X5	T42.3X6
anesthetic (intravenous)	T41.1X1	T41.1X2	T41.1X3	T41.1X4	T41.1X5	T41.1X6
Barium (carbonate) (chloride) (sulfite)	T57.8X1	T57.8X2	T57.8X3	T57.8X4	—	—
diagnostic agent	T50.8X1	T50.8X2	T50.8X3	T50.8X4	T50.8X5	T50.8X6
pesticide	T60.4X1	T60.4X2	T60.4X3	T60.4X4	—	—
rodenticide	T60.4X1	T60.4X2	T60.4X3	T60.4X4	—	—
sulfate (medicinal)	T50.8X1	T50.8X2	T50.8X3	T50.8X4	T50.8X5	T50.8X6
Barrier cream	T49.3X1	T49.3X2	T49.3X3	T49.3X4	T49.3X5	T49.3X6
Basic fuchsin	T49.0X1	T49.0X2	T49.0X3	T49.0X4	T49.0X5	T49.0X6
Battery acid or fluid	T54.2X1	T54.2X2	T54.2X3	T54.2X4	—	—
Bay rum	T51.8X1	T51.8X2	T51.8X3	T51.8X4	—	—
BCG (vaccine)	T50.A91	T50.A92	T50.A93	T50.A94	T50.A95	T50.A96
BCNU	T45.1X1	T45.1X2	T45.1X3	T45.1X4	T45.1X5	T45.1X6
Bearsfoot	T62.2X1	T62.2X2	T62.2X3	T62.2X4	—	—
Beclamide	T42.6X1	T42.6X2	T42.6X3	T42.6X4	T42.6X5	T42.6X6
Beclomethasone	T44.5X1	T44.5X2	T44.5X3	T44.5X4	T44.5X5	T44.5X6
Bee (sting) (venom)	T63.441	T63.442	T63.443	T63.444	—	—
Befunolol	T49.5X1	T49.5X2	T49.5X3	T49.5X4	T49.5X5	T49.5X6
Bekanamycin	T36.5X1	T36.5X2	T36.5X3	T36.5X4	T36.5X5	T36.5X6
Belladonna — *see also Nightshade*						
alkaloids	T44.3X1	T44.3X2	T44.3X3	T44.3X4	T44.3X5	T44.3X6
extract	T44.3X1	T44.3X2	T44.3X3	T44.3X4	T44.3X5	T44.3X6
herb	T44.3X1	T44.3X2	T44.3X3	T44.3X4	T44.3X5	T44.3X6
Bemegride	T50.7X1	T50.7X2	T50.7X3	T50.7X4	T50.7X5	T50.7X6
Benactyzine	T44.3X1	T44.3X2	T44.3X3	T44.3X4	T44.3X5	T44.3X6
Benadryl	T45.0X1	T45.0X2	T45.0X3	T45.0X4	T45.0X5	T45.0X6
Benaprizine	T44.3X1	T44.3X2	T44.3X3	T44.3X4	T44.3X5	T44.3X6
Benazepril	T46.4X1	T46.4X2	T46.4X3	T46.4X4	T46.4X5	T46.4X6
Bencyclane	T46.7X1	T46.7X2	T46.7X3	T46.7X4	T46.7X5	T46.7X6
Bendazol	T46.3X1	T46.3X2	T46.3X3	T46.3X4	T46.3X5	T46.3X6
Bendrofluazide	T50.2X1	T50.2X2	T50.2X3	T50.2X4	T50.2X5	T50.2X6
Bendroflumethiazide	T50.2X1	T50.2X2	T50.2X3	T50.2X4	T50.2X5	T50.2X6
Benemid	T50.4X1	T50.4X2	T50.4X3	T50.4X4	T50.4X5	T50.4X6
Benethamine penicillin	T36.0X1	T36.0X2	T36.0X3	T36.0X4	T36.0X5	T36.0X6
Benisone	T49.0X1	T49.0X2	T49.0X3	T49.0X4	T49.0X5	T49.0X6

Substance	Poisoning, Accidental (Unintentional)	Poisoning, Intentional Self-Harm	Poisoning, Assault	Poisoning, Undetermined	Adverse Effect	Underdosing
Benexate	T47.1X1	T47.1X2	T47.1X3	T47.1X4	T47.1X5	T47.1X6
Benfluorex	T46.6X1	T46.6X2	T46.6X3	T46.6X4	T46.6X5	T46.6X6
Benfotiamine	T45.2X1	T45.2X2	T45.2X3	T45.2X4	T45.2X5	T45.2X6
Benomyl	T60.0X1	T60.0X2	T60.0X3	T60.0X4	—	—
Benoquin	T49.8X1	T49.8X2	T49.8X3	T49.8X4	T49.8X5	T49.8X6
Benoxinate	T41.3X1	T41.3X2	T41.3X3	T41.3X4	T41.3X5	T41.3X6
Benperidol	T43.4X1	T43.4X2	T43.4X3	T43.4X4	T43.4X5	T43.4X6
Benproperine	T48.3X1	T48.3X2	T48.3X3	T48.3X4	T48.3X5	T48.3X6
Benserazide	T42.8X1	T42.8X2	T42.8X3	T42.8X4	T42.8X5	T42.8X6
Bentazepam	T42.4X1	T42.4X2	T42.4X3	T42.4X4	T42.4X5	T42.4X6
Bentiromide	T50.8X1	T50.8X2	T50.8X3	T50.8X4	T50.8X5	T50.8X6
Bentonite	T49.3X1	T49.3X2	T49.3X3	T49.3X4	T49.3X5	T49.3X6
Benzalbutyramide	T46.6X1	T46.6X2	T46.6X3	T46.6X4	T46.6X5	T46.6X6
Benzalkonium (chloride)	T49.0X1	T49.0X2	T49.0X3	T49.0X4	T49.0X5	T49.0X6
ophthalmic preparation	T49.5X1	T49.5X2	T49.5X3	T49.5X4	T49.5X5	T49.5X6
Benzamine	T41.3X1	T41.3X2	T41.3X3	T41.3X4	T41.3X5	T41.3X6
lactate	T49.1X1	T49.1X2	T49.1X3	T49.1X4	T49.1X5	T49.1X6
Benzamidosalicylate (calcium)	T37.1X1	T37.1X2	T37.1X3	T37.1X4	T37.1X5	T37.1X6
Benzamphetamine	T50.5X1	T50.5X2	T50.5X3	T50.5X4	T50.5X5	T50.5X6
Benzapril hydrochloride	T46.5X1	T46.5X2	T46.5X3	T46.5X4	T46.5X5	T46.5X6
Benzathine benzylpenicillin	T36.0X1	T36.0X2	T36.0X3	T36.0X4	T36.0X5	T36.0X6
Benzathine penicillin	T36.0X1	T36.0X2	T36.0X3	T36.0X4	T36.0X5	T36.0X6
Benzatropine	T42.8X1	T42.8X2	T42.8X3	T42.8X4	T42.8X5	T42.8X6
Benzbromarone	T50.4X1	T50.4X2	T50.4X3	T50.4X4	T50.4X5	T50.4X6
Benzcarbimine	T45.1X1	T45.1X2	T45.1X3	T45.1X4	T45.1X5	T45.1X6
Benzedrex	T44.991	T44.992	T44.993	T44.994	T44.995	T44.996
Benzedrine (amphetamine)	T43.621	T43.622	T43.623	T43.624	T43.625	T43.626
Benzenamine	T65.3X1	T65.3X2	T65.3X3	T65.3X4	—	—
Benzene	T52.1X1	T52.1X2	T52.1X3	T52.1X4	—	—
homologues (acetyl) (dimethyl) (methyl) (solvent)	T52.2X1	T52.2X2	T52.2X3	T52.2X4	—	—
Benzethonium (chloride)	T49.0X1	T49.0X2	T49.0X3	T49.0X4	T49.0X5	T49.0X6
Benzfetamine	T50.5X1	T50.5X2	T50.5X3	T50.5X4	T50.5X5	T50.5X6
Benzhexol	T44.3X1	T44.3X2	T44.3X3	T44.3X4	T44.3X5	T44.3X6
Benzhydramine (chloride)	T45.0X1	T45.0X2	T45.0X3	T45.0X4	T45.0X5	T45.0X6
Benzidine	T65.891	T65.892	T65.893	T65.894	—	—
Benzilonium bromide	T44.3X1	T44.3X2	T44.3X3	T44.3X4	T44.3X5	T44.3X6
Benzimidazole	T60.3X1	T60.3X2	T60.3X3	T60.3X4	—	—
Benzin(e)—*see Ligroin*						
Benziodarone	T46.3X1	T46.3X2	T46.3X3	T46.3X4	T46.3X5	T46.3X6
Benznidazole	T37.3X1	T37.3X2	T37.3X3	T37.3X4	T37.3X5	T37.3X6
Benzocaine	T41.3X1	T41.3X2	T41.3X3	T41.3X4	T41.3X5	T41.3X6

Substance	Poisoning, Accidental (Unintentional)	Poisoning, Intentional Self-Harm	Poisoning, Assault	Poisoning, Undetermined	Adverse Effect	Underdosing
Benzoctamine	T43.0X1	T43.0X2	T43.0X3	T43.0X4	T43.0X5	T43.0X6
Benzodiapin	T42.4X1	T42.4X2	T42.4X3	T42.4X4	T42.4X5	T42.4X6
Benzodiazepine NEC	T42.4X1	T42.4X2	T42.4X3	T42.4X4	T42.4X5	T42.4X6
Benzoic acid	T49.0X1	T49.0X2	T49.0X3	T49.0X4	T49.0X5	T49.0X6
with salicylic acid	T49.0X1	T49.0X2	T49.0X3	T49.0X4	T49.0X5	T49.0X6
Benzoin (tincture)	T48.5X1	T48.5X2	T48.5X3	T48.5X4	T48.5X5	T48.5X6
Benzol (benzene)	T52.1X1	T52.1X2	T52.1X3	T52.1X4	—	—
vapor	T52.0X1	T52.0X2	T52.0X3	T52.0X4	—	—
Benzomorphan	T40.2X1	T40.2X2	T40.2X3	T40.2X4	T40.2X5	T40.2X6
Benzonatate	T48.3X1	T48.3X2	T48.3X3	T48.3X4	T48.3X5	T48.3X6
Benzophenones	T49.3X1	T49.3X2	T49.3X3	T49.3X4	T49.3X5	T49.3X6
Benzopyrone	T46.991	T46.992	T46.993	T46.994	T46.995	T46.996
Benzothiadiazides	T50.2X1	T50.2X2	T50.2X3	T50.2X4	T50.2X5	T50.2X6
Benzoxonium chloride	T49.0X1	T49.0X2	T49.0X3	T49.0X4	T49.0X5	T49.0X6
Benzoyl peroxide	T49.0X1	T49.0X2	T49.0X3	T49.0X4	T49.0X5	T49.0X6
Benzoylpas calcium	T37.1X1	T37.1X2	T37.1X3	T37.1X4	T37.1X5	T37.1X6
Benzperidin	T43.591	T43.592	T43.593	T43.594	T43.595	T43.596
Benzperidol	T43.591	T43.592	T43.593	T43.594	T43.595	T43.596
Benzphetamine	T50.5X1	T50.5X2	T50.5X3	T50.5X4	T50.5X5	T50.5X6
Benzpyrinium bromide	T44.1X1	T44.1X2	T44.1X3	T44.1X4	T44.1X5	T44.1X6
Benzquinamide	T45.0X1	T45.0X2	T45.0X3	T45.0X4	T45.0X5	T45.0X6
Benzthiazide	T50.2X1	T50.2X2	T50.2X3	T50.2X4	T50.2X5	T50.2X6
Benztropine						
anticholinergic	T44.3X1	T44.3X2	T44.3X3	T44.3X4	T44.3X5	T44.3X6
antiparkinson	T42.8X1	T42.8X2	T42.8X3	T42.8X4	T42.8X5	T42.8X6
Benzydamine	T49.0X1	T49.0X2	T49.0X3	T49.0X4	T49.0X5	T49.0X6
Benzyl						
acetate	T52.8X1	T52.8X2	T52.8X3	T52.8X4	—	—
alcohol	T49.0X1	T49.0X2	T49.0X3	T49.0X4	T49.0X5	T49.0X6
benzoate	T49.0X1	T49.0X2	T49.0X3	T49.0X4	T49.0X5	T49.0X6
Benzoic acid	T49.0X1	T49.0X2	T49.0X3	T49.0X4	T49.0X5	T49.0X6
morphine	T40.2X1	T40.2X2	T40.2X3	T40.2X4	—	—
nicotinate	T46.6X1	T46.6X2	T46.6X3	T46.6X4	T46.6X5	T46.6X6
penicillin	T36.0X1	T36.0X2	T36.0X3	T36.0X4	T36.0X5	T36.0X6
Benzylhydrochlorthia-zide	T50.2X1	T50.2X2	T50.2X3	T50.2X4	T50.2X5	T50.2X6
Benzylpenicillin	T36.0X1	T36.0X2	T36.0X3	T36.0X4	T36.0X5	T36.0X6
Benzylthiouracil	T38.2X1	T38.2X2	T38.2X3	T38.2X4	T38.2X5	T38.2X6
Bephenium hydroxy-naphthoate	T37.4X1	T37.4X2	T37.4X3	T37.4X4	T37.4X5	T37.4X6
Bepridil	T46.1X1	T46.1X2	T46.1X3	T46.1X4	T46.1X5	T46.1X6
Bergamot oil	T65.891	T65.892	T65.893	T65.894	—	—
Bergapten	T50.991	T50.992	T50.993	T50.994	T50.995	T50.996
Berries, poisonous	T62.1X1	T62.1X2	T62.1X3	T62.1X4	—	—

Substance	Poisoning, Accidental (Unintentional)	Poisoning, Intentional Self-Harm	Poisoning, Assault	Poisoning, Undetermined	Adverse Effect	Underdosing
Beryllium (compounds)	T56.7X1	T56.7X2	T56.7X3	T56.7X4	—	—
b-acetyldigoxin	T46.ØX1	T46.ØX2	T46.ØX3	T46.ØX4	T46.ØX5	T46.ØX6
beta adrenergic blocking agent, heart	T44.7X1	T44.7X2	T44.7X3	T44.7X4	T44.7X5	T44.7X6
b-benzalbutyramide	T46.6X1	T46.6X2	T46.6X3	T46.6X4	T46.6X5	T46.6X6
Betacarotene	T45.2X1	T45.2X2	T45.2X3	T45.2X4	T45.2X5	T45.2X6
b-eucaine	T49.1X1	T49.1X2	T49.1X3	T49.1X4	T49.1X5	T49.1X6
Beta-Chlor	T42.6X1	T42.6X2	T42.6X3	T42.6X4	T42.6X5	T42.6X6
b-galactosidase	T47.5X1	T47.5X2	T47.5X3	T47.5X4	T47.5X5	T47.5X6
Betahistine	T46.7X1	T46.7X2	T46.7X3	T46.7X4	T46.7X5	T46.7X6
Betaine	T47.5X1	T47.5X2	T47.5X3	T47.5X4	T47.5X5	T47.5X6
Betamethasone	T49.ØX1	T49.ØX2	T49.ØX3	T49.ØX4	T49.ØX5	T49.ØX6
topical	T49.ØX1	T49.ØX2	T49.ØX3	T49.ØX4	T49.ØX5	T49.ØX6
Betamicin	T36.8X1	T36.8X2	T36.8X3	T36.8X4	T36.8X5	T36.8X6
Betanidine	T46.5X1	T46.5X2	T46.5X3	T46.5X4	T46.5X5	T46.5X6
b-sitosterol(s)	T46.6X1	T46.6X2	T46.6X3	T46.6X4	T46.6X5	T46.6X6
Betaxolol	T44.7X1	T44.7X2	T44.7X3	T44.7X4	T44.7X5	T44.7X6
Betazole	T5Ø.8X1	T5Ø.8X2	T5Ø.8X3	T5Ø.8X4	T5Ø.8X5	T5Ø.8X6
Bethanechol	T44.1X1	T44.1X2	T44.1X3	T44.1X4	T44.1X5	T44.1X6
chloride	T44.1X1	T44.1X2	T44.1X3	T44.1X4	T44.1X5	T44.1X6
Bethanidine	T46.5X1	T46.5X2	T46.5X3	T46.5X4	T46.5X5	T46.5X6
Betoxycaine	T41.3X1	T41.3X2	T41.3X3	T41.3X4	T41.3X5	T41.3X6
Betula oil	T49.3X1	T49.3X2	T49.3X3	T49.3X4	T49.3X5	T49.3X6
Bevantolol	T44.7X1	T44.7X2	T44.7X3	T44.7X4	T44.7X5	T44.7X6
Bevonium metilsulfate	T44.3X1	T44.3X2	T44.3X3	T44.3X4	T44.3X5	T44.3X6
Bezafibrate	T46.6X1	T46.6X2	T46.6X3	T46.6X4	T46.6X5	T46.6X6
Bezitramide	T4Ø.4X1	T4Ø.4X2	T4Ø.4X3	T4Ø.4X4	T4Ø.4X5	T4Ø.4X6
BHA	T5Ø.991	T5Ø.992	T5Ø.993	T5Ø.994	T5Ø.995	T5Ø.996
Bhang	T4Ø.7X1	T4Ø.7X2	T4Ø.7X3	T4Ø.7X4	T4Ø.7X5	T4Ø.7X6
BHC (medicinal)	T49.ØX1	T49.ØX2	T49.ØX3	T49.ØX4	T49.ØX5	T49.ØX6
nonmedicinal (vapor)	T53.6X1	T53.6X2	T53.6X3	T53.6X4	—	—
Bialamicol	T37.3X1	T37.3X2	T37.3X3	T37.3X4	T37.3X5	T37.3X6
Bibenzonium bromide	T48.3X1	T48.3X2	T48.3X3	T48.3X4	T48.3X5	T48.3X6
Bibrocathol	T49.5X1	T49.5X2	T49.5X3	T49.5X4	T49.5X5	T49.5X6
Bichloride of mercury — *see Mercury, chloride*						
Bichromates (calcium) (potassium) (sodium) (crystals)	T57.8X1	T57.8X2	T57.8X3	T57.8X4	—	—
fumes	T56.2X1	T56.2X2	T56.2X3	T56.2X4	—	—
Biclotymol	T49.6X1	T49.6X2	T49.6X3	T49.6X4	T49.6X5	T49.6X6
Bicucculine	T5Ø.7X1	T5Ø.7X2	T5Ø.7X3	T5Ø.7X4	T5Ø.7X5	T5Ø.7X6
Bifemelane	T43.291	T43.292	T43.293	T43.294	T43.295	T43.296
Biguanide derivatives, oral	T38.3X1	T38.3X2	T38.3X3	T38.3X4	T38.3X5	T38.3X6
Biligrafin	T5Ø.8X1	T5Ø.8X2	T5Ø.8X3	T5Ø.8X4	T5Ø.8X5	T5Ø.8X6
Bile salts	T47.5X1	T47.5X2	T47.5X3	T47.5X4	T47.5X5	T47.5X6
Bilopaque	T5Ø.8X1	T5Ø.8X2	T5Ø.8X3	T5Ø.8X4	T5Ø.8X5	T5Ø.8X6
Binifibrate	T46.6X1	T46.6X2	T46.6X3	T46.6X4	T46.6X5	T46.6X6
Binitrobenzol	T65.3X1	T65.3X2	T65.3X3	T65.3X4	—	—
Bioflavonoid(s)	T46.991	T46.992	T46.993	T46.994	T46.995	T46.996
Biological substance NEC	T5Ø.9Ø1	T5Ø.9Ø2	T5Ø.9Ø3	T5Ø.9Ø4	T5Ø.9Ø5	T5Ø.9Ø6
Biotin	T45.2X1	T45.2X2	T45.2X3	T45.2X4	T45.2X5	T45.2X6
Biperiden	T44.3X1	T44.3X2	T44.3X3	T44.3X4	T44.3X5	T44.3X6
Bisacodyl	T47.2X1	T47.2X2	T47.2X3	T47.2X4	T47.2X5	T47.2X6
Bisbentiamine	T45.2X1	T45.2X2	T45.2X3	T45.2X4	T45.2X5	T45.2X6
Bisbutiamine	T45.2X1	T45.2X2	T45.2X3	T45.2X4	T45.2X5	T45.2X6
Bisdequalinium (salts) (diacetate)	T49.6X1	T49.6X2	T49.6X3	T49.6X4	T49.6X5	T49.6X6
Bishydroxycoumarin	T45.511	T45.512	T45.513	T45.514	T45.515	T45.516
Bismarsen	T37.8X1	T37.8X2	T37.8X3	T37.8X4	T37.8X5	T37.8X6
Bismuth salts	T47.6X1	T47.6X2	T47.6X3	T47.6X4	T47.6X5	T47.6X6
aluminate	T47.1X1	T47.1X2	T47.1X3	T47.1X4	T47.1X5	T47.1X6
anti-infectives	T37.8X1	T37.8X2	T37.8X3	T37.8X4	T37.8X5	T37.8X6
formic iodide	T49.ØX1	T49.ØX2	T49.ØX3	T49.ØX4	T49.ØX5	T49.ØX6
glycolylarsenate	T49.ØX1	T49.ØX2	T49.ØX3	T49.ØX4	T49.ØX5	T49.ØX6
nonmedicinal (compounds) NEC	T65.91	T65.92	T65.93	T65.94	—	—
subcarbonate	T47.6X1	T47.6X2	T47.6X3	T47.6X4	T47.6X5	T47.6X6
subsalicylate	T37.8X1	T37.8X2	T37.8X3	T37.8X4	T37.8X5	T37.8X6
sulfarsphenamine	T37.8X1	T37.8X2	T37.8X3	T37.8X4	T37.8X5	T37.8X6
Bisoprolol	T44.7X1	T44.7X2	T44.7X3	T44.7X4	T44.7X5	T44.7X6
Bisoxatin	T47.2X1	T47.2X2	T47.2X3	T47.2X4	T47.2X5	T47.2X6
Bisulepin (hydrochloride)	T45.ØX1	T45.ØX2	T45.ØX3	T45.ØX4	T45.ØX5	T45.ØX6
Bithionol	T37.8X1	T37.8X2	T37.8X3	T37.8X4	T37.8X5	T37.8X6
anthelminthic	T37.4X1	T37.4X2	T37.4X3	T37.4X4	T37.4X5	T37.4X6
Bitolterol	T48.6X1	T48.6X2	T48.6X3	T48.6X4	T48.6X5	T48.6X6
Bitoscanate	T37.4X1	T37.4X2	T37.4X3	T37.4X4	T37.4X5	T37.4X6
Bitter almond oil	T62.8X1	T62.8X2	T62.8X3	T62.8X4	—	—
Bittersweet	T62.2X1	T62.2X2	T62.2X3	T62.2X4	—	—
Black						
flag	T6Ø.91	T6Ø.92	T6Ø.93	T6Ø.94	—	—
henbane	T62.2X1	T62.2X2	T62.2X3	T62.2X4	—	—
leaf (4Ø)	T6Ø.91	T6Ø.92	T6Ø.93	T6Ø.94	—	—
widow spider (bite)	T63.311	T63.312	T63.313	T63.314	—	—
antivenin	T5Ø.Z11	T5Ø.Z12	T5Ø.Z13	T5Ø.Z14	T5Ø.Z15	T5Ø.Z16
Blast furnace gas (carbon monoxide from)	T58.8X1	T58.8X2	T58.8X3	T58.8X4	—	—
Bleach	T54.91	T54.92	T54.93	T54.94	—	—

Substance	Poisoning, Accidental (Unintentional)	Poisoning, Intentional Self-Harm	Poisoning, Assault	Poisoning, Undetermined	Adverse Effect	Underdosing
Bleaching agent (medicinal)	T49.4X1	T49.4X2	T49.4X3	T49.4X4	T49.4X5	T49.4X6
Bleomycin	T45.1X1	T45.1X2	T45.1X3	T45.1X4	T45.1X5	T45.1X6
Blockain	T41.3X1	T41.3X2	T41.3X3	T41.3X4	T41.3X5	T41.3X6
infiltration (subcutaneous)	T41.3X1	T41.3X2	T41.3X3	T41.3X4	T41.3X5	T41.3X6
nerve block (peripheral) (plexus)	T41.3X1	T41.3X2	T41.3X3	T41.3X4	T41.3X5	T41.3X6
topical (surface)	T41.3X1	T41.3X2	T41.3X3	T41.3X4	T41.3X5	T41.3X6
Blockers, calcium channel	T46.1X1	T46.1X2	T46.1X3	T46.1X4	T46.1X5	T46.1X6
Blood (derivatives) (natural) (plasma) (whole)	T45.8X1	T45.8X2	T45.8X3	T45.8X4	T45.8X5	T45.8X6
dried	T45.8X1	T45.8X2	T45.8X3	T45.8X4	T45.8X5	T45.8X6
drug affecting NEC	T45.91	T45.92	T45.93	T45.94	T45.95	T45.96
expander NEC	T45.8X1	T45.8X2	T45.8X3	T45.8X4	T45.8X5	T45.8X6
fraction NEC	T45.8X1	T45.8X2	T45.8X3	T45.8X4	T45.8X5	T45.8X6
substitute (macromolecular)	T45.8X1	T45.8X2	T45.8X3	T45.8X4	T45.8X5	T45.8X6
Blue velvet	T40.2X1	T40.2X2	T40.2X3	T40.2X4	—	—
Bone meal	T62.8X1	T62.8X2	T62.8X3	T62.8X4	—	—
Bonine	T45.0X1	T45.0X2	T45.0X3	T45.0X4	T45.0X5	T45.0X6
Bopindolol	T44.7X1	T44.7X2	T44.7X3	T44.7X4	T44.7X5	T44.7X6
Boracic acid	T49.0X1	T49.0X2	T49.0X3	T49.0X4	T49.0X5	T49.0X6
ENT agent	T49.6X1	T49.6X2	T49.6X3	T49.6X4	T49.6X5	T49.6X6
ophthalmic preparation	T49.5X1	T49.5X2	T49.5X3	T49.5X4	T49.5X5	T49.5X6
Borane complex	T57.8X1	T57.8X2	T57.8X3	T57.8X4	—	—
Borate(s)	T57.8X1	T57.8X2	T57.8X3	T57.8X4	—	—
buffer	T50.991	T50.992	T50.993	T50.994	T50.995	T50.996
cleanser	T54.91	T54.92	T54.93	T54.94	—	—
sodium	T57.8X1	T57.8X2	T57.8X3	T57.8X4	—	—
Borax (cleanser)	T54.91	T54.92	T54.93	T54.94	—	—
Bordeaux mixture	T60.3X1	T60.3X2	T60.3X3	T60.3X4	—	—
Boric acid	T49.0X1	T49.0X2	T49.0X3	T49.0X4	T49.0X5	T49.0X6
ENT agent	T49.6X1	T49.6X2	T49.6X3	T49.6X4	T49.6X5	T49.6X6
ophthalmic preparation	T49.5X1	T49.5X2	T49.5X3	T49.5X4	T49.5X5	T49.5X6
Bornaprine	T44.3X1	T44.3X2	T44.3X3	T44.3X4	T44.3X5	T44.3X6
Boron	T57.8X1	T57.8X2	T57.8X3	T57.8X4	—	—
hydride NEC	T57.8X1	T57.8X2	T57.8X3	T57.8X4	—	—
fumes or gas	T57.8X1	T57.8X2	T57.8X3	T57.8X4	—	—
trifluoride	T59.891	T59.892	T59.893	T59.894	—	—
Botox	T48.291	T48.292	T48.293	T48.294	T48.295	T48.296
Botulinus anti-toxin (type A, B)	T50.Z11	T50.Z12	T50.Z13	T50.Z14	T50.Z15	T50.Z16
Brake fluid vapor	T59.891	T59.892	T59.893	T59.894	—	—
Brallobarbital	T42.3X1	T42.3X2	T42.3X3	T42.3X4	T42.3X5	T42.3X6
Bran (wheat)	T47.4X1	T47.4X2	T47.4X3	T47.4X4	T47.4X5	T47.4X6
Brass (fumes)	T56.891	T56.892	T56.893	T56.894	—	—

Substance	Poisoning, Accidental (Unintentional)	Poisoning, Intentional Self-Harm	Poisoning, Assault	Poisoning, Undetermined	Adverse Effect	Underdosing
Brasso	T52.0X1	T52.0X2	T52.0X3	T52.0X4	—	—
Bretylium tosilate	T46.2X1	T46.2X2	T46.2X3	T46.2X4	T46.2X5	T46.2X6
Brevital (sodium)	T41.1X1	T41.1X2	T41.1X3	T41.1X4	T41.1X5	T41.1X6
Brinase	T45.3X1	T45.3X2	T45.3X3	T45.3X4	T45.3X5	T45.3X6
British antilewisite	T45.8X1	T45.8X2	T45.8X3	T45.8X4	T45.8X5	T45.8X6
Brodifacoum	T60.4X1	T60.4X2	T60.4X3	T60.4X4	—	—
Bromal (hydrate)	T42.6X1	T42.6X2	T42.6X3	T42.6X4	T42.6X5	T42.6X6
Bromazepam	T42.4X1	T42.4X2	T42.4X3	T42.4X4	T42.4X5	T42.4X6
Bromazine	T45.0X1	T45.0X2	T45.0X3	T45.0X4	T45.0X5	T45.0X6
Brombenzylcyanide	T59.3X1	T59.3X2	T59.3X3	T59.3X4	—	—
Bromelains	T45.3X1	T45.3X2	T45.3X3	T45.3X4	T45.3X5	T45.3X6
Bromethalin	T60.4X1	T60.4X2	T60.4X3	T60.4X4	—	—
Bromhexine	T48.4X1	T48.4X2	T48.4X3	T48.4X4	T48.4X5	T48.4X6
Bromide salts	T42.6X1	T42.6X2	T42.6X3	T42.6X4	T42.6X5	T42.6X6
Bromindione	T45.511	T45.512	T45.513	T45.514	T45.515	T45.516
Bromine						
compounds (medicinal)	T42.6X1	T42.6X2	T42.6X3	T42.6X4	T42.6X5	T42.6X6
sedative	T42.6X1	T42.6X2	T42.6X3	T42.6X4	T42.6X5	T42.6X6
vapor	T59.891	T59.892	T59.893	T59.894	—	—
Bromisovalum	T42.6X1	T42.6X2	T42.6X3	T42.6X4	T42.6X5	T42.6X6
Bromisoval	T42.6X1	T42.6X2	T42.6X3	T42.6X4	T42.6X5	T42.6X6
Bromobenzylcyanide	T59.3X1	T59.3X2	T59.3X3	T59.3X4	—	—
Bromochlorosalicylani-lide	T49.0X1	T49.0X2	T49.0X3	T49.0X4	T49.0X5	T49.0X6
Bromocriptine	T42.8X1	T42.8X2	T42.8X3	T42.8X4	T42.8X5	T42.8X6
Bromodiphenhydramine	T45.0X1	T45.0X2	T45.0X3	T45.0X4	T45.0X5	T45.0X6
Bromoform	T42.6X1	T42.6X2	T42.6X3	T42.6X4	T42.6X5	T42.6X6
Bromophenol blue reagent	T50.991	T50.992	T50.993	T50.994	T50.995	T50.996
Bromopride	T47.8X1	T47.8X2	T47.8X3	T47.8X4	T47.8X5	T47.8X6
Bromosalicylchloranitide	T49.0X1	T49.0X2	T49.0X3	T49.0X4	T49.0X5	T49.0X6
Bromosalicylhydroxamic acid	T37.1X1	T37.1X2	T37.1X3	T37.1X4	T37.1X5	T37.1X6
Bromo-seltzer	T39.1X1	T39.1X2	T39.1X3	T39.1X4	T39.1X5	T39.1X6
Bromoxynil	T60.3X1	T60.3X2	T60.3X3	T60.3X4	—	—
Bromperidol	T43.4X1	T43.4X2	T43.4X3	T43.4X4	T43.4X5	T43.4X6
Brompheniramine	T45.0X1	T45.0X2	T45.0X3	T45.0X4	T45.0X5	T45.0X6
Bromsulfophthalein	T50.8X1	T50.8X2	T50.8X3	T50.8X4	T50.8X5	T50.8X6
Bromural	T42.6X1	T42.6X2	T42.6X3	T42.6X4	T42.6X5	T42.6X6
Bromvaletone	T42.6X1	T42.6X2	T42.6X3	T42.6X4	T42.6X5	T42.6X6
Bronchodilator NEC	T48.6X1	T48.6X2	T48.6X3	T48.6X4	T48.6X5	T48.6X6
Brotizolam	T42.4X1	T42.4X2	T42.4X3	T42.4X4	T42.4X5	T42.4X6
Brovincamine	T46.7X1	T46.7X2	T46.7X3	T46.7X4	T46.7X5	T46.7X6
Brown spider (bite) (venom)	T63.391	T63.392	T63.393	T63.394	—	—

◀ New ⟸ Revised ~~deleted~~ Deleted

TABLE OF DRUGS AND CHEMICALS

Substance	Poisoning, Accidental (Unintentional)	Poisoning, Intentional Self-Harm	Poisoning, Assault	Poisoning, Undetermined	Adverse Effect	Underdosing
Brown recluse spider (bite) (venom)	T63.331	T63.332	T63.333	T63.334	—	—
Broxaterol	T48.6X1	T48.6X2	T48.6X3	T48.6X4	T48.6X5	T48.6X6
Broxuridine	T45.1X1	T45.1X2	T45.1X3	T45.1X4	T45.1X5	T45.1X6
Broxyquinoline	T37.8X1	T37.8X2	T37.8X3	T37.8X4	T37.8X5	T37.8X6
Bruceine	T48.291	T48.292	T48.293	T48.294	T48.295	T48.296
Brucia	T62.2X1	T62.2X2	T62.2X3	T62.2X4	—	—
Brucine	T65.1X1	T65.1X2	T65.1X3	T65.1X4	—	—
Brunswick green — *see Copper*						
Bruten — *see Ibuprofen*						
Bryonia	T47.2X1	T47.2X2	T47.2X3	T47.2X4	T47.2X5	T47.2X6
Buclizine	T45.ØX1	T45.ØX2	T45.ØX3	T45.ØX4	T45.ØX5	T45.ØX6
Buclosamide	T49.ØX1	T49.ØX2	T49.ØX3	T49.ØX4	T49.ØX5	T49.ØX6
Budesonide	T44.5X1	T44.5X2	T44.5X3	T44.5X4	T44.5X5	T44.5X6
Budralazine	T46.5X1	T46.5X2	T46.5X3	T46.5X4	T46.5X5	T46.5X6
Bufferin	T39.Ø11	T39.Ø12	T39.Ø13	T39.Ø14	T39.Ø15	T39.Ø16
Buflomedil	T46.7X1	T46.7X2	T46.7X3	T46.7X4	T46.7X5	T46.7X6
Buformin	T38.3X1	T38.3X2	T38.3X3	T38.3X4	T38.3X5	T38.3X6
Bufotenine	T4Ø.991	T4Ø.992	T4Ø.993	T4Ø.994	—	—
Bufrolin	T48.6X1	T48.6X2	T48.6X3	T48.6X4	T48.6X5	T48.6X6
Bufylline	T48.6X1	T48.6X2	T48.6X3	T48.6X4	T48.6X5	T48.6X6
Bulk filler	T5Ø.5X1	T5Ø.5X2	T5Ø.5X3	T5Ø.5X4	T5Ø.5X5	T5Ø.5X6
cathartic	T47.4X1	T47.4X2	T47.4X3	T47.4X4	T47.4X5	T47.4X6
Bumetanide	T5Ø.1X1	T5Ø.1X2	T5Ø.1X3	T5Ø.1X4	T5Ø.1X5	T5Ø.1X6
Bunaftine	T46.2X1	T46.2X2	T46.2X3	T46.2X4	T46.2X5	T46.2X6
Bunamiodyl	T5Ø.8X1	T5Ø.8X2	T5Ø.8X3	T5Ø.8X4	T5Ø.8X5	T5Ø.8X6
Bunazosin	T44.6X1	T44.6X2	T44.6X3	T44.6X4	T44.6X5	T44.6X6
Bunitrolol	T44.7X1	T44.7X2	T44.7X3	T44.7X4	T44.7X5	T44.7X6
Buphenine	T46.7X1	T46.7X2	T46.7X3	T46.7X4	T46.7X5	T46.7X6
Bupivacaine	T41.3X1	T41.3X2	T41.3X3	T41.3X4	T41.3X5	T41.3X6
infiltration (subcutaneous)	T41.3X1	T41.3X2	T41.3X3	T41.3X4	T41.3X5	T41.3X6
nerve block (peripheral) (plexus)	T41.3X1	T41.3X2	T41.3X3	T41.3X4	T41.3X5	T41.3X6
spinal	T41.3X1	T41.3X2	T41.3X3	T41.3X4	T41.3X5	T41.3X6
Bupranolol	T44.7X1	T44.7X2	T44.7X3	T44.7X4	T44.7X5	T44.7X6
Buprenorphine	T4Ø.4X1	T4Ø.4X2	T4Ø.4X3	T4Ø.4X4	T4Ø.4X5	T4Ø.4X6
Bupropion	T43.291	T43.292	T43.293	T43.294	T43.295	T43.296
Burimamide	T47.1X1	T47.1X2	T47.1X3	T47.1X4	T47.1X5	T47.1X6
Buserelin	T38.891	T38.892	T38.893	T38.894	T38.895	T38.896
Buspirone	T43.591	T43.592	T43.593	T43.594	T43.595	T43.596
Busulfan, busulphan	T45.1X1	T45.1X2	T45.1X3	T45.1X4	T45.1X5	T45.1X6
Butabarbital (sodium)	T42.3X1	T42.3X2	T42.3X3	T42.3X4	T42.3X5	T42.3X6
Butabarbitone	T42.3X1	T42.3X2	T42.3X3	T42.3X4	T42.3X5	T42.3X6
Butabarpal	T42.3X1	T42.3X2	T42.3X3	T42.3X4	T42.3X5	T42.3X6
Butacaine	T41.3X1	T41.3X2	T41.3X3	T41.3X4	T41.3X5	T41.3X6
Butalamine	T46.7X1	T46.7X2	T46.7X3	T46.7X4	T46.7X5	T46.7X6
Butalbital	T42.3X1	T42.3X2	T42.3X3	T42.3X4	T42.3X5	T42.3X6
Butallylonal	T42.3X1	T42.3X2	T42.3X3	T42.3X4	T42.3X5	T42.3X6
Butamben	T41.3X1	T41.3X2	T41.3X3	T41.3X4	T41.3X5	T41.3X6
Butamirate	T48.3X1	T48.3X2	T48.3X3	T48.3X4	T48.3X5	T48.3X6
Butane (distributed in mobile container)	T59.891	T59.892	T59.893	T59.894	—	—
distributed through pipes	T59.891	T59.892	T59.893	T59.894	—	—
incomplete combustion	T58.11	T58.12	T58.13	T58.14	—	—
Butanilicaine	T41.3X1	T41.3X2	T41.3X3	T41.3X4	T41.3X5	T41.3X6
Butanol	T51.3X1	T51.3X2	T51.3X3	T51.3X4	—	—
Butanone, 2-butanone	T52.4X1	T52.4X2	T52.4X3	T52.4X4	—	—
Butantrone	T49.4X1	T49.4X2	T49.4X3	T49.4X4	T49.4X5	T49.4X6
Butaperazine	T43.3X1	T43.3X2	T43.3X3	T43.3X4	T43.3X5	T43.3X6
Butazolidin	T39.2X1	T39.2X2	T39.2X3	T39.2X4	T39.2X5	T39.2X6
Butetamate	T48.6X1	T48.6X2	T48.6X3	T48.6X4	T48.6X5	T48.6X6
Butethal	T42.3X1	T42.3X2	T42.3X3	T42.3X4	T42.3X5	T42.3X6
Butethamate	T44.3X1	T44.3X2	T44.3X3	T44.3X4	T44.3X5	T44.3X6
Buthalitone (sodium)	T41.1X1	T41.1X2	T41.1X3	T41.1X4	T41.1X5	T41.1X6
Butisol (sodium)	T42.3X1	T42.3X2	T42.3X3	T42.3X4	T42.3X5	T42.3X6
Butizide	T5Ø.2X1	T5Ø.2X2	T5Ø.2X3	T5Ø.2X4	T5Ø.2X5	T5Ø.2X6
Butobarbital	T42.3X1	T42.3X2	T42.3X3	T42.3X4	T42.3X5	T42.3X6
sodium	T42.3X1	T42.3X2	T42.3X3	T42.3X4	T42.3X5	T42.3X6
Butobarbitone	T42.3X1	T42.3X2	T42.3X3	T42.3X4	T42.3X5	T42.3X6
Butoconazole (nitrate)	T49.ØX1	T49.ØX2	T49.ØX3	T49.ØX4	T49.ØX5	T49.ØX6
Butorphanol	T4Ø.4X1	T4Ø.4X2	T4Ø.4X3	T4Ø.4X4	T4Ø.4X5	T4Ø.4X6
Butriptyline	T43.Ø11	T43.Ø12	T43.Ø13	T43.Ø14	T43.Ø15	T43.Ø16
Butropium bromide	T44.3X1	T44.3X2	T44.3X3	T44.3X4	T44.3X5	T44.3X6
Buttercups	T62.2X1	T62.2X2	T62.2X3	T62.2X4	—	—
Butter of antimony — *see Antimony*						
Butyl						
acetate (secondary)	T52.8X1	T52.8X2	T52.8X3	T52.8X4	—	—
alcohol	T51.3X1	T51.3X2	T51.3X3	T51.3X4	—	—
aminobenzoate	T41.3X1	T41.3X2	T41.3X3	T41.3X4	T41.3X5	T41.3X6
butyrate	T52.8X1	T52.8X2	T52.8X3	T52.8X4	—	—
carbinol	T51.3X1	T51.3X2	T51.3X3	T51.3X4	—	—
carbitol	T52.3X1	T52.3X2	T52.3X3	T52.3X4	—	—
cellosolve	T52.3X1	T52.3X2	T52.3X3	T52.3X4	—	—
chloral (hydrate)	T42.6X1	T42.6X2	T42.6X3	T42.6X4	T42.6X5	T42.6X6
formate	T52.8X1	T52.8X2	T52.8X3	T52.8X4	—	—

Substance	Poisoning, Accidental (Unintentional)	Poisoning, Intentional Self-Harm	Poisoning, Assault	Poisoning, Undetermined	Adverse Effect	Underdosing
Butyl *(Continued)*						
lactate	T52.8X1	T52.8X2	T52.8X3	T52.8X4	—	—
propionate	T52.8X1	T52.8X2	T52.8X3	T52.8X4	—	—
scopolamine bromide	T44.3X1	T44.3X2	T44.3X3	T44.3X4	T44.3X5	T44.3X6
thiobarbital sodium	T41.1X1	T41.1X2	T41.1X3	T41.1X4	T41.1X5	T41.1X6
Butylated hydroxy-anisole	T5Ø.991	T5Ø.992	T5Ø.993	T5Ø.994	T5Ø.995	T5Ø.996
Butylchloral hydrate	T42.6X1	T42.6X2	T42.6X3	T42.6X4	T42.6X5	T42.6X6
Butyltoluene	T52.2X1	T52.2X2	T52.2X3	T52.2X4	—	—
Butyn	T41.3X1	T41.3X2	T41.3X3	T41.3X4	T41.3X5	T41.3X6
Butyrophenone (-based tranquilizers)	T43.4X1	T43.4X2	T43.4X3	T43.4X4	T43.4X5	T43.4X6
C						
Cabergoline	T42.8X1	T42.8X2	T42.8X3	T42.8X4	T42.8X5	T42.8X6
Cacodyl, cacodylic acid	T57.ØX1	T57.ØX2	T57.ØX3	T57.ØX4	—	—
Cactinomycin	T45.1X1	T45.1X2	T45.1X3	T45.1X4	T45.1X5	T45.1X6
Cade oil	T49.4X1	T49.4X2	T49.4X3	T49.4X4	T49.4X5	T49.4X6
Cadexomer iodine	T49.ØX1	T49.ØX2	T49.ØX3	T49.ØX4	T49.ØX5	T49.ØX6
Cadmium (chloride) (fumes) (oxide)	T56.3X1	T56.3X2	T56.3X3	T56.3X4	—	—
sulfide (medicinal) NEC	T49.4X1	T49.4X2	T49.4X3	T49.4X4	T49.4X5	T49.4X6
Cadralazine	T46.5X1	T46.5X2	T46.5X3	T46.5X4	T46.5X5	T46.5X6
Caffeine	T43.611	T43.612	T43.613	T43.614	T43.615	T43.616
Calabar bean	T62.2X1	T62.2X2	T62.2X3	T62.2X4	—	—
Caladium seguinum	T62.2X1	T62.2X2	T62.2X3	T62.2X4	—	—
Calamine (lotion)	T49.3X1	T49.3X2	T49.3X3	T49.3X4	T49.3X5	T49.3X6
Calcifediol	T45.2X1	T45.2X2	T45.2X3	T45.2X4	T45.2X5	T45.2X6
Calciferol	T45.2X1	T45.2X2	T45.2X3	T45.2X4	T45.2X5	T45.2X6
Calcitonin	T5Ø.991	T5Ø.992	T5Ø.993	T5Ø.994	T5Ø.995	T5Ø.996
Calcitriol	T45.2X1	T45.2X2	T45.2X3	T45.2X4	T45.2X5	T45.2X6
Calcium	T5Ø.3X1	T5Ø.3X2	T5Ø.3X3	T5Ø.3X4	T5Ø.3X5	T5Ø.3X6
actylsalicylate	T39.Ø11	T39.Ø12	T39.Ø13	T39.Ø14	T39.Ø15	T39.Ø16
benzamidosalicylate	T37.1X1	T37.1X2	T37.1X3	T37.1X4	T37.1X5	T37.1X6
bromide	T42.6X1	T42.6X2	T42.6X3	T42.6X4	T42.6X5	T42.6X6
bromolactobionate	T42.6X1	T42.6X2	T42.6X3	T42.6X4	T42.6X5	T42.6X6
carbaspirin	T39.Ø11	T39.Ø12	T39.Ø13	T39.Ø14	T39.Ø15	T39.Ø16
carbimide	T5Ø.6X1	T5Ø.6X2	T5Ø.6X3	T5Ø.6X4	T5Ø.6X5	T5Ø.6X6
carbonate	T47.1X1	T47.1X2	T47.1X3	T47.1X4	T47.1X5	T47.1X6
chloride	T5Ø.991	T5Ø.992	T5Ø.993	T5Ø.994	T5Ø.995	T5Ø.996
anhydrous	T5Ø.991	T5Ø.992	T5Ø.993	T5Ø.994	T5Ø.995	T5Ø.996
cyanide	T57.8X1	T57.8X2	T57.8X3	T57.8X4	—	—
dioctyl sulfosuccinate	T47.4X1	T47.4X2	T47.4X3	T47.4X4	T47.4X5	T47.4X6
disodium edathamil	T45.8X1	T45.8X2	T45.8X3	T45.8X4	T45.8X5	T45.8X6

Substance	Poisoning, Accidental (Unintentional)	Poisoning, Intentional Self-Harm	Poisoning, Assault	Poisoning, Undetermined	Adverse Effect	Underdosing
Calcium *(Continued)*						
disodium edetate	T45.8X1	T45.8X2	T45.8X3	T45.8X4	T45.8X5	T45.8X6
dobesilate	T46.991	T46.992	T46.993	T46.994	T46.995	T46.996
EDTA	T45.8X1	T45.8X2	T45.8X3	T45.8X4	T45.8X5	T45.8X6
ferrous citrate	T45.4X1	T45.4X2	T45.4X3	T45.4X4	T45.4X5	T45.4X6
folinate	T45.8X1	T45.8X2	T45.8X3	T45.8X4	T45.8X5	T45.8X6
glubionate	T5Ø.3X1	T5Ø.3X2	T5Ø.3X3	T5Ø.3X4	T5Ø.3X5	T5Ø.3X6
gluconate	T5Ø.3X1	T5Ø.3X2	T5Ø.3X3	T5Ø.3X4	T5Ø.3X5	T5Ø.3X6
gluconogalactogluconate	T5Ø.3X1	T5Ø.3X2	T5Ø.3X3	T5Ø.3X4	T5Ø.3X5	T5Ø.3X6
hydrate, hydroxide	T54.3X1	T54.3X2	T54.3X3	T54.3X4	—	—
hypochlorite	T54.3X1	T54.3X2	T54.3X3	T54.3X4	—	—
iodide	T48.4X1	T48.4X2	T48.4X3	T48.4X4	T48.4X5	T48.4X6
ipodate	T5Ø.8X1	T5Ø.8X2	T5Ø.8X3	T5Ø.8X4	T5Ø.8X5	T5Ø.8X6
lactate	T5Ø.3X1	T5Ø.3X2	T5Ø.3X3	T5Ø.3X4	T5Ø.3X5	T5Ø.3X6
leucovorin	T45.8X1	T45.8X2	T45.8X3	T45.8X4	T45.8X5	T45.8X6
mandelate	T37.91	T37.92	T37.93	T37.94	T37.95	T37.96
oxide	T54.3X1	T54.3X2	T54.3X3	T54.3X4	—	—
pantothenate	T45.2X1	T45.2X2	T45.2X3	T45.2X4	T45.2X5	T45.2X6
phosphate	T5Ø.3X1	T5Ø.3X2	T5Ø.3X3	T5Ø.3X4	T5Ø.3X5	T5Ø.3X6
salicylate	T39.Ø91	T39.Ø92	T39.Ø93	T39.Ø94	T39.Ø95	T39.Ø96
salts	T5Ø.3X1	T5Ø.3X2	T5Ø.3X3	T5Ø.3X4	T5Ø.3X5	T5Ø.3X6
Calculus-dissolving drug	T5Ø.991	T5Ø.992	T5Ø.993	T5Ø.994	T5Ø.995	T5Ø.996
Calomel	T49.ØX1	T49.ØX2	T49.ØX3	T49.ØX4	T49.ØX5	T49.ØX6
Caloric agent	T5Ø.3X1	T5Ø.3X2	T5Ø.3X3	T5Ø.3X4	T5Ø.3X5	T5Ø.3X6
Calusterone	T38.7X1	T38.7X2	T38.7X3	T38.7X4	T38.7X5	T38.7X6
Camazepam	T42.4X1	T42.4X2	T42.4X3	T42.4X4	T42.4X5	T42.4X6
Camomile	T49.ØX1	T49.ØX2	T49.ØX3	T49.ØX4	T49.ØX5	T49.ØX6
Camoquin	T37.2X1	T37.2X2	T37.2X3	T37.2X4	T37.2X5	T37.2X6
Camphor						
insecticide	T6Ø.2X1	T6Ø.2X2	T6Ø.2X3	T6Ø.2X4	—	—
medicinal	T49.8X1	T49.8X2	T49.8X3	T49.8X4	T49.8X5	T49.8X6
Camylofin	T44.3X1	T44.3X2	T44.3X3	T44.3X4	T44.3X5	T44.3X6
Cancer chemotherapy drug regimen	T45.1X1	T45.1X2	T45.1X3	T45.1X4	T45.1X5	T45.1X6
Candeptin	T49.ØX1	T49.ØX2	T49.ØX3	T49.ØX4	T49.ØX5	T49.ØX6
Candicidin	T49.ØX1	T49.ØX2	T49.ØX3	T49.ØX4	T49.ØX5	T49.ØX6
Cannabinol	T4Ø.7X1	T4Ø.7X2	T4Ø.7X3	T4Ø.7X4	T4Ø.7X5	T4Ø.7X6
Cannabis (derivatives)	T4Ø.7X1	T4Ø.7X2	T4Ø.7X3	T4Ø.7X4	T4Ø.7X5	T4Ø.7X6
Canned heat	T51.1X1	T51.1X2	T51.1X3	T51.1X4	—	—
Canrenoic acid	T5Ø.ØX1	T5Ø.ØX2	T5Ø.ØX3	T5Ø.ØX4	T5Ø.ØX5	T5Ø.ØX6
Canrenone	T5Ø.ØX1	T5Ø.ØX2	T5Ø.ØX3	T5Ø.ØX4	T5Ø.ØX5	T5Ø.ØX6
Cantharides, cantharidin, cantharis	T49.8X1	T49.8X2	T49.8X3	T49.8X4	T49.8X5	T49.8X6

◀ New ⬅ Revised ~~deleted~~ Deleted

Substance	Poisoning, Accidental (Unintentional)	Poisoning, Intentional Self-Harm	Poisoning, Assault	Poisoning, Undetermined	Adverse Effect	Underdosing
Canthaxanthin	T5Ø.991	T5Ø.992	T5Ø.993	T5Ø.994	T5Ø.995	T5Ø.996
Capillary-active drug NEC	T46.9Ø1	T46.9Ø2	T46.9Ø3	T46.9Ø4	T46.9Ø5	T46.9Ø6
Capreomycin	T36.8X1	T36.8X2	T36.8X3	T36.8X4	T36.8X5	T36.8X6
Capsicum	T49.4X1	T49.4X2	T49.4X3	T49.4X4	T49.4X5	T49.4X6
Captafol	T6Ø.3X1	T6Ø.3X2	T6Ø.3X3	T6Ø.3X4	—	—
Captan	T6Ø.3X1	T6Ø.3X2	T6Ø.3X3	T6Ø.3X4	—	—
Captodiame, captodiamine	T43.591	T43.592	T43.593	T43.594	T43.595	T43.596
Captopril	T46.4X1	T46.4X2	T46.4X3	T46.4X4	T46.4X5	T46.4X6
Caramiphen	T44.3X1	T44.3X2	T44.3X3	T44.3X4	T44.3X5	T44.3X6
Carazolol	T44.7X1	T44.7X2	T44.7X3	T44.7X4	T44.7X5	T44.7X6
Carbachol	T44.1X1	T44.1X2	T44.1X3	T44.1X4	T44.1X5	T44.1X6
Carbacrylamine (resin)	T5Ø.3X1	T5Ø.3X2	T5Ø.3X3	T5Ø.3X4	T5Ø.3X5	T5Ø.3X6
Carbamate (insecticide)	T6Ø.ØX1	T6Ø.ØX2	T6Ø.ØX3	T6Ø.ØX4	—	—
Carbamate (sedative)	T42.6X1	T42.6X2	T42.6X3	T42.6X4	T42.6X5	T42.6X6
herbicide	T6Ø.ØX1	T6Ø.ØX2	T6Ø.ØX3	T6Ø.ØX4	—	—
insecticide	T6Ø.ØX1	T6Ø.ØX2	T6Ø.ØX3	T6Ø.ØX4	—	—
Carbamazepine	T42.1X1	T42.1X2	T42.1X3	T42.1X4	T42.1X5	T42.1X6
Carbamide	T47.3X1	T47.3X2	T47.3X3	T47.3X4	T47.3X5	T47.3X6
peroxide	T49.ØX1	T49.ØX2	T49.ØX3	T49.ØX4	T49.ØX5	T49.ØX6
topical	T49.8X1	T49.8X2	T49.8X3	T49.8X4	T49.8X5	T49.8X6
Carbamylcholine chloride	T44.1X1	T44.1X2	T44.1X3	T44.1X4	T44.1X5	T44.1X6
Carbaril	T6Ø.ØX1	T6Ø.ØX2	T6Ø.ØX3	T6Ø.ØX4	—	—
Carbarsone	T37.3X1	T37.3X2	T37.3X3	T37.3X4	T37.3X5	T37.3X6
Carbaryl	T6Ø.ØX1	T6Ø.ØX2	T6Ø.ØX3	T6Ø.ØX4	—	—
Carbaspirin	T39.Ø11	T39.Ø12	T39.Ø13	T39.Ø14	T39.Ø15	T39.Ø16
Carbazochrome (salicylate) (sodium sulfonate)	T49.4X1	T49.4X2	T49.4X3	T49.4X4	T49.4X5	T49.4X6
Carbenicillin	T36.ØX1	T36.ØX2	T36.ØX3	T36.ØX4	T36.ØX5	T36.ØX6
Carbenoxolone	T47.1X1	T47.1X2	T47.1X3	T47.1X4	T47.1X5	T47.1X6
Carbetapentane	T48.3X1	T48.3X2	T48.3X3	T48.3X4	T48.3X5	T48.3X6
Carbethyl salicylate	T39.Ø91	T39.Ø92	T39.Ø93	T39.Ø94	T39.Ø95	T39.Ø96
Carbidopa (with levodopa)	T42.8X1	T42.8X2	T42.8X3	T42.8X4	T42.8X5	T42.8X6
Carbimazole	T38.2X1	T38.2X2	T38.2X3	T38.2X4	T38.2X5	T38.2X6
Carbinol	T51.1X1	T51.1X2	T51.1X3	T51.1X4	—	—
Carbinoxamine	T45.ØX1	T45.ØX2	T45.ØX3	T45.ØX4	T45.ØX5	T45.ØX6
Carbiphene	T39.8X1	T39.8X2	T39.8X3	T39.8X4	T39.8X5	T39.8X6
Carbitol	T52.3X1	T52.3X2	T52.3X3	T52.3X4	—	—
Carbocaine	T41.3X1	T41.3X2	T41.3X3	T41.3X4	T41.3X5	T41.3X6
infiltration (subcutaneous)	T41.3X1	T41.3X2	T41.3X3	T41.3X4	T41.3X5	T41.3X6
nerve block (peripheral) (plexus)	T41.3X1	T41.3X2	T41.3X3	T41.3X4	T41.3X5	T41.3X6
topical (surface)	T41.3X1	T41.3X2	T41.3X3	T41.3X4	T41.3X5	T41.3X6
Carbo medicinalis	T47.6X1	T47.6X2	T47.6X3	T47.6X4	T47.6X5	T47.6X6

Substance	Poisoning, Accidental (Unintentional)	Poisoning, Intentional Self-Harm	Poisoning, Assault	Poisoning, Undetermined	Adverse Effect	Underdosing
Carbomycin	T36.8X1	T36.8X2	T36.8X3	T36.8X4	T36.8X5	T36.8X6
Carbocisteine	T48.4X1	T48.4X2	T48.4X3	T48.4X4	T48.4X5	T48.4X6
Carbocromen	T46.3X1	T46.3X2	T46.3X3	T46.3X4	T46.3X5	T46.3X6
Carbol fuchsin	T49.ØX1	T49.ØX2	T49.ØX3	T49.ØX4	T49.ØX5	T49.ØX6
Carbolic acid — *see also Phenol*	T54.ØX1	T54.ØX2	T54.ØX3	T54.ØX4	—	—
Carbolonium (bromide)	T48.1X1	T48.1X2	T48.1X3	T48.1X4	T48.1X5	T48.1X6
Carbon						
bisulfide (liquid)	T65.4X1	T65.4X2	T65.4X3	T65.4X4	—	—
vapor	T65.4X1	T65.4X2	T65.4X3	T65.4X4	—	—
dioxide (gas)	T59.7X1	T59.7X2	T59.7X3	T59.7X4	—	—
medicinal	T41.5X1	T41.5X2	T41.5X3	T41.5X4	T41.5X5	T41.5X6
nonmedicinal	T59.7X1	T59.7X2	T59.7X3	T59.7X4	—	—
snow	T49.4X1	T49.4X2	T49.4X3	T49.4X4	T49.4X5	T49.4X6
disulfide (liquid)	T65.4X1	T65.4X2	T65.4X3	T65.4X4	—	—
vapor	T65.4X1	T65.4X2	T65.4X3	T65.4X4	—	—
monoxide (from incomplete combustion)	T58.91	T58.92	T58.93	T58.94	—	—
blast furnace gas	T58.8X1	T58.8X2	T58.8X3	T58.8X4	—	—
butane (distributed in mobile container)	T58.11	T58.12	T58.13	T58.14	—	—
distributed through pipes	T58.11	T58.12	T58.13	T58.14	—	—
charcoal fumes	T58.2X1	T58.2X2	T58.2X3	T58.2X4	—	—
coal	T58.2X1	T58.2X2	T58.2X3	T58.2X4		
coke (in domestic stoves, fireplaces)	T58.2X1	T58.2X2	T58.2X3	T58.2X4	—	—
gas (piped)	T58.11	T58.12	T58.13	T58.14	—	—
solid (in domestic stoves, fireplaces)	T58.2X1	T58.2X2	T58.2X3	T58.2X4	—	—
exhaust gas (motor) not in transit	T58.Ø1	T58.Ø2	T58.Ø3	T58.Ø4	—	—
combustion engine, any not in watercraft	T58.Ø1	T58.Ø2	T58.Ø3	T58.Ø4	—	—
farm tractor, not in transit	T58.Ø1	T58.Ø2	T58.Ø3	T58.Ø4	—	—
gas engine	T58.Ø1	T58.Ø2	T58.Ø3	T58.Ø4	—	—
motor pump	T58.Ø1	T58.Ø2	T58.Ø3	T58.Ø4	—	—
motor vehicle, not in transit	T58.Ø1	T58.Ø2	T58.Ø3	T58.Ø4	—	—
fuel (in domestic use)	T58.2X1	T58.2X2	T58.2X3	T58.2X4	—	—
gas (piped)	T58.11	T58.12	T58.13	T58.14	—	—
in mobile container	T58.11	T58.12	T58.13	T58.14	—	—
utility	T58.11	T58.12	T58.13	T58.14	—	—
in mobile container	T58.11	T58.12	T58.13	T58.14	—	—
piped (natural)	T58.11	T58.12	T58.13	T58.14	—	—

Substance	Poisoning, Accidental (Unintentional)	Poisoning, Intentional Self-Harm	Poisoning, Assault	Poisoning, Undetermined	Adverse Effect	Underdosing
Carbon *(Continued)*						
monoxide *(Continued)*						
illuminating gas	T58.11	T58.12	T58.13	T58.14	—	—
industrial fuels or gases, any	T58.8X1	T58.8X2	T58.8X3	T58.8X4	—	—
kerosene (in domestic stoves, fireplaces)	T58.2X1	T58.2X2	T58.2X3	T58.2X4	—	—
kiln gas or vapor	T58.8X1	T58.8X2	T58.8X3	T58.8X4	—	—
motor exhaust gas, not in transit	T58.Ø1	T58.Ø2	T58.Ø3	T58.Ø4	—	—
piped gas (manufactured) (natural)	T58.11	T58.12	T58.13	T58.14	—	—
producer gas	T58.8X1	T58.8X2	T58.8X3	T58.8X4	—	—
propane (distributed in mobile container)	T58.11	T58.12	T58.13	T58.14	—	—
distributed through pipes	T58.11	T58.12	T58.13	T58.14	—	—
specified source NEC	T58.8X1	T58.8X2	T58.8X3	T58.8X4	—	—
stove gas	T58.11	T58.12	T58.13	T58.14	—	—
piped	T58.11	T58.12	T58.13	T58.14	—	—
utility gas	T58.11	T58.12	T58.13	T58.14	—	—
piped	T58.11	T58.12	T58.13	T58.14	—	—
water gas	T58.11	T58.12	T58.13	T58.14	—	—
wood (in domestic stoves, fireplaces)	T58.2X1	T58.2X2	T58.2X3	T58.2X4	—	—
tetrachloride (vapor) NEC	T53.ØX1	T53.ØX2	T53.ØX3	T53.ØX4	—	—
liquid (cleansing agent) NEC	T53.ØX1	T53.ØX2	T53.ØX3	T53.ØX4	—	—
solvent	T53.ØX1	T53.ØX2	T53.ØX3	T53.ØX4	—	—
Carbonic acid gas	T59.7X1	T59.7X2	T59.7X3	T59.7X4	—	—
anhydrase inhibitor NEC	T5Ø.2X1	T5Ø.2X2	T5Ø.2X3	T5Ø.2X4	T5Ø.2X5	T5Ø.2X6
Carbophenothion	T6Ø.ØX1	T6Ø.ØX2	T6Ø.ØX3	T6Ø.ØX4	—	—
Carboplatin	T45.1X1	T45.1X2	T45.1X3	T45.1X4	T45.1X5	T45.1X6
Carboprost	T48.ØX1	T48.ØX2	T48.ØX3	T48.ØX4	T48.ØX5	T48.ØX6
Carboquone	T45.1X1	T45.1X2	T45.1X3	T45.1X4	T45.1X5	T45.1X6
Carbowax	T49.3X1	T49.3X2	T49.3X3	T49.3X4	T49.3X5	T49.3X6
Carboxymethyl-cellulose	T47.4X1	T47.4X2	T47.4X3	T47.4X4	T47.4X5	T47.4X6
S-Carboxymethyl-cysteine	T48.4X1	T48.4X2	T48.4X3	T48.4X4	T48.4X5	T48.4X6
Carbrital	T42.3X1	T42.3X2	T42.3X3	T42.3X4	T42.3X5	T42.3X6
Carbromal	T42.6X1	T42.6X2	T42.6X3	T42.6X4	T42.6X5	T42.6X6
Carbutamide	T38.3X1	T38.3X2	T38.3X3	T38.3X4	T38.3X5	T38.3X6
Carbuterol	T48.6X1	T48.6X2	T48.6X3	T48.6X4	T48.6X5	T48.6X6
Cardiac						
depressants	T46.2X1	T46.2X2	T46.2X3	T46.2X4	T46.2X5	T46.2X6
rhythm regulator	T46.2X1	T46.2X2	T46.2X3	T46.2X4	T46.2X5	T46.2X6
specified NEC	T46.2X1	T46.2X2	T46.2X3	T46.2X4	T46.2X5	T46.2X6

Substance	Poisoning, Accidental (Unintentional)	Poisoning, Intentional Self-Harm	Poisoning, Assault	Poisoning, Undetermined	Adverse Effect	Underdosing
Cardiografin	T5Ø.8X1	T5Ø.8X2	T5Ø.8X3	T5Ø.8X4	T5Ø.8X5	T5Ø.8X6
Cardio-green	T5Ø.8X1	T5Ø.8X2	T5Ø.8X3	T5Ø.8X4	T5Ø.8X5	T5Ø.8X6
Cardiotonic (glycoside) NEC	T46.ØX1	T46.ØX2	T46.ØX3	T46.ØX4	T46.ØX5	T46.ØX6
Cardiovascular drug NEC	T46.9Ø1	T46.9Ø2	T46.9Ø3	T46.9Ø4	T46.9Ø5	T46.9Ø6
Cardrase	T5Ø.2X1	T5Ø.2X2	T5Ø.2X3	T5Ø.2X4	T5Ø.2X5	T5Ø.2X6
Carfusin	T49.ØX1	T49.ØX2	T49.ØX3	T49.ØX4	T49.ØX5	T49.ØX6
Carfecillin	T36.ØX1	T36.ØX2	T36.ØX3	T36.ØX4	T36.ØX5	T36.ØX6
Carfenazine	T43.3X1	T43.3X2	T43.3X3	T43.3X4	T43.3X5	T43.3X6
Carindacillin	T36.ØX1	T36.ØX2	T36.ØX3	T36.ØX4	T36.ØX5	T36.ØX6
Carisoprodol	T42.8X1	T42.8X2	T42.8X3	T42.8X4	T42.8X5	T42.8X6
Carmellose	T47.4X1	T47.4X2	T47.4X3	T47.4X4	T47.4X5	T47.4X6
Carminative	T47.5X1	T47.5X2	T47.5X3	T47.5X4	T47.5X5	T47.5X6
Carmofur	T45.1X1	T45.1X2	T45.1X3	T45.1X4	T45.1X5	T45.1X6
Carmustine	T45.1X1	T45.1X2	T45.1X3	T45.1X4	T45.1X5	T45.1X6
Carotene	T45.2X1	T45.2X2	T45.2X3	T45.2X4	T45.2X5	T45.2X6
Carphenazine	T43.3X1	T43.3X2	T43.3X3	T43.3X4	T43.3X5	T43.3X6
Carpipramine	T42.4X1	T42.4X2	T42.4X3	T42.4X4	T42.4X5	T42.4X6
Carprofen	T39.311	T39.312	T39.313	T39.314	T39.315	T39.316
Carpronium chloride	T44.3X1	T44.3X2	T44.3X3	T44.3X4	T44.3X5	T44.3X6
Carrageenan	T47.8X1	T47.8X2	T47.8X3	T47.8X4	T47.8X5	T47.8X6
Carteolol	T44.7X1	T44.7X2	T44.7X3	T44.7X4	T44.7X5	T44.7X6
Carter's Little Pills	T47.2X1	T47.2X2	T47.2X3	T47.2X4	T47.2X5	T47.2X6
Cascara (sagrada)	T47.2X1	T47.2X2	T47.2X3	T47.2X4	T47.2X5	T47.2X6
Cassava	T62.2X1	T62.2X2	T62.2X3	T62.2X4	—	—
Castellani's paint	T49.ØX1	T49.ØX2	T49.ØX3	T49.ØX4	T49.ØX5	T49.ØX6
Castor						
bean	T62.2X1	T62.2X2	T62.2X3	T62.2X4	—	—
oil	T47.2X1	T47.2X2	T47.2X3	T47.2X4	T47.2X5	T47.2X6
Catalase	T45.3X1	T45.3X2	T45.3X3	T45.3X4	T45.3X5	T45.3X6
Caterpillar (sting)	T63.431	T63.432	T63.433	T63.434	—	—
Catha (edulis) (tea)	T43.691	T43.692	T43.693	T43.694	—	—
Cathartic NEC	T47.4X1	T47.4X2	T47.4X3	T47.4X4	T47.4X5	T47.4X6
anthacene derivative	T47.2X1	T47.2X2	T47.2X3	T47.2X4	T47.2X5	T47.2X6
bulk	T47.4X1	T47.4X2	T47.4X3	T47.4X4	T47.4X5	T47.4X6
contact	T47.2X1	T47.2X2	T47.2X3	T47.2X4	T47.2X5	T47.2X6
emollient NEC	T47.4X1	T47.4X2	T47.4X3	T47.4X4	T47.4X5	T47.4X6
irritant NEC	T47.2X1	T47.2X2	T47.2X3	T47.2X4	T47.2X5	T47.2X6
mucilage	T47.4X1	T47.4X2	T47.4X3	T47.4X4	T47.4X5	T47.4X6
saline	T47.3X1	T47.3X2	T47.3X3	T47.3X4	T47.3X5	T47.3X6
vegetable	T47.2X1	T47.2X2	T47.2X3	T47.2X4	T47.2X5	T47.2X6
Cathine	T5Ø.5X1	T5Ø.5X2	T5Ø.5X3	T5Ø.5X4	T5Ø.5X5	T5Ø.5X6
Cathomycin	T36.8X1	T36.8X2	T36.8X3	T36.8X4	T36.8X5	T36.8X6

Substance	Poisoning, Accidental (Unintentional)	Poisoning, Intentional Self-Harm	Poisoning, Assault	Poisoning, Undetermined	Adverse Effect	Underdosing
Cation exchange resin	T50.3X1	T50.3X2	T50.3X3	T50.3X4	T50.3X5	T50.3X6
Caustic(s) NEC	T54.91	T54.92	T54.93	T54.94	—	—
alkali	T54.3X1	T54.3X2	T54.3X3	T54.3X4	—	—
hydroxide	T54.3X1	T54.3X2	T54.3X3	T54.3X4	—	—
potash	T54.3X1	T54.3X2	T54.3X3	T54.3X4	—	—
soda	T54.3X1	T54.3X2	T54.3X3	T54.3X4	—	—
specified NEC	T54.91	T54.92	T54.93	T54.94	—	—
Ceepryn	T49.0X1	T49.0X2	T49.0X3	T49.0X4	T49.0X5	T49.0X6
ENT agent	T49.6X1	T49.6X2	T49.6X3	T49.6X4	T49.6X5	T49.6X6
lozenges	T49.6X1	T49.6X2	T49.6X3	T49.6X4	T49.6X5	T49.6X6
Cefacetrile	T36.1X1	T36.1X2	T36.1X3	T36.1X4	T36.1X5	T36.1X6
Cefaclor	T36.1X1	T36.1X2	T36.1X3	T36.1X4	T36.1X5	T36.1X6
Cefadroxil	T36.1X1	T36.1X2	T36.1X3	T36.1X4	T36.1X5	T36.1X6
Cefalexin	T36.1X1	T36.1X2	T36.1X3	T36.1X4	T36.1X5	T36.1X6
Cefaloglycin	T36.1X1	T36.1X2	T36.1X3	T36.1X4	T36.1X5	T36.1X6
Cefaloridine	T36.1X1	T36.1X2	T36.1X3	T36.1X4	T36.1X5	T36.1X6
Cefalosporins	T36.1X1	T36.1X2	T36.1X3	T36.1X4	T36.1X5	T36.1X6
Cefalotin	T36.1X1	T36.1X2	T36.1X3	T36.1X4	T36.1X5	T36.1X6
Cefamandole	T36.1X1	T36.1X2	T36.1X3	T36.1X4	T36.1X5	T36.1X6
Cefamycin antibiotic	T36.1X1	T36.1X2	T36.1X3	T36.1X4	T36.1X5	T36.1X6
Cefapirin	T36.1X1	T36.1X2	T36.1X3	T36.1X4	T36.1X5	T36.1X6
Cefatrizine	T36.1X1	T36.1X2	T36.1X3	T36.1X4	T36.1X5	T36.1X6
Cefazedone	T36.1X1	T36.1X2	T36.1X3	T36.1X4	T36.1X5	T36.1X6
Cefazolin	T36.1X1	T36.1X2	T36.1X3	T36.1X4	T36.1X5	T36.1X6
Cefbuperazone	T36.1X1	T36.1X2	T36.1X3	T36.1X4	T36.1X5	T36.1X6
Cefetamet	T36.1X1	T36.1X2	T36.1X3	T36.1X4	T36.1X5	T36.1X6
Cefixime	T36.1X1	T36.1X2	T36.1X3	T36.1X4	T36.1X5	T36.1X6
Cefmenoxime	T36.1X1	T36.1X2	T36.1X3	T36.1X4	T36.1X5	T36.1X6
Cefmetazole	T36.1X1	T36.1X2	T36.1X3	T36.1X4	T36.1X5	T36.1X6
Cefminox	T36.1X1	T36.1X2	T36.1X3	T36.1X4	T36.1X5	T36.1X6
Cefonicid	T36.1X1	T36.1X2	T36.1X3	T36.1X4	T36.1X5	T36.1X6
Cefoperazone	T36.1X1	T36.1X2	T36.1X3	T36.1X4	T36.1X5	T36.1X6
Ceforanide	T36.1X1	T36.1X2	T36.1X3	T36.1X4	T36.1X5	T36.1X6
Cefotaxime	T36.1X1	T36.1X2	T36.1X3	T36.1X4	T36.1X5	T36.1X6
Cefotetan	T36.1X1	T36.1X2	T36.1X3	T36.1X4	T36.1X5	T36.1X6
Cefotiam	T36.1X1	T36.1X2	T36.1X3	T36.1X4	T36.1X5	T36.1X6
Cefoxitin	T36.1X1	T36.1X2	T36.1X3	T36.1X4	T36.1X5	T36.1X6
Cefpimizole	T36.1X1	T36.1X2	T36.1X3	T36.1X4	T36.1X5	T36.1X6
Cefpiramide	T36.1X1	T36.1X2	T36.1X3	T36.1X4	T36.1X5	T36.1X6
Cefradine	T36.1X1	T36.1X2	T36.1X3	T36.1X4	T36.1X5	T36.1X6
Cefroxadine	T36.1X1	T36.1X2	T36.1X3	T36.1X4	T36.1X5	T36.1X6
Cefsulodin	T36.1X1	T36.1X2	T36.1X3	T36.1X4	T36.1X5	T36.1X6
Ceftazidime	T36.1X1	T36.1X2	T36.1X3	T36.1X4	T36.1X5	T36.1X6
Cefteram	T36.1X1	T36.1X2	T36.1X3	T36.1X4	T36.1X5	T36.1X6
Ceftezole	T36.1X1	T36.1X2	T36.1X3	T36.1X4	T36.1X5	T36.1X6
Ceftizoxime	T36.1X1	T36.1X2	T36.1X3	T36.1X4	T36.1X5	T36.1X6
Ceftriaxone	T36.1X1	T36.1X2	T36.1X3	T36.1X4	T36.1X5	T36.1X6
Cefuroxime	T36.1X1	T36.1X2	T36.1X3	T36.1X4	T36.1X5	T36.1X6
Cefuzonam	T36.1X1	T36.1X2	T36.1X3	T36.1X4	T36.1X5	T36.1X6
Celestone	T38.0X1	T38.0X2	T38.0X3	T38.0X4	T38.0X5	T38.0X6
topical	T49.0X1	T49.0X2	T49.0X3	T49.0X4	T49.0X5	T49.0X6
Celiprolol	T44.7X1	T44.7X2	T44.7X3	T44.7X4	T44.7X5	T44.7X6
Cellosolve	T52.91	T52.92	T52.93	T52.94	—	—
Cell stimulants and proliferants	T49.8X1	T49.8X2	T49.8X3	T49.8X4	T49.8X5	T49.8X6
Cellulose						
cathartic	T47.4X1	T47.4X2	T47.4X3	T47.4X4	T47.4X5	T47.4X6
hydroxyethyl	T47.4X1	T47.4X2	T47.4X3	T47.4X4	T47.4X5	T47.4X6
nitrates (topical)	T49.3X1	T49.3X2	T49.3X3	T49.3X4	T49.3X5	T49.3X6
oxidized	T49.4X1	T49.4X2	T49.4X3	T49.4X4	T49.4X5	T49.4X6
Centipede (bite)	T63.411	T63.412	T63.413	T63.414	—	—
Central nervous system						
depressants	T42.71	T42.72	T42.73	T42.74	T42.75	T42.76
anesthetic (general) NEC	T41.201	T41.202	T41.203	T41.204	T41.205	T41.206
gases NEC	T41.0X1	T41.0X2	T41.0X3	T41.0X4	T41.0X5	T41.0X6
intravenous	T41.1X1	T41.1X2	T41.1X3	T41.1X4	T41.1X5	T41.1X6
barbiturates	T42.3X1	T42.3X2	T42.3X3	T42.3X4	T42.3X5	T42.3X6
benzodiazepines	T42.4X1	T42.4X2	T42.4X3	T42.4X4	T42.4X5	T42.4X6
bromides	T42.6X1	T42.6X2	T42.6X3	T42.6X4	T42.6X5	T42.6X6
cannabis sativa	T40.7X1	T40.7X2	T40.7X3	T40.7X4	T40.7X5	T40.7X6
chloral hydrate	T42.6X1	T42.6X2	T42.6X3	T42.6X4	T42.6X5	T42.6X6
ethanol	T51.0X1	T51.0X2	T51.0X3	T51.0X4	—	—
hallucinogenics	T40.901	T40.902	T40.903	T40.904	T40.905	T40.906
hypnotics	T42.71	T42.72	T42.73	T42.74	T42.75	T42.76
specified NEC	T42.6X1	T42.6X2	T42.6X3	T42.6X4	T42.6X5	T42.6X6
muscle relaxants	T42.8X1	T42.8X2	T42.8X3	T42.8X4	T42.8X5	T42.8X6
paraldehyde	T42.6X1	T42.6X2	T42.6X3	T42.6X4	T42.6X5	T42.6X6
sedatives; sedative-hypnotics	T42.71	T42.72	T42.73	T42.74	T42.75	T42.76
mixed NEC	T42.6X1	T42.6X2	T42.6X3	T42.6X4	T42.6X5	T42.6X6
specified NEC	T42.6X1	T42.6X2	T42.6X3	T42.6X4	T42.6X5	T42.6X6
muscle-tone depressants	T42.8X1	T42.8X2	T42.8X3	T42.8X4	T42.8X5	T42.8X6
stimulants	T43.601	T43.602	T43.603	T43.604	T43.605	T43.606
amphetamines	T43.621	T43.622	T43.623	T43.624	T43.625	T43.626
analeptics	T50.7X1	T50.7X2	T50.7X3	T50.7X4	T50.7X5	T50.7X6

Substance	Poisoning, Accidental (Unintentional)	Poisoning, Intentional Self-Harm	Poisoning, Assault	Poisoning, Undetermined	Adverse Effect	Underdosing
Central nervous system *(Continued)*						
stimulants *(Continued)*						
antidepressants	T43.201	T43.202	T43.203	T43.204	T43.205	T43.206
opiate antagonists	T50.7X1	T50.7X2	T50.7X3	T50.7X4	T50.7X5	T50.7X6
specified NEC	T43.691	T43.692	T43.693	T43.694	T43.695	T43.696
Cephalexin	T36.1X1	T36.1X2	T36.1X3	T36.1X4	T36.1X5	T36.1X6
Cephaloglycin	T36.1X1	T36.1X2	T36.1X3	T36.1X4	T36.1X5	T36.1X6
Cephaloridine	T36.1X1	T36.1X2	T36.1X3	T36.1X4	T36.1X5	T36.1X6
Cephalosporins	T36.1X1	T36.1X2	T36.1X3	T36.1X4	T36.1X5	T36.1X6
N (adicillin)	T36.0X1	T36.0X2	T36.0X3	T36.0X4	T36.0X5	T36.0X6
Cephalothin	T36.1X1	T36.1X2	T36.1X3	T36.1X4	T36.1X5	T36.1X6
Cephalotin	T36.1X1	T36.1X2	T36.1X3	T36.1X4	T36.1X5	T36.1X6
Cephradine	T36.1X1	T36.1X2	T36.1X3	T36.1X4	T36.1X5	T36.1X6
Cerbera (odallam)	T62.2X1	T62.2X2	T62.2X3	T62.2X4	—	—
Cerberin	T46.0X1	T46.0X2	T46.0X3	T46.0X4	T46.0X5	T46.0X6
Cerebral stimulants	T43.601	T43.602	T43.603	T43.604	T43.605	T43.606
psychotherapeutic	T43.601	T43.602	T43.603	T43.604	T43.605	T43.606
specified NEC	T43.691	T43.692	T43.693	T43.694	T43.695	T43.696
Cerium oxalate	T45.0X1	T45.0X2	T45.0X3	T45.0X4	T45.0X5	T45.0X6
Cerous oxalate	T45.0X1	T45.0X2	T45.0X3	T45.0X4	T45.0X5	T45.0X6
Ceruletide	T50.8X1	T50.8X2	T50.8X3	T50.8X4	T50.8X5	T50.8X6
Cetalkonium (chloride)	T49.0X1	T49.0X2	T49.0X3	T49.0X4	T49.0X5	T49.0X6
Cethexonium chloride	T49.0X1	T49.0X2	T49.0X3	T49.0X4	T49.0X5	T49.0X6
Cetiedil	T46.7X1	T46.7X2	T46.7X3	T46.7X4	T46.7X5	T46.7X6
Cetirizine	T45.0X1	T45.0X2	T45.0X3	T45.0X4	T45.0X5	T45.0X6
Cetomacrogol	T50.991	T50.992	T50.993	T50.994	T50.995	T50.996
Cetotiamine	T45.2X1	T45.2X2	T45.2X3	T45.2X4	T45.2X5	T45.2X6
Cetoxime	T45.0X1	T45.0X2	T45.0X3	T45.0X4	T45.0X5	T45.0X6
Cetraxate	T47.1X1	T47.1X2	T47.1X3	T47.1X4	T47.1X5	T47.1X6
Cetrimide	T49.0X1	T49.0X2	T49.0X3	T49.0X4	T49.0X5	T49.0X6
Cetrimonium (bromide)	T49.0X1	T49.0X2	T49.0X3	T49.0X4	T49.0X5	T49.0X6
Cetylpyridinium chloride	T49.0X1	T49.0X2	T49.0X3	T49.0X4	T49.0X5	T49.0X6
ENT agent	T49.6X1	T49.6X2	T49.6X3	T49.6X4	T49.6X5	T49.6X6
lozenges	T49.6X1	T49.6X2	T49.6X3	T49.6X4	T49.6X5	T49.6X6
Cevadillasee Sabadilla						
Cevitamic acid	T45.2X1	T45.2X2	T45.2X3	T45.2X4	T45.2X5	T45.2X6
Chalk, precipitated	T47.1X1	T47.1X2	T47.1X3	T47.1X4	T47.1X5	T47.1X6
Chamomile	T49.0X1	T49.0X2	T49.0X3	T49.0X4	T49.0X5	T49.0X6
Ch'an su	T46.0X1	T46.0X2	T46.0X3	T46.0X4	T46.0X5	T46.0X6
Charcoal	T47.6X1	T47.6X2	T47.6X3	T47.6X4	T47.6X5	T47.6X6
activated—*see also Charcoal, medicinal*	T47.6X1	T47.6X2	T47.6X3	T47.6X4	T47.6X5	T47.6X6
Charcoal *(Continued)*						
fumes (Carbon monoxide)	T58.2X1	T58.2X2	T58.2X3	T58.2X4	—	—
industrial	T58.8X1	T58.8X2	T58.8X3	T58.8X4	—	—
medicinal (activated)	T47.6X1	T47.6X2	T47.6X3	T47.6X4	T47.6X5	T47.6X6
antidiarrheal	T47.6X1	T47.6X2	T47.6X3	T47.6X4	T47.6X5	T47.6X6
poison control	T47.8X1	T47.8X2	T47.8X3	T47.8X4	T47.8X5	T47.8X6
specified use other than for diarrhea	T47.8X1	T47.8X2	T47.8X3	T47.8X4	T47.8X5	T47.8X6
topical	T49.8X1	T49.8X2	T49.8X3	T49.8X4	T49.8X5	T49.8X6
Chaulmosulfone	T37.1X1	T37.1X2	T37.1X3	T37.1X4	T37.1X5	T37.1X6
Chelating agent NEC	T50.6X1	T50.6X2	T50.6X3	T50.6X4	T50.6X5	T50.6X6
Chelidonium majus	T62.2X1	T62.2X2	T62.2X3	T62.2X4	—	—
Chemical substance NEC	T65.91	T65.92	T65.93	T65.94	—	—
Chenodeoxycholic acid	T47.5X1	T47.5X2	T47.5X3	T47.5X4	T47.5X5	T47.5X6
Chenodiol	T47.5X1	T47.5X2	T47.5X3	T47.5X4	T47.5X5	T47.5X6
Chenopodium	T37.4X1	T37.4X2	T37.4X3	T37.4X4	T37.4X5	T37.4X6
Cherry laurel	T62.2X1	T62.2X2	T62.2X3	T62.2X4	—	—
Chinidin(e)	T46.2X1	T46.2X2	T46.2X3	T46.2X4	T46.2X5	T46.2X6
Chiniofon	T37.8X1	T37.8X2	T37.8X3	T37.8X4	T37.8X5	T37.8X6
Chlophedianol	T48.3X1	T48.3X2	T48.3X3	T48.3X4	T48.3X5	T48.3X6
Chloral	T42.6X1	T42.6X2	T42.6X3	T42.6X4	T42.6X5	T42.6X6
derivative	T42.6X1	T42.6X2	T42.6X3	T42.6X4	T42.6X5	T42.6X6
hydrate	T42.6X1	T42.6X2	T42.6X3	T42.6X4	T42.6X5	T42.6X6
Chloralamide	T42.6X1	T42.6X2	T42.6X3	T42.6X4	T42.6X5	T42.6X6
Chloralodol	T42.6X1	T42.6X2	T42.6X3	T42.6X4	T42.6X5	T42.6X6
Chloralose	T60.4X1	T60.4X2	T60.4X3	T60.4X4	—	—
Chlorambucil	T45.1X1	T45.1X2	T45.1X3	T45.1X4	T45.1X5	T45.1X6
Chloramine	T57.8X1	T57.8X2	T57.8X3	T57.8X4	—	—
T	T49.0X1	T49.0X2	T49.0X3	T49.0X4	T49.0X5	T49.0X6
topical	T49.0X1	T49.0X2	T49.0X3	T49.0X4	T49.0X5	T49.0X6
Chloramphenicol	T36.2X1	T36.2X2	T36.2X3	T36.2X4	T36.2X5	T36.2X6
ENT agent	T49.6X1	T49.6X2	T49.6X3	T49.6X4	T49.6X5	T49.6X6
ophthalmic preparation	T49.5X1	T49.5X2	T49.5X3	T49.5X4	T49.5X5	T49.5X6
topical NEC	T49.0X1	T49.0X2	T49.0X3	T49.0X4	T49.0X5	T49.0X6
Chlorate (potassium) (sodium) NEC	T60.3X1	T60.3X2	T60.3X3	T60.3X4	—	—
herbicide	T60.3X1	T60.3X2	T60.3X3	T60.3X4	—	—
Chlorazanil	T50.2X1	T50.2X2	T50.2X3	T50.2X4	T50.2X5	T50.2X6
Chlorbenzene, chlorbenzol	T53.7X1	T53.7X2	T53.7X3	T53.7X4	—	—
Chlorbenzoxamine	T44.3X1	T44.3X2	T44.3X3	T44.3X4	T44.3X5	T44.3X6
Chlorbutol	T42.6X1	T42.6X2	T42.6X3	T42.6X4	T42.6X5	T42.6X6
Chlorcyclizine	T45.0X1	T45.0X2	T45.0X3	T45.0X4	T45.0X5	T45.0X6

Substance	Poisoning, Accidental (Unintentional)	Poisoning, Intentional Self-Harm	Poisoning, Assault	Poisoning, Undetermined	Adverse Effect	Underdosing
Chlordan(e) (dust)	T60.1X1	T60.1X2	T60.1X3	T60.1X4	—	—
Chlordantoin	T49.0X1	T49.0X2	T49.0X3	T49.0X4	T49.0X5	T49.0X6
Chlordiazepoxide	T42.4X1	T42.4X2	T42.4X3	T42.4X4	T42.4X5	T42.4X6
Chlordiethyl benzamide	T49.3X1	T49.3X2	T49.3X3	T49.3X4	T49.3X5	T49.3X6
Chloresium	T49.8X1	T49.8X2	T49.8X3	T49.8X4	T49.8X5	T49.8X6
Chlorethiazol	T42.6X1	T42.6X2	T42.6X3	T42.6X4	T42.6X5	T42.6X6
Chlorethyl — *see Ethyl chloride*						
Chloretone	T42.6X1	T42.6X2	T42.6X3	T42.6X4	T42.6X5	T42.6X6
Chlorex	T53.6X1	T53.6X2	T53.6X3	T53.6X4	—	—
insecticide	T60.1X1	T60.1X2	T60.1X3	T60.1X4	—	—
Chlorfenvinphos	T60.0X1	T60.0X2	T60.0X3	T60.0X4	—	—
Chlorhexadol	T42.6X1	T42.6X2	T42.6X3	T42.6X4	T42.6X5	T42.6X6
Chlorhexamide	T45.1X1	T45.1X2	T45.1X3	T45.1X4	T45.1X5	T45.1X6
Chlorhexidine	T49.0X1	T49.0X2	T49.0X3	T49.0X4	T49.0X5	T49.0X6
Chlorhydroxyquinolin	T49.0X1	T49.0X2	T49.0X3	T49.0X4	T49.0X5	T49.0X6
Chloride of lime (bleach)	T54.3X1	T54.3X2	T54.3X3	T54.3X4	—	—
Chlorimipramine	T43.011	T43.012	T43.013	T43.014	T43.015	T43.016
Chlorinated						
camphene	T53.6X1	T53.6X2	T53.6X3	T53.6X4	—	—
diphenyl	T53.7X1	T53.7X2	T53.7X3	T53.7X4	—	—
hydrocarbons NEC	T53.91	T53.92	T53.93	T53.94	—	—
solvents	T53.91	T53.92	T53.93	T53.94	—	—
lime (bleach)	T54.3X1	T54.3X2	T54.3X3	T54.3X4	—	—
and boric acid solution	T49.0X1	T49.0X2	T49.0X3	T49.0X4	T49.0X5	T49.0X6
naphthalene (insecticide)	T60.1X1	T60.1X2	T60.1X3	T60.1X4	—	—
industrial (non-pesticide)	T53.7X1	T53.7X2	T53.7X3	T53.7X4	—	—
pesticide NEC	T60.8X1	T60.8X2	T60.8X3	T60.8X4	—	—
soda — *see also sodium hypochlorite*						
solution	T49.0X1	T49.0X2	T49.0X3	T49.0X4	T49.0X5	T49.0X6
Chlorine (fumes) (gas)	T59.4X1	T59.4X2	T59.4X3	T59.4X4	—	—
bleach	T54.3X1	T54.3X2	T54.3X3	T54.3X4	—	—
compound gas NEC	T59.4X1	T59.4X2	T59.4X3	T59.4X4	—	—
disinfectant	T59.4X1	T59.4X2	T59.4X3	T59.4X4	—	—
releasing agents NEC	T59.4X1	T59.4X2	T59.4X3	T59.4X4	—	—
Chlorisondamine chloride	T46.991	T46.992	T46.993	T46.994	T46.995	T46.996
Chlormadinone	T38.5X1	T38.5X2	T38.5X3	T38.5X4	T38.5X5	T38.5X6
Chlormephos	T60.0X1	T60.0X2	T60.0X3	T60.0X4	—	—
Chlormerodrin	T50.2X1	T50.2X2	T50.2X3	T50.2X4	T50.2X5	T50.2X6
Chlormethiazole	T42.6X1	T42.6X2	T42.6X3	T42.6X4	T42.6X5	T42.6X6
Chlormethine	T45.1X1	T45.1X2	T45.1X3	T45.1X4	T45.1X5	T45.1X6
Chlormethylenecycline	T36.4X1	T36.4X2	T36.4X3	T36.4X4	T36.4X5	T36.4X6
Chlormezanone	T42.6X1	T42.6X2	T42.6X3	T42.6X4	T42.6X5	T42.6X6
Chloroacetic acid	T60.3X1	T60.3X2	T60.3X3	T60.3X4	—	—
Chloroacetone	T59.3X1	T59.3X2	T59.3X3	T59.3X4	—	—
Chloroacetophenone	T59.3X1	T59.3X2	T59.3X3	T59.3X4	—	—
Chloroaniline	T53.7X1	T53.7X2	T53.7X3	T53.7X4	—	—
Chlorobenzene, chlorobenzol	T53.7X1	T53.7X2	T53.7X3	T53.7X4	—	—
Chlorobromomethane (fire extinguisher)	T53.6X1	T53.6X2	T53.6X3	T53.6X4	—	—
Chlorobutanol	T49.0X1	T49.0X2	T49.0X3	T49.0X4	T49.0X5	T49.0X6
Chlorocresol	T49.0X1	T49.0X2	T49.0X3	T49.0X4	T49.0X5	T49.0X6
Chlorodehydro-methyltestosterone	T38.7X1	T38.7X2	T38.7X3	T38.7X4	T38.7X5	T38.7X6
Chlorodinitrobenzene	T53.7X1	T53.7X2	T53.7X3	T53.7X4	—	—
dust or vapor	T53.7X1	T53.7X2	T53.7X3	T53.7X4	—	—
Chlorodiphenyl	T53.7X1	T53.7X2	T53.7X3	T53.7X4	—	—
Chloroethane — *see Ethyl chloride*						
Chloroethylene	T53.6X1	T53.6X2	T53.6X3	T53.6X4	—	—
Chlorofluorocarbons	T53.5X1	T53.5X2	T53.5X3	T53.5X4	—	—
Chloroform (fumes) (vapor)	T53.1X1	T53.1X2	T53.1X3	T53.1X4	—	—
anesthetic	T41.0X1	T41.0X2	T41.0X3	T41.0X4	T41.0X5	T41.0X6
solvent	T53.1X1	T53.1X2	T53.1X3	T53.1X4	—	—
water, concentrated	T41.0X1	T41.0X2	T41.0X3	T41.0X4	T41.0X5	T41.0X6
Chloroguanide	T37.2X1	T37.2X2	T37.2X3	T37.2X4	T37.2X5	T37.2X6
Chloromycetin	T36.2X1	T36.2X2	T36.2X3	T36.2X4	T36.2X5	T36.2X6
ENT agent	T49.6X1	T49.6X2	T49.6X3	T49.6X4	T49.6X5	T49.6X6
ophthalmic preparation	T49.5X1	T49.5X2	T49.5X3	T49.5X4	T49.5X5	T49.5X6
otic solution	T49.6X1	T49.6X2	T49.6X3	T49.6X4	T49.6X5	T49.6X6
topical NEC	T49.0X1	T49.0X2	T49.0X3	T49.0X4	T49.0X5	T49.0X6
Chloronitrobenzene	T53.7X1	T53.7X2	T53.7X3	T53.7X4	—	—
dust or vapor	T53.7X1	T53.7X2	T53.7X3	T53.7X4	—	—
Chlorophacinone	T60.4X1	T60.4X2	T60.4X3	T60.4X4	—	—
Chlorophenol	T53.7X1	T53.7X2	T53.7X3	T53.7X4	—	—
Chlorophenothane	T60.1X1	T60.1X2	T60.1X3	T60.1X4	—	—
Chlorophyll	T50.991	T50.992	T50.993	T50.994	T50.995	T50.996
Chloropicrin (fumes)	T53.6X1	T53.6X2	T53.6X3	T53.6X4	—	—
fumigant	T60.8X1	T60.8X2	T60.8X3	T60.8X4	—	—
fungicide	T60.3X1	T60.3X2	T60.3X3	T60.3X4	—	—
pesticide	T60.8X1	T60.8X2	T60.8X3	T60.8X4	—	—
Chloroprocaine	T41.3X1	T41.3X2	T41.3X3	T41.3X4	T41.3X5	T41.3X6
infiltration (subcutaneous)	T41.3X1	T41.3X2	T41.3X3	T41.3X4	T41.3X5	T41.3X6
nerve block (peripheral) (plexus)	T41.3X1	T41.3X2	T41.3X3	T41.3X4	T41.3X5	T41.3X6
spinal	T41.3X1	T41.3X2	T41.3X3	T41.3X4	T41.3X5	T41.3X6

Substance	Poisoning, Accidental (Unintentional)	Poisoning, Intentional Self-Harm	Poisoning, Assault	Poisoning, Undetermined	Adverse Effect	Underdosing
Chloroptic	T49.5X1	T49.5X2	T49.5X3	T49.5X4	T49.5X5	T49.5X6
Chloropurine	T45.1X1	T45.1X2	T45.1X3	T45.1X4	T45.1X5	T45.1X6
Chloropyramine	T45.0X1	T45.0X2	T45.0X3	T45.0X4	T45.0X5	T45.0X6
Chloropyrifos	T60.0X1	T60.0X2	T60.0X3	T60.0X4	—	—
Chloropyrilene	T45.0X1	T45.0X2	T45.0X3	T45.0X4	T45.0X5	T45.0X6
Chloroquine	T37.2X1	T37.2X2	T37.2X3	T37.2X4	T37.2X5	T37.2X6
Chlorothalonil	T60.3X1	T60.3X2	T60.3X3	T60.3X4	—	—
Chlorothen	T45.0X1	T45.0X2	T45.0X3	T45.0X4	T45.0X5	T45.0X6
Chlorothiazide	T50.2X1	T50.2X2	T50.2X3	T50.2X4	T50.2X5	T50.2X6
Chlorothymol	T49.4X1	T49.4X2	T49.4X3	T49.4X4	T49.4X5	T49.4X6
Chlorotrianisene	T38.5X1	T38.5X2	T38.5X3	T38.5X4	T38.5X5	T38.5X6
Chlorovinyldichloro-arsine, not in war	T57.0X1	T57.0X2	T57.0X3	T57.0X4	—	—
Chloroxine	T49.4X1	T49.4X2	T49.4X3	T49.4X4	T49.4X5	T49.4X6
Chloroxylenol	T49.0X1	T49.0X2	T49.0X3	T49.0X4	T49.0X5	T49.0X6
Chlorphenamine	T45.0X1	T45.0X2	T45.0X3	T45.0X4	T45.0X5	T45.0X6
Chlorphenesin	T42.8X1	T42.8X2	T42.8X3	T42.8X4	T42.8X5	T42.8X6
topical (antifungal)	T49.0X1	T49.0X2	T49.0X3	T49.0X4	T49.0X5	T49.0X6
Chlorpheniramine	T45.0X1	T45.0X2	T45.0X3	T45.0X4	T45.0X5	T45.0X6
Chlorphenoxamine	T45.0X1	T45.0X2	T45.0X3	T45.0X4	T45.0X5	T45.0X6
Chlorphentermine	T50.5X1	T50.5X2	T50.5X3	T50.5X4	T50.5X5	T50.5X6
Chlorprocaine — *see Chloroprocaine*						
Chlorproguanil	T37.2X1	T37.2X2	T37.2X3	T37.2X4	T37.2X5	T37.2X6
Chlorpromazine	T43.3X1	T43.3X2	T43.3X3	T43.3X4	T43.3X5	T43.3X6
Chlorpropamide	T38.3X1	T38.3X2	T38.3X3	T38.3X4	T38.3X5	T38.3X6
Chlorprothixene	T43.4X1	T43.4X2	T43.4X3	T43.4X4	T43.4X5	T43.4X6
Chlorquinaldol	T49.0X1	T49.0X2	T49.0X3	T49.0X4	T49.0X5	T49.0X6
Chlorquinol	T49.0X1	T49.0X2	T49.0X3	T49.0X4	T49.0X5	T49.0X6
Chlortalidone	T50.2X1	T50.2X2	T50.2X3	T50.2X4	T50.2X5	T50.2X6
Chlortetracycline	T36.4X1	T36.4X2	T36.4X3	T36.4X4	T36.4X5	T36.4X6
Chlorthalidone	T50.2X1	T50.2X2	T50.2X3	T50.2X4	T50.2X5	T50.2X6
Chlorthiophos	T60.0X1	T60.0X2	T60.0X3	T60.0X4	—	—
Chlorotrianisene	T38.5X1	T38.5X2	T38.5X3	T38.5X4	T38.5X5	T38.5X6
Chlor-Trimeton	T45.0X1	T45.0X2	T45.0X3	T45.0X4	T45.0X5	T45.0X6
Chlorthion	T60.0X1	T60.0X2	T60.0X3	T60.0X4	—	—
Chlorzoxazone	T42.8X1	T42.8X2	T42.8X3	T42.8X4	T42.8X5	T42.8X6
Choke damp	T59.7X1	T59.7X2	T59.7X3	T59.7X4	—	—
Cholagogues	T47.5X1	T47.5X2	T47.5X3	T47.5X4	T47.5X5	T47.5X6
Cholebrine	T50.8X1	T50.8X2	T50.8X3	T50.8X4	T50.8X5	T50.8X6
Cholecalciferol	T45.2X1	T45.2X2	T45.2X3	T45.2X4	T45.2X5	T45.2X6
Cholecystokinin	T50.8X1	T50.8X2	T50.8X3	T50.8X4	T50.8X5	T50.8X6
Cholera vaccine	T50.A91	T50.A92	T50.A93	T50.A94	T50.A95	T50.A96

Substance	Poisoning, Accidental (Unintentional)	Poisoning, Intentional Self-Harm	Poisoning, Assault	Poisoning, Undetermined	Adverse Effect	Underdosing
Choleretic	T47.5X1	T47.5X2	T47.5X3	T47.5X4	T47.5X5	T47.5X6
Cholesterol-lowering agents	T46.6X1	T46.6X2	T46.6X3	T46.6X4	T46.6X5	T46.6X6
Cholestyramine (resin)	T46.6X1	T46.6X2	T46.6X3	T46.6X4	T46.6X5	T46.6X6
Cholic acid	T47.5X1	T47.5X2	T47.5X3	T47.5X4	T47.5X5	T47.5X6
Choline	T48.6X1	T48.6X2	T48.6X3	T48.6X4	T48.6X5	T48.6X6
chloride	T50.991	T50.992	T50.993	T50.994	T50.995	T50.996
dihydrogen citrate	T50.991	T50.992	T50.993	T50.994	T50.995	T50.996
salicylate	T39.091	T39.092	T39.093	T39.094	T39.095	T39.096
theophyllinate	T48.6X1	T48.6X2	T48.6X3	T48.6X4	T48.6X5	T48.6X6
Cholinergic (drug) NEC	T44.1X1	T44.1X2	T44.1X3	T44.1X4	T44.1X5	T44.1X6
muscle tone enhancer	T44.1X1	T44.1X2	T44.1X3	T44.1X4	T44.1X5	T44.1X6
organophosphorus	T44.0X1	T44.0X2	T44.0X3	T44.0X4	T44.0X5	T44.0X6
insecticide	T60.0X1	T60.0X2	T60.0X3	T60.0X4	—	—
nerve gas	T59.891	T59.892	T59.893	T59.894	—	—
trimethyl ammonium propanediol	T44.1X1	T44.1X2	T44.1X3	T44.1X4	T44.1X5	T44.1X6
Cholinesterase reactivator	T50.6X1	T50.6X2	T50.6X3	T50.6X4	T50.6X5	T50.6X6
Cholografin	T50.8X1	T50.8X2	T50.8X3	T50.8X4	T50.8X5	T50.8X6
Chorionic gonadotropin	T38.891	T38.892	T38.893	T38.894	T38.895	T38.896
Chromate	T56.2X1	T56.2X2	T56.2X3	T56.2X4	—	—
dust or mist	T56.2X1	T56.2X2	T56.2X3	T56.2X4	—	—
lead — *see also lead*	T56.0X1	T56.0X2	T56.0X3	T56.0X4	—	—
paint	T56.0X1	T56.0X2	T56.0X3	T56.0X4	—	—
Chromic						
acid	T56.2X1	T56.2X2	T56.2X3	T56.2X4	—	—
dust or mist	T56.2X1	T56.2X2	T56.2X3	T56.2X4	—	—
phosphate 32P	T45.1X1	T45.1X2	T45.1X3	T45.1X4	T45.1X5	T45.1X6
Chromium	T56.2X1	T56.2X2	T56.2X3	T56.2X4	—	—
compounds — *see Chromate*						
sesquioxide	T50.8X1	T50.8X2	T50.8X3	T50.8X4	T50.8X5	T50.8X6
Chromomycin A3	T45.1X1	T45.1X2	T45.1X3	T45.1X4	T45.1X5	T45.1X6
Chromonar	T46.3X1	T46.3X2	T46.3X3	T46.3X4	T46.3X5	T46.3X6
Chromyl chloride	T56.2X1	T56.2X2	T56.2X3	T56.2X4	—	—
Chrysarobin	T49.4X1	T49.4X2	T49.4X3	T49.4X4	T49.4X5	T49.4X6
Chrysazin	T47.2X1	T47.2X2	T47.2X3	T47.2X4	T47.2X5	T47.2X6
Chymar	T45.3X1	T45.3X2	T45.3X3	T45.3X4	T45.3X5	T45.3X6
ophthalmic preparation	T49.5X1	T49.5X2	T49.5X3	T49.5X4	T49.5X5	T49.5X6
Chymopapain	T45.3X1	T45.3X2	T45.3X3	T45.3X4	T45.3X5	T45.3X6
Chymotrypsin	T45.3X1	T45.3X2	T45.3X3	T45.3X4	T45.3X5	T45.3X6
ophthalmic preparation	T49.5X1	T49.5X2	T49.5X3	T49.5X4	T49.5X5	T49.5X6
Cianidanol	T50.991	T50.992	T50.993	T50.994	T50.995	T50.996
Cianopramine	T43.011	T43.012	T43.013	T43.014	T43.015	T43.016
Cibenzoline	T46.2X1	T46.2X2	T46.2X3	T46.2X4	T46.2X5	T46.2X6

◀ New ⬅ Revised ~~deleted~~ Deleted

Substance	Poisoning, Accidental (Unintentional)	Poisoning, Intentional Self-Harm	Poisoning, Assault	Poisoning, Undetermined	Adverse Effect	Underdosing
Ciclacillin	T36.ØX1	T36.ØX2	T36.ØX3	T36.ØX4	T36.ØX5	T36.ØX6
Ciclobarbital—*see Hexobarbital*						
Ciclonicate	T46.7X1	T46.7X2	T46.7X3	T46.7X4	T46.7X5	T46.7X6
Ciclopirox (olamine)	T49.ØX1	T49.ØX2	T49.ØX3	T49.ØX4	T49.ØX5	T49.ØX6
Ciclosporin	T45.1X1	T45.1X2	T45.1X3	T45.1X4	T45.1X5	T45.1X6
Cicuta maculata or virosa	T62.2X1	T62.2X2	T62.2X3	T62.2X4	—	—
Cicutoxin	T62.2X1	T62.2X2	T62.2X3	T62.2X4	—	—
Cigarette lighter fluid	T52.ØX1	T52.ØX2	T52.ØX3	T52.ØX4	—	—
Cigarettes (tobacco)	T65.221	T65.222	T65.223	T65.224	—	—
Ciguatoxin	T61.Ø1	T61.Ø2	T61.Ø3	T61.Ø4	—	—
Cilazapril	T46.4X1	T46.4X2	T46.4X3	T46.4X4	T46.4X5	T46.4X6
Cimetidine	T47.ØX1	T47.ØX2	T47.ØX3	T47.ØX4	T47.ØX5	T47.ØX6
Cimetropium bromide	T44.3X1	T44.3X2	T44.3X3	T44.3X4	T44.3X5	T44.3X6
Cinchocaine	T41.3X1	T41.3X2	T41.3X3	T41.3X4	T41.3X5	T41.3X6
topical (surface)	T41.3X1	T41.3X2	T41.3X3	T41.3X4	T41.3X5	T41.3X6
Cinchona	T37.2X1	T37.2X2	T37.2X3	T37.2X4	T37.2X5	T37.2X6
Cinchonine alkaloids	T37.2X1	T37.2X2	T37.2X3	T37.2X4	T37.2X5	T37.2X6
Cinchophen	T5Ø.4X1	T5Ø.4X2	T5Ø.4X3	T5Ø.4X4	T5Ø.4X5	T5Ø.4X6
Cinepazide	T46.7X1	T46.7X2	T46.7X3	T46.7X4	T46.7X5	T46.7X6
Cinnamedrine	T48.5X1	T48.5X2	T48.5X3	T48.5X4	T48.5X5	T48.5X6
Cinnarizine	T45.ØX1	T45.ØX2	T45.ØX3	T45.ØX4	T45.ØX5	T45.ØX6
Cinoxacin	T37.8X1	T37.8X2	T37.8X3	T37.8X4	T37.8X5	T37.8X6
Ciprofibrate	T46.6X1	T46.6X2	T46.6X3	T46.6X4	T46.6X5	T46.6X6
Ciprofloxacin	T36.8X1	T36.8X2	T36.8X3	T36.8X4	T36.8X5	T36.8X6
Cisapride	T47.8X1	T47.8X2	T47.8X3	T47.8X4	T47.8X5	T47.8X6
Cisplatin	T45.1X1	T45.1X2	T45.1X3	T45.1X4	T45.1X5	T45.1X6
Citalopram	T43.221	T43.222	T43.223	T43.224	T43.225	T43.226
Citanest	T41.3X1	T41.3X2	T41.3X3	T41.3X4	T41.3X5	T41.3X6
infiltration (subcutaneous)	T41.3X1	T41.3X2	T41.3X3	T41.3X4	T41.3X5	T41.3X6
nerve block (peripheral) (plexus)	T41.3X1	T41.3X2	T41.3X3	T41.3X4	T41.3X5	T41.3X6
Citric acid	T47.5X1	T47.5X2	T47.5X3	T47.5X4	T47.5X5	T47.5X6
Citrovorum (factor)	T45.8X1	T45.8X2	T45.8X3	T45.8X4	T45.8X5	T45.8X6
Claviceps purpurea	T62.2X1	T62.2X2	T62.2X3	T62.2X4	—	—
Clavulanic acid	T36.1X1	T36.1X2	T36.1X3	T36.1X4	T36.1X5	T36.1X6
Cleaner, cleansing agent, type not specified	T65.891	T65.892	T65.893	T65.894	—	—
of paint or varnish	T52.91	T52.92	T52.93	T52.94	—	—
specified type NEC	T65.891	T65.892	T65.893	T65.894	—	—
Clebopride	T47.8X1	T47.8X2	T47.8X3	T47.8X4	T47.8X5	T47.8X6
Clefamide	T37.3X1	T37.3X2	T37.3X3	T37.3X4	T37.3X5	T37.3X6
Clemastine	T45.ØX1	T45.ØX2	T45.ØX3	T45.ØX4	T45.ØX5	T45.ØX6
Clematis vitalba	T62.2X1	T62.2X2	T62.2X3	T62.2X4	—	—
Clemizole	T45.ØX1	T45.ØX2	T45.ØX3	T45.ØX4	T45.ØX5	T45.ØX6
penicillin	T36.ØX1	T36.ØX2	T36.ØX3	T36.ØX4	T36.ØX5	T36.ØX6
Clenbuterol	T48.6X1	T48.6X2	T48.6X3	T48.6X4	T48.6X5	T48.6X6
Clidinium bromide	T44.3X1	T44.3X2	T44.3X3	T44.3X4	T44.3X5	T44.3X6
Clindamycin	T36.8X1	T36.8X2	T36.8X3	T36.8X4	T36.8X5	T36.8X6
Clinofibrate	T46.6X1	T46.6X2	T46.6X3	T46.6X4	T46.6X5	T46.6X6
Clioquinol	T37.8X1	T37.8X2	T37.8X3	T37.8X4	T37.8X5	T37.8X6
Cliradon	T4Ø.2X1	T4Ø.2X2	T4Ø.2X3	T4Ø.2X4	—	—
Clobazam	T42.4X1	T42.4X2	T42.4X3	T42.4X4	T42.4X5	T42.4X6
Clobenzorex	T5Ø.5X1	T5Ø.5X2	T5Ø.5X3	T5Ø.5X4	T5Ø.5X5	T5Ø.5X6
Clobetasol	T49.ØX1	T49.ØX2	T49.ØX3	T49.ØX4	T49.ØX5	T49.ØX6
Clobetasone	T49.ØX1	T49.ØX2	T49.ØX3	T49.ØX4	T49.ØX5	T49.ØX6
Clobutinol	T48.3X1	T48.3X2	T48.3X3	T48.3X4	T48.3X5	T48.3X6
Clocapramine	T43.ØX1	T43.ØX2	T43.ØX3	T43.ØX4	T43.ØX5	T43.ØX6
Clocortolone	T38.ØX1	T38.ØX2	T38.ØX3	T38.ØX4	T38.ØX5	T38.ØX6
Clodantoin	T49.ØX1	T49.ØX2	T49.ØX3	T49.ØX4	T49.ØX5	T49.ØX6
Clodronic acid	T5Ø.991	T5Ø.992	T5Ø.993	T5Ø.994	T5Ø.995	T5Ø.996
Clofazimine	T37.1X1	T37.1X2	T37.1X3	T37.1X4	T37.1X5	T37.1X6
Clofedanol	T48.3X1	T48.3X2	T48.3X3	T48.3X4	T48.3X5	T48.3X6
Clofenamide	T5Ø.2X1	T5Ø.2X2	T5Ø.2X3	T5Ø.2X4	T5Ø.2X5	T5Ø.2X6
Clofenotane	T49.ØX1	T49.ØX2	T49.ØX3	T49.ØX4	T49.ØX5	T49.ØX6
Clofezone	T39.2X1	T39.2X2	T39.2X3	T39.2X4	T39.2X5	T39.2X6
Clofibrate	T46.6X1	T46.6X2	T46.6X3	T46.6X4	T46.6X5	T46.6X6
Clofibride	T46.6X1	T46.6X2	T46.6X3	T46.6X4	T46.6X5	T46.6X6
Cloforex	T5Ø.5X1	T5Ø.5X2	T5Ø.5X3	T5Ø.5X4	T5Ø.5X5	T5Ø.5X6
Clomacran	T43.ØX1	T43.ØX2	T43.ØX3	T43.ØX4	T43.ØX5	T43.ØX6
Clomethiazole	T42.6X1	T42.6X2	T42.6X3	T42.6X4	T42.6X5	T42.6X6
Clometocillin	T36.ØX1	T36.ØX2	T36.ØX3	T36.ØX4	T36.ØX5	T36.ØX6
Clomifene	T38.5X1	T38.5X2	T38.5X3	T38.5X4	T38.5X5	T38.5X6
Clomiphene	T38.5X1	T38.5X2	T38.5X3	T38.5X4	T38.5X5	T38.5X6
Clomipramine	T43.Ø11	T43.Ø12	T43.Ø13	T43.Ø14	T43.Ø15	T43.Ø16
Clomocycline	T36.4X1	T36.4X2	T36.4X3	T36.4X4	T36.4X5	T36.4X6
Clonazepam	T42.4X1	T42.4X2	T42.4X3	T42.4X4	T42.4X5	T42.4X6
Clonidine	T46.5X1	T46.5X2	T46.5X3	T46.5X4	T46.5X5	T46.5X6
Clonixin	T39.8X1	T39.8X2	T39.8X3	T39.8X4	T39.8X5	T39.8X6
Clopamide	T5Ø.2X1	T5Ø.2X2	T5Ø.2X3	T5Ø.2X4	T5Ø.2X5	T5Ø.2X6
Clopenthixol	T43.4X1	T43.4X2	T43.4X3	T43.4X4	T43.4X5	T43.4X6
Cloperastine	T48.3X1	T48.3X2	T48.3X3	T48.3X4	T48.3X5	T48.3X6
Clophedianol	T48.3X1	T48.3X2	T48.3X3	T48.3X4	T48.3X5	T48.3X6
Cloponone	T36.2X1	T36.2X2	T36.2X3	T36.2X4	T36.2X5	T36.2X6
Cloprednol	T38.ØX1	T38.ØX2	T38.ØX3	T38.ØX4	T38.ØX5	T38.ØX6
Cloral betaine	T42.6X1	T42.6X2	T42.6X3	T42.6X4	T42.6X5	T42.6X6

Substance	Poisoning, Accidental (Unintentional)	Poisoning, Intentional Self-Harm	Poisoning, Assault	Poisoning, Undetermined	Adverse Effect	Underdosing
Cloramfenicol	T36.2X1	T36.2X2	T36.2X3	T36.2X4	T36.2X5	T36.2X6
Clorazepate (dipotassium)	T42.4X1	T42.4X2	T42.4X3	T42.4X4	T42.4X5	T42.4X6
Clorexolone	T50.2X1	T50.2X2	T50.2X3	T50.2X4	T50.2X5	T50.2X6
Clorox (bleach)	T54.91	T54.92	T54.93	T54.94	—	—
Clorfenamine	T45.0X1	T45.0X2	T45.0X3	T45.0X4	T45.0X5	T45.0X6
Clorgiline	T43.1X1	T43.1X2	T43.1X3	T43.1X4	T43.1X5	T43.1X6
Clorotepine	T44.3X1	T44.3X2	T44.3X3	T44.3X4	T44.3X5	T44.3X6
Clorprenaline	T48.6X1	T48.6X2	T48.6X3	T48.6X4	T48.6X5	T48.6X6
Clortermine	T50.5X1	T50.5X2	T50.5X3	T50.5X4	T50.5X5	T50.5X6
Clotiapine	T43.591	T43.592	T43.593	T43.594	T43.595	T43.596
Clotiazepam	T42.4X1	T42.4X2	T42.4X3	T42.4X4	T42.4X5	T42.4X6
Clotibric acid	T46.6X1	T46.6X2	T46.6X3	T46.6X4	T46.6X5	T46.6X6
Clotrimazole	T49.0X1	T49.0X2	T49.0X3	T49.0X4	T49.0X5	T49.0X6
Cloxacillin	T36.0X1	T36.0X2	T36.0X3	T36.0X4	T36.0X5	T36.0X6
Cloxazolam	T42.4X1	T42.4X2	T42.4X3	T42.4X4	T42.4X5	T42.4X6
Cloxiquine	T49.0X1	T49.0X2	T49.0X3	T49.0X4	T49.0X5	T49.0X6
Clozapine	T42.4X1	T42.4X2	T42.4X3	T42.4X4	T42.4X5	T42.4X6
Coagulant NEC	T45.7X1	T45.7X2	T45.7X3	T45.7X4	T45.7X5	T45.7X6
Coal (carbon monoxide from) — *see also Carbon, monoxide, coal*	T58.2X1	T58.2X2	T58.2X3	T58.2X4	—	—
oil — *see Kerosene*						
tar	T49.1X1	T49.1X2	T49.1X3	T49.1X4	T49.1X5	T49.1X6
fumes	T59.891	T59.892	T59.893	T59.894	—	—
medicinal (ointment)	T49.4X1	T49.4X2	T49.4X3	T49.4X4	T49.4X5	T49.4X6
analgesics NEC	T39.2X1	T39.2X2	T39.2X3	T39.2X4	T39.2X5	T39.2X6
naphtha (solvent)	T52.0X1	T52.0X2	T52.0X3	T52.0X4		
Cobalamine	T45.2X1	T45.2X2	T45.2X3	T45.2X4	T45.2X5	T45.2X6
Cobalt (nonmedicinal) (fumes) (industrial)	T56.891	T56.892	T56.893	T56.894		
medicinal (trace) (chloride)	T45.8X1	T45.8X2	T45.8X3	T45.8X4	T45.8X5	T45.8X6
Cobra (venom)	T63.041	T63.042	T63.043	T63.044		
Coca (leaf)	T40.5X1	T40.5X2	T40.5X3	T40.5X4	T40.5X5	T40.5X6
Cocaine	T40.5X1	T40.5X2	T40.5X3	T40.5X4	T40.5X5	T40.5X6
topical anesthetic	T41.3X1	T41.3X2	T41.3X3	T41.3X4	T41.3X5	T41.3X6
Cocarboxylase	T45.3X1	T45.3X2	T45.3X3	T45.3X4	T45.3X5	T45.3X6
Coccidioidin	T50.8X1	T50.8X2	T50.8X3	T50.8X4	T50.8X5	T50.8X6
Cocculus indicus	T62.1X1	T62.1X2	T62.1X3	T62.1X4		
Cochineal	T65.6X1	T65.6X2	T65.6X3	T65.6X4		
medicinal products	T50.991	T50.992	T50.993	T50.994	T50.995	T50.996
Codeine	T40.2X1	T40.2X2	T40.2X3	T40.2X4	T40.2X5	T40.2X6
Cod-liver oil	T45.2X1	T45.2X2	T45.2X3	T45.2X4	T45.2X5	T45.2X6

Substance	Poisoning, Accidental (Unintentional)	Poisoning, Intentional Self-Harm	Poisoning, Assault	Poisoning, Undetermined	Adverse Effect	Underdosing
Coenzyme A	T50.991	T50.992	T50.993	T50.994	T50.995	T50.996
Coffee	T62.8X1	T62.8X2	T62.8X3	T62.8X4	—	—
Cogalactoisomerase	T50.991	T50.992	T50.993	T50.994	T50.995	T50.996
Cogentin	T44.3X1	T44.3X2	T44.3X3	T44.3X4	T44.3X5	T44.3X6
Coke fumes or gas (carbon monoxide)	T58.2X1	T58.2X2	T58.2X3	T58.2X4	—	—
industrial use	T58.8X1	T58.8X2	T58.8X3	T58.8X4	—	—
Colace	T47.4X1	T47.4X2	T47.4X3	T47.4X4	T47.4X5	T47.4X6
Colaspase	T45.1X1	T45.1X2	T45.1X3	T45.1X4	T45.1X5	T45.1X6
Colchicine	T50.4X1	T50.4X2	T50.4X3	T50.4X4	T50.4X5	T50.4X6
Colchicum	T62.2X1	T62.2X2	T62.2X3	T62.2X4	—	—
Cold cream	T49.3X1	T49.3X2	T49.3X3	T49.3X4	T49.3X5	T49.3X6
Colecalciferol	T45.2X1	T45.2X2	T45.2X3	T45.2X4	T45.2X5	T45.2X6
Colestipol	T46.6X1	T46.6X2	T46.6X3	T46.6X4	T46.6X5	T46.6X6
Colestyramine	T46.6X1	T46.6X2	T46.6X3	T46.6X4	T46.6X5	T46.6X6
Colimycin	T36.8X1	T36.8X2	T36.8X3	T36.8X4	T36.8X5	T36.8X6
Colistimethate	T36.8X1	T36.8X2	T36.8X3	T36.8X4	T36.8X5	T36.8X6
Colistin	T36.8X1	T36.8X2	T36.8X3	T36.8X4	T36.8X5	T36.8X6
sulfate (eye preparation)	T49.5X1	T49.5X2	T49.5X3	T49.5X4	T49.5X5	T49.5X6
Collagen	T50.991	T50.992	T50.993	T50.994	T50.995	T50.996
Collagenase	T49.4X1	T49.4X2	T49.4X3	T49.4X4	T49.4X5	T49.4X6
Collodion	T49.3X1	T49.3X2	T49.3X3	T49.3X4	T49.3X5	T49.3X6
Colocynth	T47.2X1	T47.2X2	T47.2X3	T47.2X4	T47.2X5	T47.2X6
Colophony adhesive	T49.3X1	T49.3X2	T49.3X3	T49.3X4	T49.3X5	T49.3X6
Colorant — *see also Dye*	T50.991	T50.992	T50.993	T50.994	T50.995	T50.996
Coloring matter — *see Dye(s)*						
Combustion gas (after combustion) — *see Carbon, monoxide*						
prior to combustion	T59.891	T59.892	T59.893	T59.894	—	—
Compazine	T43.3X1	T43.3X2	T43.3X3	T43.3X4	T43.3X5	T43.3X6
Compound						
42 (warfarin)	T60.4X1	T60.4X2	T60.4X3	T60.4X4	—	—
269 (endrin)	T60.1X1	T60.1X2	T60.1X3	T60.1X4	—	—
497 (dieldrin)	T60.1X1	T60.1X2	T60.1X3	T60.1X4	—	—
1080 (sodium fluoroacetate)	T60.4X1	T60.4X2	T60.4X3	T60.4X4	—	—
3422 (parathion)	T60.0X1	T60.0X2	T60.0X3	T60.0X4	—	—
3911 (phorate)	T60.0X1	T60.0X2	T60.0X3	T60.0X4	—	—
3956 (toxaphene)	T60.1X1	T60.1X2	T60.1X3	T60.1X4	—	—
4049 (malathion)	T60.0X1	T60.0X2	T60.0X3	T60.0X4	—	—
4069 (malathion)	T60.0X1	T60.0X2	T60.0X3	T60.0X4	—	—
4124 (dicapthon)	T60.0X1	T60.0X2	T60.0X3	T60.0X4	—	—

Substance	Poisoning, Accidental (Unintentional)	Poisoning, Intentional Self-Harm	Poisoning, Assault	Poisoning, Undetermined	Adverse Effect	Underdosing
Compound *(Continued)*						
E (cortisone)	T38.ØX1	T38.ØX2	T38.ØX3	T38.ØX4	T38.ØX5	T38.ØX6
F (hydrocortisone)	T38.ØX1	T38.ØX2	T38.ØX3	T38.ØX4	T38.ØX5	T38.ØX6
Congener, anabolic	T38.7X1	T38.7X2	T38.7X3	T38.7X4	T38.7X5	T38.7X6
Congo red	T5Ø.8X1	T5Ø.8X2	T5Ø.8X3	T5Ø.8X4	T5Ø.8X5	T5Ø.8X6
Coniine, conine	T62.2X1	T62.2X2	T62.2X3	T62.2X4	—	—
Conium (maculatum)	T62.2X1	T62.2X2	T62.2X3	T62.2X4	—	—
Conjugated estrogenic substances	T38.5X1	T38.5X2	T38.5X3	T38.5X4	T38.5X5	T38.5X6
Contac	T48.5X1	T48.5X2	T48.5X3	T48.5X4	T48.5X5	T48.5X6
Contact lens solution	T49.5X1	T49.5X2	T49.5X3	T49.5X4	T49.5X5	T49.5X6
Contraceptive (oral)	T38.4X1	T38.4X2	T38.4X3	T38.4X4	T38.4X5	T38.4X6
vaginal	T49.8X1	T49.8X2	T49.8X3	T49.8X4	T49.8X5	T49.8X6
Contrast medium, radiography	T5Ø.8X1	T5Ø.8X2	T5Ø.8X3	T5Ø.8X4	T5Ø.8X5	T5Ø.8X6
Convallaria glycosides	T46.ØX1	T46.ØX2	T46.ØX3	T46.ØX4	T46.ØX5	T46.ØX6
Convallaria majalis	T62.2X1	T62.2X2	T62.2X3	T62.2X4	—	—
berry	T62.1X1	T62.1X2	T62.1X3	T62.1X4	—	—
Copper (dust) (fumes) (nonmedicinal) NEC	T56.4X1	T56.4X2	T56.4X3	T56.4X4	—	—
arsenate, arsenite	T57.ØX1	T57.ØX2	T57.ØX3	T57.ØX4	—	—
insecticide	T6Ø.2X1	T6Ø.2X2	T6Ø.2X3	T6Ø.2X4	—	—
emetic	T47.7X1	T47.7X2	T47.7X3	T47.7X4	T47.7X5	T47.7X6
fungicide	T6Ø.3X1	T6Ø.3X2	T6Ø.3X3	T6Ø.3X4	—	—
gluconate	T49.ØX1	T49.ØX2	T49.ØX3	T49.ØX4	T49.ØX5	T49.ØX6
insecticide	T6Ø.2X1	T6Ø.2X2	T6Ø.2X3	T6Ø.2X4	—	—
medicinal (trace)	T45.8X1	T45.8X2	T45.8X3	T45.8X4	T45.8X5	T45.8X6
oleate	T49.ØX1	T49.ØX2	T49.ØX3	T49.ØX4	T49.ØX5	T49.ØX6
sulfate	T56.4X1	T56.4X2	T56.4X3	T56.4X4	—	—
cupric	T56.4X1	T56.4X2	T56.4X3	T56.4X4	—	—
fungicide	T6Ø.3X1	T6Ø.3X2	T6Ø.3X3	T6Ø.3X4	—	—
medicinal						
ear	T49.6X1	T49.6X2	T49.6X3	T49.6X4	T49.6X5	T49.6X6
emetic	T47.7X1	T47.7X2	T47.7X3	T47.7X4	T47.7X5	T47.7X6
eye	T49.5X1	T49.5X2	T49.5X3	T49.5X4	T49.5X5	T49.5X6
cuprous	T56.4X1	T56.4X2	T56.4X3	T56.4X4	—	—
fungicide	T6Ø.3X1	T6Ø.3X2	T6Ø.3X3	T6Ø.3X4	—	—
medicinal						
ear	T49.6X1	T49.6X2	T49.6X3	T49.6X4	T49.6X5	T49.6X6
emetic	T47.7X1	T47.7X2	T47.7X3	T47.7X4	T47.7X5	T47.7X6
eye	T49.5X1	T49.5X2	T49.5X3	T49.5X4	T49.5X5	T49.5X6
Copperhead snake (bite) (venom)	T63.Ø61	T63.Ø62	T63.Ø63	T63.Ø64	—	—
Coral (sting)	T63.691	T63.692	T63.693	T63.694	—	—
snake (bite) (venom)	T63.Ø21	T63.Ø22	T63.Ø23	T63.Ø24	—	—

Substance	Poisoning, Accidental (Unintentional)	Poisoning, Intentional Self-Harm	Poisoning, Assault	Poisoning, Undetermined	Adverse Effect	Underdosing
Corbadrine	T49.6X1	T49.6X2	T49.6X3	T49.6X4	T49.6X5	T49.6X6
Cordran	T49.ØX1	T49.ØX2	T49.ØX3	T49.ØX4	T49.ØX5	T49.ØX6
Cordite	T65.891	T65.892	T65.893	T65.894	—	—
vapor	T59.891	T59.892	T59.893	T59.894	—	—
Corn cures	T49.4X1	T49.4X2	T49.4X3	T49.4X4	T49.4X5	T49.4X6
Cornhusker's lotion	T49.3X1	T49.3X2	T49.3X3	T49.3X4	T49.3X5	T49.3X6
Corn starch	T49.3X1	T49.3X2	T49.3X3	T49.3X4	T49.3X5	T49.3X6
Coronary vasodilator NEC	T46.3X1	T46.3X2	T46.3X3	T46.3X4	T46.3X5	T46.3X6
Corrosive NEC	T54.91	T54.92	T54.93	T54.94	—	—
acid NEC	T54.2X1	T54.2X2	T54.2X3	T54.2X4	—	—
aromatics	T54.1X1	T54.1X2	T54.1X3	T54.1X4	—	—
disinfectant	T54.1X1	T54.1X2	T54.1X3	T54.1X4	—	—
fumes NEC	T54.91	T54.92	T54.93	T54.94	—	—
specified NEC	T54.91	T54.92	T54.93	T54.94	—	—
sublimate	T56.1X1	T56.1X2	T56.1X3	T56.1X4	—	—
Cortate	T38.ØX1	T38.ØX2	T38.ØX3	T38.ØX4	T38.ØX5	T38.ØX6
Cort-Dome	T38.ØX1	T38.ØX2	T38.ØX3	T38.ØX4	T38.ØX5	T38.ØX6
ENT agent	T49.6X1	T49.6X2	T49.6X3	T49.6X4	T49.6X5	T49.6X6
ophthalmic preparation	T49.5X1	T49.5X2	T49.5X3	T49.5X4	T49.5X5	T49.5X6
topical NEC	T49.ØX1	T49.ØX2	T49.ØX3	T49.ØX4	T49.ØX5	T49.ØX6
Cortef	T38.ØX1	T38.ØX2	T38.ØX3	T38.ØX4	T38.ØX5	T38.ØX6
ENT agent	T49.6X1	T49.6X2	T49.6X3	T49.6X4	T49.6X5	T49.6X6
ophthalmic preparation	T49.5X1	T49.5X2	T49.5X3	T49.5X4	T49.5X5	T49.5X6
topical NEC	T49.ØX1	T49.ØX2	T49.ØX3	T49.ØX4	T49.ØX5	T49.ØX6
Corticosteroid	T38.ØX1	T38.ØX2	T38.ØX3	T38.ØX4	T38.ØX5	T38.ØX6
ENT agent	T49.6X1	T49.6X2	T49.6X3	T49.6X4	T49.6X5	T49.6X6
mineral	T5Ø.ØX1	T5Ø.ØX2	T5Ø.ØX3	T5Ø.ØX4	T5Ø.ØX5	T5Ø.ØX6
ophthalmic	T49.5X1	T49.5X2	T49.5X3	T49.5X4	T49.5X5	T49.5X6
topical NEC	T49.ØX1	T49.ØX2	T49.ØX3	T49.ØX4	T49.ØX5	T49.ØX6
Corticotropin	T38.811	T38.812	T38.813	T38.814	T38.815	T38.816
Cortisol	T49.ØX1	T49.ØX2	T49.ØX3	T49.ØX4	T49.ØX5	T49.ØX6
ENT agent	T49.6X1	T49.6X2	T49.6X3	T49.6X4	T49.6X5	T49.6X6
ophthalmic preparation	T49.5X1	T49.5X2	T49.5X3	T49.5X4	T49.5X5	T49.5X6
topical NEC	T49.ØX1	T49.ØX2	T49.ØX3	T49.ØX4	T49.ØX5	T49.ØX6
Cortisone (acetate)	T38.ØX1	T38.ØX2	T38.ØX3	T38.ØX4	T38.ØX5	T38.ØX6
ENT agent	T49.6X1	T49.6X2	T49.6X3	T49.6X4	T49.6X5	T49.6X6
ophthalmic preparation	T49.5X1	T49.5X2	T49.5X3	T49.5X4	T49.5X5	T49.5X6
topical NEC	T49.ØX1	T49.ØX2	T49.ØX3	T49.ØX4	T49.ØX5	T49.ØX6
Cortivazol	T38.ØX1	T38.ØX2	T38.ØX3	T38.ØX4	T38.ØX5	T38.ØX6
Cortogen	T38.ØX1	T38.ØX2	T38.ØX3	T38.ØX4	T38.ØX5	T38.ØX6
ENT agent	T49.6X1	T49.6X2	T49.6X3	T49.6X4	T49.6X5	T49.6X6
ophthalmic preparation	T49.5X1	T49.5X2	T49.5X3	T49.5X4	T49.5X5	T49.5X6

Substance	Poisoning, Accidental (Unintentional)	Poisoning, Intentional Self-Harm	Poisoning, Assault	Poisoning, Undetermined	Adverse Effect	Underdosing
Cortone	T38.0X1	T38.0X2	T38.0X3	T38.0X4	T38.0X5	T38.0X6
ENT agent	T49.6X1	T49.6X2	T49.6X3	T49.6X4	T49.6X5	T49.6X6
ophthalmic preparation	T49.5X1	T49.5X2	T49.5X3	T49.5X4	T49.5X5	T49.5X6
Cortril	T38.0X1	T38.0X2	T38.0X3	T38.0X4	T38.0X5	T38.0X6
ENT agent	T49.6X1	T49.6X2	T49.6X3	T49.6X4	T49.6X5	T49.6X6
ophthalmic preparation	T49.5X1	T49.5X2	T49.5X3	T49.5X4	T49.5X5	T49.5X6
topical NEC	T49.0X1	T49.0X2	T49.0X3	T49.0X4	T49.0X5	T49.0X6
Corynebacterium parvum	T45.1X1	T45.1X2	T45.1X3	T45.1X4	T45.1X5	T45.1X6
Cosmetic preparation	T49.8X1	T49.8X2	T49.8X3	T49.8X4	T49.8X5	T49.8X6
Cosmetics	T49.8X1	T49.8X2	T49.8X3	T49.8X4	T49.8X5	T49.8X6
Cosyntropin	T38.811	T38.812	T38.813	T38.814	T38.815	T38.816
Cotarnine	T45.7X1	T45.7X2	T45.7X3	T45.7X4	T45.7X5	T45.7X6
Co-trimoxazole	T36.8X1	T36.8X2	T36.8X3	T36.8X4	T36.8X5	T36.8X6
Cottonseed oil	T49.3X1	T49.3X2	T49.3X3	T49.3X4	T49.3X5	T49.3X6
Cough mixture (syrup)	T48.4X1	T48.4X2	T48.4X3	T48.4X4	T48.4X5	T48.4X6
containing opiates	T40.2X1	T40.2X2	T40.2X3	T40.2X4	T40.2X5	T40.2X6
expectorants	T48.4X1	T48.4X2	T48.4X3	T48.4X4	T48.4X5	T48.4X6
Coumadin	T45.511	T45.512	T45.513	T45.514	T45.515	T45.516
rodenticide	T60.4X1	T60.4X2	T60.4X3	T60.4X4	—	—
Coumaphos	T60.0X1	T60.0X2	T60.0X3	T60.0X4	—	—
Coumarin	T45.511	T45.512	T45.513	T45.514	T45.515	T45.516
Coumetarol	T45.511	T45.512	T45.513	T45.514	T45.515	T45.516
Cowbane	T62.2X1	T62.2X2	T62.2X3	T62.2X4	—	—
Cozyme	T45.2X1	T45.2X2	T45.2X3	T45.2X4	T45.2X5	T45.2X6
Crack	T40.5X1	T40.5X2	T40.5X3	T40.5X4	—	—
Crataegus extract	T46.0X1	T46.0X2	T46.0X3	T46.0X4	T46.0X5	T46.0X6
Creolin	T54.1X1	T54.1X2	T54.1X3	T54.1X4	—	—
disinfectant	T54.1X1	T54.1X2	T54.1X3	T54.1X4	—	—
Creosol (compound)	T49.0X1	T49.0X2	T49.0X3	T49.0X4	T49.0X5	T49.0X6
Creosote (coal tar) (beechwood)	T49.0X1	T49.0X2	T49.0X3	T49.0X4	T49.0X5	T49.0X6
medicinal (expectorant)	T48.4X1	T48.4X2	T48.4X3	T48.4X4	T48.4X5	T48.4X6
syrup	T48.4X1	T48.4X2	T48.4X3	T48.4X4	T48.4X5	T48.4X6
Cresol(s)	T49.0X1	T49.0X2	T49.0X3	T49.0X4	T49.0X5	T49.0X6
and soap solution	T49.0X1	T49.0X2	T49.0X3	T49.0X4	T49.0X5	T49.0X6
Cresyl acetate	T49.0X1	T49.0X2	T49.0X3	T49.0X4	T49.0X5	T49.0X6
Cresylic acid	T49.0X1	T49.0X2	T49.0X3	T49.0X4	T49.0X5	T49.0X6
Crimidine	T60.4X1	T60.4X2	T60.4X3	T60.4X4	—	—
Croconazole	T37.8X1	T37.8X2	T37.8X3	T37.8X4	T37.8X5	T37.8X6
Cromoglicic acid	T48.6X1	T48.6X2	T48.6X3	T48.6X4	T48.6X5	T48.6X6
Cromolyn	T48.6X1	T48.6X2	T48.6X3	T48.6X4	T48.6X5	T48.6X6
Cromonar	T46.3X1	T46.3X2	T46.3X3	T46.3X4	T46.3X5	T46.3X6

Substance	Poisoning, Accidental (Unintentional)	Poisoning, Intentional Self-Harm	Poisoning, Assault	Poisoning, Undetermined	Adverse Effect	Underdosing
Cropropamide	T39.8X1	T39.8X2	T39.8X3	T39.8X4	T39.8X5	T39.8X6
with crotethamide	T50.7X1	T50.7X2	T50.7X3	T50.7X4	T50.7X5	T50.7X6
Crotamiton	T49.0X1	T49.0X2	T49.0X3	T49.0X4	T49.0X5	T49.0X6
Crotethamide	T39.8X1	T39.8X2	T39.8X3	T39.8X4	T39.8X5	T39.8X6
with cropropamide	T50.7X1	T50.7X2	T50.7X3	T50.7X4	T50.7X5	T50.7X6
Croton (oil)	T47.2X1	T47.2X2	T47.2X3	T47.2X4	T47.2X5	T47.2X6
chloral	T42.6X1	T42.6X2	T42.6X3	T42.6X4	T42.6X5	T42.6X6
Crude oil	T52.0X1	T52.0X2	T52.0X3	T52.0X4	—	—
Cryogenine	T39.8X1	T39.8X2	T39.8X3	T39.8X4	T39.8X5	T39.8X6
Cryolite (vapor)	T60.1X1	T60.1X2	T60.1X3	T60.1X4	—	—
insecticide	T60.1X1	T60.1X2	T60.1X3	T60.1X4	—	—
Cryptenamine (tannates)	T46.5X1	T46.5X2	T46.5X3	T46.5X4	T46.5X5	T46.5X6
Crystal violet	T49.0X1	T49.0X2	T49.0X3	T49.0X4	T49.0X5	T49.0X6
Cuckoopint	T62.2X1	T62.2X2	T62.2X3	T62.2X4	—	—
Cumetharol	T45.511	T45.512	T45.513	T45.514	T45.515	T45.516
Cupric						
acetate	T60.3X1	T60.3X2	T60.3X3	T60.3X4	—	—
acetoarsenite	T57.0X1	T57.0X2	T57.0X3	T57.0X4	—	—
arsenate	T57.0X1	T57.0X2	T57.0X3	T57.0X4	—	—
gluconate	T49.0X1	T49.0X2	T49.0X3	T49.0X4	T49.0X5	T49.0X6
oleate	T49.0X1	T49.0X2	T49.0X3	T49.0X4	T49.0X5	T49.0X6
sulfate	T56.4X1	T56.4X2	T56.4X3	T56.4X4	—	—
Cuprous sulfate — *see also Copper sulfate*	T56.4X1	T56.4X2	T56.4X3	T56.4X4	—	—
Curare, curarine	T48.1X1	T48.1X2	T48.1X3	T48.1X4	T48.1X5	T48.1X6
Cyamemazine	T43.3X1	T43.3X2	T43.3X3	T43.3X4	T43.3X5	T43.3X6
Cyamopsis tetragono-loba	T46.6X1	T46.6X2	T46.6X3	T46.6X4	T46.6X5	T46.6X6
Cyanacetyl hydrazide	T37.1X1	T37.1X2	T37.1X3	T37.1X4	T37.1X5	T37.1X6
Cyanic acid (gas)	T59.891	T59.892	T59.893	T59.894	—	—
Cyanide(s) (compounds) (potassium) (sodium) NEC	T65.0X1	T65.0X2	T65.0X3	T65.0X4	—	—
dust or gas (inhalation) NEC	T57.3X1	T57.3X2	T57.3X3	T57.3X4	—	—
fumigant	T65.0X1	T65.0X2	T65.0X3	T65.0X4	—	—
hydrogen	T57.3X1	T57.3X2	T57.3X3	T57.3X4	—	—
mercuric — *see Mercury*						
pesticide (dust) (fumes)	T65.0X1	T65.0X2	T65.0X3	T65.0X4	—	—
Cyanoacrylate adhesive	T49.3X1	T49.3X2	T49.3X3	T49.3X4	T49.3X5	T49.3X6
Cyanocobalamin	T45.8X1	T45.8X2	T45.8X3	T45.8X4	T45.8X5	T45.8X6
Cyanogen (chloride) (gas) NEC	T59.891	T59.892	T59.893	T59.894	—	—
Cyclacillin	T36.0X1	T36.0X2	T36.0X3	T36.0X4	T36.0X5	T36.0X6
Cyclaine	T41.3X1	T41.3X2	T41.3X3	T41.3X4	T41.3X5	T41.3X6
Cyclamate	T50.991	T50.992	T50.993	T50.994	T50.995	T50.996

◀ New ◀▮▮▮ Revised ~~deleted~~ Deleted

Substance	Poisoning, Accidental (Unintentional)	Poisoning, Intentional Self-Harm	Poisoning, Assault	Poisoning, Undetermined	Adverse Effect	Underdosing
Cyclamen europaeum	T62.2X1	T62.2X2	T62.2X3	T62.2X4	—	—
Cyclandelate	T46.7X1	T46.7X2	T46.7X3	T46.7X4	T46.7X5	T46.7X6
Cyclazocine	T5Ø.7X1	T5Ø.7X2	T5Ø.7X3	T5Ø.7X4	T5Ø.7X5	T5Ø.7X6
Cyclizine	T45.ØX1	T45.ØX2	T45.ØX3	T45.ØX4	T45.ØX5	T45.ØX6
Cyclobarbital	T42.3X1	T42.3X2	T42.3X3	T42.3X4	T42.3X5	T42.3X6
Cyclobarbitone	T42.3X1	T42.3X2	T42.3X3	T42.3X4	T42.3X5	T42.3X6
Cyclobenzaprine	T48.1X1	T48.1X2	T48.1X3	T48.1X4	T48.1X5	T48.1X6
Cyclodrine	T44.3X1	T44.3X2	T44.3X3	T44.3X4	T44.3X5	T44.3X6
Cycloguanil embonate	T37.2X1	T37.2X2	T37.2X3	T37.2X4	T37.2X5	T37.2X6
Cycloheptadiene	T43.291	T43.292	T43.293	T43.294	T43.295	T43.296
Cyclohexane	T52.8X1	T52.8X2	T52.8X3	T52.8X4	—	—
Cyclohexanol	T51.8X1	T51.8X2	T51.8X3	T51.8X4	—	—
Cyclohexanone	T52.4X1	T52.4X2	T52.4X3	T52.4X4	—	—
Cycloheximide	T6Ø.3X1	T6Ø.3X2	T6Ø.3X3	T6Ø.3X4	—	—
Cyclohexyl acetate	T52.8X1	T52.8X2	T52.8X3	T52.8X4	—	—
Cycloleucin	T45.1X1	T45.1X2	T45.1X3	T45.1X4	T45.1X5	T45.1X6
Cyclomethycaine	T41.3X1	T41.3X2	T41.3X3	T41.3X4	T41.3X5	T41.3X6
Cyclopentamine	T44.4X1	T44.4X2	T44.4X3	T44.4X4	T44.4X5	T44.4X6
Cyclopenthiazide	T5Ø.2X1	T5Ø.2X2	T5Ø.2X3	T5Ø.2X4	T5Ø.2X5	T5Ø.2X6
Cyclopentolate	T44.3X1	T44.3X2	T44.3X3	T44.3X4	T44.3X5	T44.3X6
Cyclophosphamide	T45.1X1	T45.1X2	T45.1X3	T45.1X4	T45.1X5	T45.1X6
Cycloplegic drug	T49.5X1	T49.5X2	T49.5X3	T49.5X4	T49.5X5	T49.5X6
Cyclopropane	T41.291	T41.292	T41.293	T41.294	T41.295	T41.296
Cyclopyrabital	T39.8X1	T39.8X2	T39.8X3	T39.8X4	T39.8X5	T39.8X6
Cycloserine	T37.1X1	T37.1X2	T37.1X3	T37.1X4	T37.1X5	T37.1X6
Cyclosporin	T45.1X1	T45.1X2	T45.1X3	T45.1X4	T45.1X5	T45.1X6
Cyclothiazide	T5Ø.2X1	T5Ø.2X2	T5Ø.2X3	T5Ø.2X4	T5Ø.2X5	T5Ø.2X6
Cycrimine	T44.3X1	T44.3X2	T44.3X3	T44.3X4	T44.3X5	T44.3X6
Cyhalothrin	T6Ø.1X1	T6Ø.1X2	T6Ø.1X3	T6Ø.1X4	—	—
Cymarin	T46.ØX1	T46.ØX2	T46.ØX3	T46.ØX4	T46.ØX5	T46.ØX6
Cypermethrin	T6Ø.1X1	T6Ø.1X2	T6Ø.1X3	T6Ø.1X4	—	—
Cyphenothrin	T6Ø.2X1	T6Ø.2X2	T6Ø.2X3	T6Ø.2X4	—	—
Cyproheptadine	T45.ØX1	T45.ØX2	T45.ØX3	T45.ØX4	T45.ØX5	T45.ØX6
Cyprolidol	T43.291	T43.292	T43.293	T43.294	T43.295	T43.296
Cyproterone	T38.6X1	T38.6X2	T38.6X3	T38.6X4	T38.6X5	T38.6X6
Cysteamine	T5Ø.6X1	T5Ø.6X2	T5Ø.6X3	T5Ø.6X4	T5Ø.6X5	T5Ø.6X6
Cytarabine	T45.1X1	T45.1X2	T45.1X3	T45.1X4	T45.1X5	T45.1X6
Cytisus						
laburnum	T62.2X1	T62.2X2	T62.2X3	T62.2X4	—	—
scoparius	T62.2X1	T62.2X2	T62.2X3	T62.2X4	—	—
Cytochrome C	T47.5X1	T47.5X2	T47.5X3	T47.5X4	T47.5X5	T47.5X6
Cytomel	T38.1X1	T38.1X2	T38.1X3	T38.1X4	T38.1X5	T38.1X6

Substance	Poisoning, Accidental (Unintentional)	Poisoning, Intentional Self-Harm	Poisoning, Assault	Poisoning, Undetermined	Adverse Effect	Underdosing
Cytosine arabinoside	T45.1X1	T45.1X2	T45.1X3	T45.1X4	T45.1X5	T45.1X6
Cytoxan	T45.1X1	T45.1X2	T45.1X3	T45.1X4	T45.1X5	T45.1X6
Cytozyme	T45.7X1	T45.7X2	T45.7X3	T45.7X4	T45.7X5	T45.7X6
2,4-D	T6Ø.3X1	T6Ø.3X2	T6Ø.3X3	T6Ø.3X4	—	—
D						
Dacarbazine	T45.1X1	T45.1X2	T45.1X3	T45.1X4	T45.1X5	T45.1X6
Dactinomycin	T45.1X1	T45.1X2	T45.1X3	T45.1X4	T45.1X5	T45.1X6
DADPS	T37.1X1	T37.1X2	T37.1X3	T37.1X4	T37.1X5	T37.1X6
Dakin's solution	T49.ØX1	T49.ØX2	T49.ØX3	T49.ØX4	T49.ØX5	T49.ØX6
Dalapon (sodium)	T6Ø.3X1	T6Ø.3X2	T6Ø.3X3	T6Ø.3X4	—	—
Dalmane	T42.4X1	T42.4X2	T42.4X3	T42.4X4	T42.4X5	T42.4X6
Danazol	T38.6X1	T38.6X2	T38.6X3	T38.6X4	T38.6X5	T38.6X6
Danilone	T45.511	T45.512	T45.513	T45.514	T45.515	T45.516
Danthron	T47.2X1	T47.2X2	T47.2X3	T47.2X4	T47.2X5	T47.2X6
Dantrolene	T42.8X1	T42.8X2	T42.8X3	T42.8X4	T42.8X5	T42.8X6
Dantron	T47.2X1	T47.2X2	T47.2X3	T47.2X4	T47.2X5	T47.2X6
Daphne (gnidium) (mezereum)	T62.2X1	T62.2X2	T62.2X3	T62.2X4	—	—
berry	T62.1X1	T62.1X2	T62.1X3	T62.1X4	—	—
Dapsone	T37.1X1	T37.1X2	T37.1X3	T37.1X4	T37.1X5	T37.1X6
Daraprim	T37.2X1	T37.2X2	T37.2X3	T37.2X4	T37.2X5	T37.2X6
Darnel	T62.2X1	T62.2X2	T62.2X3	T62.2X4	—	—
Darvon	T39.8X1	T39.8X2	T39.8X3	T39.8X4	T39.8X5	T39.8X6
Daunomycin	T45.1X1	T45.1X2	T45.1X3	T45.1X4	T45.1X5	T45.1X6
Daunorubicin	T45.1X1	T45.1X2	T45.1X3	T45.1X4	T45.1X5	T45.1X6
DBI	T38.3X1	T38.3X2	T38.3X3	T38.3X4	T38.3X5	T38.3X6
D-Con	T6Ø.91	T6Ø.92	T6Ø.93	T6Ø.94	—	—
insecticide	T6Ø.2X1	T6Ø.2X2	T6Ø.2X3	T6Ø.2X4	—	—
rodenticide	T6Ø.4X1	T6Ø.4X2	T6Ø.4X3	T6Ø.4X4	—	—
DDAVP	T38.891	T38.892	T38.893	T38.894	T38.895	T38.896
DDE (bis(chlorophenyl)-dichloroethylene)	T6Ø.2X1	T6Ø.2X2	T6Ø.2X3	T6Ø.2X4	—	—
DDS	T37.1X1	T37.1X2	T37.1X3	T37.1X4	T37.1X5	T37.1X6
DDT (dust)	T6Ø.1X1	T6Ø.1X2	T6Ø.1X3	T6Ø.1X4	—	—
Deadly nightshade — *see also Belladonna*	T62.2X1	T62.2X2	T62.2X3	T62.2X4	—	—
berry	T62.1X1	T62.1X2	T62.1X3	T62.1X4	—	—
Deamino-D-arginine vasopressin	T38.891	T38.892	T38.893	T38.894	T38.895	T38.896
Deanol (aceglumate)	T5Ø.991	T5Ø.992	T5Ø.993	T5Ø.994	T5Ø.995	T5Ø.996
Debrisoquine	T46.5X1	T46.5X2	T46.5X3	T46.5X4	T46.5X5	T46.5X6
Decaborane	T57.8X1	T57.8X2	T57.8X3	T57.8X4	—	—
fumes	T59.891	T59.892	T59.893	T59.894	—	—

Substance	Poisoning, Accidental (Unintentional)	Poisoning, Intentional Self-Harm	Poisoning, Assault	Poisoning, Undetermined	Adverse Effect	Underdosing
Decadron	T38.ØX1	T38.ØX2	T38.ØX3	T38.ØX4	T38.ØX5	T38.ØX6
ENT agent	T49.6X1	T49.6X2	T49.6X3	T49.6X4	T49.6X5	T49.6X6
ophthalmic preparation	T49.5X1	T49.5X2	T49.5X3	T49.5X4	T49.5X5	T49.5X6
topical NEC	T49.ØX1	T49.ØX2	T49.ØX3	T49.ØX4	T49.ØX5	T49.ØX6
Decahydronaphthalene	T52.8X1	T52.8X2	T52.8X3	T52.8X4	—	—
Decalin	T52.8X1	T52.8X2	T52.8X3	T52.8X4	—	—
Decamethonium (bromide)	T48.1X1	T48.1X2	T48.1X3	T48.1X4	T48.1X5	T48.1X6
Decholin	T47.5X1	T47.5X2	T47.5X3	T47.5X4	T47.5X5	T47.5X6
Declomycin	T36.4X1	T36.4X2	T36.4X3	T36.4X4	T36.4X5	T36.4X6
Decongestant, nasal (mucosa)	T48.5X1	T48.5X2	T48.5X3	T48.5X4	T48.5X5	T48.5X6
combination	T48.5X1	T48.5X2	T48.5X3	T48.5X4	T48.5X5	T48.5X6
Deet	T6Ø.8X1	T6Ø.8X2	T6Ø.8X3	T6Ø.8X4	—	—
Deferoxamine	T45.8X1	T45.8X2	T45.8X3	T45.8X4	T45.8X5	T45.8X6
Deflazacort	T38.ØX1	T38.ØX2	T38.ØX3	T38.ØX4	T38.ØX5	T38.ØX6
Deglycyrrhizinized extract of licorice	T48.4X1	T48.4X2	T48.4X3	T48.4X4	T48.4X5	T48.4X6
Dehydrocholic acid	T47.5X1	T47.5X2	T47.5X3	T47.5X4	T47.5X5	T47.5X6
Dehydroemetine	T37.3X1	T37.3X2	T37.3X3	T37.3X4	T37.3X5	T37.3X6
Dekalin	T52.8X1	T52.8X2	T52.8X3	T52.8X4	—	—
Delalutin	T38.5X1	T38.5X2	T38.5X3	T38.5X4	T38.5X5	T38.5X6
Delphinium	T62.2X1	T62.2X2	T62.2X3	T62.2X4	—	—
Deltasone	T38.ØX1	T38.ØX2	T38.ØX3	T38.ØX4	T38.ØX5	T38.ØX6
Deltra	T38.ØX1	T38.ØX2	T38.ØX3	T38.ØX4	T38.ØX5	T38.ØX6
Delvinal	T42.3X1	T42.3X2	T42.3X3	T42.3X4	T42.3X5	T42.3X6
Delorazepam	T42.4X1	T42.4X2	T42.4X3	T42.4X4	T42.4X5	T42.4X6
Deltamethrin	T6Ø.1X1	T6Ø.1X2	T6Ø.1X3	T6Ø.1X4	—	—
Demecarium (bromide)	T49.5X1	T49.5X2	T49.5X3	T49.5X4	T49.5X5	T49.5X6
Demeclocycline	T36.4X1	T36.4X2	T36.4X3	T36.4X4	T36.4X5	T36.4X6
Demecolcine	T45.1X1	T45.1X2	T45.1X3	T45.1X4	T45.1X5	T45.1X6
Demegestone	T38.5X1	T38.5X2	T38.5X3	T38.5X4	T38.5X5	T38.5X6
Demelanizing agents	T49.8X1	T49.8X2	T49.8X3	T49.8X4	T49.8X5	T49.8X6
Demephion -O and -S	T6Ø.ØX1	T6Ø.ØX2	T6Ø.ØX3	T6Ø.ØX4	—	—
Demerol	T4Ø.2X1	T4Ø.2X2	T4Ø.2X3	T4Ø.2X4	T4Ø.2X5	T4Ø.2X6
Demethylchlortetracycline	T36.4X1	T36.4X2	T36.4X3	T36.4X4	T36.4X5	T36.4X6
Demethyltetracycline	T36.4X1	T36.4X2	T36.4X3	T36.4X4	T36.4X5	T36.4X6
Demeton -O and -S	T6Ø.ØX1	T6Ø.ØX2	T6Ø.ØX3	T6Ø.ØX4	—	—
Demulcent (external)	T49.3X1	T49.3X2	T49.3X3	T49.3X4	T49.3X5	T49.3X6
specified NEC	T49.3X1	T49.3X2	T49.3X3	T49.3X4	T49.3X5	T49.3X6
Demulen	T38.4X1	T38.4X2	T38.4X3	T38.4X4	T38.4X5	T38.4X6
Denatured alcohol	T51.ØX1	T51.ØX2	T51.ØX3	T51.ØX4	—	—
Dendrid	T49.5X1	T49.5X2	T49.5X3	T49.5X4	T49.5X5	T49.5X6
Dental drug, topical application NEC	T49.7X1	T49.7X2	T49.7X3	T49.7X4	T49.7X5	T49.7X6
Dentifrice	T49.7X1	T49.7X2	T49.7X3	T49.7X4	T49.7X5	T49.7X6
Deodorant spray (feminine hygiene)	T49.8X1	T49.8X2	T49.8X3	T49.8X4	T49.8X5	T49.8X6
Deoxycortone	T5Ø.ØX1	T5Ø.ØX2	T5Ø.ØX3	T5Ø.ØX4	T5Ø.ØX5	T5Ø.ØX6
2-Deoxy-5-fluorouridine	T45.1X1	T45.1X2	T45.1X3	T45.1X4	T45.1X5	T45.1X6
5-Deoxy-5-fluorouridine	T45.1X1	T45.1X2	T45.1X3	T45.1X4	T45.1X5	T45.1X6
Deoxyribonuclease (pancreatic)	T45.3X1	T45.3X2	T45.3X3	T45.3X4	T45.3X5	T45.3X6
Depilatory	T49.4X1	T49.4X2	T49.4X3	T49.4X4	T49.4X5	T49.4X6
Deprenalin	T42.8X1	T42.8X2	T42.8X3	T42.8X4	T42.8X5	T42.8X6
Deprenyl	T42.8X1	T42.8X2	T42.8X3	T42.8X4	T42.8X5	T42.8X6
Depressant, appetite	T5Ø.5X1	T5Ø.5X2	T5Ø.5X3	T5Ø.5X4	T5Ø.5X5	T5Ø.5X6
Depressant						
appetite, central	T5Ø.5X1	T5Ø.5X2	T5Ø.5X3	T5Ø.5X4	T5Ø.5X5	T5Ø.5X6
cardiac	T46.2X1	T46.2X2	T46.2X3	T46.2X4	T46.2X5	T46.2X6
central nervous system (anesthetic) — *see also Central nervous system, depressants*	T42.71	T42.72	T42.73	T42.74	T42.75	T42.76
general anesthetic	T41.2Ø1	T41.2Ø2	T41.2Ø3	T41.2Ø4	T41.2Ø5	T41.2Ø6
muscle tone	T42.8X1	T42.8X2	T42.8X3	T42.8X4	T42.8X5	T42.8X6
muscle tone, central	T42.8X1	T42.8X2	T42.8X3	T42.8X4	T42.8X5	T42.8X6
psychotherapeutic	T43.5Ø1	T43.5Ø2	T43.5Ø3	T43.5Ø4	T43.5Ø5	T43.5Ø6
Deptropine	T45.ØX1	T45.ØX2	T45.ØX3	T45.ØX4	T45.ØX5	T45.ØX6
Dequalinium (chloride)	T49.ØX1	T49.ØX2	T49.ØX3	T49.ØX4	T49.ØX5	T49.ØX6
Derris root	T6Ø.2X1	T6Ø.2X2	T6Ø.2X3	T6Ø.2X4	—	—
Deserpidine	T43.Ø11	T43.Ø12	T43.Ø13	T43.Ø14	T43.Ø15	T43.Ø16
Desferrioxamine	T45.8X1	T45.8X2	T45.8X3	T45.8X4	T45.8X5	T45.8X6
Desipramine	T43.ØX1	T43.ØX2	T43.ØX3	T43.ØX4	T43.ØX5	T43.ØX6
Deslanoside	T46.ØX1	T46.ØX2	T46.ØX3	T46.ØX4	T46.ØX5	T46.ØX6
Desloughing agent	T49.4X1	T49.4X2	T49.4X3	T49.4X4	T49.4X5	T49.4X6
Desmethylimipramine	T43.Ø11	T43.Ø12	T43.Ø13	T43.Ø14	T43.Ø15	T43.Ø16
Desmopressin	T38.891	T38.892	T38.893	T38.894	T38.895	T38.896
Desocodeine	T4Ø.2X1	T4Ø.2X2	T4Ø.2X3	T4Ø.2X4	T4Ø.2X5	T4Ø.2X6
Desogestrel	T38.5X1	T38.5X2	T38.5X3	T38.5X4	T38.5X5	T38.5X6
Desomorphine	T4Ø.2X1	T4Ø.2X2	T4Ø.2X3	T4Ø.2X4	—	—
Desonide	T49.ØX1	T49.ØX2	T49.ØX3	T49.ØX4	T49.ØX5	T49.ØX6
Desoximetasone	T49.ØX1	T49.ØX2	T49.ØX3	T49.ØX4	T49.ØX5	T49.ØX6
Desoxycorticosteroid	T5Ø.ØX1	T5Ø.ØX2	T5Ø.ØX3	T5Ø.ØX4	T5Ø.ØX5	T5Ø.ØX6
Desoxycortone	T5Ø.ØX1	T5Ø.ØX2	T5Ø.ØX3	T5Ø.ØX4	T5Ø.ØX5	T5Ø.ØX6
Desoxyephedrine	T43.621	T43.622	T43.623	T43.624	T43.625	T43.626
Detaxtran	T46.6X1	T46.6X2	T46.6X3	T46.6X4	T46.6X5	T46.6X6
Detergent	T49.2X1	T49.2X2	T49.2X3	T49.2X4	T49.2X5	T49.2X6
external medication	T49.2X1	T49.2X2	T49.2X3	T49.2X4	T49.2X5	T49.2X6
local	T49.2X1	T49.2X2	T49.2X3	T49.2X4	T49.2X5	T49.2X6

Substance	Poisoning, Accidental (Unintentional)	Poisoning, Intentional Self-Harm	Poisoning, Assault	Poisoning, Undetermined	Adverse Effect	Underdosing
Detergent *(Continued)*						
medicinal	T49.2X1	T49.2X2	T49.2X3	T49.2X4	T49.2X5	T49.2X6
nonmedicinal	T55.1X1	T55.1X2	T55.1X3	T55.1X4	—	—
specified NEC	T55.1X1	T55.1X2	T55.1X3	T55.1X4	T55.1X5	T55.1X6
Deterrent, alcohol	T50.6X1	T50.6X2	T50.6X3	T50.6X4	T50.6X5	T50.6X6
Detoxifying agent	T50.6X1	T50.6X2	T50.6X3	T50.6X4	T50.6X5	T50.6X6
Detrothyronine	T38.1X1	T38.1X2	T38.1X3	T38.1X4	T38.1X5	T38.1X6
Dettol (external medication)	T49.0X1	T49.0X2	T49.0X3	T49.0X4	T49.0X5	T49.0X6
Dexamethasone	T38.0X1	T38.0X2	T38.0X3	T38.0X4	T38.0X5	T38.0X6
ENT agent	T49.6X1	T49.6X2	T49.6X3	T49.6X4	T49.6X5	T49.6X6
ophthalmic preparation	T49.5X1	T49.5X2	T49.5X3	T49.5X4	T49.5X5	T49.5X6
topical NEC	T49.0X1	T49.0X2	T49.0X3	T49.0X4	T49.0X5	T49.0X6
Dexamfetamine	T43.621	T43.622	T43.623	T43.624	T43.625	T43.626
Dexamphetamine	T43.621	T43.622	T43.623	T43.624	T43.625	T43.626
Dexbrompheniramine	T45.0X1	T45.0X2	T45.0X3	T45.0X4	T45.0X5	T45.0X6
Dexchlorpheniramine	T45.0X1	T45.0X2	T45.0X3	T45.0X4	T45.0X5	T45.0X6
Dexedrine	T43.621	T43.622	T43.623	T43.624	T43.625	T43.626
Dexetimide	T44.3X1	T44.3X2	T44.3X3	T44.3X4	T44.3X5	T44.3X6
Dexfenfluramine	T50.5X1	T50.5X2	T50.5X3	T50.5X4	T50.5X5	T50.5X6
Dexpanthenol	T45.2X1	T45.2X2	T45.2X3	T45.2X4	T45.2X5	T45.2X6
Dextran (40) (70) (150)	T45.8X1	T45.8X2	T45.8X3	T45.8X4	T45.8X5	T45.8X6
Dextriferron	T45.4X1	T45.4X2	T45.4X3	T45.4X4	T45.4X5	T45.4X6
Dextroamphetamine	T43.621	T43.622	T43.623	T43.624	T43.625	T43.626
Dextro calcium pantothenate	T45.2X1	T45.2X2	T45.2X3	T45.2X4	T45.2X5	T45.2X6
Dextromethorphan	T48.3X1	T48.3X2	T48.3X3	T48.3X4	T48.3X5	T48.3X6
Dextromoramide	T40.4X1	T40.4X2	T40.4X3	T40.4X4	—	—
topical	T49.8X1	T49.8X2	T49.8X3	T49.8X4	T49.8X5	T49.8X6
Dextro pantothenyl alcohol	T45.2X1	T45.2X2	T45.2X3	T45.2X4	T45.2X5	T45.2X6
Dextropropoxyphene	T40.4X1	T40.4X2	T40.4X3	T40.4X4	T40.4X5	T40.4X6
Dextrorphan	T40.2X1	T40.2X2	T40.2X3	T40.2X4	T40.2X5	T40.2X6
Dextrose	T50.3X1	T50.3X2	T50.3X3	T50.3X4	T50.3X5	T50.3X6
concentrated solution, intravenous	T46.8X1	T46.8X2	T46.8X3	T46.8X4	T46.8X5	T46.8X6
Dextrothyroxin	T38.1X1	T38.1X2	T38.1X3	T38.1X4	T38.1X5	T38.1X6
Dextrothyroxine sodium	T38.1X1	T38.1X2	T38.1X3	T38.1X4	T38.1X5	T38.1X6
DFP	T44.0X1	T44.0X2	T44.0X3	T44.0X4	T44.0X5	T44.0X6
DHE	T37.3X1	T37.3X2	T37.3X3	T37.3X4	T37.3X5	T37.3X6
45	T46.5X1	T46.5X2	T46.5X3	T46.5X4	T46.5X5	T46.5X6
Diabinese	T38.3X1	T38.3X2	T38.3X3	T38.3X4	T38.3X5	T38.3X6
Diacetone alcohol	T52.4X1	T52.4X2	T52.4X3	T52.4X4	—	—
Diacetyl monoxime	T50.991	T50.992	T50.993	T50.994	—	—
Diacetylmorphine	T40.1X1	T40.1X2	T40.1X3	T40.1X4	—	—

Substance	Poisoning, Accidental (Unintentional)	Poisoning, Intentional Self-Harm	Poisoning, Assault	Poisoning, Undetermined	Adverse Effect	Underdosing
Diachylon plaster	T49.4X1	T49.4X2	T49.4X3	T49.4X4	T49.4X5	T49.4X6
Diaethylstilboestrolum	T38.5X1	T38.5X2	T38.5X3	T38.5X4	T38.5X5	T38.5X6
Diagnostic agent NEC	T50.8X1	T50.8X2	T50.8X3	T50.8X4	T50.8X5	T50.8X6
Dial (soap)	T49.2X1	T49.2X2	T49.2X3	T49.2X4	T49.2X5	T49.2X6
sedative	T42.3X1	T42.3X2	T42.3X3	T42.3X4	T42.3X5	T42.3X6
Dialkyl carbonate	T52.91	T52.92	T52.93	T52.94	—	—
Diallylbarbituric acid	T42.3X1	T42.3X2	T42.3X3	T42.3X4	T42.3X5	T42.3X6
Diallymal	T42.3X1	T42.3X2	T42.3X3	T42.3X4	T42.3X5	T42.3X6
Dialysis solution (intraperitoneal)	T50.3X1	T50.3X2	T50.3X3	T50.3X4	T50.3X5	T50.3X6
Diaminodiphenylsulfone	T37.1X1	T37.1X2	T37.1X3	T37.1X4	T37.1X5	T37.1X6
Diamorphine	T40.1X1	T40.1X2	T40.1X3	T40.1X4	—	—
Diamox	T50.2X1	T50.2X2	T50.2X3	T50.2X4	T50.2X5	T50.2X6
Diamthazole	T49.0X1	T49.0X2	T49.0X3	T49.0X4	T49.0X5	T49.0X6
Dianthone	T47.2X1	T47.2X2	T47.2X3	T47.2X4	T47.2X5	T47.2X6
Diaphenylsulfone	T37.0X1	T37.0X2	T37.0X3	T37.0X4	T37.0X5	T37.0X6
Diasone (sodium)	T37.1X1	T37.1X2	T37.1X3	T37.1X4	T37.1X5	T37.1X6
Diastase	T47.5X1	T47.5X2	T47.5X3	T47.5X4	T47.5X5	T47.5X6
Diatrizoate	T50.8X1	T50.8X2	T50.8X3	T50.8X4	T50.8X5	T50.8X6
Diazepam	T42.4X1	T42.4X2	T42.4X3	T42.4X4	T42.4X5	T42.4X6
Diazinon	T60.0X1	T60.0X2	T60.0X3	T60.0X4	—	—
Diazomethane (gas)	T59.891	T59.892	T59.893	T59.894	—	—
Diazoxide	T46.5X1	T46.5X2	T46.5X3	T46.5X4	T46.5X5	T46.5X6
Dibekacin	T36.5X1	T36.5X2	T36.5X3	T36.5X4	T36.5X5	T36.5X6
Dibenamine	T44.6X1	T44.6X2	T44.6X3	T44.6X4	T44.6X5	T44.6X6
Dibenzepin	T43.011	T43.012	T43.013	T43.014	T43.015	T43.016
Dibenzheptropine	T45.0X1	T45.0X2	T45.0X3	T45.0X4	T45.0X5	T45.0X6
Dibenzyline	T44.6X1	T44.6X2	T44.6X3	T44.6X4	T44.6X5	T44.6X6
Diborane (gas)	T59.891	T59.892	T59.893	T59.894	—	—
Dibromochloropropane	T60.8X1	T60.8X2	T60.8X3	T60.8X4	—	—
Dibromodulcitol	T45.1X1	T45.1X2	T45.1X3	T45.1X4	T45.1X5	T45.1X6
Dibromoethane	T53.6X1	T53.6X2	T53.6X3	T53.6X4	—	—
Dibromomannitol	T45.1X1	T45.1X2	T45.1X3	T45.1X4	T45.1X5	T45.1X6
Dibromopropamidine isethionate	T49.0X1	T49.0X2	T49.0X3	T49.0X4	T49.0X5	T49.0X6
Dibrompropamidine	T49.0X1	T49.0X2	T49.0X3	T49.0X4	T49.0X5	T49.0X6
Dibucaine	T41.3X1	T41.3X2	T41.3X3	T41.3X4	T41.3X5	T41.3X6
topical (surface)	T41.3X1	T41.3X2	T41.3X3	T41.3X4	T41.3X5	T41.3X6
Dibunate sodium	T48.3X1	T48.3X2	T48.3X3	T48.3X4	T48.3X5	T48.3X6
Dibutoline sulfate	T44.3X1	T44.3X2	T44.3X3	T44.3X4	T44.3X5	T44.3X6
Dicamba	T60.3X1	T60.3X2	T60.3X3	T60.3X4	—	—
Dicapthon	T60.0X1	T60.0X2	T60.0X3	T60.0X4	—	—
Dichlobenil	T60.3X1	T60.3X2	T60.3X3	T60.3X4	—	—
Dichlone	T60.3X1	T60.3X2	T60.3X3	T60.3X4	—	—

Substance	Poisoning, Accidental (Unintentional)	Poisoning, Intentional Self-Harm	Poisoning, Assault	Poisoning, Undetermined	Adverse Effect	Underdosing
Dichloralphenozone	T42.6X1	T42.6X2	T42.6X3	T42.6X4	T42.6X5	T42.6X6
Dichlorbenzidine	T65.3X1	T65.3X2	T65.3X3	T65.3X4	—	—
Dichlorhydrin	T52.8X1	T52.8X2	T52.8X3	T52.8X4	—	—
Dichlorhydroxyquinoline	T37.8X1	T37.8X2	T37.8X3	T37.8X4	T37.8X5	T37.8X6
Dichlorobenzene	T53.7X1	T53.7X2	T53.7X3	T53.7X4	—	—
Dichlorobenzyl alcohol	T49.6X1	T49.6X2	T49.6X3	T49.6X4	T49.6X5	T49.6X6
Dichlorodifluoromethane	T53.5X1	T53.5X2	T53.5X3	T53.5X4	—	—
Dichloroethane	T52.8X1	T52.8X2	T52.8X3	T52.8X4	—	—
Sym-Dichloroethyl ether	T53.6X1	T53.6X2	T53.6X3	T53.6X4	—	—
Dichloroethyl sulfide, not in war	T59.891	T59.892	T59.893	T59.894	—	—
Dichloroethylene	T53.6X1	T53.6X2	T53.6X3	T53.6X4	—	—
Dichloroformoxine, not in war	T59.891	T59.892	T59.893	T59.894	—	—
Dichlorohydrin, alpha-dichlorohydrin	T52.8X1	T52.8X2	T52.8X3	T52.8X4	—	—
Dichloromethane (solvent)	T53.4X1	T53.4X2	T53.4X3	T53.4X4	—	—
vapor	T53.4X1	T53.4X2	T53.4X3	T53.4X4	—	—
Dichloronaphthoquinone	T60.3X1	T60.3X2	T60.3X3	T60.3X4	—	—
Dichlorophen	T37.4X1	T37.4X2	T37.4X3	T37.4X4	T37.4X5	T37.4X6
2,4-Dichlorophenoxy-acetic acid	T60.3X1	T60.3X2	T60.3X3	T60.3X4	—	—
Dichloropropene	T60.3X1	T60.3X2	T60.3X3	T60.3X4	—	—
Dichloropropionic acid	T60.3X1	T60.3X2	T60.3X3	T60.3X4	—	—
Dichlorphenamide	T50.2X1	T50.2X2	T50.2X3	T50.2X4	T50.2X5	T50.2X6
Dichlorvos	T60.0X1	T60.0X2	T60.0X3	T60.0X4	—	—
Diclofenac	T39.391	T39.392	T39.393	T39.394	T39.395	T39.396
Diclofenamide	T50.2X1	T50.2X2	T50.2X3	T50.2X4	T50.2X5	T50.2X6
Diclofensine	T43.291	T43.292	T43.293	T43.294	T43.295	T43.296
Diclonixine	T39.8X1	T39.8X2	T39.8X3	T39.8X4	T39.8X5	T39.8X6
Dicloxacillin	T36.0X1	T36.0X2	T36.0X3	T36.0X4	T36.0X5	T36.0X6
Dicophane	T49.0X1	T49.0X2	T49.0X3	T49.0X4	T49.0X5	T49.0X6
Dicoumarol, dicoumarin, dicumarol	T45.511	T45.512	T45.513	T45.514	T45.515	T45.516
Dicrotophos	T60.0X1	T60.0X2	T60.0X3	T60.0X4	—	—
Dicyanogen (gas)	T65.0X1	T65.0X2	T65.0X3	T65.0X4	—	—
Dicyclomine	T44.3X1	T44.3X2	T44.3X3	T44.3X4	T44.3X5	T44.3X6
Dicycloverine	T44.3X1	T44.3X2	T44.3X3	T44.3X4	T44.3X5	T44.3X6
Dideoxycytidine	T37.5X1	T37.5X2	T37.5X3	T37.5X4	T37.5X5	T37.5X6
Dideoxyinosine	T37.5X1	T37.5X2	T37.5X3	T37.5X4	T37.5X5	T37.5X6
Dieldrin (vapor)	T60.1X1	T60.1X2	T60.1X3	T60.1X4	—	—
Diemal	T42.3X1	T42.3X2	T42.3X3	T42.3X4	T42.3X5	T42.3X6
Dienestrol	T38.5X1	T38.5X2	T38.5X3	T38.5X4	T38.5X5	T38.5X6
Dienoestrol	T38.5X1	T38.5X2	T38.5X3	T38.5X4	T38.5X5	T38.5X6
Dietetic drug NEC	T50.901	T50.902	T50.903	T50.904	T50.905	T50.906
Diethazine	T42.8X1	T42.8X2	T42.8X3	T42.8X4	T42.8X5	T42.8X6
Diethyl						
barbituric acid	T42.3X1	T42.3X2	T42.3X3	T42.3X4	T42.3X5	T42.3X6
carbamazine	T37.4X1	T37.4X2	T37.4X3	T37.4X4	T37.4X5	T37.4X6
carbinol	T51.3X1	T51.3X2	T51.3X3	T51.3X4	—	—
carbonate	T52.8X1	T52.8X2	T52.8X3	T52.8X4	—	—
ether (vapor) — *see also* ether	T41.0X1	T41.0X2	T41.0X3	T41.0X4	T41.0X5	T41.0X6
oxide	T52.8X1	T52.8X2	T52.8X3	T52.8X4	—	—
propion	T50.5X1	T50.5X2	T50.5X3	T50.5X4	T50.5X5	T50.5X6
stilbestrol	T38.5X1	T38.5X2	T38.5X3	T38.5X4	T38.5X5	T38.5X6
toluamide (nonmedicinal)	T60.8X1	T60.8X2	T60.8X3	T60.8X4	—	—
medicinal	T49.3X1	T49.3X2	T49.3X3	T49.3X4	T49.3X5	T49.3X6
Diethylcarbamazine	T37.4X1	T37.4X2	T37.4X3	T37.4X4	T37.4X5	T37.4X6
Diethylene						
dioxide	T52.8X1	T52.8X2	T52.8X3	T52.8X4	—	—
glycol (monoacetate) (monobutyl ether) (monoethyl ether)	T52.3X1	T52.3X2	T52.3X3	T52.3X4	—	—
Diethylhexylphthalate	T65.891	T65.892	T65.893	T65.894	—	—
Diethylpropion	T50.5X1	T50.5X2	T50.5X3	T50.5X4	T50.5X5	T50.5X6
Diethylstilbestrol	T38.5X1	T38.5X2	T38.5X3	T38.5X4	T38.5X5	T38.5X6
Diethylstilboestrol	T38.5X1	T38.5X2	T38.5X3	T38.5X4	T38.5X5	T38.5X6
Diethylsulfone-diethylmethane	T42.6X1	T42.6X2	T42.6X3	T42.6X4	T42.6X5	T42.6X6
Diethyltoluamide	T49.0X1	T49.0X2	T49.0X3	T49.0X4	T49.0X5	T49.0X6
Diethyltryptamine (DET)	T40.991	T40.992	T40.993	T40.994	—	—
Difebarbamate	T42.3X1	T42.3X2	T42.3X3	T42.3X4	T42.3X5	T42.3X6
Difencloxazine	T40.2X1	T40.2X2	T40.2X3	T40.2X4	T40.2X5	T40.2X6
Difenidol	T45.0X1	T45.0X2	T45.0X3	T45.0X4	T45.0X5	T45.0X6
Difenoxin	T47.6X1	T47.6X2	T47.6X3	T47.6X4	T47.6X5	T47.6X6
Difetarsone	T37.3X1	T37.3X2	T37.3X3	T37.3X4	T37.3X5	T37.3X6
Diffusin	T45.3X1	T45.3X2	T45.3X3	T45.3X4	T45.3X5	T45.3X6
Diflorasone	T49.0X1	T49.0X2	T49.0X3	T49.0X4	T49.0X5	T49.0X6
Diflubenzuron	T60.1X1	T60.1X2	T60.1X3	T60.1X4	—	—
Diflos	T44.0X1	T44.0X2	T44.0X3	T44.0X4	T44.0X5	T44.0X6
Diflucortolone	T49.0X1	T49.0X2	T49.0X3	T49.0X4	T49.0X5	T49.0X6
Diflunisal	T39.091	T39.092	T39.093	T39.094	T39.095	T39.096
Difluoromethyldopa	T42.8X1	T42.8X2	T42.8X3	T42.8X4	T42.8X5	T42.8X6
Difluorophate	T44.0X1	T44.0X2	T44.0X3	T44.0X4	T44.0X5	T44.0X6
Digestant NEC	T47.5X1	T47.5X2	T47.5X3	T47.5X4	T47.5X5	T47.5X6
Digitalin(e)	T46.0X1	T46.0X2	T46.0X3	T46.0X4	T46.0X5	T46.0X6
Digitalis (leaf) (glycoside)	T46.0X1	T46.0X2	T46.0X3	T46.0X4	T46.0X5	T46.0X6
lanata	T46.0X1	T46.0X2	T46.0X3	T46.0X4	T46.0X5	T46.0X6
purpurea	T46.0X1	T46.0X2	T46.0X3	T46.0X4	T46.0X5	T46.0X6
Digitoxin	T46.0X1	T46.0X2	T46.0X3	T46.0X4	T46.0X5	T46.0X6

TABLE OF DRUGS AND CHEMICALS

◀ New ⬅ Revised ~~deleted~~ Deleted

Substance	Poisoning, Accidental (Unintentional)	Poisoning, Intentional Self-Harm	Poisoning, Assault	Poisoning, Undetermined	Adverse Effect	Underdosing
Digitoxose	T46.0X1	T46.0X2	T46.0X3	T46.0X4	T46.0X5	T46.0X6
Digoxin	T46.0X1	T46.0X2	T46.0X3	T46.0X4	T46.0X5	T46.0X6
Digoxine	T46.0X1	T46.0X2	T46.0X3	T46.0X4	T46.0X5	T46.0X6
Dihydralazine	T46.5X1	T46.5X2	T46.5X3	T46.5X4	T46.5X5	T46.5X6
Dihydrazine	T46.5X1	T46.5X2	T46.5X3	T46.5X4	T46.5X5	T46.5X6
Dihydrocodeinone	T40.2X1	T40.2X2	T40.2X3	T40.2X4	T40.2X5	T40.2X6
Dihydroergocornine	T46.7X1	T46.7X2	T46.7X3	T46.7X4	T46.7X5	T46.7X6
Dihydroergocristine (mesilate)	T46.7X1	T46.7X2	T46.7X3	T46.7X4	T46.7X5	T46.7X6
Dihydroergokryptine	T46.7X1	T46.7X2	T46.7X3	T46.7X4	T46.7X5	T46.7X6
Dihydroergotamine	T46.5X1	T46.5X2	T46.5X3	T46.5X4	T46.5X5	T46.5X6
Dihydroergotoxine	T46.7X1	T46.7X2	T46.7X3	T46.7X4	T46.7X5	T46.7X6
mesilate	T46.7X1	T46.7X2	T46.7X3	T46.7X4	T46.7X5	T46.7X6
Dihydrohydroxycodein-one	T40.2X1	T40.2X2	T40.2X3	T40.2X4	T40.2X5	T40.2X6
Dihydrohydroxymorphinone	T40.2X1	T40.2X2	T40.2X3	T40.2X4	T40.2X5	T40.2X6
Dihydroisocodeine	T40.2X1	T40.2X2	T40.2X3	T40.2X4	T40.2X5	T40.2X6
Dihydromorphine	T40.2X1	T40.2X2	T40.2X3	T40.2X4	—	—
Dihydromorphinone	T40.2X1	T40.2X2	T40.2X3	T40.2X4	T40.2X5	T40.2X6
Dihydrostreptomycin	T36.5X1	T36.5X2	T36.5X3	T36.5X4	T36.5X5	T36.5X6
Dihydrotachysterol	T45.2X1	T45.2X2	T45.2X3	T45.2X4	T45.2X5	T45.2X6
Dihydroxyaluminum aminoacetate	T47.1X1	T47.1X2	T47.1X3	T47.1X4	T47.1X5	T47.1X6
Dihydroxyaluminum sodium carbonate	T47.1X1	T47.1X2	T47.1X3	T47.1X4	T47.1X5	T47.1X6
Dihydroxyanthraquinone	T47.2X1	T47.2X2	T47.2X3	T47.2X4	T47.2X5	T47.2X6
Dihydroxycodeinone	T40.2X1	T40.2X2	T40.2X3	T40.2X4	T40.2X5	T40.2X6
Dihydroxypropyl theophylline	T50.2X1	T50.2X2	T50.2X3	T50.2X4	T50.2X5	T50.2X6
Diiodohydroxyquin	T37.8X1	T37.8X2	T37.8X3	T37.8X4	T37.8X5	T37.8X6
topical	T49.0X1	T49.0X2	T49.0X3	T49.0X4	T49.0X5	T49.0X6
Diiodohydroxyquinoline	T37.8X1	T37.8X2	T37.8X3	T37.8X4	T37.8X5	T37.8X6
Diiodotyrosine	T38.2X1	T38.2X2	T38.2X3	T38.2X4	T38.2X5	T38.2X6
Diisopromine	T44.3X1	T44.3X2	T44.3X3	T44.3X4	T44.3X5	T44.3X6
Diisopropylamine	T46.3X1	T46.3X2	T46.3X3	T46.3X4	T46.3X5	T46.3X6
Diisopropylfluorophosphonate	T44.0X1	T44.0X2	T44.0X3	T44.0X4	T44.0X5	T44.0X6
Dilantin	T42.0X1	T42.0X2	T42.0X3	T42.0X4	T42.0X5	T42.0X6
Dilaudid	T40.2X1	T40.2X2	T40.2X3	T40.2X4	T40.2X5	T40.2X6
Dilazep	T46.3X1	T46.3X2	T46.3X3	T46.3X4	T46.3X5	T46.3X6
Dill	T47.5X1	T47.5X2	T47.5X3	T47.5X4	T47.5X5	T47.5X6
Diloxanide	T37.3X1	T37.3X2	T37.3X3	T37.3X4	T37.3X5	T37.3X6
Diltiazem	T46.1X1	T46.1X2	T46.1X3	T46.1X4	T46.1X5	T46.1X6
Dimazole	T49.0X1	T49.0X2	T49.0X3	T49.0X4	T49.0X5	T49.0X6
Dimefline	T50.7X1	T50.7X2	T50.7X3	T50.7X4	T50.7X5	T50.7X6
Dimefox	T60.0X1	T60.0X2	T60.0X3	T60.0X4	—	—

Substance	Poisoning, Accidental (Unintentional)	Poisoning, Intentional Self-Harm	Poisoning, Assault	Poisoning, Undetermined	Adverse Effect	Underdosing
Dimemorfan	T48.3X1	T48.3X2	T48.3X3	T48.3X4	T48.3X5	T48.3X6
Dimenhydrinate	T45.0X1	T45.0X2	T45.0X3	T45.0X4	T45.0X5	T45.0X6
Dimercaprol (British anti-lewisite)	T45.8X1	T45.8X2	T45.8X3	T45.8X4	T45.8X5	T45.8X6
Dimercaptopropanol	T45.8X1	T45.8X2	T45.8X3	T45.8X4	T45.8X5	T45.8X6
Dimestrol	T38.5X1	T38.5X2	T38.5X3	T38.5X4	T38.5X5	T38.5X6
Dimetane	T45.0X1	T45.0X2	T45.0X3	T45.0X4	T45.0X5	T45.0X6
Dimethicone	T47.1X1	T47.1X2	T47.1X3	T47.1X4	T47.1X5	T47.1X6
Dimethindene	T45.0X1	T45.0X2	T45.0X3	T45.0X4	T45.0X5	T45.0X6
Dimethisoquin	T49.1X1	T49.1X2	T49.1X3	T49.1X4	T49.1X5	T49.1X6
Dimethisterone	T38.5X1	T38.5X2	T38.5X3	T38.5X4	T38.5X5	T38.5X6
Dimethoate	T60.0X1	T60.0X2	T60.0X3	T60.0X4	—	—
Dimethocaine	T41.3X1	T41.3X2	T41.3X3	T41.3X4	T41.3X5	T41.3X6
Dimethoxanate	T48.3X1	T48.3X2	T48.3X3	T48.3X4	T48.3X5	T48.3X6
Dimethyl						
arsine, arsinic acid	T57.0X1	T57.0X2	T57.0X3	T57.0X4	—	—
carbinol	T51.2X1	T51.2X2	T51.2X3	T51.2X4	—	—
carbonate	T52.8X1	T52.8X2	T52.8X3	T52.8X4	—	—
diguanide	T38.3X1	T38.3X2	T38.3X3	T38.3X4	T38.3X5	T38.3X6
ketone	T52.4X1	T52.4X2	T52.4X3	T52.4X4	—	—
vapor	T52.4X1	T52.4X2	T52.4X3	T52.4X4	—	—
meperidine	T40.2X1	T40.2X2	T40.2X3	T40.2X4	T40.2X5	T40.2X6
parathion	T60.0X1	T60.0X2	T60.0X3	T60.0X4	—	—
phthlate	T49.3X1	T49.3X2	T49.3X3	T49.3X4	T49.3X5	T49.3X6
polysiloxane	T47.8X1	T47.8X2	T47.8X3	T47.8X4	T47.8X5	T47.8X6
sulfate (fumes)	T59.891	T59.892	T59.893	T59.894	—	—
liquid	T65.891	T65.892	T65.893	T65.894	—	—
sulfoxide (nonmedicinal)	T52.8X1	T52.8X2	T52.8X3	T52.8X4	—	—
medicinal	T49.4X1	T49.4X2	T49.4X3	T49.4X4	T49.4X5	T49.4X6
tryptamine	T40.991	T40.992	T40.993	T40.994	—	—
tubocurarine	T48.1X1	T48.1X2	T48.1X3	T48.1X4	T48.1X5	T48.1X6
Dimethylamine sulfate	T49.4X1	T49.4X2	T49.4X3	T49.4X4	T49.4X5	T49.4X6
Dimethylformamide	T52.8X1	T52.8X2	T52.8X3	T52.8X4	—	—
Dimethyltubocurarinium chloride	T48.1X1	T48.1X2	T48.1X3	T48.1X4	T48.1X5	T48.1X6
Dimeticone	T47.1X1	T47.1X2	T47.1X3	T47.1X4	T47.1X5	T47.1X6
Dimetilan	T60.0X1	T60.0X2	T60.0X3	T60.0X4	—	—
Dimetindene	T45.0X1	T45.0X2	T45.0X3	T45.0X4	T45.0X5	T45.0X6
Dimetotiazine	T43.3X1	T43.3X2	T43.3X3	T43.3X4	T43.3X5	T43.3X6
Dimorpholamine	T50.7X1	T50.7X2	T50.7X3	T50.7X4	T50.7X5	T50.7X6
Dimoxyline	T46.3X1	T46.3X2	T46.3X3	T46.3X4	T46.3X5	T46.3X6
Dinitrobenzene	T65.3X1	T65.3X2	T65.3X3	T65.3X4	—	—
vapor	T59.891	T59.892	T59.893	T59.894	—	—

Substance	Poisoning, Accidental (Unintentional)	Poisoning, Intentional Self-Harm	Poisoning, Assault	Poisoning, Undetermined	Adverse Effect	Underdosing
Dinitrobenzol	T65.3X1	T65.3X2	T65.3X3	T65.3X4	—	—
vapor	T59.891	T59.892	T59.893	T59.894	—	—
Dinitrobutylphenol	T65.3X1	T65.3X2	T65.3X3	T65.3X4	—	—
Dinitro (-ortho-)cresol (pesticide) (spray)	T65.3X1	T65.3X2	T65.3X3	T65.3X4	—	—
Dinitrocyclohexylphenol	T65.3X1	T65.3X2	T65.3X3	T65.3X4	—	—
Dinitrophenol	T65.3X1	T65.3X2	T65.3X3	T65.3X4	—	—
Dinoprost	T48.0X1	T48.0X2	T48.0X3	T48.0X4	T48.0X5	T48.0X6
Dinoprostone	T48.0X1	T48.0X2	T48.0X3	T48.0X4	T48.0X5	T48.0X6
Dinoseb	T60.3X1	T60.3X2	T60.3X3	T60.3X4	—	—
Dioctyl sulfosuccinate (calcium) (sodium)	T47.4X1	T47.4X2	T47.4X3	T47.4X4	T47.4X5	T47.4X6
Diodone	T50.8X1	T50.8X2	T50.8X3	T50.8X4	T50.8X5	T50.8X6
Diodoquin	T37.8X1	T37.8X2	T37.8X3	T37.8X4	T37.8X5	T37.8X6
Dionin	T40.2X1	T40.2X2	T40.2X3	T40.2X4	T40.2X5	T40.2X6
Diosmin	T46.991	T46.992	T46.993	T46.994	T46.995	T46.996
Dioxane	T52.8X1	T52.8X2	T52.8X3	T52.8X4	—	—
Dioxathion	T60.0X1	T60.0X2	T60.0X3	T60.0X4	—	—
Dioxin	T53.7X1	T53.7X2	T53.7X3	T53.7X4	—	—
Dioxopromethazine	T43.3X1	T43.3X2	T43.3X3	T43.3X4	T43.3X5	T43.3X6
Dioxyline	T46.3X1	T46.3X2	T46.3X3	T46.3X4	T46.3X5	T46.3X6
Dipentene	T52.8X1	T52.8X2	T52.8X3	T52.8X4	—	—
Diperodon	T41.3X1	T41.3X2	T41.3X3	T41.3X4	T41.3X5	T41.3X6
Diphacinone	T60.4X1	T60.4X2	T60.4X3	T60.4X4	—	—
Diphemanil	T44.3X1	T44.3X2	T44.3X3	T44.3X4	T44.3X5	T44.3X6
metilsulfate	T44.3X1	T44.3X2	T44.3X3	T44.3X4	T44.3X5	T44.3X6
Diphenadione	T45.511	T45.512	T45.513	T45.514	T45.515	T45.516
rodenticide	T60.4X1	T60.4X2	T60.4X3	T60.4X4	—	—
Diphenhydramine	T45.0X1	T45.0X2	T45.0X3	T45.0X4	T45.0X5	T45.0X6
Diphenidol	T45.0X1	T45.0X2	T45.0X3	T45.0X4	T45.0X5	T45.0X6
Diphenoxylate	T47.6X1	T47.6X2	T47.6X3	T47.6X4	T47.6X5	T47.6X6
Diphenylamine	T65.3X1	T65.3X2	T65.3X3	T65.3X4	—	—
Diphenylbutazone	T39.2X1	T39.2X2	T39.2X3	T39.2X4	T39.2X5	T39.2X6
Diphenylchloroarsine, not in war	T57.0X1	T57.0X2	T57.0X3	T57.0X4	—	—
Diphenylhydantoin	T42.0X1	T42.0X2	T42.0X3	T42.0X4	T42.0X5	T42.0X6
Diphenylmethane dye	T52.1X1	T52.1X2	T52.1X3	T52.1X4	—	—
Diphenylpyraline	T45.0X1	T45.0X2	T45.0X3	T45.0X4	T45.0X5	T45.0X6
Diphtheria						
antitoxin	T50.Z11	T50.Z12	T50.Z13	T50.Z14	T50.Z15	T50.Z16
toxoid	T50.A91	T50.A92	T50.A93	T50.A94	T50.A95	T50.A96
with tetanus toxoid	T50.A21	T50.A22	T50.A23	T50.A24	T50.A25	T50.A26
with pertussis component	T50.A11	T50.A12	T50.A13	T50.A14	T50.A15	T50.A16
Diphtheria *(Continued)*						
vaccine (combination)	T50.A91	T50.A92	T50.A93	T50.A94	T50.A95	T50.A96
combination						
including pertussis	T50.A11	T50.A12	T50.A13	T50.A14	T50.A15	T50.A16
without pertussis	T50.A21	T50.A22	T50.A23	T50.A24	T50.A25	T50.A26
Diphylline	T50.2X1	T50.2X2	T50.2X3	T50.2X4	T50.2X5	T50.2X6
Dipipanone	T40.4X1	T40.4X2	T40.4X3	T40.4X4	—	—
Dipivefrine	T49.5X1	T49.5X2	T49.5X3	T49.5X4	T49.5X5	T49.5X6
Diplovax	T50.B91	T50.B92	T50.B93	T50.B94	T50.B95	T50.B96
Diprophylline	T50.2X1	T50.2X2	T50.2X3	T50.2X4	T50.2X5	T50.2X6
Dipropyline	T48.291	T48.292	T48.293	T48.294	T48.295	T48.296
Dipyridamole	T46.3X1	T46.3X2	T46.3X3	T46.3X4	T46.3X5	T46.3X6
Dipyrone	T39.2X1	T39.2X2	T39.2X3	T39.2X4	T39.2X5	T39.2X6
Diquat (dibromide)	T60.3X1	T60.3X2	T60.3X3	T60.3X4	—	—
Disinfectant	T65.891	T65.892	T65.893	T65.894	—	—
alkaline	T54.3X1	T54.3X2	T54.3X3	T54.3X4	—	—
aromatic	T54.1X1	T54.1X2	T54.1X3	T54.1X4	—	—
intestinal	T37.8X1	T37.8X2	T37.8X3	T37.8X4	T37.8X5	T37.8X6
Disipal	T42.8X1	T42.8X2	T42.8X3	T42.8X4	T42.8X5	T42.8X6
Disodium edetate	T50.6X1	T50.6X2	T50.6X3	T50.6X4	T50.6X5	T50.6X6
Disoprofol	T41.291	T41.292	T41.293	T41.294	T41.295	T41.296
Disopyramide	T46.2X1	T46.2X2	T46.2X3	T46.2X4	T46.2X5	T46.2X6
Distigmine (bromide)	T44.0X1	T44.0X2	T44.0X3	T44.0X4	T44.0X5	T44.0X6
Disulfamide	T50.2X1	T50.2X2	T50.2X3	T50.2X4	T50.2X5	T50.2X6
Disulfanilamide	T37.0X1	T37.0X2	T37.0X3	T37.0X4	T37.0X5	T37.0X6
Disulfiram	T50.6X1	T50.6X2	T50.6X3	T50.6X4	T50.6X5	T50.6X6
Disulfoton	T60.0X1	T60.0X2	T60.0X3	T60.0X4	—	—
Dithiazanine iodide	T37.4X1	T37.4X2	T37.4X3	T37.4X4	T37.4X5	T37.4X6
Dithiocarbamate	T60.0X1	T60.0X2	T60.0X3	T60.0X4	—	—
Dithranol	T49.4X1	T49.4X2	T49.4X3	T49.4X4	T49.4X5	T49.4X6
Diucardin	T50.2X1	T50.2X2	T50.2X3	T50.2X4	T50.2X5	T50.2X6
Diupres	T50.2X1	T50.2X2	T50.2X3	T50.2X4	T50.2X5	T50.2X6
Diuretic NEC	T50.2X1	T50.2X2	T50.2X3	T50.2X4	T50.2X5	T50.2X6
benzothiadiazine	T50.2X1	T50.2X2	T50.2X3	T50.2X4	T50.2X5	T50.2X6
carbonic acid anhydrase inhibitors	T50.2X1	T50.2X2	T50.2X3	T50.2X4	T50.2X5	T50.2X6
furfuryl NEC	T50.2X1	T50.2X2	T50.2X3	T50.2X4	T50.2X5	T50.2X6
loop (high-ceiling)	T50.1X1	T50.1X2	T50.1X3	T50.1X4	T50.1X5	T50.1X6
mercurial NEC	T50.2X1	T50.2X2	T50.2X3	T50.2X4	T50.2X5	T50.2X6
osmotic	T50.2X1	T50.2X2	T50.2X3	T50.2X4	T50.2X5	T50.2X6
purine NEC	T50.2X1	T50.2X2	T50.2X3	T50.2X4	T50.2X5	T50.2X6
saluretic NEC	T50.2X1	T50.2X2	T50.2X3	T50.2X4	T50.2X5	T50.2X6

◀ New ⇐ Revised ~~deleted~~ Deleted

Substance	Poisoning, Accidental (Unintentional)	Poisoning, Intentional Self-Harm	Poisoning, Assault	Poisoning, Undetermined	Adverse Effect	Underdosing
Diuretic NEC *(Continued)*						
sulfonamide	T50.2X1	T50.2X2	T50.2X3	T50.2X4	T50.2X5	T50.2X6
thiazide NEC	T50.2X1	T50.2X2	T50.2X3	T50.2X4	T50.2X5	T50.2X6
xanthine	T50.2X1	T50.2X2	T50.2X3	T50.2X4	T50.2X5	T50.2X6
Diurgin	T50.2X1	T50.2X2	T50.2X3	T50.2X4	T50.2X5	T50.2X6
Diuril	T50.2X1	T50.2X2	T50.2X3	T50.2X4	T50.2X5	T50.2X6
Diuron	T60.3X1	T60.3X2	T60.3X3	T60.3X4	—	—
Divalproex	T42.6X1	T42.6X2	T42.6X3	T42.6X4	T42.6X5	T42.6X6
Divinyl ether	T41.0X1	T41.0X2	T41.0X3	T41.0X4	T41.0X5	T41.0X6
Dixanthogen	T49.0X1	T49.0X2	T49.0X3	T49.0X4	T49.0X5	T49.0X6
Dixyrazine	T43.3X1	T43.3X2	T43.3X3	T43.3X4	T43.3X5	T43.3X6
D-lysergic acid diethylamide	T40.8X1	T40.8X2	T40.8X3	T40.8X4	—	—
DMCT	T36.4X1	T36.4X2	T36.4X3	T36.4X4	T36.4X5	T36.4X6
DMSO — *see Dimethyl sulfoxide*						
DNBP	T60.3X1	T60.3X2	T60.3X3	T60.3X4	—	—
DNOC	T65.3X1	T65.3X2	T65.3X3	T65.3X4	—	—
DOCA	T38.0X1	T38.0X2	T38.0X3	T38.0X4	T38.0X5	T38.0X6
Dobutamine	T44.5X1	T44.5X2	T44.5X3	T44.5X4	T44.5X5	T44.5X6
Docusate sodium	T47.4X1	T47.4X2	T47.4X3	T47.4X4	T47.4X5	T47.4X6
Dodicin	T49.0X1	T49.0X2	T49.0X3	T49.0X4	T49.0X5	T49.0X6
Dofamium chloride	T49.0X1	T49.0X2	T49.0X3	T49.0X4	T49.0X5	T49.0X6
Dolophine	T40.3X1	T40.3X2	T40.3X3	T40.3X4	T40.3X5	T40.3X6
Doloxene	T39.8X1	T39.8X2	T39.8X3	T39.8X4	T39.8X5	T39.8X6
Domestic gas (after combustion) — *see Gas, utility*						
prior to combustion	T59.891	T59.892	T59.893	T59.894	—	—
Domiodol	T48.4X1	T48.4X2	T48.4X3	T48.4X4	T48.4X5	T48.4X6
Domiphen (bromide)	T49.0X1	T49.0X2	T49.0X3	T49.0X4	T49.0X5	T49.0X6
Domperidone	T45.0X1	T45.0X2	T45.0X3	T45.0X4	T45.0X5	T45.0X6
Dopa	T42.8X1	T42.8X2	T42.8X3	T42.8X4	T42.8X5	T42.8X6
Dopamine	T44.991	T44.992	T44.993	T44.994	T44.995	T44.996
Doriden	T42.6X1	T42.6X2	T42.6X3	T42.6X4	T42.6X5	T42.6X6
Dormiral	T42.3X1	T42.3X2	T42.3X3	T42.3X4	T42.3X5	T42.3X6
Dormison	T42.6X1	T42.6X2	T42.6X3	T42.6X4	T42.6X5	T42.6X6
Dornase	T48.4X1	T48.4X2	T48.4X3	T48.4X4	T48.4X5	T48.4X6
Dorsacaine	T41.3X1	T41.3X2	T41.3X3	T41.3X4	T41.3X5	T41.3X6
Dosulepin	T43.011	T43.012	T43.013	T43.014	T43.015	T43.016
Dothiepin	T43.011	T43.012	T43.013	T43.014	T43.015	T43.016
Doxantrazole	T48.6X1	T48.6X2	T48.6X3	T48.6X4	T48.6X5	T48.6X6
Doxapram	T50.7X1	T50.7X2	T50.7X3	T50.7X4	T50.7X5	T50.7X6
Doxazosin	T44.6X1	T44.6X2	T44.6X3	T44.6X4	T44.6X5	T44.6X6
Doxepin	T43.011	T43.012	T43.013	T43.014	T43.015	T43.016

Substance	Poisoning, Accidental (Unintentional)	Poisoning, Intentional Self-Harm	Poisoning, Assault	Poisoning, Undetermined	Adverse Effect	Underdosing
Doxifluridine	T45.1X1	T45.1X2	T45.1X3	T45.1X4	T45.1X5	T45.1X6
Doxorubicin	T45.1X1	T45.1X2	T45.1X3	T45.1X4	T45.1X5	T45.1X6
Doxycycline	T36.4X1	T36.4X2	T36.4X3	T36.4X4	T36.4X5	T36.4X6
Doxylamine	T45.0X1	T45.0X2	T45.0X3	T45.0X4	T45.0X5	T45.0X6
Dramamine	T45.0X1	T45.0X2	T45.0X3	T45.0X4	T45.0X5	T45.0X6
Drano (drain cleaner)	T54.3X1	T54.3X2	T54.3X3	T54.3X4	—	—
Dressing, live pulp	T49.7X1	T49.7X2	T49.7X3	T49.7X4	T49.7X5	T49.7X6
Drocode	T40.2X1	T40.2X2	T40.2X3	T40.2X4	T40.2X5	T40.2X6
Dromoran	T40.2X1	T40.2X2	T40.2X3	T40.2X4	T40.2X5	T40.2X6
Dromostanolone	T38.7X1	T38.7X2	T38.7X3	T38.7X4	T38.7X5	T38.7X6
Dronabinol	T40.7X1	T40.7X2	T40.7X3	T40.7X4	T40.7X5	T40.7X6
Droperidol	T43.591	T43.592	T43.593	T43.594	T43.595	T43.596
Dropropizine	T48.3X1	T48.3X2	T48.3X3	T48.3X4	T48.3X5	T48.3X6
Drostanolone	T38.7X1	T38.7X2	T38.7X3	T38.7X4	T38.7X5	T38.7X6
Drotaverine	T44.3X1	T44.3X2	T44.3X3	T44.3X4	T44.3X5	T44.3X6
Drotrecogin alfa	T45.511	T45.512	T45.513	T45.514	T45.515	T45.516
Drug NEC	T50.901	T50.902	T50.903	T50.904	T50.905	T50.906
specified NEC	T50.991	T50.992	T50.993	T50.994	T50.995	T50.996
DTIC	T45.1X1	T45.1X2	T45.1X3	T45.1X4	T45.1X5	T45.1X6
Duboisine	T44.3X1	T44.3X2	T44.3X3	T44.3X4	T44.3X5	T44.3X6
Dulcolax	T47.2X1	T47.2X2	T47.2X3	T47.2X4	T47.2X5	T47.2X6
Duponol (C) (EP)	T49.2X1	T49.2X2	T49.2X3	T49.2X4	T49.2X5	T49.2X6
Durabolin	T38.7X1	T38.7X2	T38.7X3	T38.7X4	T38.7X5	T38.7X6
Dyclone	T41.3X1	T41.3X2	T41.3X3	T41.3X4	T41.3X5	T41.3X6
Dyclonine	T41.3X1	T41.3X2	T41.3X3	T41.3X4	T41.3X5	T41.3X6
Dydrogesterone	T38.5X1	T38.5X2	T38.5X3	T38.5X4	T38.5X5	T38.5X6
Dye NEC	T65.6X1	T65.6X2	T65.6X3	T65.6X4	—	—
antiseptic	T49.0X1	T49.0X2	T49.0X3	T49.0X4	T49.0X5	T49.0X6
diagnostic agents	T50.8X1	T50.8X2	T50.8X3	T50.8X4	T50.8X5	T50.8X6
pharmaceutical NEC	T50.901	T50.902	T50.903	T50.904	T50.905	T50.906
Dyflos	T44.0X1	T44.0X2	T44.0X3	T44.0X4	T44.0X5	T44.0X6
Dymelor	T38.3X1	T38.3X2	T38.3X3	T38.3X4	T38.3X5	T38.3X6
Dynamite	T65.3X1	T65.3X2	T65.3X3	T65.3X4	—	—
fumes	T59.891	T59.892	T59.893	T59.894	—	—
Dyphylline	T44.3X1	T44.3X2	T44.3X3	T44.3X4	T44.3X5	T44.3X6
E						
Ear drug NEC	T49.6X1	T49.6X2	T49.6X3	T49.6X4	T49.6X5	T49.6X6
Ear preparations	T49.6X1	T49.6X2	T49.6X3	T49.6X4	T49.6X5	T49.6X6
Econazole	T49.0X1	T49.0X2	T49.0X3	T49.0X4	T49.0X5	T49.0X6
Ecothiopate iodide	T49.5X1	T49.5X2	T49.5X3	T49.5X4	T49.5X5	T49.5X6
Echothiophate, echothiopate, ecothiopate	T49.5X1	T49.5X2	T49.5X3	T49.5X4	T49.5X5	T49.5X6

Substance	Poisoning, Accidental (Unintentional)	Poisoning, Intentional Self-Harm	Poisoning, Assault	Poisoning, Undetermined	Adverse Effect	Underdosing
Ecstasy	T43.621	T43.622	T43.623	T43.624	T43.625	T43.626
Ectylurea	T42.6X1	T42.6X2	T42.6X3	T42.6X4	T42.6X5	T42.6X6
Edathamil disodium	T45.8X1	T45.8X2	T45.8X3	T45.8X4	T45.8X5	T45.8X6
Edecrin	T50.1X1	T50.1X2	T50.1X3	T50.1X4	T50.1X5	T50.1X6
Edetate, disodium (calcium)	T45.8X1	T45.8X2	T45.8X3	T45.8X4	T45.8X5	T45.8X6
Edoxudine	T49.5X1	T49.5X2	T49.5X3	T49.5X4	T49.5X5	T49.5X6
Edrophonium	T44.0X1	T44.0X2	T44.0X3	T44.0X4	T44.0X5	T44.0X6
chloride	T44.0X1	T44.0X2	T44.0X3	T44.0X4	T44.0X5	T44.0X6
EDTA	T50.6X1	T50.6X2	T50.6X3	T50.6X4	T50.6X5	T50.6X6
Eflornithine	T37.2X1	T37.2X2	T37.2X3	T37.2X4	T37.2X5	T37.2X6
Efloxate	T46.3X1	T46.3X2	T46.3X3	T46.3X4	T46.3X5	T46.3X6
Elase	T49.8X1	T49.8X2	T49.8X3	T49.8X4	T49.8X5	T49.8X6
Elastase	T47.5X1	T47.5X2	T47.5X3	T47.5X4	T47.5X5	T47.5X6
Elaterium	T47.2X1	T47.2X2	T47.2X3	T47.2X4	T47.2X5	T47.2X6
Elcatonin	T50.991	T50.992	T50.993	T50.994	T50.995	T50.996
Elder	T62.2X1	T62.2X2	T62.2X3	T62.2X4	—	—
berry (unripe)	T62.1X1	T62.1X2	T62.1X3	T62.1X4	—	—
Electrolyte balance drug	T50.3X1	T50.3X2	T50.3X3	T50.3X4	T50.3X5	T50.3X6
Electrolytes NEC	T50.3X1	T50.3X2	T50.3X3	T50.3X4	T50.3X5	T50.3X6
Electrolytic agent NEC	T50.3X1	T50.3X2	T50.3X3	T50.3X4	T50.3X5	T50.3X6
Elemental diet	T50.901	T50.902	T50.903	T50.904	T50.905	T50.906
Elliptinium acetate	T45.1X1	T45.1X2	T45.1X3	T45.1X4	T45.1X5	T45.1X6
Embramine	T45.0X1	T45.0X2	T45.0X3	T45.0X4	T45.0X5	T45.0X6
Emepronium (salts)	T44.3X1	T44.3X2	T44.3X3	T44.3X4	T44.3X5	T44.3X6
bromide	T44.3X1	T44.3X2	T44.3X3	T44.3X4	T44.3X5	T44.3X6
Emetic NEC	T47.7X1	T47.7X2	T47.7X3	T47.7X4	T47.7X5	T47.7X6
Emetine	T37.3X1	T37.3X2	T37.3X3	T37.3X4	T37.3X5	T37.3X6
Emollient NEC	T49.3X1	T49.3X2	T49.3X3	T49.3X4	T49.3X5	T49.3X6
Emorfazone	T39.8X1	T39.8X2	T39.8X3	T39.8X4	T39.8X5	T39.8X6
Emylcamate	T43.591	T43.592	T43.593	T43.594	T43.595	T43.596
Enalapril	T46.4X1	T46.4X2	T46.4X3	T46.4X4	T46.4X5	T46.4X6
Enalaprilat	T46.4X1	T46.4X2	T46.4X3	T46.4X4	T46.4X5	T46.4X6
Encainide	T46.2X1	T46.2X2	T46.2X3	T46.2X4	T46.2X5	T46.2X6
Endocaine	T41.3X1	T41.3X2	T41.3X3	T41.3X4	T41.3X5	T41.3X6
Endosulfan	T60.2X1	T60.2X2	T60.2X3	T60.2X4	—	—
Endothall	T60.3X1	T60.3X2	T60.3X3	T60.3X4	—	—
Endralazine	T46.5X1	T46.5X2	T46.5X3	T46.5X4	T46.5X5	T46.5X6
Endrin	T60.1X1	T60.1X2	T60.1X3	T60.1X4	—	—
Enflurane	T41.0X1	T41.0X2	T41.0X3	T41.0X4	T41.0X5	T41.0X6
Enhexymal	T42.3X1	T42.3X2	T42.3X3	T42.3X4	T42.3X5	T42.3X6
Enocitabine	T45.1X1	T45.1X2	T45.1X3	T45.1X4	T45.1X5	T45.1X6
Enovid	T38.4X1	T38.4X2	T38.4X3	T38.4X4	T38.4X5	T38.4X6

Substance	Poisoning, Accidental (Unintentional)	Poisoning, Intentional Self-Harm	Poisoning, Assault	Poisoning, Undetermined	Adverse Effect	Underdosing
Enoxacin	T36.8X1	T36.8X2	T36.8X3	T36.8X4	T36.8X5	T36.8X6
Enoxaparin (sodium)	T45.511	T45.512	T45.513	T45.514	T45.515	T45.516
Enpiprazole	T43.591	T43.592	T43.593	T43.594	T43.595	T43.596
Enprofylline	T48.6X1	T48.6X2	T48.6X3	T48.6X4	T48.6X5	T48.6X6
Enprostil	T47.1X1	T47.1X2	T47.1X3	T47.1X4	T47.1X5	T47.1X6
ENT preparations (anti-infectives)	T49.6X1	T49.6X2	T49.6X3	T49.6X4	T49.6X5	T49.6X6
Enviomycin	T36.8X1	T36.8X2	T36.8X3	T36.8X4	T36.8X5	T36.8X6
Enzodase	T45.3X1	T45.3X2	T45.3X3	T45.3X4	T45.3X5	T45.3X6
Enzyme NEC	T45.3X1	T45.3X2	T45.3X3	T45.3X4	T45.3X5	T45.3X6
depolymerizing	T49.8X1	T49.8X2	T49.8X3	T49.8X4	T49.8X5	T49.8X6
fibrolytic	T45.3X1	T45.3X2	T45.3X3	T45.3X4	T45.3X5	T45.3X6
gastric	T47.5X1	T47.5X2	T47.5X3	T47.5X4	T47.5X5	T47.5X6
intestinal	T47.5X1	T47.5X2	T47.5X3	T47.5X4	T47.5X5	T47.5X6
local action	T49.4X1	T49.4X2	T49.4X3	T49.4X4	T49.4X5	T49.4X6
proteolytic	T49.4X1	T49.4X2	T49.4X3	T49.4X4	T49.4X5	T49.4X6
thrombolytic	T45.3X1	T45.3X2	T45.3X3	T45.3X4	T45.3X5	T45.3X6
EPAB	T41.3X1	T41.3X2	T41.3X3	T41.3X4	T41.3X5	T41.3X6
Epanutin	T42.0X1	T42.0X2	T42.0X3	T42.0X4	T42.0X5	T42.0X6
Ephedra	T44.991	T44.992	T44.993	T44.994	T44.995	T44.996
Ephedrine	T44.991	T44.992	T44.993	T44.994	T44.995	T44.996
Epichlorhydrin, epichlorohydrin	T52.8X1	T52.8X2	T52.8X3	T52.8X4	—	—
Epicillin	T36.0X1	T36.0X2	T36.0X3	T36.0X4	T36.0X5	T36.0X6
Epiestriol	T38.5X1	T38.5X2	T38.5X3	T38.5X4	T38.5X5	T38.5X6
Epilim — *see Sodium valproate*						
Epimestrol	T38.5X1	T38.5X2	T38.5X3	T38.5X4	T38.5X5	T38.5X6
Epinephrine	T44.5X1	T44.5X2	T44.5X3	T44.5X4	T44.5X5	T44.5X6
Epirubicin	T45.1X1	T45.1X2	T45.1X3	T45.1X4	T45.1X5	T45.1X6
Epitiostanol	T38.7X1	T38.7X2	T38.7X3	T38.7X4	T38.7X5	T38.7X6
Epitizide	T50.2X1	T50.2X2	T50.2X3	T50.2X4	T50.2X5	T50.2X6
EPN	T60.0X1	T60.0X2	T60.0X3	T60.0X4	—	—
EPO	T45.8X1	T45.8X2	T45.8X3	T45.8X4	T45.8X5	T45.8X6
Epoetin alpha	T45.8X1	T45.8X2	T45.8X3	T45.8X4	T45.8X5	T45.8X6
Epomediol	T50.991	T50.992	T50.993	T50.994	T50.995	T50.996
Epoprostenol	T45.521	T45.522	T45.523	T45.524	T45.525	T45.526
Epoxy resin	T65.891	T65.892	T65.893	T65.894	—	—
Eprazinone	T48.4X1	T48.4X2	T48.4X3	T48.4X4	T48.4X5	T48.4X6
Epsilon amino-caproic acid	T45.621	T45.622	T45.623	T45.624	T45.625	T45.626
Epsom salt	T47.3X1	T47.3X2	T47.3X3	T47.3X4	T47.3X5	T47.3X6
Eptazocine	T40.4X1	T40.4X2	T40.4X3	T40.4X4	T40.4X5	T40.4X6
Equanil	T43.591	T43.592	T43.593	T43.594	T43.595	T43.596
Equisetum	T62.2X1	T62.2X2	T62.2X3	T62.2X4	—	—
diuretic	T50.2X1	T50.2X2	T50.2X3	T50.2X4	T50.2X5	T50.2X6

Substance	Poisoning, Accidental (Unintentional)	Poisoning, Intentional Self-Harm	Poisoning, Assault	Poisoning, Undetermined	Adverse Effect	Underdosing
Ergobasine	T48.ØX1	T48.ØX2	T48.ØX3	T48.ØX4	T48.ØX5	T48.ØX6
Ergocalciferol	T45.2X1	T45.2X2	T45.2X3	T45.2X4	T45.2X5	T45.2X6
Ergoloid mesylates	T46.7X1	T46.7X2	T46.7X3	T46.7X4	T46.7X5	T46.7X6
Ergometrine	T48.ØX1	T48.ØX2	T48.ØX3	T48.ØX4	T48.ØX5	T48.ØX6
Ergonovine	T48.ØX1	T48.ØX2	T48.ØX3	T48.ØX4	T48.ØX5	T48.ØX6
Ergot NEC	T64.81	T64.82	T64.83	T64.84	—	—
derivative	T48.ØX1	T48.ØX2	T48.ØX3	T48.ØX4	T48.ØX5	T48.ØX6
medicinal (alkaloids)	T48.ØX1	T48.ØX2	T48.ØX3	T48.ØX4	T48.ØX5	T48.ØX6
prepared	T48.ØX1	T48.ØX2	T48.ØX3	T48.ØX4	T48.ØX5	T48.ØX6
Ergotamine	T46.5X1	T46.5X2	T46.5X3	T46.5X4	T46.5X5	T46.5X6
Ergotocine	T48.ØX1	T48.ØX2	T48.ØX3	T48.ØX4	T48.ØX5	T48.ØX6
Ergotrate	T48.ØX1	T48.ØX2	T48.ØX3	T48.ØX4	T48.ØX5	T48.ØX6
Eritrityl tetranitrate	T46.3X1	T46.3X2	T46.3X3	T46.3X4	T46.3X5	T46.3X6
Erythrityl tetranitrate	T46.3X1	T46.3X2	T46.3X3	T46.3X4	T46.3X5	T46.3X6
Erythrol tetranitrate	T46.3X1	T46.3X2	T46.3X3	T46.3X4	T46.3X5	T46.3X6
Erythromycin (salts)	T36.3X1	T36.3X2	T36.3X3	T36.3X4	T36.3X5	T36.3X6
ophthalmic preparation	T49.5X1	T49.5X2	T49.5X3	T49.5X4	T49.5X5	T49.5X6
topical NEC	T49.ØX1	T49.ØX2	T49.ØX3	T49.ØX4	T49.ØX5	T49.ØX6
Erythropoietin	T45.8X1	T45.8X2	T45.8X3	T45.8X4	T45.8X5	T45.8X6
human	T45.8X1	T45.8X2	T45.8X3	T45.8X4	T45.8X5	T45.8X6
Escin	T46.991	T46.992	T46.993	T46.994	T46.995	T46.996
Esculin	T45.2X1	T45.2X2	T45.2X3	T45.2X4	T45.2X5	T45.2X6
Esculoside	T45.2X1	T45.2X2	T45.2X3	T45.2X4	T45.2X5	T45.2X6
ESDT (ether-soluble tar distillate)	T49.1X1	T49.1X2	T49.1X3	T49.1X4	T49.1X5	T49.1X6
Eserine	T49.5X1	T49.5X2	T49.5X3	T49.5X4	T49.5X5	T49.5X6
Esflurbiprofen	T39.311	T39.312	T39.313	T39.314	T39.315	T39.316
Eskabarb	T42.3X1	T42.3X2	T42.3X3	T42.3X4	T42.3X5	T42.3X6
Eskalith	T43.8X1	T43.8X2	T43.8X3	T43.8X4	T43.8X5	T43.8X6
Esmolol	T44.7X1	T44.7X2	T44.7X3	T44.7X4	T44.7X5	T44.7X6
Estanozolol	T38.7X1	T38.7X2	T38.7X3	T38.7X4	T38.7X5	T38.7X6
Estazolam	T42.4X1	T42.4X2	T42.4X3	T42.4X4	T42.4X5	T42.4X6
Estradiol	T38.5X1	T38.5X2	T38.5X3	T38.5X4	T38.5X5	T38.5X6
with testosterone	T38.7X1	T38.7X2	T38.7X3	T38.7X4	T38.7X5	T38.7X6
benzoate	T38.5X1	T38.5X2	T38.5X3	T38.5X4	T38.5X5	T38.5X6
Estramustine	T45.1X1	T45.1X2	T45.1X3	T45.1X4	T45.1X5	T45.1X6
Estriol	T38.5X1	T38.5X2	T38.5X3	T38.5X4	T38.5X5	T38.5X6
Estrogen	T38.5X1	T38.5X2	T38.5X3	T38.5X4	T38.5X5	T38.5X6
with progesterone	T38.5X1	T38.5X2	T38.5X3	T38.5X4	T38.5X5	T38.5X6
conjugated	T38.5X1	T38.5X2	T38.5X3	T38.5X4	T38.5X5	T38.5X6
Estrone	T38.5X1	T38.5X2	T38.5X3	T38.5X4	T38.5X5	T38.5X6
Estropipate	T38.5X1	T38.5X2	T38.5X3	T38.5X4	T38.5X5	T38.5X6

Substance	Poisoning, Accidental (Unintentional)	Poisoning, Intentional Self-Harm	Poisoning, Assault	Poisoning, Undetermined	Adverse Effect	Underdosing
Etacrynate sodium	T5Ø.1X1	T5Ø.1X2	T5Ø.1X3	T5Ø.1X4	T5Ø.1X5	T5Ø.1X6
Etacrynic acid	T5Ø.1X1	T5Ø.1X2	T5Ø.1X3	T5Ø.1X4	T5Ø.1X5	T5Ø.1X6
Etafedrine	T48.6X1	T48.6X2	T48.6X3	T48.6X4	T48.6X5	T48.6X6
Etafenone	T46.3X1	T46.3X2	T46.3X3	T46.3X4	T46.3X5	T46.3X6
Etambutol	T37.1X1	T37.1X2	T37.1X3	T37.1X4	T37.1X5	T37.1X6
Etamiphyllin	T48.6X1	T48.6X2	T48.6X3	T48.6X4	T48.6X5	T48.6X6
Etamivan	T5Ø.7X1	T5Ø.7X2	T5Ø.7X3	T5Ø.7X4	T5Ø.7X5	T5Ø.7X6
Etamsylate	T45.7X1	T45.7X2	T45.7X3	T45.7X4	T45.7X5	T45.7X6
Etebenecid	T5Ø.4X1	T5Ø.4X2	T5Ø.4X3	T5Ø.4X4	T5Ø.4X5	T5Ø.4X6
Ethacridine	T49.ØX1	T49.ØX2	T49.ØX3	T49.ØX4	T49.ØX5	T49.ØX6
Ethacrynic acid	T5Ø.1X1	T5Ø.1X2	T5Ø.1X3	T5Ø.1X4	T5Ø.1X5	T5Ø.1X6
Ethadione	T42.2X1	T42.2X2	T42.2X3	T42.2X4	T42.2X5	T42.2X6
Ethambutol	T37.1X1	T37.1X2	T37.1X3	T37.1X4	T37.1X5	T37.1X6
Ethamide	T5Ø.2X1	T5Ø.2X2	T5Ø.2X3	T5Ø.2X4	T5Ø.2X5	T5Ø.2X6
Ethamivan	T5Ø.7X1	T5Ø.7X2	T5Ø.7X3	T5Ø.7X4	T5Ø.7X5	T5Ø.7X6
Ethamsylate	T45.7X1	T45.7X2	T45.7X3	T45.7X4	T45.7X5	T45.7X6
Ethanol	T51.ØX1	T51.ØX2	T51.ØX3	T51.ØX4	—	—
beverage	T51.ØX1	T51.ØX2	T51.ØX3	T51.ØX4	—	—
Ethanolamine oleate	T46.8X1	T46.8X2	T46.8X3	T46.8X4	T46.8X5	T46.8X6
Ethaverine	T44.3X1	T44.3X2	T44.3X3	T44.3X4	T44.3X5	T44.3X6
Ethchlorvynol	T42.6X1	T42.6X2	T42.6X3	T42.6X4	T42.6X5	T42.6X6
Ethebenecid	T5Ø.4X1	T5Ø.4X2	T5Ø.4X3	T5Ø.4X4	T5Ø.4X5	T5Ø.4X6
Ether (vapor)	T41.ØX1	T41.ØX2	T41.ØX3	T41.ØX4	T41.ØX5	T41.ØX6
anesthetic	T41.ØX1	T41.ØX2	T41.ØX3	T41.ØX4	T41.ØX5	T41.ØX6
divinyl	T41.ØX1	T41.ØX2	T41.ØX3	T41.ØX4	T41.ØX5	T41.ØX6
ethyl (medicinal)	T41.ØX1	T41.ØX2	T41.ØX3	T41.ØX4	T41.ØX5	T41.ØX6
nonmedicinal	T52.8X1	T52.8X2	T52.8X3	T52.8X4	—	—
petroleum—*see Ligroin*						
solvent	T52.8X1	T52.8X2	T52.8X3	T52.8X4	—	—
Ethiazide	T5Ø.2X1	T5Ø.2X2	T5Ø.2X3	T5Ø.2X4	T5Ø.2X5	T5Ø.2X6
Ethidium chloride (vapor)	T59.891	T59.892	T59.893	T59.894	—	—
Ethinamate	T42.6X1	T42.6X2	T42.6X3	T42.6X4	T42.6X5	T42.6X6
Ethinylestradiol, ethinyloestradiol	T38.5X1	T38.5X2	T38.5X3	T38.5X4	T38.5X5	T38.5X6
with						
levonorgestrel	T38.4X1	T38.4X2	T38.4X3	T38.4X4	T38.4X5	T38.4X6
norethisterone	T38.4X1	T38.4X2	T38.4X3	T38.4X4	T38.4X5	T38.4X6
Ethiodized oil (131 I)	T5Ø.8X1	T5Ø.8X2	T5Ø.8X3	T5Ø.8X4	T5Ø.8X5	T5Ø.8X6
Ethion	T6Ø.ØX1	T6Ø.ØX2	T6Ø.ØX3	T6Ø.ØX4	—	—
Ethionamide	T37.1X1	T37.1X2	T37.1X3	T37.1X4	T37.1X5	T37.1X6
Ethioniamide	T37.1X1	T37.1X2	T37.1X3	T37.1X4	T37.1X5	T37.1X6
Ethisterone	T38.5X1	T38.5X2	T38.5X3	T38.5X4	T38.5X5	T38.5X6
Ethobral	T42.3X1	T42.3X2	T42.3X3	T42.3X4	T42.3X5	T42.3X6

Substance	Poisoning, Accidental (Unintentional)	Poisoning, Intentional Self-Harm	Poisoning, Assault	Poisoning, Undetermined	Adverse Effect	Underdosing
Ethocaine (infiltration) (topical)	T41.3X1	T41.3X2	T41.3X3	T41.3X4	T41.3X5	T41.3X6
nerve block (peripheral) (plexus)	T41.3X1	T41.3X2	T41.3X3	T41.3X4	T41.3X5	T41.3X6
spinal	T41.3X1	T41.3X2	T41.3X3	T41.3X4	T41.3X5	T41.3X6
Ethoheptazine	T40.4X1	T40.4X2	T40.4X3	T40.4X4	T40.4X5	T40.4X6
Ethopropazine	T44.3X1	T44.3X2	T44.3X3	T44.3X4	T44.3X5	T44.3X6
Ethosuximide	T42.2X1	T42.2X2	T42.2X3	T42.2X4	T42.2X5	T42.2X6
Ethotoin	T42.0X1	T42.0X2	T42.0X3	T42.0X4	T42.0X5	T42.0X6
Ethoxazene	T37.91	T37.92	T37.93	T37.94	T37.95	T37.96
Ethoxazorutoside	T46.991	T46.992	T46.993	T46.994	T46.995	T46.996
2-Ethoxyethanol	T52.3X1	T52.3X2	T52.3X3	T52.3X4	—	—
Ethoxzolamide	T50.2X1	T50.2X2	T50.2X3	T50.2X4	T50.2X5	T50.2X6
Ethyl						
acetate	T52.8X1	T52.8X2	T52.8X3	T52.8X4	—	—
alcohol	T51.0X1	T51.0X2	T51.0X3	T51.0X4	—	—
beverage	T51.0X1	T51.0X2	T51.0X3	T51.0X4	—	—
aldehyde (vapor)	T59.891	T59.892	T59.893	T59.894	—	—
liquid	T52.8X1	T52.8X2	T52.8X3	T52.8X4	—	—
aminobenzoate	T41.3X1	T41.3X2	T41.3X3	T41.3X4	T41.3X5	T41.3X6
aminophenothiazine	T43.3X1	T43.3X2	T43.3X3	T43.3X4	T43.3X5	T43.3X6
benzoate	T52.8X1	T52.8X2	T52.8X3	T52.8X4	—	—
biscoumacetate	T45.511	T45.512	T45.513	T45.514	T45.515	T45.516
bromide (anesthetic)	T41.0X1	T41.0X2	T41.0X3	T41.0X4	T41.0X5	T41.0X6
carbamate	T45.1X1	T45.1X2	T45.1X3	T45.1X4	T45.1X5	T45.1X6
carbinol	T51.3X1	T51.3X2	T51.3X3	T51.3X4	—	—
carbonate	T52.8X1	T52.8X2	T52.8X3	T52.8X4	—	—
chaulmoograte	T37.1X1	T37.1X2	T37.1X3	T37.1X4	T37.1X5	T37.1X6
chloride (anesthetic)	T41.0X1	T41.0X2	T41.0X3	T41.0X4	T41.0X5	T41.0X6
anesthetic (local)	T41.3X1	T41.3X2	T41.3X3	T41.3X4	T41.3X5	T41.3X6
inhaled	T41.0X1	T41.0X2	T41.0X3	T41.0X4	T41.0X5	T41.0X6
local	T49.4X1	T49.4X2	T49.4X3	T49.4X4	T49.4X5	T49.4X6
solvent	T53.6X1	T53.6X2	T53.6X3	T53.6X4	—	—
dibunate	T48.3X1	T48.3X2	T48.3X3	T48.3X4	T48.3X5	T48.3X6
dichloroarsine (vapor)	T57.0X1	T57.0X2	T57.0X3	T57.0X4	—	—
estranol	T38.7X1	T38.7X2	T38.7X3	T38.7X4	T38.7X5	T38.7X6
ether — *see also* ether	T52.8X1	T52.8X2	T52.8X3	T52.8X4	—	—
formate NEC (solvent)	T52.0X1	T52.0X2	T52.0X3	T52.0X4	—	—
fumarate	T49.4X1	T49.4X2	T49.4X3	T49.4X4	T49.4X5	T49.4X6
hydroxyisobutyrate NEC (solvent)	T52.8X1	T52.8X2	T52.8X3	T52.8X4	—	—
iodoacetate	T59.3X1	T59.3X2	T59.3X3	T59.3X4	—	—
lactate NEC (solvent)	T52.8X1	T52.8X2	T52.8X3	T52.8X4	—	—
loflazepate	T42.4X1	T42.4X2	T42.4X3	T42.4X4	T42.4X5	T42.4X6

Substance	Poisoning, Accidental (Unintentional)	Poisoning, Intentional Self-Harm	Poisoning, Assault	Poisoning, Undetermined	Adverse Effect	Underdosing
Ethyl *(Continued)*						
mercuric chloride	T56.1X1	T56.1X2	T56.1X3	T56.1X4	—	—
methylcarbinol	T51.8X1	T51.8X2	T51.8X3	T51.8X4	—	—
morphine	T40.2X1	T40.2X2	T40.2X3	T40.2X4	T40.2X5	T40.2X6
noradrenaline	T48.6X1	T48.6X2	T48.6X3	T48.6X4	T48.6X5	T48.6X6
oxybutyrate NEC (solvent)	T52.8X1	T52.8X2	T52.8X3	T52.8X4	—	—
Ethylene (gas)	T59.891	T59.892	T59.893	T59.894	—	—
anesthetic (general)	T41.0X1	T41.0X2	T41.0X3	T41.0X4	T41.0X5	T41.0X6
chlorohydrin	T52.8X1	T52.8X2	T52.8X3	T52.8X4	—	—
vapor	T53.6X1	T53.6X2	T53.6X3	T53.6X4	—	—
dichloride	T52.8X1	T52.8X2	T52.8X3	T52.8X4	—	—
vapor	T53.6X1	T53.6X2	T53.6X3	T53.6X4	—	—
dinitrate	T52.3X1	T52.3X2	T52.3X3	T52.3X4	—	—
glycol(s)	T52.8X1	T52.8X2	T52.8X3	T52.8X4	—	—
dinitrate	T52.3X1	T52.3X2	T52.3X3	T52.3X4	—	—
monobutyl ether	T52.3X1	T52.3X2	T52.3X3	T52.3X4	—	—
imine	T54.1X1	T54.1X2	T54.1X3	T54.1X4	—	—
oxide (fumigant) (nonmedicinal)	T59.891	T59.892	T59.893	T59.894	—	—
medicinal	T49.0X1	T49.0X2	T49.0X3	T49.0X4	T49.0X5	T49.0X6
Ethylenediamine theophylline	T48.6X1	T48.6X2	T48.6X3	T48.6X4	T48.6X5	T48.6X6
Ethylenediaminetetra-acetic acid	T50.6X1	T50.6X2	T50.6X3	T50.6X4	T50.6X5	T50.6X6
Ethylenedinitrilotetra-acetate	T50.6X1	T50.6X2	T50.6X3	T50.6X4	T50.6X5	T50.6X6
Ethylestrenol	T38.7X1	T38.7X2	T38.7X3	T38.7X4	T38.7X5	T38.7X6
Ethylhydroxycellulose	T47.4X1	T47.4X2	T47.4X3	T47.4X4	T47.4X5	T47.4X6
Ethylidene						
chloride NEC	T53.6X1	T53.6X2	T53.6X3	T53.6X4	—	—
diacetate	T60.3X1	T60.3X2	T60.3X3	T60.3X4	—	—
dicoumarin	T45.511	T45.512	T45.513	T45.514	T45.515	T45.516
dicoumarol	T45.511	T45.512	T45.513	T45.514	T45.515	T45.516
diethyl ether	T52.0X1	T52.0X2	T52.0X3	T52.0X4	—	—
Ethylmorphine	T40.2X1	T40.2X2	T40.2X3	T40.2X4	T40.2X5	T40.2X6
Ethylnorepinephrine	T48.6X1	T48.6X2	T48.6X3	T48.6X4	T48.6X5	T48.6X6
Ethylparachlorophen-oxyisobutyrate	T46.6X1	T46.6X2	T46.6X3	T46.6X4	T46.6X5	T46.6X6
Ethynodiol	T38.4X1	T38.4X2	T38.4X3	T38.4X4	T38.4X5	T38.4X6
with mestranol diacetate	T38.4X1	T38.4X2	T38.4X3	T38.4X4	T38.4X5	T38.4X6
Etidocaine	T41.3X1	T41.3X2	T41.3X3	T41.3X4	T41.3X5	T41.3X6
infiltration (subcutaneous)	T41.3X1	T41.3X2	T41.3X3	T41.3X4	T41.3X5	T41.3X6
nerve (peripheral) (plexus)	T41.3X1	T41.3X2	T41.3X3	T41.3X4	T41.3X5	T41.3X6
Etidronate	T50.991	T50.992	T50.993	T50.994	T50.995	T50.996
Etidronic acid (disodium salt)	T50.991	T50.992	T50.993	T50.994	T50.995	T50.996
Etifoxine	T42.6X1	T42.6X2	T42.6X3	T42.6X4	T42.6X5	T42.6X6

◀ New ⟸ Revised ~~deleted~~ Deleted

Substance	Poisoning, Accidental (Unintentional)	Poisoning, Intentional Self-Harm	Poisoning, Assault	Poisoning, Undetermined	Adverse Effect	Underdosing
Etilefrine	T44.4X1	T44.4X2	T44.4X3	T44.4X4	T44.4X5	T44.4X6
Etilfen	T42.3X1	T42.3X2	T42.3X3	T42.3X4	T42.3X5	T42.3X6
Etinodiol	T38.4X1	T38.4X2	T38.4X3	T38.4X4	T38.4X5	T38.4X6
Etiroxate	T46.6X1	T46.6X2	T46.6X3	T46.6X4	T46.6X5	T46.6X6
Etizolam	T42.4X1	T42.4X2	T42.4X3	T42.4X4	T42.4X5	T42.4X6
Etodolac	T39.391	T39.392	T39.393	T39.394	T39.395	T39.396
Etofamide	T37.3X1	T37.3X2	T37.3X3	T37.3X4	T37.3X5	T37.3X6
Etofibrate	T46.6X1	T46.6X2	T46.6X3	T46.6X4	T46.6X5	T46.6X6
Etofylline	T46.7X1	T46.7X2	T46.7X3	T46.7X4	T46.7X5	T46.7X6
clofibrate	T46.6X1	T46.6X2	T46.6X3	T46.6X4	T46.6X5	T46.6X6
Etoglucid	T45.1X1	T45.1X2	T45.1X3	T45.1X4	T45.1X5	T45.1X6
Etomidate	T41.1X1	T41.1X2	T41.1X3	T41.1X4	T41.1X5	T41.1X6
Etomide	T39.8X1	T39.8X2	T39.8X3	T39.8X4	T39.8X5	T39.8X6
Etomidoline	T44.3X1	T44.3X2	T44.3X3	T44.3X4	T44.3X5	T44.3X6
Etoposide	T45.1X1	T45.1X2	T45.1X3	T45.1X4	T45.1X5	T45.1X6
Etorphine	T40.2X1	T40.2X2	T40.2X3	T40.2X4	T40.2X5	T40.2X6
Etoval	T42.3X1	T42.3X2	T42.3X3	T42.3X4	T42.3X5	T42.3X6
Etozolin	T50.1X1	T50.1X2	T50.1X3	T50.1X4	T50.1X5	T50.1X6
Etretinate	T50.991	T50.992	T50.993	T50.994	T50.995	T50.996
Etryptamine	T43.691	T43.692	T43.693	T43.694	T43.695	T43.696
Etybenzatropine	T44.3X1	T44.3X2	T44.3X3	T44.3X4	T44.3X5	T44.3X6
Etynodiol	T38.4X1	T38.4X2	T38.4X3	T38.4X4	T38.4X5	T38.4X6
Eucaine	T41.3X1	T41.3X2	T41.3X3	T41.3X4	T41.3X5	T41.3X6
Eucalyptus oil	T49.7X1	T49.7X2	T49.7X3	T49.7X4	T49.7X5	T49.7X6
Eucatropine	T49.5X1	T49.5X2	T49.5X3	T49.5X4	T49.5X5	T49.5X6
Eucodal	T40.2X1	T40.2X2	T40.2X3	T40.2X4	T40.2X5	T40.2X6
Euneryl	T42.3X1	T42.3X2	T42.3X3	T42.3X4	T42.3X5	T42.3X6
Euphthalmine	T44.3X1	T44.3X2	T44.3X3	T44.3X4	T44.3X5	T44.3X6
Eurax	T49.0X1	T49.0X2	T49.0X3	T49.0X4	T49.0X5	T49.0X6
Euresol	T49.4X1	T49.4X2	T49.4X3	T49.4X4	T49.4X5	T49.4X6
Euthroid	T38.1X1	T38.1X2	T38.1X3	T38.1X4	T38.1X5	T38.1X6
Evans blue	T50.8X1	T50.8X2	T50.8X3	T50.8X4	T50.8X5	T50.8X6
Evipal	T42.3X1	T42.3X2	T42.3X3	T42.3X4	T42.3X5	T42.3X6
sodium	T41.1X1	T41.1X2	T41.1X3	T41.1X4	T41.1X5	T41.1X6
Evipan	T42.3X1	T42.3X2	T42.3X3	T42.3X4	T42.3X5	T42.3X6
sodium	T41.1X1	T41.1X2	T41.1X3	T41.1X4	T41.1X5	T41.1X6
Exalamide	T49.0X1	T49.0X2	T49.0X3	T49.0X4	T49.0X5	T49.0X6
Exalgin	T39.1X1	T39.1X2	T39.1X3	T39.1X4	T39.1X5	T39.1X6
Excipients, pharmaceutical	T50.901	T50.902	T50.903	T50.904	T50.905	T50.906
Exhaust gas (engine) (motor vehicle)	T58.01	T58.02	T58.03	T58.04	—	—
Ex-Lax (phenolphthalein)	T47.2X1	T47.2X2	T47.2X3	T47.2X4	T47.2X5	T47.2X6
Expectorant NEC	T48.4X1	T48.4X2	T48.4X3	T48.4X4	T48.4X5	T48.4X6
Extended insulin zinc suspension	T38.3X1	T38.3X2	T38.3X3	T38.3X4	T38.3X5	T38.3X6
External medications (skin) (mucous membrane)	T49.91	T49.92	T49.93	T49.94	T49.95	T49.96
dental agent	T49.7X1	T49.7X2	T49.7X3	T49.7X4	T49.7X5	T49.7X6
ENT agent	T49.6X1	T49.6X2	T49.6X3	T49.6X4	T49.6X5	T49.6X6
ophthalmic preparation	T49.5X1	T49.5X2	T49.5X3	T49.5X4	T49.5X5	T49.5X6
specified NEC	T49.8X1	T49.8X2	T49.8X3	T49.8X4	T49.8X5	T49.8X6
Extrapyramidal antagonist NEC	T44.3X1	T44.3X2	T44.3X3	T44.3X4	T44.3X5	T44.3X6
Eye agents (anti-infective)	T49.5X1	T49.5X2	T49.5X3	T49.5X4	T49.5X5	T49.5X6
Eye drug NEC	T49.5X1	T49.5X2	T49.5X3	T49.5X4	T49.5X5	T49.5X6
F						
FAC (fluorouracil + doxorubicin + cyclophosphamide)	T45.1X1	T45.1X2	T45.1X3	T45.1X4	T45.1X5	T45.1X6
Factor						
I (fibrinogen)	T45.8X1	T45.8X2	T45.8X3	T45.8X4	T45.8X5	T45.8X6
III (thromboplastin)	T45.8X1	T45.8X2	T45.8X3	T45.8X4	T45.8X5	T45.8X6
VIII (antihemophilic Factor) (Concentrate)	T45.8X1	T45.8X2	T45.8X3	T45.8X4	T45.8X5	T45.8X6
IX complex	T45.7X1	T45.7X2	T45.7X3	T45.7X4	T45.7X5	T45.7X6
human	T45.8X1	T45.8X2	T45.8X3	T45.8X4	T45.8X5	T45.8X6
Famotidine	T47.0X1	T47.0X2	T47.0X3	T47.0X4	T47.0X5	T47.0X6
Fat suspension, intravenous	T50.991	T50.992	T50.993	T50.994	T50.995	T50.996
Fazadinium bromide	T48.1X1	T48.1X2	T48.1X3	T48.1X4	T48.1X5	T48.1X6
Febarbamate	T42.3X1	T42.3X2	T42.3X3	T42.3X4	T42.3X5	T42.3X6
Fecal softener	T47.4X1	T47.4X2	T47.4X3	T47.4X4	T47.4X5	T47.4X6
Fedrilate	T48.3X1	T48.3X2	T48.3X3	T48.3X4	T48.3X5	T48.3X6
Felodipine	T46.1X1	T46.1X2	T46.1X3	T46.1X4	T46.1X5	T46.1X6
Felypressin	T38.891	T38.892	T38.893	T38.894	T38.895	T38.896
Femoxetine	T43.221	T43.222	T43.223	T43.224	T43.225	T43.226
Fenalcomine	T46.3X1	T46.3X2	T46.3X3	T46.3X4	T46.3X5	T46.3X6
Fenamisal	T37.1X1	T37.1X2	T37.1X3	T37.1X4	T37.1X5	T37.1X6
Fenazone	T39.2X1	T39.2X2	T39.2X3	T39.2X4	T39.2X5	T39.2X6
Fenbendazole	T37.4X1	T37.4X2	T37.4X3	T37.4X4	T37.4X5	T37.4X6
Fenbutrazate	T50.5X1	T50.5X2	T50.5X3	T50.5X4	T50.5X5	T50.5X6
Fencamfamine	T43.691	T43.692	T43.693	T43.694	T43.695	T43.696
Fendiline	T46.1X1	T46.1X2	T46.1X3	T46.1X4	T46.1X5	T46.1X6
Fenetylline	T43.691	T43.692	T43.693	T43.694	T43.695	T43.696
Fenflumizole	T39.391	T39.392	T39.393	T39.394	T39.395	T39.396
Fenfluramine	T50.5X1	T50.5X2	T50.5X3	T50.5X4	T50.5X5	T50.5X6
Fenobarbital	T42.3X1	T42.3X2	T42.3X3	T42.3X4	T42.3X5	T42.3X6
Fenofibrate	T46.6X1	T46.6X2	T46.6X3	T46.6X4	T46.6X5	T46.6X6
Fenoprofen	T39.311	T39.312	T39.313	T39.314	T39.315	T39.316
Fenoterol	T48.6X1	T48.6X2	T48.6X3	T48.6X4	T48.6X5	T48.6X6

Substance	Poisoning, Accidental (Unintentional)	Poisoning, Intentional Self-Harm	Poisoning, Assault	Poisoning, Undetermined	Adverse Effect	Underdosing
Fenoverine	T44.3X1	T44.3X2	T44.3X3	T44.3X4	T44.3X5	T44.3X6
Fenoxazoline	T48.5X1	T48.5X2	T48.5X3	T48.5X4	T48.5X5	T48.5X6
Fenproporex	T50.5X1	T50.5X2	T50.5X3	T50.5X4	T50.5X5	T50.5X6
Fenquizone	T50.2X1	T50.2X2	T50.2X3	T50.2X4	T50.2X5	T50.2X6
Fentanyl	T40.4X1	T40.4X2	T40.4X3	T40.4X4	T40.4X5	T40.4X6
Fentazin	T43.3X1	T43.3X2	T43.3X3	T43.3X4	T43.3X5	T43.3X6
Fenthion	T60.0X1	T60.0X2	T60.0X3	T60.0X4	—	—
Fenticlor	T49.0X1	T49.0X2	T49.0X3	T49.0X4	T49.0X5	T49.0X6
Fenylbutazone	T39.2X1	T39.2X2	T39.2X3	T39.2X4	T39.2X5	T39.2X6
Feprazone	T39.2X1	T39.2X2	T39.2X3	T39.2X4	T39.2X5	T39.2X6
Fer de lance (bite) (venom)	T63.061	T63.062	T63.063	T63.064	—	—
Ferric — *see also Iron*						
chloride	T45.4X1	T45.4X2	T45.4X3	T45.4X4	T45.4X5	T45.4X6
citrate	T45.4X1	T45.4X2	T45.4X3	T45.4X4	T45.4X5	T45.4X6
hydroxide						
colloidal	T45.4X1	T45.4X2	T45.4X3	T45.4X4	T45.4X5	T45.4X6
polymaltose	T45.4X1	T45.4X2	T45.4X3	T45.4X4	T45.4X5	T45.4X6
pyrophosphate	T45.4X1	T45.4X2	T45.4X3	T45.4X4	T45.4X5	T45.4X6
Ferritin	T45.4X1	T45.4X2	T45.4X3	T45.4X4	T45.4X5	T45.4X6
Ferrocholinate	T45.4X1	T45.4X2	T45.4X3	T45.4X4	T45.4X5	T45.4X6
Ferrodextrane	T45.4X1	T45.4X2	T45.4X3	T45.4X4	T45.4X5	T45.4X6
Ferropolimaler	T45.4X1	T45.4X2	T45.4X3	T45.4X4	T45.4X5	T45.4X6
Ferrous — *see also Iron*						
phosphate	T45.4X1	T45.4X2	T45.4X3	T45.4X4	T45.4X5	T45.4X6
salt	T45.4X1	T45.4X2	T45.4X3	T45.4X4	T45.4X5	T45.4X6
with folic acid	T45.4X1	T45.4X2	T45.4X3	T45.4X4	T45.4X5	T45.4X6
Ferrous fumerate, gluconate, lactate, salt NEC, sulfate (medicinal)	T45.4X1	T45.4X2	T45.4X3	T45.4X4	T45.4X5	T45.4X6
Ferrovanadium (fumes)	T59.891	T59.892	T59.893	T59.894	—	—
Ferrum — *see Iron*						
Fertilizers NEC	T65.891	T65.892	T65.893	T65.894	—	—
with herbicide mixture	T60.3X1	T60.3X2	T60.3X3	T60.3X4	—	—
Fetoxilate	T47.6X1	T47.6X2	T47.6X3	T47.6X4	T47.6X5	T47.6X6
Fiber, dietary	T47.4X1	T47.4X2	T47.4X3	T47.4X4	T47.4X5	T47.4X6
Fibrinogen (human)	T45.8X1	T45.8X2	T45.8X3	T45.8X4	T45.8X5	T45.8X6
Fibrinolysin (human)	T45.691	T45.692	T45.693	T45.694	T45.695	T45.696
Fibrinolysis						
affecting drug	T45.601	T45.602	T45.603	T45.604	T45.605	T45.606
inhibitor NEC	T45.621	T45.622	T45.623	T45.624	T45.625	T45.626
Fibrinolytic drug	T45.611	T45.612	T45.613	T45.614	T45.615	T45.616
Filix mas	T37.4X1	T37.4X2	T37.4X3	T37.4X4	T37.4X5	T37.4X6
Filtering cream	T49.3X1	T49.3X2	T49.3X3	T49.3X4	T49.3X5	T49.3X6
Fiorinal	T39.011	T39.012	T39.013	T39.014	T39.015	T39.016
Firedamp	T59.891	T59.892	T59.893	T59.894	—	—
Fish, noxious, nonbacterial	T61.91	T61.92	T61.93	T61.94	—	—
ciguatera	T61.01	T61.02	T61.03	T61.04	—	—
scombroid	T61.11	T61.12	T61.13	T61.14	—	—
shell	T61.781	T61.782	T61.783	T61.784	—	—
specified NEC	T61.771	T61.772	T61.773	T61.774	—	—
Flagyl	T37.3X1	T37.3X2	T37.3X3	T37.3X4	T37.3X5	T37.3X6
Flavine adenine dinucleotide	T45.2X1	T45.2X2	T45.2X3	T45.2X4	T45.2X5	T45.2X6
Flavodic acid	T46.991	T46.992	T46.993	T46.994	T46.995	T46.996
Flavoxate	T44.3X1	T44.3X2	T44.3X3	T44.3X4	T44.3X5	T44.3X6
Flaxedil	T48.1X1	T48.1X2	T48.1X3	T48.1X4	T48.1X5	T48.1X6
Flaxseed (medicinal)	T49.3X1	T49.3X2	T49.3X3	T49.3X4	T49.3X5	T49.3X6
Flecainide	T46.2X1	T46.2X2	T46.2X3	T46.2X4	T46.2X5	T46.2X6
Fleroxacin	T36.8X1	T36.8X2	T36.8X3	T36.8X4	T36.8X5	T36.8X6
Floctafenine	T39.8X1	T39.8X2	T39.8X3	T39.8X4	T39.8X5	T39.8X6
Flomax	T44.6X1	T44.6X2	T44.6X3	T44.6X4	T44.6X5	T44.6X6
Flomoxef	T36.1X1	T36.1X2	T36.1X3	T36.1X4	T36.1X5	T36.1X6
Flopropione	T44.3X1	T44.3X2	T44.3X3	T44.3X4	T44.3X5	T44.3X6
Florantyrone	T47.5X1	T47.5X2	T47.5X3	T47.5X4	T47.5X5	T47.5X6
Floraquin	T37.8X1	T37.8X2	T37.8X3	T37.8X4	T37.8X5	T37.8X6
Florinef	T38.0X1	T38.0X2	T38.0X3	T38.0X4	T38.0X5	T38.0X6
ENT agent	T49.6X1	T49.6X2	T49.6X3	T49.6X4	T49.6X5	T49.6X6
ophthalmic preparation	T49.5X1	T49.5X2	T49.5X3	T49.5X4	T49.5X5	T49.5X6
topical NEC	T49.0X1	T49.0X2	T49.0X3	T49.0X4	T49.0X5	T49.0X6
Flowers of sulfur	T49.4X1	T49.4X2	T49.4X3	T49.4X4	T49.4X5	T49.4X6
Floxuridine	T45.1X1	T45.1X2	T45.1X3	T45.1X4	T45.1X5	T45.1X6
Fluanisone	T43.4X1	T43.4X2	T43.4X3	T43.4X4	T43.4X5	T43.4X6
Flubendazole	T37.4X1	T37.4X2	T37.4X3	T37.4X4	T37.4X5	T37.4X6
Fluclorolone acetonide	T49.0X1	T49.0X2	T49.0X3	T49.0X4	T49.0X5	T49.0X6
Flucloxacillin	T36.0X1	T36.0X2	T36.0X3	T36.0X4	T36.0X5	T36.0X6
Fluconazole	T37.8X1	T37.8X2	T37.8X3	T37.8X4	T37.8X5	T37.8X6
Flucytosine	T37.8X1	T37.8X2	T37.8X3	T37.8X4	T37.8X5	T37.8X6
Fludeoxyglucose (18F)	T50.8X1	T50.8X2	T50.8X3	T50.8X4	T50.8X5	T50.8X6
Fludiazepam	T42.4X1	T42.4X2	T42.4X3	T42.4X4	T42.4X5	T42.4X6
Fludrocortisone	T50.0X1	T50.0X2	T50.0X3	T50.0X4	T50.0X5	T50.0X6
ENT agent	T49.6X1	T49.6X2	T49.6X3	T49.6X4	T49.6X5	T49.6X6
ophthalmic preparation	T49.5X1	T49.5X2	T49.5X3	T49.5X4	T49.5X5	T49.5X6
topical NEC	T49.0X1	T49.0X2	T49.0X3	T49.0X4	T49.0X5	T49.0X6
Fludroxycortide	T49.0X1	T49.0X2	T49.0X3	T49.0X4	T49.0X5	T49.0X6
Flufenamic acid	T39.391	T39.392	T39.393	T39.394	T39.395	T39.396
Fluindione	T45.511	T45.512	T45.513	T45.514	T45.515	T45.516

TABLE OF DRUGS AND CHEMICALS

Substance	Poisoning, Accidental (Unintentional)	Poisoning, Intentional Self-Harm	Poisoning, Assault	Poisoning, Undetermined	Adverse Effect	Underdosing
Flumequine	T37.8X1	T37.8X2	T37.8X3	T37.8X4	T37.8X5	T37.8X6
Flumethasone	T49.ØX1	T49.ØX2	T49.ØX3	T49.ØX4	T49.ØX5	T49.ØX6
Flumethiazide	T5Ø.2X1	T5Ø.2X2	T5Ø.2X3	T5Ø.2X4	T5Ø.2X5	T5Ø.2X6
Flumidin	T37.5X1	T37.5X2	T37.5X3	T37.5X4	T37.5X5	T37.5X6
Flunarizine	T46.7X1	T46.7X2	T46.7X3	T46.7X4	T46.7X5	T46.7X6
Flunidazole	T37.8X1	T37.8X2	T37.8X3	T37.8X4	T37.8X5	T37.8X6
Flunisolide	T48.6X1	T48.6X2	T48.6X3	T48.6X4	T48.6X5	T48.6X6
Flunitrazepam	T42.4X1	T42.4X2	T42.4X3	T42.4X4	T42.4X5	T42.4X6
Fluocinolone (acetonide)	T49.ØX1	T49.ØX2	T49.ØX3	T49.ØX4	T49.ØX5	T49.ØX6
Fluocinonide	T49.ØX1	T49.ØX2	T49.ØX3	T49.ØX4	T49.ØX5	T49.ØX6
Fluocortin (butyl)	T49.ØX1	T49.ØX2	T49.ØX3	T49.ØX4	T49.ØX5	T49.ØX6
Fluocortolone	T49.ØX1	T49.ØX2	T49.ØX3	T49.ØX4	T49.ØX5	T49.ØX6
Fluohydrocortisone	T38.ØX1	T38.ØX2	T38.ØX3	T38.ØX4	T38.ØX5	T38.ØX6
ENT agent	T49.6X1	T49.6X2	T49.6X3	T49.6X4	T49.6X5	T49.6X6
ophthalmic preparation	T49.5X1	T49.5X2	T49.5X3	T49.5X4	T49.5X5	T49.5X6
topical NEC	T49.ØX1	T49.ØX2	T49.ØX3	T49.ØX4	T49.ØX5	T49.ØX6
Fluonid	T49.ØX1	T49.ØX2	T49.ØX3	T49.ØX4	T49.ØX5	T49.ØX6
Fluopromazine	T43.3X1	T43.3X2	T43.3X3	T43.3X4	T43.3X5	T43.3X6
Fluoroacetate	T6Ø.8X1	T6Ø.8X2	T6Ø.8X3	T6Ø.8X4	—	—
Fluorescein	T5Ø.8X1	T5Ø.8X2	T5Ø.8X3	T5Ø.8X4	T5Ø.8X5	T5Ø.8X6
Fluorhydrocortisone	T5Ø.ØX1	T5Ø.ØX2	T5Ø.ØX3	T5Ø.ØX4	T5Ø.ØX5	T5Ø.ØX6
Fluoride (nonmedicinal) (pesticide) (sodium) NEC	T6Ø.8X1	T6Ø.8X2	T6Ø.8X3	T6Ø.8X4	—	—
hydrogen — *see Hydrofluoric acid*						
medicinal NEC	T5Ø.991	T5Ø.992	T5Ø.993	T5Ø.994	T5Ø.995	T5Ø.996
dental use	T49.7X1	T49.7X2	T49.7X3	T49.7X4	T49.7X5	T49.7X6
not pesticide NEC	T54.91	T54.92	T54.93	T54.94	—	—
stannous	T49.7X1	T49.7X2	T49.7X3	T49.7X4	T49.7X5	T49.7X6
Fluorinated corticosteroids	T38.ØX1	T38.ØX2	T38.ØX3	T38.ØX4	T38.ØX5	T38.ØX6
Fluorine (gas)	T59.5X1	T59.5X2	T59.5X3	T59.5X4	—	—
salt — *see Fluoride(s)*						
Fluoristan	T49.7X1	T49.7X2	T49.7X3	T49.7X4	T49.7X5	T49.7X6
Fluormetholone	T49.ØX1	T49.ØX2	T49.ØX3	T49.ØX4	T49.ØX5	T49.ØX6
Fluoroacetate	T6Ø.8X1	T6Ø.8X2	T6Ø.8X3	T6Ø.8X4	—	—
Fluorocarbon monomer	T53.6X1	T53.6X2	T53.6X3	T53.6X4	—	—
Fluorocytosine	T37.8X1	T37.8X2	T37.8X3	T37.8X4	T37.8X5	T37.8X6
Fluorodeoxyuridine	T45.1X1	T45.1X2	T45.1X3	T45.1X4	T45.1X5	T45.1X6
Fluorometholone	T49.ØX1	T49.ØX2	T49.ØX3	T49.ØX4	T49.ØX5	T49.ØX6
ophthalmic preparation	T49.5X1	T49.5X2	T49.5X3	T49.5X4	T49.5X5	T49.5X6
Fluorophosphate insecticide	T6Ø.ØX1	T6Ø.ØX2	T6Ø.ØX3	T6Ø.ØX4	—	—
Fluorosol	T46.3X1	T46.3X2	T46.3X3	T46.3X4	T46.3X5	T46.3X6
Fluorouracil	T45.1X1	T45.1X2	T45.1X3	T45.1X4	T45.1X5	T45.1X6

Substance	Poisoning, Accidental (Unintentional)	Poisoning, Intentional Self-Harm	Poisoning, Assault	Poisoning, Undetermined	Adverse Effect	Underdosing
Fluorphenylalanine	T49.5X1	T49.5X2	T49.5X3	T49.5X4	T49.5X5	T49.5X6
Fluothane	T41.ØX1	T41.ØX2	T41.ØX3	T41.ØX4	T41.ØX5	T41.ØX6
Fluoxetine	T43.221	T43.222	T43.223	T43.224	T43.225	T43.226
Fluoxymesterone	T38.7X1	T38.7X2	T38.7X3	T38.7X4	T38.7X5	T38.7X6
Flupenthixol	T43.4X1	T43.4X2	T43.4X3	T43.4X4	T43.4X5	T43.4X6
Flupentixol	T43.4X1	T43.4X2	T43.4X3	T43.4X4	T43.4X5	T43.4X6
Fluphenazine	T43.3X1	T43.3X2	T43.3X3	T43.3X4	T43.3X5	T43.3X6
Fluprednidene	T49.ØX1	T49.ØX2	T49.ØX3	T49.ØX4	T49.ØX5	T49.ØX6
Fluprednisolone	T38.ØX1	T38.ØX2	T38.ØX3	T38.ØX4	T38.ØX5	T38.ØX6
Fluradoline	T39.8X1	T39.8X2	T39.8X3	T39.8X4	T39.8X5	T39.8X6
Flurandrenolide	T49.ØX1	T49.ØX2	T49.ØX3	T49.ØX4	T49.ØX5	T49.ØX6
Flurandrenolone	T49.ØX1	T49.ØX2	T49.ØX3	T49.ØX4	T49.ØX5	T49.ØX6
Flurazepam	T42.4X1	T42.4X2	T42.4X3	T42.4X4	T42.4X5	T42.4X6
Flurbiprofen	T39.311	T39.312	T39.313	T39.314	T39.315	T39.316
Flurobate	T49.ØX1	T49.ØX2	T49.ØX3	T49.ØX4	T49.ØX5	T49.ØX6
Flurotyl	T43.291	T43.292	T43.293	T43.294	T43.295	T43.296
Fluroxene	T41.ØX1	T41.ØX2	T41.ØX3	T41.ØX4	T41.ØX5	T41.ØX6
Fluspirilene	T43.591	T43.592	T43.593	T43.594	T43.595	T43.596
Flutamide	T38.6X1	T38.6X2	T38.6X3	T38.6X4	T38.6X5	T38.6X6
Flutazolam	T42.4X1	T42.4X2	T42.4X3	T42.4X4	T42.4X5	T42.4X6
Fluticasone propionate	T49.1X1	T49.1X2	T49.1X3	T49.1X4	T49.1X5	T49.1X6
Flutoprazepam	T42.4X1	T42.4X2	T42.4X3	T42.4X4	T42.4X5	T42.4X6
Flutropium bromide	T48.6X1	T48.6X2	T48.6X3	T48.6X4	T48.6X5	T48.6X6
Fluvoxamine	T43.221	T43.222	T43.223	T43.224	T43.225	T43.226
Folacin	T45.8X1	T45.8X2	T45.8X3	T45.8X4	T45.8X5	T45.8X6
Folic acid	T45.8X1	T45.8X2	T45.8X3	T45.8X4	T45.8X5	T45.8X6
with ferrous salt	T45.2X1	T45.2X2	T45.2X3	T45.2X4	T45.2X5	T45.2X6
antagonist	T45.1X1	T45.1X2	T45.1X3	T45.1X4	T45.1X5	T45.1X6
Folinic acid	T45.8X1	T45.8X2	T45.8X3	T45.8X4	T45.8X5	T45.8X6
Folium stramoniae	T48.6X1	T48.6X2	T48.6X3	T48.6X4	T48.6X5	T48.6X6
Follicle-stimulating hormone, human	T38.811	T38.812	T38.813	T38.814	T38.815	T38.816
Folpet	T6Ø.3X1	T6Ø.3X2	T6Ø.3X3	T6Ø.3X4	—	—
Fominoben	T48.3X1	T48.3X2	T48.3X3	T48.3X4	T48.3X5	T48.3X6
Food, foodstuffs, noxious, nonbacterial, NEC	T62.91	T62.92	T62.93	T62.94	—	—
berries	T62.1X1	T62.1X2	T62.1X3	T62.1X4	—	—
fish — *see also Fish*	T61.91	T61.92	T61.93	T61.94	—	—
mushrooms	T62.ØX1	T62.ØX2	T62.ØX3	T62.ØX4	—	—
plants	T62.2X1	T62.2X2	T62.2X3	T62.2X4	—	—
seafood	T61.91	T61.92	T61.93	T61.94	—	—
specified NEC	T61.8X1	T61.8X2	T61.8X3	T61.8X4	—	—
seeds	T62.2X1	T62.2X2	T62.2X3	T62.2X4	—	—

TABLE OF DRUGS AND CHEMICALS

Substance	Poisoning, Accidental (Unintentional)	Poisoning, Intentional Self-Harm	Poisoning, Assault	Poisoning, Undetermined	Adverse Effect	Underdosing
Food, foodstuffs, noxious, nonbacterial, NEC *(Continued)*						
shellfish	T61.781	T61.782	T61.783	T61.784	—	—
specified NEC	T62.8X1	T62.8X2	T62.8X3	T62.8X4	—	—
Fool's parsley	T62.2X1	T62.2X2	T62.2X3	T62.2X4	—	—
Formaldehyde (solution), gas or vapor	T59.2X1	T59.2X2	T59.2X3	T59.2X4	—	—
fungicide	T60.3X1	T60.3X2	T60.3X3	T60.3X4	—	—
Formalin	T59.2X1	T59.2X2	T59.2X3	T59.2X4	—	—
fungicide	T60.3X1	T60.3X2	T60.3X3	T60.3X4	—	—
vapor	T59.2X1	T59.2X2	T59.2X3	T59.2X4	—	—
Formic acid	T54.2X1	T54.2X2	T54.2X3	T54.2X4	—	—
vapor	T59.891	T59.892	T59.893	T59.894	—	—
Foscarnet sodium	T37.5X1	T37.5X2	T37.5X3	T37.5X4	T37.5X5	T37.5X6
Fosfestrol	T38.5X1	T38.5X2	T38.5X3	T38.5X4	T38.5X5	T38.5X6
Fosfomycin	T36.8X1	T36.8X2	T36.8X3	T36.8X4	T36.8X5	T36.8X6
Fosfonet sodium	T37.5X1	T37.5X2	T37.5X3	T37.5X4	T37.5X5	T37.5X6
Fosinopril	T46.4X1	T46.4X2	T46.4X3	T46.4X4	T46.4X5	T46.4X6
sodium	T46.4X1	T46.4X2	T46.4X3	T46.4X4	T46.4X5	T46.4X6
Fowler's solution	T57.0X1	T57.0X2	T57.0X3	T57.0X4	—	—
Foxglove	T62.2X1	T62.2X2	T62.2X3	T62.2X4	—	—
Framycetin	T36.5X1	T36.5X2	T36.5X3	T36.5X4	T36.5X5	T36.5X6
Frangula	T47.2X1	T47.2X2	T47.2X3	T47.2X4	T47.2X5	T47.2X6
extract	T47.2X1	T47.2X2	T47.2X3	T47.2X4	T47.2X5	T47.2X6
Frei antigen	T50.8X1	T50.8X2	T50.8X3	T50.8X4	T50.8X5	T50.8X6
Freon	T53.5X1	T53.5X2	T53.5X3	T53.5X4	—	—
Fructose	T50.3X1	T50.3X2	T50.3X3	T50.3X4	T50.3X5	T50.3X6
Frusemide	T50.1X1	T50.1X2	T50.1X3	T50.1X4	T50.1X5	T50.1X6
FSH	T38.811	T38.812	T38.813	T38.814	T38.815	T38.816
Ftorafur	T45.1X1	T45.1X2	T45.1X3	T45.1X4	T45.1X5	T45.1X6
Fuel						
automobile	T52.0X1	T52.0X2	T52.0X3	T52.0X4	—	—
exhaust gas, not in transit	T58.01	T58.02	T58.03	T58.04	—	—
vapor NEC	T52.0X1	T52.0X2	T52.0X3	T52.0X4	—	—
gas (domestic use) — *see also Carbon, monoxide, fuel, utility*	T59.891	T59.892	T59.893	T59.894	—	—
utility	T59.891	T59.892	T59.893	T59.894	—	—
in mobile container	T59.891	T59.892	T59.893	T59.894	—	—
incomplete combustion of — *see Carbon, monoxide, fuel, utility*						
piped (natural)	T59.891	T59.892	T59.893	T59.894	—	—
industrial, incomplete combustion	T58.8X1	T58.8X2	T58.8X3	T58.8X4	—	—

Substance	Poisoning, Accidental (Unintentional)	Poisoning, Intentional Self-Harm	Poisoning, Assault	Poisoning, Undetermined	Adverse Effect	Underdosing
Fugillin	T36.8X1	T36.8X2	T36.8X3	T36.8X4	T36.8X5	T36.8X6
Fulminate of mercury	T56.1X1	T56.1X2	T56.1X3	T56.1X4	—	—
Fulvicin	T36.7X1	T36.7X2	T36.7X3	T36.7X4	T36.7X5	T36.7X6
Fumadil	T36.8X1	T36.8X2	T36.8X3	T36.8X4	T36.8X5	T36.8X6
Fumagillin	T36.8X1	T36.8X2	T36.8X3	T36.8X4	T36.8X5	T36.8X6
Fumaric acid	T49.4X1	T49.4X2	T49.4X3	T49.4X4	T49.4X5	T49.4X6
Fumes (from)	T59.91	T59.92	T59.93	T59.94	—	—
carbon monoxide — *see Carbon, monoxide*						
charcoal (domestic use) — *see Charcoal, fumes*						
chloroform — *see Chloroform*						
coke (in domestic stoves, fireplaces) — *see Coke, fumes*						
corrosive NEC	T54.91	T54.92	T54.93	T54.94	—	—
ether — *see ether*						
freons	T53.5X1	T53.5X2	T53.5X3	T53.5X4	—	—
hydrocarbons	T59.891	T59.892	T59.893	T59.894	—	—
petroleum (liquefied)	T59.891	T59.892	T59.893	T59.894	—	—
distributed through pipes (pure or mixed with air)	T59.891	T59.892	T59.893	T59.894	—	—
lead — *see lead*						
metal — *see Metals, or the specified metal*						
nitrogen dioxide	T59.0X1	T59.0X2	T59.0X3	T59.0X4	—	—
pesticides — *see Pesticides*						
petroleum (liquefied)	T59.891	T59.892	T59.893	T59.894	—	—
distributed through pipes (pure or mixed with air)	T59.891	T59.892	T59.893	T59.894	—	—
polyester	T59.891	T59.892	T59.893	T59.894	—	—
specified source NEC — *see also substance specified*	T59.891	T59.892	T59.893	T59.894	—	—
sulfur dioxide	T59.1X1	T59.1X2	T59.1X3	T59.1X4	—	—
Fumigant NEC	T60.91	T60.92	T60.93	T60.94	—	—
Fungi, noxious, used as food	T62.0X1	T62.0X2	T62.0X3	T62.0X4	—	—
Fungicide NEC (nonmedicinal)	T60.3X1	T60.3X2	T60.3X3	T60.3X4	—	—
Fungizone	T36.7X1	T36.7X2	T36.7X3	T36.7X4	T36.7X5	T36.7X6
topical	T49.0X1	T49.0X2	T49.0X3	T49.0X4	T49.0X5	T49.0X6
Furacin	T49.0X1	T49.0X2	T49.0X3	T49.0X4	T49.0X5	T49.0X6
Furadantin	T37.91	T37.92	T37.93	T37.94	T37.95	T37.96
Furazolidone	T37.8X1	T37.8X2	T37.8X3	T37.8X4	T37.8X5	T37.8X6
Furazolium chloride	T49.0X1	T49.0X2	T49.0X3	T49.0X4	T49.0X5	T49.0X6
Furfural	T52.8X1	T52.8X2	T52.8X3	T52.8X4	—	—

Substance	Poisoning, Accidental (Unintentional)	Poisoning, Intentional Self-Harm	Poisoning, Assault	Poisoning, Undetermined	Adverse Effect	Underdosing
Furnace (coal burning) (domestic), gas from industrial	T58.2X1	T58.2X2	T58.2X3	T58.2X4	—	—
industrial	T58.8X1	T58.8X2	T58.8X3	T58.8X4	—	—
Furniture polish	T65.891	T65.892	T65.893	T65.894	—	—
Furosemide	T5Ø.1X1	T5Ø.1X2	T5Ø.1X3	T5Ø.1X4	T5Ø.1X5	T5Ø.1X6
Furoxone	T37.91	T37.92	T37.93	T37.94	T37.95	T37.96
Fursultiamine	T45.2X1	T45.2X2	T45.2X3	T45.2X4	T45.2X5	T45.2X6
Fusafungine	T36.8X1	T36.8X2	T36.8X3	T36.8X4	T36.8X5	T36.8X6
Fusel oil (any) (amyl) (butyl) (propyl), vapor	T51.3X1	T51.3X2	T51.3X3	T51.3X4	—	—
Fusidate (ethanolamine) (sodium)	T36.8X1	T36.8X2	T36.8X3	T36.8X4	T36.8X5	T36.8X6
Fusidic acid	T36.8X1	T36.8X2	T36.8X3	T36.8X4	T36.8X5	T36.8X6
Fytic acid, nonasodium	T5Ø.6X1	T5Ø.6X2	T5Ø.6X3	T5Ø.6X4	T5Ø.6X5	T5Ø.6X6
G						
GABA	T43.8X1	T43.8X2	T43.8X3	T43.8X4	T43.8X5	T43.8X6
Gadopentetic acid	T5Ø.8X1	T5Ø.8X2	T5Ø.8X3	T5Ø.8X4	T5Ø.8X5	T5Ø.8X6
Galactose	T5Ø.3X1	T5Ø.3X2	T5Ø.3X3	T5Ø.3X4	T5Ø.3X5	T5Ø.3X6
b-Galactosidase	T47.5X1	T47.5X2	T47.5X3	T47.5X4	T47.5X5	T47.5X6
Galantamine	T44.ØX1	T44.ØX2	T44.ØX3	T44.ØX4	T44.ØX5	T44.ØX6
Gallamine (triethiodide)	T48.1X1	T48.1X2	T48.1X3	T48.1X4	T48.1X5	T48.1X6
Gallium citrate	T5Ø.991	T5Ø.992	T5Ø.993	T5Ø.994	T5Ø.995	T5Ø.996
Gallopamil	T46.1X1	T46.1X2	T46.1X3	T46.1X4	T46.1X5	T46.1X6
Gamboge	T47.2X1	T47.2X2	T47.2X3	T47.2X4	T47.2X5	T47.2X6
Gamimune	T5Ø.Z11	T5Ø.Z12	T5Ø.Z13	T5Ø.Z14	T5Ø.Z15	T5Ø.Z16
Gamma-aminobutyric acid	T43.8X1	T43.8X2	T43.8X3	T43.8X4	T43.8X5	T43.8X6
Gamma-benzene hexachloride (medicinal)	T49.ØX1	T49.ØX2	T49.ØX3	T49.ØX4	T49.ØX5	T49.ØX6
nonmedicinal, vapor	T53.6X1	T53.6X2	T53.6X3	T53.6X4	—	—
Gamma-BHC (medicinal) — *see also Gamma-benzene hexachloride*	T49.ØX1	T49.ØX2	T49.ØX3	T49.ØX4	T49.ØX5	T49.ØX6
Gamma globulin	T5Ø.Z11	T5Ø.Z12	T5Ø.Z13	T5Ø.Z14	T5Ø.Z15	T5Ø.Z16
Gamulin	T5Ø.Z11	T5Ø.Z12	T5Ø.Z13	T5Ø.Z14	T5Ø.Z15	T5Ø.Z16
Ganciclovir (sodium)	T37.5X1	T37.5X2	T37.5X3	T37.5X4	T37.5X5	T37.5X6
Ganglionic blocking drug NEC	T44.2X1	T44.2X2	T44.2X3	T44.2X4	T44.2X5	T44.2X6
specified NEC	T44.2X1	T44.2X2	T44.2X3	T44.2X4	T44.2X5	T44.2X6
Ganja	T4Ø.7X1	T4Ø.7X2	T4Ø.7X3	T4Ø.7X4	T4Ø.7X5	T4Ø.7X6
Garamycin	T36.5X1	T36.5X2	T36.5X3	T36.5X4	T36.5X5	T36.5X6
ophthalmic preparation	T49.5X1	T49.5X2	T49.5X3	T49.5X4	T49.5X5	T49.5X6
topical NEC	T49.ØX1	T49.ØX2	T49.ØX3	T49.ØX4	T49.ØX5	T49.ØX6
Gardenal	T42.3X1	T42.3X2	T42.3X3	T42.3X4	T42.3X5	T42.3X6
Gardepanyl	T42.3X1	T42.3X2	T42.3X3	T42.3X4	T42.3X5	T42.3X6

Substance	Poisoning, Accidental (Unintentional)	Poisoning, Intentional Self-Harm	Poisoning, Assault	Poisoning, Undetermined	Adverse Effect	Underdosing
Gas	T59.91	T59.92	T59.93	T59.94	—	—
acetylene	T59.891	T59.892	T59.893	T59.894	—	—
incomplete combustion of	T58.11	T58.12	T58.13	T58.14	—	—
air contaminants, source or type not specified	T59.91	T59.92	T59.93	T59.94	—	—
anesthetic	T41.ØX1	T41.ØX2	T41.ØX3	T41.ØX4	T41.ØX5	T41.ØX6
blast furnace	T58.8X1	T58.8X2	T58.8X3	T58.8X4	—	—
butane — *see butane*						
carbon monoxide — *see Carbon, monoxide*						
chlorine	T59.4X1	T59.4X2	T59.4X3	T59.4X4	—	—
coal	T58.2X1	T58.2X2	T58.2X3	T58.2X4	—	—
cyanide	T57.3X1	T57.3X2	T57.3X3	T57.3X4	—	—
dicyanogen	T65.ØX1	T65.ØX2	T65.ØX3	T65.ØX4	—	—
domestic — *see Domestic gas*	T57.91	T57.92	T57.93	T57.94	—	—
exhaust	T57.91	T57.92	T57.93	T57.94	—	—
from utility (for cooking, heating, or lighting) (after combustion) — *see Carbon, monoxide, fuel, utility*						
prior to combustion	T59.891	T59.892	T59.893	T59.894	—	—
from wood or coal-burning stove or fireplace	T57.91	T57.92	T57.93	T57.94	—	—
fuel (domestic use) (after combustion) — *see also Carbon, monoxide, fuel*	T57.91	T57.92	T57.93	T57.94	—	—
industrial use	T58.8X1	T58.8X2	T58.8X3	T58.8X4	—	—
prior to combustion	T59.891	T59.892	T59.893	T59.894	—	—
utility	T59.891	T59.892	T59.893	T59.894	—	—
in mobile container	T59.891	T59.892	T59.893	T59.894	—	—
incomplete combustion of — *see Carbon, monoxide, fuel, utility*						
piped (natural)	T59.891	T59.892	T59.893	T59.894	—	—
garage	T58.Ø1	T58.Ø2	T58.Ø3	T58.Ø4	—	—
hydrocarbon NEC	T59.891	T59.892	T59.893	T59.894	—	—
incomplete combustion of — *see Carbon, monoxide, fuel, utility*						
liquefied — *see butane*						
piped	T59.891	T59.892	T59.893	T59.894	—	—
hydrocyanic acid	T65.ØX1	T65.ØX2	T65.ØX3	T65.ØX4	—	—

Substance	Poisoning, Accidental (Unintentional)	Poisoning, Intentional Self-Harm	Poisoning, Assault	Poisoning, Undetermined	Adverse Effect	Underdosing
Gas *(Continued)*						
illuminating (after combustion)	T58.11	T58.12	T58.13	T58.14	—	—
prior to combustion	T59.891	T59.892	T59.893	T59.894	—	—
incomplete combustion, any — *see Carbon, monoxide*						
kiln	T58.8X1	T58.8X2	T58.8X3	T58.8X4	—	—
lacrimogenic	T59.3X1	T59.3X2	T59.3X3	T59.3X4	—	—
liquefied petroleum — *see butane*						
marsh	T59.891	T59.892	T59.893	T59.894	—	—
motor exhaust, not in transit	T58.01	T58.02	T58.03	T58.04	—	—
mustard, not in war	T59.891	T59.892	T59.893	T59.894	—	—
natural	T59.891	T59.892	T59.893	T59.894	—	—
nerve, not in war	T59.91	T59.92	T59.93	T59.94	—	—
oil	T52.0X1	T52.0X2	T52.0X3	T52.0X4	—	—
petroleum (liquefied) (distributed in mobile containers)	T59.891	T59.892	T59.893	T59.894	—	—
piped (pure or mixed with air)	T59.891	T59.892	T59.893	T59.894	—	—
piped (manufactured) (natural) NEC	T59.891	T59.892	T59.893	T59.894	—	—
producer	T58.8X1	T58.8X2	T58.8X3	T58.8X4	—	—
propane — *see propane*						
refrigerant (chlorofluoro-carbon)	T53.5X1	T53.5X2	T53.5X3	T53.5X4	—	—
not chlorofluoro-carbon	T59.891	T59.892	T59.893	T59.894	—	—
sewer	T59.91	T59.92	T59.93	T59.94	—	—
specified source NEC	T59.91	T59.92	T59.93	T59.94	—	—
stove (after combustion)	T58.11	T58.12	T58.13	T58.14	—	—
tear	T59.3X1	T59.3X2	T59.3X3	T59.3X4	—	—
therapeutic	T41.5X1	T41.5X2	T41.5X3	T41.5X4	T41.5X5	T41.5X6
utility (for cooking, heating, or lighting) (piped) NEC	T59.891	T59.892	T59.893	T59.894	—	—
in mobile container	T59.891	T59.892	T59.893	T59.894	—	—
incomplete combustion of — *see Carbon, monoxide, fuel, utility*						
piped (natural)	T59.891	T59.892	T59.893	T59.894	—	—
water	T58.11	T58.12	T58.13	T58.14	—	—
incomplete combustion of — *see Carbon, monoxide, fuel, utility*						
Gaseous substance — *see Gas*						
Gasoline	T52.0X1	T52.0X2	T52.0X3	T52.0X4	—	—
vapor	T52.0X1	T52.0X2	T52.0X3	T52.0X4	—	—
Gastric enzymes	T47.5X1	T47.5X2	T47.5X3	T47.5X4	T47.5X5	T47.5X6
Gastrografin	T50.8X1	T50.8X2	T50.8X3	T50.8X4	T50.8X5	T50.8X6
Gastrointestinal drug	T47.91	T47.92	T47.93	T47.94	T47.95	T47.96
biological	T47.8X1	T47.8X2	T47.8X3	T47.8X4	T47.8X5	T47.8X6
specified NEC	T47.8X1	T47.8X2	T47.8X3	T47.8X4	T47.8X5	T47.8X6
Gaultheria procumbens	T62.2X1	T62.2X2	T62.2X3	T62.2X4	—	—
Gelatin (intravenous)	T45.8X1	T45.8X2	T45.8X3	T45.8X4	T45.8X5	T45.8X6
absorbable (sponge)	T45.7X1	T45.7X2	T45.7X3	T45.7X4	T45.7X5	T45.7X6
Gefarnate	T44.3X1	T44.3X2	T44.3X3	T44.3X4	T44.3X5	T44.3X6
Gelfilm	T49.8X1	T49.8X2	T49.8X3	T49.8X4	T49.8X5	T49.8X6
Gelfoam	T45.7X1	T45.7X2	T45.7X3	T45.7X4	T45.7X5	T45.7X6
Gelsemine	T50.991	T50.992	T50.993	T50.994	T50.995	T50.996
Gelsemium (sempervirens)	T62.2X1	T62.2X2	T62.2X3	T62.2X4	—	—
Gemeprost	T48.0X1	T48.0X2	T48.0X3	T48.0X4	T48.0X5	T48.0X6
Gemfibrozil	T46.6X1	T46.6X2	T46.6X3	T46.6X4	T46.6X5	T46.6X6
Gemonil	T42.3X1	T42.3X2	T42.3X3	T42.3X4	T42.3X5	T42.3X6
Gentamicin	T36.5X1	T36.5X2	T36.5X3	T36.5X4	T36.5X5	T36.5X6
ophthalmic preparation	T49.5X1	T49.5X2	T49.5X3	T49.5X4	T49.5X5	T49.5X6
topical NEC	T49.0X1	T49.0X2	T49.0X3	T49.0X4	T49.0X5	T49.0X6
Gentian	T47.5X1	T47.5X2	T47.5X3	T47.5X4	T47.5X5	T47.5X6
violet	T49.0X1	T49.0X2	T49.0X3	T49.0X4	T49.0X5	T49.0X6
Gepefrine	T44.4X1	T44.4X2	T44.4X3	T44.4X4	T44.4X5	T44.4X6
Gestonorone caproate	T38.5X1	T38.5X2	T38.5X3	T38.5X4	T38.5X5	T38.5X6
Gexane	T49.0X1	T49.0X2	T49.0X3	T49.0X4	T49.0X5	T49.0X6
Gila monster (venom)	T63.111	T63.112	T63.113	T63.114	—	—
Ginger	T47.5X1	T47.5X2	T47.5X3	T47.5X4	T47.5X5	T47.5X6
Jamaica — *see Jamaica, ginger*						
Gitalin	T46.0X1	T46.0X2	T46.0X3	T46.0X4	T46.0X5	T46.0X6
amorphous	T46.0X1	T46.0X2	T46.0X3	T46.0X4	T46.0X5	T46.0X6
Gitaloxin	T46.0X1	T46.0X2	T46.0X3	T46.0X4	T46.0X5	T46.0X6
Gitoxin	T46.0X1	T46.0X2	T46.0X3	T46.0X4	T46.0X5	T46.0X6
Glafenine	T39.8X1	T39.8X2	T39.8X3	T39.8X4	T39.8X5	T39.8X6
Glandular extract (medicinal) NEC	T50.Z91	T50.Z92	T50.Z93	T50.Z94	T50.Z95	T50.Z96
Glaucarubin	T37.3X1	T37.3X2	T37.3X3	T37.3X4	T37.3X5	T37.3X6
Glibenclamide	T38.3X1	T38.3X2	T38.3X3	T38.3X4	T38.3X5	T38.3X6
Glibornuride	T38.3X1	T38.3X2	T38.3X3	T38.3X4	T38.3X5	T38.3X6
Gliclazide	T38.3X1	T38.3X2	T38.3X3	T38.3X4	T38.3X5	T38.3X6
Glimidine	T38.3X1	T38.3X2	T38.3X3	T38.3X4	T38.3X5	T38.3X6

Substance	Poisoning, Accidental (Unintentional)	Poisoning, Intentional Self-Harm	Poisoning, Assault	Poisoning, Undetermined	Adverse Effect	Underdosing
Glipizide	T38.3X1	T38.3X2	T38.3X3	T38.3X4	T38.3X5	T38.3X6
Gliquidone	T38.3X1	T38.3X2	T38.3X3	T38.3X4	T38.3X5	T38.3X6
Glisolamide	T38.3X1	T38.3X2	T38.3X3	T38.3X4	T38.3X5	T38.3X6
Glisoxepide	T38.3X1	T38.3X2	T38.3X3	T38.3X4	T38.3X5	T38.3X6
Globin zinc insulin	T38.3X1	T38.3X2	T38.3X3	T38.3X4	T38.3X5	T38.3X6
Globulin						
antilymphocytic	T5Ø.Z11	T5Ø.Z12	T5Ø.Z13	T5Ø.Z14	T5Ø.Z15	T5Ø.Z16
antirhesus	T5Ø.Z11	T5Ø.Z12	T5Ø.Z13	T5Ø.Z14	T5Ø.Z15	T5Ø.Z16
antivenin	T5Ø.Z11	T5Ø.Z12	T5Ø.Z13	T5Ø.Z14	T5Ø.Z15	T5Ø.Z16
antiviral	T5Ø.Z11	T5Ø.Z12	T5Ø.Z13	T5Ø.Z14	T5Ø.Z15	T5Ø.Z16
Glucagon	T38.3X1	T38.3X2	T38.3X3	T38.3X4	T38.3X5	T38.3X6
Glucocorticoids	T38.ØX1	T38.ØX2	T38.ØX3	T38.ØX4	T38.ØX5	T38.ØX6
Glucocorticosteroid	T38.ØX1	T38.ØX2	T38.ØX3	T38.ØX4	T38.ØX5	T38.ØX6
Gluconic acid	T5Ø.991	T5Ø.992	T5Ø.993	T5Ø.994	T5Ø.995	T5Ø.996
Glucosamine sulfate	T39.4X1	T39.4X2	T39.4X3	T39.4X4	T39.4X5	T39.4X6
Glucose	T5Ø.3X1	T5Ø.3X2	T5Ø.3X3	T5Ø.3X4	T5Ø.3X5	T5Ø.3X6
with sodium chloride	T5Ø.3X1	T5Ø.3X2	T5Ø.3X3	T5Ø.3X4	T5Ø.3X5	T5Ø.3X6
Glucosulfone sodium	T37.1X1	T37.1X2	T37.1X3	T37.1X4	T37.1X5	T37.1X6
Glucurolactone	T47.8X1	T47.8X2	T47.8X3	T47.8X4	T47.8X5	T47.8X6
Glue NEC	T52.8X1	T52.8X2	T52.8X3	T52.8X4	—	—
Glutamic acid	T47.5X1	T47.5X2	T47.5X3	T47.5X4	T47.5X5	T47.5X6
Glutaral (medicinal)	T49.ØX1	T49.ØX2	T49.ØX3	T49.ØX4	T49.ØX5	T49.ØX6
nonmedicinal	T65.891	T65.892	T65.893	T65.894	—	—
Glutaraldehyde (nonmedicinal)	T65.891	T65.892	T65.893	T65.894	—	—
medicinal	T49.ØX1	T49.ØX2	T49.ØX3	T49.ØX4	T49.ØX5	T49.ØX6
Glutathione	T5Ø.6X1	T5Ø.6X2	T5Ø.6X3	T5Ø.6X4	T5Ø.6X5	T5Ø.6X6
Glutethimide	T42.6X1	T42.6X2	T42.6X3	T42.6X4	T42.6X5	T42.6X6
Glyburide	T38.3X1	T38.3X2	T38.3X3	T38.3X4	T38.3X5	T38.3X6
Glycerin	T47.4X1	T47.4X2	T47.4X3	T47.4X4	T47.4X5	T47.4X6
Glycerol	T47.4X1	T47.4X2	T47.4X3	T47.4X4	T47.4X5	T47.4X6
borax	T49.6X1	T49.6X2	T49.6X3	T49.6X4	T49.6X5	T49.6X6
intravenous	T5Ø.3X1	T5Ø.3X2	T5Ø.3X3	T5Ø.3X4	T5Ø.3X5	T5Ø.3X6
iodinated	T48.4X1	T48.4X2	T48.4X3	T48.4X4	T48.4X5	T48.4X6
Glycerophosphate	T5Ø.991	T5Ø.992	T5Ø.993	T5Ø.994	T5Ø.995	T5Ø.996
Glyceryl						
guaiacolate	T48.4X1	T48.4X2	T48.4X3	T48.4X4	T48.4X5	T48.4X6
nitrate	T46.3X1	T46.3X2	T46.3X3	T46.3X4	T46.3X5	T46.3X6
triacetate (topical)	T49.ØX1	T49.ØX2	T49.ØX3	T49.ØX4	T49.ØX5	T49.ØX6
trinitrate	T46.3X1	T46.3X2	T46.3X3	T46.3X4	T46.3X5	T46.3X6
Glycine	T5Ø.3X1	T5Ø.3X2	T5Ø.3X3	T5Ø.3X4	T5Ø.3X5	T5Ø.3X6
Glyclopyramide	T38.3X1	T38.3X2	T38.3X3	T38.3X4	T38.3X5	T38.3X6
Glycobiarsol	T37.3X1	T37.3X2	T37.3X3	T37.3X4	T37.3X5	T37.3X6
Glycols (ether)	T52.3X1	T52.3X2	T52.3X3	T52.3X4	—	—
Glyconiazide	T37.1X1	T37.1X2	T37.1X3	T37.1X4	T37.1X5	T37.1X6
Glycopyrrolate	T44.3X1	T44.3X2	T44.3X3	T44.3X4	T44.3X5	T44.3X6
Glycopyrronium	T44.3X1	T44.3X2	T44.3X3	T44.3X4	T44.3X5	T44.3X6
bromide	T44.3X1	T44.3X2	T44.3X3	T44.3X4	T44.3X5	T44.3X6
Glycoside, cardiac (stimulant)	T46.ØX1	T46.ØX2	T46.ØX3	T46.ØX4	T46.ØX5	T46.ØX6
Glycyclamide	T38.3X1	T38.3X2	T38.3X3	T38.3X4	T38.3X5	T38.3X6
Glycyrrhiza extract	T48.4X1	T48.4X2	T48.4X3	T48.4X4	T48.4X5	T48.4X6
Glycyrrhizic acid	T48.4X1	T48.4X2	T48.4X3	T48.4X4	T48.4X5	T48.4X6
Glycyrrhizinate potassium	T48.4X1	T48.4X2	T48.4X3	T48.4X4	T48.4X5	T48.4X6
Glymidine sodium	T38.3X1	T38.3X2	T38.3X3	T38.3X4	T38.3X5	T38.3X6
Glyphosate	T6Ø.3X1	T6Ø.3X2	T6Ø.3X3	T6Ø.3X4	—	—
Glyphylline	T48.6X1	T48.6X2	T48.6X3	T48.6X4	T48.6X5	T48.6X6
Gold						
colloidal (198Au)	T45.1X1	T45.1X2	T45.1X3	T45.1X4	T45.1X5	T45.1X6
salts	T39.4X1	T39.4X2	T39.4X3	T39.4X4	T39.4X5	T39.4X6
Golden sulfide of antimony	T56.891	T56.892	T56.893	T56.894	—	—
Goldylocks	T62.2X1	T62.2X2	T62.2X3	T62.2X4	—	—
Gonadal tissue extract	T38.9Ø1	T38.9Ø2	T38.9Ø3	T38.9Ø4	T38.9Ø5	T38.9Ø6
female	T38.5X1	T38.5X2	T38.5X3	T38.5X4	T38.5X5	T38.5X6
male	T38.7X1	T38.7X2	T38.7X3	T38.7X4	T38.7X5	T38.7X6
Gonadorelin	T38.891	T38.892	T38.893	T38.894	T38.895	T38.896
Gonadotropin	T38.891	T38.892	T38.893	T38.894	T38.895	T38.896
chorionic	T38.891	T38.892	T38.893	T38.894	T38.895	T38.896
pituitary	T38.811	T38.812	T38.813	T38.814	T38.815	T38.816
Goserelin	T45.1X1	T45.1X2	T45.1X3	T45.1X4	T45.1X5	T45.1X6
Grain alcohol	T51.ØX1	T51.ØX2	T51.ØX3	T51.ØX4	—	—
Gramicidin	T49.ØX1	T49.ØX2	T49.ØX3	T49.ØX4	T49.ØX5	T49.ØX6
Granisetron	T45.ØX1	T45.ØX2	T45.ØX3	T45.ØX4	T45.ØX5	T45.ØX6
Gratiola officinalis	T62.2X1	T62.2X2	T62.2X3	T62.2X4	—	—
Grease	T65.891	T65.892	T65.893	T65.894	—	—
Green hellebore	T62.2X1	T62.2X2	T62.2X3	T62.2X4	—	—
Green soap	T49.2X1	T49.2X2	T49.2X3	T49.2X4	T49.2X5	T49.2X6
Grifulvin	T36.7X1	T36.7X2	T36.7X3	T36.7X4	T36.7X5	T36.7X6
Griseofulvin	T36.7X1	T36.7X2	T36.7X3	T36.7X4	T36.7X5	T36.7X6
Growth hormone	T38.811	T38.812	T38.813	T38.814	T38.815	T38.816
Guaiacol derivatives	T48.4X1	T48.4X2	T48.4X3	T48.4X4	T48.4X5	T48.4X6
Guaiac reagent	T5Ø.991	T5Ø.992	T5Ø.993	T5Ø.994	T5Ø.995	T5Ø.996
Guaifenesin	T48.4X1	T48.4X2	T48.4X3	T48.4X4	T48.4X5	T48.4X6
Guaimesal	T48.4X1	T48.4X2	T48.4X3	T48.4X4	T48.4X5	T48.4X6
Guaiphenesin	T48.4X1	T48.4X2	T48.4X3	T48.4X4	T48.4X5	T48.4X6
Guamecycline	T36.4X1	T36.4X2	T36.4X3	T36.4X4	T36.4X5	T36.4X6

Substance	Poisoning, Accidental (Unintentional)	Poisoning, Intentional Self-Harm	Poisoning, Assault	Poisoning, Undetermined	Adverse Effect	Underdosing
Guanabenz	T46.5X1	T46.5X2	T46.5X3	T46.5X4	T46.5X5	T46.5X6
Guanacline	T46.5X1	T46.5X2	T46.5X3	T46.5X4	T46.5X5	T46.5X6
Guanadrel	T46.5X1	T46.5X2	T46.5X3	T46.5X4	T46.5X5	T46.5X6
Guanatol	T37.2X1	T37.2X2	T37.2X3	T37.2X4	T37.2X5	T37.2X6
Guanethidine	T46.5X1	T46.5X2	T46.5X3	T46.5X4	T46.5X5	T46.5X6
Guanfacine	T46.5X1	T46.5X2	T46.5X3	T46.5X4	T46.5X5	T46.5X6
Guano	T65.891	T65.892	T65.893	T65.894	—	—
Guanochlor	T46.5X1	T46.5X2	T46.5X3	T46.5X4	T46.5X5	T46.5X6
Guanoclor	T46.5X1	T46.5X2	T46.5X3	T46.5X4	T46.5X5	T46.5X6
Guanoctine	T46.5X1	T46.5X2	T46.5X3	T46.5X4	T46.5X5	T46.5X6
Guanoxabenz	T46.5X1	T46.5X2	T46.5X3	T46.5X4	T46.5X5	T46.5X6
Guanoxan	T46.5X1	T46.5X2	T46.5X3	T46.5X4	T46.5X5	T46.5X6
Guar gum (medicinal)	T46.6X1	T46.6X2	T46.6X3	T46.6X4	T46.6X5	T46.6X6
H						
Hachimycin	T36.7X1	T36.7X2	T36.7X3	T36.7X4	T36.7X5	T36.7X6
Hair						
dye	T49.4X1	T49.4X2	T49.4X3	T49.4X4	T49.4X5	T49.4X6
preparation NEC	T49.4X1	T49.4X2	T49.4X3	T49.4X4	T49.4X5	T49.4X6
Halazepam	T42.4X1	T42.4X2	T42.4X3	T42.4X4	T42.4X5	T42.4X6
Halcinolone	T49.ØX1	T49.ØX2	T49.ØX3	T49.ØX4	T49.ØX5	T49.ØX6
Halcinonide	T49.ØX1	T49.ØX2	T49.ØX3	T49.ØX4	T49.ØX5	T49.ØX6
Halethazole	T49.ØX1	T49.ØX2	T49.ØX3	T49.ØX4	T49.ØX5	T49.ØX6
Hallucinogen NEC	T4Ø.9Ø1	T4Ø.9Ø2	T4Ø.9Ø3	T4Ø.9Ø4	T4Ø.9Ø5	T4Ø.9Ø6
Halofantrine	T37.2X1	T37.2X2	T37.2X3	T37.2X4	T37.2X5	T37.2X6
Halofenate	T46.6X1	T46.6X2	T46.6X3	T46.6X4	T46.6X5	T46.6X6
Halometasone	T49.ØX1	T49.ØX2	T49.ØX3	T49.ØX4	T49.ØX5	T49.ØX6
Haloperidol	T43.4X1	T43.4X2	T43.4X3	T43.4X4	T43.4X5	T43.4X6
Haloprogin	T49.ØX1	T49.ØX2	T49.ØX3	T49.ØX4	T49.ØX5	T49.ØX6
Halotex	T49.ØX1	T49.ØX2	T49.ØX3	T49.ØX4	T49.ØX5	T49.ØX6
Halothane	T41.ØX1	T41.ØX2	T41.ØX3	T41.ØX4	T41.ØX5	T41.ØX6
Haloxazolam	T42.4X1	T42.4X2	T42.4X3	T42.4X4	T42.4X5	T42.4X6
Halquinols	T49.ØX1	T49.ØX2	T49.ØX3	T49.ØX4	T49.ØX5	T49.ØX6
Hamamelis	T49.2X1	T49.2X2	T49.2X3	T49.2X4	T49.2X5	T49.2X6
Haptendextran	T45.8X1	T45.8X2	T45.8X3	T45.8X4	T45.8X5	T45.8X6
Harmonyl	T46.5X1	T46.5X2	T46.5X3	T46.5X4	T46.5X5	T46.5X6
Hartmann's solution	T5Ø.3X1	T5Ø.3X2	T5Ø.3X3	T5Ø.3X4	T5Ø.3X5	T5Ø.3X6
Hashish	T4Ø.7X1	T4Ø.7X2	T4Ø.7X3	T4Ø.7X4	T4Ø.7X5	T4Ø.7X6
Hawaiian Woodrose seeds	T4Ø.991	T4Ø.992	T4Ø.993	T4Ø.994	—	—
HCB	T6Ø.3X1	T6Ø.3X2	T6Ø.3X3	T6Ø.3X4	—	—
HCH	T53.6X1	T53.6X2	T53.6X3	T53.6X4	—	—
medicinal	T49.ØX1	T49.ØX2	T49.ØX3	T49.ØX4	T49.ØX5	T49.ØX6
HCN	T57.3X1	T57.3X2	T57.3X3	T57.3X4	—	—
Headache cures, drugs, powders NEC	T5Ø.9Ø1	T5Ø.9Ø2	T5Ø.9Ø3	T5Ø.9Ø4	T5Ø.9Ø5	T5Ø.9Ø6
Heavenly Blue (morning glory)	T4Ø.991	T4Ø.992	T4Ø.993	T4Ø.994	—	—
Heavy metal antidote	T45.8X1	T45.8X2	T45.8X3	T45.8X4	T45.8X5	T45.8X6
Hedaquinium	T49.ØX1	T49.ØX2	T49.ØX3	T49.ØX4	T49.ØX5	T49.ØX6
Hedge hyssop	T62.2X1	T62.2X2	T62.2X3	T62.2X4	—	—
Heet	T49.8X1	T49.8X2	T49.8X3	T49.8X4	T49.8X5	T49.8X6
Helium	T48.991	T48.992	T48.993	T48.994	T48.995	T48.996
Helenin	T37.4X1	T37.4X2	T37.4X3	T37.4X4	T37.4X5	T37.4X6
Hellebore (black) (green) (white)	T62.2X1	T62.2X2	T62.2X3	T62.2X4	—	—
Helium (nonmedicinal) NEC	T59.891	T59.892	T59.893	T59.894	—	—
medicinal	T48.991	T48.992	T48.993	T48.994	T48.995	T48.996
Hematin	T45.8X1	T45.8X2	T45.8X3	T45.8X4	T45.8X5	T45.8X6
Hematinic preparation	T45.8X1	T45.8X2	T45.8X3	T45.8X4	T45.8X5	T45.8X6
Hemlock	T62.2X1	T62.2X2	T62.2X3	T62.2X4	—	—
Hemostatic	T45.621	T45.622	T45.623	T45.624	T45.625	T45.626
drug, systemic	T45.621	T45.622	T45.623	T45.624	T45.625	T45.626
Hemostyptic	T49.4X1	T49.4X2	T49.4X3	T49.4X4	T49.4X5	T49.4X6
Henbane	T62.2X1	T62.2X2	T62.2X3	T62.2X4	—	—
Heparin (sodium)	T45.511	T45.512	T45.513	T45.514	T45.515	T45.516
action reverser	T45.7X1	T45.7X2	T45.7X3	T45.7X4	T45.7X5	T45.7X6
Heparin-fraction	T45.511	T45.512	T45.513	T45.514	T45.515	T45.516
Heparinoid (systemic)	T45.511	T45.512	T45.513	T45.514	T45.515	T45.516
Hepatic secretion stimulant	T47.8X1	T47.8X2	T47.8X3	T47.8X4	T47.8X5	T47.8X6
Hepatitis B						
immune globulin	T5Ø.Z11	T5Ø.Z12	T5Ø.Z13	T5Ø.Z14	T5Ø.Z15	T5Ø.Z16
vaccine	T5Ø.B91	T5Ø.B92	T5Ø.B93	T5Ø.B94	T5Ø.B95	T5Ø.B96
Hepronicate	T46.7X1	T46.7X2	T46.7X3	T46.7X4	T46.7X5	T46.7X6
Heptabarb	T42.3X1	T42.3X2	T42.3X3	T42.3X4	T42.3X5	T42.3X6
Heptabarbitone	T42.3X1	T42.3X2	T42.3X3	T42.3X4	T42.3X5	T42.3X6
Heptabarbital	T42.3X1	T42.3X2	T42.3X3	T42.3X4	T42.3X5	T42.3X6
Heptachlor	T6Ø.1X1	T6Ø.1X2	T6Ø.1X3	T6Ø.1X4	—	—
Heptalgin	T4Ø.2X1	T4Ø.2X2	T4Ø.2X3	T4Ø.2X4	T4Ø.2X5	T4Ø.2X6
Heptaminol	T46.3X1	T46.3X2	T46.3X3	T46.3X4	T46.3X5	T46.3X6
Herbicide NEC	T6Ø.3X1	T6Ø.3X2	T6Ø.3X3	T6Ø.3X4	—	—
Heroin	T4Ø.1X1	T4Ø.1X2	T4Ø.1X3	T4Ø.1X4	—	—
Herplex	T49.5X1	T49.5X2	T49.5X3	T49.5X4	T49.5X5	T49.5X6
HES	T45.8X1	T45.8X2	T45.8X3	T45.8X4	T45.8X5	T45.8X6
Hesperidin	T46.991	T46.992	T46.993	T46.994	T46.995	T46.996
Hetacillin	T36.ØX1	T36.ØX2	T36.ØX3	T36.ØX4	T36.ØX5	T36.ØX6

Substance	Poisoning, Accidental (Unintentional)	Poisoning, Intentional Self-Harm	Poisoning, Assault	Poisoning, Undetermined	Adverse Effect	Underdosing
Hetastarch	T45.8X1	T45.8X2	T45.8X3	T45.8X4	T45.8X5	T45.8X6
HETP	T6Ø.ØX1	T6Ø.ØX2	T6Ø.ØX3	T6Ø.ØX4	—	—
Hexachlorobenzene (vapor)	T6Ø.3X1	T6Ø.3X2	T6Ø.3X3	T6Ø.3X4	—	—
Hexachlorocyclohexane	T53.6X1	T53.6X2	T53.6X3	T53.6X4	—	—
Hexachlorophene	T49.ØX1	T49.ØX2	T49.ØX3	T49.ØX4	T49.ØX5	T49.ØX6
Hexadiline	T46.3X1	T46.3X2	T46.3X3	T46.3X4	T46.3X5	T46.3X6
Hexadimethrine (bromide)	T45.7X1	T45.7X2	T45.7X3	T45.7X4	T45.7X5	T45.7X6
Hexadylamine	T46.3X1	T46.3X2	T46.3X3	T46.3X4	T46.3X5	T46.3X6
Hexaethyl tetraphosphate	T6Ø.ØX1	T6Ø.ØX2	T6Ø.ØX3	T6Ø.ØX4	—	—
Hexafluorenium bromide	T48.1X1	T48.1X2	T48.1X3	T48.1X4	T48.1X5	T48.1X6
Hexafluorodiethyl ether	T43.291	T43.292	T43.293	T43.294	T43.295	T43.296
Hexafluronium (bromide)	T48.1X1	T48.1X2	T48.1X3	T48.1X4	T48.1X5	T48.1X6
Hexahydrobenzol	T52.8X1	T52.8X2	T52.8X3	T52.8X4	—	—
Hexahydrocresol(s)	T51.8X1	T51.8X2	T51.8X3	T51.8X4	—	—
arsenide	T57.ØX1	T57.ØX2	T57.ØX3	T57.ØX4	—	—
arseniurated	T57.ØX1	T57.ØX2	T57.ØX3	T57.ØX4	—	—
cyanide	T57.3X1	T57.3X2	T57.3X3	T57.3X4	—	—
gas	T59.891	T59.892	T59.893	T59.894	—	—
Fluoride (liquid)	T57.8X1	T57.8X2	T57.8X3	T57.8X4	—	—
vapor	T59.891	T59.892	T59.893	T59.894	—	—
phophorated	T6Ø.ØX1	T6Ø.ØX2	T6Ø.ØX3	T6Ø.ØX4	—	—
sulfate	T57.8X1	T57.8X2	T57.8X3	T57.8X4	—	—
sulfide (gas)	T59.6X1	T59.6X2	T59.6X3	T59.6X4	—	—
arseniurated	T57.ØX1	T57.ØX2	T57.ØX3	T57.ØX4	—	—
sulfurated	T57.8X1	T57.8X2	T57.8X3	T57.8X4	—	—
Hexahydrophenol	T51.8X1	T51.8X2	T51.8X3	T51.8X4	—	—
Hexa-germ	T49.2X1	T49.2X2	T49.2X3	T49.2X4	T49.2X5	T49.2X6
Hexalen	T51.8X1	T51.8X2	T51.8X3	T51.8X4	—	—
Hexamethonium bromide	T44.2X1	T44.2X2	T44.2X3	T44.2X4	T44.2X5	T44.2X6
Hexamethylene	T52.8X1	T52.8X2	T52.8X3	T52.8X4	—	—
Hexamethylmelamine	T45.1X1	T45.1X2	T45.1X3	T45.1X4	T45.1X5	T45.1X6
Hexamidine	T49.ØX1	T49.ØX2	T49.ØX3	T49.ØX4	T49.ØX5	T49.ØX6
Hexamine (mandelate)	T37.8X1	T37.8X2	T37.8X3	T37.8X4	T37.8X5	T37.8X6
Hexanone, 2-hexanone	T52.4X1	T52.4X2	T52.4X3	T52.4X4	—	—
Hexanuorenium	T48.1X1	T48.1X2	T48.1X3	T48.1X4	T48.1X5	T48.1X6
Hexapropymate	T42.6X1	T42.6X2	T42.6X3	T42.6X4	T42.6X5	T42.6X6
Hexasonium iodide	T44.3X1	T44.3X2	T44.3X3	T44.3X4	T44.3X5	T44.3X6
Hexcarbacholine bromide	T48.1X1	T48.1X2	T48.1X3	T48.1X4	T48.1X5	T48.1X6
Hexemal	T42.3X1	T42.3X2	T42.3X3	T42.3X4	T42.3X5	T42.3X6
Hexestrol	T38.5X1	T38.5X2	T38.5X3	T38.5X4	T38.5X5	T38.5X6
Hexethal (sodium)	T42.3X1	T42.3X2	T42.3X3	T42.3X4	T42.3X5	T42.3X6
Hexetidine	T37.8X1	T37.8X2	T37.8X3	T37.8X4	T37.8X5	T37.8X6

Substance	Poisoning, Accidental (Unintentional)	Poisoning, Intentional Self-Harm	Poisoning, Assault	Poisoning, Undetermined	Adverse Effect	Underdosing
Hexobarbital	T42.3X1	T42.3X2	T42.3X3	T42.3X4	T42.3X5	T42.3X6
rectal	T41.291	T41.292	T41.293	T41.294	T41.295	T41.296
sodium	T41.1X1	T41.1X2	T41.1X3	T41.1X4	T41.1X5	T41.1X6
Hexobendine	T46.3X1	T46.3X2	T46.3X3	T46.3X4	T46.3X5	T46.3X6
Hexocyclium	T44.3X1	T44.3X2	T44.3X3	T44.3X4	T44.3X5	T44.3X6
metilsulfate	T44.3X1	T44.3X2	T44.3X3	T44.3X4	T44.3X5	T44.3X6
Hexoestrol	T38.5X1	T38.5X2	T38.5X3	T38.5X4	T38.5X5	T38.5X6
Hexone	T52.4X1	T52.4X2	T52.4X3	T52.4X4	—	—
Hexoprenaline	T48.6X1	T48.6X2	T48.6X3	T48.6X4	T48.6X5	T48.6X6
Hexylcaine	T41.3X1	T41.3X2	T41.3X3	T41.3X4	T41.3X5	T41.3X6
Hexylresorcinol	T52.2X1	T52.2X2	T52.2X3	T52.2X4	—	—
HGH (human growth hormone)	T38.811	T38.812	T38.813	T38.814	T38.815	T38.816
Hinkle's pills	T47.2X1	T47.2X2	T47.2X3	T47.2X4	T47.2X5	T47.2X6
Histalog	T5Ø.8X1	T5Ø.8X2	T5Ø.8X3	T5Ø.8X4	T5Ø.8X5	T5Ø.8X6
Histamine (phosphate)	T5Ø.8X1	T5Ø.8X2	T5Ø.8X3	T5Ø.8X4	T5Ø.8X5	T5Ø.8X6
Histoplasmin	T5Ø.8X1	T5Ø.8X2	T5Ø.8X3	T5Ø.8X4	T5Ø.8X5	T5Ø.8X6
Holly berries	T62.2X1	T62.2X2	T62.2X3	T62.2X4	—	—
Homatropine	T44.3X1	T44.3X2	T44.3X3	T44.3X4	T44.3X5	T44.3X6
methylbromide	T44.3X1	T44.3X2	T44.3X3	T44.3X4	T44.3X5	T44.3X6
Homochlorcyclizine	T45.ØX1	T45.ØX2	T45.ØX3	T45.ØX4	T45.ØX5	T45.ØX6
Homosalate	T49.3X1	T49.3X2	T49.3X3	T49.3X4	T49.3X5	T49.3X6
Homo-tet	T5Ø.Z11	T5Ø.Z12	T5Ø.Z13	T5Ø.Z14	T5Ø.Z15	T5Ø.Z16
Hormone	T38.8Ø1	T38.8Ø2	T38.8Ø3	T38.8Ø4	T38.8Ø5	T38.8Ø6
adrenal cortical steroids	T38.ØX1	T38.ØX2	T38.ØX3	T38.ØX4	T38.ØX5	T38.ØX6
androgenic	T38.7X1	T38.7X2	T38.7X3	T38.7X4	T38.7X5	T38.7X6
anterior pituitary NEC	T38.811	T38.812	T38.813	T38.814	T38.815	T38.816
antidiabetic agents	T38.3X1	T38.3X2	T38.3X3	T38.3X4	T38.3X5	T38.3X6
antidiuretic	T38.891	T38.892	T38.893	T38.894	T38.895	T38.896
cancer therapy	T45.1X1	T45.1X2	T45.1X3	T45.1X4	T45.1X5	T45.1X6
follicle stimulating	T38.811	T38.812	T38.813	T38.814	T38.815	T38.816
gonadotropic	T38.891	T38.892	T38.893	T38.894	T38.895	T38.896
pituitary	T38.811	T38.812	T38.813	T38.814	T38.815	T38.816
growth	T38.811	T38.812	T38.813	T38.814	T38.815	T38.816
luteinizing	T38.811	T38.812	T38.813	T38.814	T38.815	T38.816
ovarian	T38.5X1	T38.5X2	T38.5X3	T38.5X4	T38.5X5	T38.5X6
oxytocic	T48.ØX1	T48.ØX2	T48.ØX3	T48.ØX4	T48.ØX5	T48.ØX6
parathyroid (derivatives)	T5Ø.991	T5Ø.992	T5Ø.993	T5Ø.994	T5Ø.995	T5Ø.996
pituitary (posterior) NEC	T38.891	T38.892	T38.893	T38.894	T38.895	T38.896
anterior	T38.811	T38.812	T38.813	T38.814	T38.815	T38.816
specified, NEC	T38.891	T38.892	T38.893	T38.894	T38.895	T38.896
thyroid	T38.1X1	T38.1X2	T38.1X3	T38.1X4	T38.1X5	T38.1X6
Hornet (sting)	T63.451	T63.452	T63.453	T63.454	—	—

Substance	Poisoning, Accidental (Unintentional)	Poisoning, Intentional Self-Harm	Poisoning, Assault	Poisoning, Undetermined	Adverse Effect	Underdosing
Horse anti-human lymphocytic serum	T5Ø.Z11	T5Ø.Z12	T5Ø.Z13	T5Ø.Z14	T5Ø.Z15	T5Ø.Z16
Horticulture agent NEC	T65.91	T65.92	T65.93	T65.94	—	—
with pesticide	T6Ø.91	T6Ø.92	T6Ø.93	T6Ø.94	—	—
Human						
albumin	T45.8X1	T45.8X2	T45.8X3	T45.8X4	T45.8X5	T45.8X6
growth hormone (HGH)	T38.811	T38.812	T38.813	T38.814	T38.815	T38.816
immune serum	T5Ø.Z11	T5Ø.Z12	T5Ø.Z13	T5Ø.Z14	T5Ø.Z15	T5Ø.Z16
Hyaluronidase	T45.3X1	T45.3X2	T45.3X3	T45.3X4	T45.3X5	T45.3X6
Hyazyme	T45.3X1	T45.3X2	T45.3X3	T45.3X4	T45.3X5	T45.3X6
Hycodan	T4Ø.2X1	T4Ø.2X2	T4Ø.2X3	T4Ø.2X4	T4Ø.2X5	T4Ø.2X6
Hydantoin derivative NEC	T42.ØX1	T42.ØX2	T42.ØX3	T42.ØX4	T42.ØX5	T42.ØX6
Hydeltra	T38.ØX1	T38.ØX2	T38.ØX3	T38.ØX4	T38.ØX5	T38.ØX6
Hydergine	T44.6X1	T44.6X2	T44.6X3	T44.6X4	T44.6X5	T44.6X6
Hydrabamine penicillin	T36.ØX1	T36.ØX2	T36.ØX3	T36.ØX4	T36.ØX5	T36.ØX6
Hydralazine	T46.5X1	T46.5X2	T46.5X3	T46.5X4	T46.5X5	T46.5X6
Hydrargaphen	T49.ØX1	T49.ØX2	T49.ØX3	T49.ØX4	T49.ØX5	T49.ØX6
Hydrargyri amino-chloridum	T49.ØX1	T49.ØX2	T49.ØX3	T49.ØX4	T49.ØX5	T49.ØX6
Hydrastine	T48.291	T48.292	T48.293	T48.294	T48.295	T48.296
Hydrazine	T54.1X1	T54.1X2	T54.1X3	T54.1X4	—	—
monoamine oxidase inhibitors	T43.1X1	T43.1X2	T43.1X3	T43.1X4	T43.1X5	T43.1X6
Hydrazoic acid, azides	T54.2X1	T54.2X2	T54.2X3	T54.2X4	—	—
Hydriodic acid	T48.4X1	T48.4X2	T48.4X3	T48.4X4	T48.4X5	T48.4X6
Hydrocarbon gas	T59.891	T59.892	T59.893	T59.894	—	—
incomplete combustion of — *see Carbon, monoxide, fuel, utility*						
liquefied (mobile container)	T59.891	T59.892	T59.893	T59.894	—	—
piped (natural)	T59.891	T59.892	T59.893	T59.894	—	—
Hydrochloric acid (liquid)	T54.2X1	T54.2X2	T54.2X3	T54.2X4	—	—
medicinal (digestant)	T47.5X1	T47.5X2	T47.5X3	T47.5X4	T47.5X5	T47.5X6
vapor	T59.891	T59.892	T59.893	T59.894	—	—
Hydrochlorothiazide	T5Ø.2X1	T5Ø.2X2	T5Ø.2X3	T5Ø.2X4	T5Ø.2X5	T5Ø.2X6
Hydrocodone	T4Ø.2X1	T4Ø.2X2	T4Ø.2X3	T4Ø.2X4	T4Ø.2X5	T4Ø.2X6
Hydrocortisone (derivatives)	T38.ØX1	T38.ØX2	T38.ØX3	T38.ØX4	T38.ØX5	T38.ØX6
aceponate	T49.ØX1	T49.ØX2	T49.ØX3	T49.ØX4	T49.ØX5	T49.ØX6
ENT agent	T49.6X1	T49.6X2	T49.6X3	T49.6X4	T49.6X5	T49.6X6
ophthalmic preparation	T49.5X1	T49.5X2	T49.5X3	T49.5X4	T49.5X5	T49.5X6
topical NEC	T49.ØX1	T49.ØX2	T49.ØX3	T49.ØX4	T49.ØX5	T49.ØX6
Hydrocortone	T38.ØX1	T38.ØX2	T38.ØX3	T38.ØX4	T38.ØX5	T38.ØX6
ENT agent	T49.6X1	T49.6X2	T49.6X3	T49.6X4	T49.6X5	T49.6X6
ophthalmic preparation	T49.5X1	T49.5X2	T49.5X3	T49.5X4	T49.5X5	T49.5X6
topical NEC	T49.ØX1	T49.ØX2	T49.ØX3	T49.ØX4	T49.ØX5	T49.ØX6

Substance	Poisoning, Accidental (Unintentional)	Poisoning, Intentional Self-Harm	Poisoning, Assault	Poisoning, Undetermined	Adverse Effect	Underdosing
Hydrocyanic acid (liquid)	T57.3X1	T57.3X2	T57.3X3	T57.3X4	—	—
gas	T65.ØX1	T65.ØX2	T65.ØX3	T65.ØX4	—	—
Hydroflumethiazide	T5Ø.2X1	T5Ø.2X2	T5Ø.2X3	T5Ø.2X4	T5Ø.2X5	T5Ø.2X6
Hydrofluoric acid (liquid)	T54.2X1	T54.2X2	T54.2X3	T54.2X4	—	—
vapor	T59.891	T59.892	T59.893	T59.894	—	—
Hydrogen	T59.891	T59.892	T59.893	T59.894	—	—
arsenide	T57.ØX1	T57.ØX2	T57.ØX3	T57.ØX4	—	—
arseniureted	T57.ØX1	T57.ØX2	T57.ØX3	T57.ØX4	—	—
chloride	T57.8X1	T57.8X2	T57.8X3	T57.8X4	—	—
cyanide (salts)	T57.3X1	T57.3X2	T57.3X3	T57.3X4	—	—
gas	T57.3X1	T57.3X2	T57.3X3	T57.3X4	—	—
Fluoride	T59.5X1	T59.5X2	T59.5X3	T59.5X4	—	—
vapor	T59.5X1	T59.5X2	T59.5X3	T59.5X4	—	—
peroxide	T49.ØX1	T49.ØX2	T49.ØX3	T49.ØX4	T49.ØX5	T49.ØX6
phosphureted	T57.1X1	T57.1X2	T57.1X3	T57.1X4	—	—
sulfide	T59.6X1	T59.6X2	T59.6X3	T59.6X4	—	—
arseniureted	T57.ØX1	T57.ØX2	T57.ØX3	T57.ØX4	—	—
sulfureted	T59.6X1	T59.6X2	T59.6X3	T59.6X4	—	—
Hydromethylpyridine	T46.7X1	T46.7X2	T46.7X3	T46.7X4	T46.7X5	T46.7X6
Hydromorphinol	T4Ø.2X1	T4Ø.2X2	T4Ø.2X3	T4Ø.2X4	—	—
Hydromorphinone	T4Ø.2X1	T4Ø.2X2	T4Ø.2X3	T4Ø.2X4	T4Ø.2X5	T4Ø.2X6
Hydromorphone	T4Ø.2X1	T4Ø.2X2	T4Ø.2X3	T4Ø.2X4	T4Ø.2X5	T4Ø.2X6
Hydromox	T5Ø.2X1	T5Ø.2X2	T5Ø.2X3	T5Ø.2X4	T5Ø.2X5	T5Ø.2X6
Hydrophilic lotion	T49.3X1	T49.3X2	T49.3X3	T49.3X4	T49.3X5	T49.3X6
Hydroquinidine	T46.2X1	T46.2X2	T46.2X3	T46.2X4	T46.2X5	T46.2X6
Hydroquinone	T52.2X1	T52.2X2	T52.2X3	T52.2X4	—	—
vapor	T59.891	T59.892	T59.893	T59.894	—	—
Hydrosulfuric acid (gas)	T59.6X1	T59.6X2	T59.6X3	T59.6X4	—	—
Hydrotalcite	T47.1X1	T47.1X2	T47.1X3	T47.1X4	T47.1X5	T47.1X6
Hydrous wool fat	T49.3X1	T49.3X2	T49.3X3	T49.3X4	T49.3X5	T49.3X6
Hydroxide, caustic	T54.3X1	T54.3X2	T54.3X3	T54.3X4	—	—
Hydroxocobalamin	T45.8X1	T45.8X2	T45.8X3	T45.8X4	T45.8X5	T45.8X6
Hydroxyamphetamine	T49.5X1	T49.5X2	T49.5X3	T49.5X4	T49.5X5	T49.5X6
Hydroxycarbamide	T45.1X1	T45.1X2	T45.1X3	T45.1X4	T45.1X5	T45.1X6
Hydroxychloroquine	T37.8X1	T37.8X2	T37.8X3	T37.8X4	T37.8X5	T37.8X6
Hydroxydihydrocodeinone	T4Ø.2X1	T4Ø.2X2	T4Ø.2X3	T4Ø.2X4	T4Ø.2X5	T4Ø.2X6
Hydroxyestrone	T38.5X1	T38.5X2	T38.5X3	T38.5X4	T38.5X5	T38.5X6
Hydroxyethyl starch	T45.8X1	T45.8X2	T45.8X3	T45.8X4	T45.8X5	T45.8X6
Hydroxymethylpentanone	T52.4X1	T52.4X2	T52.4X3	T52.4X4	—	—
Hydroxyphenamate	T43.591	T43.592	T43.593	T43.594	T43.595	T43.596
Hydroxyphenylbutazone	T39.2X1	T39.2X2	T39.2X3	T39.2X4	T39.2X5	T39.2X6

Substance	Poisoning, Accidental (Unintentional)	Poisoning, Intentional Self-Harm	Poisoning, Assault	Poisoning, Undetermined	Adverse Effect	Underdosing
Hydroxyprogesterone	T38.5X1	T38.5X2	T38.5X3	T38.5X4	T38.5X5	T38.5X6
caproate	T38.5X1	T38.5X2	T38.5X3	T38.5X4	T38.5X5	T38.5X6
Hydroxyquinoline (derivatives) NEC	T37.8X1	T37.8X2	T37.8X3	T37.8X4	T37.8X5	T37.8X6
Hydroxystilbamidine	T37.3X1	T37.3X2	T37.3X3	T37.3X4	T37.3X5	T37.3X6
Hydroxytoluene (nonmedicinal)	T54.ØX1	T54.ØX2	T54.ØX3	T54.ØX4	—	—
medicinal	T49.ØX1	T49.ØX2	T49.ØX3	T49.ØX4	T49.ØX5	T49.ØX6
Hydroxyurea	T45.1X1	T45.1X2	T45.1X3	T45.1X4	T45.1X5	T45.1X6
Hydroxyzine	T43.591	T43.592	T43.593	T43.594	T43.595	T43.596
Hyoscine	T44.3X1	T44.3X2	T44.3X3	T44.3X4	T44.3X5	T44.3X6
Hyoscyamine	T44.3X1	T44.3X2	T44.3X3	T44.3X4	T44.3X5	T44.3X6
Hyoscyamus	T44.3X1	T44.3X2	T44.3X3	T44.3X4	T44.3X5	T44.3X6
dry extract	T44.3X1	T44.3X2	T44.3X3	T44.3X4	T44.3X5	T44.3X6
Hypaque	T5Ø.8X1	T5Ø.8X2	T5Ø.8X3	T5Ø.8X4	T5Ø.8X5	T5Ø.8X6
Hypertussis	T5Ø.Z11	T5Ø.Z12	T5Ø.Z13	T5Ø.Z14	T5Ø.Z15	T5Ø.Z16
Hypnotic	T42.71	T42.72	T42.73	T42.74	T42.75	T42.76
anticonvulsant	T42.71	T42.72	T42.73	T42.74	T42.75	T42.76
specified NEC	T42.6X1	T42.6X2	T42.6X3	T42.6X4	T42.6X5	T42.6X6
Hypochlorite	T49.ØX1	T49.ØX2	T49.ØX3	T49.ØX4	T49.ØX5	T49.ØX6
Hypophysis, posterior	T38.891	T38.892	T38.893	T38.894	T38.895	T38.896
Hypotensive NEC	T46.5X1	T46.5X2	T46.5X3	T46.5X4	T46.5X5	T46.5X6
Hypromellose	T49.5X1	T49.5X2	T49.5X3	T49.5X4	T49.5X5	T49.5X6
I						
Ibacitabine	T37.5X1	T37.5X2	T37.5X3	T37.5X4	T37.5X5	T37.5X6
Ibopamine	T44.991	T44.992	T44.993	T44.994	T44.995	T44.996
Ibufenac	T39.311	T39.312	T39.313	T39.314	T39.315	T39.316
Ibuprofen	T39.311	T39.312	T39.313	T39.314	T39.315	T39.316
Ibuproxam	T39.311	T39.312	T39.313	T39.314	T39.315	T39.316
Ibuterol	T48.6X1	T48.6X2	T48.6X3	T48.6X4	T48.6X5	T48.6X6
Ichthammol	T49.ØX1	T49.ØX2	T49.ØX3	T49.ØX4	T49.ØX5	T49.ØX6
Ichthyol	T49.4X1	T49.4X2	T49.4X3	T49.4X4	T49.4X5	T49.4X6
Idarubicin	T45.1X1	T45.1X2	T45.1X3	T45.1X4	T45.1X5	T45.1X6
Idrocilamide	T42.8X1	T42.8X2	T42.8X3	T42.8X4	T42.8X5	T42.8X6
Ifenprodil	T46.7X1	T46.7X2	T46.7X3	T46.7X4	T46.7X5	T46.7X6
Ifosfamide	T45.1X1	T45.1X2	T45.1X3	T45.1X4	T45.1X5	T45.1X6
Iletin	T38.3X1	T38.3X2	T38.3X3	T38.3X4	T38.3X5	T38.3X6
Ilex	T62.2X1	T62.2X2	T62.2X3	T62.2X4	—	—
Illuminating gas (after combustion)	T58.11	T58.12	T58.13	T58.14	—	—
prior to combustion	T59.891	T59.892	T59.893	T59.894	—	—
Ilopan	T45.2X1	T45.2X2	T45.2X3	T45.2X4	T45.2X5	T45.2X6
Iloprost	T46.7X1	T46.7X2	T46.7X3	T46.7X4	T46.7X5	T46.7X6

Substance	Poisoning, Accidental (Unintentional)	Poisoning, Intentional Self-Harm	Poisoning, Assault	Poisoning, Undetermined	Adverse Effect	Underdosing
Ilotycin	T36.3X1	T36.3X2	T36.3X3	T36.3X4	T36.3X5	T36.3X6
ophthalmic preparation	T49.5X1	T49.5X2	T49.5X3	T49.5X4	T49.5X5	T49.5X6
topical NEC	T49.ØX1	T49.ØX2	T49.ØX3	T49.ØX4	T49.ØX5	T49.ØX6
Imidazole-4-carboxamide	T45.1X1	T45.1X2	T45.1X3	T45.1X4	T45.1X5	T45.1X6
Imipenem	T36.ØX1	T36.ØX2	T36.ØX3	T36.ØX4	T36.ØX5	T36.ØX6
Imipramine	T43.Ø11	T43.Ø12	T43.Ø13	T43.Ø14	T43.Ø15	T43.Ø16
Iminostilbene	T42.1X1	T42.1X2	T42.1X3	T42.1X4	T42.1X5	T42.1X6
Immu-G	T5Ø.Z11	T5Ø.Z12	T5Ø.Z13	T5Ø.Z14	T5Ø.Z15	T5Ø.Z16
Immuglobin	T5Ø.Z11	T5Ø.Z12	T5Ø.Z13	T5Ø.Z14	T5Ø.Z15	T5Ø.Z16
Immune						
globulin	T5Ø.Z11	T5Ø.Z12	T5Ø.Z13	T5Ø.Z14	T5Ø.Z15	T5Ø.Z16
serum globulin	T5Ø.Z11	T5Ø.Z12	T5Ø.Z13	T5Ø.Z14	T5Ø.Z15	T5Ø.Z16
Immunoglobin human (intravenous) (normal)	T5Ø.Z11	T5Ø.Z12	T5Ø.Z13	T5Ø.Z14	T5Ø.Z15	T5Ø.Z16
unmodified	T5Ø.Z11	T5Ø.Z12	T5Ø.Z13	T5Ø.Z14	T5Ø.Z15	T5Ø.Z16
Immunosuppressive drug	T45.1X1	T45.1X2	T45.1X3	T45.1X4	T45.1X5	T45.1X6
Immu-tetanus	T5Ø.Z11	T5Ø.Z12	T5Ø.Z13	T5Ø.Z14	T5Ø.Z15	T5Ø.Z16
Indalpine	T43.221	T43.222	T43.223	T43.224	T43.225	T43.226
Indanazoline	T48.5X1	T48.5X2	T48.5X3	T48.5X4	T48.5X5	T48.5X6
Indandione (derivatives)	T45.511	T45.512	T45.513	T45.514	T45.515	T45.516
Indapamide	T46.5X1	T46.5X2	T46.5X3	T46.5X4	T46.5X5	T46.5X6
Indendione (derivatives)	T45.511	T45.512	T45.513	T45.514	T45.515	T45.516
Indenolol	T44.7X1	T44.7X2	T44.7X3	T44.7X4	T44.7X5	T44.7X6
Inderal	T44.7X1	T44.7X2	T44.7X3	T44.7X4	T44.7X5	T44.7X6
Indian						
hemp	T4Ø.7X1	T4Ø.7X2	T4Ø.7X3	T4Ø.7X4	T4Ø.7X5	T4Ø.7X6
tobacco	T62.2X1	T62.2X2	T62.2X3	T62.2X4	—	—
Indigo carmine	T5Ø.8X1	T5Ø.8X2	T5Ø.8X3	T5Ø.8X4	T5Ø.8X5	T5Ø.8X6
Indobufen	T45.521	T45.522	T45.523	T45.524	T45.525	T45.526
Indocin	T39.2X1	T39.2X2	T39.2X3	T39.2X4	T39.2X5	T39.2X6
Indocyanine green	T5Ø.8X1	T5Ø.8X2	T5Ø.8X3	T5Ø.8X4	T5Ø.8X5	T5Ø.8X6
Indometacin	T39.391	T39.392	T39.393	T39.394	T39.395	T39.396
Indomethacin	T39.391	T39.392	T39.393	T39.394	T39.395	T39.396
farnesil	T39.4X1	T39.4X2	T39.4X3	T39.4X4	T39.4X5	T39.4X6
Indoramin	T44.6X1	T44.6X2	T44.6X3	T44.6X4	T44.6X5	T44.6X6
Industrial						
alcohol	T51.ØX1	T51.ØX2	T51.ØX3	T51.ØX4	—	—
fumes	T59.891	T59.892	T59.893	T59.894	—	—
solvents (fumes) (vapors)	T52.91	T52.92	T52.93	T52.94	—	—
Influenza vaccine	T5Ø.B91	T5Ø.B92	T5Ø.B93	T5Ø.B94	T5Ø.B95	T5Ø.B96
Ingested substance NEC	T65.91	T65.92	T65.93	T65.94	—	—
INH	T37.1X1	T37.1X2	T37.1X3	T37.1X4	T37.1X5	T37.1X6

Substance	Poisoning, Accidental (Unintentional)	Poisoning, Intentional Self-Harm	Poisoning, Assault	Poisoning, Undetermined	Adverse Effect	Underdosing
Inhalation, gas (noxious) — *see Gas*						
Inhibitor						
angiotensin-converting enzyme	T46.4X1	T46.4X2	T46.4X3	T46.4X4	T46.4X5	T46.4X6
carbonic anhydrase	T5Ø.2X1	T5Ø.2X2	T5Ø.2X3	T5Ø.2X4	T5Ø.2X5	T5Ø.2X6
fibrinolysis	T45.621	T45.622	T45.623	T45.624	T45.625	T45.626
monoamine oxidase NEC	T43.1X1	T43.1X2	T43.1X3	T43.1X4	T43.1X5	T43.1X6
hydrazine	T43.1X1	T43.1X2	T43.1X3	T43.1X4	T43.1X5	T43.1X6
postsynaptic	T43.8X1	T43.8X2	T43.8X3	T43.8X4	T43.8X5	T43.8X6
prothrombin synthesis	T45.511	T45.512	T45.513	T45.514	T45.515	T45.516
Ink	T65.891	T65.892	T65.893	T65.894	—	—
Inorganic substance NEC	T57.91	T57.92	T57.93	T57.94	—	—
Inosine pranobex	T37.5X1	T37.5X2	T37.5X3	T37.5X4	T37.5X5	T37.5X6
Inositol	T5Ø.991	T5Ø.992	T5Ø.993	T5Ø.994	T5Ø.995	T5Ø.996
nicotinate	T46.7X1	T46.7X2	T46.7X3	T46.7X4	T46.7X5	T46.7X6
Inproquone	T45.1X1	T45.1X2	T45.1X3	T45.1X4	T45.1X5	T45.1X6
Insect (sting), venomous	T63.481	T63.482	T63.483	T63.484	—	—
ant	T63.421	T63.422	T63.423	T63.424	—	—
bee	T63.441	T63.442	T63.443	T63.444	—	—
caterpillar	T63.431	T63.432	T63.433	T63.434	—	—
hornet	T63.451	T63.452	T63.453	T63.454	—	—
wasp	T63.461	T63.462	T63.463	T63.464	—	—
Insecticide NEC	T6Ø.91	T6Ø.92	T6Ø.93	T6Ø.94	—	—
carbamate	T6Ø.ØX1	T6Ø.ØX2	T6Ø.ØX3	T6Ø.ØX4	—	—
chlorinated	T6Ø.1X1	T6Ø.1X2	T6Ø.1X3	T6Ø.1X4	—	—
mixed	T6Ø.91	T6Ø.92	T6Ø.93	T6Ø.94	—	—
organochlorine	T6Ø.1X1	T6Ø.1X2	T6Ø.1X3	T6Ø.1X4	—	—
organophosphorus	T6Ø.ØX1	T6Ø.ØX2	T6Ø.ØX3	T6Ø.ØX4	—	—
Insular tissue extract	T38.3X1	T38.3X2	T38.3X3	T38.3X4	T38.3X5	T38.3X6
Insulin (amorphous) (globin) (isophane) (Lente) (NPH) (Semilente) (Ultralente)	T38.3X1	T38.3X2	T38.3X3	T38.3X4	T38.3X5	T38.3X6
defalan	T38.3X1	T38.3X2	T38.3X3	T38.3X4	T38.3X5	T38.3X6
human	T38.3X1	T38.3X2	T38.3X3	T38.3X4	T38.3X5	T38.3X6
injection, soluble	T38.3X1	T38.3X2	T38.3X3	T38.3X4	T38.3X5	T38.3X6
biphasic	T38.3X1	T38.3X2	T38.3X3	T38.3X4	T38.3X5	T38.3X6
intermediate acting	T38.3X1	T38.3X2	T38.3X3	T38.3X4	T38.3X5	T38.3X6
protamine zinc	T38.3X1	T38.3X2	T38.3X3	T38.3X4	T38.3X5	T38.3X6
slow acting	T38.3X1	T38.3X2	T38.3X3	T38.3X4	T38.3X5	T38.3X6
zinc						
protamine injection	T38.3X1	T38.3X2	T38.3X3	T38.3X4	T38.3X5	T38.3X6
suspension (amorphous) (crystalline)	T38.3X1	T38.3X2	T38.3X3	T38.3X4	T38.3X5	T38.3X6

Substance	Poisoning, Accidental (Unintentional)	Poisoning, Intentional Self-Harm	Poisoning, Assault	Poisoning, Undetermined	Adverse Effect	Underdosing
Interferon (alpha) (beta) (gamma)	T37.5X1	T37.5X2	T37.5X3	T37.5X4	T37.5X5	T37.5X6
Intestinal motility control drug	T47.6X1	T47.6X2	T47.6X3	T47.6X4	T47.6X5	T47.6X6
biological	T47.8X1	T47.8X2	T47.8X3	T47.8X4	T47.8X5	T47.8X6
Intranarcon	T41.1X1	T41.1X2	T41.1X3	T41.1X4	T41.1X5	T41.1X6
Intravenous						
amino acids	T5Ø.991	T5Ø.992	T5Ø.993	T5Ø.994	T5Ø.995	T5Ø.996
fat suspension	T5Ø.991	T5Ø.992	T5Ø.993	T5Ø.994	T5Ø.995	T5Ø.996
Inulin	T5Ø.8X1	T5Ø.8X2	T5Ø.8X3	T5Ø.8X4	T5Ø.8X5	T5Ø.8X6
Invert sugar	T5Ø.3X1	T5Ø.3X2	T5Ø.3X3	T5Ø.3X4	T5Ø.3X5	T5Ø.3X6
Inza — *see Naproxen*						
Iobenzamic acid	T5Ø.8X1	T5Ø.8X2	T5Ø.8X3	T5Ø.8X4	T5Ø.8X5	T5Ø.8X6
Iocarmic acid	T5Ø.8X1	T5Ø.8X2	T5Ø.8X3	T5Ø.8X4	T5Ø.8X5	T5Ø.8X6
Iocetamic acid	T5Ø.8X1	T5Ø.8X2	T5Ø.8X3	T5Ø.8X4	T5Ø.8X5	T5Ø.8X6
Iodamide	T5Ø.8X1	T5Ø.8X2	T5Ø.8X3	T5Ø.8X4	T5Ø.8X5	T5Ø.8X6
Iodide NEC — *see also Iodine*	T49.ØX1	T49.ØX2	T49.ØX3	T49.ØX4	T49.ØX5	T49.ØX6
mercury (ointment)	T49.ØX1	T49.ØX2	T49.ØX3	T49.ØX4	T49.ØX5	T49.ØX6
methylate	T49.ØX1	T49.ØX2	T49.ØX3	T49.ØX4	T49.ØX5	T49.ØX6
potassium (expectorant) NEC	T48.4X1	T48.4X2	T48.4X3	T48.4X4	T48.4X5	T48.4X6
Iodinated						
contrast medium	T5Ø.8X1	T5Ø.8X2	T5Ø.8X3	T5Ø.8X4	T5Ø.8X5	T5Ø.8X6
glycerol	T48.4X1	T48.4X2	T48.4X3	T48.4X4	T48.4X5	T48.4X6
human serum albumin (131I)	T5Ø.8X1	T5Ø.8X2	T5Ø.8X3	T5Ø.8X4	T5Ø.8X5	T5Ø.8X6
Iodine (antiseptic, external) (tincture) NEC	T49.ØX1	T49.ØX2	T49.ØX3	T49.ØX4	T49.ØX5	T49.ØX6
125 — *see also Radiation sickness, and Exposure to radioactivce isotopes*	T5Ø.8X1	T5Ø.8X2	T5Ø.8X3	T5Ø.8X4	T5Ø.8X5	T5Ø.8X6
therapeutic	T5Ø.991	T5Ø.992	T5Ø.993	T5Ø.994	T5Ø.995	T5Ø.996
131 — *see also Radiation sickness, and Exposure to radioactivce isotopes*	T5Ø.8X1	T5Ø.8X2	T5Ø.8X3	T5Ø.8X4	T5Ø.8X5	T5Ø.8X6
therapeutic	T38.2X1	T38.2X2	T38.2X3	T38.2X4	T38.2X5	T38.2X6
diagnostic	T5Ø.8X1	T5Ø.8X2	T5Ø.8X3	T5Ø.8X4	T5Ø.8X5	T5Ø.8X6
for thyroid conditions (antithyroid)	T38.2X1	T38.2X2	T38.2X3	T38.2X4	T38.2X5	T38.2X6
solution	T49.ØX1	T49.ØX2	T49.ØX3	T49.ØX4	T49.ØX5	T49.ØX6
vapor	T59.891	T59.892	T59.893	T59.894	—	—
Iodipamide	T5Ø.8X1	T5Ø.8X2	T5Ø.8X3	T5Ø.8X4	T5Ø.8X5	T5Ø.8X6
Iodized (poppy seed) oil	T5Ø.8X1	T5Ø.8X2	T5Ø.8X3	T5Ø.8X4	T5Ø.8X5	T5Ø.8X6
Iodobismitol	T37.8X1	T37.8X2	T37.8X3	T37.8X4	T37.8X5	T37.8X6
Iodochlorhydroxyquin	T37.8X1	T37.8X2	T37.8X3	T37.8X4	T37.8X5	T37.8X6
topical	T49.ØX1	T49.ØX2	T49.ØX3	T49.ØX4	T49.ØX5	T49.ØX6
Iodochlorhydroxyquino-line	T37.8X1	T37.8X2	T37.8X3	T37.8X4	T37.8X5	T37.8X6
Iodocholesterol (131I)	T5Ø.8X1	T5Ø.8X2	T5Ø.8X3	T5Ø.8X4	T5Ø.8X5	T5Ø.8X6

Substance	Poisoning, Accidental (Unintentional)	Poisoning, Intentional Self-Harm	Poisoning, Assault	Poisoning, Undetermined	Adverse Effect	Underdosing
Iodoform	T49.ØX1	T49.ØX2	T49.ØX3	T49.ØX4	T49.ØX5	T49.ØX6
Iodohippuric acid	T5Ø.8X1	T5Ø.8X2	T5Ø.8X3	T5Ø.8X4	T5Ø.8X5	T5Ø.8X6
Iodopanoic acid	T5Ø.8X1	T5Ø.8X2	T5Ø.8X3	T5Ø.8X4	T5Ø.8X5	T5Ø.8X6
Iodophthalein (sodium)	T5Ø.8X1	T5Ø.8X2	T5Ø.8X3	T5Ø.8X4	T5Ø.8X5	T5Ø.8X6
Iodopyracet	T5Ø.8X1	T5Ø.8X2	T5Ø.8X3	T5Ø.8X4	T5Ø.8X5	T5Ø.8X6
Iodoquinol	T37.8X1	T37.8X2	T37.8X3	T37.8X4	T37.8X5	T37.8X6
Iodoxamic acid	T5Ø.8X1	T5Ø.8X2	T5Ø.8X3	T5Ø.8X4	T5Ø.8X5	T5Ø.8X6
Iofendylate	T5Ø.8X1	T5Ø.8X2	T5Ø.8X3	T5Ø.8X4	T5Ø.8X5	T5Ø.8X6
Ioglycamic acid	T5Ø.8X1	T5Ø.8X2	T5Ø.8X3	T5Ø.8X4	T5Ø.8X5	T5Ø.8X6
Iohexol	T5Ø.8X1	T5Ø.8X2	T5Ø.8X3	T5Ø.8X4	T5Ø.8X5	T5Ø.8X6
Ion exchange resin						
anion	T47.8X1	T47.8X2	T47.8X3	T47.8X4	T47.8X5	T47.8X6
cation	T5Ø.3X1	T5Ø.3X2	T5Ø.3X3	T5Ø.3X4	T5Ø.3X5	T5Ø.3X6
cholestyramine	T46.6X1	T46.6X2	T46.6X3	T46.6X4	T46.6X5	T46.6X6
intestinal	T47.8X1	T47.8X2	T47.8X3	T47.8X4	T47.8X5	T47.8X6
Iopamidol	T5Ø.8X1	T5Ø.8X2	T5Ø.8X3	T5Ø.8X4	T5Ø.8X5	T5Ø.8X6
Iopanoic acid	T5Ø.8X1	T5Ø.8X2	T5Ø.8X3	T5Ø.8X4	T5Ø.8X5	T5Ø.8X6
Iophenoic acid	T5Ø.8X1	T5Ø.8X2	T5Ø.8X3	T5Ø.8X4	T5Ø.8X5	T5Ø.8X6
Iopodate, sodium	T5Ø.8X1	T5Ø.8X2	T5Ø.8X3	T5Ø.8X4	T5Ø.8X5	T5Ø.8X6
Iopodic acid	T5Ø.8X1	T5Ø.8X2	T5Ø.8X3	T5Ø.8X4	T5Ø.8X5	T5Ø.8X6
Iopromide	T5Ø.8X1	T5Ø.8X2	T5Ø.8X3	T5Ø.8X4	T5Ø.8X5	T5Ø.8X6
Iopydol	T5Ø.8X1	T5Ø.8X2	T5Ø.8X3	T5Ø.8X4	T5Ø.8X5	T5Ø.8X6
Iotalamic acid	T5Ø.8X1	T5Ø.8X2	T5Ø.8X3	T5Ø.8X4	T5Ø.8X5	T5Ø.8X6
Iothalamate	T5Ø.8X1	T5Ø.8X2	T5Ø.8X3	T5Ø.8X4	T5Ø.8X5	T5Ø.8X6
Iothiouracil	T38.2X1	T38.2X2	T38.2X3	T38.2X4	T38.2X5	T38.2X6
Iotrol	T5Ø.8X1	T5Ø.8X2	T5Ø.8X3	T5Ø.8X4	T5Ø.8X5	T5Ø.8X6
Iotrolan	T5Ø.8X1	T5Ø.8X2	T5Ø.8X3	T5Ø.8X4	T5Ø.8X5	T5Ø.8X6
Iotroxate	T5Ø.8X1	T5Ø.8X2	T5Ø.8X3	T5Ø.8X4	T5Ø.8X5	T5Ø.8X6
Iotroxic acid	T5Ø.8X1	T5Ø.8X2	T5Ø.8X3	T5Ø.8X4	T5Ø.8X5	T5Ø.8X6
Ioversol	T5Ø.8X1	T5Ø.8X2	T5Ø.8X3	T5Ø.8X4	T5Ø.8X5	T5Ø.8X6
Ioxaglate	T5Ø.8X1	T5Ø.8X2	T5Ø.8X3	T5Ø.8X4	T5Ø.8X5	T5Ø.8X6
Ioxaglic acid	T5Ø.8X1	T5Ø.8X2	T5Ø.8X3	T5Ø.8X4	T5Ø.8X5	T5Ø.8X6
Ioxitalamic acid	T5Ø.8X1	T5Ø.8X2	T5Ø.8X3	T5Ø.8X4	T5Ø.8X5	T5Ø.8X6
Ipecac	T47.7X1	T47.7X2	T47.7X3	T47.7X4	T47.7X5	T47.7X6
Ipecacuanha	T48.4X1	T48.4X2	T48.4X3	T48.4X4	T48.4X5	T48.4X6
Ipodate, calcium	T5Ø.8X1	T5Ø.8X2	T5Ø.8X3	T5Ø.8X4	T5Ø.8X5	T5Ø.8X6
Ipral	T42.3X1	T42.3X2	T42.3X3	T42.3X4	T42.3X5	T42.3X6
Ipratropium (bromide)	T48.6X1	T48.6X2	T48.6X3	T48.6X4	T48.6X5	T48.6X6
Ipriflavone	T46.3X1	T46.3X2	T46.3X3	T46.3X4	T46.3X5	T46.3X6
Iprindole	T43.Ø11	T43.Ø12	T43.Ø13	T43.Ø14	T43.Ø15	T43.Ø16
Iproclozide	T43.1X1	T43.1X2	T43.1X3	T43.1X4	T43.1X5	T43.1X6
Iprofenin	T5Ø.8X1	T5Ø.8X2	T5Ø.8X3	T5Ø.8X4	T5Ø.8X5	T5Ø.8X6

Substance	Poisoning, Accidental (Unintentional)	Poisoning, Intentional Self-Harm	Poisoning, Assault	Poisoning, Undetermined	Adverse Effect	Underdosing
Iproheptine	T49.2X1	T49.2X2	T49.2X3	T49.2X4	T49.2X5	T49.2X6
Iproniazid	T43.1X1	T43.1X2	T43.1X3	T43.1X4	T43.1X5	T43.1X6
Iproplatin	T45.1X1	T45.1X2	T45.1X3	T45.1X4	T45.1X5	T45.1X6
Iproveratril	T46.1X1	T46.1X2	T46.1X3	T46.1X4	T46.1X5	T46.1X6
Iron (compounds) (medicinal) NEC	T45.4X1	T45.4X2	T45.4X3	T45.4X4	T45.4X5	T45.4X6
ammonium	T45.4X1	T45.4X2	T45.4X3	T45.4X4	T45.4X5	T45.4X6
dextran injection	T45.4X1	T45.4X2	T45.4X3	T45.4X4	T45.4X5	T45.4X6
nonmedicinal	T56.891	T56.892	T56.893	T56.894	—	—
salts	T45.4X1	T45.4X2	T45.4X3	T45.4X4	T45.4X5	T45.4X6
sorbitex	T45.4X1	T45.4X2	T45.4X3	T45.4X4	T45.4X5	T45.4X6
sorbitol citric acid complex	T45.4X1	T45.4X2	T45.4X3	T45.4X4	T45.4X5	T45.4X6
Irrigating fluid (vaginal)	T49.8X1	T49.8X2	T49.8X3	T49.8X4	T49.8X5	T49.8X6
eye	T49.5X1	T49.5X2	T49.5X3	T49.5X4	T49.5X5	T49.5X6
Isepamicin	T36.5X1	T36.5X2	T36.5X3	T36.5X4	T36.5X5	T36.5X6
Isoaminile (citrate)	T48.3X1	T48.3X2	T48.3X3	T48.3X4	T48.3X5	T48.3X6
Isoamyl nitrite	T46.3X1	T46.3X2	T46.3X3	T46.3X4	T46.3X5	T46.3X6
Isobenzan	T6Ø.1X1	T6Ø.1X2	T6Ø.1X3	T6Ø.1X4	—	—
Isobutyl acetate	T52.8X1	T52.8X2	T52.8X3	T52.8X4	—	—
Isocarboxazid	T43.1X1	T43.1X2	T43.1X3	T43.1X4	T43.1X5	T43.1X6
Isoconazole	T49.ØX1	T49.ØX2	T49.ØX3	T49.ØX4	T49.ØX5	T49.ØX6
Isocyanate	T65.ØX1	T65.ØX2	T65.ØX3	T65.ØX4	—	—
Isoephedrine	T44.991	T44.992	T44.993	T44.994	T44.995	T44.996
Isoetarine	T48.6X1	T48.6X2	T48.6X3	T48.6X4	T48.6X5	T48.6X6
Isoethadione	T42.2X1	T42.2X2	T42.2X3	T42.2X4	T42.2X5	T42.2X6
Isoetharine	T44.5X1	T44.5X2	T44.5X3	T44.5X4	T44.5X5	T44.5X6
Isoflurane	T41.ØX1	T41.ØX2	T41.ØX3	T41.ØX4	T41.ØX5	T41.ØX6
Isoflurophate	T44.ØX1	T44.ØX2	T44.ØX3	T44.ØX4	T44.ØX5	T44.ØX6
Isomaltose, ferric complex	T45.4X1	T45.4X2	T45.4X3	T45.4X4	T45.4X5	T45.4X6
Isometheptene	T44.3X1	T44.3X2	T44.3X3	T44.3X4	T44.3X5	T44.3X6
Isoniazid	T37.1X1	T37.1X2	T37.1X3	T37.1X4	T37.1X5	T37.1X6
with						
rifampicin	T36.6X1	T36.6X2	T36.6X3	T36.6X4	T36.6X5	T36.6X6
thioacetazone	T37.1X1	T37.1X2	T37.1X3	T37.1X4	T37.1X5	T37.1X6
Isonicotinic acid hydrazide	T37.1X1	T37.1X2	T37.1X3	T37.1X4	T37.1X5	T37.1X6
Isonipecaine	T4Ø.4X1	T4Ø.4X2	T4Ø.4X3	T4Ø.4X4	T4Ø.4X5	T4Ø.4X6
Isopentaquine	T37.2X1	T37.2X2	T37.2X3	T37.2X4	T37.2X5	T37.2X6
Isophane insulin	T38.3X1	T38.3X2	T38.3X3	T38.3X4	T38.3X5	T38.3X6
Isophorone	T65.891	T65.892	T65.893	T65.894	—	—
Isophosphamide	T45.1X1	T45.1X2	T45.1X3	T45.1X4	T45.1X5	T45.1X6
Isopregnenone	T38.5X1	T38.5X2	T38.5X3	T38.5X4	T38.5X5	T38.5X6
Isoprenaline	T48.6X1	T48.6X2	T48.6X3	T48.6X4	T48.6X5	T48.6X6
Isopromethazine	T43.3X1	T43.3X2	T43.3X3	T43.3X4	T43.3X5	T43.3X6

Substance	Poisoning, Accidental (Unintentional)	Poisoning, Intentional Self-Harm	Poisoning, Assault	Poisoning, Undetermined	Adverse Effect	Underdosing
Isopropamide	T44.3X1	T44.3X2	T44.3X3	T44.3X4	T44.3X5	T44.3X6
iodide	T44.3X1	T44.3X2	T44.3X3	T44.3X4	T44.3X5	T44.3X6
Isopropanol	T51.2X1	T51.2X2	T51.2X3	T51.2X4	—	—
Isopropyl						
acetate	T52.8X1	T52.8X2	T52.8X3	T52.8X4	—	—
alcohol	T51.2X1	T51.2X2	T51.2X3	T51.2X4	—	—
medicinal	T49.4X1	T49.4X2	T49.4X3	T49.4X4	T49.4X5	T49.4X6
ether	T52.8X1	T52.8X2	T52.8X3	T52.8X4	—	—
Isopropylaminophena-zone	T39.2X1	T39.2X2	T39.2X3	T39.2X4	T39.2X5	T39.2X6
Isoproterenol	T48.6X1	T48.6X2	T48.6X3	T48.6X4	T48.6X5	T48.6X6
Isosorbide dinitrate	T46.3X1	T46.3X2	T46.3X3	T46.3X4	T46.3X5	T46.3X6
Isothipendyl	T45.ØX1	T45.ØX2	T45.ØX3	T45.ØX4	T45.ØX5	T45.ØX6
Isotretinoin	T5Ø.991	T5Ø.992	T5Ø.993	T5Ø.994	T5Ø.995	T5Ø.996
Isoxazolyl penicillin	T36.ØX1	T36.ØX2	T36.ØX3	T36.ØX4	T36.ØX5	T36.ØX6
Isoxicam	T39.391	T39.392	T39.393	T39.394	T39.395	T39.396
Isoxsuprine	T46.7X1	T46.7X2	T46.7X3	T46.7X4	T46.7X5	T46.7X6
Ispagula	T47.4X1	T47.4X2	T47.4X3	T47.4X4	T47.4X5	T47.4X6
husk	T47.4X1	T47.4X2	T47.4X3	T47.4X4	T47.4X5	T47.4X6
Isradipine	T46.1X1	T46.1X2	T46.1X3	T46.1X4	T46.1X5	T46.1X6
I-thyroxine sodium	T38.1X1	T38.1X2	T38.1X3	T38.1X4	T38.1X5	T38.1X6
Itraconazole	T37.8X1	T37.8X2	T37.8X3	T37.8X4	T37.8X5	T37.8X6
Itramin tosilate	T46.3X1	T46.3X2	T46.3X3	T46.3X4	T46.3X5	T46.3X6
Ivermectin	T37.4X1	T37.4X2	T37.4X3	T37.4X4	T37.4X5	T37.4X6
Izoniazid	T37.1X1	T37.1X2	T37.1X3	T37.1X4	T37.1X5	T37.1X6
with thioacetazone	T37.1X1	T37.1X2	T37.1X3	T37.1X4	T37.1X5	T37.1X6
J						
Jalap	T47.2X1	T47.2X2	T47.2X3	T47.2X4	T47.2X5	T47.2X6
Jamaica						
dogwood (bark)	T39.8X1	T39.8X2	T39.8X3	T39.8X4	T39.8X5	T39.8X6
ginger	T65.891	T65.892	T65.893	T65.894	—	—
root	T62.2X1	T62.2X2	T62.2X3	T62.2X4	—	—
Jatropha	T62.2X1	T62.2X2	T62.2X3	T62.2X4	—	—
curcas	T62.2X1	T62.2X2	T62.2X3	T62.2X4	—	—
Jectofer	T45.4X1	T45.4X2	T45.4X3	T45.4X4	T45.4X5	T45.4X6
Jellyfish (sting)	T63.621	T63.622	T63.623	T63.624	—	—
Jequirity (bean)	T62.2X1	T62.2X2	T62.2X3	T62.2X4	—	—
Jimson weed (stramonium)	T62.2X1	T62.2X2	T62.2X3	T62.2X4	—	—
seeds	T62.2X1	T62.2X2	T62.2X3	T62.2X4	—	—
Josamycin	T36.3X1	T36.3X2	T36.3X3	T36.3X4	T36.3X5	T36.3X6
Juniper tar	T49.1X1	T49.1X2	T49.1X3	T49.1X4	T49.1X5	T49.1X6

Substance	Poisoning, Accidental (Unintentional)	Poisoning, Intentional Self-Harm	Poisoning, Assault	Poisoning, Undetermined	Adverse Effect	Underdosing
K						
Kallidinogenase	T46.7X1	T46.7X2	T46.7X3	T46.7X4	T46.7X5	T46.7X6
Kallikrein	T46.7X1	T46.7X2	T46.7X3	T46.7X4	T46.7X5	T46.7X6
Kanamycin	T36.5X1	T36.5X2	T36.5X3	T36.5X4	T36.5X5	T36.5X6
Kantrex	T36.5X1	T36.5X2	T36.5X3	T36.5X4	T36.5X5	T36.5X6
Kaolin	T47.6X1	T47.6X2	T47.6X3	T47.6X4	T47.6X5	T47.6X6
light	T47.6X1	T47.6X2	T47.6X3	T47.6X4	T47.6X5	T47.6X6
Karaya (gum)	T47.4X1	T47.4X2	T47.4X3	T47.4X4	T47.4X5	T47.4X6
Kebuzone	T39.2X1	T39.2X2	T39.2X3	T39.2X4	T39.2X5	T39.2X6
Kelevan	T6Ø.1X1	T6Ø.1X2	T6Ø.1X3	T6Ø.1X4	—	—
Kemithal	T41.1X1	T41.1X2	T41.1X3	T41.1X4	T41.1X5	T41.1X6
Kenacort	T38.ØX1	T38.ØX2	T38.ØX3	T38.ØX4	T38.ØX5	T38.ØX6
Keratolytic drug NEC	T49.4X1	T49.4X2	T49.4X3	T49.4X4	T49.4X5	T49.4X6
anthracene	T49.4X1	T49.4X2	T49.4X3	T49.4X4	T49.4X5	T49.4X6
Keratoplastic NEC	T49.4X1	T49.4X2	T49.4X3	T49.4X4	T49.4X5	T49.4X6
Kerosene, kerosine (fuel) (solvent) NEC	T52.ØX1	T52.ØX2	T52.ØX3	T52.ØX4	—	—
insecticide	T52.ØX1	T52.ØX2	T52.ØX3	T52.ØX4	—	—
vapor	T52.ØX1	T52.ØX2	T52.ØX3	T52.ØX4	—	—
Ketamine	T41.291	T41.292	T41.293	T41.294	T41.295	T41.296
Ketazolam	T42.4X1	T42.4X2	T42.4X3	T42.4X4	T42.4X5	T42.4X6
Ketazon	T39.2X1	T39.2X2	T39.2X3	T39.2X4	T39.2X5	T39.2X6
Ketobemidone	T4Ø.4X1	T4Ø.4X2	T4Ø.4X3	T4Ø.4X4	—	—
Ketoconazole	T49.ØX1	T49.ØX2	T49.ØX3	T49.ØX4	T49.ØX5	T49.ØX6
Ketols	T52.4X1	T52.4X2	T52.4X3	T52.4X4	—	—
Ketone oils	T52.4X1	T52.4X2	T52.4X3	T52.4X4	—	—
Ketoprofen	T39.311	T39.312	T39.313	T39.314	T39.315	T39.316
Ketorolac	T39.8X1	T39.8X2	T39.8X3	T39.8X4	T39.8X5	T39.8X6
Ketotifen	T45.ØX1	T45.ØX2	T45.ØX3	T45.ØX4	T45.ØX5	T45.ØX6
Khat	T43.691	T43.692	T43.693	T43.694	—	—
Khellin	T46.3X1	T46.3X2	T46.3X3	T46.3X4	T46.3X5	T46.3X6
Khelloside	T46.3X1	T46.3X2	T46.3X3	T46.3X4	T46.3X5	T46.3X6
Kiln gas or vapor (carbon monoxide)	T58.8X1	T58.8X2	T58.8X3	T58.8X4	—	—
Kitasamycin	T36.3X1	T36.3X2	T36.3X3	T36.3X4	T36.3X5	T36.3X6
Konsyl	T47.4X1	T47.4X2	T47.4X3	T47.4X4	T47.4X5	T47.4X6
Kosam seed	T62.2X1	T62.2X2	T62.2X3	T62.2X4	—	—
Krait (venom)	T63.Ø91	T63.Ø92	T63.Ø93	T63.Ø94	—	—
Kwell (insecticide)	T6Ø.1X1	T6Ø.1X2	T6Ø.1X3	T6Ø.1X4	—	—
anti-infective (topical)	T49.ØX1	T49.ØX2	T49.ØX3	T49.ØX4	T49.ØX5	T49.ØX6

◀ New ⟸ Revised ~~deleted~~ Deleted

Substance	Poisoning, Accidental (Unintentional)	Poisoning, Intentional Self-Harm	Poisoning, Assault	Poisoning, Undetermined	Adverse Effect	Underdosing
L						
Labetalol	T44.8X1	T44.8X2	T44.8X3	T44.8X4	T44.8X5	T44.8X6
Laburnum (seeds)	T62.2X1	T62.2X2	T62.2X3	T62.2X4	—	—
leaves	T62.2X1	T62.2X2	T62.2X3	T62.2X4	—	—
Lachesine	T49.5X1	T49.5X2	T49.5X3	T49.5X4	T49.5X5	T49.5X6
Lacidipine	T46.5X1	T46.5X2	T46.5X3	T46.5X4	T46.5X5	T46.5X6
Lacquer	T65.6X1	T65.6X2	T65.6X3	T65.6X4	—	—
Lacrimogenic gas	T59.3X1	T59.3X2	T59.3X3	T59.3X4	—	—
Lactated potassic saline	T50.3X1	T50.3X2	T50.3X3	T50.3X4	T50.3X5	T50.3X6
Lactic acid	T49.8X1	T49.8X2	T49.8X3	T49.8X4	T49.8X5	T49.8X6
Lactobacillus						
acidophilus	T47.6X1	T47.6X2	T47.6X3	T47.6X4	T47.6X5	T47.6X6
compound	T47.6X1	T47.6X2	T47.6X3	T47.6X4	T47.6X5	T47.6X6
bifidus, lyophilized	T47.6X1	T47.6X2	T47.6X3	T47.6X4	T47.6X5	T47.6X6
bulgaricus	T47.6X1	T47.6X2	T47.6X3	T47.6X4	T47.6X5	T47.6X6
sporogenes	T47.6X1	T47.6X2	T47.6X3	T47.6X4	T47.6X5	T47.6X6
Lactoflavin	T45.2X1	T45.2X2	T45.2X3	T45.2X4	T45.2X5	T45.2X6
Lactose (as excipient)	T50.901	T50.902	T50.903	T50.904	T50.905	T50.906
Lactuca (virosa) (extract)	T42.6X1	T42.6X2	T42.6X3	T42.6X4	T42.6X5	T42.6X6
Lactucarium	T42.6X1	T42.6X2	T42.6X3	T42.6X4	T42.6X5	T42.6X6
Lactulose	T47.3X1	T47.3X2	T47.3X3	T47.3X4	T47.3X5	T47.3X6
Laevo — *see Levo-*						
Lanatosides	T46.0X1	T46.0X2	T46.0X3	T46.0X4	T46.0X5	T46.0X6
Lanolin	T49.3X1	T49.3X2	T49.3X3	T49.3X4	T49.3X5	T49.3X6
Largactil	T43.3X1	T43.3X2	T43.3X3	T43.3X4	T43.3X5	T43.3X6
Larkspur	T62.2X1	T62.2X2	T62.2X3	T62.2X4	—	—
Laroxyl	T43.011	T43.012	T43.013	T43.014	T43.015	T43.016
Lassar's paste	T49.4X1	T49.4X2	T49.4X3	T49.4X4	T49.4X5	T49.4X6
Lasix	T50.1X1	T50.1X2	T50.1X3	T50.1X4	T50.1X5	T50.1X6
Latamoxef	T36.1X1	T36.1X2	T36.1X3	T36.1X4	T36.1X5	T36.1X6
Latex	T65.811	T65.812	T65.813	T65.814	—	—
Lathyrus (seed)	T62.2X1	T62.2X2	T62.2X3	T62.2X4	—	—
Laudanum	T40.0X1	T40.0X2	T40.0X3	T40.0X4	T40.0X5	T40.0X6
Laudexium	T48.1X1	T48.1X2	T48.1X3	T48.1X4	T48.1X5	T48.1X6
Laughing gas	T41.0X1	T41.0X2	T41.0X3	T41.0X4	T41.0X5	T41.0X6
Laurel, black or cherry	T62.2X1	T62.2X2	T62.2X3	T62.2X4	—	—
Laurolinium	T49.0X1	T49.0X2	T49.0X3	T49.0X4	T49.0X5	T49.0X6
Lauryl sulfoacetate	T49.2X1	T49.2X2	T49.2X3	T49.2X4	T49.2X5	T49.2X6
Laxative NEC	T47.4X1	T47.4X2	T47.4X3	T47.4X4	T47.4X5	T47.4X6
osmotic	T47.3X1	T47.3X2	T47.3X3	T47.3X4	T47.3X5	T47.3X6
saline	T47.3X1	T47.3X2	T47.3X3	T47.3X4	T47.3X5	T47.3X6
stimulant	T47.2X1	T47.2X2	T47.2X3	T47.2X4	T47.2X5	T47.2X6
L-dopa	T42.8X1	T42.8X2	T42.8X3	T42.8X4	T42.8X5	T42.8X6
Lead (dust) (fumes) (vapor) NEC	T56.0X1	T56.0X2	T56.0X3	T56.0X4	—	—
acetate	T49.2X1	T49.2X2	T49.2X3	T49.2X4	T49.2X5	T49.2X6
alkyl (fuel additive)	T56.0X1	T56.0X2	T56.0X3	T56.0X4	—	—
anti-infectives	T37.8X1	T37.8X2	T37.8X3	T37.8X4	T37.8X5	T37.8X6
antiknock compound (tetraethyl)	T56.0X1	T56.0X2	T56.0X3	T56.0X4	—	—
arsenate, arsenite (dust) (herbicide) (insecticide) (vapor)	T57.0X1	T57.0X2	T57.0X3	T57.0X4	—	—
carbonate	T56.0X1	T56.0X2	T56.0X3	T56.0X4	—	—
paint	T56.0X1	T56.0X2	T56.0X3	T56.0X4	—	—
chromate	T56.0X1	T56.0X2	T56.0X3	T56.0X4	—	—
paint	T56.0X1	T56.0X2	T56.0X3	T56.0X4	—	—
dioxide	T56.0X1	T56.0X2	T56.0X3	T56.0X4	—	—
inorganic	T56.0X1	T56.0X2	T56.0X3	T56.0X4	—	—
iodide	T56.0X1	T56.0X2	T56.0X3	T56.0X4	—	—
pigment (paint)	T56.0X1	T56.0X2	T56.0X3	T56.0X4	—	—
monoxide (dust)	T56.0X1	T56.0X2	T56.0X3	T56.0X4	—	—
paint	T56.0X1	T56.0X2	T56.0X3	T56.0X4	—	—
organic	T56.0X1	T56.0X2	T56.0X3	T56.0X4	—	—
oxide	T56.0X1	T56.0X2	T56.0X3	T56.0X4	—	—
paint	T56.0X1	T56.0X2	T56.0X3	T56.0X4	—	—
paint	T56.0X1	T56.0X2	T56.0X3	T56.0X4	—	—
salts	T56.0X1	T56.0X2	T56.0X3	T56.0X4	—	—
specified compound NEC	T56.0X1	T56.0X2	T56.0X3	T56.0X4	—	—
tetra-ethyl	T56.0X1	T56.0X2	T56.0X3	T56.0X4	—	—
Lebanese red	T40.7X1	T40.7X2	T40.7X3	T40.7X4	T40.7X5	T40.7X6
Lefetamine	T39.8X1	T39.8X2	T39.8X3	T39.8X4	T39.8X5	T39.8X6
Lenperone	T43.4X1	T43.4X2	T43.4X3	T43.4X4	T43.4X5	T43.4X6
Lente lietin (insulin)	T38.3X1	T38.3X2	T38.3X3	T38.3X4	T38.3X5	T38.3X6
Leptazol	T50.7X1	T50.7X2	T50.7X3	T50.7X4	T50.7X5	T50.7X6
Leptophos	T60.0X1	T60.0X2	T60.0X3	T60.0X4	—	—
Leritine	T40.2X1	T40.2X2	T40.2X3	T40.2X4	T40.2X5	T40.2X6
Letosteine	T48.4X1	T48.4X2	T48.4X3	T48.4X4	T48.4X5	T48.4X6
Letter	T38.1X1	T38.1X2	T38.1X3	T38.1X4	T38.1X5	T38.1X6
Lettuce opium	T42.6X1	T42.6X2	T42.6X3	T42.6X4	T42.6X5	T42.6X6
Leucinocaine	T41.3X1	T41.3X2	T41.3X3	T41.3X4	T41.3X5	T41.3X6

Substance	Poisoning, Accidental (Unintentional)	Poisoning, Intentional Self-Harm	Poisoning, Assault	Poisoning, Undetermined	Adverse Effect	Underdosing
Leucocianidol	T46.991	T46.992	T46.993	T46.994	T46.995	T46.996
Leucovorin (factor)	T45.8X1	T45.8X2	T45.8X3	T45.8X4	T45.8X5	T45.8X6
Leukeran	T45.1X1	T45.1X2	T45.1X3	T45.1X4	T45.1X5	T45.1X6
Leuprolide	T38.891	T38.892	T38.893	T38.894	T38.895	T38.896
Levalbuterol	T48.6X1	T48.6X2	T48.6X3	T48.6X4	T48.6X5	T48.6X6
Levallorphan	T50.7X1	T50.7X2	T50.7X3	T50.7X4	T50.7X5	T50.7X6
Levamisole	T37.4X1	T37.4X2	T37.4X3	T37.4X4	T37.4X5	T37.4X6
Levanil	T42.6X1	T42.6X2	T42.6X3	T42.6X4	T42.6X5	T42.6X6
Levarterenol	T44.4X1	T44.4X2	T44.4X3	T44.4X4	T44.4X5	T44.4X6
Levdropropizine	T48.3X1	T48.3X2	T48.3X3	T48.3X4	T48.3X5	T48.3X6
Levobunolol	T49.5X1	T49.5X2	T49.5X3	T49.5X4	T49.5X5	T49.5X6
Levocabastine (hydrochloride)	T45.0X1	T45.0X2	T45.0X3	T45.0X4	T45.0X5	T45.0X6
Levocarnitine	T50.991	T50.992	T50.993	T50.994	T50.995	T50.996
Levodopa	T42.8X1	T42.8X2	T42.8X3	T42.8X4	T42.8X5	T42.8X6
with carbidopa	T42.8X1	T42.8X2	T42.8X3	T42.8X4	T42.8X5	T42.8X6
Levo-dromoran	T40.2X1	T40.2X2	T40.2X3	T40.2X4	T40.2X5	T40.2X6
Levoglutamide	T50.991	T50.992	T50.993	T50.994	T50.995	T50.996
Levoid	T38.1X1	T38.1X2	T38.1X3	T38.1X4	T38.1X5	T38.1X6
Levo-iso-methadone	T40.3X1	T40.3X2	T40.3X3	T40.3X4	T40.3X5	T40.3X6
Levomepromazine	T43.3X1	T43.3X2	T43.3X3	T43.3X4	T43.3X5	T43.3X6
Levonordefrin	T49.6X1	T49.6X2	T49.6X3	T49.6X4	T49.6X5	T49.6X6
Levonorgestrel	T38.4X1	T38.4X2	T38.4X3	T38.4X4	T38.4X5	T38.4X6
with ethinylestradiol	T38.5X1	T38.5X2	T38.5X3	T38.5X4	T38.5X5	T38.5X6
Levopromazine	T43.3X1	T43.3X2	T43.3X3	T43.3X4	T43.3X5	T43.3X6
Levoprome	T42.6X1	T42.6X2	T42.6X3	T42.6X4	T42.6X5	T42.6X6
Levopropoxyphene	T40.4X1	T40.4X2	T40.4X3	T40.4X4	T40.4X5	T40.4X6
Levopropylhexedrine	T50.5X1	T50.5X2	T50.5X3	T50.5X4	T50.5X5	T50.5X6
Levoproxyphylline	T48.6X1	T48.6X2	T48.6X3	T48.6X4	T48.6X5	T48.6X6
Levorphanol	T40.4X1	T40.4X2	T40.4X3	T40.4X4	T40.4X5	T40.4X6
Levothyroxine	T38.1X1	T38.1X2	T38.1X3	T38.1X4	T38.1X5	T38.1X6
sodium	T38.1X1	T38.1X2	T38.1X3	T38.1X4	T38.1X5	T38.1X6
Levsin	T44.3X1	T44.3X2	T44.3X3	T44.3X4	T44.3X5	T44.3X6
Levulose	T50.3X1	T50.3X2	T50.3X3	T50.3X4	T50.3X5	T50.3X6
Lewisite (gas), not in war	T57.0X1	T57.0X2	T57.0X3	T57.0X4	—	—
Librium	T42.4X1	T42.4X2	T42.4X3	T42.4X4	T42.4X5	T42.4X6
Lidex	T49.0X1	T49.0X2	T49.0X3	T49.0X4	T49.0X5	T49.0X6
Lidocaine	T41.3X1	T41.3X2	T41.3X3	T41.3X4	T41.3X5	T41.3X6
regional	T41.3X1	T41.3X2	T41.3X3	T41.3X4	T41.3X5	T41.3X6
spinal	T41.3X1	T41.3X2	T41.3X3	T41.3X4	T41.3X5	T41.3X6
Lidofenin	T50.8X1	T50.8X2	T50.8X3	T50.8X4	T50.8X5	T50.8X6
Lidoflazine	T46.1X1	T46.1X2	T46.1X3	T46.1X4	T46.1X5	T46.1X6
Lighter fluid	T52.0X1	T52.0X2	T52.0X3	T52.0X4	—	—

Substance	Poisoning, Accidental (Unintentional)	Poisoning, Intentional Self-Harm	Poisoning, Assault	Poisoning, Undetermined	Adverse Effect	Underdosing
Lignin hemicellulose	T47.6X1	T47.6X2	T47.6X3	T47.6X4	T47.6X5	T47.6X6
Lignocaine	T41.3X1	T41.3X2	T41.3X3	T41.3X4	T41.3X5	T41.3X6
regional	T41.3X1	T41.3X2	T41.3X3	T41.3X4	T41.3X5	T41.3X6
spinal	T41.3X1	T41.3X2	T41.3X3	T41.3X4	T41.3X5	T41.3X6
Ligroin(e) (solvent)	T52.0X1	T52.0X2	T52.0X3	T52.0X4	—	—
vapor	T59.891	T59.892	T59.893	T59.894	—	—
Ligustrum vulgare	T62.2X1	T62.2X2	T62.2X3	T62.2X4	—	—
Lily of the valley	T62.2X1	T62.2X2	T62.2X3	T62.2X4	—	—
Lime (chloride)	T54.3X1	T54.3X2	T54.3X3	T54.3X4	—	—
Limonene	T52.8X1	T52.8X2	T52.8X3	T52.8X4	—	—
Lincomycin	T36.8X1	T36.8X2	T36.8X3	T36.8X4	T36.8X5	T36.8X6
Lindane (insecticide) (nonmedicinal) (vapor)	T53.6X1	T53.6X2	T53.6X3	T53.6X4	—	—
medicinal	T49.0X1	T49.0X2	T49.0X3	T49.0X4	T49.0X5	T49.0X6
Liniments NEC	T49.91	T49.92	T49.93	T49.94	T49.95	T49.96
Linoleic acid	T46.6X1	T46.6X2	T46.6X3	T46.6X4	T46.6X5	T46.6X6
Linolenic acid	T46.6X1	T46.6X2	T46.6X3	T46.6X4	T46.6X5	T46.6X6
Linseed	T47.4X1	T47.4X2	T47.4X3	T47.4X4	T47.4X5	T47.4X6
Liothyronine	T38.1X1	T38.1X2	T38.1X3	T38.1X4	T38.1X5	T38.1X6
Liotrix	T38.1X1	T38.1X2	T38.1X3	T38.1X4	T38.1X5	T38.1X6
Lipancreatin	T47.5X1	T47.5X2	T47.5X3	T47.5X4	T47.5X5	T47.5X6
Lipo-alprostadil	T46.7X1	T46.7X2	T46.7X3	T46.7X4	T46.7X5	T46.7X6
Lipo-Lutin	T38.5X1	T38.5X2	T38.5X3	T38.5X4	T38.5X5	T38.5X6
Lipotropic drug NEC	T50.901	T50.902	T50.903	T50.904	T50.905	T50.906
Liquefied petroleum gases	T59.891	T59.892	T59.893	T59.894	—	—
piped (pure or mixed with air)	T59.891	T59.892	T59.893	T59.894	—	—
Liquid						
paraffin	T47.4X1	T47.4X2	T47.4X3	T47.4X4	T47.4X5	T47.4X6
petrolatum	T47.4X1	T47.4X2	T47.4X3	T47.4X4	T47.4X5	T47.4X6
topical	T49.3X1	T49.3X2	T49.3X3	T49.3X4	T49.3X5	T49.3X6
specified NEC	T65.891	T65.892	T65.893	T65.894	—	—
substance	T65.91	T65.92	T65.93	T65.94	—	—
Liquor creosolis compositus	T65.891	T65.892	T65.893	T65.894	—	—
Liquorice	T48.4X1	T48.4X2	T48.4X3	T48.4X4	T48.4X5	T48.4X6
extract	T47.8X1	T47.8X2	T47.8X3	T47.8X4	T47.8X5	T47.8X6
Lirugen	T50.991	T50.992	T50.993	T50.994	T50.995	T50.996
Lisinopril	T46.4X1	T46.4X2	T46.4X3	T46.4X4	T46.4X5	T46.4X6
Lisuride	T42.8X1	T42.8X2	T42.8X3	T42.8X4	T42.8X5	T42.8X6
Lithane	T43.8X1	T43.8X2	T43.8X3	T43.8X4	T43.8X5	T43.8X6
Lithium	T56.891	T56.892	T56.893	T56.894	—	—
gluconate	T43.591	T43.592	T43.593	T43.594	T43.595	T43.596
salts (carbonate)	T43.591	T43.592	T43.593	T43.594	T43.595	T43.596

Substance	Poisoning, Accidental (Unintentional)	Poisoning, Intentional Self-Harm	Poisoning, Assault	Poisoning, Undetermined	Adverse Effect	Underdosing
Lithonate	T43.8X1	T43.8X2	T43.8X3	T43.8X4	T43.8X5	T43.8X6
Liver						
extract	T45.8X1	T45.8X2	T45.8X3	T45.8X4	T45.8X5	T45.8X6
for parenteral use	T45.8X1	T45.8X2	T45.8X3	T45.8X4	T45.8X5	T45.8X6
fraction 1	T45.8X1	T45.8X2	T45.8X3	T45.8X4	T45.8X5	T45.8X6
hydrolysate	T45.8X1	T45.8X2	T45.8X3	T45.8X4	T45.8X5	T45.8X6
Lizard (bite) (venom)	T63.121	T63.122	T63.123	T63.124	—	—
LMD	T45.8X1	T45.8X2	T45.8X3	T45.8X4	T45.8X5	T45.8X6
Lobelia	T62.2X1	T62.2X2	T62.2X3	T62.2X4	—	—
Lobeline	T5Ø.7X1	T5Ø.7X2	T5Ø.7X3	T5Ø.7X4	T5Ø.7X5	T5Ø.7X6
Local action drug NEC	T49.8X1	T49.8X2	T49.8X3	T49.8X4	T49.8X5	T49.8X6
Locorten	T49.ØX1	T49.ØX2	T49.ØX3	T49.ØX4	T49.ØX5	T49.ØX6
Lofepramine	T43.Ø11	T43.Ø12	T43.Ø13	T43.Ø14	T43.Ø15	T43.Ø16
Lolium temulentum	T62.2X1	T62.2X2	T62.2X3	T62.2X4	—	—
Lomotil	T47.6X1	T47.6X2	T47.6X3	T47.6X4	T47.6X5	T47.6X6
Lomustine	T45.1X1	T45.1X2	T45.1X3	T45.1X4	T45.1X5	T45.1X6
Lonidamine	T45.1X1	T45.1X2	T45.1X3	T45.1X4	T45.1X5	T45.1X6
Loperamide	T47.6X1	T47.6X2	T47.6X3	T47.6X4	T47.6X5	T47.6X6
Loprazolam	T42.4X1	T42.4X2	T42.4X3	T42.4X4	T42.4X5	T42.4X6
Lorajmine	T46.2X1	T46.2X2	T46.2X3	T46.2X4	T46.2X5	T46.2X6
Loratidine	T45.ØX1	T45.ØX2	T45.ØX3	T45.ØX4	T45.ØX5	T45.ØX6
Lorazepam	T42.4X1	T42.4X2	T42.4X3	T42.4X4	T42.4X5	T42.4X6
Lorcainide	T46.2X1	T46.2X2	T46.2X3	T46.2X4	T46.2X5	T46.2X6
Lormetazepam	T42.4X1	T42.4X2	T42.4X3	T42.4X4	T42.4X5	T42.4X6
Lotions NEC	T49.91	T49.92	T49.93	T49.94	T49.95	T49.96
Lotusate	T42.3X1	T42.3X2	T42.3X3	T42.3X4	T42.3X5	T42.3X6
Lovastatin	T46.6X1	T46.6X2	T46.6X3	T46.6X4	T46.6X5	T46.6X6
Loxapine	T43.591	T43.592	T43.593	T43.594	T43.595	T43.596
Lowila	T49.2X1	T49.2X2	T49.2X3	T49.2X4	T49.2X5	T49.2X6
Lozenges (throat)	T49.6X1	T49.6X2	T49.6X3	T49.6X4	T49.6X5	T49.6X6
LSD	T4Ø.8X1	T4Ø.8X2	T4Ø.8X3	T4Ø.8X4	—	—
L-Tryptophan — *see amino acid*						
Lubricant, eye	T49.5X1	T49.5X2	T49.5X3	T49.5X4	T49.5X5	T49.5X6
Lubricating oil NEC	T52.ØX1	T52.ØX2	T52.ØX3	T52.ØX4	—	—
Lucanthone	T37.4X1	T37.4X2	T37.4X3	T37.4X4	T37.4X5	T37.4X6
Luminal	T42.3X1	T42.3X2	T42.3X3	T42.3X4	T42.3X5	T42.3X6
Lung irritant (gas) NEC	T59.91	T59.92	T59.93	T59.94	—	—
Luteinizing hormone	T38.811	T38.812	T38.813	T38.814	T38.815	T38.816
Lutocylol	T38.5X1	T38.5X2	T38.5X3	T38.5X4	T38.5X5	T38.5X6
Lutromone	T38.5X1	T38.5X2	T38.5X3	T38.5X4	T38.5X5	T38.5X6
Lututrin	T48.291	T48.292	T48.293	T48.294	T48.295	T48.296
Lye (Concentrated)	T54.3X1	T54.3X2	T54.3X3	T54.3X4	—	—

Substance	Poisoning, Accidental (Unintentional)	Poisoning, Intentional Self-Harm	Poisoning, Assault	Poisoning, Undetermined	Adverse Effect	Underdosing
Lygranum (skin test)	T5Ø.8X1	T5Ø.8X2	T5Ø.8X3	T5Ø.8X4	T5Ø.8X5	T5Ø.8X6
Lymecycline	T36.4X1	T36.4X2	T36.4X3	T36.4X4	T36.4X5	T36.4X6
Lymphogranuloma venereum antigen	T5Ø.8X1	T5Ø.8X2	T5Ø.8X3	T5Ø.8X4	T5Ø.8X5	T5Ø.8X6
Lynestrenol	T38.4X1	T38.4X2	T38.4X3	T38.4X4	T38.4X5	T38.4X6
Lypressin	T38.891	T38.892	T38.893	T38.894	T38.895	T38.896
Lyovac Sodium Edecrin	T5Ø.1X1	T5Ø.1X2	T5Ø.1X3	T5Ø.1X4	T5Ø.1X5	T5Ø.1X6
Lysergic acid diethylamide	T4Ø.8X1	T4Ø.8X2	T4Ø.8X3	T4Ø.8X4	—	—
Lysergide	T4Ø.8X1	T4Ø.8X2	T4Ø.8X3	T4Ø.8X4	—	—
Lysine vasopressin	T38.891	T38.892	T38.893	T38.894	T38.895	T38.896
Lysol	T54.1X1	T54.1X2	T54.1X3	T54.1X4	—	—
Lysozyme	T49.ØX1	T49.ØX2	T49.ØX3	T49.ØX4	T49.ØX5	T49.ØX6
Lytta (vitatta)	T49.8X1	T49.8X2	T49.8X3	T49.8X4	T49.8X5	T49.8X6
M						
Mace	T59.3X1	T59.3X2	T59.3X3	T59.3X4	—	—
Macrogol	T5Ø.991	T5Ø.992	T5Ø.993	T5Ø.994	T5Ø.995	T5Ø.996
Macrolide						
anabolic drug	T38.7X1	T38.7X2	T38.7X3	T38.7X4	T38.7X5	T38.7X6
antibiotic	T36.3X1	T36.3X2	T36.3X3	T36.3X4	T36.3X5	T36.3X6
Mafenide	T49.ØX1	T49.ØX2	T49.ØX3	T49.ØX4	T49.ØX5	T49.ØX6
Magaldrate	T47.1X1	T47.1X2	T47.1X3	T47.1X4	T47.1X5	T47.1X6
Magic mushroom	T4Ø.991	T4Ø.992	T4Ø.993	T4Ø.994	—	—
Magnamycin	T36.8X1	T36.8X2	T36.8X3	T36.8X4	T36.8X5	T36.8X6
Magnesia magma	T47.1X1	T47.1X2	T47.1X3	T47.1X4	T47.1X5	T47.1X6
Magnesium NEC	T56.891	T56.892	T56.893	T56.894	—	—
carbonate	T47.1X1	T47.1X2	T47.1X3	T47.1X4	T47.1X5	T47.1X6
citrate	T47.4X1	T47.4X2	T47.4X3	T47.4X4	T47.4X5	T47.4X6
hydroxide	T47.1X1	T47.1X2	T47.1X3	T47.1X4	T47.1X5	T47.1X6
oxide	T47.1X1	T47.1X2	T47.1X3	T47.1X4	T47.1X5	T47.1X6
peroxide	T49.ØX1	T49.ØX2	T49.ØX3	T49.ØX4	T49.ØX5	T49.ØX6
salicylate	T39.Ø91	T39.Ø92	T39.Ø93	T39.Ø94	T39.Ø95	T39.Ø96
silicofluoride	T5Ø.3X1	T5Ø.3X2	T5Ø.3X3	T5Ø.3X4	T5Ø.3X5	T5Ø.3X6
sulfate	T47.4X1	T47.4X2	T47.4X3	T47.4X4	T47.4X5	T47.4X6
thiosulfate	T45.ØX1	T45.ØX2	T45.ØX3	T45.ØX4	T45.ØX5	T45.ØX6
trisilicate	T47.1X1	T47.1X2	T47.1X3	T47.1X4	T47.1X5	T47.1X6
Malathion (medicinal)	T49.ØX1	T49.ØX2	T49.ØX3	T49.ØX4	T49.ØX5	T49.ØX6
insecticide	T6Ø.ØX1	T6Ø.ØX2	T6Ø.ØX3	T6Ø.ØX4	—	—
Male fern extract	T37.4X1	T37.4X2	T37.4X3	T37.4X4	T37.4X5	T37.4X6
M-AMSA	T45.1X1	T45.1X2	T45.1X3	T45.1X4	T45.1X5	T45.1X6
Mandelic acid	T37.8X1	T37.8X2	T37.8X3	T37.8X4	T37.8X5	T37.8X6
Manganese (dioxide) (salts)	T57.2X1	T57.2X2	T57.2X3	T57.2X4	—	—
medicinal	T5Ø.991	T5Ø.992	T5Ø.993	T5Ø.994	T5Ø.995	T5Ø.996

Substance	Poisoning, Accidental (Unintentional)	Poisoning, Intentional Self-Harm	Poisoning, Assault	Poisoning, Undetermined	Adverse Effect	Underdosing
Mannitol	T47.3X1	T47.3X2	T47.3X3	T47.3X4	T47.3X5	T47.3X6
hexanitrate	T46.3X1	T46.3X2	T46.3X3	T46.3X4	T46.3X5	T46.3X6
Mannomustine	T45.1X1	T45.1X2	T45.1X3	T45.1X4	T45.1X5	T45.1X6
MAO inhibitors	T43.1X1	T43.1X2	T43.1X3	T43.1X4	T43.1X5	T43.1X6
Mapharsen	T37.8X1	T37.8X2	T37.8X3	T37.8X4	T37.8X5	T37.8X6
Maphenide	T49.0X1	T49.0X2	T49.0X3	T49.0X4	T49.0X5	T49.0X6
Maprotiline	T43.021	T43.022	T43.023	T43.024	T43.025	T43.026
Marcaine	T41.3X1	T41.3X2	T41.3X3	T41.3X4	T41.3X5	T41.3X6
infiltration (subcutaneous)	T41.3X1	T41.3X2	T41.3X3	T41.3X4	T41.3X5	T41.3X6
nerve block (peripheral) (plexus)	T41.3X1	T41.3X2	T41.3X3	T41.3X4	T41.3X5	T41.3X6
Marezine	T45.0X1	T45.0X2	T45.0X3	T45.0X4	T45.0X5	T45.0X6
Marihuana	T40.7X1	T40.7X2	T40.7X3	T40.7X4	T40.7X5	T40.7X6
Marijuana	T40.7X1	T40.7X2	T40.7X3	T40.7X4	T40.7X5	T40.7X6
Marine (sting)	T63.691	T63.692	T63.693	T63.694	—	—
animals (sting)	T63.691	T63.692	T63.693	T63.694	—	—
plants (sting)	T63.711	T63.712	T63.713	T63.714	—	—
Marplan	T43.1X1	T43.1X2	T43.1X3	T43.1X4	T43.1X5	T43.1X6
Marsh gas	T59.891	T59.892	T59.893	T59.894	—	—
Marsilid	T43.1X1	T43.1X2	T43.1X3	T43.1X4	T43.1X5	T43.1X6
Matulane	T45.1X1	T45.1X2	T45.1X3	T45.1X4	T45.1X5	T45.1X6
Mazindol	T50.5X1	T50.5X2	T50.5X3	T50.5X4	T50.5X5	T50.5X6
MCPA	T60.3X1	T60.3X2	T60.3X3	T60.3X4	—	—
MDMA	T43.621	T43.622	T43.623	T43.624	T43.625	T43.626
Meadow saffron	T62.2X1	T62.2X2	T62.2X3	T62.2X4	—	—
Measles virus vaccine (attenuated)	T50.B91	T50.B92	T50.B93	T50.B94	T50.B95	T50.B96
Meat, noxious	T62.8X1	T62.8X2	T62.8X3	T62.8X4	—	—
Meballymal	T42.3X1	T42.3X2	T42.3X3	T42.3X4	T42.3X5	T42.3X6
Mebanazine	T43.1X1	T43.1X2	T43.1X3	T43.1X4	T43.1X5	T43.1X6
Mebaral	T42.3X1	T42.3X2	T42.3X3	T42.3X4	T42.3X5	T42.3X6
Mebendazole	T37.4X1	T37.4X2	T37.4X3	T37.4X4	T37.4X5	T37.4X6
Mebeverine	T44.3X1	T44.3X2	T44.3X3	T44.3X4	T44.3X5	T44.3X6
Mebhydrolin	T45.0X1	T45.0X2	T45.0X3	T45.0X4	T45.0X5	T45.0X6
Mebumal	T42.3X1	T42.3X2	T42.3X3	T42.3X4	T42.3X5	T42.3X6
Mebutamate	T43.591	T43.592	T43.593	T43.594	T43.595	T43.596
Mecamylamine	T44.2X1	T44.2X2	T44.2X3	T44.2X4	T44.2X5	T44.2X6
Mechlorethamine	T45.1X1	T45.1X2	T45.1X3	T45.1X4	T45.1X5	T45.1X6
Mecillinam	T36.0X1	T36.0X2	T36.0X3	T36.0X4	T36.0X5	T36.0X6
Meclizine (hydrochloride)	T45.0X1	T45.0X2	T45.0X3	T45.0X4	T45.0X5	T45.0X6
Meclocycline	T36.4X1	T36.4X2	T36.4X3	T36.4X4	T36.4X5	T36.4X6
Meclofenamate	T39.391	T39.392	T39.393	T39.394	T39.395	T39.396
Meclofenamic acid	T39.391	T39.392	T39.393	T39.394	T39.395	T39.396
Meclofenoxate	T43.691	T43.692	T43.693	T43.694	T43.695	T43.696
Meclozine	T45.0X1	T45.0X2	T45.0X3	T45.0X4	T45.0X5	T45.0X6
Mecobalamin	T45.8X1	T45.8X2	T45.8X3	T45.8X4	T45.8X5	T45.8X6
Mecoprop	T60.3X1	T60.3X2	T60.3X3	T60.3X4	—	—
Mecrilate	T49.3X1	T49.3X2	T49.3X3	T49.3X4	T49.3X5	T49.3X6
Mecysteine	T48.4X1	T48.4X2	T48.4X3	T48.4X4	T48.4X5	T48.4X6
Medazepam	T42.4X1	T42.4X2	T42.4X3	T42.4X4	T42.4X5	T42.4X6
Medicament NEC	T50.901	T50.902	T50.903	T50.904	T50.905	T50.906
Medinal	T42.3X1	T42.3X2	T42.3X3	T42.3X4	T42.3X5	T42.3X6
Medomin	T42.3X1	T42.3X2	T42.3X3	T42.3X4	T42.3X5	T42.3X6
Medrogestone	T38.5X1	T38.5X2	T38.5X3	T38.5X4	T38.5X5	T38.5X6
Medroxalol	T44.8X1	T44.8X2	T44.8X3	T44.8X4	T44.8X5	T44.8X6
Medroxyprogesterone acetate (depot)	T38.5X1	T38.5X2	T38.5X3	T38.5X4	T38.5X5	T38.5X6
Medrysone	T49.0X1	T49.0X2	T49.0X3	T49.0X4	T49.0X5	T49.0X6
Mefenamic acid	T39.391	T39.392	T39.393	T39.394	T39.395	T39.396
Mefenorex	T50.5X1	T50.5X2	T50.5X3	T50.5X4	T50.5X5	T50.5X6
Mefloquine	T37.2X1	T37.2X2	T37.2X3	T37.2X4	T37.2X5	T37.2X6
Mefruside	T50.2X1	T50.2X2	T50.2X3	T50.2X4	T50.2X5	T50.2X6
Megahallucinogen	T40.901	T40.902	T40.903	T40.904	T40.905	T40.906
Megestrol	T38.5X1	T38.5X2	T38.5X3	T38.5X4	T38.5X5	T38.5X6
Meglumine						
antimoniate	T37.8X1	T37.8X2	T37.8X3	T37.8X4	T37.8X5	T37.8X6
diatrizoate	T50.8X1	T50.8X2	T50.8X3	T50.8X4	T50.8X5	T50.8X6
iodipamide	T50.8X1	T50.8X2	T50.8X3	T50.8X4	T50.8X5	T50.8X6
iotroxate	T50.8X1	T50.8X2	T50.8X3	T50.8X4	T50.8X5	T50.8X6
MEK (methyl ethyl ketone)	T52.4X1	T52.4X2	T52.4X3	T52.4X4	—	—
Meladrazine	T44.3X1	T44.3X2	T44.3X3	T44.3X4	T44.3X5	T44.3X6
Meladinin	T49.3X1	T49.3X2	T49.3X3	T49.3X4	T49.3X5	T49.3X6
Melaleuca alternifolia oil	T49.0X1	T49.0X2	T49.0X3	T49.0X4	T49.0X5	T49.0X6
Melanizing agents	T49.3X1	T49.3X2	T49.3X3	T49.3X4	T49.3X5	T49.3X6
Melanocyte-stimulating hormone	T38.891	T38.892	T38.893	T38.894	T38.895	T38.896
Melarsonyl potassium	T37.3X1	T37.3X2	T37.3X3	T37.3X4	T37.3X5	T37.3X6
Melarsoprol	T37.3X1	T37.3X2	T37.3X3	T37.3X4	T37.3X5	T37.3X6
Melia azedarach	T62.2X1	T62.2X2	T62.2X3	T62.2X4	—	—
Melitracen	T43.011	T43.012	T43.013	T43.014	T43.015	T43.016
Mellaril	T43.3X1	T43.3X2	T43.3X3	T43.3X4	T43.3X5	T43.3X6
Meloxine	T49.3X1	T49.3X2	T49.3X3	T49.3X4	T49.3X5	T49.3X6
Melperone	T43.4X1	T43.4X2	T43.4X3	T43.4X4	T43.4X5	T43.4X6
Melphalan	T45.1X1	T45.1X2	T45.1X3	T45.1X4	T45.1X5	T45.1X6
Memantine	T43.8X1	T43.8X2	T43.8X3	T43.8X4	T43.8X5	T43.8X6

Substance	Poisoning, Accidental (Unintentional)	Poisoning, Intentional Self-Harm	Poisoning, Assault	Poisoning, Undetermined	Adverse Effect	Underdosing
Menadiol	T45.7X1	T45.7X2	T45.7X3	T45.7X4	T45.7X5	T45.7X6
sodium sulfate	T45.7X1	T45.7X2	T45.7X3	T45.7X4	T45.7X5	T45.7X6
Menadione	T45.7X1	T45.7X2	T45.7X3	T45.7X4	T45.7X5	T45.7X6
sodium bisulfite	T45.7X1	T45.7X2	T45.7X3	T45.7X4	T45.7X5	T45.7X6
Menaphthone	T45.7X1	T45.7X2	T45.7X3	T45.7X4	T45.7X5	T45.7X6
Menaquinone	T45.7X1	T45.7X2	T45.7X3	T45.7X4	T45.7X5	T45.7X6
Menatetrenone	T45.7X1	T45.7X2	T45.7X3	T45.7X4	T45.7X5	T45.7X6
Meningococcal vaccine	T5Ø.A91	T5Ø.A92	T5Ø.A93	T5Ø.A94	T5Ø.A95	T5Ø.A96
Menningovax (-AC) (-C)	T5Ø.A91	T5Ø.A92	T5Ø.A93	T5Ø.A94	T5Ø.A95	T5Ø.A96
Menotropins	T38.811	T38.812	T38.813	T38.814	T38.815	T38.816
Menthol	T48.5X1	T48.5X2	T48.5X3	T48.5X4	T48.5X5	T48.5X6
Mepacrine	T37.2X1	T37.2X2	T37.2X3	T37.2X4	T37.2X5	T37.2X6
Meparfynol	T42.6X1	T42.6X2	T42.6X3	T42.6X4	T42.6X5	T42.6X6
Mepartricin	T36.7X1	T36.7X2	T36.7X3	T36.7X4	T36.7X5	T36.7X6
Mepazine	T43.3X1	T43.3X2	T43.3X3	T43.3X4	T43.3X5	T43.3X6
Mepenzolate	T44.3X1	T44.3X2	T44.3X3	T44.3X4	T44.3X5	T44.3X6
bromide	T44.3X1	T44.3X2	T44.3X3	T44.3X4	T44.3X5	T44.3X6
Meperidine	T4Ø.4X1	T4Ø.4X2	T4Ø.4X3	T4Ø.4X4	T4Ø.4X5	T4Ø.4X6
Mephebarbital	T42.3X1	T42.3X2	T42.3X3	T42.3X4	T42.3X5	T42.3X6
Mephenamin(e)	T42.8X1	T42.8X2	T42.8X3	T42.8X4	T42.8X5	T42.8X6
Mephenesin	T42.8X1	T42.8X2	T42.8X3	T42.8X4	T42.8X5	T42.8X6
Mephenhydramine	T45.ØX1	T45.ØX2	T45.ØX3	T45.ØX4	T45.ØX5	T45.ØX6
Mephenoxalone	T42.8X1	T42.8X2	T42.8X3	T42.8X4	T42.8X5	T42.8X6
Mephentermine	T44.991	T44.992	T44.993	T44.994	T44.995	T44.996
Mephenytoin	T42.ØX1	T42.ØX2	T42.ØX3	T42.ØX4	T42.ØX5	T42.ØX6
with phenobarbital	T42.3X1	T42.3X2	T42.3X3	T42.3X4	T42.3X5	T42.3X6
Mephobarbital	T42.3X1	T42.3X2	T42.3X3	T42.3X4	T42.3X5	T42.3X6
Mephosfolan	T6Ø.ØX1	T6Ø.ØX2	T6Ø.ØX3	T6Ø.ØX4	—	—
Mepindolol	T44.7X1	T44.7X2	T44.7X3	T44.7X4	T44.7X5	T44.7X6
Mepiperphenidol	T44.3X1	T44.3X2	T44.3X3	T44.3X4	T44.3X5	T44.3X6
Mepitiostane	T38.7X1	T38.7X2	T38.7X3	T38.7X4	T38.7X5	T38.7X6
Mepivacaine	T41.3X1	T41.3X2	T41.3X3	T41.3X4	T41.3X5	T41.3X6
epidural	T41.3X1	T41.3X2	T41.3X3	T41.3X4	T41.3X5	T41.3X6
Meprednisone	T38.ØX1	T38.ØX2	T38.ØX3	T38.ØX4	T38.ØX5	T38.ØX6
Meprobam	T43.591	T43.592	T43.593	T43.594	T43.595	T43.596
Meprobamate	T43.591	T43.592	T43.593	T43.594	T43.595	T43.596
Meproscillarin	T46.ØX1	T46.ØX2	T46.ØX3	T46.ØX4	T46.ØX5	T46.ØX6
Meprylcaine	T41.3X1	T41.3X2	T41.3X3	T41.3X4	T41.3X5	T41.3X6
Meptazinol	T39.8X1	T39.8X2	T39.8X3	T39.8X4	T39.8X5	T39.8X6
Mepyramine	T45.ØX1	T45.ØX2	T45.ØX3	T45.ØX4	T45.ØX5	T45.ØX6
Mequitazine	T43.3X1	T43.3X2	T43.3X3	T43.3X4	T43.3X5	T43.3X6
Meralluride	T5Ø.2X1	T5Ø.2X2	T5Ø.2X3	T5Ø.2X4	T5Ø.2X5	T5Ø.2X6

Substance	Poisoning, Accidental (Unintentional)	Poisoning, Intentional Self-Harm	Poisoning, Assault	Poisoning, Undetermined	Adverse Effect	Underdosing
Merbaphen	T5Ø.2X1	T5Ø.2X2	T5Ø.2X3	T5Ø.2X4	T5Ø.2X5	T5Ø.2X6
Merbromin	T49.ØX1	T49.ØX2	T49.ØX3	T49.ØX4	T49.ØX5	T49.ØX6
Mercaptobenzothiazole salts	T49.ØX1	T49.ØX2	T49.ØX3	T49.ØX4	T49.ØX5	T49.ØX6
Mercaptomerin	T5Ø.2X1	T5Ø.2X2	T5Ø.2X3	T5Ø.2X4	T5Ø.2X5	T5Ø.2X6
Mercaptopurine	T45.1X1	T45.1X2	T45.1X3	T45.1X4	T45.1X5	T45.1X6
Mercumatilin	T5Ø.2X1	T5Ø.2X2	T5Ø.2X3	T5Ø.2X4	T5Ø.2X5	T5Ø.2X6
Mercuramide	T5Ø.2X1	T5Ø.2X2	T5Ø.2X3	T5Ø.2X4	T5Ø.2X5	T5Ø.2X6
Mercurochrome	T49.ØX1	T49.ØX2	T49.ØX3	T49.ØX4	T49.ØX5	T49.ØX6
Mercurophylline	T5Ø.2X1	T5Ø.2X2	T5Ø.2X3	T5Ø.2X4	T5Ø.2X5	T5Ø.2X6
Mercury, mercurial, mercuric, mercurous (compounds) (cyanide) (fumes) (nonmedicinal) (vapor) NEC	T56.1X1	T56.1X2	T56.1X3	T56.1X4	—	—
ammoniated	T49.ØX1	T49.ØX2	T49.ØX3	T49.ØX4	T49.ØX5	T49.ØX6
anti-infective						
local	T49.ØX1	T49.ØX2	T49.ØX3	T49.ØX4	T49.ØX5	T49.ØX6
systemic	T37.8X1	T37.8X2	T37.8X3	T37.8X4	T37.8X5	T37.8X6
topical	T49.ØX1	T49.ØX2	T49.ØX3	T49.ØX4	T49.ØX5	T49.ØX6
chloride (ammoniated)	T49.ØX1	T49.ØX2	T49.ØX3	T49.ØX4	T49.ØX5	T49.ØX6
fungicide	T56.1X1	T56.1X2	T56.1X3	T56.1X4	—	—
diuretic NEC	T5Ø.2X1	T5Ø.2X2	T5Ø.2X3	T5Ø.2X4	T5Ø.2X5	T5Ø.2X6
fungicide	T56.1X1	T56.1X2	T56.1X3	T56.1X4	—	—
organic (fungicide)	T56.1X1	T56.1X2	T56.1X3	T56.1X4	—	—
oxide, yellow	T49.ØX1	T49.ØX2	T49.ØX3	T49.ØX4	T49.ØX5	T49.ØX6
Mersalyl	T5Ø.2X1	T5Ø.2X2	T5Ø.2X3	T5Ø.2X4	T5Ø.2X5	T5Ø.2X6
Merthiolate	T49.ØX1	T49.ØX2	T49.ØX3	T49.ØX4	T49.ØX5	T49.ØX6
ophthalmic preparation	T49.5X1	T49.5X2	T49.5X3	T49.5X4	T49.5X5	T49.5X6
Meruvax	T5Ø.B91	T5Ø.B92	T5Ø.B93	T5Ø.B94	T5Ø.B95	T5Ø.B96
Mesalazine	T47.8X1	T47.8X2	T47.8X3	T47.8X4	T47.8X5	T47.8X6
Mescal buttons	T4Ø.991	T4Ø.992	T4Ø.993	T4Ø.994	—	—
Mescaline	T4Ø.991	T4Ø.992	T4Ø.993	T4Ø.994	—	—
Mesna	T48.4X1	T48.4X2	T48.4X3	T48.4X4	T48.4X5	T48.4X6
Mesoglycan	T46.6X1	T46.6X2	T46.6X3	T46.6X4	T46.6X5	T46.6X6
Mesoridazine	T43.3X1	T43.3X2	T43.3X3	T43.3X4	T43.3X5	T43.3X6
Mestanolone	T38.7X1	T38.7X2	T38.7X3	T38.7X4	T38.7X5	T38.7X6
Mesterolone	T38.7X1	T38.7X2	T38.7X3	T38.7X4	T38.7X5	T38.7X6
Mestranol	T38.5X1	T38.5X2	T38.5X3	T38.5X4	T38.5X5	T38.5X6
Mesulergine	T42.8X1	T42.8X2	T42.8X3	T42.8X4	T42.8X5	T42.8X6
Mesulfen	T49.ØX1	T49.ØX2	T49.ØX3	T49.ØX4	T49.ØX5	T49.ØX6
Mesuximide	T42.2X1	T42.2X2	T42.2X3	T42.2X4	T42.2X5	T42.2X6
Metabutethamine	T41.3X1	T41.3X2	T41.3X3	T41.3X4	T41.3X5	T41.3X6
Metactesylacetate	T49.ØX1	T49.ØX2	T49.ØX3	T49.ØX4	T49.ØX5	T49.ØX6

Substance	Poisoning, Accidental (Unintentional)	Poisoning, Intentional Self-Harm	Poisoning, Assault	Poisoning, Undetermined	Adverse Effect	Underdosing
Metacycline	T36.4X1	T36.4X2	T36.4X3	T36.4X4	T36.4X5	T36.4X6
Metaldehyde (snail killer) NEC	T6Ø.8X1	T6Ø.8X2	T6Ø.8X3	T6Ø.8X4	—	—
Metals (heavy) (nonmedicinal)	T56.91	T56.92	T56.93	T56.94	—	—
dust, fumes, or vapor NEC	T56.91	T56.92	T56.93	T56.94	—	—
light NEC	T56.91	T56.92	T56.93	T56.94	—	—
dust, fumes, or vapor NEC	T56.91	T56.92	T56.93	T56.94	—	—
specified NEC	T56.891	T56.892	T56.893	T56.894	—	—
thallium	T56.811	T56.812	T56.813	T56.814	—	—
Metamfetamine	T43.621	T43.622	T43.623	T43.624	T43.625	T43.626
Metamizole sodium	T39.2X1	T39.2X2	T39.2X3	T39.2X4	T39.2X5	T39.2X6
Metampicillin	T36.ØX1	T36.ØX2	T36.ØX3	T36.ØX4	T36.ØX5	T36.ØX6
Metamucil	T47.4X1	T47.4X2	T47.4X3	T47.4X4	T47.4X5	T47.4X6
Metaphen	T49.ØX1	T49.ØX2	T49.ØX3	T49.ØX4	T49.ØX5	T49.ØX6
Metandienone	T38.7X1	T38.7X2	T38.7X3	T38.7X4	T38.7X5	T38.7X6
Metandrostenolone	T38.7X1	T38.7X2	T38.7X3	T38.7X4	T38.7X5	T38.7X6
Metaphos	T6Ø.ØX1	T6Ø.ØX2	T6Ø.ØX3	T6Ø.ØX4	—	—
Metapramine	T43.Ø11	T43.Ø12	T43.Ø13	T43.Ø14	T43.Ø15	T43.Ø16
Metaproterenol	T48.291	T48.292	T48.293	T48.294	T48.295	T48.296
Metaraminol	T44.4X1	T44.4X2	T44.4X3	T44.4X4	T44.4X5	T44.4X6
Metaxalone	T42.8X1	T42.8X2	T42.8X3	T42.8X4	T42.8X5	T42.8X6
Metenolone	T38.7X1	T38.7X2	T38.7X3	T38.7X4	T38.7X5	T38.7X6
Metergoline	T42.8X1	T42.8X2	T42.8X3	T42.8X4	T42.8X5	T42.8X6
Metescufylline	T46.991	T46.992	T46.993	T46.994	T46.995	T46.996
Metetoin	T42.ØX1	T42.ØX2	T42.ØX3	T42.ØX4	T42.ØX5	T42.ØX6
Metformin	T38.3X1	T38.3X2	T38.3X3	T38.3X4	T38.3X5	T38.3X6
Methacholine	T44.1X1	T44.1X2	T44.1X3	T44.1X4	T44.1X5	T44.1X6
Methacycline	T36.4X1	T36.4X2	T36.4X3	T36.4X4	T36.4X5	T36.4X6
Methadone	T4Ø.3X1	T4Ø.3X2	T4Ø.3X3	T4Ø.3X4	T4Ø.3X5	T4Ø.3X6
Methallenestril	T38.5X1	T38.5X2	T38.5X3	T38.5X4	T38.5X5	T38.5X6
Methallenoestril	T38.5X1	T38.5X2	T38.5X3	T38.5X4	T38.5X5	T38.5X6
Methamphetamine	T43.621	T43.622	T43.623	T43.624	T43.625	T43.626
Methampyrone	T39.2X1	T39.2X2	T39.2X3	T39.2X4	T39.2X5	T39.2X6
Methandienone	T38.7X1	T38.7X2	T38.7X3	T38.7X4	T38.7X5	T38.7X6
Methandriol	T38.7X1	T38.7X2	T38.7X3	T38.7X4	T38.7X5	T38.7X6
Methandrostenolone	T38.7X1	T38.7X2	T38.7X3	T38.7X4	T38.7X5	T38.7X6
Methane	T59.891	T59.892	T59.893	T59.894	—	—
Methanethiol	T59.891	T59.892	T59.893	T59.894	—	—
Methaniazide	T37.1X1	T37.1X2	T37.1X3	T37.1X4	T37.1X5	T37.1X6
Methanol (vapor)	T51.1X1	T51.1X2	T51.1X3	T51.1X4	—	—
Methantheline	T44.3X1	T44.3X2	T44.3X3	T44.3X4	T44.3X5	T44.3X6
Methanthelinium bromide	T44.3X1	T44.3X2	T44.3X3	T44.3X4	T44.3X5	T44.3X6
Methaphenilene	T45.ØX1	T45.ØX2	T45.ØX3	T45.ØX4	T45.ØX5	T45.ØX6

Substance	Poisoning, Accidental (Unintentional)	Poisoning, Intentional Self-Harm	Poisoning, Assault	Poisoning, Undetermined	Adverse Effect	Underdosing
Methapyrilene	T45.ØX1	T45.ØX2	T45.ØX3	T45.ØX4	T45.ØX5	T45.ØX6
Methaqualone (compound)	T42.6X1	T42.6X2	T42.6X3	T42.6X4	T42.6X5	T42.6X6
Metharbital	T42.3X1	T42.3X2	T42.3X3	T42.3X4	T42.3X5	T42.3X6
Methazolamide	T5Ø.2X1	T5Ø.2X2	T5Ø.2X3	T5Ø.2X4	T5Ø.2X5	T5Ø.2X6
Methdilazine	T43.3X1	T43.3X2	T43.3X3	T43.3X4	T43.3X5	T43.3X6
Methedrine	T43.621	T43.622	T43.623	T43.624	T43.625	T43.626
Methenamine (mandelate)	T37.8X1	T37.8X2	T37.8X3	T37.8X4	T37.8X5	T37.8X6
Methenolone	T38.7X1	T38.7X2	T38.7X3	T38.7X4	T38.7X5	T38.7X6
Methergine	T48.ØX1	T48.ØX2	T48.ØX3	T48.ØX4	T48.ØX5	T48.ØX6
Methetoin	T42.ØX1	T42.ØX2	T42.ØX3	T42.ØX4	T42.ØX5	T42.ØX6
Methiacil	T38.2X1	T38.2X2	T38.2X3	T38.2X4	T38.2X5	T38.2X6
Methicillin	T36.ØX1	T36.ØX2	T36.ØX3	T36.ØX4	T36.ØX5	T36.ØX6
Methimazole	T38.2X1	T38.2X2	T38.2X3	T38.2X4	T38.2X5	T38.2X6
Methiodal sodium	T5Ø.8X1	T5Ø.8X2	T5Ø.8X3	T5Ø.8X4	T5Ø.8X5	T5Ø.8X6
Methionine	T5Ø.991	T5Ø.992	T5Ø.993	T5Ø.994	T5Ø.995	T5Ø.996
Methisazone	T37.5X1	T37.5X2	T37.5X3	T37.5X4	T37.5X5	T37.5X6
Methisoprinol	T37.5X1	T37.5X2	T37.5X3	T37.5X4	T37.5X5	T37.5X6
Methitural	T42.3X1	T42.3X2	T42.3X3	T42.3X4	T42.3X5	T42.3X6
Methixene	T44.3X1	T44.3X2	T44.3X3	T44.3X4	T44.3X5	T44.3X6
Methobarbital, methobarbitone	T42.3X1	T42.3X2	T42.3X3	T42.3X4	T42.3X5	T42.3X6
Methocarbamol	T42.8X1	T42.8X2	T42.8X3	T42.8X4	T42.8X5	T42.8X6
skeletal muscle relaxant	T48.1X1	T48.1X2	T48.1X3	T48.1X4	T48.1X5	T48.1X6
Methohexital	T41.1X1	T41.1X2	T41.1X3	T41.1X4	T41.1X5	T41.1X6
Methohexitone	T41.1X1	T41.1X2	T41.1X3	T41.1X4	T41.1X5	T41.1X6
Methoin	T42.ØX1	T42.ØX2	T42.ØX3	T42.ØX4	T42.ØX5	T42.ØX6
Methopholine	T39.8X1	T39.8X2	T39.8X3	T39.8X4	T39.8X5	T39.8X6
Methopromazine	T43.3X1	T43.3X2	T43.3X3	T43.3X4	T43.3X5	T43.3X6
Methorate	T48.3X1	T48.3X2	T48.3X3	T48.3X4	T48.3X5	T48.3X6
Methoserpidine	T46.5X1	T46.5X2	T46.5X3	T46.5X4	T46.5X5	T46.5X6
Methotrexate	T45.1X1	T45.1X2	T45.1X3	T45.1X4	T45.1X5	T45.1X6
Methotrimeprazine	T43.3X1	T43.3X2	T43.3X3	T43.3X4	T43.3X5	T43.3X6
Methoxa-Dome	T49.3X1	T49.3X2	T49.3X3	T49.3X4	T49.3X5	T49.3X6
Methoxamine	T44.4X1	T44.4X2	T44.4X3	T44.4X4	T44.4X5	T44.4X6
Methoxsalen	T5Ø.991	T5Ø.992	T5Ø.993	T5Ø.994	T5Ø.995	T5Ø.996
Methoxyaniline	T65.3X1	T65.3X2	T65.3X3	T65.3X4	—	—
Methoxybenzyl penicillin	T36.ØX1	T36.ØX2	T36.ØX3	T36.ØX4	T36.ØX5	T36.ØX6
Methoxychlor	T53.7X1	T53.7X2	T53.7X3	T53.7X4	—	—
Methoxy-DDT	T53.7X1	T53.7X2	T53.7X3	T53.7X4	—	—
2-Methoxyethanol	T52.3X1	T52.3X2	T52.3X3	T52.3X4	—	—
Methoxyflurane	T41.ØX1	T41.ØX2	T41.ØX3	T41.ØX4	T41.ØX5	T41.ØX6
Methoxyphenamine	T48.6X1	T48.6X2	T48.6X3	T48.6X4	T48.6X5	T48.6X6
Methoxypromazine	T43.3X1	T43.3X2	T43.3X3	T43.3X4	T43.3X5	T43.3X6

Substance	Poisoning, Accidental (Unintentional)	Poisoning, Intentional Self-Harm	Poisoning, Assault	Poisoning, Undetermined	Adverse Effect	Underdosing
5-Methoxypsoralen (5-MOP)	T50.991	T50.992	T50.993	T50.994	T50.995	T50.996
8-Methoxypsoralen (8-MOP)	T50.991	T50.992	T50.993	T50.994	T50.995	T50.996
Methscopolamine bromide	T44.3X1	T44.3X2	T44.3X3	T44.3X4	T44.3X5	T44.3X6
Methsuximide	T42.2X1	T42.2X2	T42.2X3	T42.2X4	T42.2X5	T42.2X6
Methyclothiazide	T50.2X1	T50.2X2	T50.2X3	T50.2X4	T50.2X5	T50.2X6
Methyl						
acetate	T52.4X1	T52.4X2	T52.4X3	T52.4X4	—	—
acetone	T52.4X1	T52.4X2	T52.4X3	T52.4X4	—	—
acrylate	T65.891	T65.892	T65.893	T65.894	—	—
alcohol	T51.1X1	T51.1X2	T51.1X3	T51.1X4	—	—
aminophenol	T65.3X1	T65.3X2	T65.3X3	T65.3X4	—	—
amphetamine	T43.621	T43.622	T43.623	T43.624	T43.625	T43.626
androstanolone	T38.7X1	T38.7X2	T38.7X3	T38.7X4	T38.7X5	T38.7X6
atropine	T44.3X1	T44.3X2	T44.3X3	T44.3X4	T44.3X5	T44.3X6
benzene	T52.2X1	T52.2X2	T52.2X3	T52.2X4	—	—
benzoate	T52.8X1	T52.8X2	T52.8X3	T52.8X4	—	—
benzol	T52.2X1	T52.2X2	T52.2X3	T52.2X4	—	—
bromide (gas)	T59.891	T59.892	T59.893	T59.894	—	—
fumigant	T60.8X1	T60.8X2	T60.8X3	T60.8X4	—	—
butanol	T51.3X1	T51.3X2	T51.3X3	T51.3X4	—	—
carbinol	T51.1X1	T51.1X2	T51.1X3	T51.1X4	—	—
carbonate	T52.8X1	T52.8X2	T52.8X3	T52.8X4	—	—
CCNU	T45.1X1	T45.1X2	T45.1X3	T45.1X4	T45.1X5	T45.1X6
cellosolve	T52.91	T52.92	T52.93	T52.94	—	—
cellulose	T47.4X1	T47.4X2	T47.4X3	T47.4X4	T47.4X5	T47.4X6
chloride (gas)	T59.891	T59.892	T59.893	T59.894	—	—
chloroformate	T59.3X1	T59.3X2	T59.3X3	T59.3X4	—	—
cyclohexane	T52.8X1	T52.8X2	T52.8X3	T52.8X4	—	—
cyclohexanol	T51.8X1	T51.8X2	T51.8X3	T51.8X4	—	—
cyclohexanone	T52.8X1	T52.8X2	T52.8X3	T52.8X4	—	—
cyclohexyl acetate	T52.8X1	T52.8X2	T52.8X3	T52.8X4	—	—
demeton	T60.0X1	T60.0X2	T60.0X3	T60.0X4	—	—
dihydromorphinone	T40.2X1	T40.2X2	T40.2X3	T40.2X4	T40.2X5	T40.2X6
ergometrine	T48.0X1	T48.0X2	T48.0X3	T48.0X4	T48.0X5	T48.0X6
ergonovine	T48.0X1	T48.0X2	T48.0X3	T48.0X4	T48.0X5	T48.0X6
ethyl ketone	T52.4X1	T52.4X2	T52.4X3	T52.4X4	—	—
glucamine antimonate	T37.8X1	T37.8X2	T37.8X3	T37.8X4	T37.8X5	T37.8X6
hydrazine	T65.891	T65.892	T65.893	T65.894	—	—
iodide	T65.891	T65.892	T65.893	T65.894	—	—
isobutyl ketone	T52.4X1	T52.4X2	T52.4X3	T52.4X4	—	—
isothiocyanate	T60.3X1	T60.3X2	T60.3X3	T60.3X4	—	—
mercaptan	T59.891	T59.892	T59.893	T59.894	—	—
Methyl *(Continued)*						
morphine NEC	T40.2X1	T40.2X2	T40.2X3	T40.2X4	T40.2X5	T40.2X6
nicotinate	T49.4X1	T49.4X2	T49.4X3	T49.4X4	T49.4X5	T49.4X6
paraben	T49.0X1	T49.0X2	T49.0X3	T49.0X4	T49.0X5	T49.0X6
parafynol	T42.6X1	T42.6X2	T42.6X3	T42.6X4	T42.6X5	T42.6X6
parathion	T60.0X1	T60.0X2	T60.0X3	T60.0X4	—	—
peridol	T43.4X1	T43.4X2	T43.4X3	T43.4X4	T43.4X5	T43.4X6
phenidate	T43.631	T43.632	T43.633	T43.634	T43.635	T43.636
prednisolone	T38.0X1	T38.0X2	T38.0X3	T38.0X4	T38.0X5	T38.0X6
ENT agent	T49.6X1	T49.6X2	T49.6X3	T49.6X4	T49.6X5	T49.6X6
ophthalmic preparation	T49.5X1	T49.5X2	T49.5X3	T49.5X4	T49.5X5	T49.5X6
topical NEC	T49.0X1	T49.0X2	T49.0X3	T49.0X4	T49.0X5	T49.0X6
propylcarbinol	T51.3X1	T51.3X2	T51.3X3	T51.3X4	—	—
rosaniline NEC	T49.0X1	T49.0X2	T49.0X3	T49.0X4	T49.0X5	T49.0X6
salicylate	T49.2X1	T49.2X2	T49.2X3	T49.2X4	T49.2X5	T49.2X6
sulfate (fumes)	T59.891	T59.892	T59.893	T59.894	—	—
liquid	T52.8X1	T52.8X2	T52.8X3	T52.8X4	—	—
sulfonal	T42.6X1	T42.6X2	T42.6X3	T42.6X4	T42.6X5	T42.6X6
testosterone	T38.7X1	T38.7X2	T38.7X3	T38.7X4	T38.7X5	T38.7X6
thiouracil	T38.2X1	T38.2X2	T38.2X3	T38.2X4	T38.2X5	T38.2X6
Methylamphetamine	T43.621	T43.622	T43.623	T43.624	T43.625	T43.626
Methylated spirit	T51.1X1	T51.1X2	T51.1X3	T51.1X4	—	—
Methylatropine nitrate	T44.3X1	T44.3X2	T44.3X3	T44.3X4	T44.3X5	T44.3X6
Methylbenactyzium bromide	T44.3X1	T44.3X2	T44.3X3	T44.3X4	T44.3X5	T44.3X6
Methylbenzethonium chloride	T49.0X1	T49.0X2	T49.0X3	T49.0X4	T49.0X5	T49.0X6
Methylcellulose	T47.4X1	T47.4X2	T47.4X3	T47.4X4	T47.4X5	T47.4X6
laxative	T47.4X1	T47.4X2	T47.4X3	T47.4X4	T47.4X5	T47.4X6
Methylchlorophenoxy-acetic acid	T60.3X1	T60.3X2	T60.3X3	T60.3X4	—	—
Methyldopa	T46.5X1	T46.5X2	T46.5X3	T46.5X4	T46.5X5	T46.5X6
Methyldopate	T46.5X1	T46.5X2	T46.5X3	T46.5X4	T46.5X5	T46.5X6
Methylene						
blue	T50.6X1	T50.6X2	T50.6X3	T50.6X4	T50.6X5	T50.6X6
chloride or dichloride (solvent) NEC	T53.4X1	T53.4X2	T53.4X3	T53.4X4	—	—
Methylenedioxyamphet-amine	T43.621	T43.622	T43.623	T43.624	T43.625	T43.626
Methylenedioxymethamphetamine	T43.621	T43.622	T43.623	T43.624	T43.625	T43.626
Methylergometrine	T48.0X1	T48.0X2	T48.0X3	T48.0X4	T48.0X5	T48.0X6
Methylergonovine	T48.0X1	T48.0X2	T48.0X3	T48.0X4	T48.0X5	T48.0X6
Methylestrenolone	T38.5X1	T38.5X2	T38.5X3	T38.5X4	T38.5X5	T38.5X6
Methylethyl cellulose	T50.991	T50.992	T50.993	T50.994	T50.995	T50.996
Methylhexabital	T42.3X1	T42.3X2	T42.3X3	T42.3X4	T42.3X5	T42.3X6
Methylmorphine	T40.2X1	T40.2X2	T40.2X3	T40.2X4	T40.2X5	T40.2X6

Substance	Poisoning, Accidental (Unintentional)	Poisoning, Intentional Self-Harm	Poisoning, Assault	Poisoning, Undetermined	Adverse Effect	Underdosing
Methylparaben (ophthalmic)	T49.5X1	T49.5X2	T49.5X3	T49.5X4	T49.5X5	T49.5X6
Methylparafynol	T42.6X1	T42.6X2	T42.6X3	T42.6X4	T42.6X5	T42.6X6
Methylpentynol, methylpenthynol	T42.6X1	T42.6X2	T42.6X3	T42.6X4	T42.6X5	T42.6X6
Methylphenidate	T43.631	T43.632	T43.633	T43.634	T43.635	T43.636
Methylphenobarbital	T42.3X1	T42.3X2	T42.3X3	T42.3X4	T42.3X5	T42.3X6
Methylpolysiloxane	T47.1X1	T47.1X2	T47.1X3	T47.1X4	T47.1X5	T47.1X6
Methylprednisolone — *see Methyl, prednisolone*						
Methylrosaniline	T49.0X1	T49.0X2	T49.0X3	T49.0X4	T49.0X5	T49.0X6
Methylrosanilinium chloride	T49.0X1	T49.0X2	T49.0X3	T49.0X4	T49.0X5	T49.0X6
Methyltestosterone	T38.7X1	T38.7X2	T38.7X3	T38.7X4	T38.7X5	T38.7X6
Methylthionine chloride	T50.6X1	T50.6X2	T50.6X3	T50.6X4	T50.6X5	T50.6X6
Methylthioninium chloride	T50.6X1	T50.6X2	T50.6X3	T50.6X4	T50.6X5	T50.6X6
Methylthiouracil	T38.2X1	T38.2X2	T38.2X3	T38.2X4	T38.2X5	T38.2X6
Methyprylon	T42.6X1	T42.6X2	T42.6X3	T42.6X4	T42.6X5	T42.6X6
Methysergide	T46.5X1	T46.5X2	T46.5X3	T46.5X4	T46.5X5	T46.5X6
Metiamide	T47.1X1	T47.1X2	T47.1X3	T47.1X4	T47.1X5	T47.1X6
Meticillin	T36.0X1	T36.0X2	T36.0X3	T36.0X4	T36.0X5	T36.0X6
Meticrane	T50.2X1	T50.2X2	T50.2X3	T50.2X4	T50.2X5	T50.2X6
Metildigoxin	T46.0X1	T46.0X2	T46.0X3	T46.0X4	T46.0X5	T46.0X6
Metipranolol	T49.5X1	T49.5X2	T49.5X3	T49.5X4	T49.5X5	T49.5X6
Metirosine	T46.5X1	T46.5X2	T46.5X3	T46.5X4	T46.5X5	T46.5X6
Metisazone	T37.5X1	T37.5X2	T37.5X3	T37.5X4	T37.5X5	T37.5X6
Metixene	T44.3X1	T44.3X2	T44.3X3	T44.3X4	T44.3X5	T44.3X6
Metizoline	T48.5X1	T48.5X2	T48.5X3	T48.5X4	T48.5X5	T48.5X6
Metoclopramide	T45.0X1	T45.0X2	T45.0X3	T45.0X4	T45.0X5	T45.0X6
Metofenazate	T43.3X1	T43.3X2	T43.3X3	T43.3X4	T43.3X5	T43.3X6
Metofoline	T39.8X1	T39.8X2	T39.8X3	T39.8X4	T39.8X5	T39.8X6
Metolazone	T50.2X1	T50.2X2	T50.2X3	T50.2X4	T50.2X5	T50.2X6
Metopon	T40.2X1	T40.2X2	T40.2X3	T40.2X4	T40.2X5	T40.2X6
Metoprine	T45.1X1	T45.1X2	T45.1X3	T45.1X4	T45.1X5	T45.1X6
Metoprolol	T44.7X1	T44.7X2	T44.7X3	T44.7X4	T44.7X5	T44.7X6
Metrifonate	T60.0X1	T60.0X2	T60.0X3	T60.0X4	—	—
Metrizamide	T50.8X1	T50.8X2	T50.8X3	T50.8X4	T50.8X5	T50.8X6
Metrizoic acid	T50.8X1	T50.8X2	T50.8X3	T50.8X4	T50.8X5	T50.8X6
Metronidazole	T37.8X1	T37.8X2	T37.8X3	T37.8X4	T37.8X5	T37.8X6
Metycaine	T41.3X1	T41.3X2	T41.3X3	T41.3X4	T41.3X5	T41.3X6
infiltration (subcutaneous)	T41.3X1	T41.3X2	T41.3X3	T41.3X4	T41.3X5	T41.3X6
nerve block (peripheral) (plexus)	T41.3X1	T41.3X2	T41.3X3	T41.3X4	T41.3X5	T41.3X6
topical (surface)	T41.3X1	T41.3X2	T41.3X3	T41.3X4	T41.3X5	T41.3X6
Metyrapone	T50.8X1	T50.8X2	T50.8X3	T50.8X4	T50.8X5	T50.8X6
Mevinphos	T60.0X1	T60.0X2	T60.0X3	T60.0X4	—	—

Substance	Poisoning, Accidental (Unintentional)	Poisoning, Intentional Self-Harm	Poisoning, Assault	Poisoning, Undetermined	Adverse Effect	Underdosing
Mexazolam	T42.4X1	T42.4X2	T42.4X3	T42.4X4	T42.4X5	T42.4X6
Mexenone	T49.3X1	T49.3X2	T49.3X3	T49.3X4	T49.3X5	T49.3X6
Mexiletine	T46.2X1	T46.2X2	T46.2X3	T46.2X4	T46.2X5	T46.2X6
Mezereon	T62.2X1	T62.2X2	T62.2X3	T62.2X4	—	—
berries	T62.1X1	T62.1X2	T62.1X3	T62.1X4	—	—
Mezlocillin	T36.0X1	T36.0X2	T36.0X3	T36.0X4	T36.0X5	T36.0X6
Mianserin	T43.021	T43.022	T43.023	T43.024	T43.025	T43.026
Micatin	T49.0X1	T49.0X2	T49.0X3	T49.0X4	T49.0X5	T49.0X6
Miconazole	T49.0X1	T49.0X2	T49.0X3	T49.0X4	T49.0X5	T49.0X6
Micronomicin	T36.5X1	T36.5X2	T36.5X3	T36.5X4	T36.5X5	T36.5X6
Midazolam	T42.4X1	T42.4X2	T42.4X3	T42.4X4	T42.4X5	T42.4X6
Midecamycin	T36.3X1	T36.3X2	T36.3X3	T36.3X4	T36.3X5	T36.3X6
Mifepristone	T38.6X1	T38.6X2	T38.6X3	T38.6X4	T38.6X5	T38.6X6
Milk of magnesia	T47.1X1	T47.1X2	T47.1X3	T47.1X4	T47.1X5	T47.1X6
Millipede (tropical) (venomous)	T63.411	T63.412	T63.413	T63.414	—	—
Miltown	T43.591	T43.592	T43.593	T43.594	T43.595	T43.596
Milverine	T44.3X1	T44.3X2	T44.3X3	T44.3X4	T44.3X5	T44.3X6
Minaprine	T43.291	T43.292	T43.293	T43.294	T43.295	T43.296
Minaxolone	T41.291	T41.292	T41.293	T41.294	T41.295	T41.296
Mineral						
acids	T54.2X1	T54.2X2	T54.2X3	T54.2X4	—	—
oil (laxative) (medicinal)	T47.4X1	T47.4X2	T47.4X3	T47.4X4	T47.4X5	T47.4X6
emulsion	T47.2X1	T47.2X2	T47.2X3	T47.2X4	T47.2X5	T47.2X6
nonmedicinal	T52.0X1	T52.0X2	T52.0X3	T52.0X4	—	—
topical	T49.3X1	T49.3X2	T49.3X3	T49.3X4	T49.3X5	T49.3X6
salt NEC	T50.3X1	T50.3X2	T50.3X3	T50.3X4	T50.3X5	T50.3X6
spirits	T52.0X1	T52.0X2	T52.0X3	T52.0X4	—	—
Mineralocorticosteroid	T50.0X1	T50.0X2	T50.0X3	T50.0X4	T50.0X5	T50.0X6
Minocycline	T36.4X1	T36.4X2	T36.4X3	T36.4X4	T36.4X5	T36.4X6
Minoxidil	T46.7X1	T46.7X2	T46.7X3	T46.7X4	T46.7X5	T46.7X6
Miokamycin	T36.3X1	T36.3X2	T36.3X3	T36.3X4	T36.3X5	T36.3X6
Miotic drug	T49.5X1	T49.5X2	T49.5X3	T49.5X4	T49.5X5	T49.5X6
Mipafox	T60.0X1	T60.0X2	T60.0X3	T60.0X4	—	—
Mirex	T60.1X1	T60.1X2	T60.1X3	T60.1X4	—	—
Mirtazapine	T43.021	T43.022	T43.023	T43.024	T43.025	T43.026
Misonidazole	T37.3X1	T37.3X2	T37.3X3	T37.3X4	T37.3X5	T37.3X6
Misoprostol	T47.1X1	T47.1X2	T47.1X3	T47.1X4	T47.1X5	T47.1X6
Mithramycin	T45.1X1	T45.1X2	T45.1X3	T45.1X4	T45.1X5	T45.1X6
Mitobronitol	T45.1X1	T45.1X2	T45.1X3	T45.1X4	T45.1X5	T45.1X6
Mitoguazone	T45.1X1	T45.1X2	T45.1X3	T45.1X4	T45.1X5	T45.1X6
Mitolactol	T45.1X1	T45.1X2	T45.1X3	T45.1X4	T45.1X5	T45.1X6
Mitomycin	T45.1X1	T45.1X2	T45.1X3	T45.1X4	T45.1X5	T45.1X6

Substance	Poisoning, Accidental (Unintentional)	Poisoning, Intentional Self-Harm	Poisoning, Assault	Poisoning, Undetermined	Adverse Effect	Underdosing
Mitopodozide	T45.1X1	T45.1X2	T45.1X3	T45.1X4	T45.1X5	T45.1X6
Mitotane	T45.1X1	T45.1X2	T45.1X3	T45.1X4	T45.1X5	T45.1X6
Mitoxantrone	T45.1X1	T45.1X2	T45.1X3	T45.1X4	T45.1X5	T45.1X6
Mivacurium chloride	T48.1X1	T48.1X2	T48.1X3	T48.1X4	T48.1X5	T48.1X6
Miyari bacteria	T47.6X1	T47.6X2	T47.6X3	T47.6X4	T47.6X5	T47.6X6
Moclobemide	T43.1X1	T43.1X2	T43.1X3	T43.1X4	T43.1X5	T43.1X6
Moderil	T46.5X1	T46.5X2	T46.5X3	T46.5X4	T46.5X5	T46.5X6
Mofebutazone	T39.2X1	T39.2X2	T39.2X3	T39.2X4	T39.2X5	T39.2X6
Mogadon — *see Nitrazepam*						
Molindone	T43.591	T43.592	T43.593	T43.594	T43.595	T43.596
Molsidomine	T46.3X1	T46.3X2	T46.3X3	T46.3X4	T46.3X5	T46.3X6
Mometasone	T49.ØX1	T49.ØX2	T49.ØX3	T49.ØX4	T49.ØX5	T49.ØX6
Monistat	T49.ØX1	T49.ØX2	T49.ØX3	T49.ØX4	T49.ØX5	T49.ØX6
Monkshood	T62.2X1	T62.2X2	T62.2X3	T62.2X4	—	—
Monoamine oxidase inhibitor NEC	T43.1X1	T43.1X2	T43.1X3	T43.1X4	T43.1X5	T43.1X6
hydrazine	T43.1X1	T43.1X2	T43.1X3	T43.1X4	T43.1X5	T43.1X6
Monobenzone	T49.4X1	T49.4X2	T49.4X3	T49.4X4	T49.4X5	T49.4X6
Monochloroacetic acid	T6Ø.3X1	T6Ø.3X2	T6Ø.3X3	T6Ø.3X4	—	—
Monochlorobenzene	T53.7X1	T53.7X2	T53.7X3	T53.7X4	—	—
Monoethanolamine	T46.8X1	T46.8X2	T46.8X3	T46.8X4	T46.8X5	T46.8X6
oleate	T46.8X1	T46.8X2	T46.8X3	T46.8X4	T46.8X5	T46.8X6
Monooctanoin	T5Ø.991	T5Ø.992	T5Ø.993	T5Ø.994	T5Ø.995	T5Ø.996
Monophenylbutazone	T39.2X1	T39.2X2	T39.2X3	T39.2X4	T39.2X5	T39.2X6
Monosodium glutamate	T65.891	T65.892	T65.893	T65.894	—	—
Monosulfiram	T49.ØX1	T49.ØX2	T49.ØX3	T49.ØX4	T49.ØX5	T49.ØX6
Monoxide, carbon — *see Carbon, monoxide*	T57.91	T57.92	T57.93	T57.94	—	—
Monoxidine hydrochloride	T46.1X1	T46.1X2	T46.1X3	T46.1X4	T46.1X5	T46.1X6
Monuron	T6Ø.3X1	T6Ø.3X2	T6Ø.3X3	T6Ø.3X4	—	—
Moperone	T43.4X1	T43.4X2	T43.4X3	T43.4X4	T43.4X5	T43.4X6
Mopidamol	T45.1X1	T45.1X2	T45.1X3	T45.1X4	T45.1X5	T45.1X6
MOPP (mechlorethamine + vincristine + prednisone + procarbazine)	T45.1X1	T45.1X2	T45.1X3	T45.1X4	T45.1X5	T45.1X6
Morfin	T4Ø.2X1	T4Ø.2X2	T4Ø.2X3	T4Ø.2X4	T4Ø.2X5	T4Ø.2X6
Morinamide	T37.1X1	T37.1X2	T37.1X3	T37.1X4	T37.1X5	T37.1X6
Morning glory seeds	T4Ø.991	T4Ø.992	T4Ø.993	T4Ø.994	—	—
Moroxydine	T37.5X1	T37.5X2	T37.5X3	T37.5X4	T37.5X5	T37.5X6
Morphazinamide	T37.1X1	T37.1X2	T37.1X3	T37.1X4	T37.1X5	T37.1X6
Morphine	T4Ø.2X1	T4Ø.2X2	T4Ø.2X3	T4Ø.2X4	T4Ø.2X5	T4Ø.2X6
antagonist	T5Ø.7X1	T5Ø.7X2	T5Ø.7X3	T5Ø.7X4	T5Ø.7X5	T5Ø.7X6
Morpholinylethylmorphine	T4Ø.2X1	T4Ø.2X2	T4Ø.2X3	T4Ø.2X4	—	—
Morsuximide	T42.2X1	T42.2X2	T42.2X3	T42.2X4	T42.2X5	T42.2X6
Mosapramine	T43.591	T43.592	T43.593	T43.594	T43.595	T43.596
Moth balls — *see also Pesticides*	T6Ø.2X1	T6Ø.2X2	T6Ø.2X3	T6Ø.2X4	—	—
naphthalene	T6Ø.2X1	T6Ø.2X2	T6Ø.2X3	T6Ø.2X4	—	—
paradichlorobenzene	T6Ø.1X1	T6Ø.1X2	T6Ø.1X3	T6Ø.1X4	—	—
Motor exhaust gas	T58.Ø1	T58.Ø2	T58.Ø3	T58.Ø4	—	—
Mouthwash (antiseptic) (zinc chloride)	T49.6X1	T49.6X2	T49.6X3	T49.6X4	T49.6X5	T49.6X6
Moxastine	T45.ØX1	T45.ØX2	T45.ØX3	T45.ØX4	T45.ØX5	T45.ØX6
Moxaverine	T44.3X1	T44.3X2	T44.3X3	T44.3X4	T44.3X5	T44.3X6
Moxifensine	T43.291	T43.292	T43.293	T43.294	T43.295	T43.296
Moxisylyte	T46.7X1	T46.7X2	T46.7X3	T46.7X4	T46.7X5	T46.7X6
Mucilage, plant	T47.4X1	T47.4X2	T47.4X3	T47.4X4	T47.4X5	T47.4X6
Mucolytic drug	T48.4X1	T48.4X2	T48.4X3	T48.4X4	T48.4X5	T48.4X6
Mucomyst	T48.4X1	T48.4X2	T48.4X3	T48.4X4	T48.4X5	T48.4X6
Mucous membrane agents (external)	T49.91	T49.92	T49.93	T49.94	T49.95	T49.96
specified NEC	T49.8X1	T49.8X2	T49.8X3	T49.8X4	T49.8X5	T49.8X6
Mumps						
immune globulin (human)	T5Ø.Z11	T5Ø.Z12	T5Ø.Z13	T5Ø.Z14	T5Ø.Z15	T5Ø.Z16
skin test antigen	T5Ø.8X1	T5Ø.8X2	T5Ø.8X3	T5Ø.8X4	T5Ø.8X5	T5Ø.8X6
vaccine	T5Ø.B91	T5Ø.B92	T5Ø.B93	T5Ø.B94	T5Ø.B95	T5Ø.B96
Mumpsvax	T5Ø.B91	T5Ø.B92	T5Ø.B93	T5Ø.B94	T5Ø.B95	T5Ø.B96
Mupirocin	T49.ØX1	T49.ØX2	T49.ØX3	T49.ØX4	T49.ØX5	T49.ØX6
Muriatic acid — *see Hydrochloric acid*						
Muromonab-CD3	T45.1X1	T45.1X2	T45.1X3	T45.1X4	T45.1X5	T45.1X6
Muscle relaxant — *see Relaxant, muscle*						
Muscle-action drug NEC	T48.2Ø1	T48.2Ø2	T48.2Ø3	T48.2Ø4	T48.2Ø5	T48.2Ø6
Muscle affecting agents NEC	T48.2Ø1	T48.2Ø2	T48.2Ø3	T48.2Ø4	T48.2Ø5	T48.2Ø6
oxytocic	T48.ØX1	T48.ØX2	T48.ØX3	T48.ØX4	T48.ØX5	T48.ØX6
relaxants	T48.2Ø1	T48.2Ø2	T48.2Ø3	T48.2Ø4	T48.2Ø5	T48.2Ø6
central nervous system	T42.8X1	T42.8X2	T42.8X3	T42.8X4	T42.8X5	T42.8X6
skeletal	T48.1X1	T48.1X2	T48.1X3	T48.1X4	T48.1X5	T48.1X6
smooth	T44.3X1	T44.3X2	T44.3X3	T44.3X4	T44.3X5	T44.3X6
Muscle-tone depressant, central NEC	T42.8X1	T42.8X2	T42.8X3	T42.8X4	T42.8X5	T42.8X6
specified NEC	T42.8X1	T42.8X2	T42.8X3	T42.8X4	T42.8X5	T42.8X6
Mushroom, noxious	T62.ØX1	T62.ØX2	T62.ØX3	T62.ØX4	—	—
Mussel, noxious	T61.781	T61.782	T61.783	T61.784	—	—
Mustard (emetic)	T47.7X1	T47.7X2	T47.7X3	T47.7X4	T47.7X5	T47.7X6
black	T47.7X1	T47.7X2	T47.7X3	T47.7X4	T47.7X5	T47.7X6
gas, not in war	T59.91	T59.92	T59.93	T59.94	—	—
nitrogen	T45.1X1	T45.1X2	T45.1X3	T45.1X4	T45.1X5	T45.1X6

Substance	Poisoning, Accidental (Unintentional)	Poisoning, Intentional Self-Harm	Poisoning, Assault	Poisoning, Undetermined	Adverse Effect	Underdosing
Mustine	T45.1X1	T45.1X2	T45.1X3	T45.1X4	T45.1X5	T45.1X6
M-vac	T45.1X1	T45.1X2	T45.1X3	T45.1X4	T45.1X5	T45.1X6
Mycifradin	T36.5X1	T36.5X2	T36.5X3	T36.5X4	T36.5X5	T36.5X6
topical	T49.ØX1	T49.ØX2	T49.ØX3	T49.ØX4	T49.ØX5	T49.ØX6
Mycitracin	T36.8X1	T36.8X2	T36.8X3	T36.8X4	T36.8X5	T36.8X6
ophthalmic preparation	T49.5X1	T49.5X2	T49.5X3	T49.5X4	T49.5X5	T49.5X6
Mycostatin	T36.7X1	T36.7X2	T36.7X3	T36.7X4	T36.7X5	T36.7X6
topical	T49.ØX1	T49.ØX2	T49.ØX3	T49.ØX4	T49.ØX5	T49.ØX6
Mycotoxins	T64.81	T64.82	T64.83	T64.84	—	—
aflatoxin	T64.Ø1	T64.Ø2	T64.Ø3	T64.Ø4	—	—
specified NEC	T64.81	T64.82	T64.83	T64.84	—	—
Mydriacyl	T44.3X1	T44.3X2	T44.3X3	T44.3X4	T44.3X5	T44.3X6
Mydriatic drug	T49.5X1	T49.5X2	T49.5X3	T49.5X4	T49.5X5	T49.5X6
Myelobromal	T45.1X1	T45.1X2	T45.1X3	T45.1X4	T45.1X5	T45.1X6
Myleran	T45.1X1	T45.1X2	T45.1X3	T45.1X4	T45.1X5	T45.1X6
Myochrysin(e)	T39.2X1	T39.2X2	T39.2X3	T39.2X4	T39.2X5	T39.2X6
Myoneural blocking agents	T48.1X1	T48.1X2	T48.1X3	T48.1X4	T48.1X5	T48.1X6
Myralact	T49.ØX1	T49.ØX2	T49.ØX3	T49.ØX4	T49.ØX5	T49.ØX6
Myristica fragrans	T62.2X1	T62.2X2	T62.2X3	T62.2X4	—	—
Myristicin	T65.891	T65.892	T65.893	T65.894	—	—
Mysoline	T42.3X1	T42.3X2	T42.3X3	T42.3X4	T42.3X5	T42.3X6

N

Substance	Poisoning, Accidental (Unintentional)	Poisoning, Intentional Self-Harm	Poisoning, Assault	Poisoning, Undetermined	Adverse Effect	Underdosing
Nabilone	T4Ø.7X1	T4Ø.7X2	T4Ø.7X3	T4Ø.7X4	T4Ø.7X5	T4Ø.7X6
Nabumetone	T39.391	T39.392	T39.393	T39.394	T39.395	T39.396
Nadolol	T44.7X1	T44.7X2	T44.7X3	T44.7X4	T44.7X5	T44.7X6
Nafcillin	T36.ØX1	T36.ØX2	T36.ØX3	T36.ØX4	T36.ØX5	T36.ØX6
Nafoxidine	T38.6X1	T38.6X2	T38.6X3	T38.6X4	T38.6X5	T38.6X6
Naftazone	T46.991	T46.992	T46.993	T46.994	T46.995	T46.996
Naftidrofuryl (oxalate)	T46.7X1	T46.7X2	T46.7X3	T46.7X4	T46.7X5	T46.7X6
Naftifine	T49.ØX1	T49.ØX2	T49.ØX3	T49.ØX4	T49.ØX5	T49.ØX6
Nail polish remover	T52.91	T52.92	T52.93	T52.94	—	—
Nalbuphine	T4Ø.4X1	T4Ø.4X2	T4Ø.4X3	T4Ø.4X4	T4Ø.4X5	T4Ø.4X6
Naled	T6Ø.ØX1	T6Ø.ØX2	T6Ø.ØX3	T6Ø.ØX4	—	—
Nalidixic acid	T37.8X1	T37.8X2	T37.8X3	T37.8X4	T37.8X5	T37.8X6
Nalorphine	T5Ø.7X1	T5Ø.7X2	T5Ø.7X3	T5Ø.7X4	T5Ø.7X5	T5Ø.7X6
Naloxone	T5Ø.7X1	T5Ø.7X2	T5Ø.7X3	T5Ø.7X4	T5Ø.7X5	T5Ø.7X6
Naltrexone	T5Ø.7X1	T5Ø.7X2	T5Ø.7X3	T5Ø.7X4	T5Ø.7X5	T5Ø.7X6
Namenda	T43.8X1	T43.8X2	T43.8X3	T43.8X4	T43.8X5	T43.8X6
Nandrolone	T38.7X1	T38.7X2	T38.7X3	T38.7X4	T38.7X5	T38.7X6
Naphazoline	T48.5X1	T48.5X2	T48.5X3	T48.5X4	T48.5X5	T48.5X6

Substance	Poisoning, Accidental (Unintentional)	Poisoning, Intentional Self-Harm	Poisoning, Assault	Poisoning, Undetermined	Adverse Effect	Underdosing
Naphtha (painters') (petroleum)	T52.ØX1	T52.ØX2	T52.ØX3	T52.ØX4	—	—
solvent	T52.ØX1	T52.ØX2	T52.ØX3	T52.ØX4	—	—
vapor	T52.ØX1	T52.ØX2	T52.ØX3	T52.ØX4	—	—
Naphthalene (non-chlorinated)	T6Ø.2X1	T6Ø.2X2	T6Ø.2X3	T6Ø.2X4	—	—
chlorinated	T6Ø.1X1	T6Ø.1X2	T6Ø.1X3	T6Ø.1X4	—	—
vapor	T6Ø.1X1	T6Ø.1X2	T6Ø.1X3	T6Ø.1X4	—	—
insecticide or moth repellent	T6Ø.2X1	T6Ø.2X2	T6Ø.2X3	T6Ø.2X4	—	—
chlorinated	T6Ø.1X1	T6Ø.1X2	T6Ø.1X3	T6Ø.1X4	—	—
vapor	T6Ø.2X1	T6Ø.2X2	T6Ø.2X3	T6Ø.2X4	—	—
chlorinated	T6Ø.1X1	T6Ø.1X2	T6Ø.1X3	T6Ø.1X4	—	—
Naphthol	T65.891	T65.892	T65.893	T65.894	—	—
Naphthylamine	T65.891	T65.892	T65.893	T65.894	—	—
Naphthylthiourea (ANTU)	T6Ø.4X1	T6Ø.4X2	T6Ø.4X3	T6Ø.4X4	—	—
Naprosyn — *see Naproxen*						
Naproxen	T39.311	T39.312	T39.313	T39.314	T39.315	T39.316
Narcotic (drug)	T4Ø.6Ø1	T4Ø.6Ø2	T4Ø.6Ø3	T4Ø.6Ø4	T4Ø.6Ø5	T4Ø.6Ø6
analgesic NEC	T4Ø.6Ø1	T4Ø.6Ø2	T4Ø.6Ø3	T4Ø.6Ø4	T4Ø.6Ø5	T4Ø.6Ø6
antagonist	T5Ø.7X1	T5Ø.7X2	T5Ø.7X3	T5Ø.7X4	T5Ø.7X5	T5Ø.7X6
specified NEC	T4Ø.691	T4Ø.692	T4Ø.693	T4Ø.694	T4Ø.695	T4Ø.696
synthetic	T4Ø.4X1	T4Ø.4X2	T4Ø.4X3	T4Ø.4X4	T4Ø.4X5	T4Ø.4X6
Narcotine	T48.3X1	T48.3X2	T48.3X3	T48.3X4	T48.3X5	T48.3X6
Nardil	T43.1X1	T43.1X2	T43.1X3	T43.1X4	T43.1X5	T43.1X6
Nasal drug NEC	T49.6X1	T49.6X2	T49.6X3	T49.6X4	T49.6X5	T49.6X6
Natamycin	T49.ØX1	T49.ØX2	T49.ØX3	T49.ØX4	T49.ØX5	T49.ØX6
Natrium cyanide — *see Cyanide(s)*						
Natural gas	T59.891	T59.892	T59.893	T59.894	—	—
incomplete combustion	T57.91	T57.92	T57.93	T57.94	—	—
Natural						
blood (product)	T45.8X1	T45.8X2	T45.8X3	T45.8X4	T45.8X5	T45.8X6
gas (piped)	T59.891	T59.892	T59.893	T59.894	—	—
incomplete combustion	T58.11	T58.12	T58.13	T58.14	—	—
Nealbarbital	T42.3X1	T42.3X2	T42.3X3	T42.3X4	T42.3X5	T42.3X6
Nectadon	T48.3X1	T48.3X2	T48.3X3	T48.3X4	T48.3X5	T48.3X6
Nedocromil	T48.6X1	T48.6X2	T48.6X3	T48.6X4	T48.6X5	T48.6X6
Nefopam	T39.8X1	T39.8X2	T39.8X3	T39.8X4	T39.8X5	T39.8X6
Nematocyst (sting)	T63.691	T63.692	T63.693	T63.694	—	—
Nembutal	T42.3X1	T42.3X2	T42.3X3	T42.3X4	T42.3X5	T42.3X6
Nemonapride	T43.591	T43.592	T43.593	T43.594	T43.595	T43.596
Neoarsphenamine	T37.8X1	T37.8X2	T37.8X3	T37.8X4	T37.8X5	T37.8X6

Substance	Poisoning, Accidental (Unintentional)	Poisoning, Intentional Self-Harm	Poisoning, Assault	Poisoning, Undetermined	Adverse Effect	Underdosing
Neocinchophen	T50.4X1	T50.4X2	T50.4X3	T50.4X4	T50.4X5	T50.4X6
Neomycin (derivatives)	T36.5X1	T36.5X2	T36.5X3	T36.5X4	T36.5X5	T36.5X6
with						
bacitracin	T49.0X1	T49.0X2	T49.0X3	T49.0X4	T49.0X5	T49.0X6
neostigmine	T44.0X1	T44.0X2	T44.0X3	T44.0X4	T44.0X5	T44.0X6
ENT agent	T49.6X1	T49.6X2	T49.6X3	T49.6X4	T49.6X5	T49.6X6
ophthalmic preparation	T49.5X1	T49.5X2	T49.5X3	T49.5X4	T49.5X5	T49.5X6
topical NEC	T49.0X1	T49.0X2	T49.0X3	T49.0X4	T49.0X5	T49.0X6
Neonal	T42.3X1	T42.3X2	T42.3X3	T42.3X4	T42.3X5	T42.3X6
Neoprontosil	T37.0X1	T37.0X2	T37.0X3	T37.0X4	T37.0X5	T37.0X6
Neosalvarsan	T37.8X1	T37.8X2	T37.8X3	T37.8X4	T37.8X5	T37.8X6
Neosilversalvarsan	T37.8X1	T37.8X2	T37.8X3	T37.8X4	T37.8X5	T37.8X6
Neosporin	T36.8X1	T36.8X2	T36.8X3	T36.8X4	T36.8X5	T36.8X6
ENT agent	T49.6X1	T49.6X2	T49.6X3	T49.6X4	T49.6X5	T49.6X6
opthalmic preparation	T49.5X1	T49.5X2	T49.5X3	T49.5X4	T49.5X5	T49.5X6
topical NEC	T49.0X1	T49.0X2	T49.0X3	T49.0X4	T49.0X5	T49.0X6
Neostigmine bromide	T44.0X1	T44.0X2	T44.0X3	T44.0X4	T44.0X5	T44.0X6
Neraval	T42.3X1	T42.3X2	T42.3X3	T42.3X4	T42.3X5	T42.3X6
Neravan	T42.3X1	T42.3X2	T42.3X3	T42.3X4	T42.3X5	T42.3X6
Nerium oleander	T62.2X1	T62.2X2	T62.2X3	T62.2X4	—	—
Nerve gas, not in war	T59.91	T59.92	T59.93	T59.94	—	—
Nesacaine	T41.3X1	T41.3X2	T41.3X3	T41.3X4	T41.3X5	T41.3X6
infiltration (subcutaneous)	T41.3X1	T41.3X2	T41.3X3	T41.3X4	T41.3X5	T41.3X6
nerve block (peripheral) (plexus)	T41.3X1	T41.3X2	T41.3X3	T41.3X4	T41.3X5	T41.3X6
Netilmicin	T36.5X1	T36.5X2	T36.5X3	T36.5X4	T36.5X5	T36.5X6
Neurobarb	T42.3X1	T42.3X2	T42.3X3	T42.3X4	T42.3X5	T42.3X6
Neuroleptic drug NEC	T43.501	T43.502	T43.503	T43.504	T43.505	T43.506
Neuromuscular blocking drug	T48.1X1	T48.1X2	T48.1X3	T48.1X4	T48.1X5	T48.1X6
Neutral insulin injection	T38.3X1	T38.3X2	T38.3X3	T38.3X4	T38.3X5	T38.3X6
Neutral spirits	T51.0X1	T51.0X2	T51.0X3	T51.0X4	—	—
beverage	T51.0X1	T51.0X2	T51.0X3	T51.0X4	—	—
Niacin	T46.7X1	T46.7X2	T46.7X3	T46.7X4	T46.7X5	T46.7X6
Niacinamide	T45.2X1	T45.2X2	T45.2X3	T45.2X4	T45.2X5	T45.2X6
Nialamide	T43.1X1	T43.1X2	T43.1X3	T43.1X4	T43.1X5	T43.1X6
Niaprazine	T42.6X1	T42.6X2	T42.6X3	T42.6X4	T42.6X5	T42.6X6
Nicametate	T46.7X1	T46.7X2	T46.7X3	T46.7X4	T46.7X5	T46.7X6
Nicardipine	T46.1X1	T46.1X2	T46.1X3	T46.1X4	T46.1X5	T46.1X6
Nicergoline	T46.7X1	T46.7X2	T46.7X3	T46.7X4	T46.7X5	T46.7X6
Nickel (carbonyl) (tetra-carbonyl) (fumes) (vapor)	T56.891	T56.892	T56.893	T56.894	—	—

Substance	Poisoning, Accidental (Unintentional)	Poisoning, Intentional Self-Harm	Poisoning, Assault	Poisoning, Undetermined	Adverse Effect	Underdosing
Nickelocene	T56.891	T56.892	T56.893	T56.894	—	—
Niclosamide	T37.4X1	T37.4X2	T37.4X3	T37.4X4	T37.4X5	T37.4X6
Nicofuranose	T46.7X1	T46.7X2	T46.7X3	T46.7X4	T46.7X5	T46.7X6
Nicomorphine	T40.2X1	T40.2X2	T40.2X3	T40.2X4	—	—
Nicorandil	T46.3X1	T46.3X2	T46.3X3	T46.3X4	T46.3X5	T46.3X6
Nicotiana (plant)	T62.2X1	T62.2X2	T62.2X3	T62.2X4	—	—
Nicotinamide	T45.2X1	T45.2X2	T45.2X3	T45.2X4	T45.2X5	T45.2X6
Nicotine (insecticide) (spray) (sulfate) NEC	T60.2X1	T60.2X2	T60.2X3	T60.2X4	—	—
from tobacco	T65.291	T65.292	T65.293	T65.294	—	—
cigarettes	T65.221	T65.222	T65.223	T65.224	—	—
not insecticide	T65.291	T65.292	T65.293	T65.294	—	—
Nicotinic acid	T46.7X1	T46.7X2	T46.7X3	T46.7X4	T46.7X5	T46.7X6
Nicotinyl alcohol	T46.7X1	T46.7X2	T46.7X3	T46.7X4	T46.7X5	T46.7X6
Nicoumalone	T45.511	T45.512	T45.513	T45.514	T45.515	T45.516
Nifedipine	T46.1X1	T46.1X2	T46.1X3	T46.1X4	T46.1X5	T46.1X6
Nifenazone	T39.2X1	T39.2X2	T39.2X3	T39.2X4	T39.2X5	T39.2X6
Nifuraldezone	T37.91	T37.92	T37.93	T37.94	T37.95	T37.96
Nifuratel	T37.8X1	T37.8X2	T37.8X3	T37.8X4	T37.8X5	T37.8X6
Nifurtimox	T37.3X1	T37.3X2	T37.3X3	T37.3X4	T37.3X5	T37.3X6
Nifurtoinol	T37.8X1	T37.8X2	T37.8X3	T37.8X4	T37.8X5	T37.8X6
Nightshade, deadly (solanum)—*see also Belladonna*	T62.2X1	T62.2X2	T62.2X3	T62.2X4	—	—
berry	T62.1X1	T62.1X2	T62.1X3	T62.1X4	—	—
Nikethamide	T50.7X1	T50.7X2	T50.7X3	T50.7X4	T50.7X5	T50.7X6
Nilstat	T36.7X1	T36.7X2	T36.7X3	T36.7X4	T36.7X5	T36.7X6
topical	T49.0X1	T49.0X2	T49.0X3	T49.0X4	T49.0X5	T49.0X6
Nilutamide	T38.6X1	T38.6X2	T38.6X3	T38.6X4	T38.6X5	T38.6X6
Nimesulide	T39.391	T39.392	T39.393	T39.394	T39.395	T39.396
Nimetazepam	T42.4X1	T42.4X2	T42.4X3	T42.4X4	T42.4X5	T42.4X6
Nimodipine	T46.1X1	T46.1X2	T46.1X3	T46.1X4	T46.1X5	T46.1X6
Nimorazole	T37.3X1	T37.3X2	T37.3X3	T37.3X4	T37.3X5	T37.3X6
Nimustine	T45.1X1	T45.1X2	T45.1X3	T45.1X4	T45.1X5	T45.1X6
Niridazole	T37.4X1	T37.4X2	T37.4X3	T37.4X4	T37.4X5	T37.4X6
Nisentil	T40.2X1	T40.2X2	T40.2X3	T40.2X4	T40.2X5	T40.2X6
Nisoldipine	T46.1X1	T46.1X2	T46.1X3	T46.1X4	T46.1X5	T46.1X6
Nitramine	T65.3X1	T65.3X2	T65.3X3	T65.3X4	—	—
Nitrate, organic	T46.3X1	T46.3X2	T46.3X3	T46.3X4	T46.3X5	T46.3X6
Nitrazepam	T42.4X1	T42.4X2	T42.4X3	T42.4X4	T42.4X5	T42.4X6
Nitrefazole	T50.6X1	T50.6X2	T50.6X3	T50.6X4	T50.6X5	T50.6X6
Nitrendipine	T46.1X1	T46.1X2	T46.1X3	T46.1X4	T46.1X5	T46.1X6

Substance	Poisoning, Accidental (Unintentional)	Poisoning, Intentional Self-Harm	Poisoning, Assault	Poisoning, Undetermined	Adverse Effect	Underdosing
Nitric						
acid (liquid)	T54.2X1	T54.2X2	T54.2X3	T54.2X4	—	—
vapor	T59.891	T59.892	T59.893	T59.894	—	—
oxide (gas)	T59.ØX1	T59.ØX2	T59.ØX3	T59.ØX4	—	—
Nitrimidazine	T37.3X1	T37.3X2	T37.3X3	T37.3X4	T37.3X5	T37.3X6
Nitrite, amyl (medicinal) (vapor)	T46.3X1	T46.3X2	T46.3X3	T46.3X4	T46.3X5	T46.3X6
Nitroaniline	T65.3X1	T65.3X2	T65.3X3	T65.3X4	—	—
vapor	T59.891	T59.892	T59.893	T59.894	—	—
Nitrobenzene, nitrobenzol	T65.3X1	T65.3X2	T65.3X3	T65.3X4	—	—
vapor	T65.3X1	T65.3X2	T65.3X3	T65.3X4	—	—
Nitrocellulose	T65.891	T65.892	T65.893	T65.894	—	—
lacquer	T65.891	T65.892	T65.893	T65.894	—	—
Nitrodiphenyl	T65.3X1	T65.3X2	T65.3X3	T65.3X4	—	—
Nitrofural	T49.ØX1	T49.ØX2	T49.ØX3	T49.ØX4	T49.ØX5	T49.ØX6
Nitrofurantoin	T37.8X1	T37.8X2	T37.8X3	T37.8X4	T37.8X5	T37.8X6
Nitrofurazone	T49.ØX1	T49.ØX2	T49.ØX3	T49.ØX4	T49.ØX5	T49.ØX6
Nitrogen	T59.ØX1	T59.ØX2	T59.ØX3	T59.ØX4	—	—
mustard	T45.1X1	T45.1X2	T45.1X3	T45.1X4	T45.1X5	T45.1X6
Nitroglycerin, nitro-glycerol (medicinal)	T46.3X1	T46.3X2	T46.3X3	T46.3X4	T46.3X5	T46.3X6
nonmedicinal	T65.5X1	T65.5X2	T65.5X3	T65.5X4	—	—
fumes	T65.5X1	T65.5X2	T65.5X3	T65.5X4	—	—
Nitroglycol	T52.3X1	T52.3X2	T52.3X3	T52.3X4	—	—
Nitrohydrochloric acid	T54.2X1	T54.2X2	T54.2X3	T54.2X4	—	—
Nitromersol	T49.ØX1	T49.ØX2	T49.ØX3	T49.ØX4	T49.ØX5	T49.ØX6
Nitronaphthalene	T65.891	T65.892	T65.893	T65.894	—	—
Nitrophenol	T54.ØX1	T54.ØX2	T54.ØX3	T54.ØX4	—	—
Nitropropane	T52.8X1	T52.8X2	T52.8X3	T52.8X4	—	—
Nitroprusside	T46.5X1	T46.5X2	T46.5X3	T46.5X4	T46.5X5	T46.5X6
Nitrosodimethylamine	T65.3X1	T65.3X2	T65.3X3	T65.3X4	—	—
Nitrothiazol	T37.4X1	T37.4X2	T37.4X3	T37.4X4	T37.4X5	T37.4X6
Nitrotoluene, nitrotoluol	T65.3X1	T65.3X2	T65.3X3	T65.3X4	—	—
vapor	T65.3X1	T65.3X2	T65.3X3	T65.3X4	—	—
Nitrous						
acid (liquid)	T54.2X1	T54.2X2	T54.2X3	T54.2X4	—	—
fumes	T59.891	T59.892	T59.893	T59.894	—	—
ether spirit	T46.3X1	T46.3X2	T46.3X3	T46.3X4	T46.3X5	T46.3X6
oxide	T41.ØX1	T41.ØX2	T41.ØX3	T41.ØX4	T41.ØX5	T41.ØX6
Nitroxoline	T37.8X1	T37.8X2	T37.8X3	T37.8X4	T37.8X5	T37.8X6
Nitrozone	T49.ØX1	T49.ØX2	T49.ØX3	T49.ØX4	T49.ØX5	T49.ØX6
Nizatidine	T47.ØX1	T47.ØX2	T47.ØX3	T47.ØX4	T47.ØX5	T47.ØX6
Nizofenone	T43.8X1	T43.8X2	T43.8X3	T43.8X4	T43.8X5	T43.8X6
Noctec	T42.6X1	T42.6X2	T42.6X3	T42.6X4	T42.6X5	T42.6X6
Noludar	T42.6X1	T42.6X2	T42.6X3	T42.6X4	T42.6X5	T42.6X6
Noptil	T42.3X1	T42.3X2	T42.3X3	T42.3X4	T42.3X5	T42.3X6
Nomegestrol	T38.5X1	T38.5X2	T38.5X3	T38.5X4	T38.5X5	T38.5X6
Nomifensine	T43.291	T43.292	T43.293	T43.294	T43.295	T43.296
Nonoxinol	T49.8X1	T49.8X2	T49.8X3	T49.8X4	T49.8X5	T49.8X6
Nonylphenoxy (polyethoxy-ethanol)	T49.8X1	T49.8X2	T49.8X3	T49.8X4	T49.8X5	T49.8X6
Noptil	T42.3X1	T42.3X2	T42.3X3	T42.3X4	T42.3X5	T42.3X6
Noradrenaline	T44.4X1	T44.4X2	T44.4X3	T44.4X4	T44.4X5	T44.4X6
Noramidopyrine	T39.2X1	T39.2X2	T39.2X3	T39.2X4	T39.2X5	T39.2X6
methanesulfonate sodium	T39.2X1	T39.2X2	T39.2X3	T39.2X4	T39.2X5	T39.2X6
Norbormide	T6Ø.4X1	T6Ø.4X2	T6Ø.4X3	T6Ø.4X4	—	—
Nordazepam	T42.4X1	T42.4X2	T42.4X3	T42.4X4	T42.4X5	T42.4X6
Norepinephrine	T44.4X1	T44.4X2	T44.4X3	T44.4X4	T44.4X5	T44.4X6
Norethandrolone	T38.7X1	T38.7X2	T38.7X3	T38.7X4	T38.7X5	T38.7X6
Norethindrone	T38.4X1	T38.4X2	T38.4X3	T38.4X4	T38.4X5	T38.4X6
Norethisterone (acetate) (enantate)	T38.4X1	T38.4X2	T38.4X3	T38.4X4	T38.4X5	T38.4X6
with ethinylestradiol	T38.5X1	T38.5X2	T38.5X3	T38.5X4	T38.5X5	T38.5X6
Noretynodrel	T38.5X1	T38.5X2	T38.5X3	T38.5X4	T38.5X5	T38.5X6
Norfenefrine	T44.4X1	T44.4X2	T44.4X3	T44.4X4	T44.4X5	T44.4X6
Norfloxacin	T36.8X1	T36.8X2	T36.8X3	T36.8X4	T36.8X5	T36.8X6
Norgestrel	T38.4X1	T38.4X2	T38.4X3	T38.4X4	T38.4X5	T38.4X6
Norgestrienone	T38.4X1	T38.4X2	T38.4X3	T38.4X4	T38.4X5	T38.4X6
Norlestrin	T38.4X1	T38.4X2	T38.4X3	T38.4X4	T38.4X5	T38.4X6
Norlutin	T38.4X1	T38.4X2	T38.4X3	T38.4X4	T38.4X5	T38.4X6
Normal serum albumin (human), salt-poor	T45.8X1	T45.8X2	T45.8X3	T45.8X4	T45.8X5	T45.8X6
Normethandrone	T38.5X1	T38.5X2	T38.5X3	T38.5X4	T38.5X5	T38.5X6
Normison — *see Benzodiazepines*						
Normorphine	T4Ø.2X1	T4Ø.2X2	T4Ø.2X3	T4Ø.2X4	—	—
Norpseudoephedrine	T5Ø.5X1	T5Ø.5X2	T5Ø.5X3	T5Ø.5X4	T5Ø.5X5	T5Ø.5X6
Nortestosterone (furanpropionate)	T38.7X1	T38.7X2	T38.7X3	T38.7X4	T38.7X5	T38.7X6
Nortriptyline	T43.Ø11	T43.Ø12	T43.Ø13	T43.Ø14	T43.Ø15	T43.Ø16
Noscapine	T48.3X1	T48.3X2	T48.3X3	T48.3X4	T48.3X5	T48.3X6
Nose preparations	T49.6X1	T49.6X2	T49.6X3	T49.6X4	T49.6X5	T49.6X6
Novobiocin	T36.5X1	T36.5X2	T36.5X3	T36.5X4	T36.5X5	T36.5X6
Novocain (infiltration) (topical)	T41.3X1	T41.3X2	T41.3X3	T41.3X4	T41.3X5	T41.3X6
nerve block (peripheral) (plexus)	T41.3X1	T41.3X2	T41.3X3	T41.3X4	T41.3X5	T41.3X6
spinal	T41.3X1	T41.3X2	T41.3X3	T41.3X4	T41.3X5	T41.3X6

Substance	Poisoning, Accidental (Unintentional)	Poisoning, Intentional Self-Harm	Poisoning, Assault	Poisoning, Undetermined	Adverse Effect	Underdosing
Noxious foodstuff	T62.91	T62.92	T62.93	T62.94	—	—
specified NEC	T62.8X1	T62.8X2	T62.8X3	T62.8X4	—	—
Noxiptiline	T43.011	T43.012	T43.013	T43.014	T43.015	T43.016
Noxytiolin	T49.0X1	T49.0X2	T49.0X3	T49.0X4	T49.0X5	T49.0X6
NPH Iletin (insulin)	T38.3X1	T38.3X2	T38.3X3	T38.3X4	T38.3X5	T38.3X6
Numorphan	T40.2X1	T40.2X2	T40.2X3	T40.2X4	T40.2X5	T40.2X6
Nunol	T42.3X1	T42.3X2	T42.3X3	T42.3X4	T42.3X5	T42.3X6
Nupercaine (spinal anesthetic)	T41.3X1	T41.3X2	T41.3X3	T41.3X4	T41.3X5	T41.3X6
topical (surface)	T41.3X1	T41.3X2	T41.3X3	T41.3X4	T41.3X5	T41.3X6
Nutmeg oil (liniment)	T49.3X1	T49.3X2	T49.3X3	T49.3X4	T49.3X5	T49.3X6
Nutritional supplement	T50.901	T50.902	T50.903	T50.904	T50.905	T50.906
Nux vomica	T65.1X1	T65.1X2	T65.1X3	T65.1X4	—	—
Nydrazid	T37.1X1	T37.1X2	T37.1X3	T37.1X4	T37.1X5	T37.1X6
Nylidrin	T46.7X1	T46.7X2	T46.7X3	T46.7X4	T46.7X5	T46.7X6
Nystatin	T36.7X1	T36.7X2	T36.7X3	T36.7X4	T36.7X5	T36.7X6
topical	T49.0X1	T49.0X2	T49.0X3	T49.0X4	T49.0X5	T49.0X6
Nytol	T45.0X1	T45.0X2	T45.0X3	T45.0X4	T45.0X5	T45.0X6
O						
Obidoxime chloride	T50.6X1	T50.6X2	T50.6X3	T50.6X4	T50.6X5	T50.6X6
Octafonium (chloride)	T49.3X1	T49.3X2	T49.3X3	T49.3X4	T49.3X5	T49.3X6
Octamethyl pyrophosphoramide	T60.0X1	T60.0X2	T60.0X3	T60.0X4	—	—
Octanoin	T50.991	T50.992	T50.993	T50.994	T50.995	T50.996
Octatropine methylbromide	T44.3X1	T44.3X2	T44.3X3	T44.3X4	T44.3X5	T44.3X6
Octotiamine	T45.2X1	T45.2X2	T45.2X3	T45.2X4	T45.2X5	T45.2X6
Octoxinol (9)	T49.8X1	T49.8X2	T49.8X3	T49.8X4	T49.8X5	T49.8X6
Octreotide	T38.991	T38.992	T38.993	T38.994	T38.995	T38.996
Octyl nitrite	T46.3X1	T46.3X2	T46.3X3	T46.3X4	T46.3X5	T46.3X6
Oestradiol	T38.5X1	T38.5X2	T38.5X3	T38.5X4	T38.5X5	T38.5X6
Oestriol	T38.5X1	T38.5X2	T38.5X3	T38.5X4	T38.5X5	T38.5X6
Oestrogen	T38.5X1	T38.5X2	T38.5X3	T38.5X4	T38.5X5	T38.5X6
Oestrone	T38.5X1	T38.5X2	T38.5X3	T38.5X4	T38.5X5	T38.5X6
Ofloxacin	T36.8X1	T36.8X2	T36.8X3	T36.8X4	T36.8X5	T36.8X6
Oil (of)	T65.891	T65.892	T65.893	T65.894	—	—
bitter almond	T62.8X1	T62.8X2	T62.8X3	T62.8X4	—	—
cloves	T49.7X1	T49.7X2	T49.7X3	T49.7X4	T49.7X5	T49.7X6
colors	T65.6X1	T65.6X2	T65.6X3	T65.6X4	—	—
fumes	T59.891	T59.892	T59.893	T59.894	—	—
lubricating	T52.0X1	T52.0X2	T52.0X3	T52.0X4	—	—
Niobe	T52.8X1	T52.8X2	T52.8X3	T52.8X4	—	—

Substance	Poisoning, Accidental (Unintentional)	Poisoning, Intentional Self-Harm	Poisoning, Assault	Poisoning, Undetermined	Adverse Effect	Underdosing
Oil (of) *(Continued)*						
vitriol (liquid)	T54.2X1	T54.2X2	T54.2X3	T54.2X4	—	—
fumes	T54.2X1	T54.2X2	T54.2X3	T54.2X4	—	—
wintergreen (bitter) NEC	T49.3X1	T49.3X2	T49.3X3	T49.3X4	T49.3X5	T49.3X6
Oily preparation (for skin)	T49.3X1	T49.3X2	T49.3X3	T49.3X4	T49.3X5	T49.3X6
Ointment NEC	T49.3X1	T49.3X2	T49.3X3	T49.3X4	T49.3X5	T49.3X6
Olanzapine	T43.591	T43.592	T43.593	T43.594	T43.595	T43.596
Oleander	T62.2X1	T62.2X2	T62.2X3	T62.2X4	—	—
Oleandomycin	T36.3X1	T36.3X2	T36.3X3	T36.3X4	T36.3X5	T36.3X6
Oleandrin	T46.0X1	T46.0X2	T46.0X3	T46.0X4	T46.0X5	T46.0X6
Oleic acid	T46.6X1	T46.6X2	T46.6X3	T46.6X4	T46.6X5	T46.6X6
Oleovitamin A	T45.2X1	T45.2X2	T45.2X3	T45.2X4	T45.2X5	T45.2X6
Oleum ricini	T47.2X1	T47.2X2	T47.2X3	T47.2X4	T47.2X5	T47.2X6
Olive oil (medicinal) NEC	T47.4X1	T47.4X2	T47.4X3	T47.4X4	T47.4X5	T47.4X6
Olivomycin	T45.1X1	T45.1X2	T45.1X3	T45.1X4	T45.1X5	T45.1X6
Olsalazine	T47.8X1	T47.8X2	T47.8X3	T47.8X4	T47.8X5	T47.8X6
Omeprazole	T47.1X1	T47.1X2	T47.1X3	T47.1X4	T47.1X5	T47.1X6
OMPA	T60.0X1	T60.0X2	T60.0X3	T60.0X4	—	—
Ondansetron	T45.0X1	T45.0X2	T45.0X3	T45.0X4	T45.0X5	T45.0X6
Oncovin	T45.1X1	T45.1X2	T45.1X3	T45.1X4	T45.1X5	T45.1X6
Ophthaine	T41.3X1	T41.3X2	T41.3X3	T41.3X4	T41.3X5	T41.3X6
Ophthetic	T41.3X1	T41.3X2	T41.3X3	T41.3X4	T41.3X5	T41.3X6
Opiate NEC	T40.601	T40.602	T40.603	T40.604	T40.605	T40.606
antagonists	T50.7X1	T50.7X2	T50.7X3	T50.7X4	T50.7X5	T50.7X6
Opioid NEC	T40.2X1	T40.2X2	T40.2X3	T40.2X4	T40.2X5	T40.2X6
Opipramol	T43.011	T43.012	T43.013	T43.014	T43.015	T43.016
Opium alkaloids (total)	T40.0X1	T40.0X2	T40.0X3	T40.0X4	T40.0X5	T40.0X6
standardized powdered	T40.0X1	T40.0X2	T40.0X3	T40.0X4	T40.0X5	T40.0X6
tincture (camphorated)	T40.0X1	T40.0X2	T40.0X3	T40.0X4	T40.0X5	T40.0X6
Oracon	T38.4X1	T38.4X2	T38.4X3	T38.4X4	T38.4X5	T38.4X6
Oragrafin	T50.8X1	T50.8X2	T50.8X3	T50.8X4	T50.8X5	T50.8X6
Oral contraceptives	T38.4X1	T38.4X2	T38.4X3	T38.4X4	T38.4X5	T38.4X6
Oral rehydration salts	T50.3X1	T50.3X2	T50.3X3	T50.3X4	T50.3X5	T50.3X6
Orazamide	T50.991	T50.992	T50.993	T50.994	T50.995	T50.996
Orciprenaline	T48.291	T48.292	T48.293	T48.294	T48.295	T48.296
Organidin	T48.4X1	T48.4X2	T48.4X3	T48.4X4	T48.4X5	T48.4X6
Organonitrate NEC	T46.3X1	T46.3X2	T46.3X3	T46.3X4	T46.3X5	T46.3X6
Organophosphates	T60.0X1	T60.0X2	T60.0X3	T60.0X4	—	—
Orimune	T50.B91	T50.B92	T50.B93	T50.B94	T50.B95	T50.B96
Orinase	T38.3X1	T38.3X2	T38.3X3	T38.3X4	T38.3X5	T38.3X6
Ormeloxifene	T38.6X1	T38.6X2	T38.6X3	T38.6X4	T38.6X5	T38.6X6

Substance	Poisoning, Accidental (Unintentional)	Poisoning, Intentional Self-Harm	Poisoning, Assault	Poisoning, Undetermined	Adverse Effect	Underdosing
Ornidazole	T37.3X1	T37.3X2	T37.3X3	T37.3X4	T37.3X5	T37.3X6
Ornithine aspartate	T5Ø.991	T5Ø.992	T5Ø.993	T5Ø.994	T5Ø.995	T5Ø.996
Ornoprostil	T47.1X1	T47.1X2	T47.1X3	T47.1X4	T47.1X5	T47.1X6
Orphenadrine (hydrochloride)	T42.8X1	T42.8X2	T42.8X3	T42.8X4	T42.8X5	T42.8X6
Ortal (sodium)	T42.3X1	T42.3X2	T42.3X3	T42.3X4	T42.3X5	T42.3X6
Orthoboric acid	T49.ØX1	T49.ØX2	T49.ØX3	T49.ØX4	T49.ØX5	T49.ØX6
ENT agent	T49.6X1	T49.6X2	T49.6X3	T49.6X4	T49.6X5	T49.6X6
ophthalmic preparation	T49.5X1	T49.5X2	T49.5X3	T49.5X4	T49.5X5	T49.5X6
Orthocaine	T41.3X1	T41.3X2	T41.3X3	T41.3X4	T41.3X5	T41.3X6
Orthodichlorobenzene	T53.7X1	T53.7X2	T53.7X3	T53.7X4	—	—
Ortho-Novum	T38.4X1	T38.4X2	T38.4X3	T38.4X4	T38.4X5	T38.4X6
Orthotolidine (reagent)	T54.2X1	T54.2X2	T54.2X3	T54.2X4	—	—
Osmic acid (liquid)	T54.2X1	T54.2X2	T54.2X3	T54.2X4	—	—
fumes	T54.2X1	T54.2X2	T54.2X3	T54.2X4	—	—
Osmotic diuretics	T5Ø.2X1	T5Ø.2X2	T5Ø.2X3	T5Ø.2X4	T5Ø.2X5	T5Ø.2X6
Otilonium bromide	T44.3X1	T44.3X2	T44.3X3	T44.3X4	T44.3X5	T44.3X6
Otorhinolaryngological drug NEC	T49.6X1	T49.6X2	T49.6X3	T49.6X4	T49.6X5	T49.6X6
Ouabain(e)	T46.ØX1	T46.ØX2	T46.ØX3	T46.ØX4	T46.ØX5	T46.ØX6
Ovarian						
hormone	T38.5X1	T38.5X2	T38.5X3	T38.5X4	T38.5X5	T38.5X6
stimulant	T38.5X1	T38.5X2	T38.5X3	T38.5X4	T38.5X5	T38.5X6
Ovral	T38.4X1	T38.4X2	T38.4X3	T38.4X4	T38.4X5	T38.4X6
Ovulen	T38.4X1	T38.4X2	T38.4X3	T38.4X4	T38.4X5	T38.4X6
Oxacillin	T36.ØX1	T36.ØX2	T36.ØX3	T36.ØX4	T36.ØX5	T36.ØX6
Oxalic acid	T54.2X1	T54.2X2	T54.2X3	T54.2X4	—	—
ammonium salt	T5Ø.991	T5Ø.992	T5Ø.993	T5Ø.994	T5Ø.995	T5Ø.996
Oxamniquine	T37.4X1	T37.4X2	T37.4X3	T37.4X4	T37.4X5	T37.4X6
Oxanamide	T43.591	T43.592	T43.593	T43.594	T43.595	T43.596
Oxandrolone	T38.7X1	T38.7X2	T38.7X3	T38.7X4	T38.7X5	T38.7X6
Oxantel	T37.4X1	T37.4X2	T37.4X3	T37.4X4	T37.4X5	T37.4X6
Oxapium iodide	T44.3X1	T44.3X2	T44.3X3	T44.3X4	T44.3X5	T44.3X6
Oxaprotiline	T43.Ø21	T43.Ø22	T43.Ø23	T43.Ø24	T43.Ø25	T43.Ø26
Oxaprozin	T39.311	T39.312	T39.313	T39.314	T39.315	T39.316
Oxatomide	T45.ØX1	T45.ØX2	T45.ØX3	T45.ØX4	T45.ØX5	T45.ØX6
Oxazepam	T42.4X1	T42.4X2	T42.4X3	T42.4X4	T42.4X5	T42.4X6
Oxazimedrine	T5Ø.5X1	T5Ø.5X2	T5Ø.5X3	T5Ø.5X4	T5Ø.5X5	T5Ø.5X6
Oxazolam	T42.4X1	T42.4X2	T42.4X3	T42.4X4	T42.4X5	T42.4X6
Oxazolidine derivatives	T42.2X1	T42.2X2	T42.2X3	T42.2X4	T42.2X5	T42.2X6
Oxazolidinedione (derivative)	T42.2X1	T42.2X2	T42.2X3	T42.2X4	T42.2X5	T42.2X6
Ox bile extract	T47.5X1	T47.5X2	T47.5X3	T47.5X4	T47.5X5	T47.5X6
Oxcarbazepine	T42.1X1	T42.1X2	T42.1X3	T42.1X4	T42.1X5	T42.1X6
Oxedrine	T44.4X1	T44.4X2	T44.4X3	T44.4X4	T44.4X5	T44.4X6

Substance	Poisoning, Accidental (Unintentional)	Poisoning, Intentional Self-Harm	Poisoning, Assault	Poisoning, Undetermined	Adverse Effect	Underdosing
Oxeladin (citrate)	T48.3X1	T48.3X2	T48.3X3	T48.3X4	T48.3X5	T48.3X6
Oxendolone	T38.5X1	T38.5X2	T38.5X3	T38.5X4	T38.5X5	T38.5X6
Oxetacaine	T41.3X1	T41.3X2	T41.3X3	T41.3X4	T41.3X5	T41.3X6
Oxethazine	T41.3X1	T41.3X2	T41.3X3	T41.3X4	T41.3X5	T41.3X6
Oxetorone	T39.8X1	T39.8X2	T39.8X3	T39.8X4	T39.8X5	T39.8X6
Oxiconazole	T49.ØX1	T49.ØX2	T49.ØX3	T49.ØX4	T49.ØX5	T49.ØX6
Oxidizing agent NEC	T54.91	T54.92	T54.93	T54.94	—	—
Oxipurinol	T5Ø.4X1	T5Ø.4X2	T5Ø.4X3	T5Ø.4X4	T5Ø.4X5	T5Ø.4X6
Oxitriptan	T43.291	T43.292	T43.293	T43.294	T43.295	T43.296
Oxitropium bromide	T48.6X1	T48.6X2	T48.6X3	T48.6X4	T48.6X5	T48.6X6
Oxodipine	T46.1X1	T46.1X2	T46.1X3	T46.1X4	T46.1X5	T46.1X6
Oxolamine	T48.3X1	T48.3X2	T48.3X3	T48.3X4	T48.3X5	T48.3X6
Oxolinic acid	T37.8X1	T37.8X2	T37.8X3	T37.8X4	T37.8X5	T37.8X6
Oxomemazine	T43.3X1	T43.3X2	T43.3X3	T43.3X4	T43.3X5	T43.3X6
Oxophenarsine	T37.3X1	T37.3X2	T37.3X3	T37.3X4	T37.3X5	T37.3X6
Oxprenolol	T44.7X1	T44.7X2	T44.7X3	T44.7X4	T44.7X5	T44.7X6
Oxsoralen	T49.3X1	T49.3X2	T49.3X3	T49.3X4	T49.3X5	T49.3X6
Oxtriphylline	T48.6X1	T48.6X2	T48.6X3	T48.6X4	T48.6X5	T48.6X6
Oxybate sodium	T41.291	T41.292	T41.293	T41.294	T41.295	T41.296
Oxybuprocaine	T41.3X1	T41.3X2	T41.3X3	T41.3X4	T41.3X5	T41.3X6
Oxybutynin	T44.3X1	T44.3X2	T44.3X3	T44.3X4	T44.3X5	T44.3X6
Oxychlorosene	T49.ØX1	T49.ØX2	T49.ØX3	T49.ØX4	T49.ØX5	T49.ØX6
Oxycodone	T4Ø.2X1	T4Ø.2X2	T4Ø.2X3	T4Ø.2X4	T4Ø.2X5	T4Ø.2X6
Oxyfedrine	T46.3X1	T46.3X2	T46.3X3	T46.3X4	T46.3X5	T46.3X6
Oxygen	T41.5X1	T41.5X2	T41.5X3	T41.5X4	T41.5X5	T41.5X6
Oxylone	T49.ØX1	T49.ØX2	T49.ØX3	T49.ØX4	T49.ØX5	T49.ØX6
ophthalmic preparation	T49.5X1	T49.5X2	T49.5X3	T49.5X4	T49.5X5	T49.5X6
Oxymesterone	T38.7X1	T38.7X2	T38.7X3	T38.7X4	T38.7X5	T38.7X6
Oxymetazoline	T48.5X1	T48.5X2	T48.5X3	T48.5X4	T48.5X5	T48.5X6
Oxymetholone	T38.7X1	T38.7X2	T38.7X3	T38.7X4	T38.7X5	T38.7X6
Oxymorphone	T4Ø.2X1	T4Ø.2X2	T4Ø.2X3	T4Ø.2X4	T4Ø.2X5	T4Ø.2X6
Oxypertine	T43.591	T43.592	T43.593	T43.594	T43.595	T43.596
Oxyphenbutazone	T39.2X1	T39.2X2	T39.2X3	T39.2X4	T39.2X5	T39.2X6
Oxyphencyclimine	T44.3X1	T44.3X2	T44.3X3	T44.3X4	T44.3X5	T44.3X6
Oxyphenisatine	T47.2X1	T47.2X2	T47.2X3	T47.2X4	T47.2X5	T47.2X6
Oxyphenonium bromide	T44.3X1	T44.3X2	T44.3X3	T44.3X4	T44.3X5	T44.3X6
Oxypolygelatin	T45.8X1	T45.8X2	T45.8X3	T45.8X4	T45.8X5	T45.8X6
Oxyquinoline (derivatives)	T37.8X1	T37.8X2	T37.8X3	T37.8X4	T37.8X5	T37.8X6
Oxytetracycline	T36.4X1	T36.4X2	T36.4X3	T36.4X4	T36.4X5	T36.4X6
Oxytocic drug NEC	T48.ØX1	T48.ØX2	T48.ØX3	T48.ØX4	T48.ØX5	T48.ØX6
Oxytocin (synthetic)	T48.ØX1	T48.ØX2	T48.ØX3	T48.ØX4	T48.ØX5	T48.ØX6
Ozone	T59.891	T59.892	T59.893	T59.894	—	—

Substance	Poisoning, Accidental (Unintentional)	Poisoning, Intentional Self-Harm	Poisoning, Assault	Poisoning, Undetermined	Adverse Effect	Underdosing
P						
PABA	T49.3X1	T49.3X2	T49.3X3	T49.3X4	T49.3X5	T49.3X6
Packed red cells	T45.8X1	T45.8X2	T45.8X3	T45.8X4	T45.8X5	T45.8X6
Padimate	T49.3X1	T49.3X2	T49.3X3	T49.3X4	T49.3X5	T49.3X6
Paint NEC	T65.6X1	T65.6X2	T65.6X3	T65.6X4	—	—
cleaner	T52.91	T52.92	T52.93	T52.94	—	—
fumes NEC	T59.891	T59.892	T59.893	T59.894	—	—
lead (fumes)	T56.ØX1	T56.ØX2	T56.ØX3	T56.ØX4	—	—
solvent NEC	T52.8X1	T52.8X2	T52.8X3	T52.8X4	—	—
stripper	T52.8X1	T52.8X2	T52.8X3	T52.8X4	—	—
Palfium	T4Ø.2X1	T4Ø.2X2	T4Ø.2X3	T4Ø.2X4	—	—
Palm kernel oil	T5Ø.991	T5Ø.992	T5Ø.993	T5Ø.994	T5Ø.995	T5Ø.996
Paludrine	T37.2X1	T37.2X2	T37.2X3	T37.2X4	T37.2X5	T37.2X6
PAM (pralidoxime)	T5Ø.6X1	T5Ø.6X2	T5Ø.6X3	T5Ø.6X4	T5Ø.6X5	T5Ø.6X6
Pamaquine (naphthoute)	T37.2X1	T37.2X2	T37.2X3	T37.2X4	T37.2X5	T37.2X6
Panadol	T39.1X1	T39.1X2	T39.1X3	T39.1X4	T39.1X5	T39.1X6
Pancreatic						
digestive secretion stimulant	T47.8X1	T47.8X2	T47.8X3	T47.8X4	T47.8X5	T47.8X6
dornase	T45.3X1	T45.3X2	T45.3X3	T45.3X4	T45.3X5	T45.3X6
Pancreatin	T47.5X1	T47.5X2	T47.5X3	T47.5X4	T47.5X5	T47.5X6
Pancrelipase	T47.5X1	T47.5X2	T47.5X3	T47.5X4	T47.5X5	T47.5X6
Pancuronium (bromide)	T48.1X1	T48.1X2	T48.1X3	T48.1X4	T48.1X5	T48.1X6
Pangamic acid	T45.2X1	T45.2X2	T45.2X3	T45.2X4	T45.2X5	T45.2X6
Panthenol	T45.2X1	T45.2X2	T45.2X3	T45.2X4	T45.2X5	T45.2X6
topical	T49.8X1	T49.8X2	T49.8X3	T49.8X4	T49.8X5	T49.8X6
Pantopon	T4Ø.ØX1	T4Ø.ØX2	T4Ø.ØX3	T4Ø.ØX4	T4Ø.ØX5	T4Ø.ØX6
Pantothenic acid	T45.2X1	T45.2X2	T45.2X3	T45.2X4	T45.2X5	T45.2X6
Panwarfin	T45.511	T45.512	T45.513	T45.514	T45.515	T45.516
Papain	T47.5X1	T47.5X2	T47.5X3	T47.5X4	T47.5X5	T47.5X6
digestant	T47.5X1	T47.5X2	T47.5X3	T47.5X4	T47.5X5	T47.5X6
Papaveretum	T4Ø.ØX1	T4Ø.ØX2	T4Ø.ØX3	T4Ø.ØX4	T4Ø.ØX5	T4Ø.ØX6
Papaverine	T44.3X1	T44.3X2	T44.3X3	T44.3X4	T44.3X5	T44.3X6
Para-acetamidophenol	T39.1X1	T39.1X2	T39.1X3	T39.1X4	T39.1X5	T39.1X6
Para-aminobenzoic acid	T49.3X1	T49.3X2	T49.3X3	T49.3X4	T49.3X5	T49.3X6
Para-aminophenol derivatives	T39.1X1	T39.1X2	T39.1X3	T39.1X4	T39.1X5	T39.1X6
Para-aminosalicylic acid	T37.1X1	T37.1X2	T37.1X3	T37.1X4	T37.1X5	T37.1X6
Paracetaldehyde	T42.6X1	T42.6X2	T42.6X3	T42.6X4	T42.6X5	T42.6X6
Paracetamol	T39.1X1	T39.1X2	T39.1X3	T39.1X4	T39.1X5	T39.1X6
Parachlorophenol (camphorated)	T49.ØX1	T49.ØX2	T49.ØX3	T49.ØX4	T49.ØX5	T49.ØX6
Paracodin	T4Ø.2X1	T4Ø.2X2	T4Ø.2X3	T4Ø.2X4	T4Ø.2X5	T4Ø.2X6
Paradione	T42.2X1	T42.2X2	T42.2X3	T42.2X4	T42.2X5	T42.2X6
Paraffin(s) (wax)	T52.ØX1	T52.ØX2	T52.ØX3	T52.ØX4	—	—
liquid (medicinal)	T47.4X1	T47.4X2	T47.4X3	T47.4X4	T47.4X5	T47.4X6
nonmedicinal	T52.ØX1	T52.ØX2	T52.ØX3	T52.ØX4	—	—
Paraformaldehyde	T6Ø.3X1	T6Ø.3X2	T6Ø.3X3	T6Ø.3X4	—	—
Paraldehyde	T42.6X1	T42.6X2	T42.6X3	T42.6X4	T42.6X5	T42.6X6
Paramethadione	T42.2X1	T42.2X2	T42.2X3	T42.2X4	T42.2X5	T42.2X6
Paramethasone	T38.ØX1	T38.ØX2	T38.ØX3	T38.ØX4	T38.ØX5	T38.ØX6
acetate	T49.ØX1	T49.ØX2	T49.ØX3	T49.ØX4	T49.ØX5	T49.ØX6
Paraoxon	T6Ø.ØX1	T6Ø.ØX2	T6Ø.ØX3	T6Ø.ØX4	—	—
Paraquat	T6Ø.3X1	T6Ø.3X2	T6Ø.3X3	T6Ø.3X4	—	—
Parasympatholytic NEC	T44.3X1	T44.3X2	T44.3X3	T44.3X4	T44.3X5	T44.3X6
Parasympathomimetic drug NEC	T44.1X1	T44.1X2	T44.1X3	T44.1X4	T44.1X5	T44.1X6
Parathion	T6Ø.ØX1	T6Ø.ØX2	T6Ø.ØX3	T6Ø.ØX4	—	—
Parathormone	T5Ø.991	T5Ø.992	T5Ø.993	T5Ø.994	T5Ø.995	T5Ø.996
Parathyroid extract	T5Ø.991	T5Ø.992	T5Ø.993	T5Ø.994	T5Ø.995	T5Ø.996
Paratyphoid vaccine	T5Ø.A91	T5Ø.A92	T5Ø.A93	T5Ø.A94	T5Ø.A95	T5Ø.A96
Paredrine	T44.4X1	T44.4X2	T44.4X3	T44.4X4	T44.4X5	T44.4X6
Paregoric	T4Ø.ØX1	T4Ø.ØX2	T4Ø.ØX3	T4Ø.ØX4	T4Ø.ØX5	T4Ø.ØX6
Pargyline	T46.5X1	T46.5X2	T46.5X3	T46.5X4	T46.5X5	T46.5X6
Paris green	T57.ØX1	T57.ØX2	T57.ØX3	T57.ØX4	—	—
insecticide	T57.ØX1	T57.ØX2	T57.ØX3	T57.ØX4	—	—
Parnate	T43.1X1	T43.1X2	T43.1X3	T43.1X4	T43.1X5	T43.1X6
Paromomycin	T36.5X1	T36.5X2	T36.5X3	T36.5X4	T36.5X5	T36.5X6
Paroxypropione	T45.1X1	T45.1X2	T45.1X3	T45.1X4	T45.1X5	T45.1X6
Parzone	T4Ø.2X1	T4Ø.2X2	T4Ø.2X3	T4Ø.2X4	T4Ø.2X5	T4Ø.2X6
PAS	T37.1X1	T37.1X2	T37.1X3	T37.1X4	T37.1X5	T37.1X6
Pasiniazid	T37.1X1	T37.1X2	T37.1X3	T37.1X4	T37.1X5	T37.1X6
PBB (polybrominated biphenyls)	T65.891	T65.892	T65.893	T65.894	—	—
PCB	T65.891	T65.892	T65.893	T65.894	—	—
PCP						
meaning pentachlorophenol	T6Ø.1X1	T6Ø.1X2	T6Ø.1X3	T6Ø.1X4	—	—
fungicide	T6Ø.3X1	T6Ø.3X2	T6Ø.3X3	T6Ø.3X4	—	—
herbicide	T6Ø.3X1	T6Ø.3X2	T6Ø.3X3	T6Ø.3X4	—	—
insecticide	T6Ø.1X1	T6Ø.1X2	T6Ø.1X3	T6Ø.1X4	—	—
meaning phencyclidine	T4Ø.991	T4Ø.992	T4Ø.993	T4Ø.994	—	—
Peach kernel oil (emulsion)	T47.4X1	T47.4X2	T47.4X3	T47.4X4	T47.4X5	T47.4X6
Peanut oil (emulsion) NEC	T47.4X1	T47.4X2	T47.4X3	T47.4X4	T47.4X5	T47.4X6
topical	T49.3X1	T49.3X2	T49.3X3	T49.3X4	T49.3X5	T49.3X6
Pearly Gates (morning glory seeds)	T4Ø.991	T4Ø.992	T4Ø.993	T4Ø.994	—	—
Pecazine	T43.3X1	T43.3X2	T43.3X3	T43.3X4	T43.3X5	T43.3X6
Pectin	T47.6X1	T47.6X2	T47.6X3	T47.6X4	T47.6X5	T47.6X6

TABLE OF DRUGS AND CHEMICALS

Substance	Poisoning, Accidental (Unintentional)	Poisoning, Intentional Self-Harm	Poisoning, Assault	Poisoning, Undetermined	Adverse Effect	Underdosing
Pefloxacin	T37.8X1	T37.8X2	T37.8X3	T37.8X4	T37.8X5	T37.8X6
Pegademase, bovine	T5Ø.Z91	T5Ø.Z92	T5Ø.Z93	T5Ø.Z94	T5Ø.Z95	T5Ø.Z96
Pelletierine tannate	T37.4X1	T37.4X2	T37.4X3	T37.4X4	T37.4X5	T37.4X6
Pemirolast (potassium)	T48.6X1	T48.6X2	T48.6X3	T48.6X4	T48.6X5	T48.6X6
Pemoline	T5Ø.7X1	T5Ø.7X2	T5Ø.7X3	T5Ø.7X4	T5Ø.7X5	T5Ø.7X6
Pempidine	T44.2X1	T44.2X2	T44.2X3	T44.2X4	T44.2X5	T44.2X6
Penamecillin	T36.ØX1	T36.ØX2	T36.ØX3	T36.ØX4	T36.ØX5	T36.ØX6
Penbutolol	T44.7X1	T44.7X2	T44.7X3	T44.7X4	T44.7X5	T44.7X6
Penethamate	T36.ØX1	T36.ØX2	T36.ØX3	T36.ØX4	T36.ØX5	T36.ØX6
Penfluridol	T43.591	T43.592	T43.593	T43.594	T43.595	T43.596
Penflutizide	T5Ø.2X1	T5Ø.2X2	T5Ø.2X3	T5Ø.2X4	T5Ø.2X5	T5Ø.2X6
Pengitoxin	T46.ØX1	T46.ØX2	T46.ØX3	T46.ØX4	T46.ØX5	T46.ØX6
Penicillamine	T5Ø.6X1	T5Ø.6X2	T5Ø.6X3	T5Ø.6X4	T5Ø.6X5	T5Ø.6X6
Penicillin (any)	T36.ØX1	T36.ØX2	T36.ØX3	T36.ØX4	T36.ØX5	T36.ØX6
Penicillinase	T45.3X1	T45.3X2	T45.3X3	T45.3X4	T45.3X5	T45.3X6
Penicilloyl polylysine	T5Ø.8X1	T5Ø.8X2	T5Ø.8X3	T5Ø.8X4	T5Ø.8X5	T5Ø.8X6
Penimepicycline	T36.4X1	T36.4X2	T36.4X3	T36.4X4	T36.4X5	T36.4X6
Pentachloroethane	T53.6X1	T53.6X2	T53.6X3	T53.6X4	—	—
Pentachloronaphthalene	T53.7X1	T53.7X2	T53.7X3	T53.7X4	—	—
Pentachlorophenol (pesticide)	T6Ø.1X1	T6Ø.1X2	T6Ø.1X3	T6Ø.1X4	—	—
fungicide	T6Ø.3X1	T6Ø.3X2	T6Ø.3X3	T6Ø.3X4	—	—
herbicide	T6Ø.3X1	T6Ø.3X2	T6Ø.3X3	T6Ø.3X4	—	—
insecticide	T6Ø.1X1	T6Ø.1X2	T6Ø.1X3	T6Ø.1X4	—	—
Pentaerythritol tetranitrate	T46.3X1	T46.3X2	T46.3X3	T46.3X4	T46.3X5	T46.3X6
Pentaerythritol	T46.3X1	T46.3X2	T46.3X3	T46.3X4	T46.3X5	T46.3X6
chloral	T42.6X1	T42.6X2	T42.6X3	T42.6X4	T42.6X5	T42.6X6
tetranitrate NEC	T46.3X1	T46.3X2	T46.3X3	T46.3X4	T46.3X5	T46.3X6
Pentagastrin	T5Ø.8X1	T5Ø.8X2	T5Ø.8X3	T5Ø.8X4	T5Ø.8X5	T5Ø.8X6
Pentalin	T53.6X1	T53.6X2	T53.6X3	T53.6X4	—	—
Pentamethonium bromide	T44.2X1	T44.2X2	T44.2X3	T44.2X4	T44.2X5	T44.2X6
Pentamidine	T37.3X1	T37.3X2	T37.3X3	T37.3X4	T37.3X5	T37.3X6
Pentanol	T51.3X1	T51.3X2	T51.3X3	T51.3X4	—	—
Pentapyrrolinium (bitartrate)	T44.2X1	T44.2X2	T44.2X3	T44.2X4	T44.2X5	T44.2X6
Pentaquine	T37.2X1	T37.2X2	T37.2X3	T37.2X4	T37.2X5	T37.2X6
Pentazocine	T4Ø.4X1	T4Ø.4X2	T4Ø.4X3	T4Ø.4X4	T4Ø.4X5	T4Ø.4X6
Pentetrazole	T5Ø.7X1	T5Ø.7X2	T5Ø.7X3	T5Ø.7X4	T5Ø.7X5	T5Ø.7X6
Penthienate bromide	T44.3X1	T44.3X2	T44.3X3	T44.3X4	T44.3X5	T44.3X6
Pentifylline	T46.7X1	T46.7X2	T46.7X3	T46.7X4	T46.7X5	T46.7X6
Pentobarbital	T42.3X1	T42.3X2	T42.3X3	T42.3X4	T42.3X5	T42.3X6
sodium	T42.3X1	T42.3X2	T42.3X3	T42.3X4	T42.3X5	T42.3X6
Pentobarbitone	T42.3X1	T42.3X2	T42.3X3	T42.3X4	T42.3X5	T42.3X6
Pentolonium tartrate	T44.2X1	T44.2X2	T44.2X3	T44.2X4	T44.2X5	T44.2X6

Substance	Poisoning, Accidental (Unintentional)	Poisoning, Intentional Self-Harm	Poisoning, Assault	Poisoning, Undetermined	Adverse Effect	Underdosing
Pentosan polysulfate (sodium)	T39.8X1	T39.8X2	T39.8X3	T39.8X4	T39.8X5	T39.8X6
Pentostatin	T45.1X1	T45.1X2	T45.1X3	T45.1X4	T45.1X5	T45.1X6
Pentothal	T41.1X1	T41.1X2	T41.1X3	T41.1X4	T41.1X5	T41.1X6
Pentoxifylline	T46.7X1	T46.7X2	T46.7X3	T46.7X4	T46.7X5	T46.7X6
Pentoxyverine	T48.3X1	T48.3X2	T48.3X3	T48.3X4	T48.3X5	T48.3X6
Pentrinat	T46.3X1	T46.3X2	T46.3X3	T46.3X4	T46.3X5	T46.3X6
Pentylenetetrazole	T5Ø.7X1	T5Ø.7X2	T5Ø.7X3	T5Ø.7X4	T5Ø.7X5	T5Ø.7X6
Pentylsalicylamide	T37.1X1	T37.1X2	T37.1X3	T37.1X4	T37.1X5	T37.1X6
Pentymal	T42.3X1	T42.3X2	T42.3X3	T42.3X4	T42.3X5	T42.3X6
Peplomycin	T45.1X1	T45.1X2	T45.1X3	T45.1X4	T45.1X5	T45.1X6
Peppermint (oil)	T47.5X1	T47.5X2	T47.5X3	T47.5X4	T47.5X5	T47.5X6
Pepsin	T47.5X1	T47.5X2	T47.5X3	T47.5X4	T47.5X5	T47.5X6
digestant	T47.5X1	T47.5X2	T47.5X3	T47.5X4	T47.5X5	T47.5X6
Pepstatin	T47.1X1	T47.1X2	T47.1X3	T47.1X4	T47.1X5	T47.1X6
Peptavlon	T5Ø.8X1	T5Ø.8X2	T5Ø.8X3	T5Ø.8X4	T5Ø.8X5	T5Ø.8X6
Perazine	T43.3X1	T43.3X2	T43.3X3	T43.3X4	T43.3X5	T43.3X6
Percaine (spinal)	T41.3X1	T41.3X2	T41.3X3	T41.3X4	T41.3X5	T41.3X6
topical (surface)	T41.3X1	T41.3X2	T41.3X3	T41.3X4	T41.3X5	T41.3X6
Perchloroethylene	T53.3X1	T53.3X2	T53.3X3	T53.3X4	—	—
medicinal	T37.4X1	T37.4X2	T37.4X3	T37.4X4	T37.4X5	T37.4X6
vapor	T53.3X1	T53.3X2	T53.3X3	T53.3X4	—	—
Percodan	T4Ø.2X1	T4Ø.2X2	T4Ø.2X3	T4Ø.2X4	T4Ø.2X5	T4Ø.2X6
Percogesic — *see also acetaminophen*	T45.ØX1	T45.ØX2	T45.ØX3	T45.ØX4	T45.ØX5	T45.ØX6
Percorten	T38.ØX1	T38.ØX2	T38.ØX3	T38.ØX4	T38.ØX5	T38.ØX6
Pergolide	T42.8X1	T42.8X2	T42.8X3	T42.8X4	T42.8X5	T42.8X6
Pergonal	T38.811	T38.812	T38.813	T38.814	T38.815	T38.816
Perhexilene	T46.3X1	T46.3X2	T46.3X3	T46.3X4	T46.3X5	T46.3X6
Perhexiline (maleate)	T46.3X1	T46.3X2	T46.3X3	T46.3X4	T46.3X5	T46.3X6
Periactin	T45.ØX1	T45.ØX2	T45.ØX3	T45.ØX4	T45.ØX5	T45.ØX6
Periciazine	T43.3X1	T43.3X2	T43.3X3	T43.3X4	T43.3X5	T43.3X6
Periclor	T42.6X1	T42.6X2	T42.6X3	T42.6X4	T42.6X5	T42.6X6
Perindopril	T46.4X1	T46.4X2	T46.4X3	T46.4X4	T46.4X5	T46.4X6
Perisoxal	T39.8X1	T39.8X2	T39.8X3	T39.8X4	T39.8X5	T39.8X6
Peritrate	T46.3X1	T46.3X2	T46.3X3	T46.3X4	T46.3X5	T46.3X6
Peritoneal dialysis solution	T5Ø.3X1	T5Ø.3X2	T5Ø.3X3	T5Ø.3X4	T5Ø.3X5	T5Ø.3X6
Perlapine	T42.4X1	T42.4X2	T42.4X3	T42.4X4	T42.4X5	T42.4X6
Permanganate	T65.891	T65.892	T65.893	T65.894	—	—
Permethrin	T6Ø.1X1	T6Ø.1X2	T6Ø.1X3	T6Ø.1X4	—	—
Pernocton	T42.3X1	T42.3X2	T42.3X3	T42.3X4	T42.3X5	T42.3X6
Pernoston	T42.3X1	T42.3X2	T42.3X3	T42.3X4	T42.3X5	T42.3X6
Peronine	T4Ø.2X1	T4Ø.2X2	T4Ø.2X3	T4Ø.2X4	—	—
Perphenazine	T43.3X1	T43.3X2	T43.3X3	T43.3X4	T43.3X5	T43.3X6

Substance	Poisoning, Accidental (Unintentional)	Poisoning, Intentional Self-Harm	Poisoning, Assault	Poisoning, Undetermined	Adverse Effect	Underdosing
Pertofrane	T43.Ø11	T43.Ø12	T43.Ø13	T43.Ø14	T43.Ø15	T43.Ø16
Pertussis						
immune serum (human)	T5Ø.Z11	T5Ø.Z12	T5Ø.Z13	T5Ø.Z14	T5Ø.Z15	T5Ø.Z16
vaccine (with diphtheria toxoid) (with tetanus toxoid)	T5Ø.A11	T5Ø.A12	T5Ø.A13	T5Ø.A14	T5Ø.A15	T5Ø.A16
Peruvian balsam	T49.ØX1	T49.ØX2	T49.ØX3	T49.ØX4	T49.ØX5	T49.ØX6
Peruvoside	T46.ØX1	T46.ØX2	T46.ØX3	T46.ØX4	T46.ØX5	T46.ØX6
Pesticide (dust) (fumes) (vapor) NEC	T6Ø.91	T6Ø.92	T6Ø.93	T6Ø.94	—	—
arsenic	T57.ØX1	T57.ØX2	T57.ØX3	T57.ØX4	—	—
chlorinated	T6Ø.1X1	T6Ø.1X2	T6Ø.1X3	T6Ø.1X4	—	—
cyanide	T65.ØX1	T65.ØX2	T65.ØX3	T65.ØX4	—	—
kerosene	T52.ØX1	T52.ØX2	T52.ØX3	T52.ØX4	—	—
mixture (of compounds)	T6Ø.91	T6Ø.92	T6Ø.93	T6Ø.94	—	—
naphthalene	T6Ø.2X1	T6Ø.2X2	T6Ø.2X3	T6Ø.2X4	—	—
organochlorine (compounds)	T6Ø.1X1	T6Ø.1X2	T6Ø.1X3	T6Ø.1X4	—	—
petroleum (distillate) (products) NEC	T6Ø.8X1	T6Ø.8X2	T6Ø.8X3	T6Ø.8X4	—	—
specified ingredient NEC	T6Ø.8X1.	T6Ø.8X2	T6Ø.8X3	T6Ø.8X4	—	—
strychnine	T65.1X1	T65.1X2	T65.1X3	T65.1X4	—	—
thallium	T6Ø.4X1	T6Ø.4X2	T6Ø.4X3	T6Ø.4X4	—	—
Pethidine	T4Ø.4X1	T4Ø.4X2	T4Ø.4X3	T4Ø.4X4	T4Ø.4X5	T4Ø.4X6
Petrichloral	T42.6X1	T42.6X2	T42.6X3	T42.6X4	T42.6X5	T42.6X6
Petrol	T52.ØX1	T52.ØX2	T52.ØX3	T52.ØX4	—	—
vapor	T52.ØX1	T52.ØX2	T52.ØX3	T52.ØX4	—	—
Petrolatum	T49.3X1	T49.3X2	T49.3X3	T49.3X4	T49.3X5	T49.3X6
hydrophilic	T49.3X1	T49.3X2	T49.3X3	T49.3X4	T49.3X5	T49.3X6
liquid	T47.4X1	T47.4X2	T47.4X3	T47.4X4	T47.4X5	T47.4X6
topical	T49.3X1	T49.3X2	T49.3X3	T49.3X4	T49.3X5	T49.3X6
nonmedicinal	T52.ØX1	T52.ØX2	T52.ØX3	T52.ØX4	—	—
red veterinary	T49.3X1	T49.3X2	T49.3X3	T49.3X4	T49.3X5	T49.3X6
white	T49.3X1	T49.3X2	T49.3X3	T49.3X4	T49.3X5	T49.3X6
Petroleum (products) NEC	T52.ØX1	T52.ØX2	T52.ØX3	T52.ØX4	—	—
benzine(s) — *see Ligroin*						
ether — *see Ligroin*						
jelly — *see Petrolatum*						
naphtha — *see Ligroin*						
pesticide	T6Ø.8X1	T6Ø.8X2	T6Ø.8X3	T6Ø.8X4	—	—
solids	T52.ØX1	T52.ØX2	T52.ØX3	T52.ØX4	—	—
solvents	T52.ØX1	T52.ØX2	T52.ØX3	T52.ØX4	—	—
vapor	T52.ØX1	T52.ØX2	T52.ØX3	T52.ØX4	—	—
Peyote	T4Ø.991	T4Ø.992	T4Ø.993	T4Ø.994	—	—
Phanodorm, phanodorn	T42.3X1	T42.3X2	T42.3X3	T42.3X4	T42.3X5	T42.3X6
Phanquinone	T37.3X1	T37.3X2	T37.3X3	T37.3X4	T37.3X5	T37.3X6
Phanquone	T37.3X1	T37.3X2	T37.3X3	T37.3X4	T37.3X5	T37.3X6
Pharmaceutical						
adjunct NEC	T5Ø.9Ø1	T5Ø.9Ø2	T5Ø.9Ø3	T5Ø.9Ø4	T5Ø.9Ø5	T5Ø.9Ø6
excipient NEC	T5Ø.9Ø1	T5Ø.9Ø2	T5Ø.9Ø3	T5Ø.9Ø4	T5Ø.9Ø5	T5Ø.9Ø6
sweetener	T5Ø.9Ø1	T5Ø.9Ø2	T5Ø.9Ø3	T5Ø.9Ø4	T5Ø.9Ø5	T5Ø.9Ø6
viscous agent	T5Ø.9Ø1	T5Ø.9Ø2	T5Ø.9Ø3	T5Ø.9Ø4	T5Ø.9Ø5	T5Ø.9Ø6
Phemitone	T42.3X1	T42.3X2	T42.3X3	T42.3X4	T42.3X5	T42.3X6
Phenacaine	T41.3X1	T41.3X2	T41.3X3	T41.3X4	T41.3X5	T41.3X6
Phenacemide	T42.6X1	T42.6X2	T42.6X3	T42.6X4	T42.6X5	T42.6X6
Phenacetin	T39.1X1	T39.1X2	T39.1X3	T39.1X4	T39.1X5	T39.1X6
Phenadoxone	T4Ø.2X1	T4Ø.2X2	T4Ø.2X3	T4Ø.2X4	—	—
Phenaglycodol	T43.591	T43.592	T43.593	T43.594	T43.595	T43.596
Phenantoin	T42.ØX1	T42.ØX2	T42.ØX3	T42.ØX4	T42.ØX5	T42.ØX6
Phenaphthazine reagent	T5Ø.991	T5Ø.992	T5Ø.993	T5Ø.994	T5Ø.995	T5Ø.996
Phenazocine	T4Ø.4X1	T4Ø.4X2	T4Ø.4X3	T4Ø.4X4	T4Ø.4X5	T4Ø.4X6
Phenazone	T39.2X1	T39.2X2	T39.2X3	T39.2X4	T39.2X5	T39.2X6
Phenazopyridine	T39.8X1	T39.8X2	T39.8X3	T39.8X4	T39.8X5	T39.8X6
Phenbenicillin	T36.ØX1	T36.ØX2	T36.ØX3	T36.ØX4	T36.ØX5	T36.ØX6
Phenbutrazate	T5Ø.5X1	T5Ø.5X2	T5Ø.5X3	T5Ø.5X4	T5Ø.5X5	T5Ø.5X6
Phencyclidine	T4Ø.991	T4Ø.992	T4Ø.993	T4Ø.994	T4Ø.995	T4Ø.996
Phendimetrazine	T5Ø.5X1	T5Ø.5X2	T5Ø.5X3	T5Ø.5X4	T5Ø.5X5	T5Ø.5X6
Phenelzine	T43.1X1	T43.1X2	T43.1X3	T43.1X4	T43.1X5	T43.1X6
Phenemal	T42.3X1	T42.3X2	T42.3X3	T42.3X4	T42.3X5	T42.3X6
Phenergan	T42.6X1	T42.6X2	T42.6X3	T42.6X4	T42.6X5	T42.6X6
Pheneticillin	T36.ØX1	T36.ØX2	T36.ØX3	T36.ØX4	T36.ØX5	T36.ØX6
Pheneturide	T42.6X1	T42.6X2	T42.6X3	T42.6X4	T42.6X5	T42.6X6
Phenformin	T38.3X1	T38.3X2	T38.3X3	T38.3X4	T38.3X5	T38.3X6
Phenglutarimide	T44.3X1	T44.3X2	T44.3X3	T44.3X4	T44.3X5	T44.3X6
Phenicarbazide	T39.8X1	T39.8X2	T39.8X3	T39.8X4	T39.8X5	T39.8X6
Phenindamine	T45.ØX1	T45.ØX2	T45.ØX3	T45.ØX4	T45.ØX5	T45.ØX6
Phenindione	T45.511	T45.512	T45.513	T45.514	T45.515	T45.516
Pheniprazine	T43.1X1	T43.1X2	T43.1X3	T43.1X4	T43.1X5	T43.1X6
Pheniramine	T45.ØX1	T45.ØX2	T45.ØX3	T45.ØX4	T45.ØX5	T45.ØX6
Phenisatin	T47.2X1	T47.2X2	T47.2X3	T47.2X4	T47.2X5	T47.2X6
Phenmetrazine	T5Ø.5X1	T5Ø.5X2	T5Ø.5X3	T5Ø.5X4	T5Ø.5X5	T5Ø.5X6
Phenobal	T42.3X1	T42.3X2	T42.3X3	T42.3X4	T42.3X5	T42.3X6
Phenobarbital	T42.3X1	T42.3X2	T42.3X3	T42.3X4	T42.3X5	T42.3X6
with						
mephenytoin	T42.3X1	T42.3X2	T42.3X3	T42.3X4	T42.3X5	T42.3X6
phenytoin	T42.3X1	T42.3X2	T42.3X3	T42.3X4	T42.3X5	T42.3X6
sodium	T42.3X1	T42.3X2	T42.3X3	T42.3X4	T42.3X5	T42.3X6

Substance	Poisoning, Accidental (Unintentional)	Poisoning, Intentional Self-Harm	Poisoning, Assault	Poisoning, Undetermined	Adverse Effect	Underdosing
Phenobarbitone	T42.3X1	T42.3X2	T42.3X3	T42.3X4	T42.3X5	T42.3X6
Phenobutiodil	T50.8X1	T50.8X2	T50.8X3	T50.8X4	T50.8X5	T50.8X6
Phenoctide	T49.0X1	T49.0X2	T49.0X3	T49.0X4	T49.0X5	T49.0X6
Phenol	T49.0X1	T49.0X2	T49.0X3	T49.0X4	T49.0X5	T49.0X6
disinfectant	T54.0X1	T54.0X2	T54.0X3	T54.0X4	—	—
in oil injection	T46.8X1	T46.8X2	T46.8X3	T46.8X4	T46.8X5	T46.8X6
medicinal	T49.1X1	T49.1X2	T49.1X3	T49.1X4	T49.1X5	T49.1X6
nonmedicinal NEC	T54.0X1	T54.0X2	T54.0X3	T54.0X4	—	—
pesticide	T60.8X1	T60.8X2	T60.8X3	T60.8X4	—	—
red	T50.8X1	T50.8X2	T50.8X3	T50.8X4	T50.8X5	T50.8X6
Phenolic preparation	T49.1X1	T49.1X2	T49.1X3	T49.1X4	T49.1X5	T49.1X6
Phenolphthalein	T47.2X1	T47.2X2	T47.2X3	T47.2X4	T47.2X5	T47.2X6
Phenolsulfonphthalein	T50.8X1	T50.8X2	T50.8X3	T50.8X4	T50.8X5	T50.8X6
Phenomorphan	T40.2X1	T40.2X2	T40.2X3	T40.2X4	—	—
Phenonyl	T42.3X1	T42.3X2	T42.3X3	T42.3X4	T42.3X5	T42.3X6
Phenoperidine	T40.4X1	T40.4X2	T40.4X3	T40.4X4	—	—
Phenopyrazone	T46.991	T46.992	T46.993	T46.994	T46.995	T46.996
Phenoquin	T50.4X1	T50.4X2	T50.4X3	T50.4X4	T50.4X5	T50.4X6
Phenothiazine (psychotropic) NEC	T43.3X1	T43.3X2	T43.3X3	T43.3X4	T43.3X5	T43.3X6
insecticide	T60.2X1	T60.2X2	T60.2X3	T60.2X4	—	—
Phenothrin	T49.0X1	T49.0X2	T49.0X3	T49.0X4	T49.0X5	T49.0X6
Phenoxybenzamine	T46.7X1	T46.7X2	T46.7X3	T46.7X4	T46.7X5	T46.7X6
Phenoxyethanol	T49.0X1	T49.0X2	T49.0X3	T49.0X4	T49.0X5	T49.0X6
Phenoxymethyl penicillin	T36.0X1	T36.0X2	T36.0X3	T36.0X4	T36.0X5	T36.0X6
Phenprobamate	T42.8X1	T42.8X2	T42.8X3	T42.8X4	T42.8X5	T42.8X6
Phenprocoumon	T45.511	T45.512	T45.513	T45.514	T45.515	T45.516
Phensuximide	T42.2X1	T42.2X2	T42.2X3	T42.2X4	T42.2X5	T42.2X6
Phentermine	T50.5X1	T50.5X2	T50.5X3	T50.5X4	T50.5X5	T50.5X6
Phenthicillin	T36.0X1	T36.0X2	T36.0X3	T36.0X4	T36.0X5	T36.0X6
Phentolamine	T46.7X1	T46.7X2	T46.7X3	T46.7X4	T46.7X5	T46.7X6
Phenyl						
butazone	T39.2X1	T39.2X2	T39.2X3	T39.2X4	T39.2X5	T39.2X6
enediamine	T65.3X1	T65.3X2	T65.3X3	T65.3X4	—	—
hydrazine	T65.3X1	T65.3X2	T65.3X3	T65.3X4	—	—
antineoplastic	T45.1X1	T45.1X2	T45.1X3	T45.1X4	T45.1X5	T45.1X6
mercuric compounds — *see Mercury*						
salicylate	T49.3X1	T49.3X2	T49.3X3	T49.3X4	T49.3X5	T49.3X6
Phenylalanine mustard	T45.1X1	T45.1X2	T45.1X3	T45.1X4	T45.1X5	T45.1X6
Phenylbutazone	T39.2X1	T39.2X2	T39.2X3	T39.2X4	T39.2X5	T39.2X6
Phenylenediamine	T65.3X1	T65.3X2	T65.3X3	T65.3X4	—	—
Phenylephrine	T44.4X1	T44.4X2	T44.4X3	T44.4X4	T44.4X5	T44.4X6

Substance	Poisoning, Accidental (Unintentional)	Poisoning, Intentional Self-Harm	Poisoning, Assault	Poisoning, Undetermined	Adverse Effect	Underdosing
Phenylethylbiguanide	T38.3X1	T38.3X2	T38.3X3	T38.3X4	T38.3X5	T38.3X6
Phenylmercuric						
acetate	T49.0X1	T49.0X2	T49.0X3	T49.0X4	T49.0X5	T49.0X6
borate	T49.0X1	T49.0X2	T49.0X3	T49.0X4	T49.0X5	T49.0X6
nitrate	T49.0X1	T49.0X2	T49.0X3	T49.0X4	T49.0X5	T49.0X6
Phenylmethylbarbitone	T42.3X1	T42.3X2	T42.3X3	T42.3X4	T42.3X5	T42.3X6
Phenylpropanol	T47.5X1	T47.5X2	T47.5X3	T47.5X4	T47.5X5	T47.5X6
Phenylpropanolamine	T44.991	T44.992	T44.993	T44.994	T44.995	T44.996
Phenylsulfthion	T60.0X1	T60.0X2	T60.0X3	T60.0X4	—	—
Phenyltoloxamine	T45.0X1	T45.0X2	T45.0X3	T45.0X4	T45.0X5	T45.0X6
Phenyramidol, phenyramidon	T39.8X1	T39.8X2	T39.8X3	T39.8X4	T39.8X5	T39.8X6
Phenytoin	T42.0X1	T42.0X2	T42.0X3	T42.0X4	T42.0X5	T42.0X6
with Phenobarbital	T42.3X1	T42.3X2	T42.3X3	T42.3X4	T42.3X5	T42.3X6
pHisoHex	T49.2X1	T49.2X2	T49.2X3	T49.2X4	T49.2X5	T49.2X6
Pholcodine	T48.3X1	T48.3X2	T48.3X3	T48.3X4	T48.3X5	T48.3X6
Pholedrine	T46.991	T46.992	T46.993	T46.994	T46.995	T46.996
Phorate	T60.0X1	T60.0X2	T60.0X3	T60.0X4	—	—
Phosdrin	T60.0X1	T60.0X2	T60.0X3	T60.0X4	—	—
Phosfolan	T60.0X1	T60.0X2	T60.0X3	T60.0X4	—	—
Phosgene (gas)	T59.891	T59.892	T59.893	T59.894	—	—
Phosphamidon	T60.0X1	T60.0X2	T60.0X3	T60.0X4	—	—
Phosphate	T65.891	T65.892	T65.893	T65.894	—	—
laxative	T47.4X1	T47.4X2	T47.4X3	T47.4X4	T47.4X5	T47.4X6
organic	T60.0X1	T60.0X2	T60.0X3	T60.0X4	—	—
solvent	T52.91	T52.92	T52.93	T52.94	—	—
tricresyl	T65.891	T65.892	T65.893	T65.894	—	—
Phosphine	T57.1X1	T57.1X2	T57.1X3	T57.1X4	—	—
fumigant	T57.1X1	T57.1X2	T57.1X3	T57.1X4	—	—
Phospholine	T49.5X1	T49.5X2	T49.5X3	T49.5X4	T49.5X5	T49.5X6
Phosphoric acid	T54.2X1	T54.2X2	T54.2X3	T54.2X4	—	—
Phosphorus (compound) NEC	T57.1X1	T57.1X2	T57.1X3	T57.1X4	—	—
pesticide	T60.0X1	T60.0X2	T60.0X3	T60.0X4	—	—
Phthalates	T65.891	T65.892	T65.893	T65.894	—	—
Phthalic anhydride	T65.891	T65.892	T65.893	T65.894	—	—
Phthalimidoglutarimide	T42.6X1	T42.6X2	T42.6X3	T42.6X4	T42.6X5	T42.6X6
Phthalylsulfathiazole	T37.0X1	T37.0X2	T37.0X3	T37.0X4	T37.0X5	T37.0X6
Phylloquinone	T45.7X1	T45.7X2	T45.7X3	T45.7X4	T45.7X5	T45.7X6
Physeptone	T40.3X1	T40.3X2	T40.3X3	T40.3X4	T40.3X5	T40.3X6
Physostigma venenosum	T62.2X1	T62.2X2	T62.2X3	T62.2X4	—	—
Physostigmine	T49.5X1	T49.5X2	T49.5X3	T49.5X4	T49.5X5	T49.5X6
Phytolacca decandra	T62.2X1	T62.2X2	T62.2X3	T62.2X4	—	—
berries	T62.1X1	T62.1X2	T62.1X3	T62.1X4	—	—

◀ New ⬅ Revised ~~deleted~~ Deleted

Substance	Poisoning, Accidental (Unintentional)	Poisoning, Intentional Self-Harm	Poisoning, Assault	Poisoning, Undetermined	Adverse Effect	Underdosing
Phytomenadione	T45.7X1	T45.7X2	T45.7X3	T45.7X4	T45.7X5	T45.7X6
Phytonadione	T45.7X1	T45.7X2	T45.7X3	T45.7X4	T45.7X5	T45.7X6
Picoperine	T48.3X1	T48.3X2	T48.3X3	T48.3X4	T48.3X5	T48.3X6
Picosulfate (sodium)	T47.2X1	T47.2X2	T47.2X3	T47.2X4	T47.2X5	T47.2X6
Picric (acid)	T54.2X1	T54.2X2	T54.2X3	T54.2X4	—	—
Picrotoxin	T50.7X1	T50.7X2	T50.7X3	T50.7X4	T50.7X5	T50.7X6
Piketoprofen	T49.0X1	T49.0X2	T49.0X3	T49.0X4	T49.0X5	T49.0X6
Pilocarpine	T44.1X1	T44.1X2	T44.1X3	T44.1X4	T44.1X5	T44.1X6
Pilocarpus (jaborandi) extract	T44.1X1	T44.1X2	T44.1X3	T44.1X4	T44.1X5	T44.1X6
Pilsicainide (hydrochloride)	T46.2X1	T46.2X2	T46.2X3	T46.2X4	T46.2X5	T46.2X6
Pimaricin	T36.7X1	T36.7X2	T36.7X3	T36.7X4	T36.7X5	T36.7X6
Pimeclone	T50.7X1	T50.7X2	T50.7X3	T50.7X4	T50.7X5	T50.7X6
Pimelic ketone	T52.8X1	T52.8X2	T52.8X3	T52.8X4	—	—
Pimethixene	T45.0X1	T45.0X2	T45.0X3	T45.0X4	T45.0X5	T45.0X6
Piminodine	T40.2X1	T40.2X2	T40.2X3	T40.2X4	T40.2X5	T40.2X6
Pimozide	T43.591	T43.592	T43.593	T43.594	T43.595	T43.596
Pinacidil	T46.5X1	T46.5X2	T46.5X3	T46.5X4	T46.5X5	T46.5X6
Pinaverium bromide	T44.3X1	T44.3X2	T44.3X3	T44.3X4	T44.3X5	T44.3X6
Pinazepam	T42.4X1	T42.4X2	T42.4X3	T42.4X4	T42.4X5	T42.4X6
Pindolol	T44.7X1	T44.7X2	T44.7X3	T44.7X4	T44.7X5	T44.7X6
Pindone	T60.4X1	T60.4X2	T60.4X3	T60.4X4	—	—
Pine oil (disinfectant)	T65.891	T65.892	T65.893	T65.894	—	—
Pinkroot	T37.4X1	T37.4X2	T37.4X3	T37.4X4	T37.4X5	T37.4X6
Pipadone	T40.2X1	T40.2X2	T40.2X3	T40.2X4	—	—
Pipamazine	T45.0X1	T45.0X2	T45.0X3	T45.0X4	T45.0X5	T45.0X6
Pipamperone	T43.4X1	T43.4X2	T43.4X3	T43.4X4	T43.4X5	T43.4X6
Pipazetate	T48.3X1	T48.3X2	T48.3X3	T48.3X4	T48.3X5	T48.3X6
Pipemidic acid	T37.8X1	T37.8X2	T37.8X3	T37.8X4	T37.8X5	T37.8X6
Pipenzolate bromide	T44.3X1	T44.3X2	T44.3X3	T44.3X4	T44.3X5	T44.3X6
Piperacetazine	T43.3X1	T43.3X2	T43.3X3	T43.3X4	T43.3X5	T43.3X6
Piperacillin	T36.0X1	T36.0X2	T36.0X3	T36.0X4	T36.0X5	T36.0X6
Piperazine	T37.4X1	T37.4X2	T37.4X3	T37.4X4	T37.4X5	T37.4X6
estrone sulfate	T38.5X1	T38.5X2	T38.5X3	T38.5X4	T38.5X5	T38.5X6
Piper cubeba	T62.2X1	T62.2X2	T62.2X3	T62.2X4	—	—
Piperidione	T48.3X1	T48.3X2	T48.3X3	T48.3X4	—	—
Piperidolate	T44.3X1	T44.3X2	T44.3X3	T44.3X4	T44.3X5	T44.3X6
Piperocaine	T41.3X1	T41.3X2	T41.3X3	T41.3X4	T41.3X5	T41.3X6
infiltration (subcutaneous)	T41.3X1	T41.3X2	T41.3X3	T41.3X4	T41.3X5	T41.3X6
nerve block (peripheral) (plexus)	T41.3X1	T41.3X2	T41.3X3	T41.3X4	T41.3X5	T41.3X6
topical (surface)	T41.3X1	T41.3X2	T41.3X3	T41.3X4	T41.3X5	T41.3X6
Piperonyl butoxide	T60.8X1	T60.8X2	T60.8X3	T60.8X4	—	—
Pipethanate	T44.3X1	T44.3X2	T44.3X3	T44.3X4	T44.3X5	T44.3X6

Substance	Poisoning, Accidental (Unintentional)	Poisoning, Intentional Self-Harm	Poisoning, Assault	Poisoning, Undetermined	Adverse Effect	Underdosing
Pipobroman	T45.1X1	T45.1X2	T45.1X3	T45.1X4	T45.1X5	T45.1X6
Pipofezine	T43.0X1	T43.0X2	T43.0X3	T43.0X4	T43.0X5	T43.0X6
Pipotiazine	T43.3X1	T43.3X2	T43.3X3	T43.3X4	T43.3X5	T43.3X6
Pipoxizine	T45.0X1	T45.0X2	T45.0X3	T45.0X4	T45.0X5	T45.0X6
Pipradrol	T43.691	T43.692	T43.693	T43.694	T43.695	T43.696
Piprinhydrinate	T45.0X1	T45.0X2	T45.0X3	T45.0X4	T45.0X5	T45.0X6
Pirarubicin	T45.1X1	T45.1X2	T45.1X3	T45.1X4	T45.1X5	T45.1X6
Pirazinamide	T37.1X1	T37.1X2	T37.1X3	T37.1X4	T37.1X5	T37.1X6
Pirbuterol	T48.6X1	T48.6X2	T48.6X3	T48.6X4	T48.6X5	T48.6X6
Pirenzepine	T47.1X1	T47.1X2	T47.1X3	T47.1X4	T47.1X5	T47.1X6
Piretanide	T50.1X1	T50.1X2	T50.1X3	T50.1X4	T50.1X5	T50.1X6
Piribedil	T42.8X1	T42.8X2	T42.8X3	T42.8X4	T42.8X5	T42.8X6
Piridoxilate	T46.3X1	T46.3X2	T46.3X3	T46.3X4	T46.3X5	T46.3X6
Piritramide	T40.4X1	T40.4X2	T40.4X3	T40.4X4	—	—
Pirlindole	T43.0X1	T43.0X2	T43.0X3	T43.0X4	T43.0X5	T43.0X6
Piromidic acid	T37.8X1	T37.8X2	T37.8X3	T37.8X4	T37.8X5	T37.8X6
Piroxicam	T39.391	T39.392	T39.393	T39.394	T39.395	T39.396
beta-cyclodextrin complex	T39.8X1	T39.8X2	T39.8X3	T39.8X4	T39.8X5	T39.8X6
Pirozadil	T46.6X1	T46.6X2	T46.6X3	T46.6X4	T46.6X5	T46.6X6
Piscidia (bark) (erythrina)	T39.8X1	T39.8X2	T39.8X3	T39.8X4	T39.8X5	T39.8X6
Pitch	T65.891	T65.892	T65.893	T65.894	—	—
Pitkin's solution	T41.3X1	T41.3X2	T41.3X3	T41.3X4	T41.3X5	T41.3X6
Pitocin	T48.0X1	T48.0X2	T48.0X3	T48.0X4	T48.0X5	T48.0X6
Pitressin (tannate)	T38.891	T38.892	T38.893	T38.894	T38.895	T38.896
Pituitary extracts (posterior)	T38.891	T38.892	T38.893	T38.894	T38.895	T38.896
anterior	T38.811	T38.812	T38.813	T38.814	T38.815	T38.816
Pituitrin	T38.891	T38.892	T38.893	T38.894	T38.895	T38.896
Pivampicillin	T36.0X1	T36.0X2	T36.0X3	T36.0X4	T36.0X5	T36.0X6
Pivmecillinam	T36.0X1	T36.0X2	T36.0X3	T36.0X4	T36.0X5	T36.0X6
Placental hormone	T38.891	T38.892	T38.893	T38.894	T38.895	T38.896
Placidyl	T42.6X1	T42.6X2	T42.6X3	T42.6X4	T42.6X5	T42.6X6
Plague vaccine	T50.A91	T50.A92	T50.A93	T50.A94	T50.A95	T50.A96
Plant						
food or fertilizer NEC	T65.891	T65.892	T65.893	T65.894	—	—
containing herbicide	T60.3X1	T60.3X2	T60.3X3	T60.3X4	—	—
noxious, used as food	T62.2X1	T62.2X2	T62.2X3	T62.2X4	—	—
berries	T62.1X1	T62.1X2	T62.1X3	T62.1X4	—	—
seeds	T62.2X1	T62.2X2	T62.2X3	T62.2X4	—	—
specified type NEC	T62.2X1	T62.2X2	T62.2X3	T62.2X4	—	—
Plasma	T45.8X1	T45.8X2	T45.8X3	T45.8X4	T45.8X5	T45.8X6
expander NEC	T45.8X1	T45.8X2	T45.8X3	T45.8X4	T45.8X5	T45.8X6
protein fraction (human)	T45.8X1	T45.8X2	T45.8X3	T45.8X4	T45.8X5	T45.8X6

Substance	Poisoning, Accidental (Unintentional)	Poisoning, Intentional Self-Harm	Poisoning, Assault	Poisoning, Undetermined	Adverse Effect	Underdosing
Plasmanate	T45.8X1	T45.8X2	T45.8X3	T45.8X4	T45.8X5	T45.8X6
Plasminogen (tissue) activator	T45.611	T45.612	T45.613	T45.614	T45.615	T45.616
Plaster dressing	T49.3X1	T49.3X2	T49.3X3	T49.3X4	T49.3X5	T49.3X6
Plastic dressing	T49.3X1	T49.3X2	T49.3X3	T49.3X4	T49.3X5	T49.3X6
Plegicil	T43.3X1	T43.3X2	T43.3X3	T43.3X4	T43.3X5	T43.3X6
Plicamycin	T45.1X1	T45.1X2	T45.1X3	T45.1X4	T45.1X5	T45.1X6
Podophyllotoxin	T49.8X1	T49.8X2	T49.8X3	T49.8X4	T49.8X5	T49.8X6
Podophyllum (resin)	T49.4X1	T49.4X2	T49.4X3	T49.4X4	T49.4X5	T49.4X6
Poison NEC	T65.91	T65.92	T65.93	T65.94	—	—
Poisonous berries	T62.1X1	T62.1X2	T62.1X3	T62.1X4	—	—
Pokeweed (any part)	T62.2X1	T62.2X2	T62.2X3	T62.2X4	—	—
Poldine metilsulfate	T44.3X1	T44.3X2	T44.3X3	T44.3X4	T44.3X5	T44.3X6
Polidexide (sulfate)	T46.6X1	T46.6X2	T46.6X3	T46.6X4	T46.6X5	T46.6X6
Polidocanol	T46.8X1	T46.8X2	T46.8X3	T46.8X4	T46.8X5	T46.8X6
Poliomyelitis vaccine	T50.B91	T50.B92	T50.B93	T50.B94	T50.B95	T50.B96
Polish (car) (floor) (furniture) (metal) (porcelain) (silver)	T65.891	T65.892	T65.893	T65.894	—	—
abrasive	T65.891	T65.892	T65.893	T65.894	—	—
porcelain	T65.891	T65.892	T65.893	T65.894	—	—
Poloxalkol	T47.4X1	T47.4X2	T47.4X3	T47.4X4	T47.4X5	T47.4X6
Poloxamer	T47.4X1	T47.4X2	T47.4X3	T47.4X4	T47.4X5	T47.4X6
Polyaminostyrene resins	T50.3X1	T50.3X2	T50.3X3	T50.3X4	T50.3X5	T50.3X6
Polycarbophil	T47.4X1	T47.4X2	T47.4X3	T47.4X4	T47.4X5	T47.4X6
Polychlorinated biphenyl	T65.891	T65.892	T65.893	T65.894	—	—
Polycycline	T36.4X1	T36.4X2	T36.4X3	T36.4X4	T36.4X5	T36.4X6
Polyester fumes	T59.891	T59.892	T59.893	T59.894	—	—
Polyester resin hardener	T52.91	T52.92	T52.93	T52.94	—	—
fumes	T59.891	T59.892	T59.893	T59.894	—	—
Polyestradiol phosphate	T38.5X1	T38.5X2	T38.5X3	T38.5X4	T38.5X5	T38.5X6
Polyethanolamine alkyl sulfate	T49.2X1	T49.2X2	T49.2X3	T49.2X4	T49.2X5	T49.2X6
Polyethylene adhesive	T49.3X1	T49.3X2	T49.3X3	T49.3X4	T49.3X5	T49.3X6
Polyferose	T45.4X1	T45.4X2	T45.4X3	T45.4X4	T45.4X5	T45.4X6
Polygeline	T45.8X1	T45.8X2	T45.8X3	T45.8X4	T45.8X5	T45.8X6
Polymyxin	T36.8X1	T36.8X2	T36.8X3	T36.8X4	T36.8X5	T36.8X6
B	T36.8X1	T36.8X2	T36.8X3	T36.8X4	T36.8X5	T36.8X6
ENT agent	T49.6X1	T49.6X2	T49.6X3	T49.6X4	T49.6X5	T49.6X6
ophthalmic preparation	T49.5X1	T49.5X2	T49.5X3	T49.5X4	T49.5X5	T49.5X6
topical NEC	T49.0X1	T49.0X2	T49.0X3	T49.0X4	T49.0X5	T49.0X6
E sulfate (eye preparation)	T49.5X1	T49.5X2	T49.5X3	T49.5X4	T49.5X5	T49.5X6
Polynoxylin	T49.0X1	T49.0X2	T49.0X3	T49.0X4	T49.0X5	T49.0X6
Polyoestradiol phosphate	T38.5X1	T38.5X2	T38.5X3	T38.5X4	T38.5X5	T38.5X6
Polyoxymethyleneurea	T49.0X1	T49.0X2	T49.0X3	T49.0X4	T49.0X5	T49.0X6

Substance	Poisoning, Accidental (Unintentional)	Poisoning, Intentional Self-Harm	Poisoning, Assault	Poisoning, Undetermined	Adverse Effect	Underdosing
Polysilane	T47.8X1	T47.8X2	T47.8X3	T47.8X4	T47.8X5	T47.8X6
Polytetrafluoroethylene (inhaled)	T59.891	T59.892	T59.893	T59.894	—	—
Polythiazide	T50.2X1	T50.2X2	T50.2X3	T50.2X4	T50.2X5	T50.2X6
Polyvidone	T45.8X1	T45.8X2	T45.8X3	T45.8X4	T45.8X5	T45.8X6
Polyvinylpyrrolidone	T45.8X1	T45.8X2	T45.8X3	T45.8X4	T45.8X5	T45.8X6
Pontocaine (hydrochloride) (infiltration) (topical)	T41.3X1	T41.3X2	T41.3X3	T41.3X4	T41.3X5	T41.3X6
nerve block (peripheral) (plexus)	T41.3X1	T41.3X2	T41.3X3	T41.3X4	T41.3X5	T41.3X6
spinal	T41.3X1	T41.3X2	T41.3X3	T41.3X4	T41.3X5	T41.3X6
Porfiromycin	T45.1X1	T45.1X2	T45.1X3	T45.1X4	T45.1X5	T45.1X6
Posterior pituitary hormone NEC	T38.891	T38.892	T38.893	T38.894	T38.895	T38.896
Pot	T40.7X1	T40.7X2	T40.7X3	T40.7X4	T40.7X5	T40.7X6
Potash (caustic)	T54.3X1	T54.3X2	T54.3X3	T54.3X4	—	—
Potassic saline injection (lactated)	T50.3X1	T50.3X2	T50.3X3	T50.3X4	T50.3X5	T50.3X6
Potassium (salts) NEC	T50.3X1	T50.3X2	T50.3X3	T50.3X4	T50.3X5	T50.3X6
aminobenzoate	T45.8X1	T45.8X2	T45.8X3	T45.8X4	T45.8X5	T45.8X6
aminosalicylate	T37.1X1	T37.1X2	T37.1X3	T37.1X4	T37.1X5	T37.1X6
antimony 'tartrate'	T37.8X1	T37.8X2	T37.8X3	T37.8X4	T37.8X5	T37.8X6
arsenite (solution)	T57.0X1	T57.0X2	T57.0X3	T57.0X4	—	—
bichromate	T56.2X1	T56.2X2	T56.2X3	T56.2X4	—	—
bisulfate	T47.3X1	T47.3X2	T47.3X3	T47.3X4	T47.3X5	T47.3X6
bromide	T42.6X1	T42.6X2	T42.6X3	T42.6X4	T42.6X5	T42.6X6
canrenoate	T50.0X1	T50.0X2	T50.0X3	T50.0X4	T50.0X5	T50.0X6
carbonate	T54.3X1	T54.3X2	T54.3X3	T54.3X4	—	—
chlorate NEC	T65.891	T65.892	T65.893	T65.894	—	—
chloride	T50.3X1	T50.3X2	T50.3X3	T50.3X4	T50.3X5	T50.3X6
citrate	T50.991	T50.992	T50.993	T50.994	T50.995	T50.996
cyanide	T65.0X1	T65.0X2	T65.0X3	T65.0X4	—	—
ferric hexacyanoferrate (medicinal)	T50.6X1	T50.6X2	T50.6X3	T50.6X4	T50.6X5	T50.6X6
nonmedicinal	T65.891	T65.892	T65.893	T65.894	—	—
Fluoride	T57.8X1	T57.8X2	T57.8X3	T57.8X4	—	—
glucaldrate	T47.1X1	T47.1X2	T47.1X3	T47.1X4	T47.1X5	T47.1X6
hydroxide	T54.3X1	T54.3X2	T54.3X3	T54.3X4	—	—
iodate	T49.0X1	T49.0X2	T49.0X3	T49.0X4	T49.0X5	T49.0X6
iodide	T48.4X1	T48.4X2	T48.4X3	T48.4X4	T48.4X5	T48.4X6
nitrate	T57.8X1	T57.8X2	T57.8X3	T57.8X4	—	—
oxalate	T65.891	T65.892	T65.893	T65.894	—	—
perchlorate (nonmedicinal) NEC	T65.891	T65.892	T65.893	T65.894	—	—
antithyroid	T38.2X1	T38.2X2	T38.2X3	T38.2X4	T38.2X5	T38.2X6
medicinal	T38.2X1	T38.2X2	T38.2X3	T38.2X4	T38.2X5	T38.2X6

Substance	Poisoning, Accidental (Unintentional)	Poisoning, Intentional Self-Harm	Poisoning, Assault	Poisoning, Undetermined	Adverse Effect	Underdosing
Permanganate (nonmedicinal)	T65.891	T65.892	T65.893	T65.894	—	—
medicinal	T49.0X1	T49.0X2	T49.0X3	T49.0X4	T49.0X5	T49.0X6
sulfate	T47.2X1	T47.2X2	T47.2X3	T47.2X4	T47.2X5	T47.2X6
Potassium-removing resin	T50.3X1	T50.3X2	T50.3X3	T50.3X4	T50.3X5	T50.3X6
Potassium-retaining drug	T50.3X1	T50.3X2	T50.3X3	T50.3X4	T50.3X5	T50.3X6
Povidone	T45.8X1	T45.8X2	T45.8X3	T45.8X4	T45.8X5	T45.8X6
iodine	T49.0X1	T49.0X2	T49.0X3	T49.0X4	T49.0X5	T49.0X6
Practolol	T44.7X1	T44.7X2	T44.7X3	T44.7X4	T44.7X5	T44.7X6
Prajmalium bitartrate	T46.2X1	T46.2X2	T46.2X3	T46.2X4	T46.2X5	T46.2X6
Pralidoxime (iodide)	T50.6X1	T50.6X2	T50.6X3	T50.6X4	T50.6X5	T50.6X6
chloride	T50.6X1	T50.6X2	T50.6X3	T50.6X4	T50.6X5	T50.6X6
Pramiverine	T44.3X1	T44.3X2	T44.3X3	T44.3X4	T44.3X5	T44.3X6
Pramocaine	T49.1X1	T49.1X2	T49.1X3	T49.1X4	T49.1X5	T49.1X6
Pramoxine	T49.1X1	T49.1X2	T49.1X3	T49.1X4	T49.1X5	T49.1X6
Prasterone	T38.7X1	T38.7X2	T38.7X3	T38.7X4	T38.7X5	T38.7X6
Pravastatin	T46.6X1	T46.6X2	T46.6X3	T46.6X4	T46.6X5	T46.6X6
Prazepam	T42.4X1	T42.4X2	T42.4X3	T42.4X4	T42.4X5	T42.4X6
Praziquantel	T37.4X1	T37.4X2	T37.4X3	T37.4X4	T37.4X5	T37.4X6
Prazitone	T43.291	T43.292	T43.293	T43.294	T43.295	T43.296
Prazosin	T44.6X1	T44.6X2	T44.6X3	T44.6X4	T44.6X5	T44.6X6
Prednicarbate	T49.0X1	T49.0X2	T49.0X3	T49.0X4	T49.0X5	T49.0X6
Prednimustine	T45.1X1	T45.1X2	T45.1X3	T45.1X4	T45.1X5	T45.1X6
Prednisolone	T38.0X1	T38.0X2	T38.0X3	T38.0X4	T38.0X5	T38.0X6
ENT agent	T49.6X1	T49.6X2	T49.6X3	T49.6X4	T49.6X5	T49.6X6
ophthalmic preparation	T49.5X1	T49.5X2	T49.5X3	T49.5X4	T49.5X5	T49.5X6
steaglate	T49.0X1	T49.0X2	T49.0X3	T49.0X4	T49.0X5	T49.0X6
topical NEC	T49.0X1	T49.0X2	T49.0X3	T49.0X4	T49.0X5	T49.0X6
Prednisone	T38.0X1	T38.0X2	T38.0X3	T38.0X4	T38.0X5	T38.0X6
Prednylidene	T38.0X1	T38.0X2	T38.0X3	T38.0X4	T38.0X5	T38.0X6
Pregnandiol	T38.5X1	T38.5X2	T38.5X3	T38.5X4	T38.5X5	T38.5X6
Pregneninolone	T38.5X1	T38.5X2	T38.5X3	T38.5X4	T38.5X5	T38.5X6
Preludin	T43.691	T43.692	T43.693	T43.694	T43.695	T43.696
Premarin	T38.5X1	T38.5X2	T38.5X3	T38.5X4	T38.5X5	T38.5X6
Premedication anesthetic	T41.201	T41.202	T41.203	T41.204	T41.205	T41.206
Prenalterol	T44.5X1	T44.5X2	T44.5X3	T44.5X4	T44.5X5	T44.5X6
Prenoxdiazine	T48.3X1	T48.3X2	T48.3X3	T48.3X4	T48.3X5	T48.3X6
Prenylamine	T46.3X1	T46.3X2	T46.3X3	T46.3X4	T46.3X5	T46.3X6
Preparation, local	T49.4X1	T49.4X2	T49.4X3	T49.4X4	T49.4X5	T49.4X6
Preparation H	T49.8X1	T49.8X2	T49.8X3	T49.8X4	T49.8X5	T49.8X6
Preservative (nonmedicinal)	T65.891	T65.892	T65.893	T65.894	—	—
medicinal	T50.901	T50.902	T50.903	T50.904	T50.905	T50.906
wood	T60.91	T60.92	T60.93	T60.94	—	—

Substance	Poisoning, Accidental (Unintentional)	Poisoning, Intentional Self-Harm	Poisoning, Assault	Poisoning, Undetermined	Adverse Effect	Underdosing
Prethcamide	T50.7X1	T50.7X2	T50.7X3	T50.7X4	T50.7X5	T50.7X6
Pride of China	T62.2X1	T62.2X2	T62.2X3	T62.2X4	—	—
Pridinol	T44.3X1	T44.3X2	T44.3X3	T44.3X4	T44.3X5	T44.3X6
Prifinium bromide	T44.3X1	T44.3X2	T44.3X3	T44.3X4	T44.3X5	T44.3X6
Prilocaine	T41.3X1	T41.3X2	T41.3X3	T41.3X4	T41.3X5	T41.3X6
infiltration (subcutaneous)	T41.3X1	T41.3X2	T41.3X3	T41.3X4	T41.3X5	T41.3X6
nerve block (peripheral) (plexus)	T41.3X1	T41.3X2	T41.3X3	T41.3X4	T41.3X5	T41.3X6
regional	T41.3X1	T41.3X2	T41.3X3	T41.3X4	T41.3X5	T41.3X6
Primaquine	T37.2X1	T37.2X2	T37.2X3	T37.2X4	T37.2X5	T37.2X6
Primidone	T42.6X1	T42.6X2	T42.6X3	T42.6X4	T42.6X5	T42.6X6
Primula (veris)	T62.2X1	T62.2X2	T62.2X3	T62.2X4	—	—
Prinadol	T40.2X1	T40.2X2	T40.2X3	T40.2X4	T40.2X5	T40.2X6
Priscol, Priscoline	T44.6X1	T44.6X2	T44.6X3	T44.6X4	T44.6X5	T44.6X6
Pristinamycin	T36.3X1	T36.3X2	T36.3X3	T36.3X4	T36.3X5	T36.3X6
Privet	T62.2X1	T62.2X2	T62.2X3	T62.2X4	—	—
berries	T62.1X1	T62.1X2	T62.1X3	T62.1X4	—	—
Privine	T44.4X1	T44.4X2	T44.4X3	T44.4X4	T44.4X5	T44.4X6
Pro-Banthine	T44.3X1	T44.3X2	T44.3X3	T44.3X4	T44.3X5	T44.3X6
Probarbital	T42.3X1	T42.3X2	T42.3X3	T42.3X4	T42.3X5	T42.3X6
Probenecid	T50.4X1	T50.4X2	T50.4X3	T50.4X4	T50.4X5	T50.4X6
Probucol	T46.6X1	T46.6X2	T46.6X3	T46.6X4	T46.6X5	T46.6X6
Procainamide	T46.2X1	T46.2X2	T46.2X3	T46.2X4	T46.2X5	T46.2X6
Procaine	T41.3X1	T41.3X2	T41.3X3	T41.3X4	T41.3X5	T41.3X6
benzylpenicillin	T36.0X1	T36.0X2	T36.0X3	T36.0X4	T36.0X5	T36.0X6
nerve block (periphreal) (plexus)	T41.3X1	T41.3X2	T41.3X3	T41.3X4	T41.3X5	T41.3X6
penicillin G	T36.0X1	T36.0X2	T36.0X3	T36.0X4	T36.0X5	T36.0X6
regional	T41.3X1	T41.3X2	T41.3X3	T41.3X4	T41.3X5	T41.3X6
spinal	T41.3X1	T41.3X2	T41.3X3	T41.3X4	T41.3X5	T41.3X6
Procalmidol	T43.591	T43.592	T43.593	T43.594	T43.595	T43.596
Procarbazine	T45.1X1	T45.1X2	T45.1X3	T45.1X4	T45.1X5	T45.1X6
Procaterol	T44.5X1	T44.5X2	T44.5X3	T44.5X4	T44.5X5	T44.5X6
Prochlorperazine	T43.3X1	T43.3X2	T43.3X3	T43.3X4	T43.3X5	T43.3X6
Procyclidine	T44.3X1	T44.3X2	T44.3X3	T44.3X4	T44.3X5	T44.3X6
Producer gas	T58.8X1	T58.8X2	T58.8X3	T58.8X4	—	—
Profadol	T40.4X1	T40.4X2	T40.4X3	T40.4X4	T40.4X5	T40.4X6
Profenamine	T44.3X1	T44.3X2	T44.3X3	T44.3X4	T44.3X5	T44.3X6
Profenil	T44.3X1	T44.3X2	T44.3X3	T44.3X4	T44.3X5	T44.3X6
Proflavine	T49.0X1	T49.0X2	T49.0X3	T49.0X4	T49.0X5	T49.0X6
Progabide	T42.6X1	T42.6X2	T42.6X3	T42.6X4	T42.6X5	T42.6X6
Progestin	T38.5X1	T38.5X2	T38.5X3	T38.5X4	T38.5X5	T38.5X6
oral contraceptive	T38.4X1	T38.4X2	T38.4X3	T38.4X4	T38.4X5	T38.4X6

Substance	Poisoning, Accidental (Unintentional)	Poisoning, Intentional Self-Harm	Poisoning, Assault	Poisoning, Undetermined	Adverse Effect	Underdosing
Progesterone	T38.5X1	T38.5X2	T38.5X3	T38.5X4	T38.5X5	T38.5X6
Progestogen NEC	T38.5X1	T38.5X2	T38.5X3	T38.5X4	T38.5X5	T38.5X6
Progestone	T38.5X1	T38.5X2	T38.5X3	T38.5X4	T38.5X5	T38.5X6
Proglumide	T47.1X1	T47.1X2	T47.1X3	T47.1X4	T47.1X5	T47.1X6
Proguanil	T37.2X1	T37.2X2	T37.2X3	T37.2X4	T37.2X5	T37.2X6
Prolactin	T38.811	T38.812	T38.813	T38.814	T38.815	T38.816
Prolintane	T43.691	T43.692	T43.693	T43.694	T43.695	T43.696
Proloid	T38.1X1	T38.1X2	T38.1X3	T38.1X4	T38.1X5	T38.1X6
Proluton	T38.5X1	T38.5X2	T38.5X3	T38.5X4	T38.5X5	T38.5X6
Promacetin	T37.1X1	T37.1X2	T37.1X3	T37.1X4	T37.1X5	T37.1X6
Promazine	T43.3X1	T43.3X2	T43.3X3	T43.3X4	T43.3X5	T43.3X6
Promedol	T40.2X1	T40.2X2	T40.2X3	T40.2X4	—	—
Promegestone	T38.5X1	T38.5X2	T38.5X3	T38.5X4	T38.5X5	T38.5X6
Promethazine (teoclate)	T43.3X1	T43.3X2	T43.3X3	T43.3X4	T43.3X5	T43.3X6
Promin	T37.1X1	T37.1X2	T37.1X3	T37.1X4	T37.1X5	T37.1X6
Pronase	T45.3X1	T45.3X2	T45.3X3	T45.3X4	T45.3X5	T45.3X6
Pronestyl (hydrochloride)	T46.2X1	T46.2X2	T46.2X3	T46.2X4	T46.2X5	T46.2X6
Pronetalol	T44.7X1	T44.7X2	T44.7X3	T44.7X4	T44.7X5	T44.7X6
Prontosil	T37.0X1	T37.0X2	T37.0X3	T37.0X4	T37.0X5	T37.0X6
Propachlor	T60.3X1	T60.3X2	T60.3X3	T60.3X4	—	—
Propafenone	T46.2X1	T46.2X2	T46.2X3	T46.2X4	T46.2X5	T46.2X6
Propallylonal	T42.3X1	T42.3X2	T42.3X3	T42.3X4	T42.3X5	T42.3X6
Propamidine	T49.0X1	T49.0X2	T49.0X3	T49.0X4	T49.0X5	T49.0X6
Propane (distributed in mobile container)	T59.891	T59.892	T59.893	T59.894	—	—
distributed through pipes	T59.891	T59.892	T59.893	T59.894	—	—
incomplete combustion	T57.11	T57.12	T57.13	T57.14	—	—
Propanidid	T41.291	T41.292	T41.293	T41.294	T41.295	T41.296
Propanil	T60.3X1	T60.3X2	T60.3X3	T60.3X4	—	—
1-Propanol	T51.3X1	T51.3X2	T51.3X3	T51.3X4	—	—
2-Propanol	T51.2X1	T51.2X2	T51.2X3	T51.2X4	—	—
Propantheline	T44.3X1	T44.3X2	T44.3X3	T44.3X4	T44.3X5	T44.3X6
bromide	T44.3X1	T44.3X2	T44.3X3	T44.3X4	T44.3X5	T44.3X6
Proparacaine	T41.3X1	T41.3X2	T41.3X3	T41.3X4	T41.3X5	T41.3X6
Propatylnitrate	T46.3X1	T46.3X2	T46.3X3	T46.3X4	T46.3X5	T46.3X6
Propicillin	T36.0X1	T36.0X2	T36.0X3	T36.0X4	T36.0X5	T36.0X6
Propiolactone	T49.0X1	T49.0X2	T49.0X3	T49.0X4	T49.0X5	T49.0X6
Propiomazine	T45.0X1	T45.0X2	T45.0X3	T45.0X4	T45.0X5	T45.0X6
~~Propionaldehyde (medicinal)~~	~~T42.6X1~~	~~T42.6X2~~	~~T42.6X3~~	~~T42.6X4~~	~~T42.6X5~~	~~T42.6X6~~
Propionaldehyde (medicinal)	T42.6X1	T42.6X2	T42.6X3	T42.6X4	T42.6X5	T42.6X6 ◄
Propionate (calcium) (sodium)	T49.0X1	T49.0X2	T49.0X3	T49.0X4	T49.0X5	T49.0X6
Propion gel	T49.0X1	T49.0X2	T49.0X3	T49.0X4	T49.0X5	T49.0X6

Substance	Poisoning, Accidental (Unintentional)	Poisoning, Intentional Self-Harm	Poisoning, Assault	Poisoning, Undetermined	Adverse Effect	Underdosing
Propitocaine	T41.3X1	T41.3X2	T41.3X3	T41.3X4	T41.3X5	T41.3X6
infiltration (subcutaneous)	T41.3X1	T41.3X2	T41.3X3	T41.3X4	T41.3X5	T41.3X6
nerve block (peripheral) (plexus)	T41.3X1	T41.3X2	T41.3X3	T41.3X4	T41.3X5	T41.3X6
Propofol	T41.291	T41.292	T41.293	T41.294	T41.295	T41.296
Propoxur	T60.0X1	T60.0X2	T60.0X3	T60.0X4	—	—
Propoxycaine	T41.3X1	T41.3X2	T41.3X3	T41.3X4	T41.3X5	T41.3X6
infiltration (subcutaneous)	T41.3X1	T41.3X2	T41.3X3	T41.3X4	T41.3X5	T41.3X6
nerve block (peripheral) (plexus)	T41.3X1	T41.3X2	T41.3X3	T41.3X4	T41.3X5	T41.3X6
topical (surface)	T41.3X1	T41.3X2	T41.3X3	T41.3X4	T41.3X5	T41.3X6
Propoxyphene	T40.4X1	T40.4X2	T40.4X3	T40.4X4	T40.4X5	T40.4X6
Propranolol	T44.7X1	T44.7X2	T44.7X3	T44.7X4	T44.7X5	T44.7X6
Propyl						
alcohol	T51.3X1	T51.3X2	T51.3X3	T51.3X4	—	—
carbinol	T51.3X1	T51.3X2	T51.3X3	T51.3X4	—	—
hexadrine	T44.4X1	T44.4X2	T44.4X3	T44.4X4	T44.4X5	T44.4X6
iodone	T50.8X1	T50.8X2	T50.8X3	T50.8X4	T50.8X5	T50.8X6
thiouracil	T38.2X1	T38.2X2	T38.2X3	T38.2X4	T38.2X5	T38.2X6
Propylaminophenothiazine	T43.3X1	T43.3X2	T43.3X3	T43.3X4	T43.3X5	T43.3X6
Propylene	T59.891	T59.892	T59.893	T59.894	—	—
Propylhexedrine	T48.5X1	T48.5X2	T48.5X3	T48.5X4	T48.5X5	T48.5X6
Propyliodone	T50.8X1	T50.8X2	T50.8X3	T50.8X4	T50.8X5	T50.8X6
Propylthiouracil	T38.2X1	T38.2X2	T38.2X3	T38.2X4	T38.2X5	T38.2X6
Propylparaben (ophthalmic)	T49.5X1	T49.5X2	T49.5X3	T49.5X4	T49.5X5	T49.5X6
Propyphenazone	T39.2X1	T39.2X2	T39.2X3	T39.2X4	T39.2X5	T39.2X6
Proquazone	T39.391	T39.392	T39.393	T39.394	T39.395	T39.396
Proscillaridin	T46.0X1	T46.0X2	T46.0X3	T46.0X4	T46.0X5	T46.0X6
Prostacyclin	T45.521	T45.522	T45.523	T45.524	T45.525	T45.526
Prostaglandin (I2)	T45.521	T45.522	T45.523	T45.524	T45.525	T45.526
E1	T46.7X1	T46.7X2	T46.7X3	T46.7X4	T46.7X5	T46.7X6
E2	T48.0X1	T48.0X2	T48.0X3	T48.0X4	T48.0X5	T48.0X6
F2 alpha	T48.0X1	T48.0X2	T48.0X3	T48.0X4	T48.0X5	T48.0X6
Prostigmin	T44.0X1	T44.0X2	T44.0X3	T44.0X4	T44.0X5	T44.0X6
Prosultiamine	T45.2X1	T45.2X2	T45.2X3	T45.2X4	T45.2X5	T45.2X6
Protamine sulfate	T45.7X1	T45.7X2	T45.7X3	T45.7X4	T45.7X5	T45.7X6
zinc insulin	T38.3X1	T38.3X2	T38.3X3	T38.3X4	T38.3X5	T38.3X6
Protease	T47.5X1	T47.5X2	T47.5X3	T47.5X4	T47.5X5	T47.5X6
Protectant, skin NEC	T49.3X1	T49.3X2	T49.3X3	T49.3X4	T49.3X5	T49.3X6
Protein hydrolysate	T50.991	T50.992	T50.993	T50.994	T50.995	T50.996
Prothiaden — *see Dothiepin hydrochloride*						
Prothionamide	T37.1X1	T37.1X2	T37.1X3	T37.1X4	T37.1X5	T37.1X6

◄ New ◄||| Revised ~~deleted~~ Deleted

Substance	Poisoning, Accidental (Unintentional)	Poisoning, Intentional Self-Harm	Poisoning, Assault	Poisoning, Undetermined	Adverse Effect	Underdosing
Prothipendyl	T43.591	T43.592	T43.593	T43.594	T43.595	T43.596
Prothoate	T60.0X1	T60.0X2	T60.0X3	T60.0X4	—	—
Prothrombin						
activator	T45.7X1	T45.7X2	T45.7X3	T45.7X4	T45.7X5	T45.7X6
synthesis inhibitor	T45.511	T45.512	T45.513	T45.514	T45.515	T45.516
Protionamide	T37.1X1	T37.1X2	T37.1X3	T37.1X4	T37.1X5	T37.1X6
Protirelin	T38.891	T38.892	T38.893	T38.894	T38.895	T38.896
Protokylol	T48.6X1	T48.6X2	T48.6X3	T48.6X4	T48.6X5	T48.6X6
Protopam	T50.6X1	T50.6X2	T50.6X3	T50.6X4	T50.6X5	T50.6X6
Protoveratrine(s) (A) (B)	T46.5X1	T46.5X2	T46.5X3	T46.5X4	T46.5X5	T46.5X6
Protriptyline	T43.011	T43.012	T43.013	T43.014	T43.015	T43.016
Provera	T38.5X1	T38.5X2	T38.5X3	T38.5X4	T38.5X5	T38.5X6
Provitamin A	T45.2X1	T45.2X2	T45.2X3	T45.2X4	T45.2X5	T45.2X6
Proxibarbal	T42.3X1	T42.3X2	T42.3X3	T42.3X4	T42.3X5	T42.3X6
Proxymetacaine	T41.3X1	T41.3X2	T41.3X3	T41.3X4	T41.3X5	T41.3X6
Proxyphylline	T48.6X1	T48.6X2	T48.6X3	T48.6X4	T48.6X5	T48.6X6
Prozac — *see Fluoxetine hydrochloride*						
Prunus						
laurocerasus	T62.2X1	T62.2X2	T62.2X3	T62.2X4	—	—
virginiana	T62.2X1	T62.2X2	T62.2X3	T62.2X4	—	—
Prussian blue						
commercial	T65.891	T65.892	T65.893	T65.894	—	—
therapeutic	T50.6X1	T50.6X2	T50.6X3	T50.6X4	T50.6X5	T50.6X6
Prussic acid	T65.0X1	T65.0X2	T65.0X3	T65.0X4	—	—
vapor	T57.3X1	T57.3X2	T57.3X3	T57.3X4	—	—
Pseudoephedrine	T44.991	T44.992	T44.993	T44.994	T44.995	T44.996
Psilocin	T40.991	T40.992	T40.993	T40.994	—	—
Psilocybin	T40.991	T40.992	T40.993	T40.994	—	—
Psilocybine	T40.991	T40.992	T40.993	T40.994	—	—
Psoralene (nonmedicinal)	T65.891	T65.892	T65.893	T65.894	—	—
Psoralens (medicinal)	T50.991	T50.992	T50.993	T50.994	T50.995	T50.996
PSP (phenolsulfonphthalein)	T50.8X1	T50.8X2	T50.8X3	T50.8X4	T50.8X5	T50.8X6
Psychodysleptic drug NEC	T40.901	T40.902	T40.903	T40.904	T40.905	T40.906
Psychostimulant	T43.601	T43.602	T43.603	T43.604	T43.605	T43.606
amphetamine	T43.621	T43.622	T43.623	T43.624	T43.625	T43.626
caffeine	T43.611	T43.612	T43.613	T43.614	T43.615	T43.616
methylphenidate	T43.631	T43.632	T43.633	T43.634	T43.635	T43.636
specified NEC	T43.691	T43.692	T43.693	T43.694	T43.695	T43.696
Psychotherapeutic drug NEC	T43.91	T43.92	T43.93	T43.94	T43.95	T43.96
antidepressants — *see also Antidepressant*	T43.201	T43.202	T43.203	T43.204	T43.205	T43.206

Substance	Poisoning, Accidental (Unintentional)	Poisoning, Intentional Self-Harm	Poisoning, Assault	Poisoning, Undetermined	Adverse Effect	Underdosing
Psychotherapeutic drug NEC *(Continued)*						
specified NEC	T43.8X1	T43.8X2	T43.8X3	T43.8X4	T43.8X5	T43.8X6
tranquilizers NEC	T43.501	T43.502	T43.503	T43.504	T43.505	T43.506
Psychotomimetic agents	T40.901	T40.902	T40.903	T40.904	T40.905	T40.906
Psychotropic drug NEC	T43.91	T43.92	T43.93	T43.94	T43.95	T43.96
specified NEC	T43.8X1	T43.8X2	T43.8X3	T43.8X4	T43.8X5	T43.8X6
Psyllium hydrophilic mucilloid	T47.4X1	T47.4X2	T47.4X3	T47.4X4	T47.4X5	T47.4X6
Pteroylglutamic acid	T45.8X1	T45.8X2	T45.8X3	T45.8X4	T45.8X5	T45.8X6
Pteroyltriglutamate	T45.1X1	T45.1X2	T45.1X3	T45.1X4	T45.1X5	T45.1X6
PTFE — *see Polytetrafluoroethylene*						
Pulp						
devitalizing paste	T49.7X1	T49.7X2	T49.7X3	T49.7X4	T49.7X5	T49.7X6
dressing	T49.7X1	T49.7X2	T49.7X3	T49.7X4	T49.7X5	T49.7X6
Pulsatilla	T62.2X1	T62.2X2	T62.2X3	T62.2X4	—	—
Pumpkin seed extract	T37.4X1	T37.4X2	T37.4X3	T37.4X4	T37.4X5	T37.4X6
Purex (bleach)	T54.91	T54.92	T54.93	T54.94	—	—
Purgative NEC — *see also Cathartic*	T47.4X1	T47.4X2	T47.4X3	T47.4X4	T47.4X5	T47.4X6
Purine analogue (antineoplastic)	T45.1X1	T45.1X2	T45.1X3	T45.1X4	T45.1X5	T45.1X6
Purine diuretics	T50.2X1	T50.2X2	T50.2X3	T50.2X4	T50.2X5	T50.2X6
Purinethol	T45.1X1	T45.1X2	T45.1X3	T45.1X4	T45.1X5	T45.1X6
PVP	T45.8X1	T45.8X2	T45.8X3	T45.8X4	T45.8X5	T45.8X6
Pyrabital	T39.8X1	T39.8X2	T39.8X3	T39.8X4	T39.8X5	T39.8X6
Pyramidon	T39.2X1	T39.2X2	T39.2X3	T39.2X4	T39.2X5	T39.2X6
Pyrantel	T37.4X1	T37.4X2	T37.4X3	T37.4X4	T37.4X5	T37.4X6
Pyrathiazine	T45.0X1	T45.0X2	T45.0X3	T45.0X4	T45.0X5	T45.0X6
Pyrazinamide	T37.1X1	T37.1X2	T37.1X3	T37.1X4	T37.1X5	T37.1X6
Pyrazinoic acid (amide)	T37.1X1	T37.1X2	T37.1X3	T37.1X4	T37.1X5	T37.1X6
Pyrazole (derivatives)	T39.2X1	T39.2X2	T39.2X3	T39.2X4	T39.2X5	T39.2X6
Pyrazolone analgesic NEC	T39.2X1	T39.2X2	T39.2X3	T39.2X4	T39.2X5	T39.2X6
Pyrethrin, pyrethrum (nonmedicinal)	T60.2X1	T60.2X2	T60.2X3	T60.2X4	—	—
Pyrethrum extract	T49.0X1	T49.0X2	T49.0X3	T49.0X4	T49.0X5	T49.0X6
Pyribenzamine	T45.0X1	T45.0X2	T45.0X3	T45.0X4	T45.0X5	T45.0X6
Pyridine	T52.8X1	T52.8X2	T52.8X3	T52.8X4	—	—
aldoxime methiodide	T50.6X1	T50.6X2	T50.6X3	T50.6X4	T50.6X5	T50.6X6
aldoxime methyl chloride	T50.6X1	T50.6X2	T50.6X3	T50.6X4	T50.6X5	T50.6X6
vapor	T59.891	T59.892	T59.893	T59.894	—	—
Pyridium	T39.8X1	T39.8X2	T39.8X3	T39.8X4	T39.8X5	T39.8X6
Pyridostigmine bromide	T44.0X1	T44.0X2	T44.0X3	T44.0X4	T44.0X5	T44.0X6
Pyridoxal phosphate	T45.2X1	T45.2X2	T45.2X3	T45.2X4	T45.2X5	T45.2X6

Substance	Poisoning, Accidental (Unintentional)	Poisoning, Intentional Self-Harm	Poisoning, Assault	Poisoning, Undetermined	Adverse Effect	Underdosing
Pyridoxine	T45.2X1	T45.2X2	T45.2X3	T45.2X4	T45.2X5	T45.2X6
Pyrilamine	T45.ØX1	T45.ØX2	T45.ØX3	T45.ØX4	T45.ØX5	T45.ØX6
Pyrimethamine	T37.2X1	T37.2X2	T37.2X3	T37.2X4	T37.2X5	T37.2X6
with sulfadoxine	T37.2X1	T37.2X2	T37.2X3	T37.2X4	T37.2X5	T37.2X6
Pyrimidine antagonist	T45.1X1	T45.1X2	T45.1X3	T45.1X4	T45.1X5	T45.1X6
Pyriminil	T6Ø.4X1	T6Ø.4X2	T6Ø.4X3	T6Ø.4X4	—	—
Pyrithione zinc	T49.4X1	T49.4X2	T49.4X3	T49.4X4	T49.4X5	T49.4X6
Pyrithyldione	T42.6X1	T42.6X2	T42.6X3	T42.6X4	T42.6X5	T42.6X6
Pyrogallic acid	T49.ØX1	T49.ØX2	T49.ØX3	T49.ØX4	T49.ØX5	T49.ØX6
Pyrogallol	T49.ØX1	T49.ØX2	T49.ØX3	T49.ØX4	T49.ØX5	T49.ØX6
Pyroxylin	T49.3X1	T49.3X2	T49.3X3	T49.3X4	T49.3X5	T49.3X6
Pyrrobutamine	T45.ØX1	T45.ØX2	T45.ØX3	T45.ØX4	T45.ØX5	T45.ØX6
Pyrrolizidine alkaloids	T62.8X1	T62.8X2	T62.8X3	T62.8X4	—	—
Pyrvinium chloride	T37.4X1	T37.4X2	T37.4X3	T37.4X4	T37.4X5	T37.4X6
PZI	T38.3X1	T38.3X2	T38.3X3	T38.3X4	T38.3X5	T38.3X6
Q						
Quaalude	T42.6X1	T42.6X2	T42.6X3	T42.6X4	T42.6X5	T42.6X6
Quarternary ammonium						
anti-infective	T49.ØX1	T49.ØX2	T49.ØX3	T49.ØX4	T49.ØX5	T49.ØX6
ganglion blocking	T44.2X1	T44.2X2	T44.2X3	T44.2X4	T44.2X5	T44.2X6
parasympatholytic	T44.3X1	T44.3X2	T44.3X3	T44.3X4	T44.3X5	T44.3X6
Quazepam	T42.4X1	T42.4X2	T42.4X3	T42.4X4	T42.4X5	T42.4X6
Quicklime	T54.3X1	T54.3X2	T54.3X3	T54.3X4	—	—
Quillaja extract	T48.4X1	T48.4X2	T48.4X3	T48.4X4	T48.4X5	T48.4X6
Quinacrine	T37.2X1	T37.2X2	T37.2X3	T37.2X4	T37.2X5	T37.2X6
Quinaglute	T46.2X1	T46.2X2	T46.2X3	T46.2X4	T46.2X5	T46.2X6
Quinalbarbital	T42.3X1	T42.3X2	T42.3X3	T42.3X4	T42.3X5	T42.3X6
Quinalbarbitone sodium	T42.3X1	T42.3X2	T42.3X3	T42.3X4	T42.3X5	T42.3X6
Quinalphos	T6Ø.ØX1	T6Ø.ØX2	T6Ø.ØX3	T6Ø.ØX4	—	—
Quinapril	T46.4X1	T46.4X2	T46.4X3	T46.4X4	T46.4X5	T46.4X6
Quinestradiol	T38.5X1	T38.5X2	T38.5X3	T38.5X4	T38.5X5	T38.5X6
Quinestradol	T38.5X1	T38.5X2	T38.5X3	T38.5X4	T38.5X5	T38.5X6
Quinestrol	T38.5X1	T38.5X2	T38.5X3	T38.5X4	T38.5X5	T38.5X6
Quinethazone	T5Ø.2X1	T5Ø.2X2	T5Ø.2X3	T5Ø.2X4	T5Ø.2X5	T5Ø.2X6
Quingestanol	T38.4X1	T38.4X2	T38.4X3	T38.4X4	T38.4X5	T38.4X6
Quinidine	T46.2X1	T46.2X2	T46.2X3	T46.2X4	T46.2X5	T46.2X6
Quinine	T37.2X1	T37.2X2	T37.2X3	T37.2X4	T37.2X5	T37.2X6
Quiniobine	T37.8X1	T37.8X2	T37.8X3	T37.8X4	T37.8X5	T37.8X6
Quinisocaine	T49.1X1	T49.1X2	T49.1X3	T49.1X4	T49.1X5	T49.1X6
Quinocide	T37.2X1	T37.2X2	T37.2X3	T37.2X4	T37.2X5	T37.2X6
Quinoline (derivatives) NEC	T37.8X1	T37.8X2	T37.8X3	T37.8X4	T37.8X5	T37.8X6
Quinupramine	T43.Ø11	T43.Ø12	T43.Ø13	T43.Ø14	T43.Ø15	T43.Ø16
Quotane	T41.3X1	T41.3X2	T41.3X3	T41.3X4	T41.3X5	T41.3X6
R						
Rabies						
immune globulin (human)	T5Ø.Z11	T5Ø.Z12	T5Ø.Z13	T5Ø.Z14	T5Ø.Z15	T5Ø.Z16
vaccine	T5Ø.B91	T5Ø.B92	T5Ø.B93	T5Ø.B94	T5Ø.B95	T5Ø.B96
Racemoramide	T4Ø.2X1	T4Ø.2X2	T4Ø.2X3	T4Ø.2X4	—	—
Racemorphan	T4Ø.2X1	T4Ø.2X2	T4Ø.2X3	T4Ø.2X4	T4Ø.2X5	T4Ø.2X6
Racepinefrin	T44.5X1	T44.5X2	T44.5X3	T44.5X4	T44.5X5	T44.5X6
Raclopride	T43.591	T43.592	T43.593	T43.594	T43.595	T43.596
Radiator alcohol	T51.1X1	T51.1X2	T51.1X3	T51.1X4	—	—
Radioactive drug NEC	T5Ø.8X1	T5Ø.8X2	T5Ø.8X3	T5Ø.8X4	T5Ø.8X5	T5Ø.8X6
Radio-opaque (drugs) (materials)	T5Ø.8X1	T5Ø.8X2	T5Ø.8X3	T5Ø.8X4	T5Ø.8X5	T5Ø.8X6
Ramifenazone	T39.2X1	T39.2X2	T39.2X3	T39.2X4	T39.2X5	T39.2X6
Ramipril	T46.4X1	T46.4X2	T46.4X3	T46.4X4	T46.4X5	T46.4X6
Ranitidine	T47.ØX1	T47.ØX2	T47.ØX3	T47.ØX4	T47.ØX5	T47.ØX6
Ranunculus	T62.2X1	T62.2X2	T62.2X3	T62.2X4	—	—
Rat poison NEC	T6Ø.4X1	T6Ø.4X2	T6Ø.4X3	T6Ø.4X4	—	—
Rattlesnake (venom)	T63.Ø11	T63.Ø12	T63.Ø13	T63.Ø14	—	—
Raubasine	T46.7X1	T46.7X2	T46.7X3	T46.7X4	T46.7X5	T46.7X6
Raudixin	T46.5X1	T46.5X2	T46.5X3	T46.5X4	T46.5X5	T46.5X6
Rautensin	T46.5X1	T46.5X2	T46.5X3	T46.5X4	T46.5X5	T46.5X6
Rautina	T46.5X1	T46.5X2	T46.5X3	T46.5X4	T46.5X5	T46.5X6
Rautotal	T46.5X1	T46.5X2	T46.5X3	T46.5X4	T46.5X5	T46.5X6
Rauwiloid	T46.5X1	T46.5X2	T46.5X3	T46.5X4	T46.5X5	T46.5X6
Rauwoldin	T46.5X1	T46.5X2	T46.5X3	T46.5X4	T46.5X5	T46.5X6
Rauwolfia (alkaloids)	T46.5X1	T46.5X2	T46.5X3	T46.5X4	T46.5X5	T46.5X6
Razoxane	T45.1X1	T45.1X2	T45.1X3	T45.1X4	T45.1X5	T45.1X6
Realgar	T57.ØX1	T57.ØX2	T57.ØX3	T57.ØX4	—	—
Recombinant (R) — *see specific protein*						
Red blood cells, packed	T45.8X1	T45.8X2	T45.8X3	T45.8X4	T45.8X5	T45.8X6
Red squill (scilliroside)	T6Ø.4X1	T6Ø.4X2	T6Ø.4X3	T6Ø.4X4	—	—
Reducing agent, industrial NEC	T65.891	T65.892	T65.893	T65.894	—	—
Refrigerant gas (chlorofluoro-carbon)	T53.5X1	T53.5X2	T53.5X3	T53.5X4	—	—
not chlorofluoro-carbon	T59.891	T59.892	T59.893	T59.894	—	—
Regroton	T5Ø.2X1	T5Ø.2X2	T5Ø.2X3	T5Ø.2X4	T5Ø.2X5	T5Ø.2X6
Rehydration salts (oral)	T5Ø.3X1	T5Ø.3X2	T5Ø.3X3	T5Ø.3X4	T5Ø.3X5	T5Ø.3X6
Rela	T42.8X1	T42.8X2	T42.8X3	T42.8X4	T42.8X5	T42.8X6

Substance	Poisoning, Accidental (Unintentional)	Poisoning, Intentional Self-Harm	Poisoning, Assault	Poisoning, Undetermined	Adverse Effect	Underdosing
Relaxant, muscle						
anesthetic	T48.1X1	T48.1X2	T48.1X3	T48.1X4	T48.1X5	T48.1X6
central nervous system	T42.8X1	T42.8X2	T42.8X3	T42.8X4	T42.8X5	T42.8X6
skeletal NEC	T48.1X1	T48.1X2	T48.1X3	T48.1X4	T48.1X5	T48.1X6
smooth NEC	T44.3X1	T44.3X2	T44.3X3	T44.3X4	T44.3X5	T44.3X6
Remoxipride	T43.591	T43.592	T43.593	T43.594	T43.595	T43.596
Renese	T5Ø.2X1	T5Ø.2X2	T5Ø.2X3	T5Ø.2X4	T5Ø.2X5	T5Ø.2X6
Renografin	T5Ø.8X1	T5Ø.8X2	T5Ø.8X3	T5Ø.8X4	T5Ø.8X5	T5Ø.8X6
Replacement solution	T5Ø.3X1	T5Ø.3X2	T5Ø.3X3	T5Ø.3X4	T5Ø.3X5	T5Ø.3X6
Reproterol	T48.6X1	T48.6X2	T48.6X3	T48.6X4	T48.6X5	T48.6X6
Rescinnamine	T46.5X1	T46.5X2	T46.5X3	T46.5X4	T46.5X5	T46.5X6
Reserpin(e)	T46.5X1	T46.5X2	T46.5X3	T46.5X4	T46.5X5	T46.5X6
Resorcin, resorcinol (nonmedicinal)	T65.891	T65.892	T65.893	T65.894	—	—
medicinal	T49.4X1	T49.4X2	T49.4X3	T49.4X4	T49.4X5	T49.4X6
Respaire	T48.4X1	T48.4X2	T48.4X3	T48.4X4	T48.4X5	T48.4X6
Respiratory drug NEC	T48.9Ø1	T48.9Ø2	T48.9Ø3	T48.9Ø4	T48.9Ø5	T48.9Ø6
antiasthmatic NEC	T48.6X1	T48.6X2	T48.6X3	T48.6X4	T48.6X5	T48.6X6
anti-common-cold NEC	T48.5X1	T48.5X2	T48.5X3	T48.5X4	T48.5X5	T48.5X6
expectorant NEC	T48.4X1	T48.4X2	T48.4X3	T48.4X4	T48.4X5	T48.4X6
stimulant	T48.9Ø1	T48.9Ø2	T48.9Ø3	T48.9Ø4	T48.9Ø5	T48.9Ø6
Retinoic acid	T49.ØX1	T49.ØX2	T49.ØX3	T49.ØX4	T49.ØX5	T49.ØX6
Retinol	T45.2X1	T45.2X2	T45.2X3	T45.2X4	T45.2X5	T45.2X6
Rh (D) immune globulin (human)	T5Ø.Z11	T5Ø.Z12	T5Ø.Z13	T5Ø.Z14	T5Ø.Z15	T5Ø.Z16
Rhodine	T39.Ø11	T39.Ø12	T39.Ø13	T39.Ø14	T39.Ø15	T39.Ø16
RhoGAM	T5Ø.Z11	T5Ø.Z12	T5Ø.Z13	T5Ø.Z14	T5Ø.Z15	T5Ø.Z16
Rhubarb						
dry extract	T47.2X1	T47.2X2	T47.2X3	T47.2X4	T47.2X5	T47.2X6
tincture, compound	T47.2X1	T47.2X2	T47.2X3	T47.2X4	T47.2X5	T47.2X6
Ribavirin	T37.5X1	T37.5X2	T37.5X3	T37.5X4	T37.5X5	T37.5X6
Riboflavin	T45.2X1	T45.2X2	T45.2X3	T45.2X4	T45.2X5	T45.2X6
Ribostamycin	T36.5X1	T36.5X2	T36.5X3	T36.5X4	T36.5X5	T36.5X6
Ricin	T62.2X1	T62.2X2	T62.2X3	T62.2X4	—	—
Ricinus communis	T62.2X1	T62.2X2	T62.2X3	T62.2X4	—	—
Rickettsial vaccine NEC	T5Ø.A91	T5Ø.A92	T5Ø.A93	T5Ø.A94	T5Ø.A95	T5Ø.A96
Rifabutin	T36.6X1	T36.6X2	T36.6X3	T36.6X4	T36.6X5	T36.6X6
Rifamide	T36.6X1	T36.6X2	T36.6X3	T36.6X4	T36.6X5	T36.6X6
Rifampicin	T36.6X1	T36.6X2	T36.6X3	T36.6X4	T36.6X5	T36.6X6
with isoniazid	T37.1X1	T37.1X2	T37.1X3	T37.1X4	T37.1X5	T37.1X6
Rifampin	T36.6X1	T36.6X2	T36.6X3	T36.6X4	T36.6X5	T36.6X6
Rifamycin	T36.6X1	T36.6X2	T36.6X3	T36.6X4	T36.6X5	T36.6X6
Rifaximin	T36.6X1	T36.6X2	T36.6X3	T36.6X4	T36.6X5	T36.6X6
Rimantadine	T37.5X1	T37.5X2	T37.5X3	T37.5X4	T37.5X5	T37.5X6
Rimazolium metilsulfate	T39.8X1	T39.8X2	T39.8X3	T39.8X4	T39.8X5	T39.8X6
Rimifon	T37.1X1	T37.1X2	T37.1X3	T37.1X4	T37.1X5	T37.1X6
Rimiterol	T48.6X1	T48.6X2	T48.6X3	T48.6X4	T48.6X5	T48.6X6
Ringer (lactate) solution	T5Ø.3X1	T5Ø.3X2	T5Ø.3X3	T5Ø.3X4	T5Ø.3X5	T5Ø.3X6
Ristocetin	T36.8X1	T36.8X2	T36.8X3	T36.8X4	T36.8X5	T36.8X6
Ritalin	T43.631	T43.632	T43.633	T43.634	T43.635	T43.636
Ritodrine	T44.5X1	T44.5X2	T44.5X3	T44.5X4	T44.5X5	T44.5X6
Roach killer — *see Insecticide*						
Rociverine	T44.3X1	T44.3X2	T44.3X3	T44.3X4	T44.3X5	T44.3X6
Rocky Mountain spotted fever vaccine	T5Ø.A91	T5Ø.A92	T5Ø.A93	T5Ø.A94	T5Ø.A95	T5Ø.A96
Rodenticide NEC	T6Ø.4X1	T6Ø.4X2	T6Ø.4X3	T6Ø.4X4	—	—
Rohypnol	T42.4X1	T42.4X2	T42.4X3	T42.4X4	T42.4X5	T42.4X6
Rokitamycin	T36.3X1	T36.3X2	T36.3X3	T36.3X4	T36.3X5	T36.3X6
Rolaids	T47.1X1	T47.1X2	T47.1X3	T47.1X4	T47.1X5	T47.1X6
Rolitetracycline	T36.4X1	T36.4X2	T36.4X3	T36.4X4	T36.4X5	T36.4X6
Romilar	T48.3X1	T48.3X2	T48.3X3	T48.3X4	T48.3X5	T48.3X6
Ronifibrate	T46.6X1	T46.6X2	T46.6X3	T46.6X4	T46.6X5	T46.6X6
Rosaprostol	T47.1X1	T47.1X2	T47.1X3	T47.1X4	T47.1X5	T47.1X6
Rose bengal sodium (131I)	T5Ø.8X1	T5Ø.8X2	T5Ø.8X3	T5Ø.8X4	T5Ø.8X5	T5Ø.8X6
Rose water ointment	T49.3X1	T49.3X2	T49.3X3	T49.3X4	T49.3X5	T49.3X6
Rosoxacin	T37.8X1	T37.8X2	T37.8X3	T37.8X4	T37.8X5	T37.8X6
Rotenone	T6Ø.2X1	T6Ø.2X2	T6Ø.2X3	T6Ø.2X4	—	—
Rotoxamine	T45.ØX1	T45.ØX2	T45.ØX3	T45.ØX4	T45.ØX5	T45.ØX6
Rough-on-rats	T6Ø.4X1	T6Ø.4X2	T6Ø.4X3	T6Ø.4X4	—	—
Roxatidine	T47.ØX1	T47.ØX2	T47.ØX3	T47.ØX4	T47.ØX5	T47.ØX6
Roxithromycin	T36.3X1	T36.3X2	T36.3X3	T36.3X4	T36.3X5	T36.3X6
Rt-PA	T45.611	T45.612	T45.613	T45.614	T45.615	T45.616
Rubbing alcohol	T51.2X1	T51.2X2	T51.2X3	T51.2X4	—	—
Rubefacient	T49.4X1	T49.4X2	T49.4X3	T49.4X4	T49.4X5	T49.4X6
Rubella vaccine	T5Ø.B91	T5Ø.B92	T5Ø.B93	T5Ø.B94	T5Ø.B95	T5Ø.B96
Rubelogen	T5Ø.B91	T5Ø.B92	T5Ø.B93	T5Ø.B94	T5Ø.B95	T5Ø.B96
Rubeovax	T5Ø.991	T5Ø.992	T5Ø.993	T5Ø.994	T5Ø.995	T5Ø.996
Rubidium chloride Rb82	T5Ø.8X1	T5Ø.8X2	T5Ø.8X3	T5Ø.8X4	T5Ø.8X5	T5Ø.8X6
Rubidomycin	T45.1X1	T45.1X2	T45.1X3	T45.1X4	T45.1X5	T45.1X6
Rue	T62.2X1	T62.2X2	T62.2X3	T62.2X4	—	—
Rufocromomycin	T45.1X1	T45.1X2	T45.1X3	T45.1X4	T45.1X5	T45.1X6
Russel's viper venin	T45.7X1	T45.7X2	T45.7X3	T45.7X4	T45.7X5	T45.7X6
Ruta (graveolens)	T62.2X1	T62.2X2	T62.2X3	T62.2X4	—	—
Rutinum	T46.991	T46.992	T46.993	T46.994	T46.995	T46.996
Rutoside	T46.991	T46.992	T46.993	T46.994	T46.995	T46.996

Substance	Poisoning, Accidental (Unintentional)	Poisoning, Intentional Self-Harm	Poisoning, Assault	Poisoning, Undetermined	Adverse Effect	Underdosing
S						
Sabadilla (plant)	T62.2X1	T62.2X2	T62.2X3	T62.2X4	—	—
pesticide	T60.2X1	T60.2X2	T60.2X3	T60.2X4	—	—
Saccharated iron oxide	T45.8X1	T45.8X2	T45.8X3	T45.8X4	T45.8X5	T45.8X6
Saccharin	T50.901	T50.902	T50.903	T50.904	T50.905	T50.906
Saccharomyces boulardii	T47.6X1	T47.6X2	T47.6X3	T47.6X4	T47.6X5	T47.6X6
Safflower oil	T46.6X1	T46.6X2	T46.6X3	T46.6X4	T46.6X5	T46.6X6
Safrazine	T43.1X1	T43.1X2	T43.1X3	T43.1X4	T43.1X5	T43.1X6
Salazosulfapyridine	T37.0X1	T37.0X2	T37.0X3	T37.0X4	T37.0X5	T37.0X6
Salbutamol	T48.6X1	T48.6X2	T48.6X3	T48.6X4	T48.6X5	T48.6X6
Salicylamide	T39.091	T39.092	T39.093	T39.094	T39.095	T39.096
Salicylate NEC	T39.091	T39.092	T39.093	T39.094	T39.095	T39.096
methyl	T49.3X1	T49.3X2	T49.3X3	T49.3X4	T49.3X5	T49.3X6
theobromine calcium	T50.2X1	T50.2X2	T50.2X3	T50.2X4	T50.2X5	T50.2X6
Salicylazosulfapyridine	T37.0X1	T37.0X2	T37.0X3	T37.0X4	T37.0X5	T37.0X6
Salicylhydroxamic acid	T49.0X1	T49.0X2	T49.0X3	T49.0X4	T49.0X5	T49.0X6
Salicylic acid	T49.4X1	T49.4X2	T49.4X3	T49.4X4	T49.4X5	T49.4X6
with benzoic acid	T49.4X1	T49.4X2	T49.4X3	T49.4X4	T49.4X5	T49.4X6
congeners	T39.091	T39.092	T39.093	T39.094	T39.095	T39.096
derivative	T39.091	T39.092	T39.093	T39.094	T39.095	T39.096
salts	T39.091	T39.092	T39.093	T39.094	T39.095	T39.096
Salinazid	T37.1X1	T37.1X2	T37.1X3	T37.1X4	T37.1X5	T37.1X6
Salmeterol	T48.6X1	T48.6X2	T48.6X3	T48.6X4	T48.6X5	T48.6X6
Salol	T49.3X1	T49.3X2	T49.3X3	T49.3X4	T49.3X5	T49.3X6
Salsalate	T39.091	T39.092	T39.093	T39.094	T39.095	T39.096
Salt substitute	T50.901	T50.902	T50.903	T50.904	T50.905	T50.906
Salt-replacing drug	T50.901	T50.902	T50.903	T50.904	T50.905	T50.906
Salt-retaining mineralocorticoid	T50.0X1	T50.0X2	T50.0X3	T50.0X4	T50.0X5	T50.0X6
Saluretic NEC	T50.2X1	T50.2X2	T50.2X3	T50.2X4	T50.2X5	T50.2X6
Saluron	T50.2X1	T50.2X2	T50.2X3	T50.2X4	T50.2X5	T50.2X6
Salvarsan 606 (neosilver) (silver)	T37.8X1	T37.8X2	T37.8X3	T37.8X4	T37.8X5	T37.8X6
Sambucus canadensis	T62.2X1	T62.2X2	T62.2X3	T62.2X4	—	—
berry	T62.1X1	T62.1X2	T62.1X3	T62.1X4	—	—
Sandril	T46.5X1	T46.5X2	T46.5X3	T46.5X4	T46.5X5	T46.5X6
Sanguinaria canadensis	T62.2X1	T62.2X2	T62.2X3	T62.2X4	—	—
Saniflush (cleaner)	T54.2X1	T54.2X2	T54.2X3	T54.2X4	—	—
Santonin	T37.4X1	T37.4X2	T37.4X3	T37.4X4	T37.4X5	T37.4X6
Santyl	T49.8X1	T49.8X2	T49.8X3	T49.8X4	T49.8X5	T49.8X6
Saralasin	T46.5X1	T46.5X2	T46.5X3	T46.5X4	T46.5X5	T46.5X6
Sarcolysin	T45.1X1	T45.1X2	T45.1X3	T45.1X4	T45.1X5	T45.1X6
Sarkomycin	T45.1X1	T45.1X2	T45.1X3	T45.1X4	T45.1X5	T45.1X6
Saroten	T43.011	T43.012	T43.013	T43.014	T43.015	T43.016
Saturnine — *see Lead*						
Savin (oil)	T49.4X1	T49.4X2	T49.4X3	T49.4X4	T49.4X5	T49.4X6
Scammony	T47.2X1	T47.2X2	T47.2X3	T47.2X4	T47.2X5	T47.2X6
Scarlet red	T49.8X1	T49.8X2	T49.8X3	T49.8X4	T49.8X5	T49.8X6
Scheele's green	T57.0X1	T57.0X2	T57.0X3	T57.0X4	—	—
insecticide	T57.0X1	T57.0X2	T57.0X3	T57.0X4	—	—
Schizontozide (blood) (tissue)	T37.2X1	T37.2X2	T37.2X3	T37.2X4	T37.2X5	T37.2X6
Schradan	T60.0X1	T60.0X2	T60.0X3	T60.0X4	—	—
Schweinfurth green	T57.0X1	T57.0X2	T57.0X3	T57.0X4	—	—
insecticide	T57.0X1	T57.0X2	T57.0X3	T57.0X4	—	—
Scilla, rat poison	T60.4X1	T60.4X2	T60.4X3	T60.4X4	—	—
Scillaren	T60.4X1	T60.4X2	T60.4X3	T60.4X4	—	—
Sclerosing agent	T46.8X1	T46.8X2	T46.8X3	T46.8X4	T46.8X5	T46.8X6
Scombrotoxin	T61.11	T61.12	T61.13	T61.14	—	—
Scopolamine	T44.3X1	T44.3X2	T44.3X3	T44.3X4	T44.3X5	T44.3X6
Scopolia extract	T44.3X1	T44.3X2	T44.3X3	T44.3X4	T44.3X5	T44.3X6
Scouring powder	T65.891	T65.892	T65.893	T65.894	—	—
Sea						
anemone (sting)	T63.631	T63.632	T63.633	T63.634	—	—
cucumber (sting)	T63.691	T63.692	T63.693	T63.694	—	—
snake (bite) (venom)	T63.091	T63.092	T63.093	T63.094	—	—
urchin spine (puncture)	T63.691	T63.692	T63.693	T63.694	—	—
Seafood	T61.91	T61.92	T61.93	T61.94	—	—
specified NEC	T61.8X1	T61.8X2	T61.8X3	T61.8X4	—	—
Secbutabarbital	T42.3X1	T42.3X2	T42.3X3	T42.3X4	T42.3X5	T42.3X6
Secbutabarbitone	T42.3X1	T42.3X2	T42.3X3	T42.3X4	T42.3X5	T42.3X6
Secnidazole	T37.3X1	T37.3X2	T37.3X3	T37.3X4	T37.3X5	T37.3X6
Secobarbital	T42.3X1	T42.3X2	T42.3X3	T42.3X4	T42.3X5	T42.3X6
Seconal	T42.3X1	T42.3X2	T42.3X3	T42.3X4	T42.3X5	T42.3X6
Secretin	T50.8X1	T50.8X2	T50.8X3	T50.8X4	T50.8X5	T50.8X6
Sedative NEC	T42.71	T42.72	T42.73	T42.74	T42.75	T42.76
mixed NEC	T42.6X1	T42.6X2	T42.6X3	T42.6X4	T42.6X5	T42.6X6
Sedormid	T42.6X1	T42.6X2	T42.6X3	T42.6X4	T42.6X5	T42.6X6
Seed disinfectant or dressing	T60.8X1	T60.8X2	T60.8X3	T60.8X4	—	—
Seeds (poisonous)	T62.2X1	T62.2X2	T62.2X3	T62.2X4	—	—
Selegiline	T42.8X1	T42.8X2	T42.8X3	T42.8X4	T42.8X5	T42.8X6
Selenium NEC	T56.891	T56.892	T56.893	T56.894	—	—
disulfide or sulfide	T49.4X1	T49.4X2	T49.4X3	T49.4X4	T49.4X5	T49.4X6
fumes	T59.891	T59.892	T59.893	T59.894	—	—
sulfide	T49.4X1	T49.4X2	T49.4X3	T49.4X4	T49.4X5	T49.4X6
Selenomethionine (75Se)	T50.8X1	T50.8X2	T50.8X3	T50.8X4	T50.8X5	T50.8X6
Selsun	T49.4X1	T49.4X2	T49.4X3	T49.4X4	T49.4X5	T49.4X6

◀ New ⟵ Revised ~~deleted~~ Deleted

Substance	Poisoning, Accidental (Unintentional)	Poisoning, Intentional Self-Harm	Poisoning, Assault	Poisoning, Undetermined	Adverse Effect	Underdosing
Semustine	T45.1X1	T45.1X2	T45.1X3	T45.1X4	T45.1X5	T45.1X6
Senega syrup	T48.4X1	T48.4X2	T48.4X3	T48.4X4	T48.4X5	T48.4X6
Senna	T47.2X1	T47.2X2	T47.2X3	T47.2X4	T47.2X5	T47.2X6
Sennoside A+B	T47.2X1	T47.2X2	T47.2X3	T47.2X4	T47.2X5	T47.2X6
Septisol	T49.2X1	T49.2X2	T49.2X3	T49.2X4	T49.2X5	T49.2X6
Seractide	T38.811	T38.812	T38.813	T38.814	T38.815	T38.816
Serax	T42.4X1	T42.4X2	T42.4X3	T42.4X4	T42.4X5	T42.4X6
Serenesil	T42.6X1	T42.6X2	T42.6X3	T42.6X4	T42.6X5	T42.6X6
Serenium (hydrochloride)	T37.91	T37.92	T37.93	T37.94	T37.95	T37.96
Serepax — *see Oxazepam*						
Sermorelin	T38.891	T38.892	T38.893	T38.894	T38.895	T38.896
Sernyl	T41.1X1	T41.1X2	T41.1X3	T41.1X4	T41.1X5	T41.1X6
Serotonin	T50.991	T50.992	T50.993	T50.994	T50.995	T50.996
Serpasil	T46.5X1	T46.5X2	T46.5X3	T46.5X4	T46.5X5	T46.5X6
Serrapeptase	T45.3X1	T45.3X2	T45.3X3	T45.3X4	T45.3X5	T45.3X6
Serum						
antibotulinus	T50.Z11	T50.Z12	T50.Z13	T50.Z14	T50.Z15	T50.Z16
anticytotoxic	T50.Z11	T50.Z12	T50.Z13	T50.Z14	T50.Z15	T50.Z16
antidiphtheria	T50.Z11	T50.Z12	T50.Z13	T50.Z14	T50.Z15	T50.Z16
antimeningococcus	T50.Z11	T50.Z12	T50.Z13	T50.Z14	T50.Z15	T50.Z16
anti-Rh	T50.Z11	T50.Z12	T50.Z13	T50.Z14	T50.Z15	T50.Z16
anti-snake-bite	T50.Z11	T50.Z12	T50.Z13	T50.Z14	T50.Z15	T50.Z16
antitetanic	T50.Z11	T50.Z12	T50.Z13	T50.Z14	T50.Z15	T50.Z16
antitoxic	T50.Z11	T50.Z12	T50.Z13	T50.Z14	T50.Z15	T50.Z16
complement (inhibitor)	T45.8X1	T45.8X2	T45.8X3	T45.8X4	T45.8X5	T45.8X6
convalescent	T50.Z11	T50.Z12	T50.Z13	T50.Z14	T50.Z15	T50.Z16
hemolytic complement	T45.8X1	T45.8X2	T45.8X3	T45.8X4	T45.8X5	T45.8X6
immune (human)	T50.Z11	T50.Z12	T50.Z13	T50.Z14	T50.Z15	T50.Z16
protective NEC	T50.Z11	T50.Z12	T50.Z13	T50.Z14	T50.Z15	T50.Z16
Setastine	T45.0X1	T45.0X2	T45.0X3	T45.0X4	T45.0X5	T45.0X6
Setoperone	T43.591	T43.592	T43.593	T43.594	T43.595	T43.596
Sewer gas	T59.91	T59.92	T59.93	T59.94	—	—
Shampoo	T55.0X1	T55.0X2	T55.0X3	T55.0X4	—	—
Shellfish, noxious, nonbacterial	T61.781	T61.782	T61.783	T61.784	—	—
Sildenafil	T46.7X1	T46.7X2	T46.7X3	T46.7X4	T46.7X5	T46.7X6
Silibinin	T50.991	T50.992	T50.993	T50.994	T50.995	T50.996
Silicone NEC	T65.891	T65.892	T65.893	T65.894	—	—
medicinal	T49.3X1	T49.3X2	T49.3X3	T49.3X4	T49.3X5	T49.3X6
Silvadene	T49.0X1	T49.0X2	T49.0X3	T49.0X4	T49.0X5	T49.0X6
Silver	T49.0X1	T49.0X2	T49.0X3	T49.0X4	T49.0X5	T49.0X6
anti-infectives	T49.0X1	T49.0X2	T49.0X3	T49.0X4	T49.0X5	T49.0X6
arsphenamine	T37.8X1	T37.8X2	T37.8X3	T37.8X4	T37.8X5	T37.8X6
Silver *(Continued)*						
colloidal	T49.0X1	T49.0X2	T49.0X3	T49.0X4	T49.0X5	T49.0X6
nitrate	T49.0X1	T49.0X2	T49.0X3	T49.0X4	T49.0X5	T49.0X6
ophthalmic preparation	T49.5X1	T49.5X2	T49.5X3	T49.5X4	T49.5X5	T49.5X6
toughened (keratolytic)	T49.4X1	T49.4X2	T49.4X3	T49.4X4	T49.4X5	T49.4X6
nonmedicinal (dust)	T56.891	T56.892	T56.893	T56.894	—	—
protein	T49.5X1	T49.5X2	T49.5X3	T49.5X4	T49.5X5	T49.5X6
salvarsan	T37.8X1	T37.8X2	T37.8X3	T37.8X4	T37.8X5	T37.8X6
sulfadiazine	T49.4X1	T49.4X2	T49.4X3	T49.4X4	T49.4X5	T49.4X6
Silymarin	T50.991	T50.992	T50.993	T50.994	T50.995	T50.996
Simaldrate	T47.1X1	T47.1X2	T47.1X3	T47.1X4	T47.1X5	T47.1X6
Simazine	T60.3X1	T60.3X2	T60.3X3	T60.3X4	—	—
Simethicone	T47.1X1	T47.1X2	T47.1X3	T47.1X4	T47.1X5	T47.1X6
Simfibrate	T46.6X1	T46.6X2	T46.6X3	T46.6X4	T46.6X5	T46.6X6
Simvastatin	T46.6X1	T46.6X2	T46.6X3	T46.6X4	T46.6X5	T46.6X6
Sincalide	T50.8X1	T50.8X2	T50.8X3	T50.8X4	T50.8X5	T50.8X6
Sinequan	T43.011	T43.012	T43.013	T43.014	T43.015	T43.016
Singoserp	T46.5X1	T46.5X2	T46.5X3	T46.5X4	T46.5X5	T46.5X6
Sintrom	T45.511	T45.512	T45.513	T45.514	T45.515	T45.516
Sisomicin	T36.5X1	T36.5X2	T36.5X3	T36.5X4	T36.5X5	T36.5X6
Sitosterols	T46.6X1	T46.6X2	T46.6X3	T46.6X4	T46.6X5	T46.6X6
Skeletal muscle relaxants	T48.1X1	T48.1X2	T48.1X3	T48.1X4	T48.1X5	T48.1X6
Skin						
agents (external)	T49.91	T49.92	T49.93	T49.94	T49.95	T49.96
specified NEC	T49.8X1	T49.8X2	T49.8X3	T49.8X4	T49.8X5	T49.8X6
test antigen	T50.8X1	T50.8X2	T50.8X3	T50.8X4	T50.8X5	T50.8X6
Sleep-eze	T45.0X1	T45.0X2	T45.0X3	T45.0X4	T45.0X5	T45.0X6
Sleeping draught, pill	T42.71	T42.72	T42.73	T42.74	T42.75	T42.76
Smallpox vaccine	T50.B11	T50.B12	T50.B13	T50.B14	T50.B15	T50.B16
Smelter fumes NEC	T56.91	T56.92	T56.93	T56.94	—	—
Smog	T59.1X1	T59.1X2	T59.1X3	T59.1X4	—	—
Smoke NEC	T59.811	T59.812	T59.813	T59.814	—	—
Smooth muscle relaxant	T44.3X1	T44.3X2	T44.3X3	T44.3X4	T44.3X5	T44.3X6
Snail killer NEC	T60.8X1	T60.8X2	T60.8X3	T60.8X4	—	—
Snake venom or bite	T63.001	T63.002	T63.003	T63.004	—	—
hemocoagulase	T45.7X1	T45.7X2	T45.7X3	T45.7X4	T45.7X5	T45.7X6
Snuff	T65.211	T65.212	T65.213	T65.214	—	—
Soap (powder) (product)	T55.0X1	T55.0X2	T55.0X3	T55.0X4	—	—
enema	T47.4X1	T47.4X2	T47.4X3	T47.4X4	T47.4X5	T47.4X6
medicinal, soft	T49.2X1	T49.2X2	T49.2X3	T49.2X4	T49.2X5	T49.2X6
superfatted	T49.2X1	T49.2X2	T49.2X3	T49.2X4	T49.2X5	T49.2X6
Sobrerol	T48.4X1	T48.4X2	T48.4X3	T48.4X4	T48.4X5	T48.4X6

Substance	Poisoning, Accidental (Unintentional)	Poisoning, Intentional Self-Harm	Poisoning, Assault	Poisoning, Undetermined	Adverse Effect	Underdosing
Soda (caustic)	T54.3X1	T54.3X2	T54.3X3	T54.3X4	—	—
bicarb	T47.1X1	T47.1X2	T47.1X3	T47.1X4	T47.1X5	T47.1X6
chlorinated — *see Sodium, hypochlorite*						
Sodium						
acetosulfone	T37.1X1	T37.1X2	T37.1X3	T37.1X4	T37.1X5	T37.1X6
acetrizoate	T5Ø.8X1	T5Ø.8X2	T5Ø.8X3	T5Ø.8X4	T5Ø.8X5	T5Ø.8X6
acid phosphate	T5Ø.3X1	T5Ø.3X2	T5Ø.3X3	T5Ø.3X4	T5Ø.3X5	T5Ø.3X6
alginate	T47.8X1	T47.8X2	T47.8X3	T47.8X4	T47.8X5	T47.8X6
amidotrizoate	T5Ø.8X1	T5Ø.8X2	T5Ø.8X3	T5Ø.8X4	T5Ø.8X5	T5Ø.8X6
aminopterin	T45.1X1	T45.1X2	T45.1X3	T45.1X4	T45.1X5	T45.1X6
amylosulfate	T47.8X1	T47.8X2	T47.8X3	T47.8X4	T47.8X5	T47.8X6
amytal	T42.3X1	T42.3X2	T42.3X3	T42.3X4	T42.3X5	T42.3X6
antimony gluconate	T37.3X1	T37.3X2	T37.3X3	T37.3X4	T37.3X5	T37.3X6
arsenate	T57.ØX1	T57.ØX2	T57.ØX3	T57.ØX4	—	—
aurothiomalate	T39.4X1	T39.4X2	T39.4X3	T39.4X4	T39.4X5	T39.4X6
aurothiosulfate	T39.4X1	T39.4X2	T39.4X3	T39.4X4	T39.4X5	T39.4X6
barbiturate	T42.3X1	T42.3X2	T42.3X3	T42.3X4	T42.3X5	T42.3X6
basic phosphate	T47.4X1	T47.4X2	T47.4X3	T47.4X4	T47.4X5	T47.4X6
bicarbonate	T47.1X1	T47.1X2	T47.1X3	T47.1X4	T47.1X5	T47.1X6
bichromate	T57.8X1	T57.8X2	T57.8X3	T57.8X4	—	—
biphosphate	T5Ø.3X1	T5Ø.3X2	T5Ø.3X3	T5Ø.3X4	T5Ø.3X5	T5Ø.3X6
bisulfate	T65.891	T65.892	T65.893	T65.894	—	—
borate						
cleanser	T57.8X1	T57.8X2	T57.8X3	T57.8X4	—	—
eye	T49.5X1	T49.5X2	T49.5X3	T49.5X4	T49.5X5	T49.5X6
therapeutic	T49.8X1	T49.8X2	T49.8X3	T49.8X4	T49.8X5	T49.8X6
bromide	T42.6X1	T42.6X2	T42.6X3	T42.6X4	T42.6X5	T42.6X6
cacodylate (nonmedicinal) NEC	T5Ø.8X1	T5Ø.8X2	T5Ø.8X3	T5Ø.8X4	T5Ø.8X5	T5Ø.8X6
anti-infective	T37.8X1	T37.8X2	T37.8X3	T37.8X4	T37.8X5	T37.8X6
herbicide	T6Ø.3X1	T6Ø.3X2	T6Ø.3X3	T6Ø.3X4	—	—
calcium edetate	T45.8X1	T45.8X2	T45.8X3	T45.8X4	T45.8X5	T45.8X6
carbonate NEC	T54.3X1	T54.3X2	T54.3X3	T54.3X4	—	—
chlorate NEC	T65.891	T65.892	T65.893	T65.894	—	—
herbicide	T54.91	T54.92	T54.93	T54.94	—	—
chloride	T5Ø.3X1	T5Ø.3X2	T5Ø.3X3	T5Ø.3X4	T5Ø.3X5	T5Ø.3X6
with glucose	T5Ø.3X1	T5Ø.3X2	T5Ø.3X3	T5Ø.3X4	T5Ø.3X5	T5Ø.3X6
chromate	T65.891	T65.892	T65.893	T65.894	—	—
citrate	T5Ø.991	T5Ø.992	T5Ø.993	T5Ø.994	T5Ø.995	T5Ø.996
cromoglicate	T48.6X1	T48.6X2	T48.6X3	T48.6X4	T48.6X5	T48.6X6
cyanide	T65.ØX1	T65.ØX2	T65.ØX3	T65.ØX4	—	—
cyclamate	T5Ø.3X1	T5Ø.3X2	T5Ø.3X3	T5Ø.3X4	T5Ø.3X5	T5Ø.3X6
Sodium *(Continued)*						
dehydrocholate	T45.8X1	T45.8X2	T45.8X3	T45.8X4	T45.8X5	T45.8X6
diatrizoate	T5Ø.8X1	T5Ø.8X2	T5Ø.8X3	T5Ø.8X4	T5Ø.8X5	T5Ø.8X6
dibunate	T48.4X1	T48.4X2	T48.4X3	T48.4X4	T48.4X5	T48.4X6
dioctyl sulfosuccinate	T47.4X1	T47.4X2	T47.4X3	T47.4X4	T47.4X5	T47.4X6
dipantoyl ferrate	T45.8X1	T45.8X2	T45.8X3	T45.8X4	T45.8X5	T45.8X6
edetate	T45.8X1	T45.8X2	T45.8X3	T45.8X4	T45.8X5	T45.8X6
ethacrynate	T5Ø.1X1	T5Ø.1X2	T5Ø.1X3	T5Ø.1X4	T5Ø.1X5	T5Ø.1X6
feredetate	T45.8X1	T45.8X2	T45.8X3	T45.8X4	T45.8X5	T45.8X6
Fluoride — *see Fluoride*						
fluoroacetate (dust) (pesticide)	T6Ø.4X1	T6Ø.4X2	T6Ø.4X3	T6Ø.4X4	—	—
free salt	T5Ø.3X1	T5Ø.3X2	T5Ø.3X3	T5Ø.3X4	T5Ø.3X5	T5Ø.3X6
fusidate	T36.8X1	T36.8X2	T36.8X3	T36.8X4	T36.8X5	T36.8X6
glucaldrate	T47.1X1	T47.1X2	T47.1X3	T47.1X4	T47.1X5	T47.1X6
glucosulfone	T37.1X1	T37.1X2	T37.1X3	T37.1X4	T37.1X5	T37.1X6
glutamate	T45.8X1	T45.8X2	T45.8X3	T45.8X4	T45.8X5	T45.8X6
hydrogen carbonate	T5Ø.3X1	T5Ø.3X2	T5Ø.3X3	T5Ø.3X4	T5Ø.3X5	T5Ø.3X6
hydroxide	T54.3X1	T54.3X2	T54.3X3	T54.3X4	—	—
hypochlorite (bleach) NEC	T54.3X1	T54.3X2	T54.3X3	T54.3X4	—	—
disinfectant	T54.3X1	T54.3X2	T54.3X3	T54.3X4	—	—
medicinal (anti-infective) (external)	T49.ØX1	T49.ØX2	T49.ØX3	T49.ØX4	T49.ØX5	T49.ØX6
vapor	T54.3X1	T54.3X2	T54.3X3	T54.3X4	—	—
hyposulfite	T49.ØX1	T49.ØX2	T49.ØX3	T49.ØX4	T49.ØX5	T49.ØX6
indigotin disulfonate	T5Ø.8X1	T5Ø.8X2	T5Ø.8X3	T5Ø.8X4	T5Ø.8X5	T5Ø.8X6
iodide	T5Ø.991	T5Ø.992	T5Ø.993	T5Ø.994	T5Ø.995	T5Ø.996
I-131	T5Ø.8X1	T5Ø.8X2	T5Ø.8X3	T5Ø.8X4	T5Ø.8X5	T5Ø.8X6
therapeutic	T38.2X1	T38.2X2	T38.2X3	T38.2X4	T38.2X5	T38.2X6
iodohippurate (131I)	T5Ø.8X1	T5Ø.8X2	T5Ø.8X3	T5Ø.8X4	T5Ø.8X5	T5Ø.8X6
iopodate	T5Ø.8X1	T5Ø.8X2	T5Ø.8X3	T5Ø.8X4	T5Ø.8X5	T5Ø.8X6
iothalamate	T5Ø.8X1	T5Ø.8X2	T5Ø.8X3	T5Ø.8X4	T5Ø.8X5	T5Ø.8X6
iron edetate	T45.4X1	T45.4X2	T45.4X3	T45.4X4	T45.4X5	T45.4X6
lactate (compound solution)	T45.8X1	T45.8X2	T45.8X3	T45.8X4	T45.8X5	T45.8X6
lauryl (sulfate)	T49.2X1	T49.2X2	T49.2X3	T49.2X4	T49.2X5	T49.2X6
(L)-triiodothyronine	T38.1X1	T38.1X2	T38.1X3	T38.1X4	T38.1X5	T38.1X6
magnesium citrate	T5Ø.991	T5Ø.992	T5Ø.993	T5Ø.994	T5Ø.995	T5Ø.996
mersalate	T5Ø.2X1	T5Ø.2X2	T5Ø.2X3	T5Ø.2X4	T5Ø.2X5	T5Ø.2X6
metasilicate	T65.891	T65.892	T65.893	T65.894	—	—
metrizoate	T5Ø.8X1	T5Ø.8X2	T5Ø.8X3	T5Ø.8X4	T5Ø.8X5	T5Ø.8X6
monofluoroacetate (pesticide)	T6Ø.1X1	T6Ø.1X2	T6Ø.1X3	T6Ø.1X4	—	—
morrhuate	T46.8X1	T46.8X2	T46.8X3	T46.8X4	T46.8X5	T46.8X6
nafcillin	T36.ØX1	T36.ØX2	T36.ØX3	T36.ØX4	T36.ØX5	T36.ØX6

◀ New ◀ Revised ~~deleted~~ Deleted

Substance	Poisoning, Accidental (Unintentional)	Poisoning, Intentional Self-Harm	Poisoning, Assault	Poisoning, Undetermined	Adverse Effect	Underdosing
Sodium *(Continued)*						
nitrate (oxidizing agent)	T65.891	T65.892	T65.893	T65.894	—	—
nitrite	T50.6X1	T50.6X2	T50.6X3	T50.6X4	T50.6X5	T50.6X6
nitroferricyanide	T46.5X1	T46.5X2	T46.5X3	T46.5X4	T46.5X5	T46.5X6
nitroprusside	T46.5X1	T46.5X2	T46.5X3	T46.5X4	T46.5X5	T46.5X6
oxalate	T65.891	T65.892	T65.893	T65.894	—	—
oxide/peroxide	T65.891	T65.892	T65.893	T65.894	—	—
oxybate	T41.291	T41.292	T41.293	T41.294	T41.295	T41.296
para-aminohippurate	T50.8X1	T50.8X2	T50.8X3	T50.8X4	T50.8X5	T50.8X6
perborate (nonmedicinal) NEC	T65.891	T65.892	T65.893	T65.894	—	—
medicinal	T49.0X1	T49.0X2	T49.0X3	T49.0X4	T49.0X5	T49.0X6
soap	T55.0X1	T55.0X2	T55.0X3	T55.0X4	—	—
percarbonate — *see Sodium, perborate*						
pertechnetate Tc99m	T50.8X1	T50.8X2	T50.8X3	T50.8X4	T50.8X5	T50.8X6
phosphate						
cellulose	T45.8X1	T45.8X2	T45.8X3	T45.8X4	T45.8X5	T45.8X6
dibasic	T47.2X1	T47.2X2	T47.2X3	T47.2X4	T47.2X5	T47.2X6
monobasic	T47.2X1	T47.2X2	T47.2X3	T47.2X4	T47.2X5	T47.2X6
phytate	T50.6X1	T50.6X2	T50.6X3	T50.6X4	T50.6X5	T50.6X6
picosulfate	T47.2X1	T47.2X2	T47.2X3	T47.2X4	T47.2X5	T47.2X6
polyhydroxyaluminium monocarbonate	T47.1X1	T47.1X2	T47.1X3	T47.1X4	T47.1X5	T47.1X6
polystyrene sulfonate	T50.3X1	T50.3X2	T50.3X3	T50.3X4	T50.3X5	T50.3X6
propionate	T49.0X1	T49.0X2	T49.0X3	T49.0X4	T49.0X5	T49.0X6
propyl hydroxybenzoate	T50.991	T50.992	T50.993	T50.994	T50.995	T50.996
psylliate	T46.8X1	T46.8X2	T46.8X3	T46.8X4	T46.8X5	T46.8X6
removing resins	T50.3X1	T50.3X2	T50.3X3	T50.3X4	T50.3X5	T50.3X6
salicylate	T39.091	T39.092	T39.093	T39.094	T39.095	T39.096
salt NEC	T50.3X1	T50.3X2	T50.3X3	T50.3X4	T50.3X5	T50.3X6
selenate	T60.2X1	T60.2X2	T60.2X3	T60.2X4	—	—
stibogluconate	T37.3X1	T37.3X2	T37.3X3	T37.3X4	T37.3X5	T37.3X6
sulfate	T47.4X1	T47.4X2	T47.4X3	T47.4X4	T47.4X5	T47.4X6
sulfoxone	T37.1X1	T37.1X2	T37.1X3	T37.1X4	T37.1X5	T37.1X6
tetradecyl sulfate	T46.8X1	T46.8X2	T46.8X3	T46.8X4	T46.8X5	T46.8X6
thiopental	T41.1X1	T41.1X2	T41.1X3	T41.1X4	T41.1X5	T41.1X6
thiosalicylate	T39.091	T39.092	T39.093	T39.094	T39.095	T39.096
thiosulfate	T50.6X1	T50.6X2	T50.6X3	T50.6X4	T50.6X5	T50.6X6
tolbutamide	T38.3X1	T38.3X2	T38.3X3	T38.3X4	T38.3X5	T38.3X6
l-triiodothyronine	T38.1X1	T38.1X2	T38.1X3	T38.1X4	T38.1X5	T38.1X6
tyropanoate	T50.8X1	T50.8X2	T50.8X3	T50.8X4	T50.8X5	T50.8X6
valproate	T42.6X1	T42.6X2	T42.6X3	T42.6X4	T42.6X5	T42.6X6
versenate	T50.6X1	T50.6X2	T50.6X3	T50.6X4	T50.6X5	T50.6X6

Substance	Poisoning, Accidental (Unintentional)	Poisoning, Intentional Self-Harm	Poisoning, Assault	Poisoning, Undetermined	Adverse Effect	Underdosing
Sodium-free salt	T50.901	T50.902	T50.903	T50.904	T50.905	T50.906
Sodium-removing resin	T50.3X1	T50.3X2	T50.3X3	T50.3X4	T50.3X5	T50.3X6
Soft soap	T55.0X1	T55.0X2	T55.0X3	T55.0X4	—	—
Solanine	T62.2X1	T62.2X2	T62.2X3	T62.2X4	—	—
berries	T62.1X1	T62.1X2	T62.1X3	T62.1X4	—	—
Solanum dulcamara	T62.2X1	T62.2X2	T62.2X3	T62.2X4	—	—
berries	T62.1X1	T62.1X2	T62.1X3	T62.1X4	—	—
Solapsone	T37.1X1	T37.1X2	T37.1X3	T37.1X4	T37.1X5	T37.1X6
Solar lotion	T49.3X1	T49.3X2	T49.3X3	T49.3X4	T49.3X5	T49.3X6
Solasulfone	T37.1X1	T37.1X2	T37.1X3	T37.1X4	T37.1X5	T37.1X6
Soldering fluid	T65.891	T65.892	T65.893	T65.894	—	—
Solid substance	T65.91	T65.92	T65.93	T65.94	—	—
specified NEC	T65.891	T65.892	T65.893	T65.894	—	—
Solvent, industrial NEC	T52.91	T52.92	T52.93	T52.94	—	—
naphtha	T52.0X1	T52.0X2	T52.0X3	T52.0X4	—	—
petroleum	T52.0X1	T52.0X2	T52.0X3	T52.0X4	—	—
specified NEC	T52.8X1	T52.8X2	T52.8X3	T52.8X4	—	—
Soma	T42.8X1	T42.8X2	T42.8X3	T42.8X4	T42.8X5	T42.8X6
Somatorelin	T38.891	T38.892	T38.893	T38.894	T38.895	T38.896
Somatostatin	T38.991	T38.992	T38.993	T38.994	T38.995	T38.996
Somatotropin	T38.811	T38.812	T38.813	T38.814	T38.815	T38.816
Somatrem	T38.811	T38.812	T38.813	T38.814	T38.815	T38.816
Somatropin	T38.811	T38.812	T38.813	T38.814	T38.815	T38.816
Sominex	T45.0X1	T45.0X2	T45.0X3	T45.0X4	T45.0X5	T45.0X6
Somnos	T42.6X1	T42.6X2	T42.6X3	T42.6X4	T42.6X5	T42.6X6
Somonal	T42.3X1	T42.3X2	T42.3X3	T42.3X4	T42.3X5	T42.3X6
Soneryl	T42.3X1	T42.3X2	T42.3X3	T42.3X4	T42.3X5	T42.3X6
Soothing syrup	T50.901	T50.902	T50.903	T50.904	T50.905	T50.906
Sopor	T42.6X1	T42.6X2	T42.6X3	T42.6X4	T42.6X5	T42.6X6
Soporific	T42.71	T42.72	T42.73	T42.74	T42.75	T42.76
Soporific drug	T42.71	T42.72	T42.73	T42.74	T42.75	T42.76
specified type NEC	T42.6X1	T42.6X2	T42.6X3	T42.6X4	T42.6X5	T42.6X6
Sorbide nitrate	T46.3X1	T46.3X2	T46.3X3	T46.3X4	T46.3X5	T46.3X6
Sorbitol	T47.4X1	T47.4X2	T47.4X3	T47.4X4	T47.4X5	T47.4X6
Sotalol	T44.7X1	T44.7X2	T44.7X3	T44.7X4	T44.7X5	T44.7X6
Sotradecol	T46.8X1	T46.8X2	T46.8X3	T46.8X4	T46.8X5	T46.8X6
Soysterol	T46.6X1	T46.6X2	T46.6X3	T46.6X4	T46.6X5	T46.6X6
Spacoline	T44.3X1	T44.3X2	T44.3X3	T44.3X4	T44.3X5	T44.3X6
Spanish fly	T49.8X1	T49.8X2	T49.8X3	T49.8X4	T49.8X5	T49.8X6
Sparine	T43.3X1	T43.3X2	T43.3X3	T43.3X4	T43.3X5	T43.3X6
Sparteine	T48.0X1	T48.0X2	T48.0X3	T48.0X4	T48.0X5	T48.0X6

Substance	Poisoning, Accidental (Unintentional)	Poisoning, Intentional Self-Harm	Poisoning, Assault	Poisoning, Undetermined	Adverse Effect	Underdosing
Spasmolytic						
anticholinergics	T44.3X1	T44.3X2	T44.3X3	T44.3X4	T44.3X5	T44.3X6
autonomic	T44.3X1	T44.3X2	T44.3X3	T44.3X4	T44.3X5	T44.3X6
bronchial NEC	T48.6X1	T48.6X2	T48.6X3	T48.6X4	T48.6X5	T48.6X6
quaternary ammonium	T44.3X1	T44.3X2	T44.3X3	T44.3X4	T44.3X5	T44.3X6
skeletal muscle NEC	T48.1X1	T48.1X2	T48.1X3	T48.1X4	T48.1X5	T48.1X6
Spectinomycin	T36.5X1	T36.5X2	T36.5X3	T36.5X4	T36.5X5	T36.5X6
Speed	T43.621	T43.622	T43.623	T43.624	T43.625	T43.626
Spermicide	T49.8X1	T49.8X2	T49.8X3	T49.8X4	T49.8X5	T49.8X6
Spider (bite) (venom)	T63.391	T63.392	T63.393	T63.394	—	—
antivenin	T5Ø.Z11	T5Ø.Z12	T5Ø.Z13	T5Ø.Z14	T5Ø.Z15	T5Ø.Z16
Spigelia (root)	T37.4X1	T37.4X2	T37.4X3	T37.4X4	T37.4X5	T37.4X6
Spindle inactivator	T5Ø.4X1	T5Ø.4X2	T5Ø.4X3	T5Ø.4X4	T5Ø.4X5	T5Ø.4X6
Spiperone	T43.4X1	T43.4X2	T43.4X3	T43.4X4	T43.4X5	T43.4X6
Spiramycin	T36.3X1	T36.3X2	T36.3X3	T36.3X4	T36.3X5	T36.3X6
Spirapril	T46.4X1	T46.4X2	T46.4X3	T46.4X4	T46.4X5	T46.4X6
Spirilene	T43.591	T43.592	T43.593	T43.594	T43.595	T43.596
Spirit(s) (neutral) NEC	T51.ØX1	T51.ØX2	T51.ØX3	T51.ØX4	—	—
beverage	T51.ØX1	T51.ØX2	T51.ØX3	T51.ØX4	—	—
industrial	T51.ØX1	T51.ØX2	T51.ØX3	T51.ØX4	—	—
mineral	T52.ØX1	T52.ØX2	T52.ØX3	T52.ØX4	—	—
of salt — *see Hydrochloric acid*						
surgical	T51.ØX1	T51.ØX2	T51.ØX3	T51.ØX4	—	—
Spironolactone	T5Ø.ØX1	T5Ø.ØX2	T5Ø.ØX3	T5Ø.ØX4	T5Ø.ØX5	T5Ø.ØX6
Spiroperidol	T43.4X1	T43.4X2	T43.4X3	T43.4X4	T43.4X5	T43.4X6
Sponge, absorbable (gelatin)	T45.7X1	T45.7X2	T45.7X3	T45.7X4	T45.7X5	T45.7X6
Sporostacin	T49.ØX1	T49.ØX2	T49.ØX3	T49.ØX4	T49.ØX5	T49.ØX6
Spray (aerosol)	T65.91	T65.92	T65.93	T65.94	—	—
cosmetic	T65.891	T65.892	T65.893	T65.894	—	—
medicinal NEC	T5Ø.901	T5Ø.902	T5Ø.903	T5Ø.904	T5Ø.905	T5Ø.906
pesticides — *see Pesticides*						
specified content — *see specific substance*						
Spurge flax	T62.2X1	T62.2X2	T62.2X3	T62.2X4	—	—
Spurges	T62.2X1	T62.2X2	T62.2X3	T62.2X4	—	—
Sputum viscosity-lowering drug	T48.4X1	T48.4X2	T48.4X3	T48.4X4	T48.4X5	T48.4X6
Squill	T46.ØX1	T46.ØX2	T46.ØX3	T46.ØX4	T46.ØX5	T46.ØX6
rat poison	T6Ø.4X1	T6Ø.4X2	T6Ø.4X3	T6Ø.4X4	—	—
Squirting cucumber (cathartic)	T47.2X1	T47.2X2	T47.2X3	T47.2X4	T47.2X5	T47.2X6
Stains	T65.6X1	T65.6X2	T65.6X3	T65.6X4	—	—
Stannous fluoride	T49.7X1	T49.7X2	T49.7X3	T49.7X4	T49.7X5	T49.7X6
Stanolone	T38.7X1	T38.7X2	T38.7X3	T38.7X4	T38.7X5	T38.7X6
Stanozolol	T38.7X1	T38.7X2	T38.7X3	T38.7X4	T38.7X5	T38.7X6
Staphisagria or stavesacre (pediculicide)	T49.ØX1	T49.ØX2	T49.ØX3	T49.ØX4	T49.ØX5	T49.ØX6
Starch	T5Ø.901	T5Ø.902	T5Ø.903	T5Ø.904	T5Ø.905	T5Ø.906
Stelazine	T43.3X1	T43.3X2	T43.3X3	T43.3X4	T43.3X5	T43.3X6
Stemetil	T43.3X1	T43.3X2	T43.3X3	T43.3X4	T43.3X5	T43.3X6
Stepronin	T48.4X1	T48.4X2	T48.4X3	T48.4X4	T48.4X5	T48.4X6
Sterculia	T47.4X1	T47.4X2	T47.4X3	T47.4X4	T47.4X5	T47.4X6
Sternutator gas	T59.891	T59.892	T59.893	T59.894	—	—
Steroid	T38.ØX1	T38.ØX2	T38.ØX3	T38.ØX4	T38.ØX5	T38.ØX6
anabolic	T38.7X1	T38.7X2	T38.7X3	T38.7X4	T38.7X5	T38.7X6
androgenic	T38.7X1	T38.7X2	T38.7X3	T38.7X4	T38.7X5	T38.7X6
antineoplastic, hormone	T38.7X1	T38.7X2	T38.7X3	T38.7X4	T38.7X5	T38.7X6
estrogen	T38.5X1	T38.5X2	T38.5X3	T38.5X4	T38.5X5	T38.5X6
ENT agent	T49.6X1	T49.6X2	T49.6X3	T49.6X4	T49.6X5	T49.6X6
ophthalmic preparation	T49.5X1	T49.5X2	T49.5X3	T49.5X4	T49.5X5	T49.5X6
topical NEC	T49.ØX1	T49.ØX2	T49.ØX3	T49.ØX4	T49.ØX5	T49.ØX6
Stibine	T56.891	T56.892	T56.893	T56.894	—	—
Stibogluconate	T37.3X1	T37.3X2	T37.3X3	T37.3X4	T37.3X5	T37.3X6
Stibophen	T37.4X1	T37.4X2	T37.4X3	T37.4X4	T37.4X5	T37.4X6
Stilbamidine (isetionate)	T37.3X1	T37.3X2	T37.3X3	T37.3X4	T37.3X5	T37.3X6
Stilbestrol	T38.5X1	T38.5X2	T38.5X3	T38.5X4	T38.5X5	T38.5X6
Stilboestrol	T38.5X1	T38.5X2	T38.5X3	T38.5X4	T38.5X5	T38.5X6
Stimulant						
central nervous system — *see also Psychostimulant*	T43.6Ø1	T43.6Ø2	T43.6Ø3	T43.6Ø4	T43.6Ø5	T43.6Ø6
analeptics	T5Ø.7X1	T5Ø.7X2	T5Ø.7X3	T5Ø.7X4	T5Ø.7X5	T5Ø.7X6
opiate antagonist	T5Ø.7X1	T5Ø.7X2	T5Ø.7X3	T5Ø.7X4	T5Ø.7X5	T5Ø.7X6
psychotherapeutic NEC — *see also Psychotherapeutic drug*	T43.6Ø1	T43.6Ø2	T43.6Ø3	T43.6Ø4	T43.6Ø5	T43.6Ø6
specified NEC	T43.691	T43.692	T43.693	T43.694	T43.695	T43.696
respiratory	T48.901	T48.902	T48.903	T48.904	T48.905	T48.906
Stone-dissolving drug	T5Ø.901	T5Ø.902	T5Ø.903	T5Ø.904	T5Ø.905	T5Ø.906
Storage battery (cells) (acid)	T54.2X1	T54.2X2	T54.2X3	T54.2X4	—	—
Stovaine	T41.3X1	T41.3X2	T41.3X3	T41.3X4	T41.3X5	T41.3X6
infiltration (subcutaneous)	T41.3X1	T41.3X2	T41.3X3	T41.3X4	T41.3X5	T41.3X6
nerve block (peripheral) (plexus)	T41.3X1	T41.3X2	T41.3X3	T41.3X4	T41.3X5	T41.3X6
spinal	T41.3X1	T41.3X2	T41.3X3	T41.3X4	T41.3X5	T41.3X6
topical (surface)	T41.3X1	T41.3X2	T41.3X3	T41.3X4	T41.3X5	T41.3X6
Stovarsal	T37.8X1	T37.8X2	T37.8X3	T37.8X4	T37.8X5	T37.8X6
Stove gas — *see Gas, stove*	T57.91	T57.92	T57.93	T57.94	—	—

◄ New ◄▮▮ Revised ~~deleted~~ Deleted

Substance	Poisoning, Accidental (Unintentional)	Poisoning, Intentional Self-Harm	Poisoning, Assault	Poisoning, Undetermined	Adverse Effect	Underdosing
Stoxil	T49.5X1	T49.5X2	T49.5X3	T49.5X4	T49.5X5	T49.5X6
Stramonium	T48.6X1	T48.6X2	T48.6X3	T48.6X4	T48.6X5	T48.6X6
natural state	T62.2X1	T62.2X2	T62.2X3	T62.2X4	—	—
Streptodornase	T45.3X1	T45.3X2	T45.3X3	T45.3X4	T45.3X5	T45.3X6
Streptoduocin	T36.5X1	T36.5X2	T36.5X3	T36.5X4	T36.5X5	T36.5X6
Streptokinase	T45.611	T45.612	T45.613	T45.614	T45.615	T45.616
Streptomycin (derivative)	T36.5X1	T36.5X2	T36.5X3	T36.5X4	T36.5X5	T36.5X6
Streptonivicin	T36.5X1	T36.5X2	T36.5X3	T36.5X4	T36.5X5	T36.5X6
Streptovarycin	T36.5X1	T36.5X2	T36.5X3	T36.5X4	T36.5X5	T36.5X6
Streptozocin	T45.1X1	T45.1X2	T45.1X3	T45.1X4	T45.1X5	T45.1X6
Streptozotocin	T45.1X1	T45.1X2	T45.1X3	T45.1X4	T45.1X5	T45.1X6
Stripper (paint) (solvent)	T52.8X1	T52.8X2	T52.8X3	T52.8X4	—	—
Strobane	T60.1X1	T60.1X2	T60.1X3	T60.1X4	—	—
Strofantina	T46.0X1	T46.0X2	T46.0X3	T46.0X4	T46.0X5	T46.0X6
Strophanthin (g) (k)	T46.0X1	T46.0X2	T46.0X3	T46.0X4	T46.0X5	T46.0X6
Strophanthus	T46.0X1	T46.0X2	T46.0X3	T46.0X4	T46.0X5	T46.0X6
Strophantin	T46.0X1	T46.0X2	T46.0X3	T46.0X4	T46.0X5	T46.0X6
Strophantin-g	T46.0X1	T46.0X2	T46.0X3	T46.0X4	T46.0X5	T46.0X6
Strychnine (nonmedicinal) (pesticide) (salts)	T65.1X1	T65.1X2	T65.1X3	T65.1X4	—	—
medicinal	T48.291	T48.292	T48.293	T48.294	T48.295	T48.296
Strychnos (ignatii) — *see Strychnine*						
Styramate	T42.8X1	T42.8X2	T42.8X3	T42.8X4	T42.8X5	T42.8X6
Styrene	T65.891	T65.892	T65.893	T65.894	—	—
Succinimide, antiepileptic or anticonvulsant	T42.2X1	T42.2X2	T42.2X3	T42.2X4	T42.2X5	T42.2X6
mercuric — *see Mercury*						
Succinylcholine	T48.1X1	T48.1X2	T48.1X3	T48.1X4	T48.1X5	T48.1X6
Succinylsulfathiazole	T37.0X1	T37.0X2	T37.0X3	T37.0X4	T37.0X5	T37.0X6
Sucralfate	T47.1X1	T47.1X2	T47.1X3	T47.1X4	T47.1X5	T47.1X6
Sucrose	T50.3X1	T50.3X2	T50.3X3	T50.3X4	T50.3X5	T50.3X6
Sufentanil	T40.4X1	T40.4X2	T40.4X3	T40.4X4	T40.4X5	T40.4X6
Sulbactam	T36.0X1	T36.0X2	T36.0X3	T36.0X4	T36.0X5	T36.0X6
Sulbenicillin	T36.0X1	T36.0X2	T36.0X3	T36.0X4	T36.0X5	T36.0X6
Sulbentine	T49.0X1	T49.0X2	T49.0X3	T49.0X4	T49.0X5	T49.0X6
Sulfacetamide	T49.0X1	T49.0X2	T49.0X3	T49.0X4	T49.0X5	T49.0X6
ophthalmic preparation	T49.5X1	T49.5X2	T49.5X3	T49.5X4	T49.5X5	T49.5X6
Sulfachlorpyridazine	T37.0X1	T37.0X2	T37.0X3	T37.0X4	T37.0X5	T37.0X6
Sulfacitine	T37.0X1	T37.0X2	T37.0X3	T37.0X4	T37.0X5	T37.0X6
Sulfadiasulfone sodium	T37.0X1	T37.0X2	T37.0X3	T37.0X4	T37.0X5	T37.0X6
Sulfadiazine	T37.0X1	T37.0X2	T37.0X3	T37.0X4	T37.0X5	T37.0X6
silver (topical)	T49.0X1	T49.0X2	T49.0X3	T49.0X4	T49.0X5	T49.0X6
Sulfadimethoxine	T37.0X1	T37.0X2	T37.0X3	T37.0X4	T37.0X5	T37.0X6
Sulfadimidine	T37.0X1	T37.0X2	T37.0X3	T37.0X4	T37.0X5	T37.0X6
Sulfadoxine	T37.0X1	T37.0X2	T37.0X3	T37.0X4	T37.0X5	T37.0X6
with pyrimethamine	T37.2X1	T37.2X2	T37.2X3	T37.2X4	T37.2X5	T37.2X6
Sulfaethidole	T37.0X1	T37.0X2	T37.0X3	T37.0X4	T37.0X5	T37.0X6
Sulfafurazole	T37.0X1	T37.0X2	T37.0X3	T37.0X4	T37.0X5	T37.0X6
Sulfaguanidine	T37.0X1	T37.0X2	T37.0X3	T37.0X4	T37.0X5	T37.0X6
Sulfalene	T37.0X1	T37.0X2	T37.0X3	T37.0X4	T37.0X5	T37.0X6
Sulfaloxate	T37.0X1	T37.0X2	T37.0X3	T37.0X4	T37.0X5	T37.0X6
Sulfaloxic acid	T37.0X1	T37.0X2	T37.0X3	T37.0X4	T37.0X5	T37.0X6
Sulfamazone	T39.2X1	T39.2X2	T39.2X3	T39.2X4	T39.2X5	T39.2X6
Sulfamerazine	T37.0X1	T37.0X2	T37.0X3	T37.0X4	T37.0X5	T37.0X6
Sulfameter	T37.0X1	T37.0X2	T37.0X3	T37.0X4	T37.0X5	T37.0X6
Sulfamethazine	T37.0X1	T37.0X2	T37.0X3	T37.0X4	T37.0X5	T37.0X6
Sulfamethizole	T37.0X1	T37.0X2	T37.0X3	T37.0X4	T37.0X5	T37.0X6
Sulfamethoxazole	T37.0X1	T37.0X2	T37.0X3	T37.0X4	T37.0X5	T37.0X6
with trimethoprim	T36.8X1	T36.8X2	T36.8X3	T36.8X4	T36.8X5	T36.8X6
Sulfamethoxydiazine	T37.0X1	T37.0X2	T37.0X3	T37.0X4	T37.0X5	T37.0X6
Sulfamethoxypyridazine	T37.0X1	T37.0X2	T37.0X3	T37.0X4	T37.0X5	T37.0X6
Sulfamethylthiazole	T37.0X1	T37.0X2	T37.0X3	T37.0X4	T37.0X5	T37.0X6
Sulfametoxydiazine	T37.0X1	T37.0X2	T37.0X3	T37.0X4	T37.0X5	T37.0X6
Sulfamidopyrine	T39.2X1	T39.2X2	T39.2X3	T39.2X4	T39.2X5	T39.2X6
Sulfamonomethoxine	T37.0X1	T37.0X2	T37.0X3	T37.0X4	T37.0X5	T37.0X6
Sulfamoxole	T37.0X1	T37.0X2	T37.0X3	T37.0X4	T37.0X5	T37.0X6
Sulfamylon	T49.0X1	T49.0X2	T49.0X3	T49.0X4	T49.0X5	T49.0X6
Sulfan blue (diagnostic dye)	T50.8X1	T50.8X2	T50.8X3	T50.8X4	T50.8X5	T50.8X6
Sulfanilamide	T37.0X1	T37.0X2	T37.0X3	T37.0X4	T37.0X5	T37.0X6
Sulfanilylguanidine	T37.0X1	T37.0X2	T37.0X3	T37.0X4	T37.0X5	T37.0X6
Sulfaperin	T37.0X1	T37.0X2	T37.0X3	T37.0X4	T37.0X5	T37.0X6
Sulfaphenazole	T37.0X1	T37.0X2	T37.0X3	T37.0X4	T37.0X5	T37.0X6
Sulfaphenylthiazole	T37.0X1	T37.0X2	T37.0X3	T37.0X4	T37.0X5	T37.0X6
Sulfaproxyline	T37.0X1	T37.0X2	T37.0X3	T37.0X4	T37.0X5	T37.0X6
Sulfapyridine	T37.0X1	T37.0X2	T37.0X3	T37.0X4	T37.0X5	T37.0X6
Sulfapyrimidine	T37.0X1	T37.0X2	T37.0X3	T37.0X4	T37.0X5	T37.0X6
Sulfarsphenamine	T37.8X1	T37.8X2	T37.8X3	T37.8X4	T37.8X5	T37.8X6
Sulfasalazine	T37.0X1	T37.0X2	T37.0X3	T37.0X4	T37.0X5	T37.0X6
Sulfasuxidine	T37.0X1	T37.0X2	T37.0X3	T37.0X4	T37.0X5	T37.0X6
Sulfasymazine	T37.0X1	T37.0X2	T37.0X3	T37.0X4	T37.0X5	T37.0X6
Sulfated amylopectin	T47.8X1	T47.8X2	T47.8X3	T47.8X4	T47.8X5	T47.8X6
Sulfathiazole	T37.0X1	T37.0X2	T37.0X3	T37.0X4	T37.0X5	T37.0X6
Sulfatostearate	T49.2X1	T49.2X2	T49.2X3	T49.2X4	T49.2X5	T49.2X6
Sulfinpyrazone	T50.4X1	T50.4X2	T50.4X3	T50.4X4	T50.4X5	T50.4X6

Substance	Poisoning, Accidental (Unintentional)	Poisoning, Intentional Self-Harm	Poisoning, Assault	Poisoning, Undetermined	Adverse Effect	Underdosing
Sulfiram	T49.0X1	T49.0X2	T49.0X3	T49.0X4	T49.0X5	T49.0X6
Sulfisomidine	T37.0X1	T37.0X2	T37.0X3	T37.0X4	T37.0X5	T37.0X6
Sulfisoxazole	T37.0X1	T37.0X2	T37.0X3	T37.0X4	T37.0X5	T37.0X6
ophthalmic preparation	T49.5X1	T49.5X2	T49.5X3	T49.5X4	T49.5X5	T49.5X6
Sulfobromophthalein (sodium)	T50.8X1	T50.8X2	T50.8X3	T50.8X4	T50.8X5	T50.8X6
Sulfobromphthalein	T50.8X1	T50.8X2	T50.8X3	T50.8X4	T50.8X5	T50.8X6
Sulfogaiacol	T48.4X1	T48.4X2	T48.4X3	T48.4X4	T48.4X5	T48.4X6
Sulfomyxin	T36.8X1	T36.8X2	T36.8X3	T36.8X4	T36.8X5	T36.8X6
Sulfonal	T42.6X1	T42.6X2	T42.6X3	T42.6X4	T42.6X5	T42.6X6
Sulfonamide NEC	T37.0X1	T37.0X2	T37.0X3	T37.0X4	T37.0X5	T37.0X6
eye	T49.5X1	T49.5X2	T49.5X3	T49.5X4	T49.5X5	T49.5X6
Sulfonazide	T37.1X1	T37.1X2	T37.1X3	T37.1X4	T37.1X5	T37.1X6
Sulfones	T37.1X1	T37.1X2	T37.1X3	T37.1X4	T37.1X5	T37.1X6
Sulfonethylmethane	T42.6X1	T42.6X2	T42.6X3	T42.6X4	T42.6X5	T42.6X6
Sulfonmethane	T42.6X1	T42.6X2	T42.6X3	T42.6X4	T42.6X5	T42.6X6
Sulfonphthal, sulfonphthol	T50.8X1	T50.8X2	T50.8X3	T50.8X4	T50.8X5	T50.8X6
Sulfonylurea derivatives, oral	T38.3X1	T38.3X2	T38.3X3	T38.3X4	T38.3X5	T38.3X6
Sulforidazine	T43.3X1	T43.3X2	T43.3X3	T43.3X4	T43.3X5	T43.3X6
Sulfoxone	T37.1X1	T37.1X2	T37.1X3	T37.1X4	T37.1X5	T37.1X6
Sulfur, sulfurated, sulfuric, sulfurous, sulfuryl (compounds NEC) (medicinal)	T49.4X1	T49.4X2	T49.4X3	T49.4X4	T49.4X5	T49.4X6
acid	T54.2X1	T54.2X2	T54.2X3	T54.2X4	—	—
dioxide (gas)	T59.1X1	T59.1X2	T59.1X3	T59.1X4	—	—
ether — *see Ether(s)*						
hydrogen	T59.6X1	T59.6X2	T59.6X3	T59.6X4	—	—
medicinal (keratolytic) (ointment) NEC	T49.4X1	T49.4X2	T49.4X3	T49.4X4	T49.4X5	T49.4X6
ointment	T49.0X1	T49.0X2	T49.0X3	T49.0X4	T49.0X5	T49.0X6
pesticide (vapor)	T60.91	T60.92	T60.93	T60.94	—	—
vapor NEC	T59.891	T59.892	T59.893	T59.894	—	—
Sulfuric acid	T54.2X1	T54.2X2	T54.2X3	T54.2X4	—	—
Sulglicotide	T47.1X1	T47.1X2	T47.1X3	T47.1X4	T47.1X5	T47.1X6
Sulindac	T39.391	T39.392	T39.393	T39.394	T39.395	T39.396
Sulisatin	T47.2X1	T47.2X2	T47.2X3	T47.2X4	T47.2X5	T47.2X6
Sulisobenzone	T49.3X1	T49.3X2	T49.3X3	T49.3X4	T49.3X5	T49.3X6
Sulkowitch's reagent	T50.8X1	T50.8X2	T50.8X3	T50.8X4	T50.8X5	T50.8X6
Sulmetozine	T44.3X1	T44.3X2	T44.3X3	T44.3X4	T44.3X5	T44.3X6
Suloctidil	T46.7X1	T46.7X2	T46.7X3	T46.7X4	T46.7X5	T46.7X6
Sulph — *see also Sulf-*						
Sulphadiazine	T37.0X1	T37.0X2	T37.0X3	T37.0X4	T37.0X5	T37.0X6

Substance	Poisoning, Accidental (Unintentional)	Poisoning, Intentional Self-Harm	Poisoning, Assault	Poisoning, Undetermined	Adverse Effect	Underdosing
Sulphadimethoxine	T37.0X1	T37.0X2	T37.0X3	T37.0X4	T37.0X5	T37.0X6
Sulphadimidine	T37.0X1	T37.0X2	T37.0X3	T37.0X4	T37.0X5	T37.0X6
Sulphadione	T37.1X1	T37.1X2	T37.1X3	T37.1X4	T37.1X5	T37.1X6
Sulphafurazole	T37.0X1	T37.0X2	T37.0X3	T37.0X4	T37.0X5	T37.0X6
Sulphamethizole	T37.0X1	T37.0X2	T37.0X3	T37.0X4	T37.0X5	T37.0X6
Sulphamethoxazole	T37.0X1	T37.0X2	T37.0X3	T37.0X4	T37.0X5	T37.0X6
Sulphan blue	T50.8X1	T50.8X2	T50.8X3	T50.8X4	T50.8X5	T50.8X6
Sulphaphenazole	T37.0X1	T37.0X2	T37.0X3	T37.0X4	T37.0X5	T37.0X6
Sulphapyridine	T37.0X1	T37.0X2	T37.0X3	T37.0X4	T37.0X5	T37.0X6
Sulphasalazine	T37.0X1	T37.0X2	T37.0X3	T37.0X4	T37.0X5	T37.0X6
Sulphinpyrazone	T50.4X1	T50.4X2	T50.4X3	T50.4X4	T50.4X5	T50.4X6
Sulpiride	T43.591	T43.592	T43.593	T43.594	T43.595	T43.596
Sulprostone	T48.0X1	T48.0X2	T48.0X3	T48.0X4	T48.0X5	T48.0X6
Sulpyrine	T39.2X1	T39.2X2	T39.2X3	T39.2X4	T39.2X5	T39.2X6
Sultamicillin	T36.0X1	T36.0X2	T36.0X3	T36.0X4	T36.0X5	T36.0X6
Sulthiame	T42.6X1	T42.6X2	T42.6X3	T42.6X4	T42.6X5	T42.6X6
Sultiame	T42.6X1	T42.6X2	T42.6X3	T42.6X4	T42.6X5	T42.6X6
Sultopride	T43.591	T43.592	T43.593	T43.594	T43.595	T43.596
Sumatriptan	T39.8X1	T39.8X2	T39.8X3	T39.8X4	T39.8X5	T39.8X6
Sunflower seed oil	T46.6X1	T46.6X2	T46.6X3	T46.6X4	T46.6X5	T46.6X6
Superinone	T48.4X1	T48.4X2	T48.4X3	T48.4X4	T48.4X5	T48.4X6
Suprofen	T39.311	T39.312	T39.313	T39.314	T39.315	T39.316
Suramin (sodium)	T37.4X1	T37.4X2	T37.4X3	T37.4X4	T37.4X5	T37.4X6
Surfacaine	T41.3X1	T41.3X2	T41.3X3	T41.3X4	T41.3X5	T41.3X6
Surital	T41.1X1	T41.1X2	T41.1X3	T41.1X4	T41.1X5	T41.1X6
Sutilains	T45.3X1	T45.3X2	T45.3X3	T45.3X4	T45.3X5	T45.3X6
Suxamethonium (chloride)	T48.1X1	T48.1X2	T48.1X3	T48.1X4	T48.1X5	T48.1X6
Suxethonium (chloride)	T48.1X1	T48.1X2	T48.1X3	T48.1X4	T48.1X5	T48.1X6
Suxibuzone	T39.2X1	T39.2X2	T39.2X3	T39.2X4	T39.2X5	T39.2X6
Sweet oil (birch)	T49.3X1	T49.3X2	T49.3X3	T49.3X4	T49.3X5	T49.3X6
Sweet niter spirit	T46.3X1	T46.3X2	T46.3X3	T46.3X4	T46.3X5	T46.3X6
Sweetener	T50.901	T50.902	T50.903	T50.904	T50.905	T50.906
Sym-dichloroethyl ether	T53.6X1	T53.6X2	T53.6X3	T53.6X4	—	—
Sympatholytic NEC	T44.8X1	T44.8X2	T44.8X3	T44.8X4	T44.8X5	T44.8X6
haloalkylamine	T44.8X1	T44.8X2	T44.8X3	T44.8X4	T44.8X5	T44.8X6
Sympathomimetic NEC	T44.901	T44.902	T44.903	T44.904	T44.905	T44.906
anti-common-cold	T48.5X1	T48.5X2	T48.5X3	T48.5X4	T48.5X5	T48.5X6
bronchodilator	T48.6X1	T48.6X2	T48.6X3	T48.6X4	T48.6X5	T48.6X6
specified NEC	T44.991	T44.992	T44.993	T44.994	T44.995	T44.996
Synagis	T50.B91	T50.B92	T50.B93	T50.B94	T50.B95	T50.B96
Synalar	T49.0X1	T49.0X2	T49.0X3	T49.0X4	T49.0X5	T49.0X6
Synthroid	T38.1X1	T38.1X2	T38.1X3	T38.1X4	T38.1X5	T38.1X6

◀ New ◀▮▮▮ Revised ~~deleted~~ Deleted

Substance	Poisoning, Accidental (Unintentional)	Poisoning, Intentional Self-Harm	Poisoning, Assault	Poisoning, Undetermined	Adverse Effect	Underdosing
Syntocinon	T48.ØX1	T48.ØX2	T48.ØX3	T48.ØX4	T48.ØX5	T48.ØX6
Syrosingopine	T46.5X1	T46.5X2	T46.5X3	T46.5X4	T46.5X5	T46.5X6
Systemic drug	T45.91	T45.92	T45.93	T45.94	T45.95	T45.96
specified NEC	T45.8X1	T45.8X2	T45.8X3	T45.8X4	T45.8X5	T45.8X6
2,4,5-T	T6Ø.3X1	T6Ø.3X2	T6Ø.3X3	T6Ø.3X4	—	—
T						
Tablets — *see also specified substance*	T5Ø.9Ø1	T5Ø.9Ø2	T5Ø.9Ø3	T5Ø.9Ø4	T5Ø.9Ø5	T5Ø.9Ø6
Tace	T38.5X1	T38.5X2	T38.5X3	T38.5X4	T38.5X5	T38.5X6
Tacrine	T44.ØX1	T44.ØX2	T44.ØX3	T44.ØX4	T44.ØX5	T44.ØX6
Tadalafil	T46.7X1	T46.7X2	T46.7X3	T46.7X4	T46.7X5	T46.7X6
Talampicillin	T36.ØX1	T36.ØX2	T36.ØX3	T36.ØX4	T36.ØX5	T36.ØX6
Talbutal	T42.3X1	T42.3X2	T42.3X3	T42.3X4	T42.3X5	T42.3X6
Talc powder	T49.3X1	T49.3X2	T49.3X3	T49.3X4	T49.3X5	T49.3X6
Talcum	T49.3X1	T49.3X2	T49.3X3	T49.3X4	T49.3X5	T49.3X6
Taleranol	T38.6X1	T38.6X2	T38.6X3	T38.6X4	T38.6X5	T38.6X6
Tamoxifen	T38.6X1	T38.6X2	T38.6X3	T38.6X4	T38.6X5	T38.6X6
Tamsulosin	T44.6X1	T44.6X2	T44.6X3	T44.6X4	T44.6X5	T44.6X6
Tandearil, tanderil	T39.2X1	T39.2X2	T39.2X3	T39.2X4	T39.2X5	T39.2X6
Tannic acid	T49.2X1	T49.2X2	T49.2X3	T49.2X4	T49.2X5	T49.2X6
medicinal (astringent)	T49.2X1	T49.2X2	T49.2X3	T49.2X4	T49.2X5	T49.2X6
Tannin — *see Tannic acid*						
Tansy	T62.2X1	T62.2X2	T62.2X3	T62.2X4	—	—
TAO	T36.3X1	T36.3X2	T36.3X3	T36.3X4	T36.3X5	T36.3X6
Tapazole	T38.2X1	T38.2X2	T38.2X3	T38.2X4	T38.2X5	T38.2X6
Tar NEC	T52.ØX1	T52.ØX2	T52.ØX3	T52.ØX4	—	—
camphor	T6Ø.1X1	T6Ø.1X2	T6Ø.1X3	T6Ø.1X4	—	—
distillate	T49.1X1	T49.1X2	T49.1X3	T49.1X4	T49.1X5	T49.1X6
fumes	T59.891	T59.892	T59.893	T59.894	—	—
medicinal	T49.1X1	T49.1X2	T49.1X3	T49.1X4	T49.1X5	T49.1X6
ointment	T49.1X1	T49.1X2	T49.1X3	T49.1X4	T49.1X5	T49.1X6
Taractan	T43.591	T43.592	T43.593	T43.594	T43.595	T43.596
Tarantula (venomous)	T63.321	T63.322	T63.323	T63.324	—	—
Tartar emetic	T37.8X1	T37.8X2	T37.8X3	T37.8X4	T37.8X5	T37.8X6
Tartaric acid	T65.891	T65.892	T65.893	T65.894	—	—
Tartrated antimony (anti-infective)	T37.8X1	T37.8X2	T37.8X3	T37.8X4	T37.8X5	T37.8X6
Tartrate, laxative	T47.4X1	T47.4X2	T47.4X3	T47.4X4	T47.4X5	T47.4X6
Tauromustine	T45.1X1	T45.1X2	T45.1X3	T45.1X4	T45.1X5	T45.1X6
TCA — *see Trichloroacetic acid*						
TCDD	T53.7X1	T53.7X2	T53.7X3	T53.7X4	—	—
TDI (vapor)	T65.ØX1	T65.ØX2	T65.ØX3	T65.ØX4	—	—

Substance	Poisoning, Accidental (Unintentional)	Poisoning, Intentional Self-Harm	Poisoning, Assault	Poisoning, Undetermined	Adverse Effect	Underdosing
Tear						
gas	T59.3X1	T59.3X2	T59.3X3	T59.3X4	—	—
solution	T49.5X1	T49.5X2	T49.5X3	T49.5X4	T49.5X5	T49.5X6
Teclothiazide	T5Ø.2X1	T5Ø.2X2	T5Ø.2X3	T5Ø.2X4	T5Ø.2X5	T5Ø.2X6
Teclozan	T37.3X1	T37.3X2	T37.3X3	T37.3X4	T37.3X5	T37.3X6
Tegafur	T45.1X1	T45.1X2	T45.1X3	T45.1X4	T45.1X5	T45.1X6
Tegretol	T42.1X1	T42.1X2	T42.1X3	T42.1X4	T42.1X5	T42.1X6
Teicoplanin	T36.8X1	T36.8X2	T36.8X3	T36.8X4	T36.8X5	T36.8X6
Telepaque	T5Ø.8X1	T5Ø.8X2	T5Ø.8X3	T5Ø.8X4	T5Ø.8X5	T5Ø.8X6
Tellurium	T56.891	T56.892	T56.893	T56.894	—	—
fumes	T56.891	T56.892	T56.893	T56.894	—	—
TEM	T45.1X1	T45.1X2	T45.1X3	T45.1X4	T45.1X5	T45.1X6
Temazepam	T42.4X1	T42.4X2	T42.4X3	T42.4X4	T42.4X5	T42.4X6
Temocillin	T36.ØX1	T36.ØX2	T36.ØX3	T36.ØX4	T36.ØX5	T36.ØX6
Tenamfetamine	T43.621	T43.622	T43.623	T43.624	T43.625	T43.626
Teniposide	T45.1X1	T45.1X2	T45.1X3	T45.1X4	T45.1X5	T45.1X6
Tenitramine	T46.3X1	T46.3X2	T46.3X3	T46.3X4	T46.3X5	T46.3X6
Tenoglicin	T48.4X1	T48.4X2	T48.4X3	T48.4X4	T48.4X5	T48.4X6
Tenonitrozole	T37.3X1	T37.3X2	T37.3X3	T37.3X4	T37.3X5	T37.3X6
Tenoxicam	T39.391	T39.392	T39.393	T39.394	T39.395	T39.396
TEPA	T45.1X1	T45.1X2	T45.1X3	T45.1X4	T45.1X5	T45.1X6
TEPP	T6Ø.ØX1	T6Ø.ØX2	T6Ø.ØX3	T6Ø.ØX4	—	—
Teprotide	T46.5X1	T46.5X2	T46.5X3	T46.5X4	T46.5X5	T46.5X6
Terazosin	T44.6X1	T44.6X2	T44.6X3	T44.6X4	T44.6X5	T44.6X6
Terbufos	T6Ø.ØX1	T6Ø.ØX2	T6Ø.ØX3	T6Ø.ØX4	—	—
Terbutaline	T48.6X1	T48.6X2	T48.6X3	T48.6X4	T48.6X5	T48.6X6
Terconazole	T49.ØX1	T49.ØX2	T49.ØX3	T49.ØX4	T49.ØX5	T49.ØX6
Terfenadine	T45.ØX1	T45.ØX2	T45.ØX3	T45.ØX4	T45.ØX5	T45.ØX6
Teriparatide (acetate)	T5Ø.991	T5Ø.992	T5Ø.993	T5Ø.994	T5Ø.995	T5Ø.996
Terizidone	T37.1X1	T37.1X2	T37.1X3	T37.1X4	T37.1X5	T37.1X6
Terlipressin	T38.891	T38.892	T38.893	T38.894	T38.895	T38.896
Terodiline	T46.3X1	T46.3X2	T46.3X3	T46.3X4	T46.3X5	T46.3X6
Teroxalene	T37.4X1	T37.4X2	T37.4X3	T37.4X4	T37.4X5	T37.4X6
Terpin(cis) hydrate	T48.4X1	T48.4X2	T48.4X3	T48.4X4	T48.4X5	T48.4X6
Terramycin	T36.4X1	T36.4X2	T36.4X3	T36.4X4	T36.4X5	T36.4X6
Tertatolol	T44.7X1	T44.7X2	T44.7X3	T44.7X4	T44.7X5	T44.7X6
Tessalon	T48.3X1	T48.3X2	T48.3X3	T48.3X4	T48.3X5	T48.3X6
Testolactone	T38.7X1	T38.7X2	T38.7X3	T38.7X4	T38.7X5	T38.7X6
Testosterone	T38.7X1	T38.7X2	T38.7X3	T38.7X4	T38.7X5	T38.7X6
Tetanus toxoid or vaccine	T5Ø.A91	T5Ø.A92	T5Ø.A93	T5Ø.A94	T5Ø.A95	T5Ø.A96
antitoxin	T5Ø.Z11	T5Ø.Z12	T5Ø.Z13	T5Ø.Z14	T5Ø.Z15	T5Ø.Z16
immune globulin (human)	T5Ø.Z11	T5Ø.Z12	T5Ø.Z13	T5Ø.Z14	T5Ø.Z15	T5Ø.Z16

Substance	Poisoning, Accidental (Unintentional)	Poisoning, Intentional Self-Harm	Poisoning, Assault	Poisoning, Undetermined	Adverse Effect	Underdosing
Tetanus toxoid or vaccine *(Continued)*						
toxoid	T5Ø.A91	T5Ø.A92	T5Ø.A93	T5Ø.A94	T5Ø.A95	T5Ø.A96
with diphtheria toxoid	T5Ø.A21	T5Ø.A22	T5Ø.A23	T5Ø.A24	T5Ø.A25	T5Ø.A26
with pertussis	T5Ø.A11	T5Ø.A12	T5Ø.A13	T5Ø.A14	T5Ø.A15	T5Ø.A16
Tetrabenazine	T43.591	T43.592	T43.593	T43.594	T43.595	T43.596
Tetracaine	T41.3X1	T41.3X2	T41.3X3	T41.3X4	T41.3X5	T41.3X6
nerve block (peripheral) (plexus)	T41.3X1	T41.3X2	T41.3X3	T41.3X4	T41.3X5	T41.3X6
regional	T41.3X1	T41.3X2	T41.3X3	T41.3X4	T41.3X5	T41.3X6
spinal	T41.3X1	T41.3X2	T41.3X3	T41.3X4	T41.3X5	T41.3X6
Tetrachlorethylene — *see Tetrachloroethylene*						
Tetrachlormethiazide	T5Ø.2X1	T5Ø.2X2	T5Ø.2X3	T5Ø.2X4	T5Ø.2X5	T5Ø.2X6
2,3,7,8-Tetrachlorodibenzo-p-dioxin	T53.7X1	T53.7X2	T53.7X3	T53.7X4	—	—
Tetrachloroethane	T53.6X1	T53.6X2	T53.6X3	T53.6X4	—	—
vapor	T53.6X1	T53.6X2	T53.6X3	T53.6X4	—	—
paint or varnish	T53.6X1	T53.6X2	T53.6X3	T53.6X4	—	—
Tetrachloroethylene (liquid)	T53.3X1	T53.3X2	T53.3X3	T53.3X4	—	—
medicinal	T37.4X1	T37.4X2	T37.4X3	T37.4X4	T37.4X5	T37.4X6
vapor	T53.3X1	T53.3X2	T53.3X3	T53.3X4	—	—
Tetrachloromethane — *see Carbon tetrachloride*						
Tetracosactide	T38.811	T38.812	T38.813	T38.814	T38.815	T38.816
Tetracosactrin	T38.811	T38.812	T38.813	T38.814	T38.815	T38.816
Tetracycline	T36.4X1	T36.4X2	T36.4X3	T36.4X4	T36.4X5	T36.4X6
ophthalmic preparation	T49.5X1	T49.5X2	T49.5X3	T49.5X4	T49.5X5	T49.5X6
topical NEC	T49.ØX1	T49.ØX2	T49.ØX3	T49.ØX4	T49.ØX5	T49.ØX6
Tetradifon	T6Ø.8X1	T6Ø.8X2	T6Ø.8X3	T6Ø.8X4	—	—
Tetradotoxin	T61.771	T61.772	T61.773	T61.774	—	—
Tetraethyl						
lead	T56.ØX1	T56.ØX2	T56.ØX3	T56.ØX4	—	—
pyrophosphate	T6Ø.ØX1	T6Ø.ØX2	T6Ø.ØX3	T6Ø.ØX4	—	—
Tetraethylammonium chloride	T44.2X1	T44.2X2	T44.2X3	T44.2X4	T44.2X5	T44.2X6
Tetraethylthiuram disulfide	T5Ø.6X1	T5Ø.6X2	T5Ø.6X3	T5Ø.6X4	T5Ø.6X5	T5Ø.6X6
Tetrahydroaminoacridine	T44.ØX1	T44.ØX2	T44.ØX3	T44.ØX4	T44.ØX5	T44.ØX6
Tetrahydrocannabinol	T4Ø.7X1	T4Ø.7X2	T4Ø.7X3	T4Ø.7X4	T4Ø.7X5	T4Ø.7X6
Tetrahydrofuran	T52.8X1	T52.8X2	T52.8X3	T52.8X4	—	—
Tetrahydronaphthalene	T52.8X1	T52.8X2	T52.8X3	T52.8X4	—	—
Tetrahydrozoline	T49.5X1	T49.5X2	T49.5X3	T49.5X4	T49.5X5	T49.5X6
Tetralin	T52.8X1	T52.8X2	T52.8X3	T52.8X4	—	—
Tetramethrin	T6Ø.2X1	T6Ø.2X2	T6Ø.2X3	T6Ø.2X4	—	—

Substance	Poisoning, Accidental (Unintentional)	Poisoning, Intentional Self-Harm	Poisoning, Assault	Poisoning, Undetermined	Adverse Effect	Underdosing
Tetramethylthiuram (disulfide) NEC	T6Ø.3X1	T6Ø.3X2	T6Ø.3X3	T6Ø.3X4	—	—
medicinal	T49.ØX1	T49.ØX2	T49.ØX3	T49.ØX4	T49.ØX5	T49.ØX6
Tetramisole	T37.4X1	T37.4X2	T37.4X3	T37.4X4	T37.4X5	T37.4X6
Tetranicotinoyl fructose	T46.7X1	T46.7X2	T46.7X3	T46.7X4	T46.7X5	T46.7X6
Tetronal	T42.6X1	T42.6X2	T42.6X3	T42.6X4	T42.6X5	T42.6X6
Tetrazepam	T42.4X1	T42.4X2	T42.4X3	T42.4X4	T42.4X5	T42.4X6
Tetryl	T65.3X1	T65.3X2	T65.3X3	T65.3X4	—	—
Tetrylammonium chloride	T44.2X1	T44.2X2	T44.2X3	T44.2X4	T44.2X5	T44.2X6
Tetryzoline	T49.5X1	T49.5X2	T49.5X3	T49.5X4	T49.5X5	T49.5X6
Thalidomide	T45.1X1	T45.1X2	T45.1X3	T45.1X4	T45.1X5	T45.1X6
Thallium (compounds) (dust) NEC	T56.811	T56.812	T56.813	T56.814	—	—
pesticide	T6Ø.4X1	T6Ø.4X2	T6Ø.4X3	T6Ø.4X4	—	—
THC	T4Ø.7X1	T4Ø.7X2	T4Ø.7X3	T4Ø.7X4	T4Ø.7X5	T4Ø.7X6
Thebacon	T48.3X1	T48.3X2	T48.3X3	T48.3X4	T48.3X5	T48.3X6
Thebaine	T4Ø.2X1	T4Ø.2X2	T4Ø.2X3	T4Ø.2X4	T4Ø.2X5	T4Ø.2X6
Thenoic acid	T49.6X1	T49.6X2	T49.6X3	T49.6X4	T49.6X5	T49.6X6
Thenyldiamine	T45.ØX1	T45.ØX2	T45.ØX3	T45.ØX4	T45.ØX5	T45.ØX6
Theobromine (calcium salicylate)	T48.6X1	T48.6X2	T48.6X3	T48.6X4	T48.6X5	T48.6X6
sodium salicylate	T48.6X1	T48.6X2	T48.6X3	T48.6X4	T48.6X5	T48.6X6
Theophyllamine	T48.6X1	T48.6X2	T48.6X3	T48.6X4	T48.6X5	T48.6X6
Theophylline	T48.6X1	T48.6X2	T48.6X3	T48.6X4	T48.6X5	T48.6X6
aminobenzoic acid	T48.6X1	T48.6X2	T48.6X3	T48.6X4	T48.6X5	T48.6X6
ethylenediamine	T48.6X1	T48.6X2	T48.6X3	T48.6X4	T48.6X5	T48.6X6
piperazine p-amino-benzoate	T48.6X1	T48.6X2	T48.6X3	T48.6X4	T48.6X5	T48.6X6
Thiabendazole	T37.4X1	T37.4X2	T37.4X3	T37.4X4	T37.4X5	T37.4X6
Thialbarbital	T41.1X1	T41.1X2	T41.1X3	T41.1X4	T41.1X5	T41.1X6
Thiamazole	T38.2X1	T38.2X2	T38.2X3	T38.2X4	T38.2X5	T38.2X6
Thiambutosine	T37.1X1	T37.1X2	T37.1X3	T37.1X4	T37.1X5	T37.1X6
Thiamine	T45.2X1	T45.2X2	T45.2X3	T45.2X4	T45.2X5	T45.2X6
Thiamphenicol	T36.2X1	T36.2X2	T36.2X3	T36.2X4	T36.2X5	T36.2X6
Thiamylal	T41.1X1	T41.1X2	T41.1X3	T41.1X4	T41.1X5	T41.1X6
sodium	T41.1X1	T41.1X2	T41.1X3	T41.1X4	T41.1X5	T41.1X6
Thiazesim	T43.291	T43.292	T43.293	T43.294	T43.295	T43.296
Thiazides (diuretics)	T5Ø.2X1	T5Ø.2X2	T5Ø.2X3	T5Ø.2X4	T5Ø.2X5	T5Ø.2X6
Thiazinamium metilsulfate	T43.3X1	T43.3X2	T43.3X3	T43.3X4	T43.3X5	T43.3X6
Thiethylperazine	T43.3X1	T43.3X2	T43.3X3	T43.3X4	T43.3X5	T43.3X6
Thimerosal	T49.ØX1	T49.ØX2	T49.ØX3	T49.ØX4	T49.ØX5	T49.ØX6
ophthalmic preparation	T49.5X1	T49.5X2	T49.5X3	T49.5X4	T49.5X5	T49.5X6
Thioacetazone	T37.1X1	T37.1X2	T37.1X3	T37.1X4	T37.1X5	T37.1X6
with isoniazid	T37.1X1	T37.1X2	T37.1X3	T37.1X4	T37.1X5	T37.1X6
Thiobarbital sodium	T41.1X1	T41.1X2	T41.1X3	T41.1X4	T41.1X5	T41.1X6

Substance	Poisoning, Accidental (Unintentional)	Poisoning, Intentional Self-Harm	Poisoning, Assault	Poisoning, Undetermined	Adverse Effect	Underdosing
Thiobarbiturate anesthetic	T41.1X1	T41.1X2	T41.1X3	T41.1X4	T41.1X5	T41.1X6
Thiobismol	T37.8X1	T37.8X2	T37.8X3	T37.8X4	T37.8X5	T37.8X6
Thiobutabarbital sodium	T41.1X1	T41.1X2	T41.1X3	T41.1X4	T41.1X5	T41.1X6
Thiocarbamate (insecticide)	T60.0X1	T60.0X2	T60.0X3	T60.0X4	—	—
Thiocarbamide	T38.2X1	T38.2X2	T38.2X3	T38.2X4	T38.2X5	T38.2X6
Thiocarbarsone	T37.8X1	T37.8X2	T37.8X3	T37.8X4	T37.8X5	T37.8X6
Thiocarlide	T37.1X1	T37.1X2	T37.1X3	T37.1X4	T37.1X5	T37.1X6
Thioctamide	T50.991	T50.992	T50.993	T50.994	T50.995	T50.996
Thioctic acid	T50.991	T50.992	T50.993	T50.994	T50.995	T50.996
Thiofos	T60.0X1	T60.0X2	T60.0X3	T60.0X4	—	—
Thioglycolate	T49.4X1	T49.4X2	T49.4X3	T49.4X4	T49.4X5	T49.4X6
Thioglycolic acid	T65.891	T65.892	T65.893	T65.894	—	—
Thioguanine	T45.1X1	T45.1X2	T45.1X3	T45.1X4	T45.1X5	T45.1X6
Thiomercaptomerin	T50.2X1	T50.2X2	T50.2X3	T50.2X4	T50.2X5	T50.2X6
Thiomerin	T50.2X1	T50.2X2	T50.2X3	T50.2X4	T50.2X5	T50.2X6
Thiomersal	T49.0X1	T49.0X2	T49.0X3	T49.0X4	T49.0X5	T49.0X6
Thionazin	T60.0X1	T60.0X2	T60.0X3	T60.0X4	—	—
Thiopental (sodium)	T41.1X1	T41.1X2	T41.1X3	T41.1X4	T41.1X5	T41.1X6
Thiopentone (sodium)	T41.1X1	T41.1X2	T41.1X3	T41.1X4	T41.1X5	T41.1X6
Thiopropazate	T43.3X1	T43.3X2	T43.3X3	T43.3X4	T43.3X5	T43.3X6
Thioproperazine	T43.3X1	T43.3X2	T43.3X3	T43.3X4	T43.3X5	T43.3X6
Thioridazine	T43.3X1	T43.3X2	T43.3X3	T43.3X4	T43.3X5	T43.3X6
Thiosinamine	T49.3X1	T49.3X2	T49.3X3	T49.3X4	T49.3X5	T49.3X6
Thiotepa	T45.1X1	T45.1X2	T45.1X3	T45.1X4	T45.1X5	T45.1X6
Thiothixene	T43.4X1	T43.4X2	T43.4X3	T43.4X4	T43.4X5	T43.4X6
Thiouracil (benzyl) (methyl) (propyl)	T38.2X1	T38.2X2	T38.2X3	T38.2X4	T38.2X5	T38.2X6
Thiourea	T38.2X1	T38.2X2	T38.2X3	T38.2X4	T38.2X5	T38.2X6
Thiphenamil	T44.3X1	T44.3X2	T44.3X3	T44.3X4	T44.3X5	T44.3X6
Thiram	T60.3X1	T60.3X2	T60.3X3	T60.3X4	—	—
medicinal	T49.2X1	T49.2X2	T49.2X3	T49.2X4	T49.2X5	T49.2X6
Thonzylamine (systemic)	T45.0X1	T45.0X2	T45.0X3	T45.0X4	T45.0X5	T45.0X6
mucosal decongestant	T48.5X1	T48.5X2	T48.5X3	T48.5X4	T48.5X5	T48.5X6
Thorazine	T43.3X1	T43.3X2	T43.3X3	T43.3X4	T43.3X5	T43.3X6
Thorium dioxide suspension	T50.8X1	T50.8X2	T50.8X3	T50.8X4	T50.8X5	T50.8X6
Thornapple	T62.2X1	T62.2X2	T62.2X3	T62.2X4	—	—
Throat drug NEC	T49.6X1	T49.6X2	T49.6X3	T49.6X4	T49.6X5	T49.6X6
Thrombin	T45.7X1	T45.7X2	T45.7X3	T45.7X4	T45.7X5	T45.7X6
Thrombolysin	T45.611	T45.612	T45.613	T45.614	T45.615	T45.616
Thromboplastin	T45.7X1	T45.7X2	T45.7X3	T45.7X4	T45.7X5	T45.7X6
Thurfyl nicotinate	T46.7X1	T46.7X2	T46.7X3	T46.7X4	T46.7X5	T46.7X6
Thymol	T49.0X1	T49.0X2	T49.0X3	T49.0X4	T49.0X5	T49.0X6

Substance	Poisoning, Accidental (Unintentional)	Poisoning, Intentional Self-Harm	Poisoning, Assault	Poisoning, Undetermined	Adverse Effect	Underdosing
Thymopentin	T37.5X1	T37.5X2	T37.5X3	T37.5X4	T37.5X5	T37.5X6
Thymoxamine	T46.7X1	T46.7X2	T46.7X3	T46.7X4	T46.7X5	T46.7X6
Thymus extract	T38.891	T38.892	T38.893	T38.894	T38.895	T38.896
Thyreotrophic hormone	T38.811	T38.812	T38.813	T38.814	T38.815	T38.816
Thyroglobulin	T38.1X1	T38.1X2	T38.1X3	T38.1X4	T38.1X5	T38.1X6
Thyroid (hormone)	T38.1X1	T38.1X2	T38.1X3	T38.1X4	T38.1X5	T38.1X6
Thyrolar	T38.1X1	T38.1X2	T38.1X3	T38.1X4	T38.1X5	T38.1X6
Thyrotrophin	T38.811	T38.812	T38.813	T38.814	T38.815	T38.816
Thyrotropic hormone	T38.811	T38.812	T38.813	T38.814	T38.815	T38.816
Thyroxine	T38.1X1	T38.1X2	T38.1X3	T38.1X4	T38.1X5	T38.1X6
Tiabendazole	T37.4X1	T37.4X2	T37.4X3	T37.4X4	T37.4X5	T37.4X6
Tiamizide	T50.2X1	T50.2X2	T50.2X3	T50.2X4	T50.2X5	T50.2X6
Tianeptine	T43.291	T43.292	T43.293	T43.294	T43.295	T43.296
Tiapamil	T46.1X1	T46.1X2	T46.1X3	T46.1X4	T46.1X5	T46.1X6
Tiapride	T43.591	T43.592	T43.593	T43.594	T43.595	T43.596
Tiaprofenic acid	T39.311	T39.312	T39.313	T39.314	T39.315	T39.316
Tiaramide	T39.8X1	T39.8X2	T39.8X3	T39.8X4	T39.8X5	T39.8X6
Ticarcillin	T36.0X1	T36.0X2	T36.0X3	T36.0X4	T36.0X5	T36.0X6
Ticlatone	T49.0X1	T49.0X2	T49.0X3	T49.0X4	T49.0X5	T49.0X6
Ticlopidine	T45.521	T45.522	T45.523	T45.524	T45.525	T45.526
Ticrynafen	T50.1X1	T50.1X2	T50.1X3	T50.1X4	T50.1X5	T50.1X6
Tidiacic	T50.991	T50.992	T50.993	T50.994	T50.995	T50.996
Tiemonium	T44.3X1	T44.3X2	T44.3X3	T44.3X4	T44.3X5	T44.3X6
iodide	T44.3X1	T44.3X2	T44.3X3	T44.3X4	T44.3X5	T44.3X6
Tienilic acid	T50.1X1	T50.1X2	T50.1X3	T50.1X4	T50.1X5	T50.1X6
Tifenamil	T44.3X1	T44.3X2	T44.3X3	T44.3X4	T44.3X5	T44.3X6
Tigan	T45.0X1	T45.0X2	T45.0X3	T45.0X4	T45.0X5	T45.0X6
Tigloidine	T44.3X1	T44.3X2	T44.3X3	T44.3X4	T44.3X5	T44.3X6
Tilactase	T47.5X1	T47.5X2	T47.5X3	T47.5X4	T47.5X5	T47.5X6
Tiletamine	T41.291	T41.292	T41.293	T41.294	T41.295	T41.296
Tilidine	T40.4X1	T40.4X2	T40.4X3	T40.4X4	—	—
Timepidium bromide	T44.3X1	T44.3X2	T44.3X3	T44.3X4	T44.3X5	T44.3X6
Timiperone	T43.4X1	T43.4X2	T43.4X3	T43.4X4	T43.4X5	T43.4X6
Timolol	T44.7X1	T44.7X2	T44.7X3	T44.7X4	T44.7X5	T44.7X6
Tin (chloride) (dust) (oxide) NEC	T56.6X1	T56.6X2	T56.6X3	T56.6X4	—	—
anti-infectives	T37.8X1	T37.8X2	T37.8X3	T37.8X4	T37.8X5	T37.8X6
Tincture, iodine — *see Iodine*						
Tindal	T43.3X1	T43.3X2	T43.3X3	T43.3X4	T43.3X5	T43.3X6
Tinidazole	T37.3X1	T37.3X2	T37.3X3	T37.3X4	T37.3X5	T37.3X6
Tinoridine	T39.8X1	T39.8X2	T39.8X3	T39.8X4	T39.8X5	T39.8X6
Tiocarlide	T37.1X1	T37.1X2	T37.1X3	T37.1X4	T37.1X5	T37.1X6
Tioclomarol	T45.511	T45.512	T45.513	T45.514	T45.515	T45.516

Substance	Poisoning, Accidental (Unintentional)	Poisoning, Intentional Self-Harm	Poisoning, Assault	Poisoning, Undetermined	Adverse Effect	Underdosing
Tioconazole	T49.ØX1	T49.ØX2	T49.ØX3	T49.ØX4	T49.ØX5	T49.ØX6
Tioguanine	T45.1X1	T45.1X2	T45.1X3	T45.1X4	T45.1X5	T45.1X6
Tiopronin	T5Ø.991	T5Ø.992	T5Ø.993	T5Ø.994	T5Ø.995	T5Ø.996
Tiotixene	T43.4X1	T43.4X2	T43.4X3	T43.4X4	T43.4X5	T43.4X6
Tioxolone	T49.4X1	T49.4X2	T49.4X3	T49.4X4	T49.4X5	T49.4X6
Tipepidine	T48.3X1	T48.3X2	T48.3X3	T48.3X4	T48.3X5	T48.3X6
Tiquizium bromide	T44.3X1	T44.3X2	T44.3X3	T44.3X4	T44.3X5	T44.3X6
Tiratricol	T38.1X1	T38.1X2	T38.1X3	T38.1X4	T38.1X5	T38.1X6
Tisopurine	T5Ø.4X1	T5Ø.4X2	T5Ø.4X3	T5Ø.4X4	T5Ø.4X5	T5Ø.4X6
Titanium (compounds) (vapor)	T56.891	T56.892	T56.893	T56.894	—	—
dioxide	T49.3X1	T49.3X2	T49.3X3	T49.3X4	T49.3X5	T49.3X6
ointment	T49.3X1	T49.3X2	T49.3X3	T49.3X4	T49.3X5	T49.3X6
oxide	T49.3X1	T49.3X2	T49.3X3	T49.3X4	T49.3X5	T49.3X6
tetrachloride	T56.891	T56.892	T56.893	T56.894	—	—
Titanocene	T56.891	T56.892	T56.893	T56.894	—	—
Titroid	T38.1X1	T38.1X2	T38.1X3	T38.1X4	T38.1X5	T38.1X6
Tizanidine	T42.8X1	T42.8X2	T42.8X3	T42.8X4	T42.8X5	T42.8X6
TMTD	T6Ø.3X1	T6Ø.3X2	T6Ø.3X3	T6Ø.3X4	—	—
TNT (fumes)	T65.3X1	T65.3X2	T65.3X3	T65.3X4	—	—
Toadstool	T62.ØX1	T62.ØX2	T62.ØX3	T62.ØX4	—	—
Tobacco NEC	T65.291	T65.292	T65.293	T65.294	—	—
cigarettes	T65.221	T65.222	T65.223	T65.224	—	—
Indian	T62.2X1	T62.2X2	T62.2X3	T62.2X4	—	—
smoke, second-hand	T65.221	T65.222	T65.223	T65.224	—	—
Tobramycin	T36.5X1	T36.5X2	T36.5X3	T36.5X4	T36.5X5	T36.5X6
Tocainide	T46.2X1	T46.2X2	T46.2X3	T46.2X4	T46.2X5	T46.2X6
Tocoferol	T45.2X1	T45.2X2	T45.2X3	T45.2X4	T45.2X5	T45.2X6
Tocopherol	T45.2X1	T45.2X2	T45.2X3	T45.2X4	T45.2X5	T45.2X6
acetate	T45.2X1	T45.2X2	T45.2X3	T45.2X4	T45.2X5	T45.2X6
Tocosamine	T48.ØX1	T48.ØX2	T48.ØX3	T48.ØX4	T48.ØX5	T48.ØX6
Todralazine	T46.5X1	T46.5X2	T46.5X3	T46.5X4	T46.5X5	T46.5X6
Tofisopam	T42.4X1	T42.4X2	T42.4X3	T42.4X4	T42.4X5	T42.4X6
Tofranil	T43.Ø11	T43.Ø12	T43.Ø13	T43.Ø14	T43.Ø15	T43.Ø16
Toilet deodorizer	T65.891	T65.892	T65.893	T65.894	—	—
Tolamolol	T44.7X1	T44.7X2	T44.7X3	T44.7X4	T44.7X5	T44.7X6
Tolazamide	T38.3X1	T38.3X2	T38.3X3	T38.3X4	T38.3X5	T38.3X6
Tolazoline	T46.7X1	T46.7X2	T46.7X3	T46.7X4	T46.7X5	T46.7X6
Tolbutamide (sodium)	T38.3X1	T38.3X2	T38.3X3	T38.3X4	T38.3X5	T38.3X6
Tolciclate	T49.ØX1	T49.ØX2	T49.ØX3	T49.ØX4	T49.ØX5	T49.ØX6
Tolmetin	T39.391	T39.392	T39.393	T39.394	T39.395	T39.396
Tolnaftate	T49.ØX1	T49.ØX2	T49.ØX3	T49.ØX4	T49.ØX5	T49.ØX6
Tolonidine	T46.5X1	T46.5X2	T46.5X3	T46.5X4	T46.5X5	T46.5X6
Toloxatone	T42.6X1	T42.6X2	T42.6X3	T42.6X4	T42.6X5	T42.6X6
Tolperisone	T44.3X1	T44.3X2	T44.3X3	T44.3X4	T44.3X5	T44.3X6
Tolserol	T42.8X1	T42.8X2	T42.8X3	T42.8X4	T42.8X5	T42.8X6
Toluene (liquid)	T52.2X1	T52.2X2	T52.2X3	T52.2X4	—	—
diisocyanate	T65.ØX1	T65.ØX2	T65.ØX3	T65.ØX4	—	—
Toluidine	T65.891	T65.892	T65.893	T65.894	—	—
vapor	T59.891	T59.892	T59.893	T59.894	—	—
Toluol (liquid)	T52.2X1	T52.2X2	T52.2X3	T52.2X4	—	—
vapor	T52.2X1	T52.2X2	T52.2X3	T52.2X4	—	—
Toluylenediamine	T65.3X1	T65.3X2	T65.3X3	T65.3X4	—	—
Tolylene-2,4-diisocyanate	T65.ØX1	T65.ØX2	T65.ØX3	T65.ØX4	—	—
Tonic NEC	T5Ø.9Ø1	T5Ø.9Ø2	T5Ø.9Ø3	T5Ø.9Ø4	T5Ø.9Ø5	T5Ø.9Ø6
Topical action drug NEC	T49.91	T49.92	T49.93	T49.94	T49.95	T49.96
ear, nose or throat	T49.6X1	T49.6X2	T49.6X3	T49.6X4	T49.6X5	T49.6X6
eye	T49.5X1	T49.5X2	T49.5X3	T49.5X4	T49.5X5	T49.5X6
skin	T49.91	T49.92	T49.93	T49.94	T49.95	T49.96
specified NEC	T49.8X1	T49.8X2	T49.8X3	T49.8X4	T49.8X5	T49.8X6
Toquizine	T44.3X1	T44.3X2	T44.3X3	T44.3X4	T44.3X5	T44.3X6
Toremifene	T38.6X1	T38.6X2	T38.6X3	T38.6X4	T38.6X5	T38.6X6
Tosylchloramide sodium	T49.8X1	T49.8X2	T49.8X3	T49.8X4	T49.8X5	T49.8X6
Toxaphene (dust) (spray)	T6Ø.1X1	T6Ø.1X2	T6Ø.1X3	T6Ø.1X4	—	—
Toxin, diphtheria (Schick Test)	T5Ø.8X1	T5Ø.8X2	T5Ø.8X3	T5Ø.8X4	T5Ø.8X5	T5Ø.8X6
Toxoid						
combined	T5Ø.A21	T5Ø.A22	T5Ø.A23	T5Ø.A24	T5Ø.A25	T5Ø.A26
diphtheria	T5Ø.A91	T5Ø.A92	T5Ø.A93	T5Ø.A94	T5Ø.A95	T5Ø.A96
tetanus	T5Ø.A91	T5Ø.A92	T5Ø.A93	T5Ø.A94	T5Ø.A95	T5Ø.A96
Trace element NEC	T45.8X1	T45.8X2	T45.8X3	T45.8X4	T45.8X5	T45.8X6
Tractor fuel NEC	T52.ØX1	T52.ØX2	T52.ØX3	T52.ØX4	—	—
Tragacanth	T5Ø.991	T5Ø.992	T5Ø.993	T5Ø.994	T5Ø.995	T5Ø.996
Tramadol	T4Ø.4X1	T4Ø.4X2	T4Ø.4X3	T4Ø.4X4	T4Ø.4X5	T4Ø.4X6
Tramazoline	T48.5X1	T48.5X2	T48.5X3	T48.5X4	T48.5X5	T48.5X6
Tranexamic acid	T45.621	T45.622	T45.623	T45.624	T45.625	T45.626
Tranilast	T45.ØX1	T45.ØX2	T45.ØX3	T45.ØX4	T45.ØX5	T45.ØX6
Tranquilizer NEC	T43.5Ø1	T43.5Ø2	T43.5Ø3	T43.5Ø4	T43.5Ø5	T43.5Ø6
with hypnotic or sedative	T42.6X1	T42.6X2	T42.6X3	T42.6X4	T42.6X5	T42.6X6
benzodiazepine NEC	T42.4X1	T42.4X2	T42.4X3	T42.4X4	T42.4X5	T42.4X6
butyrophenone NEC	T43.4X1	T43.4X2	T43.4X3	T43.4X4	T43.4X5	T43.4X6
carbamate	T43.591	T43.592	T43.593	T43.594	T43.595	T43.596
dimethylamine	T43.3X1	T43.3X2	T43.3X3	T43.3X4	T43.3X5	T43.3X6
ethylamine	T43.3X1	T43.3X2	T43.3X3	T43.3X4	T43.3X5	T43.3X6
hydroxyzine	T43.591	T43.592	T43.593	T43.594	T43.595	T43.596
major NEC	T43.5Ø1	T43.5Ø2	T43.5Ø3	T43.5Ø4	T43.5Ø5	T43.5Ø6

Substance	Poisoning, Accidental (Unintentional)	Poisoning, Intentional Self-Harm	Poisoning, Assault	Poisoning, Undetermined	Adverse Effect	Underdosing
Tranquilizer NEC *(Continued)*						
penothiazine NEC	T43.3X1	T43.3X2	T43.3X3	T43.3X4	T43.3X5	T43.3X6
phenothiazine-based	T43.3X1	T43.3X2	T43.3X3	T43.3X4	T43.3X5	T43.3X6
piperazine NEC	T43.3X1	T43.3X2	T43.3X3	T43.3X4	T43.3X5	T43.3X6
piperidine	T43.3X1	T43.3X2	T43.3X3	T43.3X4	T43.3X5	T43.3X6
propylamine	T43.3X1	T43.3X2	T43.3X3	T43.3X4	T43.3X5	T43.3X6
specified NEC	T43.591	T43.592	T43.593	T43.594	T43.595	T43.596
thioxanthene NEC	T43.591	T43.592	T43.593	T43.594	T43.595	T43.596
Tranxene	T42.4X1	T42.4X2	T42.4X3	T42.4X4	T42.4X5	T42.4X6
Tranylcypromine	T43.1X1	T43.1X2	T43.1X3	T43.1X4	T43.1X5	T43.1X6
Trapidil	T46.3X1	T46.3X2	T46.3X3	T46.3X4	T46.3X5	T46.3X6
Trasentine	T44.3X1	T44.3X2	T44.3X3	T44.3X4	T44.3X5	T44.3X6
Travert	T50.3X1	T50.3X2	T50.3X3	T50.3X4	T50.3X5	T50.3X6
Trazodone	T43.211	T43.212	T43.213	T43.214	T43.215	T43.216
Trecator	T37.1X1	T37.1X2	T37.1X3	T37.1X4	T37.1X5	T37.1X6
Treosulfan	T45.1X1	T45.1X2	T45.1X3	T45.1X4	T45.1X5	T45.1X6
Tretamine	T45.1X1	T45.1X2	T45.1X3	T45.1X4	T45.1X5	T45.1X6
Tretinoin	T49.0X1	T49.0X2	T49.0X3	T49.0X4	T49.0X5	T49.0X6
Tretoquinol	T48.6X1	T48.6X2	T48.6X3	T48.6X4	T48.6X5	T48.6X6
Triacetin	T49.0X1	T49.0X2	T49.0X3	T49.0X4	T49.0X5	T49.0X6
Triacetoxyanthracene	T49.4X1	T49.4X2	T49.4X3	T49.4X4	T49.4X5	T49.4X6
Triacetyloleandomycin	T36.3X1	T36.3X2	T36.3X3	T36.3X4	T36.3X5	T36.3X6
Triamcinolone	T49.0X1	T49.0X2	T49.0X3	T49.0X4	T49.0X5	T49.0X6
ENT agent	T49.6X1	T49.6X2	T49.6X3	T49.6X4	T49.6X5	T49.6X6
hexacetonide	T49.0X1	T49.0X2	T49.0X3	T49.0X4	T49.0X5	T49.0X6
ophthalmic preparation	T49.5X1	T49.5X2	T49.5X3	T49.5X4	T49.5X5	T49.5X6
topical NEC	T49.0X1	T49.0X2	T49.0X3	T49.0X4	T49.0X5	T49.0X6
Triampyzine	T44.3X1	T44.3X2	T44.3X3	T44.3X4	T44.3X5	T44.3X6
Triamterene	T50.2X1	T50.2X2	T50.2X3	T50.2X4	T50.2X5	T50.2X6
Triazine (herbicide)	T60.3X1	T60.3X2	T60.3X3	T60.3X4	—	—
Triaziquone	T45.1X1	T45.1X2	T45.1X3	T45.1X4	T45.1X5	T45.1X6
Triazolam	T42.4X1	T42.4X2	T42.4X3	T42.4X4	T42.4X5	T42.4X6
Triazole (herbicide)	T60.3X1	T60.3X2	T60.3X3	T60.3X4	—	—
Tribenoside	T46.991	T46.992	T46.993	T46.994	T46.995	T46.996
Tribromacetaldehyde	T42.6X1	T42.6X2	T42.6X3	T42.6X4	T42.6X5	T42.6X6
Tribromoethanol, rectal	T41.291	T41.292	T41.293	T41.294	T41.295	T41.296
Tribromomethane	T42.6X1	T42.6X2	T42.6X3	T42.6X4	T42.6X5	T42.6X6
Trichlorethane	T53.2X1	T53.2X2	T53.2X3	T53.2X4	—	—
Trichlorethylene	T53.2X1	T53.2X2	T53.2X3	T53.2X4	—	—
Trichlorfon	T60.0X1	T60.0X2	T60.0X3	T60.0X4	—	—
Trichlormethiazide	T50.2X1	T50.2X2	T50.2X3	T50.2X4	T50.2X5	T50.2X6
Trichlormethine	T45.1X1	T45.1X2	T45.1X3	T45.1X4	T45.1X5	T45.1X6

Substance	Poisoning, Accidental (Unintentional)	Poisoning, Intentional Self-Harm	Poisoning, Assault	Poisoning, Undetermined	Adverse Effect	Underdosing
Trichloroacetic acid, Trichloracetic acid	T54.2X1	T54.2X2	T54.2X3	T54.2X4	—	—
medicinal	T49.4X1	T49.4X2	T49.4X3	T49.4X4	T49.4X5	T49.4X6
Trichloroethane	T53.2X1	T53.2X2	T53.2X3	T53.2X4	—	—
Trichloroethanol	T42.6X1	T42.6X2	T42.6X3	T42.6X4	T42.6X5	T42.6X6
Trichloroethylene (liquid) (vapor)	T53.2X1	T53.2X2	T53.2X3	T53.2X4	—	—
anesthetic (gas)	T41.0X1	T41.0X2	T41.0X3	T41.0X4	T41.0X5	T41.0X6
vapor NEC	T53.2X1	T53.2X2	T53.2X3	T53.2X4	—	—
Trichloroethyl phosphate	T42.6X1	T42.6X2	T42.6X3	T42.6X4	T42.6X5	T42.6X6
Trichlorofluoromethane NEC	T53.5X1	T53.5X2	T53.5X3	T53.5X4	—	—
Trichloronate	T60.0X1	T60.0X2	T60.0X3	T60.0X4	—	—
2,4,5-Trichlorophen-oxyacetic acid	T60.3X1	T60.3X2	T60.3X3	T60.3X4	—	—
Trichloropropane	T53.6X1	T53.6X2	T53.6X3	T53.6X4	—	—
Trichlorotriethylamine	T45.1X1	T45.1X2	T45.1X3	T45.1X4	T45.1X5	T45.1X6
Trichomonacldes NEC	T37.3X1	T37.3X2	T37.3X3	T37.3X4	T37.3X5	T37.3X6
Trichomycin	T36.7X1	T36.7X2	T36.7X3	T36.7X4	T36.7X5	T36.7X6
Triclobisonium chloride	T49.0X1	T49.0X2	T49.0X3	T49.0X4	T49.0X5	T49.0X6
Triclocarban	T49.0X1	T49.0X2	T49.0X3	T49.0X4	T49.0X5	T49.0X6
Triclofos	T42.6X1	T42.6X2	T42.6X3	T42.6X4	T42.6X5	T42.6X6
Triclosan	T49.0X1	T49.0X2	T49.0X3	T49.0X4	T49.0X5	T49.0X6
Tricresyl phosphate	T65.891	T65.892	T65.893	T65.894	—	—
solvent	T52.91	T52.92	T52.93	T52.94	—	—
Tricyclamol chloride	T44.3X1	T44.3X2	T44.3X3	T44.3X4	T44.3X5	T44.3X6
Tridesilon	T49.0X1	T49.0X2	T49.0X3	T49.0X4	T49.0X5	T49.0X6
Tridihexethyl iodide	T44.3X1	T44.3X2	T44.3X3	T44.3X4	T44.3X5	T44.3X6
Tridione	T42.2X1	T42.2X2	T42.2X3	T42.2X4	T42.2X5	T42.2X6
Trientine	T45.8X1	T45.8X2	T45.8X3	T45.8X4	T45.8X5	T45.8X6
Triethanolamine NEC	T54.3X1	T54.3X2	T54.3X3	T54.3X4	—	—
detergent	T54.3X1	T54.3X2	T54.3X3	T54.3X4	—	—
trinitrate (biphosphate)	T46.3X1	T46.3X2	T46.3X3	T46.3X4	T46.3X5	T46.3X6
Triethanomelamine	T45.1X1	T45.1X2	T45.1X3	T45.1X4	T45.1X5	T45.1X6
Triethylenemelamine	T45.1X1	T45.1X2	T45.1X3	T45.1X4	T45.1X5	T45.1X6
Triethylenephosphoramide	T45.1X1	T45.1X2	T45.1X3	T45.1X4	T45.1X5	T45.1X6
Triethylenethiophosphoramide	T45.1X1	T45.1X2	T45.1X3	T45.1X4	T45.1X5	T45.1X6
Trifluoperazine	T43.3X1	T43.3X2	T43.3X3	T43.3X4	T43.3X5	T43.3X6
Trifluoroethyl vinyl ether	T41.0X1	T41.0X2	T41.0X3	T41.0X4	T41.0X5	T41.0X6
Trifluperidol	T43.4X1	T43.4X2	T43.4X3	T43.4X4	T43.4X5	T43.4X6
Triflupromazine	T43.3X1	T43.3X2	T43.3X3	T43.3X4	T43.3X5	T43.3X6
Trifluridine	T37.5X1	T37.5X2	T37.5X3	T37.5X4	T37.5X5	T37.5X6
Triflusal	T45.521	T45.522	T45.523	T45.524	T45.525	T45.526
Trihexyphenidyl	T44.3X1	T44.3X2	T44.3X3	T44.3X4	T44.3X5	T44.3X6
Triiodothyronine	T38.1X1	T38.1X2	T38.1X3	T38.1X4	T38.1X5	T38.1X6

Substance	Poisoning, Accidental (Unintentional)	Poisoning, Intentional Self-Harm	Poisoning, Assault	Poisoning, Undetermined	Adverse Effect	Underdosing
Trilene	T41.0X1	T41.0X2	T41.0X3	T41.0X4	T41.0X5	T41.0X6
Trilostane	T38.991	T38.992	T38.993	T38.994	T38.995	T38.996
Trimebutine	T44.3X1	T44.3X2	T44.3X3	T44.3X4	T44.3X5	T44.3X6
Trimecaine	T41.3X1	T41.3X2	T41.3X3	T41.3X4	T41.3X5	T41.3X6
Trimeprazine (tartrate)	T44.3X1	T44.3X2	T44.3X3	T44.3X4	T44.3X5	T44.3X6
Trimetaphan camsilate	T44.2X1	T44.2X2	T44.2X3	T44.2X4	T44.2X5	T44.2X6
Trimetazidine	T46.7X1	T46.7X2	T46.7X3	T46.7X4	T46.7X5	T46.7X6
Trimethadione	T42.2X1	T42.2X2	T42.2X3	T42.2X4	T42.2X5	T42.2X6
Trimethaphan	T44.2X1	T44.2X2	T44.2X3	T44.2X4	T44.2X5	T44.2X6
Trimethidinium	T44.2X1	T44.2X2	T44.2X3	T44.2X4	T44.2X5	T44.2X6
Trimethobenzamide	T45.0X1	T45.0X2	T45.0X3	T45.0X4	T45.0X5	T45.0X6
Trimethoprim	T37.8X1	T37.8X2	T37.8X3	T37.8X4	T37.8X5	T37.8X6
with sulfamethoxazole	T36.8X1	T36.8X2	T36.8X3	T36.8X4	T36.8X5	T36.8X6
Trimethylcarbinol	T51.3X1	T51.3X2	T51.3X3	T51.3X4	—	—
Trimethylpsoralen	T49.3X1	T49.3X2	T49.3X3	T49.3X4	T49.3X5	T49.3X6
Trimeton	T45.0X1	T45.0X2	T45.0X3	T45.0X4	T45.0X5	T45.0X6
Trimetrexate	T45.1X1	T45.1X2	T45.1X3	T45.1X4	T45.1X5	T45.1X6
Trimipramine	T43.011	T43.012	T43.013	T43.014	T43.015	T43.016
Trimustine	T45.1X1	T45.1X2	T45.1X3	T45.1X4	T45.1X5	T45.1X6
Trinitrine	T46.3X1	T46.3X2	T46.3X3	T46.3X4	T46.3X5	T46.3X6
Trinitrobenzol	T65.3X1	T65.3X2	T65.3X3	T65.3X4	—	—
Trinitrophenol	T65.3X1	T65.3X2	T65.3X3	T65.3X4	—	—
Trinitrotoluene (fumes)	T65.3X1	T65.3X2	T65.3X3	T65.3X4	—	—
Trional	T42.6X1	T42.6X2	T42.6X3	T42.6X4	T42.6X5	T42.6X6
Triorthocresyl phosphate	T65.891	T65.892	T65.893	T65.894	—	—
Trioxide of arsenic	T57.0X1	T57.0X2	T57.0X3	T57.0X4	—	—
Trioxysalen	T49.4X1	T49.4X2	T49.4X3	T49.4X4	T49.4X5	T49.4X6
Tripamide	T50.2X1	T50.2X2	T50.2X3	T50.2X4	T50.2X5	T50.2X6
Triparanol	T46.6X1	T46.6X2	T46.6X3	T46.6X4	T46.6X5	T46.6X6
Tripelennamine	T45.0X1	T45.0X2	T45.0X3	T45.0X4	T45.0X5	T45.0X6
Triperiden	T44.3X1	T44.3X2	T44.3X3	T44.3X4	T44.3X5	T44.3X6
Triperidol	T43.4X1	T43.4X2	T43.4X3	T43.4X4	T43.4X5	T43.4X6
Triphenylphosphate	T65.891	T65.892	T65.893	T65.894	—	—
Triple						
bromides	T42.6X1	T42.6X2	T42.6X3	T42.6X4	T42.6X5	T42.6X6
carbonate	T47.1X1	T47.1X2	T47.1X3	T47.1X4	T47.1X5	T47.1X6
vaccine						
DPT	T50.A11	T50.A12	T50.A13	T50.A14	T50.A15	T50.A16
including pertussis	T50.A11	T50.A12	T50.A13	T50.A14	T50.A15	T50.A16
MMR	T50.B91	T50.B92	—	—	—	—
Triprolidine	T45.0X1	T45.0X2	T45.0X3	T45.0X4	T45.0X5	T45.0X6
Trisodium hydrogen edetate	T50.6X1	T50.6X2	T50.6X3	T50.6X4	T50.6X5	T50.6X6

Substance	Poisoning, Accidental (Unintentional)	Poisoning, Intentional Self-Harm	Poisoning, Assault	Poisoning, Undetermined	Adverse Effect	Underdosing
Trisoralen	T49.3X1	T49.3X2	T49.3X3	T49.3X4	T49.3X5	T49.3X6
Trisulfapyrimidines	T37.0X1	T37.0X2	T37.0X3	T37.0X4	T37.0X5	T37.0X6
Trithiozine	T44.3X1	T44.3X2	T44.3X3	T44.3X4	T44.3X5	T44.3X6
Tritiozine	T44.3X1	T44.3X2	T44.3X3	T44.3X4	T44.3X5	T44.3X6
Tritoqualine	T45.0X1	T45.0X2	T45.0X3	T45.0X4	T45.0X5	T45.0X6
Trofosfamide	T45.1X1	T45.1X2	T45.1X3	T45.1X4	T45.1X5	T45.1X6
Troleandomycin	T36.3X1	T36.3X2	T36.3X3	T36.3X4	T36.3X5	T36.3X6
Trolnitrate (phosphate)	T46.3X1	T46.3X2	T46.3X3	T46.3X4	T46.3X5	T46.3X6
Tromantadine	T37.5X1	T37.5X2	T37.5X3	T37.5X4	T37.5X5	T37.5X6
Trometamol	T50.2X1	T50.2X2	T50.2X3	T50.2X4	T50.2X5	T50.2X6
Tromethamine	T50.2X1	T50.2X2	T50.2X3	T50.2X4	T50.2X5	T50.2X6
Tronothane	T41.3X1	T41.3X2	T41.3X3	T41.3X4	T41.3X5	T41.3X6
Tropacine	T44.3X1	T44.3X2	T44.3X3	T44.3X4	T44.3X5	T44.3X6
Tropatepine	T44.3X1	T44.3X2	T44.3X3	T44.3X4	T44.3X5	T44.3X6
Tropicamide	T44.3X1	T44.3X2	T44.3X3	T44.3X4	T44.3X5	T44.3X6
Trospium chloride	T44.3X1	T44.3X2	T44.3X3	T44.3X4	T44.3X5	T44.3X6
Troxerutin	T46.991	T46.992	T46.993	T46.994	T46.995	T46.996
Troxidone	T42.2X1	T42.2X2	T42.2X3	T42.2X4	T42.2X5	T42.2X6
Tryparsamide	T37.3X1	T37.3X2	T37.3X3	T37.3X4	T37.3X5	T37.3X6
Trypsin	T45.3X1	T45.3X2	T45.3X3	T45.3X4	T45.3X5	T45.3X6
Tryptizol	T43.011	T43.012	T43.013	T43.014	T43.015	T43.016
TSH	T38.811	T38.812	T38.813	T38.814	T38.815	T38.816
Tuaminoheptane	T48.5X1	T48.5X2	T48.5X3	T48.5X4	T48.5X5	T48.5X6
Tuberculin, purified protein derivative (PPD)	T50.8X1	T50.8X2	T50.8X3	T50.8X4	T50.8X5	T50.8X6
Tubocurare	T48.1X1	T48.1X2	T48.1X3	T48.1X4	T48.1X5	T48.1X6
Tubocurarine (chloride)	T48.1X1	T48.1X2	T48.1X3	T48.1X4	T48.1X5	T48.1X6
Tulobuterol	T48.6X1	T48.6X2	T48.6X3	T48.6X4	T48.6X5	T48.6X6
Turpentine (spirits of)	T52.8X1	T52.8X2	T52.8X3	T52.8X4	—	—
vapor	T52.8X1	T52.8X2	T52.8X3	T52.8X4	—	—
Tybamate	T43.591	T43.592	T43.593	T43.594	T43.595	T43.596
Tyloxapol	T48.4X1	T48.4X2	T48.4X3	T48.4X4	T48.4X5	T48.4X6
Tymazoline	T48.5X1	T48.5X2	T48.5X3	T48.5X4	T48.5X5	T48.5X6
Typhoid-paratyphoid vaccine	T50.A91	T50.A92	T50.A93	T50.A94	T50.A95	T50.A96
Typhus vaccine	T50.A91	T50.A92	T50.A93	T50.A94	T50.A95	T50.A96
Tyropanoate	T50.8X1	T50.8X2	T50.8X3	T50.8X4	T50.8X5	T50.8X6
Tyrothricin	T49.6X1	T49.6X2	T49.6X3	T49.6X4	T49.6X5	T49.6X6
ENT agent	T49.6X1	T49.6X2	T49.6X3	T49.6X4	T49.6X5	T49.6X6
ophthalmic preparation	T49.5X1	T49.5X2	T49.5X3	T49.5X4	T49.5X5	T49.5X6
U						
Ufenamate	T39.391	T39.392	T39.393	T39.394	T39.395	T39.396
Ultraviolet light protectant	T49.3X1	T49.3X2	T49.3X3	T49.3X4	T49.3X5	T49.3X6

◀ New ⬅ Revised ~~deleted~~ Deleted

Substance	Poisoning, Accidental (Unintentional)	Poisoning, Intentional Self-Harm	Poisoning, Assault	Poisoning, Undetermined	Adverse Effect	Underdosing
Undecenoic acid	T49.0X1	T49.0X2	T49.0X3	T49.0X4	T49.0X5	T49.0X6
Undecoylium	T49.0X1	T49.0X2	T49.0X3	T49.0X4	T49.0X5	T49.0X6
Undecylenic acid (derivatives)	T49.0X1	T49.0X2	T49.0X3	T49.0X4	T49.0X5	T49.0X6
Unna's boot	T49.3X1	T49.3X2	T49.3X3	T49.3X4	T49.3X5	T49.3X6
Unsaturated fatty acid	T46.6X1	T46.6X2	T46.6X3	T46.6X4	T46.6X5	T46.6X6
Uracil mustard	T45.1X1	T45.1X2	T45.1X3	T45.1X4	T45.1X5	T45.1X6
Uramustine	T45.1X1	T45.1X2	T45.1X3	T45.1X4	T45.1X5	T45.1X6
Urapidil	T46.5X1	T46.5X2	T46.5X3	T46.5X4	T46.5X5	T46.5X6
Urari	T48.1X1	T48.1X2	T48.1X3	T48.1X4	T48.1X5	T48.1X6
Urate oxidase	T50.4X1	T50.4X2	T50.4X3	T50.4X4	T50.4X5	T50.4X6
Urea	T47.3X1	T47.3X2	T47.3X3	T47.3X4	T47.3X5	T47.3X6
peroxide	T49.0X1	T49.0X2	T49.0X3	T49.0X4	T49.0X5	T49.0X6
stibamine	T37.4X1	T37.4X2	T37.4X3	T37.4X4	T37.4X5	T37.4X6
topical	T49.8X1	T49.8X2	T49.8X3	T49.8X4	T49.8X5	T49.8X6
Urethane	T45.1X1	T45.1X2	T45.1X3	T45.1X4	T45.1X5	T45.1X6
Urginea (maritima) (scilla) — *see Squill*						
Uric acid metabolism drug NEC	T50.4X1	T50.4X2	T50.4X3	T50.4X4	T50.4X5	T50.4X6
Uricosuric agent	T50.4X1	T50.4X2	T50.4X3	T50.4X4	T50.4X5	T50.4X6
Urinary anti-infective	T37.8X1	T37.8X2	T37.8X3	T37.8X4	T37.8X5	T37.8X6
Urofollitropin	T38.811	T38.812	T38.813	T38.814	T38.815	T38.816
Urokinase	T45.611	T45.612	T45.613	T45.614	T45.615	T45.616
Urokon	T50.8X1	T50.8X2	T50.8X3	T50.8X4	T50.8X5	T50.8X6
Ursodeoxycholic acid	T50.991	T50.992	T50.993	T50.994	T50.995	T50.996
Ursodiol	T50.991	T50.992	T50.993	T50.994	T50.995	T50.996
Urtica	T62.2X1	T62.2X2	T62.2X3	T62.2X4	—	—
Utility gas — *see Gas, utility*						
V						
Vaccine NEC	T50.Z91	T50.Z92	T50.Z93	T50.Z94	T50.Z95	T50.Z96
antineoplastic	T50.Z91	T50.Z92	T50.Z93	T50.Z94	T50.Z95	T50.Z96
bacterial NEC	T50.A91	T50.A92	T50.A93	T50.A94	T50.A95	T50.A96
with						
other bacterial component	T50.A91	T50.A92	T50.A93	T50.A94	T50.A95	T50.A96
pertussis component	T50.A91	T50.A92	T50.A93	T50.A94	T50.A95	T50.A96
viral-rickettsial component	T50.A91	T50.A92	T50.A93	T50.A94	T50.A95	T50.A96
mixed NEC	T50.A91	T50.A92	T50.A93	T50.A94	T50.A95	T50.A96
BCG	T50.A91	T50.A92	T50.A93	T50.A94	T50.A95	T50.A96
cholera	T50.A91	T50.A92	T50.A93	T50.A94	T50.A95	T50.A96
diphtheria	T50.A91	T50.A92	T50.A93	T50.A94	T50.A95	T50.A96
with tetanus	T50.A21	T50.A22	T50.A23	T50.A24	T50.A25	T50.A26
and pertussis	T50.A11	T50.A12	T50.A13	T50.A14	T50.A15	T50.A16
Vaccine NEC *(Continued)*						
influenza	T50.B91	T50.B92	T50.B93	T50.B94	T50.B95	T50.B96
measles	T50.B91	T50.B92	T50.B93	T50.B94	T50.B95	T50.B96
with mumps and rubella	T50.B91	T50.B92	T50.B93	T50.B94	T50.B95	T50.B96
meningococcal	T50.A91	T50.A92	T50.A93	T50.A94	T50.A95	T50.A96
mumps	T50.B91	T50.B92	T50.B93	T50.B94	T50.B95	T50.B96
paratyphoid	T50.A91	T50.A92	T50.A93	T50.A94	T50.A95	T50.A96
pertussis	T50.A11	T50.A12	T50.A13	T50.A14	T50.A15	T50.A16
with diphtheria	T50.A11	T50.A12	T50.A13	T50.A14	T50.A15	T50.A16
and tetanus	T50.A11	T50.A12	T50.A13	T50.A14	T50.A15	T50.A16
plague	T50.A91	T50.A92	T50.A93	T50.A94	T50.A95	T50.A96
poliomyelitis	T50.B91	T50.B92	T50.B93	T50.B94	T50.B95	T50.B96
poliovirus	T50.B91	T50.B92	T50.B93	T50.B94	T50.B95	T50.B96
rabies	T50.B91	T50.B92	T50.B93	T50.B94	T50.B95	T50.B96
respiratory syncytial virus	T50.B91	T50.B92	T50.B93	T50.B94	T50.B95	T50.B96
rickettsial NEC	T50.A91	T50.A92	T50.A93	T50.A94	T50.A95	T50.A96
with						
bacterial component	T50.A21	T50.A22	T50.A23	T50.A24	T50.A25	T50.A26
Rocky Mountain spotted fever	T50.A91	T50.A92	T50.A93	T50.A94	T50.A95	T50.A96
rubella	T50.B91	T50.B92	T50.B93	T50.B94	T50.B95	T50.B96
sabin oral	T50.B91	T50.B92	T50.B93	T50.B94	T50.B95	T50.B96
smallpox	T50.B11	T50.B12	T50.B13	T50.B14	T50.B15	T50.B16
TAB	T50.A91	T50.A92	T50.A93	T50.A94	T50.A95	T50.A96
tetanus	T50.A91	T50.A92	T50.A93	T50.A94	T50.A95	T50.A96
typhoid	T50.A91	T50.A92	T50.A93	T50.A94	T50.A95	T50.A96
typhus	T50.A91	T50.A92	T50.A93	T50.A94	T50.A95	T50.A96
viral NEC	T50.B91	T50.B92	T50.B93	T50.B94	T50.B95	T50.B96
yellow fever	T50.B91	T50.B92	T50.B93	T50.B94	T50.B95	T50.B96
Vaccinia immune globulin	T50.Z11	T50.Z12	T50.Z13	T50.Z14	T50.Z15	T50.Z16
Vaginal contraceptives	T49.8X1	T49.8X2	T49.8X3	T49.8X4	T49.8X5	T49.8X6
Valerian						
root	T42.6X1	T42.6X2	T42.6X3	T42.6X4	T42.6X5	T42.6X6
tincture	T42.6X1	T42.6X2	T42.6X3	T42.6X4	T42.6X5	T42.6X6
Valethamate bromide	T44.3X1	T44.3X2	T44.3X3	T44.3X4	T44.3X5	T44.3X6
Valisone	T49.0X1	T49.0X2	T49.0X3	T49.0X4	T49.0X5	T49.0X6
Valium	T42.4X1	T42.4X2	T42.4X3	T42.4X4	T42.4X5	T42.4X6
Valmid	T42.6X1	T42.6X2	T42.6X3	T42.6X4	T42.6X5	T42.6X6
Valnoctamide	T42.6X1	T42.6X2	T42.6X3	T42.6X4	T42.6X5	T42.6X6
Valproate (sodium)	T42.6X1	T42.6X2	T42.6X3	T42.6X4	T42.6X5	T42.6X6
Valproic acid	T42.6X1	T42.6X2	T42.6X3	T42.6X4	T42.6X5	T42.6X6
Valpromide	T42.6X1	T42.6X2	T42.6X3	T42.6X4	T42.6X5	T42.6X6
Vanadium	T56.891	T56.892	T56.893	T56.894	—	—

Substance	Poisoning, Accidental (Unintentional)	Poisoning, Intentional Self-Harm	Poisoning, Assault	Poisoning, Undetermined	Adverse Effect	Underdosing
Vancomycin	T36.8X1	T36.8X2	T36.8X3	T36.8X4	T36.8X5	T36.8X6
Vapor — *see also* Gas	T59.91	T59.92	T59.93	T59.94	—	—
kiln (carbon monoxide)	T58.8X1	T58.8X2	T58.8X3	T58.8X4	—	—
lead — *see lead*						
specified source NEC	T59.891	T59.892	T59.893	T59.894	—	—
Vardenafil	T46.7X1	T46.7X2	T46.7X3	T46.7X4	T46.7X5	T46.7X6
Varicose reduction drug	T46.8X1	T46.8X2	T46.8X3	T46.8X4	T46.8X5	T46.8X6
Varnish	T65.4X1	T65.4X2	T65.4X3	T65.4X4	—	—
cleaner	T52.91	T52.92	T52.93	T52.94	—	—
Vaseline	T49.3X1	T49.3X2	T49.3X3	T49.3X4	T49.3X5	T49.3X6
Vasodilan	T46.7X1	T46.7X2	T46.7X3	T46.7X4	T46.7X5	T46.7X6
Vasodilator						
coronary NEC	T46.3X1	T46.3X2	T46.3X3	T46.3X4	T46.3X5	T46.3X6
peripheral NEC	T46.7X1	T46.7X2	T46.7X3	T46.7X4	T46.7X5	T46.7X6
Vasopressin	T38.891	T38.892	T38.893	T38.894	T38.895	T38.896
Vasopressor drugs	T38.891	T38.892	T38.893	T38.894	T38.895	T38.896
Vecuronium bromide	T48.1X1	T48.1X2	T48.1X3	T48.1X4	T48.1X5	T48.1X6
Vegetable extract, astringent	T49.2X1	T49.2X2	T49.2X3	T49.2X4	T49.2X5	T49.2X6
Venlafaxine	T43.211	T43.212	T43.213	T43.214	T43.215	T43.216
Venom, venomous (bite) (sting)	T63.91	T63.92	T63.93	T63.94	—	—
amphibian NEC	T63.831	T63.832	T63.833	T63.834	—	—
animal NEC	T63.891	T63.892	T63.893	T63.894	—	—
ant	T63.421	T63.422	T63.423	T63.424	—	—
arthropod NEC	T63.481	T63.482	T63.483	T63.484	—	—
bee	T63.441	T63.442	T63.443	T63.444	—	—
centipede	T63.411	T63.412	T63.413	T63.414	—	—
fish	T63.591	T63.592	T63.593	T63.594	—	—
frog	T63.811	T63.812	T63.813	T63.814	—	—
hornet	T63.451	T63.452	T63.453	T63.454	—	—
insect NEC	T63.481	T63.482	T63.483	T63.484	—	—
lizard	T63.121	T63.122	T63.123	T63.124	—	—
marine						
animals	T63.691	T63.692	T63.693	T63.694	—	—
bluebottle	T63.611	T63.612	T63.613	T63.614	—	—
jellyfish NEC	T63.621	T63.622	T63.623	T63.624	—	—
Portugese Man-o-war	T63.611	T63.612	T63.613	T63.614	—	—
sea anemone	T63.631	T63.632	T63.633	T63.634	—	—
specified NEC	T63.691	T63.692	T63.693	T63.694	—	—
fish	T63.591	T63.592	T63.593	T63.594	—	—
plants	T63.711	T63.712	T63.713	T63.714	—	—
sting ray	T63.511	T63.512	T63.513	T63.514	—	—
Venom, venomous *(Continued)*						
millipede (tropical)	T63.411	T63.412	T63.413	T63.414	—	—
plant NEC	T63.791	T63.792	T63.793	T63.794	—	—
marine	T63.711	T63.712	T63.713	T63.714	—	—
reptile	T63.191	T63.192	T63.193	T63.194	—	—
gila monster	T63.111	T63.112	T63.113	T63.114	—	—
lizard NEC	T63.121	T63.122	T63.123	T63.124	—	—
scorpion	T63.2X1	T63.2X2	T63.2X3	T63.2X4	—	—
snake	T63.001	T63.002	T63.003	T63.004	—	—
African NEC	T63.081	T63.082	T63.083	T63.084	—	—
American (North) (South) NEC	T63.061	T63.062	T63.063	T63.064	—	—
Asian	T63.081	T63.082	T63.083	T63.084	—	—
Australian	T63.071	T63.072	T63.073	T63.074	—	—
cobra	T63.041	T63.042	T63.043	T63.044	—	—
coral snake	T63.021	T63.022	T63.023	T63.024	—	—
rattlesnake	T63.011	T63.012	T63.013	T63.014	—	—
specified NEC	T63.091	T63.092	T63.093	T63.094	—	—
taipan	T63.031	T63.032	T63.033	T63.034	—	—
specified NEC	T63.891	T63.892	T63.893	T63.894	—	—
spider	T63.301	T63.302	T63.303	T63.304	—	—
black widow	T63.311	T63.312	T63.313	T63.314	—	—
brown recluse	T63.331	T63.332	T63.333	T63.334	—	—
specified NEC	T63.391	T63.392	T63.393	T63.394	—	—
tarantula	T63.321	T63.322	T63.323	T63.324	—	—
sting ray	T63.511	T63.512	T63.513	T63.514	—	—
toad	T63.821	T63.822	T63.823	T63.824	—	—
wasp	T63.461	T63.462	T63.463	T63.464	—	—
Venous sclerosing drug NEC	T46.8X1	T46.8X2	T46.8X3	T46.8X4	T46.8X5	T46.8X6
Ventolin — *see Albuterol*						
Verapamil	T46.1X1	T46.1X2	T46.1X3	T46.1X4	T46.1X5	T46.1X6
Veramon	T42.3X1	T42.3X2	T42.3X3	T42.3X4	T42.3X5	T42.3X6
Veratrine	T46.5X1	T46.5X2	T46.5X3	T46.5X4	T46.5X5	T46.5X6
Veratrum						
album	T62.2X1	T62.2X2	T62.2X3	T62.2X4	—	—
alkaloids	T46.5X1	T46.5X2	T46.5X3	T46.5X4	T46.5X5	T46.5X6
viride	T62.2X1	T62.2X2	T62.2X3	T62.2X4	—	—
Verdigris	T60.3X1	T60.3X2	T60.3X3	T60.3X4	—	—
Veronal	T42.3X1	T42.3X2	T42.3X3	T42.3X4	T42.3X5	T42.3X6
Veroxil	T37.4X1	T37.4X2	T37.4X3	T37.4X4	T37.4X5	T37.4X6
Versenate	T50.6X1	T50.6X2	T50.6X3	T50.6X4	T50.6X5	T50.6X6

Substance	Poisoning, Accidental (Unintentional)	Poisoning, Intentional Self-Harm	Poisoning, Assault	Poisoning, Undetermined	Adverse Effect	Underdosing
Versidyne	T39.8X1	T39.8X2	T39.8X3	T39.8X4	T39.8X5	T39.8X6
Vetrabutine	T48.0X1	T48.0X2	T48.0X3	T48.0X4	T48.0X5	T48.0X6
Vidarabine	T37.5X1	T37.5X2	T37.5X3	T37.5X4	T37.5X5	T37.5X6
Vienna						
green	T57.0X1	T57.0X2	T57.0X3	T57.0X4	—	—
insecticide	T60.2X1	T60.2X2	T60.2X3	T60.2X4	—	—
red	T57.0X1	T57.0X2	T57.0X3	T57.0X4	—	—
pharmaceutical dye	T50.991	T50.992	T50.993	T50.994	T50.995	T50.996
Vigabatrin	T42.6X1	T42.6X2	T42.6X3	T42.6X4	T42.6X5	T42.6X6
Viloxazine	T43.291	T43.292	T43.293	T43.294	T43.295	T43.296
Viminol	T39.8X1	T39.8X2	T39.8X3	T39.8X4	T39.8X5	T39.8X6
Vinbarbital, vinbarbitone	T42.3X1	T42.3X2	T42.3X3	T42.3X4	T42.3X5	T42.3X6
Vinblastine	T45.1X1	T45.1X2	T45.1X3	T45.1X4	T45.1X5	T45.1X6
Vinburnine	T46.7X1	T46.7X2	T46.7X3	T46.7X4	T46.7X5	T46.7X6
Vincamine	T45.1X1	T45.1X2	T45.1X3	T45.1X4	T45.1X5	T45.1X6
Vincristine	T45.1X1	T45.1X2	T45.1X3	T45.1X4	T45.1X5	T45.1X6
Vindesine	T45.1X1	T45.1X2	T45.1X3	T45.1X4	T45.1X5	T45.1X6
Vinesthene, vinethene	T41.0X1	T41.0X2	T41.0X3	T41.0X4	T41.0X5	T41.0X6
Vinorelbine tartrate	T45.1X1	T45.1X2	T45.1X3	T45.1X4	T45.1X5	T45.1X6
Vinpocetine	T46.7X1	T46.7X2	T46.7X3	T46.7X4	T46.7X5	T46.7X6
Vinyl						
acetate	T65.891	T65.892	T65.893	T65.894	—	—
bital	T42.3X1	T42.3X2	T42.3X3	T42.3X4	T42.3X5	T42.3X6
bromide	T65.891	T65.892	T65.893	T65.894	—	—
chloride	T59.891	T59.892	T59.893	T59.894	—	—
ether	T41.0X1	T41.0X2	T41.0X3	T41.0X4	T41.0X5	T41.0X6
Vinylbital	T42.3X1	T42.3X2	T42.3X3	T42.3X4	T42.3X5	T42.3X6
Vinylidene chloride	T65.891	T65.892	T65.893	T65.894	—	—
Vioform	T37.8X1	T37.8X2	T37.8X3	T37.8X4	T37.8X5	T37.8X6
topical	T49.0X1	T49.0X2	T49.0X3	T49.0X4	T49.0X5	T49.0X6
Viomycin	T36.8X1	T36.8X2	T36.8X3	T36.8X4	T36.8X5	T36.8X6
Viosterol	T45.2X1	T45.2X2	T45.2X3	T45.2X4	T45.2X5	T45.2X6
Viper (venom)	T63.091	T63.092	T63.093	T63.094	—	—
Viprynium	T37.4X1	T37.4X2	T37.4X3	T37.4X4	T37.4X5	T37.4X6
Viquidil	T46.7X1	T46.7X2	T46.7X3	T46.7X4	T46.7X5	T46.7X6
Viral vaccine NEC	T50.B91	T50.B92	T50.B93	T50.B94	T50.B95	T50.B96
Virginiamycin	T36.8X1	T36.8X2	T36.8X3	T36.8X4	T36.8X5	T36.8X6
Virugon	T37.5X1	T37.5X2	T37.5X3	T37.5X4	T37.5X5	T37.5X6
Viscous agent	T50.901	T50.902	T50.903	T50.904	T50.905	T50.906
Visine	T49.5X1	T49.5X2	T49.5X3	T49.5X4	T49.5X5	T49.5X6
Visnadine	T46.3X1	T46.3X2	T46.3X3	T46.3X4	T46.3X5	T46.3X6

Substance	Poisoning, Accidental (Unintentional)	Poisoning, Intentional Self-Harm	Poisoning, Assault	Poisoning, Undetermined	Adverse Effect	Underdosing
Vitamin NEC	T45.2X1	T45.2X2	T45.2X3	T45.2X4	T45.2X5	T45.2X6
A	T45.2X1	T45.2X2	T45.2X3	T45.2X4	T45.2X5	T45.2X6
B NEC	T45.2X1	T45.2X2	T45.2X3	T45.2X4	T45.2X5	T45.2X6
nicotinic acid	T46.7X1	T46.7X2	T46.7X3	T46.7X4	T46.7X5	T46.7X6
B1	T45.2X1	T45.2X2	T45.2X3	T45.2X4	T45.2X5	T45.2X6
B2	T45.2X1	T45.2X2	T45.2X3	T45.2X4	T45.2X5	T45.2X6
B6	T45.2X1	T45.2X2	T45.2X3	T45.2X4	T45.2X5	T45.2X6
B12	T45.2X1	T45.2X2	T45.2X3	T45.2X4	T45.2X5	T45.2X6
B15	T45.2X1	T45.2X2	T45.2X3	T45.2X4	T45.2X5	T45.2X6
C	T45.2X1	T45.2X2	T45.2X3	T45.2X4	T45.2X5	T45.2X6
D	T45.2X1	T45.2X2	T45.2X3	T45.2X4	T45.2X5	T45.2X6
D2	T45.2X1	T45.2X2	T45.2X3	T45.2X4	T45.2X5	T45.2X6
D3	T45.2X1	T45.2X2	T45.2X3	T45.2X4	T45.2X5	T45.2X6
E	T45.2X1	T45.2X2	T45.2X3	T45.2X4	T45.2X5	T45.2X6
E acetate	T45.2X1	T45.2X2	T45.2X3	T45.2X4	T45.2X5	T45.2X6
hematopoietic	T45.8X1	T45.8X2	T45.8X3	T45.8X4	T45.8X5	T45.8X6
K NEC	T45.7X1	T45.7X2	T45.7X3	T45.7X4	T45.7X5	T45.7X6
K1	T45.7X1	T45.7X2	T45.7X3	T45.7X4	T45.7X5	T45.7X6
K2	T45.7X1	T45.7X2	T45.7X3	T45.7X4	T45.7X5	T45.7X6
PP	T45.2X1	T45.2X2	T45.2X3	T45.2X4	T45.2X5	T45.2X6
ulceroprotectant	T47.1X1	T47.1X2	T47.1X3	T47.1X4	T47.1X5	T47.1X6
Vleminckx's solution	T49.4X1	T49.4X2	T49.4X3	T49.4X4	T49.4X5	T49.4X6
Voltaren — *see Diclofenac sodium*						
W						
Warfarin	T45.511	T45.512	T45.513	T45.514	T45.515	T45.516
rodenticide	T60.4X1	T60.4X2	T60.4X3	T60.4X4	—	—
sodium	T60.4X1	T60.4X2	T60.4X3	T60.4X4	—	—
Wasp (sting)	T63.461	T63.462	T63.463	T63.464	—	—
Water						
balance drug	T50.3X1	T50.3X2	T50.3X3	T50.3X4	T50.3X5	T50.3X6
distilled	T50.3X1	T50.3X2	T50.3X3	T50.3X4	T50.3X5	T50.3X6
gas — *see Gas, water*						
incomplete combustion of — *see Carbon, monoxide, fuel, utility*						
hemlock	T62.2X1	T62.2X2	T62.2X3	T62.2X4	—	—
moccasin (venom)	T63.061	T63.062	T63.063	T63.064	—	—
purified	T50.3X1	T50.3X2	T50.3X3	T50.3X4	T50.3X5	T50.3X6
Wax (paraffin) (petroleum)	T52.0X1	T52.0X2	T52.0X3	T52.0X4	—	—
automobile	T65.891	T65.892	T65.893	T65.894	—	—
floor	T52.0X1	T52.0X2	T52.0X3	T52.0X4	—	—

Substance	Poisoning, Accidental (Unintentional)	Poisoning, Intentional Self-Harm	Poisoning, Assault	Poisoning, Undetermined	Adverse Effect	Underdosing
Weed killers NEC	T6Ø.3X1	T6Ø.3X2	T6Ø.3X3	T6Ø.3X4	—	—
Welldorm	T42.6X1	T42.6X2	T42.6X3	T42.6X4	T42.6X5	T42.6X6
White						
arsenic	T57.ØX1	T57.ØX2	T57.ØX3	T57.ØX4	—	—
hellebore	T62.2X1	T62.2X2	T62.2X3	T62.2X4	—	—
lotion (keratolytic)	T49.4X1	T49.4X2	T49.4X3	T49.4X4	T49.4X5	T49.4X6
spirit	T52.ØX1	T52.ØX2	T52.ØX3	T52.ØX4	—	—
Whitewash	T65.891	T65.892	T65.893	T65.894	—	—
Whole blood (human)	T45.8X1	T45.8X2	T45.8X3	T45.8X4	T45.8X5	T45.8X6
Wild						
black cherry	T62.2X1	T62.2X2	T62.2X3	T62.2X4	—	—
poisonous plants NEC	T62.2X1	T62.2X2	T62.2X3	T62.2X4	—	—
Window cleaning fluid	T65.891	T65.892	T65.893	T65.894	—	—
Wintergreen (oil)	T49.3X1	T49.3X2	T49.3X3	T49.3X4	T49.3X5	T49.3X6
Wisterine	T62.2X1	T62.2X2	T62.2X3	T62.2X4	—	—
Witch hazel	T49.2X1	T49.2X2	T49.2X3	T49.2X4	T49.2X5	T49.2X6
Wood alcohol or spirit	T51.1X1	T51.1X2	T51.1X3	T51.1X4	—	—
Wool fat (hydrous)	T49.3X1	T49.3X2	T49.3X3	T49.3X4	T49.3X5	T49.3X6
Woorali	T48.1X1	T48.1X2	T48.1X3	T48.1X4	T48.1X5	T48.1X6
Wormseed, American	T37.4X1	T37.4X2	T37.4X3	T37.4X4	T37.4X5	T37.4X6
X						
Xamoterol	T44.5X1	T44.5X2	T44.5X3	T44.5X4	T44.5X5	T44.5X6
Xanthine diuretics	T5Ø.2X1	T5Ø.2X2	T5Ø.2X3	T5Ø.2X4	T5Ø.2X5	T5Ø.2X6
Xanthinol nicotinate	T46.7X1	T46.7X2	T46.7X3	T46.7X4	T46.7X5	T46.7X6
Xanthotoxin	T49.3X1	T49.3X2	T49.3X3	T49.3X4	T49.3X5	T49.3X6
Xantinol nicotinate	T46.7X1	T46.7X2	T46.7X3	T46.7X4	T46.7X5	T46.7X6
Xantocillin	T36.ØX1	T36.ØX2	T36.ØX3	T36.ØX4	T36.ØX5	T36.ØX6
Xenon (127Xe) (133Xe)	T5Ø.8X1	T5Ø.8X2	T5Ø.8X3	T5Ø.8X4	T5Ø.8X5	T5Ø.8X6
Xenysalate	T49.4X1	T49.4X2	T49.4X3	T49.4X4	T49.4X5	T49.4X6
Xibornol	T37.8X1	T37.8X2	T37.8X3	T37.8X4	T37.8X5	T37.8X6
Xigris	T45.511	T45.512	T45.513	T45.514	T45.515	T45.516
Xipamide	T5Ø.2X1	T5Ø.2X2	T5Ø.2X3	T5Ø.2X4	T5Ø.2X5	T5Ø.2X6
Xylene (vapor)	T52.2X1	T52.2X2	T52.2X3	T52.2X4	—	—
Xylocaine (infiltration) (topical)	T41.3X1	T41.3X2	T41.3X3	T41.3X4	T41.3X5	T41.3X6
nerve block (peripheral) (plexus)	T41.3X1	T41.3X2	T41.3X3	T41.3X4	T41.3X5	T41.3X6
spinal	T41.3X1	T41.3X2	T41.3X3	T41.3X4	T41.3X5	T41.3X6
Xylol (vapor)	T52.2X1	T52.2X2	T52.2X3	T52.2X4	—	—
Xylometazoline	T48.5X1	T48.5X2	T48.5X3	T48.5X4	T48.5X5	T48.5X6

Substance	Poisoning, Accidental (Unintentional)	Poisoning, Intentional Self-Harm	Poisoning, Assault	Poisoning, Undetermined	Adverse Effect	Underdosing
Y						
Yeast	T45.2X1	T45.2X2	T45.2X3	T45.2X4	T45.2X5	T45.2X6
dried	T45.2X1	T45.2X2	T45.2X3	T45.2X4	T45.2X5	T45.2X6
Yellow						
fever vaccine	T5Ø.B91	T5Ø.B92	T5Ø.B93	T5Ø.B94	T5Ø.B95	T5Ø.B96
jasmine	T62.2X1	T62.2X2	T62.2X3	T62.2X4	—	—
phenolphthalein	T47.2X1	T47.2X2	T47.2X3	T47.2X4	T47.2X5	T47.2X6
Yew	T62.2X1	T62.2X2	T62.2X3	T62.2X4	—	—
Yohimbic acid	T4Ø.991	T4Ø.992	T4Ø.993	T4Ø.994	T4Ø.995	T4Ø.996
Z						
Zactane	T39.8X1	T39.8X2	T39.8X3	T39.8X4	T39.8X5	T39.8X6
Zalcitabine	T37.5X1	T37.5X2	T37.5X3	T37.5X4	T37.5X5	T37.5X6
Zaroxolyn	T5Ø.2X1	T5Ø.2X2	T5Ø.2X3	T5Ø.2X4	T5Ø.2X5	T5Ø.2X6
Zephiran (topical)	T49.ØX1	T49.ØX2	T49.ØX3	T49.ØX4	T49.ØX5	T49.ØX6
ophthalmic preparation	T49.5X1	T49.5X2	T49.5X3	T49.5X4	T49.5X5	T49.5X6
Zeranol	T38.7X1	T38.7X2	T38.7X3	T38.7X4	T38.7X5	T38.7X6
Zerone	T51.1X1	T51.1X2	T51.1X3	T51.1X4	—	—
Zidovudine	T37.5X1	T37.5X2	T37.5X3	T37.5X4	T37.5X5	T37.5X6
Zimeldine	T43.221	T43.222	T43.223	T43.224	T43.225	T43.226
Zinc (compounds) (fumes) (vapor) NEC	T56.5X1	T56.5X2	T56.5X3	T56.5X4	—	—
anti-infectives	T49.ØX1	T49.ØX2	T49.ØX3	T49.ØX4	T49.ØX5	T49.ØX6
antivaricose	T46.8X1	T46.8X2	T46.8X3	T46.8X4	T46.8X5	T46.8X6
bacitracin	T49.ØX1	T49.ØX2	T49.ØX3	T49.ØX4	T49.ØX5	T49.ØX6
chloride (mouthwash)	T49.6X1	T49.6X2	T49.6X3	T49.6X4	T49.6X5	T49.6X6
chromate	T56.5X1	T56.5X2	T56.5X3	T56.5X4	—	—
gelatin	T49.3X1	T49.3X2	T49.3X3	T49.3X4	T49.3X5	T49.3X6
oxide	T49.3X1	T49.3X2	T49.3X3	T49.3X4	T49.3X5	T49.3X6
plaster	T49.3X1	T49.3X2	T49.3X3	T49.3X4	T49.3X5	T49.3X6
peroxide	T49.ØX1	T49.ØX2	T49.ØX3	T49.ØX4	T49.ØX5	T49.ØX6
pesticides	T56.5X1	T56.5X2	T56.5X3	T56.5X4	—	—
phosphide	T6Ø.4X1	T6Ø.4X2	T6Ø.4X3	T6Ø.4X4	—	—
pyrithionate	T49.4X1	T49.4X2	T49.4X3	T49.4X4	T49.4X5	T49.4X6
stearate	T49.3X1	T49.3X2	T49.3X3	T49.3X4	T49.3X5	T49.3X6
sulfate	T49.5X1	T49.5X2	T49.5X3	T49.5X4	T49.5X5	T49.5X6
ENT agent	T49.6X1	T49.6X2	T49.6X3	T49.6X4	T49.6X5	T49.6X6
ophthalmic solution	T49.5X1	T49.5X2	T49.5X3	T49.5X4	T49.5X5	T49.5X6
topical NEC	T49.ØX1	T49.ØX2	T49.ØX3	T49.ØX4	T49.ØX5	T49.ØX6
undecylenate	T49.ØX1	T49.ØX2	T49.ØX3	T49.ØX4	T49.ØX5	T49.ØX6

Substance	Poisoning, Accidental (Unintentional)	Poisoning, Intentional Self-Harm	Poisoning, Assault	Poisoning, Undetermined	Adverse Effect	Underdosing
Zineb	T60.0X1	T60.0X2	T60.0X3	T60.0X4	—	—
Zinostatin	T45.1X1	T45.1X2	T45.1X3	T45.1X4	T45.1X5	T45.1X6
Zipeprol	T48.3X1	T48.3X2	T48.3X3	T48.3X4	T48.3X5	T48.3X6
Zofenopril	T46.4X1	T46.4X2	T46.4X3	T46.4X4	T46.4X5	T46.4X6
Zolpidem	T42.6X1	T42.6X2	T42.6X3	T42.6X4	T42.6X5	T42.6X6
Zomepirac	T39.391	T39.392	T39.393	T39.394	T39.395	T39.396
Zopiclone	T42.6X1	T42.6X2	T42.6X3	T42.6X4	T42.6X5	T42.6X6
Zorubicin	T45.1X1	T45.1X2	T45.1X3	T45.1X4	T45.1X5	T45.1X6
Zotepine	T43.591	T43.592	T43.593	T43.594	T43.595	T43.596
Zovant	T45.511	T45.512	T45.513	T45.514	T45.515	T45.516
Zoxazolamine	T42.8X1	T42.8X2	T42.8X3	T42.8X4	T42.8X5	T42.8X6
Zuclopenthixol	T43.4X1	T43.4X2	T43.4X3	T43.4X4	T43.4X5	T43.4X6
Zygadenus (venenosus)	T62.2X1	T62.2X2	T62.2X3	T62.2X4	—	—
Zyprexa	T43.591	T43.592	T43.593	T43.594	T43.595	T43.596

External Cause of Injuries Index

ICD-10-CM EXTERNAL CAUSE OF INJURIES INDEX

A

Abandonment (causing exposure to weather conditions) (with intent to injure or kill) NEC X58
Abuse (adult) (child) (mental) (physical) (sexual) X58
Accident (to) X58
aircraft (in transit) (powered) —*see also* Accident, transport, aircraft
due to, caused by cataclysm —*see* Forces of nature, by type
animal-drawn vehicle —*see* Accident, transport, animal-drawn vehicle occupant
animal-rider —*see* Accident, transport, animal-rider
automobile —*see* Accident, transport, car occupant
bare foot water skiier V94.4
boat, boating —*see also* Accident, watercraft
striking swimmer
powered V94.11
unpowered V94.12
bus —*see* Accident, transport, bus occupant
cable car, not on rails V98.0
on rails —*see* Accident, transport, streetcar occupant
car —*see* Accident, transport, car occupant
caused by, due to
animal NEC W64
chain hoist W24.0
cold (excessive) —*see* Exposure, cold
corrosive liquid, substance —*see* Table of Drugs and Chemicals (Revised)
cutting or piercing instrument —*see* Contact, with, by type of instrument
drive belt W24.0
electric
current —*see* Exposure, electric current
motor —*see also* Contact, with, by type of machine W31.3
current (of) W86.8
environmental factor NEC X58
explosive material —*see* Explosion
fire, flames —*see* Exposure, fire
firearm missile —*see* Discharge, firearm by type
heat (excessive) —*see* Heat
hot —*see* Contact, with, hot
ignition —*see* Ignition
lifting device W24.0
lightning —*see* subcategory T75.0
causing fire —*see* Exposure, fire
machine, machinery —*see* Contact, with, by type of machine
natural factor NEC X58
pulley (block) W24.0
radiation —*see* Radiation
steam X13.1
inhalation X13.0
pipe X16
thunderbolt —*see* subcategory T75.0
causing fire —*see* Exposure, fire
transmission device W24.1
coach —*see* Accident, transport, bus occupant
coal car —*see* Accident, transport, industrial vehicle occupant
diving —*see also* Fall, into, water
with
drowning or submersion —*see* Drowning
forklift —*see* Accident, transport, industrial vehicle occupant
heavy transport vehicle NOS —*see* Accident, transport, truck occupant
ice yacht V98.2

Accident *(Continued)*
in
medical, surgical procedure
as, or due to misadventure —*see* Misadventure
causing an abnormal reaction or later complication without mention of misadventure —*see also* Complication of or following, by type of procedure Y84.9
land yacht V98.1
late effect of —*see* W00-X58 with 7th character S
logging car —*see* Accident, transport, industrial vehicle occupant
machine, machinery —*see also* Contact, with, by type of machine
on board watercraft V93.69
explosion —*see* Explosion, in, watercraft
fire —*see* Burn, on board watercraft
powered craft V93.63
ferry boat V93.61
fishing boat V93.62
jetskis V93.63
liner V93.61
merchant ship V93.60
passenger ship V93.61
sailboat V93.64
mine tram —*see* Accident, transport, industrial vehicle occupant
mobility scooter (motorized) —*see* Accident, transport, pedestrian, conveyance, specified type NEC
motor scooter —*see* Accident, transport, motorcyclist
motor vehicle NOS (traffic) —*see also* Accident, transport V89.2
nontraffic V89.0
three-wheeled NOS —*see* Accident, transport, three-wheeled motor vehicle occupant
motorcycle NOS —*see* Accident, transport, motorcyclist
nonmotor vehicle NOS (nontraffic) —*see also* Accident, transport V89.1
traffic NOS V89.3
nontraffic (victim's mode of transport NOS) V88.9
collision (between) V88.7
bus and truck V88.5
car and:
bus V88.3
pickup V88.2
three-wheeled motor vehicle V88.0
train V88.6
truck V88.4
two-wheeled motor vehicle V88.0
van V88.2
specified vehicle NEC and:
three-wheeled motor vehicle V88.1
two-wheeled motor vehicle V88.1
known mode of transport —*see* Accident, transport, by type of vehicle
noncollision V88.8
on board watercraft V93.89
powered craft V93.83
ferry boat V93.81
fishing boat V93.82
jetskis V93.83
liner V93.81
merchant ship V93.80
passenger ship V93.81
unpowered craft V93.88
canoe V93.85
inflatable V93.86
in tow
recreational V94.31
specified NEC V94.32
kayak V93.85

Accident *(Continued)*
on board watercraft *(Continued)*
unpowered craft *(Continued)*
sailboat V93.84
surf-board V93.88
water skis V93.87
windsurfer V93.88
parachutist V97.29
entangled in object V97.21
injured on landing V97.22
pedal cycle —*see* Accident, transport, pedal cyclist
pedestrian (on foot)
with
another pedestrian W51
with fall W03
due to ice or snow W00.0
on pedestrian conveyance NEC V00.09
roller skater (in-line) V00.01
skate boarder V00.02
transport vehicle —*see* Accident, transport
on pedestrian conveyance —*see* Accident, transport, pedestrian, conveyance
pick-up truck or van —*see* Accident, transport, pickup truck occupant
quarry truck —*see* Accident, transport, industrial vehicle occupant
railway vehicle (any) (in motion) —*see* Accident, transport, railway vehicle occupant
due to cataclysm —*see* Forces of nature, by type
scooter (non-motorized) —*see* Accident, transport, pedestrian, conveyance, scooter
sequelae of —*see* W00-X58 with 7th character S
skateboard —*see* Accident, transport, pedestrian, conveyance, skateboard
ski (ing) —*see* Accident, transport, pedestrian, conveyance
lift V98.3
specified cause NEC X58
streetcar —*see* Accident, transport, streetcar occupant
traffic (victim's mode of transport NOS) V87.9
collision (between) V87.7
bus and truck V87.5
car and:
bus V87.3
pickup V87.2
three-wheeled motor vehicle V87.0
train V87.6
truck V87.4
two-wheeled motor vehicle V87.0
van V87.2
specified vehicle NEC and:
three-wheeled motor vehicle V87.1
two-wheeled motor vehicle V87.1
known mode of transport —*see* Accident, transport, by type of vehicle
noncollision V87.8
transport (involving injury to) V99
18 wheeler —*see* Accident, transport, truck occupant
agricultural vehicle occupant (nontraffic) V84.9
driver V84.5
hanger-on V84.7
passenger V84.6
traffic V84.3
driver V84.0
hanger-on V84.2
passenger V84.1
while boarding or alighting V84.4

A

A

- **Accident** *(Continued)*
  - transport *(Continued)*
    - bus occupant *(Continued)*
      - driver *(Continued)*
        - collision *(Continued)*
          - motor vehicle NOS (traffic) V79.40
            - nontraffic V79.00
            - specified type NEC (traffic) V79.49
              - nontraffic V79.09
          - pedal cycle (traffic) V71.5
            - nontraffic V71.0
          - pickup truck (traffic) V73.5
            - nontraffic V73.0
          - railway vehicle (traffic) V75.5
            - nontraffic V75.0
          - specified vehicle NEC (traffic) V76.5
            - nontraffic V76.0
          - stationary object (traffic) V77.5
            - nontraffic V77.0
          - streetcar (traffic) V76.5
            - nontraffic V76.0
          - three wheeled motor vehicle (traffic) V72.5
            - nontraffic V72.0
          - truck (traffic) V74.5
            - nontraffic V74.0
          - two wheeled motor vehicle (traffic) V72.5
            - nontraffic V72.0
          - van (traffic) V73.5
            - nontraffic V73.0
        - noncollision accident (traffic) V78.5
          - nontraffic V78.0
      - hanger-on
        - collision (with)
          - animal (traffic) V70.7
            - being ridden (traffic) V76.7
              - nontraffic V76.2
            - nontraffic V70.2
          - animal-drawn vehicle (traffic) V76.7
            - nontraffic V76.2
          - bus (traffic) V74.7
            - nontraffic V74.2
          - car (traffic) V73.7
            - nontraffic V73.2
          - pedal cycle (traffic) V71.7
            - nontraffic V71.2
          - pickup truck (traffic) V73.7
            - nontraffic V73.2
          - railway vehicle (traffic) V75.7
            - nontraffic V75.2
          - specified vehicle NEC (traffic) V76.7
            - nontraffic V76.2
          - stationary object (traffic) V77.7
            - nontraffic V77.2
          - streetcar (traffic) V76.7
            - nontraffic V76.2
          - three wheeled motor vehicle (traffic) V72.7
            - nontraffic V72.2
          - truck (traffic) V74.7
            - nontraffic V74.2
          - two wheeled motor vehicle (traffic) V72.7
            - nontraffic V72.2
          - van (traffic) V73.7
            - nontraffic V73.2
        - noncollision accident (traffic) V78.7
          - nontraffic V78.2
      - noncollision accident (traffic) V78.9
        - nontraffic V78.3
        - while boarding or alighting V78.4
      - nontraffic V79.3
      - passenger
        - collision (with)
          - animal (traffic) V70.6
            - being ridden (traffic) V76.6
              - nontraffic V76.1
            - nontraffic V70.1

- **Accident** *(Continued)*
  - transport *(Continued)*
    - bus occupant *(Continued)*
      - passenger *(Continued)*
        - collision *(Continued)*
          - animal-drawn vehicle (traffic) V76.6
            - nontraffic V76.1
          - bus (traffic) V74.6
            - nontraffic V74.1
          - car (traffic) V73.6
            - nontraffic V73.1
          - motor vehicle NOS (traffic) V79.50
            - nontraffic V79.10
            - specified type NEC (traffic) V79.59
              - nontraffic V79.19
          - pedal cycle (traffic) V71.6
            - nontraffic V71.1
          - pickup truck (traffic) V73.6
            - nontraffic V73.1
          - railway vehicle (traffic) V75.6
            - nontraffic V75.1
          - specified vehicle NEC (traffic) V76.6
            - nontraffic V76.1
          - stationary object (traffic) V77.6
            - nontraffic V77.1
          - streetcar (traffic) V76.6
            - nontraffic V76.1
          - three wheeled motor vehicle (traffic) V72.6
            - nontraffic V72.1
          - truck (traffic) V74.6
            - nontraffic V74.1
          - two wheeled motor vehicle (traffic) V72.6
            - nontraffic V72.1
          - van (traffic) V73.6
            - nontraffic V73.1
        - noncollision accident (traffic) V78.6
          - nontraffic V78.1
      - specified type NEC V79.88
        - military vehicle V79.81
    - cable car, not on rails V98.0
      - on rails —*see* Accident, transport, streetcar occupant
    - car occupant V49.9
      - ambulance occupant —*see* Accident, transport, ambulance occupant
      - collision (with)
        - animal (traffic) V40.9
          - being ridden (traffic) V46.9
            - nontraffic V46.3
            - while boarding or alighting V46.4
          - nontraffic V40.3
          - while boarding or alighting V40.4
        - animal-drawn vehicle (traffic) V46.9
          - nontraffic V46.3
          - while boarding or alighting V46.4
        - bus (traffic) V44.9
          - nontraffic V44.3
          - while boarding or alighting V44.4
        - car (traffic) V43.92
          - nontraffic V43.32
          - while boarding or alighting V43.42
        - motor vehicle NOS (traffic) V49.60
          - nontraffic V49.20
          - specified type NEC (traffic) V49.69
            - nontraffic V49.29
        - pedal cycle (traffic) V41.9
          - nontraffic V41.3
          - while boarding or alighting V41.4
        - pickup truck (traffic) V43.93
          - nontraffic V43.33
          - while boarding or alighting V43.43
        - railway vehicle (traffic) V45.9
          - nontraffic V45.3
          - while boarding or alighting V45.4
        - specified vehicle NEC (traffic) V46.9
          - nontraffic V46.3
          - while boarding or alighting V46.4

- **Accident** *(Continued)*
  - transport *(Continued)*
    - car occupant *(Continued)*
      - collision *(Continued)*
        - sport utility vehicle (traffic) V43.91
          - nontraffic V43.31
          - while boarding or alighting V43.41
        - stationary object (traffic) V47.92
          - nontraffic V47.32
          - while boarding or alighting V47.4
        - streetcar (traffic) V46.9
          - nontraffic V46.3
          - while boarding or alighting V46.4
        - three wheeled motor vehicle (traffic) V42.9
          - nontraffic V42.3
          - while boarding or alighting V42.4
        - truck (traffic) V44.9
          - nontraffic V44.3
          - while boarding or alighting V44.4
        - two wheeled motor vehicle (traffic) V42.9
          - nontraffic V42.3
          - while boarding or alighting V42.4
        - van (traffic) V43.94
          - nontraffic V43.34
          - while boarding or alighting V43.44
      - driver
        - collision (with)
          - animal (traffic) V40.5
            - being ridden (traffic) V46.5
              - nontraffic V46.0
            - nontraffic V40.0
          - animal-drawn vehicle (traffic) V46.5
            - nontraffic V46.0
          - bus (traffic) V44.5
            - nontraffic V44.0
          - car (traffic) V43.52
            - nontraffic V43.02
          - motor vehicle NOS (traffic) V49.40
            - nontraffic V49.00
            - specified type NEC (traffic) V49.49
              - nontraffic V49.09
          - pedal cycle (traffic) V41.5
            - nontraffic V41.0
          - pickup truck (traffic) V43.53
            - nontraffic V43.03
          - railway vehicle (traffic) V45.5
            - nontraffic V45.0
          - specified vehicle NEC (traffic) V46.5
            - nontraffic V46.0
          - sport utility vehicle (traffic) V43.51
            - nontraffic V43.01
          - stationary object (traffic) V47.52
            - nontraffic V47.02
          - streetcar (traffic) V46.5
            - nontraffic V46.0
          - three wheeled motor vehicle (traffic) V42.5
            - nontraffic V42.0
          - truck (traffic) V44.5
            - nontraffic V44.0
          - two wheeled motor vehicle (traffic) V42.5
            - nontraffic V42.0
          - van (traffic) V43.54
            - nontraffic V43.04
        - noncollision accident (traffic) V48.5
          - nontraffic V48.0
      - hanger-on
        - collision (with)
          - animal (traffic) V40.7
            - being ridden (traffic) V46.7
              - nontraffic V46.2
            - nontraffic V40.2
          - animal-drawn vehicle (traffic) V46.7
            - nontraffic V46.2
          - bus (traffic) V44.7
            - nontraffic V44.2

- **Accident** *(Continued)*
  - transport *(Continued)*
    - car occupant *(Continued)*
      - hanger-on *(Continued)*
        - collision *(Continued)*
          - car (traffic) V43.72
            - nontraffic V43.22
          - pedal cycle (traffic) V41.7
            - nontraffic V41.2
          - pickup truck (traffic) V43.73
            - nontraffic V43.23
          - railway vehicle (traffic) V45.7
            - nontraffic V45.2
          - specified vehicle NEC (traffic) V46.7
            - nontraffic V46.2
          - sport utility vehicle (traffic) V43.71
            - nontraffic V43.21
          - stationary object (traffic) V47.7
            - nontraffic V47.2
          - streetcar (traffic) V46.7
            - nontraffic V46.2
          - three wheeled motor vehicle (traffic) V42.7
            - nontraffic V42.2
          - truck (traffic) V44.7
            - nontraffic V44.2
          - two wheeled motor vehicle (traffic) V42.7
            - nontraffic V42.2
          - van (traffic) V43.74
            - nontraffic V43.24
        - noncollision accident (traffic) V48.7
          - nontraffic V48.2
      - noncollision accident (traffic) V48.9
        - nontraffic V48.3
        - while boarding or alighting V48.4
      - nontraffic V49.3
      - passenger
        - collision (with)
          - animal (traffic) V40.6
            - being ridden (traffic) V46.6
              - nontraffic V46.1
            - nontraffic V40.1
          - animal-drawn vehicle (traffic) V46.6
            - nontraffic V46.1
          - bus (traffic) V44.6
            - nontraffic V44.1
          - car (traffic) V43.62
            - nontraffic V43.12
          - motor vehicle NOS (traffic) V49.50
            - nontraffic V49.10
            - specified type NEC (traffic) V49.59
              - nontraffic V49.19
          - pedal cycle (traffic) V41.6
            - nontraffic V41.1
          - pickup truck (traffic) V43.63
            - nontraffic V43.13
          - railway vehicle (traffic) V45.6
            - nontraffic V45.1
          - specified vehicle NEC (traffic) V46.6
            - nontraffic V46.1
          - sport utility vehicle (traffic) V43.61
            - nontraffic V43.11
          - stationary object (traffic) V47.62
            - nontraffic V47.12
          - streetcar (traffic) V46.6
            - nontraffic V46.1
          - three wheeled motor vehicle (traffic) V42.6
            - nontraffic V42.1
          - truck (traffic) V44.6
            - nontraffic V44.1
          - two wheeled motor vehicle (traffic) V42.6
            - nontraffic V42.1
          - van (traffic) V43.64
            - nontraffic V43.14
        - noncollision accident (traffic) V48.6
          - nontraffic V48.1
      - specified type NEC V49.88
      - military vehicle V49.81

- **Accident** *(Continued)*
  - transport *(Continued)*
    - coal car —*see* Accident, transport, industrial vehicle occupant
    - construction vehicle occupant (nontraffic) V85.9
      - driver V85.5
      - hanger-on V85.7
      - passenger V85.6
      - traffic V85.3
        - driver V85.0
        - hanger-on V85.2
        - passenger V85.1
      - while boarding or alighting V85.4
    - dirt bike rider —*see* Accident, transport, all-terrain vehicle occupant
    - due to cataclysm —*see* Forces of nature, by type
    - dune buggy occupant (nontraffic) V86.93
      - driver V86.53
      - hanger-on V86.73
      - passenger V86.63
      - traffic V86.33
        - driver V86.03
        - hanger-on V86.23
        - passenger V86.13
      - while boarding or alighting V86.43
    - forklift —*see* Accident, transport, industrial vehicle occupant
    - go cart —*see* Accident, transport, all-terrain vehicle occupant
    - golf cart —*see* Accident, transport, all-terrain vehicle occupant
    - heavy transport vehicle occupant —*see* Accident, transport, truck occupant
    - ice yacht V98.2
    - industrial vehicle occupant (nontraffic) V83.9
      - driver V83.5
      - hanger-on V83.7
      - passenger V83.6
      - traffic V83.3
        - driver V83.0
        - hanger-on V83.2
        - passenger V83.1
      - while boarding or alighting V83.4
    - interurban electric car —*see* Accident, transport, streetcar
    - land yacht V98.1
    - logging car —*see* Accident, transport, industrial vehicle occupant
    - military vehicle occupant (traffic) V86.34
      - driver V86.04
      - hanger-on V86.24
      - nontraffic V86.94
        - driver V86.54
        - hanger-on V86.74
        - passenger V86.64
      - passenger V86.14
      - while boarding or alighting V86.44
    - mine tram —*see* Accident, transport, industrial vehicle occupant
    - motor vehicle NEC occupant (traffic) V89.2 ⬅
      - ~~driver V86.09~~
      - ~~hanger-on V86.29~~
      - ~~nontraffic V86.99~~
        - ~~driver V86.59~~
        - ~~hanger-on V86.79~~
        - ~~passenger V86.69~~
      - ~~passenger V86.19~~
      - ~~while boarding or alighting V86.49~~
    - motorcoach —*see* Accident, transport, bus occupant
    - motorcyclist V29.9
      - collision (with)
        - animal (traffic) V20.9
          - being ridden (traffic) V26.9
            - nontraffic V26.2
            - while boarding or alighting V26.3
          - nontraffic V20.2
          - while boarding or alighting V20.3

- **Accident** *(Continued)*
  - transport *(Continued)*
    - motorcyclist *(Continued)*
      - collision *(Continued)*
        - animal-drawn vehicle (traffic) V26.9
          - nontraffic V26.2
          - while boarding or alighting V26.3
        - bus (traffic) V24.9
          - nontraffic V24.2
          - while boarding or alighting V24.3
        - car (traffic) V23.9
          - nontraffic V23.2
          - while boarding or alighting V23.3
        - motor vehicle NOS (traffic) V29.60
          - nontraffic V29.20
          - specified type NEC (traffic) V29.69
            - nontraffic V29.29
        - pedal cycle (traffic) V21.9
          - nontraffic V21.2
          - while boarding or alighting V21.3
        - pickup truck (traffic) V23.9
          - nontraffic V23.2
          - while boarding or alighting V23.3
        - railway vehicle (traffic) V25.9
          - nontraffic V25.2
          - while boarding or alighting V25.3
        - specified vehicle NEC (traffic) V26.9
          - nontraffic V26.2
          - while boarding or alighting V26.3
        - stationary object (traffic) V27.9
          - nontraffic V27.2
          - while boarding or alighting V27.3
        - streetcar (traffic) V26.9
          - nontraffic V26.2
          - while boarding or alighting V26.3
        - three wheeled motor vehicle (traffic) V22.9
          - nontraffic V22.2
          - while boarding or alighting V22.3
        - truck (traffic) V24.9
          - nontraffic V24.2
          - while boarding or alighting V24.3
        - two wheeled motor vehicle (traffic) V22.9
          - nontraffic V22.2
          - while boarding or alighting V22.3
        - van (traffic) V23.9
          - nontraffic V23.2
          - while boarding or alighting V23.3
      - driver
        - collision (with)
          - animal (traffic) V20.4
            - being ridden (traffic) V26.4
              - nontraffic V26.0
            - nontraffic V20.0
          - animal-drawn vehicle (traffic) V26.4
            - nontraffic V26.0
          - bus (traffic) V24.4
            - nontraffic V24.0
          - car (traffic) V23.4
            - nontraffic V23.0
          - motor vehicle NOS (traffic) V29.40
            - nontraffic V29.00
            - specified type NEC (traffic) V29.49
              - nontraffic V29.09
          - pedal cycle (traffic) V21.4
            - nontraffic V21.0
          - pickup truck (traffic) V23.4
            - nontraffic V23.0
          - railway vehicle (traffic) V25.4
            - nontraffic V25.0
          - specified vehicle NEC (traffic) V26.4
            - nontraffic V26.0
          - stationary object (traffic) V27.4
            - nontraffic V27.0
          - streetcar (traffic) V26.4
            - nontraffic V26.0
          - three wheeled motor vehicle (traffic) V22.4
            - nontraffic V22.0

A

◄ New ⬅ Revised ~~deleted~~ Deleted

- **Accident** *(Continued)*
  - transport *(Continued)*
    - motorcyclist *(Continued)*
      - driver *(Continued)*
        - collision *(Continued)*
          - truck (traffic) V24.4
            - nontraffic V24.Ø
          - two wheeled motor vehicle (traffic) V22.4
            - nontraffic V22.Ø
          - van (traffic) V23.4
            - nontraffic V23.Ø
        - noncollision accident (traffic) V28.4
          - nontraffic V28.Ø
      - noncollision accident (traffic) V28.9
        - nontraffic V28.2
        - while boarding or alighting V28.3
      - nontraffic V29.3
      - passenger
        - collision (with)
          - animal (traffic) V2Ø.5
            - being ridden (traffic) V26.5
              - nontraffic V26.1
            - nontraffic V2Ø.1
          - animal-drawn vehicle (traffic) V26.5
            - nontraffic V26.1
          - bus (traffic) V24.5
            - nontraffic V24.1
          - car (traffic) V23.5
            - nontraffic V23.1
          - motor vehicle NOS (traffic) V29.5Ø
            - nontraffic V29.1Ø
            - specified type NEC (traffic) V29.59
              - nontraffic V29.19
          - pedal cycle (traffic) V21.5
            - nontraffic V21.1
          - pickup truck (traffic) V23.5
            - nontraffic V23.1
          - railway vehicle (traffic) V25.5
            - nontraffic V25.1
          - specified vehicle NEC (traffic) V26.5
            - nontraffic V26.1
          - stationary object (traffic) V27.5
            - nontraffic V27.1
          - streetcar (traffic) V26.5
            - nontraffic V26.1
          - three wheeled motor vehicle (traffic) V22.5
            - nontraffic V22.1
          - truck (traffic) V24.5
            - nontraffic V24.1
          - two wheeled motor vehicle (traffic) V22.5
            - nontraffic V22.1
          - van (traffic) V23.5
            - nontraffic V23.1
        - noncollision accident (traffic) V28.5
          - nontraffic V28.1
      - specified type NEC V29.88
        - military vehicle V29.81
    - occupant (of)
      - aircraft (powered) V95.9
        - fixed wing
          - commercial —*see* Accident, transport, aircraft, occupant, powered, fixed wing, commercial
          - private —*see* Accident, transport, aircraft, occupant, powered, fixed wing, private
        - nonpowered V96.9
        - specified NEC V95.8
      - airport battery-powered vehicle —*see* Accident, transport, industrial vehicle occupant
      - all-terrain vehicle (ATV) —*see* Accident, transport, all-terrain vehicle occupant

- **Accident** *(Continued)*
  - transport *(Continued)*
    - occupant *(Continued)*
      - animal-drawn vehicle —*see* Accident, transport, animal-drawn vehicle occupant
      - automobile —*see* Accident, transport, car occupant
      - balloon V96.ØØ
      - battery-powered vehicle —*see* Accident, transport, industrial vehicle occupant
      - bicycle —*see* Accident, transport, pedal cyclist
        - motorized —*see* Accident, transport, motorcycle rider
      - boat NEC —*see* Accident, watercraft
      - bulldozer —*see* Accident, transport, construction vehicle occupant
      - bus —*see* Accident, transport, bus occupant
      - cable car (on rails) —*see also* Accident, transport, streetcar occupant
        - not on rails V98.Ø
      - car —*see also* Accident, transport, car occupant
        - cable (on rails) —*see also* Accident, transport, streetcar occupant
          - not on rails V98.Ø
      - coach —*see* Accident, transport, bus occupant
      - coal-car —*see* Accident, transport, industrial vehicle occupant
      - digger —*see* Accident, transport, construction vehicle occupant
      - dump truck —*see* Accident, transport, construction vehicle occupant
      - earth-leveler —*see* Accident, transport, construction vehicle occupant
      - farm machinery (self-propelled) —*see* Accident, transport, agricultural vehicle occupant
      - forklift —*see* Accident, transport, industrial vehicle occupant
      - glider (unpowered) V96.2Ø
        - hang V96.1Ø
        - powered (microlight) (ultralight) —*see* Accident, transport, aircraft, occupant, powered, glider
      - glider (unpowered) NEC V96.2Ø
      - hang-glider V96.1Ø
      - harvester —*see* Accident, transport, agricultural vehicle occupant
      - heavy (transport) vehicle —*see* Accident, transport, truck occupant
      - helicopter —*see* Accident, transport, aircraft, occupant, helicopter
      - ice-yacht V98.2
      - kite (carrying person) V96.8
      - land-yacht V98.1
      - logging car —*see* Accident, transport, industrial vehicle occupant
      - mechanical shovel —*see* Accident, transport, construction vehicle occupant
      - microlight —*see* Accident, transport, aircraft, occupant, powered, glider
      - minibus —*see* Accident, transport, pickup truck occupant (Revised)
      - minivan —*see* Accident, transport, pickup truck occupant (Revised)
      - moped —*see* Accident, transport, motorcycle
      - motor scooter —*see* Accident, transport, motorcycle
      - motorcycle (with sidecar) —*see* Accident, transport, motorcycle
      - pedal cycle —*see also* Accident, transport, pedal cyclist
      - pick-up (truck) —*see* Accident, transport, pickup truck occupant

- **Accident** *(Continued)*
  - transport *(Continued)*
    - occupant *(Continued)*
      - railway (train) (vehicle) (subterranean) (elevated) —*see* Accident, transport, railway vehicle occupant
      - rickshaw —*see* Accident, transport, pedal cycle
        - pedal driven —*see* Accident, transport, pedal cyclist
      - road-roller —*see* Accident, transport, construction vehicle occupant
      - ship NOS V94.9
      - ski-lift (chair) (gondola) V98.3
      - snowmobile —*see* Accident, transport, snowmobile occupant
      - spacecraft, spaceship —*see* Accident, transport, aircraft, occupant, spacecraft
      - sport utility vehicle —*see* Accident, transport, pickup truck occupant (Revised)
      - streetcar (interurban) (operating on public street or highway) —*see* Accident, transport, streetcar occupant
      - SUV —*see* Accident, transport, pickup truck occupant (Revised)
      - téléférique V98.Ø
      - three-wheeled vehicle (motorized) —*see also* Accident, transport, three-wheeled motor vehicle occupant
        - nonmotorized —*see* Accident, transport, pedal cycle
      - tractor (farm) (and trailer) —*see* Accident, transport, agricultural vehicle occupant
      - train —*see* Accident, transport, railway vehicle occupant
      - tram —*see* Accident, transport, streetcar occupant
        - in mine or quarry —*see* Accident, transport, industrial vehicle occupant
      - tricycle —*see* Accident, transport, pedal cycle
        - motorized —*see* Accident, transport, three-wheeled motor vehicle
      - trolley —*see* Accident, transport, streetcar occupant
        - in mine or quarry —*see* Accident, transport, industrial vehicle occupant
      - tub, in mine or quarry —*see* Accident, transport, industrial vehicle occupant
      - ultralight —*see* Accident, transport, aircraft, occupant, powered, glider
      - van —*see* Accident, transport, van occupant
      - vehicle NEC V89.9
        - heavy transport —*see* Accident, transport, truck occupant
        - motor (traffic) NEC V89.2
          - nontraffic NEC V89.Ø
      - watercraft NOS V94.9
        - causing drowning —*see* Drowning, resulting from accident to boat (New)
  - parachutist V97.29
    - after accident to aircraft —*see* Accident, transport, aircraft
    - entangled in object V97.21
    - injured on landing V97.22
  - pedal cyclist V19.9
    - collision (with)
      - animal (traffic) V1Ø.9
        - being ridden (traffic) V16.9
          - nontraffic V16.2
          - while boarding or alighting V16.3
        - nontraffic V1Ø.2
        - while boarding or alighting V1Ø.3

A

Accident *(Continued)*
transport *(Continued)*
pedal cyclist *(Continued)*
collision *(Continued)*
animal-drawn vehicle (traffic) V16.9
nontraffic V16.2
while boarding or alighting V16.3
bus (traffic) V14.9
nontraffic V14.2
while boarding or alighting V14.3
car (traffic) V13.9
nontraffic V13.2
while boarding or alighting V13.3
motor vehicle NOS (traffic) V19.60
nontraffic V19.20
specified type NEC (traffic) V19.69
nontraffic V19.29
pedal cycle (traffic) V11.9
nontraffic V11.2
while boarding or alighting V11.3
pickup truck (traffic) V13.9
nontraffic V13.2
while boarding or alighting V13.3
railway vehicle (traffic) V15.9
nontraffic V15.2
while boarding or alighting V15.3
specified vehicle NEC (traffic) V16.9
nontraffic V16.2
while boarding or alighting V16.3
stationary object (traffic) V17.9
nontraffic V17.2
while boarding or alighting V17.3
streetcar (traffic) V16.9
nontraffic V16.2
while boarding or alighting V16.3
three wheeled motor vehicle (traffic) V12.9
nontraffic V12.2
while boarding or alighting V12.3
truck (traffic) V14.9
nontraffic V14.2
while boarding or alighting V14.3
two wheeled motor vehicle (traffic) V12.9
nontraffic V12.2
while boarding or alighting V12.3
van (traffic) V13.9
nontraffic V13.2
while boarding or alighting V13.3
driver
collision (with)
animal (traffic) V10.4
being ridden (traffic) V16.4
nontraffic V16.0
nontraffic V10.0
animal-drawn vehicle (traffic) V16.4
nontraffic V16.0
bus (traffic) V14.4
nontraffic V14.0
car (traffic) V13.4
nontraffic V13.0
motor vehicle NOS (traffic) V19.40
nontraffic V19.00
specified type NEC (traffic) V19.49
nontraffic V19.09
pedal cycle (traffic) V11.4
nontraffic V11.0
pickup truck (traffic) V13.4
nontraffic V13.0
railway vehicle (traffic) V15.4
nontraffic V15.0
specified vehicle NEC (traffic) V16.4
nontraffic V16.0
stationary object (traffic) V17.4
nontraffic V17.0
streetcar (traffic) V16.4
nontraffic V16.0
three wheeled motor vehicle (traffic) V12.4
nontraffic V12.0

Accident *(Continued)*
transport *(Continued)*
pedal cyclist *(Continued)*
driver *(Continued)*
collision *(Continued)*
truck (traffic) V14.4
nontraffic V14.0
two wheeled motor vehicle (traffic) V12.4
nontraffic V12.0
van (traffic) V13.4
nontraffic V13.0
noncollision accident (traffic) V18.4
nontraffic V18.0
noncollision accident (traffic) V18.9
nontraffic V18.2
while boarding or alighting V18.3
nontraffic V19.3
passenger
collision (with)
animal (traffic) V10.5
being ridden (traffic) V16.5
nontraffic V16.1
nontraffic V10.1
animal-drawn vehicle (traffic) V16.5
nontraffic V16.1
bus (traffic) V14.5
nontraffic V14.1
car (traffic) V13.5
nontraffic V13.1
motor vehicle NOS (traffic) V19.50
nontraffic V19.10
specified type NEC (traffic) V19.59
nontraffic V19.19
pedal cycle (traffic) V11.5
nontraffic V11.1
pickup truck (traffic) V13.5
nontraffic V13.1
railway vehicle (traffic) V15.5
nontraffic V15.1
specified vehicle NEC (traffic) V16.5
nontraffic V16.1
stationary object (traffic) V17.5
nontraffic V17.1
streetcar (traffic) V16.5
nontraffic V16.1
three wheeled motor vehicle (traffic) V12.5
nontraffic V12.1
truck (traffic) V14.5
nontraffic V14.1
two wheeled motor vehicle (traffic) V12.5
nontraffic V12.1
van (traffic) V13.5
nontraffic V13.1
noncollision accident (traffic) V18.5
nontraffic V18.1
specified type NEC V19.88
military vehicle V19.81
pedestrian
conveyance (occupant) V09.9
babystroller V00.828
collision (with) V09.9
animal being ridden or animal drawn vehicle V06.99
nontraffic V06.09
traffic V06.19
bus or heavy transport V04.99
nontraffic V04.09
traffic V04.19
car V03.99
nontraffic V03.09
traffic V03.19
pedal cycle V01.99
nontraffic V01.09
traffic V01.19
pick-up truck or van V03.99
nontraffic V03.09
traffic V03.19

Accident *(Continued)*
transport *(Continued)*
pedestrian *(Continued)*
conveyance *(Continued)*
babystroller *(Continued)*
collision *(Continued)*
railway (train) (vehicle) V05.99
nontraffic V05.09
traffic V05.19
stationary object V00.822
streetcar V06.99
nontraffic V06.09
traffic V06.19
two- or three-wheeled motor vehicle V02.99
nontraffic V02.09
traffic V02.19
vehicle V09.9
animal-drawn V06.99
nontraffic V06.09
traffic V06.19
motor
nontraffic V09.00
traffic V09.20
fall V00.821
nontraffic V09.1
involving motor vehicle NEC V09.00
traffic V09.3
involving motor vehicle NEC V09.20
flat-bottomed NEC V00.388
collision (with) V09.9
animal being ridden or animal drawn vehicle V06.99
nontraffic V06.09
traffic V06.19
bus or heavy transport V04.99
nontraffic V04.09
traffic V04.19
car V03.99
nontraffic V03.09
traffic V03.19
pedal cycle V01.99
nontraffic V01.09
traffic V01.19
pick-up truck or van V03.99
nontraffic V03.09
traffic V03.19
railway (train) (vehicle) V05.99
nontraffic V05.09
traffic V05.19
stationary object V00.382
streetcar V06.99
nontraffic V06.09
traffic V06.19
two-or three-wheeled motor vehicle V02.99
nontraffic V02.09
traffic V02.19
vehicle V09.9
animal-drawn V06.99
nontraffic V06.09
traffic V06.19
motor
nontraffic V09.00
traffic V09.20
fall V00.381
nontraffic V09.1
involving motor vehicle NEC V09.00
snow
board —*see* Accident, transport, pedestrian, conveyance, snow board
ski —*see* Accident, transport, pedestrian, conveyance, skis (snow)
traffic V09.3
involving motor vehicle NEC V09.20

A

Accident *(Continued)*
transport *(Continued)*
pedestrian *(Continued)*
conveyance *(Continued)*
specified type NEC *(Continued)*
collision *(Continued)*
bus or heavy transport V04.99
nontraffic V04.09
traffic V04.19
car V03.99
nontraffic V03.09
traffic V03.19
pedal cycle V01.99
nontraffic V01.09
traffic V01.19
pick-up truck or van V03.99
nontraffic V03.09
traffic V03.19
railway (train) (vehicle) V05.99
nontraffic V05.09
traffic V05.19
stationary object V00.892
streetcar V06.99
nontraffic V06.09
traffic V06.19
two- or three-wheeled motor vehicle V02.99
nontraffic V02.09
traffic V02.19
vehicle V09.9
animal-drawn V06.99
nontraffic V06.09
traffic V06.19
motor
nontraffic V09.00
traffic V09.20
fall V00.891
nontraffic V09.1
involving motor vehicle NEC V09.00
traffic V09.3
involving motor vehicle NEC V09.20
traffic V09.3
involving motor vehicle V09.20
military V09.21
specified type NEC V09.29
wheelchair (powered) V00.818
collision (with) V09.9
animal being ridden or animal drawn vehicle V06.99
nontraffic V06.09
traffic V06.19
bus or heavy transport V04.99
nontraffic V04.09
traffic V04.19
car V03.99
nontraffic V03.09
traffic V03.19
pedal cycle V01.99
nontraffic V01.09
traffic V01.19
pick-up truck or van V03.99
nontraffic V03.09
traffic V03.19
railway (train) (vehicle) V05.99
nontraffic V05.09
traffic V05.19
stationary object V00.812
streetcar V06.99
nontraffic V06.09
traffic V06.19
two- or three-wheeled motor vehicle V02.99
nontraffic V02.09
traffic V02.19

Accident *(Continued)*
transport *(Continued)*
pedestrian *(Continued)*
conveyance *(Continued)*
wheelchair *(Continued)*
collision *(Continued)*
vehicle V09.9
animal-drawn V06.99
nontraffic V06.09
traffic V06.19
motor
nontraffic V09.00
traffic V09.20
fall V00.811
nontraffic V09.1
involving motor vehicle NEC V09.00
traffic V09.3
involving motor vehicle NEC V09.20
wheeled shoe V00.158
colliding with stationary object V00.152
fall V00.151
on foot —*see also* Accident, pedestrian
collision (with)
animal being ridden or animal drawn vehicle V06.90
nontraffic V06.00
traffic V06.10
bus or heavy transport V04.90
nontraffic V04.00
traffic V04.10
car V03.90
nontraffic V03.00
traffic V03.10
pedal cycle V01.90
nontraffic V01.00
traffic V01.10
pick-up truck or van V03.90
nontraffic V03.00
traffic V03.10
railway (train) (vehicle) V05.90
nontraffic V05.00
traffic V05.10
streetcar V06.90
nontraffic V06.00
traffic V06.10
two- or three-wheeled motor vehicle V02.90
nontraffic V02.00
traffic V02.10
vehicle V09.9
animal-drawn V06.90
nontraffic V06.00
traffic V06.10
motor
nontraffic V09.00
traffic V09.20
nontraffic V09.1
involving motor vehicle V09.00
military V09.01
specified type NEC V09.09
traffic V09.3
involving motor vehicle V09.20
military V09.21
specified type NEC V09.29
person NEC (unknown way or transportation) V99
collision (between)
bus (with)
heavy transport vehicle (traffic) V87.5
nontraffic V88.5
car (with)
nontraffic V88.5
bus (traffic) V87.3
nontraffic V88.3
heavy transport vehicle (traffic) V87.4
nontraffic V88.4

Accident *(Continued)*
transport *(Continued)*
person NEC *(Continued)*
collision *(Continued)*
car *(Continued)*
pick-up truck or van (traffic) V87.2
nontraffic V88.2
train or railway vehicle (traffic) V87.6
nontraffic V88.6
two- or three-wheeled motor vehicle (traffic) V87.0
nontraffic V88.0
motor vehicle (traffic) NEC V87.7
nontraffic V88.7
two- or three-wheeled vehicle (with) (traffic)
motor vehicle NEC V87.1
nontraffic V88.1
nonmotor vehicle (collision) (noncollision) (traffic) V87.9
nontraffic V88.9
pickup truck occupant V59.9
collision (with)
animal (traffic) V50.9
being ridden (traffic) V56.9
nontraffic V56.3
while boarding or alighting V56.4
nontraffic V50.3
while boarding or alighting V50.4
animal-drawn vehicle (traffic) V56.9
nontraffic V56.3
while boarding or alighting V56.4
bus (traffic) V54.9
nontraffic V54.3
while boarding or alighting V54.4
car (traffic) V53.9
nontraffic V53.3
while boarding or alighting V53.4
motor vehicle NOS (traffic) V59.60
nontraffic V59.20
specified type NEC (traffic) V59.69
nontraffic V59.29
pedal cycle (traffic) V51.9
nontraffic V51.3
while boarding or alighting V51.4
pickup truck (traffic) V53.9
nontraffic V53.3
while boarding or alighting V53.4
railway vehicle (traffic) V55.9
nontraffic V55.3
while boarding or alighting V55.4
specified vehicle NEC (traffic) V56.9
nontraffic V56.3
while boarding or alighting V56.4
stationary object (traffic) V57.9
nontraffic V57.3
while boarding or alighting V57.4
streetcar (traffic) V56.9
nontraffic V56.3
while boarding or alighting V56.4
three wheeled motor vehicle (traffic) V52.9
nontraffic V52.3
while boarding or alighting V52.4
truck (traffic) V54.9
nontraffic V54.3
while boarding or alighting V54.4
two wheeled motor vehicle (traffic) V52.9
nontraffic V52.3
while boarding or alighting V52.4
van (traffic) V53.9
nontraffic V53.3
while boarding or alighting V53.4
driver
collision (with)
animal (traffic) V50.5
being ridden (traffic) V56.5
nontraffic V56.0
nontraffic V50.0

A

A

A

◀ New ⟸ Revised ~~deleted~~ Deleted

Accident *(Continued)*
transport *(Continued)*
truck occupant *(Continued)*
driver *(Continued)*
collision *(Continued)*
pedal cycle (traffic) V61.5
nontraffic V61.0
pickup truck (traffic) V63.5
nontraffic V63.0
railway vehicle (traffic) V65.5
nontraffic V65.0
specified vehicle NEC (traffic) V66.5
nontraffic V66.0
stationary object (traffic) V67.5
nontraffic V67.0
streetcar (traffic) V66.5
nontraffic V66.0
three wheeled motor vehicle (traffic) V62.5
nontraffic V62.0
truck (traffic) V64.5
nontraffic V64.0
two wheeled motor vehicle (traffic) V62.5
nontraffic V62.0
van (traffic) V63.5
nontraffic V63.0
noncollision accident (traffic) V68.5
nontraffic V68.0
dump —*see* Accident, transport, construction vehicle occupant
hanger-on
collision (with)
animal (traffic) V60.7
being ridden (traffic) V66.7
nontraffic V66.2
nontraffic V60.2
animal-drawn vehicle (traffic) V66.7
nontraffic V66.2
bus (traffic) V64.7
nontraffic V64.2
car (traffic) V63.7
nontraffic V63.2
pedal cycle (traffic) V61.7
nontraffic V61.2
pickup truck (traffic) V63.7
nontraffic V63.2
railway vehicle (traffic) V65.7
nontraffic V65.2
specified vehicle NEC (traffic) V66.7
nontraffic V66.2
stationary object (traffic) V67.7
nontraffic V67.2
streetcar (traffic) V66.7
nontraffic V66.2
three wheeled motor vehicle (traffic) V62.7
nontraffic V62.2
truck (traffic) V64.7
nontraffic V64.2
two wheeled motor vehicle (traffic) V62.7
nontraffic V62.2
van (traffic) V63.7
nontraffic V63.2
noncollision accident (traffic) V68.7
nontraffic V68.2
noncollision accident (traffic) V68.9
nontraffic V68.3
while boarding or alighting V68.4
nontraffic V69.3
passenger
collision (with)
animal (traffic) V60.6
being ridden (traffic) V66.6
nontraffic V66.1
nontraffic V60.1
animal-drawn vehicle (traffic) V66.6
nontraffic V66.1
bus (traffic) V64.6
nontraffic V64.1

Accident *(Continued)*
transport *(Continued)*
truck occupant *(Continued)*
passenger *(Continued)*
collision *(Continued)*
car (traffic) V63.6
nontraffic V63.1
motor vehicle NOS (traffic) V69.50
nontraffic V69.10
specified type NEC (traffic) V69.59
nontraffic V69.19
pedal cycle (traffic) V61.6
nontraffic V61.1
pickup truck (traffic) V63.6
nontraffic V63.1
railway vehicle (traffic) V65.6
nontraffic V65.1
specified vehicle NEC (traffic) V66.6
nontraffic V66.1
stationary object (traffic) V67.6
nontraffic V67.1
streetcar (traffic) V66.6
nontraffic V66.1
three wheeled motor vehicle (traffic) V62.6
nontraffic V62.1
truck (traffic) V64.6
nontraffic V64.1
two wheeled motor vehicle (traffic) V62.6
nontraffic V62.1
van (traffic) V63.6
nontraffic V63.1
noncollision accident (traffic) V68.6
nontraffic V68.1
pickup —*see* Accident, transport, pickup truck occupant
specified type NEC V69.88
military vehicle V69.81
van occupant V59.9
collision (with)
animal (traffic) V50.9
being ridden (traffic) V56.9
nontraffic V56.3
while boarding or alighting V56.4
nontraffic V50.3
while boarding or alighting V50.4
animal-drawn vehicle (traffic) V56.9
nontraffic V56.3
while boarding or alighting V56.4
bus (traffic) V54.9
nontraffic V54.3
while boarding or alighting V54.4
car (traffic) V53.9
nontraffic V53.3
while boarding or alighting V53.4
motor vehicle NOS (traffic) V59.60
nontraffic V59.20
specified type NEC (traffic) V59.69
nontraffic V59.29
pedal cycle (traffic) V51.9
nontraffic V51.3
while boarding or alighting V51.4
pickup truck (traffic) V53.9
nontraffic V53.3
while boarding or alighting V53.4
railway vehicle (traffic) V55.9
nontraffic V55.3
while boarding or alighting V55.4
specified vehicle NEC (traffic) V56.9
nontraffic V56.3
while boarding or alighting V56.4
stationary object (traffic) V57.9
nontraffic V57.3
while boarding or alighting V57.4
streetcar (traffic) V56.9
nontraffic V56.3
while boarding or alighting V56.4

Accident *(Continued)*
transport *(Continued)*
van occupant *(Continued)*
collision *(Continued)*
three wheeled motor vehicle (traffic) V52.9
nontraffic V52.3
while boarding or alighting V52.4
truck (traffic) V54.9
nontraffic V54.3
while boarding or alighting V54.4
two wheeled motor vehicle (traffic) V52.9
nontraffic V52.3
while boarding or alighting V52.4
van (traffic) V53.9
nontraffic V53.3
while boarding or alighting V53.4
driver
collision (with)
animal (traffic) V50.5
being ridden (traffic) V56.5
nontraffic V56.0
nontraffic V50.0
animal-drawn vehicle (traffic) V56.5
nontraffic V56.0
bus (traffic) V54.5
nontraffic V54.0
car (traffic) V53.5
nontraffic V53.0
motor vehicle NOS (traffic) V59.40
nontraffic V59.00
specified type NEC (traffic) V59.49
nontraffic V59.09
pedal cycle (traffic) V51.5
nontraffic V51.0
pickup truck (traffic) V53.5
nontraffic V53.0
railway vehicle (traffic) V55.5
nontraffic V55.0
specified vehicle NEC (traffic) V56.5
nontraffic V56.0
stationary object (traffic) V57.5
nontraffic V57.0
streetcar (traffic) V56.5
nontraffic V56.0
three wheeled motor vehicle (traffic) V52.5
nontraffic V52.0
truck (traffic) V54.5
nontraffic V54.0
two wheeled motor vehicle (traffic) V52.5
nontraffic V52.0
van (traffic) V53.5
nontraffic V53.0
noncollision accident (traffic) V58.5
nontraffic V58.0
hanger-on
collision (with)
animal (traffic) V50.7
being ridden (traffic) V56.7
nontraffic V56.2
nontraffic V50.2
animal-drawn vehicle (traffic) V56.7
nontraffic V56.2
bus (traffic) V54.7
nontraffic V54.2
car (traffic) V53.7
nontraffic V53.2
pedal cycle (traffic) V51.7
nontraffic V51.2
pickup truck (traffic) V53.7
nontraffic V53.2
railway vehicle (traffic) V55.7
nontraffic V55.2
specified vehicle NEC (traffic) V56.7
nontraffic V56.2
stationary object (traffic) V57.7
nontraffic V57.2

A

Accident *(Continued)*
transport *(Continued)*
van occupant *(Continued)*
hanger-on *(Continued)*
collision *(Continued)*
streetcar (traffic) V56.7
nontraffic V56.2
three wheeled motor vehicle (traffic) V52.7
nontraffic V52.2
truck (traffic) V54.7
nontraffic V54.2
two wheeled motor vehicle (traffic) V52.7
nontraffic V52.2
van (traffic) V53.7
nontraffic V53.2
noncollision accident (traffic) V58.7
nontraffic V58.2
noncollision accident (traffic) V58.9
nontraffic V58.3
while boarding or alighting V58.4
nontraffic V59.3
passenger
collision (with)
animal (traffic) V50.6
being ridden (traffic) V56.6
nontraffic V56.1
nontraffic V50.1
animal-drawn vehicle (traffic) V56.6
nontraffic V56.1
bus (traffic) V54.6
nontraffic V54.1
car (traffic) V53.6
nontraffic V53.1
motor vehicle NOS (traffic) V59.50
nontraffic V59.10
specified type NEC (traffic) V59.59
nontraffic V59.19
pedal cycle (traffic) V51.6
nontraffic V51.1
pickup truck (traffic) V53.6
nontraffic V53.1
railway vehicle (traffic) V55.6
nontraffic V55.1
specified vehicle NEC (traffic) V56.6
nontraffic V56.1
stationary object (traffic) V57.6
nontraffic V57.1
streetcar (traffic) V56.6
nontraffic V56.1
three wheeled motor vehicle (traffic) V52.6
nontraffic V52.1
truck (traffic) V54.6
nontraffic V54.1
two wheeled motor vehicle (traffic) V52.6
nontraffic V52.1
van (traffic) V53.6
nontraffic V53.1
noncollision accident (traffic) V58.6
nontraffic V58.1
specified type NEC V59.88
military vehicle V59.81
watercraft occupant —*see* Accident, watercraft
vehicle NEC V89.9
animal-drawn NEC —*see* Accident, transport, animal-drawn vehicle occupant
special
agricultural —*see* Accident, transport, agricultural vehicle occupant
construction —*see* Accident, transport, construction vehicle occupant
industrial —*see* Accident, transport, industrial vehicle occupant
three-wheeled NEC (motorized) —*see* Accident, transport, three-wheeled motor vehicle occupant

Accident *(Continued)*
watercraft V94.9
causing
drowning —*see* Drowning, due to, accident to, watercraft ◀
injury NEC V91.89
crushed between craft and object V91.19
powered craft V91.13
ferry boat V91.11
fishing boat V91.12
jetskis V91.13
liner V91.11
merchant ship V91.10
passenger ship V91.11
unpowered craft V91.18
canoe V91.15
inflatable V91.16
kayak V91.15
sailboat V91.14
surf-board V91.18
windsurfer V91.18
fall on board V91.29
powered craft V91.23
ferry boat V91.21
fishing boat V91.22
jetskis V91.23
liner V91.21
merchant ship V91.20
passenger ship V91.21
unpowered craft
canoe V91.25
inflatable V91.26
kayak V91.25
sailboat V91.24
fire on board causing burn V91.09
powered craft V91.03
ferry boat V91.01
fishing boat V91.02
jetskis V91.03
liner V91.01
merchant ship V91.00
passenger ship V91.01
unpowered craft V91.08
canoe V91.05
inflatable V91.06
kayak V91.05
sailboat V91.04
surf-board V91.08
water skis V91.07
windsurfer V91.08
hit by falling object V91.39
powered craft V91.33
ferry boat V91.31
fishing boat V91.32
jetskis V91.33
liner V91.31
merchant ship V91.30
passenger ship V91.31
unpowered craft V91.38
canoe V91.35
inflatable V91.36
kayak V91.35
sailboat V91.34
surf-board V91.38
water skis V91.37
windsurfer V91.38
specified type NEC V91.89
powered craft V91.83
ferry boat V91.81
fishing boat V91.82
jetskis V91.83
liner V91.81
merchant ship V91.80
passenger ship V91.81
unpowered craft V91.88
canoe V91.85
inflatable V91.86
kayak V91.85
sailboat V91.84
surf-board V91.88

Accident *(Continued)*
watercraft *(Continued)*
causing *(Continued)*
injury NEC *(Continued)*
specified type NEC *(Continued)*
unpowered craft *(Continued)*
water skis V91.87
windsurfer V91.88
due to, caused by cataclysm —*see* Forces of nature, by type
military NEC V94.818
with civilian watercraft V94.810
civilian in water injured by V94.811
nonpowered, struck by
nonpowered vessel V94.22
powered vessel V94.21
specified type NEC V94.89
striking swimmer
powered V94.11
unpowered V94.12
Acid throwing (assault) Y08.89
Activity (involving) (of victim at time of event) Y93.9
aerobic and step exercise (class) Y93.A3
alpine skiing Y93.23
animal care NEC Y93.K9
arts and handcrafts NEC Y93.D9
athletics NEC Y93.79
athletics played as a team or group NEC Y93.69
athletics played individually NEC Y93.59
baking Y93.G3
ballet Y93.41
barbells Y93.B3
BASE (Building, Antenna, Span, Earth) jumping Y93.33
baseball Y93.64
basketball Y93.67
bathing (personal) Y93.E1
beach volleyball Y93.68
bike riding Y93.55
blackout game Y93.85 ◀
boogie boarding Y93.18
bowling Y93.54
boxing Y93.71
brass instrument playing Y93.J4
building construction Y93.H3
bungee jumping Y93.34
calisthenics Y93.A2
canoeing (in calm and turbulent water) Y93.16
capture the flag Y93.6A
cardiorespiratory exercise NEC Y93.A9
caregiving (providing) NEC Y93.F9
bathing Y93.F1
lifting Y93.F2
cellular
communication device Y93.C2
telephone Y93.C2
challenge course Y93.A5
cheerleading Y93.45
choking game Y93.85 ◀
circuit training Y93.A4
cleaning
floor Y93.E5
climbing NEC Y93.39
mountain Y93.31
rock Y93.31
wall Y93.31
clothing care and maintenance NEC Y93.E9
combatives Y93.75
computer
keyboarding Y93.C1
technology NEC Y93.C9
confidence course Y93.A5
construction (building) Y93.H3
cooking and baking Y93.G3
cool down exercises Y93.A2
cricket Y93.69
crocheting Y93.D1
cross country skiing Y93.24
dancing (all types) Y93.41

Activity *(Continued)*
digging
dirt Y93.H1
dirt digging Y93.H1
dishwashing Y93.G1
diving (platform) (springboard) Y93.12
underwater Y93.15
dodge ball Y93.6A
downhill skiing Y93.23
drum playing Y93.J2
dumbbells Y93.B3
electronic
devices NEC Y93.C9
hand held interactive Y93.C2
game playing (using) (with)
interactive device Y93.C2
keyboard or other stationary device Y93.C1
elliptical machine Y93.A1
exercise (s)
machines ((primarily) for)
cardiorespiratory conditioning Y93.A1
muscle strengthening Y93.B1
muscle strengthening (non-machine) NEC Y93.B9
external motion NEC Y93.I9
rollercoaster Y93.I1
fainting game Y93.85 ◀
field hockey Y93.65
figure skating (pairs) (singles) Y93.21
flag football Y93.62
floor mopping and cleaning Y93.E5
food preparation and clean up Y93.G1
football (American) NOS Y93.61
flag Y93.62
tackle Y93.61
touch Y93.62
four square Y93.6A
free weights Y93.B3
frisbee (ultimate) Y93.74
furniture
building Y93.D3
finishing Y93.D3
repair Y93.D3
game playing (electronic)
using interactive device Y93.C2
using keyboard or other stationary device Y93.C1
gardening Y93.H2
golf Y93.53
grass drills Y93.A6
grilling and smoking food Y93.G2
grooming and shearing an animal Y93.K3
guerilla drills Y93.A6
gymnastics (rhythmic) Y93.43
hand held interactive electronic device Y93.C2
handball Y93.73
handcrafts NEC Y93.D9
hang gliding Y93.35
hiking (on level or elevated terrain) Y93.Ø1
hockey (ice) Y93.22
field Y93.65
horseback riding Y93.52
household (interior) maintenance NEC Y93.E9
ice NEC Y93.29
dancing Y93.21
hockey Y93.22
skating Y93.21
inline roller skating Y93.51
ironing Y93.E4
judo Y93.75
jumping (off) NEC Y93.39
BASE (Building, Antenna, Span, Earth) Y93.33
bungee Y93.34
jacks Y93.A2
rope Y93.56
jumping jacks Y93.A2
jumping rope Y93.56
karate Y93.75

Activity *(Continued)*
kayaking (in calm and turbulent water) Y93.16
keyboarding (computer) Y93.C1
kickball Y93.6A
knitting Y93.D1
lacrosse Y93.65
land maintenance NEC Y93.H9
landscaping Y93.H2
laundry Y93.E2
machines (exercise)
primarily for cardiorespiratory conditioning Y93.A1
primarily for muscle strengthening Y93.B1
maintenance
exterior building NEC Y93.H9
household (interior) NEC Y93.E9
land Y93.H9
property Y93.H9
marching (on level or elevated terrain) Y93.Ø1
martial arts Y93.75
microwave oven Y93.G3
milking an animal Y93.K2
mopping (floor) Y93.E5
mountain climbing Y93.31
muscle strengthening
exercises (non-machine) NEC Y93.B9
machines Y93.B1
musical keyboard (electronic) playing Y93.J1
nordic skiing Y93.24
obstacle course Y93.A5
oven (microwave) Y93.G3
packing up and unpacking in moving to a new residence Y93.E6
parasailing Y93.19
pass out game Y93.85 ◀
percussion instrument playing NEC Y93.J2
personal
bathing and showering Y93.E1
hygiene NEC Y93.E8
showering Y93.E1
physical games generally associated with school recess, summer camp and children Y93.6A
physical training NEC Y93.A9
piano playing Y93.J1
pilates Y93.B4
platform diving Y93.12
playing musical instrument
brass instrument Y93.J4
drum Y93.J2
musical keyboard (electronic) Y93.J1
percussion instrument NEC Y93.J2
piano Y93.J1
string instrument Y93.J3
winds instrument Y93.J4
property maintenance
exterior NEC Y93.H9
interior NEC Y93.E9
pruning (garden and lawn) Y93.H2
pull-ups Y93.B2
push-ups Y93.B2
racquetball Y93.73
rafting (in calm and turbulent water) Y93.16
raking (leaves) Y93.H1
rappelling Y93.32
refereeing a sports activity Y93.81
residential relocation Y93.E6
rhythmic gymnastics Y93.43
rhythmic movement NEC Y93.49
riding
horseback Y93.52
rollercoaster Y93.I1
rock climbing Y93.31
roller skating (inline) Y93.51
rollercoaster riding Y93.I1
rough housing and horseplay Y93.83
rowing (in calm and turbulent water) Y93.16
rugby Y93.63
SCUBA diving Y93.15
sewing Y93.D2

Activity *(Continued)*
shoveling Y93.H1
dirt Y93.H1
snow Y93.H1
showering (personal) Y93.E1
sit-ups Y93.B2
skateboarding Y93.51
skating (ice) Y93.21
roller Y93.51
skiing (alpine) (downhill) Y93.23
cross country Y93.24
nordic Y93.24
water Y93.17
sledding (snow) Y93.23
sleeping (sleep) Y93.84
smoking and grilling food Y93.G2
snorkeling Y93.15
snow NEC Y93.29
boarding Y93.23
shoveling Y93.H1
sledding Y93.23
tubing Y93.23
soccer Y93.66
softball Y93.64
specified NEC Y93.89
spectator at an event Y93.82
sports NEC Y93.79
sports played as a team or group NEC Y93.69
sports played individually NEC Y93.59
springboard diving Y93.12
squash Y93.73
stationary bike Y93.A1
step (stepping) exercise (class) Y93.A3
stepper machine Y93.A1
stove Y93.G3
string instrument playing Y93.J3
surfing Y93.18
wind Y93.18
swimming Y93.11
tackle football Y93.61
tap dancing Y93.41
tennis Y93.73
tobogganing Y93.23
touch football Y93.62
track and field events (non-running) Y93.57
running Y93.Ø2
trampoline Y93.44
treadmill Y93.A1
trimming shrubs Y93.H2
tubing (in calm and turbulent water) Y93.16
snow Y93.23
ultimate frisbee Y93.74
underwater diving Y93.15
unpacking in moving to a new residence Y93.E6
use of stove, oven and microwave oven Y93.G3
vacuuming Y93.E3
volleyball (beach) (court) Y93.68
wake boarding Y93.17
walking (on level or elevated terrain) Y93.Ø1
an animal Y93.K1
walking an animal Y93.K1
wall climbing Y93.31
warm up and cool down exercises Y93.A2
water NEC Y93.19
aerobics Y93.14
craft NEC Y93.19
exercise Y93.14
polo Y93.13
skiing Y93.17
sliding Y93.18
survival training and testing Y93.19
weeding (garden and lawn) Y93.H2
wind instrument playing Y93.J4
windsurfing Y93.18
wrestling Y93.72
yoga Y93.42
Adverse effect of drugs —*see* Table of Drugs and Chemicals

A

Aerosinusitis —*see* Air, pressure
After-effect, late —*see* Sequelae
Air
- blast in war operations —*see* War operations, air blast
- pressure
  - change, rapid
    - during
      - ascent W94.29
        - while (in) (surfacing from)
          - aircraft W94.23
          - deep water diving W94.21
          - underground W94.22
      - descent W94.39
        - in
          - aircraft W94.31
          - water W94.32
  - high, prolonged W94.Ø
  - low, prolonged W94.12
    - due to residence or long visit at high altitude W94.11

Alpine sickness W94.11
Altitude sickness W94.11
Anaphylactic shock, anaphylaxis —*see* Table of Drugs and Chemicals ⬅
Andes disease W94.11
Arachnidism, arachnoidism X58
Arson (with intent to injure or kill) X97
Asphyxia, asphyxiation
- by
  - food (bone) (seed) —*see* categories T17 and T18
  - gas —*see also* Table of Drugs and Chemicals ⬅
    - legal
      - execution —*see* Legal, intervention, gas
      - intervention —*see* Legal, intervention, gas
- from
  - fire —*see also* Exposure, fire
    - in war operations —*see* War operations, fire
  - ignition —*see* Ignition
  - vomitus T17.81
- in war operations —*see* War operations, restriction of airway

Aspiration
- food (any type) (into respiratory tract) (with asphyxia, obstruction respiratory tract, suffocation) —*see* categories T17 and T18
- foreign body —*see* Foreign body, aspiration
- vomitus (with asphyxia, obstruction respiratory tract, suffocation) T17.81

Assassination (attempt) —*see* Assault
Assault (homicidal) (by) (in) YØ9
- arson X97
- bite (of human being) YØ4.1
- bodily force YØ4.8
  - bite YØ4.1
  - bumping into YØ4.2
  - sexual —*see* subcategories T74.Ø, T76.Ø
  - unarmed fight YØ4.Ø

Assault *(Continued)*
- bomb X96.9
  - antipersonnel X96.Ø
  - fertilizer X96.3
  - gasoline X96.1
  - letter X96.2
  - petrol X96.1
  - pipe X96.3
  - specified NEC X96.8
- brawl (hand) (fists) (foot) (unarmed) YØ4.Ø
- burning, burns (by fire) NEC X97
  - acid YØ8.89
  - caustic, corrosive substance YØ8.89
  - chemical from swallowing caustic, corrosive substance —*see* Table of Drugs and Chemicals ⬅
  - cigarette(s) X97
  - hot object X98.9
    - fluid NEC X98.2
    - household appliance X98.3
    - specified NEC X98.8
    - steam X98.Ø
    - tap water X98.1
    - vapors X98.Ø
  - scalding —*see* Assault, burning
  - steam X98.Ø
  - vitriol YØ8.89
- caustic, corrosive substance (gas) YØ8.89
- crashing of
  - aircraft YØ8.81
  - motor vehicle YØ3.8
    - pushed in front of YØ2.Ø
    - run over YØ3.Ø
    - specified NEC YØ3.8
- cutting or piercing instrument X99.9
  - dagger X99.2
  - glass X99.Ø
  - knife X99.1
  - specified NEC X99.8
  - sword X99.2
- dagger X99.2
- drowning (in) X92.9
  - bathtub X92.Ø
  - natural water X92.3
  - specified NEC X92.8
  - swimming pool X92.1
    - following fall X92.2
- dynamite X96.8
- explosive (s) (material) X96.9
- fight (hand) (fists) (foot) (unarmed) YØ4.Ø
  - with weapon —*see* Assault, by type of weapon
- fire X97
- firearm X95.9
  - airgun X95.Ø1
  - handgun X93
  - hunting rifle X94.1
  - larger X94.9
    - specified NEC X94.8
  - machine gun X94.2
  - shotgun X94.Ø
  - specified NEC X95.8

Assault *(Continued)*
- from high place YØ1
- gunshot (wound) NEC —*see* Assault, firearm, by type
- incendiary device X97
- injury YØ9
  - to child due to criminal abortion attempt NEC YØ8.89
- knife X99.1
- late effect of —*see* X92-YØ8 with 7th character S
- placing before moving object NEC YØ2.8
  - motor vehicle YØ2.Ø
- poisoning —*see* categories T36-T65 with 7th character S
- puncture, any part of body —*see* Assault, cutting or piercing instrument
- pushing
  - before moving object NEC YØ2.8
    - motor vehicle YØ2.Ø
    - subway train YØ2.1
    - train YØ2.1
- rape T74.2-
- scalding —*see* Assault, burning
- sequelae of —*see* X92-YØ8 with 7th character S
- sexual (by bodily force) T74.2-
- shooting —*see* Assault, firearm
- specified means NEC YØ8.89
- stab, any part of body —*see* Assault, cutting or piercing instrument
- steam X98.Ø
- striking against
  - other person YØ4.2
  - sports equipment YØ8.Ø9
    - baseball bat YØ8.Ø2
    - hockey stick YØ8.Ø1
- struck by
  - sports equipment YØ8.Ø9
    - baseball bat YØ8.Ø2
    - hockey stick YØ8.Ø1
- submersion —*see* Assault, drowning
- violence YØ9
- weapon YØ9
  - blunt YØØ
  - cutting or piercing —*see* Assault, cutting or piercing instrument
  - firearm —*see* Assault, firearm
- wound YØ9
  - cutting —*see* Assault, cutting or piercing instrument
  - gunshot —*see* Assault, firearm
  - knife X99.1
  - piercing —*see* Assault, cutting or piercing instrument
  - puncture —*see* Assault, cutting or piercing instrument
  - stab —*see* Assault, cutting or piercing instrument

Attack by mammals NEC W55.89
Avalanche —*see* Landslide ◀
Aviator's disease —*see* Air, pressure

A

B

- **Barotitis, barodontalgia, barosinusitis, barotrauma** (otitic) (sinus) —*see* Air, pressure
- **Battered** (baby) (child) (person) (syndrome) X58
- **Bayonet wound** W26.1
  - in
    - legal intervention —*see* Legal, intervention, sharp object, bayonet
    - war operations —*see* War operations, combat
  - stated as undetermined whether accidental or intentional Y28.8
  - suicide (attempt) X78.2
- **Bean in nose** —*see* categories T17 and T18
- **Bed set on fire NEC** —*see* Exposure, fire, uncontrolled, building, bed
- **Beheading** (by guillotine)
  - homicide X99.9
  - legal execution —*see* Legal, intervention
- **Bending, injury in** (prolonged) (static) X50.1 ⬅
- **Bends** —*see* Air, pressure, change
- **Bite, bitten by**
  - alligator W58.01
  - arthropod (nonvenomous) NEC W57
  - bull W55.21
  - cat W55.01
  - cow W55.21
  - crocodile W58.11
  - dog W54.0
  - goat W55.31
  - hoof stock NEC W55.31
  - horse W55.11
  - human being (accidentally) W50.3
    - with intent to injure or kill Y04.1
    - as, or caused by, a crowd or human stampede (with fall) W52
    - assault Y04.1
    - homicide (attempt) Y04.1
    - in
      - fight Y04.1
  - insect (nonvenomous) W57
  - lizard (nonvenomous) W59.01
  - mammal NEC W55.81
    - marine W56.31 ◀
  - marine animal (nonvenomous) W56.81
  - millipede W57
  - moray eel W56.51
  - mouse W53.01
  - person (s) (accidentally) W50.3
    - with intent to injure or kill Y04.1
    - as, or caused by, a crowd or human stampede (with fall) W52
    - assault Y04.1
    - homicide (attempt) Y04.1
    - in
      - fight Y04.1
  - pig W55.41
  - raccoon W55.51
  - rat W53.11
  - reptile W59.81
    - lizard W59.01
    - snake W59.11
    - turtle W59.21
      - terrestrial W59.81
  - rodent W53.81
    - mouse W53.01
    - rat W53.11
    - specified NEC W53.81
    - squirrel W53.21
  - shark W56.41
  - sheep W55.31
  - snake (nonvenomous) W59.11
  - spider (nonvenomous) W57
  - squirrel W53.21
- **Blast** (air) **in war operations** —*see* War operations, blast
- **Blizzard** X37.2
- **Blood alcohol level** Y90.9
  - 20-39mg/100ml Y90.1
  - 40-59mg/100ml Y90.2
  - 60-79mg/100ml Y90.3
  - 80-99mg/100ml Y90.4
  - 100-119mg/100ml Y90.5
  - 120-199mg/100ml Y90.6
  - 200-239mg/100ml Y90.7
  - less than 20mg/100ml Y90.0
  - presence in blood, level not specified Y90.9
- **Blow** X58
  - by law-enforcing agent, police (on duty) —*see* Legal, intervention, manhandling
    - blunt object —*see* Legal, intervention, blunt object
- **Blowing up** —*see* Explosion
- **Brawl** (hand) (fists) (foot) Y04.0
- **Breakage** (accidental) (part of)
  - ladder (causing fall) W11
  - scaffolding (causing fall) W12
- **Broken**
  - glass, contact with —*see* Contact, with, glass
  - power line (causing electric shock) W85
- **Bumping against, into** (accidentally)
  - object NEC W22.8
    - with fall —*see* Fall, due to, bumping against, object
    - caused by crowd or human stampede (with fall) W52
    - sports equipment W21.9
  - person (s) W51
    - with fall W03
      - due to ice or snow W00.0
    - assault Y04.2
    - caused by, a crowd or human stampede (with fall) W52
    - homicide (attempt) Y04.2
  - sports equipment W21.9
- **Burn, burned, burning** (accidental) (by) (from) (on)
  - acid NEC —*see* Table of Drugs and Chemicals ⬅
  - bed linen —*see* Exposure, fire, uncontrolled, in building, bed
  - blowtorch X08.8
    - with ignition of clothing NEC X06.2
      - nightwear X05
  - bonfire, campfire (controlled) —*see also* Exposure, fire, controlled, not in building
    - uncontrolled —*see* Exposure, fire, uncontrolled, not in building
  - candle X08.8
    - with ignition of clothing NEC X06.2
      - nightwear X05
  - caustic liquid, substance (external) (internal) NEC —*see* Table of Drugs and Chemicals ⬅
  - chemical (external) (internal) —*see also* Table of Drugs and Chemicals ⬅
    - in war operations —*see* War operations, fire
  - cigar (s) or cigarette (s) X08.8
    - with ignition of clothing NEC X06.2
      - nightwear X05
  - clothes, clothing NEC (from controlled fire) X06.2
    - with conflagration —*see* Exposure, fire, uncontrolled, building
      - not in building or structure —*see* Exposure, fire, uncontrolled, not in building
  - cooker (hot) X15.8
    - stated as undetermined whether accidental or intentional Y27.3
    - suicide (attempt) X77.3
  - electric blanket X16
  - engine (hot) X17
  - fire, flames —*see* Exposure, fire
  - flare, Very pistol —*see* Discharge, firearm NEC

Burn, burned, burning *(Continued)*

- heat
  - from appliance (electrical) (household) X15.8
    - cooker X15.8
    - hotplate X15.2
    - kettle X15.8
    - light bulb X15.8
    - saucepan X15.3
    - skillet X15.3
    - stated as undetermined whether accidental or intentional Y27.3
    - stove X15.0
    - suicide (attempt) X77.3
    - toaster X15.1
  - in local application or packing during medical or surgical procedure Y63.5
- heating
  - appliance, radiator or pipe X16
- homicide (attempt) —*see* Assault, burning
- hot
  - air X14.1
  - cooker X15.8
  - drink X10.0
  - engine X17
  - fat X10.2
  - fluid NEC X12
  - food X10.1
  - gases X14.1
  - heating appliance X16
  - household appliance NEC X15.8
  - kettle X15.8
  - liquid NEC X12
  - machinery X17
  - metal (molten) (liquid) NEC X18
  - object (not producing fire or flames) NEC X19
  - oil (cooking) X10.2
  - pipe (s) X16
  - radiator X16
  - saucepan (glass) (metal) X15.3
  - stove (kitchen) X15.0
  - substance NEC X19
    - caustic or corrosive NEC —*see* Table of Drugs and Chemicals ⬅
  - toaster X15.1
  - tool X17
  - vapor X13.1
  - water (tap) —*see* Contact, with, hot, tap water
- hotplate X15.2
  - suicide (attempt) X77.3
- ignition —*see* Ignition
- in war operations —*see* War operations, fire
- inflicted by other person X97
  - by hot objects, hot vapor, and steam —*see* Assault, burning, hot object
- internal, from swallowed caustic, corrosive liquid, substance —*see* Table of Drugs and Chemicals ⬅
- iron (hot) X15.8
  - stated as undetermined whether accidental or intentional Y27.3
  - suicide (attempt) X77.3
- kettle (hot) X15.8
  - stated as undetermined whether accidental or intentional Y27.3
  - suicide (attempt) X77.3
- lamp (flame) X08.8
  - with ignition of clothing NEC X06.2
    - nightwear X05
- lighter (cigar) (cigarette) X08.8
  - with ignition of clothing NEC X06.2
    - nightwear X05
- lightning —*see* subcategory T75.0
  - causing fire —*see* Exposure, fire
- liquid (boiling) (hot) NEC X12
  - stated as undetermined whether accidental or intentional Y27.2
  - suicide (attempt) X77.2

B

C

Caisson disease —*see* Air, pressure, change
Campfire (exposure to) (controlled) —*see also* Exposure, fire, controlled, not in building
  uncontrolled —*see* Exposure, fire, uncontrolled, not in building
Capital punishment (any means) —*see* Legal, intervention
Car sickness T75.3
Casualty (not due to war) NEC X58
  war —*see* War operations
Cat
  bite W55.Ø1
  scratch W55.Ø3
Cataclysm, cataclysmic (any injury) NEC —*see* Forces of nature
Catching fire —*see* Exposure, fire
Caught
  between
    folding object W23.Ø
    objects (moving) (stationary and moving) W23.Ø
      and machinery —*see* Contact, with, by type of machine
      stationary W23.1
    sliding door and door frame W23.Ø
  by, in
    machinery (moving parts of) —*see* Contact, with, by type of machine
    washing-machine wringer W23.Ø
  under packing crate (due to losing grip) W23.1
Cave-in caused by cataclysmic earth surface movement or eruption —*see* Landslide
Change(s) in air pressure —*see* Air, pressure, change
Choked, choking (on) (any object except food or vomitus)
  food (bone) (seed) —*see* categories T17 and T18
  vomitus T17.81-
Civil insurrection —*see* War operations
Cloudburst (any injury) X37.8
Cold, exposure to (accidental) (excessive) (extreme) (natural) (place) **NEC** —*see* Exposure, cold
Collapse
  building W2Ø.1
    burning (uncontrolled fire) XØØ.2
  dam or man-made structure (causing earth movement) X36.Ø
  machinery —*see* Contact, with, by type of machine
  structure W2Ø.1
    burning (uncontrolled fire) XØØ.2
Collision (accidental) **NEC** —*see also* Accident, transport V89.9
  pedestrian W51
    with fall WØ3
      due to ice or snow WØØ.Ø
      involving pedestrian conveyance —*see* Accident, transport, pedestrian, conveyance
    and
      crowd or human stampede (with fall) W52
      object W22.8
        with fall —*see* Fall, due to, bumping against, object
  person (s) —*see* Collision, pedestrian
  transport vehicle NEC V89.9
    and
      avalanche, fallen or not moving —*see* Accident, transport
        falling or moving —*see* Landslide ◀
      landslide, fallen or not moving —*see* Accident, transport
        falling or moving —*see* Landslide

Collision NEC *(Continued)*
  transport vehicle NEC *(Continued)*
    due to cataclysm —*see* Forces of nature, by type
    intentional, purposeful suicide (attempt) —*see* Suicide, collision
Combustion, spontaneous —*see* Ignition
Complication (delayed) **of or following** (medical or surgical procedure) Y84.9
  with misadventure —*see* Misadventure
  amputation of limb (s) Y83.5
  anastomosis (arteriovenous) (blood vessel) (gastrojejunal) (tendon) (natural or artificial material) Y83.2
  aspiration (of fluid) Y84.4
    tissue Y84.8
  biopsy Y84.8
  blood
    sampling Y84.7
    transfusion
      procedure Y84.8
  bypass Y83.2
  catheterization (urinary) Y84.6
    cardiac Y84.Ø
  colostomy Y83.3
  cystostomy Y83.3
  dialysis (kidney) Y84.1
  drug —*see* Table of Drugs and Chemicals ⬅
  due to misadventure —*see* Misadventure
  duodenostomy Y83.3
  electroshock therapy Y84.3
  external stoma, creation of Y83.3
  formation of external stoma Y83.3
  gastrostomy Y83.3
  graft Y83.2
  hypothermia (medically-induced) Y84.8
  implant, implantation (of)
    artificial
      internal device (cardiac pacemaker) (electrodes in brain) (heart valve prosthesis) (orthopedic) Y83.1
      material or tissue (for anastomosis or bypass) Y83.2
        with creation of external stoma Y83.3
    natural tissues (for anastomosis or bypass) Y83.2
      with creation of external stoma Y83.3
  infusion
    procedure Y84.8
  injection —*see* Table of Drugs and Chemicals ⬅
    procedure Y84.8
  insertion of gastric or duodenal sound Y84.5
  insulin-shock therapy Y84.3
  paracentesis (abdominal) (thoracic) (aspirative) Y84.4
  procedures other than surgical operation —*see* Complication of or following, by type of procedure
  radiological procedure or therapy Y84.2
  removal of organ (partial) (total) NEC Y83.6
  sampling
    blood Y84.7
    fluid NEC Y84.4
    tissue Y84.8
  shock therapy Y84.3
  surgical operation NEC —*see also* Complication of or following, by type of operation Y83.9
    reconstructive NEC Y83.4
      with
        anastomosis, bypass or graft Y83.2
        formation of external stoma Y83.3
    specified NEC Y83.8
  transfusion —*see also* Table of Drugs and Chemicals ⬅
    procedure Y84.8
  transplant, transplantation (heart) (kidney) (liver) (whole organ, any) Y83.Ø
    partial organ Y83.4
  ureterostomy Y83.3

Complication of or following *(Continued)*
  vaccination —*see also* Table of Drugs and Chemicals ⬅
    procedure Y84.8
Compression
  divers' squeeze —*see* Air, pressure, change
  trachea by
    food (lodged in esophagus) —*see* categories T17 and T18
    vomitus (lodged in esophagus) T17.81-
Conflagration —*see* Exposure, fire, uncontrolled
Constriction (external)
  hair W49.Ø1
  jewelry W49.Ø4
  ring W49.Ø4
  rubber band W49.Ø3
  specified item NEC W49.Ø9
  string W49.Ø2
  thread W49.Ø2
Contact (accidental)
  with
    abrasive wheel (metalworking) W31.1
    alligator W58.Ø9
      bite W58.Ø1
      crushing W58.Ø3
      strike W58.Ø2
    amphibian W62.9
      frog W62.Ø
      toad W62.1
    animal (nonvenomous) NEC W64
      marine W56.89
        bite W56.81
        dolphin —*see* Contact, with, dolphin
        fish NEC —*see* Contact, with, fish
        mammal —*see* Contact, with, mammal, marine
        orca —*see* Contact, with, orca
        sea lion —*see* Contact, with, sea lion
        shark —*see* Contact, with, shark
        strike W56.82
    animate mechanical force NEC W64
    arrow W21.89
      not thrown, projected or falling W45.8
    arthropods (nonvenomous) W57
    axe W27.Ø
    band-saw (industrial) W31.2
    bayonet —*see* Bayonet wound
    bee (s) X58
    bench-saw (industrial) W31.2
    bird W61.99
      bite W61.91
      chicken —*see* Contact, with, chicken
      duck —*see* Contact, with, duck
      goose —*see* Contact, with, goose
      macaw —*see* Contact, with, macaw
      parrot —*see* Contact, with, parrot
      psittacine —*see* Contact, with, psittacine
      strike W61.92
      turkey —*see* Contact, with, turkey
    blender W29.Ø
    boiling water X12
      stated as undetermined whether accidental or intentional Y27.2
      suicide (attempt) X77.2
    bore, earth-drilling or mining (land) (seabed) W31.Ø
    buffalo —*see* Contact, with, hoof stock NEC
    bull W55.29
      bite W55.21
      gored W55.22
      strike W55.22
    bumper cars W31.81
    camel —*see* Contact, with, hoof stock NEC
    can
      lid W26.8 ⬅
      opener W27.4
        powered W29.Ø
    cat W55.Ø9
      bite W55.Ø1
      scratch W55.Ø3
    caterpillar (venomous) X58

C

Contact *(Continued)*
with *(Continued)*
centipede (venomous) X58
chain
hoist W24.Ø
agricultural operations W3Ø.89
saw W29.3
chicken W61.39
peck W61.33
strike W61.32
chisel W27.Ø
circular saw W31.2
cobra X58
combine (harvester) W3Ø.Ø
conveyer belt W24.1
cooker (hot) X15.8
stated as undetermined whether accidental or intentional Y27.3
suicide (attempt) X77.3
coral X58
cotton gin W31.82
cow W55.29
bite W55.21
strike W55.22
crane W24.Ø
agricultural operations W3Ø.89
crocodile W58.19
bite W58.11
crushing W58.13
strike W58.12
dagger W26.1
stated as undetermined whether accidental or intentional Y28.2
suicide (attempt) X78.2
dairy equipment W31.82
dart W21.89
not thrown, projected or falling W45.8
deer —*see* Contact, with, hoof stock NEC
derrick W24.Ø
agricultural operations W3Ø.89
hay W3Ø.2
dog W54.8
bite W54.Ø
strike W54.1
dolphin W56.Ø9
bite W56.Ø1
strike W56.Ø2
donkey —*see* Contact, with, hoof stock NEC
drill (powered) W29.8
earth (land) (seabed) W31.Ø
nonpowered W27.8
drive belt W24.Ø
agricultural operations W3Ø.89
dry ice —*see* Exposure, cold, man-made
dryer (clothes) (powered) (spin) W29.2
duck W61.69
bite W61.61
strike W61.62
earth(-)
drilling machine (industrial) W31.Ø
scraping machine in stationary use W31.83
edge of stiff paper W26.2 ◄
electric
beater W29.Ø
blanket X16
fan W29.2
commercial W31.82
knife W29.1
mixer W29.Ø
elevator (building) W24.Ø
agricultural operations W3Ø.89
grain W3Ø.3
engine (s), hot NEC X17
excavating machine W31.Ø
farm machine W3Ø.9
feces —*see* Contact, with, by type of animal
fer de lance X58

Contact *(Continued)*
with *(Continued)*
fish W56.59
bite W56.51
shark —*see* Contact, with, shark
strike W56.52
flying horses W31.81
forging (metalworking) machine W31.1
fork W27.4
forklift (truck) W24.Ø
agricultural operations W3Ø.89
frog W62.Ø
garden
cultivator (powered) W29.3
riding W3Ø.89
fork W27.1
gas turbine W31.3
Gila monster X58
giraffe —*see* Contact, with, hoof stock NEC
glass (sharp) (broken) W25
with subsequent fall W18.Ø2
assault X99.Ø
due to fall —*see* Fall, by type
stated as undetermined whether accidental or intentional Y28. Ø
suicide (attempt) X78.Ø
goat W55.39
bite W55.31
strike W55.32
goose W61.59
bite W61.51
strike W61.52
hand
saw W27.Ø
tool (not powered) NEC W27.8
powered W29.8
harvester W3Ø.Ø
hay-derrick W3Ø.2
heat NEC X19
from appliance (electrical) (household) —*see* Contact, with, hot, household appliance
heating appliance X16
heating
appliance (hot) X16
pad (electric) X16
hedge-trimmer (powered) W29.3
hoe W27.1
hoist (chain) (shaft) NEC W24.Ø
agricultural W3Ø.89
hoof stock NEC W55.39
bite W55.31
strike W55.32
hornet (s) X58
horse W55.19
bite W55.11
strike W55.12
hot
air X14.1
inhalation X14.Ø
cooker X15.8
drinks X1Ø.Ø
engine X17
fats X1Ø.2
fluids NEC X12
assault X98.2
suicide (attempt) X77.2
undetermined whether accidental or intentional Y27.2
food X1Ø.1
gases X14.1
inhalation X14.Ø
heating appliance X16
household appliance X15.8
assault X98.3
cooker X15.8
hotplate X15.2
kettle X15.8
light bulb X15.8

Contact *(Continued)*
with *(Continued)*
hot *(Continued)*
household appliance *(Continued)*
object NEC X19
assault X98.8
stated as undetermined whether accidental or intentional Y27.9
suicide (attempt) X77.8
saucepan X15.3
skillet X15.3
stated as undetermined whether accidental or intentional Y27.3
stove X15.Ø
suicide (attempt) X77.3
toaster X15.1
kettle X15.8
light bulb X15.8
liquid NEC —*see also* Burn X12 ◄
drinks X1Ø.Ø
stated as undetermined whether accidental or intentional Y27.2
suicide (attempt) X77.2
tap water X11.8
stated as undetermined whether accidental or intentional Y27.1
suicide (attempt) X77.1
machinery X17
metal (molten) (liquid) NEC X18
object (not producing fire or flames) NEC X19
oil (cooking) X1Ø.2
pipe X16
plate X15.2
radiator X16
saucepan (glass) (metal) X15.3
skillet X15.3
stove (kitchen) X15.Ø
substance NEC X19
tap-water X11.8
assault X98.1
heated on stove X12
stated as undetermined whether accidental or intentional Y27.2
suicide (attempt) X77.2
in bathtub X11.Ø
running X11.1
stated as undetermined whether accidental or intentional Y27.1
suicide (attempt) X77.1
toaster X15.1
tool X17
vapors X13.1
inhalation X13.Ø
water (tap) X11.8
boiling X12
stated as undetermined whether accidental or intentional Y27.2
suicide (attempt) X77.2
heated on stove X12
stated as undetermined whether accidental or intentional Y27.2
suicide (attempt) X77.2
in bathtub X11.Ø
running X11.1
stated as undetermined whether accidental or intentional Y27.1
suicide (attempt) X77.1
hotplate X15.2
ice-pick W27.4
insect (nonvenomous) NEC W57
kettle (hot) X15.8
knife W26.Ø
assault X99.1
electric W29.1
stated as undetermined whether accidental or intentional Y28.1
suicide (attempt) X78.1
lathe (metalworking) W31.1
turnings W45.8
woodworking W31.2

Contact *(Continued)*
with *(Continued)*
lawnmower (powered) (ridden) W28
causing electrocution W86.8
suicide (attempt) X83.1
unpowered W27.1
lift, lifting (devices) W24.Ø
agricultural operations W3Ø.89
shaft W24.Ø
liquefied gas —*see* Exposure, cold, man-made
liquid air, hydrogen, nitrogen —*see* Exposure, cold, man-made
lizard (nonvenomous) W59.Ø9
bite W59.Ø1
strike W59.Ø2
llama —*see* Contact, with, hoof stock NEC
macaw W61.19
bite W61.11
strike W61.12
machine, machinery W31.9
abrasive wheel W31.1
agricultural including animal-powered W3Ø.9
combine harvester W3Ø.Ø
grain storage elevator W3Ø.3
hay derrick W3Ø.2
power take-off device W3Ø.1
reaper W3Ø.Ø
specified NEC W3Ø.89
thresher W3Ø.Ø
transport vehicle, stationary W3Ø.81
band saw W31.2
bench saw W31.2
circular saw W31.2
commercial NEC W31.82
drilling, metal (industrial) W31.1
earth-drilling W31.Ø
earthmoving or scraping W31.89
excavating W31.89
forging machine W31.1
gas turbine W31.3
hot X17
internal combustion engine W31.3
land drill W31.Ø
lathe W31.1
lifting (devices) W24.Ø
metal drill W31.1
metalworking (industrial) W31.1
milling, metal W31.1
mining W31.Ø
molding W31.2
overhead plane W31.2
power press, metal W31.1
prime mover W31.3
printing W31.89
radial saw W31.2
recreational W31.81
roller-coaster W31.81
rolling mill, metal W31.1
sander W31.2
seabed drill W31.Ø
shaft
hoist W31.Ø
lift W31.Ø
specified NEC W31.89
spinning W31.89
steam engine W31.3
transmission W24.1
undercutter W31.Ø
water driven turbine W31.3
weaving W31.89
woodworking or forming (industrial) W31.2
mammal (feces) (urine) W55.89
bull —*see* Contact, with, bull
cat —*see* Contact, with, cat
cow —*see* Contact, with, cow
goat —*see* Contact, with, goat
hoof stock —*see* Contact, with, hoof stock

Contact *(Continued)*
with *(Continued)*
mammal *(Continued)*
horse —*see* Contact, with, horse
marine W56.39
dolphin —*see* Contact, with, dolphin
orca —*see* Contact, with, orca
sea lion —*see* Contact, with, sea lion
specified NEC W56.39
bite W56.31
strike W56.32
pig —*see* Contact, with, pig
raccoon —*see* Contact, with, raccoon
rodent —*see* Contact, with, rodent
sheep —*see* Contact, with, sheep
specified NEC W55.89
bite W55.81
strike W55.82
marine
animal W56.89
bite W56.81
dolphin —*see* Contact, with, dolphin
fish NEC —*see* Contact, with, fish
mammal —*see* Contact, with, mammal, marine
orca —*see* Contact, with, orca
sea lion —*see* Contact, with, sea lion
shark —*see* Contact, with, shark
strike W56.82
meat
grinder (domestic) W29.Ø
industrial W31.82
nonpowered W27.4
slicer (domestic) W29.Ø
industrial W31.82
merry go round W31.81
metal, (hot) (liquid) (molten) NEC X18
millipede W57
nail W45.Ø
gun W29.4
needle (sewing) W27.3
hypodermic W46.Ø
contaminated W46.1
object (blunt) NEC
hot NEC X19
legal intervention —*see* Legal, intervention, blunt object
sharp NEC W45.8
inflicted by other person NEC W45.8
stated as
intentional homicide (attempt) —*see* Assault, cutting or piercing instrument
legal intervention —*see* Legal, intervention, sharp object
self-inflicted X78.9
orca W56.29
bite W56.21
strike W56.22
overhead plane W31.2
paper (as sharp object) W26.2 ⬅ (Revised)
paper-cutter W27.5
parrot W61.Ø9
bite W61.Ø1
strike W61.Ø2
pig W55.49
bite W55.41
strike W55.42
pipe, hot X16
pitchfork W27.1
plane (metal) (wood) W27.Ø
overhead W31.2
plant thorns, spines, sharp leaves or other mechanisms W6Ø
powered
garden cultivator W29.3
household appliance, implement, or machine W29.8
saw (industrial) W31.2
hand W29.8
printing machine W31.89

Contact *(Continued)*
with *(Continued)*
psittacine bird W61.29
bite W61.21
macaw —*see* Contact, with, macaw ⬅ (Revised)
parrot —*see* Contact, with, parrot
strike W61.22
pulley (block) (transmission) W24.Ø
agricultural operations W3Ø.89
raccoon W55.59
bite W55.51
strike W55.52
radial-saw (industrial) W31.2
radiator (hot) X16
rake W27.1
rattlesnake X58
reaper W3Ø.Ø
reptile W59.89
lizard —*see* Contact, with, lizard
snake —*see* Contact, with, snake
specified NEC W59.89
bite W59.81
crushing W59.83
strike W59.82
turtle —*see* Contact, with, turtle
rivet gun (powered) W29.4
road scraper —*see* Accident, transport, construction vehicle
rodent (feces) (urine) W53.89
bite W53.81
mouse W53.Ø9
bite W53.Ø1
rat W53.19
bite W53.11
specified NEC W53.89
bite W53.81
squirrel W53.29
bite W53.21
roller coaster W31.81
rope NEC W24.Ø
agricultural operations W3Ø.89
saliva —*see* Contact, with, by type of animal
sander W29.8
industrial W31.2
saucepan (hot) (glass) (metal) X15.3
saw W27.Ø
band (industrial) W31.2
bench (industrial) W31.2
chain W29.3
hand W27.Ø
sawing machine, metal W31.1
scissors W27.2
scorpion X58
screwdriver W27.Ø
powered W29.8
sea
anemone, cucumber or urchin (spine) X58
lion W56.19
bite W56.11
strike W56.12
serpent —*see* Contact, with, snake, by type
sewing-machine (electric) (powered) W29.2
not powered W27.8
shaft (hoist) (lift) (transmission) NEC W24.Ø
agricultural W3Ø.89
shark W56.49
bite W56.41
strike W56.42
sharp object(s) W26.9 ◀ (New)
specified NEC W26.8 ◀ (New)
shears (hand) W27.2
powered (industrial) W31.1
domestic W29.2
sheep W55.39
bite W55.31
strike W55.32
shovel W27.8
steam —*see* Accident, transport, construction vehicle

C

Contact *(Continued)*
  with *(Continued)*
    snake (nonvenomous) W59.19
      bite W59.11
      crushing W59.13
      strike W59.12
    spade W27.1
    spider (venomous) X58
    spin-drier W29.2
    spinning machine W31.89
    splinter W45.8
    sports equipment W21.9
    staple gun (powered) W29.8
    steam X13.1
      engine W31.3
      inhalation X13.Ø
      pipe X16
      shovel W31.89
    stove (hot) (kitchen) X15.Ø
    substance, hot NEC X19
      molten (metal) X18
    sword W26.1
      assault X99.2
      stated as undetermined whether accidental or intentional Y28.2
      suicide (attempt) X78.2
    tarantula X58
    thresher W3Ø.Ø
    tin can lid W26.8 ⇐
    toad W62.1
    toaster (hot) X15.1
    tool W27.8
      hand (not powered) W27.8
        auger W27.Ø
        axe W27.Ø
        can opener W27.4
        chisel W27.Ø
        fork W27.4
        garden W27.1
        handsaw W27.Ø
        hoe W27.1
        ice-pick W27.4
        kitchen utensil W27.4
        manual
          lawn mower W27.1
          sewing machine W27.8
        meat grinder W27.4
        needle (sewing) W27.3
          hypodermic W46.Ø
            contaminated W46.1
        paper cutter W27.5
        pitchfork W27.1
        rake W27.1
        scissors W27.2
        screwdriver W27.Ø
        specified NEC W27.8
        workbench W27.Ø
      hot X17
      powered W29.8
        blender W29.Ø
          commercial W31.82
        can opener W29.Ø
          commercial W31.82
        chainsaw W29.3
        clothes dryer W29.2
          commercial W31.82
        dishwasher W29.2
          commercial W31.82
        edger W29.3
        electric fan W29.2
          commercial W31.82
        electric knife W29.1
        food processor W29.Ø
          commercial W31.82
        garbage disposal W29.Ø
          commercial W31.82

Contact *(Continued)*
  with *(Continued)*
    tool *(Continued)*
      powered *(Continued)*
        garden tool W29.3
        hedge trimmer W29.3
        ice maker W29.Ø
          commercial W31.82
        kitchen appliance W29.Ø
          commercial W31.82
        lawn mower W28
        meat grinder W29.Ø
          commercial W31.82
        mixer W29.Ø
          commercial W31.82
        rototiller W29.3
        sewing machine W29.2
          commercial W31.82
        washing machine W29.2
          commercial W31.82
    transmission device (belt, cable, chain, gear, pinion, shaft) W24.1
      agricultural operations W3Ø.89
    turbine (gas) (water-driven) W31.3
    turkey W61.49
      peck W61.43
      strike W61.42
    turtle (nonvenomous) W59.29
      bite W59.21
      strike W59.22
      terrestrial W59.89
        bite W59.81
        crushing W59.83
        strike W59.82
    under-cutter W31.Ø
    urine —*see* Contact, with, by type of animal
    vehicle
      agricultural use (transport) —*see* Accident, transport, agricultural vehicle
        not on public highway W3Ø.81
      industrial use (transport) —*see* Accident, transport, industrial vehicle
        not on public highway W31.83
      off-road use (transport) —*see* Accident, transport, all-terrain or off-road vehicle
        not on public highway W31.83
      special construction use (transport) —*see* Accident, transport, construction vehicle
        not on public highway W31.83
    venomous
      animal X58
      arthropods X58
      lizard X58
      marine animal NEC X58
      marine plant NEC X58
      millipedes (tropical) X58
      plant (s) X58
      snake X58
      spider X58
    viper X58
    washing-machine (powered) W29.2
    wasp X58
    weaving-machine W31.89
    winch W24.Ø
      agricultural operations W3Ø.89
    wire NEC W24.Ø
      agricultural operations W3Ø.89
    wood slivers W45.8
    yellow jacket X58
    zebra —*see* Contact, with, hoof stock NEC
  pressure X5Ø.9 ◀
  stress X5Ø.9 ◀
Coup de soleil X32

Crash
  aircraft (in transit) (powered) V95.9
    balloon V96.Ø1
    fixed wing NEC (private) V95.21
      commercial V95.31
    glider V96.21
      hang V96.11
      powered V95.11
    helicopter V95.Ø1
    in war operations —*see* War operations, destruction of aircraft
    microlight V95.11
    nonpowered V96.9
      specified NEC V96.8
    powered NEC V95.8
    stated as
      homicide (attempt) YØ8.81
      suicide (attempt) X83.Ø
    ultralight V95.11
  spacecraft V95.41
  transport vehicle NEC —*see also* Accident, transport V89.9
    homicide (attempt) YØ3.8
    motor NEC (traffic) V89.2
      homicide (attempt) YØ3.8
      suicide (attempt) —*see* Suicide, collision
Cruelty (mental) (physical) (sexual) X58
Crushed (accidentally) X58
  between objects (moving) (stationary and moving) W23.Ø
    stationary W23.1
  by
    alligator W58.Ø3
    avalanche NEC —*see* Landslide ◀
    cave-in W2Ø.Ø
      caused by cataclysmic earth surface movement —*see* Landslide ◀
    crocodile W58.13
    crowd or human stampede W52
    falling
      aircraft V97.39
        in war operations —*see* War operations, destruction of aircraft
      earth, material W2Ø.Ø
        caused by cataclysmic earth surface movement —*see* Landslide
      object NEC W2Ø.8
    landslide NEC —*see* Landslide ◀
    lizard (nonvenomous) W59.Ø9
    machinery —*see* Contact, with, by type of machine
    reptile NEC W59.89
    snake (nonvenomous) W59.13
  in
    machinery —*see* Contact, with, by type of machine
Cut, cutting (any part of body) (accidental) —*see also* Contact, with, by object or machine
  during medical or surgical treatment as misadventure —*see* Index to Diseases and Injuries, Complications ⇐
  homicide (attempt) —*see* Assault, cutting or piercing instrument
  inflicted by other person —*see* Assault, cutting or piercing instrument
  legal
    execution —*see* Legal, intervention
    intervention —*see* Legal, intervention, sharp object
  machine NEC —*see also* Contact, with, by type of machine W31.9
  self-inflicted —*see* Suicide, cutting or piercing instrument
  suicide (attempt) —*see* Suicide, cutting or piercing instrument
Cyclone (any injury) X37.1

◀ New ⇐ Revised ~~deleted~~ Deleted

D

D

- **Drowning** *(Continued)*
  - due to *(Continued)*
    - accident *(Continued)*
      - watercraft *(Continued)*
        - sinking *(Continued)*
          - unpowered V90.18
            - canoe V90.15
            - inflatable V90.16
            - kayak V90.15
            - sailboat V90.14
          - specified type NEC V90.89
            - powered V90.83
              - fishing boat V90.82
              - jetskis V90.83
              - merchant ship V90.80
              - passenger ship V90.81
            - unpowered V90.88
              - canoe V90.85
              - inflatable V90.86
              - kayak V90.85
              - sailboat V90.84
              - water skis V90.87
    - avalanche —*see* Landslide ◀
    - cataclysmic
      - earth surface movement NEC —*see* Forces of nature, earth movement ◀
      - storm —*see* Forces of nature, cataclysmic storm ◀
    - cloudburst X37.8
    - cyclone X37.1
    - fall overboard (from) V92.09
      - powered craft V92.03
        - ferry boat V92.01
        - fishing boat V92.02
        - jetskis V92.03
        - liner V92.01
        - merchant ship V92.00
        - passenger ship V92.01
      - resulting from
        - accident to watercraft —*see* Drowning, due to, accident to, watercraft
        - being washed overboard (from) V92.29
          - powered craft V92.23
            - ferry boat V92.21
            - fishing boat V92.22
            - jetskis V92.23
            - liner V92.21
            - merchant ship V92.20
            - passenger ship V92.21
          - unpowered craft V92.28
            - canoe V92.25
            - inflatable V92.26
            - kayak V92.25
            - sailboat V92.24
            - surf-board V92.28
            - water skis V92.27
            - windsurfer V92.28
        - motion of watercraft V92.19
          - powered craft V92.13
            - ferry boat V92.11
            - fishing boat V92.12
            - jetskis V92.13
            - liner V92.11
            - merchant ship V92.10
            - passenger ship V92.11
          - unpowered craft
            - canoe V92.15
            - inflatable V92.16
            - kayak V92.15
            - sailboat V92.14
      - unpowered craft V92.08
        - canoe V92.05
        - inflatable V92.06
        - kayak V92.05

- **Drowning** *(Continued)*
  - due to *(Continued)*
    - fall overboard *(Continued)*
      - unpowered craft *(Continued)*
        - sailboat V92.04
        - surf-board V92.08
        - water skis V92.07
        - windsurfer V92.08
    - hurricane X37.0
    - jumping into water from watercraft (involved in accident) —*see also* Drowning, due to, accident to, watercraft
      - without accident to or on watercraft W16.711
    - tidal wave NEC —*see* Forces of nature, tidal wave ◀
    - torrential rain X37.8
  - following
    - fall
      - into
        - bathtub W16.211
        - bucket W16.221
        - fountain —*see* Drowning, following, fall, into, water, specified NEC
        - quarry —*see* Drowning, following, fall, into, water, specified NEC
        - reservoir —*see* Drowning, following, fall, into, water, specified NEC
        - swimming-pool W16.011
          - stated as undetermined whether accidental or intentional Y21.3
          - striking
            - bottom W16.021
            - wall W16.031
          - suicide (attempt) X71.2
        - water NOS W16.41
          - natural (lake) (open sea) (river) (stream) (pond) W16.111
            - striking
              - bottom W16.121
              - side W16.131
          - specified NEC W16.311
            - striking
              - bottom W16.321
              - wall W16.331
      - overboard NEC —*see* Drowning, due to, fall overboard
    - jump or dive
      - from boat W16.711
        - striking bottom W16.721
      - into
        - fountain —*see* Drowning, following, jump or dive, into, water, specified NEC
        - quarry —*see* Drowning, following, jump or dive, into, water, specified NEC
        - reservoir —*see* Drowning, following, jump or dive, into, water, specified NEC
        - swimming-pool W16.511
          - striking
            - bottom W16.521
            - wall W16.531
          - suicide (attempt) X71.2
        - water NOS W16.91
          - natural (lake) (open sea) (river) (stream) (pond) W16.611
          - specified NEC W16.811
            - striking
              - bottom W16.821
              - wall W16.831
          - striking bottom W16.621

- **Drowning** *(Continued)*
  - homicide (attempt) X92.9
  - in
    - bathtub (accidental) W65
      - assault X92.0
      - following fall W16.211
        - stated as undetermined whether accidental or intentional Y21.1
      - stated as undetermined whether accidental or intentional Y21.0
      - suicide (attempt) X71.0
    - lake —*see* Drowning, in, natural water
    - natural water (lake) (open sea) (river) (stream) (pond) W69
      - assault X92.3
      - following
        - dive or jump W16.611
          - striking bottom W16.621
        - fall W16.111
          - striking
            - bottom W16.121
            - side W16.131
      - stated as undetermined whether accidental or intentional Y21.4
      - suicide (attempt) X71.3
    - quarry —*see* Drowning, in, specified place NEC
    - quenching tank —*see* Drowning, in, specified place NEC
    - reservoir —*see* Drowning, in, specified place NEC
    - river —*see* Drowning, in, natural water
    - sea —*see* Drowning, in, natural water
    - specified place NEC W73
      - assault X92.8
      - following
        - dive or jump W16.811
          - striking
            - bottom W16.821
            - wall W16.831
        - fall W16.311
          - striking
            - bottom W16.321
            - wall W16.331
      - stated as undetermined whether accidental or intentional Y21.8
      - suicide (attempt) X71.8
    - stream —*see* Drowning, in, natural water
    - swimming-pool W67
      - assault X92.1
        - following fall X92.2
      - following
        - dive or jump W16.511
          - striking
            - bottom W16.521
            - wall W16.531
        - fall W16.011
          - striking
            - bottom W16.021
            - wall W16.031
      - stated as undetermined whether accidental or intentional Y21.2
        - following fall Y21.3
      - suicide (attempt) X71.1
        - following fall X71.2
    - war operations —*see* War operations, restriction of airway
  - resulting from accident to watercraft —*see* Drowning, due to, accident, watercraft
  - self-inflicted X71.9
  - stated as undetermined whether accidental or intentional Y21.9
  - suicide (attempt) X71.9

E

Earth (surface) movement NEC —*see* Forces of nature, earth movement
Earth falling (on) W20.0
caused by cataclysmic earth surface movement or eruption —*see* Landslide
Earthquake (any injury) X34
Effect (s) (adverse) of
air pressure (any) —*see* Air, pressure
cold, excessive (exposure to) —*see* Exposure, cold
heat (excessive) —*see* Heat
hot place (weather) —*see* Heat
insolation X30
late —*see* Sequelae
motion —*see* Motion
nuclear explosion or weapon in war operations —*see* War operations, nuclear weapon
radiation —*see* Radiation
travel —*see* Travel
Electric shock (accidental) (by) (in) —*see* Exposure, electric current
Electrocution (accidental) —*see* Exposure, electric current
Endotracheal tube wrongly placed during anesthetic procedure Y65.3
Entanglement
in
bed linen, causing suffocation —*see* category T71
wheel of pedal cycle V19.88
Entry of foreign body or material —*see* Foreign body
Environmental pollution related condition —*see* Z57
Execution, legal (any method) —*see* Legal, intervention
Exhaustion
cold —*see* Exposure, cold
due to excessive exertion —*see also* Overexertion X50.9
heat —*see* Heat
Explosion (accidental) (of) (with secondary fire) W40.9
acetylene W40.1
aerosol can W36.1
air tank (compressed) (in machinery) W36.2
aircraft (in transit) (powered) NEC V95.9
balloon V96.05
fixed wing NEC (private) V95.25
commercial V95.35
glider V96.25
hang V96.15
powered V95.15
helicopter V95.05
in war operations —*see* War operations, destruction of aircraft
microlight V95.15
nonpowered V96.9
specified NEC V96.8
powered NEC V95.8
stated as
homicide (attempt) Y03.8
suicide (attempt) X83.0
ultralight V95.15
anesthetic gas in operating room W40.1
antipersonnel bomb W40.8
assault X96.0
homicide (attempt) X96.0
suicide (attempt) X75
assault X96.9
bicycle tire W37.0
blasting (cap) (materials) W40.0
boiler (machinery), not on transport vehicle W35
on watercraft —*see* Explosion, in, watercraft
butane W40.1
caused by other person X96.9
coal gas W40.1

Explosion (*Continued*)
detonator W40.0
dump (munitions) W40.8
dynamite W40.0
in
assault X96.8
homicide (attempt) X96.8
legal intervention
injuring
bystander Y35.112
law enforcement personnel Y35.111
suspect Y35.113
suicide (attempt) X75
explosive (material) W40.9
gas W40.1
in blasting operation W40.0
specified NEC W40.8
in
assault X96.8
homicide (attempt) X96.8
legal intervention
injuring
bystander Y35.192
law enforcement personnel Y35.191
suspect Y35.193
suicide (attempt) X75
factory (munitions) W40.8
fertilizer bomb W40.8
assault X96.3
homicide (attempt) X96.3
suicide (attempt) X75
fire-damp W40.1
firearm (parts) NEC W34.19
airgun W34.110
BB gun W34.110
gas, air or spring-operated gun NEC W34.118
handgun W32.1
hunting rifle W33.12
larger firearm W33.10
specified NEC W33.19
machine gun W33.13
paintball gun W34.111
pellet gun W34.110
shotgun W33.11
Very pistol [flare] W34.19
fireworks W39
gas (coal) (explosive) W40.1
cylinder W36.9
aerosol can W36.1
air tank W36.2
pressurized W36.3
specified NEC W36.8
gasoline (fumes) (tank) not in moving motor vehicle W40.1
bomb W40.8
assault X96.1
homicide (attempt) X96.1
suicide (attempt) X75
in motor vehicle —*see* Accident, transport, by type of vehicle
grain store W40.8
grenade W40.8
in
assault X96.8
homicide (attempt) X96.8
legal intervention
injuring
bystander Y35.192
law enforcement personnel Y35.191
suspect Y35.193
suicide (attempt) X75
handgun (parts) —*see* Explosion, firearm, handgun (parts)
homicide (attempt) X96.9
antipersonnel bomb —*see* Explosion, antipersonnel bomb
fertilizer bomb —*see* Explosion, fertilizer bomb

Explosion (*Continued*)
homicide (*Continued*)
gasoline bomb —*see* Explosion, gasoline bomb
letter bomb —*see* Explosion, letter bomb
pipe bomb —*see* Explosion, pipe bomb
specified NEC X96.8
hose, pressurized W37.8
hot water heater, tank (in machinery) W35
on watercraft —*see* Explosion, in, watercraft
in, on
dump W40.8
factory W40.8
mine (of explosive gases) NEC W40.1
watercraft V93.59
powered craft V93.53
ferry boat V93.51
fishing boat V93.52
jetskis V93.53
liner V93.51
merchant ship V93.50
passenger ship V93.51
sailboat V93.54
letter bomb W40.8
assault X96.2
homicide (attempt) X96.2
suicide (attempt) X75
machinery —*see also* Contact, with, by type of machine
on board watercraft —*see* Explosion, in, watercraft
pressure vessel —*see* Explosion, by type of vessel
methane W40.1
mine W40.1
missile NEC W40.8
mortar bomb W40.8
in
assault X96.8
homicide (attempt) X96.8
legal intervention
injuring
bystander Y35.192
law enforcement personnel Y35.191
suspect Y35.193
suicide (attempt) X75
munitions (dump) (factory) W40.8
pipe, pressurized W37.8
bomb W40.8
assault X96.4
homicide (attempt) X96.4
suicide (attempt) X75
pressure, pressurized
cooker W38
gas tank (in machinery) W36.3
hose W37.8
pipe W37.8
specified device NEC W38
tire W37.8
bicycle W37.0
vessel (in machinery) W38
propane W40.1
self-inflicted X75
shell (artillery) NEC W40.8
during war operations —*see* War operations, explosion
in
legal intervention
injuring
bystander Y35.122
law enforcement personnel Y35.121
suspect Y35.123
war —*see* War operations, explosion
spacecraft V95.45
stated as undetermined whether accidental or intentional Y25
steam or water lines (in machinery) W37.8
stove W40.9
suicide (attempt) X75

E

- **Explosion** *(Continued)*
  - tire, pressurized W37.8
    - bicycle W37.0
  - undetermined whether accidental or intentional Y25
  - vehicle tire NEC W37.8
    - bicycle W37.0
  - war operations —*see* War operations, explosion
- **Exposure** (to) X58
  - air pressure change —*see* Air, pressure
  - cold (accidental) (excessive) (extreme) (natural) (place) X31
    - assault Y08.89
    - due to
      - man-made conditions W93.8
        - dry ice (contact) W93.01
          - inhalation W93.02
        - liquid air (contact) (hydrogen) (nitrogen) W93.11
          - inhalation W93.12
        - refrigeration unit (deep freeze) W93.2
        - suicide (attempt) X83.2
      - weather (conditions) X31
    - homicide (attempt) Y08.89
    - self-inflicted X83.2
  - due to abandonment or neglect X58
  - electric current W86.8
    - appliance (faulty) W86.8
      - domestic W86.0
    - caused by other person Y08.89
    - conductor (faulty) W86.1
    - control apparatus (faulty) W86.1
    - electric power generating plant, distribution station W86.1
    - electroshock gun —*see* Exposure, electric current, taser
    - high-voltage cable W85
    - homicide (attempt) Y08.89
    - legal execution —*see* Legal, intervention, specified means NEC
    - lightning —*see* subcategory T75.0
    - live rail W86.8
    - misadventure in medical or surgical procedure in electroshock therapy Y63.4
    - motor (electric) (faulty) W86.8
      - domestic W86.0
    - self-inflicted X83.1
    - specified NEC W86.8
      - domestic W86.0
    - stun gun —*see* Exposure, electric current, taser
    - suicide (attempt) X83.1
    - taser W86.8
      - assault Y08.89
      - legal intervention —*see* category Y35
      - self-harm (intentional) X83.8
      - undetermined intent Y33
    - third rail W86.8
    - transformer (faulty) W86.1
    - transmission lines W85
  - environmental tobacco smoke X58
  - excessive
    - cold —*see* Exposure, cold
    - heat (natural) NEC X30
      - man-made W92
  - factor (s) NOS X58
    - environmental NEC X58
      - man-made NEC W99
      - natural NEC —*see* Forces of nature ◀
    - specified NEC X58
  - fire, flames (accidental) X08.8
    - assault X97
    - campfire —*see* Exposure, fire, controlled, not in building
    - controlled (in)
      - with ignition (of) clothing —*see also* Ignition, clothes X06.2
        - nightwear X05

- **Exposure** *(Continued)*
  - fire, flames *(Continued)*
    - controlled *(Continued)*
      - bonfire —*see* Exposure, fire, controlled, not in building
      - brazier (in building or structure) —*see also* Exposure, fire, controlled, building
        - not in building or structure —*see* Exposure, fire, controlled, not in building
      - building or structure X02.0
        - with
          - fall from building X02.3
          - from building X02.5
          - injury due to building collapse X02.2
          - smoke inhalation X02.1
        - hit by object from building X02.4
        - specified mode of injury NEC X02.8
      - fireplace, furnace or stove —*see* Exposure, fire, controlled, building
      - not in building or structure X03.0
        - with
          - fall X03.3
          - smoke inhalation X03.1
        - hit by object X03.4
        - specified mode of injury NEC X03.8
      - trash —*see* Exposure, fire, controlled, not in building
    - fireplace —*see* Exposure, fire, controlled, building
    - fittings or furniture (in building or structure) (uncontrolled) —*see* Exposure, fire, uncontrolled, building
    - forest (uncontrolled) —*see* Exposure, fire, uncontrolled, not in building
    - grass (uncontrolled) —*see* Exposure, fire, uncontrolled, not in building
    - hay (uncontrolled) —*see* Exposure, fire, uncontrolled, not in building
    - homicide (attempt) X97
    - ignition of highly flammable material X04
    - in, of, on, starting in
      - machinery —*see* Contact, with, by type of machine
      - motor vehicle (in motion) —*see also* Accident, transport, occupant by type of vehicle V87.8
        - with collision —*see* Collision
      - railway rolling stock, train, vehicle V81.81
        - with collision —*see* Accident, transport, railway vehicle occupant
      - street car (in motion) V82.8
        - with collision —*see* Accident, transport, streetcar occupant
      - transport vehicle NEC —*see also* Accident, transport
        - with collision —*see* Collision
      - war operations —*see also* War operations, fire
        - from nuclear explosion —*see* War operations, nuclear weapons
      - watercraft (in transit) (not in transit) V91.09
        - localized —*see* Burn, on board watercraft, due to, fire on board
        - powered craft V91.03
          - ferry boat V91.01
          - fishing boat V91.02
          - jet skis V91.03
          - liner V91.01
          - merchant ship V91.00
          - passenger ship V91.01
        - unpowered craft V91.08
          - canoe V91.05
          - inflatable V91.06
          - kayak V91.05
          - sailboat V91.04

- **Exposure** *(Continued)*
  - fire, flames *(Continued)*
    - in, of, on, starting in *(Continued)*
      - watercraft *(Continued)*
        - unpowered craft *(Continued)*
          - surf-board V91.08
          - waterskis V91.07
          - windsurfer V91.08
    - lumber (uncontrolled) —*see* Exposure, fire, uncontrolled, not in building
    - mine (uncontrolled) —*see* Exposure, fire, uncontrolled, not in building
    - prairie (uncontrolled) —*see* Exposure, fire, uncontrolled, not in building
    - resulting from
      - explosion —*see* Explosion
      - lightning X08.8
    - self-inflicted X76
    - specified NEC X08.8
    - started by other person X97
    - stated as undetermined whether accidental or intentional Y26
    - stove —*see* Exposure, fire, controlled, building
    - suicide (attempt) X76
    - tunnel (uncontrolled) —*see* Exposure, fire, uncontrolled, not in building
    - uncontrolled
      - in building or structure X00.0
        - with
          - fall from building X00.3
          - injury due to building collapse X00.2
          - jump from building X00.5
          - smoke inhalation X00.1
        - bed X08.00
          - due to
            - cigarette X08.01
            - specified material NEC X08.09
        - furniture NEC X08.20
          - due to
            - cigarette X08.21
            - specified material NEC X08.29
        - hit by object from building X00.4
        - sofa X08.10
          - due to
            - cigarette X08.11
            - specified material NEC X08.19
        - specified mode of injury NEC X00.8
      - not in building or structure (any) X01.0
        - with
          - fall X01.3
          - smoke inhalation X01.1
        - hit by object X01.4
        - specified mode of injury NEC X01.8
    - undetermined whether accidental or intentional Y26
  - forces of nature NEC —*see* Forces of nature ◀
  - G-forces (abnormal) W49.9
  - gravitational forces (abnormal) W49.9
  - heat (natural) NEC —*see* Heat
  - high-pressure jet (hydraulic) (pneumatic) W49.9
  - hydraulic jet W49.9
  - inanimate mechanical force W49.9
  - jet, high-pressure (hydraulic) (pneumatic) W49.9
  - lightning —*see* subcategory T75.0
    - causing fire —*see* Exposure, fire
  - mechanical forces NEC W49.9
    - animate NEC W64
    - inanimate NEC W49.9
  - noise W42.9
    - supersonic W42.0
  - noxious substance —*see* Table of Drugs and Chemicals ⬅
  - pneumatic jet W49.9

E

Exposure *(Continued)*
prolonged in deep-freeze unit or refrigerator W93.2
radiation *—see* Radiation
smoke *—see also* Exposure, fire
tobacco, second hand Z77.22
specified factors NEC X58
sunlight X32
man-made (sun lamp) W89.8
tanning bed W89.1
supersonic waves W42.Ø
transmission line (s), electric W85
vibration W49.9

Exposure *(Continued)*
waves
infrasound W49.9
sound W42.9
supersonic W42.Ø
weather NEC *—see* Forces of nature ◀
External cause status Y99.9
child assisting in compensated work for family Y99.8
civilian activity done for financial or other compensation Y99.Ø
civilian activity done for income or pay Y99.Ø

External cause status *(Continued)*
family member assisting in compensated work for other family member Y99.8
hobby not done for income Y99.8
leisure activity Y99.8
military activity Y99.1
off-duty activity of military personnel Y99.8
recreation or sport not for income or while a student Y99.8
specified NEC Y99.8
student activity Y99.8
volunteer activity Y99.2

E

F

- **Factors, supplemental**
  - alcohol
    - blood level
      - less than 20mg/100ml Y90.0
      - presence in blood, level not specified Y90.9
      - 20-39mg/100ml Y90.1
      - 40-59mg/100ml Y90.2
      - 60-79mg/100ml Y90.3
      - 80-99mg/100ml Y90.4
      - 100-119mg/100ml Y90.5
      - 120-199mg/100ml Y90.6
      - 200-239mg/100ml Y90.7
      - 240mg/100ml or more Y90.8
    - presence in blood, but level not specified Y90.9
  - environmental-pollution-related condition —*see* Z57
  - nosocomial condition Y95
  - work-related condition Y99.0
- **Failure**
  - in suture or ligature during surgical procedure Y65.2
  - mechanical, of instrument or apparatus (any) (during any medical or surgical procedure) Y65.8
  - sterile precautions (during medical and surgical care) —*see* Misadventure, failure, sterile precautions, by type of procedure
  - to
    - introduce tube or instrument Y65.4
      - endotracheal tube during anesthesia Y65.3
    - make curve (transport vehicle) NEC —*see* Accident, transport
    - remove tube or instrument Y65.4
- **Fall, falling** (accidental) W19
  - building W20.1
    - burning (uncontrolled fire) X00.3
  - down
    - embankment W17.81
    - escalator W10.0
    - hill W17.81
    - ladder W11
    - ramp W10.2
    - stairs, steps W10.9
  - due to
    - bumping against
      - object W18.00
        - sharp glass W18.02
        - specified NEC W18.09
        - sports equipment W18.01
      - person W03
        - due to ice or snow W00.0
        - on pedestrian conveyance —*see* Accident, transport, pedestrian, conveyance
    - collision with another person W03
      - due to ice or snow W00.0
      - involving pedestrian conveyance —*see* Accident, transport, pedestrian, conveyance
    - grocery cart tipping over W17.82
    - ice or snow W00.9
      - from one level to another W00.2
        - on stairs or steps W00.1
      - involving pedestrian conveyance —*see* Accident, transport, pedestrian, conveyance
      - on same level W00.0
    - slipping (on moving sidewalk) W01.0
      - with subsequent striking against object W01.10
        - furniture W01.190
        - sharp object W01.119
          - glass W01.110
          - power tool or machine W01.111
          - specified NEC W01.118
        - specified NEC W01.198

- **Fall, falling** *(Continued)*
  - due to *(Continued)*
    - striking against
      - object W18.00
        - sharp glass W18.02
        - specified NEC W18.09
        - sports equipment W18.01
      - person W03
        - due to ice or snow W00.0
        - on pedestrian conveyance —*see* Accident, transport, pedestrian, conveyance
  - earth (with asphyxia or suffocation (by pressure)) —*see* Earth, falling
  - from, off, out of
    - aircraft NEC (with accident to aircraft NEC) V97.0
      - while boarding or alighting V97.1
    - balcony W13.0
    - bed W06
    - boat, ship, watercraft NEC (with drowning or submersion) —*see* Drowning, due to, fall overboard
      - with hitting bottom or object V94.0
    - bridge W13.1
    - building W13.9
      - burning (uncontrolled fire) X00.3
    - cavity W17.2
    - chair W07
    - cherry picker W17.89
    - cliff W15
    - dock W17.4
    - embankment W17.81
    - escalator W10.0
    - flagpole W13.8
    - furniture NEC W08
    - grocery cart W17.82
    - haystack W17.89
    - high place NEC W17.89
      - stated as undetermined whether accidental or intentional Y30
    - hole W17.2
    - incline W10.2
    - ladder W11
    - lifting device W17.89
    - machine, machinery —*see also* Contact, with, by type of machine
      - not in operation W17.89
    - manhole W17.1
    - mobile elevated work platform [MEWP] W17.89
    - motorized mobility scooter W05.2
    - one level to another NEC W17.89
      - intentional, purposeful, suicide (attempt) X80
      - stated as undetermined whether accidental or intentional Y30
    - pit W17.2
    - playground equipment W09.8
      - jungle gym W09.2
      - slide W09.0
      - swing W09.1
    - quarry W17.89
    - railing W13.9
    - ramp W10.2
    - roof W13.2
    - scaffolding W12
    - scooter (nonmotorized) W05.1
      - motorized mobility W05.2
    - sky lift W17.89
    - stairs, steps W10.9
      - curb W10.1
      - due to ice or snow W00.1
      - escalator W10.0
      - incline W10.2
      - ramp W10.2
      - sidewalk curb W10.1
      - specified NEC W10.8
    - stepladder W11
    - storm drain W17.1

- **Fall, falling** *(Continued)*
  - from, off, out of *(Continued)*
    - streetcar NEC V82.6
      - with antecedent collision —*see* Accident, transport, streetcar occupant
      - while boarding or alighting V82.4
    - structure NEC W13.8
      - burning (uncontrolled fire) X00.3
    - table W08
    - toilet W18.11
      - with subsequent striking against object W18.12
    - train NEC V81.6
      - during derailment (without antecedent collision) V81.7
        - with antecedent collision —*see* Accident, transport, railway vehicle occupant
      - while boarding or alighting V81.4
    - transport vehicle after collision —*see* Accident, transport, by type of vehicle, collision
    - tree W14
    - vehicle (in motion) NEC —*see also* Accident, transport V89.9
      - motor NEC —*see also* Accident, transport, occupant, by type of vehicle V87.8
      - stationary W17.89
        - while boarding or alighting —*see* Accident, transport, by type of vehicle, while boarding or alighting ◀
    - viaduct W13.8
    - wall W13.8
    - watercraft —*see also* Drowning, due to, fall overboard
      - with hitting bottom or object V94.0
    - well W17.0
    - wheelchair, non-moving W05.0
      - powered —*see* Accident, transport, pedestrian, conveyance occupant, specified type NEC
    - window W13.4
  - in, on
    - aircraft NEC V97.0
      - with accident to aircraft V97.0
      - while boarding or alighting V97.1
    - bathtub (empty) W18.2
      - filled W16.212
        - causing drowning W16.211
    - escalator W10.0
    - incline W10.2
    - ladder W11
    - machine, machinery —*see* Contact, with, by type of machine
    - object, edged, pointed or sharp (with cut) —*see* Fall, by type
    - playground equipment W09.8
      - jungle gym W09.2
      - slide W09.0
      - swing W09.1
    - ramp W10.2
    - scaffolding W12
    - shower W18.2
      - causing drowning W16.211
    - staircase, stairs, steps W10.9
      - curb W10.1
      - due to ice or snow W00.1
      - escalator W10.0
      - incline W10.2
      - specified NEC W10.8
    - streetcar (without antecedent collision) V82.5
      - with antecedent collision —*see* Accident, transport, streetcar occupant
      - while boarding or alighting V82.4

◀ New ⬅ Revised ~~deleted~~ Deleted

Forces of nature *(Continued)*
radiation (natural) X39.Ø8
radon X39.Ø1
radon X39.Ø1
specified force NEC X39.8
storm surge X37.Ø
structure collapse causing
earth movement
X36.Ø
sunlight X32
tidal wave X37.41
due to
earthquake X37.41
landslide X37.43
storm X37.42
volcanic eruption X37.41
tornado X37.1

Forces of nature *(Continued)*
tsunami X37.41
twister X37.1
typhoon X37.Ø
volcanic eruption X35
Foreign body ◀
aspiration - *see* Index to Diseases and Injuries, Foreign body, respitory tract ◀
embedded in skin W45 ◀
entering through skin W45.8 ◀
can lid W26.2 ◀
nail W45.Ø ◀
paper W26.2 ◀
specified NEC 45.8 ◀
splinter W45.8 ◀

Forest fire (exposure to) —*see* Exposure, fire, uncontrolled, not in building
Found injured X58
from exposure (to) —*see* Exposure
on
highway, road(way), street V89.9
railway right of way V81.9
Fracture (circumstances unknown or unspecified) X58
due to specified cause NEC X58
Freezing —*see* Exposure, cold
Frostbite X31
due to man-made conditions —*see* Exposure, cold, man-made
Frozen —*see* Exposure, cold

G

Gored by bull W55.22
Gunshot wound W34.ØØ

H

Hailstones, injured by X39.8
Hanged herself or himself —*see* Hanging, self-inflicted
Hanging (accidental) —*see also* category T71
legal execution —*see* Legal, intervention, specified means NEC
Heat (effects of) (excessive) X3Ø
due to
man-made conditions W92
on board watercraft V93.29
fishing boat V93.22
merchant ship V93.2Ø
passenger ship V93.21
sailboat V93.24
specified powered craft NEC V93.23
weather (conditions) X3Ø

Heat *(Continued)*
from
electric heating apparatus causing burning X16
nuclear explosion in war operations —*see* War operations, nuclear weapons
inappropriate in local application or packing in medical or surgical procedure Y63.5
Hemorrhage
delayed following medical or surgical treatment without mention of misadventure —*see* Index to Diseases and Injuries, Complication(s) ⬅
during medical or surgical treatment as misadventure —*see* Index to Diseases and Injuries, Complication(s) ⬅

High
altitude (effects) —*see* Air, pressure, low
level of radioactivity, effects —*see* Radiation
pressure (effects) —*see* Air, pressure, high
temperature, effects —*see* Heat
Hit, hitting (accidental) by —*see* Struck by
Hitting against —*see* Striking against
Homicide (attempt) (justifiable) —*see* Assault
Hot
place, effects —*see also* Heat
weather, effects X3Ø
House fire (uncontrolled) —*see* Exposure, fire, uncontrolled, building
Humidity, causing problem X39.8
Hunger X58
Hurricane (any injury) X37.Ø
Hypobarism, hypobaropathy —*see* Air, pressure, low

I

Ictus
caloris —*see also* Heat
solaris X3Ø
Ignition (accidental) —*see also* Exposure, fire X08.8
anesthetic gas in operating room W4Ø.1
apparel XØ6.2
from highly flammable material XØ4
nightwear XØ5
bed linen (sheets) (spreads) (pillows) (mattress) —*see* Exposure, fire, uncontrolled, building, bed
benzine XØ4
clothes, clothing NEC (from controlled fire) XØ6.2
from
highly flammable material XØ4
ether XØ4
in operating room W4Ø.1
explosive material —*see* Explosion
gasoline XØ4
jewelry (plastic) (any) XØ6.Ø
kerosene XØ4
material
explosive —*see* Explosion
highly flammable with secondary explosion XØ4
nightwear XØ5
paraffin XØ4
petrol XØ4
Immersion (accidental) —*see also* Drowning
hand or foot due to cold (excessive) X31
Implantation of quills of porcupine W55.89
Inanition (from) (hunger) X58
thirst X58.8
Inappropriate operation performed
correct operation on wrong side or body part (wrong side) (wrong site) Y65.53
operation intended for another patient done on wrong patient Y65.52
wrong operation performed on correct patient Y65.51
Inattention after, at birth (homicidal intent) (infanticidal intent) X58
Incident, adverse
device
anesthesiology Y7Ø.8
accessory Y7Ø.2
diagnostic Y7Ø.Ø
miscellaneous Y7Ø.8
monitoring Y7Ø.Ø
prosthetic Y7Ø.2
rehabilitative Y7Ø.1
surgical Y7Ø.3
therapeutic Y7Ø.1
cardiovascular Y71.8
accessory Y71.2
diagnostic Y71.Ø
miscellaneous Y71.8
monitoring Y71.Ø
prosthetic Y71.2
rehabilitative Y71.1
surgical Y71.3
therapeutic Y71.1
gastroenterology Y73.8
accessory Y73.2
diagnostic Y73.Ø
miscellaneous Y73.8
monitoring Y73.Ø
prosthetic Y73.2
rehabilitative Y73.1
surgical Y73.3
therapeutic Y73.1
general
hospital Y74.8
accessory Y74.2
diagnostic Y74.Ø

Incident, adverse *(Continued)*
device *(Continued)*
general *(Continued)*
hospital *(Continued)*
miscellaneous Y74.8
monitoring Y74.Ø
prosthetic Y74.2
rehabilitative Y74.1
surgical Y74.3
therapeutic Y74.1
surgical Y81.8
accessory Y81.2
diagnostic Y81.Ø
miscellaneous Y81.8
monitoring Y81.Ø
prosthetic Y81.2
rehabilitative Y81.1
surgical Y81.3
therapeutic Y81.1
gynecological Y76.8
accessory Y76.2
diagnostic Y76.Ø
miscellaneous Y76.8
monitoring Y76.Ø
prosthetic Y76.2
rehabilitative Y76.1
surgical Y76.3
therapeutic Y76.1
medical Y82.9
specified type NEC Y82.8
neurological Y75.8
accessory Y75.2
diagnostic Y75.Ø
miscellaneous Y75.8
monitoring Y75.Ø
prosthetic Y75.2
rehabilitative Y75.1
surgical Y75.3
therapeutic Y75.1
obstetrical Y76.8
accessory Y76.2
diagnostic Y76.Ø
miscellaneous Y76.8
monitoring Y76.Ø
prosthetic Y76.2
rehabilitative Y76.1
surgical Y76.3
therapeutic Y76.1
ophthalmic Y77.8
accessory Y77.2
diagnostic Y77.Ø
miscellaneous Y77.8
monitoring Y77.Ø
prosthetic Y77.2
rehabilitative Y77.1
surgical Y77.3
therapeutic Y77.1
orthopedic Y79.8
accessory Y79.2
diagnostic Y79.Ø
miscellaneous Y79.8
monitoring Y79.Ø
prosthetic Y79.2
rehabilitative Y79.1
surgical Y79.3
therapeutic Y79.1
otorhinolaryngological Y72.8
accessory Y72.2
diagnostic Y72.Ø
miscellaneous Y72.8
monitoring Y72.Ø
prosthetic Y72.2
rehabilitative Y72.1
surgical Y72.3
therapeutic Y72.1
personal use Y74.8
accessory Y74.2
diagnostic Y74.Ø
miscellaneous Y74.8
monitoring Y74.Ø
prosthetic Y74.2

Incident, adverse *(Continued)*
device *(Continued)*
personal use *(Continued)*
rehabilitative Y74.1
surgical Y74.3
therapeutic Y74.1
physical medicine Y8Ø.8
accessory Y8Ø.2
diagnostic Y8Ø.Ø
miscellaneous Y8Ø.8
monitoring Y8Ø.Ø
prosthetic Y8Ø.2
rehabilitative Y8Ø.1
surgical Y8Ø.3
therapeutic Y8Ø.1
plastic surgical Y81.8
accessory Y81.2
diagnostic Y81.Ø
miscellaneous Y81.8
monitoring Y81.Ø
prosthetic Y81.2
rehabilitative Y81.1
surgical Y81.3
therapeutic Y81.1
radiological Y78.8
accessory Y78.2
diagnostic Y78.Ø
miscellaneous Y78.8
monitoring Y78.Ø
prosthetic Y78.2
rehabilitative Y78.1
surgical Y78.3
therapeutic Y78.1
urology Y73.8
accessory Y73.2
diagnostic Y73.Ø
miscellaneous Y73.8
monitoring Y73.Ø
prosthetic Y73.2
rehabilitative Y73.1
surgical Y73.3
therapeutic Y73.1
Incineration (accidental) —*see* Exposure, fire
Infanticide —*see* Assault
Infrasound waves (causing injury) W49.9
Ingestion
foreign body (causing injury) (with obstruction) —*see* Foreign body, alimentary canal
poisonous
plant (s) X58
substance NEC —*see* Table of Drugs and Chemicals ⬅
Inhalation
excessively cold substance, man-made —*see* Exposure, cold, man-made
food (any type) (into respiratory tract) (with asphyxia, obstruction respiratory tract, suffocation) —*see* categories T17 and T18
foreign body —*see* Foreign body, aspiration
gastric contents (with asphyxia, obstruction respiratory passage, suffocation) T17.81-
hot air or gases X14.Ø
liquid air, hydrogen, nitrogen W93.12
suicide (attempt) X83.2
steam X13.Ø
assault X98.Ø
stated as undetermined whether accidental or intentional Y27.Ø
suicide (attempt) X77.Ø
toxic gas —*see* Table of Drugs and Chemicals ⬅
vomitus (with asphyxia, obstruction respiratory passage, suffocation)T17.81-
Injury, injured (accidental(ly)) **NOS** X58
by, caused by, from
assault —*see* Assault
law-enforcing agent, police, in course of legal intervention —*see* Legal intervention
suicide (attempt) X83.8

- **Injury, injured NOS** *(Continued)*
  - due to, in
    - civil insurrection —*see* War operations
    - fight —*see also* Assault, fight Y04.0
    - war operations —*see* War operations
  - homicide —*see also* Assault Y09
  - inflicted (by)
    - in course of arrest (attempted), suppression of disturbance, maintenance of order, by law-enforcing agents —*see* Legal intervention

- **Injury, injured NOS** *(Continued)*
  - inflicted *(Continued)*
    - other person
      - stated as
        - accidental X58
        - intentional, homicide (attempt) —*see* Assault
        - undetermined whether accidental or intentional Y33
    - purposely (inflicted) by other person (s) —*see* Assault
  - self-inflicted X83.8
    - stated as accidental X58
  - specified cause NEC X58

- **Injury, injured NOS** *(Continued)*
  - undetermined whether accidental or intentional Y33
- **Insolation, effects** X30
- **Insufficient nourishment** X58
- **Interruption of respiration** (by)
  - food (lodged in esophagus) —*see* categories T17 and T18
  - vomitus (lodged in esophagus) T17.81-
- **Intervention, legal** —*see* Legal intervention
- **Intoxication**
  - drug —*see* Table of Drugs and Chemicals ⬅
  - poison —*see* Table of Drugs and Chemicals ⬅

J

- **Jammed** (accidentally)
  - between objects (moving) (stationary and moving) W23.0
  - stationary W23.1
- **Jumped, jumping**
  - before moving object NEC X81.8
    - motor vehicle X81.0
    - subway train X81.1
    - train X81.1
    - undetermined whether accidental or intentional Y31
  - from
    - boat (into water) voluntarily, without accident (to or on boat) W16.712
      - with
        - accident to or on boat —*see* Accident, watercraft
        - drowning or submersion W16.711
          - suicide (attempt) X71.3

- **Jumped, jumping** *(Continued)*
  - from *(Continued)*
    - boat voluntarily, without accident *(Continued)*
      - striking bottom W16.722
        - causing drowning W16.721
    - building —*see also* Jumped, from, high place W13.9
      - burning (uncontrolled fire) X00.5
    - high place NEC W17.89
      - suicide (attempt) X80
      - undetermined whether accidental or intentional Y30
    - structure —*see also* Jumped, from, high place W13.9
      - burning (uncontrolled fire) X00.5
  - into water W16.92
    - causing drowning W16.91
    - from, off watercraft —*see* Jumped, from, boat

- **Jumped, jumping** *(Continued)*
  - into water *(Continued)*
    - in
      - natural body W16.612
        - causing drowning W16.611
        - striking bottom W16.622
          - causing drowning W16.621
      - specified place NEC W16.812
        - causing drowning W16.811
        - striking
          - bottom W16.822
            - causing drowning W16.821
          - wall W16.832
            - causing drowning W16.831
      - swimming pool W16.512
        - causing drowning W16.511
        - striking
          - bottom W16.522
            - causing drowning W16.521
          - wall W16.532
            - causing drowning W16.531
    - suicide (attempt) X71.3

K

- **Kicked by**
  - animal NEC W55.82
  - person (s) (accidentally) W50.1
    - with intent to injure or kill Y04.0
    - as, or caused by, a crowd or human stampede (with fall) W52
    - assault Y04.0
    - homicide (attempt) Y04.0
    - in
      - fight Y04.0
      - legal intervention
        - injuring
          - bystander Y35.812
          - law enforcement personnel Y35.811
          - suspect Y35.813
- ~~Kicking against~~
  - ~~object W22.8~~
    - ~~sports equipment W21.9~~
    - ~~stationary W22.09~~
      - ~~sports equipment W21.89~~
  - ~~person —see Striking against, person~~
  - ~~sports equipment W21.9~~

- **Kicking** ◀
  - against ◀
    - object W22.8 ◀
      - sports equipment W21.9 ◀
      - stationary W22.09 ◀
        - sports equipment W21.89 ◀
    - person —*see* Striking against, person ◀
    - sports equipment W21.9 ◀
  - carpet stretcher with knee X50.3 ◀
- **Killed, killing** (accidentally) **NOS** —*see also* Injury X58
  - in
    - action —*see* War operations
    - brawl, fight (hand) (fists) (foot) Y04.0
      - by weapon —*see also* Assault
        - cutting, piercing —*see* Assault, cutting or piercing instrument
        - firearm —*see* Discharge, firearm, by type, homicide

- **Killed, killing NOS** *(Continued)*
  - self
    - stated as
      - accident NOS X58
      - suicide —*see* Suicide
      - undetermined whether accidental or intentional Y33
- **Kneeling** (prolonged) (static) X50.1 ◀
- **Knocked down** (accidentally) (by) **NOS** X58
  - animal (not being ridden) NEC —*see also* Struck by, by type of animal
  - crowd or human stampede W52
  - person W51
    - in brawl, fight Y04.0
  - transport vehicle NEC —*see also* Accident, transport V09.9

◀ New ⬅ Revised ~~deleted~~ Deleted

L

- **Laceration NEC** —*see* Injury
- **Lack of**
  - care (helpless person) (infant) (newborn) X58
  - food except as result of abandonment or neglect X58
    - due to abandonment or neglect X58
  - water except as result of transport accident X58
    - due to transport accident —*see* Accident, transport, by type ◀
  - helpless person, infant, newborn X58
- **Landslide** (falling on transport vehicle) X36.1
  - caused by collapse of man-made structure X36.0
- **Late effect** —*see* Sequelae
- **Legal**
  - execution (any method) —*see* Legal, intervention
  - intervention (by)
    - baton —*see* Legal, intervention, blunt object, baton
    - bayonet —*see* Legal, intervention, sharp object, bayonet
    - blow —*see* Legal, intervention, manhandling
    - blunt object
      - baton
        - injuring
          - bystander Y35.312
          - law enforcement personnel Y35.311
          - suspect Y35.313
      - injuring
        - bystander Y35.302
        - law enforcement personnel Y35.301
        - suspect Y35.303
      - specified NEC
        - injuring
          - bystander Y35.392
          - law enforcement personnel Y35.391
          - suspect Y35.393
      - stave
        - injuring
          - bystander Y35.392
          - law enforcement personnel Y35.391
          - suspect Y35.393
    - bomb —*see* Legal, intervention, explosive
    - cutting or piercing instrument —*see* Legal, intervention, sharp object
    - dynamite —*see* Legal, intervention, explosive, dynamite
    - explosive (s)
      - dynamite
        - injuring
          - bystander Y35.112
          - law enforcement personnel Y35.111
          - suspect Y35.113
      - grenade
        - injuring
          - bystander Y35.192
          - law enforcement personnel Y35.191
          - suspect Y35.193
      - injuring
        - bystander Y35.102
        - law enforcement personnel Y35.101
        - suspect Y35.103

Legal *(Continued)*
- intervention *(Continued)*
  - explosive *(Continued)*
    - mortar bomb
      - injuring
        - bystander Y35.192
        - law enforcement personnel Y35.191
        - suspect Y35.193
    - shell
      - injuring
        - bystander Y35.122
        - law enforcement personnel Y35.121
        - suspect Y35.123
    - specified NEC
      - injuring
        - bystander Y35.192
        - law enforcement personnel Y35.191
        - suspect Y35.193
  - firearm (s) (discharge)
    - handgun
      - injuring
        - bystander Y35.022
        - law enforcement personnel Y35.021
        - suspect Y35.023
    - injuring
      - bystander Y35.002
      - law enforcement personnel Y35.001
      - suspect Y35.003
    - machine gun
      - injuring
        - bystander Y35.012
        - law enforcement personnel Y35.011
        - suspect Y35.013
    - rifle pellet
      - injuring
        - bystander Y35.032
        - law enforcement personnel Y35.031
        - suspect Y35.033
    - rubber bullet
      - injuring
        - bystander Y35.042
        - law enforcement personnel Y35.041
        - suspect Y35.043
    - shotgun —*see* Legal, intervention, firearm, specified NEC
    - specified NEC
      - injuring
        - bystander Y35.092
        - law enforcement personnel Y35.091
        - suspect Y35.093
  - gas (asphyxiation) (poisoning)
    - injuring
      - bystander Y35.202
      - law enforcement personnel Y35.201
      - suspect Y35.203
    - specified NEC
      - injuring
        - bystander Y35.292
        - law enforcement personnel Y35.291
        - suspect Y35.293
    - tear gas
      - injuring
        - bystander Y35.212
        - law enforcement personnel Y35.211
        - suspect Y35.213

Legal *(Continued)*
- intervention *(Continued)*
  - grenade —*see* Legal, intervention, explosive, grenade
  - injuring
    - bystander Y35.92
    - law enforcement personnel Y35.91
    - suspect Y35.93
  - late effect (of) —*see* with 7th character S Y35
  - manhandling
    - injuring
      - bystander Y35.812
      - law enforcement personnel Y35.811
      - suspect Y35.813
  - sequelae (of) —*see* with 7th character S Y35
  - sharp objects
    - bayonet
      - injuring
        - bystander Y35.412
        - law enforcement personnel Y35.411
        - suspect Y35.413
    - injuring
      - bystander Y35.402
      - law enforcement personnel Y35.401
      - suspect Y35.403
    - specified NEC
      - injuring
        - bystander Y35.492
        - law enforcement personnel Y35.491
        - suspect Y35.493
  - specified means NEC
    - injuring
      - bystander Y35.892
      - law enforcement personnel Y35.891
      - suspect Y35.893
  - stabbing —*see* Legal, intervention, sharp object
  - stave —*see* Legal, intervention, blunt object, stave
  - tear gas —*see* Legal, intervention, gas, tear gas
  - truncheon —*see* Legal, intervention, blunt object, stave
- **Lifting** —*see also* Overexertion ◀
  - heavy objects X50.0 ◀
  - weights X50.0 ◀
- **Lightning** (shock) (stroke) (struck by) —*see* subcategory T75.0
  - causing fire —*see* Exposure, fire
- **Loss of control** (transport vehicle) **NEC** —*see* Accident, transport
- **Lost at sea NOS** —*see* Drowning, due to, fall overboard
- **Low**
  - pressure (effects) —*see* Air, pressure, low
  - temperature (effects) —*see* Exposure, cold
- **Lying before train, vehicle or other moving object** X81.8
  - subway train X81.1
  - train X81.1
  - undetermined whether accidental or intentional Y31
- **Lynching** —*see* Assault

L

M

Malfunction (mechanism or component) (of)
firearm
airgun W34.1Ø
BB gun W34.11Ø
gas, air or spring-operated gun NEC W34.118
handgun W32.1
hunting rifle W33.12
larger firearm W33.1Ø
specified NEC W33.19
machine gun W33.13
paintball gun W34.111
pellet gun W34.11Ø
shotgun W33.11
specified NEC W34.19
Very pistol [flare] W34.19
handgun —*see* Malfunction, firearm, handgun
Maltreatment —*see* Perpetrator
Mangled (accidentally) **NOS** X58
Manhandling (in brawl, fight) YØ4.Ø
legal intervention —*see* Legal, intervention, manhandling
Manslaughter (nonaccidental) —*see* Assault
Mauled by animal NEC W55.89
Medical procedure, complication of (delayed or as an abnormal reaction without mention of misadventure) —*see* Complication of or following, by specified type of procedure
due to or as a result of misadventure —*see* Misadventure
Melting (due to fire) —*see also* Exposure, fire
apparel NEC XØ6.3
clothes, clothing NEC XØ6.3
nightwear XØ5
fittings or furniture (burning building) (uncontrolled fire) XØØ.8
nightwear XØ5
plastic jewelry XØ6.1
Mental cruelty X58
Military operations (injuries to military and civilians occuring during peacetime on military property and during routine military exercises and operations) (by) (from) (involving) Y37.9Ø-
air blast Y37.2Ø-
aircraft
destruction —*see* Military operations, destruction of aircraft
airway restriction —*see* Military operations, restriction of airways
asphyxiation —*see* Military operations, restriction of airways
biological weapons Y37.6X-
blast Y37.2Ø-
blast fragments Y37.2Ø-
blast wave Y37.2Ø-
blast wind Y37.2Ø-
bomb Y37.2Ø-
dirty Y37.5Ø-
gasoline Y37.31-
incendiary Y37.31-
petrol Y37.31-
bullet Y37.43-
incendiary Y37.32-
rubber Y37.41-
chemical weapons Y37.7X-
combat
hand to hand (unarmed) combat Y37.44-
using blunt or piercing object Y37.45-
conflagration —*see* Military operations, fire
conventional warfare NEC Y37.49-
depth-charge Y37.Ø1-
destruction of aircraft Y37.1Ø-
due to
air to air missile Y37.11-
collision with other aircraft Y37.12-

Military operations *(Continued)*
destruction of aircraft *(Continued)*
due to *(Continued)*
detonation (accidental) of onboard munitions and explosives Y37.14-
enemy fire or explosives Y37.11-
explosive placed on aircraft Y37.11-
onboard fire Y37.13-
rocket propelled grenade [RPG] Y37.11-
small arms fire Y37.11-
surface to air missile Y37.11-
specified NEC Y37.19-
detonation (accidental) of
onboard marine weapons Y37.Ø5-
own munitions or munitions launch device Y37.24-
dirty bomb Y37.5Ø-
explosion (of) Y37.2Ø-
aerial bomb Y37.21-
bomb NOS —*see also* Military operations, bomb (s) Y37.2Ø-
fragments Y37.2Ø-
grenade Y37.29-
guided missile Y37.22-
improvised explosive device [IED] (person-borne) (roadside) (vehicle-borne) Y37.23-
land mine Y37.29-
marine mine (at sea) (in harbor) Y37.Ø2-
marine weapon Y37.ØØ-
specified NEC Y37.Ø9-
own munitions or munitions launch device (accidental) Y37.24-
sea-based artillery shell Y37.Ø3-
specified NEC Y37.29-
torpedo Y37.Ø4-
fire Y37.3Ø-
specified NEC Y37.39-
firearms
discharge Y37.43-
pellets Y37.42-
flamethrower Y37.33-
fragments (from) (of)
improvised explosive device [IED] (person-borne) (roadside) (vehicle-borne) Y37.26-
munitions Y37.25-
specified NEC Y37.29-
weapons Y37.27-
friendly fire Y37.92-
hand to hand (unarmed) combat Y37.44-
hot substances —*see* Military operations, fire
incendiary bullet Y37.32-
nuclear weapon (effects of) Y37.5Ø-
acute radiation exposure Y37.54-
blast pressure Y37.51-
direct blast Y37.51-
direct heat Y37.53-
fallout exposure Y37.54-
fireball Y37.53-
indirect blast (struck or crushed by blast debris) (being thrown by blast) Y37.52-
ionizing radiation (immediate exposure) Y37.54-
nuclear radiation Y37.54-
radiation
ionizing (immediate exposure) Y37.54-
nuclear Y37.54-
thermal Y37.53-
secondary effects Y37.54-
specified NEC Y37.59-
thermal radiation Y37.53-
restriction of air (airway)
intentional Y37.46-
unintentional Y37.47-
rubber bullets Y37.41-
shrapnel NOS Y37.29-
suffocation —*see* Military operations, restriction of airways
unconventional warfare NEC Y37.7X-

Military operations *(Continued)*
underwater blast NOS Y37.ØØ-
warfare
conventional NEC Y37.49-
unconventional NEC Y37.7X-
weapon of mass destruction [WMD] Y37.91-
weapons
biological weapons Y37.6X-
chemical Y37.7X-
nuclear (effects of) Y37.5Ø-
acute radiation exposure Y37.54-
blast pressure Y37.51-
direct blast Y37.51-
direct heat Y37.53-
fallout exposure Y37.54-
fireball Y37.53-
~~indirect blast (struck or crushed by blast debris) (being thrown by blast) Y37.52-~~
radiation
ionizing (immediate exposure) Y37.54-
nuclear Y37.54-
thermal Y37.53-
secondary effects Y37.54-
specified NEC Y37.59-
of mass destruction [WMD] Y37.91-
Misadventure (s) to patient (s) during surgical or medical care Y69
contaminated medical or biological substance (blood, drug, fluid) Y64.9
administered (by) NEC Y64.9
immunization Y64.1
infusion Y64.Ø
injection Y64.1
specified means NEC Y64.8
transfusion Y64.Ø
vaccination Y64.1
excessive amount of blood or other fluid during transfusion or infusion Y63.Ø
failure
in dosage Y63.9
electroshock therapy Y63.4
inappropriate temperature (too hot or too cold) in local application and packing Y63.5
infusion
excessive amount of fluid Y63.Ø
incorrect dilution of fluid Y63.1
insulin-shock therapy Y63.4
nonadministration of necessary drug or biological substance Y63.6 ⬅
overdose —*see* Table of Drugs and Chemicals ⬅
radiation, in therapy Y63.2
radiation
overdose Y63.2
specified procedure NEC Y63.8
transfusion
excessive amount of blood Y63.Ø
mechanical, of instrument or apparatus (any) (during any procedure) Y65.8
sterile precautions (during procedure) Y62.9
aspiration of fluid or tissue (by puncture or catheterization, except heart) Y62.6
biopsy (except needle aspiration) Y62.8
needle (aspirating) Y62.6
blood sampling Y62.6
catheterization Y62.6
heart Y62.5
dialysis (kidney) Y62.2
endoscopic examination Y62.4
enema Y62.8
immunization Y62.3
infusion Y62.1
injection Y62.3
needle biopsy Y62.6
paracentesis (abdominal) (thoracic) Y62.6
perfusion Y62.2

◀ New ⬅ Revised ~~deleted~~ Deleted

Misadventure (s) to patient (s) during surgical or medical care *(Continued)*
  failure *(Continued)*
    sterile precautions *(Continued)*
      puncture (lumbar) Y62.6
      removal of catheter or packing Y62.8
      specified procedure NEC Y62.8
      surgical operation Y62.Ø
      transfusion Y62.1
      vaccination Y62.3
    suture or ligature during surgical procedure Y65.2
    to introduce or to remove tube or instrument —*see* Failure, to ◀
  hemorrhage —*see* Index to Diseases and Injuries, Complication(s) ⬅
  inadvertent exposure of patient to radiation Y63.3
  inappropriate
    operation performed —*see* Inappropriate operation performed
    temperature (too hot or too cold) in local application or packing Y63.5

Misadventure (s) to patient (s) during surgical or medical care *(Continued)*
  infusion —*see also* Misadventure, by type, infusion Y69
    excessive amount of fluid Y63.Ø
    incorrect dilution of fluid Y63.1
    wrong fluid Y65.1
  mismatched blood in transfusion Y65.Ø
  nonadministration of necessary drug or biological substance Y63.6 ⬅
  overdose —*see* Table of Drugs and Chemicals ⬅
    radiation (in therapy) Y63.2
  perforation —*see* Index to Diseases and Injuries, Complication(s) ⬅
  performance of inappropriate operation —*see* Inappropriate operation performed
  puncture —*see* Index to Diseases and Injuries, Complication(s) ⬅
  specified type NEC Y65.8
    failure
      suture or ligature during surgical operation Y65.2
      to introduce or to remove tube or instrument —*see* Failure, to ◀
    infusion of wrong fluid Y65.1

Misadventure (s) to patient (s) during surgical or medical care *(Continued)*
  specified type NEC *(Continued)*
    performance of inappropriate operation —*see* Inappropriate operation performed
    transfusion of mismatched blood Y65.Ø
    wrong
      fluid in infusion Y65.1
      placement of endotracheal tube during anesthetic procedure Y65.3
  transfusion —*see* Misadventure, by type, transfusion
    excessive amount of blood Y63.Ø
    mismatched blood Y65.Ø
  wrong
    drug given in error —*see* Table of Drugs and Chemicals ⬅
    fluid in infusion Y65.1
    placement of endotracheal tube during anesthetic procedure Y65.3
Mismatched blood in transfusion Y65.Ø
Motion sickness T75.3
Mountain sickness W94.11
Mudslide (of cataclysmic nature) —*see* Landslide
Murder (attempt) —*see* Assault

M, N, & O

N

Nail ◀
  contact with W45.Ø ◀
    gun W29.4 ◀
  embedded in skin W45.Ø ◀
~~Nail, contact with W45.0~~
  ~~gun W29.4~~
Neglect (criminal) (homicidal intent) X58
Noise (causing injury) (pollution) W42.9
  supersonic W42.Ø
Nonadministration (of)
  drug or biological substance (necessary) Y63.6 ⬅
  surgical and medical care Y66
Nosocomial condition Y95

O

Object
  falling
    from, in, on, hitting
      machinery —*see* Contact, with, by type of machine
  set in motion by
    accidental explosion or rupture of pressure vessel W38
    firearm —*see* Discharge, firearm, by type
    machine (ry) —*see* Contact, with, by type of machine
Overdose (drug) —*see* Table of Drugs and Chemicals ⬅
  radiation Y63.2
Overexertion X5Ø.9 ⬅
  from ◀
    prolonged static or awkward postures X5Ø.1 ◀
    repetitive movements X5Ø.3 ◀
    specified strenuous movements or postures NEC X5Ø.9 ◀
    strenuous movement or load X5Ø.Ø ◀
Overexposure (accidental) (to)
  cold —*see also* Exposure, cold X31
    due to man-made conditions —*see* Exposure, cold, man-made
  heat —*see also* Heat X3Ø
  radiation —*see* Radiation
  radioactivity W88.Ø
  sun (sunburn) X32
Overexposure *(Continued)*
  weather NEC —*see* Forces of nature ◀
  wind NEC —*see* Forces of nature ◀
Overheated —*see* Heat
Overturning (accidental)
  machinery —*see* Contact, with, by type of machine
  transport vehicle NEC —*see also* Accident, transport V89.9
  watercraft (causing drowning, submersion) —*see also* Drowning, due to, accident to, watercraft, overturning
    causing injury except drowning or submersion —*see* Accident, watercraft, causing, injury NEC ◀

P

- **Parachute descent** (voluntary) (without accident to aircraft) V97.29
  - due to accident to aircraft —*see* Accident, transport, aircraft
- **Pecked by bird** W61.99
- **Perforation during medical or surgical treatment as misadventure** —*see* Index to Diseases and Injuries, Complication(s) ⟸
- **Perpetrator, perpetration, of assault, maltreatment and neglect (by)** Y07.9
  - boyfriend Y07.03
  - brother Y07.410
    - stepbrother Y07.435
  - coach Y07.53
  - cousin
    - female Y07.491
    - male Y07.490
  - daycare provider Y07.519
    - at-home
      - adult care Y07.512
      - childcare Y07.510
    - care center
      - adult care Y07.513
      - childcare Y07.511
  - family member NEC Y07.499
  - father Y07.11
    - adoptive Y07.13
    - foster Y07.420
    - stepfather Y07.430
  - foster father Y07.420
  - foster mother Y07.421
  - girl friend Y07.04
  - healthcare provider Y07.529
    - mental health Y07.521
    - specified NEC Y07.528
  - husband Y07.01
  - instructor Y07.53
  - mother Y07.12
    - adoptive Y07.14
    - foster Y07.421
    - stepmother Y07.433
  - nonfamily member Y07.50
    - specified NEC Y07.59
  - nurse Y07.528
  - occupational therapist Y07.528
  - partner of parent
    - female Y07.434
    - male Y07.432
  - physical therapist Y07.528
  - sister Y07.411
  - speech therapist Y07.528
  - stepbrother Y07.435
  - stepfather Y07.430
  - stepmother Y07.433
  - stepsister Y07.436
  - teacher Y07.53
  - wife Y07.02
- **Piercing** —*see* Contact, with, by type of object or machine
- **Pinched**
  - between objects (moving) (stationary and moving) W23.0
    - stationary W23.1
- **Pinned under machine** (ry) —*see* Contact, with, by type of machine
- **Place of occurrence** Y92.9
  - abandoned house Y92.89
  - airplane Y92.813
  - airport Y92.520
  - ambulatory health services establishment NEC Y92.538
  - ambulatory surgery center Y92.530
  - amusement park Y92.831
  - apartment (co-op) —*see* Place of occurrence, residence, apartment
  - assembly hall Y92.29
  - bank Y92.510
  - barn Y92.71
  - baseball field Y92.320

Place of occurrence *(Continued)*

  - basketball court Y92.310
  - beach Y92.832
  - boarding house —*see* Place of occurrence, residence, boarding house
  - boat Y92.814
  - bowling alley Y92.39
  - bridge Y92.89
  - building under construction Y92.61
  - bus Y92.811
    - station Y92.521
  - cafe Y92.511
  - campsite Y92.833
  - campus —*see* Place of occurrence, school
  - canal Y92.89
  - car Y92.810
  - casino Y92.59
  - children's home —*see* Place of occurrence, residence, institutional, orphanage
  - church Y92.22
  - cinema Y92.26
  - clubhouse Y92.29
  - coal pit Y92.64
  - college (community) Y92.214
  - condominium —*see* Place of occurrence, residence, apartment
  - construction area —*see* Place of occurrence, industrial and construction area
  - convalescent home —*see* Place of occurrence, residence, institutional, nursing home
  - court-house Y92.240
  - cricket ground Y92.328
  - cultural building Y92.258
    - art gallery Y92.250
    - museum Y92.251
    - music hall Y92.252
    - opera house Y92.253
    - specified NEC Y92.258
    - theater Y92.254
  - dancehall Y92.252
  - day nursery Y92.210
  - dentist office Y92.531
  - derelict house Y92.89
  - desert Y92.820
  - dock NOS Y92.89
  - dockyard Y92.62
  - doctor's office Y92.531
  - dormitory —*see* Place of occurrence, residence, institutional, school dormitory
  - dry dock Y92.62
  - factory (building) (premises) Y92.63
  - farm (land under cultivation) (outbuildings) Y92.79
    - barn Y92.71
    - chicken coop Y92.72
    - field Y92.73
    - hen house Y92.72
    - house —*see* Place of occurrence, residence, house
    - orchard Y92.74
    - specified NEC Y92.79
  - football field Y92.321
  - forest Y92.821
  - freeway Y92.411
  - gallery Y92.250
  - garage (commercial) Y92.59
    - boarding house Y92.044
    - military base Y92.135
    - mobile home Y92.025
    - nursing home Y92.124
    - orphanage Y92.114
    - private house Y92.015
    - reform school Y92.155
  - gas station Y92.524
  - gasworks Y92.69
  - golf course Y92.39
  - gravel pit Y92.64
  - grocery Y92.512
  - gymnasium Y92.39
  - handball court Y92.318
  - harbor Y92.89

Place of occurrence *(Continued)*

  - harness racing course Y92.39
  - healthcare provider office Y92.531
  - highway (interstate) Y92.411
  - hill Y92.828
  - hockey rink Y92.330
  - home —*see* Place of occurrence, residence
  - hospice —*see* Place of occurrence, residence, institutional, nursing home
  - hospital Y92.239
    - cafeteria Y92.233
    - corridor Y92.232
    - operating room Y92.234
    - patient
      - bathroom Y92.231
      - room Y92.230
    - specified NEC Y92.238
  - hotel Y92.59
  - house —*see also* Place of occurrence, residence
    - abandoned Y92.89
    - under construction Y92.61
  - industrial and construction area (yard) Y92.69
    - building under construction Y92.61
    - dock Y92.62
    - dry dock Y92.62
    - factory Y92.63
    - gasworks Y92.69
    - mine Y92.64
    - oil rig Y92.65
    - pit Y92.64
    - power station Y92.69
    - shipyard Y92.62
    - specified NEC Y92.69
    - tunnel under construction Y92.69
    - workshop Y92.69
  - kindergarten Y92.211
  - lacrosse field Y92.328
  - lake Y92.828
  - library Y92.241
  - mall Y92.59
  - market Y92.512
  - marsh Y92.828
  - military
    - base —*see* Place of occurrence, residence, institutional, military base
    - training ground Y92.84
  - mine Y92.64
  - mosque Y92.22
  - motel Y92.59
  - motorway (interstate) Y92.411
  - mountain Y92.828
  - movie-house Y92.26
  - museum Y92.251
  - music-hall Y92.252
  - not applicable Y92.9
  - nuclear power station Y92.69
  - nursing home —*see* Place of occurrence, residence, institutional, nursing home
  - office building Y92.59
  - offshore installation Y92.65
  - oil rig Y92.65
  - old people's home —*see* Place of occurrence, residence, institutional, specified NEC
  - opera-house Y92.253
  - orphanage —*see* Place of occurrence, residence, institutional, orphanage
  - outpatient surgery center Y92.530
  - park (public) Y92.830
    - amusement Y92.831
  - parking garage Y92.89
    - lot Y92.481
  - pavement Y92.480
  - physician office Y92.531
  - polo field Y92.328
  - pond Y92.828
  - post office Y92.242
  - power station Y92.69
  - prairie Y92.828
  - prison —*see* Place of occurrence, residence, institutional, prison

- **Place of occurrence** *(Continued)*
  - public
    - administration building Y92.248
      - city hall Y92.243
      - courthouse Y92.240
      - library Y92.241
      - post office Y92.242
      - specified NEC Y92.248
    - building NEC Y92.29
    - hall Y92.29
    - place NOS Y92.89
  - race course Y92.39
  - radio station Y92.59
  - railway line (bridge) Y92.85
  - ranch (outbuildings) —*see* Place of occurrence, farm
  - recreation area Y92.838
    - amusement park Y92.831
    - beach Y92.832
    - campsite Y92.833
    - park (public) Y92.830
    - seashore Y92.832
    - specified NEC Y92.838
  - reform school —*see* Place of occurrence, residence, institutional, reform school
  - religious institution Y92.22
  - residence (non-institutional) (private) Y92.009
    - apartment Y92.039
      - bathroom Y92.031
      - bedroom Y92.032
      - kitchen Y92.030
      - specified NEC Y92.038
    - bathroom Y92.002
    - bedroom Y92.003
    - boarding house Y92.049
      - bathroom Y92.041
      - bedroom Y92.042
      - driveway Y92.043
      - garage Y92.044
      - garden Y92.046
      - kitchen Y92.040
      - specified NEC Y92.048
      - swimming pool Y92.045
      - yard Y92.046
    - dining room Y92.001
    - garden Y92.007
    - home Y92.009
    - house, single family Y92.019
      - bathroom Y92.012
      - bedroom Y92.013
      - dining room Y92.011
      - driveway Y92.014
      - garage Y92.015
      - garden Y92.017
      - kitchen Y92.010
      - specified NEC Y92.018
      - swimming pool Y92.016
      - yard Y92.017
    - institutional Y92.10
      - children's home —*see* Place of occurrence, residence, institutional, orphanage
      - hospice —*see* Place of occurrence, residence, institutional, nursing home
      - military base Y92.139
        - barracks Y92.133
        - garage Y92.135
        - garden Y92.137
        - kitchen Y92.130
        - mess hall Y92.131
        - specified NEC Y92.138
        - swimming pool Y92.136
        - yard Y92.137
      - nursing home Y92.129
        - bathroom Y92.121
        - bedroom Y92.122
        - driveway Y92.123
        - garage Y92.124
        - garden Y92.126
        - kitchen Y92.120

- **Place of occurrence** *(Continued)*
  - residence *(Continued)*
    - institutional *(Continued)*
      - nursing home *(Continued)*
        - specified NEC Y92.128
        - swimming pool Y92.125
        - yard Y92.126
      - orphanage Y92.119
        - bathroom Y92.111
        - bedroom Y92.112
        - driveway Y92.113
        - garage Y92.114
        - garden Y92.116
        - kitchen Y92.110
        - specified NEC Y92.118
        - swimming pool Y92.115
        - yard Y92.116
      - prison Y92.149
        - bathroom Y92.142
        - cell Y92.143
        - courtyard Y92.147
        - dining room Y92.141
        - kitchen Y92.140
        - specified NEC Y92.148
        - swimming pool Y92.146
      - reform school Y92.159
        - bathroom Y92.152
        - bedroom Y92.153
        - dining room Y92.151
        - driveway Y92.154
        - garage Y92.155
        - garden Y92.157
        - kitchen Y92.150
        - specified NEC Y92.158
        - swimming pool Y92.156
        - yard Y92.157
      - school dormitory Y92.169
        - bathroom Y92.162
        - bedroom Y92.163
        - dining room Y92.161
        - kitchen Y92.160
        - specified NEC Y92.168
      - specified NEC Y92.199
        - bathroom Y92.192
        - bedroom Y92.193
        - dining room Y92.191
        - driveway Y92.194
        - garage Y92.195
        - garden Y92.197
        - kitchen Y92.190
        - specified NEC Y92.198
        - swimming pool Y92.196
        - yard Y92.197
    - kitchen Y92.000
    - mobile home Y92.029
      - bathroom Y92.022
      - bedroom Y92.023
      - dining room Y92.021
      - driveway Y92.024
      - garage Y92.025
      - garden Y92.027
      - kitchen Y92.020
      - specified NEC Y92.028
      - swimming pool Y92.026
      - yard Y92.027
    - specified place in residence NEC Y92.008 ⬅
    - specified residence type NEC Y92.099
      - bathroom Y92.091
      - bedroom Y92.092
      - driveway Y92.093
      - garage Y92.094
      - garden Y92.096
      - kitchen Y92.090
      - specified NEC Y92.098
      - swimming pool Y92.095
      - yard Y92.096
  - restaurant Y92.511
  - riding school Y92.39
  - river Y92.828
  - road Y92.488
  - rodeo ring Y92.39

- **Place of occurrence** *(Continued)*
  - rugby field Y92.328
  - same day surgery center Y92.530
  - sand pit Y92.64
  - school (private) (public) (state) Y92.219
    - college Y92.214
    - daycare center Y92.210
    - elementary school Y92.211
    - high school Y92.213
    - kindergarten Y92.211
    - middle school Y92.212
    - specified NEC Y92.218
    - trace school Y92.215
    - university Y92.214
    - vocational school Y92.215
  - sea (shore) Y92.832
  - senior citizen center Y92.29
  - service area
    - airport Y92.520
    - bus station Y92.521
    - gas station Y92.524
    - highway rest stop Y92.523
    - railway station Y92.522
  - shipyard Y92.62
  - shop(commercial) Y92.513
  - sidewalk Y92.480
  - silo Y92.79
  - skating rink (roller) Y92.331
    - ice Y92.330
  - slaughter house Y92.86
  - soccer field Y92.322
  - specified place NEC Y92.89
  - sports area Y92.39
    - athletic
      - court Y92.318
        - basketball Y92.310
        - specified NEC Y92.318
        - squash Y92.311
        - tennis Y92.312
      - field Y92.328
        - baseball Y92.320
        - cricket ground Y92.328
        - football Y92.321
        - hockey Y92.328
        - soccer Y92.322
        - specified NEC Y92.328
    - golf course Y92.39
    - gymnasium Y92.39
    - riding school Y92.39
    - skating rink (roller) Y92.331
      - ice Y92.330
    - stadium Y92.39
    - swimming pool Y92.34
  - squash court Y92.311
  - stadium Y92.39
  - steeplechasing course Y92.39
  - store Y92.512
  - stream Y92.828
  - street and highway Y92.410
    - bike path Y92.482
    - freeway Y92.411
    - highway ramp Y92.415
    - interstate highway Y92.411
    - local residential or business street Y92.414
    - motorway Y92.411
    - parking lot Y92.481
    - parkway Y92.412
    - sidewalk Y92.480
    - specified NEC Y92.488
    - state road Y92.413
  - subway car Y92.816
  - supermarket Y92.512
  - swamp Y92.828
  - swimming pool (public) Y92.34
    - private (at) Y92.095
      - boarding house Y92.045
      - military base Y92.136
      - mobile home Y92.026
      - nursing home Y92.125
      - orphanage Y92.115

Place of occurrence *(Continued)*
swimming pool *(Continued)*
private *(Continued)*
prison Y92.146
reform school Y92.156
single family residence Y92.016
synagogue Y92.22
television station Y92.59
tennis court Y92.312
theater Y92.254
trade area Y92.59
bank Y92.510
cafe Y92.511
casino Y92.59
garage Y92.59
hotel Y92.59
market Y92.512
office building Y92.59
radio station Y92.59
restaurant Y92.511
shop Y92.513
shopping mall Y92.59
store Y92.512
supermarket Y92.512
television station Y92.59
warehouse Y92.59
trailer park, residential —*see* Place of occurrence, residence, mobile home
trailer site NOS Y92.89
train Y92.815
station Y92.522
truck Y92.812
tunnel under construction Y92. 69
university Y92.214
urgent (health) care center Y92.532
vehicle (transport) Y92.818
airplane Y92.813
boat Y92.814
bus Y92.811
car Y92.810
specified NEC Y92.818
subway car Y92.816
train Y92.815
truck Y92.812
warehouse Y92.59
water reservoir Y92.89
wilderness area Y92.828
desert Y92.820
forest Y92.821
marsh Y92.828
mountain Y92.828
prairie Y92.828
specified NEC Y92.828
swamp Y92.828
workshop Y92.69
yard, private Y92.096
boarding house Y92.046
mobile home Y92.027
single family house Y92.017

Place of occurrence *(Continued)*
youth center Y92.29
zoo (zoological garden) Y92.834
Plumbism —*see* Table of Drugs and Chemicals, lead ◄
Poisoning (accidental) (by) —*see also* Table of Drugs and Chemicals ◄
by plant, thorns, spines, sharp leaves or other mechanisms NEC X58
carbon monoxide
generated by
motor vehicle —*see* Accident, transport
watercraft (in transit) (not in transit) V93.89
ferry boat V93.81
fishing boat V93.82
jet skis V93.83
liner V93.81
merchant ship V93.80
passenger ship V93.81
powered craft NEC V93.83
caused by injection of poisons into skin by plant thorns, spines, sharp leaves X58
marine or sea plants (venomous) X58
exhaust gas
generated by
motor vehicle —*see* Accident, transport
watercraft (in transit) (not in transit) V93.89
ferry boat V93.81
fishing boat V93.82
jet skis V93.83
liner V93.81
merchant ship V93.80
passenger ship V93.81
powered craft NEC V93.83
fumes or smoke due to
explosion —*see also* Explosion W40.9
fire —*see* Exposure, fire
ignition —*see* Ignition
gas
in legal intervention —*see* Legal, intervention, gas
legal execution —*see* Legal, intervention, gas
in war operations —*see* War operations
legal
execution —*see* Legal, intervention, gas
intervention
by gas —*see* Legal, intervention, gas
other specified means —*see* Legal, intervention, specified means NEC
Powder burn (by) (from)
airgun W34.110
BB gun W34.110
firearm NEC W34.19
gas, air or spring-operated gun NEC W34.118
handgun W32.1
hunting rifle W33.12

Powder burn *(Continued)*
larger firearm W33.10
specified NEC W33.19
machine gun W33.13
paintball gun W34.111
pellet gun W34.110
shotgun W33.11
Very pistol [flare] W34.19
Premature cessation (of) surgical and medical care Y66
Privation (food) (water) X58
Procedure (operation)
correct, on wrong side or body part (wrong side) (wrong site) Y65.53
intended for another patient done on wrong patient Y65.52
performed on patient not scheduled for surgery Y65.52
performed on wrong patient Y65.52
wrong, performed on correct patient Y65.51
Prolonged
sitting in transport vehicle —*see* Travel, by type of vehicle
stay in
high altitude as cause of anoxia, barodontalgia, barotitis or hypoxia W94.11
weightless environment X52
Pulling, excessive —*see also* Overexertion X50.9 ◄
Puncture, puncturing —*see also* Contact, with, by type of object or machine
by
plant thorns, spines, sharp leaves or other mechanisms NEC W60
during medical or surgical treatment as misadventure —*see* Index to Diseases and Injuries, Complication(s) ◄
Pushed, pushing (accidental) (injury in) ◄
by other person (s) (accidental) W51
with fall W03
due to ice or snow W00.0
as, or caused by, a crowd or human stampede (with fall) W52
before moving object NEC Y02.8
motor vehicle Y02.0
subway train Y02.1
train Y02.1
from
high place NEC
in accidental circumstances W17.89
stated as
intentional, homicide (attempt) Y01
undetermined whether accidental or intentional Y30
transport vehicle NEC —*see also* Accident, transport V89.9
stated as
intentional, homicide (attempt) Y08.89
overexertion X50.9 ◄

P

R

- **Radiation** (exposure to)
  - arc lamps W89.Ø
  - atomic power plant (malfunction) NEC W88.1
  - complication of or abnormal reaction to medical radiotherapy Y84.2
  - electromagnetic, ionizing W88.Ø
  - gamma rays W88.1
  - in
    - war operations (from or following nuclear explosion) —*see also* War operations
  - inadvertent exposure of patient (receiving test or therapy) Y63.3
  - infrared (heaters and lamps) W9Ø.1
    - excessive heat from W92
  - ionized, ionizing (particles, artificially accelerated)
    - radioisotopes W88.1
    - specified NEC W88.8
    - x-rays W88.Ø
  - isotopes, radioactive —*see* Radiation, radioactive isotopes
  - laser (s) W9Ø.2
    - in war operations —*see* War operations
    - misadventure in medical care Y63.2
  - light sources (man-made visible and ultraviolet) W89.9
    - natural X32
    - specified NEC W89.8
    - tanning bed W89.1
    - welding light W89.Ø
  - man-made visible light W89.9
    - specified NEC W89.8
    - tanning bed W89.1
    - welding light W89.Ø
  - microwave W9Ø.8
  - misadventure in medical or surgical procedure Y63.2
  - natural NEC X39.Ø8
    - radon X39.Ø1
  - overdose (in medical or surgical procedure) Y63.2
  - radar W9Ø.Ø
  - radioactive isotopes (any) W88.1
    - atomic power plant malfunction W88.1
    - misadventure in medical or surgical treatment Y63.2
  - radiofrequency W9Ø.Ø
  - radium NEC W88.1
  - sun X32
  - ultraviolet (light) (man-made) W89.9
    - natural X32
    - specified NEC W89.8
    - tanning bed W89.1
    - welding light W89.Ø
  - welding arc, torch, or light W89.Ø
    - excessive heat from W92
  - x-rays (hard) (soft) W88.Ø
- **Range disease** W94.11
- **Rape** (attempted) T74.2-
- **Rat bite** W53.11
- **Reaching** (prolonged) (static) X5Ø.1 ◀
- **Reaction, abnormal to medical procedure** —*see also* Complication of or following, by type of procedure Y84.9
  - with misadventure —*see* Misadventure
  - biologicals —*see* Table of Drugs and Chemicals ⬅
  - drugs —*see* Table of Drugs and Chemicals ⬅
  - vaccine —*see* Table of Drugs and Chemicals ⬅
- **Recoil**
  - airgun W34.11Ø
  - BB gun W34.11Ø
  - firearm NEC W34.19
  - gas, air or spring-operated gun NEC W34.118
  - handgun W32.1
  - hunting rifle W33.12
  - larger firearm W33.1Ø
    - specified NEC W33.19
  - machine gun W33.13
  - paintball gun W34.111
  - pellet W34.11Ø
  - shotgun W33.11
  - Very pistol [flare] W34.19
- **Reduction in**
  - atmospheric pressure —*see* Air, pressure, change
- **Rock falling on or hitting** (accidentally) (person) W2Ø.8
  - in cave-in W2Ø.Ø
- **Run over** (accidentally) (by)
  - animal (not being ridden) NEC W55.89
  - machinery —*see* Contact, with, by specified type of machine
  - transport vehicle NEC —*see also* Accident, transport VØ9.9
    - intentional homicide (attempt) YØ3.Ø
    - motor NEC VØ9.2Ø
      - intentional homicide (attempt) YØ3.Ø
- **Running**
  - before moving object X81.8
    - motor vehicle X81.Ø
- **Running off, away**
  - animal (being ridden) —*see also* Accident, transport V8Ø.918
    - not being ridden W55.89
  - animal-drawn vehicle NEC —*see also* Accident, transport V8Ø.928
  - highway, road(way), street
    - transport vehicle NEC —*see also* Accident, transport V89.9
- **Rupture pressurized devices** —*see* Explosion, by type of device

R

S

Saturnism —*see* Table of Drugs and Chemicals, lead ⬅
Scald, scalding (accidental) (by) (from) (in) X19
air (hot) X14.1
gases (hot) X14.1
homicide (attempt) —*see* Assault, burning, hot object
inflicted by other person
stated as intentional, homicide (attempt) —*see* Assault, burning, hot object
liquid (boiling) (hot) NEC X12
stated as undetermined whether accidental or intentional Y27.2
suicide (attempt) X77.2
local application of externally applied substance in medical or surgical care Y63.5
metal (molten) (liquid) (hot) NEC X18
self-inflicted X77.9
stated as undetermined whether accidental or intentional Y27.8
steam X13.1
assault X98.Ø
stated as undetermined whether accidental or intentional Y27.Ø
suicide (attempt) X77.Ø
suicide (attempt) X77.9
vapor (hot) X13.1
assault X98.Ø
stated as undetermined whether accidental or intentional Y27.Ø
suicide (attempt) X77.Ø
Scratched by
cat W55.Ø3
person (s) (accidentally) W5Ø.4
with intent to injure or kill YØ4.Ø
as, or caused by, a crowd or human stampede (with fall) W52
assault YØ4.Ø
homicide (attempt) YØ4.Ø
in
fight YØ4.Ø
legal intervention
injuring
bystander Y35.892
law enforcement personnel Y35.891
suspect Y35.893
Seasickness T75.3
Self-harm NEC —*see also* External cause by type, undetermined whether accidental or intentional
intentional —*see* Suicide
poisoning NEC —*see* Table of drugs and biologicals, accident
Self-inflicted (injury) **NEC** —*see also* External cause by type, undetermined whether accidental or intentional
intentional —*see* Suicide
poisoning NEC —*see* Table of drugs and biologicals, accident
Sequelae (of)
accident NEC —*see* WØØ-X58 with 7th character S
assault (homicidal) (any means) —*see* X92-YØ8 with 7th character S
homicide, attempt (any means) —*see* X92-YØ8 with 7th character S
injury undetermined whether accidentally or purposely inflicted —*see* Y21-Y33 with 7th character S
intentional self-harm (classifiable to X71-X83) —*see* X71-X83 with 7th character S
legal intervention (*see* with 7th character S Y35)
motor vehicle accident —*see* VØØ-V99 with 7th character S
suicide, attempt (any means) —*see* X71-X83 with 7th character S

Sequelae *(Continued)*
transport accident —*see* VØØ-V99 with 7th character S
war operations —*see* War operations
Shock
electric —*see* Exposure, electric current
from electric appliance (any) (faulty) W86.8
domestic W86.Ø
suicide (attempt) X83.1
Shooting, shot (accidental (ly)) —*see also* Discharge, firearm, by type
herself or himself —*see* Discharge, firearm by type, self-inflicted
homicide (attempt) —*see* Discharge, firearm by type, homicide
in war operations —*see* War operations
inflicted by other person —*see* Discharge, firearm by type, homicide
accidental —*see* Discharge, firearm, by type of firearm
legal
execution —*see* Legal, intervention, firearm
intervention —*see* Legal, intervention, firearm
self-inflicted —*see* Discharge, firearm by type, suicide
accidental —*see* Discharge, firearm, by type of firearm
suicide (attempt) —*see* Discharge, firearm by type, suicide
Shoving (accidentally) **by other person** —*see* Pushed, by other person ⬅
Sickness
alpine W94.11
motion —*see* Motion
mountain W94.11
Sinking (accidental)
watercraft (causing drowning, submersion) —*see also* Drowning, due to, accident to, watercraft, sinking
causing injury except drowning or submersion —*see* Accident, watercraft, causing, injury NEC ◀
Siriasis X32
Sitting (prolonged) (static) X5Ø.1 ◀
Slashed wrists —*see* Cut, self-inflicted
Slipping (accidental) (on same level) (with fall) WØ1.Ø
without fall W18.4Ø
due to
specified NEC W18.49
stepping from one level to another W18.43
stepping into hole or opening W18.42
stepping on object W18.41
on
ice WØØ.Ø
with skates —*see* Accident, transport, pedestrian, conveyance
mud WØ1.Ø
oil WØ1.Ø
snow WØØ.Ø
with skis —*see* Accident, transport, pedestrian, conveyance
surface (slippery) (wet) NEC WØ1.Ø
Sliver, wood, contact with W45.8
Smoldering (due to fire) —*see* Exposure, fire
Sodomy (attempted) **by force** T74.2-
Sound waves (causing injury) W42.9
supersonic W42.Ø
Splinter, contact with W45.8
Stab, stabbing —*see* Cut ◀
Standing (prolonged) (static) X5Ø.1 ◀
Starvation X58
Status of external cause Y99.9
child assisting in compensated work for family Y99.8
civilian activity done for financial or other compensation Y99.Ø
civilian activity done for income or pay Y99.Ø

Status of external cause *(Continued)*
family member assisting in compensated work for other family member Y99.8
hobby not done for income Y99.8
leisure activity Y99.8
military activity Y99.1
off-duty activity of military personnel Y99.8
recreation or sport not for income or while a student Y99.8
specified NEC Y99.8
student activity Y99.8
volunteer activity Y99.2
Stepped on
by
animal (not being ridden) NEC W55.89
crowd or human stampede W52
person W5Ø.Ø
Stepping on
object W22.8
with fall W18.31
sports equipment W21.9
stationary W22.Ø9
sports equipment W21.89
person W51
by crowd or human stampede W52
sports equipment W21.9
Sting
arthropod, nonvenomous W57
insect, nonvenomous W57
Storm (cataclysmic) —*see* Forces of nature, cataclysmic storm ⬅
Straining, excessive —*see also* Overexertion X5Ø.9 ⬅
Strangling —*see* Strangulation
Strangulation (accidental) —*see* category T71
Strenuous movements —*see also* Overexertion X5Ø.9 ⬅
Striking against
airbag (automobile) W22.1Ø
driver side W22.11
front passenger side W22.12
specified NEC W22.19
bottom when
diving or jumping into water (in) W16.822
causing drowning W16.821
from boat W16.722
causing drowning W16.721
natural body W16.622
causing drowning W16.821
swimming pool W16.522
causing drowning W16.521
falling into water (in) W16.322
causing drowning W16.321
fountain —*see* Striking against, bottom when, falling into water, specified NEC
natural body W16.122
causing drowning W16.121
reservoir —*see* Striking against, bottom when, falling into water, specified NEC
specified NEC W16.322
causing drowning W16.321
swimming pool W16.Ø22
causing drowning W16.Ø21
diving board (swimming-pool) W21.4
object W22.8
with
drowning or submersion —*see* Drowning
fall —*see* Fall, due to, bumping against, object
caused by crowd or human stampede (with fall) W52
furniture W22.Ø3
lamppost W22.Ø2
sports equipment W21.9
stationary W22.Ø9
sports equipment W21.89
wall W22.Ø1

Striking against *(Continued)*
person (s) W51
with fall W03
due to ice or snow WØØ.Ø
as, or caused by, a crowd or human stampede (with fall) W52
assault YØ4.2
homicide (attempt) YØ4.2
sports equipment W21.9
wall (when) W22.Ø1
diving or jumping into water (in) W16.832
causing drowning W16.831
swimming pool W16.532
causing drowning W16.531
falling into water (in) W16.332
causing drowning W16.331
fountain —*see* Striking against, wall when, falling into water, specified NEC
natural body W16.132
causing drowning W16.131
reservoir —*see* Striking against, wall when, falling into water, specified NEC
specified NEC W16.332
causing drowning W16.331
swimming pool W16.Ø32
causing drowning W16.Ø31
swimming pool (when) W22.Ø42
causing drowning W22.Ø41
diving or jumping into water W16.532
causing drowning W16.531
falling into water W16.Ø32
causing drowning W16.Ø31

Struck (accidentally) by
airbag (automobile) W22.1Ø
driver side W22.11
front passenger side W22.12
specified NEC W22.19
alligator W58.Ø2
animal (not being ridden) NEC W55.89
avalanche —*see* Landslide ◀
ball (hit) (thrown) W21.ØØ
assault YØ8.Ø9
baseball W21.Ø3
basketball W21.Ø5
football W21.Ø1
golf ball W21.Ø4
football W21.Ø1
soccer W21.Ø2
softball W21.Ø7
specified NEC W21.Ø9
volleyball W21.Ø6
bat or racquet
baseball bat W21.11
assault YØ8.Ø2
golf club W21.13
assault YØ8.Ø9
specified NEC W21.19
assault YØ8.Ø9
tennis racquet W21.12
assault YØ8.Ø9
bullet —*see also* Discharge, firearm by type
in war operations —*see* War operations
crocodile W58.12
dog W54.1
flare, Very pistol —*see* Discharge, firearm NEC
hailstones X39.8
hockey (ice)
field
puck W21.221
stick W21.211
puck W21.22Ø
stick W21.21Ø
assault YØ8.Ø1
landslide —*see* Landslide ◀
law-enforcement agent (on duty) —*see* Legal, intervention, manhandling
with blunt object —*see* Legal, intervention, blunt object

Struck by *(Continued)*
lightning —*see* subcategory T75.Ø
causing fire —*see* Exposure, fire
machine —*see* Contact, with, by type of machine
mammal NEC W55.89
marine W56.32
marine animal W56.82
missile
firearm —*see* Discharge, firearm by type
in war operations —*see* War operations, missile
object W22.8
blunt W22.8
assault YØØ
suicide (attempt) X79
undetermined whether accidental or intentional Y29
falling W2Ø.8
from, in, on
building W2Ø.1
burning (uncontrolled fire) XØØ.4
cataclysmic
earth surface movement NEC —*see* Landslide ◀
storm —*see* Forces of nature, cataclysmic storm ◀
cave-in W2Ø.Ø
earthquake X34
machine (in operation) —*see* Contact, with, by type of machine
structure W2Ø.1
burning XØØ.4
transport vehicle (in motion) —*see* Accident, transport, by type of vehicle
watercraft V93.49
due to
accident to craft V91.39
powered craft V91.33
ferry boat V91.31
fishing boat V91.32
jetskis V91.33
liner V91.31
merchant ship V91.3Ø
passenger ship V91.31
unpowered craft V91.38
canoe V91.35
inflatable V91.36
kayak V91.35
sailboat V91.34
surf-board V91.38
windsurfer V91.38
powered craft V93.43
ferry boat V93.41
fishing boat V93.42
jetskis V93.43
liner V93.41
merchant ship V93.4Ø
passenger ship V93.41
unpowered craft V93.48
sailboat V93.44
surf-board V93.48
windsurfer V93.48
moving NEC W2Ø.8
projected W2Ø.8
assault YØØ
in sports W21.9
assault YØ8.Ø9
ball W21.ØØ
baseball W21.Ø3
basketball W21.Ø5
football W21.Ø1
golf ball W21.Ø4
soccer W21.Ø2
softball W21.Ø7
specified NEC W21.Ø9
volleyball W21.Ø6
bat or racquet
baseball bat W21.11
assault YØ8.Ø2

Struck by *(Continued)*
object *(Continued)*
projected *(Continued)*
in sports *(Continued)*
bat or racquet *(Continued)*
golf club W21.13
assault YØ8.Ø9-
specified NEC W21.19
assault YØ8.Ø9
tennis racquet W21.12
assault YØ8.Ø9
hockey (ice)
field
puck W21.221
stick W21.211
puck W21.22Ø
stick W21.21Ø
assault YØ8.Ø1
specified NEC W21.89
set in motion by explosion —*see* Explosion
thrown W2Ø.8
assault YØØ
in sports W21.9
assault YØ8.Ø9
ball W21.ØØ
baseball W21.Ø3
basketball W21.Ø5
football W21.Ø1
golf ball W21.Ø4
soccer W21.Ø2
soft ball W21.Ø7
specified NEC W21.Ø9
volleyball W21.Ø6
bat or racquet
baseball bat W21.11
assault YØ8.Ø2
golf club W21.13
assault YØ8.Ø9
specified NEC W21.19
assault YØ8.Ø9
tennis racquet W21.12
assault YØ8.Ø9
hockey (ice)
field
puck W21.221
stick W21.211
puck W21.22Ø
stick W21.21Ø
assault YØ8.Ø1
specified NEC W21.89
other person (s) W5Ø.Ø
with
blunt object W22.8
intentional, homicide (attempt) YØØ
sports equipment W21.9
undetermined whether accidental or intentional Y29
fall WØ3
due to ice or snow WØØ.Ø
as, or caused by, a crowd or human stampede (with fall) W52
assault YØ4.2
homicide (attempt) YØ4.2
in legal intervention
injuring
bystander Y35.812
law enforcement personnel Y35.811
suspect Y35.813
sports equipment W21.9
police (on duty) —*see* Legal, intervention, manhandling
with blunt object —*see* Legal, intervention, blunt object
sports equipment W21.9
assault YØ8.Ø9
ball W21.ØØ
baseball W21.Ø3
basketball W21.Ø5
football W21.Ø1
golf ball W21.Ø4
soccer W21.Ø2

S

Struck by *(Continued)*
sports equipment *(Continued)*
ball *(Continued)*
soft ball W21.07
specified NEC W21.09
volleyball W21.06
bat or racquet
baseball bat W21.11
assault Y08.02
golf club W21.13
assault Y08.09
specified NEC W21.19
tennis racquet W21.12
assault Y08.09
cleats (shoe) W21.31
foot wear NEC W21.39
football helmet W21.81
hockey (ice)
field
puck W21.221
stick W21.211
puck W21.220
stick W21.210
assault Y08.01
skate blades W21.32
specified NEC W21.89
assault Y08.09
thunderbolt —*see* subcategory T75.0
causing fire —*see* Exposure, fire
transport vehicle NEC —*see also* Accident, transport V09.9
intentional, homicide (attempt) Y03.0
motor NEC —*see also* Accident, transport V09.20
homicide Y03.0
vehicle (transport) NEC —*see* Accident, transport, by type of vehicle
stationary (falling from jack, hydraulic lift, ramp) W20.8

Stumbling
without fall W18.40
due to
specified NEC W18.49
stepping from one level to another W18.43
stepping into hole or opening W18.42
stepping on object W18.41
over
animal NEC W01.0
with fall W18.09
carpet, rug or (small) object W22.8
with fall W18.09
person W51
with fall W03
due to ice or snow W00.0

Submersion (accidental) —*see* Drowning

Suffocation (accidental) (by external means) (by pressure) (mechanical) —*see also* category T71
due to, by
avalanche —*see* Landslide
explosion —*see* Explosion
fire —*see* Exposure, fire
food, any type (aspiration) (ingestion) (inhalation) —*see* categories T17 and T18
ignition —*see* Ignition
landslide —*see* Landslide
machine (ry) —*see* Contact, with, by type of machine
vomitus (aspiration) (inhalation) T17.81-
in
burning building X00.8

Suicide, suicidal (attempted) (by) X83.8
blunt object X79
burning, burns X76
hot object X77.9
fluid NEC X77.2
household appliance X77.3
specified NEC X77.8
steam X77.0
tap water X77.1
vapors X77.0
caustic substance —*see* Table of Drugs and Chemicals ⬅
cold, extreme X83.2
collision of motor vehicle with
motor vehicle X82.0
specified NEC X82.8
train X82.1
tree X82.2
crashing of aircraft X83.0
cut (any part of body) X78.9
cutting or piercing instrument X78.9
dagger X78.2
glass X78.0
knife X78.1
specified NEC X78.8
sword X78.2
drowning (in) X71.9
bathtub X71.0
natural water X71.3
specified NEC X71.8
swimming pool X71.1
following fall X71.2
electrocution X83.1
explosive (s) (material) X75
fire, flames X76
firearm X74.9
airgun X74.01
handgun X72

Suicide, suicidal *(Continued)*
firearm *(Continued)*
hunting rifle X73.1
larger X73.9
specified NEC X73.8
machine gun X73.2
shotgun X73.0
specified NEC X74.8
hanging X83.8
hot object —*see* Suicide, burning, hot object
jumping
before moving object X81.8
motor vehicle X81.0
subway train X81.1
train X81.1
from high place X80
late effect of attempt —*see* X71-X83 with 7th character S
lying before moving object, train, vehicle X81.8
poisoning —*see* Table of Drugs and Chemicals ⬅
puncture (any part of body) —*see* Suicide, cutting or piercing instrument
scald —*see* Suicide, burning, hot object
sequelae of attempt —*see* X71-X83 with 7th character S
sharp object (any) —*see* Suicide, cutting or piercing instrument
shooting —*see* Suicide, firearm
specified means NEC X83.8
stab (any part of body) —*see* Suicide, cutting or piercing instrument
steam, hot vapors X77.0
strangulation X83.8
submersion —*see* Suicide, drowning
suffocation X83.8
wound NEC X83.8

Sunstroke X32

Supersonic waves (causing injury) W42.0

Surgical procedure, complication of (delayed or as an abnormal reaction without mention of misadventure) —*see also* Complication of or following, by type of procedure
due to or as a result of misadventure —*see* Misadventure

Swallowed, swallowing
foreign body —*see* Foreign body, alimentary canal
poison —*see* Table of Drugs and Chemicals
substance
caustic or corrosive —*see* Table of Drugs and Chemicals
poisonous —*see* Table of Drugs and Chemicals

S

T

Tackle in sport WØ3
Terrorism (involving) Y38.8Ø
- biological weapons Y38.6X-
- chemical weapons Y38.7X-
- conflagration Y38.3X-
- drowning and submersion Y38.89- ◀
- explosion Y38.2X-
  - destruction of aircraft Y38.1X-
  - marine weapons Y38.ØX-
- fire Y38.3X-
- firearms Y38.4X-
- hot substances Y38.3X- ⬅
- lasers Y38.89- ◀
- nuclear weapons Y38.5X-
- piercing or stabbing instruments Y38.89- ◀
- secondary effects Y38.9X- ◀
- specified method NEC Y38.89- ⬅
- suicide bomber Y38.81- ◀

Thirst X58
Threat to breathing
- aspiration —*see* Aspiration
- due to cave-in, falling earth or substance NEC —*see* category T71

Thrown (accidentally)
- against part (any) of or object in transport vehicle (in motion) NEC —*see also* Accident, transport
- from
  - high place, homicide (attempt) YØ1
  - machinery —*see* Contact, with, by type of machine
  - transport vehicle NEC —*see also* Accident, transport V89.9
- off —*see* Thrown, from

Thunderbolt —*see* subcategory T75.Ø
- causing fire —*see* Exposure, fire

Tidal wave (any injury) NEC —*see* Forces of nature, tidal wave ⬅
Took
- overdose (drug) —*see* Table of Drugs and Chemicals ⬅
- poison —*see* Table of Drugs and Chemicals ⬅

Tornado (any injury) X37.1
Torrential rain (any injury) X37.8
Torture X58
Trampled by animal NEC W55.89
Trapped (accidentally)
- between objects (moving) (stationary and moving) —*see* Caught
- by part (any) of
  - motorcycle V29.88
  - pedal cycle V19.88
  - transport vehicle NEC —*see also* Accident, transport V89.9

Travel (effects) (sickness) T75.3
Tree falling on or hitting (accidentally) (person) W2Ø.8
Tripping
- without fall W18.4Ø
  - due to
    - specified NEC W18.49
    - stepping from one level to another W18.43
    - stepping into hole or opening W18.42
    - stepping on object W18.41
- over
  - animal WØ1.Ø
    - with fall WØ1.Ø
  - carpet, rug or (small) object W22.8
    - with fall W18.Ø9
  - person W51
    - with fall WØ3
      - due to ice or snow WØØ.Ø

Twisted by person (s) (accidentally) W5Ø.2
- with intent to injure or kill YØ4.Ø
- as, or caused by, a crowd or human stampede (with fall) W52
- assault YØ4.Ø
- homicide (attempt) YØ4.Ø
- in
  - fight YØ4.Ø
  - legal intervention —*see* Legal, intervention, manhandling

Twisting (prolonged) (static) X5Ø.1 ◀

U

Underdosing of necessary drugs, medicaments or biological substances Y63.6 ⬅
Undetermined intent (contact) (exposure)
- automobile collision Y32
- blunt object Y29
- drowning (submersion) (in) Y21.9
  - bathtub Y21.Ø
    - after fall Y21.1
  - natural water (lake) (ocean) (pond) (river) (stream) Y21.4
  - specified place NEC Y21.8
  - swimming pool Y21.2
    - after fall Y21.3
- explosive material Y25
- fall, jump or push from high place Y3Ø
- falling, lying or running before moving object Y31
- fire Y26
- firearm discharge Y24.9
  - airgun (BB) (pellet) Y24.Ø
  - handgun (pistol) (revolver) Y22
  - hunting rifle Y23.1
  - larger Y23.9
    - hunting rifle Y23.1
    - machine gun Y23.3
    - military Y23.2
    - shotgun Y23.Ø
    - specified type NEC Y23.8
  - machine gun Y23.3
  - military Y23.2
  - shotgun Y23.Ø
  - specified type NEC Y24.8
  - Very pistol Y24.8
- hot object Y27.9
  - fluid NEC Y27.2
  - household appliance Y27.3
  - specified object NEC Y27.8
  - steam Y27.Ø
  - tap water Y27.1
  - vapor Y27.Ø
- jump, fall or push from high place Y3Ø
- lying, falling or running before moving object Y31
- motor vehicle crash Y32
- push, fall or jump from high place Y3Ø
- running, falling or lying before moving object Y31
- sharp object Y28.9
  - dagger Y28.2
  - glass Y28.Ø
  - knife Y28.1
  - specified object NEC Y28.8
  - sword Y28.2
- smoke Y26
- specified event NEC Y33

Use of hand as hammer X5Ø.3 ◀

V

Vibration (causing injury) W49.9
Victim (of)
- avalanche —*see* Landslide ◀
- earth movements NEC —*see* Forces of nature, earth movement ◀
- earthquake X34
- flood —*see* Flood ◀
- landslide —*see* Landslide ◀
- lightning —*see* subcategory T75.Ø
  - causing fire —*see* Exposure, fire
- storm (cataclysmic) NEC —*see* Forces of nature, cataclysmic storm ◀
- volcanic eruption X35

Volcanic eruption (any injury) X35
Vomitus, gastric contents in air passages (with asphyxia, obstruction or suffocation) T17.81-

W

- **Walked into stationary object** (any) W22.Ø9
  - furniture W22.Ø3
  - lamppost W22.Ø2
  - wall W22.Ø1
- **War operations** (injuries to military personnel and civilians during war, civil insurrection and peacekeeping missions) (by) (from) (involving) Y36.9Ø-
  - after cessation of hostilities Y36.89-
    - explosion (of)
      - bomb placed during war operations Y36.82-
      - mine placed during war operations Y36.81-
    - specified NEC Y36.88-
  - air blast Y36.2Ø-
  - aircraft
    - destruction —*see* War operations, destruction of aircraft
  - airway restriction —*see* War operations, restriction of airways
  - asphyxiation —*see* War operations, restriction of airways
  - biological weapons Y36.6X-
  - blast Y36.2Ø-
  - blast fragments Y36.2Ø-
  - blast wave Y36.2Ø-
  - blast wind Y36.2Ø-
  - bomb Y36.2Ø-
    - dirty Y36.5Ø-
    - gasoline Y36.31-
    - incendiary Y36.31-
    - petrol Y36.31-
  - bullet Y36.43-
    - incendiary Y36.32-
    - rubber Y36.41-
  - chemical weapons Y36.7X-
  - combat
    - hand to hand (unarmed) combat Y36.44-
    - using blunt or piercing object Y36.45-
  - conflagration —*see* War operations, fire
  - conventional warfare NEC Y36.49-
  - depth-charge Y36.Ø1-
  - destruction of aircraft Y36.1Ø-
    - due to
      - air to air missile Y36.11-
      - collision with other aircraft Y36.12-
      - detonation (accidental) of onboard munitions and explosives Y36.14-
      - enemy fire or explosives Y36.11-
      - explosive placed on aircraft Y36.11-
      - onboard fire Y36.13-
      - rocket propelled grenade [RPG] Y36.11-
      - small arms fire Y36.11-
      - surface to air missile Y36.11-
    - specified NEC Y36.19-
  - detonation (accidental) of
    - onboard marine weapons Y36.Ø5-
    - own munitions or munitions launch device Y36.24-

War operations *(Continued)*

  - dirty bomb Y36.5Ø-
  - explosion (of) Y36.2Ø-
    - aerial bomb Y36.21-
    - after cessation of hostilities
      - bomb placed during war operations Y36.82-
      - mine placed during war operations Y36.81-
    - bomb NOS —*see also* War operations, bomb (s) Y36.2Ø-
    - fragments Y36.2Ø-
    - grenade Y36.29-
    - guided missile Y36.22-
    - improvised explosive device [IED] (person-borne) (roadside) (vehicle-borne) Y36.23-
    - land mine Y36.29-
    - marine mine (at sea) (in harbor) Y36.Ø2-
    - marine weapon Y36.ØØ-
      - specified NEC Y36.Ø9-
    - own munitions or munitions launch device (accidental) Y36.24-
    - sea-based artillery shell Y36.Ø3-
    - specified NEC Y36.29-
    - torpedo Y36.Ø4-
  - fire Y36.3Ø-
    - specified NEC Y36.39-
  - firearms
    - discharge Y36.43-
    - pellets Y36.42-
  - flamethrower Y36.33-
  - fragments (from) (of)
    - improvised explosive device [IED] (person-borne) (roadside) (vehicle-borne) Y36.26-
    - munitions Y36.25-
    - specified NEC Y36.29-
    - weapons Y36.27-
  - friendly fire Y36.92
  - hand to hand (unarmed) combat Y36.44-
  - hot substances —*see* War operations, fire
  - incendiary bullet Y36.32-
  - nuclear weapon (effects of) Y36.5Ø-
    - acute radiation exposure Y36.54-
    - blast pressure Y36.51-
    - direct blast Y36.51-
    - direct heat Y36.53-
    - fallout exposure Y36.54-
    - fireball Y36.53-
    - indirect blast (struck or crushed by blast debris) (being thrown by blast) Y36.52-
    - ionizing radiation (immediate exposure) Y36.54-
    - nuclear radiation Y36.54-
    - radiation
      - ionizing (immediate exposure) Y36.54-

War operations *(Continued)*

  - nuclear weapon *(Continued)*
    - radiation *(Continued)*
      - nuclear Y36.54-
      - thermal Y36.53-
    - secondary effects Y36.54-
    - specified NEC Y36.59-
    - thermal radiation Y36.53-
  - restriction of air (airway)
    - intentional Y36.46-
    - unintentional Y36.47-
  - rubber bullets Y36.41-
  - shrapnel NOS Y36.29-
  - suffocation —*see* War operations, restriction of airways
  - unconventional warfare NEC Y36.7X-
  - underwater blast NOS Y36.ØØ-
  - warfare
    - conventional NEC Y36.49-
    - unconventional NEC Y36.7X-
  - weapon of mass destruction [WMD] Y36.91
  - weapons
    - biological weapons Y36.6X-
    - chemical Y36.7X-
    - nuclear (effects of) Y36.5Ø-
      - acute radiation exposure Y36.54-
      - blast pressure Y36.51-
      - direct blast Y36.51-
      - direct heat Y36.53-
      - fallout exposure Y36.54-
      - fireball Y36.53-
      - ~~indirect blast (struck or crushed by blast debris) (being thrown by blast) Y36.52-~~
      - radiation
        - ionizing (immediate exposure) Y36.54-
        - nuclear Y36.54-
        - thermal Y36.53-
      - secondary effects Y36.54-
      - specified NEC Y36.59-
    - of mass destruction [WMD] Y36.91-
- **Washed**
  - away by flood —*see* Flood
  - off road by storm (transport vehicle) —*see* Forces of nature, cataclysmic storm
- **Weather exposure NEC** —*see* Forces of nature
- **Weightlessness** (causing injury) (effects of) (in spacecraft, real or simulated) X52
- **Work related condition** Y99.Ø
- **Wound** (accidental) NEC —*see also* Injury X58
  - battle —*see also* War operations Y36.9Ø
  - gunshot —*see* Discharge, firearm by type
- **Wreck transport vehicle NEC** —*see also* Accident, transport V89.9
- **Wrong**
  - device implanted into correct surgical site Y65.51
  - fluid in infusion Y65.1
  - patient, procedure performed on Y65.52
  - procedure (operation) on correct patient Y65.51

PART III

ICD-10-CM Tabular List of Diseases and Injuries

CHAPTER 1

CERTAIN INFECTIOUS AND PARASITIC DISEASES (AØØ-B99)

OGCR Chapter-Specific Coding Guidelines

1. **Chapter 1: Certain Infectious and Parasitic Diseases (AØØ-B99)**

a. Human Immunodeficiency Virus (HIV) Infections

1) Code only confirmed cases

Code only confirmed cases of HIV infection/illness. This is an exception to the hospital inpatient guideline Section II, H.

In this context, "confirmation" does not require documentation of positive serology or culture for HIV; the provider's diagnostic statement that the patient is HIV positive, or has an HIV-related illness is sufficient.

2) Selection and sequencing of HIV codes

(a) Patient admitted for HIV-related condition

If a patient is admitted for an HIV-related condition, the principal diagnosis should be B2Ø, Human immunodeficiency virus [HIV] disease followed by additional diagnosis codes for all reported HIV-related conditions.

(b) Patient with HIV disease admitted for unrelated condition

If a patient with HIV disease is admitted for an unrelated condition (such as a traumatic injury), the code for the unrelated condition (e.g., the nature of injury code) should be the principal diagnosis. Other diagnoses would be B2Ø followed by additional diagnosis codes for all reported HIV-related conditions.

(c) Whether the patient is newly diagnosed

Whether the patient is newly diagnosed or has had previous admissions/encounters for HIV conditions is irrelevant to the sequencing decision.

(d) Asymptomatic human immunodeficiency virus

Z21, Asymptomatic human immunodeficiency virus [HIV] infection status, is to be applied when the patient without any documentation of symptoms is listed as being "HIV positive," "known HIV," "HIV test positive," or similar terminology. Do not use this code if the term "AIDS" is used or if the patient is treated for any HIV-related illness or is described as having any condition(s) resulting from his/her HIV positive status; use B2Ø in these cases.

(e) Patients with inconclusive HIV serology

Patients with inconclusive HIV serology, but no definitive diagnosis or manifestations of the illness, may be assigned code R75, Inconclusive laboratory evidence of human immunodeficiency virus [HIV].

(f) Previously diagnosed HIV-related illness

Patients with any known prior diagnosis of an HIV-related illness should be coded to B2Ø. Once a patient has developed an HIV-related illness, the patient should always be assigned code B2Ø on every subsequent admission/encounter. Patients previously diagnosed with any HIV illness (B2Ø) should never be assigned to R75 or Z21, Asymptomatic human immunodeficiency virus [HIV] infection status.

(g) HIV Infection in Pregnancy, Childbirth and the Puerperium

During pregnancy, childbirth or the puerperium, a patient admitted (or presenting for a health care encounter) because of an HIV-related illness should receive a principal diagnosis code of O98.7-, Human immunodeficiency [HIV] disease complicating pregnancy, childbirth and the puerperium, followed by B2Ø and the code(s) for the HIV-related illness(es). Codes from Chapter 15 always take sequencing priority.

Patients with asymptomatic HIV infection status admitted (or presenting for a health care encounter) during pregnancy, childbirth, or the puerperium should receive codes of O98.7- and Z21.

(h) Encounters for testing for HIV

If a patient is being seen to determine his/her HIV status, use code Z11.4, Encounter for screening for human immunodeficiency virus [HIV]. Use additional codes for any associated high risk behavior.

If a patient with signs or symptoms is being seen for HIV testing, code the signs and symptoms. An additional counseling code Z71.7, Human immunodeficiency virus [HIV] counseling, may be used if counseling is provided during the encounter for the test.

When a patient returns to be informed of his/her HIV test results and the test result is negative, use code Z71.7, Human immunodeficiency virus [HIV] counseling.

If the results are positive, see previous guidelines and assign codes as appropriate.

b. Infectious agents as the cause of diseases classified to other chapters

Certain infections are classified in chapters other than Chapter 1 and no organism is identified as part of the infection code. In these instances, it is necessary to use an additional code from Chapter 1 to identify the organism. A code from category B95, Streptococcus, Staphylococcus, and Enterococcus as the cause of diseases classified to other chapters, B96, Other bacterial agents as the cause of diseases classified to other chapters, or B97, Viral agents as the cause of diseases classified to other chapters, is to be used as an additional code to identify the organism. An instructional note will be found at the infection code advising that an additional organism code is required.

c. Infections resistant to antibiotics

Many bacterial infections are resistant to current antibiotics. It is necessary to identify all infections documented as antibiotic resistant. Assign a code from category Z16, Resistance to antimicrobial drugs, following the infection code only if the infection code does not identify drug resistance.

d. Sepsis, Severe Sepsis, and Septic Shock

1) Coding of Sepsis and Severe Sepsis

(a) Sepsis

For a diagnosis of sepsis, assign the appropriate code for the underlying systemic infection. If the type of infection or causal organism is not further specified, assign code A41.9, Sepsis, unspecified organism.

A code from subcategory R65.2, Severe sepsis, should not be assigned unless severe sepsis or an associated acute organ dysfunction is documented.

(i) Negative or inconclusive blood cultures and sepsis
Negative or inconclusive blood cultures do not preclude a diagnosis of sepsis in patients with clinical evidence of the condition, however, the provider should be queried.

(ii) Urosepsis
The term urosepsis is a nonspecific term. It is not to be considered synonymous with sepsis. It has no default code in the Alphabetic Index. Should a provider use this term, he/she must be queried for clarification.

(iii) Sepsis with organ dysfunction
If a patient has sepsis and associated acute organ dysfunction or multiple organ dysfunction (MOD), follow the instructions for coding severe sepsis.

(iv) Acute organ dysfunction that is not clearly associated with the sepsis
If a patient has sepsis and an acute organ dysfunction, but the medical record documentation indicates that the acute organ dysfunction is related to a medical condition other than the sepsis, do not assign a code from subcategory R65.2, Severe sepsis. An acute organ dysfunction must be associated with the sepsis in order to assign the severe sepsis code. If the documentation is not clear as to whether an acute organ dysfunction is related to the sepsis or another medical condition, query the provider.

(b) Severe sepsis

The coding of severe sepsis requires a minimum of 2 codes: first a code for the underlying systemic infection, followed by a code from subcategory R65.2, Severe sepsis. If the causal organism is not documented, assign code A41.9, Sepsis, unspecified organism, for the infection. Additional code(s) for the associated acute organ dysfunction are also required.

Due to the complex nature of severe sepsis, some cases may require querying the provider prior to assignment of the codes.

2) Septic shock

(a) Septic shock generally refers to circulatory failure associated with severe sepsis, and therefore, it represents a type of acute organ dysfunction.

For all cases of septic shock, the code for the systemic infection should be sequenced first, followed by code R65.21, Severe sepsis with septic shock or code T81.12, Postprocedural septic shock. Any additional codes for the other acute organ dysfunctions should also be assigned. As noted in the sequencing instructions in the Tabular List, the code for septic shock cannot be assigned as a principal diagnosis.

3) Sequencing of severe sepsis

If severe sepsis is present on admission, and meets the definition of principal diagnosis, the underlying systemic infection should be assigned as principal diagnosis followed by the appropriate code from subcategory R65.2 as required by the sequencing rules in the Tabular List. A code from subcategory R65.2 can never be assigned as a principal diagnosis.

When severe sepsis develops during an encounter (it was not present on admission) the underlying systemic infection and the appropriate code from subcategory R65.2 should be assigned as secondary diagnoses.

Severe sepsis may be present on admission but the diagnosis may not be confirmed until sometime after admission. If the documentation is not clear whether severe sepsis was present on admission, the provider should be queried.

4) Sepsis and severe sepsis with a localized infection

If the reason for admission is both sepsis or severe sepsis and a localized infection, such as pneumonia or cellulitis, a code(s) for the underlying systemic infection should be assigned first and the code for the localized infection should be assigned as a secondary diagnosis. If the patient has severe sepsis, a code from subcategory R65.2 should also be assigned as a secondary diagnosis. If the patient is admitted with a localized infection, such as pneumonia, and sepsis/severe sepsis doesn't develop until after admission, the localized infection should be assigned first, followed by the appropriate sepsis/severe sepsis codes.

5) Sepsis due to a postprocedural infection

(a) Documentation of causal relationship

As with all postprocedural complications, code assignment is based on the provider's documentation of the relationship between the infection and the procedure.

(b) Sepsis due to a postprocedural infection

For such cases, the postprocedural infection code, such as, T8Ø.2, Infections following infusion, transfusion, and therapeutic injection, T81.4, Infection following a procedure, T88.Ø, Infection following immunization, or O86.Ø, Infection of obstetric surgical wound, should be coded first, followed by the code for the specific infection. If the patient has severe sepsis the appropriate code from subcategory R65.2 should also be assigned with the additional code(s) for any acute organ dysfunction.

(c) Postprocedural infection and postprocedural septic shock

In cases where a postprocedural infection has occurred and has resulted in severe sepsis the code for the precipitating complication such as code T81.4, Infection following a procedure, or O86.Ø, Infection of obstetrical surgical wound should be coded first followed by code R65.2Ø, Severe sepsis without septic shock. A Code for the systemic infection should also be assigned.

If a postprocedural infection has resulted in postprocedural septic shock, the code for the precipitating complication such as code T81.4, Infection following a procedure, or O86.Ø, Infection of obstetrical surgical wound should be coded first followed by code T81.12-, Postprocedural septic shock. A code for the systemic infection should also be assigned.

6) Sepsis and severe sepsis associated with a noninfectious process (condition)

In some cases a noninfectious process (condition), such as trauma, may lead to an infection which can result in sepsis or severe sepsis. If sepsis or severe sepsis is documented as associated with a noninfectious condition, such as a burn or serious injury, and this condition meets the definition for principal diagnosis, the code for the noninfectious condition should be sequenced first, followed by the code for the resulting infection. If severe sepsis is present, a code from subcategory R65.2 should also be assigned with any associated organ dysfunction(s) codes. It is not necessary to assign a code from subcategory R65.1, Systemic inflammatory response syndrome (SIRS) of non-infectious origin, for these cases.

If the infection meets the definition of principal diagnosis it should be sequenced before the non-infectious condition. When both the associated non-infectious condition and the infection meet the definition of principal diagnosis either may be assigned as principal diagnosis.

Only one code from category R65, Symptoms and signs specifically associated with systemic inflammation and infection, should be assigned. Therefore, when a non-infectious condition leads to an infection resulting in severe sepsis, assign the appropriate code from subcategory R65.2, Severe sepsis. Do not additionally assign a code from subcategory R65.1, Systemic inflammatory response syndrome (SIRS) of non-infectious origin.

See Section I.C.18. SIRS due to non-infectious process

7) Sepsis and septic shock complicating abortion, pregnancy, childbirth, and the puerperium

See Section I.C.15. Sepsis and septic shock complicating abortion, pregnancy, childbirth and the puerperium

8) Newborn sepsis

See Section I.C.16. f. Bacterial sepsis of Newborn

e. Methicillin Resistant Staphylococcus aureus (MRSA) Conditions

1) Selection and sequencing of MRSA codes

(a) Combination codes for MRSA infection

When a patient is diagnosed with an infection that is due to methicillin resistant *Staphylococcus aureus* (MRSA), and that infection has a combination code that includes the causal organism (e.g., sepsis, pneumonia) assign the appropriate combination code for the condition (e.g., code A41.Ø2, Sepsis due to Methicillin resistant Staphylococcus aureus or code J15.212, Pneumonia due to Methicillin resistant Staphylococcus aureus). Do not assign code B95.62, Methicillin resistant Staphylococcus aureus infection as the cause of diseases classified elsewhere, as an additional code because the combination code includes the type of infection and the MRSA organism. Do not assign a code from subcategory Z16.11, Resistance to penicillins, as an additional diagnosis.

See Section C.1. for instructions on coding and sequencing of sepsis and severe sepsis.

(b) Other codes for MRSA infection

When there is documentation of a current infection (e.g., wound infection, stitch abscess, urinary tract infection) due to MRSA, and that infection does not have a combination code that includes the causal organism, assign the appropriate code to identify the condition along with code B95.62, Methicillin resistant Staphylococcus aureus infection as the cause of diseases classified elsewhere for the MRSA infection. Do not assign a code from subcategory Z16.11, Resistance to penicillins.

(c) Methicillin susceptible Staphylococcus aureus (MSSA) and MRSA colonization

The condition or state of being colonized or carrying MSSA or MRSA is called colonization or carriage, while an individual person is described as being colonized or being a carrier. Colonization means that MSSA or MSRA is present on or in the body without necessarily causing illness. A positive MRSA colonization test might be documented by the provider as "MRSA screen positive" or "MRSA nasal swab positive".

Assign code Z22.322, Carrier or suspected carrier of Methicillin resistant Staphylococcus aureus, for patients documented as having MRSA colonization. Assign code Z22.321, Carrier or suspected carrier of Methicillin susceptible Staphylococcus aureus, for patient documented as having MSSA colonization. Colonization is not necessarily indicative of a disease process or as the cause of a specific condition the patient may have unless documented as such by the provider.

(d) MRSA colonization and infection

If a patient is documented as having both MRSA colonization and infection during a hospital admission, code Z22.322, Carrier or suspected carrier of Methicillin resistant Staphylococcus aureus, and a code for the MRSA infection may both be assigned.

f. Zika virus infections

1) Code only confirmed cases

Code only a confirmed diagnosis of Zika virus (A92.5, Zika virus disease) as documented by the provider. This is an exception to the hospital inpatient guideline Section II, H.

In this context, "confirmation" does not require documentation of the type of test performed; the physician's diagnostic statement that the condition is confirmed is sufficient. This code should be assigned regardless of the stated mode of transmission.

If the provider documents "suspected", "possible" or "probable" Zika, do not assign code A92.5. Assign a code(s) explaining the reason for encounter (such as fever, rash, or joint pain) or Z2Ø.828, Contact with and (suspected) exposure to other viral communicable diseases.

CHAPTER 1

CERTAIN INFECTIOUS AND PARASITIC DISEASES (A00-B99)

Includes diseases generally recognized as communicable or transmissible

Use additional code to identify resistance to antimicrobial drugs (Z16.-)

Excludes1 certain localized infections - see body system-related chapters

Excludes2 carrier or suspected carrier of infectious disease (Z22.-)
infectious and parasitic diseases complicating pregnancy, childbirth and the puerperium (O98.-)
infectious and parasitic diseases specific to the perinatal period (P35-P39)
influenza and other acute respiratory infections (J00-J22)

This chapter contains the following blocks:

A00-A09	Intestinal infectious diseases
A15-A19	Tuberculosis
A20-A28	Certain zoonotic bacterial diseases
A30-A49	Other bacterial diseases
A50-A64	Infections with a predominantly sexual mode of transmission
A65-A69	Other spirochetal diseases
A70-A74	Other diseases caused by chlamydiae
A75-A79	Rickettsioses
A80-A89	Viral and prion infections of the central nervous system
A90-A99	Arthropod-borne viral fevers and viral hemorrhagic fevers
B00-B09	Viral infections characterized by skin and mucous membrane lesions
B10	Other human herpesviruses
B15-B19	Viral hepatitis
B20	Human immunodeficiency virus [HIV] disease
B25-B34	Other viral diseases
B35-B49	Mycoses
B50-B64	Protozoal diseases
B65-B83	Helminthiases
B85-B89	Pediculosis, acariasis and other infestations
B90-B94	Sequelae of infectious and parasitic diseases
B95-B97	Bacterial and viral infectious agents
B99	Other infectious diseases

INTESTINAL INFECTIOUS DISEASES (A00-A09)

● **A00 Cholera**
A serious, often deadly, infectious disease of the small intestine

A00.0 Cholera due to Vibrio cholerae 01, biovar cholerae
Classical cholera

A00.1 Cholera due to Vibrio cholerae 01, biovar eltor
Cholera eltor

A00.9 Cholera, unspecified

● **A01 Typhoid and paratyphoid fevers**
Caused by Salmonella typhi and Salmonella paratyphi A, B, and C bacteria

● **A01.0 Typhoid fever**
Infection due to Salmonella typhi

A01.00 Typhoid fever, unspecified

A01.01 Typhoid meningitis

A01.02 Typhoid fever with heart involvement
Typhoid endocarditis
Typhoid myocarditis

A01.03 Typhoid pneumonia

A01.04 Typhoid arthritis

A01.05 Typhoid osteomyelitis

A01.09 Typhoid fever with other complications

A01.1 Paratyphoid fever A

A01.2 Paratyphoid fever B

A01.3 Paratyphoid fever C

A01.4 Paratyphoid fever, unspecified
Infection due to Salmonella paratyphi NOS

● **A02 Other salmonella infections**

Includes infection or foodborne intoxication due to any Salmonella species other than S. typhi and S. paratyphi

A02.0 Salmonella enteritis
Salmonellosis

A02.1 Salmonella sepsis

● **A02.2 Localized salmonella infections**

A02.20 Localized salmonella infection, unspecified
Specified in the documentation as localized, but unspecified as to type

A02.21 Salmonella meningitis
Specified as localized in the meninges

A02.22 Salmonella pneumonia
Specified as localized in the lungs

A02.23 Salmonella arthritis
Specified as localized in the joints

A02.24 Salmonella osteomyelitis
Specified as localized in bone

A02.25 Salmonella pyelonephritis
Salmonella tubulo-interstitial nephropathy

A02.29 Salmonella with other localized infection
Specified as localized (because it is still under localized heading) but does not assign into any of the above codes

A02.8 Other specified salmonella infections
Any specified salmonella infection which does NOT assign into any of the above codes (not specified as localized)

A02.9 Salmonella infection, unspecified
Unspecified in the documentation as to specific type of salmonella

● **A03 Shigellosis**
An infectious disease caused by bacteria (Shigella)

A03.0 Shigellosis due to Shigella dysenteriae
Group A shigellosis [Shiga-Kruse dysentery]

A03.1 Shigellosis due to Shigella flexneri
Group B shigellosis

A03.2 Shigellosis due to Shigella boydii
Group C shigellosis

A03.3 Shigellosis due to Shigella sonnei
Group D shigellosis

A03.8 Other shigellosis

A03.9 Shigellosis, unspecified
Bacillary dysentery NOS

Item 1-1 Salmonella is a bacterium that lives in the intestines of fowl and mammals and can spread to humans through improper food preparation and cooking. Salmonellosis is an infection with the bacterium. Symptoms include diarrhea, fever, and abdominal cramps 12 to 72 hours after infection. The illness usually lasts 4 to 7 days, and most persons recover without treatment. The diarrhea may be so severe that the patient needs to be hospitalized. Patients with immunocompromised systems in chronic, ill health are more likely to have the infection invade their bloodstream with life-threatening results. For example, patients with sickle cell disease are more prone to salmonella osteomyelitis than others.

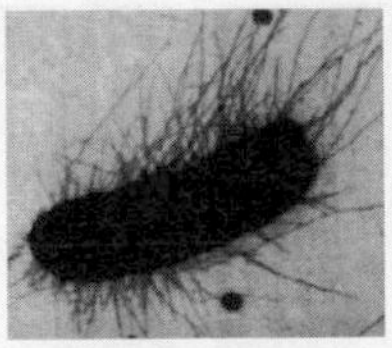

Figure 1-1 Electron micrograph of escherichia coli (E. coli) expressing P fimbriae. (From Mandell, Bennett, & Dolin: Principles and Practice of Infectious Diseases, ed 7, Churchill Livingstone, An Imprint of Elsevier, 2009)

Item 1-2 ***Escherichia coli [E. coli]*** is a gram-negative bacterium found in the intestinal tracts of humans and animals and is usually nonpathogenic. Pathogenic strains can cause diarrhea or pyogenic (pus-producing) infections. Can be a threat to food safety.

● **AØ4 Other bacterial intestinal infections**
Excludes1 bacterial foodborne intoxications, NEC (AØ5.-)
tuberculous enteritis (A18.32)

AØ4.Ø Enteropathogenic Escherichia coli infection
Pertaining to or producing intestinal disease

AØ4.1 Enterotoxigenic Escherichia coli infection
Producing or containing intestinal toxin

AØ4.2 Enteroinvasive Escherichia coli infection
Capable of penetrating and spreading through intestinal mucosal epithelium

AØ4.3 Enterohemorrhagic Escherichia coli infection
Causing bloody diarrhea, resulting from microorganisms

AØ4.4 Other intestinal Escherichia coli infections
Escherichia coli enteritis NOS

AØ4.5 Campylobacter enteritis
Spiral shaped bacterium

AØ4.6 Enteritis due to Yersinia enterocolitica
Excludes1 extraintestinal yersiniosis (A28.2)
Transmitted by infected food /water and person-to-person contact, affecting intestinal tract

AØ4.7 Enterocolitis due to Clostridium difficile
Foodborne intoxication by Clostridium difficile
Pseudomembraneous colitis
Marked by fibrinous deposit (false membrane) with enmeshed necrotic cells

AØ4.8 Other specified bacterial intestinal infections

AØ4.9 Bacterial intestinal infection, unspecified
Bacterial enteritis NOS

● **AØ5 Other bacterial foodborne intoxications, not elsewhere classified**
Excludes1 Clostridium difficile foodborne intoxication and infection (AØ4.7)
Escherichia coli infection (AØ4.Ø-AØ4.4)
listeriosis (A32.-)
salmonella foodborne intoxication and infection (AØ2.-)
toxic effect of noxious foodstuffs (T61-T62)

AØ5.Ø Foodborne staphylococcal intoxication

AØ5.1 Botulism food poisoning
Botulism NOS
Classical foodborne intoxication due to Clostridium botulinum
Excludes1 infant botulism (A48.51)
wound botulism (A48.52)

AØ5.2 Foodborne Clostridium perfringens [Clostridium welchii] intoxication
Type A causes gas gangrene and necrotizing colitis; major cause of food poisoning in humans
Enteritis necroticans
Pig-bel

AØ5.3 Foodborne Vibrio parahaemolyticus intoxication
Organism that survives only in high salt environment (halophilic), major cause of gastroenteritis due to consumption of raw or improperly cooked fish/seafood

AØ5.4 Foodborne Bacillus cereus intoxication
Spore-forming species commonly found in soil, causes food poisoning from formation of intestinal toxins in contaminated foods

AØ5.5 Foodborne Vibrio vulnificus intoxication
Species that survives in high salt environment (halophilic) with infection by eating raw seafood causes septicemia and cellulitis

AØ5.8 Other specified bacterial foodborne intoxications

AØ5.9 Bacterial foodborne intoxication, unspecified

● **AØ6 Amebiasis**
An intestinal illness caused by the microscopic parasite Entamoeba histolytica
Includes infection due to Entamoeba histolytica
Excludes1 other protozoal intestinal diseases (AØ7.-)
Excludes2 acanthamebiasis (B6Ø.1-)
Naegleriasis (B6Ø.2)

AØ6.Ø Acute amebic dysentery
Acute amebiasis
Intestinal amebiasis NOS

AØ6.1 Chronic intestinal amebiasis

AØ6.2 Amebic nondysenteric colitis
Pertaining to single cell microorganism

AØ6.3 Ameboma of intestine
Tumorlike mass produced by localized inflammation often in intestine
Ameboma NOS

AØ6.4 Amebic liver abscess
Hepatic amebiasis

AØ6.5 Amebic lung abscess
Amebic abscess of lung (and liver)

AØ6.6 Amebic brain abscess
Amebic abscess of brain (and liver) (and lung)

AØ6.7 Cutaneous amebiasis

● **AØ6.8 Amebic infection of other sites**

AØ6.81 Amebic cystitis

AØ6.82 Other amebic genitourinary infections
Amebic balanitis
Amebic vesiculitis
Amebic vulvovaginitis

AØ6.89 Other amebic infections
Amebic appendicitis
Amebic splenic abscess

AØ6.9 Amebiasis, unspecified

● **AØ7 Other protozoal intestinal diseases**

AØ7.Ø Balantidiasis
Balantidial dysentery
Infection by protozoa that may cause diarrhea and dysentery, with ulceration of colonic mucous membranes

AØ7.1 Giardiasis [lambliasis]
Common infection in small intestine spread by contaminated food, water, or direct person-to-person contact

AØ7.2 Cryptosporidiosis
Human infection with protozoa usually seen as self-limited diarrhea in those who work with cattle

AØ7.3 Isosporiasis
Human intestinal disease caused by protozoa
Infection due to Isospora belli and Isospora hominis
Intestinal coccidiosis
Isosporosis

AØ7.4 Cyclosporiasis
Infection by protozoa with most common species infecting humans being C cayetanensis

A07.8 **Other specified protozoal intestinal diseases**
Intestinal microsporidiosis
Intestinal trichomoniasis
Sarcocystosis
Sarcosporidiosis

A07.9 **Protozoal intestinal disease, unspecified**
Flagellate diarrhea
Protozoal colitis
Protozoal diarrhea
Protozoal dysentery

● **A08 Viral and other specified intestinal infections**
Excludes1 influenza with involvement of gastrointestinal tract (J09.X3, J10.2, J11.2)

A08.0 **Rotaviral enteritis**

● A08.1 **Acute gastroenteropathy due to Norwalk agent and other small round viruses**

A08.11 **Acute gastroenteropathy due to Norwalk agent**
Acute gastroenteropathy due to Norovirus
Acute gastroenteropathy due to Norwalk-like agent

A08.19 **Acute gastroenteropathy due to other small round viruses**
Acute gastroenteropathy due to small round virus [SRV] NOS

A08.2 **Adenoviral enteritis**

● A08.3 **Other viral enteritis**

A08.31 **Calicivirus enteritis**

A08.32 **Astrovirus enteritis**

A08.39 **Other viral enteritis**
Coxsackie virus enteritis
Echovirus enteritis
Enterovirus enteritis NEC
Torovirus enteritis

A08.4 **Viral intestinal infection, unspecified**
Viral enteritis NOS
Viral gastroenteritis NOS
Viral gastroenteropathy NOS

A08.8 **Other specified intestinal infections**

A09 Infectious gastroenteritis and colitis, unspecified
Infectious colitis NOS
Infectious enteritis NOS
Infectious gastroenteritis NOS
Excludes1 colitis NOS (K52.9)
diarrhea NOS (R19.7)
enteritis NOS (K52.9)
gastroenteritis NOS (K52.9)
noninfective gastroenteritis and colitis, unspecified (K52.9)

TUBERCULOSIS (A15-A19)

Includes infections due to Mycobacterium tuberculosis and Mycobacterium bovis

Excludes1 congenital tuberculosis (P37.0)
nonspecific reaction to test for tuberculosis without active tuberculosis (R76.1-)
pneumoconiosis associated with tuberculosis, any type in A15 (J65)
positive PPD (R76.11)
positive tuberculin skin test without active tuberculosis (R76.11)
sequelae of tuberculosis (B90.-)
silicotuberculosis (J65)

● **A15 Respiratory tuberculosis**

A15.0 **Tuberculosis of lung**
Tuberculous bronchiectasis
Chronic dilatation of bronchi
Tuberculous fibrosis of lung
Tuberculous pneumonia
Tuberculous pneumothorax

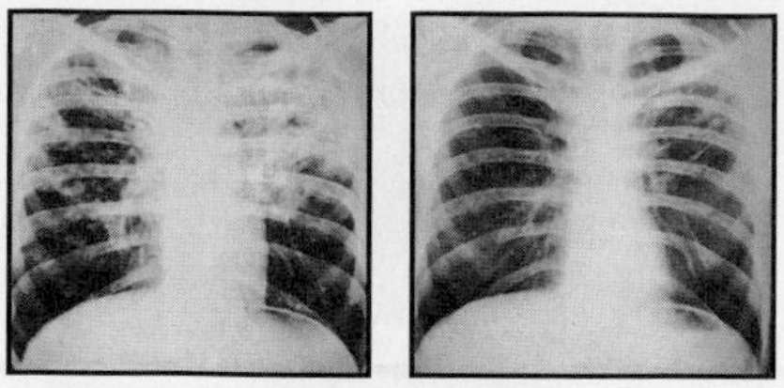

Figure 1-2 Far advanced bilateral pulmonary tuberculosis before and after 8 months of treatment with streptomycin, PAS, and isoniazid. (From Hinshaw HC, Garland LH: Diseases of the Chest, ed 4, Philadelphia, WB Saunders, 1980)

Item 1–3 Tuberculosis is a common and deadly infectious disease caused by the *Mycobacterium tuberculosis* organism. The first tuberculosis infection is called the **primary infection** and most commonly attacks the lungs but can affect the central nervous system, lymphatic system, circulatory system, genitourinary system, bones, joints, and even the skin. A **Ghon** lesion is the **initial lesion.** A **secondary lesion** occurs when the tubercle bacilli are carried to other areas.

Item 1–4 Although it primarily affects the lungs, the bacteria ***Mycobacterium tuberculosis*** can travel from the pulmonary circulation to virtually any organ in the body, much as a cancer metastasizes to a secondary site. If the immune system becomes compromised by age or disease, what would otherwise be a self-limiting primary tuberculosis in the lungs will develop in other organs. These are known as extrapulmonary sites.

A15.4 **Tuberculosis of intrathoracic lymph nodes**
Tuberculosis of hilar lymph nodes
Tuberculosis of mediastinal lymph nodes
Tuberculosis of tracheobronchial lymph nodes
Excludes1 tuberculosis specified as primary (A15.7)

A15.5 **Tuberculosis of larynx, trachea and bronchus**
Tuberculosis of bronchus
Tuberculosis of glottis
Tuberculosis of larynx
Tuberculosis of trachea

A15.6 **Tuberculous pleurisy**
Tuberculosis of pleura
Tuberculous empyema
Excludes1 primary respiratory tuberculosis (A15.7)

A15.7 **Primary respiratory tuberculosis**

A15.8 **Other respiratory tuberculosis**
Mediastinal tuberculosis
Nasopharyngeal tuberculosis
Tuberculosis of nose
Tuberculosis of sinus [any nasal]

A15.9 **Respiratory tuberculosis unspecified**

● **A17 Tuberculosis of nervous system**

A17.0 **Tuberculous meningitis**
Tuberculosis of meninges (cerebral) (spinal)
Tuberculous leptomeningitis
Excludes1 tuberculous meningoencephalitis (A17.82)

A17.1 **Meningeal tuberculoma**
Tuberculoma of meninges (cerebral) (spinal)
Excludes2 tuberculoma of brain and spinal cord (A17.81)

● **A17.8 Other tuberculosis of nervous system**

A17.81 Tuberculoma of brain and spinal cord
Tuberculous abscess of brain and spinal cord

A17.82 Tuberculous meningoencephalitis
Inflammation of brain and meninges; AKA cerebromeningitis and encephalomeningitis
Tuberculous myelitis

A17.83 Tuberculous neuritis
Tuberculous mononeuropathy

A17.89 Other tuberculosis of nervous system
Tuberculous polyneuropathy

A17.9 Tuberculosis of nervous system, unspecified

● **A18 Tuberculosis of other organs**

● **A18.0 Tuberculosis of bones and joints**

A18.01 Tuberculosis of spine
Pott's disease or curvature of spine
Tuberculous arthritis
Tuberculous osteomyelitis of spine
Tuberculous spondylitis

A18.02 Tuberculous arthritis of other joints
Tuberculosis of hip (joint)
Tuberculosis of knee (joint)

A18.03 Tuberculosis of other bones
Tuberculous mastoiditis
Tuberculous osteomyelitis

A18.09 Other musculoskeletal tuberculosis
Tuberculous myositis
Tuberculous synovitis
Tuberculous tenosynovitis

● **A18.1 Tuberculosis of genitourinary system**

A18.10 Tuberculosis of genitourinary system, unspecified

A18.11 Tuberculosis of kidney and ureter

A18.12 Tuberculosis of bladder

A18.13 Tuberculosis of other urinary organs
Tuberculous urethritis

A18.14 Tuberculosis of prostate

A18.15 Tuberculosis of other male genital organs

A18.16 Tuberculosis of cervix

A18.17 Tuberculous female pelvic inflammatory disease
Tuberculous endometritis
Tuberculous oophoritis and salpingitis
Oophoritis = inflammation of ovary
Salpingitis = inflammation of fallopian tube

A18.18 Tuberculosis of other female genital organs
Tuberculous ulceration of vulva

A18.2 Tuberculous peripheral lymphadenopathy
Tuberculous adenitis
Excludes2 tuberculosis of bronchial and mediastinal lymph nodes (A15.4)
tuberculosis of mesenteric and retroperitoneal lymph nodes (A18.39)
tuberculous tracheobronchial adenopathy (A15.4)

● **A18.3 Tuberculosis of intestines, peritoneum and mesenteric glands**

A18.31 Tuberculous peritonitis
Tuberculous ascites

A18.32 Tuberculous enteritis
Tuberculosis of anus and rectum
Tuberculosis of intestine (large) (small)

A18.39 Retroperitoneal tuberculosis
Tuberculosis of mesenteric glands
Tuberculosis of retroperitoneal (lymph glands)

A18.4 Tuberculosis of skin and subcutaneous tissue
Erythema induratum, tuberculous
Lupus excedens
Lupus vulgaris NOS
Lupus vulgaris of eyelid
Cutaneous tuberculosis characterized by reddish brown plaque on skin surrounded by papules and nodules
Scrofuloderma
Type of cutaneous tuberculosis, with direct extension of tuberculosis into skin from underlying structures; AKA tuberculosis colliquativa
Tuberculosis of external ear
Excludes2 lupus erythematosus (L93.-)
lupus NOS (M32.9)
systemic (M32.-)

● **A18.5 Tuberculosis of eye**
Excludes2 lupus vulgaris of eyelid (A18.4)

A18.50 Tuberculosis of eye, unspecified

A18.51 Tuberculous episcleritis
Inflammation of episclera and adjacent tissues

A18.52 Tuberculous keratitis
Tuberculous interstitial keratitis
Tuberculous keratoconjunctivitis (interstitial) (phlyctenular)
Inflammation of cornea and conjunctiva

A18.53 Tuberculous chorioretinitis
Inflammation of choroid and retina; retinochoroiditis

A18.54 Tuberculous iridocyclitis
Inflammation of iris and ciliary body

A18.59 Other tuberculosis of eye
Tuberculous conjunctivitis

A18.6 Tuberculosis of (inner) (middle) ear
Tuberculous otitis media
Excludes2 tuberculosis of external ear (A18.4)
tuberculous mastoiditis (A18.03)

A18.7 Tuberculosis of adrenal glands
Tuberculous Addison's disease

● **A18.8 Tuberculosis of other specified organs**

A18.81 Tuberculosis of thyroid gland

A18.82 Tuberculosis of other endocrine glands
Tuberculosis of pituitary gland
Tuberculosis of thymus gland

A18.83 Tuberculosis of digestive tract organs, not elsewhere classified
Excludes1 tuberculosis of intestine (A18.32)

A18.84 Tuberculosis of heart
Tuberculous cardiomyopathy
Tuberculous endocarditis
Tuberculous myocarditis
Tuberculous pericarditis

A18.85 Tuberculosis of spleen

A18.89 Tuberculosis of other sites
Tuberculosis of muscle
Tuberculous cerebral arteritis

● **A19 Miliary tuberculosis**
Includes disseminated tuberculosis
generalized tuberculosis
tuberculous polyserositis

A19.0 Acute miliary tuberculosis of a single specified site

A19.1 Acute miliary tuberculosis of multiple sites

A19.2 Acute miliary tuberculosis, unspecified

A19.8 Other miliary tuberculosis

A19.9 Miliary tuberculosis, unspecified

Item 1-5 Miliary tuberculosis can be a life-threatening condition. If a tuberculous lesion enters a blood vessel, immense dissemination of tuberculous organisms can occur if the immune system is weak. High-risk populations—children under 4 years of age, the elderly, or the immunocompromised—are particularly prone to this type of infection. The lesions will have a millet seedlike appearance on chest x-ray. Bronchial washings and biopsy may aid in diagnosis.

CHAPTER 1 (A00-B99)

CERTAIN ZOONOTIC BACTERIAL DISEASES (A20-A28)

● **A20 Plague**
Infectious disease caused by a Yersinia pestis bacterium, transmitted by a rodent flea bite or handling of infected animal
Includes infection due to Yersinia pestis
- **A20.0 Bubonic plague**
- **A20.1 Cellulocutaneous plague**
  Skin and subcutaneous tissue plague
- **A20.2 Pneumonic plague**
- **A20.3 Plague meningitis**
- **A20.7 Septicemic plague**
- **A20.8 Other forms of plague**
  Abortive plague
  Asymptomatic plague
  Pestis minor
  Systemic bacterial disease
- **A20.9 Plague, unspecified**

● **A21 Tularemia**
Caused by Francisella tularensis bacterium found in rodents, rabbits, and hares and transmitted to humans by contact with infected animal tissues or by ticks, biting flies, or mosquitoes
Includes deer-fly fever
infection due to Francisella tularensis
rabbit fever
- **A21.0 Ulceroglandular tularemia**
  Most common form of tularemia in humans is painful, swollen, erythematous papule at point of inoculation that ruptures to form shallow ulcer
- **A21.1 Oculoglandular tularemia**
  Primary site of entry is conjunctival sac, results in granulomatous corneal lesions
  Ophthalmic tularemia
- **A21.2 Pulmonary tularemia**
- **A21.3 Gastrointestinal tularemia**
  Abdominal tularemia
- **A21.7 Generalized tularemia**
- **A21.8 Other forms of tularemia**
- **A21.9 Tularemia, unspecified**

● **A22 Anthrax**
An acute infectious disease caused by the spore-forming Bacillus anthracis; occurs in humans exposed to infected animals or tissue from infected animals
Includes infection due to Bacillus anthracis
- **A22.0 Cutaneous anthrax**
  Malignant carbuncle
  Malignant pustule
- **A22.1 Pulmonary anthrax**
  Inhalation anthrax
  Ragpicker's disease
  Woolsorter's disease
- **A22.2 Gastrointestinal anthrax**
- **A22.7 Anthrax sepsis**
  Infectious bacterial disease
- **A22.8 Other forms of anthrax**
  Anthrax meningitis
- **A22.9 Anthrax, unspecified**

Item 1-6 Brucellosis: An infectious disease caused by the bacterium Brucella. Humans are infected by contact with contaminated animals or animal products. In humans brucellosis symptoms that are similar to the flu include fever, sweats, headaches, back pains, and physical weakness. Severe infections of the central nervous system or lining of the heart may occur. Brucellosis can also cause chronic symptoms that include recurrent fevers, joint pain, and fatigue.

● **A23 Brucellosis**
Includes Malta fever
Mediterranean fever
undulant fever
- **A23.0 Brucellosis due to Brucella melitensis**
  Resulting in flu-like symptoms that may lead to chronic symptoms that include recurrent fevers, joint pain, and fatigue
- **A23.1 Brucellosis due to Brucella abortus**
  Most common cause of brucellosis in humans; AKA Bang bacillus
- **A23.2 Brucellosis due to Brucella suis**
  Species found primarily in pigs, rabbits, and reindeer
- **A23.3 Brucellosis due to Brucella canis**
  Species that causes respiratory tract infection in humans
- **A23.8 Other brucellosis**
- **A23.9 Brucellosis, unspecified**

● **A24 Glanders and melioidosis**
Infection, usually of rodents, which spreads to other animals and humans, caused by Burkholderia pseudomallei through break in skin contaminated with infested soil or water
- **A24.0 Glanders**
  Infection due to Pseudomonas mallei
  Malleus
- **A24.1 Acute and fulminating melioidosis**
  Melioidosis pneumonia
  Melioidosis sepsis
- **A24.2 Subacute and chronic melioidosis**
- **A24.3 Other melioidosis**
- **A24.9 Melioidosis, unspecified**
  Infection due to Pseudomonas pseudomallei NOS
  Whitmore's disease

● **A25 Rat-bite fevers**
RBF, infectious disease caused by Streptobacillus moniliformis or Spirillum minus.
- **A25.0 Spirillosis**
  Any disease condition caused by spirilla
  Sodoku
- **A25.1 Streptobacillosis**
  Acute, febrile human illness caused by bacteria transmitted by rats in most cases, passed from rodent to human via rodent's urine or mucous secretions; AKA rat fever
  Epidemic arthritic erythema
  Haverhill fever
  Streptobacillary rat-bite fever
- **A25.9 Rat-bite fever, unspecified**

● **A26 Erysipeloid**
Infection with Erysipelothrix rhusiopathiae, occurring often as occupational disease resulting from handling infected fish, shellfish, meat, or poultry
- **A26.0 Cutaneous erysipeloid**
  Erythema migrans
- **A26.7 Erysipelothrix sepsis**
- **A26.8 Other forms of erysipeloid**
- **A26.9 Erysipeloid, unspecified**

● **A27 Leptospirosis**
Occurs most commonly in the tropics
A27.0 Leptospirosis icterohemorrhagica
Leptospiral or spirochetal jaundice (hemorrhagic)
Weil's disease
● **A27.8 Other forms of leptospirosis**
A27.81 Aseptic meningitis in leptospirosis
A27.89 Other forms of leptospirosis
A27.9 Leptospirosis, unspecified

● **A28 Other zoonotic bacterial diseases, not elsewhere classified**
A28.0 Pasteurellosis
Infection of humans or other animals by species of Pasteurella
A28.1 Cat-scratch disease
Cat-scratch fever
A28.2 Extraintestinal yersiniosis
Infection from Yersinia enterocolitica; *AKA enteric yersiniosis, intestinal yersiniosis, Yersinia enteritis*
Excludes1 enteritis due to Yersinia enterocolitica (A04.6)
plague (A20.-)
A28.8 Other specified zoonotic bacterial diseases, not elsewhere classified
A28.9 Zoonotic bacterial disease, unspecified

OTHER BACTERIAL DISEASES (A30-A49)

● **A30 Leprosy [Hansen's disease]**
Chronic infectious disease attacking the skin, peripheral nerves, and mucous membranes
Includes infection due to Mycobacterium leprae
Excludes1 sequelae of leprosy (B92)
A30.0 Indeterminate leprosy
I leprosy
A30.1 Tuberculoid leprosy
TT leprosy
A30.2 Borderline tuberculoid leprosy
BT leprosy
A30.3 Borderline leprosy
BB leprosy
A30.4 Borderline lepromatous leprosy
BL leprosy
A30.5 Lepromatous leprosy
LL leprosy
A30.8 Other forms of leprosy
A30.9 Leprosy, unspecified

● **A31 Infection due to other mycobacteria**
Excludes2 leprosy (A30.-)
tuberculosis (A15-A19)
A31.0 Pulmonary mycobacterial infection
Infection due to Mycobacterium avium
Infection due to Mycobacterium intracellulare [Battey bacillus]
Infection due to Mycobacterium kansasii
A31.1 Cutaneous mycobacterial infection
Buruli ulcer
Infection due to Mycobacterium marinum
Infection due to Mycobacterium ulcerans
A31.2 Disseminated mycobacterium avium-intracellulare complex (DMAC)
MAC sepsis
A31.8 Other mycobacterial infections
A31.9 Mycobacterial infection, unspecified
Atypical mycobacterial infection NOS
Mycobacteriosis NOS

● **A32 Listeriosis**
Infection caused by Listeria monocytogenes
Includes listerial foodborne infection
Excludes1 neonatal (disseminated) listeriosis (P37.2)
A32.0 Cutaneous listeriosis
● **A32.1 Listerial meningitis and meningoencephalitis**
A32.11 Listerial meningitis
A32.12 Listerial meningoencephalitis
A32.7 Listerial sepsis
● **A32.8 Other forms of listeriosis**
A32.81 Oculoglandular listeriosis
Primary infection site is conjunctival sac, which if untreated may result in perforation of cornea and optic atrophy
A32.82 Listerial endocarditis
Exudative and proliferative inflammatory condition of endocardium caused by listeria bacteria
A32.89 Other forms of listeriosis
Listerial cerebral arteritis
A32.9 Listeriosis, unspecified

A33 Tetanus neonatorum
Neonate = newborn

A34 Obstetrical tetanus

A35 Other tetanus
Tetanus NOS
Excludes1 tetanus neonatorum (A33)
obstetrical tetanus (A34)

● **A36 Diphtheria**
A36.0 Pharyngeal diphtheria
Diphtheritic membranous angina
Tonsillar diphtheria
A36.1 Nasopharyngeal diphtheria
A36.2 Laryngeal diphtheria
Diphtheritic laryngotracheitis
A36.3 Cutaneous diphtheria
Excludes2 erythrasma (L08.1)
● **A36.8 Other diphtheria**
A36.81 Diphtheritic cardiomyopathy
Diphtheritic myocarditis
A36.82 Diphtheritic radiculomyelitis
A36.83 Diphtheritic polyneuritis
A36.84 Diphtheritic tubulo-interstitial nephropathy
A36.85 Diphtheritic cystitis
A36.86 Diphtheritic conjunctivitis
A36.89 Other diphtheritic complications
Diphtheritic peritonitis
A36.9 Diphtheria, unspecified

Item 1-7 Diptheria: A highly contagious bacterial disease that results in the formation of an adherent membrane in the throat that may lead to suffocation. In its most poisonous form, it attacks the heart and lungs. It is spread by direct physical contact or breathing the aerosolized secretions of infected individuals. The exact location is specified in the codes.

● **A37 Whooping cough**
Pertussis is a highly contagious disease caused by the bacterium Bordetella pertussis and results in a whooping sounding cough.
● **A37.0 Whooping cough due to Bordetella pertussis**
A37.00 Whooping cough due to Bordetella pertussis without pneumonia
A37.01 Whooping cough due to Bordetella pertussis with pneumonia
● **A37.1 Whooping cough due to Bordetella parapertussis**
A37.10 Whooping cough due to Bordetella parapertussis without pneumonia
A37.11 Whooping cough due to Bordetella parapertussis with pneumonia
● **A37.8 Whooping cough due to other Bordetella species**
A37.80 Whooping cough due to other Bordetella species without pneumonia
A37.81 Whooping cough due to other Bordetella species with pneumonia
● **A37.9 Whooping cough, unspecified species**
A37.90 Whooping cough, unspecified species without pneumonia
A37.91 Whooping cough, unspecified species with pneumonia

● **A38 Scarlet fever**
Most commonly caused by the bacteria Streptococcus pneumoniae and Neisseria meningitides
Includes scarlatina
Excludes2 streptococcal sore throat (J02.0)
A38.0 Scarlet fever with otitis media
A38.1 Scarlet fever with myocarditis
A38.8 Scarlet fever with other complications
A38.9 Scarlet fever, uncomplicated
Scarlet fever, NOS

● **A39 Meningococcal infection**
Most commonly caused by the bacteria Streptococcus pneumoniae and Neisseria meningitides
A39.0 Meningococcal meningitis
A39.1 Waterhouse-Friderichsen syndrome
Fulminating complication of meningococcemia
Meningococcal hemorrhagic adrenalitis
Meningococcic adrenal syndrome
A39.2 Acute meningococcemia
A39.3 Chronic meningococcemia
A39.4 Meningococcemia, unspecified
● **A39.5 Meningococcal heart disease**
A39.50 Meningococcal carditis, unspecified
A39.51 Meningococcal endocarditis
A39.52 Meningococcal myocarditis
A39.53 Meningococcal pericarditis
● **A39.8 Other meningococcal infections**
A39.81 Meningococcal encephalitis
A39.82 Meningococcal retrobulbar neuritis
Optic neuritis in portion of optic nerve posterior to eyeball; AKA postocular optic neuritis
A39.83 Meningococcal arthritis
A39.84 Postmeningococcal arthritis
A39.89 Other meningococcal infections
Meningococcal conjunctivitis
A39.9 Meningococcal infection, unspecified
Meningococcal disease NOS

● **A40 Streptococcal sepsis**
Code first
postprocedural streptococcal sepsis (T81.4-) ◀
streptococcal sepsis during labor (O75.3)
streptococcal sepsis following abortion or ectopic or molar pregnancy (O03-O07, O08.0)
streptococcal sepsis following immunization (T88.0)
streptococcal sepsis following infusion, transfusion or therapeutic injection (T80.2-)
Excludes1 neonatal (P36.0-P36.1)
puerperal sepsis (O85)
sepsis due to Streptococcus, group D (A41.81)
A40.0 Sepsis due to streptococcus, group A
A40.1 Sepsis due to streptococcus, group B
A40.3 Sepsis due to Streptococcus pneumoniae
Pneumococcal sepsis
A40.8 Other streptococcal sepsis
A40.9 Streptococcal sepsis, unspecified

● **A41 Other sepsis**
Code first
postprocedural sepsis (T81.4-) ◀
sepsis during labor (O75.3)
sepsis following abortion, ectopic or molar pregnancy (O03-O07, O08.0)
sepsis following immunization (T88.0)
sepsis following infusion, transfusion or therapeutic injection (T80.2-)
Excludes1 bacteremia NOS (R78.81)
neonatal (P36.-)
puerperal sepsis (O85)
~~sepsis NOS (A41.9)~~
streptococcal sepsis (A40.-)
Excludes2 sepsis (due to) (in) actinomycotic (A42.7)
sepsis (due to) (in) anthrax (A22.7)
sepsis (due to) (in) candidal (B37.7)
sepsis (due to) (in) Erysipelothrix (A26.7)
sepsis (due to) (in) extraintestinal yersiniosis (A28.2)
sepsis (due to) (in) gonococcal (A54.86)
sepsis (due to) (in) herpesviral (B00.7)
sepsis (due to) (in) listerial (A32.7)
sepsis (due to) (in) melioidosis (A24.1)
sepsis (due to) (in) meningococcal (A39.2-A39.4)
sepsis (due to) (in) plague (A20.7)
sepsis (due to) (in) tularemia (A21.7)
toxic shock syndrome (A48.3)
● **A41.0 Sepsis due to Staphylococcus aureus**
A41.01 Sepsis due to Methicillin susceptible Staphylococcus aureus
MSSA sepsis
Staphylococcus aureus sepsis NOS
A41.02 Sepsis due to Methicillin resistant Staphylococcus aureus
A41.1 Sepsis due to other specified staphylococcus
Coagulase negative staphylococcus sepsis
A41.2 Sepsis due to unspecified staphylococcus
A41.3 Sepsis due to Hemophilus influenzae
A41.4 Sepsis due to anaerobes
Excludes1 gas gangrene (A48.0)
● **A41.5 Sepsis due to other Gram-negative organisms**
A41.50 Gram-negative sepsis, unspecified
Gram-negative sepsis NOS
A41.51 Sepsis due to Escherichia coli [E. coli]
A41.52 Sepsis due to Pseudomonas
Pseudomonas aeroginosa
A41.53 Sepsis due to Serratia
A41.59 Other Gram-negative sepsis

● **A41.8 Other specified sepsis**
A41.81 Sepsis due to Enterococcus
A41.89 Other specified sepsis
A41.9 Sepsis, unspecified organism
Septicemia NOS

● **A42 Actinomycosis**
Excludes1 actinomycetoma (B47.1)
A42.Ø Pulmonary actinomycosis
A42.1 Abdominal actinomycosis
A42.2 Cervicofacial actinomycosis
A42.7 Actinomycotic sepsis
● **A42.8 Other forms of actinomycosis**
A42.81 Actinomycotic meningitis
A42.82 Actinomycotic encephalitis
A42.89 Other forms of actinomycosis
A42.9 Actinomycosis, unspecified

● **A43 Nocardiosis**
A43.Ø Pulmonary nocardiosis
A43.1 Cutaneous nocardiosis
A43.8 Other forms of nocardiosis
A43.9 Nocardiosis, unspecified

● **A44 Bartonellosis**
A44.Ø Systemic bartonellosis
Oroya fever
A44.1 Cutaneous and mucocutaneous bartonellosis
Verruga peruana
A44.8 Other forms of bartonellosis
A44.9 Bartonellosis, unspecified

A46 Erysipelas
Excludes1 postpartum or puerperal erysipelas (O86.89)

● **A48 Other bacterial diseases, not elsewhere classified**
Excludes1 actinomycetoma (B47.1)
A48.Ø Gas gangrene
Clostridial cellulitis
Clostridial myonecrosis
A48.1 Legionnaires' disease
A48.2 Nonpneumonic Legionnaires' disease [Pontiac fever]
A48.3 Toxic shock syndrome
Use additional code to identify the organism (B95, B96)
Excludes1 endotoxic shock NOS (R57.8)
sepsis NOS (A41.9)
A48.4 Brazilian purpuric fever
Systemic Hemophilus aegyptius infection
● **A48.5 Other specified botulism**
Non-foodborne intoxication due to toxins of Clostridium botulinum [C. botulinum]
Excludes1 food poisoning due to toxins of Clostridium botulinum (AØ5.1)
A48.51 Infant botulism
A48.52 Wound botulism
Non-foodborne botulism NOS
Use additional code for associated wound
A48.8 Other specified bacterial diseases

Item 1-8 Gas gangrene is a necrotizing subcutaneous infection that will cause tissue death. Patients with poor circulation (e.g., diabetes, peripheral nephropathy) will have low oxygen content in their tissues (hypoxia), which allows the Clostridium bacteria to flourish. Gas gangrene often occurs at the site of a surgical wound or trauma. Onset is sudden and dramatic. Treatment can include debridement, amputation, and/or hyperbaric oxygen treatments.

● **A49 Bacterial infection of unspecified site**
Excludes1 bacterial agents as the cause of diseases classified elsewhere (B95-B96)
chlamydial infection NOS (A74.9)
meningococcal infection NOS (A39.9)
rickettsial infection NOS (A79.9)
spirochetal infection NOS (A69.9)
● **A49.Ø Staphylococcal infection, unspecified site**
A49.Ø1 Methicillin susceptible Staphylococcus aureus infection, unspecified site
Methicillin susceptible Staphylococcus aureus (MSSA) infection
Staphylococcus aureus infection NOS
A49.Ø2 Methicillin resistant Staphylococcus aureus infection, unspecified site
Methicillin resistant Staphylococcus aureus (MRSA) infection
A49.1 Streptococcal infection, unspecified site
A49.2 Hemophilus influenzae infection, unspecified site
Any of seven bacterium of genus Haemophilus
A49.3 Mycoplasma infection, unspecified site
Bacterium of class Mollicutes, unusual group of bacteria distinguished by absence of cell wall
A49.8 Other bacterial infections of unspecified site
A49.9 Bacterial infection, unspecified
Excludes1 bacteremia NOS (R78.81)

INFECTIONS WITH A PREDOMINANTLY SEXUAL MODE OF TRANSMISSION (A5Ø-A64)

Excludes1 human immunodeficiency virus [HIV] disease (B2Ø)
nonspecific and nongonococcal urethritis (N34.1)
Reiter's disease (MØ2.3-)

● **A5Ø Congenital syphilis**
● **A5Ø.Ø Early congenital syphilis, symptomatic**
Any congenital syphilitic condition specified as early or manifest less than two years after birth
A5Ø.Ø1 Early congenital syphilitic oculopathy
A5Ø.Ø2 Early congenital syphilitic osteochondropathy
A5Ø.Ø3 Early congenital syphilitic pharyngitis
Early congenital syphilitic laryngitis
A5Ø.Ø4 Early congenital syphilitic pneumonia
A5Ø.Ø5 Early congenital syphilitic rhinitis
A5Ø.Ø6 Early cutaneous congenital syphilis
A5Ø.Ø7 Early mucocutaneous congenital syphilis
A5Ø.Ø8 Early visceral congenital syphilis
A5Ø.Ø9 Other early congenital syphilis, symptomatic

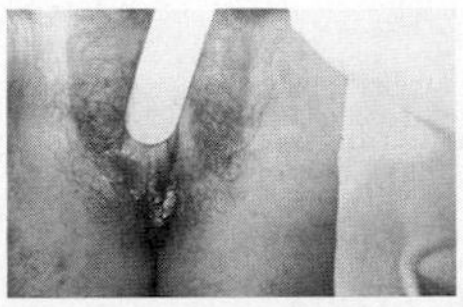

Figure 1-3 Chancre of primary syphilis. (From Mandell, Bennett, & Dolin: Principles and Practice of Infectious Diseases, ed 7, Churchill Livingstone, An Imprint of Elsevier, 2009)

Item 1-9 Syphilis, also known as lues, is the most serious of the venereal diseases caused by *Treponema pallidum*. The **primary** stage is characterized by an ulceration known as **chancre,** which usually appears on the genitals but can also develop on the anus, lips, tonsils, breasts, or fingers. Syphilis is easy to cure in its early stages. A single intramuscular injection of penicillin will usually cure a person who has had syphilis for less than a year.

The **secondary** stage is characterized by a rash that can affect any area of the body. **Latent** syphilis is divided into **early,** which is diagnosed within two years of infection, and **late,** which is diagnosed two years or more after infection. Additional doses of penicillin or another antibiotic are needed to treat someone who has had syphilis for longer than a year. For those allergic to penicillin, there are other antibiotic treatments. **Congenital** syphilis is also labeled **early** or **late** based on the time of diagnosis.

A50.1 Early congenital syphilis, latent
Congenital syphilis without clinical manifestations, with positive serological reaction and negative spinal fluid test, less than two years after birth

A50.2 Early congenital syphilis, unspecified
Congenital syphilis NOS less than two years after birth

● **A50.3 Late congenital syphilitic oculopathy**
Excludes1 Hutchinson's triad (A50.53)

A50.30 Late congenital syphilitic oculopathy, unspecified

A50.31 Late congenital syphilitic interstitial keratitis

A50.32 Late congenital syphilitic chorioretinitis

A50.39 Other late congenital syphilitic oculopathy

● **A50.4 Late congenital neurosyphilis [juvenile neurosyphilis]**
Use additional code to identify any associated mental disorder
Excludes1 Hutchinson's triad (A50.53)

A50.40 Late congenital neurosyphilis, unspecified
Juvenile neurosyphilis NOS

A50.41 Late congenital syphilitic meningitis

A50.42 Late congenital syphilitic encephalitis

A50.43 Late congenital syphilitic polyneuropathy

A50.44 Late congenital syphilitic optic nerve atrophy

A50.45 Juvenile general paresis
Dementia paralytica juvenilis
Juvenile tabetoparetic neurosyphilis

A50.49 Other late congenital neurosyphilis
Juvenile tabes dorsalis

● **A50.5 Other late congenital syphilis, symptomatic**
Any congenital syphilitic condition specified as late or manifest two years or more after birth

A50.51 Clutton's joints

A50.52 Hutchinson's teeth

A50.53 Hutchinson's triad

A50.54 Late congenital cardiovascular syphilis

A50.55 Late congenital syphilitic arthropathy

A50.56 Late congenital syphilitic osteochondropathy

A50.57 Syphilitic saddle nose

A50.59 Other late congenital syphilis, symptomatic

A50.6 Late congenital syphilis, latent
Congenital syphilis without clinical manifestations, with positive serological reaction and negative spinal fluid test, two years or more after birth.

A50.7 Late congenital syphilis, unspecified
Congenital syphilis NOS two years or more after birth.

A50.9 Congenital syphilis, unspecified

● **A51 Early syphilis**

A51.0 Primary genital syphilis
Syphilitic chancre NOS

A51.1 Primary anal syphilis

A51.2 Primary syphilis of other sites

● **A51.3 Secondary syphilis of skin and mucous membranes**

A51.31 Condyloma latum

A51.32 Syphilitic alopecia

A51.39 Other secondary syphilis of skin
Syphilitic leukoderma
Syphilitic mucous patch
Excludes1 late syphilitic leukoderma (A52.79)

● **A51.4 Other secondary syphilis**

A51.41 Secondary syphilitic meningitis

A51.42 Secondary syphilitic female pelvic disease

A51.43 Secondary syphilitic oculopathy
Secondary syphilitic chorioretinitis
Secondary syphilitic iridocyclitis, iritis
Secondary syphilitic uveitis

A51.44 Secondary syphilitic nephritis

A51.45 Secondary syphilitic hepatitis

A51.46 Secondary syphilitic osteopathy

A51.49 Other secondary syphilitic conditions
Secondary syphilitic lymphadenopathy
Secondary syphilitic myositis

A51.5 Early syphilis, latent
Syphilis (acquired) without clinical manifestations, with positive serological reaction and negative spinal fluid test, less than two years after infection.

A51.9 Early syphilis, unspecified

● **A52 Late syphilis**

● **A52.0 Cardiovascular and cerebrovascular syphilis**

A52.00 Cardiovascular syphilis, unspecified

A52.01 Syphilitic aneurysm of aorta

A52.02 Syphilitic aortitis

A52.03 Syphilitic endocarditis
Syphilitic aortic valve incompetence or stenosis
Syphilitic mitral valve stenosis
Syphilitic pulmonary valve regurgitation

A52.04 Syphilitic cerebral arteritis

A52.05 Other cerebrovascular syphilis
Syphilitic cerebral aneurysm (ruptured) (non-ruptured)
Syphilitic cerebral thrombosis

A52.06 Other syphilitic heart involvement
Syphilitic coronary artery disease
Syphilitic myocarditis
Syphilitic pericarditis

A52.09 Other cardiovascular syphilis

● **A52.1 Symptomatic neurosyphilis**

A52.10 Symptomatic neurosyphilis, unspecified

A52.11 Tabes dorsalis
Cognitive decline with progressive degeneration of posterior columns, roots, and ganglia of spinal cord, occur 15-20 years after initial infection of syphilis; AKA Duchenne disease
Locomotor ataxia (progressive)
Tabetic neurosyphilis

A52.12 Other cerebrospinal syphilis

A52.13 Late syphilitic meningitis

A52.14 Late syphilitic encephalitis

A52.15 Late syphilitic neuropathy
Late syphilitic acoustic neuritis
Late syphilitic optic (nerve) atrophy
Late syphilitic polyneuropathy
Late syphilitic retrobulbar neuritis

A52.16 Charcôt's arthropathy (tabetic)
Progressive musculoskeletal condition characterized by joint dislocation, fractures, and deformities, results in progressive destruction of bone and soft tissue of weight-bearing joints

A52.17 General paresis
Chronic meningoencephalitis results in loss of cortical function, or progressive dementia and generalized paralysis, occurring 10-20 years after initial infection of syphilis; AKA Bayle disease, dementia paralytica, paralytic dementiaparetic neurosyphilis, syphilitic meningoencephalitis
Dementia paralytica

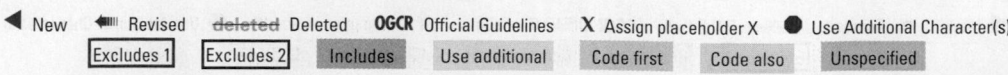

A52.19 Other symptomatic neurosyphilis
Syphilitic parkinsonism

A52.2 Asymptomatic neurosyphilis

A52.3 Neurosyphilis, unspecified
Gumma (syphilitic)
Destructive lesions of syphilis
Syphilis (late)
Syphiloma

● **A52.7 Other symptomatic late syphilis**

A52.71 Late syphilitic oculopathy
Late syphilitic chorioretinitis
Late syphilitic episcleritis

A52.72 Syphilis of lung and bronchus

A52.73 Symptomatic late syphilis of other respiratory organs

A52.74 Syphilis of liver and other viscera
Late syphilitic peritonitis

A52.75 Syphilis of kidney and ureter
Syphilitic glomerular disease

A52.76 Other genitourinary symptomatic late syphilis
Late syphilitic female pelvic inflammatory disease

A52.77 Syphilis of bone and joint

A52.78 Syphilis of other musculoskeletal tissue
Late syphilitic bursitis
Syphilis [stage unspecified] of bursa
Syphilis [stage unspecified] of muscle
Syphilis [stage unspecified] of synovium
Syphilis [stage unspecified] of tendon

A52.79 Other symptomatic late syphilis
Late syphilitic leukoderma
Syphilis of adrenal gland
Syphilis of pituitary gland
Syphilis of thyroid gland
Syphilitic splenomegaly
Excludes1 syphilitic leukoderma (secondary) (A51.39)

A52.8 Late syphilis, latent
Syphilis (acquired) without clinical manifestations, with positive serological reaction and negative spinal fluid test, two years or more after infection

A52.9 Late syphilis, unspecified

● **A53 Other and unspecified syphilis**

A53.Ø Latent syphilis, unspecified as early or late
Latent syphilis NOS
Positive serological reaction for syphilis

A53.9 Syphilis, unspecified
Infection due to Treponema pallidum NOS
Syphilis (acquired) NOS
Excludes1 syphilis NOS under two years of age (A5Ø.2)

● **A54 Gonococcal infection**

● **A54.Ø Gonococcal infection of lower genitourinary tract without periurethral or accessory gland abscess**
Excludes1 gonococcal infection with genitourinary gland abscess (A54.1)
gonococcal infection with periurethral abscess (A54.1)

A54.ØØ Gonococcal infection of lower genitourinary tract, unspecified

A54.Ø1 Gonococcal cystitis and urethritis, unspecified

A54.Ø2 Gonococcal vulvovaginitis, unspecified

A54.Ø3 Gonococcal cervicitis, unspecified

A54.Ø9 Other gonococcal infection of lower genitourinary tract

A54.1 Gonococcal infection of lower genitourinary tract with periurethral and accessory gland abscess
Gonococcal Bartholin's gland abscess

Item 1-10 An STD (sexually transmitted disease) caused by **Neisseria gonorrhoeae** that flourishes in the warm, moist areas of the reproductive tract. Untreated gonorrhea spreads to other parts of the body, causing inflammation of the testes or prostate or pelvic inflammatory disease (PID).

● **A54.2 Gonococcal pelviperitonitis and other gonococcal genitourinary infection**

A54.21 Gonococcal infection of kidney and ureter

A54.22 Gonococcal prostatitis

A54.23 Gonococcal infection of other male genital organs
Gonococcal epididymitis
Gonococcal orchitis

A54.24 Gonococcal female pelvic inflammatory disease
Gonococcal pelviperitonitis
Excludes1 gonococcal peritonitis (A54.85)

A54.29 Other gonococcal genitourinary infections

● **A54.3 Gonococcal infection of eye**

A54.3Ø Gonococcal infection of eye, unspecified

A54.31 Gonococcal conjunctivitis
Form of bacterial conjunctivitis contracted by newborns during delivery; AKA neonatal conjunctivitis
Ophthalmia neonatorum due to gonococcus

A54.32 Gonococcal iridocyclitis
Inflammation of iris and of ciliary body due to gonococcal infection

A54.33 Gonococcal keratitis
Inflammation of cornea due to gonococcal infection; AKA keratoconjunctivitis, keratopathy

A54.39 Other gonococcal eye infection
Gonococcal endophthalmia

● **A54.4 Gonococcal infection of musculoskeletal system**

A54.4Ø Gonococcal infection of musculoskeletal system, unspecified

A54.41 Gonococcal spondylopathy
Disorder of vertebrae due to gonococcal infection; AKA rachiopathy

A54.42 Gonococcal arthritis
Excludes2 gonococcal infection of spine (A54.41)

A54.43 Gonococcal osteomyelitis
Excludes2 gonococcal infection of spine (A54.41)

A54.49 Gonococcal infection of other musculoskeletal tissue
Gonococcal bursitis
Gonococcal myositis
Gonococcal synovitis
Gonococcal tenosynovitis

A54.5 Gonococcal pharyngitis

A54.6 Gonococcal infection of anus and rectum

● **A54.8 Other gonococcal infections**

A54.81 Gonococcal meningitis

A54.82 Gonococcal brain abscess

A54.83 Gonococcal heart infection
Gonococcal endocarditis
Gonococcal myocarditis
Gonococcal pericarditis

A54.84 Gonococcal pneumonia

A54.85 Gonococcal peritonitis
Excludes1 gonococcal pelviperitonitis (A54.24)

A54.86 Gonococcal sepsis

A54.89 Other gonococcal infections
Gonococcal keratoderma
Gonococcal lymphadenitis

A54.9 Gonococcal infection, unspecified

A55 Chlamydial lymphogranuloma (venereum)
Climatic or tropical bubo
Durand-Nicolas-Favre disease
Esthiomene
Lymphogranuloma inguinale

● **A56 Other sexually transmitted chlamydial diseases**
Includes sexually transmitted diseases due to Chlamydia trachomatis
Excludes1 neonatal chlamydial conjunctivitis (P39.1)
neonatal chlamydial pneumonia (P23.1)
Excludes2 chlamydial lymphogranuloma (A55)
conditions classified to A74.-

● **A56.0 Chlamydial infection of lower genitourinary tract**
A56.00 Chlamydial infection of lower genitourinary tract, unspecified
A56.01 Chlamydial cystitis and urethritis
A56.02 Chlamydial vulvovaginitis
A56.09 Other chlamydial infection of lower genitourinary tract
Chlamydial cervicitis

● **A56.1 Chlamydial infection of pelviperitoneum and other genitourinary organs**
A56.11 Chlamydial female pelvic inflammatory disease
A56.19 Other chlamydial genitourinary infection
Chlamydial epididymitis
Chlamydial orchitis
A56.2 Chlamydial infection of genitourinary tract, unspecified
A56.3 Chlamydial infection of anus and rectum
A56.4 Chlamydial infection of pharynx
A56.8 Sexually transmitted chlamydial infection of other sites

A57 Chancroid
Ulcus molle
Sexually transmitted infection caused by bacteria, Haemophilus ducreyi

A58 Granuloma inguinale
Chronic, progressive, ulcerative granulomatous disease
Donovanosis

● **A59 Trichomoniasis**
Excludes2 intestinal trichomoniasis (A07.8)
A common STD caused by a parasite, Trichomonas vaginalis

● **A59.0 Urogenital trichomoniasis**
A59.00 Urogenital trichomoniasis, unspecified
Fluor (vaginalis) due to Trichomonas
Leukorrhea (vaginalis) due to Trichomonas
A59.01 Trichomonal vulvovaginitis
A59.02 Trichomonal prostatitis
A59.03 Trichomonal cystitis and urethritis
A59.09 Other urogenital trichomoniasis
Common sexually transmitted disease (STD) caused by single-celled protozoan parasite; AKA trich
Trichomonas cervicitis
A59.8 Trichomoniasis of other sites
A59.9 Trichomoniasis, unspecified

● **A60 Anogenital herpesviral [herpes simplex] infections**
● **A60.0 Herpesviral infection of genitalia and urogenital tract**
A60.00 Herpesviral infection of urogenital system, unspecified
A60.01 Herpesviral infection of penis
A60.02 Herpesviral infection of other male genital organs
A60.03 Herpesviral cervicitis
A60.04 Herpesviral vulvovaginitis
Herpesviral [herpes simplex] ulceration
Herpesviral [herpes simplex] vaginitis
Herpesviral [herpes simplex] vulvitis
A60.09 Herpesviral infection of other urogenital tract
A60.1 Herpesviral infection of perianal skin and rectum
A60.9 Anogenital herpesviral infection, unspecified

● **A63 Other predominantly sexually transmitted diseases, not elsewhere classified**
Excludes2 molluscum contagiosum (B08.1)
papilloma of cervix (D26.0)
A63.0 Anogenital (venereal) warts
Anogenital warts due to (human) papillomavirus [HPV]
Condyloma acuminatum
A63.8 Other specified predominantly sexually transmitted diseases

A64 Unspecified sexually transmitted disease

OTHER SPIROCHETAL DISEASES (A65-A69)

Excludes2 leptospirosis (A27.-)
syphilis (A50-A53)

A65 Nonvenereal syphilis
Bejel
Endemic syphilis
Njovera

● **A66 Yaws**
Endemic, infectious, tropical disease caused by spirochete, spread by direct contact; AKA frambesia, framboesia, frambesia tropica
Includes bouba
frambesia (tropica)
pian
A66.0 Initial lesions of yaws
Chancre of yaws
Frambesia, initial or primary
Initial frambesial ulcer
Mother yaw
A66.1 Multiple papillomata and wet crab yaws
Frambesioma
Pianoma
Plantar or palmar papilloma of yaws
A66.2 Other early skin lesions of yaws
Cutaneous yaws, less than five years after infection
Early yaws (cutaneous)(macular)(maculopapular)(micropapular)(papular)
Frambeside of early yaws
A66.3 Hyperkeratosis of yaws
Hypertrophy of stratum corneum of skin in which there are small, hard, verrucous scales
Ghoul hand
Hyperkeratosis, palmar or plantar (early) (late) due to yaws
Worm-eaten soles
A66.4 Gummata and ulcers of yaws
Small, rubbery granuloma with necrotic center and inflamed characteristic of advanced stage of syphilis; AKA syphiloma
Gummatous frambeside
Nodular late yaws (ulcerated)
A66.5 Gangosa
Manifestation of yaws that develops in the soft palate and spreads eroding bone, cartilage, and soft tissue
Rhinopharyngitis mutilans
A66.6 Bone and joint lesions of yaws
Yaws ganglion
Yaws goundou
Yaws gumma, bone
Yaws gummatous osteitis or periostitis
Yaws hydrarthrosis
Yaws osteitis
Yaws periostitis (hypertrophic)

CHAPTER 1 (A00-B99)

A66.7 Other manifestations of yaws
Juxta-articular nodules of yaws
Mucosal yaws

A66.8 Latent yaws
Yaws without clinical manifestations, with positive serology

A66.9 Yaws, unspecified

● **A67 Pinta [carate]**
Group of nonvenereal diseases caused by Treponema species

A67.0 Primary lesions of pinta
Chancre (primary) of pinta
Papule (primary) of pinta

A67.1 Intermediate lesions of pinta
Erythematous plaques of pinta
Hyperchromic lesions of pinta
Hyperkeratosis of pinta
Pintids

A67.2 Late lesions of pinta
Achromic skin lesions of pinta
Cicatricial skin lesions of pinta
Dyschromic skin lesions of pinta

A67.3 Mixed lesions of pinta
Achromic with hyperchromic skin lesions of pinta [carate]

A67.9 Pinta, unspecified

● **A68 Relapsing fevers**
Includes recurrent fever
Excludes2 Lyme disease (A69.2-)

A68.0 Louse-borne relapsing fever
Relapsing fever due to Borrelia recurrentis

A68.1 Tick-borne relapsing fever
Relapsing fever due to any Borrelia species other than Borrelia recurrentis

A68.9 Relapsing fever, unspecified

● **A69 Other spirochetal infections**

A69.0 Necrotizing ulcerative stomatitis
Cancrum oris
Fusospirochetal gangrene
Noma
Stomatitis gangrenosa

A69.1 Other Vincent's infections
Fusospirochetal pharyngitis
Necrotizing ulcerative (acute) gingivitis
Necrotizing ulcerative (acute) gingivostomatitis
Spirochetal stomatitis
Trench mouth
Vincent's angina
Vincent's gingivitis

● **A69.2 Lyme disease**
Erythema chronicum migrans due to Borrelia burgdorferi

A69.20 Lyme disease, unspecified

A69.21 Meningitis due to Lyme disease

A69.22 Other neurologic disorders in Lyme disease
Cranial neuritis
Meningoencephalitis
Polyneuropathy

A69.23 Arthritis due to Lyme disease

A69.29 Other conditions associated with Lyme disease
Myopericarditis due to Lyme disease

A69.8 Other specified spirochetal infections

A69.9 Spirochetal infection, unspecified

Item 1-11 Cancrum oris, also known as **noma** or **gangrenous stomatitis,** begins as an ulcer of the gingiva and results in a progressive gangrenous process.

OTHER DISEASES CAUSED BY CHLAMYDIAE (A70-A74)

Excludes1 sexually transmitted chlamydial diseases (A55-A56)

A70 Chlamydia psittaci infections
Ornithosis
Parrot fever
Psittacosis

● **A71 Trachoma**
Excludes1 sequelae of trachoma (B94.0)

A71.0 Initial stage of trachoma
Trachoma dubium

A71.1 Active stage of trachoma
Granular conjunctivitis (trachomatous)
Trachomatous follicular conjunctivitis
Trachomatous pannus

A71.9 Trachoma, unspecified

● **A74 Other diseases caused by chlamydiae**
Excludes1 neonatal chlamydial conjunctivitis (P39.1)
neonatal chlamydial pneumonia (P23.1)
Reiter's disease (M02.3-)
sexually transmitted chlamydial diseases (A55-A56)
Excludes2 chlamydial pneumonia (J16.0)

A74.0 Chlamydial conjunctivitis
Paratrachoma

● **A74.8 Other chlamydial diseases**

A74.81 Chlamydial peritonitis

A74.89 Other chlamydial diseases

A74.9 Chlamydial infection, unspecified
Chlamydiosis NOS

RICKETTSIOSES (A75-A79)

● **A75 Typhus fever**
Excludes1 rickettsiosis due to Ehrlichia sennetsu (A79.81)

A75.0 Epidemic louse-borne typhus fever due to Rickettsia prowazekii
Organisms transmitted between humans via louse
Classical typhus (fever)
Epidemic (louse-borne) typhus

A75.1 Recrudescent typhus [Brill's disease]
Brill-Zinsser disease

A75.2 Typhus fever due to Rickettsia typhi
Murine (flea-borne) typhus

A75.3 Typhus fever due to Rickettsia tsutsugamushi
Scrub (mite-borne) typhus
Tsutsugamushi fever

A75.9 Typhus fever, unspecified
Typhus (fever) NOS

Item 1-12 Rickettsioses are diseases spread from ticks, lice, fleas, or mites to humans.

Typhus is spread to humans chiefly by the fleas of rats.

Endemic identifies a disease as being present in low numbers of humans at all times, whereas **epidemic** identifies a disease as being present in high numbers of humans at a specific time. Morbidity (death) is higher in epidemic diseases.

Brill's disease, also known as **Brill-Zinsser disease,** is spread from human to human by body lice and also from the lice of flying squirrels. **Scrub typhus** is spread in the same ways as Brill's disease.

Malaria is spread to humans by mosquitoes.

● **A77 Spotted fever [tick-borne rickettsioses]**

A77.0 Spotted fever due to Rickettsia rickettsii
Rocky Mountain spotted fever
Sao Paulo fever

A77.1 Spotted fever due to Rickettsia conorii
African tick typhus
Boutonneuse fever
India tick typhus
Kenya tick typhus
Marseilles fever
Mediterranean tick fever

A77.2 Spotted fever due to Rickettsia siberica
North Asian tick fever
Siberian tick typhus

A77.3 Spotted fever due to Rickettsia australis
Queensland tick typhus

● **A77.4 Ehrlichiosis**
Type of tick-borne fever caused by bacteria infection
Excludes1 Rickettsiosis due to Ehrlichia sennetsu (A79.81)

A77.40 Ehrlichiosis, unspecified

A77.41 Ehrlichiosis chafeensis [E. chafeensis]

A77.49 Other ehrlichiosis

A77.8 Other spotted fevers

A77.9 Spotted fever, unspecified
Tick-borne typhus NOS

A78 Q fever
Infection due to Coxiella burnetii
Nine Mile fever
Quadrilateral fever

● **A79 Other rickettsioses**

A79.0 Trench fever
Quintan fever
Wolhynian fever

A79.1 Rickettsialpox due to Rickettsia akari
Kew Garden fever
Vesicular rickettsiosis

● **A79.8 Other specified rickettsioses**

A79.81 Rickettsiosis due to Ehrlichia sennetsu

A79.89 Other specified rickettsioses

A79.9 Rickettsiosis, unspecified
Rickettsial infection NOS

VIRAL AND PRION INFECTIONS OF THE CENTRAL NERVOUS SYSTEM (A80-A89)

Excludes1 postpolio syndrome (G14)
sequelae of poliomyelitis (B91)
sequelae of viral encephalitis (B94.1)

● **A80 Acute poliomyelitis**

A80.0 Acute paralytic poliomyelitis, vaccine-associated

A80.1 Acute paralytic poliomyelitis, wild virus, imported

A80.2 Acute paralytic poliomyelitis, wild virus, indigenous

● **A80.3 Acute paralytic poliomyelitis, other and unspecified**

A80.30 Acute paralytic poliomyelitis, unspecified

A80.39 Other acute paralytic poliomyelitis

A80.4 Acute nonparalytic poliomyelitis

A80.9 Acute poliomyelitis, unspecified

Item 1-13 Acute Poliomyelitis: Also called infantile paralysis and is caused by the poliovirus, which enters the body orally and infects the intestinal wall and then enters the blood stream and central nervous system, causing muscle weakness and paralysis. This disease has been nearly eradicated with the polio vaccine.

● **A81 Atypical virus infections of central nervous system**
Includes diseases of the central nervous system caused by prions
Use additional code to identify:
dementia with behavioral disturbance (F02.81)
dementia without behavioral disturbance (F02.80)

● **A81.0 Creutzfeldt-Jakob disease**

A81.00 Creutzfeldt-Jakob disease, unspecified
Jakob-Creutzfeldt disease, unspecified

A81.01 Variant Creutzfeldt-Jakob disease
vCJD

A81.09 Other Creutzfeldt-Jakob disease
CJD
Familial Creutzfeldt-Jakob disease
Iatrogenic Creutzfeldt-Jakob disease
Sporadic Creutzfeldt-Jakob disease
Subacute spongiform encephalopathy (with dementia)

A81.1 Subacute sclerosing panencephalitis
Type of viral encephalitis that causes parenchymatous lesions in gray and white matter of brain
Dawson's inclusion body encephalitis
Van Bogaert's sclerosing leukoencephalopathy

A81.2 Progressive multifocal leukoencephalopathy
Group of diseases affecting white matter of brain
Multifocal leukoencephalopathy NOS

● **A81.8 Other atypical virus infections of central nervous system**

A81.81 Kuru

A81.82 Gerstmann-Sträussler-Scheinker syndrome
GSS syndrome

A81.83 Fatal familial insomnia
FFI

A81.89 Other atypical virus infections of central nervous system

A81.9 Atypical virus infection of central nervous system, unspecified
Prion diseases of the central nervous system NOS

● **A82 Rabies**
Viral disease affecting the central nervous system and transmitted from infected mammals to man.

A82.0 Sylvatic rabies

A82.1 Urban rabies

A82.9 Rabies, unspecified

● **A83 Mosquito-borne viral encephalitis**
Inflammation of the brain caused most commonly by Herpes Simplex virus.
Includes mosquito-borne viral meningoencephalitis
Excludes2 Venezuelan equine encephalitis (A92.2)
West Nile fever (A92.3-)
West Nile virus (A92.3-)

A83.0 Japanese encephalitis

A83.1 Western equine encephalitis

A83.2 Eastern equine encephalitis

A83.3 St. Louis encephalitis

A83.4 Australian encephalitis
Kunjin virus disease

A83.5 California encephalitis
California meningoencephalitis
La Crosse encephalitis

A83.6 Rocio virus disease
Mosquito-borne virus

A83.8 Other mosquito-borne viral encephalitis

A83.9 Mosquito-borne viral encephalitis, unspecified

CHAPTER 1 (A00-B99)

Item 1-14 Encephalitis is an inflammation of the brain most often caused by a virus but may also be caused by a bacteria and most commonly transmitted by a mosquito. **Myelitis** is an inflammation of the spinal cord that may disrupt CNS function. Untreated myelitis may rapidly lead to permanent damage to the spinal cord. **Encephalomyelitis** is a general term for an inflammation of the brain and spinal cord.

● **A84 Tick-borne viral encephalitis**
Includes tick-borne viral meningoencephalitis
A84.Ø Far Eastern tick-borne encephalitis [Russian spring-summer encephalitis]
A84.1 Central European tick-borne encephalitis
A84.8 Other tick-borne viral encephalitis
Louping ill
Powassan virus disease
A84.9 Tick-borne viral encephalitis, unspecified

● **A85 Other viral encephalitis, not elsewhere classified**
Includes specified viral encephalomyelitis NEC
specified viral meningoencephalitis NEC
Excludes1 benign myalgic encephalomyelitis (G93.3)
encephalitis due to cytomegalovirus (B25.8)
encephalitis due to herpesvirus NEC (B1Ø.Ø-)
encephalitis due to herpesvirus [herpes simplex] (BØØ.4)
encephalitis due to measles virus (BØ5.Ø)
encephalitis due to mumps virus (B26.2)
encephalitis due to poliomyelitis virus (A8Ø.-)
encephalitis due to zoster (BØ2.Ø)
lymphocytic choriomeningitis (A87.2)
A85.Ø Enteroviral encephalitis
Enteroviral encephalomyelitis
A85.1 Adenoviral encephalitis
Adenoviral meningoencephalitis
A85.2 Arthropod-borne viral encephalitis, unspecified
Excludes1 West nile virus with encephalitis (A92.31)
A85.8 Other specified viral encephalitis
Encephalitis lethargica
Von Economo-Cruchet disease

A86 Unspecified viral encephalitis
Viral encephalomyelitis NOS
Viral meningoencephalitis NOS

● **A87 Viral meningitis**
Excludes1 meningitis due to herpesvirus [herpes simplex] (BØØ.3)
meningitis due to measles virus (BØ5.1)
meningitis due to mumps virus (B26.1)
meningitis due to poliomyelitis virus (A8Ø.-)
meningitis due to zoster (BØ2.1)
A87.Ø Enteroviral meningitis
Group of common viruses responsible for the majority of viral meningitis
Coxsackievirus meningitis
Echovirus meningitis
A87.1 Adenoviral meningitis
A87.2 Lymphocytic choriomeningitis
Lymphocytic meningoencephalitis
A87.8 Other viral meningitis
A87.9 Viral meningitis, unspecified

● **A88 Other viral infections of central nervous system, not elsewhere classified**
Excludes1 viral encephalitis NOS (A86)
viral meningitis NOS (A87.9)
A88.Ø Enteroviral exanthematous fever [Boston exanthem]
Infectious skin eruption
A88.1 Epidemic vertigo
A88.8 Other specified viral infections of central nervous system

A89 Unspecified viral infection of central nervous system

ARTHROPOD-BORNE VIRAL FEVERS AND VIRAL HEMORRHAGIC FEVERS (A9Ø-A99)

A9Ø Dengue fever [classical dengue]
Acute, self-limited disease, characterized by fever, prostration, severe muscle pains, headache, rash, lymphadenopathy, and leukopenia, caused by dengue virus; AKA breakbone, dandy
Excludes1 dengue hemorrhagic fever (A91)

A91 Dengue hemorrhagic fever
Serious follow-up to regular dengue, with symptoms of hemorrhage

● **A92 Other mosquito-borne viral fevers**
Excludes1 Ross River disease (B33.1)
A92.Ø Chikungunya virus disease
Transmitted by mosquitoes
Chikungunya (hemorrhagic) fever
A92.1 O'nyong-nyong fever
Acute, nonfatal febrile disease transmitted by mosquitoes, which clinically resembles dengue and chikungunya
A92.2 Venezuelan equine fever
Venezuelan equine encephalitis
Venezuelan equine encephalomyelitis virus disease
● **A92.3 West Nile virus infection**
West Nile fever
A92.3Ø West Nile virus infection, unspecified
West Nile fever NOS
West Nile fever without complications
West Nile virus NOS
A92.31 West Nile virus infection with encephalitis
West Nile encephalitis
West Nile encephalomyelitis
A92.32 West Nile virus infection with other neurologic manifestation
Use additional code to specify the neurologic manifestation
A92.39 West Nile virus infection with other complications
Use additional code to specify the other conditions
A92.4 Rift Valley fever
A92.5 Zika virus disease ◀
Zika virus fever ◀
Zika virus infection ◀
Zika NOS ◀
A92.8 Other specified mosquito-borne viral fevers
A92.9 Mosquito-borne viral fever, unspecified

OGCR Section I. C.1.f.

Certain Infectious and Parasitic Diseases (AØØ-B99)

Zika virus infections

Code only confirmed cases

Code only a confirmed diagnosis of Zika virus (A92.5, Zika virus disease) as documented by the provider. This is an exception to the hospital inpatient guideline Section II, H.

In this context, "confirmation" does not require documentation of the type of test performed; the physician's diagnostic statement that the condition is confirmed is sufficient. This code should be assigned regardless of the stated mode of transmission.

If the provider documents "suspected", "possible" or "probable" Zika, do not assign code A92.5. Assign a code(s) explaining the reason for encounter (such as fever, rash, or joint pain) or Z2Ø.828, Contact with and (suspected) exposure to other viral communicable diseases.

● **A93 Other arthropod-borne viral fevers, not elsewhere classified**
A93.0 Oropouche virus disease
Tropical viral infection
Oropouche fever
A93.1 Sandfly fever
Pappataci fever
Phlebotomus fever
A93.2 Colorado tick fever
A93.8 Other specified arthropod-borne viral fevers
Piry virus disease
Vesicular stomatitis virus disease [Indiana fever]

A94 Unspecified arthropod-borne viral fever
Arboviral fever NOS
Arbovirus infection NOS

● **A95 Yellow fever**
Acute infectious disease transmitted by mosquitoes
A95.0 Sylvatic yellow fever
Jungle yellow fever
A95.1 Urban yellow fever
A95.9 Yellow fever, unspecified

● **A96 Arenaviral hemorrhagic fever**
Virus that causes various hemorrhagic fevers
A96.0 Junin hemorrhagic fever
Argentinian hemorrhagic fever
A96.1 Machupo hemorrhagic fever
Transmitted by contact with infected rodents
Bolivian hemorrhagic fever
A96.2 Lassa fever
Acute type of hemorrhagic fever caused by contact with disease carrying mouse or person
A96.8 Other arenaviral hemorrhagic fevers
A96.9 Arenaviral hemorrhagic fever, unspecified

● **A98 Other viral hemorrhagic fevers, not elsewhere classified**
Excludes1 chikungunya hemorrhagic fever (A92.0)
dengue hemorrhagic fever (A91)
A98.0 Crimean-Congo hemorrhagic fever
Virus transmitted by ticks and contact with blood, secretions, or fluids from infected humans or animals
Central Asian hemorrhagic fever
A98.1 Omsk hemorrhagic fever
Transmitted to humans by bites of infected ticks or contact with infected muskrats
A98.2 Kyasanur Forest disease
Transmitted via infected monkeys, voles, ticks
A98.3 Marburg virus disease
Rare, acute, often fatal type of hemorrhagic fever
A98.4 Ebola virus disease
A98.5 Hemorrhagic fever with renal syndrome
Epidemic hemorrhagic fever
Korean hemorrhagic fever
Russian hemorrhagic fever
Hantaan virus disease
Hantavirus disease with renal manifestations
Nephropathia epidemica
Songo fever
Excludes1 hantavirus (cardio)-pulmonary syndrome (B33.4)
A98.8 Other specified viral hemorrhagic fevers

A99 Unspecified viral hemorrhagic fever

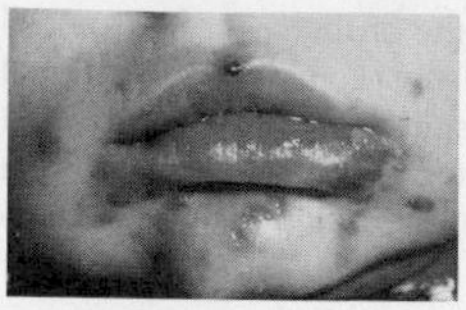

Figure 1-4 Primary herpes simplex in and around the mouth. The infection is usually acquired from siblings or parents and is readily transmitted to other direct contacts. (From Forbes, Jackson: Colour Atlas and Text of Clinical Medicine, International Edition, Mosby, 2002)

Item 1-15 Herpes is a viral disease for which there is no cure. There are two types of the herpes simplex virus: **Type I** causes **cold sores** or **fever blisters,** and **Type II** causes **genital herpes.** The virus can be spread from a sore on the lips to the genitals or from the genitals to the lips.

VIRAL INFECTIONS CHARACTERIZED BY SKIN AND MUCOUS MEMBRANE LESIONS (B00-B09)

● **B00 Herpesviral [herpes simplex] infections**
Excludes1 congenital herpesviral infections (P35.2)
Excludes2 anogenital herpesviral infection (A60.-)
gammaherpesviral mononucleosis (B27.0-)
herpangina (B08.5)
B00.0 Eczema herpeticum
Cutaneous eruption caused by herpes simplex virus (HSV) type 1, HSV-2, coxsackievirus A16, or vaccinia virus
Kaposi's varicelliform eruption
B00.1 Herpesviral vesicular dermatitis
Vesicle formation; characteristics include formation of blisters and scabs on feet and legs
Herpes simplex facialis
Herpes simplex labialis
Herpes simplex otitis externa
Vesicular dermatitis of ear
Vesicular dermatitis of lip
B00.2 Herpesviral gingivostomatitis and pharyngotonsillitis
Inflammation involving both gingivae and oral mucosa
Herpesviral pharyngitis
Inflammation of pharynx and tonsils; AKA tonsillopharyngitis
B00.3 Herpesviral meningitis
B00.4 Herpesviral encephalitis
Herpesviral meningoencephalitis
Simian B disease
Excludes1 herpesviral encephalitis due to herpesvirus 6 and 7 (B10.01, B10.09)
non-simplex herpesviral encephalitis (B10.0-)
● **B00.5 Herpesviral ocular disease**
B00.50 Herpesviral ocular disease, unspecified
B00.51 Herpesviral iridocyclitis
Herpesviral iritis
Herpesviral uveitis, anterior
B00.52 Herpesviral keratitis
Herpesviral keratoconjunctivitis
B00.53 Herpesviral conjunctivitis
B00.59 Other herpesviral disease of eye
Herpesviral dermatitis of eyelid
B00.7 Disseminated herpesviral disease
Herpesviral sepsis
● **B00.8 Other forms of herpesviral infections**
B00.81 Herpesviral hepatitis
B00.82 Herpes simplex myelitis
B00.89 Other herpesviral infection
Herpesviral whitlow
B00.9 Herpesviral infection, unspecified
Herpes simplex infection NOS

CHAPTER 1 (A00-B99)

Item 1-16 Zoster: Also known as ***shingles*** and is caused by the same virus as chickenpox. After exposure, the virus lies dormant in nerve tissue and is activated by factors including aging, stress, suppression of the immune system, and certain medication. It begins as a unilateral rash that leads to blisters and sores on the skin. It may involve the nerve pathways of the eye, forehead, nose, and eyelids and may be very painful with long-term systemic effects.

● **BØ1 Varicella [chickenpox]**
Very contagious disease caused by the varicella zoster virus that results in an itchy outbreak of skin blisters (varicella). The same virus causes shingles (zoster).

BØ1.Ø Varicella meningitis

● **BØ1.1 Varicella encephalitis, myelitis and encephalomyelitis**
Postchickenpox encephalitis, myelitis and encephalomyelitis

BØ1.11 Varicella encephalitis and encephalomyelitis
Postchickenpox encephalitis and encephalomyelitis

BØ1.12 Varicella myelitis
Postchickenpox myelitis

BØ1.2 Varicella pneumonia

● **BØ1.8 Varicella with other complications**

BØ1.81 Varicella keratitis

BØ1.89 Other varicella complications

BØ1.9 Varicella without complication
Varicella NOS

● **BØ2 Zoster [herpes zoster]**
Includes shingles
zona

BØ2.Ø Zoster encephalitis
Zoster meningoencephalitis

BØ2.1 Zoster meningitis

● **BØ2.2 Zoster with other nervous system involvement**

BØ2.21 Postherpetic geniculate ganglionitis

BØ2.22 Postherpetic trigeminal neuralgia

BØ2.23 Postherpetic polyneuropathy

BØ2.24 Postherpetic myelitis
Herpes zoster myelitis

BØ2.29 Other postherpetic nervous system involvement
Postherpetic radiculopathy

● **BØ2.3 Zoster ocular disease**

BØ2.3Ø Zoster ocular disease, unspecified

BØ2.31 Zoster conjunctivitis

BØ2.32 Zoster iridocyclitis

BØ2.33 Zoster keratitis
Herpes zoster keratoconjunctivitis

BØ2.34 Zoster scleritis

BØ2.39 Other herpes zoster eye disease
Zoster blepharitis

BØ2.7 Disseminated zoster

BØ2.8 Zoster with other complications
Herpes zoster otitis externa

BØ2.9 Zoster without complications
Zoster NOS

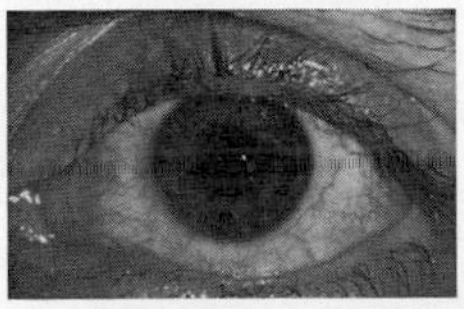

Figure 1-5 Photograph of eyelids with marginal blepharitis. (From Mandell, Bennett, & Dolin: Principles and Practice of Infectious Diseases, ed 7, Churchill Livingstone, An Imprint of Elsevier, 2009)

Item 1-17 Blepharitis is a common condition in which the eyelid is swollen and yellow scaling and conjunctivitis develop. Usually the hair on the scalp and brow is involved.

BØ3 Smallpox
Note: In 198Ø the 33rd World Health Assembly declared that smallpox had been eradicated. The classification is maintained for surveillance purposes.

BØ4 Monkeypox
Disease occurring in captive monkeys and other mammals that may be transmitted to humans, clinically similar to smallpox

● **BØ5 Measles**
Includes morbilli
Excludes1 subacute sclerosing panencephalitis (A81.1)

BØ5.Ø Measles complicated by encephalitis
Postmeasles encephalitis

BØ5.1 Measles complicated by meningitis
Postmeasles meningitis

BØ5.2 Measles complicated by pneumonia
Postmeasles pneumonia

BØ5.3 Measles complicated by otitis media
Postmeasles otitis media

BØ5.4 Measles with intestinal complications

● **BØ5.8 Measles with other complications**

BØ5.81 Measles keratitis and keratoconjunctivitis

BØ5.89 Other measles complications

BØ5.9 Measles without complication
Measles NOS

● **BØ6 Rubella [German measles]**
Excludes1 congenital rubella (P35.Ø)

● **BØ6.Ø Rubella with neurological complications**

BØ6.ØØ Rubella with neurological complication, unspecified

BØ6.Ø1 Rubella encephalitis
Rubella meningoencephalitis

BØ6.Ø2 Rubella meningitis

BØ6.Ø9 Other neurological complications of rubella

● **BØ6.8 Rubella with other complications**

BØ6.81 Rubella pneumonia

BØ6.82 Rubella arthritis

BØ6.89 Other rubella complications

BØ6.9 Rubella without complication
Rubella NOS

● **BØ7 Viral warts**
Includes verruca simplex
verruca vulgaris
viral warts due to human papillomavirus
Excludes2 anogenital (venereal) warts (A63.Ø)
papilloma of bladder (D41.4)
papilloma of cervix (D26.Ø)
papilloma larynx (D14.1)

BØ7.Ø Plantar wart
Verruca plantaris

BØ7.8 Other viral warts
Common wart
Flat wart
Verruca plana

BØ7.9 Viral wart, unspecified

● **B08 Other viral infections characterized by skin and mucous membrane lesions, not elsewhere classified**
Excludes1 vesicular stomatitis virus disease (A93.8)

● **B08.0 Other orthopoxvirus infections**
Excludes2 monkeypox (B04)

● **B08.01 Cowpox and vaccinia not from vaccine**
B08.010 Cowpox
B08.011 Vaccinia not from vaccine
Excludes1 vaccinia (from vaccination) (generalized) (T88.1)

B08.02 Orf virus disease
Contagious pustular dermatitis
Ecthyma contagiosum

B08.03 Pseudocowpox [milker's node]
B08.04 Paravaccinia, unspecified
B08.09 Other orthopoxvirus infections
Orthopoxvirus infection NOS

B08.1 Molluscum contagiosum
Various skin diseases characterized by soft, rounded, cutaneous lesions

● **B08.2 Exanthema subitum [sixth disease] Roseola infantum**
Acute, short-lived high fever in infants and young children followed by a rash mainly on the trunk, caused by human herpesvirus 6

B08.20 Exanthema subitum [sixth disease], unspecified Roseola infantum, unspecified
B08.21 Exanthema subitum [sixth disease] due to human herpesvirus 6 Roseola infantum due to human herpesvirus 6
Virus results in sudden rash; infection results in lifelong persistence
B08.22 Exanthema subitum [sixth disease] due to human herpesvirus 7 Roseola infantum due to human herpesvirus 7

B08.3 Erythema infectiosum [fifth disease]
Moderately contagious, epidemic disease in children caused by B19 virus; onset of rash that begins as redness of cheeks, later there is rash on trunk and limbs; when this fades, there may be central clearing that leaves lacelike pattern

B08.4 Enteroviral vesicular stomatitis with exanthem
Hand, foot and mouth disease
Check your documentation—this code is HAND, foot, and mouth disease. Code B08.8 is foot and mouth disease.

B08.5 Enteroviral vesicular pharyngitis
Herpangina

● **B08.6 Parapoxvirus infections**
B08.60 Parapoxvirus infection, unspecified
B08.61 Bovine stomatitis
B08.62 Sealpox
B08.69 Other parapoxvirus infections

● **B08.7 Yatapoxvirus infections**
B08.70 Yatapoxvirus infection, unspecified
B08.71 Tanapox virus disease
B08.72 Yaba pox virus disease
Yaba monkey tumor disease
B08.79 Other yatapoxvirus infections

B08.8 Other specified viral infections characterized by skin and mucous membrane lesions
Enteroviral lymphonodular pharyngitis
Foot-and-mouth disease
Check your documentation. Code B08.4 is for HAND, foot, and mouth disease.
Poxvirus NEC

B09 Unspecified viral infection characterized by skin and mucous membrane lesions
Viral enanthema NOS
Viral exanthema NOS

OTHER HUMAN HERPESVIRUSES (B10)

● **B10 Other human herpesviruses**
Excludes2 cytomegalovirus (B25.9)
Epstein-Barr virus (B27.0-)
herpes NOS (B00.9)
herpes simplex (B00.-)
herpes zoster (B02.-)
human herpesvirus NOS (B00.-)
human herpesvirus 1 and 2 (B00.-)
human herpesvirus 3 (B01.-, B02.-)
human herpesvirus 4 (B27.0-)
human herpesvirus 5 (B25.-)
varicella (B01.-)
zoster (B02.-)

● **B10.0 Other human herpesvirus encephalitis**
Excludes2 herpes encephalitis NOS (B00.4)
herpes simplex encephalitis (B00.4)
human herpesvirus encephalitis (B00.4)
simian B herpes virus encephalitis (B00.4)

B10.01 Human herpesvirus 6 encephalitis
Sudden rash or roseola
B10.09 Other human herpesvirus encephalitis
Human herpesvirus 7 encephalitis
Virus closely related to human herpesvirus 6, but not known to cause any disease

● **B10.8 Other human herpesvirus infection**
B10.81 Human herpesvirus 6 infection
Causative agent of exanthema subitum that results in sudden rash
B10.82 Human herpesvirus 7 infection
Closely related to human herpesvirus 6, but not known cause any disease
B10.89 Other human herpesvirus infection
Human herpesvirus 8 infection
May be the cause of Kaposi sarcoma, a malignant tumor
Kaposi's sarcoma-associated herpesvirus infection

VIRAL HEPATITIS (B15-B19)

Excludes1 sequelae of viral hepatitis (B94.2)
Excludes2 cytomegaloviral hepatitis (B25.1)
herpesviral [herpes simplex] hepatitis (B00.81)

● **B15 Acute hepatitis A**
B15.0 Hepatitis A with hepatic coma
B15.9 Hepatitis A without hepatic coma
Hepatitis A (acute) (viral) NOS

● **B17 Other acute viral hepatitis**
B17.0 Acute delta-(super) infection of hepatitis B carrier
● **B17.1 Acute hepatitis C**
B17.10 Acute hepatitis C without hepatic coma
Acute hepatitis C NOS
B17.11 Acute hepatitis C with hepatic coma
B17.2 Acute hepatitis E
B17.8 Other specified acute viral hepatitis
Hepatitis non-A non-B (acute) (viral) NEC
B17.9 Acute viral hepatitis, unspecified
Acute hepatitis NOS
Acute infectious hepatitis NOS ◄

CHAPTER 1 (A00-B99)

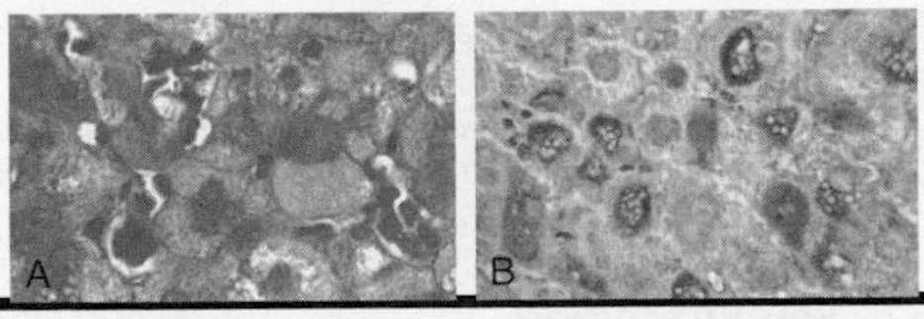

Figure 1-6 Hepatitis B viral infection. **A.** Liver parenchyma showing hepatocytes with diffuse granular cytoplasm, so-called ground glass hepatocytes (H&E). **B.** Immunoperoxidase stains from the same case, showing cytoplasmic inclusions of viral particles. (From Kumar: Robbins and Cotran: Pathologic Basis of Disease, ed 8, Saunders, An Imprint of Elsevier, 2009)

Item 1-18 **Hepatitis A (HAV)** was formerly called epidemic, infectious, short-incubation, or acute catarrhal jaundice hepatitis. The primary transmission mode is the oral–fecal route. **Hepatitis B (HBV)** was formerly called long-incubation period, serum, or homologous serum hepatitis. Transmission modes are through blood from infected persons and from body fluids of infected mother to neonate. **Hepatitis C (HCV),** caused by the hepatitis C virus, is primarily transfusion associated. **Hepatitis D (HDV),** also called delta hepatitis, is caused by the hepatitis D virus in patients formerly or currently infected with hepatitis B. **Hepatitis E (HEV)** is also called enterically transmitted non-A, non-B hepatitis. The primary transmission mode is the oral–fecal route, usually through contaminated water.

● **B18 Chronic viral hepatitis**
Includes Carrier of viral hepatitis ◀
B18.Ø Chronic viral hepatitis B with delta-agent
B18.1 Chronic viral hepatitis B without delta-agent
Carrier of viral hepatitis B ◀
Chronic (viral) hepatitis B
B18.2 Chronic viral hepatitis C
Carrier of viral hepatitis C ◀
B18.8 Other chronic viral hepatitis
Carrier of other viral hepatitis ◀
B18.9 Chronic viral hepatitis, unspecified
Carrier of unspecified viral hepatitis ◀

● **B19 Unspecified viral hepatitis**
B19.Ø Unspecified viral hepatitis with hepatic coma
● **B19.1 Unspecified viral hepatitis B**
B19.1Ø Unspecified viral hepatitis B without hepatic coma
Unspecified viral hepatitis B NOS
B19.11 Unspecified viral hepatitis B with hepatic coma
● **B19.2 Unspecified viral hepatitis C**
B19.2Ø Unspecified viral hepatitis C without hepatic coma
Viral hepatitis C NOS
B19.21 Unspecified viral hepatitis C with hepatic coma
B19.9 Unspecified viral hepatitis without hepatic coma
Viral hepatitis NOS

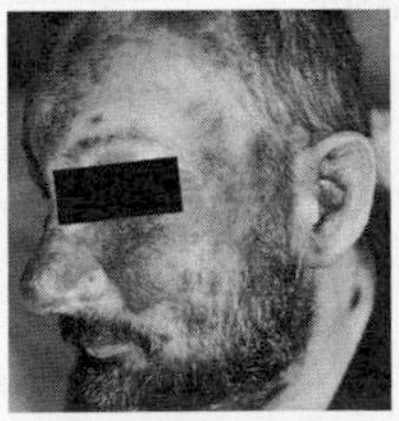

Figure 1-7 Kaposi's sarcoma. There are large confluent hyperpigmented patch-stage lesions with lymphedema. (From Cohen & Powderly: Infectious Diseases, ed 3, Mosby, An Imprint of Elsevier, 2010)

Item 1-19 **AIDS** (acquired immune deficiency syndrome) is caused by **HIV** (human immunodeficiency virus). HIV affects certain white blood cells (T-4 lymphocytes) and destroys the ability of the cells to fight infections, making patients susceptible to a host of infectious diseases (e.g., ***Pneumocystis carinii pneumonia (PCP), Kaposi's sarcoma,*** and ***lymphoma). AIDS-related complex (ARC)*** is an early stage of AIDS in which tests for HIV are positive but the symptoms are mild.

OGCR Section I. C.1.a

Certain Infectious and Parasitic Diseases (AØØ-B99)

a. Human Immunodeficiency Virus (HIV) Infections

1) Code only confirmed cases

Code only confirmed cases of HIV infection illness. This is an exception to the hospital inpatient guideline Section II, H.

In this context, "confirmation" does not require documentation of positive serology or culture for HIV; the provider's diagnostic statement that the patient is HIV positive, or has an HIV-related illness is sufficient.

HUMAN IMMUNODEFICIENCY VIRUS [HIV] DISEASE (B2Ø)

B2Ø Human immunodeficiency virus [HIV] disease
Includes acquired immune deficiency syndrome [AIDS]
AIDS-related complex [ARC]
HIV infection, symptomatic
Code first Human immunodeficiency virus [HIV] disease complicating pregnancy, childbirth and the puerperium, if applicable (O98.7-)
Use additional code(s) to identify all manifestations of HIV infection
Excludes1 asymptomatic human immunodeficiency virus [HIV] infection status (Z21)
exposure to HIV virus (Z2Ø.6)
inconclusive serologic evidence of HIV (R75)

OTHER VIRAL DISEASES (B25-B34)

● **B25 Cytomegaloviral disease**
AKA: HCMV or Human Herpesvirus 5 (HHV-5)
Excludes1 congenital cytomegalovirus infection (P35.1)
cytomegaloviral mononucleosis (B27.1-)
B25.Ø Cytomegaloviral pneumonitis
B25.1 Cytomegaloviral hepatitis
B25.2 Cytomegaloviral pancreatitis
B25.8 Other cytomegaloviral diseases
Cytomegaloviral encephalitis
B25.9 Cytomegaloviral disease, unspecified

● **B26 Mumps**
Includes epidemic parotitis
infectious parotitis
Acute, contagious, viral disease
B26.Ø Mumps orchitis
B26.1 Mumps meningitis
B26.2 Mumps encephalitis
B26.3 Mumps pancreatitis
● **B26.8 Mumps with other complications**
B26.81 Mumps hepatitis
B26.82 Mumps myocarditis
B26.83 Mumps nephritis
B26.84 Mumps polyneuropathy
B26.85 Mumps arthritis
B26.89 Other mumps complications
B26.9 Mumps without complication
Mumps NOS
Mumps parotitis NOS

CHAPTER 1 (AØØ-B99)

● **B27 Infectious mononucleosis**
Includes glandular fever
monocytic angina
Pfeiffer's disease

● **B27.0 Gammaherpesviral mononucleosis**
AKA: Pfeiffer's disease, infective mononucleosis
Mononucleosis due to Epstein-Barr virus

B27.00 Gammaherpesviral mononucleosis without complication
Infective mononucleosis

B27.01 Gammaherpesviral mononucleosis with polyneuropathy

B27.02 Gammaherpesviral mononucleosis with meningitis

B27.09 Gammaherpesviral mononucleosis with other complications
Hepatomegaly in gammaherpesviral mononucleosis

● **B27.1 Cytomegaloviral mononucleosis**
Infectious disease resembling infectious mononucleosis

B27.10 Cytomegaloviral mononucleosis without complications

B27.11 Cytomegaloviral mononucleosis with polyneuropathy

B27.12 Cytomegaloviral mononucleosis with meningitis

B27.19 Cytomegaloviral mononucleosis with other complication
Hepatomegaly in cytomegaloviral mononucleosis

● **B27.8 Other infectious mononucleosis**

B27.80 Other infectious mononucleosis without complication

B27.81 Other infectious mononucleosis with polyneuropathy

B27.82 Other infectious mononucleosis with meningitis

B27.89 Other infectious mononucleosis with other complication
Hepatomegaly in other infectious mononucleosis

● **B27.9 Infectious mononucleosis, unspecified**

B27.90 Infectious mononucleosis, unspecified without complication

B27.91 Infectious mononucleosis, unspecified with polyneuropathy

B27.92 Infectious mononucleosis, unspecified with meningitis

B27.99 Infectious mononucleosis, unspecified with other complication
Hepatomegaly in unspecified infectious mononucleosis

● **B30 Viral conjunctivitis**
Excludes1 herpesviral [herpes simplex] ocular disease (B00.5)
ocular zoster (B02.3)

B30.0 Keratoconjunctivitis due to adenovirus
Epidemic keratoconjunctivitis
Shipyard eye

B30.1 Conjunctivitis due to adenovirus
Acute adenoviral follicular conjunctivitis
Swimming-pool conjunctivitis

B30.2 Viral pharyngoconjunctivitis

B30.3 Acute epidemic hemorrhagic conjunctivitis (enteroviral)
Conjunctivitis due to coxsackievirus 24
Conjunctivitis due to enterovirus 70
Hemorrhagic conjunctivitis (acute)(epidemic)

B30.8 Other viral conjunctivitis
Newcastle conjunctivitis

B30.9 Viral conjunctivitis, unspecified

● **B33 Other viral diseases, not elsewhere classified**

B33.0 Epidemic myalgia
Acute infectious disease, caused by group A coxsackie viruses or other enteroviruses with symptoms that include sudden pain in chest or upper abdomen with fever
Bornholm disease

B33.1 Ross River disease
Epidemic polyarthritis and exanthema
Ross River fever

● **B33.2 Viral carditis**
Coxsackie (virus) carditis

B33.20 Viral carditis, unspecified

B33.21 Viral endocarditis

B33.22 Viral myocarditis

B33.23 Viral pericarditis

B33.24 Viral cardiomyopathy

B33.3 Retrovirus infections, not elsewhere classified
Retrovirus infection NOS

B33.4 Hantavirus (cardio)-pulmonary syndrome [HPS] [HCPS]
Hantavirus disease with pulmonary manifestations
Sin nombre virus disease
Use additional code to identify any associated acute kidney failure (N17.9)
Excludes1 hantavirus disease with renal manifestations (A98.5)
hemorrhagic fever with renal manifestations (A98.5)

B33.8 Other specified viral diseases
Excludes1 anogenital human papillomavirus infection (A63.0)
viral warts due to human papillomavirus infection (B07)

● **B34 Viral infection of unspecified site**
Excludes1 anogenital human papillomavirus infection (A63.0)
cytomegaloviral disease NOS (B25.9)
herpesvirus [herpes simplex] infection NOS (B00.9)
retrovirus infection NOS (B33.3)
viral agents as the cause of diseases classified elsewhere (B97.-)
viral warts due to human papillomavirus infection (B07)

B34.0 Adenovirus infection, unspecified

B34.1 Enterovirus infection, unspecified
Intestinal tract infection
Coxsackievirus infection NOS
Echovirus infection NOS

B34.2 Coronavirus infection, unspecified
Excludes1 pneumonia due to SARS-associated coronavirus (J12.81)

B34.3 Parvovirus infection, unspecified

B34.4 Papovavirus infection, unspecified

B34.8 Other viral infections of unspecified site

B34.9 Viral infection, unspecified
Viremia NOS

MYCOSES (B35-B49)

Excludes2 hypersensitivity pneumonitis due to organic dust (J67.-)
mycosis fungoides (C84.0-)

● **B35 Dermatophytosis**
AKA tinea or ringworm
Includes favus
infections due to species of Epidermophyton, Micro-sporum and Trichophyton
tinea, any type except those in B36.-

B35.0 Tinea barbae and tinea capitis
Beard ringworm
Kerion
Scalp ringworm
Sycosis, mycotic

B35.1 Tinea unguium
White patches or pits on surface or edges of nails, followed by infection under nail plate
Dermatophytic onychia
Dermatophytosis of nail
Onychomycosis
Ringworm of nails

B35.2 Tinea manuum
Tinea of hands
Dermatophytosis of hand
Hand ringworm

B35.3 Tinea pedis
Tinea affecting feet
Athlete's foot
Dermatophytosis of foot
Foot ringworm

B35.4 Tinea corporis
Infecting skin areas other than hands
Ringworm of the body

B35.5 Tinea imbricata
Chronic tropical tinea corporis; AKA Oriental ringworm, tinea inguinalis, tinea cruris
Tokelau

B35.6 Tinea cruris
In groin or perineal area, spreading to adjacent regions; AKA jock itch, eczema marginatum, ringworm of groin, or t inguinalis
Dhobi itch
Groin ringworm
Jock itch

B35.8 Other dermatophytoses
Disseminated dermatophytosis
Granulomatous dermatophytosis

B35.9 Dermatophytosis, unspecified
Ringworm NOS

● **B36 Other superficial mycoses**

B36.0 Pityriasis versicolor
Common, chronic, symptomless disorder that includes macular patches of various sizes and shapes; AKA liver spots
Tinea flava
Tinea versicolor

B36.1 Tinea nigra
Minor fungal infection, with dark lesions, usually on skin of hands
Keratomycosis nigricans palmaris
Microsporosis nigra
Pityriasis nigra

B36.2 White piedra
White to light brown nodules on hair of beard, axilla, or groin; AKA trichosporosis
Tinea blanca

B36.3 Black piedra
Characterized by small black or brown nodules on shafts of scalp hair

B36.8 Other specified superficial mycoses

B36.9 Superficial mycosis, unspecified

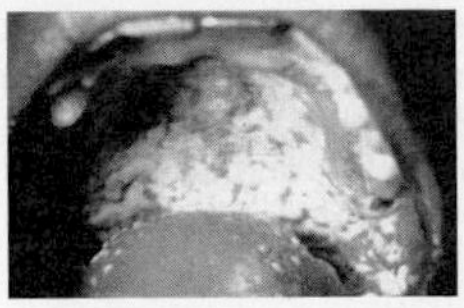

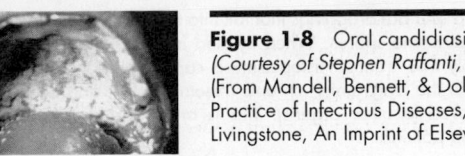

Figure 1-8 Oral candidiasis (thrush). *(Courtesy of Stephen Raffanti, MD, MPH.)* (From Mandell, Bennett, & Dolin: Principles and Practice of Infectious Diseases, ed 7, Churchill Livingstone, An Imprint of Elsevier, 2009)

Item 1-20 Candidiasis, also called oidiomycosis or moniliasis, is a fungal infection. It most often appears on moist cutaneous areas of the body but can also be responsible for a variety of systemic infections such as endocarditis, meningitis, arthritis, and myositis. Antifungal medications cure most yeast infections.

● **B37 Candidiasis**
Includes candidosis
moniliasis
Excludes1 neonatal candidiasis (P37.5)

B37.0 Candidal stomatitis
Oral thrush

B37.1 Pulmonary candidiasis
Candidal bronchitis
Candidal pneumonia

B37.2 Candidiasis of skin and nail
Candidal onychia
Candidal paronychia
Excludes2 diaper dermatitis (L22)

B37.3 Candidiasis of vulva and vagina
Candidal vulvovaginitis
Monilial vulvovaginitis
Vaginal thrush

● **B37.4 Candidiasis of other urogenital sites**

B37.41 Candidal cystitis and urethritis

B37.42 Candidal balanitis
Male condition only

B37.49 Other urogenital candidiasis
Candidal pyelonephritis

B37.5 Candidal meningitis

B37.6 Candidal endocarditis

B37.7 Candidal sepsis
Disseminated candidiasis systemic candidiasis

● **B37.8 Candidiasis of other sites**

B37.81 Candidal esophagitis

B37.82 Candidal enteritis
Candidal proctitis

B37.83 Candidal cheilitis
Inflammation affecting lip

B37.84 Candidal otitis externa
Inflammation of external auditory canal

B37.89 Other sites of candidiasis
Infection manifested by invasive candidiasis
Candidal osteomyelitis

B37.9 Candidiasis, unspecified
Thrush NOS

● **B38 Coccidioidomycosis**
Fungal disease; AKA coccidioidosis, coccidioidal granuloma, Posadas, or Posadas-Wernicke disease

B38.0 Acute pulmonary coccidioidomycosis

B38.1 Chronic pulmonary coccidioidomycosis

B38.2 Pulmonary coccidioidomycosis, unspecified

B38.3 Cutaneous coccidioidomycosis

B38.4 Coccidioidomycosis meningitis

B38.7 Disseminated coccidioidomycosis
Generalized coccidioidomycosis

● **B38.8 Other forms of coccidioidomycosis**

B38.81 Prostatic coccidioidomycosis

B38.89 Other forms of coccidioidomycosis

B38.9 Coccidioidomycosis, unspecified

Item 1–21 Bird and bat droppings that fall into the soil give rise to a fungus that can spread airborne spores. When inhaled into the lungs, these spores divide and multiply into lesions. Histoplasmosis capsulatum takes three forms: primary (lodged in the lungs only), chronic (resembles TB), and disseminated (infection has moved to other organs). This is an opportunistic infection in immunosuppressed patients.

● **B39 Histoplasmosis**
Infection resulting from inhalation or ingestion of spores; AKA Darling disease
Code first associated AIDS (B20)
Use additional code for any associated manifestations, such as:
endocarditis (I39)
meningitis (G02)
pericarditis (I32)
retinitits (H32)

B39.0 Acute pulmonary histoplasmosis capsulati
B39.1 Chronic pulmonary histoplasmosis capsulati
B39.2 Pulmonary histoplasmosis capsulati, unspecified
B39.3 Disseminated histoplasmosis capsulati
Generalized histoplasmosis capsulati
B39.4 Histoplasmosis capsulati, unspecified
American histoplasmosis
B39.5 Histoplasmosis duboisii
African histoplasmosis
B39.9 Histoplasmosis, unspecified

● **B40 Blastomycosis**
Rare and potentially fatal infection caused by inhaling fungus found in moist soil in temperate climates.
Excludes1 Brazilian blastomycosis (B41.-)
keloidal blastomycosis (B48.0)

B40.0 Acute pulmonary blastomycosis
B40.1 Chronic pulmonary blastomycosis
B40.2 Pulmonary blastomycosis, unspecified
B40.3 Cutaneous blastomycosis
B40.7 Disseminated blastomycosis
Generalized blastomycosis
● **B40.8 Other forms of blastomycosis**
B40.81 Blastomycotic meningoencephalitis
Meningomyelitis due to blastomycosis
B40.89 Other forms of blastomycosis
B40.9 Blastomycosis, unspecified

● **B41 Paracoccidioidomycosis**
Fungal infection usually chronic that begins in lungs, spreads to mucocutaneous areas which may extend to skin, tonsils, gastrointestinal lymphatics, liver, and spleen; AKA Almeida or Lutz-Splendore-Almeida disease, Brazilian or South American blastomycosis, or paracoccidioidal granuloma
Includes Brazilian blastomycosis
Lutz' disease

B41.0 Pulmonary paracoccidioidomycosis
B41.7 Disseminated paracoccidioidomycosis
Generalized paracoccidioidomycosis
B41.8 Other forms of paracoccidioidomycosis
B41.9 Paracoccidioidomycosis, unspecified

● **B42 Sporotrichosis**
Chronic fungal infection with nodular lesions
B42.0 Pulmonary sporotrichosis
B42.1 Lymphocutaneous sporotrichosis
B42.7 Disseminated sporotrichosis
Generalized sporotrichosis
● **B42.8 Other forms of sporotrichosis**
B42.81 Cerebral sporotrichosis
Meningitis due to sporotrichosis
B42.82 Sporotrichosis arthritis
B42.89 Other forms of sporotrichosis
B42.9 Sporotrichosis, unspecified

● **B43 Chromomycosis and pheomycotic abscess**
Chronic fungal infection of skin, initiated at site of puncture affecting lower limb or foot (mossy foot)
B43.0 Cutaneous chromomycosis
Dermatitis verrucosa
B43.1 Pheomycotic brain abscess
Cerebral chromomycosis
B43.2 Subcutaneous pheomycotic abscess and cyst
B43.8 Other forms of chromomycosis
B43.9 Chromomycosis, unspecified

● **B44 Aspergillosis**
Infection marked by inflammatory lesions in skin, ear, orbit, nasal sinuses, lungs, and occasionally bones and meninges
Includes aspergilloma

B44.0 Invasive pulmonary aspergillosis
B44.1 Other pulmonary aspergillosis
B44.2 Tonsillar aspergillosis
B44.7 Disseminated aspergillosis
Generalized aspergillosis
● **B44.8 Other forms of aspergillosis**
B44.81 Allergic bronchopulmonary aspergillosis
B44.89 Other forms of aspergillosis
B44.9 Aspergillosis, unspecified

● **B45 Cryptococcosis**
Infection in the immunocompromised and fatal if left untreated; AKA torulosis, Buschke, or Busse-Buschke disease
B45.0 Pulmonary cryptococcosis
B45.1 Cerebral cryptococcosis
Cryptococcal meningitis
Cryptococcosis meningocerebralis
B45.2 Cutaneous cryptococcosis
B45.3 Osseous cryptococcosis
B45.7 Disseminated cryptococcosis
Generalized cryptococcosis
B45.8 Other forms of cryptococcosis
B45.9 Cryptococcosis, unspecified

● **B46 Zygomycosis**
Fungal infections including subcutaneous lesions and infection of sinuses, brain, or lungs
B46.0 Pulmonary mucormycosis
Fungal infection affecting lung
B46.1 Rhinocerebral mucormycosis
B46.2 Gastrointestinal mucormycosis
B46.3 Cutaneous mucormycosis
Subcutaneous mucormycosis
B46.4 Disseminated mucormycosis
Generalized mucormycosis
B46.5 Mucormycosis, unspecified
B46.8 Other zygomycoses
Entomophthoromycosis
B46.9 Zygomycosis, unspecified
Phycomycosis NOS

● **B47 Mycetoma**
Slow progressive, destructive fungal infection of cutaneous and subcutaneous tissues, fascia, and bone, primarily seen in foot (Madura foot) or leg
B47.0 Eumycetoma
Madura foot, mycotic Maduromycosis
B47.1 Actinomycetoma
B47.9 Mycetoma, unspecified
Madura foot NOS

● **B48 Other mycoses, not elsewhere classified**

B48.0 Lobomycosis
Infection with symptoms of red, smooth, hard cutaneous nodules resembling keloids
Keloidal blastomycosis
Lobo's disease

B48.1 Rhinosporidiosis
Chronic, localized granulomatous fungal infection, affecting mucocutaneous tissues, usually of nose characterized by polyps, papillomas, and wartlike lesions

B48.2 Allescheriasis
Fungal infection
Infection due to Pseudallescheria boydii
Excludes1 eumycetoma (B47.0)

B48.3 Geotrichosis
Fungal infection usually of bronchi, lungs, mouth, or intestinal tract
Geotrichum stomatitis

B48.4 Penicillosis
Fungal infection

B48.8 Other specified mycoses
Adiaspiromycosis
Infection of tissue and organs by Alternaria
Infection of tissue and organs by Drechslera
Infection of tissue and organs by Fusarium
Infection of tissue and organs by saprophytic fungi NEC

B49 Unspecified mycosis
Fungemia NOS

PROTOZOAL DISEASES (B50-B64)

Excludes1 amebiasis (A06.-)
other protozoal intestinal diseases (A07.-)

● **B50 Plasmodium falciparum malaria**
Severe form of malaria that can be fatal
Includes mixed infections of Plasmodium falciparum with any other Plasmodium species

B50.0 Plasmodium falciparum malaria with cerebral complications
Cerebral malaria NOS

B50.8 Other severe and complicated Plasmodium falciparum malaria
Severe or complicated Plasmodium falciparum malaria NOS

B50.9 Plasmodium falciparum malaria, unspecified

● **B51 Plasmodium vivax malaria**
Includes mixed infections of Plasmodium vivax with other Plasmodium species, except Plasmodium falciparum
Excludes1 plasmodium vivav with Plasmodium falciparum (B50.-)

B51.0 Plasmodium vivax malaria with rupture of spleen
B51.8 Plasmodium vivax malaria with other complications
B51.9 Plasmodium vivax malaria without complication
Plasmodium vivax malaria NOS

● **B52 Plasmodium malariae malaria**
Causes fever that recurs at approximately three-day intervals (quartan fever), longer than two-day (tertian) intervals of other malarial parasites
Includes mixed infections of Plasmodium malariae with other Plasmodium species, except Plasmodium falciparum and Plasmodium vivax
Excludes1 plasmodium falciparum (B50.-)
plasmodium vivax (B51.-)

B52.0 Plasmodium malariae malaria with nephropathy
B52.8 Plasmodium malariae malaria with other complications
B52.9 Plasmodium malariae malaria without complication
Plasmodium malariae malaria NOS

● **B53 Other specified malaria**

B53.0 Plasmodium ovale malaria
Least diagnosed type of malaria spread by female mosquitoes of rare species
Excludes1 plasmodium ovale with Plasmodium falciparum (B50.-)
plasmodium ovale with Plasmodium malariae (B52.-)
plasmodium ovale with Plasmodium vivax (B51.-)

B53.1 Malaria due to simian plasmodia
Malaria-like disease (parasite infection)
Excludes1 malaria due to simian plasmodia with Plasmodium falciparum (B50.-)
malaria due to simian plasmodia with Plasmodium malariae (B52.-)
malaria due to simian plasmodia with Plasmodium ovale (B53.0)
malaria due to simian plasmodia with Plasmodium vivax (B51.-)

B53.8 Other malaria, not elsewhere classified

B54 Unspecified malaria

● **B55 Leishmaniasis**
Protozoal infection

B55.0 Visceral leishmaniasis
Kala-azar
Post-kala-azar dermal leishmaniasis

B55.1 Cutaneous leishmaniasis
B55.2 Mucocutaneous leishmaniasis
B55.9 Leishmaniasis, unspecified

● **B56 African trypanosomiasis**
Human African trypanosomiasis (HAT) is transmitted by fly bites

B56.0 Gambiense trypanosomiasis
Infection due to Trypanosoma brucei gambiense
West African sleeping sickness

B56.1 Rhodesiense trypanosomiasis
East African sleeping sickness
Infection due to Trypanosoma brucei rhodesiense

B56.9 African trypanosomiasis, unspecified
Sleeping sickness NOS

● **B57 Chagas' disease**
Tropical parasitic disease
Includes American trypanosomiasis
infection due to Trypanosoma cruzi

B57.0 Acute Chagas' disease with heart involvement
Acute Chagas' disease with myocarditis

B57.1 Acute Chagas' disease without heart involvement
Acute Chagas' disease NOS

B57.2 Chagas' disease (chronic) with heart involvement
American trypanosomiasis NOS
Chagas' disease (chronic) NOS
Chagas' disease (chronic) with myocarditis
Trypanosomiasis NOS

● **B57.3 Chagas' disease (chronic) with digestive system involvement**

B57.30 Chagas' disease with digestive system involvement, unspecified
B57.31 Megaesophagus in Chagas' disease
B57.32 Megacolon in Chagas' disease
B57.39 Other digestive system involvement in Chagas' disease

● **B57.4 Chagas' disease (chronic) with nervous system involvement**

B57.40 Chagas' disease with nervous system involvement, unspecified
B57.41 Meningitis in Chagas' disease
B57.42 Meningoencephalitis in Chagas' disease
B57.49 Other nervous system involvement in Chagas' disease

B57.5 Chagas' disease (chronic) with other organ involvement

Item 1–22 Toxoplasmosis is caused by the protozoa **Toxoplasma gondii,** of which the house cat can be a host. Human infection occurs when contact is made with materials containing the pathogen, such as feces, contaminated soil, or ingestion of infected lamb, goat, or pork. Of the infected, very few have symptoms because a healthy person's immune system keeps the parasite from causing illness. When the immune system is compromised, symptoms may occur. Clinical symptoms include flu-like symptoms, but the disease progresses to include the eyes and the brain in babies.

● **B58 Toxoplasmosis**
Infection by protozoon transmitted in cysts in feces of cats
Includes infection due to Toxoplasma gondii
Excludes1 congenital toxoplasmosis (P37.1)

● **B58.0 Toxoplasma oculopathy**
B58.00 Toxoplasma oculopathy, unspecified
B58.01 Toxoplasma chorioretinitis
B58.09 Other toxoplasma oculopathy
Toxoplasma uveitis
B58.1 Toxoplasma hepatitis
B58.2 Toxoplasma meningoencephalitis
B58.3 Pulmonary toxoplasmosis
● **B58.8 Toxoplasmosis with other organ involvement**
B58.81 Toxoplasma myocarditis
B58.82 Toxoplasma myositis
B58.83 Toxoplasma tubulo-interstitial nephropathy
Toxoplasma pyelonephritis
B58.89 Toxoplasmosis with other organ involvement
B58.9 Toxoplasmosis, unspecified

B59 Pneumocystosis
Caused by fungus
Pneumonia due to Pneumocystis carinii
Pneumonia due to Pneumocystis jiroveci

● **B60 Other protozoal diseases, not elsewhere classified**
Excludes1 cryptosporidiosis (A07.2)
intestinal microsporidiosis (A07.8)
isosporiasis (A07.3)
B60.0 Babesiosis
Tickborne disease caused by microscopic organisms
Piroplasmosis
● **B60.1 Acanthamebiasis**
B60.10 Acanthamebiasis, unspecified
B60.11 Meningoencephalitis due to Acanthamoeba (culbertsoni)
B60.12 Conjunctivitis due to Acanthamoeba
B60.13 Keratoconjunctivitis due to Acanthamoeba
B60.19 Other acanthamebic disease
B60.2 Naegleriasis
Infection with microscopic organisms
Primary amebic meningoencephalitis
B60.8 Other specified protozoal diseases
Microsporidiosis

B64 Unspecified protozoal disease

HELMINTHIASES (B65-B83)

Diseases or infestations caused by parasitic worms

● **B65 Schistosomiasis [bilharziasis]**
Infection with flukes (flat parasitic worms)
Includes snail fever
B65.0 Schistosomiasis due to Schistosoma haematobium [urinary schistosomiasis]
B65.1 Schistosomiasis due to Schistosoma mansoni [intestinal schistosomiasis]
B65.2 Schistosomiasis due to Schistosoma japonicum
Asiatic schistosomiasis
B65.3 Cercarial dermatitis
Swimmer's itch
B65.8 Other schistosomiasis
Infection due to Schistosoma intercalatum
Infection due to Schistosoma mattheei
Infection due to Schistosoma mekongi
B65.9 Schistosomiasis, unspecified

● **B66 Other fluke infections**
Trematode (parasitic worms)
B66.0 Opisthorchiasis
Infection due to cat liver fluke
Infection due to Opisthorchis (felineus)(viverrini)
B66.1 Clonorchiasis
Chinese liver fluke disease
Infection due to Clonorchis sinensis
Oriental liver fluke disease
B66.2 Dicroceliasis
Liver fluke
Infection due to Dicrocoelium dendriticum
Lancet fluke infection
B66.3 Fascioliasis
Infection due to Fasciola gigantica
Infection due to Fasciola hepatica
Infection due to Fasciola indica
Sheep liver fluke disease
B66.4 Paragonimiasis
Infection due to Paragonimus species
Lung fluke disease
Pulmonary distomiasis
B66.5 Fasciolopsiasis
Largest intestinal fluke in humans
Infection due to Fasciolopsis buski
Intestinal distomiasis
B66.8 Other specified fluke infections
Echinostomiasis
Heterophyiasis
Metagonimiasis
Nanophyetiasis
Watsoniasis
B66.9 Fluke infection, unspecified

● **B67 Echinococcosis**
Larval forms of tapeworms usually of liver or lungs
Includes hydatidosis
B67.0 Echinococcus granulosus infection of liver
B67.1 Echinococcus granulosus infection of lung
B67.2 Echinococcus granulosus infection of bone
● **B67.3 Echinococcus granulosus infection, other and multiple sites**
B67.31 Echinococcus granulosus infection, thyroid gland
B67.32 Echinococcus granulosus infection, multiple sites
B67.39 Echinococcus granulosus infection, other sites
B67.4 Echinococcus granulosus infection, unspecified
Dog tapeworm (infection)
B67.5 Echinococcus multilocularis infection of liver

Item 1–23 Echinococcosis: Also known as hydatid disease; is caused by Echinococcus granulosus, E. multilocularis, and E. vogeli tapeworms; and is contracted from infected food. Found in southern South America, the Mediterranean, the Middle East, central Asia, and Africa and uncommon in the United States but has been reported in California, New Mexico, Arizona and Utah. The disease is treated with medication over a long course as it is resistive.

- **B67.6 Echinococcus multilocularis infection, other and multiple sites**
  - **B67.61 Echinococcus multilocularis infection, multiple sites**
  - **B67.69 Echinococcus multilocularis infection, other sites**
- **B67.7 Echinococcus multilocularis infection, unspecified**
- **B67.8 Echinococcosis, unspecified, of liver**
- **B67.9 Echinococcosis, other and unspecified**
  - **B67.90 Echinococcosis, unspecified**
    Echinococcosis NOS
  - **B67.99 Other echinococcosis**

B68 Taeniasis
Intestinal tapeworm (cestode) infection from raw or undercooked meat of infected animal
Excludes1 cysticercosis (B69.-)
- **B68.0 Taenia solium taeniasis**
  Pork tapeworm (infection)
- **B68.1 Taenia saginata taeniasis**
  Beef tapeworm (infection)
  Infection due to adult tapeworm Taenia saginata
- **B68.9 Taeniasis, unspecified**

B69 Cysticercosis
Systemic illness caused by the larvae of pork tapeworm
Includes cysticerciasis infection due to larval form of Taenia solium
- **B69.0 Cysticercosis of central nervous system**
- **B69.1 Cysticercosis of eye**
- **B69.8 Cysticercosis of other sites**
  - **B69.81 Myositis in cysticercosis**
  - **B69.89 Cysticercosis of other sites**
- **B69.9 Cysticercosis, unspecified**

B70 Diphyllobothriasis and sparganosis
Infection with tapeworms seen most often from inadequately cooked fish
- **B70.0 Diphyllobothriasis**
  Diphyllobothrium (adult) (latum) (pacificum) infection
  Fish tapeworm (infection)
  Excludes2 larval diphyllobothriasis (B70.1)
- **B70.1 Sparganosis**
  Infection with migrating tapeworm larvae, which invade subcutaneous tissues, causing inflammation and fibrosis that resembles cellulitis
  Infection due to Sparganum (mansoni) (proliferum)
  Infection due to Spirometra larva
  Larval diphyllobothriasis
  Spirometrosis

B71 Other cestode infections
- **B71.0 Hymenolepiasis**
  Intestinal infestation with tapeworms
  Dwarf tapeworm infection
  Rat tapeworm (infection)
- **B71.1 Dipylidiasis**
  Infection with tapeworm common to dogs and cats and seen in children having close contact with infected pets
- **B71.8 Other specified cestode infections**
  Infection by the larval stage of a tapeworm, usually through fruit or vegetables
  Coenurosis
- **B71.9 Cestode infection, unspecified**
  Tapeworm (infection) NOS

B72 Dracunculiasis
Infection with roundworms
Includes guinea worm infection
infection due to Dracunculus medinensis

B73 Onchocerciasis
Infection with parasitic worm
Includes onchocerca volvulus infection
onchocercosis
river blindness
- **B73.0 Onchocerciasis with eye disease**
  - **B73.00 Onchocerciasis with eye involvement, unspecified**
  - **B73.01 Onchocerciasis with endophthalmitis**
  - **B73.02 Onchocerciasis with glaucoma**
  - **B73.09 Onchocerciasis with other eye involvement**
    Infestation of eyelid due to onchocerciasis
- **B73.1 Onchocerciasis without eye disease**

B74 Filariasis
Infestation with slender threadlike worms
Excludes2 onchocerciasis (B73)
tropical (pulmonary) eosinophilia NOS (J82)
- **B74.0 Filariasis due to Wuchereria bancrofti**
  Bancroftian elephantiasis
  Bancroftian filariasis
- **B74.1 Filariasis due to Brugia malayi**
- **B74.2 Filariasis due to Brugia timori**
- **B74.3 Loiasis**
  Infection with round worms growing in subcutaneous connective tissue
  Calabar swelling
  Eyeworm disease of Africa
  Loa loa infection
- **B74.4 Mansonelliasis**
  Infection with filarial parasite
  Infection due to Mansonella ozzardi
  Infection due to Mansonella perstans
  Infection due to Mansonella streptocerca
- **B74.8 Other filariases**
  Dirofilariasis
- **B74.9 Filariasis, unspecified**

B75 Trichinellosis
Infestation with parasitic roundworms ingested in undercooked contaminated meat
Includes infection due to Trichinella species trichiniasis

B76 Hookworm diseases
Occurs in hot, humid parts of world where larvae are soil borne, enter digestive tract through skin of feet/legs or in contaminated food/water; AKA ground itch
Includes uncinariasis
- **B76.0 Ancylostomiasis**
  Infection due to Ancylostoma species
- **B76.1 Necatoriasis**
  Infection due to Necator americanus
- **B76.8 Other hookworm diseases**
- **B76.9 Hookworm disease, unspecified**
  Cutaneous larva migrans NOS

B77 Ascariasis
Infection by roundworm in small intestine
Includes ascaridiasis
roundworm infection
- **B77.0 Ascariasis with intestinal complications**
- **B77.8 Ascariasis with other complications**
  - **B77.81 Ascariasis pneumonia**
  - **B77.89 Ascariasis with other complications**
- **B77.9 Ascariasis, unspecified**

● **B78 Strongyloidiasis**
Infection with adult female roundworms
Excludes1 trichostrongyliasis (B81.2)
B78.Ø Intestinal strongyloidiasis
B78.1 Cutaneous strongyloidiasis
B78.7 Disseminated strongyloidiasis
B78.9 Strongyloidiasis, unspecified

B79 Trichuriasis
Intestinal infection with roundworms
Includes trichocephaliasis
whipworm (disease)(infection)

B8Ø Enterobiasis
Intestinal infection with pinworms
Includes oxyuriasis
pinworm infection
threadworm infection

● **B81 Other intestinal helminthiases, not elsewhere classified**
Diseases or infestations caused by parasitic worms
Excludes1 angiostrongyliasis due to Parastrongylus cantonensis (B83.2)
B81.Ø Anisakiasis
Roundworm infection via contaminated undercooked infected fish or marine mammals
Infection due to Anisakis larva
B81.1 Intestinal capillariasis
Infestation with of parasites (nematodes)
Capillariasis NOS
Infection due to Capillaria philippinensis
Excludes2 hepatic capillariasis (B83.8)
B81.2 Trichostrongyliasis
B81.3 Intestinal angiostrongyliasis
Angiostrongyliasis due to Parastrongylus costaricensis
B81.4 Mixed intestinal helminthiases
Infection due to intestinal helminths classified to more than one of the categories B65.Ø-B81.3 and B81.8
Mixed helminthiasis NOS
B81.8 Other specified intestinal helminthiases
Infection due to Oesophagostomum species [esophagostomiasis]
Infection due to Ternidens diminutus [ternidensiasis]

● **B82 Unspecified intestinal parasitism**
B82.Ø Intestinal helminthiasis, unspecified
Infected with worms
B82.9 Intestinal parasitism, unspecified

● **B83 Other helminthiases**
Caused by parasitic worms
Excludes1 capillariasis NOS (B81.1)
Excludes2 intestinal capillariasis (B81.1)
B83.Ø Visceral larva migrans
Prolonged migration of nematode larvae
Toxocariasis
B83.1 Gnathostomiasis
Infection with nematode occurring from ingested undercooked fish contaminated with larvae; larvae migrate to subcutaneous tissue or deeper tissues, results are abscesses
Wandering swelling
B83.2 Angiostrongyliasis due to Parastrongylus cantonensis
Nematode infection caused by eating contaminated raw snails, slugs, or paratenic hosts such as prawns or crabs; larval worms migrate to central nervous system resulting in eosinophilic meningitis
Eosinophilic meningoencephalitis due to Parastrongylus cantonensis
Excludes2 intestinal angiostrongyliasis (B81.3)
B83.3 Syngamiasis
Infestation with gapeworm from turkey, pheasant, guinea fowl, goose, and wild birds
Syngamosis
B83.4 Internal hirudiniasis
Infestation by leeches
Excludes2 external hirudiniasis (B88.3)
B83.8 Other specified helminthiases
Parasitic worm infestation
Acanthocephaliasis
Gongylonemiasis
Hepatic capillariasis
Metastrongyliasis
Thelaziasis
B83.9 Helminthiasis, unspecified
Worms NOS
Excludes1 intestinal helminthiasis NOS (B82.Ø)

PEDICULOSIS, ACARIASIS AND OTHER INFESTATIONS (B85-B89)

● **B85 Pediculosis and phthiriasis**
Infestation of lice
B85.Ø Pediculosis due to Pediculus humanus capitis
Head-louse infestation
B85.1 Pediculosis due to Pediculus humanus corporis
Body-louse infestation
B85.2 Pediculosis, unspecified
B85.3 Phthiriasis
Crab or pubic lice
Infestation by crab-louse
Infestation by Phthirus pubis
B85.4 Mixed pediculosis and phthiriasis
Infestation classifiable to more than one of the categories B85.Ø-B85.3

B86 Scabies
Sarcoptic itch
Contagious dermatitis caused by mites

● **B87 Myiasis**
Infestation by fly maggots
Includes infestation by larva of flies
B87.Ø Cutaneous myiasis
Creeping myiasis
B87.1 Wound myiasis
Traumatic myiasis
B87.2 Ocular myiasis
B87.3 Nasopharyngeal myiasis
Laryngeal myiasis
B87.4 Aural myiasis
● **B87.8 Myiasis of other sites**
B87.81 Genitourinary myiasis
B87.82 Intestinal myiasis
B87.89 Myiasis of other sites
B87.9 Myiasis, unspecified

CHAPTER 1 (AØØ-B99)

● **B88 Other infestations**

B88.0 Other acariasis
Acarine dermatitis
Dermatitis due to Demodex species
Dermatitis due to Dermanyssus gallinae
Dermatitis due to Liponyssoides sanguineus
Trombiculosis
Excludes2 scabies (B86)

B88.1 Tungiasis [sandflea infestation]
Inflammatory skin disease caused by infestation of fleas

B88.2 Other arthropod infestations
Scarabiasis

B88.3 External hirudiniasis
Leech infestation NOS
Excludes2 internal hirudiniasis (B83.4)

B88.8 Other specified infestations
Infection of topical fresh water fish parasite
Ichthyoparasitism due to Vandellia cirrhosa
Linguatulosis
Porocephaliasis

B88.9 Infestation, unspecified
Infestation (skin) NOS
Infestation by mites NOS
Skin parasites NOS

B89 Unspecified parasitic disease

SEQUELAE OF INFECTIOUS AND PARASITIC DISEASES (B90-B94)

Note: Categories B90-B94 are to be used to indicate conditions in categories A00-B89 as the cause of sequelae, which are themselves classified elsewhere. The 'sequelae' include conditions specified as such; they also include residuals of diseases classifiable to the above categories if there is evidence that the disease itself is no longer present. Codes from these categories are not to be used for chronic infections. Code chronic current infections to active infectious disease as appropriate.

Code first condition resulting from (sequela) the infectious or parasitic disease

● **B90 Sequelae of tuberculosis**
Condition resulting from tuberculosis

B90.0 Sequelae of central nervous system tuberculosis

B90.1 Sequelae of genitourinary tuberculosis

B90.2 Sequelae of tuberculosis of bones and joints

B90.8 Sequelae of tuberculosis of other organs
Excludes2 sequelae of respiratory tuberculosis (B90.9)

B90.9 Sequelae of respiratory and unspecified tuberculosis
Sequelae of tuberculosis NOS

B91 Sequelae of poliomyelitis
Excludes1 postpolio syndrome (G14)

B92 Sequelae of leprosy

● **B94 Sequelae of other and unspecified infectious and parasitic diseases**

B94.0 Sequelae of trachoma

B94.1 Sequelae of viral encephalitis

B94.2 Sequelae of viral hepatitis

B94.8 Sequelae of other specified infectious and parasitic diseases

B94.9 Sequelae of unspecified infectious and parasitic disease

OGCR Section I.C.1.b

Certain infectious and parasitic diseases

Infectious agents as the cause of diseases classified to other chapters

Certain infections are classified in chapters other than Chapter 1 and no organism is identified as part of the infection code. In these instances, it is necessary to use an additional code from Chapter 1 to identify the organism. A code from category B95, Streptococcus, Staphylococcus, and Enterococcus as the cause of diseases classified to other chapters, B96, Other bacterial agents as the cause of diseases classified to other chapters, or B97, Viral agents as the cause of diseases classified to other chapters, is to be used as an additional code to identify the organism. An instructional note will be found at the infection code advising that an additional organism code is required.

BACTERIAL AND VIRAL INFECTIOUS AGENTS (B95-B97)

Note: These categories are provided for use as supplementary or additional codes to identify the infectious agent(s) in diseases classified elsewhere.
Code the disease first, then the bacterium. Do not report codes from B95-B97 for sepsis.

● **B95 Streptococcus, Staphylococcus, and Enterococcus as the cause of diseases classified elsewhere**

B95.0 Streptococcus, group A, as the cause of diseases classified elsewhere

B95.1 Streptococcus, group B, as the cause of diseases classified elsewhere

B95.2 Enterococcus as the cause of diseases classified elsewhere

B95.3 Streptococcus pneumoniae as the cause of diseases classified elsewhere

B95.4 Other streptococcus as the cause of diseases classified elsewhere

B95.5 Unspecified streptococcus as the cause of diseases classified elsewhere

● **B95.6 Staphylococcus aureus as the cause of diseases classified elsewhere**

B95.61 Methicillin susceptible Staphylococcus aureus infection as the cause of diseases classified elsewhere
Methicillin susceptible Staphylococcus aureus (MSSA) infection as the cause of diseases classified elsewhere
Staphylococcus aureus infection NOS as the cause of diseases classified elsewhere

B95.62 Methicillin resistant Staphylococcus aureus infection as the cause of diseases classified elsewhere
Methicillin resistant staphylococcus aureus (MRSA) infection as the cause of diseases classified elsewhere

B95.7 Other staphylococcus as the cause of diseases classified elsewhere

B95.8 Unspecified staphylococcus as the cause of diseases classified elsewhere

● **B96 Other bacterial agents as the cause of diseases classified elsewhere**

B96.0 Mycoplasma pneumoniae [M. pneumoniae] as the cause of diseases classified elsewhere
Pleuro-pneumonia-like-organism [PPLO]

B96.1 Klebsiella pneumoniae [K. pneumoniae] as the cause of diseases classified elsewhere

CHAPTER 1 (A00-B99)

● **B96.2** **Escherichia coli [E. coli] as the cause of diseases classified elsewhere**

B96.20 **Unspecified Escherichia coli [E. coli] as the cause of diseases classified elsewhere**
Escherichia coli [E. coli] NOS

B96.21 **Shiga toxin-producing Escherichia coli [E. coli] (STEC) O157 as the cause of diseases classified elsewhere**
E. coli O157:H- (nonmotile) with confirmation of Shiga toxin
E. coli O157 with confirmation of Shiga toxin when H antigen is unknown, or is not H7
O157:H7 Escherichia coli [E.coli] with or without confirmation of Shiga toxin-production
Shiga toxin-producing Escherichia coli [E.coli] O157:H7 with or without confirmation of Shiga toxin-production
STEC O157:H7 with or without confirmation of Shiga toxin-production

B96.22 **Other specified Shiga toxin-producing Escherichia coli [E. coli] (STEC) as the cause of diseases classified elsewhere**
Non-O157 Shiga toxin-producing Escherichia coli [E.coli]
Non-O157 Shiga toxin-producing Escherichia coli [E.coli] with known O group

B96.23 **Unspecified Shiga toxin-producing Escherichia coli [E. coli] (STEC) as the cause of diseases classified elsewhere**
Shiga toxin-producing Escherichia coli [E. coli] with unspecified O group
STEC NOS

B96.29 **Other Escherichia coli [E. coli] as the cause of diseases classified elsewhere**
Non-Shiga toxin-producing E. coli

B96.3 **Hemophilus influenzae [H. influenzae] as the cause of diseases classified elsewhere**

B96.4 **Proteus (mirabilis) (morganii) as the cause of diseases classified elsewhere**

B96.5 **Pseudomonas (aeruginosa) (mallei) (pseudomallei) as the cause of diseases classified elsewhere**

B96.6 **Bacteroides fragilis [B. fragilis] as the cause of diseases classified elsewhere**

B96.7 **Clostridium perfringens [C. perfringens] as the cause of diseases classified elsewhere**

● **B96.8** **Other specified bacterial agents as the cause of diseases classified elsewhere**

B96.81 **Helicobacter pylori [H. pylori] as the cause of diseases classified elsewhere**

B96.82 **Vibrio vulnificus as the cause of diseases classified elsewhere**

B96.89 **Other specified bacterial agents as the cause of diseases classified elsewhere**

● **B97** **Viral agents as the cause of diseases classified elsewhere**

B97.0 **Adenovirus as the cause of diseases classified elsewhere**

● **B97.1** **Enterovirus as the cause of diseases classified elsewhere**

B97.10 **Unspecified enterovirus as the cause of diseases classified elsewhere**

B97.11 **Coxsackievirus as the cause of diseases classified elsewhere**

B97.12 **Echovirus as the cause of diseases classified elsewhere**

B97.19 **Other enterovirus as the cause of diseases classified elsewhere**

Item 1–24 **Retrovirus** develops by copying its RNA, genetic materials, into the DNA, which then produces new virus particles. It is from the Retroviridae virus family. **Human T-cell lymphotropic virus, Type I (HTLV-I)** is also called human T-cell leukemia virus, Type I, and is a retrovirus thought to cause T-cell leukemia/lymphoma. **Human T-cell lymphotropic virus, Type II (HTLV-II),** is also called human T-cell leukemia virus, Type II, and is a retrovirus associated with hematologic disorders.

HIV-2 is one of the serotypes of HIV and is usually confined to West Africa, whereas HIV-**1** is found worldwide.

● **B97.2** **Coronavirus as the cause of diseases classified elsewhere**

B97.21 **SARS-associated coronavirus as the cause of diseases classified elsewhere**
Excludes1 pneumonia due to SARS-associated coronavirus (J12.81)

B97.29 **Other coronavirus as the cause of diseases classified elsewhere**

● **B97.3** **Retrovirus as the cause of diseases classified elsewhere**
Excludes1 human immunodeficiency virus [HIV] disease (B20)

B97.30 **Unspecified retrovirus as the cause of diseases classified elsewhere**

B97.31 **Lentivirus as the cause of diseases classified elsewhere**

B97.32 **Oncovirus as the cause of diseases classified elsewhere**

B97.33 **Human T-cell lymphotrophic virus, type I [HTLV-I] as the cause of diseases classified elsewhere**

B97.34 **Human T-cell lymphotrophic virus, type II [HTLV-II] as the cause of diseases classified elsewhere**

B97.35 **Human immunodeficiency virus, type 2 [HIV 2] as the cause of diseases classified elsewhere**

B97.39 **Other retrovirus as the cause of diseases classified elsewhere**

B97.4 **Respiratory syncytial virus as the cause of diseases classified elsewhere**

B97.5 **Reovirus as the cause of diseases classified elsewhere**

B97.6 **Parvovirus as the cause of diseases classified elsewhere**

B97.7 **Papillomavirus as the cause of diseases classified elsewhere**

● **B97.8** **Other viral agents as the cause of diseases classified elsewhere**

B97.81 **Human metapneumovirus as the cause of diseases classified elsewhere**

B97.89 **Other viral agents as the cause of diseases classified elsewhere**

OTHER INFECTIOUS DISEASES (B99)

● **B99** Other and unspecified infectious diseases

B99.8 Other infectious disease

B99.9 Unspecified infectious disease

CHAPTER 2

NEOPLASMS (C00-D49)

OGCR Chapter-Specific Coding Guidelines

2. Chapter 2: Neoplasms (C00-D49)

General guidelines

Chapter 2 of the ICD-10-CM contains the codes for most benign and all malignant neoplasms. Certain benign neoplasms, such as prostatic adenomas, may be found in the specific body system chapters. To properly code a neoplasm it is necessary to determine from the record if the neoplasm is benign, in-situ, malignant, or of uncertain histologic behavior. If malignant, any secondary (metastatic) sites should also be determined.

Primary malignant neoplasms overlapping site boundaries

A primary malignant neoplasm that overlaps two or more contiguous (next to each other) sites should be classified to the subcategory/code .8 ('overlapping lesion'), unless the combination is specifically indexed elsewhere. For multiple neoplasms of the same site that are not contiguous such as tumors in different quadrants of the same breast, codes for each site should be assigned.

Malignant neoplasm of ectopic tissue

Malignant neoplasms of ectopic tissue are to be coded to the site of origin mentioned, e.g., ectopic pancreatic malignant neoplasms involving the stomach are coded to pancreas, unspecified (C25.9).

The neoplasm table in the Alphabetic Index should be referenced first. However, if the histological term is documented, that term should be referenced first, rather than going immediately to the Neoplasm Table, in order to determine which column in the Neoplasm Table is appropriate. For example, if the documentation indicates "adenoma," refer to the term in the Alphabetic Index to review the entries under this term and the instructional note to "see also neoplasm, by site, benign." The table provides the proper code based on the type of neoplasm and the site. It is important to select the proper column in the table that corresponds to the type of neoplasm. The Tabular List should then be referenced to verify that the correct code has been selected from the table and that a more specific site code does not exist.

See Section I.C.21. Factors influencing health status and contact with health services, Status, for information regarding Z15.0, codes for genetic susceptibility to cancer.

a. Treatment directed at the malignancy

If the treatment is directed at the malignancy, designate the malignancy as the principal diagnosis.

The only exception to this guideline is if a patient admission/encounter is solely for the administration of chemotherapy, immunotherapy or radiation therapy, assign the appropriate Z51.— code as the first-listed or principal diagnosis, and the diagnosis or problem for which the service is being performed as a secondary diagnosis.

b. Treatment of secondary site

When a patient is admitted because of a primary neoplasm with metastasis and treatment is directed toward the secondary site only, the secondary neoplasm is designated as the principal diagnosis even though the primary malignancy is still present.

c. Coding and sequencing of complications

Coding and sequencing of complications associated with the malignancies or with the therapy thereof are subject to the following guidelines:

1) Anemia associated with malignancy

When admission/encounter is for management of an anemia associated with the malignancy, and the treatment is only for anemia, the appropriate code for the malignancy is sequenced as the principal or first-listed diagnosis followed by the appropriate code for the anemia (such as code D63.0, Anemia in neoplastic disease).

2) Anemia associated with chemotherapy, immunotherapy and radiation therapy

When the admission/encounter is for management of an anemia associated with an adverse effect of the administration of chemotherapy or immunotherapy and the only treatment is for the anemia, the anemia code is sequenced first followed by the appropriate codes for the neoplasm and the adverse effect (T45.1X5, Adverse effect of antineoplastic and immunosuppressive drugs).

When the admission/encounter is for management of an anemia associated with an adverse effect of radiotherapy, the anemia code should be sequenced first, followed by the appropriate neoplasm code and code Y84.2, Radiological procedure and radiotherapy as the cause of abnormal reaction of the patient, or of later complication, without mention of misadventure at the time of the procedure.

3) Management of dehydration due to the malignancy

When the admission/encounter is for management of dehydration due to the malignancy and only the dehydration is being treated (intravenous rehydration), the dehydration is sequenced first, followed by the code(s) for the malignancy.

4) Treatment of a complication resulting from a surgical procedure

When the admission/encounter is for treatment of a complication resulting from a surgical procedure, designate the complication as the principal or first-listed diagnosis if treatment is directed at resolving the complication.

d. Primary malignancy previously excised

When a primary malignancy has been previously excised or eradicated from its site and there is no further treatment directed to that site and there is no evidence of any existing primary malignancy, a code from category Z85, Personal history of malignant neoplasm, should be used to indicate the former site of the malignancy. Any mention of extension, invasion, or metastasis to another site is coded as a secondary malignant neoplasm to that site. The secondary site may be the principal or first-listed with the Z85 code used as a secondary code.

e. Admissions/Encounters involving chemotherapy, immunotherapy and radiation therapy

1) Episode of care involves surgical removal of neoplasm

When an episode of care involves the surgical removal of a neoplasm, primary or secondary site, followed by adjunct chemotherapy or radiation treatment during the same episode of care, the code for the neoplasm should be assigned as principal or first-listed diagnosis.

2) Patient admission/encounter solely for administration of chemotherapy, immunotherapy and radiation therapy

If a patient admission/encounter is solely for the administration of chemotherapy, immunotherapy or radiation therapy assign code Z51.0, Encounter for antineoplastic radiation therapy, or Z51.11, Encounter for antineoplastic chemotherapy, or Z51.12, Encounter for antineoplastic immunotherapy as the first-listed or principal diagnosis. If a patient receives more than one of these therapies during the same admission more than one of these codes may be assigned, in any sequence.

The malignancy for which the therapy is being administered should be assigned as a secondary diagnosis.

3) Patient admitted for radiation therapy, chemotherapy or immunotherapy and develops complications

When a patient is admitted for the purpose of radiotherapy, immunotherapy or chemotherapy and develops complications such as uncontrolled nausea and vomiting or dehydration, the principal or first-listed diagnosis is Z51.0, Encounter for antineoplastic radiation therapy, or Z51.11, Encounter for antineoplastic chemotherapy, or Z51.12, Encounter for antineoplastic immunotherapy followed by any codes for the complications.

f. Admission/encounter to determine extent of malignancy

When the reason for admission/encounter is to determine the extent of the malignancy, or for a procedure such as paracentesis or thoracentesis, the primary malignancy or appropriate metastatic site is designated as the principal or first-listed diagnosis, even though chemotherapy or radiotherapy is administered.

g. Symptoms, signs, and abnormal findings listed in Chapter 18 associated with neoplasms

Symptoms, signs, and ill-defined conditions listed in Chapter 18 characteristic of, or associated with, an existing primary or secondary site malignancy cannot be used to replace the malignancy as principal or first-listed diagnosis, regardless of the number of admissions or encounters for treatment and care of the neoplasm.

See section I.C.21. Factors influencing health status and contact with health services, Encounter for prophylactic organ removal.

h. Admission/encounter for pain control/management
See Section I.C.6. for information on coding admission/encounter for pain control/management.

i. Malignancy in two or more noncontiguous sites
A patient may have more than one malignant tumor in the same organ. These tumors may represent different primaries or metastatic disease, depending on the site. Should the documentation be unclear, the provider should be queried as to the status of each tumor so that the correct codes can be assigned.

j. Disseminated malignant neoplasm, unspecified
Code C80.0, Disseminated malignant neoplasm, unspecified, is for use only in those cases where the patient has advanced metastatic disease and no known primary or secondary sites are specified. It should not be used in place of assigning codes for the primary site and all known secondary sites.

k. Malignant neoplasm without specification of site
Code C80.1, Malignant (primary) neoplasm, unspecified, equates to Cancer, unspecified. This code should only be used when no determination can be made as to the primary site of a malignancy. This code should rarely be used in the inpatient setting.

l. Sequencing of neoplasm codes

1) Encounter for treatment of primary malignancy
If the reason for the encounter is for treatment of a primary malignancy, assign the malignancy as the principal/first-listed diagnosis. The primary site is to be sequenced first, followed by any metastatic sites.

2) Encounter for treatment of secondary malignancy
When an encounter is for a primary malignancy with metastasis and treatment is directed toward the metastatic (secondary) site(s) only, the metastatic site(s) is designated as the principal/first-listed diagnosis. The primary malignancy is coded as an additional code.

3) Malignant neoplasm in a pregnant patient
When a pregnant woman has a malignant neoplasm, a code from subcategory O9A.1-, Malignant neoplasm complicating pregnancy, childbirth, and the puerperium, should be sequenced first, followed by the appropriate code from Chapter 2 to indicate the type of neoplasm.

4) Encounter for complication associated with a neoplasm
When an encounter is for management of a complication associated with a neoplasm, such as dehydration, and the treatment is only for the complication, the complication is coded first, followed by the appropriate code(s) for the neoplasm.

The exception to this guideline is anemia. When the admission/encounter is for management of an anemia associated with the malignancy, and the treatment is only for anemia, the appropriate code for the malignancy is sequenced as the principal or first-listed diagnosis followed by code D63.0, Anemia in neoplastic disease.

5) Complication from surgical procedure for treatment of a neoplasm
When an encounter is for treatment of a complication resulting from a surgical procedure performed for the treatment of the neoplasm, designate the complication as the principal/first-listed diagnosis. See guideline regarding the coding of a current malignancy versus personal history to determine if the code for the neoplasm should also be assigned.

6) Pathologic fracture due to a neoplasm
When an encounter is for a pathological fracture due to a neoplasm, and the focus of treatment is the fracture, a code from subcategory M84.5, Pathological fracture in neoplastic disease, should be sequenced first, followed by the code for the neoplasm.

If the focus of treatment is the neoplasm with an associated pathological fracture, the neoplasm code should be sequenced first, followed by a code from M84.5 for the pathological fracture.

m. Current malignancy versus personal history of malignancy
When a primary malignancy has been excised but further treatment, such as an additional surgery for the malignancy, radiation therapy or chemotherapy is directed to that site, the primary malignancy code should be used until treatment is completed.

When a primary malignancy has been previously excised or eradicated from its site, there is no further treatment (of the malignancy) directed to that site, and there is no evidence of any existing primary malignancy, a code from category Z85, Personal history of malignant neoplasm, should be used to indicate the former site of the malignancy.

See Section I.C.21. Factors influencing health status and contact with health services, History (of)

n. Leukemia, Multiple Myeloma, and Malignant Plasma Cell Neoplasms in remission versus personal history
The categories for leukemia, and category C90, Multiple myeloma and malignant plasma cell neoplasms, have codes indicating whether or not the leukemia has achieved remission. There are also codes Z85.6, Personal history of leukemia, and Z85.79, Personal history of other malignant neoplasms of lymphoid, hematopoietic and related tissues. If the documentation is unclear, as to whether the leukemia has achieved remission, the provider should be queried.

See Section I.C.21. Factors influencing health status and contact with health services, History (of)

o. Aftercare following surgery for neoplasm
See Section I.C.21. Factors influencing health status and contact with health services, Aftercare

p. Follow-up care for completed treatment of a malignancy
See Section I.C.21. Factors influencing health status and contact with health services, Follow-up

q. Prophylactic organ removal for prevention of malignancy
See Section I.C. 21, Factors influencing health status and contact with health services, Prophylactic organ removal

r. Malignant neoplasm associated with transplanted organ
A malignant neoplasm of a transplanted organ should be coded as a transplant complication. Assign first the appropriate code from category T86.-, Complications of transplanted organs and tissue, followed by code C80.2, Malignant neoplasm associated with transplanted organ. Use an additional code for the specific malignancy.

Item 2–1 Neoplasm: Neo = new, plasm = growth, development, formation. This new growth (mass, tumor) can be malignant or benign, which is confirmed by the pathology report. Do not assign a code to a neoplasm until you review the pathology report. Certain CPT codes will specify benign or malignant lesion, so be certain the diagnosis code supports the procedure code.

CHAPTER 2

NEOPLASMS (CØØ-D49)

This chapter contains the following blocks:

CØØ-C14	Malignant neoplasms of lip, oral cavity and pharynx
C15-C26	Malignant neoplasms of digestive organs
C3Ø-C39	Malignant neoplasms of respiratory and intrathoracic organs
C4Ø-C41	Malignant neoplasms of bone and articular cartilage
C43-C44	Melanoma and other malignant neoplasms of skin
C45-C49	Malignant neoplasms of mesothelial and soft tissue
C5Ø	Malignant neoplasms of breast
C51-C58	Malignant neoplasms of female genital organs
C6Ø-C63	Malignant neoplasms of male genital organs
C64-C68	Malignant neoplasms of urinary tract
C69-C72	Malignant neoplasms of eye, brain and other parts of central nervous system
C73-C75	Malignant neoplasms of thyroid and other endocrine glands
C7A	Malignant neuroendocrine tumors
C7B	Secondary neuroendocrine tumors
C76-C8Ø	Malignant neoplasms of ill-defined, other secondary and unspecified sites
C81-C96	Malignant neoplasms of lymphoid, hematopoietic and related tissue
DØØ-DØ9	In situ neoplasms
D1Ø-D36	Benign neoplasms, except benign neuroendocrine tumors
D3A	Benign neuroendocrine tumors
D37-D48	Neoplasms of uncertain behavior, polycythemia vera and myelodysplastic syndromes
D49	Neoplasms of unspecified behavior

Notes: Functional activity

All neoplasms are classified in this chapter, whether they are functionally active or not. An additional code from Chapter 4 may be used, to identify functional activity associated with any neoplasm.

Morphology [Histology]

Chapter 2 classifies neoplasms primarily by site (topography), with broad groupings for behavior, malignant, in situ, benign, etc. The Table of Neoplasms should be used to identify the correct topography code. In a few cases, such as for malignant melanoma and certain neuroendocrine tumors, the morphology (histologic type) is included in the category and codes.

Primary malignant neoplasms overlapping site boundaries

A primary malignant neoplasm that overlaps two or more contiguous (next to each other) sites should be classified to the subcategory/code .8 ('overlapping lesion'), unless the combination is specifically indexed elsewhere. For multiple neoplasms of the same site that are not contiguous, such as tumors in different quadrants of the same breast, codes for each site should be assigned.

Malignant neoplasm of ectopic tissue

Malignant neoplasms of ectopic tissue are to be coded to the site mentioned, e.g., ectopic pancreatic malignant neoplasms are coded to pancreas, unspecified (C25.9).

MALIGNANT NEOPLASMS (CØØ-C96)

MALIGNANT NEOPLASMS, STATED OR PRESUMED TO BE PRIMARY (OF SPECIFIED SITES), AND CERTAIN SPECIFIED HISTOLOGIES, EXCEPT NEUROENDOCRINE, AND OF LYMPHOID, HEMATOPOIETIC AND RELATED TISSUE (CØØ-C75)

MALIGNANT NEOPLASMS OF LIP, ORAL CAVITY AND PHARYNX (CØØ-C14)

● **CØØ Malignant neoplasm of lip**

Use additional code to identify:
- alcohol abuse and dependence (F1Ø.-)
- history of tobacco dependence (Z87.891) ◄
- tobacco dependence (F17.-)
- tobacco use (Z72.Ø)

Excludes1 malignant melanoma of lip (C43.Ø)
Merkel cell carcinoma of lip (C4A.Ø)
other and unspecified malignant neoplasm of skin of lip (C44.Ø-)

CØØ.Ø Malignant neoplasm of external upper lip
Malignant neoplasm of lipstick area of upper lip
Malignant neoplasm of upper lip NOS
Malignant neoplasm of vermilion border of upper lip

CØØ.1 Malignant neoplasm of external lower lip
Malignant neoplasm of lower lip NOS
Malignant neoplasm of lipstick area of lower lip
Malignant neoplasm of vermilion border of lower lip

CØØ.2 Malignant neoplasm of external lip, unspecified
Malignant neoplasm of vermilion border of lip NOS

CØØ.3 Malignant neoplasm of upper lip, inner aspect
Malignant neoplasm of buccal aspect of upper lip
Malignant neoplasm of frenulum of upper lip
Malignant neoplasm of mucosa of upper lip
Malignant neoplasm of oral aspect of upper lip

CØØ.4 Malignant neoplasm of lower lip, inner aspect
Malignant neoplasm of buccal aspect of lower lip
Malignant neoplasm of frenulum of lower lip
Malignant neoplasm of mucosa of lower lip
Malignant neoplasm of oral aspect of lower lip

CØØ.5 Malignant neoplasm of lip, unspecified, inner aspect
Malignant neoplasm of buccal aspect of lip, unspecified
Malignant neoplasm of frenulum of lip, unspecified
Malignant neoplasm of mucosa of lip, unspecified
Malignant neoplasm of oral aspect of lip, unspecified

CØØ.6 Malignant neoplasm of commissure of lip, unspecified
Commissure: Site of union of corresponding parts

CØØ.8 Malignant neoplasm of overlapping sites of lip

CØØ.9 Malignant neoplasm of lip, unspecified

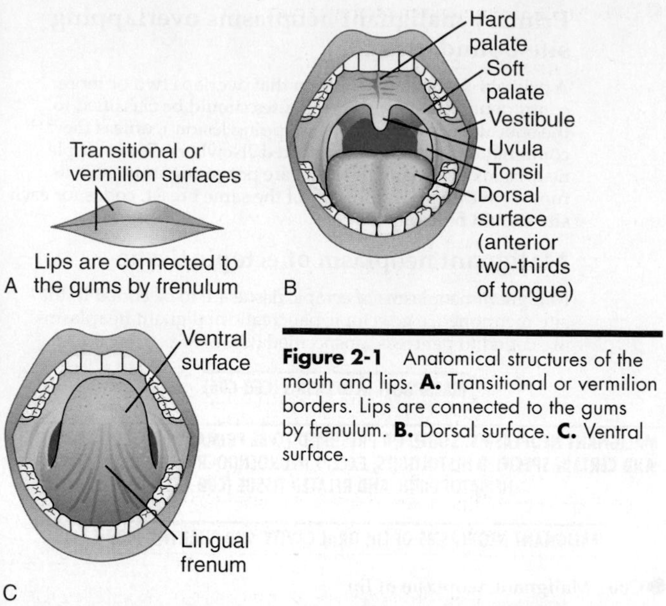

Figure 2-1 Anatomical structures of the mouth and lips. **A.** Transitional or vermilion borders. Lips are connected to the gums by frenulum. **B.** Dorsal surface. **C.** Ventral surface.

C01 Malignant neoplasm of base of tongue
Malignant neoplasm of dorsal surface of base of tongue
Malignant neoplasm of fixed part of tongue NOS
Malignant neoplasm of posterior third of tongue
Use additional code to identify:
alcohol abuse and dependence (F10.-)
history of tobacco dependence (Z87.891) ◄
tobacco dependence (F17.-)
tobacco use (Z72.0)

● **C02 Malignant neoplasm of other and unspecified parts of tongue**
Use additional code to identify:
alcohol abuse and dependence (F10.-)
history of tobacco dependence (Z87.891) ◄
tobacco dependence (F17.-)
tobacco use (Z72.0)

C02.0 Malignant neoplasm of dorsal surface of tongue
Malignant neoplasm of anterior two-thirds of tongue, dorsal surface
Excludes2 malignant neoplasm of dorsal surface of base of tongue (C01)

C02.1 Malignant neoplasm of border of tongue
Malignant neoplasm of tip of tongue

C02.2 Malignant neoplasm of ventral surface of tongue
Malignant neoplasm of anterior two-thirds of tongue, ventral surface
Malignant neoplasm of frenulum linguae

C02.3 Malignant neoplasm of anterior two-thirds of tongue, part unspecified
Malignant neoplasm of middle third of tongue NOS
Malignant neoplasm of mobile part of tongue NOS

C02.4 Malignant neoplasm of lingual tonsil
Lingual tonsil: Aggregation of lymph follicles at root of tongue
Excludes2 malignant neoplasm of tonsil NOS (C09.9)

C02.8 Malignant neoplasm of overlapping sites of tongue
Malignant neoplasm of two or more contiguous sites of tongue

C02.9 Malignant neoplasm of tongue, unspecified

● **C03 Malignant neoplasm of gum**
Includes malignant neoplasm of alveolar (ridge) mucosa
malignant neoplasm of gingiva
Use additional code to identify:
alcohol abuse and dependence (F10.-)
history of tobacco dependence (Z87.891) ◄
tobacco dependence (F17.-)
tobacco use (Z72.0)
Excludes2 malignant odontogenic neoplasms (C41.0-C41.1)

C03.0 Malignant neoplasm of upper gum

C03.1 Malignant neoplasm of lower gum

C03.9 Malignant neoplasm of gum, unspecified

● **C04 Malignant neoplasm of floor of mouth**
Use additional code to identify:
alcohol abuse and dependence (F10.-)
history of tobacco dependence (Z87.891) ◄
tobacco dependence (F17.-)
tobacco use (Z72.0)

C04.0 Malignant neoplasm of anterior floor of mouth
Malignant neoplasm of anterior to the premolar-canine junction

C04.1 Malignant neoplasm of lateral floor of mouth

C04.8 Malignant neoplasm of overlapping sites of floor of mouth

C04.9 Malignant neoplasm of floor of mouth, unspecified

● **C05 Malignant neoplasm of palate**
Use additional code to identify:
alcohol abuse and dependence (F10.-)
history of tobacco dependence (Z87.891) ◄
tobacco dependence (F17.-)
tobacco use (Z72.0)
Excludes1 Kaposi's sarcoma of palate (C46.2)

C05.0 Malignant neoplasm of hard palate

C05.1 Malignant neoplasm of soft palate
Excludes2 malignant neoplasm of nasopharyngeal surface of soft palate (C11.3)

C05.2 Malignant neoplasm of uvula

C05.8 Malignant neoplasm of overlapping sites of palate

C05.9 Malignant neoplasm of palate, unspecified
Malignant neoplasm of roof of mouth

● **C06 Malignant neoplasm of other and unspecified parts of mouth**
Use additional code to identify:
alcohol abuse and dependence (F10.-)
history of tobacco dependence (Z87.891) ◄
tobacco dependence (F17.-)
tobacco use (Z72.0)

C06.0 Malignant neoplasm of cheek mucosa
Malignant neoplasm of buccal mucosa NOS
Malignant neoplasm of internal cheek

C06.1 Malignant neoplasm of vestibule of mouth
Malignant neoplasm of buccal sulcus (upper) (lower)
Malignant neoplasm of labial sulcus (upper) (lower)

C06.2 Malignant neoplasm of retromolar area

● **C06.8 Malignant neoplasm of overlapping sites of other and unspecified parts of mouth**

C06.80 Malignant neoplasm of overlapping sites of unspecified parts of mouth

C06.89 Malignant neoplasm of overlapping sites of other parts of mouth 'book leaf' neoplasm [ventral surface of tongue and floor of mouth]

C06.9 Malignant neoplasm of mouth, unspecified
Malignant neoplasm of minor salivary gland, unspecified site
Malignant neoplasm of oral cavity NOS

CHAPTER 2 (C00-D49)

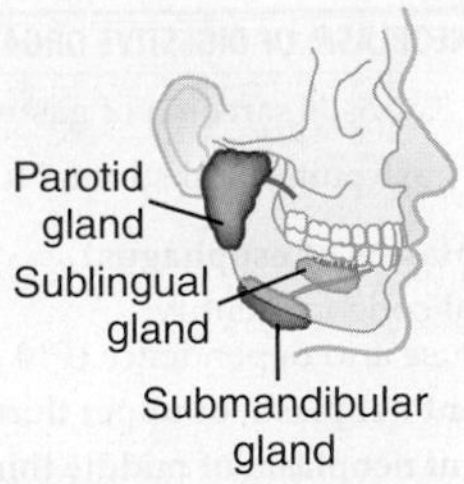

Figure 2-2 Major salivary glands.

CØ7 Malignant neoplasm of parotid gland
Use additional code to identify:
alcohol abuse and dependence (F1Ø.-)
exposure to environmental tobacco smoke (Z77.22)
exposure to tobacco smoke in the perinatal period (P96.81)
history of tobacco dependence (Z87.891)
occupational exposure to environmental tobacco smoke (Z57.31)
tobacco dependence (F17.-)
tobacco use (Z72.Ø)

● **CØ8 Malignant neoplasm of other and unspecified major salivary glands**
Includes malignant neoplasm of salivary ducts
Use additional code to identify:
alcohol abuse and dependence (F1Ø.-)
exposure to environmental tobacco smoke (Z77.22)
exposure to tobacco smoke in the perinatal period (P96.81)
history of tobacco dependence (Z87.891)
occupational exposure to environmental tobacco smoke (Z57.31)
tobacco dependence (F17.-)
tobacco use (Z72.Ø)
Excludes1 malignant neoplasms of specified minor salivary glands which are classified according to their anatomical location
Excludes2 malignant neoplasms of minor salivary glands NOS (CØ6.9)
malignant neoplasm of parotid gland (CØ7)

CØ8.Ø Malignant neoplasm of submandibular gland
Malignant neoplasm of submaxillary gland

CØ8.1 Malignant neoplasm of sublingual gland

CØ8.9 Malignant neoplasm of major salivary gland, unspecified
Malignant neoplasm of salivary gland (major) NOS

★**(See Plate 61 on page NAP-25.)**

● **CØ9 Malignant neoplasm of tonsil**
Use additional code to identify:
alcohol abuse and dependence (F1Ø.-)
exposure to environmental tobacco smoke (Z77.22)
exposure to tobacco smoke in the perinatal period (P96.81)
history of tobacco dependence (Z87.891)
occupational exposure to environmental tobacco smoke (Z57.31)
tobacco dependence (F17.-)
tobacco use (Z72.Ø)
Excludes2 malignant neoplasm of lingual tonsil (CØ2.4)
malignant neoplasm of pharyngeal tonsil (C11.1)

CØ9.Ø Malignant neoplasm of tonsillar fossa
Surface of palatine (two masses of lymphatic tissue on sides of throat) tonsils

CØ9.1 Malignant neoplasm of tonsillar pillar (anterior) (posterior)
Extension from palatine (two masses of lymphatic tissue on sides of throat) tonsils

CØ9.8 Malignant neoplasm of overlapping sites of tonsil

CØ9.9 Malignant neoplasm of tonsil, unspecified
Malignant neoplasm of tonsil NOS
Malignant neoplasm of faucial tonsils
Malignant neoplasm of palatine tonsils

● **C1Ø Malignant neoplasm of oropharynx**
Area of throat at back of mouth
Use additional code to identify:
alcohol abuse and dependence (F1Ø.-)
exposure to environmental tobacco smoke (Z77.22)
exposure to tobacco smoke in the perinatal period (P96.81)
history of tobacco dependence (Z87.891)
occupational exposure to environmental tobacco smoke (Z57.31)
tobacco dependence (F17.-)
tobacco use (Z72.Ø)
Excludes2 malignant neoplasm of tonsil (CØ9.-)

C1Ø.Ø Malignant neoplasm of vallecula
Vallecula, depression or furrow

C1Ø.1 Malignant neoplasm of anterior surface of epiglottis
Malignant neoplasm of epiglottis, free border [margin]
Malignant neoplasm of glossoepiglottic fold(s)
Excludes2 malignant neoplasm of epiglottis (suprahyoid portion) NOS (C32.1)

C1Ø.2 Malignant neoplasm of lateral wall of oropharynx

C1Ø.3 Malignant neoplasm of posterior wall of oropharynx

C1Ø.4 Malignant neoplasm of branchial cleft
Congenital slitlike openings formed between branchial arches pharyngeal groove
Malignant neoplasm of branchial cyst [site of neoplasm]

C1Ø.8 Malignant neoplasm of overlapping sites of oropharynx
Malignant neoplasm of junctional region of oropharynx

C1Ø.9 Malignant neoplasm of oropharynx, unspecified

● **C11 Malignant neoplasm of nasopharynx**
Use additional code to identify:
exposure to environmental tobacco smoke (Z77.22)
exposure to tobacco smoke in the perinatal period (P96.81)
history of tobacco dependence (Z87.891)
occupational exposure to environmental tobacco smoke (Z57.31)
tobacco dependence (F17.-)
tobacco use (Z72.Ø)

C11.Ø Malignant neoplasm of superior wall of nasopharynx
Part of pharynx that lies above soft palate
Malignant neoplasm of roof of nasopharynx

C11.1 Malignant neoplasm of posterior wall of nasopharynx
Malignant neoplasm of adenoid
Malignant neoplasm of pharyngeal tonsil

C11.2 Malignant neoplasm of lateral wall of nasopharynx
Malignant neoplasm of fossa of Rosenmüller
Malignant neoplasm of opening of auditory tube
Malignant neoplasm of pharyngeal recess

C11.3 Malignant neoplasm of anterior wall of nasopharynx
Malignant neoplasm of floor of nasopharynx
Malignant neoplasm of nasopharyngeal (anterior) (posterior) surface of soft palate
Malignant neoplasm of posterior margin of nasal choana
Malignant neoplasm of posterior margin of nasal septum

C11.8 Malignant neoplasm of overlapping sites of nasopharynx

C11.9 Malignant neoplasm of nasopharynx, unspecified
Malignant neoplasm of nasopharyngeal wall NOS

C12 Malignant neoplasm of pyriform sinus
Malignant neoplasm of pyriform fossa
Use additional code to identify:
exposure to environmental tobacco smoke (Z77.22)
exposure to tobacco smoke in the perinatal period (P96.81)
history of tobacco dependence (Z87.891)
occupational exposure to environmental tobacco smoke (Z57.31)
tobacco dependence (F17.-)
tobacco use (Z72.0)

● **C13 Malignant neoplasm of hypopharynx**
Use additional code to identify:
exposure to environmental tobacco smoke (Z77.22)
exposure to tobacco smoke in the perinatal period (P96.81)
history of tobacco dependence (Z87.891) ⬅
occupational exposure to environmental tobacco smoke (Z57.31)
tobacco dependence (F17.-)
tobacco use (Z72.Ø)
Excludes2 malignant neoplasm of pyriform sinus (C12)

C13.Ø Malignant neoplasm of postcricoid region
Behind the cricoid cartilage of neck

C13.1 Malignant neoplasm of aryepiglottic fold, hypopharyngeal aspect
Arytenoepiglottic fold, triangular opening between side of epiglottis and apex of arytenoid cartilage
Malignant neoplasm of aryepiglottic fold, marginal zone
Malignant neoplasm of aryepiglottic fold NOS
Malignant neoplasm of interarytenoid fold, marginal zone
Malignant neoplasm of interarytenoid fold NOS
Excludes2 malignant neoplasm of aryepiglottic fold or interarytenoid fold, laryngeal aspect (C32.1)

C13.2 Malignant neoplasm of posterior wall of hypopharynx

C13.8 Malignant neoplasm of overlapping sites of hypopharynx

C13.9 Malignant neoplasm of hypopharynx, unspecified
Malignant neoplasm of hypopharyngeal wall NOS

● **C14 Malignant neoplasm of other and ill-defined sites in the lip, oral cavity and pharynx**
Use additional code to identify:
alcohol abuse and dependence (F1Ø.-)
exposure to environmental tobacco smoke (Z77.22)
exposure to tobacco smoke in the perinatal period (P96.81)
history of tobacco dependence (Z87.891) ⬅
occupational exposure to environmental tobacco smoke (Z57.31)
tobacco dependence (F17.-)
tobacco use (Z72.Ø)
Excludes1 malignant neoplasm of oral cavity NOS (CØ6.9)

C14.Ø Malignant neoplasm of pharynx, unspecified

C14.2 Malignant neoplasm of Waldeyer's ring

C14.8 Malignant neoplasm of overlapping sites of lip, oral cavity and pharynx
Primary malignant neoplasm of two or more contiguous sites of lip, oral cavity and pharynx
Excludes1 'book leaf' neoplasm [ventral surface of tongue and floor of mouth] (CØ6.89)

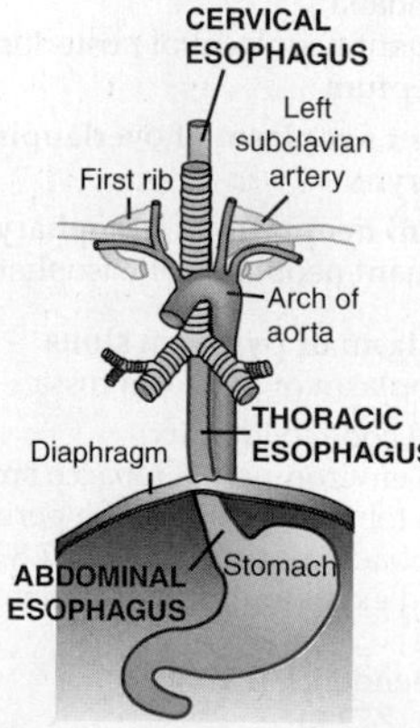

Figure 2-3 The esophagus is the muscular tube that connects the pharynx and the stomach. The 1Ø inch (25 cm) long esophagus is divided into three parts: **cervical, thoracic,** and **abdominal.**

MALIGNANT NEOPLASM OF DIGESTIVE ORGANS (C15-C26)

Excludes1 Kaposi's sarcoma of gastrointestinal sites (C46.4)
Excludes2 gastrointestinal stromal tumors (C49.A-) ◀

● **C15 Malignant neoplasms of esophagus**
Use additional code to identify:
alcohol abuse and dependence (F1Ø.-)

C15.3 Malignant neoplasm of upper third of esophagus

C15.4 Malignant neoplasm of middle third of esophagus

C15.5 Malignant neoplasm of lower third of esophagus
Excludes1 malignant neoplasm of cardio-esophageal junction (C16.Ø)

C15.8 Malignant neoplasm of overlapping sites of esophagus

C15.9 Malignant neoplasm of esophagus, unspecified

● **C16 Malignant neoplasm of stomach**
Use additional code to identify:
alcohol abuse and dependence (F1Ø.-)
Excludes2 malignant carcinoid tumor of the stomach (C7A.Ø92)

C16.Ø Malignant neoplasm of cardia
Malignant neoplasm of cardiac orifice
Malignant neoplasm of cardio-esophageal junction
Malignant neoplasm of esophagus and stomach
Malignant neoplasm of gastro-esophageal junction

C16.1 Malignant neoplasm of fundus of stomach

C16.2 Malignant neoplasm of body of stomach

C16.3 Malignant neoplasm of pyloric antrum
Malignant neoplasm of gastric antrum

C16.4 Malignant neoplasm of pylorus
Malignant neoplasm of prepylorus
Malignant neoplasm of pyloric canal

C16.5 Malignant neoplasm of lesser curvature of stomach, unspecified
Malignant neoplasm of lesser curvature of stomach, not classifiable to C16.1-C16.4

C16.6 Malignant neoplasm of greater curvature of stomach, unspecified
Malignant neoplasm of greater curvature of stomach, not classifiable to C16.Ø-C16.4

C16.8 Malignant neoplasm of overlapping sites of stomach

C16.9 Malignant neoplasm of stomach, unspecified
Gastric cancer NOS

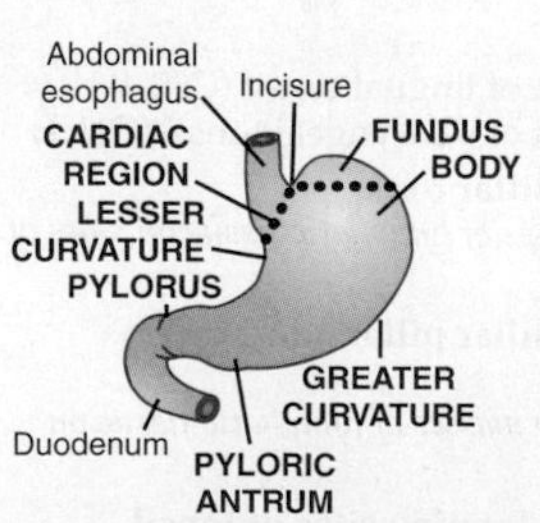

Figure 2-4 Parts of the stomach.

Item 2-2 The esophagus opens into the stomach through the **cardiac orifice,** also called the **cardioesophageal junction.** The **cardia** is adjacent to the cardiac orifice. The stomach widens into the **greater** and **lesser curvatures.** The **pyloric antrum** precedes the **pylorus,** which opens to the duodenum.

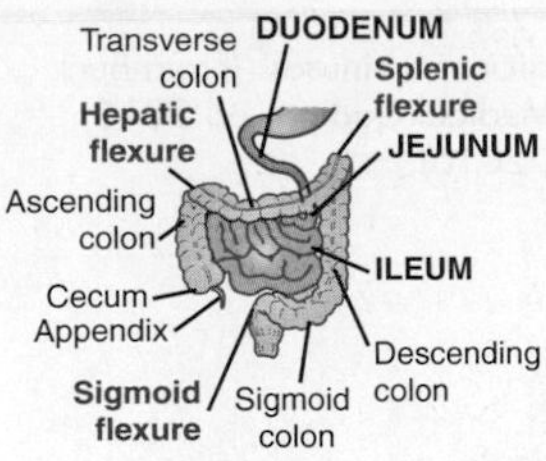

Figure 2-5 Small intestine and colon.

● **C17 Malignant neoplasm of small intestine**
Excludes1 malignant carcinoid tumor of the small intestine (C7A.Ø1)

C17.Ø Malignant neoplasm of duodenum
First or proximal portion of small intestine, extending from pylorus to jejunum

C17.1 Malignant neoplasm of jejunum
Second section of small intestine, extending from duodenum to ileum

C17.2 Malignant neoplasm of ileum
Distal and longest portion of small intestine, extending from jejunum to cecum
Excludes1 malignant neoplasm of ileocecal valve (C18.Ø)

C17.3 Meckel's diverticulum, malignant
Appendage of ileum
Excludes1 Meckel's diverticulum, congenital (Q43.Ø)

C17.8 Malignant neoplasm of overlapping sites of small intestine

C17.9 Malignant neoplasm of small intestine, unspecified

● **C18 Malignant neoplasm of colon**
Excludes1 malignant carcinoid tumors of the colon (C7A.Ø2)

C18.Ø Malignant neoplasm of cecum
First section of large intestine
Malignant neoplasm of ileocecal valve

C18.1 Malignant neoplasm of appendix
Blind ended tube connected to the cecum; AKA vermiform appendix

C18.2 Malignant neoplasm of ascending colon
Ascending colon is between cecum and right colic flexure

C18.3 Malignant neoplasm of hepatic flexure
A flexure is a bending in a structure or organ. Note the three flexures illustrated in Figure 2–5.

C18.4 Malignant neoplasm of transverse colon
Portion of colon that runs transversely across upper part of abdomen, between right and left colic flexures

C18.5 Malignant neoplasm of splenic flexure
Bend at junction of transverse and descending colon

C18.6 Malignant neoplasm of descending colon
Portion between left colic flexure and sigmoid colon at pelvic brim; AKA iliac colon

C18.7 Malignant neoplasm of sigmoid colon
S-shaped part of colon extending from pelvic brim to third segment of sacrum
Malignant neoplasm of sigmoid (flexure)
Excludes1 malignant neoplasm of rectosigmoid junction (C19)

C18.8 Malignant neoplasm of overlapping sites of colon

C18.9 Malignant neoplasm of colon, unspecified
Malignant neoplasm of large intestine NOS

C19 Malignant neoplasm of rectosigmoid junction
Malignant neoplasm of colon with rectum
Malignant neoplasm of rectosigmoid (colon)
Excludes1 malignant carcinoid tumors of the colon (C7A.Ø2-)

C2Ø Malignant neoplasm of rectum
Malignant neoplasm of rectal ampulla
Excludes1 malignant carcinoid tumor of the rectum (C7A.Ø26)

● **C21 Malignant neoplasm of anus and anal canal**
Excludes2 malignant carcinoid tumors of the colon (C7A.Ø2-)
malignant melanoma of anal margin (C43.51)
malignant melanoma of anal skin (C43.51)
malignant melanoma of perianal skin (C43.51)
other and unspecified malignant neoplasm of anal margin (C44.5ØØ, C44.51Ø, C44.52Ø, C44.59Ø)
other and unspecified malignant neoplasm of anal skin (C44.5ØØ, C44.51Ø, C44.52Ø, C44.59Ø)
other and unspecified malignant neoplasm of perianal skin (C44.5ØØ, C44.51Ø, C44.52Ø, C44.59Ø)

C21.Ø Malignant neoplasm of anus, unspecified

C21.1 Malignant neoplasm of anal canal
Terminal part of large intestine
Malignant neoplasm of anal sphincter

C21.2 Malignant neoplasm of cloacogenic zone

C21.8 Malignant neoplasm of overlapping sites of rectum, anus and anal canal
Malignant neoplasm of anorectal junction
Malignant neoplasm of anorectum
Primary malignant neoplasm of two or more contiguous sites of rectum, anus and anal canal

● **C22 Malignant neoplasm of liver and intrahepatic bile ducts**
Intrahepatic: Within liver
Use additional code to identify:
alcohol abuse and dependence (F1Ø.-)
hepatitis B (B16.-, B18.Ø-B18.1) hepatitis C (B17.1-, B18.2)
Excludes1 malignant neoplasm of biliary tract NOS (C24.9)
secondary malignant neoplasm of liver and intrahepatic bile duct (C78.7)

C22.Ø Liver cell carcinoma
Hepatocellular carcinoma
Hepatoma

C22.1 Intrahepatic bile duct carcinoma
Cholangiocarcinoma
Adenocarcinoma (cancer that originates in glandular tissue) arising from epithelium of intrahepatic bile ducts
Excludes1 malignant neoplasm of hepatic duct (C24.Ø)

C22.2 Hepatoblastoma
Malignant intrahepatic tumor

C22.3 Angiosarcoma of liver
Kupffer cell sarcoma

C22.4 Other sarcomas of liver

C22.7 Other specified carcinomas of liver

C22.8 Malignant neoplasm of liver, primary, unspecified as to type

C22.9 Malignant neoplasm of liver, not specified as primary or secondary

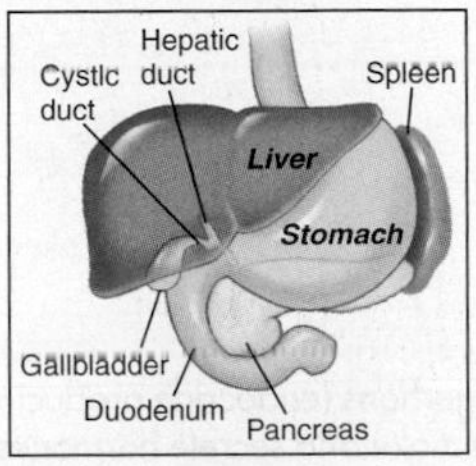

Figure 2-6 Diagram of liver, gallbladder, hepatic duct, pancreas, and spleen. (From Thibodeau and Patton: Anatomy and Physiology, ed 7, Mosby, 2010)

C23 Malignant neoplasm of gallbladder

● **C24 Malignant neoplasm of other and unspecified parts of biliary tract**

Excludes1 malignant neoplasm of intrahepatic bile duct (C22.1)

C24.0 Malignant neoplasm of extrahepatic bile duct

Extrahepatic = outside the liver

Malignant neoplasm of biliary duct or passage NOS
Malignant neoplasm of common bile duct
Malignant neoplasm of cystic duct
Malignant neoplasm of hepatic duct

C24.1 Malignant neoplasm of ampulla of Vater

Union of pancreatic duct and common bile duct

C24.8 Malignant neoplasm of overlapping sites of biliary tract

Malignant neoplasm involving both intrahepatic and extrahepatic bile ducts
Primary malignant neoplasm of two or more contiguous sites of biliary tract

C24.9 Malignant neoplasm of biliary tract, unspecified

● **C25 Malignant neoplasm of pancreas**

Check documentation for specific site.

Code also exocrine pancreatic insufficiency (K86.81) ◀

Use additional code to identify:
alcohol abuse and dependence (F10.-)

C25.0 Malignant neoplasm of head of pancreas

C25.1 Malignant neoplasm of body of pancreas

C25.2 Malignant neoplasm of tail of pancreas

C25.3 Malignant neoplasm of pancreatic duct

C25.4 Malignant neoplasm of endocrine pancreas

Malignant neoplasm of islets of Langerhans

That part of the pancreas that acts as endocrine gland and consists of islets of Langerhans

Use additional code to identify any functional activity.

C25.7 Malignant neoplasm of other parts of pancreas

Malignant neoplasm of neck of pancreas

C25.8 Malignant neoplasm of overlapping sites of pancreas

C25.9 Malignant neoplasm of pancreas, unspecified

● **C26 Malignant neoplasm of other and ill-defined digestive organs**

Excludes1 malignant neoplasm of peritoneum and retroperitoneum (C48.-)

C26.0 Malignant neoplasm of intestinal tract, part unspecified

Malignant neoplasm of intestine NOS

C26.1 Malignant neoplasm of spleen

Excludes1 Hodgkin lymphoma (C81.-)
non-Hodgkin lymphoma (C82-C85)

C26.9 Malignant neoplasm of ill-defined sites within the digestive system

Malignant neoplasm of alimentary canal or tract NOS
Malignant neoplasm of gastrointestinal tract NOS

Excludes1 malignant neoplasm of abdominal NOS (C76.2)
malignant neoplasm of intra-abdominal NOS (C76.2)

Item 2–3 Islets of Langerhans (endocrine producing cells comprising 1% to 2% of the pancreatic mass) make and secrete hormones that regulate the body's production of insulin, glucagon, and stomach acid. Breakdown of the insulin-producing cells can cause diabetes mellitus. Islet cell tumors can be benign or malignant and include glucagonomas, insulinomas, gastrinomas, and neuroendocrine tumor. The neoplasm table must be consulted for the correct neoplasm code.

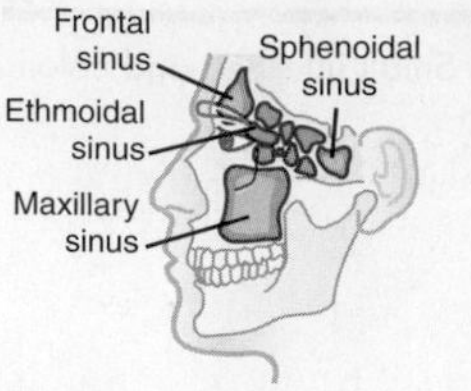

Figure 2-7 Paranasal sinuses. (From Buck CJ: Step-by-Step Medical Coding, ed 2016, St. Louis, Elsevier, 2016)

MALIGNANT NEOPLASMS OF RESPIRATORY AND INTRATHORACIC ORGANS (C30-C39)

Includes malignant neoplasm of middle ear
Excludes1 mesothelioma (C45.-)

● **C30 Malignant neoplasm of nasal cavity and middle ear**

C30.0 Malignant neoplasm of nasal cavity

Malignant neoplasm of cartilage of nose
Malignant neoplasm of nasal concha
Malignant neoplasm of internal nose
Malignant neoplasm of septum of nose
Malignant neoplasm of vestibule of nose

Anterior part of nasal cavity

Excludes1 malignant neoplasm of nasal bone (C41.0)
malignant neoplasm of nose NOS (C76.0)
malignant neoplasm of olfactory bulb (C72.2-)
malignant neoplasm of posterior margin of nasal septum and choana (C11.3)
malignant melanoma of skin of nose (C43.31)
malignant neoplasm of turbinates (C41.0)
other and unspecified malignant neoplasm of skin of nose C44.301, C44.311, C44.321, C44.391)

C30.1 Malignant neoplasm of middle ear

Malignant neoplasm of antrum tympanicum

Boney cavity or chamber

Malignant neoplasm of auditory tube
Malignant neoplasm of eustachian tube
Malignant neoplasm of inner ear
Malignant neoplasm of mastoid air cells
Malignant neoplasm of tympanic cavity

Excludes1 malignant neoplasm of auricular canal (external) (C43.2-, C44.2-)
malignant neoplasm of bone of ear (meatus) (C41.0)
malignant neoplasm of cartilage of ear (C49.0)
malignant melanoma of skin of (external) ear (C43.2-)
other and unspecified malignant neoplasm of skin of (external) ear (C44.2-)

● **C31 Malignant neoplasm of accessory sinuses**

Paired sinuses in bones of face

C31.0 Malignant neoplasm of maxillary sinus

Malignant neoplasm of antrum (Highmore) (maxillary)

C31.1 Malignant neoplasm of ethmoidal sinus

C31.2 Malignant neoplasm of frontal sinus

C31.3 Malignant neoplasm of sphenoid sinus

C31.8 Malignant neoplasm of overlapping sites of accessory sinuses

C31.9 Malignant neoplasm of accessory sinus, unspecified

● C32 Malignant neoplasm of larynx

Use additional code to identify:
alcohol abuse and dependence (F10.-)
exposure to environmental tobacco smoke (Z77.22)
exposure to tobacco smoke in the perinatal period (P96.81)
history of tobacco dependence (Z87.891) ◄
occupational exposure to environmental tobacco smoke (Z57.31)
tobacco dependence (F17.-)
tobacco use (Z72.0)

C32.0 Malignant neoplasm of glottis

Vocal apparatus of larynx, consisting of true vocal cords (plicae vocales) and opening between them (rima glottidis)

Malignant neoplasm of intrinsic larynx
Malignant neoplasm of laryngeal commissure (anterior) (posterior)
Malignant neoplasm of vocal cord (true) NOS

***True** vocal cords ("lower vocal folds") produce vocalization when air from the lungs passes between them. Check your documentation. Code C32.1 is for malignant neoplasm of the **false** vocal cords.*

C32.1 Malignant neoplasm of supraglottis

Area of pharynx above glottis

Malignant neoplasm of aryepiglottic fold or interarytenoid fold, laryngeal aspect
Malignant neoplasm of epiglottis (suprahyoid portion) NOS
Malignant neoplasm of extrinsic larynx
Malignant neoplasm of false vocal cord

***False** vocal cords ("upper vocal folds") are not involved in vocalization. Check your documentation. Code C32.0 is for true vocal cords.*

Malignant neoplasm of posterior (laryngeal) surface of epiglottis
Malignant neoplasm of ventricular bands

Excludes2 malignant neoplasm of anterior surface of epiglottis (C10.1)
malignant neoplasm of aryepiglottic fold or interarytenoid fold, hypopharyngeal aspect (C13.1)
malignant neoplasm of aryepiglottic fold or interarytenoid fold, marginal zone (C13.1)
malignant neoplasm of aryepiglottic fold or interarytenoid fold NOS (C13.1)

C32.2 Malignant neoplasm of subglottis

Lowest part of larynx from just below vocal cords down to top of trachea

C32.3 Malignant neoplasm of laryngeal cartilage

Cartilages of larynx, including cricoid, thyroid, and epiglottic, and two each of arytenoid, corniculate, and cuneiform

C32.8 Malignant neoplasm of overlapping sites of larynx

C32.9 Malignant neoplasm of larynx, unspecified

C33 Malignant neoplasm of trachea

Use additional code to identify:
exposure to environmental tobacco smoke (Z77.22)
exposure to tobacco smoke in the perinatal period (P96.81)
history of tobacco dependence (Z87.891) ◄
occupational exposure to environmental tobacco smoke (Z57.31)
tobacco dependence (F17.-)
tobacco use (Z72.0)

● C34 Malignant neoplasm of bronchus and lung

Use additional code to identify:
exposure to environmental tobacco smoke (Z77.22)
exposure to tobacco smoke in the perinatal period (P96.81)
history of tobacco dependence (Z87.891) ◄
occupational exposure to environmental tobacco smoke (Z57.31)
tobacco dependence (F17.-)
tobacco use (Z72.0)

Excludes1 Kaposi's sarcoma of lung (C46.5-)
malignant carcinoid tumor of the bronchus and lung (C7A.090)

● C34.0 Malignant neoplasm of main bronchus

Malignant neoplasm of carina
Ridgelike structure
Malignant neoplasm of hilus (of lung)
Anatomic depression or pit

C34.00 Malignant neoplasm of unspecified main bronchus

C34.01 Malignant neoplasm of right main bronchus

C34.02 Malignant neoplasm of left main bronchus

● C34.1 Malignant neoplasm of upper lobe, bronchus or lung

C34.10 Malignant neoplasm of unspecified bronchus or lung

C34.11 Malignant neoplasm of upper lobe, right bronchus or lung

C34.12 Malignant neoplasm of upper lobe, left bronchus or lung

C34.2 Malignant neoplasm of middle lobe, bronchus or lung

● C34.3 Malignant neoplasm of lower lobe, bronchus or lung

C34.30 Malignant neoplasm of lower lobe, unspecified bronchus or lung

C34.31 Malignant neoplasm of lower lobe, right bronchus or lung

C34.32 Malignant neoplasm of lower lobe, left bronchus or lung

● C34.8 Malignant neoplasm of overlapping sites of bronchus and lung

C34.80 Malignant neoplasm of overlapping sites of unspecified bronchus and lung

C34.81 Malignant neoplasm of overlapping sites of right bronchus and lung

C34.82 Malignant neoplasm of overlapping sites of left bronchus and lung

● C34.9 Malignant neoplasm of unspecified part of bronchus or lung

C34.90 Malignant neoplasm of unspecified part of unspecified bronchus or lung

Lung cancer NOS

C34.91 Malignant neoplasm of unspecified part of right bronchus or lung

C34.92 Malignant neoplasm of unspecified part of left bronchus or lung

C37 Malignant neoplasm of thymus

Excludes1 malignant carcinoid tumor of the thymus (C7A.091)

CHAPTER 2 (C00-D49)

● **C38 Malignant neoplasm of heart, mediastinum and pleura**

Excludes1 mesothelioma (C45.-)

C38.0 Malignant neoplasm of heart

Malignant neoplasm of pericardium

Excludes1 malignant neoplasm of great vessels (C49.3)

C38.1 Malignant neoplasm of anterior mediastinum

C38.2 Malignant neoplasm of posterior mediastinum

C38.3 Malignant neoplasm of mediastinum, part unspecified

C38.4 Malignant neoplasm of pleura

C38.8 Malignant neoplasm of overlapping sites of heart, mediastinum and pleura

Pleura are comprised of serous membrane that lines the thoracic cavity (parietal) and covers the lungs (visceral).

● **C39 Malignant neoplasm of other and ill-defined sites in the respiratory system and intrathoracic organs**

Intrathoracic: within thorax/chest

Use additional code to identify:

exposure to environmental tobacco smoke (Z77.22)
exposure to tobacco smoke in the perinatal period (P96.81)
history of tobacco dependence (Z87.891) ⇐
occupational exposure to environmental tobacco smoke (Z57.31)
tobacco dependence (F17.-)
tobacco use (Z72.0)

Excludes1 intrathoracic malignant neoplasm NOS (C76.1)
thoracic malignant neoplasm NOS (C76.1)

C39.0 Malignant neoplasm of upper respiratory tract, part unspecified

C39.9 Malignant neoplasm of lower respiratory tract, part unspecified

Malignant neoplasm of respiratory tract NOS

MALIGNANT NEOPLASMS OF BONE AND ARTICULAR CARTILAGE (C40-C41)

Includes malignant neoplasm of cartilage (articular) (joint)
malignant neoplasm of periosteum

Excludes1 malignant neoplasm of bone marrow NOS (C96.9)
malignant neoplasm of synovia (C49.-)

● **C40 Malignant neoplasm of bone and articular cartilage of limbs**

Use additional code to identify major osseous defect, if applicable (M89.7-)

● **C40.0 Malignant neoplasm of scapula and long bones of upper limb**

C40.00 Malignant neoplasm of scapula and long bones of unspecified upper limb

C40.01 Malignant neoplasm of scapula and long bones of right upper limb

C40.02 Malignant neoplasm of scapula and long bones of left upper limb

● **C40.1 Malignant neoplasm of short bones of upper limb**

C40.10 Malignant neoplasm of short bones of unspecified upper limb

C40.11 Malignant neoplasm of short bones of right upper limb

C40.12 Malignant neoplasm of short bones of left upper limb

● **C40.2 Malignant neoplasm of long bones of lower limb**

C40.20 Malignant neoplasm of long bones of unspecified lower limb

C40.21 Malignant neoplasm of long bones of right lower limb

C40.22 Malignant neoplasm of long bones of left lower limb

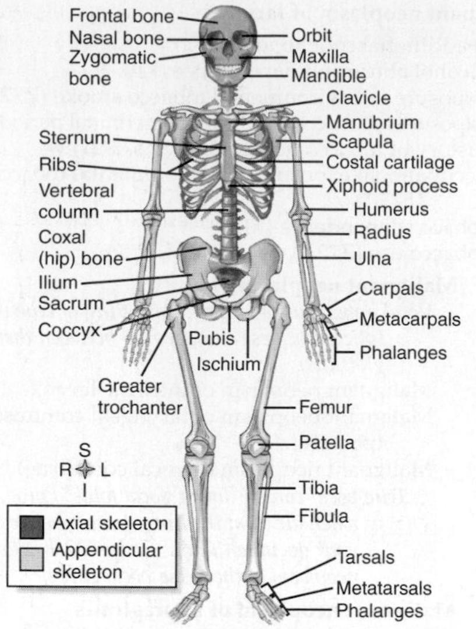

Figure 2-8 Diagram of skeleton of trunk and limbs with bones labeled. (From Thibodeau and Patton: Anatomy and Physiology, ed 7, Mosby, 2010)

● **C40.3 Malignant neoplasm of short bones of lower limb**

C40.30 Malignant neoplasm of short bones of unspecified lower limb

C40.31 Malignant neoplasm of short bones of right lower limb

C40.32 Malignant neoplasm of short bones of left lower limb

● **C40.8 Malignant neoplasm of overlapping sites of bone and articular cartilage of limb**

C40.80 Malignant neoplasm of overlapping sites of bone and articular cartilage of unspecified limb

C40.81 Malignant neoplasm of overlapping sites of bone and articular cartilage of right limb

C40.82 Malignant neoplasm of overlapping sites of bone and articular cartilage of left limb

● **C40.9 Malignant neoplasm of unspecified bones and articular cartilage of limb**

C40.90 Malignant neoplasm of unspecified bones and articular cartilage of unspecified limb

C40.91 Malignant neoplasm of unspecified bones and articular cartilage of right limb

C40.92 Malignant neoplasm of unspecified bones and articular cartilage of left limb

● **C41 Malignant neoplasm of bone and articular cartilage of other and unspecified sites**

Excludes1 malignant neoplasm of bones of limbs (C40.-)
malignant neoplasm of cartilage of ear (C49.0)
malignant neoplasm of cartilage of eyelid (C49.0)
malignant neoplasm of cartilage of larynx (C32.3)
malignant neoplasm of cartilage of limbs (C40.-)
malignant neoplasm of cartilage of nose (C30.0)

C41.0 Malignant neoplasm of bones of skull and face

Malignant neoplasm of maxilla (superior)
Malignant neoplasm of orbital bone

Excludes2 carcinoma, any type except intraosseous or odontogenic of:
maxillary sinus (C31.0)
upper jaw (C03.0)
malignant neoplasm of jaw bone (lower) (C41.1)

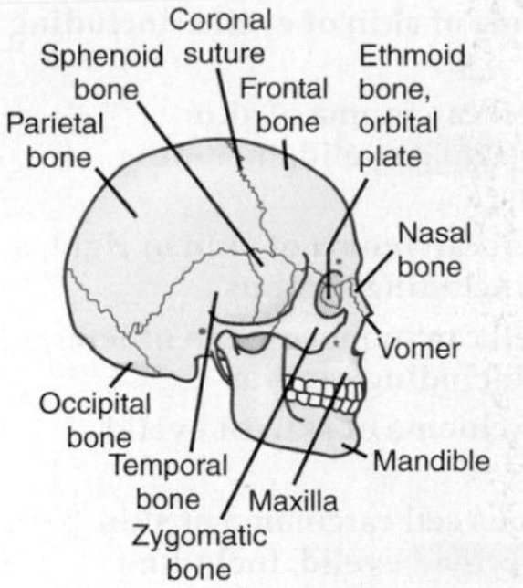

Figure 2-9 Bones of the skull.

C41.1 Malignant neoplasm of mandible
Malignant neoplasm of inferior maxilla
Malignant neoplasm of lower jaw bone
Excludes2 carcinoma, any type except intraosseous or odontogenic of:
jaw NOS (CØ3.9)
lower (CØ3.1)
malignant neoplasm of upper jaw bone (C41.Ø)

C41.2 Malignant neoplasm of vertebral column
Excludes1 malignant neoplasm of sacrum and coccyx (C41.4)

C41.3 Malignant neoplasm of ribs, sternum and clavicle

C41.4 Malignant neoplasm of pelvic bones, sacrum and coccyx

C41.9 Malignant neoplasm of bone and articular cartilage, unspecified

MELANOMA AND OTHER MALIGNANT NEOPLASMS OF SKIN (C43-C44)

● **C43 Malignant melanoma of skin**
Excludes1 melanoma in situ (DØ3.-)
Excludes2 malignant melanoma of skin of genital organs (C51-C52, C6Ø.-, C63.-)
Merkel cell carcinoma (C4A.-)
sites other than skin-code to malignant neoplasm of the site

C43.Ø Malignant melanoma of lip
Excludes1 malignant neoplasm of vermilion border of lip (CØØ.Ø-CØØ.2)

● **C43.1 Malignant melanoma of eyelid, including canthus**
Canthus: Either corner of eye where upper and lower eyelids meet

C43.1Ø Malignant melanoma of unspecified eyelid, including canthus

C43.11 Malignant melanoma of right eyelid, including canthus

C43.12 Malignant melanoma of left eyelid, including canthus

● **C43.2 Malignant melanoma of ear and external auricular canal**

C43.2Ø Malignant melanoma of unspecified ear and external auricular canal

C43.21 Malignant melanoma of right ear and external auricular canal

C43.22 Malignant melanoma of left ear and external auricular canal

● **C43.3 Malignant melanoma of other and unspecified parts of face**

C43.3Ø Malignant melanoma of unspecified part of face

C43.31 Malignant melanoma of nose

C43.39 Malignant melanoma of other parts of face

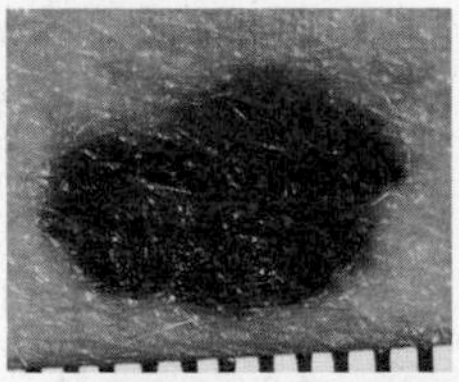

Figure 2-10 Malignant melanoma of skin. (From Goldman: Cecil Textbook of Medicine, ed 22, Saunders, 2004)

Item 2–4 Malignant melanoma is a serious form of skin cancer that affects the melanocytes (pigment-forming cells) and is caused by ultraviolet (UV) rays from the sun that damage skin. It is most commonly seen in the 4Ø- to 6Ø-year-olds with fair skin, blue or green eyes, and red or blond hair who sunburn easily.

Melanoma can spread very rapidly and is the most deadly form of skin cancer. It is less common than other types of skin cancer. The rate of melanoma is increasing and currently is the leading cause of death from skin disease.

C43.4 Malignant melanoma of scalp and neck

● **C43.5 Malignant melanoma of trunk**
Excludes2 malignant neoplasm of anus NOS (C21.Ø)
malignant neoplasm of scrotum (C63.2)

C43.51 Malignant melanoma of anal skin
Malignant melanoma of anal margin
Malignant melanoma of perianal skin

C43.52 Malignant melanoma of skin of breast

C43.59 Malignant melanoma of other part of trunk

● **C43.6 Malignant melanoma of upper limb, including shoulder**

C43.6Ø Malignant melanoma of upper limb, including shoulder, unspecified side

C43.61 Malignant melanoma of right upper limb, including shoulder

C43.62 Malignant melanoma of left upper limb, including shoulder

● **C43.7 Malignant melanoma of lower limb, including hip**

C43.7Ø Malignant melanoma of unspecified lower limb, including hip

C43.71 Malignant melanoma of right lower limb, including hip

C43.72 Malignant melanoma of left lower limb, including hip

C43.8 Malignant melanoma of overlapping sites of skin

C43.9 Malignant melanoma of skin, unspecified
Malignant melanoma of unspecified site of skin
Melanoma (malignant) NOS

● **C4A Merkel cell carcinoma**

C4A.Ø Merkel cell carcinoma of lip
Excludes1 malignant neoplasm of vermilion border of lip (CØØ.Ø-CØØ.2)

● **C4A.1 Merkel cell carcinoma of eyelid, including canthus**

C4A.1Ø Merkel cell carcinoma of unspecified eyelid, including canthus

C4A.11 Merkel cell carcinoma of right eyelid, including canthus

C4A.12 Merkel cell carcinoma of left eyelid, including canthus

● **C4A.2 Merkel cell carcinoma of ear and external auricular canal**

C4A.2Ø Merkel cell carcinoma of unspecified ear and external auricular canal

C4A.21 Merkel cell carcinoma of right ear and external auricular canal

C4A.22 Merkel cell carcinoma of left ear and external auricular canal

● C4A.3 Merkel cell carcinoma of other and unspecified parts of face
C4A.30 Merkel cell carcinoma of unspecified part of face
C4A.31 Merkel cell carcinoma of nose
C4A.39 Merkel cell carcinoma of other parts of face
C4A.4 Merkel cell carcinoma of scalp and neck
● C4A.5 Merkel cell carcinoma of trunk
Excludes2 malignant neoplasm of anus NOS (C21.Ø)
malignant neoplasm of scrotum (C63.2)
C4A.51 Merkel cell carcinoma of anal skin
Merkel cell carcinoma of anal margin
Merkel cell carcinoma of perianal skin
C4A.52 Merkel cell carcinoma of skin of breast
C4A.59 Merkel cell carcinoma of other part of trunk
● C4A.6 Merkel cell carcinoma of upper limb, including shoulder
C4A.6Ø Merkel cell carcinoma of unspecified upper limb, including shoulder
C4A.61 Merkel cell carcinoma of right upper limb, including shoulder
C4A.62 Merkel cell carcinoma of left upper limb, including shoulder
● C4A.7 Merkel cell carcinoma of lower limb, including hip
C4A.7Ø Merkel cell carcinoma of unspecified lower limb, including hip
C4A.71 Merkel cell carcinoma of right lower limb, including hip
C4A.72 Merkel cell carcinoma of left lower limb, including hip
C4A.8 Merkel cell carcinoma of overlapping sites
C4A.9 Merkel cell carcinoma, unspecified
Merkel cell carcinoma of unspecified site
Merkel cell carcinoma NOS

● C44 Other and unspecified malignant neoplasm of skin
Includes malignant neoplasm of sebaceous glands
malignant neoplasm of sweat glands
Excludes1 Kaposi's sarcoma of skin (C46.Ø)
malignant melanoma of skin (C43.-)
malignant neoplasm of skin of genital organs (C51-C52, C6Ø.-, C63.2)
Merkel cell carcinoma (C4A.-)
● C44.Ø Other and unspecified malignant neoplasm of skin of lip
Excludes1 malignant neoplasm of lip (CØØ.-)
C44.ØØ Unspecified malignant neoplasm of skin of lip
C44.Ø1 Basal cell carcinoma of skin of lip
C44.Ø2 Squamous cell carcinoma of skin of lip
C44.Ø9 Other specified malignant neoplasm of skin of lip
● C44.1 Other and unspecified malignant neoplasm of skin of eyelid, including canthus
Excludes1 connective tissue of eyelid (C49.Ø)
● C44.1Ø Unspecified malignant neoplasm of skin of eyelid, including canthus
C44.1Ø1 Unspecified malignant neoplasm of skin of unspecified eyelid, including canthus
C44.1Ø2 Unspecified malignant neoplasm of skin of right eyelid, including canthus
C44.1Ø9 Unspecified malignant neoplasm of skin of left eyelid, including canthus
● C44.11 Basal cell carcinoma of skin of eyelid, including canthus
C44.111 Basal cell carcinoma of skin of unspecified eyelid, including canthus
C44.112 Basal cell carcinoma of skin of right eyelid, including canthus
C44.119 Basal cell carcinoma of skin of left eyelid, including canthus
● C44.12 Squamous cell carcinoma of skin of eyelid, including canthus
C44.121 Squamous cell carcinoma of skin of unspecified eyelid, including canthus
C44.122 Squamous cell carcinoma of skin of right eyelid, including canthus
C44.129 Squamous cell carcinoma of skin of left eyelid, including canthus
● C44.19 Other specified malignant neoplasm of skin of eyelid, including canthus
C44.191 Other specified malignant neoplasm of skin of unspecified eyelid, including canthus
C44.192 Other specified malignant neoplasm of skin of right eyelid, including canthus
C44.199 Other specified malignant neoplasm of skin of left eyelid, including canthus
● C44.2 Other and unspecified malignant neoplasm of skin of ear and external auricular canal
Excludes1 connective tissue of ear (C49.Ø)
● C44.2Ø Unspecified malignant neoplasm of skin of ear and external auricular canal
C44.2Ø1 Unspecified malignant neoplasm of skin of unspecified ear and external auricular canal
C44.2Ø2 Unspecified malignant neoplasm of skin of right ear and external auricular canal
C44.2Ø9 Unspecified malignant neoplasm of skin of left ear and external auricular canal
● C44.21 Basal cell carcinoma of skin of ear and external auricular canal
C44.211 Basal cell carcinoma of skin of unspecified ear and external auricular canal
C44.212 Basal cell carcinoma of skin of right ear and external auricular canal
C44.219 Basal cell carcinoma of skin of left ear and external auricular canal
● C44.22 Squamous cell carcinoma of skin of ear and external auricular canal
C44.221 Squamous cell carcinoma of skin of unspecified ear and external auricular canal
C44.222 Squamous cell carcinoma of skin of right ear and external auricular canal
C44.229 Squamous cell carcinoma of skin of left ear and external auricular canal
● C44.29 Other specified malignant neoplasm of skin of ear and external auricular canal
C44.291 Other specified malignant neoplasm of skin of unspecified ear and external auricular canal
C44.292 Other specified malignant neoplasm of skin of right ear and external auricular canal
C44.299 Other specified malignant neoplasm of skin of left ear and external auricular canal

● C44.3 Other and unspecified malignant neoplasm of skin of other and unspecified parts of face
● C44.30 Unspecified malignant neoplasm of skin of other and unspecified parts of face
C44.300 Unspecified malignant neoplasm of skin of unspecified part of face
C44.301 Unspecified malignant neoplasm of skin of nose
C44.309 Unspecified malignant neoplasm of skin of other parts of face
● C44.31 Basal cell carcinoma of skin of other and unspecified parts of face
C44.310 Basal cell carcinoma of skin of unspecified parts of face
C44.311 Basal cell carcinoma of skin of nose
C44.319 Basal cell carcinoma of skin of other parts of face
● C44.32 Squamous cell carcinoma of skin of other and unspecified parts of face
C44.320 Squamous cell carcinoma of skin of unspecified parts of face
C44.321 Squamous cell carcinoma of skin of nose
C44.329 Squamous cell carcinoma of skin of other parts of face
● C44.39 Other specified malignant neoplasm of skin of other and unspecified parts of face
C44.390 Other specified malignant neoplasm of skin of unspecified parts of face
C44.391 Other specified malignant neoplasm of skin of nose
C44.399 Other specified malignant neoplasm of skin of other parts of face
● C44.4 Other and unspecified malignant neoplasm of skin of scalp and neck
C44.40 Unspecified malignant neoplasm of skin of scalp and neck
C44.41 Basal cell carcinoma of skin of scalp and neck
C44.42 Squamous cell carcinoma of skin of scalp and neck
C44.49 Other specified malignant neoplasm of skin of scalp and neck
● C44.5 Other and unspecified malignant neoplasm of skin of trunk
Excludes1 anus NOS (C21.0)
scrotum (C63.2)
● C44.50 Unspecified malignant neoplasm of skin of trunk
C44.500 Unspecified malignant neoplasm of anal skin
Unspecified malignant neoplasm of anal margin
Unspecified malignant neoplasm of perianal skin
C44.501 Unspecified malignant neoplasm of skin of breast
C44.509 Unspecified malignant neoplasm of skin of other part of trunk
● C44.51 Basal cell carcinoma of skin of trunk
C44.510 Basal cell carcinoma of anal skin
Basal cell carcinoma of anal margin
Basal cell carcinoma of perianal skin
C44.511 Basal cell carcinoma of skin of breast
C44.519 Basal cell carcinoma of skin of other part of trunk
● C44.52 Squamous cell carcinoma of skin of trunk
C44.520 Squamous cell carcinoma of anal skin
Squamous cell carcinoma of anal margin
Squamous cell carcinoma of perianal skin
C44.521 Squamous cell carcinoma of skin of breast
C44.529 Squamous cell carcinoma of skin of other part of trunk
● C44.59 Other specified malignant neoplasm of skin of trunk
C44.590 Other specified malignant neoplasm of anal skin
Other specified malignant neoplasm of anal margin
Other specified malignant neoplasm of perianal skin
C44.591 Other specified malignant neoplasm of skin of breast
C44.599 Other specified malignant neoplasm of skin of other part of trunk
● C44.6 Other and unspecified malignant neoplasm of skin of upper limb, including shoulder
● C44.60 Unspecified malignant neoplasm of skin of upper limb, including shoulder
C44.601 Unspecified malignant neoplasm of skin of unspecified upper limb, including shoulder
C44.602 Unspecified malignant neoplasm of skin of right upper limb, including shoulder
C44.609 Unspecified malignant neoplasm of skin of left upper limb, including shoulder
● C44.61 Basal cell carcinoma of skin of upper limb, including shoulder
C44.611 Basal cell carcinoma of skin of unspecified upper limb, including shoulder
C44.612 Basal cell carcinoma of skin of right upper limb, including shoulder
C44.619 Basal cell carcinoma of skin of left upper limb, including shoulder
● C44.62 Squamous cell carcinoma of skin of upper limb, including shoulder
C44.621 Squamous cell carcinoma of skin of unspecified upper limb, including shoulder
C44.622 Squamous cell carcinoma of skin of right upper limb, including shoulder
C44.629 Squamous cell carcinoma of skin of left upper limb, including shoulder
● C44.69 Other specified malignant neoplasm of skin of upper limb, including shoulder
C44.691 Other specified malignant neoplasm of skin of unspecified upper limb, including shoulder
C44.692 Other specified malignant neoplasm of skin of right upper limb, including shoulder
C44.699 Other specified malignant neoplasm of skin of left upper limb, including shoulder

CHAPTER 2 (C00-D49)

● **C44.7 Other and unspecified malignant neoplasm of skin of lower limb, including hip**

● **C44.7Ø Unspecified malignant neoplasm of skin of lower limb, including hip**

C44.7Ø1 Unspecified malignant neoplasm of skin of unspecified lower limb, including hip

C44.7Ø2 Unspecified malignant neoplasm of skin of right lower limb, including hip

C44.7Ø9 Unspecified malignant neoplasm of skin of left lower limb, including hip

● **C44.71 Basal cell carcinoma of skin of lower limb, including hip**

C44.711 Basal cell carcinoma of skin of unspecified lower limb, including hip

C44.712 Basal cell carcinoma of skin of right lower limb, including hip

C44.719 Basal cell carcinoma of skin of left lower limb, including hip

● **C44.72 Squamous cell carcinoma of skin of lower limb, including hip**

C44.721 Squamous cell carcinoma of skin of unspecified lower limb, including hip

C44.722 Squamous cell carcinoma of skin of right lower limb, including hip

C44.729 Squamous cell carcinoma of skin of left lower limb, including hip

● **C44.79 Other specified malignant neoplasm of skin of lower limb, including hip**

C44.791 Other specified malignant neoplasm of skin of unspecified lower limb, including hip

C44.792 Other specified malignant neoplasm of skin of right lower limb, including hip

C44.799 Other specified malignant neoplasm of skin of left lower limb, including hip

● **C44.8 Other and unspecified malignant neoplasm of overlapping sites of skin**

C44.8Ø Unspecified malignant neoplasm of overlapping sites of skin

C44.81 Basal cell carcinoma of overlapping sites of skin

C44.82 Squamous cell carcinoma of overlapping sites of skin

C44.89 Other specified malignant neoplasm of overlapping sites of skin

● **C44.9 Other and unspecified malignant neoplasm of skin, unspecified**

C44.9Ø Unspecified malignant neoplasm of skin, unspecified

Malignant neoplasm of unspecified site of skin

C44.91 Basal cell carcinoma of skin, unspecified

C44.92 Squamous cell carcinoma of skin, unspecified

C44.99 Other specified malignant neoplasm of skin, unspecified

MALIGNANT NEOPLASMS OF MESOTHELIAL AND SOFT TISSUE (C45-C49)

● **C45 Mesothelioma**

Malignant cells develop in protective lining that covers internal organs (mesothelium) caused by exposure to asbestos

C45.Ø Mesothelioma of pleura

Excludes1 other malignant neoplasm of pleura (C38.4)

C45.1 Mesothelioma of peritoneum

Mesothelioma of cul-de-sac
Mesothelioma of mesentery
Mesothelioma of mesocolon
Mesothelioma of omentum
Mesothelioma of peritoneum (parietal) (pelvic)

Excludes1 other malignant neoplasm of soft tissue of peritoneum (C48.-)

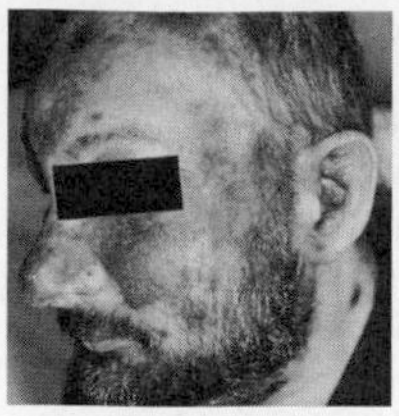

Figure 2-11 Kaposi's sarcoma. There are large confluent hyperpigmented patch-stage lesions with lymphedema. (From Cohen & Powderly: Infectious Diseases, ed 3, Mosby, An Imprint of Elsevier, 2010)

Item 2-5 Kaposi's sarcoma is a cancer that causes patches of abnormal tissue to grow under the skin; in the lining of the mouth, nose, and throat; or in other organs, often beginning and spreading to other organs. Patients who have had organ transplants or patients with AIDS are at high risk for this malignancy.

C45.2 Mesothelioma of pericardium

Excludes1 other malignant neoplasm of pericardium (C38.Ø)

C45.7 Mesothelioma of other sites

C45.9 Mesothelioma, unspecified

● **C46 Kaposi's sarcoma**

Code first any human immunodeficiency virus [HIV] disease (B2Ø)

C46.Ø Kaposi's sarcoma of skin

C46.1 Kaposi's sarcoma of soft tissue

Kaposi's sarcoma of blood vessel
Kaposi's sarcoma of connective tissue
Kaposi's sarcoma of fascia
Kaposi's sarcoma of ligament
Kaposi's sarcoma of lymphatic(s) NEC
Kaposi's sarcoma of muscle

Excludes2 Kaposi's sarcoma of lymph glands and nodes (C46.3)

C46.2 Kaposi's sarcoma of palate

C46.3 Kaposi's sarcoma of lymph nodes

C46.4 Kaposi's sarcoma of gastrointestinal sites

● **C46.5 Kaposi's sarcoma of lung**

C46.5Ø Kaposi's sarcoma of unspecified lung

C46.51 Kaposi's sarcoma of right lung

C46.52 Kaposi's sarcoma of left lung

C46.7 Kaposi's sarcoma of other sites

C46.9 Kaposi's sarcoma, unspecified

Kaposi's sarcoma of unspecified site

● **C47 Malignant neoplasm of peripheral nerves and autonomic nervous system**

Includes malignant neoplasm of sympathetic and parasympathetic nerves and ganglia

Excludes1 Kaposi's sarcoma of soft tissue (C46.1)

C47.Ø Malignant neoplasm of peripheral nerves of head, face and neck

Excludes1 malignant neoplasm of peripheral nerves of orbit (C69.6-)

● **C47.1 Malignant neoplasm of peripheral nerves of upper limb, including shoulder**

C47.1Ø Malignant neoplasm of peripheral nerves of unspecified upper limb, including shoulder

C47.11 Malignant neoplasm of peripheral nerves of right upper limb, including shoulder

C47.12 Malignant neoplasm of peripheral nerves of left upper limb, including shoulder

● **C47.2 Malignant neoplasm of peripheral nerves of lower limb, including hip**

C47.2Ø Malignant neoplasm of peripheral nerves of unspecified lower limb, including hip

C47.21 Malignant neoplasm of peripheral nerves of right lower limb, including hip

C47.22 Malignant neoplasm of peripheral nerves of left lower limb, including hip

C47.3 Malignant neoplasm of peripheral nerves of thorax
C47.4 Malignant neoplasm of peripheral nerves of abdomen
C47.5 Malignant neoplasm of peripheral nerves of pelvis
C47.6 Malignant neoplasm of peripheral nerves of trunk, unspecified
Malignant neoplasm of peripheral nerves of unspecified part of trunk
C47.8 Malignant neoplasm of overlapping sites of peripheral nerves and autonomic nervous system
C47.9 Malignant neoplasm of peripheral nerves and autonomic nervous system, unspecified
Malignant neoplasm of unspecified site of peripheral nerves and autonomic nervous system

● **C48 Malignant neoplasm of retroperitoneum and peritoneum**
Excludes1 Kaposi's sarcoma of connective tissue (C46.1)
mesothelioma (C45.-)
C48.0 Malignant neoplasm of retroperitoneum
Behind/outside of peritoneum
C48.1 Malignant neoplasm of specified parts of peritoneum
Serous membrane lining abdominopelvic walls and covering viscera
Malignant neoplasm of cul-de-sac
Malignant neoplasm of mesentery
Malignant neoplasm of mesocolon
Malignant neoplasm of omentum
Malignant neoplasm of parietal peritoneum
Malignant neoplasm of pelvic peritoneum
C48.2 Malignant neoplasm of peritoneum, unspecified
C48.8 Malignant neoplasm of overlapping sites of retroperitoneum and peritoneum

● **C49 Malignant neoplasm of other connective and soft tissue**
Includes malignant neoplasm of blood vessel
malignant neoplasm of bursa
malignant neoplasm of cartilage
malignant neoplasm of fascia
malignant neoplasm of fat
malignant neoplasm of ligament, except uterine
malignant neoplasm of lymphatic vessel
malignant neoplasm of muscle
malignant neoplasm of synovia
malignant neoplasm of tendon (sheath)
Excludes1 malignant neoplasm of cartilage (of):
articular (C40-C41)
larynx (C32.3)
nose (C30.0)
malignant neoplasm of connective tissue of breast (C50.-)
Excludes2 Kaposi's sarcoma of soft tissue (C46.1)
malignant neoplasm of heart (C38.0)
malignant neoplasm of peripheral nerves and autonomic nervous system (C47.-)
malignant neoplasm of peritoneum (C48.2)
malignant neoplasm of retroperitoneum (C48.0)
malignant neoplasm of uterine ligament (C57.3)
mesothelioma (C45.-)
C49.0 Malignant neoplasm of connective and soft tissue of head, face and neck
Malignant neoplasm of connective tissue of ear
Malignant neoplasm of connective tissue of eyelid
Excludes1 connective tissue of orbit (C69.6-)
● **C49.1 Malignant neoplasm of connective and soft tissue of upper limb, including shoulder**
C49.10 Malignant neoplasm of connective and soft tissue of unspecified upper limb, including shoulder
C49.11 Malignant neoplasm of connective and soft tissue of right upper limb, including shoulder
C49.12 Malignant neoplasm of connective and soft tissue of left upper limb, including shoulder
● **C49.2 Malignant neoplasm of connective and soft tissue of lower limb, including hip**
C49.20 Malignant neoplasm of connective and soft tissue of unspecified lower limb, including hip
C49.21 Malignant neoplasm of connective and soft tissue of right lower limb, including hip
C49.22 Malignant neoplasm of connective and soft tissue of left lower limb, including hip
C49.3 Malignant neoplasm of connective and soft tissue of thorax
Malignant neoplasm of axilla
Malignant neoplasm of diaphragm
Malignant neoplasm of great vessels
Excludes1 malignant neoplasm of breast (C50.-)
malignant neoplasm of heart (C38.0)
malignant neoplasm of mediastinum (C38.1-C38.3)
malignant neoplasm of thymus (C37)
C49.4 Malignant neoplasm of connective and soft tissue of abdomen
Malignant neoplasm of abdominal wall
Malignant neoplasm of hypochondrium
C49.5 Malignant neoplasm of connective and soft tissue of pelvis
Malignant neoplasm of buttock
Malignant neoplasm of groin
Malignant neoplasm of perineum
C49.6 Malignant neoplasm of connective and soft tissue of trunk, unspecified
Malignant neoplasm of back NOS
C49.8 Malignant neoplasm of overlapping sites of connective and soft tissue
Primary malignant neoplasm of two or more contiguous sites of connective and soft tissue
C49.9 Malignant neoplasm of connective and soft tissue, unspecified
● **C49.A Gastrointestinal stromal tumor** ◀
C49.A0 Gastrointestinal stromal tumor, unspecified site ◀
C49.A1 Gastrointestinal stromal tumor of esophagus ◀
C49.A2 Gastrointestinal stromal tumor of stomach ◀
C49.A3 Gastrointestinal stromal tumor of small intestine ◀
C49.A4 Gastrointestinal stromal tumor of large intestine ◀
C49.A5 Gastrointestinal stromal tumor of rectum ◀
C49.A9 Gastrointestinal stromal tumor of other sites ◀

MALIGNANT NEOPLASMS OF BREAST (C50)

● **C50 Malignant neoplasm of breast**
Includes connective tissue of breast
Paget's disease of breast
Paget's disease of nipple
Intraductal carcinoma of breast characterized by eczema-like inflammatory skin changes
Use additional code to identify estrogen receptor status (Z17.0, Z17.1)
Excludes1 skin of breast (C44.501, C44.511, C44.521, C44.591)
● **C50.0 Malignant neoplasm of nipple and areola**
● **C50.01 Malignant neoplasm of nipple and areola, female**
C50.011 Malignant neoplasm of nipple and areola, right female breast
C50.012 Malignant neoplasm of nipple and areola, left female breast
C50.019 Malignant neoplasm of nipple and areola, unspecified female breast

CHAPTER 2 (C00-D49)

● **C5Ø.Ø2** **Malignant neoplasm of nipple and areola, male**
- **C5Ø.Ø21** Malignant neoplasm of nipple and areola, right male breast
- **C5Ø.Ø22** Malignant neoplasm of nipple and areola, left male breast
- **C5Ø.Ø29** Malignant neoplasm of nipple and areola, unspecified male breast

● **C5Ø.1** **Malignant neoplasm of central portion of breast**

● **C5Ø.11** **Malignant neoplasm of central portion of breast, female**
- **C5Ø.111** Malignant neoplasm of central portion of right female breast
- **C5Ø.112** Malignant neoplasm of central portion of left female breast
- **C5Ø.119** Malignant neoplasm of central portion of unspecified female breast

● **C5Ø.12** **Malignant neoplasm of central portion of breast, male**
- **C5Ø.121** Malignant neoplasm of central portion of right male breast
- **C5Ø.122** Malignant neoplasm of central portion of left male breast
- **C5Ø.129** Malignant neoplasm of central portion of unspecified male breast

● **C5Ø.2** **Malignant neoplasm of upper-inner quadrant of breast**

● **C5Ø.21** **Malignant neoplasm of upper-inner quadrant of breast, female**
- **C5Ø.211** Malignant neoplasm of upper-inner quadrant of right female breast
- **C5Ø.212** Malignant neoplasm of upper-inner quadrant of left female breast
- **C5Ø.219** Malignant neoplasm of upper-inner quadrant of unspecified female breast

● **C5Ø.22** **Malignant neoplasm of upper-inner quadrant of breast, male**
- **C5Ø.221** Malignant neoplasm of upper-inner quadrant of right male breast
- **C5Ø.222** Malignant neoplasm of upper-inner quadrant of left male breast
- **C5Ø.229** Malignant neoplasm of upper-inner quadrant of unspecified male breast

● **C5Ø.3** **Malignant neoplasm of lower-inner quadrant of breast**

● **C5Ø.31** **Malignant neoplasm of lower-inner quadrant of breast, female**
- **C5Ø.311** Malignant neoplasm of lower-inner quadrant of right female breast
- **C5Ø.312** Malignant neoplasm of lower-inner quadrant of left female breast
- **C5Ø.319** Malignant neoplasm of lower-inner quadrant of unspecified female breast

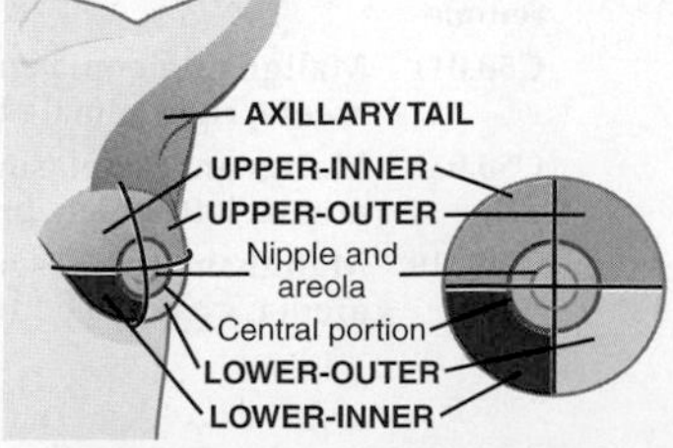

Figure 2-12 Female breast quadrants and axillary tail.

● **C5Ø.32** **Malignant neoplasm of lower-inner quadrant of breast, male**
- **C5Ø.321** Malignant neoplasm of lower-inner quadrant of right male breast
- **C5Ø.322** Malignant neoplasm of lower-inner quadrant of left male breast
- **C5Ø.329** Malignant neoplasm of lower-inner quadrant of unspecified male breast

● **C5Ø.4** **Malignant neoplasm of upper-outer quadrant of breast**

● **C5Ø.41** **Malignant neoplasm of upper-outer quadrant of breast, female**
- **C5Ø.411** Malignant neoplasm of upper-outer quadrant of right female breast
- **C5Ø.412** Malignant neoplasm of upper-outer quadrant of left female breast
- **C5Ø.419** Malignant neoplasm of upper-outer quadrant of unspecified female breast

● **C5Ø.42** **Malignant neoplasm of upper-outer quadrant of breast, male**
- **C5Ø.421** Malignant neoplasm of upper-outer quadrant of right male breast
- **C5Ø.422** Malignant neoplasm of upper-outer quadrant of left male breast
- **C5Ø.429** Malignant neoplasm of upper-outer quadrant of unspecified male breast

● **C5Ø.5** **Malignant neoplasm of lower-outer quadrant of breast**

● **C5Ø.51** **Malignant neoplasm of lower-outer quadrant of breast, female**
- **C5Ø.511** Malignant neoplasm of lower-outer quadrant of right female breast
- **C5Ø.512** Malignant neoplasm of lower-outer quadrant of left female breast
- **C5Ø.519** Malignant neoplasm of lower-outer quadrant of unspecified female breast

● **C5Ø.52** **Malignant neoplasm of lower-outer quadrant of breast, male**
- **C5Ø.521** Malignant neoplasm of lower-outer quadrant of right male breast
- **C5Ø.522** Malignant neoplasm of lower-outer quadrant of left male breast
- **C5Ø.529** Malignant neoplasm of lower-outer quadrant of unspecified male breast

● **C5Ø.6** **Malignant neoplasm of axillary tail of breast**

● **C5Ø.61** **Malignant neoplasm of axillary tail of breast, female**
- **C5Ø.611** Malignant neoplasm of axillary tail of right female breast
- **C5Ø.612** Malignant neoplasm of axillary tail of left female breast
- **C5Ø.619** Malignant neoplasm of axillary tail of unspecified female breast

● **C5Ø.62** **Malignant neoplasm of axillary tail of breast, male**
- **C5Ø.621** Malignant neoplasm of axillary tail of right male breast
- **C5Ø.622** Malignant neoplasm of axillary tail of left male breast
- **C5Ø.629** Malignant neoplasm of axillary tail of unspecified male breast

● **C5Ø.8** **Malignant neoplasm of overlapping sites of breast**

● **C5Ø.81** **Malignant neoplasm of overlapping sites of breast, female**
- **C5Ø.811** Malignant neoplasm of overlapping sites of right female breast
- **C5Ø.812** Malignant neoplasm of overlapping sites of left female breast
- **C5Ø.819** Malignant neoplasm of overlapping sites of unspecified female breast

● **C50.82 Malignant neoplasm of overlapping sites of breast, male**
- **C50.821 Malignant neoplasm of overlapping sites of right male breast**
- **C50.822 Malignant neoplasm of overlapping sites of left male breast**
- **C50.829 Malignant neoplasm of overlapping sites of unspecified male breast**

● **C50.9 Malignant neoplasm of breast of unspecified site**

● **C50.91 Malignant neoplasm of breast of unspecified site, female**
- **C50.911 Malignant neoplasm of unspecified site of right female breast**
- **C50.912 Malignant neoplasm of unspecified site of left female breast**
- **C50.919 Malignant neoplasm of unspecified site of unspecified female breast**

● **C50.92 Malignant neoplasm of breast of unspecified site, male**
- **C50.921 Malignant neoplasm of unspecified site of right male breast**
- **C50.922 Malignant neoplasm of unspecified site of left male breast**
- **C50.929 Malignant neoplasm of unspecified site of unspecified male breast**

MALIGNANT NEOPLASMS OF FEMALE GENITAL ORGANS (C51-C58)

Includes malignant neoplasm of skin of female genital organs

● **C51 Malignant neoplasm of vulva**

Excludes1 carcinoma in situ of vulva (D07.1)

C51.0 Malignant neoplasm of labium majus
Outer folds of skin external female genitalia
Malignant neoplasm of Bartholin's [greater vestibular] gland

C51.1 Malignant neoplasm of labium minus
Two inner folds surrounding vulva in female genitalia

C51.2 Malignant neoplasm of clitoris

C51.8 Malignant neoplasm of overlapping sites of vulva

C51.9 Malignant neoplasm of vulva, unspecified
Malignant neoplasm of external female genitalia NOS
Malignant neoplasm of pudendum

C52 Malignant neoplasm of vagina

Excludes1 carcinoma in situ of vagina (D07.2)

● **C53 Malignant neoplasm of cervix uteri**

Excludes1 carcinoma in situ of cervix uteri (D06.-)

C53.0 Malignant neoplasm of endocervix
Inside the cervix

C53.1 Malignant neoplasm of exocervix
Outside the cervix

C53.8 Malignant neoplasm of overlapping sites of cervix uteri

C53.9 Malignant neoplasm of cervix uteri, unspecified

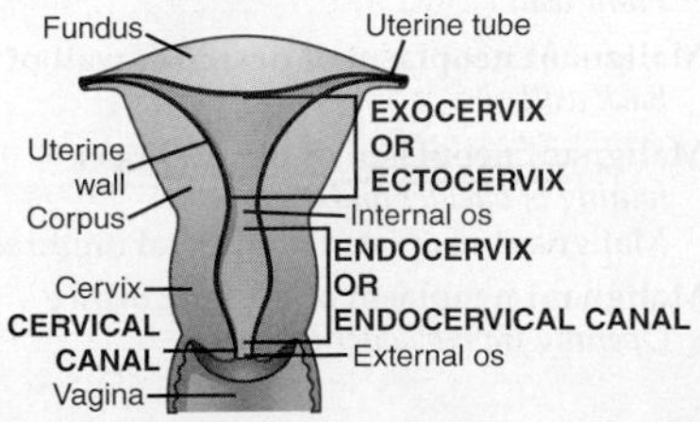

Figure 2-13 Cervix uteri.

● **C54 Malignant neoplasm of corpus uteri**

C54.0 Malignant neoplasm of isthmus uteri
Constricted part of uterus between cervix and body
Malignant neoplasm of lower uterine segment

C54.1 Malignant neoplasm of endometrium
Lining of uterus

C54.2 Malignant neoplasm of myometrium
Middle layer of uterine wall consisting of smooth muscle supporting stromal and vascular tissue

C54.3 Malignant neoplasm of fundus uteri
Top rounded portion of uterus

C54.8 Malignant neoplasm of overlapping sites of corpus uteri
Main body of uterus

C54.9 Malignant neoplasm of corpus uteri, unspecified

C55 Malignant neoplasm of uterus, part unspecified

● **C56 Malignant neoplasm of ovary**

Use additional code to identify any functional activity

- **C56.1 Malignant neoplasm of right ovary**
- **C56.2 Malignant neoplasm of left ovary**
- **C56.9 Malignant neoplasm of unspecified ovary**

● **C57 Malignant neoplasm of other and unspecified female genital organs**

● **C57.0 Malignant neoplasm of fallopian tube**
Malignant neoplasm of oviduct
Malignant neoplasm of uterine tube
- **C57.00 Malignant neoplasm of unspecified fallopian tube**
- **C57.01 Malignant neoplasm of right fallopian tube**
- **C57.02 Malignant neoplasm of left fallopian tube**

● **C57.1 Malignant neoplasm of broad ligament**
- **C57.10 Malignant neoplasm of unspecified broad ligament**
- **C57.11 Malignant neoplasm of right broad ligament**
- **C57.12 Malignant neoplasm of left broad ligament**

● **C57.2 Malignant neoplasm of round ligament**
- **C57.20 Malignant neoplasm of unspecified round ligament**
- **C57.21 Malignant neoplasm of right round ligament**
- **C57.22 Malignant neoplasm of left round ligament**

C57.3 Malignant neoplasm of parametrium
Malignant neoplasm of uterine ligament NOS

C57.4 Malignant neoplasm of uterine adnexa, unspecified

C57.7 Malignant neoplasm of other specified female genital organs
Malignant neoplasm of wolffian body or duct

C57.8 Malignant neoplasm of overlapping sites of female genital organs
Primary malignant neoplasm of two or more contiguous sites of the female genital organs whose point of origin cannot be determined
Primary tubo-ovarian malignant neoplasm whose point of origin cannot be determined
Primary utero-ovarian malignant neoplasm whose point of origin cannot be determined

C57.9 Malignant neoplasm of female genital organ, unspecified
Malignant neoplasm of female genitourinary tract NOS

C58 Malignant neoplasm of placenta

Includes: choriocarcinoma NOS
chorionepithelioma NOS

Excludes1: chorioadenoma (destruens) (D39.2)
hydatidiform mole NOS (OØ1.9)
invasive hydatidiform mole (D39.2)
male choriocarcinoma NOS (C62.9-)
malignant hydatidiform mole (D39.2)

MALIGNANT NEOPLASMS OF MALE GENITAL ORGANS (C6Ø-C63)

Includes: malignant neoplasm of skin of male genital organs

● **C6Ø Malignant neoplasm of penis**

C6Ø.Ø Malignant neoplasm of prepuce
Malignant neoplasm of foreskin

C6Ø.1 Malignant neoplasm of glans penis

C6Ø.2 Malignant neoplasm of body of penis
Malignant neoplasm of corpus cavernosum

C6Ø.8 Malignant neoplasm of overlapping sites of penis

C6Ø.9 Malignant neoplasm of penis, unspecified
Malignant neoplasm of skin of penis NOS

C61 Malignant neoplasm of prostate

Use additional code to identify: ◀
hormone sensitivity status (Z19.1-Z19.2) ◀
rising PSA following treatment for malignant neoplasm of prostate (R97.21) ◀

Excludes1: malignant neoplasm of seminal vesicle (C63.7)

● **C62 Malignant neoplasm of testis**

Use additional code to identify any functional activity.

● **C62.Ø Malignant neoplasm of undescended testis**
Malignant neoplasm of ectopic testis
Malignant neoplasm of retained testis

C62.ØØ Malignant neoplasm of unspecified undescended testis

C62.Ø1 Malignant neoplasm of undescended right testis

C62.Ø2 Malignant neoplasm of undescended left testis

● **C62.1 Malignant neoplasm of descended testis**
Malignant neoplasm of scrotal testis

C62.1Ø Malignant neoplasm of unspecified descended testis, unspecified side

C62.11 Malignant neoplasm of descended right testis

C62.12 Malignant neoplasm of descended left testis

● **C62.9 Malignant neoplasm of testis, unspecified whether descended or undescended**

C62.9Ø Malignant neoplasm of unspecified testis, unspecified whether descended or undescended
Malignant neoplasm of testis NOS

C62.91 Malignant neoplasm of right testis, unspecified whether descended or undescended

C62.92 Malignant neoplasm of left testis, unspecified whether descended or undescended

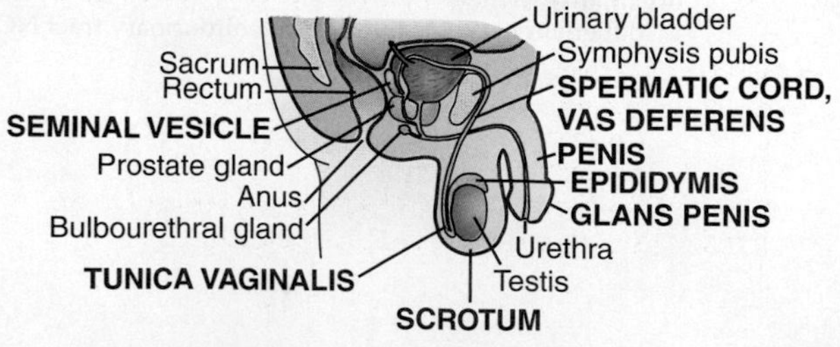

Figure 2-14 Penis and other male genital organs.

● **C63 Malignant neoplasm of other and unspecified male genital organs**

● **C63.Ø Malignant neoplasm of epididymis**

C63.ØØ Malignant neoplasm of unspecified epididymis

C63.Ø1 Malignant neoplasm of right epididymis

C63.Ø2 Malignant neoplasm of left epididymis

● **C63.1 Malignant neoplasm of spermatic cord**

C63.1Ø Malignant neoplasm of unspecified spermatic cord

C63.11 Malignant neoplasm of right spermatic cord

C63.12 Malignant neoplasm of left spermatic cord

C63.2 Malignant neoplasm of scrotum
Malignant neoplasm of skin of scrotum

C63.7 Malignant neoplasm of other specified male genital organs
Malignant neoplasm of seminal vesicle
Malignant neoplasm of tunica vaginalis

C63.8 Malignant neoplasm of overlapping sites of male genital organs
Primary malignant neoplasm of two or more contiguous sites of male genital organs whose point of origin cannot be determined

C63.9 Malignant neoplasm of male genital organ, unspecified
Malignant neoplasm of male genitourinary tract NOS

MALIGNANT NEOPLASMS OF URINARY TRACT (C64-C68)

● **C64 Malignant neoplasm of kidney, except renal pelvis**

Excludes1: malignant carcinoid tumor of the kidney (C7A.Ø93)
malignant neoplasm of renal calyces (C65.-)
malignant neoplasm of renal pelvis (C65.-)

C64.1 Malignant neoplasm of right kidney, except renal pelvis

C64.2 Malignant neoplasm of left kidney, except renal pelvis

C64.9 Malignant neoplasm of unspecified kidney, except renal pelvis

● **C65 Malignant neoplasm of renal pelvis**

Includes: malignant neoplasm of pelviureteric junction
malignant neoplasm of renal calyces

C65.1 Malignant neoplasm of right renal pelvis

C65.2 Malignant neoplasm of left renal pelvis

C65.9 Malignant neoplasm of unspecified renal pelvis

● **C66 Malignant neoplasm of ureter**

Excludes1: malignant neoplasm of ureteric orifice of bladder (C67.6)

C66.1 Malignant neoplasm of right ureter

C66.2 Malignant neoplasm of left ureter

C66.9 Malignant neoplasm of unspecified ureter

● **C67 Malignant neoplasm of bladder**

C67.Ø Malignant neoplasm of trigone of bladder
Triangular area formed by three openings in the floor of urinary bladder

C67.1 Malignant neoplasm of dome of bladder
Vaulted roof

C67.2 Malignant neoplasm of lateral wall of bladder
Side walls

C67.3 Malignant neoplasm of anterior wall of bladder
Front wall

C67.4 Malignant neoplasm of posterior wall of bladder
Back wall

C67.5 Malignant neoplasm of bladder neck
Joining of bladder and urethra
Malignant neoplasm of internal urethral orifice

C67.6 Malignant neoplasm of ureteric orifice
Opening from bladder to ureters

C67.7 Malignant neoplasm of urachus
Embryonic canal that connects the urinary bladder with the structure that forms the umbilical cord (allantois)

C67.8 Malignant neoplasm of overlapping sites of bladder

C67.9 Malignant neoplasm of bladder, unspecified

● **C68 Malignant neoplasm of other and unspecified urinary organs**
Excludes1 malignant neoplasm of female genitourinary tract NOS (C57.9)
malignant neoplasm of male genitourinary tract NOS (C63.9)

C68.Ø Malignant neoplasm of urethra
Excludes1 malignant neoplasm of urethral orifice of bladder (C67.5)

C68.1 Malignant neoplasm of paraurethral glands
Group of glands of female urethra drained by paraurethral ducts; AKA Skene glands, female prostate

C68.8 Malignant neoplasm of overlapping sites of urinary organs
Primary malignant neoplasm of two or more contiguous sites of urinary organs whose point of origin cannot be determined

C68.9 Malignant neoplasm of urinary organ, unspecified
Malignant neoplasm of urinary system NOS

MALIGNANT NEOPLASMS OF EYE, BRAIN AND OTHER PARTS OF CENTRAL NERVOUS SYSTEM (C69-C72)

● **C69 Malignant neoplasm of eye and adnexa**
Excludes1 malignant neoplasm of connective tissue of eyelid (C49.Ø)
malignant neoplasm of eyelid (skin) (C43.1-, C44.1-)
malignant neoplasm of optic nerve (C72.3-)

● **C69.Ø Malignant neoplasm of conjunctiva**
C69.ØØ Malignant neoplasm of unspecified conjunctiva
C69.Ø1 Malignant neoplasm of right conjunctiva
C69.Ø2 Malignant neoplasm of left conjunctiva

● **C69.1 Malignant neoplasm of cornea**
C69.1Ø Malignant neoplasm of unspecified cornea
C69.11 Malignant neoplasm of right cornea
C69.12 Malignant neoplasm of left cornea

● **C69.2 Malignant neoplasm of retina**
Excludes1 dark area on retina (D49.81)
neoplasm of unspecified behavior of retina and choroid (D49.81)
retinal freckle (D49.81)
C69.2Ø Malignant neoplasm of unspecified retina
C69.21 Malignant neoplasm of right retina
C69.22 Malignant neoplasm of left retina

● **C69.3 Malignant neoplasm of choroid**
C69.3Ø Malignant neoplasm of unspecified choroid
C69.31 Malignant neoplasm of right choroid
C69.32 Malignant neoplasm of left choroid

● **C69.4 Malignant neoplasm of ciliary body**
C69.4Ø Malignant neoplasm of unspecified ciliary body
C69.41 Malignant neoplasm of right ciliary body
C69.42 Malignant neoplasm of left ciliary body

● **C69.5 Malignant neoplasm of lacrimal gland and duct**
Malignant neoplasm of lacrimal sac
Malignant neoplasm of nasolacrimal duct
C69.5Ø Malignant neoplasm of unspecified lacrimal gland and duct
C69.51 Malignant neoplasm of right lacrimal gland and duct
C69.52 Malignant neoplasm of left lacrimal gland and duct

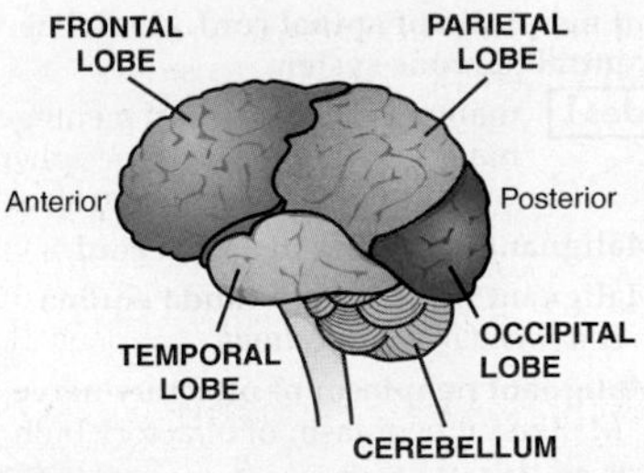

Figure 2-15 The brain.

● **C69.6 Malignant neoplasm of orbit**
Malignant neoplasm of connective tissue of orbit
Malignant neoplasm of extraocular muscle
Malignant neoplasm of peripheral nerves of orbit
Malignant neoplasm of retrobulbar tissue
Malignant neoplasm of retro-ocular tissue
Excludes1 malignant neoplasm of orbital bone (C41.Ø)
C69.6Ø Malignant neoplasm of unspecified orbit
C69.61 Malignant neoplasm of right orbit
C69.62 Malignant neoplasm of left orbit

● **C69.8 Malignant neoplasm of overlapping sites of eye and adnexa**
C69.8Ø Malignant neoplasm of overlapping sites of unspecified eye and adnexa
C69.81 Malignant neoplasm of overlapping sites of right eye and adnexa
C69.82 Malignant neoplasm of overlapping sites of left eye and adnexa

● **C69.9 Malignant neoplasm of unspecified site of eye**
Malignant neoplasm of eyeball
C69.9Ø Malignant neoplasm of unspecified site of unspecified eye
C69.91 Malignant neoplasm of unspecified site of right eye
C69.92 Malignant neoplasm of unspecified site of left eye

● **C7Ø Malignant neoplasm of meninges**
C7Ø.Ø Malignant neoplasm of cerebral meninges
C7Ø.1 Malignant neoplasm of spinal meninges
C7Ø.9 Malignant neoplasm of meninges, unspecified

● **C71 Malignant neoplasm of brain**
Excludes1 malignant neoplasm of cranial nerves (C72.2-C72.5)
retrobulbar malignant neoplasm (C69.6-)

C71.Ø Malignant neoplasm of cerebrum, except lobes and ventricles
Malignant neoplasm of supratentorial NOS
C71.1 Malignant neoplasm of frontal lobe
C71.2 Malignant neoplasm of temporal lobe
C71.3 Malignant neoplasm of parietal lobe
C71.4 Malignant neoplasm of occipital lobe
C71.5 Malignant neoplasm of cerebral ventricle
Excludes1 malignant neoplasm of fourth cerebral ventricle (C71.7)
C71.6 Malignant neoplasm of cerebellum
C71.7 Malignant neoplasm of brain stem
Malignant neoplasm of fourth cerebral ventricle
Infratentorial malignant neoplasm NOS
C71.8 Malignant neoplasm of overlapping sites of brain
C71.9 Malignant neoplasm of brain, unspecified

● C72 Malignant neoplasm of spinal cord, cranial nerves and other parts of central nervous system

Excludes1 malignant neoplasm of meninges (C7Ø.-)
malignant neoplasm of peripheral nerves and autonomic nervous system (C47.-)

C72.Ø Malignant neoplasm of spinal cord

C72.1 Malignant neoplasm of cauda equina
Lower end of spinal column

● C72.2 Malignant neoplasm of olfactory nerve
Malignant neoplasm of olfactory bulb

C72.2Ø Malignant neoplasm of unspecified olfactory nerve

C72.21 Malignant neoplasm of right olfactory nerve

C72.22 Malignant neoplasm of left olfactory nerve

● C72.3 Malignant neoplasm of optic nerve

C72.3Ø Malignant neoplasm of unspecified optic nerve

C72.31 Malignant neoplasm of right optic nerve

C72.32 Malignant neoplasm of left optic nerve

● C72.4 Malignant neoplasm of acoustic nerve

C72.4Ø Malignant neoplasm of unspecified acoustic nerve

C72.41 Malignant neoplasm of right acoustic nerve

C72.42 Malignant neoplasm of left acoustic nerve

● C72.5 Malignant neoplasm of other and unspecified cranial nerves

C72.5Ø Malignant neoplasm of unspecified cranial nerve
Malignant neoplasm of cranial nerve NOS

C72.59 Malignant neoplasm of other cranial nerves

C72.9 Malignant neoplasm of central nervous system, unspecified
Malignant neoplasm of unspecified site of central nervous system
Malignant neoplasm of nervous system NOS

MALIGNANT NEOPLASMS OF THYROID AND OTHER ENDOCRINE GLANDS (C73-C75)

C73 Malignant neoplasm of thyroid gland
Use additional code to identify any functional activity

● C74 Malignant neoplasm of adrenal gland

● C74.Ø Malignant neoplasm of cortex of adrenal gland

C74.ØØ Malignant neoplasm of cortex of unspecified adrenal gland

C74.Ø1 Malignant neoplasm of cortex of right adrenal gland

C74.Ø2 Malignant neoplasm of cortex of left adrenal gland

● C74.1 Malignant neoplasm of medulla of adrenal gland
Pair of glands situated on top of or above each kidney ("suprarenal")

C74.1Ø Malignant neoplasm of medulla of unspecified adrenal gland

C74.11 Malignant neoplasm of medulla of right adrenal gland

C74.12 Malignant neoplasm of medulla of left adrenal gland

● C74.9 Malignant neoplasm of unspecified part of adrenal gland

C74.9Ø Malignant neoplasm of unspecified part of unspecified adrenal gland

C74.91 Malignant neoplasm of unspecified part of right adrenal gland

C74.92 Malignant neoplasm of unspecified part of left adrenal gland

● C75 Malignant neoplasm of other endocrine glands and related structures

Excludes1 malignant carcinoid tumors (C7A.Ø-)
malignant neoplasm of adrenal gland (C74.-)
malignant neoplasm of endocrine pancreas (C25.4)
malignant neoplasm of islets of Langerhans (C25.4)
malignant neoplasm of ovary (C56.-)
malignant neoplasm of testis (C62.-)
malignant neoplasm of thymus (C37)
malignant neoplasm of thyroid gland (C73)
malignant neuroendocrine tumors (C7A.-)

C75.Ø Malignant neoplasm of parathyroid gland

C75.1 Malignant neoplasm of pituitary gland

C75.2 Malignant neoplasm of craniopharyngeal duct

C75.3 Malignant neoplasm of pineal gland

C75.4 Malignant neoplasm of carotid body

C75.5 Malignant neoplasm of aortic body and other paraganglia

C75.8 Malignant neoplasm with pluriglandular involvement, unspecified

C75.9 Malignant neoplasm of endocrine gland, unspecified

MALIGNANT NEUROENDOCRINE TUMORS (C7A)

● C7A Malignant neuroendocrine tumors

Code also any associated multiple endocrine neoplasia [MEN] syndromes (E31.2-)
Use additional code to identify any associated endocrine syndrome, such as:
carcinoid syndrome (E34.Ø)

Excludes2 malignant pancreatic islet cell tumors (C25.4)
Merkel cell carcinoma (C4A.-)

● C7A.Ø Malignant carcinoid tumors

C7A.ØØ Malignant carcinoid tumor of unspecified site

● C7A.Ø1 Malignant carcinoid tumors of the small intestine

C7A.Ø1Ø Malignant carcinoid tumor of the duodenum

C7A.Ø11 Malignant carcinoid tumor of the jejunum

C7A.Ø12 Malignant carcinoid tumor of the ileum

C7A.Ø19 Malignant carcinoid tumor of the small intestine, unspecified portion

● C7A.Ø2 Malignant carcinoid tumors of the appendix, large intestine, and rectum

C7A.Ø2Ø Malignant carcinoid tumor of the appendix

C7A.Ø21 Malignant carcinoid tumor of the cecum

C7A.Ø22 Malignant carcinoid tumor of the ascending colon

C7A.Ø23 Malignant carcinoid tumor of the transverse colon

C7A.Ø24 Malignant carcinoid tumor of the descending colon

C7A.Ø25 Malignant carcinoid tumor of the sigmoid colon

C7A.Ø26 Malignant carcinoid tumor of the rectum

C7A.Ø29 Malignant carcinoid tumor of the large intestine, unspecified portion
Malignant carcinoid tumor of the colon NOS

CHAPTER 2 (CØØ-D49)

● **C7A.09 Malignant carcinoid tumors of other sites**

C7A.090 Malignant carcinoid tumor of the bronchus and lung

C7A.091 Malignant carcinoid tumor of the thymus

C7A.092 Malignant carcinoid tumor of the stomach

C7A.093 Malignant carcinoid tumor of the kidney

C7A.094 Malignant carcinoid tumor of the foregut, unspecified ⟸

C7A.095 Malignant carcinoid tumor of the midgut, unspecified ⟸

C7A.096 Malignant carcinoid tumor of the hindgut, unspecified ⟸

C7A.098 Malignant carcinoid tumors of other sites

C7A.1 Malignant poorly differentiated neuroendocrine tumors

Malignant poorly differentiated neuroendocrine tumor NOS

Malignant poorly differentiated neuroendocrine carcinoma, any site

High grade neuroendocrine carcinoma, any site

C7A.8 Other malignant neuroendocrine tumors

Secondary neuroendocrine tumors (C7B)

SECONDARY NEUROENDOCRINE TUMORS (C7B)

● **C7B Secondary neuroendocrine tumors**

Use additional code to identify any functional activity

● **C7B.0 Secondary carcinoid tumors**

C7B.00 Secondary carcinoid tumors, unspecified site

C7B.01 Secondary carcinoid tumors of distant lymph nodes

C7B.02 Secondary carcinoid tumors of liver

C7B.03 Secondary carcinoid tumors of bone

C7B.04 Secondary carcinoid tumors of peritoneum

Mesentary metastasis of carcinoid tumor

C7B.09 Secondary carcinoid tumors of other sites

C7B.1 Secondary Merkel cell carcinoma

Merkel cell carcinoma nodal presentation

Merkel cell carcinoma visceral metastatic presentation

C7B.8 Other secondary neuroendocrine tumors

MALIGNANT NEOPLASMS OF ILL-DEFINED, OTHER SECONDARY AND UNSPECIFIED SITES (C76-C80)

● **C76 Malignant neoplasm of other and ill-defined sites**

Excludes1 malignant neoplasm of female genitourinary tract NOS (C57.9)
malignant neoplasm of male genitourinary tract NOS (C63.9)
malignant neoplasm of lymphoid, hematopoietic and related tissue (C81-C96)
malignant neoplasm of skin (C44.-)
malignant neoplasm of unspecified site NOS (C80.1)

C76.0 Malignant neoplasm of head, face and neck

Malignant neoplasm of cheek NOS

Malignant neoplasm of nose NOS

C76.1 Malignant neoplasm of thorax

Intrathoracic malignant neoplasm NOS

Malignant neoplasm of axilla NOS

Thoracic malignant neoplasm NOS

C76.2 Malignant neoplasm of abdomen

C76.3 Malignant neoplasm of pelvis

Malignant neoplasm of groin NOS

Malignant neoplasm of sites overlapping systems within the pelvis

Rectovaginal (septum) malignant neoplasm

Between rectum and vagina

Rectovesical (septum) malignant neoplasm

Between rectum and urinary bladder; AKA vesicorectal

● **C76.4 Malignant neoplasm of upper limb**

C76.40 Malignant neoplasm of unspecified upper limb

C76.41 Malignant neoplasm of right upper limb

C76.42 Malignant neoplasm of left upper limb

● **C76.5 Malignant neoplasm of lower limb**

C76.50 Malignant neoplasm of unspecified lower limb

C76.51 Malignant neoplasm of right lower limb

C76.52 Malignant neoplasm of left lower limb

C76.8 Malignant neoplasm of other specified ill-defined sites

Malignant neoplasm of overlapping ill-defined sites

● **C77 Secondary and unspecified malignant neoplasm of lymph nodes**

Excludes1 malignant neoplasm of lymph nodes, specified as primary (C81-C86, C88, C96.-)
mesentary metastasis of carcinoid tumor (C7B.04)
secondary carcinoid tumors of distant lymph nodes (C7B.01)

C77.0 Secondary and unspecified malignant neoplasm of lymph nodes of head, face and neck

Secondary and unspecified malignant neoplasm of supraclavicular lymph nodes

C77.1 Secondary and unspecified malignant neoplasm of intrathoracic lymph nodes

C77.2 Secondary and unspecified malignant neoplasm of intra-abdominal lymph nodes

C77.3 Secondary and unspecified malignant neoplasm of axilla and upper limb lymph nodes

Secondary and unspecified malignant neoplasm of pectoral lymph nodes

C77.4 Secondary and unspecified malignant neoplasm of inguinal and lower limb lymph nodes

C77.5 Secondary and unspecified malignant neoplasm of intrapelvic lymph nodes

C77.8 Secondary and unspecified malignant neoplasm of lymph nodes of multiple regions

C77.9 Secondary and unspecified malignant neoplasm of lymph node, unspecified

● **C78 Secondary malignant neoplasm of respiratory and digestive organs**

Excludes1 secondary carcinoid tumors of liver (C7B.02)
secondary carcinoid tumors of peritoneum (C7B.04)

Excludes2 lymph node metastases (C77.0) ◀

● **C78.0 Secondary malignant neoplasm of lung**

C78.00 Secondary malignant neoplasm of unspecified lung

C78.01 Secondary malignant neoplasm of right lung

C78.02 Secondary malignant neoplasm of left lung

C78.1 Secondary malignant neoplasm of mediastinum

Thoracic cavity between pleural cavities

C78.2 Secondary malignant neoplasm of pleura

Serous membrane covering lungs and lining thoracic cavity

● **C78.3 Secondary malignant neoplasm of other and unspecified respiratory organs**

C78.30 Secondary malignant neoplasm of unspecified respiratory organ

C78.39 Secondary malignant neoplasm of other respiratory organs

CHAPTER 2 (C00-D49)

Item 2–6 The adrenal glands are a pair of glands situated on top of or above each kidney ("suprarenal") and chiefly responsible for regulating the stress response through the synthesis of corticosteroids and catecholamines, including cortisol and adrenaline.

C78.4 **Secondary malignant neoplasm of small intestine**

C78.5 **Secondary malignant neoplasm of large intestine and rectum**

C78.6 **Secondary malignant neoplasm of retroperitoneum and peritoneum**

C78.7 **Secondary malignant neoplasm of liver and intrahepatic bile duct**

● **C78.8** **Secondary malignant neoplasm of other and unspecified digestive organs**

C78.80 **Secondary malignant neoplasm of unspecified digestive organ**

C78.89 **Secondary malignant neoplasm of other digestive organs**

Code also exocrine pancreatic insufficiency (K86.81) ◀

● **C79** **Secondary malignant neoplasm of other and unspecified sites**

Excludes1 secondary carcinoid tumors (C7B.-)
secondary neuroendocrine tumors (C7B.-)

Excludes2 lymph node metastases (C77.0) ◀

● **C79.0** **Secondary malignant neoplasm of kidney and renal pelvis**

C79.00 **Secondary malignant neoplasm of unspecified kidney and renal pelvis**

C79.01 **Secondary malignant neoplasm of right kidney and renal pelvis**

C79.02 **Secondary malignant neoplasm of left kidney and renal pelvis**

● **C79.1** **Secondary malignant neoplasm of bladder and other and unspecified urinary organs**

C79.10 **Secondary malignant neoplasm of unspecified urinary organs**

C79.11 **Secondary malignant neoplasm of bladder**

C79.19 **Secondary malignant neoplasm of other urinary organs**

C79.2 **Secondary malignant neoplasm of skin**

Excludes1 secondary Merkel cell carcinoma (C7B.1)

● **C79.3** **Secondary malignant neoplasm of brain and cerebral meninges**

C79.31 **Secondary malignant neoplasm of brain**

C79.32 **Secondary malignant neoplasm of cerebral meninges**

● **C79.4** **Secondary malignant neoplasm of other and unspecified parts of nervous system**

C79.40 **Secondary malignant neoplasm of unspecified part of nervous system**

C79.49 **Secondary malignant neoplasm of other parts of nervous system**

● **C79.5** **Secondary malignant neoplasm of bone and bone marrow**

Excludes1 secondary carcinoid tumors of bone (C7B.03)

C79.51 **Secondary malignant neoplasm of bone**

C79.52 **Secondary malignant neoplasm of bone marrow**

● **C79.6** **Secondary malignant neoplasm of ovary**

C79.60 **Secondary malignant neoplasm of unspecified ovary**

C79.61 **Secondary malignant neoplasm of right ovary**

C79.62 **Secondary malignant neoplasm of left ovary**

● **C79.7** **Secondary malignant neoplasm of adrenal gland**

C79.70 **Secondary malignant neoplasm of unspecified adrenal gland**

C79.71 **Secondary malignant neoplasm of right adrenal gland**

C79.72 **Secondary malignant neoplasm of left adrenal gland**

● **C79.8** **Secondary malignant neoplasm of other specified sites**

C79.81 **Secondary malignant neoplasm of breast**

C79.82 **Secondary malignant neoplasm of genital organs**

C79.89 **Secondary malignant neoplasm of other specified sites**

C79.9 **Secondary malignant neoplasm of unspecified site**

Metastatic cancer NOS
Metastatic disease NOS

Excludes1 carcinomatosis NOS (C80.0)
generalized cancer NOS (C80.0)
malignant (primary) neoplasm of unspecified site (C80.1)

OGCR Section I.C.2.j and k

Disseminated malignant neoplasm, unspecified

j. Code C80.0, Disseminated malignant neoplasm, unspecified, is for use only in those cases where the patient has advanced metastatic disease and no known primary or secondary sites are specified. It should not be used in place of assigning codes for the primary site and all known secondary sites.

Malignant neoplasm without specification of site

k. Code C80.1, Malignant (primary) neoplasm, unspecified, equates to Cancer, unspecified. This code should only be used when no determination can be made as to the primary site of a malignancy. This code should rarely be used in the inpatient setting.

● **C80** **Malignant neoplasm without specification of site**

Excludes1 malignant carcinoid tumor of unspecified site (C7A.00)
malignant neoplasm of specified multiple sites- code to each site

C80.0 **Disseminated malignant neoplasm, unspecified**

Carcinomatosis NOS
Generalized cancer, unspecified site (primary) (secondary)
Generalized malignancy, unspecified site (primary) (secondary)

C80.1 **Malignant (primary) neoplasm, unspecified**

Cancer NOS
Cancer unspecified site (primary)
Carcinoma unspecified site (primary)
Malignancy unspecified site (primary)

Excludes1 secondary malignant neoplasm of unspecified site (C79.9)

C80.2 **Malignant neoplasm associated with transplanted organ**

Code first complication of transplanted organ (T86.-)

Use additional code to identify the specific malignancy

CHAPTER 2 (C00-D49)

★ **(See Plate 315 on page NAP-1.)**

MALIGNANT NEOPLASMS OF LYMPHOID, HEMATOPOIETIC AND RELATED TISSUE (C81-C96)

Excludes2 Kaposi's sarcoma of lymph nodes (C46.3)
secondary and unspecified neoplasm of lymph nodes (C77.-)
secondary neoplasm of bone marrow (C79.52)
secondary neoplasm of spleen (C78.89)

● **C81 Hodgkin lymphoma**
Form of malignant lymphoma with four types, nodular sclerosis, mixed cellularity, lymphocyte depleted, and lymphocyte predominant
Excludes1 personal history of Hodgkin lymphoma (Z85.71)

● **C81.0 Nodular lymphocyte predominant Hodgkin lymphoma**
Least aggressive, least common, typically no symptoms
Lymphocytic-histiocytic predominance Hodgkin's disease

- **C81.00** Nodular lymphocyte predominant Hodgkin lymphoma, unspecified site
- **C81.01** Nodular lymphocyte predominant Hodgkin lymphoma, lymph nodes of head, face, and neck
- **C81.02** Nodular lymphocyte predominant Hodgkin lymphoma, intrathoracic lymph nodes
- **C81.03** Nodular lymphocyte predominant Hodgkin lymphoma, intra-abdominal lymph nodes
- **C81.04** Nodular lymphocyte predominant Hodgkin lymphoma, lymph nodes of axilla and upper limb
- **C81.05** Nodular lymphocyte predominant Hodgkin lymphoma, lymph nodes of inguinal region and lower limb
- **C81.06** Nodular lymphocyte predominant Hodgkin lymphoma, intrapelvic lymph nodes
- **C81.07** Nodular lymphocyte predominant Hodgkin lymphoma, spleen
- **C81.08** Nodular lymphocyte predominant Hodgkin lymphoma, lymph nodes of multiple sites
- **C81.09** Nodular lymphocyte predominant Hodgkin lymphoma, extranodal and solid organ sites

● **C81.1 Nodular sclerosis Hodgkin lymphoma** ⬅
Nodular sclerosis classical Hodgkin lymphoma ◀
Moderately aggressive; most common in young adults

- **C81.10** Nodular sclerosis Hodgkin lymphoma, unspecified site ⬅
- **C81.11** Nodular sclerosis Hodgkin lymphoma, lymph nodes of head, face, and neck ⬅
- **C81.12** Nodular sclerosis Hodgkin lymphoma, intrathoracic lymph nodes ⬅
- **C81.13** Nodular sclerosis Hodgkin lymphoma, intra-abdominal lymph nodes ⬅
- **C81.14** Nodular sclerosis Hodgkin lymphoma, lymph nodes of axilla and upper limb ⬅
- **C81.15** Nodular sclerosis Hodgkin lymphoma, lymph nodes of inguinal region and lower limb ⬅
- **C81.16** Nodular sclerosis Hodgkin lymphoma, intrapelvic lymph nodes ⬅
- **C81.17** Nodular sclerosis Hodgkin lymphoma, spleen ⬅
- **C81.18** Nodular sclerosis Hodgkin lymphoma, lymph nodes of multiple sites ⬅
- **C81.19** Nodular sclerosis Hodgkin lymphoma, extranodal and solid organ sites ⬅

● **C81.2 Mixed cellularity Hodgkin lymphoma** ⬅
Mixed cellularity classical Hodgkin lymphoma ◀
A type of Hodgkin's that is moderately aggressive with mixed cell types

- **C81.20** Mixed cellularity Hodgkin lymphoma, unspecified site ⬅
- **C81.21** Mixed cellularity Hodgkin lymphoma, lymph nodes of head, face, and neck ⬅
- **C81.22** Mixed cellularity Hodgkin lymphoma, intrathoracic lymph nodes ⬅
- **C81.23** Mixed cellularity Hodgkin lymphoma, intra-abdominal lymph nodes ⬅
- **C81.24** Mixed cellularity Hodgkin lymphoma, lymph nodes of axilla and upper limb ⬅
- **C81.25** Mixed cellularity Hodgkin lymphoma, lymph nodes of inguinal region and lower limb ⬅
- **C81.26** Mixed cellularity Hodgkin lymphoma, intrapelvic lymph nodes ⬅
- **C81.27** Mixed cellularity Hodgkin lymphoma, spleen ⬅
- **C81.28** Mixed cellularity Hodgkin lymphoma, lymph nodes of multiple sites ⬅
- **C81.29** Mixed cellularity Hodgkin lymphoma, extranodal and solid organ sites ⬅

● **C81.3 Lymphocyte depleted Hodgkin lymphoma** ⬅
Lymphocyte depleted classical Hodgkin lymphoma ◀
Most aggressive type with poor prognosis

- **C81.30** Lymphocyte depleted Hodgkin lymphoma, unspecified site ⬅
- **C81.31** Lymphocyte depleted Hodgkin lymphoma, lymph nodes of head, face, and neck ⬅
- **C81.32** Lymphocyte depleted Hodgkin lymphoma, intrathoracic lymph nodes ⬅
- **C81.33** Lymphocyte depleted Hodgkin lymphoma, intra-abdominal lymph nodes ⬅
- **C81.34** Lymphocyte depleted Hodgkin lymphoma, lymph nodes of axilla and upper limb ⬅
- **C81.35** Lymphocyte depleted Hodgkin lymphoma, lymph nodes of inguinal region and lower limb ⬅
- **C81.36** Lymphocyte depleted Hodgkin lymphoma, intrapelvic lymph nodes ⬅
- **C81.37** Lymphocyte depleted Hodgkin lymphoma, spleen ⬅
- **C81.38** Lymphocyte depleted Hodgkin lymphoma, lymph nodes of multiple sites ⬅
- **C81.39** Lymphocyte depleted Hodgkin lymphoma, extranodal and solid organ sites ⬅

● **C81.4 Lymphocyte-rich Hodgkin lymphoma** ⬅
Lymphocyte-rich classical Hodgkin lymphoma ◀
Excludes1 nodular lymphocyte predominant Hodgkin lymphoma (C81.0-)

- **C81.40** Lymphocyte-rich Hodgkin lymphoma, unspecified site ⬅
- **C81.41** Lymphocyte-rich Hodgkin lymphoma, lymph nodes of head, face, and neck ⬅
- **C81.42** Lymphocyte-rich Hodgkin lymphoma, intrathoracic lymph nodes ⬅
- **C81.43** Lymphocyte-rich Hodgkin lymphoma, intra-abdominal lymph nodes ⬅
- **C81.44** Lymphocyte-rich Hodgkin lymphoma, lymph nodes of axilla and upper limb ⬅
- **C81.45** Lymphocyte-rich Hodgkin lymphoma, lymph nodes of inguinal region and lower limb ⬅
- **C81.46** Lymphocyte-rich Hodgkin lymphoma, intrapelvic lymph nodes ⬅
- **C81.47** Lymphocyte-rich Hodgkin lymphoma, spleen ⬅
- **C81.48** Lymphocyte-rich Hodgkin lymphoma, lymph nodes of multiple sites ⬅
- **C81.49** Lymphocyte-rich Hodgkin lymphoma, extranodal and solid organ sites ⬅

● C81.7 Other Hodgkin lymphoma
Classical Hodgkin lymphoma NOS
Other classical Hodgkin lymphoma

C81.70 Other Hodgkin lymphoma, unspecified site
C81.71 Other Hodgkin lymphoma, lymph nodes of head, face, and neck
C81.72 Other Hodgkin lymphoma, intrathoracic lymph nodes
C81.73 Other Hodgkin lymphoma, intra-abdominal lymph nodes
C81.74 Other Hodgkin lymphoma, lymph nodes of axilla and upper limb
C81.75 Other Hodgkin lymphoma, lymph nodes of inguinal region and lower limb
C81.76 Other Hodgkin lymphoma, intrapelvic lymph nodes
C81.77 Other Hodgkin lymphoma, spleen
C81.78 Other Hodgkin lymphoma, lymph nodes of multiple sites
C81.79 Other Hodgkin lymphoma, extranodal and solid organ sites

● C81.9 Hodgkin lymphoma, unspecified
C81.90 Hodgkin lymphoma, unspecified, unspecified site
C81.91 Hodgkin lymphoma, unspecified, lymph nodes of head, face, and neck
C81.92 Hodgkin lymphoma, unspecified, intrathoracic lymph nodes
C81.93 Hodgkin lymphoma, unspecified, intra-abdominal lymph nodes
C81.94 Hodgkin lymphoma, unspecified, lymph nodes of axilla and upper limb
C81.95 Hodgkin lymphoma, unspecified, lymph nodes of inguinal region and lower limb
C81.96 Hodgkin lymphoma, unspecified, intrapelvic lymph nodes
C81.97 Hodgkin lymphoma, unspecified, spleen
C81.98 Hodgkin lymphoma, unspecified, lymph nodes of multiple sites
C81.99 Hodgkin lymphoma, unspecified, extranodal and solid organ sites

● C82 Follicular lymphoma
Group of malignant lymphomas

Includes follicular lymphoma with or without diffuse areas

Excludes1 mature T/NK-cell lymphomas (C84.-)
personal history of non-Hodgkin lymphoma (Z85.72)

● C82.0 Follicular lymphoma grade I
C82.00 Follicular lymphoma grade I, unspecified site
C82.01 Follicular lymphoma grade I, lymph nodes of head, face, and neck
C82.02 Follicular lymphoma grade I, intrathoracic lymph nodes
C82.03 Follicular lymphoma grade I, intra-abdominal lymph nodes
C82.04 Follicular lymphoma grade I, lymph nodes of axilla and upper limb
C82.05 Follicular lymphoma grade I, lymph nodes of inguinal region and lower limb
C82.06 Follicular lymphoma grade I, intrapelvic lymph nodes
C82.07 Follicular lymphoma grade I, spleen
C82.08 Follicular lymphoma grade I, lymph nodes of multiple sites
C82.09 Follicular lymphoma grade I, extranodal and solid organ sites

● C82.1 Follicular lymphoma grade II
C82.10 Follicular lymphoma grade II, unspecified site
C82.11 Follicular lymphoma grade II, lymph nodes of head, face, and neck
C82.12 Follicular lymphoma grade II, intrathoracic lymph nodes
C82.13 Follicular lymphoma grade II, intra-abdominal lymph nodes
C82.14 Follicular lymphoma grade II, lymph nodes of axilla and upper limb
C82.15 Follicular lymphoma grade II, lymph nodes of inguinal region and lower limb
C82.16 Follicular lymphoma grade II, intrapelvic lymph nodes
C82.17 Follicular lymphoma grade II, spleen
C82.18 Follicular lymphoma grade II, lymph nodes of multiple sites
C82.19 Follicular lymphoma grade II, extranodal and solid organ sites

● C82.2 Follicular lymphoma grade III, unspecified
C82.20 Follicular lymphoma grade III, unspecified, unspecified site
C82.21 Follicular lymphoma grade III, unspecified, lymph nodes of head, face, and neck
C82.22 Follicular lymphoma grade III, unspecified, intrathoracic lymph nodes
C82.23 Follicular lymphoma grade III, unspecified, intra-abdominal lymph nodes
C82.24 Follicular lymphoma grade III, unspecified, lymph nodes of axilla and upper limb
C82.25 Follicular lymphoma grade III, unspecified, lymph nodes of inguinal region and lower limb
C82.26 Follicular lymphoma grade III, unspecified, intrapelvic lymph nodes
C82.27 Follicular lymphoma grade III, unspecified, spleen
C82.28 Follicular lymphoma grade III, unspecified, lymph nodes of multiple sites
C82.29 Follicular lymphoma grade III, unspecified, extranodal and solid organ sites

● C82.3 Follicular lymphoma grade IIIa
C82.30 Follicular lymphoma grade IIIa, unspecified site
C82.31 Follicular lymphoma grade IIIa, lymph nodes of head, face, and neck
C82.32 Follicular lymphoma grade IIIa, intrathoracic lymph nodes
C82.33 Follicular lymphoma grade IIIa, intra-abdominal lymph nodes
C82.34 Follicular lymphoma grade IIIa, lymph nodes of axilla and upper limb
C82.35 Follicular lymphoma grade IIIa, lymph nodes of inguinal region and lower limb
C82.36 Follicular lymphoma grade IIIa, intrapelvic lymph nodes
C82.37 Follicular lymphoma grade IIIa, spleen
C82.38 Follicular lymphoma grade IIIa, lymph nodes of multiple sites
C82.39 Follicular lymphoma grade IIIa, extranodal and solid organ sites

● **C82.4 Follicular lymphoma grade IIIb**
- C82.40 Follicular lymphoma grade IIIb, unspecified site
- C82.41 Follicular lymphoma grade IIIb, lymph nodes of head, face, and neck
- C82.42 Follicular lymphoma grade IIIb, intrathoracic lymph nodes
- C82.43 Follicular lymphoma grade IIIb, intra-abdominal lymph nodes
- C82.44 Follicular lymphoma grade IIIb, lymph nodes of axilla and upper limb
- C82.45 Follicular lymphoma grade IIIb, lymph nodes of inguinal region and lower limb
- C82.46 Follicular lymphoma grade IIIb, intrapelvic lymph nodes
- C82.47 Follicular lymphoma grade IIIb, spleen
- C82.48 Follicular lymphoma grade IIIb, lymph nodes of multiple sites
- C82.49 Follicular lymphoma grade IIIb, extranodal and solid organ sites

● **C82.5 Diffuse follicle center lymphoma**
- C82.50 Diffuse follicle center lymphoma, unspecified site
- C82.51 Diffuse follicle center lymphoma, lymph nodes of head, face, and neck
- C82.52 Diffuse follicle center lymphoma, intrathoracic lymph nodes
- C82.53 Diffuse follicle center lymphoma, intra-abdominal lymph nodes
- C82.54 Diffuse follicle center lymphoma, lymph nodes of axilla and upper limb
- C82.55 Diffuse follicle center lymphoma, lymph nodes of inguinal region and lower limb
- C82.56 Diffuse follicle center lymphoma, intrapelvic lymph nodes
- C82.57 Diffuse follicle center lymphoma, spleen
- C82.58 Diffuse follicle center lymphoma, lymph nodes of multiple sites
- C82.59 Diffuse follicle center lymphoma, extranodal and solid organ sites

● **C82.6 Cutaneous follicle center lymphoma**
- C82.60 Cutaneous follicle center lymphoma, unspecified site
- C82.61 Cutaneous follicle center lymphoma, lymph nodes of head, face, and neck
- C82.62 Cutaneous follicle center lymphoma, intrathoracic lymph nodes
- C82.63 Cutaneous follicle center lymphoma, intra-abdominal lymph nodes
- C82.64 Cutaneous follicle center lymphoma, lymph nodes of axilla and upper limb
- C82.65 Cutaneous follicle center lymphoma, lymph nodes of inguinal region and lower limb
- C82.66 Cutaneous follicle center lymphoma, intrapelvic lymph nodes
- C82.67 Cutaneous follicle center lymphoma, spleen
- C82.68 Cutaneous follicle center lymphoma, lymph nodes of multiple sites
- C82.69 Cutaneous follicle center lymphoma, extranodal and solid organ sites

● **C82.8 Other types of follicular lymphoma**
- C82.80 Other types of follicular lymphoma, unspecified site
- C82.81 Other types of follicular lymphoma, lymph nodes of head, face, and neck
- C82.82 Other types of follicular lymphoma, intrathoracic lymph nodes
- C82.83 Other types of follicular lymphoma, intra-abdominal lymph nodes
- C82.84 Other types of follicular lymphoma, lymph nodes of axilla and upper limb
- C82.85 Other types of follicular lymphoma, lymph nodes of inguinal region and lower limb
- C82.86 Other types of follicular lymphoma, intrapelvic lymph nodes
- C82.87 Other types of follicular lymphoma, spleen
- C82.88 Other types of follicular lymphoma, lymph nodes of multiple sites
- C82.89 Other types of follicular lymphoma, extranodal and solid organ sites

● **C82.9 Follicular lymphoma, unspecified**
- C82.90 Follicular lymphoma, unspecified, unspecified site
- C82.91 Follicular lymphoma, unspecified, lymph nodes of head, face, and neck
- C82.92 Follicular lymphoma, unspecified, intrathoracic lymph nodes
- C82.93 Follicular lymphoma, unspecified, intra-abdominal lymph nodes
- C82.94 Follicular lymphoma, unspecified, lymph nodes of axilla and upper limb
- C82.95 Follicular lymphoma, unspecified, lymph nodes of inguinal region and lower limb
- C82.96 Follicular lymphoma, unspecified, intrapelvic lymph nodes
- C82.97 Follicular lymphoma, unspecified, spleen
- C82.98 Follicular lymphoma, unspecified, lymph nodes of multiple sites
- C82.99 Follicular lymphoma, unspecified, extranodal and solid organ sites

● **C83 Non-follicular lymphoma**

Excludes1 personal history of non-Hodgkin lymphoma (Z85.72)

● **C83.0 Small cell B-cell lymphoma**

Lymphoplasmacytic lymphoma
Nodal marginal zone lymphoma
Non-leukemic variant of B-CLL
Splenic marginal zone lymphoma

Excludes1 chronic lymphocytic leukemia (C91.1)
mature T/NK-cell lymphomas (C84.-)
Waldenström macroglobulinemia (C88.0)

- C83.00 Small cell B-cell lymphoma, unspecified site
- C83.01 Small cell B-cell lymphoma, lymph nodes of head, face, and neck
- C83.02 Small cell B-cell lymphoma, intrathoracic lymph nodes
- C83.03 Small cell B-cell lymphoma, intra-abdominal lymph nodes
- C83.04 Small cell B-cell lymphoma, lymph nodes of axilla and upper limb
- C83.05 Small cell B-cell lymphoma, lymph nodes of inguinal region and lower limb
- C83.06 Small cell B-cell lymphoma, intrapelvic lymph nodes
- C83.07 Small cell B-cell lymphoma, spleen
- C83.08 Small cell B-cell lymphoma, lymph nodes of multiple sites
- C83.09 Small cell B-cell lymphoma, extranodal and solid organ sites

CHAPTER 2 (C00-D49)

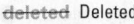

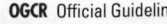

● **C83.1 Mantle cell lymphoma**
Centrocytic lymphoma
Malignant lymphomatous polyposis
C83.10 Mantle cell lymphoma, unspecified site
C83.11 Mantle cell lymphoma, lymph nodes of head, face, and neck
C83.12 Mantle cell lymphoma, intrathoracic lymph nodes
C83.13 Mantle cell lymphoma, intra-abdominal lymph nodes
C83.14 Mantle cell lymphoma, lymph nodes of axilla and upper limb
C83.15 Mantle cell lymphoma, lymph nodes of inguinal region and lower limb
C83.16 Mantle cell lymphoma, intrapelvic lymph nodes
C83.17 Mantle cell lymphoma, spleen
C83.18 Mantle cell lymphoma, lymph nodes of multiple sites
C83.19 Mantle cell lymphoma, extranodal and solid organ sites

● **C83.3 Diffuse large B-cell lymphoma**
Anaplastic diffuse large B-cell lymphoma
CD3Ø-positive diffuse large B-cell lymphoma
Centroblastic diffuse large B-cell lymphoma
Diffuse large B-cell lymphoma, subtype not specified
Immunoblastic diffuse large B-cell lymphoma
Plasmablastic diffuse large B-cell lymphoma
Diffuse large B-cell lymphoma, subtype not specified
T-cell rich diffuse large B-cell lymphoma
Excludes1 mediastinal (thymic) large B-cell lymphoma (C85.2-)
mature T/NK-cell lymphomas (C84.-)
C83.3Ø Diffuse large B-cell lymphoma, unspecified site
C83.31 Diffuse large B-cell lymphoma, lymph nodes of head, face, and neck
C83.32 Diffuse large B-cell lymphoma, intrathoracic lymph nodes
C83.33 Diffuse large B-cell lymphoma, intra-abdominal lymph nodes
C83.34 Diffuse large B-cell lymphoma, lymph nodes of axilla and upper limb
C83.35 Diffuse large B-cell lymphoma, lymph nodes of inguinal region and lower limb
C83.36 Diffuse large B-cell lymphoma, intrapelvic lymph nodes
C83.37 Diffuse large B-cell lymphoma, spleen
C83.38 Diffuse large B-cell lymphoma, lymph nodes of multiple sites
C83.39 Diffuse large B-cell lymphoma, extranodal and solid organ sites

● **C83.5 Lymphoblastic (diffuse) lymphoma**
Highly malignant type of non-Hodgkin lymphoma with diffuse infiltration
B-precursor lymphoma
Lymphoblastic B-cell lymphoma
Lymphoblastic lymphoma NOS
Lymphoblastic T-cell lymphoma
T-precursor lymphoma
C83.5Ø Lymphoblastic (diffuse) lymphoma, unspecified site
C83.51 Lymphoblastic (diffuse) lymphoma, lymph nodes of head, face, and neck
C83.52 Lymphoblastic (diffuse) lymphoma, intrathoracic lymph nodes
C83.53 Lymphoblastic (diffuse) lymphoma, intra-abdominal lymph nodes
C83.54 Lymphoblastic (diffuse) lymphoma, lymph nodes of axilla and upper limb
C83.55 Lymphoblastic (diffuse) lymphoma, lymph nodes of inguinal region and lower limb
C83.56 Lymphoblastic (diffuse) lymphoma, intrapelvic lymph nodes
C83.57 Lymphoblastic (diffuse) lymphoma, spleen
C83.58 Lymphoblastic (diffuse) lymphoma, lymph nodes of multiple sites
C83.59 Lymphoblastic (diffuse) lymphoma, extranodal and solid organ sites

● **C83.7 Burkitt lymphoma**
Form of small cell lymphoma
Atypical Burkitt lymphoma
Burkitt-like lymphoma
Excludes1 mature B-cell leukemia Burkitt type (C91.A-)
C83.7Ø Burkitt lymphoma, unspecified site
C83.71 Burkitt lymphoma, lymph nodes of head, face, and neck
C83.72 Burkitt lymphoma, intrathoracic lymph nodes
C83.73 Burkitt lymphoma, intra-abdominal lymph nodes
C83.74 Burkitt lymphoma, lymph nodes of axilla and upper limb
C83.75 Burkitt lymphoma, lymph nodes of inguinal region and lower limb
C83.76 Burkitt lymphoma, intrapelvic lymph nodes
C83.77 Burkitt lymphoma, spleen
C83.78 Burkitt lymphoma, lymph nodes of multiple sites
C83.79 Burkitt lymphoma, extranodal and solid organ sites

● **C83.8 Other non-follicular lymphoma**
Intravascular large B-cell lymphoma
Lymphoid granulomatosis
Primary effusion B-cell lymphoma
Excludes1 mediastinal (thymic) large B-cell lymphoma (C85.2-)
T-cell rich B-cell lymphoma (C83.3-)
C83.8Ø Other non-follicular lymphoma, unspecified site
C83.81 Other non-follicular lymphoma, lymph nodes of head, face, and neck
C83.82 Other non-follicular lymphoma, intrathoracic lymph nodes
C83.83 Other non-follicular lymphoma, intra-abdominal lymph nodes
C83.84 Other non-follicular lymphoma, lymph nodes of axilla and upper limb
C83.85 Other non-follicular lymphoma, lymph nodes of inguinal region and lower limb
C83.86 Other non-follicular lymphoma, intrapelvic lymph nodes
C83.87 Other non-follicular lymphoma, spleen
C83.88 Other non-follicular lymphoma, lymph nodes of multiple sites
C83.89 Other non-follicular lymphoma, extranodal and solid organ sites

● C83.9 Non-follicular (diffuse) lymphoma, unspecified
- C83.90 Non-follicular (diffuse) lymphoma, unspecified, unspecified site
- C83.91 Non-follicular (diffuse) lymphoma, unspecified, lymph nodes of head, face, and neck
- C83.92 Non-follicular (diffuse) lymphoma, unspecified, intrathoracic lymph nodes
- C83.93 Non-follicular (diffuse) lymphoma, unspecified, intra-abdominal lymph nodes
- C83.94 Non-follicular (diffuse) lymphoma, unspecified, lymph nodes of axilla and upper limb
- C83.95 Non-follicular (diffuse) lymphoma, unspecified, lymph nodes of inguinal region and lower limb
- C83.96 Non-follicular (diffuse) lymphoma, unspecified, intrapelvic lymph nodes
- C83.97 Non-follicular (diffuse) lymphoma, unspecified, spleen
- C83.98 Non-follicular (diffuse) lymphoma, unspecified, lymph nodes of multiple sites
- C83.99 Non-follicular (diffuse) lymphoma, unspecified, extranodal and solid organ sites

● C84 Mature T/NK-cell lymphomas

Excludes1 personal history of non-Hodgkin lymphoma (Z85.72)

● C84.0 Mycosis fungoides

Chronic or rapidly progressive form of cutaneous T-cell lymphoma; AKA granuloma fungoides

Excludes1 peripheral T-cell lymphoma, not classified (C84.4-)

- C84.00 Mycosis fungoides, unspecified site
- C84.01 Mycosis fungoides, lymph nodes of head, face, and neck
- C84.02 Mycosis fungoides, intrathoracic lymph nodes
- C84.03 Mycosis fungoides, intra-abdominal lymph nodes
- C84.04 Mycosis fungoides, lymph nodes of axilla and upper limb
- C84.05 Mycosis fungoides, lymph nodes of inguinal region and lower limb
- C84.06 Mycosis fungoides, intrapelvic lymph nodes
- C84.07 Mycosis fungoides, spleen
- C84.08 Mycosis fungoides, lymph nodes of multiple sites
- C84.09 Mycosis fungoides, extranodal and solid organ sites

● C84.1 Sézary disease

Type of cutaneous lymphoma affecting T-cells

- C84.10 Sézary disease, unspecified site
- C84.11 Sézary disease, lymph nodes of head, face, and neck
- C84.12 Sézary disease, intrathoracic lymph nodes
- C84.13 Sézary disease, intra-abdominal lymph nodes
- C84.14 Sézary disease, lymph nodes of axilla and upper limb
- C84.15 Sézary disease, lymph nodes of inguinal region and lower limb
- C84.16 Sézary disease, intrapelvic lymph nodes
- C84.17 Sézary disease, spleen
- C84.18 Sézary disease, lymph nodes of multiple sites
- C84.19 Sézary disease, extranodal and solid organ sites

Item 2-7 Lymphosarcoma, also known as malignant lymphoma, is a cancer of the lymph system exhibiting abnormal cells encompassing an entire lymph node creating a diffuse pattern without any definite organization. Diffuse pattern lymphoma has a more unfavorable survival outlook than those with a follicular or nodular pattern. Reticulosarcoma is the most common aggressive form of non-Hodgkin's lymphoma.

● C84.4 Peripheral T-cell lymphoma, not classified

Diverse group of blood carcinomas originating from T-cells, requiring aggressive chemotherapy

Lennert's lymphoma
Lymphoepithelioid lymphoma
Mature T-cell lymphoma, not elsewhere classified

- C84.40 Peripheral T-cell lymphoma, not classified, unspecified site
- C84.41 Peripheral T-cell lymphoma, not classified, lymph nodes of head, face, and neck
- C84.42 Peripheral T-cell lymphoma, not classified, intrathoracic lymph nodes
- C84.43 Peripheral T-cell lymphoma, not classified, intra-abdominal lymph nodes
- C84.44 Peripheral T-cell lymphoma, not classified, lymph nodes of axilla and upper limb
- C84.45 Peripheral T-cell lymphoma, not classified, lymph nodes of inguinal region and lower limb
- C84.46 Peripheral T-cell lymphoma, not classified, intrapelvic lymph nodes
- C84.47 Peripheral T-cell lymphoma, not classified, spleen
- C84.48 Peripheral T-cell lymphoma, not classified, lymph nodes of multiple sites
- C84.49 Peripheral T-cell lymphoma, not classified, extranodal and solid organ sites

● C84.6 Anaplastic large cell lymphoma, ALK-positive

Anaplastic large cell lymphoma, CD30-positive

- C84.60 Anaplastic large cell lymphoma, ALK-positive, unspecified site
- C84.61 Anaplastic large cell lymphoma, ALK-positive, lymph nodes of head, face, and neck
- C84.62 Anaplastic large cell lymphoma, ALK-positive, intrathoracic lymph nodes
- C84.63 Anaplastic large cell lymphoma, ALK-positive, intra-abdominal lymph nodes
- C84.64 Anaplastic large cell lymphoma, ALK-positive, lymph nodes of axilla and upper limb
- C84.65 Anaplastic large cell lymphoma, ALK-positive, lymph nodes of inguinal region and lower limb
- C84.66 Anaplastic large cell lymphoma, ALK-positive, intrapelvic lymph nodes
- C84.67 Anaplastic large cell lymphoma, ALK-positive, spleen
- C84.68 Anaplastic large cell lymphoma, ALK-positive, lymph nodes of multiple sites
- C84.69 Anaplastic large cell lymphoma, ALK-positive, extranodal and solid organ sites

● C84.7 Anaplastic large cell lymphoma, ALK-negative

Excludes1 primary cutaneous CD30-positive T-cell proliferations (C86.6-)

- C84.70 Anaplastic large cell lymphoma, ALK-negative, unspecified site
- C84.71 Anaplastic large cell lymphoma, ALK-negative, lymph nodes of head, face, and neck
- C84.72 Anaplastic large cell lymphoma, ALK-negative, intrathoracic lymph nodes
- C84.73 Anaplastic large cell lymphoma, ALK-negative, intra-abdominal lymph nodes
- C84.74 Anaplastic large cell lymphoma, ALK-negative, lymph nodes of axilla and upper limb
- C84.75 Anaplastic large cell lymphoma, ALK-negative, lymph nodes of inguinal region and lower limb
- C84.76 Anaplastic large cell lymphoma, ALK-negative, intrapelvic lymph nodes
- C84.77 Anaplastic large cell lymphoma, ALK-negative, spleen
- C84.78 Anaplastic large cell lymphoma, ALK-negative, lymph nodes of multiple sites
- C84.79 Anaplastic large cell lymphoma, ALK-negative, extranodal and solid organ sites

● C84.A Cutaneous T-cell lymphoma, unspecified
C84.A0 Cutaneous T-cell lymphoma, unspecified, unspecified site
C84.A1 Cutaneous T-cell lymphoma, unspecified lymph nodes of head, face, and neck
C84.A2 Cutaneous T-cell lymphoma, unspecified, intrathoracic lymph nodes
C84.A3 Cutaneous T-cell lymphoma, unspecified, intra-abdominal lymph nodes
C84.A4 Cutaneous T-cell lymphoma, unspecified, lymph nodes of axilla and upper limb
C84.A5 Cutaneous T-cell lymphoma, unspecified, lymph nodes of inguinal region and lower limb
C84.A6 Cutaneous T-cell lymphoma, unspecified, intrapelvic lymph nodes
C84.A7 Cutaneous T-cell lymphoma, unspecified, spleen
C84.A8 Cutaneous T-cell lymphoma, unspecified, lymph nodes of multiple sites
C84.A9 Cutaneous T-cell lymphoma, unspecified, extranodal and solid organ sites

● C84.Z Other mature T/NK-cell lymphomas
Note: If T-cell lineage or involvement is mentioned in conjunction with a specific lymphoma, code to the more specific description.
Excludes1 angioimmunoblastic T-cell lymphoma (C86.5)
blastic NK-cell lymphoma (C86.4)
enteropathy-type T-cell lymphoma (C86.2)
extranodal NK-cell lymphoma, nasal type (C86.0)
hepatosplenic T-cell lymphoma (C86.1)
primary cutaneous CD30-positive T-cell proliferations (C86.6)
subcutaneous panniculitis-like T-cell lymphoma (C86.3)
T-cell leukemia (C91.1-)
C84.Z0 Other mature T/NK-cell lymphomas, unspecified site
C84.Z1 Other mature T/NK-cell lymphomas, lymph nodes of head, face, and neck
C84.Z2 Other mature T/NK-cell lymphomas, intrathoracic lymph nodes
C84.Z3 Other mature T/NK-cell lymphomas, intra-abdominal lymph nodes
C84.Z4 Other mature T/NK-cell lymphomas, lymph nodes of axilla and upper limb
C84.Z5 Other mature T/NK-cell lymphomas, lymph nodes of inguinal region and lower limb
C84.Z6 Other mature T/NK-cell lymphomas, intrapelvic lymph nodes
C84.Z7 Other mature T/NK-cell lymphomas, spleen
C84.Z8 Other mature T/NK-cell lymphomas, lymph nodes of multiple sites
C84.Z9 Other mature T/NK-cell lymphomas, extranodal and solid organ sites

● C84.9 Mature T/NK-cell lymphomas, unspecified
NK/T cell lymphoma NOS
Excludes1 mature T-cell lymphoma, not elsewhere classified (C84.4-)
C84.90 Mature T/NK-cell lymphomas, unspecified, unspecified site
C84.91 Mature T/NK-cell lymphomas, unspecified, lymph nodes of head, face, and neck
C84.92 Mature T/NK-cell lymphomas, unspecified, intrathoracic lymph nodes
C84.93 Mature T/NK-cell lymphomas, unspecified, intra-abdominal lymph nodes
C84.94 Mature T/NK-cell lymphomas, unspecified, lymph nodes of axilla and upper limb
C84.95 Mature T/NK-cell lymphomas, unspecified, lymph nodes of inguinal region and lower limb
C84.96 Mature T/NK-cell lymphomas, unspecified, intrapelvic lymph nodes
C84.97 Mature T/NK-cell lymphomas, unspecified, spleen
C84.98 Mature T/NK-cell lymphomas, unspecified, lymph nodes of multiple sites
C84.99 Mature T/NK-cell lymphomas, unspecified, extranodal and solid organ sites

● C85 Other specified and unspecified types of non-Hodgkin lymphoma
Excludes1 other specified types of T/NK-cell lymphoma (C86.-)
personal history of non-Hodgkin lymphoma (Z85.72)

● C85.1 Unspecified B-cell lymphoma
Note: If B-cell lineage or involvement is mentioned in conjunction with a specific lymphoma, code to the more specific description.
C85.10 Unspecified B-cell lymphoma, unspecified site
C85.11 Unspecified B-cell lymphoma, lymph nodes of head, face, and neck
C85.12 Unspecified B-cell lymphoma, intrathoracic lymph nodes
C85.13 Unspecified B-cell lymphoma, intra-abdominal lymph nodes
C85.14 Unspecified B-cell lymphoma, lymph nodes of axilla and upper limb
C85.15 Unspecified B-cell lymphoma, lymph nodes of inguinal region and lower limb
C85.16 Unspecified B-cell lymphoma, intrapelvic lymph nodes
C85.17 Unspecified B-cell lymphoma, spleen
C85.18 Unspecified B-cell lymphoma, lymph nodes of multiple sites
C85.19 Unspecified B-cell lymphoma, extranodal and solid organ sites

● C85.2 Mediastinal (thymic) large B-cell lymphoma
C85.20 Mediastinal (thymic) large B-cell lymphoma, unspecified site
C85.21 Mediastinal (thymic) large B-cell lymphoma, lymph nodes of head, face, and neck
C85.22 Mediastinal (thymic) large B-cell lymphoma, intrathoracic lymph nodes
C85.23 Mediastinal (thymic) large B-cell lymphoma, intra-abdominal lymph nodes
C85.24 Mediastinal (thymic) large B-cell lymphoma, lymph nodes of axilla and upper limb
C85.25 Mediastinal (thymic) large B-cell lymphoma, lymph nodes of inguinal region and lower limb
C85.26 Mediastinal (thymic) large B-cell lymphoma, intrapelvic lymph nodes
C85.27 Mediastinal (thymic) large B-cell lymphoma, spleen
C85.28 Mediastinal (thymic) large B-cell lymphoma, lymph nodes of multiple sites
C85.29 Mediastinal (thymic) large B-cell lymphoma, extranodal and solid organ sites

● **C85.8 Other specified types of non-Hodgkin lymphoma**

C85.80 Other specified types of non-Hodgkin lymphoma, unspecified site

C85.81 Other specified types of non-Hodgkin lymphoma, lymph nodes of head, face, and neck

C85.82 Other specified types of non-Hodgkin lymphoma, intrathoracic lymph nodes

C85.83 Other specified types of non-Hodgkin lymphoma, intra-abdominal lymph nodes

C85.84 Other specified types of non-Hodgkin lymphoma, lymph nodes of axilla and upper limb

C85.85 Other specified types of non-Hodgkin lymphoma, lymph nodes of inguinal region and lower limb

C85.86 Other specified types of non-Hodgkin lymphoma, intrapelvic lymph nodes

C85.87 Other specified types of non-Hodgkin lymphoma, spleen

C85.88 Other specified types of non-Hodgkin lymphoma, lymph nodes of multiple sites

C85.89 Other specified types of non-Hodgkin lymphoma, extranodal and solid organ sites

● **C85.9 Non-Hodgkin lymphoma, unspecified**

Lymphoma NOS
Malignant lymphoma NOS
Non-Hodgkin lymphoma NOS

C85.90 Non-Hodgkin lymphoma, unspecified, unspecified site

C85.91 Non-Hodgkin lymphoma, unspecified, lymph nodes of head, face, and neck

C85.92 Non-Hodgkin lymphoma, unspecified, intrathoracic lymph nodes

C85.93 Non-Hodgkin lymphoma, unspecified, intra-abdominal lymph nodes

C85.94 Non-Hodgkin lymphoma, unspecified, lymph nodes of axilla and upper limb

C85.95 Non-Hodgkin lymphoma, unspecified, lymph nodes of inguinal region and lower limb

C85.96 Non-Hodgkin lymphoma, unspecified, intrapelvic lymph nodes

C85.97 Non-Hodgkin lymphoma, unspecified, spleen

C85.98 Non-Hodgkin lymphoma, unspecified, lymph nodes of multiple sites

C85.99 Non-Hodgkin lymphoma, unspecified, extranodal and solid organ sites

● **C86 Other specified types of T/NK-cell lymphoma**

Excludes1 anaplastic large cell lymphoma, ALK negative (C84.7-)
anaplastic large cell lymphoma, ALK positive (C84.6-)
mature T/NK-cell lymphomas (C84.-)
other specified types of non-Hodgkin lymphoma (C85.8-)

C86.0 Extranodal NK/T-cell lymphoma, nasal type

C86.1 Hepatosplenic T-cell lymphoma

Alpha-beta and gamma delta types

C86.2 Enteropathy-type (intestinal) T-cell lymphoma

Enteropathy associated T-cell lymphoma

C86.3 Subcutaneous panniculitis-like T-cell lymphoma

C86.4 Blastic NK-cell lymphoma

C86.5 Angioimmunoblastic T-cell lymphoma

Angioimmunoblastic lymphadenopathy with dysproteinemia (AILD)

C86.6 Primary cutaneous CD30-positive T-cell proliferations

Lymphomatoid papulosis
Primary cutaneous anaplastic large cell lymphoma
Primary cutaneous CD30-positive large T-cell lymphoma

● **C88 Malignant immunoproliferative diseases and certain other B-cell lymphomas**

Diseases involving immune system

Excludes1 B-cell lymphoma, unspecified (C85.1-)
personal history of other malignant neoplasms of lymphoid, hematopoietic and related tissues (Z85.79)

C88.0 Waldenström's macroglobulinemia

Lymphoplasmacytic lymphoma with IgM-production
Macroglobulinemia (idiopathic) (primary)

Excludes1 small cell B-cell lymphoma (C83.0)

C88.2 Heavy chain disease

Franklin disease
Gamma heavy chain disease
Mu heavy chain disease

C88.3 Immunoproliferative small intestinal disease

Alpha heavy chain disease
Mediterranean lymphoma

C88.4 Extranodal marginal zone B-cell lymphoma of mucosa-associated lymphoid tissue [MALT-lymphoma]

Lymphoma of skin-associated lymphoid tissue [SALT-lymphoma]
Lymphoma of bronchial-associated lymphoid tissue [BALT-lymphoma]

Excludes1 high malignant (diffuse large B-cell) lymphoma (C83.3-)

C88.8 Other malignant immunoproliferative diseases

C88.9 Malignant immunoproliferative disease, unspecified

Immunoproliferative disease NOS

● **C90 Multiple myeloma and malignant plasma cell neoplasms**

Excludes1 personal history of other malignant neoplasms of lymphoid, hematopoietic and related tissues (Z85.79)

● **C90.0 Multiple myeloma**

Kahler's disease
Medullary plasmacytoma
Myelomatosis
Plasma cell myeloma

Excludes1 solitary myeloma (C90.3-)
solitary plasmacytoma (C90.3-)

C90.00 Multiple myeloma not having achieved remission

Multiple myeloma with failed remission
Multiple myeloma NOS

C90.01 Multiple myeloma in remission

C90.02 Multiple myeloma in relapse

● **C90.1 Plasma cell leukemia**

Rare type of acute leukemia

Plasmacytic leukemia

C90.10 Plasma cell leukemia not having achieved remission

Plasma cell leukemia with failed remission
Plasma cell leukemia NOS

C90.11 Plasma cell leukemia in remission

C90.12 Plasma cell leukemia in relapse

● **C90.2 Extramedullary plasmacytoma**

Malignant monoclonal plasma cell tumor growing in soft tissue; AKA plasma cell dyscrasias

C90.20 Extramedullary plasmacytoma not having achieved remission

Extramedullary plasmacytoma with failed remission
Extramedullary plasmacytoma NOS

C90.21 Extramedullary plasmacytoma in remission

C90.22 Extramedullary plasmacytoma in relapse

Item 2–8 Multiple myeloma is a cancer of a plasma cell (a type of white blood cell) and is an incurable but treatable disease. Immunoproliferative neoplasm is a term for diseases (mostly cancers) in which the immune system cells proliferate.

● **C90.3 Solitary plasmacytoma**
Localized malignant plasma cell tumor NOS
Plasmacytoma NOS
Solitary myeloma

C90.30 Solitary plasmacytoma not having achieved remission
Solitary plasmacytoma with failed remission
Solitary plasmacytoma NOS

C90.31 Solitary plasmacytoma in remission

C90.32 Solitary plasmacytoma in relapse

● **C91 Lymphoid leukemia**
Type of leukemia affecting circulating cells of lymphoid origin
Excludes1 personal history of leukemia (Z85.6)

● **C91.0 Acute lymphoblastic leukemia [ALL]**
Note: Code C91.0 should only be used for T-cell and B-cell precusor leukemia

C91.00 Acute lymphoblastic leukemia not having achieved remission
Acute lymphoblastic leukemia with failed remission
Acute lymphoblastic leukemia NOS

C91.01 Acute lymphoblastic leukemia, in remission

C91.02 Acute lymphoblastic leukemia, in relapse

● **C91.1 Chronic lymphocytic leukemia of B-cell type**
Lymphoplasmacytic leukemia
Richter syndrome
Excludes1 lymphoplasmacytic lymphoma (C83.0-)

C91.10 Chronic lymphocytic leukemia of B-cell type not having achieved remission
Chronic lymphocytic leukemia of B-cell type with failed remission
Chronic lymphocytic leukemia of B-cell type NOS

C91.11 Chronic lymphocytic leukemia of B-cell type in remission

C91.12 Chronic lymphocytic leukemia of B-cell type in relapse

● **C91.3 Prolymphocytic leukemia of B-cell type**
Chronic leukemia with symptoms of large number of circulating lymphocytes

C91.30 Prolymphocytic leukemia of B-cell type not having achieved remission
Prolymphocytic leukemia of B-cell type with failed remission
Prolymphocytic leukemia of B-cell type NOS

C91.31 Prolymphocytic leukemia of B-cell type, in remission

C91.32 Prolymphocytic leukemia of B-cell type, in relapse

● **C91.4 Hairy cell leukemia**
Chronic leukemia with splenomegaly and excessive number of abnormal large mononuclear cells covered by hairlike villi
Leukemic reticuloendotheliosis

C91.40 Hairy cell leukemia not having achieved remission
Hairy cell leukemia with failed remission
Hairy cell leukemia NOS

C91.41 Hairy cell leukemia, in remission

C91.42 Hairy cell leukemia, in relapse

Item 2–9 Leukemia is a cancer (acute or chronic) of the blood-forming tissues of the bone marrow. Blood cells all start out as stem cells. They mature and become red cells, white cells, or platelets. There are three main types of leukocytes (white cells that fight infection): monocytes, lymphocytes, and granulocytes. **Acute monocytic leukemia** (AML) affects monocytes. **Acute lymphoid leukemia** (ALL) affects lymphocytes, and **acute myeloid leukemia** (AML) affects cells that typically develop into white blood cells (not lymphocytes), though it may develop in other blood cells.

● **C91.5 Adult T-cell lymphoma/leukemia (HTLV-1-associated)**
Acute variant of adult T-cell lymphoma/leukemia (HTLV-1-associated)
Chronic variant of adult T-cell lymphoma/leukemia (HTLV-1-associated)
Lymphomatoid variant of adult T-cell lymphoma/leukemia (HTLV-1-associated)
Smouldering variant of adult T-cell lymphoma/leukemia (HTLV-1-associated)

C91.50 Adult T-cell lymphoma/leukemia (HTLV-1-associated) not having achieved remission
Adult T-cell lymphoma/leukemia (HTLV-1-associated) with failed remission
Adult T-cell lymphoma/leukemia (HTLV-1-associated) NOS

C91.51 Adult T-cell lymphoma/leukemia (HTLV-1-associated), in remission

C91.52 Adult T-cell lymphoma/leukemia (HTLV-1-associated), in relapse

● **C91.6 Prolymphocytic leukemia of T-cell type**

C91.60 Prolymphocytic leukemia of T-cell type not having achieved remission
Prolymphocytic leukemia of T-cell type with failed remission
Prolymphocytic leukemia of T-cell type NOS

C91.61 Prolymphocytic leukemia of T-cell type, in remission

C91.62 Prolymphocytic leukemia of T-cell type, in relapse

● **C91.A Mature B-cell leukemia Burkitt-type**
Excludes1 Burkitt lymphoma (C83.7-)

C91.A0 Mature B-cell leukemia Burkitt-type not having achieved remission
Mature B-cell leukemia Burkitt-type with failed remission
Mature B-cell leukemia Burkitt-type NOS

C91.A1 Mature B-cell leukemia Burkitt-type, in remission

C91.A2 Mature B-cell leukemia Burkitt-type, in relapse

● **C91.Z Other lymphoid leukemia**
T-cell large granular lymphocytic leukemia (associated with rheumatoid arthritis)

C91.Z0 Other lymphoid leukemia not having achieved remission
Other lymphoid leukemia with failed remission
Other lymphoid leukemia NOS

C91.Z1 Other lymphoid leukemia, in remission

C91.Z2 Other lymphoid leukemia, in relapse

● **C91.9 Lymphoid leukemia, unspecified**

C91.90 Lymphoid leukemia, unspecified not having achieved remission
Lymphoid leukemia with failed remission
Lymphoid leukemia NOS

C91.91 Lymphoid leukemia, unspecified, in remission

C91.92 Lymphoid leukemia, unspecified, in relapse

● **C92 Myeloid leukemia**

Includes granulocytic leukemia
myelogenous leukemia

Excludes1 personal history of leukemia (Z85.6)

● **C92.0 Acute myeloblastic leukemia**
Acute myeloblastic leukemia, minimal differentiation
Acute myeloblastic leukemia (with maturation)
Acute myeloblastic leukemia 1/ETO
Acute myeloblastic leukemia MØ
Acute myeloblastic leukemia M1
Acute myeloblastic leukemia M2
Acute myeloblastic leukemia with t(8;21)
Acute myeloblastic leukemia (without a FAB classification) NOS
Refractory anemia with excess blasts in transformation [RAEB T]

Excludes1 acute exacerbation of chronic myeloid leukemia (C92.10)
refractory anemia with excess of blasts not in transformation (D46.2-)

C92.00 Acute myeloblastic leukemia, not having achieved remission
Acute myeloblastic leukemia with failed remission
Acute myeloblastic leukemia NOS

C92.01 Acute myeloblastic leukemia, in remission

C92.02 Acute myeloblastic leukemia, in relapse

● **C92.1 Chronic myeloid leukemia, BCR/ABL-positive**
Chronic myelogenous leukemia, Philadelphia chromosome (Ph1) positive
Chronic myelogenous leukemia, t(9;22) (q34;q11)
Chronic myelogenous leukemia with crisis of blast cells

Excludes1 atypical chronic myeloid leukemia BCR/ABL-negative (C92.2-)
chronic myelomonocytic leukemia (C93.1-)
chronic myeloproliferative disease (D47.1)

C92.10 Chronic myeloid leukemia, BCR/ABL-positive, not having achieved remission
Chronic myeloid leukemia, BCR/ABL-positive with failed remission
Chronic myeloid leukemia, BCR/ABL-positive NOS

C92.11 Chronic myeloid leukemia, BCR/ABL-positive, in remission

C92.12 Chronic myeloid leukemia, BCR/ABL-positive, in relapse

● **C92.2 Atypical chronic myeloid leukemia, BCR/ABL-negative**

C92.20 Atypical chronic myeloid leukemia, BCR/ABL-negative, not having achieved remission
Atypical chronic myeloid leukemia, BCR/ABL-negative with failed remission
Atypical chronic myeloid leukemia, BCR/ABL-negative NOS

C92.21 Atypical chronic myeloid leukemia, BCR/ABL-negative, in remission

C92.22 Atypical chronic myeloid leukemia, BCR/ABL-negative, in relapse

● **C92.3 Myeloid sarcoma**
A malignant tumor of immature myeloid cells
Chloroma
Granulocytic sarcoma

C92.30 Myeloid sarcoma, not having achieved remission
Myeloid sarcoma with failed remission
Myeloid sarcoma NOS

C92.31 Myeloid sarcoma, in remission

C92.32 Myeloid sarcoma, in relapse

● **C92.4 Acute promyelocytic leukemia**
AML M3
AML Me with t(15;17) and variants

C92.40 Acute promyelocytic leukemia, not having achieved remission
Acute promyelocytic leukemia with failed remission
Acute promyelocytic leukemia NOS

C92.41 Acute promyelocytic leukemia, in remission

C92.42 Acute promyelocytic leukemia, in relapse

● **C92.5 Acute myelomonocytic leukemia**
AML M4
AML M4 Eo with inv(16) or t(16;16)

C92.50 Acute myelomonocytic leukemia, not having achieved remission
Acute myelomonocytic leukemia with failed remission
Acute myelomonocytic leukemia NOS

C92.51 Acute myelomonocytic leukemia, in remission

C92.52 Acute myelomonocytic leukemia, in relapse

● **C92.6 Acute myeloid leukemia with 11q23-abnormality**
Acute myeloid leukemia with variation of MLL-gene

C92.60 Acute myeloid leukemia with 11q23-abnormality not having achieved remission
Acute myeloid leukemia with 11q23-abnormality with failed remission
Acute myeloid leukemia with 11q23-abnormality NOS

C92.61 Acute myeloid leukemia with 11q23-abnormality in remission

C92.62 Acute myeloid leukemia with 11q23-abnormality in relapse

● **C92.A Acute myeloid leukemia with multilineage dysplasia**
Acute myeloid leukemia with dysplasia of remaining hematopoesis and/or myelodysplastic disease in its history

C92.A0 Acute myeloid leukemia with multilineage dysplasia, not having achieved remission
Acute myeloid leukemia with multilineage dysplasia with failed remission
Acute myeloid leukemia with multilineage dysplasia NOS

C92.A1 Acute myeloid leukemia with multilineage dysplasia, in remission

C92.A2 Acute myeloid leukemia with multilineage dysplasia, in relapse

● **C92.Z Other myeloid leukemia**

C92.Z0 Other myeloid leukemia not having achieved remission
Myeloid leukemia NEC with failed remission
Myeloid leukemia NEC

C92.Z1 Other myeloid leukemia, in remission

C92.Z2 Other myeloid leukemia, in relapse

● **C92.9 Myeloid leukemia, unspecified**

C92.90 Myeloid leukemia, unspecified, not having achieved remission
Myeloid leukemia, unspecified with failed remission
Myeloid leukemia, unspecified NOS

C92.91 Myeloid leukemia, unspecified in remission

C92.92 Myeloid leukemia, unspecified in relapse

CHAPTER 2 (C00-D49)

● **C93 Monocytic leukemia**

Includes monocytoid leukemia

Excludes1 personal history of leukemia (Z85.6)

● **C93.0 Acute monoblastic/monocytic leukemia**

AML M5
AML M5a
AML M5b

C93.00 Acute monoblastic/monocytic leukemia, not having achieved remission

Acute monoblastic/monocytic leukemia with failed remission
Acute monoblastic/monocytic leukemia NOS

C93.01 Acute monoblastic/monocytic leukemia, in remission

C93.02 Acute monoblastic/monocytic leukemia, in relapse

● **C93.1 Chronic myelomonocytic leukemia**

Chronic monocytic leukemia
CMML-1
CMML-2
CMML with eosinophilia

C93.10 Chronic myelomonocytic leukemia not having achieved remission

Chronic myelomonocytic leukemia with failed remission
Chronic myelomonocytic leukemia NOS

C93.11 Chronic myelomonocytic leukemia, in remission

C93.12 Chronic myelomonocytic leukemia, in relapse

● **C93.3 Juvenile myelomonocytic leukemia**

C93.30 Juvenile myelomonocytic leukemia, not having achieved remission

Juvenile myelomonocytic leukemia with failed remission
Juvenile myelomonocytic leukemia NOS

C93.31 Juvenile myelomonocytic leukemia, in remission

C93.32 Juvenile myelomonocytic leukemia, in relapse

● **C93.Z Other monocytic leukemia**

C93.Z0 Other monocytic leukemia, not having achieved remission

Other monocytic leukemia NOS

C93.Z1 Other monocytic leukemia, in remission

C93.Z2 Other monocytic leukemia, in relapse

● **C93.9 Monocytic leukemia, unspecified**

C93.90 Monocytic leukemia, unspecified, not having achieved remission

Monocytic leukemia, unspecified with failed remission
Monocytic leukemia, unspecified NOS

C93.91 Monocytic leukemia, unspecified in remission

C93.92 Monocytic leukemia, unspecified in relapse

● **C94 Other leukemias of specified cell type**

Excludes1 leukemic reticuloendotheliosis (C91.4-)
myelodysplastic syndromes (D46.-)
personal history of leukemia (Z85.6)
plasma cell leukemia (C90.1-)

● **C94.0 Acute erythroid leukemia**

Acute myeloid leukemia M6(a)(b)
Erythroleukemia

C94.00 Acute erythroid leukemia, not having achieved remission

Acute erythroid leukemia with failed remission
Acute erythroid leukemia NOS

C94.01 Acute erythroid leukemia, in remission

C94.02 Acute erythroid leukemia, in relapse

● **C94.2 Acute megakaryoblastic leukemia**

Acute myeloid leukemia M7
Acute megakaryocytic leukemia

C94.20 Acute megakaryoblastic leukemia not having achieved remission

Acute megakaryoblastic leukemia with failed remission ◀
Acute megakaryoblastic leukemia NOS

C94.21 Acute megakaryoblastic leukemia, in remission

C94.22 Acute megakaryoblastic leukemia, in relapse

● **C94.3 Mast cell leukemia**

C94.30 Mast cell leukemia not having achieved remission

Mast cell leukemia with failed remission
Mast cell leukemia NOS

C94.31 Mast cell leukemia, in remission

C94.32 Mast cell leukemia, in relapse

● **C94.4 Acute panmyelosis with myelofibrosis**

Acute myelofibrosis

Excludes1 myelofibrosis NOS (D75.81)
secondary myelofibrosis NOS (D75.81)

C94.40 Acute panmyelosis with myelofibrosis not having achieved remission

Acute myelofibrosis NOS
Acute panmyelosis with myelofibrosis with failed remission
Acute panmyelosis NOS

C94.41 Acute panmyelosis with myelofibrosis, in remission

C94.42 Acute panmyelosis with myelofibrosis, in relapse

C94.6 Myelodysplastic disease, not classified

Myeloproliferative disease, not classified

● **C94.8 Other specified leukemias**

Aggressive NK-cell leukemia
Acute basophilic leukemia

C94.80 Other specified leukemias not having achieved remission

Other specified leukemia with failed remission
Other specified leukemias NOS

C94.81 Other specified leukemias, in remission

C94.82 Other specified leukemias, in relapse

● **C95 Leukemia of unspecified cell type**

Excludes1 personal history of leukemia (Z85.6)

● **C95.0 Acute leukemia of unspecified cell type**

Acute bilineal leukemia
Acute mixed lineage leukemia
Biphenotypic acute leukemia
Stem cell leukemia of unclear lineage

Excludes1 acute exacerbation of unspecified chronic leukemia (C95.10)

C95.00 Acute leukemia of unspecified cell type not having achieved remission

Acute leukemia of unspecified cell type with failed remission
Acute leukemia NOS

C95.01 Acute leukemia of unspecified cell type, in remission

C95.02 Acute leukemia of unspecified cell type, in relapse

● **C95.1 Chronic leukemia of unspecified cell type**

C95.10 Chronic leukemia of unspecified cell type not having achieved remission

Chronic leukemia of unspecified cell type with failed remission
Chronic leukemia NOS

C95.11 Chronic leukemia of unspecified cell type, in remission

C95.12 Chronic leukemia of unspecified cell type, in relapse

● C95.9 **Leukemia, unspecified**

C95.90 **Leukemia, unspecified not having achieved remission**
Leukemia, unspecified with failed remission
Leukemia NOS

C95.91 **Leukemia, unspecified, in remission**

C95.92 **Leukemia, unspecified, in relapse**

● C96 **Other and unspecified malignant neoplasms of lymphoid, hematopoietic and related tissue**
Excludes1 personal history of other malignant neoplasms of lymphoid, hematopoietic and related tissues (Z85.79)

C96.0 **Multifocal and multisystemic (disseminated) Langerhans-cell histiocytosis**
Histiocytosis X, multisystemic
Letterer-Siwe disease
Excludes1 adult pulmonary Langerhans cell histiocytosis (J84.82)
multifocal and unisystemic Langerhans-cell histiocytosis (C96.5)
unifocal Langerhans-cell histiocytosis (C96.6)

C96.2 **Malignant mast cell tumor**
Aggressive systemic mastocytosis
Mast cell sarcoma
Excludes1 indolent mastocytosis (D47.0)
mast cell leukemia (C94.30)
mastocytosis (congenital) (cutaneous) (Q82.2)

C96.4 **Sarcoma of dendritic cells (accessory cells)**
Follicular dendritic cell sarcoma
Interdigitating dendritic cell sarcoma
Langerhans cell sarcoma

C96.5 **Multifocal and unisystemic Langerhans-cell histiocytosis**
Hand-Schüller-Christian disease
Histiocytosis X, multifocal
Excludes1 multifocal and multisystemic (disseminated) Langerhans-cell histiocytosis (C96.0)
unifocal Langerhans-cell histiocytosis (C96.6)

C96.6 **Unifocal Langerhans-cell histiocytosis**
Eosinophilic granuloma
Histiocytosis X, unifocal
Histiocytosis X NOS
Langerhans-cell histiocytosis NOS
Excludes1 multifocal and multisysemic (disseminated) Langerhans-cell histiocytosis (C96.0)
multifocal and unisystemic Langerhans-cell histiocytosis (C96.5)

C96.A **Histiocytic sarcoma**
Malignant histiocytosis

C96.Z **Other specified malignant neoplasms of lymphoid, hematopoietic and related tissue**

C96.9 **Malignant neoplasm of lymphoid, hematopoietic and related tissue, unspecified**

IN SITU NEOPLASMS (D00-D09)

In situ is carcinoma involving cells in localized tissues that has not spread to nearby tissues

Includes Bowen's disease
erythroplasia
grade III intraepithelial neoplasia
Queyrat's erythroplasia

● D00 **Carcinoma in situ of oral cavity, esophagus and stomach**
Excludes1 melanoma in situ (D03.-)

● D00.0 **Carcinoma in situ of lip, oral cavity and pharynx**
Use additional code to identify:
exposure to environmental tobacco smoke (Z77.22)
exposure to tobacco smoke in the perinatal period (P96.81)
history of tobacco dependence (Z87.891) ⬅
occupational exposure to environmental tobacco smoke (Z57.31)
tobacco dependence (F17.-)
tobacco use (Z72.0)
Excludes1 carcinoma in situ of aryepiglottic fold or interarytenoid fold, laryngeal aspect (D02.0)
carcinoma in situ of epiglottis NOS (D02.0)
carcinoma in situ of epiglottis suprahyoid portion (D02.0)
carcinoma in situ of skin of lip (D03.0, D04.0)

D00.00 **Carcinoma in situ of oral cavity, unspecified site**

D00.01 **Carcinoma in situ of labial mucosa and vermilion border**

D00.02 **Carcinoma in situ of buccal mucosa**

D00.03 **Carcinoma in situ of gingiva and edentulous alveolar ridge**

D00.04 **Carcinoma in situ of soft palate**

D00.05 **Carcinoma in situ of hard palate**

D00.06 **Carcinoma in situ of floor of mouth**

D00.07 **Carcinoma in situ of tongue**

D00.08 **Carcinoma in situ of pharynx**
Carcinoma in situ of aryepiglottic fold NOS
Carcinoma in situ of hypopharyngeal aspect of aryepiglottic fold
Carcinoma in situ of marginal zone of aryepiglottic fold

D00.1 **Carcinoma in situ of esophagus**

D00.2 **Carcinoma in situ of stomach**

● D01 **Carcinoma in situ of other and unspecified digestive organs**
Excludes1 melanoma in situ (D03.-)

D01.0 **Carcinoma in situ of colon**
Excludes1 carcinoma in situ of rectosigmoid junction (D01.1)

D01.1 **Carcinoma in situ of rectosigmoid junction**

D01.2 **Carcinoma in situ of rectum**

D01.3 **Carcinoma in situ of anus and anal canal**
Anal intraepithelial neoplasia III [AIN III] ◀
Severe dysplasia of anus ◀
Excludes1 anal intraepithelial neoplasia I and II [AIN I and AIN II] (K62.82) ◀
carcinoma in situ of anal margin (D04.5)
carcinoma in situ of anal skin (D04.5)
carcinoma in situ of perianal skin (D04.5)

● D01.4 **Carcinoma in situ of other and unspecified parts of intestine**
Excludes1 carcinoma in situ of ampulla of Vater (D01.5)

D01.40 **Carcinoma in situ of unspecified part of intestine**

D01.49 **Carcinoma in situ of other parts of intestine**

D01.5 Carcinoma in situ of liver, gallbladder and bile ducts
Carcinoma in situ of ampulla of Vater

D01.7 Carcinoma in situ of other specified digestive organs
Carcinoma in situ of pancreas

D01.9 Carcinoma in situ of digestive organ, unspecified

● **D02 Carcinoma in situ of middle ear and respiratory system**
Use additional code to identify:
- exposure to environmental tobacco smoke (Z77.22)
- exposure to tobacco smoke in the perinatal period (P96.81)
- history of tobacco dependence (Z87.891) ◄
- occupational exposure to environmental tobacco smoke (Z57.31)
- tobacco dependence (F17.-)
- tobacco use (Z72.0)

Excludes1 melanoma in situ (D03.-)

D02.0 Carcinoma in situ of larynx
Carcinoma in situ of aryepiglottic fold or interarytenoid fold, laryngeal aspect
Carcinoma in situ of epiglottis (suprahyoid portion)
Excludes1 carcinoma in situ of aryepiglottic fold or interarytenoid fold NOS (D00.08)
carcinoma in situ of hypopharyngeal aspect (D00.08)
carcinoma in situ of marginal zone (D00.08)

D02.1 Carcinoma in situ of trachea

● **D02.2 Carcinoma in situ of bronchus and lung**
D02.20 Carcinoma in situ of unspecified bronchus and lung
D02.21 Carcinoma in situ of right bronchus and lung
D02.22 Carcinoma in situ of left bronchus and lung

D02.3 Carcinoma in situ of other parts of respiratory system
Carcinoma in situ of accessory sinuses
Carcinoma in situ of middle ear
Carcinoma in situ of nasal cavities
Excludes1 carcinoma in situ of ear (external) (skin) (D04.2-)
carcinoma in situ of nose NOS (D09.8)
carcinoma in situ of skin of nose (D04.3)

D02.4 Carcinoma in situ of respiratory system, unspecified

● **D03 Melanoma in situ**

D03.0 Melanoma in situ of lip

● **D03.1 Melanoma in situ of eyelid, including canthus**
D03.10 Melanoma in situ of unspecified eyelid, including canthus
D03.11 Melanoma in situ of right eyelid, including canthus
D03.12 Melanoma in situ of left eyelid, including canthus

● **D03.2 Melanoma in situ of ear and external auricular canal**
D03.20 Melanoma in situ of unspecified ear and external auricular canal
D03.21 Melanoma in situ of right ear and external auricular canal
D03.22 Melanoma in situ of left ear and external auricular canal

● **D03.3 Melanoma in situ of other and unspecified parts of face**
D03.30 Melanoma in situ of unspecified part of face
D03.39 Melanoma in situ of other parts of face

D03.4 Melanoma in situ of scalp and neck

● **D03.5 Melanoma in situ of trunk**
D03.51 Melanoma in situ of anal skin
Melanoma in situ of anal margin
Melanoma in situ of perianal skin
D03.52 Melanoma in situ of breast (skin) (soft tissue)
D03.59 Melanoma in situ of other part of trunk

● **D03.6 Melanoma in situ of upper limb, including shoulder**
D03.60 Melanoma in situ of unspecified upper limb, including shoulder
D03.61 Melanoma in situ of right upper limb, including shoulder
D03.62 Melanoma in situ of left upper limb, including shoulder

● **D03.7 Melanoma in situ of lower limb, including hip**
D03.70 Melanoma in situ of unspecified lower limb, including hip
D03.71 Melanoma in situ of right lower limb, including hip
D03.72 Melanoma in situ of left lower limb, including hip

D03.8 Melanoma in situ of other sites
Melanoma in situ of scrotum
Excludes1 carcinoma in situ of scrotum (D07.61)

D03.9 Melanoma in situ, unspecified

● **D04 Carcinoma in situ of skin**
Excludes1 erythroplasia of Queyrat (penis) NOS (D07.4)
melanoma in situ (D03.-)

D04.0 Carcinoma in situ of skin of lip
Excludes1 carcinoma in situ of vermilion border of lip (D00.01)

● **D04.1 Carcinoma in situ of skin of eyelid, including canthus**
D04.10 Carcinoma in situ of skin of unspecified eyelid, including canthus
D04.11 Carcinoma in situ of skin of right eyelid, including canthus
D04.12 Carcinoma in situ of skin of left eyelid, including canthus

● **D04.2 Carcinoma in situ of skin of ear and external auricular canal**
D04.20 Carcinoma in situ of skin of unspecified ear and external auricular canal
D04.21 Carcinoma in situ of skin of right ear and external auricular canal
D04.22 Carcinoma in situ of skin of left ear and external auricular canal

● **D04.3 Carcinoma in situ of skin of other and unspecified parts of face**
D04.30 Carcinoma in situ of skin of unspecified part of face
D04.39 Carcinoma in situ of skin of other parts of face

D04.4 Carcinoma in situ of skin of scalp and neck

D04.5 Carcinoma in situ of skin of trunk
Carcinoma in situ of anal margin
Carcinoma in situ of anal skin
Carcinoma in situ of perianal skin
Carcinoma in situ of skin of breast
Excludes1 carcinoma in situ of anus NOS (D01.3)
carcinoma in situ of scrotum (D07.61)
carcinoma in situ of skin of genital organs (D07.-)

● **D04.6 Carcinoma in situ of skin of upper limb, including shoulder**
D04.60 Carcinoma in situ of skin of unspecified upper limb, including shoulder
D04.61 Carcinoma in situ of skin of right upper limb, including shoulder
D04.62 Carcinoma in situ of skin of left upper limb, including shoulder

CHAPTER 2 (C00-D49)

◄ New ◄ Revised ~~deleted~~ Deleted OGCR Official Guidelines X Assign placeholder X ● Use Additional Character(s)
Excludes 1 Excludes 2 Includes Use additional Code first Code also Unspecified

● **D04.7 Carcinoma in situ of skin of lower limb, including hip**
- **D04.70 Carcinoma in situ of skin of unspecified lower limb, including hip**
- **D04.71 Carcinoma in situ of skin of right lower limb, including hip**
- **D04.72 Carcinoma in situ of skin of left lower limb, including hip**

D04.8 Carcinoma in situ of skin of other sites

D04.9 Carcinoma in situ of skin, unspecified

● **D05 Carcinoma in situ of breast**

Excludes1 carcinoma in situ of skin of breast (D04.5)
melanoma in situ of breast (skin) (D03.5)
Paget's disease of breast or nipple (C50.-)

● **D05.0 Lobular carcinoma in situ of breast**
- **D05.00 Lobular carcinoma in situ of unspecified breast**
- **D05.01 Lobular carcinoma in situ of right breast**
- **D05.02 Lobular carcinoma in situ of left breast**

● **D05.1 Intraductal carcinoma in situ of breast**
- **D05.10 Intraductal carcinoma in situ of unspecified breast**
- **D05.11 Intraductal carcinoma in situ of right breast**
- **D05.12 Intraductal carcinoma in situ of left breast**

● **D05.8 Other specified type of carcinoma in situ of breast**
- **D05.80 Other specified type of carcinoma in situ of unspecified breast**
- **D05.81 Other specified type of carcinoma in situ of right breast**
- **D05.82 Other specified type of carcinoma in situ of left breast**

● **D05.9 Unspecified type of carcinoma in situ of breast**
- **D05.90 Unspecified type of carcinoma in situ of unspecified breast**
- **D05.91 Unspecified type of carcinoma in situ of right breast**
- **D05.92 Unspecified type of carcinoma in situ of left breast**

● **D06 Carcinoma in situ of cervix uteri**

Includes cervical adenocarcinoma in situ
cervical intraepithelial glandular neoplasia
cervical intraepithelial neoplasia III [CIN III]
severe dysplasia of cervix uteri

Excludes1 cervical intraepithelial neoplasia II [CIN II] (N87.1)
cytologic evidence of malignancy of cervix without histologic confirmation (R87.614)
high grade squamous intraepithelial lesion (HGSIL) of cervix (R87.613)
melanoma in situ of cervix (D03.5)
moderate cervical dysplasia (N87.1)

D06.0 Carcinoma in situ of endocervix

D06.1 Carcinoma in situ of exocervix

D06.7 Carcinoma in situ of other parts of cervix

D06.9 Carcinoma in situ of cervix, unspecified

● **D07 Carcinoma in situ of other and unspecified genital organs**

Excludes1 melanoma in situ of trunk (D03.5)

D07.0 Carcinoma in situ of endometrium

D07.1 Carcinoma in situ of vulva
Severe dysplasia of vulva
Vulvar intraepithelial neoplasia III [VIN III]
Excludes1 moderate dysplasia of vulva (N90.1)
vulvar intraepithelial neoplasia II [VIN II] (N90.1)

D07.2 Carcinoma in situ of vagina
Severe dysplasia of vagina
Vaginal intraepithelial neoplasia III [VIN III]
Excludes1 moderate dysplasia of vagina (N89.1)
vaginal intraepithelial neoplasia II [VIN II] (N89.1)

● **D07.3 Carcinoma in situ of other and unspecified female genital organs**
- **D07.30 Carcinoma in situ of unspecified female genital organs**
- **D07.39 Carcinoma in situ of other female genital organs**

D07.4 Carcinoma in situ of penis
Erythroplasia of Queyrat NOS

D07.5 Carcinoma in situ of prostate
Prostatic intraepithelial neoplasia III (PIN III)
Severe dysplasia of prostate
Excludes1 dysplasia (mild) (moderate) of prostate (N42.3-) ⟸
prostatic intraepithelial neoplasia II [PIN II] (N42.3-) ◀

● **D07.6 Carcinoma in situ of other and unspecified male genital organs**
- **D07.60 Carcinoma in situ of unspecified male genital organs**
- **D07.61 Carcinoma in situ of scrotum**
- **D07.69 Carcinoma in situ of other male genital organs**

● **D09 Carcinoma in situ of other and unspecified sites**

Excludes1 melanoma in situ (D03.-)

D09.0 Carcinoma in situ of bladder

● **D09.1 Carcinoma in situ of other and unspecified urinary organs**
- **D09.10 Carcinoma in situ of unspecified urinary organ**
- **D09.19 Carcinoma in situ of other urinary organs**

● **D09.2 Carcinoma in situ of eye**
Excludes1 carcinoma in situ of skin of eyelid (D04.1-)
- **D09.20 Carcinoma in situ of unspecified eye**
- **D09.21 Carcinoma in situ of right eye**
- **D09.22 Carcinoma in situ of left eye**

D09.3 Carcinoma in situ of thyroid and other endocrine glands
Excludes1 carcinoma in situ of endocrine pancreas (D01.7)
carcinoma in situ of ovary (D07.39)
carcinoma in situ of testis (D07.69)

D09.8 Carcinoma in situ of other specified sites

D09.9 Carcinoma in situ, unspecified

BENIGN NEOPLASMS, EXCEPT BENIGN NEUROENDOCRINE TUMORS (D10-D36)

● **D10 Benign neoplasm of mouth and pharynx**

D10.0 Benign neoplasm of lip
Benign neoplasm of lip (frenulum) (inner aspect) (mucosa) (vermilion border)
Excludes1 benign neoplasm of skin of lip (D22.0, D23.0)

D10.1 Benign neoplasm of tongue
Benign neoplasm of lingual tonsil

D10.2 Benign neoplasm of floor of mouth

● **D10.3 Benign neoplasm of other and unspecified parts of mouth** ⟸
- **D10.30 Benign neoplasm of unspecified part of mouth**
- **D10.39 Benign neoplasm of other parts of mouth**
  Benign neoplasm of minor salivary gland NOS
  Excludes1 benign odontogenic neoplasms (D16.4-D16.5)
  benign neoplasm of mucosa of lip (D10.0)
  benign neoplasm of nasopharyngeal surface of soft palate (D10.6)

◀ New ⟸ Revised ~~deleted~~ Deleted OGCR Official Guidelines X Assign placeholder X ● Use Additional Character(s)
Excludes 1 | Excludes 2 | Includes | Use additional | Code first | Code also | Unspecified

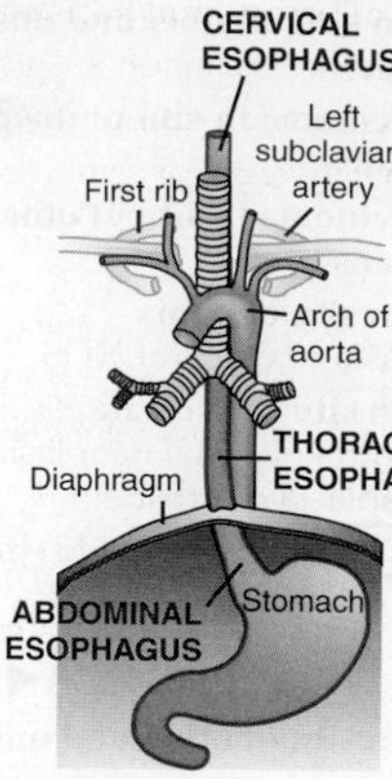

Figure 2-16 The esophagus is the muscular tube that connects the pharynx and the stomach. The 10 inch (25 cm) long esophagus is divided into three parts: **cervical, thoracic,** and **abdominal.**

D10.4 Benign neoplasm of tonsil
Benign neoplasm of tonsil (faucial) (palatine)
Excludes1 benign neoplasm of lingual tonsil (D10.1)
benign neoplasm of pharyngeal tonsil (D10.6)
benign neoplasm of tonsillar fossa (D10.5)
benign neoplasm of tonsillar pillars (D10.5)

D10.5 Benign neoplasm of other parts of oropharynx
Division of pharynx lying between soft palate and upper edge of epiglottis
Benign neoplasm of epiglottis, anterior aspect
Benign neoplasm of tonsillar fossa
Benign neoplasm of tonsillar pillars
Benign neoplasm of vallecula
Excludes1 benign neoplasm of epiglottis NOS (D14.1)
benign neoplasm of epiglottis, suprahyoid portion (D14.1)

D10.6 Benign neoplasm of nasopharynx
Segment of pharynx that lies above soft palate
Benign neoplasm of pharyngeal tonsil
Benign neoplasm of posterior margin of septum and choanae

D10.7 Benign neoplasm of hypopharynx
Segment of pharynx that lies below upper edge of epiglottis and opens into larynx and esophagus

D10.9 Benign neoplasm of pharynx, unspecified

● **D11 Benign neoplasm of major salivary glands**
Excludes1 benign neoplasms of specified minor salivary glands which are classified according to their anatomical location
benign neoplasms of minor salivary glands NOS (D10.39)

D11.0 Benign neoplasm of parotid gland

D11.7 Benign neoplasm of other major salivary glands
Benign neoplasm of sublingual salivary gland
Benign neoplasm of submandibular salivary gland

D11.9 Benign neoplasm of major salivary gland, unspecified

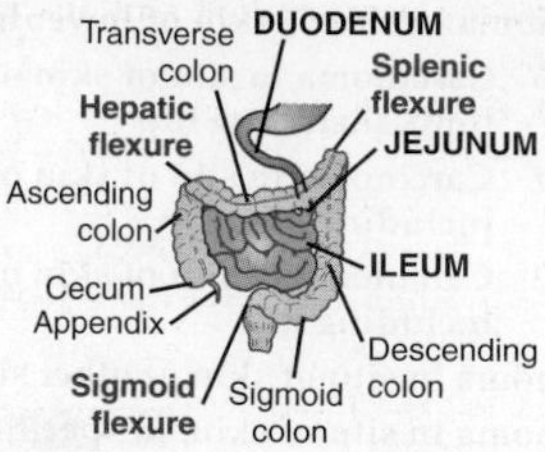

Figure 2-17 Small intestine and colon.

● **D12 Benign neoplasm of colon, rectum, anus and anal canal**
Excludes1 benign carcinoid tumors of the large intestine, and rectum (D3A.02-)

D12.0 Benign neoplasm of cecum
Benign neoplasm of ileocecal valve

D12.1 Benign neoplasm of appendix
Excludes1 benign carcinoid tumor of the appendix (D3A.020)

D12.2 Benign neoplasm of ascending colon

D12.3 Benign neoplasm of transverse colon
Benign neoplasm of hepatic flexure
Benign neoplasm of splenic flexure
Flexure is a bending in a structure or organ. Note the three flexures illustrated in Figure 2–17. Hepatic = liver, sigmoid = colon, splenic = spleen.

D12.4 Benign neoplasm of descending colon

D12.5 Benign neoplasm of sigmoid colon

D12.6 Benign neoplasm of colon, unspecified
Adenomatosis of colon
Benign neoplasm of large intestine NOS
Polyposis (hereditary) of colon
Excludes1 inflammatory polyp of colon (K51.4-)
polyp of colon NOS (K63.5)

D12.7 Benign neoplasm of rectosigmoid junction
Angle where sigmoid colon becomes rectum

D12.8 Benign neoplasm of rectum
Excludes1 benign carcinoid tumor of the rectum (D3A.026)

D12.9 Benign neoplasm of anus and anal canal
Benign neoplasm of anus NOS
Excludes1 benign neoplasm of anal margin (D22.5, D23.5)
benign neoplasm of anal skin (D22.5, D23.5)
benign neoplasm of perianal skin (D22.5, D23.5)

● **D13 Benign neoplasm of other and ill-defined parts of digestive system**
Excludes1 benign stromal tumors of digestive system (D21.4)

D13.0 Benign neoplasm of esophagus

D13.1 Benign neoplasm of stomach
Excludes1 benign carcinoid tumor of the stomach (D3A.092)

D13.2 Benign neoplasm of duodenum
Excludes1 benign carcinoid tumor of the duodenum (D3A.010)

● **D13.3 Benign neoplasm of other and unspecified parts of small intestine**
Excludes1 benign carcinoid tumors of the small intestine (D3A.01-)
benign neoplasm of ileocecal valve (D12.0)
D13.30 Benign neoplasm of unspecified part of small intestine
D13.39 Benign neoplasm of other parts of small intestine
D13.4 Benign neoplasm of liver
Benign neoplasm of intrahepatic bile ducts
D13.5 Benign neoplasm of extrahepatic bile ducts
Extensions of common hepatic bile duct (tube that collects bile from liver)
D13.6 Benign neoplasm of pancreas
Excludes1 benign neoplasm of endocrine pancreas (D13.7)
D13.7 Benign neoplasm of endocrine pancreas
Pancreatic islets: Cells scattered throughout pancreas
Islet cell tumor
Benign neoplasm of islets of Langerhans
Use additional code to identify any functional activity.
D13.9 Benign neoplasm of ill-defined sites within the digestive system
Benign neoplasm of digestive system NOS
Benign neoplasm of intestine NOS
Benign neoplasm of spleen

● **D14 Benign neoplasm of middle ear and respiratory system**
D14.0 Benign neoplasm of middle ear, nasal cavity and accessory sinuses
Benign neoplasm of cartilage of nose
Excludes1 benign neoplasm of auricular canal (external) (D22.2-, D23.2-)
benign neoplasm of bone of ear (D16.4)
benign neoplasm of bone of nose (D16.4)
benign neoplasm of cartilage of ear (D21.0)
benign neoplasm of ear (external) (skin) (D22.2-, D23.2-)
benign neoplasm of nose NOS (D36.7)
benign neoplasm of skin of nose (D22.39, D23.39)
benign neoplasm of olfactory bulb (D33.3)
benign neoplasm of posterior margin of septum and choanae (D10.6)
polyp of accessory sinus (J33.8)
polyp of ear (middle) (H74.4)
polyp of nasal (cavity) (J33.-)
D14.1 Benign neoplasm of larynx
Adenomatous polyp of larynx
Benign neoplasm of epiglottis (suprahyoid portion)
Horseshoe shaped bone in anterior midline of neck between chin and thyroid cartilage
Excludes1 benign neoplasm of epiglottis, anterior aspect (D10.5)
polyp (nonadenomatous) of vocal cord or larynx (J38.1)
D14.2 Benign neoplasm of trachea
● **D14.3 Benign neoplasm of bronchus and lung**
Excludes1 benign carcinoid tumor of the bronchus and lung (D3A.090)
D14.30 Benign neoplasm of unspecified bronchus and lung
D14.31 Benign neoplasm of right bronchus and lung
D14.32 Benign neoplasm of left bronchus and lung
D14.4 Benign neoplasm of respiratory system, unspecified

● **D15 Benign neoplasm of other and unspecified intrathoracic organs**
Excludes1 benign neoplasm of mesothelial tissue (D19.-)
D15.0 Benign neoplasm of thymus
Excludes1 benign carcinoid tumor of the thymus (D3A.091)
D15.1 Benign neoplasm of heart
Excludes1 benign neoplasm of great vessels (D21.3)
D15.2 Benign neoplasm of mediastinum
D15.7 Benign neoplasm of other specified intrathoracic organs
D15.9 Benign neoplasm of intrathoracic organ, unspecified

● **D16 Benign neoplasm of bone and articular cartilage**
Excludes1 benign neoplasm of connective tissue of ear (D21.0)
benign neoplasm of connective tissue of eyelid (D21.0)
benign neoplasm of connective tissue of larynx (D14.1)
benign neoplasm of connective tissue of nose (D14.0)
benign neoplasm of synovia (D21.-)
● **D16.0 Benign neoplasm of scapula and long bones of upper limb**
D16.00 Benign neoplasm of scapula and long bones of unspecified upper limb
D16.01 Benign neoplasm of scapula and long bones of right upper limb
D16.02 Benign neoplasm of scapula and long bones of left upper limb
● **D16.1 Benign neoplasm of short bones of upper limb**
D16.10 Benign neoplasm of short bones of unspecified upper limb
D16.11 Benign neoplasm of short bones of right upper limb
D16.12 Benign neoplasm of short bones of left upper limb
● **D16.2 Benign neoplasm of long bones of lower limb**
D16.20 Benign neoplasm of long bones of unspecified lower limb
D16.21 Benign neoplasm of long bones of right lower limb
D16.22 Benign neoplasm of long bones of left lower limb
● **D16.3 Benign neoplasm of short bones of lower limb**
D16.30 Benign neoplasm of short bones of unspecified lower limb
D16.31 Benign neoplasm of short bones of right lower limb
D16.32 Benign neoplasm of short bones of left lower limb
D16.4 Benign neoplasm of bones of skull and face
Benign neoplasm of maxilla (superior)
Benign neoplasm of orbital bone
Cavity or socket of skull in which eye and its appendages are located
Keratocyst of maxilla
Keratocystic odontogenic tumor of maxilla
Excludes2 benign neoplasm of lower jaw bone (D16.5) ◄
D16.5 Benign neoplasm of lower jaw bone
Keratocyst of mandible
Keratocystic odontogenic tumor of mandible
D16.6 Benign neoplasm of vertebral column
Excludes1 benign neoplasm of sacrum and coccyx (D16.8)
D16.7 Benign neoplasm of ribs, sternum and clavicle
D16.8 Benign neoplasm of pelvic bones, sacrum and coccyx
D16.9 Benign neoplasm of bone and articular cartilage, unspecified

CHAPTER 2 (C00-D49)

● **D17 Benign lipomatous neoplasm**
Slow-growing benign tumors (rubbery masses) of mature fat cells enclosed in a thin fibrous capsule

D17.0 Benign lipomatous neoplasm of skin and subcutaneous tissue of head, face and neck

D17.1 Benign lipomatous neoplasm of skin and subcutaneous tissue of trunk

● **D17.2 Benign lipomatous neoplasm of skin and subcutaneous tissue of limb**

D17.20 Benign lipomatous neoplasm of skin and subcutaneous tissue of unspecified limb

D17.21 Benign lipomatous neoplasm of skin and subcutaneous tissue of right arm

D17.22 Benign lipomatous neoplasm of skin and subcutaneous tissue of left arm

D17.23 Benign lipomatous neoplasm of skin and subcutaneous tissue of right leg

D17.24 Benign lipomatous neoplasm of skin and subcutaneous tissue of left leg

● **D17.3 Benign lipomatous neoplasm of skin and subcutaneous tissue of other and unspecified sites**

D17.30 Benign lipomatous neoplasm of skin and subcutaneous tissue of unspecified sites

D17.39 Benign lipomatous neoplasm of skin and subcutaneous tissue of other sites

D17.4 Benign lipomatous neoplasm of intrathoracic organs

D17.5 Benign lipomatous neoplasm of intra-abdominal organs

Excludes1 benign lipomatous neoplasm of peritoneum and retroperitoneum (D17.79)

D17.6 Benign lipomatous neoplasm of spermatic cord

● **D17.7 Benign lipomatous neoplasm of other sites**

D17.71 Benign lipomatous neoplasm of kidney

D17.72 Benign lipomatous neoplasm of other genitourinary organ

D17.79 Benign lipomatous neoplasm of other sites
Benign lipomatous neoplasm of peritoneum
Benign lipomatous neoplasm of retroperitoneum

D17.9 Benign lipomatous neoplasm, unspecified
Lipoma NOS

● **D18 Hemangioma and lymphangioma, any site**

Excludes1 benign neoplasm of glomus jugulare (D35.6)
blue or pigmented nevus (D22.-)
nevus NOS (D22.-)
vascular nevus (Q82.5)

● **D18.0 Hemangioma**
Common type of vascular malformation
Angioma NOS
Cavernous nevus

D18.00 Hemangioma unspecified site

D18.01 Hemangioma of skin and subcutaneous tissue

D18.02 Hemangioma of intracranial structures

D18.03 Hemangioma of intra-abdominal structures

D18.09 Hemangioma of other sites

D18.1 Lymphangioma, any site

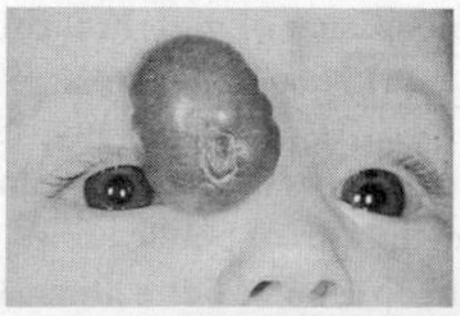

Figure 2-18 Hemangioma of skin and subcutaneous tissue. (From Yanoff: Ophthalmology, ed 3, Mosby, Inc., 2008)

Item 2-10 Hemangiomas are abnormally dense collections of dilated capillaries that occur on the skin or in internal organs. Hemangiomas are both deep and superficial and undergo a rapid growth phase when the size increases rapidly, followed by a rest phase, in which the tumor changes very little, followed by an involutional phase in which the tumor begins to and can disappear altogether. **Lymphangiomas** or cystic hygroma are benign collections of overgrown lymph vessels and, although rare, may occur anywhere but most commonly on the head and neck of children and infants. Visceral organs, lungs, and gastrointestinal tract may also be involved.

● **D19 Benign neoplasm of mesothelial tissue**
Mesothelial tissue is the membrane lining several body cavities

D19.0 Benign neoplasm of mesothelial tissue of pleura

D19.1 Benign neoplasm of mesothelial tissue of peritoneum

D19.7 Benign neoplasm of mesothelial tissue of other sites

D19.9 Benign neoplasm of mesothelial tissue, unspecified
Benign mesothelioma NOS

● **D20 Benign neoplasm of soft tissue of retroperitoneum and peritoneum**

Excludes1 benign lipomatous neoplasm of peritoneum and retroperitoneum (D17.79)
benign neoplasm of mesothelial tissue (D19.-)

D20.0 Benign neoplasm of soft tissue of retroperitoneum

D20.1 Benign neoplasm of soft tissue of peritoneum

● **D21 Other benign neoplasms of connective and other soft tissue**

Includes benign neoplasm of blood vessel
benign neoplasm of bursa
benign neoplasm of cartilage
benign neoplasm of fascia
benign neoplasm of fat
benign neoplasm of ligament, except uterine
benign neoplasm of lymphatic channel
benign neoplasm of muscle
benign neoplasm of synovia
benign neoplasm of tendon (sheath)
benign stromal tumors

Excludes1 benign neoplasm of articular cartilage (D16.-)
benign neoplasm of cartilage of larynx (D14.1)
benign neoplasm of cartilage of nose (D14.0)
benign neoplasm of connective tissue of breast (D24.-)
benign neoplasm of peripheral nerves and autonomic nervous system (D36.1-)
benign neoplasm of peritoneum (D20.1)
benign neoplasm of retroperitoneum (D20.0)
benign neoplasm of uterine ligament, any (D28.2)
benign neoplasm of vascular tissue (D18.-)
hemangioma (D18.0-)
lipomatous neoplasm (D17.-)
lymphangioma (D18.1)
uterine leiomyoma (D25.-)

D21.0 Benign neoplasm of connective and other soft tissue of head, face and neck
Benign neoplasm of connective tissue of ear
Benign neoplasm of connective tissue of eyelid

Excludes1 benign neoplasm of connective tissue of orbit (D31.6-)

● **D21.1 Benign neoplasm of connective and other soft tissue of upper limb, including shoulder**

D21.10 Benign neoplasm of connective and other soft tissue of unspecified upper limb, including shoulder

D21.11 Benign neoplasm of connective and other soft tissue of right upper limb, including shoulder

D21.12 Benign neoplasm of connective and other soft tissue of left upper limb, including shoulder

● **D21.2 Benign neoplasm of connective and other soft tissue of lower limb, including hip**
  - **D21.20 Benign neoplasm of connective and other soft tissue of unspecified lower limb, including hip**
  - **D21.21 Benign neoplasm of connective and other soft tissue of right lower limb, including hip**
  - **D21.22 Benign neoplasm of connective and other soft tissue of left lower limb, including hip**

D21.3 Benign neoplasm of connective and other soft tissue of thorax
Benign neoplasm of axilla
Benign neoplasm of diaphragm
Benign neoplasm of great vessels
Excludes1 benign neoplasm of heart (D15.1)
benign neoplasm of mediastinum (D15.2)
benign neoplasm of thymus (D15.0)

D21.4 Benign neoplasm of connective and other soft tissue of abdomen Benign stromal tumors of abdomen

D21.5 Benign neoplasm of connective and other soft tissue of pelvis
Excludes1 benign neoplasm of any uterine ligament (D28.2)
uterine leiomyoma (D25.-)

D21.6 Benign neoplasm of connective and other soft tissue of trunk, unspecified
Benign neoplasm of back NOS

D21.9 Benign neoplasm of connective and other soft tissue, unspecified

● **D22 Melanocytic nevi**
Includes atypical nevus
blue hairy pigmented nevus
nevus NOS

D22.0 Melanocytic nevi of lip
Skin lesions composed of nests of nevus cells with macules/papules

● **D22.1 Melanocytic nevi of eyelid, including canthus**
  - **D22.10 Melanocytic nevi of unspecified eyelid, including canthus**
  - **D22.11 Melanocytic nevi of right eyelid, including canthus**
  - **D22.12 Melanocytic nevi of left eyelid, including canthus**

● **D22.2 Melanocytic nevi of ear and external auricular canal**
  - **D22.20 Melanocytic nevi of unspecified ear and external auricular canal**
  - **D22.21 Melanocytic nevi of right ear and external auricular canal**
  - **D22.22 Melanocytic nevi of left ear and external auricular canal**

● **D22.3 Melanocytic nevi of other and unspecified parts of face**
  - **D22.30 Melanocytic nevi of unspecified part of face**
  - **D22.39 Melanocytic nevi of other parts of face**

D22.4 Melanocytic nevi of scalp and neck

D22.5 Melanocytic nevi of trunk
Melanocytic nevi of anal margin
Melanocytic nevi of anal skin
Melanocytic nevi of perianal skin
Melanocytic nevi of skin of breast

● **D22.6 Melanocytic nevi of upper limb, including shoulder**
  - **D22.60 Melanocytic nevi of unspecified upper limb, including shoulder**
  - **D22.61 Melanocytic nevi of right upper limb, including shoulder**
  - **D22.62 Melanocytic nevi of left upper limb, including shoulder**

● **D22.7 Melanocytic nevi of lower limb, including hip**
  - **D22.70 Melanocytic nevi of unspecified lower limb, including hip**
  - **D22.71 Melanocytic nevi of right lower limb, including hip**
  - **D22.72 Melanocytic nevi of left lower limb, including hip**

D22.9 Melanocytic nevi, unspecified

● **D23 Other benign neoplasms of skin**
Includes benign neoplasm of hair follicles
benign neoplasm of sebaceous glands
benign neoplasm of sweat glands
Excludes1 benign lipomatous neoplasms of skin (D17.0-D17.3)
melanocytic nevi (D22.-)

D23.0 Other benign neoplasm of skin of lip
Excludes1 benign neoplasm of vermilion border of lip (D10.0)

● **D23.1 Other benign neoplasm of skin of eyelid, including canthus**
  - **D23.10 Other benign neoplasm of skin unspecified of eyelid, including canthus**
  - **D23.11 Other benign neoplasm of skin of right eyelid, including canthus**
  - **D23.12 Other benign neoplasm of skin of left eyelid, including canthus**

● **D23.2 Other benign neoplasm of skin of ear and external auricular canal**
  - **D23.20 Other benign neoplasm of skin of unspecified ear and external auricular canal**
  - **D23.21 Other benign neoplasm of skin of right ear and external auricular canal**
  - **D23.22 Other benign neoplasm of skin of left ear and external auricular canal**

● **D23.3 Other benign neoplasm of skin of other and unspecified parts of face**
  - **D23.30 Other benign neoplasm of skin of unspecified part of face**
  - **D23.39 Other benign neoplasm of skin of other parts of face**

D23.4 Other benign neoplasm of skin of scalp and neck

D23.5 Other benign neoplasm of skin of trunk
Other benign neoplasm of anal margin
Other benign neoplasm of anal skin
Other benign neoplasm of perianal skin
Other benign neoplasm of skin of breast
Excludes1 benign neoplasm of anus NOS (D12.9)

● **D23.6 Other benign neoplasm of skin of upper limb, including shoulder**
  - **D23.60 Other benign neoplasm of skin of unspecified upper limb, including shoulder**
  - **D23.61 Other benign neoplasm of skin of right upper limb, including shoulder**
  - **D23.62 Other benign neoplasm of skin of left upper limb, including shoulder**

● **D23.7 Other benign neoplasm of skin of lower limb, including hip**
  - **D23.70 Other benign neoplasm of skin of unspecified lower limb, including hip**
  - **D23.71 Other benign neoplasm of skin of right lower limb, including hip**
  - **D23.72 Other benign neoplasm of skin of left lower limb, including hip**

D23.9 Other benign neoplasm of skin, unspecified

CHAPTER 2 (C00-D49)

● **D24 Benign neoplasm of breast**

Includes benign neoplasm of connective tissue of breast
benign neoplasm of soft parts of breast
fibroadenoma of breast

Excludes2 adenofibrosis of breast (N6Ø.2)
benign cyst of breast (N6Ø.-)
benign mammary dysplasia (N6Ø.-)
benign neoplasm of skin of breast (D22.5, D23.5)
fibrocystic disease of breast (N6Ø.-)

D24.1 Benign neoplasm of right breast

D24.2 Benign neoplasm of left breast

D24.9 Benign neoplasm of unspecified breast

● **D25 Leiomyoma of uterus**

Benign tumors or nodules of the uterine wall

Includes uterine fibroid
uterine fibromyoma
uterine myoma

D25.Ø Submucous leiomyoma of uterus

D25.1 Intramural leiomyoma of uterus
Interstitial leiomyoma of uterus

D25.2 Subserosal leiomyoma of uterus
Subperitoneal leiomyoma of uterus

D25.9 Leiomyoma of uterus, unspecified

● **D26 Other benign neoplasms of uterus**

D26.Ø Other benign neoplasm of cervix uteri

D26.1 Other benign neoplasm of corpus uteri

D26.7 Other benign neoplasm of other parts of uterus

D26.9 Other benign neoplasm of uterus, unspecified

● **D27 Benign neoplasm of ovary**

Use additional code to identify any functional activity.

Excludes2 corpus albicans cyst (N83.2-)
corpus luteum cyst (N83.1-)
endometrial cyst (N8Ø.1)
follicular (atretic) cyst (N83.Ø-)
graafian follicle cyst (N83.Ø-)
ovarian cyst NEC (N83.2-)
ovarian retention cyst (N83.2-)

D27.Ø Benign neoplasm of right ovary

D27.1 Benign neoplasm of left ovary

D27.9 Benign neoplasm of unspecified ovary

● **D28 Benign neoplasm of other and unspecified female genital organs**

Includes adenomatous polyp
benign neoplasm of skin of female genital organs
benign teratoma

Excludes1 epoophoron cyst (Q5Ø.5)
fimbrial cyst (Q5Ø.4)
Gartner's duct cyst (Q52.4)
parovarian cyst (Q5Ø.5)

D28.Ø Benign neoplasm of vulva

D28.1 Benign neoplasm of vagina

D28.2 Benign neoplasm of uterine tubes and ligaments
Benign neoplasm of fallopian tube
Benign neoplasm of uterine ligament (broad) (round)

D28.7 Benign neoplasm of other specified female genital organs

D28.9 Benign neoplasm of female genital organ, unspecified

Item 2–11 Teratoma: terat = monster, oma = mass, tumor. Alternate terms: dermoid cyst of the ovary, ovarian teratoma. Teratomas are neoplasms and arise from germ cells (ovaries in female and testes in male) and can be benign or malignant. Teratomas have been known to contain hair, nails, and teeth, giving them a bizarre ("monster") appearance.

● **D29 Benign neoplasm of male genital organs**

Includes benign neoplasm of skin of male genital organs

D29.Ø Benign neoplasm of penis

D29.1 Benign neoplasm of prostate

Excludes1 enlarged prostate (N4Ø.-)

● **D29.2 Benign neoplasm of testis**

Use additional code to identify any functional activity.

D29.20 Benign neoplasm of unspecified testis

D29.21 Benign neoplasm of right testis

D29.22 Benign neoplasm of left testis

● **D29.3 Benign neoplasm of epididymis**

D29.3Ø Benign neoplasm of unspecified epididymis

D29.31 Benign neoplasm of right epididymis

D29.32 Benign neoplasm of left epididymis

D29.4 Benign neoplasm of scrotum
Benign neoplasm of skin of scrotum

D29.8 Benign neoplasm of other specified male genital organs
Benign neoplasm of seminal vesicle
Benign neoplasm of spermatic cord
Benign neoplasm of tunica vaginalis

D29.9 Benign neoplasm of male genital organ, unspecified

● **D3Ø Benign neoplasm of urinary organs**

● **D3Ø.Ø Benign neoplasm of kidney**

Excludes1 benign carcinoid tumor of the kidney (D3A.Ø93)
benign neoplasm of renal calyces (D3Ø.1-)
benign neoplasm of renal pelvis (D3Ø.1-)

D3Ø.ØØ Benign neoplasm of unspecified kidney

D3Ø.Ø1 Benign neoplasm of right kidney

D3Ø.Ø2 Benign neoplasm of left kidney

● **D3Ø.1 Benign neoplasm of renal pelvis**

D3Ø.1Ø Benign neoplasm of unspecified renal pelvis

D3Ø.11 Benign neoplasm of right renal pelvis

D3Ø.12 Benign neoplasm of left renal pelvis

● **D3Ø.2 Benign neoplasm of ureter**

Excludes1 benign neoplasm of ureteric orifice of bladder (D3Ø.3)

D3Ø.2Ø Benign neoplasm of unspecified ureter

D3Ø.21 Benign neoplasm of right ureter

D3Ø.22 Benign neoplasm of left ureter

D3Ø.3 Benign neoplasm of bladder
Benign neoplasm of ureteric orifice of bladder
Benign neoplasm of urethral orifice of bladder

D3Ø.4 Benign neoplasm of urethra

Excludes1 benign neoplasm of urethral orifice of bladder (D3Ø.3)

D3Ø.8 Benign neoplasm of other specified urinary organs
Benign neoplasm of paraurethral glands

D3Ø.9 Benign neoplasm of urinary organ, unspecified
Benign neoplasm of urinary system NOS

● **D31 Benign neoplasm of eye and adnexa**

Excludes1 benign neoplasm of connective tissue of eyelid (D21.Ø)
benign neoplasm of optic nerve (D33.3)
benign neoplasm of skin of eyelid (D22.1-, D23.1-)

● **D31.Ø Benign neoplasm of conjunctiva**

D31.ØØ Benign neoplasm of unspecified conjunctiva

D31.Ø1 Benign neoplasm of right conjunctiva

D31.Ø2 Benign neoplasm of left conjunctiva

● **D31.1 Benign neoplasm of cornea**

D31.1Ø Benign neoplasm of unspecified cornea

D31.11 Benign neoplasm of right cornea

D31.12 Benign neoplasm of left cornea

● D31.2 **Benign neoplasm of retina**
Excludes1 dark area on retina (D49.81)
hemangioma of retina (D49.81)
neoplasm of unspecified behavior of retina and choroid (D49.81)
retinal freckle (D49.81)
D31.20 **Benign neoplasm of unspecified retina**
D31.21 **Benign neoplasm of right retina**
D31.22 **Benign neoplasm of left retina**

● D31.3 **Benign neoplasm of choroid**
D31.30 **Benign neoplasm of unspecified choroid**
D31.31 **Benign neoplasm of right choroid**
D31.32 **Benign neoplasm of left choroid**

● D31.4 **Benign neoplasm of ciliary body**
D31.40 **Benign neoplasm of unspecified ciliary body**
D31.41 **Benign neoplasm of right ciliary body**
D31.42 **Benign neoplasm of left ciliary body**

● D31.5 **Benign neoplasm of lacrimal gland and duct**
Benign neoplasm of lacrimal sac
Benign neoplasm of nasolacrimal duct
D31.50 **Benign neoplasm of unspecified lacrimal gland and duct**
D31.51 **Benign neoplasm of right lacrimal gland and duct**
D31.52 **Benign neoplasm of left lacrimal gland and duct**

● D31.6 **Benign neoplasm of unspecified site of orbit**
Benign neoplasm of connective tissue of orbit
Benign neoplasm of extraocular muscle
Benign neoplasm of peripheral nerves of orbit
Benign neoplasm of retrobulbar tissue
Benign neoplasm of retro-ocular tissue
Excludes1 benign neoplasm of orbital bone (D16.4)
D31.60 **Benign neoplasm of unspecified site of unspecified orbit**
D31.61 **Benign neoplasm of unspecified site of right orbit**
D31.62 **Benign neoplasm of unspecified site of left orbit**

● D31.9 **Benign neoplasm of unspecified part of eye**
Benign neoplasm of eyeball
D31.90 **Benign neoplasm of unspecified part of unspecified eye**
D31.91 **Benign neoplasm of unspecified part of right eye**
D31.92 **Benign neoplasm of unspecified part of left eye**

● D32 **Benign neoplasm of meninges**
D32.0 **Benign neoplasm of cerebral meninges**
D32.1 **Benign neoplasm of spinal meninges**
D32.9 **Benign neoplasm of meninges, unspecified**
Meningioma NOS

● D33 **Benign neoplasm of brain and other parts of central nervous system**
Excludes1 angioma (D18.0-)
benign neoplasm of meninges (D32.-)
benign neoplasm of peripheral nerves and autonomic nervous system (D36.1-)
hemangioma (D18.0-)
neurofibromatosis (Q85.0-)
retro-ocular benign neoplasm (D31.6-)
D33.0 **Benign neoplasm of brain, supratentorial**
Benign neoplasm of cerebral ventricle
Benign neoplasm of cerebrum
Benign neoplasm of frontal lobe
Benign neoplasm of occipital lobe
Benign neoplasm of parietal lobe
Benign neoplasm of temporal lobe
Excludes1 benign neoplasm of fourth ventricle (D33.1)
D33.1 **Benign neoplasm of brain, infratentorial**
Benign neoplasm of brain stem
Benign neoplasm of cerebellum
Benign neoplasm of fourth ventricle
D33.2 **Benign neoplasm of brain, unspecified**
D33.3 **Benign neoplasm of cranial nerves**
Benign neoplasm of olfactory bulb
D33.4 **Benign neoplasm of spinal cord**
D33.7 **Benign neoplasm of other specified parts of central nervous system**
D33.9 **Benign neoplasm of central nervous system, unspecified**
Benign neoplasm of nervous system (central) NOS

D34 **Benign neoplasm of thyroid gland**
Use additional code to identify any functional activity.

● D35 **Benign neoplasm of other and unspecified endocrine glands**
Use additional code to identify any functional activity.
Excludes1 benign neoplasm of endocrine pancreas (D13.7)
benign neoplasm of ovary (D27.-)
benign neoplasm of testis (D29.2.-)
benign neoplasm of thymus (D15.0)

● D35.0 **Benign neoplasm of adrenal gland**
D35.00 **Benign neoplasm of unspecified adrenal gland**
D35.01 **Benign neoplasm of right adrenal gland**
D35.02 **Benign neoplasm of left adrenal gland**
D35.1 **Benign neoplasm of parathyroid gland**
D35.2 **Benign neoplasm of pituitary gland**
D35.3 **Benign neoplasm of craniopharyngeal duct**
D35.4 **Benign neoplasm of pineal gland**
D35.5 **Benign neoplasm of carotid body**
D35.6 **Benign neoplasm of aortic body and other paraganglia**
Benign tumor of glomus jugulare
D35.7 **Benign neoplasm of other specified endocrine glands**
D35.9 **Benign neoplasm of endocrine gland, unspecified**
Benign neoplasm of unspecified endocrine gland

● D36 **Benign neoplasm of other and unspecified sites**
D36.0 **Benign neoplasm of lymph nodes**
Excludes1 lymphangioma (D18.1)

● D36.1 **Benign neoplasm of peripheral nerves and autonomic nervous system**
Excludes1 benign neoplasm of peripheral nerves of orbit (D31.6-)
neurofibromatosis (Q85.0-)
D36.10 **Benign neoplasm of peripheral nerves and autonomic nervous system, unspecified**
D36.11 **Benign neoplasm of peripheral nerves and autonomic nervous system of face, head, and neck**
D36.12 **Benign neoplasm of peripheral nerves and autonomic nervous system, upper limb, including shoulder**
D36.13 **Benign neoplasm of peripheral nerves and autonomic nervous system of lower limb, including hip**
D36.14 **Benign neoplasm of peripheral nerves and autonomic nervous system of thorax**
D36.15 **Benign neoplasm of peripheral nerves and autonomic nervous system of abdomen**
D36.16 **Benign neoplasm of peripheral nerves and autonomic nervous system of pelvis**
D36.17 **Benign neoplasm of peripheral nerves and autonomic nervous system of trunk, unspecified**
D36.7 **Benign neoplasm of other specified sites**
Benign neoplasm of nose NOS
D36.9 **Benign neoplasm, unspecified site**

BENIGN NEUROENDOCRINE TUMORS (D3A)

● **D3A Benign neuroendocrine tumors**

Code also any associated multiple endocrine neoplasia [MEN] syndromes (E31.2-)

Use additional code to identify any associated endocrine syndrome, such as:
carcinoid syndrome (E34.0)

Excludes2 benign pancreatic islet cell tumors (D13.7)

● **D3A.0 Benign carcinoid tumors**

D3A.00 Benign carcinoid tumor of unspecified site
Carcinoid tumor NOS

● **D3A.01 Benign carcinoid tumors of the small intestine**

D3A.010 Benign carcinoid tumor of the duodenum

D3A.011 Benign carcinoid tumor of the jejunum

D3A.012 Benign carcinoid tumor of the ileum

D3A.019 Benign carcinoid tumor of the small intestine, unspecified portion

● **D3A.02 Benign carcinoid tumors of the appendix, large intestine, and rectum**

D3A.020 Benign carcinoid tumor of the appendix

D3A.021 Benign carcinoid tumor of the cecum

D3A.022 Benign carcinoid tumor of the ascending colon

D3A.023 Benign carcinoid tumor of the transverse colon

D3A.024 Benign carcinoid tumor of the descending colon

D3A.025 Benign carcinoid tumor of the sigmoid colon

D3A.026 Benign carcinoid tumor of the rectum

D3A.029 Benign carcinoid tumor of the large intestine, unspecified portion
Benign carcinoid tumor of the colon NOS

● **D3A.09 Benign carcinoid tumors of other sites**

D3A.090 Benign carcinoid tumor of the bronchus and lung

D3A.091 Benign carcinoid tumor of the thymus

D3A.092 Benign carcinoid tumor of the stomach

D3A.093 Benign carcinoid tumor of the kidney

D3A.094 Benign carcinoid tumor of the foregut, unspecified (Revised)

D3A.095 Benign carcinoid tumor of the midgut, unspecified (Revised)

D3A.096 Benign carcinoid tumor of the hindgut, unspecified (Revised)

D3A.098 Benign carcinoid tumors of other sites

D3A.8 Other benign neuroendocrine tumors
Neuroendocrine tumor NOS

NEOPLASMS OF UNCERTAIN BEHAVIOR, POLYCYTHEMIA VERA AND MYELODYSPLASTIC SYNDROMES (D37-D48)

Note: Categories D37-D44, and D48 classify by site neoplasms of uncertain behavior, i.e., histologic confirmation whether the neoplasm is malignant or benign cannot be made.

Excludes1 neoplasms of unspecified behavior (D49.-)

● **D37 Neoplasm of uncertain behavior of oral cavity and digestive organs**

Excludes1 stromal tumors of uncertain behavior of digestive system (D48.1)

● **D37.0 Neoplasm of uncertain behavior of lip, oral cavity and pharynx**

Excludes1 neoplasm of uncertain behavior of aryepiglottic fold or interarytenoid fold, laryngeal aspect (D38.0)
neoplasm of uncertain behavior of epiglottis NOS (D38.0)
neoplasm of uncertain behavior of skin of lip (D48.5)
neoplasm of uncertain behavior of suprahyoid portion of epiglottis (D38.0)

D37.01 Neoplasm of uncertain behavior of lip
Neoplasm of uncertain behavior of vermilion border of lip

D37.02 Neoplasm of uncertain behavior of tongue

● **D37.03 Neoplasm of uncertain behavior of the major salivary glands**

D37.030 Neoplasm of uncertain behavior of the parotid salivary glands

D37.031 Neoplasm of uncertain behavior of the sublingual salivary glands

D37.032 Neoplasm of uncertain behavior of the submandibular salivary glands

D37.039 Neoplasm of uncertain behavior of the major salivary glands, unspecified

D37.04 Neoplasm of uncertain behavior of the minor salivary glands
Neoplasm of uncertain behavior of submucosal salivary glands of lip
Neoplasm of uncertain behavior of submucosal salivary glands of cheek
Neoplasm of uncertain behavior of submucosal salivary glands of hard palate
Neoplasm of uncertain behavior of submucosal salivary glands of soft palate

D37.05 Neoplasm of uncertain behavior of pharynx
Neoplasm of uncertain behavior of aryepiglottic fold of pharynx NOS
Neoplasm of uncertain behavior of hypopharyngeal aspect of aryepiglottic fold of pharynx
Neoplasm of uncertain behavior of marginal zone of aryepiglottic fold of pharynx

D37.09 Neoplasm of uncertain behavior of other specified sites of the oral cavity

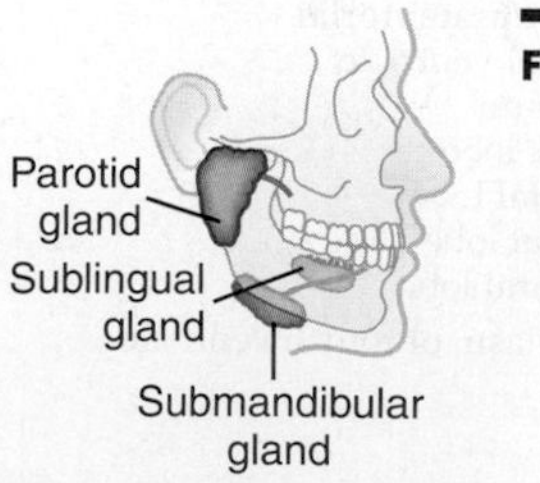

Figure 2-19 Major salivary glands.

D37.1 **Neoplasm of uncertain behavior of stomach**
D37.2 **Neoplasm of uncertain behavior of small intestine**
D37.3 **Neoplasm of uncertain behavior of appendix**
D37.4 **Neoplasm of uncertain behavior of colon**
D37.5 **Neoplasm of uncertain behavior of rectum**
Neoplasm of uncertain behavior of rectosigmoid junction
Rectosigmoid junction: Angle where sigmoid colon becomes rectum
D37.6 **Neoplasm of uncertain behavior of liver, gallbladder and bile ducts**
Neoplasm of uncertain behavior of ampulla of Vater
Ampulla of Vater: Enlarged segment of ducts from liver and pancreas at entry point to small intestine
D37.8 **Neoplasm of uncertain behavior of other specified digestive organs**
Neoplasm of uncertain behavior of anal canal
Neoplasm of uncertain behavior of anal sphincter
Neoplasm of uncertain behavior of anus NOS
Neoplasm of uncertain behavior of esophagus
Neoplasm of uncertain behavior of intestine NOS
Neoplasm of uncertain behavior of pancreas
Excludes1 neoplasm of uncertain behavior of anal margin (D48.5)
neoplasm of uncertain behavior of anal skin (D48.5)
neoplasm of uncertain behavior of perianal skin (D48.5)
D37.9 **Neoplasm of uncertain behavior of digestive organ, unspecified**

● D38 **Neoplasm of uncertain behavior of middle ear and respiratory and intrathoracic organs**
Excludes1 neoplasm of uncertain behavior of heart (D48.7)
D38.0 **Neoplasm of uncertain behavior of larynx**
Neoplasm of uncertain behavior of aryepiglottic fold or interarytenoid fold, laryngeal aspect
Neoplasm of uncertain behavior of epiglottis (suprahyoid portion)
Excludes1 neoplasm of uncertain behavior of aryepiglottic fold or interarytenoid fold NOS (D37.05)
neoplasm of uncertain behavior of hypopharyngeal aspect of aryepiglottic fold (D37.05)
neoplasm of uncertain behavior of marginal zone of aryepiglottic fold (D37.05)
D38.1 **Neoplasm of uncertain behavior of trachea, bronchus and lung**
D38.2 **Neoplasm of uncertain behavior of pleura**
D38.3 **Neoplasm of uncertain behavior of mediastinum**
D38.4 **Neoplasm of uncertain behavior of thymus**
D38.5 **Neoplasm of uncertain behavior of other respiratory organs**
Neoplasm of uncertain behavior of accessory sinuses
Neoplasm of uncertain behavior of cartilage of nose
Neoplasm of uncertain behavior of middle ear
Neoplasm of uncertain behavior of nasal cavities
Excludes1 neoplasm of uncertain behavior of ear (external) (skin) (D48.5)
neoplasm of uncertain behavior of nose NOS (D48.7)
neoplasm of uncertain behavior of skin of nose (D48.5)
D38.6 **Neoplasm of uncertain behavior of respiratory organ, unspecified**

● D39 **Neoplasm of uncertain behavior of female genital organs**
D39.0 **Neoplasm of uncertain behavior of uterus**
● D39.1 **Neoplasm of uncertain behavior of ovary**
Use additional code to identify any functional activity.
D39.10 **Neoplasm of uncertain behavior of unspecified ovary**
D39.11 **Neoplasm of uncertain behavior of right ovary**
D39.12 **Neoplasm of uncertain behavior of left ovary**
D39.2 **Neoplasm of uncertain behavior of placenta**
Chorioadenoma destruens
Invasive hydatidiform mole
Malignant hydatidiform mole
Excludes1 hydatidiform mole NOS (O01.9)
D39.8 **Neoplasm of uncertain behavior of other specified female genital organs**
Neoplasm of uncertain behavior of skin of female genital organs
D39.9 **Neoplasm of uncertain behavior of female genital organ, unspecified**

● D40 **Neoplasm of uncertain behavior of male genital organs**
D40.0 **Neoplasm of uncertain behavior of prostate**
● D40.1 **Neoplasm of uncertain behavior of testis**
D40.10 **Neoplasm of uncertain behavior of unspecified testis**
D40.11 **Neoplasm of uncertain behavior of right testis**
D40.12 **Neoplasm of uncertain behavior of left testis**
D40.8 **Neoplasm of uncertain behavior of other specified male genital organs**
Neoplasm of uncertain behavior of skin of male genital organs
D40.9 **Neoplasm of uncertain behavior of male genital organ, unspecified**

● D41 **Neoplasm of uncertain behavior of urinary organs**
● D41.0 **Neoplasm of uncertain behavior of kidney**
Excludes1 neoplasm of uncertain behavior of renal pelvis (D41.1-)
D41.00 **Neoplasm of uncertain behavior of unspecified kidney**
D41.01 **Neoplasm of uncertain behavior of right kidney**
D41.02 **Neoplasm of uncertain behavior of left kidney**
● D41.1 **Neoplasm of uncertain behavior of renal pelvis**
D41.10 **Neoplasm of uncertain behavior of unspecified renal pelvis**
D41.11 **Neoplasm of uncertain behavior of right renal pelvis**
D41.12 **Neoplasm of uncertain behavior of left renal pelvis**
● D41.2 **Neoplasm of uncertain behavior of ureter**
D41.20 **Neoplasm of uncertain behavior of unspecified ureter**
D41.21 **Neoplasm of uncertain behavior of right ureter**
D41.22 **Neoplasm of uncertain behavior of left ureter**
D41.3 **Neoplasm of uncertain behavior of urethra**
D41.4 **Neoplasm of uncertain behavior of bladder**
D41.8 **Neoplasm of uncertain behavior of other specified urinary organs**
D41.9 **Neoplasm of uncertain behavior of unspecified urinary organ**

CHAPTER 2 (C00-D49)

● **D42 Neoplasm of uncertain behavior of meninges**

D42.0 Neoplasm of uncertain behavior of cerebral meninges

D42.1 Neoplasm of uncertain behavior of spinal meninges

D42.9 Neoplasm of uncertain behavior of meninges, unspecified

● **D43 Neoplasm of uncertain behavior of brain and central nervous system**

Excludes1 neoplasm of uncertain behavior of peripheral nerves and autonomic nervous system (D48.2)

D43.0 Neoplasm of uncertain behavior of brain, supratentorial

Superior to tentorium of cerebellum

Neoplasm of uncertain behavior of cerebral ventricle
Neoplasm of uncertain behavior of cerebrum
Neoplasm of uncertain behavior of frontal lobe
Neoplasm of uncertain behavior of occipital lobe
Neoplasm of uncertain behavior of parietal lobe
Neoplasm of uncertain behavior of temporal lobe

Excludes1 neoplasm of uncertain behavior of fourth ventricle (D43.1)

D43.1 Neoplasm of uncertain behavior of brain, infratentorial

Beneath the tentorium of cerebellum

Neoplasm of uncertain behavior of brain stem
Neoplasm of uncertain behavior of cerebellum
Neoplasm of uncertain behavior of fourth ventricle

D43.2 Neoplasm of uncertain behavior of brain, unspecified

D43.3 Neoplasm of uncertain behavior of cranial nerves

D43.4 Neoplasm of uncertain behavior of spinal cord

D43.8 Neoplasm of uncertain behavior of other specified parts of central nervous system

D43.9 Neoplasm of uncertain behavior of central nervous system, unspecified

Neoplasm of uncertain behavior of nervous system (central) NOS

● **D44 Neoplasm of uncertain behavior of endocrine glands**

Excludes1 multiple endocrine adenomatosis (E31.2-)
multiple endocrine neoplasia (E31.2-)
neoplasm of uncertain behavior of endocrine pancreas (D37.8)
neoplasm of uncertain behavior of ovary (D39.1-)
neoplasm of uncertain behavior of testis (D40.1-)
neoplasm of uncertain behavior of thymus (D38.4)

D44.0 Neoplasm of uncertain behavior of thyroid gland

● **D44.1 Neoplasm of uncertain behavior of adrenal gland**

Use additional code to identify any functional activity.

D44.10 Neoplasm of uncertain behavior of unspecified adrenal gland

D44.11 Neoplasm of uncertain behavior of right adrenal gland

D44.12 Neoplasm of uncertain behavior of left adrenal gland

D44.2 Neoplasm of uncertain behavior of parathyroid gland

D44.3 Neoplasm of uncertain behavior of pituitary gland

Use additional code to identify any functional activity.

D44.4 Neoplasm of uncertain behavior of craniopharyngeal duct

D44.5 Neoplasm of uncertain behavior of pineal gland

D44.6 Neoplasm of uncertain behavior of carotid body

D44.7 Neoplasm of uncertain behavior of aortic body and other paraganglia

D44.9 Neoplasm of uncertain behavior of unspecified endocrine gland

D45 Polycythemia vera

Excludes1 familial polycythemia (D75.0)
secondary polycythemia (D75.1)

Primary polycythemia. Secondary polycythemia is D75.1. Check your documentation. Polycythemia is caused by too many red blood cells, which increase the thickness of blood (viscosity). This can cause engorgement of the spleen (splenomegaly) with extra RBCs and potential clot formation.

● **D46 Myelodysplastic syndromes**

Use additional code for adverse effect, if applicable, to identify drug (T36-T50 with fifth or sixth character 5)

Excludes2 drug-induced aplastic anemia (D61.1)

D46.0 Refractory anemia without ring sideroblasts, so stated

Refractory anemia without sideroblasts, without excess of blasts

D46.1 Refractory anemia with ring sideroblasts RARS

● **D46.2 Refractory anemia with excess of blasts [RAEB]** (Revised)

Form of myelodysplasia with increased immature white blood cells (blasts) in bone marrow

D46.20 Refractory anemia with excess of blasts, unspecified RAEB NOS

D46.21 Refractory anemia with excess of blasts 1 RAEB 1

Bone marrow disease which results in insufficient RBCs (anemia) in which level of blasts is less than 10%

D46.22 Refractory anemia with excess of blasts 2 RAEB 2

Bone marrow disease manifested by insufficient numbers of RBCs (anemia) with level of blasts 10-20%

D46.A Refractory cytopenia with multilineage dysplasia

D46.B Refractory cytopenia with multilineage dysplasia and ring sideroblasts

RCMD RS

D46.C Myelodysplastic syndrome with isolated del(5q) chromosomal abnormality

Myelodysplastic syndrome with 5q deletion
5q minus syndrome NOS

D46.4 Refractory anemia, unspecified

D46.Z Other myelodysplastic syndromes

Excludes1 chronic myelomonocytic leukemia (C93.1-)

D46.9 Myelodysplastic syndrome, unspecified

Myelodysplasia NOS

● **D47 Other neoplasms of uncertain behavior of lymphoid, hematopoietic and related tissue**

D47.0 Histiocytic and mast cell tumors of uncertain behavior

Indolent systemic mastocytosis
Mast cell tumor NOS
Mastocytoma NOS

Excludes1 malignant mast cell tumor (C96.2)
mastocytosis (congenital) (cutaneous) (Q82.2)

D47.1 Chronic myeloproliferative disease

Chronic neutrophilic leukemia
Myeloproliferative disease, unspecified

Excludes1 atypical chronic myeloid leukemia BCR/ABL-negative (C92.2-)
chronic myeloid leukemia BCR/ABL-positive (C92.1-)
myelofibrosis NOS (D75.81)
myelophthisic anemia (D61.82)
myelophthisis (D61.82)
secondary myelofibrosis NOS (D75.81)

D47.2 Monoclonal gammopathy

Monoclonal gammopathy of undetermined significance [MGUS]

D47.3 Essential (hemorrhagic) thrombocythemia

Essential thrombocytosis
Idiopathic hemorrhagic thrombocythemia

D47.4 Osteomyelofibrosis
Chronic idiopathic myelofibrosis
Myelofibrosis (idiopathic) (with myeloid metaplasia)
Myelosclerosis (megakaryocytic) with myeloid metaplasia
Secondary myelofibrosis in myeloproliferative disease
Excludes1 acute myelofibrosis (C94.4-)

● **D47.Z Other specified neoplasms of uncertain behavior of lymphoid, hematopoietic and related tissue**

D47.Z1 Post-transplant lymphoproliferative disorder (PTLD)
Code first *complications of transplanted organs and tissue (T86.-)*

D47.Z2 Castleman disease ◀
Code also if applicable human herpesvirus 8 infection (B10.89) ◀
Excludes2 Kaposi's sarcoma (C46-) ◀

D47.Z9 Other specified neoplasms of uncertain behavior of lymphoid, hematopoietic and related tissue
Histiocytic tumors of uncertain behavior

D47.9 Neoplasm of uncertain behavior of lymphoid, hematopoietic and related tissue, unspecified
Lymphoproliferative disease NOS

● **D48 Neoplasm of uncertain behavior of other and unspecified sites**
Excludes1 neurofibromatosis (nonmalignant) (Q85.0-)

D48.0 Neoplasm of uncertain behavior of bone and articular cartilage
Excludes1 neoplasm of uncertain behavior of cartilage of ear (D48.1)
neoplasm of uncertain behavior of cartilage of larynx (D38.0)
neoplasm of uncertain behavior of cartilage of nose (D38.5)
neoplasm of uncertain behavior of connective tissue of eyelid (D48.1)
neoplasm of uncertain behavior of synovia (D48.1)

D48.1 Neoplasm of uncertain behavior of connective and other soft tissue
Neoplasm of uncertain behavior of connective tissue of ear
Neoplasm of uncertain behavior of connective tissue of eyelid
Stromal tumors of uncertain behavior of digestive system
Excludes1 neoplasm of uncertain behavior of articular cartilage (D48.0)
neoplasm of uncertain behavior of cartilage of larynx (D38.0)
neoplasm of uncertain behavior of cartilage of nose (D38.5)
neoplasm of uncertain behavior of connective tissue of breast (D48.6-)

D48.2 Neoplasm of uncertain behavior of peripheral nerves and autonomic nervous system
Excludes1 neoplasm of uncertain behavior of peripheral nerves of orbit (D48.7)

D48.3 Neoplasm of uncertain behavior of retroperitoneum

D48.4 Neoplasm of uncertain behavior of peritoneum

D48.5 Neoplasm of uncertain behavior of skin
Neoplasm of uncertain behavior of anal margin
Neoplasm of uncertain behavior of anal skin
Neoplasm of uncertain behavior of perianal skin
Neoplasm of uncertain behavior of skin of breast
Excludes1 neoplasm of uncertain behavior of anus NOS (D37.8)
neoplasm of uncertain behavior of skin of genital organs (D39.8, D40.8)
neoplasm of uncertain behavior of vermilion border of lip (D37.0)

● **D48.6 Neoplasm of uncertain behavior of breast**
Neoplasm of uncertain behavior of connective tissue of breast
Cystosarcoma phyllodes
Excludes1 neoplasm of uncertain behavior of skin of breast (D48.5)

D48.60 Neoplasm of uncertain behavior of unspecified breast

D48.61 Neoplasm of uncertain behavior of right breast

D48.62 Neoplasm of uncertain behavior of left breast

D48.7 Neoplasm of uncertain behavior of other specified sites
Neoplasm of uncertain behavior of eye
Neoplasm of uncertain behavior of heart
Neoplasm of uncertain behavior of peripheral nerves of orbit
Excludes1 neoplasm of uncertain behavior of connective tissue (D48.1)
neoplasm of uncertain behavior of skin of eyelid (D48.5)

D48.9 Neoplasm of uncertain behavior, unspecified

● **D49 Neoplasms of unspecified behavior**
Note: Category D49 classifies by site neoplasms of unspecified morphology and behavior. The term 'mass,' unless otherwise stated, is not to be regarded as a neoplastic growth.
Includes 'growth' NOS
neoplasm NOS
new growth NOS
tumor NOS
Excludes1 neoplasms of uncertain behavior (D37-D44, D48)

D49.0 Neoplasm of unspecified behavior of digestive system
Excludes1 neoplasm of unspecified behavior of margin of anus (D49.2)
neoplasm of unspecified behavior of perianal skin (D49.2)
neoplasm of unspecified behavior of skin of anus (D49.2)

D49.1 Neoplasm of unspecified behavior of respiratory system

D49.2 Neoplasm of unspecified behavior of bone, soft tissue, and skin
Excludes1 neoplasm of unspecified behavior of anal canal (D49.0)
neoplasm of unspecified behavior of anus NOS (D49.0)
neoplasm of unspecified behavior of bone marrow (D49.89)
neoplasm of unspecified behavior of cartilage of larynx (D49.1)
neoplasm of unspecified behavior of cartilage of nose (D49.1)
neoplasm of unspecified behavior of connective tissue of breast (D49.3)
neoplasm of unspecified behavior of skin of genital organs (D49.59) ⇐
neoplasm of unspecified behavior of vermilion border of lip (D49.0)

D49.3 Neoplasm of unspecified behavior of breast
Excludes1 neoplasm of unspecified behavior of skin of breast (D49.2)

D49.4 Neoplasm of unspecified behavior of bladder

● D49.5 Neoplasm of unspecified behavior of other genitourinary organs

● D49.51 Neoplasm of unspecified behavior of kidney ◀

D49.511 Neoplasm of unspecified behavior of right kidney ◀

D49.512 Neoplasm of unspecified behavior of left kidney ◀

D49.519 Neoplasm of unspecified behavior of unspecified kidney ◀

D49.59 Neoplasm of unspecified behavior of other genitourinary organ ◀

D49.6 Neoplasm of unspecified behavior of brain

Excludes1 neoplasm of unspecified behavior of cerebral meninges (D49.7)
neoplasm of unspecified behavior of cranial nerves (D49.7)

D49.7 Neoplasm of unspecified behavior of endocrine glands and other parts of nervous system

Excludes1 neoplasm of unspecified behavior of peripheral, sympathetic, and parasympathetic nerves and ganglia (D49.2)

● D49.8 Neoplasm of unspecified behavior of other specified sites

Excludes1 neoplasm of unspecified behavior of eyelid (skin) (D49.2)
neoplasm of unspecified behavior of eyelid cartilage (D49.2)
neoplasm of unspecified behavior of great vessels (D49.2)
neoplasm of unspecified behavior of optic nerve (D49.7)

D49.81 Neoplasm of unspecified behavior of retina and choroid

Dark area on retina
Retinal freckle

D49.89 Neoplasm of unspecified behavior of other specified sites

D49.9 Neoplasm of unspecified behavior of unspecified site

CHAPTER 2 (C00-D49)

OGCR Chapter-Specific Coding Guidelines

3. **Chapter 3: Disease of the blood and blood-forming organs and certain disorders involving the immune mechanism (D5Ø-D89)**
Reserved for future guideline expansion

CHAPTER 3

DISEASES OF THE BLOOD AND BLOOD-FORMING ORGANS AND CERTAIN DISORDERS INVOLVING THE IMMUNE MECHANISM (D5Ø-D89)

Excludes2 autoimmune disease (systemic) NOS (M35.9)
certain conditions originating in the perinatal period (PØØ-P96)
complications of pregnancy, childbirth and the puerperium (OØØ-O9A)
congenital malformations, deformations and chromosomal abnormalities (QØØ-Q99)
endocrine, nutritional and metabolic diseases (EØØ-E88)
human immunodeficiency virus [HIV] disease (B2Ø)
injury, poisoning and certain other consequences of external causes (SØØ-T88)
neoplasms (CØØ-D49)
symptoms, signs and abnormal clinical and laboratory findings, not elsewhere classified (RØØ-R94)

This chapter contains the following blocks:

D5Ø-D53	Nutritional anemias
D55-D59	Hemolytic anemias
D6Ø-D64	Aplastic and other anemias and other bone marrow failure syndromes
D65-D69	Coagulation defects, purpura and other hemorrhagic conditions
D7Ø-D77	Other disorders of blood and blood-forming organs
D78	Intraoperative and postprocedural complications of the spleen
D8Ø-D89	Certain disorders involving the immune mechanism

NUTRITIONAL ANEMIAS (D5Ø-D53)

● **D5Ø Iron deficiency anemia**
A disease characterized by a decrease in the number of red cells (hemoglobin) in the blood.
Includes asiderotic anemia
hypochromic anemia

D5Ø.Ø Iron deficiency anemia secondary to blood loss (chronic)
Posthemorrhagic anemia (chronic)
Excludes1 acute posthemorrhagic anemia (D62)
congenital anemia from fetal blood loss (P61.3)

D5Ø.1 Sideropenic dysphagia
Web-like growth of membranes in throat that makes swallowing difficult
Kelly-Paterson syndrome
Plummer-Vinson syndrome

D5Ø.8 Other iron deficiency anemias
Iron deficiency anemia due to inadequate dietary iron intake

D5Ø.9 Iron deficiency anemia, unspecified

● **D51 Vitamin B12 deficiency anemia**
Excludes1 vitamin B12 deficiency (E53.8)

D51.Ø Vitamin B12 deficiency anemia due to intrinsic factor deficiency
Addison anemia
Biermer anemia
Pernicious (congenital) anemia
Congenital intrinsic factor deficiency

D51.1 Vitamin B12 deficiency anemia due to selective vitamin B12 malabsorption with proteinuria
Imerslund (Gräsbeck) syndrome
Megaloblastic hereditary anemia

D51.2 Transcobalamin II deficiency

D51.3 Other dietary vitamin B12 deficiency anemia
Vegan anemia

D51.8 Other vitamin B12 deficiency anemias

D51.9 Vitamin B12 deficiency anemia, unspecified

● **D52 Folate deficiency anemia**
Excludes1 folate deficiency without anemia (E53.8)

D52.Ø Dietary folate deficiency anemia
Nutritional megaloblastic anemia

D52.1 Drug-induced folate deficiency anemia
Use additional code for adverse effect, if applicable, to identify drug (T36-T5Ø with fifth or sixth character 5)

D52.8 Other folate deficiency anemias

D52.9 Folate deficiency anemia, unspecified
Folic acid deficiency anemia NOS

● **D53 Other nutritional anemias**
Includes megaloblastic anemia unresponsive to vitamin B12 or folate therapy

D53.Ø Protein deficiency anemia
Amino-acid deficiency anemia
Orotaciduric anemia
Excludes1 Lesch-Nyhan syndrome (E79.1)

D53.1 Other megaloblastic anemias, not elsewhere classified
Megaloblastic anemia NOS
Excludes1 Di Guglielmo's disease (C94.Ø)

D53.2 Scorbutic anemia
Anemia resulting from deficiency of ascorbic acid (vitamin C)
Excludes1 scurvy (E54)

D53.8 Other specified nutritional anemias
Anemia associated with deficiency of copper
Anemia associated with deficiency of molybdenum
Anemia associated with deficiency of zinc
Excludes1 nutritional deficiencies without anemia, such as:
copper deficiency NOS (E61.Ø)
molybdenum deficiency NOS (E61.5)
zinc deficiency NOS (E6Ø)

D53.9 Nutritional anemia, unspecified
Simple chronic anemia
Excludes1 anemia NOS (D64.9)

CHAPTER 3 (D5Ø-D89)

HEMOLYTIC ANEMIAS (D55-D59)

● **D55 Anemia due to enzyme disorders**

Excludes1 drug-induced enzyme deficiency anemia (D59.2)

D55.0 Anemia due to glucose-6-phosphate dehydrogenase [G6PD] deficiency
Favism
G6PD deficiency anemia

D55.1 Anemia due to other disorders of glutathione metabolism
Anemia (due to) enzyme deficiencies, except G6PD, related to the hexose monophosphate [HMP] shunt pathway
Anemia (due to) hemolytic nonspherocytic (hereditary), type I

D55.2 Anemia due to disorders of glycolytic enzymes
Hemolytic nonspherocytic (hereditary) anemia, type II
Hexokinase deficiency anemia
Pyruvate kinase [PK] deficiency anemia
Triose-phosphate isomerase deficiency anemia
Excludes1 disorders of glycolysis not associated with anemia (E74.8)

D55.3 Anemia due to disorders of nucleotide metabolism

D55.8 Other anemias due to enzyme disorders

D55.9 Anemia due to enzyme disorder, unspecified

● **D56 Thalassemia**

Hereditary disorders characterized by low production of hemoglobin or excessive destruction of red blood cells

Excludes1 sickle-cell thalassemia (D57.4-)

D56.0 Alpha thalassemia
Alpha thalassemia major
Hemoglobin H Constant Spring
Hemoglobin H disease
Hydrops fetalis due to alpha thalassemia
Severe alpha thalassemia
Triple gene defect alpha thalassemia
Use additional code, if applicable, for hydrops fetalis due to alpha thalassemia (P56.99)
Excludes1 alpha thalassemia trait or minor (D56.3)
asymptomatic alpha thalassemia (D56.3)
hydrops fetalis due to isoimmunization (P56.0)
hydrops fetalis not due to immune hemolysis (P83.2)

D56.1 Beta thalassemia
Beta thalassemia major
Cooley's anemia
Homozygous beta thalassemia
Severe beta thalassemia
Thalassemia intermedia
Thalassemia major
Excludes1 beta thalassemia minor (D56.3)
beta thalassemia trait (D56.3)
delta-beta thalassemia (D56.2)
hemoglobin E-beta thalassemia (D56.5)
sickle-cell beta thalassemia (D57.4-)

D56.2 Delta-beta thalassemia
Homozygous delta-beta thalassemia
Excludes1 delta-beta thalassemia minor (D56.3)
delta-beta thalassemia trait (D56.3)

D56.3 Thalassemia minor
Genetic disorders that have in common defective production of hemoglobin
Alpha thalassemia minor
Alpha thalassemia silent carrier
Alpha thalassemia trait
Beta thalassemia minor
Beta thalassemia trait
Delta-beta thalassemia minor
Delta-beta thalassemia trait
Thalassemia trait NOS
Excludes1 alpha thalassemia (D56.0)
beta thalassemia (D56.1)
delta-beta thalassemia (D56.2)
hemoglobin E-beta thalassemia (D56.5)
sickle-cell trait (D57.3)

D56.4 Hereditary persistence of fetal hemoglobin [HPFH]
Persistent production of hemoglobin

D56.5 Hemoglobin E-beta thalassemia
Excludes1 beta thalassemia (D56.1)
beta thalassemia minor (D56.3)
beta thalassemia trait (D56.3)
delta-beta thalassemia (D56.2)
delta-beta thalassemia trait (D56.3)
hemoglobin E disease (D58.2)
other hemoglobinopathies (D58.2)
sickle-cell beta thalassemia (D57.4-)

D56.8 Other thalassemias
Dominant thalassemia
Hemoglobin C thalassemia
Mixed thalassemia
Thalassemia with other hemoglobinopathy
Excludes1 hemoglobin C disease (D58.2)
hemoglobin E disease (D58.2)
other hemoglobinopathies (D58.2)
sickle cell anemia (D57.-)
sickle-cell thalassemia (D57.4)

D56.9 Thalassemia, unspecified
Mediterranean anemia (with other hemoglobinopathy)

● **D57 Sickle-cell disorders**

Inherited disease in which red blood cells, normally disc-shaped, become crescent shaped

Use additional code for any associated fever (R50.81)

Excludes1 other hemoglobinopathies (D58.-)

● **D57.0 Hb-SS disease with crisis**
Sickle-cell disease NOS with crisis
Hb-SS disease with vasoocclusive pain

D57.00 Hb-SS disease with crisis, unspecified

D57.01 Hb-SS disease with acute chest syndrome

D57.02 Hb-SS disease with splenic sequestration

D57.1 Sickle-cell disease without crisis Hb-SS disease without crisis
Sickle-cell anemia NOS
Sickle-cell disease NOS
Sickle-cell disorder NOS

● **D57.2 Sickle-cell/Hb-C disease**
Hb-SC disease
Hb-S/Hb-C disease

D57.20 Sickle-cell/Hb-C disease without crisis

● **D57.21 Sickle-cell/Hb-C disease with crisis**

D57.211 Sickle-cell/Hb-C disease with acute chest syndrome

D57.212 Sickle-cell/Hb-C disease with splenic sequestration

D57.219 Sickle-cell/Hb-C disease with crisis, unspecified
Sickle-cell/Hb-C disease with crisis NOS

D57.3 Sickle-cell trait
Hb-S trait
Heterozygous hemoglobin S

● **D57.4 Sickle-cell thalassemia**
Sickle-cell beta thalassemia
Thalassemia Hb-S disease

D57.40 Sickle-cell thalassemia without crisis
Microdrepanocytosis
Sickle-cell thalassemia NOS

● **D57.41 Sickle-cell thalassemia with crisis**
Sickle-cell "crisis" is precipitated when abnormally crescent-shaped red blood cells form clots and interrupt blood flow to major organs, causing severe pain and organ damage.
Sickle-cell thalassemia with vasoocclusive pain

D57.411 Sickle-cell thalassemia with acute chest syndrome

D57.412 Sickle-cell thalassemia with splenic sequestration

D57.419 Sickle-cell thalassemia with crisis, unspecified
Sickle-cell thalassemia with crisis NOS

● **D57.8 Other sickle-cell disorders**
Hb-SD disease
Hb-SE disease

D57.80 Other sickle-cell disorders without crisis

● **D57.81 Other sickle-cell disorders with crisis**

D57.811 Other sickle-cell disorders with acute chest syndrome

D57.812 Other sickle-cell disorders with splenic sequestration

D57.819 Other sickle-cell disorders with crisis, unspecified
Other sickle-cell disorders with crisis NOS

● **D58 Other hereditary hemolytic anemias**
Genetic condition in which bone marrow is unable to compensate for premature destruction of red blood cells
Excludes1 hemolytic anemia of the newborn (P55.-)

D58.0 Hereditary spherocytosis
Presence of spherocytes (spherically shaped red blood cells)
Acholuric (familial) jaundice
Congenital (spherocytic) hemolytic icterus
Minkowski-Chauffard syndrome

D58.1 Hereditary elliptocytosis
Presence of large numbers of elliptocytes in blood
Elliptocytosis (congenital)
Ovalocytosis (congenital) (hereditary)

D58.2 Other hemoglobinopathies
Abnormal hemoglobin NOS
Congenital Heinz body anemia
Hb-C disease
Hb-D disease
Hb-E disease
Hemoglobinopathy NOS
Unstable hemoglobin hemolytic disease
Excludes1 familial polycythemia (D75.0)
Hb-M disease (D74.0)
hemoglobin E-beta thalassemia (D56.5)
hereditary persistence of fetal hemoglobin [HPFH] (D56.4)
high-altitude polycythemia (D75.1)
methemoglobinemia (D74.-)
other hemoglobinopathies with thalassemia (D56.8)

D58.8 Other specified hereditary hemolytic anemias
Stomatocytosis

D58.9 Hereditary hemolytic anemia, unspecified

● **D59 Acquired hemolytic anemia**

D59.0 Drug-induced autoimmune hemolytic anemia
Use additional code for adverse effect, if applicable, to identify drug (T36-T50 with fifth or sixth character 5)

D59.1 Other autoimmune hemolytic anemias
Autoimmune hemolytic disease (cold type) (warm type)
Chronic cold hemagglutinin disease
Cold agglutinin disease
Cold agglutinin hemoglobinuria
Cold type (secondary) (symptomatic) hemolytic anemia
Warm type (secondary) (symptomatic) hemolytic anemia
Excludes1 Evans syndrome (D69.41)
hemolytic disease of newborn (P55.-)
paroxysmal cold hemoglobinuria (D59.6)

D59.2 Drug-induced nonautoimmune hemolytic anemia
Drug-induced enzyme deficiency anemia
Use additional code for adverse effect, if applicable, to identify drug (T36-T50 with fifth or sixth character 5)

D59.3 Hemolytic-uremic syndrome
Use additional code to identify associated:
E. coli infection (B96.2-)
Pneumococcal pneumonia (J13)
Shigella dysenteriae (A03.9)

D59.4 Other nonautoimmune hemolytic anemias
Mechanical hemolytic anemia
Microangiopathic hemolytic anemia
Toxic hemolytic anemia

D59.5 Paroxysmal nocturnal hemoglobinuria [Marchiafava-Micheli]
Excludes1 hemoglobinuria NOS (R82.3)

D59.6 Hemoglobinuria due to hemolysis from other external causes
Hemoglobinuria from exertion
March hemoglobinuria
Paroxysmal cold hemoglobinuria
Use additional code (Chapter 20) to identify external cause
Excludes1 hemoglobinuria NOS (R82.3)

D59.8 Other acquired hemolytic anemias

D59.9 Acquired hemolytic anemia, unspecified
Idiopathic hemolytic anemia, chronic

APLASTIC AND OTHER ANEMIAS AND OTHER BONE MARROW FAILURE SYNDROMES (D60-D64)

● **D60 Acquired pure red cell aplasia [erythroblastopenia]**
Deficiency of erythroblasts
Includes red cell aplasia (acquired) (adult) (with thymoma)
Excludes1 congenital red cell aplasia (D61.01)

D60.0 Chronic acquired pure red cell aplasia
Lack of development of blood cell

D60.1 Transient acquired pure red cell aplasia

D60.8 Other acquired pure red cell aplasias

D60.9 Acquired pure red cell aplasia, unspecified

● **D61 Other aplastic anemias and other bone marrow failure syndromes**
Excludes1 neutropenia (D70.-)

● **D61.0 Constitutional aplastic anemia**
Condition where bone marrow is unable to produce blood cells

D61.01 Constitutional (pure) red blood cell aplasia
Blackfan-Diamond syndrome
Congenital (pure) red cell aplasia
Familial hypoplastic anemia
Primary (pure) red cell aplasia
Red cell (pure) aplasia of infants
Excludes1 acquired red cell aplasia (D60.9)

D61.09 Other constitutional aplastic anemia
Fanconi's anemia
Pancytopenia with malformations

CHAPTER 3 (D50-D89)

D61.1 Drug-induced aplastic anemia

Use additional code for adverse effect, if applicable, to identify drug (T36-T5Ø with fifth or sixth character 5)

D61.2 Aplastic anemia due to other external agents

Code first*, if applicable, toxic effects of substances chiefly nonmedicinal as to source (T51-T65)*

D61.3 Idiopathic aplastic anemia

● **D61.8 Other specified aplastic anemias and other bone marrow failure syndromes**

● **D61.81 Pancytopenia**

Marked deficiency of all the blood elements: Red blood cells (erythrocytes), white blood cells (leukocytes), and platelets (thrombocytes). Check laboratory results.

Excludes1 pancytopenia (due to) (with) aplastic anemia (D61.9)
pancytopenia (due to) (with) bone marrow infiltration (D61.82)
pancytopenia (due to) (with) congenital (pure) red cell aplasia (D61.Ø1)
pancytopenia (due to) (with) hairy cell leukemia (C91.4-)
pancytopenia (due to) (with) human immunodeficiency virus disease (B2Ø.-)
pancytopenia (due to) (with) leukoerythroblastic anemia (D61.82)
pancytopenia (due to) (with) myeloproliferative disease (D47.1)

Excludes2 pancytopenia (due to) (with) myelodysplastic syndromes (D46.-) ◀

D61.81Ø Antineoplastic chemotherapy induced pancytopenia

Excludes2 aplastic anemia due to antineoplastic chemotherapy (D61.1)

D61.811 Other drug-induced pancytopenia

Excludes2 aplastic anemia due to drugs (D61.1)

D61.818 Other pancytopenia

D61.82 Myelophthisis

Leukoerythroblastic anemia
Myelophthisic anemia
Panmyelophthisis

Code also the underlying disorder, such as:
malignant neoplasm of breast (C5Ø.-)
tuberculosis (A15.-)

Excludes1 idiopathic myelofibrosis (D47.1)
myelofibrosis NOS (D75.81)
myelofibrosis with myeloid metaplasia (D47.4)
primary myelofibrosis (D47.1)
secondary myelofibrosis (D75.81)

D61.89 Other specified aplastic anemias and other bone marrow failure syndromes

D61.9 Aplastic anemia, unspecified

Hypoplastic anemia NOS
Medullary hypoplasia

D62 Acute posthemorrhagic anemia

Excludes1 anemia due to chronic blood loss (D5Ø.Ø)
blood loss anemia NOS (D5Ø.Ø)
congenital anemia from fetal blood loss (P61.3)

● **D63 Anemia in chronic diseases classified elsewhere**

D63.Ø Anemia in neoplastic disease

Code first *neoplasm (CØØ-D49)*

Excludes1 anemia due to antineoplastic chemotherapy (D64.81)
aplastic anemia due to antineoplastic chemotherapy (D61.1)

OGCR Section I.C.2.e.2.

2) Anemia associated with chemotherapy, immunotherapy and radiation therapy

When the admission/encounter is for management of an anemia associated with an adverse effect of the administration of chemotherapy or immunotherapy and the only treatment is for the anemia, the anemia code is sequenced first followed by the appropriate codes for the neoplasm and the adverse effect (T45.1X5, Adverse effect of antineoplastic and immunosuppressive drugs).

D63.1 Anemia in chronic kidney disease

Erythropoietin resistant anemia (EPO resistant anemia)

Code first *underlying chronic kidney disease (CKD) (N18.-)*

D63.8 Anemia in other chronic diseases classified elsewhere

Code first *underlying disease, such as:*
diphyllobothriasis (B7Ø.Ø)
hookworm disease (B76.Ø-B76.9)
hypothyroidism (EØØ.Ø-EØ3.9)
malaria (B5Ø.Ø-B54)
symptomatic late syphilis (A52.79)
tuberculosis (A18.89)

● **D64 Other anemias**

Excludes1 refractory anemia (D46.-)
refractory anemia with excess blasts in transformation [RAEB T] (C92.Ø-)

D64.Ø Hereditary sideroblastic anemia

Abnormal production RBCs (erythrocytes)
Sex-linked hypochromic sideroblastic anemia

D64.1 Secondary sideroblastic anemia due to disease

Code first *underlying disease*

D64.2 Secondary sideroblastic anemia due to drugs and toxins

Code first *poisoning due to drug or toxin, if applicable (T36-T65 with fifth or sixth character 1-4 or 6)*

Use additional code for adverse effect, if applicable, to identify drug (T36-T5Ø with fifth or sixth character 5)

D64.3 Other sideroblastic anemias

Sideroblastic anemia NOS
Pyridoxine-responsive sideroblastic anemia NEC

D64.4 Congenital dyserythropoietic anemia

Any of several rare hereditary anemias, mostly types of macrocytic anemia
Dyshematopoietic anemia (congenital)

Excludes1 Blackfan-Diamond syndrome (D61.Ø1)
Di Guglielmo's disease (C94.Ø)

● **D64.8 Other specified anemias**

D64.81 Anemia due to antineoplastic chemotherapy

Antineoplastic chemotherapy induced anemia

Excludes1 aplastic anemia due to antineoplastic chemotherapy (D61.1)

Excludes2 anemia in neoplastic disease (D63.Ø) ◀

D64.89 Other specified anemias

Infantile pseudoleukemia

D64.9 Anemia, unspecified

COAGULATION DEFECTS, PURPURA AND OTHER HEMORRHAGIC CONDITIONS (D65-D69)

D65 Disseminated intravascular coagulation [defibrination syndrome]
Blood clots form and consume all coagulation proteins and platelets and disrupt normal coagulation, resulting in abnormal bleeding
Afibrinogenemia, acquired
Consumption coagulopathy
Diffuse or disseminated intravascular coagulation [DIC]
Fibrinolytic hemorrhage, acquired
Fibrinolytic purpura
Purpura fulminans
Excludes1 disseminated intravascular coagulation (complicating):
abortion or ectopic or molar pregnancy (O00-O07, O08.1)
in newborn (P60)
pregnancy, childbirth and the puerperium (O45.0, O46.0, O67.0, O72.3)

D66 Hereditary factor VIII deficiency
Inherited coagulation disorder carried by females but most often affecting males
Classical hemophilia
Deficiency factor VIII (with functional defect)
Hemophilia NOS
Hemophilia A
Excludes1 factor VIII deficiency with vascular defect (D68.0)

D67 Hereditary factor IX deficiency
Christmas disease
Factor IX deficiency (with functional defect)
Hemophilia B
Plasma thromboplastin component [PTC] deficiency

● **D68 Other coagulation defects**
Excludes1 abnormal coagulation profile (R79.1)
coagulation defects complicating abortion or ectopic or molar pregnancy (O00-O07, O08.1)
coagulation defects complicating pregnancy, childbirth and the puerperium (O45.0, O46.0, O67.0, O72.3)

D68.0 Von Willebrand's disease
Congenital bleeding disorder
Angiohemophilia
Factor VIII deficiency with vascular defect
Vascular hemophilia
Excludes1 capillary fragility (hereditary) (D69.8)
factor VIII deficiency NOS (D66)
factor VIII deficiency with functional defect (D66)

D68.1 Hereditary factor XI deficiency
Deficiency of blood coagulation resulting in systemic blood-clotting defect
Hemophilia C
Plasma thromboplastin antecedent [PTA] deficiency
Rosenthal's disease

D68.2 Hereditary deficiency of other clotting factors
Blood clotting disorders caused by hereditary deficiencies of one or more clotting factors
AC globulin deficiency
Congenital afibrinogenemia
Deficiency of factor I [fibrinogen]
Deficiency of factor II [prothrombin]
Deficiency of factor V [labile]
Deficiency of factor VII [stable]
Deficiency of factor X [Stuart-Prower]
Deficiency of factor XII [Hageman]
Deficiency of factor XIII [fibrin stabilizing]
Dysfibrinogenemia (congenital)
Hypoproconvertinemia
Owren's disease
Proaccelerin deficiency

● **D68.3 Hemorrhagic disorder due to circulating anticoagulants**
Blood clotting disorders caused by anticoagulants (warfarin and heparin)

● **D68.31 Hemorrhagic disorder due to intrinsic circulating anticoagulants, antibodies, or inhibitors**

D68.311 Acquired hemophilia
Autoimmune hemophilia
Autoimmune inhibitors to clotting factors
Secondary hemophilia

D68.312 Antiphospholipid antibody with hemorrhagic disorder
Lupus anticoagulant (LAC) with hemorrhagic disorder
Systemic lupus erythematosus [SLE] inhibitor with hemorrhagic disorder
Excludes1 antiphospholipid antibody, finding without diagnosis (R76.0)
antiphospholipid antibody syndrome (D68.61)
antiphospholipid antibody with hypercoagulable state (D68.61)
lupus anticoagulant (LAC) finding without diagnosis (R76.0)
lupus anticoagulant (LAC) with hypercoagulable state (D68.62)
systemic lupus erythematosus [SLE] inhibitor finding without diagnosis (R76.0)
systemic lupus erythematosus [SLE] inhibitor with hypercoagulable state (D68.62)

D68.318 Other hemorrhagic disorder due to intrinsic circulating anticoagulants, antibodies, or inhibitors
Antithromboplastinemia
Antithromboplastinogenemia
Hemorrhagic disorder due to intrinsic increase in antithrombin
Hemorrhagic disorder due to intrinsic increase in anti-VIIIa
Hemorrhagic disorder due to intrinsic increase in anti-IXa
Hemorrhagic disorder due to intrinsic increase in anti-XIa

D68.32 Hemorrhagic disorder due to extrinsic circulating anticoagulants
Drug-induced hemorrhagic disorder
Hemorrhagic disorder due to increase in anti-IIa
Hemorrhagic disorder due to increase in anti-Xa
Hyperheparinemia
Use additional code for adverse effect, if applicable, to identify drug (T45.515, T45.525)

CHAPTER 3 (D50-D89)

D68.4 Acquired coagulation factor deficiency
Deficiency of coagulation factor due to liver disease
Deficiency of coagulation factor due to vitamin K deficiency
Excludes1 vitamin K deficiency of newborn (P53)

● **D68.5 Primary thrombophilia**
AKA idiopathic thrombocytopenia, may be acquired or congenital and is a common cause of coagulation disorders.
Primary hypercoagulable states
Excludes1 antiphospholipid syndrome (D68.61)
lupus anticoagulant (D68.62)
secondary activated protein C resistance (D68.69)
secondary antiphospholipid antibody syndrome (D68.69)
secondary lupus anticoagulant with hypercoagulable state (D68.69)
secondary systemic lupus erythematosus [SLE] inhibitor with hypercoagulable state (D68.69)
systemic lupus erythematosus [SLE] inhibitor finding without diagnosis (R76.Ø)
systemic lupus erythematosus [SLE] inhibitor with hemorrhagic disorder (D68.312)
thrombotic thrombocytopenic purpura (M31.1)

D68.51 Activated protein C resistance
Factor V Leiden mutation

D68.52 Prothrombin gene mutation

D68.59 Other primary thrombophilia
Antithrombin III deficiency
Hypercoagulable state NOS
Primary hypercoagulable state NEC
Primary thrombophilia NEC
Protein C deficiency
Protein S deficiency
Thrombophilia NOS

● **D68.6 Other thrombophilia**
Other hypercoagulable states
Excludes1 diffuse or disseminated intravascular coagulation [DIC] (D65)
heparin induced thrombocytopenia (HIT) (D75.82)
hyperhomocysteinemia (E72.11)

D68.61 Antiphospholipid syndrome
Anticardiolipin syndrome
Antiphospholipid antibody syndrome
Excludes1 anti-phospholipid antibody, finding without diagnosis (R76.Ø)
anti-phospholipid antibody with hemorrhagic disorder (D68.312)
lupus anticoagulant syndrome (D68.62)

D68.62 Lupus anticoagulant syndrome
Lupus anticoagulant
Presence of systemic lupus erythematosus [SLE] inhibitor
Excludes1 anticardiolipin syndrome (D68.61)
antiphospholipid syndrome (D68.61)
lupus anticoagulant (LAC) finding without diagnosis (R76.Ø) ◄
lupus anticoagulant (LAC) with hemorrhagic disorder (D68.312)

D68.69 Other thrombophilia
Hypercoagulable states NEC
Secondary hypercoagulable state NOS

D68.8 Other specified coagulation defects
Excludes1 hemorrhagic disease of newborn (P53)

D68.9 Coagulation defect, unspecified

● **D69 Purpura and other hemorrhagic conditions**
Group of conditions characterized by small hemorrhages in skin, mucous membranes, or serosal surfaces
Excludes1 benign hypergammaglobulinemic purpura (D89.Ø)
cryoglobulinemic purpura (D89.1)
essential (hemorrhagic) thrombocythemia (D47.3)
hemorrhagic thrombocythemia (D47.3)
purpura fulminans (D65)
thrombotic thrombocytopenic purpura (M31.1)
Waldenström hypergammaglobulinemic purpura (D89.Ø)

D69.Ø Allergic purpura
Allergic vasculitis
Nonthrombocytopenic hemorrhagic purpura
Nonthrombocytopenic idiopathic purpura
Purpura anaphylactoid
Purpura Henoch(-Schönlein)
Purpura rheumatica
Vascular purpura
Excludes1 thrombocytopenic hemorrhagic purpura (D69.3)

D69.1 Qualitative platelet defects
Bernard-Soulier [giant platelet] syndrome
Glanzmann's disease
Grey platelet syndrome
Thromboasthenia (hemorrhagic) (hereditary)
Thrombocytopathy
Excludes1 von Willebrand's disease (D68.Ø)

D69.2 Other nonthrombocytopenic purpura
Purpura NOS
Purpura simplex
Senile purpura

D69.3 Immune thrombocytopenic purpura
Hemorrhagic (thrombocytopenic) purpura
Idiopathic thrombocytopenic purpura
Tidal platelet dysgenesis

● **D69.4 Other primary thrombocytopenia**
Excludes1 transient neonatal thrombocytopenia (P61.Ø)
Wiskott-Aldrich syndrome (D82.Ø)

D69.41 Evans syndrome
Acquired hemolytic anemia and thrombocytopenia

D69.42 Congenital and hereditary thrombocytopenia purpura
Congenital thrombocytopenia
Hereditary thrombocytopenia
Code first congential or hereditary disorder, such as:
thrombocytopenia with absent radius (TAR syndrome) (Q87.2)

D69.49 Other primary thrombocytopenia
Megakaryocytic hypoplasia
Primary thrombocytopenia NOS

● **D69.5 Secondary thrombocytopenia**
Acquired reduction of number of platelets required for blood clotting
Excludes1 heparin induced thrombocytopenia (HIT) (D75.82)
transient thrombocytopenia of newborn (P61.Ø)

D69.51 Posttransfusion purpura
Posttransfusion purpura from whole blood (fresh) or blood products PTP

D69.59 Other secondary thrombocytopenia

D69.6 Thrombocytopenia, unspecified

D69.8 Other specified hemorrhagic conditions
Capillary fragility (hereditary)
Vascular pseudohemophilia

D69.9 Hemorrhagic condition, unspecified

OTHER DISORDERS OF BLOOD AND BLOOD-FORMING ORGANS (D70-D77)

● **D70 Neutropenia**
Decrease in number of neutrophils (type of white blood cell)
Includes agranulocytosis
decreased absolute neurophile count (ANC)
Use additional code for any associated:
fever (R50.81)
mucositis (J34.81, K12.3-, K92.81, N76.81)
Excludes1 neutropenic splenomegaly (D73.81)
transient neonatal neutropenia (P61.5)

D70.0 Congenital agranulocytosis
Reduced numbers of neutrophils (type of white blood cell)
Congenital neutropenia
Infantile genetic agranulocytosis
Kostmann's disease

D70.1 Agranulocytosis secondary to cancer chemotherapy
Decreased numbers of granulocytes (type of white blood cell)
Code also *underlying neoplasm*
Use additional code for adverse effect, if applicable, to identify drug (T45.1X5)

D70.2 Other drug-induced agranulocytosis
Use additional code for adverse effect, if applicable, to identify drug (T36-T50 with fifth or sixth character 5)

D70.3 Neutropenia due to infection

D70.4 Cyclic neutropenia
Chronic neutropenia (low number of type of white blood cell)
Cyclic hematopoiesis
Periodic neutropenia

D70.8 Other neutropenia

D70.9 Neutropenia, unspecified

D71 Functional disorders of polymorphonuclear neutrophils
Polymorphonuclear: varying shapes of nucleus; AKA PMNs
Cell membrane receptor complex [CR3] defect
Chronic (childhood) granulomatous disease
Congenital dysphagocytosis
Progressive septic granulomatosis

● **D72 Other disorders of white blood cells**
Excludes1 basophilia (D72.824)
immunity disorders (D80-D89)
neutropenia (D70)
preleukemia (syndrome) (D46.9)

D72.0 Genetic anomalies of leukocytes
Alder (granulation) (granulocyte) anomaly
Alder syndrome
Hereditary leukocytic hypersegmentation
Hereditary leukocytic hyposegmentation
Hereditary leukomelanopathy
May-Hegglin (granulation) (granulocyte) anomaly
May-Hegglin syndrome
Pelger-Huët (granulation) (granulocyte) anomaly
Pelger-Huët syndrome
Excludes1 Chédiak (-Steinbrinck)-Higashi syndrome (E70.330)

D72.1 Eosinophilia
Formation and accumulation of high number of white cells in blood/tissue
Allergic eosinophilia
Hereditary eosinophilia
Excludes1 Löffler's syndrome (J82)
pulmonary eosinophilia (J82)

● **D72.8 Other specified disorders of white blood cells**
Excludes1 leukemia (C91-C95)

● **D72.81 Decreased white blood cell count**
Excludes1 neutropenia (D70.-)

D72.810 Lymphocytopenia
Decreased lymphocytes
Reduction in number of lympho cytes in blood

D72.818 Other decreased white blood cell count
Basophilic leukopenia
Eosinophilic leukopenia
Monocytopenia
Other decreased leukocytes
Plasmacytopenia

D72.819 Decreased white blood cell count, unspecified
Decreased leukocytes, unspecified
Leukocytopenia, unspecified
Leukopenia
Excludes1 malignant leukopenia (D70.9)

● **D72.82 Elevated white blood cell count**
Excludes1 eosinophilia (D72.1)

D72.820 Lymphocytosis (symptomatic)
Elevated lymphocytes
Excess of normal lymphocytes

D72.821 Monocytosis (symptomatic)
Excludes1 infectious mononucleosis (B27.-)

D72.822 Plasmacytosis
Presence of excess plasma cells

D72.823 Leukemoid reaction
Basophilic leukemoid reaction
Leukemoid reaction NOS
Lymphocytic leukemoid reaction
Monocytic leukemoid reaction
Myelocytic leukemoid reaction
Neutrophilic leukemoid reaction

D72.824 Basophilia
Increase of basophils in blood

D72.825 Bandemia
Bandemia without diagnosis of specific infection
Excess number of band cells (immature white blood cells) released by bone marrow
Excludes1 confirmed infection -code to infection
leukemia (C91.-, C92.-, C93.-, C94.-, C95.-)

D72.828 Other elevated white blood cell count

D72.829 Elevated white blood cell count, unspecified
Elevated leukocytes, unspecified
Leukocytosis, unspecified

D72.89 Other specified disorders of white blood cells
Abnormality of white blood cells NEC

D72.9 Disorder of white blood cells, unspecified
Abnormal leukocyte differential NOS

● **D73 Diseases of spleen**

D73.0 Hyposplenism
Diminished functioning of spleen
Atrophy of spleen
Excludes1 asplenia (congenital) (Q89.01)
postsurgical absence of spleen (Z90.81)

D73.1 Hypersplenism
Accelerated function of spleen
Excludes1 neutropenic splenomegaly (D73.81)
primary splenic neutropenia (D73.81)
splenitis, splenomegaly in late syphilis (A52.79)
splenitis, splenomegaly in tuberculosis (A18.85)
splenomegaly NOS (R16.1)
splenomegaly congenital (Q89.0)

CHAPTER 3 (D50-D89)

D73.2 Chronic congestive splenomegaly
Enlargement of spleen

D73.3 Abscess of spleen

D73.4 Cyst of spleen

D73.5 Infarction of spleen
Splenic rupture, nontraumatic
Torsion of spleen
Excludes1 rupture of spleen due to Plasmodium vivax malaria (B51.Ø)
traumatic rupture of spleen (S36.Ø3-)

● **D73.8 Other diseases of spleen**

D73.81 Neutropenic splenomegaly
Werner-Schultz disease
Enlarged spleen responding to inadequate number of neutrophils

D73.89 Other diseases of spleen
Fibrosis of spleen NOS
Perisplenitis
Splenitis NOS

D73.9 Disease of spleen, unspecified

● **D74 Methemoglobinemia**
Excessive methemoglobin (form of hemoglobin)

D74.Ø Congenital methemoglobinemia
Congenital NADH-methemoglobin reductase deficiency
Hemoglobin-M [Hb-M] disease
Methemoglobinemia, hereditary

D74.8 Other methemoglobinemias
Acquired methemoglobinemia (with sulfhemoglobinemia)
Toxic methemoglobinemia

D74.9 Methemoglobinemia, unspecified

● **D75 Other and unspecified diseases of blood and blood-forming organs**
Excludes2 acute lymphadenitis (LØ4.-)
chronic lymphadenitis (I88.1)
enlarged lymph nodes (R59.-)
hypergammaglobulinemia NOS (D89.2)
lymphadenitis NOS (I88.9)
mesenteric lymphadenitis (acute) (chronic) (I88.Ø)

D75.Ø Familial erythrocytosis
Genetic mutation of gene that results in increased circulating RBCs
Benign polycythemia
Familial polycythemia
Excludes1 hereditary ovalocytosis (D58.1)

D75.1 Secondary polycythemia
Increase in total red cell mass
Acquired polycythemia
Emotional polycythemia
Erythrocytosis NOS
Hypoxemic polycythemia
Nephrogenous polycythemia
Polycythemia due to erythropoietin
Polycythemia due to fall in plasma volume
Polycythemia due to high altitude
Polycythemia due to stress
Polycythemia NOS
Relative polycythemia
Excludes1 polycythemia neonatorum (P61.1)
polycythemia vera (D45)

● **D75.8 Other specified diseases of blood and blood-forming organs**

D75.81 Myelofibrosis
Replacing bone marrow by fibrous tissue
Myelofibrosis NOS
Secondary myelofibrosis NOS
Code first the underlying disorder, such as:
malignant neoplasm of breast (C5Ø.-)
Use additional code, if applicable, for associated therapy-related myelodysplastic syndrome (D46.-)
Use additional code for adverse effect, if applicable, to identify drug (T45.1X5)
Excludes1 acute myelofibrosis (C94.4-)
idiopathic myelofibrosis (D47.1)
leukoerythroblastic anemia (D61.82)
myelofibrosis with myeloid metaplasia (D47.4)
myelophthisic anemia (D61.82)
myelophthisis (D61.82)
primary myelofibrosis (D47.1)

D75.82 Heparin induced thrombocytopenia (HIT)

D75.89 Other specified diseases of blood and blood-forming organs

D75.9 Disease of blood and blood-forming organs, unspecified

● **D76 Other specified diseases with participation of lymphoreticular and reticulohistiocytic tissue**
Excludes1 (Abt-) Letterer-Siwe disease (C96.Ø)
eosinophilic granuloma (C96.6)
Hand-Schüller-Christian disease (C96.5)
histiocytic medullary reticulosis (C96.9) ◀
histiocytic sarcoma (C96.A)
histiocytosis X, multifocal (C96.5)
histiocytosis X, unifocal (C96.6)
Langerhans-cell histiocytosis, multifocal (C96.5)
Langerhans-cell histiocytosis NOS (C96.6)
Langerhans-cell histiocytosis, unifocal (C96.6)
leukemic reticuloendotheliosis (C91.4-) ◀
lipomelanotic reticulosis (I89.8) ◀
malignant histiocytosis (C96.A)
malignant reticulosis (C86.Ø) ◀
nonlipid reticuloendotheliosis (C96.Ø) ◀

D76.1 Hemophagocytic lymphohistiocytosis
Familial hemophagocytic reticulosis
Histiocytoses of mononuclear phagocytes

D76.2 Hemophagocytic syndrome, infection-associated
Use additional code to identify infectious agent or disease.

D76.3 Other histiocytosis syndromes
Reticulohistiocytoma (giant-cell)
Sinus histiocytosis with massive lymphadenopathy
Xanthogranuloma

D77 Other disorders of blood and blood-forming organs in diseases classified elsewhere
Code first underlying disease, such as:
amyloidosis (E85.-)
congenital early syphilis (A5Ø.Ø)
echinococcosis (B67.Ø-B67.9)
malaria (B5Ø.Ø-B54)
schistosomiasis [bilharziasis] (B65.Ø-B65.9)
vitamin C deficiency (E54)
Excludes1 rupture of spleen due to Plasmodium vivax malaria (B51.Ø)
splenitis, splenomegaly in late syphilis (A52.79)
splenitis, splenomegaly in tuberculosis (A18.85)

INTRAOPERATIVE AND POSTPROCEDURAL COMPLICATIONS OF THE SPLEEN (D78)

● **D78 Intraoperative and postprocedural complications of the spleen**

● **D78.0 Intraoperative hemorrhage and hematoma of the spleen complicating a procedure**

Excludes1 intraoperative hemorrhage and hematoma of the spleen due to accidental puncture or laceration during a procedure (D78.1-)

D78.01 Intraoperative hemorrhage and hematoma of the spleen complicating a procedure on the spleen

D78.02 Intraoperative hemorrhage and hematoma of the spleen complicating other procedure

● **D78.1 Accidental puncture and laceration of the spleen during a procedure**

D78.11 Accidental puncture and laceration of the spleen during a procedure on the spleen

D78.12 Accidental puncture and laceration of the spleen during other procedure

● **D78.2 Postprocedural hemorrhage of the spleen following a procedure** (Revised)

D78.21 Postprocedural hemorrhage of the spleen following a procedure on the spleen (Revised)

D78.22 Postprocedural hemorrhage of the spleen following other procedure (Revised)

● **D78.3 Postprocedural hematoma and seroma of the spleen following a procedure** ◀

D78.31 Postprocedural hematoma of the spleen following a procedure on the spleen ◀

D78.32 Postprocedural hematoma of the spleen following other procedure ◀

D78.33 Postprocedural seroma of the spleen following a procedure on the spleen ◀

D78.34 Postprocedural seroma of the spleen following other procedure ◀

● **D78.8 Other intraoperative and postprocedural complications of the spleen**

Use additional code, if applicable, to further specify disorder

D78.81 Other intraoperative complications of the spleen

D78.89 Other postprocedural complications of the spleen

CERTAIN DISORDERS INVOLVING THE IMMUNE MECHANISM (D80-D89)

Includes defects in the complement system
immunodeficiency disorders, except human immunodeficiency virus [HIV] disease
sarcoidosis

Excludes1 autoimmune disease (systemic) NOS (M35.9)
functional disorders of polymorphonuclear neutrophils (D71)
human immunodeficiency virus [HIV] disease (B20)

● **D80 Immunodeficiency with predominantly antibody defects**

D80.0 Hereditary hypogammaglobulinemia
Autosomal recessive agammaglobulinemia (Swiss type)
X-linked agammaglobulinemia [Bruton] (with growth hormone deficiency)

D80.1 Nonfamilial hypogammaglobulinemia
Abnormally low levels of all classes of immunoglobulins
Agammaglobulinemia with immunoglobulin-bearing B-lymphocytes
Common variable agammaglobulinemia [CVAgamma]
Hypogammaglobulinemia NOS

D80.2 Selective deficiency of immunoglobulin A [IgA]

D80.3 Selective deficiency of immunoglobulin G [IgG] subclasses

D80.4 Selective deficiency of immunoglobulin M [IgM]

D80.5 Immunodeficiency with increased immunoglobulin M [IgM]

D80.6 Antibody deficiency with near-normal immunoglobulins or with hyperimmunoglobulinemia
Abnormally high levels of immunoglobulins in serum

D80.7 Transient hypogammaglobulinemia of infancy

D80.8 Other immunodeficiencies with predominantly antibody defects
Kappa light chain deficiency

D80.9 Immunodeficiency with predominantly antibody defects, unspecified

● **D81 Combined immunodeficiencies**

Excludes1 autosomal recessive agammaglobulinemia (Swiss type) (D80.0)

D81.0 Severe combined immunodeficiency [SCID] with reticular dysgenesis

D81.1 Severe combined immunodeficiency [SCID] with low T- and B-cell numbers

D81.2 Severe combined immunodeficiency [SCID] with low or normal B-cell numbers

D81.3 Adenosine deaminase [ADA] deficiency

D81.4 Nezelof's syndrome

D81.5 Purine nucleoside phosphorylase [PNP] deficiency

D81.6 Major histocompatibility complex class I deficiency
Bare lymphocyte syndrome

D81.7 Major histocompatibility complex class II deficiency

● **D81.8 Other combined immunodeficiencies**

● **D81.81 Biotin-dependent carboxylase deficiency**
Multiple carboxylase deficiency

Excludes1 biotin-dependent carboxylase deficiency due to dietary deficiency of biotin (E53.8)

D81.810 Biotinidase deficiency

D81.818 Other biotin-dependent carboxylase deficiency
Holocarboxylase synthetase deficiency
Other multiple carboxylase deficiency

D81.819 Biotin-dependent carboxylase deficiency, unspecified
Multiple carboxylase deficiency, unspecified

D81.89 Other combined immunodeficiencies

D81.9 Combined immunodeficiency, unspecified
Severe combined immunodeficiency disorder [SCID] NOS

● **D82 Immunodeficiency associated with other major defects**

Excludes1 ataxia telangiectasia [Louis-Bar] (G11.3)

D82.0 Wiskott-Aldrich syndrome
X-linked immunodeficiency
Immunodeficiency with thrombocytopenia and eczema

D82.1 Di George's syndrome
Congenital disorder with defective development of third and fourth pharyngeal pouches
Pharyngeal pouch syndrome
Thymic alymphoplasia
Thymic aplasia or hypoplasia with immunodeficiency

D82.2 Immunodeficiency with short-limbed stature

D82.3 Immunodeficiency following hereditary defective response to Epstein-Barr virus
X-linked lymphoproliferative disease

D82.4 Hyperimmunoglobulin E [IgE] syndrome
Suspected genetic defect that produces high levels of antibody immunoglobulin (IgE) that causes skin and lung infections and eczema

D82.8 Immunodeficiency associated with other specified major defects

D82.9 Immunodeficiency associated with major defect, unspecified

CHAPTER 3 (D50-D89)

Item 3-1 Sarcoidosis: A symptom of an inflammation producing tiny lumps of cells (granulomas) in various organs, most commonly the lungs and lymph nodes, that affect organ function. Cause is unknown occurring primarily in 2Ø- to 4Ø-year-olds, African-American, especially women, and those of Asian, German, Irish, Scandinavian, and Puerto Rican heritage.

● **D83 Common variable immunodeficiency**
- **D83.Ø Common variable immunodeficiency with predominant abnormalities of B-cell numbers and function**
- **D83.1 Common variable immunodeficiency with predominant immunoregulatory T-cell disorders**
- **D83.2 Common variable immunodeficiency with autoantibodies to B- or T-cells**
- **D83.8 Other common variable immunodeficiencies**
- **D83.9 Common variable immunodeficiency, unspecified**

● **D84 Other immunodeficiencies**
- **D84.Ø Lymphocyte function antigen-1 [LFA-1] defect**
- **D84.1 Defects in the complement system**
  - C1 esterase inhibitor [C1-INH] deficiency
- **D84.8 Other specified immunodeficiencies**
- **D84.9 Immunodeficiency, unspecified**

● **D86 Sarcoidosis**
- **D86.Ø Sarcoidosis of lung**
- **D86.1 Sarcoidosis of lymph nodes**
- **D86.2 Sarcoidosis of lung with sarcoidosis of lymph nodes**
- **D86.3 Sarcoidosis of skin**
- ● **D86.8 Sarcoidosis of other sites**
  - **D86.81 Sarcoid meningitis**
  - **D86.82 Multiple cranial nerve palsies in sarcoidosis**
  - **D86.83 Sarcoid iridocyclitis**
    - *Rare large tumor with irregular surface of iris*
  - **D86.84 Sarcoid pyelonephritis**
    - *Systemic disease of unknown etiology characterized by chronic granulomatous inflammation with tissue destruction of pelvis kidney*
    - Tubulo-interstitial nephropathy in sarcoidosis
  - **D86.85 Sarcoid myocarditis**
  - **D86.86 Sarcoid arthropathy**
    - Polyarthritis in sarcoidosis
  - **D86.87 Sarcoid myositis**
    - *Granumloma of muscle*
  - **D86.89 Sarcoidosis of other sites**
    - Hepatic granuloma
    - Uveoparotid fever [Heerfordt]
- **D86.9 Sarcoidosis, unspecified**

● **D89 Other disorders involving the immune mechanism, not elsewhere classified**

Excludes1 hyperglobulinemia NOS (R77.1)
monoclonal gammopathy (of undetermined significance) (D47.2)

Excludes2 transplant failure and rejection (T86.-)

- **D89.Ø Polyclonal hypergammaglobulinemia**
  - Benign hypergammaglobulinemic purpura
  - Polyclonal gammopathy NOS
- **D89.1 Cryoglobulinemia**
  - *Cryoglobulin (proteins) in blood that precipitate temperatures below 98.6° F; usually symptomatic of underlying disease*
  - Cryoglobulinemic purpura
  - Cryoglobulinemic vasculitis
  - Essential cryoglobulinemia
  - Idiopathic cryoglobulinemia
  - Mixed cryoglobulinemia
  - Primary cryoglobulinemia
  - Secondary cryoglobulinemia
- **D89.2 Hypergammaglobulinemia, unspecified**
- **D89.3 Immune reconstitution syndrome**
  - Immune reconstitution inflammatory syndrome [IRIS]
  - Use additional code for adverse effect, if applicable, to identify drug (T36-T5Ø with fifth or sixth character 5)
- ● **D89.4 Mast cell activation syndrome and related disorders** ◀

  Excludes1 aggressive systemic mastocytosis (C96.2) ◀
  cutaneous mastocytosis (Q82.2) ◀
  indolent systemic mastocytosis (D47.Ø) ◀
  malignant mastocytoma (C96.2) ◀
  mast cell leukemia (C94.3-) ◀
  mastocytoma (D47.Ø) ◀
  systemic mastocytosis associated with a clonal hematologic non-mast cell lineage disease (SM-AHNMD) (D47.Ø) ◀

  - **D89.40 Mast cell activation, unspecified** ◀
    - Mast cell activation disorder, unspecified ◀
    - Mast cell activation syndrome, NOS ◀
  - **D89.41 Monoclonal mast cell activation syndrome** ◀
  - **D89.42 Idiopathic mast cell activation syndrome** ◀
  - **D89.43 Secondary mast cell activation** ◀
    - Secondary mast cell activation syndrome ◀
    - Code also underlying etiology, if known ◀
  - **D89.49 Other mast cell activation disorder** ◀
    - Other mast cell activation syndrome ◀
- ● **D89.8 Other specified disorders involving the immune mechanism, not elsewhere classified**
  - ● **D89.81 Graft-versus-host disease**
    - Code first *underlying cause, such as:*
      complications of transplanted organs and tissue (T86.-)
      complications of blood transfusion (T8Ø.89)
    - Use additional code to identify associated manifestations, such as:
      desquamative dermatitis (L3Ø.8)
      diarrhea (R19.7)
      elevated bilirubin (R17)
      hair loss (L65.9)
    - **D89.81Ø Acute graft-versus-host disease**
    - **D89.811 Chronic graft-versus-host disease**
    - **D89.812 Acute on chronic graft-versus-host disease**
    - **D89.813 Graft-versus-host disease, unspecified**
  - **D89.82 Autoimmune lymphoproliferative syndrome [ALPS]**
  - **D89.89 Other specified disorders involving the immune mechanism, not elsewhere classified**

    Excludes1 human immunodeficiency virus disease (B2Ø)
- **D89.9 Disorder involving the immune mechanism, unspecified**
  - Immune disease NOS

CHAPTER 4

ENDOCRINE, NUTRITIONAL AND METABOLIC DISEASES (EØØ-E89)

OGCR Chapter-Specific Coding Guidelines

4. Chapter 4: Endocrine, Nutritional, and Metabolic Diseases (EØØ-E89)

a. Diabetes mellitus

The diabetes mellitus codes are combination codes that include the type of diabetes mellitus, the body system affected, and the complications affecting that body system. As many codes within a particular category as are necessary to describe all of the complications of the disease may be used. They should be sequenced based on the reason for a particular encounter. Assign as many codes from categories EØ8 – E13 as needed to identify all of the associated conditions that the patient has.

1) Type of diabetes

The age of a patient is not the sole determining factor, though most type 1 diabetics develop the condition before reaching puberty. For this reason type 1 diabetes mellitus is also referred to as juvenile diabetes.

2) Type of diabetes mellitus not documented

If the type of diabetes mellitus is not documented in the medical record the default is E11.-, Type 2 diabetes mellitus.

3) Diabetes mellitus and the use of insulin oral hypoglycemics

If the documentation in a medical record does not indicate the type of diabetes but does indicate that the patient uses insulin, code E11, Type 2 diabetes mellitus, should be assigned. Code Z79.4, Long-term (current) use of insulin **or Z79.84, Long term (current) use of oral hypoglycemic drugs,** should also be assigned to indicate that the patient uses insulin **or hypoglycemic drugs**. Code Z79.4 should not be assigned if insulin is given temporarily to bring a type 2 patient's blood sugar under control during an encounter.

4) Diabetes mellitus in pregnancy and gestational diabetes

See Section I.C.15. Diabetes mellitus in pregnancy.
See Section I.C.15. Gestational (pregnancy induced) diabetes

5) Complications due to insulin pump malfunction

(a) Underdose of insulin due to insulin pump failure

An underdose of insulin due to an insulin pump failure should be assigned to a code from subcategory T85.6, Mechanical complication of other specified internal and external prosthetic devices, implants and grafts, that specifies the type of pump malfunction, as the principal or first-listed code, followed by code T38.3X6-, Underdosing of insulin and oral hypoglycemic [antidiabetic] drugs. Additional codes for the type of diabetes mellitus and any associated complications due to the underdosing should also be assigned.

(b) Overdose of insulin due to insulin pump failure

The principal or first-listed code for an encounter due to an insulin pump malfunction resulting in an overdose of insulin, should also be T85.6-, Mechanical complication of other specified internal and external prosthetic devices, implants and grafts, followed by code T38.3X1-, Poisoning by insulin and oral hypoglycemic [antidiabetic] drugs, accidental (unintentional).

6) Secondary diabetes mellitus

Codes under categories EØ8, Diabetes mellitus due to underlying condition, EØ9, Drug or chemical induced diabetes mellitus and E13, Other specified diabetes mellitus, identify complications/manifestations associated with secondary diabetes mellitus. Secondary diabetes is always caused by another condition or event (e.g., cystic fibrosis, malignant neoplasm of pancreas, pancreatectomy, adverse effect of drug, or poisoning).

(a) Secondary diabetes mellitus and the use of insulin or hypoglycemic drugs

For patients who routinely use insulin **or hypoglycemic drugs,** code Z79.4, Long-term (current) use of insulin **or Z79.84, Long term (current) use of oral hypoglycemic drugs,** should also be assigned. Code Z79.4 should not be assigned if insulin is given temporarily to bring a patient's blood sugar under control during an encounter.

(b) Assigning and sequencing secondary diabetes codes and its causes

The sequencing of the secondary diabetes codes in relationship to codes for the cause of the diabetes is based on the Tabular List instructions for categories EØ8, EØ9 and E13.

(i) Secondary diabetes mellitus due to pancreatectomy For postpancreatectomy diabetes mellitus (lack of insulin due to the surgical removal of all or part of the pancreas), assign code E89.1, Postprocedural hypoinsulinemia. Assign a code from category E13 and a code from subcategory Z9Ø.41-, Acquired absence of pancreas, as additional codes.

(ii) Secondary diabetes due to drugs Secondary diabetes may be caused by an adverse effect of correctly administered medications, poisoning or sequela of poisoning.

See section I.C.19.e for coding of adverse effects and poisoning, and section I.C.2Ø for external cause code reporting.

CHAPTER 4 (EØØ-E9Ø)

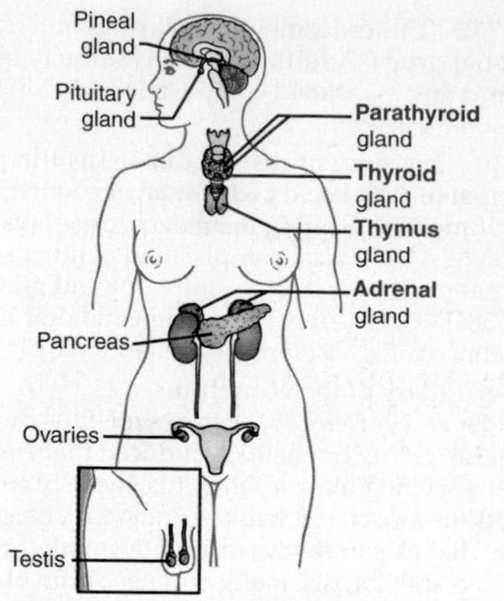

Figure 4-1 The endocrine system. (From Buck CJ: Step-by-Step Medical Coding, ed 2016, St. Louis, Elsevier, 2016)

CHAPTER 4

ENDOCRINE, NUTRITIONAL AND METABOLIC DISEASES (EØØ-E89)

All neoplasms, whether functionally active or not, are classified in Chapter 2. Appropriate codes in this chapter (i.e., EØ5.8, EØ7.Ø, E16-E31, E34.-) may be used as additional codes to indicate either functional activity by neoplasms and ectopic endocrine tissue or hyperfunction and hypofunction of endocrine glands associated with neoplasms and other conditions classified elsewhere.

Excludes1 transitory endocrine and metabolic disorders specific to newborn (P7Ø-P74)

This chapter contains the following blocks:

EØØ-EØ7	Disorders of thyroid gland
EØ8-E13	Diabetes mellitus
E15-E16	Other disorders of glucose regulation and pancreatic internal secretion
E2Ø-E35	Disorders of other endocrine glands
E36	Intraoperative complications of endocrine system
E4Ø-E46	Malnutrition
E5Ø-E64	Other nutritional deficiencies
E65-E68	Overweight, obesity and other hyperalimentation
E7Ø-E88	Metabolic disorders
E89	Postprocedural endocrine and metabolic complications and disorders, not elsewhere classified

DISORDERS OF THYROID GLAND (EØØ-EØ7)

● **EØØ Congenital iodine-deficiency syndrome**

Use additional code (F7Ø-F79) to identify associated intellectual disabilities.

Excludes1 subclinical iodine-deficiency hypothyroidism (EØ2)

EØØ.Ø Congenital iodine-deficiency syndrome, neurological type
Endemic cretinism, neurological type

EØØ.1 Congenital iodine-deficiency syndrome, myxedematous type
Dry, waxy type of swelling (nonpitting edema) with abnormal deposits of mucin in skin (mucinosis) and other tissues
Endemic hypothyroid cretinism
Endemic cretinism, myxedematous type

EØØ.2 Congenital iodine-deficiency syndrome, mixed type
Endemic cretinism, mixed type

EØØ.9 Congenital iodine-deficiency syndrome, unspecified
Congenital iodine-deficiency hypothyroidism NOS
Endemic cretinism NOS

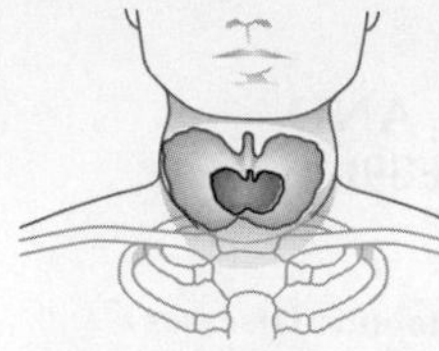

Figure 4-2 Goiter is an enlargement of the thyroid gland.

Item 4-1 Simple goiter indicates no nodules are present. The most common type of goiter is a **diffuse colloidal,** also called a **nontoxic** or **endemic** goiter.

● **EØ1 Iodine-deficiency related thyroid disorders and allied conditions**

Excludes1 congenital iodine-deficiency syndrome (EØØ.-)
subclinical iodine-deficiency hypothyroidism (EØ2)

EØ1.Ø Iodine-deficiency related diffuse (endemic) goiter
Thyroid gland is enlarged

EØ1.1 Iodine-deficiency related multinodular (endemic) goiter
Iodine-deficiency related nodular goiter

EØ1.2 Iodine-deficiency related (endemic) goiter, unspecified
Endemic goiter NOS

EØ1.8 Other iodine-deficiency related thyroid disorders and allied conditions
Acquired iodine-deficiency hypothyroidism NOS

EØ2 Subclinical iodine-deficiency hypothyroidism

● **EØ3 Other hypothyroidism**

Excludes1 iodine-deficiency related hypothyroidism (EØØ-EØ2)
postprocedural hypothyroidism (E89.Ø)

EØ3.Ø Congenital hypothyroidism with diffuse goiter
Congenital parenchymatous goiter (nontoxic)
Congenital goiter (nontoxic) NOS

Excludes1 transitory congenital goiter with normal function (P72.Ø)

EØ3.1 Congenital hypothyroidism without goiter
Aplasia of thyroid (with myxedema)
Congenital atrophy of thyroid
Congenital hypothyroidism NOS

EØ3.2 Hypothyroidism due to medicaments and other exogenous substances
Code first poisoning due to drug or toxin, if applicable (T36-T65 with fifth or sixth character 1-4 or 6)
Use additional code for adverse effect, if applicable, to identify drug (T36-T5Ø with fifth or sixth character 5)

EØ3.3 Postinfectious hypothyroidism

EØ3.4 Atrophy of thyroid (acquired)

Excludes1 congenital atrophy of thyroid (EØ3.1)

EØ3.5 Myxedema coma
Often fatal complication of long-term hypothyroidism

EØ3.8 Other specified hypothyroidism

EØ3.9 Hypothyroidism, unspecified
Myxedema NOS

Item 4-2 Hypothyroidism is a condition in which there are insufficient levels of thyroxine. **Cretinism** is congenital hypothyroidism, which can result in mental and physical retardation.

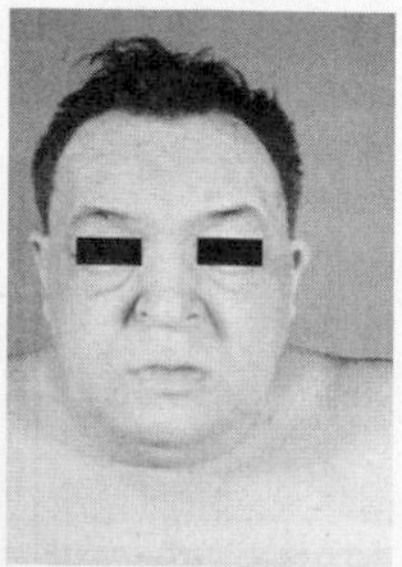

Figure 4-3 Typical appearance of patients with moderately severe primary hypothyroidism or myxedema. (From Larsen: Williams Textbook of Endocrinology, ed 10, Saunders, An Imprint of Elsevier, 2003)

● **E04 Other nontoxic goiter**

Excludes1 congenital goiter (NOS) (diffuse) (parenchymatous) (E03.0)
iodine-deficiency related goiter (E00-E02)

E04.0 Nontoxic diffuse goiter
Thyroid gland is enlarged
Diffuse (colloid) nontoxic goiter
Simple nontoxic goiter

E04.1 Nontoxic single thyroid nodule
Colloid nodule (cystic) (thyroid)
Nontoxic uninodular goiter
Thyroid (cystic) nodule NOS

E04.2 Nontoxic multinodular goiter
Enlarged thyroid gland with multiple nodules
Cystic goiter NOS
Multinodular (cystic) goiter NOS

E04.8 Other specified nontoxic goiter

E04.9 Nontoxic goiter, unspecified
Goiter NOS
Nodular goiter (nontoxic) NOS

● **E05 Thyrotoxicosis [hyperthyroidism]**
Enlarged thyroid gland with multiple nodules

Excludes1 chronic thyroiditis with transient thyrotoxicosis (E06.2)
neonatal thyrotoxicosis (P72.1)

● **E05.0 Thyrotoxicosis with diffuse goiter**
Exophthalmic or toxic goiter NOS
Graves' disease
Toxic diffuse goiter

E05.00 Thyrotoxicosis with diffuse goiter without thyrotoxic crisis or storm

E05.01 Thyrotoxicosis with diffuse goiter with thyrotoxic crisis or storm

● **E05.1 Thyrotoxicosis with toxic single thyroid nodule**
Thyrotoxicosis with toxic uninodular goiter

E05.10 Thyrotoxicosis with toxic single thyroid nodule without thyrotoxic crisis or storm

E05.11 Thyrotoxicosis with toxic single thyroid nodule with thyrotoxic crisis or storm

● **E05.2 Thyrotoxicosis with toxic multinodular goiter**
Toxic nodular goiter NOS

E05.20 Thyrotoxicosis with toxic multinodular goiter without thyrotoxic crisis or storm

E05.21 Thyrotoxicosis with toxic multinodular goiter with thyrotoxic crisis or storm

● **E05.3 Thyrotoxicosis from ectopic thyroid tissue**

E05.30 Thyrotoxicosis from ectopic thyroid tissue without thyrotoxic crisis or storm

E05.31 Thyrotoxicosis from ectopic thyroid tissue with thyrotoxic crisis or storm

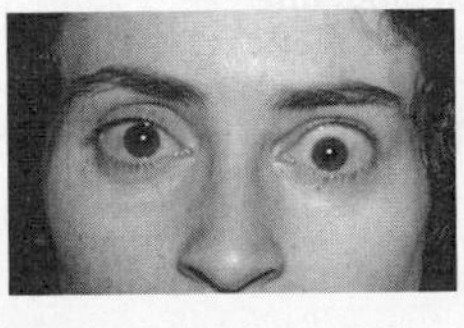

Figure 4-4 Graves' disease. In Graves' disease, exophthalmos often looks more pronounced than it actually is because of the extreme lid retraction that may occur. This patient, for instance, had minimal proptosis of the left eye but marked lid retraction.

(Courtesy Dr. HG Scheie. From Yanoff M, Fine BS: Ocular Pathology, ed 6, St. Louis, Mosby, 2008)

Item 4–3 Thyrotoxicosis is a condition caused by excessive amounts of the thyroid hormone thyroxine production or hyperthyroidism. **Graves' disease is associated with hyperthyroidism** (known as **Basedow's disease** in Europe).

● **E05.4 Thyrotoxicosis factitia**

E05.40 Thyrotoxicosis factitia without thyrotoxic crisis or storm

E05.41 Thyrotoxicosis factitia with thyrotoxic crisis or storm

● **E05.8 Other thyrotoxicosis**
Overproduction of thyroid-stimulating hormone

E05.80 Other thyrotoxicosis without thyrotoxic crisis or storm

E05.81 Other thyrotoxicosis with thyrotoxic crisis or storm

● **E05.9 Thyrotoxicosis, unspecified**
Hyperthyroidism NOS

E05.90 Thyrotoxicosis, unspecified without thyrotoxic crisis or storm

E05.91 Thyrotoxicosis, unspecified with thyrotoxic crisis or storm

● **E06 Thyroiditis**
An inflammation of the thyroid gland which results in an inability to convert iodine into thyroid hormone

Excludes1 postpartum thyroiditis (O90.5)

E06.0 Acute thyroiditis
Abscess of thyroid
Pyogenic thyroiditis
Suppurative thyroiditis
Use additional code (B95-B97) to identify infectious agent.

E06.1 Subacute thyroiditis
Inflammation of thyroid gland following viral upper respiratory infection
de Quervain thyroiditis
Giant-cell thyroiditis
Granulomatous thyroiditis
Nonsuppurative thyroiditis
Viral thyroiditis

Excludes1 autoimmune thyroiditis (E06.3)

E06.2 Chronic thyroiditis with transient thyrotoxicosis
Chronic inflammation of thyroid gland with intermittent overproduction of thyroid hormone

Excludes1 autoimmune thyroiditis (E06.3)

E06.3 Autoimmune thyroiditis
Hashimoto's thyroiditis
Hashitoxicosis (transient)
Lymphadenoid goiter
Lymphocytic thyroiditis
Struma lymphomatosa

E06.4 Drug-induced thyroiditis
Use additional code for adverse effect, if applicable, to identify drug (T36-T50 with fifth or sixth character 5)

E06.5 Other chronic thyroiditis
Chronic fibrous thyroiditis
Chronic thyroiditis NOS
Ligneous thyroiditis
Riedel thyroiditis

E06.9 Thyroiditis, unspecified

● **E07 Other disorders of thyroid**

E07.0 Hypersecretion of calcitonin
C-cell hyperplasia of thyroid
Hypersecretion of thyrocalcitonin

E07.1 Dyshormogenetic goiter
Group of several types of goiter resulting from enzyme defects in hormone synthesis
Familial dyshormogenetic goiter
Pendred's syndrome
Excludes1 transitory congenital goiter with normal function (P72.0)

● **E07.8 Other specified disorders of thyroid**

E07.81 Sick-euthyroid syndrome
Euthyroid sick-syndrome

E07.89 Other specified disorders of thyroid
Abnormality of thyroid-binding globulin
Hemorrhage of thyroid
Infarction of thyroid

E07.9 Disorder of thyroid, unspecified

OGCR Section I.C.4.a

Diabetes mellitus

The diabetes mellitus codes are combination codes that include the type of diabetes mellitus, body system affected, and the complications affecting that body system. As many codes within a particular category as are necessary to describe all of the complications of the disease may be used. They should be sequenced based on the reason for a particular visit. Assign as many codes from categories E08–E13 as needed to identify all of the associated conditions that the patient has.

DIABETES MELLITUS (E08-E13)

A metabolic disease that results in persistent hyperglycemia.

● **E08 Diabetes mellitus due to underlying condition**
Code first the underlying condition, such as:
congenital rubella (P35.0)
Cushing's syndrome (E24.-)
cystic fibrosis (E84.-)
malignant neoplasm (C00-C96)
malnutrition (E40-E46)
pancreatitis and other diseases of the pancreas (K85-K86.-)
Use additional code to identify control using: (Revised)
insulin (Z79.4) ◀
oral antidiabetic drugs (Z79.84) ◀
oral hypoglycemic drugs (Z79.84) ◀
Excludes1 drug or chemical induced diabetes mellitus (E09.-)
gestational diabetes (O24.4-)
neonatal diabetes mellitus (P70.2)
postpancreatectomy diabetes mellitus (E13.-)
postprocedural diabetes mellitus (E13.-)
secondary diabetes mellitus NEC (E13.-)
type 1 diabetes mellitus (E10.-)
type 2 diabetes mellitus (E11.-)

● **E08.0 Diabetes mellitus due to underlying condition with hyperosmolarity**

E08.00 Diabetes mellitus due to underlying condition with hyperosmolarity without nonketotic hyperglycemic-hyperosmolar coma (NKHHC)

E08.01 Diabetes mellitus due to underlying condition with hyperosmolarity with coma

● **E08.1 Diabetes mellitus due to underlying condition with ketoacidosis**

E08.10 Diabetes mellitus due to underlying condition with ketoacidosis without coma

E08.11 Diabetes mellitus due to underlying condition with ketoacidosis with coma

● **E08.2 Diabetes mellitus due to underlying condition with kidney complications**

E08.21 Diabetes mellitus due to underlying condition with diabetic nephropathy
Diabetes mellitus due to underlying condition with intercapillary glomerulosclerosis
Diabetes mellitus due to underlying condition with intracapillary glomerulonephrosis
Diabetes mellitus due to underlying condition with Kimmelstiel-Wilson disease

E08.22 Diabetes mellitus due to underlying condition with diabetic chronic kidney disease
Use additional code to identify stage of chronic kidney disease (N18.1-N18.6)

E08.29 Diabetes mellitus due to underlying condition with other diabetic kidney complication
Renal tubular degeneration in diabetes mellitus due to underlying condition

● **E08.3 Diabetes mellitus due to underlying condition with ophthalmic complications**
Changes in blood vessels of retina in which blood vessels swell and leak fluid into retinal surface.

● **E08.31 Diabetes mellitus due to underlying condition with unspecified diabetic retinopathy**

E08.311 Diabetes mellitus due to underlying condition with unspecified diabetic retinopathy with macular edema

E08.319 Diabetes mellitus due to underlying condition with unspecified diabetic retinopathy without macular edema

● **E08.32 Diabetes mellitus due to underlying condition with mild nonproliferative diabetic retinopathy**
Diabetes mellitus due to underlying condition with nonproliferative diabetic retinopathy NOS
One of the following 7th characters is to be assigned to codes in subcategory E08.32 to designate laterality of the disease: ◀

1	right eye ◀
2	left eye ◀
3	bilateral ◀
9	unspecified eye ◀

● **E08.321 Diabetes mellitus due to underlying condition with mild nonproliferative diabetic retinopathy with macular edema**

● **E08.329 Diabetes mellitus due to underlying condition with mild nonproliferative diabetic retinopathy without macular edema**

● **E08.33 Diabetes mellitus due to underlying condition with moderate nonproliferative diabetic retinopathy**
One of the following 7th characters is to be assigned to codes in subcategory E08.33 to designate laterality of the disease: ◀

1	right eye ◀
2	left eye ◀
3	bilateral ◀
9	unspecified eye ◀

● **E08.331 Diabetes mellitus due to underlying condition with moderate nonproliferative diabetic retinopathy with macular edema**

● **E08.339 Diabetes mellitus due to underlying condition with moderate nonproliferative diabetic retinopathy without macular edema**

● E08.34 **Diabetes mellitus due to underlying condition with severe nonproliferative diabetic retinopathy**

One of the following 7th characters is to be assigned to codes in subcategory E08.34 to designate laterality of the disease: ◀

1	right eye ◀
2	left eye ◀
3	bilateral ◀
9	unspecified eye ◀

● E08.341 **Diabetes mellitus due to underlying condition with severe nonproliferative diabetic retinopathy with macular edema**

● E08.349 **Diabetes mellitus due to underlying condition with severe nonproliferative diabetic retinopathy without macular edema**

● E08.35 **Diabetes mellitus due to underlying condition with proliferative diabetic retinopathy**

One of the following 7th characters is to be assigned to codes in subcategory E08.35 to designate laterality of the disease: ◀

1	right eye ◀
2	left eye ◀
3	bilateral ◀
9	unspecified eye ◀

● E08.351 **Diabetes mellitus due to underlying condition with proliferative diabetic retinopathy with macular edema**

● E08.352 **Diabetes mellitus due to underlying condition with proliferative diabetic retinopathy with traction retinal detachment involving the macula** ◀

● E08.353 **Diabetes mellitus due to underlying condition with proliferative diabetic retinopathy with traction retinal detachment not involving the macula** ◀

● E08.354 **Diabetes mellitus due to underlying condition with proliferative diabetic retinopathy with combined traction retinal detachment and rhegmatogenous retinal detachment** ◀

● E08.355 **Diabetes mellitus due to underlying condition with stable proliferative diabetic retinopathy** ◀

● E08.359 **Diabetes mellitus due to underlying condition with proliferative diabetic retinopathy without macular edema**

E08.36 **Diabetes mellitus due to underlying condition with diabetic cataract**

X● E08.37 **Diabetes mellitus due to underlying condition with diabetic macular edema, resolved following treatment** ◀

One of the following 7th characters is to be assigned to code E08.37 to designate laterality of the disease: ◀

1	right eye ◀
2	left eye ◀
3	bilateral ◀
9	unspecified eye ◀

E08.39 **Diabetes mellitus due to underlying condition with other diabetic ophthalmic complication**

Use additional code to identify manifestation, such as:
diabetic glaucoma (H40-H42)

● E08.4 **Diabetes mellitus due to underlying condition with neurological complications**

E08.40 **Diabetes mellitus due to underlying condition with diabetic neuropathy, unspecified**

E08.41 **Diabetes mellitus due to underlying condition with diabetic mononeuropathy**

E08.42 **Diabetes mellitus due to underlying condition with diabetic polyneuropathy**
Diabetes mellitus due to underlying condition with diabetic neuralgia

E08.43 **Diabetes mellitus due to underlying condition with diabetic autonomic (poly)neuropathy**
Diabetes mellitus due to underlying condition with diabetic gastroparesis

E08.44 **Diabetes mellitus due to underlying condition with diabetic amyotrophy**

E08.49 **Diabetes mellitus due to underlying condition with other diabetic neurological complication**

● E08.5 **Diabetes mellitus due to underlying condition with circulatory complications**

E08.51 **Diabetes mellitus due to underlying condition with diabetic peripheral angiopathy without gangrene**

E08.52 **Diabetes mellitus due to underlying condition with diabetic peripheral angiopathy with gangrene**
Diabetes mellitus due to underlying condition with diabetic gangrene

E08.59 **Diabetes mellitus due to underlying condition with other circulatory complications**

● E08.6 **Diabetes mellitus due to underlying condition with other specified complications**

● E08.61 **Diabetes mellitus due to underlying condition with diabetic arthropathy**

E08.610 **Diabetes mellitus due to underlying condition with diabetic neuropathic arthropathy**
Diabetes mellitus due to underlying condition with Charcôt's joints

E08.618 **Diabetes mellitus due to underlying condition with other diabetic arthropathy**

● E08.62 **Diabetes mellitus due to underlying condition with skin complications**

E08.620 **Diabetes mellitus due to underlying condition with diabetic dermatitis**
Diabetes mellitus due to underlying condition with diabetic necrobiosis lipoidica

E08.621 **Diabetes mellitus due to underlying condition with foot ulcer**
Use additional code to identify site of ulcer (L97.4-, L97.5-)

E08.622 **Diabetes mellitus due to underlying condition with other skin ulcer**
Use additional code to identify site of ulcer (L97.1-L97.9, L98.41-L98.49)

E08.628 **Diabetes mellitus due to underlying condition with other skin complications**

● E08.63 **Diabetes mellitus due to underlying condition with oral complications**

E08.630 **Diabetes mellitus due to underlying condition with periodontal disease**

E08.638 **Diabetes mellitus due to underlying condition with other oral complications**

● **E08.64 Diabetes mellitus due to underlying condition with hypoglycemia**

E08.641 Diabetes mellitus due to underlying condition with hypoglycemia with coma

E08.649 Diabetes mellitus due to underlying condition with hypoglycemia without coma

E08.65 Diabetes mellitus due to underlying condition with hyperglycemia

E08.69 Diabetes mellitus due to underlying condition with other specified complication

Use additional code to identify complication

E08.8 Diabetes mellitus due to underlying condition with unspecified complications

E08.9 Diabetes mellitus due to underlying condition without complications

● **E09 Drug or chemical induced diabetes mellitus**

Code first poisoning due to drug or toxin, if applicable (T36-T65 with fifth or sixth character 1-4 or 6)

Use additional code for adverse effect, if applicable, to identify drug (T36-T50 with fifth or sixth character 5)

Use additional code to identify control using: ◀
- insulin (Z79.4) ◀
- oral antidiabetic drugs (Z79.84) ◀
- oral hypoglycemic drugs (Z79.84) ◀

Excludes1 diabetes mellitus due to underlying condition (E08.-)
- gestational diabetes (O24.4-)
- neonatal diabetes mellitus (P70.2)
- postpancreatectomy diabetes mellitus (E13.-)
- postprocedural diabetes mellitus (E13.-)
- secondary diabetes mellitus NEC (E13.-)
- type 1 diabetes mellitus (E10.-)
- type 2 diabetes mellitus (E11.-)

● **E09.0 Drug or chemical induced diabetes mellitus with hyperosmolarity**

E09.00 Drug or chemical induced diabetes mellitus with hyperosmolarity without nonketotic hyperglycemic-hyperosmolar coma (NKHHC)

E09.01 Drug or chemical induced diabetes mellitus with hyperosmolarity with coma

● **E09.1 Drug or chemical induced diabetes mellitus with ketoacidosis**

E09.10 Drug or chemical induced diabetes mellitus with ketoacidosis without coma

E09.11 Drug or chemical induced diabetes mellitus with ketoacidosis with coma

● **E09.2 Drug or chemical induced diabetes mellitus with kidney complications**

E09.21 Drug or chemical induced diabetes mellitus with diabetic nephropathy

Drug or chemical induced diabetes mellitus with intercapillary glomerulosclerosis

Drug or chemical induced diabetes mellitus with intracapillary glomerulonephrosis

Drug or chemical induced diabetes mellitus with Kimmelstiel-Wilson disease

E09.22 Drug or chemical induced diabetes mellitus with diabetic chronic kidney disease

Use additional code to identify stage of chronic kidney disease (N18.1-N18.6)

E09.29 Drug or chemical induced diabetes mellitus with other diabetic kidney complication

Drug or chemical induced diabetes mellitus with renal tubular degeneration

● **E09.3 Drug or chemical induced diabetes mellitus with ophthalmic complications**

● **E09.31 Drug or chemical induced diabetes mellitus with unspecified diabetic retinopathy**

E09.311 Drug or chemical induced diabetes mellitus with unspecified diabetic retinopathy with macular edema

E09.319 Drug or chemical induced diabetes mellitus with unspecified diabetic retinopathy without macular edema

● **E09.32 Drug or chemical induced diabetes mellitus with mild nonproliferative diabetic retinopathy**

Drug or chemical induced diabetes mellitus with nonproliferative diabetic retinopathy NOS

One of the following 7th characters is to be assigned to codes in subcategory E09.32 to designate laterality of the disease: ◀

1	right eye ◀
2	left eye ◀
3	bilateral ◀
9	unspecified eye ◀

● **E09.321 Drug or chemical induced diabetes mellitus with mild nonproliferative diabetic retinopathy with macular edema**

● **E09.329 Drug or chemical induced diabetes mellitus with mild nonproliferative diabetic retinopathy without macular edema**

● **E09.33 Drug or chemical induced diabetes mellitus with moderate nonproliferative diabetic retinopathy**

One of the following 7th characters is to be assigned to codes in subcategory E09.33 to designate laterality of the disease: ◀

1	right eye ◀
2	left eye ◀
3	bilateral ◀
9	unspecified eye ◀

● **E09.331 Drug or chemical induced diabetes mellitus with moderate nonproliferative diabetic retinopathy with macular edema**

● **E09.339 Drug or chemical induced diabetes mellitus with moderate nonproliferative diabetic retinopathy without macular edema**

● **E09.34 Drug or chemical induced diabetes mellitus with severe nonproliferative diabetic retinopathy**

One of the following 7th characters is to be assigned to codes in subcategory E09.34 to designate laterality of the disease: ◀

1	right eye ◀
2	left eye ◀
3	bilateral ◀
9	unspecified eye ◀

● **E09.341 Drug or chemical induced diabetes mellitus with severe nonproliferative diabetic retinopathy with macular edema**

● **E09.349 Drug or chemical induced diabetes mellitus with severe nonproliferative diabetic retinopathy without macular edema**

● EØ9.35 **Drug or chemical induced diabetes mellitus with proliferative diabetic retinopathy**

One of the following 7th characters is to be assigned to codes in subcategory EØ9.35 to designate laterality of the disease: ◀

1	right eye ◀
2	left eye ◀
3	bilateral ◀
9	unspecified eye ◀

● EØ9.351 **Drug or chemical induced diabetes mellitus with proliferative diabetic retinopathy with macular edema**

● EØ9.352 **Drug or chemical induced diabetes mellitus with proliferative diabetic retinopathy with traction retinal detachment involving the macula** ◀

● EØ9.353 **Drug or chemical induced diabetes mellitus with proliferative diabetic retinopathy with traction retinal detachment not involving the macula** ◀

● EØ9.354 **Drug or chemical induced diabetes mellitus with proliferative diabetic retinopathy with combined traction retinal detachment and rhegmatogenous retinal detachment** ◀

● EØ9.355 **Drug or chemical induced diabetes mellitus with stable proliferative diabetic retinopathy** ◀

● EØ9.359 **Drug or chemical induced diabetes mellitus with proliferative diabetic retinopathy without macular edema**

EØ9.36 **Drug or chemical induced diabetes mellitus with diabetic cataract**

X● EØ9.37 **Drug or chemical induced diabetes mellitus with diabetic macular edema, resolved following treatment** ◀

One of the following 7th characters is to be assigned to code EØ9.37 to designate laterality of the disease: ◀

1	right eye ◀
2	left eye ◀
3	bilateral ◀
9	unspecified eye ◀

EØ9.39 **Drug or chemical induced diabetes mellitus with other diabetic ophthalmic complication**

Use additional code to identify manifestation, such as:
diabetic glaucoma (H4Ø-H42)

● EØ9.4 **Drug or chemical induced diabetes mellitus with neurological complications**

EØ9.4Ø **Drug or chemical induced diabetes mellitus with neurological complications with diabetic neuropathy, unspecified**

EØ9.41 **Drug or chemical induced diabetes mellitus with neurological complications with diabetic mononeuropathy**

EØ9.42 **Drug or chemical induced diabetes mellitus with neurological complications with diabetic polyneuropathy**

Drug or chemical induced diabetes mellitus with diabetic neuralgia

EØ9.43 **Drug or chemical induced diabetes mellitus with neurological complications with diabetic autonomic (poly)neuropathy**

Drug or chemical induced diabetes mellitus with diabetic gastroparesis

EØ9.44 **Drug or chemical induced diabetes mellitus with neurological complications with diabetic amyotrophy**

EØ9.49 **Drug or chemical induced diabetes mellitus with neurological complications with other diabetic neurological complication**

● EØ9.5 **Drug or chemical induced diabetes mellitus with circulatory complications**

EØ9.51 **Drug or chemical induced diabetes mellitus with diabetic peripheral angiopathy without gangrene**

EØ9.52 **Drug or chemical induced diabetes mellitus with diabetic peripheral angiopathy with gangrene**

Drug or chemical induced diabetes mellitus with diabetic gangrene

EØ9.59 **Drug or chemical induced diabetes mellitus with other circulatory complications**

● EØ9.6 **Drug or chemical induced diabetes mellitus with other specified complications**

● EØ9.61 **Drug or chemical induced diabetes mellitus with diabetic arthropathy**

EØ9.61Ø **Drug or chemical induced diabetes mellitus with diabetic neuropathic arthropathy**

Drug or chemical induced diabetes mellitus with Charcôt's joints

Progressive degeneration of weight-bearing joint

EØ9.618 **Drug or chemical induced diabetes mellitus with other diabetic arthropathy**

● EØ9.62 **Drug or chemical induced diabetes mellitus with skin complications**

EØ9.62Ø **Drug or chemical induced diabetes mellitus with diabetic dermatitis**

Drug or chemical induced diabetes mellitus with diabetic necrobiosis lipoidica

Necrotizing skin condition

EØ9.621 **Drug or chemical induced diabetes mellitus with foot ulcer**

Use additional code to identify site of ulcer (L97.4-, L97.5-)

EØ9.622 **Drug or chemical induced diabetes mellitus with other skin ulcer**

Use additional code to identify site of ulcer (L97.1-L97.9, L98.41-L98.49)

EØ9.628 **Drug or chemical induced diabetes mellitus with other skin complications**

● EØ9.63 **Drug or chemical induced diabetes mellitus with oral complications**

EØ9.63Ø **Drug or chemical induced diabetes mellitus with periodontal disease**

EØ9.638 **Drug or chemical induced diabetes mellitus with other oral complications**

● EØ9.64 **Drug or chemical induced diabetes mellitus with hypoglycemia**

EØ9.641 **Drug or chemical induced diabetes mellitus with hypoglycemia with coma**

EØ9.649 **Drug or chemical induced diabetes mellitus with hypoglycemia without coma**

EØ9.65 **Drug or chemical induced diabetes mellitus with hyperglycemia**

EØ9.69 **Drug or chemical induced diabetes mellitus with other specified complication**

Use additional code to identify complication

EØ9.8 **Drug or chemical induced diabetes mellitus with unspecified complications**

EØ9.9 **Drug or chemical induced diabetes mellitus without complications**

● **E1Ø Type 1 diabetes mellitus**

Includes brittle diabetes (mellitus)
diabetes (mellitus) due to autoimmune process
diabetes (mellitus) due to immune mediated pancreatic islet beta-cell destruction
idiopathic diabetes (mellitus)
juvenile onset diabetes (mellitus)
ketosis-prone diabetes (mellitus)

Excludes1 diabetes mellitus due to underlying condition (EØ8.-)
drug or chemical induced diabetes mellitus (EØ9.-)
gestational diabetes (O24.4-)
hyperglycemia NOS (R73.9)
neonatal diabetes mellitus (P7Ø.2)
postpancreatectomy diabetes mellitus (E13.-)
postprocedural diabetes mellitus (E13.-)
secondary diabetes mellitus NEC (E13.-)
type 2 diabetes mellitus (E11.-)

● **E1Ø.1 Type 1 diabetes mellitus with ketoacidosis**
Acidosis accompanied by accumulation of ketone bodies (ketosis) in body tissues and fluids

E1Ø.1Ø Type 1 diabetes mellitus with ketoacidosis without coma

E1Ø.11 Type 1 diabetes mellitus with ketoacidosis with coma

● **E1Ø.2 Type 1 diabetes mellitus with kidney complications**

E1Ø.21 Type 1 diabetes mellitus with diabetic nephropathy
Type 1 diabetes mellitus with intercapillary glomerulosclerosis
Type 1 diabetes mellitus with intracapillary glomerulonephrosis
Type 1 diabetes mellitus with Kimmelstiel-Wilson disease

E1Ø.22 Type 1 diabetes mellitus with diabetic chronic kidney disease
Use additional code to identify stage of chronic kidney disease (N18.1-N18.6)

E1Ø.29 Type 1 diabetes mellitus with other diabetic kidney complication
Type 1 diabetes mellitus with renal tubular degeneration

● **E1Ø.3 Type 1 diabetes mellitus with ophthalmic complications**

● **E1Ø.31 Type 1 diabetes mellitus with unspecified diabetic retinopathy**

E1Ø.311 Type 1 diabetes mellitus with unspecified diabetic retinopathy with macular edema

E1Ø.319 Type 1 diabetes mellitus with unspecified diabetic retinopathy without macular edema

● **E1Ø.32 Type 1 diabetes mellitus with mild nonproliferative diabetic retinopathy**
Type 1 diabetes mellitus with nonproliferative diabetic retinopathy NOS
One of the following 7th characters is to be assigned to codes in subcategory E1Ø.32 to designate laterality of the disease: ◄

1 right eye ◄
2 left eye ◄
3 bilateral ◄
9 unspecified eye ◄

● **E1Ø.321 Type 1 diabetes mellitus with mild nonproliferative diabetic retinopathy with macular edema**

● **E1Ø.329 Type 1 diabetes mellitus with mild nonproliferative diabetic retinopathy without macular edema**

● **E1Ø.33 Type 1 diabetes mellitus with moderate nonproliferative diabetic retinopathy**
One of the following 7th characters is to be assigned to codes in subcategory E1Ø.33 to designate laterality of the disease: ◄

1 right eye ◄
2 left eye ◄
3 bilateral ◄
9 unspecified eye ◄

● **E1Ø.331 Type 1 diabetes mellitus with moderate nonproliferative diabetic retinopathy with macular edema**

● **E1Ø.339 Type 1 diabetes mellitus with moderate nonproliferative diabetic retinopathy without macular edema**

● **E1Ø.34 Type 1 diabetes mellitus with severe nonproliferative diabetic retinopathy**
One of the following 7th characters is to be assigned to codes in subcategory E1Ø.34 to designate laterality of the disease: ◄

1 right eye ◄
2 left eye ◄
3 bilateral ◄
9 unspecified eye ◄

● **E1Ø.341 Type 1 diabetes mellitus with severe nonproliferative diabetic retinopathy with macular edema**

● **E1Ø.349 Type 1 diabetes mellitus with severe nonproliferative diabetic retinopathy without macular edema**

● **E1Ø.35 Type 1 diabetes mellitus with proliferative diabetic retinopathy**
One of the following 7th characters is to be assigned to codes in subcategory E1Ø.35 to designate laterality of the disease: ◄

1 right eye ◄
2 left eye ◄
3 bilateral ◄
9 unspecified eye ◄

● **E1Ø.351 Type 1 diabetes mellitus with proliferative diabetic retinopathy with macular edema**

● **E1Ø.352 Type 1 diabetes mellitus with proliferative diabetic retinopathy with traction retinal detachment involving the macula** ◄

● **E1Ø.353 Type 1 diabetes mellitus with proliferative diabetic retinopathy with traction retinal detachment not involving the macula** ◄

● **E1Ø.354 Type 1 diabetes mellitus with proliferative diabetic retinopathy with combined traction retinal detachment and rhegmatogenous retinal detachment** ◄

● **E1Ø.355 Type 1 diabetes mellitus with stable proliferative diabetic retinopathy** ◄

● **E1Ø.359 Type 1 diabetes mellitus with proliferative diabetic retinopathy without macular edema**

E10.36 Type 1 diabetes mellitus with diabetic cataract

X● **E10.37 Type 1 diabetes mellitus with diabetic macular edema, resolved following treatment** ◀

One of the following 7th characters is to be assigned to code E10.37 to designate laterality of the disease: ◀

1	right eye ◀
2	left eye ◀
3	bilateral ◀
9	unspecified eye ◀

E10.39 Type 1 diabetes mellitus with other diabetic ophthalmic complication

Use additional code to identify manifestation, such as:
diabetic glaucoma (H40-H42)

● **E10.4 Type 1 diabetes mellitus with neurological complications**

E10.40 Type 1 diabetes mellitus with diabetic neuropathy, unspecified

E10.41 Type 1 diabetes mellitus with diabetic mononeuropathy

E10.42 Type 1 diabetes mellitus with diabetic polyneuropathy

Type 1 diabetes mellitus with diabetic neuralgia

E10.43 Type 1 diabetes mellitus with diabetic autonomic (poly)neuropathy

Type 1 diabetes mellitus with diabetic gastroparesis

E10.44 Type 1 diabetes mellitus with diabetic amyotrophy

E10.49 Type 1 diabetes mellitus with other diabetic neurological complication

● **E10.5 Type 1 diabetes mellitus with circulatory complications**

E10.51 Type 1 diabetes mellitus with diabetic peripheral angiopathy without gangrene

E10.52 Type 1 diabetes mellitus with diabetic peripheral angiopathy with gangrene

Type 1 diabetes mellitus with diabetic gangrene

E10.59 Type 1 diabetes mellitus with other circulatory complications

● **E10.6 Type 1 diabetes mellitus with other specified complications**

● **E10.61 Type 1 diabetes mellitus with diabetic arthropathy**

E10.610 Type 1 diabetes mellitus with diabetic neuropathic arthropathy

Type 1 diabetes mellitus with Charcôt's joints

E10.618 Type 1 diabetes mellitus with other diabetic arthropathy

● **E10.62 Type 1 diabetes mellitus with skin complications**

E10.620 Type 1 diabetes mellitus with diabetic dermatitis

Type 1 diabetes mellitus with diabetic necrobiosis lipoidica

E10.621 Type 1 diabetes mellitus with foot ulcer

Use additional code to identify site of ulcer (L97.4-, L97.5-)

E10.622 Type 1 diabetes mellitus with other skin ulcer

Use additional code to identify site of ulcer (L97.1-L97.9, L98.41-L98.49)

E10.628 Type 1 diabetes mellitus with other skin complications

● **E10.63 Type 1 diabetes mellitus with oral complications**

E10.630 Type 1 diabetes mellitus with periodontal disease

E10.638 Type 1 diabetes mellitus with other oral complications

● **E10.64 Type 1 diabetes mellitus with hypoglycemia**

E10.641 Type 1 diabetes mellitus with hypoglycemia with coma

E10.649 Type 1 diabetes mellitus with hypoglycemia without coma

E10.65 Type 1 diabetes mellitus with hyperglycemia

E10.69 Type 1 diabetes mellitus with other specified complication

Use additional code to identify complication
Use this code with E10.65 to report hyperosmolarity in a Type 1 patient

E10.8 Type 1 diabetes mellitus with unspecified complications

E10.9 Type 1 diabetes mellitus without complications

● **E11 Type 2 diabetes mellitus**

Includes diabetes (mellitus) due to insulin secretory defect
diabetes NOS
insulin resistant diabetes (mellitus)

Use additional code to identify control using: ⬅
insulin (Z79.4) ◀
oral antidiabetic drugs (Z79.84) ◀
oral hypoglycemic drugs (Z79.84) ◀

Excludes1 diabetes mellitus due to underlying condition (E08.-)
drug or chemical induced diabetes mellitus (E09.-)
gestational diabetes (O24.4-)
neonatal diabetes mellitus (P70.2)
postpancreatectomy diabetes mellitus (E13.-)
postprocedural diabetes mellitus (E13.-)
secondary diabetes mellitus NEC (E13.-)
type 1 diabetes mellitus (E10.-)

● **E11.0 Type 2 diabetes mellitus with hyperosmolarity**

E11.00 Type 2 diabetes mellitus with hyperosmolarity without nonketotic hyperglycemic-hyperosmolar coma (NKHHC)

E11.01 Type 2 diabetes mellitus with hyperosmolarity with coma

● **E11.2 Type 2 diabetes mellitus with kidney complications**

E11.21 Type 2 diabetes mellitus with diabetic nephropathy

Type 2 diabetes mellitus with intercapillary glomerulosclerosis
Type 2 diabetes mellitus with intracapillary glomerulonephrosis
Type 2 diabetes mellitus with Kimmelstiel-Wilson disease

E11.22 Type 2 diabetes mellitus with diabetic chronic kidney disease

Use additional code to identify stage of chronic kidney disease (N18.1-N18.6)

E11.29 Type 2 diabetes mellitus with other diabetic kidney complication

Type 2 diabetes mellitus with renal tubular degeneration

CHAPTER 4 (E00-E90)

● E11.3 **Type 2 diabetes mellitus with ophthalmic complications**

● E11.31 **Type 2 diabetes mellitus with unspecified diabetic retinopathy**

E11.311 **Type 2 diabetes mellitus with unspecified diabetic retinopathy with macular edema**

E11.319 **Type 2 diabetes mellitus with unspecified diabetic retinopathy without macular edema**

● E11.32 **Type 2 diabetes mellitus with mild nonproliferative diabetic retinopathy**

Type 2 diabetes mellitus with nonproliferative diabetic retinopathy NOS

One of the following 7th characters is to be assigned to codes in subcategory E11.32 to designate laterality of the disease: ◀

1	right eye ◀
2	left eye ◀
3	bilateral ◀
9	unspecified eye ◀

● E11.321 **Type 2 diabetes mellitus with mild nonproliferative diabetic retinopathy with macular edema**

● E11.329 **Type 2 diabetes mellitus with mild nonproliferative diabetic retinopathy without macular edema**

● E11.33 **Type 2 diabetes mellitus with moderate nonproliferative diabetic retinopathy**

One of the following 7th characters is to be assigned to codes in subcategory E11.33 to designate laterality of the disease: ◀

1	right eye ◀
2	left eye ◀
3	bilateral ◀
9	unspecified eye ◀

● E11.331 **Type 2 diabetes mellitus with moderate nonproliferative diabetic retinopathy with macular edema**

● E11.339 **Type 2 diabetes mellitus with moderate nonproliferative diabetic retinopathy without macular edema**

● E11.34 **Type 2 diabetes mellitus with severe nonproliferative diabetic retinopathy**

One of the following 7th characters is to be assigned to codes in subcategory E11.34 to designate laterality of the disease: ◀

1	right eye ◀
2	left eye ◀
3	bilateral ◀
9	unspecified eye ◀

● E11.341 **Type 2 diabetes mellitus with severe nonproliferative diabetic retinopathy with macular edema**

● E11.349 **Type 2 diabetes mellitus with severe nonproliferative diabetic retinopathy without macular edema**

● E11.35 **Type 2 diabetes mellitus with proliferative diabetic retinopathy**

One of the following 7th characters is to be assigned to codes in subcategory E11.35 to designate laterality of the disease: ◀

1	right eye ◀
2	left eye ◀
3	bilateral ◀
9	unspecified eye ◀

● E11.351 **Type 2 diabetes mellitus with proliferative diabetic retinopathy with macular edema**

● E11.352 **Type 2 diabetes mellitus with proliferative diabetic retinopathy with traction retinal detachment involving the macula** ◀

● E11.353 **Type 2 diabetes mellitus with proliferative diabetic retinopathy with traction retinal detachment not involving the macula** ◀

● E11.354 **Type 2 diabetes mellitus with proliferative diabetic retinopathy with combined traction retinal detachment and rhegmatogenous retinal detachment** ◀

● E11.355 **Type 2 diabetes mellitus with stable proliferative diabetic retinopathy** ◀

● E11.359 **Type 2 diabetes mellitus with proliferative diabetic retinopathy without macular edema**

E11.36 **Type 2 diabetes mellitus with diabetic cataract**

X● E11.37 **Type 2 diabetes mellitus with diabetic macular edema, resolved following treatment** ◀

One of the following 7th characters is to be assigned to code E11.37 to designate laterality of the disease: ◀

1	right eye ◀
2	left eye ◀
3	bilateral ◀
9	unspecified eye ◀

E11.39 **Type 2 diabetes mellitus with other diabetic ophthalmic complication**

Use additional code to identify manifestation, such as:

diabetic glaucoma (H40-H42)

● E11.4 **Type 2 diabetes mellitus with neurological complications**

E11.40 **Type 2 diabetes mellitus with diabetic neuropathy, unspecified**

E11.41 **Type 2 diabetes mellitus with diabetic mononeuropathy**

E11.42 **Type 2 diabetes mellitus with diabetic polyneuropathy**

Type 2 diabetes mellitus with diabetic neuralgia

E11.43 **Type 2 diabetes mellitus with diabetic autonomic (poly)neuropathy**

Type 2 diabetes mellitus with diabetic gastroparesis

E11.44 **Type 2 diabetes mellitus with diabetic amyotrophy**

E11.49 **Type 2 diabetes mellitus with other diabetic neurological complication**

CHAPTER 4 (E00-E90)

◀ New ⬅ Revised ~~deleted~~ Deleted OGCR Official Guidelines X Assign placeholder X ● Use Additional Character(s)

Excludes 1 | Excludes 2 | Includes | Use additional | Code first | Code also | Unspecified

● **E11.5 Type 2 diabetes mellitus with circulatory complications**

E11.51 Type 2 diabetes mellitus with diabetic peripheral angiopathy without gangrene

E11.52 Type 2 diabetes mellitus with diabetic peripheral angiopathy with gangrene

Type 2 diabetes mellitus with diabetic gangrene

E11.59 Type 2 diabetes mellitus with other circulatory complications

● **E11.6 Type 2 diabetes mellitus with other specified complications**

● **E11.61 Type 2 diabetes mellitus with diabetic arthropathy**

E11.610 Type 2 diabetes mellitus with diabetic neuropathic arthropathy

Type 2 diabetes mellitus with Charcôt's joints

E11.618 Type 2 diabetes mellitus with other diabetic arthropathy

● **E11.62 Type 2 diabetes mellitus with skin complications**

E11.620 Type 2 diabetes mellitus with diabetic dermatitis

Type 2 diabetes mellitus with diabetic necrobiosis lipoidica

E11.621 Type 2 diabetes mellitus with foot ulcer

Use additional code to identify site of ulcer (L97.4-, L97.5-)

E11.622 Type 2 diabetes mellitus with other skin ulcer

Use additional code to identify site of ulcer (L97.1-L97.9, L98.41-L98.49)

E11.628 Type 2 diabetes mellitus with other skin complications

● **E11.63 Type 2 diabetes mellitus with oral complications**

E11.630 Type 2 diabetes mellitus with periodontal disease

E11.638 Type 2 diabetes mellitus with other oral complications

● **E11.64 Type 2 diabetes mellitus with hypoglycemia**

E11.641 Type 2 diabetes mellitus with hypoglycemia with coma

E11.649 Type 2 diabetes mellitus with hypoglycemia without coma

E11.65 Type 2 diabetes mellitus with hyperglycemia

E11.69 Type 2 diabetes mellitus with other specified complication

Use additional code to identify complication

Use this code with E11.65 to report DKA in a Type 2 patient

E11.8 Type 2 diabetes mellitus with unspecified complications

E11.9 Type 2 diabetes mellitus without complications

● **E13 Other specified diabetes mellitus**

Includes diabetes mellitus due to genetic defects of beta-cell function
diabetes mellitus due to genetic defects in insulin action
postpancreatectomy diabetes mellitus
postprocedural diabetes mellitus
secondary diabetes mellitus NEC

Use additional code to identify control using: ◄
insulin (Z79.4) ◄
oral antidiabetic drugs (Z79.84) ◄
oral hypoglycemic drugs (Z79.84) ◄

Excludes1 diabetes (mellitus) due to autoimmune process (E10.-)
diabetes (mellitus) due to immune mediated pancreatic islet beta-cell destruction (E10.-)
diabetes mellitus due to underlying condition (E08.-)
drug or chemical induced diabetes mellitus (E09.-)
gestational diabetes (O24.4-)
neonatal diabetes mellitus (P70.2)
type 1 diabetes mellitus (E10.-) ◄
type 2 diabetes mellitus (E11.-)

● **E13.0 Other specified diabetes mellitus with hyperosmolarity**

E13.00 Other specified diabetes mellitus with hyperosmolarity without nonketotic hyperglycemic-hyperosmolar coma (NKHHC)

E13.01 Other specified diabetes mellitus with hyperosmolarity with coma

● **E13.1 Other specified diabetes mellitus with ketoacidosis**

E13.10 Other specified diabetes mellitus with ketoacidosis without coma

E13.11 Other specified diabetes mellitus with ketoacidosis with coma

● **E13.2 Other specified diabetes mellitus with kidney complications**

E13.21 Other specified diabetes mellitus with diabetic nephropathy

Other specified diabetes mellitus with intercapillary glomerulosclerosis
Other specified diabetes mellitus with intracapillary glomerulonephrosis
Other specified diabetes mellitus with Kimmelstiel-Wilson disease

E13.22 Other specified diabetes mellitus with diabetic chronic kidney disease

Use additional code to identify stage of chronic kidney disease (N18.1-N18.6)

E13.29 Other specified diabetes mellitus with other diabetic kidney complication

Other specified diabetes mellitus with renal tubular degeneration

● **E13.3 Other specified diabetes mellitus with ophthalmic complications**

● **E13.31 Other specified diabetes mellitus with unspecified diabetic retinopathy**

E13.311 Other specified diabetes mellitus with unspecified diabetic retinopathy with macular edema

E13.319 Other specified diabetes mellitus with unspecified diabetic retinopathy without macular edema

● **E13.32 Other specified diabetes mellitus with mild nonproliferative diabetic retinopathy**
Other specified diabetes mellitus with nonproliferative diabetic retinopathy NOS
One of the following 7th characters is to be assigned to codes in subcategory E13.32 to designate laterality of the disease: ◀

1	right eye ◀
2	left eye ◀
3	bilateral ◀
9	unspecified eye ◀

● **E13.321 Other specified diabetes mellitus with mild nonproliferative diabetic retinopathy with macular edema**

● **E13.329 Other specified diabetes mellitus with mild nonproliferative diabetic retinopathy without macular edema**

● **E13.33 Other specified diabetes mellitus with moderate nonproliferative diabetic retinopathy**
One of the following 7th characters is to be assigned to codes in subcategory E13.33 to designate laterality of the disease: ◀

1	right eye ◀
2	left eye ◀
3	bilateral ◀
9	unspecified eye ◀

● **E13.331 Other specified diabetes mellitus with moderate nonproliferative diabetic retinopathy with macular edema**

● **E13.339 Other specified diabetes mellitus with moderate nonproliferative diabetic retinopathy without macular edema**

● **E13.34 Other specified diabetes mellitus with severe nonproliferative diabetic retinopathy**
One of the following 7th characters is to be assigned to codes in subcategory E13.34 to designate laterality of the disease: ◀

1	right eye ◀
2	left eye ◀
3	bilateral ◀
9	unspecified eye ◀

● **E13.341 Other specified diabetes mellitus with severe nonproliferative diabetic retinopathy with macular edema**

● **E13.349 Other specified diabetes mellitus with severe nonproliferative diabetic retinopathy without macular edema**

● **E13.35 Other specified diabetes mellitus with proliferative diabetic retinopathy**
One of the following 7th characters is to be assigned to codes in subcategory E13.35 to designate laterality of the disease: ◀

1	right eye ◀
2	left eye ◀
3	bilateral ◀
9	unspecified eye ◀

● **E13.351 Other specified diabetes mellitus with proliferative diabetic retinopathy with macular edema**

● **E13.352 Other specified diabetes mellitus with proliferative diabetic retinopathy with traction retinal detachment involving the macula** ◀

● **E13.353 Other specified diabetes mellitus with proliferative diabetic retinopathy with traction retinal detachment not involving the macula** ◀

● **E13.354 Other specified diabetes mellitus with proliferative diabetic retinopathy with combined traction retinal detachment and rhegmatogenous retinal detachment** ◀

● **E13.355 Other specified diabetes mellitus with stable proliferative diabetic retinopathy** ◀

● **E13.359 Other specified diabetes mellitus with proliferative diabetic retinopathy without macular edema**

E13.36 Other specified diabetes mellitus with diabetic cataract

X● **E13.37 Other specified diabetes mellitus with diabetic macular edema, resolved following treatment**
One of the following 7th characters is to be assigned to code E13.37 to designate laterality of the disease: ◀

1	right eye ◀
2	left eye ◀
3	bilateral ◀
9	unspecified eye ◀

E13.39 Other specified diabetes mellitus with other diabetic ophthalmic complication
Use additional code to identify manifestation, such as:
diabetic glaucoma (H40-H42)

● **E13.4 Other specified diabetes mellitus with neurological complications**

E13.40 Other specified diabetes mellitus with diabetic neuropathy, unspecified

E13.41 Other specified diabetes mellitus with diabetic mononeuropathy

E13.42 Other specified diabetes mellitus with diabetic polyneuropathy
Other specified diabetes mellitus with diabetic neuralgia

E13.43 Other specified diabetes mellitus with diabetic autonomic (poly)neuropathy
Other specified diabetes mellitus with diabetic gastroparesis

E13.44 Other specified diabetes mellitus with diabetic amyotrophy

E13.49 Other specified diabetes mellitus with other diabetic neurological complication

● **E13.5 Other specified diabetes mellitus with circulatory complications**

E13.51 Other specified diabetes mellitus with diabetic peripheral angiopathy without gangrene

E13.52 Other specified diabetes mellitus with diabetic peripheral angiopathy with gangrene
Other specified diabetes mellitus with diabetic gangrene

E13.59 Other specified diabetes mellitus with other circulatory complications

● **E13.6 Other specified diabetes mellitus with other specified complications**

● **E13.61 Other specified diabetes mellitus with diabetic arthropathy**

E13.610 Other specified diabetes mellitus with diabetic neuropathic arthropathy
Other specified diabetes mellitus with Charcôt's joints

E13.618 Other specified diabetes mellitus with other diabetic arthropathy

● **E13.62 Other specified diabetes mellitus with skin complications**

E13.620 Other specified diabetes mellitus with diabetic dermatitis

Other specified diabetes mellitus with diabetic necrobiosis lipoidica

E13.621 Other specified diabetes mellitus with foot ulcer

Use additional code to identify site of ulcer (L97.4-, L97.5-)

E13.622 Other specified diabetes mellitus with other skin ulcer

Use additional code to identify site of ulcer (L97.1-L97.9, L98.41-L98.49)

E13.628 Other specified diabetes mellitus with other skin complications

● **E13.63 Other specified diabetes mellitus with oral complications**

E13.630 Other specified diabetes mellitus with periodontal disease

E13.638 Other specified diabetes mellitus with other oral complications

● **E13.64 Other specified diabetes mellitus with hypoglycemia**

E13.641 Other specified diabetes mellitus with hypoglycemia with coma

E13.649 Other specified diabetes mellitus with hypoglycemia without coma

E13.65 Other specified diabetes mellitus with hyperglycemia

E13.69 Other specified diabetes mellitus with other specified complication

Use additional code to identify complication

E13.8 Other specified diabetes mellitus with unspecified complications

E13.9 Other specified diabetes mellitus without complications

OTHER DISORDERS OF GLUCOSE REGULATION AND PANCREATIC INTERNAL SECRETION (E15-E16)

E15 Nondiabetic hypoglycemic coma

Includes drug-induced insulin coma in nondiabetic
hyperinsulinism with hypoglycemic coma
hypoglycemic coma NOS

● **E16 Other disorders of pancreatic internal secretion**

E16.0 Drug-induced hypoglycemia without coma

Excludes1 diabetes with hypoglycemia without coma (E09.692) ◄

Use additional code for adverse effect, if applicable, to identify drug (T36-T50 with fifth or sixth character 5)

E16.1 Other hypoglycemia

Functional hyperinsulinism
Functional nonhyperinsulinemic hypoglycemia
Hyperinsulinism NOS
Hyperplasia of pancreatic islet beta cells NOS

Excludes1 diabetes with hypoglycemia (E08.649, E10.649, E11.649, E13.649) ◄
hypoglycemia in infant of diabetic mother (P70.1)
neonatal hypoglycemia (P70.4)

E16.2 Hypoglycemia, unspecified

Excludes1 diabetes with hypoglycemia (E08.649, E10.649, E11.649, E13.649) ◄

E16.3 Increased secretion of glucagon

Hyperplasia of pancreatic endocrine cells with glucagon excess

E16.4 Increased secretion of gastrin

Hypergastrinemia
Hyperplasia of pancreatic endocrine cells with gastrin excess
Zollinger-Ellison syndrome

E16.8 Other specified disorders of pancreatic internal secretion

Increased secretion from endocrine pancreas of growth hormone-releasing hormone
Increased secretion from endocrine pancreas of pancreatic polypeptide
Increased secretion from endocrine pancreas of somatostatin
Increased secretion from endocrine pancreas of vasoactive-intestinal polypeptide

E16.9 Disorder of pancreatic internal secretion, unspecified

Islet-cell hyperplasia NOS
Pancreatic endocrine cell hyperplasia NOS

DISORDERS OF OTHER ENDOCRINE GLANDS (E20-E35)

Excludes1 galactorrhea (N64.3)
gynecomastia (N62)

● **E20 Hypoparathyroidism**

Greatly reduced function of parathyroid glands; AKA parathyroid insufficiency

Excludes1 Di George's syndrome (D82.1)
postprocedural hypoparathyroidism (E89.2)
tetany NOS (R29.0)
transitory neonatal hypoparathyroidism (P71.4)

E20.0 Idiopathic hypoparathyroidism

Rare condition, unknown cause; short dwarf-like with round face

E20.1 Pseudohypoparathyroidism

Hereditary condition resembling hypoparathyroidism, but caused by inability to respond to parathyroid hormone

E20.8 Other hypoparathyroidism

E20.9 Hypoparathyroidism, unspecified

Parathyroid tetany

● **E21 Hyperparathyroidism and other disorders of parathyroid gland**

Excludes1 adult osteomalacia (M83.-)
ectopic hyperparathyroidism (E34.2)
familial hypocalciuric hypercalcemia (E83.52)
hungry bone syndrome (E83.81)
infantile and juvenile osteomalacia (E55.0)

E21.0 Primary hyperparathyroidism

Hyperplasia of parathyroid
Osteitis fibrosa cystica generalisata [von Recklinghausen's disease of bone]

E21.1 Secondary hyperparathyroidism, not elsewhere classified

Excludes1 secondary hyperparathyroidism of renal origin (N25.81)

E21.2 Other hyperparathyroidism

Tertiary hyperparathyroidism

Excludes1 familial hypocalciuric hypercalcemia (E83.52)

E21.3 Hyperparathyroidism, unspecified

E21.4 Other specified disorders of parathyroid gland

E21.5 Disorder of parathyroid gland, unspecified

Item 4–4 Hyperparathyroidism is an overactive parathyroid gland that secretes excessive parathormone, causing increased levels of circulating calcium. This results in a loss of calcium in the bone (osteoporosis).

Hypoparathyroidism is an underactive parathyroid gland that results in decreased levels of circulating calcium. The primary manifestation is **tetany,** a continuous muscle spasm.

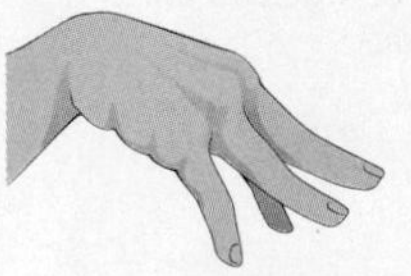

Figure 4-5 Tetany caused by hypoparathyroidism.

Item 4–5 Hyperadrenalism is overactivity of the adrenal cortex, which secretes corticosteroid hormones. Excessive glucocorticoid hormone results in hyperglycemia **(Cushing's syndrome),** and excessive aldosterone results in **Conn's syndrome. Adrenogenital syndrome** is the result of excessive secretion of androgens, male hormones, which stimulates premature sexual development. **Hypoadrenalism, Addison's disease,** is a condition in which the adrenal glands atrophy.

● **E22 Hyperfunction of pituitary gland**
 Excludes1 Cushing's syndrome (E24.-)
 Nelson's syndrome (E24.1)
 overproduction of ACTH not associated with Cushing's disease (E27.Ø)
 overproduction of pituitary ACTH (E24.Ø)
 overproduction of thyroid-stimulating hormone (EØ5.8-)

E22.Ø Acromegaly and pituitary gigantism
 Chronic disease caused by hypersecretion of growth hormone
 Overproduction of growth hormone
 Excludes1 constitutional gigantism (E34.4)
 constitutional tall stature (E34.4)
 increased secretion from endocrine pancreas of growth hormone-releasing hormone (E16.8)

E22.1 Hyperprolactinemia
 Increased levels of prolactin
 Use additional code for adverse effect, if applicable, to identify drug (T36-T5Ø with fifth or sixth character 5)

E22.2 Syndrome of inappropriate secretion of antidiuretic hormone

E22.8 Other hyperfunction of pituitary gland
 Central precocious puberty

E22.9 Hyperfunction of pituitary gland, unspecified

● **E23 Hypofunction and other disorders of the pituitary gland**
 Includes the listed conditions whether the disorder is in the pituitary or the hypothalamus
 Excludes1 postprocedural hypopituitarism (E89.3)

E23.Ø Hypopituitarism
 Fertile eunuch syndrome
 Hypogonadotropic hypogonadism
 Idiopathic growth hormone deficiency
 Isolated deficiency of gonadotropin
 Isolated deficiency of growth hormone
 Isolated deficiency of pituitary hormone
 Kallmann's syndrome
 Lorain-Levi short stature
 Necrosis of pituitary gland (postpartum)
 Panhypopituitarism
 Pituitary cachexia
 Pituitary insufficiency NOS
 Pituitary short stature
 Sheehan's syndrome
 Simmonds' disease

E23.1 Drug-induced hypopituitarism
 Use additional code for adverse effect, if applicable, to identify drug (T36-T5Ø with fifth or sixth character 5)

E23.2 Diabetes insipidus
 Excludes1 nephrogenic diabetes insipidus (N25.1)

E23.3 Hypothalamic dysfunction, not elsewhere classified
 Excludes1 Prader-Willi syndrome (Q87.1)
 Russell-Silver syndrome (Q87.1)

E23.6 Other disorders of pituitary gland
 Abscess of pituitary
 Adiposogenital dystrophy

E23.7 Disorder of pituitary gland, unspecified

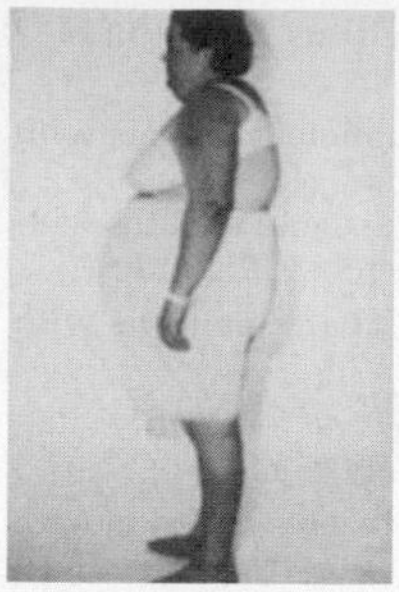

Figure 4-6 Centripetal and generalized obesity and dorsal kyphosis in a 3Ø-year-old woman with Cushing's disease. (From Larsen: Williams Textbook of Endocrinology, ed 10, Saunders, An Imprint of Elsevier, 2003)

● **E24 Cushing's syndrome**
 Excludes1 congenital adrenal hyperplasia (E25.Ø)

E24.Ø Pituitary-dependent Cushing's disease
 Overproduction of pituitary ACTH
 Pituitary-dependent hypercorticalism

E24.1 Nelson's syndrome

E24.2 Drug-induced Cushing's syndrome
 Use additional code for adverse effect, if applicable, to identify drug (T36-T5Ø with fifth or sixth character 5)

E24.3 Ectopic ACTH syndrome

E24.4 Alcohol-induced pseudo-Cushing's syndrome

E24.8 Other Cushing's syndrome

E24.9 Cushing's syndrome, unspecified

● **E25 Adrenogenital disorders**
 Disorder of production of steroid hormone in adrenal gland
 Includes adrenogenital syndromes, virilizing or feminizing, whether acquired or due to adrenal hyperplasia consequent on inborn enzyme defects in hormone synthesis
 female adrenal pseudohermaphroditism
 female heterosexual precocious pseudopuberty
 male isosexual precocious pseudopuberty
 male macrogenitosomia praecox
 male sexual precocity with adrenal hyperplasia
 male virilization (female)
 Excludes1 indeterminate sex and pseudohermaphroditism (Q56)
 chromosomal abnormalities (Q9Ø-Q99)

E25.Ø Congenital adrenogenital disorders associated with enzyme deficiency
 Congenital adrenal hyperplasia
 21-Hydroxylase deficiency
 Salt-losing congenital adrenal hyperplasia

E25.8 Other adrenogenital disorders
 Idiopathic adrenogenital disorder
 Use additional code for adverse effect, if applicable, to identify drug (T36-T5Ø with fifth or sixth character 5)

E25.9 Adrenogenital disorder, unspecified
 Adrenogenital syndrome NOS

● **E26 Hyperaldosteronism**
 Abnormality of electrolyte metabolism caused by excessive secretion of aldosterone

● **E26.Ø Primary hyperaldosteronism**

E26.Ø1 Conn's syndrome
 Code also adrenal adenoma (D35.Ø-)

E26.Ø2 Glucocorticoid-remediable aldosteronism
 Familial aldosteronism type I

E26.Ø9 Other primary hyperaldosteronism
 Primary aldosteronism due to adrenal hyperplasia (bilateral)

E26.1 Secondary hyperaldosteronism

● **E26.8 Other hyperaldosteronism**

E26.81 Bartter's syndrome

E26.89 Other hyperaldosteronism

E26.9 Hyperaldosteronism, unspecified
Aldosteronism NOS
Hyperaldosteronism NOS

● **E27 Other disorders of adrenal gland**

E27.0 Other adrenocortical overactivity
Overproduction of ACTH, not associated with Cushing's disease
Premature adrenarche
Excludes1 Cushing's syndrome (E24.-)

E27.1 Primary adrenocortical insufficiency
Addison's disease
Autoimmune adrenalitis
Excludes1 Addison only phenotype adrenoleukodystrophy (E71.528)
amyloidosis (E85.-)
tuberculous Addison's disease (A18.7)
Waterhouse-Friderichsen syndrome (A39.1)

E27.2 Addisonian crisis
Acute onset of adrenocortical insufficiency
Adrenal crisis
Adrenocortical crisis

E27.3 Drug-induced adrenocortical insufficiency
Use additional code for adverse effect, if applicable, to identify drug (T36-T50 with fifth or sixth character 5)

● **E27.4 Other and unspecified adrenocortical insufficiency**
Excludes1 adrenoleukodystrophy [Addison-Schilder] (E71.528)
Waterhouse-Friderichsen syndrome (A39.1)

E27.40 Unspecified adrenocortical insufficiency
Adrenocortical insufficiency NOS
Hypoaldosteronism

E27.49 Other adrenocortical insufficiency
Adrenal hemorrhage
Adrenal infarction

E27.5 Adrenomedullary hyperfunction
Adrenomedullary hyperplasia
Catecholamine hypersecretion

E27.8 Other specified disorders of adrenal gland
Abnormality of cortisol-binding globulin

E27.9 Disorder of adrenal gland, unspecified

● **E28 Ovarian dysfunction**
Excludes1 isolated gonadotropin deficiency (E23.0)
postprocedural ovarian failure (E89.4-)

E28.0 Estrogen excess
Use additional code for adverse effect, if applicable, to identify drug (T36-T50 with fifth or sixth character 5)

E28.1 Androgen excess
Hypersecretion of ovarian androgens
Use additional code for adverse effect, if applicable, to identify drug (T36-T50 with fifth or sixth character 5)

E28.2 Polycystic ovarian syndrome
Sclerocystic ovary syndrome
Stein-Leventhal syndrome

● **E28.3 Primary ovarian failure**
Excludes1 pure gonadal dysgenesis (Q99.1)
Turner's syndrome (Q96.-)

● **E28.31 Premature menopause**

E28.310 Symptomatic premature menopause
Symptoms such as flushing, sleeplessness, headache, lack of concentration, associated with premature menopause

E28.319 Asymptomatic premature menopause
Premature menopause NOS

E28.39 Other primary ovarian failure
Decreased estrogen
Resistant ovary syndrome

E28.8 Other ovarian dysfunction
Ovarian hyperfunction NOS
Excludes1 postprocedural ovarian failure (E89.4-)

E28.9 Ovarian dysfunction, unspecified

● **E29 Testicular dysfunction**
Excludes1 androgen insensitivity syndrome (E34.5-)
azoospermia or oligospermia NOS (N46.0-N46.1)
isolated gonadotropin deficiency (E23.0)
Klinefelter's syndrome (Q98.0-Q98.1, Q98.4) ◄

E29.0 Testicular hyperfunction
Hypersecretion of testicular hormones

E29.1 Testicular hypofunction
Defective biosynthesis of testicular androgen NOS
5-delta-Reductase deficiency (with male pseudohermaphroditism)
Testicular hypogonadism NOS
Use additional code for adverse effect, if applicable, to identify drug (T36-T50 with fifth or sixth character 5)
Excludes1 postprocedural testicular hypofunction (E89.5)

E29.8 Other testicular dysfunction

E29.9 Testicular dysfunction, unspecified

● **E30 Disorders of puberty, not elsewhere classified**

E30.0 Delayed puberty
Constitutional delay of puberty
Delayed sexual development

E30.1 Precocious puberty
Sexual maturation at earlier age than normal, or before age 8 in girls and 9 in boys, usually hormonal; AKA sexual precocity or pubertas praecox
Precocious menstruation
Excludes1 Albright (-McCune) (-Sternberg) syndrome (Q78.1)
central precocious puberty (E22.8)
congenital adrenal hyperplasia (E25.0)
female heterosexual precocious pseudopuberty (E25.-)
male isosexual precocious pseudopuberty (E25.-)

E30.8 Other disorders of puberty
Premature thelarche

E30.9 Disorder of puberty, unspecified

CHAPTER 4 (E00-E90)

● **E31 Polyglandular dysfunction**

Excludes1 ataxia telangiectasia [Louis-Bar] (G11.3)
dystrophia myotonica [Steinert] (G71.11)
pseudohypoparathyroidism (E20.1)

E31.0 Autoimmune polyglandular failure
Schmidt's syndrome

E31.1 Polyglandular hyperfunction
Excludes1 multiple endocrine adenomatosis (E31.2-)
multiple endocrine neoplasia (E31.2-)

● **E31.2 Multiple endocrine neoplasia [MEN] syndromes**
Adenomatous hyperplasia and malignant tumors in endocrine glands
Multiple endocrine adenomatosis
Code also any associated malignancies and other conditions associated with the syndromes

E31.20 Multiple endocrine neoplasia [MEN] syndrome, unspecified
Multiple endocrine adenomatosis NOS
Multiple endocrine neoplasia [MEN] syndrome NOS

E31.21 Multiple endocrine neoplasia [MEN] type I
Wermer's syndrome

E31.22 Multiple endocrine neoplasia [MEN] type IIA
Sipple's syndrome

E31.23 Multiple endocrine neoplasia [MEN] type IIB

E31.8 Other polyglandular dysfunction

E31.9 Polyglandular dysfunction, unspecified

● **E32 Diseases of thymus**

Excludes1 aplasia or hypoplasia of thymus with immunodeficiency (D82.1)
myasthenia gravis (G70.0)

E32.0 Persistent hyperplasia of thymus
Hypertrophy of thymus

E32.1 Abscess of thymus

E32.8 Other diseases of thymus
Excludes1 aplasia or hypoplasia with immunodeficiency (D82.1)
thymoma (D15.0)

E32.9 Disease of thymus, unspecified

● **E34 Other endocrine disorders**

Excludes1 pseudohypoparathyroidism (E20.1)

E34.0 Carcinoid syndrome
Note: May be used as an additional code to identify functional activity associated with a carcinoid tumor.

E34.1 Other hypersecretion of intestinal hormones

E34.2 Ectopic hormone secretion, not elsewhere classified
Excludes1 ectopic ACTH syndrome (E24.3)

E34.3 Short stature due to endocrine disorder
Constitutional short stature
Laron-type short stature
Excludes1 achondroplastic short stature (Q77.4)
hypochondroplastic short stature (Q77.4)
nutritional short stature (E45)
pituitary short stature (E23.0)
progeria (E34.8)
renal short stature (N25.0)
Russell-Silver syndrome (Q87.1)
short-limbed stature with immunodeficiency (D82.2)
short stature in specific dysmorphic syndromes - code to syndrome - see Alphabetical Index
short stature NOS (R62.52)

E34.4 Constitutional tall stature
Constitutional gigantism

● **E34.5 Androgen insensitivity syndrome**

E34.50 Androgen insensitivity syndrome, unspecified
Androgen insensitivity NOS

E34.51 Complete androgen insensitivity syndrome
Complete androgen insensitivity
de Quervain syndrome
Goldberg-Maxwell syndrome

E34.52 Partial androgen insensitivity syndrome
Partial androgen insensitivity
Reifenstein syndrome

E34.8 Other specified endocrine disorders
Pineal gland dysfunction
Progeria
Excludes2 pseudohypoparathyroidism (E20.1)

E34.9 Endocrine disorder, unspecified
Endocrine disturbance NOS
Hormone disturbance NOS

E35 Disorders of endocrine glands in diseases classified elsewhere

Code first underlying disease, such as:
late congenital syphilis of thymus gland [Dubois disease] (A50.5)
Use additional code, if applicable, to identify:
sequelae of tuberculosis of other organs (B90.8)
Excludes1 Echinococcus granulosus infection of thyroid gland (B67.3)
meningococcal hemorrhagic adrenalitis (A39.1)
syphilis of endocrine gland (A52.79)
tuberculosis of adrenal gland, except calcification (A18.7)
tuberculosis of endocrine gland NEC (A18.82)
tuberculosis of thyroid gland (A18.81)
Waterhouse-Friderichsen syndrome (A39.1)

INTRAOPERATIVE COMPLICATIONS OF ENDOCRINE SYSTEM (E36)

● **E36 Intraoperative complications of endocrine system**

Excludes2 postprocedural endocrine and metabolic complications and disorders, not elsewhere classified (E89.-)

● **E36.0 Intraoperative hemorrhage and hematoma of an endocrine system organ or structure complicating a procedure**
Excludes1 intraoperative hemorrhage and hematoma of an endocrine system organ or structure due to accidental puncture or laceration during a procedure (E36.1-)

E36.01 Intraoperative hemorrhage and hematoma of an endocrine system organ or structure complicating an endocrine system procedure

E36.02 Intraoperative hemorrhage and hematoma of an endocrine system organ or structure complicating other procedure

● **E36.1 Accidental puncture and laceration of an endocrine system organ or structure during a procedure**

E36.11 Accidental puncture and laceration of an endocrine system organ or structure during an endocrine system procedure

E36.12 Accidental puncture and laceration of an endocrine system organ or structure during other procedure

E36.8 Other intraoperative complications of endocrine system
Use additional code, if applicable, to further specify disorder

MALNUTRITION (E4Ø-E46)

Excludes1 intestinal malabsorption (K9Ø.-)
sequelae of protein-calorie malnutrition (E64.Ø)
Excludes2 nutritional anemias (D5Ø-D53)
starvation (T73.Ø)

E4Ø Kwashiorkor
Malnutrition produced by severe protein deficiency
Severe malnutrition with nutritional edema with dyspigmentation of skin and hair
Excludes1 marasmic kwashiorkor (E42)

E41 Nutritional marasmus
Severe malnutrition with marasmus
Excludes1 marasmic kwashiorkor (E42)

E42 Marasmic kwashiorkor
Severe protein malnutrition
Intermediate form severe protein-calorie malnutrition
Severe protein-calorie malnutrition with signs of both kwashiorkor and marasmus

E43 Unspecified severe protein-calorie malnutrition
Starvation edema

● **E44 Protein-calorie malnutrition of moderate and mild degree**
E44.Ø Moderate protein-calorie malnutrition
E44.1 Mild protein-calorie malnutrition

E45 Retarded development following protein-calorie malnutrition
Nutritional short stature
Nutritional stunting
Physical retardation due to malnutrition

E46 Unspecified protein-calorie malnutrition
Malnutrition NOS
Protein-calorie imbalance NOS
Excludes1 nutritional deficiency NOS (E63.9)

OTHER NUTRITIONAL DEFICIENCIES (E5Ø-E64)

Excludes2 nutritional anemias (D5Ø-D53)

● **E5Ø Vitamin A deficiency**
Excludes1 sequelae of vitamin A deficiency (E64.1)
E5Ø.Ø Vitamin A deficiency with conjunctival xerosis
E5Ø.1 Vitamin A deficiency with Bitot's spot and conjunctival xerosis
Bitot's spot in the young child
E5Ø.2 Vitamin A deficiency with corneal xerosis
E5Ø.3 Vitamin A deficiency with corneal ulceration and xerosis
E5Ø.4 Vitamin A deficiency with keratomalacia
Eye disorder that results in dry cornea caused by vitamin A deficiency
E5Ø.5 Vitamin A deficiency with night blindness
E5Ø.6 Vitamin A deficiency with xerophthalmic scars of cornea
Abnormal dryness and thickening of conjunctiva and cornea due to vitamin A deficiency
E5Ø.7 Other ocular manifestations of vitamin A deficiency
Xerophthalmia NOS
E5Ø.8 Other manifestations of vitamin A deficiency
Follicular keratosis
Xeroderma
E5Ø.9 Vitamin A deficiency, unspecified
Hypovitaminosis A NOS

● **E51 Thiamine deficiency**
Excludes1 sequelae of thiamine deficiency (E64.8)
● **E51.1 Beriberi**
E51.11 Dry beriberi
Thiamine deficiency with nervous system manifestation most often caused by excessive alcohol consumption
Beriberi NOS
Beriberi with polyneuropathy
E51.12 Wet beriberi
Thiamine deficiency with cardiovascular manifestation most often caused by excessive alcohol consumption
Beriberi with cardiovascular manifestations
Cardiovascular beriberi
Shoshin disease
E51.2 Wernicke's encephalopathy
Acute disease of brain due to thiamine deficiency most often associated with excessive alcohol consumption
E51.8 Other manifestations of thiamine deficiency
E51.9 Thiamine deficiency, unspecified

E52 Niacin deficiency [pellagra]
Niacin (-tryptophan) deficiency
Nicotinamide deficiency
Pellagra (alcoholic)
Excludes1 sequelae of niacin deficiency (E64.8)

● **E53 Deficiency of other B group vitamins**
Excludes1 sequelae of vitamin B deficiency (E64.8)
E53.Ø Riboflavin deficiency
Ariboflavinosis
Vitamin B2 deficiency
E53.1 Pyridoxine deficiency
Vitamin B6 deficiency
Excludes1 pyridoxine-responsive sideroblastic anemia (D64.3)
E53.8 Deficiency of other specified B group vitamins
Biotin deficiency
Cyanocobalamin deficiency
Folate deficiency
Folic acid deficiency
Pantothenic acid deficiency
Vitamin B12 deficiency
Excludes1 folate deficiency anemia (D52.-)
vitamin B12 deficiency anemia (D51.-)
E53.9 Vitamin B deficiency, unspecified

Item 4–6 Bitot's spots are the result of a buildup of keratin debris found on the superficial surface the conjunctiva; oval, triangular, or irregular in shape; and a sign of vitamin A deficiency and associated with night blindness. The disease may progress to **keratomalacia,** which can result in eventual prolapse of the iris and loss of the lens.

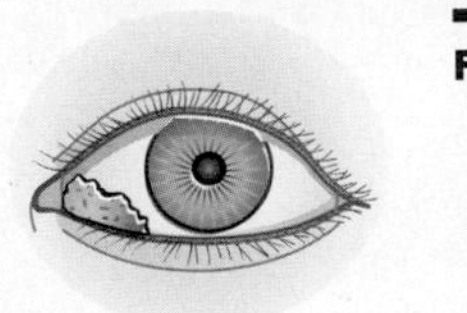

Figure 4-7 Bitot's spot on the conjunctiva.

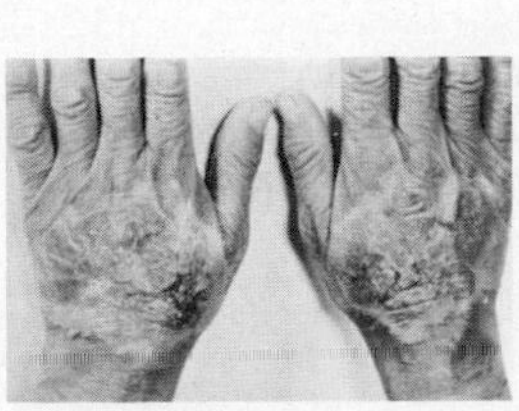

Figure 4-8 The sharply demarcated, characteristic scaling dermatitis of pellagra. (From Kumar: Robbins and Cotran: Pathologic Basis of Disease, ed 8, Saunders, An Imprint of Elsevier, 2009)

Item 4–7 Pellagra is associated with a deficiency of niacin and its precursor, **tryptophan.** Characteristics of the condition include diarrhea, dermatitis on exposed skin surfaces, dementia, and death. It is prevalent in developing countries where nutrition is inadequate. **Beriberi** is associated with thiamine deficiency.

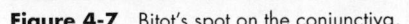

E54 Ascorbic acid deficiency
Deficiency of vitamin C
Scurvy
Excludes1 scorbutic anemia (D53.2)
sequelae of vitamin C deficiency (E64.2)

● **E55 Vitamin D deficiency**
Excludes1 adult osteomalacia (M83.-)
osteoporosis (M8Ø.-)
sequelae of rickets (E64.3)

E55.Ø Rickets, active
Infantile osteomalacia
Juvenile osteomalacia
Softening of bone
Excludes1 celiac rickets (K9Ø.Ø)
Crohn's rickets (K5Ø.-)
hereditary vitamin D-dependent rickets (E83.32)
inactive rickets (E64.3)
renal rickets (N25.Ø)
sequelae of rickets (E64.3)
vitamin D-resistant rickets (E83.31)

E55.9 Vitamin D deficiency, unspecified
Avitaminosis D

● **E56 Other vitamin deficiencies**
Excludes1 sequelae of other vitamin deficiencies (E64.8)

E56.Ø Deficiency of vitamin E
E56.1 Deficiency of vitamin K
Excludes1 deficiency of coagulation factor due to vitamin K deficiency (D68.4)
vitamin K deficiency of newborn (P53)
E56.8 Deficiency of other vitamins
E56.9 Vitamin deficiency, unspecified

E58 Dietary calcium deficiency
Excludes1 disorders of calcium metabolism (E83.5-)
sequelae of calcium deficiency (E64.8)

E59 Dietary selenium deficiency
Keshan disease
Excludes1 sequelae of selenium deficiency (E64.8)

E6Ø Dietary zinc deficiency

● **E61 Deficiency of other nutrient elements**
Use additional code for adverse effect, if applicable, to identify drug (T36-T5Ø with fifth or sixth character 5)
Excludes1 disorders of mineral metabolism (E83.-)
iodine deficiency related thyroid disorders (EØØ-EØ2)
sequelae of malnutrition and other nutritional deficiencies (E64.-)

E61.Ø Copper deficiency
E61.1 Iron deficiency
Excludes1 iron deficiency anemia (D5Ø.-)
E61.2 Magnesium deficiency
E61.3 Manganese deficiency
E61.4 Chromium deficiency
E61.5 Molybdenum deficiency
E61.6 Vanadium deficiency
E61.7 Deficiency of multiple nutrient elements
E61.8 Deficiency of other specified nutrient elements
E61.9 Deficiency of nutrient element, unspecified

● **E63 Other nutritional deficiencies**
Excludes1 dehydration (E86.Ø)
failure to thrive, adult (R62.7)
failure to thrive, child (R62.51)
feeding problems in newborn (P92.-)
sequelae of malnutrition and other nutritional deficiencies (E64.-)

E63.Ø Essential fatty acid [EFA] deficiency
E63.1 Imbalance of constituents of food intake
E63.8 Other specified nutritional deficiencies
E63.9 Nutritional deficiency, unspecified

● **E64 Sequelae of malnutrition and other nutritional deficiencies**
Pathological condition resulting from disease, injury, or other trauma
Note: This category is to be used to indicate conditions in categories E43, E44, E46, E5Ø-E63 as the cause of sequelae, which are themselves classified elsewhere. The 'sequelae' include conditions specified as such; they also include the late effects of diseases classifiable to the above categories if the disease itself is no longer present
Code first condition resulting from (sequela) of malnutrition and other nutritional deficiencies

E64.Ø Sequelae of protein-calorie malnutrition
Excludes2 retarded development following protein-calorie malnutrition (E45)
E64.1 Sequelae of vitamin A deficiency
E64.2 Sequelae of vitamin C deficiency
E64.3 Sequelae of rickets
E64.8 Sequelae of other nutritional deficiencies
E64.9 Sequelae of unspecified nutritional deficiency

OVERWEIGHT, OBESITY AND OTHER HYPERALIMENTATION (E65-E68)

E65 Localized adiposity
Fat pad

● **E66 Overweight and obesity**
Code first obesity complicating pregnancy, childbirth and the puerperium, if applicable (O99.21-)
Use additional code to identify body mass index (BMI), if known (Z68.-)
Excludes1 adiposogenital dystrophy (E23.6)
lipomatosis NOS (E88.2)
lipomatosis dolorosa [Dercum] (E88.2)
Prader-Willi syndrome (Q87.1)

● **E66.Ø Obesity due to excess calories**
E66.Ø1 Morbid (severe) obesity due to excess calories
Excludes1 morbid (severe) obesity with alveolar hypoventilation (E66.2)
E66.Ø9 Other obesity due to excess calories

E66.1 Drug-induced obesity
Use additional code for adverse effect, if applicable, to identify drug (T36-T5Ø with fifth or sixth character 5)

E66.2 Morbid (severe) obesity with alveolar hypoventilation
Uncommon condition of unknown cause leading to inadequate ventilation in lungs, even though lungs and airways are normal
Obesity hypoventilation syndrome (OHS) ◀
Pickwickian syndrome

E66.3 Overweight
E66.8 Other obesity
E66.9 Obesity, unspecified
Obesity NOS

◀ New ◀ Revised ~~deleted~~ Deleted OGCR Official Guidelines X Assign placeholder X ● Use Additional Character(s)
Excludes1 Excludes2 Includes Use additional Code first Code also Unspecified

CHAPTER 4 (EØØ-E9Ø)

● **E67 Other hyperalimentation**
Ingestion of more than optimal amount of nutrients
Excludes1 hyperalimentation NOS (R63.2)
sequelae of hyperalimentation (E68)
E67.0 Hypervitaminosis A
E67.1 Hypercarotinemia
E67.2 Megavitamin-B6 syndrome
E67.3 Hypervitaminosis D
E67.8 Other specified hyperalimentation

E68 Sequelae of hyperalimentation
Code first condition resulting from (sequela) of hyperalimentation

METABOLIC DISORDERS (E70-E88)

Excludes1 androgen insensitivity syndrome (E34.5-)
congenital adrenal hyperplasia (E25.0)
Ehlers-Danlos syndrome (Q79.6)
hemolytic anemias attributable to enzyme disorders (D55.-)
Marfan's syndrome (Q87.4)
5-alpha-reductase deficiency (E29.1)

● **E70 Disorders of aromatic amino-acid metabolism**
E70.0 Classical phenylketonuria
Inherited disorder that increases to harmful levels amino acid phenylalanine
E70.1 Other hyperphenylalaninemias
● **E70.2 Disorders of tyrosine metabolism**
Excludes1 transitory tyrosinemia of newborn (P74.5)
E70.20 Disorder of tyrosine metabolism, unspecified
Tyrosine: Nonessential amino acid occurring in most proteins
E70.21 Tyrosinemia
Congenital amino acid metabolism
Hypertyrosinemia
E70.29 Other disorders of tyrosine metabolism
Alkaptonuria
Ochronosis
● **E70.3 Albinism**
Congenital condition of reduced or absent pigment in eyes, skin, and hair
E70.30 Albinism, unspecified
● **E70.31 Ocular albinism**
E70.310 X-linked ocular albinism
E70.311 Autosomal recessive ocular albinism
E70.318 Other ocular albinism
E70.319 Ocular albinism, unspecified
● **E70.32 Oculocutaneous albinism**
Partial or total lack of melanin pigment in eyes
Excludes1 Chediak-Higashi syndrome (E70.330)
Hermansky-Pudlak syndrome (E70.331)
E70.320 Tyrosinase negative oculocutaneous albinism
Albinism I
Oculocutaneous albinism ty-neg
E70.321 Tyrosinase positive oculocutaneous albinism
Albinism II
Oculocutaneous albinism ty-pos
E70.328 Other oculocutaneous albinism
Cross syndrome
E70.329 Oculocutaneous albinism, unspecified
● **E70.33 Albinism with hematologic abnormality**
E70.330 Chediak-Higashi syndrome
E70.331 Hermansky-Pudlak syndrome
E70.338 Other albinism with hematologic abnormality
E70.339 Albinism with hematologic abnormality, unspecified
E70.39 Other specified albinism
Piebaldism
● **E70.4 Disorders of histidine metabolism**
E70.40 Disorders of histidine metabolism, unspecified
E70.41 Histidinemia
E70.49 Other disorders of histidine metabolism
E70.5 Disorders of tryptophan metabolism
E70.8 Other disorders of aromatic amino-acid metabolism
E70.9 Disorder of aromatic amino-acid metabolism, unspecified

● **E71 Disorders of branched-chain amino-acid metabolism and fatty-acid metabolism**
E71.0 Maple-syrup-urine disease
Due to defect in amino acid catabolism, causing severe ketoacidosis with smell of maple syrup in urine and on body
● **E71.1 Other disorders of branched-chain amino-acid metabolism**
● **E71.11 Branched-chain organic acidurias**
E71.110 Isovaleric acidemia
E71.111 3-methylglutaconic aciduria
E71.118 Other branched-chain organic acidurias
● **E71.12 Disorders of propionate metabolism**
E71.120 Methylmalonic acidemia
E71.121 Propionic acidemia
E71.128 Other disorders of propionate metabolism
E71.19 Other disorders of branched-chain amino-acid metabolism
Hyperleucine-isoleucinemia
Hypervalinemia
E71.2 Disorder of branched-chain amino-acid metabolism, unspecified
● **E71.3 Disorders of fatty-acid metabolism**
Excludes1 peroxisomal disorders (E71.5)
Refsum's disease (G60.1)
Schilder's disease (G37.0)
Excludes2 carnitine deficiency due to inborn error of metabolism (E71.42)
E71.30 Disorder of fatty-acid metabolism, unspecified
● **E71.31 Disorders of fatty-acid oxidation**
E71.310 Long chain/very long chain acyl CoA dehydrogenase deficiency
LCAD
VLCAD
E71.311 Medium chain acyl CoA dehydrogenase deficiency
MCAD
E71.312 Short chain acyl CoA dehydrogenase deficiency
SCAD
E71.313 Glutaric aciduria type II
Glutaric aciduria type II A
Glutaric aciduria type II B
Glutaric aciduria type II C
Excludes1 glutaric aciduria (type 1) NOS (E72.3)
E71.314 Muscle carnitine palmitoyltransferase deficiency
E71.318 Other disorders of fatty-acid oxidation
E71.32 Disorders of ketone metabolism
E71.39 Other disorders of fatty-acid metabolism

● **E71.4 Disorders of carnitine metabolism**
Excludes1 muscle carnitine palmitoyltransferase deficiency (E71.314)

E71.40 Disorder of carnitine metabolism, unspecified

E71.41 Primary carnitine deficiency

E71.42 Carnitine deficiency due to inborn errors of metabolism
Code also associated inborn error or metabolism

E71.43 Iatrogenic carnitine deficiency
Iatrogenic: Outcomes from activity of physicians
Carnitine deficiency due to hemodialysis
Carnitine deficiency due to Valproic acid therapy

● **E71.44 Other secondary carnitine deficiency**

E71.440 Ruvalcaba-Myhre-Smith syndrome

E71.448 Other secondary carnitine deficiency

● **E71.5 Peroxisomal disorders**
Class of conditions which lead to disorders of lipid metabolism
Excludes1 Schilder's disease (G37.0)

E71.50 Peroxisomal disorder, unspecified

● **E71.51 Disorders of peroxisome biogenesis**
Group 1 peroxisomal disorders
Excludes1 Refsum's disease (G60.1)

E71.510 Zellweger syndrome

E71.511 Neonatal adrenoleukodystrophy
Excludes1 X-linked adrenoleukodystrophy (E71.42-)

E71.518 Other disorders of peroxisome biogenesis

● **E71.52 X-linked adrenoleukodystrophy**

E71.520 Childhood cerebral X-linked adrenoleukodystrophy

E71.521 Adolescent X-linked adrenoleukodystrophy

E71.522 Adrenomyeloneuropathy

E71.528 Other X-linked adrenoleukodystrophy
Addison only phenotype adrenoleukodystrophy
Addison-Schilder adrenoleukodystrophy

E71.529 X-linked adrenoleukodystrophy, unspecified type

E71.53 Other group 2 peroxisomal disorders

● **E71.54 Other peroxisomal disorders**

E71.540 Rhizomelic chondrodysplasia punctata
Rare, severe, inherited disorder with limb shortening, bone and cartilage abnormalities, abnormal facial appearance, severe mental retardation, psychomotor retardation, and cataracts
Excludes1 chondrodysplasia punctata NOS (Q77.3)

E71.541 Zellweger-like syndrome

E71.542 Other group 3 peroxisomal disorders

E71.548 Other peroxisomal disorders

● **E72 Other disorders of amino-acid metabolism**
Excludes1 disorders of:
aromatic amino-acid metabolism (E70.-)
branched-chain amino-acid metabolism (E71.0-E71.2)
fatty-acid metabolism (E71.3)
purine and pyrimidine metabolism (E79.-)
gout (M1A.-, M10.-)

● **E72.0 Disorders of amino-acid transport**
Excludes1 disorders of tryptophan metabolism (E70.5)

E72.00 Disorders of amino-acid transport, unspecified

E72.01 Cystinuria
Hereditary aminoaciduria due to impairment of renal transport with predominant symptom of urinary cystine calculi

E72.02 Hartnup's disease
Inborn error of metabolism

E72.03 Lowe's syndrome
X-linked disorder with rickets, hydrophthalmia, congenital glaucoma, cataracts, mental retardation, and renal tubule dysfunction
Use additional code for associated glaucoma (H42)

E72.04 Cystinosis
Genetic disease with excessive depostits of amino acid cystine in cells
Fanconi (-de Toni) (-Debré) syndrome with cystinosis
Excludes1 Fanconi (-de Toni) (-Debré) syndrome without cystinosis (E72.09)

E72.09 Other disorders of amino-acid transport
Fanconi (-de Toni) (-Debré) syndrome, unspecified

● **E72.1 Disorders of sulfur-bearing amino-acid metabolism**
Excludes1 cystinosis (E72.04)
cystinuria (E72.01)
transcobalamin II deficiency (D51.2)

E72.10 Disorders of sulfur-bearing amino-acid metabolism, unspecified

E72.11 Homocystinuria
Cystathionine synthase deficiency

E72.12 Methylenetetrahydrofolate reductase deficiency

E72.19 Other disorders of sulfur-bearing amino-acid metabolism
Cystathioninuria
Methioninemia
Sulfite oxidase deficiency

● **E72.2 Disorders of urea cycle metabolism**
Excludes1 disorders of ornithine metabolism (E72.4)

E72.20 Disorder of urea cycle metabolism, unspecified
Hyperammonemia
Elevated levels of ammonia
Excludes1 hyperammonemia-hyperornithinemia-homocitrullinemia syndrome E72.4
transient hyperammonemia of newborn (P74.6)

E72.21 Argininemia
Disorder in which deficiency of enzyme arginase causes build up of arginine and ammonia in blood

E72.22 Arginosuccinic aciduria
Gene disorder of urea cycle resulting accumulation of ammonia

E72.23 Citrullinemia
Urea cycle disorder that causes ammonia and other toxic substances to accumulate in blood

E72.29 Other disorders of urea cycle metabolism

◄ New ◄ Revised ~~deleted~~ Deleted OGCR Official Guidelines X Assign placeholder X ● Use Additional Character(s)
Excludes 1 | Excludes 2 | Includes | Use additional | Code first | Code also | Unspecified

CHAPTER 4 (E00-E90)

E72.3 Disorders of lysine and hydroxylysine metabolism
Glutaric aciduria NOS
Glutaric aciduria (type I)
Hydroxylysinemia
Hyperlysinemia
Excludes1 glutaric aciduria type II (E71.313)
Refsum's disease (G60.1)
Zellweger syndrome (E71.510)

E72.4 Disorders of ornithine metabolism
Hyperammonemia-Hyperornithinemia-Homocitrullinemia syndrome
Ornithinemia (types I, II)
Ornithine transcarbamylase deficiency
Excludes1 hereditary choroidal dystrophy (H31.2-)

● **E72.5 Disorders of glycine metabolism**
E72.50 Disorder of glycine metabolism, unspecified
E72.51 Non-ketotic hyperglycinemia
E72.52 Trimethylaminuria
E72.53 Hyperoxaluria
Oxalosis
Oxaluria
E72.59 Other disorders of glycine metabolism
D-glycericacidemia
Hyperhydroxyprolinemia
Hyperprolinemia (types I, II)
Sarcosinemia

E72.8 Other specified disorders of amino-acid metabolism
Disorders of beta-amino-acid metabolism
Disorders of gamma-glutamyl cycle

E72.9 Disorder of amino-acid metabolism, unspecified

● **E73 Lactose intolerance**
Intolerance for lactose, due to inherited deficiency of lactase activity in intestinal mucosa
E73.0 Congenital lactase deficiency
E73.1 Secondary lactase deficiency
E73.8 Other lactose intolerance
E73.9 Lactose intolerance, unspecified

● **E74 Other disorders of carbohydrate metabolism**
Excludes1 diabetes mellitus (E08-E13)
hypoglycemia NOS (E16.2)
increased secretion of glucagon (E16.3)
mucopolysaccharidosis (E76.0-E76.3)

● **E74.0 Glycogen storage disease**
E74.00 Glycogen storage disease, unspecified
E74.01 von Gierke's disease
Type I glycogen storage disease
E74.02 Pompe disease
Cardiac glycogenosis
Type II glycogen storage disease
E74.03 Cori disease
Forbes' disease
Type III glycogen storage disease
E74.04 McArdle disease
Type V glycogen storage disease
E74.09 Other glycogen storage disease
Andersen disease
Hers disease
Tauri disease
Glycogen storage disease, types 0, IV, VI-XI
Liver phosphorylase deficiency
Muscle phosphofructokinase deficiency

● **E74.1 Disorders of fructose metabolism**
Excludes1 muscle phosphofructokinase deficiency (E74.09)
E74.10 Disorder of fructose metabolism, unspecified
E74.11 Essential fructosuria
Fructokinase deficiency
E74.12 Hereditary fructose intolerance
Fructosemia
E74.19 Other disorders of fructose metabolism
Fructose-1, 6-diphosphatase deficiency

● **E74.2 Disorders of galactose metabolism**
E74.20 Disorders of galactose metabolism, unspecified
E74.21 Galactosemia
Genetic disorders resulting from defective simple sugar (galactose) metabolism
E74.29 Other disorders of galactose metabolism
Galactokinase deficiency

● **E74.3 Other disorders of intestinal carbohydrate absorption**
Excludes2 lactose intolerance (E73.-)
E74.31 Sucrase-isomaltase deficiency
Deficiency in metabolism in intestinal mucosa results in malabsorption of sucrose and starch
E74.39 Other disorders of intestinal carbohydrate absorption
Disorder of intestinal carbohydrate absorption NOS
Glucose-galactose malabsorption
Sucrase deficiency

E74.4 Disorders of pyruvate metabolism and gluconeogenesis
Deficiency of phosphoenolpyruvate carboxykinase
Deficiency of pyruvate carboxylase
Deficiency of pyruvate dehydrogenase
Excludes1 disorders of pyruvate metabolism and gluconeogenesis with anemia (D55.-)
Leigh's syndrome (G31.82)

E74.8 Other specified disorders of carbohydrate metabolism
Essential pentosuria
Renal glycosuria

E74.9 Disorder of carbohydrate metabolism, unspecified

● **E75 Disorders of sphingolipid metabolism and other lipid storage disorders**
Excludes1 mucolipidosis, types I-III (E77.0-E77.1)
Refsum's disease (G60.1)

● **E75.0 GM2 gangliosidosis**
Rare metabolic disorder that causes destruction of nerve cells of brain and spinal cord
E75.00 GM2 gangliosidosis, unspecified
E75.01 Sandhoff disease
E75.02 Tay-Sachs disease
E75.09 Other GM2 gangliosidosis
Adult GM2 gangliosidosis
Juvenile GM2 gangliosidosis

● **E75.1 Other and unspecified gangliosidosis**
E75.10 Unspecified gangliosidosis
Gangliosidosis NOS
E75.11 Mucolipidosis IV
Disorder with symptoms of psychomotor retardation and severe visual impairment
E75.19 Other gangliosidosis
GM1 gangliosidosis
GM3 gangliosidosis

CHAPTER 4 (E00-E90)

Item 4–8 Leukodystrophy is characterized by degeneration and/or failure of the myelin formation of the central nervous system and sometimes of the peripheral nervous system. The disease is inherited and progressive.

● **E75.2 Other sphingolipidosis**
Lysosomal (a particle in a cytoplasm cell that contains digestive enzymes) storage diseases with symptoms of abnormal storage of amino acids
Excludes1 adrenoleukodystrophy [Addison-Schilder] (E71.528)
E75.21 Fabry (-Anderson) disease
E75.22 Gaucher disease
E75.23 Krabbe disease
● **E75.24 Niemann-Pick disease**
E75.240 Niemann-Pick disease type A
E75.241 Niemann-Pick disease type B
E75.242 Niemann-Pick disease type C
E75.243 Niemann-Pick disease type D
E75.248 Other Niemann-Pick disease
E75.249 Niemann-Pick disease, unspecified
E75.25 Metachromatic leukodystrophy
E75.29 Other sphingolipidosis
Farber's syndrome
Sulfatase deficiency
Sulfatide lipidosis
E75.3 Sphingolipidosis, unspecified
E75.4 Neuronal ceroid lipofuscinosis
Batten disease
Bielschowsky-Jansky disease
Kufs disease
Spielmeyer-Vogt disease
E75.5 Other lipid storage disorders
Cerebrotendinous cholesterosis [van Bogaert-Scherer-Epstein]
Wolman's disease
E75.6 Lipid storage disorder, unspecified

● **E76 Disorders of glycosaminoglycan metabolism**
● **E76.0 Mucopolysaccharidosis, type I**
Inborn metabolic disorder of enzymes that break down carbohydrates
E76.01 Hurler's syndrome
E76.02 Hurler-Scheie syndrome
E76.03 Scheie's syndrome
E76.1 Mucopolysaccharidosis, type II
Inborn metabolic disorder of enzymes that break down carbohydrates occurs in 2-4 year old males
Hunter's syndrome
● **E76.2 Other mucopolysaccharidoses**
● **E76.21 Morquio mucopolysaccharidoses**
E76.210 Morquio A mucopolysaccharidoses
Classic Morquio syndrome
Morquio syndrome A
Mucopolysaccharidosis, type IVA
E76.211 Morquio B mucopolysaccharidoses
Morquio-like mucopolysaccharidoses
Morquio-like syndrome
Morquio syndrome B
Mucopolysaccharidosis, type IVB
E76.219 Morquio mucopolysaccharidoses, unspecified
Morquio syndrome
Mucopolysaccharidosis, type IV
E76.22 Sanfilippo mucopolysaccharidoses
Mucopolysaccharidosis, type III (A) (B) (C) (D)
Sanfilippo A syndrome
Sanfilippo B syndrome
Sanfilippo C syndrome
Sanfilippo D syndrome
E76.29 Other mucopolysaccharidoses
beta-Glucuronidase deficiency
Maroteaux-Lamy (mild) (severe) syndrome
Mucopolysaccharidosis, types VI, VII
E76.3 Mucopolysaccharidosis, unspecified
E76.8 Other disorders of glucosaminoglycan metabolism
E76.9 Glucosaminoglycan metabolism disorder, unspecified

● **E77 Disorders of glycoprotein metabolism**
E77.0 Defects in post-translational modification of lysosomal enzymes
Mucolipidosis II [I-cell disease]
Mucolipidosis III [pseudo-Hurler polydystrophy]
E77.1 Defects in glycoprotein degradation
Aspartylglucosaminuria
Fucosidosis
Mannosidosis
Sialidosis [mucolipidosis I]
E77.8 Other disorders of glycoprotein metabolism
E77.9 Disorder of glycoprotein metabolism, unspecified

● **E78 Disorders of lipoprotein metabolism and other lipidemias**
Excludes1 sphingolipidosis (E75.0-E75.3)
● **E78.0 Pure hypercholesterolemia**
~~Familial hypercholesterolemia~~
~~Hyperlipidemia, Group A~~
E78.00 Pure hypercholesterolemia, unspecified ◀
Fredrickson's hyperlipoproteinemia, type IIa ◀
Hyperbetalipoproteinemia ◀
Low-density-lipoprotein-type [LDL] hyperlipoproteinemia ◀
E78.01 Familial hypercholesterolemia ◀
E78.1 Pure hyperglyceridemia
Elevated fasting triglycerides
Endogenous hyperglyceridemia
Fredrickson's hyperlipoproteinemia, type IV
Hyperlipidemia, group B
Hyperprebetalipoproteinemia
Very-low-density-lipoprotein-type [VLDL] hyperlipoproteinemia
E78.2 Mixed hyperlipidemia
Broad- or floating-betalipoproteinemia
Combined hyperlipidemia NOS
Elevated cholesterol with elevated triglycerides NEC
Fredrickson's hyperlipoproteinemia, type IIb or III
Hyperbetalipoproteinemia with prebetalipoproteinemia
Hypercholesteremia with endogenous hyperglyceridemia
Hyperlipidemia, group C
Tubo-eruptive xanthoma
Xanthoma tuberosum
Excludes1 cerebrotendinous cholesterosis [van Bogaert-Scherer-Epstein] (E75.5)
familial combined hyperlipidemia (E78.4)
E78.3 Hyperchylomicronemia
Chylomicron retention disease
Fredrickson's hyperlipoproteinemia, type I or V
Hyperlipidemia, group D
Mixed hyperglyceridemia
E78.4 Other hyperlipidemia
Familial combined hyperlipidemia

E78.5 **Hyperlipidemia, unspecified**
E78.6 **Lipoprotein deficiency**
Abetalipoproteinemia
Depressed HDL cholesterol
High-density lipoprotein deficiency
Hypoalphalipoproteinemia
Hypobetalipoproteinemia (familial)
Lecithin cholesterol acyltransferase deficiency
Tangier disease
● E78.7 **Disorders of bile acid and cholesterol metabolism**
Excludes1 Niemann-Pick disease type C (E75.242)
E78.70 **Disorder of bile acid and cholesterol metabolism, unspecified**
E78.71 **Barth syndrome**
E78.72 **Smith-Lemli-Opitz syndrome**
E78.79 **Other disorders of bile acid and cholesterol metabolism**
● E78.8 **Other disorders of lipoprotein metabolism**
E78.81 **Lipoid dermatoarthritis**
E78.89 **Other lipoprotein metabolism disorders**
E78.9 **Disorder of lipoprotein metabolism, unspecified**

● E79 **Disorders of purine and pyrimidine metabolism**
Purines, along with pyrimidines, signal RNA and DNA production
Excludes1 Ataxia-telangiectasia (Q87.1)
Bloom's syndrome (Q82.8)
Cockayne's syndrome (Q87.1)
calculus of kidney (N20.0)
combined immunodeficiency disorders (D81.-)
Fanconi's anemia (D61.09)
gout (M1A.-, M10.-)
orotaciduric anemia (D53.0)
progeria (E34.8)
Werner's syndrome (E34.8)
xeroderma pigmentosum (Q82.1)
E79.0 **Hyperuricemia without signs of inflammatory arthritis and tophaceous disease**
Asymptomatic hyperuricemia
E79.1 **Lesch-Nyhan syndrome**
HGPRT deficiency
E79.2 **Myoadenylate deaminase deficiency**
E79.8 **Other disorders of purine and pyrimidine metabolism**
Hereditary xanthinuria
E79.9 **Disorder of purine and pyrimidine metabolism, unspecified**

● E80 **Disorders of porphyrin and bilirubin metabolism**
Group of chemical compounds in RBC's that combine with iron to form heme
Includes defects of catalase and peroxidase
E80.0 **Hereditary erythropoietic porphyria**
Congenital erythropoietic porphyria
Erythropoietic protoporphyria
E80.1 **Porphyria cutanea tarda**
● E80.2 **Other and unspecified porphyria**
E80.20 **Unspecified porphyria**
Porphyria NOS
E80.21 **Acute intermittent (hepatic) porphyria**
E80.29 **Other porphyria**
Hereditary coproporphyria
E80.3 **Defects of catalase and peroxidase**
Acatalasia [Takahara]
E80.4 **Gilbert syndrome**
E80.5 **Crigler-Najjar syndrome**
E80.6 **Other disorders of bilirubin metabolism**
Dubin-Johnson syndrome
Rotor's syndrome
E80.7 **Disorder of bilirubin metabolism, unspecified**

● E83 **Disorders of mineral metabolism**
Excludes1 dietary mineral deficiency (E58-E61)
parathyroid disorders (E20-E21)
vitamin D deficiency (E55.-)
● E83.0 **Disorders of copper metabolism**
E83.00 **Disorder of copper metabolism, unspecified**
E83.01 **Wilson's disease**
Code also associated Kayser Fleischer ring (H18.04-)
E83.09 **Other disorders of copper metabolism**
Menkes' (kinky hair) (steely hair) disease
● E83.1 **Disorders of iron metabolism**
Excludes1 iron deficiency anemia (D50.-)
sideroblastic anemia (D64.0-D64.3)
E83.10 **Disorder of iron metabolism, unspecified**
● E83.11 **Hemochromatosis**
E83.110 **Hereditary hemochromatosis**
Bronzed diabetes
Pigmentary cirrhosis (of liver)
Primary (hereditary) hemochromatosis
E83.111 **Hemochromatosis due to repeated red blood cell transfusions**
Iron overload due to repeated red blood cell transfusions
Transfusion (red blood cell) associated hemochromatosis
E83.118 **Other hemochromatosis**
E83.119 **Hemochromatosis, unspecified**
E83.19 **Other disorders of iron metabolism**
Use additional code, if applicable, for idiopathic pulmonary hemosiderosis (J84.03)
E83.2 **Disorders of zinc metabolism**
Acrodermatitis enteropathica
● E83.3 **Disorders of phosphorus metabolism and phosphatases**
Excludes1 adult osteomalacia (M83.-)
osteoporosis (M80.-)
E83.30 **Disorder of phosphorus metabolism, unspecified**
E83.31 **Familial hypophosphatemia**
Vitamin D-resistant osteomalacia
Vitamin D-resistant rickets
Excludes1 vitamin D-deficiency rickets (E55.0)
E83.32 **Hereditary vitamin D-dependent rickets (type 1) (type 2)**
25-hydroxyvitamin D 1-alpha-hydroxylase deficiency
Pseudovitamin D deficiency
Vitamin D receptor defect
E83.39 **Other disorders of phosphorus metabolism**
Acid phosphatase deficiency
Hypophosphatasia
● E83.4 **Disorders of magnesium metabolism**
E83.40 **Disorders of magnesium metabolism, unspecified**
E83.41 **Hypermagnesemia**
E83.42 **Hypomagnesemia**
E83.49 **Other disorders of magnesium metabolism**
● E83.5 **Disorders of calcium metabolism**
Excludes1 chondrocalcinosis (M11.1-M11.2)
hungry bone syndrome (E83.81)
hyperparathyroidism (E21.0-E21.3)
E83.50 **Unspecified disorder of calcium metabolism**
E83.51 **Hypocalcemia**
E83.52 **Hypercalcemia**
Familial hypocalciuric hypercalcemia
E83.59 **Other disorders of calcium metabolism**
Idiopathic hypercalciuria

CHAPTER 4 (E00-E90)

- ● **E83.8 Other disorders of mineral metabolism**
  - **E83.81 Hungry bone syndrome**
  - **E83.89 Other disorders of mineral metabolism**
- **E83.9 Disorder of mineral metabolism, unspecified**

● **E84 Cystic fibrosis**

Includes mucoviscidosis

Code also exocrine pancreatic insufficiency (K86.81) ◀

- **E84.0 Cystic fibrosis with pulmonary manifestations**
  - Use additional code to identify any infectious organism present, such as:
  - Pseudomonas (B96.5)
- ● **E84.1 Cystic fibrosis with intestinal manifestations**
  - **E84.11 Meconium ileus in cystic fibrosis**
    - Excludes1 meconium ileus not due to cystic fibrosis (P76.0)
  - **E84.19 Cystic fibrosis with other intestinal manifestations**
    - Distal intestinal obstruction syndrome
- **E84.8 Cystic fibrosis with other manifestations**
- **E84.9 Cystic fibrosis, unspecified**

● **E85 Amyloidosis**

A disorder resulting from the abnormal deposition of a particular protein (amyloid) into tissues of the body

Excludes1 Alzheimer's disease (G30.0-)

- **E85.0 Non-neuropathic heredofamilial amyloidosis**
  - ~~Familial Mediterranean fever~~
  - Hereditary amyloid nephropathy
- **E85.1 Neuropathic heredofamilial amyloidosis**
  - Amyloid polyneuropathy (Portuguese)
- **E85.2 Heredofamilial amyloidosis, unspecified**
- **E85.3 Secondary systemic amyloidosis**
  - Hemodialysis-associated amyloidosis
- **E85.4 Organ-limited amyloidosis**
  - Localized amyloidosis
- **E85.8 Other amyloidosis**
- **E85.9 Amyloidosis, unspecified**

● **E86 Volume depletion**

Excludes1 dehydration of newborn (P74.1)
hypovolemic shock NOS (R57.1)
postprocedural hypovolemic shock (T81.19)
traumatic hypovolemic shock (T79.4)

Use additional code(s) for any associated disorders of electrolyte and acid-base balance (E87.-) ◀

- **E86.0 Dehydration**
  - *Excessive loss of body water*
- **E86.1 Hypovolemia**
  - *Diminished volume of circulating blood*
  - Depletion of volume of plasma
- **E86.9 Volume depletion, unspecified**

Item 4–9 Circulating fluid volume is regulated by the amount of water and sodium ingested, excreted by the kidneys into the urine, and lost through the gastrointestinal tract, lungs, and skin. To maintain blood volume within a normal range, the kidneys regulate the amount of water and sodium lost into the urine. Too much **(fluid overload)** or too little fluid volume **(volume depletion)** will affect blood pressure. Severe cases of vomiting, diarrhea, bleeding, and burns (fluid loss through exposed burn surface area) can contribute to fluid loss. Internal body environment must maintain a precise balance (homeostasis) between too much fluid and too little fluid. This complex balancing mechanism is critical to good health.

● **E87 Other disorders of fluid, electrolyte and acid-base balance**

Excludes1 diabetes insipidus (E23.2)
electrolyte imbalance associated with hyperemesis gravidarum (O21.1)
electrolyte imbalance following ectopic or molar pregnancy (O08.5)
familial periodic paralysis (G72.3)

- **E87.0 Hyperosmolality and hypernatremia**
  - Sodium [Na] excess
  - Sodium [Na] overload
- **E87.1 Hypo-osmolality and hyponatremia**
  - Sodium [Na] deficiency
  - Excludes1 syndrome of inappropriate secretion of antidiuretic hormone (E22.2)
- **E87.2 Acidosis**
  - Acidosis NOS
  - Lactic acidosis
  - Metabolic acidosis
  - Respiratory acidosis
  - Excludes1 diabetic acidosis - see categories E08-E10, E13 with ketoacidosis
- **E87.3 Alkalosis**
  - Alkalosis NOS
  - Metabolic alkalosis
  - Respiratory alkalosis
- **E87.4 Mixed disorder of acid-base balance**
- **E87.5 Hyperkalemia**
  - Potassium [K] excess
  - Potassium [K] overload
- **E87.6 Hypokalemia**
  - Potassium [K] deficiency
- ● **E87.7 Fluid overload**
  - Excludes1 edema NOS (R60.9)
    fluid retention (R60.9)
  - **E87.70 Fluid overload, unspecified**
  - **E87.71 Transfusion associated circulatory overload**
    - Fluid overload due to transfusion (blood) (blood components) TACO
  - **E87.79 Other fluid overload**
- **E87.8 Other disorders of electrolyte and fluid balance, not elsewhere classified**
  - Electrolyte imbalance NOS
  - Hyperchloremia
  - Hypochloremia

● **E88 Other and unspecified metabolic disorders**

Use additional codes for associated conditions

Excludes1 histiocytosis X (chronic) (C96.6)

- ● **E88.0 Disorders of plasma-protein metabolism, not elsewhere classified**
  - Excludes1 disorder of lipoprotein metabolism (E78.-)
    monoclonal gammopathy (of undetermined significance) (D47.2)
    polyclonal hypergammaglobulinemia (D89.0)
    Waldenström macroglobulinemia (C88.0)
  - **E88.01 Alpha-1-antitrypsin deficiency AAT deficiency**
  - **E88.09 Other disorders of plasma-protein metabolism, not elsewhere classified**
    - Bisalbuminemia
- **E88.1 Lipodystrophy, not elsewhere classified**
  - *Defective fat metabolism resulting in absence of subcutaneous fat*
  - Lipodystrophy NOS
  - Excludes1 Whipple's disease (K90.81)
- **E88.2 Lipomatosis, not elsewhere classified**
  - *Abnormal tumorlike accumulations of fat in tissue*
  - Lipomatosis NOS
  - Lipomatosis (Check) dolorosa [Dercum]

◀ New ◀ Revised ~~deleted~~ Deleted OGCR Official Guidelines X Assign placeholder X ● Use Additional Character(s)
Excludes1 Excludes2 Includes Use additional Code first Code also Unspecified

E88.3 Tumor lysis syndrome
Tumor lysis syndrome (spontaneous)
Tumor lysis syndrome following antineoplastic drug chemotherapy
Use additional code for adverse effect, if applicable, to identify drug (T45.1X5)

● **E88.4 Mitochondrial metabolism disorders**
Congenital disorder of metabolism
Excludes1 disorders of pyruvate metabolism (E74.4)
Kearns-Sayre syndrome (H49.81)
Leber's disease (H47.22)
Leigh's encephalopathy (G31.82)
Mitochondrial myopathy, NEC (G71.3)
Reye's syndrome (G93.7)

E88.40 Mitochondrial metabolism disorder, unspecified

E88.41 MELAS syndrome
Mitochondrial myopathy, encephalopathy, lactic acidosis and stroke-like episodes

E88.42 MERRF syndrome
Myoclonic epilepsy associated with ragged-red fibers
Code also progressive myoclonic epilepsy (G40.3-) ⬅

E88.49 Other mitochondrial metabolism disorders

● **E88.8 Other specified metabolic disorders**

E88.81 Metabolic syndrome
Dysmetabolic syndrome X
Use additional codes for associated manifestations, such as:
obesity (E66.-)

E88.89 Other specified metabolic disorders
Launois-Bensaude adenolipomatosis
Excludes1 adult pulmonary Langerhans cell histiocytosis (J84.82)

E88.9 Metabolic disorder, unspecified

POSTPROCEDURAL ENDOCRINE AND METABOLIC COMPLICATIONS AND DISORDERS, NOT ELSEWHERE CLASSIFIED (E89)

● **E89 Postprocedural endocrine and metabolic complications and disorders, not elsewhere classified**
Excludes2 intraoperative complications of endocrine system organ or structure (E36.0-, E36.1-, E36.8)

E89.0 Postprocedural hypothyroidism
Postirradiation hypothyroidism
Postsurgical hypothyroidism

E89.1 Postprocedural hypoinsulinemia
Postpancreatectomy hyperglycemia
Postsurgical hypoinsulinemia
Use additional code, if applicable, to identify:
acquired absence of pancreas (Z90.41-)
diabetes mellitus (postpancreatectomy) (postprocedural) (E13.-)
insulin use (Z79.4)
Excludes1 transient postprocedural hyperglycemia (R73.9)
transient postprocedural hypoglycemia (E16.2)

E89.2 Postprocedural hypoparathyroidism
Parathyroprival tetany

E89.3 Postprocedural hypopituitarism
Postirradiation hypopituitarism

● **E89.4 Postprocedural ovarian failure**

E89.40 Asymptomatic postprocedural ovarian failure
Postprocedural ovarian failure NOS

E89.41 Symptomatic postprocedural ovarian failure
Symptoms such as flushing, sleeplessness, headache, lack of concentration, associated with postprocedural menopause

E89.5 Postprocedural testicular hypofunction

E89.6 Postprocedural adrenocortical (-medullary) hypofunction

● **E89.8 Other postprocedural endocrine and metabolic complications and disorders**

● **E89.81 Postprocedural hemorrhage of an endocrine system organ or structure following a procedure** ⬅

E89.810 Postprocedural hemorrhage of an endocrine system organ or structure following an endocrine system procedure ⬅

E89.811 Postprocedural hemorrhage of an endocrine system organ or structure following other procedure ⬅

● **E89.82 Postprocedural hematoma and seroma of an endocrine system organ or structure** ◀

E89.820 Postprocedural hematoma of an endocrine system organ or structure following an endocrine system procedure ◀

E89.821 Postprocedural hematoma of an endocrine system organ or structure following other procedure ◀

E89.822 Postprocedural seroma of an endocrine system organ or structure following an endocrine system procedure ◀

E89.823 Postprocedural seroma of an endocrine system organ or structure following other procedure ◀

E89.89 Other postprocedural endocrine and metabolic complications and disorders
Use additional code, if applicable, to further specify disorder

CHAPTER 4 (E00-E90)

CHAPTER 5

MENTAL, BEHAVIORAL AND NEURODEVELOPMENTAL DISORDERS (FØ1-F99)

OGCR Chapter-Specific Coding Guidelines

5. **Chapter 5: Mental, Behavioral and Neurodevelopmental disorders (FØ1 – F99)**

a. Pain disorders related to psychological factors

Assign code F45.41, for pain that is exclusively related to psychological disorders. As indicated by the Excludes 1 note under category G89, a code from category G89 should not be assigned with code F45.41

Code F45.42, Pain disorders with related psychological factors, should be used with a code from category G89, Pain, not elsewhere classified, if there is documentation of a psychological component for a patient with acute or chronic pain.

See Section I.C.6. Pain

c. Mental and behavioral disorders due to psychoactive substance use

1) In Remission

Selection of codes for "in remission" for categories F1Ø-F19, Mental and behavioral disorders due to psychoactive substance use (categories F1Ø-F19 with -.21) requires the provider's clinical judgment. The appropriate codes for "in remission" are assigned only on the basis of provider documentation (as defined in the Official Guidelines for Coding and Reporting).

2) Psychoactive Substance Use, Abuse And Dependence

When the provider documentation refers to use, abuse and dependence of the same substance (e.g. alcohol, opioid, cannabis, etc.), only one code should be assigned to identify the pattern of use based on the following hierarchy:

- If both use and abuse are documented, assign only the code for abuse
- If both abuse and dependence are documented, assign only the code for dependence
- If use, abuse and dependence are all documented, assign only the code for dependence
- If both use and dependence are documented, assign only the code for dependence.

3) Psychoactive Substance Use

As with all other diagnoses, the codes for psychoactive substance use (F1Ø.9-, F11.9-, F12.9-, F13.9-, F14.9-, F15.9-, F16.9-) should only be assigned based on provider documentation and when they meet the definition of a reportable diagnosis (see Section III, Reporting Additional Diagnoses). The codes are to be used only when the psychoactive substance use is associated with a mental or behavioral disorder, and such a relationship is documented by the provider.

CHAPTER 5

MENTAL, BEHAVIORAL AND NEURODEVELOPMENTAL DISORDERS (FØ1-F99)

Includes disorders of psychological development

Excludes2 symptoms, signs and abnormal clinical laboratory findings, not elsewhere classified (RØØ-R99)

This chapter contains the following blocks:

FØ1-FØ9	Mental disorders due to known physiological conditions
F1Ø-F19	Mental and behavioral disorders due to psychoactive substance use
F2Ø-F29	Schizophrenia, schizotypal, delusional, and other non-mood psychotic disorders
F3Ø-F39	Mood [affective] disorders
F4Ø-F48	Anxiety, dissociative, stress-related, somatoform and other nonpsychotic mental disorders
F5Ø-F59	Behavioral syndromes associated with physiological disturbances and physical factors
F6Ø-F69	Disorders of adult personality and behavior
F7Ø-F79	Intellectual disabilities
F8Ø-F89	Pervasive and specific developmental disorders
F9Ø-F98	Behavioral and emotional disorders with onset usually occurring in childhood and adolescence
F99	Unspecified mental disorder

MENTAL DISORDERS DUE TO KNOWN PHYSIOLOGICAL CONDITIONS (FØ1-FØ9)

This block comprises a range of mental disorders grouped together on the basis of their having in common a demonstrable etiology in cerebral disease, brain injury, or other insult leading to cerebral dysfunction. The dysfunction may be primary, as in diseases, injuries, and insults that affect the brain directly and selectively; or secondary, as in systemic diseases and disorders that attack the brain only as one of the multiple organs or systems of the body that are involved.

● **FØ1 Vascular dementia**

Vascular dementia as a result of infarction of the brain due to vascular disease, including hypertensive cerebrovascular disease.

Includes arteriosclerotic dementia

Code first *the underlying physiological condition or sequelae of cerebrovascular disease.*

● **FØ1.5 Vascular dementia**

FØ1.5Ø Vascular dementia without behavioral disturbance

Major neurocognitive disorder without behavioral disturbance ◀

FØ1.51 Vascular dementia with behavioral disturbance

Major neurocognitive disorder due to vascular disease, with behavioral disturbance ◀

Major neurocognitive disorder with aggressive behavior ◀

Major neurocognitive disorder with combative behavior ◀

Major neurocognitive disorder with violent behavior ◀

Vascular dementia with aggressive behavior

Vascular dementia with combative behavior

Vascular dementia with violent behavior

Use additional code, if applicable, to identify wandering in vascular dementia (Z91.83)

● FØ2 **Dementia in other diseases classified elsewhere**
Code first the underlying physiological condition, such as:
Alzheimer's (G3Ø.-)
cerebral lipidosis (E75.4)
Creutzfeldt-Jakob disease (A81.Ø-)
dementia with Lewy bodies (G31.83)
dementia with Parkinsonism (G31.83) ◀
epilepsy and recurrent seizures (G4Ø.-)
frontotemporal dementia (G31.Ø9)
hepatolenticular degeneration (E83.Ø)
human immunodeficiency virus [HIV] disease (B2Ø)
Huntington's disease (G1Ø) ◀
hypercalcemia (E83.52)
hypothyroidism, acquired (EØØ-EØ3.-)
intoxications (T36-T65)
Jakob-Creutzfeldt disease (A81.Ø-)
multiple sclerosis (G35)
neurosyphilis (A52.17)
niacin deficiency [pellagra] (E52)
Parkinson's disease (G2Ø)
Pick's disease (G31.Ø1)
polyarteritis nodosa (M3Ø.Ø)
prion disease (A81.9) ◀
systemic lupus erythematosus (M32.-)
traumatic brain injury (SØ6.-) ◀
trypanosomiasis (B56.-, B57.-)
vitamin B deficiency (E53.8)

Includes Major neurocognitive disorder in other diseases classified elsewhere ◀

Excludes2 dementia in alcohol and psychoactive substance disorders (F1Ø-F19, with .17, .27, .97)
vascular dementia (FØ1.5-)

● FØ2.8 **Dementia in other diseases classified elsewhere**

FØ2.8Ø **Dementia in other diseases classified elsewhere without behavioral disturbance**
Dementia in other diseases classified elsewhere NOS
Major neurocognitive disorder in other diseases classified elsewhere ◀

FØ2.81 **Dementia in other diseases classified elsewhere with behavioral disturbance**
Dementia in other diseases classified elsewhere with aggressive behavior
Dementia in other diseases classified elsewhere with combative behavior
Dementia in other diseases classified elsewhere with violent behavior
Major neurocognitive disorder in other diseases classified elsewhere with aggressive behavior ◀
Major neurocognitive disorder in other diseases classified elsewhere with combative behavior ◀
Major neurocognitive disorder in other diseases classified elsewhere with violent behavior ◀
Use additional code, if applicable, to identify wandering in dementia in conditions classified elsewhere (Z91.83)

Item 5-1 Psychosis was a term formerly applied to any mental disorder but is now restricted to disturbances of a great magnitude in which there is a personality disintegration and loss of contact with reality.

● FØ3 **Unspecified dementia**
Presenile dementia NOS
Presenile psychosis NOS
Primary degenerative dementia NOS
Senile dementia NOS
Senile dementia depressed or paranoid type
Senile psychosis NOS

Excludes1 senility NOS (R41.81)

Excludes2 mild memory disturbance due to known physiological condition (FØ6.8)
senile dementia with delirium or acute confusional state (FØ5)

● FØ3.9 **Unspecified dementia**

FØ3.9Ø **Unspecified dementia without behavioral disturbance**
Dementia NOS

FØ3.91 **Unspecified dementia with behavioral disturbance**
Unspecified dementia with aggressive behavior
Unspecified dementia with combative behavior
Unspecified dementia with violent behavior
Use additional code, if applicable, to identify wandering in unspecified dementia (Z91.83)

FØ4 **Amnestic disorder due to known physiological condition**
Korsakov's psychosis or syndrome, nonalcoholic
Code first the underlying physiological condition

Excludes1 amnesia NOS (R41.3)
anterograde amnesia (R41.1)
dissociative amnesia (F44.Ø)
retrograde amnesia (R41.2)

Excludes2 alcohol-induced or unspecified Korsakov's syndrome (F1Ø.26, F1Ø.96)
Korsakov's syndrome induced by other psychoactive substances (F13.26, F13.96, F19.16, F19.26, F19.96)

FØ5 **Delirium due to known physiological condition**
Acute or subacute brain syndrome
Acute or subacute confusional state (nonalcoholic)
Acute or subacute infective psychosis
Acute or subacute organic reaction
Acute or subacute psycho-organic syndrome
Delirium of mixed etiology
Delirium superimposed on dementia
Sundowning
Code first the underlying physiological condition

Excludes1 delirium NOS (R41.Ø)

Excludes2 delirium tremens alcohol-induced or unspecified (F1Ø.231, F1Ø.921)

CHAPTER 5 (FØ1-F99)

● **F06 Other mental disorders due to known physiological condition**

Includes mental disorders due to endocrine disorder
mental disorders due to exogenous hormone
mental disorders due to exogenous toxic substance
mental disorders due to primary cerebral disease
mental disorders due to somatic illness
mental disorders due to systemic disease affecting the brain

Code first the underlying physiological condition

Excludes1 unspecified dementia (F03)

Excludes2 delirium due to known physiological condition (F05)
dementia as classified in F01-F02
other mental disorders associated with alcohol and other psychoactive substances (F10-F19)

F06.0 Psychotic disorder with hallucinations due to known physiological condition

Organic hallucinatory state (nonalcoholic)

Excludes2 hallucinations and perceptual disturbance induced by alcohol and other psychoactive substances (F10-F19 with .151, .251, .951)
schizophrenia (F20.-)

F06.1 Catatonic disorder due to known physiological condition

Catatonia associated with another mental disorder ◀
Catatonia NOS ◀

Excludes1 catatonic stupor (R40.1)
stupor NOS (R40.1)

Excludes2 catatonic schizophrenia (F20.2)
dissociative stupor (F44.2)

F06.2 Psychotic disorder with delusions due to known physiological condition

Paranoid and paranoid-hallucinatory organic states
Schizophrenia-like psychosis in epilepsy

Excludes2 alcohol and drug-induced psychotic disorder (F10-F19 with .150, .250, .950)
brief psychotic disorder (F23)
delusional disorder (F22)
schizophrenia (F20.-)

● **F06.3 Mood disorder due to known physiological condition**

Excludes2 mood disorders due to alcohol and other psychoactive substances (F10-F19 with .14, .24, .94)
mood disorders, not due to known physiological condition or unspecified (F30-F39)

F06.30 Mood disorder due to known physiological condition, unspecified

F06.31 Mood disorder due to known physiological condition with depressive features

F06.32 Mood disorder due to known physiological condition with major depressive-like episode

F06.33 Mood disorder due to known physiological condition with manic features

F06.34 Mood disorder due to known physiological condition with mixed features

F06.4 Anxiety disorder due to known physiological condition

Excludes2 anxiety disorders due to alcohol and other psychoactive substances (F10-F19 with .180, .280, .980)
anxiety disorders, not due to known physiological condition or unspecified (F40.-, F41.-)

F06.8 Other specified mental disorders due to known physiological condition

Epileptic psychosis NOS
Organic dissociative disorder
Organic emotionally labile [asthenic] disorder

● **F07 Personality and behavioral disorders due to known physiological condition**

Code first the underlying physiological condition

F07.0 Personality change due to known physiological condition

Frontal lobe syndrome
Limbic epilepsy personality syndrome
Lobotomy syndrome
Organic personality disorder
Organic pseudopsychopathic personality
Organic pseudoretarded personality
Postleucotomy syndrome

Code first underlying physiological condition

Excludes1 mild cognitive impairment (G31.84)
postconcussional syndrome (F07.81)
postencephalitic syndrome (F07.89)
signs and symptoms involving emotional state (R45.-)

Excludes2 specific personality disorder (F60.-)

● **F07.8 Other personality and behavioral disorders due to known physiological condition**

F07.81 Postconcussional syndrome

Postcontusional syndrome (encephalopathy)
Post-traumatic brain syndrome, nonpsychotic

Use additional code to identify associated post-traumatic headache, if applicable (G44.3-)

Excludes1 current concussion (brain) (S06.0-)
postencephalitic syndrome (F07.89)

F07.89 Other personality and behavioral disorders due to known physiological condition

Postencephalitic syndrome
Damage to temporal brain lobes with memory loss and abnormal behavior
Right hemispheric organic affective disorder

F07.9 Unspecified personality and behavioral disorder due to known physiological condition

Organic psychosyndrome
Due to exposure to organic solvents

F09 Unspecified mental disorder due to known physiological condition

Mental disorder NOS due to known physiological condition
Organic brain syndrome NOS
Organic mental disorder NOS
Organic psychosis NOS
Symptomatic psychosis NOS

Code first the underlying physiological condition

Excludes1 psychosis NOS (F29)

MENTAL AND BEHAVIORAL DISORDERS DUE TO PSYCHOACTIVE SUBSTANCE USE (F10-F19)

● **F10 Alcohol related disorders**

Use additional code for blood alcohol level, if applicable (Y90.-)

● **F10.1 Alcohol abuse**

Excludes1 alcohol dependence (F10.2-)
alcohol use, unspecified (F10.9-)

F10.10 Alcohol abuse, uncomplicated

Alcohol use disorder, mild ◀

● **F10.12 Alcohol abuse with intoxication**

F10.120 Alcohol abuse with intoxication, uncomplicated

F10.121 Alcohol abuse with intoxication, delirium

F10.129 Alcohol abuse with intoxication, unspecified

F10.14 Alcohol abuse with alcohol-induced mood disorder
Alcohol use disorder, mild, with alcohol-induced bipolar or related disorder ◀
Alcohol use disorder, mild, with alcohol-induced depressive disorder ◀

● **F10.15 Alcohol abuse with alcohol-induced psychotic disorder**
F10.150 Alcohol abuse with alcohol-induced psychotic disorder with delusions
F10.151 Alcohol abuse with alcohol-induced psychotic disorder with hallucinations
F10.159 Alcohol abuse with alcohol-induced psychotic disorder, unspecified

● **F10.18 Alcohol abuse with other alcohol-induced disorders**
F10.180 Alcohol abuse with alcohol-induced anxiety disorder
F10.181 Alcohol abuse with alcohol-induced sexual dysfunction
F10.182 Alcohol abuse with alcohol-induced sleep disorder
F10.188 Alcohol abuse with other alcohol-induced disorder

F10.19 Alcohol abuse with unspecified alcohol-induced disorder

● **F10.2 Alcohol dependence**
Excludes1 alcohol abuse (F10.1-)
alcohol use, unspecified (F10.9-)
Excludes2 toxic effect of alcohol (T51.0-)

F10.20 Alcohol dependence, uncomplicated
Alcohol use disorder, moderate ◀
Alcohol use disorder, severe ◀

F10.21 Alcohol dependence, in remission

● **F10.22 Alcohol dependence with intoxication**
Acute drunkenness (in alcoholism)
Excludes2 alcohol dependence with withdrawal (F10.23-) ◀
F10.220 Alcohol dependence with intoxication, uncomplicated
F10.221 Alcohol dependence with intoxication delirium
F10.229 Alcohol dependence with intoxication, unspecified

● **F10.23 Alcohol dependence with withdrawal**
Excludes2 alcohol dependence with intoxication (F10.22-) ◀
F10.230 Alcohol dependence with withdrawal, uncomplicated
F10.231 Alcohol dependence with withdrawal delirium
F10.232 Alcohol dependence with withdrawal with perceptual disturbance
F10.239 Alcohol dependence with withdrawal, unspecified

F10.24 Alcohol dependence with alcohol-induced mood disorder
Alcohol use disorder, moderate, with alcohol-induced bipolar or related disorder ◀
Alcohol use disorder, moderate, with alcohol-induced depressive disorder ◀
Alcohol use disorder, severe, with alcohol-induced bipolar or related disorder ◀
Alcohol use disorder, severe, with alcohol-induced depressive disorder ◀

● **F10.25 Alcohol dependence with alcohol-induced psychotic disorder**
F10.250 Alcohol dependence with alcohol-induced psychotic disorder with delusions
F10.251 Alcohol dependence with alcohol-induced psychotic disorder with hallucinations
F10.259 Alcohol dependence with alcohol-induced psychotic disorder, unspecified

F10.26 Alcohol dependence with alcohol-induced persisting amnestic disorder
Alcohol use disorder, moderate, with alcohol-induced major neurocognitive disorder, amnestic-confabulatory type ◀
Alcohol use disorder, severe, with alcohol-induced major neurocognitive disorder, amnestic-confabulatory type ◀

F10.27 Alcohol dependence with alcohol-induced persisting dementia
Alcohol use disorder, moderate, with alcohol-induced major neurocognitive disorder, nonamnestic-confabulatory type ◀
Alcohol use disorder, severe, with alcohol-induced major neurocognitive disorder, nonamnestic-confabulatory type ◀

● **F10.28 Alcohol dependence with other alcohol-induced disorders**
F10.280 Alcohol dependence with alcohol-induced anxiety disorder
F10.281 Alcohol dependence with alcohol-induced sexual dysfunction
F10.282 Alcohol dependence with alcohol-induced sleep disorder
F10.288 Alcohol dependence with other alcohol-induced disorder
Alcohol use disorder, moderate, with alcohol-induced mild neurocognitive disorder ◀
Alcohol use disorder, severe, with alcohol-induced mild neurocognitive disorder ◀

F10.29 Alcohol dependence with unspecified alcohol-induced disorder

● **F10.9 Alcohol use, unspecified**
Excludes1 alcohol abuse (F10.1-)
alcohol dependence (F10.2-)

● **F10.92 Alcohol use, unspecified with intoxication**
F10.920 Alcohol use, unspecified with intoxication, uncomplicated
F10.921 Alcohol use, unspecified with intoxication delirium
F10.929 Alcohol use, unspecified with intoxication, unspecified

F10.94 Alcohol use, unspecified with alcohol-induced mood disorder
Alcohol-induced bipolar or related disorder, without use disorder ◀
Alcohol-induced depressive disorder, without use disorder ◀

CHAPTER 5 (F01-F99)

● **F10.95 Alcohol use, unspecified with alcohol-induced psychotic disorder**

F10.950 Alcohol use, unspecified with alcohol-induced psychotic disorder with delusions

F10.951 Alcohol use, unspecified with alcohol-induced psychotic disorder with hallucinations

F10.959 Alcohol use, unspecified with alcohol-induced psychotic disorder, unspecified
Alcohol-induced psychotic disorder without use disorder ◀

F10.96 Alcohol use, unspecified with alcohol-induced persisting amnestic disorder
Alcohol-induced major neurocognitive disorder, amnestic-confabulatory type, without use disorder ◀

F10.97 Alcohol use, unspecified with alcohol-induced persisting dementia
Alcohol-induced major neurocognitive disorder, nonamnestic-confabulatory type, without use disorder ◀

● **F10.98 Alcohol use, unspecified with other alcohol-induced disorders**

F10.980 Alcohol use, unspecified with alcohol-induced anxiety disorder
Alcohol-induced anxiety disorder, without use disorder ◀

F10.981 Alcohol use, unspecified with alcohol-induced sexual dysfunction
Alcohol-induced sexual dysfunction, without use disorder ◀

F10.982 Alcohol use, unspecified with alcohol-induced sleep disorder
Alcohol-induced sleep disorder, without use disorder ◀

F10.988 Alcohol use, unspecified with other alcohol-induced disorder
Alcohol-induced mild neurocognitive disorder, without use disorder ◀

F10.99 Alcohol use, unspecified with unspecified alcohol-induced disorder

● **F11 Opioid related disorders**

● **F11.1 Opioid abuse**

Excludes1 opioid dependence (F11.2-)
opioid use, unspecified (F11.9-)

F11.10 Opioid abuse, uncomplicated
Opioid use disorder, mild ◀

● **F11.12 Opioid abuse with intoxication**

F11.120 Opioid abuse with intoxication, uncomplicated

F11.121 Opioid abuse with intoxication delirium

F11.122 Opioid abuse with intoxication with perceptual disturbance

F11.129 Opioid abuse with intoxication, unspecified

F11.14 Opioid abuse with opioid-induced mood disorder
Opioid use disorder, mild, with opioid-induced depressive disorder ◀

● **F11.15 Opioid abuse with opioid-induced psychotic disorder**

F11.150 Opioid abuse with opioid-induced psychotic disorder with delusions

F11.151 Opioid abuse with opioid-induced psychotic disorder with hallucinations

F11.159 Opioid abuse with opioid-induced psychotic disorder, unspecified

● **F11.18 Opioid abuse with other opioid-induced disorder**

F11.181 Opioid abuse with opioid-induced sexual dysfunction

F11.182 Opioid abuse with opioid-induced sleep disorder

F11.188 Opioid abuse with other opioid-induced disorder

F11.19 Opioid abuse with unspecified opioid-induced disorder

● **F11.2 Opioid dependence**

Excludes1 opioid abuse (F11.1-)
opioid use, unspecified (F11.9-)

Excludes2 opioid poisoning (T40.0--T40.2-)

F11.20 Opioid dependence, uncomplicated
Opioid use disorder, moderate ◀
Opioid use disorder, severe ◀

F11.21 Opioid dependence, in remission

● **F11.22 Opioid dependence with intoxication**

Excludes1 opioid dependence with withdrawal (F11.23)

F11.220 Opioid dependence with intoxication, uncomplicated

F11.221 Opioid dependence with intoxication delirium

F11.222 Opioid dependence with intoxication with perceptual disturbance

F11.229 Opioid dependence with intoxication, unspecified

F11.23 Opioid dependence with withdrawal

Excludes1 opioid dependence with intoxication (F11.22-)

F11.24 Opioid dependence with opioid-induced mood disorder
Opioid use disorder, moderate, with opioid-induced depressive disorder ◀

● **F11.25 Opioid dependence with opioid-induced psychotic disorder**

F11.250 Opioid dependence with opioid-induced psychotic disorder with delusions

F11.251 Opioid dependence with opioid-induced psychotic disorder with hallucinations

F11.259 Opioid dependence with opioid-induced psychotic disorder, unspecified

● **F11.28 Opioid dependence with other opioid-induced disorder**

F11.281 Opioid dependence with opioid-induced sexual dysfunction

F11.282 Opioid dependence with opioid-induced sleep disorder

F11.288 Opioid dependence with other opioid-induced disorder

F11.29 Opioid dependence with unspecified opioid-induced disorder

CHAPTER 5 (F01-F99)

● F11.9 Opioid use, unspecified
Excludes1 opioid abuse (F11.1-)
opioid dependence (F11.2-)
F11.90 Opioid use, unspecified, uncomplicated
● F11.92 Opioid use, unspecified with intoxication
Excludes1 opioid use, unspecified with withdrawal (F11.93)
F11.920 Opioid use, unspecified with intoxication, uncomplicated
F11.921 Opioid use, unspecified with intoxication delirium
Opioid-induced delirium ◀
F11.922 Opioid use, unspecified with intoxication with perceptual disturbance
F11.929 Opioid use, unspecified with intoxication, unspecified
F11.93 Opioid use, unspecified with withdrawal
Excludes1 opioid use, unspecified with intoxication (F11.92-)
F11.94 Opioid use, unspecified with opioid-induced mood disorder
Opioid-induced depressive disorder, without use disorder ◀
● F11.95 Opioid use, unspecified with opioid-induced psychotic disorder
F11.950 Opioid use, unspecified with opioid-induced psychotic disorder with delusions
F11.951 Opioid use, unspecified with opioid-induced psychotic disorder with hallucinations
F11.959 Opioid use, unspecified with opioid-induced psychotic disorder, unspecified
● F11.98 Opioid use, unspecified with other specified opioid-induced disorder
F11.981 Opioid use, unspecified with opioid-induced sexual dysfunction
Opioid-induced sexual dysfunction, without use disorder ◀
F11.982 Opioid use, unspecified with opioid-induced sleep disorder
Opioid-induced sleep disorder, without use disorder ◀
F11.988 Opioid use, unspecified with other opioid-induced disorder
Opioid-induced anxiety disorder, without use disorder ◀
F11.99 Opioid use, unspecified with unspecified opioid-induced disorder

● F12 Cannabis related disorders
Includes marijuana
● F12.1 Cannabis abuse
Excludes1 cannabis dependence (F12.2-)
cannabis use, unspecified (F12.9-)
F12.10 Cannabis abuse, uncomplicated
Cannabis use disorder, mild ◀
● F12.12 Cannabis abuse with intoxication
F12.120 Cannabis abuse with intoxication, uncomplicated
F12.121 Cannabis abuse with intoxication delirium
F12.122 Cannabis abuse with intoxication with perceptual disturbance
F12.129 Cannabis abuse with intoxication, unspecified
● F12.15 Cannabis abuse with psychotic disorder
F12.150 Cannabis abuse with psychotic disorder with delusions
F12.151 Cannabis abuse with psychotic disorder with hallucinations
F12.159 Cannabis abuse with psychotic disorder, unspecified
● F12.18 Cannabis abuse with other cannabis-induced disorder
F12.180 Cannabis abuse with cannabis-induced anxiety disorder
F12.188 Cannabis abuse with other cannabis-induced disorder
Cannabis use disorder, mild, with cannabis-induced sleep disorder ◀
F12.19 Cannabis abuse with unspecified cannabis-induced disorder
● F12.2 Cannabis dependence
Excludes1 cannabis abuse (F12.1-)
cannabis use, unspecified (F12.9-)
Excludes2 cannabis poisoning (T40.7-)
F12.20 Cannabis dependence, uncomplicated
Cannabis use disorder, moderate ◀
Cannabis use disorder, severe ◀
F12.21 Cannabis dependence, in remission
● F12.22 Cannabis dependence with intoxication
F12.220 Cannabis dependence with intoxication, uncomplicated
F12.221 Cannabis dependence with intoxication delirium
F12.222 Cannabis dependence with intoxication with perceptual disturbance
F12.229 Cannabis dependence with intoxication, unspecified
● F12.25 Cannabis dependence with psychotic disorder
F12.250 Cannabis dependence with psychotic disorder with delusions
F12.251 Cannabis dependence with psychotic disorder with hallucinations
F12.259 Cannabis dependence with psychotic disorder, unspecified
● F12.28 Cannabis dependence with other cannabis-induced disorder
F12.280 Cannabis dependence with cannabis-induced anxiety disorder
F12.288 Cannabis dependence with other cannabis-induced disorder
Cannabis use disorder, moderate, with cannabis-induced sleep disorder ◀
Cannabis use disorder, severe, with cannabis-induced sleep disorder ◀
Cannabis withdrawal ◀
F12.29 Cannabis dependence with unspecified cannabis-induced disorder
● F12.9 Cannabis use, unspecified
Excludes1 cannabis abuse (F12.1-)
cannabis dependence (F12.2-)
F12.90 Cannabis use, unspecified, uncomplicated
● F12.92 Cannabis use, unspecified with intoxication
F12.920 Cannabis use, unspecified with intoxication, uncomplicated
F12.921 Cannabis use, unspecified with intoxication delirium
F12.922 Cannabis use, unspecified with intoxication with perceptual disturbance
F12.929 Cannabis use, unspecified with intoxication, unspecified

F12.95 Cannabis use, unspecified with psychotic disorder
F12.950 Cannabis use, unspecified with psychotic disorder with delusions
F12.951 Cannabis use, unspecified with psychotic disorder with hallucinations
F12.959 Cannabis use, unspecified with psychotic disorder, unspecified
Cannabis-induced psychotic disorder, without use disorder ◀
F12.98 Cannabis use, unspecified with other cannabis-induced disorder
F12.980 Cannabis use, unspecified with anxiety disorder
Cannabis-induced anxiety disorder, without use disorder ◀
F12.988 Cannabis use, unspecified with other cannabis-induced disorder
Cannabis-induced sleep disorder, without use disorder ◀
F12.99 Cannabis use, unspecified with unspecified cannabis-induced disorder

F13 Sedative, hypnotic, or anxiolytic related disorders
F13.1 Sedative, hypnotic or anxiolytic-related abuse
Excludes1 sedative, hypnotic or anxiolytic-related dependence (F13.2-)
sedative, hypnotic, or anxiolytic use, unspecified (F13.9-)
F13.10 Sedative, hypnotic or anxiolytic abuse, uncomplicated
Sedative, hypnotic, or anxiolytic use disorder, mild ◀
F13.12 Sedative, hypnotic or anxiolytic abuse with intoxication
F13.120 Sedative, hypnotic or anxiolytic abuse with intoxication, uncomplicated
F13.121 Sedative, hypnotic or anxiolytic abuse with intoxication delirium
F13.129 Sedative, hypnotic or anxiolytic abuse with intoxication, unspecified
F13.14 Sedative, hypnotic or anxiolytic abuse with sedative, hypnotic or anxiolytic-induced mood disorder
Sedative, hypnotic, or anxiolytic use disorder, mild, with sedative, hypnotic, or anxiolytic-induced bipolar or related disorder ◀
Sedative, hypnotic, or anxiolytic use disorder, mild, with sedative, hypnotic, or anxiolytic-induced depressive disorder ◀
F13.15 Sedative, hypnotic or anxiolytic abuse with sedative, hypnotic or anxiolytic-induced psychotic disorder
F13.150 Sedative, hypnotic or anxiolytic abuse with sedative, hypnotic or anxiolytic-induced psychotic disorder with delusions
F13.151 Sedative, hypnotic or anxiolytic abuse with sedative, hypnotic or anxiolytic-induced psychotic disorder with hallucinations
F13.159 Sedative, hypnotic or anxiolytic abuse with sedative, hypnotic or anxiolytic-induced psychotic disorder, unspecified
F13.18 Sedative, hypnotic or anxiolytic abuse with other sedative, hypnotic or anxiolytic-induced disorders
F13.180 Sedative, hypnotic or anxiolytic abuse with sedative, hypnotic or anxiolytic-induced anxiety disorder
F13.181 Sedative, hypnotic or anxiolytic abuse with sedative, hypnotic or anxiolytic-induced sexual dysfunction
F13.182 Sedative, hypnotic or anxiolytic abuse with sedative, hypnotic or anxiolytic-induced sleep disorder
F13.188 Sedative, hypnotic or anxiolytic abuse with other sedative, hypnotic or anxiolytic-induced disorder
F13.19 Sedative, hypnotic or anxiolytic abuse with unspecified sedative, hypnotic or anxiolytic-induced disorder
F13.2 Sedative, hypnotic or anxiolytic-related dependence
Excludes1 sedative, hypnotic or anxiolytic-related abuse (F13.1-)
sedative, hypnotic, or anxiolytic use, unspecified (F13.9-)
Excludes2 sedative, hypnotic, or anxiolytic poisoning (T42.-)
F13.20 Sedative, hypnotic or anxiolytic dependence, uncomplicated
F13.21 Sedative, hypnotic or anxiolytic dependence, in remission
F13.22 Sedative, hypnotic or anxiolytic dependence with intoxication
Excludes1 sedative, hypnotic or anxiolytic dependence with withdrawal (F13.23-)
F13.220 Sedative, hypnotic or anxiolytic dependence with intoxication, uncomplicated
F13.221 Sedative, hypnotic or anxiolytic dependence with intoxication delirium
F13.229 Sedative, hypnotic or anxiolytic dependence with intoxication, unspecified
F13.23 Sedative, hypnotic or anxiolytic dependence with withdrawal
Sedative, hypnotic, or anxiolytic use disorder, moderate ◀
Sedative, hypnotic, or anxiolytic use disorder, severe ◀
Excludes1 sedative, hypnotic or anxiolytic dependence with intoxication (F13.22-)
F13.230 Sedative, hypnotic or anxiolytic dependence with withdrawal, uncomplicated
F13.231 Sedative, hypnotic or anxiolytic dependence with withdrawal delirium
F13.232 Sedative, hypnotic or anxiolytic dependence with withdrawal with perceptual disturbance
Sedative, hypnotic, or anxiolytic withdrawal with perceptual disturbances ◀
F13.239 Sedative, hypnotic or anxiolytic dependence with withdrawal, unspecified
Sedative, hypnotic, or anxiolytic withdrawal without perceptual disturbances ◀

F13.24 Sedative, hypnotic or anxiolytic dependence with sedative, hypnotic or anxiolytic-induced mood disorder
Sedative, hypnotic, or anxiolytic use disorder, moderate, with sedative, hypnotic, or anxiolytic-induced bipolar or related disorder ◀
Sedative, hypnotic, or anxiolytic use disorder, moderate, with sedative, hypnotic, or anxiolytic-induced depressive disorder ◀
Sedative, hypnotic, or anxiolytic use disorder, severe, with sedative, hypnotic, or anxiolytic-induced bipolar or related disorder ◀
Sedative, hypnotic, or anxiolytic use disorder, severe, with sedative, hypnotic, or anxiolytic-induced depressive disorder ◀

● **F13.25 Sedative, hypnotic or anxiolytic dependence with sedative, hypnotic or anxiolytic-induced psychotic disorder**
F13.250 Sedative, hypnotic or anxiolytic dependence with sedative, hypnotic or anxiolytic-induced psychotic disorder with delusions
F13.251 Sedative, hypnotic or anxiolytic dependence with sedative, hypnotic or anxiolytic-induced psychotic disorder with hallucinations
F13.259 Sedative, hypnotic or anxiolytic dependence with sedative, hypnotic or anxiolytic-induced psychotic disorder, unspecified

F13.26 Sedative, hypnotic or anxiolytic dependence with sedative, hypnotic or anxiolytic-induced persisting amnestic disorder

F13.27 Sedative, hypnotic or anxiolytic dependence with sedative, hypnotic or anxiolytic-induced persisting dementia
Sedative, hypnotic, or anxiolytic use disorder, moderate, with sedative, hypnotic, or anxiolytic-induced major neurocognitive disorder ◀
Sedative, hypnotic, or anxiolytic use disorder, severe, with sedative, hypnotic, or anxiolytic-induced major neurocognitive disorder ◀

● **F13.28 Sedative, hypnotic or anxiolytic dependence with other sedative, hypnotic or anxiolytic-induced disorders**
F13.280 Sedative, hypnotic or anxiolytic dependence with sedative, hypnotic or anxiolytic-induced anxiety disorder
F13.281 Sedative, hypnotic or anxiolytic dependence with sedative, hypnotic or anxiolytic-induced sexual dysfunction
F13.282 Sedative, hypnotic or anxiolytic dependence with sedative, hypnotic or anxiolytic-induced sleep disorder
F13.288 Sedative, hypnotic or anxiolytic dependence with other sedative, hypnotic or anxiolytic-induced disorder
Sedative, hypnotic, or anxiolytic use disorder, moderate, with sedative, hypnotic, or anxiolytic-induced mild neurocognitive disorder ◀
Sedative, hypnotic, or anxiolytic use disorder, severe, with sedative, hypnotic, or anxiolytic-induced mild neurocognitive disorder ◀

F13.29 Sedative, hypnotic or anxiolytic dependence with unspecified sedative, hypnotic or anxiolytic-induced disorder

● **F13.9 Sedative, hypnotic or anxiolytic-related use, unspecified**
Excludes1 sedative, hypnotic or anxiolytic-related abuse (F13.1-)
sedative, hypnotic or anxiolytic-related dependence (F13.2-)

F13.90 Sedative, hypnotic, or anxiolytic use, unspecified, uncomplicated

● **F13.92 Sedative, hypnotic or anxiolytic use, unspecified with intoxication**
Excludes1 sedative, hypnotic or anxiolytic use, unspecified with withdrawal (F13.93-)
F13.920 Sedative, hypnotic or anxiolytic use, unspecified with intoxication, uncomplicated
F13.921 Sedative, hypnotic or anxiolytic use, unspecified with intoxication delirium
Sedative, hypnotic, or anxiolytic-induced delirium ◀
F13.929 Sedative, hypnotic or anxiolytic use, unspecified with intoxication, unspecified

● **F13.93 Sedative, hypnotic or anxiolytic use, unspecified with withdrawal**
Excludes1 sedative, hypnotic or anxiolytic use, unspecified with intoxication (F13.92-)
F13.930 Sedative, hypnotic or anxiolytic use, unspecified with withdrawal, uncomplicated
F13.931 Sedative, hypnotic or anxiolytic use, unspecified with withdrawal delirium
F13.932 Sedative, hypnotic or anxiolytic use, unspecified with withdrawal with perceptual disturbances
F13.939 Sedative, hypnotic or anxiolytic use, unspecified with withdrawal, unspecified

F13.94 Sedative, hypnotic or anxiolytic use, unspecified with sedative, hypnotic or anxiolytic-induced mood disorder
Sedative, hypnotic, or anxiolytic-induced bipolar or related disorder, without use disorder ◀
Sedative, hypnotic, or anxiolytic-induced depressive disorder, without use disorder ◀

● **F13.95 Sedative, hypnotic or anxiolytic use, unspecified with sedative, hypnotic or anxiolytic-induced psychotic disorder**
F13.950 Sedative, hypnotic or anxiolytic use, unspecified with sedative, hypnotic or anxiolytic-induced psychotic disorder with delusions
F13.951 Sedative, hypnotic or anxiolytic use, unspecified with sedative, hypnotic or anxiolytic-induced psychotic disorder with hallucinations
F13.959 Sedative, hypnotic or anxiolytic use, unspecified with sedative, hypnotic or anxiolytic-induced psychotic disorder, unspecified
Sedative, hypnotic, or anxiolytic-induced psychotic disorder, without use disorder ◀

CHAPTER 5 (F01-F99)

F13.96 **Sedative, hypnotic or anxiolytic use, unspecified with sedative, hypnotic or anxiolytic-induced persisting amnestic disorder**

F13.97 **Sedative, hypnotic or anxiolytic use, unspecified with sedative, hypnotic or anxiolytic-induced persisting dementia**
Sedative, hypnotic, or anxiolytic-induced major neurocognitive disorder, without use disorder ◀

● F13.98 **Sedative, hypnotic or anxiolytic use, unspecified with other sedative, hypnotic or anxiolytic-induced disorders**

F13.980 **Sedative, hypnotic or anxiolytic use, unspecified with sedative, hypnotic or anxiolytic-induced anxiety disorder**
Sedative, hypnotic, or anxiolytic-induced anxiety disorder, without use disorder ◀

F13.981 **Sedative, hypnotic or anxiolytic use, unspecified with sedative, hypnotic or anxiolytic-induced sexual dysfunction**
Sedative, hypnotic, or anxiolytic-induced sexual dysfunction disorder, without use disorder ◀

F13.982 **Sedative, hypnotic or anxiolytic use, unspecified with sedative, hypnotic or anxiolytic-induced sleep disorder**
Sedative, hypnotic, or anxiolytic-induced sleep disorder, without use disorder ◀

F13.988 **Sedative, hypnotic or anxiolytic use, unspecified with other sedative, hypnotic or anxiolytic-induced disorder**
Sedative, hypnotic, or anxiolytic-induced mild neurocognitive disorder ◀

F13.99 **Sedative, hypnotic or anxiolytic use, unspecified with unspecified sedative, hypnotic or anxiolytic-induced disorder**

● F14 **Cocaine related disorders**
Excludes2 other stimulant-related disorders (F15.-)

● F14.1 **Cocaine abuse**
Excludes1 cocaine dependence (F14.2-)
cocaine use, unspecified (F14.9-)

F14.10 **Cocaine abuse, uncomplicated**
Cocaine use disorder, mild ◀

● F14.12 **Cocaine abuse with intoxication**

F14.120 **Cocaine abuse with intoxication, uncomplicated**

F14.121 **Cocaine abuse with intoxication with delirium**

F14.122 **Cocaine abuse with intoxication with perceptual disturbance**

F14.129 **Cocaine abuse with intoxication, unspecified**

F14.14 **Cocaine abuse with cocaine-induced mood disorder**
Cocaine use disorder, mild, with cocaine-induced bipolar or related disorder ◀
Cocaine use disorder, mild, with cocaine-induced depressive disorder ◀

● F14.15 **Cocaine abuse with cocaine-induced psychotic disorder**

F14.150 **Cocaine abuse with cocaine-induced psychotic disorder with delusions**

F14.151 **Cocaine abuse with cocaine-induced psychotic disorder with hallucinations**

F14.159 **Cocaine abuse with cocaine-induced psychotic disorder, unspecified**

● F14.18 **Cocaine abuse with other cocaine-induced disorder**

F14.180 **Cocaine abuse with cocaine-induced anxiety disorder**

F14.181 **Cocaine abuse with cocaine-induced sexual dysfunction**

F14.182 **Cocaine abuse with cocaine-induced sleep disorder**

F14.188 **Cocaine abuse with other cocaine-induced disorder**
Cocaine use disorder, mild, with cocaine-induced obsessive-compulsive or related disorder ◀

F14.19 **Cocaine abuse with unspecified cocaine-induced disorder**

● F14.2 **Cocaine dependence**
Excludes1 cocaine abuse (F14.1-)
cocaine use, unspecified (F14.9-)
Excludes2 cocaine poisoning (T40.5-)

F14.20 **Cocaine dependence, uncomplicated**
Cocaine use disorder, moderate ◀
Cocaine use disorder, severe ◀

F14.21 **Cocaine dependence, in remission**

● F14.22 **Cocaine dependence with intoxication**
Excludes1 cocaine dependence with withdrawal (F14.23)

F14.220 **Cocaine dependence with intoxication, uncomplicated**

F14.221 **Cocaine dependence with intoxication delirium**

F14.222 **Cocaine dependence with intoxication with perceptual disturbance**

F14.229 **Cocaine dependence with intoxication, unspecified**

F14.23 **Cocaine dependence with withdrawal**
Excludes1 cocaine dependence with intoxication (F14.22-)

F14.24 **Cocaine dependence with cocaine-induced mood disorder**
Cocaine use disorder, moderate, with cocaine-induced bipolar or related disorder ◀
Cocaine use disorder, moderate, with cocaine-induced depressive disorder ◀
Cocaine use disorder, severe, with cocaine-induced bipolar or related disorder ◀
Cocaine use disorder, severe, with cocaine-induced depressive disorder ◀

● F14.25 **Cocaine dependence with cocaine-induced psychotic disorder**

F14.250 **Cocaine dependence with cocaine-induced psychotic disorder with delusions**

F14.251 **Cocaine dependence with cocaine-induced psychotic disorder with hallucinations**

F14.259 **Cocaine dependence with cocaine-induced psychotic disorder, unspecified**

● F14.28 Cocaine dependence with other cocaine-induced disorder

F14.280 Cocaine dependence with cocaine-induced anxiety disorder

F14.281 Cocaine dependence with cocaine-induced sexual dysfunction

F14.282 Cocaine dependence with cocaine-induced sleep disorder

F14.288 Cocaine dependence with other cocaine-induced disorder
Cocaine use disorder, moderate, with cocaine-induced obsessive-compulsive or related disorder ◀
Cocaine use disorder, severe, with cocaine-induced obsessive-compulsive or related disorder ◀

F14.29 Cocaine dependence with unspecified cocaine-induced disorder

● F14.9 Cocaine use, unspecified
Excludes1 cocaine abuse (F14.1-)
cocaine dependence (F14.2-)

F14.90 Cocaine use, unspecified, uncomplicated

● F14.92 Cocaine use, unspecified with intoxication

F14.920 Cocaine use, unspecified with intoxication, uncomplicated

F14.921 Cocaine use, unspecified with intoxication delirium

F14.922 Cocaine use, unspecified with intoxication with perceptual disturbance

F14.929 Cocaine use, unspecified with intoxication, unspecified

F14.94 Cocaine use, unspecified with cocaine-induced mood disorder
Cocaine-induced bipolar or related disorder, without use disorder ◀
Cocaine-induced depressive disorder, without use disorder ◀

● F14.95 Cocaine use, unspecified with cocaine-induced psychotic disorder

F14.950 Cocaine use, unspecified with cocaine-induced psychotic disorder with delusions

F14.951 Cocaine use, unspecified with cocaine-induced psychotic disorder with hallucinations

F14.959 Cocaine use, unspecified with cocaine-induced psychotic disorder, unspecified
Cocaine-induced psychotic disorder, without use disorder ◀

● F14.98 Cocaine use, unspecified with other specified cocaine-induced disorder

F14.980 Cocaine use, unspecified with cocaine-induced anxiety disorder
Cocaine-induced anxiety disorder, without use disorder ◀

F14.981 Cocaine use, unspecified with cocaine-induced sexual dysfunction
Cocaine-induced sexual dysfunction, without use disorder ◀

F14.982 Cocaine use, unspecified with cocaine-induced sleep disorder
Cocaine-induced sleep disorder, without use disorder ◀

F14.988 Cocaine use, unspecified with other cocaine-induced disorder
Cocaine-induced obsessive-compulsive or related disorder ◀

F14.99 Cocaine use, unspecified with unspecified cocaine-induced disorder

● F15 Other stimulant related disorders
Includes amphetamine-related disorders
caffeine
Excludes2 cocaine-related disorders (F14.-)

● F15.1 Other stimulant abuse
Excludes1 other stimulant dependence (F15.2-)
other stimulant use, unspecified (F15.9-)

F15.10 Other stimulant abuse, uncomplicated
Amphetamine type substance use disorder, mild ◀
Other or unspecified stimulant use disorder, mild ◀

● F15.12 Other stimulant abuse with intoxication

F15.120 Other stimulant abuse with intoxication, uncomplicated

F15.121 Other stimulant abuse with intoxication delirium

F15.122 Other stimulant abuse with intoxication with perceptual disturbance
Amphetamine or other stimulant use disorder, mild, with amphetamine or other stimulant intoxication, with perceptual disturbances ◀

F15.129 Other stimulant abuse with intoxication, unspecified
Amphetamine or other stimulant use disorder, mild, with amphetamine or other stimulant intoxication, without perceptual disturbances ◀

F15.14 Other stimulant abuse with stimulant-induced mood disorder
Amphetamine or other stimulant use disorder, mild, with amphetamine or other stimulant-induced bipolar or related disorder ◀
Amphetamine or other stimulant use disorder, mild, with amphetamine or other stimulant-induced depressive disorder ◀

● F15.15 Other stimulant abuse with stimulant-induced psychotic disorder

F15.150 Other stimulant abuse with stimulant-induced psychotic disorder with delusions

F15.151 Other stimulant abuse with stimulant-induced psychotic disorder with hallucinations

F15.159 Other stimulant abuse with stimulant-induced psychotic disorder, unspecified

● F15.18 Other stimulant abuse with other stimulant-induced disorder

F15.180 Other stimulant abuse with stimulant-induced anxiety disorder

F15.181 Other stimulant abuse with stimulant-induced sexual dysfunction

F15.182 Other stimulant abuse with stimulant-induced sleep disorder

F15.188 Other stimulant abuse with other stimulant-induced disorder
Amphetamine or other stimulant use disorder, mild, with amphetamine or other stimulant-induced obsessive-compulsive or related disorder ◀

F15.19 Other stimulant abuse with unspecified stimulant-induced disorder

CHAPTER 5 (F01-F99)

● **F15.2 Other stimulant dependence**
Excludes1 other stimulant abuse (F15.1-)
other stimulant use, unspecified (F15.9-)

F15.20 Other stimulant dependence, uncomplicated
Amphetamine type substance use disorder, moderate ◀
Amphetamine type substance use disorder, severe ◀
Other or unspecified stimulant use disorder, moderate ◀
Other or unspecified stimulant use disorder, severe ◀

F15.21 Other stimulant dependence, in remission

● **F15.22 Other stimulant dependence with intoxication**
Excludes1 other stimulant dependence with withdrawal (F15.23)

F15.220 Other stimulant dependence with intoxication, uncomplicated

F15.221 Other stimulant dependence with intoxication delirium

F15.222 Other stimulant dependence with intoxication with perceptual disturbance
Amphetamine or other stimulant use disorder, moderate, with amphetamine or other stimulant intoxication, with perceptual disturbances ◀
Amphetamine or other stimulant use disorder, severe, with amphetamine or other stimulant intoxication, with perceptual disturbances ◀

F15.229 Other stimulant dependence with intoxication, unspecified
Amphetamine or other stimulant use disorder, moderate, with amphetamine or other stimulant intoxication, without perceptual disturbances ◀
Amphetamine or other stimulant use disorder, severe, with amphetamine or other stimulant intoxication, without perceptual disturbances ◀

F15.23 Other stimulant dependence with withdrawal
Amphetamine or other stimulant withdrawal ◀
Excludes1 other stimulant dependence with intoxication (F15.22-)

F15.24 Other stimulant dependence with stimulant-induced mood disorder
Amphetamine or other stimulant use disorder, moderate, with amphetamine or other stimulant-induced bipolar or related disorder ◀
Amphetamine or other stimulant use disorder, moderate, with amphetamine or other stimulant-induced depressive disorder ◀
Amphetamine or other stimulant use disorder, severe, with amphetamine or other stimulant-induced bipolar or related disorder ◀
Amphetamine or other stimulant use disorder, severe, with amphetamine or other stimulant-induced depressive disorder ◀

● **F15.25 Other stimulant dependence with stimulant-induced psychotic disorder**

F15.250 Other stimulant dependence with stimulant-induced psychotic disorder with delusions

F15.251 Other stimulant dependence with stimulant-induced psychotic disorder with hallucinations

F15.259 Other stimulant dependence with stimulant-induced psychotic disorder, unspecified

● **F15.28 Other stimulant dependence with other stimulant-induced disorder**

F15.280 Other stimulant dependence with stimulant-induced anxiety disorder

F15.281 Other stimulant dependence with stimulant-induced sexual dysfunction

F15.282 Other stimulant dependence with stimulant-induced sleep disorder

F15.288 Other stimulant dependence with other stimulant-induced disorder
Amphetamine or other stimulant use disorder, moderate, with amphetamine or other stimulant-induced obsessive-compulsive or related disorder ◀
Amphetamine or other stimulant use disorder, severe, with amphetamine or other stimulant-induced obsessive-compulsive or related disorder ◀

F15.29 Other stimulant dependence with unspecified stimulant-induced disorder

● **F15.9 Other stimulant use, unspecified**
Excludes1 other stimulant abuse (F15.1-)
other stimulant dependence (F15.2-)

F15.90 Other stimulant use, unspecified, uncomplicated

● **F15.92 Other stimulant use, unspecified with intoxication**
Excludes1 other stimulant use, unspecified with withdrawal (F15.93)

F15.920 Other stimulant use, unspecified with intoxication, uncomplicated

F15.921 Other stimulant use, unspecified with intoxication delirium
Amphetamine or other stimulant-induced delirium ◀

F15.922 Other stimulant use, unspecified with intoxication with perceptual disturbance

F15.929 Other stimulant use, unspecified with intoxication, unspecified
Caffeine intoxication ◀

F15.93 Other stimulant use, unspecified with withdrawal
Caffeine withdrawal ◀
Excludes1 other stimulant use, unspecified with intoxication (F15.92-)

F15.94 Other stimulant use, unspecified with stimulant-induced mood disorder
Amphetamine or other stimulant-induced bipolar or related disorder, without use disorder ◀
Amphetamine or other stimulant-induced depressive disorder, without use disorder ◀

● F15.95 **Other stimulant use, unspecified with stimulant-induced psychotic disorder**

F15.950 **Other stimulant use, unspecified with stimulant-induced psychotic disorder with delusions**

F15.951 **Other stimulant use, unspecified with stimulant-induced psychotic disorder with hallucinations**

F15.959 **Other stimulant use, unspecified with stimulant-induced psychotic disorder, unspecified**
Amphetamine or other stimulant-induced psychotic disorder, without use disorder ◀

● F15.98 **Other stimulant use, unspecified with other stimulant-induced disorder**

F15.980 **Other stimulant use, unspecified with stimulant-induced anxiety disorder**
Amphetamine or other stimulant-induced anxiety disorder, without use disorder ◀
Caffeine-induced anxiety disorder, without use disorder ◀

F15.981 **Other stimulant use, unspecified with stimulant-induced sexual dysfunction**
Amphetamine or other stimulant-induced sexual dysfunction, without use disorder ◀

F15.982 **Other stimulant use, unspecified with stimulant-induced sleep disorder**
Amphetamine or other stimulant-induced sleep disorder, without use disorder ◀
Caffeine-induced sleep disorder, without use disorder ◀

F15.988 **Other stimulant use, unspecified with other stimulant-induced disorder**
Amphetamine or other stimulant-induced obsessive-compulsive or related disorder, without use disorder ◀

F15.99 **Other stimulant use, unspecified with unspecified stimulant-induced disorder**

● F16 **Hallucinogen related disorders**

Includes ecstasy
PCP
phencyclidine

● F16.1 **Hallucinogen abuse**

Excludes1 hallucinogen dependence (F16.2-)
hallucinogen use, unspecified (F16.9-)

F16.10 **Hallucinogen abuse, uncomplicated**
Other hallucinogen use disorder, mild ◀
Phencyclidine use disorder, mild ◀

● F16.12 **Hallucinogen abuse with intoxication**

F16.120 **Hallucinogen abuse with intoxication, uncomplicated**

F16.121 **Hallucinogen abuse with intoxication with delirium**

F16.122 **Hallucinogen abuse with intoxication with perceptual disturbance**

F16.129 **Hallucinogen abuse with intoxication, unspecified**

F16.14 **Hallucinogen abuse with hallucinogen-induced mood disorder**
Other hallucinogen use disorder, mild, with other hallucinogen-induced bipolar or related disorder ◀
Other hallucinogen use disorder, mild, with other hallucinogen-induced depressive disorder ◀
Phencyclidine use disorder, mild, with phencyclidine-induced bipolar or related disorder ◀
Phencyclidine use disorder, mild, with phencyclidine-induced depressive disorder ◀

● F16.15 **Hallucinogen abuse with hallucinogen-induced psychotic disorder**

F16.150 **Hallucinogen abuse with hallucinogen-induced psychotic disorder with delusions**

F16.151 **Hallucinogen abuse with hallucinogen-induced psychotic disorder with hallucinations**

F16.159 **Hallucinogen abuse with hallucinogen-induced psychotic disorder, unspecified**

● F16.18 **Hallucinogen abuse with other hallucinogen-induced disorder**

F16.180 **Hallucinogen abuse with hallucinogen-induced anxiety disorder**

F16.183 **Hallucinogen abuse with hallucinogen persisting perception disorder (flashbacks)**

F16.188 **Hallucinogen abuse with other hallucinogen-induced disorder**

F16.19 **Hallucinogen abuse with unspecified hallucinogen-induced disorder**

● F16.2 **Hallucinogen dependence**

Excludes1 hallucinogen abuse (F16.1-)
hallucinogen use, unspecified (F16.9-)

F16.20 **Hallucinogen dependence, uncomplicated**
Other hallucinogen use disorder, moderate ◀
Other hallucinogen use disorder, severe ◀
Phencyclidine use disorder, moderate ◀
Phencyclidine use disorder, severe ◀

F16.21 **Hallucinogen dependence, in remission**

● F16.22 **Hallucinogen dependence with intoxication**

F16.220 **Hallucinogen dependence with intoxication, uncomplicated**

F16.221 **Hallucinogen dependence with intoxication with delirium**

F16.229 **Hallucinogen dependence with intoxication, unspecified**

F16.24 **Hallucinogen dependence with hallucinogen-induced mood disorder**
Other hallucinogen use disorder, moderate, with other hallucinogen-induced bipolar or related disorder ◀
Other hallucinogen use disorder, moderate, with other hallucinogen-induced depressive disorder ◀
Other hallucinogen use disorder, severe, with other hallucinogen-induced bipolar or related disorder ◀
Other hallucinogen use disorder, severe, with other hallucinogen-induced depressive disorder ◀
Phencyclidine use disorder, moderate, with phencyclidine-induced bipolar or related disorder ◀
Phencyclidine use disorder, moderate, with phencyclidine-induced depressive disorder ◀
Phencyclidine use disorder, severe, with phencyclidine-induced bipolar or related disorder ◀
Phencyclidine use disorder, severe, with phencyclidine-induced depressive disorder ◀

CHAPTER 5 (F01-F99)

● F16.25 Hallucinogen dependence with hallucinogen-induced psychotic disorder

F16.250 Hallucinogen dependence with hallucinogen-induced psychotic disorder with delusions

F16.251 Hallucinogen dependence with hallucinogen-induced psychotic disorder with hallucinations

F16.259 Hallucinogen dependence with hallucinogen-induced psychotic disorder, unspecified

● F16.28 Hallucinogen dependence with other hallucinogen-induced disorder

F16.280 Hallucinogen dependence with hallucinogen-induced anxiety disorder

F16.283 Hallucinogen dependence with hallucinogen persisting perception disorder (flashbacks)

F16.288 Hallucinogen dependence with other hallucinogen-induced disorder

F16.29 Hallucinogen dependence with unspecified hallucinogen-induced disorder

● F16.9 Hallucinogen use, unspecified

Excludes1 hallucinogen abuse (F16.1-)
hallucinogen dependence (F16.2-)

F16.90 Hallucinogen use, unspecified, uncomplicated

● F16.92 Hallucinogen use, unspecified with intoxication

F16.920 Hallucinogen use, unspecified with intoxication, uncomplicated

F16.921 Hallucinogen use, unspecified with intoxication with delirium
Other hallucinogen intoxication delirium ◀

F16.929 Hallucinogen use, unspecified with intoxication, unspecified

F16.94 Hallucinogen use, unspecified with hallucinogen-induced mood disorder
Other hallucinogen-induced bipolar or related disorder, without use disorder ◀
Other hallucinogen-induced depressive disorder, without use disorder ◀
Phencyclidine-induced bipolar or related disorder, without use disorder ◀
Phencyclidine-induced depressive disorder, without use disorder ◀

● F16.95 Hallucinogen use, unspecified with hallucinogen-induced psychotic disorder

F16.950 Hallucinogen use, unspecified with hallucinogen-induced psychotic disorder with delusions

F16.951 Hallucinogen use, unspecified with hallucinogen-induced psychotic disorder with hallucinations

F16.959 Hallucinogen use, unspecified with hallucinogen-induced psychotic disorder, unspecified
Other hallucinogen-induced psychotic disorder, without use disorder ◀
Phencyclidine-induced psychotic disorder, without use disorder ◀

● F16.98 Hallucinogen use, unspecified with other specified hallucinogen-induced disorder

F16.980 Hallucinogen use, unspecified with hallucinogen-induced anxiety disorder
Other hallucinogen-induced anxiety disorder, without use disorder ◀
Phencyclidine-induced anxiety disorder, without use disorder ◀

F16.983 Hallucinogen use, unspecified with hallucinogen persisting perception disorder (flashbacks)

F16.988 Hallucinogen use, unspecified with other hallucinogen-induced disorder

F16.99 Hallucinogen use, unspecified with unspecified hallucinogen-induced disorder

● F17 Nicotine dependence

Excludes1 history of tobacco dependence (Z87.891)
tobacco use NOS (Z72.0)

Excludes2 tobacco use (smoking) during pregnancy, childbirth and the puerperium (O99.33-)
toxic effect of nicotine (T65.2-)

● F17.2 Nicotine dependence

● F17.20 Nicotine dependence, unspecified

F17.200 Nicotine dependence, unspecified, uncomplicated
Tobacco use disorder, mild ◀
Tobacco use disorder, moderate ◀
Tobacco use disorder, severe ◀

F17.201 Nicotine dependence, unspecified, in remission

F17.203 Nicotine dependence unspecified, with withdrawal
Tobacco withdrawal ◀

F17.208 Nicotine dependence, unspecified, with other nicotine-induced disorders

F17.209 Nicotine dependence, unspecified, with unspecified nicotine-induced disorders

● F17.21 Nicotine dependence, cigarettes

F17.210 Nicotine dependence, cigarettes, uncomplicated

F17.211 Nicotine dependence, cigarettes, in remission

F17.213 Nicotine dependence, cigarettes, with withdrawal

F17.218 Nicotine dependence, cigarettes, with other nicotine-induced disorders

F17.219 Nicotine dependence, cigarettes, with unspecified nicotine-induced disorders

● F17.22 Nicotine dependence, chewing tobacco

F17.220 Nicotine dependence, chewing tobacco, uncomplicated

F17.221 Nicotine dependence, chewing tobacco, in remission

F17.223 Nicotine dependence, chewing tobacco, with withdrawal

F17.228 Nicotine dependence, chewing tobacco, with other nicotine-induced disorders

F17.229 Nicotine dependence, chewing tobacco, with unspecified nicotine-induced disorders

● F17.29 Nicotine dependence, other tobacco product

F17.290 Nicotine dependence, other tobacco product, uncomplicated

F17.291 Nicotine dependence, other tobacco product, in remission

F17.293 Nicotine dependence, other tobacco product, with withdrawal

F17.298 Nicotine dependence, other tobacco product, with other nicotine-induced disorders

F17.299 Nicotine dependence, other tobacco product, with unspecified nicotine-induced disorders

● **F18 Inhalant related disorders**
Includes volatile solvents

● **F18.1 Inhalant abuse**
Excludes1 inhalant dependence (F18.2-)
inhalant use, unspecified (F18.9-)

F18.10 Inhalant abuse, uncomplicated
Inhalant use disorder, mild ◀

● **F18.12 Inhalant abuse with intoxication**
F18.120 Inhalant abuse with intoxication, uncomplicated
F18.121 Inhalant abuse with intoxication delirium
F18.129 Inhalant abuse with intoxication, unspecified

F18.14 Inhalant abuse with inhalant-induced mood disorder
Inhalant use disorder, mild, with inhalant-induced depressive disorder ◀

● **F18.15 Inhalant abuse with inhalant-induced psychotic disorder**
F18.150 Inhalant abuse with inhalant-induced psychotic disorder with delusions
F18.151 Inhalant abuse with inhalant-induced psychotic disorder with hallucinations
F18.159 Inhalant abuse with inhalant-induced psychotic disorder, unspecified

F18.17 Inhalant abuse with inhalant-induced dementia
Inhalant use disorder, mild, with inhalant-induced major neurocognitive disorder ◀

● **F18.18 Inhalant abuse with other inhalant-induced disorders**
F18.180 Inhalant abuse with inhalant-induced anxiety disorder
F18.188 Inhalant abuse with other inhalant-induced disorder
Inhalant use disorder, mild, with inhalant-induced mild neurocognitive disorder ◀

F18.19 Inhalant abuse with unspecified inhalant-induced disorder

● **F18.2 Inhalant dependence**
Excludes1 inhalant abuse (F18.1-)
inhalant use, unspecified (F18.9-)

F18.20 Inhalant dependence, uncomplicated
Inhalant use disorder, moderate ◀
Inhalant use disorder, severe ◀

F18.21 Inhalant dependence, in remission

● **F18.22 Inhalant dependence with intoxication**
F18.220 Inhalant dependence with intoxication, uncomplicated
F18.221 Inhalant dependence with intoxication delirium
F18.229 Inhalant dependence with intoxication, unspecified

F18.24 Inhalant dependence with inhalant-induced mood disorder
Inhalant use disorder, moderate, with inhalant-induced depressive disorder ◀
Inhalant use disorder, severe, with inhalant-induced depressive disorder ◀

● **F18.25 Inhalant dependence with inhalant-induced psychotic disorder**
F18.250 Inhalant dependence with inhalant-induced psychotic disorder with delusions
F18.251 Inhalant dependence with inhalant-induced psychotic disorder with hallucinations
F18.259 Inhalant dependence with inhalant-induced psychotic disorder, unspecified

F18.27 Inhalant dependence with inhalant-induced dementia
Inhalant use disorder, moderate, with inhalant-induced major neurocognitive disorder ◀
Inhalant use disorder, severe, with inhalant-induced major neurocognitive disorder ◀

● **F18.28 Inhalant dependence with other inhalant-induced disorders**
F18.280 Inhalant dependence with inhalant-induced anxiety disorder
F18.288 Inhalant dependence with other inhalant-induced disorder
Inhalant use disorder, moderate, with inhalant-induced mild neurocognitive disorder ◀
Inhalant use disorder, severe, with inhalant-induced mild neurocognitive disorder ◀

F18.29 Inhalant dependence with unspecified inhalant-induced disorder

● **F18.9 Inhalant use, unspecified**
Excludes1 inhalant abuse (F18.1-)
inhalant dependence (F18.2-)

F18.90 Inhalant use, unspecified, uncomplicated

● **F18.92 Inhalant use, unspecified with intoxication**
F18.920 Inhalant use, unspecified with intoxication, uncomplicated
F18.921 Inhalant use, unspecified with intoxication with delirium
F18.929 Inhalant use, unspecified with intoxication, unspecified

F18.94 Inhalant use, unspecified with inhalant-induced mood disorder
Inhalant-induced depressive disorder ◀

● **F18.95 Inhalant use, unspecified with inhalant-induced psychotic disorder**
F18.950 Inhalant use, unspecified with inhalant-induced psychotic disorder with delusions
F18.951 Inhalant use, unspecified with inhalant-induced psychotic disorder with hallucinations
F18.959 Inhalant use, unspecified with inhalant-induced psychotic disorder, unspecified

F18.97 Inhalant use, unspecified with inhalant-induced persisting dementia
Inhalant-induced major neurocognitive disorder ◀

● **F18.98 Inhalant use, unspecified with other inhalant-induced disorders**
F18.980 Inhalant use, unspecified with inhalant-induced anxiety disorder
F18.988 Inhalant use, unspecified with other inhalant-induced disorder
Inhalant-induced mild neurocognitive disorder ◀

F18.99 Inhalant use, unspecified with unspecified inhalant-induced disorder

● **F19 Other psychoactive substance related disorders**

Includes polysubstance drug use (indiscriminate drug use)

● **F19.1 Other psychoactive substance abuse**

Excludes1 other psychoactive substance dependence (F19.2-)
other psychoactive substance use, unspecified (F19.9-)

F19.10 Other psychoactive substance abuse, uncomplicated
Other (or unknown) substance use disorder, mild ◀

● **F19.12 Other psychoactive substance abuse with intoxication**

F19.120 Other psychoactive substance abuse with intoxication, uncomplicated

F19.121 Other psychoactive substance abuse with intoxication delirium

F19.122 Other psychoactive substance abuse with intoxication with perceptual disturbances

F19.129 Other psychoactive substance abuse with intoxication, unspecified

F19.14 Other psychoactive substance abuse with psychoactive substance-induced mood disorder
Other (or unknown) substance use disorder, mild, with other (or unknown) substance-induced bipolar or related disorder ◀
Other (or unknown) substance use disorder, mild, with other (or unknown) substance-induced depressive disorder ◀

● **F19.15 Other psychoactive substance abuse with psychoactive substance-induced psychotic disorder**

F19.150 Other psychoactive substance abuse with psychoactive substance-induced psychotic disorder with delusions

F19.151 Other psychoactive substance abuse with psychoactive substance-induced psychotic disorder with hallucinations

F19.159 Other psychoactive substance abuse with psychoactive substance-induced psychotic disorder, unspecified

F19.16 Other psychoactive substance abuse with psychoactive substance-induced persisting amnestic disorder

F19.17 Other psychoactive substance abuse with psychoactive substance-induced persisting dementia
Other (or unknown) substance use disorder, mild, with other (or unknown) substance-induced major neurocognitive disorder ◀

● **F19.18 Other psychoactive substance abuse with other psychoactive substance-induced disorders**

F19.180 Other psychoactive substance abuse with psychoactive substance-induced anxiety disorder

F19.181 Other psychoactive substance abuse with psychoactive substance-induced sexual dysfunction

F19.182 Other psychoactive substance abuse with psychoactive substance-induced sleep disorder

F19.188 Other psychoactive substance abuse with other psychoactive substance-induced disorder
Other (or unknown) substance use disorder, mild, with other (or unknown) substance-induced mild neurocognitive disorder ◀
Other (or unknown) substance use disorder, mild, with other (or unknown) substance-induced obsessive-compulsive or related disorder ◀

F19.19 Other psychoactive substance abuse with unspecified psychoactive substance-induced disorder

● **F19.2 Other psychoactive substance dependence**

Excludes1 other psychoactive substance abuse (F19.1-)
other psychoactive substance use, unspecified (F19.9-)

F19.20 Other psychoactive substance dependence, uncomplicated
Other (or unknown) substance use disorder, moderate ◀
Other (or unknown) substance use disorder, severe ◀

F19.21 Other psychoactive substance dependence, in remission

● **F19.22 Other psychoactive substance dependence with intoxication**

Excludes1 other psychoactive substance dependence with withdrawal (F19.23-)

F19.220 Other psychoactive substance dependence with intoxication, uncomplicated

F19.221 Other psychoactive substance dependence with intoxication delirium

F19.222 Other psychoactive substance dependence with intoxication with perceptual disturbance

F19.229 Other psychoactive substance dependence with intoxication, unspecified

● **F19.23 Other psychoactive substance dependence with withdrawal**

Excludes1 other psychoactive substance dependence with intoxication (F19.22-)

F19.230 Other psychoactive substance dependence with withdrawal, uncomplicated

F19.231 Other psychoactive substance dependence with withdrawal delirium

F19.232 **Other psychoactive substance dependence with withdrawal with perceptual disturbance**

F19.239 **Other psychoactive substance dependence with withdrawal, unspecified**

F19.24 **Other psychoactive substance dependence with psychoactive substance-induced mood disorder**
Other (or unknown) substance use disorder, moderate, with other (or unknown) substance-induced bipolar or related disorder ◀
Other (or unknown) substance use disorder, moderate, with other (or unknown) substance-induced depressive disorder ◀
Other (or unknown) substance use disorder, severe, with other (or unknown) substance-induced bipolar or related disorder ◀
Other (or unknown) substance use disorder, severe, with other (or unknown) substance-induced depressive disorder ◀

● F19.25 **Other psychoactive substance dependence with psychoactive substance-induced psychotic disorder**

F19.250 **Other psychoactive substance dependence with psychoactive substance-induced psychotic disorder with delusions**

F19.251 **Other psychoactive substance dependence with psychoactive substance-induced psychotic disorder with hallucinations**

F19.259 **Other psychoactive substance dependence with psychoactive substance-induced psychotic disorder, unspecified**

F19.26 **Other psychoactive substance dependence with psychoactive substance-induced persisting amnestic disorder**

F19.27 **Other psychoactive substance dependence with psychoactive substance-induced persisting dementia**
Other (or unknown) substance use disorder, moderate, with other (or unknown) substance-induced major neurocognitive disorder ◀
Other (or unknown) substance use disorder, severe, with other (or unknown) substance-induced major neurocognitive disorder ◀

● F19.28 **Other psychoactive substance dependence with other psychoactive substance-induced disorders**

F19.280 **Other psychoactive substance dependence with psychoactive substance-induced anxiety disorder**

F19.281 **Other psychoactive substance dependence with psychoactive substance-induced sexual dysfunction**

F19.282 **Other psychoactive substance dependence with psychoactive substance-induced sleep disorder**

F19.288 **Other psychoactive substance dependence with other psychoactive substance-induced disorder**
Other (or unknown) substance use disorder, moderate, with other (or unknown) substance-induced mild neurocognitive disorder ◀
Other (or unknown) substance use disorder, severe, with other (or unknown) substance-induced mild neurocognitive disorder ◀
Other (or unknown) substance use disorder, moderate, with other (or unknown) substance-induced obsessive-compulsive or related disorder ◀
Other (or unknown) substance use disorder, severe, with other (or unknown) substance-induced obsessive-compulsive or related disorder ◀

F19.29 **Other psychoactive substance dependence with unspecified psychoactive substance-induced disorder**

● F19.9 **Other psychoactive substance use, unspecified**
Excludes1 other psychoactive substance abuse (F19.1-)
other psychoactive substance dependence (F19.2-)

F19.90 **Other psychoactive substance use, unspecified, uncomplicated**

● F19.92 **Other psychoactive substance use, unspecified with intoxication**
Excludes1 other psychoactive substance use, unspecified with withdrawal (F19.93)

F19.920 **Other psychoactive substance use, unspecified with intoxication, uncomplicated**

F19.921 **Other psychoactive substance use, unspecified with intoxication with delirium**
Other (or unknown) substance-induced delirium ◀

F19.922 **Other psychoactive substance use, unspecified with intoxication with perceptual disturbance**

F19.929 **Other psychoactive substance use, unspecified with intoxication, unspecified**

● F19.93 **Other psychoactive substance use, unspecified with withdrawal**
Excludes1 other psychoactive substance use, unspecified with intoxication (F19.92-)

F19.930 **Other psychoactive substance use, unspecified with withdrawal, uncomplicated**

F19.931 **Other psychoactive substance use, unspecified with withdrawal delirium**

F19.932 **Other psychoactive substance use, unspecified with withdrawal with perceptual disturbance**

F19.939 **Other psychoactive substance use, unspecified with withdrawal, unspecified**

CHAPTER 5 (FØ1-F99)

F19.94 Other psychoactive substance use, unspecified with psychoactive substance-induced mood disorder
Other (or unknown) substance-induced bipolar or related disorder, without use disorder ◀
Other (or unknown) substance-induced depressive disorder, without use disorder ◀

● **F19.95 Other psychoactive substance use, unspecified with psychoactive substance-induced psychotic disorder**

F19.950 Other psychoactive substance use, unspecified with psychoactive substance-induced psychotic disorder with delusions

F19.951 Other psychoactive substance use, unspecified with psychoactive substance-induced psychotic disorder with hallucinations

F19.959 Other psychoactive substance use, unspecified with psychoactive substance-induced psychotic disorder, unspecified
Other or unknown substance-induced psychotic disorder, without use disorder ◀

F19.96 Other psychoactive substance use, unspecified with psychoactive substance-induced persisting amnestic disorder

F19.97 Other psychoactive substance use, unspecified with psychoactive substance-induced persisting dementia
Other (or unknown) substance-induced major neurocognitive disorder, without use disorder ◀

● **F19.98 Other psychoactive substance use, unspecified with other psychoactive substance-induced disorders**

F19.980 Other psychoactive substance use, unspecified with psychoactive substance-induced anxiety disorder
Other (or unknown) substance-induced anxiety disorder, without use disorder ◀

F19.981 Other psychoactive substance use, unspecified with psychoactive substance-induced sexual dysfunction
Other (or unknown) substance-induced sexual dysfunction, without use disorder ◀

F19.982 Other psychoactive substance use, unspecified with psychoactive substance-induced sleep disorder
Other (or unknown) substance-induced sleep disorder, without use disorder ◀

F19.988 Other psychoactive substance use, unspecified with other psychoactive substance-induced disorder
Other (or unknown) substance-induced mild neurocognitive disorder, without use disorder ◀
Other (or unknown) substance-induced obsessive-compulsive or related disorder, without use disorder ◀

F19.99 Other psychoactive substance use, unspecified with unspecified psychoactive substance-induced disorder

SCHIZOPHRENIA, SCHIZOTYPAL, DELUSIONAL, AND OTHER NON-MOOD PSYCHOTIC DISORDERS (F2Ø-F29)

● **F2Ø Schizophrenia**
Personality disorders characterized by multiple mental and behavioral irregularities (may exhibit disorganized thinking, delusions, and auditory hallucinations)

Excludes1 brief psychotic disorder (F23)
cyclic schizophrenia (F25.Ø)
mood [affective] disorders with psychotic symptoms (F3Ø.2, F31.2, F31.5, F31.64, F32.3, F33.3)
schizoaffective disorder (F25.-)
schizophrenic reaction NOS (F23)

Excludes2 schizophrenic reaction in:
alcoholism (F1Ø.15-, F1Ø.25-, F1Ø.95-)
brain disease (FØ6.2)
epilepsy (FØ6.2)
psychoactive drug use (F11-F19 with .15, .25, .95)
schizotypal disorder (F21)

F2Ø.Ø Paranoid schizophrenia
Paraphrenic schizophrenia
Excludes1 involutional paranoid state (F22)
paranoia (F22)

F2Ø.1 Disorganized schizophrenia
Hebephrenic schizophrenia
Hebephrenia

F2Ø.2 Catatonic schizophrenia
Schizophrenic catalepsy
Schizophrenic catatonia
Schizophrenic flexibilitas cerea
Excludes1 catatonic stupor (R4Ø.1)

F2Ø.3 Undifferentiated schizophrenia
Atypical schizophrenia
Excludes1 acute schizophrenia-like psychotic disorder (F23)
Excludes2 post-schizophrenic depression (F32.89) ⬅

F2Ø.5 Residual schizophrenia
Restzustand (schizophrenic)
Schizophrenic residual state

● **F2Ø.8 Other schizophrenia**

F2Ø.81 Schizophreniform disorder
Schizophreniform psychosis NOS

F2Ø.89 Other schizophrenia
Cenesthopathic schizophrenia
Simple schizophrenia

F2Ø.9 Schizophrenia, unspecified

F21 Schizotypal disorder
Personality disorder characterized by need for social isolation, odd behavior and thinking, and often unconventional beliefs
Borderline schizophrenia
Latent schizophrenia
Latent schizophrenic reaction
Prepsychotic schizophrenia
Prodromal schizophrenia
Pseudoneurotic schizophrenia
Pseudopsychopathic schizophrenia
Schizotypal personality disorder
Excludes2 Asperger's syndrome (F84.5)
schizoid personality disorder (F6Ø.1)

CHAPTER 5 (FØ1-F99)

F22 Delusional disorders
Delusional dysmorphophobia
Involutional paranoid state
Paranoia
Paranoia querulans
Paranoid psychosis
Paranoid state
Paraphrenia (late)
Sensitiver Beziehungswahn
Excludes1 mood [affective] disorders with psychotic symptoms (F30.2, F31.2, F31.5, F31.64, F32.3, F33.3)
paranoid schizophrenia (F20.0)
Excludes2 paranoid personality disorder (F60.0)
paranoid psychosis, psychogenic (F23)
paranoid reaction (F23)

F23 Brief psychotic disorder
Paranoid reaction
Psychogenic paranoid psychosis
Excludes2 mood [affective] disorders with psychotic symptoms (F30.2, F31.2, F31.5, F31.64, F32.3, F33.3)

F24 Shared psychotic disorder
Folie à deux
Induced paranoid disorder
Induced psychotic disorder

● **F25 Schizoaffective disorders**
Mental disorder exhibiting major depressive episode, manic episode, or mixed episode occurs with symptoms of schizophrenia, and mood disorder
Excludes1 mood [affective] disorders with psychotic symptoms (F30.2, F31.2, F31.5, F31.64, F32.3, F33.3)
schizophrenia (F20.-)

F25.0 Schizoaffective disorder, bipolar type
Cyclic schizophrenia
Schizoaffective disorder, manic type
Schizoaffective disorder, mixed type
Schizoaffective psychosis, bipolar type
Schizophreniform psychosis, manic type

F25.1 Schizoaffective disorder, depressive type
Schizoaffective psychosis, depressive type
Schizophreniform psychosis, depressive type

F25.8 Other schizoaffective disorders

F25.9 Schizoaffective disorder, unspecified
Schizoaffective psychosis NOS

F28 Other psychotic disorder not due to a substance or known physiological condition
Chronic hallucinatory psychosis

F29 Unspecified psychosis not due to a substance or known physiological condition
Psychosis NOS
Excludes1 mental disorder NOS (F99)
unspecified mental disorder due to known physiological condition (F09)

MOOD [AFFECTIVE] DISORDERS (F30-F39)

● **F30 Manic episode**
Elevated, expansive, or irritable mood
Includes bipolar disorder, single manic episode
mixed affective episode
Excludes1 bipolar disorder (F31.-)
major depressive disorder, single episode (F32.-)
major depressive disorder, recurrent (F33.-)

● **F30.1 Manic episode without psychotic symptoms**

F30.10 Manic episode without psychotic symptoms, unspecified

F30.11 Manic episode without psychotic symptoms, mild

F30.12 Manic episode without psychotic symptoms, moderate

F30.13 Manic episode, severe, without psychotic symptoms

F30.2 Manic episode, severe with psychotic symptoms
Manic stupor
Mania with mood-congruent psychotic symptoms
Mania with mood-incongruent psychotic symptoms

F30.3 Manic episode in partial remission

F30.4 Manic episode in full remission

F30.8 Other manic episodes
Abnormality of mood resembling mania but less intense
Hypomania

F30.9 Manic episode, unspecified
Mania NOS

● **F31 Bipolar disorder**
Mood disorders with history of manic, mixed, or hypomanic episodes
Includes manic-depressive illness
manic-depressive psychosis
manic-depressive reaction
Excludes1 bipolar disorder, single manic episode (F30.-)
major depressive disorder, single episode (F32.-)
major depressive disorder, recurrent (F33.-)
Excludes2 cyclothymia (F34.0)

F31.0 Bipolar disorder, current episode hypomanic

● **F31.1 Bipolar disorder, current episode manic without psychotic features**

F31.10 Bipolar disorder, current episode manic without psychotic features, unspecified

F31.11 Bipolar disorder, current episode manic without psychotic features, mild

F31.12 Bipolar disorder, current episode manic without psychotic features, moderate

F31.13 Bipolar disorder, current episode manic without psychotic features, severe

F31.2 Bipolar disorder, current episode manic severe with psychotic features
Bipolar disorder, current episode manic with mood-congruent psychotic symptoms
Bipolar disorder, current episode manic with mood-incongruent psychotic symptoms

● **F31.3 Bipolar disorder, current episode depressed, mild or moderate severity**

F31.30 Bipolar disorder, current episode depressed, mild or moderate severity, unspecified

F31.31 Bipolar disorder, current episode depressed, mild

F31.32 Bipolar disorder, current episode depressed, moderate

F31.4 Bipolar disorder, current episode depressed, severe, without psychotic features

F31.5 Bipolar disorder, current episode depressed, severe, with psychotic features
Bipolar disorder, current episode depressed with mood-incongruent psychotic symptoms
Bipolar disorder, current episode depressed with mood-congruent psychotic symptoms

● **F31.6 Bipolar disorder, current episode mixed**

F31.60 Bipolar disorder, current episode mixed, unspecified

F31.61 Bipolar disorder, current episode mixed, mild

F31.62 Bipolar disorder, current episode mixed, moderate

F31.63 Bipolar disorder, current episode mixed, severe, without psychotic features

F31.64 Bipolar disorder, current episode mixed, severe, with psychotic features
Bipolar disorder, current episode mixed with mood-congruent psychotic symptoms
Bipolar disorder, current episode mixed with mood-incongruent psychotic symptoms

● F31.7 **Bipolar disorder, currently in remission**
- F31.70 **Bipolar disorder, currently in remission, most recent episode unspecified**
- F31.71 **Bipolar disorder, in partial remission, most recent episode hypomanic**
- F31.72 **Bipolar disorder, in full remission, most recent episode hypomanic**
- F31.73 **Bipolar disorder, in partial remission, most recent episode manic**
- F31.74 **Bipolar disorder, in full remission, most recent episode manic**
- F31.75 **Bipolar disorder, in partial remission, most recent episode depressed**
- F31.76 **Bipolar disorder, in full remission, most recent episode depressed**
- F31.77 **Bipolar disorder, in partial remission, most recent episode mixed**
- F31.78 **Bipolar disorder, in full remission, most recent episode mixed**

● F31.8 **Other bipolar disorders**
- F31.81 **Bipolar II disorder**
- F31.89 **Other bipolar disorder**
  - Recurrent manic episodes NOS

F31.9 **Bipolar disorder, unspecified**

● F32 **Major depressive disorder, single episode**

Includes single episode of agitated depression
single episode of depressive reaction
single episode of major depression
single episode of psychogenic depression
single episode of reactive depression
single episode of vital depression

Excludes1 bipolar disorder (F31.-)
manic episode (F3Ø.-)
recurrent depressive disorder (F33.-)

Excludes2 adjustment disorder (F43.2)

- F32.Ø **Major depressive disorder, single episode, mild**
- F32.1 **Major depressive disorder, single episode, moderate**
- F32.2 **Major depressive disorder, single episode, severe without psychotic features**
- F32.3 **Major depressive disorder, single episode, severe with psychotic features**
  - Single episode of major depression with mood-congruent psychotic symptoms
  - Single episode of major depression with mood-incongruent psychotic symptoms
  - Single episode of major depression with psychotic symptoms
  - Single episode of psychogenic depressive psychosis
  - Single episode of psychotic depression
  - Single episode of reactive depressive psychosis
- F32.4 **Major depressive disorder, single episode, in partial remission**
- F32.5 **Major depressive disorder, single episode, in full remission**

● F32.8 **Other depressive episodes**
- F32.81 **Premenstrual dysphoric disorder** ◀
  - **Excludes1** premenstrual tension syndrome (N94.3) ◀
- F32.89 **Other specified depressive episodes** ◀
  - Atypical depression ◀
  - Post-schizophrenic depression ◀
  - Single episode of 'masked' depression NOS ◀

F32.9 **Major depressive disorder, single episode, unspecified**
- Depression NOS
- Depressive disorder NOS
- Major depression NOS

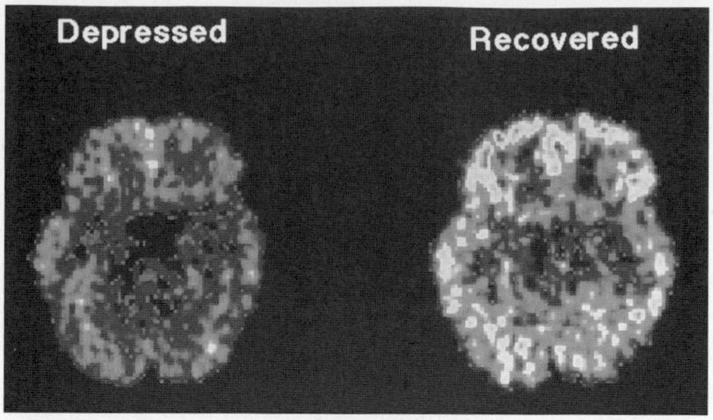

Figure 5-1 PET scan of depressed individual's brain before and after recovery. (From Fortinash KM: Psychiatric Mental Health Nursing, ed 4, St. Louis, Mosby, 2008)

● F33 **Major depressive disorder, recurrent**

Includes recurrent episodes of depressive reaction
recurrent episodes of endogenous depression
recurrent episodes of major depression
recurrent episodes of psychogenic depression
recurrent episodes of reactive depression
recurrent episodes of seasonal depressive disorder
recurrent episodes of vital depression

Excludes1 bipolar disorder (F31.-)
manic episode (F3Ø.-)

- F33.Ø **Major depressive disorder, recurrent, mild**
- F33.1 **Major depressive disorder, recurrent, moderate**
- F33.2 **Major depressive disorder, recurrent severe without psychotic features**
- F33.3 **Major depressive disorder, recurrent, severe with psychotic symptoms**
  - Endogenous depression with psychotic symptoms
  - Recurrent severe episodes of major depression with mood-congruent psychotic symptoms
  - Recurrent severe episodes of major depression with mood-incongruent psychotic symptoms
  - Recurrent severe episodes of major depression with psychotic symptoms
  - Recurrent severe episodes of psychogenic depressive psychosis
  - Recurrent severe episodes of psychotic depression
  - Recurrent severe episodes of reactive depressive psychosis

● F33.4 **Major depressive disorder, recurrent, in remission**
- F33.4Ø **Major depressive disorder, recurrent, in remission, unspecified**
- F33.41 **Major depressive disorder, recurrent, in partial remission**
- F33.42 **Major depressive disorder, recurrent, in full remission**

F33.8 **Other recurrent depressive disorders**
- Recurrent brief depressive episodes

F33.9 **Major depressive disorder, recurrent, unspecified**
- Monopolar depression NOS

● **F34 Persistent mood [affective] disorders**

F34.0 Cyclothymic disorder
Affective personality disorder
Cycloid personality
Cyclothymia
Cyclothymic personality

F34.1 Dysthymic disorder
Depressive neurosis
Depressive personality disorder
Dysthymia
Neurotic depression
Persistent anxiety depression
Persistent depressive disorder ◀
Excludes2 anxiety depression (mild or not persistent) (F41.8)

● **F34.8 Other persistent mood [affective] disorders**
F34.81 Disruptive mood dysregulation disorder ◀
F34.89 Other specified persistent mood disorders ◀

F34.9 Persistent mood [affective] disorder, unspecified

F39 Unspecified mood [affective] disorder
Affective psychosis NOS

ANXIETY, DISSOCIATIVE, STRESS-RELATED, SOMATOFORM AND OTHER NONPSYCHOTIC MENTAL DISORDERS (F40-F48)

● **F40 Phobic anxiety disorders**
Irrational fear with avoidance of the feared subject, activity, or situation even though the individual knows that the reaction is excessive

● **F40.0 Agoraphobia**
Intense, irrational fear of open spaces
F40.00 Agoraphobia, unspecified
F40.01 Agoraphobia with panic disorder
Panic disorder with agoraphobia
Excludes1 panic disorder without agoraphobia (F41.0)
F40.02 Agoraphobia without panic disorder

● **F40.1 Social phobias**
Anthropophobia
Social anxiety disorder of childhood
Social neurosis
F40.10 Social phobia, unspecified
F40.11 Social phobia, generalized

● **F40.2 Specific (isolated) phobias**
Excludes2 dysmorphophobia (nondelusional) (F45.22)
nosophobia (F45.22)

● **F40.21 Animal type phobia**
F40.210 Arachnophobia
Fear of spiders
F40.218 Other animal type phobia

● **F40.22 Natural environment type phobia**
F40.220 Fear of thunderstorms
F40.228 Other natural environment type phobia

● **F40.23 Blood, injection, injury type phobia**
F40.230 Fear of blood
F40.231 Fear of injections and transfusions
F40.232 Fear of other medical care
F40.233 Fear of injury

● **F40.24 Situational type phobia**
F40.240 Claustrophobia
Fear of closed spaces
F40.241 Acrophobia
Fear of heights
F40.242 Fear of bridges
F40.243 Fear of flying
F40.248 Other situational type phobia

● **F40.29 Other specified phobia**
F40.290 Androphobia
Fear of men
F40.291 Gynephobia
Fear of women
F40.298 Other specified phobia

F40.8 Other phobic anxiety disorders
Phobic anxiety disorder of childhood

F40.9 Phobic anxiety disorder, unspecified
Phobia NOS
Phobic state NOS

● **F41 Other anxiety disorders**
Excludes2 anxiety in:
acute stress reaction (F43.0)
transient adjustment reaction (F43.2)
neurasthenia (F48.8)
psychophysiologic disorders (F45.-)
separation anxiety (F93.0)

F41.0 Panic disorder [episodic paroxysmal anxiety] without agoraphobia
Panic attack
Panic state
Excludes1 panic disorder with agoraphobia (F40.01)

F41.1 Generalized anxiety disorder
Anxiety neurosis
Anxiety reaction
Anxiety state
Overanxious disorder
Excludes2 neurasthenia (F48.8)

F41.3 Other mixed anxiety disorders

F41.8 Other specified anxiety disorders
Anxiety depression (mild or not persistent)
Anxiety hysteria
Mixed anxiety and depressive disorder

F41.9 Anxiety disorder, unspecified
Anxiety NOS

● **F42 Obsessive-compulsive disorder**
Anxiety disorder with recurrent obsessions or compulsions
Excludes2 obsessive-compulsive personality (disorder) (F60.5)
obsessive-compulsive symptoms occurring in depression (F32-F33)
obsessive-compulsive symptoms occurring in schizophrenia (F20.-)

F42.2 Mixed obsessional thoughts and acts ◀
F42.3 Hoarding disorder ◀
F42.4 Excoriation (skin-picking) disorder ◀
Excludes1 factitial dermatitis (L98.1) ◀
other specified behavioral and emotional disorders with onset usually occurring in early childhood and adolescence (F98.8) ◀

F42.8 Other obsessive-compulsive disorder ◀
Anancastic neurosis ◀
Obsessive-compulsive neurosis ◀

F42.9 Obsessive-compulsive disorder, unspecified ◀

● **F43 Reaction to severe stress and adjustment disorders**

F43.0 Acute stress reaction
Acute crisis reaction
Acute reaction to stress
Combat and operational stress reaction
Combat fatigue
Crisis state
Psychic shock

● **F43.1 Post-traumatic stress disorder (PTSD)**
Traumatic neurosis
F43.10 Post-traumatic stress disorder, unspecified
F43.11 Post-traumatic stress disorder, acute
F43.12 Post-traumatic stress disorder, chronic

● F43.2 **Adjustment disorders**
Culture shock
Grief reaction
Hospitalism in children
Excludes2 separation anxiety disorder of childhood (F93.Ø)

F43.2Ø **Adjustment disorder, unspecified**
F43.21 **Adjustment disorder with depressed mood**
F43.22 **Adjustment disorder with anxiety**
F43.23 **Adjustment disorder with mixed anxiety and depressed mood**
F43.24 **Adjustment disorder with disturbance of conduct**
F43.25 **Adjustment disorder with mixed disturbance of emotions and conduct**
F43.29 **Adjustment disorder with other symptoms**

F43.8 **Other reactions to severe stress**
Other specified trauma and stressor-related disorder ◀

F43.9 **Reaction to severe stress, unspecified**
Trauma and stressor-related disorder, NOS ◀

● F44 **Dissociative and conversion disorders**
Includes conversion hysteria
conversion reaction
hysteria
hysterical psychosis
Excludes2 malingering [conscious simulation] (Z76.5)

F44.Ø **Dissociative amnesia**
Sudden loss of memory for personal information
Excludes1 amnesia NOS (R41.3)
anterograde amnesia (R41.1)
dissociative amnesia with dissociative fugue (F44.1) ◀
retrograde amnesia (R41.2)
Excludes2 alcohol-or other psychoactive substance-induced amnestic disorder (F1Ø, F13, F19 with .26, .96)
amnestic disorder due to known physiological condition (FØ4)
postictal amnesia in epilepsy (G4Ø.-)

F44.1 **Dissociative fugue**
Characterized by episode of sudden, unexpected travel with amnesia for past and partial to total confusion about identity or assumption of new identity
Dissociative amnesia with dissociative fugue ◀
Excludes2 postictal fugue in epilepsy (G4Ø.-)

F44.2 **Dissociative stupor**
Profound diminution or absence of voluntary movement and responsiveness to external stimuli
Excludes1 catatonic stupor (R4Ø.1)
stupor NOS (R4Ø.1)
Excludes2 catatonic disorder due to known physiological condition (FØ6.1)
depressive stupor (F32, F33)
manic stupor (F3Ø, F31)

F44.4 **Conversion disorder with motor symptom or deficit**
Dissociative motor disorders
Psychogenic aphonia
Psychogenic dysphonia

F44.5 **Conversion disorder with seizures or convulsions**
Dissociative convulsions

F44.6 **Conversion disorder with sensory symptom or deficit**
Dissociative anesthesia and sensory loss
Psychogenic deafness

F44.7 **Conversion disorder with mixed symptom presentation**

● F44.8 **Other dissociative and conversion disorders**
F44.81 **Dissociative identity disorder**
Multiple personality disorder
F44.89 **Other dissociative and conversion disorders**
Ganser's syndrome
Psychogenic confusion
Psychogenic twilight state
Trance and possession disorders

F44.9 **Dissociative and conversion disorder, unspecified**
Dissociative disorder NOS

OGCR Section I.C.5.a

> Pain disorders related to psychological factors
> Assign code F45.41, for pain that is exclusively psychological. Code F45.41, Pain disorder exclusively related to psychological factors, should be used following the appropriate code from category G89, Pain, not elsewhere classified, if there is documentation of a psychological component for a patient with acute or chronic pain.
> *See Section I.C.6. Pain*

● F45 **Somatoform disorders**
Mental disorders characterized by symptoms suggesting general medical condition
Excludes2 dissociative and conversion disorders (F44.-)
factitious disorders (F68.1-)
hair-plucking (F63.3)
lalling (F8Ø.Ø)
lisping (F8Ø.Ø)
malingering [conscious simulation] (Z76.5)
nail-biting (F98.8)
psychological or behavioral factors associated with disorders or diseases classified elsewhere (F54)
sexual dysfunction, not due to a substance or known physiological condition (F52.-)
thumb-sucking (F98.8)
tic disorders (in childhood and adolescence) (F95.-)
Tourette's syndrome (F95.2)
trichotillomania (F63.3)

F45.Ø **Somatization disorder**
Briquet's disorder
Multiple psychosomatic disorder

F45.1 **Undifferentiated somatoform disorder**
Somatic symptom disorder ◀
Undifferentiated psychosomatic disorder

● F45.2 **Hypochondriacal disorders**
Persistent, unrealistic preoccupation with possibility of having serious disease
Excludes2 delusional dysmorphophobia (F22)
fixed delusions about bodily functions or shape (F22)

F45.2Ø **Hypochondriacal disorder, unspecified**
F45.21 **Hypochondriasis**
Hypochondriacal neurosis
Illness anxiety disorder ◀
F45.22 **Body dysmorphic disorder**
Dysmorphophobia (nondelusional)
Nosophobia
F45.29 **Other hypochondriacal disorders**

● F45.4 **Pain disorders related to psychological factors**
Excludes1 pain NOS (R52)
F45.41 **Pain disorder exclusively related to psychological factors**
Somatoform pain disorder (persistent)
F45.42 **Pain disorder with related psychological factors**
Code also associated acute or chronic pain (G89.-)

F45.8 Other somatoform disorders
Psychogenic dysmenorrhea
Psychogenic dysphagia, including 'globus hystericus'
Psychogenic pruritus
Psychogenic torticollis
Somatoform autonomic dysfunction
Teeth grinding
Excludes1 sleep related teeth grinding (G47.63)

F45.9 Somatoform disorder, unspecified
Psychosomatic disorder NOS

● **F48 Other nonpsychotic mental disorders**

F48.1 Depersonalization-derealization syndrome

F48.2 Pseudobulbar affect
Involuntary emotional expression disorder
Code first underlying cause, if known, such as:
amyotrophic lateral sclerosis (G12.21)
multiple sclerosis (G35)
sequelae of cerebrovascular disease (I69.-)
sequelae of traumatic intracranial injury (S06.-)

F48.8 Other specified nonpsychotic mental disorders
Dhat syndrome
Neurasthenia
Occupational neurosis, including writer's cramp
Psychasthenia
Psychasthenic neurosis
Psychogenic syncope

F48.9 Nonpsychotic mental disorder, unspecified
Neurosis NOS

BEHAVIORAL SYNDROMES ASSOCIATED WITH PHYSIOLOGICAL DISTURBANCES AND PHYSICAL FACTORS (F50-F59)

● **F50 Eating disorders**
Excludes1 anorexia NOS (R63.0)
feeding difficulties (R63.3)
polyphagia (R63.2)
Excludes2 feeding disorder in infancy or childhood (F98.2-)

● **F50.0 Anorexia nervosa**
Excludes1 loss of appetite (R63.0)
psychogenic loss of appetite (F50.89) (Revised)

F50.00 Anorexia nervosa, unspecified

F50.01 Anorexia nervosa, restricting type

F50.02 Anorexia nervosa, binge eating/purging type
Excludes1 bulimia nervosa (F50.2)

F50.2 Bulimia nervosa
Bulimia NOS
Hyperorexia nervosa
Excludes1 anorexia nervosa, binge eating/purging type (F50.02)

● **F50.8 Other eating disorders**
Excludes2 pica of infancy and childhood (F98.3)

F50.81 Binge eating disorder ◀

F50.89 Other specified eating disorder ◀
Pica in adults ◀
Psychogenic loss of appetite ◀

F50.9 Eating disorder, unspecified
Atypical anorexia nervosa
Atypical bulimia nervosa

● **F51 Sleep disorders not due to a substance or known physiological condition**
Excludes2 organic sleep disorders (G47.-)

● **F51.0 Insomnia not due to a substance or known physiological condition**
Excludes2 alcohol related insomnia (F10.182, F10.282, F10.982)
drug-related insomnia (F11.182, F11.282, F11.982, F13.182, F13.282, F13.982, F14.182, F14.282, F14.982, F15.182, F15.282, F15.982, F19.182, F19.282, F19.982)
insomnia NOS (G47.0-)
insomnia due to known physiological condition (G47.0-)
organic insomnia (G47.0-)
sleep deprivation (Z72.820)

F51.01 Primary insomnia
Idiopathic insomnia

F51.02 Adjustment insomnia

F51.03 Paradoxical insomnia

F51.04 Psychophysiologic insomnia

F51.05 Insomnia due to other mental disorder
Code also associated mental disorder

F51.09 Other insomnia not due to a substance or known physiological condition

● **F51.1 Hypersomnia not due to a substance or known physiological condition**
Hypersomnia: Excessive sleeping/sleepiness
Excludes2 alcohol related hypersomnia (F10.182, F10.282, F10.982)
drug-related hypersomnia (F11.182, F11.282, F11.982, F13.182, F13.282, F13.982, F14.182, F14.282, F14.982, F15.182, F15.282, F15.982, F19.182, F19.282, F19.982)
hypersomnia NOS (G47.10)
hypersomnia due to known physiological condition (G47.10)
idiopathic hypersomnia (G47.11, G47.12)
narcolepsy (G47.4-)

F51.11 Primary hypersomnia

F51.12 Insufficient sleep syndrome
Excludes1 sleep deprivation (Z72.820)

F51.13 Hypersomnia due to other mental disorder
Code also associated mental disorder

F51.19 Other hypersomnia not due to a substance or known physiological condition

F51.3 Sleepwalking [somnambulism]

F51.4 Sleep terrors [night terrors]

F51.5 Nightmare disorder
Dream anxiety disorder

F51.8 Other sleep disorders not due to a substance or known physiological condition

F51.9 Sleep disorder not due to a substance or known physiological condition, unspecified
Emotional sleep disorder NOS

CHAPTER 5 (F01-F99)

● **F52 Sexual dysfunction not due to a substance or known physiological condition**

Excludes2 Dhat syndrome (F48.8)

F52.0 Hypoactive sexual desire disorder

Total loss of feeling of sexual pleasure

Lack or loss of sexual desire

Sexual anhedonia ◀

Excludes1 decreased libido (R68.82)

F52.1 Sexual aversion disorder

Sexual aversion and lack of sexual enjoyment

● **F52.2 Sexual arousal disorders**

Failure of genital response

F52.21 Male erectile disorder

Psychogenic impotence

Excludes1 impotence of organic origin (N52.-)

impotence NOS (N52.-)

F52.22 Female sexual arousal disorder

~~Frigidity~~

● **F52.3 Orgasmic disorder**

Inhibited orgasm

Psychogenic anorgasmy

F52.31 Female orgasmic disorder

F52.32 Male orgasmic disorder

Delayed ejaculation ◀

F52.4 Premature ejaculation

F52.5 Vaginismus not due to a substance or known physiological condition

Psychogenic vaginismus

Excludes2 vaginismus (due to a known physiological condition) (N94.2)

F52.6 Dyspareunia not due to a substance or known physiological condition

Dyspareunia: Difficult or painful sexual intercourse

Genito-pelvic pain penetration disorder ◀

Psychogenic dyspareunia

Excludes2 dyspareunia (due to a known physiological condition) (N94.1-) ⬅

F52.8 Other sexual dysfunction not due to a substance or known physiological condition

Excessive sexual drive

Nymphomania

Satyriasis

F52.9 Unspecified sexual dysfunction not due to a substance or known physiological condition

Sexual dysfunction NOS

F53 Puerperal psychosis

Postpartum depression

Acute mental illness with sudden onset following childbirth with symptoms of affective psychosis, disorientation, and confusion are prevalent

Excludes1 mood disorders with psychotic features (F30.2, F31.2, F31.5, F31.64, F32.3, F33.3)

postpartum dysphoria (O90.6)

psychosis in schizophrenia, schizotypal, delusional, and other psychotic disorders (F20-F29)

F54 Psychological and behavioral factors associated with disorders or diseases classified elsewhere

Psychological factors affecting physical conditions

Code first *the associated physical disorder, such as:*

asthma (J45.-)

dermatitis (L23-L25)

gastric ulcer (K25.-)

mucous colitis (K58.-)

ulcerative colitis (K51.-)

urticaria (L50.-)

Excludes2 tension-type headache (G44.2)

● **F55 Abuse of non-psychoactive substances**

Excludes2 abuse of psychoactive substances (F10-F19)

F55.0 Abuse of antacids

F55.1 Abuse of herbal or folk remedies

F55.2 Abuse of laxatives

F55.3 Abuse of steroids or hormones

F55.4 Abuse of vitamins

F55.8 Abuse of other non-psychoactive substances

F59 Unspecified behavioral syndromes associated with physiological disturbances and physical factors

Psychogenic physiological dysfunction NOS

DISORDERS OF ADULT PERSONALITY AND BEHAVIOR (F60-F69)

● **F60 Specific personality disorders**

Long-term patterns of thoughts and behaviors causing serious problems with relationships and work.

F60.0 Paranoid personality disorder

Hostile, devious, and combative response to disappointments

Expansive paranoid personality (disorder)

Fanatic personality (disorder)

Querulant personality (disorder)

Paranoid personality (disorder)

Sensitive paranoid personality (disorder)

Excludes2 paranoia (F22)

paranoia querulans (F22)

paranoid psychosis (F22)

paranoid schizophrenia (F20.0)

paranoid state (F22)

F60.1 Schizoid personality disorder

Detachment from social relationships with minimal emotional experiences and expressions

Excludes2 Asperger's syndrome (F84.5)

delusional disorder (F22)

schizoid disorder of childhood (F84.5)

schizophrenia (F20.-)

schizotypal disorder (F21)

F60.2 Antisocial personality disorder

Continuous and chronic antisocial behavior

Amoral personality (disorder)

Asocial personality (disorder)

Dissocial personality disorder

Psychopathic personality (disorder)

Sociopathic personality (disorder)

Excludes1 conduct disorders (F91.-)

Excludes2 borderline personality disorder (F60.3)

F60.3 Borderline personality disorder

Instability of mood, self-image or sense of self, and interpersonal relationships

Aggressive personality (disorder)

Emotionally unstable personality disorder

Explosive personality (disorder)

Excludes2 antisocial personality disorder (F60.2)

F60.4 Histrionic personality disorder

Personality disorder with excessive emotional and attention-seeking behavior

Hysterical personality (disorder)

Psychoinfantile personality (disorder)

F60.5 Obsessive-compulsive personality disorder

Anankastic personality (disorder)

Compulsive personality (disorder)

Obsessional personality (disorder)

Excludes2 obsessive-compulsive disorder (F42-) ⬅

F60.6 Avoidant personality disorder

Anxious personality disorder

F60.7 Dependent personality disorder

Asthenic personality (disorder)

Inadequate personality (disorder)

Passive personality (disorder)

● **F60.8 Other specific personality disorders**

F60.81 Narcissistic personality disorder

Vanity, conceit, egotism or indifference to plight of others

F60.89 Other specific personality disorders

Eccentric personality disorder
'Haltlose' type personality disorder
Immature personality disorder
Passive-aggressive personality disorder
Psychoneurotic personality disorder
Self-defeating personality disorder

F60.9 Personality disorder, unspecified

Character disorder NOS
Character neurosis NOS
Pathological personality NOS

● **F63 Impulse disorders**

Excludes2 habitual excessive use of alcohol or psychoactive substances (F10-F19)
impulse disorders involving sexual behavior (F65.-)

F63.0 Pathological gambling

Compulsive gambling

Excludes1 gambling and betting NOS (Z72.6)

Excludes2 excessive gambling by manic patients (F30, F31)
gambling in antisocial personality disorder (F60.2)

F63.1 Pyromania

Pathological fire-setting

Excludes2 fire-setting (by) (in):
adult with antisocial personality disorder (F60.2)
alcohol or psychoactive substance intoxication (F10-F19)
conduct disorders (F91.-)
mental disorders due to known physiological condition (F01-F09)
schizophrenia (F20.-)

F63.2 Kleptomania

Pathological stealing

Excludes1 shoplifting as the reason for observation for suspected mental disorder (Z03.8)

Excludes2 depressive disorder with stealing (F31-F33)
stealing due to underlying mental condition-code to mental condition
stealing in mental disorders due to known physiological condition (F01-F09)

F63.3 Trichotillomania

Hair plucking

Excludes2 other stereotyped movement disorder (F98.4)

● **F63.8 Other impulse disorders**

F63.81 Intermittent explosive disorder

F63.89 Other impulse disorders

F63.9 Impulse disorder, unspecified

Impulse control disorder NOS

● **F64 Gender identity disorders**

F64.0 Transsexualism ◀

Gender identity disorder in adolescence and adulthood ◀
Gender dysphoria in adolescents and adults ◀

F64.1 Dual role transvestism (Revised)

Use additional code to identify sex reassignment status (Z87.890)

Excludes1 gender identity disorder in childhood (F64.2)

Excludes2 fetishistic transvestism (F65.1)

F64.2 Gender identity disorder of childhood

Gender dysphoria in children ◀

Excludes1 gender identity disorder in adolescence and adulthood (F64.0) (Revised)

Excludes2 sexual maturation disorder (F66)

F64.8 Other gender identity disorders

F64.9 Gender identity disorder, unspecified

Gender-role disorder NOS

● **F65 Paraphilias**

F65.0 Fetishism

Intense sexual urges and arousing fantasies using inanimate objects

F65.1 Transvestic fetishism

Intense sexual urges, arousal, or orgasm associated with fantasized/actual cross-dressing

Fetishistic transvestism

F65.2 Exhibitionism

F65.3 Voyeurism

Sexual urges or arousal involving real or fantasized observation of unsuspecting people who are naked, disrobing, or engaging in sexual activity

F65.4 Pedophilia

● **F65.5 Sadomasochism**

F65.50 Sadomasochism, unspecified

F65.51 Sexual masochism

F65.52 Sexual sadism

● **F65.8 Other paraphilias**

F65.81 Frotteurism

Sexual arousal or orgasm is achieved by rubbing up against another person (or fantasies of), in crowded place with unsuspecting victim

F65.89 Other paraphilias

Necrophilia

F65.9 Paraphilia, unspecified

Sexual deviation NOS

F66 Other sexual disorders

Sexual maturation disorder
Sexual relationship disorder

● **F68 Other disorders of adult personality and behavior**

● **F68.1 Factitious disorder**

Compensation neurosis
Elaboration of physical symptoms for psychological reasons
Hospital hopper syndrome
Münchhausen's syndrome
Peregrinating patient

Excludes2 factitial dermatitis (L98.1)
person feigning illness (with obvious motivation) (Z76.5)

F68.10 Factitious disorder, unspecified

F68.11 Factitious disorder with predominantly psychological signs and symptoms

F68.12 Factitious disorder with predominantly physical signs and symptoms

F68.13 Factitious disorder with combined psychological and physical signs and symptoms

F68.8 Other specified disorders of adult personality and behavior

F69 Unspecified disorder of adult personality and behavior

CHAPTER 5 (F01-F99)

INTELLECTUAL DISABILITIES (F70-F79)

Code first any associated physical or developmental disorders

Excludes1 borderline intellectual functioning, IQ above 70 to 84 (R41.83)

F70 Mild intellectual disabilities
IQ level 50-55 to approximately 70
Mild mental subnormality

F71 Moderate intellectual disabilities
IQ level 35-40 to 50-55
Moderate mental subnormality

F72 Severe intellectual disabilities
IQ 20-25 to 35-40
Severe mental subnormality

F73 Profound intellectual disabilities
IQ level below 20-25
Profound mental subnormality

F78 Other intellectual disabilities

F79 Unspecified intellectual disabilities
Mental deficiency NOS
Mental subnormality NOS

PERVASIVE AND SPECIFIC DEVELOPMENTAL DISORDERS (F80-F89)

● **F80 Specific developmental disorders of speech and language**

F80.0 Phonological disorder
Communication disorder of unknown cause, characterized by failure to use age-appropriate sounds
Dyslalia
Functional speech articulation disorder
Lalling
Lisping
Phonological developmental disorder
Speech articulation developmental disorder
Speech-sound disorder ◀

Excludes1 speech articulation impairment due to aphasia NOS (R47.01)
speech articulation impairment due to apraxia (R48.2)

Excludes2 speech articulation impairment due to hearing loss (F80.4)
speech articulation impairment due to intellectual disabilities (F70-F79)
speech articulation impairment with expressive language developmental disorder (F80.1)
speech articulation impairment with mixed receptive expressive language developmental disorder (F80.2)

F80.1 Expressive language disorder
Developmental dysphasia or aphasia, expressive type

Excludes1 mixed receptive-expressive language disorder (F80.2)
dysphasia and aphasia NOS (R47.-)

Excludes2 acquired aphasia with epilepsy [Landau-Kleffner] (G40.80-)
intellectual disabilities (F70-F79)
pervasive developmental disorders (F84.-)
selective mutism (F94.0)

F80.2 Mixed receptive-expressive language disorder
Developmental dysphasia or aphasia, receptive type
Developmental Wernicke's aphasia

Excludes1 central auditory processing disorder (H93.25)
dysphasia or aphasia NOS (R47.-)
expressive language disorder (F80.1)
expressive type dysphasia or aphasia (F80.1)
word deafness (H93.25)

Excludes2 acquired aphasia with epilepsy [Landau-Kleffner] (G40.80-)
intellectual disabilities (F70-F79)
pervasive developmental disorders (F84.-)
selective mutism (F94.0)

F80.4 Speech and language development delay due to hearing loss
Code also type of hearing loss (H90.-, H91.-)

● **F80.8 Other developmental disorders of speech or language**

F80.81 Childhood onset fluency disorder
Cluttering NOS
Stuttering NOS

Excludes1 adult onset fluency disorder (F98.5)
fluency disorder in conditions classified elsewhere (R47.82)
fluency disorder (stuttering) following cerebrovascular disease (I69. with final characters -23)

F80.82 Social pragmatic communication disorder ◀

Excludes1 Asperger's syndrome (F84.5) ◀
autistic disorder (F84.0) ◀

F80.89 Other developmental disorders of speech and language

F80.9 Developmental disorder of speech and language, unspecified
Communication disorder NOS
Language disorder NOS

● **F81 Specific developmental disorders of scholastic skills**

F81.0 Specific reading disorder
'Backward reading'
Developmental dyslexia
Specific reading retardation

Excludes1 alexia NOS (R48.0)
dyslexia NOS (R48.0)

F81.2 Mathematics disorder
Developmental acalculia
Developmental arithmetical disorder
Developmental Gerstmann's syndrome

Excludes1 acalculia NOS (R48.8)

Excludes2 arithmetical difficulties associated with a reading disorder (F81.0)
arithmetical difficulties associated with a spelling disorder (F81.81)
arithmetical difficulties due to inadequate teaching (Z55.8)

● **F81.8 Other developmental disorders of scholastic skills**

F81.81 Disorder of written expression
Specific spelling disorder

F81.89 Other developmental disorders of scholastic skills

F81.9 Developmental disorder of scholastic skills, unspecified
Knowledge acquisition disability NOS
Learning disability NOS
Learning disorder NOS

F82 Specific developmental disorder of motor function
Clumsy child syndrome
Developmental coordination disorder
Developmental dyspraxia
Excludes1 abnormalities of gait and mobility (R26.-)
lack of coordination (R27.-)
Excludes2 lack of coordination secondary to intellectual disabilities (F70-F79)

● **F84 Pervasive developmental disorders**
Use additional code to identify any associated medical condition and intellectual disabilities.

F84.0 Autistic disorder
Autism spectrum disorder ◀
Infantile autism
Infantile psychosis
Kanner's syndrome
Excludes1 Asperger's syndrome (F84.5)

F84.2 Rett's syndrome
Neurodevelopmental disorder
Excludes1 Asperger's syndrome (F84.5)
Autistic disorder (F84.0)
other childhood disintegrative disorder (F84.3)

F84.3 Other childhood disintegrative disorder
Dementia infantilis
At least two years of normal development followed by significant loss of language abilities, social skills, bowel/bladder control, motor skills
Disintegrative psychosis
Heller's syndrome
At least two years of normal development followed by significant loss of language abilities, social skills, bowel/bladder control, motor skills
Symbiotic psychosis
Abnormal relationship to mothering figure, characterized by intense separation anxiety, severe regression, giving up of useful speech, and autism
Use additional code to identify any associated neurological condition.
Excludes1 Asperger's syndrome (F84.5)
Autistic disorder (F84.0)
Rett's syndrome (F84.2)

F84.5 Asperger's syndrome
Developmental disorder
Asperger's disorder
Autistic psychopathy
Schizoid disorder of childhood

F84.8 Other pervasive developmental disorders
Overactive disorder associated with intellectual disabilities and stereotyped movements

F84.9 Pervasive developmental disorder, unspecified
Atypical autism

F88 Other disorders of psychological development
Developmental agnosia
Global developmental delay ◀
Other specified neurodevelopmental disorder ◀

F89 Unspecified disorder of psychological development
Developmental disorder NOS
Neurodevelopmental disorder NOS ◀

BEHAVIORAL AND EMOTIONAL DISORDERS WITH ONSET USUALLY OCCURRING IN CHILDHOOD AND ADOLESCENCE (F90-F98)

Note: Codes within categories F90-F98 may be used regardless of the age of a patient. These disorders generally have onset within the childhood or adolescent years, but may continue throughout life or not be diagnosed until adulthood.

● **F90 Attention-deficit hyperactivity disorders**
Attention deficit disorder with hyperactivity=ADHD
Includes attention deficit disorder with hyperactivity
attention deficit syndrome with hyperactivity
Excludes2 anxiety disorders (F40.-, F41.-)
mood [affective] disorders (F30-F39)
pervasive developmental disorders (F84.-)
schizophrenia (F20.-)

F90.0 Attention-deficit hyperactivity disorder, predominantly inattentive type

F90.1 Attention-deficit hyperactivity disorder, predominantly hyperactive type

F90.2 Attention-deficit hyperactivity disorder, combined type

F90.8 Attention-deficit hyperactivity disorder, other type

F90.9 Attention-deficit hyperactivity disorder, unspecified type
Attention-deficit hyperactivity disorder of childhood or adolescence NOS
Attention-deficit hyperactivity disorder NOS

● **F91 Conduct disorders**
Childhood/adolescence disruptive behavior disorder
Excludes1 antisocial behavior (Z72.81-)
antisocial personality disorder (F60.2)
Excludes2 conduct problems associated with attention-deficit hyperactivity disorder (F90.-)
mood [affective] disorders (F30-F39)
pervasive developmental disorders (F84.-)
schizophrenia (F20.-)

F91.0 Conduct disorder confined to family context

F91.1 Conduct disorder, childhood-onset type
Unsocialized conduct disorder
Conduct disorder, solitary aggressive type
Unsocialized aggressive disorder

F91.2 Conduct disorder, adolescent-onset type
Socialized conduct disorder
Conduct disorder, group type

F91.3 Oppositional defiant disorder

F91.8 Other conduct disorders
Other specified conduct disorder ◀
Other specified disruptive disorder ◀

F91.9 Conduct disorder, unspecified
Behavioral disorder NOS
Conduct disorder NOS
Disruptive behavior disorder NOS
Disruptive disorder NOS ◀

● **F93 Emotional disorders with onset specific to childhood**

F93.0 Separation anxiety disorder of childhood
Excludes2 mood [affective] disorders (F30-F39)
nonpsychotic mental disorders (F40-F48)
phobic anxiety disorder of childhood (F40.8)
social phobia (F40.1)

F93.8 Other childhood emotional disorders
Identity disorder
Excludes2 gender identity disorder of childhood (F64.2)

F93.9 Childhood emotional disorder, unspecified

CHAPTER 5 (F01-F99)

● **F94 Disorders of social functioning with onset specific to childhood and adolescence**

F94.Ø Selective mutism
Elective mutism
Excludes2 pervasive developmental disorders (F84.-)
schizophrenia (F2Ø.-)
specific developmental disorders of speech and language (F8Ø.-)
transient mutism as part of separation anxiety in young children (F93.Ø)

F94.1 Reactive attachment disorder of childhood
Use additional code to identify any associated failure to thrive or growth retardation
Excludes1 disinhibited attachment disorder of childhood (F94.2)
normal variation in pattern of selective attachment
Excludes2 Asperger's syndrome (F84.5)
maltreatment syndromes (T74.-)
sexual or physical abuse in childhood, resulting in psychosocial problems (Z62.81-)

F94.2 Disinhibited attachment disorder of childhood
Affectionless psychopathy
Institutional syndrome
Excludes1 reactive attachment disorder of childhood (F94.1)
Excludes2 Asperger's syndrome (F84.5)
attention-deficit hyperactivity disorders (F9Ø.-)
hospitalism in children (F43.2-)

F94.8 Other childhood disorders of social functioning

F94.9 Childhood disorder of social functioning, unspecified

● **F95 Tic disorder**
Involuntary twitch

F95.Ø Transient tic disorder
Provisional tic disorder ◀

F95.1 Chronic motor or vocal tic disorder

F95.2 Tourette's disorder
Combined vocal and multiple motor tic disorder [de la Tourette]
Tourette's syndrome

F95.8 Other tic disorders

F95.9 Tic disorder, unspecified
Tic NOS

● **F98 Other behavioral and emotional disorders with onset usually occurring in childhood and adolescence**
Excludes2 breath-holding spells (RØ6.89)
gender identity disorder of childhood (F64.2)
Kleine-Levin syndrome (G47.13)
obsessive-compulsive disorder (F42-) ◀
sleep disorders not due to a substance or known physiological condition (F51.-)

F98.Ø Enuresis not due to a substance or known physiological condition
Enuresis: Urinary incontinence
Enuresis (primary) (secondary) of nonorganic origin
Functional enuresis
Psychogenic enuresis
Urinary incontinence of nonorganic origin
Excludes1 enuresis NOS (R32)

F98.1 Encopresis not due to a substance or known physiological condition
Encopresis: Fecal incontinence
Functional encopresis
Incontinence of feces of nonorganic origin
Psychogenic encopresis
Use additional code to identify the cause of any coexisting constipation.
Excludes1 encopresis NOS (R15.-)

● **F98.2 Other feeding disorders of infancy and childhood**
Excludes1 feeding difficulties (R63.3)
Excludes2 anorexia nervosa and other eating disorders (F5Ø.-)
feeding problems of newborn (P92.-)
pica of infancy or childhood (F98.3)

F98.21 Rumination disorder of infancy

F98.29 Other feeding disorders of infancy and early childhood

F98.3 Pica of infancy and childhood
Craving and eating substances such as paint, clay, or dirt to replace a nutritional deficit in the body.

F98.4 Stereotyped movement disorders
Stereotype/habit disorder
Excludes1 abnormal involuntary movements (R25.-)
Excludes2 compulsions in obsessive-compulsive disorder (F42-) ◀
hair plucking (F63.3)
movement disorders of organic origin (G2Ø-G25)
nail-biting (F98.8)
nose-picking (F98.8)
stereotypies that are part of a broader psychiatric condition (FØ1-F95)
thumb-sucking (F98.8)
tic disorders (F95.-)
trichotillomania (F63.3)

F98.5 Adult onset fluency disorder
Excludes1 childhood onset fluency disorder (F8Ø.81)
dysphasia (R47.Ø2)
fluency disorder in conditions classified elsewhere (R47.82)
fluency disorder (stuttering) following cerebrovascular disease (I69. with final characters -23)
tic disorders (F95.-)

F98.8 Other specified behavioral and emotional disorders with onset usually occurring in childhood and adolescence
Excessive masturbation
Nail-biting
Nose-picking
Thumb-sucking

F98.9 Unspecified behavioral and emotional disorders with onset usually occurring in childhood and adolescence

UNSPECIFIED MENTAL DISORDER (F99)

F99 Mental disorder, not otherwise specified
Mental illness NOS
Excludes1 unspecified mental disorder due to known physiological condition (FØ9)

Item 5–2 Enuresis: Bed wetting by children at night. Causes can be either psychological or medical (diabetes, urinary tract infections, or abnormalities). **Encopresis:** Overflow incontinence of bowels sometimes resulting from chronic constipation or fecal impaction. Check the documentation for additional diagnoses.

CHAPTER 6

DISEASES OF THE NERVOUS SYSTEM (GØØ-G99)

OGCR Chapter-Specific Coding Guidelines

6. Chapter 6: Diseases of the Nervous System (GØØ-G99)

a. Dominant/nondominant side

Codes from category G81, Hemiplegia and hemiparesis, and subcategories, G83.1, Monoplegia of lower limb, G83.2, Monoplegia of upper limb, and G83.3, Monoplegia, unspecified, identify whether the dominant or nondominant side is affected. Should the affected side be documented, but not specified as dominant or nondominant, and the classification system does not indicate a default, code selection is as follows:

- For ambidextrous patients, the default should be dominant.
- If the left side is affected, the default is non-dominant.
- If the right side is affected, the default is dominant.

b. Pain - Category G89

1) General coding information

Codes in category G89, Pain, not elsewhere classified, may be used in conjunction with codes from other categories and chapters to provide more detail about acute or chronic pain and neoplasm-related pain, unless otherwise indicated below.

If the pain is not specified as acute or chronic, post-thoracotomy, postprocedural, or neoplasm-related, do not assign codes from category G89.

A code from category G89 should not be assigned if the underlying (definitive) diagnosis is known, unless the reason for the encounter is pain control/management and not management of the underlying condition.

When an admission or encounter is for a procedure aimed at treating the underlying condition (e.g., spinal fusion, kyphoplasty), a code for the underlying condition (e.g., vertebral fracture, spinal stenosis) should be assigned as the principal diagnosis. No code from category G89 should be assigned.

(a) Category G89 Codes as Principal or First-Listed Diagnosis

Category G89 codes are acceptable as principal diagnosis or the first-listed code:

- When pain control or pain management is the reason for the admission/encounter (e.g., a patient with displaced intervertebral disc, nerve impingement and severe back pain presents for injection of steroid into the spinal canal). The underlying cause of the pain should be reported as an additional diagnosis, if known.
- When a patient is admitted for the insertion of a neurostimulator for pain control, assign the appropriate pain code as the principal or first-listed diagnosis. When an admission or encounter is for a procedure aimed at treating the underlying condition and a neurostimulator is inserted for pain control during the same admission/encounter, a code for the underlying condition should be assigned as the principal diagnosis and the appropriate pain code should be assigned as a secondary diagnosis.

(b) Use of Category G89 Codes in Conjunction with Site Specific Pain Codes

(i) Assigning Category G89 and Site-Specific Pain Codes

Codes from category G89 may be used in conjunction with codes that identify the site of pain (including codes from chapter 18) if the category G89 code provides additional information. For example, if the code describes the site of the pain, but does not fully describe whether the pain is acute or chronic, then both codes should be assigned.

(ii) Sequencing of Category G89 Codes with Site-Specific Pain Codes

The sequencing of category G89 codes with site-specific pain codes (including chapter 18 codes), is dependent on the circumstances of the encounter/admission as follows:

- If the encounter is for pain control or pain management, assign the code from category G89 followed by the code identifying the specific site of pain (e.g., encounter for pain management for acute neck pain from trauma is assigned code G89.11, Acute pain due to trauma, followed by code M54.2, Cervicalgia, to identify the site of pain).
- If the encounter is for any other reason except pain control or pain management, and a related definitive diagnosis has not been established (confirmed) by the provider, assign the code for the specific site of pain first, followed by the appropriate code from category G89.

2) Pain due to devices, implants and grafts

See Section I.C.19. Pain due to medical devices

3) Postoperative Pain

The provider's documentation should be used to guide the coding of postoperative pain, as well as *Section III. Reporting Additional Diagnoses* and *Section IV. Diagnostic Coding and Reporting in the Outpatient Setting.*

The default for post-thoracotomy and other postoperative pain not specified as acute or chronic is the code for the acute form.

Routine or expected postoperative pain immediately after surgery should not be coded.

(a) Postoperative pain not associated with specific postoperative complication

Postoperative pain not associated with a specific postoperative complication is assigned to the appropriate postoperative pain code in category G89.

(b) Postoperative pain associated with specific postoperative complication

Postoperative pain associated with a specific postoperative complication (such as painful wire sutures) is assigned to the appropriate code(s) found in Chapter 19, Injury, poisoning, and certain other consequences of external causes. If appropriate, use additional code(s) from category G89 to identify acute or chronic pain (G89.18 or G89.28).

4) Chronic pain

Chronic pain is classified to subcategory G89.2. There is no time frame defining when pain becomes chronic pain. The provider's documentation should be used to guide use of these codes.

5) Neoplasm Related Pain

Code G89.3 is assigned to pain documented as being related, associated or due to cancer, primary or secondary malignancy, or tumor. This code is assigned regardless of whether the pain is acute or chronic.

This code may be assigned as the principal or first-listed code when the stated reason for the admission/encounter is documented as pain control/pain management. The underlying neoplasm should be reported as an additional diagnosis.

When the reason for the admission/encounter is management of the neoplasm and the pain associated with the neoplasm is also documented, code G89.3 may be assigned as an additional diagnosis. It is not necessary to assign an additional code for the site of the pain.

See Section I.C.2 for instructions on the sequencing of neoplasms for all other stated reasons for the admission/encounter (except for pain control/pain management).

6) Chronic pain syndrome

Central pain syndrome (G89.Ø) and chronic pain syndrome (G89.4) are different than the term "chronic pain," and therefore codes should only be used when the provider has specifically documented this condition.

See Section I.C.5. Pain disorders related to psychological factors

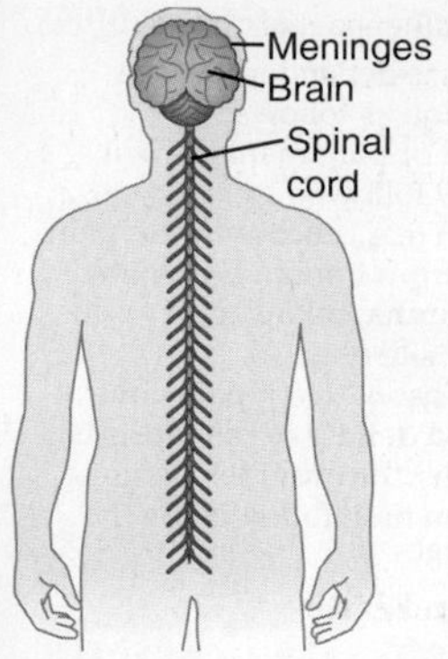

Figure 6-1 The brain and spinal cord make up the central nervous system.

Item 6–1 The two major classifications of the nervous system are the peripheral nervous system and the central nervous system (CNS). The central nervous system is comprised of the brain and the spinal cord. The peripheral nervous system is comprised of the parasympathetic and sympathetic systems. **Encephalitis** is the swelling of the brain. **Meningitis** is swelling of the covering of the brain, the meninges. Types and causes of brain infections are:

Type	Cause
purulent	bacterial
aseptic/abacterial	viral
chronic meningitis	mycobacterial and fungal

CHAPTER 6

DISEASES OF THE NERVOUS SYSTEM (GØØ-G99)

Excludes2 certain conditions originating in the perinatal period (PØ4-P96)
certain infectious and parasitic diseases (AØØ-B99)
complications of pregnancy, childbirth and the puerperium (OØØ-O9A)
congenital malformations, deformations, and chromosomal abnormalities (QØØ-Q99)
endocrine, nutritional and metabolic diseases (EØØ-E88)
injury, poisoning and certain other consequences of external causes (SØØ-T88)
neoplasms (CØØ-D49)
symptoms, signs and abnormal clinical and laboratory findings, not elsewhere classified (RØØ-R94)

This chapter contains the following blocks:

GØØ-GØ9	Inflammatory diseases of the central nervous system
G1Ø-G14	Systemic atrophies primarily affecting the central nervous system
G2Ø-G26	Extrapyramidal and movement disorders
G3Ø-G32	Other degenerative diseases of the nervous system
G35-G37	Demyelinating diseases of the central nervous system
G4Ø-G47	Episodic and paroxysmal disorders
G5Ø-G59	Nerve, nerve root and plexus disorders
G6Ø-G65	Polyneuropathies and other disorders of the peripheral nervous system
G7Ø-G73	Diseases of myoneural junction and muscle
G8Ø-G83	Cerebral palsy and other paralytic syndromes
G89-G99	Other disorders of the nervous system

INFLAMMATORY DISEASES OF THE CENTRAL NERVOUS SYSTEM (GØØ-GØ9)

● **GØØ Bacterial meningitis, not elsewhere classified**
An infection of the cerebrospinal fluid surrounding the spinal cord and brain.
Includes bacterial arachnoiditis
bacterial leptomeningitis
bacterial meningitis
bacterial pachymeningitis
Excludes1 bacterial:
meningoencephalitis (GØ4.2)
meningomyelitis (GØ4.2)

GØØ.Ø Hemophilus meningitis
Meningitis due to Hemophilus influenzae

GØØ.1 Pneumococcal meningitis
Meningitis due to Streptococcal pneumoniae ◀

GØØ.2 Streptococcal meningitis
Use additional code to further identify organism (B95.Ø-B95.5)

GØØ.3 Staphylococcal meningitis
Use additional code to further identify organism (B95.61-B95.8)

GØØ.8 Other bacterial meningitis
Meningitis due to Escherichia coli
Meningitis due to Friedländer bacillus
Meningitis due to Klebsiella
Use additional code to further identify organism (B96.-)

GØØ.9 Bacterial meningitis, unspecified
Meningitis due to gram-negative bacteria, unspecified
Purulent meningitis NOS
Pyogenic meningitis NOS
Suppurative meningitis NOS

GØ1 Meningitis in bacterial diseases classified elsewhere
Code first underlying disease
Excludes1 meningitis (in):
gonococcal (A54.81)
leptospirosis (A27.81)
listeriosis (A32.11)
Lyme disease (A69.21)
meningococcal (A39.Ø)
neurosyphilis (A52.13)
tuberculosis (A17.Ø)
meningoencephalitis and meningomyelitis in bacterial diseases classified elsewhere (GØ5)

GØ2 Meningitis in other infectious and parasitic diseases classified elsewhere
Code first underlying disease, such as:
African trypanosomiasis (B56.-)
poliovirus infection (A8Ø.-)
Excludes1 candidal meningitis (B37.5)
coccidioidomycosis meningitis (B38.4)
cryptococcal meningitis (B45.1)
herpesviral [herpes simplex] meningitis (BØØ.3)
infectious mononucleosis complicated by meningitis (B27.- with fourth character 2)
measles complicated by meningitis (BØ5.1)
meningoencephalitis and meningomyelitis in other infectious and parasitic diseases classified elsewhere (GØ5)
mumps meningitis (B26.1)
rubella meningitis (BØ6.Ø2)
varicella [chickenpox] meningitis (BØ1.Ø)
zoster meningitis (BØ2.1)

● **G03 Meningitis due to other and unspecified causes**
Includes arachnoiditis NOS
leptomeningitis NOS
meningitis NOS
pachymeningitis NOS
Excludes1 meningoencephalitis (G04.-)
meningomyelitis (G04.-)

G03.0 Nonpyogenic meningitis
Aseptic meningitis
Nonbacterial meningitis

G03.1 Chronic meningitis

G03.2 Benign recurrent meningitis [Mollaret]

G03.8 Meningitis due to other specified causes

G03.9 Meningitis, unspecified
Arachnoiditis (spinal) NOS

● **G04 Encephalitis, myelitis and encephalomyelitis**
Includes acute ascending myelitis
meningoencephalitis
meningomyelitis
Excludes1 encephalopathy NOS (G93.40)
other noninfectious acute disseminated encephalomyelitis (noninfectious ADEM) (G04.81)
Excludes2 acute transverse myelitis (G37.3-)
alcoholic encephalopathy (G31.2)
benign myalgic encephalomyelitis (G93.3)
multiple sclerosis (G35)
subacute necrotizing myelitis (G37.4)
toxic encephalitis (G92)
toxic encephalopathy (G92)

● **G04.0 Acute disseminated encephalitis and encephalomyelitis (ADEM)**
Excludes1 acute necrotizing hemorrhagic encephalopathy (G04.3-)

G04.00 Acute disseminated encephalitis and encephalomyelitis, unspecified

G04.01 Postinfectious acute disseminated encephalitis and encephalomyelitis (postinfectious ADEM)
Excludes1 post chickenpox encephalitis (B01.1)
post measles encephalitis (B05.0)
post measles myelitis (B05.1)

G04.02 Postimmunization acute disseminated encephalitis, myelitis and encephalomyelitis
Encephalitis, post immunization
Encephalomyelitis, post immunization
Use additional code to identify the vaccine (T50.A-, T50.B-, T50.Z-)

G04.1 Tropical spastic paraplegia

G04.2 Bacterial meningoencephalitis and meningomyelitis, not elsewhere classified

● **G04.3 Acute necrotizing hemorrhagic encephalopathy**
Sudden and severe CNS disease with pathology of hemorrhages and necrosis of white matter
Excludes1 acute disseminated encephalitis and encephalomyelitis (G04.0-)

G04.30 Acute necrotizing hemorrhagic encephalopathy, unspecified

G04.31 Postinfectious acute necrotizing hemorrhagic encephalopathy

G04.32 Postimmunization acute necrotizing hemorrhagic encephalopathy
Use additional code to identify vaccine (T50.A-, T50.B-, T50.Z-)

G04.39 Other acute necrotizing hemorrhagic encephalopathy
Code also underlying etiology, if applicable

● **G04.8 Other encephalitis, myelitis and encephalomyelitis**
Code also any associated seizure (G40.-, R56.9)

G04.81 Other encephalitis and encephalomyelitis
Noninfectious acute disseminated encephalomyelitis (noninfectious ADEM)

G04.89 Other myelitis

● **G04.9 Encephalitis, myelitis and encephalomyelitis, unspecified**

G04.90 Encephalitis and encephalomyelitis, unspecified
Ventriculitis (cerebral) NOS

G04.91 Myelitis, unspecified

● **G05 Encephalitis, myelitis and encephalomyelitis in diseases classified elsewhere**
Code first underlying disease, such as:
human immunodeficiency virus [HIV] disease (B20)
poliovirus (A80.-)
suppurative otitis media (H66.01-H66.4)
trichinellosis (B75)
Excludes1 adenoviral encephalitis, myelitis and encephalomyelitis (A85.1)
congenital toxoplasmosis encephalitis, myelitis and encephalomyelitis (P37.1)
cytomegaloviral encephalitis, myelitis and encephalomyelitis (B25.8)
encephalitis, myelitis and encephalomyelitis (in) measles (B05.0)
encephalitis, myelitis and encephalomyelitis (in) systemic lupus erythematosus (M32.19)
enteroviral encephalitis, myelitis and encephalomyelitis (A85.0)
herpesviral [herpes simplex] encephalitis, myelitis and encephalomyelitis (B00.4)
listerial encephalitis, myelitis and encephalomyelitis (A32.12)
meningococcal encephalitis, myelitis and encephalomyelitis (A39.81)
mumps encephalitis, myelitis and encephalomyelitis (B26.2)
postchickenpox encephalitis, myelitis and encephalomyelitis (B01.1-)
rubella encephalitis, myelitis and encephalomyelitis (B06.01)
toxoplasmosis encephalitis, myelitis and encephalomyelitis (B58.2)
zoster encephalitis, myelitis and encephalomyelitis (B02.0)

G05.3 Encephalitis and encephalomyelitis in diseases classified elsewhere
Meningoencephalitis in diseases classified elsewhere

G05.4 Myelitis in diseases classified elsewhere
Meningomyelitis in diseases classified elsewhere

● **G06 Intracranial and intraspinal abscess and granuloma**
An accumulation of pus in either the brain or spinal cord
Use additional code (B95-B97) to identify infectious agent.

G06.0 Intracranial abscess and granuloma
Brain [any part] abscess (embolic)
Cerebellar abscess (embolic)
Cerebral abscess (embolic)
Intracranial epidural abscess or granuloma
Intracranial extradural abscess or granuloma
Intracranial subdural abscess or granuloma
Otogenic abscess (embolic)
Excludes1 tuberculous intracranial abscess and granuloma (A17.81)

G06.1 Intraspinal abscess and granuloma
Abscess (embolic) of spinal cord [any part]
Intraspinal epidural abscess or granuloma
Intraspinal extradural abscess or granuloma
Intraspinal subdural abscess or granuloma
Excludes1 tuberculous intraspinal abscess and granuloma (A17.81)

G06.2 Extradural and subdural abscess, unspecified

G07 Intracranial and intraspinal abscess and granuloma in diseases classified elsewhere

Code first underlying disease, such as:
schistosomiasis granuloma of brain (B65.-)

Excludes1 abscess of brain:
amebic (A06.6)
chromomycotic (B43.1)
gonococcal (A54.82)
tuberculous (A17.81)
tuberculoma of meninges (A17.1)

G08 Intracranial and intraspinal phlebitis and thrombophlebitis

Septic embolism of intracranial or intraspinal venous sinuses and veins
Septic endophlebitis of intracranial or intraspinal venous sinuses and veins
Septic phlebitis of intracranial or intraspinal venous sinuses and veins
Septic thrombophlebitis of intracranial or intraspinal venous sinuses and veins
Septic thrombosis of intracranial or intraspinal venous sinuses and veins

Excludes1 intracranial phlebitis and thrombophlebitis complicating:
abortion, ectopic or molar pregnancy (O00-O07, O08.7)
pregnancy, childbirth and the puerperium (O22.5, O87.3)
nonpyogenic intracranial phlebitis and thrombophlebitis (I67.6)

Excludes2 intracranial phlebitis and thrombophlebitis complicating nonpyogenic intraspinal phlebitis and thrombophlebitis (G95.1)

G09 Sequelae of inflammatory diseases of central nervous system

Note: Category G09 is to be used to indicate conditions whose primary classification is to G00-G08 as the cause of sequelae, themselves classifiable elsewhere. The 'sequelae' include conditions specified as residuals.

Code first condition resulting from (sequela) of inflammatory diseases of central nervous system

SYSTEMIC ATROPHIES PRIMARILY AFFECTING THE CENTRAL NERVOUS SYSTEM (G10-G14)

G10 Huntington's disease

Genetic disease with degeneration of cells of the nervous system, including brain
Huntington's chorea
Huntington's dementia

● **G11 Hereditary ataxia**

Genetic neurological disorder affecting coordination

Excludes2 cerebral palsy (G80.-)
hereditary and idiopathic neuropathy (G60.-)
metabolic disorders (E70-E88)

G11.0 Congenital nonprogressive ataxia

G11.1 Early-onset cerebellar ataxia
Early-onset cerebellar ataxia with essential tremor
Early-onset cerebellar ataxia with myoclonus [Hunt's ataxia]
Early-onset cerebellar ataxia with retained tendon reflexes
Friedreich's ataxia (autosomal recessive)
X-linked recessive spinocerebellar ataxia

G11.2 Late-onset cerebellar ataxia

G11.3 Cerebellar ataxia with defective DNA repair
Ataxia telangiectasia [Louis-Bar]

Excludes2 Cockayne's syndrome (Q87.1)
other disorders of purine and pyrimidine metabolism (E79.-)
xeroderma pigmentosum (Q82.1)

G11.4 Hereditary spastic paraplegia

G11.8 Other hereditary ataxias

G11.9 Hereditary ataxia, unspecified
Hereditary cerebellar ataxia NOS
Hereditary cerebellar degeneration
Hereditary cerebellar disease
Hereditary cerebellar syndrome

● **G12 Spinal muscular atrophy and related syndromes**

G12.0 Infantile spinal muscular atrophy, type I [Werdnig-Hoffman]

G12.1 Other inherited spinal muscular atrophy
Adult form spinal muscular atrophy
Childhood form, type II spinal muscular atrophy
Distal spinal muscular atrophy
Juvenile form, type III spinal muscular atrophy [Kugelberg-Welander]
Progressive bulbar palsy of childhood [Fazio-Londe]
Scapuloperoneal form spinal muscular atrophy

● **G12.2 Motor neuron disease**
Progressive disease of motor neurons that carry impluses to muscles to move

G12.20 Motor neuron disease, unspecified

G12.21 Amyotrophic lateral sclerosis
Lou Gehrig's disease (ALS)
Progressive spinal muscle atrophy

G12.22 Progressive bulbar palsy

G12.29 Other motor neuron disease
Familial motor neuron disease
Primary lateral sclerosis

G12.8 Other spinal muscular atrophies and related syndromes

G12.9 Spinal muscular atrophy, unspecified

● **G13 Systemic atrophies primarily affecting central nervous system in diseases classified elsewhere**

G13.0 Paraneoplastic neuromyopathy and neuropathy
Carcinomatous neuromyopathy
Sensorial paraneoplastic neuropathy [Denny Brown]
Code first underlying neoplasm (C00-D49)

G13.1 Other systemic atrophy primarily affecting central nervous system in neoplastic disease
Paraneoplastic limbic encephalopathy
Code first underlying neoplasm (C00-D49)

G13.2 Systemic atrophy primarily affecting the central nervous system in myxedema
Code first underlying disease, such as:
hypothyroidism (E03.-)
myxedematous congenital iodine deficiency (E00.1)

G13.8 Systemic atrophy primarily affecting central nervous system in other diseases classified elsewhere
Code first underlying disease

G14 Postpolio syndrome

Includes Postpolio myelitic syndrome

Excludes1 sequelae of poliomyelitis (B91)

EXTRAPYRAMIDAL AND MOVEMENT DISORDERS (G20-G26)

G20 Parkinson's disease

Progressive disease of the nervous system that affects muscle coordination
Hemiparkinsonism
Idiopathic Parkinsonism or Parkinson's disease
Paralysis agitans
Parkinsonism or Parkinson's disease NOS
Primary Parkinsonism or Parkinson's disease

Excludes1 dementia with Parkinsonism (G31.83)

Item 6–2 Huntington's chorea is an inherited degenerative disorder of the central nervous system and is characterized by ceaseless, jerky movements and progressive cognitive and behavioral deterioration.

● **G21 Secondary parkinsonism**
Symptoms of Parkinson's caused by medicines, illness, or other nervous system disorder
Excludes1 dementia with Parkinsonism (G31.83)
Huntington's disease (G1Ø)
Shy-Drager syndrome (G9Ø.3)
syphilitic Parkinsonism (A52.19)

G21.Ø Malignant neuroleptic syndrome
Use additional code for adverse effect, if applicable, to identify drug (T43.3X5, T43.4X5, T43.5Ø5, T43.595)
Excludes1 neuroleptic induced parkinsonism (G21.11)

● **G21.1 Other drug-induced secondary parkinsonism**

G21.11 Neuroleptic induced parkinsonism
Use additional code for adverse effect, if applicable, to identify drug (T43.3X5, T43.4X5, T43.5Ø5, T43.595)
Excludes1 malignant neuroleptic syndrome (G21.Ø)

G21.19 Other drug induced secondary parkinsonism
Use additional code for adverse effect, if applicable, to identify drug (T36-T5Ø with fifth or sixth character 5)

G21.2 Secondary parkinsonism due to other external agents
Code first (T51-T65) to identify external agent

G21.3 Postencephalitic parkinsonism

G21.4 Vascular parkinsonism

G21.8 Other secondary parkinsonism

G21.9 Secondary parkinsonism, unspecified

● **G23 Other degenerative diseases of basal ganglia**
Excludes2 multi-system degeneration of the autonomic nervous system (G9Ø.3)

G23.Ø Hallervorden-Spatz disease
Pigmentary pallidal degeneration

G23.1 Progressive supranuclear ophthalmoplegia [Steele-Richardson-Olszewski]
Progressive supranuclear palsy

G23.2 Striatonigral degeneration

G23.8 Other specified degenerative diseases of basal ganglia
Calcification of basal ganglia

G23.9 Degenerative disease of basal ganglia, unspecified

● **G24 Dystonia**
Involuntary movements
Includes dyskinesia
Excludes2 athetoid cerebral palsy (G8Ø.3)

● **G24.Ø Drug induced dystonia**
Use additional code for adverse effect, if applicable, to identify drug (T36-T5Ø with fifth or sixth character 5)

G24.Ø1 Drug induced subacute dyskinesia
Drug induced blepharospasm
Drug induced orofacial dyskinesia
Neuroleptic induced tardive dyskinesia
Tardive dyskinesia

G24.Ø2 Drug induced acute dystonia
Acute dystonic reaction to drugs
Neuroleptic induced acute dystonia

G24.Ø9 Other drug induced dystonia

G24.1 Genetic torsion dystonia
Dystonia deformans progressiva
Dystonia musculorum deformans
Familial torsion dystonia
Idiopathic familial dystonia
Idiopathic (torsion) dystonia NOS
(Schwalbe-) Ziehen-Oppenheim disease

G24.2 Idiopathic nonfamilial dystonia

G24.3 Spasmodic torticollis
Head tilts toward one side and chin is elevated and turned toward opposite side (wry neck)
Excludes1 congenital torticollis (Q68.Ø)
hysterical torticollis (F44.4)
ocular torticollis (R29.891)
psychogenic torticollis (F45.8)
torticollis NOS (M43.6)
traumatic recurrent torticollis (S13.4)

G24.4 Idiopathic orofacial dystonia
Orofacial dyskinesia
Excludes1 drug induced orofacial dyskinesia (G24.Ø1)

G24.5 Blepharospasm
Tonic spasm of orbicularis oculi muscle, producing closure of eyelids
Excludes1 drug induced blepharospasm (G24.Ø1)

G24.8 Other dystonia
Acquired torsion dystonia NOS

G24.9 Dystonia, unspecified
Dyskinesia NOS

● **G25 Other extrapyramidal and movement disorders**
Extrapyramidal: Other than pyramidal tracts
Excludes2 sleep related movement disorders (G47.6-)

G25.Ø Essential tremor
Familial tremor
Excludes1 tremor NOS (R25.1)

G25.1 Drug-induced tremor
Use additional code for adverse effect, if applicable, to identify drug (T36-T5Ø with fifth or sixth character 5)

G25.2 Other specified forms of tremor
Intention tremor

G25.3 Myoclonus
Shocklike contractions muscle(s)
Drug-induced myoclonus
Palatal myoclonus
Use additional code for adverse effect, if applicable, to identify drug (T36-T5Ø with fifth or sixth character 5)
Excludes1 facial myokymia (G51.4)
myoclonic epilepsy (G4Ø.-)

G25.4 Drug-induced chorea
Use additional code for adverse effect, if applicable, to identify drug (T36-T5Ø with fifth or sixth character 5)

G25.5 Other chorea
Continual, involuntary, jerky, movements
Chorea NOS
Excludes1 chorea NOS with heart involvement (IØ2.Ø)
Huntington's chorea (G1Ø)
rheumatic chorea (IØ2.-)
Sydenham's chorea (IØ2.-)

● **G25.6 Drug induced tics and other tics of organic origin**

G25.61 Drug induced tics
Use additional code for adverse effect, if applicable, to identify drug (T36-T5Ø with fifth or sixth character 5)

G25.69 Other tics of organic origin
Excludes1 habit spasm (F95.9)
tic NOS (F95.9)
Tourette's syndrome (F95.2)

● **G25.7 Other and unspecified drug induced movement disorders**
Use additional code for adverse effect, if applicable, to identify drug (T36-T5Ø with fifth or sixth character 5)
G25.7Ø Drug induced movement disorder, unspecified
G25.71 Drug induced akathisia
Drug induced acathisia
Neuroleptic induced acute akathisia
G25.79 Other drug induced movement disorders

● **G25.8 Other specified extrapyramidal and movement disorders**
G25.81 Restless legs syndrome
G25.82 Stiff-man syndrome
G25.83 Benign shuddering attacks
G25.89 Other specified extrapyramidal and movement disorders

G25.9 Extrapyramidal and movement disorder, unspecified

G26 Extrapyramidal and movement disorders in diseases classified elsewhere
Code first underlying disease

OTHER DEGENERATIVE DISEASES OF THE NERVOUS SYSTEM (G3Ø-G32)

● **G3Ø Alzheimer's disease**
Progressive central neurodegenerative disorder
Includes Alzheimer's dementia senile and presenile forms
Use additional code to identify:
delirium, if applicable (FØ5)
dementia with behavioral disturbance (FØ2.81)
dementia without behavioral disturbance (FØ2.8Ø)
Excludes1 senile degeneration of brain NEC (G31.1)
senile dementia NOS (FØ3)
senility NOS (R41.81)
G3Ø.Ø Alzheimer's disease with early onset
G3Ø.1 Alzheimer's disease with late onset
G3Ø.8 Other Alzheimer's disease
G3Ø.9 Alzheimer's disease, unspecified

● **G31 Other degenerative diseases of nervous system, not elsewhere classified**
Use additional code to identify:
dementia with behavioral disturbance (FØ2.81)
dementia without behavioral disturbance (FØ2.8Ø)
Excludes2 Reye's syndrome (G93.7)

● **G31.Ø Frontotemporal dementia**
G31.Ø1 Pick's disease
Primary progressive aphasia
Progressive isolated aphasia
G31.Ø9 Other frontotemporal dementia
Frontal dementia

G31.1 Senile degeneration of brain, not elsewhere classified
Excludes1 Alzheimer's disease (G3Ø.-)
senility NOS (R41.81)

G31.2 Degeneration of nervous system due to alcohol
Alcoholic cerebellar ataxia
Alcoholic cerebellar degeneration
Alcoholic cerebral degeneration
Alcoholic encephalopathy
Dysfunction of the autonomic nervous system due to alcohol
Code also associated alcoholism (F1Ø.-)

● **G31.8 Other specified degenerative diseases of nervous system**
G31.81 Alpers' disease
Rare neuronal degeneration of cerebral cortex disease of young children
Grey-matter degeneration
G31.82 Leigh's disease
Rare neurometabolic disorder that affects central nervous system
Subacute necrotizing encephalopathy
G31.83 Dementia with Lewy bodies
Closely allied to Parkinson's Disease
Dementia with Parkinsonism
Lewy body dementia
Lewy body disease
G31.84 Mild cognitive impairment, so stated
Excludes1 age related cognitive decline (R41.81)
altered mental status (R41.82)
cerebral degeneration (G31.9)
change in mental status (R41.82)
cognitive deficits following (sequelae of) cerebral hemorrhage or infarction (I69.Ø1-, I69.11-, I69.21-, I69.31-, I69.81-, I69.91-) ◄
cognitive impairment due to intracranial or head injury (SØ6.-)
dementia (FØ1.-, FØ2.-, FØ3)
mild memory disturbance (FØ6.8)
neurologic neglect syndrome (R41.4)
personality change, nonpsychotic (F68.8)
G31.85 Corticobasal degeneration
G31.89 Other specified degenerative diseases of nervous system

G31.9 Degenerative disease of nervous system, unspecified

● **G32 Other degenerative disorders of nervous system in diseases classified elsewhere**
G32.Ø Subacute combined degeneration of spinal cord in diseases classified elsewhere
Dana-Putnam syndrome
Sclerosis of spinal cord (combined) (dorsolateral) (posterolateral)
Code first underlying disease, such as:
anemia (D51.9)
dietary (D51.3)
pernicious (D51.Ø)
vitamin B12 deficiency (E53.8)
Excludes1 syphilitic combined degeneration of spinal cord (A52.11)

● **G32.8 Other specified degenerative disorders of nervous system in diseases classified elsewhere**
Code first underlying disease, such as:
amyloidosis cerebral degeneration (E85.-)
cerebral degeneration (due to) hypothyroidism (EØØ.Ø-EØ3.9)
cerebral degeneration (due to) neoplasm (CØØ-D49)
cerebral degeneration (due to) vitamin B deficiency, except thiamine (E52-E53.-)
Excludes1 superior hemorrhagic polioencephalitis [Wernicke's encephalopathy] (E51.2)
G32.81 Cerebellar ataxia in diseases classified elsewhere
Code first underlying disease, such as:
celiac disease (with gluten ataxia) (K9Ø.Ø)
cerebellar ataxia (in) neoplastic disease (paraneoplastic cerebellar degeneration) (CØØ-D49)
non-celiac gluten ataxia (M35.9)
Excludes1 systemic atrophy primarily affecting the central nervous system in alcoholic cerebellar ataxia (G31.2)
systemic atrophy primarily affecting the central nervous system in myxedema (G13.2)
G32.89 Other specified degenerative disorders of nervous system in diseases classified elsewhere
Degenerative encephalopathy in diseases classified elsewhere

DEMYELINATING DISEASES OF THE CENTRAL NERVOUS SYSTEM (G35-G37)

G35 Multiple sclerosis
Destruction of central nervous system; four types: relapsing remitting, secondary progressive, primary progressive, and progressive relapsing
Disseminated multiple sclerosis
Generalized multiple sclerosis
Multiple sclerosis NOS
Multiple sclerosis of brain stem
Multiple sclerosis of cord

● **G36 Other acute disseminated demyelination**
Excludes1 postinfectious encephalitis and encephalomyelitis NOS (G04.01)

G36.0 Neuromyelitis optica [Devic]
Inflammatory disorder in which immune system attacks optic nerves and spinal cord producing inflammation of optic nerve (optic neuritis) and spinal cord (myelitis)
Demyelination in optic neuritis
Excludes1 optic neuritis NOS (H46)

G36.1 Acute and subacute hemorrhagic leukoencephalitis [Hurst]

G36.8 Other specified acute disseminated demyelination

G36.9 Acute disseminated demyelination, unspecified

● **G37 Other demyelinating diseases of central nervous system**
Destruction of central nervous system

G37.0 Diffuse sclerosis of central nervous system
Periaxial encephalitis
Schilder's disease
Excludes1 X linked adrenoleukodystrophy (E71.52-)

G37.1 Central demyelination of corpus callosum

G37.2 Central pontine myelinolysis

G37.3 Acute transverse myelitis in demyelinating disease of central nervous system
Acute transverse myelitis NOS
Acute transverse myelopathy
Excludes1 multiple sclerosis (G35)
neuromyelitis optica [Devic] (G36.0)

G37.4 Subacute necrotizing myelitis of central nervous system

G37.5 Concentric sclerosis [Baló] of central nervous system

G37.8 Other specified demyelinating diseases of central nervous system

G37.9 Demyelinating disease of central nervous system, unspecified

Item 6–3 Multiple sclerosis (MS) is a nervous system disease affecting the brain and spinal cord by damaging the myelin sheath surrounding and protecting nerve cells. The damage slows down/blocks messages between the brain and body. Symptoms are: visual disturbances, muscle weakness, coordination and balance issues, numbness, prickling, thinking and memory problems. The cause is unknown, though it is thought that it may be an autoimmune disease. It affects women more than men, between 20 and 40 years of age. MS can be mild, but it may cause the loss of ability to write, walk, and speak. There is no cure, but medication may slow or control symptoms.

EPISODIC AND PAROXYSMAL DISORDERS (G40-G47)

● **G40 Epilepsy and recurrent seizures**
Note: The following terms are to be considered equivalent to intractable: pharmacoresistant (pharmacologically resistant), treatment resistant, refractory (medically) and poorly controlled
Excludes1 conversion disorder with seizures (F44.5)
convulsions NOS (R56.9)
post traumatic seizures (R56.1)
seizure (convulsive) NOS (R56.9)
seizure of newborn (P90)
Excludes2 hippocampal sclerosis (G93.81) ◀
mesial temporal sclerosis (G93.81) ◀
temporal sclerosis (G93.81) ◀
Todd's paralysis (G83.84) ◀

● **G40.0 Localization-related (focal) (partial) idiopathic epilepsy and epileptic syndromes with seizures of localized onset**
Benign childhood epilepsy with centrotemporal EEG spikes
Childhood epilepsy with occipital EEG paroxysms
Excludes1 adult onset localization-related epilepsy (G40.1-, G40.2-)

● **G40.00 Localization-related (focal) (partial) idiopathic epilepsy and epileptic syndromes with seizures of localized onset, not intractable**
Localization-related (focal) (partial) idiopathic epilepsy and epileptic syndromes with seizures of localized onset without intractability

G40.001 Localization-related (focal) (partial) idiopathic epilepsy and epileptic syndromes with seizures of localized onset, not intractable, with status epilepticus

G40.009 Localization-related (focal) (partial) idiopathic epilepsy and epileptic syndromes with seizures of localized onset, not intractable, without status epilepticus
Localization-related (focal) (partial) idiopathic epilepsy and epileptic syndromes with seizures of localized onset NOS

● **G40.01 Localization-related (focal) (partial) idiopathic epilepsy and epileptic syndromes with seizures of localized onset, intractable**

G40.011 Localization-related (focal) (partial) idiopathic epilepsy and epileptic syndromes with seizures of localized onset, intractable, with status epilepticus

G40.019 Localization-related (focal) (partial) idiopathic epilepsy and epileptic syndromes with seizures of localized onset, intractable, without status epilepticus

CHAPTER 6 (G00-G99)

● G40.1 **Localization-related (focal) (partial) symptomatic epilepsy and epileptic syndromes with simple partial seizures**
Attacks without alteration of consciousness
Epilepsia partialis continua [Kozhevnikof]
Simple partial seizures developing into secondarily generalized seizures

● G40.10 **Localization-related (focal) (partial) symptomatic epilepsy and epileptic syndromes with simple partial seizures, not intractable**
Localization-related (focal) (partial) symptomatic epilepsy and epileptic syndromes with simple partial seizures without intractability

G40.101 **Localization-related (focal) (partial) symptomatic epilepsy and epileptic syndromes with simple partial seizures, not intractable, with status epilepticus**

G40.109 **Localization-related (focal) (partial) symptomatic epilepsy and epileptic syndromes with simple partial seizures, not intractable, without status epilepticus**
Localization-related (focal) (partial) symptomatic epilepsy and epileptic syndromes with simple partial seizures NOS

● G40.11 **Localization-related (focal) (partial) symptomatic epilepsy and epileptic syndromes with simple partial seizures, intractable**

G40.111 **Localization-related (focal) (partial) symptomatic epilepsy and epileptic syndromes with simple partial seizures, intractable, with status epilepticus**

G40.119 **Localization-related (focal) (partial) symptomatic epilepsy and epileptic syndromes with simple partial seizures, intractable, without status epilepticus**

● G40.2 **Localization-related (focal) (partial) symptomatic epilepsy and epileptic syndromes with complex partial seizures**
Attacks with alteration of consciousness, often with automatisms
Complex partial seizures developing into secondarily generalized seizures

● G40.20 **Localization-related (focal) (partial) symptomatic epilepsy and epileptic syndromes with complex partial seizures, not intractable**
Localization-related (focal) (partial) symptomatic epilepsy and epileptic syndromes with complex partial seizures without intractability

G40.201 **Localization-related (focal) (partial) symptomatic epilepsy and epileptic syndromes with complex partial seizures, not intractable, with status epilepticus**

G40.209 **Localization-related (focal) (partial) symptomatic epilepsy and epileptic syndromes with complex partial seizures, not intractable, without status epilepticus**
Localization-related (focal) (partial) symptomatic epilepsy and epileptic syndromes with complex partial seizures NOS

● G40.21 **Localization-related (focal) (partial) symptomatic epilepsy and epileptic syndromes with complex partial seizures, intractable**

G40.211 **Localization-related (focal) (partial) symptomatic epilepsy and epileptic syndromes with complex partial seizures, intractable, with status epilepticus**

G40.219 **Localization-related (focal) (partial) symptomatic epilepsy and epileptic syndromes with complex partial seizures, intractable, without status epilepticus**

● G40.3 **Generalized idiopathic epilepsy and epileptic syndromes**
Code also MERRF syndrome, if applicable (E88.42)

● G40.30 **Generalized idiopathic epilepsy and epileptic syndromes, not intractable**
Generalized idiopathic epilepsy and epileptic syndromes without intractability

G40.301 **Generalized idiopathic epilepsy and epileptic syndromes, not intractable, with status epilepticus**

G40.309 **Generalized idiopathic epilepsy and epileptic syndromes, not intractable, without status epilepticus**
Generalized idiopathic epilepsy and epileptic syndromes NOS

● G40.31 **Generalized idiopathic epilepsy and epileptic syndromes, intractable**

G40.311 **Generalized idiopathic epilepsy and epileptic syndromes, intractable, with status epilepticus**

G40.319 **Generalized idiopathic epilepsy and epileptic syndromes, intractable, without status epilepticus**

● G40.A **Absence epileptic syndrome**
Childhood absence epilepsy [pyknolepsy]
Juvenile absence epilepsy
Absence epileptic syndrome, NOS

● G40.A0 **Absence epileptic syndrome, not intractable**

G40.A01 **Absence epileptic syndrome, not intractable, with status epilepticus**

G40.A09 **Absence epileptic syndrome, not intractable, without status epilepticus**

● G40.A1 **Absence epileptic syndrome, intractable**

G40.A11 **Absence epileptic syndrome, intractable, with status epilepticus**

G40.A19 **Absence epileptic syndrome, intractable, without status epilepticus**

● G40.B **Juvenile myoclonic epilepsy [impulsive petit mal]**

● G40.B0 **Juvenile myoclonic epilepsy, not intractable**

G40.B01 **Juvenile myoclonic epilepsy, not intractable, with status epilepticus**

G40.B09 **Juvenile myoclonic epilepsy, not intractable, without status epilepticus**

● G40.B1 **Juvenile myoclonic epilepsy, intractable**

G40.B11 **Juvenile myoclonic epilepsy, intractable, with status epilepticus**

G40.B19 **Juvenile myoclonic epilepsy, intractable, without status epilepticus**

● **G40.4 Other generalized epilepsy and epileptic syndromes**
Epilepsy with grand mal seizures on awakening
Epilepsy with myoclonic absences
Epilepsy with myoclonic-astatic seizures
Grand mal seizure NOS
Nonspecific atonic epileptic seizures
Nonspecific clonic epileptic seizures
Nonspecific myoclonic epileptic seizures
Nonspecific tonic epileptic seizures
Nonspecific tonic-clonic epileptic seizures
Symptomatic early myoclonic encephalopathy

● **G40.40 Other generalized epilepsy and epileptic syndromes, not intractable**
Other generalized epilepsy and epileptic syndromes without intractability
Other generalized epilepsy and epileptic syndromes NOS

G40.401 Other generalized epilepsy and epileptic syndromes, not intractable, with status epilepticus

G40.409 Other generalized epilepsy and epileptic syndromes, not intractable, without status epilepticus

● **G40.41 Other generalized epilepsy and epileptic syndromes, intractable**

G40.411 Other generalized epilepsy and epileptic syndromes, intractable, with status epilepticus

G40.419 Other generalized epilepsy and epileptic syndromes, intractable, without status epilepticus

● **G40.5 Epileptic seizures related to external causes**
Epileptic seizures related to alcohol
Epileptic seizures related to drugs
Epileptic seizures related to hormonal changes
Epileptic seizures related to sleep deprivation
Epileptic seizures related to stress

Code also, if applicable, associated epilepsy and recurrent seizures (G40.-)

Use additional code for adverse effect, if applicable, to identify drug (T36-T50 with fifth or sixth character 5)

● **G40.50 Epileptic seizures related to external causes, not intractable**

G40.501 Epileptic seizures related to external causes, not intractable, with status epilepticus

G40.509 Epileptic seizures related to external causes, not intractable, without status epilepticus
Epileptic seizures related to external causes, NOS

● **G40.8 Other epilepsy and recurrent seizures**
Epilepsies and epileptic syndromes undetermined as to whether they are focal or generalized
Landau-Kleffner syndrome

● **G40.80 Other epilepsy**

G40.801 Other epilepsy, not intractable, with status epilepticus
Other epilepsy without intractability with status epilepticus

G40.802 Other epilepsy, not intractable, without status epilepticus
Other epilepsy NOS
Other epilepsy without intractability without status epilepticus

G40.803 Other epilepsy, intractable, with status epilepticus

G40.804 Other epilepsy, intractable, without status epilepticus

● **G40.81 Lennox-Gastaut syndrome**

G40.811 Lennox-Gastaut syndrome, not intractable, with status epilepticus

G40.812 Lennox-Gastaut syndrome, not intractable, without status epilepticus

G40.813 Lennox-Gastaut syndrome, intractable, with status epilepticus

G40.814 Lennox-Gastaut syndrome, intractable, without status epilepticus

● **G40.82 Epileptic spasms**
Infantile spasms
Salaam attacks
West's syndrome

G40.821 Epileptic spasms, not intractable, with status epilepticus

G40.822 Epileptic spasms, not intractable, without status epilepticus

G40.823 Epileptic spasms, intractable, with status epilepticus

G40.824 Epileptic spasms, intractable, without status epilepticus

G40.89 Other seizures

Excludes1 post traumatic seizures (R56.1)
recurrent seizures NOS (G40.909)
seizure NOS (R56.9)

● **G40.9 Epilepsy, unspecified**

● **G40.90 Epilepsy, unspecified, not intractable**
Epilepsy, unspecified, without intractability

G40.901 Epilepsy, unspecified, not intractable, with status epilepticus

G40.909 Epilepsy, unspecified, not intractable, without status epilepticus
Epilepsy NOS
Epileptic convulsions NOS
Epileptic fits NOS
Epileptic seizures NOS
Recurrent seizures NOS
Seizure disorder NOS

● **G40.91 Epilepsy, unspecified, intractable**
Intractable seizure disorder NOS

G40.911 Epilepsy, unspecified, intractable, with status epilepticus

G40.919 Epilepsy, unspecified, intractable, without status epilepticus

● **G43 Migraine**

Note: The following terms are to be considered equivalent to intractable: pharmacoresistant (pharmacologically resistant), treatment resistant, refractory (medically) and poorly controlled

Use additional code for adverse effect, if applicable, to identify drug (T36-T50 with fifth or sixth character 5)

Excludes1 headache NOS (R51)
lower half migraine (G44.00)

Excludes2 headache syndromes (G44.-)

● **G43.0 Migraine without aura**
Neurological disorder, generally recurring headaches without early symptom (aura)
Common migraine

Excludes1 chronic migraine without aura (G43.7-)

● **G43.00 Migraine without aura, not intractable**
Neurological disorder, generally recurring headaches without early symptom (aura); resistant to cure, relief, or control
Migraine without aura without mention of refractory migraine

G43.001 Migraine without aura, not intractable, with status migrainosus

G43.009 Migraine without aura, not intractable, without status migrainosus
Migraine without aura NOS

◄ New ⟸ Revised ~~deleted~~ Deleted OGCR Official Guidelines X Assign placeholder X ● Use Additional Character(s)
Excludes 1 Excludes 2 Includes Use additional Code first Code also Unspecified

CHAPTER 6 (G00-G99)

Item 6–4 Migraine headache is described as an intense pulsing or throbbing pain in one area of the head. It can be accompanied by extreme sensitivity to light (photophobic) and sound and is three times more common in women than in men. Symptoms include nausea and vomiting. Research indicates migraine headaches are caused by inherited abnormalities in genes that control the activities of certain cell populations in the brain.

● **G43.01 Migraine without aura, intractable**
Intractable migraine: Not easily cured or managed; relentless pain from a migraine
Migraine without aura with refractory migraine

G43.011 Migraine without aura, intractable, with status migrainosus

G43.019 Migraine without aura, intractable, without status migrainosus

● **G43.1 Migraine with aura**
Basilar migraine
Classical migraine
Migraine equivalents
Migraine preceded or accompanied by transient focal neurological phenomena
Migraine triggered seizures
Migraine with acute-onset aura
Migraine with aura without headache (migraine equivalents)
Migraine with prolonged aura
Migraine with typical aura
Retinal migraine
Code also any associated seizure (G40.-, R56.9)
Excludes1 persistent migraine aura (G43.5-, G43.6-)

● **G43.10 Migraine with aura, not intractable**
Migraine with aura without mention of refractory migraine

G43.101 Migraine with aura, not intractable, with status migrainosus

G43.109 Migraine with aura, not intractable, without status migrainosus
Migraine with aura NOS

● **G43.11 Migraine with aura, intractable**
Migraine with aura with refractory migraine

G43.111 Migraine with aura, intractable, with status migrainosus

G43.119 Migraine with aura, intractable, without status migrainosus

● **G43.4 Hemiplegic migraine**
Inherited migraine disorder causing temporary paralysis of one side of body followed by severe headache and nausea
Familial migraine
Sporadic migraine

● **G43.40 Hemiplegic migraine, not intractable**
Hemiplegic migraine without refractory migraine

G43.401 Hemiplegic migraine, not intractable, with status migrainosus

G43.409 Hemiplegic migraine, not intractable, without status migrainosus
Hemiplegic migraine NOS

● **G43.41 Hemiplegic migraine, intractable**
Hemiplegic migraine with refractory migraine

G43.411 Hemiplegic migraine, intractable, with status migrainosus

G43.419 Hemiplegic migraine, intractable, without status migrainosus

● **G43.5 Persistent migraine aura without cerebral infarction**

● **G43.50 Persistent migraine aura without cerebral infarction, not intractable**
Persistent migraine aura without cerebral infarction, without refractory migraine

G43.501 Persistent migraine aura without cerebral infarction, not intractable, with status migrainosus

G43.509 Persistent migraine aura without cerebral infarction, not intractable, without status migrainosus
Persistent migraine aura NOS

● **G43.51 Persistent migraine aura without cerebral infarction, intractable**
Persistent migraine aura without cerebral infarction, with refractory migraine

G43.511 Persistent migraine aura without cerebral infarction, intractable, with status migrainosus

G43.519 Persistent migraine aura without cerebral infarction, intractable, without status migrainosus

● **G43.6 Persistent migraine aura with cerebral infarction**
Visual, motor, or psychic disturbances, paresthesias, and related neurologic abnormalities accompanying migraine
Code also the type of cerebral infarction (I63.-)

● **G43.60 Persistent migraine aura with cerebral infarction, not intractable**
Persistent migraine aura with cerebral infarction, without refractory migraine

G43.601 Persistent migraine aura with cerebral infarction, not intractable, with status migrainosus

G43.609 Persistent migraine aura with cerebral infarction, not intractable, without status migrainosus

● **G43.61 Persistent migraine aura with cerebral infarction, intractable**
Persistent migraine aura with cerebral infarction, with refractory migraine

G43.611 Persistent migraine aura with cerebral infarction, intractable, with status migrainosus

G43.619 Persistent migraine aura with cerebral infarction, intractable, without status migrainosus

● **G43.7 Chronic migraine without aura**
Transformed migraine
Excludes1 migraine without aura (G43.0-)

● **G43.70 Chronic migraine without aura, not intractable**
Chronic migraine without aura, without refractory migraine

G43.701 Chronic migraine without aura, not intractable, with status migrainosus

G43.709 Chronic migraine without aura, not intractable, without status migrainosus
Chronic migraine without aura NOS

● **G43.71 Chronic migraine without aura, intractable**
Chronic migraine without aura, with refractory migraine

G43.711 Chronic migraine without aura, intractable, with status migrainosus

G43.719 Chronic migraine without aura, intractable, without status migrainosus

● G43.A Cyclical vomiting
G43.A0 **Cyclical vomiting, not intractable**
Cyclical vomiting, without refractory migraine
G43.A1 **Cyclical vomiting, intractable**
Cyclical vomiting, with refractory migraine

● G43.B Ophthalmoplegic migraine
G43.B0 **Ophthalmoplegic migraine, not intractable**
Ophthalmoplegic migraine, without refractory migraine
G43.B1 **Ophthalmoplegic migraine, intractable**
Ophthalmoplegic migraine, with refractory migraine

● G43.C Periodic headache syndromes in child or adult
G43.C0 **Periodic headache syndromes in child or adult, not intractable**
Periodic headache syndromes in child or adult, without refractory migraine
G43.C1 **Periodic headache syndromes in child or adult, intractable**
Periodic headache syndromes in child or adult, with refractory migraine

● G43.D Abdominal migraine
G43.D0 **Abdominal migraine, not intractable**
Abdominal migraine, without refractory migraine
G43.D1 **Abdominal migraine, intractable**
Abdominal migraine, with refractory migraine

● G43.8 Other migraine
● G43.80 **Other migraine, not intractable**
Other migraine, without refractory migraine
G43.801 **Other migraine, not intractable, with status migrainosus**
G43.809 **Other migraine, not intractable, without status migrainosus**
● G43.81 **Other migraine, intractable**
Other migraine, with refractory migraine
G43.811 **Other migraine, intractable, with status migrainosus**
G43.819 **Other migraine, intractable, without status migrainosus**
● G43.82 **Menstrual migraine, not intractable**
Menstrual headache, not intractable
Menstrual migraine, without refractory migraine
Menstrually related migraine, not intractable
Pre-menstrual headache, not intractable
Pre-menstrual migraine, not intractable
Pure menstrual migraine, not intractable
Code also associated premenstrual tension syndrome (N94.3)
G43.821 **Menstrual migraine, not intractable, with status migrainosus**
G43.829 **Menstrual migraine, not intractable, without status migrainosus**
Menstrual migraine NOS
● G43.83 **Menstrual migraine, intractable**
Menstrual headache, intractable
Menstrual migraine, with refractory migraine
Menstrually related migraine, intractable
Pre-menstrual headache, intractable
Pre-menstrual migraine, intractable
Pure menstrual migraine, intractable
Code also associated premenstrual tension syndrome (N94.3)
G43.831 **Menstrual migraine, intractable, with status migrainosus**
G43.839 **Menstrual migraine, intractable, without status migrainosus**

● G43.9 Migraine, unspecified
● G43.90 **Migraine, unspecified, not intractable**
Migraine, unspecified, without refractory migraine
G43.901 **Migraine, unspecified, not intractable, with status migrainosus**
Status migrainosus NOS
G43.909 **Migraine, unspecified, not intractable, without status migrainosus**
Migraine NOS
● G43.91 **Migraine, unspecified, intractable**
Migraine, unspecified, with refractory migraine
G43.911 **Migraine, unspecified, intractable, with status migrainosus**
G43.919 **Migraine, unspecified, intractable, without status migrainosus**

● G44 Other headache syndromes
Excludes1 headache NOS (R51)
Excludes2 atypical facial pain (G50.1)
headache due to lumbar puncture (G97.1)
migraines (G43.-)
trigeminal neuralgia (G50.0)

● G44.0 **Cluster headaches and other trigeminal autonomic cephalgias (TAC)**
● G44.00 **Cluster headache syndrome, unspecified**
Ciliary neuralgia
Cluster headache NOS
Histamine cephalgia
Lower half migraine
Migrainous neuralgia
G44.001 **Cluster headache syndrome, unspecified, intractable**
G44.009 **Cluster headache syndrome, unspecified, not intractable**
Cluster headache syndrome NOS
● G44.01 **Episodic cluster headache**
G44.011 **Episodic cluster headache, intractable**
G44.019 **Episodic cluster headache, not intractable**
Episodic cluster headache NOS
● G44.02 **Chronic cluster headache**
G44.021 **Chronic cluster headache, intractable**
G44.029 **Chronic cluster headache, not intractable**
Chronic cluster headache NOS
● G44.03 **Episodic paroxysmal hemicrania**
Paroxysmal hemicrania NOS
G44.031 **Episodic paroxysmal hemicrania, intractable**
G44.039 **Episodic paroxysmal hemicrania, not intractable**
Episodic paroxysmal hemicrania NOS
● G44.04 **Chronic paroxysmal hemicrania**
Unilateral headache
G44.041 **Chronic paroxysmal hemicrania, intractable**
G44.049 **Chronic paroxysmal hemicrania, not intractable**
Chronic paroxysmal hemicrania NOS

● G44.05 **Short lasting unilateral neuralgiform headache with conjunctival injection and tearing (SUNCT)**
- G44.051 **Short lasting unilateral neuralgiform headache with conjunctival injection and tearing (SUNCT), intractable**
- G44.059 **Short lasting unilateral neuralgiform headache with conjunctival injection and tearing (SUNCT), not intractable**
  - Short lasting unilateral neuralgiform headache with conjunctival injection and tearing (SUNCT) NOS

● G44.09 **Other trigeminal autonomic cephalgias (TAC)**
Cluster headaches
- G44.091 **Other trigeminal autonomic cephalgias (TAC), intractable**
- G44.099 **Other trigeminal autonomic cephalgias (TAC), not intractable**

G44.1 **Vascular headache, not elsewhere classified**
Excludes2 cluster headache (G44.0)
complicated headache syndromes (G44.5-)
drug-induced headache (G44.4-)
migraine (G43.-)
other specified headache syndromes (G44.8-)
post-traumatic headache (G44.3-)
tension-type headache (G44.2-)

● G44.2 **Tension-type headache**

● G44.20 **Tension-type headache, unspecified**
- G44.201 **Tension-type headache, unspecified, intractable**
- G44.209 **Tension-type headache, unspecified, not intractable**
  - Tension headache NOS

● G44.21 **Episodic tension-type headache**
- G44.211 **Episodic tension-type headache, intractable**
- G44.219 **Episodic tension-type headache, not intractable**
  - Episodic tension-type headache NOS

● G44.22 **Chronic tension-type headache**
- G44.221 **Chronic tension-type headache, intractable**
- G44.229 **Chronic tension-type headache, not intractable**
  - Chronic tension-type headache NOS

● G44.3 **Post-traumatic headache**

● G44.30 **Post-traumatic headache, unspecified**
- G44.301 **Post-traumatic headache, unspecified, intractable**
- G44.309 **Post-traumatic headache, unspecified, not intractable**
  - Post-traumatic headache NOS

● G44.31 **Acute post-traumatic headache**
- G44.311 **Acute post-traumatic headache, intractable**
- G44.319 **Acute post-traumatic headache, not intractable**
  - Acute post-traumatic headache NOS

● G44.32 **Chronic post-traumatic headache**
- G44.321 **Chronic post-traumatic headache, intractable**
- G44.329 **Chronic post-traumatic headache, not intractable**
  - Chronic post-traumatic headache NOS

● G44.4 **Drug-induced headache, not elsewhere classified**
Medication overuse headache
Use additional code for adverse effect, if applicable, to identify drug (T36-T50 with fifth or sixth character 5)
- G44.40 **Drug-induced headache, not elsewhere classified, not intractable**
- G44.41 **Drug-induced headache, not elsewhere classified, intractable**

● G44.5 **Complicated headache syndromes**
- G44.51 **Hemicrania continua**
  - *Persistent unilateral headache*
- G44.52 **New daily persistent headache (NDPH)**
- G44.53 **Primary thunderclap headache**
- G44.59 **Other complicated headache syndrome**

● G44.8 **Other specified headache syndromes**
- G44.81 **Hypnic headache**
  - *Benign primary headaches*
- G44.82 **Headache associated with sexual activity**
  - Orgasmic headache
  - Preorgasmic headache
- G44.83 **Primary cough headache**
- G44.84 **Primary exertional headache**
- G44.85 **Primary stabbing headache**
- G44.89 **Other headache syndrome**

● G45 **Transient cerebral ischemic attacks and related syndromes**
Excludes1 neonatal cerebral ischemia (P91.0)
transient retinal artery occlusion (H34.0-)
- G45.0 **Vertebro-basilar artery syndrome**
- G45.1 **Carotid artery syndrome (hemispheric)**
- G45.2 **Multiple and bilateral precerebral artery syndromes**
- G45.3 **Amaurosis fugax**
  - *Transient visual loss in one eye*
- G45.4 **Transient global amnesia**
  - *Episode of short-term memory loss, nonrecurrent, lasting few hours*
  - **Excludes1** amnesia NOS (R41.3)
- G45.8 **Other transient cerebral ischemic attacks and related syndromes**
- G45.9 **Transient cerebral ischemic attack, unspecified**
  - Spasm of cerebral artery
  - TIA
  - Transient cerebral ischemia NOS

● G46 **Vascular syndromes of brain in cerebrovascular diseases**
Code first *underlying cerebrovascular disease (I60-I69)*
- G46.0 **Middle cerebral artery syndrome**
- G46.1 **Anterior cerebral artery syndrome**
- G46.2 **Posterior cerebral artery syndrome**
- G46.3 **Brain stem stroke syndrome**
  - Benedikt syndrome
  - Claude syndrome
  - Foville syndrome
  - Millard-Gubler syndrome
  - Wallenberg syndrome
  - Weber syndrome
- G46.4 **Cerebellar stroke syndrome**
- G46.5 **Pure motor lacunar syndrome**
  - *Occlusion of single deep penetrating artery*
- G46.6 **Pure sensory lacunar syndrome**
- G46.7 **Other lacunar syndromes**
- G46.8 **Other vascular syndromes of brain in cerebrovascular diseases**

● G47 Sleep disorders

Excludes2 nightmares (F51.5)
nonorganic sleep disorders (F51.-)
sleep terrors (F51.4)
sleepwalking (F51.3)

● G47.0 Insomnia

Excludes2 alcohol related insomnia (F10.182, F10.282, F10.982)
drug-related insomnia (F11.182, F11.282, F11.982, F13.182, F13.282, F13.982, F14.182, F14.282, F14.982, F15.182, F15.282, F15.982, F19.182, F19.282, F19.982)
idiopathic insomnia (F51.01)
insomnia due to a mental disorder (F51.05)
insomnia not due to a substance or known physiological condition (F51.0-)
nonorganic insomnia (F51.0-)
primary insomnia (F51.01)
sleep apnea (G47.3-)

G47.00 Insomnia, unspecified
Insomnia NOS

G47.01 Insomnia due to medical condition
Code also associated medical condition

G47.09 Other insomnia

● G47.1 Hypersomnia

Excludes2 alcohol-related hypersomnia (F10.182, F10.282, F10.982)
drug-related hypersomnia (F11.182, F11.282, F11.982, F13.182, F13.282, F13.982, F14.182, F14.282, F14.982, F15.182, F15.282, F15.982, F19.182, F19.282, F19.982)
hypersomnia due to a mental disorder (F51.13)
hypersomnia not due to a substance or known physiological condition (F51.1-)
primary hypersomnia (F51.11)
sleep apnea (G47.3-)

G47.10 Hypersomnia, unspecified
Hypersomnia NOS

G47.11 Idiopathic hypersomnia with long sleep time
Idiopathic hypersomnia NOS

G47.12 Idiopathic hypersomnia without long sleep time

G47.13 Recurrent hypersomnia
Kleine-Levin syndrome
Menstrual related hypersomnia

G47.14 Hypersomnia due to medical condition
Code also associated medical condition

G47.19 Other hypersomnia

● G47.2 Circadian rhythm sleep disorders
Disorders of the sleep wake schedule
Inversion of nyctohemeral rhythm
Inversion of sleep rhythm

G47.20 Circadian rhythm sleep disorder, unspecified type
Sleep wake schedule disorder NOS

G47.21 Circadian rhythm sleep disorder, delayed sleep phase type
Delayed sleep phase syndrome

G47.22 Circadian rhythm sleep disorder, advanced sleep phase type

G47.23 Circadian rhythm sleep disorder, irregular sleep wake type
Irregular sleep-wake pattern

G47.24 Circadian rhythm sleep disorder, free running type

G47.25 Circadian rhythm sleep disorder, jet lag type

G47.26 Circadian rhythm sleep disorder, shift work type

G47.27 Circadian rhythm sleep disorder in conditions classified elsewhere
Code first underlying condition

G47.29 Other circadian rhythm sleep disorder

● G47.3 Sleep apnea
Characterized by episodes in which breathing stops during sleep
Code also any associated underlying condition

Excludes1 apnea NOS (R06.81)
Cheyne-Stokes breathing (R06.3)
pickwickian syndrome (E66.2)
sleep apnea of newborn (P28.3)

G47.30 Sleep apnea, unspecified
Sleep apnea NOS

G47.31 Primary central sleep apnea

G47.32 High altitude periodic breathing

G47.33 Obstructive sleep apnea (adult) (pediatric)
Excludes1 obstructive sleep apnea of newborn (P28.3)

G47.34 Idiopathic sleep related nonobstructive alveolar hypoventilation
Sleep related hypoxia

G47.35 Congenital central alveolar hypoventilation syndrome

G47.36 Sleep related hypoventilation in conditions classified elsewhere
Sleep related hypoxemia in conditions classified elsewhere
Code first underlying condition

G47.37 Central sleep apnea in conditions classified elsewhere
Code first underlying condition

G47.39 Other sleep apnea

● G47.4 Narcolepsy and cataplexy
***Cataplexy** is a disorder evidenced by seizures including minor slacking of the facial muscles to complete collapse and often affects people who have **narcolepsy**, a disorder in which there is great difficulty remaining awake during the daytime.*

● G47.41 Narcolepsy

G47.411 Narcolepsy with cataplexy

G47.419 Narcolepsy without cataplexy
Narcolepsy NOS

● G47.42 Narcolepsy in conditions classified elsewhere
Code first underlying condition

G47.421 Narcolepsy in conditions classified elsewhere with cataplexy

G47.429 Narcolepsy in conditions classified elsewhere without cataplexy

● G47.5 Parasomnia

Excludes1 alcohol induced parasomnia (F10.182, F10.282, F10.982)
drug induced parasomnia (F11.182, F11.282, F11.982, F13.182, F13.282, F13.982, F14.182, F14.282, F14.982, F15.182, F15.282, F15.982, F19.182, F19.282, F19.982)
parasomnia not due to a substance or known physiological condition (F51.8)

G47.50 Parasomnia, unspecified
Parasomnia NOS

G47.51 Confusional arousals

G47.52 REM sleep behavior disorder

G47.53 Recurrent isolated sleep paralysis

G47.54 Parasomnia in conditions classified elsewhere
Code first underlying condition

G47.59 Other parasomnia

CHAPTER 6 (G00-G99)

G47.6 Sleep related movement disorders
Excludes2 restless legs syndrome (G25.81)
G47.61 Periodic limb movement disorder
Periodic limb movement disorder
G47.62 Sleep related leg cramps
G47.63 Sleep related bruxism
Excludes1 psychogenic bruxism (F45.8)
G47.69 Other sleep related movement disorders
G47.8 Other sleep disorders
G47.9 Sleep disorder, unspecified
Sleep disorder NOS

★ **(See Plate 118 on page NAP-6.)**

NERVE, NERVE ROOT AND PLEXUS DISORDERS (G50-G59)

Excludes1 current traumatic nerve, nerve root and plexus disorders - see Injury, nerve by body region
neuralgia NOS (M79.2)
neuritis NOS (M79.2)
peripheral neuritis in pregnancy (O26.82-)
radiculitis NOS (M54.1-)

G50 Disorders of trigeminal nerve
Includes disorders of 5th cranial nerve
G50.0 Trigeminal neuralgia
Syndrome of paroxysmal facial pain
Tic douloureux
G50.1 Atypical facial pain
G50.8 Other disorders of trigeminal nerve
G50.9 Disorder of trigeminal nerve, unspecified

G51 Facial nerve disorders
Includes disorders of 7th cranial nerve
G51.0 Bell's palsy
Facial palsy
G51.1 Geniculate ganglionitis
Rare disorder with symptoms of severe pain deep in ear, spreading to ear canal, outer ear, mastoid or eye regions
Excludes1 postherpetic geniculate ganglionitis (B02.21)
G51.2 Melkersson's syndrome
Melkersson-Rosenthal syndrome
G51.3 Clonic hemifacial spasm
G51.4 Facial myokymia
Involuntary facial muscle movement
G51.8 Other disorders of facial nerve
G51.9 Disorder of facial nerve, unspecified

G52 Disorders of other cranial nerves
Excludes2 disorders of acoustic [8th] nerve (H93.3)
disorders of optic [2nd] nerve (H46, H47.0)
paralytic strabismus due to nerve palsy (H49.0-H49.2)
G52.0 Disorders of olfactory nerve
Disorders of 1st cranial nerve
G52.1 Disorders of glossopharyngeal nerve
Disorder of 9th cranial nerve
Glossopharyngeal neuralgia
G52.2 Disorders of vagus nerve
Disorders of pneumogastric [10th] nerve
G52.3 Disorders of hypoglossal nerve
Disorders of 12th cranial nerve

Item 6-5 Trigeminal neuralgia, tic douloureux, is a pain syndrome diagnosed from the patient's history alone. The condition is characterized by pain and a brief facial spasm or tic. Pain is unilateral and follows the sensory distribution of cranial nerve V, typically radiating to the maxillary (V2) or mandibular (V3) area.

Item 6-6 The most common facial nerve disorder is **Bell's Palsy,** which occurs suddenly and results in facial drooping unilaterally. This disorder is the result of a reaction to a virus that causes the facial nerve in the ear to swell resulting in pressure in the bony canal.

G52.7 Disorders of multiple cranial nerves
Polyneuritis cranialis
G52.8 Disorders of other specified cranial nerves
G52.9 Cranial nerve disorder, unspecified

G53 Cranial nerve disorders in diseases classified elsewhere
Code first underlying disease, such as:
neoplasm (C00-D49)
Excludes1 multiple cranial nerve palsy in sarcoidosis (D86.82)
multiple cranial nerve palsy in syphilis (A52.15)
postherpetic geniculate ganglionitis (B02.21)
postherpetic trigeminal neuralgia (B02.22)

G54 Nerve root and plexus disorders
Raiculopathy (nerve root disorder) caused by pressure on nerve root, most common cause is herniation of intervertebral disk. Plexus disorders (plexopathies) are due to compression or injury.
Excludes1 current traumatic nerve root and plexus disorders - see nerve injury by body region
intervertebral disc disorders (M50-M51)
neuralgia or neuritis NOS (M79.2)
neuritis or radiculitis brachial NOS (M54.13)
neuritis or radiculitis lumbar NOS (M54.16)
neuritis or radiculitis lumbosacral NOS (M54.17)
neuritis or radiculitis thoracic NOS (M54.14)
radiculitis NOS (M54.10)
radiculopathy NOS (M54.10)
spondylosis (M47.-)
G54.0 Brachial plexus disorders
Thoracic outlet syndrome
G54.1 Lumbosacral plexus disorders
G54.2 Cervical root disorders, not elsewhere classified
G54.3 Thoracic root disorders, not elsewhere classified
G54.4 Lumbosacral root disorders, not elsewhere classified
G54.5 Neuralgic amyotrophy
Parsonage-Aldren-Turner syndrome
Shoulder-girdle neuritis
Excludes1 neuralgic amyotrophy in diabetes mellitus (E08-E13 with .44)
G54.6 Phantom limb syndrome with pain
Sensations (cramping, itching) in a limb that no longer exists
G54.7 Phantom limb syndrome without pain
Phantom limb syndrome NOS
G54.8 Other nerve root and plexus disorders
G54.9 Nerve root and plexus disorder, unspecified

G55 Nerve root and plexus compressions in diseases classified elsewhere
Code first underlying disease, such as:
neoplasm (C00-D49)
Excludes1 nerve root compression (due to) (in) ankylosing spondylitis (M45.-)
nerve root compression (due to) (in)dorsopathies (M53.-, M54.-)
nerve root compression (due to) (in)intervertebral disc disorders (M50.1.-, M51.1.-)
nerve root compression (due to) (in) spondylopathies (M46.-, M48.-)

★ **(See Plates 472 and 473 on pages NAP-8 and NAP-9.)**

G56 Mononeuropathies of upper limb
Excludes1 current traumatic nerve disorder - see nerve injury by body region
G56.0 Carpal tunnel syndrome
G56.00 Carpal tunnel syndrome, unspecified upper limb
G56.01 Carpal tunnel syndrome, right upper limb
G56.02 Carpal tunnel syndrome, left upper limb
G56.03 Carpal tunnel syndrome, bilateral upper limbs ◀

● **G56.1 Other lesions of median nerve**
- **G56.1Ø Other lesions of median nerve, unspecified side**
- **G56.11 Other lesions of median nerve, right upper limb**
- **G56.12 Other lesions of median nerve, left upper limb**
- **G56.13 Other lesions of median nerve, bilateral upper limbs** ◀

● **G56.2 Lesion of ulnar nerve**
Tardy ulnar nerve palsy
- **G56.2Ø Lesion of ulnar nerve, unspecified upper limb**
- **G56.21 Lesion of ulnar nerve, right upper limb**
- **G56.22 Lesion of ulnar nerve, left upper limb**
- **G56.23 Lesion of ulnar nerve, bilateral upper limbs** ◀

● **G56.3 Lesion of radial nerve**
- **G56.3Ø Lesion of radial nerve, unspecified upper limb**
- **G56.31 Lesion of radial nerve, right upper limb**
- **G56.32 Lesion of radial nerve, left upper limb**
- **G56.33 Lesion of radial nerve, bilateral upper limbs** ◀

● **G56.4 Causalgia of upper limb**
Intense burning pain and sensitivity to slight touch
Complex regional pain syndrome II of upper limb
Excludes1 complex regional pain syndrome I of lower limb (G9Ø.52-)
complex regional pain syndrome I of upper limb (G9Ø.51-)
complex regional pain syndrome II of lower limb (G57.7-)
reflex sympathetic dystrophy of lower limb (G9Ø.52-)
reflex sympathetic dystrophy (G9Ø.51-)
- **G56.4Ø Causalgia of unspecified upper limb**
- **G56.41 Causalgia of right upper limb**
- **G56.42 Causalgia of left upper limb**
- **G56.43 Causalgia of bilateral upper limbs** ◀

● **G56.8 Other specified mononeuropathies of upper limb**
Disease of a single nerve
Interdigital neuroma of upper limb
- **G56.8Ø Other specified mononeuropathies of unspecified upper limb**
- **G56.81 Other specified mononeuropathies of right upper limb**
- **G56.82 Other specified mononeuropathies of left upper limb**
- **G56.83 Other specified mononeuropathies of bilateral upper limbs** ◀

● **G56.9 Unspecified mononeuropathy of upper limb**
Disease of a single nerve
- **G56.9Ø Unspecified mononeuropathy of unspecified upper limb**
- **G56.91 Unspecified mononeuropathy of right upper limb**
- **G56.92 Unspecified mononeuropathy of left upper limb**
- **G56.93 Unspecified mononeuropathy of bilateral upper limbs** ◀

● G57 Mononeuropathies of lower limb
Excludes1 current traumatic nerve disorder - see nerve injury by body region

★ **(See Plates 544 and 545 on pages NAP-10 and NAP-11.)**

● **G57.Ø Lesion of sciatic nerve**
Excludes1 sciatica NOS (M54.3-)
Excludes2 sciatica attributed to intervertebral disc disorder (M51.1.-)
- **G57.ØØ Lesion of sciatic nerve, unspecified lower limb**
- **G57.Ø1 Lesion of sciatic nerve, right lower limb**
- **G57.Ø2 Lesion of sciatic nerve, left lower limb**
- **G57.Ø3 Lesion of sciatic nerve, bilateral lower limbs** ◀

● **G57.1 Meralgia paresthetica**
Numbness or pain in outer thigh caused by injury to nerve
Lateral cutaneous nerve of thigh syndrome
- **G57.1Ø Meralgia paresthetica, unspecified lower limb**
- **G57.11 Meralgia paresthetica, right lower limb**
- **G57.12 Meralgia paresthetica, left lower limb**
- **G57.13 Meralgia paresthetica, bilateral lower limbs** ◀

● **G57.2 Lesion of femoral nerve**
- **G57.2Ø Lesion of femoral nerve, unspecified lower limb**
- **G57.21 Lesion of femoral nerve, right lower limb**
- **G57.22 Lesion of femoral nerve, left lower limb**
- **G57.23 Lesion of femoral nerve, bilateral lower limbs** ◀

● **G57.3 Lesion of lateral popliteal nerve**
Peroneal nerve palsy
- **G57.3Ø Lesion of lateral popliteal nerve, unspecified lower limb**
- **G57.31 Lesion of lateral popliteal nerve, right lower limb**
- **G57.32 Lesion of lateral popliteal nerve, left lower limb**
- **G57.33 Lesion of lateral popliteal nerve, bilateral lower limbs** ◀

● **G57.4 Lesion of medial popliteal nerve**
- **G57.4Ø Lesion of medial popliteal nerve, unspecified lower limb**
- **G57.41 Lesion of medial popliteal nerve, right lower limb**
- **G57.42 Lesion of medial popliteal nerve, left lower limb**
- **G57.43 Lesion of medial popliteal nerve, bilateral lower limbs** ◀

● **G57.5 Tarsal tunnel syndrome**
- **G57.5Ø Tarsal tunnel syndrome, unspecified lower limb**
- **G57.51 Tarsal tunnel syndrome, right lower limb**
- **G57.52 Tarsal tunnel syndrome, left lower limb**
- **G57.53 Tarsal tunnel syndrome, bilateral lower limbs** ◀

● **G57.6 Lesion of plantar nerve**
Morton's metatarsalgia
- **G57.6Ø Lesion of plantar nerve, unspecified lower limb**
- **G57.61 Lesion of plantar nerve, right lower limb**
- **G57.62 Lesion of plantar nerve, left lower limb**
- **G57.63 Lesion of plantar nerve, bilateral lower limbs** ◀

● **G57.7 Causalgia of lower limb**
Complex regional pain syndrome II of lower limb
Excludes1 complex regional pain syndrome I of lower limb (G9Ø.52-)
complex regional pain syndrome I of upper limb (G9Ø.51-)
complex regional pain syndrome II of upper limb (G56.4-)
reflex sympathetic dystrophy of lower limb (G9Ø.52-)
reflex sympathetic dystrophy of upper limb (G9Ø.51-)
- **G57.7Ø Causalgia of unspecified lower limb**
- **G57.71 Causalgia of right lower limb**
- **G57.72 Causalgia of left lower limb**
- **G57.73 Causalgia of bilateral lower limbs** ◀

● **G57.8 Other specified mononeuropathies of lower limb**
Interdigital neuroma of lower limb
- **G57.8Ø Other specified mononeuropathies of unspecified lower limb**
- **G57.81 Other specified mononeuropathies of right lower limb**
- **G57.82 Other specified mononeuropathies of left lower limb**
- **G57.83 Other specified mononeuropathies of bilateral lower limbs** ◀

●G57.9 Unspecified mononeuropathy of lower limb
- G57.90 Unspecified mononeuropathy of unspecified lower limb
- G57.91 Unspecified mononeuropathy of right lower limb
- G57.92 Unspecified mononeuropathy of left lower limb
- G57.93 Unspecified mononeuropathy of bilateral lower limbs ◀

●G58 Other mononeuropathies
- G58.0 Intercostal neuropathy
- G58.7 Mononeuritis multiplex
- G58.8 Other specified mononeuropathies
- G58.9 Mononeuropathy, unspecified

G59 Mononeuropathy in diseases classified elsewhere

Code first underlying disease

Excludes1 diabetic mononeuropathy (E08-E13 with .41)
syphilitic nerve paralysis (A52.19)
syphilitic neuritis (A52.15)
tuberculous mononeuropathy (A17.83)

POLYNEUROPATHIES AND OTHER DISORDERS OF THE PERIPHERAL NERVOUS SYSTEM (G60-G65)

Excludes1 neuralgia NOS (M79.2)
neuritis NOS (M79.2)
peripheral neuritis in pregnancy (O26.82-)
radiculitis NOS (M54.10)

●G60 Hereditary and idiopathic neuropathy
- G60.0 Hereditary motor and sensory neuropathy
  - Charcot-Marie-Tooth disease
  - Déjerine-Sottas disease
  - Hereditary motor and sensory neuropathy, types I-IV
  - Hypertrophic neuropathy of infancy
  - Peroneal muscular atrophy (axonal type) (hypertrophic type)
  - Roussy-Lévy syndrome
- G60.1 Refsum's disease
  - *Genetic disorder affecting fatty acid metabolism*
  - Infantile Refsum disease
- G60.2 Neuropathy in association with hereditary ataxia

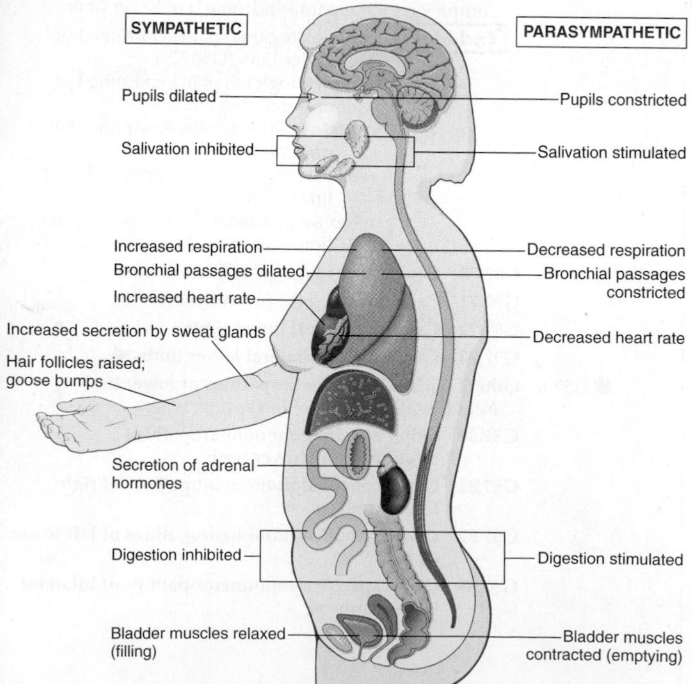

Item 6–7 The **peripheral nervous system** consists of 31 pairs of spinal nerves, 12 pairs of cranial nerves, and the autonomic nerves, which are divided into the parasympathetic and sympathetic nerves. The cranial nerves are: olfactory (I), optic (II), oculomotor (III), trochlear (IV), trigeminal (V), abducens (VI), facial (VII), vestibulocochlear (VIII), glossopharyngeal (IX), vagus (X), accessory (XI), and hypoglossal (XII).

- G60.3 Idiopathic progressive neuropathy
- G60.8 Other hereditary and idiopathic neuropathies
  - Dominantly inherited sensory neuropathy
  - Morvan's disease
  - Nelaton's syndrome
  - Recessively inherited sensory neuropathy
- G60.9 Hereditary and idiopathic neuropathy, unspecified

●G61 Inflammatory polyneuropathy
- G61.0 Guillain-Barré syndrome
  - *Autoimmune disease affecting peripheral nervous system*
  - Acute (post-)infective polyneuritis
  - Miller Fisher Syndrome
- G61.1 Serum neuropathy
  - Use additional code for adverse effect, if applicable, to identify serum (T50.-)
- ●G61.8 Other inflammatory polyneuropathies
  - G61.81 Chronic inflammatory demyelinating polyneuritis
  - G61.82 Multifocal motor neuropathy ◀
    - MMN ◀
  - G61.89 Other inflammatory polyneuropathies
- G61.9 Inflammatory polyneuropathy, unspecified

●G62 Other and unspecified polyneuropathies
- G62.0 Drug-induced polyneuropathy
  - Use additional code for adverse effect, if applicable, to identify drug (T36-T50 with fifth or sixth character 5)
- G62.1 Alcoholic polyneuropathy
  - *Malfunction of many peripheral nerves throughout the body*
- G62.2 Polyneuropathy due to other toxic agents
  - *Code first (T51-T65) to identify toxic agent*

Figure 6-2 Actions of parasympathetic and sympathetic nerves. (From Chabner: The Language of Medicine, ed 9, St. Louis, Saunders, 2011)

● G62.8 **Other specified polyneuropathies**
G62.81 **Critical illness polyneuropathy**
Acute motor neuropathy
G62.82 **Radiation-induced polyneuropathy**
Use additional external cause code (W88-W90, X39.0-) to identify cause
G62.89 **Other specified polyneuropathies**
G62.9 **Polyneuropathy, unspecified**
Neuropathy NOS

G63 **Polyneuropathy in diseases classified elsewhere**
Code first *underlying disease, such as:*
amyloidosis (E85.-)
endocrine disease, except diabetes (E00-E07, E15-E16, E20-E34)
metabolic diseases (E70-E88)
neoplasm (C00-D49)
nutritional deficiency (E40-E64)
Excludes1 polyneuropathy (in):
diabetes mellitus (E08-E13 with .42)
diphtheria (A36.83)
infectious mononucleosis (B27.0-B27.9 with 1)
Lyme disease (A69.22)
mumps (B26.84)
postherpetic (B02.23)
rheumatoid arthritis (M05.33)
scleroderma (M34.83)
systemic lupus erythematosus (M32.19)

G64 **Other disorders of peripheral nervous system**
Disorder of peripheral nervous system NOS

● G65 **Sequelae of inflammatory and toxic polyneuropathies**
Code first *condition resulting from (sequela) of inflammatory and toxic polyneuropathies*
G65.0 **Sequelae of Guillain-Barré syndrome**
G65.1 **Sequelae of other inflammatory polyneuropathy**
G65.2 **Sequelae of toxic polyneuropathy**

DISEASES OF MYONEURAL JUNCTION AND MUSCLE (G70-G73)

● G70 **Myasthenia gravis and other myoneural disorders**
Excludes1 botulism (A05.1, A48.51-A48.52)
transient neonatal myasthenia gravis (P94.0)
● G70.0 **Myasthenia gravis**
Acquired and results in fatigable muscle weakness exacerbated by activity and improved with rest
G70.00 **Myasthenia gravis without (acute) exacerbation**
Myasthenia gravis NOS
G70.01 **Myasthenia gravis with (acute) exacerbation**
Myasthenia gravis in crisis
G70.1 **Toxic myoneural disorders**
Dysfunction at junction of muscle and motor nerve (myoneural junction)
Code first *(T51-T65) to identify toxic agent*
G70.2 **Congenital and developmental myasthenia**
● G70.8 **Other specified myoneural disorders**
G70.80 **Lambert-Eaton syndrome, unspecified**
Lambert-Eaton syndrome NOS
G70.81 **Lambert-Eaton syndrome in disease classified elsewhere**
Code first *underlying disease*
Excludes1 Lambert-Eaton syndrome in neoplastic disease (G73.1)
G70.89 **Other specified myoneural disorders**
G70.9 **Myoneural disorder, unspecified**

Item 6–8 Muscular dystrophies (MD) are a group of rare inherited muscle diseases. Voluntary muscles become progressively weaker. In the late stages of MD, fat and connective tissue replace muscle fibers. In some types of muscular dystrophy, heart muscles, other involuntary muscles, and other organs are affected. **Myopathies** is a general term for neuromuscular diseases in which the muscle fibers dysfunction for any one of many reasons, resulting in muscular weakness.

● G71 **Primary disorders of muscles**
Excludes2 arthrogryposis multiplex congenita (Q74.3)
metabolic disorders (E70-E88)
myositis (M60.-)
G71.0 **Muscular dystrophy**
Autosomal recessive, childhood type, muscular dystrophy resembling Duchenne or Becker muscular dystrophy
Benign [Becker] muscular dystrophy
Benign scapuloperoneal muscular dystrophy with early contractures [Emery-Dreifuss]
Congenital muscular dystrophy NOS
Congenital muscular dystrophy with specific morphological abnormalities of the muscle fiber
Distal muscular dystrophy
Facioscapulohumeral muscular dystrophy
Limb-girdle muscular dystrophy
Ocular muscular dystrophy
Oculopharyngeal muscular dystrophy
Scapuloperoneal muscular dystrophy
Severe [Duchenne] muscular dystrophy
● G71.1 **Myotonic disorders**
Inherited disorder that affects muscles tone
G71.11 **Myotonic muscular dystrophy**
Dystrophia myotonica [Steinert]
Myotonia atrophica
Myotonic dystrophy
Proximal myotonic myopathy (PROMM)
Steinert disease
G71.12 **Myotonia congenita**
Acetazolamide responsive myotonia congenita
Dominant myotonia congenita [Thomsen disease]
Myotonia levior
Recessive myotonia congenita [Becker disease]
G71.13 **Myotonic chondrodystrophy**
Chondrodystrophic myotonia
Congenital myotonic chondrodystrophy
Schwartz-Jampel disease
G71.14 **Drug induced myotonia**
Use additional code for adverse effect, if applicable, to identify drug (T36-T50 with fifth or sixth character 5)
G71.19 **Other specified myotonic disorders**
Myotonia fluctuans
Myotonia permanens
Neuromyotonia [Isaacs]
Paramyotonia congenita (of von Eulenburg)
Pseudomyotonia
Symptomatic myotonia
G71.2 **Congenital myopathies**
Central core disease
Fiber-type disproportion
Minicore disease
Multicore disease
Myotubular (centronuclear) myopathy
Nemaline myopathy
Excludes1 arthrogryposis multiplex congenita (Q74.3)

G71.3 Mitochondrial myopathy, not elsewhere classified
Myopathies associated with increased number of enlarged, often abnormal, mitochondria in muscle fibers
Excludes1 Kearns-Sayre syndrome (H49.81)
Leber's disease (H47.21)
Leigh's encephalopathy (G31.82)
mitochondrial metabolism disorders (E88.4.-)
Reye's syndrome (G93.7)

G71.8 Other primary disorders of muscles

G71.9 Primary disorder of muscle, unspecified
Hereditary myopathy NOS

● **G72 Other and unspecified myopathies**
Excludes1 arthrogryposis multiplex congenita (Q74.3)
dermatopolymyositis (M33.-)
ischemic infarction of muscle (M62.2-)
myositis (M60.-)
polymyositis (M33.2.-)

G72.0 Drug-induced myopathy
Use additional code for adverse effect, if applicable, to identify drug (T36-T50 with fifth or sixth character 5)

G72.1 Alcoholic myopathy
Use additional code to identify alcoholism (F10.-)

G72.2 Myopathy due to other toxic agents
Code first (T51-T65) to identify toxic agent

G72.3 Periodic paralysis
Familial periodic paralysis
Hyperkalemic periodic paralysis (familial)
Hypokalemic periodic paralysis (familial)
Myotonic periodic paralysis (familial)
Normokalemic paralysis (familial)
Potassium sensitive periodic paralysis
Excludes1 paramyotonia congenita (of von Eulenburg) (G71.19)

● **G72.4 Inflammatory and immune myopathies, not elsewhere classified**

G72.41 Inclusion body myositis [IBM]

G72.49 Other inflammatory and immune myopathies, not elsewhere classified
Inflammatory myopathy NOS

● **G72.8 Other specified myopathies**

G72.81 Critical illness myopathy
Acute necrotizing myopathy
Acute quadriplegic myopathy
Intensive care (ICU) myopathy
Myopathy of critical illness

G72.89 Other specified myopathies

G72.9 Myopathy, unspecified

● **G73 Disorders of myoneural junction and muscle in diseases classified elsewhere**

G73.1 Lambert-Eaton syndrome in neoplastic disease
Rare autoimmune disorder affecting calcium channels of nerve-muscle (neuromuscular) junction
Code first underlying neoplasm (C00-D49)
Excludes1 Lambert-Eaton syndrome not associated with neoplasm (G70.80-G70.81)

G73.3 Myasthenic syndromes in other diseases classified elsewhere
Code first underlying disease, such as:
neoplasm (C00-D49)
thyrotoxicosis (E05.-)

G73.7 Myopathy in diseases classified elsewhere
Code first underlying disease, such as:
hyperparathyroidism (E21.0, E21.3)
hypoparathyroidism (E20.-)
glycogen storage disease (E74.0)
lipid storage disorders (E75.-)
Excludes1 myopathy in:
rheumatoid arthritis (M05.32)
sarcoidosis (D86.87)
scleroderma (M34.82)
sicca syndrome [Sjögren] (M35.03)
systemic lupus erythematosus (M32.19)

CEREBRAL PALSY AND OTHER PARALYTIC SYNDROMES (G80-G83)

● **G80 Cerebral palsy**
Excludes1 hereditary spastic paraplegia (G11.4)

G80.0 Spastic quadriplegic cerebral palsy
Congenital spastic paralysis (cerebral)

G80.1 Spastic diplegic cerebral palsy
Spastic cerebral palsy NOS

G80.2 Spastic hemiplegic cerebral palsy

G80.3 Athetoid cerebral palsy
Result of damage to cerebellum or basal ganglia responsible for processing neuromuscular signals
Double athetosis (syndrome)
Dyskinetic cerebral palsy
Dystonic cerebral palsy
Vogt disease

G80.4 Ataxic cerebral palsy
Poor muscle tone and coordination

G80.8 Other cerebral palsy
Mixed cerebral palsy syndromes

G80.9 Cerebral palsy, unspecified
Cerebral palsy NOS

OGCR Section I.C.6.a.

Dominant/nondominant side

Codes from category G81, Hemiplegia and hemiparesis, and subcategories, G83.1, Monoplegia of lower limb, G83.2, Monoplegia of upper limb, and G83.3, Monoplegia, unspecified, identify whether the dominant and nondominant side is affected. Should the affected side be documented, but not specified as dominant or nondominant, and the classification system does not indicate a default, code selection is as follows:

- For ambidextrous patients, the default should be dominant.
- If the left side is affected, the default is non-dominant.
- If the right side is affected, the default is dominant.

● **G81 Hemiplegia and hemiparesis**
Note: This category is to be used only when hemiplegia (complete)(incomplete) is reported without further specification, or is stated to be old or longstanding but of unspecified cause. The category is also for use in multiple coding to identify these types of hemiplegia resulting from any cause.
Excludes1 congenital cerebral palsy (G80.-)
hemiplegia and hemiparesis due to sequela of cerebrovascular disease (I69.05-, I69.15-, I69.25-, I69.35-, I69.85-, I69.95-)

● **G81.0 Flaccid hemiplegia**
Paralysis of half of body with loss of tone of muscles of paralyzed part and absence of tendon reflexes

G81.00 Flaccid hemiplegia affecting unspecified side

G81.01 Flaccid hemiplegia affecting right dominant side

G81.02 Flaccid hemiplegia affecting left dominant side

G81.03 Flaccid hemiplegia affecting right nondominant side

G81.04 Flaccid hemiplegia affecting left nondominant side

CHAPTER 6 (G00-G99)

Item 6–9 **Hemiplegia** is complete paralysis of one side of the body—arm, leg, and trunk. **Hemiparesis** is a generalized weakness or incomplete paralysis of one side of the body. If most activities (eating, writing) are performed with the right hand, the right is the dominant side, and the left is the nondominant side. **Quadriplegia,** also called tetraplegia, is the complete paralysis of all four limbs. **Quadriparesis** is the incomplete paralysis of all four limbs. Nerve damage in C1–C4 is associated with lower limb paralysis, and C5–C7 damage is associated with upper limb paralysis. **Diplegia** is the paralysis of the upper limbs. **Monoplegia** is the complete paralysis of one limb.

● **G81.1 Spastic hemiplegia**
Paralysis of half of body with spasticity of muscles of paralyzed part and increased tendon reflexes
G81.10 Spastic hemiplegia affecting unspecified side
G81.11 Spastic hemiplegia affecting right dominant side
G81.12 Spastic hemiplegia affecting left dominant side
G81.13 Spastic hemiplegia affecting right nondominant side
G81.14 Spastic hemiplegia affecting left nondominant side

● **G81.9 Hemiplegia, unspecified**
G81.90 Hemiplegia, unspecified affecting unspecified side
G81.91 Hemiplegia, unspecified affecting right dominant side
G81.92 Hemiplegia, unspecified affecting left dominant side
G81.93 Hemiplegia, unspecified affecting right nondominant side
G81.94 Hemiplegia, unspecified affecting left nondominant side

● **G82 Paraplegia (paraparesis) and quadriplegia (quadriparesis)**
Note: This category is to be used only when the listed conditions are reported without further specification, or are stated to be old or longstanding but of unspecified cause. The category is also for use in multiple coding to identify these conditions resulting from any cause.
Excludes1 congenital cerebral palsy (G80.-)
functional quadriplegia (R53.2)
hysterical paralysis (F44.4)

● **G82.2 Paraplegia**
Paralysis of both lower limbs NOS
Paraparesis (lower) NOS
Paraplegia (lower) NOS
G82.20 Paraplegia, unspecified
G82.21 Paraplegia, complete
G82.22 Paraplegia, incomplete

● **G82.5 Quadriplegia**
Paralysis of all limbs; AKA tetraplegia
G82.50 Quadriplegia, unspecified
G82.51 Quadriplegia, C1-C4 complete
G82.52 Quadriplegia, C1-C4 incomplete
G82.53 Quadriplegia, C5-C7 complete
G82.54 Quadriplegia, C5-C7 incomplete

● **G83 Other paralytic syndromes**
Note: This category is to be used only when the listed conditions are reported without further specification, or are stated to be old or longstanding but of unspecified cause. The category is also for use in multiple coding to identify these conditions resulting from any cause.
Includes paralysis (complete) (incomplete), except as in G80-G82

G83.0 Diplegia of upper limbs
Paralysis affecting limbs on both sides; AKA bilateral paralysis
Diplegia (upper)
Paralysis of both upper limbs

● **G83.1 Monoplegia of lower limb**
Paralysis of limb on one side
Paralysis of lower limb
Excludes1 monoplegia of lower limbs due to sequela of cerebrovascular disease (I69.04-, I69.14-, I69.24-, I69.34-, I69.84-, I69.94-)
G83.10 Monoplegia of lower limb affecting unspecified side
G83.11 Monoplegia of lower limb affecting right dominant side
G83.12 Monoplegia of lower limb affecting left dominant side
G83.13 Monoplegia of lower limb affecting right nondominant side
G83.14 Monoplegia of lower limb affecting left nondominant side

● **G83.2 Monoplegia of upper limb**
Paralysis of upper limb
Excludes1 monoplegia of upper limbs due to sequela of cerebrovascular disease (I69.03-, I69.13-, I69.23-, I69.33-, I69.83-, I69.93-)
G83.20 Monoplegia of upper limb affecting unspecified side
G83.21 Monoplegia of upper limb affecting right dominant side
G83.22 Monoplegia of upper limb affecting left dominant side
G83.23 Monoplegia of upper limb affecting right nondominant side
G83.24 Monoplegia of upper limb affecting left nondominant side

● **G83.3 Monoplegia, unspecified**
G83.30 Monoplegia, unspecified affecting unspecified side
G83.31 Monoplegia, unspecified affecting right dominant side
G83.32 Monoplegia, unspecified affecting left dominant side
G83.33 Monoplegia, unspecified affecting right nondominant side
G83.34 Monoplegia, unspecified affecting left nondominant side

G83.4 Cauda equina syndrome
Aching pain due to compression of spinal nerve roots
Neurogenic bladder due to cauda equina syndrome
Excludes1 cord bladder NOS (G95.89)
neurogenic bladder NOS (N31.9)

G83.5 Locked-in state

● **G83.8 Other specified paralytic syndromes**
Excludes1 paralytic syndromes due to current spinal cord injury-code to spinal cord injury (S14, S24, S34)
G83.81 Brown-Séquard syndrome
G83.82 Anterior cord syndrome
G83.83 Posterior cord syndrome
G83.84 Todd's paralysis (postepileptic)
G83.89 Other specified paralytic syndromes

G83.9 Paralytic syndrome, unspecified

CHAPTER 6 (G00-G99)

OTHER DISORDERS OF THE NERVOUS SYSTEM (G89-G99)

● **G89 Pain, not elsewhere classified**

Code also related psychological factors associated with pain (F45.42)

Excludes1 generalized pain NOS (R52)
pain disorders exclusively related to psychological factors (F45.41)
pain NOS (R52)

Excludes2 atypical face pain (G50.1)
headache syndromes (G44.-)
localized pain, unspecified type - code to pain by site, such as:
abdomen pain (R10.-)
back pain (M54.9)
breast pain (N64.4)
chest pain (R07.1-R07.9)
ear pain (H92.0-)
eye pain (H57.1)
headache (R51)
joint pain (M25.5-)
limb pain (M79.6-)
lumbar region pain (M54.5)
painful urination (R30.9)
pelvic and perineal pain (R10.2)
shoulder pain (M25.51-)
spine pain (M54.-)
throat pain (R07.0)
tongue pain (K14.6)
tooth pain (K08.8)
renal colic (N23)
migraines (G43.-)
myalgia (M79.1)
pain from prosthetic devices, implants, and grafts (T82.84, T83.84, T84.84, T85.84-) ⬅
phantom limb syndrome with pain (G54.6)
vulvar vestibulitis (N94.810)
vulvodynia (N94.81-)

G89.0 Central pain syndrome
Neurological condition causing intractable pain resulting from damage to CNS
Déjérine-Roussy syndrome
Myelopathic pain syndrome
Thalamic pain syndrome (hyperesthetic)

● **G89.1 Acute pain, not elsewhere classified**

G89.11 Acute pain due to trauma

G89.12 Acute post-thoracotomy pain
Post-thoracotomy pain NOS

G89.18 Other acute postprocedural pain
Postoperative pain NOS
Postprocedural pain NOS

● **G89.2 Chronic pain, not elsewhere classified**

Excludes1 causalgia, lower limb (G57.7-)
causalgia, upper limb (G56.4-)
central pain syndrome (G89.0)
chronic pain syndrome (G89.4)
complex regional pain syndrome II, lower limb (G57.7-)
complex regional pain syndrome II, upper limb (G56.4-)
neoplasm related chronic pain (G89.3)
reflex sympathetic dystrophy (G90.5-)

G89.21 Chronic pain due to trauma

G89.22 Chronic post-thoracotomy pain

G89.28 Other chronic postprocedural pain
Other chronic postoperative pain

G89.29 Other chronic pain

G89.3 Neoplasm related pain (acute) (chronic)
Cancer associated pain
Pain due to malignancy (primary) (secondary)
Tumor associated pain

G89.4 Chronic pain syndrome
Chronic pain associated with significant psychosocial dysfunction

● **G90 Disorders of autonomic nervous system**

Excludes1 dysfunction of the autonomic nervous system due to alcohol (G31.2)

● **G90.0 Idiopathic peripheral autonomic neuropathy**

G90.01 Carotid sinus syncope
Carotid sinus syndrome

G90.09 Other idiopathic peripheral autonomic neuropathy
Idiopathic peripheral autonomic neuropathy NOS

G90.1 Familial dysautonomia [Riley-Day]
Inherited disorder that affects nerve function

G90.2 Horner's syndrome
Due to damage of the sympathetic nervous system
Bernard(-Horner) syndrome
Cervical sympathetic dystrophy or paralysis

G90.3 Multi-system degeneration of the autonomic nervous system
Neurogenic orthostatic hypotension [Shy-Drager]

Excludes1 orthostatic hypotension NOS (I95.1)

G90.4 Autonomic dysreflexia
Syndrome resulting from lesions of spinal cord
Use additional code to identify the cause, such as:
fecal impaction (K56.41)
pressure ulcer (pressure area) (L89.-)
urinary tract infection (N39.0)

● **G90.5 Complex regional pain syndrome I (CRPS I)**
Reflex sympathetic dystrophy

Excludes1 causalgia of lower limb (G57.7-)
causalgia of upper limb (G56.4-)
complex regional pain syndrome II of lower limb (G57.7-)
complex regional pain syndrome II of upper limb (G56.4-)

G90.50 Complex regional pain syndrome I, unspecified

● **G90.51 Complex regional pain syndrome I of upper limb**

G90.511 Complex regional pain syndrome I of right upper limb

G90.512 Complex regional pain syndrome I of left upper limb

G90.513 Complex regional pain syndrome I of upper limb, bilateral

G90.519 Complex regional pain syndrome I of unspecified upper limb

● **G90.52 Complex regional pain syndrome I of lower limb**

G90.521 Complex regional pain syndrome I of right lower limb

G90.522 Complex regional pain syndrome I of left lower limb

G90.523 Complex regional pain syndrome I of lower limb, bilateral

G90.529 Complex regional pain syndrome I of unspecified lower limb

G90.59 Complex regional pain syndrome I of other specified site

G90.8 Other disorders of autonomic nervous system

G90.9 Disorder of the autonomic nervous system, unspecified

● **G91 Hydrocephalus**
Dilatation of cerebral ventricles, accompanied by accumulation of cerebrospinal fluid
Includes acquired hydrocephalus
Excludes1 Arnold-Chiari syndrome with hydrocephalus (Q07.-)
congenital hydrocephalus (Q03.-)
spina bifida with hydrocephalus (Q05.-)

G91.0 Communicating hydrocephalus
Secondary normal pressure hydrocephalus

G91.1 Obstructive hydrocephalus

G91.2 (Idiopathic) normal pressure hydrocephalus
Normal pressure hydrocephalus NOS

G91.3 Post-traumatic hydrocephalus, unspecified

G91.4 Hydrocephalus in diseases classified elsewhere
Code first underlying condition, such as:
congenital syphilis (A50.4-)
neoplasm (C00-D49)
Excludes1 hydrocephalus due to congenital toxoplasmosis (P37.1)

G91.8 Other hydrocephalus

G91.9 Hydrocephalus, unspecified

G92 Toxic encephalopathy
Disorder or disease of brain caused by chemicals
Toxic encephalitis
Toxic metabolic encephalopathy
Code first (T51-T65) to identify toxic agent

● **G93 Other disorders of brain**

G93.0 Cerebral cysts
Arachnoid cyst
Porencephalic cyst, acquired
Excludes1 acquired periventricular cysts of newborn (P91.1)
congenital cerebral cysts (Q04.6)

G93.1 Anoxic brain damage, not elsewhere classified
Permanent brain damage by lack of oxygen perfusion through brain tissues.
Excludes1 cerebral anoxia due to anesthesia during labor and delivery (O74.3)
cerebral anoxia due to anesthesia during the puerperium (O89.2)
neonatal anoxia (P84)

G93.2 Benign intracranial hypertension
Excludes1 hypertensive encephalopathy (I67.4)

G93.3 Postviral fatigue syndrome
Benign myalgic encephalomyelitis
Excludes1 chronic fatigue syndrome NOS (R53.82)

● **G93.4 Other and unspecified encephalopathy**
Excludes1 alcoholic encephalopathy (G31.2)
encephalopathy in diseases classified elsewhere (G94)
hypertensive encephalopathy (I67.4)
toxic (metabolic) encephalopathy (G92)

G93.40 Encephalopathy, unspecified

G93.41 Metabolic encephalopathy
Septic encephalopathy

G93.49 Other encephalopathy
Encephalopathy NEC

G93.5 Compression of brain
Arnold-Chiari type 1 compression of brain
Compression of brain (stem)
Herniation of brain (stem)
Excludes1 diffuse traumatic compression of brain (S06.2-)
focal traumatic compression of brain (S06.3-)

G93.6 Cerebral edema
Excludes1 cerebral edema due to birth injury (P11.0)
traumatic cerebral edema (S06.1-)

G93.7 Reye's syndrome
Life-threatening neurological condition, usually follows viral illness
Code first (T39.0-), if salicylates-induced

● **G93.8 Other specified disorders of brain**

G93.81 Temporal sclerosis
Hippocampal sclerosis
Mesial temporal sclerosis

G93.82 Brain death

G93.89 Other specified disorders of brain
Postradiation encephalopathy

G93.9 Disorder of brain, unspecified

G94 Other disorders of brain in diseases classified elsewhere
Code first underlying disease
Excludes1 encephalopathy in congenital syphilis (A50.49)
encephalopathy in influenza (J09.X9, J10.81, J11.81)
encephalopathy in syphilis (A52.19)
hydrocephalus in diseases classified elsewhere (G91.4)

● **G95 Other and unspecified diseases of spinal cord**
Excludes2 myelitis (G04.-)

G95.0 Syringomyelia and syringobulbia

● **G95.1 Vascular myelopathies**
Excludes2 intraspinal phlebitis and thrombophlebitis, except non-pyogenic (G08)

G95.11 Acute infarction of spinal cord (embolic) (nonembolic)
Anoxia of spinal cord
Arterial thrombosis of spinal cord

G95.19 Other vascular myelopathies
Edema of spinal cord
Hematomyelia
Nonpyogenic intraspinal phlebitis and thrombophlebitis
Subacute necrotic myelopathy

● **G95.2 Other and unspecified cord compression**

G95.20 Unspecified cord compression

G95.29 Other cord compression

● **G95.8 Other specified diseases of spinal cord**
Excludes1 neurogenic bladder NOS (N31.9)
neurogenic bladder due to cauda equina syndrome (G83.4)
neuromuscular dysfunction of bladder without spinal cord lesion (N31.-)

G95.81 Conus medullaris syndrome
Damage to gray matter and/or nerve roots in lower end of spinal cord

G95.89 Other specified diseases of spinal cord
Cord bladder NOS
Drug-induced myelopathy
Radiation-induced myelopathy
Excludes1 myelopathy NOS (G95.9)

G95.9 Disease of spinal cord, unspecified
Myelopathy NOS

● G96 Other disorders of central nervous system

G96.Ø Cerebrospinal fluid leak

Excludes1 cerebrospinal fluid leak from spinal puncture (G97.Ø)

● G96.1 Disorders of meninges, not elsewhere classified

G96.11 Dural tear

Excludes1 accidental puncture or laceration of dura during a procedure (G97.41)

G96.12 Meningeal adhesions (cerebral) (spinal)

G96.19 Other disorders of meninges, not elsewhere classified

G96.8 Other specified disorders of central nervous system

G96.9 Disorder of central nervous system, unspecified

● G97 Intraoperative and postprocedural complications and disorders of nervous system, not elsewhere classified

Excludes2 intraoperative and postprocedural cerebrovascular infarction (I97.81-, I97.82-)

G97.Ø Cerebrospinal fluid leak from spinal puncture

G97.1 Other reaction to spinal and lumbar puncture
Headache due to lumbar puncture

G97.2 Intracranial hypotension following ventricular shunting

● G97.3 Intraoperative hemorrhage and hematoma of a nervous system organ or structure complicating a procedure

Excludes1 intraoperative hemorrhage and hematoma of a nervous system organ or structure due to accidental puncture and laceration during a procedure (G97.4-)

G97.31 Intraoperative hemorrhage and hematoma of a nervous system organ or structure complicating a nervous system procedure

G97.32 Intraoperative hemorrhage and hematoma of a nervous system organ or structure complicating other procedure

● G97.4 Accidental puncture and laceration of a nervous system organ or structure during a procedure

G97.41 Accidental puncture or laceration of dura during a procedure
Incidental (inadvertent) durotomy

G97.48 Accidental puncture and laceration of other nervous system organ or structure during a nervous system procedure

G97.49 Accidental puncture and laceration of other nervous system organ or structure during other procedure

● G97.5 Postprocedural hemorrhage of a nervous system organ or structure following a procedure ⬅

G97.51 Postprocedural hemorrhage of a nervous system organ or structure following a nervous system procedure ⬅

G97.52 Postprocedural hemorrhage of a nervous system organ or structure following other procedure ⬅

● G97.6 Postprocedural hematoma and seroma of a nervous system organ or structure following a procedure ◀

G97.61 Postprocedural hematoma of a nervous system organ or structure following a nervous system procedure ◀

G97.62 Postprocedural hematoma of a nervous system organ or structure following other procedure ◀

G97.63 Postprocedural seroma of a nervous system organ or structure following a nervous system procedure ◀

G97.64 Postprocedural seroma of a nervous system organ or structure following other procedure ◀

● G97.8 Other intraoperative and postprocedural complications and disorders of nervous system

Use additional code to further specify disorder

G97.81 Other intraoperative complications of nervous system

G97.82 Other postprocedural complications and disorders of nervous system

● G98 Other disorders of nervous system not elsewhere classified

Includes nervous system disorder NOS

G98.Ø Neurogenic arthritis, not elsewhere classified
Nonsyphilitic neurogenic arthropathy NEC
Nonsyphilitic neurogenic spondylopathy NEC

Excludes1 spondylopathy (in):
syringomyelia and syringobulbia (G95.Ø)
tabes dorsalis (A52.11)

G98.8 Other disorders of nervous system
Nervous system disorder NOS

● G99 Other disorders of nervous system in diseases classified elsewhere

G99.Ø Autonomic neuropathy in diseases classified elsewhere

Code first underlying disease, such as:
amyloidosis (E85.-)
gout (M1A.-, M1Ø.-)
hyperthyroidism (EØ5.-)

Excludes1 diabetic autonomic neuropathy (EØ8-E13 with .43)

G99.2 Myelopathy in diseases classified elsewhere

Code first underlying disease, such as:
neoplasm (CØØ-D49)

Excludes1 myelopathy in:
intervertebral disease (M5Ø.Ø-, M51.Ø-)
spondylosis (M47.Ø-, M47.1-)

G99.8 Other specified disorders of nervous system in diseases classified elsewhere

Code first underlying disorder, such as:
amyloidosis (E85.-)
avitaminosis (E56.9)

Excludes1 nervous system involvement in:
cysticercosis (B69.Ø)
rubella (BØ6.Ø-)
syphilis (A52.1-)

CHAPTER 6 (GØØ-G99)

CHAPTER 7

DISEASES OF THE EYE AND ADNEXA (H00-H59)

OGCR Chapter-Specific Coding Guidelines

7. Chapter 7: Diseases of the Eye and Adnexa (H00-H59)

a. Glaucoma

1) **Assigning Glaucoma Codes**

Assign as many codes from category H40, Glaucoma, as needed to identify the type of glaucoma, the affected eye, and the glaucoma stage.

2) **Bilateral glaucoma with same type and stage**

When a patient has bilateral glaucoma and both eyes are documented as being the same type and stage, and there is a code for bilateral glaucoma, report only the code for the type of glaucoma, bilateral, with the seventh character for the stage.

When a patient has bilateral glaucoma and both eyes are documented as being the same type and stage, and the classification does not provide a code for bilateral glaucoma (i.e. subcategories H40.10, H40.11 and H40.20) report only one code for the type of glaucoma with the appropriate seventh character for the stage.

3) **Bilateral glaucoma stage with different types or stages**

When a patient has bilateral glaucoma and each eye is documented as having a different type or stage, and the classification distinguishes laterality, assign the appropriate code for each eye rather than the code for bilateral glaucoma.

When a patient has bilateral glaucoma and each eye is documented as having a different type, and the classification does not distinguish laterality (i.e. subcategories H40.10, H40.11 and H40.20), assign one code for each type of glaucoma with the appropriate seventh character for the stage.

When a patient has bilateral glaucoma and each eye is documented as having the same type, but different stage, and the classification does not distinguish laterality (i.e. subcategories H40.10, H40.11 and H40.20), assign a code for the type of glaucoma for each eye with the seventh character for the specific glaucoma stage documented for each eye.

4) **Patient admitted with glaucoma and stage evolves during the admission**

If a patient is admitted with glaucoma and the stage progresses during the admission, assign the code for highest stage documented.

5) **Indeterminate stage glaucoma**

Assignment of the seventh character "4" for "indeterminate stage" should be based on the clinical documentation. The seventh character "4" is used for glaucomas whose stage cannot be clinically determined. This seventh character should not be confused with the seventh character "0", unspecified, which should be assigned when there is no documentation regarding the stage of the glaucoma.

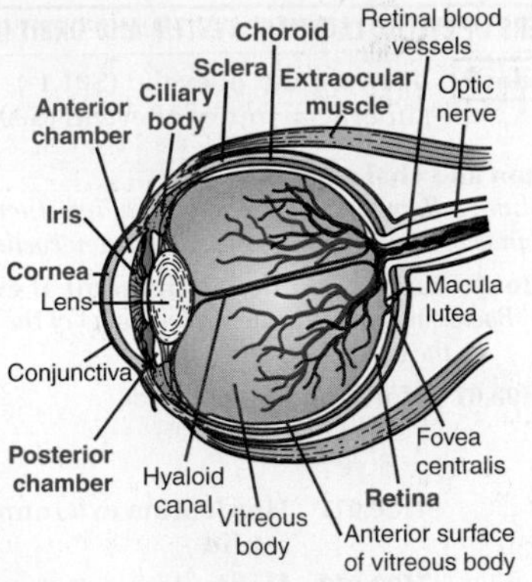

Figure 7–1 Eye and ocular adnexa. (From Buck CJ: Step-by-Step Medical Coding, ed 2016, St. Louis, Elsevier, 2016)

★**(See Plate 87 on page NAP-15.)**

CHAPTER 7

DISEASES OF THE EYE AND ADNEXA (H00-H59)

Note: Use an external cause code following the code for the eye condition, if applicable, to identify the cause of the eye condition

Excludes2 certain conditions originating in the perinatal period (P04-P96)
certain infectious and parasitic diseases (A00-B99)
complications of pregnancy, childbirth and the puerperium (O00-O9A)
congenital malformations, deformations, and chromosomal abnormalities (Q00-Q99)
diabetes mellitus related eye conditions (E09.3-, E10.3-, E11.3-, E13.3-)
endocrine, nutritional and metabolic diseases (E00-E88)
injury (trauma) of eye and orbit (S05.-)
injury, poisoning and certain other consequences of external causes (S00-T88)
neoplasms (C00-D49)
symptoms, signs and abnormal clinical and laboratory findings, not elsewhere classified (R00-R94)
syphilis related eye disorders (A50.01, A50.3-, A51.43, A52.71)

This chapter contains the following blocks:

H00-H05	Disorders of eyelid, lacrimal system and orbit
H10-H11	Disorders of conjunctiva
H15-H22	Disorders of sclera, cornea, iris and ciliary body
H25-H28	Disorders of lens
H30-H36	Disorders of choroid and retina
H40-H42	Glaucoma
H43-H44	Disorders of vitreous body and globe
H46-H47	Disorders of optic nerve and visual pathways
H49-H52	Disorders of ocular muscles, binocular movement, accommodation and refraction
H53-H54	Visual disturbances and blindness
H55-H57	Other disorders of eye and adnexa
H59	Intraoperative and postprocedural complications and disorders of eye and adnexa, not elsewhere classified

DISORDERS OF EYELID, LACRIMAL SYSTEM AND ORBIT (H00-H05)

Excludes2 open wound of eyelid (S01.1-)
superficial injury of eyelid (S00.1-, S00.2-)

● **H00 Hordeolum and chalazion**
Hordeolum: inflammatory staphylococcal infection of sebaceous glands of eyelids; AKA stye. Chalazion: eyelid mass

● **H00.0 Hordeolum (externum) (internum) of eyelid**
Bacterial infection (staphylococcus) of the sebaceous gland of the eyelid (stye)

● **H00.01 Hordeolum externum**
Hordeolum NOS
Stye

- **H00.011 Hordeolum externum right upper eyelid**
- **H00.012 Hordeolum externum right lower eyelid**
- **H00.013 Hordeolum externum right eye, unspecified eyelid**
- **H00.014 Hordeolum externum left upper eyelid**
- **H00.015 Hordeolum externum left lower eyelid**
- **H00.016 Hordeolum externum left eye, unspecified eyelid**
- **H00.019 Hordeolum externum unspecified eye, unspecified eyelid**

● **H00.02 Hordeolum internum**
Infection of meibomian gland

- **H00.021 Hordeolum internum right upper eyelid**
- **H00.022 Hordeolum internum right lower eyelid**
- **H00.023 Hordeolum internum right eye, unspecified eyelid**
- **H00.024 Hordeolum internum left upper eyelid**
- **H00.025 Hordeolum internum left lower eyelid**
- **H00.026 Hordeolum internum left eye, unspecified eyelid**
- **H00.029 Hordeolum internum unspecified eye, unspecified eyelid**

● **H00.03 Abscess of eyelid**
Furuncle of eyelid

- **H00.031 Abscess of right upper eyelid**
- **H00.032 Abscess of right lower eyelid**
- **H00.033 Abscess of eyelid right eye, unspecified eyelid**
- **H00.034 Abscess of left upper eyelid**
- **H00.035 Abscess of left lower eyelid**
- **H00.036 Abscess of eyelid left eye, unspecified eyelid**
- **H00.039 Abscess of eyelid unspecified eye, unspecified eyelid**

● **H00.1 Chalazion**
Often caused by accumulation of meibomian gland secretions resulting from a blockage of duct.
Meibomian (gland) cyst

Excludes2 infected meibomian gland (H00.02-)

- **H00.11 Chalazion right upper eyelid**
- **H00.12 Chalazion right lower eyelid**
- **H00.13 Chalazion right eye, unspecified eyelid**
- **H00.14 Chalazion left upper eyelid**
- **H00.15 Chalazion left lower eyelid**
- **H00.16 Chalazion left eye, unspecified eyelid**
- **H00.19 Chalazion unspecified eye, unspecified eyelid**

● **H01 Other inflammation of eyelid**

● **H01.0 Blepharitis**
Inflammation of eyelids

Excludes1 blepharoconjunctivitis (H10.5-)

● **H01.00 Unspecified blepharitis**

- **H01.001 Unspecified blepharitis right upper eyelid**
- **H01.002 Unspecified blepharitis right lower eyelid**
- **H01.003 Unspecified blepharitis right eye, unspecified eyelid**
- **H01.004 Unspecified blepharitis left upper eyelid**
- **H01.005 Unspecified blepharitis left lower eyelid**
- **H01.006 Unspecified blepharitis left eye, unspecified eyelid**
- **H01.009 Unspecified blepharitis unspecified eye, unspecified eyelid**

● **H01.01 Ulcerative blepharitis**

- **H01.011 Ulcerative blepharitis right upper eyelid**
- **H01.012 Ulcerative blepharitis right lower eyelid**
- **H01.013 Ulcerative blepharitis right eye, unspecified eyelid**
- **H01.014 Ulcerative blepharitis left upper eyelid**
- **H01.015 Ulcerative blepharitis left lower eyelid**
- **H01.016 Ulcerative blepharitis left eye, unspecified eyelid**
- **H01.019 Ulcerative blepharitis unspecified eye, unspecified eyelid**

● **H01.02 Squamous blepharitis**

- **H01.021 Squamous blepharitis right upper eyelid**
- **H01.022 Squamous blepharitis right lower eyelid**
- **H01.023 Squamous blepharitis right eye, unspecified eyelid**
- **H01.024 Squamous blepharitis left upper eyelid**
- **H01.025 Squamous blepharitis left lower eyelid**
- **H01.026 Squamous blepharitis left eye, unspecified eyelid**
- **H01.029 Squamous blepharitis unspecified eye, unspecified eyelid**

● **H01.1 Noninfectious dermatoses of eyelid**

● **H01.11 Allergic dermatitis of eyelid**
Contact dermatitis of eyelid

- **H01.111 Allergic dermatitis of right upper eyelid**
- **H01.112 Allergic dermatitis of right lower eyelid**
- **H01.113 Allergic dermatitis of right eye, unspecified eyelid**
- **H01.114 Allergic dermatitis of left upper eyelid**
- **H01.115 Allergic dermatitis of left lower eyelid**
- **H01.116 Allergic dermatitis of left eye, unspecified eyelid**
- **H01.119 Allergic dermatitis of unspecified eye, unspecified eyelid**

- ● H01.12 Discoid lupus erythematosus of eyelid
  - H01.121 Discoid lupus erythematosus of right upper eyelid
  - H01.122 Discoid lupus erythematosus of right lower eyelid
  - H01.123 Discoid lupus erythematosus of right eye, unspecified eyelid
  - H01.124 Discoid lupus erythematosus of left upper eyelid
  - H01.125 Discoid lupus erythematosus of left lower eyelid
  - H01.126 Discoid lupus erythematosus of left eye, unspecified eyelid
  - H01.129 Discoid lupus erythematosus of unspecified eye, unspecified eyelid
- ● H01.13 Eczematous dermatitis of eyelid
  - H01.131 Eczematous dermatitis of right upper eyelid
  - H01.132 Eczematous dermatitis of right lower eyelid
  - H01.133 Eczematous dermatitis of right eye, unspecified eyelid
  - H01.134 Eczematous dermatitis of left upper eyelid
  - H01.135 Eczematous dermatitis of left lower eyelid
  - H01.136 Eczematous dermatitis of left eye, unspecified eyelid
  - H01.139 Eczematous dermatitis of unspecified eye, unspecified eyelid
- ● H01.14 Xeroderma of eyelid
  Abnormally dry
  - H01.141 Xeroderma of right upper eyelid
  - H01.142 Xeroderma of right lower eyelid
  - H01.143 Xeroderma of right eye, unspecified eyelid
  - H01.144 Xeroderma of left upper eyelid
  - H01.145 Xeroderma of left lower eyelid
  - H01.146 Xeroderma of left eye, unspecified eyelid
  - H01.149 Xeroderma of unspecified eye, unspecified eyelid
- H01.8 Other specified inflammations of eyelid
- H01.9 Unspecified inflammation of eyelid
  Inflammation of eyelid NOS

● **H02 Other disorders of eyelid**
Turning inward (inversion) of eyelid margin and ingrowing eyelashes
Excludes1 congenital malformations of eyelid (Q10.0-Q10.3)

- ● H02.0 Entropion and trichiasis of eyelid
  - ● H02.00 Unspecified entropion of eyelid
    - H02.001 Unspecified entropion of right upper eyelid
    - H02.002 Unspecified entropion of right lower eyelid
    - H02.003 Unspecified entropion of right eye, unspecified eyelid
    - H02.004 Unspecified entropion of left upper eyelid
    - H02.005 Unspecified entropion of left lower eyelid
    - H02.006 Unspecified entropion of left eye, unspecified eyelid
    - H02.009 Unspecified entropion of unspecified eye, unspecified eyelid
  - ● H02.01 Cicatricial entropion of eyelid
    Scar
    - H02.011 Cicatricial entropion of right upper eyelid
    - H02.012 Cicatricial entropion of right lower eyelid
    - H02.013 Cicatricial entropion of right eye, unspecified eyelid
    - H02.014 Cicatricial entropion of left upper eyelid
    - H02.015 Cicatricial entropion of left lower eyelid
    - H02.016 Cicatricial entropion of left eye, unspecified eyelid
    - H02.019 Cicatricial entropion of unspecified eye, unspecified eyelid
  - ● H02.02 Mechanical entropion of eyelid
    Turning inward (inversion) of eyelid margin due to lack of support
    - H02.021 Mechanical entropion of right upper eyelid
    - H02.022 Mechanical entropion of right lower eyelid
    - H02.023 Mechanical entropion of right eye, unspecified eyelid
    - H02.024 Mechanical entropion of left upper eyelid
    - H02.025 Mechanical entropion of left lower eyelid
    - H02.026 Mechanical entropion of left eye, unspecified eyelid
    - H02.029 Mechanical entropion of unspecified eye, unspecified eyelid
  - ● H02.03 Senile entropion of eyelid
    Turning inward (inversion) of eyelid margin due to aging
    - H02.031 Senile entropion of right upper eyelid
    - H02.032 Senile entropion of right lower eyelid
    - H02.033 Senile entropion of right eye, unspecified eyelid
    - H02.034 Senile entropion of left upper eyelid
    - H02.035 Senile entropion of left lower eyelid
    - H02.036 Senile entropion of left eye, unspecified eyelid
    - H02.039 Senile entropion of unspecified eye, unspecified eyelid
  - ● H02.04 Spastic entropion of eyelid
    Turning inward (inversion) of eyelid margin caused by spasm of muscle
    - H02.041 Spastic entropion of right upper eyelid
    - H02.042 Spastic entropion of right lower eyelid
    - H02.043 Spastic entropion of right eye, unspecified eyelid
    - H02.044 Spastic entropion of left upper eyelid
    - H02.045 Spastic entropion of left lower eyelid
    - H02.046 Spastic entropion of left eye, unspecified eyelid
    - H02.049 Spastic entropion of unspecified eye, unspecified eyelid

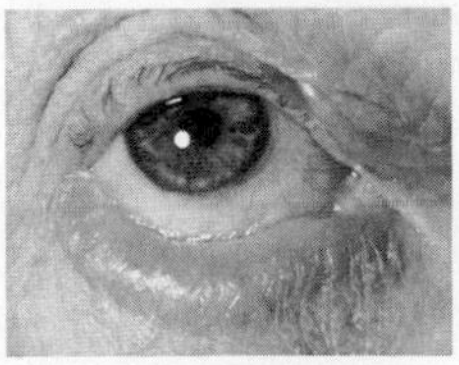

Figure 7-2 Right lower eyelid entropion. Note the inward rotation of the tarsal plate about the horizontal axis and the resultant contact between the mucocutaneous junction and ocular surface. (From Yanoff: Ophthalmology, ed 3, Mosby, Inc., 2008)

● **H02.05 Trichiasis without entropian**
Ingrowing hairs of eyelashes
H02.051 Trichiasis without entropian right upper eyelid
H02.052 Trichiasis without entropian right lower eyelid
H02.053 Trichiasis without entropian right eye, unspecified eyelid
H02.054 Trichiasis without entropian left upper eyelid
H02.055 Trichiasis without entropian left lower eyelid
H02.056 Trichiasis without entropian left eye, unspecified eyelid
H02.059 Trichiasis without entropian unspecified eye, unspecified eyelid

● **H02.1 Ectropion of eyelid**
Eversion (pulling away) of eyelid

● **H02.10 Unspecified ectropion of eyelid**
H02.101 Unspecified ectropion of right upper eyelid
H02.102 Unspecified ectropion of right lower eyelid
H02.103 Unspecified ectropion of right eye, unspecified eyelid
H02.104 Unspecified ectropion of left upper eyelid
H02.105 Unspecified ectropion of left lower eyelid
H02.106 Unspecified ectropion of left eye, unspecified eyelid
H02.109 Unspecified ectropion of unspecified eye, unspecified eyelid

● **H02.11 Cicatricial ectropion of eyelid**
Pulling of eyelid down and away from eye due to scar or tightening
H02.111 Cicatricial ectropion of right upper eyelid
H02.112 Cicatricial ectropion of right lower eyelid
H02.113 Cicatricial ectropion of right eye, unspecified eyelid
H02.114 Cicatricial ectropion of left upper eyelid
H02.115 Cicatricial ectropion of left lower eyelid
H02.116 Cicatricial ectropion of left eye, unspecified eyelid
H02.119 Cicatricial ectropion of unspecified eye, unspecified eyelid

● **H02.12 Mechanical ectropion of eyelid**
Eversion (pulling away) of eyelid due to lack of support
H02.121 Mechanical ectropion of right upper eyelid
H02.122 Mechanical ectropion of right lower eyelid
H02.123 Mechanical ectropion of right eye, unspecified eyelid
H02.124 Mechanical ectropion of left upper eyelid
H02.125 Mechanical ectropion of left lower eyelid
H02.126 Mechanical ectropion of left eye, unspecified eyelid
H02.129 Mechanical ectropion of unspecified eye, unspecified eyelid

● **H02.13 Senile ectropion of eyelid**
Eversion (pulling away) of eyelid due to age
H02.131 Senile ectropion of right upper eyelid
H02.132 Senile ectropion of right lower eyelid
H02.133 Senile ectropion of right eye, unspecified eyelid
H02.134 Senile ectropion of left upper eyelid
H02.135 Senile ectropion of left lower eyelid
H02.136 Senile ectropion of left eye, unspecified eyelid
H02.139 Senile ectropion of unspecified eye, unspecified eyelid

● **H02.14 Spastic ectropion of eyelid**
Eversion (pulling away) of eyelid due to tonic muscle spasm
H02.141 Spastic ectropion of right upper eyelid
H02.142 Spastic ectropion of right lower eyelid
H02.143 Spastic ectropion of right eye, unspecified eyelid
H02.144 Spastic ectropion of left upper eyelid
H02.145 Spastic ectropion of left lower eyelid
H02.146 Spastic ectropion of left eye, unspecified eyelid
H02.149 Spastic ectropion of unspecified eye, unspecified eyelid

● **H02.2 Lagophthalmos**
Condition in which eye cannot completely close

● **H02.20 Unspecified lagophthalmos**
H02.201 Unspecified lagophthalmos right upper eyelid
H02.202 Unspecified lagophthalmos right lower eyelid
H02.203 Unspecified lagophthalmos right eye, unspecified eyelid
H02.204 Unspecified lagophthalmos left upper eyelid
H02.205 Unspecified lagophthalmos left lower eyelid
H02.206 Unspecified lagophthalmos left eye, unspecified eyelid
H02.209 Unspecified lagophthalmos unspecified eye, unspecified eyelid

● **H02.21 Cicatricial lagophthalmos**
Upper or lower eyelid does not close due to scar or tightening
H02.211 Cicatricial lagophthalmos right upper eyelid
H02.212 Cicatricial lagophthalmos right lower eyelid
H02.213 Cicatricial lagophthalmos right eye, unspecified eyelid
H02.214 Cicatricial lagophthalmos left upper eyelid
H02.215 Cicatricial lagophthalmos left lower eyelid
H02.216 Cicatricial lagophthalmos left eye, unspecified eyelid
H02.219 Cicatricial lagophthalmos unspecified eye, unspecified eyelid

CHAPTER 7 (H00-H59)

● H02.22 Mechanical lagophthalmos
Inability to close lids due to structural disorder
H02.221 Mechanical lagophthalmos right upper eyelid
H02.222 Mechanical lagophthalmos right lower eyelid
H02.223 Mechanical lagophthalmos right eye, unspecified eyelid
H02.224 Mechanical lagophthalmos left upper eyelid
H02.225 Mechanical lagophthalmos left lower eyelid
H02.226 Mechanical lagophthalmos left eye, unspecified eyelid
H02.229 Mechanical lagophthalmos unspecified eye, unspecified eyelid

● H02.23 Paralytic lagophthalmos
Eyelids do not close due to paralysis
H02.231 Paralytic lagophthalmos right upper eyelid
H02.232 Paralytic lagophthalmos right lower eyelid
H02.233 Paralytic lagophthalmos right eye, unspecified eyelid
H02.234 Paralytic lagophthalmos left upper eyelid
H02.235 Paralytic lagophthalmos left lower eyelid
H02.236 Paralytic lagophthalmos left eye, unspecified eyelid
H02.239 Paralytic lagophthalmos unspecified eye, unspecified eyelid

★ **(See Plate 81, middle, on page NAP-17.)**

● H02.3 Blepharochalasis
Relaxation of skin of eyelid, due to atrophy of intercellular tissue
Pseudoptosis
H02.30 Blepharochalasis unspecified eye, unspecified eyelid
H02.31 Blepharochalasis right upper eyelid
H02.32 Blepharochalasis right lower eyelid
H02.33 Blepharochalasis right eye, unspecified eyelid
H02.34 Blepharochalasis left upper eyelid
H02.35 Blepharochalasis left lower eyelid
H02.36 Blepharochalasis left eye, unspecified eyelid

● H02.4 Ptosis of eyelid
Falling forward, drooping, sagging of eyelid

● H02.40 Unspecified ptosis of eyelid
H02.401 Unspecified ptosis of right eyelid
H02.402 Unspecified ptosis of left eyelid
H02.403 Unspecified ptosis of bilateral eyelids
H02.409 Unspecified ptosis of unspecified eyelid

● H02.41 Mechanical ptosis of eyelid
H02.411 Mechanical ptosis of right eyelid
H02.412 Mechanical ptosis of left eyelid
H02.413 Mechanical ptosis of bilateral eyelids
H02.419 Mechanical ptosis of unspecified eyelid

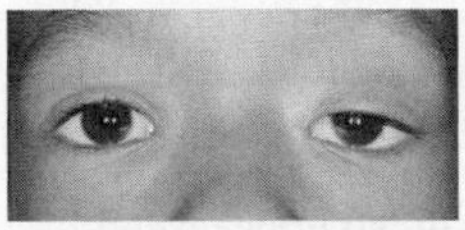

Figure 7-3 Ptosis of eyelid. (From Yanoff: Ophthalmology, ed 3, Mosby, Inc., 2008)

Item 7-1 Ptosis of eyelid is drooping of the upper eyelid over the pupil when the eyes are fully opened resulting from nerve or muscle damage, which may require surgical correction.

● H02.42 Myogenic ptosis of eyelid
H02.421 Myogenic ptosis of right eyelid
H02.422 Myogenic ptosis of left eyelid
H02.423 Myogenic ptosis of bilateral eyelids
H02.429 Myogenic ptosis of unspecified eyelid

● H02.43 Paralytic ptosis of eyelid
Neurogenic ptosis of eyelid
H02.431 Paralytic ptosis of right eyelid
H02.432 Paralytic ptosis of left eyelid
H02.433 Paralytic ptosis of bilateral eyelids
H02.439 Paralytic ptosis unspecified eyelid

● H02.5 Other disorders affecting eyelid function
Excludes2 blepharospasm (G24.5)
organic tic (G25.69)
psychogenic tic (F95.-)

● H02.51 Abnormal innervation syndrome
H02.511 Abnormal innervation syndrome right upper eyelid
H02.512 Abnormal innervation syndrome right lower eyelid
H02.513 Abnormal innervation syndrome right eye, unspecified eyelid
H02.514 Abnormal innervation syndrome left upper eyelid
H02.515 Abnormal innervation syndrome left lower eyelid
H02.516 Abnormal innervation syndrome left eye, unspecified eyelid
H02.519 Abnormal innervation syndrome unspecified eye, unspecified eyelid

● H02.52 Blepharophimosis
Drooping of eyelid with reduced lid size
Ankyloblepharon
H02.521 Blepharophimosis right upper eyelid
H02.522 Blepharophimosis right lower eyelid
H02.523 Blepharophimosis right eye, unspecified eyelid
H02.524 Blepharophimosis left upper eyelid
H02.525 Blepharophimosis left lower eyelid
H02.526 Blepharophimosis left eye, unspecified eyelid
H02.529 Blepharophimosis unspecified eye, unspecified lid

● H02.53 Eyelid retraction
Eyelid lag
H02.531 Eyelid retraction right upper eyelid
H02.532 Eyelid retraction right lower eyelid
H02.533 Eyelid retraction right eye, unspecified eyelid
H02.534 Eyelid retraction left upper eyelid
H02.535 Eyelid retraction left lower eyelid
H02.536 Eyelid retraction left eye, unspecified eyelid
H02.539 Eyelid retraction unspecified eye, unspecified lid

H02.59 Other disorders affecting eyelid function
Deficient blink reflex
Sensory disorders

● **H02.6** Xanthelasma of eyelid
Yellow-to-orange patches or pimples clustered together on eyelid
- **H02.60** Xanthelasma of unspecified eye, unspecified eyelid
- **H02.61** Xanthelasma of right upper eyelid
- **H02.62** Xanthelasma of right lower eyelid
- **H02.63** Xanthelasma of right eye, unspecified eyelid
- **H02.64** Xanthelasma of left upper eyelid
- **H02.65** Xanthelasma of left lower eyelid
- **H02.66** Xanthelasma of left eye, unspecified eyelid

● **H02.7** Other and unspecified degenerative disorders of eyelid and periocular area
- **H02.70** Unspecified degenerative disorders of eyelid and periocular area

● **H02.71** Chloasma of eyelid and periocular area
Dyspigmentation of eyelid
Hyperpigmentation of eyelid
- **H02.711** Chloasma of right upper eyelid and periocular area
- **H02.712** Chloasma of right lower eyelid and periocular area
- **H02.713** Chloasma of right eye, unspecified eyelid and periocular area
- **H02.714** Chloasma of left upper eyelid and periocular area
- **H02.715** Chloasma of left lower eyelid and periocular area
- **H02.716** Chloasma of left eye, unspecified eyelid and periocular area
- **H02.719** Chloasma of unspecified eye, unspecified eyelid and periocular area

● **H02.72** Madarosis of eyelid and periocular area
Loss of eyelashes and/or eyebrows
Hypotrichosis of eyelid
- **H02.721** Madarosis of right upper eyelid and periocular area
- **H02.722** Madarosis of right lower eyelid and periocular area
- **H02.723** Madarosis of right eye, unspecified eyelid and periocular area
- **H02.724** Madarosis of left upper eyelid and periocular area
- **H02.725** Madarosis of left lower eyelid and periocular area
- **H02.726** Madarosis of left eye, unspecified eyelid and periocular area
- **H02.729** Madarosis of unspecified eye, unspecified eyelid and periocular area

● **H02.73** Vitiligo of eyelid and periocular area
Skin pigmentation disease characterized by white patches
Hypopigmentation of eyelid
- **H02.731** Vitiligo of right upper eyelid and periocular area
- **H02.732** Vitiligo of right lower eyelid and periocular area
- **H02.733** Vitiligo of right eye, unspecified eyelid and periocular area
- **H02.734** Vitiligo of left upper eyelid and periocular area
- **H02.735** Vitiligo of left lower eyelid and periocular area
- **H02.736** Vitiligo of left eye, unspecified eyelid and periocular area
- **H02.739** Vitiligo of unspecified eye, unspecified eyelid and periocular area

H02.79 Other degenerative disorders of eyelid and periocular area

● **H02.8** Other specified disorders of eyelid

● **H02.81** Retained foreign body in eyelid
Use additional code to identify the type of retained foreign body (Z18.-)
Excludes1 laceration of eyelid with foreign body (S01.12-)
retained intraocular foreign body (H44.6-, H44.7-)
superficial foreign body of eyelid and periocular area (S00.25-)
- **H02.811** Retained foreign body in right upper eyelid
- **H02.812** Retained foreign body in right lower eyelid
- **H02.813** Retained foreign body in right eye, unspecified eyelid
- **H02.814** Retained foreign body in left upper eyelid
- **H02.815** Retained foreign body in left lower eyelid
- **H02.816** Retained foreign body in left eye, unspecified eyelid
- **H02.819** Retained foreign body in unspecified eye, unspecified eyelid

● **H02.82** Cysts of eyelid
Sebaceous cyst of eyelid
- **H02.821** Cysts of right upper eyelid
- **H02.822** Cysts of right lower eyelid
- **H02.823** Cysts of right eye, unspecified eyelid
- **H02.824** Cysts of left upper eyelid
- **H02.825** Cysts of left lower eyelid
- **H02.826** Cysts of left eye, unspecified eyelid
- **H02.829** Cysts of unspecified eye, unspecified eyelid

● **H02.83** Dermatochalasis of eyelid
Skin is inelastic and hangs loosely in folds
- **H02.831** Dermatochalasis of right upper eyelid
- **H02.832** Dermatochalasis of right lower eyelid
- **H02.833** Dermatochalasis of right eye, unspecified eyelid
- **H02.834** Dermatochalasis of left upper eyelid
- **H02.835** Dermatochalasis of left lower eyelid
- **H02.836** Dermatochalasis of left eye, unspecified eyelid
- **H02.839** Dermatochalasis of unspecified eye, unspecified eyelid

● **H02.84** Edema of eyelid
Hyperemia of eyelid
- **H02.841** Edema of right upper eyelid
- **H02.842** Edema of right lower eyelid
- **H02.843** Edema of right eye, unspecified eyelid
- **H02.844** Edema of left upper eyelid
- **H02.845** Edema of left lower eyelid
- **H02.846** Edema of left eye, unspecified eyelid
- **H02.849** Edema of unspecified eye, unspecified eyelid

● **H02.85** Elephantiasis of eyelid
Massive secondary lymphedema with hypertrophy of skin and subcutaneous tissues (pachyderma)
- **H02.851** Elephantiasis of right upper eyelid
- **H02.852** Elephantiasis of right lower eyelid
- **H02.853** Elephantiasis of right eye, unspecified eyelid
- **H02.854** Elephantiasis of left upper eyelid
- **H02.855** Elephantiasis of left lower eyelid

H02.856 Elephantiasis of left eye, unspecified eyelid
H02.859 Elephantiasis of unspecified eye, unspecified eyelid

● H02.86 Hypertrichosis of eyelid
Excessive growth of hair
H02.861 Hypertrichosis of right upper eyelid
H02.862 Hypertrichosis of right lower eyelid
H02.863 Hypertrichosis of right eye, unspecified eyelid
H02.864 Hypertrichosis of left upper eyelid
H02.865 Hypertrichosis of left lower eyelid
H02.866 Hypertrichosis of left eye, unspecified eyelid
H02.869 Hypertrichosis of unspecified eye, unspecified eyelid

● H02.87 Vascular anomalies of eyelid
H02.871 Vascular anomalies of right upper eyelid
H02.872 Vascular anomalies of right lower eyelid
H02.873 Vascular anomalies of right eye, unspecified eyelid
H02.874 Vascular anomalies of left upper eyelid
H02.875 Vascular anomalies of left lower eyelid
H02.876 Vascular anomalies of left eye, unspecified eyelid
H02.879 Vascular anomalies of unspecified eye, unspecified eyelid

H02.89 Other specified disorders of eyelid
Hemorrhage of eyelid

H02.9 Unspecified disorder of eyelid
Disorder of eyelid NOS

● H04 Disorders of lacrimal system
Excludes1 congenital malformations of lacrimal system (Q10.4-Q10.6)

● H04.0 Dacryoadenitis
Inflammation of lacrimal gland

● H04.00 Unspecified dacryoadenitis
H04.001 Unspecified dacryoadenitis, right lacrimal gland
H04.002 Unspecified dacryoadenitis, left lacrimal gland
H04.003 Unspecified dacryoadenitis, bilateral lacrimal glands
H04.009 Unspecified dacryoadenitis, unspecified lacrimal gland

● H04.01 Acute dacryoadenitis
H04.011 Acute dacryoadenitis, right lacrimal gland
H04.012 Acute dacryoadenitis, left lacrimal gland
H04.013 Acute dacryoadenitis, bilateral lacrimal glands
H04.019 Acute dacryoadenitis, unspecified lacrimal gland

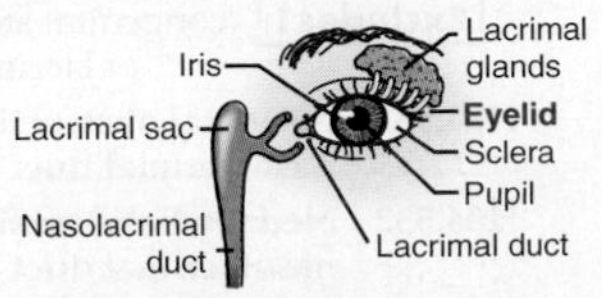

Figure 7-4 Lacrimal apparatus. (From Buck CJ: Step-by-Step Medical Coding, 2016, St. Louis, Elsevier, 2016)

★ **(See Plate 82 on page NAP-19.)**

● H04.02 Chronic dacryoadenitis
H04.021 Chronic dacryoadenitis, right lacrimal gland
H04.022 Chronic dacryoadenitis, left lacrimal gland
H04.023 Chronic dacryoadenitis, bilateral lacrimal gland
H04.029 Chronic dacryoadenitis, unspecified lacrimal gland

● H04.03 Chronic enlargement of lacrimal gland
H04.031 Chronic enlargement of right lacrimal gland
H04.032 Chronic enlargement of left lacrimal gland
H04.033 Chronic enlargement of bilateral lacrimal glands
H04.039 Chronic enlargement of unspecified lacrimal gland

● H04.1 Other disorders of lacrimal gland

● H04.11 Dacryops
Watery eye or distention of lacrimal duct due to fluid
H04.111 Dacryops of right lacrimal gland
H04.112 Dacryops of left lacrimal gland
H04.113 Dacryops of bilateral lacrimal glands
H04.119 Dacryops of unspecified lacrimal gland

● H04.12 Dry eye syndrome
Tear film insufficiency, NOS
H04.121 Dry eye syndrome of right lacrimal gland
H04.122 Dry eye syndrome of left lacrimal gland
H04.123 Dry eye syndrome of bilateral lacrimal glands
H04.129 Dry eye syndrome of unspecified lacrimal gland

● H04.13 Lacrimal cyst
Lacrimal cystic degeneration
H04.131 Lacrimal cyst right lacrimal gland
H04.132 Lacrimal cyst left lacrimal gland
H04.133 Lacrimal cyst bilateral lacrimal glands
H04.139 Lacrimal cyst unspecified lacrimal gland

● H04.14 Primary lacrimal gland atrophy
H04.141 Primary lacrimal gland atrophy, right lacrimal gland
H04.142 Primary lacrimal gland atrophy, left lacrimal gland
H04.143 Primary lacrimal gland atrophy, bilateral lacrimal glands
H04.149 Primary lacrimal gland atrophy, unspecified lacrimal gland

● H04.15 Secondary lacrimal gland atrophy
H04.151 Secondary lacrimal gland atrophy, right lacrimal gland
H04.152 Secondary lacrimal gland atrophy, left lacrimal gland
H04.153 Secondary lacrimal gland atrophy, bilateral lacrimal glands
H04.159 Secondary lacrimal gland atrophy, unspecified lacrimal gland

● H04.16 Lacrimal gland dislocation
H04.161 Lacrimal gland dislocation, right lacrimal gland
H04.162 Lacrimal gland dislocation, left lacrimal gland

CHAPTER 7 (H00-H59)

H04.163 Lacrimal gland dislocation, bilateral lacrimal glands
H04.169 Lacrimal gland dislocation, unspecified lacrimal gland
H04.19 Other specified disorders of lacrimal gland
● **H04.2** Epiphora
Overflow of tears due to stricture of lacrimal passages; AKA lacrimation
● **H04.20** Unspecified epiphora
H04.201 Unspecified epiphora, right lacrimal gland
H04.202 Unspecified epiphora, left lacrimal gland
H04.203 Unspecified epiphora, bilateral lacrimal glands
H04.209 Unspecified epiphora, unspecified lacrimal gland
● **H04.21** Epiphora due to excess lacrimation
H04.211 Epiphora due to excess lacrimation, right lacrimal gland
H04.212 Epiphora due to excess lacrimation, left lacrimal gland
H04.213 Epiphora due to excess lacrimation, bilateral lacrimal glands
H04.219 Epiphora due to excess lacrimation, unspecified lacrimal gland
● **H04.22** Epiphora due to insufficient drainage
H04.221 Epiphora due to insufficient drainage, right lacrimal gland
H04.222 Epiphora due to insufficient drainage, left lacrimal gland
H04.223 Epiphora due to insufficient drainage, bilateral lacrimal glands
H04.229 Epiphora due to insufficient drainage, unspecified lacrimal gland
● **H04.3** Acute and unspecified inflammation of lacrimal passages
Excludes1 neonatal dacryocystitis (P39.1)
● **H04.30** Unspecified dacryocystitis
H04.301 Unspecified dacryocystitis of right lacrimal passage
H04.302 Unspecified dacryocystitis of left lacrimal passage
H04.303 Unspecified dacryocystitis of bilateral lacrimal passages
H04.309 Unspecified dacryocystitis of unspecified lacrimal passage
● **H04.31** Phlegmonous dacryocystitis
Cellulitis of lacrimal sac
H04.311 Phlegmonous dacryocystitis of right lacrimal passage
H04.312 Phlegmonous dacryocystitis of left lacrimal passage
H04.313 Phlegmonous dacryocystitis of bilateral lacrimal passages
H04.319 Phlegmonous dacryocystitis of unspecified lacrimal passage
● **H04.32** Acute dacryocystitis
Acute dacryopericystitis
H04.321 Acute dacryocystitis of right lacrimal passage
H04.322 Acute dacryocystitis of left lacrimal passage
H04.323 Acute dacryocystitis of bilateral lacrimal passages
H04.329 Acute dacryocystitis of unspecified lacrimal passage
● **H04.33** Acute lacrimal canaliculitis
H04.331 Acute lacrimal canaliculitis of right lacrimal passage
H04.332 Acute lacrimal canaliculitis of left lacrimal passage
H04.333 Acute lacrimal canaliculitis of bilateral lacrimal passages
H04.339 Acute lacrimal canaliculitis of unspecified lacrimal passage
● **H04.4** Chronic inflammation of lacrimal passages
● **H04.41** Chronic dacryocystitis
Inflammation of lacrimal sac
H04.411 Chronic dacryocystitis of right lacrimal passage
H04.412 Chronic dacryocystitis of left lacrimal passage
H04.413 Chronic dacryocystitis of bilateral lacrimal passages
H04.419 Chronic dacryocystitis of unspecified lacrimal passage
● **H04.42** Chronic lacrimal canaliculitis
Inflammation of lacrimal ducts
H04.421 Chronic lacrimal canaliculitis of right lacrimal passage
H04.422 Chronic lacrimal canaliculitis of left lacrimal passage
H04.423 Chronic lacrimal canaliculitis of bilateral lacrimal passages
H04.429 Chronic lacrimal canaliculitis of unspecified lacrimal passage
● **H04.43** Chronic lacrimal mucocele
Accumulation of mucous secretion
H04.431 Chronic lacrimal mucocele of right lacrimal passage
H04.432 Chronic lacrimal mucocele of left lacrimal passage
H04.433 Chronic lacrimal mucocele of bilateral lacrimal passages
H04.439 Chronic lacrimal mucocele of unspecified lacrimal passage
● **H04.5** Stenosis and insufficiency of lacrimal passages
● **H04.51** Dacryolith
Concretion in lacrimal sac/duct; AKA lacrimal calculus
H04.511 Dacryolith of right lacrimal passage
H04.512 Dacryolith of left lacrimal passage
H04.513 Dacryolith of bilateral lacrimal passages
H04.519 Dacryolith of unspecified lacrimal passage
● **H04.52** Eversion of lacrimal punctum
Turning out of lacrimal drainage opening
H04.521 Eversion of right lacrimal punctum
H04.522 Eversion of left lacrimal punctum
H04.523 Eversion of bilateral lacrimal punctum
H04.529 Eversion of unspecified lacrimal punctum
● **H04.53** Neonatal obstruction of nasolacrimal duct
Excludes1 congenital stenosis and stricture of lacrimal duct (Q10.5)
H04.531 Neonatal obstruction of right nasolacrimal duct
H04.532 Neonatal obstruction of left nasolacrimal duct
H04.533 Neonatal obstruction of bilateral nasolacrimal duct
H04.539 Neonatal obstruction of unspecified nasolacrimal duct

●H04.54 Stenosis of lacrimal canaliculi
- H04.541 Stenosis of right lacrimal canaliculi
- H04.542 Stenosis of left lacrimal canaliculi
- H04.543 Stenosis of bilateral lacrimal canaliculi
- H04.549 Stenosis of unspecified lacrimal canaliculi

●H04.55 Acquired stenosis of nasolacrimal duct
- H04.551 Acquired stenosis of right nasolacrimal duct
- H04.552 Acquired stenosis of left nasolacrimal duct
- H04.553 Acquired stenosis of bilateral nasolacrimal duct
- H04.559 Acquired stenosis of unspecified nasolacrimal duct

●H04.56 Stenosis of lacrimal punctum
- H04.561 Stenosis of right lacrimal punctum
- H04.562 Stenosis of left lacrimal punctum
- H04.563 Stenosis of bilateral lacrimal punctum
- H04.569 Stenosis of unspecified lacrimal punctum

●H04.57 Stenosis of lacrimal sac
- H04.571 Stenosis of right lacrimal sac
- H04.572 Stenosis of left lacrimal sac
- H04.573 Stenosis of bilateral lacrimal sac
- H04.579 Stenosis of unspecified lacrimal sac

●H04.6 Other changes of lacrimal passages

●H04.61 Lacrimal fistula
- H04.611 Lacrimal fistula right lacrimal passage
- H04.612 Lacrimal fistula left lacrimal passage
- H04.613 Lacrimal fistula bilateral lacrimal passages
- H04.619 Lacrimal fistula unspecified lacrimal passage

H04.69 Other changes of lacrimal passages

●H04.8 Other disorders of lacrimal system

●H04.81 Granuloma of lacrimal passages
Inflammatory response due to infectious or noninfectious agents
- H04.811 Granuloma of right lacrimal passage
- H04.812 Granuloma of left lacrimal passage
- H04.813 Granuloma of bilateral lacrimal passages
- H04.819 Granuloma of unspecified lacrimal passage

H04.89 Other disorders of lacrimal system

H04.9 Disorder of lacrimal system, unspecified

●H05 Disorders of orbit

Excludes1 congenital malformation of orbit (Q10.7)

●H05.0 Acute inflammation of orbit

H05.00 Unspecified acute inflammation of orbit

●H05.01 Cellulitis of orbit
Infection of soft tissue of orbit
Abscess of orbit
- H05.011 Cellulitis of right orbit
- H05.012 Cellulitis of left orbit
- H05.013 Cellulitis of bilateral orbits
- H05.019 Cellulitis of unspecified orbit

●H05.02 Osteomyelitis of orbit
Infection of boney orbit of eye
- H05.021 Osteomyelitis of right orbit
- H05.022 Osteomyelitis of left orbit
- H05.023 Osteomyelitis of bilateral orbits
- H05.029 Osteomyelitis of unspecified orbit

●H05.03 Periostitis of orbit
Inflammation of periosteum (membrane covering bone surface)
- H05.031 Periostitis of right orbit
- H05.032 Periostitis of left orbit
- H05.033 Periostitis of bilateral orbits
- H05.039 Periostitis of unspecified orbit

●H05.04 Tenonitis of orbit
Inflammation of tenon capsule (space enclosing fascia of Tenon between eyeball and fat of orbit)
- H05.041 Tenonitis of right orbit
- H05.042 Tenonitis of left orbit
- H05.043 Tenonitis of bilateral orbits
- H05.049 Tenonitis of unspecified orbit

●H05.1 Chronic inflammatory disorders of orbit

H05.10 Unspecified chronic inflammatory disorders of orbit

●H05.11 Granuloma of orbit
Pseudotumor (inflammatory) of orbit
- H05.111 Granuloma of right orbit
- H05.112 Granuloma of left orbit
- H05.113 Granuloma of bilateral orbits
- H05.119 Granuloma of unspecified orbit

●H05.12 Orbital myositis
Inflammation of extraocular muscles of orbit
- H05.121 Orbital myositis, right orbit
- H05.122 Orbital myositis, left orbit
- H05.123 Orbital myositis, bilateral
- H05.129 Orbital myositis, unspecified orbit

●H05.2 Exophthalmic conditions
Bulging eyes

H05.20 Unspecified exophthalmos

●H05.21 Displacement (lateral) of globe
- H05.211 Displacement (lateral) of globe, right eye
- H05.212 Displacement (lateral) of globe, left eye
- H05.213 Displacement (lateral) of globe, bilateral
- H05.219 Displacement (lateral) of globe, unspecified eye

●H05.22 Edema of orbit
Orbital congestion
- H05.221 Edema of right orbit
- H05.222 Edema of left orbit
- H05.223 Edema of bilateral orbit
- H05.229 Edema of unspecified orbit

●H05.23 Hemorrhage of orbit
- H05.231 Hemorrhage of right orbit
- H05.232 Hemorrhage of left orbit
- H05.233 Hemorrhage of bilateral orbit
- H05.239 Hemorrhage of unspecified orbit

CHAPTER 7 (H00-H59)

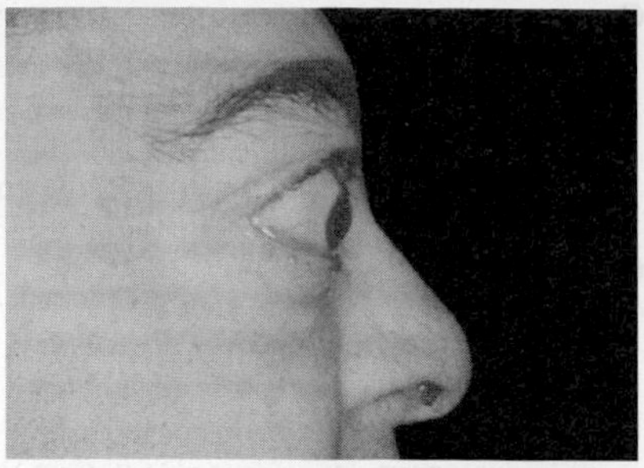

Figure 7-5 Exophthalmos. (From Stein: The Ophthalmic Assistant: Fundamentals and Clinical Practice, ed 6, London, Mosby, 1994)

● **HØ5.24 Constant exophthalmos**
Constant bulging eyes, often symptom of Graves disease
HØ5.241 Constant exophthalmos, right eye
HØ5.242 Constant exophthalmos, left eye
HØ5.243 Constant exophthalmos, bilateral
HØ5.249 Constant exophthalmos, unspecified eye

● **HØ5.25 Intermittent exophthalmos**
Intermittent bulging eye occurring with bending forward or sharp turning of head
HØ5.251 Intermittent exophthalmos, right eye
HØ5.252 Intermittent exophthalmos, left eye
HØ5.253 Intermittent exophthalmos, bilateral
HØ5.259 Intermittent exophthalmos, unspecified eye

● **HØ5.26 Pulsating exophthalmos**
Bulging eyes with pulsation and bruit, often due to aneurysm pushing eye forward
HØ5.261 Pulsating exophthalmos, right eye
HØ5.262 Pulsating exophthalmos, left eye
HØ5.263 Pulsating exophthalmos, bilateral
HØ5.269 Pulsating exophthalmos, unspecified eye

● **HØ5.3 Deformity of orbit**
Excludes1 congenital deformity of orbit (Q1Ø.7)
hypertelorism (Q75.2)

HØ5.3Ø Unspecified deformity of orbit

● **HØ5.31 Atrophy of orbit**
HØ5.311 Atrophy of right orbit
HØ5.312 Atrophy of left orbit
HØ5.313 Atrophy of bilateral orbit
HØ5.319 Atrophy of unspecified orbit

● **HØ5.32 Deformity of orbit due to bone disease**
Code also associated bone disease
HØ5.321 Deformity of right orbit due to bone disease
HØ5.322 Deformity of left orbit due to bone disease
HØ5.323 Deformity of bilateral orbits due to bone disease
HØ5.329 Deformity of unspecified orbit due to bone disease

● **HØ5.33 Deformity of orbit due to trauma or surgery**
HØ5.331 Deformity of right orbit due to trauma or surgery
HØ5.332 Deformity of left orbit due to trauma or surgery
HØ5.333 Deformity of bilateral orbits due to trauma or surgery
HØ5.339 Deformity of unspecified orbit due to trauma or surgery

● **HØ5.34 Enlargement of orbit**
HØ5.341 Enlargement of right orbit
HØ5.342 Enlargement of left orbit
HØ5.343 Enlargement of bilateral orbits
HØ5.349 Enlargement of unspecified orbit

● **HØ5.35 Exostosis of orbit**
HØ5.351 Exostosis of right orbit
HØ5.352 Exostosis of left orbit
HØ5.353 Exostosis of bilateral orbits
HØ5.359 Exostosis of unspecified orbit

● **HØ5.4 Enophthalmos**
Recessed eyeball into orbit

● **HØ5.4Ø Unspecified enophthalmos**
HØ5.4Ø1 Unspecified enophthalmos, right eye
HØ5.4Ø2 Unspecified enophthalmos, left eye
HØ5.4Ø3 Unspecified enophthalmos, bilateral
HØ5.4Ø9 Unspecified enophthalmos, unspecified eye

● **HØ5.41 Enophthalmos due to atrophy of orbital tissue**
HØ5.411 Enophthalmos due to atrophy of orbital tissue, right eye
HØ5.412 Enophthalmos due to atrophy of orbital tissue, left eye
HØ5.413 Enophthalmos due to atrophy of orbital tissue, bilateral
HØ5.419 Enophthalmos due to atrophy of orbital tissue, unspecified eye

● **HØ5.42 Enophthalmos due to trauma or surgery**
HØ5.421 Enophthalmos due to trauma or surgery, right eye
HØ5.422 Enophthalmos due to trauma or surgery, left eye
HØ5.423 Enophthalmos due to trauma or surgery, bilateral
HØ5.429 Enophthalmos due to trauma or surgery, unspecified eye

● **HØ5.5 Retained (old) foreign body following penetrating wound of orbit**
Retrobulbar foreign body
Use additional code to identify the type of retained foreign body (Z18.-)
Excludes1 current penetrating wound of orbit (SØ5.4-)
Excludes2 retained foreign body of eyelid (HØ2.81-)
retained intraocular foreign body (H44.6-, H44.7-)

HØ5.5Ø Retained (old) foreign body following penetrating wound of unspecified orbit
HØ5.51 Retained (old) foreign body following penetrating wound of right orbit
HØ5.52 Retained (old) foreign body following penetrating wound of left orbit
HØ5.53 Retained (old) foreign body following penetrating wound of bilateral orbits

● **HØ5.8 Other disorders of orbit**

● **HØ5.81 Cyst of orbit**
Encephalocele of orbit
HØ5.811 Cyst of right orbit
HØ5.812 Cyst of left orbit
HØ5.813 Cyst of bilateral orbits
HØ5.819 Cyst of unspecified orbit

- H05.82 Myopathy of extraocular muscles
  Weakness of muscles of eye
  - H05.821 Myopathy of extraocular muscles, right orbit
  - H05.822 Myopathy of extraocular muscles, left orbit
  - H05.823 Myopathy of extraocular muscles, bilateral
  - H05.829 Myopathy of extraocular muscles, unspecified orbit
- H05.89 Other disorders of orbit

H05.9 Unspecified disorder of orbit

DISORDERS OF CONJUNCTIVA (H10-H11)

★(See Plate 81, upper, on page NAP-18.)

● H10 Conjunctivitis
Inflammation of membrane of the inside of the eyelid or on surface of eye (conjunctiva)
Excludes1 keratoconjunctivitis (H16.2-)

- ● H10.0 Mucopurulent conjunctivitis
  - ● H10.01 Acute follicular conjunctivitis
    - H10.011 Acute follicular conjunctivitis, right eye
    - H10.012 Acute follicular conjunctivitis, left eye
    - H10.013 Acute follicular conjunctivitis, bilateral
    - H10.019 Acute follicular conjunctivitis, unspecified eye
  - ● H10.02 Other mucopurulent conjunctivitis
    - H10.021 Other mucopurulent conjunctivitis, right eye
    - H10.022 Other mucopurulent conjunctivitis, left eye
    - H10.023 Other mucopurulent conjunctivitis, bilateral
    - H10.029 Other mucopurulent conjunctivitis, unspecified eye
- ● H10.1 Acute atopic conjunctivitis
  Acute papillary conjunctivitis
  - H10.10 Acute atopic conjunctivitis, unspecified eye
  - H10.11 Acute atopic conjunctivitis, right eye
  - H10.12 Acute atopic conjunctivitis, left eye
  - H10.13 Acute atopic conjunctivitis, bilateral
- ● H10.2 Other acute conjunctivitis
  - ● H10.21 Acute toxic conjunctivitis
    Acute chemical conjunctivitis
    Code first (T51-T65) to identify chemical and intent
    Excludes1 burn and corrosion of eye and adnexa (T26.-)
    - H10.211 Acute toxic conjunctivitis, right eye
    - H10.212 Acute toxic conjunctivitis, left eye
    - H10.213 Acute toxic conjunctivitis, bilateral
    - H10.219 Acute toxic conjunctivitis, unspecified eye
  - ● H10.22 Pseudomembranous conjunctivitis
    - H10.221 Pseudomembranous conjunctivitis, right eye
    - H10.222 Pseudomembranous conjunctivitis, left eye
    - H10.223 Pseudomembranous conjunctivitis, bilateral
    - H10.229 Pseudomembranous conjunctivitis, unspecified eye
  - ● H10.23 Serous conjunctivitis, except viral
    Excludes1 viral conjunctivitis (B30.-)
    - H10.231 Serous conjunctivitis, except viral, right eye
    - H10.232 Serous conjunctivitis, except viral, left eye
    - H10.233 Serous conjunctivitis, except viral, bilateral
    - H10.239 Serous conjunctivitis, except viral, unspecified eye
- ● H10.3 Unspecified acute conjunctivitis
  Excludes1 ophthalmia neonatorum NOS (P39.1)
  - H10.30 Unspecified acute conjunctivitis, unspecified eye
  - H10.31 Unspecified acute conjunctivitis, right eye
  - H10.32 Unspecified acute conjunctivitis, left eye
  - H10.33 Unspecified acute conjunctivitis, bilateral
- ● H10.4 Chronic conjunctivitis
  - ● H10.40 Unspecified chronic conjunctivitis
    - H10.401 Unspecified chronic conjunctivitis, right eye
    - H10.402 Unspecified chronic conjunctivitis, left eye
    - H10.403 Unspecified chronic conjunctivitis, bilateral
    - H10.409 Unspecified chronic conjunctivitis, unspecified eye
  - ● H10.41 Chronic giant papillary conjunctivitis
    Inflammation of membrane of the inside of the eyelid or on surface of eye often associated with contact lens wear
    - H10.411 Chronic giant papillary conjunctivitis, right eye
    - H10.412 Chronic giant papillary conjunctivitis, left eye
    - H10.413 Chronic giant papillary conjunctivitis, bilateral
    - H10.419 Chronic giant papillary conjunctivitis, unspecified eye
  - ● H10.42 Simple chronic conjunctivitis
    - H10.421 Simple chronic conjunctivitis, right eye
    - H10.422 Simple chronic conjunctivitis, left eye
    - H10.423 Simple chronic conjunctivitis, bilateral
    - H10.429 Simple chronic conjunctivitis, unspecified eye
  - ● H10.43 Chronic follicular conjunctivitis
    Inflammation of membrane of the inside of the eyelid or on surface of eye due to topical medications or infection
    - H10.431 Chronic follicular conjunctivitis, right eye
    - H10.432 Chronic follicular conjunctivitis, left eye
    - H10.433 Chronic follicular conjunctivitis, bilateral
    - H10.439 Chronic follicular conjunctivitis, unspecified eye
  - H10.44 Vernal conjunctivitis
    Affecting children, especially boys in which there are flattened papules with thick, gelatinous exudate on conjunctivae on inside of upper lid
    Excludes1 vernal keratoconjunctivitis with limbar and corneal involvement (H16.26-)
  - H10.45 Other chronic allergic conjunctivitis

CHAPTER 7 (H00-H59)

● H10.5 Blepharoconjunctivitis
Inflammation of eyelids and conjunctiva
● H10.50 Unspecified blepharoconjunctivitis
H10.501 Unspecified blepharoconjunctivitis, right eye
H10.502 Unspecified blepharoconjunctivitis, left eye
H10.503 Unspecified blepharoconjunctivitis, bilateral
H10.509 Unspecified blepharoconjunctivitis, unspecified eye
● H10.51 Ligneous conjunctivitis
H10.511 Ligneous conjunctivitis, right eye
H10.512 Ligneous conjunctivitis, left eye
H10.513 Ligneous conjunctivitis, bilateral
H10.519 Ligneous conjunctivitis, unspecified eye
● H10.52 Angular blepharoconjunctivitis
H10.521 Angular blepharoconjunctivitis, right eye
H10.522 Angular blepharoconjunctivitis, left eye
H10.523 Angular blepharoconjunctivitis, bilateral
H10.529 Angular blepharoconjunctivitis, unspecified eye
● H10.53 Contact blepharoconjunctivitis
H10.531 Contact blepharoconjunctivitis, right eye
H10.532 Contact blepharoconjunctivitis, left eye
H10.533 Contact blepharoconjunctivitis, bilateral
H10.539 Contact blepharoconjunctivitis, unspecified eye
● H10.8 Other conjunctivitis
● H10.81 Pingueculitis
Inflammation of a yellow, raised thickening on the white of the eye associated with chronic dry eyes
Excludes1 pinguecula (H11.15-)
H10.811 Pingueculitis, right eye
H10.812 Pingueculitis, left eye
H10.813 Pingueculitis, bilateral
H10.819 Pingueculitis, unspecified eye
H10.89 Other conjunctivitis
H10.9 Unspecified conjunctivitis
● H11 Other disorders of conjunctiva
Excludes1 keratoconjunctivitis (H16.2-)
● H11.0 Pterygium of eye
Excludes1 pseudopterygium (H11.81-)
● H11.00 Unspecified pterygium of eye
H11.001 Unspecified pterygium of right eye
H11.002 Unspecified pterygium of left eye
H11.003 Unspecified pterygium of eye, bilateral
H11.009 Unspecified pterygium of unspecified eye
● H11.01 Amyloid pterygium
H11.011 Amyloid pterygium of right eye
H11.012 Amyloid pterygium of left eye
H11.013 Amyloid pterygium of eye, bilateral
H11.019 Amyloid pterygium of unspecified eye

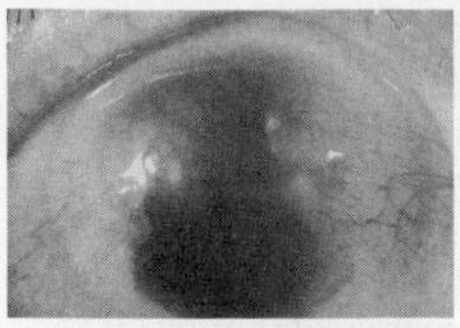

Figure 7-6 Double pterygium. Note both nasal and temporal pterygia in a 57-year-old farmer. (From Yanoff: Ophthalmology, ed 3, Mosby, Inc., 2008)

Item 7-2 Pterygium is Greek for batlike. The condition is characterized by a membrane that extends from the limbus to the center of the cornea and resembles a wing.

● H11.02 Central pterygium of eye
H11.021 Central pterygium of right eye
H11.022 Central pterygium of left eye
H11.023 Central pterygium of eye, bilateral
H11.029 Central pterygium of unspecified eye
● H11.03 Double pterygium of eye
H11.031 Double pterygium of right eye
H11.032 Double pterygium of left eye
H11.033 Double pterygium of eye, bilateral
H11.039 Double pterygium of unspecified eye
● H11.04 Peripheral pterygium of eye, stationary
H11.041 Peripheral pterygium, stationary, right eye
H11.042 Peripheral pterygium, stationary, left eye
H11.043 Peripheral pterygium, stationary, bilateral
H11.049 Peripheral pterygium, stationary, unspecified eye
● H11.05 Peripheral pterygium of eye, progressive
H11.051 Peripheral pterygium, progressive, right eye
H11.052 Peripheral pterygium, progressive, left eye
H11.053 Peripheral pterygium, progressive, bilateral
H11.059 Peripheral pterygium, progressive, unspecified eye
● H11.06 Recurrent pterygium of eye
H11.061 Recurrent pterygium of right eye
H11.062 Recurrent pterygium of left eye
H11.063 Recurrent pterygium of eye, bilateral
H11.069 Recurrent pterygium of unspecified eye
● H11.1 Conjunctival degenerations and deposits
Excludes2 pseudopterygium (H11.81)
H11.10 Unspecified conjunctival degenerations
● H11.11 Conjunctival deposits
H11.111 Conjunctival deposits, right eye
H11.112 Conjunctival deposits, left eye
H11.113 Conjunctival deposits, bilateral
H11.119 Conjunctival deposits, unspecified eye
● H11.12 Conjunctival concretions
White to yellow nodules within or beneath conjunctiva
H11.121 Conjunctival concretions, right eye
H11.122 Conjunctival concretions, left eye
H11.123 Conjunctival concretions, bilateral
H11.129 Conjunctival concretions, unspecified eye
● H11.13 Conjunctival pigmentations
Conjunctival argyrosis [argyria]
H11.131 Conjunctival pigmentations, right eye
H11.132 Conjunctival pigmentations, left eye
H11.133 Conjunctival pigmentations, bilateral
H11.139 Conjunctival pigmentations, unspecified eye

● H11.14 Conjunctival xerosis, unspecified
Excludes1 xerosis of conjunctiva due to vitamin A deficiency (E50.0, E50.1)
H11.141 Conjunctival xerosis, unspecified, right eye
H11.142 Conjunctival xerosis, unspecified, left eye
H11.143 Conjunctival xerosis, unspecified, bilateral
H11.149 Conjunctival xerosis, unspecified, unspecified eye

● H11.15 Pinguecula
Yellowish spot near sclerocorneal junction, usually on nasal side; associated with aging
Excludes1 pingueculitis (H10.81-)
H11.151 Pinguecula, right eye
H11.152 Pinguecula, left eye
H11.153 Pinguecula, bilateral
H11.159 Pinguecula, unspecified eye

● H11.2 Conjunctival scars
● H11.21 Conjunctival adhesions and strands (localized)
H11.211 Conjunctival adhesions and strands (localized), right eye
H11.212 Conjunctival adhesions and strands (localized), left eye
H11.213 Conjunctival adhesions and strands (localized), bilateral
H11.219 Conjunctival adhesions and strands (localized), unspecified eye

● H11.22 Conjunctival granuloma
H11.221 Conjunctival granuloma, right eye
H11.222 Conjunctival granuloma, left eye
H11.223 Conjunctival granuloma, bilateral
H11.229 Conjunctival granuloma, unspecified

● H11.23 Symblepharon
Adhesion between tarsal conjunctiva and bulbar conjunctiva
H11.231 Symblepharon, right eye
H11.232 Symblepharon, left eye
H11.233 Symblepharon, bilateral
H11.239 Symblepharon, unspecified eye

● H11.24 Scarring of conjunctiva
H11.241 Scarring of conjunctiva, right eye
H11.242 Scarring of conjunctiva, left eye
H11.243 Scarring of conjunctiva, bilateral
H11.249 Scarring of conjunctiva, unspecified eye

● H11.3 Conjunctival hemorrhage
Subconjunctival hemorrhage
H11.30 Conjunctival hemorrhage, unspecified eye
H11.31 Conjunctival hemorrhage, right eye
H11.32 Conjunctival hemorrhage, left eye
H11.33 Conjunctival hemorrhage, bilateral

● H11.4 Other conjunctival vascular disorders and cysts
● H11.41 Vascular abnormalities of conjunctiva
Conjunctival aneurysm
H11.411 Vascular abnormalities of conjunctiva, right eye
H11.412 Vascular abnormalities of conjunctiva, left eye
H11.413 Vascular abnormalities of conjunctiva, bilateral
H11.419 Vascular abnormalities of conjunctiva, unspecified eye

● H11.42 Conjunctival edema
H11.421 Conjunctival edema, right eye
H11.422 Conjunctival edema, left eye
H11.423 Conjunctival edema, bilateral
H11.429 Conjunctival edema, unspecified eye

● H11.43 Conjunctival hyperemia
H11.431 Conjunctival hyperemia, right eye
H11.432 Conjunctival hyperemia, left eye
H11.433 Conjunctival hyperemia, bilateral
H11.439 Conjunctival hyperemia, unspecified eye

● H11.44 Conjunctival cysts
H11.441 Conjunctival cysts, right eye
H11.442 Conjunctival cysts, left eye
H11.443 Conjunctival cysts, bilateral
H11.449 Conjunctival cysts, unspecified eye

● H11.8 Other specified disorders of conjunctiva
● H11.81 Pseudopterygium of conjunctiva
Conjunctival scar attached to cornea
H11.811 Pseudopterygium of conjunctiva, right eye
H11.812 Pseudopterygium of conjunctiva, left eye
H11.813 Pseudopterygium of conjunctiva, bilateral
H11.819 Pseudopterygium of conjunctiva, unspecified eye

● H11.82 Conjunctivochalasis
Conjunctiva bulges over eyelid margin or covers lower punctum
H11.821 Conjunctivochalasis, right eye
H11.822 Conjunctivochalasis, left eye
H11.823 Conjunctivochalasis, bilateral
H11.829 Conjunctivochalasis, unspecified eye

H11.89 Other specified disorders of conjunctiva

H11.9 Unspecified disorder of conjunctiva

DISORDERS OF SCLERA, CORNEA, IRIS AND CILIARY BODY (H15-H22)

● H15 Disorders of sclera
● H15.0 Scleritis
Inflammation of the white (sclera and episclera) of the eye.
● H15.00 Unspecified scleritis
H15.001 Unspecified scleritis, right eye
H15.002 Unspecified scleritis, left eye
H15.003 Unspecified scleritis, bilateral
H15.009 Unspecified scleritis, unspecified eye

● H15.01 Anterior scleritis
H15.011 Anterior scleritis, right eye
H15.012 Anterior scleritis, left eye
H15.013 Anterior scleritis, bilateral
H15.019 Anterior scleritis, unspecified eye

● H15.02 Brawny scleritis
Swelling around the cornea that is gelantinous in appearance
H15.021 Brawny scleritis, right eye
H15.022 Brawny scleritis, left eye
H15.023 Brawny scleritis, bilateral
H15.029 Brawny scleritis, unspecified eye

● H15.03 Posterior scleritis
Sclerotenonitis
H15.031 Posterior scleritis, right eye
H15.032 Posterior scleritis, left eye
H15.033 Posterior scleritis, bilateral
H15.039 Posterior scleritis, unspecified eye

● H15.Ø4 Scleritis with corneal involvement
- H15.Ø41 Scleritis with corneal involvement, right eye
- H15.Ø42 Scleritis with corneal involvement, left eye
- H15.Ø43 Scleritis with corneal involvement, bilateral
- H15.Ø49 Scleritis with corneal involvement, unspecified eye

● H15.Ø5 Scleromalacia perforans

Necrotic without inflammation; usually associated with rheumatoid arthritis

- H15.Ø51 Scleromalacia perforans, right eye
- H15.Ø52 Scleromalacia perforans, left eye
- H15.Ø53 Scleromalacia perforans, bilateral
- H15.Ø59 Scleromalacia perforans, unspecified eye

● H15.Ø9 Other scleritis

Scleral abscess

- H15.Ø91 Other scleritis, right eye
- H15.Ø92 Other scleritis, left eye
- H15.Ø93 Other scleritis, bilateral
- H15.Ø99 Other scleritis, unspecified eye

● H15.1 Episcleritis

Inflammation of the white (sclera and episclera) of the eye.

● H15.1Ø Unspecified episcleritis
- H15.1Ø1 Unspecified episcleritis, right eye
- H15.1Ø2 Unspecified episcleritis, left eye
- H15.1Ø3 Unspecified episcleritis, bilateral
- H15.1Ø9 Unspecified episcleritis, unspecified eye

● H15.11 Episcleritis periodica fugax

Transient, recurrent inflammation of portion of episclera (connective tissue on the surface of the sclera)

- H15.111 Episcleritis periodica fugax, right eye
- H15.112 Episcleritis periodica fugax, left eye
- H15.113 Episcleritis periodica fugax, bilateral
- H15.119 Episcleritis periodica fugax, unspecified eye

● H15.12 Nodular episcleritis

Characterized by tender, localized, moveable nodule within inflamed area

- H15.121 Nodular episcleritis, right eye
- H15.122 Nodular episcleritis, left eye
- H15.123 Nodular episcleritis, bilateral
- H15.129 Nodular episcleritis, unspecified eye

● H15.8 Other disorders of sclera

Excludes2 blue sclera (Q13.5)
degenerative myopia (H44.2-)

● H15.81 Equatorial staphyloma
- H15.811 Equatorial staphyloma, right eye
- H15.812 Equatorial staphyloma, left eye
- H15.813 Equatorial staphyloma, bilateral
- H15.819 Equatorial staphyloma, unspecified eye

● H15.82 Localized anterior staphyloma
- H15.821 Localized anterior staphyloma, right eye
- H15.822 Localized anterior staphyloma, left eye
- H15.823 Localized anterior staphyloma, bilateral
- H15.829 Localized anterior staphyloma, unspecified eye

● H15.83 Staphyloma posticum
- H15.831 Staphyloma posticum, right eye
- H15.832 Staphyloma posticum, left eye
- H15.833 Staphyloma posticum, bilateral
- H15.839 Staphyloma posticum, unspecified eye

● H15.84 Scleral ectasia
- H15.841 Scleral ectasia, right eye
- H15.842 Scleral ectasia, left eye
- H15.843 Scleral ectasia, bilateral
- H15.849 Scleral ectasia, unspecified eye

● H15.85 Ring staphyloma
- H15.851 Ring staphyloma, right eye
- H15.852 Ring staphyloma, left eye
- H15.853 Ring staphyloma, bilateral
- H15.859 Ring staphyloma, unspecified eye

H15.89 Other disorders of sclera

H15.9 Unspecified disorder of sclera

● H16 Keratitis

● H16.Ø Corneal ulcer

● H16.ØØ Unspecified corneal ulcer
- H16.ØØ1 Unspecified corneal ulcer, right eye
- H16.ØØ2 Unspecified corneal ulcer, left eye
- H16.ØØ3 Unspecified corneal ulcer, bilateral
- H16.ØØ9 Unspecified corneal ulcer, unspecified eye

● H16.Ø1 Central corneal ulcer
- H16.Ø11 Central corneal ulcer, right eye
- H16.Ø12 Central corneal ulcer, left eye
- H16.Ø13 Central corneal ulcer, bilateral
- H16.Ø19 Central corneal ulcer, unspecified eye

● H16.Ø2 Ring corneal ulcer
- H16.Ø21 Ring corneal ulcer, right eye
- H16.Ø22 Ring corneal ulcer, left eye
- H16.Ø23 Ring corneal ulcer, bilateral
- H16.Ø29 Ring corneal ulcer, unspecified eye

● H16.Ø3 Corneal ulcer with hypopyon
- H16.Ø31 Corneal ulcer with hypopyon, right eye
- H16.Ø32 Corneal ulcer with hypopyon, left eye
- H16.Ø33 Corneal ulcer with hypopyon, bilateral
- H16.Ø39 Corneal ulcer with hypopyon, unspecified eye

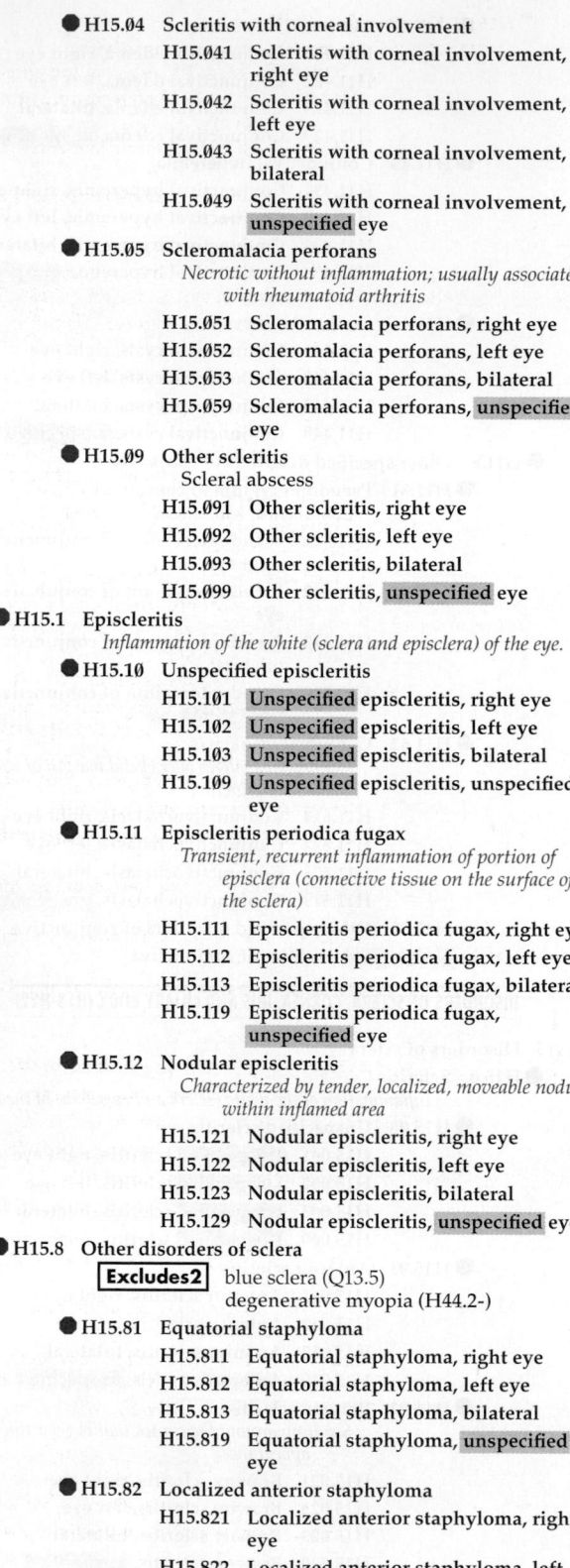

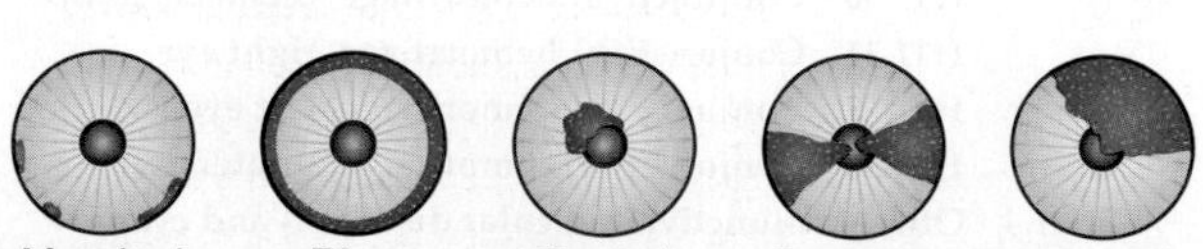

Figure 7-7 Corneal ulcers: marginal, ring, central corneal, rosacea, and Mooren's.

Item 7–3 An infected ulcer is usually called a **serpiginous** or **hypopyon** ulcer which is a pus sac in the anterior chamber of the eye. **Marginal** ulcers are usually asymptomatic, not primary, and are often superficial and simple. More severe marginal ulcers spread to form a ring ulcer. **Ring** ulcers can extend around the entire corneal periphery. **Central corneal** ulcers develop when there is an abrasion to the epithelium and an infection develops in the eroded area. The **pyocyaneal** ulcer is the most serious corneal infection, which, if left untreated, can lead to loss of the eye.

- H16.04 Marginal corneal ulcer
  - H16.041 Marginal corneal ulcer, right eye
  - H16.042 Marginal corneal ulcer, left eye
  - H16.043 Marginal corneal ulcer, bilateral
  - H16.049 Marginal corneal ulcer, unspecified eye
- H16.05 Mooren's corneal ulcer
  - H16.051 Mooren's corneal ulcer, right eye
  - H16.052 Mooren's corneal ulcer, left eye
  - H16.053 Mooren's corneal ulcer, bilateral
  - H16.059 Mooren's corneal ulcer, unspecified eye
- H16.06 Mycotic corneal ulcer
  - H16.061 Mycotic corneal ulcer, right eye
  - H16.062 Mycotic corneal ulcer, left eye
  - H16.063 Mycotic corneal ulcer, bilateral
  - H16.069 Mycotic corneal ulcer, unspecified eye
- H16.07 Perforated corneal ulcer
  - H16.071 Perforated corneal ulcer, right eye
  - H16.072 Perforated corneal ulcer, left eye
  - H16.073 Perforated corneal ulcer, bilateral
  - H16.079 Perforated corneal ulcer, unspecified eye

H16.1 Other and unspecified superficial keratitis without conjunctivitis

- H16.10 Unspecified superficial keratitis
  - H16.101 Unspecified superficial keratitis, right eye
  - H16.102 Unspecified superficial keratitis, left eye
  - H16.103 Unspecified superficial keratitis, bilateral
  - H16.109 Unspecified superficial keratitis, unspecified eye
- H16.11 Macular keratitis
  - Areolar keratitis
  - Nummular keratitis
  - Stellate keratitis
  - Striate keratitis
  - H16.111 Macular keratitis, right eye
  - H16.112 Macular keratitis, left eye
  - H16.113 Macular keratitis, bilateral
  - H16.119 Macular keratitis, unspecified eye
- H16.12 Filamentary keratitis
  - H16.121 Filamentary keratitis, right eye
  - H16.122 Filamentary keratitis, left eye
  - H16.123 Filamentary keratitis, bilateral
  - H16.129 Filamentary keratitis, unspecified eye
- H16.13 Photokeratitis
  - Snow blindness
  - Welders' keratitis
  - H16.131 Photokeratitis, right eye
  - H16.132 Photokeratitis, left eye
  - H16.133 Photokeratitis, bilateral
  - H16.139 Photokeratitis, unspecified eye
- H16.14 Punctate keratitis
  - H16.141 Punctate keratitis, right eye
  - H16.142 Punctate keratitis, left eye
  - H16.143 Punctate keratitis, bilateral
  - H16.149 Punctate keratitis, unspecified eye

H16.2 Keratoconjunctivitis

- H16.20 Unspecified keratoconjunctivitis
  - Superficial keratitis with conjunctivitis NOS
  - H16.201 Unspecified keratoconjunctivitis, right eye
  - H16.202 Unspecified keratoconjunctivitis, left eye
  - H16.203 Unspecified keratoconjunctivitis, bilateral
  - H16.209 Unspecified keratoconjunctivitis, unspecified eye
- H16.21 Exposure keratoconjunctivitis
  - H16.211 Exposure keratoconjunctivitis, right eye
  - H16.212 Exposure keratoconjunctivitis, left eye
  - H16.213 Exposure keratoconjunctivitis, bilateral
  - H16.219 Exposure keratoconjunctivitis, unspecified eye
- H16.22 Keratoconjunctivitis sicca, not specified as Sjögren's
  - **Excludes1** Sjogren's syndrome (M35.01)
  - H16.221 Keratoconjunctivitis sicca, not specified as Sjögren's, right eye
  - H16.222 Keratoconjunctivitis sicca, not specified as Sjögren's, left eye
  - H16.223 Keratoconjunctivitis sicca, not specified as Sjögren's, bilateral
  - H16.229 Keratoconjunctivitis sicca, not specified as Sjögren's, unspecified eye
- H16.23 Neurotrophic keratoconjunctivitis
  - H16.231 Neurotrophic keratoconjunctivitis, right eye
  - H16.232 Neurotrophic keratoconjunctivitis, left eye
  - H16.233 Neurotrophic keratoconjunctivitis, bilateral
  - H16.239 Neurotrophic keratoconjunctivitis, unspecified eye
- H16.24 Ophthalmia nodosa
  - H16.241 Ophthalmia nodosa, right eye
  - H16.242 Ophthalmia nodosa, left eye
  - H16.243 Ophthalmia nodosa, bilateral
  - H16.249 Ophthalmia nodosa, unspecified eye
- H16.25 Phlyctenular keratoconjunctivitis
  - H16.251 Phlyctenular keratoconjunctivitis, right eye
  - H16.252 Phlyctenular keratoconjunctivitis, left eye
  - H16.253 Phlyctenular keratoconjunctivitis, bilateral
  - H16.259 Phlyctenular keratoconjunctivitis, unspecified eye
- H16.26 Vernal keratoconjunctivitis, with limbar and corneal involvement
  - **Excludes1** vernal conjunctivitis without limbar and corneal involvement (H10.44)
  - H16.261 Vernal keratoconjunctivitis, with limbar and corneal involvement, right eye
  - H16.262 Vernal keratoconjunctivitis, with limbar and corneal involvement, left eye

CHAPTER 7 (H00-H59)

H16.263 Vernal keratoconjunctivitis, with limbar and corneal involvement, bilateral
H16.269 Vernal keratoconjunctivitis, with limbar and corneal involvement, unspecified eye
● H16.29 Other keratoconjunctivitis
H16.291 Other keratoconjunctivitis, right eye
H16.292 Other keratoconjunctivitis, left eye
H16.293 Other keratoconjunctivitis, bilateral
H16.299 Other keratoconjunctivitis, unspecified eye
● H16.3 Interstitial and deep keratitis
● H16.3Ø Unspecified interstitial keratitis
H16.3Ø1 Unspecified interstitial keratitis, right eye
H16.3Ø2 Unspecified interstitial keratitis, left eye
H16.3Ø3 Unspecified interstitial keratitis, bilateral
H16.3Ø9 Unspecified interstitial keratitis, unspecified eye
● H16.31 Corneal abscess
H16.311 Corneal abscess, right eye
H16.312 Corneal abscess, left eye
H16.313 Corneal abscess, bilateral
H16.319 Corneal abscess, unspecified eye
● H16.32 Diffuse interstitial keratitis
Cogan's syndrome
H16.321 Diffuse interstitial keratitis, right eye
H16.322 Diffuse interstitial keratitis, left eye
H16.323 Diffuse interstitial keratitis, bilateral
H16.329 Diffuse interstitial keratitis, unspecified eye
● H16.33 Sclerosing keratitis
H16.331 Sclerosing keratitis, right eye
H16.332 Sclerosing keratitis, left eye
H16.333 Sclerosing keratitis, bilateral
H16.339 Sclerosing keratitis, unspecified eye
● H16.39 Other interstitial and deep keratitis
H16.391 Other interstitial and deep keratitis, right eye
H16.392 Other interstitial and deep keratitis, left eye
H16.393 Other interstitial and deep keratitis, bilateral
H16.399 Other interstitial and deep keratitis, unspecified eye
● H16.4 Corneal neovascularization
● H16.4Ø Unspecified corneal neovascularization
H16.4Ø1 Unspecified corneal neovascularization, right eye
H16.4Ø2 Unspecified corneal neovascularization, left eye
H16.4Ø3 Unspecified corneal neovascularization, bilateral
H16.4Ø9 Unspecified corneal neovascularization, unspecified eye
● H16.41 Ghost vessels (corneal)
H16.411 Ghost vessels (corneal), right eye
H16.412 Ghost vessels (corneal), left eye
H16.413 Ghost vessels (corneal), bilateral
H16.419 Ghost vessels (corneal), unspecified eye

● H16.42 Pannus (corneal)
H16.421 Pannus (corneal), right eye
H16.422 Pannus (corneal), left eye
H16.423 Pannus (corneal), bilateral
H16.429 Pannus (corneal), unspecified eye
● H16.43 Localized vascularization of cornea
H16.431 Localized vascularization of cornea, right eye
H16.432 Localized vascularization of cornea, left eye
H16.433 Localized vascularization of cornea, bilateral
H16.439 Localized vascularization of cornea, unspecified eye
● H16.44 Deep vascularization of cornea
H16.441 Deep vascularization of cornea, right eye
H16.442 Deep vascularization of cornea, left eye
H16.443 Deep vascularization of cornea, bilateral
H16.449 Deep vascularization of cornea, unspecified eye
H16.8 Other keratitis
H16.9 Unspecified keratitis
● H17 Corneal scars and opacities
● H17.Ø Adherent leukoma
H17.ØØ Adherent leukoma, unspecified eye
H17.Ø1 Adherent leukoma, right eye
H17.Ø2 Adherent leukoma, left eye
H17.Ø3 Adherent leukoma, bilateral
● H17.1 Central corneal opacity
H17.1Ø Central corneal opacity, unspecified eye
H17.11 Central corneal opacity, right eye
H17.12 Central corneal opacity, left eye
H17.13 Central corneal opacity, bilateral
● H17.8 Other corneal scars and opacities
● H17.81 Minor opacity of cornea
Corneal nebula
H17.811 Minor opacity of cornea, right eye
H17.812 Minor opacity of cornea, left eye
H17.813 Minor opacity of cornea, bilateral
H17.819 Minor opacity of cornea, unspecified eye
● H17.82 Peripheral opacity of cornea
H17.821 Peripheral opacity of cornea, right eye
H17.822 Peripheral opacity of cornea, left eye
H17.823 Peripheral opacity of cornea, bilateral
H17.829 Peripheral opacity of cornea, unspecified eye
H17.89 Other corneal scars and opacities
H17.9 Unspecified corneal scar and opacity
● H18 Other disorders of cornea
● H18.Ø Corneal pigmentations and deposits
● H18.ØØ Unspecified corneal deposit
H18.ØØ1 Unspecified corneal deposit, right eye
H18.ØØ2 Unspecified corneal deposit, left eye
H18.ØØ3 Unspecified corneal deposit, bilateral
H18.ØØ9 Unspecified corneal deposit, unspecified eye
● H18.Ø1 Anterior corneal pigmentations
Staehli's line
H18.Ø11 Anterior corneal pigmentations, right eye
H18.Ø12 Anterior corneal pigmentations, left eye

H18.013 Anterior corneal pigmentations, bilateral
H18.019 Anterior corneal pigmentations, unspecified eye

● H18.02 Argentous corneal deposits
H18.021 Argentous corneal deposits, right eye
H18.022 Argentous corneal deposits, left eye
H18.023 Argentous corneal deposits, bilateral
H18.029 Argentous corneal deposits, unspecified eye

● H18.03 Corneal deposits in metabolic disorders
Code also associated metabolic disorder
H18.031 Corneal deposits in metabolic disorders, right eye
H18.032 Corneal deposits in metabolic disorders, left eye
H18.033 Corneal deposits in metabolic disorders, bilateral
H18.039 Corneal deposits in metabolic disorders, unspecified eye

● H18.04 Kayser-Fleischer ring
Code also associated Wilson's disease (E83.01)
H18.041 Kayser-Fleischer ring, right eye
H18.042 Kayser-Fleischer ring, left eye
H18.043 Kayser-Fleischer ring, bilateral
H18.049 Kayser-Fleischer ring, unspecified eye

● H18.05 Posterior corneal pigmentations
Krukenberg's spindle
H18.051 Posterior corneal pigmentations, right eye
H18.052 Posterior corneal pigmentations, left eye
H18.053 Posterior corneal pigmentations, bilateral
H18.059 Posterior corneal pigmentations, unspecified eye

● H18.06 Stromal corneal pigmentations
Hematocornea
H18.061 Stromal corneal pigmentations, right eye
H18.062 Stromal corneal pigmentations, left eye
H18.063 Stromal corneal pigmentations, bilateral
H18.069 Stromal corneal pigmentations, unspecified eye

● H18.1 Bullous keratopathy
H18.10 Bullous keratopathy, unspecified eye
H18.11 Bullous keratopathy, right eye
H18.12 Bullous keratopathy, left eye
H18.13 Bullous keratopathy, bilateral

● H18.2 Other and unspecified corneal edema
H18.20 Unspecified corneal edema

● H18.21 Corneal edema secondary to contact lens
Excludes2 other corneal disorders due to contact lens (H18.82-)
H18.211 Corneal edema secondary to contact lens, right eye
H18.212 Corneal edema secondary to contact lens, left eye
H18.213 Corneal edema secondary to contact lens, bilateral
H18.219 Corneal edema secondary to contact lens, unspecified eye

● H18.22 Idiopathic corneal edema
H18.221 Idiopathic corneal edema, right eye
H18.222 Idiopathic corneal edema, left eye
H18.223 Idiopathic corneal edema, bilateral
H18.229 Idiopathic corneal edema, unspecified eye

● H18.23 Secondary corneal edema
H18.231 Secondary corneal edema, right eye
H18.232 Secondary corneal edema, left eye
H18.233 Secondary corneal edema, bilateral
H18.239 Secondary corneal edema, unspecified eye

● H18.3 Changes of corneal membranes
H18.30 Unspecified corneal membrane change

● H18.31 Folds and rupture in Bowman's membrane
H18.311 Folds and rupture in Bowman's membrane, right eye
H18.312 Folds and rupture in Bowman's membrane, left eye
H18.313 Folds and rupture in Bowman's membrane, bilateral
H18.319 Folds and rupture in Bowman's membrane, unspecified eye

● H18.32 Folds in Descemet's membrane
H18.321 Folds in Descemet's membrane, right eye
H18.322 Folds in Descemet's membrane, left eye
H18.323 Folds in Descemet's membrane, bilateral
H18.329 Folds in Descemet's membrane, unspecified eye

● H18.33 Rupture in Descemet's membrane
H18.331 Rupture in Descemet's membrane, right eye
H18.332 Rupture in Descemet's membrane, left eye
H18.333 Rupture in Descemet's membrane, bilateral
H18.339 Rupture in Descemet's membrane, unspecified eye

● H18.4 Corneal degeneration
Excludes1 Mooren's ulcer (H16.0-)
recurrent erosion of cornea (H18.83-)
H18.40 Unspecified corneal degeneration

● H18.41 Arcus senilis
Senile corneal changes
H18.411 Arcus senilis, right eye
H18.412 Arcus senilis, left eye
H18.413 Arcus senilis, bilateral
H18.419 Arcus senilis, unspecified eye

● H18.42 Band keratopathy
H18.421 Band keratopathy, right eye
H18.422 Band keratopathy, left eye
H18.423 Band keratopathy, bilateral
H18.429 Band keratopathy, unspecified eye
H18.43 Other calcerous corneal degeneration

● H18.44 Keratomalacia
Excludes1 keratomalacia due to vitamin A deficiency (E50.4)
H18.441 Keratomalacia, right eye
H18.442 Keratomalacia, left eye
H18.443 Keratomalacia, bilateral
H18.449 Keratomalacia, unspecified eye

CHAPTER 7 (H00-H59)

● H18.45 Nodular corneal degeneration
H18.451 Nodular corneal degeneration, right eye
H18.452 Nodular corneal degeneration, left eye
H18.453 Nodular corneal degeneration, bilateral
H18.459 Nodular corneal degeneration, unspecified eye

● H18.46 Peripheral corneal degeneration
H18.461 Peripheral corneal degeneration, right eye
H18.462 Peripheral corneal degeneration, left eye
H18.463 Peripheral corneal degeneration, bilateral
H18.469 Peripheral corneal degeneration, unspecified eye

H18.49 Other corneal degeneration

● H18.5 Hereditary corneal dystrophies
H18.5Ø Unspecified hereditary corneal dystrophies
H18.51 Endothelial corneal dystrophy
Fuchs' dystrophy
H18.52 Epithelial (juvenile) corneal dystrophy
H18.53 Granular corneal dystrophy
H18.54 Lattice corneal dystrophy
H18.55 Macular corneal dystrophy
H18.59 Other hereditary corneal dystrophies

● H18.6 Keratoconus
● H18.6Ø Keratoconus, unspecified
H18.6Ø1 Keratoconus, unspecified, right eye
H18.6Ø2 Keratoconus, unspecified, left eye
H18.6Ø3 Keratoconus, unspecified, bilateral
H18.6Ø9 Keratoconus, unspecified, unspecified eye

● H18.61 Keratoconus, stable
H18.611 Keratoconus, stable, right eye
H18.612 Keratoconus, stable, left eye
H18.613 Keratoconus, stable, bilateral
H18.619 Keratoconus, stable, unspecified eye

● H18.62 Keratoconus, unstable
Acute hydrops
H18.621 Keratoconus, unstable, right eye
H18.622 Keratoconus, unstable, left eye
H18.623 Keratoconus, unstable, bilateral
H18.629 Keratoconus, unstable, unspecified eye

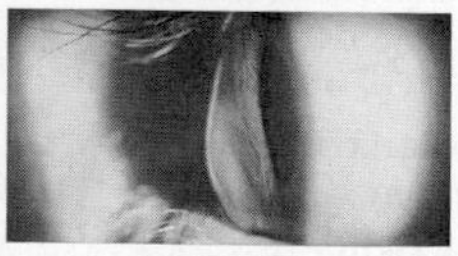

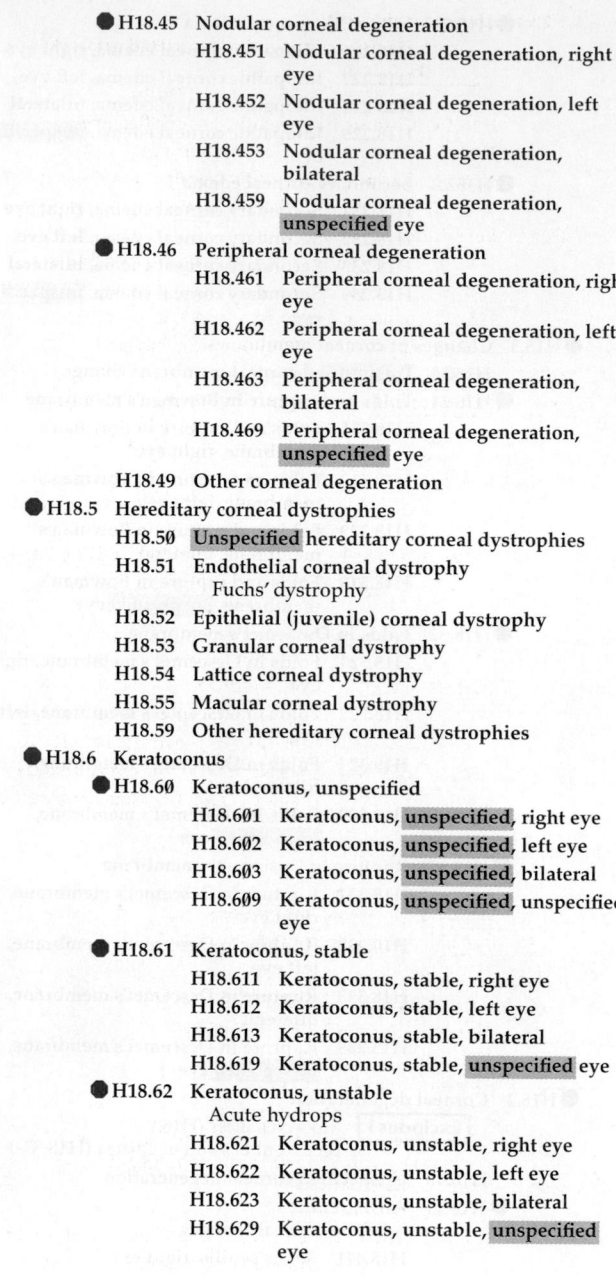

Figure 7-8 Lateral view of the displacement of the cone apex in keratoconus. (From Yanoff: Ophthalmology, ed 3, Mosby, Inc., 2008)

Item 7–4 Keratoconus results in corneal degeneration that begins in childhood, gradually changes the cornea from a round to cone shape, decreasing visual acuity. Treatment includes contact lenses. In severe cases the need for corneal transplant may be the treatment of choice; however, newer technologies may use high frequency radio energy to shrink the edges of the cornea, pulling the central area back to a more normal shape. It can help delay or avoid the need for a corneal transplantation.

● H18.7 Other and unspecified corneal deformities
Excludes1 congenital malformations of cornea (Q13.3-Q13.4)
H18.7Ø Unspecified corneal deformity

● H18.71 Corneal ectasia
H18.711 Corneal ectasia, right eye
H18.712 Corneal ectasia, left eye
H18.713 Corneal ectasia, bilateral
H18.719 Corneal ectasia, unspecified eye

● H18.72 Corneal staphyloma
H18.721 Corneal staphyloma, right eye
H18.722 Corneal staphyloma, left eye
H18.723 Corneal staphyloma, bilateral
H18.729 Corneal staphyloma, unspecified eye

● H18.73 Descemetocele
H18.731 Descemetocele, right eye
H18.732 Descemetocele, left eye
H18.733 Descemetocele, bilateral
H18.739 Descemetocele, unspecified eye

● H18.79 Other corneal deformities
H18.791 Other corneal deformities, right eye
H18.792 Other corneal deformities, left eye
H18.793 Other corneal deformities, bilateral
H18.799 Other corneal deformities, unspecified eye

● H18.8 Other specified disorders of cornea
● H18.81 Anesthesia and hypoesthesia of cornea
H18.811 Anesthesia and hypoesthesia of cornea, right eye
H18.812 Anesthesia and hypoesthesia of cornea, left eye
H18.813 Anesthesia and hypoesthesia of cornea, bilateral
H18.819 Anesthesia and hypoesthesia of cornea, unspecified eye

● H18.82 Corneal disorder due to contact lens
Excludes2 corneal edema due to contact lens (H18.21-)
H18.821 Corneal disorder due to contact lens, right eye
H18.822 Corneal disorder due to contact lens, left eye
H18.823 Corneal disorder due to contact lens, bilateral
H18.829 Corneal disorder due to contact lens, unspecified eye

● H18.83 Recurrent erosion of cornea
H18.831 Recurrent erosion of cornea, right eye
H18.832 Recurrent erosion of cornea, left eye
H18.833 Recurrent erosion of cornea, bilateral
H18.839 Recurrent erosion of cornea, unspecified eye

● H18.89 Other specified disorders of cornea
H18.891 Other specified disorders of cornea, right eye
H18.892 Other specified disorders of cornea, left eye
H18.893 Other specified disorders of cornea, bilateral
H18.899 Other specified disorders of cornea, unspecified eye

H18.9 Unspecified disorder of cornea

● H20 Iridocyclitis

● H20.0 Acute and subacute iridocyclitis
Acute anterior uveitis
Acute cyclitis
Acute iritis
Subacute anterior uveitis
Subacute cyclitis
Subacute iritis

Excludes1 iridocyclitis, iritis, uveitis (due to) (in) diabetes mellitus (E08-E13 with .39)
iridocyclitis, iritis, uveitis (due to) (in) diphtheria (A36.89)
iridocyclitis, iritis, uveitis (due to) (in) gonococcal (A54.32)
iridocyclitis, iritis, uveitis (due to) (in) herpes (simplex) (B00.51)
iridocyclitis, iritis, uveitis (due to) (in) herpes zoster (B02.32)
iridocyclitis, iritis, uveitis (due to) (in) late congenital syphilis (A50.39)
iridocyclitis, iritis, uveitis (due to) (in) late syphilis (A52.71)
iridocyclitis, iritis, uveitis (due to) (in) sarcoidosis (D86.83)
iridocyclitis, iritis, uveitis (due to) (in) syphilis (A51.43)
iridocyclitis, iritis, uveitis (due to) (in) toxoplasmosis (B58.09)
iridocyclitis, iritis, uveitis (due to) (in) tuberculosis (A18.54)

H20.00 Unspecified acute and subacute iridocyclitis

● H20.01 Primary iridocyclitis
H20.011 Primary iridocyclitis, right eye
H20.012 Primary iridocyclitis, left eye
H20.013 Primary iridocyclitis, bilateral
H20.019 Primary iridocyclitis, unspecified eye

● H20.02 Recurrent acute iridocyclitis
H20.021 Recurrent acute iridocyclitis, right eye
H20.022 Recurrent acute iridocyclitis, left eye
H20.023 Recurrent acute iridocyclitis, bilateral
H20.029 Recurrent acute iridocyclitis, unspecified eye

● H20.03 Secondary infectious iridocyclitis
H20.031 Secondary infectious iridocyclitis, right eye
H20.032 Secondary infectious iridocyclitis, left eye
H20.033 Secondary infectious iridocyclitis, bilateral
H20.039 Secondary infectious iridocyclitis, unspecified eye

● H20.04 Secondary noninfectious iridocyclitis
H20.041 Secondary noninfectious iridocyclitis, right eye
H20.042 Secondary noninfectious iridocyclitis, left eye
H20.043 Secondary noninfectious iridocyclitis, bilateral
H20.049 Secondary noninfectious iridocyclitis, unspecified eye

● H20.05 Hypopyon
H20.051 Hypopyon, right eye
H20.052 Hypopyon, left eye
H20.053 Hypopyon, bilateral
H20.059 Hypopyon, unspecified eye

● H20.1 Chronic iridocyclitis
Use additional code for any associated cataract (H26.21-)

Excludes2 posterior cyclitis (H30.2-)

H20.10 Chronic iridocyclitis, unspecified eye
H20.11 Chronic iridocyclitis, right eye
H20.12 Chronic iridocyclitis, left eye
H20.13 Chronic iridocyclitis, bilateral

● H20.2 Lens-induced iridocyclitis
H20.20 Lens-induced iridocyclitis, unspecified eye
H20.21 Lens-induced iridocyclitis, right eye
H20.22 Lens-induced iridocyclitis, left eye
H20.23 Lens-induced iridocyclitis, bilateral

● H20.8 Other iridocyclitis

Excludes2 glaucomatocyclitis crises (H40.4-)
posterior cyclitis (H30.2-)
sympathetic uveitis (H44.13-)

● H20.81 Fuchs' heterochromic cyclitis
H20.811 Fuchs' heterochromic cyclitis, right eye
H20.812 Fuchs' heterochromic cyclitis, left eye
H20.813 Fuchs' heterochromic cyclitis, bilateral
H20.819 Fuchs' heterochromic cyclitis, unspecified eye

● H20.82 Vogt-Koyanagi syndrome
H20.821 Vogt-Koyanagi syndrome, right eye
H20.822 Vogt-Koyanagi syndrome, left eye
H20.823 Vogt-Koyanagi syndrome, bilateral
H20.829 Vogt-Koyanagi syndrome, unspecified eye

H20.9 Unspecified iridocyclitis
Uveitis NOS

● H21 Other disorders of iris and ciliary body

Excludes2 sympathetic uveitis (H44.1-)

● H21.0 Hyphema

Excludes1 traumatic hyphema (S05.1-)

H21.00 Hyphema, unspecified eye
H21.01 Hyphema, right eye
H21.02 Hyphema, left eye
H21.03 Hyphema, bilateral

● H21.1 Other vascular disorders of iris and ciliary body
Neovascularization of iris or ciliary body
Rubeosis iridis
Rubeosis of iris

● H21.1X Other vascular disorders of iris and ciliary body
H21.1X1 Other vascular disorders of iris and ciliary body, right eye
H21.1X2 Other vascular disorders of iris and ciliary body, left eye
H21.1X3 Other vascular disorders of iris and ciliary body, bilateral
H21.1X9 Other vascular disorders of iris and ciliary body, unspecified eye

● H21.2 Degeneration of iris and ciliary body

● H21.21 Degeneration of chamber angle
H21.211 Degeneration of chamber angle, right eye
H21.212 Degeneration of chamber angle, left eye
H21.213 Degeneration of chamber angle, bilateral
H21.219 Degeneration of chamber angle, unspecified eye

CHAPTER 7 (H00-H59)

● H21.22 Degeneration of ciliary body
H21.221 Degeneration of ciliary body, right eye
H21.222 Degeneration of ciliary body, left eye
H21.223 Degeneration of ciliary body, bilateral
H21.229 Degeneration of ciliary body, unspecified eye

● H21.23 Degeneration of iris (pigmentary)
Translucency of iris
H21.231 Degeneration of iris (pigmentary), right eye
H21.232 Degeneration of iris (pigmentary), left eye
H21.233 Degeneration of iris (pigmentary), bilateral
H21.239 Degeneration of iris (pigmentary), unspecified eye

● H21.24 Degeneration of pupillary margin
H21.241 Degeneration of pupillary margin, right eye
H21.242 Degeneration of pupillary margin, left eye
H21.243 Degeneration of pupillary margin, bilateral
H21.249 Degeneration of pupillary margin, unspecified eye

● H21.25 Iridoschisis
H21.251 Iridoschisis, right eye
H21.252 Iridoschisis, left eye
H21.253 Iridoschisis, bilateral
H21.259 Iridoschisis, unspecified eye

● H21.26 Iris atrophy (essential) (progressive)
H21.261 Iris atrophy (essential) (progressive), right eye
H21.262 Iris atrophy (essential) (progressive), left eye
H21.263 Iris atrophy (essential) (progressive), bilateral
H21.269 Iris atrophy (essential) (progressive), unspecified eye

● H21.27 Miotic pupillary cyst
H21.271 Miotic pupillary cyst, right eye
H21.272 Miotic pupillary cyst, left eye
H21.273 Miotic pupillary cyst, bilateral
H21.279 Miotic pupillary cyst, unspecified eye

H21.29 Other iris atrophy

● H21.3 Cyst of iris, ciliary body and anterior chamber
Excludes2 miotic pupillary cyst (H21.27-)

● H21.30 Idiopathic cysts of iris, ciliary body or anterior chamber
Cyst of iris, ciliary body or anterior chamber NOS
H21.301 Idiopathic cysts of iris, ciliary body or anterior chamber, right eye
H21.302 Idiopathic cysts of iris, ciliary body or anterior chamber, left eye
H21.303 Idiopathic cysts of iris, ciliary body or anterior chamber, bilateral
H21.309 Idiopathic cysts of iris, ciliary body or anterior chamber, unspecified eye

● H21.31 Exudative cysts of iris or anterior chamber
H21.311 Exudative cysts of iris or anterior chamber, right eye
H21.312 Exudative cysts of iris or anterior chamber, left eye
H21.313 Exudative cysts of iris or anterior chamber, bilateral
H21.319 Exudative cysts of iris or anterior chamber, unspecified eye

● H21.32 Implantation cysts of iris, ciliary body or anterior chamber
H21.321 Implantation cysts of iris, ciliary body or anterior chamber, right eye
H21.322 Implantation cysts of iris, ciliary body or anterior chamber, left eye
H21.323 Implantation cysts of iris, ciliary body or anterior chamber, bilateral
H21.329 Implantation cysts of iris, ciliary body or anterior chamber, unspecified eye

● H21.33 Parasitic cyst of iris, ciliary body or anterior chamber
H21.331 Parasitic cyst of iris, ciliary body or anterior chamber, right eye
H21.332 Parasitic cyst of iris, ciliary body or anterior chamber, left eye
H21.333 Parasitic cyst of iris, ciliary body or anterior chamber, bilateral
H21.339 Parasitic cyst of iris, ciliary body or anterior chamber, unspecified eye

● H21.34 Primary cyst of pars plana
H21.341 Primary cyst of pars plana, right eye
H21.342 Primary cyst of pars plana, left eye
H21.343 Primary cyst of pars plana, bilateral
H21.349 Primary cyst of pars plana, unspecified eye

● H21.35 Exudative cyst of pars plana
H21.351 Exudative cyst of pars plana, right eye
H21.352 Exudative cyst of pars plana, left eye
H21.353 Exudative cyst of pars plana, bilateral
H21.359 Exudative cyst of pars plana, unspecified eye

● H21.4 Pupillary membranes
Iris bombé
Pupillary occlusion
Pupillary seclusion
Excludes1 congenital pupillary membranes (Q13.8)
H21.40 Pupillary membranes, unspecified eye
H21.41 Pupillary membranes, right eye
H21.42 Pupillary membranes, left eye
H21.43 Pupillary membranes, bilateral

● H21.5 Other and unspecified adhesions and disruptions of iris and ciliary body
Excludes1 corectopia (Q13.2)

● H21.50 Unspecified adhesions of iris
Synechia (iris) NOS
H21.501 Unspecified adhesions of iris, right eye
H21.502 Unspecified adhesions of iris, left eye
H21.503 Unspecified adhesions of iris, bilateral
H21.509 Unspecified adhesions of iris and ciliary body, unspecified eye

● H21.51 Anterior synechiae (iris)
H21.511 Anterior synechiae (iris), right eye
H21.512 Anterior synechiae (iris), left eye
H21.513 Anterior synechiae (iris), bilateral
H21.519 Anterior synechiae (iris), unspecified eye

● H21.52 Goniosynechiae
H21.521 Goniosynechiae, right eye
H21.522 Goniosynechiae, left eye
H21.523 Goniosynechiae, bilateral
H21.529 Goniosynechiae, unspecified eye

● H21.53 Iridodialysis
- H21.531 Iridodialysis, right eye
- H21.532 Iridodialysis, left eye
- H21.533 Iridodialysis, bilateral
- H21.539 Iridodialysis, unspecified eye

● H21.54 Posterior synechiae (iris)
- H21.541 Posterior synechiae (iris), right eye
- H21.542 Posterior synechiae (iris), left eye
- H21.543 Posterior synechiae (iris), bilateral
- H21.549 Posterior synechiae (iris), unspecified eye

● H21.55 Recession of chamber angle
- H21.551 Recession of chamber angle, right eye
- H21.552 Recession of chamber angle, left eye
- H21.553 Recession of chamber angle, bilateral
- H21.559 Recession of chamber angle, unspecified eye

● H21.56 Pupillary abnormalities
Deformed pupil
Ectopic pupil
Rupture of sphincter, pupil
Excludes1 congenital deformity of pupil (Q13.2-)
- H21.561 Pupillary abnormality, right eye
- H21.562 Pupillary abnormality, left eye
- H21.563 Pupillary abnormality, bilateral
- H21.569 Pupillary abnormality, unspecified eye

● H21.8 Other specified disorders of iris and ciliary body
- H21.81 Floppy iris syndrome
  Intraoperative floppy iris syndrome (IFIS)
  Use additional code for adverse effect, if applicable, to identify drug (T36-T5Ø with fifth or sixth character 5)
- H21.82 Plateau iris syndrome (post-iridectomy) (postprocedural)
- H21.89 Other specified disorders of iris and ciliary body

H21.9 Unspecified disorder of iris and ciliary body

H22 Disorders of iris and ciliary body in diseases classified elsewhere
Code first underlying disease, such as:
gout (M1A.-, M1Ø.-)
leprosy (A3Ø.-)
parasitic disease (B89)

DISORDERS OF LENS (H25-H28)

● H25 Age-related cataract
Senile cataract
Excludes2 capsular glaucoma with pseudoexfoliation of lens (H4Ø.1-)

● H25.Ø Age-related incipient cataract

● H25.Ø1 Cortical age-related cataract
- H25.Ø11 Cortical age-related cataract, right eye
- H25.Ø12 Cortical age-related cataract, left eye
- H25.Ø13 Cortical age-related cataract, bilateral
- H25.Ø19 Cortical age-related cataract, unspecified eye

● H25.Ø3 Anterior subcapsular polar age-related cataract
- H25.Ø31 Anterior subcapsular polar age-related cataract, right eye
- H25.Ø32 Anterior subcapsular polar age-related cataract, left eye
- H25.Ø33 Anterior subcapsular polar age-related cataract, bilateral
- H25.Ø39 Anterior subcapsular polar age-related cataract, unspecified eye

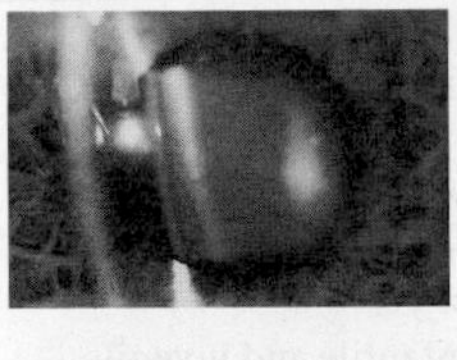

Figure 7-9 Age-related cataract. Nuclear sclerosis and cortical lens opacities are present. (From Yanoff: Ophthalmology, ed 3, Mosby, Inc., 2008)

Item 7–5 Senile cataracts are linked to the aging process. The most common area for the formation of a cataract is the cortical area of the lens. **Polar cataracts** can be either anterior or posterior. **Anterior polar cataracts** are more common and are small, white, capsular cataracts located on the anterior portion of the lens. **Total cataracts,** also called **complete** or **mature,** cause an opacity of all fibers of the lens. **Hypermature** describes a mature cataract with a swollen, milky cortex that covers the entire lens. **Immature,** also called **incipient,** cataracts have a clear cortex and are only slightly opaque. Treatment for all cataracts is the removal of the lens.

● H25.Ø4 Posterior subcapsular polar age-related cataract
- H25.Ø41 Posterior subcapsular polar age-related cataract, right eye
- H25.Ø42 Posterior subcapsular polar age-related cataract, left eye
- H25.Ø43 Posterior subcapsular polar age-related cataract, bilateral
- H25.Ø49 Posterior subcapsular polar age-related cataract, unspecified eye

● H25.Ø9 Other age-related incipient cataract
Coronary age-related cataract
Punctate age-related cataract
Water clefts
- H25.Ø91 Other age-related incipient cataract, right eye
- H25.Ø92 Other age-related incipient cataract, left eye
- H25.Ø93 Other age-related incipient cataract, bilateral
- H25.Ø99 Other age-related incipient cataract, unspecified eye

● H25.1 Age-related nuclear cataract
Cataracta brunescens
Nuclear sclerosis cataract
- H25.1Ø Age-related nuclear cataract, unspecified eye
- H25.11 Age-related nuclear cataract, right eye
- H25.12 Age-related nuclear cataract, left eye
- H25.13 Age-related nuclear cataract, bilateral

● H25.2 Age-related cataract, morgagnian type
Age-related hypermature cataract
- H25.2Ø Age-related cataract, morgagnian type, unspecified eye
- H25.21 Age-related cataract, morgagnian type, right eye
- H25.22 Age-related cataract, morgagnian type, left eye
- H25.23 Age-related cataract, morgagnian type, bilateral

● H25.8 Other age-related cataract

● H25.81 Combined forms of age-related cataract
- H25.811 Combined forms of age-related cataract, right eye
- H25.812 Combined forms of age-related cataract, left eye
- H25.813 Combined forms of age-related cataract, bilateral
- H25.819 Combined forms of age-related cataract, unspecified eye

H25.89 Other age-related cataract

H25.9 Unspecified age-related cataract

● H26 Other cataract
Excludes1 congenital cataract (Q12.0)
● H26.0 Infantile and juvenile cataract
● H26.00 Unspecified infantile and juvenile cataract
H26.001 Unspecified infantile and juvenile cataract, right eye
H26.002 Unspecified infantile and juvenile cataract, left eye
H26.003 Unspecified infantile and juvenile cataract, bilateral
H26.009 Unspecified infantile and juvenile cataract, unspecified eye
● H26.01 Infantile and juvenile cortical, lamellar, or zonular cataract
H26.011 Infantile and juvenile cortical, lamellar, or zonular cataract, right eye
H26.012 Infantile and juvenile cortical, lamellar, or zonular cataract, left eye
H26.013 Infantile and juvenile cortical, lamellar, or zonular cataract, bilateral
H26.019 Infantile and juvenile cortical, lamellar, or zonular cataract, unspecified eye
● H26.03 Infantile and juvenile nuclear cataract
H26.031 Infantile and juvenile nuclear cataract, right eye
H26.032 Infantile and juvenile nuclear cataract, left eye
H26.033 Infantile and juvenile nuclear cataract, bilateral
H26.039 Infantile and juvenile nuclear cataract, unspecified eye
● H26.04 Anterior subcapsular polar infantile and juvenile cataract
H26.041 Anterior subcapsular polar infantile and juvenile cataract, right eye
H26.042 Anterior subcapsular polar infantile and juvenile cataract, left eye
H26.043 Anterior subcapsular polar infantile and juvenile cataract, bilateral
H26.049 Anterior subcapsular polar infantile and juvenile cataract, unspecified eye
● H26.05 Posterior subcapsular polar infantile and juvenile cataract
H26.051 Posterior subcapsular polar infantile and juvenile cataract, right eye
H26.052 Posterior subcapsular polar infantile and juvenile cataract, left eye
H26.053 Posterior subcapsular polar infantile and juvenile cataract, bilateral
H26.059 Posterior subcapsular polar infantile and juvenile cataract, unspecified eye
● H26.06 Combined forms of infantile and juvenile cataract
H26.061 Combined forms of infantile and juvenile cataract, right eye
H26.062 Combined forms of infantile and juvenile cataract, left eye
H26.063 Combined forms of infantile and juvenile cataract bilateral
H26.069 Combined forms of infantile and juvenile cataract, unspecified eye
H26.09 Other infantile and juvenile cataract

● H26.1 Traumatic cataract
Use additional code (Chapter 20) to identify external cause
● H26.10 Unspecified traumatic cataract
H26.101 Unspecified traumatic cataract, right eye
H26.102 Unspecified traumatic cataract, left eye
H26.103 Unspecified traumatic cataract, bilateral
H26.109 Unspecified traumatic cataract, unspecified eye
● H26.11 Localized traumatic opacities
H26.111 Localized traumatic opacities, right eye
H26.112 Localized traumatic opacities, left eye
H26.113 Localized traumatic opacities, bilateral
H26.119 Localized traumatic opacities, unspecified eye
● H26.12 Partially resolved traumatic cataract
H26.121 Partially resolved traumatic cataract, right eye
H26.122 Partially resolved traumatic cataract, left eye
H26.123 Partially resolved traumatic cataract, bilateral
H26.129 Partially resolved traumatic cataract, unspecified eye
● H26.13 Total traumatic cataract
H26.131 Total traumatic cataract, right eye
H26.132 Total traumatic cataract, left eye
H26.133 Total traumatic cataract, bilateral
H26.139 Total traumatic cataract, unspecified eye
● H26.2 Complicated cataract
H26.20 Unspecified complicated cataract
Cataracta complicata NOS
● H26.21 Cataract with neovascularization
Code also associated condition, such as:
chronic iridocyclitis (H20.1-)
H26.211 Cataract with neovascularization, right eye
H26.212 Cataract with neovascularization, left eye
H26.213 Cataract with neovascularization, bilateral
H26.219 Cataract with neovascularization, unspecified eye
● H26.22 Cataract secondary to ocular disorders (degenerative) (inflammatory)
Code also associated ocular disorder
H26.221 Cataract secondary to ocular disorders (degenerative) (inflammatory), right eye
H26.222 Cataract secondary to ocular disorders (degenerative) (inflammatory), left eye
H26.223 Cataract secondary to ocular disorders (degenerative) (inflammatory), bilateral
H26.229 Cataract secondary to ocular disorders (degenerative) (inflammatory), unspecified eye
● H26.23 Glaucomatous flecks (subcapsular)
Code first *underlying glaucoma (H40-H42)*
H26.231 Glaucomatous flecks (subcapsular), right eye
H26.232 Glaucomatous flecks (subcapsular), left eye

H26.233 Glaucomatous flecks (subcapsular), bilateral
H26.239 Glaucomatous flecks (subcapsular), unspecified eye

● **H26.3 Drug-induced cataract**
Toxic cataract
Use additional code for adverse effect, if applicable, to identify drug (T36-T50 with fifth or sixth character 5)
H26.30 Drug-induced cataract, unspecified eye
H26.31 Drug-induced cataract, right eye
H26.32 Drug-induced cataract, left eye
H26.33 Drug-induced cataract, bilateral

● **H26.4 Secondary cataract**
H26.40 Unspecified secondary cataract
● H26.41 Soemmering's ring
H26.411 Soemmering's ring, right eye
H26.412 Soemmering's ring, left eye
H26.413 Soemmering's ring, bilateral
H26.419 Soemmering's ring, unspecified eye
● H26.49 Other secondary cataract
H26.491 Other secondary cataract, right eye
H26.492 Other secondary cataract, left eye
H26.493 Other secondary cataract, bilateral
H26.499 Other secondary cataract, unspecified eye

H26.8 Other specified cataract
H26.9 Unspecified cataract

● **H27 Other disorders of lens**
Excludes1 congenital lens malformations (Q12.-)
mechanical complications of intraocular lens implant (T85.2)
pseudophakia (Z96.1)

● **H27.0 Aphakia**
Acquired absence of lens
Acquired aphakia
Aphakia due to trauma
Excludes1 cataract extraction status (Z98.4-)
congenital absence of lens (Q12.3)
congenital aphakia (Q12.3)
H27.00 Aphakia, unspecified eye
H27.01 Aphakia, right eye
H27.02 Aphakia, left eye
H27.03 Aphakia, bilateral

● **H27.1 Dislocation of lens**
H27.10 Unspecified dislocation of lens
● H27.11 Subluxation of lens
H27.111 Subluxation of lens, right eye
H27.112 Subluxation of lens, left eye
H27.113 Subluxation of lens, bilateral
H27.119 Subluxation of lens, unspecified eye
● H27.12 Anterior dislocation of lens
H27.121 Anterior dislocation of lens, right eye
H27.122 Anterior dislocation of lens, left eye
H27.123 Anterior dislocation of lens, bilateral
H27.129 Anterior dislocation of lens, unspecified eye
● H27.13 Posterior dislocation of lens
H27.131 Posterior dislocation of lens, right eye
H27.132 Posterior dislocation of lens, left eye
H27.133 Posterior dislocation of lens, bilateral
H27.139 Posterior dislocation of lens, unspecified eye

H27.8 Other specified disorders of lens
H27.9 Unspecified disorder of lens

H28 Cataract in diseases classified elsewhere
Code first underlying disease, such as:
hypoparathyroidism (E20.-)
myotonia (G71.1-)
myxedema (E03.-)
protein-calorie malnutrition (E40-E46)
Excludes1 cataract in diabetes mellitus (E08.36, E09.36, E10.36, E11.36, E13.36)

DISORDERS OF CHOROID AND RETINA (H30-H36)

★(See Plate 90 on page NAP-16.)

● **H30 Chorioretinal inflammation**

● **H30.0 Focal chorioretinal inflammation**
Focal chorioretinitis
Focal choroiditis
Focal retinitis
Focal retinochoroiditis
● H30.00 Unspecified focal chorioretinal inflammation
Focal chorioretinitis NOS
Focal choroiditis NOS
Focal retinitis NOS
Focal retinochoroiditis NOS
H30.001 Unspecified focal chorioretinal inflammation, right eye
H30.002 Unspecified focal chorioretinal inflammation, left eye
H30.003 Unspecified focal chorioretinal inflammation, bilateral
H30.009 Unspecified focal chorioretinal inflammation, unspecified eye
● H30.01 Focal chorioretinal inflammation, juxtapapillary
H30.011 Focal chorioretinal inflammation, juxtapapillary, right eye
H30.012 Focal chorioretinal inflammation, juxtapapillary, left eye
H30.013 Focal chorioretinal inflammation, juxtapapillary, bilateral
H30.019 Focal chorioretinal inflammation, juxtapapillary, unspecified eye
● H30.02 Focal chorioretinal inflammation of posterior pole
H30.021 Focal chorioretinal inflammation of posterior pole, right eye
H30.022 Focal chorioretinal inflammation of posterior pole, left eye
H30.023 Focal chorioretinal inflammation of posterior pole, bilateral
H30.029 Focal chorioretinal inflammation of posterior pole, unspecified eye
● H30.03 Focal chorioretinal inflammation, peripheral
H30.031 Focal chorioretinal inflammation, peripheral, right eye
H30.032 Focal chorioretinal inflammation, peripheral, left eye
H30.033 Focal chorioretinal inflammation, peripheral, bilateral
H30.039 Focal chorioretinal inflammation, peripheral, unspecified eye
● H30.04 Focal chorioretinal inflammation, macular or paramacular
H30.041 Focal chorioretinal inflammation, macular or paramacular, right eye
H30.042 Focal chorioretinal inflammation, macular or paramacular, left eye
H30.043 Focal chorioretinal inflammation, macular or paramacular, bilateral
H30.049 Focal chorioretinal inflammation, macular or paramacular, unspecified eye

● H30.1 Disseminated chorioretinal inflammation
Disseminated chorioretinitis
Disseminated choroiditis
Disseminated retinitis
Disseminated retinochoroiditis
Excludes2 exudative retinopathy (H35.02-)

● H30.10 Unspecified disseminated chorioretinal inflammation
Disseminated chorioretinitis NOS
Disseminated choroiditis NOS
Disseminated retinitis NOS
Disseminated retinochoroiditis NOS
H30.101 Unspecified disseminated chorioretinal inflammation, right eye
H30.102 Unspecified disseminated chorioretinal inflammation, left eye
H30.103 Unspecified disseminated chorioretinal inflammation, bilateral
H30.109 Unspecified disseminated chorioretinal inflammation, unspecified eye

● H30.11 Disseminated chorioretinal inflammation of posterior pole
H30.111 Disseminated chorioretinal inflammation of posterior pole, right eye
H30.112 Disseminated chorioretinal inflammation of posterior pole, left eye
H30.113 Disseminated chorioretinal inflammation of posterior pole, bilateral
H30.119 Disseminated chorioretinal inflammation of posterior pole, unspecified eye

● H30.12 Disseminated chorioretinal inflammation, peripheral
H30.121 Disseminated chorioretinal inflammation, peripheral right eye
H30.122 Disseminated chorioretinal inflammation, peripheral, left eye
H30.123 Disseminated chorioretinal inflammation, peripheral, bilateral
H30.129 Disseminated chorioretinal inflammation, peripheral, unspecified eye

● H30.13 Disseminated chorioretinal inflammation, generalized
H30.131 Disseminated chorioretinal inflammation, generalized, right eye
H30.132 Disseminated chorioretinal inflammation, generalized, left eye
H30.133 Disseminated chorioretinal inflammation, generalized, bilateral
H30.139 Disseminated chorioretinal inflammation, generalized, unspecified eye

● H30.14 Acute posterior multifocal placoid pigment epitheliopathy
H30.141 Acute posterior multifocal placoid pigment epitheliopathy, right eye
H30.142 Acute posterior multifocal placoid pigment epitheliopathy, left eye
H30.143 Acute posterior multifocal placoid pigment epitheliopathy, bilateral
H30.149 Acute posterior multifocal placoid pigment epitheliopathy, unspecified eye

● H30.2 Posterior cyclitis
Pars planitis
H30.20 Posterior cyclitis, unspecified eye
H30.21 Posterior cyclitis, right eye
H30.22 Posterior cyclitis, left eye
H30.23 Posterior cyclitis, bilateral

● H30.8 Other chorioretinal inflammations

● H30.81 Harada's disease
H30.811 Harada's disease, right eye
H30.812 Harada's disease, left eye
H30.813 Harada's disease, bilateral
H30.819 Harada's disease, unspecified eye

● H30.89 Other chorioretinal inflammations
H30.891 Other chorioretinal inflammations, right eye
H30.892 Other chorioretinal inflammations, left eye
H30.893 Other chorioretinal inflammations, bilateral
H30.899 Other chorioretinal inflammations, unspecified eye

● H30.9 Unspecified chorioretinal inflammation
Chorioretinitis NOS
Choroiditis NOS
Neuroretinitis NOS
Retinitis NOS
Retinochoroiditis NOS
H30.90 Unspecified chorioretinal inflammation, unspecified eye
H30.91 Unspecified chorioretinal inflammation, right eye
H30.92 Unspecified chorioretinal inflammation, left eye
H30.93 Unspecified chorioretinal inflammation, bilateral

● H31 Other disorders of choroid

● H31.0 Chorioretinal scars
Excludes2 postsurgical chorioretinal scars (H59.81-)

● H31.00 Unspecified chorioretinal scars
H31.001 Unspecified chorioretinal scars, right eye
H31.002 Unspecified chorioretinal scars, left eye
H31.003 Unspecified chorioretinal scars, bilateral
H31.009 Unspecified chorioretinal scars, unspecified eye

● H31.01 Macula scars of posterior pole (postinflammatory) (post-traumatic)
Excludes1 postprocedural chorioretinal scar (H59.81-)
H31.011 Macula scars of posterior pole (postinflammatory) (post-traumatic), right eye
H31.012 Macula scars of posterior pole (postinflammatory) (post-traumatic), left eye
H31.013 Macula scars of posterior pole (postinflammatory) (post-traumatic), bilateral
H31.019 Macula scars of posterior pole (postinflammatory) (post-traumatic), unspecified eye

● H31.02 Solar retinopathy
H31.021 Solar retinopathy, right eye
H31.022 Solar retinopathy, left eye
H31.023 Solar retinopathy, bilateral
H31.029 Solar retinopathy, unspecified eye
● H31.09 Other chorioretinal scars
H31.091 Other chorioretinal scars, right eye
H31.092 Other chorioretinal scars, left eye
H31.093 Other chorioretinal scars, bilateral
H31.099 Other chorioretinal scars, unspecified eye
● H31.1 Choroidal degeneration
Excludes2 angioid streaks of macula (H35.33)
● H31.10 Unspecified choroidal degeneration
Choroidal sclerosis NOS
H31.101 Choroidal degeneration, unspecified, right eye
H31.102 Choroidal degeneration, unspecified, left eye
H31.103 Choroidal degeneration, unspecified, bilateral
H31.109 Choroidal degeneration, unspecified, unspecified eye
● H31.11 Age-related choroidal atrophy
H31.111 Age-related choroidal atrophy, right eye
H31.112 Age-related choroidal atrophy, left eye
H31.113 Age-related choroidal atrophy, bilateral
H31.119 Age-related choroidal atrophy, unspecified eye
● H31.12 Diffuse secondary atrophy of choroid
H31.121 Diffuse secondary atrophy of choroid, right eye
H31.122 Diffuse secondary atrophy of choroid, left eye
H31.123 Diffuse secondary atrophy of choroid, bilateral
H31.129 Diffuse secondary atrophy of choroid, unspecified eye
● H31.2 Hereditary choroidal dystrophy
Excludes2 hyperornithinemia (E72.4)
ornithinemia (E72.4)
H31.20 Hereditary choroidal dystrophy, unspecified
H31.21 Choroideremia
H31.22 Choroidal dystrophy (central areolar) (generalized) (peripapillary)
H31.23 Gyrate atrophy, choroid
H31.29 Other hereditary choroidal dystrophy
● H31.3 Choroidal hemorrhage and rupture
● H31.30 Unspecified choroidal hemorrhage
H31.301 Unspecified choroidal hemorrhage, right eye
H31.302 Unspecified choroidal hemorrhage, left eye
H31.303 Unspecified choroidal hemorrhage, bilateral
H31.309 Unspecified choroidal hemorrhage, unspecified eye
● H31.31 Expulsive choroidal hemorrhage
H31.311 Expulsive choroidal hemorrhage, right eye
H31.312 Expulsive choroidal hemorrhage, left eye
H31.313 Expulsive choroidal hemorrhage, bilateral
H31.319 Expulsive choroidal hemorrhage, unspecified eye
● H31.32 Choroidal rupture
H31.321 Choroidal rupture, right eye
H31.322 Choroidal rupture, left eye
H31.323 Choroidal rupture, bilateral
H31.329 Choroidal rupture, unspecified eye
● H31.4 Choroidal detachment
● H31.40 Unspecified choroidal detachment
H31.401 Unspecified choroidal detachment, right eye
H31.402 Unspecified choroidal detachment, left eye
H31.403 Unspecified choroidal detachment, bilateral
H31.409 Unspecified choroidal detachment, unspecified eye
● H31.41 Hemorrhagic choroidal detachment
H31.411 Hemorrhagic choroidal detachment, right eye
H31.412 Hemorrhagic choroidal detachment, left eye
H31.413 Hemorrhagic choroidal detachment, bilateral
H31.419 Hemorrhagic choroidal detachment, unspecified eye
● H31.42 Serous choroidal detachment
H31.421 Serous choroidal detachment, right eye
H31.422 Serous choroidal detachment, left eye
H31.423 Serous choroidal detachment, bilateral
H31.429 Serous choroidal detachment, unspecified eye
H31.8 Other specified disorders of choroid
H31.9 Unspecified disorder of choroid
H32 Chorioretinal disorders in diseases classified elsewhere
Code first underlying disease, such as:
congenital toxoplasmosis (P37.1)
histoplasmosis (B39.-)
leprosy (A30.-)
Excludes1 chorioretinitis (in):
toxoplasmosis (acquired) (B58.01)
tuberculosis (A18.53)
● H33 Retinal detachments and breaks
Excludes1 detachment of retinal pigment epithelium (H35.72-, H35.73-)
● H33.0 Retinal detachment with retinal break
Rhegmatogenous retinal detachment
Excludes1 serous retinal detachment (without retinal break) (H33.2-)
● H33.00 Unspecified retinal detachment with retinal break
H33.001 Unspecified retinal detachment with retinal break, right eye
H33.002 Unspecified retinal detachment with retinal break, left eye
H33.003 Unspecified retinal detachment with retinal break, bilateral
H33.009 Unspecified retinal detachment with retinal break, unspecified eye

CHAPTER 7 (H00-H59)

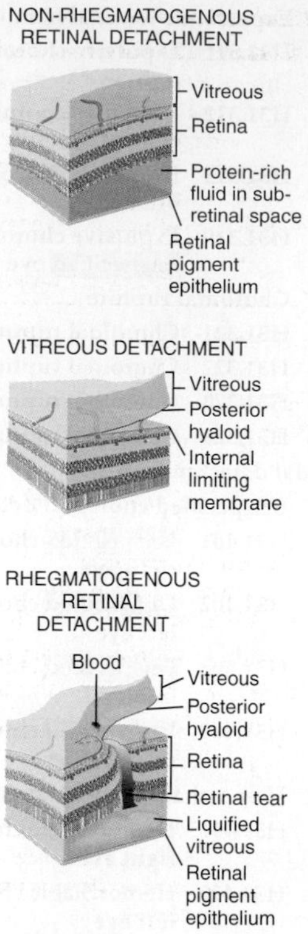

Figure 7-10 Retinal detachment. (From Kumar: Robbins and Cotran: Pathologic Basis of Disease, ed 7, Saunders, 2005)

Item 7-6 Retinal detachments and defects are conditions of the eye in which the retina separates from the underlying tissue. Initial detachment may be localized, requiring rapid treatment (medical emergency) to avoid the entire retina from detaching which leads to vision loss and blindness.

● **H33.Ø1 Retinal detachment with single break**
- **H33.Ø11 Retinal detachment with single break, right eye**
- **H33.Ø12 Retinal detachment with single break, left eye**
- **H33.Ø13 Retinal detachment with single break, bilateral**
- **H33.Ø19 Retinal detachment with single break, unspecified eye**

● **H33.Ø2 Retinal detachment with multiple breaks**
- **H33.Ø21 Retinal detachment with multiple breaks, right eye**
- **H33.Ø22 Retinal detachment with multiple breaks, left eye**
- **H33.Ø23 Retinal detachment with multiple breaks, bilateral**
- **H33.Ø29 Retinal detachment with multiple breaks, unspecified eye**

● **H33.Ø3 Retinal detachment with giant retinal tear**
- **H33.Ø31 Retinal detachment with giant retinal tear, right eye**
- **H33.Ø32 Retinal detachment with giant retinal tear, left eye**
- **H33.Ø33 Retinal detachment with giant retinal tear, bilateral**
- **H33.Ø39 Retinal detachment with giant retinal tear, unspecified eye**

● **H33.Ø4 Retinal detachment with retinal dialysis**
- **H33.Ø41 Retinal detachment with retinal dialysis, right eye**
- **H33.Ø42 Retinal detachment with retinal dialysis, left eye**
- **H33.Ø43 Retinal detachment with retinal dialysis, bilateral**
- **H33.Ø49 Retinal detachment with retinal dialysis, unspecified eye**

● **H33.Ø5 Total retinal detachment**
- **H33.Ø51 Total retinal detachment, right eye**
- **H33.Ø52 Total retinal detachment, left eye**
- **H33.Ø53 Total retinal detachment, bilateral**
- **H33.Ø59 Total retinal detachment, unspecified eye**

● **H33.1 Retinoschisis and retinal cysts**

Excludes1 congenital retinoschisis (Q14.1)
microcystoid degeneration of retina (H35.42-)

● **H33.1Ø Unspecified retinoschisis**
- **H33.1Ø1 Unspecified retinoschisis, right eye**
- **H33.1Ø2 Unspecified retinoschisis, left eye**
- **H33.1Ø3 Unspecified retinoschisis, bilateral**
- **H33.1Ø9 Unspecified retinoschisis, unspecified eye**

● **H33.11 Cyst of ora serrata**
- **H33.111 Cyst of ora serrata, right eye**
- **H33.112 Cyst of ora serrata, left eye**
- **H33.113 Cyst of ora serrata, bilateral**
- **H33.119 Cyst of ora serrata, unspecified eye**

● **H33.12 Parasitic cyst of retina**
- **H33.121 Parasitic cyst of retina, right eye**
- **H33.122 Parasitic cyst of retina, left eye**
- **H33.123 Parasitic cyst of retina, bilateral**
- **H33.129 Parasitic cyst of retina, unspecified eye**

● **H33.19 Other retinoschisis and retinal cysts**
Pseudocyst of retina
- **H33.191 Other retinoschisis and retinal cysts, right eye**
- **H33.192 Other retinoschisis and retinal cysts, left eye**
- **H33.193 Other retinoschisis and retinal cysts, bilateral**
- **H33.199 Other retinoschisis and retinal cysts, unspecified eye**

● **H33.2 Serous retinal detachment**
Retinal detachment NOS
Retinal detachment without retinal break

Excludes1 central serous chorioretinopathy (H35.71-)

- **H33.2Ø Serous retinal detachment, unspecified eye**
- **H33.21 Serous retinal detachment, right eye**
- **H33.22 Serous retinal detachment, left eye**
- **H33.23 Serous retinal detachment, bilateral**

● **H33.3 Retinal breaks without detachment**

Excludes1 chorioretinal scars after surgery for detachment (H59.81-)
peripheral retinal degeneration without break (H35.4-)

● **H33.3Ø Unspecified retinal break**
- **H33.3Ø1 Unspecified retinal break, right eye**
- **H33.3Ø2 Unspecified retinal break, left eye**
- **H33.3Ø3 Unspecified retinal break, bilateral**
- **H33.3Ø9 Unspecified retinal break, unspecified eye**

● H33.31 Horseshoe tear of retina without detachment
Operculum of retina without detachment
H33.311 Horseshoe tear of retina without detachment, right eye
H33.312 Horseshoe tear of retina without detachment, left eye
H33.313 Horseshoe tear of retina without detachment, bilateral
H33.319 Horseshoe tear of retina without detachment, unspecified eye
● H33.32 Round hole of retina without detachment
H33.321 Round hole, right eye
H33.322 Round hole, left eye
H33.323 Round hole, bilateral
H33.329 Round hole, unspecified eye
● H33.33 Multiple defects of retina without detachment
H33.331 Multiple defects of retina without detachment, right eye
H33.332 Multiple defects of retina without detachment, left eye
H33.333 Multiple defects of retina without detachment, bilateral
H33.339 Multiple defects of retina without detachment, unspecified eye
● H33.4 Traction detachment of retina
Proliferative vitreo-retinopathy with retinal detachment
H33.40 Traction detachment of retina, unspecified eye
H33.41 Traction detachment of retina, right eye
H33.42 Traction detachment of retina, left eye
H33.43 Traction detachment of retina, bilateral
H33.8 Other retinal detachments

● **H34 Retinal vascular occlusions**
Blockage in vessel of the retina
Excludes1 amaurosis fugax (G45.3)
● H34.0 Transient retinal artery occlusion
H34.00 Transient retinal artery occlusion, unspecified eye
H34.01 Transient retinal artery occlusion, right eye
H34.02 Transient retinal artery occlusion, left eye
H34.03 Transient retinal artery occlusion, bilateral
● H34.1 Central retinal artery occlusion
H34.10 Central retinal artery occlusion, unspecified eye
H34.11 Central retinal artery occlusion, right eye
H34.12 Central retinal artery occlusion, left eye
H34.13 Central retinal artery occlusion, bilateral
● H34.2 Other retinal artery occlusions
● H34.21 Partial retinal artery occlusion
Hollenhorst's plaque
Retinal microembolism
H34.211 Partial retinal artery occlusion, right eye
H34.212 Partial retinal artery occlusion, left eye
H34.213 Partial retinal artery occlusion, bilateral
H34.219 Partial retinal artery occlusion, unspecified eye
● H34.23 Retinal artery branch occlusion
H34.231 Retinal artery branch occlusion, right eye
H34.232 Retinal artery branch occlusion, left eye
H34.233 Retinal artery branch occlusion, bilateral
H34.239 Retinal artery branch occlusion, unspecified eye
● H34.8 Other retinal vascular occlusions
● H34.81 Central retinal vein occlusion
One of the following 7th characters is to be assigned to codes in subcategory H34.81 to designate the severity of the occlusion: ◀

0 with macular edema ◀
1 with retinal neovascularization ◀
2 stable ◀
Old central retinal vein occlusion ◀

● H34.811 Central retinal vein occlusion, right eye
● H34.812 Central retinal vein occlusion, left eye
● H34.813 Central retinal vein occlusion, bilateral
● H34.819 Central retinal vein occlusion, unspecified eye
● H34.82 Venous engorgement
Incipient retinal vein occlusion
Partial retinal vein occlusion
H34.821 Venous engorgement, right eye
H34.822 Venous engorgement, left eye
H34.823 Venous engorgement, bilateral
H34.829 Venous engorgement, unspecified eye
● H34.83 Tributary (branch) retinal vein occlusion
One of the following 7th characters is to be assigned to codes in subcategory H34.83 to designate the severity of the occlusion: ◀

0 with macular edema ◀
1 with retinal neovascularization ◀
2 stable ◀
Old tributary (branch) retinal vein occlusion ◀

● H34.831 Tributary (branch) retinal vein occlusion, right eye
● H34.832 Tributary (branch) retinal vein occlusion, left eye
● H34.833 Tributary (branch) retinal vein occlusion, bilateral
● H34.839 Tributary (branch) retinal vein occlusion, unspecified eye
H34.9 Unspecified retinal vascular occlusion

● **H35 Other retinal disorders**
Excludes2 diabetic retinal disorders (E08.311-E08.359, E09.311-E09.359, E10.311-E10.359, E11.311-E11.359, E13.311-E13.359)
● H35.0 Background retinopathy and retinal vascular changes
Code also any associated hypertension (I10.-)
OGCR Section I. C.9.a.5.
Hypertensive Retinopathy
Subcategory H35.0, Background retinopathy and retinal vascular changes, should be used with a code from category I10–I15, Hypertensive disease to include the systemic hypertension. The sequencing is based on the reason for the encounter.
H35.00 Unspecified background retinopathy
● H35.01 Changes in retinal vascular appearance
Retinal vascular sheathing
H35.011 Changes in retinal vascular appearance, right eye
H35.012 Changes in retinal vascular appearance, left eye
H35.013 Changes in retinal vascular appearance, bilateral
H35.019 Changes in retinal vascular appearance, unspecified eye

CHAPTER 7 (H00-H59)

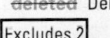

◀ New ◀ Revised ~~deleted~~ Deleted **OGCR** Official Guidelines **X** Assign placeholder X ● Use Additional Character(s)
Excludes 1 Excludes 2 Includes Use additional Code first Code also Unspecified

- ● H35.02 Exudative retinopathy
  - Coats retinopathy
  - H35.021 Exudative retinopathy, right eye
  - H35.022 Exudative retinopathy, left eye
  - H35.023 Exudative retinopathy, bilateral
  - H35.029 Exudative retinopathy, unspecified eye
- ● H35.03 Hypertensive retinopathy
  - H35.031 Hypertensive retinopathy, right eye
  - H35.032 Hypertensive retinopathy, left eye
  - H35.033 Hypertensive retinopathy, bilateral
  - H35.039 Hypertensive retinopathy, unspecified eye
- ● H35.04 Retinal micro-aneurysms, unspecified
  - H35.041 Retinal micro-aneurysms, unspecified, right eye
  - H35.042 Retinal micro-aneurysms, unspecified, left eye
  - H35.043 Retinal micro-aneurysms, unspecified, bilateral
  - H35.049 Retinal micro-aneurysms, unspecified, unspecified eye
- ● H35.05 Retinal neovascularization, unspecified
  - H35.051 Retinal neovascularization, unspecified, right eye
  - H35.052 Retinal neovascularization, unspecified, left eye
  - H35.053 Retinal neovascularization, unspecified, bilateral
  - H35.059 Retinal neovascularization, unspecified, unspecified eye
- ● H35.06 Retinal vasculitis
  - Eales disease
  - Retinal perivasculitis
  - H35.061 Retinal vasculitis, right eye
  - H35.062 Retinal vasculitis, left eye
  - H35.063 Retinal vasculitis, bilateral
  - H35.069 Retinal vasculitis, unspecified eye
- ● H35.07 Retinal telangiectasis
  - H35.071 Retinal telangiectasis, right eye
  - H35.072 Retinal telangiectasis, left eye
  - H35.073 Retinal telangiectasis, bilateral
  - H35.079 Retinal telangiectasis, unspecified eye
- H35.09 Other intraretinal microvascular abnormalities
  - Retinal varices

● H35.1 Retinopathy of prematurity

- ● H35.10 Retinopathy of prematurity, unspecified
  - Retinopathy of prematurity NOS
  - H35.101 Retinopathy of prematurity, unspecified, right eye
  - H35.102 Retinopathy of prematurity, unspecified, left eye
  - H35.103 Retinopathy of prematurity, unspecified, bilateral
  - H35.109 Retinopathy of prematurity, unspecified, unspecified eye
- ● H35.11 Retinopathy of prematurity, stage 0
  - H35.111 Retinopathy of prematurity, stage 0, right eye
  - H35.112 Retinopathy of prematurity, stage 0, left eye
  - H35.113 Retinopathy of prematurity, stage 0, bilateral
  - H35.119 Retinopathy of prematurity, stage 0, unspecified eye
- ● H35.12 Retinopathy of prematurity, stage 1
  - H35.121 Retinopathy of prematurity, stage 1, right eye
  - H35.122 Retinopathy of prematurity, stage 1, left eye
  - H35.123 Retinopathy of prematurity, stage 1, bilateral
  - H35.129 Retinopathy of prematurity, stage 1, unspecified eye
- ● H35.13 Retinopathy of prematurity, stage 2
  - H35.131 Retinopathy of prematurity, stage 2, right eye
  - H35.132 Retinopathy of prematurity, stage 2, left eye
  - H35.133 Retinopathy of prematurity, stage 2, bilateral
  - H35.139 Retinopathy of prematurity, stage 2, unspecified eye
- ● H35.14 Retinopathy of prematurity, stage 3
  - H35.141 Retinopathy of prematurity, stage 3, right eye
  - H35.142 Retinopathy of prematurity, stage 3, left eye
  - H35.143 Retinopathy of prematurity, stage 3, bilateral
  - H35.149 Retinopathy of prematurity, stage 3, unspecified eye
- ● H35.15 Retinopathy of prematurity, stage 4
  - H35.151 Retinopathy of prematurity, stage 4, right eye
  - H35.152 Retinopathy of prematurity, stage 4, left eye
  - H35.153 Retinopathy of prematurity, stage 4, bilateral
  - H35.159 Retinopathy of prematurity, stage 4, unspecified eye
- ● H35.16 Retinopathy of prematurity, stage 5
  - H35.161 Retinopathy of prematurity, stage 5, right eye
  - H35.162 Retinopathy of prematurity, stage 5, left eye
  - H35.163 Retinopathy of prematurity, stage 5, bilateral
  - H35.169 Retinopathy of prematurity, stage 5, unspecified eye
- ● H35.17 Retrolental fibroplasia
  - H35.171 Retrolental fibroplasia, right eye
  - H35.172 Retrolental fibroplasia, left eye
  - H35.173 Retrolental fibroplasia, bilateral
  - H35.179 Retrolental fibroplasia, unspecified eye

● H35.2 Other non-diabetic proliferative retinopathy

- Proliferative vitreo-retinopathy
- **Excludes1** proliferative vitreo-retinopathy with retinal detachment (H33.4-)
- H35.20 Other non-diabetic proliferative retinopathy, unspecified eye
- H35.21 Other non-diabetic proliferative retinopathy, right eye
- H35.22 Other non-diabetic proliferative retinopathy, left eye
- H35.23 Other non-diabetic proliferative retinopathy, bilateral

Item 7–7 Macular degeneration is typically age-related, chronic, and is evidenced by deterioration of the macula (the part of the retina that provides for central field vision), resulting in blurred vision or a blind spot in the center of visual field while not affecting peripheral vision.

● **H35.3 Degeneration of macula and posterior pole**

H35.30 Unspecified macular degeneration
Age-related macular degeneration

● **H35.31 Nonexudative age-related macular degeneration**
Atrophic age-related macular degeneration
Dry age-related macular degeneration ◄
One of the following 7th characters is to be assigned to codes in subcategory H35.31 to designate the stage of the disease: ◄

0	stage unspecified ◄
1	early dry stage ◄
2	intermediate dry stage ◄
3	advanced atrophic without subfoveal involvement ◄ advanced dry stage ◄
4	advanced atrophic with subfoveal involvement ◄

● **H35.311 Nonexudative age-related macular degeneration, right eye** ◄
● **H35.312 Nonexudative age-related macular degeneration, left eye** ◄
● **H35.313 Nonexudative age-related macular degeneration, bilateral** ◄
● **H35.319 Nonexudative age-related macular degeneration, unspecified eye** ◄

● **H35.32 Exudative age-related macular degeneration**
Wet age-related macular degeneration ◄
One of the following 7th characters is to be assigned to codes in subcategory H35.32 to designate the stage of the disease: ◄

0	stage unspecified ◄
1	with active choroidal neovascularization ◄
2	with inactive choroidal neovascularization ◄ with involuted or regressed neovascularization ◄
3	with inactive scar ◄

● **H35.321 Exudative age-related macular degeneration, right eye** ◄
● **H35.322 Exudative age-related macular degeneration, left eye** ◄
● **H35.323 Exudative age-related macular degeneration, bilateral** ◄
● **H35.329 Exudative age-related macular degeneration, unspecified eye** ◄

H35.33 Angioid streaks of macula

● **H35.34 Macular cyst, hole, or pseudohole**
H35.341 Macular cyst, hole, or pseudohole, right eye
H35.342 Macular cyst, hole, or pseudohole, left eye
H35.343 Macular cyst, hole, or pseudohole, bilateral
H35.349 Macular cyst, hole, or pseudohole, unspecified eye

● **H35.35 Cystoid macular degeneration**
Excludes1 cystoid macular edema following cataract surgery (H59.03-)
H35.351 Cystoid macular degeneration, right eye
H35.352 Cystoid macular degeneration, left eye
H35.353 Cystoid macular degeneration, bilateral
H35.359 Cystoid macular degeneration, unspecified eye

● **H35.36 Drusen (degenerative) of macula**
H35.361 Drusen (degenerative) of macula, right eye
H35.362 Drusen (degenerative) of macula, left eye
H35.363 Drusen (degenerative) of macula, bilateral
H35.369 Drusen (degenerative) of macula, unspecified eye

● **H35.37 Puckering of macula**
H35.371 Puckering of macula, right eye
H35.372 Puckering of macula, left eye
H35.373 Puckering of macula, bilateral
H35.379 Puckering of macula, unspecified eye

● **H35.38 Toxic maculopathy**
Code first poisoning due to drug or toxin, if applicable (T36-T65 with fifth or sixth character 1-4 or 6)
Use additional code for adverse effect, if applicable, to identify drug (T36-T50 with fifth or sixth character 5)
H35.381 Toxic maculopathy, right eye
H35.382 Toxic maculopathy, left eye
H35.383 Toxic maculopathy, bilateral
H35.389 Toxic maculopathy, unspecified eye

● **H35.4 Peripheral retinal degeneration**
Excludes1 hereditary retinal degeneration (dystrophy) (H35.5-)
peripheral retinal degeneration with retinal break (H33.3-)

H35.40 Unspecified peripheral retinal degeneration

● **H35.41 Lattice degeneration of retina**
Palisade degeneration of retina
H35.411 Lattice degeneration of retina, right eye
H35.412 Lattice degeneration of retina, left eye
H35.413 Lattice degeneration of retina, bilateral
H35.419 Lattice degeneration of retina, unspecified eye

● **H35.42 Microcystoid degeneration of retina**
H35.421 Microcystoid degeneration of retina, right eye
H35.422 Microcystoid degeneration of retina, left eye
H35.423 Microcystoid degeneration of retina, bilateral
H35.429 Microcystoid degeneration of retina, unspecified eye

CHAPTER 7 (H00-H59)

● H35.43 Paving stone degeneration of retina
H35.431 Paving stone degeneration of retina, right eye
H35.432 Paving stone degeneration of retina, left eye
H35.433 Paving stone degeneration of retina, bilateral
H35.439 Paving stone degeneration of retina, unspecified eye
● H35.44 Age-related reticular degeneration of retina
H35.441 Age-related reticular degeneration of retina, right eye
H35.442 Age-related reticular degeneration of retina, left eye
H35.443 Age-related reticular degeneration of retina, bilateral
H35.449 Age-related reticular degeneration of retina, unspecified eye
● H35.45 Secondary pigmentary degeneration
H35.451 Secondary pigmentary degeneration, right eye
H35.452 Secondary pigmentary degeneration, left eye
H35.453 Secondary pigmentary degeneration, bilateral
H35.459 Secondary pigmentary degeneration, unspecified eye
● H35.46 Secondary vitreoretinal degeneration
H35.461 Secondary vitreoretinal degeneration, right eye
H35.462 Secondary vitreoretinal degeneration, left eye
H35.463 Secondary vitreoretinal degeneration, bilateral
H35.469 Secondary vitreoretinal degeneration, unspecified eye
● H35.5 Hereditary retinal dystrophy
Excludes1 dystrophies primarily involving Bruch's membrane (H31.1-)
H35.50 Unspecified hereditary retinal dystrophy
H35.51 Vitreoretinal dystrophy
H35.52 Pigmentary retinal dystrophy
Albipunctate retinal dystrophy
Retinitis pigmentosa
Tapetoretinal dystrophy
H35.53 Other dystrophies primarily involving the sensory retina
Stargardt's disease
H35.54 Dystrophies primarily involving the retinal pigment epithelium
Vitelliform retinal dystrophy
● H35.6 Retinal hemorrhage
H35.60 Retinal hemorrhage, unspecified eye
H35.61 Retinal hemorrhage, right eye
H35.62 Retinal hemorrhage, left eye
H35.63 Retinal hemorrhage, bilateral
● H35.7 Separation of retinal layers
Excludes1 retinal detachment (serous) (H33.2-)
rhegmatogenous retinal detachment (H33.0-)
H35.70 Unspecified separation of retinal layers
● H35.71 Central serous chorioretinopathy
H35.711 Central serous chorioretinopathy, right eye
H35.712 Central serous chorioretinopathy, left eye
H35.713 Central serous chorioretinopathy, bilateral
H35.719 Central serous chorioretinopathy, unspecified eye
● H35.72 Serous detachment of retinal pigment epithelium
H35.721 Serous detachment of retinal pigment epithelium, right eye
H35.722 Serous detachment of retinal pigment epithelium, left eye
H35.723 Serous detachment of retinal pigment epithelium, bilateral
H35.729 Serous detachment of retinal pigment epithelium, unspecified eye
● H35.73 Hemorrhagic detachment of retinal pigment epithelium
H35.731 Hemorrhagic detachment of retinal pigment epithelium, right eye
H35.732 Hemorrhagic detachment of retinal pigment epithelium, left eye
H35.733 Hemorrhagic detachment of retinal pigment epithelium, bilateral
H35.739 Hemorrhagic detachment of retinal pigment epithelium, unspecified eye
● H35.8 Other specified retinal disorders
Excludes2 retinal hemorrhage (H35.6-)
H35.81 Retinal edema
Retinal cotton wool spots
H35.82 Retinal ischemia
H35.89 Other specified retinal disorders
H35.9 Unspecified retinal disorder
H36 Retinal disorders in diseases classified elsewhere
Code first underlying disease, such as:
lipid storage disorders (E75.-)
sickle-cell disorders (D57.-)
Excludes1 arteriosclerotic retinopathy (H35.0-)
diabetic retinopathy (E08.3-, E09.3-, E10.3-, E11.3-, E13.3-)

GLAUCOMA (H40-H42)

● H40 Glaucoma
Intraocular pressure (IOP) that is too high results from too much aqueous humor and because of excess production or inadequate drainage, optic nerve damage and vision loss may occur.
Excludes1 absolute glaucoma (H44.51-)
congenital glaucoma (Q15.0)
traumatic glaucoma due to birth injury (P15.3)
● H40.0 Glaucoma suspect
● H40.00 Preglaucoma, unspecified
H40.001 Preglaucoma, unspecified, right eye
H40.002 Preglaucoma, unspecified, left eye
H40.003 Preglaucoma, unspecified, bilateral
H40.009 Preglaucoma, unspecified, unspecified eye
● H40.01 Open angle with borderline findings, low risk
Open angle, low risk
H40.011 Open angle with borderline findings, low risk, right eye
H40.012 Open angle with borderline findings, low risk, left eye
H40.013 Open angle with borderline findings, low risk, bilateral
H40.019 Open angle with borderline findings, low risk, unspecified eye

CHAPTER 7 (H00-H59)

● H40.02 Open angle with borderline findings, high risk
Open angle, high risk
H40.021 Open angle with borderline findings, high risk, right eye
H40.022 Open angle with borderline findings, high risk, left eye
H40.023 Open angle with borderline findings, high risk, bilateral
H40.029 Open angle with borderline findings, high risk, unspecified eye

● H40.03 Anatomical narrow angle
Primary angle closure suspect
H40.031 Anatomical narrow angle, right eye
H40.032 Anatomical narrow angle, left eye
H40.033 Anatomical narrow angle, bilateral
H40.039 Anatomical narrow angle, unspecified eye

● H40.04 Steroid responder
H40.041 Steroid responder, right eye
H40.042 Steroid responder, left eye
H40.043 Steroid responder, bilateral
H40.049 Steroid responder, unspecified eye

● H40.05 Ocular hypertension
H40.051 Ocular hypertension, right eye
H40.052 Ocular hypertension, left eye
H40.053 Ocular hypertension, bilateral
H40.059 Ocular hypertension, unspecified eye

● H40.06 Primary angle closure without glaucoma damage
H40.061 Primary angle closure without glaucoma damage, right eye
H40.062 Primary angle closure without glaucoma damage, left eye
H40.063 Primary angle closure without glaucoma damage, bilateral
H40.069 Primary angle closure without glaucoma damage, unspecified eye

● H40.1 Open-angle glaucoma

X ● H40.10 Unspecified open-angle glaucoma
One of the following 7th characters is to be assigned to code H40.10 to designate the stage of glaucoma

0	stage unspecified
1	mild stage
2	moderate stage
3	severe stage
4	indeterminate stage

● H40.11 Primary open-angle glaucoma
Chronic simple glaucoma
One of the following 7th characters is to be assigned to each code in subcategory H40.11 to designate the stage of glaucoma

0	stage unspecified
1	mild stage
2	moderate stage
3	severe stage
4	indeterminate stage

● H40.111 Primary open-angle glaucoma, right eye ◀
● H40.112 Primary open-angle glaucoma, left eye ◀
● H40.113 Primary open-angle glaucoma, bilateral ◀
● H40.119 Primary open-angle glaucoma, unspecified eye ◀

● H40.12 Low-tension glaucoma
One of the following 7th characters is to be assigned to each code in subcategory H40.12 to designate the stage of glaucoma

0	stage unspecified
1	mild stage
2	moderate stage
3	severe stage
4	indeterminate stage

● H40.121 Low-tension glaucoma, right eye
● H40.122 Low-tension glaucoma, left eye
● H40.123 Low-tension glaucoma, bilateral
● H40.129 Low-tension glaucoma, unspecified eye

● H40.13 Pigmentary glaucoma
One of the following 7th characters is to be assigned to each code in subcategory H40.13 to designate the stage of glaucoma

0	stage unspecified
1	mild stage
2	moderate stage
3	severe stage
4	indeterminate stage

● H40.131 Pigmentary glaucoma, right eye
● H40.132 Pigmentary glaucoma, left eye
● H40.133 Pigmentary glaucoma, bilateral
● H40.139 Pigmentary glaucoma, unspecified eye

● H40.14 Capsular glaucoma with pseudoexfoliation of lens
One of the following 7th characters is to be assigned to each code in subcategory H40.14 to designate the stage of glaucoma

0	stage unspecified
1	mild stage
2	moderate stage
3	severe stage
4	indeterminate stage

● H40.141 Capsular glaucoma with pseudoexfoliation of lens, right eye
● H40.142 Capsular glaucoma with pseudoexfoliation of lens, left eye
● H40.143 Capsular glaucoma with pseudoexfoliation of lens, bilateral
● H40.149 Capsular glaucoma with pseudoexfoliation of lens, unspecified eye

● H40.15 Residual stage of open-angle glaucoma
H40.151 Residual stage of open-angle glaucoma, right eye
H40.152 Residual stage of open-angle glaucoma, left eye
H40.153 Residual stage of open-angle glaucoma, bilateral
H40.159 Residual stage of open-angle glaucoma, unspecified eye

● H40.2 Primary angle-closure glaucoma
Excludes1 aqueous misdirection (H40.83-)
malignant glaucoma (H40.83-)

X● H40.20 Unspecified primary angle-closure glaucoma
One of the following 7th characters is to be assigned to code H40.20 to designate the stage of glaucoma

0	stage unspecified
1	mild stage
2	moderate stage
3	severe stage
4	indeterminate stage

● H40.21 Acute angle-closure glaucoma
Acute angle-closure glaucoma attack
Acute angle-closure glaucoma crisis

H40.211 Acute angle-closure glaucoma, right eye

H40.212 Acute angle-closure glaucoma, left eye

H40.213 Acute angle-closure glaucoma, bilateral

H40.219 Acute angle-closure glaucoma, unspecified eye

● H40.22 Chronic angle-closure glaucoma
Chronic primary angle closure glaucoma
One of the following 7th characters is to be assigned to each code in subcategory H40.22 to designate the stage of glaucoma

0	stage unspecified
1	mild stage
2	moderate stage
3	severe stage
4	indeterminate stage

● H40.221 Chronic angle-closure glaucoma, right eye

● H40.222 Chronic angle-closure glaucoma, left eye

● H40.223 Chronic angle-closure glaucoma, bilateral

● H40.229 Chronic angle-closure glaucoma, unspecified eye

● H40.23 Intermittent angle-closure glaucoma

H40.231 Intermittent angle-closure glaucoma, right eye

H40.232 Intermittent angle-closure glaucoma, left eye

H40.233 Intermittent angle-closure glaucoma, bilateral

H40.239 Intermittent angle-closure glaucoma, unspecified eye

● H40.24 Residual stage of angle-closure glaucoma

H40.241 Residual stage of angle-closure glaucoma, right eye

H40.242 Residual stage of angle-closure glaucoma, left eye

H40.243 Residual stage of angle-closure glaucoma, bilateral

H40.249 Residual stage of angle-closure glaucoma, unspecified eye

● H40.3 Glaucoma secondary to eye trauma
Code also underlying condition
One of the following 7th characters is to be assigned to each code in subcategory H40.3 to designate the stage of glaucoma

0	stage unspecified
1	mild stage
2	moderate stage
3	severe stage
4	indeterminate stage

X● H40.30 Glaucoma secondary to eye trauma, unspecified eye

X● H40.31 Glaucoma secondary to eye trauma, right eye

X● H40.32 Glaucoma secondary to eye trauma, left eye

X● H40.33 Glaucoma secondary to eye trauma, bilateral

● H40.4 Glaucoma secondary to eye inflammation
Code also underlying condition
One of the following 7th characters is to be assigned to each code in subcategory H40.4 to designate the stage of glaucoma

0	stage unspecified
1	mild stage
2	moderate stage
3	severe stage
4	indeterminate stage

X● H40.40 Glaucoma secondary to eye inflammation, unspecified eye

X● H40.41 Glaucoma secondary to eye inflammation, right eye

X● H40.42 Glaucoma secondary to eye inflammation, left eye

X● H40.43 Glaucoma secondary to eye inflammation, bilateral

● H40.5 Glaucoma secondary to other eye disorders
Code also underlying eye disorder
One of the following 7th characters is to be assigned to each code in subcategory H40.5 to designate the stage of glaucoma

0	stage unspecified
1	mild stage
2	moderate stage
3	severe stage
4	indeterminate stage

X● H40.50 Glaucoma secondary to other eye disorders, unspecified eye

X● H40.51 Glaucoma secondary to other eye disorders, right eye

X● H40.52 Glaucoma secondary to other eye disorders, left eye

X● H40.53 Glaucoma secondary to other eye disorders, bilateral

● H40.6 Glaucoma secondary to drugs
Use additional code for adverse effect, if applicable, to identify drug (T36-T50 with fifth or sixth character 5)
One of the following 7th characters is to be assigned to each code in subcategory H40.6 to designate the stage of glaucoma

0	stage unspecified
1	mild stage
2	moderate stage
3	severe stage
4	indeterminate stage

X● H40.60 Glaucoma secondary to drugs, unspecified eye
X● H40.61 Glaucoma secondary to drugs, right eye
X● H40.62 Glaucoma secondary to drugs, left eye
X● H40.63 Glaucoma secondary to drugs, bilateral
● H40.8 Other glaucoma
● H40.81 Glaucoma with increased episcleral venous pressure
H40.811 Glaucoma with increased episcleral venous pressure, right eye
H40.812 Glaucoma with increased episcleral venous pressure, left eye
H40.813 Glaucoma with increased episcleral venous pressure, bilateral
H40.819 Glaucoma with increased episcleral venous pressure, unspecified eye
● H40.82 Hypersecretion glaucoma
H40.821 Hypersecretion glaucoma, right eye
H40.822 Hypersecretion glaucoma, left eye
H40.823 Hypersecretion glaucoma, bilateral
H40.829 Hypersecretion glaucoma, unspecified eye
● H40.83 Aqueous misdirection
Malignant glaucoma
H40.831 Aqueous misdirection, right eye
H40.832 Aqueous misdirection, left eye
H40.833 Aqueous misdirection, bilateral
H40.839 Aqueous misdirection, unspecified eye
H40.89 Other specified glaucoma
H40.9 Unspecified glaucoma

H42 Glaucoma in diseases classified elsewhere
Code first underlying condition, such as:
amyloidosis (E85.-)
aniridia (Q13.1)
Lowe's syndrome (E72.03)
Reiger's anomaly (Q13.81)
specified metabolic disorder (E70-E88)
Excludes1 glaucoma (in) onchocerciasis (B73.02) ◄
glaucoma (in) syphilis (A52.71) ◄
glaucoma (in) tuberculous (A18.59) ◄
Excludes2 glaucoma (in) diabetes mellitus (E08.39, E09.39, E10.39, E11.39, E13.39) ◄

DISORDERS OF VITREOUS BODY AND GLOBE (H43-H44)

● H43 Disorders of vitreous body
● H43.0 Vitreous prolapse
Excludes1 vitreous syndrome following cataract surgery (H59.0-)
traumatic vitreous prolapse (S05.2-)
H43.00 Vitreous prolapse, unspecified eye
H43.01 Vitreous prolapse, right eye
H43.02 Vitreous prolapse, left eye
H43.03 Vitreous prolapse, bilateral
● H43.1 Vitreous hemorrhage
H43.10 Vitreous hemorrhage, unspecified eye
H43.11 Vitreous hemorrhage, right eye
H43.12 Vitreous hemorrhage, left eye
H43.13 Vitreous hemorrhage, bilateral
● H43.2 Crystalline deposits in vitreous body
H43.20 Crystalline deposits in vitreous body, unspecified eye
H43.21 Crystalline deposits in vitreous body, right eye
H43.22 Crystalline deposits in vitreous body, left eye
H43.23 Crystalline deposits in vitreous body, bilateral
● H43.3 Other vitreous opacities
● H43.31 Vitreous membranes and strands
H43.311 Vitreous membranes and strands, right eye
H43.312 Vitreous membranes and strands, left eye
H43.313 Vitreous membranes and strands, bilateral
H43.319 Vitreous membranes and strands, unspecified eye
● H43.39 Other vitreous opacities
Vitreous floaters
Small clumps of cells that float in the vitreous of the eye, appearing as black specks or dots in the field of vision and common in the aging eye.
H43.391 Other vitreous opacities, right eye
H43.392 Other vitreous opacities, left eye
H43.393 Other vitreous opacities, bilateral
H43.399 Other vitreous opacities, unspecified eye
● H43.8 Other disorders of vitreous body
Excludes1 proliferative vitreo-retinopathy with retinal detachment (H33.4)
Excludes2 vitreous abscess (H44.02-)
● H43.81 Vitreous degeneration
Vitreous detachment
H43.811 Vitreous degeneration, right eye
H43.812 Vitreous degeneration, left eye
H43.813 Vitreous degeneration, bilateral
H43.819 Vitreous degeneration, unspecified eye
● H43.82 Vitreomacular adhesion
Vitreomacular traction
H43.821 Vitreomacular adhesion, right eye
H43.822 Vitreomacular adhesion, left eye
H43.823 Vitreomacular adhesion, bilateral
H43.829 Vitreomacular adhesion, unspecified eye
H43.89 Other disorders of vitreous body
H43.9 Unspecified disorder of vitreous body

CHAPTER 7 (H00-H59)

● H44 Disorders of globe
Includes disorders affecting multiple structures of eye
● H44.0 Purulent endophthalmitis
Use additional code to identify organism
Excludes1 bleb associated endophthalmitis (H59.4-)
● H44.00 Unspecified purulent endophthalmitis
H44.001 Unspecified purulent endophthalmitis, right eye
H44.002 Unspecified purulent endophthalmitis, left eye
H44.003 Unspecified purulent endophthalmitis, bilateral
H44.009 Unspecified purulent endophthalmitis, unspecified eye
● H44.01 Panophthalmitis (acute)
H44.011 Panophthalmitis (acute), right eye
H44.012 Panophthalmitis (acute), left eye
H44.013 Panophthalmitis (acute), bilateral
H44.019 Panophthalmitis (acute), unspecified eye
● H44.02 Vitreous abscess (chronic)
H44.021 Vitreous abscess (chronic), right eye
H44.022 Vitreous abscess (chronic), left eye
H44.023 Vitreous abscess (chronic), bilateral
H44.029 Vitreous abscess (chronic), unspecified eye
● H44.1 Other endophthalmitis
Excludes1 bleb associated endophthalmitis (H59.4-)
Excludes2 ophthalmia nodosa (H16.2-)
● H44.11 Panuveitis
H44.111 Panuveitis, right eye
H44.112 Panuveitis, left eye
H44.113 Panuveitis, bilateral
H44.119 Panuveitis, unspecified eye
● H44.12 Parasitic endophthalmitis, unspecified
H44.121 Parasitic endophthalmitis, unspecified, right eye
H44.122 Parasitic endophthalmitis, unspecified, left eye
H44.123 Parasitic endophthalmitis, unspecified, bilateral
H44.129 Parasitic endophthalmitis, unspecified, unspecified eye
● H44.13 Sympathetic uveitis
H44.131 Sympathetic uveitis, right eye
H44.132 Sympathetic uveitis, left eye
H44.133 Sympathetic uveitis, bilateral
H44.139 Sympathetic uveitis, unspecified eye
H44.19 Other endophthalmitis
● H44.2 Degenerative myopia
Malignant myopia
H44.20 Degenerative myopia, unspecified eye
H44.21 Degenerative myopia, right eye
H44.22 Degenerative myopia, left eye
H44.23 Degenerative myopia, bilateral
● H44.3 Other and unspecified degenerative disorders of globe
H44.30 Unspecified degenerative disorder of globe
● H44.31 Chalcosis
H44.311 Chalcosis, right eye
H44.312 Chalcosis, left eye
H44.313 Chalcosis, bilateral
H44.319 Chalcosis, unspecified eye
● H44.32 Siderosis of eye
H44.321 Siderosis of eye, right eye
H44.322 Siderosis of eye, left eye
H44.323 Siderosis of eye, bilateral
H44.329 Siderosis of eye, unspecified eye
● H44.39 Other degenerative disorders of globe
H44.391 Other degenerative disorders of globe, right eye
H44.392 Other degenerative disorders of globe, left eye
H44.393 Other degenerative disorders of globe, bilateral
H44.399 Other degenerative disorders of globe, unspecified eye
● H44.4 Hypotony of eye
H44.40 Unspecified hypotony of eye
● H44.41 Flat anterior chamber hypotony of eye
H44.411 Flat anterior chamber hypotony of right eye
H44.412 Flat anterior chamber hypotony of left eye
H44.413 Flat anterior chamber hypotony of eye, bilateral
H44.419 Flat anterior chamber hypotony of unspecified eye
● H44.42 Hypotony of eye due to ocular fistula
H44.421 Hypotony of right eye due to ocular fistula
H44.422 Hypotony of left eye due to ocular fistula
H44.423 Hypotony of eye due to ocular fistula, bilateral
H44.429 Hypotony of unspecified eye due to ocular fistula
● H44.43 Hypotony of eye due to other ocular disorders
H44.431 Hypotony of eye due to other ocular disorders, right eye
H44.432 Hypotony of eye due to other ocular disorders, left eye
H44.433 Hypotony of eye due to other ocular disorders, bilateral
H44.439 Hypotony of eye due to other ocular disorders, unspecified eye
● H44.44 Primary hypotony of eye
H44.441 Primary hypotony of right eye
H44.442 Primary hypotony of left eye
H44.443 Primary hypotony of eye, bilateral
H44.449 Primary hypotony of unspecified eye
● H44.5 Degenerated conditions of globe
H44.50 Unspecified degenerated conditions of globe
● H44.51 Absolute glaucoma
H44.511 Absolute glaucoma, right eye
H44.512 Absolute glaucoma, left eye
H44.513 Absolute glaucoma, bilateral
H44.519 Absolute glaucoma, unspecified eye
● H44.52 Atrophy of globe
Phthisis bulbi
H44.521 Atrophy of globe, right eye
H44.522 Atrophy of globe, left eye
H44.523 Atrophy of globe, bilateral
H44.529 Atrophy of globe, unspecified eye
● H44.53 Leucocoria
H44.531 Leucocoria, right eye
H44.532 Leucocoria, left eye
H44.533 Leucocoria, bilateral
H44.539 Leucocoria, unspecified eye

● H44.6 Retained (old) intraocular foreign body, magnetic
Use additional code to identify magnetic foreign body (Z18.11)
Excludes1 current intraocular foreign body (SØ5.-)
Excludes2 retained foreign body in eyelid (HØ2.81-)
retained (old) foreign body following penetrating wound of orbit (HØ5.5-)
retained (old) intraocular foreign body, nonmagnetic (H44.7-)

● H44.6Ø Unspecified retained (old) intraocular foreign body, magnetic
H44.6Ø1 Unspecified retained (old) intraocular foreign body, magnetic, right eye
H44.6Ø2 Unspecified retained (old) intraocular foreign body, magnetic, left eye
H44.6Ø3 Unspecified retained (old) intraocular foreign body, magnetic, bilateral
H44.6Ø9 Unspecified retained (old) intraocular foreign body, magnetic, unspecified eye

● H44.61 Retained (old) magnetic foreign body in anterior chamber
H44.611 Retained (old) magnetic foreign body in anterior chamber, right eye
H44.612 Retained (old) magnetic foreign body in anterior chamber, left eye
H44.613 Retained (old) magnetic foreign body in anterior chamber, bilateral
H44.619 Retained (old) magnetic foreign body in anterior chamber, unspecified eye

● H44.62 Retained (old) magnetic foreign body in iris or ciliary body
H44.621 Retained (old) magnetic foreign body in iris or ciliary body, right eye
H44.622 Retained (old) magnetic foreign body in iris or ciliary body, left eye
H44.623 Retained (old) magnetic foreign body in iris or ciliary body, bilateral
H44.629 Retained (old) magnetic foreign body in iris or ciliary body, unspecified eye

● H44.63 Retained (old) magnetic foreign body in lens
H44.631 Retained (old) magnetic foreign body in lens, right eye
H44.632 Retained (old) magnetic foreign body in lens, left eye
H44.633 Retained (old) magnetic foreign body in lens, bilateral
H44.639 Retained (old) magnetic foreign body in lens, unspecified eye

● H44.64 Retained (old) magnetic foreign body in posterior wall of globe
H44.641 Retained (old) magnetic foreign body in posterior wall of globe, right eye
H44.642 Retained (old) magnetic foreign body in posterior wall of globe, left eye
H44.643 Retained (old) magnetic foreign body in posterior wall of globe, bilateral
H44.649 Retained (old) magnetic foreign body in posterior wall of globe, unspecified eye

● H44.65 Retained (old) magnetic foreign body in vitreous body
H44.651 Retained (old) magnetic foreign body in vitreous body, right eye
H44.652 Retained (old) magnetic foreign body in vitreous body, left eye
H44.653 Retained (old) magnetic foreign body in vitreous body, bilateral
H44.659 Retained (old) magnetic foreign body in vitreous body, unspecified eye

● H44.69 Retained (old) intraocular foreign body, magnetic, in other or multiple sites
H44.691 Retained (old) intraocular foreign body, magnetic, in other or multiple sites, right eye
H44.692 Retained (old) intraocular foreign body, magnetic, in other or multiple sites, left eye
H44.693 Retained (old) intraocular foreign body, magnetic, in other or multiple sites, bilateral
H44.699 Retained (old) intraocular foreign body, magnetic, in other or multiple sites, unspecified eye

● H44.7 Retained (old) intraocular foreign body, nonmagnetic
Use additional code to identify nonmagnetic foreign body (Z18.Ø1-Z18.1Ø, Z18.12, Z18.2-Z18.9)
Excludes1 current intraocular foreign body (SØ5.-)
Excludes2 retained foreign body in eyelid (HØ2.81-)
retained (old) foreign body following penetrating wound of orbit (HØ5.5-)
retained (old) intraocular foreign body, magnetic (H44.6-)

● H44.7Ø Unspecified retained (old) intraocular foreign body, nonmagnetic
H44.7Ø1 Unspecified retained (old) intraocular foreign body, nonmagnetic, right eye
H44.7Ø2 Unspecified retained (old) intraocular foreign body, nonmagnetic, left eye
H44.7Ø3 Unspecified retained (old) intraocular foreign body, nonmagnetic, bilateral
H44.7Ø9 Unspecified retained (old) intraocular foreign body, nonmagnetic, unspecified eye
Retained (old) intraocular foreign body NOS

● H44.71 Retained (nonmagnetic) (old) foreign body in anterior chamber
H44.711 Retained (nonmagnetic) (old) foreign body in anterior chamber, right eye
H44.712 Retained (nonmagnetic) (old) foreign body in anterior chamber, left eye
H44.713 Retained (nonmagnetic) (old) foreign body in anterior chamber, bilateral
H44.719 Retained (nonmagnetic) (old) foreign body in anterior chamber, unspecified eye

● H44.72 Retained (nonmagnetic) (old) foreign body in iris or ciliary body
H44.721 Retained (nonmagnetic) (old) foreign body in iris or ciliary body, right eye
H44.722 Retained (nonmagnetic) (old) foreign body in iris or ciliary body, left eye
H44.723 Retained (nonmagnetic) (old) foreign body in iris or ciliary body, bilateral
H44.729 Retained (nonmagnetic) (old) foreign body in iris or ciliary body, unspecified eye

CHAPTER 7 (HØØ-H59)

● H44.73 Retained (nonmagnetic) (old) foreign body in lens
- H44.731 Retained (nonmagnetic) (old) foreign body in lens, right eye
- H44.732 Retained (nonmagnetic) (old) foreign body in lens, left eye
- H44.733 Retained (nonmagnetic) (old) foreign body in lens, bilateral
- H44.739 Retained (nonmagnetic) (old) foreign body in lens, unspecified eye

● H44.74 Retained (nonmagnetic) (old) foreign body in posterior wall of globe
- H44.741 Retained (nonmagnetic) (old) foreign body in posterior wall of globe, right eye
- H44.742 Retained (nonmagnetic) (old) foreign body in posterior wall of globe, left eye
- H44.743 Retained (nonmagnetic) (old) foreign body in posterior wall of globe, bilateral
- H44.749 Retained (nonmagnetic) (old) foreign body in posterior wall of globe, unspecified eye

● H44.75 Retained (nonmagnetic) (old) foreign body in vitreous body
- H44.751 Retained (nonmagnetic) (old) foreign body in vitreous body, right eye
- H44.752 Retained (nonmagnetic) (old) foreign body in vitreous body, left eye
- H44.753 Retained (nonmagnetic) (old) foreign body in vitreous body, bilateral
- H44.759 Retained (nonmagnetic) (old) foreign body in vitreous body, unspecified eye

● H44.79 Retained (old) intraocular foreign body, nonmagnetic, in other or multiple sites
- H44.791 Retained (old) intraocular foreign body, nonmagnetic, in other or multiple sites, right eye
- H44.792 Retained (old) intraocular foreign body, nonmagnetic, in other or multiple sites, left eye
- H44.793 Retained (old) intraocular foreign body, nonmagnetic, in other or multiple sites, bilateral
- H44.799 Retained (old) intraocular foreign body, nonmagnetic, in other or multiple sites, unspecified eye

● H44.8 Other disorders of globe

● H44.81 Hemophthalmos
- H44.811 Hemophthalmos, right eye
- H44.812 Hemophthalmos, left eye
- H44.813 Hemophthalmos, bilateral
- H44.819 Hemophthalmos, unspecified eye

● H44.82 Luxation of globe
- H44.821 Luxation of globe, right eye
- H44.822 Luxation of globe, left eye
- H44.823 Luxation of globe, bilateral
- H44.829 Luxation of globe, unspecified eye

H44.89 Other disorders of globe

H44.9 Unspecified disorder of globe

★ (See Plate 86 on page NAP-7.)

DISORDERS OF OPTIC NERVE AND VISUAL PATHWAYS (H46-H47)

● H46 Optic neuritis

Excludes2 ischemic optic neuropathy (H47.01-)
neuromyelitis optica [Devic] (G36.0)

● H46.0 Optic papillitis
- H46.00 Optic papillitis, unspecified eye
- H46.01 Optic papillitis, right eye
- H46.02 Optic papillitis, left eye
- H46.03 Optic papillitis, bilateral

● H46.1 Retrobulbar neuritis

Retrobulbar neuritis NOS

Excludes1 syphilitic retrobulbar neuritis (A52.15)
- H46.10 Retrobulbar neuritis, unspecified eye
- H46.11 Retrobulbar neuritis, right eye
- H46.12 Retrobulbar neuritis, left eye
- H46.13 Retrobulbar neuritis, bilateral

H46.2 Nutritional optic neuropathy

H46.3 Toxic optic neuropathy

Code first (T51-T65) to identify cause

H46.8 Other optic neuritis

H46.9 Unspecified optic neuritis

● H47 Other disorders of optic [2nd] nerve and visual pathways

● H47.0 Disorders of optic nerve, not elsewhere classified

● H47.01 Ischemic optic neuropathy
- H47.011 Ischemic optic neuropathy, right eye
- H47.012 Ischemic optic neuropathy, left eye
- H47.013 Ischemic optic neuropathy, bilateral
- H47.019 Ischemic optic neuropathy, unspecified eye

● H47.02 Hemorrhage in optic nerve sheath
- H47.021 Hemorrhage in optic nerve sheath, right eye
- H47.022 Hemorrhage in optic nerve sheath, left eye
- H47.023 Hemorrhage in optic nerve sheath, bilateral
- H47.029 Hemorrhage in optic nerve sheath, unspecified eye

● H47.03 Optic nerve hypoplasia
- H47.031 Optic nerve hypoplasia, right eye
- H47.032 Optic nerve hypoplasia, left eye
- H47.033 Optic nerve hypoplasia, bilateral
- H47.039 Optic nerve hypoplasia, unspecified eye

● H47.09 Other disorders of optic nerve, not elsewhere classified

Compression of optic nerve
- H47.091 Other disorders of optic nerve, not elsewhere classified, right eye
- H47.092 Other disorders of optic nerve, not elsewhere classified, left eye
- H47.093 Other disorders of optic nerve, not elsewhere classified, bilateral
- H47.099 Other disorders of optic nerve, not elsewhere classified, unspecified eye

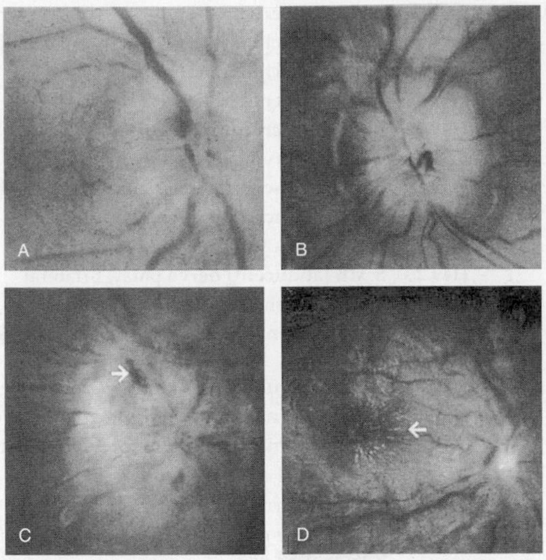

Figure 7-11 Papilledema. (From Behrma: Nelson Textbook of Pediatrics, ed 17, Saunders, 2004)

Item 7–8 Papilledema is swelling of the optic disc caused by increased intracranial pressure. It is most often bilateral and occurs quickly (hours) or over weeks of time. It is a common symptom of a brain tumor. The term should not be used to describe optic disc swelling with underlying infectious, infiltrative, or inflammatory etiologies.

● **H47.1 Papilledema**
- **H47.10 Unspecified papilledema**
- **H47.11 Papilledema associated with increased intracranial pressure**
- **H47.12 Papilledema associated with decreased ocular pressure**
- **H47.13 Papilledema associated with retinal disorder**
- ● **H47.14 Foster-Kennedy syndrome**
  - **H47.141 Foster-Kennedy syndrome, right eye**
  - **H47.142 Foster-Kennedy syndrome, left eye**
  - **H47.143 Foster-Kennedy syndrome, bilateral**
  - **H47.149 Foster-Kennedy syndrome, unspecified eye**

● **H47.2 Optic atrophy**
- **H47.20 Unspecified optic atrophy**
- ● **H47.21 Primary optic atrophy**
  - **H47.211 Primary optic atrophy, right eye**
  - **H47.212 Primary optic atrophy, left eye**
  - **H47.213 Primary optic atrophy, bilateral**
  - **H47.219 Primary optic atrophy, unspecified eye**
- **H47.22 Hereditary optic atrophy**
  - Leber's optic atrophy
- ● **H47.23 Glaucomatous optic atrophy**
  - **H47.231 Glaucomatous optic atrophy, right eye**
  - **H47.232 Glaucomatous optic atrophy, left eye**
  - **H47.233 Glaucomatous optic atrophy, bilateral**
  - **H47.239 Glaucomatous optic atrophy, unspecified eye**
- ● **H47.29 Other optic atrophy**
  - Temporal pallor of optic disc
  - **H47.291 Other optic atrophy, right eye**
  - **H47.292 Other optic atrophy, left eye**
  - **H47.293 Other optic atrophy, bilateral**
  - **H47.299 Other optic atrophy, unspecified eye**

● **H47.3 Other disorders of optic disc**
- ● **H47.31 Coloboma of optic disc**
  - **H47.311 Coloboma of optic disc, right eye**
  - **H47.312 Coloboma of optic disc, left eye**
  - **H47.313 Coloboma of optic disc, bilateral**
  - **H47.319 Coloboma of optic disc, unspecified eye**
- ● **H47.32 Drusen of optic disc**
  - **H47.321 Drusen of optic disc, right eye**
  - **H47.322 Drusen of optic disc, left eye**
  - **H47.323 Drusen of optic disc, bilateral**
  - **H47.329 Drusen of optic disc, unspecified eye**
- ● **H47.33 Pseudopapilledema of optic disc**
  - **H47.331 Pseudopapilledema of optic disc, right eye**
  - **H47.332 Pseudopapilledema of optic disc, left eye**
  - **H47.333 Pseudopapilledema of optic disc, bilateral**
  - **H47.339 Pseudopapilledema of optic disc, unspecified eye**
- ● **H47.39 Other disorders of optic disc**
  - **H47.391 Other disorders of optic disc, right eye**
  - **H47.392 Other disorders of optic disc, left eye**
  - **H47.393 Other disorders of optic disc, bilateral**
  - **H47.399 Other disorders of optic disc, unspecified eye**

● **H47.4 Disorders of optic chiasm**
- Code also underlying condition
- **H47.41 Disorders of optic chiasm in (due to) inflammatory disorders**
- **H47.42 Disorders of optic chiasm in (due to) neoplasm**
- **H47.43 Disorders of optic chiasm in (due to) vascular disorders**
- **H47.49 Disorders of optic chiasm in (due to) other disorders**

● **H47.5 Disorders of other visual pathways**
- Disorders of optic tracts, geniculate nuclei and optic radiations
- Code also underlying condition
- ● **H47.51 Disorders of visual pathways in (due to) inflammatory disorders**
  - **H47.511 Disorders of visual pathways in (due to) inflammatory disorders, right side**
  - **H47.512 Disorders of visual pathways in (due to) inflammatory disorders, left side**
  - **H47.519 Disorders of visual pathways in (due to) inflammatory disorders, unspecified side**
- ● **H47.52 Disorders of visual pathways in (due to) neoplasm**
  - **H47.521 Disorders of visual pathways in (due to) neoplasm, right side**
  - **H47.522 Disorders of visual pathways in (due to) neoplasm, left side**
  - **H47.529 Disorders of visual pathways in (due to) neoplasm, unspecified side**
- ● **H47.53 Disorders of visual pathways in (due to) vascular disorders**
  - **H47.531 Disorders of visual pathways in (due to) vascular disorders, right side**
  - **H47.532 Disorders of visual pathways in (due to) vascular disorders, left side**
  - **H47.539 Disorders of visual pathways in (due to) vascular disorders, unspecified side**

● H47.6 Disorders of visual cortex
Code also underlying condition
Excludes1 injury to visual cortex SØ4.Ø4

● H47.61 Cortical blindness
- H47.611 Cortical blindness, right side of brain
- H47.612 Cortical blindness, left side of brain
- H47.619 Cortical blindness, unspecified side of brain

● H47.62 Disorders of visual cortex in (due to) inflammatory disorders
- H47.621 Disorders of visual cortex in (due to) inflammatory disorders, right side of brain
- H47.622 Disorders of visual cortex in (due to) inflammatory disorders, left side of brain
- H47.629 Disorders of visual cortex in (due to) inflammatory disorders, unspecified side of brain

● H47.63 Disorders of visual cortex in (due to) neoplasm
- H47.631 Disorders of visual cortex in (due to) neoplasm, right side of brain
- H47.632 Disorders of visual cortex in (due to) neoplasm, left side of brain
- H47.639 Disorders of visual cortex in (due to) neoplasm, unspecified side of brain

● H47.64 Disorders of visual cortex in (due to) vascular disorders
- H47.641 Disorders of visual cortex in (due to) vascular disorders, right side of brain
- H47.642 Disorders of visual cortex in (due to) vascular disorders, left side of brain
- H47.649 Disorders of visual cortex in (due to) vascular disorders, unspecified side of brain

H47.9 Unspecified disorder of visual pathways

DISORDERS OF OCULAR MUSCLES, BINOCULAR MOVEMENT, ACCOMMODATION AND REFRACTION (H49-H52)

Excludes2 nystagmus and other irregular eye movements (H55)

● H49 Paralytic strabismus
Excludes2 internal ophthalmoplegia (H52.51-)
internuclear ophthalmoplegia (H51.2-)
progressive supranuclear ophthalmoplegia (G23.1)

● H49.Ø Third [oculomotor] nerve palsy
- H49.ØØ Third [oculomotor] nerve palsy, unspecified eye
- H49.Ø1 Third [oculomotor] nerve palsy, right eye
- H49.Ø2 Third [oculomotor] nerve palsy, left eye
- H49.Ø3 Third [oculomotor] nerve palsy, bilateral

Item 7–9 Strabismus or esotropia (crossed eyes) is a condition of the extraocular eye muscles, resulting in an inability of the eyes to focus and also affects depth perception.

A

B

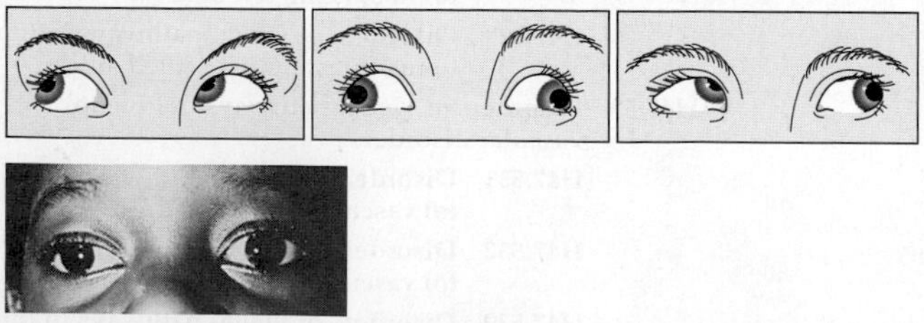

Figure 7-12 **A.** Image of strabismus. **B.** Exotropia. (**A** from Yanoff: Ophthalmology, ed 3, Mosby, Inc., 2008. **B** from Rakel: Textbook of Family Practice, ed 7, Saunders, 2007)

● H49.1 Fourth [trochlear] nerve palsy
- H49.1Ø Fourth [trochlear] nerve palsy, unspecified eye
- H49.11 Fourth [trochlear] nerve palsy, right eye
- H49.12 Fourth [trochlear] nerve palsy, left eye
- H49.13 Fourth [trochlear] nerve palsy, bilateral

● H49.2 Sixth [abducent] nerve palsy
- H49.2Ø Sixth [abducent] nerve palsy, unspecified eye
- H49.21 Sixth [abducent] nerve palsy, right eye
- H49.22 Sixth [abducent] nerve palsy, left eye
- H49.23 Sixth [abducent] nerve palsy, bilateral

● H49.3 Total (external) ophthalmoplegia
- H49.3Ø Total (external) ophthalmoplegia, unspecified eye
- H49.31 Total (external) ophthalmoplegia, right eye
- H49.32 Total (external) ophthalmoplegia, left eye
- H49.33 Total (external) ophthalmoplegia, bilateral

● H49.4 Progressive external ophthalmoplegia
Excludes1 Kearns-Sayre syndrome (H49.81-)
- H49.4Ø Progressive external ophthalmoplegia, unspecified eye
- H49.41 Progressive external ophthalmoplegia, right eye
- H49.42 Progressive external ophthalmoplegia, left eye
- H49.43 Progressive external ophthalmoplegia, bilateral

● H49.8 Other paralytic strabismus

● H49.81 Kearns-Sayre syndrome
Progressive external ophthalmoplegia with pigmentary retinopathy
Use additional code for other manifestation, such as:
heart block (I45.9)
- H49.811 Kearns-Sayre syndrome, right eye
- H49.812 Kearns-Sayre syndrome, left eye
- H49.813 Kearns-Sayre syndrome, bilateral
- H49.819 Kearns-Sayre syndrome, unspecified eye

● H49.88 Other paralytic strabismus
External ophthalmoplegia NOS
- H49.881 Other paralytic strabismus, right eye
- H49.882 Other paralytic strabismus, left eye
- H49.883 Other paralytic strabismus, bilateral
- H49.889 Other paralytic strabismus, unspecified eye

H49.9 Unspecified paralytic strabismus

● H5Ø Other strabismus

● H5Ø.Ø Esotropia
Convergent concomitant strabismus
Excludes1 intermittent esotropia (H5Ø.31-, H5Ø.32)
- H5Ø.ØØ Unspecified esotropia

● H5Ø.Ø1 Monocular esotropia
- H5Ø.Ø11 Monocular esotropia, right eye
- H5Ø.Ø12 Monocular esotropia, left eye

● H5Ø.Ø2 Monocular esotropia with A pattern
- H5Ø.Ø21 Monocular esotropia with A pattern, right eye
- H5Ø.Ø22 Monocular esotropia with A pattern, left eye

● H5Ø.Ø3 Monocular esotropia with V pattern
- H5Ø.Ø31 Monocular esotropia with V pattern, right eye
- H5Ø.Ø32 Monocular esotropia with V pattern, left eye

● H50.04 Monocular esotropia with other noncomitancies
H50.041 Monocular esotropia with other noncomitancies, right eye
H50.042 Monocular esotropia with other noncomitancies, left eye
H50.05 Alternating esotropia
H50.06 Alternating esotropia with A pattern
H50.07 Alternating esotropia with V pattern
H50.08 Alternating esotropia with other noncomitancies

● H50.1 Exotropia
Misalignment in which one eye deviates outward (away from nose) while the other fixates normally
Divergent concomitant strabismus
Excludes1 intermittent exotropia (H50.33-, H50.34)
H50.10 Unspecified exotropia
● H50.11 Monocular exotropia
H50.111 Monocular exotropia, right eye
H50.112 Monocular exotropia, left eye
● H50.12 Monocular exotropia with A pattern
H50.121 Monocular exotropia with A pattern, right eye
H50.122 Monocular exotropia with A pattern, left eye
● H50.13 Monocular exotropia with V pattern
H50.131 Monocular exotropia with V pattern, right eye
H50.132 Monocular exotropia with V pattern, left eye
● H50.14 Monocular exotropia with other noncomitancies
H50.141 Monocular exotropia with other noncomitancies, right eye
H50.142 Monocular exotropia with other noncomitancies, left eye
H50.15 Alternating exotropia
H50.16 Alternating exotropia with A pattern
H50.17 Alternating exotropia with V pattern
H50.18 Alternating exotropia with other noncomitancies

● H50.2 Vertical strabismus
Hypertropia
H50.21 Vertical strabismus, right eye
H50.22 Vertical strabismus, left eye

● H50.3 Intermittent heterotropia
Displacement of an organ or part of an organ from its normal position
H50.30 Unspecified intermittent heterotropia
● H50.31 Intermittent monocular esotropia
H50.311 Intermittent monocular esotropia, right eye
H50.312 Intermittent monocular esotropia, left eye
H50.32 Intermittent alternating esotropia
● H50.33 Intermittent monocular exotropia
H50.331 Intermittent monocular exotropia, right eye
H50.332 Intermittent monocular exotropia, left eye
H50.34 Intermittent alternating exotropia

● H50.4 Other and unspecified heterotropia
H50.40 Unspecified heterotropia
● H50.41 Cyclotropia
H50.411 Cyclotropia, right eye
H50.412 Cyclotropia, left eye
H50.42 Monofixation syndrome
H50.43 Accommodative component in esotropia

● H50.5 Heterophoria
One or both eyes wander away from the position where both eyes are looking together in the same direction
H50.50 Unspecified heterophoria
H50.51 Esophoria
Eye deviates inward (toward the nose)
H50.52 Exophoria
Eye deviates outward (toward the ear)
H50.53 Vertical heterophoria
H50.54 Cyclophoria
H50.55 Alternating heterophoria

● H50.6 Mechanical strabismus
H50.60 Mechanical strabismus, unspecified
● H50.61 Brown's sheath syndrome
H50.611 Brown's sheath syndrome, right eye
H50.612 Brown's sheath syndrome, left eye
H50.69 Other mechanical strabismus
Strabismus due to adhesions
Traumatic limitation of duction of eye muscle

● H50.8 Other specified strabismus
● H50.81 Duane's syndrome
H50.811 Duane's syndrome, right eye
H50.812 Duane's syndrome, left eye
H50.89 Other specified strabismus

H50.9 Unspecified strabismus

● H51 Other disorders of binocular movement
H51.0 Palsy (spasm) of conjugate gaze
● H51.1 Convergence insufficiency and excess
H51.11 Convergence insufficiency
H51.12 Convergence excess
● H51.2 Internuclear ophthalmoplegia
H51.20 Internuclear ophthalmoplegia, unspecified eye
H51.21 Internuclear ophthalmoplegia, right eye
H51.22 Internuclear ophthalmoplegia, left eye
H51.23 Internuclear ophthalmoplegia, bilateral
H51.8 Other specified disorders of binocular movement
H51.9 Unspecified disorder of binocular movement

● H52 Disorders of refraction and accommodation
● H52.0 Hypermetropia
H52.00 Hypermetropia, unspecified eye
H52.01 Hypermetropia, right eye
H52.02 Hypermetropia, left eye
H52.03 Hypermetropia, bilateral
● H52.1 Myopia
Excludes1 degenerative myopia (H44.2-)
H52.10 Myopia, unspecified eye
H52.11 Myopia, right eye
H52.12 Myopia, left eye
H52.13 Myopia, bilateral

CHAPTER 7 (H00-H59)

Item 7-10 Disorders of refraction: **Hypermetropia,** or farsightedness, means focus at a distance is adequate but not on close objects. **Myopia** is near-sightedness or short-sightedness and means the focus on nearby objects is clear but distant objects appear blurred. **Astigmatism** is warping of the curvature of the cornea so light rays entering do not meet a single focal point, resulting in a distorted image. **Anisometropia** is unequal refractive power in which one eye may be myopic (near-sighted) and the other hyperopic (far-sighted). **Presbyopia** is the loss of focus on near objects, which occurs with age because the lens loses elasticity.

● H52.2 Astigmatism
- ● H52.20 Unspecified astigmatism
  - H52.201 Unspecified astigmatism, right eye
  - H52.202 Unspecified astigmatism, left eye
  - H52.203 Unspecified astigmatism, bilateral
  - H52.209 Unspecified astigmatism, unspecified eye
- ● H52.21 Irregular astigmatism
  - H52.211 Irregular astigmatism, right eye
  - H52.212 Irregular astigmatism, left eye
  - H52.213 Irregular astigmatism, bilateral
  - H52.219 Irregular astigmatism, unspecified eye
- ● H52.22 Regular astigmatism
  - H52.221 Regular astigmatism, right eye
  - H52.222 Regular astigmatism, left eye
  - H52.223 Regular astigmatism, bilateral
  - H52.229 Regular astigmatism, unspecified eye

● H52.3 Anisometropia and aniseikonia
- H52.31 Anisometropia
- H52.32 Aniseikonia

H52.4 Presbyopia

● H52.5 Disorders of accommodation
- ● H52.51 Internal ophthalmoplegia (complete) (total)
  - H52.511 Internal ophthalmoplegia (complete) (total), right eye
  - H52.512 Internal ophthalmoplegia (complete) (total), left eye
  - H52.513 Internal ophthalmoplegia (complete) (total), bilateral
  - H52.519 Internal ophthalmoplegia (complete) (total), unspecified eye
- ● H52.52 Paresis of accommodation
  - H52.521 Paresis of accommodation, right eye
  - H52.522 Paresis of accommodation, left eye
  - H52.523 Paresis of accommodation, bilateral
  - H52.529 Paresis of accommodation, unspecified eye
- ● H52.53 Spasm of accommodation
  - H52.531 Spasm of accommodation, right eye
  - H52.532 Spasm of accommodation, left eye
  - H52.533 Spasm of accommodation, bilateral
  - H52.539 Spasm of accommodation, unspecified eye

H52.6 Other disorders of refraction

H52.7 Unspecified disorder of refraction

VISUAL DISTURBANCES AND BLINDNESS (H53-H54)

● H53 Visual disturbances
- ● H53.0 Amblyopia ex anopsia
  - **Excludes1** amblyopia due to vitamin A deficiency (E50.5)
  - ● H53.00 Unspecified amblyopia
    - H53.001 Unspecified amblyopia, right eye
    - H53.002 Unspecified amblyopia, left eye
    - H53.003 Unspecified amblyopia, bilateral
    - H53.009 Unspecified amblyopia, unspecified eye
  - ● H53.01 Deprivation amblyopia
    - H53.011 Deprivation amblyopia, right eye
    - H53.012 Deprivation amblyopia, left eye
    - H53.013 Deprivation amblyopia, bilateral
    - H53.019 Deprivation amblyopia, unspecified eye
  - ● H53.02 Refractive amblyopia
    - H53.021 Refractive amblyopia, right eye
    - H53.022 Refractive amblyopia, left eye
    - H53.023 Refractive amblyopia, bilateral
    - H53.029 Refractive amblyopia, unspecified eye
  - ● H53.03 Strabismic amblyopia
    - **Excludes1** strabismus (H50.-)
    - H53.031 Strabismic amblyopia, right eye
    - H53.032 Strabismic amblyopia, left eye
    - H53.033 Strabismic amblyopia, bilateral
    - H53.039 Strabismic amblyopia, unspecified eye
  - ● H53.04 Amblyopia suspect ◀
    - H53.041 Amblyopia suspect, right eye ◀
    - H53.042 Amblyopia suspect, left eye ◀
    - H53.043 Amblyopia suspect, bilateral ◀
    - H53.049 Amblyopia suspect, unspecified eye ◀
- ● H53.1 Subjective visual disturbances
  - **Excludes1** subjective visual disturbances due to vitamin A deficiency (E50.5)
    visual hallucinations (R44.1)
  - H53.10 Unspecified subjective visual disturbances
  - H53.11 Day blindness
    Hemeralopia
  - ● H53.12 Transient visual loss
    Scintillating scotoma
    - **Excludes1** amaurosis fugax (G45.3-)
      transient retinal artery occlusion (H34.0-)
    - H53.121 Transient visual loss, right eye
    - H53.122 Transient visual loss, left eye
    - H53.123 Transient visual loss, bilateral
    - H53.129 Transient visual loss, unspecified eye
  - ● H53.13 Sudden visual loss
    - H53.131 Sudden visual loss, right eye
    - H53.132 Sudden visual loss, left eye
    - H53.133 Sudden visual loss, bilateral
    - H53.139 Sudden visual loss, unspecified eye

CHAPTER 7 (H00-H59)

● H53.14 Visual discomfort
Asthenopia
Photophobia
H53.141 Visual discomfort, right eye
H53.142 Visual discomfort, left eye
H53.143 Visual discomfort, bilateral
H53.149 Visual discomfort, unspecified
H53.15 Visual distortions of shape and size
Metamorphopsia
H53.16 Psychophysical visual disturbances
H53.19 Other subjective visual disturbances
Visual halos
H53.2 Diplopia
Double vision
● H53.3 Other and unspecified disorders of binocular vision
H53.30 Unspecified disorder of binocular vision
H53.31 Abnormal retinal correspondence
H53.32 Fusion with defective stereopsis
H53.33 Simultaneous visual perception without fusion
H53.34 Suppression of binocular vision
● H53.4 Visual field defects
H53.40 Unspecified visual field defects
● H53.41 Scotoma involving central area
Central scotoma
H53.411 Scotoma involving central area, right eye
H53.412 Scotoma involving central area, left eye
H53.413 Scotoma involving central area, bilateral
H53.419 Scotoma involving central area, unspecified eye
● H53.42 Scotoma of blind spot area
Enlarged blind spot
H53.421 Scotoma of blind spot area, right eye
H53.422 Scotoma of blind spot area, left eye
H53.423 Scotoma of blind spot area, bilateral
H53.429 Scotoma of blind spot area, unspecified eye
● H53.43 Sector or arcuate defects
Arcuate scotoma
Bjerrum scotoma
H53.431 Sector or arcuate defects, right eye
H53.432 Sector or arcuate defects, left eye
H53.433 Sector or arcuate defects, bilateral
H53.439 Sector or arcuate defects, unspecified eye
● H53.45 Other localized visual field defect
Peripheral visual field defect
Ring scotoma NOS
Scotoma NOS
H53.451 Other localized visual field defect, right eye
H53.452 Other localized visual field defect, left eye
H53.453 Other localized visual field defect, bilateral
H53.459 Other localized visual field defect, unspecified eye
● H53.46 Homonymous bilateral field defects
Homonymous hemianopia
Homonymous hemianopsia
Quadrant anopia
Quadrant anopsia
H53.461 Homonymous bilateral field defects, right side
H53.462 Homonymous bilateral field defects, left side
H53.469 Homonymous bilateral field defects, unspecified side
Homonymous bilateral field defects NOS
H53.47 Heteronymous bilateral field defects
Heteronymous hemianop(s)ia
● H53.48 Generalized contraction of visual field
H53.481 Generalized contraction of visual field, right eye
H53.482 Generalized contraction of visual field, left eye
H53.483 Generalized contraction of visual field, bilateral
H53.489 Generalized contraction of visual field, unspecified eye
● H53.5 Color vision deficiencies
Color blindness
Excludes2 day blindness (H53.11)
H53.50 Unspecified color vision deficiencies
Color blindness NOS
H53.51 Achromatopsia
H53.52 Acquired color vision deficiency
H53.53 Deuteranomaly
Deuteranopia
H53.54 Protanomaly
Protanopia
H53.55 Tritanomaly
Tritanopia
H53.59 Other color vision deficiencies
● H53.6 Night blindness
Excludes1 night blindness due to vitamin A deficiency (E50.5)
H53.60 Unspecified night blindness
H53.61 Abnormal dark adaptation curve
H53.62 Acquired night blindness
H53.63 Congenital night blindness
H53.69 Other night blindness
● H53.7 Vision sensitivity deficiencies
H53.71 Glare sensitivity
H53.72 Impaired contrast sensitivity
H53.8 Other visual disturbances
H53.9 Unspecified visual disturbance

CHAPTER 7 (H00-H59)

● **H54 Blindness and low vision**

Note: For definition of visual impairment categories see table below.

Code first any associated underlying cause of the blindness

Excludes1 amaurosis fugax (G45.3)

H54.Ø Blindness, both eyes
Visual impairment categories 3, 4, 5 in both eyes.

● **H54.1 Blindness, one eye, low vision other eye**
Visual impairment categories 3, 4, 5 in one eye, with categories 1 or 2 in the other eye.

H54.1Ø Blindness, one eye, low vision other eye, unspecified eyes

H54.11 Blindness, right eye, low vision left eye

H54.12 Blindness, left eye, low vision right eye

H54.2 Low vision, both eyes
Visual impairment categories 1 or 2 in both eyes.

H54.3 Unqualified visual loss, both eyes
Visual impairment category 9 in both eyes.

● **H54.4 Blindness, one eye**
Visual impairment categories 3, 4, 5 in one eye [normal vision in other eye]

H54.4Ø Blindness, one eye, unspecified eye

H54.41 Blindness, right eye, normal vision left eye

H54.42 Blindness, left eye, normal vision right eye

● **H54.5 Low vision, one eye**
Visual impairment categories 1 or 2 in one eye [normal vision in other eye].

H54.5Ø Low vision, one eye, unspecified eye

H54.51 Low vision, right eye, normal vision left eye

H54.52 Low vision, left eye, normal vision right eye

● **H54.6 Unqualified visual loss, one eye**
Visual impairment category 9 in one eye [normal vision in other eye].

H54.6Ø Unqualified visual loss, one eye, unspecified

H54.61 Unqualified visual loss, right eye, normal vision left eye

H54.62 Unqualified visual loss, left eye, normal vision right eye

H54.7 Unspecified visual loss
Visual impairment category 9 NOS

H54.8 Legal blindness, as defined in USA
Blindness NOS according to USA definition

Excludes1 legal blindness with specification of impairment level (H54.Ø-H54.7)

Note: The table below gives a classification of severity of visual impairment recommended by a WHO Study Group on the Prevention of Blindness, Geneva, 6-1Ø November 1972.

The term 'low vision' in category H54 comprises categories 1 and 2 of the table, the term 'blindness' categories 3, 4 and 5, and the term 'unqualified visual loss' category 9.

If the extent of the visual field is taken into account, patients with a field no greater than 1Ø but greater than 5 around central fixation should be placed in category 3 and patients with a field no greater than 5 around central fixation should be placed in category 4, even if the central acuity is not impaired.

(Document 5Ø8 compliance requires all cells in the following table to be filled.)

Category of visual impairment	Visual acuity with best possible correction	
	Maximum less than:	Minimum equal to or better than:
—	6/18	6/6Ø
3/1Ø (Ø.3)	1/1Ø (Ø.1)	—
2Ø/7Ø	2Ø/2ØØ	—
—	6/6Ø	3/6Ø
1/1Ø (Ø.1)	1/2Ø (Ø.Ø5)	—
2Ø/2ØØ	2Ø/4ØØ	—
—	3/6Ø	1/6Ø (finger counting at one meter)
1/2Ø (Ø.Ø5)	1/5Ø (Ø.Ø2)	—
2Ø/4ØØ	5/3ØØ (2Ø/12ØØ)	—
—	1/6Ø (finger counting at one meter)	Light perception
1/5Ø (Ø.Ø2)	—	—
5/3ØØ	—	—
—	No light perception	—
—	Undetermined or unspecified	—

OTHER DISORDERS OF EYE AND ADNEXA (H55-H57)

● **H55 Nystagmus and other irregular eye movements**

● **H55.Ø Nystagmus**
Rapid, involuntary movements of the eyes in the horizontal or vertical direction

H55.ØØ Unspecified nystagmus

H55.Ø1 Congenital nystagmus

H55.Ø2 Latent nystagmus

H55.Ø3 Visual deprivation nystagmus

H55.Ø4 Dissociated nystagmus

H55.Ø9 Other forms of nystagmus

● **H55.8 Other irregular eye movements**

H55.81 Saccadic eye movements

H55.89 Other irregular eye movements

● **H57 Other disorders of eye and adnexa**

● **H57.Ø Anomalies of pupillary function**

H57.ØØ Unspecified anomaly of pupillary function

H57.Ø1 Argyll Robertson pupil, atypical

Excludes1 syphilitic Argyll Robertson pupil (A52.19)

H57.Ø2 Anisocoria

H57.Ø3 Miosis

H57.Ø4 Mydriasis

● **H57.Ø5 Tonic pupil**

H57.Ø51 Tonic pupil, right eye

H57.Ø52 Tonic pupil, left eye

H57.Ø53 Tonic pupil, bilateral

H57.Ø59 Tonic pupil, unspecified eye

H57.Ø9 Other anomalies of pupillary function

● **H57.1 Ocular pain**

H57.1Ø Ocular pain, unspecified eye

H57.11 Ocular pain, right eye

H57.12 Ocular pain, left eye

H57.13 Ocular pain, bilateral

H57.8 Other specified disorders of eye and adnexa

H57.9 Unspecified disorder of eye and adnexa

INTRAOPERATIVE AND POSTPROCEDURAL COMPLICATIONS AND DISORDERS OF EYE AND ADNEXA, NOT ELSEWHERE CLASSIFIED (H59)

● **H59 Intraoperative and postprocedural complications and disorders of eye and adnexa, not elsewhere classified**

Excludes1 mechanical complication of intraocular lens (T85.2)
mechanical complication of other ocular prosthetic devices, implants and grafts (T85.3)
pseudophakia (Z96.1)
secondary cataracts (H26.4-)

● **H59.0 Disorders of the eye following cataract surgery**

● **H59.01 Keratopathy (bullous aphakic) following cataract surgery**
Vitreal corneal syndrome
Vitreous (touch) syndrome

H59.011 Keratopathy (bullous aphakic) following cataract surgery, right eye

H59.012 Keratopathy (bullous aphakic) following cataract surgery, left eye

H59.013 Keratopathy (bullous aphakic) following cataract surgery, bilateral

H59.019 Keratopathy (bullous aphakic) following cataract surgery, unspecified eye

● **H59.02 Cataract (lens) fragments in eye following cataract surgery**

H59.021 Cataract (lens) fragments in eye following cataract surgery, right eye

H59.022 Cataract (lens) fragments in eye following cataract surgery, left eye

H59.023 Cataract (lens) fragments in eye following cataract surgery, bilateral

H59.029 Cataract (lens) fragments in eye following cataract surgery, unspecified eye

● **H59.03 Cystoid macular edema following cataract surgery**

H59.031 Cystoid macular edema following cataract surgery, right eye

H59.032 Cystoid macular edema following cataract surgery, left eye

H59.033 Cystoid macular edema following cataract surgery, bilateral

H59.039 Cystoid macular edema following cataract surgery, unspecified eye

● **H59.09 Other disorders of the eye following cataract surgery**

H59.091 Other disorders of the right eye following cataract surgery

H59.092 Other disorders of the left eye following cataract surgery

H59.093 Other disorders of the eye following cataract surgery, bilateral

H59.099 Other disorders of unspecified eye following cataract surgery

● **H59.1 Intraoperative hemorrhage and hematoma of eye and adnexa complicating a procedure**

Excludes1 intraoperative hemorrhage and hematoma of eye and adnexa due to accidental puncture or laceration during a procedure (H59.2-)

● **H59.11 Intraoperative hemorrhage and hematoma of eye and adnexa complicating an ophthalmic procedure**

H59.111 Intraoperative hemorrhage and hematoma of right eye and adnexa complicating an ophthalmic procedure

H59.112 Intraoperative hemorrhage and hematoma of left eye and adnexa complicating an ophthalmic procedure

H59.113 Intraoperative hemorrhage and hematoma of eye and adnexa complicating an ophthalmic procedure, bilateral

H59.119 Intraoperative hemorrhage and hematoma of unspecified eye and adnexa complicating an ophthalmic procedure

● **H59.12 Intraoperative hemorrhage and hematoma of eye and adnexa complicating other procedure**

H59.121 Intraoperative hemorrhage and hematoma of right eye and adnexa complicating other procedure

H59.122 Intraoperative hemorrhage and hematoma of left eye and adnexa complicating other procedure

H59.123 Intraoperative hemorrhage and hematoma of eye and adnexa complicating other procedure, bilateral

H59.129 Intraoperative hemorrhage and hematoma of unspecified eye and adnexa complicating other procedure

● **H59.2 Accidental puncture and laceration of eye and adnexa during a procedure**

● **H59.21 Accidental puncture and laceration of eye and adnexa during an ophthalmic procedure**

H59.211 Accidental puncture and laceration of right eye and adnexa during an ophthalmic procedure

H59.212 Accidental puncture and laceration of left eye and adnexa during an ophthalmic procedure

H59.213 Accidental puncture and laceration of eye and adnexa during an ophthalmic procedure, bilateral

H59.219 Accidental puncture and laceration of unspecified eye and adnexa during an ophthalmic procedure

● **H59.22 Accidental puncture and laceration of eye and adnexa during other procedure**

H59.221 Accidental puncture and laceration of right eye and adnexa during other procedure

H59.222 Accidental puncture and laceration of left eye and adnexa during other procedure

H59.223 Accidental puncture and laceration of eye and adnexa during other procedure, bilateral

H59.229 Accidental puncture and laceration of unspecified eye and adnexa during other procedure

CHAPTER 7 (H00-H59)

● H59.3 Postprocedural hemorrhage, hematoma, and seroma of eye and adnexa following other procedure
● H59.31 Postprocedural hemorrhage of eye and adnexa following an ophthalmic procedure
H59.311 Postprocedural hemorrhage of right eye and adnexa following an ophthalmic procedure
H59.312 Postprocedural hemorrhage of left eye and adnexa following an ophthalmic procedure
H59.313 Postprocedural hemorrhage of eye and adnexa following an ophthalmic procedure, bilateral
H59.319 Postprocedural hemorrhage of unspecified eye and adnexa following an ophthalmic procedure
● H59.32 Postprocedural hemorrhage of eye and adnexa following other procedure
H59.321 Postprocedural hemorrhage of right eye and adnexa following other procedure
H59.322 Postprocedural hemorrhage of left eye and adnexa following other procedure
H59.323 Postprocedural hemorrhage of eye and adnexa following other procedure, bilateral
H59.329 Postprocedural hemorrhage of unspecified eye and adnexa following other procedure
● H59.33 Postprocedural hematoma of eye and adnexa following an ophthalmic procedure ◀
H59.331 Postprocedural hematoma of right eye and adnexa following an ophthalmic procedure ◀
H59.332 Postprocedural hematoma of left eye and adnexa following an ophthalmic procedure ◀
H59.333 Postprocedural hematoma of eye and adnexa following an ophthalmic procedure, bilateral ◀
H59.339 Postprocedural hematoma of unspecified eye and adnexa following an ophthalmic procedure ◀
● H59.34 Postprocedural hematoma of eye and adnexa following other procedure ◀
H59.341 Postprocedural hematoma of right eye and adnexa following other procedure ◀
H59.342 Postprocedural hematoma of left eye and adnexa following other procedure ◀
H59.343 Postprocedural hematoma of eye and adnexa following other procedure, bilateral ◀
H59.349 Postprocedural hematoma of unspecified eye and adnexa following other procedure ◀
● H59.35 Postprocedural seroma of eye and adnexa following an ophthalmic procedure ◀
H59.351 Postprocedural seroma of right eye and adnexa following an ophthalmic procedure ◀
H59.352 Postprocedural seroma of left eye and adnexa following an ophthalmic procedure ◀
H59.353 Postprocedural seroma of eye and adnexa following an ophthalmic procedure, bilateral ◀
H59.359 Postprocedural seroma of unspecified eye and adnexa following an ophthalmic procedure ◀
● H59.36 Postprocedural seroma of eye and adnexa following other procedure ◀
H59.361 Postprocedural seroma of right eye and adnexa following other procedure ◀
H59.362 Postprocedural seroma of left eye and adnexa following other procedure ◀
H59.363 Postprocedural seroma of eye and adnexa following other procedure, bilateral ◀
H59.369 Postprocedural seroma of unspecified eye and adnexa following other procedure ◀
● H59.4 Inflammation (infection) of postprocedural bleb
Postprocedural blebitis
Excludes1 filtering (vitreous) bleb after glaucoma surgery status (Z98.83)
H59.40 Inflammation (infection) of postprocedural bleb, unspecified
H59.41 Inflammation (infection) of postprocedural bleb, stage 1
H59.42 Inflammation (infection) of postprocedural bleb, stage 2
H59.43 Inflammation (infection) of postprocedural bleb, stage 3
Bleb endophthalmitis
● H59.8 Other intraoperative and postprocedural complications and disorders of eye and adnexa, not elsewhere classified
● H59.81 Chorioretinal scars after surgery for detachment
H59.811 Chorioretinal scars after surgery for detachment, right eye
H59.812 Chorioretinal scars after surgery for detachment, left eye
H59.813 Chorioretinal scars after surgery for detachment, bilateral
H59.819 Chorioretinal scars after surgery for detachment, unspecified eye
H59.88 Other intraoperative complications of eye and adnexa, not elsewhere classified
H59.89 Other postprocedural complications and disorders of eye and adnexa, not elsewhere classified

CHAPTER 8

DISEASES OF THE EAR AND MASTOID PROCESS (H60-H95)

OGCR Chapter-Specific Coding Guidelines

8. Chapter 8: Diseases of the Ear and Mastoid Process (H60-H95)
Reserved for future guideline expansion

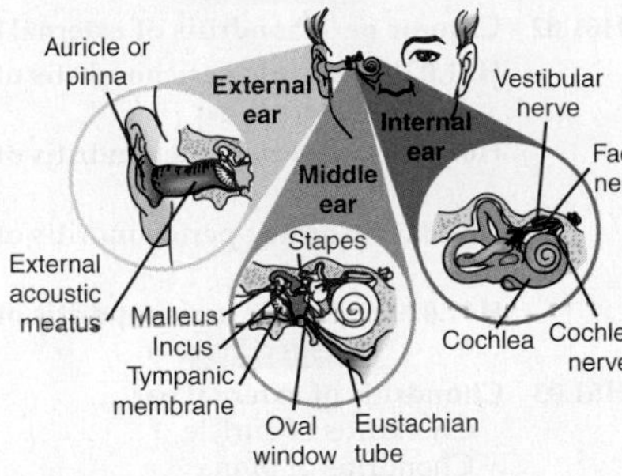

Figure 8-1 Auditory system. (From Buck CJ: Step-by-Step Medical Coding, ed 2016, St. Louis, Elsevier, 2016)

★**(See Plate 92 on page NAP-20.)**

CHAPTER 8

DISEASES OF THE EAR AND MASTOID PROCESS (H60-H95)

Note: Use an external cause code following the code for the ear condition, if applicable, to identify the cause of the ear condition

Excludes2 certain conditions originating in the perinatal period (P04-P96)
certain infectious and parasitic diseases (A00-B99)
complications of pregnancy, childbirth and the puerperium (O00-O9A)
congenital malformations, deformations and chromosomal abnormalities (Q00-Q99)
endocrine, nutritional and metabolic diseases (E00-E88)
injury, poisoning and certain other consequences of external causes (S00-T88)
neoplasms (C00-D49)
symptoms, signs and abnormal clinical and laboratory findings, not elsewhere classified (R00-R94)

This chapter contains the following blocks:

H60-H62	Diseases of external ear
H65-H75	Diseases of middle ear and mastoid
H80-H83	Diseases of inner ear
H90-H94	Other disorders of ear
H95	Intraoperative and postprocedural complications and disorders of ear and mastoid process, not elsewhere classified

DISEASES OF EXTERNAL EAR (H60-H62)

● **H60 Otitis externa**

● **H60.0 Abscess of external ear**
Boil of external ear
Carbuncle of auricle or external auditory canal
Furuncle of external ear

H60.00 Abscess of external ear, unspecified ear
H60.01 Abscess of right external ear
H60.02 Abscess of left external ear
H60.03 Abscess of external ear, bilateral

● **H60.1 Cellulitis of external ear**
Cellulitis of auricle
Cellulitis of external auditory canal

H60.10 Cellulitis of external ear, unspecified ear
H60.11 Cellulitis of right external ear
H60.12 Cellulitis of left external ear
H60.13 Cellulitis of external ear, bilateral

● **H60.2 Malignant otitis externa**

H60.20 Malignant otitis externa, unspecified ear
H60.21 Malignant otitis externa, right ear
H60.22 Malignant otitis externa, left ear
H60.23 Malignant otitis externa, bilateral

● **H60.3 Other infective otitis externa**

● **H60.31 Diffuse otitis externa**

H60.311 Diffuse otitis externa, right ear
H60.312 Diffuse otitis externa, left ear
H60.313 Diffuse otitis externa, bilateral
H60.319 Diffuse otitis externa, unspecified ear

● **H60.32 Hemorrhagic otitis externa**

H60.321 Hemorrhagic otitis externa, right ear
H60.322 Hemorrhagic otitis externa, left ear
H60.323 Hemorrhagic otitis externa, bilateral
H60.329 Hemorrhagic otitis externa, unspecified ear

● **H60.33 Swimmer's ear**

H60.331 Swimmer's ear, right ear
H60.332 Swimmer's ear, left ear
H60.333 Swimmer's ear, bilateral
H60.339 Swimmer's ear, unspecified ear

● **H60.39 Other infective otitis externa**

H60.391 Other infective otitis externa, right ear
H60.392 Other infective otitis externa, left ear
H60.393 Other infective otitis externa, bilateral
H60.399 Other infective otitis externa, unspecified ear

● **H60.4 Cholesteatoma of external ear**
Keratosis obturans of external ear (canal)

Excludes2 cholesteatoma of middle ear (H71.-)
recurrent cholesteatoma of postmastoidectomy cavity (H95.0-)

H60.40 Cholesteatoma of external ear, unspecified ear
H60.41 Cholesteatoma of right external ear
H60.42 Cholesteatoma of left external ear
H60.43 Cholesteatoma of external ear, bilateral

● **H60.5 Acute noninfective otitis externa**

● **H60.50 Unspecified acute noninfective otitis externa**
Acute otitis externa NOS

H60.501 Unspecified acute noninfective otitis externa, right ear
H60.502 Unspecified acute noninfective otitis externa, left ear
H60.503 Unspecified acute noninfective otitis externa, bilateral
H60.509 Unspecified acute noninfective otitis externa, unspecified ear

● **H60.51 Acute actinic otitis externa**

H60.511 Acute actinic otitis externa, right ear
H60.512 Acute actinic otitis externa, left ear
H60.513 Acute actinic otitis externa, bilateral
H60.519 Acute actinic otitis externa, unspecified ear

CHAPTER 8 (H60-H95)

● H60.52 Acute chemical otitis externa
- H60.521 Acute chemical otitis externa, right ear
- H60.522 Acute chemical otitis externa, left ear
- H60.523 Acute chemical otitis externa, bilateral
- H60.529 Acute chemical otitis externa, unspecified ear

● H60.53 Acute contact otitis externa
- H60.531 Acute contact otitis externa, right ear
- H60.532 Acute contact otitis externa, left ear
- H60.533 Acute contact otitis externa, bilateral
- H60.539 Acute contact otitis externa, unspecified ear

● H60.54 Acute eczematoid otitis externa
- H60.541 Acute eczematoid otitis externa, right ear
- H60.542 Acute eczematoid otitis externa, left ear
- H60.543 Acute eczematoid otitis externa, bilateral
- H60.549 Acute eczematoid otitis externa, unspecified ear

● H60.55 Acute reactive otitis externa
- H60.551 Acute reactive otitis externa, right ear
- H60.552 Acute reactive otitis externa, left ear
- H60.553 Acute reactive otitis externa, bilateral
- H60.559 Acute reactive otitis externa, unspecified ear

● H60.59 Other noninfective acute otitis externa
- H60.591 Other noninfective acute otitis externa, right ear
- H60.592 Other noninfective acute otitis externa, left ear
- H60.593 Other noninfective acute otitis externa, bilateral
- H60.599 Other noninfective acute otitis externa, unspecified ear

● H60.6 Unspecified chronic otitis externa
- H60.60 Unspecified chronic otitis externa, unspecified ear
- H60.61 Unspecified chronic otitis externa, right ear
- H60.62 Unspecified chronic otitis externa, left ear
- H60.63 Unspecified chronic otitis externa, bilateral

● H60.8 Other otitis externa

● H60.8X Other otitis externa
- H60.8X1 Other otitis externa, right ear
- H60.8X2 Other otitis externa, left ear
- H60.8X3 Other otitis externa, bilateral
- H60.8X9 Other otitis externa, unspecified ear

● H60.9 Unspecified otitis externa
- H60.90 Unspecified otitis externa, unspecified ear
- H60.91 Unspecified otitis externa, right ear
- H60.92 Unspecified otitis externa, left ear
- H60.93 Unspecified otitis externa, bilateral

● H61 Other disorders of external ear

● H61.0 Chondritis and perichondritis of external ear
Chondrodermatitis nodularis chronica helicis
Perichondritis of auricle
Perichondritis of pinna

● H61.00 Unspecified perichondritis of external ear
- H61.001 Unspecified perichondritis of right external ear
- H61.002 Unspecified perichondritis of left external ear
- H61.003 Unspecified perichondritis of external ear, bilateral
- H61.009 Unspecified perichondritis of external ear, unspecified ear

● H61.01 Acute perichondritis of external ear
- H61.011 Acute perichondritis of right external ear
- H61.012 Acute perichondritis of left external ear
- H61.013 Acute perichondritis of external ear, bilateral
- H61.019 Acute perichondritis of external ear, unspecified ear

● H61.02 Chronic perichondritis of external ear
- H61.021 Chronic perichondritis of right external ear
- H61.022 Chronic perichondritis of left external ear
- H61.023 Chronic perichondritis of external ear, bilateral
- H61.029 Chronic perichondritis of external ear, unspecified ear

● H61.03 Chondritis of external ear
Chondritis of auricle
Chondritis of pinna
- H61.031 Chondritis of right external ear
- H61.032 Chondritis of left external ear
- H61.033 Chondritis of external ear, bilateral
- H61.039 Chondritis of external ear, unspecified ear

● H61.1 Noninfective disorders of pinna
Excludes2 cauliflower ear (M95.1-)
gouty tophi of ear (M1A.-)

● H61.10 Unspecified noninfective disorders of pinna
Disorder of pinna NOS
- H61.101 Unspecified noninfective disorders of pinna, right ear
- H61.102 Unspecified noninfective disorders of pinna, left ear
- H61.103 Unspecified noninfective disorders of pinna, bilateral
- H61.109 Unspecified noninfective disorders of pinna, unspecified ear

● H61.11 Acquired deformity of pinna
Acquired deformity of auricle
Excludes2 cauliflower ear (M95.1-)
- H61.111 Acquired deformity of pinna, right ear
- H61.112 Acquired deformity of pinna, left ear
- H61.113 Acquired deformity of pinna, bilateral
- H61.119 Acquired deformity of pinna, unspecified ear

● H61.12 Hematoma of pinna
Hematoma of auricle
- H61.121 Hematoma of pinna, right ear
- H61.122 Hematoma of pinna, left ear
- H61.123 Hematoma of pinna, bilateral
- H61.129 Hematoma of pinna, unspecified ear

● H61.19 Other noninfective disorders of pinna
- H61.191 Noninfective disorders of pinna, right ear
- H61.192 Noninfective disorders of pinna, left ear
- H61.193 Noninfective disorders of pinna, bilateral
- H61.199 Noninfective disorders of pinna, unspecified ear

● **H61.2 Impacted cerumen**
Wax in ear
H61.20 Impacted cerumen, unspecified ear
H61.21 Impacted cerumen, right ear
H61.22 Impacted cerumen, left ear
H61.23 Impacted cerumen, bilateral

● **H61.3 Acquired stenosis of external ear canal**
Collapse of external ear canal
Excludes1 postprocedural stenosis of external ear canal (H95.81-)

● **H61.30** Acquired stenosis of external ear canal, unspecified
H61.301 Acquired stenosis of right external ear canal, unspecified
H61.302 Acquired stenosis of left external ear canal, unspecified
H61.303 Acquired stenosis of external ear canal, unspecified, bilateral
H61.309 Acquired stenosis of external ear canal, unspecified, unspecified ear

● **H61.31** Acquired stenosis of external ear canal secondary to trauma
H61.311 Acquired stenosis of right external ear canal secondary to trauma
H61.312 Acquired stenosis of left external ear canal secondary to trauma
H61.313 Acquired stenosis of external ear canal secondary to trauma, bilateral
H61.319 Acquired stenosis of external ear canal secondary to trauma, unspecified ear

● **H61.32** Acquired stenosis of external ear canal secondary to inflammation and infection
H61.321 Acquired stenosis of right external ear canal secondary to inflammation and infection
H61.322 Acquired stenosis of left external ear canal secondary to inflammation and infection
H61.323 Acquired stenosis of external ear canal secondary to inflammation and infection, bilateral
H61.329 Acquired stenosis of external ear canal secondary to inflammation and infection, unspecified ear

● **H61.39** Other acquired stenosis of external ear canal
H61.391 Other acquired stenosis of right external ear canal
H61.392 Other acquired stenosis of left external ear canal
H61.393 Other acquired stenosis of external ear canal, bilateral
H61.399 Other acquired stenosis of external ear canal, unspecified ear

● **H61.8 Other specified disorders of external ear**

● **H61.81** Exostosis of external canal
H61.811 Exostosis of right external canal
H61.812 Exostosis of left external canal
H61.813 Exostosis of external canal, bilateral
H61.819 Exostosis of external canal, unspecified ear

● **H61.89** Other specified disorders of external ear
H61.891 Other specified disorders of right external ear
H61.892 Other specified disorders of left external ear
H61.893 Other specified disorders of external ear, bilateral
H61.899 Other specified disorders of external ear, unspecified ear

● **H61.9 Disorder of external ear, unspecified**
H61.90 Disorder of external ear, unspecified, unspecified ear
H61.91 Disorder of right external ear, unspecified
H61.92 Disorder of left external ear, unspecified
H61.93 Disorder of external ear, unspecified, bilateral

● **H62 Disorders of external ear in diseases classified elsewhere**

● **H62.4 Otitis externa in other diseases classified elsewhere**
Code first underlying disease, such as:
erysipelas (A46)
impetigo (L01.0)
Excludes1 otitis externa (in):
candidiasis (B37.84)
herpes viral [herpes simplex] (B00.1)
herpes zoster (B02.8)
H62.40 Otitis externa in other diseases classified elsewhere, unspecified ear
H62.41 Otitis externa in other diseases classified elsewhere, right ear
H62.42 Otitis externa in other diseases classified elsewhere, left ear
H62.43 Otitis externa in other diseases classified elsewhere, bilateral

● **H62.8 Other disorders of external ear in diseases classified elsewhere**
Code first underlying disease, such as:
gout (M1A.-, M10.-)

● **H62.8X** Other disorders of external ear in diseases classified elsewhere
H62.8X1 Other disorders of right external ear in diseases classified elsewhere
H62.8X2 Other disorders of left external ear in diseases classified elsewhere
H62.8X3 Other disorders of external ear in diseases classified elsewhere, bilateral
H62.8X9 Other disorders of external ear in diseases classified elsewhere, unspecified ear

DISEASES OF MIDDLE EAR AND MASTOID (H65-H75)

★**(See Plate 94 on page NAP-21.)**

● **H65 Nonsuppurative otitis media**
Bacterial or viral infection or inflammation of the middle ear; may result in fluid accumulation with pain and temporary hearing loss.
Includes nonsuppurative otitis media with myringitis
Use additional code for any associated perforated tympanic membrane (H72.-)
Use additional code to identify:
exposure to environmental tobacco smoke (Z77.22)
exposure to tobacco smoke in the perinatal period (P96.81)
history of tobacco dependence (Z87.891) ◄
occupational exposure to environmental tobacco smoke (Z57.31)
tobacco dependence (F17.-)
tobacco use (Z72.0)

● **H65.0 Acute serous otitis media**
Acute and subacute secretory otitis
H65.00 Acute serous otitis media, unspecified ear
H65.01 Acute serous otitis media, right ear
H65.02 Acute serous otitis media, left ear
H65.03 Acute serous otitis media, bilateral
H65.04 Acute serous otitis media, recurrent, right ear
H65.05 Acute serous otitis media, recurrent, left ear
H65.06 Acute serous otitis media, recurrent, bilateral
H65.07 Acute serous otitis media, recurrent, unspecified ear

CHAPTER 8 (H60-H95)

● **H65.1 Other acute nonsuppurative otitis media**
Excludes1 otitic barotrauma (T70.0)
otitis media (acute) NOS (H66.9)

● **H65.11 Acute and subacute allergic otitis media (mucoid) (sanguinous) (serous)**
H65.111 Acute and subacute allergic otitis media (mucoid) (sanguinous) (serous), right ear
H65.112 Acute and subacute allergic otitis media (mucoid) (sanguinous) (serous), left ear
H65.113 Acute and subacute allergic otitis media (mucoid) (sanguinous) (serous), bilateral
H65.114 Acute and subacute allergic otitis media (mucoid) (sanguinous) (serous), recurrent, right ear
H65.115 Acute and subacute allergic otitis media (mucoid) (sanguinous) (serous), recurrent, left ear
H65.116 Acute and subacute allergic otitis media (mucoid) (sanguinous) (serous), recurrent, bilateral
H65.117 Acute and subacute allergic otitis media (mucoid) (sanguinous) (serous), recurrent, unspecified ear
H65.119 Acute and subacute allergic otitis media (mucoid) (sanguinous) (serous), unspecified ear

● **H65.19 Other acute nonsuppurative otitis media**
Acute and subacute mucoid otitis media
Acute and subacute nonsuppurative otitis media NOS
Acute and subacute sanguinous otitis media
Acute and subacute seromucinous otitis media
H65.191 Other acute nonsuppurative otitis media, right ear
H65.192 Other acute nonsuppurative otitis media, left ear
H65.193 Other acute nonsuppurative otitis media, bilateral
H65.194 Other acute nonsuppurative otitis media, recurrent, right ear
H65.195 Other acute nonsuppurative otitis media, recurrent, left ear
H65.196 Other acute nonsuppurative otitis media, recurrent, bilateral
H65.197 Other acute nonsuppurative otitis media recurrent, unspecified ear
H65.199 Other acute nonsuppurative otitis media, unspecified ear

● **H65.2 Chronic serous otitis media**
Chronic tubotympanal catarrh
H65.20 Chronic serous otitis media, unspecified ear
H65.21 Chronic serous otitis media, right ear
H65.22 Chronic serous otitis media, left ear
H65.23 Chronic serous otitis media, bilateral

● **H65.3 Chronic mucoid otitis media**
Chronic mucinous otitis media
Chronic secretory otitis media
Chronic transudative otitis media
Glue ear
Excludes1 adhesive middle ear disease (H74.1)
H65.30 Chronic mucoid otitis media, unspecified ear
H65.31 Chronic mucoid otitis media, right ear
H65.32 Chronic mucoid otitis media, left ear
H65.33 Chronic mucoid otitis media, bilateral

● **H65.4 Other chronic nonsuppurative otitis media**

● **H65.41 Chronic allergic otitis media**
H65.411 Chronic allergic otitis media, right ear
H65.412 Chronic allergic otitis media, left ear
H65.413 Chronic allergic otitis media, bilateral
H65.419 Chronic allergic otitis media, unspecified ear

● **H65.49 Other chronic nonsuppurative otitis media**
Chronic exudative otitis media
Chronic nonsuppurative otitis media NOS
Chronic otitis media with effusion (nonpurulent)
Chronic seromucinous otitis media
H65.491 Other chronic nonsuppurative otitis media, right ear
H65.492 Other chronic nonsuppurative otitis media, left ear
H65.493 Other chronic nonsuppurative otitis media, bilateral
H65.499 Other chronic nonsuppurative otitis media, unspecified ear

● **H65.9 Unspecified nonsuppurative otitis media**
Allergic otitis media NOS
Catarrhal otitis media NOS
Exudative otitis media NOS
Mucoid otitis media NOS
Otitis media with effusion (nonpurulent) NOS
Secretory otitis media NOS
Seromucinous otitis media NOS
Serous otitis media NOS
Transudative otitis media NOS
H65.90 Unspecified nonsuppurative otitis media, unspecified ear
H65.91 Unspecified nonsuppurative otitis media, right ear
H65.92 Unspecified nonsuppurative otitis media, left ear
H65.93 Unspecified nonsuppurative otitis media, bilateral

● **H66 Suppurative and unspecified otitis media**
Suppurative: Discharging pus
Includes suppurative and unspecified otitis media with myringitis
Use additional code to identify:
exposure to environmental tobacco smoke (Z77.22)
exposure to tobacco smoke in the perinatal period (P96.81)
history of tobacco dependence (Z87.891)
occupational exposure to environmental tobacco smoke (Z57.31)
tobacco dependence (F17.-)
tobacco use (Z72.0)

● **H66.0 Acute suppurative otitis media**

● **H66.00 Acute suppurative otitis media without spontaneous rupture of ear drum**
H66.001 Acute suppurative otitis media without spontaneous rupture of ear drum, right ear
H66.002 Acute suppurative otitis media without spontaneous rupture of ear drum, left ear
H66.003 Acute suppurative otitis media without spontaneous rupture of ear drum, bilateral
H66.004 Acute suppurative otitis media without spontaneous rupture of ear drum, recurrent, right ear
H66.005 Acute suppurative otitis media without spontaneous rupture of ear drum, recurrent, left ear
H66.006 Acute suppurative otitis media without spontaneous rupture of ear drum, recurrent, bilateral

H66.007 Acute suppurative otitis media without spontaneous rupture of ear drum, recurrent, unspecified ear

H66.009 Acute suppurative otitis media without spontaneous rupture of ear drum, unspecified ear

● H66.01 Acute suppurative otitis media with spontaneous rupture of ear drum

H66.011 Acute suppurative otitis media with spontaneous rupture of ear drum, right ear

H66.012 Acute suppurative otitis media with spontaneous rupture of ear drum, left ear

H66.013 Acute suppurative otitis media with spontaneous rupture of ear drum, bilateral

H66.014 Acute suppurative otitis media with spontaneous rupture of ear drum, recurrent, right ear

H66.015 Acute suppurative otitis media with spontaneous rupture of ear drum, recurrent, left ear

H66.016 Acute suppurative otitis media with spontaneous rupture of ear drum, recurrent, bilateral

H66.017 Acute suppurative otitis media with spontaneous rupture of ear drum, recurrent, unspecified ear

H66.019 Acute suppurative otitis media with spontaneous rupture of ear drum, unspecified ear

● H66.1 Chronic tubotympanic suppurative otitis media

Benign chronic suppurative otitis media

Chronic tubotympanic disease

Use additional code for any associated perforated tympanic membrane (H72.-)

H66.10 Chronic tubotympanic suppurative otitis media, unspecified

H66.11 Chronic tubotympanic suppurative otitis media, right ear

H66.12 Chronic tubotympanic suppurative otitis media, left ear

H66.13 Chronic tubotympanic suppurative otitis media, bilateral

● H66.2 Chronic atticoantral suppurative otitis media

Chronic atticoantral disease

Use additional code for any associated perforated tympanic membrane (H72.-)

H66.20 Chronic atticoantral suppurative otitis media, unspecified ear

H66.21 Chronic atticoantral suppurative otitis media, right ear

H66.22 Chronic atticoantral suppurative otitis media, left ear

H66.23 Chronic atticoantral suppurative otitis media, bilateral

● H66.3 Other chronic suppurative otitis media

Chronic suppurative otitis media NOS

Use additional code for any associated perforated tympanic membrane (H72.-)

Excludes1 tuberculous otitis media (A18.6)

● H66.3X Other chronic suppurative otitis media

H66.3X1 Other chronic suppurative otitis media, right ear

H66.3X2 Other chronic suppurative otitis media, left ear

H66.3X3 Other chronic suppurative otitis media, bilateral

H66.3X9 Other chronic suppurative otitis media, unspecified ear

● H66.4 Suppurative otitis media, unspecified

Purulent otitis media NOS

Use additional code for any associated perforated tympanic membrane (H72.-)

H66.40 Suppurative otitis media, unspecified, unspecified ear

H66.41 Suppurative otitis media, unspecified, right ear

H66.42 Suppurative otitis media, unspecified, left ear

H66.43 Suppurative otitis media, unspecified, bilateral

● H66.9 Otitis media, unspecified

Otitis media NOS

Acute otitis media NOS

Chronic otitis media NOS

Use additional code for any associated perforated tympanic membrane (H72.-)

H66.90 Otitis media, unspecified, unspecified ear

H66.91 Otitis media, unspecified, right ear

H66.92 Otitis media, unspecified, left ear

H66.93 Otitis media, unspecified, bilateral

● H67 Otitis media in diseases classified elsewhere

Code first underlying disease, such as:

viral disease NEC (B00-B34)

Use additional code for any associated perforated tympanic membrane (H72.-)

Excludes1 otitis media in:

influenza (J09.X9, J10.83, J11.83)

measles (B05.3)

scarlet fever (A38.0)

tuberculosis (A18.6)

H67.1 Otitis media in diseases classified elsewhere, right ear

H67.2 Otitis media in diseases classified elsewhere, left ear

H67.3 Otitis media in diseases classified elsewhere, bilateral

H67.9 Otitis media in diseases classified elsewhere, unspecified ear

● H68 Eustachian salpingitis and obstruction

● H68.0 Eustachian salpingitis

● H68.00 Unspecified Eustachian salpingitis

H68.001 Unspecified Eustachian salpingitis, right ear

H68.002 Unspecified Eustachian salpingitis, left ear

H68.003 Unspecified Eustachian salpingitis, bilateral

H68.009 Unspecified Eustachian salpingitis, unspecified ear

● H68.01 Acute Eustachian salpingitis

H68.011 Acute Eustachian salpingitis, right ear

H68.012 Acute Eustachian salpingitis, left ear

H68.013 Acute Eustachian salpingitis, bilateral

H68.019 Acute Eustachian salpingitis, unspecified ear

● H68.02 Chronic Eustachian salpingitis

H68.021 Chronic Eustachian salpingitis, right ear

H68.022 Chronic Eustachian salpingitis, left ear

H68.023 Chronic Eustachian salpingitis, bilateral

H68.029 Chronic Eustachian salpingitis, unspecified ear

CHAPTER 8 (H60-H95)

● H68.1 Obstruction of Eustachian tube
Stenosis of Eustachian tube
Stricture of Eustachian tube
● H68.10 Unspecified obstruction of Eustachian tube
H68.101 Unspecified obstruction of Eustachian tube, right ear
H68.102 Unspecified obstruction of Eustachian tube, left ear
H68.103 Unspecified obstruction of Eustachian tube, bilateral
H68.109 Unspecified obstruction of Eustachian tube, unspecified ear
● H68.11 Osseous obstruction of Eustachian tube
H68.111 Osseous obstruction of Eustachian tube, right ear
H68.112 Osseous obstruction of Eustachian tube, left ear
H68.113 Osseous obstruction of Eustachian tube, bilateral
H68.119 Osseous obstruction of Eustachian tube, unspecified ear
● H68.12 Intrinsic cartilagenous obstruction of Eustachian tube
H68.121 Intrinsic cartilagenous obstruction of Eustachian tube, right ear
H68.122 Intrinsic cartilagenous obstruction of Eustachian tube, left ear
H68.123 Intrinsic cartilagenous obstruction of Eustachian tube, bilateral
H68.129 Intrinsic cartilagenous obstruction of Eustachian tube, unspecified ear
● H68.13 Extrinsic cartilagenous obstruction of Eustachian tube
Compression of Eustachian tube
H68.131 Extrinsic cartilagenous obstruction of Eustachian tube, right ear
H68.132 Extrinsic cartilagenous obstruction of Eustachian tube, left ear
H68.133 Extrinsic cartilagenous obstruction of Eustachian tube, bilateral
H68.139 Extrinsic cartilagenous obstruction of Eustachian tube, unspecified ear

● H69 Other and unspecified disorders of Eustachian tube
● H69.0 Patulous Eustachian tube
H69.00 Patulous Eustachian tube, unspecified ear
H69.01 Patulous Eustachian tube, right ear
H69.02 Patulous Eustachian tube, left ear
H69.03 Patulous Eustachian tube, bilateral
● H69.8 Other specified disorders of Eustachian tube
H69.80 Other specified disorders of Eustachian tube, unspecified ear
H69.81 Other specified disorders of Eustachian tube, right ear
H69.82 Other specified disorders of Eustachian tube, left ear
H69.83 Other specified disorders of Eustachian tube, bilateral
● H69.9 Unspecified Eustachian tube disorder
H69.90 Unspecified Eustachian tube disorder, unspecified ear
H69.91 Unspecified Eustachian tube disorder, right ear
H69.92 Unspecified Eustachian tube disorder, left ear
H69.93 Unspecified Eustachian tube disorder, bilateral

● H70 Mastoiditis and related conditions
● H70.0 Acute mastoiditis
Abscess of mastoid
Empyema of mastoid
● H70.00 Acute mastoiditis without complications
H70.001 Acute mastoiditis without complications, right ear
H70.002 Acute mastoiditis without complications, left ear
H70.003 Acute mastoiditis without complications, bilateral
H70.009 Acute mastoiditis without complications, unspecified ear
● H70.01 Subperiosteal abscess of mastoid
H70.011 Subperiosteal abscess of mastoid, right ear
H70.012 Subperiosteal abscess of mastoid, left ear
H70.013 Subperiosteal abscess of mastoid, bilateral
H70.019 Subperiosteal abscess of mastoid, unspecified ear
● H70.09 Acute mastoiditis with other complications
H70.091 Acute mastoiditis with other complications, right ear
H70.092 Acute mastoiditis with other complications, left ear
H70.093 Acute mastoiditis with other complications, bilateral
H70.099 Acute mastoiditis with other complications, unspecified ear
● H70.1 Chronic mastoiditis
Caries of mastoid
Fistula of mastoid
Excludes1 tuberculous mastoiditis (A18.03)
H70.10 Chronic mastoiditis, unspecified ear
H70.11 Chronic mastoiditis, right ear
H70.12 Chronic mastoiditis, left ear
H70.13 Chronic mastoiditis, bilateral
● H70.2 Petrositis
Inflammation of petrous bone
● H70.20 Unspecified petrositis
H70.201 Unspecified petrositis, right ear
H70.202 Unspecified petrositis, left ear
H70.203 Unspecified petrositis, bilateral
H70.209 Unspecified petrositis, unspecified ear
● H70.21 Acute petrositis
H70.211 Acute petrositis, right ear
H70.212 Acute petrositis, left ear
H70.213 Acute petrositis, bilateral
H70.219 Acute petrositis, unspecified ear
● H70.22 Chronic petrositis
H70.221 Chronic petrositis, right ear
H70.222 Chronic petrositis, left ear
H70.223 Chronic petrositis, bilateral
H70.229 Chronic petrositis, unspecified ear

Item 8–1 Mastoiditis is an infection of the portion of the temporal bone of the skull that is behind the ear (mastoid process) caused by an untreated otitis media, leading to an infection of the surrounding structures which may include the brain.

● **H70.8** Other mastoiditis and related conditions
Excludes1 preauricular sinus and cyst (Q18.1)
sinus, fistula, and cyst of branchial cleft (Q18.0)

● **H70.81** Postauricular fistula
H70.811 Postauricular fistula, right ear
H70.812 Postauricular fistula, left ear
H70.813 Postauricular fistula, bilateral
H70.819 Postauricular fistula, unspecified ear

● **H70.89** Other mastoiditis and related conditions
H70.891 Other mastoiditis and related conditions, right ear
H70.892 Other mastoiditis and related conditions, left ear
H70.893 Other mastoiditis and related conditions, bilateral
H70.899 Other mastoiditis and related conditions, unspecified ear

● **H70.9** Unspecified mastoiditis
H70.90 Unspecified mastoiditis, unspecified ear
H70.91 Unspecified mastoiditis, right ear
H70.92 Unspecified mastoiditis, left ear
H70.93 Unspecified mastoiditis, bilateral

● **H71** Cholesteatoma of middle ear
Excludes2 cholesteatoma of external ear (H60.4-)
recurrent cholesteatoma of postmastoidectomy cavity (H95.0-)

● **H71.0** Cholesteatoma of attic
H71.00 Cholesteatoma of attic, unspecified ear
H71.01 Cholesteatoma of attic, right ear
H71.02 Cholesteatoma of attic, left ear
H71.03 Cholesteatoma of attic, bilateral

● **H71.1** Cholesteatoma of tympanum
H71.10 Cholesteatoma of tympanum, unspecified ear
H71.11 Cholesteatoma of tympanum, right ear
H71.12 Cholesteatoma of tympanum, left ear
H71.13 Cholesteatoma of tympanum, bilateral

● **H71.2** Cholesteatoma of mastoid
H71.20 Cholesteatoma of mastoid, unspecified ear
H71.21 Cholesteatoma of mastoid, right ear
H71.22 Cholesteatoma of mastoid, left ear
H71.23 Cholesteatoma of mastoid, bilateral

● **H71.3** Diffuse cholesteatosis
H71.30 Diffuse cholesteatosis, unspecified ear
H71.31 Diffuse cholesteatosis, right ear
H71.32 Diffuse cholesteatosis, left ear
H71.33 Diffuse cholesteatosis, bilateral

● **H71.9** Unspecified cholesteatoma
H71.90 Unspecified cholesteatoma, unspecified ear
H71.91 Unspecified cholesteatoma, right ear
H71.92 Unspecified cholesteatoma, left ear
H71.93 Unspecified cholesteatoma, bilateral

★(See Plate 93 on page NAP-21.)

● **H72** Perforation of tympanic membrane
Hole or rupture in ear drum
Includes persistent post-traumatic perforation of ear drum
postinflammatory perforation of ear drum
Code first any associated otitis media (H65.-, H66.1-, H66.2-, H66.3-, H66.4-, H66.9-, H67.-)
Excludes1 acute suppurative otitis media with rupture of the tympanic membrane (H66.01-)
traumatic rupture of ear drum (S09.2-)

● **H72.0** Central perforation of tympanic membrane
H72.00 Central perforation of tympanic membrane, unspecified ear
H72.01 Central perforation of tympanic membrane, right ear
H72.02 Central perforation of tympanic membrane, left ear
H72.03 Central perforation of tympanic membrane, bilateral

● **H72.1** Attic perforation of tympanic membrane
Perforation of pars flaccida
H72.10 Attic perforation of tympanic membrane, unspecified ear
H72.11 Attic perforation of tympanic membrane, right ear
H72.12 Attic perforation of tympanic membrane, left ear
H72.13 Attic perforation of tympanic membrane, bilateral

● **H72.2** Other marginal perforations of tympanic membrane
● **H72.2X** Other marginal perforations of tympanic membrane
H72.2X1 Other marginal perforations of tympanic membrane, right ear
H72.2X2 Other marginal perforations of tympanic membrane, left ear
H72.2X3 Other marginal perforations of tympanic membrane, bilateral
H72.2X9 Other marginal perforations of tympanic membrane, unspecified ear

● **H72.8** Other perforations of tympanic membrane
● **H72.81** Multiple perforations of tympanic membrane
H72.811 Multiple perforations of tympanic membrane, right ear
H72.812 Multiple perforations of tympanic membrane, left ear
H72.813 Multiple perforations of tympanic membrane, bilateral
H72.819 Multiple perforations of tympanic membrane, unspecified ear

● **H72.82** Total perforations of tympanic membrane
H72.821 Total perforations of tympanic membrane, right ear
H72.822 Total perforations of tympanic membrane, left ear
H72.823 Total perforations of tympanic membrane, bilateral
H72.829 Total perforations of tympanic membrane, unspecified ear

● **H72.9** Unspecified perforation of tympanic membrane
H72.90 Unspecified perforation of tympanic membrane, unspecified ear
H72.91 Unspecified perforation of tympanic membrane, right ear
H72.92 Unspecified perforation of tympanic membrane, left ear
H72.93 Unspecified perforation of tympanic membrane, bilateral

CHAPTER 8 (H60-H95)

- H73 Other disorders of tympanic membrane
  - H73.0 Acute myringitis
    - Excludes1 acute myringitis with otitis media (H65, H66)
    - H73.00 Unspecified acute myringitis
      - Acute tympanitis NOS
      - H73.001 Acute myringitis, right ear
      - H73.002 Acute myringitis, left ear
      - H73.003 Acute myringitis, bilateral
      - H73.009 Acute myringitis, unspecified ear
    - H73.01 Bullous myringitis
      - H73.011 Bullous myringitis, right ear
      - H73.012 Bullous myringitis, left ear
      - H73.013 Bullous myringitis, bilateral
      - H73.019 Bullous myringitis, unspecified ear
    - H73.09 Other acute myringitis
      - H73.091 Other acute myringitis, right ear
      - H73.092 Other acute myringitis, left ear
      - H73.093 Other acute myringitis, bilateral
      - H73.099 Other acute myringitis, unspecified ear
  - H73.1 Chronic myringitis
    - Chronic tympanitis
    - Excludes1 chronic myringitis with otitis media (H65, H66)
    - H73.10 Chronic myringitis, unspecified ear
    - H73.11 Chronic myringitis, right ear
    - H73.12 Chronic myringitis, left ear
    - H73.13 Chronic myringitis, bilateral
  - H73.2 Unspecified myringitis
    - H73.20 Unspecified myringitis, unspecified ear
    - H73.21 Unspecified myringitis, right ear
    - H73.22 Unspecified myringitis, left ear
    - H73.23 Unspecified myringitis, bilateral
  - H73.8 Other specified disorders of tympanic membrane
    - H73.81 Atrophic flaccid tympanic membrane
      - H73.811 Atrophic flaccid tympanic membrane, right ear
      - H73.812 Atrophic flaccid tympanic membrane, left ear
      - H73.813 Atrophic flaccid tympanic membrane, bilateral
      - H73.819 Atrophic flaccid tympanic membrane, unspecified ear
    - H73.82 Atrophic nonflaccid tympanic membrane
      - H73.821 Atrophic nonflaccid tympanic membrane, right ear
      - H73.822 Atrophic nonflaccid tympanic membrane, left ear
      - H73.823 Atrophic nonflaccid tympanic membrane, bilateral
      - H73.829 Atrophic nonflaccid tympanic membrane, unspecified ear
    - H73.89 Other specified disorders of tympanic membrane
      - H73.891 Other specified disorders of tympanic membrane, right ear
      - H73.892 Other specified disorders of tympanic membrane, left ear
      - H73.893 Other specified disorders of tympanic membrane, bilateral
      - H73.899 Other specified disorders of tympanic membrane, unspecified ear
  - H73.9 Unspecified disorder of tympanic membrane
    - H73.90 Unspecified disorder of tympanic membrane, unspecified ear
    - H73.91 Unspecified disorder of tympanic membrane, right ear
    - H73.92 Unspecified disorder of tympanic membrane, left ear
    - H73.93 Unspecified disorder of tympanic membrane, bilateral
- H74 Other disorders of middle ear mastoid
  - Excludes2 mastoiditis (H70.-)
  - H74.0 Tympanosclerosis
    - H74.01 Tympanosclerosis, right ear
    - H74.02 Tympanosclerosis, left ear
    - H74.03 Tympanosclerosis, bilateral
    - H74.09 Tympanosclerosis, unspecified ear
  - H74.1 Adhesive middle ear disease
    - Adhesive otitis
    - Excludes1 glue ear (H65.3-)
    - H74.11 Adhesive right middle ear disease
    - H74.12 Adhesive left middle ear disease
    - H74.13 Adhesive middle ear disease, bilateral
    - H74.19 Adhesive middle ear disease, unspecified ear
  - H74.2 Discontinuity and dislocation of ear ossicles
    - H74.20 Discontinuity and dislocation of ear ossicles, unspecified ear
    - H74.21 Discontinuity and dislocation of right ear ossicles
    - H74.22 Discontinuity and dislocation of left ear ossicles
    - H74.23 Discontinuity and dislocation of ear ossicles, bilateral
  - H74.3 Other acquired abnormalities of ear ossicles
    - H74.31 Ankylosis of ear ossicles
      - H74.311 Ankylosis of ear ossicles, right ear
      - H74.312 Ankylosis of ear ossicles, left ear
      - H74.313 Ankylosis of ear ossicles, bilateral
      - H74.319 Ankylosis of ear ossicles, unspecified ear
    - H74.32 Partial loss of ear ossicles
      - H74.321 Partial loss of ear ossicles, right ear
      - H74.322 Partial loss of ear ossicles, left ear
      - H74.323 Partial loss of ear ossicles, bilateral
      - H74.329 Partial loss of ear ossicles, unspecified ear
    - H74.39 Other acquired abnormalities of ear ossicles
      - H74.391 Other acquired abnormalities of right ear ossicles
      - H74.392 Other acquired abnormalities of left ear ossicles
      - H74.393 Other acquired abnormalities of ear ossicles, bilateral
      - H74.399 Other acquired abnormalities of ear ossicles, unspecified ear
  - H74.4 Polyp of middle ear
    - H74.40 Polyp of middle ear, unspecified ear
    - H74.41 Polyp of right middle ear
    - H74.42 Polyp of left middle ear
    - H74.43 Polyp of middle ear, bilateral

● H74.8 Other specified disorders of middle ear and mastoid
● H74.8X Other specified disorders of middle ear and mastoid
H74.8X1 Other specified disorders of right middle ear and mastoid
H74.8X2 Other specified disorders of left middle ear and mastoid
H74.8X3 Other specified disorders of middle ear and mastoid, bilateral
H74.8X9 Other specified disorders of middle ear and mastoid, unspecified ear
● H74.9 Unspecified disorder of middle ear and mastoid
H74.90 Unspecified disorder of middle ear and mastoid, unspecified ear
H74.91 Unspecified disorder of right middle ear and mastoid
H74.92 Unspecified disorder of left middle ear and mastoid
H74.93 Unspecified disorder of middle ear and mastoid, bilateral

● H75 Other disorders of middle ear and mastoid in diseases classified elsewhere
Code first underlying disease
● H75.0 Mastoiditis in infectious and parasitic diseases classified elsewhere
Excludes1 mastoiditis (in):
syphilis (A52.77)
tuberculosis (A18.03)
H75.00 Mastoiditis in infectious and parasitic diseases classified elsewhere, unspecified ear
H75.01 Mastoiditis in infectious and parasitic diseases classified elsewhere, right ear
H75.02 Mastoiditis in infectious and parasitic diseases classified elsewhere, left ear
H75.03 Mastoiditis in infectious and parasitic diseases classified elsewhere, bilateral
● H75.8 Other specified disorders of middle ear and mastoid in diseases classified elsewhere
H75.80 Other specified disorders of middle ear and mastoid in diseases classified elsewhere, unspecified ear
H75.81 Other specified disorders of right middle ear and mastoid in diseases classified elsewhere
H75.82 Other specified disorders of left middle ear and mastoid in diseases classified elsewhere
H75.83 Other specified disorders of middle ear and mastoid in diseases classified elsewhere, bilateral

DISEASES OF INNER EAR (H80-H83)

★(See Plate 95 on page NAP-21.)

● H80 Otosclerosis
Inherited middle ear spongelike bone growth causing hearing loss
Includes Otospongiosis
● H80.0 Otosclerosis involving oval window, nonobliterative
H80.00 Otosclerosis involving oval window, nonobliterative, unspecified ear
H80.01 Otosclerosis involving oval window, nonobliterative, right ear
H80.02 Otosclerosis involving oval window, nonobliterative, left ear
H80.03 Otosclerosis involving oval window, nonobliterative, bilateral
● H80.1 Otosclerosis involving oval window, obliterative
H80.10 Otosclerosis involving oval window, obliterative, unspecified ear
H80.11 Otosclerosis involving oval window, obliterative, right ear
H80.12 Otosclerosis involving oval window, obliterative, left ear
H80.13 Otosclerosis involving oval window, obliterative, bilateral
● H80.2 Cochlear otosclerosis
Otosclerosis involving otic capsule
Otosclerosis involving round window
H80.20 Cochlear otosclerosis, unspecified ear
H80.21 Cochlear otosclerosis, right ear
H80.22 Cochlear otosclerosis, left ear
H80.23 Cochlear otosclerosis, bilateral
● H80.8 Other otosclerosis
H80.80 Other otosclerosis, unspecified ear
H80.81 Other otosclerosis, right ear
H80.82 Other otosclerosis, left ear
H80.83 Other otosclerosis, bilateral
● H80.9 Unspecified otosclerosis
H80.90 Unspecified otosclerosis, unspecified ear
H80.91 Unspecified otosclerosis, right ear
H80.92 Unspecified otosclerosis, left ear
H80.93 Unspecified otosclerosis, bilateral

● H81 Disorders of vestibular function
Excludes1 epidemic vertigo (A88.1)
vertigo NOS (R42)
● H81.0 Ménière's disease
Vestibular disorder that produces recurring symptoms including severe and intermittent hearing loss including the feeling of ear pressure or pain
Labyrinthine hydrops
Ménière's syndrome or vertigo
H81.01 Ménière's disease, right ear
H81.02 Ménière's disease, left ear
H81.03 Ménière's disease, bilateral
H81.09 Ménière's disease, unspecified ear
● H81.1 Benign paroxysmal vertigo
H81.10 Benign paroxysmal vertigo, unspecified ear
H81.11 Benign paroxysmal vertigo, right ear
H81.12 Benign paroxysmal vertigo, left ear
H81.13 Benign paroxysmal vertigo, bilateral
● H81.2 Vestibular neuronitis
H81.20 Vestibular neuronitis, unspecified ear
H81.21 Vestibular neuronitis, right ear
H81.22 Vestibular neuronitis, left ear
H81.23 Vestibular neuronitis, bilateral
● H81.3 Other peripheral vertigo
● H81.31 Aural vertigo
H81.311 Aural vertigo, right ear
H81.312 Aural vertigo, left ear
H81.313 Aural vertigo, bilateral
H81.319 Aural vertigo, unspecified ear
● H81.39 Other peripheral vertigo
Lermoyez' syndrome
Otogenic vertigo
Peripheral vertigo NOS
H81.391 Other peripheral vertigo, right ear
H81.392 Other peripheral vertigo, left ear
H81.393 Other peripheral vertigo, bilateral
H81.399 Other peripheral vertigo, unspecified ear

CHAPTER 8 (H60-H95)

● H81.4 Vertigo of central origin
Central positional nystagmus
H81.41 Vertigo of central origin, right ear
H81.42 Vertigo of central origin, left ear
H81.43 Vertigo of central origin, bilateral
H81.49 Vertigo of central origin, unspecified ear

● H81.8 Other disorders of vestibular function
● H81.8X Other disorders of vestibular function
H81.8X1 Other disorders of vestibular function, right ear
H81.8X2 Other disorders of vestibular function, left ear
H81.8X3 Other disorders of vestibular function, bilateral
H81.8X9 Other disorders of vestibular function, unspecified ear

● H81.9 Unspecified disorder of vestibular function
Vertiginous syndrome NOS
H81.90 Unspecified disorder of vestibular function, unspecified ear
H81.91 Unspecified disorder of vestibular function, right ear
H81.92 Unspecified disorder of vestibular function, left ear
H81.93 Unspecified disorder of vestibular function, bilateral

● H82 Vertiginous syndromes in diseases classified elsewhere
Code first underlying disease
Excludes1 epidemic vertigo (A88.1)
H82.1 Vertiginous syndromes in diseases classified elsewhere, right ear
H82.2 Vertiginous syndromes in diseases classified elsewhere, left ear
H82.3 Vertiginous syndromes in diseases classified elsewhere, bilateral
H82.9 Vertiginous syndromes in diseases classified elsewhere, unspecified ear

● H83 Other diseases of inner ear
● H83.0 Labyrinthitis
Balance disorder that follows URI or head injury
H83.01 Labyrinthitis, right ear
H83.02 Labyrinthitis, left ear
H83.03 Labyrinthitis, bilateral
H83.09 Labyrinthitis, unspecified ear

● H83.1 Labyrinthine fistula
H83.11 Labyrinthine fistula, right ear
H83.12 Labyrinthine fistula, left ear
H83.13 Labyrinthine fistula, bilateral
H83.19 Labyrinthine fistula, unspecified ear

● H83.2 Labyrinthine dysfunction
Labyrinthine hypersensitivity
Labyrinthine hypofunction
Labyrinthine loss of function
● H83.2X Labyrinthine dysfunction
H83.2X1 Labyrinthine dysfunction, right ear
H83.2X2 Labyrinthine dysfunction, left ear
H83.2X3 Labyrinthine dysfunction, bilateral
H83.2X9 Labyrinthine dysfunction, unspecified ear

● H83.3 Noise effects on inner ear
Acoustic trauma of inner ear
Noise-induced hearing loss of inner ear
● H83.3X Noise effects on inner ear
H83.3X1 Noise effects on right inner ear
H83.3X2 Noise effects on left inner ear
H83.3X3 Noise effects on inner ear, bilateral
H83.3X9 Noise effects on inner ear, unspecified ear

● H83.8 Other specified diseases of inner ear
● H83.8X Other specified diseases of inner ear
H83.8X1 Other specified diseases of right inner ear
H83.8X2 Other specified diseases of left inner ear
H83.8X3 Other specified diseases of inner ear, bilateral
H83.8X9 Other specified diseases of inner ear, unspecified ear

● H83.9 Unspecified disease of inner ear
H83.90 Unspecified disease of inner ear, unspecified ear
H83.91 Unspecified disease of right inner ear
H83.92 Unspecified disease of left inner ear
H83.93 Unspecified disease of inner ear, bilateral

OTHER DISORDERS OF EAR (H90-H94)

● H90 Conductive and sensorineural hearing loss
Excludes1 deaf nonspeaking NEC (H91.3)
deafness NOS (H91.9-)
hearing loss NOS (H91.9-)
noise-induced hearing loss (H83.3-)
ototoxic hearing loss (H91.0-)
sudden (idiopathic) hearing loss (H91.2-)
H90.0 Conductive hearing loss, bilateral
● H90.1 Conductive hearing loss, unilateral with unrestricted hearing on the contralateral side
H90.11 Conductive hearing loss, unilateral, right ear, with unrestricted hearing on the contralateral side
H90.12 Conductive hearing loss, unilateral, left ear, with unrestricted hearing on the contralateral side
H90.2 Conductive hearing loss, unspecified
Conductive deafness NOS
H90.3 Sensorineural hearing loss, bilateral
● H90.4 Sensorineural hearing loss, unilateral with unrestricted hearing on the contralateral side
H90.41 Sensorineural hearing loss, unilateral, right ear, with unrestricted hearing on the contralateral side
H90.42 Sensorineural hearing loss, unilateral, left ear, with unrestricted hearing on the contralateral side
H90.5 Unspecified sensorineural hearing loss
Central hearing loss NOS
Congenital deafness NOS
Neural hearing loss NOS
Perceptive hearing loss NOS
Sensorineural deafness NOS
Sensory hearing loss NOS
Excludes1 abnormal auditory perception (H93.2-)
psychogenic deafness (F44.6)
H90.6 Mixed conductive and sensorineural hearing loss, bilateral

● **H90.7** **Mixed conductive and sensorineural hearing loss, unilateral with unrestricted hearing on the contralateral side**

H90.71 **Mixed conductive and sensorineural hearing loss, unilateral, right ear, with unrestricted hearing on the contralateral side**

H90.72 **Mixed conductive and sensorineural hearing loss, unilateral, left ear, with unrestricted hearing on the contralateral side**

H90.8 **Mixed conductive and sensorineural hearing loss, unspecified**

● **H90.A** **Conductive and sensorineural hearing loss with restricted hearing on the contralateral side** ◀

● **H90.A1** **Conductive hearing loss, unilateral, with restricted hearing on the contralateral side** ◀

H90.A11 **Conductive hearing loss, unilateral, right ear with restricted hearing on the contralateral side** ◀

H90.A12 **Conductive hearing loss, unilateral, left ear with restricted hearing on the contralateral side** ◀

● **H90.A2** **Sensorineural hearing loss, unilateral, with restricted hearing on the contralateral side** ◀

H90.A21 **Sensorineural hearing loss, unilateral, right ear, with restricted hearing on the contralateral side** ◀

H90.A22 **Sensorineural hearing loss, unilateral, left ear, with restricted hearing on the contralateral side** ◀

● **H90.A3** **Mixed conductive and sensorineural hearing loss, unilateral with restricted hearing on the contralateral side** ◀

H90.A31 **Mixed conductive and sensorineural hearing loss, unilateral, right ear with restricted hearing on the contralateral side** ◀

H90.A32 **Mixed conductive and sensorineural hearing loss, unilateral, left ear with restricted hearing on the contralateral side** ◀

● **H91** **Other and unspecified hearing loss**

Excludes1 abnormal auditory perception (H93.2-)
hearing loss as classified in H90.-
impacted cerumen (H61.2-)
noise-induced hearing loss (H83.3-)
psychogenic deafness (F44.6)
transient ischemic deafness (H93.01-)

● **H91.0** **Ototoxic hearing loss**

Code first poisoning due to drug or toxin, if applicable (T36-T65 with fifth or sixth character 1-4 or 6)

Use additional code for adverse effect, if applicable, to identify drug (T36-T50 with fifth or sixth character 5)

H91.01 **Ototoxic hearing loss, right ear**

H91.02 **Ototoxic hearing loss, left ear**

H91.03 **Ototoxic hearing loss, bilateral**

H91.09 **Ototoxic hearing loss, unspecified ear**

● **H91.1** **Presbycusis**

Presbyacusia

H91.10 **Presbycusis, unspecified ear**

H91.11 **Presbycusis, right ear**

H91.12 **Presbycusis, left ear**

H91.13 **Presbycusis, bilateral**

● **H91.2** **Sudden idiopathic hearing loss**

Sudden hearing loss NOS

H91.20 **Sudden idiopathic hearing loss, unspecified ear**

H91.21 **Sudden idiopathic hearing loss, right ear**

H91.22 **Sudden idiopathic hearing loss, left ear**

H91.23 **Sudden idiopathic hearing loss, bilateral**

H91.3 **Deaf nonspeaking, not elsewhere classified**

● **H91.8** **Other specified hearing loss**

● **H91.8X** **Other specified hearing loss**

H91.8X1 **Other specified hearing loss, right ear**

H91.8X2 **Other specified hearing loss, left ear**

H91.8X3 **Other specified hearing loss, bilateral**

H91.8X9 **Other specified hearing loss, unspecified ear**

● **H91.9** **Unspecified hearing loss**

Deafness NOS
High frequency deafness
Low frequency deafness

H91.90 **Unspecified hearing loss, unspecified ear**

H91.91 **Unspecified hearing loss, right ear**

H91.92 **Unspecified hearing loss, left ear**

H91.93 **Unspecified hearing loss, bilateral**

● **H92** **Otalgia and effusion of ear**

● **H92.0** **Otalgia**

H92.01 **Otalgia, right ear**

H92.02 **Otalgia, left ear**

H92.03 **Otalgia, bilateral**

H92.09 **Otalgia, unspecified ear**

● **H92.1** **Otorrhea**

Excludes1 leakage of cerebrospinal fluid through ear (G96.0)

H92.10 **Otorrhea, unspecified ear**

H92.11 **Otorrhea, right ear**

H92.12 **Otorrhea, left ear**

H92.13 **Otorrhea, bilateral**

● **H92.2** **Otorrhagia**

Excludes1 traumatic otorrhagia - code to injury

H92.20 **Otorrhagia, unspecified ear**

H92.21 **Otorrhagia, right ear**

H92.22 **Otorrhagia, left ear**

H92.23 **Otorrhagia, bilateral**

● **H93** **Other disorders of ear, not elsewhere classified**

● **H93.0** **Degenerative and vascular disorders of ear**

Excludes1 presbycusis (H91.1)

● **H93.01** **Transient ischemic deafness**

H93.011 **Transient ischemic deafness, right ear**

H93.012 **Transient ischemic deafness, left ear**

H93.013 **Transient ischemic deafness, bilateral**

H93.019 **Transient ischemic deafness, unspecified ear**

● **H93.09** **Unspecified degenerative and vascular disorders of ear**

H93.091 **Unspecified degenerative and vascular disorders of right ear**

H93.092 **Unspecified degenerative and vascular disorders of left ear**

H93.093 **Unspecified degenerative and vascular disorders of ear, bilateral**

H93.099 **Unspecified degenerative and vascular disorders of unspecified ear**

CHAPTER 8 (H60-H95)

● H93.1 Tinnitus
Perception of sound (ringing, buzzing, humming, whistling tunes, or singing)
H93.11 Tinnitus, right ear
H93.12 Tinnitus, left ear
H93.13 Tinnitus, bilateral
H93.19 Tinnitus, unspecified ear

● H93.A Pulsatile tinnitus ◀
H93.A1 Pulsatile tinnitus, right ear ◀
H93.A2 Pulsatile tinnitus, left ear ◀
H93.A3 Pulsatile tinnitus, bilateral ◀
H93.A9 Pulsatile tinnitus, unspecified ear ◀

● H93.2 Other abnormal auditory perceptions
Excludes2 auditory hallucinations (R44.Ø)

● H93.21 Auditory recruitment
H93.211 Auditory recruitment, right ear
H93.212 Auditory recruitment, left ear
H93.213 Auditory recruitment, bilateral
H93.219 Auditory recruitment, unspecified ear

● H93.22 Diplacusis
H93.221 Diplacusis, right ear
H93.222 Diplacusis, left ear
H93.223 Diplacusis, bilateral
H93.229 Diplacusis, unspecified ear

● H93.23 Hyperacusis
H93.231 Hyperacusis, right ear
H93.232 Hyperacusis, left ear
H93.233 Hyperacusis, bilateral
H93.239 Hyperacusis, unspecified ear

● H93.24 Temporary auditory threshold shift
H93.241 Temporary auditory threshold shift, right ear
H93.242 Temporary auditory threshold shift, left ear
H93.243 Temporary auditory threshold shift, bilateral
H93.249 Temporary auditory threshold shift, unspecified ear

H93.25 Central auditory processing disorder
Congenital auditory imperception
Word deafness
Excludes1 mixed receptive-expressive language disorder (F8Ø.2)

● H93.29 Other abnormal auditory perceptions
H93.291 Other abnormal auditory perceptions, right ear
H93.292 Other abnormal auditory perceptions, left ear
H93.293 Other abnormal auditory perceptions, bilateral
H93.299 Other abnormal auditory perceptions, unspecified ear

● H93.3 Disorders of acoustic nerve
Disorder of 8th cranial nerve
Excludes1 acoustic neuroma (D33.3)
syphilitic acoustic neuritis (A52.15)

● H93.3X Disorders of acoustic nerve
H93.3X1 Disorders of right acoustic nerve
H93.3X2 Disorders of left acoustic nerve
H93.3X3 Disorders of bilateral acoustic nerves
H93.3X9 Disorders of unspecified acoustic nerve

● H93.8 Other specified disorders of ear

● H93.8X Other specified disorders of ear
H93.8X1 Other specified disorders of right ear
H93.8X2 Other specified disorders of left ear
H93.8X3 Other specified disorders of ear, bilateral
H93.8X9 Other specified disorders of ear, unspecified ear

● H93.9 Unspecified disorder of ear
H93.9Ø Unspecified disorder of ear, unspecified ear
H93.91 Unspecified disorder of right ear
H93.92 Unspecified disorder of left ear
H93.93 Unspecified disorder of ear, bilateral

● H94 Other disorders of ear in diseases classified elsewhere

● H94.Ø Acoustic neuritis in infectious and parasitic diseases classified elsewhere
Code first underlying disease, such as:
parasitic disease (B65-B89)
Excludes1 acoustic neuritis (in):
herpes zoster (BØ2.29)
syphilis (A52.15)
H94.ØØ Acoustic neuritis in infectious and parasitic diseases classified elsewhere, unspecified ear
H94.Ø1 Acoustic neuritis in infectious and parasitic diseases classified elsewhere, right ear
H94.Ø2 Acoustic neuritis in infectious and parasitic diseases classified elsewhere, left ear
H94.Ø3 Acoustic neuritis in infectious and parasitic diseases classified elsewhere, bilateral

● H94.8 Other specified disorders of ear in diseases classified elsewhere
Code first underlying disease, such as:
congenital syphilis (A5Ø.Ø)
Excludes1 aural myiasis (B87.4)
syphilitic labyrinthitis (A52.79)
H94.8Ø Other specified disorders of ear in diseases classified elsewhere, unspecified ear
H94.81 Other specified disorders of right ear in diseases classified elsewhere
H94.82 Other specified disorders of left ear in diseases classified elsewhere
H94.83 Other specified disorders of ear in diseases classified elsewhere, bilateral

● H95 Intraoperative and postprocedural complications and disorders of ear and mastoid process, not elsewhere classified

● H95.Ø Recurrent cholesteatoma of postmastoidectomy cavity
H95.ØØ Recurrent cholesteatoma of postmastoidectomy cavity, unspecified ear
H95.Ø1 Recurrent cholesteatoma of postmastoidectomy cavity, right ear
H95.Ø2 Recurrent cholesteatoma of postmastoidectomy cavity, left ear
H95.Ø3 Recurrent cholesteatoma of postmastoidectomy cavity, bilateral ears

● **H95.1 Other disorders of ear and mastoid process following mastoidectomy**

● **H95.11 Chronic inflammation of postmastoidectomy cavity**

H95.111 Chronic inflammation of postmastoidectomy cavity, right ear

H95.112 Chronic inflammation of postmastoidectomy cavity, left ear

H95.113 Chronic inflammation of postmastoidectomy cavity, bilateral ears

H95.119 Chronic inflammation of postmastoidectomy cavity, unspecified ear

● **H95.12 Granulation of postmastoidectomy cavity**

H95.121 Granulation of postmastoidectomy cavity, right ear

H95.122 Granulation of postmastoidectomy cavity, left ear

H95.123 Granulation of postmastoidectomy cavity, bilateral ears

H95.129 Granulation of postmastoidectomy cavity, unspecified ear

● **H95.13 Mucosal cyst of postmastoidectomy cavity**

H95.131 Mucosal cyst of postmastoidectomy cavity, right ear

H95.132 Mucosal cyst of postmastoidectomy cavity, left ear

H95.133 Mucosal cyst of postmastoidectomy cavity, bilateral ears

H95.139 Mucosal cyst of postmastoidectomy cavity, unspecified ear

● **H95.19 Other disorders following mastoidectomy**

H95.191 Other disorders following mastoidectomy, right ear

H95.192 Other disorders following mastoidectomy, left ear

H95.193 Other disorders following mastoidectomy, bilateral ears

H95.199 Other disorders following mastoidectomy, unspecified ear

● **H95.2 Intraoperative hemorrhage and hematoma of ear and mastoid process complicating a procedure**

Excludes1 intraoperative hemorrhage and hematoma of ear and mastoid process due to accidental puncture or laceration during a procedure (H95.3-)

H95.21 Intraoperative hemorrhage and hematoma of ear and mastoid process complicating a procedure on the ear and mastoid process

H95.22 Intraoperative hemorrhage and hematoma of ear and mastoid process complicating other procedure

● **H95.3 Accidental puncture and laceration of ear and mastoid process during a procedure**

H95.31 Accidental puncture and laceration of the ear and mastoid process during a procedure on the ear and mastoid process

H95.32 Accidental puncture and laceration of the ear and mastoid process during other procedure

● **H95.4 Postprocedural hemorrhage of ear and mastoid process following a procedure** (Revised)

H95.41 Postprocedural hemorrhage of ear and mastoid process following a procedure on the ear and mastoid process (Revised)

H95.42 Postprocedural hemorrhage of ear and mastoid process following other procedure (Revised)

● **H95.5 Postprocedural hematoma and seroma of ear and mastoid process following a procedure** ◀

H95.51 Postprocedural hematoma of ear and mastoid process following a procedure on the ear and mastoid process ◀

H95.52 Postprocedural hematoma of ear and mastoid process following other procedure ◀

H95.53 Postprocedural seroma of ear and mastoid process following a procedure on the ear and mastoid process ◀

H95.54 Postprocedural seroma of ear and mastoid process following other procedure ◀

● **H95.8 Other intraoperative and postprocedural complications and disorders of the ear and mastoid process, not elsewhere classified**

Excludes2 postprocedural complications and disorders following mastoidectomy (H95.Ø-, H95.1-)

● **H95.81 Postprocedural stenosis of external ear canal**

H95.811 Postprocedural stenosis of right external ear canal

H95.812 Postprocedural stenosis of left external ear canal

H95.813 Postprocedural stenosis of external ear canal, bilateral

H95.819 Postprocedural stenosis of unspecified external ear canal

H95.88 Other intraoperative complications and disorders of the ear and mastoid process, not elsewhere classified

Use additional code, if applicable, to further specify disorder

H95.89 Other postprocedural complications and disorders of the ear and mastoid process, not elsewhere classified

Use additional code, if applicable, to further specify disorder

◀ New ⬅ Revised ~~deleted~~ Deleted OGCR Official Guidelines X Assign placeholder X ● Use Additional Character(s)

Excludes 1 | Excludes 2 | Includes | Use additional | Code first | Code also | Unspecified

CHAPTER 8 (H6Ø-H95)

CHAPTER 9 DISEASES OF THE CIRCULATORY SYSTEM (IØØ-I99)

OGCR Chapter-Specific Coding Guidelines

9. Chapter 9: Diseases of the Circulatory System (IØØ-I99)

a. Hypertension

The classification presumes a causal relationship between hypertension and heart involvement and between hypertension and kidney involvement, as the two conditions are linked by the term "with" in the Alphabetic Index. These conditions should be coded as related even in the absence of provider documentation explicitly linking them, unless the documentation clearly states the conditions are unrelated.

For hypertension and conditions not specifically linked by relational terms such as "with," "associated with" or "due to" in the classification, provider documentation must link the conditions in order to code them as related.

1) Hypertension with Heart Disease

Hypertension with heart conditions classified to I5Ø.- or I51.4-I51.9, are assigned to, a code from category I11, Hypertensive heart disease. Use an additional code from category I5Ø, Heart failure, to identify the type of heart failure in those patients with heart failure.

The same heart conditions (I5Ø.-, I51.4-I51.9) with hypertension, are coded separately **if the provider has specifically documented a different cause**. Sequence according to the circumstances of the admission/encounter.

2) Hypertensive Chronic Kidney Disease

Assign codes from category I12, Hypertensive chronic kidney disease, when both hypertension and a condition classifiable to category N18, Chronic kidney disease (CKD), are present. **CKD should not be coded as hypertensive if the physician has specifically documented a different cause.**

The appropriate code from category N18 should be used as a secondary code with a code from category I12 to identify the stage of chronic kidney disease.

See Section I.C.14. Chronic kidney disease.

If a patient has hypertensive chronic kidney disease and acute renal failure, an additional code for the acute renal failure is required.

3) Hypertensive Heart and Chronic Kidney Disease

Assign codes from combination category I13, Hypertensive heart and chronic kidney disease, when **there is hypertension with both heart and kidney involvement.** If heart failure is present, assign an additional code from category I5Ø to identify the type of heart failure.

The appropriate code from category N18, Chronic kidney disease, should be used as a secondary code with a code from category I13 to identify the stage of chronic kidney disease.

See Section I.C.14. Chronic kidney disease.

The codes in category I13, Hypertensive heart and chronic kidney disease, are combination codes that include hypertension, heart disease and chronic kidney disease. The Includes note at I13 specifies that the conditions included at I11 and I12 are included together in I13. If a patient has hypertension, heart disease and chronic kidney disease then a code from I13 should be used, not individual codes for hypertension, heart disease and chronic kidney disease, or codes from I11 or I12.

For patients with both acute renal failure and chronic kidney disease an additional code for acute renal failure is required.

4) Hypertensive Cerebrovascular Disease

For hypertensive cerebrovascular disease, first assign the appropriate code from categories I6Ø-I69, followed by the appropriate hypertension code.

5) Hypertensive Retinopathy

Subcategory H35.Ø, Background retinopathy and retinal vascular changes, should be used with a code from category I1Ø – I15, Hypertensive disease to include the systemic hypertension. The sequencing is based on the reason for the encounter.

6) Hypertension, Secondary

Secondary hypertension is due to an underlying condition. Two codes are required: one to identify the underlying etiology and one from category I15 to identify the hypertension. Sequencing of codes is determined by the reason for admission/encounter.

7) Hypertension, Transient

Assign code RØ3.Ø, Elevated blood pressure reading without diagnosis of hypertension, unless patient has an established diagnosis of hypertension. Assign code O13.-, Gestational [pregnancy-induced] hypertension without significant proteinuria, or O14.-, Pre-eclampsia, for transient hypertension of pregnancy.

8) Hypertension, Controlled

This diagnostic statement usually refers to an existing state of hypertension under control by therapy. Assign the appropriate code from categories I1Ø-I15, Hypertensive diseases.

9) Hypertension, Uncontrolled

Uncontrolled hypertension may refer to untreated hypertension or hypertension not responding to current therapeutic regimen. In either case, assign the appropriate code from categories I1Ø-I15, Hypertensive diseases.

10) Hypertensive Crisis

Assign a code from category I16, Hypertensive crisis, for documented hypertensive urgency, hypertensive emergency or unspecified hypertensive crisis. Code also any identified hypertensive disease (I1Ø-I15). The sequencing is based on the reason for the encounter.

b. Atherosclerotic Coronary Artery Disease and Angina

ICD-10-CM has combination codes for atherosclerotic heart disease with angina pectoris. The subcategories for these codes are I25.11, Atherosclerotic heart disease of native coronary artery with angina pectoris and I25.7, Atherosclerosis of coronary artery bypass graft(s) and coronary artery of transplanted heart with angina pectoris.

When using one of these combination codes it is not necessary to use an additional code for angina pectoris. A causal relationship can be assumed in a patient with both atherosclerosis and angina pectoris, unless the documentation indicates the angina is due to something other than the atherosclerosis.

If a patient with coronary artery disease is admitted due to an acute myocardial infarction (AMI), the AMI should be sequenced before the coronary artery disease.

See Section I.C.9. Acute myocardial infarction (AMI)

c. Intraoperative and Postprocedural Cerebrovascular Accident

Medical record documentation should clearly specify the cause-and-effect relationship between the medical intervention and the cerebrovascular accident in order to assign a code for intraoperative or postprocedural cerebrovascular accident.

Proper code assignment depends on whether it was an infarction or hemorrhage and whether it occurred intraoperatively or postoperatively. If it was a cerebral hemorrhage, code assignment depends on the type of procedure performed.

d. Sequelae of Cerebrovascular Disease

1) Category I69, Sequelae of Cerebrovascular disease

Category I69 is used to indicate conditions classifiable to categories I6Ø-I67 as the causes of sequela (neurologic deficits), themselves classified elsewhere. These "late effects" include neurologic deficits that persist after initial onset of conditions classifiable to categories I6Ø-I67. The neurologic deficits caused by cerebrovascular disease may be present from the onset or may arise at any time after the onset of the condition classifiable to categories I6Ø-I67.

Codes from category I69, Sequelae of cerebrovascular disease, that specify hemiplegia, hemiparesis and monoplegia identify whether the dominant or nondominant side is affected. Should the affected side be documented, but not specified as dominant or nondominant, and the classification system does not indicate a default, code selection is as follows:

- For ambidextrous patients, the default should be dominant.
- If the left side is affected, the default is non-dominant.
- If the right side is affected, the default is dominant.

2) Codes from category I69 with codes from I60-I67
Codes from category I69 may be assigned on a health care record with codes from I60-I67, if the patient has a current cerebrovascular disease and deficits from an old cerebrovascular disease.

3) Codes from category I69 and Personal history of transient ischemic attack (TIA) and cerebral infarction (Z86.73)
Codes from category I69 should not be assigned if the patient does not have neurologic deficits.

See Section I.C.21. 4. History (of) for use of personal history codes

e. Acute myocardial infarction (AMI)

1) ST elevation myocardial infarction (STEMI) and non ST elevation myocardial infarction (NSTEMI)
The ICD-10-CM codes for acute myocardial infarction (AMI) identify the site, such as anterolateral wall or true posterior wall. Subcategories I21.0-I21.2 and code I21.3 are used for ST elevation myocardial infarction (STEMI). Code I21.4, Non-ST elevation (NSTEMI) myocardial infarction, is used for non ST elevation myocardial infarction (NSTEMI) and nontransmural MIs.

If NSTEMI evolves to STEMI, assign the STEMI code. If STEMI converts to NSTEMI due to thrombolytic therapy, it is still coded as STEMI.

For encounters occurring while the myocardial infarction is equal to, or less than, four weeks old, including transfers to another acute setting or a postacute setting, and the myocardial infarction **meets the definition for "other diagnoses" (see Section III, Reporting Additional Diagnoses)**, codes from category I21 may continue to be reported. For encounters after the 4 week time frame and the patient is still receiving care related to the myocardial infarction, the appropriate aftercare code should be assigned, rather than a code from category I21. For old or healed myocardial infarctions not requiring further care, code I25.2, Old myocardial infarction, may be assigned.

2) Acute myocardial infarction, unspecified
Code I21.3, ST elevation (STEMI) myocardial infarction of unspecified site, is the default for unspecified acute myocardial infarction. If only STEMI or transmural MI without the site is documented, assign code I21.3.

3) AMI documented as nontransmural or subendocardial but site provided
If an AMI is documented as nontransmural or subendocardial, but the site is provided, it is still coded as a subendocardial AMI.

See Section I.C.21.3 for information on coding status post administration of tPA in a different facility within the last 24 hours.

4) Subsequent acute myocardial infarction
A code from category I22, Subsequent ST elevation (STEMI) and non ST elevation (NSTEMI) myocardial infarction, is to be used when a patient who has suffered an AMI has a new AMI within the 4 week time frame of the initial AMI. A code from category I22 must be used in conjunction with a code from category I21. The sequencing of the I22 and I21 codes depends on the circumstances of the encounter.

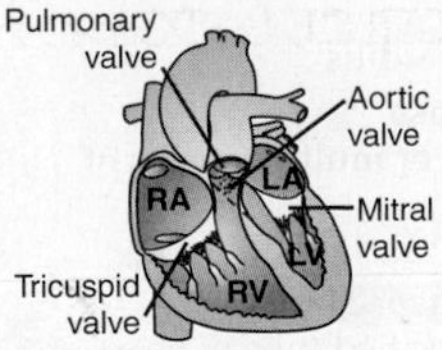

Figure 9-1 Cardiovascular valves.

Item 9–1 Rheumatic fever is the inflammation of the valve(s) of the heart, usually the mitral or aortic, which leads to valve damage. Rheumatic heart inflammations are usually **pericarditis** (sac surrounding heart), **endocarditis** (heart cavity), or **myocarditis** (heart muscle).

CHAPTER 9 DISEASES OF THE CIRCULATORY SYSTEM (I00-I99)

Excludes2 certain conditions originating in the perinatal period (P04-P96)
certain infectious and parasitic diseases (A00-B99)
complications of pregnancy, childbirth and the puerperium (O00-O9A)
congenital malformations, deformations, and chromosomal abnormalities (Q00-Q99)
endocrine, nutritional and metabolic diseases (E00-E88)
injury, poisoning and certain other consequences of external causes (S00-T88)
neoplasms (C00-D49)
symptoms, signs and abnormal clinical and laboratory findings, not elsewhere classified (R00-R94)
systemic connective tissue disorders (M30-M36)
transient cerebral ischemic attacks and related syndromes (G45.-)

This chapter contains the following blocks:

I00-I02	Acute rheumatic fever
I05-I09	Chronic rheumatic heart diseases
I10-I16	Hypertensive diseases ⟸
I20-I25	Ischemic heart diseases
I26-I28	Pulmonary heart disease and diseases of pulmonary circulation
I30-I52	Other forms of heart disease
I60-I69	Cerebrovascular diseases
I70-I79	Diseases of arteries, arterioles and capillaries
I80-I89	Diseases of veins, lymphatic vessels and lymph nodes, not elsewhere classified
I95-I99	Other and unspecified disorders of the circulatory system

ACUTE RHEUMATIC FEVER (I00-I02)

I00 Rheumatic fever without heart involvement
Includes arthritis, rheumatic, acute or subacute
Excludes1 rheumatic fever with heart involvement (I01.0-I01.9)

● **I01 Rheumatic fever with heart involvement**
Excludes1 chronic diseases of rheumatic origin (I05-I09) unless rheumatic fever is also present or there is evidence of reactivation or activity of the rheumatic process.

I01.0 Acute rheumatic pericarditis
Any condition in I00 with pericarditis
Rheumatic pericarditis (acute)
Excludes1 acute pericarditis not specified as rheumatic (I30.-)

I01.1 Acute rheumatic endocarditis
Any condition in I00 with endocarditis or valvulitis
Acute rheumatic valvulitis

Item 9–2 Rheumatic chorea, also called Sydenham's, juvenile, minor, simple, or St. Vitus' dance, is a major symptom of rheumatic fever and is characterized by ceaseless, involuntary, jerky, purposeless movements.

I01.2 Acute rheumatic myocarditis
Any condition in I00 with myocarditis

I01.8 Other acute rheumatic heart disease
Any condition in I00 with other or multiple types of heart involvement
Acute rheumatic pancarditis

I01.9 Acute rheumatic heart disease, unspecified
Any condition in I00 with unspecified type of heart involvement
Rheumatic carditis, acute
Rheumatic heart disease, active or acute

● **I02 Rheumatic chorea**
Includes Sydenham's chorea
Excludes1 chorea NOS (G25.5)
Huntington's chorea (G10)

I02.0 Rheumatic chorea with heart involvement
Chorea NOS with heart involvement
Rheumatic chorea with heart involvement of any type classifiable under I01.-

I02.9 Rheumatic chorea without heart involvement
Rheumatic chorea NOS

CHRONIC RHEUMATIC HEART DISEASES (I05-I09)

● **I05 Rheumatic mitral valve diseases**
Includes conditions classifiable to both I05.0 and I05.2-I05.9, whether specified as rheumatic or not
Excludes1 mitral valve disease specified as nonrheumatic (I34.-)
mitral valve disease with aortic and/or tricuspid valve involvement (I08.-)

I05.0 Rheumatic mitral stenosis
Mitral (valve) obstruction (rheumatic)

I05.1 Rheumatic mitral insufficiency
Rheumatic mitral incompetence
Rheumatic mitral regurgitation
Excludes1 mitral insufficiency not specified as rheumatic (I34.0)

I05.2 Rheumatic mitral stenosis with insufficiency
Rheumatic mitral stenosis with incompetence or regurgitation

I05.8 Other rheumatic mitral valve diseases
Rheumatic mitral (valve) failure

I05.9 Rheumatic mitral valve disease, unspecified
Rheumatic mitral (valve) disorder (chronic) NOS

● **I06 Rheumatic aortic valve diseases**
Excludes1 aortic valve disease not specified as rheumatic (I35.-)
aortic valve disease with mitral and/or tricuspid valve involvement (I08.-)

I06.0 Rheumatic aortic stenosis
Rheumatic aortic (valve) obstruction

I06.1 Rheumatic aortic insufficiency
Rheumatic aortic incompetence
Rheumatic aortic regurgitation

I06.8 Other rheumatic aortic valve diseases

I06.9 Rheumatic aortic valve disease, unspecified
Rheumatic aortic (valve) disease NOS

★**(See Plate 244 on page NAP-30.)**

I06.2 Rheumatic aortic stenosis with insufficiency
Rheumatic aortic stenosis with incompetence or regurgitation

Item 9–3 Mitral stenosis is the narrowing of the mitral valve separating the left atrium from the left ventricle. **Mitral insufficiency** is the improper closure of the mitral valve which may lead to enlargement (hypertrophy) of the left atrium.

Item 9–4 Aortic stenosis is the narrowing of the aortic valve located between the left ventricle and the aorta. **Aortic insufficiency** is the improper closure of the aortic valve which may lead to enlargement (hypertrophy) of the left ventricle.

● **I07 Rheumatic tricuspid valve diseases**
Includes rheumatic tricuspid valve diseases specified as rheumatic or unspecified
Excludes1 tricuspid valve disease specified as nonrheumatic (I36.-)
tricuspid valve disease with aortic and/or mitral valve involvement (I08.-)

I07.0 Rheumatic tricuspid stenosis
Tricuspid (valve) stenosis (rheumatic)

I07.1 Rheumatic tricuspid insufficiency
Tricuspid (valve) insufficiency (rheumatic)

I07.2 Rheumatic tricuspid stenosis and insufficiency

I07.8 Other rheumatic tricuspid valve diseases

I07.9 Rheumatic tricuspid valve disease, unspecified
Rheumatic tricuspid valve disorder NOS

● **I08 Multiple valve diseases**
Includes multiple valve diseases specified as rheumatic or unspecified
Excludes1 endocarditis, valve unspecified (I38)
multiple valve disease specified a nonrheumatic (I34.-, I35.-, I36.-, I37.-, I38.-, Q22.-, Q23.-, Q24.8-)
rheumatic valve disease NOS (I09.1)

I08.0 Rheumatic disorders of both mitral and aortic valves
Involvement of both mitral and aortic valves specified as rheumatic or unspecified

I08.1 Rheumatic disorders of both mitral and tricuspid valves

I08.2 Rheumatic disorders of both aortic and tricuspid valves

I08.3 Combined rheumatic disorders of mitral, aortic and tricuspid valves

I08.8 Other rheumatic multiple valve diseases

I08.9 Rheumatic multiple valve disease, unspecified

● **I09 Other rheumatic heart diseases**

I09.0 Rheumatic myocarditis
Excludes1 myocarditis not specified as rheumatic (I51.4)

I09.1 Rheumatic diseases of endocardium, valve unspecified
Rheumatic endocarditis (chronic)
Rheumatic valvulitis (chronic)
Excludes1 endocarditis, valve unspecified (I38)

I09.2 Chronic rheumatic pericarditis
Adherent pericardium, rheumatic
Chronic rheumatic mediastinopericarditis
Chronic rheumatic myopericarditis
Excludes1 chronic pericarditis not specified as rheumatic (I31.-)

● **I09.8 Other specified rheumatic heart diseases**

I09.81 Rheumatic heart failure
Use additional code to identify type of heart failure (I50.-)

I09.89 Other specified rheumatic heart diseases
Rheumatic disease of pulmonary valve

I09.9 Rheumatic heart disease, unspecified
Rheumatic carditis
Excludes1 rheumatoid carditis (M05.31)

Item 9–5 Hypertension is caused by high arterial blood pressure in the arteries. **Essential, primary,** or **idiopathic** hypertension occurs without identifiable organic cause. **Secondary** hypertension is that which has an organic cause. **Malignant** hypertension is severely elevated blood pressure. **Benign** hypertension is mildly elevated blood pressure.

HYPERTENSIVE DISEASES (I10-I16) ◀═

Use additional code to identify:
exposure to environmental tobacco smoke (Z77.22)
history of tobacco dependence (Z87.891) ◀═
occupational exposure to environmental tobacco smoke (Z57.31)
tobacco dependence (F17.-)
tobacco use (Z72.0)

Excludes1 neonatal hypertension (P29.2)
primary pulmonary hypertension (I27.0)

Excludes2 hypertensive disease complicating pregnancy, childbirth and the puerperium (O10-O11, O13-O16) ◀

I10 Essential (primary) hypertension

Includes high blood pressure
hypertension (arterial) (benign) (essential) (malignant) (primary) (systemic)

Excludes1 hypertensive disease complicating pregnancy, childbirth and the puerperium (O10-O11, O13-O16)

Excludes2 essential (primary) hypertension involving vessels of brain (I60-I69)
essential (primary) hypertension involving vessels of eye (H35.0-)

● **I11 Hypertensive heart disease**

Includes any condition in I51.4-I51.9 due to hypertension

I11.0 Hypertensive heart disease with heart failure
Hypertensive heart failure
Use additional code to identify type of heart failure (I50.-)

I11.9 Hypertensive heart disease without heart failure
Hypertensive heart disease NOS

OGCR Section I.C.9.a.2

Hypertensive Chronic Kidney Disease

Assign codes from category I12, Hypertensive chronic kidney disease, when both hypertension and a condition classifiable to category N18, Chronic kidney disease (CKD), are present. **CKD should not be coded as hypertensive if the physician has specifically documented a different cause.**

The appropriate code from category N18 should be used as a secondary code with a code from category I12 to identify the stage of chronic kidney disease.

See Section I.C.14. Chronic kidney disease.

If a patient has hypertensive chronic kidney disease and acute renal failure, an additional code for the acute renal failure is required.

● **I12 Hypertensive chronic kidney disease**

Includes any condition in N18 and N26 - due to hypertension
arteriosclerosis of kidney
arteriosclerotic nephritis (chronic) (interstitial)
hypertensive nephropathy
nephrosclerosis

Excludes1 hypertension due to kidney disease (I15.0, I15.1)
renovascular hypertension (I15.0)
secondary hypertension (I15.-)

Excludes2 acute kidney failure (N17.-)

I12.0 Hypertensive chronic kidney disease with stage 5 chronic kidney disease or end stage renal disease
Use additional code to identify the stage of chronic kidney disease (N18.5, N18.6)

I12.9 Hypertensive chronic kidney disease with stage 1 through stage 4 chronic kidney disease, or unspecified chronic kidney disease
Hypertensive chronic kidney disease NOS
Hypertensive renal disease NOS
Use additional code to identify the stage of chronic kidney disease (N18.1-N18.4, N18.9)

OGCR Section I.c.9.a.3

Hypertensive Heart and Chronic Kidney Disease

Assign codes from combination category I13, Hypertensive heart and chronic kidney disease, when **there is hypertension with both heart and kidney involvement.** If heart failure is present, assign an additional code from category I50 to identify the type of heart failure.

The appropriate code from category N18, Chronic kidney disease, should be used as a secondary code with a code from category I13 to identify the stage of chronic kidney disease.

See Section I.C.14. Chronic kidney disease.

The codes in category I13, Hypertensive heart and chronic kidney disease, are combination codes that include hypertension, heart disease and chronic kidney disease. The Includes note at I13 specifies that the conditions included at I11 and I12 are included together in I13. If a patient has hypertension, heart disease and chronic kidney disease then a code from I13 should be used, not individual codes for hypertension, heart disease and chronic kidney disease, or codes from I11 or I12.

For patients with both acute renal failure and chronic kidney disease an additional code for acute renal failure is required.

● **I13 Hypertensive heart and chronic kidney disease**

Includes any condition in I11.- with any condition in I12.-
cardiorenal disease
cardiovascular renal disease

I13.0 Hypertensive heart and chronic kidney disease with heart failure and stage 1 through stage 4 chronic kidney disease, or unspecified chronic kidney disease
Use additional code to identify type of heart failure (I50.-)
Use additional code to identify stage of chronic kidney disease (N18.1-N18.4, N18.9)

● **I13.1 Hypertensive heart and chronic kidney disease without heart failure**

I13.10 Hypertensive heart and chronic kidney disease without heart failure, with stage 1 through stage 4 chronic kidney disease, or unspecified chronic kidney disease
Hypertensive heart disease and hypertensive chronic kidney disease NOS
Use additional code to identify the stage of chronic kidney disease (N18.1-N18.4, N18.9)

I13.11 Hypertensive heart and chronic kidney disease without heart failure, with stage 5 chronic kidney disease, or end stage renal disease
Use additional code to identify the stage of chronic kidney disease (N18.5, N18.6)

I13.2 Hypertensive heart and chronic kidney disease with heart failure and with stage 5 chronic kidney disease, or end stage renal disease
Use additional code to identify type of heart failure (I50.-)
Use additional code to identify the stage of chronic kidney disease (N18.5, N18.6)

CHAPTER 9 (I00-I99)

OGCR Section I.9.a.6

Hypertension, Secondary

Secondary hypertension is due to an underlying condition. Two codes are required: one to identify the underlying etiology and one from category I15 to identify the hypertension. Sequencing of codes is determined by the reason for admission/encounter.

● **I15 Secondary hypertension**

Code also underlying condition

Excludes1 postprocedural hypertension (I97.3)

Excludes2 secondary hypertension involving vessels of brain (I60-I69)

secondary hypertension involving vessels of eye (H35.0-)

I15.0 Renovascular hypertension

I15.1 Hypertension secondary to other renal disorders

I15.2 Hypertension secondary to endocrine disorders

I15.8 Other secondary hypertension

I15.9 Secondary hypertension, unspecified

● **I16 Hypertensive crisis** ◀

Code also any identified hypertensive disease (I10-I15) ◀

I16.0 Hypertensive urgency ◀

I16.1 Hypertensive emergency ◀

I16.9 Hypertensive crisis, unspecified ◀

ISCHEMIC HEART DISEASES (I20-I25)

Use additional code to identify presence of hypertension (I10-I16) ⬅

● **I20 Angina pectoris**

Chest pain/discomfort due to lack of oxygen to the heart muscle. Principal symptom of myocardial infarction.

Use additional code to identify:

exposure to environmental tobacco smoke (Z77.22)

history of tobacco dependence (Z87.891) ⬅

occupational exposure to environmental tobacco smoke (Z57.31)

tobacco dependence (F17.-)

tobacco use (Z72.0)

Excludes1 angina pectoris with atherosclerotic heart disease of native coronary arteries (I25.1-)

atherosclerosis of coronary artery bypass graft(s) and coronary artery of transplanted heart with angina pectoris (I25.7-)

postinfarction angina (I23.7)

I20.0 Unstable angina

Accelerated angina

Crescendo angina

De novo effort angina

Intermediate coronary syndrome

Preinfarction syndrome

Worsening effort angina

I20.1 Angina pectoris with documented spasm

Angiospastic angina

Prinzmetal angina

Spasm-induced angina

Variant angina

I20.8 Other forms of angina pectoris

Angina equivalent

Angina of effort

Coronary slow flow syndrome

Stable angina ◀

Stenocardia

Use additional code(s) for symptoms associated with angina equivalent

I20.9 Angina pectoris, unspecified

Angina NOS

Anginal syndrome

Cardiac angina

Ischemic chest pain

I21 ST elevation (STEMI) and non-ST elevation (NSTEMI) myocardial infarction

Includes cardiac infarction

coronary (artery) embolism

coronary (artery) occlusion

coronary (artery) rupture

coronary (artery) thrombosis

infarction of heart, myocardium, or ventricle

myocardial infarction specified as acute or with a stated duration of 4 weeks (28 days) or less from onset

Use additional code, if applicable, to identify:

exposure to environmental tobacco smoke (Z77.22)

history of tobacco dependence (Z87.891) ⬅

occupational exposure to environmental tobacco smoke (Z57.31)

status post administration of tPA (rtPA) in a different facility within the last 24 hours prior to admission to current facility (Z92.82)

tobacco dependence (F17.-)

tobacco use (Z72.0)

Excludes2 old myocardial infarction (I25.2)

postmyocardial infarction syndrome (I24.1)

subsequent myocardial infarction (I22.-)

● **I21.0 ST elevation (STEMI) myocardial infarction of anterior wall**

I21.01 ST elevation (STEMI) myocardial infarction involving left main coronary artery

I21.02 ST elevation (STEMI) myocardial infarction involving left anterior descending coronary artery

ST elevation (STEMI) myocardial infarction involving diagonal coronary artery

I21.09 ST elevation (STEMI) myocardial infarction involving other coronary artery of anterior wall

Acute transmural myocardial infarction of anterior wall

Anteroapical transmural (Q wave) infarction (acute)

Anterolateral transmural (Q wave) infarction (acute)

Anteroseptal transmural (Q wave) infarction (acute)

Transmural (Q wave) infarction (acute) (of) anterior (wall) NOS

● I21.1 **ST elevation (STEMI) myocardial infarction of inferior wall**

I21.11 **ST elevation (STEMI) myocardial infarction involving right coronary artery**
Inferoposterior transmural (Q wave) infarction (acute)

I21.19 **ST elevation (STEMI) myocardial infarction involving other coronary artery of inferior wall**
Acute transmural myocardial infarction of inferior wall
Inferolateral transmural (Q wave) infarction (acute)
Transmural (Q wave) infarction (acute) (of) diaphragmatic wall
Transmural (Q wave) infarction (acute) (of) inferior (wall) NOS

Excludes2 ST elevation (STEMI) myocardial infarction involving left circumflex coronary artery (I21.21)

● I21.2 **ST elevation (STEMI) myocardial infarction of other sites**

I21.21 **ST elevation (STEMI) myocardial infarction involving left circumflex coronary artery**
ST elevation (STEMI) myocardial infarction involving oblique marginal coronary artery

I21.29 **ST elevation (STEMI) myocardial infarction involving other sites**
Acute transmural myocardial infarction of other sites
Apical-lateral transmural (Q wave) infarction (acute)
Basal-lateral transmural (Q wave) infarction (acute)
High lateral transmural (Q wave) infarction (acute)
Lateral (wall) NOS transmural (Q wave) infarction (acute)
Posterior (true) transmural (Q wave) infarction (acute)
Posterobasal transmural (Q wave) infarction (acute)
Posterolateral transmural (Q wave) infarction (acute)
Posteroseptal transmural (Q wave) infarction (acute)
Septal transmural (Q wave) infarction (acute) NOS

OGCR Section I.c.9.e.2

Acute myocardial infarction, unspecified
Code I21.3, ST elevation (STEMI) myocordial infarction of unspecified site, is the default for unspecified acute myocardial infarction. If only STEMI or transmural MI without the site is documented, assign I21.3.

I21.3 **ST elevation (STEMI) myocardial infarction of unspecified site**
Acute transmural myocardial infarction of unspecified site
Myocardial infarction (acute) NOS
Transmural (Q wave) myocardial infarction NOS

I21.4 **Non-ST elevation (NSTEMI) myocardial infarction**
Acute subendocardial myocardial infarction
Non-Q wave myocardial infarction NOS
Nontransmural myocardial infarction NOS

● I22 **Subsequent ST elevation (STEMI) and non-ST elevation (NSTEMI) myocardial infarction**

Includes acute myocardial infarction occurring within four weeks (28 days) of a previous acute myocardial infarction, regardless of site
cardiac infarction
coronary (artery) embolism
coronary (artery) occlusion
coronary (artery) rupture
coronary (artery) thrombosis
infarction of heart, myocardium, or ventricle
recurrent myocardial infarction
reinfarction of myocardium
rupture of heart, myocardium, or ventricle

Use additional code, if applicable, to identify:
exposure to environmental tobacco smoke (Z77.22)
history of tobacco dependence (Z87.891) ◄
occupational exposure to environmental tobacco smoke (Z57.31)
status post administration of tPA (rtPA) in a different facility within the last 24 hours prior to admission to current facility (Z92.82)
tobacco dependence (F17.-)
tobacco use (Z72.0)

I22.0 **Subsequent ST elevation (STEMI) myocardial infarction of anterior wall**
Subsequent acute transmural myocardial infarction of anterior wall
Subsequent transmural (Q wave) infarction (acute)(of) anterior (wall) NOS
Subsequent anteroapical transmural (Q wave) infarction (acute)
Subsequent anterolateral transmural (Q wave) infarction (acute)
Subsequent anteroseptal transmural (Q wave) infarction (acute)

I22.1 **Subsequent ST elevation (STEMI) myocardial infarction of inferior wall**
Subsequent acute transmural myocardial infarction of inferior wall
Subsequent transmural (Q wave) infarction (acute)(of) diaphragmatic wall
Subsequent transmural (Q wave) infarction (acute)(of) inferior (wall) NOS
Subsequent inferolateral transmural (Q wave) infarction (acute)
Subsequent inferoposterior transmural (Q wave) infarction (acute)

I22.2 **Subsequent non-ST elevation (NSTEMI) myocardial infarction**
Subsequent acute subendocardial myocardial infarction
Subsequent non-Q wave myocardial infarction NOS
Subsequent nontransmural myocardial infarction NOS

I22.8 **Subsequent ST elevation (STEMI) myocardial infarction of other sites**
Subsequent acute transmural myocardial infarction of other sites
Subsequent apical-lateral transmural (Q wave) myocardial infarction (acute)
Subsequent basal-lateral transmural (Q wave) myocardial infarction (acute)
Subsequent high lateral transmural (Q wave) myocardial infarction (acute)
Subsequent transmural (Q wave) myocardial infarction (acute)(of) lateral (wall) NOS
Subsequent posterior (true) transmural (Q wave) myocardial infarction (acute)
Subsequent posterobasal transmural (Q wave) myocardial infarction (acute)
Subsequent posterolateral transmural (Q wave) myocardial infarction (acute)
Subsequent posteroseptal transmural (Q wave) myocardial infarction (acute)
Subsequent septal NOS transmural (Q wave) myocardial infarction (acute)

CHAPTER 9 (I00-I99)

I22.9 **Subsequent ST elevation (STEMI) myocardial infarction of unspecified site**
Subsequent acute myocardial infarction of unspecified site
Subsequent myocardial infarction (acute) NOS

● I23 **Certain current complications following ST elevation (STEMI) and non-ST elevation (NSTEMI) myocardial infarction (within the 28 day period)**

I23.0 **Hemopericardium as current complication following acute myocardial infarction**
Excludes1 hemopericardium not specified as current complication following acute myocardial infarction (I31.2)

I23.1 **Atrial septal defect as current complication following acute myocardial infarction**
Excludes1 acquired atrial septal defect not specified as current complication following acute myocardial infarction (I51.0)

I23.2 **Ventricular septal defect as current complication following acute myocardial infarction**
Excludes1 acquired ventricular septal defect not specified as current complication following acute myocardial infarction (I51.0)

I23.3 **Rupture of cardiac wall without hemopericardium as current complication following acute myocardial infarction**

I23.4 **Rupture of chordae tendineae as current complication following acute myocardial infarction**
Excludes1 rupture of chordae tendineae not specified as current complication following acute myocardial infarction (I51.1)

I23.5 **Rupture of papillary muscle as current complication following acute myocardial infarction**
Excludes1 rupture of papillary muscle not specified as current complication following acute myocardial infarction (I51.2)

I23.6 **Thrombosis of atrium, auricular appendage, and ventricle as current complications following acute myocardial infarction**
Excludes1 thrombosis of atrium, auricular appendage, and ventricle not specified as current complication following acute myocardial infarction (I51.3)

I23.7 **Postinfarction angina**

I23.8 **Other current complications following acute myocardial infarction**

● I24 **Other acute ischemic heart diseases**
Excludes1 angina pectoris (I20.-)
transient myocardial ischemia in newborn (P29.4)

I24.0 **Acute coronary thrombosis not resulting in myocardial infarction**
Acute coronary (artery) (vein) embolism not resulting in myocardial infarction
Acute coronary (artery) (vein) occlusion not resulting in myocardial infarction
Acute coronary (artery) (vein) thromboembolism not resulting in myocardial infarction
Excludes1 atherosclerotic heart disease (I25.1-)

I24.1 **Dressler's syndrome**
Postmyocardial infarction syndrome
Excludes1 postinfarction angina (I23.7)

I24.8 **Other forms of acute ischemic heart disease**

I24.9 **Acute ischemic heart disease, unspecified**
Excludes1 ischemic heart disease (chronic) NOS (I25.9)

● I25 **Chronic ischemic heart disease**
Use additional code to identify:
chronic total occlusion of coronary artery (I25.82)
exposure to environmental tobacco smoke (Z77.22)
history of tobacco dependence (Z87.891) ◄
occupational exposure to environmental tobacco smoke (Z57.31)
tobacco dependence (F17.-)
tobacco use (Z72.0)

★**(See Plates 218 and 219 on pages NAP-26 and NAP-27.)**

● I25.1 **Atherosclerotic heart disease of native coronary artery**
Disease in which fatty deposits form on the walls of arteries
Atherosclerotic cardiovascular disease
Coronary (artery) atheroma
Coronary (artery) atherosclerosis
Coronary (artery) disease
Coronary (artery) sclerosis
Use additional code, if applicable, to identify:
coronary atherosclerosis due to calcified coronary lesion (I25.84)
coronary atherosclerosis due to lipid rich plaque (I25.83)
Excludes2 atheroembolism (I75.-)
atherosclerosis of coronary artery bypass graft(s) and transplanted heart (I25.7-)

I25.10 **Atherosclerotic heart disease of native coronary artery without angina pectoris**
Atherosclerotic heart disease NOS

OGCR See Section I.9.b.

Atherosclerotic Coronary Artery Disease and Angina

ICD-10-CM has combination codes for atherosclerotic heart disease with angina pectoris. The subcategories for these codes are I25.11, Atherosclerotic heart disease of native coronary artery with angina pectoris and I25.7, Atherosclerosis of coronary artery bypass graft(s) and coronary artery of transplanted heart with angina pectoris.

When using one of these combination codes it is not necessary to use an additional code for angina pectoris. A causal relationship can be assumed in a patient with both atherosclerosis and angina pectoris, unless the documentation indicates the angina is due to something other than the atherosclerosis.

If a patient with coronary artery disease is admitted due to an acute myocardial infarction (AMI), the AMI should be sequenced before the coronary artery disease.

See Section I.C.9. Acute myocardial infarction (AMI)

● I25.11 **Atherosclerotic heart disease of native coronary artery with angina pectoris**

I25.110 **Atherosclerotic heart disease of native coronary artery with unstable angina pectoris**
Excludes1 unstable angina without atherosclerotic heart disease (I20.0)

I25.111 **Atherosclerotic heart disease of native coronary artery with angina pectoris with documented spasm**
Excludes1 angina pectoris with documented spasm without atherosclerotic heart disease (I20.1)

◄ New ◄ Revised ~~deleted~~ Deleted OGCR Official Guidelines X Assign placeholder X ● Use Additional Character(s)
Excludes 1 Excludes 2 Includes Use additional Code first Code also Unspecified

Item 9–6 Classification is based on the location of the atherosclerosis. **"Of native coronary artery"** indicates the atherosclerosis is within an original heart artery. **"Of autologous vein bypass graft"** indicates that the atherosclerosis is within a vein graft that was taken from within the patient. **"Of nonautologous biological bypass graft"** indicates the atherosclerosis is within a vessel grafted from other than the patient. **"Of artery bypass graft"** indicates the atherosclerosis is within an artery that was grafted from within the patient.

Figure 9-2 Atherosclerotic plaque.

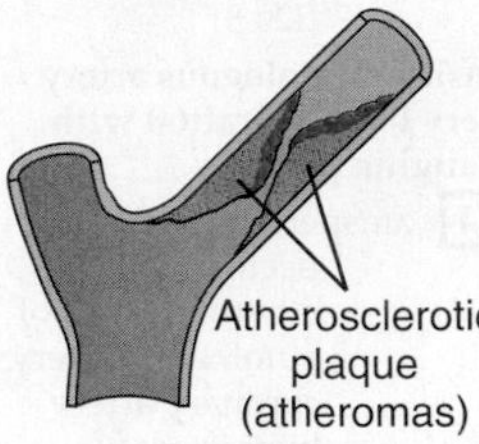

I25.118 Atherosclerotic heart disease of native coronary artery with other forms of angina pectoris
Excludes1 other forms of angina pectoris without atherosclerotic heart disease (I2Ø.8)

I25.119 Atherosclerotic heart disease of native coronary artery with unspecified angina pectoris
Atherosclerotic heart disease with angina NOS
Atherosclerotic heart disease with ischemic chest pain
Excludes1 unspecified angina pectoris without atherosclerotic heart disease (I2Ø.9)

I25.2 Old myocardial infarction
Healed myocardial infarction
Past myocardial infarction diagnosed by ECG or other investigation, but currently presenting no symptoms

I25.3 Aneurysm of heart
Mural aneurysm
Ventricular aneurysm

● **I25.4 Coronary artery aneurysm and dissection**

I25.41 Coronary artery aneurysm
Coronary arteriovenous fistula, acquired
Excludes1 congenital coronary (artery) aneurysm (Q24.5)

I25.42 Coronary artery dissection

I25.5 Ischemic cardiomyopathy
Excludes2 coronary atherosclerosis (I25.1-, I25.7-)

I25.6 Silent myocardial ischemia

● **I25.7 Atherosclerosis of coronary artery bypass graft(s) and coronary artery of transplanted heart with angina pectoris**
Use additional code, if applicable, to identify:
coronary atherosclerosis due to calcified coronary lesion (I25.84)
coronary atherosclerosis due to lipid rich plaque (I25.83)
Excludes1 atherosclerosis of bypass graft(s) of transplanted heart without angina pectoris (I25.812)
atherosclerosis of coronary artery bypass graft(s) without angina pectoris (I25.81Ø)
atherosclerosis of native coronary artery of transplanted heart without angina pectoris (I25.811)
embolism or thrombus of coronary artery bypass graft(s) (T82.8-)

● **I25.7Ø Atherosclerosis of coronary artery bypass graft(s), unspecified, with angina pectoris**

I25.7ØØ Atherosclerosis of coronary artery bypass graft(s), unspecified, with unstable angina pectoris
Excludes1 unstable angina pectoris without atherosclerosis of coronary artery bypass graft (I2Ø.Ø)

I25.7Ø1 Atherosclerosis of coronary artery bypass graft(s), unspecified, with angina pectoris with documented spasm
Excludes1 angina pectoris with documented spasm without atherosclerosis of coronary artery bypass graft (I2Ø.1)

I25.7Ø8 Atherosclerosis of coronary artery bypass graft(s), unspecified, with other forms of angina pectoris
Excludes1 other forms of angina pectoris without atherosclerosis of coronary artery bypass graft (I2Ø.8)

I25.7Ø9 Atherosclerosis of coronary artery bypass graft(s), unspecified, with unspecified angina pectoris
Excludes1 unspecified angina pectoris without atherosclerosis of coronary artery bypass graft (I2Ø.9)

CHAPTER 9 (IØØ-I99)

● **I25.71 Atherosclerosis of autologous vein coronary artery bypass graft(s) with angina pectoris**

I25.710 Atherosclerosis of autologous vein coronary artery bypass graft(s) with unstable angina pectoris

Excludes1 unstable angina without atherosclerosis of autologous vein coronary artery bypass graft(s) (I2Ø.Ø)

I25.711 Atherosclerosis of autologous vein coronary artery bypass graft(s) with angina pectoris with documented spasm

Excludes1 angina pectoris with documented spasm without atherosclerosis of autologous vein coronary artery bypass graft(s) (I2Ø.1)

I25.718 Atherosclerosis of autologous vein coronary artery bypass graft(s) with other forms of angina pectoris

Excludes1 other forms of angina pectoris without atherosclerosis of autologous vein coronary artery bypass graft(s) (I2Ø.8)

I25.719 Atherosclerosis of autologous vein coronary artery bypass graft(s) with unspecified angina pectoris

Excludes1 unspecified angina pectoris without atherosclerosis of autologous vein coronary artery bypass graft(s) (I2Ø.9)

● **I25.72 Atherosclerosis of autologous artery coronary artery bypass graft(s) with angina pectoris**

Atherosclerosis of internal mammary artery graft with angina pectoris

I25.72Ø Atherosclerosis of autologous artery coronary artery bypass graft(s) with unstable angina pectoris

Excludes1 unstable angina without atherosclerosis of autologous artery coronary artery bypass graft(s) (I2Ø.Ø)

I25.721 Atherosclerosis of autologous artery coronary artery bypass graft(s) with angina pectoris with documented spasm

Excludes1 angina pectoris with documented spasm without atherosclerosis of autologous artery coronary artery bypass graft(s) (I2Ø.1)

I25.728 Atherosclerosis of autologous artery coronary artery bypass graft(s) with other forms of angina pectoris

Excludes1 other forms of angina pectoris without atherosclerosis of autologous artery coronary artery bypass graft(s) (I2Ø.8)

I25.729 Atherosclerosis of autologous artery coronary artery bypass graft(s) with unspecified angina pectoris

Excludes1 unspecified angina pectoris without atherosclerosis of autologous artery coronary artery bypass graft(s) (I2Ø.9)

● **I25.73 Atherosclerosis of nonautologous biological coronary artery bypass graft(s) with angina pectoris**

I25.73Ø Atherosclerosis of nonautologous biological coronary artery bypass graft(s) with unstable angina pectoris

Excludes1 unstable angina without atherosclerosis of nonautologous biological coronary artery bypass graft(s) (I2Ø.Ø)

I25.731 Atherosclerosis of nonautologous biological coronary artery bypass graft(s) with angina pectoris with documented spasm

Excludes1 angina pectoris with documented spasm without atherosclerosis of nonautologous biological coronary artery bypass graft(s) (I2Ø.1)

I25.738 Atherosclerosis of nonautologous biological coronary artery bypass graft(s) with other forms of angina pectoris

Excludes1 other forms of angina pectoris without atherosclerosis of nonautologous biological coronary artery bypass graft(s) (I2Ø.8)

I25.739 Atherosclerosis of nonautologous biological coronary artery bypass graft(s) with unspecified angina pectoris

Excludes1 unspecified angina pectoris without atherosclerosis of nonautologous biological coronary artery bypass graft(s) (I2Ø.9)

● **I25.75 Atherosclerosis of native coronary artery of transplanted heart with angina pectoris**

Excludes1 atherosclerosis of native coronary artery of transplanted heart without angina pectoris (I25.811)

I25.750 Atherosclerosis of native coronary artery of transplanted heart with unstable angina

I25.751 Atherosclerosis of native coronary artery of transplanted heart with angina pectoris with documented spasm

I25.758 Atherosclerosis of native coronary artery of transplanted heart with other forms of angina pectoris

I25.759 Atherosclerosis of native coronary artery of transplanted heart with unspecified angina pectoris

● **I25.76 Atherosclerosis of bypass graft of coronary artery of transplanted heart with angina pectoris**

Excludes1 atherosclerosis of bypass graft of coronary artery of transplanted heart without angina pectoris (I25.812)

I25.760 Atherosclerosis of bypass graft of coronary artery of transplanted heart with unstable angina

I25.761 Atherosclerosis of bypass graft of coronary artery of transplanted heart with angina pectoris with documented spasm

I25.768 Atherosclerosis of bypass graft of coronary artery of transplanted heart with other forms of angina pectoris

I25.769 Atherosclerosis of bypass graft of coronary artery of transplanted heart with unspecified angina pectoris

● **I25.79 Atherosclerosis of other coronary artery bypass graft(s) with angina pectoris**

I25.790 Atherosclerosis of other coronary artery bypass graft(s) with unstable angina pectoris

Excludes1 unstable angina without atherosclerosis of other coronary artery bypass graft(s) (I20.0)

I25.791 Atherosclerosis of other coronary artery bypass graft(s) with angina pectoris with documented spasm

Excludes1 angina pectoris with documented spasm without atherosclerosis of other coronary artery bypass graft(s) (I20.1)

I25.798 Atherosclerosis of other coronary artery bypass graft(s) with other forms of angina pectoris

Excludes1 other forms of angina pectoris without atherosclerosis of other coronary artery bypass graft(s) (I20.8)

I25.799 Atherosclerosis of other coronary artery bypass graft(s) with unspecified angina pectoris

Excludes1 unspecified angina pectoris without atherosclerosis of other coronary artery bypass graft(s) (I20.9)

● **I25.8 Other forms of chronic ischemic heart disease**

● **I25.81 Atherosclerosis of other coronary vessels without angina pectoris**

Use additional code, if applicable, to identify:
coronary atherosclerosis due to calcified coronary lesion (I25.84)
coronary atherosclerosis due to lipid rich plaque (I25.83)

Excludes1 atherosclerotic heart disease of native coronary artery without angina pectoris (I25.10)

I25.810 Atherosclerosis of coronary artery bypass graft(s) without angina pectoris

Atherosclerosis of coronary artery bypass graft NOS

Excludes1 atherosclerosis of coronary bypass graft(s) with angina pectoris (I25.70- -I25.73-, I25.79-)

I25.811 Atherosclerosis of native coronary artery of transplanted heart without angina pectoris

Atherosclerosis of native coronary artery of transplanted heart NOS

Excludes1 atherosclerosis of native coronary artery of transplanted heart with angina pectoris (I25.75-)

I25.812 Atherosclerosis of bypass graft of coronary artery of transplanted heart without angina pectoris

Atherosclerosis of bypass graft of transplanted heart NOS

Excludes1 atherosclerosis of bypass graft of transplanted heart with angina pectoris (I25.76)

I25.82 Chronic total occlusion of coronary artery

Complete occlusion of coronary artery
Total occlusion of coronary artery

Code first coronary atherosclerosis (I25.1-, I25.7-, I25.81-)

Excludes1 acute coronary occulsion with myocardial infarction (I21.-, I22.-)
acute coronary occulsion without myocardial infarction (I24.0)

I25.83 Coronary atherosclerosis due to lipid rich plaque

Code first coronary atherosclerosis (I25.1-, I25.7-, I25.81-)

CHAPTER 9 (I00-I99)

I25.84 **Coronary atherosclerosis due to calcified coronary lesion**
Coronary atherosclerosis due to severely calcified coronary lesion
Code first *coronary atherosclerosis (I25.1-, I25.7-, I25.81-)*

I25.89 **Other forms of chronic ischemic heart disease**

I25.9 **Chronic ischemic heart disease, unspecified**
Ischemic heart disease (chronic) NOS

PULMONARY HEART DISEASE AND DISEASES OF PULMONARY CIRCULATION (I26-I28)

● I26 **Pulmonary embolism**
Includes pulmonary (acute)(artery)(vein) infarction
pulmonary (acute)(artery)(vein) thromboembolism
pulmonary (acute)(artery)(vein) thrombosis
Excludes2 chronic pulmonary embolism (I27.82)
personal history of pulmonary embolism (Z86.711)
pulmonary embolism due to trauma (T79.0, T79.1)
pulmonary embolism due to complications of surgical and medical care (T80.0, T81.7-, T82.8-)
pulmonary embolism complicating abortion, ectopic or molar pregnancy (O00-O07, O08.2)
pulmonary embolism complicating pregnancy, childbirth and the puerperium (O88.-)
septic (non-pulmonary) arterial embolism (I76)

● I26.0 **Pulmonary embolism with acute cor pulmonale**

I26.01 **Septic pulmonary embolism with acute cor pulmonale**
Code first *underlying infection*

I26.02 **Saddle embolus of pulmonary artery with acute cor pulmonale**

I26.09 **Other pulmonary embolism with acute cor pulmonale**
Acute cor pulmonale NOS

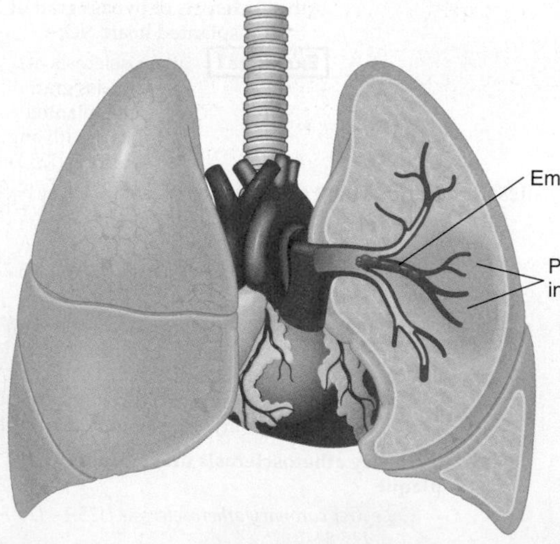

Figure 9-3 Pulmonary Embolism. (From Chabner: The Language of Medicine, ed 8, St. Louis, Saunders, 2007)

Item 9-7 Pulmonary heart disease or **cor pulmonale** is right ventricle hypertrophy or RVH as a result of a respiratory disorder increasing back flow pressure to the right ventricle. Left untreated, cor pulmonale leads to right-heart failure and death.

● I26.9 **Pulmonary embolism without acute cor pulmonale**

I26.90 **Septic pulmonary embolism without acute cor pulmonale**
Code first *underlying infection*

I26.92 **Saddle embolus of pulmonary artery without acute cor pulmonale**

I26.99 **Other pulmonary embolism without acute cor pulmonale**
Acute pulmonary embolism NOS
Pulmonary embolism NOS

● I27 **Other pulmonary heart diseases**

I27.0 **Primary pulmonary hypertension**
Excludes1 pulmonary hypertension NOS (I27.2)
secondary pulmonary hypertension (I27.2)

I27.1 **Kyphoscoliotic heart disease**

I27.2 **Other secondary pulmonary hypertension**
Pulmonary hypertension NOS
Code also associated underlying condition

● I27.8 **Other specified pulmonary heart diseases**

I27.81 **Cor pulmonale (chronic)**
Cor pulmonale NOS
Excludes1 acute cor pulmonale (I26.0-)

I27.82 **Chronic pulmonary embolism**
Use additional code, if applicable, for associated long-term (current) use of anticoagulants (Z79.01)
Excludes1 personal history of pulmonary embolism (Z86.711)

I27.89 **Other specified pulmonary heart diseases**
Eisenmenger's complex
Eisenmenger's syndrome
Excludes1 Eisenmenger's defect (Q21.8)

I27.9 **Pulmonary heart disease, unspecified**
Chronic cardiopulmonary disease

● I28 **Other diseases of pulmonary vessels**

I28.0 **Arteriovenous fistula of pulmonary vessels**
Excludes1 congenital arteriovenous fistula (Q25.72)

I28.1 **Aneurysm of pulmonary artery**
Excludes1 congenital aneurysm (Q25.79)
congenital arteriovenous aneurysm (Q25.72)

I28.8 **Other diseases of pulmonary vessels**
Pulmonary arteritis
Pulmonary endarteritis
Rupture of pulmonary vessels
Stenosis of pulmonary vessels
Stricture of pulmonary vessels

I28.9 **Disease of pulmonary vessels, unspecified**

OTHER FORMS OF HEART DISEASE (I3Ø-I52)

● **I3Ø Acute pericarditis**
Inflammation of pericardium (sac surrounding the heart) caused by an infection
Includes acute mediastinopericarditis
acute myopericarditis
acute pericardial effusion
acute pleuropericarditis
acute pneumopericarditis
Excludes1 Dressler's syndrome (I24.1)
rheumatic pericarditis (acute) (IØ1.Ø)

I3Ø.Ø Acute nonspecific idiopathic pericarditis

I3Ø.1 Infective pericarditis
Pneumococcal pericarditis
Pneumopyopericardium
Purulent pericarditis
Pyopericarditis
Pyopericardium
Pyopneumopericardium
Staphylococcal pericarditis
Streptococcal pericarditis
Suppurative pericarditis
Viral pericarditis
Use additional code (B95-B97) to identify infectious agent

I3Ø.8 Other forms of acute pericarditis

I3Ø.9 Acute pericarditis, unspecified

● **I31 Other diseases of pericardium**
Excludes1 diseases of pericardium specified as rheumatic (IØ9.2)
postcardiotomy syndrome (I97.Ø)
traumatic injury to pericardium (S26.-)

I31.Ø Chronic adhesive pericarditis
Accretio cordis
Adherent pericardium
Adhesive mediastinopericarditis

I31.1 Chronic constrictive pericarditis
Concretio cordis
Pericardial calcification

I31.2 Hemopericardium, not elsewhere classified
Excludes1 hemopericardium as current complication following acute myocardial infarction (I23.Ø)

I31.3 Pericardial effusion (noninflammatory)
Chylopericardium
Excludes1 acute pericardial effusion (I3Ø.9)

I31.4 Cardiac tamponade
Code first underlying cause

I31.8 Other specified diseases of pericardium
Epicardial plaques
Focal pericardial adhesions

I31.9 Disease of pericardium, unspecified
Pericarditis (chronic) NOS

I32 Pericarditis in diseases classified elsewhere
Code first underlying disease
Excludes1 pericarditis (in):
coxsackie (virus) (B33.23)
gonococcal (A54.83)
meningococcal (A39.53)
rheumatoid (arthritis) (MØ5.31)
syphilitic (A52.Ø6)
systemic lupus erythematosus (M32.12)
tuberculosis (A18.84)

● **I33 Acute and subacute endocarditis**
Inflammation/infection of lining of heart, affecting heart valves including replacement valves and is usually caused by a bacterial infection
Excludes1 acute rheumatic endocarditis (IØ1.1)
endocarditis NOS (I38)

I33.Ø Acute and subacute infective endocarditis
Bacterial endocarditis (acute) (subacute)
Infective endocarditis (acute) (subacute) NOS
Endocarditis lenta (acute) (subacute)
Malignant endocarditis (acute) (subacute)
Purulent endocarditis (acute) (subacute)
Septic endocarditis (acute) (subacute)
Ulcerative endocarditis (acute) (subacute)
Vegetative endocarditis (acute) (subacute)
Use additional code (B95-B97) to identify infectious agent

I33.9 Acute and subacute endocarditis, unspecified
Acute endocarditis NOS
Acute myoendocarditis NOS
Acute periendocarditis NOS
Subacute endocarditis NOS
Subacute myoendocarditis NOS
Subacute periendocarditis NOS

● **I34 Nonrheumatic mitral valve disorders**
Excludes1 mitral valve disease (IØ5.9)
mitral valve failure (IØ5.8)
mitral valve stenosis (IØ5.Ø)
mitral valve disorder of unspecified cause with diseases of aortic and/or tricuspid valve(s) (IØ8.-)
mitral valve disorder of unspecified cause with mitral stenosis or obstruction (IØ5.Ø)
mitral valve disorder specified as congenital (Q23.2, Q23.3)
mitral valve disorder specified as rheumatic (IØ5.-)

I34.Ø Nonrheumatic mitral (valve) insufficiency
Nonrheumatic mitral (valve) incompetence NOS
Nonrheumatic mitral (valve) regurgitation NOS

I34.1 Nonrheumatic mitral (valve) prolapse
Floppy nonrheumatic mitral valve syndrome
Excludes1 Marfan's syndrome (Q87.4-)

I34.2 Nonrheumatic mitral (valve) stenosis

I34.8 Other nonrheumatic mitral valve disorders

I34.9 Nonrheumatic mitral valve disorder, unspecified

● **I35 Nonrheumatic aortic valve disorders**
Excludes1 aortic valve disorder of unspecified cause but with diseases of mitral and/or tricuspid valve(s) (IØ8.-)
aortic valve disorder specified as congenital (Q23.Ø, Q23.1)
aortic valve disorder specified as rheumatic (IØ6.-)
hypertrophic subaortic stenosis (I42.1)

I35.Ø Nonrheumatic aortic (valve) stenosis

I35.1 Nonrheumatic aortic (valve) insufficiency
Nonrheumatic aortic (valve) incompetence NOS
Nonrheumatic aortic (valve) regurgitation NOS

I35.2 Nonrheumatic aortic (valve) stenosis with insufficiency

I35.8 Other nonrheumatic aortic valve disorders

I35.9 Nonrheumatic aortic valve disorder, unspecified

CHAPTER 9 (IØØ-I99)

● **I36 Nonrheumatic tricuspid valve disorders**

Excludes1 tricuspid valve disorders of unspecified cause (I07.-)
tricuspid valve disorders specified as congenital (Q22.4, Q22.8, Q22.9)
tricuspid valve disorders specified as rheumatic (I07.-)
tricuspid valve disorders with aortic and/or mitral valve involvement (I08.-)

I36.0 Nonrheumatic tricuspid (valve) stenosis

I36.1 Nonrheumatic tricuspid (valve) insufficiency
Nonrheumatic tricuspid (valve) incompetence
Nonrheumatic tricuspid (valve) regurgitation

I36.2 Nonrheumatic tricuspid (valve) stenosis with insufficiency

I36.8 Other nonrheumatic tricuspid valve disorders

I36.9 Nonrheumatic tricuspid valve disorder, unspecified

● **I37 Nonrheumatic pulmonary valve disorders**

Excludes1 pulmonary valve disorder specified as congenital (Q22.1, Q22.2, Q22.3)
pulmonary valve disorder specified as rheumatic (I09.89)

I37.0 Nonrheumatic pulmonary valve stenosis

I37.1 Nonrheumatic pulmonary valve insufficiency
Nonrheumatic pulmonary valve incompetence
Nonrheumatic pulmonary valve regurgitation

I37.2 Nonrheumatic pulmonary valve stenosis with insufficiency

I37.8 Other nonrheumatic pulmonary valve disorders

I37.9 Nonrheumatic pulmonary valve disorder, unspecified

I38 Endocarditis, valve unspecified

Includes endocarditis (chronic) NOS
valvular incompetence NOS
valvular insufficiency NOS
valvular regurgitation NOS
valvular stenosis NOS
valvulitis (chronic) NOS

Excludes1 congenital insufficiency of cardiac valve NOS (Q24.8)
congenital stenosis of cardiac valve NOS (Q24.8)
endocardial fibroelastosis (I42.4)
endocarditis specified as rheumatic (I09.1)

I39 Endocarditis and heart valve disorders in diseases classified elsewhere

Code first underlying disease, such as:
Q fever (A78)

Excludes1 endocardial involvement in:
candidiasis (B37.6)
gonococcal infection (A54.83)
Libman-Sacks disease (M32.11)
listerosis (A32.82)
meningococcal infection (A39.51)
rheumatoid arthritis (M05.31)
syphilis (A52.03)
tuberculosis (A18.84)
typhoid fever (A01.02)

● **I40 Acute myocarditis**

Inflammation of heart muscle due to infection (viral/bacterial)

Includes subacute myocarditis

Excludes1 acute rheumatic myocarditis (I01.2)

I40.0 Infective myocarditis
Septic myocarditis
Use additional code (B95-B97) to identify infectious agent

I40.1 Isolated myocarditis
Fiedler's myocarditis
Giant cell myocarditis
Idiopathic myocarditis

I40.8 Other acute myocarditis

I40.9 Acute myocarditis, unspecified

I41 Myocarditis in diseases classified elsewhere

Code first underlying disease, such as:
typhus (A75.0-A75.9)

Excludes1 myocarditis (in):
Chagas' disease (chronic) (B57.2)
acute (B57.0)
coxsackie (virus) infection (B33.22)
diphtheritic (A36.81)
gonococcal (A54.83)
influenzal (J09.X9, J10.82, J11.82)
meningococcal (A39.52)
mumps (B26.82)
rheumatoid arthritis (M05.31)
sarcoid (D86.85)
syphilis (A52.06)
toxoplasmosis (B58.81)
tuberculous (A18.84)

● **I42 Cardiomyopathy**

Disease of the heart muscle resulting in an abnormally enlarged, weakened, thickened, and/or stiffened muscles

Includes myocardiopathy

Code first pre-existing cardiomyopathy complicating pregnancy and puerperium (O99.4)

Excludes2 ischemic cardiomyopathy (I25.5) ◀
peripartum cardiomyopathy (O90.3) ◀
ventricular hypertrophy (I51.7)

I42.0 Dilated cardiomyopathy
Congestive cardiomyopathy

I42.1 Obstructive hypertrophic cardiomyopathy
Hypertrophic subaortic stenosis (idiopathic)

I42.2 Other hypertrophic cardiomyopathy
Nonobstructive hypertrophic cardiomyopathy

I42.3 Endomyocardial (eosinophilic) disease
Endomyocardial (tropical) fibrosis
Löffler's endocarditis

I42.4 Endocardial fibroelastosis
Congenital cardiomyopathy
Elastomyofibrosis

I42.5 Other restrictive cardiomyopathy
Constrictive cardiomyopathy NOS

I42.6 Alcoholic cardiomyopathy
Code also presence of alcoholism (F10.-)

I42.7 Cardiomyopathy due to drug and external agent
Code first poisoning due to drug or toxin, if applicable (T36-T65 with fifth or sixth character 1-4 or 6)
Use additional code for adverse effect, if applicable, to identify drug (T36-T50 with fifth or sixth character 5)

I42.8 Other cardiomyopathies

I42.9 Cardiomyopathy, unspecified
Cardiomyopathy (primary) (secondary) NOS

I43 Cardiomyopathy in diseases classified elsewhere

Code first underlying disease, such as:
amyloidosis (E85.-)
glycogen storage disease (E74.0)
gout (M10.0-)
thyrotoxicosis (E05.0-E05.9-)

Excludes1 cardiomyopathy (in):
coxsackie (virus) (B33.24)
diphtheria (A36.81)
sarcoidosis (D86.85)
tuberculosis (A18.84)

CHAPTER 9 (I00-I99)

● **I44 Atrioventricular and left bundle-branch block**
Conduction problem resulting in arrhythmias/dysrhythmias due to a lack of electrical impulses being transmitted normally through the heart

I44.0 Atrioventricular block, first degree

I44.1 Atrioventricular block, second degree
Atrioventricular block, type I and II
Möbitz block, type I and II
Second degree block, type I and II
Wenckebach's block

I44.2 Atrioventricular block, complete
Complete heart block NOS
Third degree block

● **I44.3 Other and unspecified atrioventricular block**
Atrioventricular block NOS

I44.30 Unspecified atrioventricular block

I44.39 Other atrioventricular block

I44.4 Left anterior fascicular block

I44.5 Left posterior fascicular block

● **I44.6 Other and unspecified fascicular block**

I44.60 Unspecified fascicular block
Left bundle-branch hemiblock NOS

I44.69 Other fascicular block

I44.7 Left bundle-branch block, unspecified

● **I45 Other conduction disorders**

I45.0 Right fascicular block

● **I45.1 Other and unspecified right bundle-branch block**

I45.10 Unspecified right bundle-branch block
Right bundle-branch block NOS

I45.19 Other right bundle-branch block

I45.2 Bifascicular block

I45.3 Trifascicular block

I45.4 Nonspecific intraventricular block
Bundle-branch block NOS

I45.5 Other specified heart block
Sinoatrial block
Sinoauricular block

Excludes1 heart block NOS (I45.9)

I45.6 Pre-excitation syndrome
Accelerated atrioventricular conduction
Accessory atrioventricular conduction
Anomalous atrioventricular excitation
Lown-Ganong-Levine syndrome
Pre-excitation atrioventricular conduction
Wolff-Parkinson-White syndrome

● **I45.8 Other specified conduction disorders**

I45.81 Long QT syndrome

I45.89 Other specified conduction disorders
Atrioventricular [AV] dissociation
Interference dissociation
Isorhythmic dissociation
Nonparoxysmal AV nodal tachycardia

I45.9 Conduction disorder, unspecified
Heart block NOS
Stokes-Adams syndrome

● **I46 Cardiac arrest**

Excludes1 cardiogenic shock (R57.0)

I46.2 Cardiac arrest due to underlying cardiac condition
Code first underlying cardiac condition

I46.8 Cardiac arrest due to other underlying condition
Code first underlying condition

I46.9 Cardiac arrest, cause unspecified

● **I47 Paroxysmal tachycardia**
Code first tachycardia complicating:
abortion or ectopic or molar pregnancy (O00-O07, O08.8)
obstetric surgery and procedures (O75.4)

Excludes1 tachycardia NOS (R00.0)
sinoauricular tachycardia NOS (R00.0)
sinus [sinusal] tachycardia NOS (R00.0)

I47.0 Re-entry ventricular arrhythmia

I47.1 Supraventricular tachycardia
Atrial (paroxysmal) tachycardia
Atrioventricular [AV] (paroxysmal) tachycardia
Atrioventricular re-entrant (nodal) tachycardia [AVNRT] [AVRT]
Junctional (paroxysmal) tachycardia
Nodal (paroxysmal) tachycardia

I47.2 Ventricular tachycardia

I47.9 Paroxysmal tachycardia, unspecified
Bouveret (-Hoffman) syndrome

● **I48 Atrial fibrillation and flutter**
Most common abnormal heart rhythm (arrhythmia) presenting as irregular, rapid beating (tachycardia) of the heart's upper chamber.

I48.0 Paroxysmal atrial fibrillation

I48.1 Persistent atrial fibrillation
Rapid contractions of the upper heart chamber

I48.2 Chronic atrial fibrillation
Permanent atrial fibrillation

I48.3 Typical atrial flutter
Type I atrial flutter

I48.4 Atypical atrial flutter
Type II atrial flutter

● **I48.9 Unspecified atrial fibrillation and atrial flutter**

I48.91 Unspecified atrial fibrillation

I48.92 Unspecified atrial flutter

● **I49 Other cardiac arrhythmias**
Code first cardiac arrhythmia complicating:
abortion or ectopic or molar pregnancy (O00-O07, O08.8)
obstetric surgery and procedures (O75.4)

Excludes1 bradycardia NOS (R00.1)
neonatal dysrhythmia (P29.1-)
sinoatrial bradycardia (R00.1)
sinus bradycardia (R00.1)
vagal bradycardia (R00.1)

● **I49.0 Ventricular fibrillation and flutter**

I49.01 Ventricular fibrillation

I49.02 Ventricular flutter

I49.1 Atrial premature depolarization
Atrial premature beats

I49.2 Junctional premature depolarization

I49.3 Ventricular premature depolarization

● **I49.4 Other and unspecified premature depolarization**

I49.40 Unspecified premature depolarization
Premature beats NOS

I49.49 Other premature depolarization
Ectopic beats
Extrasystoles
Extrasystolic arrhythmias
Premature contractions

I49.5 Sick sinus syndrome
Tachycardia-bradycardia syndrome

I49.8 Other specified cardiac arrhythmias
Coronary sinus rhythm disorder
Ectopic rhythm disorder
Nodal rhythm disorder

I49.9 Cardiac arrhythmia, unspecified
Arrhythmia (cardiac) NOS

● I5Ø **Heart failure**
Code first *heart failure complicating abortion or ectopic or molar pregnancy (OØØ-OØ7, OØ8.8)*
heart failure due to hypertension (I11.Ø)
heart failure due to hypertension with chronic kidney disease (I13.-)
heart failure following surgery (I97.13-)
obstetric surgery and procedures (O75.4)
rheumatic heart failure (IØ9.81)
Excludes1 neonatal cardiac failure (P29.Ø)
Excludes2 cardiac arrest (I46.-) ◀

I5Ø.1 **Left ventricular failure**
Cardiac asthma
Edema of lung with heart disease NOS
Edema of lung with heart failure
Left heart failure
Pulmonary edema with heart disease NOS
Pulmonary edema with heart failure
Excludes1 edema of lung without heart disease or heart failure (J81.-)
pulmonary edema without heart disease or failure (J81.-)

● I5Ø.2 **Systolic (congestive) heart failure**
Excludes1 combined systolic (congestive) and diastolic (congestive) heart failure (I5Ø.4-)

I5Ø.2Ø **Unspecified systolic (congestive) heart failure**
I5Ø.21 **Acute systolic (congestive) heart failure**
Presenting a short and relatively severe episode
I5Ø.22 **Chronic systolic (congestive) heart failure**
Long-lasting, presenting over time
I5Ø.23 **Acute on chronic systolic (congestive) heart failure**
Combination code. What was a chronic condition now has an acute exacerbation (to make more severe).

● I5Ø.3 **Diastolic (congestive) heart failure**
Excludes1 combined systolic (congestive) and diastolic (congestive) heart failure (I5Ø.4-)

I5Ø.3Ø **Unspecified diastolic (congestive) heart failure**
I5Ø.31 **Acute diastolic (congestive) heart failure**
I5Ø.32 **Chronic diastolic (congestive) heart failure**
I5Ø.33 **Acute on chronic diastolic (congestive) heart failure**

● I5Ø.4 **Combined systolic (congestive) and diastolic (congestive) heart failure**
I5Ø.4Ø **Unspecified combined systolic (congestive) and diastolic (congestive) heart failure**
I5Ø.41 **Acute combined systolic (congestive) and diastolic (congestive) heart failure**
I5Ø.42 **Chronic combined systolic (congestive) and diastolic (congestive) heart failure**
I5Ø.43 **Acute on chronic combined systolic (congestive) and diastolic (congestive) heart failure**

I5Ø.9 **Heart failure, unspecified**
Biventricular (heart) failure NOS
Cardiac, heart or myocardial failure NOS
Congestive heart disease
Congestive heart failure NOS
Right ventricular failure (secondary to left heart failure)
Excludes2 fluid overload (E87.7Ø) ◀

Item 9–8 Congestive heart failure (CHF) is a condition in which the left ventricle of the heart cannot pump enough blood to the body. The blood flow from the heart slows or returns to the heart from the venous system back flow resulting in congestion (fluid accumulation) particularly in the abdomen. Most commonly, fluid collects in the lungs and results in shortness of breath, especially when in a reclining position.

● I51 **Complications and ill-defined descriptions of heart disease**
Excludes1 any condition in I51.4-I51.9 due to hypertension (I11.-)
any condition in I51.4-I51.9 due to hypertension and chronic kidney disease (I13.-)
heart disease specified as rheumatic (IØØ-IØ9)

I51.Ø **Cardiac septal defect, acquired**
Acquired septal atrial defect (old)
Acquired septal auricular defect (old)
Acquired septal ventricular defect (old)
Excludes1 cardiac septal defect as current complication following acute myocardial infarction (I23.1, I23.2)

I51.1 **Rupture of chordae tendineae, not elsewhere classified**
Excludes1 rupture of chordae tendineae as current complication following acute myocardial infarction (I23.4)

I51.2 **Rupture of papillary muscle, not elsewhere classified**
Excludes1 rupture of papillary muscle as current complication following acute myocardial infarction (I23.5)

I51.3 **Intracardiac thrombosis, not elsewhere classified**
Apical thrombosis (old)
Atrial thrombosis (old)
Auricular thrombosis (old)
Mural thrombosis (old)
Ventricular thrombosis (old)
Excludes1 intracardiac thrombosis as current complication following acute myocardial infarction (I23.6)

I51.4 **Myocarditis, unspecified**
Chronic (interstitial) myocarditis
Myocardial fibrosis
Myocarditis NOS
Excludes1 acute or subacute myocarditis (I4Ø.-)

I51.5 **Myocardial degeneration**
Fatty degeneration of heart or myocardium
Myocardial disease
Senile degeneration of heart or myocardium

I51.7 **Cardiomegaly**
Cardiac dilatation
Cardiac hypertrophy
Ventricular dilatation

● I51.8 **Other ill-defined heart diseases**
I51.81 **Takotsubo syndrome**
Reversible left ventricular dysfunction following sudden emotional stress
Stress induced cardiomyopathy
Takotsubo cardiomyopathy
Transient left ventricular apical ballooning syndrome
I51.89 **Other ill-defined heart diseases**
Carditis (acute)(chronic)
Pancarditis (acute)(chronic)

I51.9 **Heart disease, unspecified**

I52 **Other heart disorders in diseases classified elsewhere**
Code first *underlying disease, such as:*
congenital syphilis (A5Ø.5)
mucopolysaccharidosis (E76.3)
schistosomiasis (B65.Ø-B65.9)
Excludes1 heart disease (in):
gonococcal infection (A54.83)
meningococcal infection (A39.5Ø)
rheumatoid arthritis (MØ5.31)
syphilis (A52.Ø6)

CHAPTER 9 (IØØ-I99)

CEREBROVASCULAR DISEASES (I60-I69)

Use additional code to identify presence of:
- alcohol abuse and dependence (F10.-)
- exposure to environmental tobacco smoke (Z77.22)
- history of tobacco dependence (Z87.891) ⬅ (Revised)
- hypertension (I10-I15)
- occupational exposure to environmental tobacco smoke (Z57.31)
- tobacco dependence (F17.-)
- tobacco use (Z72.0)

Excludes1 transient cerebral ischemic attacks and related syndromes (G45.-)
traumatic intracranial hemorrhage (S06.-)

● **I60 Nontraumatic subarachnoid hemorrhage**

Includes ruptured cerebral aneurysm
Excludes1 syphilitic ruptured cerebral aneurysm (A52.05)
Excludes2 sequelae of subarachnoid hemorrhage (I69.0-) ◀

● **I60.0 Nontraumatic subarachnoid hemorrhage from carotid siphon and bifurcation**
- **I60.00 Nontraumatic subarachnoid hemorrhage from unspecified carotid siphon and bifurcation**
- **I60.01 Nontraumatic subarachnoid hemorrhage from right carotid siphon and bifurcation**
- **I60.02 Nontraumatic subarachnoid hemorrhage from left carotid siphon and bifurcation**

● **I60.1 Nontraumatic subarachnoid hemorrhage from middle cerebral artery**
- **I60.10 Nontraumatic subarachnoid hemorrhage from unspecified middle cerebral artery**
- **I60.11 Nontraumatic subarachnoid hemorrhage from right middle cerebral artery**
- **I60.12 Nontraumatic subarachnoid hemorrhage from left middle cerebral artery**

I60.2 Nontraumatic subarachnoid hemorrhage from anterior communicating artery
- ~~I60.20 Nontraumatic subarachnoid hemorrhage from unspecified anterior communicating artery~~
- ~~I60.21 Nontraumatic subarachnoid hemorrhage from right anterior communicating artery~~
- ~~I60.22 Nontraumatic subarachnoid hemorrhage from left anterior communicating artery~~

● **I60.3 Nontraumatic subarachnoid hemorrhage from posterior communicating artery**
- **I60.30 Nontraumatic subarachnoid hemorrhage from unspecified posterior communicating artery**
- **I60.31 Nontraumatic subarachnoid hemorrhage from right posterior communicating artery**
- **I60.32 Nontraumatic subarachnoid hemorrhage from left posterior communicating artery**

I60.4 Nontraumatic subarachnoid hemorrhage from basilar artery

● **I60.5 Nontraumatic subarachnoid hemorrhage from vertebral artery**
- **I60.50 Nontraumatic subarachnoid hemorrhage from unspecified vertebral artery**
- **I60.51 Nontraumatic subarachnoid hemorrhage from right vertebral artery**
- **I60.52 Nontraumatic subarachnoid hemorrhage from left vertebral artery**

I60.6 Nontraumatic subarachnoid hemorrhage from other intracranial arteries

I60.7 Nontraumatic subarachnoid hemorrhage from unspecified intracranial artery
Ruptured (congenital) berry aneurysm
Ruptured (congenital) cerebral aneurysm
Subarachnoid hemorrhage (nontraumatic) from cerebral artery NOS
Subarachnoid hemorrhage (nontraumatic) from communicating artery NOS
Excludes1 berry aneurysm, nonruptured (I67.1)

I60.8 Other nontraumatic subarachnoid hemorrhage
Meningeal hemorrhage
Rupture of cerebral arteriovenous malformation

I60.9 Nontraumatic subarachnoid hemorrhage, unspecified

● **I61 Nontraumatic intracerebral hemorrhage**

Excludes2 sequelae of intracerebral hemorrhage (I69.1-) ◀

I61.0 Nontraumatic intracerebral hemorrhage in hemisphere, subcortical
Deep intracerebral hemorrhage (nontraumatic)

I61.1 Nontraumatic intracerebral hemorrhage in hemisphere, cortical
Cerebral lobe hemorrhage (nontraumatic)
Superficial intracerebral hemorrhage (nontraumatic)

I61.2 Nontraumatic intracerebral hemorrhage in hemisphere, unspecified
I61.3 Nontraumatic intracerebral hemorrhage in brain stem
I61.4 Nontraumatic intracerebral hemorrhage in cerebellum
I61.5 Nontraumatic intracerebral hemorrhage, intraventricular
I61.6 Nontraumatic intracerebral hemorrhage, multiple localized
I61.8 Other nontraumatic intracerebral hemorrhage
I61.9 Nontraumatic intracerebral hemorrhage, unspecified

● **I62 Other and unspecified nontraumatic intracranial hemorrhage**

Excludes2 sequelae of intracranial hemorrhage (I69.2) ◀

● **I62.0 Nontraumatic subdural hemorrhage**
- **I62.00 Nontraumatic subdural hemorrhage, unspecified**
- **I62.01 Nontraumatic acute subdural hemorrhage**
- **I62.02 Nontraumatic subacute subdural hemorrhage**
- **I62.03 Nontraumatic chronic subdural hemorrhage**

I62.1 Nontraumatic extradural hemorrhage
Nontraumatic epidural hemorrhage

I62.9 Nontraumatic intracranial hemorrhage, unspecified

★**(See Plate 141 on page NAP-28.)**

● **I63 Cerebral infarction**

Includes occlusion and stenosis of cerebral and precerebral arteries, resulting in cerebral infarction

Use additional code, if applicable, to identify status post administration of tPA (rtPA) in a different facility within the last 24 hours prior to admission to current facility (Z92.82)

Use additional code, if known, to indicate National Institutes of Health Stroke Scale (NIHSS) score (R29.7-) ◀

Excludes2 sequelae of cerebral infarction (I69.3-) ◀

● **I63.0 Cerebral infarction due to thrombosis of precerebral arteries**
- **I63.00 Cerebral infarction due to thrombosis of unspecified precerebral artery**
- ● **I63.01 Cerebral infarction due to thrombosis of vertebral artery**
  - **I63.011 Cerebral infarction due to thrombosis of right vertebral artery**
  - **I63.012 Cerebral infarction due to thrombosis of left vertebral artery**
  - **I63.013 Cerebral infarction due to thrombosis of bilateral vertebral arteries** ◀
  - **I63.019 Cerebral infarction due to thrombosis of unspecified vertebral artery**

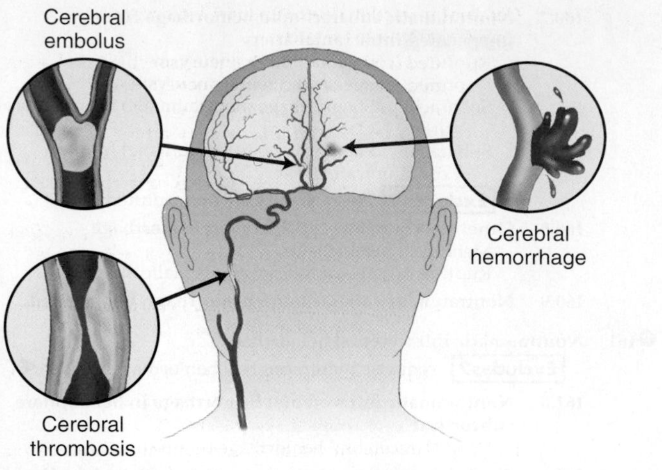

Figure 9-4 Events causing a stroke. (From Shiland: Mastering Healthcare Terminology, ed 1, St. Louis, Mosby, 2003)

I63.Ø2 Cerebral infarction due to thrombosis of basilar artery

● **I63.Ø3** Cerebral infarction due to thrombosis of carotid artery

I63.Ø31 Cerebral infarction due to thrombosis of right carotid artery

I63.Ø32 Cerebral infarction due to thrombosis of left carotid artery

I63.Ø33 Cerebral infarction due to thrombosis of bilateral carotid arteries ◀

I63.Ø39 Cerebral infarction due to thrombosis of unspecified carotid artery

I63.Ø9 Cerebral infarction due to thrombosis of other precerebral artery

● **I63.1** Cerebral infarction due to embolism of precerebral arteries

I63.1Ø Cerebral infarction due to embolism of unspecified precerebral artery

● **I63.11** Cerebral infarction due to embolism of vertebral artery

I63.111 Cerebral infarction due to embolism of right vertebral artery

I63.112 Cerebral infarction due to embolism of left vertebral artery

I63.113 Cerebral infarction due to embolism of bilateral vertebral arteries ◀

I63.119 Cerebral infarction due to embolism of unspecified vertebral artery

I63.12 Cerebral infarction due to embolism of basilar artery

● **I63.13** Cerebral infarction due to embolism of carotid artery

I63.131 Cerebral infarction due to embolism of right carotid artery

I63.132 Cerebral infarction due to embolism of left carotid artery

I63.133 Cerebral infarction due to embolism of bilateral carotid arteries ◀

I63.139 Cerebral infarction due to embolism of unspecified carotid artery

I63.19 Cerebral infarction due to embolism of other precerebral artery

● **I63.2** Cerebral infarction due to unspecified occlusion or stenosis of precerebral arteries

I63.2Ø Cerebral infarction due to unspecified occlusion or stenosis of unspecified precerebral arteries

● **I63.21** Cerebral infarction due to unspecified occlusion or stenosis of vertebral arteries

I63.211 Cerebral infarction due to unspecified occlusion or stenosis of right vertebral arteries

I63.212 Cerebral infarction due to unspecified occlusion or stenosis of left vertebral arteries

I63.213 Cerebral infarction due to unspecified occlusion or stenosis of bilateral vertebral arteries ◀

I63.219 Cerebral infarction due to unspecified occlusion or stenosis of unspecified vertebral arteries

I63.22 Cerebral infarction due to unspecified occlusion or stenosis of basilar arteries

● **I63.23** Cerebral infarction due to unspecified occlusion or stenosis of carotid arteries

I63.231 Cerebral infarction due to unspecified occlusion or stenosis of right carotid arteries

I63.232 Cerebral infarction due to unspecified occlusion or stenosis of left carotid arteries

I63.233 Cerebral infarction due to unspecified occlusion or stenosis of bilateral carotid arteries ◀

I63.239 Cerebral infarction due to unspecified occlusion or stenosis of unspecified carotid arteries

I63.29 Cerebral infarction due to unspecified occlusion or stenosis of other precerebral arteries

● **I63.3** Cerebral infarction due to thrombosis of cerebral arteries

I63.3Ø Cerebral infarction due to thrombosis of unspecified cerebral artery

● **I63.31** Cerebral infarction due to thrombosis of middle cerebral artery

I63.311 Cerebral infarction due to thrombosis of right middle cerebral artery

I63.312 Cerebral infarction due to thrombosis of left middle cerebral artery

I63.313 Cerebral infarction due to thrombosis of bilateral middle cerebral arteries ◀

I63.319 Cerebral infarction due to thrombosis of unspecified middle cerebral artery

● **I63.32** Cerebral infarction due to thrombosis of anterior cerebral artery

I63.321 Cerebral infarction due to thrombosis of right anterior cerebral artery

I63.322 Cerebral infarction due to thrombosis of left anterior cerebral artery

I63.323 Cerebral infarction due to thrombosis of bilateral anterior arteries ◀

I63.329 Cerebral infarction due to thrombosis of unspecified anterior cerebral artery

● **I63.33** Cerebral infarction due to thrombosis of posterior cerebral artery

I63.331 Cerebral infarction due to thrombosis of right posterior cerebral artery

I63.332 Cerebral infarction due to thrombosis of left posterior cerebral artery

I63.333 Cerebral infarction to thrombosis of bilateral posterior arteries ◀

I63.339 Cerebral infarction due to thrombosis of unspecified posterior cerebral artery

● I63.34 Cerebral infarction due to thrombosis of cerebellar artery
I63.341 Cerebral infarction due to thrombosis of right cerebellar artery
I63.342 Cerebral infarction due to thrombosis of left cerebellar artery
I63.343 Cerebral infarction to thrombosis of bilateral cerebellar arteries ◀
I63.349 Cerebral infarction due to thrombosis of unspecified cerebellar artery
I63.39 Cerebral infarction due to thrombosis of other cerebral artery
● I63.4 Cerebral infarction due to embolism of cerebral arteries
I63.40 Cerebral infarction due to embolism of unspecified cerebral artery
● I63.41 Cerebral infarction due to embolism of middle cerebral artery
I63.411 Cerebral infarction due to embolism of right middle cerebral artery
I63.412 Cerebral infarction due to embolism of left middle cerebral artery
I63.413 Cerebral infarction due to embolism of bilateral middle cerebral arteries ◀
I63.419 Cerebral infarction due to embolism of unspecified middle cerebral artery
● I63.42 Cerebral infarction due to embolism of anterior cerebral artery
I63.421 Cerebral infarction due to embolism of right anterior cerebral artery
I63.422 Cerebral infarction due to embolism of left anterior cerebral artery
I63.423 Cerebral infarction due to embolism of bilateral anterior cerebral arteries ◀
I63.429 Cerebral infarction due to embolism of unspecified anterior cerebral artery
● I63.43 Cerebral infarction due to embolism of posterior cerebral artery
I63.431 Cerebral infarction due to embolism of right posterior cerebral artery
I63.432 Cerebral infarction due to embolism of left posterior cerebral artery
I63.433 Cerebral infarction due to embolism of bilateral posterior cerebral arteries ◀
I63.439 Cerebral infarction due to embolism of unspecified posterior cerebral artery
● I63.44 Cerebral infarction due to embolism of cerebellar artery
I63.441 Cerebral infarction due to embolism of right cerebellar artery
I63.442 Cerebral infarction due to embolism of left cerebellar artery
I63.443 Cerebral infarction due to embolism of bilateral cerebellar arteries ◀
I63.449 Cerebral infarction due to embolism of unspecified cerebellar artery
I63.49 Cerebral infarction due to embolism of other cerebral artery
● I63.5 Cerebral infarction due to unspecified occlusion or stenosis of cerebral arteries
I63.50 Cerebral infarction due to unspecified occlusion or stenosis of unspecified cerebral artery
● I63.51 Cerebral infarction due to unspecified occlusion or stenosis of middle cerebral artery
I63.511 Cerebral infarction due to unspecified occlusion or stenosis of right middle cerebral artery
I63.512 Cerebral infarction due to unspecified occlusion or stenosis of left middle cerebral artery
I63.513 Cerebral infarction due to unspecified occlusion or stenosis of bilateral middle arteries ◀
I63.519 Cerebral infarction due to unspecified occlusion or stenosis of unspecified middle cerebral artery
● I63.52 Cerebral infarction due to unspecified occlusion or stenosis of anterior cerebral artery
I63.521 Cerebral infarction due to unspecified occlusion or stenosis of right anterior cerebral artery
I63.522 Cerebral infarction due to unspecified occlusion or stenosis of left anterior cerebral artery
I63.523 Cerebral infarction due to unspecified occlusion or stenosis of bilateral anterior arteries ◀
I63.529 Cerebral infarction due to unspecified occlusion or stenosis of unspecified anterior cerebral artery
● I63.53 Cerebral infarction due to unspecified occlusion or stenosis of posterior cerebral artery
I63.531 Cerebral infarction due to unspecified occlusion or stenosis of right posterior cerebral artery
I63.532 Cerebral infarction due to unspecified occlusion or stenosis of left posterior cerebral artery
I63.533 Cerebral infarction due to unspecified occlusion or stenosis of bilateral posterior arteries ◀
I63.539 Cerebral infarction due to unspecified occlusion or stenosis of unspecified posterior cerebral artery
● I63.54 Cerebral infarction due to unspecified occlusion or stenosis of cerebellar artery
I63.541 Cerebral infarction due to unspecified occlusion or stenosis of right cerebellar artery
I63.542 Cerebral infarction due to unspecified occlusion or stenosis of left cerebellar artery
I63.543 Cerebral infarction due to unspecified occlusion or stenosis of bilateral cerebellar arteries ◀
I63.549 Cerebral infarction due to unspecified occlusion or stenosis of unspecified cerebellar artery
I63.59 Cerebral infarction due to unspecified occlusion or stenosis of other cerebral artery
I63.6 Cerebral infarction due to cerebral venous thrombosis, nonpyogenic
I63.8 Other cerebral infarction
I63.9 Cerebral infarction, unspecified
Stroke NOS

● I65 **Occlusion and stenosis of precerebral arteries, not resulting in cerebral infarction**

Includes embolism of precerebral artery
narrowing of precerebral artery
obstruction (complete) (partial) of precerebral artery
thrombosis of precerebral artery

Excludes1 insufficiency, NOS, of precerebral artery (G45.-)
insufficiency of precerebral arteries causing cerebral infarction (I63.Ø-I63.2)

● I65.Ø **Occlusion and stenosis of vertebral artery**

I65.Ø1 **Occlusion and stenosis of right vertebral artery**

I65.Ø2 **Occlusion and stenosis of left vertebral artery**

I65.Ø3 **Occlusion and stenosis of bilateral vertebral arteries**

I65.Ø9 **Occlusion and stenosis of unspecified vertebral artery**

I65.1 **Occlusion and stenosis of basilar artery**

● I65.2 **Occlusion and stenosis of carotid artery**

I65.21 **Occlusion and stenosis of right carotid artery**

I65.22 **Occlusion and stenosis of left carotid artery**

I65.23 **Occlusion and stenosis of bilateral carotid arteries**

I65.29 **Occlusion and stenosis of unspecified carotid artery**

I65.8 **Occlusion and stenosis of other precerebral arteries**

I65.9 **Occlusion and stenosis of unspecified precerebral artery**
Occlusion and stenosis of precerebral artery NOS

● I66 **Occlusion and stenosis of cerebral arteries, not resulting in cerebral infarction**

Includes embolism of cerebral artery
narrowing of cerebral artery
obstruction (complete) (partial) of cerebral artery
thrombosis of cerebral artery

Excludes1 occlusion and stenosis of cerebral artery causing cerebral infarction (I63.3-I63.5)

● I66.Ø **Occlusion and stenosis of middle cerebral artery**

I66.Ø1 **Occlusion and stenosis of right middle cerebral artery**

I66.Ø2 **Occlusion and stenosis of left middle cerebral artery**

I66.Ø3 **Occlusion and stenosis of bilateral middle cerebral arteries**

I66.Ø9 **Occlusion and stenosis of unspecified middle cerebral artery**

● I66.1 **Occlusion and stenosis of anterior cerebral artery**

I66.11 **Occlusion and stenosis of right anterior cerebral artery**

I66.12 **Occlusion and stenosis of left anterior cerebral artery**

I66.13 **Occlusion and stenosis of bilateral anterior cerebral arteries**

I66.19 **Occlusion and stenosis of unspecified anterior cerebral artery**

● I66.2 **Occlusion and stenosis of posterior cerebral artery**

I66.21 **Occlusion and stenosis of right posterior cerebral artery**

I66.22 **Occlusion and stenosis of left posterior cerebral artery**

I66.23 **Occlusion and stenosis of bilateral posterior cerebral arteries**

I66.29 **Occlusion and stenosis of unspecified posterior cerebral artery**

I66.3 **Occlusion and stenosis of cerebellar arteries**

I66.8 **Occlusion and stenosis of other cerebral arteries**
Occlusion and stenosis of perforating arteries

I66.9 **Occlusion and stenosis of unspecified cerebral artery**

● I67 **Other cerebrovascular diseases**

Excludes2 sequelae of the listed conditions (I69.8) ◀

I67.Ø **Dissection of cerebral arteries, nonruptured**

Excludes1 ruptured cerebral arteries (I6Ø.7)

I67.1 **Cerebral aneurysm, nonruptured**
Cerebral aneurysm NOS
Cerebral arteriovenous fistula, acquired
Internal carotid artery aneurysm, intracranial portion
Internal carotid artery aneurysm, NOS

Excludes1 congenital cerebral aneurysm, nonruptured (Q28.-)
ruptured cerebral aneurysm (I6Ø.7)

I67.2 **Cerebral atherosclerosis**
Atheroma of cerebral and precerebral arteries

I67.3 **Progressive vascular leukoencephalopathy**
Binswanger's disease

I67.4 **Hypertensive encephalopathy**

I67.5 **Moyamoya disease**

I67.6 **Nonpyogenic thrombosis of intracranial venous system**
Nonpyogenic thrombosis of cerebral vein
Nonpyogenic thrombosis of intracranial venous sinus

Excludes1 nonpyogenic thrombosis of intracranial venous system causing infarction (I63.6)

I67.7 **Cerebral arteritis, not elsewhere classified**
Granulomatous angiitis of the nervous system

Excludes1 allergic granulomatous angiitis (M3Ø.1)

● I67.8 **Other specified cerebrovascular diseases**

I67.81 **Acute cerebrovascular insufficiency**
Acute cerebrovascular insufficiency unspecified as to location or reversibility

I67.82 **Cerebral ischemia**
Chronic cerebral ischemia

I67.83 **Posterior reversible encephalopathy syndrome**
PRES

● I67.84 **Cerebral vasospasm and vasoconstriction**

I67.841 **Reversible cerebrovascular vasoconstriction syndrome**
Call-Fleming syndrome
Code first underlying condition, if applicable, such as eclampsia (O15.ØØ-O15.9)

I67.848 **Other cerebrovascular vasospasm and vasoconstriction**

I67.89 **Other cerebrovascular disease**

I67.9 **Cerebrovascular disease, unspecified**

● I68 **Cerebrovascular disorders in diseases classified elsewhere**

I68.Ø **Cerebral amyloid angiopathy**
Code first underlying amyloidosis (E85.-)

I68.2 **Cerebral arteritis in other diseases classified elsewhere**
Code first underlying disease

Excludes1 cerebral arteritis (in):
listerosis (A32.89)
systemic lupus erythematosus (M32.19)
syphilis (A52.Ø4)
tuberculosis (A18.89)

I68.8 **Other cerebrovascular disorders in diseases classified elsewhere**
Code first underlying disease

Excludes1 syphilitic cerebral aneurysm (A52.Ø5)

CHAPTER 9 (IØØ-I99)

◀ New ⟸ Revised ~~deleted~~ Deleted OGCR Official Guidelines X Assign placeholder X ● Use Additional Character(s)
Excludes 1 Excludes 2 Includes Use additional Code first Code also Unspecified

OGCR Section I.c.9.d.

Sequelae of Cerebrovascular Disease

1) Category I69, Sequelae of Cerebrovascular disease

Category 169 is used to indicate conditions classifiable to categories I60-I67 as the causes of sequela (neurologic deficits), themselves classified elsewhere. These "late effects" include neurologic deficits that persist after initial onset of conditions classifiable to categories I60-I67. The neurologic deficits caused by cerebrovascular disease may be present from the onset of may arise at any time after the onset of the condition classifiable to categories I60-I67.

Codes from category I69, Sequelae of cerebrovascular disease, that specify hemiplegia, hemiparesis and monoplegia identify whether the dominant or nondominant side is affected. Should the affected side be documented, but not specified as dominant or nondominant, and the classification system does not indicate a default, code selection is as follows:

For ambidextrous patients, the default should be dominant.

If the left side is affected, the default is non-dominant.

If the right side is affected, the default is dominant.

2) Codes from category I69 with codes from I60-I67

Codes from category I69 may be assigned on a health care record with codes from I60-I67, if the patient has a current cerebrovascular disease and deficits from an old cerebrovascular disease.

● **I69 Sequelae of cerebrovascular disease**

Note: Category I69 is to be used to indicate conditions in I60-I67 as the cause of sequelae. The 'sequelae' include conditions specified as such or as residuals which may occur at any time after the onset of the causal condition.

Excludes1 personal history of cerebral infarction without residual deficit (Z86.73)
personal history of prolonged reversible ischemic neurologic deficit (PRIND) (Z86.73)
personal history of reversible ischemic neurologcial deficit (RIND) (Z86.73)
sequelae of traumatic intracranial injury (S06.-)
transient ischemic attack (TIA) (G45.9)

● **I69.0 Sequelae of nontraumatic subarachnoid hemorrhage**

I69.00 Unspecified sequelae of nontraumatic subarachnoid hemorrhage

● **I69.01 Cognitive deficits following nontraumatic subarachnoid hemorrhage**

I69.010 Attention and concentration deficit following nontraumatic subarachnoid hemorrhage ◀

I69.011 Memory deficit following nontraumatic subarachnoid hemorrhage ◀

I69.012 Visuospatial deficit and spatial neglect following nontraumatic subarachnoid hemorrhage ◀

I69.013 Psychomotor deficit following nontraumatic subarachnoid hemorrhage ◀

I69.014 Frontal lobe and executive function deficit following nontraumatic subarachnoid hemorrhage ◀

I69.015 Cognitive social or emotional deficit following nontraumatic subarachnoid hemorrhage ◀

I69.018 Other symptoms and signs involving cognitive functions following nontraumatic subarachnoid hemorrhage ◀

I69.019 Unspecified symptoms and signs involving cognitive functions following nontraumatic subarachnoid hemorrhage ◀

● **I69.02 Speech and language deficits following nontraumatic subarachnoid hemorrhage**

I69.020 Aphasia following nontraumatic subarachnoid hemorrhage

I69.021 Dysphasia following nontraumatic subarachnoid hemorrhage

I69.022 Dysarthria following nontraumatic subarachnoid hemorrhage

I69.023 Fluency disorder following nontraumatic subarachnoid hemorrhage

Stuttering following nontraumatic subarachnoid hemorrhage

I69.028 Other speech and language deficits following nontraumatic subarachnoid hemorrhage

● **I69.03 Monoplegia of upper limb following nontraumatic subarachnoid hemorrhage**

I69.031 Monoplegia of upper limb following nontraumatic subarachnoid hemorrhage affecting right dominant side

I69.032 Monoplegia of upper limb following nontraumatic subarachnoid hemorrhage affecting left dominant side

I69.033 Monoplegia of upper limb following nontraumatic subarachnoid hemorrhage affecting right non-dominant side

I69.034 Monoplegia of upper limb following nontraumatic subarachnoid hemorrhage affecting left non-dominant side

I69.039 Monoplegia of upper limb following nontraumatic subarachnoid hemorrhage affecting unspecified side

● **I69.04 Monoplegia of lower limb following nontraumatic subarachnoid hemorrhage**

I69.041 Monoplegia of lower limb following nontraumatic subarachnoid hemorrhage affecting right dominant side

I69.042 Monoplegia of lower limb following nontraumatic subarachnoid hemorrhage affecting left dominant side

I69.043 Monoplegia of lower limb following nontraumatic subarachnoid hemorrhage affecting right non-dominant side

I69.044 Monoplegia of lower limb following nontraumatic subarachnoid hemorrhage affecting left non-dominant side

I69.049 Monoplegia of lower limb following nontraumatic subarachnoid hemorrhage affecting unspecified side

CHAPTER 9 (I00-I99)

● I69.05 **Hemiplegia and hemiparesis following nontraumatic subarachnoid hemorrhage**

I69.051 **Hemiplegia and hemiparesis following nontraumatic subarachnoid hemorrhage affecting right dominant side**

I69.052 **Hemiplegia and hemiparesis following nontraumatic subarachnoid hemorrhage affecting left dominant side**

I69.053 **Hemiplegia and hemiparesis following nontraumatic subarachnoid hemorrhage affecting right non-dominant side**

I69.054 **Hemiplegia and hemiparesis following nontraumatic subarachnoid hemorrhage affecting left non-dominant side**

I69.059 **Hemiplegia and hemiparesis following nontraumatic subarachnoid hemorrhage affecting unspecified side**

● I69.06 **Other paralytic syndrome following nontraumatic subarachnoid hemorrhage**

Use additional code to identify type of paralytic syndrome, such as:
locked-in state (G83.5)
quadriplegia (G82.5-)

Excludes1 hemiplegia/hemiparesis following nontraumatic subarachnoid hemorrhage (I69.05-)
monoplegia of lower limb following nontraumatic subarachnoid hemorrhage (I69.04-)
monoplegia of upper limb following nontraumatic subarachnoid hemorrhage (I69.03-)

I69.061 **Other paralytic syndrome following nontraumatic subarachnoid hemorrhage affecting right dominant side**

I69.062 **Other paralytic syndrome following nontraumatic subarachnoid hemorrhage affecting left dominant side**

I69.063 **Other paralytic syndrome following nontraumatic subarachnoid hemorrhage affecting right non-dominant side**

I69.064 **Other paralytic syndrome following nontraumatic subarachnoid hemorrhage affecting left non-dominant side**

I69.065 **Other paralytic syndrome following nontraumatic subarachnoid hemorrhage, bilateral**

I69.069 **Other paralytic syndrome following nontraumatic subarachnoid hemorrhage affecting unspecified side**

● I69.09 **Other sequelae of nontraumatic subarachnoid hemorrhage**

I69.090 **Apraxia following nontraumatic subarachnoid hemorrhage**

I69.091 **Dysphagia following nontraumatic subarachnoid hemorrhage**

Use additional code to identify the type of dysphagia, if known (R13.1-)

I69.092 **Facial weakness following nontraumatic subarachnoid hemorrhage**

Facial droop following nontraumatic subarachnoid hemorrhage

I69.093 **Ataxia following nontraumatic subarachnoid hemorrhage**

I69.098 **Other sequelae following nontraumatic subarachnoid hemorrhage**

Alterations of sensation following nontraumatic subarachnoid hemorrhage
Disturbance of vision following nontraumatic subarachnoid hemorrhage

Use additional code to identify the sequelae

● I69.1 **Sequelae of nontraumatic intracerebral hemorrhage**

I69.10 **Unspecified sequelae of nontraumatic intracerebral hemorrhage**

● I69.11 **Cognitive deficits following nontraumatic intracerebral hemorrhage**

I69.110 **Attention and concentration deficit following nontraumatic intracerebral hemorrhage** ◀

I69.111 **Memory deficit following nontraumatic intracerebral hemorrhage** ◀

I69.112 **Visuospatial deficit and spatial neglect following nontraumatic intracerebral hemorrhage** ◀

I69.113 **Psychomotor deficit following nontraumatic intracerebral hemorrhage** ◀

I69.114 **Frontal lobe and executive function deficit following nontraumatic intracerebral hemorrhage** ◀

I69.115 **Cognitive social or emotional deficit following nontraumatic intracerebral hemorrhage** ◀

I69.118 **Other symptoms and signs involving cognitive functions following nontraumatic intracerebral hemorrhage** ◀

I69.119 **Unspecified symptoms and signs involving cognitive functions following nontraumatic intracerebral hemorrhage** ◀

● I69.12 **Speech and language deficits following nontraumatic intracerebral hemorrhage**

I69.120 **Aphasia following nontraumatic intracerebral hemorrhage**

I69.121 **Dysphasia following nontraumatic intracerebral hemorrhage**

I69.122 **Dysarthria following nontraumatic intracerebral hemorrhage**

I69.123 **Fluency disorder following nontraumatic intracerebral hemorrhage**

Stuttering following nontraumatic intracerebral hemorrhage ⟸

I69.128 **Other speech and language deficits following nontraumatic intracerebral hemorrhage**

● **I69.13 Monoplegia of upper limb following nontraumatic intracerebral hemorrhage**

I69.131 Monoplegia of upper limb following nontraumatic intracerebral hemorrhage affecting right dominant side

I69.132 Monoplegia of upper limb following nontraumatic intracerebral hemorrhage affecting left dominant side

I69.133 Monoplegia of upper limb following nontraumatic intracerebral hemorrhage affecting right non-dominant side

I69.134 Monoplegia of upper limb following nontraumatic intracerebral hemorrhage affecting left non-dominant side

I69.139 Monoplegia of upper limb following nontraumatic intracerebral hemorrhage affecting unspecified side

● **I69.14 Monoplegia of lower limb following nontraumatic intracerebral hemorrhage**

I69.141 Monoplegia of lower limb following nontraumatic intracerebral hemorrhage affecting right dominant side

I69.142 Monoplegia of lower limb following nontraumatic intracerebral hemorrhage affecting left dominant side

I69.143 Monoplegia of lower limb following nontraumatic intracerebral hemorrhage affecting right non-dominant side

I69.144 Monoplegia of lower limb following nontraumatic intracerebral hemorrhage affecting left non-dominant side

I69.149 Monoplegia of lower limb following nontraumatic intracerebral hemorrhage affecting unspecified side

● **I69.15 Hemiplegia and hemiparesis following nontraumatic intracerebral hemorrhage**

I69.151 Hemiplegia and hemiparesis following nontraumatic intracerebral hemorrhage affecting right dominant side

I69.152 Hemiplegia and hemiparesis following nontraumatic intracerebral hemorrhage affecting left dominant side

I69.153 Hemiplegia and hemiparesis following nontraumatic intracerebral hemorrhage affecting right non-dominant side

I69.154 Hemiplegia and hemiparesis following nontraumatic intracerebral hemorrhage affecting left non-dominant side

I69.159 Hemiplegia and hemiparesis following nontraumatic intracerebral hemorrhage affecting unspecified side

● **I69.16 Other paralytic syndrome following nontraumatic intracerebral hemorrhage**

Use additional code to identify type of paralytic syndrome, such as:
- locked-in state (G83.5)
- quadriplegia (G82.5-)

Excludes1 hemiplegia/hemiparesis following nontraumatic intracerebral hemorrhage (I69.15-)
monoplegia of lower limb following nontraumatic intracerebral hemorrhage (I69.14-)
monoplegia of upper limb following nontraumatic intracerebral hemorrhage (I69.13-)

I69.161 Other paralytic syndrome following nontraumatic intracerebral hemorrhage affecting right dominant side

I69.162 Other paralytic syndrome following nontraumatic intracerebral hemorrhage affecting left dominant side

I69.163 Other paralytic syndrome following nontraumatic intracerebral hemorrhage affecting right non-dominant side

I69.164 Other paralytic syndrome following nontraumatic intracerebral hemorrhage affecting left non-dominant side

I69.165 Other paralytic syndrome following nontraumatic intracerebral hemorrhage, bilateral

I69.169 Other paralytic syndrome following nontraumatic intracerebral hemorrhage affecting unspecified side

● **I69.19 Other sequelae of nontraumatic intracerebral hemorrhage**

I69.190 Apraxia following nontraumatic intracerebral hemorrhage

I69.191 Dysphagia following nontraumatic intracerebral hemorrhage

Use additional code to identify the type of dysphagia, if known (R13.1-)

I69.192 Facial weakness following nontraumatic intracerebral hemorrhage

Facial droop following nontraumatic intracerebral hemorrhage

I69.193 Ataxia following nontraumatic intracerebral hemorrhage

I69.198 Other sequelae of nontraumatic intracerebral hemorrhage

Alteration of sensations following nontraumatic intracerebral hemorrhage
Disturbance of vision following nontraumatic intracerebral hemorrhage

Use additional code to identify the sequelae

CHAPTER 9 (I00-I99)

● I69.2 Sequelae of other nontraumatic intracranial hemorrhage
I69.20 Unspecified sequelae of other nontraumatic intracranial hemorrhage
● I69.21 Cognitive deficits following other nontraumatic intracranial hemorrhage
I69.210 Attention and concentration deficit following other nontraumatic intracranial hemorrhage ◀
I69.211 Memory deficit following other nontraumatic intracranial hemorrhage ◀
I69.212 Visuospatial deficit and spatial neglect following other nontraumatic intracranial hemorrhage ◀
I69.213 Psychomotor deficit following other nontraumatic intracranial hemorrhage ◀
I69.214 Frontal lobe and executive function deficit following other nontraumatic intracranial hemorrhage ◀
I69.215 Cognitive social or emotional deficit following other nontraumatic intracranial hemorrhage ◀
I69.218 Other symptoms and signs involving cognitive functions following other nontraumatic intracranial hemorrhage ◀
I69.219 Unspecified symptoms and signs involving cognitive functions following other nontraumatic intracranial hemorrhage ◀
● I69.22 Speech and language deficits following other nontraumatic intracranial hemorrhage
I69.220 Aphasia following other nontraumatic intracranial hemorrhage
I69.221 Dysphasia following other nontraumatic intracranial hemorrhage
I69.222 Dysarthria following other nontraumatic intracranial hemorrhage
I69.223 Fluency disorder following other nontraumatic intracranial hemorrhage
Stuttering following other nontraumatic intracranial hemorrhage ◀
I69.228 Other speech and language deficits following other nontraumatic intracranial hemorrhage
● I69.23 Monoplegia of upper limb following other nontraumatic intracranial hemorrhage
I69.231 Monoplegia of upper limb following other nontraumatic intracranial hemorrhage affecting right dominant side
I69.232 Monoplegia of upper limb following other nontraumatic intracranial hemorrhage affecting left dominant side
I69.233 Monoplegia of upper limb following other nontraumatic intracranial hemorrhage affecting right non-dominant side
I69.234 Monoplegia of upper limb following other nontraumatic intracranial hemorrhage affecting left non-dominant side
I69.239 Monoplegia of upper limb following other nontraumatic intracranial hemorrhage affecting unspecified side
● I69.24 Monoplegia of lower limb following other nontraumatic intracranial hemorrhage
I69.241 Monoplegia of lower limb following other nontraumatic intracranial hemorrhage affecting right dominant side
I69.242 Monoplegia of lower limb following other nontraumatic intracranial hemorrhage affecting left dominant side
I69.243 Monoplegia of lower limb following other nontraumatic intracranial hemorrhage affecting right non-dominant side
I69.244 Monoplegia of lower limb following other nontraumatic intracranial hemorrhage affecting left non-dominant side
I69.249 Monoplegia of lower limb following other nontraumatic intracranial hemorrhage affecting unspecified side
● I69.25 Hemiplegia and hemiparesis following other nontraumatic intracranial hemorrhage
I69.251 Hemiplegia and hemiparesis following other nontraumatic intracranial hemorrhage affecting right dominant side
I69.252 Hemiplegia and hemiparesis following other nontraumatic intracranial hemorrhage affecting left dominant side
I69.253 Hemiplegia and hemiparesis following other nontraumatic intracranial hemorrhage affecting right non-dominant side
I69.254 Hemiplegia and hemiparesis following other nontraumatic intracranial hemorrhage affecting left non-dominant side
I69.259 Hemiplegia and hemiparesis following other nontraumatic intracranial hemorrhage affecting unspecified side
● I69.26 Other paralytic syndrome following other nontraumatic intracranial hemorrhage
Use additional code to identify type of paralytic syndrome, such as:
locked-in state (G83.5)
quadriplegia (G82.5-)
Excludes1 hemiplegia/hemiparesis following other nontraumatic intracranial hemorrhage (I69.25-)
monoplegia of lower limb following other nontraumatic intracranial hemorrhage (I69.24-)
monoplegia of upper limb following other nontraumatic intracranial hemorrhage (I69.23-)
I69.261 Other paralytic syndrome following other nontraumatic intracranial hemorrhage affecting right dominant side
I69.262 Other paralytic syndrome following other nontraumatic intracranial hemorrhage affecting left dominant side

I69.263 Other paralytic syndrome following other nontraumatic intracranial hemorrhage affecting right non-dominant side

I69.264 Other paralytic syndrome following other nontraumatic intracranial hemorrhage affecting left non-dominant side

I69.265 Other paralytic syndrome following other nontraumatic intracranial hemorrhage, bilateral

I69.269 Other paralytic syndrome following other nontraumatic intracranial hemorrhage affecting unspecified side

● I69.29 Other sequelae of other nontraumatic intracranial hemorrhage

I69.290 Apraxia following other nontraumatic intracranial hemorrhage

I69.291 Dysphagia following other nontraumatic intracranial hemorrhage

Use additional code to identify the type of dysphagia, if known (R13.1-)

I69.292 Facial weakness following other nontraumatic intracranial hemorrhage

Facial droop following other nontraumatic intracranial hemorrhage

I69.293 Ataxia following other nontraumatic intracranial hemorrhage

I69.298 Other sequelae of other nontraumatic intracranial hemorrhage

Alteration of sensation following other nontraumatic intracranial hemorrhage

Disturbance of vision following other nontraumatic intracranial hemorrhage

Use additional code to identify the sequelae

● I69.3 Sequelae of cerebral infarction

Sequelae of stroke NOS

I69.30 Unspecified sequelae of cerebral infarction

● I69.31 Cognitive deficits following cerebral infarction

I69.310 Attention and concentration deficit following cerebral infarction ◀

I69.311 Memory deficit following cerebral infarction ◀

I69.312 Visuospatial deficit and spatial neglect following cerebral infarction ◀

I69.313 Psychomotor deficit following cerebral infarction ◀

I69.314 Frontal lobe and executive function deficit following cerebral infarction ◀

I69.315 Cognitive social or emotional deficit following cerebral infarction ◀

I69.318 Other symptoms and signs involving cognitive functions following cerebral infarction ◀

I69.319 Unspecified symptoms and signs involving cognitive functions following cerebral infarction ◀

● I69.32 Speech and language deficits following cerebral infarction

I69.320 Aphasia following cerebral infarction

I69.321 Dysphasia following cerebral infarction

I69.322 Dysarthria following cerebral infarction

I69.323 Fluency disorder following cerebral infarction

Stuttering following cerebral infarction ◀▬

I69.328 Other speech and language deficits following cerebral infarction

● I69.33 Monoplegia of upper limb following cerebral infarction

I69.331 Monoplegia of upper limb following cerebral infarction affecting right dominant side

I69.332 Monoplegia of upper limb following cerebral infarction affecting left dominant side

I69.333 Monoplegia of upper limb following cerebral infarction affecting right non-dominant side

I69.334 Monoplegia of upper limb following cerebral infarction affecting left non-dominant side

I69.339 Monoplegia of upper limb following cerebral infarction affecting unspecified side

● I69.34 Monoplegia of lower limb following cerebral infarction

I69.341 Monoplegia of lower limb following cerebral infarction affecting right dominant side

I69.342 Monoplegia of lower limb following cerebral infarction affecting left dominant side

I69.343 Monoplegia of lower limb following cerebral infarction affecting right non-dominant side

I69.344 Monoplegia of lower limb following cerebral infarction affecting left non-dominant side

I69.349 Monoplegia of lower limb following cerebral infarction affecting unspecified side

● I69.35 Hemiplegia and hemiparesis following cerebral infarction

I69.351 Hemiplegia and hemiparesis following cerebral infarction affecting right dominant side

I69.352 Hemiplegia and hemiparesis following cerebral infarction affecting left dominant side

I69.353 Hemiplegia and hemiparesis following cerebral infarction affecting right non-dominant side

I69.354 Hemiplegia and hemiparesis following cerebral infarction affecting left non-dominant side

I69.359 Hemiplegia and hemiparesis following cerebral infarction affecting unspecified side

● I69.36 Other paralytic syndrome following cerebral infarction

Use additional code to identify type of paralytic syndrome, such as:
locked-in state (G83.5)
quadriplegia (G82.5-)

Excludes1 hemiplegia/hemiparesis following cerebral infarction (I69.35-)
monoplegia of lower limb following cerebral infarction (I69.34-)
monoplegia of upper limb following cerebral infarction (I69.33-)

I69.361 **Other paralytic syndrome following cerebral infarction affecting right dominant side**

I69.362 **Other paralytic syndrome following cerebral infarction affecting left dominant side**

I69.363 **Other paralytic syndrome following cerebral infarction affecting right non-dominant side**

I69.364 **Other paralytic syndrome following cerebral infarction affecting left non-dominant side**

I69.365 **Other paralytic syndrome following cerebral infarction, bilateral**

I69.369 **Other paralytic syndrome following cerebral infarction affecting unspecified side**

● I69.39 **Other sequelae of cerebral infarction**

I69.390 **Apraxia following cerebral infarction**

I69.391 **Dysphagia following cerebral infarction**

Use additional code to identify the type of dysphagia, if known (R13.1-)

I69.392 **Facial weakness following cerebral infarction**

Facial droop following cerebral infarction

I69.393 **Ataxia following cerebral infarction**

I69.398 **Other sequelae of cerebral infarction**

Alteration of sensation following cerebral infarction
Disturbance of vision following cerebral infarction

Use additional code to identify the sequelae

● I69.8 **Sequelae of other cerebrovascular diseases**

Excludes1 sequelae of traumatic intracranial injury (S06.-)

I69.80 **Unspecified sequelae of other cerebrovascular disease**

● I69.81 **Cognitive deficits following other cerebrovascular disease**

I69.810 **Attention and concentration deficit following other cerebrovascular disease** ◀

I69.811 **Memory deficit following other cerebrovascular disease** ◀

I69.812 **Visuospatial deficit and spatial neglect following other cerebrovascular disease** ◀

I69.813 **Psychomotor deficit following other cerebrovascular disease** ◀

I69.814 **Frontal lobe and executive function deficit following other cerebrovascular disease** ◀

I69.815 **Cognitive social or emotional deficit following other cerebrovascular disease** ◀

I69.818 **Other symptoms and signs involving cognitive functions following other cerebrovascular disease** ◀

I69.819 **Unspecified symptoms and signs involving cognitive functions following other cerebrovascular disease** ◀

● I69.82 **Speech and language deficits following other cerebrovascular disease**

I69.820 **Aphasia following other cerebrovascular disease**

I69.821 **Dysphasia following other cerebrovascular disease**

I69.822 **Dysarthria following other cerebrovascular disease**

I69.823 **Fluency disorder following other cerebrovascular disease**

Stuttering following other cerebrovascular disease ⬅

I69.828 **Other speech and language deficits following other cerebrovascular disease**

● I69.83 **Monoplegia of upper limb following other cerebrovascular disease**

I69.831 **Monoplegia of upper limb following other cerebrovascular disease affecting right dominant side**

I69.832 **Monoplegia of upper limb following other cerebrovascular disease affecting left dominant side**

I69.833 **Monoplegia of upper limb following other cerebrovascular disease affecting right non-dominant side**

I69.834 **Monoplegia of upper limb following other cerebrovascular disease affecting left non-dominant side**

I69.839 **Monoplegia of upper limb following other cerebrovascular disease affecting unspecified side**

● I69.84 **Monoplegia of lower limb following other cerebrovascular disease**

I69.841 **Monoplegia of lower limb following other cerebrovascular disease affecting right dominant side**

I69.842 **Monoplegia of lower limb following other cerebrovascular disease affecting left dominant side**

I69.843 **Monoplegia of lower limb following other cerebrovascular disease affecting right non-dominant side**

I69.844 **Monoplegia of lower limb following other cerebrovascular disease affecting left non-dominant side**

I69.849 **Monoplegia of lower limb following other cerebrovascular disease affecting unspecified side**

● I69.85 **Hemiplegia and hemiparesis following other cerebrovascular disease**

I69.851 **Hemiplegia and hemiparesis following other cerebrovascular disease affecting right dominant side**

I69.852 **Hemiplegia and hemiparesis following other cerebrovascular disease affecting left dominant side**

I69.853 **Hemiplegia and hemiparesis following other cerebrovascular disease affecting right non-dominant side**

I69.854 Hemiplegia and hemiparesis following other cerebrovascular disease affecting left non-dominant side

I69.859 Hemiplegia and hemiparesis following other cerebrovascular disease affecting unspecified side

● **I69.86 Other paralytic syndrome following other cerebrovascular disease**

Use additional code to identify type of paralytic syndrome, such as:
locked-in state (G83.5)
quadriplegia (G82.5-)

Excludes1 hemiplegia/hemiparesis following other cerebrovascular disease (I69.85-)
monoplegia of lower limb following other cerebrovascular disease (I69.84-)
monoplegia of upper limb following other cerebrovascular disease (I69.83-)

I69.861 Other paralytic syndrome following other cerebrovascular disease affecting right dominant side

I69.862 Other paralytic syndrome following other cerebrovascular disease affecting left dominant side

I69.863 Other paralytic syndrome following other cerebrovascular disease affecting right non-dominant side

I69.864 Other paralytic syndrome following other cerebrovascular disease affecting left non-dominant side

I69.865 Other paralytic syndrome following other cerebrovascular disease, bilateral

I69.869 Other paralytic syndrome following other cerebrovascular disease affecting unspecified side

● **I69.89 Other sequelae of other cerebrovascular disease**

I69.890 Apraxia following other cerebrovascular disease

I69.891 Dysphagia following other cerebrovascular disease

Use additional code to identify the type of dysphagia, if known (R13.1-)

I69.892 Facial weakness following other cerebrovascular disease

Facial droop following other cerebrovascular disease

I69.893 Ataxia following other cerebrovascular disease

I69.898 Other sequelae of other cerebrovascular disease

Alteration of sensation following other cerebrovascular disease
Disturbance of vision following other cerebrovascular disease

Use additional code to identify the sequelae

● **I69.9 Sequelae of unspecified cerebrovascular diseases**

Excludes1 sequelae of stroke (I69.3)
sequelae of traumatic intracranial injury (S06.-)

I69.90 Unspecified sequelae of unspecified cerebrovascular disease

● **I69.91 Cognitive deficits following unspecified cerebrovascular disease**

I69.910 Attention and concentration deficit following unspecified cerebrovascular disease ◀

I69.911 Memory deficit following unspecified cerebrovascular disease ◀

I69.912 Visuospatial deficit and spatial neglect following unspecified cerebrovascular disease ◀

I69.913 Psychomotor deficit following unspecified cerebrovascular disease ◀

I69.914 Frontal lobe and executive function deficit following unspecified cerebrovascular disease ◀

I69.915 Cognitive social or emotional deficit following unspecified cerebrovascular disease ◀

I69.918 Other symptoms and signs involving cognitive functions following unspecified cerebrovascular disease ◀

I69.919 Unspecified symptoms and signs involving cognitive functions following unspecified cerebrovascular disease ◀

● **I69.92 Speech and language deficits following unspecified cerebrovascular disease**

I69.920 Aphasia following unspecified cerebrovascular disease

I69.921 Dysphasia following unspecified cerebrovascular disease

I69.922 Dysarthria following unspecified cerebrovascular disease

I69.923 Fluency disorder following unspecified cerebrovascular disease

Stuttering following unspecified cerebrovascular disease ⬅

I69.928 Other speech and language deficits following unspecified cerebrovascular disease

● **I69.93 Monoplegia of upper limb following unspecified cerebrovascular disease**

I69.931 Monoplegia of upper limb following unspecified cerebrovascular disease affecting right dominant side

I69.932 Monoplegia of upper limb following unspecified cerebrovascular disease affecting left dominant side

I69.933 Monoplegia of upper limb following unspecified cerebrovascular disease affecting right non-dominant side

I69.934 Monoplegia of upper limb following unspecified cerebrovascular disease affecting left non-dominant side

I69.939 Monoplegia of upper limb following unspecified cerebrovascular disease affecting unspecified side

● **I69.94 Monoplegia of lower limb following unspecified cerebrovascular disease**

I69.941 Monoplegia of lower limb following unspecified cerebrovascular disease affecting right dominant side

I69.942 Monoplegia of lower limb following unspecified cerebrovascular disease affecting left dominant side

I69.943 Monoplegia of lower limb following unspecified cerebrovascular disease affecting right non-dominant side

I69.944 Monoplegia of lower limb following unspecified cerebrovascular disease affecting left non-dominant side

I69.949 Monoplegia of lower limb following unspecified cerebrovascular disease affecting unspecified side

● **I69.95 Hemiplegia and hemiparesis following unspecified cerebrovascular disease**

I69.951 Hemiplegia and hemiparesis following unspecified cerebrovascular disease affecting right dominant side

I69.952 Hemiplegia and hemiparesis following unspecified cerebrovascular disease affecting left dominant side

I69.953 Hemiplegia and hemiparesis following unspecified cerebrovascular disease affecting right non-dominant side

I69.954 Hemiplegia and hemiparesis following unspecified cerebrovascular disease affecting left non-dominant side

I69.959 Hemiplegia and hemiparesis following unspecified cerebrovascular disease affecting unspecified side

● **I69.96 Other paralytic syndrome following unspecified cerebrovascular disease**

Use additional code to identify type of paralytic syndrome, such as:
- locked-in state (G83.5)
- quadriplegia (G82.5-)

Excludes1 hemiplegia/hemiparesis following unspecified cerebrovascular disease (I69.95-)
monoplegia of lower limb following unspecified cerebrovascular disease (I69.94-)
monoplegia of upper limb following unspecified cerebrovascular disease (I69.93-)

I69.961 Other paralytic syndrome following unspecified cerebrovascular disease affecting right dominant side

I69.962 Other paralytic syndrome following unspecified cerebrovascular disease affecting left dominant side

I69.963 Other paralytic syndrome following unspecified cerebrovascular disease affecting right non-dominant side

I69.964 Other paralytic syndrome following unspecified cerebrovascular disease affecting left non-dominant side

I69.965 Other paralytic syndrome following unspecified cerebrovascular disease, bilateral

I69.969 Other paralytic syndrome following unspecified cerebrovascular disease affecting unspecified side

● **I69.99 Other sequelae of unspecified cerebrovascular disease**

I69.990 Apraxia following unspecified cerebrovascular disease

I69.991 Dysphagia following unspecified cerebrovascular disease

Use additional code to identify the type of dysphagia, if known (R13.1-)

I69.992 Facial weakness following unspecified cerebrovascular disease

Facial droop following unspecified cerebrovascular disease

I69.993 Ataxia following unspecified cerebrovascular disease

I69.998 Other sequelae following unspecified cerebrovascular disease

Alteration in sensation following unspecified cerebrovascular disease
Disturbance of vision following unspecified cerebrovascular disease

Use additional code to identify the sequelae

DISEASES OF ARTERIES, ARTERIOLES AND CAPILLARIES (I70-I79)

● **I70 Atherosclerosis**

Includes arteriolosclerosis
arterial degeneration
arteriosclerosis
arteriosclerotic vascular disease
arteriovascular degeneration
atheroma
endarteritis deformans or obliterans
senile arteritis
senile endarteritis
vascular degeneration

Use additional code to identify:
- exposure to environmental tobacco smoke (Z77.22)
- history of tobacco dependence (Z87.891) ◀
- occupational exposure to environmental tobacco smoke (Z57.31)
- tobacco dependence (F17.-)
- tobacco use (Z72.0)

Excludes2 arteriosclerotic cardiovascular disease (I25.1-)
arteriosclerotic heart disease (I25.1-)
atheroembolism (I75.-)
cerebral atherosclerosis (I67.2)
coronary atherosclerosis (I25.1-)
mesenteric atherosclerosis (K55.1)
precerebral atherosclerosis (I67.2)
primary pulmonary atherosclerosis (I27.0)

I70.0 Atherosclerosis of aorta

I70.1 Atherosclerosis of renal artery

Goldblatt's kidney

Excludes2 atherosclerosis of renal arterioles (I12.-)

CHAPTER 9 (I00-I99)

★(See Plates 500, 501, and 502 on pages NAP-12 – NAP-14.)

● **I70.2 Atherosclerosis of native arteries of the extremities**
Mönckeberg's (medial) sclerosis
Use additional code, if applicable, to identify chronic total occlusion of artery of extremity (I70.92)
Excludes2 atherosclerosis of bypass graft of extremities (I70.30-I70.79)

● **I70.20 Unspecified atherosclerosis of native arteries of extremities**

I70.201 Unspecified **atherosclerosis of native arteries of extremities, right leg**

I70.202 Unspecified **atherosclerosis of native arteries of extremities, left leg**

I70.203 Unspecified **atherosclerosis of native arteries of extremities, bilateral legs**

I70.208 Unspecified **atherosclerosis of native arteries of extremities, other extremity**

I70.209 Unspecified **atherosclerosis of native arteries of extremities, unspecified extremity**

● **I70.21 Atherosclerosis of native arteries of extremities with intermittent claudication**

I70.211 Atherosclerosis of native arteries of extremities with intermittent claudication, right leg

I70.212 Atherosclerosis of native arteries of extremities with intermittent claudication, left leg

I70.213 Atherosclerosis of native arteries of extremities with intermittent claudication, bilateral legs

I70.218 Atherosclerosis of native arteries of extremities with intermittent claudication, other extremity

I70.219 Atherosclerosis of native arteries of extremities with intermittent claudication, unspecified extremity

● **I70.22 Atherosclerosis of native arteries of extremities with rest pain**
Includes any condition classifiable to I70.21-

I70.221 Atherosclerosis of native arteries of extremities with rest pain, right leg

I70.222 Atherosclerosis of native arteries of extremities with rest pain, left leg

I70.223 Atherosclerosis of native arteries of extremities with rest pain, bilateral legs

I70.228 Atherosclerosis of native arteries of extremities with rest pain, other extremity

I70.229 Atherosclerosis of native arteries of extremities with rest pain, unspecified extremity

● **I70.23 Atherosclerosis of native arteries of right leg with ulceration**
Includes any condition classifiable to I70.211 and I70.221
Use additional code to identify severity of ulcer (L97.-)

I70.231 Atherosclerosis of native arteries of right leg with ulceration of thigh

I70.232 Atherosclerosis of native arteries of right leg with ulceration of calf

I70.233 Atherosclerosis of native arteries of right leg with ulceration of ankle

I70.234 Atherosclerosis of native arteries of right leg with ulceration of heel and midfoot
Atherosclerosis of native arteries of right leg with ulceration of plantar surface of midfoot

I70.235 Atherosclerosis of native arteries of right leg with ulceration of other part of foot
Atherosclerosis of native arteries of right leg extremities with ulceration of toe

I70.238 Atherosclerosis of native arteries of right leg with ulceration of other part of lower right leg

I70.239 Atherosclerosis of native arteries of right leg with ulceration of unspecified site

● **I70.24 Atherosclerosis of native arteries of left leg with ulceration**
Includes any condition classifiable to I70.212 and I70.222
Use additional code to identify severity of ulcer (L97.-)

I70.241 Atherosclerosis of native arteries of left leg with ulceration of thigh

I70.242 Atherosclerosis of native arteries of left leg with ulceration of calf

I70.243 Atherosclerosis of native arteries of left leg with ulceration of ankle

I70.244 Atherosclerosis of native arteries of left leg with ulceration of heel and midfoot
Atherosclerosis of native arteries of left leg with ulceration of plantar surface of midfoot

I70.245 Atherosclerosis of native arteries of left leg with ulceration of other part of foot
Atherosclerosis of native arteries of left leg extremities with ulceration of toe

I70.248 Atherosclerosis of native arteries of left leg with ulceration of other part of lower left leg

I70.249 Atherosclerosis of native arteries of left leg with ulceration of unspecified site

I70.25 Atherosclerosis of native arteries of other extremities with ulceration
Includes any condition classifiable to I70.218 and I70.228
Use additional code to identify the severity of the ulcer (L98.49-)

CHAPTER 9 (I00-I99)

● I70.26 **Atherosclerosis of native arteries of extremities with gangrene**

Includes any condition classifiable to I70.21-, I70.22-, I70.23-, I70.24-, and I70.25-

Use additional code to identify the severity of any ulcer (L97.-, L98.49-), if applicable

I70.261 **Atherosclerosis of native arteries of extremities with gangrene, right leg**

I70.262 **Atherosclerosis of native arteries of extremities with gangrene, left leg**

I70.263 **Atherosclerosis of native arteries of extremities with gangrene, bilateral legs**

I70.268 **Atherosclerosis of native arteries of extremities with gangrene, other extremity**

I70.269 **Atherosclerosis of native arteries of extremities with gangrene, unspecified extremity**

● I70.29 **Other atherosclerosis of native arteries of extremities**

I70.291 **Other atherosclerosis of native arteries of extremities, right leg**

I70.292 **Other atherosclerosis of native arteries of extremities, left leg**

I70.293 **Other atherosclerosis of native arteries of extremities, bilateral legs**

I70.298 **Other atherosclerosis of native arteries of extremities, other extremity**

I70.299 **Other atherosclerosis of native arteries of extremities, unspecified extremity**

● I70.3 **Atherosclerosis of unspecified type of bypass graft(s) of the extremities**

Use additional code, if applicable, to identify chronic total occlusion of artery of extremity (I70.92)

Excludes1 embolism or thrombus of bypass graft(s) of extremities (T82.8-)

● I70.30 **Unspecified atherosclerosis of unspecified type of bypass graft(s) of the extremities**

70.301 **Unspecified atherosclerosis of unspecified type of bypass graft(s) of the extremities, right leg**

I70.302 **Unspecified atherosclerosis of unspecified type of bypass graft(s) of the extremities, left leg**

I70.303 **Unspecified atherosclerosis of unspecified type of bypass graft(s) of the extremities, bilateral legs**

I70.308 **Unspecified atherosclerosis of unspecified type of bypass graft(s) of the extremities, other extremity**

I70.309 **Unspecified atherosclerosis of unspecified type of bypass graft(s) of the extremities, unspecified extremity**

● I70.31 **Atherosclerosis of unspecified type of bypass graft(s) of the extremities with intermittent claudication**

I70.311 **Atherosclerosis of unspecified type of bypass graft(s) of the extremities with intermittent claudication, right leg**

I70.312 **Atherosclerosis of unspecified type of bypass graft(s) of the extremities with intermittent claudication, left leg**

I70.313 **Atherosclerosis of unspecified type of bypass graft(s) of the extremities with intermittent claudication, bilateral legs**

I70.318 **Atherosclerosis of unspecified type of bypass graft(s) of the extremities with intermittent claudication, other extremity**

I70.319 **Atherosclerosis of unspecified type of bypass graft(s) of the extremities with intermittent claudication, unspecified extremity**

● I70.32 **Atherosclerosis of unspecified type of bypass graft(s) of the extremities with rest pain**

Includes any condition classifiable to I70.31-

I70.321 **Atherosclerosis of unspecified type of bypass graft(s) of the extremities with rest pain, right leg**

I70.322 **Atherosclerosis of unspecified type of bypass graft(s) of the extremities with rest pain, left leg**

I70.323 **Atherosclerosis of unspecified type of bypass graft(s) of the extremities with rest pain, bilateral legs**

I70.328 **Atherosclerosis of unspecified type of bypass graft(s) of the extremities with rest pain, other extremity**

I70.329 **Atherosclerosis of unspecified type of bypass graft(s) of the extremities with rest pain, unspecified extremity**

● I70.33 **Atherosclerosis of unspecified type of bypass graft(s) of the right leg with ulceration**

Includes any condition classifiable to I70.311 and I70.321

Use additional code to identify severity of ulcer (L97.-)

I70.331 **Atherosclerosis of unspecified type of bypass graft(s) of the right leg with ulceration of thigh**

I70.332 **Atherosclerosis of unspecified type of bypass graft(s) of the right leg with ulceration of calf**

I70.333 **Atherosclerosis of unspecified type of bypass graft(s) of the right leg with ulceration of ankle**

I70.334 **Atherosclerosis of unspecified type of bypass graft(s) of the right leg with ulceration of heel and midfoot**

Atherosclerosis of unspecified type of bypass graft(s) of right leg with ulceration of plantar surface of midfoot

I70.335 **Atherosclerosis of unspecified type of bypass graft(s) of the right leg with ulceration of other part of foot**

Atherosclerosis of unspecified type of bypass graft(s) of the right leg with ulceration of toe

I70.338 **Atherosclerosis of unspecified type of bypass graft(s) of the right leg with ulceration of other part of lower leg**

I70.339 **Atherosclerosis of unspecified type of bypass graft(s) of the right leg with ulceration of unspecified site**

● **I70.34 Atherosclerosis of unspecified type of bypass graft(s) of the left leg with ulceration**

Includes any condition classifiable to I70.312 and I70.322

Use additional code to identify severity of ulcer (L97.-)

I70.341 Atherosclerosis of unspecified type of bypass graft(s) of the left leg with ulceration of thigh

I70.342 Atherosclerosis of unspecified type of bypass graft(s) of the left leg with ulceration of calf

I70.343 Atherosclerosis of unspecified type of bypass graft(s) of the left leg with ulceration of ankle

I70.344 Atherosclerosis of unspecified type of bypass graft(s) of the left leg with ulceration of heel and midfoot

Atherosclerosis of unspecified type of bypass graft(s) of left leg with ulceration of plantar surface of midfoot

I70.345 Atherosclerosis of unspecified type of bypass graft(s) of the left leg with ulceration of other part of foot

Atherosclerosis of unspecified type of bypass graft(s) of the left leg with ulceration of toe

I70.348 Atherosclerosis of unspecified type of bypass graft(s) of the left leg with ulceration of other part of lower leg

I70.349 Atherosclerosis of unspecified type of bypass graft(s) of the left leg with ulceration of unspecified site

I70.35 Atherosclerosis of unspecified type of bypass graft(s) of other extremity with ulceration

Includes any condition classifiable to I70.318 and I70.328

Use additional code to identify severity of ulcer (L98.49-)

● **I70.36 Atherosclerosis of unspecified type of bypass graft(s) of the extremities with gangrene**

Includes any condition classifiable to I70.31-, I70.32-, I70.33-, I70.34-, I70.35

Use additional code to identify the severity of any ulcer (L97.-, L98.49-), if applicable

I70.361 Atherosclerosis of unspecified type of bypass graft(s) of the extremities with gangrene, right leg

I70.362 Atherosclerosis of unspecified type of bypass graft(s) of the extremities with gangrene, left leg

I70.363 Atherosclerosis of unspecified type of bypass graft(s) of the extremities with gangrene, bilateral legs

I70.368 Atherosclerosis of unspecified type of bypass graft(s) of the extremities with gangrene, other extremity

I70.369 Atherosclerosis of unspecified type of bypass graft(s) of the extremities with gangrene, unspecified extremity

● **I70.39 Other atherosclerosis of unspecified type of bypass graft(s) of the extremities**

I70.391 Other atherosclerosis of unspecified type of bypass graft(s) of the extremities, right leg

I70.392 Other atherosclerosis of unspecified type of bypass graft(s) of the extremities, left leg

I70.393 Other atherosclerosis of unspecified type of bypass graft(s) of the extremities, bilateral legs

I70.398 Other atherosclerosis of unspecified type of bypass graft(s) of the extremities, other extremity

I70.399 Other atherosclerosis of unspecified type of bypass graft(s) of the extremities, unspecified extremity

● **I70.4 Atherosclerosis of autologous vein bypass graft(s) of the extremities**

Use additional code, if applicable, to identify chronic total occlusion of artery of extremity (I70.92)

● **I70.40 Unspecified atherosclerosis of autologous vein bypass graft(s) of the extremities**

I70.401 Unspecified atherosclerosis of autologous vein bypass graft(s) of the extremities, right leg

I70.402 Unspecified atherosclerosis of autologous vein bypass graft(s) of the extremities, left leg

I70.403 Unspecified atherosclerosis of autologous vein bypass graft(s) of the extremities, bilateral legs

I70.408 Unspecified atherosclerosis of autologous vein bypass graft(s) of the extremities, other extremity

I70.409 Unspecified atherosclerosis of autologous vein bypass graft(s) of the extremities, unspecified extremity

● **I70.41 Atherosclerosis of autologous vein bypass graft(s) of the extremities with intermittent claudication**

I70.411 Atherosclerosis of autologous vein bypass graft(s) of the extremities with intermittent claudication, right leg

I70.412 Atherosclerosis of autologous vein bypass graft(s) of the extremities with intermittent claudication, left leg

I70.413 Atherosclerosis of autologous vein bypass graft(s) of the extremities with intermittent claudication, bilateral legs

I70.418 Atherosclerosis of autologous vein bypass graft(s) of the extremities with intermittent claudication, other extremity

I70.419 Atherosclerosis of autologous vein bypass graft(s) of the extremities with intermittent claudication, unspecified extremity

● **I70.42 Atherosclerosis of autologous vein bypass graft(s) of the extremities with rest pain**

Includes any condition classifiable to I70.41-

I70.421 Atherosclerosis of autologous vein bypass graft(s) of the extremities with rest pain, right leg

I70.422 Atherosclerosis of autologous vein bypass graft(s) of the extremities with rest pain, left leg

I70.423 Atherosclerosis of autologous vein bypass graft(s) of the extremities with rest pain, bilateral legs

I70.428 Atherosclerosis of autologous vein bypass graft(s) of the extremities with rest pain, other extremity

I70.429 Atherosclerosis of autologous vein bypass graft(s) of the extremities with rest pain, unspecified extremity

CHAPTER 9 (I00-I99)

I70.43 Atherosclerosis of autologous vein bypass graft(s) of the right leg with ulceration

Includes any condition classifiable to I70.411 and I70.421

Use additional code to identify severity of ulcer (L97.-)

I70.431 Atherosclerosis of autologous vein bypass graft(s) of the right leg with ulceration of thigh

I70.432 Atherosclerosis of autologous vein bypass graft(s) of the right leg with ulceration of calf

I70.433 Atherosclerosis of autologous vein bypass graft(s) of the right leg with ulceration of ankle

I70.434 Atherosclerosis of autologous vein bypass graft(s) of the right leg with ulceration of heel and midfoot

Atherosclerosis of autologous vein bypass graft(s) of right leg with ulceration of plantar surface of midfoot

I70.435 Atherosclerosis of autologous vein bypass graft(s) of the right leg with ulceration of other part of foot

Atherosclerosis of autologous vein bypass graft(s) of right leg with ulceration of toe

I70.438 Atherosclerosis of autologous vein bypass graft(s) of the right leg with ulceration of other part of lower leg

I70.439 Atherosclerosis of autologous vein bypass graft(s) of the right leg with ulceration of unspecified site

I70.44 Atherosclerosis of autologous vein bypass graft(s) of the left leg with ulceration

Includes any condition classifiable to I70.412 and I70.422

Use additional code to identify severity of ulcer (L97.-)

I70.441 Atherosclerosis of autologous vein bypass graft(s) of the left leg with ulceration of thigh

I70.442 Atherosclerosis of autologous vein bypass graft(s) of the left leg with ulceration of calf

I70.443 Atherosclerosis of autologous vein bypass graft(s) of the left leg with ulceration of ankle

I70.444 Atherosclerosis of autologous vein bypass graft(s) of the left leg with ulceration of heel and midfoot

Atherosclerosis of autologous vein bypass graft(s) of left leg with ulceration of plantar surface of midfoot

I70.445 Atherosclerosis of autologous vein bypass graft(s) of the left leg with ulceration of other part of foot

Atherosclerosis of autologous vein bypass graft(s) of left leg with ulceration of toe

I70.448 Atherosclerosis of autologous vein bypass graft(s) of the left leg with ulceration of other part of lower leg

I70.449 Atherosclerosis of autologous vein bypass graft(s) of the left leg with ulceration of unspecified site

I70.45 Atherosclerosis of autologous vein bypass graft(s) of other extremity with ulceration

Includes any condition classifiable to I70.418, I70.428, and I70.438

Use additional code to identify severity of ulcer (L98.49-)

I70.46 Atherosclerosis of autologous vein bypass graft(s) of the extremities with gangrene

Includes any condition classifiable to I70.41-, I70.42-, and I70.43-, I70.44-, I70.45

Use additional code to identify the severity of any ulcer (L97.-, L98.49-), if applicable

I70.461 Atherosclerosis of autologous vein bypass graft(s) of the extremities with gangrene, right leg

I70.462 Atherosclerosis of autologous vein bypass graft(s) of the extremities with gangrene, left leg

I70.463 Atherosclerosis of autologous vein bypass graft(s) of the extremities with gangrene, bilateral legs

I70.468 Atherosclerosis of autologous vein bypass graft(s) of the extremities with gangrene, other extremity

I70.469 Atherosclerosis of autologous vein bypass graft(s) of the extremities with gangrene, unspecified extremity

I70.49 Other atherosclerosis of autologous vein bypass graft(s) of the extremities

I70.491 Other atherosclerosis of autologous vein bypass graft(s) of the extremities, right leg

I70.492 Other atherosclerosis of autologous vein bypass graft(s) of the extremities, left leg

I70.493 Other atherosclerosis of autologous vein bypass graft(s) of the extremities, bilateral legs

I70.498 Other atherosclerosis of autologous vein bypass graft(s) of the extremities, other extremity

I70.499 Other atherosclerosis of autologous vein bypass graft(s) of the extremities, unspecified extremity

I70.5 Atherosclerosis of nonautologous biological bypass graft(s) of the extremities

Use additional code, if applicable, to identify chronic total occlusion of artery of extremity (I70.92)

I70.50 Unspecified atherosclerosis of nonautologous biological bypass graft(s) of the extremities

I70.501 Unspecified atherosclerosis of nonautologous biological bypass graft(s) of the extremities, right leg

I70.502 Unspecified atherosclerosis of nonautologous biological bypass graft(s) of the extremities, left leg

I70.503 Unspecified atherosclerosis of nonautologous biological bypass graft(s) of the extremities, bilateral legs

I70.508 Unspecified atherosclerosis of nonautologous biological bypass graft(s) of the extremities, other extremity

I70.509 Unspecified atherosclerosis of nonautologous biological bypass graft(s) of the extremities, unspecified extremity

● **I70.51 Atherosclerosis of nonautologous biological bypass graft(s) of the extremities intermittent claudication**

I70.511 Atherosclerosis of nonautologous biological bypass graft(s) of the extremities with intermittent claudication, right leg

I70.512 Atherosclerosis of nonautologous biological bypass graft(s) of the extremities with intermittent claudication, left leg

I70.513 Atherosclerosis of nonautologous biological bypass graft(s) of the extremities with intermittent claudication, bilateral legs

I70.518 Atherosclerosis of nonautologous biological bypass graft(s) of the extremities with intermittent claudication, other extremity

I70.519 Atherosclerosis of nonautologous biological bypass graft(s) of the extremities with intermittent claudication, unspecified extremity

● **I70.52 Atherosclerosis of nonautologous biological bypass graft(s) of the extremities with rest pain**

Includes any condition classifiable to I70.51-

I70.521 Atherosclerosis of nonautologous biological bypass graft(s) of the extremities with rest pain, right leg

I70.522 Atherosclerosis of nonautologous biological bypass graft(s) of the extremities with rest pain, left leg

I70.523 Atherosclerosis of nonautologous biological bypass graft(s) of the extremities with rest pain, bilateral legs

I70.528 Atherosclerosis of nonautologous biological bypass graft(s) of the extremities with rest pain, other extremity

I70.529 Atherosclerosis of nonautologous biological bypass graft(s) of the extremities with rest pain, unspecified extremity

● **I70.53 Atherosclerosis of nonautologous biological bypass graft(s) of the right leg with ulceration**

Includes any condition classifiable to I70.511 and I70.521

Use additional code to identify severity of ulcer (L97.-)

I70.531 Atherosclerosis of nonautologous biological bypass graft(s) of the right leg with ulceration of thigh

I70.532 Atherosclerosis of nonautologous biological bypass graft(s) of the right leg with ulceration of calf

I70.533 Atherosclerosis of nonautologous biological bypass graft(s) of the right leg with ulceration of ankle

I70.534 Atherosclerosis of nonautologous biological bypass graft(s) of the right leg with ulceration of heel and midfoot

Atherosclerosis of nonautologous biological bypass graft(s) of right leg with ulceration of plantar surface of midfoot

I70.535 Atherosclerosis of nonautologous biological bypass graft(s) of the right leg with ulceration of other part of foot

Atherosclerosis of nonautologous biological bypass graft(s) of the right leg with ulceration of toe

I70.538 Atherosclerosis of nonautologous biological bypass graft(s) of the right leg with ulceration of other part of lower leg

I70.539 Atherosclerosis of nonautologous biological bypass graft(s) of the right leg with ulceration of unspecified site

● **I70.54 Atherosclerosis of nonautologous biological bypass graft(s) of the left leg with ulceration**

Includes any condition classifiable to I70.512 and I70.522

Use additional code to identify severity of ulcer (L97.-)

I70.541 Atherosclerosis of nonautologous biological bypass graft(s) of the left leg with ulceration of thigh

I70.542 Atherosclerosis of nonautologous biological bypass graft(s) of the left leg with ulceration of calf

I70.543 Atherosclerosis of nonautologous biological bypass graft(s) of the left leg with ulceration of ankle

I70.544 Atherosclerosis of nonautologous biological bypass graft(s) of the left leg with ulceration of heel and midfoot

Atherosclerosis of nonautologous biological bypass graft(s) of left leg with ulceration of plantar surface of midfoot

I70.545 Atherosclerosis of nonautologous biological bypass graft(s) of the left leg with ulceration of other part of foot

Atherosclerosis of nonautologous biological bypass graft(s) of the left leg with ulceration of toe

I70.548 Atherosclerosis of nonautologous biological bypass graft(s) of the left leg with ulceration of other part of lower leg

I70.549 Atherosclerosis of nonautologous biological bypass graft(s) of the left leg with ulceration of unspecified site

I70.55 Atherosclerosis of nonautologous biological bypass graft(s) of other extremity with ulceration

Includes any condition classifiable to I70.518, I70.528, and I70.538

Use additional code to identify severity of ulcer (L98.49)

● I70.56 **Atherosclerosis of nonautologous biological bypass graft(s) of the extremities with gangrene**
Includes any condition classifiable to I70.51-, I70.52-, and I70.53-, I70.54-, I70.55
Use additional code to identify the severity of any ulcer (L97.-, L98.49-), if applicable

I70.561 **Atherosclerosis of nonautologous biological bypass graft(s) of the extremities with gangrene, right leg**

I70.562 **Atherosclerosis of nonautologous biological bypass graft(s) of the extremities with gangrene, left leg**

I70.563 **Atherosclerosis of nonautologous biological bypass graft(s) of the extremities with gangrene, bilateral legs**

I70.568 **Atherosclerosis of nonautologous biological bypass graft(s) of the extremities with gangrene, other extremity**

I70.569 **Atherosclerosis of nonautologous biological bypass graft(s) of the extremities with gangrene, unspecified extremity**

● I70.59 **Other atherosclerosis of nonautologous biological bypass graft(s) of the extremities**

I70.591 **Other atherosclerosis of nonautologous biological bypass graft(s) of the extremities, right leg**

I70.592 **Other atherosclerosis of nonautologous biological bypass graft(s) of the extremities, left leg**

I70.593 **Other atherosclerosis of nonautologous biological bypass graft(s) of the extremities, bilateral legs**

I70.598 **Other atherosclerosis of nonautologous biological bypass graft(s) of the extremities, other extremity**

I70.599 **Other atherosclerosis of nonautologous biological bypass graft(s) of the extremities, unspecified extremity**

● I70.6 **Atherosclerosis of nonbiological bypass graft(s) of the extremities**
Use additional code, if applicable, to identify chronic total occlusion of artery of extremity (I70.92)

● I70.60 **Unspecified atherosclerosis of nonbiological bypass graft(s) of the extremities**

I70.601 **Unspecified atherosclerosis of nonbiological bypass graft(s) of the extremities, right leg**

I70.602 **Unspecified atherosclerosis of nonbiological bypass graft(s) of the extremities, left leg**

I70.603 **Unspecified atherosclerosis of nonbiological bypass graft(s) of the extremities, bilateral legs**

I70.608 **Unspecified atherosclerosis of nonbiological bypass graft(s) of the extremities, other extremity**

I70.609 **Unspecified atherosclerosis of nonbiological bypass graft(s) of the extremities, unspecified extremity**

● I70.61 **Atherosclerosis of nonbiological bypass graft(s) of the extremities with intermittent claudication**

I70.611 **Atherosclerosis of nonbiological bypass graft(s) of the extremities with intermittent claudication, right leg**

I70.612 **Atherosclerosis of nonbiological bypass graft(s) of the extremities with intermittent claudication, left leg**

I70.613 **Atherosclerosis of nonbiological bypass graft(s) of the extremities with intermittent claudication, bilateral legs**

I70.618 **Atherosclerosis of nonbiological bypass graft(s) of the extremities with intermittent claudication, other extremity**

I70.619 **Atherosclerosis of nonbiological bypass graft(s) of the extremities with intermittent claudication, unspecified extremity**

● I70.62 **Atherosclerosis of nonbiological bypass graft(s) of the extremities with rest pain**
Includes any condition classifiable to I70.61-

I70.621 **Atherosclerosis of nonbiological bypass graft(s) of the extremities with rest pain, right leg**

I70.622 **Atherosclerosis of nonbiological bypass graft(s) of the extremities with rest pain, left leg**

I70.623 **Atherosclerosis of nonbiological bypass graft(s) of the extremities with rest pain, bilateral legs**

I70.628 **Atherosclerosis of nonbiological bypass graft(s) of the extremities with rest pain, other extremity**

I70.629 **Atherosclerosis of nonbiological bypass graft(s) of the extremities with rest pain, unspecified extremity**

● I70.63 **Atherosclerosis of nonbiological bypass graft(s) of the right leg with ulceration**
Includes any condition classifiable to I70.611 and I70.621
Use additional code to identify severity of ulcer (L97.-)

I70.631 **Atherosclerosis of nonbiological bypass graft(s) of the right leg with ulceration of thigh**

I70.632 **Atherosclerosis of nonbiological bypass graft(s) of the right leg with ulceration of calf**

I70.633 **Atherosclerosis of nonbiological bypass graft(s) of the right leg with ulceration of ankle**

I70.634 **Atherosclerosis of nonbiological bypass graft(s) of the right leg with ulceration of heel and midfoot**
Atherosclerosis of nonbiological bypass graft(s) of right leg with ulceration of plantar surface of midfoot

I70.635 **Atherosclerosis of nonbiological bypass graft(s) of the right leg with ulceration of other part of foot**
Atherosclerosis of nonbiological bypass graft(s) of the right leg with ulceration of toe

I70.638 **Atherosclerosis of nonbiological bypass graft(s) of the right leg with ulceration of other part of lower leg**

I70.639 **Atherosclerosis of nonbiological bypass graft(s) of the right leg with ulceration of unspecified site**

● **I70.64 Atherosclerosis of nonbiological bypass graft(s) of the left leg with ulceration**
Includes any condition classifiable to I70.612 and I70.622
Use additional code to identify severity of ulcer (L97.-)
I70.641 Atherosclerosis of nonbiological bypass graft(s) of the left leg with ulceration of thigh
I70.642 Atherosclerosis of nonbiological bypass graft(s) of the left leg with ulceration of calf
I70.643 Atherosclerosis of nonbiological bypass graft(s) of the left leg with ulceration of ankle
I70.644 Atherosclerosis of nonbiological bypass graft(s) of the left leg with ulceration of heel and midfoot
Atherosclerosis of nonbiological bypass graft(s) of left leg with ulceration of plantar surface of midfoot
I70.645 Atherosclerosis of nonbiological bypass graft(s) of the left leg with ulceration of other part of foot
Atherosclerosis of nonbiological bypass graft(s) of the left leg with ulceration of toe
I70.648 Atherosclerosis of nonbiological bypass graft(s) of the left leg with ulceration of other part of lower leg
I70.649 Atherosclerosis of nonbiological bypass graft(s) of the left leg with ulceration of unspecified site

I70.65 Atherosclerosis of nonbiological bypass graft(s) of other extremity with ulceration
Includes any condition classifiable to I70.618 and I70.628
Use additional code to identify severity of ulcer (L98.49-)

● **I70.66 Atherosclerosis of nonbiological bypass graft(s) of the extremities with gangrene**
Includes any condition classifiable to I70.61-, I70.62-, I70.63-, I70.64-, I70.65
Use additional code to identify the severity of any ulcer (L97.-, L98.49-), if applicable
I70.661 Atherosclerosis of nonbiological bypass graft(s) of the extremities with gangrene, right leg
I70.662 Atherosclerosis of nonbiological bypass graft(s) of the extremities with gangrene, left leg
I70.663 Atherosclerosis of nonbiological bypass graft(s) of the extremities with gangrene, bilateral legs
I70.668 Atherosclerosis of nonbiological bypass graft(s) of the extremities with gangrene, other extremity
I70.669 Atherosclerosis of nonbiological bypass graft(s) of the extremities with gangrene, unspecified extremity

● **I70.69 Other atherosclerosis of nonbiological bypass graft(s) of the extremities**
I70.691 Other atherosclerosis of nonbiological bypass graft(s) of the extremities, right leg
I70.692 Other atherosclerosis of nonbiological bypass graft(s) of the extremities, left leg
I70.693 Other atherosclerosis of nonbiological bypass graft(s) of the extremities, bilateral legs
I70.698 Other atherosclerosis of nonbiological bypass graft(s) of the extremities, other extremity
I70.699 Other atherosclerosis of nonbiological bypass graft(s) of the extremities, unspecified extremity

● **I70.7 Atherosclerosis of other type of bypass graft(s) of the extremities**
Use additional code, if applicable, to identify chronic total occlusion of artery of extremity (I70.92)

● **I70.70 Unspecified atherosclerosis of other type of bypass graft(s) of the extremities**
I70.701 Unspecified atherosclerosis of other type of bypass graft(s) of the extremities, right leg
I70.702 Unspecified atherosclerosis of other type of bypass graft(s) of the extremities, left leg
I70.703 Unspecified atherosclerosis of other type of bypass graft(s) of the extremities, bilateral legs
I70.708 Unspecified atherosclerosis of other type of bypass graft(s) of the extremities, other extremity
I70.709 Unspecified atherosclerosis of other type of bypass graft(s) of the extremities, unspecified extremity

● **I70.71 Atherosclerosis of other type of bypass graft(s) of the extremities with intermittent claudication**
I70.711 Atherosclerosis of other type of bypass graft(s) of the extremities with intermittent claudication, right leg
I70.712 Atherosclerosis of other type of bypass graft(s) of the extremities with intermittent claudication, left leg
I70.713 Atherosclerosis of other type of bypass graft(s) of the extremities with intermittent claudication, bilateral legs
I70.718 Atherosclerosis of other type of bypass graft(s) of the extremities with intermittent claudication, other extremity
I70.719 Atherosclerosis of other type of bypass graft(s) of the extremities with intermittent claudication, unspecified extremity

● **I70.72 Atherosclerosis of other type of bypass graft(s) of the extremities with rest pain**
Includes any condition classifiable to I70.71-
I70.721 Atherosclerosis of other type of bypass graft(s) of the extremities with rest pain, right leg
I70.722 Atherosclerosis of other type of bypass graft(s) of the extremities with rest pain, left leg
I70.723 Atherosclerosis of other type of bypass graft(s) of the extremities with rest pain, bilateral legs
I70.728 Atherosclerosis of other type of bypass graft(s) of the extremities with rest pain, other extremity
I70.729 Atherosclerosis of other type of bypass graft(s) of the extremities with rest pain, unspecified extremity

CHAPTER 9 (I00-I99)

● **I70.73 Atherosclerosis of other type of bypass graft(s) of the right leg with ulceration**

Includes any condition classifiable to I70.711 and I70.721

Use additional code to identify severity of ulcer (L97.-)

I70.731 Atherosclerosis of other type of bypass graft(s) of the right leg with ulceration of thigh

I70.732 Atherosclerosis of other type of bypass graft(s) of the right leg with ulceration of calf

I70.733 Atherosclerosis of other type of bypass graft(s) of the right leg with ulceration of ankle

I70.734 Atherosclerosis of other type of bypass graft(s) of the right leg with ulceration of heel and midfoot

Atherosclerosis of other type of bypass graft(s) of right leg with ulceration of plantar surface of midfoot

I70.735 Atherosclerosis of other type of bypass graft(s) of the right leg with ulceration of other part of foot

Atherosclerosis of other type of bypass graft(s) of right leg with ulceration of toe

I70.738 Atherosclerosis of other type of bypass graft(s) of the right leg with ulceration of other part of lower leg

I70.739 Atherosclerosis of other type of bypass graft(s) of the right leg with ulceration of unspecified site

● **I70.74 Atherosclerosis of other type of bypass graft(s) of the left leg with ulceration**

Includes any condition classifiable to I70.712 and I70.722

Use additional code to identify severity of ulcer (L97.-)

I70.741 Atherosclerosis of other type of bypass graft(s) of the left leg with ulceration of thigh

I70.742 Atherosclerosis of other type of bypass graft(s) of the left leg with ulceration of calf

I70.743 Atherosclerosis of other type of bypass graft(s) of the left leg with ulceration of ankle

I70.744 Atherosclerosis of other type of bypass graft(s) of the left leg with ulceration of heel and midfoot

Atherosclerosis of other type of bypass graft(s) of left leg with ulceration of plantar surface of midfoot

I70.745 Atherosclerosis of other type of bypass graft(s) of the left leg with ulceration of other part of foot

Atherosclerosis of other type of bypass graft(s) of left leg with ulceration of toe

I70.748 Atherosclerosis of other type of bypass graft(s) of the left leg with ulceration of other part of lower leg

I70.749 Atherosclerosis of other type of bypass graft(s) of the left leg with ulceration of unspecified site

I70.75 Atherosclerosis of other type of bypass graft(s) of other extremity with ulceration

Includes any condition classifiable to I70.718 and I70.728

Use additional code to identify severity of ulcer (L98.49)

● **I70.76 Atherosclerosis of other type of bypass graft(s) of the extremities with gangrene**

Includes any condition classifiable to I70.71-, I70.72-, I70.73-, I70.74-, I70.75

Use additional code to identify the severity of any ulcer (L97.-, L98.49-), if applicable

I70.761 Atherosclerosis of other type of bypass graft(s) of the extremities with gangrene, right leg

I70.762 Atherosclerosis of other type of bypass graft(s) of the extremities with gangrene, left leg

I70.763 Atherosclerosis of other type of bypass graft(s) of the extremities with gangrene, bilateral legs

I70.768 Atherosclerosis of other type of bypass graft(s) of the extremities with gangrene, other extremity

I70.769 Atherosclerosis of other type of bypass graft(s) of the extremities with gangrene, unspecified extremity

● **I70.79 Other atherosclerosis of other type of bypass graft(s) of the extremities**

I70.791 Other atherosclerosis of other type of bypass graft(s) of the extremities, right leg

I70.792 Other atherosclerosis of other type of bypass graft(s) of the extremities, left leg

I70.793 Other atherosclerosis of other type of bypass graft(s) of the extremities, bilateral legs

I70.798 Other atherosclerosis of other type of bypass graft(s) of the extremities, other extremity

I70.799 Other atherosclerosis of other type of bypass graft(s) of the extremities, unspecified extremity

I70.8 Atherosclerosis of other arteries

● **I70.9 Other and unspecified atherosclerosis**

I70.90 Unspecified atherosclerosis

I70.91 Generalized atherosclerosis

I70.92 Chronic total occlusion of artery of the extremities

Complete occlusion of artery of the extremities
Total occlusion of artery of the extremities

Code first *atherosclerosis of arteries of the extremities (I70.2-, I70.3-, I70.4-, I70.5-, I70.6-, I70.7-)*

● I71 Aortic aneurysm and dissection
Excludes1 aortic ectasia (I77.81-)
syphilitic aortic aneurysm (A52.01)
traumatic aortic aneurysm (S25.09, S35.09)

● I71.0 Dissection of aorta
I71.00 Dissection of unspecified site of aorta
I71.01 Dissection of thoracic aorta
I71.02 Dissection of abdominal aorta
I71.03 Dissection of thoracoabdominal aorta
I71.1 Thoracic aortic aneurysm, ruptured
I71.2 Thoracic aortic aneurysm, without rupture
I71.3 Abdominal aortic aneurysm, ruptured
I71.4 Abdominal aortic aneurysm, without rupture
I71.5 Thoracoabdominal aortic aneurysm, ruptured
I71.6 Thoracoabdominal aortic aneurysm, without rupture
I71.8 Aortic aneurysm of unspecified site, ruptured
Rupture of aorta NOS
I71.9 Aortic aneurysm of unspecified site, without rupture
Aneurysm of aorta
Dilatation of aorta
Hyaline necrosis of aorta

● I72 Other aneurysm
Includes aneurysm (cirsoid) (false) (ruptured)
Excludes2 acquired aneurysm (I77.0)
aneurysm (of) aorta (I71.-)
aneurysm (of) arteriovenous NOS (Q27.3-)
carotid artery dissection (I77.71)
cerebral (nonruptured) aneurysm (I67.1)
coronary aneurysm (I25.4)
coronary artery dissection (I25.42)
dissection of artery NEC (I77.79)
dissection of precerebral artery, congenital (nonruptured) (Q28.1) ◀
heart aneurysm (I25.3)
iliac artery dissection (I77.72)
pulmonary artery aneurysm (I28.1)
renal artery dissection (I77.73)
retinal aneurysm (H35.0)
ruptured cerebral aneurysm (I60.7)
varicose aneurysm (I77.0)
vertebral artery dissection (I77.74)

I72.0 Aneurysm of carotid artery
Aneurysm of common carotid artery
Aneurysm of external carotid artery
Aneurysm of internal carotid artery, extracranial portion
Excludes1 aneurysm of internal carotid artery, intracranial portion (I67.1)
aneurysm of internal carotid artery NOS (I67.1)
I72.1 Aneurysm of artery of upper extremity
I72.2 Aneurysm of renal artery
I72.3 Aneurysm of iliac artery
I72.4 Aneurysm of artery of lower extremity
I72.5 Aneurysm of other precerebral arteries ◀
Aneurysm of basilar artery (trunk) ◀
Excludes2 aneurysm of carotid artery (I72.0) ◀
aneurysm of vertebral artery (I72.6) ◀
dissection of carotid artery (I77.71) ◀
dissection of other precerebral arteries (I77.75) ◀
dissection of vertebral artery (I77.74) ◀
I72.6 Aneurysm of vertebral artery ◀
Excludes2 dissection of vertebral artery (I77.74) ◀
I72.8 Aneurysm of other specified arteries
I72.9 Aneurysm of unspecified site

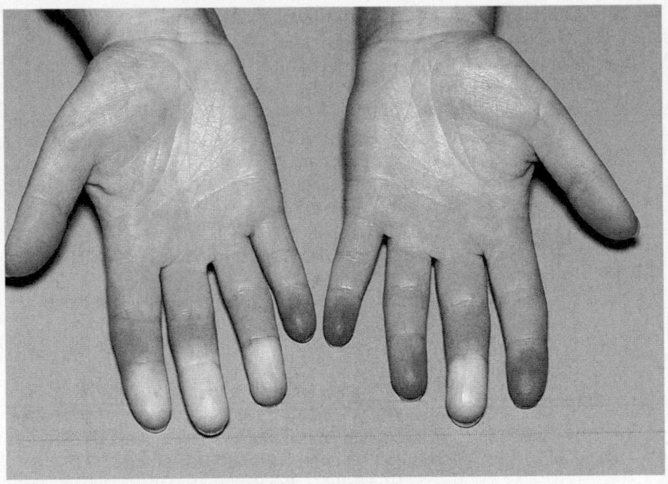

Figure 9-5 Raynaud's syndrome. (From Hallett: Comprehensive Vascular and Endovascular Surgery, ed 2, Philadelphia, Mosby Ltd., 2010)

● I73 Other peripheral vascular diseases
Excludes2 chilblains (T69.1)
frostbite (T33-T34)
immersion hand or foot (T69.0-)
spasm of cerebral artery (G45.9)

● I73.0 Raynaud's syndrome
Diminishing oxygen supply to fingers, toes, nose, and ears when exposed to temperature changes or stress
Raynaud's disease
Raynaud's phenomenon (secondary)
I73.00 Raynaud's syndrome without gangrene
I73.01 Raynaud's syndrome with gangrene
I73.1 Thromboangiitis obliterans [Buerger's disease]
Inflammatory occlusive disease resulting in poor circulation to the legs, feet, and sometimes the hands due to progressive inflammatory narrowing and eventually obliteration of the small arteries
● I73.8 Other specified peripheral vascular diseases
Excludes1 diabetic (peripheral) angiopathy (E08-E13 with .51-.52)
I73.81 Erythromelalgia
I73.89 Other specified peripheral vascular diseases
Acrocyanosis
Erythrocyanosis
Simple acroparesthesia [Schultze's type]
Vasomotor acroparesthesia [Nothnagel's type]
I73.9 Peripheral vascular disease, unspecified
Intermittent claudication
Peripheral angiopathy NOS
Spasm of artery
Excludes1 atherosclerosis of the extremities (I70.2--I70.7-)

CHAPTER 9 (I00-I99)

● **I74 Arterial embolism and thrombosis**

Includes embolic infarction
embolic occlusion
thrombotic infarction
thrombotic occlusion

Code first embolism and thrombosis complicating abortion or ectopic or molar pregnancy (O00-O07, O08.2)
embolism and thrombosis complicating pregnancy, childbirth and the puerperium (O88.-)

Excludes2 atheroembolism (I75.-)
basilar embolism and thrombosis (I63.0-I63.2, I65.1)
carotid embolism and thrombosis (I63.0-I63.2, I65.2)
cerebral embolism and thrombosis (I63.3-I63.5, I66.-)
coronary embolism and thrombosis (I21-I25)
mesenteric embolism and thrombosis (K55.0-) ◄
ophthalmic embolism and thrombosis (H34.-)
precerebral embolism and thrombosis NOS (I63.0-I63.2, I65.9)
pulmonary embolism and thrombosis (I26.-)
renal embolism and thrombosis (N28.0)
retinal embolism and thrombosis (H34.-)
septic embolism and thrombosis (I76)
vertebral embolism and thrombosis (I63.0-I63.2, I65.0)

● **I74.0 Embolism and thrombosis of abdominal aorta**

I74.01 Saddle embolus of abdominal aorta

I74.09 Other arterial embolism and thrombosis of abdominal aorta
Aortic bifurcation syndrome
Aortoiliac obstruction
Leriche's syndrome

● **I74.1 Embolism and thrombosis of other and unspecified parts of aorta**

I74.10 Embolism and thrombosis of unspecified parts of aorta

I74.11 Embolism and thrombosis of thoracic aorta

I74.19 Embolism and thrombosis of other parts of aorta

I74.2 Embolism and thrombosis of arteries of the upper extremities

I74.3 Embolism and thrombosis of arteries of the lower extremities

I74.4 Embolism and thrombosis of arteries of extremities, unspecified
Peripheral arterial embolism NOS

I74.5 Embolism and thrombosis of iliac artery

I74.8 Embolism and thrombosis of other arteries

I74.9 Embolism and thrombosis of unspecified artery

Item 9–9 An **embolus** is a mass of undissolved matter present in the blood that is transported by the blood current. A **thrombus** is a blood clot that occludes or shuts off a vessel. When a thrombus is dislodged, it becomes an embolus.

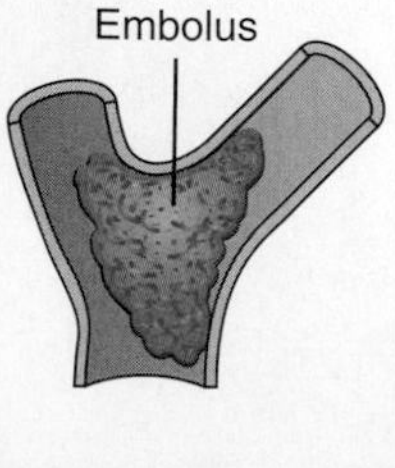

Figure 9-6 An arterial embolus.

● **I75 Atheroembolism**

Includes atherothrombotic microembolism
cholesterol embolism

● **I75.0 Atheroembolism of extremities**

● **I75.01 Atheroembolism of upper extremity**

I75.011 Atheroembolism of right upper extremity

I75.012 Atheroembolism of left upper extremity

I75.013 Atheroembolism of bilateral upper extremities

I75.019 Atheroembolism of unspecified upper extremity

● **I75.02 Atheroembolism of lower extremity**

I75.021 Atheroembolism of right lower extremity

I75.022 Atheroembolism of left lower extremity

I75.023 Atheroembolism of bilateral lower extremities

I75.029 Atheroembolism of unspecified lower extremity

● **I75.8 Atheroembolism of other sites**

I75.81 Atheroembolism of kidney
Use additional code for any associated acute kidney failure and chronic kidney disease (N17.-, N18.-)

I75.89 Atheroembolism of other site

I76 Septic arterial embolism

Code first underlying infection, such as:
infective endocarditis (I33.0)
lung abscess (J85.-)

Use additional code to identify the site of the embolism (I74.-)

Excludes2 septic pulmonary embolism (I26.01, I26.90)

● **I77 Other disorders of arteries and arterioles**

Excludes2 collagen (vascular) diseases (M30-M36)
hypersensitivity angiitis (M31.0)
pulmonary artery (I28.-)

I77.0 Arteriovenous fistula, acquired
Aneurysmal varix
Arteriovenous aneurysm, acquired

Excludes1 arteriovenous aneurysm NOS (Q27.3-)
presence of arteriovenous shunt (fistula) for dialysis (Z99.2)
traumatic - see injury of blood vessel by body region

Excludes2 cerebral (I67.1)
coronary (I25.4)

I77.1 Stricture of artery
Narrowing of artery

I77.2 Rupture of artery
Erosion of artery
Fistula of artery
Ulcer of artery

Excludes1 traumatic rupture of artery - see injury of blood vessel by body region

I77.3 Arterial fibromuscular dysplasia
Fibromuscular hyperplasia (of) carotid artery
Fibromuscular hyperplasia (of) renal artery

I77.4 Celiac artery compression syndrome

I77.5 Necrosis of artery

I77.6 Arteritis, unspecified
Aortitis NOS
Endarteritis NOS
Excludes1 arteritis or endarteritis:
aortic arch (M31.4)
cerebral NEC (I67.7)
coronary (I25.89)
deformans (I70.-)
giant cell (M31.5., M31.6)
obliterans (I70.-)
senile (I70.-)

● **I77.7 Other arterial dissection**
Excludes2 dissection of aorta (I71.0-)
dissection of coronary artery (I25.42)

I77.70 Dissection of unspecified artery ◀

I77.71 Dissection of carotid artery

I77.72 Dissection of iliac artery

I77.73 Dissection of renal artery

I77.74 Dissection of vertebral artery
Excludes2 aneurysm of vertebral artery (I72.6) ◀

I77.75 Dissection of other precerebral arteries ◀
Dissection of basilar artery (trunk) ◀
Excludes2 aneurysm of carotid artery (I72.0) ◀
aneurysm of other precerebral arteries (I72.5) ◀
aneurysm of vertebral artery (I72.6) ◀
dissection of carotid artery (I77.71) ◀
dissection of vertebral artery (I77.74) ◀

I77.76 Dissection of artery of upper extremity ◀

I77.77 Dissection of artery of lower extremity ◀

I77.79 Dissection of other specified artery ⬅

● **I77.8 Other specified disorders of arteries and arterioles**

I77.81 Aortic ectasia
Ectasis aorta
Excludes1 aortic aneurysm and dissection (I71.0-)

I77.810 Thoracic aortic ectasia

I77.811 Abdominal aortic ectasia

I77.812 Thoracoabdominal aortic ectasia

I77.819 Aortic ectasia, unspecified site

I77.89 Other specified disorders of arteries and arterioles

I77.9 Disorder of arteries and arterioles, unspecified

● **I78 Diseases of capillaries**

I78.0 Hereditary hemorrhagic telangiectasia
Rendu-Osler-Weber disease

I78.1 Nevus, non-neoplastic
Araneus nevus
Spider nevus
Senile nevus
Stellar nevus
Excludes1 nevus NOS (D22.-)
vascular NOS (Q82.5)
Excludes2 blue nevus (D22.-)
flammeus nevus (Q82.5)
hairy nevus (D22.-)
melanocytic nevus (D22.-)
pigmented nevus (D22.-)
portwine nevus (Q82.5)
sanguineous nevus (Q82.5)
strawberry nevus (Q82.5)
verrucous nevus (Q82.5)

I78.8 Other diseases of capillaries

I78.9 Disease of capillaries, unspecified

● **I79 Disorders of arteries, arterioles and capillaries in diseases classified elsewhere**

I79.0 Aneurysm of aorta in diseases classified elsewhere
Code first *underlying disease*
Excludes1 syphilitic aneurysm (A52.01)

I79.1 Aortitis in diseases classified elsewhere
Code first *underlying disease*
Excludes1 syphilitic aortitis (A52.02)

I79.8 Other disorders of arteries, arterioles and capillaries in diseases classified elsewhere
Code first *underlying disease, such as:*
amyloidosis (E85.-)
Excludes1 diabetic (peripheral) angiopathy (E08-E13 with .51-.52)
syphilitic endarteritis (A52.09)
tuberculous endarteritis (A18.89)

DISEASES OF VEINS, LYMPHATIC VESSELS AND LYMPH NODES, NOT ELSEWHERE CLASSIFIED (I80-I89)

● **I80 Phlebitis and thrombophlebitis**
Inflammation of a vein with infiltration of walls (phlebitis).
Includes endophlebitis
inflammation, vein
periphlebitis
suppurative phlebitis
Code first phlebitis and thrombophlebitis complicating abortion, ectopic or molar pregnancy (O00-O07, O08.7)
phlebitis and thrombophlebitis complicating pregnancy, childbirth and the puerperium (O22.-, O87.-)
Excludes1 venous embolism and thrombosis of lower extremities (I82.4-, I82.5-, I82.81-)

● **I80.0 Phlebitis and thrombophlebitis of superficial vessels of lower extremities**
Phlebitis and thrombophlebitis of femoropopliteal vein

I80.00 Phlebitis and thrombophlebitis of superficial vessels of unspecified lower extremity

I80.01 Phlebitis and thrombophlebitis of superficial vessels of right lower extremity

I80.02 Phlebitis and thrombophlebitis of superficial vessels of left lower extremity

I80.03 Phlebitis and thrombophlebitis of superficial vessels of lower extremities, bilateral

CHAPTER 9 (I00-I99)

● I80.1 **Phlebitis and thrombophlebitis of femoral vein**
- I80.10 **Phlebitis and thrombophlebitis of unspecified femoral vein**
- I80.11 **Phlebitis and thrombophlebitis of right femoral vein**
- I80.12 **Phlebitis and thrombophlebitis of left femoral vein**
- I80.13 **Phlebitis and thrombophlebitis of femoral vein, bilateral**

● I80.2 **Phlebitis and thrombophlebitis of other and unspecified deep vessels of lower extremities**

● I80.20 **Phlebitis and thrombophlebitis of unspecified deep vessels of lower extremities**
- I80.201 **Phlebitis and thrombophlebitis of unspecified deep vessels of right lower extremity**
- I80.202 **Phlebitis and thrombophlebitis of unspecified deep vessels of left lower extremity**
- I80.203 **Phlebitis and thrombophlebitis of unspecified deep vessels of lower extremities, bilateral**
- I80.209 **Phlebitis and thrombophlebitis of unspecified deep vessels of unspecified lower extremity**

● I80.21 **Phlebitis and thrombophlebitis of iliac vein**
- I80.211 **Phlebitis and thrombophlebitis of right iliac vein**
- I80.212 **Phlebitis and thrombophlebitis of left iliac vein**
- I80.213 **Phlebitis and thrombophlebitis of iliac vein, bilateral**
- I80.219 **Phlebitis and thrombophlebitis of unspecified iliac vein**

● I80.22 **Phlebitis and thrombophlebitis of popliteal vein**
- I80.221 **Phlebitis and thrombophlebitis of right popliteal vein**
- I80.222 **Phlebitis and thrombophlebitis of left popliteal vein**
- I80.223 **Phlebitis and thrombophlebitis of popliteal vein, bilateral**
- I80.229 **Phlebitis and thrombophlebitis of unspecified popliteal vein**

● I80.23 **Phlebitis and thrombophlebitis of tibial vein**
- I80.231 **Phlebitis and thrombophlebitis of right tibial vein**
- I80.232 **Phlebitis and thrombophlebitis of left tibial vein**
- I80.233 **Phlebitis and thrombophlebitis of tibial vein, bilateral**
- I80.239 **Phlebitis and thrombophlebitis of unspecified tibial vein**

● I80.29 **Phlebitis and thrombophlebitis of other deep vessels of lower extremities**
- I80.291 **Phlebitis and thrombophlebitis of other deep vessels of right lower extremity**
- I80.292 **Phlebitis and thrombophlebitis of other deep vessels of left lower extremity**
- I80.293 **Phlebitis and thrombophlebitis of other deep vessels of lower extremity, bilateral**
- I80.299 **Phlebitis and thrombophlebitis of other deep vessels of unspecified lower extremity**

I80.3 **Phlebitis and thrombophlebitis of lower extremities, unspecified**

I80.8 **Phlebitis and thrombophlebitis of other sites**

I80.9 **Phlebitis and thrombophlebitis of unspecified site**

I81 **Portal vein thrombosis**
Portal (vein) obstruction
Excludes2 hepatic vein thrombosis (I82.0)
phlebitis of portal vein (K75.1)

● I82 **Other venous embolism and thrombosis**
Code first venous embolism and thrombosis complicating:
abortion, ectopic or molar pregnancy (O00-O07, O08.7)
pregnancy, childbirth and the puerperium (O22.-, O87.-)
Excludes2 venous embolism and thrombosis (of):
cerebral (I63.6, I67.6)
coronary (I21-I25)
intracranial and intraspinal, septic or NOS (G08)
intracranial, nonpyogenic (I67.6)
intraspinal, nonpyogenic (G95.1)
mesenteric (K55.0-) ◀
portal (I81)
pulmonary (I26.-)

I82.0 **Budd-Chiari syndrome**
Hepatic vein thrombosis

I82.1 **Thrombophlebitis migrans**
"White leg" is the other term to describe a migrating thrombus.

● I82.2 **Embolism and thrombosis of vena cava and other thoracic veins**

● I82.21 **Embolism and thrombosis of superior vena cava**
- I82.210 **Acute embolism and thrombosis of superior vena cava**
  Embolism and thrombosis of superior vena cava NOS
- I82.211 **Chronic embolism and thrombosis of superior vena cava**

● I82.22 **Embolism and thrombosis of inferior vena cava**
- I82.220 **Acute embolism and thrombosis of inferior vena cava**
  Embolism and thrombosis of inferior vena cava NOS
- I82.221 **Chronic embolism and thrombosis of inferior vena cava**

● I82.29 **Embolism and thrombosis of other thoracic veins**
Embolism and thrombosis of brachiocephalic (innominate) vein
- I82.290 **Acute embolism and thrombosis of other thoracic veins**
- I82.291 **Chronic embolism and thrombosis of other thoracic veins**

I82.3 **Embolism and thrombosis of renal vein**

● I82.4 **Acute embolism and thrombosis of deep veins of lower extremity**

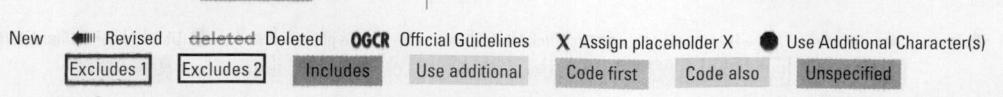

I82.40 **Acute embolism and thrombosis of unspecified deep veins of lower extremity**
Deep vein thrombosis NOS
DVT NOS
Excludes1 acute embolism and thrombosis of unspecified deep veins of distal lower extremity (I82.4Z-)
acute embolism and thrombosis of unspecified deep veins of proximal lower extremity (I82.4Y-)
- I82.401 **Acute embolism and thrombosis of unspecified deep veins of right lower extremity**
- I82.402 **Acute embolism and thrombosis of unspecified deep veins of left lower extremity**
- I82.403 **Acute embolism and thrombosis of unspecified deep veins of lower extremity, bilateral**
- I82.409 **Acute embolism and thrombosis of unspecified deep veins of unspecified lower extremity**

● I82.41 Acute embolism and thrombosis of femoral vein
- I82.411 Acute embolism and thrombosis of right femoral vein
- I82.412 Acute embolism and thrombosis of left femoral vein
- I82.413 Acute embolism and thrombosis of femoral vein, bilateral
- I82.419 Acute embolism and thrombosis of unspecified femoral vein

● I82.42 Acute embolism and thrombosis of iliac vein
- I82.421 Acute embolism and thrombosis of right iliac vein
- I82.422 Acute embolism and thrombosis of left iliac vein
- I82.423 Acute embolism and thrombosis of iliac vein, bilateral
- I82.429 Acute embolism and thrombosis of unspecified iliac vein

● I82.43 Acute embolism and thrombosis of popliteal vein
- I82.431 Acute embolism and thrombosis of right popliteal vein
- I82.432 Acute embolism and thrombosis of left popliteal vein
- I82.433 Acute embolism and thrombosis of popliteal vein, bilateral
- I82.439 Acute embolism and thrombosis of unspecified popliteal vein

● I82.44 Acute embolism and thrombosis of tibial vein
- I82.441 Acute embolism and thrombosis of right tibial vein
- I82.442 Acute embolism and thrombosis of left tibial vein
- I82.443 Acute embolism and thrombosis of tibial vein, bilateral
- I82.449 Acute embolism and thrombosis of unspecified tibial vein

● I82.49 Acute embolism and thrombosis of other specified deep vein of lower extremity
- I82.491 Acute embolism and thrombosis of other specified deep vein of right lower extremity
- I82.492 Acute embolism and thrombosis of other specified deep vein of left lower extremity
- I82.493 Acute embolism and thrombosis of other specified deep vein of lower extremity, bilateral
- I82.499 Acute embolism and thrombosis of other specified deep vein of unspecified lower extremity

● I82.4Y Acute embolism and thrombosis of unspecified deep veins of proximal lower extremity

Acute embolism and thrombosis of deep vein of thigh NOS

Acute embolism and thrombosis of deep vein of upper leg NOS
- I82.4Y1 Acute embolism and thrombosis of unspecified deep veins of right proximal lower extremity
- I82.4Y2 Acute embolism and thrombosis of unspecified deep veins of left proximal lower extremity
- I82.4Y3 Acute embolism and thrombosis of unspecified deep veins of proximal lower extremity, bilateral
- I82.4Y9 Acute embolism and thrombosis of unspecified deep veins of unspecified proximal lower extremity

● I82.4Z Acute embolism and thrombosis of unspecified deep veins of distal lower extremity

Acute embolism and thrombosis of deep vein of calf NOS

Acute embolism and thrombosis of deep vein of lower leg NOS
- I82.4Z1 Acute embolism and thrombosis of unspecified deep veins of right distal lower extremity
- I82.4Z2 Acute embolism and thrombosis of unspecified deep veins of left distal lower extremity
- I82.4Z3 Acute embolism and thrombosis of unspecified deep veins of distal lower extremity, bilateral
- I82.4Z9 Acute embolism and thrombosis of unspecified deep veins of unspecified distal lower extremity

● I82.5 Chronic embolism and thrombosis of deep veins of lower extremity

Use additional code, if applicable, for associated long-term (current) use of anticoagulants (Z79.01)

Excludes1 personal history of venous embolism and thrombosis (Z86.718)

● I82.50 Chronic embolism and thrombosis of unspecified deep veins of lower extremity

Excludes1 chronic embolism and thrombosis of unspecified deep veins of distal lower extremity (I82.5Z-)

chronic embolism and thrombosis of unspecified deep veins of proximal lower extremity (I82.5Y-)
- I82.501 Chronic embolism and thrombosis of unspecified deep veins of right lower extremity
- I82.502 Chronic embolism and thrombosis of unspecified deep veins of left lower extremity
- I82.503 Chronic embolism and thrombosis of unspecified deep veins of lower extremity, bilateral
- I82.509 Chronic embolism and thrombosis of unspecified deep veins of unspecified lower extremity

● I82.51 Chronic embolism and thrombosis of femoral vein
- I82.511 Chronic embolism and thrombosis of right femoral vein
- I82.512 Chronic embolism and thrombosis of left femoral vein
- I82.513 Chronic embolism and thrombosis of femoral vein, bilateral
- I82.519 Chronic embolism and thrombosis of unspecified femoral vein

● I82.52 Chronic embolism and thrombosis of iliac vein
- I82.521 Chronic embolism and thrombosis of right iliac vein
- I82.522 Chronic embolism and thrombosis of left iliac vein
- I82.523 Chronic embolism and thrombosis of iliac vein, bilateral
- I82.529 Chronic embolism and thrombosis of unspecified iliac vein

CHAPTER 9 (I00-I99)

Item 9–10 Varicose/Varicosities (varix = singular, varices = plural): Enlarged, engorged, tortuous, twisted vascular vessels (veins, arteries, lymphatics). As such, the condition can present in various parts of the body, although the most familiar locations are the lower extremities. A common complication of varices is thrombophlebitis. Varicosities of the anus and rectum are called hemorrhoids.

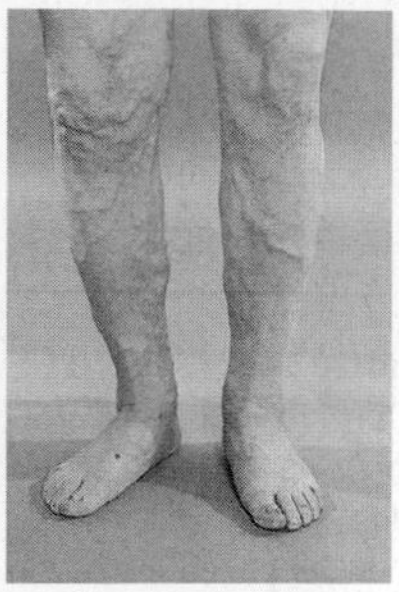

Figure 9-7 Varicose veins of the legs. (From Goldman: Cecil Medicine, ed 23, Saunders, 2008)

● **I82.53 Chronic embolism and thrombosis of popliteal vein**
- **I82.531 Chronic embolism and thrombosis of right popliteal vein**
- **I82.532 Chronic embolism and thrombosis of left popliteal vein**
- **I82.533 Chronic embolism and thrombosis of popliteal vein, bilateral**
- **I82.539 Chronic embolism and thrombosis of unspecified popliteal vein**

● **I82.54 Chronic embolism and thrombosis of tibial vein**
- **I82.541 Chronic embolism and thrombosis of right tibial vein**
- **I82.542 Chronic embolism and thrombosis of left tibial vein**
- **I82.543 Chronic embolism and thrombosis of tibial vein, bilateral**
- **I82.549 Chronic embolism and thrombosis of unspecified tibial vein**

● **I82.59 Chronic embolism and thrombosis of other specified deep vein of lower extremity**
- **I82.591 Chronic embolism and thrombosis of other specified deep vein of right lower extremity**
- **I82.592 Chronic embolism and thrombosis of other specified deep vein of left lower extremity**
- **I82.593 Chronic embolism and thrombosis of other specified deep vein of lower extremity, bilateral**
- **I82.599 Chronic embolism and thrombosis of other specified deep vein of unspecified lower extremity**

● **I82.5Y Chronic embolism and thrombosis of unspecified deep veins of proximal lower extremity**

Chronic embolism and thrombosis of deep veins of thigh NOS

Chronic embolism and thrombosis of deep veins of upper leg NOS
- **I82.5Y1 Chronic embolism and thrombosis of unspecified deep veins of right proximal lower extremity**
- **I82.5Y2 Chronic embolism and thrombosis of unspecified deep veins of left proximal lower extremity**
- **I82.5Y3 Chronic embolism and thrombosis of unspecified deep veins of proximal lower extremity, bilateral**
- **I82.5Y9 Chronic embolism and thrombosis of unspecified deep veins of unspecified proximal lower extremity**

● **I82.5Z Chronic embolism and thrombosis of unspecified deep veins of distal lower extremity**

Chronic embolism and thrombosis of deep veins of calf NOS

Chronic embolism and thrombosis of deep veins of lower leg NOS
- **I82.5Z1 Chronic embolism and thrombosis of unspecified deep veins of right distal lower extremity**
- **I82.5Z2 Chronic embolism and thrombosis of unspecified deep veins of left distal lower extremity**
- **I82.5Z3 Chronic embolism and thrombosis of unspecified deep veins of distal lower extremity, bilateral**
- **I82.5Z9 Chronic embolism and thrombosis of unspecified deep veins of unspecified distal lower extremity**

● **I82.6 Acute embolism and thrombosis of veins of upper extremity**

● **I82.6Ø Acute embolism and thrombosis of unspecified veins of upper extremity**
- **I82.6Ø1 Acute embolism and thrombosis of unspecified veins of right upper extremity**
- **I82.6Ø2 Acute embolism and thrombosis of unspecified veins of left upper extremity**
- **I82.6Ø3 Acute embolism and thrombosis of unspecified veins of upper extremity, bilateral**
- **I82.6Ø9 Acute embolism and thrombosis of unspecified veins of unspecified upper extremity**

● **I82.61 Acute embolism and thrombosis of superficial veins of upper extremity**

Acute embolism and thrombosis of antecubital vein

Acute embolism and thrombosis of basilic vein

Acute embolism and thrombosis of cephalic vein
- **I82.611 Acute embolism and thrombosis of superficial veins of right upper extremity**
- **I82.612 Acute embolism and thrombosis of superficial veins of left upper extremity**
- **I82.613 Acute embolism and thrombosis of superficial veins of upper extremity, bilateral**
- **I82.619 Acute embolism and thrombosis of superficial veins of unspecified upper extremity**

● **I82.62 Acute embolism and thrombosis of deep veins of upper extremity**

Acute embolism and thrombosis of brachial vein

Acute embolism and thrombosis of radial vein

Acute embolism and thrombosis of ulnar vein
- **I82.621 Acute embolism and thrombosis of deep veins of right upper extremity**
- **I82.622 Acute embolism and thrombosis of deep veins of left upper extremity**
- **I82.623 Acute embolism and thrombosis of deep veins of upper extremity, bilateral**
- **I82.629 Acute embolism and thrombosis of deep veins of unspecified upper extremity**

● **I82.7 Chronic embolism and thrombosis of veins of upper extremity**

Use additional code, if applicable, for associated long-term (current) use of anticoagulants (Z79.01)

Excludes1 personal history of venous embolism and thrombosis (Z86.718)

● **I82.70 Chronic embolism and thrombosis of unspecified veins of upper extremity**

I82.701 Chronic embolism and thrombosis of unspecified veins of right upper extremity

I82.702 Chronic embolism and thrombosis of unspecified veins of left upper extremity

I82.703 Chronic embolism and thrombosis of unspecified veins of upper extremity, bilateral

I82.709 Chronic embolism and thrombosis of unspecified veins of unspecified upper extremity

● **I82.71 Chronic embolism and thrombosis of superficial veins of upper extremity**

Chronic embolism and thrombosis of antecubital vein

Chronic embolism and thrombosis of basilic vein

Chronic embolism and thrombosis of cephalic vein

I82.711 Chronic embolism and thrombosis of superficial veins of right upper extremity

I82.712 Chronic embolism and thrombosis of superficial veins of left upper extremity

I82.713 Chronic embolism and thrombosis of superficial veins of upper extremity, bilateral

I82.719 Chronic embolism and thrombosis of superficial veins of unspecified upper extremity

● **I82.72 Chronic embolism and thrombosis of deep veins of upper extremity**

Chronic embolism and thrombosis of brachial vein

Chronic embolism and thrombosis of radial vein

Chronic embolism and thrombosis of ulnar vein

I82.721 Chronic embolism and thrombosis of deep veins of right upper extremity

I82.722 Chronic embolism and thrombosis of deep veins of left upper extremity

I82.723 Chronic embolism and thrombosis of deep veins of upper extremity, bilateral

I82.729 Chronic embolism and thrombosis of deep veins of unspecified upper extremity

● **I82.A Embolism and thrombosis of axillary vein**

● **I82.A1 Acute embolism and thrombosis of axillary vein**

I82.A11 Acute embolism and thrombosis of right axillary vein

I82.A12 Acute embolism and thrombosis of left axillary vein

I82.A13 Acute embolism and thrombosis of axillary vein, bilateral

I82.A19 Acute embolism and thrombosis of unspecified axillary vein

● **I82.A2 Chronic embolism and thrombosis of axillary vein**

I82.A21 Chronic embolism and thrombosis of right axillary vein

I82.A22 Chronic embolism and thrombosis of left axillary vein

I82.A23 Chronic embolism and thrombosis of axillary vein, bilateral

I82.A29 Chronic embolism and thrombosis of unspecified axillary vein

● **I82.B Embolism and thrombosis of subclavian vein**

● **I82.B1 Acute embolism and thrombosis of subclavian vein**

I82.B11 Acute embolism and thrombosis of right subclavian vein

I82.B12 Acute embolism and thrombosis of left subclavian vein

I82.B13 Acute embolism and thrombosis of subclavian vein, bilateral

I82.B19 Acute embolism and thrombosis of unspecified subclavian vein

● **I82.B2 Chronic embolism and thrombosis of subclavian vein**

I82.B21 Chronic embolism and thrombosis of right subclavian vein

I82.B22 Chronic embolism and thrombosis of left subclavian vein

I82.B23 Chronic embolism and thrombosis of subclavian vein, bilateral

I82.B29 Chronic embolism and thrombosis of unspecified subclavian vein

● **I82.C Embolism and thrombosis of internal jugular vein**

● **I82.C1 Acute embolism and thrombosis of internal jugular vein**

I82.C11 Acute embolism and thrombosis of right internal jugular vein

I82.C12 Acute embolism and thrombosis of left internal jugular vein

I82.C13 Acute embolism and thrombosis of internal jugular vein, bilateral

I82.C19 Acute embolism and thrombosis of unspecified internal jugular vein

● **I82.C2 Chronic embolism and thrombosis of internal jugular vein**

I82.C21 Chronic embolism and thrombosis of right internal jugular vein

I82.C22 Chronic embolism and thrombosis of left internal jugular vein

I82.C23 Chronic embolism and thrombosis of internal jugular vein, bilateral

I82.C29 Chronic embolism and thrombosis of unspecified internal jugular vein

● **I82.8 Embolism and thrombosis of other specified veins**

Use additional code, if applicable, for associated long-term (current) use of anticoagulants (Z79.01)

● **I82.81 Embolism and thrombosis of superficial veins of lower extremities**

Embolism and thrombosis of saphenous vein (greater) (lesser)

I82.811 Embolism and thrombosis of superficial veins of right lower extremities

I82.812 Embolism and thrombosis of superficial veins of left lower extremities

I82.813 Embolism and thrombosis of superficial veins of lower extremities, bilateral

I82.819 Embolism and thrombosis of superficial veins of unspecified lower extremities

● I82.89 **Embolism and thrombosis of other specified veins**
- I82.890 **Acute embolism and thrombosis of other specified veins**
- I82.891 **Chronic embolism and thrombosis of other specified veins**

● I82.9 **Embolism and thrombosis of unspecified vein**
- I82.90 **Acute embolism and thrombosis of unspecified vein**
  - Embolism of vein NOS
  - Thrombosis (vein) NOS
- I82.91 **Chronic embolism and thrombosis of unspecified vein**

● I83 **Varicose veins of lower extremities**

Excludes1 varicose veins complicating pregnancy (O22.0-)
varicose veins complicating the puerperium (O87.4)

● I83.0 **Varicose veins of lower extremities with ulcer**

Use additional code to identify severity of ulcer (L97.-)

● I83.00 **Varicose veins of unspecified lower extremity with ulcer**
- I83.001 **Varicose veins of unspecified lower extremity with ulcer of thigh**
- I83.002 **Varicose veins of unspecified lower extremity with ulcer of calf**
- I83.003 **Varicose veins of unspecified lower extremity with ulcer of ankle**
- I83.004 **Varicose veins of unspecified lower extremity with ulcer of heel and midfoot**
  - Varicose veins of unspecified lower extremity with ulcer of plantar surface of midfoot
- I83.005 **Varicose veins of unspecified lower extremity with ulcer other part of foot**
  - Varicose veins of unspecified lower extremity with ulcer of toe
- I83.008 **Varicose veins of unspecified lower extremity with ulcer other part of lower leg**
- I83.009 **Varicose veins of unspecified lower extremity with ulcer of unspecified site**

● I83.01 **Varicose veins of right lower extremity with ulcer**
- I83.011 **Varicose veins of right lower extremity with ulcer of thigh**
- I83.012 **Varicose veins of right lower extremity with ulcer of calf**
- I83.013 **Varicose veins of right lower extremity with ulcer of ankle**
- I83.014 **Varicose veins of right lower extremity with ulcer of heel and midfoot**
  - Varicose veins of right lower extremity with ulcer of plantar surface of midfoot
- I83.015 **Varicose veins of right lower extremity with ulcer other part of foot**
  - Varicose veins of right lower extremity with ulcer of toe
- I83.018 **Varicose veins of right lower extremity with ulcer other part of lower leg**
- I83.019 **Varicose veins of right lower extremity with ulcer of unspecified site**

● I83.02 **Varicose veins of left lower extremity with ulcer**
- I83.021 **Varicose veins of left lower extremity with ulcer of thigh**
- I83.022 **Varicose veins of left lower extremity with ulcer of calf**
- I83.023 **Varicose veins of left lower extremity with ulcer of ankle**
- I83.024 **Varicose veins of left lower extremity with ulcer of heel and midfoot**
  - Varicose veins of left lower extremity with ulcer of plantar surface of midfoot
- I83.025 **Varicose veins of left lower extremity with ulcer other part of foot**
  - Varicose veins of left lower extremity with ulcer of toe
- I83.028 **Varicose veins of left lower extremity with ulcer other part of lower leg**
- I83.029 **Varicose veins of left lower extremity with ulcer of unspecified site**

● I83.1 **Varicose veins of lower extremities with inflammation**

~~Stasis dermatitis~~
- I83.10 **Varicose veins of unspecified lower extremity with inflammation**
- I83.11 **Varicose veins of right lower extremity with inflammation**
- I83.12 **Varicose veins of left lower extremity with inflammation**

● I83.2 **Varicose veins of lower extremities with both ulcer and inflammation**

Use additional code to identify severity of ulcer (L97.-)

● I83.20 **Varicose veins of unspecified lower extremity with both ulcer and inflammation**
- I83.201 **Varicose veins of unspecified lower extremity with both ulcer of thigh and inflammation**
- I83.202 **Varicose veins of unspecified lower extremity with both ulcer of calf and inflammation**
- I83.203 **Varicose veins of unspecified lower extremity with both ulcer of ankle and inflammation**
- I83.204 **Varicose veins of unspecified lower extremity with both ulcer of heel and midfoot and inflammation**
  - Varicose veins of unspecified lower extremity with both ulcer of plantar surface of midfoot and inflammation
- I83.205 **Varicose veins of unspecified lower extremity with both ulcer other part of foot and inflammation**
  - Varicose veins of unspecified lower extremity with both ulcer of toe and inflammation
- I83.208 **Varicose veins of unspecified lower extremity with both ulcer of other part of lower extremity and inflammation**
- I83.209 **Varicose veins of unspecified lower extremity with both ulcer of unspecified site and inflammation**

● I83.21 **Varicose veins of right lower extremity with both ulcer and inflammation**
- I83.211 **Varicose veins of right lower extremity with both ulcer of thigh and inflammation**
- I83.212 **Varicose veins of right lower extremity with both ulcer of calf and inflammation**
- I83.213 **Varicose veins of right lower extremity with both ulcer of ankle and inflammation**
- I83.214 **Varicose veins of right lower extremity with both ulcer of heel and midfoot and inflammation**
  Varicose veins of right lower extremity with both ulcer of plantar surface of midfoot and inflammation
- I83.215 **Varicose veins of right lower extremity with both ulcer other part of foot and inflammation**
  Varicose veins of right lower extremity with both ulcer of toe and inflammation
- I83.218 **Varicose veins of right lower extremity with both ulcer of other part of lower extremity and inflammation**
- I83.219 **Varicose veins of right lower extremity with both ulcer of unspecified site and inflammation**

● I83.22 **Varicose veins of left lower extremity with both ulcer and inflammation**
- I83.221 **Varicose veins of left lower extremity with both ulcer of thigh and inflammation**
- I83.222 **Varicose veins of left lower extremity with both ulcer of calf and inflammation**
- I83.223 **Varicose veins of left lower extremity with both ulcer of ankle and inflammation**
- I83.224 **Varicose veins of left lower extremity with both ulcer of heel and midfoot and inflammation**
  Varicose veins of left lower extremity with both ulcer of plantar surface of midfoot and inflammation
- I83.225 **Varicose veins of left lower extremity with both ulcer other part of foot and inflammation**
  Varicose veins of left lower extremity with both ulcer of toe and inflammation
- I83.228 **Varicose veins of left lower extremity with both ulcer of other part of lower extremity and inflammation**
- I83.229 **Varicose veins of left lower extremity with both ulcer of unspecified site and inflammation**

● I83.8 **Varicose veins of lower extremities with other complications**

● I83.81 **Varicose veins of lower extremities with pain**
- I83.811 **Varicose veins of right lower extremities with pain**
- I83.812 **Varicose veins of left lower extremities with pain**
- I83.813 **Varicose veins of bilateral lower extremities with pain**
- I83.819 **Varicose veins of unspecified lower extremities with pain**

● I83.89 **Varicose veins of lower extremities with other complications**
  Varicose veins of lower extremities with edema
  Varicose veins of lower extremities with swelling
- I83.891 **Varicose veins of right lower extremities with other complications**
- I83.892 **Varicose veins of left lower extremities with other complications**
- I83.893 **Varicose veins of bilateral lower extremities with other complications**
- I83.899 **Varicose veins of unspecified lower extremities with other complications**

● I83.9 **Asymptomatic varicose veins of lower extremities**
  Phlebectasia of lower extremities
  Varicose veins of lower extremities
  Varix of lower extremities
- I83.90 **Asymptomatic varicose veins of unspecified lower extremity**
  Varicose veins NOS
- I83.91 **Asymptomatic varicose veins of right lower extremity**
- I83.92 **Asymptomatic varicose veins of left lower extremity**
- I83.93 **Asymptomatic varicose veins of bilateral lower extremities**

● I85 **Esophageal varices**
  Use additional code to identify:
  alcohol abuse and dependence (F10.-)

● I85.0 **Esophageal varices**
  Idiopathic esophageal varices
  Primary esophageal varices
- I85.00 **Esophageal varices without bleeding**
  Esophageal varices NOS
- I85.01 **Esophageal varices with bleeding**

● I85.1 **Secondary esophageal varices**
  Esophageal varices secondary to alcoholic liver disease
  Esophageal varices secondary to cirrhosis of liver
  Esophageal varices secondary to schistosomiasis
  Esophageal varices secondary to toxic liver disease
  Code first underlying disease
- I85.10 **Secondary esophageal varices without bleeding**
- I85.11 **Secondary esophageal varices with bleeding**

● I86 **Varicose veins of other sites**
  Excludes1 varicose veins of unspecified site (I83.9-)
  Excludes2 retinal varices (H35.0-)
- I86.0 **Sublingual varices**
- I86.1 **Scrotal varices**
  Varicocele
- I86.2 **Pelvic varices**
- I86.3 **Vulval varices**
  Excludes1 vulval varices complicating childbirth and the puerperium (O87.8)
  vulval varices complicating pregnancy (O22.1-)
- I86.4 **Gastric varices**
- I86.8 **Varicose veins of other specified sites**
  Varicose ulcer of nasal septum

CHAPTER 9 (I00-I99)

● I87 **Other disorders of veins**

● I87.Ø **Postthrombotic syndrome**

Chronic venous hypertension due to deep vein thrombosis

Postphlebitic syndrome

Excludes1 chronic venous hypertension without deep vein thrombosis (I87.3-)

● I87.ØØ **Postthrombotic syndrome without complications**

Asymptomatic Postthrombotic syndrome

I87.ØØ1 **Postthrombotic syndrome without complications of right lower extremity**

I87.ØØ2 **Postthrombotic syndrome without complications of left lower extremity**

I87.ØØ3 **Postthrombotic syndrome without complications of bilateral lower extremity**

I87.ØØ9 **Postthrombotic syndrome without complications of unspecified extremity**

Postthrombotic syndrome NOS

● I87.Ø1 **Postthrombotic syndrome with ulcer**

Use additional code to specify site and severity of ulcer (L97.-)

I87.Ø11 **Postthrombotic syndrome with ulcer of right lower extremity**

I87.Ø12 **Postthrombotic syndrome with ulcer of left lower extremity**

I87.Ø13 **Postthrombotic syndrome with ulcer of bilateral lower extremity**

I87.Ø19 **Postthrombotic syndrome with ulcer of unspecified lower extremity**

● I87.Ø2 **Postthrombotic syndrome with inflammation**

I87.Ø21 **Postthrombotic syndrome with inflammation of right lower extremity**

I87.Ø22 **Postthrombotic syndrome with inflammation of left lower extremity**

I87.Ø23 **Postthrombotic syndrome with inflammation of bilateral lower extremity**

I87.Ø29 **Postthrombotic syndrome with inflammation of unspecified lower extremity**

● I87.Ø3 **Postthrombotic syndrome with ulcer and inflammation**

Use additional code to specify site and severity of ulcer (L97.-)

I87.Ø31 **Postthrombotic syndrome with ulcer and inflammation of right lower extremity**

I87.Ø32 **Postthrombotic syndrome with ulcer and inflammation of left lower extremity**

I87.Ø33 **Postthrombotic syndrome with ulcer and inflammation of bilateral lower extremity**

I87.Ø39 **Postthrombotic syndrome with ulcer and inflammation of unspecified lower extremity**

● I87.Ø9 **Postthrombotic syndrome with other complications**

I87.Ø91 **Postthrombotic syndrome with other complications of right lower extremity**

I87.Ø92 **Postthrombotic syndrome with other complications of left lower extremity**

I87.Ø93 **Postthrombotic syndrome with other complications of bilateral lower extremity**

I87.Ø99 **Postthrombotic syndrome with other complications of unspecified lower extremity**

I87.1 **Compression of vein**

Stricture of vein

Vena cava syndrome (inferior) (superior)

Excludes2 compression of pulmonary vein (I28.8)

I87.2 **Venous insufficiency (chronic) (peripheral)**

Stasis dermatitis ◀

Excludes1 stasis dermatitis with varicose veins of lower extremities (I83.1-, I83.2-) ◀

● I87.3 **Chronic venous hypertension (idiopathic)**

Stasis edema

Excludes1 chronic venous hypertension due to deep vein thrombosis (I87.Ø-)

varicose veins of lower extremities (I83.-)

● I87.3Ø **Chronic venous hypertension (idiopathic) without complications**

Asymptomatic chronic venous hypertension (idiopathic)

I87.3Ø1 **Chronic venous hypertension (idiopathic) without complications of right lower extremity**

I87.3Ø2 **Chronic venous hypertension (idiopathic) without complications of left lower extremity**

I87.3Ø3 **Chronic venous hypertension (idiopathic) without complications of bilateral lower extremity**

I87.3Ø9 **Chronic venous hypertension (idiopathic) without complications of unspecified lower extremity**

Chronic venous hypertension NOS

● I87.31 **Chronic venous hypertension (idiopathic) with ulcer**

Use additional code to specify site and severity of ulcer (L97.-)

I87.311 **Chronic venous hypertension (idiopathic) with ulcer of right lower extremity**

I87.312 **Chronic venous hypertension (idiopathic) with ulcer of left lower extremity**

I87.313 **Chronic venous hypertension (idiopathic) with ulcer of bilateral lower extremity**

I87.319 **Chronic venous hypertension (idiopathic) with ulcer of unspecified lower extremity**

● **I87.32 Chronic venous hypertension (idiopathic) with inflammation**

I87.321 Chronic venous hypertension (idiopathic) with inflammation of right lower extremity

I87.322 Chronic venous hypertension (idiopathic) with inflammation of left lower extremity

I87.323 Chronic venous hypertension (idiopathic) with inflammation of bilateral lower extremity

I87.329 Chronic venous hypertension (idiopathic) with inflammation of unspecified lower extremity

● **I87.33 Chronic venous hypertension (idiopathic) with ulcer and inflammation**

Use additional code to specify site and severity of ulcer (L97.-)

I87.331 Chronic venous hypertension (idiopathic) with ulcer and inflammation of right lower extremity

I87.332 Chronic venous hypertension (idiopathic) with ulcer and inflammation of left lower extremity

I87.333 Chronic venous hypertension (idiopathic) with ulcer and inflammation of bilateral lower extremity

I87.339 Chronic venous hypertension (idiopathic) with ulcer and inflammation of unspecified lower extremity

● **I87.39 Chronic venous hypertension (idiopathic) with other complications**

I87.391 Chronic venous hypertension (idiopathic) with other complications of right lower extremity

I87.392 Chronic venous hypertension (idiopathic) with other complications of left lower extremity

I87.393 Chronic venous hypertension (idiopathic) with other complications of bilateral lower extremity

I87.399 Chronic venous hypertension (idiopathic) with other complications of unspecified lower extremity

I87.8 Other specified disorders of veins

Phlebosclerosis

Venofibrosis

I87.9 Disorder of vein, unspecified

● **I88 Nonspecific lymphadenitis**

Excludes1 acute lymphadenitis, except mesenteric (L04.-)

enlarged lymph nodes NOS (R59.-)

human immunodeficiency virus [HIV] disease resulting in generalized lymphadenopathy (B20)

I88.0 Nonspecific mesenteric lymphadenitis

Mesenteric lymphadenitis (acute)(chronic)

I88.1 Chronic lymphadenitis, except mesenteric

Adenitis

Lymphadenitis

I88.8 Other nonspecific lymphadenitis

I88.9 Nonspecific lymphadenitis, unspecified

Lymphadenitis NOS

● **I89 Other noninfective disorders of lymphatic vessels and lymph nodes**

Excludes1 chylocele, tunica vaginalis (nonfilarial) NOS (N50.89) ◄

enlarged lymph nodes NOS (R59.-)

filarial chylocele (B74.-)

hereditary lymphedema (Q82.0)

I89.0 Lymphedema, not elsewhere classified

Elephantiasis (nonfilarial) NOS

Lymphangiectasis

Obliteration, lymphatic vessel

Praecox lymphedema

Secondary lymphedema

Excludes1 postmastectomy lymphedema (I97.2)

I89.1 Lymphangitis

Chronic lymphangitis

Lymphangitis NOS

Subacute lymphangitis

Excludes1 acute lymphangitis (L03.-)

I89.8 Other specified noninfective disorders of lymphatic vessels and lymph nodes

Chylocele (nonfilarial)

Chylous ascites

Chylous cyst

Lipomelanotic reticulosis

Lymph node or vessel fistula

Lymph node or vessel infarction

Lymph node or vessel rupture

I89.9 Noninfective disorder of lymphatic vessels and lymph nodes, unspecified

Disease of lymphatic vessels NOS

OTHER AND UNSPECIFIED DISORDERS OF THE CIRCULATORY SYSTEM (I95-I99)

● **I95 Hypotension**

Subnormal arterial blood pressure

Excludes1 cardiovascular collapse (R57.9)

maternal hypotension syndrome (O26.5-)

nonspecific low blood pressure reading NOS (R03.1)

I95.0 Idiopathic hypotension

I95.1 Orthostatic hypotension

Hypotension, postural

Moving from a sitting or reclining position to a standing position precipitates a sudden drop in blood pressure (hypotension).

Excludes1 neurogenic orthostatic hypotension [Shy-Drager] (G90.3)

orthostatic hypotension due to drugs (I95.2)

I95.2 Hypotension due to drugs

Orthostatic hypotension due to drugs

Use additional code for adverse effect, if applicable, to identify drug (T36-T50 with fifth or sixth character 5)

I95.3 Hypotension of hemodialysis

Intra-dialytic hypotension

● **I95.8 Other hypotension**

I95.81 Postprocedural hypotension

I95.89 Other hypotension

Chronic hypotension

I95.9 Hypotension, unspecified

CHAPTER 9 (I00-I99)

I96 Gangrene, not elsewhere classified
Gangrenous cellulitis
Excludes1 gangrene in atherosclerosis of native arteries of the extremities (I7Ø.26)
gangrene of certain specified sites - *see* Alphabetical Index
gangrene in diabetes mellitus (EØ8-E13 with .52)
gangrene in hernia (K4Ø.1, K4Ø.4, K41.1, K41.4, K42.1, K43.1-, K44.1, K45.1, K46.1)
gangrene in other peripheral vascular diseases (I73.-)
gas gangrene (A48.Ø)
pyoderma gangrenosum (L88)

● I97 Intraoperative and postprocedural complications and disorders of circulatory system, not elsewhere classified
Excludes2 postprocedural shock (T81.1-)

I97.Ø Postcardiotomy syndrome

● I97.1 Other postprocedural cardiac functional disturbances
Excludes2 acute pulmonary insufficiency following thoracic surgery (J95.1)
intraoperative cardiac functional disturbances (I97.7-)

● I97.11 Postprocedural cardiac insufficiency
I97.11Ø Postprocedural cardiac insufficiency following cardiac surgery
I97.111 Postprocedural cardiac insufficiency following other surgery

● I97.12 Postprocedural cardiac arrest
I97.12Ø Postprocedural cardiac arrest following cardiac surgery
I97.121 Postprocedural cardiac arrest following other surgery

● I97.13 Postprocedural heart failure
Use additional code to identify the heart failure (I5Ø.-)
I97.13Ø Postprocedural heart failure following cardiac surgery
I97.131 Postprocedural heart failure following other surgery

● I97.19 Other postprocedural cardiac functional disturbances
Use additional code, if applicable, to further specify disorder
I97.19Ø Other postprocedural cardiac functional disturbances following cardiac surgery
I97.191 Other postprocedural cardiac functional disturbances following other surgery

I97.2 Postmastectomy lymphedema syndrome
Elephantiasis due to mastectomy
Obliteration of lymphatic vessels

I97.3 Postprocedural hypertension

● I97.4 Intraoperative hemorrhage and hematoma of a circulatory system organ or structure complicating a procedure
Excludes1 intraoperative hemorrhage and hematoma of a circulatory system organ or structure due to accidental puncture and laceration during a procedure (I97.5-)
Excludes2 intraoperative cerebrovascular hemorrhage complicating a procedure (G97.3-)

● I97.41 Intraoperative hemorrhage and hematoma of a circulatory system organ or structure complicating a circulatory system procedure
I97.41Ø Intraoperative hemorrhage and hematoma of a circulatory system organ or structure complicating a cardiac catheterization
I97.411 Intraoperative hemorrhage and hematoma of a circulatory system organ or structure complicating a cardiac bypass
I97.418 Intraoperative hemorrhage and hematoma of a circulatory system organ or structure complicating other circulatory system procedure

I97.42 Intraoperative hemorrhage and hematoma of a circulatory system organ or structure complicating other procedure

● I97.5 Accidental puncture and laceration of a circulatory system organ or structure during a procedure
Excludes2 accidental puncture and laceration of brain during a procedure (G97.4-)

I97.51 Accidental puncture and laceration of a circulatory system organ or structure during a circulatory system procedure
I97.52 Accidental puncture and laceration of a circulatory system organ or structure during other procedure

● I97.6 Postprocedural hemorrhage, hematoma and seroma of a circulatory system organ or structure following a procedure
Excludes2 postprocedural cerebrovascular hemorrhage complicating a procedure (G97.5-)

● I97.61 Postprocedural hemorrhage of a circulatory system organ or structure following a circulatory system procedure
I97.61Ø Postprocedural hemorrhage of a circulatory system organ or structure following a cardiac catheterization
I97.611 Postprocedural hemorrhage of a circulatory system organ or structure following cardiac bypass
I97.618 Postprocedural hemorrhage of a circulatory system organ or structure following other circulatory system procedure

CHAPTER 9 (IØØ-I99)

● I97.62 **Postprocedural hemorrhage, hematoma and seroma of a circulatory system organ or structure following other procedure**

I97.620 **Postprocedural hemorrhage of a circulatory system organ or structure following other procedure** ◀

I97.621 **Postprocedural hematoma of a circulatory system organ or structure following other procedure** ◀

I97.622 **Postprocedural seroma of a circulatory system organ or structure following other procedure** ◀

● I97.63 **Postprocedural hematoma of a circulatory system organ or structure following a circulatory system procedure** ◀

I97.630 **Postprocedural hematoma of a circulatory system organ or structure following a cardiac catheterization** ◀

I97.631 **Postprocedural hematoma of a circulatory system organ or structure following cardiac bypass** ◀

I97.638 **Postprocedural hematoma of a circulatory system organ or structure following other circulatory system procedure** ◀

● I97.64 **Postprocedural seroma of a circulatory system organ or structure following a circulatory system procedure** ◀

I97.640 **Postprocedural seroma of a circulatory system organ or structure following a cardiac catheterization** ◀

I97.641 **Postprocedural seroma of a circulatory system organ or structure following cardiac bypass** ◀

I97.648 **Postprocedural seroma of a circulatory system organ or structure following other circulatory system procedure** ◀

● I97.7 **Intraoperative cardiac functional disturbances**

Excludes2 acute pulmonary insufficiency following thoracic surgery (J95.1)
postprocedural cardiac functional disturbances (I97.1-)

● I97.71 **Intraoperative cardiac arrest**

I97.710 **Intraoperative cardiac arrest during cardiac surgery**

I97.711 **Intraoperative cardiac arrest during other surgery**

● I97.79 **Other intraoperative cardiac functional disturbances**

Use additional code, if applicable, to further specify disorder

I97.790 **Other intraoperative cardiac functional disturbances during cardiac surgery**

I97.791 **Other intraoperative cardiac functional disturbances during other surgery**

● I97.8 **Other intraoperative and postprocedural complications and disorders of the circulatory system, not elsewhere classified**

Use additional code, if applicable, to further specify disorder

● I97.81 **Intraoperative cerebrovascular infarction**

I97.810 **Intraoperative cerebrovascular infarction during cardiac surgery**

I97.811 **Intraoperative cerebrovascular infarction during other surgery**

● I97.82 **Postprocedural cerebrovascular infarction**

I97.820 **Postprocedural cerebrovascular infarction following cardiac surgery**

I97.821 **Postprocedural cerebrovascular infarction following other surgery**

I97.88 **Other intraoperative complications of the circulatory system, not elsewhere classified**

I97.89 **Other postprocedural complications and disorders of the circulatory system, not elsewhere classified**

● I99 **Other and unspecified disorders of circulatory system**

I99.8 **Other disorder of circulatory system**

I99.9 **Unspecified disorder of circulatory system**

CHAPTER 10

DISEASES OF THE RESPIRATORY SYSTEM (J00-J99)

OGCR Chapter-Specific Coding Guidelines

10. Chapter 10: Diseases of the Respiratory System (J00-J99)

a. Chronic Obstructive Pulmonary Disease [COPD] and Asthma

1) Acute exacerbation of chronic obstructive bronchitis and asthma

The codes in categories J44 and J45 distinguish between uncomplicated cases and those in acute exacerbation. An acute exacerbation is a worsening or a decompensation of a chronic condition. An acute exacerbation is not equivalent to an infection superimposed on a chronic condition, though an exacerbation may be triggered by an infection.

b. Acute Respiratory Failure

1) Acute respiratory failure as principal diagnosis

A code from subcategory J96.0, Acute respiratory failure, or subcategory J96.2, Acute and chronic respiratory failure, may be assigned as a principal diagnosis when it is the condition established after study to be chiefly responsible for occasioning the admission to the hospital, and the selection is supported by the Alphabetic Index and Tabular List. However, chapter-specific coding guidelines (such as obstetrics, poisoning, HIV, newborn) that provide sequencing direction take precedence.

2) Acute respiratory failure as secondary diagnosis

Respiratory failure may be listed as a secondary diagnosis if it occurs after admission, or if it is present on admission, but does not meet the definition of principal diagnosis.

3) Sequencing of acute respiratory failure and another acute condition

When a patient is admitted with respiratory failure and another acute condition, (e.g., myocardial infarction, cerebrovascular accident, aspiration pneumonia), the principal diagnosis will not be the same in every situation. This applies whether the other acute condition is a respiratory or nonrespiratory condition. Selection of the principal diagnosis will be dependent on the circumstances of admission. If both the respiratory failure and the other acute condition are equally responsible for occasioning the admission to the hospital, and there are no chapter-specific sequencing rules, the guideline regarding two or more diagnoses that equally meet the definition for principal diagnosis *(Section II, C.)* may be applied in these situations.

If the documentation is not clear as to whether acute respiratory failure and another condition are equally responsible for occasioning the admission, query the provider for clarification.

c. Influenza due to certain identified influenza viruses

Code only confirmed cases of influenza due to certain identified influenza viruses (category J09), and due to other identified influenza virus (category J10). This is an exception to the hospital inpatient guideline Section II, H. (Uncertain Diagnosis).

In this context, "confirmation" does not require documentation of positive laboratory testing specific for avian or other novel influenza A or other identified influenza virus. However, coding should be based on the provider's diagnostic statement that the patient has avian influenza, or other novel influenza A, for category J09, or has another particular identified strain of influenza, such as H1N1 or H3N2, but not identified as novel or variant, for category J10.

If the provider records "suspected" or "possible" or "probable" avian influenza, or novel influenza, or other identified influenza, then the appropriate influenza code from category J11, Influenza due to unidentified influenza virus, should be assigned. A code from category J09, Influenza due to certain identified influenza viruses, should not be assigned nor should a code from category J10, Influenza due to other identified influenza virus.

d. Ventilator associated Pneumonia

1) Documentation of Ventilator associated Pneumonia

As with all procedural or postprocedural complications, code assignment is based on the provider's documentation of the relationship between the condition and the procedure.

Code J95.851, Ventilator associated pneumonia, should be assigned only when the provider has documented ventilator associated pneumonia (VAP). An additional code to identify the organism (e.g., Pseudomonas aeruginosa, code B96.5) should also be assigned. Do not assign an additional code from categories J12-J18 to identify the type of pneumonia.

Code J95.851 should not be assigned for cases where the patient has pneumonia and is on a mechanical ventilator and the provider has not specifically stated that the pneumonia is ventilator-associated pneumonia. If the documentation is unclear as to whether the patient has a pneumonia that is a complication attributable to the mechanical ventilator, query the provider.

2) Ventilator associated Pneumonia Develops after Admission

A patient may be admitted with one type of pneumonia (e.g., code J13, Pneumonia due to Streptococcus pneumonia) and subsequently develop VAP. In this instance, the principal diagnosis would be the appropriate code from categories J12-J18 for the pneumonia diagnosed at the time of admission. Code J95.851, Ventilator associated pneumonia, would be assigned as an additional diagnosis when the provider has also documented the presence of ventilator associated pneumonia.

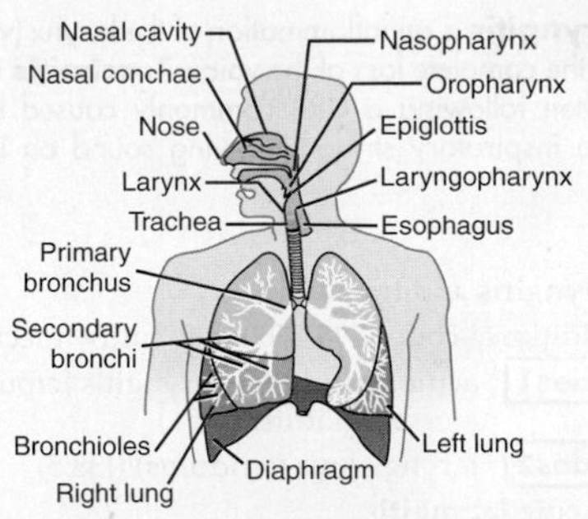

Figure 10-1 Respiratory system. (From Buck CJ: Step-by-Step Medical Coding, ed 2016, St. Louis, Elsevier, 2016)

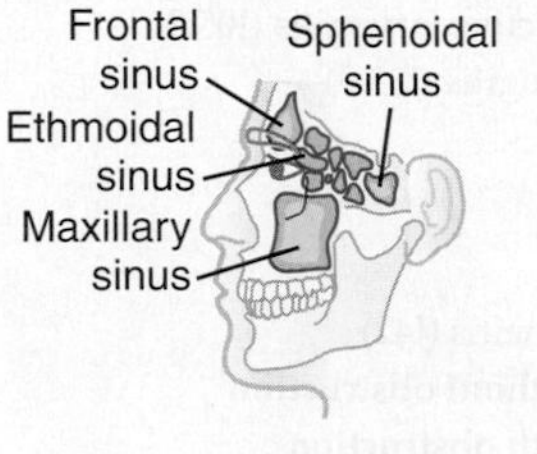

Figure 10-2 Paranasal sinuses. (From Buck CJ: Step-by-Step Medical Coding, ed 2016, St. Louis, Elsevier, 2016)

Item 10-1 Pharyngitis is painful inflammation of the pharynx (sore throat). Ninety percent of the infections are caused by a virus with the remaining being bacterial and rarely a fungus (candidiasis). Other irritants such as pollutants, chemicals, or smoke may cause similar symptoms.

CHAPTER 1Ø

DISEASES OF THE RESPIRATORY SYSTEM (JØØ-J99)

Note: When a respiratory condition is described as occurring in more than one site and is not specifically indexed, it should be classified to the lower anatomic site (e.g., tracheobronchitis to bronchitis in J4Ø).

Use additional code, where applicable, to identify:
- exposure to environmental tobacco smoke (Z77.22)
- exposure to tobacco smoke in the perinatal period (P96.81)
- history of tobacco dependence (Z87.891)
- occupational exposure to environmental tobacco smoke (Z57.31)
- tobacco dependence (F17.-)
- tobacco use (Z72.Ø)

Excludes2
- certain conditions originating in the perinatal period (PØ4-P96)
- certain infectious and parasitic diseases (AØØ-B99)
- complications of pregnancy, childbirth and the puerperium (OØØ-O99A)
- congenital malformations, deformations and chromosomal abnormalities (QØØ-Q99)
- endocrine, nutritional and metabolic diseases (EØØ-E88)
- injury, poisoning and certain other consequences of external causes (SØØ-T88)
- neoplasms (CØØ-D49)
- smoke inhalation (T59.81-)
- symptoms, signs and abnormal clinical and laboratory findings, not elsewhere classified (RØØ-R94)

This chapter contains the following blocks:

JØØ-JØ6	Acute upper respiratory infections
JØ9-J18	Influenza and pneumonia
J2Ø-J22	Other acute lower respiratory infections
J3Ø-J39	Other diseases of upper respiratory tract
J4Ø-J47	Chronic lower respiratory diseases
J6Ø-J7Ø	Lung diseases due to external agents
J8Ø-J84	Other respiratory diseases principally affecting the interstitium
J85-J86	Suppurative and necrotic conditions of the lower respiratory tract
J9Ø-J94	Other diseases of the pleura
J95	Intraoperative and postprocedural complications and disorders of respiratory system, not elsewhere classified
J96-J99	Other diseases of the respiratory system

ACUTE UPPER RESPIRATORY INFECTIONS (JØØ-JØ6)

Excludes1
- chronic obstructive pulmonary disease with acute lower respiratory infection (J44.Ø)
- influenza virus with other respiratory manifestations (JØ9.X2, J1Ø.1, J11.1)

JØØ Acute nasopharyngitis [common cold]
- Acute rhinitis
- Coryza (acute)
- Infective nasopharyngitis NOS
- Infective rhinitis
- Nasal catarrh, acute
- Nasopharyngitis NOS

Excludes1
- acute pharyngitis (JØ2.-)
- acute sore throat NOS (JØ2.9)
- pharyngitis NOS (JØ2.9)
- rhinitis NOS (J31.Ø)
- sore throat NOS (JØ2.9)

Excludes2
- allergic rhinitis (J3Ø.1-J3Ø.9)
- chronic pharyngitis (J31.2)
- chronic rhinitis (J31.Ø)
- chronic sore throat (J31.2)
- nasopharyngitis, chronic (J31.1)
- vasomotor rhinitis (J3Ø.Ø)

★**(See Plate 49 on page NAP-24.)**

● **JØ1 Acute sinusitis**

Includes
- acute abscess of sinus
- acute empyema of sinus
- acute infection of sinus
- acute inflammation of sinus
- acute suppuration of sinus

Use additional code (B95-B97) to identify infectious agent.

Excludes1 sinusitis NOS (J32.9)

Excludes2 chronic sinusitis (J32.Ø-J32.8)

● **JØ1.Ø Acute maxillary sinusitis**
Acute antritis
- **JØ1.ØØ Acute maxillary sinusitis, unspecified**
- **JØ1.Ø1 Acute recurrent maxillary sinusitis**

● **JØ1.1 Acute frontal sinusitis**
- **JØ1.1Ø Acute frontal sinusitis, unspecified**
- **JØ1.11 Acute recurrent frontal sinusitis**

● **JØ1.2 Acute ethmoidal sinusitis**
- **JØ1.2Ø Acute ethmoidal sinusitis, unspecified**
- **JØ1.21 Acute recurrent ethmoidal sinusitis**

● **JØ1.3 Acute sphenoidal sinusitis**
- **JØ1.3Ø Acute sphenoidal sinusitis, unspecified**
- **JØ1.31 Acute recurrent sphenoidal sinusitis**

● **JØ1.4 Acute pansinusitis**
- **JØ1.4Ø Acute pansinusitis, unspecified**
- **JØ1.41 Acute recurrent pansinusitis**

● **J01.8 Other acute sinusitis**

J01.80 Other acute sinusitis
Acute sinusitis involving more than one sinus but not pansinusitis

J01.81 Other acute recurrent sinusitis
Acute recurrent sinusitis involving more than one sinus but not pansinusitis

● **J01.9 Acute sinusitis, unspecified**

J01.90 Acute sinusitis, unspecified

J01.91 Acute recurrent sinusitis, unspecified

● **J02 Acute pharyngitis**

Includes acute sore throat

Excludes1 acute laryngopharyngitis (J06.0)
peritonsillar abscess (J36)
pharyngeal abscess (J39.1)
retropharyngeal abscess (J39.0)

Excludes2 chronic pharyngitis (J31.2)

J02.0 Streptococcal pharyngitis
Septic pharyngitis
Streptococcal sore throat

Excludes2 scarlet fever (A38.-)

J02.8 Acute pharyngitis due to other specified organisms
Use additional code (B95-B97) to identify infectious agent

Excludes1 pharyngitis due to coxsackie virus (B08.5)
pharyngitis due to gonococcus (A54.5)
acute pharyngitis due to herpes [simplex] virus (B00.2)
acute pharyngitis due to infectious mononucleosis (B27.-)
enteroviral vesicular pharyngitis (B08.5)

J02.9 Acute pharyngitis, unspecified
Gangrenous pharyngitis (acute)
Infective pharyngitis (acute) NOS
Pharyngitis (acute) NOS
Sore throat (acute) NOS
Suppurative pharyngitis (acute)
Ulcerative pharyngitis (acute)

● **J03 Acute tonsillitis**
Inflammation of pharyngeal tonsils caused by virus or bacteria

Excludes1 acute sore throat (J02.-)
hypertrophy of tonsils (J35.1)
peritonsillar abscess (J36)
sore throat NOS (J02.9)
streptococcal sore throat (J02.0)

Excludes2 chronic tonsillitis (J35.0)

● **J03.0 Streptococcal tonsillitis**

J03.00 Acute streptococcal tonsillitis, unspecified

J03.01 Acute recurrent streptococcal tonsillitis

● **J03.8 Acute tonsillitis due to other specified organisms**
Use additional code (B95-B97) to identify infectious agent.

Excludes1 diphtheritic tonsillitis (A36.0)
herpesviral pharyngotonsillitis (B00.2)
streptococcal tonsillitis (J03.0)
tuberculous tonsillitis (A15.8)
Vincent's tonsillitis (A69.1)

J03.80 Acute tonsillitis due to other specified organisms

J03.81 Acute recurrent tonsillitis due to other specified organisms

● **J03.9 Acute tonsillitis, unspecified**
Follicular tonsillitis (acute)
Gangrenous tonsillitis (acute)
Infective tonsillitis (acute)
Tonsillitis (acute) NOS
Ulcerative tonsillitis (acute)

J03.90 Acute tonsillitis, unspecified

J03.91 Acute recurrent tonsillitis, unspecified

Item 10–2 Laryngitis is an inflammation of the larynx (voice box) resulting in hoarse voice or the complete loss of the voice. **Tracheitis** is an inflammation of the trachea (often following a URI) commonly caused by *staphylococcus aureus* resulting in inspiratory stridor (crowing sound on inspiration) and a croup like cough.

● **J04 Acute laryngitis and tracheitis**
Use additional code (B95-B97) to identify infectious agent.

Excludes1 acute obstructive laryngitis [croup] and epiglottitis (J05.-)

Excludes2 laryngismus (stridulus) (J38.5)

J04.0 Acute laryngitis
Edematous laryngitis (acute)
Laryngitis (acute) NOS
Subglottic laryngitis (acute)
Suppurative laryngitis (acute)
Ulcerative laryngitis (acute)

Excludes1 acute obstructive laryngitis (J05.0)

Excludes2 chronic laryngitis (J37.0)

● **J04.1 Acute tracheitis**
Acute viral tracheitis
Catarrhal tracheitis (acute)
Tracheitis (acute) NOS

Excludes2 chronic tracheitis (J42)

J04.10 Acute tracheitis without obstruction

J04.11 Acute tracheitis with obstruction

J04.2 Acute laryngotracheitis
Laryngotracheitis NOS
Tracheitis (acute) with laryngitis (acute)

Excludes1 acute obstructive laryngotracheitis (J05.0)

Excludes2 chronic laryngotracheitis (J37.1)

● **J04.3 Supraglottitis, unspecified**

J04.30 Supraglottitis, unspecified, without obstruction

J04.31 Supraglottitis, unspecified, with obstruction

● **J05 Acute obstructive laryngitis [croup] and epiglottitis**
Use additional code (B95-B97) to identify infectious agent.

J05.0 Acute obstructive laryngitis [croup]
Obstructive laryngitis (acute) NOS
Obstructive laryngotracheitis NOS

● **J05.1 Acute epiglottitis**

Excludes2 epiglottitis, chronic (J37.0)

J05.10 Acute epiglottitis without obstruction
Epiglottitis NOS

J05.11 Acute epiglottitis with obstruction

● **J06 Acute upper respiratory infections of multiple and unspecified sites**

Excludes1 acute respiratory infection NOS (J22)
streptococcal pharyngitis (J02.0)

J06.0 Acute laryngopharyngitis

J06.9 Acute upper respiratory infection, unspecified
Upper respiratory disease, acute
Upper respiratory infection NOS

CHAPTER 10 (J00-J99)

◀ New ◀ Revised ~~deleted~~ Deleted OGCR Official Guidelines X Assign placeholder X ● Use Additional Character(s)
Excludes 1 | Excludes 2 | Includes | Use additional | Code first | Code also | Unspecified

INFLUENZA AND PNEUMONIA (J09-J18)

Excludes2 allergic or eosinophilic pneumonia (J82)
aspiration pneumonia NOS (J69.0)
meconium pneumonia (P24.01)
neonatal aspiration pneumonia (P24.-)
pneumonia due to solids and liquids (J69.-)
congenital pneumonia (P23.9)
lipid pneumonia (J69.1)
rheumatic pneumonia (I00)
ventilator associated pneumonia (J95.851)

● **J09 Influenza due to certain identified influenza viruses**

Excludes1 influenza due to other influenza viruses (J10.-)
influenza due to unidentified influenza virus (J11.-)
seasonal influenza due to other identified influenza virus (J10.-)
seasonal influenza due to unidentified influenza virus (J11.-)

● **J09.X Influenza due to identified novel influenza A virus**

Avian influenza
Bird influenza
Influenza A/H5N1
Influenza of other animal origin, not bird or swine
Swine influenza virus (viruses that normally cause infections in pigs)

J09.X1 Influenza due to identified novel influenza A virus with pneumonia

Code also, if applicable, associated:
lung abscess (J85.1)
other specified type of pneumonia

J09.X2 Influenza due to identified novel influenza A virus with other respiratory manifestations

Influenza due to identified novel influenza A virus NOS
Influenza due to identified novel influenza A virus with laryngitis
Influenza due to identified novel influenza A virus with pharyngitis
Influenza due to identified novel influenza A virus with upper respiratory symptoms

Use additional code, if applicable, for associated:
pleural effusion (J91.8)
sinusitis (J01.-)

J09.X3 Influenza due to identified novel influenza A virus with gastrointestinal manifestations

Influenza due to identified novel influenza A virus gastroenteritis

Excludes1 'intestinal flu' [viral gastroenteritis] (A08.-)

J09.X9 Influenza due to identified novel influenza A virus with other manifestations

Influenza due to identified novel influenza A virus with encephalopathy
Influenza due to identified novel influenza A virus with myocarditis
Influenza due to identified novel influenza A virus with otitis media

Use additional code to identify manifestation

● **J10 Influenza due to other identified influenza virus**

Excludes1 influenza due to avian influenza virus (J09.X-)
influenza due to swine flu (J09.X-)
influenza due to unidentified influenza virus (J11.-)

● **J10.0 Influenza due to other identified influenza virus with pneumonia**

Code also associated lung abscess, if applicable (J85.1)

J10.00 Influenza due to other identified influenza virus with unspecified type of pneumonia

J10.01 Influenza due to other identified influenza virus with the same other identified influenza virus pneumonia

J10.08 Influenza due to other identified influenza virus with other specified pneumonia

Code also other specified type of pneumonia

J10.1 Influenza due to other identified influenza virus with other respiratory manifestations

Influenza due to other identified influenza virus NOS
Influenza due to other identified influenza virus with laryngitis
Influenza due to other identified influenza virus with pharyngitis
Influenza due to other identified influenza virus with upper respiratory symptoms

Use additional code for associated pleural effusion, if applicable (J91.8)

Use additional code for associated sinusitis, if applicable (J01.-)

J10.2 Influenza due to other identified influenza virus with gastrointestinal manifestations

Influenza due to other identified influenza virus gastroenteritis

Excludes1 'intestinal flu' [viral gastroenteritis] (A08.-)

● **J10.8 Influenza due to other identified influenza virus with other manifestations**

J10.81 Influenza due to other identified influenza virus with encephalopathy

J10.82 Influenza due to other identified influenza virus with myocarditis

J10.83 Influenza due to other identified influenza virus with otitis media

Use additional code for any associated perforated tympanic membrane (H72.-)

J10.89 Influenza due to other identified influenza virus with other manifestations

Use additional codes to identify the manifestations

● **J11 Influenza due to unidentified influenza virus**

● **J11.0 Influenza due to unidentified influenza virus with pneumonia**

Code also associated lung abscess, if applicable (J85.1)

J11.00 Influenza due to unidentified influenza virus with unspecified type of pneumonia

Influenza with pneumonia NOS

J11.08 Influenza due to unidentified influenza virus with specified pneumonia

Code also other specified type of pneumonia

J11.1 Influenza due to unidentified influenza virus with other respiratory manifestations

Influenza NOS
Influenzal laryngitis NOS
Influenzal pharyngitis NOS
Influenza with upper respiratory symptoms NOS

Use additional code for associated pleural effusion, if applicable (J91.8)

Use additional code for associated sinusitis, if applicable (J01.-)

CHAPTER 10 (J00-J99)

J11.2 Influenza due to unidentified influenza virus with gastrointestinal manifestations
Influenza gastroenteritis NOS
Excludes1 'intestinal flu' [viral gastroenteritis] (AØ8.-)

● **J11.8 Influenza due to unidentified influenza virus with other manifestations**

J11.81 Influenza due to unidentified influenza virus with encephalopathy
Influenzal encephalopathy NOS

J11.82 Influenza due to unidentified influenza virus with myocarditis
Influenzal myocarditis NOS

J11.83 Influenza due to unidentified influenza virus with otitis media
Influenzal otitis media NOS
Use additional code for any associated perforated tympanic membrane (H72.-)

J11.89 Influenza due to unidentified influenza virus with other manifestations
Use additional codes to identify the manifestations

● **J12 Viral pneumonia, not elsewhere classified**
Includes bronchopneumonia due to viruses other than influenza viruses
Code first associated influenza, if applicable (JØ9.X1, J1Ø.Ø-, J11.Ø-)
Code also associated abscess, if applicable (J85.1)
Excludes1 aspiration pneumonia due to anesthesia during labor and delivery (O74.Ø)
aspiration pneumonia due to anesthesia during pregnancy (O29)
aspiration pneumonia due to anesthesia during puerperium (O89.Ø)
aspiration pneumonia due to solids and liquids (J69.-)
aspiration pneumonia NOS (J69.Ø)
congenital pneumonia (P23.Ø)
congenital rubella pneumonitis (P35.Ø)
interstitial pneumonia NOS (J84.9)
lipid pneumonia (J69.1)
neonatal aspiration pneumonia (P24.-)

J12.Ø Adenoviral pneumonia

J12.1 Respiratory syncytial virus pneumonia

J12.2 Parainfluenza virus pneumonia

J12.3 Human metapneumovirus pneumonia

● **J12.8 Other viral pneumonia**

J12.81 Pneumonia due to SARS-associated coronavirus
Severe acute respiratory syndrome NOS

J12.89 Other viral pneumonia

J12.9 Viral pneumonia, unspecified

J13 Pneumonia due to Streptococcus pneumoniae
Bronchopneumonia due to S. pneumoniae
Code first associated influenza, if applicable (JØ9.X1, J1Ø.Ø-, J11.Ø-)
Code also associated abscess, if applicable (J85.1)
Excludes1 congenital pneumonia due to S. pneumoniae (P23.6)
lobar pneumonia, unspecified organism (J18.1)
pneumonia due to other streptococci (J15.3-J15.4)

Item 10–3 Pneumonia is an infection of the lungs, caused by a variety of microorganisms, including viruses, most commonly the Streptococcus pneumoniae (pneumococcus) bacteria, fungi, and parasites. Pneumonia occurs when the immune system is weakened, often by a URI or influenza.

J14 Pneumonia due to Hemophilus influenzae
Bronchopneumonia due to H. influenzae
Code first associated influenza, if applicable (JØ9.X1, J1Ø.Ø-, J11.Ø-)
Code also associated abscess, if applicable (J85.1)
Excludes1 congenital pneumonia due to H. influenzae (P23.6)

● **J15 Bacterial pneumonia, not elsewhere classified**
Includes bronchopneumonia due to bacteria other than S. pneumoniae and H. influenzae
Code first associated influenza, if applicable (JØ9.X1, J1Ø.Ø-, J11.Ø-)
Code also associated abscess, if applicable (J85.1)
Excludes1 chlamydial pneumonia (J16.Ø)
congenital pneumonia (P23.-)
Legionnaires' disease (A48.1)
spirochetal pneumonia (A69.8)

J15.Ø Pneumonia due to Klebsiella pneumoniae

J15.1 Pneumonia due to Pseudomonas

● **J15.2 Pneumonia due to staphylococcus**

J15.2Ø Pneumonia due to staphylococcus, unspecified

● **J15.21 Pneumonia due to staphylococcus aureus**

J15.211 Pneumonia due to Methicillin susceptible Staphylococcus aureus
MSSA pneumonia
Pneumonia due to Staphylococcus aureus NOS

J15.212 Pneumonia due to Methicillin resistant Staphylococcus aureus

J15.29 Pneumonia due to other staphylococcus

J15.3 Pneumonia due to streptococcus, group B

J15.4 Pneumonia due to other streptococci
Excludes1 pneumonia due to streptococcus, group B (J15.3)
pneumonia due to Streptococcus pneumoniae (J13)

J15.5 Pneumonia due to Escherichia coli

J15.6 Pneumonia due to other aerobic Gram-negative bacteria
Pneumonia due to Serratia marcescens

J15.7 Pneumonia due to Mycoplasma pneumoniae

J15.8 Pneumonia due to other specified bacteria

J15.9 Unspecified bacterial pneumonia
Pneumonia due to gram-positive bacteria

● **J16 Pneumonia due to other infectious organisms, not elsewhere classified**
Code first associated influenza, if applicable (JØ9.X1, J1Ø.Ø-, J11.Ø-)
Code also associated abscess, if applicable (J85.1)
Excludes1 congenital pneumonia (P23.-)
ornithosis (A7Ø)
pneumocystosis (B59)
pneumonia NOS (J18.9)

J16.Ø Chlamydial pneumonia

J16.8 Pneumonia due to other specified infectious organisms

J17 Pneumonia in diseases classified elsewhere
Code first underlying disease, such as:
Q fever (A78)
rheumatic fever (IØØ)
schistosomiasis (B65.Ø-B65.9)

Excludes1 candidial pneumonia (B37.1)
chlamydial pneumonia (J16.Ø)
gonorrheal pneumonia (A54.84)
histoplasmosis pneumonia (B39.Ø-B39.2)
measles pneumonia (BØ5.2)
nocardiosis pneumonia (A43.Ø)
pneumocystosis (B59)
pneumonia due to Pneumocystis carinii (B59)
pneumonia due to Pneumocystis jiroveci (B59)
pneumonia in actinomycosis (A42.Ø)
pneumonia in anthrax (A22.1)
pneumonia in ascariasis (B77.81)
pneumonia in aspergillosis (B44.Ø-B44.1)
pneumonia in coccidioidomycosis (B38.Ø-B38.2)
pneumonia in cytomegalovirus disease (B25.Ø)
pneumonia in toxoplasmosis (B58.3)
rubella pneumonia (BØ6.81)
salmonella pneumonia (AØ2.22)
spirochetal infection NEC with pneumonia (A69.8)
tularemia pneumonia (A21.2)
typhoid fever with pneumonia (AØ1.Ø3)
varicella pneumonia (BØ1.2)
whooping cough with pneumonia (A37 with fifth-character 1)

● **J18 Pneumonia, unspecified organism**
Code first associated influenza, if applicable (JØ9.X1, J1Ø.Ø-, J11.Ø-)

Excludes1 abscess of lung with pneumonia (J85.1)
aspiration pneumonia due to anesthesia during labor and delivery (O74.Ø)
aspiration pneumonia due to anesthesia during pregnancy (O29)
aspiration pneumonia due to anesthesia during puerperium (O89.Ø)
aspiration pneumonia due to solids and liquids (J69.-)
aspiration pneumonia NOS (J69.Ø)
congenital pneumonia (P23.Ø)
drug-induced interstitial lung disorder (J7Ø.2-J7Ø.4)
interstitial pneumonia NOS (J84.9)
lipid pneumonia (J69.1)
neonatal aspiration pneumonia (P24.-)
pneumonitis due to external agents (J67-J7Ø)
pneumonitis due to fumes and vapors (J68.Ø)
usual interstitial pneumonia (J84.17)

J18.Ø Bronchopneumonia, unspecified organism

Excludes1 hypostatic bronchopneumonia (J18.2)
lipid pneumonia (J69.1)

Excludes2 acute bronchiolitis (J21.-)
chronic bronchiolitis (J44.9)

J18.1 Lobar pneumonia, unspecified organism

J18.2 Hypostatic pneumonia, unspecified organism
Hypostatic bronchopneumonia
Passive pneumonia

J18.8 Other pneumonia, unspecified organism

J18.9 Pneumonia, unspecified organism

OTHER ACUTE LOWER RESPIRATORY INFECTIONS (J2Ø-J22)

Excludes2 chronic obstructive pulmonary disease with acute lower respiratory infection (J44.Ø)

● **J2Ø Acute bronchitis**
Inflammation/irritation of the bronchial tubes lasting 2-3 weeks, most commonly caused by a virus

Includes acute and subacute bronchitis (with) bronchospasm
acute and subacute bronchitis (with) tracheitis
acute and subacute bronchitis (with) tracheobronchitis, acute
acute and subacute fibrinous bronchitis
acute and subacute membranous bronchitis
acute and subacute purulent bronchitis
acute and subacute septic bronchitis

Excludes1 bronchitis NOS (J4Ø)
tracheobronchitis NOS (J4Ø)

Excludes2 acute bronchitis with bronchiectasis (J47.Ø)
acute bronchitis with chronic obstructive asthma (J44.Ø)
acute bronchitis with chronic obstructive pulmonary disease (J44.Ø)
allergic bronchitis NOS (J45.9Ø9-)
bronchitis due to chemicals, fumes and vapors (J68.Ø)
chronic bronchitis NOS (J42)
chronic mucopurulent bronchitis (J41.1)
chronic obstructive bronchitis (J44.-)
chronic obstructive tracheobronchitis (J44.-)
chronic simple bronchitis (J41.Ø)
chronic tracheobronchitis (J42)

J2Ø.Ø Acute bronchitis due to Mycoplasma pneumoniae
J2Ø.1 Acute bronchitis due to Hemophilus influenzae
J2Ø.2 Acute bronchitis due to streptococcus
J2Ø.3 Acute bronchitis due to coxsackievirus
J2Ø.4 Acute bronchitis due to parainfluenza virus
J2Ø.5 Acute bronchitis due to respiratory syncytial virus
J2Ø.6 Acute bronchitis due to rhinovirus
J2Ø.7 Acute bronchitis due to echovirus
J2Ø.8 Acute bronchitis due to other specified organisms
J2Ø.9 Acute bronchitis, unspecified

● **J21 Acute bronchiolitis**
Bronchiolitis obliterans with organizing pneumonia (BOOP) inflammation of bronchioles and surrounding tissue in lung

Includes acute bronchiolitis with bronchospasm

Excludes2 respiratory bronchiolitis interstitial lung disease (J84.115)

J21.Ø Acute bronchiolitis due to respiratory syncytial virus
J21.1 Acute bronchiolitis due to human metapneumovirus
J21.8 Acute bronchiolitis due to other specified organisms
J21.9 Acute bronchiolitis, unspecified
Bronchiolitis (acute)

Excludes1 chronic bronchiolitis (J44.-)

J22 Unspecified acute lower respiratory infection
Acute (lower) respiratory (tract) infection NOS

Excludes1 upper respiratory infection (acute) (JØ6.9)

CHAPTER 1Ø (JØØ-J99)

OTHER DISEASES OF UPPER RESPIRATORY TRACT (J30-J39)

● **J30 Vasomotor and allergic rhinitis**

Includes spasmodic rhinorrhea

Excludes1 allergic rhinitis with asthma (bronchial) (J45.909)
rhinitis NOS (J31.0)

J30.0 Vasomotor rhinitis

J30.1 Allergic rhinitis due to pollen
Allergy NOS due to pollen
Hay fever
Pollinosis

J30.2 Other seasonal allergic rhinitis

J30.5 Allergic rhinitis due to food

● **J30.8 Other allergic rhinitis**

J30.81 Allergic rhinitis due to animal (cat) (dog) hair and dander

J30.89 Other allergic rhinitis
Perennial allergic rhinitis

J30.9 Allergic rhinitis, unspecified

● **J31 Chronic rhinitis, nasopharyngitis and pharyngitis**

Use additional code to identify:
exposure to environmental tobacco smoke (Z77.22)
exposure to tobacco smoke in the perinatal period (P96.81)
history of tobacco dependence (Z87.891) ◄
occupational exposure to environmental tobacco smoke (Z57.31)
tobacco dependence (F17.-)
tobacco use (Z72.0)

J31.0 Chronic rhinitis
Atrophic rhinitis (chronic)
Granulomatous rhinitis (chronic)
Hypertrophic rhinitis (chronic)
Obstructive rhinitis (chronic)
Ozena
Purulent rhinitis (chronic)
Rhinitis (chronic) NOS
Ulcerative rhinitis (chronic)

Excludes1 allergic rhinitis (J30.1-J30.9)
vasomotor rhinitis (J30.0)

J31.1 Chronic nasopharyngitis

Excludes2 acute nasopharyngitis (J00)

J31.2 Chronic pharyngitis
Chronic sore throat
Atrophic pharyngitis (chronic)
Granular pharyngitis (chronic)
Hypertrophic pharyngitis (chronic)

Excludes2 acute pharyngitis (J02.9)

● **J32 Chronic sinusitis**

Includes sinus abscess
sinus empyema
sinus infection
sinus suppuration

Use additional code to identify:
exposure to environmental tobacco smoke (Z77.22)
exposure to tobacco smoke in the perinatal period (P96.81)
history of tobacco dependence (Z87.891) ◄
infectious agent (B95-B97)
occupational exposure to environmental tobacco smoke (Z57.31)
tobacco dependence (F17.-)
tobacco use (Z72.0)

Excludes2 acute sinusitis (J01.-)

J32.0 Chronic maxillary sinusitis
Antritis (chronic)
Maxillary sinusitis NOS

J32.1 Chronic frontal sinusitis
Frontal sinusitis NOS

Item 10–4 Nasal polyps are an abnormal growth of tissue (tumor) projecting from a mucous membrane and attached to the surface by a narrow elongated stalk (pedunculated). Nasal polyps usually originate in the ethmoid sinus but also may occur in the maxillary sinus. Symptoms are nasal block, sinusitis, anosmia, and secondary infections.

J32.2 Chronic ethmoidal sinusitis
Ethmoidal sinusitis NOS

Excludes1 Woakes' ethmoiditis (J33.1)

J32.3 Chronic sphenoidal sinusitis
Sphenoidal sinusitis NOS

J32.4 Chronic pansinusitis
Pansinusitis NOS

J32.8 Other chronic sinusitis
Sinusitis (chronic) involving more than one sinus but not pansinusitis

J32.9 Chronic sinusitis, unspecified
Sinusitis (chronic) NOS

● **J33 Nasal polyp**

Use additional code to identify:
exposure to environmental tobacco smoke (Z77.22)
exposure to tobacco smoke in the perinatal period (P96.81)
history of tobacco dependence (Z87.891) ◄
occupational exposure to environmental tobacco smoke (Z57.31)
tobacco dependence (F17.-)
tobacco use (Z72.0)

Excludes1 adenomatous polyps (D14.0)

J33.0 Polyp of nasal cavity
Choanal polyp
Nasopharyngeal polyp

J33.1 Polypoid sinus degeneration
Woakes' syndrome or ethmoiditis

J33.8 Other polyp of sinus
Accessory polyp of sinus
Ethmoidal polyp of sinus
Maxillary polyp of sinus
Sphenoidal polyp of sinus

J33.9 Nasal polyp, unspecified

● **J34 Other and unspecified disorders of nose and nasal sinuses**

Excludes2 varicose ulcer of nasal septum (I86.8)

J34.0 Abscess, furuncle and carbuncle of nose
Cellulitis of nose
Necrosis of nose
Ulceration of nose

J34.1 Cyst and mucocele of nose and nasal sinus

J34.2 Deviated nasal septum
Deflection or deviation of septum (nasal) (acquired)

Excludes1 congenital deviated nasal septum (Q67.4)

J34.3 Hypertrophy of nasal turbinates

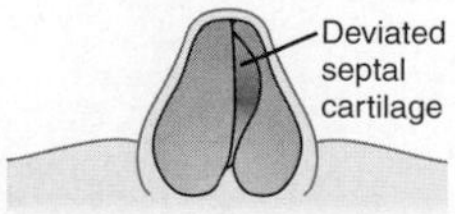

Figure 10-3 Deviated nasal septum.

Item 10–5 A **deviated nasal septum** is the displacement of the septal cartilage that separates the nares. This displacement causes obstructed air flow through the nasal passages. A child can be born with this displacement (congenital), or the condition may be acquired through trauma, such as a sports injury. Symptoms include nasal block, sinusitis, and related secondary infections. Septoplasty is surgical repair of this condition.

● **J34.8 Other specified disorders of nose and nasal sinuses**

J34.81 Nasal mucositis (ulcerative)

Code also type of associated therapy, such as:
antineoplastic and immunosuppressive drugs (T45.1X-)
radiological procedure and radiotherapy (Y84.2)

Excludes2 gastrointestinal mucositis (ulcerative) (K92.81)
mucositis (ulcerative) of vagina and vulva (N76.81)
oral mucositis (ulcerative) (K12.3-)

J34.89 Other specified disorders of nose and nasal sinuses

Perforation of nasal septum NOS
Rhinolith

J34.9 Unspecified disorder of nose and nasal sinuses

● **J35 Chronic diseases of tonsils and adenoids**

Use additional code to identify:
exposure to environmental tobacco smoke (Z77.22)
exposure to tobacco smoke in the perinatal period (P96.81)
history of tobacco dependence (Z87.891) ◄
occupational exposure to environmental tobacco smoke (Z57.31)
tobacco dependence (F17.-)
tobacco use (Z72.Ø)

● **J35.Ø Chronic tonsillitis and adenoiditis**

Excludes2 acute tonsillitis (JØ3.-)

J35.Ø1 Chronic tonsillitis

J35.Ø2 Chronic adenoiditis

J35.Ø3 Chronic tonsillitis and adenoiditis

J35.1 Hypertrophy of tonsils

Enlargement of tonsils

Excludes1 hypertrophy of tonsils with tonsillitis (J35.Ø-)

J35.2 Hypertrophy of adenoids

Enlargement of adenoids

Excludes1 hypertrophy of adenoids with adenoiditis (J35.Ø-)

J35.3 Hypertrophy of tonsils with hypertrophy of adenoids

Excludes1 hypertrophy of tonsils and adenoids with tonsillitis and adenoiditis (J35.Ø3)

J35.8 Other chronic diseases of tonsils and adenoids

Adenoid vegetations
Amygdalolith
Calculus, tonsil
Cicatrix of tonsil (and adenoid)
Tonsillar tag
Ulcer of tonsil

J35.9 Chronic disease of tonsils and adenoids, unspecified

Disease (chronic) of tonsils and adenoids NOS

J36 Peritonsillar abscess

Includes abscess of tonsil
peritonsillar cellulitis
quinsy

Use additional code (B95-B97) to identify infectious agent.

Excludes1 acute tonsillitis (JØ3.-)
chronic tonsillitis (J35.Ø)
retropharyngeal abscess (J39.Ø)
tonsillitis NOS (JØ3.9-)

● **J37 Chronic laryngitis and laryngotracheitis**

Use additional code to identify:
exposure to environmental tobacco smoke (Z77.22)
exposure to tobacco smoke in the perinatal period (P96.81)
history of tobacco dependence (Z87.891) ◄
infectious agent (B95-B97)
occupational exposure to environmental tobacco smoke (Z57.31)
tobacco dependence (F17.-)
tobacco use (Z72.Ø)

J37.Ø Chronic laryngitis

Catarrhal laryngitis
Hypertrophic laryngitis
Sicca laryngitis

Excludes2 acute laryngitis (JØ4.Ø)
obstructive (acute) laryngitis (JØ5.Ø)

J37.1 Chronic laryngotracheitis

Laryngitis, chronic, with tracheitis (chronic)
Tracheitis, chronic, with laryngitis

Excludes1 chronic tracheitis (J42)

Excludes2 acute laryngotracheitis (JØ4.2)
acute tracheitis (JØ4.1)

● **J38 Diseases of vocal cords and larynx, not elsewhere classified**

Use additional code to identify:
exposure to environmental tobacco smoke (Z77.22)
exposure to tobacco smoke in the perinatal period (P96.81)
history of tobacco dependence (Z87.891) ◄
occupational exposure to environmental tobacco smoke (Z57.31)
tobacco dependence (F17.-)
tobacco use (Z72.Ø)

Excludes1 congenital laryngeal stridor (P28.89)
obstructive laryngitis (acute) (JØ5.Ø)
postprocedural subglottic stenosis (J95.5)
stridor (RØ6.1)
ulcerative laryngitis (JØ4.Ø)

● **J38.Ø Paralysis of vocal cords and larynx**

Laryngoplegia
Paralysis of glottis

J38.ØØ Paralysis of vocal cords and larynx, unspecified

J38.Ø1 Paralysis of vocal cords and larynx, unilateral

J38.Ø2 Paralysis of vocal cords and larynx, bilateral

J38.1 Polyp of vocal cord and larynx

Excludes1 adenomatous polyps (D14.1)

J38.2 Nodules of vocal cords

Chorditis (fibrinous)(nodosa)(tuberosa)
Singer's nodes
Teacher's nodes

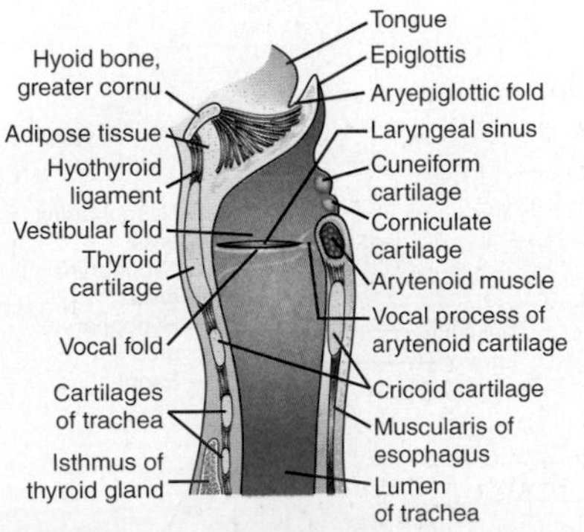

Figure 10-4 Coronal section of the larynx.

Item 10-6 The **larynx** extends from the tongue to the trachea and is divided into an upper and lower portion separated by folds. The framework of the larynx is cartilage composed of the single cricoid, thyroid, and epiglottic cartilages, and the paired arytenoid, cuneiform, and corniculate cartilages.

CHAPTER 1Ø (JØØ-J99)

J38.3 Other diseases of vocal cords
Abscess of vocal cords
Cellulitis of vocal cords
Granuloma of vocal cords
Leukokeratosis of vocal cords
Leukoplakia of vocal cords

J38.4 Edema of larynx
Edema (of) glottis
Subglottic edema
Supraglottic edema
Excludes1 acute obstructive laryngitis [croup] (JØ5.Ø)
edematous laryngitis (JØ4.Ø)

J38.5 Laryngeal spasm
Laryngismus (stridulus)

J38.6 Stenosis of larynx

J38.7 Other diseases of larynx
Abscess of larynx
Cellulitis of larynx
Disease of larynx NOS
Necrosis of larynx
Pachyderma of larynx
Perichondritis of larynx
Ulcer of larynx

● **J39 Other diseases of upper respiratory tract**
Excludes1 acute respiratory infection NOS (J22)
acute upper respiratory infection (JØ6.9)
upper respiratory inflammation due to chemicals, gases, fumes or vapors (J68.2)

J39.Ø Retropharyngeal and parapharyngeal abscess
Peripharyngeal abscess
Excludes1 peritonsillar abscess (J36)

J39.1 Other abscess of pharynx
Cellulitis of pharynx
Nasopharyngeal abscess

J39.2 Other diseases of pharynx
Cyst of pharynx
Edema of pharynx
Excludes2 chronic pharyngitis (J31.2)
ulcerative pharyngitis (JØ2.9)

J39.3 Upper respiratory tract hypersensitivity reaction, site unspecified
Excludes1 hypersensitivity reaction of upper respiratory tract, such as:
extrinsic allergic alveolitis (J67.9)
pneumoconiosis (J6Ø-J67.9)

J39.8 Other specified diseases of upper respiratory tract

J39.9 Disease of upper respiratory tract, unspecified

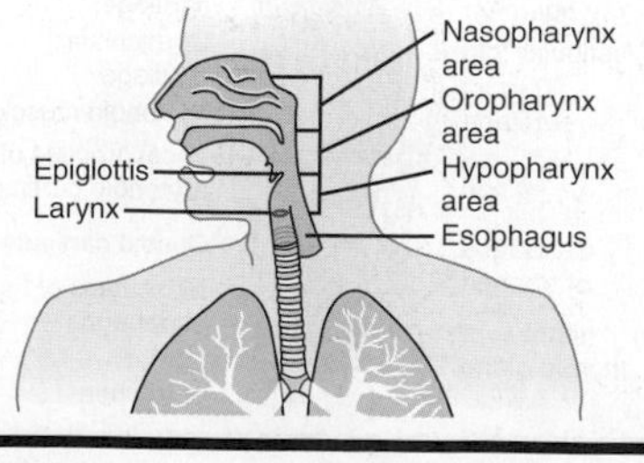

Figure 10-5 The pharynx.

Item 10-7 The **pharynx** is the passage for both food and air between the mouth and the esophagus and is divided into three areas: nasopharynx, oropharynx, and hypopharynx. The hypopharynx branches into the esophagus and the voice box.

Item 10-8 **Chronic bronchitis** is usually defined as being present in any patient who has persistent cough with sputum production for at least three months in at least two consecutive years. **Simple chronic bronchitis** is marked by a productive cough but no pathological airflow obstruction. **Chronic obstructive pulmonary disease (COPD)** is a group of conditions—bronchitis, emphysema, asthma, bronchiectasis, allergic alveolitis—marked by dyspnea. **Catarrhal** bronchitis is an acute form of bronchitis marked by profuse mucus and pus production (**mucopurulent** discharge). **Croupous** bronchitis, also known as pseudomembranous, fibrinous, plastic, exudative, or membranous, is marked by a violent cough and dyspnea.

CHRONIC LOWER RESPIRATORY DISEASES (J4Ø-J47)

Excludes1 bronchitis due to chemicals, gases, fumes and vapors (J68.Ø)
Excludes2 cystic fibrosis (E84.-)

J4Ø Bronchitis, not specified as acute or chronic
Bronchitis NOS
Catarrhal bronchitis
Bronchitis with tracheitis NOS
Tracheobronchitis NOS
Use additional code to identify:
exposure to environmental tobacco smoke (Z77.22)
exposure to tobacco smoke in the perinatal period (P96.81)
history of tobacco dependence (Z87.891)
occupational exposure to environmental tobacco smoke (Z57.31)
tobacco dependence (F17.-)
tobacco use (Z72.Ø)
Excludes1 acute bronchitis (J2Ø.-)
allergic bronchitis NOS (J45.9Ø9-)
asthmatic bronchitis NOS (J45.9-)
bronchitis due to chemicals, gases, fumes and vapors (J68.Ø)

● **J41 Simple and mucopurulent chronic bronchitis**
Use additional code to identify:
exposure to environmental tobacco smoke (Z77.22)
exposure to tobacco smoke in the perinatal period (P96.81)
history of tobacco dependence (Z87.891)
occupational exposure to environmental tobacco smoke (Z57.31)
tobacco dependence (F17.-)
tobacco use (Z72.Ø)
Excludes1 chronic bronchitis NOS (J42)
chronic obstructive bronchitis (J44.-)

J41.Ø Simple chronic bronchitis

J41.1 Mucopurulent chronic bronchitis

J41.8 Mixed simple and mucopurulent chronic bronchitis

J42 Unspecified chronic bronchitis
Chronic bronchitis NOS
Chronic tracheitis
Chronic tracheobronchitis
Use additional code to identify:
exposure to environmental tobacco smoke (Z77.22)
exposure to tobacco smoke in the perinatal period (P96.81)
history of tobacco dependence (Z87.891)
occupational exposure to environmental tobacco smoke (Z57.31)
tobacco dependence (F17.-)
tobacco use (Z72.Ø)
Excludes1 chronic asthmatic bronchitis (J44.-)
chronic bronchitis with airways obstruction (J44.-)
chronic emphysematous bronchitis (J44.-)
chronic obstructive pulmonary disease NOS (J44.9)
simple and mucopurulent chronic bronchitis (J41.-)

● **J43 Emphysema**
Use additional code to identify:
exposure to environmental tobacco smoke (Z77.22)
history of tobacco dependence (Z87.891) ⟸
occupational exposure to environmental tobacco smoke (Z57.31)
tobacco dependence (F17.-)
tobacco use (Z72.Ø)
Excludes1 compensatory emphysema (J98.3)
emphysema due to inhalation of chemicals, gases, fumes or vapors (J68.4)
emphysema with chronic (obstructive) bronchitis (J44.-)
emphysematous (obstructive) bronchitis (J44.-)
interstitial emphysema (J98.2)
mediastinal emphysema (J98.2)
neonatal interstitial emphysema (P25.Ø)
surgical (subcutaneous) emphysema (T81.82)
traumatic subcutaneous emphysema (T79.7)

J43.Ø Unilateral pulmonary emphysema [MacLeod's syndrome]
Swyer-James syndrome
Unilateral emphysema
Unilateral hyperlucent lung
Unilateral pulmonary artery functional hypoplasia
Unilateral transparency of lung

J43.1 Panlobular emphysema
Panacinar emphysema

J43.2 Centrilobular emphysema

J43.8 Other emphysema

J43.9 Emphysema, unspecified
Bullous emphysema (lung)(pulmonary)
Emphysema (lung)(pulmonary) NOS
Emphysematous bleb
Vesicular emphysema (lung)(pulmonary)

● **J44 Other chronic obstructive pulmonary disease**
Includes asthma with chronic obstructive pulmonary disease
chronic asthmatic (obstructive) bronchitis
chronic bronchitis with airways obstruction
chronic bronchitis with emphysema
chronic emphysematous bronchitis
chronic obstructive asthma
chronic obstructive bronchitis
chronic obstructive tracheobronchitis
Code also type of asthma, if applicable (J45.-)
Use additional code to identify:
exposure to environmental tobacco smoke (Z77.22)
history of tobacco dependence (Z87.891) ⟸
occupational exposure to environmental tobacco smoke (Z57.31)
tobacco dependence (F17.-)
tobacco use (Z72.Ø)
Excludes1 bronchiectasis (J47.-)
chronic bronchitis NOS (J42)
chronic simple and mucopurulent bronchitis (J41.-)
chronic tracheitis (J42)
chronic tracheobronchitis (J42)
emphysema without chronic bronchitis (J43.-)
Excludes2 lung diseases due to external agents (J6Ø-J7Ø) ◀

J44.Ø Chronic obstructive pulmonary disease with acute lower respiratory infection
Use additional code to identify the infection

J44.1 Chronic obstructive pulmonary disease with (acute) exacerbation
Decompensated COPD
Decompensated COPD with (acute) exacerbation
Excludes2 chronic obstructive pulmonary disease [COPD] with acute bronchitis (J44.Ø)

J44.9 Chronic obstructive pulmonary disease, unspecified
Chronic obstructive airway disease NOS
Chronic obstructive lung disease NOS

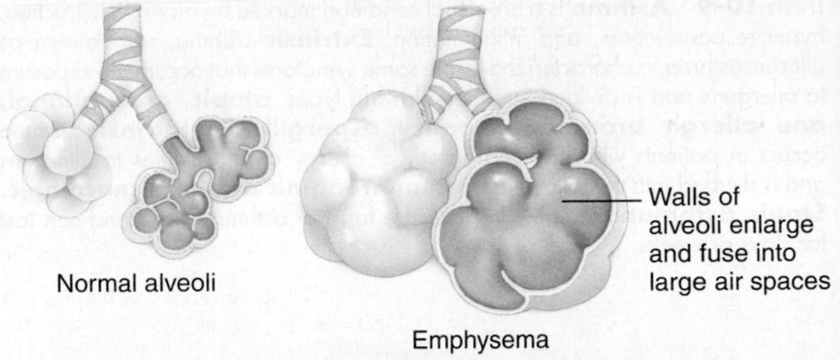

Figure 10-6 Emphysema. (From Shiland, BJ: Medical Terminology & Anatomy for ICD-10 Coding, ed 2, Mosby, 2015)

● **J45 Asthma**
Allergic (predominantly) asthma
Allergic bronchitis NOS
Allergic rhinitis with asthma
Atopic asthma
Extrinsic allergic asthma
Hay fever with asthma
Idiosyncratic asthma
Intrinsic nonallergic asthma
Nonallergic asthma
Use additional code to identify:
exposure to environmental tobacco smoke (Z77.22)
exposure to tobacco smoke in the perinatal period (P96.81)
history of tobacco dependence (Z87.891) ⟸
occupational exposure to environmental tobacco smoke (Z57.31)
tobacco dependence (F17.-)
tobacco use (Z72.Ø)
Excludes1 detergent asthma (J69.8)
eosinophilic asthma (J82)
lung diseases due to external agents (J6Ø-J7Ø)
miner's asthma (J6Ø)
wheezing NOS (RØ6.2)
wood asthma (J67.8)
Excludes2 asthma with chronic obstructive pulmonary disease (J44.9)
chronic asthmatic (obstructive) bronchitis (J44.9)
chronic obstructive asthma (J44.9)

● **J45.2 Mild intermittent asthma**
J45.2Ø Mild intermittent asthma, uncomplicated
Mild intermittent asthma NOS
J45.21 Mild intermittent asthma with (acute) exacerbation
J45.22 Mild intermittent asthma with status asthmaticus

● **J45.3 Mild persistent asthma**
J45.3Ø Mild persistent asthma, uncomplicated
Mild persistent asthma NOS
J45.31 Mild persistent asthma with (acute) exacerbation
J45.32 Mild persistent asthma with status asthmaticus

● **J45.4 Moderate persistent asthma**
J45.4Ø Moderate persistent asthma, uncomplicated
Moderate persistent asthma NOS
J45.41 Moderate persistent asthma with (acute) exacerbation
J45.42 Moderate persistent asthma with status asthmaticus

● **J45.5 Severe persistent asthma**
J45.5Ø Severe persistent asthma, uncomplicated
Severe persistent asthma NOS
J45.51 Severe persistent asthma with (acute) exacerbation
J45.52 Severe persistent asthma with status asthmaticus

Item 10–9 Asthma is a bronchial condition marked by airway obstruction, hyper-responsiveness, and inflammation. **Extrinsic** asthma, also known as allergic asthma, is characterized by the same symptoms that occur with exposure to allergens and is divided into the following types: **atopic, occupational, and allergic bronchopulmonary aspergillosis. Intrinsic** asthma occurs in patients who have no history of allergy or sensitivities to allergens and is divided into the following types: **nonreaginic and pharmacologic. Status asthmaticus** is the most severe form of asthma attack and can last for days or weeks.

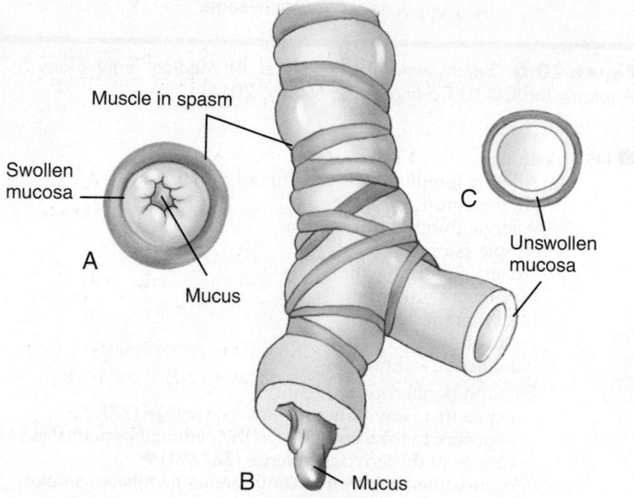

Figure 10-7 Factors causing expiratory obstruction in asthma. **A.** Cross section of a bronchiole occluded by muscle spasm, swollen mucosa, and mucus. **B.** Longitudinal section of an obstructed bronchiole. **C.** Cross-section of a clear bronchiole. (From Shiland: Mastering Healthcare Terminology, ed 1, St. Louis, Mosby, 2003)

●**J45.9 Other and unspecified asthma**

●**J45.90 Unspecified asthma**
Asthmatic bronchitis NOS
Childhood asthma NOS
Late onset asthma

J45.901 Unspecified asthma with (acute) exacerbation

J45.902 Unspecified asthma with status asthmaticus

J45.909 Unspecified asthma, uncomplicated
Asthma NOS

●**J45.99 Other asthma**

J45.990 Exercise induced bronchospasm

J45.991 Cough variant asthma

J45.998 Other asthma

●**J47 Bronchiectasis**
Includes bronchiolectasis
Use additional code to identify:
exposure to environmental tobacco smoke (Z77.22)
exposure to tobacco smoke in the perinatal period (P96.81)
history of tobacco dependence (Z87.891) ◄
occupational exposure to environmental tobacco smoke (Z57.31)
tobacco dependence (F17.-)
tobacco use (Z72.0)
Excludes1 congenital bronchiectasis (Q33.4)
tuberculous bronchiectasis (current disease) (A15.0)

J47.0 Bronchiectasis with acute lower respiratory infection
Bronchiectasis with acute bronchitis
Use additional code to identify the infection ◄

J47.1 Bronchiectasis with (acute) exacerbation

J47.9 Bronchiectasis, uncomplicated
Bronchiectasis NOS

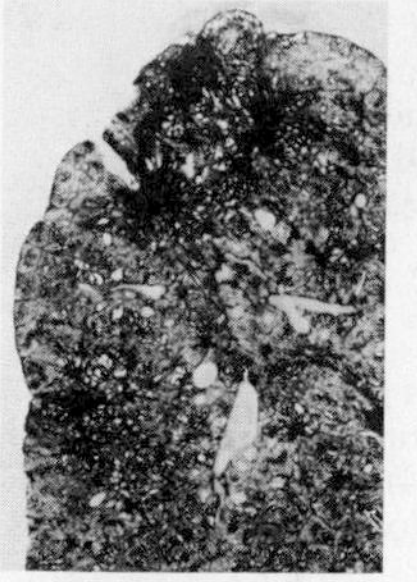

Figure 10-8 Progressive massive fibrosis superimposed on coal workers' pneumoconiosis. The large, blackened scars are located principally in the upper lobe. (From Cotran R, Kumar V, Collins T: Robbins Pathologic Basis of Disease, ed 8, Philadelphia, WB Saunders, 2009. Courtesy of Dr. Warner Laquer, Dr. Jerome Kleinerman, and the National Institute of Occupational Safety and Health, Morgantown, WV)

Item 10–10 Pneumoconiosis refers to a lung condition resulting from exposure to inorganic or organic airborne particles, such as coal dust or moldy hay, as well as chemical fumes and vapors, such as insecticides. In this condition, the lungs retain the airborne particles.

LUNG DISEASES DUE TO EXTERNAL AGENTS (J60-J70)

Excludes2 asthma (J45.-)
malignant neoplasm of bronchus and lung (C34.-)

J60 Coalworker's pneumoconiosis
Anthracosilicosis
Anthracosis
Black lung disease
Coalworker's lung
Excludes1 coalworker pneumoconiosis with tuberculosis, any type in A15 (J65)

J61 Pneumoconiosis due to asbestos and other mineral fibers
Asbestosis
Excludes1 pleural plaque with asbestosis (J92.0)
pneumoconiosis with tuberculosis, any type in A15 (J65)

●**J62 Pneumoconiosis due to dust containing silica**
Includes silicotic fibrosis (massive) of lung
Excludes1 pneumoconiosis with tuberculosis, any type in A15 (J65)

J62.0 Pneumoconiosis due to talc dust

J62.8 Pneumoconiosis due to other dust containing silica
Silicosis NOS

●**J63 Pneumoconiosis due to other inorganic dusts**
Excludes1 pneumoconiosis with tuberculosis, any type in A15 (J65)

J63.0 Aluminosis (of lung)

J63.1 Bauxite fibrosis (of lung)

J63.2 Berylliosis

J63.3 Graphite fibrosis (of lung)

J63.4 Siderosis

J63.5 Stannosis

J63.6 Pneumoconiosis due to other specified inorganic dusts

J64 Unspecified pneumoconiosis
Excludes1 pneumonoconiosis with tuberculosis, any type in A15 (J65)

J65 Pneumoconiosis associated with tuberculosis
Any condition in J60-J64 with tuberculosis, any type in A15
Silicotuberculosis

●**J66 Airway disease due to specific organic dust**
Excludes2 allergic alveolitis (J67.-)
asbestosis (J61)
bagassosis (J67.1)
farmer's lung (J67.0)
hypersensitivity pneumonitis due to organic dust (J67.-)
reactive airways dysfunction syndrome (J68.3)

J66.0 Byssinosis
Airway disease due to cotton dust

J66.1 Flax-dressers' disease

J66.2 Cannabinosis

J66.8 Airway disease due to other specific organic dusts

● **J67 Hypersensitivity pneumonitis due to organic dust**

Includes allergic alveolitis and pneumonitis due to inhaled organic dust and particles of fungal, actinomycetic or other origin

Excludes1 pneumonitis due to inhalation of chemicals, gases, fumes or vapors (J68.0)

J67.0 Farmer's lung
Harvester's lung
Haymaker's lung
Moldy hay disease

J67.1 Bagassosis
Bagasse disease
Bagasse pneumonitis

J67.2 Bird fancier's lung
Budgerigar fancier's disease or lung
Pigeon fancier's disease or lung

J67.3 Suberosis
Corkhandler's disease or lung
Corkworker's disease or lung

J67.4 Maltworker's lung
Alveolitis due to Aspergillus clavatus

J67.5 Mushroom-worker's lung

J67.6 Maple-bark-stripper's lung
Alveolitis due to Cryptostroma corticale
Cryptostromosis

J67.7 Air conditioner and humidifier lung
Allergic alveolitis due to fungal, thermophilic actinomycetes and other organisms growing in ventilation [air conditioning] systems

J67.8 Hypersensitivity pneumonitis due to other organic dusts
Cheese-washer's lung
Coffee-worker's lung
Fish-meal worker's lung
Furrier's lung
Sequoiosis

J67.9 Hypersensitivity pneumonitis due to unspecified organic dust
Allergic alveolitis (extrinsic) NOS
Hypersensitivity pneumonitis NOS

● **J68 Respiratory conditions due to inhalation of chemicals, gases, fumes and vapors**

Code first (T51-T65) to identify cause

Use additional code to identify associated respiratory conditions, such as:
acute respiratory failure (J96.0-)

J68.0 Bronchitis and pneumonitis due to chemicals, gases, fumes and vapors
Chemical bronchitis (acute)

J68.1 Pulmonary edema due to chemicals, gases, fumes and vapors
Chemical pulmonary edema (acute) (chronic)
Excludes1 pulmonary edema (acute) (chronic) NOS (J81.-)

J68.2 Upper respiratory inflammation due to chemicals, gases, fumes and vapors, not elsewhere classified

J68.3 Other acute and subacute respiratory conditions due to chemicals, gases, fumes and vapors
Reactive airways dysfunction syndrome

J68.4 Chronic respiratory conditions due to chemicals, gases, fumes and vapors
Emphysema (diffuse) (chronic) due to inhalation of chemicals, gases, fumes and vapors
Obliterative bronchiolitis (chronic) (subacute) due to inhalation of chemicals, gases, fumes and vapors
Pulmonary fibrosis (chronic) due to inhalation of chemicals, gases, fumes and vapors
Excludes1 chronic pulmonary edema due to chemicals, gases, fumes and vapors (J68.1)

J68.8 Other respiratory conditions due to chemicals, gases, fumes and vapors

J68.9 Unspecified respiratory condition due to chemicals, gases, fumes and vapors

● **J69 Pneumonitis due to solids and liquids**

Excludes1 neonatal aspiration syndromes (P24.-)
postprocedural pneumonitis (J95.4)

J69.0 Pneumonitis due to inhalation of food and vomit
Aspiration pneumonia NOS
Aspiration pneumonia (due to) food (regurgitated)
Aspiration pneumonia (due to) gastric secretions
Aspiration pneumonia (due to) milk
Aspiration pneumonia (due to) vomit
Code also any associated foreign body in respiratory tract (T17.-)
Excludes1 chemical pneumonitis due to anesthesia (J95.4)
obstetric aspiration pneumonitis (O74.0)

J69.1 Pneumonitis due to inhalation of oils and essences
Exogenous lipoid pneumonia
Lipid pneumonia NOS
Code first (T51-T65) to identify substance
Excludes1 endogenous lipoid pneumonia (J84.89)

J69.8 Pneumonitis due to inhalation of other solids and liquids
Pneumonitis due to aspiration of blood
Pneumonitis due to aspiration of detergent
Code first (T51-T65) to identify substance

● **J70 Respiratory conditions due to other external agents**

J70.0 Acute pulmonary manifestations due to radiation
Radiation pneumonitis
Use additional code (W88-W90, X39.0-) to identify the external cause

J70.1 Chronic and other pulmonary manifestations due to radiation
Fibrosis of lung following radiation
Use additional code (W88-W90, X39.0-) to identify the external cause

J70.2 Acute drug-induced interstitial lung disorders
Use additional code for adverse effect, if applicable, to identify drug (T36-T50 with fifth or sixth character 5)
Excludes1 interstitial pneumonia NOS (J84.9)
lymphoid interstitial pneumonia (J84.2)

J70.3 Chronic drug-induced interstitial lung disorders
Use additional code for adverse effect, if applicable, to identify drug (T36-T50 with fifth or sixth character 5)
Excludes1 interstitial pneumonia NOS (J84.9)
lymphoid interstitial pneumonia (J84.2)

J70.4 Drug-induced interstitial lung disorders, unspecified
Use additional code for adverse effect, if applicable, to identify drug (T36-T50 with fifth or sixth character 5)
Excludes1 interstitial pneumonia NOS (J84.9)
lymphoid interstitial pneumonia (J84.2)

J70.5 Respiratory conditions due to smoke inhalation
Smoke inhalation NOS
Excludes1 smoke inhalation due to chemicals, gases, fumes and vapors (J68.9)

J70.8 Respiratory conditions due to other specified external agents
Code first (T51-T65) to identify the external agent

J70.9 Respiratory conditions due to unspecified external agent
Code first (T51-T65) to identify the external agent

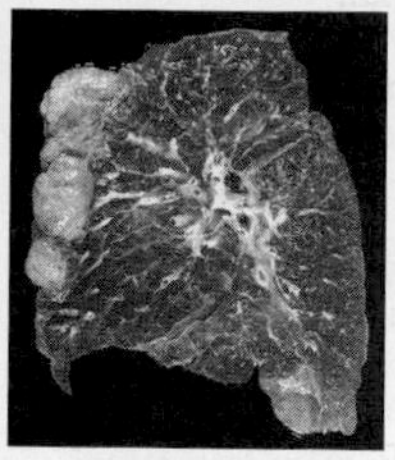

Figure 10-9 Bullous emphysema with large subpleural bullae *(upper left)*. (From Kumar: Robbins and Cotran: Pathologic Basis of Disease, ed 8, Saunders, An Imprint of Elsevier, 2009)

OTHER RESPIRATORY DISEASES PRINCIPALLY AFFECTING THE INTERSTITIUM (J80-J84)

J80 Acute respiratory distress syndrome
Acute respiratory distress syndrome in adult or child
Adult hyaline membrane disease
Excludes1 respiratory distress syndrome in newborn (perinatal) (P22.0)

● **J81 Pulmonary edema**
Use additional code to identify:
exposure to environmental tobacco smoke (Z77.22)
history of tobacco dependence (Z87.891)
occupational exposure to environmental tobacco smoke (Z57.31)
tobacco dependence (F17.-)
tobacco use (Z72.0)
Excludes1 chemical (acute) pulmonary edema (J68.1)
hypostatic pneumonia (J18.2)
passive pneumonia (J18.2)
pulmonary edema due to external agents (J60-J70)
pulmonary edema with heart disease NOS (I50.1)
pulmonary edema with heart failure (I50.1)

J81.0 Acute pulmonary edema
Acute edema of lung

J81.1 Chronic pulmonary edema
Pulmonary congestion (chronic) (passive)
Pulmonary edema NOS

J82 Pulmonary eosinophilia, not elsewhere classified
Allergic pneumonia
Eosinophilic asthma
Eosinophilic pneumonia
Löffler's pneumonia
Tropical (pulmonary) eosinophilia NOS
Excludes1 pulmonary eosinophilia due to aspergillosis (B44.-)
pulmonary eosinophilia due to drugs (J70.2-J70.4)
pulmonary eosinophilia due to specified parasitic infection (B50-B83)
pulmonary eosinophilia due to systemic connective tissue disorders (M30-M36)
pulmonary infiltrate NOS (R91.8)

● **J84 Other interstitial pulmonary diseases**
Excludes1 drug-induced interstitial lung disorders (J70.2-J70.4)
interstitial emphysema (J98.2)
lung diseases due to external agents (J60-J70)

● **J84.0 Alveolar and parieto-alveolar conditions**

J84.01 Alveolar proteinosis

J84.02 Pulmonary alveolar microlithiasis

J84.03 Idiopathic pulmonary hemosiderosis
Essential brown induration of lung
Code first underlying disease, such as:
disorders of iron metabolism (E83.1-)
Excludes1 acute idiopathic pulmonary hemorrhage in infants [AIPHI] (R04.81)

J84.09 Other alveolar and parieto-alveolar conditions

● **J84.1 Other interstitial pulmonary diseases with fibrosis**
Excludes1 pulmonary fibrosis (chronic) due to inhalation of chemicals, gases, fumes or vapors (J68.4)
pulmonary fibrosis (chronic) following radiation (J70.1)

J84.10 Pulmonary fibrosis, unspecified
Capillary fibrosis of lung
Cirrhosis of lung (chronic) NOS
Fibrosis of lung (atrophic) (chronic) (confluent) (massive) (perialveolar) (peribronchial) NOS
Induration of lung (chronic) NOS
Postinflammatory pulmonary fibrosis

● **J84.11 Idiopathic interstitial pneumonia**
Excludes1 lymphoid interstitial pneumonia (J84.2)
pneumocystis pneumonia (B59)

J84.111 Idiopathic interstitial pneumonia, not otherwise specified

J84.112 Idiopathic pulmonary fibrosis
Cryptogenic fibrosing alveolitis
Idiopathic fibrosing alveolitis

J84.113 Idiopathic non-specific interstitial pneumonitis
Excludes1 non-specific interstitial pneumonia NOS, or due to known underlying cause (J84.89)

J84.114 Acute interstitial pneumonitis
Hamman-Rich syndrome
Excludes1 pneumocystis pneumonia (B59)

J84.115 Respiratory bronchiolitis interstitial lung disease

J84.116 Cryptogenic organizing pneumonia
Excludes1 organizing pneumonia NOS, or due to known underlying cause (J84.89)

J84.117 Desquamative interstitial pneumonia

J84.17 Other interstitial pulmonary diseases with fibrosis in diseases classified elsewhere
Interstitial pneumonia (nonspecific) (usual) due to collagen vascular disease
Interstitial pneumonia (nonspecific) (usual) in diseases classified elsewhere
Organizing pneumonia due to collagen vascular disease
Organizing pneumonia in diseases classified elsewhere
Code first underlying disease, such as:
progressive systemic sclerosis (M34.0)
rheumatoid arthritis (M05.00-M06.9)
systemic lupus erythematosis (M32.0-M32.9)

J84.2 Lymphoid interstitial pneumonia
Lymphoid interstitial pneumonitis

● **J84.8 Other specified interstitial pulmonary diseases**
Excludes1 exogenous lipoid pneumonia (J69.1)
unspecified lipoid pneumonia (J69.1)

J84.81 Lymphangioleiomyomatosis
Lymphangiomyomatosis

J84.82 Adult pulmonary Langerhans cell histiocytosis
Adult PLCH

J84.83 Surfactant mutations of the lung

CHAPTER 10 (J00-J99)

● **J84.84 Other interstitial lung diseases of childhood**
- **J84.841 Neuroendocrine cell hyperplasia of infancy**
- **J84.842 Pulmonary interstitial glycogenosis**
- **J84.843 Alveolar capillary dysplasia with vein misalignment**
- **J84.848 Other interstitial lung diseases of childhood**

J84.89 Other specified interstitial pulmonary diseases
Endogenous lipoid pneumonia
Interstitial pneumonitis
Non-specific interstitial pneumonitis NOS
~~Organizing pneumonia due to known underlying cause~~
Organizing pneumonia NOS
Code first, if applicable:
poisoning due to drug or toxin (T51-T65 with fifth or sixth character to indicate intent), for toxic pneumonopathy
underlying cause of pneumonopathy, if known
Use additional code, for adverse effect, to identify drug (T36-T50 with fifth or sixth character 5), if drug-induced
Excludes1 cryptogenic organizing pneumonia (J84.116)
idiopathic non-specific interstitial pneumonitis (J84.113)
lipoid pneumonia, exogenous or unspecified (J69.1)
lymphoid interstitial pneumonia (J84.2)

J84.9 Interstitial pulmonary disease, unspecified
Interstitial pneumonia NOS

SUPPURATIVE AND NECROTIC CONDITIONS OF THE LOWER RESPIRATORY TRACT (J85-J86)

● **J85 Abscess of lung and mediastinum**
Use additional code (B95-B97) to identify infectious agent.
- **J85.0 Gangrene and necrosis of lung**
- **J85.1 Abscess of lung with pneumonia**
  Code also the type of pneumonia
- **J85.2 Abscess of lung without pneumonia**
  Abscess of lung NOS
- **J85.3 Abscess of mediastinum**

● **J86 Pyothorax**
Use additional code (B95-B97) to identify infectious agent.
Excludes1 abscess of lung (J85.-)
pyothorax due to tuberculosis (A15.6)
- **J86.0 Pyothorax with fistula**
  Bronchocutaneous fistula
  Bronchopleural fistula
  Hepatopleural fistula
  Mediastinal fistula
  Pleural fistula
  Thoracic fistula
  Any condition classifiable to J86.9 with fistula
- **J86.9 Pyothorax without fistula**
  Abscess of pleura
  Abscess of thorax
  Empyema (chest) (lung) (pleura)
  Fibrinopurulent pleurisy
  Purulent pleurisy
  Pyopneumothorax
  Septic pleurisy
  Seropurulent pleurisy
  Suppurative pleurisy

Item 10–11 Empyema is a condition in which pus accumulates in a body cavity. Empyema **with fistula** occurs when the pus passes from one cavity to another organ or structure.

OTHER DISEASES OF THE PLEURA (J90-J94)

J90 Pleural effusion, not elsewhere classified
Encysted pleurisy
Pleural effusion NOS
Pleurisy with effusion (exudative) (serous)
Excludes1 chylous (pleural) effusion (J94.0)
malignant pleural effusion (J91.0))
pleurisy NOS (R09.1)
tuberculous pleural effusion (A15.6)

● **J91 Pleural effusion in conditions classified elsewhere**
Excludes2 pleural effusion in heart failure (I50.-)
pleural effusion in systemic lupus erythematosus (M32.13)
- **J91.0 Malignant pleural effusion**
  Code first underlying neoplasm
- **J91.8 Pleural effusion in other conditions classified elsewhere**
  Code first underlying disease, such as:
  filariasis (B74.0-B74.9)
  influenza (J09.X2, J10.1, J11.1)

● **J92 Pleural plaque**
Includes pleural thickening
- **J92.0 Pleural plaque with presence of asbestos**
- **J92.9 Pleural plaque without asbestos**
  Pleural plaque NOS

● **J93 Pneumothorax and air leak**
Collapsed lung
Excludes1 congenital or perinatal pneumothorax (P25.1)
postprocedural air leak (J95.812)
postprocedural pneumothorax (J95.811)
traumatic pneumothorax (S27.0)
tuberculous (current disease) pneumothorax (A15.-)
pyopneumothorax (J86.-)
- **J93.0 Spontaneous tension pneumothorax**
  Tension pneumothorax (most serious type) occurs when air (positive pressure) collects in the pleural space
- ● **J93.1 Other spontaneous pneumothorax**
  - **J93.11 Primary spontaneous pneumothorax**
  - **J93.12 Secondary spontaneous pneumothorax**
    Code first underlying condition, such as:
    catamenial pneumothorax due to endometriosis (N80.8)
    cystic fibrosis (E84.-)
    eosinophilic pneumonia (J82)
    lymphangioleiomyomatosis (J84.81)
    malignant neoplasm of bronchus and lung (C34.-)
    Marfan's syndrome (Q87.4)
    pneumonia due to Pneumocystis carinii (B59)
    secondary malignant neoplasm of lung (C78.0-)
    spontaneous rupture of the esophagus (K22.3)
- ● **J93.8 Other pneumothorax and air leak**
  - **J93.81 Chronic pneumothorax**
  - **J93.82 Other air leak**
    Persistent air leak
  - **J93.83 Other pneumothorax**
    Acute pneumothorax
    Spontaneous pneumothorax NOS
- **J93.9 Pneumothorax, unspecified**
  Pneumothorax NOS

● J94 **Other pleural conditions**
Excludes1 pleurisy NOS (RØ9.1)
traumatic hemopneumothorax (S27.2)
traumatic hemothorax (S27.1)
tuberculous pleural conditions (current disease) (A15.-)

J94.Ø **Chylous effusion**
Chyliform effusion

J94.1 **Fibrothorax**

J94.2 **Hemothorax**
Hemopneumothorax

J94.8 **Other specified pleural conditions**
Hydropneumothorax
Hydrothorax

J94.9 **Pleural condition, unspecified**

INTRAOPERATIVE AND POSTPROCEDURAL COMPLICATIONS AND DISORDERS OF RESPIRATORY SYSTEM, NOT ELSEWHERE CLASSIFIED (J95)

● J95 **Intraoperative and postprocedural complications and disorders of respiratory system, not elsewhere classified**
Excludes2 aspiration pneumonia (J69.-)
emphysema (subcutaneous) resulting from a procedure (T81.82)
hypostatic pneumonia (J18.2)
pulmonary manifestations due to radiation (J7Ø.Ø- J7Ø.1)

● J95.Ø **Tracheostomy complications**

J95.ØØ **Unspecified tracheostomy complication**

J95.Ø1 **Hemorrhage from tracheostomy stoma**

J95.Ø2 **Infection of tracheostomy stoma**
Use additional code to identify type of infection, such as:
cellulitis of neck (LØ3.8)
sepsis (A4Ø, A41.-)

J95.Ø3 **Malfunction of tracheostomy stoma**
Mechanical complication of tracheostomy stoma
Obstruction of tracheostomy airway
Tracheal stenosis due to tracheostomy

J95.Ø4 **Tracheo-esophageal fistula following tracheostomy**

J95.Ø9 **Other tracheostomy complication**

J95.1 **Acute pulmonary insufficiency following thoracic surgery**
Excludes2 functional disturbances following cardiac surgery (I97.Ø, I97.1-)

J95.2 **Acute pulmonary insufficiency following nonthoracic surgery**
Excludes2 functional disturbances following cardiac surgery (I97.Ø, I97.1-)

J95.3 **Chronic pulmonary insufficiency following surgery**
Excludes2 functional disturbances following cardiac surgery (I97.Ø, I97.1-)

J95.4 **Chemical pneumonitis due to anesthesia**
Mendelson's syndrome
Postprocedural aspiration pneumonia
Use additional code for adverse effect, if applicable, to identify drug (T41.- with fifth or sixth character 5)
Excludes1 aspiration pneumonitis due to anesthesia complicating labor and delivery (O74.Ø)
aspiration pneumonitis due to anesthesia complicating pregnancy (O29)
aspiration pneumonitis due to anesthesia complicating the puerperium (O89.Ø1)

J95.5 **Postprocedural subglottic stenosis**

● J95.6 **Intraoperative hemorrhage and hematoma of a respiratory system organ or structure complicating a procedure**
Excludes1 intraoperative hemorrhage and hematoma of a respiratory system organ or structure due to accidental puncture and laceration during procedure (J95.7-)

J95.61 **Intraoperative hemorrhage and hematoma of a respiratory system organ or structure complicating a respiratory system procedure**

J95.62 **Intraoperative hemorrhage and hematoma of a respiratory system organ or structure complicating other procedure**

● J95.7 **Accidental puncture and laceration of a respiratory system organ or structure during a procedure**
Excludes2 postprocedural pneumothorax (J95.811)

J95.71 **Accidental puncture and laceration of a respiratory system organ or structure during a respiratory system procedure**

J95.72 **Accidental puncture and laceration of a respiratory system organ or structure during other procedure**

● J95.8 **Other intraoperative and postprocedural complications and disorders of respiratory system, not elsewhere classified**

● J95.81 **Postprocedural pneumothorax and air leak**

J95.811 **Postprocedural pneumothorax**

J95.812 **Postprocedural air leak**

● J95.82 **Postprocedural respiratory failure**
Excludes1 Respiratory failure in other conditions (J96.-)

J95.821 **Acute postprocedural respiratory failure**
Postprocedural respiratory failure NOS

J95.822 **Acute and chronic postprocedural respiratory failure**

● J95.83 **Postprocedural hemorrhage of a respiratory system organ or structure following a procedure** ◄

J95.83Ø **Postprocedural hemorrhage of a respiratory system organ or structure following a respiratory system procedure** ◄

J95.831 **Postprocedural hemorrhage of a respiratory system organ or structure following other procedure** ◄

J95.84 **Transfusion-related acute lung injury (TRALI)**

● J95.85 **Complication of respirator [ventilator]**

J95.85Ø **Mechanical complication of respirator**
Excludes1 encounter for respirator [ventilator] dependence during power failure (Z99.12)

J95.851 **Ventilator associated pneumonia**
Ventilator associated pneumonitis
Use additional code to identify the organism, if known (B95.-, B96.-, B97.-)
Excludes1 ventilator lung in newborn (P27.8)

J95.859 **Other complication of respirator [ventilator]**

CHAPTER 1Ø (JØØ-J99)

● **J95.86 Postprocedural hematoma and seroma of a respiratory system organ or structure following a procedure ◀**

J95.860 Postprocedural hematoma of a respiratory system organ or structure following a respiratory system procedure ◀

J95.861 Postprocedural hematoma of a respiratory system organ or structure following other procedure ◀

J95.862 Postprocedural seroma of a respiratory system organ or structure following a respiratory system procedure ◀

J95.863 Postprocedural seroma of a respiratory system organ or structure following other procedure ◀

J95.88 Other intraoperative complications of respiratory system, not elsewhere classified

J95.89 Other postprocedural complications and disorders of respiratory system, not elsewhere classified

Use additional code to identify disorder, such as:
aspiration pneumonia (J69.-)
bacterial or viral pneumonia (J12-J18)

Excludes2 acute pulmonary insufficiency following thoracic surgery (J95.1)
postprocedural subglottic stenosis (J95.5)

OTHER DISEASES OF THE RESPIRATORY SYSTEM (J96-J99)

● **J96 Respiratory failure, not elsewhere classified**

Excludes1 acute respiratory distress syndrome (J80)
cardiorespiratory failure (R09.2)
newborn respiratory distress syndrome (P22.0)
postprocedural respiratory failure (J95.82-)
respiratory arrest (R09.2)
respiratory arrest of newborn (P28.81)
respiratory failure of newborn (P28.5)

● **J96.0 Acute respiratory failure**

J96.00 Acute respiratory failure, unspecified whether with hypoxia or hypercapnia

J96.01 Acute respiratory failure with hypoxia

J96.02 Acute respiratory failure with hypercapnia

● **J96.1 Chronic respiratory failure**

J96.10 Chronic respiratory failure, unspecified whether with hypoxia or hypercapnia

J96.11 Chronic respiratory failure with hypoxia

J96.12 Chronic respiratory failure with hypercapnia

● **J96.2 Acute and chronic respiratory failure**

Acute on chronic respiratory failure

J96.20 Acute and chronic respiratory failure, unspecified whether with hypoxia or hypercapnia

J96.21 Acute and chronic respiratory failure with hypoxia

J96.22 Acute and chronic respiratory failure with hypercapnia

● **J96.9 Respiratory failure, unspecified**

J96.90 Respiratory failure, unspecified, unspecified whether with hypoxia or hypercapnia

J96.91 Respiratory failure, unspecified with hypoxia

J96.92 Respiratory failure, unspecified with hypercapnia

● **J98 Other respiratory disorders**

Use additional code to identify:
exposure to environmental tobacco smoke (Z77.22)
exposure to tobacco smoke in the perinatal period (P96.81)
history of tobacco dependence (Z87.891) ⬅
occupational exposure to environmental tobacco smoke (Z57.31)
tobacco dependence (F17.-)
tobacco use (Z72.0)

Excludes1 newborn apnea (P28.4)
newborn sleep apnea (P28.3)

Excludes2 apnea NOS (R06.81)
sleep apnea (G47.3-)

● **J98.0 Diseases of bronchus, not elsewhere classified**

J98.01 Acute bronchospasm

Excludes1 acute bronchiolitis with bronchospasm (J21.-)
acute bronchitis with bronchospasm (J20.-)
asthma (J45.-)
exercise induced bronchospasm (J45.990)

J98.09 Other diseases of bronchus, not elsewhere classified

Broncholithiasis
Calcification of bronchus
Stenosis of bronchus
Tracheobronchial collapse
Tracheobronchial dyskinesia
Ulcer of bronchus

● **J98.1 Pulmonary collapse**

Excludes1 therapeutic collapse of lung status (Z98.3)

J98.11 Atelectasis

Excludes1 newborn atelectasis
tuberculous atelectasis (current disease) (A15)

J98.19 Other pulmonary collapse

J98.2 Interstitial emphysema

Mediastinal emphysema

Excludes1 emphysema NOS (J43.9)
emphysema in newborn (P25.0)
surgical emphysema (subcutaneous) (T81.82)
traumatic subcutaneous emphysema (T79.7)

J98.3 Compensatory emphysema

J98.4 Other disorders of lung

Calcification of lung
Cystic lung disease (acquired)
Lung disease NOS
Pulmolithiasis

Excludes1 acute interstitial pneumonitis (J84.114)
pulmonary insufficiency following surgery (J95.1-J95.2)

CHAPTER 10 (J00-J99)

J98.5 Diseases of mediastinum, not elsewhere classified
Excludes2 abscess of mediastinum (J85.3)

J98.51 Mediastinitis
Code first underlying condition, if applicable, such as postoperative mediastinitis (T81.-)

J98.59 Other diseases of mediastinum, not elsewhere classified
Fibrosis of mediastinum
Hernia of mediastinum
Retraction of mediastinum

J98.6 Disorders of diaphragm
Diaphragmatitis
Paralysis of diaphragm
Relaxation of diaphragm
Excludes1 congenital malformation of diaphragm NEC (Q79.1)
congenital diaphragmatic hernia (Q79.0)
Excludes2 diaphragmatic hernia (K44.-)

J98.8 Other specified respiratory disorders

J98.9 Respiratory disorder, unspecified
Respiratory disease (chronic) NOS

J99 Respiratory disorders in diseases classified elsewhere
Code first underlying disease, such as:
amyloidosis (E85.-)
ankylosing spondylitis (M45)
congenital syphilis (A50.5)
cryoglobulinemia (D89.1)
early congenital syphilis (A50.0)
schistosomiasis (B65.0-B65.9)
Excludes1 respiratory disorders in:
amebiasis (A06.5)
blastomycosis (B40.0-B40.2)
candidiasis (B37.1)
coccidioidomycosis (B38.0-B38.2)
cystic fibrosis with pulmonary manifestations (E84.0)
dermatomyositis (M33.01, M33.11)
histoplasmosis (B39.0-B39.2)
late syphilis (A52.72, A52.73)
polymyositis (M33.21)
sicca syndrome (M35.02)
systemic lupus erythematosus (M32.13)
systemic sclerosis (M34.81)
Wegener's granulomatosis (M31.30-M31.31)

CHAPTER 11

DISEASES OF THE DIGESTIVE SYSTEM (K00-K95)

OGCR Chapter-Specific Coding Guidelines

11. Chapter 11: Diseases of the Digestive System (K00-K95)
Reserved for future guideline expansion

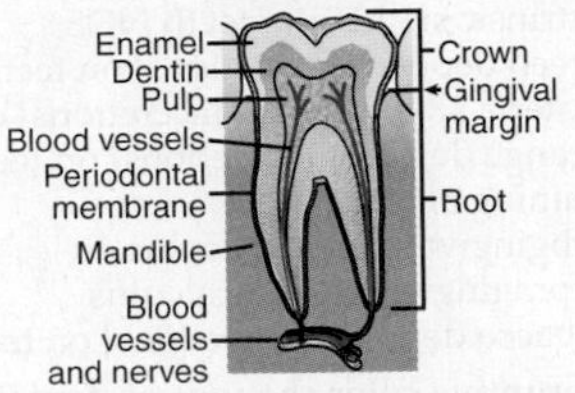

Figure 11-1 Anatomy of a tooth.

Item 11-1 **Anodontia** is the congenital absence of teeth. **Hypodontia** is partial anodontia. **Oligodontia** is the congenital absence of some teeth, whereas **supernumerary** is having more teeth than the normal number. **Mesiodens** are small extra teeth that often appear in pairs, although single small teeth are not uncommon.

CHAPTER 11

DISEASES OF THE DIGESTIVE SYSTEM (K00-K95)

Excludes2 certain conditions originating in the perinatal period (P04-P96)
certain infectious and parasitic diseases (A00-B99)
complications of pregnancy, childbirth and the puerperium (O00-O9A)
congenital malformations, deformations and chromosomal abnormalities (Q00-Q99)
endocrine, nutritional and metabolic diseases (E00-E88)
injury, poisoning and certain other consequences of external causes (S00-T88)
neoplasms (C00-D49)
symptoms, signs and abnormal clinical and laboratory findings, not elsewhere classified (R00-R94)

This chapter contains the following blocks:

K00-K14	Diseases of oral cavity and salivary glands
K20-K31	Diseases of esophagus, stomach and duodenum
K35-K38	Diseases of appendix
K40-K46	Hernia
K50-K52	Noninfective enteritis and colitis
K55-K64	Other diseases of intestines
K65-K68	Diseases of peritoneum and retroperitoneum
K70-K77	Diseases of liver
K80-K87	Disorders of gallbladder, biliary tract and pancreas
K90-K95	Other diseases of the digestive system

DISEASES OF ORAL CAVITY AND SALIVARY GLANDS (K00-K14)

● **K00 Disorders of tooth development and eruption**
Excludes2 embedded and impacted teeth (K01.-)

K00.0 Anodontia
Hypodontia
Oligodontia
Excludes1 acquired absence of teeth (K08.1-)

K00.1 Supernumerary teeth
Distomolar
Fourth molar
Mesiodens
Paramolar
Supplementary teeth
Excludes2 supernumerary roots (K00.2)

K00.2 Abnormalities of size and form of teeth
Concrescence of teeth
Fusion of teeth
Gemination of teeth
Dens evaginatus
Dens in dente
Dens invaginatus
Enamel pearls
Macrodontia
Microdontia
Peg-shaped [conical] teeth
Supernumerary roots
Taurodontism
Tuberculum paramolare
Excludes1 abnormalities of teeth due to congenital syphilis (A50.5)
tuberculum Carabelli, which is regarded as a normal variation and should not be coded

K00.3 Mottled teeth
Dental fluorosis
Mottling of enamel
Nonfluoride enamel opacities
Excludes2 deposits [accretions] on teeth (K03.6)

K00.4 Disturbances in tooth formation
Aplasia and hypoplasia of cementum
Dilaceration of tooth
Enamel hypoplasia (neonatal) (postnatal) (prenatal)
Regional odontodysplasia
Turner's tooth
Excludes1 Hutchinson's teeth and mulberry molars in congenital syphilis (A50.5)
Excludes2 mottled teeth (K00.3)

K00.5 Hereditary disturbances in tooth structure, not elsewhere classified
Amelogenesis imperfecta
Dentinogenesis imperfecta
Odontogenesis imperfecta
Dentinal dysplasia
Shell teeth

K00.6 Disturbances in tooth eruption
Dentia praecox
Natal tooth
Neonatal tooth
Premature eruption of tooth
Premature shedding of primary [deciduous] tooth
Prenatal teeth
Retained [persistent] primary tooth
Excludes2 embedded and impacted teeth (K01.-)

K00.7 Teething syndrome

K00.8 Other disorders of tooth development
Color changes during tooth formation
Intrinsic staining of teeth NOS
Excludes2 posteruptive color changes (K03.7)

K00.9 Disorder of tooth development, unspecified
Disorder of odontogenesis NOS

● **K01 Embedded and impacted teeth**
Excludes1 abnormal position of fully erupted teeth (M26.3-)

K01.0 Embedded teeth

K01.1 Impacted teeth

◄ New ◄ Revised ~~deleted~~ Deleted **OGCR** Official Guidelines X Assign placeholder X ● Use Additional Character(s)
Excludes 1 | Excludes 2 | Includes | Use additional | Code first | Code also | Unspecified

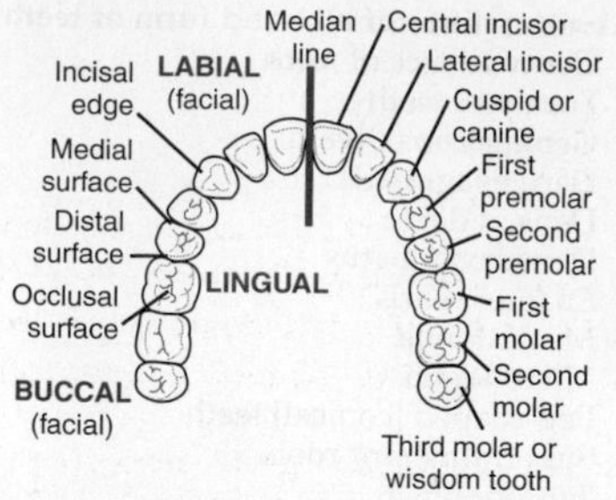

Figure 11-2 The permanent teeth within the dental arch.

Item 11-2 Each dental arch (jaw) normally contains 16 teeth. Tooth decay or **dental caries** is a disease of the enamel, dentin, and cementum of the tooth and can result in a cavity.

● **KØ2 Dental caries**
 Includes caries of dentine ◀
 dental cavities
 early childhood caries ◀
 pre-eruptive caries ◀
 recurrent caries (dentino enamel junction) (enamel) (to the pulp) ◀
 tooth decay

KØ2.3 Arrested dental caries
 Arrested coronal and root caries

● **KØ2.5 Dental caries on pit and fissure surface**
 Dental caries on chewing surface of tooth

KØ2.51 Dental caries on pit and fissure surface limited to enamel
 White spot lesions [initial caries] on pit and fissure surface of tooth

KØ2.52 Dental caries on pit and fissure surface penetrating into dentin
 Primary dental caries, cervical origin ◀

KØ2.53 Dental caries on pit and fissure surface penetrating into pulp

● **KØ2.6 Dental caries on smooth surface**

KØ2.61 Dental caries on smooth surface limited to enamel
 White spot lesions [initial caries] on smooth surface of tooth

KØ2.62 Dental caries on smooth surface penetrating into dentin

KØ2.63 Dental caries on smooth surface penetrating into pulp

KØ2.7 Dental root caries

KØ2.9 Dental caries, unspecified

● **KØ3 Other diseases of hard tissues of teeth**
 Excludes2 bruxism (F45.8)
 dental caries (KØ2.-)
 teeth-grinding NOS (F45.8)

KØ3.Ø Excessive attrition of teeth
 Approximal wear of teeth
 Occlusal wear of teeth

KØ3.1 Abrasion of teeth
 Dentifrice abrasion of teeth
 Habitual abrasion of teeth
 Occupational abrasion of teeth
 Ritual abrasion of teeth
 Traditional abrasion of teeth
 Wedge defect NOS

KØ3.2 Erosion of teeth
 Erosion of teeth due to diet
 Erosion of teeth due to drugs and medicaments
 Erosion of teeth due to persistent vomiting
 Erosion of teeth NOS
 Idiopathic erosion of teeth
 Occupational erosion of teeth

KØ3.3 Pathological resorption of teeth
 Internal granuloma of pulp
 Resorption of teeth (external)

KØ3.4 Hypercementosis
 Cementation hyperplasia

KØ3.5 Ankylosis of teeth

KØ3.6 Deposits [accretions] on teeth
 Betel deposits [accretions] on teeth
 Black deposits [accretions] on teeth
 Extrinsic staining of teeth NOS
 Green deposits [accretions] on teeth
 Materia alba deposits [accretions] on teeth
 Orange deposits [accretions] on teeth
 Staining of teeth NOS
 Subgingival dental calculus
 Supragingival dental calculus
 Tobacco deposits [accretions] on teeth

KØ3.7 Posteruptive color changes of dental hard tissues
 Excludes2 deposits [accretions] on teeth (KØ3.6)

● **KØ3.8 Other specified diseases of hard tissues of teeth**

KØ3.81 Cracked tooth
 Excludes1 asymptomatic craze lines in enamel - omit code
 broken or fractured tooth due to trauma (SØ2.5)

KØ3.89 Other specified diseases of hard tissues of teeth

KØ3.9 Disease of hard tissues of teeth, unspecified

KØ4 Diseases of pulp and periapical tissues

● **KØ4.Ø Pulpitis**
 Acute pulpitis
 Chronic (hyperplastic) (ulcerative) pulpitis

KØ4.Ø1 Reversible pulpitis ◀

KØ4.Ø2 Irreversible pulpitis ◀

KØ4.1 Necrosis of pulp
 Pulpal gangrene

KØ4.2 Pulp degeneration
 Denticles
 Pulpal calcifications
 Pulpal stones

KØ4.3 Abnormal hard tissue formation in pulp
 Secondary or irregular dentine

KØ4.4 Acute apical periodontitis of pulpal origin
 Acute apical periodontitis NOS
 Excludes1 acute periodontitis (KØ5.2-)

KØ4.5 Chronic apical periodontitis
 Apical or periapical granuloma
 Apical periodontitis NOS
 Excludes1 chronic periodontitis (KØ5.3-)

KØ4.6 Periapical abscess with sinus
 Dental abscess with sinus
 Dentoalveolar abscess with sinus

KØ4.7 Periapical abscess without sinus
 Dental abscess without sinus
 Dentoalveolar abscess without sinus
 Periapical abscess without sinus

KØ4.8 Radicular cyst
 Apical (periodontal) cyst
 Periapical cyst
 Residual radicular cyst
 Excludes2 lateral periodontal cyst (KØ9.Ø)

● **KØ4.9 Other and unspecified diseases of pulp and periapical tissues**

KØ4.9Ø Unspecified diseases of pulp and periapical tissues

KØ4.99 Other diseases of pulp and periapical tissues

Item 11–3 Acute gingivitis, also known as orilitis or ulitis, is the short-term, severe inflammation of the gums (gingiva) caused by bacteria. **Chronic gingivitis** is persistent inflammation of the gums. When the gingivitis moves into the periodontium it is called periodontitis, also known as paradentitis.

● **K05 Gingivitis and periodontal diseases**
Use additional code to identify:
alcohol abuse and dependence (F10.-)
exposure to environmental tobacco smoke (Z77.22)
exposure to tobacco smoke in the perinatal period (P96.81)
history of tobacco dependence (Z87.891)
occupational exposure to environmental tobacco smoke (Z57.31)
tobacco dependence (F17.-)
tobacco use (Z72.0)

● **K05.0 Acute gingivitis**
Excludes1 acute necrotizing ulcerative gingivitis (A69.1)
herpesviral [herpes simplex] gingivostomatitis (B00.2)

K05.00 Acute gingivitis, plaque induced
Acute gingivitis NOS
Plaque induced gingival disease ◀

K05.01 Acute gingivitis, non-plaque induced

● **K05.1 Chronic gingivitis**
Desquamative gingivitis (chronic)
Gingivitis (chronic) NOS
Hyperplastic gingivitis (chronic)
Pregnancy associated gingivitis ◀
Simple marginal gingivitis (chronic)
Ulcerative gingivitis (chronic)
Code first, if applicable, diseases of the digestive system complicating pregnancy (O99.61-) ◀

K05.10 Chronic gingivitis, plaque induced
Chronic gingivitis NOS
Gingivitis NOS

K05.11 Chronic gingivitis, non-plaque induced

● **K05.2 Aggressive periodontitis**
Acute pericoronitis
Excludes1 acute apical periodontitis (K04.4)
periapical abscess (K04.7)
periapical abscess with sinus (K04.6)

K05.20 Aggressive periodontitis, unspecified

● **K05.21 Aggressive periodontitis, localized**
Periodontal abscess

K05.211 Aggressive periodontitis, localized, slight ◀
K05.212 Aggressive periodontitis, localized, moderate ◀
K05.213 Aggressive periodontitis, localized, severe ◀
K05.219 Aggressive periodontitis, localized, unspecified severity ◀

● **K05.22 Aggressive periodontitis, generalized**
K05.221 Aggressive periodontitis, generalized, slight ◀
K05.222 Aggressive periodontitis, generalized, moderate ◀
K05.223 Aggressive periodontitis, generalized, severe ◀
K05.229 Aggressive periodontitis, generalized, unspecified severity ◀

● **K05.3 Chronic periodontitis**
Chronic pericoronitis
Complex periodontitis
Periodontitis NOS
Simplex periodontitis
Excludes1 chronic apical periodontitis (K04.5)

K05.30 Chronic periodontitis, unspecified

● **K05.31 Chronic periodontitis, localized**
K05.311 Chronic periodontitis, localized, slight ◀
K05.312 Chronic periodontitis, localized, moderate ◀
K05.313 Chronic periodontitis, localized, severe ◀
K05.319 Chronic periodontitis, localized, unspecified severity ◀

● **K05.32 Chronic periodontitis, generalized**
K05.321 Chronic periodontitis, generalized, slight ◀
K05.322 Chronic periodontitis, generalized, moderate ◀
K05.323 Chronic periodontitis, generalized, severe ◀
K05.329 Chronic periodontitis, generalized, unspecified severity ◀

K05.4 Periodontosis
Juvenile periodontosis

K05.5 Other periodontal diseases
Combined periodontic-endodontic lesion ◀
Narrow gingival width (of periodontal soft tissue) ◀
Excludes2 leukoplakia of gingiva (K13.21)

K05.6 Periodontal disease, unspecified

● **K06 Other disorders of gingiva and edentulous alveolar ridge**
Excludes2 acute gingivitis (K05.0)
atrophy of edentulous alveolar ridge (K08.2)
chronic gingivitis (K05.1)
gingivitis NOS (K05.1)

K06.0 Gingival recession
Gingival recession (generalized) (localized) (postinfective) (postprocedural)

K06.1 Gingival enlargement
Gingival fibromatosis

K06.2 Gingival and edentulous alveolar ridge lesions associated with trauma
Irritative hyperplasia of edentulous ridge [denture hyperplasia]
Use additional code (Chapter 20) to identify external cause or denture status (Z97.2)

K06.3 Horizontal alveolar bone loss ◀

K06.8 Other specified disorders of gingiva and edentulous alveolar ridge
Fibrous epulis
Flabby alveolar ridge
Giant cell epulis
Peripheral giant cell granuloma of gingiva
Pyogenic granuloma of gingiva
Vertical ridge deficiency ◀
Excludes2 gingival cyst (K09.0)

K06.9 Disorder of gingiva and edentulous alveolar ridge, unspecified

● KØ8 **Other disorders of teeth and supporting structures**
Excludes2 dentofacial anomalies [including malocclusion] (M26.-)
disorders of jaw (M27.-)

KØ8.Ø **Exfoliation of teeth due to systemic causes**
Code also underlying systemic condition

● KØ8.1 **Complete loss of teeth**
Acquired loss of teeth, complete
Excludes1 congenital absence of teeth (KØØ.Ø)
exfoliation of teeth due to systemic causes (KØ8.Ø)
partial loss of teeth (KØ8.4-)

● KØ8.1Ø **Complete loss of teeth, unspecified cause**
KØ8.1Ø1 **Complete loss of teeth, unspecified cause, class I**
KØ8.1Ø2 **Complete loss of teeth, unspecified cause, class II**
KØ8.1Ø3 **Complete loss of teeth, unspecified cause, class III**
KØ8.1Ø4 **Complete loss of teeth, unspecified cause, class IV**
KØ8.1Ø9 **Complete loss of teeth, unspecified cause, unspecified class**
Edentulism NOS

● KØ8.11 **Complete loss of teeth due to trauma**
KØ8.111 **Complete loss of teeth due to trauma, class I**
KØ8.112 **Complete loss of teeth due to trauma, class II**
KØ8.113 **Complete loss of teeth due to trauma, class III**
KØ8.114 **Complete loss of teeth due to trauma, class IV**
KØ8.119 **Complete loss of teeth due to trauma, unspecified class**

● KØ8.12 **Complete loss of teeth due to periodontal diseases**
KØ8.121 **Complete loss of teeth due to periodontal diseases, class I**
KØ8.122 **Complete loss of teeth due to periodontal diseases, class II**
KØ8.123 **Complete loss of teeth due to periodontal diseases, class III**
KØ8.124 **Complete loss of teeth due to periodontal diseases, class IV**
KØ8.129 **Complete loss of teeth due to periodontal diseases, unspecified class**

● KØ8.13 **Complete loss of teeth due to caries**
KØ8.131 **Complete loss of teeth due to caries, class I**
KØ8.132 **Complete loss of teeth due to caries, class II**
KØ8.133 **Complete loss of teeth due to caries, class III**
KØ8.134 **Complete loss of teeth due to caries, class IV**
KØ8.139 **Complete loss of teeth due to caries, unspecified class**

● KØ8.19 **Complete loss of teeth due to other specified cause**
KØ8.191 **Complete loss of teeth due to other specified cause, class I**
KØ8.192 **Complete loss of teeth due to other specified cause, class II**
KØ8.193 **Complete loss of teeth due to other specified cause, class III**
KØ8.194 **Complete loss of teeth due to other specified cause, class IV**
KØ8.199 **Complete loss of teeth due to other specified cause, unspecified class**

● KØ8.2 **Atrophy of edentulous alveolar ridge**
KØ8.2Ø **Unspecified atrophy of edentulous alveolar ridge**
Atrophy of the mandible NOS
Atrophy of the maxilla NOS
KØ8.21 **Minimal atrophy of the mandible**
Minimal atrophy of the edentulous mandible
KØ8.22 **Moderate atrophy of the mandible**
Moderate atrophy of the edentulous mandible
KØ8.23 **Severe atrophy of the mandible**
Severe atrophy of the edentulous mandible
KØ8.24 **Minimal atrophy of maxilla**
Minimal atrophy of the edentulous maxilla
KØ8.25 **Moderate atrophy of the maxilla**
Moderate atrophy of the edentulous maxilla
KØ8.26 **Severe atrophy of the maxilla**
Severe atrophy of the edentulous maxilla

KØ8.3 **Retained dental root**

● KØ8.4 **Partial loss of teeth**
Acquired loss of teeth, partial
Excludes1 complete loss of teeth (KØ8.1-)
congenital absence of teeth (KØØ.Ø)
Excludes2 exfoliation of teeth due to systemic causes (KØ8.Ø)

● KØ8.4Ø **Partial loss of teeth, unspecified cause**
KØ8.4Ø1 **Partial loss of teeth, unspecified cause, class I**
KØ8.4Ø2 **Partial loss of teeth, unspecified cause, class II**
KØ8.4Ø3 **Partial loss of teeth, unspecified cause, class III**
KØ8.4Ø4 **Partial loss of teeth, unspecified cause, class IV**
KØ8.4Ø9 **Partial loss of teeth, unspecified cause, unspecified class**
Tooth extraction status NOS

● KØ8.41 **Partial loss of teeth due to trauma**
KØ8.411 **Partial loss of teeth due to trauma, class I**
KØ8.412 **Partial loss of teeth due to trauma, class II**
KØ8.413 **Partial loss of teeth due to trauma, class III**
KØ8.414 **Partial loss of teeth due to trauma, class IV**
KØ8.419 **Partial loss of teeth due to trauma, unspecified class**

● KØ8.42 **Partial loss of teeth due to periodontal diseases**
KØ8.421 **Partial loss of teeth due to periodontal diseases, class I**
KØ8.422 **Partial loss of teeth due to periodontal diseases, class II**
KØ8.423 **Partial loss of teeth due to periodontal diseases, class III**
KØ8.424 **Partial loss of teeth due to periodontal diseases, class IV**
KØ8.429 **Partial loss of teeth due to periodontal diseases, unspecified class**

● KØ8.43 **Partial loss of teeth due to caries**
KØ8.431 **Partial loss of teeth due to caries, class I**
KØ8.432 **Partial loss of teeth due to caries, class II**
KØ8.433 **Partial loss of teeth due to caries, class III**
KØ8.434 **Partial loss of teeth due to caries, class IV**
KØ8.439 **Partial loss of teeth due to caries, unspecified class**

● **K08.49 Partial loss of teeth due to other specified cause**

K08.491 Partial loss of teeth due to other specified cause, class I

K08.492 Partial loss of teeth due to other specified cause, class II

K08.493 Partial loss of teeth due to other specified cause, class III

K08.494 Partial loss of teeth due to other specified cause, class IV

K08.499 Partial loss of teeth due to other specified cause, unspecified class

● **K08.5 Unsatisfactory restoration of tooth**
Defective bridge, crown, filling
Defective dental restoration

Excludes1 dental restoration status (Z98.811)
Excludes2 endosseous dental implant failure (M27.6-)
unsatisfactory endodontic treatment (M27.5-)

K08.50 Unsatisfactory restoration of tooth, unspecified
Defective dental restoration NOS

K08.51 Open restoration margins of tooth
Dental restoration failure of marginal integrity
Open margin on tooth restoration
Poor gingival margin to tooth restoration

K08.52 Unrepairable overhanging of dental restorative materials
Overhanging of tooth restoration

● **K08.53 Fractured dental restorative material**
Excludes1 cracked tooth (K03.81)
traumatic fracture of tooth (S02.5)

K08.530 Fractured dental restorative material without loss of material

K08.531 Fractured dental restorative material with loss of material

K08.539 Fractured dental restorative material, unspecified

K08.54 Contour of existing restoration of tooth biologically incompatible with oral health
Dental restoration failure of periodontal anatomical integrity
Unacceptable contours of existing restoration of tooth
Unacceptable morphology of existing restoration of tooth

K08.55 Allergy to existing dental restorative material
Use additional code to identify the specific type of allergy

K08.56 Poor aesthetic of existing restoration of tooth
Dental restoration aesthetically inadequate or displeasing

K08.59 Other unsatisfactory restoration of tooth
Other defective dental restoration

● **K08.8 Other specified disorders of teeth and supporting structures**

K08.81 Primary occlusal trauma ◀

K08.82 Secondary occlusal trauma ◀

K08.89 Other specified disorders of teeth and supporting structures ◀
Enlargement of alveolar ridge NOS ◀
Insufficient anatomic crown height ◀
Insufficient clinical crown length ◀
Irregular alveolar process ◀
Toothache NOS ◀

K08.9 Disorder of teeth and supporting structures, unspecified

● **K09 Cysts of oral region, not elsewhere classified**
Includes lesions showing histological features both of aneurysmal cyst and of another fibro-osseous lesion
Excludes2 cysts of jaw (M27.0-, M27.4-)
radicular cyst (K04.8)

K09.0 Developmental odontogenic cysts
Dentigerous cyst
Eruption cyst
Follicular cyst
Gingival cyst
Lateral periodontal cyst
Primordial cyst
Excludes2 keratocysts (D16.4, D16.5)
odontogenic keratocystic tumors (D16.4, D16.5)

K09.1 Developmental (nonodontogenic) cysts of oral region
Cyst (of) incisive canal
Cyst (of) palatine of papilla
Globulomaxillary cyst
Median palatal cyst
Nasoalveolar cyst
Nasolabial cyst
Nasopalatine duct cyst

K09.8 Other cysts of oral region, not elsewhere classified
Dermoid cyst
Epidermoid cyst
Lymphoepithelial cyst
Epstein's pearl

K09.9 Cyst of oral region, unspecified

★ (See Plate 61 on page NAP-25.)

● **K11 Diseases of salivary glands**
Use additional code to identify:
alcohol abuse and dependence (F10.-)
exposure to environmental tobacco smoke (Z77.22)
exposure to tobacco smoke in the perinatal period (P96.81)
history of tobacco dependence (Z87.891) ⬅
occupational exposure to environmental tobacco smoke (Z57.31)
tobacco dependence (F17.-)
tobacco use (Z72.0)

K11.0 Atrophy of salivary gland

K11.1 Hypertrophy of salivary gland

● **K11.2 Sialoadenitis**
Parotitis
Excludes1 epidemic parotitis (B26.-)
mumps (B26.-)
uveoparotid fever [Heerfordt] (D86.89)

K11.20 Sialoadenitis, unspecified

K11.21 Acute sialoadenitis
Excludes1 acute recurrent sialoadenitis (K11.22)

K11.22 Acute recurrent sialoadenitis

K11.23 Chronic sialoadenitis

Item 11–4 Atrophy is wasting away of a tissue or organ, whereas **hypertrophy** is overdevelopment or enlargement of a tissue or organ. **Sialoadenitis** is salivary gland inflammation. **Parotitis** is the inflammation of the parotid gland. In the epidemic form, parotitis is also known as mumps. **Sialolithiasis** is the formation of calculus within a salivary gland. **Mucocele** is a polyp composed of mucus.

Figure 11-3 Major salivary glands.

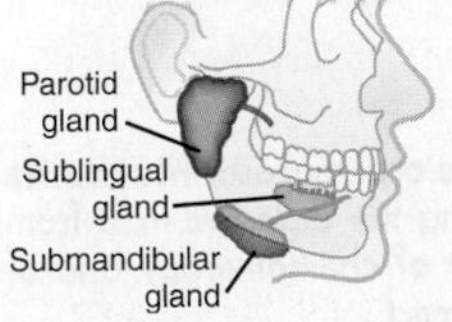

CHAPTER 11 (K00-K95)

K11.3 **Abscess of salivary gland**
K11.4 **Fistula of salivary gland**
Excludes1 congenital fistula of salivary gland (Q38.4)
K11.5 **Sialolithiasis**
Calculus of salivary gland or duct
Stone of salivary gland or duct
K11.6 **Mucocele of salivary gland**
Mucous extravasation cyst of salivary gland
Mucous retention cyst of salivary gland
Ranula
K11.7 **Disturbances of salivary secretion**
Hypoptyalism
Ptyalism
Xerostomia
Excludes2 dry mouth NOS (R68.2)
K11.8 **Other diseases of salivary glands**
Benign lymphoepithelial lesion of salivary gland
Mikulicz' disease
Necrotizing sialometaplasia
Sialectasia
Stenosis of salivary duct
Stricture of salivary duct
Excludes1 sicca syndrome [Sjögren] (M35.Ø-)
K11.9 **Disease of salivary gland, unspecified**
Sialoadenopathy NOS

● K12 **Stomatitis and related lesions**
Use additional code to identify:
alcohol abuse and dependence (F1Ø.-)
exposure to environmental tobacco smoke (Z77.22)
exposure to tobacco smoke in the perinatal period (P96.81)
history of tobacco dependence (Z87.891) ◀
occupational exposure to environmental tobacco smoke (Z57.31)
tobacco dependence (F17.-)
tobacco use (Z72.Ø)
Excludes1 cancrum oris (A69.Ø)
cheilitis (K13.Ø)
gangrenous stomatitis (A69.Ø)
herpesviral [herpes simplex] gingivostomatitis (BØØ.2)
noma (A69.Ø)
K12.Ø **Recurrent oral aphthae**
Aphthous stomatitis (major) (minor)
Bednar's aphthae
Periadenitis mucosa necrotica recurrens
Recurrent aphthous ulcer
Stomatitis herpetiformis
K12.1 **Other forms of stomatitis**
Stomatitis NOS
Denture stomatitis
Ulcerative stomatitis
Vesicular stomatitis
Excludes1 acute necrotizing ulcerative stomatitis (A69.1)
Vincent's stomatitis (A69.1)
K12.2 **Cellulitis and abscess of mouth**
Cellulitis of mouth (floor)
Submandibular abscess
Excludes2 abscess of salivary gland (K11.3)
abscess of tongue (K14.Ø)
periapical abscess (KØ4.6-KØ4.7)
periodontal abscess (KØ5.21)
peritonsillar abscess (J36)

● K12.3 **Oral mucositis (ulcerative)**
Mucositis (oral) (oropharyneal)
Excludes2 gastrointestinal mucositis (ulcerative) (K92.81)
mucositis (ulcerative) of vagina and vulva (N76.81)
nasal mucositis (ulcerative) (J34.81)
K12.3Ø **Oral mucositis (ulcerative), unspecified**
K12.31 **Oral mucositis (ulcerative) due to antineoplastic therapy**
Use additional code for adverse effect, if applicable, to identify antineoplastic and immunosuppressive drugs (T45.1X5)
Use additional code for other antineoplastic therapy, such as:
radiological procedure and radiotherapy (Y84.2)
K12.32 **Oral mucositis (ulcerative) due to other drugs**
Use additional code for adverse effect, if applicable, to identify drug (T36-T5Ø with fifth or sixth character 5)
K12.33 **Oral mucositis (ulcerative) due to radiation**
Use additional external cause code (W88-W9Ø, X39.Ø-) to identify cause
K12.39 **Other oral mucositis (ulcerative)**
Viral oral mucositis (ulcerative)

● K13 **Other diseases of lip and oral mucosa**
Includes epithelial disturbances of tongue
Use additional code to identify:
alcohol abuse and dependence (F1Ø.-)
exposure to environmental tobacco smoke (Z77.22)
exposure to tobacco smoke in the perinatal period (P96.81)
history of tobacco dependence (Z87.891) ◀
occupational exposure to environmental tobacco smoke (Z57.31)
tobacco dependence (F17.-)
tobacco use (Z72.Ø)
Excludes2 certain disorders of gingiva and edentulous alveolar ridge (KØ5-KØ6)
cysts of oral region (KØ9.-)
diseases of tongue (K14.-)
stomatitis and related lesions (K12.-)
K13.Ø **Diseases of lips**
Abscess of lips
Angular cheilitis
Cellulitis of lips
Cheilitis NOS
Cheilodynia
Cheilosis
Exfoliative cheilitis
Fistula of lips
Glandular cheilitis
Hypertrophy of lips
Perlèche NEC
Excludes1 ariboflavinosis (E53.Ø)
cheilitis due to radiation-related disorders (L55-L59)
congenital fistula of lips (Q38.Ø)
congenital hypertrophy of lips (Q18.6)
Perlèche due to candidiasis (B37.83)
Perlèche due to riboflavin deficiency (E53.Ø)
K13.1 **Cheek and lip biting**

Item 11-5 Stomatitis is the inflammation of the oral mucosa. **Mucositis** is the inflammation of the mucous membranes lining the digestive tract from the mouth to the anus. It is a common side effect of chemotherapy and of radiotherapy that involves any part of the digestive tract.

◀ New ◀ Revised ~~deleted~~ Deleted **OGCR** Official Guidelines X Assign placeholder X ● Use Additional Character(s)
Excludes1 Excludes2 Includes Use additional Code first Code also Unspecified

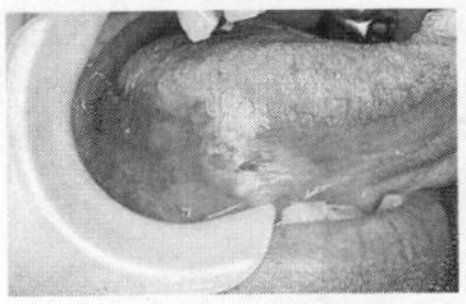

Figure 11-4 Oral leukoplakia and associated squamous carcinoma. (From Feldman: Sleisenger & Fordtran's Gastrointestinal and Liver Disease, ed 8, Saunders, An Imprint of Elsevier, 2006)

● **K13.2 Leukoplakia and other disturbances of oral epithelium, including tongue**
- **Excludes1** carcinoma in situ of oral epithelium (DØØ.Ø-)
  - hairy leukoplakia (K13.3)

K13.21 Leukoplakia of oral mucosa, including tongue
Considered precancerous and evidenced by thickened white patches of epithelium on mucous membranes
- Leukokeratosis of oral mucosa
- Leukoplakia of gingiva, lips, tongue
- **Excludes1** hairy leukoplakia (K13.3)
  - leukokeratosis nicotina palati (K13.24)

K13.22 Minimal keratinized residual ridge mucosa
- Minimal keratinization of alveolar ridge mucosa

K13.23 Excessive keratinized residual ridge mucosa
- Excessive keratinization of alveolar ridge mucosa

K13.24 Leukokeratosis nicotina palati
- Smoker's palate

K13.29 Other disturbances of oral epithelium, including tongue
- Erythroplakia of mouth or tongue
- Focal epithelial hyperplasia of mouth or tongue
- Leukoedema of mouth or tongue
- Other oral epithelium disturbances

K13.3 Hairy leukoplakia

K13.4 Granuloma and granuloma-like lesions of oral mucosa
- Eosinophilic granuloma
- Granuloma pyogenicum
- Verrucous xanthoma

K13.5 Oral submucous fibrosis
- Submucous fibrosis of tongue

K13.6 Irritative hyperplasia of oral mucosa
- **Excludes2** irritative hyperplasia of edentulous ridge [denture hyperplasia] (KØ6.2)

● **K13.7 Other and unspecified lesions of oral mucosa**

K13.70 Unspecified lesions of oral mucosa

K13.79 Other lesions of oral mucosa
- Focal oral mucinosis

★**(See Plate 58 on page NAP-23.)**

● **K14 Diseases of tongue**

Use additional code to identify:
- alcohol abuse and dependence (F1Ø.-)
- exposure to environmental tobacco smoke (Z77.22)
- history of tobacco dependence (Z87.891) (Revised)
- occupational exposure to environmental tobacco smoke (Z57.31)
- tobacco dependence (F17.-)
- tobacco use (Z72.Ø)

Excludes2
- erythroplakia (K13.29)
- focal epithelial hyperplasia (K13.29)
- leukedema of tongue (K13.29)
- leukoplakia of tongue (K13.21)
- hairy leukoplakia (K13.3)
- macroglossia (congenital) (Q38.2)
- submucous fibrosis of tongue (K13.5)

K14.Ø Glossitis
- Abscess of tongue
- Ulceration (traumatic) of tongue
- **Excludes1** atrophic glossitis (K14.4)

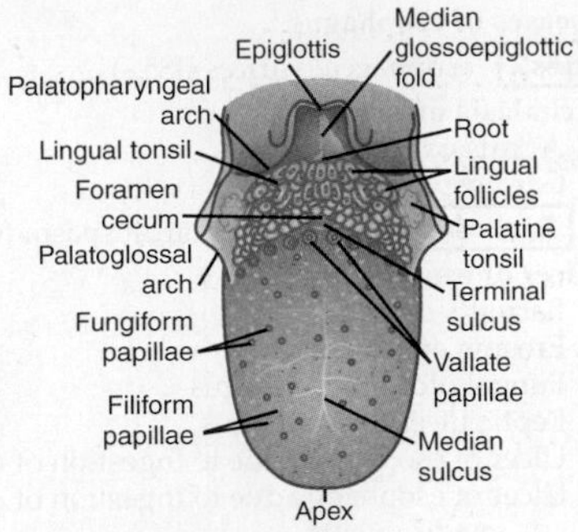

Figure 11-5 Structure of the tongue.

K14.1 Geographic tongue
- Benign migratory glossitis
- Glossitis areata exfoliativa

K14.2 Median rhomboid glossitis

K14.3 Hypertrophy of tongue papillae
- Black hairy tongue
- Coated tongue
- Hypertrophy of foliate papillae
- Lingua villosa nigra

K14.4 Atrophy of tongue papillae
- Atrophic glossitis

K14.5 Plicated tongue
- Fissured tongue
- Furrowed tongue
- Scrotal tongue
- **Excludes1** fissured tongue, congenital (Q38.3)

K14.6 Glossodynia
- Glossopyrosis
- Painful tongue

K14.8 Other diseases of tongue
- Atrophy of tongue
- Crenated tongue
- Enlargement of tongue
- Glossocele
- Glossoptosis
- Hypertrophy of tongue

K14.9 Disease of tongue, unspecified
- Glossopathy NOS

DISEASES OF ESOPHAGUS, STOMACH AND DUODENUM (K2Ø-K31)

Excludes2 hiatus hernia (K44.-)

● **K2Ø Esophagitis**

Use additional code to identify:
- alcohol abuse and dependence (F1Ø.-)

Excludes1
- erosion of esophagus (K22.1-)
- esophagitis with gastro-esophageal reflux disease (K21.Ø)
- reflux esophagitis (K21.Ø)
- ulcerative esophagitis (K22.1-)

Excludes2 eosinophilic gastritis or gastroenteritis (K52.81)

K2Ø.Ø Eosinophilic esophagitis

K2Ø.8 Other esophagitis
- Abscess of esophagus

K2Ø.9 Esophagitis, unspecified
- Esophagitis NOS

● **K21 Gastro-esophageal reflux disease**
- **Excludes1** newborn esophageal reflux (P78.83)

K21.Ø Gastro-esophageal reflux disease with esophagitis
- Reflux esophagitis

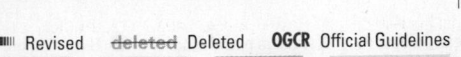

K21.9 Gastro-esophageal reflux disease without esophagitis
- Esophageal reflux NOS

● **K22 Other diseases of esophagus**
Excludes2 esophageal varices (I85.-)
K22.Ø Achalasia of cardia
Achalasia NOS
Cardiospasm
Excludes1 congenital cardiospasm (Q39.5)
● **K22.1 Ulcer of esophagus**
Barrett's ulcer
Erosion of esophagus
Fungal ulcer of esophagus
Peptic ulcer of esophagus
Ulcer of esophagus due to ingestion of chemicals
Ulcer of esophagus due to ingestion of drugs and medicaments
Ulcerative esophagitis
Code first poisoning due to drug or toxin, if applicable (T36-T65 with fifth or sixth character 1-4 or 6)
Use additional code for adverse effect, if applicable, to identify drug (T36-T5Ø with fifth or sixth character 5)
Excludes1 Barrett's esophagus (K22.87-)
K22.1Ø Ulcer of esophagus without bleeding
Ulcer of esophagus NOS
K22.11 Ulcer of esophagus with bleeding
Excludes2 bleeding esophageal varices (I85.Ø1, I85.11)
K22.2 Esophageal obstruction
Compression of esophagus
Constriction of esophagus
Stenosis of esophagus
Stricture of esophagus
Excludes1 congenital stenosis or stricture of esophagus (Q39.3)
K22.3 Perforation of esophagus
Rupture of esophagus
Excludes1 traumatic perforation of (thoracic) esophagus (S27.8-)
K22.4 Dyskinesia of esophagus
Difficulty in moving
Corkscrew esophagus
Diffuse esophageal spasm
Spasm of esophagus
Excludes1 cardiospasm (K22.Ø)
K22.5 Diverticulum of esophagus, acquired
Esophageal pouch, acquired
Excludes1 diverticulum of esophagus (congenital) (Q39.6)

Item 11-6 Esophageal reflux is the return flow of the contents of the stomach to the esophagus and is referred to as GERD and/or "heartburn." **Gastroesophageal reflux** is the return flow of the contents of the stomach and duodenum to the esophagus. **Esophageal leukoplakia** are white areas on the mucous membrane of the esophagus for which no specific cause can be identified.

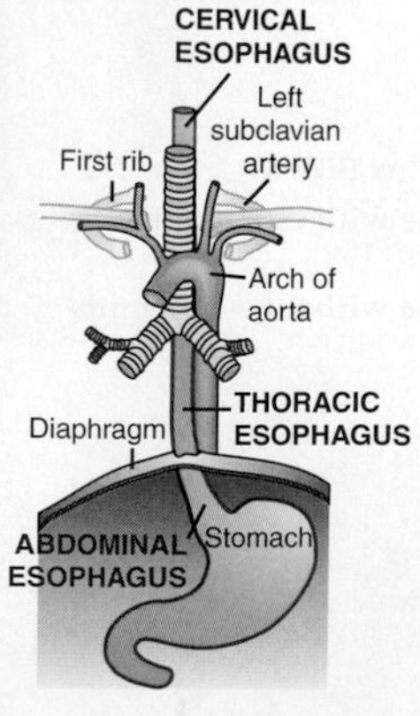

Figure 11-6 The esophagus is the muscular tube that connects the pharynx and the stomach. The 1Ø inch (25 cm) long esophagus is divided into three parts: **cervical, thoracic,** and **abdominal.**

Item 11-7 Achalasia is a condition in which the smooth muscle fibers of the esophagus do not relax. Most frequently, this condition occurs at the esophagogastric sphincter. **Cardiospasm,** also known as **megaesophagus,** is achalasia of the thoracic esophagus.

K22.6 Gastro-esophageal laceration-hemorrhage syndrome
Mallory-Weiss syndrome
● **K22.7 Barrett's esophagus**
Barrett's disease
Barrett's syndrome
Excludes1 Barrett's ulcer (K22.1)
malignant neoplasm of esophagus (C15.-)
K22.7Ø Barrett's esophagus without dysplasia
Barrett's esophagus NOS
● **K22.71 Barrett's esophagus with dysplasia**
K22.71Ø Barrett's esophagus with low grade dysplasia
K22.711 Barrett's esophagus with high grade dysplasia
K22.719 Barrett's esophagus with dysplasia, unspecified
K22.8 Other specified diseases of esophagus
Hemorrhage of esophagus NOS
Excludes2 esophageal varices (I85.-)
Paterson-Kelly syndrome (D5Ø.1)
K22.9 Disease of esophagus, unspecified
K23 Disorders of esophagus in diseases classified elsewhere
Code first underlying disease, such as:
congenital syphilis (A5Ø.5)
Excludes1 late syphilis (A52.79)
megaesophagus due to Chagas' disease (B57.31)
tuberculosis (A18.83)
● **K25 Gastric ulcer**
Includes erosion (acute) of stomach
pylorus ulcer (peptic)
stomach ulcer (peptic)
Use additional code to identify:
alcohol abuse and dependence (F1Ø.-)
Excludes1 acute gastritis (K29.Ø-)
peptic ulcer NOS (K27.-)
K25.Ø Acute gastric ulcer with hemorrhage
K25.1 Acute gastric ulcer with perforation
K25.2 Acute gastric ulcer with both hemorrhage and perforation
K25.3 Acute gastric ulcer without hemorrhage or perforation
K25.4 Chronic or unspecified gastric ulcer with hemorrhage
K25.5 Chronic or unspecified gastric ulcer with perforation
K25.6 Chronic or unspecified gastric ulcer with both hemorrhage and perforation
K25.7 Chronic gastric ulcer without hemorrhage or perforation
K25.9 Gastric ulcer, unspecified as acute or chronic, without hemorrhage or perforation

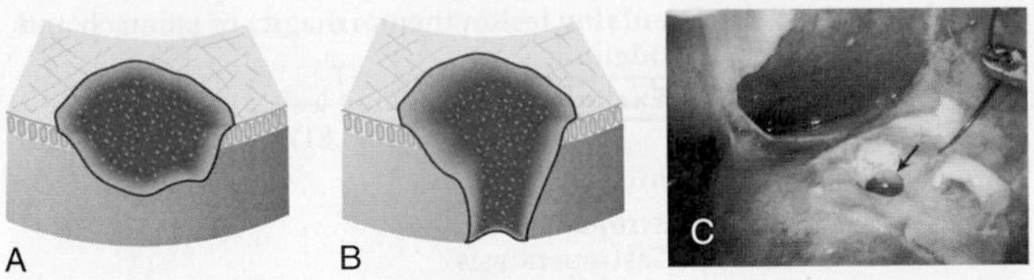

Figure 11-7 **A.** Ulcer. **B.** Perforated ulcer. **C.** Laparoscopic view of a perforated duodenal ulcer *(arrow)* with fibrinous exudate on the adjacent peritoneum. (**C** from Feldman: Sleisenger & Fordtran's Gastrointestinal and Liver Disease, ed 8, Saunders, An Imprint of Elsevier, 2006)

Item 11-8 **Gastric ulcers** are lesions of the stomach that result in the death of the tissue and a defect of the surface. **Perforated ulcers** are those in which the lesion penetrates the gastric wall, leaving a hole. **Peptic ulcers** are lesions of the stomach or the duodenum. **Peptic** refers to the gastric juice, pepsin.

● **K26 Duodenal ulcer**

Includes erosion (acute) of duodenum
duodenum ulcer (peptic)
postpyloric ulcer (peptic)

Use additional code to identify:
alcohol abuse and dependence (F1Ø.-)

Excludes1 peptic ulcer NOS (K27.-)

- **K26.Ø Acute duodenal ulcer with hemorrhage**
- **K26.1 Acute duodenal ulcer with perforation**
- **K26.2 Acute duodenal ulcer with both hemorrhage and perforation**
- **K26.3 Acute duodenal ulcer without hemorrhage or perforation**
- **K26.4 Chronic or unspecified duodenal ulcer with hemorrhage**
- **K26.5 Chronic or unspecified duodenal ulcer with perforation**
- **K26.6 Chronic or unspecified duodenal ulcer with both hemorrhage and perforation**
- **K26.7 Chronic duodenal ulcer without hemorrhage or perforation**
- **K26.9 Duodenal ulcer, unspecified as acute or chronic, without hemorrhage or perforation**

● **K27 Peptic ulcer, site unspecified**

Includes gastroduodenal ulcer NOS
peptic ulcer NOS

Use additional code to identify:
alcohol abuse and dependence (F1Ø.-)

Excludes1 peptic ulcer of newborn (P78.82)

- **K27.Ø Acute peptic ulcer, site unspecified, with hemorrhage**
- **K27.1 Acute peptic ulcer, site unspecified, with perforation**
- **K27.2 Acute peptic ulcer, site unspecified, with both hemorrhage and perforation**
- **K27.3 Acute peptic ulcer, site unspecified, without hemorrhage or perforation**
- **K27.4 Chronic or unspecified peptic ulcer, site unspecified, with hemorrhage**
- **K27.5 Chronic or unspecified peptic ulcer, site unspecified, with perforation**
- **K27.6 Chronic or unspecified peptic ulcer, site unspecified, with both hemorrhage and perforation**
- **K27.7 Chronic peptic ulcer, site unspecified, without hemorrhage or perforation**
- **K27.9 Peptic ulcer, site unspecified, unspecified as acute or chronic, without hemorrhage or perforation**

● **K28 Gastrojejunal ulcer**

Includes anastomotic ulcer (peptic) or erosion
gastrocolic ulcer (peptic) or erosion
gastrointestinal ulcer (peptic) or erosion
gastrojejunal ulcer (peptic) or erosion
jejunal ulcer (peptic) or erosion
marginal ulcer (peptic) or erosion
stomal ulcer (peptic) or erosion

Use additional code to identify:
alcohol abuse and dependence (F1Ø.-)

Excludes1 primary ulcer of small intestine (K63.3)

- **K28.Ø Acute gastrojejunal ulcer with hemorrhage**
- **K28.1 Acute gastrojejunal ulcer with perforation**
- **K28.2 Acute gastrojejunal ulcer with both hemorrhage and perforation**
- **K28.3 Acute gastrojejunal ulcer without hemorrhage or perforation**
- **K28.4 Chronic or unspecified gastrojejunal ulcer with hemorrhage**
- **K28.5 Chronic or unspecified gastrojejunal ulcer with perforation**
- **K28.6 Chronic or unspecified gastrojejunal ulcer with both hemorrhage and perforation**
- **K28.7 Chronic gastrojejunal ulcer without hemorrhage or perforation**
- **K28.9 Gastrojejunal ulcer, unspecified as acute or chronic, without hemorrhage or perforation**

● **K29 Gastritis and duodenitis**

Excludes1 eosinophilic gastritis or gastroenteritis (K52.81)
Zollinger-Ellison syndrome (E16.4)

● **K29.Ø Acute gastritis**

Use additional code to identify:
alcohol abuse and dependence (F1Ø.-)

Excludes1 erosion (acute) of stomach (K25.-)

- **K29.ØØ Acute gastritis without bleeding**
- **K29.Ø1 Acute gastritis with bleeding**

● **K29.2 Alcoholic gastritis**

Use additional code to identify:
alcohol abuse and dependence (F1Ø.-)

- **K29.2Ø Alcoholic gastritis without bleeding**
- **K29.21 Alcoholic gastritis with bleeding**

● **K29.3 Chronic superficial gastritis**

- **K29.3Ø Chronic superficial gastritis without bleeding**
- **K29.31 Chronic superficial gastritis with bleeding**

● **K29.4 Chronic atrophic gastritis**

Gastric atrophy

- **K29.4Ø Chronic atrophic gastritis without bleeding**
- **K29.41 Chronic atrophic gastritis with bleeding**

● **K29.5 Unspecified chronic gastritis**

Chronic antral gastritis
Chronic fundal gastritis

- **K29.5Ø Unspecified chronic gastritis without bleeding**
- **K29.51 Unspecified chronic gastritis with bleeding**

● **K29.6 Other gastritis**

Giant hypertrophic gastritis
Granulomatous gastritis
Ménétrier's disease

- **K29.6Ø Other gastritis without bleeding**
- **K29.61 Other gastritis with bleeding**

Item 11-9 **Gastritis** is a severe inflammation of the stomach. **Atrophic gastritis** is a chronic inflammation of the stomach that results in destruction of the cells of the mucosa of the stomach. Duodenitis is an inflammation of the duodenum, the first section of the small intestine.

● K29.7 **Gastritis, unspecified**
K29.7Ø **Gastritis, unspecified, without bleeding**
K29.71 **Gastritis, unspecified, with bleeding**
● K29.8 **Duodenitis**
K29.8Ø **Duodenitis without bleeding**
K29.81 **Duodenitis with bleeding**
● K29.9 **Gastroduodenitis, unspecified**
K29.9Ø **Gastroduodenitis, unspecified, without bleeding**
K29.91 **Gastroduodenitis, unspecified, with bleeding**

K3Ø **Functional dyspepsia**
Indigestion
Excludes1 dyspepsia NOS (R1Ø.13)
heartburn (R12)
nervous dyspepsia (F45.8)
neurotic dyspepsia (F45.8)
psychogenic dyspepsia (F45.8)

● K31 **Other diseases of stomach and duodenum**
Includes functional disorders of stomach
Excludes2 diabetic gastroparesis (EØ8.43, EØ9.43, E1Ø.43, E11.43, E13.43)
diverticulum of duodenum (K57.ØØ-K57.13)
K31.Ø **Acute dilatation of stomach**
Acute distention of stomach
K31.1 **Adult hypertrophic pyloric stenosis**
Pyloric stenosis NOS
Excludes1 congenital or infantile pyloric stenosis (Q4Ø.Ø)
K31.2 **Hourglass stricture and stenosis of stomach**
Excludes1 congenital hourglass stomach (Q4Ø.2)
hourglass contraction of stomach (K31.89)
K31.3 **Pylorospasm, not elsewhere classified**
Excludes1 congenital or infantile pylorospasm (Q4Ø.Ø)
neurotic pylorospasm (F45.8)
psychogenic pylorospasm (F45.8)
K31.4 **Gastric diverticulum**
Excludes1 congenital diverticulum of stomach (Q4Ø.2)
K31.5 **Obstruction of duodenum**
Constriction of duodenum
Duodenal ileus (chronic)
Stenosis of duodenum
Narrowing
Stricture of duodenum
Narrowing
Volvulus of duodenum
Twisting/knotting
Excludes1 congenital stenosis of duodenum (Q41.Ø)
K31.6 **Fistula of stomach and duodenum**
Gastrocolic fistula
Gastrojejunocolic fistula
K31.7 **Polyp of stomach and duodenum**
Excludes1 adenomatous polyp of stomach (D13.1)
● K31.8 **Other specified diseases of stomach and duodenum**
● K31.81 **Angiodysplasia of stomach and duodenum**
K31.811 **Angiodysplasia of stomach and duodenum with bleeding**
K31.819 **Angiodysplasia of stomach and duodenum without bleeding**
Angiodysplasia of stomach and duodenum NOS

Item 11–10 Achlorhydria, also known as gastric anacidity, is the absence of gastric acid.

K31.82 **Dieulafoy lesion (hemorrhagic) of stomach and duodenum**
Excludes2 Dieulafoy lesion of intestine (K63.81)
K31.83 **Achlorhydria**
K31.84 **Gastroparesis**
Gastroparalysis
Code first *underlying disease, if known, such as:*
anorexia nervosa (F5Ø.Ø-)
diabetes mellitus (EØ8.43, EØ9.43, E1Ø.43, E11.43, E13.43)
scleroderma (M34.-)
K31.89 **Other diseases of stomach and duodenum**
K31.9 **Disease of stomach and duodenum, unspecified**

DISEASES OF APPENDIX (K35-K38)

● K35 **Acute appendicitis**
K35.2 **Acute appendicitis with generalized peritonitis**
Appendicitis (acute) with generalized (diffuse) peritonitis following rupture or perforation of appendix
Perforated appendix NOS
Ruptured appendix NOS
K35.3 **Acute appendicitis with localized peritonitis**
Acute appendicitis with or without perforation or rupture with peritonitis NOS ◄
Acute appendicitis with or without perforation or rupture with localized peritonitis
Acute appendicitis with peritoneal abscess
● K35.8 **Other and unspecified acute appendicitis**
K35.8Ø **Unspecified acute appendicitis**
Acute appendicitis NOS
Acute appendicitis without (localized) (generalized) peritonitis
K35.89 **Other acute appendicitis**

K36 **Other appendicitis**
Chronic appendicitis
Recurrent appendicitis

K37 **Unspecified appendicitis**
Excludes1 ~~unspecified appendicitis with peritonitis (K35.2-K35.3)~~

● K38 **Other diseases of appendix**
K38.Ø **Hyperplasia of appendix**
K38.1 **Appendicular concretions**
Fecalith of appendix
Stercolith of appendix
K38.2 **Diverticulum of appendix**
K38.3 **Fistula of appendix**
K38.8 **Other specified diseases of appendix**
Intussusception of appendix
K38.9 **Disease of appendix, unspecified**

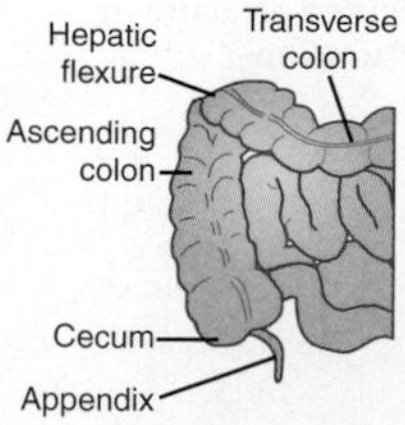

Figure 11-8 Acute appendicitis is the inflammation of the appendix, usually associated with obstruction. Most often this is a disease of adolescents and young adults.

Item 11–11 **Hernias** of the groin are the most common type, accounting for 8Ø percent of all hernias. There are two major types of inguinal hernias: indirect (oblique) affecting men only and direct. **Indirect inguinal hernias** result when the intestines emerge through the abdominal wall in an indirect fashion through the inguinal canal. **Direct inguinal hernias** penetrate through the abdominal wall in a direct fashion. **Femoral hernias** occur at the femoral ring where the femoral vessels enter the thigh and is most common in women. An abdominal wall hernia is also called a ventral or epigastric hernia and occurs in both sexes. Classification is based on location of the hernia and whether there is obstruction or gangrene.

Ventral, epigastric, or incisional hernia occurs on the abdominal surface caused by musculature weakness or a tear at a previous surgical site and is evidenced by a bulge that changes in size, becoming larger with exertion. An **incarcerated** hernia is one in which the intestines become trapped in the hernia. A **strangulated** hernia is one in which the blood supply to the intestines is lost. Hiatal hernia occurs when a loop of the stomach protrudes upward through the small opening in the diaphragm through which the esophagus passes, leaving the abdominal cavity and entering the chest. It occurs in both sexes.

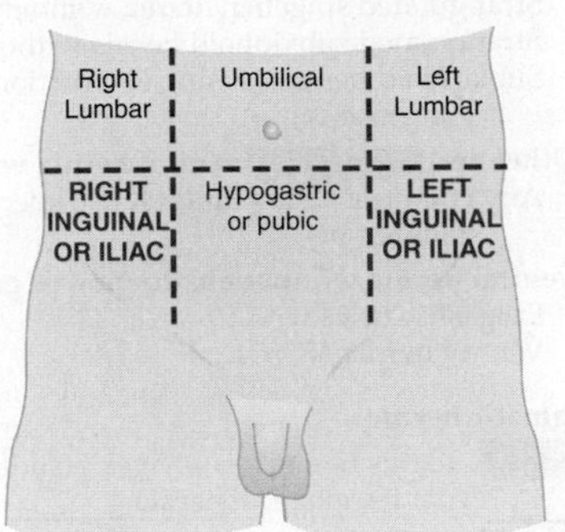

Figure 11-9 Inguinal hernias are those that are located in the inguinal or iliac areas of the abdomen.

HERNIA (K4Ø-K46)

Note: Hernia with both gangrene and obstruction is classified to hernia with gangrene.

Includes acquired hernia
congenital [except diaphragmatic or hiatus] hernia
recurrent hernia

● **K4Ø Inguinal hernia**

Includes bubonocele
direct inguinal hernia
double inguinal hernia
indirect inguinal hernia
inguinal hernia NOS
oblique inguinal hernia
scrotal hernia

● **K4Ø.Ø Bilateral inguinal hernia, with obstruction, without gangrene**
Inguinal hernia (bilateral) causing obstruction without gangrene
Incarcerated inguinal hernia (bilateral) without gangrene
Irreducible inguinal hernia (bilateral) without gangrene
Strangulated inguinal hernia (bilateral) without gangrene

K4Ø.ØØ Bilateral inguinal hernia, with obstruction, without gangrene, not specified as recurrent
Bilateral inguinal hernia, with obstruction, without gangrene NOS

K4Ø.Ø1 Bilateral inguinal hernia, with obstruction, without gangrene, recurrent

● **K4Ø.1 Bilateral inguinal hernia, with gangrene**

K4Ø.1Ø Bilateral inguinal hernia, with gangrene, not specified as recurrent
Bilateral inguinal hernia, with gangrene NOS

K4Ø.11 Bilateral inguinal hernia, with gangrene, recurrent

● **K4Ø.2 Bilateral inguinal hernia, without obstruction or gangrene**

K4Ø.2Ø Bilateral inguinal hernia, without obstruction or gangrene, not specified as recurrent
Bilateral inguinal hernia NOS

K4Ø.21 Bilateral inguinal hernia, without obstruction or gangrene, recurrent

● **K4Ø.3 Unilateral inguinal hernia, with obstruction, without gangrene**
Inguinal hernia (unilateral) causing obstruction without gangrene
Incarcerated inguinal hernia (unilateral) without gangrene
Irreducible inguinal hernia (unilateral) without gangrene
Strangulated inguinal hernia (unilateral) without gangrene

K4Ø.3Ø Unilateral inguinal hernia, with obstruction, without gangrene, not specified as recurrent
Inguinal hernia, with obstruction NOS
Unilateral inguinal hernia, with obstruction, without gangrene NOS

K4Ø.31 Unilateral inguinal hernia, with obstruction, without gangrene, recurrent

● **K4Ø.4 Unilateral inguinal hernia, with gangrene**

K4Ø.4Ø Unilateral inguinal hernia, with gangrene, not specified as recurrent
Inguinal hernia with gangrene NOS
Unilateral inguinal hernia with gangrene NOS

K4Ø.41 Unilateral inguinal hernia, with gangrene, recurrent

● **K4Ø.9 Unilateral inguinal hernia, without obstruction or gangrene**

K4Ø.9Ø Unilateral inguinal hernia, without obstruction or gangrene, not specified as recurrent
Inguinal hernia NOS
Unilateral inguinal hernia NOS

K4Ø.91 Unilateral inguinal hernia, without obstruction or gangrene, recurrent

● **K41 Femoral hernia**

● **K41.Ø Bilateral femoral hernia, with obstruction, without gangrene**
Femoral hernia (bilateral) causing obstruction, without gangrene
Incarcerated femoral hernia (bilateral), without gangrene
Irreducible femoral hernia (bilateral), without gangrene
Strangulated femoral hernia (bilateral), without gangrene

K41.ØØ Bilateral femoral hernia, with obstruction, without gangrene, not specified as recurrent
Bilateral femoral hernia, with obstruction, without gangrene NOS

K41.Ø1 Bilateral femoral hernia, with obstruction, without gangrene, recurrent

● **K41.1 Bilateral femoral hernia, with gangrene**

K41.1Ø Bilateral femoral hernia, with gangrene, not specified as recurrent
Bilateral femoral hernia, with gangrene NOS

K41.11 Bilateral femoral hernia, with gangrene, recurrent

● **K41.2 Bilateral femoral hernia, without obstruction or gangrene**

K41.2Ø Bilateral femoral hernia, without obstruction or gangrene, not specified as recurrent
Bilateral femoral hernia NOS

K41.21 Bilateral femoral hernia, without obstruction or gangrene, recurrent

● **K41.3 Unilateral femoral hernia, with obstruction, without gangrene**
Femoral hernia (unilateral) causing obstruction, without gangrene
Incarcerated femoral hernia (unilateral), without gangrene
Irreducible femoral hernia (unilateral), without gangrene
Strangulated femoral hernia (unilateral), without gangrene

K41.30 Unilateral femoral hernia, with obstruction, without gangrene, not specified as recurrent
Femoral hernia, with obstruction NOS
Unilateral femoral hernia, with obstruction NOS

K41.31 Unilateral femoral hernia, with obstruction, without gangrene, recurrent

● **K41.4 Unilateral femoral hernia, with gangrene**

K41.40 Unilateral femoral hernia, with gangrene, not specified as recurrent
Femoral hernia, with gangrene NOS
Unilateral femoral hernia, with gangrene NOS

K41.41 Unilateral femoral hernia, with gangrene, recurrent

● **K41.9 Unilateral femoral hernia, without obstruction or gangrene**

K41.90 Unilateral femoral hernia, without obstruction or gangrene, not specified as recurrent
Femoral hernia NOS
Unilateral femoral hernia NOS

K41.91 Unilateral femoral hernia, without obstruction or gangrene, recurrent

● **K42 Umbilical hernia**
Includes paraumbilical hernia
Excludes1 omphalocele (Q79.2)

K42.0 Umbilical hernia with obstruction, without gangrene
Umbilical hernia causing obstruction, without gangrene
Incarcerated umbilical hernia, without gangrene
Irreducible umbilical hernia, without gangrene
Strangulated umbilical hernia, without gangrene

K42.1 Umbilical hernia with gangrene
Gangrenous umbilical hernia

K42.9 Umbilical hernia without obstruction or gangrene
Umbilical hernia NOS

● **K43 Ventral hernia**

K43.0 Incisional hernia with obstruction, without gangrene
Incisional hernia causing obstruction, without gangrene
Incarcerated incisional hernia, without gangrene
Irreducible incisional hernia, without gangrene
Strangulated incisional hernia, without gangrene

K43.1 Incisional hernia with gangrene
Gangrenous incisional hernia

K43.2 Incisional hernia without obstruction or gangrene
Incisional hernia NOS

K43.3 Parastomal hernia with obstruction, without gangrene
Incarcerated parastomal hernia, without gangrene
Irreducible parastomal hernia, without gangrene
Parastomal hernia causing obstruction, without gangrene
Strangulated parastomal hernia, without gangrene

K43.4 Parastomal hernia with gangrene
Gangrenous parastomal hernia

K43.5 Parastomal hernia without obstruction or gangrene
Parastomal hernia NOS

K43.6 Other and unspecified ventral hernia with obstruction, without gangrene
Epigastric hernia causing obstruction, without gangrene
Hypogastric hernia causing obstruction, without gangrene
Incarcerated epigastric hernia without gangrene
Incarcerated hypogastric hernia without gangrene
Incarcerated midline hernia without gangrene
Incarcerated spigelian hernia without gangrene
Incarcerated subxiphoid hernia without gangrene
Irreducible epigastric hernia without gangrene
Irreducible hypogastric hernia without gangrene
Irreducible midline hernia without gangrene
Irreducible spigelian hernia without gangrene
Irreducible subxiphoid hernia without gangrene
Midline hernia causing obstruction, without gangrene
Spigelian hernia causing obstruction, without gangrene
Strangulated epigastric hernia without gangrene
Strangulated hypogastric hernia without gangrene
Strangulated midline hernia without gangrene
Strangulated spigelian hernia without gangrene
Strangulated subxiphoid hernia without gangrene
Subxiphoid hernia causing obstruction, without gangrene

K43.7 Other and unspecified ventral hernia with gangrene
Any condition listed under K43.6 specified as gangrenous

K43.9 Ventral hernia without obstruction or gangrene
Epigastric hernia
Ventral hernia NOS

● **K44 Diaphragmatic hernia**
Includes hiatus hernia (esophageal) (sliding)
paraesophageal hernia
Excludes1 congenital diaphragmatic hernia (Q79.0)
congenital hiatus hernia (Q40.1)

K44.0 Diaphragmatic hernia with obstruction, without gangrene
Diaphragmatic hernia causing obstruction
Incarcerated diaphragmatic hernia
Irreducible diaphragmatic hernia
Strangulated diaphragmatic hernia

K44.1 Diaphragmatic hernia with gangrene
Gangrenous diaphragmatic hernia

K44.9 Diaphragmatic hernia without obstruction or gangrene
Diaphragmatic hernia NOS

● **K45 Other abdominal hernia**
Includes abdominal hernia, specified site NEC
lumbar hernia
obturator hernia
pudendal hernia
retroperitoneal hernia
sciatic hernia

K45.0 Other specified abdominal hernia with obstruction, without gangrene
Other specified abdominal hernia causing obstruction
Other specified incarcerated abdominal hernia
Other specified irreducible abdominal hernia
Other specified strangulated abdominal hernia

K45.1 Other specified abdominal hernia with gangrene
Any condition listed under K45 specified as gangrenous

K45.8 Other specified abdominal hernia without obstruction or gangrene

● **K46 Unspecified abdominal hernia**
Includes enterocele
epiplocele
hernia NOS
interstitial hernia
intestinal hernia
intra-abdominal hernia
Excludes1 vaginal enterocele (N81.5)

K46.Ø Unspecified abdominal hernia with obstruction, without gangrene
Unspecified abdominal hernia causing obstruction
Unspecified incarcerated abdominal hernia
Unspecified irreducible abdominal hernia
Unspecified strangulated abdominal hernia

K46.1 Unspecified abdominal hernia with gangrene
Any condition listed under K46 specified as gangrenous

K46.9 Unspecified abdominal hernia without obstruction or gangrene
Abdominal hernia NOS

★**(See Plate 284 on page NAP-29.)**

NONINFECTIVE ENTERITIS AND COLITIS (K5Ø-K52)

Includes noninfective inflammatory bowel disease
Excludes1 irritable bowel syndrome (K58.-)
megacolon (K59.3-) ◄

● **K5Ø Crohn's disease [regional enteritis]**
Includes granulomatous enteritis
Use additional code to identify manifestations, such as:
pyoderma gangrenosum (L88)
Excludes1 ulcerative colitis (K51.-)

● **K5Ø.Ø Crohn's disease of small intestine**
Crohn's disease [regional enteritis] of duodenum
Crohn's disease [regional enteritis] of ileum
Crohn's disease [regional enteritis] of jejunum
Regional ileitis
Terminal ileitis
Excludes1 Crohn's disease of both small and large intestine (K5Ø.8-)

K5Ø.ØØ Crohn's disease of small intestine without complications

● **K5Ø.Ø1 Crohn's disease of small intestine with complications**
K5Ø.Ø11 Crohn's disease of small intestine with rectal bleeding
K5Ø.Ø12 Crohn's disease of small intestine with intestinal obstruction
K5Ø.Ø13 Crohn's disease of small intestine with fistula
K5Ø.Ø14 Crohn's disease of small intestine with abscess
K5Ø.Ø18 Crohn's disease of small intestine with other complication
K5Ø.Ø19 Crohn's disease of small intestine with unspecified complications

Item 11-12 Crohn's disease, also known as **regional enteritis,** is a chronic inflammatory disease of the intestines. Classification is based on location in the small (duodenum, ileum, jejunum) or large (cecum, colon, rectum, anal canal) intestine.

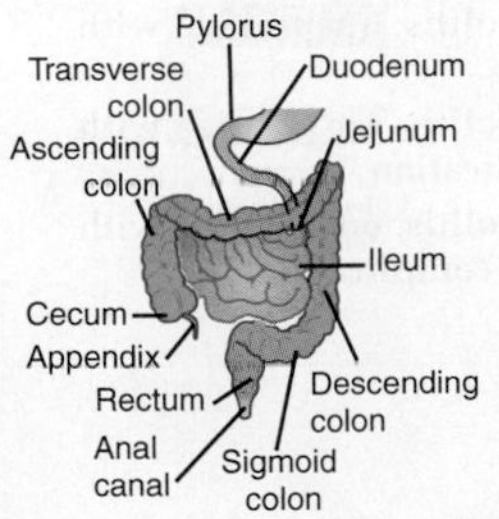

Figure 11-10 Small and large intestines.

● **K5Ø.1 Crohn's disease of large intestine**
Crohn's disease [regional enteritis] of colon
Crohn's disease [regional enteritis] of large bowel
Crohn's disease [regional enteritis] of rectum
Granulomatous colitis
Regional colitis
Excludes1 Crohn's disease of both small and large intestine (K5Ø.8)

K5Ø.1Ø Crohn's disease of large intestine without complications

● **K5Ø.11 Crohn's disease of large intestine with complications**
K5Ø.111 Crohn's disease of large intestine with rectal bleeding
K5Ø.112 Crohn's disease of large intestine with intestinal obstruction
K5Ø.113 Crohn's disease of large intestine with fistula
K5Ø.114 Crohn's disease of large intestine with abscess
K5Ø.118 Crohn's disease of large intestine with other complication
K5Ø.119 Crohn's disease of large intestine with unspecified complications

● **K5Ø.8 Crohn's disease of both small and large intestine**
K5Ø.8Ø Crohn's disease of both small and large intestine without complications

● **K5Ø.81 Crohn's disease of both small and large intestine with complications**
K5Ø.811 Crohn's disease of both small and large intestine with rectal bleeding
K5Ø.812 Crohn's disease of both small and large intestine with intestinal obstruction
K5Ø.813 Crohn's disease of both small and large intestine with fistula
K5Ø.814 Crohn's disease of both small and large intestine with abscess
K5Ø.818 Crohn's disease of both small and large intestine with other complication
K5Ø.819 Crohn's disease of both small and large intestine with unspecified complications

● **K5Ø.9 Crohn's disease, unspecified**
K5Ø.9Ø Crohn's disease, unspecified, without complications
Crohn's disease NOS
Regional enteritis NOS

● **K5Ø.91 Crohn's disease, unspecified, with complications**
K5Ø.911 Crohn's disease, unspecified, with rectal bleeding
K5Ø.912 Crohn's disease, unspecified, with intestinal obstruction
K5Ø.913 Crohn's disease, unspecified, with fistula
K5Ø.914 Crohn's disease, unspecified, with abscess
K5Ø.918 Crohn's disease, unspecified, with other complication
K5Ø.919 Crohn's disease, unspecified, with unspecified complications

Item 11–13 Ulcerative colitis attacks the colonic mucosa and forms abscesses. The disease involves the intestines. Classification is based on the location:

- Enterocolitis: large and small intestine
- Ileocolitis: ileum and colon
- Proctitis: rectum
- Proctosigmoiditis: sigmoid colon and rectum

● **K51 Ulcerative colitis**

Use additional code to identify manifestations, such as:
pyoderma gangrenosum (L88)

Excludes1 Crohn's disease [regional enteritis] (K5Ø.-)

● **K51.Ø Ulcerative (chronic) pancolitis**
Backwash ileitis

K51.ØØ Ulcerative (chronic) pancolitis without complications
Ulcerative (chronic) pancolitis NOS

● **K51.Ø1 Ulcerative (chronic) pancolitis with complications**

K51.Ø11 Ulcerative (chronic) pancolitis with rectal bleeding

K51.Ø12 Ulcerative (chronic) pancolitis with intestinal obstruction

K51.Ø13 Ulcerative (chronic) pancolitis with fistula

K51.Ø14 Ulcerative (chronic) pancolitis with abscess

K51.Ø18 Ulcerative (chronic) pancolitis with other complication

K51.Ø19 Ulcerative (chronic) pancolitis with unspecified complications

● **K51.2 Ulcerative (chronic) proctitis**

K51.2Ø Ulcerative (chronic) proctitis without complications
Ulcerative (chronic) proctitis NOS

● **K51.21 Ulcerative (chronic) proctitis with complications**

K51.211 Ulcerative (chronic) proctitis with rectal bleeding

K51.212 Ulcerative (chronic) proctitis with intestinal obstruction

K51.213 Ulcerative (chronic) proctitis with fistula

K51.214 Ulcerative (chronic) proctitis with abscess

K51.218 Ulcerative (chronic) proctitis with other complication

K51.219 Ulcerative (chronic) proctitis with unspecified complications

● **K51.3 Ulcerative (chronic) rectosigmoiditis**

K51.3Ø Ulcerative (chronic) rectosigmoiditis without complications
Ulcerative (chronic) rectosigmoiditis NOS

● **K51.31 Ulcerative (chronic) rectosigmoiditis with complications**

K51.311 Ulcerative (chronic) rectosigmoiditis with rectal bleeding

K51.312 Ulcerative (chronic) rectosigmoiditis with intestinal obstruction

K51.313 Ulcerative (chronic) rectosigmoiditis with fistula

K51.314 Ulcerative (chronic) rectosigmoiditis with abscess

K51.318 Ulcerative (chronic) rectosigmoiditis with other complication

K51.319 Ulcerative (chronic) rectosigmoiditis with unspecified complications

● **K51.4 Inflammatory polyps of colon**

Excludes1 adenomatous polyp of colon (D12.6)
polyposis of colon (D12.6)
polyps of colon NOS (K63.5)

K51.4Ø Inflammatory polyps of colon without complications
Inflammatory polyps of colon NOS

● **K51.41 Inflammatory polyps of colon with complications**

K51.411 Inflammatory polyps of colon with rectal bleeding

K51.412 Inflammatory polyps of colon with intestinal obstruction

K51.413 Inflammatory polyps of colon with fistula

K51.414 Inflammatory polyps of colon with abscess

K51.418 Inflammatory polyps of colon with other complication

K51.419 Inflammatory polyps of colon with unspecified complications

● **K51.5 Left sided colitis**
Left hemicolitis

K51.5Ø Left sided colitis without complications
Left sided colitis NOS

● **K51.51 Left sided colitis with complications**

K51.511 Left sided colitis with rectal bleeding

K51.512 Left sided colitis with intestinal obstruction

K51.513 Left sided colitis with fistula

K51.514 Left sided colitis with abscess

K51.518 Left sided colitis with other complication

K51.519 Left sided colitis with unspecified complications

● **K51.8 Other ulcerative colitis**

K51.8Ø Other ulcerative colitis without complications

● **K51.81 Other ulcerative colitis with complications**

K51.811 Other ulcerative colitis with rectal bleeding

K51.812 Other ulcerative colitis with intestinal obstruction

K51.813 Other ulcerative colitis with fistula

K51.814 Other ulcerative colitis with abscess

K51.818 Other ulcerative colitis with other complication

K51.819 Other ulcerative colitis with unspecified complications

● **K51.9 Ulcerative colitis, unspecified**

K51.9Ø Ulcerative colitis, unspecified, without complications

● **K51.91 Ulcerative colitis, unspecified, with complications**

K51.911 Ulcerative colitis, unspecified with rectal bleeding

K51.912 Ulcerative colitis, unspecified with intestinal obstruction

K51.913 Ulcerative colitis, unspecified with fistula

K51.914 Ulcerative colitis, unspecified with abscess

K51.918 Ulcerative colitis, unspecified with other complication

K51.919 Ulcerative colitis, unspecified with unspecified complications

● **K52 Other and unspecified noninfective gastroenteritis and colitis**

K52.Ø Gastroenteritis and colitis due to radiation

K52.1 Toxic gastroenteritis and colitis
Drug-induced gastroenteritis and colitis
Code first *(T51-T65) to identify toxic agent*
Use additional code for adverse effect, if applicable, to identify drug (T36-T5Ø with fifth or sixth character 5)

● **K52.2 Allergic and dietetic gastroenteritis and colitis**
Food hypersensitivity gastroenteritis or colitis
Use additional code to identify type of food allergy (Z91.Ø1-, Z91.Ø2-)
Excludes2 allergic eosinophilic colitis (K52.82) ◀
allergic eosinophilic esophagitis (K2Ø.Ø) ◀
allergic eosinophilic gastritis (K52.81) ◀
allergic eosinophilic gastroenteritis (K52.81) ◀
food protein-induced proctocolitis (K52.82) ◀

K52.21 Food protein-induced enterocolitis syndrome ◀
Use additional code for hypovolemic shock, if present (R57.1) ◀

K52.22 Food protein-induced enteropathy ◀

K52.29 Other allergic and dietetic gastroenteritis and colitis ◀
Food hypersensitivity gastroenteritis or colitis ◀
Immediate gastrointestinal hypersensitivity ◀

K52.3 Indeterminate colitis ◀
Colonic inflammatory bowel disease unclassified (IBDU) ◀
Excludes1 unspecified colitis (K52.9) ◀

● **K52.8 Other specified noninfective gastroenteritis and colitis**

K52.81 Eosinophilic gastritis or gastroenteritis
Eosinophilic enteritis
Excludes2 eosinophilic esophagitis (K2Ø.Ø) ◀

K52.82 Eosinophilic colitis
Allergic proctocolitis ◀
Food-induced eosinophilic proctocolitis ◀
Food protein-induced proctocolitis ◀
Milk protein-induced proctocolitis ◀

● **K52.83 Microscopic colitis** ◀

K52.831 Collagenous colitis ◀

K52.832 Lymphocytic colitis ◀

K52.838 Other microscopic colitis ◀

K52.839 Microscopic colitis, unspecified ◀

K52.89 Other specified noninfective gastroenteritis and colitis

K52.9 Noninfective gastroenteritis and colitis, unspecified
Colitis NOS
Enteritis NOS
Gastroenteritis NOS
Ileitis NOS
Jejunitis NOS
Sigmoiditis NOS
Excludes1 diarrhea NOS (R19.7)
functional diarrhea (K59.1)
infectious gastroenteritis and colitis NOS (AØ9)
neonatal diarrhea (noninfective) (P78.3)
psychogenic diarrhea (F45.8)

OTHER DISEASES OF INTESTINES (K55-K64)

● **K55 Vascular disorders of intestine**
Excludes1 necrotizing enterocolitis of newborn (P77.-)

● **K55.Ø Acute vascular disorders of intestine**
Infarction of appendices epiploicae
Mesenteric (artery) (vein) embolism
Mesenteric (artery) (vein) infarction
Mesenteric (artery) (vein) thrombosis

● **K55.Ø1 Acute (reversible) ischemia of small intestine** ◀

K55.Ø11 Focal (segmental) acute (reversible) ischemia of small intestine ◀

K55.Ø12 Diffuse acute (reversible) ischemia of small intestine ◀

K55.Ø19 Acute (reversible) ischemia of small intestine, extent unspecified ◀

● **K55.Ø2 Acute infarction of small intestine** ◀
Gangrene of small intestine ◀
Necrosis of small intestine ◀

K55.Ø21 Focal (segmental) acute infarction of small intestine ◀

K55.Ø22 Diffuse acute infarction of small intestine ◀

K55.Ø29 Acute infarction of small intestine, extent unspecified ◀

● **K55.Ø3 Acute (reversible) ischemia of large intestine** ◀
Acute fulminant ischemic colitis ◀
Subacute ischemic colitis ◀

K55.Ø31 Focal (segmental) acute (reversible) ischemia of large intestine ◀

K55.Ø32 Diffuse acute (reversible) ischemia of large intestine ◀

K55.Ø39 Acute (reversible) ischemia of large intestine, extent unspecified ◀

● **K55.Ø4 Acute infarction of large intestine** ◀
Gangrene of large intestine ◀
Necrosis of large intestine ◀

K55.Ø41 Focal (segmental) acute infarction of large intestine ◀

K55.Ø42 Diffuse acute infarction of large intestine ◀

K55.Ø49 Acute infarction of large intestine, extent unspecified ◀

● **K55.Ø5 Acute (reversible) ischemia of intestine, part unspecified** ◀

K55.Ø51 Focal (segmental) acute (reversible) ischemia of intestine, part unspecified ◀

K55.Ø52 Diffuse acute (reversible) ischemia of intestine, part unspecified ◀

K55.Ø59 Acute (reversible) ischemia of intestine, part and extent unspecified ◀

● **K55.Ø6 Acute infarction of intestine, part unspecified** ◀
Acute intestinal infarction ◀
Gangrene of intestine ◀
Necrosis of intestine ◀

K55.Ø61 Focal (segmental) acute infarction of intestine, part unspecified ◀

K55.Ø62 Diffuse acute infarction of intestine, part unspecified ◀

K55.Ø69 Acute infarction of intestine, part and extent unspecified ◀

K55.1 Chronic vascular disorders of intestine
Chronic ischemic colitis
Chronic ischemic enteritis
Chronic ischemic enterocolitis
Ischemic stricture of intestine
Mesenteric atherosclerosis
Mesenteric vascular insufficiency

● **K55.2 Angiodysplasia of colon**

K55.2Ø Angiodysplasia of colon without hemorrhage

K55.21 Angiodysplasia of colon with hemorrhage

● **K55.3 Necrotizing enterocolitis** ◀

Excludes1 necrotizing enterocolitis of newborn (P77.-) ◀

Excludes2 necrotizing enterocolitis due to Clostridium difficile (AØ4.7) ◀

K55.3Ø Necrotizing enterocolitis, unspecified ◀
Necrotizing enterocolitis, NOS ◀

K55.31 Stage 1 necrotizing enterocolitis ◀
Necrotizing enterocolitis without pneumatosis, without perforation ◀

K55.32 Stage 2 necrotizing enterocolitis ◀
Necrotizing enterocolitis with pneumatosis, without perforation ◀

K55.33 Stage 3 necrotizing enterocolitis ◀
Necrotizing enterocolitis with perforation ◀
Necrotizing enterocolitis with pneumatosis and perforation ◀

K55.8 Other vascular disorders of intestine

K55.9 Vascular disorder of intestine, unspecified
Ischemic colitis
Ischemic enteritis
Ischemic enterocolitis

● **K56 Paralytic ileus and intestinal obstruction without hernia**

Excludes1 congenital stricture or stenosis of intestine (Q41-Q42)
cystic fibrosis with meconium ileus (E84.11)
ischemic stricture of intestine (K55.1)
meconium ileus NOS (P76.Ø)
neonatal intestinal obstructions classifiable to P76.-
obstruction of duodenum (K31.5)
postprocedural intestinal obstruction (K91.3)
stenosis of anus or rectum (K62.4)
intestinal obstruction with hernia (K4Ø-K46)

K56.Ø Paralytic ileus
Paralysis of bowel
Paralysis of colon
Paralysis of intestine

Excludes1 gallstone ileus (K56.3)
ileus NOS (K56.7)
obstructive ileus NOS (K56.69)

K56.1 Intussusception
Intussusception or invagination of bowel
Intussusception or invagination of colon
Intussusception or invagination of intestine
Intussusception or invagination of rectum

Excludes2 intussusception of appendix (K38.8)

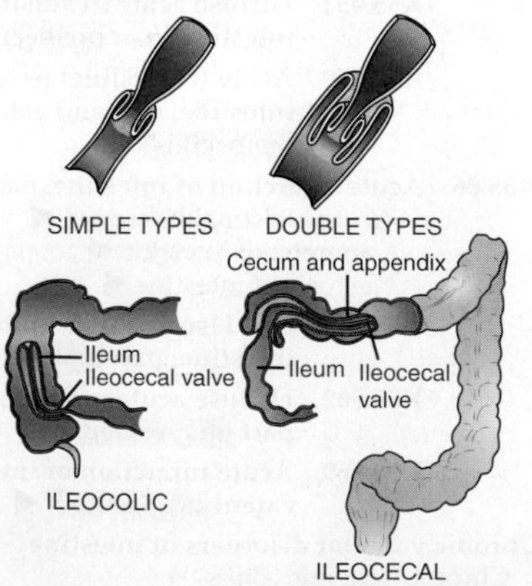

Figure 11-11 Types of intussusception.

Item 11-14 Intussusception is the prolapse (telescoping) of a part of the intestine into another adjacent part of the intestine. Intussusception may be enteric (ileoileal, jejunoileal, jejunojejunal), colic (colocolic), or intracolic (ileocecal, ileocolic).

Item 11-15 Volvulus is the twisting of a segment of the intestine, resulting in obstruction. Paralytic ileus is paralysis of the intestine. It need not be a complete paralysis, but it must prohibit the passage of food through the intestine and lead to intestinal blockage. It is a common aftermath of some types of surgery.

K56.2 Volvulus
Strangulation of colon or intestine
Torsion of colon or intestine
Twist of colon or intestine

Excludes2 volvulus of duodenum (K31.5)

K56.3 Gallstone ileus
Obstruction of intestine by gallstone

● **K56.4 Other impaction of intestine**

K56.41 Fecal impaction

Excludes1 constipation (K59.Ø-)
incomplete defecation (R15.Ø)

K56.49 Other impaction of intestine

K56.5 Intestinal adhesions [bands] with obstruction (postprocedural) (postinfection)
Abdominal hernia due to adhesions with obstruction
Peritoneal adhesions [bands] with intestinal obstruction (postprocedural) (postinfection)

● **K56.6 Other and unspecified intestinal obstruction**

K56.6Ø Unspecified intestinal obstruction Intestinal obstruction NOS

Excludes1 intestinal obstruction due to specified condition-code to condition

K56.69 Other intestinal obstruction
Enterostenosis NOS
Obstructive ileus NOS
Occlusion of colon or intestine NOS
Stenosis of colon or intestine NOS
Stricture of colon or intestine NOS

Excludes1 intestinal obstruction due to specified condition-code to condition

K56.7 Ileus, unspecified

Excludes1 obstructive ileus (K56.69)

● **K57 Diverticular disease of intestine**

Excludes1 congenital diverticulum of intestine (Q43.8)
Meckel's diverticulum (Q43.Ø)

Excludes2 diverticulum of appendix (K38.2)

● **K57.Ø Diverticulitis of small intestine with perforation and abscess**
Diverticulitis of small intestine with peritonitis

Excludes1 diverticulitis of both small and large intestine with perforation and abscess (K57.4-)

K57.ØØ Diverticulitis of small intestine with perforation and abscess without bleeding

K57.Ø1 Diverticulitis of small intestine with perforation and abscess with bleeding

● **K57.1 Diverticular disease of small intestine without perforation or abscess**

Excludes1 diverticular disease of both small and large intestine without perforation or abscess (K57.5-)

K57.1Ø Diverticulosis of small intestine without perforation or abscess without bleeding
Diverticular disease of small intestine NOS

K57.11 Diverticulosis of small intestine without perforation or abscess with bleeding

K57.12 Diverticulitis of small intestine without perforation or abscess without bleeding

K57.13 Diverticulitis of small intestine without perforation or abscess with bleeding

● **K57.2 Diverticulitis of large intestine with perforation and abscess**
Diverticulitis of colon with peritonitis
Excludes1 diverticulitis of both small and large intestine with perforation and abscess (K57.4-)

K57.2Ø Diverticulitis of large intestine with perforation and abscess without bleeding

K57.21 Diverticulitis of large intestine with perforation and abscess with bleeding

● **K57.3 Diverticular disease of large intestine without perforation or abscess**
Excludes1 diverticular disease of both small and large intestine without perforation or abscess (K57.5-)

K57.3Ø Diverticulosis of large intestine without perforation or abscess without bleeding
Diverticular disease of colon NOS

K57.31 Diverticulosis of large intestine without perforation or abscess with bleeding

K57.32 Diverticulitis of large intestine without perforation or abscess without bleeding

K57.33 Diverticulitis of large intestine without perforation or abscess with bleeding

● **K57.4 Diverticulitis of both small and large intestine with perforation and abscess**
Diverticulitis of both small and large intestine with peritonitis

K57.4Ø Diverticulitis of both small and large intestine with perforation and abscess without bleeding

K57.41 Diverticulitis of both small and large intestine with perforation and abscess with bleeding

● **K57.5 Diverticular disease of both small and large intestine without perforation or abscess**

K57.5Ø Diverticulosis of both small and large intestine without perforation or abscess without bleeding
Diverticular disease of both small and large intestine NOS

K57.51 Diverticulosis of both small and large intestine without perforation or abscess with bleeding

K57.52 Diverticulitis of both small and large intestine without perforation or abscess without bleeding

K57.53 Diverticulitis of both small and large intestine without perforation or abscess with bleeding

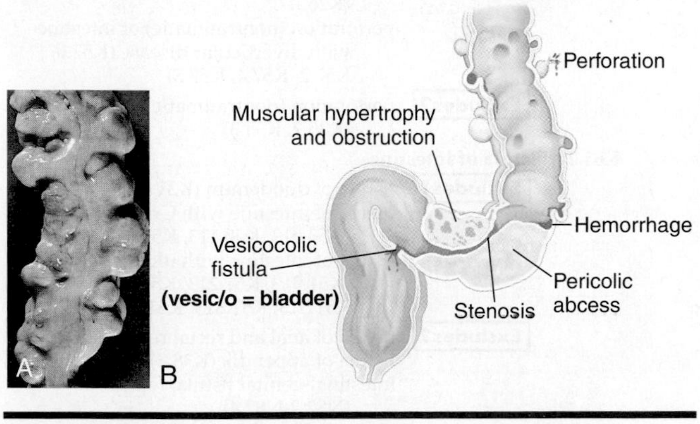

Figure 11-12 Diverticulosis. (From Shiland: Mastering Healthcare Terminology, ed 4, St. Louis, Mosby, 2012)

Item 11-16 Diverticula of the intestines are acquired herniations of the mucosa. Diverticulum (singular): Pocket or pouch that bulges outward through a weak spot (herniation) in the colon. Diverticula (plural). **Diverticulosis** is the condition of having diverticula. **Diverticulitis** is inflammation of these pouches or herniations. Classification is based on location (small intestine or colon) and whether it occurs with or without hemorrhage.

● **K57.8 Diverticulitis of intestine, part unspecified, with perforation and abscess**
Diverticulitis of intestine NOS with peritonitis

K57.8Ø Diverticulitis of intestine, part unspecified, with perforation and abscess without bleeding

K57.81 Diverticulitis of intestine, part unspecified, with perforation and abscess with bleeding

● **K57.9 Diverticular disease of intestine, part unspecified, without perforation or abscess**

K57.9Ø Diverticulosis of intestine, part unspecified, without perforation or abscess without bleeding
Diverticular disease of intestine NOS

K57.91 Diverticulosis of intestine, part unspecified, without perforation or abscess with bleeding

K57.92 Diverticulitis of intestine, part unspecified, without perforation or abscess without bleeding

K57.93 Diverticulitis of intestine, part unspecified, without perforation or abscess with bleeding

● **K58 Irritable bowel syndrome**
Includes irritable colon
spastic colon

K58.Ø Irritable bowel syndrome with diarrhea

K58.1 Irritable bowel syndrome with constipation ◀

K58.2 Mixed irritable bowel syndrome ◀

K58.8 Other irritable bowel syndrome ◀

K58.9 Irritable bowel syndrome without diarrhea
Irritable bowel syndrome NOS

● **K59 Other functional intestinal disorders**
Excludes1 change in bowel habit NOS (R19.4)
intestinal malabsorption (K9Ø.-)
psychogenic intestinal disorders (F45.8)
Excludes2 functional disorders of stomach (K31.-)

● **K59.Ø Constipation**
Use additional code for adverse effect, if applicable, to identify drug (T36-T5Ø with fifth or sixth character 5) ◀
Excludes1 fecal impaction (K56.41)
incomplete defecation (R15.Ø)

K59.ØØ Constipation, unspecified

K59.Ø1 Slow transit constipation

K59.Ø2 Outlet dysfunction constipation

K59.Ø3 Drug induced constipation ◀
Use additional code for adverse effect, if applicable, to identify drug (T36-T5Ø with fifth or sixth character 5) ◀

K59.Ø4 Chronic idiopathic constipation ◀
Functional constipation ◀

K59.Ø9 Other constipation
Chronic constipation ◀

K59.1 Functional diarrhea
Excludes1 diarrhea NOS (R19.7)
irritable bowel syndrome with diarrhea (K58.Ø)

K59.2 Neurogenic bowel, not elsewhere classified

● **K59.3 Megacolon, not elsewhere classified**
Dilatation of colon
Code first, if applicable (T51-T65) to identify toxic agent ⟸
Excludes1 congenital megacolon (aganglionic) (Q43.1)
megacolon (due to) (in) Chagas' disease (B57.32)
megacolon (due to) (in) Clostridium difficile (AØ4.7)
megacolon (due to) (in) Hirschsprung's disease (Q43.1)

K59.31 Toxic megacolon ◀

K59.39 Other megacolon ◀
Megacolon NOS ◀

Item 11–17 A **fissure** is a groove in the surface, whereas a **fistula** is an abnormal passage. An **abscess** is an accumulation of pus in a tissue cavity resulting from a bacterial or parasitic infection.

K59.4 Anal spasm
Proctalgia fugax

K59.8 Other specified functional intestinal disorders
Atony of colon Pseudo-obstruction (acute) (chronic) of intestine

K59.9 Functional intestinal disorder, unspecified

● **K60 Fissure and fistula of anal and rectal regions**
Excludes1 fissure and fistula of anal and rectal regions with abscess or cellulitis (K61.-)
Excludes2 anal sphincter tear (healed) (nontraumatic) (old) (K62.81)

K60.0 Acute anal fissure
K60.1 Chronic anal fissure
K60.2 Anal fissure, unspecified
K60.3 Anal fistula
K60.4 Rectal fistula
Fistula of rectum to skin
Excludes1 rectovaginal fistula (N82.3)
vesicorectal fistula (N32.1)

K60.5 Anorectal fistula

● **K61 Abscess of anal and rectal regions**
Includes abscess of anal and rectal regions
cellulitis of anal and rectal regions

K61.0 Anal abscess
Perianal abscess
Excludes1 intrasphincteric abscess (K61.4)

K61.1 Rectal abscess
Perirectal abscess
Excludes1 ischiorectal abscess (K61.3)

K61.2 Anorectal abscess
K61.3 Ischiorectal abscess
Abscess of ischiorectal fossa
K61.4 Intrasphincteric abscess

● **K62 Other diseases of anus and rectum**
Includes anal canal
Excludes2 colostomy and enterostomy malfunction (K94.0-, K91.4-)
fecal incontinence (R15.-)
hemorrhoids (K64.-)

K62.0 Anal polyp
K62.1 Rectal polyp
Excludes1 adenomatous polyp (D12.8)

K62.2 Anal prolapse
Prolapse of anal canal

K62.3 Rectal prolapse
Prolapse of rectal mucosa

K62.4 Stenosis of anus and rectum
Stricture of anus (sphincter)

K62.5 Hemorrhage of anus and rectum
Excludes1 gastrointestinal bleeding NOS (K92.2)
melena (K92.1)
neonatal rectal hemorrhage (P54.2)

K62.6 Ulcer of anus and rectum
Solitary ulcer of anus and rectum
Stercoral ulcer of anus and rectum
Excludes1 fissure and fistula of anus and rectum (K60.-)
ulcerative colitis (K51.-)

K62.7 Radiation proctitis
Use additional code to identify the type of radiation (W90.-)

● **K62.8 Other specified diseases of anus and rectum**
Excludes2 ulcerative proctitis (K51.2)

K62.81 Anal sphincter tear (healed) (nontraumatic) (old)
Tear of anus, nontraumatic
Use additional code for any associated fecal incontinence (R15.-)
Excludes2 anal fissure (K60.-)
anal sphincter tear (healed) (old) complicating delivery (O34.7-)
traumatic tear of anal sphincter (S31.831)

K62.82 Dysplasia of anus
Anal intraepithelial neoplasia I and II (AIN I and II) (histologically confirmed)
Dysplasia of anus NOS
Mild and moderate dysplasia of anus (histologically confirmed)
Excludes1 abnormal results from anal cytologic examination without histologic confirmation (R85.61-)
anal intraepithelial neoplasia III (D01.3)
carcinoma in situ of anus (D01.3)
HGSIL of anus (R85.613)
severe dysplasia of anus (D01.3)

K62.89 Other specified diseases of anus and rectum
Proctitis NOS
Use additional code for any associated fecal incontinence (R15.-)

K62.9 Disease of anus and rectum, unspecified

● **K63 Other diseases of intestine**

K63.0 Abscess of intestine
Excludes1 abscess of intestine with Crohn's disease (K50.014, K50.114, K50.814, K50.914)
abscess of intestine with diverticular disease (K57.0, K57.2, K57.4, K57.8)
abscess of intestine with ulcerative colitis (K51.014, K51.214, K51.314, K51.414, K51.514, K51.814, K51.914)
Excludes2 abscess of anal and rectal regions (K61.-)
abscess of appendix (K35.3)

K63.1 Perforation of intestine (nontraumatic)
Perforation (nontraumatic) of rectum
Excludes1 perforation (nontraumatic) of duodenum (K26.-)
perforation (nontraumatic) of intestine with diverticular disease (K57.0, K57.2, K57.4, K57.8)
Excludes2 perforation (nontraumatic) of appendix (K35.2, K35.3)

K63.2 Fistula of intestine
Excludes1 fistula of duodenum (K31.6)
fistula of intestine with Crohn's disease (K50.013, K50.113, K50.813, K50.913)
fistula of intestine with ulcerative colitis (K51.013, K51.213, K51.313, K51.413, K51.513, K51.813, K51.913)
Excludes2 fistula of anal and rectal regions (K60.-)
fistula of appendix (K38.3)
intestinal-genital fistula, female (N82.2-N82.4)
vesicointestinal fistula (N32.1)

K63.3 **Ulcer of intestine**
Primary ulcer of small intestine
Excludes1 duodenal ulcer (K26.-)
gastrointestinal ulcer (K28.-)
gastrojejunal ulcer (K28.-)
jejunal ulcer (K28.-)
peptic ulcer, site unspecified (K27.-)
ulcer of intestine with perforation (K63.1)
ulcer of anus or rectum (K62.6)
ulcerative colitis (K51.-)

K63.4 **Enteroptosis**

K63.5 **Polyp of colon**
Excludes1 adenomatous polyp of colon (D12.6)
inflammatory polyp of colon (K51.4-)
polyposis of colon (D12.6)

● K63.8 **Other specified diseases of intestine**
K63.81 **Dieulafoy lesion of intestine**
Excludes2 Dieulafoy lesion of stomach and duodenum (K31.82)
K63.89 **Other specified diseases of intestine**

K63.9 **Disease of intestine, unspecified**

● K64 **Hemorrhoids and perianal venous thrombosis**
Includes piles
Excludes1 hemorrhoids complicating childbirth and the puerperium (O87.2)
hemorrhoids complicating pregnancy (O22.4)

K64.0 **First degree hemorrhoids**
Grade/stage I hemorrhoids
Hemorrhoids (bleeding) without prolapse outside of anal canal

K64.1 **Second degree hemorrhoids**
Grade/stage II hemorrhoids
Hemorrhoids (bleeding) that prolapse with straining, but retract spontaneously

K64.2 **Third degree hemorrhoids**
Grade/stage III hemorrhoids
Hemorrhoids (bleeding) that prolapse with straining and require manual replacement back inside anal canal

K64.3 **Fourth degree hemorrhoids**
Grade/stage IV hemorrhoids
Hemorrhoids (bleeding) with prolapsed tissue that cannot be manually replaced

K64.4 **Residual hemorrhoidal skin tags**
External hemorrhoids, NOS
Skin tags of anus

K64.5 **Perianal venous thrombosis**
External hemorrhoids with thrombosis
Perianal hematoma
Thrombosed hemorrhoids NOS

K64.8 **Other hemorrhoids**
Internal hemorrhoids, without mention of degree
Prolapsed hemorrhoids, degree not specified

K64.9 **Unspecified hemorrhoids**
Hemorrhoids (bleeding) NOS
Hemorrhoids (bleeding) without mention of degree

Item 11–18 Peritonitis is an inflammation of the lining (peritoneum) of the abdominal cavity and surface of the intestines.

DISEASES OF PERITONEUM AND RETROPERITONEUM (K65-K68)

● K65 **Peritonitis**
Use additional code (B95-B97), to identify infectious agent
Excludes1 acute appendicitis with generalized peritonitis (K35.2)
aseptic peritonitis (T81.6)
benign paroxysmal peritonitis (E85.0)
chemical peritonitis (T81.6)
diverticulitis of both small and large intestine with peritonitis (K57.4-)
diverticulitis of colon with peritonitis (K57.2-)
diverticulitis of intestine, NOS, with peritonitis (K57.8-)
diverticulitis of small intestine with peritonitis (K57.0-)
gonococcal peritonitis (A54.85)
neonatal peritonitis (P78.0-P78.1)
pelvic peritonitis, female (N73.3-N73.5)
periodic familial peritonitis (E85.0)
peritonitis due to talc or other foreign substance (T81.6)
peritonitis in chlamydia (A74.81)
peritonitis in diphtheria (A36.89)
peritonitis in syphilis (late) (A52.74)
peritonitis in tuberculosis (A18.31)
peritonitis with or following abortion or ectopic or molar pregnancy (O00-O07, O08.0)
peritonitis with or following appendicitis (K35.-)
peritonitis with or following diverticular disease of intestine (K57.-)
puerperal peritonitis (O85)
retroperitoneal infections (K68.-)

K65.0 **Generalized (acute) peritonitis**
Pelvic peritonitis (acute), male
Subphrenic peritonitis (acute)
Suppurative peritonitis (acute)

K65.1 **Peritoneal abscess**
Abdominopelvic abscess
Abscess (of) omentum
Abscess (of) peritoneum
Mesenteric abscess
Retrocecal abscess
Subdiaphragmatic abscess
Subhepatic abscess
Subphrenic abscess

K65.2 **Spontaneous bacterial peritonitis**
Excludes1 bacterial peritonitis NOS (K65.9)

K65.3 **Choleperitonitis**
Peritonitis due to bile

K65.4 **Sclerosing mesenteritis**
Fat necrosis of peritoneum
(Idiopathic) sclerosing mesenteric fibrosis
Mesenteric lipodystrophy
Mesenteric panniculitis
Retractile mesenteritis

K65.8 **Other peritonitis**
Chronic proliferative peritonitis
Peritonitis due to urine

K65.9 **Peritonitis, unspecified**
Bacterial peritonitis NOS

Item 11-19 Retroperitoneal infections occur between the posterior parietal peritoneum and posterior abdominal wall where the kidneys, adrenal glands, ureters, duodenum, ascending colon, descending colon, pancreas, and the large vessels and nerves are located.

● **K66 Other disorders of peritoneum**

Excludes2 ascites (R18.-)
peritoneal effusion (chronic) (R18.8)

K66.Ø Peritoneal adhesions (postprocedural) (postinfection)
Adhesions (of) abdominal (wall)
Adhesions (of) diaphragm
Adhesions (of) intestine
Adhesions (of) male pelvis
Adhesions (of) omentum
Adhesions (of) stomach
Adhesive bands
Mesenteric adhesions

Excludes1 female pelvic adhesions [bands] (N73.6)
peritoneal adhesions with intestinal obstruction (K56.5)

K66.1 Hemoperitoneum

Excludes1 traumatic hemoperitoneum (S36.8-)

K66.8 Other specified disorders of peritoneum

K66.9 Disorder of peritoneum, unspecified

K67 Disorders of peritoneum in infectious diseases classified elsewhere

Code first underlying disease, such as:
congenital syphilis (A5Ø.Ø)
helminthiasis (B65.Ø-B83.9)

Excludes1 peritonitis in chlamydia (A74.81)
peritonitis in diphtheria (A36.89)
peritonitis in gonococcal (A54.85)
peritonitis in syphilis (late) (A52.74)
peritonitis in tuberculosis (A18.31)

● **K68 Disorders of retroperitoneum**

● **K68.1 Retroperitoneal abscess**

K68.11 Postprocedural retroperitoneal abscess

K68.12 Psoas muscle abscess

K68.19 Other retroperitoneal abscess

K68.9 Other disorders of retroperitoneum

DISEASES OF LIVER (K7Ø-K77)

Excludes1 jaundice NOS (R17)

Excludes2 hemochromatosis (E83.11-)
Reye's syndrome (G93.7)
viral hepatitis (B15-B19)
Wilson's disease (E83.Ø)

● **K7Ø Alcoholic liver disease**

Use additional code to identify:
alcohol abuse and dependence (F1Ø.-)

K7Ø.Ø Alcoholic fatty liver

● **K7Ø.1 Alcoholic hepatitis**

K7Ø.1Ø Alcoholic hepatitis without ascites

K7Ø.11 Alcoholic hepatitis with ascites

K7Ø.2 Alcoholic fibrosis and sclerosis of liver

● **K7Ø.3 Alcoholic cirrhosis of liver**
Alcoholic cirrhosis NOS

K7Ø.3Ø Alcoholic cirrhosis of liver without ascites

K7Ø.31 Alcoholic cirrhosis of liver with ascites

● **K7Ø.4 Alcoholic hepatic failure**
Acute alcoholic hepatic failure
Alcoholic hepatic failure NOS
Chronic alcoholic hepatic failure
Subacute alcoholic hepatic failure

K7Ø.4Ø Alcoholic hepatic failure without coma

K7Ø.41 Alcoholic hepatic failure with coma

K7Ø.9 Alcoholic liver disease, unspecified

● **K71 Toxic liver disease**

Includes drug-induced idiosyncratic (unpredictable) liver disease
drug-induced toxic (predictable) liver disease

Code first poisoning due to drug or toxin, if applicable (T36-T65 with fifth or sixth character 1-4 or 6)

Use additional code for adverse effect, if applicable, to identify drug (T36-T5Ø with fifth or sixth character 5)

Excludes2 alcoholic liver disease (K7Ø.-)
Budd-Chiari syndrome (I82.Ø)

K71.Ø Toxic liver disease with cholestasis
Cholestasis with hepatocyte injury
'Pure' cholestasis

● **K71.1 Toxic liver disease with hepatic necrosis**
Hepatic failure (acute) (chronic) due to drugs

K71.1Ø Toxic liver disease with hepatic necrosis, without coma

K71.11 Toxic liver disease with hepatic necrosis, with coma

K71.2 Toxic liver disease with acute hepatitis

K71.3 Toxic liver disease with chronic persistent hepatitis

K71.4 Toxic liver disease with chronic lobular hepatitis

● **K71.5 Toxic liver disease with chronic active hepatitis**
Toxic liver disease with lupoid hepatitis

K71.5Ø Toxic liver disease with chronic active hepatitis without ascites

K71.51 Toxic liver disease with chronic active hepatitis with ascites

K71.6 Toxic liver disease with hepatitis, not elsewhere classified

K71.7 Toxic liver disease with fibrosis and cirrhosis of liver

K71.8 Toxic liver disease with other disorders of liver
Toxic liver disease with focal nodular hyperplasia
Toxic liver disease with hepatic granulomas
Toxic liver disease with peliosis hepatis
Toxic liver disease with veno-occlusive disease of liver

K71.9 Toxic liver disease, unspecified

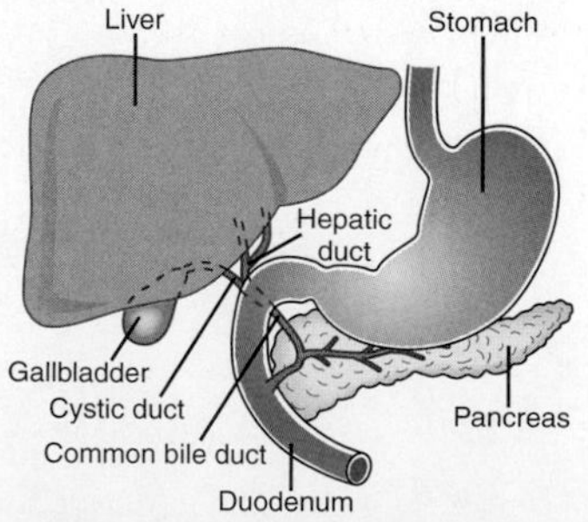

Figure 11-13 Liver and bile ducts.

Item 11-20 Cirrhosis is the progressive fibrosis of the liver resulting in loss of liver function. The main causes of cirrhosis of the liver are alcohol abuse, chronic hepatitis (inflammation of the liver), biliary disease, and excessive amounts of iron. **Alcoholic cirrhosis of the liver** is also called portal, Laënnec's, or fatty nutritional cirrhosis.

● **K72 Hepatic failure, not elsewhere classified**

Includes ~~acute hepatitis NEC, with hepatic failure~~
fulminant hepatitis NEC, with hepatic failure
hepatic encephalopathy NOS
liver (cell) necrosis with hepatic failure
malignant hepatitis NEC, with hepatic failure
yellow liver atrophy or dystrophy

Excludes1 alcoholic hepatic failure (K70.4)
hepatic failure with toxic liver disease (K71.1-)
icterus of newborn (P55-P59)
postprocedural hepatic failure (K91.82)

Excludes2 hepatic failure complicating abortion or ectopic or molar pregnancy (O00-O07, O08.8)
hepatic failure complicating pregnancy, childbirth and the puerperium (O26.6-)
viral hepatitis with hepatic coma (B15-B19) ◀

● **K72.0 Acute and subacute hepatic failure**
Acute non-viral hepatitis NOS ◀

K72.00 Acute and subacute hepatic failure without coma

K72.01 Acute and subacute hepatic failure with coma

● **K72.1 Chronic hepatic failure**

K72.10 Chronic hepatic failure without coma

K72.11 Chronic hepatic failure with coma

● **K72.9 Hepatic failure, unspecified**

K72.90 Hepatic failure, unspecified without coma

K72.91 Hepatic failure, unspecified with coma
Hepatic coma NOS

● **K73 Chronic hepatitis, not elsewhere classified**

Excludes1 alcoholic hepatitis (chronic) (K70.1-)
drug-induced hepatitis (chronic) (K71.-)
granulomatous hepatitis (chronic) NEC (K75.3)
reactive, nonspecific hepatitis (chronic) (K75.2)
viral hepatitis (chronic) (B15-B19)

K73.0 Chronic persistent hepatitis, not elsewhere classified

K73.1 Chronic lobular hepatitis, not elsewhere classified

K73.2 Chronic active hepatitis, not elsewhere classified

K73.8 Other chronic hepatitis, not elsewhere classified

K73.9 Chronic hepatitis, unspecified

● **K74 Fibrosis and cirrhosis of liver**

Code also, if applicable, viral hepatitis (acute) (chronic) (B15-B19)

Excludes1 alcoholic cirrhosis (of liver) (K70.3)
alcoholic fibrosis of liver (K70.2)
cardiac sclerosis of liver (K76.1)
cirrhosis (of liver) with toxic liver disease (K71.7)
congenital cirrhosis (of liver) (P78.81)
pigmentary cirrhosis (of liver) (E83.110)

K74.0 Hepatic fibrosis

K74.1 Hepatic sclerosis

K74.2 Hepatic fibrosis with hepatic sclerosis

K74.3 Primary biliary cirrhosis
Chronic nonsuppurative destructive cholangitis

K74.4 Secondary biliary cirrhosis

K74.5 Biliary cirrhosis, unspecified

● **K74.6 Other and unspecified cirrhosis of liver**

K74.60 Unspecified cirrhosis of liver
Cirrhosis (of liver) NOS

K74.69 Other cirrhosis of liver
Cryptogenic cirrhosis (of liver)
Macronodular cirrhosis (of liver)
Micronodular cirrhosis (of liver)
Mixed type cirrhosis (of liver)
Portal cirrhosis (of liver)
Postnecrotic cirrhosis (of liver)

● **K75 Other inflammatory liver diseases**

Excludes2 toxic liver disease (K71.-)

K75.0 Abscess of liver
Cholangitic hepatic abscess
Hematogenic hepatic abscess
Hepatic abscess NOS
Lymphogenic hepatic abscess
Pylephlebitic hepatic abscess

Excludes1 amebic liver abscess (A06.4)
cholangitis without liver abscess (K83.0)
pylephlebitis without liver abscess (K75.1)

Excludes2 acute or subacute hepatitis NOS (B17.9) ◀
acute or subacute non-viral hepatitis (K72.0) ◀
chronic hepatitis NEC (K73.8) ◀

K75.1 Phlebitis of portal vein
Pylephlebitis

Excludes1 pylephlebitic liver abscess (K75.0)

K75.2 Nonspecific reactive hepatitis

Excludes1 acute or subacute hepatitis (K72.0-)
chronic hepatitis NEC (K73.-)
viral hepatitis (B15-B19)

K75.3 Granulomatous hepatitis, not elsewhere classified

Excludes1 acute or subacute hepatitis (K72.0-)
chronic hepatitis NEC (K73.-)
viral hepatitis (B15-B19)

K75.4 Autoimmune hepatitis
Lupoid hepatitis NEC

● **K75.8 Other specified inflammatory liver diseases**

K75.81 Nonalcoholic steatohepatitis (NASH)

K75.89 Other specified inflammatory liver diseases

K75.9 Inflammatory liver disease, unspecified
Hepatitis NOS

Excludes1 acute or subacute hepatitis (K72.0-)
chronic hepatitis NEC (K73.-)
viral hepatitis (B15-B19)

● **K76 Other diseases of liver**

Excludes2 alcoholic liver disease (K70.-)
amyloid degeneration of liver (E85.-)
cystic disease of liver (congenital) (Q44.6)
hepatic vein thrombosis (I82.0)
hepatomegaly NOS (R16.0)
pigmentary cirrhosis (of liver) (E83.110)
portal vein thrombosis (I81)
toxic liver disease (K71.-)

K76.0 Fatty (change of) liver, not elsewhere classified
Nonalcoholic fatty liver disease (NAFLD)

Excludes1 nonalcoholic steatohepatitis (NASH) (K75.81)

K76.1 Chronic passive congestion of liver
Cardiac cirrhosis
Cardiac sclerosis

K76.2 Central hemorrhagic necrosis of liver

Excludes1 liver necrosis with hepatic failure (K72.-)

K76.3 Infarction of liver

K76.4 Peliosis hepatis
Hepatic angiomatosis

K76.5 Hepatic veno-occlusive disease

Excludes1 Budd-Chiari syndrome (I82.0)

K76.6 Portal hypertension
Use additional code for any associated complications, such as:
portal hypertensive gastropathy (K31.89)

K76.7 Hepatorenal syndrome

Excludes1 hepatorenal syndrome following labor and delivery (O90.4)
postprocedural hepatorenal syndrome (K91.83) ⇐

● **K76.8 Other specified diseases of liver**

K76.81 Hepatopulmonary syndrome

Code first underlying liver disease, such as:
alcoholic cirrhosis of liver (K7Ø.3-)
cirrhosis of liver without mention of alcohol (K74.6-)

K76.89 Other specified diseases of liver
Cyst (simple) of liver
Focal nodular hyperplasia of liver
Hepatoptosis

K76.9 Liver disease, unspecified

K77 Liver disorders in diseases classified elsewhere

Code first underlying disease, such as:
amyloidosis (E85.-)
congenital syphilis (A5Ø.Ø, A5Ø.5)
congenital toxoplasmosis (P37.1)
schistosomiasis (B65.Ø-B65.9)

Excludes1 alcoholic hepatitis (K7Ø.1-)
alcoholic liver disease (K7Ø.-)
cytomegaloviral hepatitis (B25.1)
herpesviral [herpes simplex] hepatitis (BØØ.81)
infectious mononucleosis with liver disease (B27.Ø-B27.9 with .9)
mumps hepatitis (B26.81)
sarcoidosis with liver disease (D86.89)
secondary syphilis with liver disease (A51.45)
syphilis (late) with liver disease (A52.74)
toxoplasmosis (acquired) hepatitis (B58.1)
tuberculosis with liver disease (A18.83)

DISORDERS OF GALLBLADDER, BILIARY TRACT AND PANCREAS (K8Ø–K87)

● **K8Ø Cholelithiasis**

Presence or formation of gallstones

Excludes1 retained cholelithiasis following cholecystectomy (K91.86)

● **K8Ø.Ø Calculus of gallbladder with acute cholecystitis**
Any condition listed in K8Ø.2 with acute cholecystitis
Check documentation for acute/chronic gallbladder/common bile duct either with or without obstruction.

K8Ø.ØØ Calculus of gallbladder with acute cholecystitis without obstruction

K8Ø.Ø1 Calculus of gallbladder with acute cholecystitis with obstruction

● **K8Ø.1 Calculus of gallbladder with other cholecystitis**

K8Ø.1Ø Calculus of gallbladder with chronic cholecystitis without obstruction
Cholelithiasis with cholecystitis NOS

K8Ø.11 Calculus of gallbladder with chronic cholecystitis with obstruction

K8Ø.12 Calculus of gallbladder with acute and chronic cholecystitis without obstruction

K8Ø.13 Calculus of gallbladder with acute and chronic cholecystitis with obstruction

K8Ø.18 Calculus of gallbladder with other cholecystitis without obstruction

K8Ø.19 Calculus of gallbladder with other cholecystitis with obstruction

● **K8Ø.2 Calculus of gallbladder without cholecystitis**
Cholecystolithiasis without cholecystitis
Cholelithiasis (without cholecystitis)
Colic (recurrent) of gallbladder (without cholecystitis)
Gallstone (impacted) of cystic duct (without cholecystitis)
Gallstone (impacted) of gallbladder (without cholecystitis)

K8Ø.2Ø Calculus of gallbladder without cholecystitis without obstruction

K8Ø.21 Calculus of gallbladder without cholecystitis with obstruction

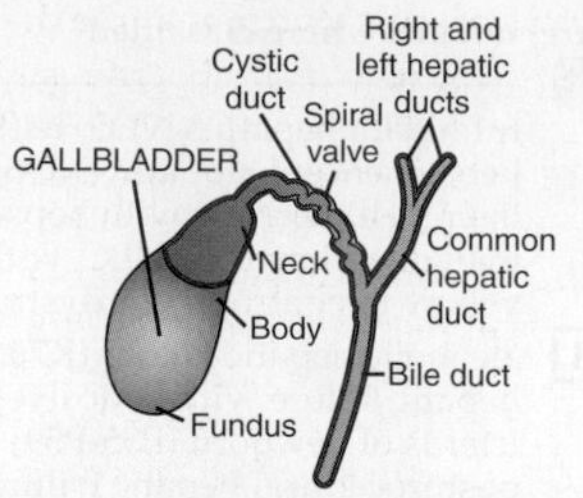

Figure 11-14 Gallbladder and bile ducts.

● **K8Ø.3 Calculus of bile duct with cholangitis**
Any condition listed in K8Ø.5 with cholangitis

K8Ø.3Ø Calculus of bile duct with cholangitis, unspecified, without obstruction

K8Ø.31 Calculus of bile duct with cholangitis, unspecified, with obstruction

K8Ø.32 Calculus of bile duct with acute cholangitis without obstruction

K8Ø.33 Calculus of bile duct with acute cholangitis with obstruction

K8Ø.34 Calculus of bile duct with chronic cholangitis without obstruction

K8Ø.35 Calculus of bile duct with chronic cholangitis with obstruction

K8Ø.36 Calculus of bile duct with acute and chronic cholangitis without obstruction

K8Ø.37 Calculus of bile duct with acute and chronic cholangitis with obstruction

● **K8Ø.4 Calculus of bile duct with cholecystitis**
Any condition listed in K8Ø.5 with cholecystitis (with cholangitis)

K8Ø.4Ø Calculus of bile duct with cholecystitis, unspecified, without obstruction

K8Ø.41 Calculus of bile duct with cholecystitis, unspecified, with obstruction

K8Ø.42 Calculus of bile duct with acute cholecystitis without obstruction

K8Ø.43 Calculus of bile duct with acute cholecystitis with obstruction

K8Ø.44 Calculus of bile duct with chronic cholecystitis without obstruction

K8Ø.45 Calculus of bile duct with chronic cholecystitis with obstruction

K8Ø.46 Calculus of bile duct with acute and chronic cholecystitis without obstruction

K8Ø.47 Calculus of bile duct with acute and chronic cholecystitis with obstruction

● **K8Ø.5 Calculus of bile duct without cholangitis or cholecystitis**
Choledocholithiasis (without cholangitis or cholecystitis)
Gallstone (impacted) of bile duct NOS (without cholangitis or cholecystitis)
Gallstone (impacted) of common duct (without cholangitis or cholecystitis)
Gallstone (impacted) of hepatic duct (without cholangitis or cholecystitis)
Hepatic cholelithiasis (without cholangitis or cholecystitis)
Hepatic colic (recurrent) (without cholangitis or cholecystitis)

K8Ø.5Ø Calculus of bile duct without cholangitis or cholecystitis without obstruction

K8Ø.51 Calculus of bile duct without cholangitis or cholecystitis with obstruction

● **K80.6 Calculus of gallbladder and bile duct with cholecystitis**
- **K80.60 Calculus of gallbladder and bile duct with cholecystitis, unspecified, without obstruction**
- **K80.61 Calculus of gallbladder and bile duct with cholecystitis, unspecified, with obstruction**
- **K80.62 Calculus of gallbladder and bile duct with acute cholecystitis without obstruction**
- **K80.63 Calculus of gallbladder and bile duct with acute cholecystitis with obstruction**
- **K80.64 Calculus of gallbladder and bile duct with chronic cholecystitis without obstruction**
- **K80.65 Calculus of gallbladder and bile duct with chronic cholecystitis with obstruction**
- **K80.66 Calculus of gallbladder and bile duct with acute and chronic cholecystitis without obstruction**
- **K80.67 Calculus of gallbladder and bile duct with acute and chronic cholecystitis with obstruction**

● **K80.7 Calculus of gallbladder and bile duct without cholecystitis**
- **K80.70 Calculus of gallbladder and bile duct without cholecystitis without obstruction**
- **K80.71 Calculus of gallbladder and bile duct without cholecystitis with obstruction**

● **K80.8 Other cholelithiasis**
- **K80.80 Other cholelithiasis without obstruction**
- **K80.81 Other cholelithiasis with obstruction**

● **K81 Cholecystitis**

Chronic or acute inflammation of the gallbladder

Excludes1 cholecystitis with cholelithiasis (K80.-)

K81.0 Acute cholecystitis

Abscess of gallbladder
Angiocholecystitis
Emphysematous (acute) cholecystitis
Empyema of gallbladder
Gangrene of gallbladder
Gangrenous cholecystitis
Suppurative cholecystitis

K81.1 Chronic cholecystitis

K81.2 Acute cholecystitis with chronic cholecystitis

K81.9 Cholecystitis, unspecified

● **K82 Other diseases of gallbladder**

Excludes1 nonvisualization of gallbladder (R93.2)
postcholecystectomy syndrome (K91.5)

K82.0 Obstruction of gallbladder

Occlusion of cystic duct or gallbladder without cholelithiasis
Stenosis of cystic duct or gallbladder without cholelithiasis
Stricture of cystic duct or gallbladder without cholelithiasis

Excludes1 obstruction of gallbladder with cholelithiasis (K80.-)

K82.1 Hydrops of gallbladder

Mucocele of gallbladder

K82.2 Perforation of gallbladder

Rupture of cystic duct or gallbladder

K82.3 Fistula of gallbladder

Cholecystocolic fistula
Cholecystoduodenal fistula

K82.4 Cholesterolosis of gallbladder

Strawberry gallbladder

Excludes1 cholesterolosis of gallbladder with cholecystitis (K81.-)
cholesterolosis of gallbladder with cholelithiasis (K80.-)

K82.8 Other specified diseases of gallbladder

Adhesions of cystic duct or gallbladder
Atrophy of cystic duct or gallbladder
Cyst of cystic duct or gallbladder
Dyskinesia of cystic duct or gallbladder
Hypertrophy of cystic duct or gallbladder
Nonfunctioning of cystic duct or gallbladder
Ulcer of cystic duct or gallbladder

K82.9 Disease of gallbladder, unspecified

● **K83 Other diseases of biliary tract**

Excludes1 postcholecystectomy syndrome (K91.5)

Excludes2 conditions involving the gallbladder (K81-K82)
conditions involving the cystic duct (K81-K82)

K83.0 Cholangitis

Ascending cholangitis	Sclerosing cholangitis
Cholangitis NOS	Secondary cholangitis
Primary cholangitis	Stenosing cholangitis
Recurrent cholangitis	Suppurative cholangitis

Excludes1 cholangitic liver abscess (K75.0)
cholangitis with choledocholithiasis (K80.3-, K80.4-)
chronic nonsuppurative destructive cholangitis (K74.3)

K83.1 Obstruction of bile duct

Occlusion of bile duct without cholelithiasis
Stenosis of bile duct without cholelithiasis
Stricture of bile duct without cholelithiasis

Excludes1 congenital obstruction of bile duct (Q44.3)
obstruction of bile duct with cholelithiasis (K80.-)

K83.2 Perforation of bile duct

Rupture of bile duct

K83.3 Fistula of bile duct

Choledochoduodenal fistula

K83.4 Spasm of sphincter of Oddi

K83.5 Biliary cyst

K83.8 Other specified diseases of biliary tract

Adhesions of biliary tract
Atrophy of biliary tract
Hypertrophy of biliary tract
Ulcer of biliary tract

K83.9 Disease of biliary tract, unspecified

● **K85 Acute pancreatitis**

Inflammatory process in which pancreatic enzymes autodigest the gland

Includes ~~abscess of pancreas~~
~~acute necrosis of pancreas~~
acute (recurrent) pancreatitis
~~gangrene of (gangrenous) pancreas~~
~~hemorrhagic pancreatitis~~
~~infective necrosis of pancreas~~
subacute pancreatitis
~~suppurative pancreatitis~~

● **K85.0 Idiopathic acute pancreatitis**
- **K85.00 Idiopathic acute pancreatitis without necrosis or infection** ◀
- **K85.01 Idiopathic acute pancreatitis with uninfected necrosis** ◀
- **K85.02 Idiopathic acute pancreatitis with infected necrosis** ◀

● **K85.1 Biliary acute pancreatitis**

Gallstone pancreatitis
- **K85.10 Biliary acute pancreatitis without necrosis or infection** ◀
- **K85.11 Biliary acute pancreatitis with uninfected necrosis** ◀
- **K85.12 Biliary acute pancreatitis with infected necrosis** ◀

● **K85.2 Alcohol induced acute pancreatitis**

Excludes2 alcohol induced chronic pancreatitis (K86.Ø)

K85.20 Alcohol induced acute pancreatitis without necrosis or infection ◀

K85.21 Alcohol induced acute pancreatitis with uninfected necrosis ◀

K85.22 Alcohol induced acute pancreatitis with infected necrosis ◀

● **K85.3 Drug induced acute pancreatitis**

Use additional code for adverse effect, if applicable, to identify drug (T36-T5Ø with fifth or sixth character 5)

Use additional code to identify drug abuse and dependence (F11.-F17.-)

K85.3Ø Drug induced acute pancreatitis without necrosis or infection ◀

K85.31 Drug induced acute pancreatitis with uninfected necrosis ◀

K85.32 Drug induced acute pancreatitis with infected necrosis ◀

● **K85.8 Other acute pancreatitis**

K85.8Ø Other acute pancreatitis without necrosis or infection ◀

K85.81 Other acute pancreatitis with uninfected necrosis ◀

K85.82 Other acute pancreatitis with infected necrosis ◀

● **K85.9 Acute pancreatitis, unspecified**

Pancreatitis NOS

K85.9Ø Acute pancreatitis without necrosis or infection, unspecified ◀

K85.91 Acute pancreatitis with uninfected necrosis, unspecified ◀

K85.92 Acute pancreatitis with infected necrosis, unspecified ◀

● **K86 Other diseases of pancreas**

Excludes2 fibrocystic disease of pancreas (E84.-)
islet cell tumor (of pancreas) (D13.7)
pancreatic steatorrhea (K9Ø.3)

K86.Ø Alcohol-induced chronic pancreatitis

Use additional code to identify:
alcohol abuse and dependence (F1Ø.-)

Code also exocrine pancreatic insufficiency (K86.81) ◀

Excludes2 alcohol induced acute pancreatitis (K85.2-) ⬅

K86.1 Other chronic pancreatitis

Chronic pancreatitis NOS
Infectious chronic pancreatitis
Recurrent chronic pancreatitis
Relapsing chronic pancreatitis

Code also exocrine pancreatic insufficiency (K86.81) ◀

K86.2 Cyst of pancreas

K86.3 Pseudocyst of pancreas

● **K86.8 Other specified diseases of pancreas**

K86.81 Exocrine pancreatic insufficiency ◀

K86.89 Other specified diseases of pancreas ◀

Aseptic pancreatic necrosis, unrelated to acute pancreatitis ◀
Atrophy of pancreas ◀
Calculus of pancreas ◀
Cirrhosis of pancreas ◀
Fibrosis of pancreas ◀
Pancreatic fat necrosis, unrelated to acute pancreatitis ◀
Pancreatic infantilism ◀
Pancreatic necrosis NOS, unrelated to acute pancreatitis ◀

K86.9 Disease of pancreas, unspecified

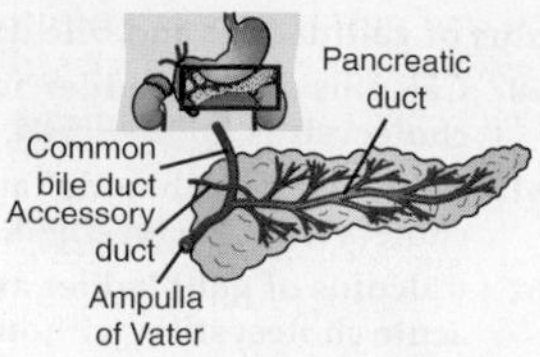

Figure 11-15 Pancreatic ductal system.

K87 Disorders of gallbladder, biliary tract and pancreas in diseases classified elsewhere

Code first underlying disease

Excludes1 cytomegaloviral pancreatitis (B25.2)
mumps pancreatitis (B26.3)
syphilitic gallbladder (A52.74)
syphilitic pancreas (A52.74)
tuberculosis of gallbladder (A18.83)
tuberculosis of pancreas (A18.83)

OTHER DISEASES OF THE DIGESTIVE SYSTEM (K9Ø-K95)

● **K9Ø Intestinal malabsorption**

Excludes1 intestinal malabsorption following gastrointestinal surgery (K91.2)

K9Ø.Ø Celiac disease

Celiac disease with steatorrhea ◀
Gluten-sensitive enteropathy
~~Idiopathic steatorrhea~~
Nontropical sprue

Use additional code for associated disorders including:
dermatitis herpetiformis (L13.Ø)
gluten ataxia (G32.81)

Code also exocrine pancreatic insufficiency (K86.81) ◀

K9Ø.1 Tropical sprue

Sprue NOS
Tropical steatorrhea

K9Ø.2 Blind loop syndrome, not elsewhere classified

Blind loop syndrome NOS

Excludes1 congenital blind loop syndrome (Q43.8)
postsurgical blind loop syndrome (K91.2)

K9Ø.3 Pancreatic steatorrhea

● **K9Ø.4 Other malabsorption due to intolerance** ⬅

Excludes2 gluten-sensitive enteropathy (K9Ø.Ø)
lactose intolerance (E73.-)

K9Ø.41 Non-celiac gluten sensitivity ◀

Gluten sensitivity NOS ◀
Non-celiac gluten sensitive enteropathy ◀

K9Ø.49 Malabsorption due to intolerance, not elsewhere classified ◀

Malabsorption due to intolerance to carbohydrate ◀
Malabsorption due to intolerance to fat ◀
Malabsorption due to intolerance to protein ◀
Malabsorption due to intolerance to starch ◀

● **K9Ø.8 Other intestinal malabsorption**

K9Ø.81 Whipple's disease

K9Ø.89 Other intestinal malabsorption

K9Ø.9 Intestinal malabsorption, unspecified

● **K91 Intraoperative and postprocedural complications and disorders of digestive system, not elsewhere classified**
Excludes2 complications of artificial opening of digestive system (K94.-)
complications of bariatric procedures (K95.-)
gastrojejunal ulcer (K28.-)
postprocedural (radiation) retroperitoneal abscess (K68.11)
radiation colitis (K52.0)
radiation gastroenteritis (K52.0)
radiation proctitis (K62.7)

K91.0 Vomiting following gastrointestinal surgery

K91.1 Postgastric surgery syndromes
Dumping syndrome
Postgastrectomy syndrome
Postvagotomy syndrome

K91.2 Postsurgical malabsorption, not elsewhere classified
Postsurgical blind loop syndrome
Excludes1 malabsorption osteomalacia in adults (M83.2)
malabsorption osteoporosis, postsurgical (M80.8-, M81.8)

K91.3 Postprocedural intestinal obstruction

K91.5 Postcholecystectomy syndrome

● **K91.6 Intraoperative hemorrhage and hematoma of a digestive system organ or structure complicating a procedure**
Excludes1 intraoperative hemorrhage and hematoma of a digestive system organ or structure due to accidental puncture and laceration during a procedure (K91.7-)

K91.61 Intraoperative hemorrhage and hematoma of a digestive system organ or structure complicating a digestive system procedure (Revised)

K91.62 Intraoperative hemorrhage and hematoma of a digestive system organ or structure complicating other procedure

● **K91.7 Accidental puncture and laceration of a digestive system organ or structure during a procedure**

K91.71 Accidental puncture and laceration of a digestive system organ or structure during a digestive system procedure

K91.72 Accidental puncture and laceration of a digestive system organ or structure during other procedure

● **K91.8 Other intraoperative and postprocedural complications and disorders of digestive system**

K91.81 Other intraoperative complications of digestive system

K91.82 Postprocedural hepatic failure

K91.83 Postprocedural hepatorenal syndrome

● **K91.84 Postprocedural hemorrhage of a digestive system organ or structure following a procedure** (Revised)

K91.840 Postprocedural hemorrhage of a digestive system organ or structure following a digestive system procedure (Revised)

K91.841 Postprocedural hemorrhage of a digestive system organ or structure following other procedure (Revised)

● **K91.85 Complications of intestinal pouch**

K91.850 Pouchitis
Inflammation of internal ileoanal pouch

K91.858 Other complications of intestinal pouch

K91.86 Retained cholelithiasis following cholecystectomy

● **K91.87 Postprocedural hematoma and seroma of a digestive system organ or structure following a procedure** (New)

K91.870 Postprocedural hematoma of a digestive system organ or structure following a digestive system procedure (New)

K91.871 Postprocedural hematoma of a digestive system organ or structure following other procedure (New)

K91.872 Postprocedural seroma of a digestive system organ or structure following a digestive system procedure (New)

K91.873 Postprocedural seroma of a digestive system organ or structure following other procedure (New)

K91.89 Other postprocedural complications and disorders of digestive system
Use additional code, if applicable, to further specify disorder
Excludes2 postprocedural retroperitoneal abscess (K68.11)

● **K92 Other diseases of digestive system**
Excludes1 neonatal gastrointestinal hemorrhage (P54.0-P54.3)

K92.0 Hematemesis

K92.1 Melena
Excludes1 occult blood in feces (R19.5)

K92.2 Gastrointestinal hemorrhage, unspecified
Gastric hemorrhage NOS
Intestinal hemorrhage NOS
Excludes1 acute hemorrhagic gastritis (K29.01)
hemorrhage of anus and rectum (K62.5)
angiodysplasia of stomach with hemorrhage (K31.811)
diverticular disease with hemorrhage (K57.-)
gastritis and duodenitis with hemorrhage (K29.-)
peptic ulcer with hemorrhage (K25-K28)

● **K92.8 Other specified diseases of the digestive system**

K92.81 Gastrointestinal mucositis (ulcerative)
Code also type of associated therapy, such as:
antineoplastic and immunosuppressive drugs (T45.1X-)
radiological procedure and radiotherapy (Y84.2)
Excludes2 mucositis (ulcerative) of vagina and vulva (N76.81)
nasal mucositis (ulcerative) (J34.81)
oral mucositis (ulcerative) (K12.3-)

K92.89 Other specified diseases of the digestive system

K92.9 Disease of digestive system, unspecified

● **K94 Complications of artificial openings of the digestive system**

● **K94.0 Colostomy complications**

K94.00 Colostomy complication, unspecified

K94.01 Colostomy hemorrhage

K94.02 Colostomy infection
Use additional code to specify type of infection, such as:
cellulitis of abdominal wall (L03.311)
sepsis (A40.-, A41.-)

K94.03 Colostomy malfunction
Mechanical complication of colostomy

K94.09 Other complications of colostomy

CHAPTER 11 (K00-K95)

● **K94.1 Enterostomy complications**

K94.10 Enterostomy complication, unspecified

K94.11 Enterostomy hemorrhage

K94.12 Enterostomy infection

Use additional code to specify type of infection, such as:
cellulitis of abdominal wall (LØ3.311)
sepsis (A4Ø.-, A41.-)

K94.13 Enterostomy malfunction

Mechanical complication of enterostomy

K94.19 Other complications of enterostomy

● **K94.2 Gastrostomy complications**

K94.2Ø Gastrostomy complication, unspecified

K94.21 Gastrostomy hemorrhage

K94.22 Gastrostomy infection

Use additional code to specify type of infection, such as:
cellulitis of abdominal wall (LØ3.311)
sepsis (A4Ø.-, A41.-)

K94.23 Gastrostomy malfunction

Mechanical complication of gastrostomy

K94.29 Other complications of gastrostomy

● **K94.3 Esophagostomy complications**

K94.3Ø Esophagostomy complications, unspecified

K94.31 Esophagostomy hemorrhage

K94.32 Esophagostomy infection

Use additional code to identify the infection

K94.33 Esophagostomy malfunction

Mechanical complication of esophagostomy

K94.39 Other complications of esophagostomy

● **K95 Complications of bariatric procedures**

● **K95.Ø Complications of gastric band procedure**

K95.Ø1 Infection due to gastric band procedure

Use additional code to specify type of infection or organism, such as:
bacterial and viral infectious agents (B95.-, B96.-)
cellulitis of abdominal wall (LØ3.311)
sepsis (A4Ø.-, A41.-)

K95.Ø9 Other complications of gastric band procedure

Use additional code, if applicable, to further specify complication

● **K95.8 Complications of other bariatric procedure**

Excludes1 complications of gastric band surgery (K95.Ø-)

K95.81 Infection due to other bariatric procedure

Use additional code to specify type of infection or organism, such as:
bacterial and viral infectious agents (B95.-, B96.-)
cellulitis of abdominal wall (LØ3.311)
sepsis (A4Ø.-, A41.-)

K95.89 Other complications of other bariatric procedure

Use additional code, if applicable, to further specify complication

CHAPTER 12

DISEASES OF THE SKIN AND SUBCUTANEOUS TISSUE (L00-L99)

OGCR Chapter-Specific Coding Guidelines

12. **Chapter 12: Diseases of the Skin and Subcutaneous Tissue (L00-L99)**

a. Pressure ulcer stage codes

1) Pressure ulcer stages

Codes from category L89, Pressure ulcer, identify the site of the pressure ulcer as well as the stage of the ulcer.

The ICD-10-CM classifies pressure ulcer stages based on severity, which is designated by stages 1-4, unspecified stage and unstageable.

Assign as many codes from category L89 as needed to identify all the pressure ulcers the patient has, if applicable.

2) Unstageable pressure ulcers

Assignment of the code for unstageable pressure ulcer (L89.--0) should be based on the clinical documentation. These codes are used for pressure ulcers whose stage cannot be clinically determined (e.g., the ulcer is covered by eschar or has been treated with a skin or muscle graft) and pressure ulcers that are documented as deep tissue injury but not documented as due to trauma. This code should not be confused with the codes for unspecified stage (L89.--9). When there is no documentation regarding the stage of the pressure ulcer, assign the appropriate code for unspecified stage (L89.--9).

3) Documented pressure ulcer stage

Assignment of the pressure ulcer stage code should be guided by clinical documentation of the stage or documentation of the terms found in the Alphabetic Index. For clinical terms describing the stage that are not found in the Alphabetic Index, and there is no documentation of the stage, the provider should be queried.

4) Patients admitted with pressure ulcers documented as healed

No code is assigned if the documentation states that the pressure ulcer is completely healed.

5) Patients admitted with pressure ulcers documented as healing

Pressure ulcers described as healing should be assigned the appropriate pressure ulcer stage code based on the documentation in the medical record. If the documentation does not provide information about the stage of the healing pressure ulcer, assign the appropriate code for unspecified stage.

If the documentation is unclear as to whether the patient has a current (new) pressure ulcer or if the patient is being treated for a healing pressure ulcer, query the provider.

For ulcers that were present on admission but healed at the time of discharge, assign the code for the site and stage of the pressure ulcer at the time of admission.

6) Patient admitted with pressure ulcer evolving into another stage during the admission

If a patient is admitted with a pressure ulcer at one stage and it progresses to a higher stage, **two separate codes should be assigned: one code for the site and stage of the ulcer on admission and a second code for the same ulcer site and the highest stage reported during the stay.**

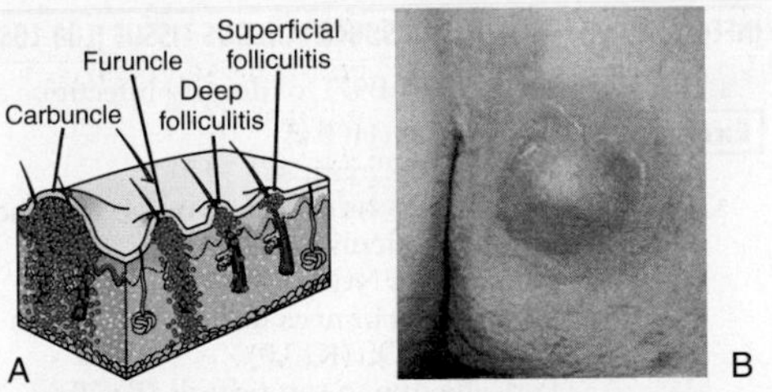

Figure 12-1 Furuncle, also known as a boil, is a staphylococcal infection. The organism enters the body through a hair follicle and so furuncles usually appear in hairy areas of the body. A cluster of furuncles is known as a carbuncle and involves infection into the deep subcutaneous fascia. These usually appear on the back and neck. (**B** from Habif: Clinical Dermatology, ed 5, Mosby, 2009)

CHAPTER 12

DISEASES OF THE SKIN AND SUBCUTANEOUS TISSUE (L00-L99)

Excludes2 certain conditions originating in the perinatal period (P04-P96)
certain infectious and parasitic diseases (A00-B99)
complications of pregnancy, childbirth and the puerperium (O00-O9A)
congenital malformations, deformations, and chromosomal abnormalities (Q00-Q99)
endocrine, nutritional and metabolic diseases (E00-E88)
lipomelanotic reticulosis (I89.8)
neoplasms (C00-D49)
symptoms, signs and abnormal clinical and laboratory findings, not elsewhere classified (R00-R94)
systemic connective tissue disorders (M30-M36)
viral warts (B07.-)

This chapter contains the following blocks:

L00-L08	Infections of the skin and subcutaneous tissue
L10-L14	Bullous disorders
L20-L30	Dermatitis and eczema
L40-L45	Papulosquamous disorders
L49-L54	Urticaria and erythema
L55-L59	Radiation-related disorders of the skin and subcutaneous tissue
L60-L75	Disorders of skin appendages
L76	Intraoperative and postprocedural complications of skin and subcutaneous tissue
L80-L99	Other disorders of the skin and subcutaneous tissue

INFECTIONS OF THE SKIN AND SUBCUTANEOUS TISSUE (LØØ-LØ8)

Use additional code (B95-B97) to identify infectious agent.

Excludes2 hordeolum (HØØ.Ø)
infective dermatitis (L3Ø.3)
local infections of skin classified in Chapter 1
lupus panniculitis (L93.2)
panniculitis NOS (M79.3)
panniculitis of neck and back (M54.Ø-)
Perlèche NOS (K13.Ø)
Perlèche due to candidiasis (B37.Ø)
Perlèche due to riboflavin deficiency (E53.Ø)
pyogenic granuloma (L98.Ø)
relapsing panniculitis [Weber-Christian] (M35.6)
viral warts (BØ7.-)
zoster (BØ2.-)

LØØ Staphylococcal scalded skin syndrome
Ritter's disease
Use additional code to identify percentage of skin exfoliation (L49.-)
Excludes1 bullous impetigo (LØ1.Ø3)
pemphigus neonatorum (LØ1.Ø3)
toxic epidermal necrolysis [Lyell] (L51.2)

● **LØ1 Impetigo**
Contagious skin infection caused by a streptococcus or staphylococcus aureus, common skin infections among children
Excludes1 impetigo herpetiformis (L4Ø.1)

● **LØ1.Ø Impetigo**
Impetigo contagiosa
Impetigo vulgaris

LØ1.ØØ Impetigo, unspecified
Impetigo NOS

LØ1.Ø1 Non-bullous impetigo

LØ1.Ø2 Bockhart's impetigo
Impetigo follicularis
Perifolliculitis NOS
Superficial pustular perifolliculitis

LØ1.Ø3 Bullous impetigo
Impetigo neonatorum
Pemphigus neonatorum
Neonate = newborn

LØ1.Ø9 Other impetigo
Ulcerative impetigo

LØ1.1 Impetiginization of other dermatoses

● **LØ2 Cutaneous abscess, furuncle and carbuncle**
Use additional code to identify organism (B95-B96)
Excludes2 abscess of anus and rectal regions (K61.-)
abscess of female genital organs (external) (N76.4)
abscess of male genital organs (external) (N48.2, N49.-)

● **LØ2.Ø Cutaneous abscess, furuncle and carbuncle of face**
Excludes2 abscess of ear, external (H6Ø.Ø)
abscess of eyelid (HØØ.Ø)
abscess of head [any part, except face] (LØ2.8)
abscess of lacrimal gland (HØ4.Ø)
abscess of lacrimal passages (HØ4.3)
abscess of mouth (K12.2)
abscess of nose (J34.Ø)
abscess of orbit (HØ5.Ø)
submandibular abscess (K12.2)

LØ2.Ø1 Cutaneous abscess of face

LØ2.Ø2 Furuncle of face
Boil of face
Folliculitis of face

LØ2.Ø3 Carbuncle of face

● **LØ2.1 Cutaneous abscess, furuncle and carbuncle of neck**

LØ2.11 Cutaneous abscess of neck

LØ2.12 Furuncle of neck
Boil of neck
Folliculitis of neck

LØ2.13 Carbuncle of neck

● **LØ2.2 Cutaneous abscess, furuncle and carbuncle of trunk**
Excludes1 non-newborn omphalitis (LØ8.82)
omphalitis of newborn (P38.-)
Excludes2 abscess of breast (N61.1) ⬅
abscess of buttocks (LØ2.3)
abscess of female external genital organs (N76.4)
abscess of male external genital organs (N48.2, N49.-)
abscess of hip (LØ2.4)

● **LØ2.21 Cutaneous abscess of trunk**

LØ2.211 Cutaneous abscess of abdominal wall

LØ2.212 Cutaneous abscess of back [any part, except buttock]

LØ2.213 Cutaneous abscess of chest wall

LØ2.214 Cutaneous abscess of groin

LØ2.215 Cutaneous abscess of perineum

LØ2.216 Cutaneous abscess of umbilicus

LØ2.219 Cutaneous abscess of trunk, unspecified

● **LØ2.22 Furuncle of trunk**
Boil of trunk
Folliculitis of trunk

LØ2.221 Furuncle of abdominal wall

LØ2.222 Furuncle of back [any part, except buttock]

LØ2.223 Furuncle of chest wall

LØ2.224 Furuncle of groin

LØ2.225 Furuncle of perineum

LØ2.226 Furuncle of umbilicus

LØ2.229 Furuncle of trunk, unspecified

● **LØ2.23 Carbuncle of trunk**

LØ2.231 Carbuncle of abdominal wall

LØ2.232 Carbuncle of back [any part, except buttock]

LØ2.233 Carbuncle of chest wall

LØ2.234 Carbuncle of groin

LØ2.235 Carbuncle of perineum

LØ2.236 Carbuncle of umbilicus

LØ2.239 Carbuncle of trunk, unspecified

● **LØ2.3 Cutaneous abscess, furuncle and carbuncle of buttock**
Excludes1 pilonidal cyst with abscess (LØ5.Ø1)

LØ2.31 Cutaneous abscess of buttock
Cutaneous abscess of gluteal region

LØ2.32 Furuncle of buttock
Boil of buttock
Folliculitis of buttock
Furuncle of gluteal region

LØ2.33 Carbuncle of buttock
Carbuncle of gluteal region

● L02.4 Cutaneous abscess, furuncle and carbuncle of limb
Excludes2 Cutaneous abscess, furuncle and carbuncle of groin (L02.214, L02.224, L02.234)
Cutaneous abscess, furuncle and carbuncle of hand (L02.5-)
Cutaneous abscess, furuncle and carbuncle of foot (L02.6-)

● L02.41 Cutaneous abscess of limb
- L02.411 Cutaneous abscess of right axilla
- L02.412 Cutaneous abscess of left axilla
- L02.413 Cutaneous abscess of right upper limb
- L02.414 Cutaneous abscess of left upper limb
- L02.415 Cutaneous abscess of right lower limb
- L02.416 Cutaneous abscess of left lower limb
- L02.419 Cutaneous abscess of limb, unspecified

● L02.42 Furuncle of limb
Boil of limb
Folliculitis of limb
- L02.421 Furuncle of right axilla
- L02.422 Furuncle of left axilla
- L02.423 Furuncle of right upper limb
- L02.424 Furuncle of left upper limb
- L02.425 Furuncle of right lower limb
- L02.426 Furuncle of left lower limb
- L02.429 Furuncle of limb, unspecified

● L02.43 Carbuncle of limb
- L02.431 Carbuncle of right axilla
- L02.432 Carbuncle of left axilla
- L02.433 Carbuncle of right upper limb
- L02.434 Carbuncle of left upper limb
- L02.435 Carbuncle of right lower limb
- L02.436 Carbuncle of left lower limb
- L02.439 Carbuncle of limb, unspecified

● L02.5 Cutaneous abscess, furuncle and carbuncle of hand

● L02.51 Cutaneous abscess of hand
- L02.511 Cutaneous abscess of right hand
- L02.512 Cutaneous abscess of left hand
- L02.519 Cutaneous abscess of unspecified hand

● L02.52 Furuncle hand
Boil of hand
Folliculitis of hand
- L02.521 Furuncle right hand
- L02.522 Furuncle left hand
- L02.529 Furuncle unspecified hand

● L02.53 Carbuncle of hand
- L02.531 Carbuncle of right hand
- L02.532 Carbuncle of left hand
- L02.539 Carbuncle of unspecified hand

● L02.6 Cutaneous abscess, furuncle and carbuncle of foot

● L02.61 Cutaneous abscess of foot
- L02.611 Cutaneous abscess of right foot
- L02.612 Cutaneous abscess of left foot
- L02.619 Cutaneous abscess of unspecified foot

● L02.62 Furuncle of foot
Boil of foot
Folliculitis of foot
- L02.621 Furuncle of right foot
- L02.622 Furuncle of left foot
- L02.629 Furuncle of unspecified foot

● L02.63 Carbuncle of foot
- L02.631 Carbuncle of right foot
- L02.632 Carbuncle of left foot
- L02.639 Carbuncle of unspecified foot

● L02.8 Cutaneous abscess, furuncle and carbuncle of other sites

● L02.81 Cutaneous abscess of other sites
- L02.811 Cutaneous abscess of head [any part, except face]
- L02.818 Cutaneous abscess of other sites

● L02.82 Furuncle of other sites
Boil of other sites
Folliculitis of other sites
- L02.821 Furuncle of head [any part, except face]
- L02.828 Furuncle of other sites

● L02.83 Carbuncle of other sites
- L02.831 Carbuncle of head [any part, except face]
- L02.838 Carbuncle of other sites

● L02.9 Cutaneous abscess, furuncle and carbuncle, unspecified
- L02.91 Cutaneous abscess, unspecified
- L02.92 Furuncle, unspecified
  Boil NOS
  Furunculosis NOS
- L02.93 Carbuncle, unspecified

● L03 Cellulitis and acute lymphangitis
Excludes2 cellulitis of anal and rectal region (K61.-)
cellulitis of external auditory canal (H60.1)
cellulitis of eyelid (H00.0)
cellulitis of female external genital organs (N76.4)
cellulitis of lacrimal apparatus (H04.3)
cellulitis of male external genital organs (N48.2, N49.-)
cellulitis of mouth (K12.2)
cellulitis of nose (J34.0)
eosinophilic cellulitis [Wells] (L98.3)
febrile neutrophilic dermatosis [Sweet] (L98.2)
lymphangitis (chronic) (subacute) (I89.1)

● L03.0 Cellulitis and acute lymphangitis of finger and toe
Infection of nail
Onychia
Paronychia
Perionychia

● L03.01 Cellulitis of finger
Felon
Whitlow
Excludes1 herpetic whitlow (B00.89)
- L03.011 Cellulitis of right finger
- L03.012 Cellulitis of left finger
- L03.019 Cellulitis of unspecified finger

● L03.02 Acute lymphangitis of finger
Hangnail with lymphangitis of finger
- L03.021 Acute lymphangitis of right finger
- L03.022 Acute lymphangitis of left finger
- L03.029 Acute lymphangitis of unspecified finger

● L03.03 Cellulitis of toe
- L03.031 Cellulitis of right toe
- L03.032 Cellulitis of left toe
- L03.039 Cellulitis of unspecified toe

● L03.04 Acute lymphangitis of toe
Hangnail with lymphangitis of toe
- L03.041 Acute lymphangitis of right toe
- L03.042 Acute lymphangitis of left toe
- L03.049 Acute lymphangitis of unspecified toe

Item 12-1 Onychia is an inflammation of the tissue surrounding the nail with pus accumulation and loss of the nail, resulting from microscopic pathogens entering through small wounds. **Paronychia** is a nail disease also known as felon or whitlow and is a bacterial or fungal infection.

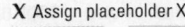

● LØ3.1 **Cellulitis and acute lymphangitis of other parts of limb**

● LØ3.11 **Cellulitis of other parts of limb**

Excludes2 cellulitis of fingers (LØ3.Ø1-)
cellulitis of toes (LØ3.Ø3-)
groin (LØ3.314)

LØ3.111 **Cellulitis of right axilla**

LØ3.112 **Cellulitis of left axilla**

LØ3.113 **Cellulitis of right upper limb**

LØ3.114 **Cellulitis of left upper limb**

LØ3.115 **Cellulitis of right lower limb**

LØ3.116 **Cellulitis of left lower limb**

LØ3.119 **Cellulitis of unspecified part of limb**

● LØ3.12 **Acute lymphangitis of other parts of limb**

Excludes2 acute lymphangitis of fingers (LØ3.2-)
acute lymphangitis of toes (LØ3.Ø4-)
acute lymphangitis of groin (LØ3.324)

LØ3.121 **Acute lymphangitis of right axilla**

LØ3.122 **Acute lymphangitis of left axilla**

LØ3.123 **Acute lymphangitis of right upper limb**

LØ3.124 **Acute lymphangitis of left upper limb**

LØ3.125 **Acute lymphangitis of right lower limb**

LØ3.126 **Acute lymphangitis of left lower limb**

LØ3.129 **Acute lymphangitis of unspecified part of limb**

● LØ3.2 **Cellulitis and acute lymphangitis of face and neck**

● LØ3.21 **Cellulitis and acute lymphangitis of face**

LØ3.211 **Cellulitis of face**

Excludes2 abscess of orbit (HØ5.Ø1-) ◀
cellulitis of ear (H6Ø.1-)
cellulitis of eyelid (HØØ.Ø-)
cellulitis of head (LØ3.81)
cellulitis of lacrimal apparatus (HØ4.3)
cellulitis of lip (K13.Ø)
cellulitis of mouth (K12.2)
cellulitis of nose (internal) (J34.Ø)
cellulitis of orbit (HØ5.Ø1-) (revised)
cellulitis of scalp (LØ3.81)

LØ3.212 **Acute lymphangitis of face**

LØ3.213 **Periorbital cellulitis** ◀
Preseptal cellulitis ◀

● LØ3.22 **Cellulitis and acute lymphangitis of neck**

LØ3.221 **Cellulitis of neck**

LØ3.222 **Acute lymphangitis of neck**

Item 12–2 Cellulitis is an acute spreading bacterial infection below the surface of the skin characterized by redness (erythema), warmth, swelling, pain, fever, chills, and enlarged lymph nodes ("swollen glands").

● LØ3.3 **Cellulitis and acute lymphangitis of trunk**

● LØ3.31 **Cellulitis of trunk**

Excludes2 cellulitis of anal and rectal regions (K61.-)
cellulitis of breast NOS (N61.Ø) (revised)
cellulitis of female external genital organs (N76.4)
cellulitis of male external genital organs (N48.2, N49.-)
omphalitis of newborn (P38.-)
puerperal cellulitis of breast (O91.2)

LØ3.311 **Cellulitis of abdominal wall**

Excludes2 cellulitis of umbilicus (LØ3.316)
cellulitis of groin (LØ3.314)

LØ3.312 **Cellulitis of back [any part except buttock]**

LØ3.313 **Cellulitis of chest wall**

LØ3.314 **Cellulitis of groin**

LØ3.315 **Cellulitis of perineum**

LØ3.316 **Cellulitis of umbilicus**

LØ3.317 **Cellulitis of buttock**

LØ3.319 **Cellulitis of trunk, unspecified**

● LØ3.32 **Acute lymphangitis of trunk**

LØ3.321 **Acute lymphangitis of abdominal wall**

LØ3.322 **Acute lymphangitis of back [any part except buttock]**

LØ3.323 **Acute lymphangitis of chest wall**

LØ3.324 **Acute lymphangitis of groin**

LØ3.325 **Acute lymphangitis of perineum**

LØ3.326 **Acute lymphangitis of umbilicus**

LØ3.327 **Acute lymphangitis of buttock**

LØ3.329 **Acute lymphangitis of trunk, unspecified**

● LØ3.8 **Cellulitis and acute lymphangitis of other sites**

● LØ3.81 **Cellulitis of other sites**

LØ3.811 **Cellulitis of head [any part, except face]**
Cellulitis of scalp

Excludes2 cellulitis of face (LØ3.211)

LØ3.818 **Cellulitis of other sites**

● LØ3.89 **Acute lymphangitis of other sites**

LØ3.891 **Acute lymphangitis of head [any part, except face]**

LØ3.898 **Acute lymphangitis of other sites**

● LØ3.9 **Cellulitis and acute lymphangitis, unspecified**

LØ3.90 **Cellulitis, unspecified**

LØ3.91 **Acute lymphangitis, unspecified**

Excludes1 lymphangitis NOS (I89.1)

Item 12–3 Abscess is a localized collection of pus in tissues or organs and is a sign of infection resulting in swelling and inflammation.

Item 12–4 Pilonidal cyst, also called a coccygeal cyst, is the result of a disorder called pilonidal disease. The cyst usually contains hair and pus.

● **LØ4 Acute lymphadenitis**
Short-term inflammation of lymph nodes which can be regionalized to involve a given area of the lymph system or systemic involving much of the body

Includes abscess (acute) of lymph nodes, except mesenteric
acute lymphadenitis, except mesenteric

Excludes1 chronic or subacute lymphadenitis, except mesenteric (I88.1)
enlarged lymph nodes (R59.-)
human immunodeficiency virus [HIV] disease resulting in generalized lymphadenopathy (B2Ø)
lymphadenitis NOS (I88.9)
nonspecific mesenteric lymphadenitis (I88.Ø)

LØ4.Ø Acute lymphadenitis of face, head and neck

LØ4.1 Acute lymphadenitis of trunk

LØ4.2 Acute lymphadenitis of upper limb
Acute lymphadenitis of axilla
Acute lymphadenitis of shoulder

LØ4.3 Acute lymphadenitis of lower limb
Acute lymphadenitis of hip
Excludes2 acute lymphadenitis of groin (LØ4.1)

LØ4.8 Acute lymphadenitis of other sites

LØ4.9 Acute lymphadenitis, unspecified

● **LØ5 Pilonidal cyst and sinus**

● **LØ5.Ø Pilonidal cyst and sinus with abscess**

LØ5.Ø1 Pilonidal cyst with abscess
Pilonidal abscess
Pilonidal dimple with abscess
Postanal dimple with abscess
Excludes2 congenital sacral dimple (Q82.6) ◀
parasacral dimple (Q82.6) ◀

LØ5.Ø2 Pilonidal sinus with abscess
Coccygeal fistula with abscess
Coccygeal sinus with abscess
Pilonidal fistula with abscess

● **LØ5.9 Pilonidal cyst and sinus without abscess**

LØ5.91 Pilonidal cyst without abscess
Pilonidal dimple
Postanal dimple
Pilonidal cyst NOS
Excludes2 congenital sacral dimple (Q82.6) ◀
parasacral dimple (Q82.6) ◀

LØ5.92 Pilonidal sinus without abscess
Coccygeal fistula
Coccygeal sinus without abscess
Pilonidal fistula

● **LØ8 Other local infections of skin and subcutaneous tissue**

LØ8.Ø Pyoderma
Dermatitis gangrenosa
Purulent dermatitis
Septic dermatitis
Suppurative dermatitis
Excludes1 pyoderma gangrenosum (L88)
pyoderma vegetans (LØ8.81)

LØ8.1 Erythrasma

● **LØ8.8 Other specified local infections of the skin and subcutaneous tissue**

LØ8.81 Pyoderma vegetans
Excludes1 pyoderma gangrenosum (L88)
pyoderma NOS (LØ8.Ø)

LØ8.82 Omphalitis not of newborn
Excludes1 omphalitis of newborn (P38.-)

LØ8.89 Other specified local infections of the skin and subcutaneous tissue

LØ8.9 Local infection of the skin and subcutaneous tissue, unspecified

BULLOUS DISORDERS (L1Ø-L14)

Excludes1 benign familial pemphigus [Hailey-Hailey] (Q82.8)
staphylococcal scalded skin syndrome (LØØ)
toxic epidermal necrolysis [Lyell] (L51.2)

● **L1Ø Pemphigus**
Excludes1 pemphigus neonatorum (LØ1.Ø3)

L1Ø.Ø Pemphigus vulgaris

L1Ø.1 Pemphigus vegetans

L1Ø.2 Pemphigus foliaceous

L1Ø.3 Brazilian pemphigus [fogo selvagem]

L1Ø.4 Pemphigus erythematosus
Senear-Usher syndrome

L1Ø.5 Drug-induced pemphigus
Use additional code for adverse effect, if applicable, to identify drug (T36-T5Ø with fifth or sixth character 5)

● **L1Ø.8 Other pemphigus**

L1Ø.81 Paraneoplastic pemphigus

L1Ø.89 Other pemphigus

L1Ø.9 Pemphigus, unspecified

● **L11 Other acantholytic disorders**

L11.Ø Acquired keratosis follicularis
Excludes1 keratosis follicularis (congenital) [Darier-White] (Q82.8)

L11.1 Transient acantholytic dermatosis [Grover]

L11.8 Other specified acantholytic disorders

L11.9 Acantholytic disorder, unspecified

● **L12 Pemphigoid**
Excludes1 herpes gestationis (O26.4-)
impetigo herpetiformis (L4Ø.1)

L12.Ø Bullous pemphigoid

L12.1 Cicatricial pemphigoid
Benign mucous membrane pemphigoid

L12.2 Chronic bullous disease of childhood
Juvenile dermatitis herpetiformis

● **L12.3 Acquired epidermolysis bullosa**
Excludes1 epidermolysis bullosa (congenital) (Q81.-)

L12.3Ø Acquired epidermolysis bullosa, unspecified

L12.31 Epidermolysis bullosa due to drug
Use additional code for adverse effect, if applicable, to identify drug (T36-T5Ø with fifth or sixth character 5)

L12.35 Other acquired epidermolysis bullosa

L12.8 Other pemphigoid

L12.9 Pemphigoid, unspecified

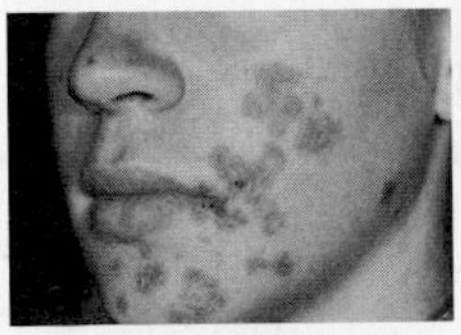

Figure 12-2 Impetigo. A thick, honey-yellow adherent crust covers the entire eroded surface. (From Habif: Clinical Dermatology, ed 4, Mosby, Inc., 2004)

● **L13 Other bullous disorders**

L13.0 Dermatitis herpetiformis
Duhring's disease
Hydroa herpetiformis
Excludes1 juvenile dermatitis herpetiformis (L12.2)
senile dermatitis herpetiformis (L12.0)

L13.1 Subcorneal pustular dermatitis
Sneddon-Wilkinson disease

L13.8 Other specified bullous disorders

L13.9 Bullous disorder, unspecified

L14 Bullous disorders in diseases classified elsewhere
Code first underlying disease

DERMATITIS AND ECZEMA (L20-L30)

Note: In this block the terms dermatitis and eczema are used synonymously and interchangeably.

Excludes2 chronic (childhood) granulomatous disease (D71)
dermatitis gangrenosa (L08.0)
dermatitis herpetiformis (L13.0)
dry skin dermatitis (L85.3)
factitial dermatitis (L98.1)
perioral dermatitis (L71.0)
radiation-related disorders of the skin and subcutaneous tissue (L55-L59)
stasis dermatitis (I87.2)

● **L20 Atopic dermatitis**

L20.0 Besnier's prurigo

● **L20.8 Other atopic dermatitis**
Excludes2 circumscribed neurodermatitis (L28.0)

L20.81 Atopic neurodermatitis
Diffuse neurodermatitis

L20.82 Flexural eczema

L20.83 Infantile (acute) (chronic) eczema

L20.84 Intrinsic (allergic) eczema

L20.89 Other atopic dermatitis

L20.9 Atopic dermatitis, unspecified

● **L21 Seborrheic dermatitis**
Excludes2 infective dermatitis (L30.3)
seborrheic keratosis (L82.-)

L21.0 Seborrhea capitis
Cradle cap

L21.1 Seborrheic infantile dermatitis

L21.8 Other seborrheic dermatitis

L21.9 Seborrheic dermatitis, unspecified
Seborrhea NOS

Item 12-5 Dermatitis herpetiformis, also known as Duhring's disease, is a systemic disease characterized by small blisters (3 to 5 mm) and occasionally large bullae (> 5 mm).

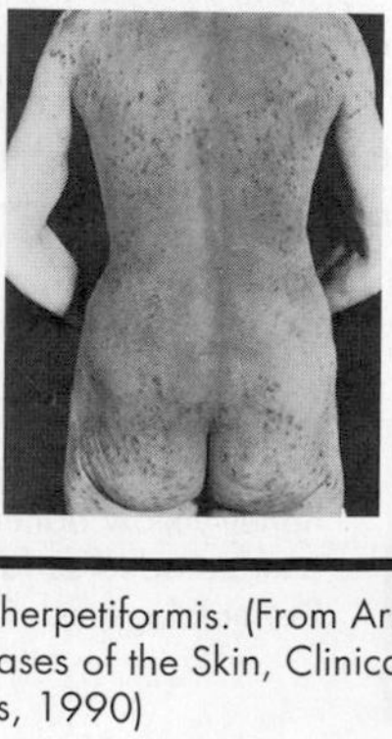

Figure 12-3 Dermatitis herpetiformis. (From Arnold HL, Odom RB, James WD: Andrews' Diseases of the Skin, Clinical Dermatology, ed 8, Philadelphia, WB Saunders, 1990)

Item 12-6 Seborrheic dermatitis is characterized by greasy, scaly, red patches and is associated with oily skin and scalp.

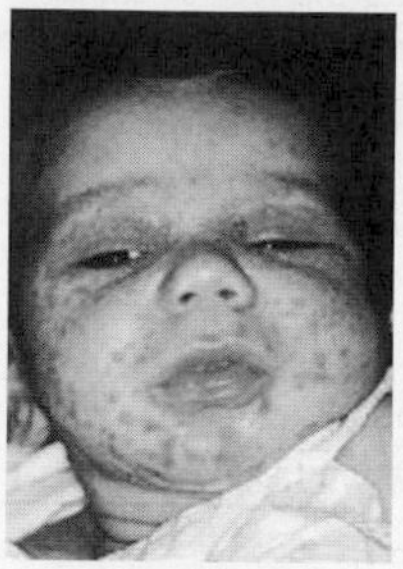

Figure 12-4 Seborrheic dermatitis. (From Cohen BA: Atlas of Pediatric Dermatology, St. Louis, Mosby, 1993)

Item 12-7 Atopic dermatitis, also known as atopic eczema, infantile eczema, disseminated neuro dermatitis, flexural eczema, and *prurigo diathesique* (Besnier), is characterized by intense itching and is often hereditary.

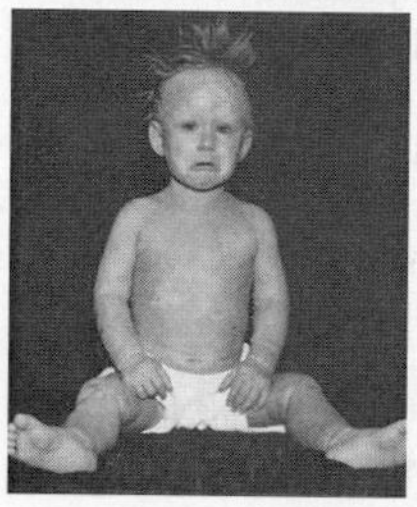

Figure 12-5 Atopic dermatitis. (From Moschella SL, Hurley HJ: Dermatology, ed 3, Philadelphia, WB Saunders, 1993)

L22 Diaper dermatitis
Diaper erythema
Diaper rash
Psoriasiform diaper rash

● **L23 Allergic contact dermatitis**
Excludes1 allergy NOS (T78.40)
contact dermatitis NOS (L25.9)
dermatitis NOS (L30.9)
Excludes2 dermatitis due to substances taken internally (L27.-)
dermatitis of eyelid (H01.1-)
diaper dermatitis (L22)
eczema of external ear (H60.5-)
irritant contact dermatitis (L24.-)
perioral dermatitis (L71.0)
radiation-related disorders of the skin and subcutaneous tissue (L55-L59)

L23.0 Allergic contact dermatitis due to metals
Allergic contact dermatitis due to chromium
Allergic contact dermatitis due to nickel

L23.1 Allergic contact dermatitis due to adhesives

L23.2 Allergic contact dermatitis due to cosmetics

L23.3 Allergic contact dermatitis due to drugs in contact with skin
Use additional code for adverse effect, if applicable, to identify drug (T36-T50 with fifth or sixth character 5)
Excludes2 dermatitis due to ingested drugs and medicaments (L27.0-L27.1)

L23.4 Allergic contact dermatitis due to dyes

L23.5 Allergic contact dermatitis due to other chemical products
Allergic contact dermatitis due to cement
Allergic contact dermatitis due to insecticide
Allergic contact dermatitis due to plastic
Allergic contact dermatitis due to rubber

L23.6 **Allergic contact dermatitis due to food in contact with the skin**
Excludes2 dermatitis due to ingested food (L27.2)
L23.7 **Allergic contact dermatitis due to plants, except food**
Excludes2 allergy NOS due to pollen (J30.1)
● L23.8 **Allergic contact dermatitis due to other agents**
L23.81 **Allergic contact dermatitis due to animal (cat) (dog) dander**
Allergic contact dermatitis due to animal (cat) (dog) hair
L23.89 **Allergic contact dermatitis due to other agents**
L23.9 **Allergic contact dermatitis, unspecified cause**
Allergic contact eczema NOS

● L24 **Irritant contact dermatitis**
Excludes1 allergy NOS (T78.40)
contact dermatitis NOS (L25.9)
dermatitis NOS (L30.9)
Excludes2 allergic contact dermatitis (L23.-)
dermatitis due to substances taken internally (L27.-)
dermatitis of eyelid (H01.1-)
diaper dermatitis (L22)
eczema of external ear (H60.5-)
perioral dermatitis (L71.0)
radiation-related disorders of the skin and subcutaneous tissue (L55-L59)
L24.0 **Irritant contact dermatitis due to detergents**
L24.1 **Irritant contact dermatitis due to oils and greases**
L24.2 **Irritant contact dermatitis due to solvents**
Irritant contact dermatitis due to chlorocompound
Irritant contact dermatitis due to cyclohexane
Irritant contact dermatitis due to ester
Irritant contact dermatitis due to glycol
Irritant contact dermatitis due to hydrocarbon
Irritant contact dermatitis due to ketone
L24.3 **Irritant contact dermatitis due to cosmetics**
L24.4 **Irritant contact dermatitis due to drugs in contact with skin**
Use additional code for adverse effect, if applicable, to identify drug (T36-T50 with fifth or sixth character 5)
L24.5 **Irritant contact dermatitis due to other chemical products**
Irritant contact dermatitis due to cement
Irritant contact dermatitis due to insecticide
Irritant contact dermatitis due to plastic
Irritant contact dermatitis due to rubber
L24.6 **Irritant contact dermatitis due to food in contact with skin**
Excludes2 dermatitis due to ingested food (L27.2)
L24.7 **Irritant contact dermatitis due to plants, except food**
Excludes2 allergy NOS to pollen (J30.1)
● L24.8 **Irritant contact dermatitis due to other agents**
L24.81 **Irritant contact dermatitis due to metals**
Irritant contact dermatitis due to chromium
Irritant contact dermatitis due to nickel
L24.89 **Irritant contact dermatitis due to other agents**
Irritant contact dermatitis due to dyes
L24.9 **Irritant contact dermatitis, unspecified cause**
Irritant contact eczema NOS

● L25 **Unspecified contact dermatitis**
Excludes1 allergic contact dermatitis (L23.-)
allergy NOS (T78.40)
dermatitis NOS (L30.9)
irritant contact dermatitis (L24.-)
Excludes2 dermatitis due to ingested substances (L27.-)
dermatitis of eyelid (H01.1-)
eczema of external ear (H60.5-)
perioral dermatitis (L71.0)
radiation-related disorders of the skin and subcutaneous tissue (L55-L59)
L25.0 **Unspecified contact dermatitis due to cosmetics**
L25.1 **Unspecified contact dermatitis due to drugs in contact with skin**
Use additional code for adverse effect, if applicable, to identify drug (T36-T50 with fifth or sixth character 5)
Excludes2 dermatitis due to ingested drugs and medicaments (L27.0-L27.1)
L25.2 **Unspecified contact dermatitis due to dyes**
L25.3 **Unspecified contact dermatitis due to other chemical products**
Unspecified contact dermatitis due to cement
Unspecified contact dermatitis due to insecticide
L25.4 **Unspecified contact dermatitis due to food in contact with skin**
Excludes2 dermatitis due to ingested food (L27.2)
L25.5 **Unspecified contact dermatitis due to plants, except food**
Excludes1 nettle rash (L50.9)
Excludes2 allergy NOS due to pollen (J30.1)
L25.8 **Unspecified contact dermatitis due to other agents**
L25.9 **Unspecified contact dermatitis, unspecified cause**
Contact dermatitis (occupational) NOS
Contact eczema (occupational) NOS

L26 **Exfoliative dermatitis**
Hebra's pityriasis
Excludes1 Ritter's disease (L00)

● L27 **Dermatitis due to substances taken internally**
Excludes1 allergy NOS (T78.40)
Excludes2 adverse food reaction, except dermatitis (T78.0-T78.1)
contact dermatitis (L23-L25)
drug photoallergic response (L56.1)
drug phototoxic response (L56.0)
urticaria (L50.-)
L27.0 **Generalized skin eruption due to drugs and medicaments taken internally**
Use additional code for adverse effect, if applicable, to identify drug (T36-T50 with fifth or sixth character 5)
L27.1 **Localized skin eruption due to drugs and medicaments taken internally**
Use additional code for adverse effect, if applicable, to identify drug (T36-T50 with fifth or sixth character 5)
L27.2 **Dermatitis due to ingested food**
Excludes2 dermatitis due to food in contact with skin (L23.6, L24.6, L25.4)
L27.8 **Dermatitis due to other substances taken internally**
L27.9 **Dermatitis due to unspecified substance taken internally**

CHAPTER 12 (L00-L99)

● L28 **Lichen simplex chronicus and prurigo**
- L28.0 **Lichen simplex chronicus**
  - Circumscribed neurodermatitis
  - Lichen NOS
- L28.1 **Prurigo nodularis**
- L28.2 **Other prurigo**
  - Prurigo NOS
  - Prurigo Hebra
  - Prurigo mitis
  - Urticaria papulosa

● L29 **Pruritus**

Excludes1 neurotic excoriation (L98.1)
psychogenic pruritus (F45.8)

- L29.0 **Pruritus ani**
- L29.1 **Pruritus scroti**
- L29.2 **Pruritus vulvae**
- L29.3 **Anogenital pruritus, unspecified**
- L29.8 **Other pruritus**
- L29.9 **Pruritus, unspecified**
  - Itch NOS

● L30 **Other and unspecified dermatitis**

Excludes2 contact dermatitis (L23-L25)
dry skin dermatitis (L85.3)
small plaque parapsoriasis (L41.3)
stasis dermatitis (I87.2) ◄

- L30.0 **Nummular dermatitis**
- L30.1 **Dyshidrosis [pompholyx]**
- L30.2 **Cutaneous autosensitization**
  - Candidid [levurid]
  - Dermatophytid
  - Eczematid
- L30.3 **Infective dermatitis**
  - Infectious eczematoid dermatitis
- L30.4 **Erythema intertrigo**
- L30.5 **Pityriasis alba**
- L30.8 **Other specified dermatitis**
- L30.9 **Dermatitis, unspecified**
  - Eczema NOS

PAPULOSQUAMOUS DISORDERS (L40-L45)

● L40 **Psoriasis**
- L40.0 **Psoriasis vulgaris**
  - Nummular psoriasis
  - Plaque psoriasis
- L40.1 **Generalized pustular psoriasis**
  - Impetigo herpetiformis
  - Von Zumbusch's disease
- L40.2 **Acrodermatitis continua**
- L40.3 **Pustulosis palmaris et plantaris**
- L40.4 **Guttate psoriasis**
- ● L40.5 **Arthropathic psoriasis**
  - L40.50 **Arthropathic psoriasis, unspecified**
  - L40.51 **Distal interphalangeal psoriatic arthropathy**
  - L40.52 **Psoriatic arthritis mutilans**
  - L40.53 **Psoriatic spondylitis**
  - L40.54 **Psoriatic juvenile arthropathy**
  - L40.59 **Other psoriatic arthropathy**
- L40.8 **Other psoriasis**
  - Flexural psoriasis
- L40.9 **Psoriasis, unspecified**

● L41 **Parapsoriasis**

Excludes1 poikiloderma vasculare atrophicans (L94.5)

- L41.0 **Pityriasis lichenoides et varioliformis acuta**
  - Mucha-Habermann disease
- L41.1 **Pityriasis lichenoides chronica**
- L41.3 **Small plaque parapsoriasis**
- L41.4 **Large plaque parapsoriasis**
- L41.5 **Retiform parapsoriasis**
- L41.8 **Other parapsoriasis**
- L41.9 **Parapsoriasis, unspecified**

L42 **Pityriasis rosea**

● L43 **Lichen planus**

Excludes1 lichen planopilaris (L66.1)

- L43.0 **Hypertrophic lichen planus**
- L43.1 **Bullous lichen planus**
- L43.2 **Lichenoid drug reaction**
  - Use additional code for adverse effect, if applicable, to identify drug (T36-T50 with fifth or sixth character 5)
- L43.3 **Subacute (active) lichen planus**
  - Lichen planus tropicus
- L43.8 **Other lichen planus**
- L43.9 **Lichen planus, unspecified**

● L44 **Other papulosquamous disorders**
- L44.0 **Pityriasis rubra pilaris**
- L44.1 **Lichen nitidus**
- L44.2 **Lichen striatus**
- L44.3 **Lichen ruber moniliformis**
- L44.4 **Infantile papular acrodermatitis [Gianotti-Crosti]**
- L44.8 **Other specified papulosquamous disorders**
- L44.9 **Papulosquamous disorder, unspecified**

L45 **Papulosquamous disorders in diseases classified elsewhere**

Code first underlying disease

URTICARIA AND ERYTHEMA (L49-L54)

Excludes1 Lyme disease (A69.2-)
rosacea (L71.-)

● L49 **Exfoliation due to erythematous conditions according to extent of body surface involved**

Code first erythematous condition causing exfoliation, such as:
Ritter's disease (L00)
(Staphylococcal) scalded skin syndrome (L00)
Stevens-Johnson syndrome (L51.1)
Stevens-Johnson syndrome-toxic epidermal necrolysis overlap syndrome (L51.3)
Toxic epidermal necrolysis (L51.2)

- L49.0 **Exfoliation due to erythematous condition involving less than 10 percent of body surface**
  - Exfoliation due to erythematous condition NOS
- L49.1 **Exfoliation due to erythematous condition involving 10-19 percent of body surface**
- L49.2 **Exfoliation due to erythematous condition involving 20-29 percent of body surface**
- L49.3 **Exfoliation due to erythematous condition involving 30-39 percent of body surface**
- L49.4 **Exfoliation due to erythematous condition involving 40-49 percent of body surface**
- L49.5 **Exfoliation due to erythematous condition involving 50-59 percent of body surface**

Item 12–8 Psoriasis is a chronic, recurrent inflammatory skin disease characterized by small patches covered with thick silvery scales. **Parapsoriasis** is a treatment-resistant erythroderma. **Pityriasis rosea** is characterized by a herald patch that is a single large lesion and that usually appears on the trunk and is followed by scattered, smaller lesions.

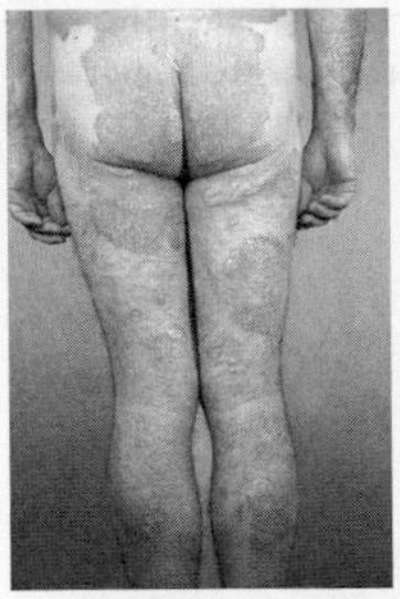

Figure 12-6 Erythematous plaques with silvery scales in a patient with psoriasis. (From Goldman: Cecil Textbook of Medicine, ed 22, Saunders, 2004)

L49.6 Exfoliation due to erythematous condition involving 60-69 percent of body surface

L49.7 Exfoliation due to erythematous condition involving 70-79 percent of body surface

L49.8 Exfoliation due to erythematous condition involving 80-89 percent of body surface

L49.9 Exfoliation due to erythematous condition involving 90 or more percent of body surface

● **L50 Urticaria**

Excludes1 allergic contact dermatitis (L23.-)
angioneurotic edema (T78.3)
giant urticaria (T78.3)
hereditary angio-edema (D84.1)
Quincke's edema (T78.3)
serum urticaria (T80.6-)
solar urticaria (L56.3)
urticaria neonatorum (P83.8)
urticaria papulosa (L28.2)
urticaria pigmentosa (Q82.2)

L50.0 Allergic urticaria

L50.1 Idiopathic urticaria

L50.2 Urticaria due to cold and heat

Excludes2 familial cold urticaria (M04.2) ◀

L50.3 Dermatographic urticaria

L50.4 Vibratory urticaria

L50.5 Cholinergic urticaria

L50.6 Contact urticaria

L50.8 Other urticaria

Chronic urticaria
Recurrent periodic urticaria

L50.9 Urticaria, unspecified

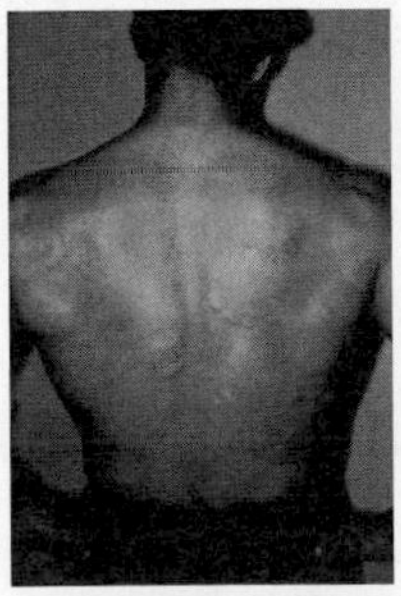

Figure 12-7 Urticaria (hives). *(Courtesy of David Effron, MD.)* (From Marx: Rosen's Emergency Medicine: Concepts and Clinical Practice, ed 6, Mosby, Inc., 2006)

Item 12-9 Urticaria is a vascular reaction in which wheals surrounded by a red halo appear and cause severe itching. The causes of urticaria or hives are extensive and varied (e.g., food, heat, cold, drugs, stress, infections).

● **L51 Erythema multiforme**

Use additional code for adverse effect, if applicable, to identify drug (T36-T50 with fifth or sixth character 5)

Use additional code to identify associated manifestations, such as:
arthropathy associated with dermatological disorders (M14.8-)
conjunctival edema (H11.42)
conjunctivitis (H10.22-)
corneal scars and opacities (H17.-)
corneal ulcer (H16.0-)
edema of eyelid (H02.84)
inflammation of eyelid (H01.8)
keratoconjunctivitis sicca (H16.22-)
mechanical lagophthalmos (H02.22-)
stomatitis (K12.-)
symblepharon (H11.23-)

Use additional code to identify percentage of skin exfoliation (L49.-)

Excludes1 staphylococcal scalded skin syndrome (L00)
Ritter's disease (L00)

L51.0 Nonbullous erythema multiforme

L51.1 Stevens-Johnson syndrome

L51.2 Toxic epidermal necrolysis [Lyell]

L51.3 Stevens-Johnson syndrome-toxic epidermal necrolysis overlap syndrome

SJS-TEN overlap syndrome

L51.8 Other erythema multiforme

L51.9 Erythema multiforme, unspecified

Erythema iris
Erythema multiforme major NOS
Erythema multiforme minor NOS
Herpes iris

L52 Erythema nodosum

Excludes1 tuberculous erythema nodosum (A18.4)

● **L53 Other erythematous conditions**

Excludes1 erythema ab igne (L59.0)
erythema due to external agents in contact with skin (L23-L25)
erythema intertrigo (L30.4)

L53.0 Toxic erythema

Code first poisoning due to drug or toxin, if applicable (T36-T65 with fifth or sixth character 1-4 or 6)

Use additional code for adverse effect, if applicable, to identify drug (T36-T50 with fifth or sixth character 5)

Excludes1 neonatal erythema toxicum (P83.1)

L53.1 Erythema annulare centrifugum

L53.2 Erythema marginatum

L53.3 Other chronic figurate erythema

L53.8 Other specified erythematous conditions

L53.9 Erythematous condition, unspecified

Erythema NOS
Erythroderma NOS

L54 Erythema in diseases classified elsewhere

Code first underlying disease

RADIATION-RELATED DISORDERS OF THE SKIN AND SUBCUTANEOUS TISSUE (L55-L59)

● **L55 Sunburn**

L55.0 Sunburn of first degree

L55.1 Sunburn of second degree

L55.2 Sunburn of third degree

L55.9 Sunburn, unspecified

CHAPTER 12 (L00-L99)

◀ New ⬅ Revised ~~deleted~~ Deleted **OGCR** Official Guidelines X Assign placeholder X ● Use Additional Character(s)
Excludes 1 | Excludes 2 | Includes | Use additional | Code first | Code also | Unspecified

● **L56 Other acute skin changes due to ultraviolet radiation**
Use additional code to identify the source of the ultraviolet radiation (W89, X32)
L56.0 Drug phototoxic response
Use additional code for adverse effect, if applicable, to identify drug (T36-T50 with fifth or sixth character 5)
L56.1 Drug photoallergic response
Use additional code for adverse effect, if applicable, to identify drug (T36-T50 with fifth or sixth character 5)
L56.2 Photocontact dermatitis [berloque dermatitis]
L56.3 Solar urticaria
L56.4 Polymorphous light eruption
L56.5 Disseminated superficial actinic porokeratosis (DSAP)
L56.8 Other specified acute skin changes due to ultraviolet radiation
L56.9 Acute skin change due to ultraviolet radiation, unspecified

● **L57 Skin changes due to chronic exposure to nonionizing radiation**
Use additional code to identify the source of the ultraviolet radiation (W89, X32)
L57.0 Actinic keratosis
Keratosis NOS
Solar keratosis
Senile keratosis
L57.1 Actinic reticuloid
L57.2 Cutis rhomboidalis nuchae
L57.3 Poikiloderma of Civatte
L57.4 Cutis laxa senilis
Elastosis senilis
L57.5 Actinic granuloma
L57.8 Other skin changes due to chronic exposure to nonionizing radiation
Farmer's skin
Solar dermatitis
Sailor's skin
L57.9 Skin changes due to chronic exposure to nonionizing radiation, unspecified

● **L58 Radiodermatitis**
Use additional code to identify the source of the radiation (W88, W90)
L58.0 Acute radiodermatitis
L58.1 Chronic radiodermatitis
L58.9 Radiodermatitis, unspecified

● **L59 Other disorders of skin and subcutaneous tissue related to radiation**
L59.0 Erythema ab igne [dermatitis ab igne]
L59.8 Other specified disorders of the skin and subcutaneous tissue related to radiation
L59.9 Disorder of the skin and subcutaneous tissue related to radiation, unspecified

DISORDERS OF SKIN APPENDAGES (L60-L75)

Excludes1 congenital malformations of integument (Q84.-)

● **L60 Nail disorders**
Excludes2 clubbing of nails (R68.3)
onychia and paronychia (L03.0-)
L60.0 Ingrowing nail
L60.1 Onycholysis
L60.2 Onychogryphosis
L60.3 Nail dystrophy
L60.4 Beau's lines
L60.5 Yellow nail syndrome
L60.8 Other nail disorders
L60.9 Nail disorder, unspecified

L62 Nail disorders in diseases classified elsewhere
Code first underlying disease, such as:
pachydermoperiostosis (M89.4-)

Item 12-10 Alopecia is lack of hair and takes many forms. The most common is male pattern alopecia, also known as **androgenetic alopecia. Telogen effluvium** is early and excessive loss of hair resulting from a trauma to the hair follicle (fever, drugs, surgery, etc.).

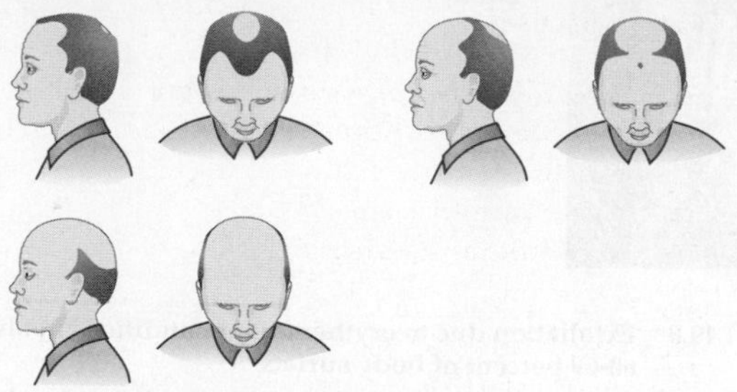

Figure 12-8 Male pattern alopecia.

● **L63 Alopecia areata**
L63.0 Alopecia (capitis) totalis
L63.1 Alopecia universalis
L63.2 Ophiasis
L63.8 Other alopecia areata
L63.9 Alopecia areata, unspecified

● **L64 Androgenic alopecia**
Includes male-pattern baldness
L64.0 Drug-induced androgenic alopecia
Use additional code for adverse effect, if applicable, to identify drug (T36-T50 with fifth or sixth character 5)
L64.8 Other androgenic alopecia
L64.9 Androgenic alopecia, unspecified

● **L65 Other nonscarring hair loss**
Use additional code for adverse effect, if applicable, to identify drug (T36-T50 with fifth or sixth character 5)
Excludes1 trichotillomania (F63.3)
L65.0 Telogen effluvium
L65.1 Anagen effluvium
L65.2 Alopecia mucinosa
L65.8 Other specified nonscarring hair loss
L65.9 Nonscarring hair loss, unspecified
Alopecia NOS

● **L66 Cicatricial alopecia [scarring hair loss]**
L66.0 Pseudopelade
L66.1 Lichen planopilaris
Follicular lichen planus
L66.2 Folliculitis decalvans
L66.3 Perifolliculitis capitis abscedens
L66.4 Folliculitis ulerythematosa reticulata
L66.8 Other cicatricial alopecia
L66.9 Cicatricial alopecia, unspecified

● **L67 Hair color and hair shaft abnormalities**
Excludes1 monilethrix (Q84.1)
pili annulati (Q84.1)
telogen effluvium (L65.0)
L67.0 Trichorrhexis nodosa
L67.1 Variations in hair color
Canities
Greyness, hair (premature)
Heterochromia of hair
Poliosis circumscripta, acquired
Poliosis NOS
L67.8 Other hair color and hair shaft abnormalities
Fragilitas crinium
L67.9 Hair color and hair shaft abnormality, unspecified

● **L68 Hypertrichosis**
  Includes excess hair
  Excludes1 congenital hypertrichosis (Q84.2)
  persistent lanugo (Q84.2)
  L68.0 Hirsutism
  Excessive growth of hair
  L68.1 Acquired hypertrichosis lanuginosa
  L68.2 Localized hypertrichosis
  L68.3 Polytrichia
  L68.8 Other hypertrichosis
  L68.9 Hypertrichosis, unspecified

● **L70 Acne**
  Excludes2 acne keloid (L73.0)
  L70.0 Acne vulgaris
  L70.1 Acne conglobata
  L70.2 Acne varioliformis
  Acne necrotica miliaris
  L70.3 Acne tropica
  L70.4 Infantile acne
  L70.5 Acné excoriée ⬅
  Acné excoriée des jeunes filles ◀
  Picker's acne
  L70.8 Other acne
  L70.9 Acne, unspecified

● **L71 Rosacea**
  Use additional code for adverse effect, if applicable, to identify drug (T36-T50 with fifth or sixth character 5)
  L71.0 Perioral dermatitis
  L71.1 Rhinophyma
  L71.8 Other rosacea
  L71.9 Rosacea, unspecified

● **L72 Follicular cysts of skin and subcutaneous tissue**
  L72.0 Epidermal cyst
  ● **L72.1 Pilar and trichodermal cyst**
    L72.11 Pilar cyst
    L72.12 Trichodermal cyst
    Trichilemmal (proliferating) cyst
  L72.3 Sebaceous cyst
  Excludes2 pilar cyst (L72.11)
  trichilemmal (proliferating) cyst (L72.12)
  L72.2 Steatocystoma multiplex
  L72.8 Other follicular cysts of the skin and subcutaneous tissue
  L72.9 Follicular cyst of the skin and subcutaneous tissue, unspecified

● **L73 Other follicular disorders**
  L73.0 Acne keloid
  L73.1 Pseudofolliculitis barbae
  L73.2 Hidradenitis suppurativa
  L73.8 Other specified follicular disorders
  Sycosis barbae
  L73.9 Follicular disorder, unspecified

● **L74 Eccrine sweat disorders**
  Excludes2 generalized hyperhidrosis (R61)
  L74.0 Miliaria rubra
  L74.1 Miliaria crystallina
  L74.2 Miliaria profunda
  Miliaria tropicalis
  L74.3 Miliaria, unspecified
  L74.4 Anhidrosis
  Hypohidrosis
  ● **L74.5 Focal hyperhidrosis**
    ● **L74.51 Primary focal hyperhidrosis**
      L74.510 Primary focal hyperhidrosis, axilla
      L74.511 Primary focal hyperhidrosis, face
      L74.512 Primary focal hyperhidrosis, palms
      L74.513 Primary focal hyperhidrosis, soles
      L74.519 Primary focal hyperhidrosis, unspecified
    L74.52 Secondary focal hyperhidrosis
    Frey's syndrome
  L74.8 Other eccrine sweat disorders
  L74.9 Eccrine sweat disorder, unspecified
  Sweat gland disorder NOS

● **L75 Apocrine sweat disorders**
  Excludes1 dyshidrosis (L30.1)
  hidradenitis suppurativa (L73.2)
  L75.0 Bromhidrosis
  L75.1 Chromhidrosis
  L75.2 Apocrine miliaria
  Fox-Fordyce disease
  L75.8 Other apocrine sweat disorders
  L75.9 Apocrine sweat disorder, unspecified
  Intraoperative and postprocedural complications of skin and subcutaneous tissue (L76)

INTRAOPERATIVE AND POSTPROCEDURAL COMPLICATIONS OF SKIN AND SUBCUTANEOUS TISSUE (L76)

● **L76 Intraoperative and postprocedural complications of skin and subcutaneous tissue**
  ● **L76.0 Intraoperative hemorrhage and hematoma of skin and subcutaneous tissue complicating a procedure**
  Excludes1 intraoperative hemorrhage and hematoma of skin and subcutaneous tissue due to accidental puncture and laceration during a procedure (L76.1-)
    L76.01 Intraoperative hemorrhage and hematoma of skin and subcutaneous tissue complicating a dermatologic procedure
    L76.02 Intraoperative hemorrhage and hematoma of skin and subcutaneous tissue complicating other procedure
  ● **L76.1 Accidental puncture and laceration of skin and subcutaneous tissue during a procedure**
    L76.11 Accidental puncture and laceration of skin and subcutaneous tissue during a dermatologic procedure
    L76.12 Accidental puncture and laceration of skin and subcutaneous tissue during other procedure
  ● **L76.2 Postprocedural hemorrhage of skin and subcutaneous tissue following a procedure** ⬅
    L76.21 Postprocedural hemorrhage of skin and subcutaneous tissue following a dermatologic procedure ⬅
    L76.22 Postprocedural hemorrhage of skin and subcutaneous tissue following other procedure ⬅
  ● **L76.3 Postprocedural hematoma and seroma of skin and subcutaneous tissue following a procedure** ◀
    L76.31 Postprocedural hematoma of skin and subcutaneous tissue following a dermatologic procedure ◀
    L76.32 Postprocedural hematoma of skin and subcutaneous tissue following other procedure ◀
    L76.33 Postprocedural seroma of skin and subcutaneous tissue following a dermatologic procedure ◀
    L76.34 Postprocedural seroma of skin and subcutaneous tissue following other procedure ◀

CHAPTER 12 (L00-L99)

● **L76.8 Other intraoperative and postprocedural complications of skin and subcutaneous tissue**

Use additional code, if applicable, to further specify disorder

L76.81 Other intraoperative complications of skin and subcutaneous tissue

L76.82 Other postprocedural complications of skin and subcutaneous tissue

OTHER DISORDERS OF THE SKIN AND SUBCUTANEOUS TISSUE (L8Ø-L99)

L8Ø Vitiligo

Excludes2 vitiligo of eyelids (HØ2.73-)
vitiligo of vulva (N9Ø.89)

● **L81 Other disorders of pigmentation**

Excludes1 birthmark NOS (Q82.5)
Peutz-Jeghers syndrome (Q85.8)

Excludes2 nevus - see Alphabetical Index

L81.Ø Postinflammatory hyperpigmentation

L81.1 Chloasma

L81.2 Freckles

L81.3 Café au lait spots

L81.4 Other melanin hyperpigmentation
Lentigo

L81.5 Leukoderma, not elsewhere classified

L81.6 Other disorders of diminished melanin formation

L81.7 Pigmented purpuric dermatosis
Angioma serpiginosum

L81.8 Other specified disorders of pigmentation
Iron pigmentation
Tattoo pigmentation

L81.9 Disorder of pigmentation, unspecified

● **L82 Seborrheic keratosis**

Includes basal cell papilloma ◀
dermatosis papulosa nigra
Leser-Trélat disease

Excludes2 seborrheic dermatitis (L21.-)

L82.Ø Inflamed seborrheic keratosis

L82.1 Other seborrheic keratosis
Seborrheic keratosis NOS

L83 Acanthosis nigricans
Confluent and reticulated papillomatosis

L84 Corns and callosities
Callus
Clavus

● **L85 Other epidermal thickening**

Excludes2 hypertrophic disorders of the skin (L91.-)

L85.Ø Acquired ichthyosis

Excludes1 congenital ichthyosis (Q8Ø.-)

L85.1 Acquired keratosis [keratoderma] palmaris et plantaris

Excludes1 inherited keratosis palmaris et plantaris (Q82.8)

L85.2 Keratosis punctata (palmaris et plantaris)

L85.3 Xerosis cutis
Dry skin dermatitis

L85.8 Other specified epidermal thickening
Cutaneous horn

L85.9 Epidermal thickening, unspecified

L86 Keratoderma in diseases classified elsewhere

Firm horny papules that have a cobblestone appearance.

Code first underlying disease, such as:
Reiter's disease (MØ2.3-)

Excludes1 gonococcal keratoderma (A54.89)
gonococcal keratosis (A54.89)
keratoderma due to vitamin A deficiency (E5Ø.8)
keratosis due to vitamin A deficiency (E5Ø.8)
xeroderma due to vitamin A deficiency (E5Ø.8)

● **L87 Transepidermal elimination disorders**

Excludes1 granuloma annulare (perforating) (L92.Ø)

L87.Ø Keratosis follicularis et parafollicularis in cutem penetrans
Kyrle disease
Hyperkeratosis follicularis penetrans

L87.1 Reactive perforating collagenosis

L87.2 Elastosis perforans serpiginosa

L87.8 Other transepidermal elimination disorders

L87.9 Transepidermal elimination disorder, unspecified

L88 Pyoderma gangrenosum
Phagedenic pyoderma

Excludes1 dermatitis gangrenosa (LØ8.Ø)

OGCR Section I.B.14.

General Coding Guidelines

Documentation for BMI, ***Depth of*** Non-pressure ulcers, Pressure Ulcer Stages, **Coma Scale, and *NIH Stroke Scale***

For the Body Mass Index (BMI), depth of non-pressure chronic ulcers, pressure ulcer stage, **coma scale, and NIH stroke scale (NIHSS) codes,** code assignment may be based on medical record documentation from clinicians who are not the patient's provider (i.e., physician or other qualified healthcare practitioner legally accountable for establishing the patient's diagnosis), since this information is typically documented by other clinicians involved in the care of the patient (e.g., a dietitian often documents the BMI, a nurse often documents the pressure ulcer stages, **and an emergency medical technician often documents the coma scale**). However, the associated diagnosis (such as overweight, obesity, **acute stroke,** or pressure ulcer) must be documented by the patient's provider. If there is conflicting medical record documentation, either from the same clinician or different clinicians, the patient's attending provider should be queried for clarification.

The BMI, **coma scale, and NHSS** codes should only be reported as secondary diagnoses.

● **L89 Pressure ulcer**

Includes bed sore
decubitus ulcer
plaster ulcer
pressure area
pressure sore

Code first any associated gangrene (I96)

Excludes2 decubitus (trophic) ulcer of cervix (uteri) (N86)
diabetic ulcers (EØ8.621, EØ8.622, EØ9.621, EØ9.622, E1Ø.621, E1Ø.622, E11.621, E11.622, E13.621, E13.622)
non-pressure chronic ulcer of skin (L97.-)
skin infections (LØØ-LØ8)
varicose ulcer (I83.Ø, I83.2)

● **L89.Ø Pressure ulcer of elbow**

● **L89.ØØ Pressure ulcer of unspecified elbow**

L89.ØØØ Pressure ulcer of unspecified elbow, unstageable

L89.ØØ1 Pressure ulcer of unspecified elbow, stage 1
Healing pressure ulcer of unspecified elbow, stage 1
Pressure pre-ulcer skin changes limited to persistent focal edema, unspecified elbow

L89.ØØ2 Pressure ulcer of unspecified elbow, stage 2
Healing pressure ulcer of unspecified elbow, stage 2
Pressure ulcer with abrasion, blister, partial thickness skin loss involving epidermis and/or dermis, unspecified elbow

L89.ØØ3 Pressure ulcer of unspecified elbow, stage 3
Healing pressure ulcer of unspecified elbow, stage 3
Pressure ulcer with full thickness skin loss involving damage or necrosis of subcutaneous tissue, unspecified elbow

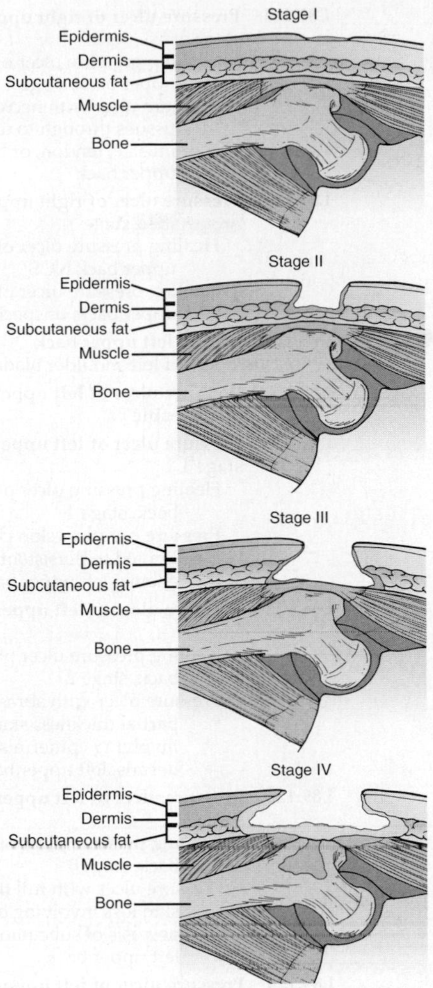

Figure 12-9 Stage I, II, III, and IV of pressure ulcers.

L89.004 Pressure ulcer of unspecified elbow, stage 4
Healing pressure ulcer of unspecified elbow, stage 4
Pressure ulcer with necrosis of soft tissues through to underlying muscle, tendon, or bone, unspecified elbow

L89.009 Pressure ulcer of unspecified elbow, unspecified stage
Healing pressure ulcer of elbow NOS
Healing pressure ulcer of unspecified elbow, unspecified stage

● **L89.01 Pressure ulcer of right elbow**

L89.010 Pressure ulcer of right elbow, unstageable

L89.011 Pressure ulcer of right elbow, stage 1
Healing pressure ulcer of right elbow, stage 1
Pressure pre-ulcer skin changes limited to persistent focal edema, right elbow

L89.012 Pressure ulcer of right elbow, stage 2
Healing pressure ulcer of right elbow, stage 2
Pressure ulcer with abrasion, blister, partial thickness skin loss involving epidermis and/or dermis, right elbow

L89.013 Pressure ulcer of right elbow, stage 3
Healing pressure ulcer of right elbow, stage 3
Pressure ulcer with full thickness skin loss involving damage or necrosis of subcutaneous tissue, right elbow

L89.014 Pressure ulcer of right elbow, stage 4
Healing pressure ulcer of right elbow, stage 4
Pressure ulcer with necrosis of soft tissues through to underlying muscle, tendon, or bone, right elbow

L89.019 Pressure ulcer of right elbow, unspecified stage
Healing pressure right of elbow NOS
Healing pressure ulcer of unspecified elbow, unspecified stage

● **L89.02 Pressure ulcer of left elbow**

L89.020 Pressure ulcer of left elbow, unstageable

L89.021 Pressure ulcer of left elbow, stage 1
Healing pressure ulcer of left elbow, stage 1
Pressure pre-ulcer skin changes limited to persistent focal edema, left elbow

L89.022 Pressure ulcer of left elbow, stage 2
Healing pressure ulcer of left elbow, stage 2
Pressure ulcer with abrasion, blister, partial thickness skin loss involving epidermis and/or dermis, left elbow

L89.023 Pressure ulcer of left elbow, stage 3
Healing pressure ulcer of left elbow, stage 3
Pressure ulcer with full thickness skin loss involving damage or necrosis of subcutaneous tissue, left elbow

L89.024 Pressure ulcer of left elbow, stage 4
Healing pressure ulcer of left elbow, stage 4
Pressure ulcer with necrosis of soft tissues through to underlying muscle, tendon, or bone, left elbow

L89.029 Pressure ulcer of left elbow, unspecified stage
Healing pressure ulcer of left of elbow NOS
Healing pressure ulcer of unspecified elbow, unspecified stage

CHAPTER 12 (L00-L99)

● L89.1 Pressure ulcer of back

● L89.10 Pressure ulcer of unspecified part of back

L89.100 Pressure ulcer of unspecified part of back, unstageable

L89.101 Pressure ulcer of unspecified part of back, stage 1
Healing pressure ulcer of unspecified part of back, stage 1
Pressure pre-ulcer skin changes limited to persistent focal edema, unspecified part of back

L89.102 Pressure ulcer of unspecified part of back, stage 2
Healing pressure ulcer of unspecified part of back, stage 2
Pressure ulcer with abrasion, blister, partial thickness skin loss involving epidermis and/or dermis, unspecified part of back

L89.103 Pressure ulcer of unspecified part of back, stage 3
Healing pressure ulcer of unspecified part of back, stage 3
Pressure ulcer with full thickness skin loss involving damage or necrosis of subcutaneous tissue, unspecified part of back

L89.104 Pressure ulcer of unspecified part of back, stage 4
Healing pressure ulcer of unspecified part of back, stage 4
Pressure ulcer with necrosis of soft tissues through to underlying muscle, tendon, or bone, unspecified part of back

L89.109 Pressure ulcer of unspecified part of back, unspecified stage
Healing pressure ulcer of unspecified part of back NOS
Healing pressure ulcer of unspecified part of back, unspecified stage

● L89.11 Pressure ulcer of right upper back
Pressure ulcer of right shoulder blade

L89.110 Pressure ulcer of right upper back, unstageable

L89.111 Pressure ulcer of right upper back, stage 1
Healing pressure ulcer of right upper back, stage 1
Pressure pre-ulcer skin changes limited to persistent focal edema, right upper back

L89.112 Pressure ulcer of right upper back, stage 2
Healing pressure ulcer of right upper back, stage 2
Pressure ulcer with abrasion, blister, partial thickness skin loss involving epidermis and/or dermis, right upper back

L89.113 Pressure ulcer of right upper back, stage 3
Healing pressure ulcer of right upper back, stage 3
Pressure ulcer with full thickness skin loss involving damage or necrosis of subcutaneous tissue, right upper back

L89.114 Pressure ulcer of right upper back, stage 4
Healing pressure ulcer of right upper back, stage 4
Pressure ulcer with necrosis of soft tissues through to underlying muscle, tendon, or bone, right upper back

L89.119 Pressure ulcer of right upper back, unspecified stage
Healing pressure ulcer of right upper back NOS
Healing pressure ulcer of right upper back, unspecified stage

● L89.12 Pressure ulcer of left upper back
Pressure ulcer of left shoulder blade

L89.120 Pressure ulcer of left upper back, unstageable

L89.121 Pressure ulcer of left upper back, stage 1
Healing pressure ulcer of left upper back, stage 1
Pressure pre-ulcer skin changes limited to persistent focal edema, left upper back

L89.122 Pressure ulcer of left upper back, stage 2
Healing pressure ulcer of left upper back, stage 2
Pressure ulcer with abrasion, blister, partial thickness skin loss involving epidermis and/or dermis, left upper back

L89.123 Pressure ulcer of left upper back, stage 3
Healing pressure ulcer of left upper back, stage 3
Pressure ulcer with full thickness skin loss involving damage or necrosis of subcutaneous tissue, left upper back

L89.124 Pressure ulcer of left upper back, stage 4
Healing pressure ulcer of left upper back, stage 4
Pressure ulcer with necrosis of soft tissues through to underlying muscle, tendon, or bone, left upper back

L89.129 Pressure ulcer of left upper back, unspecified stage
Healing pressure ulcer of left upper back NOS
Healing pressure ulcer of left upper back, unspecified stage

● L89.13 Pressure ulcer of right lower back

L89.130 Pressure ulcer of right lower back, unstageable

L89.131 Pressure ulcer of right lower back, stage 1
Healing pressure ulcer of right lower back, stage 1
Pressure pre-ulcer skin changes limited to persistent focal edema, right lower back

L89.132 Pressure ulcer of right lower back, stage 2
Healing pressure ulcer of right lower back, stage 2
Pressure ulcer with abrasion, blister, partial thickness skin loss involving epidermis and/or dermis, right lower back

L89.133 Pressure ulcer of right lower back, stage 3
Healing pressure ulcer of right lower back, stage 3
Pressure ulcer with full thickness skin loss involving damage or necrosis of subcutaneous tissue, right lower back

L89.134 Pressure ulcer of right lower back, stage 4
Healing pressure ulcer of right lower back, stage 4
Pressure ulcer with necrosis of soft tissues through to underlying muscle, tendon, or bone, right lower back

L89.139 Pressure ulcer of right lower back, unspecified stage
Healing pressure ulcer of right lower back NOS
Healing pressure ulcer of right lower back, unspecified stage

● L89.14 Pressure ulcer of left lower back

L89.14Ø Pressure ulcer of left lower back, unstageable

L89.141 Pressure ulcer of left lower back, stage 1
Healing pressure ulcer of left lower back, stage 1
Pressure pre-ulcer skin changes limited to persistent focal edema, left lower back

L89.142 Pressure ulcer of left lower back, stage 2
Healing pressure ulcer of left lower back, stage 2
Pressure ulcer with abrasion, blister, partial thickness skin loss involving epidermis and/or dermis, left lower back

L89.143 Pressure ulcer of left lower back, stage 3
Healing pressure ulcer of left lower back, stage 3
Pressure ulcer with full thickness skin loss involving damage or necrosis of subcutaneous tissue, left lower back

L89.144 Pressure ulcer of left lower back, stage 4
Healing pressure ulcer of left lower back, stage 4
Pressure ulcer with necrosis of soft tissues through to underlying muscle, tendon, or bone, left lower back

L89.149 Pressure ulcer of left lower back, unspecified stage
Healing pressure ulcer of left lower back NOS
Healing pressure ulcer of left lower back, unspecified stage

● L89.15 Pressure ulcer of sacral region
Pressure ulcer of coccyx
Pressure ulcer of tailbone

L89.15Ø Pressure ulcer of sacral region, unstageable

L89.151 Pressure ulcer of sacral region, stage 1
Healing pressure ulcer of sacral region, stage 1
Pressure pre-ulcer skin changes limited to persistent focal edema, sacral region

L89.152 Pressure ulcer of sacral region, stage 2
Healing pressure ulcer of sacral region, stage 2
Pressure ulcer with abrasion, blister, partial thickness skin loss involving epidermis and/or dermis, sacral region

L89.153 Pressure ulcer of sacral region, stage 3
Healing pressure ulcer of sacral region, stage 3
Pressure ulcer with full thickness skin loss involving damage or necrosis of subcutaneous tissue, sacral region

L89.154 Pressure ulcer of sacral region, stage 4
Healing pressure ulcer of sacral region, stage 4
Pressure ulcer with necrosis of soft tissues through to underlying muscle, tendon, or bone, sacral region

L89.159 Pressure ulcer of sacral region, unspecified stage
Healing pressure ulcer of sacral region NOS
Healing pressure ulcer of sacral region, unspecified stage

● L89.2 Pressure ulcer of hip

● L89.2Ø Pressure ulcer of unspecified hip

L89.2ØØ Pressure ulcer of unspecified hip, unstageable

L89.2Ø1 Pressure ulcer of unspecified hip, stage 1
Healing pressure ulcer of unspecified hip back, stage 1
Pressure pre-ulcer skin changes limited to persistent focal edema, unspecified hip

L89.2Ø2 Pressure ulcer of unspecified hip, stage 2
Healing pressure ulcer of unspecified hip, stage 2
Pressure ulcer with abrasion, blister, partial thickness skin loss involving epidermis and/or dermis, unspecified hip

L89.2Ø3 Pressure ulcer of unspecified hip, stage 3
Healing pressure ulcer of unspecified hip, stage 3
Pressure ulcer with full thickness skin loss involving damage or necrosis of subcutaneous tissue, unspecified hip

L89.2Ø4 Pressure ulcer of unspecified hip, stage 4
Healing pressure ulcer of unspecified hip, stage 4
Pressure ulcer with necrosis of soft tissues through to underlying muscle, tendon, or bone, unspecified hip

L89.2Ø9 Pressure ulcer of unspecified hip, unspecified stage
Healing pressure ulcer of unspecified hip NOS
Healing pressure ulcer of unspecified hip, unspecified stage

● L89.21 **Pressure ulcer of right hip**
L89.210 **Pressure ulcer of right hip, unstageable**
L89.211 **Pressure ulcer of right hip, stage 1**
Healing pressure ulcer of right hip back, stage 1
Pressure pre-ulcer skin changes limited to persistent focal edema, right hip
L89.212 **Pressure ulcer of right hip, stage 2**
Healing pressure ulcer of right hip, stage 2
Pressure ulcer with abrasion, blister, partial thickness skin loss involving epidermis and/or dermis, right hip
L89.213 **Pressure ulcer of right hip, stage 3**
Healing pressure ulcer of right hip, stage 3
Pressure ulcer with full thickness skin loss involving damage or necrosis of subcutaneous tissue, right hip
L89.214 **Pressure ulcer of right hip, stage 4**
Healing pressure ulcer of right hip, stage 4
Pressure ulcer with necrosis of soft tissues through to underlying muscle, tendon, or bone, right hip
L89.219 **Pressure ulcer of right hip, unspecified stage**
Healing pressure ulcer of right hip NOS
Healing pressure ulcer of right hip, unspecified stage

● L89.22 **Pressure ulcer of left hip**
L89.220 **Pressure ulcer of left hip, unstageable**
L89.221 **Pressure ulcer of left hip, stage 1**
Healing pressure ulcer of left hip back, stage 1
Pressure pre-ulcer skin changes limited to persistent focal edema, left hip
L89.222 **Pressure ulcer of left hip, stage 2**
Healing pressure ulcer of left hip, stage 2
Pressure ulcer with abrasion, blister, partial thickness skin loss involving epidermis and/or dermis, left hip
L89.223 **Pressure ulcer of left hip, stage 3**
Healing pressure ulcer of left hip, stage 3
Pressure ulcer with full thickness skin loss involving damage or necrosis of subcutaneous tissue, left hip
L89.224 **Pressure ulcer of left hip, stage 4**
Healing pressure ulcer of left hip, stage 4
Pressure ulcer with necrosis of soft tissues through to underlying muscle, tendon, or bone, left hip
L89.229 **Pressure ulcer of left hip, unspecified stage**
Healing pressure ulcer of left hip NOS
Healing pressure ulcer of left hip, unspecified stage

● L89.3 **Pressure ulcer of buttock**
● L89.30 **Pressure ulcer of unspecified buttock**
L89.300 **Pressure ulcer of unspecified buttock, unstageable**
L89.301 **Pressure ulcer of unspecified buttock, stage 1**
Healing pressure ulcer of unspecified buttock, stage 1
Pressure pre-ulcer skin changes limited to persistent focal edema, unspecified buttock
L89.302 **Pressure ulcer of unspecified buttock, stage 2**
Healing pressure ulcer of unspecified buttock, stage 2
Pressure ulcer with abrasion, blister, partial thickness skin loss involving epidermis and/or dermis, unspecified buttock
L89.303 **Pressure ulcer of unspecified buttock, stage 3**
Healing pressure ulcer of unspecified buttock, stage 3
Pressure ulcer with full thickness skin loss involving damage or necrosis of subcutaneous tissue, unspecified buttock
L89.304 **Pressure ulcer of unspecified buttock, stage 4**
Healing pressure ulcer of unspecified buttock, stage 4
Pressure ulcer with necrosis of soft tissues through to underlying muscle, tendon, or bone, unspecified buttock
L89.309 **Pressure ulcer of unspecified buttock, unspecified stage**
Healing pressure ulcer of unspecified buttock NOS
Healing pressure ulcer of unspecified buttock, unspecified stage

● L89.31 **Pressure ulcer of right buttock**
L89.310 **Pressure ulcer of right buttock, unstageable**
L89.311 **Pressure ulcer of right buttock, stage 1**
Healing pressure ulcer of right buttock, stage 1
Pressure pre-ulcer skin changes limited to persistent focal edema, right buttock
L89.312 **Pressure ulcer of right buttock, stage 2**
Healing pressure ulcer of right buttock, stage 2
Pressure ulcer with abrasion, blister, partial thickness skin loss involving epidermis and/or dermis, right buttock
L89.313 **Pressure ulcer of right buttock, stage 3**
Healing pressure ulcer of right buttock, stage 3
Pressure ulcer with full thickness skin loss involving damage or necrosis of subcutaneous tissue, right buttock

L89.314 Pressure ulcer of right buttock, stage 4
Healing pressure ulcer of right buttock, stage 4
Pressure ulcer with necrosis of soft tissues through to underlying muscle, tendon, or bone, right buttock

L89.319 Pressure ulcer of right buttock, unspecified stage
Healing pressure ulcer of right buttock NOS
Healing pressure ulcer of right buttock, unspecified stage

● **L89.32 Pressure ulcer of left buttock**

L89.320 Pressure ulcer of left buttock, unstageable

L89.321 Pressure ulcer of left buttock, stage 1
Healing pressure ulcer of left buttock, stage 1
Pressure pre-ulcer skin changes limited to persistent focal edema, left buttock

L89.322 Pressure ulcer of left buttock, stage 2
Healing pressure ulcer of left buttock, stage 2
Pressure ulcer with abrasion, blister, partial thickness skin loss involving epidermis and/or dermis, left buttock

L89.323 Pressure ulcer of left buttock, stage 3
Healing pressure ulcer of left buttock, stage 3
Pressure ulcer with full thickness skin loss involving damage or necrosis of subcutaneous tissue, left buttock

L89.324 Pressure ulcer of left buttock, stage 4
Healing pressure ulcer of left buttock, stage 4
Pressure ulcer with necrosis of soft tissues through to underlying muscle, tendon, or bone, left buttock

L89.329 Pressure ulcer of left buttock, unspecified stage
Healing pressure ulcer of left buttock NOS
Healing pressure ulcer of left buttock, unspecified stage

● **L89.4 Pressure ulcer of contiguous site of back, buttock and hip**

L89.40 Pressure ulcer of contiguous site of back, buttock and hip, unspecified stage
Healing pressure ulcer of contiguous site of back, buttock and hip NOS
Healing pressure ulcer of contiguous site of back, buttock and hip, unspecified stage

L89.41 Pressure ulcer of contiguous site of back, buttock and hip, stage 1
Healing pressure ulcer of contiguous site of back, buttock and hip, stage 1
Pressure pre-ulcer skin changes limited to persistent focal edema, contiguous site of back, buttock and hip

L89.42 Pressure ulcer of contiguous site of back, buttock and hip, stage 2
Healing pressure ulcer of contiguous site of back, buttock and hip, stage 2
Pressure ulcer with abrasion, blister, partial thickness skin loss involving epidermis and/or dermis, contiguous site of back, buttock and hip

L89.43 Pressure ulcer of contiguous site of back, buttock and hip, stage 3
Healing pressure ulcer of contiguous site of back, buttock and hip, stage 3
Pressure ulcer with full thickness skin loss involving damage or necrosis of subcutaneous tissue, contiguous site of back, buttock and hip

L89.44 Pressure ulcer of contiguous site of back, buttock and hip, stage 4
Healing pressure ulcer of contiguous site of back, buttock and hip, stage 4
Pressure ulcer with necrosis of soft tissues through to underlying muscle, tendon, or bone, contiguous site of back, buttock and hip

L89.45 Pressure ulcer of contiguous site of back, buttock and hip, unstageable

● **L89.5 Pressure ulcer of ankle**

● **L89.50 Pressure ulcer of unspecified ankle**

L89.500 Pressure ulcer of unspecified ankle, unstageable

L89.501 Pressure ulcer of unspecified ankle, stage 1
Healing pressure ulcer of unspecified ankle, stage 1
Pressure pre-ulcer skin changes limited to persistent focal edema, unspecified ankle

L89.502 Pressure ulcer of unspecified ankle, stage 2
Healing pressure ulcer of unspecified ankle, stage 2
Pressure ulcer with abrasion, blister, partial thickness skin loss involving epidermis and/or dermis, unspecified ankle

L89.503 Pressure ulcer of unspecified ankle, stage 3
Healing pressure ulcer of unspecified ankle, stage 3
Pressure ulcer with full thickness skin loss involving damage or necrosis of subcutaneous tissue, unspecified ankle

L89.504 Pressure ulcer of unspecified ankle, stage 4
Healing pressure ulcer of unspecified ankle, stage 4
Pressure ulcer with necrosis of soft tissues through to underlying muscle, tendon, or bone, unspecified ankle

L89.509 Pressure ulcer of unspecified ankle, unspecified stage
Healing pressure ulcer of unspecified ankle NOS
Healing pressure ulcer of unspecified ankle, unspecified stage

● **L89.51 Pressure ulcer of right ankle**

L89.510 Pressure ulcer of right ankle, unstageable

L89.511 Pressure ulcer of right ankle, stage 1
Healing pressure ulcer of right ankle, stage 1
Pressure pre-ulcer skin changes limited to persistent focal edema, right ankle

L89.512 Pressure ulcer of right ankle, stage 2
Healing pressure ulcer of right ankle, stage 2
Pressure ulcer with abrasion, blister, partial thickness skin loss involving epidermis and/or dermis, right ankle

L89.513 Pressure ulcer of right ankle, stage 3
Healing pressure ulcer of right ankle, stage 3
Pressure ulcer with full thickness skin loss involving damage or necrosis of subcutaneous tissue, right ankle

L89.514 Pressure ulcer of right ankle, stage 4
Healing pressure ulcer of right ankle, stage 4
Pressure ulcer with necrosis of soft tissues through to underlying muscle, tendon, or bone, right ankle

L89.519 Pressure ulcer of right ankle, unspecified stage
Healing pressure ulcer of right ankle NOS
Healing pressure ulcer of right ankle, unspecified stage

● **L89.52 Pressure ulcer of left ankle**

L89.520 Pressure ulcer of left ankle, unstageable

L89.521 Pressure ulcer of left ankle, stage 1
Healing pressure ulcer of left ankle, stage 1
Pressure pre-ulcer skin changes limited to persistent focal edema, left ankle ◄

L89.522 Pressure ulcer of left ankle, stage 2
Healing pressure ulcer of left ankle, stage 2
Pressure ulcer with abrasion, blister, partial thickness skin loss involving epidermis and/or dermis, left ankle

L89.523 Pressure ulcer of left ankle, stage 3
Healing pressure ulcer of left ankle, stage 3
Pressure ulcer with full thickness skin loss involving damage or necrosis of subcutaneous tissue, left ankle

L89.524 Pressure ulcer of left ankle, stage 4
Healing pressure ulcer of left ankle, stage 4
Pressure ulcer with necrosis of soft tissues through to underlying muscle, tendon, or bone, left ankle

L89.529 Pressure ulcer of left ankle, unspecified stage
Healing pressure ulcer of left ankle NOS
Healing pressure ulcer of left ankle, unspecified stage

● **L89.6 Pressure ulcer of heel**

● **L89.60 Pressure ulcer of unspecified heel**

L89.600 Pressure ulcer of unspecified heel, unstageable

L89.601 Pressure ulcer of unspecified heel, stage 1
Healing pressure ulcer of unspecified heel, stage 1
Pressure pre-ulcer skin changes limited to persistent focal edema, unspecified heel

L89.602 Pressure ulcer of unspecified heel, stage 2
Healing pressure ulcer of unspecified heel, stage 2
Pressure ulcer with abrasion, blister, partial thickness skin loss involving epidermis and/or dermis, unspecified heel

L89.603 Pressure ulcer of unspecified heel, stage 3
Healing pressure ulcer of unspecified heel, stage 3
Pressure ulcer with full thickness skin loss involving damage or necrosis of subcutaneous tissue, unspecified heel

L89.604 Pressure ulcer of unspecified heel, stage 4
Healing pressure ulcer of unspecified heel, stage 4
Pressure ulcer with necrosis of soft tissues through to underlying muscle, tendon, or bone, unspecified heel

L89.609 Pressure ulcer of unspecified heel, unspecified stage
Healing pressure ulcer of unspecified heel NOS
Healing pressure ulcer of unspecified heel, unspecified stage

● **L89.61 Pressure ulcer of right heel**

L89.610 Pressure ulcer of right heel, unstageable

L89.611 Pressure ulcer of right heel, stage 1
Healing pressure ulcer of right heel, stage 1
Pressure pre-ulcer skin changes limited to persistent focal edema, right heel

L89.612 Pressure ulcer of right heel, stage 2
Healing pressure ulcer of right heel, stage 2
Pressure ulcer with abrasion, blister, partial thickness skin loss involving epidermis and/or dermis, right heel

L89.613 Pressure ulcer of right heel, stage 3
Healing pressure ulcer of right heel, stage 3
Pressure ulcer with full thickness skin loss involving damage or necrosis of subcutaneous tissue, right heel

L89.614 Pressure ulcer of right heel, stage 4
Healing pressure ulcer of right heel, stage 4
Pressure ulcer with necrosis of soft tissues through to underlying muscle, tendon, or bone, right heel

L89.619 Pressure ulcer of right heel, unspecified stage
Healing pressure ulcer of right heel NOS
Healing pressure ulcer of unspecified heel, right stage

L89.62 Pressure ulcer of left heel

L89.620 Pressure ulcer of left heel, unstageable

L89.621 Pressure ulcer of left heel, stage 1
Healing pressure ulcer of left heel, stage 1
Pressure pre-ulcer skin changes limited to persistent focal edema, left heel

L89.622 Pressure ulcer of left heel, stage 2
Healing pressure ulcer of left heel, stage 2
Pressure ulcer with abrasion, blister, partial thickness skin loss involving epidermis and/or dermis, left heel

L89.623 Pressure ulcer of left heel, stage 3
Healing pressure ulcer of left heel, stage 3
Pressure ulcer with full thickness skin loss involving damage or necrosis of subcutaneous tissue, left heel

L89.624 Pressure ulcer of left heel, stage 4
Healing pressure ulcer of left heel, stage 4
Pressure ulcer with necrosis of soft tissues through to underlying muscle, tendon, or bone, left heel

L89.629 Pressure ulcer of left heel, unspecified stage
Healing pressure ulcer of left heel NOS
Healing pressure ulcer of left heel, unspecified stage

L89.8 Pressure ulcer of other site

L89.81 Pressure ulcer of head
Pressure ulcer of face

L89.810 Pressure ulcer of head, unstageable

L89.811 Pressure ulcer of head, stage 1
Healing pressure ulcer of head, stage 1
Pressure pre-ulcer skin changes limited to persistent focal edema, head

L89.812 Pressure ulcer of head, stage 2
Healing pressure ulcer of head, stage 2
Pressure ulcer with abrasion, blister, partial thickness skin loss involving epidermis and/or dermis, head

L89.813 Pressure ulcer of head, stage 3
Healing pressure ulcer of head, stage 3
Pressure ulcer with full thickness skin loss involving damage or necrosis of subcutaneous tissue, head

L89.814 Pressure ulcer of head, stage 4
Healing pressure ulcer of head, stage 4
Pressure ulcer with necrosis of soft tissues through to underlying muscle, tendon, or bone, head

L89.819 Pressure ulcer of head, unspecified stage
Healing pressure ulcer of head NOS
Healing pressure ulcer of head, unspecified stage

L89.89 Pressure ulcer of other site

L89.890 Pressure ulcer of other site, unstageable

L89.891 Pressure ulcer of other site, stage 1
Healing pressure ulcer of other site, stage 1
Pressure pre-ulcer skin changes limited to persistent focal edema, other site

L89.892 Pressure ulcer of other site, stage 2
Healing pressure ulcer of other site, stage 2
Pressure ulcer with abrasion, blister, partial thickness skin loss involving epidermis and/or dermis, other site

L89.893 Pressure ulcer of other site, stage 3
Healing pressure ulcer of other site, stage 3
Pressure ulcer with full thickness skin loss involving damage or necrosis of subcutaneous tissue, other site

L89.894 Pressure ulcer of other site, stage 4
Healing pressure ulcer of other site, stage 4
Pressure ulcer with necrosis of soft tissues through to underlying muscle, tendon, or bone, other site

L89.899 Pressure ulcer of other site, unspecified stage
Healing pressure ulcer of other site NOS
Healing pressure ulcer of other site, unspecified stage

L89.9 Pressure ulcer of unspecified site

L89.90 Pressure ulcer of unspecified site, unspecified stage
Healing pressure ulcer of unspecified site NOS
Healing pressure ulcer of unspecified site, unspecified stage

L89.91 Pressure ulcer of unspecified site, stage 1
Healing pressure ulcer of unspecified site, stage 1
Pressure pre-ulcer skin changes limited to persistent focal edema, unspecified site

L89.92 Pressure ulcer of unspecified site, stage 2
Healing pressure ulcer of unspecified site, stage 2
Pressure ulcer with abrasion, blister, partial thickness skin loss involving epidermis and/or dermis, unspecified site

L89.93 Pressure ulcer of unspecified site, stage 3
Healing pressure ulcer of unspecified site, stage 3
Pressure ulcer with full thickness skin loss involving damage or necrosis of subcutaneous tissue, unspecified site

L89.94 Pressure ulcer of unspecified site, stage 4
Healing pressure ulcer of unspecified site, stage 4
Pressure ulcer with necrosis of soft tissues through to underlying muscle, tendon, or bone, unspecified site

L89.95 Pressure ulcer of unspecified site, unstageable

● L90 **Atrophic disorders of skin**

L90.0 **Lichen sclerosus et atrophicus**

Excludes2 lichen sclerosus of external female genital organs (N90.4)
lichen sclerosus of external male genital organs (N48.0)

L90.1 **Anetoderma of Schweninger-Buzzi**

L90.2 **Anetoderma of Jadassohn-Pellizzari**

L90.3 **Atrophoderma of Pasini and Pierini**

L90.4 **Acrodermatitis chronica atrophicans**

L90.5 **Scar conditions and fibrosis of skin**
Adherent scar (skin)
Cicatrix
Disfigurement of skin due to scar
Fibrosis of skin NOS
Scar NOS

Excludes2 hypertrophic scar (L91.0)
keloid scar (L91.0)

L90.6 **Striae atrophicae**

L90.8 **Other atrophic disorders of skin**

L90.9 **Atrophic disorder of skin, unspecified**

● L91 **Hypertrophic disorders of skin**

L91.0 **Keloid scar**
Hypertrophic scar
Keloid

Excludes2 acne keloid (L73.0)
scar NOS (L90.5)

L91.8 **Other hypertrophic disorders of the skin**

L91.9 **Hypertrophic disorder of the skin, unspecified**

● L92 **Granulomatous disorders of skin and subcutaneous tissue**

Excludes2 actinic granuloma (L57.5)

L92.0 **Granuloma annulare**
Perforating granuloma annulare

L92.1 **Necrobiosis lipoidica, not elsewhere classified**

Excludes1 necrobiosis lipoidica associated with diabetes mellitus (E08-E13 with .620)

L92.2 **Granuloma faciale [eosinophilic granuloma of skin]**

L92.3 **Foreign body granuloma of the skin and subcutaneous tissue**

Use additional code to identify the type of retained foreign body (Z18.-)

L92.8 **Other granulomatous disorders of the skin and subcutaneous tissue**

L92.9 **Granulomatous disorder of the skin and subcutaneous tissue, unspecified**

● L93 **Lupus erythematosus**

Use additional code for adverse effect, if applicable, to identify drug (T36-T50 with fifth or sixth character 5)

Excludes1 lupus exedens (A18.4)
lupus vulgaris (A18.4)
scleroderma (M34.-)
systemic lupus erythematosus (M32.-)

L93.0 **Discoid lupus erythematosus**
Lupus erythematosus NOS

L93.1 **Subacute cutaneous lupus erythematosus**

L93.2 **Other local lupus erythematosus**
Lupus erythematosus profundus
Lupus panniculitis

Item 12–11 Scleroderma means hard skin. It is a group of diseases that causes abnormal growth of connective tissues that support the skin and organs. There are two types: localized scleroderma affecting the skin and systemic scleroderma affecting blood vessels and internal organs and the skin.

● L94 **Other localized connective tissue disorders**

Excludes1 systemic connective tissue disorders (M30-M36)

L94.0 **Localized scleroderma [morphea]**
Circumscribed scleroderma

L94.1 **Linear scleroderma**
En coup de sabre lesion

L94.2 **Calcinosis cutis**

L94.3 **Sclerodactyly**

L94.4 **Gottron's papules**

L94.5 **Poikiloderma vasculare atrophicans**

L94.6 **Ainhum**

L94.8 **Other specified localized connective tissue disorders**

L94.9 **Localized connective tissue disorder, unspecified**

● L95 **Vasculitis limited to skin, not elsewhere classified**

Excludes1 angioma serpiginosum (L81.7)
Henoch(-Schönlein) purpura (D69.0)
hypersensitivity angiitis (M31.0)
lupus panniculitis (L93.2)
panniculitis NOS (M79.3)
panniculitis of neck and back (M54.0-)
polyarteritis nodosa (M30.0)
relapsing panniculitis (M35.6)
rheumatoid vasculitis (M05.2)
serum sickness (T80.6-)
urticaria (L50.-)
Wegener's granulomatosis (M31.3-)

L95.0 **Livedoid vasculitis**
Atrophie blanche (en plaque)

L95.1 **Erythema elevatum diutinum**

L95.8 **Other vasculitis limited to the skin**

L95.9 **Vasculitis limited to the skin, unspecified**

● L97 **Non-pressure chronic ulcer of lower limb, not elsewhere classified**

Includes chronic ulcer of skin of lower limb NOS
non-healing ulcer of skin
non-infected sinus of skin
trophic ulcer NOS
tropical ulcer NOS
ulcer of skin of lower limb NOS

Code first any associated underlying condition, such as:
any associated gangrene (I96)
atherosclerosis of the lower extremities (I70.23-, I70.24-, I70.33-, I70.34-, I70.43-, I70.44-, I70.53-, I70.54-, I70.63-, I70.64-, I70.73-, I70.74-)
chronic venous hypertension (I87.31-, I87.33-)
diabetic ulcers (E08.621, E08.622, E09.621, E09.622, E10.621, E10.622, E11.621, E11.622, E13.621, E13.622)
postphlebitic syndrome (I87.01-, I87.03-)
postthrombotic syndrome (I87.01-, I87.03-)
varicose ulcer (I83.0-, I83.2-)

Excludes2 pressure ulcer (pressure area) (L89.-)
skin infections (L00-L08)
specific infections classified to A00-B99

● L97.1 **Non-pressure chronic ulcer of thigh**

● L97.10 **Non-pressure chronic ulcer of unspecified thigh**

L97.101 **Non-pressure chronic ulcer of unspecified thigh limited to breakdown of skin**

L97.102 **Non-pressure chronic ulcer of unspecified thigh with fat layer exposed**

L97.103 **Non-pressure chronic ulcer of unspecified thigh with necrosis of muscle**

L97.104 **Non-pressure chronic ulcer of unspecified thigh with necrosis of bone**

L97.109 **Non-pressure chronic ulcer of unspecified thigh with unspecified severity**

● L97.11 Non-pressure chronic ulcer of right thigh
L97.111 Non-pressure chronic ulcer of right thigh limited to breakdown of skin
L97.112 Non-pressure chronic ulcer of right thigh with fat layer exposed
L97.113 Non-pressure chronic ulcer of right thigh with necrosis of muscle
L97.114 Non-pressure chronic ulcer of right thigh with necrosis of bone
L97.119 Non-pressure chronic ulcer of right thigh with unspecified severity
● L97.12 Non-pressure chronic ulcer of left thigh
L97.121 Non-pressure chronic ulcer of left thigh limited to breakdown of skin
L97.122 Non-pressure chronic ulcer of left thigh with fat layer exposed
L97.123 Non-pressure chronic ulcer of left thigh with necrosis of muscle
L97.124 Non-pressure chronic ulcer of left thigh with necrosis of bone
L97.129 Non-pressure chronic ulcer of left thigh with unspecified severity
● L97.2 Non-pressure chronic ulcer of calf
● L97.20 Non-pressure chronic ulcer of unspecified calf
L97.201 Non-pressure chronic ulcer of unspecified calf limited to breakdown of skin
L97.202 Non-pressure chronic ulcer of unspecified calf with fat layer exposed
L97.203 Non-pressure chronic ulcer of unspecified calf with necrosis of muscle
L97.204 Non-pressure chronic ulcer of unspecified calf with necrosis of bone
L97.209 Non-pressure chronic ulcer of unspecified calf with unspecified severity
● L97.21 Non-pressure chronic ulcer of right calf
L97.211 Non-pressure chronic ulcer of right calf limited to breakdown of skin
L97.212 Non-pressure chronic ulcer of right calf with fat layer exposed
L97.213 Non-pressure chronic ulcer of right calf with necrosis of muscle
L97.214 Non-pressure chronic ulcer of right calf with necrosis of bone
L97.219 Non-pressure chronic ulcer of right calf with unspecified severity
● L97.22 Non-pressure chronic ulcer of left calf
L97.221 Non-pressure chronic ulcer of left calf limited to breakdown of skin
L97.222 Non-pressure chronic ulcer of left calf with fat layer exposed
L97.223 Non-pressure chronic ulcer of left calf with necrosis of muscle
L97.224 Non-pressure chronic ulcer of left calf with necrosis of bone
L97.229 Non-pressure chronic ulcer of left calf with unspecified severity
● L97.3 Non-pressure chronic ulcer of ankle
● L97.30 Non-pressure chronic ulcer of unspecified ankle
L97.301 Non-pressure chronic ulcer of unspecified ankle limited to breakdown of skin
L97.302 Non-pressure chronic ulcer of unspecified ankle with fat layer exposed
L97.303 Non-pressure chronic ulcer of unspecified ankle with necrosis of muscle
L97.304 Non-pressure chronic ulcer of unspecified ankle with necrosis of bone
L97.309 Non-pressure chronic ulcer of unspecified ankle with unspecified severity
● L97.31 Non-pressure chronic ulcer of right ankle
L97.311 Non-pressure chronic ulcer of right ankle limited to breakdown of skin
L97.312 Non-pressure chronic ulcer of right ankle with fat layer exposed
L97.313 Non-pressure chronic ulcer of right ankle with necrosis of muscle
L97.314 Non-pressure chronic ulcer of right ankle with necrosis of bone
L97.319 Non-pressure chronic ulcer of right ankle with unspecified severity
● L97.32 Non-pressure chronic ulcer of left ankle
L97.321 Non-pressure chronic ulcer of left ankle limited to breakdown of skin
L97.322 Non-pressure chronic ulcer of left ankle with fat layer exposed
L97.323 Non-pressure chronic ulcer of left ankle with necrosis of muscle
L97.324 Non-pressure chronic ulcer of left ankle with necrosis of bone
L97.329 Non-pressure chronic ulcer of left ankle with unspecified severity
● L97.4 Non-pressure chronic ulcer of heel and midfoot
Non-pressure chronic ulcer of plantar surface of midfoot
● L97.40 Non-pressure chronic ulcer of unspecified heel and midfoot
L97.401 Non-pressure chronic ulcer of unspecified heel and midfoot limited to breakdown of skin
L97.402 Non-pressure chronic ulcer of unspecified heel and midfoot with fat layer exposed
L97.403 Non-pressure chronic ulcer of unspecified heel and midfoot with necrosis of muscle
L97.404 Non-pressure chronic ulcer of unspecified heel and midfoot with necrosis of bone
L97.409 Non-pressure chronic ulcer of unspecified heel and midfoot with unspecified severity
● L97.41 Non-pressure chronic ulcer of right heel and midfoot
L97.411 Non-pressure chronic ulcer of right heel and midfoot limited to breakdown of skin
L97.412 Non-pressure chronic ulcer of right heel and midfoot with fat layer exposed
L97.413 Non-pressure chronic ulcer of right heel and midfoot with necrosis of muscle
L97.414 Non-pressure chronic ulcer of right heel and midfoot with necrosis of bone
L97.419 Non-pressure chronic ulcer of right heel and midfoot with unspecified severity

● L97.42 Non-pressure chronic ulcer of left heel and midfoot
L97.421 Non-pressure chronic ulcer of left heel and midfoot limited to breakdown of skin
L97.422 Non-pressure chronic ulcer of left heel and midfoot with fat layer exposed
L97.423 Non-pressure chronic ulcer of left heel and midfoot with necrosis of muscle
L97.424 Non-pressure chronic ulcer of left heel and midfoot with necrosis of bone
L97.429 Non-pressure chronic ulcer of left heel and midfoot with unspecified severity

● L97.5 Non-pressure chronic ulcer of other part of foot
Non-pressure chronic ulcer of toe

● L97.50 Non-pressure chronic ulcer of other part of unspecified foot
L97.501 Non-pressure chronic ulcer of other part of unspecified foot limited to breakdown of skin
L97.502 Non-pressure chronic ulcer of other part of unspecified foot with fat layer exposed
L97.503 Non-pressure chronic ulcer of other part of unspecified foot with necrosis of muscle
L97.504 Non-pressure chronic ulcer of other part of unspecified foot with necrosis of bone
L97.509 Non-pressure chronic ulcer of other part of unspecified foot with unspecified severity

● L97.51 Non-pressure chronic ulcer of other part of right foot
L97.511 Non-pressure chronic ulcer of other part of right foot limited to breakdown of skin
L97.512 Non-pressure chronic ulcer of other part of right foot with fat layer exposed
L97.513 Non-pressure chronic ulcer of other part of right foot with necrosis of muscle
L97.514 Non-pressure chronic ulcer of other part of right foot with necrosis of bone
L97.519 Non-pressure chronic ulcer of other part of right foot with unspecified severity

● L97.52 Non-pressure chronic ulcer of other part of left foot
L97.521 Non-pressure chronic ulcer of other part of left foot limited to breakdown of skin
L97.522 Non-pressure chronic ulcer of other part of left foot with fat layer exposed
L97.523 Non-pressure chronic ulcer of other part of left foot with necrosis of muscle
L97.524 Non-pressure chronic ulcer of other part of left foot with necrosis of bone
L97.529 Non-pressure chronic ulcer of other part of left foot with unspecified severity

● L97.8 Non-pressure chronic ulcer of other part of lower leg

● L97.80 Non-pressure chronic ulcer of other part of unspecified lower leg
L97.801 Non-pressure chronic ulcer of other part of unspecified lower leg limited to breakdown of skin
L97.802 Non-pressure chronic ulcer of other part of unspecified lower leg with fat layer exposed
L97.803 Non-pressure chronic ulcer of other part of unspecified lower leg with necrosis of muscle
L97.804 Non-pressure chronic ulcer of other part of unspecified lower leg with necrosis of bone
L97.809 Non-pressure chronic ulcer of other part of unspecified lower leg with unspecified severity

● L97.81 Non-pressure chronic ulcer of other part of right lower leg
L97.811 Non-pressure chronic ulcer of other part of right lower leg limited to breakdown of skin
L97.812 Non-pressure chronic ulcer of other part of right lower leg with fat layer exposed
L97.813 Non-pressure chronic ulcer of other part of right lower leg with necrosis of muscle
L97.814 Non-pressure chronic ulcer of other part of right lower leg with necrosis of bone
L97.819 Non-pressure chronic ulcer of other part of right lower leg with unspecified severity

● L97.82 Non-pressure chronic ulcer of other part of left lower leg
L97.821 Non-pressure chronic ulcer of other part of left lower leg limited to breakdown of skin
L97.822 Non-pressure chronic ulcer of other part of left lower leg with fat layer exposed
L97.823 Non-pressure chronic ulcer of other part of left lower leg with necrosis of muscle
L97.824 Non-pressure chronic ulcer of other part of left lower leg with necrosis of bone
L97.829 Non-pressure chronic ulcer of other part of left lower leg with unspecified severity

● L97.9 Non-pressure chronic ulcer of unspecified part of lower leg

● L97.90 Non-pressure chronic ulcer of unspecified part of unspecified lower leg
L97.901 Non-pressure chronic ulcer of unspecified part of unspecified lower leg limited to breakdown of skin
L97.902 Non-pressure chronic ulcer of unspecified part of unspecified lower leg with fat layer exposed
L97.903 Non-pressure chronic ulcer of unspecified part of unspecified lower leg with necrosis of muscle
L97.904 Non-pressure chronic ulcer of unspecified part of unspecified lower leg with necrosis of bone
L97.909 Non-pressure chronic ulcer of unspecified part of unspecified lower leg with unspecified severity

● L97.91 **Non-pressure chronic ulcer of unspecified part of right lower leg**
- L97.911 **Non-pressure chronic ulcer of unspecified part of right lower leg limited to breakdown of skin**
- L97.912 **Non-pressure chronic ulcer of unspecified part of right lower leg with fat layer exposed**
- L97.913 **Non-pressure chronic ulcer of unspecified part of right lower leg with necrosis of muscle**
- L97.914 **Non-pressure chronic ulcer of unspecified part of right lower leg with necrosis of bone**
- L97.919 **Non-pressure chronic ulcer of unspecified part of right lower leg with unspecified severity**

● L97.92 **Non-pressure chronic ulcer of unspecified part of left lower leg**
- L97.921 **Non-pressure chronic ulcer of unspecified part of left lower leg limited to breakdown of skin**
- L97.922 **Non-pressure chronic ulcer of unspecified part of left lower leg with fat layer exposed**
- L97.923 **Non-pressure chronic ulcer of unspecified part of left lower leg with necrosis of muscle**
- L97.924 **Non-pressure chronic ulcer of unspecified part of left lower leg with necrosis of bone**
- L97.929 **Non-pressure chronic ulcer of unspecified part of left lower leg with unspecified severity**

● L98 **Other disorders of skin and subcutaneous tissue, not elsewhere classified**

L98.Ø **Pyogenic granuloma**

Excludes2 pyogenic granuloma of gingiva (KØ6.8)
pyogenic granuloma of maxillary alveolar ridge (KØ4.5)
pyogenic granuloma of oral mucosa (K13.4)

L98.1 **Factitial dermatitis**
Neurotic excoriation

Excludes1 Excoriation (skin-picking) disorder (F42.4) ◀

L98.2 **Febrile neutrophilic dermatosis [Sweet]**

L98.3 **Eosinophilic cellulitis [Wells]**

● L98.4 **Non-pressure chronic ulcer of skin, not elsewhere classified**
Chronic ulcer of skin NOS
Tropical ulcer NOS
Ulcer of skin NOS

Excludes2 pressure ulcer (pressure area) (L89.-)
gangrene (I96)
skin infections (LØØ-LØ8)
specific infections classified to AØØ-B99
ulcer of lower limb NEC (L97.-)
varicose ulcer (I83.Ø-I82.2)

● L98.41 **Non-pressure chronic ulcer of buttock**
- L98.411 **Non-pressure chronic ulcer of buttock limited to breakdown of skin**
- L98.412 **Non-pressure chronic ulcer of buttock with fat layer exposed**
- L98.413 **Non-pressure chronic ulcer of buttock with necrosis of muscle**
- L98.414 **Non-pressure chronic ulcer of buttock with necrosis of bone**
- L98.419 **Non-pressure chronic ulcer of buttock with unspecified severity**

● L98.42 **Non-pressure chronic ulcer of back**
- L98.421 **Non-pressure chronic ulcer of back limited to breakdown of skin**
- L98.422 **Non-pressure chronic ulcer of back with fat layer exposed**
- L98.423 **Non-pressure chronic ulcer of back with necrosis of muscle**
- L98.424 **Non-pressure chronic ulcer of back with necrosis of bone**
- L98.429 **Non-pressure chronic ulcer of back with unspecified severity**

● L98.49 **Non-pressure chronic ulcer of skin of other sites**
Non-pressure chronic ulcer of skin NOS
- L98.491 **Non-pressure chronic ulcer of skin of other sites limited to breakdown of skin**
- L98.492 **Non-pressure chronic ulcer of skin of other sites with fat layer exposed**
- L98.493 **Non-pressure chronic ulcer of skin of other sites with necrosis of muscle**
- L98.494 **Non-pressure chronic ulcer of skin of other sites with necrosis of bone**
- L98.499 **Non-pressure chronic ulcer of skin of other sites with unspecified severity**

L98.5 **Mucinosis of the skin**
Focal mucinosis
Lichen myxedematosus
Reticular erythematous mucinosis

Excludes1 focal oral mucinosis (K13.79)
myxedema (EØ3.9)

L98.6 **Other infiltrative disorders of the skin and subcutaneous tissue**

Excludes1 hyalinosis cutis et mucosae (E78.89)

L98.7 **Excessive and redundant skin and subcutaneous tissue** ◀
Loose or sagging skin following bariatric surgery weight loss ◀
Loose or sagging skin following dietary weight loss ◀
Loose or sagging skin, NOS ◀

Excludes2 acquired excess or redundant skin of eyelid (HØ2.3-) ◀
congenital excess or redundant skin of eyelid (Q1Ø.3) ◀
skin changes due to chronic exposure to nonionizing radiation (L57.-) ◀

L98.8 **Other specified disorders of the skin and subcutaneous tissue**

L98.9 **Disorder of the skin and subcutaneous tissue, unspecified**

L99 **Other disorders of skin and subcutaneous tissue in diseases classified elsewhere**

Code first underlying disease, such as:
amyloidosis (E85.-)

Excludes1 skin disorders in diabetes (EØ8-E13 with .62)
skin disorders in gonorrhea (A54.89)
skin disorders in syphilis (A51.31, A52.79)

CHAPTER 12 (LØØ-L99)

CHAPTER 13

DISEASES OF THE MUSCULOSKELETAL SYSTEM AND CONNECTIVE TISSUE (MØØ-M99)

OGCR Chapter-Specific Coding Guidelines

13. **Chapter 13: Diseases of the Musculoskeletal System and Connective Tissue (MØØ-M99)**

a. **Site and laterality**

Most of the codes within Chapter 13 have site and laterality designations. The site represents the bone, joint or the muscle involved. For some conditions where more than one bone, joint or muscle is usually involved, such as osteoarthritis, there is a "multiple sites" code available. For categories where no multiple site code is provided and more than one bone, joint or muscle is involved, multiple codes should be used to indicate the different sites involved.

1) **Bone versus joint**

For certain conditions, the bone may be affected at the upper or lower end, (e.g., avascular necrosis of bone, M87, Osteoporosis, M8Ø, M81). Though the portion of the bone affected may be at the joint, the site designation will be the bone, not the joint.

b. **Acute traumatic versus chronic or recurrent musculoskeletal conditions**

Many musculoskeletal conditions are a result of previous injury or trauma to a site, or are recurrent conditions. Bone, joint or muscle conditions that are the result of a healed injury are usually found in chapter 13. Recurrent bone, joint or muscle conditions are also usually found in chapter 13. Any current, acute injury should be coded to the appropriate injury code from chapter 19. Chronic or recurrent conditions should generally be coded with a code from chapter 13. If it is difficult to determine from the documentation in the record which code is best to describe a condition, query the provider.

c. **Coding of Pathologic Fractures**

7th character A is for use as long as the patient is receiving active treatment for the fracture. While the patient may be seen by a new or different provider over the course of treatment for a pathological fracture, assignment of the 7th character is based on whether the patient is undergoing active treatment and not whether the provider is seeing the patient for the first time.

7th character, D is to be used for encounters after the patient has completed active treatment. The other 7th characters, listed under each subcategory in the Tabular List, are to be used for subsequent encounters for **routine care of fractures during the healing and recovery phase as well as** treatment of problems associated with the healing, such as malunions, nonunions, and sequelae.

Care for complications of surgical treatment for fracture repairs during the healing or recovery phase should be coded with the appropriate complication codes.

See Section I.C.19. Coding of traumatic fractures.

d. **Osteoporosis**

Osteoporosis is a systemic condition, meaning that all bones of the musculoskeletal system are affected. Therefore, site is not a component of the codes under category M81, Osteoporosis without current pathological fracture. The site codes under category M8Ø, Osteoporosis with current pathological fracture, identify the site of the fracture, not the osteoporosis.

1) **Osteoporosis without pathological fracture**

Category M81, Osteoporosis without current pathological fracture, is for use for patients with osteoporosis who do not currently have a pathologic fracture due to the osteoporosis, even if they have had a fracture in the past. For patients with a history of osteoporosis fractures, status code Z87.31Ø, Personal history of (healed) osteoporosis fracture, should follow the code from M81.

2) **Osteoporosis with current pathological fracture**

Category M8Ø, Osteoporosis with current pathological fracture, is for patients who have a current pathologic fracture at the time of an encounter. The codes under M8Ø identify the site of the fracture. A code from category M8Ø, not a traumatic fracture code, should be used for any patient with known osteoporosis who suffers a fracture, even if the patient had a minor fall or trauma, if that fall or trauma would not usually break a normal, healthy bone.

CHAPTER 13

DISEASES OF THE MUSCULOSKELETAL SYSTEM AND CONNECTIVE TISSUE (MØØ-M99)

Note: Use an external cause code following the code for the musculoskeletal condition, if applicable, to identify the cause of the musculoskeletal condition

Excludes2 arthropathic psoriasis (L4Ø.5-)
certain conditions originating in the perinatal period (PØ4-P96)
certain infectious and parasitic diseases (AØØ-B99)
compartment syndrome (traumatic) (T79.A-)
complications of pregnancy, childbirth and the puerperium (OØØ-O9A)
congenital malformations, deformations, and chromosomal abnormalities (QØØ-Q99)
endocrine, nutritional and metabolic diseases (EØØ-E88)
injury, poisoning and certain other consequences of external causes (SØØ-T88)
neoplasms (CØØ-D49)
symptoms, signs and abnormal clinical and laboratory findings, not elsewhere classified (RØØ-R94)

This chapter contains the following blocks:

MØØ-MØ2	Infectious arthropathies
MØ4	Autoinflammatory syndromes ◀
MØ5-M14	Inflammatory polyarthropathies
M15-M19	Osteoarthritis
M2Ø-M25	Other joint disorders
M26-M27	Dentofacial anomalies [including malocclusion] and other disorders of jaw
M3Ø-M36	Systemic connective tissue disorders
M4Ø-M43	Deforming dorsopathies
M45-M49	Spondylopathies
M5Ø-M54	Other dorsopathies
M6Ø-M63	Disorders of muscles
M65-M67	Disorders of synovium and tendon
M7Ø-M79	Other soft tissue disorders
M8Ø-M85	Disorders of bone density and structure
M86-M9Ø	Other osteopathies
M91-M94	Chondropathies
M95	Other disorders of the musculoskeletal system and connective tissue
M96	Intraoperative and postprocedural complications and disorders of musculoskeletal system, not elsewhere classified
M97	Periprosthetic fracture around internal prosthetic joint ◀
M99	Biomechanical lesions, not elsewhere classified

ARTHROPATHIES (MØØ-M25)

Includes Disorders affecting predominantly peripheral (limb) joints

INFECTIOUS ARTHROPATHIES (MØØ-MØ2)

Note: This block comprises arthropathies due to microbiological agents.

Distinction is made between the following types of etiological relationship:

a) direct infection of joint, where organisms invade synovial tissue and microbial antigen is present in the joint;

b) indirect infection, which may be of two types: a reactive arthropathy, where microbial infection of the body is established but neither organisms nor antigens can be identified in the joint, and a postinfective arthropathy, where microbial antigen is present but recovery of an organism is inconstant and evidence of local multiplication is lacking.

● MØØ Pyogenic arthritis

● MØØ.Ø Staphylococcal arthritis and polyarthritis

Use additional code (B95.61-B95.8) to identify bacterial agent

Excludes2 infection and inflammatory reaction due to internal joint prosthesis (T84.5-)

MØØ.ØØ Staphylococcal arthritis, unspecified joint

● MØØ.Ø1 Staphylococcal arthritis, shoulder

MØØ.Ø11 Staphylococcal arthritis, right shoulder

MØØ.Ø12 Staphylococcal arthritis, left shoulder

MØØ.Ø19 Staphylococcal arthritis, unspecified shoulder

● MØØ.Ø2 Staphylococcal arthritis, elbow

MØØ.Ø21 Staphylococcal arthritis, right elbow

MØØ.Ø22 Staphylococcal arthritis, left elbow

MØØ.Ø29 Staphylococcal arthritis, unspecified elbow

● MØØ.Ø3 Staphylococcal arthritis, wrist

Staphylococcal arthritis of carpal bones

MØØ.Ø31 Staphylococcal arthritis, right wrist

MØØ.Ø32 Staphylococcal arthritis, left wrist

MØØ.Ø39 Staphylococcal arthritis, unspecified wrist

● MØØ.Ø4 Staphylococcal arthritis, hand

Staphylococcal arthritis of metacarpus and phalanges

MØØ.Ø41 Staphylococcal arthritis, right hand

MØØ.Ø42 Staphylococcal arthritis, left hand

MØØ.Ø49 Staphylococcal arthritis, unspecified hand

● MØØ.Ø5 Staphylococcal arthritis, hip

MØØ.Ø51 Staphylococcal arthritis, right hip

MØØ.Ø52 Staphylococcal arthritis, left hip

MØØ.Ø59 Staphylococcal arthritis, unspecified hip

● MØØ.Ø6 Staphylococcal arthritis, knee

MØØ.Ø61 Staphylococcal arthritis, right knee

MØØ.Ø62 Staphylococcal arthritis, left knee

MØØ.Ø69 Staphylococcal arthritis, unspecified knee

● MØØ.Ø7 Staphylococcal arthritis, ankle and foot

Staphylococcal arthritis, tarsus, metatarsus and phalanges

MØØ.Ø71 Staphylococcal arthritis, right ankle and foot

MØØ.Ø72 Staphylococcal arthritis, left ankle and foot

MØØ.Ø79 Staphylococcal arthritis, unspecified ankle and foot

MØØ.Ø8 Staphylococcal arthritis, vertebrae

MØØ.Ø9 Staphylococcal polyarthritis

● MØØ.1 Pneumococcal arthritis and polyarthritis

MØØ.1Ø Pneumococcal arthritis, unspecified joint

● MØØ.11 Pneumococcal arthritis, shoulder

MØØ.111 Pneumococcal arthritis, right shoulder

MØØ.112 Pneumococcal arthritis, left shoulder

MØØ.119 Pneumococcal arthritis, unspecified shoulder

● MØØ.12 Pneumococcal arthritis, elbow

MØØ.121 Pneumococcal arthritis, right elbow

MØØ.122 Pneumococcal arthritis, left elbow

MØØ.129 Pneumococcal arthritis, unspecified elbow

● MØØ.13 Pneumococcal arthritis, wrist

Pneumococcal arthritis of carpal bones

MØØ.131 Pneumococcal arthritis, right wrist

MØØ.132 Pneumococcal arthritis, left wrist

MØØ.139 Pneumococcal arthritis, unspecified wrist

● MØØ.14 Pneumococcal arthritis, hand

Pneumococcal arthritis of metacarpus and phalanges

MØØ.141 Pneumococcal arthritis, right hand

MØØ.142 Pneumococcal arthritis, left hand

MØØ.149 Pneumococcal arthritis, unspecified hand

● MØØ.15 Pneumococcal arthritis, hip

MØØ.151 Pneumococcal arthritis, right hip

MØØ.152 Pneumococcal arthritis, left hip

MØØ.159 Pneumococcal arthritis, unspecified hip

● MØØ.16 Pneumococcal arthritis, knee

MØØ.161 Pneumococcal arthritis, right knee

MØØ.162 Pneumococcal arthritis, left knee

MØØ.169 Pneumococcal arthritis, unspecified knee

● MØØ.17 Pneumococcal arthritis, ankle and foot

Pneumococcal arthritis, tarsus, metatarsus and phalanges

MØØ.171 Pneumococcal arthritis, right ankle and foot

MØØ.172 Pneumococcal arthritis, left ankle and foot

MØØ.179 Pneumococcal arthritis, unspecified ankle and foot

MØØ.18 Pneumococcal arthritis, vertebrae

MØØ.19 Pneumococcal polyarthritis

● MØØ.2 Other streptococcal arthritis and polyarthritis

Use additional code (B95.Ø-B95.2, B95.4-B95.5) to identify bacterial agent

MØØ.2Ø Other streptococcal arthritis, unspecified joint

● MØØ.21 Other streptococcal arthritis, shoulder

MØØ.211 Other streptococcal arthritis, right shoulder

MØØ.212 Other streptococcal arthritis, left shoulder

MØØ.219 Other streptococcal arthritis, unspecified shoulder

● MØØ.22 Other streptococcal arthritis, elbow

MØØ.221 Other streptococcal arthritis, right elbow

MØØ.222 Other streptococcal arthritis, left elbow

MØØ.229 Other streptococcal arthritis, unspecified elbow

● MØØ.23 Other streptococcal arthritis, wrist

Other streptococcal arthritis of carpal bones

MØØ.231 Other streptococcal arthritis, right wrist

MØØ.232 Other streptococcal arthritis, left wrist

MØØ.239 Other streptococcal arthritis, unspecified wrist

● MØØ.24 Other streptococcal arthritis, hand

Other streptococcal arthritis metacarpus and phalanges

MØØ.241 Other streptococcal arthritis, right hand

MØØ.242 Other streptococcal arthritis, left hand

MØØ.249 Other streptococcal arthritis, unspecified hand

CHAPTER 13 (MØØ-M99)

● **MØØ.25 Other streptococcal arthritis, hip**
MØØ.251 Other streptococcal arthritis, right hip
MØØ.252 Other streptococcal arthritis, left hip
MØØ.259 Other streptococcal arthritis, unspecified hip

● **MØØ.26 Other streptococcal arthritis, knee**
MØØ.261 Other streptococcal arthritis, right knee
MØØ.262 Other streptococcal arthritis, left knee
MØØ.269 Other streptococcal arthritis, unspecified knee

● **MØØ.27 Other streptococcal arthritis, ankle and foot**
Other streptococcal arthritis, tarsus, metatarsus and phalanges
MØØ.271 Other streptococcal arthritis, right ankle and foot
MØØ.272 Other streptococcal arthritis, left ankle and foot
MØØ.279 Other streptococcal arthritis, unspecified ankle and foot

MØØ.28 Other streptococcal arthritis, vertebrae
MØØ.29 Other streptococcal polyarthritis

● **MØØ.8 Arthritis and polyarthritis due to other bacteria**
Use additional code (B96) to identify bacteria
MØØ.80 Arthritis due to other bacteria, unspecified joint

● **MØØ.81 Arthritis due to other bacteria, shoulder**
MØØ.811 Arthritis due to other bacteria, right shoulder
MØØ.812 Arthritis due to other bacteria, left shoulder
MØØ.819 Arthritis due to other bacteria, unspecified shoulder

● **MØØ.82 Arthritis due to other bacteria, elbow**
MØØ.821 Arthritis due to other bacteria, right elbow
MØØ.822 Arthritis due to other bacteria, left elbow
MØØ.829 Arthritis due to other bacteria, unspecified elbow

● **MØØ.83 Arthritis due to other bacteria, wrist**
Arthritis due to other bacteria, carpal bones
MØØ.831 Arthritis due to other bacteria, right wrist
MØØ.832 Arthritis due to other bacteria, left wrist
MØØ.839 Arthritis due to other bacteria, unspecified wrist

● **MØØ.84 Arthritis due to other bacteria, hand**
Arthritis due to other bacteria, metacarpus and phalanges
MØØ.841 Arthritis due to other bacteria, right hand
MØØ.842 Arthritis due to other bacteria, left hand
MØØ.849 Arthritis due to other bacteria, unspecified hand

● **MØØ.85 Arthritis due to other bacteria, hip**
MØØ.851 Arthritis due to other bacteria, right hip
MØØ.852 Arthritis due to other bacteria, left hip
MØØ.859 Arthritis due to other bacteria, unspecified hip

● **MØØ.86 Arthritis due to other bacteria, knee**
MØØ.861 Arthritis due to other bacteria, right knee
MØØ.862 Arthritis due to other bacteria, left knee
MØØ.869 Arthritis due to other bacteria, unspecified knee

● **MØØ.87 Arthritis due to other bacteria, ankle and foot**
Arthritis due to other bacteria, tarsus, metatarsus, and phalanges
MØØ.871 Arthritis due to other bacteria, right ankle and foot
MØØ.872 Arthritis due to other bacteria, left ankle and foot
MØØ.879 Arthritis due to other bacteria, unspecified ankle and foot

MØØ.88 Arthritis due to other bacteria, vertebrae
MØØ.89 Polyarthritis due to other bacteria

MØØ.9 Pyogenic arthritis, unspecified
Infective arthritis NOS

● **MØ1 Direct infections of joint in infectious and parasitic diseases classified elsewhere**
Code first underlying disease, such as:
leprosy [Hansen's disease] (A3Ø.-)
mycoses (B35-B49)
O'nyong-nyong fever (A92.1)
paratyphoid fever (AØ1.1-AØ1.4)

Excludes1 arthropathy in Lyme disease (A69.23)
gonococcal arthritis (A54.42)
meningococcal arthritis (A39.83)
mumps arthritis (B26.85)
postinfective arthropathy (MØ2.-)
postmeningococcal arthritis (A39.84)
reactive arthritis (MØ2.3)
rubella arthritis (BØ6.82)
sarcoidosis arthritis (D86.86)
typhoid fever arthritis (AØ1.Ø4)
tuberculosis arthritis (A18.Ø1-A18.Ø2)

● **MØ1.X Direct infection of joint in infectious and parasitic diseases classified elsewhere**
MØ1.XØ Direct infection of unspecified joint in infectious and parasitic diseases classified elsewhere

● **MØ1.X1 Direct infection of shoulder joint in infectious and parasitic diseases classified elsewhere**
MØ1.X11 Direct infection of right shoulder in infectious and parasitic diseases classified elsewhere
MØ1.X12 Direct infection of left shoulder in infectious and parasitic diseases classified elsewhere
MØ1.X19 Direct infection of unspecified shoulder in infectious and parasitic diseases classified elsewhere

● **MØ1.X2 Direct infection of elbow in infectious and parasitic diseases classified elsewhere**
MØ1.X21 Direct infection of right elbow in infectious and parasitic diseases classified elsewhere
MØ1.X22 Direct infection of left elbow in infectious and parasitic diseases classified elsewhere
MØ1.X29 Direct infection of unspecified elbow in infectious and parasitic diseases classified elsewhere

CHAPTER 13 (MØØ-M99)

● MØ1.X3 **Direct infection of wrist in infectious and parasitic diseases classified elsewhere**
Direct infection of carpal bones in infectious and parasitic diseases classified elsewhere
MØ1.X31 **Direct infection of right wrist in infectious and parasitic diseases classified elsewhere**
MØ1.X32 **Direct infection of left wrist in infectious and parasitic diseases classified elsewhere**
MØ1.X39 **Direct infection of unspecified wrist in infectious and parasitic diseases classified elsewhere**

● MØ1.X4 **Direct infection of hand in infectious and parasitic diseases classified elsewhere**
Direct infection of metacarpus and phalanges in infectious and parasitic diseases classified elsewhere
MØ1.X41 **Direct infection of right hand in infectious and parasitic diseases classified elsewhere**
MØ1.X42 **Direct infection of left hand in infectious and parasitic diseases classified elsewhere**
MØ1.X49 **Direct infection of unspecified hand in infectious and parasitic diseases classified elsewhere**

● MØ1.X5 **Direct infection of hip in infectious and parasitic diseases classified elsewhere**
MØ1.X51 **Direct infection of right hip in infectious and parasitic diseases classified elsewhere**
MØ1.X52 **Direct infection of left hip in infectious and parasitic diseases classified elsewhere**
MØ1.X59 **Direct infection of unspecified hip in infectious and parasitic diseases classified elsewhere**

● MØ1.X6 **Direct infection of knee in infectious and parasitic diseases classified elsewhere**
MØ1.X61 **Direct infection of right knee in infectious and parasitic diseases classified elsewhere**
MØ1.X62 **Direct infection of left knee in infectious and parasitic diseases classified elsewhere**
MØ1.X69 **Direct infection of unspecified knee in infectious and parasitic diseases classified elsewhere**

● MØ1.X7 **Direct infection of ankle and foot in infectious and parasitic diseases classified elsewhere**
Direct infection of tarsus, metatarsus and phalanges in infectious and parasitic diseases classified elsewhere
MØ1.X71 **Direct infection of right ankle and foot in infectious and parasitic diseases classified elsewhere**
MØ1.X72 **Direct infection of left ankle and foot in infectious and parasitic diseases classified elsewhere**
MØ1.X79 **Direct infection of unspecified ankle and foot in infectious and parasitic diseases classified elsewhere**

MØ1.X8 **Direct infection of vertebrae in infectious and parasitic diseases classified elsewhere**

MØ1.X9 **Direct infection of multiple joints in infectious and parasitic diseases classified elsewhere**

● MØ2 **Postinfective and reactive arthropathies**
Code first *underlying disease, such as:*
- congenital syphilis [Clutton's joints] (A5Ø.5)
- enteritis due to Yersinia enterocolitica (AØ4.6)
- infective endocarditis (I33.Ø)
- viral hepatitis (B15-B19)

Excludes1 Behçet's disease (M35.2)
- direct infections of joint in infectious and parasitic diseases classified elsewhere (MØ1.-)
- postmeningococcal arthritis (A39.84)
- mumps arthritis (B26.85)
- rubella arthritis (BØ6.82)
- syphilis arthritis (late) (A52.77)
- rheumatic fever (IØØ)
- tabetic arthropathy [Charcôt's] (A52.16)

● MØ2.Ø **Arthropathy following intestinal bypass**
MØ2.ØØ **Arthropathy following intestinal bypass, unspecified site**
● MØ2.Ø1 **Arthropathy following intestinal bypass, shoulder**
MØ2.Ø11 **Arthropathy following intestinal bypass, right shoulder**
MØ2.Ø12 **Arthropathy following intestinal bypass, left shoulder**
MØ2.Ø19 **Arthropathy following intestinal bypass, unspecified shoulder**
● MØ2.Ø2 **Arthropathy following intestinal bypass, elbow**
MØ2.Ø21 **Arthropathy following intestinal bypass, right elbow**
MØ2.Ø22 **Arthropathy following intestinal bypass, left elbow**
MØ2.Ø29 **Arthropathy following intestinal bypass, unspecified elbow**
● MØ2.Ø3 **Arthropathy following intestinal bypass, wrist**
Arthropathy following intestinal bypass, carpal bones
MØ2.Ø31 **Arthropathy following intestinal bypass, right wrist**
MØ2.Ø32 **Arthropathy following intestinal bypass, left wrist**
MØ2.Ø39 **Arthropathy following intestinal bypass, unspecified wrist**
● MØ2.Ø4 **Arthropathy following intestinal bypass, hand**
Arthropathy following intestinal bypass, metacarpals and phalanges
MØ2.Ø41 **Arthropathy following intestinal bypass, right hand**
MØ2.Ø42 **Arthropathy following intestinal bypass, left hand**
MØ2.Ø49 **Arthropathy following intestinal bypass, unspecified hand**
● MØ2.Ø5 **Arthropathy following intestinal bypass, hip**
MØ2.Ø51 **Arthropathy following intestinal bypass, right hip**
MØ2.Ø52 **Arthropathy following intestinal bypass, left hip**
MØ2.Ø59 **Arthropathy following intestinal bypass, unspecified hip**
● MØ2.Ø6 **Arthropathy following intestinal bypass, knee**
MØ2.Ø61 **Arthropathy following intestinal bypass, right knee**
MØ2.Ø62 **Arthropathy following intestinal bypass, left knee**
MØ2.Ø69 **Arthropathy following intestinal bypass, unspecified knee**

● M02.07 Arthropathy following intestinal bypass, ankle and foot
Arthropathy following intestinal bypass, tarsus, metatarsus and phalanges
M02.071 Arthropathy following intestinal bypass, right ankle and foot
M02.072 Arthropathy following intestinal bypass, left ankle and foot
M02.079 Arthropathy following intestinal bypass, unspecified ankle and foot
M02.08 Arthropathy following intestinal bypass, vertebrae
M02.09 Arthropathy following intestinal bypass, multiple sites

● M02.1 Postdysenteric arthropathy
M02.10 Postdysenteric arthropathy, unspecified site
● M02.11 Postdysenteric arthropathy, shoulder
M02.111 Postdysenteric arthropathy, right shoulder
M02.112 Postdysenteric arthropathy, left shoulder
M02.119 Postdysenteric arthropathy, unspecified shoulder
● M02.12 Postdysenteric arthropathy, elbow
M02.121 Postdysenteric arthropathy, right elbow
M02.122 Postdysenteric arthropathy, left elbow
M02.129 Postdysenteric arthropathy, unspecified elbow
● M02.13 Postdysenteric arthropathy, wrist
Postdysenteric arthropathy, carpal bones
M02.131 Postdysenteric arthropathy, right wrist
M02.132 Postdysenteric arthropathy, left wrist
M02.139 Postdysenteric arthropathy, unspecified wrist
● M02.14 Postdysenteric arthropathy, hand
Postdysenteric arthropathy, metacarpus and phalanges
M02.141 Postdysenteric arthropathy, right hand
M02.142 Postdysenteric arthropathy, left hand
M02.149 Postdysenteric arthropathy, unspecified hand
● M02.15 Postdysenteric arthropathy, hip
M02.151 Postdysenteric arthropathy, right hip
M02.152 Postdysenteric arthropathy, left hip
M02.159 Postdysenteric arthropathy, unspecified hip
● M02.16 Postdysenteric arthropathy, knee
M02.161 Postdysenteric arthropathy, right knee
M02.162 Postdysenteric arthropathy, left knee
M02.169 Postdysenteric arthropathy, unspecified knee
● M02.17 Postdysenteric arthropathy, ankle and foot
Postdysenteric arthropathy, tarsus, metatarsus and phalanges
M02.171 Postdysenteric arthropathy, right ankle and foot
M02.172 Postdysenteric arthropathy, left ankle and foot
M02.179 Postdysenteric arthropathy, unspecified ankle and foot
M02.18 Postdysenteric arthropathy, vertebrae
M02.19 Postdysenteric arthropathy, multiple sites

● M02.2 Postimmunization arthropathy
M02.20 Postimmunization arthropathy, unspecified site
● M02.21 Postimmunization arthropathy, shoulder
M02.211 Postimmunization arthropathy, right shoulder
M02.212 Postimmunization arthropathy, left shoulder
M02.219 Postimmunization arthropathy, unspecified shoulder
● M02.22 Postimmunization arthropathy, elbow
M02.221 Postimmunization arthropathy, right elbow
M02.222 Postimmunization arthropathy, left elbow
M02.229 Postimmunization arthropathy, unspecified elbow
● M02.23 Postimmunization arthropathy, wrist
Postimmunization arthropathy, carpal bones
M02.231 Postimmunization arthropathy, right wrist
M02.232 Postimmunization arthropathy, left wrist
M02.239 Postimmunization arthropathy, unspecified wrist
● M02.24 Postimmunization arthropathy, hand
Postimmunization arthropathy, metacarpus and phalanges
M02.241 Postimmunization arthropathy, right hand
M02.242 Postimmunization arthropathy, left hand
M02.249 Postimmunization arthropathy, unspecified hand
● M02.25 Postimmunization arthropathy, hip
M02.251 Postimmunization arthropathy, right hip
M02.252 Postimmunization arthropathy, left hip
M02.259 Postimmunization arthropathy, unspecified hip
● M02.26 Postimmunization arthropathy, knee
M02.261 Postimmunization arthropathy, right knee
M02.262 Postimmunization arthropathy, left knee
M02.269 Postimmunization arthropathy, unspecified knee
● M02.27 Postimmunization arthropathy, ankle and foot
Postimmunization arthropathy, tarsus, metatarsus and phalanges
M02.271 Postimmunization arthropathy, right ankle and foot
M02.272 Postimmunization arthropathy, left ankle and foot
M02.279 Postimmunization arthropathy, unspecified ankle and foot
M02.28 Postimmunization arthropathy, vertebrae
M02.29 Postimmunization arthropathy, multiple sites

● M02.3 Reiter's disease
Reactive arthritis
M02.30 Reiter's disease, unspecified site
● M02.31 Reiter's disease, shoulder
M02.311 Reiter's disease, right shoulder
M02.312 Reiter's disease, left shoulder
M02.319 Reiter's disease, unspecified shoulder

● M02.32 Reiter's disease, elbow
- M02.321 Reiter's disease, right elbow
- M02.322 Reiter's disease, left elbow
- M02.329 Reiter's disease, unspecified elbow

● M02.33 Reiter's disease, wrist
Reiter's disease, carpal bones
- M02.331 Reiter's disease, right wrist
- M02.332 Reiter's disease, left wrist
- M02.339 Reiter's disease, unspecified wrist

● M02.34 Reiter's disease, hand
Reiter's disease, metacarpus and phalanges
- M02.341 Reiter's disease, right hand
- M02.342 Reiter's disease, left hand
- M02.349 Reiter's disease, unspecified hand

● M02.35 Reiter's disease, hip
- M02.351 Reiter's disease, right hip
- M02.352 Reiter's disease, left hip
- M02.359 Reiter's disease, unspecified hip

● M02.36 Reiter's disease, knee
- M02.361 Reiter's disease, right knee
- M02.362 Reiter's disease, left knee
- M02.369 Reiter's disease, unspecified knee

● M02.37 Reiter's disease, ankle and foot
Reiter's disease, tarsus, metatarsus and phalanges
- M02.371 Reiter's disease, right ankle and foot
- M02.372 Reiter's disease, left ankle and foot
- M02.379 Reiter's disease, unspecified ankle and foot

M02.38 Reiter's disease, vertebrae

M02.39 Reiter's disease, multiple sites

● M02.8 Other reactive arthropathies

M02.80 Other reactive arthropathies, unspecified site

● M02.81 Other reactive arthropathies, shoulder
- M02.811 Other reactive arthropathies, right shoulder
- M02.812 Other reactive arthropathies, left shoulder
- M02.819 Other reactive arthropathies, unspecified shoulder

● M02.82 Other reactive arthropathies, elbow
- M02.821 Other reactive arthropathies, right elbow
- M02.822 Other reactive arthropathies, left elbow
- M02.829 Other reactive arthropathies, unspecified elbow

● M02.83 Other reactive arthropathies, wrist
Other reactive arthropathies, carpal bones
- M02.831 Other reactive arthropathies, right wrist
- M02.832 Other reactive arthropathies, left wrist
- M02.839 Other reactive arthropathies, unspecified wrist

● M02.84 Other reactive arthropathies, hand
Other reactive arthropathies, metacarpus and phalanges
- M02.841 Other reactive arthropathies, right hand
- M02.842 Other reactive arthropathies, left hand
- M02.849 Other reactive arthropathies, unspecified hand

● M02.85 Other reactive arthropathies, hip
- M02.851 Other reactive arthropathies, right hip
- M02.852 Other reactive arthropathies, left hip
- M02.859 Other reactive arthropathies, unspecified hip

● M02.86 Other reactive arthropathies, knee
- M02.861 Other reactive arthropathies, right knee
- M02.862 Other reactive arthropathies, left knee
- M02.869 Other reactive arthropathies, unspecified knee

● M02.87 Other reactive arthropathies, ankle and foot
Other reactive arthropathies, tarsus, metatarsus and phalanges
- M02.871 Other reactive arthropathies, right ankle and foot
- M02.872 Other reactive arthropathies, left ankle and foot
- M02.879 Other reactive arthropathies, unspecified ankle and foot

M02.88 Other reactive arthropathies, vertebrae

M02.89 Other reactive arthropathies, multiple sites

M02.9 Reactive arthropathy, unspecified

AUTOINFLAMMATORY SYNDROMES (M04) ◀

● M04 Autoinflammatory syndromes ◀

Excludes2 Crohn's disease (K50.-) ◀

M04.1 Periodic fever syndromes ◀
- Familial Mediterranean fever ◀
- Hyperimmunoglobin D syndrome ◀
- Mevalonate kinase deficiency ◀
- Tumor necrosis factor receptor associated periodic syndrome [TRAPS] ◀

M04.2 Cryopyrin-associated periodic syndromes ◀
- Chronic infantile neurological, cutaneous and articular syndrome [CINCA] ◀
- Familial cold autoinflammatory syndrome ◀
- Familial cold urticaria ◀
- Muckle-Wells syndrome ◀
- Neonatal onset multisystemic inflammatory disorder [NOMID] ◀

M04.8 Other autoinflammatory syndromes ◀
- Blau syndrome ◀
- Deficiency of interleukin 1 receptor antagonist [DIRA] ◀
- Majeed syndrome ◀
- Periodic fever, aphthous stomatitis, pharyngitis, and adenopathy syndrome [PFAPA] ◀
- Pyogenic arthritis, pyoderma gangrenosum, and acne syndrome [PAPA] ◀

M04.9 Autoinflammatory syndrome, unspecified ◀

INFLAMMATORY POLYARTHROPATHIES (M05-M14)

● M05 Rheumatoid arthritis with rheumatoid factor

Excludes1 rheumatic fever (I00)
juvenile rheumatoid arthritis (M08.-)
rheumatoid arthritis of spine (M45.-)

● M05.0 Felty's syndrome
Rheumatoid arthritis with splenoadenomegaly and leukopenia

M05.00 Felty's syndrome, unspecified site

● M05.01 Felty's syndrome, shoulder
- M05.011 Felty's syndrome, right shoulder
- M05.012 Felty's syndrome, left shoulder
- M05.019 Felty's syndrome, unspecified shoulder

CHAPTER 13 (M00-M99)

Item 13–1 Rheumatoid arthritis (RA) is a chronic systemic inflammatory autoimmune disease of undetermined etiology involving primarily the synovial membranes and articular structures of multiple joints. It can also affect other organs, including the eyes, blood vessels, heart, and lungs. The disease is often progressive. In late stages, deformity, ankylosis, and other **inflammatory polyarthropathies** develop.

● M05.02 Felty's syndrome, elbow
- M05.021 Felty's syndrome, right elbow
- M05.022 Felty's syndrome, left elbow
- M05.029 Felty's syndrome, unspecified elbow

● M05.03 Felty's syndrome, wrist
Felty's syndrome, carpal bones
- M05.031 Felty's syndrome, right wrist
- M05.032 Felty's syndrome, left wrist
- M05.039 Felty's syndrome, unspecified wrist

● M05.04 Felty's syndrome, hand
Felty's syndrome, metacarpus and phalanges
- M05.041 Felty's syndrome, right hand
- M05.042 Felty's syndrome, left hand
- M05.049 Felty's syndrome, unspecified hand

● M05.05 Felty's syndrome, hip
- M05.051 Felty's syndrome, right hip
- M05.052 Felty's syndrome, left hip
- M05.059 Felty's syndrome, unspecified hip

● M05.06 Felty's syndrome, knee
- M05.061 Felty's syndrome, right knee
- M05.062 Felty's syndrome, left knee
- M05.069 Felty's syndrome, unspecified knee

● M05.07 Felty's syndrome, ankle and foot
Felty's syndrome, tarsus, metatarsus and phalanges
- M05.071 Felty's syndrome, right ankle and foot
- M05.072 Felty's syndrome, left ankle and foot
- M05.079 Felty's syndrome, unspecified ankle and foot

M05.09 Felty's syndrome, multiple sites

● M05.1 Rheumatoid lung disease with rheumatoid arthritis

M05.10 Rheumatoid lung disease with rheumatoid arthritis of unspecified site

● M05.11 Rheumatoid lung disease with rheumatoid arthritis of shoulder
- M05.111 Rheumatoid lung disease with rheumatoid arthritis of right shoulder
- M05.112 Rheumatoid lung disease with rheumatoid arthritis of left shoulder
- M05.119 Rheumatoid lung disease with rheumatoid arthritis of unspecified shoulder

● M05.12 Rheumatoid lung disease with rheumatoid arthritis of elbow
- M05.121 Rheumatoid lung disease with rheumatoid arthritis of right elbow
- M05.122 Rheumatoid lung disease with rheumatoid arthritis of left elbow
- M05.129 Rheumatoid lung disease with rheumatoid arthritis of unspecified elbow

● M05.13 Rheumatoid lung disease with rheumatoid arthritis of wrist
Rheumatoid lung disease with rheumatoid arthritis, carpal bones
- M05.131 Rheumatoid lung disease with rheumatoid arthritis of right wrist
- M05.132 Rheumatoid lung disease with rheumatoid arthritis of left wrist
- M05.139 Rheumatoid lung disease with rheumatoid arthritis of unspecified wrist

● M05.14 Rheumatoid lung disease with rheumatoid arthritis of hand
Rheumatoid lung disease with rheumatoid arthritis, metacarpus and phalanges
- M05.141 Rheumatoid lung disease with rheumatoid arthritis of right hand
- M05.142 Rheumatoid lung disease with rheumatoid arthritis of left hand
- M05.149 Rheumatoid lung disease with rheumatoid arthritis of unspecified hand

● M05.15 Rheumatoid lung disease with rheumatoid arthritis of hip
- M05.151 Rheumatoid lung disease with rheumatoid arthritis of right hip
- M05.152 Rheumatoid lung disease with rheumatoid arthritis of left hip
- M05.159 Rheumatoid lung disease with rheumatoid arthritis of unspecified hip

● M05.16 Rheumatoid lung disease with rheumatoid arthritis of knee
- M05.161 Rheumatoid lung disease with rheumatoid arthritis of right knee
- M05.162 Rheumatoid lung disease with rheumatoid arthritis of left knee
- M05.169 Rheumatoid lung disease with rheumatoid arthritis of unspecified knee

● M05.17 Rheumatoid lung disease with rheumatoid arthritis of ankle and foot
Rheumatoid lung disease with rheumatoid arthritis, tarsus, metatarsus and phalanges
- M05.171 Rheumatoid lung disease with rheumatoid arthritis of right ankle and foot
- M05.172 Rheumatoid lung disease with rheumatoid arthritis of left ankle and foot
- M05.179 Rheumatoid lung disease with rheumatoid arthritis of unspecified ankle and foot

M05.19 Rheumatoid lung disease with rheumatoid arthritis of multiple sites

● M05.2 Rheumatoid vasculitis with rheumatoid arthritis

M05.20 Rheumatoid vasculitis with rheumatoid arthritis of unspecified site

● M05.21 Rheumatoid vasculitis with rheumatoid arthritis of shoulder
- M05.211 Rheumatoid vasculitis with rheumatoid arthritis of right shoulder
- M05.212 Rheumatoid vasculitis with rheumatoid arthritis of left shoulder
- M05.219 Rheumatoid vasculitis with rheumatoid arthritis of unspecified shoulder

● M05.22 Rheumatoid vasculitis with rheumatoid arthritis of elbow
- M05.221 Rheumatoid vasculitis with rheumatoid arthritis of right elbow
- M05.222 Rheumatoid vasculitis with rheumatoid arthritis of left elbow
- M05.229 Rheumatoid vasculitis with rheumatoid arthritis of unspecified elbow

CHAPTER 13 (M00-M99)

◀ New ◀ Revised ~~deleted~~ Deleted OGCR Official Guidelines X Assign placeholder X ● Use Additional Character(s)
Excludes 1 | Excludes 2 | Includes | Use additional | Code first | Code also | Unspecified

● **M05.23 Rheumatoid vasculitis with rheumatoid arthritis of wrist**
Rheumatoid vasculitis with rheumatoid arthritis, carpal bones
M05.231 Rheumatoid vasculitis with rheumatoid arthritis of right wrist
M05.232 Rheumatoid vasculitis with rheumatoid arthritis of left wrist
M05.239 Rheumatoid vasculitis with rheumatoid arthritis of unspecified wrist
● **M05.24 Rheumatoid vasculitis with rheumatoid arthritis of hand**
Rheumatoid vasculitis with rheumatoid arthritis, metacarpus and phalanges
M05.241 Rheumatoid vasculitis with rheumatoid arthritis of right hand
M05.242 Rheumatoid vasculitis with rheumatoid arthritis of left hand
M05.249 Rheumatoid vasculitis with rheumatoid arthritis of unspecified hand
● **M05.25 Rheumatoid vasculitis with rheumatoid arthritis of hip**
M05.251 Rheumatoid vasculitis with rheumatoid arthritis of right hip
M05.252 Rheumatoid vasculitis with rheumatoid arthritis of left hip
M05.259 Rheumatoid vasculitis with rheumatoid arthritis of unspecified hip
● **M05.26 Rheumatoid vasculitis with rheumatoid arthritis of knee**
M05.261 Rheumatoid vasculitis with rheumatoid arthritis of right knee
M05.262 Rheumatoid vasculitis with rheumatoid arthritis of left knee
M05.269 Rheumatoid vasculitis with rheumatoid arthritis of unspecified knee
● **M05.27 Rheumatoid vasculitis with rheumatoid arthritis of ankle and foot**
Rheumatoid vasculitis with rheumatoid arthritis, tarsus, metatarsus and phalanges
M05.271 Rheumatoid vasculitis with rheumatoid arthritis of right ankle and foot
M05.272 Rheumatoid vasculitis with rheumatoid arthritis of left ankle and foot
M05.279 Rheumatoid vasculitis with rheumatoid arthritis of unspecified ankle and foot
M05.29 Rheumatoid vasculitis with rheumatoid arthritis of multiple sites
● **M05.3 Rheumatoid heart disease with rheumatoid arthritis**
Rheumatoid carditis
Rheumatoid endocarditis
Rheumatoid myocarditis
Rheumatoid pericarditis
M05.30 Rheumatoid heart disease with rheumatoid arthritis of unspecified site
● **M05.31 Rheumatoid heart disease with rheumatoid arthritis of shoulder**
M05.311 Rheumatoid heart disease with rheumatoid arthritis of right shoulder
M05.312 Rheumatoid heart disease with rheumatoid arthritis of left shoulder
M05.319 Rheumatoid heart disease with rheumatoid arthritis of unspecified shoulder
● **M05.32 Rheumatoid heart disease with rheumatoid arthritis of elbow**
M05.321 Rheumatoid heart disease with rheumatoid arthritis of right elbow
M05.322 Rheumatoid heart disease with rheumatoid arthritis of left elbow
M05.329 Rheumatoid heart disease with rheumatoid arthritis of unspecified elbow
● **M05.33 Rheumatoid heart disease with rheumatoid arthritis of wrist**
Rheumatoid heart disease with rheumatoid arthritis, carpal bones
M05.331 Rheumatoid heart disease with rheumatoid arthritis of right wrist
M05.332 Rheumatoid heart disease with rheumatoid arthritis of left wrist
M05.339 Rheumatoid heart disease with rheumatoid arthritis of unspecified wrist
● **M05.34 Rheumatoid heart disease with rheumatoid arthritis of hand**
Rheumatoid heart disease with rheumatoid arthritis, metacarpus and phalanges
M05.341 Rheumatoid heart disease with rheumatoid arthritis of right hand
M05.342 Rheumatoid heart disease with rheumatoid arthritis of left hand
M05.349 Rheumatoid heart disease with rheumatoid arthritis of unspecified hand
● **M05.35 Rheumatoid heart disease with rheumatoid arthritis of hip**
M05.351 Rheumatoid heart disease with rheumatoid arthritis of right hip
M05.352 Rheumatoid heart disease with rheumatoid arthritis of left hip
M05.359 Rheumatoid heart disease with rheumatoid arthritis of unspecified hip
● **M05.36 Rheumatoid heart disease with rheumatoid arthritis of knee**
M05.361 Rheumatoid heart disease with rheumatoid arthritis of right knee
M05.362 Rheumatoid heart disease with rheumatoid arthritis of left knee
M05.369 Rheumatoid heart disease with rheumatoid arthritis of unspecified knee
● **M05.37 Rheumatoid heart disease with rheumatoid arthritis of ankle and foot**
Rheumatoid heart disease with rheumatoid arthritis, tarsus, metatarsus and phalanges
M05.371 Rheumatoid heart disease with rheumatoid arthritis of right ankle and foot
M05.372 Rheumatoid heart disease with rheumatoid arthritis of left ankle and foot
M05.379 Rheumatoid heart disease with rheumatoid arthritis of unspecified ankle and foot
M05.39 Rheumatoid heart disease with rheumatoid arthritis of multiple sites

CHAPTER 13 (M00-M99)

● M05.4 Rheumatoid myopathy with rheumatoid arthritis
M05.40 Rheumatoid myopathy with rheumatoid arthritis of unspecified site
● M05.41 Rheumatoid myopathy with rheumatoid arthritis of shoulder
M05.411 Rheumatoid myopathy with rheumatoid arthritis of right shoulder
M05.412 Rheumatoid myopathy with rheumatoid arthritis of left shoulder
M05.419 Rheumatoid myopathy with rheumatoid arthritis of unspecified shoulder
● M05.42 Rheumatoid myopathy with rheumatoid arthritis of elbow
M05.421 Rheumatoid myopathy with rheumatoid arthritis of right elbow
M05.422 Rheumatoid myopathy with rheumatoid arthritis of left elbow
M05.429 Rheumatoid myopathy with rheumatoid arthritis of unspecified elbow
● M05.43 Rheumatoid myopathy with rheumatoid arthritis of wrist
Rheumatoid myopathy with rheumatoid arthritis, carpal bones
M05.431 Rheumatoid myopathy with rheumatoid arthritis of right wrist
M05.432 Rheumatoid myopathy with rheumatoid arthritis of left wrist
M05.439 Rheumatoid myopathy with rheumatoid arthritis of unspecified wrist
● M05.44 Rheumatoid myopathy with rheumatoid arthritis of hand
Rheumatoid myopathy with rheumatoid arthritis, metacarpus and phalanges
M05.441 Rheumatoid myopathy with rheumatoid arthritis of right hand
M05.442 Rheumatoid myopathy with rheumatoid arthritis of left hand
M05.449 Rheumatoid myopathy with rheumatoid arthritis of unspecified hand
● M05.45 Rheumatoid myopathy with rheumatoid arthritis of hip
M05.451 Rheumatoid myopathy with rheumatoid arthritis of right hip
M05.452 Rheumatoid myopathy with rheumatoid arthritis of left hip
M05.459 Rheumatoid myopathy with rheumatoid arthritis of unspecified hip
● M05.46 Rheumatoid myopathy with rheumatoid arthritis of knee
M05.461 Rheumatoid myopathy with rheumatoid arthritis of right knee
M05.462 Rheumatoid myopathy with rheumatoid arthritis of left knee
M05.469 Rheumatoid myopathy with rheumatoid arthritis of unspecified knee
● M05.47 Rheumatoid myopathy with rheumatoid arthritis of ankle and foot
Rheumatoid myopathy with rheumatoid arthritis, tarsus, metatarsus and phalanges
M05.471 Rheumatoid myopathy with rheumatoid arthritis of right ankle and foot
M05.472 Rheumatoid myopathy with rheumatoid arthritis of left ankle and foot
M05.479 Rheumatoid myopathy with rheumatoid arthritis of unspecified ankle and foot
M05.49 Rheumatoid myopathy with rheumatoid arthritis of multiple sites
● M05.5 Rheumatoid polyneuropathy with rheumatoid arthritis
M05.50 Rheumatoid polyneuropathy with rheumatoid arthritis of unspecified site
● M05.51 Rheumatoid polyneuropathy with rheumatoid arthritis of shoulder
M05.511 Rheumatoid polyneuropathy with rheumatoid arthritis of right shoulder
M05.512 Rheumatoid polyneuropathy with rheumatoid arthritis of left shoulder
M05.519 Rheumatoid polyneuropathy with rheumatoid arthritis of unspecified shoulder
● M05.52 Rheumatoid polyneuropathy with rheumatoid arthritis of elbow
M05.521 Rheumatoid polyneuropathy with rheumatoid arthritis of right elbow
M05.522 Rheumatoid polyneuropathy with rheumatoid arthritis of left elbow
M05.529 Rheumatoid polyneuropathy with rheumatoid arthritis of unspecified elbow
● M05.53 Rheumatoid polyneuropathy with rheumatoid arthritis of wrist
Rheumatoid polyneuropathy with rheumatoid arthritis, carpal bones
M05.531 Rheumatoid polyneuropathy with rheumatoid arthritis of right wrist
M05.532 Rheumatoid polyneuropathy with rheumatoid arthritis of left wrist
M05.539 Rheumatoid polyneuropathy with rheumatoid arthritis of unspecified wrist
● M05.54 Rheumatoid polyneuropathy with rheumatoid arthritis of hand
Rheumatoid polyneuropathy with rheumatoid arthritis, metacarpus and phalanges
M05.541 Rheumatoid polyneuropathy with rheumatoid arthritis of right hand
M05.542 Rheumatoid polyneuropathy with rheumatoid arthritis of left hand
M05.549 Rheumatoid polyneuropathy with rheumatoid arthritis of unspecified hand
● M05.55 Rheumatoid polyneuropathy with rheumatoid arthritis of hip
M05.551 Rheumatoid polyneuropathy with rheumatoid arthritis of right hip
M05.552 Rheumatoid polyneuropathy with rheumatoid arthritis of left hip
M05.559 Rheumatoid polyneuropathy with rheumatoid arthritis of unspecified hip

● **M05.56 Rheumatoid polyneuropathy with rheumatoid arthritis of knee**

M05.561 Rheumatoid polyneuropathy with rheumatoid arthritis of right knee

M05.562 Rheumatoid polyneuropathy with rheumatoid arthritis of left knee

M05.569 Rheumatoid polyneuropathy with rheumatoid arthritis of unspecified knee

● **M05.57 Rheumatoid polyneuropathy with rheumatoid arthritis of ankle and foot**

Rheumatoid polyneuropathy with rheumatoid arthritis, tarsus, metatarsus and phalanges

M05.571 Rheumatoid polyneuropathy with rheumatoid arthritis of right ankle and foot

M05.572 Rheumatoid polyneuropathy with rheumatoid arthritis of left ankle and foot

M05.579 Rheumatoid polyneuropathy with rheumatoid arthritis of unspecified ankle and foot

M05.59 Rheumatoid polyneuropathy with rheumatoid arthritis of multiple sites

● **M05.6 Rheumatoid arthritis with involvement of other organs and systems**

M05.60 Rheumatoid arthritis of unspecified site with involvement of other organs and systems

● **M05.61 Rheumatoid arthritis of shoulder with involvement of other organs and systems**

M05.611 Rheumatoid arthritis of right shoulder with involvement of other organs and systems

M05.612 Rheumatoid arthritis of left shoulder with involvement of other organs and systems

M05.619 Rheumatoid arthritis of unspecified shoulder with involvement of other organs and systems

● **M05.62 Rheumatoid arthritis of elbow with involvement of other organs and systems**

M05.621 Rheumatoid arthritis of right elbow with involvement of other organs and systems

M05.622 Rheumatoid arthritis of left elbow with involvement of other organs and systems

M05.629 Rheumatoid arthritis of unspecified elbow with involvement of other organs and systems

● **M05.63 Rheumatoid arthritis of wrist with involvement of other organs and systems**

Rheumatoid arthritis of carpal bones with involvement of other organs and systems

M05.631 Rheumatoid arthritis of right wrist with involvement of other organs and systems

M05.632 Rheumatoid arthritis of left wrist with involvement of other organs and systems

M05.639 Rheumatoid arthritis of unspecified wrist with involvement of other organs and systems

● **M05.64 Rheumatoid arthritis of hand with involvement of other organs and systems**

Rheumatoid arthritis of metacarpus and phalanges with involvement of other organs and systems

M05.641 Rheumatoid arthritis of right hand with involvement of other organs and systems

M05.642 Rheumatoid arthritis of left hand with involvement of other organs and systems

M05.649 Rheumatoid arthritis of unspecified hand with involvement of other organs and systems

● **M05.65 Rheumatoid arthritis of hip with involvement of other organs and systems**

M05.651 Rheumatoid arthritis of right hip with involvement of other organs and systems

M05.652 Rheumatoid arthritis of left hip with involvement of other organs and systems

M05.659 Rheumatoid arthritis of unspecified hip with involvement of other organs and systems

● **M05.66 Rheumatoid arthritis of knee with involvement of other organs and systems**

M05.661 Rheumatoid arthritis of right knee with involvement of other organs and systems

M05.662 Rheumatoid arthritis of left knee with involvement of other organs and systems

M05.669 Rheumatoid arthritis of unspecified knee with involvement of other organs and systems

● **M05.67 Rheumatoid arthritis of ankle and foot with involvement of other organs and systems**

Rheumatoid arthritis of tarsus, metatarsus and phalanges with involvement of other organs and systems

M05.671 Rheumatoid arthritis of right ankle and foot with involvement of other organs and systems

M05.672 Rheumatoid arthritis of left ankle and foot with involvement of other organs and systems

M05.679 Rheumatoid arthritis of unspecified ankle and foot with involvement of other organs and systems

M05.69 Rheumatoid arthritis of multiple sites with involvement of other organs and systems

● **M05.7 Rheumatoid arthritis with rheumatoid factor without organ or systems involvement**

M05.70 Rheumatoid arthritis with rheumatoid factor of unspecified site without organ or systems involvement

● **M05.71 Rheumatoid arthritis with rheumatoid factor of shoulder without organ or systems involvement**

M05.711 Rheumatoid arthritis with rheumatoid factor of right shoulder without organ or systems involvement

M05.712 Rheumatoid arthritis with rheumatoid factor of left shoulder without organ or systems involvement

M05.719 Rheumatoid arthritis with rheumatoid factor of unspecified shoulder without organ or systems involvement

CHAPTER 13 (M00-M99)

● M05.72 Rheumatoid arthritis with rheumatoid factor of elbow without organ or systems involvement
- M05.721 Rheumatoid arthritis with rheumatoid factor of right elbow without organ or systems involvement
- M05.722 Rheumatoid arthritis with rheumatoid factor of left elbow without organ or systems involvement
- M05.729 Rheumatoid arthritis with rheumatoid factor of unspecified elbow without organ or systems involvement

● M05.73 Rheumatoid arthritis with rheumatoid factor of wrist without organ or systems involvement
- M05.731 Rheumatoid arthritis with rheumatoid factor of right wrist without organ or systems involvement
- M05.732 Rheumatoid arthritis with rheumatoid factor of left wrist without organ or systems involvement
- M05.739 Rheumatoid arthritis with rheumatoid factor of unspecified wrist without organ or systems involvement

● M05.74 Rheumatoid arthritis with rheumatoid factor of hand without organ or systems involvement
- M05.741 Rheumatoid arthritis with rheumatoid factor of right hand without organ or systems involvement
- M05.742 Rheumatoid arthritis with rheumatoid factor of left hand without organ or systems involvement
- M05.749 Rheumatoid arthritis with rheumatoid factor of unspecified hand without organ or systems involvement

● M05.75 Rheumatoid arthritis with rheumatoid factor of hip without organ or systems involvement
- M05.751 Rheumatoid arthritis with rheumatoid factor of right hip without organ or systems involvement
- M05.752 Rheumatoid arthritis with rheumatoid factor of left hip without organ or systems involvement
- M05.759 Rheumatoid arthritis with rheumatoid factor of unspecified hip without organ or systems involvement

● M05.76 Rheumatoid arthritis with rheumatoid factor of knee without organ or systems involvement
- M05.761 Rheumatoid arthritis with rheumatoid factor of right knee without organ or systems involvement
- M05.762 Rheumatoid arthritis with rheumatoid factor of left knee without organ or systems involvement
- M05.769 Rheumatoid arthritis with rheumatoid factor of unspecified knee without organ or systems involvement

● M05.77 Rheumatoid arthritis with rheumatoid factor of ankle and foot without organ or systems involvement
- M05.771 Rheumatoid arthritis with rheumatoid factor of right ankle and foot without organ or systems involvement
- M05.772 Rheumatoid arthritis with rheumatoid factor of left ankle and foot without organ or systems involvement
- M05.779 Rheumatoid arthritis with rheumatoid factor of unspecified ankle and foot without organ or systems involvement

M05.79 Rheumatoid arthritis with rheumatoid factor of multiple sites without organ or systems involvement

● M05.8 Other rheumatoid arthritis with rheumatoid factor

M05.80 Other rheumatoid arthritis with rheumatoid factor of unspecified site

● M05.81 Other rheumatoid arthritis with rheumatoid factor of shoulder
- M05.811 Other rheumatoid arthritis with rheumatoid factor of right shoulder
- M05.812 Other rheumatoid arthritis with rheumatoid factor of left shoulder
- M05.819 Other rheumatoid arthritis with rheumatoid factor of unspecified shoulder

● M05.82 Other rheumatoid arthritis with rheumatoid factor of elbow
- M05.821 Other rheumatoid arthritis with rheumatoid factor of right elbow
- M05.822 Other rheumatoid arthritis with rheumatoid factor of left elbow
- M05.829 Other rheumatoid arthritis with rheumatoid factor of unspecified elbow

● M05.83 Other rheumatoid arthritis with rheumatoid factor of wrist
- M05.831 Other rheumatoid arthritis with rheumatoid factor of right wrist
- M05.832 Other rheumatoid arthritis with rheumatoid factor of left wrist
- M05.839 Other rheumatoid arthritis with rheumatoid factor of unspecified wrist

● M05.84 Other rheumatoid arthritis with rheumatoid factor of hand
- M05.841 Other rheumatoid arthritis with rheumatoid factor of right hand
- M05.842 Other rheumatoid arthritis with rheumatoid factor of left hand
- M05.849 Other rheumatoid arthritis with rheumatoid factor of unspecified hand

● M05.85 Other rheumatoid arthritis with rheumatoid factor of hip
- M05.851 Other rheumatoid arthritis with rheumatoid factor of right hip
- M05.852 Other rheumatoid arthritis with rheumatoid factor of left hip
- M05.859 Other rheumatoid arthritis with rheumatoid factor of unspecified hip

CHAPTER 13 (M00-M99)

● M05.86 Other rheumatoid arthritis with rheumatoid factor of knee
- M05.861 Other rheumatoid arthritis with rheumatoid factor of right knee
- M05.862 Other rheumatoid arthritis with rheumatoid factor of left knee
- M05.869 Other rheumatoid arthritis with rheumatoid factor of unspecified knee

● M05.87 Other rheumatoid arthritis with rheumatoid factor of ankle and foot
- M05.871 Other rheumatoid arthritis with rheumatoid factor of right ankle and foot
- M05.872 Other rheumatoid arthritis with rheumatoid factor of left ankle and foot
- M05.879 Other rheumatoid arthritis with rheumatoid factor of unspecified ankle and foot

M05.89 Other rheumatoid arthritis with rheumatoid factor of multiple sites

M05.9 Rheumatoid arthritis with rheumatoid factor, unspecified

● M06 Other rheumatoid arthritis

● M06.0 Rheumatoid arthritis without rheumatoid factor

M06.00 Rheumatoid arthritis without rheumatoid factor, unspecified site

● M06.01 Rheumatoid arthritis without rheumatoid factor, shoulder
- M06.011 Rheumatoid arthritis without rheumatoid factor, right shoulder
- M06.012 Rheumatoid arthritis without rheumatoid factor, left shoulder
- M06.019 Rheumatoid arthritis without rheumatoid factor, unspecified shoulder

● M06.02 Rheumatoid arthritis without rheumatoid factor, elbow
- M06.021 Rheumatoid arthritis without rheumatoid factor, right elbow
- M06.022 Rheumatoid arthritis without rheumatoid factor, left elbow
- M06.029 Rheumatoid arthritis without rheumatoid factor, unspecified elbow

● M06.03 Rheumatoid arthritis without rheumatoid factor, wrist
- M06.031 Rheumatoid arthritis without rheumatoid factor, right wrist
- M06.032 Rheumatoid arthritis without rheumatoid factor, left wrist
- M06.039 Rheumatoid arthritis without rheumatoid factor, unspecified wrist

● M06.04 Rheumatoid arthritis without rheumatoid factor, hand
- M06.041 Rheumatoid arthritis without rheumatoid factor, right hand
- M06.042 Rheumatoid arthritis without rheumatoid factor, left hand
- M06.049 Rheumatoid arthritis without rheumatoid factor, unspecified hand

● M06.05 Rheumatoid arthritis without rheumatoid factor, hip
- M06.051 Rheumatoid arthritis without rheumatoid factor, right hip
- M06.052 Rheumatoid arthritis without rheumatoid factor, left hip
- M06.059 Rheumatoid arthritis without rheumatoid factor, unspecified hip

● M06.06 Rheumatoid arthritis without rheumatoid factor, knee
- M06.061 Rheumatoid arthritis without rheumatoid factor, right knee
- M06.062 Rheumatoid arthritis without rheumatoid factor, left knee
- M06.069 Rheumatoid arthritis without rheumatoid factor, unspecified knee

● M06.07 Rheumatoid arthritis without rheumatoid factor, ankle and foot
- M06.071 Rheumatoid arthritis without rheumatoid factor, right ankle and foot
- M06.072 Rheumatoid arthritis without rheumatoid factor, left ankle and foot
- M06.079 Rheumatoid arthritis without rheumatoid factor, unspecified ankle and foot

M06.08 Rheumatoid arthritis without rheumatoid factor, vertebrae

M06.09 Rheumatoid arthritis without rheumatoid factor, multiple sites

M06.1 Adult-onset Still's disease

Excludes1 Still's disease NOS (M08.2-)

● M06.2 Rheumatoid bursitis

M06.20 Rheumatoid bursitis, unspecified site

● M06.21 Rheumatoid bursitis, shoulder
- M06.211 Rheumatoid bursitis, right shoulder
- M06.212 Rheumatoid bursitis, left shoulder
- M06.219 Rheumatoid bursitis, unspecified shoulder

● M06.22 Rheumatoid bursitis, elbow
- M06.221 Rheumatoid bursitis, right elbow
- M06.222 Rheumatoid bursitis, left elbow
- M06.229 Rheumatoid bursitis, unspecified elbow

● M06.23 Rheumatoid bursltls, wrist
- M06.231 Rheumatoid bursitis, right wrist
- M06.232 Rheumatoid bursitis, left wrist
- M06.239 Rheumatoid bursitis, unspecified wrist

● M06.24 Rheumatoid bursitis, hand
- M06.241 Rheumatoid bursitis, right hand
- M06.242 Rheumatoid bursitis, left hand
- M06.249 Rheumatoid bursitis, unspecified hand

● M06.25 Rheumatoid bursitis, hip
- M06.251 Rheumatoid bursitis, right hip
- M06.252 Rheumatoid bursitis, left hip
- M06.259 Rheumatoid bursitis, unspecified hip

● M06.26 Rheumatoid bursitis, knee
- M06.261 Rheumatoid bursitis, right knee
- M06.262 Rheumatoid bursitis, left knee
- M06.269 Rheumatoid bursitis, unspecified knee

● M06.27 Rheumatoid bursitis, ankle and foot
- M06.271 Rheumatoid bursitis, right ankle and foot
- M06.272 Rheumatoid bursitis, left ankle and foot
- M06.279 Rheumatoid bursitis, unspecified ankle and foot

M06.28 Rheumatoid bursitis, vertebrae

M06.29 Rheumatoid bursitis, multiple sites

● M06.3 Rheumatoid nodule
M06.30 Rheumatoid nodule, unspecified site
● M06.31 Rheumatoid nodule, shoulder
M06.311 Rheumatoid nodule, right shoulder
M06.312 Rheumatoid nodule, left shoulder
M06.319 Rheumatoid nodule, unspecified shoulder
● M06.32 Rheumatoid nodule, elbow
M06.321 Rheumatoid nodule, right elbow
M06.322 Rheumatoid nodule, left elbow
M06.329 Rheumatoid nodule, unspecified elbow
● M06.33 Rheumatoid nodule, wrist
M06.331 Rheumatoid nodule, right wrist
M06.332 Rheumatoid nodule, left wrist
M06.339 Rheumatoid nodule, unspecified wrist
● M06.34 Rheumatoid nodule, hand
M06.341 Rheumatoid nodule, right hand
M06.342 Rheumatoid nodule, left hand
M06.349 Rheumatoid nodule, unspecified hand
● M06.35 Rheumatoid nodule, hip
M06.351 Rheumatoid nodule, right hip
M06.352 Rheumatoid nodule, left hip
M06.359 Rheumatoid nodule, unspecified hip
● M06.36 Rheumatoid nodule, knee
M06.361 Rheumatoid nodule, right knee
M06.362 Rheumatoid nodule, left knee
M06.369 Rheumatoid nodule, unspecified knee
● M06.37 Rheumatoid nodule, ankle and foot
M06.371 Rheumatoid nodule, right ankle and foot
M06.372 Rheumatoid nodule, left ankle and foot
M06.379 Rheumatoid nodule, unspecified ankle and foot
M06.38 Rheumatoid nodule, vertebrae
M06.39 Rheumatoid nodule, multiple sites
M06.4 Inflammatory polyarthropathy
Excludes1 polyarthritis NOS (M13.0)
● M06.8 Other specified rheumatoid arthritis
M06.80 Other specified rheumatoid arthritis, unspecified site
● M06.81 Other specified rheumatoid arthritis, shoulder
M06.811 Other specified rheumatoid arthritis, right shoulder
M06.812 Other specified rheumatoid arthritis, left shoulder
M06.819 Other specified rheumatoid arthritis, unspecified shoulder
● M06.82 Other specified rheumatoid arthritis, elbow
M06.821 Other specified rheumatoid arthritis, right elbow
M06.822 Other specified rheumatoid arthritis, left elbow
M06.829 Other specified rheumatoid arthritis, unspecified elbow
● M06.83 Other specified rheumatoid arthritis, wrist
M06.831 Other specified rheumatoid arthritis, right wrist
M06.832 Other specified rheumatoid arthritis, left wrist
M06.839 Other specified rheumatoid arthritis, unspecified wrist
● M06.84 Other specified rheumatoid arthritis, hand
M06.841 Other specified rheumatoid arthritis, right hand
M06.842 Other specified rheumatoid arthritis, left hand
M06.849 Other specified rheumatoid arthritis, unspecified hand
● M06.85 Other specified rheumatoid arthritis, hip
M06.851 Other specified rheumatoid arthritis, right hip
M06.852 Other specified rheumatoid arthritis, left hip
M06.859 Other specified rheumatoid arthritis, unspecified hip
● M06.86 Other specified rheumatoid arthritis, knee
M06.861 Other specified rheumatoid arthritis, right knee
M06.862 Other specified rheumatoid arthritis, left knee
M06.869 Other specified rheumatoid arthritis, unspecified knee
● M06.87 Other specified rheumatoid arthritis, ankle and foot
M06.871 Other specified rheumatoid arthritis, right ankle and foot
M06.872 Other specified rheumatoid arthritis, left ankle and foot
M06.879 Other specified rheumatoid arthritis, unspecified ankle and foot
M06.88 Other specified rheumatoid arthritis, vertebrae
M06.89 Other specified rheumatoid arthritis, multiple sites
M06.9 Rheumatoid arthritis, unspecified
● M07 Enteropathic arthropathies
Code also associated enteropathy, such as:
regional enteritis [Crohn's disease] (K50.-)
ulcerative colitis (K51.-)
Excludes1 psoriatic arthropathies (L40.5-)
● M07.6 Enteropathic arthropathies
M07.60 Enteropathic arthropathies, unspecified site
● M07.61 Enteropathic arthropathies, shoulder
M07.611 Enteropathic arthropathies, right shoulder
M07.612 Enteropathic arthropathies, left shoulder
M07.619 Enteropathic arthropathies, unspecified shoulder
● M07.62 Enteropathic arthropathies, elbow
M07.621 Enteropathic arthropathies, right elbow
M07.622 Enteropathic arthropathies, left elbow
M07.629 Enteropathic arthropathies, unspecified elbow
● M07.63 Enteropathic arthropathies, wrist
M07.631 Enteropathic arthropathies, right wrist
M07.632 Enteropathic arthropathies, left wrist
M07.639 Enteropathic arthropathies, unspecified wrist
● M07.64 Enteropathic arthropathies, hand
M07.641 Enteropathic arthropathies, right hand
M07.642 Enteropathic arthropathies, left hand
M07.649 Enteropathic arthropathies, unspecified hand

● M07.65 Enteropathic arthropathies, hip
M07.651 Enteropathic arthropathies, right hip
M07.652 Enteropathic arthropathies, left hip
M07.659 Enteropathic arthropathies, unspecified hip
● M07.66 Enteropathic arthropathies, knee
M07.661 Enteropathic arthropathies, right knee
M07.662 Enteropathic arthropathies, left knee
M07.669 Enteropathic arthropathies, unspecified knee
● M07.67 Enteropathic arthropathies, ankle and foot
M07.671 Enteropathic arthropathies, right ankle and foot
M07.672 Enteropathic arthropathies, left ankle and foot
M07.679 Enteropathic arthropathies, unspecified ankle and foot
M07.68 Enteropathic arthropathies, vertebrae
M07.69 Enteropathic arthropathies, multiple sites

● M08 Juvenile arthritis
Code also any associated underlying condition, such as:
regional enteritis [Crohn's disease] (K50.-)
ulcerative colitis (K51.-)
Excludes1 arthropathy in Whipple's disease (M14.8)
Felty's syndrome (M05.0)
juvenile dermatomyositis (M33.0-)
psoriatic juvenile arthropathy (L40.54)
● M08.0 Unspecified juvenile rheumatoid arthritis
Juvenile rheumatoid arthritis with or without rheumatoid factor
M08.00 Unspecified juvenile rheumatoid arthritis of unspecified site
● M08.01 Unspecified juvenile rheumatoid arthritis, shoulder
M08.011 Unspecified juvenile rheumatoid arthritis, right shoulder
M08.012 Unspecified juvenile rheumatoid arthritis, left shoulder
M08.019 Unspecified juvenile rheumatoid arthritis, unspecified shoulder
● M08.02 Unspecified juvenile rheumatoid arthritis of elbow
M08.021 Unspecified juvenile rheumatoid arthritis, right elbow
M08.022 Unspecified juvenile rheumatoid arthritis, left elbow
M08.029 Unspecified juvenile rheumatoid arthritis, unspecified elbow
● M08.03 Unspecified juvenile rheumatoid arthritis, wrist
M08.031 Unspecified juvenile rheumatoid arthritis, right wrist
M08.032 Unspecified juvenile rheumatoid arthritis, left wrist
M08.039 Unspecified juvenile rheumatoid arthritis, unspecified wrist
● M08.04 Unspecified juvenile rheumatoid arthritis, hand
M08.041 Unspecified juvenile rheumatoid arthritis, right hand
M08.042 Unspecified juvenile rheumatoid arthritis, left hand
M08.049 Unspecified juvenile rheumatoid arthritis, unspecified hand
● M08.05 Unspecified juvenile rheumatoid arthritis, hip
M08.051 Unspecified juvenile rheumatoid arthritis, right hip
M08.052 Unspecified juvenile rheumatoid arthritis, left hip
M08.059 Unspecified juvenile rheumatoid arthritis, unspecified hip
● M08.06 Unspecified juvenile rheumatoid arthritis, knee
M08.061 Unspecified juvenile rheumatoid arthritis, right knee
M08.062 Unspecified juvenile rheumatoid arthritis, left knee
M08.069 Unspecified juvenile rheumatoid arthritis, unspecified knee
● M08.07 Unspecified juvenile rheumatoid arthritis, ankle and foot
M08.071 Unspecified juvenile rheumatoid arthritis, right ankle and foot
M08.072 Unspecified juvenile rheumatoid arthritis, left ankle and foot
M08.079 Unspecified juvenile rheumatoid arthritis, unspecified ankle and foot
M08.08 Unspecified juvenile rheumatoid arthritis, vertebrae
M08.09 Unspecified juvenile rheumatoid arthritis, multiple sites
M08.1 Juvenile ankylosing spondylitis
Excludes1 ankylosing spondylitis in adults (M45.0-)
● M08.2 Juvenile rheumatoid arthritis with systemic onset
Still's disease NOS
Excludes1 adult-onset Still's disease (M06.1-)
M08.20 Juvenile rheumatoid arthritis with systemic onset, unspecified site
● M08.21 Juvenile rheumatoid arthritis with systemic onset, shoulder
M08.211 Juvenile rheumatoid arthritis with systemic onset, right shoulder
M08.212 Juvenile rheumatoid arthritis with systemic onset, left shoulder
M08.219 Juvenile rheumatoid arthritis with systemic onset, unspecified shoulder
● M08.22 Juvenile rheumatoid arthritis with systemic onset, elbow
M08.221 Juvenile rheumatoid arthritis with systemic onset, right elbow
M08.222 Juvenile rheumatoid arthritis with systemic onset, left elbow
M08.229 Juvenile rheumatoid arthritis with systemic onset, unspecified elbow
● M08.23 Juvenile rheumatoid arthritis with systemic onset, wrist
M08.231 Juvenile rheumatoid arthritis with systemic onset, right wrist
M08.232 Juvenile rheumatoid arthritis with systemic onset, left wrist
M08.239 Juvenile rheumatoid arthritis with systemic onset, unspecified wrist
● M08.24 Juvenile rheumatoid arthritis with systemic onset, hand
M08.241 Juvenile rheumatoid arthritis with systemic onset, right hand
M08.242 Juvenile rheumatoid arthritis with systemic onset, left hand
M08.249 Juvenile rheumatoid arthritis with systemic onset, unspecified hand
● M08.25 Juvenile rheumatoid arthritis with systemic onset, hip
M08.251 Juvenile rheumatoid arthritis with systemic onset, right hip
M08.252 Juvenile rheumatoid arthritis with systemic onset, left hip
M08.259 Juvenile rheumatoid arthritis with systemic onset, unspecified hip

- ● M08.26 Juvenile rheumatoid arthritis with systemic onset, knee
  - M08.261 Juvenile rheumatoid arthritis with systemic onset, right knee
  - M08.262 Juvenile rheumatoid arthritis with systemic onset, left knee
  - M08.269 Juvenile rheumatoid arthritis with systemic onset, unspecified knee
- ● M08.27 Juvenile rheumatoid arthritis with systemic onset, ankle and foot
  - M08.271 Juvenile rheumatoid arthritis with systemic onset, right ankle and foot
  - M08.272 Juvenile rheumatoid arthritis with systemic onset, left ankle and foot
  - M08.279 Juvenile rheumatoid arthritis with systemic onset, unspecified ankle and foot
- M08.28 Juvenile rheumatoid arthritis with systemic onset, vertebrae
- M08.29 Juvenile rheumatoid arthritis with systemic onset, multiple sites

M08.3 Juvenile rheumatoid polyarthritis (seronegative)

● M08.4 Pauciarticular juvenile rheumatoid arthritis

- M08.40 Pauciarticular juvenile rheumatoid arthritis, unspecified site
- ● M08.41 Pauciarticular juvenile rheumatoid arthritis, shoulder
  - M08.411 Pauciarticular juvenile rheumatoid arthritis, right shoulder
  - M08.412 Pauciarticular juvenile rheumatoid arthritis, left shoulder
  - M08.419 Pauciarticular juvenile rheumatoid arthritis, unspecified shoulder
- ● M08.42 Pauciarticular juvenile rheumatoid arthritis, elbow
  - M08.421 Pauciarticular juvenile rheumatoid arthritis, right elbow
  - M08.422 Pauciarticular juvenile rheumatoid arthritis, left elbow
  - M08.429 Pauciarticular juvenile rheumatoid arthritis, unspecified elbow
- ● M08.43 Pauciarticular juvenile rheumatoid arthritis, wrist
  - M08.431 Pauciarticular juvenile rheumatoid arthritis, right wrist
  - M08.432 Pauciarticular juvenile rheumatoid arthritis, left wrist
  - M08.439 Pauciarticular juvenile rheumatoid arthritis, unspecified wrist
- ● M08.44 Pauciarticular juvenile rheumatoid arthritis, hand
  - M08.441 Pauciarticular juvenile rheumatoid arthritis, right hand
  - M08.442 Pauciarticular juvenile rheumatoid arthritis, left hand
  - M08.449 Pauciarticular juvenile rheumatoid arthritis, unspecified hand
- ● M08.45 Pauciarticular juvenile rheumatoid arthritis, hip
  - M08.451 Pauciarticular juvenile rheumatoid arthritis, right hip
  - M08.452 Pauciarticular juvenile rheumatoid arthritis, left hip
  - M08.459 Pauciarticular juvenile rheumatoid arthritis, unspecified hip
- ● M08.46 Pauciarticular juvenile rheumatoid arthritis, knee
  - M08.461 Pauciarticular juvenile rheumatoid arthritis, right knee
  - M08.462 Pauciarticular juvenile rheumatoid arthritis, left knee
  - M08.469 Pauciarticular juvenile rheumatoid arthritis, unspecified knee
- ● M08.47 Pauciarticular juvenile rheumatoid arthritis, ankle and foot
  - M08.471 Pauciarticular juvenile rheumatoid arthritis, right ankle and foot
  - M08.472 Pauciarticular juvenile rheumatoid arthritis, left ankle and foot
  - M08.479 Pauciarticular juvenile rheumatoid arthritis, unspecified ankle and foot
- M08.48 Pauciarticular juvenile rheumatoid arthritis, vertebrae

● M08.8 Other juvenile arthritis

- M08.80 Other juvenile arthritis, unspecified site
- ● M08.81 Other juvenile arthritis, shoulder
  - M08.811 Other juvenile arthritis, right shoulder
  - M08.812 Other juvenile arthritis, left shoulder
  - M08.819 Other juvenile arthritis, unspecified shoulder
- ● M08.82 Other juvenile arthritis, elbow
  - M08.821 Other juvenile arthritis, right elbow
  - M08.822 Other juvenile arthritis, left elbow
  - M08.829 Other juvenile arthritis, unspecified elbow
- ● M08.83 Other juvenile arthritis, wrist
  - M08.831 Other juvenile arthritis, right wrist
  - M08.832 Other juvenile arthritis, left wrist
  - M08.839 Other juvenile arthritis, unspecified wrist
- ● M08.84 Other juvenile arthritis, hand
  - M08.841 Other juvenile arthritis, right hand
  - M08.842 Other juvenile arthritis, left hand
  - M08.849 Other juvenile arthritis, unspecified hand
- ● M08.85 Other juvenile arthritis, hip
  - M08.851 Other juvenile arthritis, right hip
  - M08.852 Other juvenile arthritis, left hip
  - M08.859 Other juvenile arthritis, unspecified hip
- ● M08.86 Other juvenile arthritis, knee
  - M08.861 Other juvenile arthritis, right knee
  - M08.862 Other juvenile arthritis, left knee
  - M08.869 Other juvenile arthritis, unspecified knee
- ● M08.87 Other juvenile arthritis, ankle and foot
  - M08.871 Other juvenile arthritis, right ankle and foot
  - M08.872 Other juvenile arthritis, left ankle and foot
  - M08.879 Other juvenile arthritis, unspecified ankle and foot
- M08.88 Other juvenile arthritis, other specified site
  - Other juvenile arthritis, vertebrae
- M08.89 Other juvenile arthritis, multiple sites

● **M08.9 Juvenile arthritis, unspecified**

Excludes1 juvenile rheumatoid arthritis, unspecified (M08.0-)

M08.90 Juvenile arthritis, unspecified, unspecified site

● **M08.91 Juvenile arthritis, unspecified, shoulder**

M08.911 Juvenile arthritis, unspecified, right shoulder

M08.912 Juvenile arthritis, unspecified, left shoulder

M08.919 Juvenile arthritis, unspecified, unspecified shoulder

● **M08.92 Juvenile arthritis, unspecified, elbow**

M08.921 Juvenile arthritis, unspecified, right elbow

M08.922 Juvenile arthritis, unspecified, left elbow

M08.929 Juvenile arthritis, unspecified, unspecified elbow

● **M08.93 Juvenile arthritis, unspecified, wrist**

M08.931 Juvenile arthritis, unspecified, right wrist

M08.932 Juvenile arthritis, unspecified, left wrist

M08.939 Juvenile arthritis, unspecified, unspecified wrist

● **M08.94 Juvenile arthritis, unspecified, hand**

M08.941 Juvenile arthritis, unspecified, right hand

M08.942 Juvenile arthritis, unspecified, left hand

M08.949 Juvenile arthritis, unspecified, unspecified hand

● **M08.95 Juvenile arthritis, unspecified, hip**

M08.951 Juvenile arthritis, unspecified, right hip

M08.952 Juvenile arthritis, unspecified, left hip

M08.959 Juvenile arthritis, unspecified, unspecified hip

● **M08.96 Juvenile arthritis, unspecified, knee**

M08.961 Juvenile arthritis, unspecified, right knee

M08.962 Juvenile arthritis, unspecified, left knee

M08.969 Juvenile arthritis, unspecified, unspecified knee

● **M08.97 Juvenile arthritis, unspecified, ankle and foot**

M08.971 Juvenile arthritis, unspecified, right ankle and foot

M08.972 Juvenile arthritis, unspecified, left ankle and foot

M08.979 Juvenile arthritis, unspecified, unspecified ankle and foot

M08.98 Juvenile arthritis, unspecified, vertebrae

M08.99 Juvenile arthritis, unspecified, multiple sites

● **M1A Chronic gout**

Use additional code to identify:
Autonomic neuropathy in diseases classified elsewhere (G99.0)
Calculus of urinary tract in diseases classified elsewhere (N22)
Cardiomyopathy in diseases classified elsewhere (I43)
Disorders of external ear in diseases classified elsewhere (H61.1-, H62.8-)
Disorders of iris and ciliary body in diseases classified elsewhere (H22)
Glomerular disorders in diseases classified elsewhere (N08)

Excludes1 gout NOS (M10.-)

Excludes2 acute gout (M10.-) ◀

The appropriate 7th character is to be added to each code from category M1A

0	without tophus (tophi)
1	with tophus (tophi)

● **M1A.0 Idiopathic chronic gout**

Chronic gouty bursitis
Primary chronic gout

X● **M1A.00 Idiopathic chronic gout, unspecified site**

● **M1A.01 Idiopathic chronic gout, shoulder**

● **M1A.011 Idiopathic chronic gout, right shoulder**

● **M1A.012 Idiopathic chronic gout, left shoulder**

● **M1A.019 Idiopathic chronic gout, unspecified shoulder**

● **M1A.02 Idiopathic chronic gout, elbow**

● **M1A.021 Idiopathic chronic gout, right elbow**

● **M1A.022 Idiopathic chronic gout, left elbow**

● **M1A.029 Idiopathic chronic gout, unspecified elbow**

● **M1A.03 Idiopathic chronic gout, wrist**

● **M1A.031 Idiopathic chronic gout, right wrist**

● **M1A.032 Idiopathic chronic gout, left wrist**

● **M1A.039 Idiopathic chronic gout, unspecified wrist**

● **M1A.04 Idiopathic chronic gout, hand**

● **M1A.041 Idiopathic chronic gout, right hand**

● **M1A.042 Idiopathic chronic gout, left hand**

● **M1A.049 Idiopathic chronic gout, unspecified hand**

● **M1A.05 Idiopathic chronic gout, hip**

● **M1A.051 Idiopathic chronic gout, right hip**

● **M1A.052 Idiopathic chronic gout, left hip**

● **M1A.059 Idiopathic chronic gout, unspecified hip**

● **M1A.06 Idiopathic chronic gout, knee**

● **M1A.061 Idiopathic chronic gout, right knee**

● **M1A.062 Idiopathic chronic gout, left knee**

● **M1A.069 Idiopathic chronic gout, unspecified knee**

● **M1A.07 Idiopathic chronic gout, ankle and foot**

● **M1A.071 Idiopathic chronic gout, right ankle and foot**

● **M1A.072 Idiopathic chronic gout, left ankle and foot**

● **M1A.079 Idiopathic chronic gout, unspecified ankle and foot**

X● **M1A.08 Idiopathic chronic gout, vertebrae**

X● **M1A.09 Idiopathic chronic gout, multiple sites**

● M1A.1 Lead-induced chronic gout
Code first toxic effects of lead and its compounds (T56.0-)
X● M1A.10 Lead-induced chronic gout, unspecified site
● M1A.11 Lead-induced chronic gout, shoulder
● M1A.111 Lead-induced chronic gout, right shoulder
● M1A.112 Lead-induced chronic gout, left shoulder
● M1A.119 Lead-induced chronic gout, unspecified shoulder
● M1A.12 Lead-induced chronic gout, elbow
● M1A.121 Lead-induced chronic gout, right elbow
● M1A.122 Lead-induced chronic gout, left elbow
● M1A.129 Lead-induced chronic gout, unspecified elbow
● M1A.13 Lead-induced chronic gout, wrist
● M1A.131 Lead-induced chronic gout, right wrist
● M1A.132 Lead-induced chronic gout, left wrist
● M1A.139 Lead-induced chronic gout, unspecified wrist
● M1A.14 Lead-induced chronic gout, hand
● M1A.141 Lead-induced chronic gout, right hand
● M1A.142 Lead-induced chronic gout, left hand
● M1A.149 Lead-induced chronic gout, unspecified hand
● M1A.15 Lead-induced chronic gout, hip
● M1A.151 Lead-induced chronic gout, right hip
● M1A.152 Lead-induced chronic gout, left hip
● M1A.159 Lead-induced chronic gout, unspecified hip
● M1A.16 Lead-induced chronic gout, knee
● M1A.161 Lead-induced chronic gout, right knee
● M1A.162 Lead-induced chronic gout, left knee
● M1A.169 Lead-induced chronic gout, unspecified knee
● M1A.17 Lead-induced chronic gout, ankle and foot
● M1A.171 Lead-induced chronic gout, right ankle and foot
● M1A.172 Lead-induced chronic gout, left ankle and foot
● M1A.179 Lead-induced chronic gout, unspecified ankle and foot
X● M1A.18 Lead-induced chronic gout, vertebrae
X● M1A.19 Lead-induced chronic gout, multiple sites
● M1A.2 Drug-induced chronic gout
Use additional code for adverse effect, if applicable, to identify drug (T36-T50 with fifth or sixth character 5)
X● M1A.20 Drug-induced chronic gout, unspecified site
● M1A.21 Drug-induced chronic gout, shoulder
● M1A.211 Drug-induced chronic gout, right shoulder
● M1A.212 Drug-induced chronic gout, left shoulder
● M1A.219 Drug-induced chronic gout, unspecified shoulder
● M1A.22 Drug-induced chronic gout, elbow
● M1A.221 Drug-induced chronic gout, right elbow
● M1A.222 Drug-induced chronic gout, left elbow
● M1A.229 Drug-induced chronic gout, unspecified elbow
● M1A.23 Drug-induced chronic gout, wrist
● M1A.231 Drug-induced chronic gout, right wrist
● M1A.232 Drug-induced chronic gout, left wrist
● M1A.239 Drug-induced chronic gout, unspecified wrist
● M1A.24 Drug-induced chronic gout, hand
● M1A.241 Drug-induced chronic gout, right hand
● M1A.242 Drug-induced chronic gout, left hand
● M1A.249 Drug-induced chronic gout, unspecified hand
● M1A.25 Drug-induced chronic gout, hip
● M1A.251 Drug-induced chronic gout, right hip
● M1A.252 Drug-induced chronic gout, left hip
● M1A.259 Drug-induced chronic gout, unspecified hip
● M1A.26 Drug-induced chronic gout, knee
● M1A.261 Drug-induced chronic gout, right knee
● M1A.262 Drug-induced chronic gout, left knee
● M1A.269 Drug-induced chronic gout, unspecified knee
● M1A.27 Drug-induced chronic gout, ankle and foot
● M1A.271 Drug-induced chronic gout, right ankle and foot
● M1A.272 Drug-induced chronic gout, left ankle and foot
● M1A.279 Drug-induced chronic gout, unspecified ankle and foot
X● M1A.28 Drug-induced chronic gout, vertebrae
X● M1A.29 Drug-induced chronic gout, multiple sites
● M1A.3 Chronic gout due to renal impairment
Code first associated renal disease
X● M1A.30 Chronic gout due to renal impairment, unspecified site
● M1A.31 Chronic gout due to renal impairment, shoulder
● M1A.311 Chronic gout due to renal impairment, right shoulder
● M1A.312 Chronic gout due to renal impairment, left shoulder
● M1A.319 Chronic gout due to renal impairment, unspecified shoulder
● M1A.32 Chronic gout due to renal impairment, elbow
● M1A.321 Chronic gout due to renal impairment, right elbow
● M1A.322 Chronic gout due to renal impairment, left elbow
● M1A.329 Chronic gout due to renal impairment, unspecified elbow
● M1A.33 Chronic gout due to renal impairment, wrist
● M1A.331 Chronic gout due to renal impairment, right wrist
● M1A.332 Chronic gout due to renal impairment, left wrist
● M1A.339 Chronic gout due to renal impairment, unspecified wrist
● M1A.34 Chronic gout due to renal impairment, hand
● M1A.341 Chronic gout due to renal impairment, right hand
● M1A.342 Chronic gout due to renal impairment, left hand
● M1A.349 Chronic gout due to renal impairment, unspecified hand

● **M1A.35 Chronic gout due to renal impairment, hip**
● **M1A.351 Chronic gout due to renal impairment, right hip**
● **M1A.352 Chronic gout due to renal impairment, left hip**
● **M1A.359 Chronic gout due to renal impairment, unspecified hip**
● **M1A.36 Chronic gout due to renal impairment, knee**
● **M1A.361 Chronic gout due to renal impairment, right knee**
● **M1A.362 Chronic gout due to renal impairment, left knee**
● **M1A.369 Chronic gout due to renal impairment, unspecified knee**
● **M1A.37 Chronic gout due to renal impairment, ankle and foot**
● **M1A.371 Chronic gout due to renal impairment, right ankle and foot**
● **M1A.372 Chronic gout due to renal impairment, left ankle and foot**
● **M1A.379 Chronic gout due to renal impairment, unspecified ankle and foot**
X● **M1A.38 Chronic gout due to renal impairment, vertebrae**
X● **M1A.39 Chronic gout due to renal impairment, multiple sites**
● **M1A.4 Other secondary chronic gout**
Code first associated condition
X● **M1A.40 Other secondary chronic gout, unspecified site**
● **M1A.41 Other secondary chronic gout, shoulder**
● **M1A.411 Other secondary chronic gout, right shoulder**
● **M1A.412 Other secondary chronic gout, left shoulder**
● **M1A.419 Other secondary chronic gout, unspecified shoulder**
● **M1A.42 Other secondary chronic gout, elbow**
● **M1A.421 Other secondary chronic gout, right elbow**
● **M1A.422 Other secondary chronic gout, left elbow**
● **M1A.429 Other secondary chronic gout, unspecified elbow**
● **M1A.43 Other secondary chronic gout, wrist**
● **M1A.431 Other secondary chronic gout, right wrist**
● **M1A.432 Other secondary chronic gout, left wrist**
● **M1A.439 Other secondary chronic gout, unspecified wrist**
● **M1A.44 Other secondary chronic gout, hand**
● **M1A.441 Other secondary chronic gout, right hand**
● **M1A.442 Other secondary chronic gout, left hand**
● **M1A.449 Other secondary chronic gout, unspecified hand**
● **M1A.45 Other secondary chronic gout, hip**
● **M1A.451 Other secondary chronic gout, right hip**
● **M1A.452 Other secondary chronic gout, left hip**
● **M1A.459 Other secondary chronic gout, unspecified hip**
● **M1A.46 Other secondary chronic gout, knee**
● **M1A.461 Other secondary chronic gout, right knee**
● **M1A.462 Other secondary chronic gout, left knee**
● **M1A.469 Other secondary chronic gout, unspecified knee**
● **M1A.47 Other secondary chronic gout, ankle and foot**
● **M1A.471 Other secondary chronic gout, right ankle and foot**
● **M1A.472 Other secondary chronic gout, left ankle and foot**
● **M1A.479 Other secondary chronic gout, unspecified ankle and foot**
X● **M1A.48 Other secondary chronic gout, vertebrae**
X● **M1A.49 Other secondary chronic gout, multiple sites**
X● **M1A.9 Chronic gout, unspecified**

● **M10 Gout**
Accumulation of uric acid that results in swollen, red, hot, painful, stiff joints
Acute gout
Gout attack
Gout flare
Podagra
Use additional code to identify:
Autonomic neuropathy in diseases classified elsewhere (G99.0)
Calculus of urinary tract in diseases classified elsewhere (N22)
Cardiomyopathy in diseases classified elsewhere (I43)
Disorders of external ear in diseases classified elsewhere (H61.1-, H62.8-)
Disorders of iris and ciliary body in diseases classified elsewhere (H22)
Glomerular disorders in diseases classified elsewhere (N08)
Excludes2 chronic gout (M1A.-) ◀
● **M10.0 Idiopathic gout**
Gouty bursitis
Primary gout
M10.00 Idiopathic gout, unspecified site
● **M10.01 Idiopathic gout, shoulder**
M10.011 Idiopathic gout, right shoulder
M10.012 Idiopathic gout, left shoulder
M10.019 Idiopathic gout, unspecified shoulder
● **M10.02 Idiopathic gout, elbow**
M10.021 Idiopathic gout, right elbow
M10.022 Idiopathic gout, left elbow
M10.029 Idiopathic gout, unspecified elbow
● **M10.03 Idiopathic gout, wrist**
M10.031 Idiopathic gout, right wrist
M10.032 Idiopathic gout, left wrist
M10.039 Idiopathic gout, unspecified wrist
● **M10.04 Idiopathic gout, hand**
M10.041 Idiopathic gout, right hand
M10.042 Idiopathic gout, left hand
M10.049 Idiopathic gout, unspecified hand
● **M10.05 Idiopathic gout, hip**
M10.051 Idiopathic gout, right hip
M10.052 Idiopathic gout, left hip
M10.059 Idiopathic gout, unspecified hip
● **M10.06 Idiopathic gout, knee**
M10.061 Idiopathic gout, right knee
M10.062 Idiopathic gout, left knee
M10.069 Idiopathic gout, unspecified knee

- M10.07 Idiopathic gout, ankle and foot
  - M10.071 Idiopathic gout, right ankle and foot
  - M10.072 Idiopathic gout, left ankle and foot
  - M10.079 Idiopathic gout, unspecified ankle and foot
- M10.08 Idiopathic gout, vertebrae
- M10.09 Idiopathic gout, multiple sites

M10.1 Lead-induced gout

Code first toxic effects of lead and its compounds (T56.0-)

- M10.10 Lead-induced gout, unspecified site
- M10.11 Lead-induced gout, shoulder
  - M10.111 Lead-induced gout, right shoulder
  - M10.112 Lead-induced gout, left shoulder
  - M10.119 Lead-induced gout, unspecified shoulder
- M10.12 Lead-induced gout, elbow
  - M10.121 Lead-induced gout, right elbow
  - M10.122 Lead-induced gout, left elbow
  - M10.129 Lead-induced gout, unspecified elbow
- M10.13 Lead-induced gout, wrist
  - M10.131 Lead-induced gout, right wrist
  - M10.132 Lead-induced gout, left wrist
  - M10.139 Lead-induced gout, unspecified wrist
- M10.14 Lead-induced gout, hand
  - M10.141 Lead-induced gout, right hand
  - M10.142 Lead-induced gout, left hand
  - M10.149 Lead-induced gout, unspecified hand
- M10.15 Lead-induced gout, hip
  - M10.151 Lead-induced gout, right hip
  - M10.152 Lead-induced gout, left hip
  - M10.159 Lead-induced gout, unspecified hip
- M10.16 Lead-induced gout, knee
  - M10.161 Lead-induced gout, right knee
  - M10.162 Lead-induced gout, left knee
  - M10.169 Lead-induced gout, unspecified knee
- M10.17 Lead-induced gout, ankle and foot
  - M10.171 Lead-induced gout, right ankle and foot
  - M10.172 Lead-induced gout, left ankle and foot
  - M10.179 Lead-induced gout, unspecified ankle and foot
- M10.18 Lead-induced gout, vertebrae
- M10.19 Lead-induced gout, multiple sites

M10.2 Drug-induced gout

Use additional code for adverse effect, if applicable, to identify drug (T36-T50 with fifth or sixth character 5)

- M10.20 Drug-induced gout, unspecified site
- M10.21 Drug-induced gout, shoulder
  - M10.211 Drug-induced gout, right shoulder
  - M10.212 Drug-induced gout, left shoulder
  - M10.219 Drug-induced gout, unspecified shoulder
- M10.22 Drug-induced gout, elbow
  - M10.221 Drug-induced gout, right elbow
  - M10.222 Drug-induced gout, left elbow
  - M10.229 Drug-induced gout, unspecified elbow
- M10.23 Drug-induced gout, wrist
  - M10.231 Drug-induced gout, right wrist
  - M10.232 Drug-induced gout, left wrist
  - M10.239 Drug-induced gout, unspecified wrist
- M10.24 Drug-induced gout, hand
  - M10.241 Drug-induced gout, right hand
  - M10.242 Drug-induced gout, left hand
  - M10.249 Drug-induced gout, unspecified hand
- M10.25 Drug-induced gout, hip
  - M10.251 Drug-induced gout, right hip
  - M10.252 Drug-induced gout, left hip
  - M10.259 Drug-induced gout, unspecified hip
- M10.26 Drug-induced gout, knee
  - M10.261 Drug-induced gout, right knee
  - M10.262 Drug-induced gout, left knee
  - M10.269 Drug-induced gout, unspecified knee
- M10.27 Drug-induced gout, ankle and foot
  - M10.271 Drug-induced gout, right ankle and foot
  - M10.272 Drug-induced gout, left ankle and foot
  - M10.279 Drug-induced gout, unspecified ankle and foot
- M10.28 Drug-induced gout, vertebrae
- M10.29 Drug-induced gout, multiple sites

M10.3 Gout due to renal impairment

Code also associated renal disease

- M10.30 Gout due to renal impairment, unspecified site
- M10.31 Gout due to renal impairment, shoulder
  - M10.311 Gout due to renal impairment, right shoulder
  - M10.312 Gout due to renal impairment, left shoulder
  - M10.319 Gout due to renal impairment, unspecified shoulder
- M10.32 Gout due to renal impairment, elbow
  - M10.321 Gout due to renal impairment, right elbow
  - M10.322 Gout due to renal impairment, left elbow
  - M10.329 Gout due to renal impairment, unspecified elbow
- M10.33 Gout due to renal impairment, wrist
  - M10.331 Gout due to renal impairment, right wrist
  - M10.332 Gout due to renal impairment, left wrist
  - M10.339 Gout due to renal impairment, unspecified wrist
- M10.34 Gout due to renal impairment, hand
  - M10.341 Gout due to renal impairment, right hand
  - M10.342 Gout due to renal impairment, left hand
  - M10.349 Gout due to renal impairment, unspecified hand
- M10.35 Gout due to renal impairment, hip
  - M10.351 Gout due to renal impairment, right hip
  - M10.352 Gout due to renal impairment, left hip
  - M10.359 Gout due to renal impairment, unspecified hip
- M10.36 Gout due to renal impairment, knee
  - M10.361 Gout due to renal impairment, right knee
  - M10.362 Gout due to renal impairment, left knee
  - M10.369 Gout due to renal impairment, unspecified knee

CHAPTER 13 (M00-M99)

New | Revised | ~~deleted~~ Deleted | OGCR Official Guidelines | X Assign placeholder X | Use Additional Character(s)

Excludes 1 | Excludes 2 | Includes | Use additional | Code first | Code also | Unspecified

● M10.37 Gout due to renal impairment, ankle and foot
M10.371 Gout due to renal impairment, right ankle and foot
M10.372 Gout due to renal impairment, left ankle and foot
M10.379 Gout due to renal impairment, unspecified ankle and foot
M10.38 Gout due to renal impairment, vertebrae
M10.39 Gout due to renal impairment, multiple sites
● M10.4 Other secondary gout
Code first associated condition
M10.40 Other secondary gout, unspecified site
● M10.41 Other secondary gout, shoulder
M10.411 Other secondary gout, right shoulder
M10.412 Other secondary gout, left shoulder
M10.419 Other secondary gout, unspecified shoulder
● M10.42 Other secondary gout, elbow
M10.421 Other secondary gout, right elbow
M10.422 Other secondary gout, left elbow
M10.429 Other secondary gout, unspecified elbow
● M10.43 Other secondary gout, wrist
M10.431 Other secondary gout, right wrist
M10.432 Other secondary gout, left wrist
M10.439 Other secondary gout, unspecified wrist
● M10.44 Other secondary gout, hand
M10.441 Other secondary gout, right hand
M10.442 Other secondary gout, left hand
M10.449 Other secondary gout, unspecified hand
● M10.45 Other secondary gout, hip
M10.451 Other secondary gout, right hip
M10.452 Other secondary gout, left hip
M10.459 Other secondary gout, unspecified hip
● M10.46 Other secondary gout, knee
M10.461 Other secondary gout, right knee
M10.462 Other secondary gout, left knee
M10.469 Other secondary gout, unspecified knee
● M10.47 Other secondary gout, ankle and foot
M10.471 Other secondary gout, right ankle and foot
M10.472 Other secondary gout, left ankle and foot
M10.479 Other secondary gout, unspecified ankle and foot
M10.48 Other secondary gout, vertebrae
M10.49 Other secondary gout, multiple sites
M10.9 Gout, unspecified
Gout NOS
● M11 Other crystal arthropathies
● M11.0 Hydroxyapatite deposition disease
M11.00 Hydroxyapatite deposition disease, unspecified site
● M11.01 Hydroxyapatite deposition disease, shoulder
M11.011 Hydroxyapatite deposition disease, right shoulder
M11.012 Hydroxyapatite deposition disease, left shoulder
M11.019 Hydroxyapatite deposition disease, unspecified shoulder
● M11.02 Hydroxyapatite deposition disease, elbow
M11.021 Hydroxyapatite deposition disease, right elbow
M11.022 Hydroxyapatite deposition disease, left elbow
M11.029 Hydroxyapatite deposition disease, unspecified elbow
● M11.03 Hydroxyapatite deposition disease, wrist
M11.031 Hydroxyapatite deposition disease, right wrist
M11.032 Hydroxyapatite deposition disease, left wrist
M11.039 Hydroxyapatite deposition disease, unspecified wrist
● M11.04 Hydroxyapatite deposition disease, hand
M11.041 Hydroxyapatite deposition disease, right hand
M11.042 Hydroxyapatite deposition disease, left hand
M11.049 Hydroxyapatite deposition disease, unspecified hand
● M11.05 Hydroxyapatite deposition disease, hip
M11.051 Hydroxyapatite deposition disease, right hip
M11.052 Hydroxyapatite deposition disease, left hip
M11.059 Hydroxyapatite deposition disease, unspecified hip
● M11.06 Hydroxyapatite deposition disease, knee
M11.061 Hydroxyapatite deposition disease, right knee
M11.062 Hydroxyapatite deposition disease, left knee
M11.069 Hydroxyapatite deposition disease, unspecified knee
● M11.07 Hydroxyapatite deposition disease, ankle and foot
M11.071 Hydroxyapatite deposition disease, right ankle and foot
M11.072 Hydroxyapatite deposition disease, left ankle and foot
M11.079 Hydroxyapatite deposition disease, unspecified ankle and foot
M11.08 Hydroxyapatite deposition disease, vertebrae
M11.09 Hydroxyapatite deposition disease, multiple sites
● M11.1 Familial chondrocalcinosis
M11.10 Familial chondrocalcinosis, unspecified site
● M11.11 Familial chondrocalcinosis, shoulder
M11.111 Familial chondrocalcinosis, right shoulder
M11.112 Familial chondrocalcinosis, left shoulder
M11.119 Familial chondrocalcinosis, unspecified shoulder
● M11.12 Familial chondrocalcinosis, elbow
M11.121 Familial chondrocalcinosis, right elbow
M11.122 Familial chondrocalcinosis, left elbow
M11.129 Familial chondrocalcinosis, unspecified elbow
● M11.13 Familial chondrocalcinosis, wrist
M11.131 Familial chondrocalcinosis, right wrist
M11.132 Familial chondrocalcinosis, left wrist
M11.139 Familial chondrocalcinosis, unspecified wrist

CHAPTER 13 (M00-M99)

● M11.14 Familial chondrocalcinosis, hand
M11.141 Familial chondrocalcinosis, right hand
M11.142 Familial chondrocalcinosis, left hand
M11.149 Familial chondrocalcinosis, unspecified hand

● M11.15 Familial chondrocalcinosis, hip
M11.151 Familial chondrocalcinosis, right hip
M11.152 Familial chondrocalcinosis, left hip
M11.159 Familial chondrocalcinosis, unspecified hip

● M11.16 Familial chondrocalcinosis, knee
M11.161 Familial chondrocalcinosis, right knee
M11.162 Familial chondrocalcinosis, left knee
M11.169 Familial chondrocalcinosis, unspecified knee

● M11.17 Familial chondrocalcinosis, ankle and foot
M11.171 Familial chondrocalcinosis, right ankle and foot
M11.172 Familial chondrocalcinosis, left ankle and foot
M11.179 Familial chondrocalcinosis, unspecified ankle and foot

M11.18 Familial chondrocalcinosis, vertebrae
M11.19 Familial chondrocalcinosis, multiple sites

● M11.2 Other chondrocalcinosis
Chondrocalcinosis NOS
M11.20 Other chondrocalcinosis, unspecified site

● M11.21 Other chondrocalcinosis, shoulder
M11.211 Other chondrocalcinosis, right shoulder
M11.212 Other chondrocalcinosis, left shoulder
M11.219 Other chondrocalcinosis, unspecified shoulder

● M11.22 Other chondrocalcinosis, elbow
M11.221 Other chondrocalcinosis, right elbow
M11.222 Other chondrocalcinosis, left elbow
M11.229 Other chondrocalcinosis, unspecified elbow

● M11.23 Other chondrocalcinosis, wrist
M11.231 Other chondrocalcinosis, right wrist
M11.232 Other chondrocalcinosis, left wrist
M11.239 Other chondrocalcinosis, unspecified wrist

● M11.24 Other chondrocalcinosis, hand
M11.241 Other chondrocalcinosis, right hand
M11.242 Other chondrocalcinosis, left hand
M11.249 Other chondrocalcinosis, unspecified hand

● M11.25 Other chondrocalcinosis, hip
M11.251 Other chondrocalcinosis, right hip
M11.252 Other chondrocalcinosis, left hip
M11.259 Other chondrocalcinosis, unspecified hip

● M11.26 Other chondrocalcinosis, knee
M11.261 Other chondrocalcinosis, right knee
M11.262 Other chondrocalcinosis, left knee
M11.269 Other chondrocalcinosis, unspecified knee

● M11.27 Other chondrocalcinosis, ankle and foot
M11.271 Other chondrocalcinosis, right ankle and foot
M11.272 Other chondrocalcinosis, left ankle and foot
M11.279 Other chondrocalcinosis, unspecified ankle and foot

M11.28 Other chondrocalcinosis, vertebrae
M11.29 Other chondrocalcinosis, multiple sites

● M11.8 Other specified crystal arthropathies
M11.80 Other specified crystal arthropathies, unspecified site

● M11.81 Other specified crystal arthropathies, shoulder
M11.811 Other specified crystal arthropathies, right shoulder
M11.812 Other specified crystal arthropathies, left shoulder
M11.819 Other specified crystal arthropathies, unspecified shoulder

● M11.82 Other specified crystal arthropathies, elbow
M11.821 Other specified crystal arthropathies, right elbow
M11.822 Other specified crystal arthropathies, left elbow
M11.829 Other specified crystal arthropathies, unspecified elbow

● M11.83 Other specified crystal arthropathies, wrist
M11.831 Other specified crystal arthropathies, right wrist
M11.832 Other specified crystal arthropathies, left wrist
M11.839 Other specified crystal arthropathies, unspecified wrist

● M11.84 Other specified crystal arthropathies, hand
M11.841 Other specified crystal arthropathies, right hand
M11.842 Other specified crystal arthropathies, left hand
M11.849 Other specified crystal arthropathies, unspecified hand

● M11.85 Other specified crystal arthropathies, hip
M11.851 Other specified crystal arthropathies, right hip
M11.852 Other specified crystal arthropathies, left hip
M11.859 Other specified crystal arthropathies, unspecified hip

● M11.86 Other specified crystal arthropathies, knee
M11.861 Other specified crystal arthropathies, right knee
M11.862 Other specified crystal arthropathies, left knee
M11.869 Other specified crystal arthropathies, unspecified knee

● M11.87 Other specified crystal arthropathies, ankle and foot
M11.871 Other specified crystal arthropathies, right ankle and foot
M11.872 Other specified crystal arthropathies, left ankle and foot
M11.879 Other specified crystal arthropathies, unspecified ankle and foot

M11.88 Other specified crystal arthropathies, vertebrae
M11.89 Other specified crystal arthropathies, multiple sites

M11.9 Crystal arthropathy, unspecified

● **M12 Other and unspecified arthropathy**
Excludes1 arthrosis (M15-M19)
cricoarytenoid arthropathy (J38.7)

● **M12.0 Chronic postrheumatic arthropathy [Jaccoud]**
M12.00 Chronic postrheumatic arthropathy [Jaccoud], unspecified site
● **M12.01 Chronic postrheumatic arthropathy [Jaccoud], shoulder**
M12.011 Chronic postrheumatic arthropathy [Jaccoud], right shoulder
M12.012 Chronic postrheumatic arthropathy [Jaccoud], left shoulder
M12.019 Chronic postrheumatic arthropathy [Jaccoud], unspecified shoulder
● **M12.02 Chronic postrheumatic arthropathy [Jaccoud], elbow**
M12.021 Chronic postrheumatic arthropathy [Jaccoud], right elbow
M12.022 Chronic postrheumatic arthropathy [Jaccoud], left elbow
M12.029 Chronic postrheumatic arthropathy [Jaccoud], unspecified elbow
● **M12.03 Chronic postrheumatic arthropathy [Jaccoud], wrist**
M12.031 Chronic postrheumatic arthropathy [Jaccoud], right wrist
M12.032 Chronic postrheumatic arthropathy [Jaccoud], left wrist
M12.039 Chronic postrheumatic arthropathy [Jaccoud], unspecified wrist
● **M12.04 Chronic postrheumatic arthropathy [Jaccoud], hand**
M12.041 Chronic postrheumatic arthropathy [Jaccoud], right hand
M12.042 Chronic postrheumatic arthropathy [Jaccoud], left hand
M12.049 Chronic postrheumatic arthropathy [Jaccoud], unspecified hand
● **M12.05 Chronic postrheumatic arthropathy [Jaccoud], hip**
M12.051 Chronic postrheumatic arthropathy [Jaccoud], right hip
M12.052 Chronic postrheumatic arthropathy [Jaccoud], left hip
M12.059 Chronic postrheumatic arthropathy [Jaccoud], unspecified hip
● **M12.06 Chronic postrheumatic arthropathy [Jaccoud], knee**
M12.061 Chronic postrheumatic arthropathy [Jaccoud], right knee
M12.062 Chronic postrheumatic arthropathy [Jaccoud], left knee
M12.069 Chronic postrheumatic arthropathy [Jaccoud], unspecified knee
● **M12.07 Chronic postrheumatic arthropathy [Jaccoud], ankle and foot**
M12.071 Chronic postrheumatic arthropathy [Jaccoud], right ankle and foot
M12.072 Chronic postrheumatic arthropathy [Jaccoud], left ankle and foot
M12.079 Chronic postrheumatic arthropathy [Jaccoud], unspecified ankle and foot
M12.08 Chronic postrheumatic arthropathy [Jaccoud], other specified site
Chronic postrheumatic arthropathy [Jaccoud], vertebrae
M12.09 Chronic postrheumatic arthropathy [Jaccoud], multiple sites

● **M12.1 Kaschin-Beck disease**
Osteochondroarthrosis deformans endemica
M12.10 Kaschin-Beck disease, unspecified site
● **M12.11 Kaschin-Beck disease, shoulder**
M12.111 Kaschin-Beck disease, right shoulder
M12.112 Kaschin-Beck disease, left shoulder
M12.119 Kaschin-Beck disease, unspecified shoulder
● **M12.12 Kaschin-Beck disease, elbow**
M12.121 Kaschin-Beck disease, right elbow
M12.122 Kaschin-Beck disease, left elbow
M12.129 Kaschin-Beck disease, unspecified elbow
● **M12.13 Kaschin-Beck disease, wrist**
M12.131 Kaschin-Beck disease, right wrist
M12.132 Kaschin-Beck disease, left wrist
M12.139 Kaschin-Beck disease, unspecified wrist
● **M12.14 Kaschin-Beck disease, hand**
M12.141 Kaschin-Beck disease, right hand
M12.142 Kaschin-Beck disease, left hand
M12.149 Kaschin-Beck disease, unspecified hand
● **M12.15 Kaschin-Beck disease, hip**
M12.151 Kaschin-Beck disease, right hip
M12.152 Kaschin-Beck disease, left hip
M12.159 Kaschin-Beck disease, unspecified hip
● **M12.16 Kaschin-Beck disease, knee**
M12.161 Kaschin-Beck disease, right knee
M12.162 Kaschin-Beck disease, left knee
M12.169 Kaschin-Beck disease, unspecified knee
● **M12.17 Kaschin-Beck disease, ankle and foot**
M12.171 Kaschin-Beck disease, right ankle and foot
M12.172 Kaschin-Beck disease, left ankle and foot
M12.179 Kaschin-Beck disease, unspecified ankle and foot
M12.18 Kaschin-Beck disease, vertebrae
M12.19 Kaschin-Beck disease, multiple sites

● **M12.2 Villonodular synovitis (pigmented)**
M12.20 Villonodular synovitis (pigmented), unspecified site
● **M12.21 Villonodular synovitis (pigmented), shoulder**
M12.211 Villonodular synovitis (pigmented), right shoulder
M12.212 Villonodular synovitis (pigmented), left shoulder
M12.219 Villonodular synovitis (pigmented), unspecified shoulder
● **M12.22 Villonodular synovitis (pigmented), elbow**
M12.221 Villonodular synovitis (pigmented), right elbow
M12.222 Villonodular synovitis (pigmented), left elbow
M12.229 Villonodular synovitis (pigmented), unspecified elbow
● **M12.23 Villonodular synovitis (pigmented), wrist**
M12.231 Villonodular synovitis (pigmented), right wrist
M12.232 Villonodular synovitis (pigmented), left wrist
M12.239 Villonodular synovitis (pigmented), unspecified wrist

● M12.24 Villonodular synovitis (pigmented), hand
M12.241 Villonodular synovitis (pigmented), right hand
M12.242 Villonodular synovitis (pigmented), left hand
M12.249 Villonodular synovitis (pigmented), unspecified hand
● M12.25 Villonodular synovitis (pigmented), hip
M12.251 Villonodular synovitis (pigmented), right hip
M12.252 Villonodular synovitis (pigmented), left hip
M12.259 Villonodular synovitis (pigmented), unspecified hip
● M12.26 Villonodular synovitis (pigmented), knee
M12.261 Villonodular synovitis (pigmented), right knee
M12.262 Villonodular synovitis (pigmented), left knee
M12.269 Villonodular synovitis (pigmented), unspecified knee
● M12.27 Villonodular synovitis (pigmented), ankle and foot
M12.271 Villonodular synovitis (pigmented), right ankle and foot
M12.272 Villonodular synovitis (pigmented), left ankle and foot
M12.279 Villonodular synovitis (pigmented), unspecified ankle and foot
M12.28 Villonodular synovitis (pigmented), other specified site
Villonodular synovitis (pigmented), vertebrae
M12.29 Villonodular synovitis (pigmented), multiple sites
● M12.3 Palindromic rheumatism
M12.30 Palindromic rheumatism, unspecified site
● M12.31 Palindromic rheumatism, shoulder
M12.311 Palindromic rheumatism, right shoulder
M12.312 Palindromic rheumatism, left shoulder
M12.319 Palindromic rheumatism, unspecified shoulder
● M12.32 Palindromic rheumatism, elbow
M12.321 Palindromic rheumatism, right elbow
M12.322 Palindromic rheumatism, left elbow
M12.329 Palindromic rheumatism, unspecified elbow
● M12.33 Palindromic rheumatism, wrist
M12.331 Palindromic rheumatism, right wrist
M12.332 Palindromic rheumatism, left wrist
M12.339 Palindromic rheumatism, unspecified wrist
● M12.34 Palindromic rheumatism, hand
M12.341 Palindromic rheumatism, right hand
M12.342 Palindromic rheumatism, left hand
M12.349 Palindromic rheumatism, unspecified hand
● M12.35 Palindromic rheumatism, hip
M12.351 Palindromic rheumatism, right hip
M12.352 Palindromic rheumatism, left hip
M12.359 Palindromic rheumatism, unspecified hip
● M12.36 Palindromic rheumatism, knee
M12.361 Palindromic rheumatism, right knee
M12.362 Palindromic rheumatism, left knee
M12.369 Palindromic rheumatism, unspecified knee
● M12.37 Palindromic rheumatism, ankle and foot
M12.371 Palindromic rheumatism, right ankle and foot
M12.372 Palindromic rheumatism, left ankle and foot
M12.379 Palindromic rheumatism, unspecified ankle and foot
M12.38 Palindromic rheumatism, other specified site
Palindromic rheumatism, vertebrae
M12.39 Palindromic rheumatism, multiple sites
● M12.4 Intermittent hydrarthrosis
M12.40 Intermittent hydrarthrosis, unspecified site
● M12.41 Intermittent hydrarthrosis, shoulder
M12.411 Intermittent hydrarthrosis, right shoulder
M12.412 Intermittent hydrarthrosis, left shoulder
M12.419 Intermittent hydrarthrosis, unspecified shoulder
● M12.42 Intermittent hydrarthrosis, elbow
M12.421 Intermittent hydrarthrosis, right elbow
M12.422 Intermittent hydrarthrosis, left elbow
M12.429 Intermittent hydrarthrosis, unspecified elbow
● M12.43 Intermittent hydrarthrosis, wrist
M12.431 Intermittent hydrarthrosis, right wrist
M12.432 Intermittent hydrarthrosis, left wrist
M12.439 Intermittent hydrarthrosis, unspecified wrist
● M12.44 Intermittent hydrarthrosis, hand
M12.441 Intermittent hydrarthrosis, right hand
M12.442 Intermittent hydrarthrosis, left hand
M12.449 Intermittent hydrarthrosis, unspecified hand
● M12.45 Intermittent hydrarthrosis, hip
M12.451 Intermittent hydrarthrosis, right hip
M12.452 Intermittent hydrarthrosis, left hip
M12.459 Intermittent hydrarthrosis, unspecified hip
● M12.46 Intermittent hydrarthrosis, knee
M12.461 Intermittent hydrarthrosis, right knee
M12.462 Intermittent hydrarthrosis, left knee
M12.469 Intermittent hydrarthrosis, unspecified knee
● M12.47 Intermittent hydrarthrosis, ankle and foot
M12.471 Intermittent hydrarthrosis, right ankle and foot
M12.472 Intermittent hydrarthrosis, left ankle and foot
M12.479 Intermittent hydrarthrosis, unspecified ankle and foot
M12.48 Intermittent hydrarthrosis, other site
M12.49 Intermittent hydrarthrosis, multiple sites

● **M12.5 Traumatic arthropathy**

Excludes1 current injury-see Alphabetic Index
post-traumatic osteoarthritis of first carpometacarpal joint (M18.2-M18.3)
post-traumatic osteoarthritis of hip (M16.4-M16.5)
post-traumatic osteoarthritis of knee (M17.2-M17.3)
post-traumatic osteoarthritis NOS (M19.1-)
post-traumatic osteoarthritis of other single joints (M19.1-)

M12.50 Traumatic arthropathy, unspecified site

● **M12.51 Traumatic arthropathy, shoulder**

M12.511 Traumatic arthropathy, right shoulder

M12.512 Traumatic arthropathy, left shoulder

M12.519 Traumatic arthropathy, unspecified shoulder

● **M12.52 Traumatic arthropathy, elbow**

M12.521 Traumatic arthropathy, right elbow

M12.522 Traumatic arthropathy, left elbow

M12.529 Traumatic arthropathy, unspecified elbow

● **M12.53 Traumatic arthropathy, wrist**

M12.531 Traumatic arthropathy, right wrist

M12.532 Traumatic arthropathy, left wrist

M12.539 Traumatic arthropathy, unspecified wrist

● **M12.54 Traumatic arthropathy, hand**

M12.541 Traumatic arthropathy, right hand

M12.542 Traumatic arthropathy, left hand

M12.549 Traumatic arthropathy, unspecified hand

● **M12.55 Traumatic arthropathy, hip**

M12.551 Traumatic arthropathy, right hip

M12.552 Traumatic arthropathy, left hip

M12.559 Traumatic arthropathy, unspecified hip

● **M12.56 Traumatic arthropathy, knee**

M12.561 Traumatic arthropathy, right knee

M12.562 Traumatic arthropathy, left knee

M12.569 Traumatic arthropathy, unspecified knee

● **M12.57 Traumatic arthropathy, ankle and foot**

M12.571 Traumatic arthropathy, right ankle and foot

M12.572 Traumatic arthropathy, left ankle and foot

M12.579 Traumatic arthropathy, unspecified ankle and foot

M12.58 Traumatic arthropathy, other specified site
Traumatic arthropathy, vertebrae

M12.59 Traumatic arthropathy, multiple sites

● **M12.8 Other specific arthropathies, not elsewhere classified**
Transient arthropathy

M12.80 Other specific arthropathies, not elsewhere classified, unspecified site

● **M12.81 Other specific arthropathies, not elsewhere classified, shoulder**

M12.811 Other specific arthropathies, not elsewhere classified, right shoulder

M12.812 Other specific arthropathies, not elsewhere classified, left shoulder

M12.819 Other specific arthropathies, not elsewhere classified, unspecified shoulder

● **M12.82 Other specific arthropathies, not elsewhere classified, elbow**

M12.821 Other specific arthropathies, not elsewhere classified, right elbow

M12.822 Other specific arthropathies, not elsewhere classified, left elbow

M12.829 Other specific arthropathies, not elsewhere classified, unspecified elbow

● **M12.83 Other specific arthropathies, not elsewhere classified, wrist**

M12.831 Other specific arthropathies, not elsewhere classified, right wrist

M12.832 Other specific arthropathies, not elsewhere classified, left wrist

M12.839 Other specific arthropathies, not elsewhere classified, unspecified wrist

● **M12.84 Other specific arthropathies, not elsewhere classified, hand**

M12.841 Other specific arthropathies, not elsewhere classified, right hand

M12.842 Other specific arthropathies, not elsewhere classified, left hand

M12.849 Other specific arthropathies, not elsewhere classified, unspecified hand

● **M12.85 Other specific arthropathies, not elsewhere classified, hip**

M12.851 Other specific arthropathies, not elsewhere classified, right hip

M12.852 Other specific arthropathies, not elsewhere classified, left hip

M12.859 Other specific arthropathies, not elsewhere classified, unspecified hip

● **M12.86 Other specific arthropathies, not elsewhere classified, knee**

M12.861 Other specific arthropathies, not elsewhere classified, right knee

M12.862 Other specific arthropathies, not elsewhere classified, left knee

M12.869 Other specific arthropathies, not elsewhere classified, unspecified knee

● **M12.87 Other specific arthropathies, not elsewhere classified, ankle and foot**

M12.871 Other specific arthropathies, not elsewhere classified, right ankle and foot

M12.872 Other specific arthropathies, not elsewhere classified, left ankle and foot

M12.879 Other specific arthropathies, not elsewhere classified, unspecified ankle and foot

M12.88 Other specific arthropathies, not elsewhere classified, other specified site
Other specific arthropathies, not elsewhere classified, vertebrae

M12.89 Other specific arthropathies, not elsewhere classified, multiple sites

M12.9 Arthropathy, unspecified

● M13 Other arthritis
Excludes1 arthrosis (M15-M19)
osteoarthritis (M15-M19)

M13.0 Polyarthritis, unspecified

● M13.1 Monoarthritis, not elsewhere classified
M13.10 Monoarthritis, not elsewhere classified, unspecified site
● M13.11 Monoarthritis, not elsewhere classified, shoulder
M13.111 Monoarthritis, not elsewhere classified, right shoulder
M13.112 Monoarthritis, not elsewhere classified, left shoulder
M13.119 Monoarthritis, not elsewhere classified, unspecified shoulder
● M13.12 Monoarthritis, not elsewhere classified, elbow
M13.121 Monoarthritis, not elsewhere classified, right elbow
M13.122 Monoarthritis, not elsewhere classified, left elbow
M13.129 Monoarthritis, not elsewhere classified, unspecified elbow
● M13.13 Monoarthritis, not elsewhere classified, wrist
M13.131 Monoarthritis, not elsewhere classified, right wrist
M13.132 Monoarthritis, not elsewhere classified, left wrist
M13.139 Monoarthritis, not elsewhere classified, unspecified wrist
● M13.14 Monoarthritis, not elsewhere classified, hand
M13.141 Monoarthritis, not elsewhere classified, right hand
M13.142 Monoarthritis, not elsewhere classified, left hand
M13.149 Monoarthritis, not elsewhere classified, unspecified hand
● M13.15 Monoarthritis, not elsewhere classified, hip
M13.151 Monoarthritis, not elsewhere classified, right hip
M13.152 Monoarthritis, not elsewhere classified, left hip
M13.159 Monoarthritis, not elsewhere classified, unspecified hip
● M13.16 Monoarthritis, not elsewhere classified, knee
M13.161 Monoarthritis, not elsewhere classified, right knee
M13.162 Monoarthritis, not elsewhere classified, left knee
M13.169 Monoarthritis, not elsewhere classified, unspecified knee
● M13.17 Monoarthritis, not elsewhere classified, ankle and foot
M13.171 Monoarthritis, not elsewhere classified, right ankle and foot
M13.172 Monoarthritis, not elsewhere classified, left ankle and foot
M13.179 Monoarthritis, not elsewhere classified, unspecified ankle and foot

● M13.8 Other specified arthritis
Allergic arthritis
Excludes1 osteoarthritis (M15-M19)
M13.80 Other specified arthritis, unspecified site
● M13.81 Other specified arthritis, shoulder
M13.811 Other specified arthritis, right shoulder
M13.812 Other specified arthritis, left shoulder
M13.819 Other specified arthritis, unspecified shoulder
● M13.82 Other specified arthritis, elbow
M13.821 Other specified arthritis, right elbow
M13.822 Other specified arthritis, left elbow
M13.829 Other specified arthritis, unspecified elbow
● M13.83 Other specified arthritis, wrist
M13.831 Other specified arthritis, right wrist
M13.832 Other specified arthritis, left wrist
M13.839 Other specified arthritis, unspecified wrist
● M13.84 Other specified arthritis, hand
M13.841 Other specified arthritis, right hand
M13.842 Other specified arthritis, left hand
M13.849 Other specified arthritis, unspecified hand
● M13.85 Other specified arthritis, hip
M13.851 Other specified arthritis, right hip
M13.852 Other specified arthritis, left hip
M13.859 Other specified arthritis, unspecified hip
● M13.86 Other specified arthritis, knee
M13.861 Other specified arthritis, right knee
M13.862 Other specified arthritis, left knee
M13.869 Other specified arthritis, unspecified knee
● M13.87 Other specified arthritis, ankle and foot
M13.871 Other specified arthritis, right ankle and foot
M13.872 Other specified arthritis, left ankle and foot
M13.879 Other specified arthritis, unspecified ankle and foot
M13.88 Other specified arthritis, other site
M13.89 Other specified arthritis, multiple sites

● M14 Arthropathies in other diseases classified elsewhere
Excludes1 arthropathy in:
diabetes mellitus (E08-E13 with .61-)
hematological disorders (M36.2-M36.3)
hypersensitivity reactions (M36.4)
neoplastic disease (M36.1)
neurosyphillis (A52.16)
sarcoidosis (D86.86)
enteropathic arthropathies (M07.0-)
juvenile psoriatic arthropathy (L40.54)
lipoid dermatoarthritis (E78.81)

● M14.6 Charcôt's joint
Neuropathic arthropathy
Excludes1 Charcôt's joint in diabetes mellitus (E08-E13 with .610)
Charcôt's joint in tabes dorsalis (A52.16)
M14.60 Charcôt's joint, unspecified site
● M14.61 Charcôt's joint, shoulder
M14.611 Charcôt's joint, right shoulder
M14.612 Charcôt's joint, left shoulder
M14.619 Charcôt's joint, unspecified shoulder
● M14.62 Charcôt's joint, elbow
M14.621 Charcôt's joint, right elbow
M14.622 Charcôt's joint, left elbow
M14.629 Charcôt's joint, unspecified elbow
● M14.63 Charcôt's joint, wrist
M14.631 Charcôt's joint, right wrist
M14.632 Charcôt's joint, left wrist
M14.639 Charcôt's joint, unspecified wrist

● M14.64 Charcôt's joint, hand
M14.641 Charcôt's joint, right hand
M14.642 Charcôt's joint, left hand
M14.649 Charcôt's joint, unspecified hand
● M14.65 Charcôt's joint, hip
M14.651 Charcôt's joint, right hip
M14.652 Charcôt's joint, left hip
M14.659 Charcôt's joint, unspecified hip
● M14.66 Charcôt's joint, knee
M14.661 Charcôt's joint, right knee
M14.662 Charcôt's joint, left knee
M14.669 Charcôt's joint, unspecified knee
● M14.67 Charcôt's joint, ankle and foot
M14.671 Charcôt's joint, right ankle and foot
M14.672 Charcôt's joint, left ankle and foot
M14.679 Charcôt's joint, unspecified ankle and foot
M14.68 Charcôt's joint, vertebrae
M14.69 Charcôt's joint, multiple sites
● M14.8 Arthropathies in other specified diseases classified elsewhere
Code first underlying disease, such as:
amyloidosis (E85.-)
erythema multiforme (L51.-)
erythema nodosum (L52)
hemochromatosis (E83.11-)
hyperparathyroidism (E21.-)
hypothyroidism (E00-E03)
sickle-cell disorders (D57.-)
thyrotoxicosis [hyperthyroidism] (E05.-)
Whipple's disease (K90.81)
M14.80 Arthropathies in other specified diseases classified elsewhere, unspecified site
● M14.81 Arthropathies in other specified diseases classified elsewhere, shoulder
M14.811 Arthropathies in other specified diseases classified elsewhere, right shoulder
M14.812 Arthropathies in other specified diseases classified elsewhere, left shoulder
M14.819 Arthropathies in other specified diseases classified elsewhere, unspecified shoulder
● M14.82 Arthropathies in other specified diseases classified elsewhere, elbow
M14.821 Arthropathies in other specified diseases classified elsewhere, right elbow
M14.822 Arthropathies in other specified diseases classified elsewhere, left elbow
M14.829 Arthropathies in other specified diseases classified elsewhere, unspecified elbow
● M14.83 Arthropathies in other specified diseases classified elsewhere, wrist
M14.831 Arthropathies in other specified diseases classified elsewhere, right wrist
M14.832 Arthropathies in other specified diseases classified elsewhere, left wrist
M14.839 Arthropathies in other specified diseases classified elsewhere, unspecified wrist
● M14.84 Arthropathies in other specified diseases classified elsewhere, hand
M14.841 Arthropathies in other specified diseases classified elsewhere, right hand
M14.842 Arthropathies in other specified diseases classified elsewhere, left hand
M14.849 Arthropathies in other specified diseases classified elsewhere, unspecified hand
● M14.85 Arthropathies in other specified diseases classified elsewhere, hip
M14.851 Arthropathies in other specified diseases classified elsewhere, right hip
M14.852 Arthropathies in other specified diseases classified elsewhere, left hip
M14.859 Arthropathies in other specified diseases classified elsewhere, unspecified hip
● M14.86 Arthropathies in other specified diseases classified elsewhere, knee
M14.861 Arthropathies in other specified diseases classified elsewhere, right knee
M14.862 Arthropathies in other specified diseases classified elsewhere, left knee
M14.869 Arthropathies in other specified diseases classified elsewhere, unspecified knee
● M14.87 Arthropathies in other specified diseases classified elsewhere, ankle and foot
M14.871 Arthropathies in other specified diseases classified elsewhere, right ankle and foot
M14.872 Arthropathies in other specified diseases classified elsewhere, left ankle and foot
M14.879 Arthropathies in other specified diseases classified elsewhere, unspecified ankle and foot
M14.88 Arthropathies in other specified diseases classified elsewhere, vertebrae
M14.89 Arthropathies in other specified diseases classified elsewhere, multiple sites

OSTEOARTHRITIS (M15-M19)

Osteoarthritis is the most common degenerative joint disease and form of arthritis that breaks down the cartilage causing pain, swelling, and reduced motion in the joints.

Excludes2 osteoarthritis of spine (M47.-)

● M15 Polyosteoarthritis
Includes arthritis of multiple sites
Excludes1 bilateral involvement of single joint (M16-M19)
M15.0 Primary generalized (osteo)arthritis
M15.1 Heberden's nodes (with arthropathy)
Interphalangeal distal osteoarthritis
M15.2 Bouchard's nodes (with arthropathy)
Juxtaphalangeal distal osteoarthritis
M15.3 Secondary multiple arthritis
Post-traumatic polyosteoarthritis
M15.4 Erosive (osteo)arthritis
M15.8 Other polyosteoarthritis
M15.9 Polyosteoarthritis, unspecified
Generalized osteoarthritis NOS

● M16 Osteoarthritis of hip
M16.0 Bilateral primary osteoarthritis of hip
● M16.1 Unilateral primary osteoarthritis of hip
Primary osteoarthritis of hip NOS
M16.10 Unilateral primary osteoarthritis, unspecified hip
M16.11 Unilateral primary osteoarthritis, right hip
M16.12 Unilateral primary osteoarthritis, left hip
M16.2 Bilateral osteoarthritis resulting from hip dysplasia
● M16.3 Unilateral osteoarthritis resulting from hip dysplasia
Dysplastic osteoarthritis of hip NOS
M16.30 Unilateral osteoarthritis resulting from hip dysplasia, unspecified hip
M16.31 Unilateral osteoarthritis resulting from hip dysplasia, right hip
M16.32 Unilateral osteoarthritis resulting from hip dysplasia, left hip
M16.4 Bilateral post-traumatic osteoarthritis of hip
● M16.5 Unilateral post-traumatic osteoarthritis of hip
Post-traumatic osteoarthritis of hip NOS
M16.50 Unilateral post-traumatic osteoarthritis, unspecified hip
M16.51 Unilateral post-traumatic osteoarthritis, right hip
M16.52 Unilateral post-traumatic osteoarthritis, left hip
M16.6 Other bilateral secondary osteoarthritis of hip
M16.7 Other unilateral secondary osteoarthritis of hip
Secondary osteoarthritis of hip NOS
M16.9 Osteoarthritis of hip, unspecified

● M17 Osteoarthritis of knee
M17.0 Bilateral primary osteoarthritis of knee
● M17.1 Unilateral primary osteoarthritis of knee
Primary osteoarthritis of knee NOS
M17.10 Unilateral primary osteoarthritis, unspecified knee
M17.11 Unilateral primary osteoarthritis, right knee
M17.12 Unilateral primary osteoarthritis, left knee
M17.2 Bilateral post-traumatic osteoarthritis of knee
● M17.3 Unilateral post-traumatic osteoarthritis of knee
Post-traumatic osteoarthritis of knee NOS
M17.30 Unilateral post-traumatic osteoarthritis, unspecified knee
M17.31 Unilateral post-traumatic osteoarthritis, right knee
M17.32 Unilateral post-traumatic osteoarthritis, left knee
M17.4 Other bilateral secondary osteoarthritis of knee
M17.5 Other unilateral secondary osteoarthritis of knee
Secondary osteoarthritis of knee NOS
M17.9 Osteoarthritis of knee, unspecified

● M18 Osteoarthritis of first carpometacarpal joint
M18.0 Bilateral primary osteoarthritis of first carpometacarpal joints
● M18.1 Unilateral primary osteoarthritis of first carpometacarpal joint
Primary osteoarthritis of first carpometacarpal joint NOS
M18.10 Unilateral primary osteoarthritis of first carpometacarpal joint, unspecified hand
M18.11 Unilateral primary osteoarthritis of first carpometacarpal joint, right hand
M18.12 Unilateral primary osteoarthritis of first carpometacarpal joint, left hand
M18.2 Bilateral post-traumatic osteoarthritis of first carpometacarpal joints
● M18.3 Unilateral post-traumatic osteoarthritis of first carpometacarpal joint
Post-traumatic osteoarthritis of first carpometacarpal joint NOS
M18.30 Unilateral post-traumatic osteoarthritis of first carpometacarpal joint, unspecified hand
M18.31 Unilateral post-traumatic osteoarthritis of first carpometacarpal joint, right hand
M18.32 Unilateral post-traumatic osteoarthritis of first carpometacarpal joint, left hand
M18.4 Other bilateral secondary osteoarthritis of first carpometacarpal joints
● M18.5 Other unilateral secondary osteoarthritis of first carpometacarpal joint
Secondary osteoarthritis of first carpometacarpal joint NOS
M18.50 Other unilateral secondary osteoarthritis of first carpometacarpal joint, unspecified hand
M18.51 Other unilateral secondary osteoarthritis of first carpometacarpal joint, right hand
M18.52 Other unilateral secondary osteoarthritis of first carpometacarpal joint, left hand
M18.9 Osteoarthritis of first carpometacarpal joint, unspecified

● M19 Other and unspecified osteoarthritis
Excludes1 polyarthritis (M15.-)
Excludes2 arthrosis of spine (M47.-)
hallux rigidus (M20.2)
osteoarthritis of spine (M47.-)
● M19.0 Primary osteoarthritis of other joints
● M19.01 Primary osteoarthritis, shoulder
M19.011 Primary osteoarthritis, right shoulder
M19.012 Primary osteoarthritis, left shoulder
M19.019 Primary osteoarthritis, unspecified shoulder
● M19.02 Primary osteoarthritis, elbow
M19.021 Primary osteoarthritis, right elbow
M19.022 Primary osteoarthritis, left elbow
M19.029 Primary osteoarthritis, unspecified elbow
● M19.03 Primary osteoarthritis, wrist
M19.031 Primary osteoarthritis, right wrist
M19.032 Primary osteoarthritis, left wrist
M19.039 Primary osteoarthritis, unspecified wrist
● M19.04 Primary osteoarthritis, hand
Excludes2 primary osteoarthritis of first carpometacarpal joint (M18.0-, M18.1-)
M19.041 Primary osteoarthritis, right hand
M19.042 Primary osteoarthritis, left hand
M19.049 Primary osteoarthritis, unspecified hand
● M19.07 Primary osteoarthritis ankle and foot
M19.071 Primary osteoarthritis, right ankle and foot
M19.072 Primary osteoarthritis, left ankle and foot
M19.079 Primary osteoarthritis, unspecified ankle and foot

● M19.1 Post-traumatic osteoarthritis of other joints
● M19.11 Post-traumatic osteoarthritis, shoulder
M19.111 Post-traumatic osteoarthritis, right shoulder
M19.112 Post-traumatic osteoarthritis, left shoulder
M19.119 Post-traumatic osteoarthritis, unspecified shoulder
● M19.12 Post-traumatic osteoarthritis, elbow
M19.121 Post-traumatic osteoarthritis, right elbow
M19.122 Post-traumatic osteoarthritis, left elbow
M19.129 Post-traumatic osteoarthritis, unspecified elbow
● M19.13 Post-traumatic osteoarthritis, wrist
M19.131 Post-traumatic osteoarthritis, right wrist
M19.132 Post-traumatic osteoarthritis, left wrist
M19.139 Post-traumatic osteoarthritis, unspecified wrist
● M19.14 Post-traumatic osteoarthritis, hand
Excludes2 post-traumatic osteoarthritis of first carpometacarpal joint (M18.2-, M18.3-)
M19.141 Post-traumatic osteoarthritis, right hand
M19.142 Post-traumatic osteoarthritis, left hand
M19.149 Post-traumatic osteoarthritis, unspecified hand
● M19.17 Post-traumatic osteoarthritis, ankle and foot
M19.171 Post-traumatic osteoarthritis, right ankle and foot
M19.172 Post-traumatic osteoarthritis, left ankle and foot
M19.179 Post-traumatic osteoarthritis, unspecified ankle and foot
● M19.2 Secondary osteoarthritis of other joints
● M19.21 Secondary osteoarthritis, shoulder
M19.211 Secondary osteoarthritis, right shoulder
M19.212 Secondary osteoarthritis, left shoulder
M19.219 Secondary osteoarthritis, unspecified shoulder
● M19.22 Secondary osteoarthritis, elbow
M19.221 Secondary osteoarthritis, right elbow
M19.222 Secondary osteoarthritis, left elbow
M19.229 Secondary osteoarthritis, unspecified elbow
● M19.23 Secondary osteoarthritis, wrist
M19.231 Secondary osteoarthritis, right wrist
M19.232 Secondary osteoarthritis, left wrist
M19.239 Secondary osteoarthritis, unspecified wrist
● M19.24 Secondary osteoarthritis, hand
M19.241 Secondary osteoarthritis, right hand
M19.242 Secondary osteoarthritis, left hand
M19.249 Secondary osteoarthritis, unspecified hand
● M19.27 Secondary osteoarthritis, ankle and foot
M19.271 Secondary osteoarthritis, right ankle and foot
M19.272 Secondary osteoarthritis, left ankle and foot
M19.279 Secondary osteoarthritis, unspecified ankle and foot
● M19.9 Osteoarthritis, unspecified site
M19.90 Unspecified osteoarthritis, unspecified site
Arthrosis NOS
Arthritis NOS
Osteoarthritis NOS
M19.91 Primary osteoarthritis, unspecified site
Primary osteoarthritis NOS
M19.92 Post-traumatic osteoarthritis, unspecified site
Post-traumatic osteoarthritis NOS
M19.93 Secondary osteoarthritis, unspecified site
Secondary osteoarthritis NOS

OTHER JOINT DISORDERS (M2Ø-M25)

Excludes2 joints of the spine (M40-M54)

● M20 Acquired deformities of fingers and toes
Excludes1 acquired absence of fingers and toes (Z89.-)
congenital absence of fingers and toes (Q71.3-, Q72.3-)
congenital deformities and malformations of fingers and toes (Q66.-, Q68-Q7Ø, Q74.-)
● M2Ø.Ø Deformity of finger(s)
Excludes1 clubbing of fingers (R68.3)
palmar fascial fibromatosis [Dupuytren] (M72.Ø)
trigger finger (M65.3)
● M2Ø.ØØ Unspecified deformity of finger(s)
M2Ø.ØØ1 Unspecified deformity of right finger(s)
M2Ø.ØØ2 Unspecified deformity of left finger(s)
M2Ø.ØØ9 Unspecified deformity of unspecified finger(s)
● M2Ø.Ø1 Mallet finger
M2Ø.Ø11 Mallet finger of right finger(s)
M2Ø.Ø12 Mallet finger of left finger(s)
M2Ø.Ø19 Mallet finger of unspecified finger(s)
● M2Ø.Ø2 Boutonnière deformity
M2Ø.Ø21 Boutonnière deformity of right finger(s)
M2Ø.Ø22 Boutonnière deformity of left finger(s)
M2Ø.Ø29 Boutonnière deformity of unspecified finger(s)
● M2Ø.Ø3 Swan-neck deformity
M2Ø.Ø31 Swan-neck deformity of right finger(s)
M2Ø.Ø32 Swan-neck deformity of left finger(s)
M2Ø.Ø39 Swan-neck deformity of unspecified finger(s)
● M2Ø.Ø9 Other deformity of finger(s)
M2Ø.Ø91 Other deformity of right finger(s)
M2Ø.Ø92 Other deformity of left finger(s)
M2Ø.Ø99 Other deformity of finger(s), unspecified finger(s)

CHAPTER 13 (MØØ-M99)

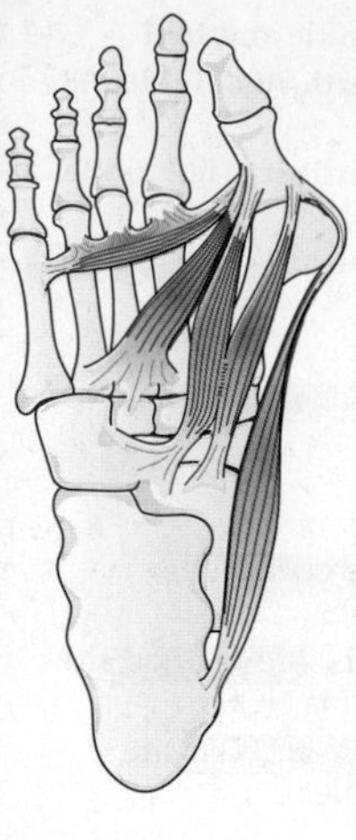

Figure 13-1 Hallux valgus or bunion.

Item 13–2 Hallux valgus or bunion is a sometimes painful structural deformity caused by an inflammation of the bursal sac at the base of the metatarsophalangeal joint (big toe). **Hallus varus** is a deviation of the great toe to the inner side of the foot or away from the next toe.

● **M20.1 Hallux valgus (acquired)**
 Excludes2 bunion (M21.6-) ◀
 M20.10 Hallux valgus (acquired), unspecified foot
 M20.11 Hallux valgus (acquired), right foot
 M20.12 Hallux valgus (acquired), left foot

● **M20.2 Hallux rigidus**
 M20.20 Hallux rigidus, unspecified foot
 M20.21 Hallux rigidus, right foot
 M20.22 Hallux rigidus, left foot

● **M20.3 Hallux varus (acquired)**
 M20.30 Hallux varus (acquired), unspecified foot
 M20.31 Hallux varus (acquired), right foot
 M20.32 Hallux varus (acquired), left foot

● **M20.4 Other hammer toe(s) (acquired)**
 M20.40 Other hammer toe(s) (acquired), unspecified foot
 M20.41 Other hammer toe(s) (acquired), right foot
 M20.42 Other hammer toe(s) (acquired), left foot

● **M20.5 Other deformities of toe(s) (acquired)**
 ● **M20.5X Other deformities of toe(s) (acquired)**
  M20.5X1 Other deformities of toe(s) (acquired), right foot
  M20.5X2 Other deformities of toe(s) (acquired), left foot
  M20.5X9 Other deformities of toe(s) (acquired), unspecified foot

● **M20.6 Acquired deformities of toe(s), unspecified**
 M20.60 Acquired deformities of toe(s), unspecified, unspecified foot
 M20.61 Acquired deformities of toe(s), unspecified, right foot
 M20.62 Acquired deformities of toe(s), unspecified, left foot

Item 13–3 Cubitus valgus is a deformity of the elbow resulting in an increased carrying angle in which the arm extends at the side and the palm faces forward, which results in the forearm and hand extended at a greater than 15 degrees.

Item 13–4 Cubitus varus is a deformity of the elbow resulting in the arm extended at the side and the palm facing forward so that the forearm and hand are held at less than 5 degrees, decreasing the carrying angle.

● **M21 Other acquired deformities of limbs**
 Excludes1 acquired absence of limb (Z89.-)
 congenital absence of limbs (Q71-Q73)
 congenital deformities and malformations of limbs (Q65-Q66, Q68-Q74)
 Excludes2 acquired deformities of fingers or toes (M20.-)
 coxa plana (M91.2)

● **M21.0 Valgus deformity, not elsewhere classified**
 Excludes1 metatarsus valgus (Q66.6)
 talipes calcaneovalgus (Q66.4)
 M21.00 Valgus deformity, not elsewhere classified, unspecified site
 ● **M21.02 Valgus deformity, not elsewhere classified, elbow**
  Cubitus valgus
  M21.021 Valgus deformity, not elsewhere classified, right elbow
  M21.022 Valgus deformity, not elsewhere classified, left elbow
  M21.029 Valgus deformity, not elsewhere classified, unspecified elbow
 ● **M21.05 Valgus deformity, not elsewhere classified, hip**
  M21.051 Valgus deformity, not elsewhere classified, right hip
  M21.052 Valgus deformity, not elsewhere classified, left hip
  M21.059 Valgus deformity, not elsewhere classified, unspecified hip
 ● **M21.06 Valgus deformity, not elsewhere classified, knee**
  Genu valgum
  Knock knee
  M21.061 Valgus deformity, not elsewhere classified, right knee
  M21.062 Valgus deformity, not elsewhere classified, left knee
  M21.069 Valgus deformity, not elsewhere classified, unspecified knee
 ● **M21.07 Valgus deformity, not elsewhere classified, ankle**
  M21.071 Valgus deformity, not elsewhere classified, right ankle
  M21.072 Valgus deformity, not elsewhere classified, left ankle
  M21.079 Valgus deformity, not elsewhere classified, unspecified ankle

● **M21.1 Varus deformity, not elsewhere classified**
 Excludes1 metatarsus varus (Q66.22) ⇐
 tibia vara (M92.5)
 M21.10 Varus deformity, not elsewhere classified, unspecified site
 ● **M21.12 Varus deformity, not elsewhere classified, elbow**
  Cubitus varus, elbow
  M21.121 Varus deformity, not elsewhere classified, right elbow
  M21.122 Varus deformity, not elsewhere classified, left elbow
  M21.129 Varus deformity, not elsewhere classified, unspecified elbow

◀ New ⇐ Revised ~~deleted~~ Deleted OGCR Official Guidelines X Assign placeholder X ● Use Additional Character(s)
Excludes 1 Excludes 2 Includes Use additional Code first Code also Unspecified

● M21.15 Varus deformity, not elsewhere classified, hip
M21.151 Varus deformity, not elsewhere classified, right hip
M21.152 Varus deformity, not elsewhere classified, left hip
M21.159 Varus deformity, not elsewhere classified, unspecified

● M21.16 Varus deformity, not elsewhere classified, knee
Bow leg
Genu varum
M21.161 Varus deformity, not elsewhere classified, right knee
M21.162 Varus deformity, not elsewhere classified, left knee
M21.169 Varus deformity, not elsewhere classified, unspecified knee

● M21.17 Varus deformity, not elsewhere classified, ankle
M21.171 Varus deformity, not elsewhere classified, right ankle
M21.172 Varus deformity, not elsewhere classified, left ankle
M21.179 Varus deformity, not elsewhere classified, unspecified ankle

● M21.2 Flexion deformity
M21.20 Flexion deformity, unspecified site

● M21.21 Flexion deformity, shoulder
M21.211 Flexion deformity, right shoulder
M21.212 Flexion deformity, left shoulder
M21.219 Flexion deformity, unspecified shoulder

● M21.22 Flexion deformity, elbow
M21.221 Flexion deformity, right elbow
M21.222 Flexion deformity, left elbow
M21.229 Flexion deformity, unspecified elbow

● M21.23 Flexion deformity, wrist
M21.231 Flexion deformity, right wrist
M21.232 Flexion deformity, left wrist
M21.239 Flexion deformity, unspecified wrist

● M21.24 Flexion deformity, finger joints
M21.241 Flexion deformity, right finger joints
M21.242 Flexion deformity, left finger joints
M21.249 Flexion deformity, unspecified finger joints

● M21.25 Flexion deformity, hip
M21.251 Flexion deformity, right hip
M21.252 Flexion deformity, left hip
M21.259 Flexion deformity, unspecified hip

● M21.26 Flexion deformity, knee
M21.261 Flexion deformity, right knee
M21.262 Flexion deformity, left knee
M21.269 Flexion deformity, unspecified knee

● M21.27 Flexion deformity, ankle and toes
M21.271 Flexion deformity, right ankle and toes
M21.272 Flexion deformity, left ankle and toes
M21.279 Flexion deformity, unspecified ankle and toes

● M21.3 Wrist or foot drop (acquired)

● M21.33 Wrist drop (acquired)
M21.331 Wrist drop, right wrist
M21.332 Wrist drop, left wrist
M21.339 Wrist drop, unspecified wrist

● M21.37 Foot drop (acquired)
M21.371 Foot drop, right foot
M21.372 Foot drop, left foot
M21.379 Foot drop, unspecified foot

● M21.4 Flat foot [pes planus] (acquired)
Excludes1 congenital pes planus (Q66.5-)
M21.40 Flat foot [pes planus] (acquired), unspecified foot
M21.41 Flat foot [pes planus] (acquired), right foot
M21.42 Flat foot [pes planus] (acquired), left foot

● M21.5 Acquired clawhand, clubhand, clawfoot and clubfoot
Excludes1 clubfoot, not specified as acquired (Q66.89)

● M21.51 Acquired clawhand
M21.511 Acquired clawhand, right hand
M21.512 Acquired clawhand, left hand
M21.519 Acquired clawhand, unspecified hand

● M21.52 Acquired clubhand
M21.521 Acquired clubhand, right hand
M21.522 Acquired clubhand, left hand
M21.529 Acquired clubhand, unspecified hand

● M21.53 Acquired clawfoot
M21.531 Acquired clawfoot, right foot
M21.532 Acquired clawfoot, left foot
M21.539 Acquired clawfoot, unspecified foot

● M21.54 Acquired clubfoot
M21.541 Acquired clubfoot, right foot
M21.542 Acquired clubfoot, left foot
M21.549 Acquired clubfoot, unspecified foot

● M21.6 Other acquired deformities of foot
Excludes2 deformities of toe (acquired) (M20.1-M20.6-) ⇐

● M21.61 Bunion ◀
M21.611 Bunion of right foot ◀
M21.612 Bunion of left foot ◀
M21.619 Bunion of unspecified foot ◀

● M21.62 Bunionette ◀
M21.621 Bunionette of right foot ◀
M21.622 Bunionette of left foot ◀
M21.629 Bunionette of unspecified foot ◀

● M21.6X Other acquired deformities of foot
M21.6X1 Other acquired deformities of right foot
M21.6X2 Other acquired deformities of left foot
M21.6X9 Other acquired deformities of unspecified foot

● M21.7 Unequal limb length (acquired)
Note: The site used should correspond to the shorter limb.
M21.70 Unequal limb length (acquired), unspecified site

● M21.72 Unequal limb length (acquired), humerus
M21.721 Unequal limb length (acquired), right humerus
M21.722 Unequal limb length (acquired), left humerus
M21.729 Unequal limb length (acquired), unspecified humerus

● M21.73 Unequal limb length (acquired), ulna and radius
M21.731 Unequal limb length (acquired), right ulna
M21.732 Unequal limb length (acquired), left ulna
M21.733 Unequal limb length (acquired), right radius
M21.734 Unequal limb length (acquired), left radius
M21.739 Unequal limb length (acquired), unspecified ulna and radius

CHAPTER 13 (M00-M99)

● M21.75 Unequal limb length (acquired), femur
M21.751 Unequal limb length (acquired), right femur
M21.752 Unequal limb length (acquired), left femur
M21.759 Unequal limb length (acquired), unspecified femur
● M21.76 Unequal limb length (acquired), tibia and fibula
M21.761 Unequal limb length (acquired), right tibia
M21.762 Unequal limb length (acquired), left tibia
M21.763 Unequal limb length (acquired), right fibula
M21.764 Unequal limb length (acquired), left fibula
M21.769 Unequal limb length (acquired), unspecified tibia and fibula
● M21.8 Other specified acquired deformities of limbs
Excludes2 coxa plana (M91.2)
M21.80 Other specified acquired deformities of unspecified limb
● M21.82 Other specified acquired deformities of upper arm
M21.821 Other specified acquired deformities of right upper arm
M21.822 Other specified acquired deformities of left upper arm
M21.829 Other specified acquired deformities of unspecified upper arm
● M21.83 Other specified acquired deformities of forearm
M21.831 Other specified acquired deformities of right forearm
M21.832 Other specified acquired deformities of left forearm
M21.839 Other specified acquired deformities of unspecified forearm
● M21.85 Other specified acquired deformities of thigh
M21.851 Other specified acquired deformities of right thigh
M21.852 Other specified acquired deformities of left thigh
M21.859 Other specified acquired deformities of unspecified thigh
● M21.86 Other specified acquired deformities of lower leg
M21.861 Other specified acquired deformities of right lower leg
M21.862 Other specified acquired deformities of left lower leg
M21.869 Other specified acquired deformities of unspecified lower leg
● M21.9 Unspecified acquired deformity of limb and hand
M21.90 Unspecified acquired deformity of unspecified limb
● M21.92 Unspecified acquired deformity of upper arm
M21.921 Unspecified acquired deformity of right upper arm
M21.922 Unspecified acquired deformity of left upper arm
M21.929 Unspecified acquired deformity of unspecified upper arm
● M21.93 Unspecified acquired deformity of forearm
M21.931 Unspecified acquired deformity of right forearm
M21.932 Unspecified acquired deformity of left forearm
M21.939 Unspecified acquired deformity of unspecified forearm
● M21.94 Unspecified acquired deformity of hand
M21.941 Unspecified acquired deformity of hand, right hand
M21.942 Unspecified acquired deformity of hand, left hand
M21.949 Unspecified acquired deformity of hand, unspecified hand
● M21.95 Unspecified acquired deformity of thigh
M21.951 Unspecified acquired deformity of right thigh
M21.952 Unspecified acquired deformity of left thigh
M21.959 Unspecified acquired deformity of unspecified thigh
● M21.96 Unspecified acquired deformity of lower leg
M21.961 Unspecified acquired deformity of right lower leg
M21.962 Unspecified acquired deformity of left lower leg
M21.969 Unspecified acquired deformity of unspecified lower leg
● M22 Disorder of patella
Excludes1 traumatic dislocation of patella (S83.0-)
● M22.0 Recurrent dislocation of patella
M22.00 Recurrent dislocation of patella, unspecified knee
M22.01 Recurrent dislocation of patella, right knee
M22.02 Recurrent dislocation of patella, left knee
● M22.1 Recurrent subluxation of patella
Incomplete dislocation of patella
M22.10 Recurrent subluxation of patella, unspecified knee
M22.11 Recurrent subluxation of patella, right knee
M22.12 Recurrent subluxation of patella, left knee
● M22.2 Patellofemoral disorders
● M22.2X Patellofemoral disorders
M22.2X1 Patellofemoral disorders, right knee
M22.2X2 Patellofemoral disorders, left knee
M22.2X9 Patellofemoral disorders, unspecified knee
● M22.3 Other derangements of patella
● M22.3X Other derangements of patella
M22.3X1 Other derangements of patella, right knee
M22.3X2 Other derangements of patella, left knee
M22.3X9 Other derangements of patella, unspecified knee
● M22.4 Chondromalacia patellae
M22.40 Chondromalacia patellae, unspecified knee
M22.41 Chondromalacia patellae, right knee
M22.42 Chondromalacia patellae, left knee
● M22.8 Other disorders of patella
● M22.8X Other disorders of patella
M22.8X1 Other disorders of patella, right knee
M22.8X2 Other disorders of patella, left knee
M22.8X9 Other disorders of patella, unspecified knee
● M22.9 Unspecified disorder of patella
M22.90 Unspecified disorder of patella, unspecified knee
M22.91 Unspecified disorder of patella, right knee
M22.92 Unspecified disorder of patella, left knee

◀ New ◀ Revised ~~deleted~~ Deleted OGCR Official Guidelines X Assign placeholder X ● Use Additional Character(s)
Excludes1 Excludes2 Includes Use additional Code first Code also Unspecified

● **M23 Internal derangement of knee**

Excludes1 ankylosis (M24.66)
current injury - see injury of knee and lower leg (S80-S89)
deformity of knee (M21.-)
osteochondritis dissecans (M93.2)
recurrent dislocation or subluxation of joints (M24.4)
recurrent dislocation or subluxation of patella (M22.0-M22.1)

● **M23.0 Cystic meniscus**

● **M23.00 Cystic meniscus, unspecified meniscus**
Cystic meniscus, unspecified lateral meniscus
Cystic meniscus, unspecified medial meniscus

M23.000 Cystic meniscus, unspecified lateral meniscus, right knee
M23.001 Cystic meniscus, unspecified lateral meniscus, left knee
M23.002 Cystic meniscus, unspecified lateral meniscus, unspecified knee
M23.003 Cystic meniscus, unspecified medial meniscus, right knee
M23.004 Cystic meniscus, unspecified medial meniscus, left knee
M23.005 Cystic meniscus, unspecified medial meniscus, unspecified knee
M23.006 Cystic meniscus, unspecified meniscus, right knee
M23.007 Cystic meniscus, unspecified meniscus, left knee
M23.009 Cystic meniscus, unspecified meniscus, unspecified knee

● **M23.01 Cystic meniscus, anterior horn of medial meniscus**

M23.011 Cystic meniscus, anterior horn of medial meniscus, right knee
M23.012 Cystic meniscus, anterior horn of medial meniscus, left knee
M23.019 Cystic meniscus, anterior horn of medial meniscus, unspecified knee

● **M23.02 Cystic meniscus, posterior horn of medial meniscus**

M23.021 Cystic meniscus, posterior horn of medial meniscus, right knee
M23.022 Cystic meniscus, posterior horn of medial meniscus, left knee
M23.029 Cystic meniscus, posterior horn of medial meniscus, unspecified knee

● **M23.03 Cystic meniscus, other medial meniscus**

M23.031 Cystic meniscus, other medial meniscus, right knee
M23.032 Cystic meniscus, other medial meniscus, left knee
M23.039 Cystic meniscus, other medial meniscus, unspecified knee

● **M23.04 Cystic meniscus, anterior horn of lateral meniscus**

M23.041 Cystic meniscus, anterior horn of lateral meniscus, right knee
M23.042 Cystic meniscus, anterior horn of lateral meniscus, left knee
M23.049 Cystic meniscus, anterior horn of lateral meniscus, unspecified knee

● **M23.05 Cystic meniscus, posterior horn of lateral meniscus**

M23.051 Cystic meniscus, posterior horn of lateral meniscus, right knee
M23.052 Cystic meniscus, posterior horn of lateral meniscus, left knee
M23.059 Cystic meniscus, posterior horn of lateral meniscus, unspecified knee

● **M23.06 Cystic meniscus, other lateral meniscus**

M23.061 Cystic meniscus, other lateral meniscus, right knee
M23.062 Cystic meniscus, other lateral meniscus, left knee
M23.069 Cystic meniscus, other lateral meniscus, unspecified knee

★(See Plate 509 on page NAP-31.)

● **M23.2 Derangement of meniscus due to old tear or injury**
Old bucket-handle tear

● **M23.20 Derangement of unspecified meniscus due to old tear or injury**
Derangement of unspecified lateral meniscus due to old tear or injury
Derangement of unspecified medial meniscus due to old tear or injury

M23.200 Derangement of unspecified lateral meniscus due to old tear or injury, right knee
M23.201 Derangement of unspecified lateral meniscus due to old tear or injury, left knee
M23.202 Derangement of unspecified lateral meniscus due to old tear or injury, unspecified knee
M23.203 Derangement of unspecified medial meniscus due to old tear or injury, right knee
M23.204 Derangement of unspecified medial meniscus due to old tear or injury, left knee
M23.205 Derangement of unspecified medial meniscus due to old tear or injury, unspecified knee
M23.206 Derangement of unspecified meniscus due to old tear or injury, right knee
M23.207 Derangement of unspecified meniscus due to old tear or injury, left knee
M23.209 Derangement of unspecified meniscus due to old tear or injury, unspecified knee

● **M23.21 Derangement of anterior horn of medial meniscus due to old tear or injury**

M23.211 Derangement of anterior horn of medial meniscus due to old tear or injury, right knee
M23.212 Derangement of anterior horn of medial meniscus due to old tear or injury, left knee
M23.219 Derangement of anterior horn of medial meniscus due to old tear or injury, unspecified knee

● **M23.22 Derangement of posterior horn of medial meniscus due to old tear or injury**

M23.221 Derangement of posterior horn of medial meniscus due to old tear or injury, right knee
M23.222 Derangement of posterior horn of medial meniscus due to old tear or injury, left knee
M23.229 Derangement of posterior horn of medial meniscus due to old tear or injury, unspecified knee

- ● **M23.23 Derangement of other medial meniscus due to old tear or injury**
  - **M23.231** Derangement of other medial meniscus due to old tear or injury, right knee
  - **M23.232** Derangement of other medial meniscus due to old tear or injury, left knee
  - **M23.239** Derangement of other medial meniscus due to old tear or injury, unspecified knee
- ● **M23.24 Derangement of anterior horn of lateral meniscus due to old tear or injury**
  - **M23.241** Derangement of anterior horn of lateral meniscus due to old tear or injury, right knee
  - **M23.242** Derangement of anterior horn of lateral meniscus due to old tear or injury, left knee
  - **M23.249** Derangement of anterior horn of lateral meniscus due to old tear or injury, unspecified knee
- ● **M23.25 Derangement of posterior horn of lateral meniscus due to old tear or injury**
  - **M23.251** Derangement of posterior horn of lateral meniscus due to old tear or injury, right knee
  - **M23.252** Derangement of posterior horn of lateral meniscus due to old tear or injury, left knee
  - **M23.259** Derangement of posterior horn of lateral meniscus due to old tear or injury, unspecified knee
- ● **M23.26 Derangement of other lateral meniscus due to old tear or injury**
  - **M23.261** Derangement of other lateral meniscus due to old tear or injury, right knee
  - **M23.262** Derangement of other lateral meniscus due to old tear or injury, left knee
  - **M23.269** Derangement of other lateral meniscus due to old tear or injury, unspecified knee

● **M23.3 Other meniscus derangements**

Degenerate meniscus
Detached meniscus
Retained meniscus

- ● **M23.30 Other meniscus derangements, unspecified meniscus**
  - Other meniscus derangements, unspecified lateral meniscus
  - Other meniscus derangements, unspecified medial meniscus
  - **M23.300** Other meniscus derangements, unspecified lateral meniscus, right knee
  - **M23.301** Other meniscus derangements, unspecified lateral meniscus, left knee
  - **M23.302** Other meniscus derangements, unspecified lateral meniscus, unspecified knee
  - **M23.303** Other meniscus derangements, unspecified medial meniscus, right knee
  - **M23.304** Other meniscus derangements, unspecified medial meniscus, left knee
  - **M23.305** Other meniscus derangements, unspecified medial meniscus, unspecified knee
  - **M23.306** Other meniscus derangements, unspecified meniscus, right knee
  - **M23.307** Other meniscus derangements, unspecified meniscus, left knee
  - **M23.309** Other meniscus derangements, unspecified meniscus, unspecified knee
- ● **M23.31 Other meniscus derangements, anterior horn of medial meniscus**
  - **M23.311** Other meniscus derangements, anterior horn of medial meniscus, right knee
  - **M23.312** Other meniscus derangements, anterior horn of medial meniscus, left knee
  - **M23.319** Other meniscus derangements, anterior horn of medial meniscus, unspecified knee
- ● **M23.32 Other meniscus derangements, posterior horn of medial meniscus**
  - **M23.321** Other meniscus derangements, posterior horn of medial meniscus, right knee
  - **M23.322** Other meniscus derangements, posterior horn of medial meniscus, left knee
  - **M23.329** Other meniscus derangements, posterior horn of medial meniscus, unspecified knee
- ● **M23.33 Other meniscus derangements, other medial meniscus**
  - **M23.331** Other meniscus derangements, other medial meniscus, right knee
  - **M23.332** Other meniscus derangements, other medial meniscus, left knee
  - **M23.339** Other meniscus derangements, other medial meniscus, unspecified knee
- ● **M23.34 Other meniscus derangements, anterior horn of lateral meniscus**
  - **M23.341** Other meniscus derangements, anterior horn of lateral meniscus, right knee
  - **M23.342** Other meniscus derangements, anterior horn of lateral meniscus, left knee
  - **M23.349** Other meniscus derangements, anterior horn of lateral meniscus, unspecified knee
- ● **M23.35 Other meniscus derangements, posterior horn of lateral meniscus**
  - **M23.351** Other meniscus derangements, posterior horn of lateral meniscus, right knee
  - **M23.352** Other meniscus derangements, posterior horn of lateral meniscus, left knee
  - **M23.359** Other meniscus derangements, posterior horn of lateral meniscus, unspecified knee
- ● **M23.36 Other meniscus derangements, other lateral meniscus**
  - **M23.361** Other meniscus derangements, other lateral meniscus, right knee
  - **M23.362** Other meniscus derangements, other lateral meniscus, left knee
  - **M23.369** Other meniscus derangements, other lateral meniscus, unspecified knee

● **M23.4 Loose body in knee**
- **M23.4Ø Loose body in knee, unspecified knee**
- **M23.41 Loose body in knee, right knee**
- **M23.42 Loose body in knee, left knee**

● **M23.5 Chronic instability of knee**
- **M23.5Ø Chronic instability of knee, unspecified knee**
- **M23.51 Chronic instability of knee, right knee**
- **M23.52 Chronic instability of knee, left knee**

● **M23.6 Other spontaneous disruption of ligament(s) of knee**

● **M23.6Ø Other spontaneous disruption of unspecified ligament of knee**
- **M23.6Ø1 Other spontaneous disruption of unspecified ligament of right knee**
- **M23.6Ø2 Other spontaneous disruption of unspecified ligament of left knee**
- **M23.6Ø9 Other spontaneous disruption of unspecified ligament of unspecified knee**

● **M23.61 Other spontaneous disruption of anterior cruciate ligament of knee**
- **M23.611 Other spontaneous disruption of anterior cruciate ligament of right knee**
- **M23.612 Other spontaneous disruption of anterior cruciate ligament of left knee**
- **M23.619 Other spontaneous disruption of anterior cruciate ligament of unspecified knee**

● **M23.62 Other spontaneous disruption of posterior cruciate ligament of knee**
- **M23.621 Other spontaneous disruption of posterior cruciate ligament of right knee**
- **M23.622 Other spontaneous disruption of posterior cruciate ligament of left knee**
- **M23.629 Other spontaneous disruption of posterior cruciate ligament of unspecified knee**

● **M23.63 Other spontaneous disruption of medial collateral ligament of knee**
- **M23.631 Other spontaneous disruption of medial collateral ligament of right knee**
- **M23.632 Other spontaneous disruption of medial collateral ligament of left knee**
- **M23.639 Other spontaneous disruption of medial collateral ligament of unspecified knee**

● **M23.64 Other spontaneous disruption of lateral collateral ligament of knee**
- **M23.641 Other spontaneous disruption of lateral collateral ligament of right knee**
- **M23.642 Other spontaneous disruption of lateral collateral ligament of left knee**
- **M23.649 Other spontaneous disruption of lateral collateral ligament of unspecified knee**

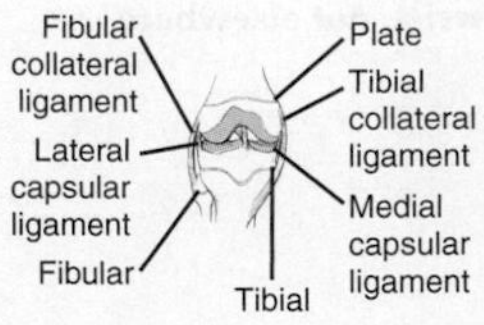

Figure 13-2 Collateral and cruciate ligament of knee. (From DeLee: DeLee and Drez's Orthopaedic Sports Medicine, ed 3, Saunders, 2009)

● **M23.67 Other spontaneous disruption of capsular ligament of knee**
- **M23.671 Other spontaneous disruption of capsular ligament of right knee**
- **M23.672 Other spontaneous disruption of capsular ligament of left knee**
- **M23.679 Other spontaneous disruption of capsular ligament of unspecified knee**

● **M23.8 Other internal derangements of knee**
Laxity of ligament of knee
Snapping knee

● **M23.8X Other internal derangements of knee**
- **M23.8X1 Other internal derangements of right knee**
- **M23.8X2 Other internal derangements of left knee**
- **M23.8X9 Other internal derangements of unspecified knee**

● **M23.9 Unspecified internal derangement of knee**
- **M23.9Ø Unspecified internal derangement of unspecified knee**
- **M23.91 Unspecified internal derangement of right knee**
- **M23.92 Unspecified internal derangement of left knee**

● **M24 Other specific joint derangements**

Excludes1 current injury - see injury of joint by body region

Excludes2 ganglion (M67.4)
snapping knee (M23.8-)
temporomandibular joint disorders (M26.6-)

● **M24.Ø Loose body in joint**

Excludes2 loose body in knee (M23.4)

- **M24.ØØ Loose body in unspecified joint**

● **M24.Ø1 Loose body in shoulder**
- **M24.Ø11 Loose body in right shoulder**
- **M24.Ø12 Loose body in left shoulder**
- **M24.Ø19 Loose body in unspecified shoulder**

● **M24.Ø2 Loose body in elbow**
- **M24.Ø21 Loose body in right elbow**
- **M24.Ø22 Loose body in left elbow**
- **M24.Ø29 Loose body in unspecified elbow**

● **M24.Ø3 Loose body in wrist**
- **M24.Ø31 Loose body in right wrist**
- **M24.Ø32 Loose body in left wrist**
- **M24.Ø39 Loose body in unspecified wrist**

● **M24.Ø4 Loose body in finger joints**
- **M24.Ø41 Loose body in right finger joint(s)**
- **M24.Ø42 Loose body in left finger joint(s)**
- **M24.Ø49 Loose body in unspecified finger joint(s)**

● **M24.Ø5 Loose body in hip**
- **M24.Ø51 Loose body in right hip**
- **M24.Ø52 Loose body in left hip**
- **M24.Ø59 Loose body in unspecified hip**

● **M24.Ø7 Loose body in ankle and toe joints**
- **M24.Ø71 Loose body in right ankle**
- **M24.Ø72 Loose body in left ankle**
- **M24.Ø73 Loose body in unspecified ankle**
- **M24.Ø74 Loose body in right toe joint(s)**
- **M24.Ø75 Loose body in left toe joint(s)**
- **M24.Ø76 Loose body in unspecified toe joints**

M24.Ø8 Loose body, other site

● **M24.1 Other articular cartilage disorders**
Excludes2 chondrocalcinosis (M11.1, M11.2-)
internal derangement of knee (M23.-)
metastatic calcification (E83.5)
ochronosis (E70.2)
M24.10 Other articular cartilage disorders, unspecified site
● **M24.11 Other articular cartilage disorders, shoulder**
M24.111 Other articular cartilage disorders, right shoulder
M24.112 Other articular cartilage disorders, left shoulder
M24.119 Other articular cartilage disorders, unspecified shoulder
● **M24.12 Other articular cartilage disorders, elbow**
M24.121 Other articular cartilage disorders, right elbow
M24.122 Other articular cartilage disorders, left elbow
M24.129 Other articular cartilage disorders, unspecified elbow
● **M24.13 Other articular cartilage disorders, wrist**
M24.131 Other articular cartilage disorders, right wrist
M24.132 Other articular cartilage disorders, left wrist
M24.139 Other articular cartilage disorders, unspecified wrist
● **M24.14 Other articular cartilage disorders, hand**
M24.141 Other articular cartilage disorders, right hand
M24.142 Other articular cartilage disorders, left hand
M24.149 Other articular cartilage disorders, unspecified hand
● **M24.15 Other articular cartilage disorders, hip**
M24.151 Other articular cartilage disorders, right hip
M24.152 Other articular cartilage disorders, left hip
M24.159 Other articular cartilage disorders, unspecified hip
● **M24.17 Other articular cartilage disorders, ankle and foot**
M24.171 Other articular cartilage disorders, right ankle
M24.172 Other articular cartilage disorders, left ankle
M24.173 Other articular cartilage disorders, unspecified ankle
M24.174 Other articular cartilage disorders, right foot
M24.175 Other articular cartilage disorders, left foot
M24.176 Other articular cartilage disorders, unspecified foot
● **M24.2 Disorder of ligament**
Instability secondary to old ligament injury
Ligamentous laxity NOS
Excludes1 familial ligamentous laxity (M35.7)
Excludes2 internal derangement of knee (M23.5-M23.89)
M24.20 Disorder of ligament, unspecified site
● **M24.21 Disorder of ligament, shoulder**
M24.211 Disorder of ligament, right shoulder
M24.212 Disorder of ligament, left shoulder
M24.219 Disorder of ligament, unspecified shoulder
● **M24.22 Disorder of ligament, elbow**
M24.221 Disorder of ligament, right elbow
M24.222 Disorder of ligament, left elbow
M24.229 Disorder of ligament, unspecified elbow
● **M24.23 Disorder of ligament, wrist**
M24.231 Disorder of ligament, right wrist
M24.232 Disorder of ligament, left wrist
M24.239 Disorder of ligament, unspecified wrist
● **M24.24 Disorder of ligament, hand**
M24.241 Disorder of ligament, right hand
M24.242 Disorder of ligament, left hand
M24.249 Disorder of ligament, unspecified hand
● **M24.25 Disorder of ligament, hip**
M24.251 Disorder of ligament, right hip
M24.252 Disorder of ligament, left hip
M24.259 Disorder of ligament, unspecified hip
● **M24.27 Disorder of ligament, ankle and foot**
M24.271 Disorder of ligament, right ankle
M24.272 Disorder of ligament, left ankle
M24.273 Disorder of ligament, unspecified ankle
M24.274 Disorder of ligament, right foot
M24.275 Disorder of ligament, left foot
M24.276 Disorder of ligament, unspecified foot
M24.28 Disorder of ligament, vertebrae
● **M24.3 Pathological dislocation of joint, not elsewhere classified**
Excludes1 congenital dislocation or displacement of joint - see congenital malformations and deformations of the musculoskeletal system (Q65-Q79)
current injury - see injury of joints and ligaments by body region
recurrent dislocation of joint (M24.4-)
M24.30 Pathological dislocation of unspecified joint, not elsewhere classified
● **M24.31 Pathological dislocation of shoulder, not elsewhere classified**
M24.311 Pathological dislocation of right shoulder, not elsewhere classified
M24.312 Pathological dislocation of left shoulder, not elsewhere classified
M24.319 Pathological dislocation of unspecified shoulder, not elsewhere classified
● **M24.32 Pathological dislocation of elbow, not elsewhere classified**
M24.321 Pathological dislocation of right elbow, not elsewhere classified
M24.322 Pathological dislocation of left elbow, not elsewhere classified
M24.329 Pathological dislocation of unspecified elbow, not elsewhere classified
● **M24.33 Pathological dislocation of wrist, not elsewhere classified**
M24.331 Pathological dislocation of right wrist, not elsewhere classified
M24.332 Pathological dislocation of left wrist, not elsewhere classified
M24.339 Pathological dislocation of unspecified wrist, not elsewhere classified

● **M24.34 Pathological dislocation of hand, not elsewhere classified**
- **M24.341 Pathological dislocation of right hand, not elsewhere classified**
- **M24.342 Pathological dislocation of left hand, not elsewhere classified**
- **M24.349 Pathological dislocation of unspecified hand, not elsewhere classified**

● **M24.35 Pathological dislocation of hip, not elsewhere classified**
- **M24.351 Pathological dislocation of right hip, not elsewhere classified**
- **M24.352 Pathological dislocation of left hip, not elsewhere classified**
- **M24.359 Pathological dislocation of unspecified hip, not elsewhere classified**

● **M24.36 Pathological dislocation of knee, not elsewhere classified**
- **M24.361 Pathological dislocation of right knee, not elsewhere classified**
- **M24.362 Pathological dislocation of left knee, not elsewhere classified**
- **M24.369 Pathological dislocation of unspecified knee, not elsewhere classified**

● **M24.37 Pathological dislocation of ankle and foot, not elsewhere classified**
- **M24.371 Pathological dislocation of right ankle, not elsewhere classified**
- **M24.372 Pathological dislocation of left ankle, not elsewhere classified**
- **M24.373 Pathological dislocation of unspecified ankle, not elsewhere classified**
- **M24.374 Pathological dislocation of right foot, not elsewhere classified**
- **M24.375 Pathological dislocation of left foot, not elsewhere classified**
- **M24.376 Pathological dislocation of unspecified foot, not elsewhere classified**

● **M24.4 Recurrent dislocation of joint**

Recurrent subluxation of joint

Excludes2 recurrent dislocation of patella (M22.Ø-M22.1)
recurrent vertebral dislocation (M43.3-, M43.4, M43.5-)

M24.4Ø Recurrent dislocation, unspecified joint

● **M24.41 Recurrent dislocation, shoulder**
- **M24.411 Recurrent dislocation, right shoulder**
- **M24.412 Recurrent dislocation, left shoulder**
- **M24.419 Recurrent dislocation, unspecified shoulder**

● **M24.42 Recurrent dislocation, elbow**
- **M24.421 Recurrent dislocation, right elbow**
- **M24.422 Recurrent dislocation, left elbow**
- **M24.429 Recurrent dislocation, unspecified elbow**

● **M24.43 Recurrent dislocation, wrist**
- **M24.431 Recurrent dislocation, right wrist**
- **M24.432 Recurrent dislocation, left wrist**
- **M24.439 Recurrent dislocation, unspecified wrist**

● **M24.44 Recurrent dislocation, hand and finger(s)**
- **M24.441 Recurrent dislocation, right hand**
- **M24.442 Recurrent dislocation, left hand**
- **M24.443 Recurrent dislocation, unspecified hand**
- **M24.444 Recurrent dislocation, right finger**
- **M24.445 Recurrent dislocation, left finger**
- **M24.446 Recurrent dislocation, unspecified finger**

● **M24.45 Recurrent dislocation, hip**
- **M24.451 Recurrent dislocation, right hip**
- **M24.452 Recurrent dislocation, left hip**
- **M24.459 Recurrent dislocation, unspecified hip**

● **M24.46 Recurrent dislocation, knee**
- **M24.461 Recurrent dislocation, right knee**
- **M24.462 Recurrent dislocation, left knee**
- **M24.469 Recurrent dislocation, unspecified knee**

● **M24.47 Recurrent dislocation, ankle, foot and toes**
- **M24.471 Recurrent dislocation, right ankle**
- **M24.472 Recurrent dislocation, left ankle**
- **M24.473 Recurrent dislocation, unspecified ankle**
- **M24.474 Recurrent dislocation, right foot**
- **M24.475 Recurrent dislocation, left foot**
- **M24.476 Recurrent dislocation, unspecified foot**
- **M24.477 Recurrent dislocation, right toe(s)**
- **M24.478 Recurrent dislocation, left toe(s)**
- **M24.479 Recurrent dislocation, unspecified toe(s)**

● **M24.5 Contracture of joint**

Excludes1 contracture of muscle without contracture of joint (M62.4-)
contracture of tendon (sheath) without contracture of joint (M62.4-)
Dupuytren's contracture (M72.Ø)

Excludes2 acquired deformities of limbs (M2Ø-M21)

M24.5Ø Contracture, unspecified joint

● **M24.51 Contracture, shoulder**
- **M24.511 Contracture, right shoulder**
- **M24.512 Contracture, left shoulder**
- **M24.519 Contracture, unspecified shoulder**

● **M24.52 Contracture, elbow**
- **M24.521 Contracture, right elbow**
- **M24.522 Contracture, left elbow**
- **M24.529 Contracture, unspecified elbow**

● **M24.53 Contracture, wrist**
- **M24.531 Contracture, right wrist**
- **M24.532 Contracture, left wrist**
- **M24.539 Contracture, unspecified wrist**

● **M24.54 Contracture, hand**
- **M24.541 Contracture, right hand**
- **M24.542 Contracture, left hand**
- **M24.549 Contracture, unspecified hand**

● **M24.55 Contracture, hip**
- **M24.551 Contracture, right hip**
- **M24.552 Contracture, left hip**
- **M24.559 Contracture, unspecified hip**

CHAPTER 13 (MØØ-M99)

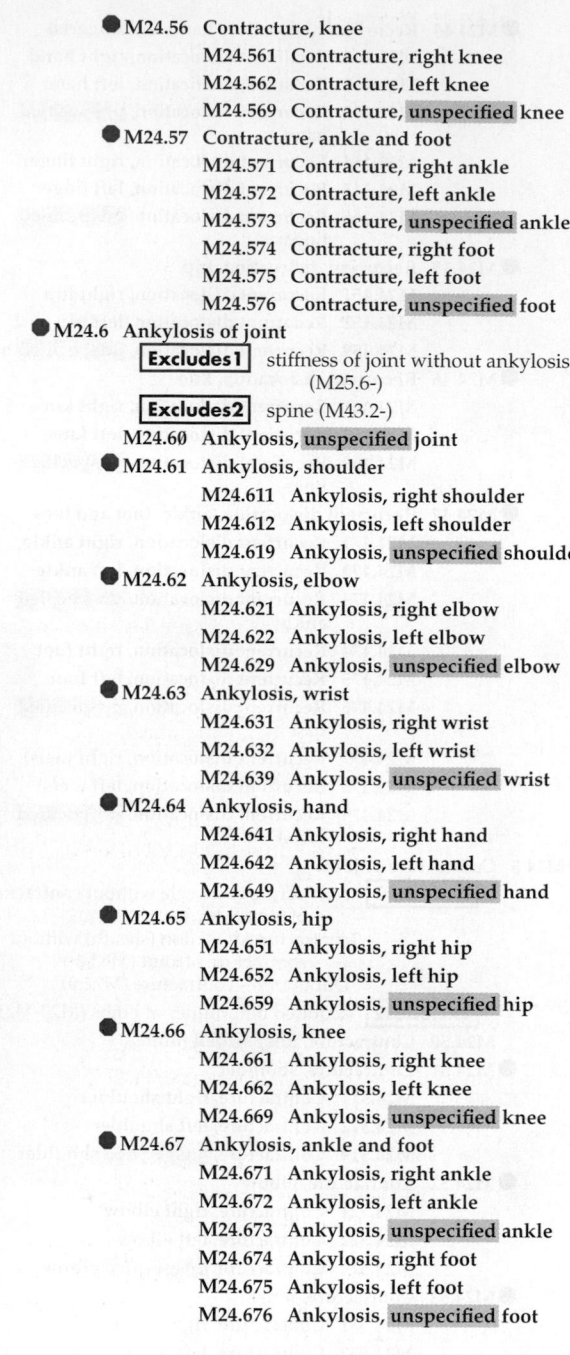

● M24.56 Contracture, knee
M24.561 Contracture, right knee
M24.562 Contracture, left knee
M24.569 Contracture, unspecified knee
● M24.57 Contracture, ankle and foot
M24.571 Contracture, right ankle
M24.572 Contracture, left ankle
M24.573 Contracture, unspecified ankle
M24.574 Contracture, right foot
M24.575 Contracture, left foot
M24.576 Contracture, unspecified foot
● M24.6 Ankylosis of joint
Excludes1 stiffness of joint without ankylosis (M25.6-)
Excludes2 spine (M43.2-)
M24.60 Ankylosis, unspecified joint
● M24.61 Ankylosis, shoulder
M24.611 Ankylosis, right shoulder
M24.612 Ankylosis, left shoulder
M24.619 Ankylosis, unspecified shoulder
● M24.62 Ankylosis, elbow
M24.621 Ankylosis, right elbow
M24.622 Ankylosis, left elbow
M24.629 Ankylosis, unspecified elbow
● M24.63 Ankylosis, wrist
M24.631 Ankylosis, right wrist
M24.632 Ankylosis, left wrist
M24.639 Ankylosis, unspecified wrist
● M24.64 Ankylosis, hand
M24.641 Ankylosis, right hand
M24.642 Ankylosis, left hand
M24.649 Ankylosis, unspecified hand
● M24.65 Ankylosis, hip
M24.651 Ankylosis, right hip
M24.652 Ankylosis, left hip
M24.659 Ankylosis, unspecified hip
● M24.66 Ankylosis, knee
M24.661 Ankylosis, right knee
M24.662 Ankylosis, left knee
M24.669 Ankylosis, unspecified knee
● M24.67 Ankylosis, ankle and foot
M24.671 Ankylosis, right ankle
M24.672 Ankylosis, left ankle
M24.673 Ankylosis, unspecified ankle
M24.674 Ankylosis, right foot
M24.675 Ankylosis, left foot
M24.676 Ankylosis, unspecified foot

Item 13–5 Ankylosis or arthrokleisis is a consolidation of a joint due to disease, injury, or surgical procedure. Spondylosis is the degeneration of the vertebral processes and formation of osteophytes and commonly occurs with age. **Spondylitis** or ankylosing spondylitis is a type of arthritis that affects the spine or backbone causing back pain and stiffness.

M24.7 Protrusio acetabuli
● M24.8 Other specific joint derangements, not elsewhere classified
Excludes2 iliotibial band syndrome (M76.3)
M24.80 Other specific joint derangements of unspecified joint, not elsewhere classified
● M24.81 Other specific joint derangements of shoulder, not elsewhere classified
M24.811 Other specific joint derangements of right shoulder, not elsewhere classified
M24.812 Other specific joint derangements of left shoulder, not elsewhere classified
M24.819 Other specific joint derangements of unspecified shoulder, not elsewhere classified
● M24.82 Other specific joint derangements of elbow, not elsewhere classified
M24.821 Other specific joint derangements of right elbow, not elsewhere classified
M24.822 Other specific joint derangements of left elbow, not elsewhere classified
M24.829 Other specific joint derangements of unspecified elbow, not elsewhere classified
● M24.83 Other specific joint derangements of wrist, not elsewhere classified
M24.831 Other specific joint derangements of right wrist, not elsewhere classified
M24.832 Other specific joint derangements of left wrist, not elsewhere classified
M24.839 Other specific joint derangements of unspecified wrist, not elsewhere classified
● M24.84 Other specific joint derangements of hand, not elsewhere classified
M24.841 Other specific joint derangements of right hand, not elsewhere classified
M24.842 Other specific joint derangements of left hand, not elsewhere classified
M24.849 Other specific joint derangements of unspecified hand, not elsewhere classified
● M24.85 Other specific joint derangements of hip, not elsewhere classified
Irritable hip
M24.851 Other specific joint derangements of right hip, not elsewhere classified
M24.852 Other specific joint derangements of left hip, not elsewhere classified
M24.859 Other specific joint derangements of unspecified hip, not elsewhere classified
● M24.87 Other specific joint derangements of ankle and foot, not elsewhere classified
M24.871 Other specific joint derangements of right ankle, not elsewhere classified
M24.872 Other specific joint derangements of left ankle, not elsewhere classified
M24.873 Other specific joint derangements of unspecified ankle, not elsewhere classified
M24.874 Other specific joint derangements of right foot, not elsewhere classified
M24.875 Other specific joint derangements left foot, not elsewhere classified
M24.876 Other specific joint derangements of unspecified foot, not elsewhere classified
M24.9 Joint derangement, unspecified

● M25 Other joint disorder, not elsewhere classified

Excludes2 abnormality of gait and mobility (R26.-)
acquired deformities of limb (M20-M21)
calcification of bursa (M71.4-)
calcification of shoulder (joint) (M75.3)
calcification of tendon (M65.2-)
difficulty in walking (R26.2)
temporomandibular joint disorder (M26.6-)

● M25.0 Hemarthrosis

Excludes1 current injury - see injury of joint by body region
hemophilic arthropathy (M36.2)

M25.00 Hemarthrosis, unspecified joint

● M25.01 Hemarthrosis, shoulder
M25.011 Hemarthrosis, right shoulder
M25.012 Hemarthrosis, left shoulder
M25.019 Hemarthrosis, unspecified shoulder

● M25.02 Hemarthrosis, elbow
M25.021 Hemarthrosis, right elbow
M25.022 Hemarthrosis, left elbow
M25.029 Hemarthrosis, unspecified elbow

● M25.03 Hemarthrosis, wrist
M25.031 Hemarthrosis, right wrist
M25.032 Hemarthrosis, left wrist
M25.039 Hemarthrosis, unspecified wrist

● M25.04 Hemarthrosis, hand
M25.041 Hemarthrosis, right hand
M25.042 Hemarthrosis, left hand
M25.049 Hemarthrosis, unspecified hand

● M25.05 Hemarthrosis, hip
M25.051 Hemarthrosis, right hip
M25.052 Hemarthrosis, left hip
M25.059 Hemarthrosis, unspecified hip

● M25.06 Hemarthrosis, knee
M25.061 Hemarthrosis, right knee
M25.062 Hemarthrosis, left knee
M25.069 Hemarthrosis, unspecified knee

● M25.07 Hemarthrosis, ankle and foot
M25.071 Hemarthrosis, right ankle
M25.072 Hemarthrosis, left ankle
M25.073 Hemarthrosis, unspecified ankle
M25.074 Hemarthrosis, right foot
M25.075 Hemarthrosis, left foot
M25.076 Hemarthrosis, unspecified foot

M25.08 Hemarthrosis, other specified site
Hemarthrosis, vertebrae

● M25.1 Fistula of joint

M25.10 Fistula, unspecified joint

● M25.11 Fistula, shoulder
M25.111 Fistula, right shoulder
M25.112 Fistula, left shoulder
M25.119 Fistula, unspecified shoulder

● M25.12 Fistula, elbow
M25.121 Fistula, right elbow
M25.122 Fistula, left elbow
M25.129 Fistula, unspecified elbow

● M25.13 Fistula, wrist
M25.131 Fistula, right wrist
M25.132 Fistula, left wrist
M25.139 Fistula, unspecified wrist

● M25.14 Fistula, hand
M25.141 Fistula, right hand
M25.142 Fistula, left hand
M25.149 Fistula, unspecified hand

● M25.15 Fistula, hip
M25.151 Fistula, right hip
M25.152 Fistula, left hip
M25.159 Fistula, unspecified hip

● M25.16 Fistula, knee
M25.161 Fistula, right knee
M25.162 Fistula, left knee
M25.169 Fistula, unspecified knee

● M25.17 Fistula, ankle and foot
M25.171 Fistula, right ankle
M25.172 Fistula, left ankle
M25.173 Fistula, unspecified ankle
M25.174 Fistula, right foot
M25.175 Fistula, left foot
M25.176 Fistula, unspecified foot

M25.18 Fistula, other specified site
Fistula, vertebrae

● M25.2 Flail joint

M25.20 Flail joint, unspecified joint

● M25.21 Flail joint, shoulder
M25.211 Flail joint, right shoulder
M25.212 Flail joint, left shoulder
M25.219 Flail joint, unspecified shoulder

● M25.22 Flail joint, elbow
M25.221 Flail joint, right elbow
M25.222 Flail joint, left elbow
M25.229 Flail joint, unspecified elbow

● M25.23 Flail joint, wrist
M25.231 Flail joint, right wrist
M25.232 Flail joint, left wrist
M25.239 Flail joint, unspecified wrist

● M25.24 Flail joint, hand
M25.241 Flail joint, right hand
M25.242 Flail joint, left hand
M25.249 Flail joint, unspecified hand

● M25.25 Flail joint, hip
M25.251 Flail joint, right hip
M25.252 Flail joint, left hip
M25.259 Flail joint, unspecified hip

● M25.26 Flail joint, knee
M25.261 Flail joint, right knee
M25.262 Flail joint, left knee
M25.269 Flail joint, unspecified knee

● M25.27 Flail joint, ankle and foot
M25.271 Flail joint, right ankle and foot
M25.272 Flail joint, left ankle and foot
M25.279 Flail joint, unspecified ankle and foot

M25.28 Flail joint, other site

● M25.3 Other instability of joint

Excludes1 instability of joint secondary to old ligament injury (M24.2-)
instability of joint secondary to removal of joint prosthesis (M96.8-)

Excludes2 spinal instabilities (M53.2-)

M25.30 Other instability, unspecified joint

● M25.31 Other instability, shoulder
M25.311 Other instability, right shoulder
M25.312 Other instability, left shoulder
M25.319 Other instability, unspecified shoulder

● M25.32 Other instability, elbow
M25.321 Other instability, right elbow
M25.322 Other instability, left elbow
M25.329 Other instability, unspecified elbow

CHAPTER 13 (M00-M99)

● M25.33 Other instability, wrist
- M25.331 Other instability, right wrist
- M25.332 Other instability, left wrist
- M25.339 Other instability, unspecified wrist

● M25.34 Other instability, hand
- M25.341 Other instability, right hand
- M25.342 Other instability, left hand
- M25.349 Other instability, unspecified hand

● M25.35 Other instability, hip
- M25.351 Other instability, right hip
- M25.352 Other instability, left hip
- M25.359 Other instability, unspecified hip

● M25.36 Other instability, knee
- M25.361 Other instability, right knee
- M25.362 Other instability, left knee
- M25.369 Other instability, unspecified knee

● M25.37 Other instability, ankle and foot
- M25.371 Other instability, right ankle
- M25.372 Other instability, left ankle
- M25.373 Other instability, unspecified ankle
- M25.374 Other instability, right foot
- M25.375 Other instability, left foot
- M25.376 Other instability, unspecified foot

● M25.4 Effusion of joint

Excludes1 hydrarthrosis in yaws (A66.6)
intermittent hydrarthrosis (M12.4-)
other infective (teno)synovitis (M65.1-)

M25.40 Effusion, unspecified joint

● M25.41 Effusion, shoulder
- M25.411 Effusion, right shoulder
- M25.412 Effusion, left shoulder
- M25.419 Effusion, unspecified shoulder

● M25.42 Effusion, elbow
- M25.421 Effusion, right elbow
- M25.422 Effusion, left elbow
- M25.429 Effusion, unspecified elbow

● M25.43 Effusion, wrist
- M25.431 Effusion, right wrist
- M25.432 Effusion, left wrist
- M25.439 Effusion, unspecified wrist

● M25.44 Effusion, hand
- M25.441 Effusion, right hand
- M25.442 Effusion, left hand
- M25.449 Effusion, unspecified hand

● M25.45 Effusion, hip
- M25.451 Effusion, right hip
- M25.452 Effusion, left hip
- M25.459 Effusion, unspecified hip

● M25.46 Effusion, knee
- M25.461 Effusion, right knee
- M25.462 Effusion, left knee
- M25.469 Effusion, unspecified knee

● M25.47 Effusion, ankle and foot
- M25.471 Effusion, right ankle
- M25.472 Effusion, left ankle
- M25.473 Effusion, unspecified ankle
- M25.474 Effusion, right foot
- M25.475 Effusion, left foot
- M25.476 Effusion, unspecified foot

M25.48 Effusion, other site

● M25.5 Pain in joint

Excludes2 pain in hand (M79.64-)
pain in fingers (M79.64-)
pain in foot (M79.67-)
pain in limb (M79.6-)
pain in toes (M79.67-)

M25.50 Pain in unspecified joint

● M25.51 Pain in shoulder
- M25.511 Pain in right shoulder
- M25.512 Pain in left shoulder
- M25.519 Pain in unspecified shoulder

● M25.52 Pain in elbow
- M25.521 Pain in right elbow
- M25.522 Pain in left elbow
- M25.529 Pain in unspecified elbow

● M25.53 Pain in wrist
- M25.531 Pain in right wrist
- M25.532 Pain in left wrist
- M25.539 Pain in unspecified wrist

● M25.54 Pain in joints of hand ◀
- M25.541 Pain in joints of right hand ◀
- M25.542 Pain in joints of left hand ◀
- M25.549 Pain in joints of unspecified hand ◀
  Pain in joints of hand NOS ◀

● M25.55 Pain in hip
- M25.551 Pain in right hip
- M25.552 Pain in left hip
- M25.559 Pain in unspecified hip

● M25.56 Pain in knee
- M25.561 Pain in right knee
- M25.562 Pain in left knee
- M25.569 Pain in unspecified knee

● M25.57 Pain in ankle and joints of foot
- M25.571 Pain in right ankle and joints of right foot
- M25.572 Pain in left ankle and joints of left foot
- M25.579 Pain in unspecified ankle and joints of unspecified foot

● M25.6 Stiffness of joint, not elsewhere classified

Excludes1 ankylosis of joint (M24.6-)
contracture of joint (M24.5-)

M25.60 Stiffness of unspecified joint, not elsewhere classified

● M25.61 Stiffness of shoulder, not elsewhere classified
- M25.611 Stiffness of right shoulder, not elsewhere classified
- M25.612 Stiffness of left shoulder, not elsewhere classified
- M25.619 Stiffness of unspecified shoulder, not elsewhere classified

● M25.62 Stiffness of elbow, not elsewhere classified
- M25.621 Stiffness of right elbow, not elsewhere classified
- M25.622 Stiffness of left elbow, not elsewhere classified
- M25.629 Stiffness of unspecified elbow, not elsewhere classified

● M25.63 Stiffness of wrist, not elsewhere classified
- M25.631 Stiffness of right wrist, not elsewhere classified
- M25.632 Stiffness of left wrist, not elsewhere classified
- M25.639 Stiffness of unspecified wrist, not elsewhere classified

● M25.64 Stiffness of hand, not elsewhere classified
M25.641 Stiffness of right hand, not elsewhere classified
M25.642 Stiffness of left hand, not elsewhere classified
M25.649 Stiffness of unspecified hand, not elsewhere classified
● M25.65 Stiffness of hip, not elsewhere classified
M25.651 Stiffness of right hip, not elsewhere classified
M25.652 Stiffness of left hip, not elsewhere classified
M25.659 Stiffness of unspecified hip, not elsewhere classified
● M25.66 Stiffness of knee, not elsewhere classified
M25.661 Stiffness of right knee, not elsewhere classified
M25.662 Stiffness of left knee, not elsewhere classified
M25.669 Stiffness of unspecified knee, not elsewhere classified
● M25.67 Stiffness of ankle and foot, not elsewhere classified
M25.671 Stiffness of right ankle, not elsewhere classified
M25.672 Stiffness of left ankle, not elsewhere classified
M25.673 Stiffness of unspecified ankle, not elsewhere classified
M25.674 Stiffness of right foot, not elsewhere classified
M25.675 Stiffness of left foot, not elsewhere classified
M25.676 Stiffness of unspecified foot, not elsewhere classified
● M25.7 Osteophyte
M25.70 Osteophyte, unspecified joint
● M25.71 Osteophyte, shoulder
M25.711 Osteophyte, right shoulder
M25.712 Osteophyte, left shoulder
M25.719 Osteophyte, unspecified shoulder
● M25.72 Osteophyte, elbow
M25.721 Osteophyte, right elbow
M25.722 Osteophyte, left elbow
M25.729 Osteophyte, unspecified elbow
● M25.73 Osteophyte, wrist
M25.731 Osteophyte, right wrist
M25.732 Osteophyte, left wrist
M25.739 Osteophyte, unspecified wrist
● M25.74 Osteophyte, hand
M25.741 Osteophyte, right hand
M25.742 Osteophyte, left hand
M25.749 Osteophyte, unspecified hand
● M25.75 Osteophyte, hip
M25.751 Osteophyte, right hip
M25.752 Osteophyte, left hip
M25.759 Osteophyte, unspecified hip
● M25.76 Osteophyte, knee
M25.761 Osteophyte, right knee
M25.762 Osteophyte, left knee
M25.769 Osteophyte, unspecified knee
● M25.77 Osteophyte, ankle and foot
M25.771 Osteophyte, right ankle
M25.772 Osteophyte, left ankle
M25.773 Osteophyte, unspecified ankle
M25.774 Osteophyte, right foot
M25.775 Osteophyte, left foot
M25.776 Osteophyte, unspecified foot
M25.78 Osteophyte, vertebrae
● M25.8 Other specified joint disorders
M25.80 Other specified joint disorders, unspecified joint
● M25.81 Other specified joint disorders, shoulder
M25.811 Other specified joint disorders, right shoulder
M25.812 Other specified joint disorders, left shoulder
M25.819 Other specified joint disorders, unspecified shoulder
● M25.82 Other specified joint disorders, elbow
M25.821 Other specified joint disorders, right elbow
M25.822 Other specified joint disorders, left elbow
M25.829 Other specified joint disorders, unspecified elbow
● M25.83 Other specified joint disorders, wrist
M25.831 Other specified joint disorders, right wrist
M25.832 Other specified joint disorders, left wrist
M25.839 Other specified joint disorders, unspecified wrist
● M25.84 Other specified joint disorders, hand
M25.841 Other specified joint disorders, right hand
M25.842 Other specified joint disorders, left hand
M25.849 Other specified joint disorders, unspecified hand
● M25.85 Other specified joint disorders, hip
M25.851 Other specified joint disorders, right hip
M25.852 Other specified joint disorders, left hip
M25.859 Other specified joint disorders, unspecified hip
● M25.86 Other specified joint disorders, knee
M25.861 Other specified joint disorders, right knee
M25.862 Other specified joint disorders, left knee
M25.869 Other specified joint disorders, unspecified knee
● M25.87 Other specified joint disorders, ankle and foot
M25.871 Other specified joint disorders, right ankle and foot
M25.872 Other specified joint disorders, left ankle and foot
M25.879 Other specified joint disorders, unspecified ankle and foot
M25.9 Joint disorder, unspecified

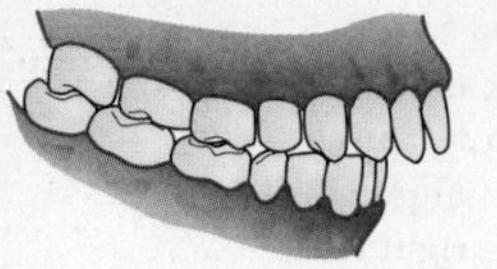

Figure 13-3 Dentofacial malocclusion.

Item 13–6 Hyperplasia is a condition of overdevelopment, whereas **hypoplasia** is a condition of underdevelopment. **Macrogenia** is overdevelopment of the chin, whereas **microgenia** is underdevelopment of the chin.

DENTOFACIAL ANOMALIES [INCLUDING MALOCCLUSION] AND OTHER DISORDERS OF JAW (M26-M27)

Excludes1 hemifacial atrophy or hypertrophy (Q67.4)
unilateral condylar hyperplasia or hypoplasia (M27.8)

● **M26 Dentofacial anomalies [including malocclusion]**

● **M26.0 Major anomalies of jaw size**

Excludes1 acromegaly (E22.0)
Robin's syndrome (Q87.0)

M26.00 Unspecified anomaly of jaw size
M26.01 Maxillary hyperplasia
M26.02 Maxillary hypoplasia
M26.03 Mandibular hyperplasia
M26.04 Mandibular hypoplasia
M26.05 Macrogenia
M26.06 Microgenia
M26.07 Excessive tuberosity of jaw
Entire maxillary tuberosity
M26.09 Other specified anomalies of jaw size

● **M26.1 Anomalies of jaw-cranial base relationship**

M26.10 Unspecified anomaly of jaw-cranial base relationship
M26.11 Maxillary asymmetry
M26.12 Other jaw asymmetry
M26.19 Other specified anomalies of jaw-cranial base relationship

● **M26.2 Anomalies of dental arch relationship**

M26.20 Unspecified anomaly of dental arch relationship

● **M26.21 Malocclusion, Angle's class**

M26.211 Malocclusion, Angle's class I
Neutro-occlusion
M26.212 Malocclusion, Angle's class II
Disto-occlusion Division I
Disto-occlusion Division II
M26.213 Malocclusion, Angle's class III
Mesio-occlusion
M26.219 Malocclusion, Angle's class, unspecified

● **M26.22 Open occlusal relationship**

M26.220 Open anterior occlusal relationship
Anterior openbite
M26.221 Open posterior occlusal relationship
Posterior openbite

M26.23 Excessive horizontal overlap
Excessive horizontal overjet
M26.24 Reverse articulation
Crossbite (anterior) (posterior)
M26.25 Anomalies of interarch distance
M26.29 Other anomalies of dental arch relationship
Midline deviation of dental arch
Overbite (excessive) deep
Overbite (excessive) horizontal
Overbite (excessive) vertical
Posterior lingual occlusion of mandibular teeth

● **M26.3 Anomalies of tooth position of fully erupted tooth or teeth**

Excludes2 embedded and impacted teeth (K01.-)

M26.30 Unspecified anomaly of tooth position of fully erupted tooth or teeth
Abnormal spacing of fully erupted tooth or teeth NOS
Displacement of fully erupted tooth or teeth NOS
Transposition of fully erupted tooth or teeth NOS
M26.31 Crowding of fully erupted teeth
M26.32 Excessive spacing of fully erupted teeth
Diastema of fully erupted tooth or teeth NOS
M26.33 Horizontal displacement of fully erupted tooth or teeth
Tipped tooth or teeth
Tipping of fully erupted tooth
M26.34 Vertical displacement of fully erupted tooth or teeth
Extruded tooth
Infraeruption of tooth or teeth
Supraeruption of tooth or teeth
M26.35 Rotation of fully erupted tooth or teeth
M26.36 Insufficient interocclusal distance of fully erupted teeth (ridge)
Lack of adequate intermaxillary vertical dimension of fully erupted teeth
M26.37 Excessive interocclusal distance of fully erupted teeth
Excessive intermaxillary vertical dimension of fully erupted teeth
Loss of occlusal vertical dimension of fully erupted teeth
M26.39 Other anomalies of tooth position of fully erupted tooth or teeth

M26.4 Malocclusion, unspecified

● **M26.5 Dentofacial functional abnormalities**

Excludes1 bruxism (F45.8)
teeth-grinding NOS (F45.8)

M26.50 Dentofacial functional abnormalities, unspecified
M26.51 Abnormal jaw closure
M26.52 Limited mandibular range of motion
M26.53 Deviation in opening and closing of the mandible
M26.54 Insufficient anterior guidance
Insufficient anterior occlusal guidance
M26.55 Centric occlusion maximum intercuspation discrepancy
Excludes1 centric occlusion NOS (M26.59)
M26.56 Non-working side interference
Balancing side interference
M26.57 Lack of posterior occlusal support
M26.59 Other dentofacial functional abnormalities
Centric occlusion (of teeth) NOS
Malocclusion due to abnormal swallowing
Malocclusion due to mouth breathing
Malocclusion due to tongue, lip or finger habits

CHAPTER 13 (M00-M99)

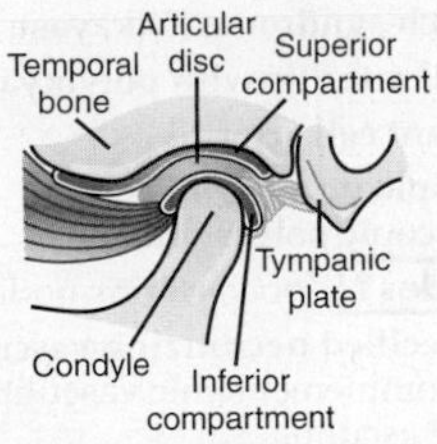

Figure 13-4 Temporomandibular joint.

Item 13–7 Dysfunction of the temporomandibular joint is termed **temporomandibular joint (TMJ) syndrome** and is characterized by pain and tenderness/spasm of the muscles of mastication, joint noise, and in the later stages, limited mandibular movement.

● **M26.6 Temporomandibular joint disorders**
Excludes2 current temporomandibular joint dislocation (SØ3.Ø)
current temporomandibular joint sprain (SØ3.4)

● **M26.6Ø Temporomandibular joint disorder, unspecified**
M26.6Ø1 Right temporomandibular joint disorder, unspecified ◀
M26.6Ø2 Left temporomandibular joint disorder, unspecified ◀
M26.6Ø3 Bilateral temporomandibular joint disorder, unspecified ◀
M26.6Ø9 Unspecified temporomandibular joint disorder, unspecified side ◀
Temporomandibular joint disorder NOS ◀

● **M26.61 Adhesions and ankylosis of temporomandibular joint**
M26.611 Adhesions and ankylosis of right temporomandibular joint ◀
M26.612 Adhesions and ankylosis of left temporomandibular joint ◀
M26.613 Adhesions and ankylosis of bilateral temporomandibular joint ◀
M26.619 Adhesions and ankylosis of temporomandibular joint, unspecified side ◀

● **M26.62 Arthralgia of temporomandibular joint**
M26.621 Arthralgia of right temporomandibular joint ◀
M26.622 Arthralgia of left temporomandibular joint ◀
M26.623 Arthralgia of bilateral temporomandibular joint ◀
M26.629 Arthralgia of temporomandibular joint, unspecified side ◀

● **M26.63 Articular disc disorder of temporomandibular joint**
M26.631 Articular disc disorder of right temporomandibular joint ◀
M26.632 Articular disc disorder of left temporomandibular joint ◀
M26.633 Articular disc disorder of bilateral temporomandibular joint ◀
M26.639 Articular disc disorder of temporomandibular joint, unspecified side ◀

M26.69 Other specified disorders of temporomandibular joint

● **M26.7 Dental alveolar anomalies**
M26.7Ø Unspecified alveolar anomaly
M26.71 Alveolar maxillary hyperplasia
M26.72 Alveolar mandibular hyperplasia
M26.73 Alveolar maxillary hypoplasia
M26.74 Alveolar mandibular hypoplasia
M26.79 Other specified alveolar anomalies

● **M26.8 Other dentofacial anomalies**
M26.81 Anterior soft tissue impingement
Anterior soft tissue impingement on teeth
M26.82 Posterior soft tissue impingement
Posterior soft tissue impingement on teeth
M26.89 Other dentofacial anomalies

M26.9 Dentofacial anomaly, unspecified

● **M27 Other diseases of jaws**

M27.Ø Developmental disorders of jaws
Latent bone cyst of jaw
Stafne's cyst
Torus mandibularis
Torus palatinus

M27.1 Giant cell granuloma, central
Giant cell granuloma NOS
Excludes1 peripheral giant cell granuloma (KØ6.8)

M27.2 Inflammatory conditions of jaws
Osteitis of jaw(s)
Osteomyelitis (neonatal) jaw(s)
Osteoradionecrosis jaw(s)
Periostitis jaw(s)
Sequestrum of jaw bone
Use additional code (W88-W9Ø, X39.Ø) to identify radiation, if radiation-induced
Excludes2 osteonecrosis of jaw due to drug (M87.18Ø)

M27.3 Alveolitis of jaws
Alveolar osteitis
Dry socket

● **M27.4 Other and unspecified cysts of jaw**
Excludes1 cysts of oral region (KØ9.-)
latent bone cyst of jaw (M27.Ø)
Stafne's cyst (M27.Ø)
M27.4Ø Unspecified cyst of jaw
Cyst of jaw NOS
M27.49 Other cysts of jaw
Aneurysmal cyst of jaw
Hemorrhagic cyst of jaw
Traumatic cyst of jaw

● **M27.5 Periradicular pathology associated with previous endodontic treatment**
M27.51 Perforation of root canal space due to endodontic treatment
M27.52 Endodontic overfill
M27.53 Endodontic underfill
M27.59 Other periradicular pathology associated with previous endodontic treatment

● **M27.6 Endosseous dental implant failure**
M27.61 Osseointegration failure of dental implant
Hemorrhagic complications of dental implant placement
Iatrogenic osseointegration failure of dental implant
Osseointegration failure of dental implant due to complications of systemic disease
Osseointegration failure of dental implant due to poor bone quality
Pre-integration failure of dental implant NOS
Pre-osseointegration failure of dental implant

M27.62 **Post-osseointegration biological failure of dental implant**
Failure of dental implant due to lack of attached gingiva
Failure of dental implant due to occlusal trauma (caused by poor prosthetic design)
Failure of dental implant due to parafunctional habits
Failure of dental implant due to periodontal infection (peri–implantitis)
Failure of dental implant due to poor oral hygiene
Iatrogenic post-osseointegration failure of dental implant
Post-osseointegration failure of dental implant due to complications of systemic disease

M27.63 **Post-osseointegration mechanical failure of dental implant**
Failure of dental prosthesis causing loss of dental implant
Fracture of dental implant
Excludes2 cracked tooth (K03.81)
fractured dental restorative material with loss of material (K08.531)
fractured dental restorative material without loss of material (K08.530)
fractured tooth (S02.5)

M27.69 **Other endosseous dental implant failure**
Dental implant failure NOS

M27.8 **Other specified diseases of jaws**
Cherubism
Exostosis
Fibrous dysplasia
Unilateral condylar hyperplasia
Unilateral condylar hypoplasia
Excludes1 jaw pain (R68.84)

M27.9 **Disease of jaws, unspecified**

SYSTEMIC CONNECTIVE TISSUE DISORDERS (M30-M36)

Includes autoimmune disease NOS
collagen (vascular) disease NOS
systemic autoimmune disease
systemic collagen (vascular) disease

Excludes1 autoimmune disease, single organ or single cell-type - code to relevant condition category

● M30 **Polyarteritis nodosa and related conditions**
Excludes1 microscopic polyarteritis (M31.7)
M30.0 **Polyarteritis nodosa**
M30.1 **Polyarteritis with lung involvement [Churg-Strauss]**
Allergic granulomatous angiitis
M30.2 **Juvenile polyarteritis**
M30.3 **Mucocutaneous lymph node syndrome [Kawasaki]**
M30.8 **Other conditions related to polyarteritis nodosa**
Polyangiitis overlap syndrome

● M31 **Other necrotizing vasculopathies**
M31.0 **Hypersensitivity angiitis**
Goodpasture's syndrome
M31.1 **Thrombotic microangiopathy**
Thrombotic thrombocytopenic purpura
M31.2 **Lethal midline granuloma**
● M31.3 **Wegener's granulomatosis**
Necrotizing respiratory granulomatosis
M31.30 **Wegener's granulomatosis without renal involvement**
Wegener's granulomatosis NOS
M31.31 **Wegener's granulomatosis with renal involvement**
M31.4 **Aortic arch syndrome [Takayasu]**
M31.5 **Giant cell arteritis with polymyalgia rheumatica**
M31.6 **Other giant cell arteritis**
M31.7 **Microscopic polyangiitis**
Microscopic polyarteritis
Excludes1 polyarteritis nodosa (M30.0)
M31.8 **Other specified necrotizing vasculopathies**
Hypocomplementemic vasculitis
Septic vasculitis
M31.9 **Necrotizing vasculopathy, unspecified**

● M32 **Systemic lupus erythematosus (SLE)**
Autoimmune inflammatory connective tissue disease of unknown cause that occurs most often in women
Excludes1 lupus erythematosus (discoid) (NOS) (L93.0)
M32.0 **Drug-induced systemic lupus erythematosus**
Use additional code for adverse effect, if applicable, to identify drug (T36-T50 with fifth or sixth character 5)
● M32.1 **Systemic lupus erythematosus with organ or system involvement**
M32.10 **Systemic lupus erythematosus, organ or system involvement unspecified**
M32.11 **Endocarditis in systemic lupus erythematosus**
Libman-Sacks disease
M32.12 **Pericarditis in systemic lupus erythematosus**
Lupus pericarditis
M32.13 **Lung involvement in systemic lupus erythematosus**
Pleural effusion due to systemic lupus erythematosus
M32.14 **Glomerular disease in systemic lupus erythematosus**
Lupus renal disease NOS
M32.15 **Tubulo-interstitial nephropathy in systemic lupus erythematosus**
M32.19 **Other organ or system involvement in systemic lupus erythematosus**
M32.8 **Other forms of systemic lupus erythematosus**
M32.9 **Systemic lupus erythematosus, unspecified**
SLE NOS
Systemic lupus erythematosus NOS
Systemic lupus erythematosus without organ involvement

● M33 **Dermatopolymyositis**
● M33.0 **Juvenile dermatopolymyositis**
M33.00 **Juvenile dermatopolymyositis, organ involvement unspecified**
M33.01 **Juvenile dermatopolymyositis with respiratory involvement**
M33.02 **Juvenile dermatopolymyositis with myopathy**
M33.09 **Juvenile dermatopolymyositis with other organ involvement**
● M33.1 **Other dermatopolymyositis**
M33.10 **Other dermatopolymyositis, organ involvement unspecified**
M33.11 **Other dermatopolymyositis with respiratory involvement**
M33.12 **Other dermatopolymyositis with myopathy**
M33.19 **Other dermatopolymyositis with other organ involvement**
● M33.2 **Polymyositis**
M33.20 **Polymyositis, organ involvement unspecified**
M33.21 **Polymyositis with respiratory involvement**
M33.22 **Polymyositis with myopathy**
M33.29 **Polymyositis with other organ involvement**

Item 13–8 Polymyalgia rheumatica is a syndrome characterized by aching and morning stiffness and is related to aging and hereditary predisposition.

● **M33.9 Dermatopolymyositis, unspecified**
- **M33.90 Dermatopolymyositis, unspecified, organ involvement unspecified**
- **M33.91 Dermatopolymyositis, unspecified with respiratory involvement**
- **M33.92 Dermatopolymyositis, unspecified with myopathy**
- **M33.99 Dermatopolymyositis, unspecified with other organ involvement**

● **M34 Systemic sclerosis [scleroderma]**
Excludes1 circumscribed scleroderma (L94.0)
neonatal scleroderma (P83.8)

M34.0 Progressive systemic sclerosis

M34.1 CR(E)ST syndrome
Combination of calcinosis, Raynaud's phenomenon, esophageal dysfunction, sclerodactyly, telangiectasia

M34.2 Systemic sclerosis induced by drug and chemical
Code first poisoning due to drug or toxin, if applicable (T36-T65 with fifth or sixth character 1-4 or 6)
Use additional code for adverse effect, if applicable, to identify drug (T36-T50 with fifth or sixth character 5)

● **M34.8 Other forms of systemic sclerosis**
- **M34.81 Systemic sclerosis with lung involvement**
- **M34.82 Systemic sclerosis with myopathy**
- **M34.83 Systemic sclerosis with polyneuropathy**
- **M34.89 Other systemic sclerosis**

M34.9 Systemic sclerosis, unspecified

● **M35 Other systemic involvement of connective tissue**
Excludes1 reactive perforating collagenosis (L87.1)

● **M35.0 Sicca syndrome [Sjögren]**
- **M35.00 Sicca syndrome, unspecified**
- **M35.01 Sicca syndrome with keratoconjunctivitis**
- **M35.02 Sicca syndrome with lung involvement**
- **M35.03 Sicca syndrome with myopathy**
- **M35.04 Sicca syndrome with tubulo-interstitial nephropathy**
  Renal tubular acidosis in sicca syndrome
- **M35.09 Sicca syndrome with other organ involvement**

M35.1 Other overlap syndromes
Mixed connective tissue disease
Excludes1 polyangiitis overlap syndrome (M30.8)

M35.2 Behçet's disease

M35.3 Polymyalgia rheumatica
Excludes1 polymyalgia rheumatica with giant cell arteritis (M31.5)

M35.4 Diffuse (eosinophilic) fasciitis

M35.5 Multifocal fibrosclerosis

M35.6 Relapsing panniculitis [Weber-Christian]
Excludes1 lupus panniculitis (L93.2)
panniculitis NOS (M79.3-)

M35.7 Hypermobility syndrome
Familial ligamentous laxity
Excludes1 Ehlers-Danlos syndrome (Q79.6)
ligamentous laxity, NOS (M24.2-)

M35.8 Other specified systemic involvement of connective tissue

M35.9 Systemic involvement of connective tissue, unspecified
Autoimmune disease (systemic) NOS
Collagen (vascular) disease NOS

● **M36 Systemic disorders of connective tissue in diseases classified elsewhere**
Excludes2 arthropathies in diseases classified elsewhere (M14.-)

M36.0 Dermato(poly)myositis in neoplastic disease
Code first underlying neoplasm (C00-D49)

M36.1 Arthropathy in neoplastic disease
Code first underlying neoplasm, such as:
leukemia (C91-C95)
malignant histiocytosis (C96.A)
multiple myeloma (C90.0)

M36.2 Hemophilic arthropathy
Hemarthrosis in hemophilic arthropathy
Code first underlying disease, such as:
factor VIII deficiency (D66)
with vascular defect (D68.0)
factor IX deficiency (D67)
hemophilia (classical) (D66)
hemophilia B (D67)
hemophilia C (D68.1)

M36.3 Arthropathy in other blood disorders

M36.4 Arthropathy in hypersensitivity reactions classified elsewhere
Code first underlying disease, such as:
Henoch (-Schönlein) purpura (D69.0)
serum sickness (T80.6-)

M36.8 Systemic disorders of connective tissue in other diseases classified elsewhere
Code first underlying disease, such as:
alkaptonuria (E70.2)
hypogammaglobulinemia (D80.-)
ochronosis (E70.2)

DORSOPATHIES (M40-M54)

DEFORMING DORSOPATHIES (M40-M43)

● **M40 Kyphosis and lordosis**
Excludes1 congenital kyphosis and lordosis (Q76.4)
kyphoscoliosis (M41.-)
postprocedural kyphosis and lordosis (M96.-)

● **M40.0 Postural kyphosis**
Excludes1 osteochondrosis of spine (M42.-)
- **M40.00 Postural kyphosis, site unspecified**
- **M40.03 Postural kyphosis, cervicothoracic region**
- **M40.04 Postural kyphosis, thoracic region**
- **M40.05 Postural kyphosis, thoracolumbar region**

● **M40.1 Other secondary kyphosis**
- **M40.10 Other secondary kyphosis, site unspecified**
- **M40.12 Other secondary kyphosis, cervical region**
- **M40.13 Other secondary kyphosis, cervicothoracic region**
- **M40.14 Other secondary kyphosis, thoracic region**
- **M40.15 Other secondary kyphosis, thoracolumbar region**

● **M40.2 Other and unspecified kyphosis**

● **M40.20 Unspecified kyphosis**
- **M40.202 Unspecified kyphosis, cervical region**
- **M40.203 Unspecified kyphosis, cervicothoracic region**
- **M40.204 Unspecified kyphosis, thoracic region**
- **M40.205 Unspecified kyphosis, thoracolumbar region**
- **M40.209 Unspecified kyphosis, site unspecified**

CHAPTER 13 (M00-M99)

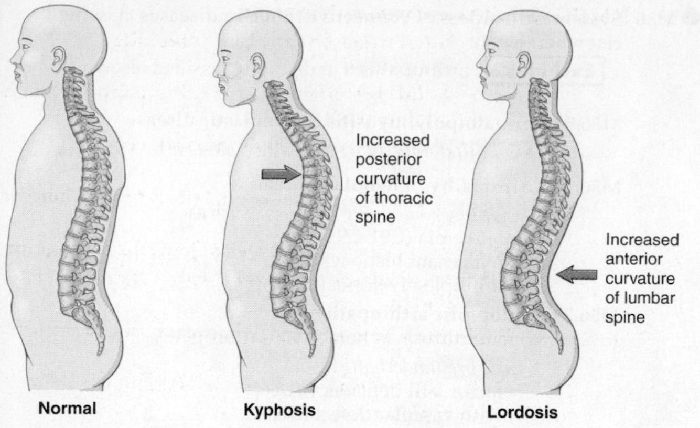

Figure 13-5 Kyphosis, Lordosis, Scoliosis. (From Chabner: The Language of Medicine, ed 8, St. Louis, Saunders, 2007)

Item 13-9 Kyphosis is an abnormal curvature of the spine. **Senile kyphosis** is a result of disc degeneration causing ossification (turning to bone). **Adolescent** or **juvenile** kyphosis is also known as **Scheuermann's disease,** a condition in which the discs of the lower thoracic spine herniate, causing the disc space to narrow and the spine to tilt forward. This condition is attributed to poor posture. Lordosis or swayback is an abnormal curvature of the spine resulting in an inward curve of the lumbar spine just above the buttocks. Scoliosis causes a sideways curve to the spine. The curves are S- or C-shaped, and it is most commonly acquired in late childhood and early teen years, when growth is fast.

● **M4Ø.29 Other kyphosis**
- **M4Ø.292 Other kyphosis, cervical region**
- **M4Ø.293 Other kyphosis, cervicothoracic region**
- **M4Ø.294 Other kyphosis, thoracic region**
- **M4Ø.295 Other kyphosis, thoracolumbar region**
- **M4Ø.299 Other kyphosis, site unspecified**

● **M4Ø.3 Flatback syndrome**
- **M4Ø.3Ø Flatback syndrome, site unspecified**
- **M4Ø.35 Flatback syndrome, thoracolumbar region**
- **M4Ø.36 Flatback syndrome, lumbar region**
- **M4Ø.37 Flatback syndrome, lumbosacral region**

● **M4Ø.4 Postural lordosis**

Abnormal increase in the normal curvature of the lumbar spine (sway back)

Acquired lordosis
- **M4Ø.4Ø Postural lordosis, site unspecified**
- **M4Ø.45 Postural lordosis, thoracolumbar region**
- **M4Ø.46 Postural lordosis, lumbar region**
- **M4Ø.47 Postural lordosis, lumbosacral region**

● **M4Ø.5 Lordosis, unspecified**
- **M4Ø.5Ø Lordosis, unspecified, site unspecified**
- **M4Ø.55 Lordosis, unspecified, thoracolumbar region**
- **M4Ø.56 Lordosis, unspecified, lumbar region**
- **M4Ø.57 Lordosis, unspecified, lumbosacral region**

● **M41 Scoliosis**

Includes kyphoscoliosis

Excludes1 congenital scoliosis NOS (Q67.5)
congenital scoliosis due to bony malformation (Q76.3)
postural congenital scoliosis (Q67.5)
kyphoscoliotic heart disease (I27.1)
postprocedural scoliosis (M96.-)

● **M41.Ø Infantile idiopathic scoliosis**
- **M41.ØØ Infantile idiopathic scoliosis, site unspecified**
- **M41.Ø2 Infantile idiopathic scoliosis, cervical region**
- **M41.Ø3 Infantile idiopathic scoliosis, cervicothoracic region**
- **M41.Ø4 Infantile idiopathic scoliosis, thoracic region**
- **M41.Ø5 Infantile idiopathic scoliosis, thoracolumbar region**
- **M41.Ø6 Infantile idiopathic scoliosis, lumbar region**
- **M41.Ø7 Infantile idiopathic scoliosis, lumbosacral region**
- **M41.Ø8 Infantile idiopathic scoliosis, sacral and sacrococcygeal region**

● **M41.1 Juvenile and adolescent idiopathic scoliosis**

● **M41.11 Juvenile idiopathic scoliosis**
- **M41.112 Juvenile idiopathic scoliosis, cervical region**
- **M41.113 Juvenile idiopathic scoliosis, cervicothoracic region**
- **M41.114 Juvenile idiopathic scoliosis, thoracic region**
- **M41.115 Juvenile idiopathic scoliosis, thoracolumbar region**
- **M41.116 Juvenile idiopathic scoliosis, lumbar region**
- **M41.117 Juvenile idiopathic scoliosis, lumbosacral region**
- **M41.119 Juvenile idiopathic scoliosis, site unspecified**

● **M41.12 Adolescent scoliosis**
- **M41.122 Adolescent idiopathic scoliosis, cervical region**
- **M41.123 Adolescent idiopathic scoliosis, cervicothoracic region**
- **M41.124 Adolescent idiopathic scoliosis, thoracic region**
- **M41.125 Adolescent idiopathic scoliosis, thoracolumbar region**
- **M41.126 Adolescent idiopathic scoliosis, lumbar region**
- **M41.127 Adolescent idiopathic scoliosis, lumbosacral region**
- **M41.129 Adolescent idiopathic scoliosis, site unspecified**

● **M41.2 Other idiopathic scoliosis**
- **M41.2Ø Other idiopathic scoliosis, site unspecified**
- **M41.22 Other idiopathic scoliosis, cervical region**
- **M41.23 Other idiopathic scoliosis, cervicothoracic region**
- **M41.24 Other idiopathic scoliosis, thoracic region**
- **M41.25 Other idiopathic scoliosis, thoracolumbar region**
- **M41.26 Other idiopathic scoliosis, lumbar region**
- **M41.27 Other idiopathic scoliosis, lumbosacral region**

● M41.3 Thoracogenic scoliosis
M41.30 Thoracogenic scoliosis, site unspecified
M41.34 Thoracogenic scoliosis, thoracic region
M41.35 Thoracogenic scoliosis, thoracolumbar region

● M41.4 Neuromuscular scoliosis
Scoliosis secondary to cerebral palsy, Friedreich's ataxia, poliomyelitis and other neuromuscular disorders
Code also underlying condition
M41.40 Neuromuscular scoliosis, site unspecified
M41.41 Neuromuscular scoliosis, occipito-atlanto-axial region
M41.42 Neuromuscular scoliosis, cervical region
M41.43 Neuromuscular scoliosis, cervicothoracic region
M41.44 Neuromuscular scoliosis, thoracic region
M41.45 Neuromuscular scoliosis, thoracolumbar region
M41.46 Neuromuscular scoliosis, lumbar region
M41.47 Neuromuscular scoliosis, lumbosacral region

● M41.5 Other secondary scoliosis
M41.50 Other secondary scoliosis, site unspecified
M41.52 Other secondary scoliosis, cervical region
M41.53 Other secondary scoliosis, cervicothoracic region
M41.54 Other secondary scoliosis, thoracic region
M41.55 Other secondary scoliosis, thoracolumbar region
M41.56 Other secondary scoliosis, lumbar region
M41.57 Other secondary scoliosis, lumbosacral region

● M41.8 Other forms of scoliosis
M41.80 Other forms of scoliosis, site unspecified
M41.82 Other forms of scoliosis, cervical region
M41.83 Other forms of scoliosis, cervicothoracic region
M41.84 Other forms of scoliosis, thoracic region
M41.85 Other forms of scoliosis, thoracolumbar region
M41.86 Other forms of scoliosis, lumbar region
M41.87 Other forms of scoliosis, lumbosacral region

M41.9 Scoliosis, unspecified

● M42 Spinal osteochondrosis

● M42.0 Juvenile osteochondrosis of spine
Calvé's disease
Scheuermann's disease
Excludes1 postural kyphosis (M40.0)
M42.00 Juvenile osteochondrosis of spine, site unspecified
M42.01 Juvenile osteochondrosis of spine, occipito-atlanto-axial region
M42.02 Juvenile osteochondrosis of spine, cervical region
M42.03 Juvenile osteochondrosis of spine, cervicothoracic region
M42.04 Juvenile osteochondrosis of spine, thoracic region
M42.05 Juvenile osteochondrosis of spine, thoracolumbar region
M42.06 Juvenile osteochondrosis of spine, lumbar region
M42.07 Juvenile osteochondrosis of spine, lumbosacral region
M42.08 Juvenile osteochondrosis of spine, sacral and sacrococcygeal region
M42.09 Juvenile osteochondrosis of spine, multiple sites in spine

● M42.1 Adult osteochondrosis of spine
M42.10 Adult osteochondrosis of spine, site unspecified
M42.11 Adult osteochondrosis of spine, occipitoatlanto-axial region
M42.12 Adult osteochondrosis of spine, cervical region
M42.13 Adult osteochondrosis of spine, cervicothoracic region
M42.14 Adult osteochondrosis of spine, thoracic region
M42.15 Adult osteochondrosis of spine, thoracolumbar region
M42.16 Adult osteochondrosis of spine, lumbar region
M42.17 Adult osteochondrosis of spine, lumbosacral region
M42.18 Adult osteochondrosis of spine, sacral and sacrococcygeal region
M42.19 Adult osteochondrosis of spine, multiple sites in spine

M42.9 Spinal osteochondrosis, unspecified

● M43 Other deforming dorsopathies
Excludes1 congenital spondylolysis and spondylolisthesis (Q76.2)
hemivertebra (Q76.3-Q76.4)
Klippel-Feil syndrome (Q76.1)
lumbarization and sacralization (Q76.4)
platyspondylisis (Q76.4)
spina bifida occulta (Q76.0)
spinal curvature in osteoporosis (M80.-)
spinal curvature in Paget's disease of bone [osteitis deformans] (M88.-)

● M43.0 Spondylolysis
Excludes1 congenital spondylolysis (Q76.2)
spondylolisthesis (M43.1)
M43.00 Spondylolysis, site unspecified
M43.01 Spondylolysis, occipito-atlanto-axial region
M43.02 Spondylolysis, cervical region
M43.03 Spondylolysis, cervicothoracic region
M43.04 Spondylolysis, thoracic region
M43.05 Spondylolysis, thoracolumbar region
M43.06 Spondylolysis, lumbar region
M43.07 Spondylolysis, lumbosacral region
M43.08 Spondylolysis, sacral and sacrococcygeal region
M43.09 Spondylolysis, multiple sites in spine

● M43.1 Spondylolisthesis
Excludes1 acute traumatic of lumbosacral region (S33.1)
acute traumatic of sites other than lumbosacral - code to Fracture, vertebra, by region
congenital spondylolisthesis (Q76.2)
M43.10 Spondylolisthesis, site unspecified
M43.11 Spondylolisthesis, occipito-atlanto-axial region
M43.12 Spondylolisthesis, cervical region
M43.13 Spondylolisthesis, cervicothoracic region
M43.14 Spondylolisthesis, thoracic region
M43.15 Spondylolisthesis, thoracolumbar region
M43.16 Spondylolisthesis, lumbar region
M43.17 Spondylolisthesis, lumbosacral region
M43.18 Spondylolisthesis, sacral and sacrococcygeal region
M43.19 Spondylolisthesis, multiple sites in spine

Item 13-10 Spondylolisthesis is a condition caused by the slipping forward of one disc over another.

● M43.2 Fusion of spine
Ankylosis of spinal joint
Excludes1 ankylosing spondylitis (M45.Ø-)
congenital fusion of spine (Q76.4)
Excludes2 arthrodesis status (Z98.1)
pseudoarthrosis after fusion or arthrodesis (M96.Ø)

M43.2Ø Fusion of spine, site unspecified
M43.21 Fusion of spine, occipito-atlanto-axial region
M43.22 Fusion of spine, cervical region
M43.23 Fusion of spine, cervicothoracic region
M43.24 Fusion of spine, thoracic region
M43.25 Fusion of spine, thoracolumbar region
M43.26 Fusion of spine, lumbar region
M43.27 Fusion of spine, lumbosacral region
M43.28 Fusion of spine, sacral and sacrococcygeal region

M43.3 Recurrent atlantoaxial dislocation with myelopathy
M43.4 Other recurrent atlantoaxial dislocation
● M43.5 Other recurrent vertebral dislocation
Excludes1 biomechanical lesions NEC (M99.-)

● M43.5X Other recurrent vertebral dislocation
M43.5X2 Other recurrent vertebral dislocation, cervical region
M43.5X3 Other recurrent vertebral dislocation, cervicothoracic region
M43.5X4 Other recurrent vertebral dislocation, thoracic region
M43.5X5 Other recurrent vertebral dislocation, thoracolumbar region
M43.5X6 Other recurrent vertebral dislocation, lumbar region
M43.5X7 Other recurrent vertebral dislocation, lumbosacral region
M43.5X8 Other recurrent vertebral dislocation, sacral and sacrococcygeal region
M43.5X9 Other recurrent vertebral dislocation, site unspecified

M43.6 Torticollis
Excludes1 congenital (sternomastoid) torticollis (Q68.Ø)
current injury - see Injury, of spine, by body region ocular torticollis (R29.891)
psychogenic torticollis (F45.8)
spasmodic torticollis (G24.3)
torticollis due to birth injury (P15.2)

● M43.8 Other specified deforming dorsopathies
Excludes2 kyphosis and lordosis (M4Ø.-)
scoliosis (M41.-)

● M43.8X Other specified deforming dorsopathies
M43.8X1 Other specified deforming dorsopathies, occipito-atlanto-axial region
M43.8X2 Other specified deforming dorsopathies, cervical region
M43.8X3 Other specified deforming dorsopathies, cervicothoracic region
M43.8X4 Other specified deforming dorsopathies, thoracic region
M43.8X5 Other specified deforming dorsopathies, thoracolumbar region
M43.8X6 Other specified deforming dorsopathies, lumbar region
M43.8X7 Other specified deforming dorsopathies, lumbosacral region
M43.8X8 Other specified deforming dorsopathies, sacral and sacrococcygeal region
M43.8X9 Other specified deforming dorsopathies, site unspecified

M43.9 Deforming dorsopathy, unspecified
Curvature of spine NOS

SPONDYLOPATHIES (M45-M49)

● M45 Ankylosing spondylitis
Rheumatoid arthritis of spine
Excludes1 arthropathy in Reiter's disease (MØ2.3-)
juvenile (ankylosing) spondylitis (MØ8.1)
Excludes2 Behçet's disease (M35.2)

M45.Ø Ankylosing spondylitis of multiple sites in spine
M45.1 Ankylosing spondylitis of occipito-atlanto-axial region
M45.2 Ankylosing spondylitis of cervical region
M45.3 Ankylosing spondylitis of cervicothoracic region
M45.4 Ankylosing spondylitis of thoracic region
M45.5 Ankylosing spondylitis of thoracolumbar region
M45.6 Ankylosing spondylitis lumbar region
M45.7 Ankylosing spondylitis of lumbosacral region
M45.8 Ankylosing spondylitis sacral and sacrococcygeal region
M45.9 Ankylosing spondylitis of unspecified sites in spine

● M46 Other inflammatory spondylopathies
● M46.Ø Spinal enthesopathy
Disorder of ligamentous or muscular attachments of spine

M46.ØØ Spinal enthesopathy, site unspecified
M46.Ø1 Spinal enthesopathy, occipito-atlanto-axial region
M46.Ø2 Spinal enthesopathy, cervical region
M46.Ø3 Spinal enthesopathy, cervicothoracic region
M46.Ø4 Spinal enthesopathy, thoracic region
M46.Ø5 Spinal enthesopathy, thoracolumbar region
M46.Ø6 Spinal enthesopathy, lumbar region
M46.Ø7 Spinal enthesopathy, lumbosacral region
M46.Ø8 Spinal enthesopathy, sacral and sacrococcygeal region
M46.Ø9 Spinal enthesopathy, multiple sites in spine

M46.1 Sacroiliitis, not elsewhere classified
● M46.2 Osteomyelitis of vertebra
M46.2Ø Osteomyelitis of vertebra, site unspecified
M46.21 Osteomyelitis of vertebra, occipito-atlanto-axial region
M46.22 Osteomyelitis of vertebra, cervical region
M46.23 Osteomyelitis of vertebra, cervicothoracic region
M46.24 Osteomyelitis of vertebra, thoracic region
M46.25 Osteomyelitis of vertebra, thoracolumbar region
M46.26 Osteomyelitis of vertebra, lumbar region
M46.27 Osteomyelitis of vertebra, lumbosacral region
M46.28 Osteomyelitis of vertebra, sacral and sacrococcygeal region

● **M46.3 Infection of intervertebral disc (pyogenic)**
Use additional code (B95-B97) to identify infectious agent
M46.30 Infection of intervertebral disc (pyogenic), site unspecified
M46.31 Infection of intervertebral disc (pyogenic), occipito-atlanto-axial region
M46.32 Infection of intervertebral disc (pyogenic), cervical region
M46.33 Infection of intervertebral disc (pyogenic), cervicothoracic region
M46.34 Infection of intervertebral disc (pyogenic), thoracic region
M46.35 Infection of intervertebral disc (pyogenic), thoracolumbar region
M46.36 Infection of intervertebral disc (pyogenic), lumbar region
M46.37 Infection of intervertebral disc (pyogenic), lumbosacral region
M46.38 Infection of intervertebral disc (pyogenic), sacral and sacrococcygeal region
M46.39 Infection of intervertebral disc (pyogenic), multiple sites in spine

● **M46.4 Discitis, unspecified**
M46.40 Discitis, unspecified, site unspecified
M46.41 Discitis, unspecified, occipito-atlanto-axial region
M46.42 Discitis, unspecified, cervical region
M46.43 Discitis, unspecified, cervicothoracic region
M46.44 Discitis, unspecified, thoracic region
M46.45 Discitis, unspecified, thoracolumbar region
M46.46 Discitis, unspecified, lumbar region
M46.47 Discitis, unspecified, lumbosacral region
M46.48 Discitis, unspecified, sacral and sacrococcygeal region
M46.49 Discitis, unspecified, multiple sites in spine

● **M46.5 Other infective spondylopathies**
M46.50 Other infective spondylopathies, site unspecified
M46.51 Other infective spondylopathies, occipitoatlanto-axial region
M46.52 Other infective spondylopathies, cervical region
M46.53 Other infective spondylopathies, cervicothoracic region
M46.54 Other infective spondylopathies, thoracic region
M46.55 Other infective spondylopathies, thoracolumbar region
M46.56 Other infective spondylopathies, lumbar region
M46.57 Other infective spondylopathies, lumbosacral region
M46.58 Other infective spondylopathies, sacral and sacrococcygeal region
M46.59 Other infective spondylopathies, multiple sites in spine

● **M46.8 Other specified inflammatory spondylopathies**
M46.80 Other specified inflammatory spondylopathies, site unspecified
M46.81 Other specified inflammatory spondylopathies, occipito-atlanto-axial region
M46.82 Other specified inflammatory spondylopathies, cervical region
M46.83 Other specified inflammatory spondylopathies, cervicothoracic region
M46.84 Other specified inflammatory spondylopathies, thoracic region
M46.85 Other specified inflammatory spondylopathies, thoracolumbar region
M46.86 Other specified inflammatory spondylopathies, lumbar region
M46.87 Other specified inflammatory spondylopathies, lumbosacral region
M46.88 Other specified inflammatory spondylopathies, sacral and sacrococcygeal region
M46.89 Other specified inflammatory spondylopathies, multiple sites in spine

● **M46.9 Unspecified inflammatory spondylopathy**
M46.90 Unspecified inflammatory spondylopathy, site unspecified
M46.91 Unspecified inflammatory spondylopathy, occipito-atlanto-axial region
M46.92 Unspecified inflammatory spondylopathy, cervical region
M46.93 Unspecified inflammatory spondylopathy, cervicothoracic region
M46.94 Unspecified inflammatory spondylopathy, thoracic region
M46.95 Unspecified inflammatory spondylopathy, thoracolumbar region
M46.96 Unspecified inflammatory spondylopathy, lumbar region
M46.97 Unspecified inflammatory spondylopathy, lumbosacral region
M46.98 Unspecified inflammatory spondylopathy, sacral and sacrococcygeal region
M46.99 Unspecified inflammatory spondylopathy, multiple sites in spine

● **M47 Spondylosis**
Includes arthrosis or osteoarthritis of spine
degeneration of facet joints

● **M47.0 Anterior spinal and vertebral artery compression syndromes**
● **M47.01 Anterior spinal artery compression syndromes**
M47.011 Anterior spinal artery compression syndromes, occipito-atlanto-axial region
M47.012 Anterior spinal artery compression syndromes, cervical region
M47.013 Anterior spinal artery compression syndromes, cervicothoracic region
M47.014 Anterior spinal artery compression syndromes, thoracic region
M47.015 Anterior spinal artery compression syndromes, thoracolumbar region
M47.016 Anterior spinal artery compression syndromes, lumbar region
M47.019 Anterior spinal artery compression syndromes, site unspecified
● **M47.02 Vertebral artery compression syndromes**
M47.021 Vertebral artery compression syndromes, occipito-atlanto-axial region
M47.022 Vertebral artery compression syndromes, cervical region
M47.029 Vertebral artery compression syndromes, site unspecified

CHAPTER 13 (M00-M99)

● M47.1 Other spondylosis with myelopathy
Spondylogenic compression of spinal cord
Excludes1 vertebral subluxation (M43.3-M43.59)
M47.10 Other spondylosis with myelopathy, site unspecified
M47.11 Other spondylosis with myelopathy, occipito-atlanto-axial region
M47.12 Other spondylosis with myelopathy, cervical region
M47.13 Other spondylosis with myelopathy, cervicothoracic region
M47.14 Other spondylosis with myelopathy, thoracic region
M47.15 Other spondylosis with myelopathy, thoracolumbar region
M47.16 Other spondylosis with myelopathy, lumbar region

● M47.2 Other spondylosis with radiculopathy
M47.20 Other spondylosis with radiculopathy, site unspecified
M47.21 Other spondylosis with radiculopathy, occipito-atlanto-axial region
M47.22 Other spondylosis with radiculopathy, cervical region
M47.23 Other spondylosis with radiculopathy, cervicothoracic region
M47.24 Other spondylosis with radiculopathy, thoracic region
M47.25 Other spondylosis with radiculopathy, thoracolumbar region
M47.26 Other spondylosis with radiculopathy, lumbar region
M47.27 Other spondylosis with radiculopathy, lumbosacral region
M47.28 Other spondylosis with radiculopathy, sacral and sacrococcygeal region

● M47.8 Other spondylosis
● M47.81 Spondylosis without myelopathy or radiculopathy
M47.811 Spondylosis without myelopathy or radiculopathy, occipito-atlanto-axial region
M47.812 Spondylosis without myelopathy or radiculopathy, cervical region
M47.813 Spondylosis without myelopathy or radiculopathy, cervicothoracic region
M47.814 Spondylosis without myelopathy or radiculopathy, thoracic region
M47.815 Spondylosis without myelopathy or radiculopathy, thoracolumbar region
M47.816 Spondylosis without myelopathy or radiculopathy, lumbar region
M47.817 Spondylosis without myelopathy or radiculopathy, lumbosacral region
M47.818 Spondylosis without myelopathy or radiculopathy, sacral and sacrococcygeal region
M47.819 Spondylosis without myelopathy or radiculopathy, site unspecified
● M47.89 Other spondylosis
M47.891 Other spondylosis, occipito-atlanto-axial region
M47.892 Other spondylosis, cervical region
M47.893 Other spondylosis, cervicothoracic region
M47.894 Other spondylosis, thoracic region
M47.895 Other spondylosis, thoracolumbar region
M47.896 Other spondylosis, lumbar region
M47.897 Other spondylosis, lumbosacral region
M47.898 Other spondylosis, sacral and sacrococcygeal region
M47.899 Other spondylosis, site unspecified
M47.9 Spondylosis, unspecified

● M48 Other spondylopathies
● M48.0 Spinal stenosis
Caudal stenosis
M48.00 Spinal stenosis, site unspecified
M48.01 Spinal stenosis, occipito-atlanto-axial region
M48.02 Spinal stenosis, cervical region
M48.03 Spinal stenosis, cervicothoracic region
M48.04 Spinal stenosis, thoracic region
M48.05 Spinal stenosis, thoracolumbar region
M48.06 Spinal stenosis, lumbar region
M48.07 Spinal stenosis, lumbosacral region
M48.08 Spinal stenosis, sacral and sacrococcygeal region

● M48.1 Ankylosing hyperostosis [Forestier]
Diffuse idiopathic skeletal hyperostosis [DISH]
M48.10 Ankylosing hyperostosis [Forestier], site unspecified
M48.11 Ankylosing hyperostosis [Forestier], occipito-atlanto-axial region
M48.12 Ankylosing hyperostosis [Forestier], cervical region
M48.13 Ankylosing hyperostosis [Forestier], cervicothoracic region
M48.14 Ankylosing hyperostosis [Forestier], thoracic region
M48.15 Ankylosing hyperostosis [Forestier], thoracolumbar region
M48.16 Ankylosing hyperostosis [Forestier], lumbar region
M48.17 Ankylosing hyperostosis [Forestier], lumbosacral region
M48.18 Ankylosing hyperostosis [Forestier], sacral and sacrococcygeal region
M48.19 Ankylosing hyperostosis [Forestier], multiple sites in spine

● M48.2 Kissing spine
M48.20 Kissing spine, site unspecified
M48.21 Kissing spine, occipito-atlanto-axial region
M48.22 Kissing spine, cervical region
M48.23 Kissing spine, cervicothoracic region
M48.24 Kissing spine, thoracic region
M48.25 Kissing spine, thoracolumbar region
M48.26 Kissing spine, lumbar region
M48.27 Kissing spine, lumbosacral region

● M48.3 Traumatic spondylopathy
M48.30 Traumatic spondylopathy, site unspecified
M48.31 Traumatic spondylopathy, occipito-atlanto-axial region
M48.32 Traumatic spondylopathy, cervical region
M48.33 Traumatic spondylopathy, cervicothoracic region
M48.34 Traumatic spondylopathy, thoracic region
M48.35 Traumatic spondylopathy, thoracolumbar region
M48.36 Traumatic spondylopathy, lumbar region
M48.37 Traumatic spondylopathy, lumbosacral region
M48.38 Traumatic spondylopathy, sacral and sacrococcygeal region

●M48.4 Fatigue fracture of vertebra
Stress fracture of vertebra
Excludes1 pathological fracture NOS (M84.4-)
pathological fracture of vertebra due to neoplasm (M84.58)
pathological fracture of vertebra due to other diagnosis (M84.68)
pathological fracture of vertebra due to osteoporosis (M8Ø.-)
traumatic fracture of vertebrae (S12.Ø-S12.3-, S22.Ø-, S32.Ø-)

The appropriate 7th character is to be added to each code from subcategory M48.4:

A	initial encounter for fracture
D	subsequent encounter for fracture with routine healing
G	subsequent encounter for fracture with delayed healing
S	sequela of fracture

X●M48.40 Fatigue fracture of vertebra, site unspecified
X●M48.41 Fatigue fracture of vertebra, occipitoatlanto-axial region
X●M48.42 Fatigue fracture of vertebra, cervical region
X●M48.43 Fatigue fracture of vertebra, cervicothoracic region
X●M48.44 Fatigue fracture of vertebra, thoracic region
X●M48.45 Fatigue fracture of vertebra, thoracolumbar region
X●M48.46 Fatigue fracture of vertebra, lumbar region
X●M48.47 Fatigue fracture of vertebra, lumbosacral region
X●M48.48 Fatigue fracture of vertebra, sacral and sacrococcygeal region

●M48.5 Collapsed vertebra, not elsewhere classified
Collapsed vertebra NOS
Compression fracture of vertebra NOS ◀
Wedging of vertebra NOS
Excludes1 current injury - see Injury of spine, by body region
fatigue fracture of vertebra (M48.4)
pathological fracture of vertebra due to neoplasm (M84.58)
pathological fracture of vertebra due to other diagnosis (M84.68)
pathological fracture of vertebra due to osteoporosis (M8Ø.-)
pathological fracture NOS (M84.4-)
stress fracture of vertebra (M48.4-)
traumatic fracture of vertebra (S12.-, S22.-, S32.-)

The appropriate 7th character is to be added to each code from subcategory M48.5:

A	initial encounter for fracture
D	subsequent encounter for fracture with routine healing
G	subsequent encounter for fracture with delayed healing
S	sequela of fracture

X●M48.5Ø Collapsed vertebra, not elsewhere classified, site unspecified
X●M48.51 Collapsed vertebra, not elsewhere classified, occipito-atlanto-axial region
X●M48.52 Collapsed vertebra, not elsewhere classified, cervical region
X●M48.53 Collapsed vertebra, not elsewhere classified, cervicothoracic region
X●M48.54 Collapsed vertebra, not elsewhere classified, thoracic region
X●M48.55 Collapsed vertebra, not elsewhere classified, thoracolumbar region
X●M48.56 Collapsed vertebra, not elsewhere classified, lumbar region
X●M48.57 Collapsed vertebra, not elsewhere classified, lumbosacral region
X●M48.58 Collapsed vertebra, not elsewhere classified, sacral and sacrococcygeal region

●M48.8 Other specified spondylopathies
Ossification of posterior longitudinal ligament
●M48.8X Other specified spondylopathies
M48.8X1 Other specified spondylopathies, occipito-atlanto-axial region
M48.8X2 Other specified spondylopathies, cervical region
M48.8X3 Other specified spondylopathies, cervicothoracic region
M48.8X4 Other specified spondylopathies, thoracic region
M48.8X5 Other specified spondylopathies, thoracolumbar region
M48.8X6 Other specified spondylopathies, lumbar region
M48.8X7 Other specified spondylopathies, lumbosacral region
M48.8X8 Other specified spondylopathies, sacral and sacrococcygeal region
M48.8X9 Other specified spondylopathies, site unspecified
M48.9 Spondylopathy, unspecified

●M49 Spondylopathies in diseases classified elsewhere
Includes curvature of spine in diseases classified elsewhere
deformity of spine in diseases classified elsewhere
kyphosis in diseases classified elsewhere
scoliosis in diseases classified elsewhere
spondylopathy in diseases classified elsewhere

Code first *underlying disease, such as:*
brucellosis (A23.-)
Charcot-Marie-Tooth disease (G6Ø.Ø)
enterobacterial infections (AØ1-AØ4)
osteitis fibrosa cystica (E21.Ø)
Excludes1 curvature of spine in tuberculosis [Pott's] (A18.Ø1)
enteropathic arthropathies (MØ7.-)
gonococcal spondylitis (A54.41)
neuropathic [tabes dorsalis] spondylitis (A52.11)
neuropathic spondylopathy in syringomyelia (G95.Ø)
neuropathic spondylopathy in tabes dorsalis (A52.11)
nonsyphilitic neuropathic spondylopathy NEC (G98.Ø)
spondylitis in syphilis (acquired) (A52.77)
tuberculous spondylitis (A18.Ø1)
typhoid fever spondylitis (AØ1.Ø5)

●M49.8 Spondylopathy in diseases classified elsewhere
M49.8Ø Spondylopathy in diseases classified elsewhere, site unspecified
M49.81 Spondylopathy in diseases classified elsewhere, occipito-atlanto-axial region
M49.82 Spondylopathy in diseases classified elsewhere, cervical region
M49.83 Spondylopathy in diseases classified elsewhere, cervicothoracic region
M49.84 Spondylopathy in diseases classified elsewhere, thoracic region
M49.85 Spondylopathy in diseases classified elsewhere, thoracolumbar region

CHAPTER 13 (MØØ-M99)

M49.86 Spondylopathy in diseases classified elsewhere, lumbar region

M49.87 Spondylopathy in diseases classified elsewhere, lumbosacral region

M49.88 Spondylopathy in diseases classified elsewhere, sacral and sacrococcygeal region

M49.89 Spondylopathy in diseases classified elsewhere, multiple sites in spine

OTHER DORSOPATHIES (M50-M54)

Excludes1 current injury - see injury of spine by body region
discitis NOS (M46.4-)

● **M50 Cervical disc disorders**

Note: Code to the most superior level of disorder.

Includes cervicothoracic disc disorders with cervicalgia
cervicothoracic disc disorders

● **M50.0 Cervical disc disorder with myelopathy**

M50.00 Cervical disc disorder with myelopathy, unspecified cervical region

M50.01 Cervical disc disorder with myelopathy, high cervical region
C2-C3 disc disorder with myelopathy
C3-C4 disc disorder with myelopathy

● **M50.02 Cervical disc disorder with myelopathy, mid-cervical region**

M50.020 Cervical disc disorder with myelopathy, mid-cervical region, unspecified level ◀

M50.021 Cervical disc disorder at C4-C5 level with myelopathy ◀
C4-C5 disc disorder with myelopathy ◀

M50.022 Cervical disc disorder at C5-C6 level with myelopathy ◀
C5-C6 disc disorder with myelopathy ◀

M50.023 Cervical disc disorder at C6-C7 level with myelopathy ◀
C6-C7 disc disorder with myelopathy ◀

M50.03 Cervical disc disorder with myelopathy, cervicothoracic region
C7-T1 disc disorder with myelopathy

● **M50.1 Cervical disc disorder with radiculopathy**

Excludes2 brachial radiculitis NOS (M54.13)

M50.10 Cervical disc disorder with radiculopathy, unspecified cervical region

M50.11 Cervical disc disorder with radiculopathy, high cervical region
C2-C3 disc disorder with radiculopathy
C3 radiculopathy due to disc disorder
C3-C4 disc disorder with radiculopathy
C4 radiculopathy due to disc disorder

● **M50.12 Cervical disc disorder with radiculopathy, mid-cervical region**

M50.120 Mid-cervical disc disorder, unspecified ◀

M50.121 Cervical disc disorder at C4-C5 level with radiculopathy ◀
C4-C5 disc disorder with radiculopathy ◀
C5 radiculopathy due to disc disorder ◀

M50.122 Cervical disc disorder at C5-C6 level with radiculopathy ◀
C5-C6 disc disorder with radiculopathy ◀
C6 radiculopathy due to disc disorder ◀

M50.123 Cervical disc disorder at C6-C7 level with radiculopathy ◀
C6-C7 disc disorder with radiculopathy ◀
C7 radiculopathy due to disc disorder ◀

M50.13 Cervical disc disorder with radiculopathy, cervicothoracic region
C7-T1 disc disorder with radiculopathy
C8 radiculopathy due to disc disorder

● **M50.2 Other cervical disc displacement**

M50.20 Other cervical disc displacement, unspecified cervical region

M50.21 Other cervical disc displacement, high cervical region
Other C2-C3 cervical disc displacement
Other C3-C4 cervical disc displacement

● **M50.22 Other cervical disc displacement, mid-cervical region**

M50.220 Other cervical disc displacement, mid-cervical region, unspecified level ◀

M50.221 Other cervical disc displacement at C4-C5 level ◀
Other C4-C5 cervical disc displacement ◀

M50.222 Other cervical disc displacement at C5-C6 level ◀
Other C5-C6 cervical disc displacement ◀

M50.223 Other cervical disc displacement at C6-C7 level ◀
Other C6-C7 cervical disc displacement ◀

M50.23 Other cervical disc displacement, cervicothoracic region
Other C7-T1 cervical disc displacement

● **M50.3 Other cervical disc degeneration**

M50.30 Other cervical disc degeneration, unspecified cervical region

M50.31 Other cervical disc degeneration, high cervical region
Other C2-C3 cervical disc degeneration
Other C3-C4 cervical disc degeneration

● **M50.32 Other cervical disc degeneration, mid-cervical region**

M50.320 Other cervical disc degeneration, mid-cervical region, unspecified level ◀

M50.321 Other cervical disc degeneration at C4-C5 level ◀
Other C4-C5 cervical disc degeneration ◀

M50.322 Other cervical disc degeneration at C5-C6 level ◀
Other C5-C6 cervical disc degeneration ◀

M50.323 Other cervical disc degeneration at C6-C7 level ◀
Other C6-C7 cervical disc degeneration ◀

M50.33 Other cervical disc degeneration, cervicothoracic region
Other C7-T1 cervical disc degeneration

● **M50.8 Other cervical disc disorders**

M50.80 Other cervical disc disorders, unspecified cervical region

M50.81 Other cervical disc disorders, high cervical region
Other C2-C3 cervical disc disorders
Other C3-C4 cervical disc disorders

● **M50.82 Other cervical disc disorders, mid-cervical region**
M50.820 Other cervical disc disorders, mid-cervical region, unspecified level ◀
M50.821 Other cervical disc disorders at C4-C5 level ◀
Other C4-C5 cervical disc disorders ◀
M50.822 Other cervical disc disorders at C5-C6 level ◀
Other C5-C6 cervical disc disorders ◀
M50.823 Other cervical disc disorders at C6-C7 level ◀
Other C6-C7 cervical disc disorders ◀
M50.83 Other cervical disc disorders, cervicothoracic region
Other C7-T1 cervical disc disorders

● **M50.9 Cervical disc disorder, unspecified**
M50.90 Cervical disc disorder, unspecified, unspecified cervical region
M50.91 Cervical disc disorder, unspecified, high cervical region
C2-C3 cervical disc disorder, unspecified
C3-C4 cervical disc disorder, unspecified
● **M50.92 Cervical disc disorder, unspecified, mid-cervical region**
M50.920 Unspecified cervical disc disorder, mid-cervical region, unspecified level ◀
M50.921 Unspecified cervical disc disorder at C4-C5 level ◀
Unspecified C4-C5 cervical disc disorder ◀
M50.922 Unspecified cervical disc disorder at C5-C6 level ◀
Unspecified C5-C6 cervical disc disorder ◀
M50.923 Unspecified cervical disc disorder at C6-C7 level ◀
Unspecified C6-C7 cervical disc disorder ◀
M50.93 Cervical disc disorder, unspecified, cervicothoracic region
C7-T1 cervical disc disorder, unspecified

● **M51 Thoracic, thoracolumbar, and lumbosacral intervertebral disc disorders**
Excludes2 cervical and cervicothoracic disc disorders (M50.-)
sacral and sacrococcygeal disorders (M53.3)

● **M51.0 Thoracic, thoracolumbar and lumbosacral intervertebral disc disorders with myelopathy**
M51.04 Intervertebral disc disorders with myelopathy, thoracic region
M51.05 Intervertebral disc disorders with myelopathy, thoracolumbar region
M51.06 Intervertebral disc disorders with myelopathy, lumbar region

● **M51.1 Thoracic, thoracolumbar and lumbosacral intervertebral disc disorders with radiculopathy**
Sciatica due to intervertebral disc disorder
Excludes1 lumbar radiculitis NOS (M54.16)
sciatica NOS (M54.3)
M51.14 Intervertebral disc disorders with radiculopathy, thoracic region
M51.15 Intervertebral disc disorders with radiculopathy, thoracolumbar region
M51.16 Intervertebral disc disorders with radiculopathy, lumbar region
M51.17 Intervertebral disc disorders with radiculopathy, lumbosacral region

● **M51.2 Other thoracic, thoracolumbar and lumbosacral intervertebral disc displacement**
Lumbago due to displacement of intervertebral disc
M51.24 Other intervertebral disc displacement, thoracic region
M51.25 Other intervertebral disc displacement, thoracolumbar region
M51.26 Other intervertebral disc displacement, lumbar region
M51.27 Other intervertebral disc displacement, lumbosacral region

● **M51.3 Other thoracic, thoracolumbar and lumbosacral intervertebral disc degeneration**
M51.34 Other intervertebral disc degeneration, thoracic region
M51.35 Other intervertebral disc degeneration, thoracolumbar region
M51.36 Other intervertebral disc degeneration, lumbar region
M51.37 Other intervertebral disc degeneration, lumbosacral region

● **M51.4 Schmorl's nodes**
M51.44 Schmorl's nodes, thoracic region
M51.45 Schmorl's nodes, thoracolumbar region
M51.46 Schmorl's nodes, lumbar region
M51.47 Schmorl's nodes, lumbosacral region

● **M51.8 Other thoracic, thoracolumbar and lumbosacral intervertebral disc disorders**
M51.84 Other intervertebral disc disorders, thoracic region
M51.85 Other intervertebral disc disorders, thoracolumbar region
M51.86 Other intervertebral disc disorders, lumbar region
M51.87 Other intervertebral disc disorders, lumbosacral region

M51.9 Unspecified thoracic, thoracolumbar and lumbosacral intervertebral disc disorder

● **M53 Other and unspecified dorsopathies, not elsewhere classified**
M53.0 Cervicocranial syndrome
Posterior cervical sympathetic syndrome
M53.1 Cervicobrachial syndrome
Excludes2 cervical disc disorder (M50.-)
thoracic outlet syndrome (G54.0)
● **M53.2 Spinal instabilities**
● **M53.2X Spinal instabilities**
M53.2X1 Spinal instabilities, occipito-atlanto-axial region
M53.2X2 Spinal instabilities, cervical region
M53.2X3 Spinal instabilities, cervicothoracic region
M53.2X4 Spinal instabilities, thoracic region
M53.2X5 Spinal instabilities, thoracolumbar region
M53.2X6 Spinal instabilities, lumbar region
M53.2X7 Spinal instabilities, lumbosacral region
M53.2X8 Spinal instabilities, sacral and sacrococcygeal region
M53.2X9 Spinal instabilities, site unspecified

CHAPTER 13 (M00-M99)

M53.3 Sacrococcygeal disorders, not elsewhere classified
Coccygodynia

● M53.8 Other specified dorsopathies
M53.80 Other specified dorsopathies, site unspecified
M53.81 Other specified dorsopathies, occipito-atlanto-axial region
M53.82 Other specified dorsopathies, cervical region
M53.83 Other specified dorsopathies, cervicothoracic region
M53.84 Other specified dorsopathies, thoracic region
M53.85 Other specified dorsopathies, thoracolumbar region
M53.86 Other specified dorsopathies, lumbar region
M53.87 Other specified dorsopathies, lumbosacral region
M53.88 Other specified dorsopathies, sacral and sacrococcygeal region

M53.9 Dorsopathy, unspecified

● M54 Dorsalgia
Excludes1 psychogenic dorsalgia (F45.41)

● M54.0 Panniculitis affecting regions of neck and back
Excludes1 lupus panniculitis (L93.2)
panniculitis NOS (M79.3)
relapsing [Weber-Christian] panniculitis (M35.6)
M54.00 Panniculitis affecting regions of neck and back, site unspecified
M54.01 Panniculitis affecting regions of neck and back, occipito-atlanto-axial region
M54.02 Panniculitis affecting regions of neck and back, cervical region
M54.03 Panniculitis affecting regions of neck and back, cervicothoracic region
M54.04 Panniculitis affecting regions of neck and back, thoracic region
M54.05 Panniculitis affecting regions of neck and back, thoracolumbar region
M54.06 Panniculitis affecting regions of neck and back, lumbar region
M54.07 Panniculitis affecting regions of neck and back, lumbosacral region
M54.08 Panniculitis affecting regions of neck and back, sacral and sacrococcygeal region
M54.09 Panniculitis affecting regions, neck and back, multiple sites in spine

● M54.1 Radiculopathy
Brachial neuritis or radiculitis NOS
Lumbar neuritis or radiculitis NOS
Lumbosacral neuritis or radiculitis NOS
Thoracic neuritis or radiculitis NOS
Radiculitis NOS
Excludes1 neuralgia and neuritis NOS (M79.2)
radiculopathy with cervical disc disorder (M50.1)
radiculopathy with lumbar and other intervertebral disc disorder (M51.1-)
radiculopathy with spondylosis (M47.2-)
M54.10 Radiculopathy, site unspecified
M54.11 Radiculopathy, occipito-atlanto-axial region
M54.12 Radiculopathy, cervical region
M54.13 Radiculopathy, cervicothoracic region
M54.14 Radiculopathy, thoracic region
M54.15 Radiculopathy, thoracolumbar region
M54.16 Radiculopathy, lumbar region
M54.17 Radiculopathy, lumbosacral region
M54.18 Radiculopathy, sacral and sacrococcygeal region

M54.2 Cervicalgia
Excludes1 cervicalgia due to intervertebral cervical disc disorder (M50.-)

● M54.3 Sciatica
Excludes1 lesion of sciatic nerve (G57.0)
sciatica due to intervertebral disc disorder (M51.1-)
sciatica with lumbago (M54.4-)
M54.30 Sciatica, unspecified side
M54.31 Sciatica, right side
M54.32 Sciatica, left side

● M54.4 Lumbago with sciatica
Excludes1 lumbago with sciatica due to intervertebral disc disorder (M51.1-)
M54.40 Lumbago with sciatica, unspecified side
M54.41 Lumbago with sciatica, right side
M54.42 Lumbago with sciatica, left side

M54.5 Low back pain
Loin pain
Lumbago NOS
Excludes1 low back strain (S39.012)
lumbago due to intervertebral disc displacement (M51.2-)
lumbago with sciatica (M54.4-)

M54.6 Pain in thoracic spine
Excludes1 pain in thoracic spine due to intervertebral disc disorder (M51.)

● M54.8 Other dorsalgia
Excludes1 dorsalgia in thoracic region (M54.6)
low back pain (M54.5)
M54.81 Occipital neuralgia
M54.89 Other dorsalgia

M54.9 Dorsalgia, unspecified
Backache NOS
Back pain NOS

SOFT TISSUE DISORDERS (M60-M79)

DISORDERS OF MUSCLES (M60-M63)

Excludes1 dermatopolymyositis (M33.-)
muscular dystrophies and myopathies (G71-G72)
myopathy in amyloidosis (E85.-)
myopathy in polyarteritis nodosa (M30.0)
myopathy in rheumatoid arthritis (M05.32)
myopathy in scleroderma (M34.-)
myopathy in Sjögren's syndrome (M35.03)
myopathy in systemic lupus erythematosus (M32.-)

● M60 Myositis
Excludes2 inclusion body myositis [IBM] (G72.41)

● M60.0 Infective myositis
Tropical pyomyositis
Use additional code (B95-B97) to identify infectious agent

● M60.00 Infective myositis, unspecified site
M60.000 Infective myositis, unspecified right arm
Infective myositis, right upper limb NOS
M60.001 Infective myositis, unspecified left arm
Infective myositis, left upper limb NOS
M60.002 Infective myositis, unspecified arm
Infective myositis, upper limb NOS

CHAPTER 13 (M00-M99)

M60.003 Infective myositis, unspecified right leg
Infective myositis, right lower limb NOS
M60.004 Infective myositis, unspecified left leg
Infective myositis, left lower limb NOS
M60.005 Infective myositis, unspecified leg
Infective myositis, lower limb NOS
M60.009 Infective myositis, unspecified site
● M60.01 Infective myositis, shoulder
M60.011 Infective myositis, right shoulder
M60.012 Infective myositis, left shoulder
M60.019 Infective myositis, unspecified shoulder
● M60.02 Infective myositis, upper arm
M60.021 Infective myositis, right upper arm
M60.022 Infective myositis, left upper arm
M60.029 Infective myositis, unspecified upper arm
● M60.03 Infective myositis, forearm
M60.031 Infective myositis, right forearm
M60.032 Infective myositis, left forearm
M60.039 Infective myositis, unspecified forearm
● M60.04 Infective myositis, hand and fingers
M60.041 Infective myositis, right hand
M60.042 Infective myositis, left hand
M60.043 Infective myositis, unspecified hand
M60.044 Infective myositis, right finger(s)
M60.045 Infective myositis, left finger(s)
M60.046 Infective myositis, unspecified finger(s)
● M60.05 Infective myositis, thigh
M60.051 Infective myositis, right thigh
M60.052 Infective myositis, left thigh
M60.059 Infective myositis, unspecified thigh
● M60.06 Infective myositis, lower leg
M60.061 Infective myositis, right lower leg
M60.062 Infective myositis, left lower leg
M60.069 Infective myositis, unspecified lower leg
● M60.07 Infective myositis, ankle, foot and toes
M60.070 Infective myositis, right ankle
M60.071 Infective myositis, left ankle
M60.072 Infective myositis, unspecified ankle
M60.073 Infective myositis, right foot
M60.074 Infective myositis, left foot
M60.075 Infective myositis, unspecified foot
M60.076 Infective myositis, right toe(s)
M60.077 Infective myositis, left toe(s)
M60.078 Infective myositis, unspecified toe(s)
M60.08 Infective myositis, other site
M60.09 Infective myositis, multiple sites
● M60.1 Interstitial myositis
M60.10 Interstitial myositis of unspecified site
● M60.11 Interstitial myositis, shoulder
M60.111 Interstitial myositis, right shoulder
M60.112 Interstitial myositis, left shoulder
M60.119 Interstitial myositis, unspecified shoulder
● M60.12 Interstitial myositis, upper arm
M60.121 Interstitial myositis, right upper arm
M60.122 Interstitial myositis, left upper arm
M60.129 Interstitial myositis, unspecified upper arm
● M60.13 Interstitial myositis, forearm
M60.131 Interstitial myositis, right forearm
M60.132 Interstitial myositis, left forearm
M60.139 Interstitial myositis, unspecified forearm
● M60.14 Interstitial myositis, hand
M60.141 Interstitial myositis, right hand
M60.142 Interstitial myositis, left hand
M60.149 Interstitial myositis, unspecified hand
● M60.15 Interstitial myositis, thigh
M60.151 Interstitial myositis, right thigh
M60.152 Interstitial myositis, left thigh
M60.159 Interstitial myositis, unspecified thigh
● M60.16 Interstitial myositis, lower leg
M60.161 Interstitial myositis, right lower leg
M60.162 Interstitial myositis, left lower leg
M60.169 Interstitial myositis, unspecified lower leg
● M60.17 Interstitial myositis, ankle and foot
M60.171 Interstitial myositis, right ankle and foot
M60.172 Interstitial myositis, left ankle and foot
M60.179 Interstitial myositis, unspecified ankle and foot
M60.18 Interstitial myositis, other site
M60.19 Interstitial myositis, multiple sites
● M60.2 Foreign body granuloma of soft tissue, not elsewhere classified
Use additional code to identify the type of retained foreign body (Z18.-)
Excludes1 foreign body granuloma of skin and subcutaneous tissue (L92.3)
M60.20 Foreign body granuloma of soft tissue, not elsewhere classified, unspecified site
● M60.21 Foreign body granuloma of soft tissue, not elsewhere classified, shoulder
M60.211 Foreign body granuloma of soft tissue, not elsewhere classified, right shoulder
M60.212 Foreign body granuloma of soft tissue, not elsewhere classified, left shoulder
M60.219 Foreign body granuloma of soft tissue, not elsewhere classified, unspecified shoulder
● M60.22 Foreign body granuloma of soft tissue, not elsewhere classified, upper arm
M60.221 Foreign body granuloma of soft tissue, not elsewhere classified, right upper arm
M60.222 Foreign body granuloma of soft tissue, not elsewhere classified, left upper arm
M60.229 Foreign body granuloma of soft tissue, not elsewhere classified, unspecified upper arm

CHAPTER 13 (M00-M99)

- M60.23 Foreign body granuloma of soft tissue, not elsewhere classified, forearm
  - M60.231 Foreign body granuloma of soft tissue, not elsewhere classified, right forearm
  - M60.232 Foreign body granuloma of soft tissue, not elsewhere classified, left forearm
  - M60.239 Foreign body granuloma of soft tissue, not elsewhere classified, unspecified forearm
- M60.24 Foreign body granuloma of soft tissue, not elsewhere classified, hand
  - M60.241 Foreign body granuloma of soft tissue, not elsewhere classified, right hand
  - M60.242 Foreign body granuloma of soft tissue, not elsewhere classified, left hand
  - M60.249 Foreign body granuloma of soft tissue, not elsewhere classified, unspecified hand
- M60.25 Foreign body granuloma of soft tissue, not elsewhere classified, thigh
  - M60.251 Foreign body granuloma of soft tissue, not elsewhere classified, right thigh
  - M60.252 Foreign body granuloma of soft tissue, not elsewhere classified, left thigh
  - M60.259 Foreign body granuloma of soft tissue, not elsewhere classified, unspecified thigh
- M60.26 Foreign body granuloma of soft tissue, not elsewhere classified, lower leg
  - M60.261 Foreign body granuloma of soft tissue, not elsewhere classified, right lower leg
  - M60.262 Foreign body granuloma of soft tissue, not elsewhere classified, left lower leg
  - M60.269 Foreign body granuloma of soft tissue, not elsewhere classified, unspecified lower leg
- M60.27 Foreign body granuloma of soft tissue, not elsewhere classified, ankle and foot
  - M60.271 Foreign body granuloma of soft tissue, not elsewhere classified, right ankle and foot
  - M60.272 Foreign body granuloma of soft tissue, not elsewhere classified, left ankle and foot
  - M60.279 Foreign body granuloma of soft tissue, not elsewhere classified, unspecified ankle and foot
- M60.28 Foreign body granuloma of soft tissue, not elsewhere classified, other site

- M60.8 Other myositis
  - M60.80 Other myositis, unspecified site
  - M60.81 Other myositis shoulder
    - M60.811 Other myositis, right shoulder
    - M60.812 Other myositis, left shoulder
    - M60.819 Other myositis, unspecified shoulder
  - M60.82 Other myositis, upper arm
    - M60.821 Other myositis, right upper arm
    - M60.822 Other myositis, left upper arm
    - M60.829 Other myositis, unspecified upper arm
  - M60.83 Other myositis, forearm
    - M60.831 Other myositis, right forearm
    - M60.832 Other myositis, left forearm
    - M60.839 Other myositis, unspecified forearm
  - M60.84 Other myositis, hand
    - M60.841 Other myositis, right hand
    - M60.842 Other myositis, left hand
    - M60.849 Other myositis, unspecified hand
  - M60.85 Other myositis, thigh
    - M60.851 Other myositis, right thigh
    - M60.852 Other myositis, left thigh
    - M60.859 Other myositis, unspecified thigh
  - M60.86 Other myositis, lower leg
    - M60.861 Other myositis, right lower leg
    - M60.862 Other myositis, left lower leg
    - M60.869 Other myositis, unspecified lower leg
  - M60.87 Other myositis, ankle and foot
    - M60.871 Other myositis, right ankle and foot
    - M60.872 Other myositis, left ankle and foot
    - M60.879 Other myositis, unspecified ankle and foot
  - M60.88 Other myositis, other site
  - M60.89 Other myositis, multiple sites
- M60.9 Myositis, unspecified

M61 Calcification and ossification of muscle

- M61.0 Myositis ossificans traumatica
  - M61.00 Myositis ossificans traumatica, unspecified site
  - M61.01 Myositis ossificans traumatica, shoulder
    - M61.011 Myositis ossificans traumatica, right shoulder
    - M61.012 Myositis ossificans traumatica, left shoulder
    - M61.019 Myositis ossificans traumatica, unspecified shoulder
  - M61.02 Myositis ossificans traumatica, upper arm
    - M61.021 Myositis ossificans traumatica, right upper arm
    - M61.022 Myositis ossificans traumatica, left upper arm
    - M61.029 Myositis ossificans traumatica, unspecified upper arm
  - M61.03 Myositis ossificans traumatica, forearm
    - M61.031 Myositis ossificans traumatica, right forearm
    - M61.032 Myositis ossificans traumatica, left forearm
    - M61.039 Myositis ossificans traumatica, unspecified forearm
  - M61.04 Myositis ossificans traumatica, hand
    - M61.041 Myositis ossificans traumatica, right hand
    - M61.042 Myositis ossificans traumatica, left hand
    - M61.049 Myositis ossificans traumatica, unspecified hand
  - M61.05 Myositis ossificans traumatica, thigh
    - M61.051 Myositis ossificans traumatica, right thigh
    - M61.052 Myositis ossificans traumatica, left thigh
    - M61.059 Myositis ossificans traumatica, unspecified thigh

● M61.06 Myositis ossificans traumatica, lower leg
M61.061 Myositis ossificans traumatica, right lower leg
M61.062 Myositis ossificans traumatica, left lower leg
M61.069 Myositis ossificans traumatica, unspecified lower leg
● M61.07 Myositis ossificans traumatica, ankle and foot
M61.071 Myositis ossificans traumatica, right ankle and foot
M61.072 Myositis ossificans traumatica, left ankle and foot
M61.079 Myositis ossificans traumatica, unspecified ankle and foot
M61.08 Myositis ossificans traumatica, other site
M61.09 Myositis ossificans traumatica, multiple sites
● M61.1 Myositis ossificans progressiva
Fibrodysplasia ossificans progressiva
M61.10 Myositis ossificans progressiva, unspecified site
● M61.11 Myositis ossificans progressiva, shoulder
M61.111 Myositis ossificans progressiva, right shoulder
M61.112 Myositis ossificans progressiva, left shoulder
M61.119 Myositis ossificans progressiva, unspecified shoulder
● M61.12 Myositis ossificans progressiva, upper arm
M61.121 Myositis ossificans progressiva, right upper arm
M61.122 Myositis ossificans progressiva, left upper arm
M61.129 Myositis ossificans progressiva, unspecified arm
● M61.13 Myositis ossificans progressiva, forearm
M61.131 Myositis ossificans progressiva, right forearm
M61.132 Myositis ossificans progressiva, left forearm
M61.139 Myositis ossificans progressiva, unspecified forearm
● M61.14 Myositis ossificans progressiva, hand and finger(s)
M61.141 Myositis ossificans progressiva, right hand
M61.142 Myositis ossificans progressiva, left hand
M61.143 Myositis ossificans progressiva, unspecified hand
M61.144 Myositis ossificans progressiva, right finger(s)
M61.145 Myositis ossificans progressiva, left finger(s)
M61.146 Myositis ossificans progressiva, unspecified finger(s)
● M61.15 Myositis ossificans progressiva, thigh
M61.151 Myositis ossificans progressiva, right thigh
M61.152 Myositis ossificans progressiva, left thigh
M61.159 Myositis ossificans progressiva, unspecified thigh
● M61.16 Myositis ossificans progressiva, lower leg
M61.161 Myositis ossificans progressiva, right lower leg
M61.162 Myositis ossificans progressiva, left lower leg
M61.169 Myositis ossificans progressiva, unspecified lower leg
● M61.17 Myositis ossificans progressiva, ankle, foot and toe(s)
M61.171 Myositis ossificans progressiva, right ankle
M61.172 Myositis ossificans progressiva, left ankle
M61.173 Myositis ossificans progressiva, unspecified ankle
M61.174 Myositis ossificans progressiva, right foot
M61.175 Myositis ossificans progressiva, left foot
M61.176 Myositis ossificans progressiva, unspecified foot
M61.177 Myositis ossificans progressiva, right toe(s)
M61.178 Myositis ossificans progressiva, left toe(s)
M61.179 Myositis ossificans progressiva, unspecified toe(s)
M61.18 Myositis ossificans progressiva, other site
M61.19 Myositis ossificans progressiva, multiple sites
● M61.2 Paralytic calcification and ossification of muscle
Myositis ossificans associated with quadriplegia or paraplegia
M61.20 Paralytic calcification and ossification of muscle, unspecified site
● M61.21 Paralytic calcification and ossification of muscle, shoulder
M61.211 Paralytic calcification and ossification of muscle, right shoulder
M61.212 Paralytic calcification and ossification of muscle, left shoulder
M61.219 Paralytic calcification and ossification of muscle, unspecified shoulder
● M61.22 Paralytic calcification and ossification of muscle, upper arm
M61.221 Paralytic calcification and ossification of muscle, right upper arm
M61.222 Paralytic calcification and ossification of muscle, left upper arm
M61.229 Paralytic calcification and ossification of muscle, unspecified upper arm
● M61.23 Paralytic calcification and ossification of muscle, forearm
M61.231 Paralytic calcification and ossification of muscle, right forearm
M61.232 Paralytic calcification and ossification of muscle, left forearm
M61.239 Paralytic calcification and ossification of muscle, unspecified forearm
● M61.24 Paralytic calcification and ossification of muscle, hand
M61.241 Paralytic calcification and ossification of muscle, right hand
M61.242 Paralytic calcification and ossification of muscle, left hand
M61.249 Paralytic calcification and ossification of muscle, unspecified hand
● M61.25 Paralytic calcification and ossification of muscle, thigh
M61.251 Paralytic calcification and ossification of muscle, right thigh
M61.252 Paralytic calcification and ossification of muscle, left thigh
M61.259 Paralytic calcification and ossification of muscle, unspecified thigh

CHAPTER 13 (M00-M99)

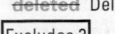

● M61.26 Paralytic calcification and ossification of muscle, lower leg
M61.261 Paralytic calcification and ossification of muscle, right lower leg
M61.262 Paralytic calcification and ossification of muscle, left lower leg
M61.269 Paralytic calcification and ossification of muscle, unspecified lower leg
● M61.27 Paralytic calcification and ossification of muscle, ankle and foot
M61.271 Paralytic calcification and ossification of muscle, right ankle and foot
M61.272 Paralytic calcification and ossification of muscle, left ankle and foot
M61.279 Paralytic calcification and ossification of muscle, unspecified ankle and foot
M61.28 Paralytic calcification and ossification of muscle, other site
M61.29 Paralytic calcification and ossification of muscle, multiple sites
● M61.3 Calcification and ossification of muscles associated with burns
Myositis ossificans associated with burns
M61.30 Calcification and ossification of muscles associated with burns, unspecified site
● M61.31 Calcification and ossification of muscles associated with burns, shoulder
M61.311 Calcification and ossification of muscles associated with burns, right shoulder
M61.312 Calcification and ossification of muscles associated with burns, left shoulder
M61.319 Calcification and ossification of muscles associated with burns, unspecified shoulder
● M61.32 Calcification and ossification of muscles associated with burns, upper arm
M61.321 Calcification and ossification of muscles associated with burns, right upper arm
M61.322 Calcification and ossification of muscles associated with burns, left upper arm
M61.329 Calcification and ossification of muscles associated with burns, unspecified upper arm
● M61.33 Calcification and ossification of muscles associated with burns, forearm
M61.331 Calcification and ossification of muscles associated with burns, right forearm
M61.332 Calcification and ossification of muscles associated with burns, left forearm
M61.339 Calcification and ossification of muscles associated with burns, unspecified forearm
● M61.34 Calcification and ossification of muscles associated with burns, hand
M61.341 Calcification and ossification of muscles associated with burns, right hand
M61.342 Calcification and ossification of muscles associated with burns, left hand
M61.349 Calcification and ossification of muscles associated with burns, unspecified hand
● M61.35 Calcification and ossification of muscles associated with burns, thigh
M61.351 Calcification and ossification of muscles associated with burns, right thigh
M61.352 Calcification and ossification of muscles associated with burns, left thigh
M61.359 Calcification and ossification of muscles associated with burns, unspecified thigh
● M61.36 Calcification and ossification of muscles associated with burns, lower leg
M61.361 Calcification and ossification of muscles associated with burns, right lower leg
M61.362 Calcification and ossification of muscles associated with burns, left lower leg
M61.369 Calcification and ossification of muscles associated with burns, unspecified lower leg
● M61.37 Calcification and ossification of muscles associated with burns, ankle and foot
M61.371 Calcification and ossification of muscles associated with burns, right ankle and foot
M61.372 Calcification and ossification of muscles associated with burns, left ankle and foot
M61.379 Calcification and ossification of muscles associated with burns, unspecified ankle and foot
M61.38 Calcification and ossification of muscles associated with burns, other site
M61.39 Calcification and ossification of muscles associated with burns, multiple sites
● M61.4 Other calcification of muscle
Excludes1 calcific tendinitis NOS (M65.2-)
calcific tendinitis of shoulder (M75.3)
M61.40 Other calcification of muscle, unspecified site
● M61.41 Other calcification of muscle, shoulder
M61.411 Other calcification of muscle, right shoulder
M61.412 Other calcification of muscle, left shoulder
M61.419 Other calcification of muscle, unspecified shoulder
● M61.42 Other calcification of muscle, upper arm
M61.421 Other calcification of muscle, right upper arm
M61.422 Other calcification of muscle, left upper arm
M61.429 Other calcification of muscle, unspecified upper arm
● M61.43 Other calcification of muscle, forearm
M61.431 Other calcification of muscle, right forearm
M61.432 Other calcification of muscle, left forearm
M61.439 Other calcification of muscle, unspecified forearm
● M61.44 Other calcification of muscle, hand
M61.441 Other calcification of muscle, right hand
M61.442 Other calcification of muscle, left hand
M61.449 Other calcification of muscle, unspecified hand

● **M61.45** Other calcification of muscle, thigh
- **M61.451** Other calcification of muscle, right thigh
- **M61.452** Other calcification of muscle, left thigh
- **M61.459** Other calcification of muscle, unspecified thigh

● **M61.46** Other calcification of muscle, lower leg
- **M61.461** Other calcification of muscle, right lower leg
- **M61.462** Other calcification of muscle, left lower leg
- **M61.469** Other calcification of muscle, unspecified lower leg

● **M61.47** Other calcification of muscle, ankle and foot
- **M61.471** Other calcification of muscle, right ankle and foot
- **M61.472** Other calcification of muscle, left ankle and foot
- **M61.479** Other calcification of muscle, unspecified ankle and foot

M61.48 Other calcification of muscle, other site

M61.49 Other calcification of muscle, multiple sites

● **M61.5** Other ossification of muscle

M61.50 Other ossification of muscle, unspecified site

● **M61.51** Other ossification of muscle, shoulder
- **M61.511** Other ossification of muscle, right shoulder
- **M61.512** Other ossification of muscle, left shoulder
- **M61.519** Other ossification of muscle, unspecified shoulder

● **M61.52** Other ossification of muscle, upper arm
- **M61.521** Other ossification of muscle, right upper arm
- **M61.522** Other ossification of muscle, left upper arm
- **M61.529** Other ossification of muscle, unspecified upper arm

● **M61.53** Other ossification of muscle, forearm
- **M61.531** Other ossification of muscle, right forearm
- **M61.532** Other ossification of muscle, left forearm
- **M61.539** Other ossification of muscle, unspecified forearm

● **M61.54** Other ossification of muscle, hand
- **M61.541** Other ossification of muscle, right hand
- **M61.542** Other ossification of muscle, left hand
- **M61.549** Other ossification of muscle, unspecified hand

● **M61.55** Other ossification of muscle, thigh
- **M61.551** Other ossification of muscle, right thigh
- **M61.552** Other ossification of muscle, left thigh
- **M61.559** Other ossification of muscle, unspecified thigh

● **M61.56** Other ossification of muscle, lower leg
- **M61.561** Other ossification of muscle, right lower leg
- **M61.562** Other ossification of muscle, left lower leg
- **M61.569** Other ossification of muscle, unspecified lower leg

● **M61.57** Other ossification of muscle, ankle and foot
- **M61.571** Other ossification of muscle, right ankle and foot
- **M61.572** Other ossification of muscle, left ankle and foot
- **M61.579** Other ossification of muscle, unspecified ankle and foot

M61.58 Other ossification of muscle, other site

M61.59 Other ossification of muscle, multiple sites

M61.9 Calcification and ossification of muscle, unspecified

● **M62** Other disorders of muscle

Excludes1 alcoholic myopathy (G72.1)
cramp and spasm (R25.2)
drug-induced myopathy (G72.Ø)
myalgia (M79.1)
stiff-man syndrome (G25.82)

Excludes2 nontraumatic hematoma of muscle (M79.81)

● **M62.Ø** Separation of muscle (nontraumatic)
Diastasis of muscle

Excludes1 diastasis recti complicating pregnancy, labor and delivery (O71.8)
traumatic separation of muscle - see strain of muscle by body region

M62.ØØ Separation of muscle (nontraumatic), unspecified site

● **M62.Ø1** Separation of muscle (nontraumatic), shoulder
- **M62.Ø11** Separation of muscle (nontraumatic), right shoulder
- **M62.Ø12** Separation of muscle (nontraumatic), left shoulder
- **M62.Ø19** Separation of muscle (nontraumatic), unspecified shoulder

● **M62.Ø2** Separation of muscle (nontraumatic), upper arm
- **M62.Ø21** Separation of muscle (nontraumatic), right upper arm
- **M62.Ø22** Separation of muscle (nontraumatic), left upper arm
- **M62.Ø29** Separation of muscle (nontraumatic), unspecified upper arm

● **M62.Ø3** Separation of muscle (nontraumatic), forearm
- **M62.Ø31** Separation of muscle (nontraumatic), right forearm
- **M62.Ø32** Separation of muscle (nontraumatic), left forearm
- **M62.Ø39** Separation of muscle (nontraumatic), unspecified forearm

● **M62.Ø4** Separation of muscle (nontraumatic), hand
- **M62.Ø41** Separation of muscle (nontraumatic), right hand
- **M62.Ø42** Separation of muscle (nontraumatic), left hand
- **M62.Ø49** Separation of muscle (nontraumatic), unspecified hand

● **M62.Ø5** Separation of muscle (nontraumatic), thigh
- **M62.Ø51** Separation of muscle (nontraumatic), right thigh
- **M62.Ø52** Separation of muscle (nontraumatic), left thigh
- **M62.Ø59** Separation of muscle (nontraumatic), unspecified thigh

● **M62.Ø6** Separation of muscle (nontraumatic), lower leg
- **M62.Ø61** Separation of muscle (nontraumatic), right lower leg
- **M62.Ø62** Separation of muscle (nontraumatic), left lower leg
- **M62.Ø69** Separation of muscle (nontraumatic), unspecified lower leg

CHAPTER 13 (MØØ-M99)

● M62.Ø7 Separation of muscle (nontraumatic), ankle and foot
M62.Ø71 Separation of muscle (nontraumatic), right ankle and foot
M62.Ø72 Separation of muscle (nontraumatic), left ankle and foot
M62.Ø79 Separation of muscle (nontraumatic), unspecified ankle and foot
M62.Ø8 Separation of muscle (nontraumatic), other site

● M62.1 Other rupture of muscle (nontraumatic)
Excludes1 traumatic rupture of muscle - see strain of muscle by body region
Excludes2 rupture of tendon (M66.-)
M62.1Ø Other rupture of muscle (nontraumatic), unspecified site
● M62.11 Other rupture of muscle (nontraumatic), shoulder
M62.111 Other rupture of muscle (nontraumatic), right shoulder
M62.112 Other rupture of muscle (nontraumatic), left shoulder
M62.119 Other rupture of muscle (nontraumatic), unspecified shoulder
● M62.12 Other rupture of muscle (nontraumatic), upper arm
M62.121 Other rupture of muscle (nontraumatic), right upper arm
M62.122 Other rupture of muscle (nontraumatic), left upper arm
M62.129 Other rupture of muscle (nontraumatic), unspecified upper arm
● M62.13 Other rupture of muscle (nontraumatic), forearm
M62.131 Other rupture of muscle (nontraumatic), right forearm
M62.132 Other rupture of muscle (nontraumatic), left forearm
M62.139 Other rupture of muscle (nontraumatic), unspecified forearm
● M62.14 Other rupture of muscle (nontraumatic), hand
M62.141 Other rupture of muscle (nontraumatic), right hand
M62.142 Other rupture of muscle (nontraumatic), left hand
M62.149 Other rupture of muscle (nontraumatic), unspecified hand
● M62.15 Other rupture of muscle (nontraumatic), thigh
M62.151 Other rupture of muscle (nontraumatic), right thigh
M62.152 Other rupture of muscle (nontraumatic), left thigh
M62.159 Other rupture of muscle (nontraumatic), unspecified thigh
● M62.16 Other rupture of muscle (nontraumatic), lower leg
M62.161 Other rupture of muscle (nontraumatic), right lower leg
M62.162 Other rupture of muscle (nontraumatic), left lower leg
M62.169 Other rupture of muscle (nontraumatic), unspecified lower leg
● M62.17 Other rupture of muscle (nontraumatic), ankle and foot
M62.171 Other rupture of muscle (nontraumatic), right ankle and foot
M62.172 Other rupture of muscle (nontraumatic), left ankle and foot
M62.179 Other rupture of muscle (nontraumatic), unspecified ankle and foot
M62.18 Other rupture of muscle (nontraumatic), other site

● M62.2 Nontraumatic ischemic infarction of muscle
Excludes1 compartment syndrome (traumatic) (T79.A-)
nontraumatic compartment syndrome (M79.A-)
traumatic ischemia of muscle (T79.6)
rhabdomyolysis (M62.82)
Volkmann's ischemic contracture (T79.6)
M62.2Ø Nontraumatic ischemic infarction of muscle, unspecified site
● M62.21 Nontraumatic ischemic infarction of muscle, shoulder
M62.211 Nontraumatic ischemic infarction of muscle, right shoulder
M62.212 Nontraumatic ischemic infarction of muscle, left shoulder
M62.219 Nontraumatic ischemic infarction of muscle, unspecified shoulder
● M62.22 Nontraumatic ischemic infarction of muscle, upper arm
M62.221 Nontraumatic ischemic infarction of muscle, right upper arm
M62.222 Nontraumatic ischemic infarction of muscle, left upper arm
M62.229 Nontraumatic ischemic infarction of muscle, unspecified upper arm
● M62.23 Nontraumatic ischemic infarction of muscle, forearm
M62.231 Nontraumatic ischemic infarction of muscle, right forearm
M62.232 Nontraumatic ischemic infarction of muscle, left forearm
M62.239 Nontraumatic ischemic infarction of muscle, unspecified forearm
● M62.24 Nontraumatic ischemic infarction of muscle, hand
M62.241 Nontraumatic ischemic infarction of muscle, right hand
M62.242 Nontraumatic ischemic infarction of muscle, left hand
M62.249 Nontraumatic ischemic infarction of muscle, unspecified hand
● M62.25 Nontraumatic ischemic infarction of muscle, thigh
M62.251 Nontraumatic ischemic infarction of muscle, right thigh
M62.252 Nontraumatic ischemic infarction of muscle, left thigh
M62.259 Nontraumatic ischemic infarction of muscle, unspecified thigh

● M62.26 Nontraumatic ischemic infarction of muscle, lower leg
M62.261 Nontraumatic ischemic infarction of muscle, right lower leg
M62.262 Nontraumatic ischemic infarction of muscle, left lower leg
M62.269 Nontraumatic ischemic infarction of muscle, unspecified lower leg
● M62.27 Nontraumatic ischemic infarction of muscle, ankle and foot
M62.271 Nontraumatic ischemic infarction of muscle, right ankle and foot
M62.272 Nontraumatic ischemic infarction of muscle, left ankle and foot
M62.279 Nontraumatic ischemic infarction of muscle, unspecified ankle and foot
M62.28 Nontraumatic ischemic infarction of muscle, other site
M62.3 Immobility syndrome (paraplegic)
M62.4 Contracture of muscle
CONTRACTURE OF TENDON (SHEATH)
Excludes1 contracture of joint (M24.5-)
M62.40 Contracture of muscle, unspecified site
● M62.41 Contracture of muscle, shoulder
M62.411 Contracture of muscle, right shoulder
M62.412 Contracture of muscle, left shoulder
M62.419 Contracture of muscle, unspecified shoulder
● M62.42 Contracture of muscle, upper arm
M62.421 Contracture of muscle, right upper arm
M62.422 Contracture of muscle, left upper arm
M62.429 Contracture of muscle, unspecified upper arm
● M62.43 Contracture of muscle, forearm
M62.431 Contracture of muscle, right forearm
M62.432 Contracture of muscle, left forearm
M62.439 Contracture of muscle, unspecified forearm
● M62.44 Contracture of muscle, hand
M62.441 Contracture of muscle, right hand
M62.442 Contracture of muscle, left hand
M62.449 Contracture of muscle, unspecified hand
● M62.45 Contracture of muscle, thigh
M62.451 Contracture of muscle, right thigh
M62.452 Contracture of muscle, left thigh
M62.459 Contracture of muscle, unspecified thigh
● M62.46 Contracture of muscle, lower leg
M62.461 Contracture of muscle, right lower leg
M62.462 Contracture of muscle, left lower leg
M62.469 Contracture of muscle, unspecified lower leg
● M62.47 Contracture of muscle, ankle and foot
M62.471 Contracture of muscle, right ankle and foot
M62.472 Contracture of muscle, left ankle and foot
M62.479 Contracture of muscle, unspecified ankle and foot
M62.48 Contracture of muscle, other site
M62.49 Contracture of muscle, multiple sites

● M62.5 Muscle wasting and atrophy, not elsewhere classified
Disuse atrophy NEC
Excludes1 neuralgic amyotrophy (G54.5)
progressive muscular atrophy (G12.29)
sarcopenia (M62.84) ◀
Excludes2 pelvic muscle wasting (N81.84)
M62.50 Muscle wasting and atrophy, not elsewhere classified, unspecified site
● M62.51 Muscle wasting and atrophy, not elsewhere classified, shoulder
M62.511 Muscle wasting and atrophy, not elsewhere classified, right shoulder
M62.512 Muscle wasting and atrophy, not elsewhere classified, left shoulder
M62.519 Muscle wasting and atrophy, not elsewhere classified, unspecified shoulder
● M62.52 Muscle wasting and atrophy, not elsewhere classified, upper arm
M62.521 Muscle wasting and atrophy, not elsewhere classified, right upper arm
M62.522 Muscle wasting and atrophy, not elsewhere classified, left upper arm
M62.529 Muscle wasting and atrophy, not elsewhere classified, unspecified upper arm
● M62.53 Muscle wasting and atrophy, not elsewhere classified, forearm
M62.531 Muscle wasting and atrophy, not elsewhere classified, right forearm
M62.532 Muscle wasting and atrophy, not elsewhere classified, left forearm
M62.539 Muscle wasting and atrophy, not elsewhere classified, unspecified forearm
● M62.54 Muscle wasting and atrophy, not elsewhere classified, hand
M62.541 Muscle wasting and atrophy, not elsewhere classified, right hand
M62.542 Muscle wasting and atrophy, not elsewhere classified, left hand
M62.549 Muscle wasting and atrophy, not elsewhere classified, unspecified hand
● M62.55 Muscle wasting and atrophy, not elsewhere classified, thigh
M62.551 Muscle wasting and atrophy, not elsewhere classified, right thigh
M62.552 Muscle wasting and atrophy, not elsewhere classified, left thigh
M62.559 Muscle wasting and atrophy, not elsewhere classified, unspecified thigh
● M62.56 Muscle wasting and atrophy, not elsewhere classified, lower leg
M62.561 Muscle wasting and atrophy, not elsewhere classified, right lower leg
M62.562 Muscle wasting and atrophy, not elsewhere classified, left lower leg
M62.569 Muscle wasting and atrophy, not elsewhere classified, unspecified lower leg

● **M62.57 Muscle wasting and atrophy, not elsewhere classified, ankle and foot**
- **M62.571 Muscle wasting and atrophy, not elsewhere classified, right ankle and foot**
- **M62.572 Muscle wasting and atrophy, not elsewhere classified, left ankle and foot**
- **M62.579 Muscle wasting and atrophy, not elsewhere classified, unspecified ankle and foot**

M62.58 Muscle wasting and atrophy, not elsewhere classified, other site

M62.59 Muscle wasting and atrophy, not elsewhere classified, multiple sites

● **M62.8 Other specified disorders of muscle**

Excludes2 nontraumatic hematoma of muscle (M79.81)

M62.81 Muscle weakness (generalized)

Excludes1 muscle weakness in sarcopenia (M62.84) ◀

M62.82 Rhabdomyolysis

Excludes1 traumatic rhabdomyolysis (T79.6)

● **M62.83 Muscle spasm**
- **M62.830 Muscle spasm of back**
- **M62.831 Muscle spasm of calf**
  - Charley-horse
- **M62.838 Other muscle spasm**

M62.84 Sarcopenia ◀

Age-related sarcopenia ◀

Code first underlying disease, if applicable, such as:
- disorders of myoneural junction and muscle disease in diseases classified elsewhere (G73.-) ◀
- other and unspecified myopathies (G72.-) ◀
- primary disorders of muscles (G71.-) ◀

M62.89 Other specified disorders of muscle

Muscle (sheath) hernia

M62.9 Disorder of muscle, unspecified

● **M63 Disorders of muscle in diseases classified elsewhere**

Code first underlying disease, such as:
- leprosy (A3Ø.-)
- neoplasm (C49.-, C79.89, D21.-, D48.1)
- schistosomiasis (B65.-)
- trichinellosis (B75)

Excludes1
- myopathy in cysticercosis (B69.81)
- myopathy in endocrine diseases (G73.7)
- myopathy in metabolic diseases (G73.7)
- myopathy in sarcoidosis (D86.87)
- myopathy in secondary syphilis (A51.49)
- myopathy in syphilis (late) (A52.78)
- myopathy in toxoplasmosis (B58.82)
- myopathy in tuberculosis (A18.Ø9)

● **M63.8 Disorders of muscle in diseases classified elsewhere**

M63.8Ø Disorders of muscle in diseases classified elsewhere, unspecified site

● **M63.81 Disorders of muscle in diseases classified elsewhere, shoulder**
- **M63.811 Disorders of muscle in diseases classified elsewhere, right shoulder**
- **M63.812 Disorders of muscle in diseases classified elsewhere, left shoulder**
- **M63.819 Disorders of muscle in diseases classified elsewhere, unspecified shoulder**

● **M63.82 Disorders of muscle in diseases classified elsewhere, upper arm**
- **M63.821 Disorders of muscle in diseases classified elsewhere, right upper arm**
- **M63.822 Disorders of muscle in diseases classified elsewhere, left upper arm**
- **M63.829 Disorders of muscle in diseases classified elsewhere, unspecified upper arm**

● **M63.83 Disorders of muscle in diseases classified elsewhere, forearm**
- **M63.831 Disorders of muscle in diseases classified elsewhere, right forearm**
- **M63.832 Disorders of muscle in diseases classified elsewhere, left forearm**
- **M63.839 Disorders of muscle in diseases classified elsewhere, unspecified forearm**

● **M63.84 Disorders of muscle in diseases classified elsewhere, hand**
- **M63.841 Disorders of muscle in diseases classified elsewhere, right hand**
- **M63.842 Disorders of muscle in diseases classified elsewhere, left hand**
- **M63.849 Disorders of muscle in diseases classified elsewhere, unspecified hand**

● **M63.85 Disorders of muscle in diseases classified elsewhere, thigh**
- **M63.851 Disorders of muscle in diseases classified elsewhere, right thigh**
- **M63.852 Disorders of muscle in diseases classified elsewhere, left thigh**
- **M63.859 Disorders of muscle in diseases classified elsewhere, unspecified thigh**

● **M63.86 Disorders of muscle in diseases classified elsewhere, lower leg**
- **M63.861 Disorders of muscle in diseases classified elsewhere, right lower leg**
- **M63.862 Disorders of muscle in diseases classified elsewhere, left lower leg**
- **M63.869 Disorders of muscle in diseases classified elsewhere, unspecified lower leg**

● **M63.87 Disorders of muscle in diseases classified elsewhere, ankle and foot**
- **M63.871 Disorders of muscle in diseases classified elsewhere, right ankle and foot**
- **M63.872 Disorders of muscle in diseases classified elsewhere, left ankle and foot**
- **M63.879 Disorders of muscle in diseases classified elsewhere, unspecified ankle and foot**

M63.88 Disorders of muscle in diseases classified elsewhere, other site

M63.89 Disorders of muscle in diseases classified elsewhere, multiple sites

Item 13–11 **Synovitis** is an inflammation of a synovial membrane resulting in pain on motion and is characterized by fluctuating swelling due to effusion in a synovial sac. **Tenosynovitis** is an inflammation of a tendon sheath and occurs most commonly in the wrists, hands, and feet. Bursitis is inflammation of a bursa (fluid filled sac) caused by repetitive use, trauma, infection, or systemic inflammatory disease. Bursae act as protectors and facilitate movement between bones and overlapping muscles (deep bursae) or between bones and tendons/skin (superficial bursae).

DISORDERS OF SYNOVIUM AND TENDON (M65-M67)

● **M65 Synovitis and tenosynovitis**

Excludes1 chronic crepitant synovitis of hand and wrist (M70.0-)
current injury - see injury of ligament or tendon by body region
soft tissue disorders related to use, overuse and pressure (M70.-)

● **M65.0 Abscess of tendon sheath**

Use additional code (B95-B96) to identify bacterial agent

M65.00 Abscess of tendon sheath, unspecified site

● **M65.01** Abscess of tendon sheath, shoulder

M65.011 Abscess of tendon sheath, right shoulder

M65.012 Abscess of tendon sheath, left shoulder

M65.019 Abscess of tendon sheath, unspecified shoulder

● **M65.02** Abscess of tendon sheath, upper arm

M65.021 Abscess of tendon sheath, right upper arm

M65.022 Abscess of tendon sheath, left upper arm

M65.029 Abscess of tendon sheath, unspecified upper arm

● **M65.03** Abscess of tendon sheath, forearm

M65.031 Abscess of tendon sheath, right forearm

M65.032 Abscess of tendon sheath, left forearm

M65.039 Abscess of tendon sheath, unspecified forearm

● **M65.04** Abscess of tendon sheath, hand

M65.041 Abscess of tendon sheath, right hand

M65.042 Abscess of tendon sheath, left hand

M65.049 Abscess of tendon sheath, unspecified hand

● **M65.05** Abscess of tendon sheath, thigh

M65.051 Abscess of tendon sheath, right thigh

M65.052 Abscess of tendon sheath, left thigh

M65.059 Abscess of tendon sheath, unspecified thigh

● **M65.06** Abscess of tendon sheath, lower leg

M65.061 Abscess of tendon sheath, right lower leg

M65.062 Abscess of tendon sheath, left lower leg

M65.069 Abscess of tendon sheath, unspecified lower leg

● **M65.07** Abscess of tendon sheath, ankle and foot

M65.071 Abscess of tendon sheath, right ankle and foot

M65.072 Abscess of tendon sheath, left ankle and foot

M65.079 Abscess of tendon sheath, unspecified ankle and foot

M65.08 Abscess of tendon sheath, other site

● **M65.1 Other infective (teno)synovitis**

M65.10 Other infective (teno)synovitis, unspecified site

● **M65.11** Other infective (teno)synovitis, shoulder

M65.111 Other infective (teno)synovitis, right shoulder

M65.112 Other infective (teno)synovitis, left shoulder

M65.119 Other infective (teno)synovitis, unspecified shoulder

● **M65.12** Other infective (teno)synovitis, elbow

M65.121 Other infective (teno)synovitis, right elbow

M65.122 Other infective (teno)synovitis, left elbow

M65.129 Other infective (teno)synovitis, unspecified elbow

● **M65.13** Other infective (teno)synovitis, wrist

M65.131 Other infective (teno)synovitis, right wrist

M65.132 Other infective (teno)synovitis, left wrist

M65.139 Other infective (teno)synovitis, unspecified wrist

● **M65.14** Other infective (teno)synovitis, hand

M65.141 Other infective (teno)synovitis, right hand

M65.142 Other infective (teno)synovitis, left hand

M65.149 Other infective (teno)synovitis, unspecified hand

● **M65.15** Other infective (teno)synovitis, hip

M65.151 Other infective (teno)synovitis, right hip

M65.152 Other infective (teno)synovitis, left hip

M65.159 Other infective (teno)synovitis, unspecified hip

● **M65.16** Other infective (teno)synovitis, knee

M65.161 Other infective (teno)synovitis, right knee

M65.162 Other infective (teno)synovitis, left knee

M65.169 Other infective (teno)synovitis, unspecified knee

● **M65.17** Other infective (teno)synovitis, ankle and foot

M65.171 Other infective (teno)synovitis, right ankle and foot

M65.172 Other infective (teno)synovitis, left ankle and foot

M65.179 Other infective (teno)synovitis, unspecified ankle and foot

M65.18 Other infective (teno)synovitis, other site

M65.19 Other infective (teno)synovitis, multiple sites

● **M65.2 Calcific tendinitis**

Excludes1 tendinitis as classified in M75-M77
calcified tendinitis of shoulder (M75.3)

M65.20 Calcific tendinitis, unspecified site

● **M65.22** Calcific tendinitis, upper arm

M65.221 Calcific tendinitis, right upper arm

M65.222 Calcific tendinitis, left upper arm

M65.229 Calcific tendinitis, unspecified upper arm

● **M65.23** Calcific tendinitis, forearm

M65.231 Calcific tendinitis, right forearm

M65.232 Calcific tendinitis, left forearm

M65.239 Calcific tendinitis, unspecified forearm

CHAPTER 13 (M00-M99)

- M65.24 Calcific tendinitis, hand
  - M65.241 Calcific tendinitis, right hand
  - M65.242 Calcific tendinitis, left hand
  - M65.249 Calcific tendinitis, unspecified hand
- M65.25 Calcific tendinitis, thigh
  - M65.251 Calcific tendinitis, right thigh
  - M65.252 Calcific tendinitis, left thigh
  - M65.259 Calcific tendinitis, unspecified thigh
- M65.26 Calcific tendinitis, lower leg
  - M65.261 Calcific tendinitis, right lower leg
  - M65.262 Calcific tendinitis, left lower leg
  - M65.269 Calcific tendinitis, unspecified lower leg
- M65.27 Calcific tendinitis, ankle and foot
  - M65.271 Calcific tendinitis, right ankle and foot
  - M65.272 Calcific tendinitis, left ankle and foot
  - M65.279 Calcific tendinitis, unspecified ankle and foot
- M65.28 Calcific tendinitis, other site
- M65.29 Calcific tendinitis, multiple sites

M65.3 Trigger finger

Nodular tendinous disease

- M65.3Ø Trigger finger, unspecified finger
- M65.31 Trigger thumb
  - M65.311 Trigger thumb, right thumb
  - M65.312 Trigger thumb, left thumb
  - M65.319 Trigger thumb, unspecified thumb
- M65.32 Trigger finger, index finger
  - M65.321 Trigger finger, right index finger
  - M65.322 Trigger finger, left index finger
  - M65.329 Trigger finger, unspecified index finger
- M65.33 Trigger finger, middle finger
  - M65.331 Trigger finger, right middle finger
  - M65.332 Trigger finger, left middle finger
  - M65.339 Trigger finger, unspecified middle finger
- M65.34 Trigger finger, ring finger
  - M65.341 Trigger finger, right ring finger
  - M65.342 Trigger finger, left ring finger
  - M65.349 Trigger finger, unspecified ring finger
- M65.35 Trigger finger, little finger
  - M65.351 Trigger finger, right little finger
  - M65.352 Trigger finger, left little finger
  - M65.359 Trigger finger, unspecified little finger

M65.4 Radial styloid tenosynovitis [de Quervain]

M65.8 Other synovitis and tenosynovitis

- M65.8Ø Other synovitis and tenosynovitis, unspecified site
- M65.81 Other synovitis and tenosynovitis, shoulder
  - M65.811 Other synovitis and tenosynovitis, right shoulder
  - M65.812 Other synovitis and tenosynovitis, left shoulder
  - M65.819 Other synovitis and tenosynovitis, unspecified shoulder
- M65.82 Other synovitis and tenosynovitis, upper arm
  - M65.821 Other synovitis and tenosynovitis, right upper arm
  - M65.822 Other synovitis and tenosynovitis, left upper arm
  - M65.829 Other synovitis and tenosynovitis, unspecified upper arm
- M65.83 Other synovitis and tenosynovitis, forearm
  - M65.831 Other synovitis and tenosynovitis, right forearm
  - M65.832 Other synovitis and tenosynovitis, left forearm
  - M65.839 Other synovitis and tenosynovitis, unspecified forearm
- M65.84 Other synovitis and tenosynovitis, hand
  - M65.841 Other synovitis and tenosynovitis, right hand
  - M65.842 Other synovitis and tenosynovitis, left hand
  - M65.849 Other synovitis and tenosynovitis, unspecified hand
- M65.85 Other synovitis and tenosynovitis, thigh
  - M65.851 Other synovitis and tenosynovitis, right thigh
  - M65.852 Other synovitis and tenosynovitis, left thigh
  - M65.859 Other synovitis and tenosynovitis, unspecified thigh
- M65.86 Other synovitis and tenosynovitis, lower leg
  - M65.861 Other synovitis and tenosynovitis, right lower leg
  - M65.862 Other synovitis and tenosynovitis, left lower leg
  - M65.869 Other synovitis and tenosynovitis, unspecified lower leg
- M65.87 Other synovitis and tenosynovitis, ankle and foot
  - M65.871 Other synovitis and tenosynovitis, right ankle and foot
  - M65.872 Other synovitis and tenosynovitis, left ankle and foot
  - M65.879 Other synovitis and tenosynovitis, unspecified ankle and foot
- M65.88 Other synovitis and tenosynovitis, other site
- M65.89 Other synovitis and tenosynovitis, multiple sites

M65.9 Synovitis and tenosynovitis, unspecified

M66 Spontaneous rupture of synovium and tendon

Includes rupture that occurs when a normal force is applied to tissues that are inferred to have less than normal strength

Excludes2 rotator cuff syndrome (M75.1-)
rupture where an abnormal force is applied to normal tissue - see injury of tendon by body region

M66.Ø Rupture of popliteal cyst

M66.1 Rupture of synovium

Rupture of synovial cyst

Excludes2 rupture of popliteal cyst (M66.Ø)

- M66.1Ø Rupture of synovium, unspecified joint
- M66.11 Rupture of synovium, shoulder
  - M66.111 Rupture of synovium, right shoulder
  - M66.112 Rupture of synovium, left shoulder
  - M66.119 Rupture of synovium, unspecified shoulder
- M66.12 Rupture of synovium, elbow
  - M66.121 Rupture of synovium, right elbow
  - M66.122 Rupture of synovium, left elbow
  - M66.129 Rupture of synovium, unspecified elbow
- M66.13 Rupture of synovium, wrist
  - M66.131 Rupture of synovium, right wrist
  - M66.132 Rupture of synovium, left wrist
  - M66.139 Rupture of synovium, unspecified wrist

CHAPTER 13 (MØØ-M99)

● M66.14 Rupture of synovium, hand and fingers
M66.141 Rupture of synovium, right hand
M66.142 Rupture of synovium, left hand
M66.143 Rupture of synovium, unspecified hand
M66.144 Rupture of synovium, right finger(s)
M66.145 Rupture of synovium, left finger(s)
M66.146 Rupture of synovium, unspecified finger(s)

● M66.15 Rupture of synovium, hip
M66.151 Rupture of synovium, right hip
M66.152 Rupture of synovium, left hip
M66.159 Rupture of synovium, unspecified hip

● M66.17 Rupture of synovium, ankle, foot and toes
M66.171 Rupture of synovium, right ankle
M66.172 Rupture of synovium, left ankle
M66.173 Rupture of synovium, unspecified ankle
M66.174 Rupture of synovium, right foot
M66.175 Rupture of synovium, left foot
M66.176 Rupture of synovium, unspecified foot
M66.177 Rupture of synovium, right toe(s)
M66.178 Rupture of synovium, left toe(s)
M66.179 Rupture of synovium, unspecified toe(s)

M66.18 Rupture of synovium, other site

● M66.2 Spontaneous rupture of extensor tendons
M66.20 Spontaneous rupture of extensor tendons, unspecified site

● M66.21 Spontaneous rupture of extensor tendons, shoulder
M66.211 Spontaneous rupture of extensor tendons, right shoulder
M66.212 Spontaneous rupture of extensor tendons, left shoulder
M66.219 Spontaneous rupture of extensor tendons, unspecified shoulder

● M66.22 Spontaneous rupture of extensor tendons, upper arm
M66.221 Spontaneous rupture of extensor tendons, right upper arm
M66.222 Spontaneous rupture of extensor tendons, left upper arm
M66.229 Spontaneous rupture of extensor tendons, unspecified upper arm

● M66.23 Spontaneous rupture of extensor tendons, forearm
M66.231 Spontaneous rupture of extensor tendons, right forearm
M66.232 Spontaneous rupture of extensor tendons, left forearm
M66.239 Spontaneous rupture of extensor tendons, unspecified forearm

● M66.24 Spontaneous rupture of extensor tendons, hand
M66.241 Spontaneous rupture of extensor tendons, right hand
M66.242 Spontaneous rupture of extensor tendons, left hand
M66.249 Spontaneous rupture of extensor tendons, unspecified hand

● M66.25 Spontaneous rupture of extensor tendons, thigh
M66.251 Spontaneous rupture of extensor tendons, right thigh
M66.252 Spontaneous rupture of extensor tendons, left thigh
M66.259 Spontaneous rupture of extensor tendons, unspecified thigh

● M66.26 Spontaneous rupture of extensor tendons, lower leg
M66.261 Spontaneous rupture of extensor tendons, right lower leg
M66.262 Spontaneous rupture of extensor tendons, left lower leg
M66.269 Spontaneous rupture of extensor tendons, unspecified lower leg

● M66.27 Spontaneous rupture of extensor tendons, ankle and foot
M66.271 Spontaneous rupture of extensor tendons, right ankle and foot
M66.272 Spontaneous rupture of extensor tendons, left ankle and foot
M66.279 Spontaneous rupture of extensor tendons, unspecified ankle and foot

M66.28 Spontaneous rupture of extensor tendons, other site
M66.29 Spontaneous rupture of extensor tendons, multiple sites

● M66.3 Spontaneous rupture of flexor tendons
M66.30 Spontaneous rupture of flexor tendons, unspecified site

● M66.31 Spontaneous rupture of flexor tendons, shoulder
M66.311 Spontaneous rupture of flexor tendons, right shoulder
M66.312 Spontaneous rupture of flexor tendons, left shoulder
M66.319 Spontaneous rupture of flexor tendons, unspecified shoulder

● M66.32 Spontaneous rupture of flexor tendons, upper arm
M66.321 Spontaneous rupture of flexor tendons, right upper arm
M66.322 Spontaneous rupture of flexor tendons, left upper arm
M66.329 Spontaneous rupture of flexor tendons, unspecified upper arm

● M66.33 Spontaneous rupture of flexor tendons, forearm
M66.331 Spontaneous rupture of flexor tendons, right forearm
M66.332 Spontaneous rupture of flexor tendons, left forearm
M66.339 Spontaneous rupture of flexor tendons, unspecified forearm

● M66.34 Spontaneous rupture of flexor tendons, hand
M66.341 Spontaneous rupture of flexor tendons, right hand
M66.342 Spontaneous rupture of flexor tendons, left hand
M66.349 Spontaneous rupture of flexor tendons, unspecified hand

● M66.35 Spontaneous rupture of flexor tendons, thigh
M66.351 Spontaneous rupture of flexor tendons, right thigh
M66.352 Spontaneous rupture of flexor tendons, left thigh
M66.359 Spontaneous rupture of flexor tendons, unspecified thigh

● M66.36 Spontaneous rupture of flexor tendons, lower leg
M66.361 Spontaneous rupture of flexor tendons, right lower leg
M66.362 Spontaneous rupture of flexor tendons, left lower leg
M66.369 Spontaneous rupture of flexor tendons, unspecified lower leg

● **M66.37 Spontaneous rupture of flexor tendons, ankle and foot**
- **M66.371 Spontaneous rupture of flexor tendons, right ankle and foot**
- **M66.372 Spontaneous rupture of flexor tendons, left ankle and foot**
- **M66.379 Spontaneous rupture of flexor tendons, unspecified ankle and foot**

M66.38 Spontaneous rupture of flexor tendons, other site

M66.39 Spontaneous rupture of flexor tendons, multiple sites

● **M66.8 Spontaneous rupture of other tendons**

M66.80 Spontaneous rupture of other tendons, unspecified site

● **M66.81 Spontaneous rupture of other tendons, shoulder**
- **M66.811 Spontaneous rupture of other tendons, right shoulder**
- **M66.812 Spontaneous rupture of other tendons, left shoulder**
- **M66.819 Spontaneous rupture of other tendons, unspecified shoulder**

● **M66.82 Spontaneous rupture of other tendons, upper arm**
- **M66.821 Spontaneous rupture of other tendons, right upper arm**
- **M66.822 Spontaneous rupture of other tendons, left upper arm**
- **M66.829 Spontaneous rupture of other tendons, unspecified upper arm**

● **M66.83 Spontaneous rupture of other tendons, forearm**
- **M66.831 Spontaneous rupture of other tendons, right forearm**
- **M66.832 Spontaneous rupture of other tendons, left forearm**
- **M66.839 Spontaneous rupture of other tendons, unspecified forearm**

● **M66.84 Spontaneous rupture of other tendons, hand**
- **M66.841 Spontaneous rupture of other tendons, right hand**
- **M66.842 Spontaneous rupture of other tendons, left hand**
- **M66.849 Spontaneous rupture of other tendons, unspecified hand**

● **M66.85 Spontaneous rupture of other tendons, thigh**
- **M66.851 Spontaneous rupture of other tendons, right thigh**
- **M66.852 Spontaneous rupture of other tendons, left thigh**
- **M66.859 Spontaneous rupture of other tendons, unspecified thigh**

● **M66.86 Spontaneous rupture of other tendons, lower leg**
- **M66.861 Spontaneous rupture of other tendons, right lower leg**
- **M66.862 Spontaneous rupture of other tendons, left lower leg**
- **M66.869 Spontaneous rupture of other tendons, unspecified lower leg**

● **M66.87 Spontaneous rupture of other tendons, ankle and foot**
- **M66.871 Spontaneous rupture of other tendons, right ankle and foot**
- **M66.872 Spontaneous rupture of other tendons, left ankle and foot**
- **M66.879 Spontaneous rupture of other tendons, unspecified ankle and foot**

M66.88 Spontaneous rupture of other tendons, other

M66.89 Spontaneous rupture of other tendons, multiple sites

M66.9 Spontaneous rupture of unspecified tendon
Rupture at musculotendinous junction, nontraumatic

● **M67 Other disorders of synovium and tendon**

Excludes1 palmar fascial fibromatosis [Dupuytren] (M72.0)
tendinitis NOS (M77.9-)
xanthomatosis localized to tendons (E78.2)

● **M67.0 Short Achilles tendon (acquired)**
- **M67.00 Short Achilles tendon (acquired), unspecified ankle**
- **M67.01 Short Achilles tendon (acquired), right ankle**
- **M67.02 Short Achilles tendon (acquired), left ankle**

● **M67.2 Synovial hypertrophy, not elsewhere classified**

Excludes1 villonodular synovitis (pigmented) (M12.2-)

M67.20 Synovial hypertrophy, not elsewhere classified, unspecified site

● **M67.21 Synovial hypertrophy, not elsewhere classified, shoulder**
- **M67.211 Synovial hypertrophy, not elsewhere classified, right shoulder**
- **M67.212 Synovial hypertrophy, not elsewhere classified, left shoulder**
- **M67.219 Synovial hypertrophy, not elsewhere classified, unspecified shoulder**

● **M67.22 Synovial hypertrophy, not elsewhere classified, upper arm**
- **M67.221 Synovial hypertrophy, not elsewhere classified, right upper arm**
- **M67.222 Synovial hypertrophy, not elsewhere classified, left upper arm**
- **M67.229 Synovial hypertrophy, not elsewhere classified, unspecified upper arm**

● **M67.23 Synovial hypertrophy, not elsewhere classified, forearm**
- **M67.231 Synovial hypertrophy, not elsewhere classified, right forearm**
- **M67.232 Synovial hypertrophy, not elsewhere classified, left forearm**
- **M67.239 Synovial hypertrophy, not elsewhere classified, unspecified forearm**

● **M67.24 Synovial hypertrophy, not elsewhere classified, hand**
- **M67.241 Synovial hypertrophy, not elsewhere classified, right hand**
- **M67.242 Synovial hypertrophy, not elsewhere classified, left hand**
- **M67.249 Synovial hypertrophy, not elsewhere classified, unspecified hand**

◀ New ◀ Revised ~~deleted~~ Deleted **OGCR** Official Guidelines **X** Assign placeholder X ● Use Additional Character(s)

Excludes 1 | Excludes 2 | Includes | Use additional | Code first | Code also | Unspecified

● **M67.25 Synovial hypertrophy, not elsewhere classified, thigh**
- **M67.251 Synovial hypertrophy, not elsewhere classified, right thigh**
- **M67.252 Synovial hypertrophy, not elsewhere classified, left thigh**
- **M67.259 Synovial hypertrophy, not elsewhere classified, unspecified thigh**

● **M67.26 Synovial hypertrophy, not elsewhere classified, lower leg**
- **M67.261 Synovial hypertrophy, not elsewhere classified, right lower leg**
- **M67.262 Synovial hypertrophy, not elsewhere classified, left lower leg**
- **M67.269 Synovial hypertrophy, not elsewhere classified, unspecified lower leg**

● **M67.27 Synovial hypertrophy, not elsewhere classified, ankle and foot**
- **M67.271 Synovial hypertrophy, not elsewhere classified, right ankle and foot**
- **M67.272 Synovial hypertrophy, not elsewhere classified, left ankle and foot**
- **M67.279 Synovial hypertrophy, not elsewhere classified, unspecified ankle and foot**

M67.28 Synovial hypertrophy, not elsewhere classified, other site

M67.29 Synovial hypertrophy, not elsewhere classified, multiple sites

● **M67.3 Transient synovitis**
Toxic synovitis
Excludes1 palindromic rheumatism (M12.3-)

M67.30 Transient synovitis, unspecified site

● **M67.31 Transient synovitis, shoulder**
- **M67.311 Transient synovitis, right shoulder**
- **M67.312 Transient synovitis, left shoulder**
- **M67.319 Transient synovitis, unspecified shoulder**

● **M67.32 Transient synovitis, elbow**
- **M67.321 Transient synovitis, right elbow**
- **M67.322 Transient synovitis, left elbow**
- **M67.329 Transient synovitis, unspecified elbow**

● **M67.33 Transient synovitis, wrist**
- **M67.331 Transient synovitis, right wrist**
- **M67.332 Transient synovitis, left wrist**
- **M67.339 Transient synovitis, unspecified wrist**

● **M67.34 Transient synovitis, hand**
- **M67.341 Transient synovitis, right hand**
- **M67.342 Transient synovitis, left hand**
- **M67.349 Transient synovitis, unspecified hand**

● **M67.35 Transient synovitis, hip**
- **M67.351 Transient synovitis, right hip**
- **M67.352 Transient synovitis, left hip**
- **M67.359 Transient synovitis, unspecified hip**

● **M67.36 Transient synovitis, knee**
- **M67.361 Transient synovitis, right knee**
- **M67.362 Transient synovitis, left knee**
- **M67.369 Transient synovitis, unspecified knee**

● **M67.37 Transient synovitis, ankle and foot**
- **M67.371 Transient synovitis, right ankle and foot**
- **M67.372 Transient synovitis, left ankle and foot**
- **M67.379 Transient synovitis, unspecified ankle and foot**

M67.38 Transient synovitis, other site

M67.39 Transient synovitis, multiple sites

● **M67.4 Ganglion**
Ganglion of joint or tendon (sheath)
Excludes1 ganglion in yaws (A66.6)
Excludes2 cyst of bursa (M71.2-M71.3)
cyst of synovium (M71.2-M71.3)

M67.40 Ganglion, unspecified site

● **M67.41 Ganglion, shoulder**
- **M67.411 Ganglion, right shoulder**
- **M67.412 Ganglion, left shoulder**
- **M67.419 Ganglion, unspecified shoulder**

● **M67.42 Ganglion, elbow**
- **M67.421 Ganglion, right elbow**
- **M67.422 Ganglion, left elbow**
- **M67.429 Ganglion, unspecified elbow**

● **M67.43 Ganglion, wrist**
- **M67.431 Ganglion, right wrist**
- **M67.432 Ganglion, left wrist**
- **M67.439 Ganglion, unspecified wrist**

● **M67.44 Ganglion, hand**
- **M67.441 Ganglion, right hand**
- **M67.442 Ganglion, left hand**
- **M67.449 Ganglion, unspecified hand**

● **M67.45 Ganglion, hip**
- **M67.451 Ganglion, right hip**
- **M67.452 Ganglion, left hip**
- **M67.459 Ganglion, unspecified hip**

● **M67.46 Ganglion, knee**
- **M67.461 Ganglion, right knee**
- **M67.462 Ganglion, left knee**
- **M67.469 Ganglion, unspecified knee**

● **M67.47 Ganglion, ankle and foot**
- **M67.471 Ganglion, right ankle and foot**
- **M67.472 Ganglion, left ankle and foot**
- **M67.479 Ganglion, unspecified ankle and foot**

M67.48 Ganglion, other site

M67.49 Ganglion, multiple sites

● **M67.5 Plica syndrome**
Plica knee

M67.50 Plica syndrome, unspecified knee

M67.51 Plica syndrome, right knee

M67.52 Plica syndrome, left knee

● **M67.8 Other specified disorders of synovium and tendon**

M67.80 Other specified disorders of synovium and tendon, unspecified site

● **M67.81 Other specified disorders of synovium and tendon, shoulder**
- **M67.811 Other specified disorders of synovium, right shoulder**
- **M67.812 Other specified disorders of synovium, left shoulder**
- **M67.813 Other specified disorders of tendon, right shoulder**
- **M67.814 Other specified disorders of tendon, left shoulder**
- **M67.819 Other specified disorders of synovium and tendon, unspecified shoulder**

CHAPTER 13 (M00-M99)

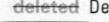

● M67.82 Other specified disorders of synovium and tendon, elbow
M67.821 Other specified disorders of synovium, right elbow
M67.822 Other specified disorders of synovium, left elbow
M67.823 Other specified disorders of tendon, right elbow
M67.824 Other specified disorders of tendon, left elbow
M67.829 Other specified disorders of synovium and tendon, unspecified elbow

● M67.83 Other specified disorders of synovium and tendon, wrist
M67.831 Other specified disorders of synovium, right wrist
M67.832 Other specified disorders of synovium, left wrist
M67.833 Other specified disorders of tendon, right wrist
M67.834 Other specified disorders of tendon, left wrist
M67.839 Other specified disorders of synovium and tendon, unspecified forearm

● M67.84 Other specified disorders of synovium and tendon, hand
M67.841 Other specified disorders of synovium, right hand
M67.842 Other specified disorders of synovium, left hand
M67.843 Other specified disorders of tendon, right hand
M67.844 Other specified disorders of tendon, left hand
M67.849 Other specified disorders of synovium and tendon, unspecified hand

● M67.85 Other specified disorders of synovium and tendon, hip
M67.851 Other specified disorders of synovium, right hip
M67.852 Other specified disorders of synovium, left hip
M67.853 Other specified disorders of tendon, right hip
M67.854 Other specified disorders of tendon, left hip
M67.859 Other specified disorders of synovium and tendon, unspecified hip

● M67.86 Other specified disorders of synovium and tendon, knee
M67.861 Other specified disorders of synovium, right knee
M67.862 Other specified disorders of synovium, left knee
M67.863 Other specified disorders of tendon, right knee
M67.864 Other specified disorders of tendon, left knee
M67.869 Other specified disorders of synovium and tendon, unspecified knee

● M67.87 Other specified disorders of synovium and tendon, ankle and foot
M67.871 Other specified disorders of synovium, right ankle and foot
M67.872 Other specified disorders of synovium, left ankle and foot
M67.873 Other specified disorders of tendon, right ankle and foot
M67.874 Other specified disorders of tendon, left ankle and foot
M67.879 Other specified disorders of synovium and tendon, unspecified ankle and foot

M67.88 Other specified disorders of synovium and tendon, other site

M67.89 Other specified disorders of synovium and tendon, multiple sites

● M67.9 Unspecified disorder of synovium and tendon

M67.90 Unspecified disorder of synovium and tendon, unspecified site

● M67.91 Unspecified disorder of synovium and tendon, shoulder
M67.911 Unspecified disorder of synovium and tendon, right shoulder
M67.912 Unspecified disorder of synovium and tendon, left shoulder
M67.919 Unspecified disorder of synovium and tendon, unspecified shoulder

● M67.92 Unspecified disorder of synovium and tendon, upper arm
M67.921 Unspecified disorder of synovium and tendon, right upper arm
M67.922 Unspecified disorder of synovium and tendon, left upper arm
M67.929 Unspecified disorder of synovium and tendon, unspecified upper arm

● M67.93 Unspecified disorder of synovium and tendon, forearm
M67.931 Unspecified disorder of synovium and tendon, right forearm
M67.932 Unspecified disorder of synovium and tendon, left forearm
M67.939 Unspecified disorder of synovium and tendon, unspecified forearm

● M67.94 Unspecified disorder of synovium and tendon, hand
M67.941 Unspecified disorder of synovium and tendon, right hand
M67.942 Unspecified disorder of synovium and tendon, left hand
M67.949 Unspecified disorder of synovium and tendon, unspecified hand

● M67.95 Unspecified disorder of synovium and tendon, thigh
M67.951 Unspecified disorder of synovium and tendon, right thigh
M67.952 Unspecified disorder of synovium and tendon, left thigh
M67.959 Unspecified disorder of synovium and tendon, unspecified thigh

● M67.96 Unspecified disorder of synovium and tendon, lower leg
M67.961 Unspecified disorder of synovium and tendon, right lower leg
M67.962 Unspecified disorder of synovium and tendon, left lower leg
M67.969 Unspecified disorder of synovium and tendon, unspecified lower leg

● M67.97 Unspecified disorder of synovium and tendon, ankle and foot
M67.971 Unspecified disorder of synovium and tendon, right ankle and foot
M67.972 Unspecified disorder of synovium and tendon, left ankle and foot
M67.979 Unspecified disorder of synovium and tendon, unspecified ankle and foot
M67.98 Unspecified disorder of synovium and tendon, other site
M67.99 Unspecified disorder of synovium and tendon, multiple sites

OTHER SOFT TISSUE DISORDERS (M70-M79)

● M70 Soft tissue disorders related to use, overuse and pressure
Includes soft tissue disorders of occupational origin
Use additional external cause code to identify activity causing disorder (Y93.-)
Excludes1 bursitis NOS (M71.9-)
Excludes2 bursitis of shoulder (M75.5)
enthesopathies (M76-M77)
pressure ulcer (pressure area) (L89.-)

● M70.0 Crepitant synovitis (acute) (chronic) of hand and wrist
● M70.03 Crepitant synovitis (acute) (chronic), wrist
M70.031 Crepitant synovitis (acute) (chronic), right wrist
M70.032 Crepitant synovitis (acute) (chronic), left wrist
M70.039 Crepitant synovitis (acute) (chronic), unspecified wrist
● M70.04 Crepitant synovitis (acute) (chronic), hand
M70.041 Crepitant synovitis (acute) (chronic), right hand
M70.042 Crepitant synovitis (acute) (chronic), left hand
M70.049 Crepitant synovitis (acute) (chronic), unspecified hand
● M70.1 Bursitis of hand
M70.10 Bursitis, unspecified hand
M70.11 Bursitis, right hand
M70.12 Bursitis, left hand
● M70.2 Olecranon bursitis
M70.20 Olecranon bursitis, unspecified elbow
M70.21 Olecranon bursitis, right elbow
M70.22 Olecranon bursitis, left elbow
● M70.3 Other bursitis of elbow
M70.30 Other bursitis of elbow, unspecified elbow
M70.31 Other bursitis of elbow, right elbow
M70.32 Other bursitis of elbow, left elbow
● M70.4 Prepatellar bursitis
M70.40 Prepatellar bursitis, unspecified knee
M70.41 Prepatellar bursitis, right knee
M70.42 Prepatellar bursitis, left knee
● M70.5 Other bursitis of knee
M70.50 Other bursitis of knee, unspecified knee
M70.51 Other bursitis of knee, right knee
M70.52 Other bursitis of knee, left knee
● M70.6 Trochanteric bursitis
Trochanteric tendinitis
M70.60 Trochanteric bursitis, unspecified hip
M70.61 Trochanteric bursitis, right hip
M70.62 Trochanteric bursitis, left hip
● M70.7 Other bursitis of hip
Ischial bursitis
M70.70 Other bursitis of hip, unspecified hip
M70.71 Other bursitis of hip, right hip
M70.72 Other bursitis of hip, left hip
● M70.8 Other soft tissue disorders related to use, overuse and pressure
M70.80 Other soft tissue disorders related to use, overuse and pressure of unspecified site
● M70.81 Other soft tissue disorders related to use, overuse and pressure of shoulder
M70.811 Other soft tissue disorders related to use, overuse and pressure, right shoulder
M70.812 Other soft tissue disorders related to use, overuse and pressure, left shoulder
M70.819 Other soft tissue disorders related to use, overuse and pressure, unspecified shoulder
● M70.82 Other soft tissue disorders related to use, overuse and pressure of upper arm
M70.821 Other soft tissue disorders related to use, overuse and pressure, right upper arm
M70.822 Other soft tissue disorders related to use, overuse and pressure, left upper arm
M70.829 Other soft tissue disorders related to use, overuse and pressure, unspecified upper arms
● M70.83 Other soft tissue disorders related to use, overuse and pressure of forearm
M70.831 Other soft tissue disorders related to use, overuse and pressure, right forearm
M70.832 Other soft tissue disorders related to use, overuse and pressure, left forearm
M70.839 Other soft tissue disorders related to use, overuse and pressure, unspecified forearm
● M70.84 Other soft tissue disorders related to use, overuse and pressure of hand
M70.841 Other soft tissue disorders related to use, overuse and pressure, right hand
M70.842 Other soft tissue disorders related to use, overuse and pressure, left hand
M70.849 Other soft tissue disorders related to use, overuse and pressure, unspecified hand
● M70.85 Other soft tissue disorders related to use, overuse and pressure of thigh
M70.851 Other soft tissue disorders related to use, overuse and pressure, right thigh
M70.852 Other soft tissue disorders related to use, overuse and pressure, left thigh
M70.859 Other soft tissue disorders related to use, overuse and pressure, unspecified thigh
● M70.86 Other soft tissue disorders related to use, overuse and pressure lower leg
M70.861 Other soft tissue disorders related to use, overuse and pressure, right lower leg
M70.862 Other soft tissue disorders related to use, overuse and pressure, left lower leg
M70.869 Other soft tissue disorders related to use, overuse and pressure, unspecified leg

CHAPTER 13 (M00-M99)

● M70.87 Other soft tissue disorders related to use, overuse and pressure of ankle and foot
M70.871 Other soft tissue disorders related to use, overuse and pressure, right ankle and foot
M70.872 Other soft tissue disorders related to use, overuse and pressure, left ankle and foot
M70.879 Other soft tissue disorders related to use, overuse and pressure, unspecified ankle and foot
M70.88 Other soft tissue disorders related to use, overuse and pressure other site
M70.89 Other soft tissue disorders related to use, overuse and pressure multiple sites

● M70.9 Unspecified soft tissue disorder related to use, overuse and pressure
M70.90 Unspecified soft tissue disorder related to use, overuse and pressure of unspecified site
● M70.91 Unspecified soft tissue disorder related to use, overuse and pressure of shoulder
M70.911 Unspecified soft tissue disorder related to use, overuse and pressure, right shoulder
M70.912 Unspecified soft tissue disorder related to use, overuse and pressure, left shoulder
M70.919 Unspecified soft tissue disorder related to use, overuse and pressure, unspecified shoulder
● M70.92 Unspecified soft tissue disorder related to use, overuse and pressure of upper arm
M70.921 Unspecified soft tissue disorder related to use, overuse and pressure, right upper arm
M70.922 Unspecified soft tissue disorder related to use, overuse and pressure, left upper arm
M70.929 Unspecified soft tissue disorder related to use, overuse and pressure, unspecified upper arm
● M70.93 Unspecified soft tissue disorder related to use, overuse and pressure of forearm
M70.931 Unspecified soft tissue disorder related to use, overuse and pressure, right forearm
M70.932 Unspecified soft tissue disorder related to use, overuse and pressure, left forearm
M70.939 Unspecified soft tissue disorder related to use, overuse and pressure, unspecified forearm
● M70.94 Unspecified soft tissue disorder related to use, overuse and pressure of hand
M70.941 Unspecified soft tissue disorder related to use, overuse and pressure, right hand
M70.942 Unspecified soft tissue disorder related to use, overuse and pressure, left hand
M70.949 Unspecified soft tissue disorder related to use, overuse and pressure, unspecified hand
● M70.95 Unspecified soft tissue disorder related to use, overuse and pressure of thigh
M70.951 Unspecified soft tissue disorder related to use, overuse and pressure, right thigh
M70.952 Unspecified soft tissue disorder related to use, overuse and pressure, left thigh
M70.959 Unspecified soft tissue disorder related to use, overuse and pressure, unspecified thigh
● M70.96 Unspecified soft tissue disorder related to use, overuse and pressure lower leg
M70.961 Unspecified soft tissue disorder related to use, overuse and pressure, right lower leg
M70.962 Unspecified soft tissue disorder related to use, overuse and pressure, left lower leg
M70.969 Unspecified soft tissue disorder related to use, overuse and pressure, unspecified lower leg
● M70.97 Unspecified soft tissue disorder related to use, overuse and pressure of ankle and foot
M70.971 Unspecified soft tissue disorder related to use, overuse and pressure, right ankle and foot
M70.972 Unspecified soft tissue disorder related to use, overuse and pressure, left ankle and foot
M70.979 Unspecified soft tissue disorder related to use, overuse and pressure, unspecified ankle and foot
M70.98 Unspecified soft tissue disorder related to use, overuse and pressure other
M70.99 Unspecified soft tissue disorder related to use, overuse and pressure multiple sites

● M71 Other bursopathies

Excludes1 bunion (M20.1)
bursitis related to use, overuse or pressure (M70.-)
enthesopathies (M76-M77)

● M71.0 Abscess of bursa
Use additional code (B95.-, B96.-) to identify causative organism
M71.00 Abscess of bursa, unspecified site
● M71.01 Abscess of bursa, shoulder
M71.011 Abscess of bursa, right shoulder
M71.012 Abscess of bursa, left shoulder
M71.019 Abscess of bursa, unspecified shoulder
● M71.02 Abscess of bursa, elbow
M71.021 Abscess of bursa, right elbow
M71.022 Abscess of bursa, left elbow
M71.029 Abscess of bursa, unspecified elbow
● M71.03 Abscess of bursa, wrist
M71.031 Abscess of bursa, right wrist
M71.032 Abscess of bursa, left wrist
M71.039 Abscess of bursa, unspecified wrist
● M71.04 Abscess of bursa, hand
M71.041 Abscess of bursa, right hand
M71.042 Abscess of bursa, left hand
M71.049 Abscess of bursa, unspecified hand

● M71.05 Abscess of bursa, hip
- M71.051 Abscess of bursa, right hip
- M71.052 Abscess of bursa, left hip
- M71.059 Abscess of bursa, unspecified hip

● M71.06 Abscess of bursa, knee
- M71.061 Abscess of bursa, right knee
- M71.062 Abscess of bursa, left knee
- M71.069 Abscess of bursa, unspecified knee

● M71.07 Abscess of bursa, ankle and foot
- M71.071 Abscess of bursa, right ankle and foot
- M71.072 Abscess of bursa, left ankle and foot
- M71.079 Abscess of bursa, unspecified ankle and foot

M71.08 Abscess of bursa, other site

M71.09 Abscess of bursa, multiple sites

● M71.1 Other infective bursitis

Use additional code (B95.-, B96.-) to identify causative organism

M71.10 Other infective bursitis, unspecified site

● M71.11 Other infective bursitis, shoulder
- M71.111 Other infective bursitis, right shoulder
- M71.112 Other infective bursitis, left shoulder
- M71.119 Other infective bursitis, unspecified shoulder

● M71.12 Other infective bursitis, elbow
- M71.121 Other infective bursitis, right elbow
- M71.122 Other infective bursitis, left elbow
- M71.129 Other infective bursitis, unspecified elbow

● M71.13 Other infective bursitis, wrist
- M71.131 Other infective bursitis, right wrist
- M71.132 Other infective bursitis, left wrist
- M71.139 Other infective bursitis, unspecified wrist

● M71.14 Other infective bursitis, hand
- M71.141 Other infective bursitis, right hand
- M71.142 Other infective bursitis, left hand
- M71.149 Other infective bursitis, unspecified hand

● M71.15 Other infective bursitis, hip
- M71.151 Other infective bursitis, right hip
- M71.152 Other infective bursitis, left hip
- M71.159 Other infective bursitis, unspecified hip

● M71.16 Other infective bursitis, knee
- M71.161 Other infective bursitis, right knee
- M71.162 Other infective bursitis, left knee
- M71.169 Other infective bursitis, unspecified knee

● M71.17 Other infective bursitis, ankle and foot
- M71.171 Other infective bursitis, right ankle and foot
- M71.172 Other infective bursitis, left ankle and foot
- M71.179 Other infective bursitis, unspecified ankle and foot

M71.18 Other infective bursitis, other site

M71.19 Other infective bursitis, multiple sites

● M71.2 Synovial cyst of popliteal space [Baker]

Popliteal space = popliteal cavity, popliteal fossa. Depression in the posterior aspect of the knee (behind the knee).

Excludes1 synovial cyst of popliteal space with rupture (M66.0)

M71.20 Synovial cyst of popliteal space [Baker], unspecified knee

M71.21 Synovial cyst of popliteal space [Baker], right knee

M71.22 Synovial cyst of popliteal space [Baker], left knee

● M71.3 Other bursal cyst

Synovial cyst NOS

Excludes1 synovial cyst with rupture (M66.1-)

M71.30 Other bursal cyst, unspecified site

● M71.31 Other bursal cyst, shoulder
- M71.311 Other bursal cyst, right shoulder
- M71.312 Other bursal cyst, left shoulder
- M71.319 Other bursal cyst, unspecified shoulder

● M71.32 Other bursal cyst, elbow
- M71.321 Other bursal cyst, right elbow
- M71.322 Other bursal cyst, left elbow
- M71.329 Other bursal cyst, unspecified elbow

● M71.33 Other bursal cyst, wrist
- M71.331 Other bursal cyst, right wrist
- M71.332 Other bursal cyst, left wrist
- M71.339 Other bursal cyst, unspecified wrist

● M71.34 Other bursal cyst, hand
- M71.341 Other bursal cyst, right hand
- M71.342 Other bursal cyst, left hand
- M71.349 Other bursal cyst, unspecified hand

● M71.35 Other bursal cyst, hip
- M71.351 Other bursal cyst, right hip
- M71.352 Other bursal cyst, left hip
- M71.359 Other bursal cyst, unspecified hip

● M71.37 Other bursal cyst, ankle and foot
- M71.371 Other bursal cyst, right ankle and foot
- M71.372 Other bursal cyst, left ankle and foot
- M71.379 Other bursal cyst, unspecified ankle and foot

M71.38 Other bursal cyst, other site

M71.39 Other bursal cyst, multiple sites

● M71.4 Calcium deposit in bursa

Excludes2 calcium deposit in bursa of shoulder (M75.3)

M71.40 Calcium deposit in bursa, unspecified site

● M71.42 Calcium deposit in bursa, elbow
- M71.421 Calcium deposit in bursa, right elbow
- M71.422 Calcium deposit in bursa, left elbow
- M71.429 Calcium deposit in bursa, unspecified elbow

● M71.43 Calcium deposit in bursa, wrist
- M71.431 Calcium deposit in bursa, right wrist
- M71.432 Calcium deposit in bursa, left wrist
- M71.439 Calcium deposit in bursa, unspecified wrist

● M71.44 Calcium deposit in bursa, hand
- M71.441 Calcium deposit in bursa, right hand
- M71.442 Calcium deposit in bursa, left hand
- M71.449 Calcium deposit in bursa, unspecified hand

● M71.45 Calcium deposit in bursa, hip
M71.451 Calcium deposit in bursa, right hip
M71.452 Calcium deposit in bursa, left hip
M71.459 Calcium deposit in bursa, unspecified hip
● M71.46 Calcium deposit in bursa, knee
M71.461 Calcium deposit in bursa, right knee
M71.462 Calcium deposit in bursa, left knee
M71.469 Calcium deposit in bursa, unspecified knee
● M71.47 Calcium deposit in bursa, ankle and foot
M71.471 Calcium deposit in bursa, right ankle and foot
M71.472 Calcium deposit in bursa, left ankle and foot
M71.479 Calcium deposit in bursa, unspecified ankle and foot
M71.48 Calcium deposit in bursa, other site
M71.49 Calcium deposit in bursa, multiple sites
● M71.5 Other bursitis, not elsewhere classified
Excludes1 bursitis NOS (M71.9-)
Excludes2 bursitis of shoulder (M75.5)
bursitis of tibial collateral [Pellegrini-Stieda] (M76.4-) ⇐
M71.50 Other bursitis, not elsewhere classified, unspecified site
● M71.52 Other bursitis, not elsewhere classified, elbow
M71.521 Other bursitis, not elsewhere classified, right elbow
M71.522 Other bursitis, not elsewhere classified, left elbow
M71.529 Other bursitis, not elsewhere classified, unspecified elbow
● M71.53 Other bursitis, not elsewhere classified, wrist
M71.531 Other bursitis, not elsewhere classified, right wrist
M71.532 Other bursitis, not elsewhere classified, left wrist
M71.539 Other bursitis, not elsewhere classified, unspecified wrist
● M71.54 Other bursitis, not elsewhere classified, hand
M71.541 Other bursitis, not elsewhere classified, right hand
M71.542 Other bursitis, not elsewhere classified, left hand
M71.549 Other bursitis, not elsewhere classified, unspecified hand
● M71.55 Other bursitis, not elsewhere classified, hip
M71.551 Other bursitis, not elsewhere classified, right hip
M71.552 Other bursitis, not elsewhere classified, left hip
M71.559 Other bursitis, not elsewhere classified, unspecified hip
● M71.56 Other bursitis, not elsewhere classified, knee
M71.561 Other bursitis, not elsewhere classified, right knee
M71.562 Other bursitis, not elsewhere classified, left knee
M71.569 Other bursitis, not elsewhere classified, unspecified knee
● M71.57 Other bursitis, not elsewhere classified, ankle and foot
M71.571 Other bursitis, not elsewhere classified, right ankle and foot
M71.572 Other bursitis, not elsewhere classified, left ankle and foot
M71.579 Other bursitis, not elsewhere classified, unspecified ankle and foot
M71.58 Other bursitis, not elsewhere classified, other site
● M71.8 Other specified bursopathies
M71.80 Other specified bursopathies, unspecified site
● M71.81 Other specified bursopathies, shoulder
M71.811 Other specified bursopathies, right shoulder
M71.812 Other specified bursopathies, left shoulder
M71.819 Other specified bursopathies, unspecified shoulder
● M71.82 Other specified bursopathies, elbow
M71.821 Other specified bursopathies, right elbow
M71.822 Other specified bursopathies, left elbow
M71.829 Other specified bursopathies, unspecified elbow
● M71.83 Other specified bursopathies, wrist
M71.831 Other specified bursopathies, right wrist
M71.832 Other specified bursopathies, left wrist
M71.839 Other specified bursopathies, unspecified wrist
● M71.84 Other specified bursopathies, hand
M71.841 Other specified bursopathies, right hand
M71.842 Other specified bursopathies, left hand
M71.849 Other specified bursopathies, unspecified hand
● M71.85 Other specified bursopathies, hip
M71.851 Other specified bursopathies, right hip
M71.852 Other specified bursopathies, left hip
M71.859 Other specified bursopathies, unspecified hip
● M71.86 Other specified bursopathies, knee
M71.861 Other specified bursopathies, right knee
M71.862 Other specified bursopathies, left knee
M71.869 Other specified bursopathies, unspecified knee
● M71.87 Other specified bursopathies, ankle and foot
M71.871 Other specified bursopathies, right ankle and foot
M71.872 Other specified bursopathies, left ankle and foot
M71.879 Other specified bursopathies, unspecified ankle and foot
M71.88 Other specified bursopathies, other site
M71.89 Other specified bursopathies, multiple sites
M71.9 Bursopathy, unspecified
Bursitis NOS

M72 Fibroblastic disorders

Excludes2 retroperitoneal fibromatosis (D48.3)

M72.0 Palmar fascial fibromatosis [Dupuytren]

M72.1 Knuckle pads

M72.2 Plantar fascial fibromatosis

Plantar fasciitis

M72.4 Pseudosarcomatous fibromatosis

Nodular fasciitis

M72.6 Necrotizing fasciitis

Use additional code (B95.-, B96.-) to identify causative organism

M72.8 Other fibroblastic disorders

Abscess of fascia
Fasciitis NEC
Other infective fasciitis

Use additional code to (B95.-, B96.-) identify causative organism

Excludes1 diffuse (eosinophilic) fasciitis (M35.4)
necrotizing fasciitis (M72.6)
nodular fasciitis (M72.4)
perirenal fasciitis NOS (N13.5)
perirenal fasciitis with infection (N13.6)
plantar fasciitis (M72.2)

M72.9 Fibroblastic disorder, unspecified

Fasciitis NOS
Fibromatosis NOS

M75 Shoulder lesions

Excludes2 shoulder-hand syndrome (M89.0-)

M75.0 Adhesive capsulitis of shoulder

Frozen shoulder
Periarthritis of shoulder

M75.00 Adhesive capsulitis of unspecified shoulder

M75.01 Adhesive capsulitis of right shoulder

M75.02 Adhesive capsulitis of left shoulder

M75.1 Rotator cuff tear or rupture, not specified as traumatic

Rotator cuff syndrome
Supraspinatus syndrome
Supraspinatus tear or rupture, not specified as traumatic

Excludes1 tear of rotator cuff, traumatic (S46.01-)

Gradual onset due to repetitive stress to rotator cuff

M75.10 Unspecified rotator cuff tear or rupture, not specified as traumatic

M75.100 Unspecified rotator cuff tear or rupture of unspecified shoulder, not specified as traumatic

M75.101 Unspecified rotator cuff tear or rupture of right shoulder, not specified as traumatic

M75.102 Unspecified rotator cuff tear or rupture of left shoulder, not specified as traumatic

M75.11 Incomplete rotator cuff tear or rupture not specified as traumatic

M75.110 Incomplete rotator cuff tear or rupture of unspecified shoulder, not specified as traumatic

M75.111 Incomplete rotator cuff tear or rupture of right shoulder, not specified as traumatic

M75.112 Incomplete rotator cuff tear or rupture of left shoulder, not specified as traumatic

M75.12 Complete rotator cuff tear or rupture not specified as traumatic

M75.120 Complete rotator cuff tear or rupture of unspecified shoulder, not specified as traumatic

M75.121 Complete rotator cuff tear or rupture of right shoulder, not specified as traumatic

M75.122 Complete rotator cuff tear or rupture of left shoulder, not specified as traumatic

M75.2 Bicipital tendinitis

M75.20 Bicipital tendinitis, unspecified shoulder

M75.21 Bicipital tendinitis, right shoulder

M75.22 Bicipital tendinitis, left shoulder

M75.3 Calcific tendinitis of shoulder

Calcified bursa of shoulder

M75.30 Calcific tendinitis of unspecified shoulder

M75.31 Calcific tendinitis of right shoulder

M75.32 Calcific tendinitis of left shoulder

M75.4 Impingement syndrome of shoulder

M75.40 Impingement syndrome of unspecified shoulder

M75.41 Impingement syndrome of right shoulder

M75.42 Impingement syndrome of left shoulder

M75.5 Bursitis of shoulder

M75.50 Bursitis of unspecified shoulder

M75.51 Bursitis of right shoulder

M75.52 Bursitis of left shoulder

M75.8 Other shoulder lesions

M75.80 Other shoulder lesions, unspecified shoulder

M75.81 Other shoulder lesions, right shoulder

M75.82 Other shoulder lesions, left shoulder

M75.9 Shoulder lesion, unspecified

M75.90 Shoulder lesion, unspecified, unspecified shoulder

M75.91 Shoulder lesion, unspecified, right shoulder

M75.92 Shoulder lesion, unspecified, left shoulder

M76 Enthesopathies, lower limb, excluding foot

Excludes2 bursitis due to use, overuse and pressure (M70.-)
enthesopathies of ankle and foot (M77.5-)

M76.0 Gluteal tendinitis

M76.00 Gluteal tendinitis, unspecified hip

M76.01 Gluteal tendinitis, right hip

M76.02 Gluteal tendinitis, left hip

M76.1 Psoas tendinitis

M76.10 Psoas tendinitis, unspecified hip

M76.11 Psoas tendinitis, right hip

M76.12 Psoas tendinitis, left hip

M76.2 Iliac crest spur

M76.20 Iliac crest spur, unspecified hip

M76.21 Iliac crest spur, right hip

M76.22 Iliac crest spur, left hip

M76.3 Iliotibial band syndrome

M76.30 Iliotibial band syndrome, unspecified leg

M76.31 Iliotibial band syndrome, right leg

M76.32 Iliotibial band syndrome, left leg

M76.4 Tibial collateral bursitis [Pellegrini-Stieda]

M76.40 Tibial collateral bursitis [Pellegrini-Stieda], unspecified leg

M76.41 Tibial collateral bursitis [Pellegrini-Stieda], right leg

M76.42 Tibial collateral bursitis [Pellegrini-Stieda], left leg

● **M76.5 Patellar tendinitis**
- **M76.50 Patellar tendinitis, unspecified knee**
- **M76.51 Patellar tendinitis, right knee**
- **M76.52 Patellar tendinitis, left knee**

● **M76.6 Achilles tendinitis**
Achilles bursitis
- **M76.60 Achilles tendinitis, unspecified leg**
- **M76.61 Achilles tendinitis, right leg**
- **M76.62 Achilles tendinitis, left leg**

● **M76.7 Peroneal tendinitis**
- **M76.70 Peroneal tendinitis, unspecified leg**
- **M76.71 Peroneal tendinitis, right leg**
- **M76.72 Peroneal tendinitis, left leg**

● **M76.8 Other specified enthesopathies of lower limb, excluding foot**

● **M76.81 Anterior tibial syndrome**
- **M76.811 Anterior tibial syndrome, right leg**
- **M76.812 Anterior tibial syndrome, left leg**
- **M76.819 Anterior tibial syndrome, unspecified leg**

● **M76.82 Posterior tibial tendinitis**
- **M76.821 Posterior tibial tendinitis, right leg**
- **M76.822 Posterior tibial tendinitis, left leg**
- **M76.829 Posterior tibial tendinitis, unspecified leg**

● **M76.89 Other specified enthesopathies of lower limb, excluding foot**
- **M76.891 Other specified enthesopathies of right lower limb, excluding foot**
- **M76.892 Other specified enthesopathies of left lower limb, excluding foot**
- **M76.899 Other specified enthesopathies of unspecified lower limb, excluding foot**

M76.9 Unspecified enthesopathy, lower limb, excluding foot

● **M77 Other enthesopathies**

Excludes1 bursitis NOS (M71.9-)

Excludes2 bursitis due to use, overuse and pressure (M7Ø.-)
osteophyte (M25.7)
spinal enthesopathy (M46.Ø-)

● **M77.Ø Medial epicondylitis**
- **M77.ØØ Medial epicondylitis, unspecified elbow**
- **M77.Ø1 Medial epicondylitis, right elbow**
- **M77.Ø2 Medial epicondylitis, left elbow**

● **M77.1 Lateral epicondylitis**
Tennis elbow
- **M77.1Ø Lateral epicondylitis, unspecified elbow**
- **M77.11 Lateral epicondylitis, right elbow**
- **M77.12 Lateral epicondylitis, left elbow**

● **M77.2 Periarthritis of wrist**
- **M77.2Ø Periarthritis, unspecified wrist**
- **M77.21 Periarthritis, right wrist**
- **M77.22 Periarthritis, left wrist**

● **M77.3 Calcaneal spur**
- **M77.3Ø Calcaneal spur, unspecified foot**
- **M77.31 Calcaneal spur, right foot**
- **M77.32 Calcaneal spur, left foot**

● **M77.4 Metatarsalgia**

Excludes1 Morton's metatarsalgia (G57.6)
- **M77.4Ø Metatarsalgia, unspecified foot**
- **M77.41 Metatarsalgia, right foot**
- **M77.42 Metatarsalgia, left foot**

● **M77.5 Other enthesopathy of foot**
- **M77.5Ø Other enthesopathy of unspecified foot**
- **M77.51 Other enthesopathy of right foot**
- **M77.52 Other enthesopathy of left foot**

M77.8 Other enthesopathies, not elsewhere classified

M77.9 Enthesopathy, unspecified
Bone spur NOS
Capsulitis NOS
Periarthritis NOS
Tendinitis NOS

● **M79 Other and unspecified soft tissue disorders, not elsewhere classified**

Excludes1 psychogenic rheumatism (F45.8)
soft tissue pain, psychogenic (F45.41)

M79.Ø Rheumatism, unspecified

Excludes1 fibromyalgia (M79.7)
palindromic rheumatism (M12.3-)

M79.1 Myalgia
Myofascial pain syndrome

Excludes1 fibromyalgia (M79.7)
myositis (M6Ø.-)

M79.2 Neuralgia and neuritis, unspecified

Excludes1 brachial radiculitis NOS (M54.1)
lumbosacral radiculitis NOS (M54.1)
mononeuropathies (G56-G58)
radiculitis NOS (M54.1)
sciatica (M54.3-M54.4)

M79.3 Panniculitis, unspecified

Excludes1 lupus panniculitis (L93.2)
neck and back panniculitis (M54.Ø-)
relapsing [Weber-Christian] panniculitis (M35.6)

M79.4 Hypertrophy of (infrapatellar) fat pad

M79.5 Residual foreign body in soft tissue

Excludes1 foreign body granuloma of skin and subcutaneous tissue (L92.3)
foreign body granuloma of soft tissue (M6Ø.2-)

● **M79.6 Pain in limb, hand, foot, fingers and toes**

Excludes2 pain in joint (M25.5-)

● **M79.6Ø Pain in limb, unspecified**
- **M79.6Ø1 Pain in right arm**
  Pain in right upper limb NOS
- **M79.6Ø2 Pain in left arm**
  Pain in left upper limb NOS
- **M79.6Ø3 Pain in arm, unspecified**
  Pain in upper limb NOS
- **M79.6Ø4 Pain in right leg**
  Pain in right lower limb NOS
- **M79.6Ø5 Pain in left leg**
  Pain in left lower limb NOS
- **M79.6Ø6 Pain in leg, unspecified**
  Pain in lower limb NOS
- **M79.6Ø9 Pain in unspecified limb**
  Pain in limb NOS

● **M79.62 Pain in upper arm**
Pain in axillary region
- **M79.621 Pain in right upper arm**
- **M79.622 Pain in left upper arm**
- **M79.629 Pain in unspecified upper arm**

● **M79.63 Pain in forearm**
- **M79.631 Pain in right forearm**
- **M79.632 Pain in left forearm**
- **M79.639 Pain in unspecified forearm**

M79.64 Pain in hand and fingers

M79.641 Pain in right hand

M79.642 Pain in left hand

M79.643 Pain in unspecified hand

M79.644 Pain in right finger(s)

M79.645 Pain in left finger(s)

M79.646 Pain in unspecified finger(s)

M79.65 Pain in thigh

M79.651 Pain in right thigh

M79.652 Pain in left thigh

M79.659 Pain in unspecified thigh

M79.66 Pain in lower leg

M79.661 Pain in right lower leg

M79.662 Pain in left lower leg

M79.669 Pain in unspecified lower leg

M79.67 Pain in foot and toes

M79.671 Pain in right foot

M79.672 Pain in left foot

M79.673 Pain in unspecified foot

M79.674 Pain in right toe(s)

M79.675 Pain in left toe(s)

M79.676 Pain in unspecified toe(s)

M79.7 Fibromyalgia
Fibromyositis
Fibrositis
Myofibrositis

M79.A Nontraumatic compartment syndrome

Code first, if applicable, associated postprocedural complication

Excludes1 compartment syndrome NOS (T79.A-)
fibromyalgia (M79.7) nontraumatic ischemic infarction of muscle (M62.2-)
traumatic compartment syndrome (T79.A-)

M79.A1 Nontraumatic compartment syndrome of upper extremity
Nontraumatic compartment syndrome of shoulder, arm, forearm, wrist, hand, and fingers

M79.A11 Nontraumatic compartment syndrome of right upper extremity

M79.A12 Nontraumatic compartment syndrome of left upper extremity

M79.A19 Nontraumatic compartment syndrome of unspecified upper extremity

M79.A2 Nontraumatic compartment syndrome of lower extremity
Nontraumatic compartment syndrome of hip, buttock, thigh, leg, foot, and toes

M79.A21 Nontraumatic compartment syndrome of right lower extremity

M79.A22 Nontraumatic compartment syndrome of left lower extremity

M79.A29 Nontraumatic compartment syndrome of unspecified lower extremity

M79.A3 Nontraumatic compartment syndrome of abdomen

M79.A9 Nontraumatic compartment syndrome of other sites

M79.8 Other specified soft tissue disorders

M79.81 Nontraumatic hematoma of soft tissue
Nontraumatic hematoma of muscle
Nontraumatic seroma of muscle and soft tissue

M79.89 Other specified soft tissue disorders
Polyalgia

M79.9 Soft tissue disorder, unspecified

OGCR See Section I.C., Chapter 13.d.

Osteoporosis

Osteoporosis is a systemic condition, meaning that all bones of the musculoskeletal system are affected. Therefore, site is not a component of the codes under category M81, Osteoporosis without current pathological fracture. The site codes under category M8Ø, Osteoporosis with current pathological fracture, identify the site of the fracture, not the osteoporosis.

1) Osteoporosis without pathological fracture

Category M81, Osteoporosis without current pathological fracture, is for use for patients with osteoporosis who do not currently have a pathologic fracture due to the osteoporosis, even if they have had a fracture in the past. For patients with a history of osteoporosis fractures, status code Z87.31Ø, Personal history of (healed) osteoporosis fracture, should follow the code from M81.

2) Osteoporosis with current pathological fracture

Category M8Ø, Osteoporosis with current pathological fracture, is for patients who have a current pathologic fracture at the time of an encounter. The codes under M8Ø identify the site of the fracture. A code from category M8Ø, not a traumatic fracture code, should be used for any patient with known osteoporosis who suffers a fracture, even if the patient had a minor fall or trauma, if that fall or trauma would not usually break a normal, healthy bone.

OSTEOPATHIES AND CHONDROPATHIES (M8Ø-M94)

DISORDERS OF BONE DENSITY AND STRUCTURE (M8Ø-M85)

M8Ø Osteoporosis with current pathological fracture

Excessive skeletal fragility (porous bone) resulting in bone fractures

Includes osteoporosis with current fragility fracture

Use additional code to identify major osseous defect, if applicable (M89.7-)

Excludes1 collapsed vertebra NOS (M48.5)
pathological fracture NOS (M84.4)
wedging of vertebra NOS (M48.5)

Excludes2 personal history of (healed) osteoporosis fracture (Z87.31Ø)

The appropriate 7th character is to be added to each code from category M8Ø:

A initial encounter for fracture
All encounters involving diagnosis and treatment
D subsequent encounter for fracture with routine healing
G subsequent encounter for fracture with delayed healing
Encounters for attention to casting or fixation devices, medication, and follow-up visits during the healing phase
K subsequent encounter for fracture with nonunion
Total failure of fracture healing
P subsequent encounter for fracture with malunion
Fracture ends do not heal together correctly.
S sequela

M8Ø.Ø Age-related osteoporosis with current pathological fracture
Involutional osteoporosis with current pathological fracture
Osteoporosis NOS with current pathological fracture
Postmenopausal osteoporosis with current pathological fracture
Senile osteoporosis with current pathological fracture

X **M8Ø.ØØ Age-related osteoporosis with current pathological fracture, unspecified site**

M8Ø.Ø1 Age-related osteoporosis with current pathological fracture, shoulder

M8Ø.Ø11 Age-related osteoporosis with current pathological fracture, right shoulder

M8Ø.Ø12 Age-related osteoporosis with current pathological fracture, left shoulder

M8Ø.Ø19 Age-related osteoporosis with current pathological fracture, unspecified shoulder

● M80.02 **Age-related osteoporosis with current pathological fracture, humerus**

● M80.021 **Age-related osteoporosis with current pathological fracture, right humerus**

● M80.022 **Age-related osteoporosis with current pathological fracture, left humerus**

● M80.029 **Age-related osteoporosis with current pathological fracture, unspecified humerus**

● M80.03 **Age-related osteoporosis with current pathological fracture, forearm**

Age-related osteoporosis with current pathological fracture of wrist

● M80.031 **Age-related osteoporosis with current pathological fracture, right forearm**

● M80.032 **Age-related osteoporosis with current pathological fracture, left forearm**

● M80.039 **Age-related osteoporosis with current pathological fracture, unspecified forearm**

● M80.04 **Age-related osteoporosis with current pathological fracture, hand**

● M80.041 **Age-related osteoporosis with current pathological fracture, right hand**

● M80.042 **Age-related osteoporosis with current pathological fracture, left hand**

● M80.049 **Age-related osteoporosis with current pathological fracture, unspecified hand**

● M80.05 **Age-related osteoporosis with current pathological fracture, femur**

Age-related osteoporosis with current pathological fracture of hip

● M80.051 **Age-related osteoporosis with current pathological fracture, right femur**

● M80.052 **Age-related osteoporosis with current pathological fracture, left femur**

● M80.059 **Age-related osteoporosis with current pathological fracture, unspecified femur**

● M80.06 **Age-related osteoporosis with current pathological fracture, lower leg**

● M80.061 **Age-related osteoporosis with current pathological fracture, right lower leg**

● M80.062 **Age-related osteoporosis with current pathological fracture, left lower leg**

● M80.069 **Age-related osteoporosis with current pathological fracture, unspecified lower leg**

● M80.07 **Age-related osteoporosis with current pathological fracture, ankle and foot**

● M80.071 **Age-related osteoporosis with current pathological fracture, right ankle and foot**

● M80.072 **Age-related osteoporosis with current pathological fracture, left ankle and foot**

● M80.079 **Age-related osteoporosis with current pathological fracture, unspecified ankle and foot**

X● M80.08 **Age-related osteoporosis with current pathological fracture, vertebra(e)**

● M80.8 **Other osteoporosis with current pathological fracture**

Drug-induced osteoporosis with current pathological fracture

Idiopathic osteoporosis with current pathological fracture

Osteoporosis of disuse with current pathological fracture

Postoophorectomy osteoporosis with current pathological fracture

Postsurgical malabsorption osteoporosis with current pathological fracture

Post-traumatic osteoporosis with current pathological fracture

Use additional code for adverse effect, if applicable, to identify drug (T36-T50 with fifth or sixth character 5)

X● M80.80 **Other osteoporosis with current pathological fracture, unspecified site**

● M80.81 **Other osteoporosis with pathological fracture, shoulder**

● M80.811 **Other osteoporosis with current pathological fracture, right shoulder**

● M80.812 **Other osteoporosis with current pathological fracture, left shoulder**

● M80.819 **Other osteoporosis with current pathological fracture, unspecified shoulder**

● M80.82 **Other osteoporosis with current pathological fracture, humerus**

● M80.821 **Other osteoporosis with current pathological fracture, right humerus**

● M80.822 **Other osteoporosis with current pathological fracture, left humerus**

● M80.829 **Other osteoporosis with current pathological fracture, unspecified humerus**

● M80.83 **Other osteoporosis with current pathological fracture, forearm**

Other osteoporosis with current pathological fracture of wrist

● M80.831 **Other osteoporosis with current pathological fracture, right forearm**

● M80.832 **Other osteoporosis with current pathological fracture, left forearm**

● M80.839 **Other osteoporosis with current pathological fracture, unspecified forearm**

● M80.84 **Other osteoporosis with current pathological fracture, hand**

● M80.841 **Other osteoporosis with current pathological fracture, right hand**

● M80.842 **Other osteoporosis with current pathological fracture, left hand**

● M80.849 **Other osteoporosis with current pathological fracture, unspecified hand**

● M80.85 **Other osteoporosis with current pathological fracture, femur**

Other osteoporosis with current pathological fracture of hip

● M80.851 **Other osteoporosis with current pathological fracture, right femur**

● M80.852 **Other osteoporosis with current pathological fracture, left femur**

● M80.859 **Other osteoporosis with current pathological fracture, unspecified femur**

● M80.86 Other osteoporosis with current pathological fracture, lower leg
- ● M80.861 Other osteoporosis with current pathological fracture, right lower leg
- ● M80.862 Other osteoporosis with current pathological fracture, left lower leg
- ● M80.869 Other osteoporosis with current pathological fracture, unspecified lower leg

● M80.87 Other osteoporosis with current pathological fracture, ankle and foot
- ● M80.871 Other osteoporosis with current pathological fracture, right ankle and foot
- ● M80.872 Other osteoporosis with current pathological fracture, left ankle and foot
- ● M80.879 Other osteoporosis with current pathological fracture, unspecified ankle and foot

X ● M80.88 Other osteoporosis with current pathological fracture, vertebra(e)

● M81 Osteoporosis without current pathological fracture

Use additional code to identify:
major osseous defect, if applicable (M89.7-)
personal history of (healed) osteoporosis fracture, if applicable (Z87.310)

Excludes1 osteoporosis with current pathological fracture (M80.-)
Sudeck's atrophy (M89.0)

M81.0 Age-related osteoporosis without current pathological fracture
Involutional osteoporosis without current pathological fracture
Osteoporosis NOS
Postmenopausal osteoporosis without current pathological fracture
Senile osteoporosis without current pathological fracture

M81.6 Localized osteoporosis [Lequesne]
Excludes1 Sudeck's atrophy (M89.0)

M81.8 Other osteoporosis without current pathological fracture
Drug-induced osteoporosis without current pathological fracture
Idiopathic osteoporosis without current pathological fracture
Osteoporosis of disuse without current pathological fracture
Postoophorectomy osteoporosis without current pathological fracture
Postsurgical malabsorption osteoporosis without current pathological fracture
Post-traumatic osteoporosis without current pathological fracture
Use additional code for adverse effect, if applicable, to identify drug (T36-T50 with fifth or sixth character 5)

● M83 Adult osteomalacia

Excludes1 infantile and juvenile osteomalacia (E55.0)
renal osteodystrophy (N25.0)
rickets (active) (E55.0)
rickets (active) sequelae (E64.3)
vitamin D-resistant osteomalacia (E83.3)
vitamin D-resistant rickets (active) (E83.3)

M83.0 Puerperal osteomalacia

M83.1 Senile osteomalacia

M83.2 Adult osteomalacia due to malabsorption
Postsurgical malabsorption osteomalacia in adults

M83.3 Adult osteomalacia due to malnutrition

M83.4 Aluminum bone disease

M83.5 Other drug-induced osteomalacia in adults
Use additional code for adverse effect, if applicable, to identify drug (T36-T50 with fifth or sixth character 5)

M83.8 Other adult osteomalacia

M83.9 Adult osteomalacia, unspecified

● M84 Disorder of continuity of bone

Excludes2 traumatic fracture of bone-see fracture, by site

● M84.3 Stress fracture
Fatigue fracture
March fracture
Stress fracture NOS
Stress reaction
Use additional external cause code(s) to identify the cause of the stress fracture

Excludes1 pathological fracture NOS (M84.4.-)
pathological fracture due to osteoporosis (M80.-)
traumatic fracture (S12.-, S22.-, S32.-, S42.-, S52.-, S62.-, S72.-, S82.-, S92.-)

Excludes2 personal history of (healed) stress (fatigue) fracture (Z87.312)
stress fracture of vertebra (M48.4-)

The appropriate 7th character is to be added to each code from subcategory M84.3:

A	initial encounter for fracture
D	subsequent encounter for fracture with routine healing
G	subsequent encounter for fracture with delayed healing
K	subsequent encounter for fracture with nonunion
P	subsequent encounter for fracture with malunion
S	sequela

X ● M84.30 Stress fracture, unspecified site

● M84.31 Stress fracture, shoulder
- ● M84.311 Stress fracture, right shoulder
- ● M84.312 Stress fracture, left shoulder
- ● M84.319 Stress fracture, unspecified shoulder

● M84.32 Stress fracture, humerus
- ● M84.321 Stress fracture, right humerus
- ● M84.322 Stress fracture, left humerus
- ● M84.329 Stress fracture, unspecified humerus

● M84.33 Stress fracture, ulna and radius
- ● M84.331 Stress fracture, right ulna
- ● M84.332 Stress fracture, left ulna
- ● M84.333 Stress fracture, right radius
- ● M84.334 Stress fracture, left radius
- ● M84.339 Stress fracture, unspecified ulna and radius

● M84.34 Stress fracture, hand and fingers
- ● M84.341 Stress fracture, right hand
- ● M84.342 Stress fracture, left hand
- ● M84.343 Stress fracture, unspecified hand
- ● M84.344 Stress fracture, right finger(s)
- ● M84.345 Stress fracture, left finger(s)
- ● M84.346 Stress fracture, unspecified finger(s)

● M84.35 Stress fracture, pelvis and femur
Stress fracture, hip
- ● M84.350 Stress fracture, pelvis
- ● M84.351 Stress fracture, right femur
- ● M84.352 Stress fracture, left femur
- ● M84.353 Stress fracture, unspecified femur
- ● M84.359 Stress fracture, hip, unspecified

CHAPTER 13 (M00-M99)

- M84.36 Stress fracture, tibia and fibula
  - M84.361 Stress fracture, right tibia
  - M84.362 Stress fracture, left tibia
  - M84.363 Stress fracture, right fibula
  - M84.364 Stress fracture, left fibula
  - M84.369 Stress fracture, unspecified tibia and fibula
- M84.37 Stress fracture, ankle, foot and toes
  - M84.371 Stress fracture, right ankle
  - M84.372 Stress fracture, left ankle
  - M84.373 Stress fracture, unspecified ankle
  - M84.374 Stress fracture, right foot
  - M84.375 Stress fracture, left foot
  - M84.376 Stress fracture, unspecified foot
  - M84.377 Stress fracture, right toe(s)
  - M84.378 Stress fracture, left toe(s)
  - M84.379 Stress fracture, unspecified toe(s)
- X M84.38 Stress fracture, other site

  Excludes2 stress fracture of vertebra (M48.4-)

M84.4 Pathological fracture, not elsewhere classified

Chronic fracture
Pathological fracture NOS

Excludes1 collapsed vertebra NEC (M48.5)
pathological fracture in neoplastic disease (M84.5-)
pathological fracture in osteoporosis (M80.-)
pathological fracture in other disease (M84.6-)
stress fracture (M84.3-)
traumatic fracture (S12.-, S22.-, S32.-, S42.-, S52.-, S62.-, S72.-, S82.-, S92.-)

Excludes2 personal history of (healed) pathological fracture (Z87.311)

The appropriate 7th character is to be added to each code from subcategory M84.4:

A	initial encounter for fracture
D	subsequent encounter for fracture with routine healing
G	subsequent encounter for fracture with delayed healing
K	subsequent encounter for fracture with nonunion
P	subsequent encounter for fracture with malunion
S	sequela

- X M84.40 Pathological fracture, unspecified site
- M84.41 Pathological fracture, shoulder
  - M84.411 Pathological fracture, right shoulder
  - M84.412 Pathological fracture, left shoulder
  - M84.419 Pathological fracture, unspecified shoulder
- M84.42 Pathological fracture, humerus
  - M84.421 Pathological fracture, right humerus
  - M84.422 Pathological fracture, left humerus
  - M84.429 Pathological fracture, unspecified humerus
- M84.43 Pathological fracture, ulna and radius
  - M84.431 Pathological fracture, right ulna
  - M84.432 Pathological fracture, left ulna
  - M84.433 Pathological fracture, right radius
  - M84.434 Pathological fracture, left radius
  - M84.439 Pathological fracture, unspecified ulna and radius
- M84.44 Pathological fracture, hand and fingers
  - M84.441 Pathological fracture, right hand
  - M84.442 Pathological fracture, left hand
  - M84.443 Pathological fracture, unspecified hand
  - M84.444 Pathological fracture, right finger(s)
  - M84.445 Pathological fracture, left finger(s)
  - M84.446 Pathological fracture, unspecified finger(s)
- M84.45 Pathological fracture, femur and pelvis
  - M84.451 Pathological fracture, right femur
  - M84.452 Pathological fracture, left femur
  - M84.453 Pathological fracture, unspecified femur
  - M84.454 Pathological fracture, pelvis
  - M84.459 Pathological fracture, hip, unspecified
- M84.46 Pathological fracture, tibia and fibula
  - M84.461 Pathological fracture, right tibia
  - M84.462 Pathological fracture, left tibia
  - M84.463 Pathological fracture, right fibula
  - M84.464 Pathological fracture, left fibula
  - M84.469 Pathological fracture, unspecified tibia and fibula
- M84.47 Pathological fracture, ankle, foot and toes
  - M84.471 Pathological fracture, right ankle
  - M84.472 Pathological fracture, left ankle
  - M84.473 Pathological fracture, unspecified ankle
  - M84.474 Pathological fracture, right foot
  - M84.475 Pathological fracture, left foot
  - M84.476 Pathological fracture, unspecified foot
  - M84.477 Pathological fracture, right toe(s)
  - M84.478 Pathological fracture, left toe(s)
  - M84.479 Pathological fracture, unspecified toe(s)
- X M84.48 Pathological fracture, other site

CHAPTER 13 (MØØ-M99)

OGCR Section I.a, Chapter 13.C.

Coding of Pathologic Fractures

7th character A is for use as long as the patient is receiving active treatment for the fracture. While the patient may be seen by a new or different provider over the course of treatment for a pathological fracture, assignment of the 7th character is based on whether the patient is undergoing active treatment and not whether the provider is seeing the patient for the first time.3. 7th character, D is to be used for encounters after the patient has completed active treatment. The other 7th characters, listed under each subcategory in the Tabular List, are to be used for subsequent encounters for **routine care of fractures during the healing and recovery phase as well as** treatment of problems associated with the healing, such as malunions, nonunions, and sequelae.

Care for complications of surgical treatment for fracture repairs during the healing or recovery phase should be coded with the appropriate complication codes.

See Section I.C.19. Coding of traumatic fractures.

● **M84.5 Pathological fracture in neoplastic disease**

Code also underlying neoplasm

The appropriate 7th character is to be added to each code from subcategory M84.5:

A	initial encounter for fracture
D	subsequent encounter for fracture with routine healing
G	subsequent encounter for fracture with delayed healing
K	subsequent encounter for fracture with nonunion
P	subsequent encounter for fracture with malunion
S	sequela

X● **M84.50 Pathological fracture in neoplastic disease, unspecified site**

● **M84.51 Pathological fracture in neoplastic disease, shoulder**

● **M84.511 Pathological fracture in neoplastic disease, right shoulder**

● **M84.512 Pathological fracture in neoplastic disease, left shoulder**

● **M84.519 Pathological fracture in neoplastic disease, unspecified shoulder**

● **M84.52 Pathological fracture in neoplastic disease, humerus**

● **M84.521 Pathological fracture in neoplastic disease, right humerus**

● **M84.522 Pathological fracture in neoplastic disease, left humerus**

● **M84.529 Pathological fracture in neoplastic disease, unspecified humerus**

● **M84.53 Pathological fracture in neoplastic disease, ulna and radius**

● **M84.531 Pathological fracture in neoplastic disease, right ulna**

● **M84.532 Pathological fracture in neoplastic disease, left ulna**

● **M84.533 Pathological fracture in neoplastic disease, right radius**

● **M84.534 Pathological fracture in neoplastic disease, left radius**

● **M84.539 Pathological fracture in neoplastic disease, unspecified ulna and radius**

● **M84.54 Pathological fracture in neoplastic disease, hand**

● **M84.541 Pathological fracture in neoplastic disease, right hand**

● **M84.542 Pathological fracture in neoplastic disease, left hand**

● **M84.549 Pathological fracture in neoplastic disease, unspecified hand**

● **M84.55 Pathological fracture in neoplastic disease, pelvis and femur**

● **M84.550 Pathological fracture in neoplastic disease, pelvis**

● **M84.551 Pathological fracture in neoplastic disease, right femur**

● **M84.552 Pathological fracture in neoplastic disease, left femur**

● **M84.553 Pathological fracture in neoplastic disease, unspecified femur**

● **M84.559 Pathological fracture in neoplastic disease, hip, unspecified**

● **M84.56 Pathological fracture in neoplastic disease, tibia and fibula**

● **M84.561 Pathological fracture in neoplastic disease, right tibia**

● **M84.562 Pathological fracture in neoplastic disease, left tibia**

● **M84.563 Pathological fracture in neoplastic disease, right fibula**

● **M84.564 Pathological fracture in neoplastic disease, left fibula**

● **M84.569 Pathological fracture in neoplastic disease, unspecified tibia and fibula**

● **M84.57 Pathological fracture in neoplastic disease, ankle and foot**

● **M84.571 Pathological fracture in neoplastic disease, right ankle**

● **M84.572 Pathological fracture in neoplastic disease, left ankle**

● **M84.573 Pathological fracture in neoplastic disease, unspecified ankle**

● **M84.574 Pathological fracture in neoplastic disease, right foot**

● **M84.575 Pathological fracture in neoplastic disease, left foot**

● **M84.576 Pathological fracture in neoplastic disease, unspecified foot**

X● **M84.58 Pathological fracture in neoplastic disease, other specified site**

Pathological fracture in neoplastic disease, vertebrae

CHAPTER 13 (M00-M99)

● M84.6 Pathological fracture in other disease
Code also underlying condition
Excludes1 pathological fracture in osteoporosis (M8Ø.-)

The appropriate 7th character is to be added to each code from subcategory M84.6:

A	initial encounter for fracture
D	subsequent encounter for fracture with routine healing
G	subsequent encounter for fracture with delayed healing
K	subsequent encounter for fracture with nonunion
P	subsequent encounter for fracture with malunion
S	sequela

X● M84.6Ø Pathological fracture in other disease, unspecified site
● M84.61 Pathological fracture in other disease, shoulder
● M84.611 Pathological fracture in other disease, right shoulder
● M84.612 Pathological fracture in other disease, left shoulder
● M84.619 Pathological fracture in other disease, unspecified shoulder
● M84.62 Pathological fracture in other disease, humerus
● M84.621 Pathological fracture in other disease, right humerus
● M84.622 Pathological fracture in other disease, left humerus
● M84.629 Pathological fracture in other disease, unspecified humerus
● M84.63 Pathological fracture in other disease, ulna and radius
● M84.631 Pathological fracture in other disease, right ulna
● M84.632 Pathological fracture in other disease, left ulna
● M84.633 Pathological fracture in other disease, right radius
● M84.634 Pathological fracture in other disease, left radius
● M84.639 Pathological fracture in other disease, unspecified ulna and radius
● M84.64 Pathological fracture in other disease, hand
● M84.641 Pathological fracture in other disease, right hand
● M84.642 Pathological fracture in other disease, left hand
● M84.649 Pathological fracture in other disease, unspecified hand
● M84.65 Pathological fracture in other disease, pelvis and femur
● M84.65Ø Pathological fracture in other disease, pelvis
● M84.651 Pathological fracture in other disease, right femur
● M84.652 Pathological fracture in other disease, left femur
● M84.653 Pathological fracture in other disease, unspecified femur
● M84.659 Pathological fracture in other disease, hip, unspecified
● M84.66 Pathological fracture in other disease, tibia and fibula
● M84.661 Pathological fracture in other disease, right tibia
● M84.662 Pathological fracture in other disease, left tibia
● M84.663 Pathological fracture in other disease, right fibula
● M84.664 Pathological fracture in other disease, left fibula
● M84.669 Pathological fracture in other disease, unspecified tibia and fibula
● M84.67 Pathological fracture in other disease, ankle and foot
● M84.671 Pathological fracture in other disease, right ankle
● M84.672 Pathological fracture in other disease, left ankle
● M84.673 Pathological fracture in other disease, unspecified ankle
● M84.674 Pathological fracture in other disease, right foot
● M84.675 Pathological fracture in other disease, left foot
● M84.676 Pathological fracture in other disease, unspecified foot
X● M84.68 Pathological fracture in other disease, other site
● M84.7 Nontraumatic fracture, not elsewhere classified ◀
● M84.75 Atypical femoral fracture ◀

The appropriate 7th character is to be added to each code from M84.75: ◀

A	initial encounter for fracture ◀
D	subsequent encounter for fracture with routine healing ◀
G	subsequent encounter for fracture with delayed healing ◀
K	subsequent encounter for fracture with nonunion ◀
P	subsequent encounter for fracture with malunion ◀
S	sequela ◀

● M84.75Ø Atypical femoral fracture, unspecified ◀
● M84.751 Incomplete atypical femoral fracture, right leg ◀
● M84.752 Incomplete atypical femoral fracture, left leg ◀
● M84.753 Incomplete atypical femoral fracture, unspecified leg ◀
● M84.754 Complete transverse atypical femoral fracture, right leg ◀
● M84.755 Complete transverse atypical femoral fracture, left leg ◀
● M84.756 Complete transverse atypical femoral fracture, unspecified leg ◀
● M84.757 Complete oblique atypical femoral fracture, right leg ◀
● M84.758 Complete oblique atypical femoral fracture, left leg ◀
● M84.759 Complete oblique atypical femoral fracture, unspecified leg ◀

● M84.8 Other disorders of continuity of bone
M84.80 Other disorders of continuity of bone, unspecified site
● M84.81 Other disorders of continuity of bone, shoulder
M84.811 Other disorders of continuity of bone, right shoulder
M84.812 Other disorders of continuity of bone, left shoulder
M84.819 Other disorders of continuity of bone, unspecified shoulder
● M84.82 Other disorders of continuity of bone, humerus
M84.821 Other disorders of continuity of bone, right humerus
M84.822 Other disorders of continuity of bone, left humerus
M84.829 Other disorders of continuity of bone, unspecified humerus
● M84.83 Other disorders of continuity of bone, ulna and radius
M84.831 Other disorders of continuity of bone, right ulna
M84.832 Other disorders of continuity of bone, left ulna
M84.833 Other disorders of continuity of bone, right radius
M84.834 Other disorders of continuity of bone, left radius
M84.839 Other disorders of continuity of bone, unspecified ulna and radius
● M84.84 Other disorders of continuity of bone, hand
M84.841 Other disorders of continuity of bone, right hand
M84.842 Other disorders of continuity of bone, left hand
M84.849 Other disorders of continuity of bone, unspecified hand
● M84.85 Other disorders of continuity of bone, pelvic region and thigh
M84.851 Other disorders of continuity of bone, right pelvic region and thigh
M84.852 Other disorders of continuity of bone, left pelvic region and thigh
M84.859 Other disorders of continuity of bone, unspecified pelvic region and thigh
● M84.86 Other disorders of continuity of bone, tibia and fibula
M84.861 Other disorders of continuity of bone, right tibia
M84.862 Other disorders of continuity of bone, left tibia
M84.863 Other disorders of continuity of bone, right fibula
M84.864 Other disorders of continuity of bone, left fibula
M84.869 Other disorders of continuity of bone, unspecified tibia and fibula
● M84.87 Other disorders of continuity of bone, ankle and foot
M84.871 Other disorders of continuity of bone, right ankle and foot
M84.872 Other disorders of continuity of bone, left ankle and foot
M84.879 Other disorders of continuity of bone, unspecified ankle and foot
M84.88 Other disorders of continuity of bone, other site
M84.9 Disorder of continuity of bone, unspecified

● M85 Other disorders of bone density and structure
Excludes1 osteogenesis imperfecta (Q78.0)
osteopetrosis (Q78.2)
osteopoikilosis (Q78.8)
polyostotic fibrous dysplasia (Q78.1)
● M85.0 Fibrous dysplasia (monostotic)
Excludes2 fibrous dysplasia of jaw (M27.8)
M85.00 Fibrous dysplasia (monostotic), unspecified site
● M85.01 Fibrous dysplasia (monostotic), shoulder
M85.011 Fibrous dysplasia (monostotic), right shoulder
M85.012 Fibrous dysplasia (monostotic), left shoulder
M85.019 Fibrous dysplasia (monostotic), unspecified shoulder
● M85.02 Fibrous dysplasia (monostotic), upper arm
M85.021 Fibrous dysplasia (monostotic), right upper arm
M85.022 Fibrous dysplasia (monostotic), left upper arm
M85.029 Fibrous dysplasia (monostotic), unspecified upper arm
● M85.03 Fibrous dysplasia (monostotic), forearm
M85.031 Fibrous dysplasia (monostotic), right forearm
M85.032 Fibrous dysplasia (monostotic), left forearm
M85.039 Fibrous dysplasia (monostotic), unspecified forearm
● M85.04 Fibrous dysplasia (monostotic), hand
M85.041 Fibrous dysplasia (monostotic), right hand
M85.042 Fibrous dysplasia (monostotic), left hand
M85.049 Fibrous dysplasia (monostotic), unspecified hand
● M85.05 Fibrous dysplasia (monostotic), thigh
M85.051 Fibrous dysplasia (monostotic), right thigh
M85.052 Fibrous dysplasia (monostotic), left thigh
M85.059 Fibrous dysplasia (monostotic), unspecified thigh
● M85.06 Fibrous dysplasia (monostotic), lower leg
M85.061 Fibrous dysplasia (monostotic), right lower leg
M85.062 Fibrous dysplasia (monostotic), left lower leg
M85.069 Fibrous dysplasia (monostotic), unspecified lower leg
● M85.07 Fibrous dysplasia (monostotic), ankle and foot
M85.071 Fibrous dysplasia (monostotic), right ankle and foot
M85.072 Fibrous dysplasia (monostotic), left ankle and foot
M85.079 Fibrous dysplasia (monostotic), unspecified ankle and foot
M85.08 Fibrous dysplasia (monostotic), other site
M85.09 Fibrous dysplasia (monostotic), multiple sites
● M85.1 Skeletal fluorosis
M85.10 Skeletal fluorosis, unspecified site
● M85.11 Skeletal fluorosis, shoulder
M85.111 Skeletal fluorosis, right shoulder
M85.112 Skeletal fluorosis, left shoulder
M85.119 Skeletal fluorosis, unspecified shoulder

- M85.12 Skeletal fluorosis, upper arm
  - M85.121 Skeletal fluorosis, right upper arm
  - M85.122 Skeletal fluorosis, left upper arm
  - M85.129 Skeletal fluorosis, unspecified upper arm
- M85.13 Skeletal fluorosis, forearm
  - M85.131 Skeletal fluorosis, right forearm
  - M85.132 Skeletal fluorosis, left forearm
  - M85.139 Skeletal fluorosis, unspecified forearm
- M85.14 Skeletal fluorosis, hand
  - M85.141 Skeletal fluorosis, right hand
  - M85.142 Skeletal fluorosis, left hand
  - M85.149 Skeletal fluorosis, unspecified hand
- M85.15 Skeletal fluorosis, thigh
  - M85.151 Skeletal fluorosis, right thigh
  - M85.152 Skeletal fluorosis, left thigh
  - M85.159 Skeletal fluorosis, unspecified thigh
- M85.16 Skeletal fluorosis, lower leg
  - M85.161 Skeletal fluorosis, right lower leg
  - M85.162 Skeletal fluorosis, left lower leg
  - M85.169 Skeletal fluorosis, unspecified lower leg
- M85.17 Skeletal fluorosis, ankle and foot
  - M85.171 Skeletal fluorosis, right ankle and foot
  - M85.172 Skeletal fluorosis, left ankle and foot
  - M85.179 Skeletal fluorosis, unspecified ankle and foot
- M85.18 Skeletal fluorosis, other site
- M85.19 Skeletal fluorosis, multiple sites

M85.2 Hyperostosis of skull

M85.3 Osteitis condensans
- M85.30 Osteitis condensans, unspecified site
- M85.31 Osteitis condensans, shoulder
  - M85.311 Osteitis condensans, right shoulder
  - M85.312 Osteitis condensans, left shoulder
  - M85.319 Osteitis condensans, unspecified shoulder
- M85.32 Osteitis condensans, upper arm
  - M85.321 Osteitis condensans, right upper arm
  - M85.322 Osteitis condensans, left upper arm
  - M85.329 Osteitis condensans, unspecified upper arm
- M85.33 Osteitis condensans, forearm
  - M85.331 Osteitis condensans, right forearm
  - M85.332 Osteitis condensans, left forearm
  - M85.339 Osteitis condensans, unspecified forearm
- M85.34 Osteitis condensans, hand
  - M85.341 Osteitis condensans, right hand
  - M85.342 Osteitis condensans, left hand
  - M85.349 Osteitis condensans, unspecified hand
- M85.35 Osteitis condensans, thigh
  - M85.351 Osteitis condensans, right thigh
  - M85.352 Osteitis condensans, left thigh
  - M85.359 Osteitis condensans, unspecified thigh
- M85.36 Osteitis condensans, lower leg
  - M85.361 Osteitis condensans, right lower leg
  - M85.362 Osteitis condensans, left lower leg
  - M85.369 Osteitis condensans, unspecified lower leg
- M85.37 Osteitis condensans, ankle and foot
  - M85.371 Osteitis condensans, right ankle and foot
  - M85.372 Osteitis condensans, left ankle and foot
  - M85.379 Osteitis condensans, unspecified ankle and foot
- M85.38 Osteitis condensans, other site
- M85.39 Osteitis condensans, multiple sites

M85.4 Solitary bone cyst

Excludes2 solitary cyst of jaw (M27.4)

- M85.40 Solitary bone cyst, unspecified site
- M85.41 Solitary bone cyst, shoulder
  - M85.411 Solitary bone cyst, right shoulder
  - M85.412 Solitary bone cyst, left shoulder
  - M85.419 Solitary bone cyst, unspecified shoulder
- M85.42 Solitary bone cyst, humerus
  - M85.421 Solitary bone cyst, right humerus
  - M85.422 Solitary bone cyst, left humerus
  - M85.429 Solitary bone cyst, unspecified humerus
- M85.43 Solitary bone cyst, ulna and radius
  - M85.431 Solitary bone cyst, right ulna and radius
  - M85.432 Solitary bone cyst, left ulna and radius
  - M85.439 Solitary bone cyst, unspecified ulna and radius
- M85.44 Solitary bone cyst, hand
  - M85.441 Solitary bone cyst, right hand
  - M85.442 Solitary bone cyst, left hand
  - M85.449 Solitary bone cyst, unspecified hand
- M85.45 Solitary bone cyst, pelvis
  - M85.451 Solitary bone cyst, right pelvis
  - M85.452 Solitary bone cyst, left pelvis
  - M85.459 Solitary bone cyst, unspecified pelvis
- M85.46 Solitary bone cyst, tibia and fibula
  - M85.461 Solitary bone cyst, right tibia and fibula
  - M85.462 Solitary bone cyst, left tibia and fibula
  - M85.469 Solitary bone cyst, unspecified tibia and fibula
- M85.47 Solitary bone cyst, ankle and foot
  - M85.471 Solitary bone cyst, right ankle and foot
  - M85.472 Solitary bone cyst, left ankle and foot
  - M85.479 Solitary bone cyst, unspecified ankle and foot
- M85.48 Solitary bone cyst, other site

M85.5 Aneurysmal bone cyst

Excludes2 aneurysmal cyst of jaw (M27.4)

- M85.50 Aneurysmal bone cyst, unspecified site
- M85.51 Aneurysmal bone cyst, shoulder
  - M85.511 Aneurysmal bone cyst, right shoulder
  - M85.512 Aneurysmal bone cyst, left shoulder
  - M85.519 Aneurysmal bone cyst, unspecified shoulder
- M85.52 Aneurysmal bone cyst, upper arm
  - M85.521 Aneurysmal bone cyst, right upper arm
  - M85.522 Aneurysmal bone cyst, left upper arm
  - M85.529 Aneurysmal bone cyst, unspecified upper arm

● M85.53 Aneurysmal bone cyst, forearm
- M85.531 Aneurysmal bone cyst, right forearm
- M85.532 Aneurysmal bone cyst, left forearm
- M85.539 Aneurysmal bone cyst, unspecified forearm

● M85.54 Aneurysmal bone cyst, hand
- M85.541 Aneurysmal bone cyst, right hand
- M85.542 Aneurysmal bone cyst, left hand
- M85.549 Aneurysmal bone cyst, unspecified hand

● M85.55 Aneurysmal bone cyst, thigh
- M85.551 Aneurysmal bone cyst, right thigh
- M85.552 Aneurysmal bone cyst, left thigh
- M85.559 Aneurysmal bone cyst, unspecified thigh

● M85.56 Aneurysmal bone cyst, lower leg
- M85.561 Aneurysmal bone cyst, right lower leg
- M85.562 Aneurysmal bone cyst, left lower leg
- M85.569 Aneurysmal bone cyst, unspecified lower leg

● M85.57 Aneurysmal bone cyst, ankle and foot
- M85.571 Aneurysmal bone cyst, right ankle and foot
- M85.572 Aneurysmal bone cyst, left ankle and foot
- M85.579 Aneurysmal bone cyst, unspecified ankle and foot

M85.58 Aneurysmal bone cyst, other site

M85.59 Aneurysmal bone cyst, multiple sites

● M85.6 Other cyst of bone

Excludes1 cyst of jaw NEC (M27.4)
osteitis fibrosa cystica generalisata [von Recklinghausen's disease of bone] (E21.Ø)

M85.6Ø Other cyst of bone, unspecified site

● M85.61 Other cyst of bone, shoulder
- M85.611 Other cyst of bone, right shoulder
- M85.612 Other cyst of bone, left shoulder
- M85.619 Other cyst of bone, unspecified shoulder

● M85.62 Other cyst of bone, upper arm
- M85.621 Other cyst of bone, right upper arm
- M85.622 Other cyst of bone, left upper arm
- M85.629 Other cyst of bone, unspecified upper arm

● M85.63 Other cyst of bone, forearm
- M85.631 Other cyst of bone, right forearm
- M85.632 Other cyst of bone, left forearm
- M85.639 Other cyst of bone, unspecified forearm

● M85.64 Other cyst of bone, hand
- M85.641 Other cyst of bone, right hand
- M85.642 Other cyst of bone, left hand
- M85.649 Other cyst of bone, unspecified hand

● M85.65 Other cyst of bone, thigh
- M85.651 Other cyst of bone, right thigh
- M85.652 Other cyst of bone, left thigh
- M85.659 Other cyst of bone, unspecified thigh

● M85.66 Other cyst of bone, lower leg
- M85.661 Other cyst of bone, right lower leg
- M85.662 Other cyst of bone, left lower leg
- M85.669 Other cyst of bone, unspecified lower leg

● M85.67 Other cyst of bone, ankle and foot
- M85.671 Other cyst of bone, right ankle and foot
- M85.672 Other cyst of bone, left ankle and foot
- M85.679 Other cyst of bone, unspecified ankle and foot

M85.68 Other cyst of bone, other site

M85.69 Other cyst of bone, multiple sites

● M85.8 Other specified disorders of bone density and structure

Hyperostosis of bones, except skull
Osteosclerosis, acquired

Excludes1 diffuse idiopathic skeletal hyperostosis [DISH] (M48.1)
osteosclerosis congenita (Q77.4)
osteosclerosis fragilitas (generalista) (Q78.2)
osteosclerosis myelofibrosis (D75.81)

M85.8Ø Other specified disorders of bone density and structure, unspecified site

● M85.81 Other specified disorders of bone density and structure, shoulder
- M85.811 Other specified disorders of bone density and structure, right shoulder
- M85.812 Other specified disorders of bone density and structure, left shoulder
- M85.819 Other specified disorders of bone density and structure, unspecified shoulder

● M85.82 Other specified disorders of bone density and structure, upper arm
- M85.821 Other specified disorders of bone density and structure, right upper arm
- M85.822 Other specified disorders of bone density and structure, left upper arm
- M85.829 Other specified disorders of bone density and structure, unspecified upper arm

● M85.83 Other specified disorders of bone density and structure, forearm
- M85.831 Other specified disorders of bone density and structure, right forearm
- M85.832 Other specified disorders of bone density and structure, left forearm
- M85.839 Other specified disorders of bone density and structure, unspecified forearm

● M85.84 Other specified disorders of bone density and structure, hand
- M85.841 Other specified disorders of bone density and structure, right hand
- M85.842 Other specified disorders of bone density and structure, left hand
- M85.849 Other specified disorders of bone density and structure, unspecified hand

● M85.85 Other specified disorders of bone density and structure, thigh
- M85.851 Other specified disorders of bone density and structure, right thigh
- M85.852 Other specified disorders of bone density and structure, left thigh
- M85.859 Other specified disorders of bone density and structure, unspecified thigh

CHAPTER 13 (MØØ-M99)

● M85.86 Other specified disorders of bone density and structure, lower leg
M85.861 Other specified disorders of bone density and structure, right lower leg
M85.862 Other specified disorders of bone density and structure, left lower leg
M85.869 Other specified disorders of bone density and structure, unspecified lower leg
● M85.87 Other specified disorders of bone density and structure, ankle and foot
M85.871 Other specified disorders of bone density and structure, right ankle and foot
M85.872 Other specified disorders of bone density and structure, left ankle and foot
M85.879 Other specified disorders of bone density and structure, unspecified ankle and foot
M85.88 Other specified disorders of bone density and structure, other site
M85.89 Other specified disorders of bone density and structure, multiple sites
M85.9 Disorder of bone density and structure, unspecified

OTHER OSTEOPATHIES (M86-M9Ø)

Excludes1 postprocedural osteopathies (M96.-)

● M86 Osteomyelitis
Use additional code (B95-B97) to identify infectious agent
Use additional code to identify major osseous defect, if applicable (M89.7-)
Excludes1 osteomyelitis due to:
echinococcus (B67.2)
gonococcus (A54.43)
salmonella (AØ2.24)
Excludes2 ostemyelitis of:
orbit (HØ5.Ø-)
petrous bone (H7Ø.2-)
vertebra (M46.2-)

● M86.Ø Acute hematogenous osteomyelitis
M86.ØØ Acute hematogenous osteomyelitis, unspecified site
● M86.Ø1 Acute hematogenous osteomyelitis, shoulder
M86.Ø11 Acute hematogenous osteomyelitis, right shoulder
M86.Ø12 Acute hematogenous osteomyelitis, left shoulder
M86.Ø19 Acute hematogenous osteomyelitis, unspecified shoulder
● M86.Ø2 Acute hematogenous osteomyelitis, humerus
M86.Ø21 Acute hematogenous osteomyelitis, right humerus
M86.Ø22 Acute hematogenous osteomyelitis, left humerus
M86.Ø29 Acute hematogenous osteomyelitis, unspecified humerus
● M86.Ø3 Acute hematogenous osteomyelitis, radius and ulna
M86.Ø31 Acute hematogenous osteomyelitis, right radius and ulna
M86.Ø32 Acute hematogenous osteomyelitis, left radius and ulna
M86.Ø39 Acute hematogenous osteomyelitis, unspecified radius and ulna

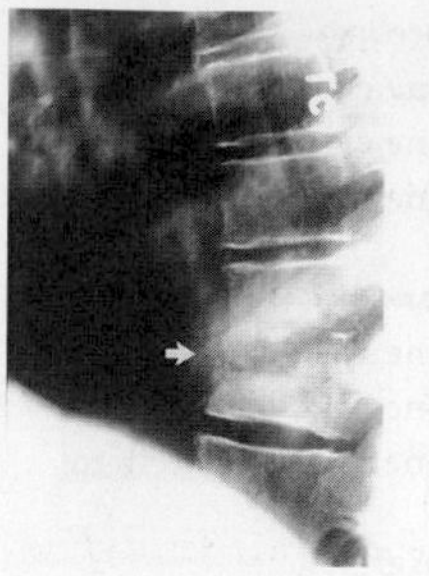

Figure 13-6 Osteomyelitis of the spine. A lateral view of the lower thoracic spine demonstrates destruction of the disk space *(arrow)* as well as destruction of the adjoining vertebral bodies. (From Mettler: Essentials of Radiology, ed 2, Saunders, An Imprint of Elsevier, 2005)

Item 13-12 Osteomyelitis is an inflammation of the bone. **Acute osteomyelitis** is a rapidly destructive, pus-producing infection capable of causing severe bone destruction. **Chronic osteomyelitis** can remain long after the initial acute episode has passed and may lead to a recurrence of the acute phase. **Brodie's abscess** is an encapsulated focal abscess that must be surgically drained. Periostitis is an inflammation of the periosteum, a dense membrane composed of fibrous connective tissue that closely wraps all bone, except those with articulating surfaces in joints, which are covered by synovial membranes.

● M86.Ø4 Acute hematogenous osteomyelitis, hand
M86.Ø41 Acute hematogenous osteomyelitis, right hand
M86.Ø42 Acute hematogenous osteomyelitis, left hand
M86.Ø49 Acute hematogenous osteomyelitis, unspecified hand
● M86.Ø5 Acute hematogenous osteomyelitis, femur
M86.Ø51 Acute hematogenous osteomyelitis, right femur
M86.Ø52 Acute hematogenous osteomyelitis, left femur
M86.Ø59 Acute hematogenous osteomyelitis, unspecified femur
● M86.Ø6 Acute hematogenous osteomyelitis, tibia and fibula
M86.Ø61 Acute hematogenous osteomyelitis, right tibia and fibula
M86.Ø62 Acute hematogenous osteomyelitis, left tibia and fibula
M86.Ø69 Acute hematogenous osteomyelitis, unspecified tibia and fibula
● M86.Ø7 Acute hematogenous osteomyelitis, ankle and foot
M86.Ø71 Acute hematogenous osteomyelitis, right ankle and foot
M86.Ø72 Acute hematogenous osteomyelitis, left ankle and foot
M86.Ø79 Acute hematogenous osteomyelitis, unspecified ankle and foot
M86.Ø8 Acute hematogenous osteomyelitis, other sites
M86.Ø9 Acute hematogenous osteomyelitis, multiple sites
● M86.1 Other acute osteomyelitis
M86.1Ø Other acute osteomyelitis, unspecified site
● M86.11 Other acute osteomyelitis, shoulder
M86.111 Other acute osteomyelitis, right shoulder
M86.112 Other acute osteomyelitis, left shoulder
M86.119 Other acute osteomyelitis, unspecified shoulder

CHAPTER 13 (MØØ-M99)

● M86.12 Other acute osteomyelitis, humerus
M86.121 Other acute osteomyelitis, right humerus
M86.122 Other acute osteomyelitis, left humerus
M86.129 Other acute osteomyelitis, unspecified humerus
● M86.13 Other acute osteomyelitis, radius and ulna
M86.131 Other acute osteomyelitis, right radius and ulna
M86.132 Other acute osteomyelitis, left radius and ulna
M86.139 Other acute osteomyelitis, unspecified radius and ulna
● M86.14 Other acute osteomyelitis, hand
M86.141 Other acute osteomyelitis, right hand
M86.142 Other acute osteomyelitis, left hand
M86.149 Other acute osteomyelitis, unspecified hand
● M86.15 Other acute osteomyelitis, femur
M86.151 Other acute osteomyelitis, right femur
M86.152 Other acute osteomyelitis, left femur
M86.159 Other acute osteomyelitis, unspecified femur
● M86.16 Other acute osteomyelitis, tibia and fibula
M86.161 Other acute osteomyelitis, right tibia and fibula
M86.162 Other acute osteomyelitis, left tibia and fibula
M86.169 Other acute osteomyelitis, unspecified tibia and fibula
● M86.17 Other acute osteomyelitis, ankle and foot
M86.171 Other acute osteomyelitis, right ankle and foot
M86.172 Other acute osteomyelitis, left ankle and foot
M86.179 Other acute osteomyelitis, unspecified ankle and foot
M86.18 Other acute osteomyelitis, other site
M86.19 Other acute osteomyelitis, multiple sites
● M86.2 Subacute osteomyelitis
M86.20 Subacute osteomyelitis, unspecified site
● M86.21 Subacute osteomyelitis, shoulder
M86.211 Subacute osteomyelitis, right shoulder
M86.212 Subacute osteomyelitis, left shoulder
M86.219 Subacute osteomyelitis, unspecified shoulder
● M86.22 Subacute osteomyelitis, humerus
M86.221 Subacute osteomyelitis, right humerus
M86.222 Subacute osteomyelitis, left humerus
M86.229 Subacute osteomyelitis, unspecified humerus
● M86.23 Subacute osteomyelitis, radius and ulna
M86.231 Subacute osteomyelitis, right radius and ulna
M86.232 Subacute osteomyelitis, left radius and ulna
M86.239 Subacute osteomyelitis, unspecified radius and ulna
● M86.24 Subacute osteomyelitis, hand
M86.241 Subacute osteomyelitis, right hand
M86.242 Subacute osteomyelitis, left hand
M86.249 Subacute osteomyelitis, unspecified hand
● M86.25 Subacute osteomyelitis, femur
M86.251 Subacute osteomyelitis, right femur
M86.252 Subacute osteomyelitis, left femur
M86.259 Subacute osteomyelitis, unspecified femur
● M86.26 Subacute osteomyelitis, tibia and fibula
M86.261 Subacute osteomyelitis, right tibia and fibula
M86.262 Subacute osteomyelitis, left tibia and fibula
M86.269 Subacute osteomyelitis, unspecified tibia and fibula
● M86.27 Subacute osteomyelitis, ankle and foot
M86.271 Subacute osteomyelitis, right ankle and foot
M86.272 Subacute osteomyelitis, left ankle and foot
M86.279 Subacute osteomyelitis, unspecified ankle and foot
M86.28 Subacute osteomyelitis, other site
M86.29 Subacute osteomyelitis, multiple sites
● M86.3 Chronic multifocal osteomyelitis
M86.30 Chronic multifocal osteomyelitis, unspecified site
● M86.31 Chronic multifocal osteomyelitis, shoulder
M86.311 Chronic multifocal osteomyelitis, right shoulder
M86.312 Chronic multifocal osteomyelitis, left shoulder
M86.319 Chronic multifocal osteomyelitis, unspecified shoulder
● M86.32 Chronic multifocal osteomyelitis, humerus
M86.321 Chronic multifocal osteomyelitis, right humerus
M86.322 Chronic multifocal osteomyelitis, left humerus
M86.329 Chronic multifocal osteomyelitis, unspecified humerus
● M86.33 Chronic multifocal osteomyelitis, radius and ulna
M86.331 Chronic multifocal osteomyelitis, right radius and ulna
M86.332 Chronic multifocal osteomyelitis, left radius and ulna
M86.339 Chronic multifocal osteomyelitis, unspecified radius and ulna
● M86.34 Chronic multifocal osteomyelitis, hand
M86.341 Chronic multifocal osteomyelitis, right hand
M86.342 Chronic multifocal osteomyelitis, left hand
M86.349 Chronic multifocal osteomyelitis, unspecified hand
● M86.35 Chronic multifocal osteomyelitis, femur
M86.351 Chronic multifocal osteomyelitis, right femur
M86.352 Chronic multifocal osteomyelitis, left femur
M86.359 Chronic multifocal osteomyelitis, unspecified femur
● M86.36 Chronic multifocal osteomyelitis, tibia and fibula
M86.361 Chronic multifocal osteomyelitis, right tibia and fibula
M86.362 Chronic multifocal osteomyelitis, left tibia and fibula
M86.369 Chronic multifocal osteomyelitis, unspecified tibia and fibula

- ● M86.37 Chronic multifocal osteomyelitis, ankle and foot
  - M86.371 Chronic multifocal osteomyelitis, right ankle and foot
  - M86.372 Chronic multifocal osteomyelitis, left ankle and foot
  - M86.379 Chronic multifocal osteomyelitis, unspecified ankle and foot
- M86.38 Chronic multifocal osteomyelitis, other site
- M86.39 Chronic multifocal osteomyelitis, multiple sites

● M86.4 Chronic osteomyelitis with draining sinus
- M86.40 Chronic osteomyelitis with draining sinus, unspecified site
- ● M86.41 Chronic osteomyelitis with draining sinus, shoulder
  - M86.411 Chronic osteomyelitis with draining sinus, right shoulder
  - M86.412 Chronic osteomyelitis with draining sinus, left shoulder
  - M86.419 Chronic osteomyelitis with draining sinus, unspecified shoulder
- ● M86.42 Chronic osteomyelitis with draining sinus, humerus
  - M86.421 Chronic osteomyelitis with draining sinus, right humerus
  - M86.422 Chronic osteomyelitis with draining sinus, left humerus
  - M86.429 Chronic osteomyelitis with draining sinus, unspecified humerus
- ● M86.43 Chronic osteomyelitis with draining sinus, radius and ulna
  - M86.431 Chronic osteomyelitis with draining sinus, right radius and ulna
  - M86.432 Chronic osteomyelitis with draining sinus, left radius and ulna
  - M86.439 Chronic osteomyelitis with draining sinus, unspecified radius and ulna
- ● M86.44 Chronic osteomyelitis with draining sinus, hand
  - M86.441 Chronic osteomyelitis with draining sinus, right hand
  - M86.442 Chronic osteomyelitis with draining sinus, left hand
  - M86.449 Chronic osteomyelitis with draining sinus, unspecified hand
- ● M86.45 Chronic osteomyelitis with draining sinus, femur
  - M86.451 Chronic osteomyelitis with draining sinus, right femur
  - M86.452 Chronic osteomyelitis with draining sinus, left femur
  - M86.459 Chronic osteomyelitis with draining sinus, unspecified femur
- ● M86.46 Chronic osteomyelitis with draining sinus, tibia and fibula
  - M86.461 Chronic osteomyelitis with draining sinus, right tibia and fibula
  - M86.462 Chronic osteomyelitis with draining sinus, left tibia and fibula
  - M86.469 Chronic osteomyelitis with draining sinus, unspecified tibia and fibula
- ● M86.47 Chronic osteomyelitis with draining sinus, ankle and foot
  - M86.471 Chronic osteomyelitis with draining sinus, right ankle and foot
  - M86.472 Chronic osteomyelitis with draining sinus, left ankle and foot
  - M86.479 Chronic osteomyelitis with draining sinus, unspecified ankle and foot
- M86.48 Chronic osteomyelitis with draining sinus, other site
- M86.49 Chronic osteomyelitis with draining sinus, multiple sites

● M86.5 Other chronic hematogenous osteomyelitis
- M86.50 Other chronic hematogenous osteomyelitis, unspecified site
- ● M86.51 Other chronic hematogenous osteomyelitis, shoulder
  - M86.511 Other chronic hematogenous osteomyelitis, right shoulder
  - M86.512 Other chronic hematogenous osteomyelitis, left shoulder
  - M86.519 Other chronic hematogenous osteomyelitis, unspecified shoulder
- ● M86.52 Other chronic hematogenous osteomyelitis, humerus
  - M86.521 Other chronic hematogenous osteomyelitis, right humerus
  - M86.522 Other chronic hematogenous osteomyelitis, left humerus
  - M86.529 Other chronic hematogenous osteomyelitis, unspecified humerus
- ● M86.53 Other chronic hematogenous osteomyelitis, radius and ulna
  - M86.531 Other chronic hematogenous osteomyelitis, right radius and ulna
  - M86.532 Other chronic hematogenous osteomyelitis, left radius and ulna
  - M86.539 Other chronic hematogenous osteomyelitis, unspecified radius and ulna
- ● M86.54 Other chronic hematogenous osteomyelitis, hand
  - M86.541 Other chronic hematogenous osteomyelitis, right hand
  - M86.542 Other chronic hematogenous osteomyelitis, left hand
  - M86.549 Other chronic hematogenous osteomyelitis, unspecified hand
- ● M86.55 Other chronic hematogenous osteomyelitis, femur
  - M86.551 Other chronic hematogenous osteomyelitis, right femur
  - M86.552 Other chronic hematogenous osteomyelitis, left femur
  - M86.559 Other chronic hematogenous osteomyelitis, unspecified femur
- ● M86.56 Other chronic hematogenous osteomyelitis, tibia and fibula
  - M86.561 Other chronic hematogenous osteomyelitis, right tibia and fibula
  - M86.562 Other chronic hematogenous osteomyelitis, left tibia and fibula
  - M86.569 Other chronic hematogenous osteomyelitis, unspecified tibia and fibula
- ● M86.57 Other chronic hematogenous osteomyelitis, ankle and foot
  - M86.571 Other chronic hematogenous osteomyelitis, right ankle and foot
  - M86.572 Other chronic hematogenous osteomyelitis, left ankle and foot
  - M86.579 Other chronic hematogenous osteomyelitis, unspecified ankle and foot
- M86.58 Other chronic hematogenous osteomyelitis, other site
- M86.59 Other chronic hematogenous osteomyelitis, multiple sites

● M86.6 Other chronic osteomyelitis
M86.60 Other chronic osteomyelitis, unspecified site
● M86.61 Other chronic osteomyelitis, shoulder
M86.611 Other chronic osteomyelitis, right shoulder
M86.612 Other chronic osteomyelitis, left shoulder
M86.619 Other chronic osteomyelitis, unspecified shoulder
● M86.62 Other chronic osteomyelitis, humerus
M86.621 Other chronic osteomyelitis, right humerus
M86.622 Other chronic osteomyelitis, left humerus
M86.629 Other chronic osteomyelitis, unspecified humerus
● M86.63 Other chronic osteomyelitis, radius and ulna
M86.631 Other chronic osteomyelitis, right radius and ulna
M86.632 Other chronic osteomyelitis, left radius and ulna
M86.639 Other chronic osteomyelitis, unspecified radius and ulna
● M86.64 Other chronic osteomyelitis, hand
M86.641 Other chronic osteomyelitis, right hand
M86.642 Other chronic osteomyelitis, left hand
M86.649 Other chronic osteomyelitis, unspecified hand
● M86.65 Other chronic osteomyelitis, thigh
M86.651 Other chronic osteomyelitis, right thigh
M86.652 Other chronic osteomyelitis, left thigh
M86.659 Other chronic osteomyelitis, unspecified thigh
● M86.66 Other chronic osteomyelitis, tibia and fibula
M86.661 Other chronic osteomyelitis, right tibia and fibula
M86.662 Other chronic osteomyelitis, left tibia and fibula
M86.669 Other chronic osteomyelitis, unspecified tibia and fibula
● M86.67 Other chronic osteomyelitis, ankle and foot
M86.671 Other chronic osteomyelitis, right ankle and foot
M86.672 Other chronic osteomyelitis, left ankle and foot
M86.679 Other chronic osteomyelitis, unspecified ankle and foot
M86.68 Other chronic osteomyelitis, other site
M86.69 Other chronic osteomyelitis, multiple sites
● M86.8 Other osteomyelitis
Brodie's abscess
● M86.8X Other osteomyelitis
M86.8X0 Other osteomyelitis, multiple sites
M86.8X1 Other osteomyelitis, shoulder
M86.8X2 Other osteomyelitis, upper arm
M86.8X3 Other osteomyelitis, forearm
M86.8X4 Other osteomyelitis, hand
M86.8X5 Other osteomyelitis, thigh
M86.8X6 Other osteomyelitis, lower leg
M86.8X7 Other osteomyelitis, ankle and foot
M86.8X8 Other osteomyelitis, other site
M86.8X9 Other osteomyelitis, unspecified sites
M86.9 Osteomyelitis, unspecified
Infection of bone NOS
Periostitis without osteomyelitis

● M87 Osteonecrosis
Includes avascular necrosis of bone
Use additional code to identify major osseous defect, if applicable (M89.7-)
Excludes1 juvenile osteonecrosis (M91-M92)
osteochondropathies (M90-M93)
● M87.0 Idiopathic aseptic necrosis of bone
M87.00 Idiopathic aseptic necrosis of unspecified bone
● M87.01 Idiopathic aseptic necrosis of shoulder
Idiopathic aseptic necrosis of clavicle and scapula
M87.011 Idiopathic aseptic necrosis of right shoulder
M87.012 Idiopathic aseptic necrosis of left shoulder
M87.019 Idiopathic aseptic necrosis of unspecified shoulder
● M87.02 Idiopathic aseptic necrosis of humerus
M87.021 Idiopathic aseptic necrosis of right humerus
M87.022 Idiopathic aseptic necrosis of left humerus
M87.029 Idiopathic aseptic necrosis of unspecified humerus
● M87.03 Idiopathic aseptic necrosis of radius, ulna and carpus
M87.031 Idiopathic aseptic necrosis of right radius
M87.032 Idiopathic aseptic necrosis of left radius
M87.033 Idiopathic aseptic necrosis of unspecified radius
M87.034 Idiopathic aseptic necrosis of right ulna
M87.035 Idiopathic aseptic necrosis of left ulna
M87.036 Idiopathic aseptic necrosis of unspecified ulna
M87.037 Idiopathic aseptic necrosis of right carpus
M87.038 Idiopathic aseptic necrosis of left carpus
M87.039 Idiopathic aseptic necrosis of unspecified carpus
● M87.04 Idiopathic aseptic necrosis of hand and fingers
Idiopathic aseptic necrosis of metacarpals and phalanges of hands
M87.041 Idiopathic aseptic necrosis of right hand
M87.042 Idiopathic aseptic necrosis of left hand
M87.043 Idiopathic aseptic necrosis of unspecified hand
M87.044 Idiopathic aseptic necrosis of right finger(s)
M87.045 Idiopathic aseptic necrosis of left finger(s)
M87.046 Idiopathic aseptic necrosis of unspecified finger(s)
● M87.05 Idiopathic aseptic necrosis of pelvis and femur
M87.050 Idiopathic aseptic necrosis of pelvis
M87.051 Idiopathic aseptic necrosis of right femur
M87.052 Idiopathic aseptic necrosis of left femur
M87.059 Idiopathic aseptic necrosis of unspecified femur
Idiopathic aseptic necrosis of hip NOS

CHAPTER 13 (M00-M99)

● M87.06 Idiopathic aseptic necrosis of tibia and fibula
M87.061 Idiopathic aseptic necrosis of right tibia
M87.062 Idiopathic aseptic necrosis of left tibia
M87.063 Idiopathic aseptic necrosis of unspecified tibia
M87.064 Idiopathic aseptic necrosis of right fibula
M87.065 Idiopathic aseptic necrosis of left fibula
M87.066 Idiopathic aseptic necrosis of unspecified fibula
● M87.07 Idiopathic aseptic necrosis of ankle, foot and toes
Idiopathic aseptic necrosis of metatarsus, tarsus, and phalanges of toes
M87.071 Idiopathic aseptic necrosis of right ankle
M87.072 Idiopathic aseptic necrosis of left ankle
M87.073 Idiopathic aseptic necrosis of unspecified ankle
M87.074 Idiopathic aseptic necrosis of right foot
M87.075 Idiopathic aseptic necrosis of left foot
M87.076 Idiopathic aseptic necrosis of unspecified foot
M87.077 Idiopathic aseptic necrosis of right toe(s)
M87.078 Idiopathic aseptic necrosis of left toe(s)
M87.079 Idiopathic aseptic necrosis of unspecified toe(s)
M87.08 Idiopathic aseptic necrosis of bone, other site
M87.09 Idiopathic aseptic necrosis of bone, multiple sites
● M87.1 Osteonecrosis due to drugs
Use additional code for adverse effect, if applicable, to identify drug (T36-T50 with fifth or sixth character 5)
M87.10 Osteonecrosis due to drugs, unspecified bone
● M87.11 Osteonecrosis due to drugs, shoulder
M87.111 Osteonecrosis due to drugs, right shoulder
M87.112 Osteonecrosis due to drugs, left shoulder
M87.119 Osteonecrosis due to drugs, unspecified shoulder
● M87.12 Osteonecrosis due to drugs, humerus
M87.121 Osteonecrosis due to drugs, right humerus
M87.122 Osteonecrosis due to drugs, left humerus
M87.129 Osteonecrosis due to drugs, unspecified humerus
● M87.13 Osteonecrosis due to drugs of radius, ulna and carpus
M87.131 Osteonecrosis due to drugs of right radius
M87.132 Osteonecrosis due to drugs of left radius
M87.133 Osteonecrosis due to drugs of unspecified radius
M87.134 Osteonecrosis due to drugs of right ulna
M87.135 Osteonecrosis due to drugs of left ulna
M87.136 Osteonecrosis due to drugs of unspecified ulna
M87.137 Osteonecrosis due to drugs of right carpus
M87.138 Osteonecrosis due to drugs of left carpus
M87.139 Osteonecrosis due to drugs of unspecified carpus
● M87.14 Osteonecrosis due to drugs, hand and fingers
M87.141 Osteonecrosis due to drugs, right hand
M87.142 Osteonecrosis due to drugs, left hand
M87.143 Osteonecrosis due to drugs, unspecified hand
M87.144 Osteonecrosis due to drugs, right finger(s)
M87.145 Osteonecrosis due to drugs, left finger(s)
M87.146 Osteonecrosis due to drugs, unspecified finger(s)
● M87.15 Osteonecrosis due to drugs, pelvis and femur
M87.150 Osteonecrosis due to drugs, pelvis
M87.151 Osteonecrosis due to drugs, right femur
M87.152 Osteonecrosis due to drugs, left femur
M87.159 Osteonecrosis due to drugs, unspecified femur
● M87.16 Osteonecrosis due to drugs, tibia and fibula
M87.161 Osteonecrosis due to drugs, right tibia
M87.162 Osteonecrosis due to drugs, left tibia
M87.163 Osteonecrosis due to drugs, unspecified tibia
M87.164 Osteonecrosis due to drugs, right fibula
M87.165 Osteonecrosis due to drugs, left fibula
M87.166 Osteonecrosis due to drugs, unspecified fibula
● M87.17 Osteonecrosis due to drugs, ankle, foot and toes
M87.171 Osteonecrosis due to drugs, right ankle
M87.172 Osteonecrosis due to drugs, left ankle
M87.173 Osteonecrosis due to drugs, unspecified ankle
M87.174 Osteonecrosis due to drugs, right foot
M87.175 Osteonecrosis due to drugs, left foot
M87.176 Osteonecrosis due to drugs, unspecified foot
M87.177 Osteonecrosis due to drugs, right toe(s)
M87.178 Osteonecrosis due to drugs, left toe(s)
M87.179 Osteonecrosis due to drugs, unspecified toe(s)
● M87.18 Osteonecrosis due to drugs, other site
M87.180 Osteonecrosis due to drugs, jaw
M87.188 Osteonecrosis due to drugs, other site
M87.19 Osteonecrosis due to drugs, multiple sites
● M87.2 Osteonecrosis due to previous trauma
M87.20 Osteonecrosis due to previous trauma, unspecified bone
● M87.21 Osteonecrosis due to previous trauma, shoulder
M87.211 Osteonecrosis due to previous trauma, right shoulder
M87.212 Osteonecrosis due to previous trauma, left shoulder
M87.219 Osteonecrosis due to previous trauma, unspecified shoulder

CHAPTER 13 (M00-M99)

● M87.22 Osteonecrosis due to previous trauma, humerus
M87.221 Osteonecrosis due to previous trauma, right humerus
M87.222 Osteonecrosis due to previous trauma, left humerus
M87.229 Osteonecrosis due to previous trauma, unspecified humerus
● M87.23 Osteonecrosis due to previous trauma of radius, ulna and carpus
M87.231 Osteonecrosis due to previous trauma of right radius
M87.232 Osteonecrosis due to previous trauma of left radius
M87.233 Osteonecrosis due to previous trauma of unspecified radius
M87.234 Osteonecrosis due to previous trauma of right ulna
M87.235 Osteonecrosis due to previous trauma of left ulna
M87.236 Osteonecrosis due to previous trauma of unspecified ulna
M87.237 Osteonecrosis due to previous trauma of right carpus
M87.238 Osteonecrosis due to previous trauma of left carpus
M87.239 Osteonecrosis due to previous trauma of unspecified carpus
● M87.24 Osteonecrosis due to previous trauma, hand and fingers
M87.241 Osteonecrosis due to previous trauma, right hand
M87.242 Osteonecrosis due to previous trauma, left hand
M87.243 Osteonecrosis due to previous trauma, unspecified hand
M87.244 Osteonecrosis due to previous trauma, right finger(s)
M87.245 Osteonecrosis due to previous trauma, left finger(s)
M87.246 Osteonecrosis due to previous trauma, unspecified finger(s)
● M87.25 Osteonecrosis due to previous trauma, pelvis and femur
M87.250 Osteonecrosis due to previous trauma, pelvis
M87.251 Osteonecrosis due to previous trauma, right femur
M87.252 Osteonecrosis due to previous trauma, left femur
M87.256 Osteonecrosis due to previous trauma, unspecified femur
● M87.26 Osteonecrosis due to previous trauma, tibia and fibula
M87.261 Osteonecrosis due to previous trauma, right tibia
M87.262 Osteonecrosis due to previous trauma, left tibia
M87.263 Osteonecrosis due to previous trauma, unspecified tibia
M87.264 Osteonecrosis due to previous trauma, right fibula
M87.265 Osteonecrosis due to previous trauma, left fibula
M87.266 Osteonecrosis due to previous trauma, unspecified fibula
● M87.27 Osteonecrosis due to previous trauma, ankle, foot and toes
M87.271 Osteonecrosis due to previous trauma, right ankle
M87.272 Osteonecrosis due to previous trauma, left ankle
M87.273 Osteonecrosis due to previous trauma, unspecified ankle
M87.274 Osteonecrosis due to previous trauma, right foot
M87.275 Osteonecrosis due to previous trauma, left foot
M87.276 Osteonecrosis due to previous trauma, unspecified foot
M87.277 Osteonecrosis due to previous trauma, right toe(s)
M87.278 Osteonecrosis due to previous trauma, left toe(s)
M87.279 Osteonecrosis due to previous trauma, unspecified toe(s)
M87.28 Osteonecrosis due to previous trauma, other site
M87.29 Osteonecrosis due to previous trauma, multiple sites
● M87.3 Other secondary osteonecrosis
M87.30 Other secondary osteonecrosis, unspecified bone
● M87.31 Other secondary osteonecrosis, shoulder
M87.311 Other secondary osteonecrosis, right shoulder
M87.312 Other secondary osteonecrosis, left shoulder
M87.319 Other secondary osteonecrosis, unspecified shoulder
● M87.32 Other secondary osteonecrosis, humerus
M87.321 Other secondary osteonecrosis, right humerus
M87.322 Other secondary osteonecrosis, left humerus
M87.329 Other secondary osteonecrosis, unspecified humerus
● M87.33 Other secondary osteonecrosis of radius, ulna and carpus
M87.331 Other secondary osteonecrosis of right radius
M87.332 Other secondary osteonecrosis of left radius
M87.333 Other secondary osteonecrosis of unspecified radius
M87.334 Other secondary osteonecrosis of right ulna
M87.335 Other secondary osteonecrosis of left ulna
M87.336 Other secondary osteonecrosis of unspecified ulna
M87.337 Other secondary osteonecrosis of right carpus
M87.338 Other secondary osteonecrosis of left carpus
M87.339 Other secondary osteonecrosis of unspecified carpus

● M87.34 Other secondary osteonecrosis, hand and fingers
M87.341 Other secondary osteonecrosis, right hand
M87.342 Other secondary osteonecrosis, left hand
M87.343 Other secondary osteonecrosis, unspecified hand
M87.344 Other secondary osteonecrosis, right finger(s)
M87.345 Other secondary osteonecrosis, left finger(s)
M87.346 Other secondary osteonecrosis, unspecified finger(s)

● M87.35 Other secondary osteonecrosis, pelvis and femur
M87.350 Other secondary osteonecrosis, pelvis
M87.351 Other secondary osteonecrosis, right femur
M87.352 Other secondary osteonecrosis, left femur
M87.353 Other secondary osteonecrosis, unspecified femur

● M87.36 Other secondary osteonecrosis, tibia and fibula
M87.361 Other secondary osteonecrosis, right tibia
M87.362 Other secondary osteonecrosis, left tibia
M87.363 Other secondary osteonecrosis, unspecified tibia
M87.364 Other secondary osteonecrosis, right fibula
M87.365 Other secondary osteonecrosis, left fibula
M87.366 Other secondary osteonecrosis, unspecified fibula

● M87.37 Other secondary osteonecrosis, ankle and foot
M87.371 Other secondary osteonecrosis, right ankle
M87.372 Other secondary osteonecrosis, left ankle
M87.373 Other secondary osteonecrosis, unspecified ankle
M87.374 Other secondary osteonecrosis, right foot
M87.375 Other secondary osteonecrosis, left foot
M87.376 Other secondary osteonecrosis, unspecified foot
M87.377 Other secondary osteonecrosis, right toe(s)
M87.378 Other secondary osteonecrosis, left toe(s)
M87.379 Other secondary osteonecrosis, unspecified toe(s)

M87.38 Other secondary osteonecrosis, other site
M87.39 Other secondary osteonecrosis, multiple sites

● M87.8 Other osteonecrosis
M87.80 Other osteonecrosis, unspecified bone

● M87.81 Other osteonecrosis, shoulder
M87.811 Other osteonecrosis, right shoulder
M87.812 Other osteonecrosis, left shoulder
M87.819 Other osteonecrosis, unspecified shoulder

● M87.82 Other osteonecrosis, humerus
M87.821 Other osteonecrosis, right humerus
M87.822 Other osteonecrosis, left humerus
M87.829 Other osteonecrosis, unspecified humerus

● M87.83 Other osteonecrosis of radius, ulna and carpus
M87.831 Other osteonecrosis of right radius
M87.832 Other osteonecrosis of left radius
M87.833 Other osteonecrosis of unspecified radius
M87.834 Other osteonecrosis of right ulna
M87.835 Other osteonecrosis of left ulna
M87.836 Other osteonecrosis of unspecified ulna
M87.837 Other osteonecrosis of right carpus
M87.838 Other osteonecrosis of left carpus
M87.839 Other osteonecrosis of unspecified carpus

● M87.84 Other osteonecrosis, hand and fingers
M87.841 Other osteonecrosis, right hand
M87.842 Other osteonecrosis, left hand
M87.843 Other osteonecrosis, unspecified hand
M87.844 Other osteonecrosis, right finger(s)
M87.845 Other osteonecrosis, left finger(s)
M87.849 Other osteonecrosis, unspecified finger(s)

● M87.85 Other osteonecrosis, pelvis and femur
M87.850 Other osteonecrosis, pelvis
M87.851 Other osteonecrosis, right femur
M87.852 Other osteonecrosis, left femur
M87.859 Other osteonecrosis, unspecified femur

● M87.86 Other osteonecrosis, tibia and fibula
M87.861 Other osteonecrosis, right tibia
M87.862 Other osteonecrosis, left tibia
M87.863 Other osteonecrosis, unspecified tibia
M87.864 Other osteonecrosis, right fibula
M87.865 Other osteonecrosis, left fibula
M87.869 Other osteonecrosis, unspecified fibula

● M87.87 Other osteonecrosis, ankle, foot and toes
M87.871 Other osteonecrosis, right ankle
M87.872 Other osteonecrosis, left ankle
M87.873 Other osteonecrosis, unspecified ankle
M87.874 Other osteonecrosis, right foot
M87.875 Other osteonecrosis, left foot
M87.876 Other osteonecrosis, unspecified foot
M87.877 Other osteonecrosis, right toe(s)
M87.878 Other osteonecrosis, left toe(s)
M87.879 Other osteonecrosis, unspecified toe(s)

M87.88 Other osteonecrosis, other site
M87.89 Other osteonecrosis, multiple sites

M87.9 Osteonecrosis, unspecified
Necrosis of bone NOS

● **M88 Osteitis deformans [Paget's disease of bone]**
Chronic disorder that results in enlarged and deformed bones. The excessive breakdown and formation of bone tissue causes bones to weaken and results in bone pain, arthritis, deformities, and fractures.
Excludes1 osteitis deformans in neoplastic disease (M90.6)

M88.0 Osteitis deformans of skull
M88.1 Osteitis deformans of vertebrae
● **M88.8 Osteitis deformans of other bones**
● **M88.81 Osteitis deformans of shoulder**
M88.811 Osteitis deformans of right shoulder
M88.812 Osteitis deformans of left shoulder
M88.819 Osteitis deformans of unspecified shoulder
● **M88.82 Osteitis deformans of upper arm**
M88.821 Osteitis deformans of right upper arm
M88.822 Osteitis deformans of left upper arm
M88.829 Osteitis deformans of unspecified upper arm
● **M88.83 Osteitis deformans of forearm**
M88.831 Osteitis deformans of right forearm
M88.832 Osteitis deformans of left forearm
M88.839 Osteitis deformans of unspecified forearm
● **M88.84 Osteitis deformans of hand**
M88.841 Osteitis deformans of right hand
M88.842 Osteitis deformans of left hand
M88.849 Osteitis deformans of unspecified hand
● **M88.85 Osteitis deformans of thigh**
M88.851 Osteitis deformans of right thigh
M88.852 Osteitis deformans of left thigh
M88.859 Osteitis deformans of unspecified thigh
● **M88.86 Osteitis deformans of lower leg**
M88.861 Osteitis deformans of right lower leg
M88.862 Osteitis deformans of left lower leg
M88.869 Osteitis deformans of unspecified lower leg
● **M88.87 Osteitis deformans of ankle and foot**
M88.871 Osteitis deformans of right ankle and foot
M88.872 Osteitis deformans of left ankle and foot
M88.879 Osteitis deformans of unspecified ankle and foot
M88.88 Osteitis deformans of other bones
Excludes2 osteitis deformans of skull (M88.0)
osteitis deformans of vertebrae (M88.1)
M88.89 Osteitis deformans of multiple sites
M88.9 Osteitis deformans of unspecified bone

● **M89 Other disorders of bone**
● **M89.0 Algoneurodystrophy**
Shoulder-hand syndrome
Sudeck's atrophy
Excludes1 causalgia, lower limb (G57.7-)
causalgia, upper limb (G56.4-)
complex regional pain syndrome II, lower limb (G57.7-)
complex regional pain syndrome II, upper limb (G56.4-)
reflex sympathetic dystrophy (G90.5-)

M89.00 Algoneurodystrophy, unspecified site
● **M89.01 Algoneurodystrophy, shoulder**
M89.011 Algoneurodystrophy, right shoulder
M89.012 Algoneurodystrophy, left shoulder
M89.019 Algoneurodystrophy, unspecified shoulder
● **M89.02 Algoneurodystrophy, upper arm**
M89.021 Algoneurodystrophy, right upper arm
M89.022 Algoneurodystrophy, left upper arm
M89.029 Algoneurodystrophy, unspecified upper arm
● **M89.03 Algoneurodystrophy, forearm**
M89.031 Algoneurodystrophy, right forearm
M89.032 Algoneurodystrophy, left forearm
M89.039 Algoneurodystrophy, unspecified forearm
● **M89.04 Algoneurodystrophy, hand**
M89.041 Algoneurodystrophy, right hand
M89.042 Algoneurodystrophy, left hand
M89.049 Algoneurodystrophy, unspecified hand
● **M89.05 Algoneurodystrophy, thigh**
M89.051 Algoneurodystrophy, right thigh
M89.052 Algoneurodystrophy, left thigh
M89.059 Algoneurodystrophy, unspecified thigh
● **M89.06 Algoneurodystrophy, lower leg**
M89.061 Algoneurodystrophy, right lower leg
M89.062 Algoneurodystrophy, left lower leg
M89.069 Algoneurodystrophy, unspecified lower leg
● **M89.07 Algoneurodystrophy, ankle and foot**
M89.071 Algoneurodystrophy, right ankle and foot
M89.072 Algoneurodystrophy, left ankle and foot
M89.079 Algoneurodystrophy, unspecified ankle and foot
M89.08 Algoneurodystrophy, other site
M89.09 Algoneurodystrophy, multiple sites

● M89.1 Physeal arrest
Arrest of growth plate
Epiphyseal arrest
Growth plate arrest

● M89.12 Physeal arrest, humerus
M89.121 Complete physeal arrest, right proximal humerus
M89.122 Complete physeal arrest, left proximal humerus
M89.123 Partial physeal arrest, right proximal humerus
M89.124 Partial physeal arrest, left proximal humerus
M89.125 Complete physeal arrest, right distal humerus
M89.126 Complete physeal arrest, left distal humerus
M89.127 Partial physeal arrest, right distal humerus
M89.128 Partial physeal arrest, left distal humerus
M89.129 Physeal arrest, humerus, unspecified

● M89.13 Physeal arrest, forearm
M89.131 Complete physeal arrest, right distal radius
M89.132 Complete physeal arrest, left distal radius
M89.133 Partial physeal arrest, right distal radius
M89.134 Partial physeal arrest, left distal radius
M89.138 Other physeal arrest of forearm
M89.139 Physeal arrest, forearm, unspecified

● M89.15 Physeal arrest, femur
M89.151 Complete physeal arrest, right proximal femur
M89.152 Complete physeal arrest, left proximal femur
M89.153 Partial physeal arrest, right proximal femur
M89.154 Partial physeal arrest, left proximal femur
M89.155 Complete physeal arrest, right distal femur
M89.156 Complete physeal arrest, left distal femur
M89.157 Partial physeal arrest, right distal femur
M89.158 Partial physeal arrest, left distal femur
M89.159 Physeal arrest, femur, unspecified

● M89.16 Physeal arrest, lower leg
M89.160 Complete physeal arrest, right proximal tibia
M89.161 Complete physeal arrest, left proximal tibia
M89.162 Partial physeal arrest, right proximal tibia
M89.163 Partial physeal arrest, left proximal tibia
M89.164 Complete physeal arrest, right distal tibia
M89.165 Complete physeal arrest, left distal tibia
M89.166 Partial physeal arrest, right distal tibia
M89.167 Partial physeal arrest, left distal tibia
M89.168 Other physeal arrest of lower leg
M89.169 Physeal arrest, lower leg, unspecified

M89.18 Physeal arrest, other site

● M89.2 Other disorders of bone development and growth
M89.20 Other disorders of bone development and growth, unspecified site

● M89.21 Other disorders of bone development and growth, shoulder
M89.211 Other disorders of bone development and growth, right shoulder
M89.212 Other disorders of bone development and growth, left shoulder
M89.219 Other disorders of bone development and growth, unspecified shoulder

● M89.22 Other disorders of bone development and growth, humerus
M89.221 Other disorders of bone development and growth, right humerus
M89.222 Other disorders of bone development and growth, left humerus
M89.229 Other disorders of bone development and growth, unspecified humerus

● M89.23 Other disorders of bone development and growth, ulna and radius
M89.231 Other disorders of bone development and growth, right ulna
M89.232 Other disorders of bone development and growth, left ulna
M89.233 Other disorders of bone development and growth, right radius
M89.234 Other disorders of bone development and growth, left radius
M89.239 Other disorders of bone development and growth, unspecified ulna and radius

● M89.24 Other disorders of bone development and growth, hand
M89.241 Other disorders of bone development and growth, right hand
M89.242 Other disorders of bone development and growth, left hand
M89.249 Other disorders of bone development and growth, unspecified hand

● M89.25 Other disorders of bone development and growth, femur
M89.251 Other disorders of bone development and growth, right femur
M89.252 Other disorders of bone development and growth, left femur
M89.259 Other disorders of bone development and growth, unspecified femur

● M89.26 Other disorders of bone development and growth, tibia and fibula
M89.261 Other disorders of bone development and growth, right tibia
M89.262 Other disorders of bone development and growth, left tibia
M89.263 Other disorders of bone development and growth, right fibula
M89.264 Other disorders of bone development and growth, left fibula
M89.269 Other disorders of bone development and growth, unspecified lower leg

● M89.27 Other disorders of bone development and growth, ankle and foot
M89.271 Other disorders of bone development and growth, right ankle and foot
M89.272 Other disorders of bone development and growth, left ankle and foot
M89.279 Other disorders of bone development and growth, unspecified ankle and foot

M89.28 Other disorders of bone development and growth, other site
M89.29 Other disorders of bone development and growth, multiple sites

● M89.3 Hypertrophy of bone
M89.30 Hypertrophy of bone, unspecified site
● M89.31 Hypertrophy of bone, shoulder
M89.311 Hypertrophy of bone, right shoulder
M89.312 Hypertrophy of bone, left shoulder
M89.319 Hypertrophy of bone, unspecified shoulder
● M89.32 Hypertrophy of bone, humerus
M89.321 Hypertrophy of bone, right humerus
M89.322 Hypertrophy of bone, left humerus
M89.329 Hypertrophy of bone, unspecified humerus
● M89.33 Hypertrophy of bone, ulna and radius
M89.331 Hypertrophy of bone, right ulna
M89.332 Hypertrophy of bone, left ulna
M89.333 Hypertrophy of bone, right radius
M89.334 Hypertrophy of bone, left radius
M89.339 Hypertrophy of bone, unspecified ulna and radius
● M89.34 Hypertrophy of bone, hand
M89.341 Hypertrophy of bone, right hand
M89.342 Hypertrophy of bone, left hand
M89.349 Hypertrophy of bone, unspecified hand
● M89.35 Hypertrophy of bone, femur
M89.351 Hypertrophy of bone, right femur
M89.352 Hypertrophy of bone, left femur
M89.359 Hypertrophy of bone, unspecified femur
● M89.36 Hypertrophy of bone, tibia and fibula
M89.361 Hypertrophy of bone, right tibia
M89.362 Hypertrophy of bone, left tibia
M89.363 Hypertrophy of bone, right fibula
M89.364 Hypertrophy of bone, left fibula
M89.369 Hypertrophy of bone, unspecified tibia and fibula
● M89.37 Hypertrophy of bone, ankle and foot
M89.371 Hypertrophy of bone, right ankle and foot
M89.372 Hypertrophy of bone, left ankle and foot
M89.379 Hypertrophy of bone, unspecified ankle and foot
M89.38 Hypertrophy of bone, other site
M89.39 Hypertrophy of bone, multiple sites

● M89.4 Other hypertrophic osteoarthropathy
Marie-Bamberger disease
Pachydermoperiostosis
M89.40 Other hypertrophic osteoarthropathy, unspecified site
● M89.41 Other hypertrophic osteoarthropathy, shoulder
M89.411 Other hypertrophic osteoarthropathy, right shoulder
M89.412 Other hypertrophic osteoarthropathy, left shoulder
M89.419 Other hypertrophic osteoarthropathy, unspecified shoulder
● M89.42 Other hypertrophic osteoarthropathy, upper arm
M89.421 Other hypertrophic osteoarthropathy, right upper arm
M89.422 Other hypertrophic osteoarthropathy, left upper arm
M89.429 Other hypertrophic osteoarthropathy, unspecified upper arm
● M89.43 Other hypertrophic osteoarthropathy, forearm
M89.431 Other hypertrophic osteoarthropathy, right forearm
M89.432 Other hypertrophic osteoarthropathy, left forearm
M89.439 Other hypertrophic osteoarthropathy, unspecified forearm
● M89.44 Other hypertrophic osteoarthropathy, hand
M89.441 Other hypertrophic osteoarthropathy, right hand
M89.442 Other hypertrophic osteoarthropathy, left hand
M89.449 Other hypertrophic osteoarthropathy, unspecified hand
● M89.45 Other hypertrophic osteoarthropathy, thigh
M89.451 Other hypertrophic osteoarthropathy, right thigh
M89.452 Other hypertrophic osteoarthropathy, left thigh
M89.459 Other hypertrophic osteoarthropathy, unspecified thigh
● M89.46 Other hypertrophic osteoarthropathy, lower leg
M89.461 Other hypertrophic osteoarthropathy, right lower leg
M89.462 Other hypertrophic osteoarthropathy, left lower leg
M89.469 Other hypertrophic osteoarthropathy, unspecified lower leg
● M89.47 Other hypertrophic osteoarthropathy, ankle and foot
M89.471 Other hypertrophic osteoarthropathy, right ankle and foot
M89.472 Other hypertrophic osteoarthropathy, left ankle and foot
M89.479 Other hypertrophic osteoarthropathy, unspecified ankle and foot
M89.48 Other hypertrophic osteoarthropathy, other site
M89.49 Other hypertrophic osteoarthropathy, multiple sites

● M89.5 Osteolysis
Use additional code to identify major osseous defect, if applicable (M89.7-)
Excludes2 periprosthetic osteolysis of internal prosthetic joint (T84.05-)
M89.50 Osteolysis, unspecified site
● M89.51 Osteolysis, shoulder
M89.511 Osteolysis, right shoulder
M89.512 Osteolysis, left shoulder
M89.519 Osteolysis, unspecified shoulder
● M89.52 Osteolysis, upper arm
M89.521 Osteolysis, right upper arm
M89.522 Osteolysis, left upper arm
M89.529 Osteolysis, unspecified upper arm
● M89.53 Osteolysis, forearm
M89.531 Osteolysis, right forearm
M89.532 Osteolysis, left forearm
M89.539 Osteolysis, unspecified forearm

● M89.54 Osteolysis, hand
M89.541 Osteolysis, right hand
M89.542 Osteolysis, left hand
M89.549 Osteolysis, unspecified hand
● M89.55 Osteolysis, thigh
M89.551 Osteolysis, right thigh
M89.552 Osteolysis, left thigh
M89.559 Osteolysis, unspecified thigh
● M89.56 Osteolysis, lower leg
M89.561 Osteolysis, right lower leg
M89.562 Osteolysis, left lower leg
M89.569 Osteolysis, unspecified lower leg
● M89.57 Osteolysis, ankle and foot
M89.571 Osteolysis, right ankle and foot
M89.572 Osteolysis, left ankle and foot
M89.579 Osteolysis, unspecified ankle and foot
M89.58 Osteolysis, other site
M89.59 Osteolysis, multiple sites
● M89.6 Osteopathy after poliomyelitis
Use additional code (B91) to identify previous poliomyelitis
Excludes1 postpolio syndrome (G14)
M89.60 Osteopathy after poliomyelitis, unspecified site
● M89.61 Osteopathy after poliomyelitis, shoulder
M89.611 Osteopathy after poliomyelitis, right shoulder
M89.612 Osteopathy after poliomyelitis, left shoulder
M89.619 Osteopathy after poliomyelitis, unspecified shoulder
● M89.62 Osteopathy after poliomyelitis, upper arm
M89.621 Osteopathy after poliomyelitis, right upper arm
M89.622 Osteopathy after poliomyelitis, left upper arm
M89.629 Osteopathy after poliomyelitis, unspecified upper arm
● M89.63 Osteopathy after poliomyelitis, forearm
M89.631 Osteopathy after poliomyelitis, right forearm
M89.632 Osteopathy after poliomyelitis, left forearm
M89.639 Osteopathy after poliomyelitis, unspecified forearm
● M89.64 Osteopathy after poliomyelitis, hand
M89.641 Osteopathy after poliomyelitis, right hand
M89.642 Osteopathy after poliomyelitis, left hand
M89.649 Osteopathy after poliomyelitis, unspecified hand
● M89.65 Osteopathy after poliomyelitis, thigh
M89.651 Osteopathy after poliomyelitis, right thigh
M89.652 Osteopathy after poliomyelitis, left thigh
M89.659 Osteopathy after poliomyelitis, unspecified thigh
● M89.66 Osteopathy after poliomyelitis, lower leg
M89.661 Osteopathy after poliomyelitis, right lower leg
M89.662 Osteopathy after poliomyelitis, left lower leg
M89.669 Osteopathy after poliomyelitis, unspecified lower leg
● M89.67 Osteopathy after poliomyelitis, ankle and foot
M89.671 Osteopathy after poliomyelitis, right ankle and foot
M89.672 Osteopathy after poliomyelitis, left ankle and foot
M89.679 Osteopathy after poliomyelitis, unspecified ankle and foot
M89.68 Osteopathy after poliomyelitis, other site
M89.69 Osteopathy after poliomyelitis, multiple sites
● M89.7 Major osseous defect
Code first *underlying disease, if known, such as:*
aseptic necrosis of bone (M87.-)
malignant neoplasm of bone (C4Ø.-)
osteolysis (M89.5)
osteomyelitis (M86.-)
osteonecrosis (M87.-)
osteoporosis (M8Ø.-, M81.-)
periprosthetic osteolysis (T84.Ø5-)
M89.7Ø Major osseous defect, unspecified site
● M89.71 Major osseous defect, shoulder region
Major osseous defect clavicle or scapula
M89.711 Major osseous defect, right shoulder region
M89.712 Major osseous defect, left shoulder region
M89.719 Major osseous defect, unspecified shoulder region
● M89.72 Major osseous defect, humerus
M89.721 Major osseous defect, right humerus
M89.722 Major osseous defect, left humerus
M89.729 Major osseous defect, unspecified humerus
● M89.73 Major osseous defect, forearm
Major osseous defect of radius and ulna
M89.731 Major osseous defect, right forearm
M89.732 Major osseous defect, left forearm
M89.739 Major osseous defect, unspecified forearm
● M89.74 Major osseous defect, hand
Major osseous defect of carpus, fingers, metacarpus
M89.741 Major osseous defect, right hand
M89.742 Major osseous defect, left hand
M89.749 Major osseous defect, unspecified hand
● M89.75 Major osseous defect, pelvic region and thigh
Major osseous defect of femur and pelvis
M89.751 Major osseous defect, right pelvic region and thigh
M89.752 Major osseous defect, left pelvic region and thigh
M89.759 Major osseous defect, unspecified pelvic region and thigh
● M89.76 Major osseous defect, lower leg
Major osseous defect of fibula and tibia
M89.761 Major osseous defect, right lower leg
M89.762 Major osseous defect, left lower leg
M89.769 Major osseous defect, unspecified lower leg
● M89.77 Major osseous defect, ankle and foot
Major osseous defect of metatarsus, tarsus, toes
M89.771 Major osseous defect, right ankle and foot
M89.772 Major osseous defect, left ankle and foot
M89.779 Major osseous defect, unspecified ankle and foot
M89.78 Major osseous defect, other site
M89.79 Major osseous defect, multiple sites

●**M89.8 Other specified disorders of bone**
Infantile cortical hyperostoses
Post-traumatic subperiosteal ossification
●**M89.8X Other specified disorders of bone**
M89.8XØ Other specified disorders of bone, multiple sites
M89.8X1 Other specified disorders of bone, shoulder
M89.8X2 Other specified disorders of bone, upper arm
M89.8X3 Other specified disorders of bone, forearm
M89.8X4 Other specified disorders of bone, hand
M89.8X5 Other specified disorders of bone, thigh
M89.8X6 Other specified disorders of bone, lower leg
M89.8X7 Other specified disorders of bone, ankle and foot
M89.8X8 Other specified disorders of bone, other site
M89.8X9 Other specified disorders of bone, unspecified site
M89.9 Disorder of bone, unspecified

●**M9Ø Osteopathies in diseases classified elsewhere**
Excludes1 osteochondritis, osteomyelitis, and osteopathy (in):
cryptococcosis (B45.3)
diabetes mellitus (EØ8-E13 with .69-)
gonococcal (A54.43)
neurogenic syphilis (A52.11)
renal osteodystrophy (N25.Ø)
salmonellosis (AØ2.24)
secondary syphilis (A51.46)
syphilis (late) (A52.77)

●**M9Ø.5 Osteonecrosis in diseases classified elsewhere**
Code first underlying disease, such as:
caisson disease (T7Ø.3)
hemoglobinopathy (D5Ø-D64)
M9Ø.5Ø Osteonecrosis in diseases classified elsewhere, unspecified site
●**M9Ø.51 Osteonecrosis in diseases classified elsewhere, shoulder**
M9Ø.511 Osteonecrosis in diseases classified elsewhere, right shoulder
M9Ø.512 Osteonecrosis in diseases classified elsewhere, left shoulder
M9Ø.519 Osteonecrosis in diseases classified elsewhere, unspecified shoulder
●**M9Ø.52 Osteonecrosis in diseases classified elsewhere, upper arm**
M9Ø.521 Osteonecrosis in diseases classified elsewhere, right upper arm
M9Ø.522 Osteonecrosis in diseases classified elsewhere, left upper arm
M9Ø.529 Osteonecrosis in diseases classified elsewhere, unspecified upper arm
●**M9Ø.53 Osteonecrosis in diseases classified elsewhere, forearm**
M9Ø.531 Osteonecrosis in diseases classified elsewhere, right forearm
M9Ø.532 Osteonecrosis in diseases classified elsewhere, left forearm
M9Ø.539 Osteonecrosis in diseases classified elsewhere, unspecified forearm
●**M9Ø.54 Osteonecrosis in diseases classified elsewhere, hand**
M9Ø.541 Osteonecrosis in diseases classified elsewhere, right hand
M9Ø.542 Osteonecrosis in diseases classified elsewhere, left hand
M9Ø.549 Osteonecrosis in diseases classified elsewhere, unspecified hand
●**M9Ø.55 Osteonecrosis in diseases classified elsewhere, thigh**
M9Ø.551 Osteonecrosis in diseases classified elsewhere, right thigh
M9Ø.552 Osteonecrosis in diseases classified elsewhere, left thigh
M9Ø.559 Osteonecrosis in diseases classified elsewhere, unspecified thigh
●**M9Ø.56 Osteonecrosis in diseases classified elsewhere, lower leg**
M9Ø.561 Osteonecrosis in diseases classified elsewhere, right lower leg
M9Ø.562 Osteonecrosis in diseases classified elsewhere, left lower leg
M9Ø.569 Osteonecrosis in diseases classified elsewhere, unspecified lower leg
●**M9Ø.57 Osteonecrosis in diseases classified elsewhere, ankle and foot**
M9Ø.571 Osteonecrosis in diseases classified elsewhere, right ankle and foot
M9Ø.572 Osteonecrosis in diseases classified elsewhere, left ankle and foot
M9Ø.579 Osteonecrosis in diseases classified elsewhere, unspecified ankle and foot
M9Ø.58 Osteonecrosis in diseases classified elsewhere, other site
M9Ø.59 Osteonecrosis in diseases classified elsewhere, multiple sites

●**M9Ø.6 Osteitis deformans in neoplastic diseases**
Osteitis deformans in malignant neoplasm of bone
Code first the neoplasm (C4Ø.-, C41.-)
Excludes1 osteitis deformans [Paget's disease of bone] (M88.-)
M9Ø.6Ø Osteitis deformans in neoplastic diseases, unspecified site
●**M9Ø.61 Osteitis deformans in neoplastic diseases, shoulder**
M9Ø.611 Osteitis deformans in neoplastic diseases, right shoulder
M9Ø.612 Osteitis deformans in neoplastic diseases, left shoulder
M9Ø.619 Osteitis deformans in neoplastic diseases, unspecified shoulder
●**M9Ø.62 Osteitis deformans in neoplastic diseases, upper arm**
M9Ø.621 Osteitis deformans in neoplastic diseases, right upper arm
M9Ø.622 Osteitis deformans in neoplastic diseases, left upper arm
M9Ø.629 Osteitis deformans in neoplastic diseases, unspecified upper arm
●**M9Ø.63 Osteitis deformans in neoplastic diseases, forearm**
M9Ø.631 Osteitis deformans in neoplastic diseases, right forearm
M9Ø.632 Osteitis deformans in neoplastic diseases, left forearm
M9Ø.639 Osteitis deformans in neoplastic diseases, unspecified forearm

● M90.64 Osteitis deformans in neoplastic diseases, hand
M90.641 Osteitis deformans in neoplastic diseases, right hand
M90.642 Osteitis deformans in neoplastic diseases, left hand
M90.649 Osteitis deformans in neoplastic diseases, unspecified hand
● M90.65 Osteitis deformans in neoplastic diseases, thigh
M90.651 Osteitis deformans in neoplastic diseases, right thigh
M90.652 Osteitis deformans in neoplastic diseases, left thigh
M90.659 Osteitis deformans in neoplastic diseases, unspecified thigh
● M90.66 Osteitis deformans in neoplastic diseases, lower leg
M90.661 Osteitis deformans in neoplastic diseases, right lower leg
M90.662 Osteitis deformans in neoplastic diseases, left lower leg
M90.669 Osteitis deformans in neoplastic diseases, unspecified lower leg
● M90.67 Osteitis deformans in neoplastic diseases, ankle and foot
M90.671 Osteitis deformans in neoplastic diseases, right ankle and foot
M90.672 Osteitis deformans in neoplastic diseases, left ankle and foot
M90.679 Osteitis deformans in neoplastic diseases, unspecified ankle and foot
M90.68 Osteitis deformans in neoplastic diseases, other site
M90.69 Osteitis deformans in neoplastic diseases, multiple sites
● M90.8 Osteopathy in diseases classified elsewhere
Code first underlying disease, such as:
rickets (E55.0)
vitamin-D-resistant rickets (E83.3)
M90.80 Osteopathy in diseases classified elsewhere, unspecified site
● M90.81 Osteopathy in diseases classified elsewhere, shoulder
M90.811 Osteopathy in diseases classified elsewhere, right shoulder
M90.812 Osteopathy in diseases classified elsewhere, left shoulder
M90.819 Osteopathy in diseases classified elsewhere, unspecified shoulder
● M90.82 Osteopathy in diseases classified elsewhere, upper arm
M90.821 Osteopathy in diseases classified elsewhere, right upper arm
M90.822 Osteopathy in diseases classified elsewhere, left upper arm
M90.829 Osteopathy in diseases classified elsewhere, unspecified upper arm
● M90.83 Osteopathy in diseases classified elsewhere, forearm
M90.831 Osteopathy in diseases classified elsewhere, right forearm
M90.832 Osteopathy in diseases classified elsewhere, left forearm
M90.839 Osteopathy in diseases classified elsewhere, unspecified forearm
● M90.84 Osteopathy in diseases classified elsewhere, hand
M90.841 Osteopathy in diseases classified elsewhere, right hand
M90.842 Osteopathy in diseases classified elsewhere, left hand
M90.849 Osteopathy in diseases classified elsewhere, unspecified hand
● M90.85 Osteopathy in diseases classified elsewhere, thigh
M90.851 Osteopathy in diseases classified elsewhere, right thigh
M90.852 Osteopathy in diseases classified elsewhere, left thigh
M90.859 Osteopathy in diseases classified elsewhere, unspecified thigh
● M90.86 Osteopathy in diseases classified elsewhere, lower leg
M90.861 Osteopathy in diseases classified elsewhere, right lower leg
M90.862 Osteopathy in diseases classified elsewhere, left lower leg
M90.869 Osteopathy in diseases classified elsewhere, unspecified lower leg
● M90.87 Osteopathy in diseases classified elsewhere, ankle and foot
M90.871 Osteopathy in diseases classified elsewhere, right ankle and foot
M90.872 Osteopathy in diseases classified elsewhere, left ankle and foot
M90.879 Osteopathy in diseases classified elsewhere, unspecified ankle and foot
M90.88 Osteopathy in diseases classified elsewhere, other site
M90.89 Osteopathy in diseases classified elsewhere, multiple sites

CHONDROPATHIES (M91-M94)

Excludes1 postprocedural chondropathies (M96.-)

● M91 Juvenile osteochondrosis of hip and pelvis
Excludes1 slipped upper femoral epiphysis (nontraumatic) (M93.0)
M91.0 Juvenile osteochondrosis of pelvis
Osteochondrosis (juvenile) of acetabulum
Osteochondrosis (juvenile) of iliac crest [Buchanan]
Osteochondrosis (juvenile) of ischiopubic synchondrosis [van Neck]
Osteochondrosis (juvenile) of symphysis pubis [Pierson]
● M91.1 Juvenile osteochondrosis of head of femur [Legg-Calvé-Perthes]
M91.10 Juvenile osteochondrosis of head of femur [Legg-Calvé-Perthes], unspecified leg
M91.11 Juvenile osteochondrosis of head of femur [Legg-Calvé-Perthes], right leg
M91.12 Juvenile osteochondrosis of head of femur [Legg-Calvé-Perthes], left leg
● M91.2 Coxa plana
Hip deformity due to previous juvenile osteochondrosis
M91.20 Coxa plana, unspecified hip
M91.21 Coxa plana, right hip
M91.22 Coxa plana, left hip
● M91.3 Pseudocoxalgia
M91.30 Pseudocoxalgia, unspecified hip
M91.31 Pseudocoxalgia, right hip
M91.32 Pseudocoxalgia, left hip

CHAPTER 13 (M00-M99)

● M91.4 Coxa magna
M91.40 Coxa magna, unspecified hip
M91.41 Coxa magna, right hip
M91.42 Coxa magna, left hip
● M91.8 Other juvenile osteochondrosis of hip and pelvis
Juvenile osteochondrosis after reduction of congenital dislocation of hip
M91.80 Other juvenile osteochondrosis of hip and pelvis, unspecified leg
M91.81 Other juvenile osteochondrosis of hip and pelvis, right leg
M91.82 Other juvenile osteochondrosis of hip and pelvis, left leg
● M91.9 Juvenile osteochondrosis of hip and pelvis, unspecified
M91.90 Juvenile osteochondrosis of hip and pelvis, unspecified, unspecified leg
M91.91 Juvenile osteochondrosis of hip and pelvis, unspecified, right leg
M91.92 Juvenile osteochondrosis of hip and pelvis, unspecified, left leg

● M92 Other juvenile osteochondrosis
● M92.0 Juvenile osteochondrosis of humerus
Osteochondrosis (juvenile) of capitulum of humerus [Panner]
Osteochondrosis (juvenile) of head of humerus [Haas]
M92.00 Juvenile osteochondrosis of humerus, unspecified arm
M92.01 Juvenile osteochondrosis of humerus, right arm
M92.02 Juvenile osteochondrosis of humerus, left arm
● M92.1 Juvenile osteochondrosis of radius and ulna
Osteochondrosis (juvenile) of lower ulna [Burns]
Osteochondrosis (juvenile) of radial head [Brailsford]
M92.10 Juvenile osteochondrosis of radius and ulna, unspecified arm
M92.11 Juvenile osteochondrosis of radius and ulna, right arm
M92.12 Juvenile osteochondrosis of radius and ulna, left arm
● M92.2 Juvenile osteochondrosis, hand
● M92.20 Unspecified juvenile osteochondrosis, hand
M92.201 Unspecified juvenile osteochondrosis, right hand
M92.202 Unspecified juvenile osteochondrosis, left hand
M92.209 Unspecified juvenile osteochondrosis, unspecified hand
● M92.21 Osteochondrosis (juvenile) of carpal lunate [Kienböck]
M92.211 Osteochondrosis (juvenile) of carpal lunate [Kienböck], right hand
M92.212 Osteochondrosis (juvenile) of carpal lunate [Kienböck], left hand
M92.219 Osteochondrosis (juvenile) of carpal lunate [Kienböck], unspecified hand
● M92.22 Osteochondrosis (juvenile) of metacarpal heads [Mauclaire]
M92.221 Osteochondrosis (juvenile) of metacarpal heads [Mauclaire], right hand
M92.222 Osteochondrosis (juvenile) of metacarpal heads [Mauclaire], left hand
M92.229 Osteochondrosis (juvenile) of metacarpal heads [Mauclaire], unspecified hand
● M92.29 Other juvenile osteochondrosis, hand
M92.291 Other juvenile osteochondrosis, right hand
M92.292 Other juvenile osteochondrosis, left hand
M92.299 Other juvenile osteochondrosis, unspecified hand
● M92.3 Other juvenile osteochondrosis, upper limb
M92.30 Other juvenile osteochondrosis, unspecified upper limb
M92.31 Other juvenile osteochondrosis, right upper limb
M92.32 Other juvenile osteochondrosis, left upper limb
● M92.4 Juvenile osteochondrosis of patella
Osteochondrosis (juvenile) of primary patellar center [Köhler]
Osteochondrosis (juvenile) of secondary patellar center [Sinding Larsen]
M92.40 Juvenile osteochondrosis of patella, unspecified knee
M92.41 Juvenile osteochondrosis of patella, right knee
M92.42 Juvenile osteochondrosis of patella, left knee
● M92.5 Juvenile osteochondrosis of tibia and fibula
Osteochondrosis (juvenile) of proximal tibia [Blount]
Osteochondrosis (juvenile) of tibial tubercle [Osgood-Schlatter]
Tibia vara
M92.50 Juvenile osteochondrosis of tibia and fibula, unspecified leg
M92.51 Juvenile osteochondrosis of tibia and fibula, right leg
M92.52 Juvenile osteochondrosis of tibia and fibula, left leg
● M92.6 Juvenile osteochondrosis of tarsus
Osteochondrosis (juvenile) of calcaneum [Sever]
Osteochondrosis (juvenile) of os tibiale externum [Haglund]
Osteochondrosis (juvenile) of talus [Diaz]
Osteochondrosis (juvenile) of tarsal navicular [Köhler]
M92.60 Juvenile osteochondrosis of tarsus, unspecified ankle
M92.61 Juvenile osteochondrosis of tarsus, right ankle
M92.62 Juvenile osteochondrosis of tarsus, left ankle
● M92.7 Juvenile osteochondrosis of metatarsus
Osteochondrosis (juvenile) of fifth metatarsus [Iselin]
Osteochondrosis (juvenile) of second metatarsus [Freiberg]
M92.70 Juvenile osteochondrosis of metatarsus, unspecified foot
M92.71 Juvenile osteochondrosis of metatarsus, right foot
M92.72 Juvenile osteochondrosis of metatarsus, left foot
M92.8 Other specified juvenile osteochondrosis
Calcaneal apophysitis
M92.9 Juvenile osteochondrosis, unspecified
Juvenile apophysitis NOS
Juvenile epiphysitis NOS
Juvenile osteochondritis NOS
Juvenile osteochondrosis NOS

CHAPTER 13 (M00-M99)

● M93 Other osteochondropathies
Excludes2 osteochondrosis of spine (M42.-)
● M93.0 Slipped upper femoral epiphysis (nontraumatic)
Use additional code for associated chondrolysis (M94.3)
● M93.00 Unspecified slipped upper femoral epiphysis (nontraumatic)
M93.001 Unspecified slipped upper femoral epiphysis (nontraumatic), right hip
M93.002 Unspecified slipped upper femoral epiphysis (nontraumatic), left hip
M93.003 Unspecified slipped upper femoral epiphysis (nontraumatic), unspecified hip
● M93.01 Acute slipped upper femoral epiphysis (nontraumatic)
M93.011 Acute slipped upper femoral epiphysis (nontraumatic), right hip
M93.012 Acute slipped upper femoral epiphysis (nontraumatic), left hip
M93.013 Acute slipped upper femoral epiphysis (nontraumatic), unspecified hip
● M93.02 Chronic slipped upper femoral epiphysis (nontraumatic)
M93.021 Chronic slipped upper femoral epiphysis (nontraumatic), right hip
M93.022 Chronic slipped upper femoral epiphysis (nontraumatic), left hip
M93.023 Chronic slipped upper femoral epiphysis (nontraumatic), unspecified hip
● M93.03 Acute on chronic slipped upper femoral epiphysis (nontraumatic)
M93.031 Acute on chronic slipped upper femoral epiphysis (nontraumatic), right hip
M93.032 Acute on chronic slipped upper femoral epiphysis (nontraumatic), left hip
M93.033 Acute on chronic slipped upper femoral epiphysis (nontraumatic), unspecified hip
M93.1 Kienböck's disease of adults
Adult osteochondrosis of carpal lunates
● M93.2 Osteochondritis dissecans
M93.20 Osteochondritis dissecans of unspecified site
● M93.21 Osteochondritis dissecans of shoulder
M93.211 Osteochondritis dissecans, right shoulder
M93.212 Osteochondritis dissecans, left shoulder
M93.219 Osteochondritis dissecans, unspecified shoulder
● M93.22 Osteochondritis dissecans of elbow
M93.221 Osteochondritis dissecans, right elbow
M93.222 Osteochondritis dissecans, left elbow
M93.229 Osteochondritis dissecans, unspecified elbow
● M93.23 Osteochondritis dissecans of wrist
M93.231 Osteochondritis dissecans, right wrist
M93.232 Osteochondritis dissecans, left wrist
M93.239 Osteochondritis dissecans, unspecified wrist
● M93.24 Osteochondritis dissecans of joints of hand
M93.241 Osteochondritis dissecans, joints of right hand
M93.242 Osteochondritis dissecans, joints of left hand
M93.249 Osteochondritis dissecans, joints of unspecified hand
● M93.25 Osteochondritis dissecans of hip
M93.251 Osteochondritis dissecans, right hip
M93.252 Osteochondritis dissecans, left hip
M93.259 Osteochondritis dissecans, unspecified hip
● M93.26 Osteochondritis dissecans knee
M93.261 Osteochondritis dissecans, right knee
M93.262 Osteochondritis dissecans, left knee
M93.269 Osteochondritis dissecans, unspecified knee
● M93.27 Osteochondritis dissecans of ankle and joints of foot
M93.271 Osteochondritis dissecans, right ankle and joints of right foot
M93.272 Osteochondritis dissecans, left ankle and joints of left foot
M93.279 Osteochondritis dissecans, unspecified ankle and joints of foot
M93.28 Osteochondritis dissecans other site
M93.29 Osteochondritis dissecans multiple sites
● M93.8 Other specified osteochondropathies
M93.80 Other specified osteochondropathies of unspecified site
● M93.81 Other specified osteochondropathies of shoulder
M93.811 Other specified osteochondropathies, right shoulder
M93.812 Other specified osteochondropathies, left shoulder
M93.819 Other specified osteochondropathies, unspecified shoulder
● M93.82 Other specified osteochondropathies of upper arm
M93.821 Other specified osteochondropathies, right upper arm
M93.822 Other specified osteochondropathies, left upper arm
M93.829 Other specified osteochondropathies, unspecified upper arm
● M93.83 Other specified osteochondropathies of forearm
M93.831 Other specified osteochondropathies, right forearm
M93.832 Other specified osteochondropathies, left forearm
M93.839 Other specified osteochondropathies, unspecified forearm
● M93.84 Other specified osteochondropathies of hand
M93.841 Other specified osteochondropathies, right hand
M93.842 Other specified osteochondropathies, left hand
M93.849 Other specified osteochondropathies, unspecified hand
● M93.85 Other specified osteochondropathies of thigh
M93.851 Other specified osteochondropathies, right thigh
M93.852 Other specified osteochondropathies, left thigh
M93.859 Other specified osteochondropathies, unspecified thigh

● M93.86 Other specified osteochondropathies lower leg
M93.861 Other specified osteochondropathies, right lower leg
M93.862 Other specified osteochondropathies, left lower leg
M93.869 Other specified osteochondropathies, unspecified lower leg
● M93.87 Other specified osteochondropathies of ankle and foot
M93.871 Other specified osteochondropathies, right ankle and foot
M93.872 Other specified osteochondropathies, left ankle and foot
M93.879 Other specified osteochondropathies, unspecified ankle and foot
M93.88 Other specified osteochondropathies other
M93.89 Other specified osteochondropathies multiple sites

M93.9 Osteochondropathy, unspecified
Apophysitis NOS
Epiphysitis NOS
Osteochondritis NOS
Osteochondrosis NOS
M93.90 Osteochondropathy, unspecified of unspecified site
● M93.91 Osteochondropathy, unspecified of shoulder
M93.911 Osteochondropathy, unspecified, right shoulder
M93.912 Osteochondropathy, unspecified, left shoulder
M93.919 Osteochondropathy, unspecified, unspecified shoulder
● M93.92 Osteochondropathy, unspecified of upper arm
M93.921 Osteochondropathy, unspecified, right upper arm
M93.922 Osteochondropathy, unspecified, left upper arm
M93.929 Osteochondropathy, unspecified, unspecified upper arm
● M93.93 Osteochondropathy, unspecified of forearm
M93.931 Osteochondropathy, unspecified, right forearm
M93.932 Osteochondropathy, unspecified, left forearm
M93.939 Osteochondropathy, unspecified, unspecified forearm
● M93.94 Osteochondropathy, unspecified of hand
M93.941 Osteochondropathy, unspecified, right hand
M93.942 Osteochondropathy, unspecified, left hand
M93.949 Osteochondropathy, unspecified, unspecified hand
● M93.95 Osteochondropathy, unspecified of thigh
M93.951 Osteochondropathy, unspecified, right thigh
M93.952 Osteochondropathy, unspecified, left thigh
M93.959 Osteochondropathy, unspecified, unspecified thigh
● M93.96 Osteochondropathy, unspecified lower leg
M93.961 Osteochondropathy, unspecified, right lower leg
M93.962 Osteochondropathy, unspecified, left lower leg
M93.969 Osteochondropathy, unspecified, unspecified lower leg
● M93.97 Osteochondropathy, unspecified of ankle and foot
M93.971 Osteochondropathy, unspecified, right ankle and foot
M93.972 Osteochondropathy, unspecified, left ankle and foot
M93.979 Osteochondropathy, unspecified, unspecified ankle and foot
M93.98 Osteochondropathy, unspecified other
M93.99 Osteochondropathy, unspecified multiple sites

● M94 Other disorders of cartilage
M94.0 Chondrocostal junction syndrome [Tietze]
Costochondritis
M94.1 Relapsing polychondritis
● M94.2 Chondromalacia
Excludes1 chondromalacia patellae (M22.4)
M94.20 Chondromalacia, unspecified site
● M94.21 Chondromalacia, shoulder
M94.211 Chondromalacia, right shoulder
M94.212 Chondromalacia, left shoulder
M94.219 Chondromalacia, unspecified shoulder
● M94.22 Chondromalacia, elbow
M94.221 Chondromalacia, right elbow
M94.222 Chondromalacia, left elbow
M94.229 Chondromalacia, unspecified elbow
● M94.23 Chondromalacia, wrist
M94.231 Chondromalacia, right wrist
M94.232 Chondromalacia, left wrist
M94.239 Chondromalacia, unspecified wrist
● M94.24 Chondromalacia, joints of hand
M94.241 Chondromalacia, joints of right hand
M94.242 Chondromalacia, joints of left hand
M94.249 Chondromalacia, joints of unspecified hand
● M94.25 Chondromalacia, hip
M94.251 Chondromalacia, right hip
M94.252 Chondromalacia, left hip
M94.259 Chondromalacia, unspecified hip
● M94.26 Chondromalacia, knee
M94.261 Chondromalacia, right knee
M94.262 Chondromalacia, left knee
M94.269 Chondromalacia, unspecified knee
● M94.27 Chondromalacia, ankle and joints of foot
M94.271 Chondromalacia, right ankle and joints of right foot
M94.272 Chondromalacia, left ankle and joints of left foot
M94.279 Chondromalacia, unspecified ankle and joints of foot
M94.28 Chondromalacia, other site
M94.29 Chondromalacia, multiple sites

● M94.3 Chondrolysis
Code first any associated slipped upper femoral epiphysis (nontraumatic) (M93.Ø-)
● M94.35 Chondrolysis, hip
M94.351 Chondrolysis, right hip
M94.352 Chondrolysis, left hip
M94.359 Chondrolysis, unspecified hip
● M94.8 Other specified disorders of cartilage
● M94.8X Other specified disorders of cartilage
M94.8XØ Other specified disorders of cartilage, multiple sites
M94.8X1 Other specified disorders of cartilage, shoulder
M94.8X2 Other specified disorders of cartilage, upper arm
M94.8X3 Other specified disorders of cartilage, forearm
M94.8X4 Other specified disorders of cartilage, hand
M94.8X5 Other specified disorders of cartilage, thigh
M94.8X6 Other specified disorders of cartilage, lower leg
M94.8X7 Other specified disorders of cartilage, ankle and foot
M94.8X8 Other specified disorders of cartilage, other site
M94.8X9 Other specified disorders of cartilage, unspecified sites
M94.9 Disorder of cartilage, unspecified

OTHER DISORDERS OF THE MUSCULOSKELETAL SYSTEM AND CONNECTIVE TISSUE (M95)

● M95 Other acquired deformities of musculoskeletal system and connective tissue
Excludes2 acquired absence of limbs and organs (Z89-Z9Ø)
acquired deformities of limbs (M2Ø-M21)
congenital malformations and deformations of the musculoskeletal system (Q65-Q79)
deforming dorsopathies (M4Ø-M43)
dentofacial anomalies [including malocclusion] (M26.-)
postprocedural musculoskeletal disorders (M96.-)
M95.Ø Acquired deformity of nose
Excludes2 deviated nasal septum (J34.2)
● M95.1 Cauliflower ear
Excludes2 other acquired deformities of ear (H61.1)
M95.1Ø Cauliflower ear, unspecified ear
M95.11 Cauliflower ear, right ear
M95.12 Cauliflower ear, left ear
M95.2 Other acquired deformity of head
M95.3 Acquired deformity of neck
M95.4 Acquired deformity of chest and rib
M95.5 Acquired deformity of pelvis
Excludes1 maternal care for known or suspected disproportion (O33.-)
M95.8 Other specified acquired deformities of musculoskeletal system
M95.9 Acquired deformity of musculoskeletal system, unspecified

INTRAOPERATIVE AND POSTPROCEDURAL COMPLICATIONS AND DISORDERS OF MUSCULOSKELETAL SYSTEM, NOT ELSEWHERE CLASSIFIED (M96)

● M96 Intraoperative and postprocedural complications and disorders of musculoskeletal system, not elsewhere classified
Excludes2 arthropathy following intestinal bypass (MØ2.Ø-)
complications of internal orthopedic prosthetic devices, implants and grafts (T84.-)
disorders associated with osteoporosis (M8Ø)
periprosthetic fracture around internal prosthetic joint (M97.-) ◀
presence of functional implants and other devices (Z96-Z97)
M96.Ø Pseudarthrosis after fusion or arthrodesis
M96.1 Postlaminectomy syndrome, not elsewhere classified
M96.2 Postradiation kyphosis
M96.3 Postlaminectomy kyphosis
M96.4 Postsurgical lordosis
M96.5 Postradiation scoliosis
● M96.6 Fracture of bone following insertion of orthopedic implant, joint prosthesis, or bone plate
Intraoperative fracture of bone during insertion of orthopedic implant, joint prosthesis, or bone plate
Excludes2 complication of internal orthopedic devices, implants or grafts (T84.-)
● M96.62 Fracture of humerus following insertion of orthopedic implant, joint prosthesis, or bone plate
M96.621 Fracture of humerus following insertion of orthopedic implant, joint prosthesis, or bone plate, right arm
M96.622 Fracture of humerus following insertion of orthopedic implant, joint prosthesis, or bone plate, left arm
M96.629 Fracture of humerus following insertion of orthopedic implant, joint prosthesis, or bone plate, unspecified arm
● M96.63 Fracture of radius or ulna following insertion of orthopedic implant, joint prosthesis, or bone plate
M96.631 Fracture of radius or ulna following insertion of orthopedic implant, joint prosthesis, or bone plate, right arm
M96.632 Fracture of radius or ulna following insertion of orthopedic implant, joint prosthesis, or bone plate, left arm
M96.639 Fracture of radius or ulna following insertion of orthopedic implant, joint prosthesis, or bone plate, unspecified arm
M96.65 Fracture of pelvis following insertion of orthopedic implant, joint prosthesis, or bone plate
● M96.66 Fracture of femur following insertion of orthopedic implant, joint prosthesis, or bone plate
M96.661 Fracture of femur following insertion of orthopedic implant, joint prosthesis, or bone plate, right leg
M96.662 Fracture of femur following insertion of orthopedic implant, joint prosthesis, or bone plate, left leg
M96.669 Fracture of femur following insertion of orthopedic implant, joint prosthesis, or bone plate, unspecified leg

● M96.67 Fracture of tibia or fibula following insertion of orthopedic implant, joint prosthesis, or bone plate
M96.671 Fracture of tibia or fibula following insertion of orthopedic implant, joint prosthesis, or bone plate, right leg
M96.672 Fracture of tibia or fibula following insertion of orthopedic implant, joint prosthesis, or bone plate, left leg
M96.679 Fracture of tibia or fibula following insertion of orthopedic implant, joint prosthesis, or bone plate, unspecified leg
M96.69 Fracture of other bone following insertion of orthopedic implant, joint prosthesis, or bone plate
● M96.8 Other intraoperative and postprocedural complications and disorders of musculoskeletal system, not elsewhere classified
● M96.81 Intraoperative hemorrhage and hematoma of a musculoskeletal structure complicating a procedure
Excludes1 intraoperative hemorrhage and hematoma of a musculoskeletal structure due to accidental puncture and laceration during a procedure (M96.82-)
M96.810 Intraoperative hemorrhage and hematoma of a musculoskeletal structure complicating a musculoskeletal system procedure
M96.811 Intraoperative hemorrhage and hematoma of a musculoskeletal structure complicating other procedure
● M96.82 Accidental puncture and laceration of a musculoskeletal structure during a procedure
M96.820 Accidental puncture and laceration of a musculoskeletal structure during a musculoskeletal system procedure
M96.821 Accidental puncture and laceration of a musculoskeletal structure during other procedure
● M96.83 Postprocedural hemorrhage of a musculoskeletal structure following a procedure
M96.830 Postprocedural hemorrhage of a musculoskeletal structure following a musculoskeletal system procedure
M96.831 Postprocedural hemorrhage of a musculoskeletal structure following other procedure
● M96.84 Postprocedural hematoma and seroma of a musculoskeletal structure following a procedure ◀
M96.840 Postprocedural hematoma of a musculoskeletal structure following a musculoskeletal system procedure ◀
M96.841 Postprocedural hematoma of a musculoskeletal structure following other procedure ◀
M96.842 Postprocedural seroma of a musculoskeletal structure following a musculoskeletal system procedure ◀
M96.843 Postprocedural seroma of a musculoskeletal structure following other procedure ◀
M96.89 Other intraoperative and postprocedural complications and disorders of the musculoskeletal system
Instability of joint secondary to removal of joint prosthesis
Use additional code, if applicable, to further specify disorder

PERIPROSTHETIC FRACTURE AROUND INTERNAL PROSTHETIC JOINT (M97) ◀

● M97 Periprosthetic fracture around internal prosthetic joint ◀
Excludes2 fracture of bone following insertion of orthopedic implant, joint prosthesis or bone plate (M96.6-) ◀
breakage (fracture) of prosthetic joint (T84.01-) ◀
The appropriate 7th character is to be added to each code from category M97: ◀

A	initial encounter ◀
D	subsequent encounter ◀
S	sequela ◀

● M97.0 Periprosthetic fracture around internal prosthetic hip joint
X● M97.01 Periprosthetic fracture around internal prosthetic right hip joint ◀
X● M97.02 Periprosthetic fracture around internal prosthetic left hip joint ◀
● M97.1 Periprosthetic fracture around internal prosthetic knee joint
X● M97.11 Periprosthetic fracture around internal prosthetic right knee joint ◀
X● M97.12 Periprosthetic fracture around internal prosthetic left knee joint ◀
● M97.2 Periprosthetic fracture around internal prosthetic ankle joint
X● M97.21 Periprosthetic fracture around internal prosthetic right ankle joint ◀
X● M97.22 Periprosthetic fracture around internal prosthetic left ankle joint ◀
● M97.3 Periprosthetic fracture around internal prosthetic shoulder joint ◀
X● M97.31 Periprosthetic fracture around internal prosthetic right shoulder joint ◀
X● M97.32 Periprosthetic fracture around internal prosthetic left shoulder joint ◀
● M97.4 Periprosthetic fracture around internal prosthetic elbow joint ◀
X● M97.41 Periprosthetic fracture around internal prosthetic right elbow joint ◀
X● M97.42 Periprosthetic fracture around internal prosthetic left elbow joint ◀
X● M97.8 Periprosthetic fracture around other internal prosthetic joint ◀
Periprosthetic fracture around internal prosthetic finger joint ◀
Periprosthetic fracture around internal prosthetic spinal joint ◀
Periprosthetic fracture around internal prosthetic toe joint ◀
Periprosthetic fracture around internal prosthetic wrist joint ◀
Use additional code to identify the joint (Z96.6-) ◀
X● M97.9 Periprosthetic fracture around unspecified internal prosthetic joint ◀

CHAPTER 13 (M00-M99)

◀ New ⟸ Revised ~~deleted~~ Deleted OGCR Official Guidelines X Assign placeholder X ● Use Additional Character(s)
Excludes1 Excludes2 Includes Use additional Code first Code also Unspecified

BIOMECHANICAL LESIONS, NOT ELSEWHERE CLASSIFIED (M99)

● M99 Biomechanical lesions, not elsewhere classified

Note: This category should not be used if the condition can be classified elsewhere.

● M99.0 Segmental and somatic dysfunction
- M99.00 Segmental and somatic dysfunction of head region
- M99.01 Segmental and somatic dysfunction of cervical region
- M99.02 Segmental and somatic dysfunction of thoracic region
- M99.03 Segmental and somatic dysfunction of lumbar region
- M99.04 Segmental and somatic dysfunction of sacral region
- M99.05 Segmental and somatic dysfunction of pelvic region
- M99.06 Segmental and somatic dysfunction of lower extremity
- M99.07 Segmental and somatic dysfunction of upper extremity
- M99.08 Segmental and somatic dysfunction of rib cage
- M99.09 Segmental and somatic dysfunction of abdomen and other regions

● M99.1 Subluxation complex (vertebral)
- M99.10 Subluxation complex (vertebral) of head region
- M99.11 Subluxation complex (vertebral) of cervical region
- M99.12 Subluxation complex (vertebral) of thoracic region
- M99.13 Subluxation complex (vertebral) of lumbar region
- M99.14 Subluxation complex (vertebral) of sacral region
- M99.15 Subluxation complex (vertebral) of pelvic region
- M99.16 Subluxation complex (vertebral) of lower extremity
- M99.17 Subluxation complex (vertebral) of upper extremity
- M99.18 Subluxation complex (vertebral) of rib cage
- M99.19 Subluxation complex (vertebral) of abdomen and other regions

● M99.2 Subluxation stenosis of neural canal
- M99.20 Subluxation stenosis of neural canal of head region
- M99.21 Subluxation stenosis of neural canal of cervical region
- M99.22 Subluxation stenosis of neural canal of thoracic region
- M99.23 Subluxation stenosis of neural canal of lumbar region
- M99.24 Subluxation stenosis of neural canal of sacral region
- M99.25 Subluxation stenosis of neural canal of pelvic region
- M99.26 Subluxation stenosis of neural canal of lower extremity
- M99.27 Subluxation stenosis of neural canal of upper extremity
- M99.28 Subluxation stenosis of neural canal of rib cage
- M99.29 Subluxation stenosis of neural canal of abdomen and other regions

● M99.3 Osseous stenosis of neural canal
- M99.30 Osseous stenosis of neural canal of head region
- M99.31 Osseous stenosis of neural canal of cervical region
- M99.32 Osseous stenosis of neural canal of thoracic region
- M99.33 Osseous stenosis of neural canal of lumbar region
- M99.34 Osseous stenosis of neural canal of sacral region
- M99.35 Osseous stenosis of neural canal of pelvic region
- M99.36 Osseous stenosis of neural canal of lower extremity
- M99.37 Osseous stenosis of neural canal of upper extremity
- M99.38 Osseous stenosis of neural canal of rib cage
- M99.39 Osseous stenosis of neural canal of abdomen and other regions

● M99.4 Connective tissue stenosis of neural canal
- M99.40 Connective tissue stenosis of neural canal of head region
- M99.41 Connective tissue stenosis of neural canal of cervical region
- M99.42 Connective tissue stenosis of neural canal of thoracic region
- M99.43 Connective tissue stenosis of neural canal of lumbar region
- M99.44 Connective tissue stenosis of neural canal of sacral region
- M99.45 Connective tissue stenosis of neural canal of pelvic region
- M99.46 Connective tissue stenosis of neural canal of lower extremity
- M99.47 Connective tissue stenosis of neural canal of upper extremity
- M99.48 Connective tissue stenosis of neural canal of rib cage
- M99.49 Connective tissue stenosis of neural canal of abdomen and other regions

● M99.5 Intervertebral disc stenosis of neural canal
- M99.50 Intervertebral disc stenosis of neural canal of head region
- M99.51 Intervertebral disc stenosis of neural canal of cervical region
- M99.52 Intervertebral disc stenosis of neural canal of thoracic region
- M99.53 Intervertebral disc stenosis of neural canal of lumbar region
- M99.54 Intervertebral disc stenosis of neural canal of sacral region
- M99.55 Intervertebral disc stenosis of neural canal of pelvic region
- M99.56 Intervertebral disc stenosis of neural canal of lower extremity
- M99.57 Intervertebral disc stenosis of neural canal of upper extremity
- M99.58 Intervertebral disc stenosis of neural canal of rib cage
- M99.59 Intervertebral disc stenosis of neural canal of abdomen and other regions

● M99.6 Osseous and subluxation stenosis of intervertebral foramina
M99.60 Osseous and subluxation stenosis of intervertebral foramina of head region
M99.61 Osseous and subluxation stenosis of intervertebral foramina of cervical region
M99.62 Osseous and subluxation stenosis of intervertebral foramina of thoracic region
M99.63 Osseous and subluxation stenosis of intervertebral foramina of lumbar region
M99.64 Osseous and subluxation stenosis of intervertebral foramina of sacral region
M99.65 Osseous and subluxation stenosis of intervertebral foramina of pelvic region
M99.66 Osseous and subluxation stenosis of intervertebral foramina of lower extremity
M99.67 Osseous and subluxation stenosis of intervertebral foramina of upper extremity
M99.68 Osseous and subluxation stenosis of intervertebral foramina of rib cage
M99.69 Osseous and subluxation stenosis of intervertebral foramina of abdomen and other regions

● M99.7 Connective tissue and disc stenosis of intervertebral foramina
M99.70 Connective tissue and disc stenosis of intervertebral foramina of head region
M99.71 Connective tissue and disc stenosis of intervertebral foramina of cervical region
M99.72 Connective tissue and disc stenosis of intervertebral foramina of thoracic region
M99.73 Connective tissue and disc stenosis of intervertebral foramina of lumbar region
M99.74 Connective tissue and disc stenosis of intervertebral foramina of sacral region
M99.75 Connective tissue and disc stenosis of intervertebral foramina of pelvic region
M99.76 Connective tissue and disc stenosis of intervertebral foramina of lower extremity
M99.77 Connective tissue and disc stenosis of intervertebral foramina of upper extremity
M99.78 Connective tissue and disc stenosis of intervertebral foramina of rib cage
M99.79 Connective tissue and disc stenosis of intervertebral foramina of abdomen and other regions

● M99.8 Other biomechanical lesions
M99.80 Other biomechanical lesions of head region
M99.81 Other biomechanical lesions of cervical region
M99.82 Other biomechanical lesions of thoracic region
M99.83 Other biomechanical lesions of lumbar region
M99.84 Other biomechanical lesions of sacral region
M99.85 Other biomechanical lesions of pelvic region
M99.86 Other biomechanical lesions of lower extremity
M99.87 Other biomechanical lesions of upper extremity
M99.88 Other biomechanical lesions of rib cage
M99.89 Other biomechanical lesions of abdomen and other regions

M99.9 Biomechanical lesion, unspecified

CHAPTER 14

DISEASES OF THE GENITOURINARY SYSTEM (NØØ-N99)

OGCR Chapter-Specific Coding Guidelines

14. Chapter 14: Diseases of Genitourinary System (NØØ-N99)

a. Chronic kidney disease

1) Stages of chronic kidney disease (CKD)

The ICD-10-CM classifies CKD based on severity. The severity of CKD is designated by stages 1-5. Stage 2, code N18.2, equates to mild CKD; stage 3, code N18.3, equates to moderate CKD; and stage 4, code N18.4, equates to severe CKD. Code N18.6, End stage renal disease (ESRD), is assigned when the provider has documented end-stage-renal disease (ESRD).

If both a stage of CKD and ESRD are documented, assign code N18.6 only.

2) Chronic kidney disease and kidney transplant status

Patients who have undergone kidney transplant may still have some form of chronic kidney disease CKD because the kidney transplant may not fully restore kidney function. Therefore, the presence of CKD alone does not constitute a transplant complication. Assign the appropriate N18 code for the patient's stage of CKD and code Z94.Ø, Kidney transplant status. If a transplant complication such as failure or rejection or other transplant complication is documented, see section I.C.19.g for information on coding complications of a kidney transplant. If the documentation is unclear as to whether the patient has a complication of the transplant, query the provider.

3) Chronic kidney disease with other conditions

Patients with CKD may also suffer from other serious conditions, most commonly diabetes mellitus and hypertension. The sequencing of the CKD code in relationship to codes for other contributing conditions is based on the conventions in the Tabular List.

See I.C.9. Hypertensive chronic kidney disease.

See I.C.19. Chronic kidney disease and kidney transplant complications.

Item 14–1 Nephritis (inflammation) or **nephropathy** (disease) **with lesion of proliferative glomerulonephritis** results from a streptococcal infection.

Nephritis (inflammation) or **nephropathy** (disease) **with lesion of membranous glomerulonephritis** is characterized by deposits along the epithelial side of the basement membrane.

Nephritis (inflammation) or **nephropathy** (disease) **with lesion of membranoproliferative glomerulonephritis** is characterized by alterations in the basement membranes of the kidney and the glomerular cells.

Nephritis (inflammation) or **nephropathy** (disease) **with lesion of rapidly progressive glomerulonephritis** is characterized by rapid and progressive decline in renal function.

Nephritis (inflammation) or **nephropathy** (disease) **with lesion of renal cortical necrosis** is characterized by death of the cortical tissues.

Nephritis (inflammation) or **nephropathy** (disease) **with lesion of renal medullary necrosis** is characterized by death of the tissues that collect urine.

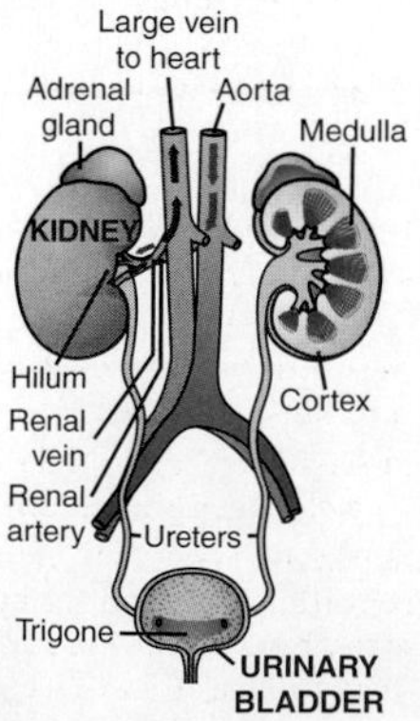

Figure 14-1 Kidneys within the urinary system.

Item 14–2 Glomerulonephritis is nephritis accompanied by inflammation of the glomeruli of the kidney, resulting in the degeneration of the glomeruli and the nephrons.

Acute glomerulonephritis primarily affects children and young adults and is usually a result of a streptococcal infection.

Proliferative glomerulonephritis is the acute form of the disease resulting from a streptococcal infection.

Rapidly progressive glomerulonephritis, also known as **crescentic** or **malignant glomerulonephritis**, is the acute form of the disease, which leads quickly to rapid and progressive decline in renal function.

CHAPTER 14

DISEASES OF THE GENITOURINARY SYSTEM (NØØ-N99)

Excludes2 certain conditions originating in the perinatal period (PØ4-P96)
certain infectious and parasitic diseases (AØØ-B99)
complications of pregnancy, childbirth and the puerperium (OØØ-O9A)
congenital malformations, deformations and chromosomal abnormalities (QØØ-Q99)
endocrine, nutritional and metabolic diseases (EØØ-E88)
injury, poisoning and certain other consequences of external causes (SØØ-T88)
neoplasms (CØØ-D49)
symptoms, signs and abnormal clinical and laboratory findings, not elsewhere classified (RØØ-R94)

This chapter contains the following blocks:

NØØ-NØ8	Glomerular diseases
N1Ø-N16	Renal tubulo-interstitial diseases
N17-N19	Acute kidney failure and chronic kidney disease
N2Ø-N23	Urolithiasis
N25-N29	Other disorders of kidney and ureter
N3Ø-N39	Other diseases of the urinary system
N4Ø-N53	Diseases of male genital organs
N6Ø-N65	Disorders of breast
N7Ø-N77	Inflammatory diseases of female pelvic organs
N8Ø-N98	Noninflammatory disorders of female genital tract
N99	Intraoperative and postprocedural complications and disorders of genitourinary system, not elsewhere classified

GLOMERULAR DISEASES (NØØ-NØ8)

Code also any associated kidney failure (N17-N19)

Excludes1 hypertensive chronic kidney disease (I12.-)

● **NØØ Acute nephritic syndrome**

Includes acute glomerular disease
acute glomerulonephritis
acute nephritis

Excludes1 acute tubulo-interstitial nephritis (N1Ø)
nephritic syndrome NOS (NØ5.-)

NØØ.Ø Acute nephritic syndrome with minor glomerular abnormality

Acute nephritic syndrome with minimal change lesion

NØØ.1 Acute nephritic syndrome with focal and segmental glomerular lesions

Acute nephritic syndrome with focal and segmental hyalinosis
Acute nephritic syndrome with focal and segmental sclerosis
Acute nephritic syndrome with focal glomerulonephritis

N00.2 Acute nephritic syndrome with diffuse membranous glomerulonephritis

N00.3 Acute nephritic syndrome with diffuse mesangial proliferative glomerulonephritis

N00.4 Acute nephritic syndrome with diffuse endocapillary proliferative glomerulonephritis

N00.5 Acute nephritic syndrome with diffuse mesangiocapillary glomerulonephritis
Acute nephritic syndrome with membranoproliferative glomerulonephritis, types 1 and 3, or NOS

N00.6 Acute nephritic syndrome with dense deposit disease
Acute nephritic syndrome with membranoproliferative glomerulonephritis, type 2

N00.7 Acute nephritic syndrome with diffuse crescentic glomerulonephritis
Acute nephritic syndrome with extracapillary glomerulonephritis

N00.8 Acute nephritic syndrome with other morphologic changes
Acute nephritic syndrome with proliferative glomerulonephritis NOS

N00.9 Acute nephritic syndrome with unspecified morphologic changes

● N01 Rapidly progressive nephritic syndrome

Includes
rapidly progressive glomerular disease
rapidly progressive glomerulonephritis
rapidly progressive nephritis

Excludes1
nephritic syndrome NOS (N05.-)

N01.0 Rapidly progressive nephritic syndrome with minor glomerular abnormality
Rapidly progressive nephritic syndrome with minimal change lesion

N01.1 Rapidly progressive nephritic syndrome with focal and segmental glomerular lesions
Rapidly progressive nephritic syndrome with focal and segmental hyalinosis
Rapidly progressive nephritic syndrome with focal and segmental sclerosis
Rapidly progressive nephritic syndrome with focal glomerulonephritis

N01.2 Rapidly progressive nephritic syndrome with diffuse membranous glomerulonephritis

N01.3 Rapidly progressive nephritic syndrome with diffuse mesangial proliferative glomerulonephritis

N01.4 Rapidly progressive nephritic syndrome with diffuse endocapillary proliferative glomerulonephritis

N01.5 Rapidly progressive nephritic syndrome with diffuse mesangiocapillary glomerulonephritis
Rapidly progressive nephritic syndrome with membranoproliferative glomerulonephritis, types 1 and 3, or NOS

N01.6 Rapidly progressive nephritic syndrome with dense deposit disease
Rapidly progressive nephritic syndrome with membranoproliferative glomerulonephritis, type 2

N01.7 Rapidly progressive nephritic syndrome with diffuse crescentic glomerulonephritis
Rapidly progressive nephritic syndrome with extracapillary glomerulonephritis

N01.8 Rapidly progressive nephritic syndrome with other morphologic changes
Rapidly progressive nephritic syndrome with proliferative glomerulonephritis NOS

N01.9 Rapidly progressive nephritic syndrome with unspecified morphologic changes

● N02 Recurrent and persistent hematuria

Excludes1
acute cystitis with hematuria (N30.01)
hematuria NOS (R31.9)
hematuria not associated with specified morphologic lesions (R31.-)

N02.0 Recurrent and persistent hematuria with minor glomerular abnormality
Recurrent and persistent hematuria with minimal change lesion

N02.1 Recurrent and persistent hematuria with focal and segmental glomerular lesions
Recurrent and persistent hematuria with focal and segmental hyalinosis
Recurrent and persistent hematuria with focal and segmental sclerosis
Recurrent and persistent hematuria with focal glomerulonephritis

N02.2 Recurrent and persistent hematuria with diffuse membranous glomerulonephritis

N02.3 Recurrent and persistent hematuria with diffuse mesangial proliferative glomerulonephritis

N02.4 Recurrent and persistent hematuria with diffuse endocapillary proliferative glomerulonephritis

N02.5 Recurrent and persistent hematuria with diffuse mesangiocapillary glomerulonephritis
Recurrent and persistent hematuria with membranoproliferative glomerulonephritis, types 1 and 3, or NOS

N02.6 Recurrent and persistent hematuria with dense deposit disease
Recurrent and persistent hematuria with membranoproliferative glomerulonephritis, type 2

N02.7 Recurrent and persistent hematuria with diffuse crescentic glomerulonephritis
Recurrent and persistent hematuria with extracapillary glomerulonephritis

N02.8 Recurrent and persistent hematuria with other morphologic changes
Recurrent and persistent hematuria with proliferative glomerulonephritis NOS

N02.9 Recurrent and persistent hematuria with unspecified morphologic changes

● N03 Chronic nephritic syndrome

Includes
chronic glomerular disease
chronic glomerulonephritis
chronic nephritis

Excludes1
chronic tubulo-interstitial nephritis (N11.-)
diffuse sclerosing glomerulonephritis (N05.8-)
nephritic syndrome NOS (N05.-)

N03.0 Chronic nephritic syndrome with minor glomerular abnormality
Chronic nephritic syndrome with minimal change lesion

N03.1 Chronic nephritic syndrome with focal and segmental glomerular lesions
Chronic nephritic syndrome with focal and segmental hyalinosis
Chronic nephritic syndrome with focal and segmental sclerosis
Chronic nephritic syndrome with focal glomerulonephritis

N03.2 Chronic nephritic syndrome with diffuse membranous glomerulonephritis

N03.3 Chronic nephritic syndrome with diffuse mesangial proliferative glomerulonephritis

N03.4 Chronic nephritic syndrome with diffuse endocapillary proliferative glomerulonephritis

N03.5 Chronic nephritic syndrome with diffuse mesangiocapillary glomerulonephritis
Chronic nephritic syndrome with membranoproliferative glomerulonephritis, types 1 and 3, or NOS

Item 14–3 Chronic glomerulonephritis (GN) persists over a period of years, with remissions and exacerbation.
Chronic GN with lesion of proliferative glomerulonephritis results from a streptococcal infection.
Chronic GN with lesion of membranous glomerulonephritis, also known as membranous nephropathy, is characterized by deposits along the epithelial side of the basement membrane.
Chronic GN with lesion of membrano-proliferative glomerulonephritis (MPGN) is a group of disorders characterized by alterations in the basement membranes of the kidney and the glomerular cells.
Chronic GN with lesion of rapidly progressive glomerulonephritis is characterized by necrosis, endothelial proliferation, and mesangial proliferation. The condition is marked by rapid and progressive decline in renal function.

N03.6 Chronic nephritic syndrome with dense deposit disease
Chronic nephritic syndrome with membranoproliferative glomerulonephritis, type 2

N03.7 Chronic nephritic syndrome with diffuse crescentic glomerulonephritis
Chronic nephritic syndrome with extracapillary glomerulonephritis

N03.8 Chronic nephritic syndrome with other morphologic changes
Chronic nephritic syndrome with proliferative glomerulonephritis NOS

N03.9 Chronic nephritic syndrome with unspecified morphologic changes

● **N04 Nephrotic syndrome**
Includes congenital nephrotic syndrome
lipoid nephrosis

N04.0 Nephrotic syndrome with minor glomerular abnormality
Nephrotic syndrome with minimal change lesion

N04.1 Nephrotic syndrome with focal and segmental glomerular lesions
Nephrotic syndrome with focal and segmental hyalinosis
Nephrotic syndrome with focal and segmental sclerosis
Nephrotic syndrome with focal glomerulonephritis

N04.2 Nephrotic syndrome with diffuse membranous glomerulonephritis

N04.3 Nephrotic syndrome with diffuse mesangial proliferative glomerulonephritis

N04.4 Nephrotic syndrome with diffuse endocapillary proliferative glomerulonephritis

N04.5 Nephrotic syndrome with diffuse mesangiocapillary glomerulonephritis
Nephrotic syndrome with membranoproliferative glomerulonephritis, types 1 and 3, or NOS

N04.6 Nephrotic syndrome with dense deposit disease
Nephrotic syndrome with membranoproliferative glomerulonephritis, type 2

N04.7 Nephrotic syndrome with diffuse crescentic glomerulonephritis
Nephrotic syndrome with extracapillary glomerulonephritis

N04.8 Nephrotic syndrome with other morphologic changes
Nephrotic syndrome with proliferative glomerulonephritis NOS

N04.9 Nephrotic syndrome with unspecified morphologic changes

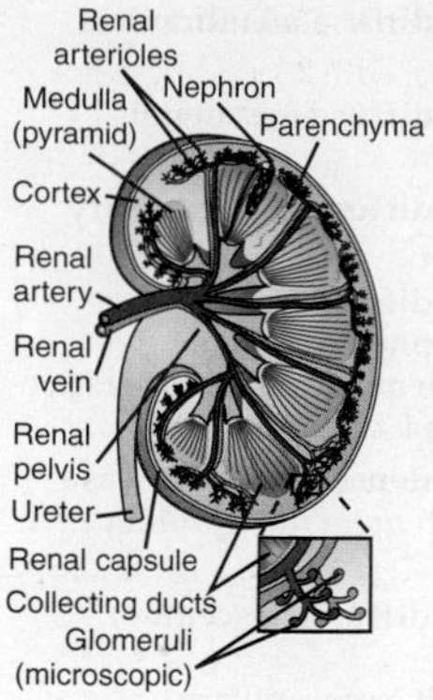

Figure 14-2 Kidney cross section.

Item 14–4 Nephrotic syndrome (NS) is marked by massive proteinuria (protein in the urine) and water retention. Patients with NS are particularly vulnerable to staphylococcal and pneumococcal infections. NS with lesion of proliferative glomerulonephritis results from a streptococcal infection. NS with lesion of membranous glomerulonephritis results in thickening of the capillary walls. NS with lesion of minimal change glomerulonephritis is usually a benign disorder that occurs mostly in children and requires electron microscopy (biopsy) to verify changes in the glomeruli.

● **N05 Unspecified nephritic syndrome**
Includes glomerular disease NOS
glomerulonephritis NOS
nephritis NOS
nephropathy NOS and renal disease NOS with morphological lesion specified in .0-.8

Excludes1 nephropathy NOS with no stated morphological lesion (N28.9)
renal disease NOS with no stated morphological lesion (N28.9)
tubulo-interstitial nephritis NOS (N12)

N05.0 Unspecified nephritic syndrome with minor glomerular abnormality
Unspecified nephritic syndrome with minimal change lesion

N05.1 Unspecified nephritic syndrome with focal and segmental glomerular lesions
Unspecified nephritic syndrome with focal and segmental hyalinosis
Unspecified nephritic syndrome with focal and segmental sclerosis
Unspecified nephritic syndrome with focal glomerulonephritis

N05.2 Unspecified nephritic syndrome with diffuse membranous glomerulonephritis

N05.3 Unspecified nephritic syndrome with diffuse mesangial proliferative glomerulonephritis

N05.4 Unspecified nephritic syndrome with diffuse endocapillary proliferative glomerulonephritis

N05.5 Unspecified nephritic syndrome with diffuse mesangiocapillary glomerulonephritis
Unspecified nephritic syndrome with membranoproliferative glomerulonephritis, types 1 and 3, or NOS

N05.6 Unspecified nephritic syndrome with dense deposit disease
Unspecified nephritic syndrome with membranoproliferative glomerulonephritis, type 2

N05.7 Unspecified nephritic syndrome with diffuse crescentic glomerulonephritis
Unspecified nephritic syndrome with extracapillary glomerulonephritis

N05.8 Unspecified nephritic syndrome with other morphologic changes
Unspecified nephritic syndrome with proliferative glomerulonephritis NOS

N05.9 Unspecified nephritic syndrome with unspecified morphologic changes

● **N06 Isolated proteinuria with specified morphological lesion**
Excludes1 proteinuria not associated with specific morphologic lesions (R80.0)

N06.0 Isolated proteinuria with minor glomerular abnormality
Isolated proteinuria with minimal change lesion

N06.1 Isolated proteinuria with focal and segmental glomerular lesions
Isolated proteinuria with focal and segmental hyalinosis
Isolated proteinuria with focal and segmental sclerosis
Isolated proteinuria with focal glomerulonephritis

N06.2 Isolated proteinuria with diffuse membranous glomerulonephritis

N06.3 Isolated proteinuria with diffuse mesangial proliferative glomerulonephritis

N06.4 Isolated proteinuria with diffuse endocapillary proliferative glomerulonephritis

N06.5 Isolated proteinuria with diffuse mesangiocapillary glomerulonephritis
Isolated proteinuria with membranoproliferative glomerulonephritis, types 1 and 3, or NOS

N06.6 Isolated proteinuria with dense deposit disease
Isolated proteinuria with membranoproliferative glomerulonephritis, type 2

N06.7 Isolated proteinuria with diffuse crescentic glomerulonephritis
Isolated proteinuria with extracapillary glomerulonephritis

N06.8 Isolated proteinuria with other morphologic lesion
Isolated proteinuria with proliferative glomerulonephritis NOS

N06.9 Isolated proteinuria with unspecified morphologic lesion

● **N07 Hereditary nephropathy, not elsewhere classified**
Excludes2 Alport's syndrome (Q87.81-)
hereditary amyloid nephropathy (E85.-)
nail patella syndrome (Q87.2)
non-neuropathic heredofamilial amyloidosis (E85.-)

N07.0 Hereditary nephropathy, not elsewhere classified with minor glomerular abnormality
Hereditary nephropathy, not elsewhere classified with minimal change lesion

N07.1 Hereditary nephropathy, not elsewhere classified with focal and segmental glomerular lesions
Hereditary nephropathy, not elsewhere classified with focal and segmental hyalinosis
Hereditary nephropathy, not elsewhere classified with focal and segmental sclerosis
Hereditary nephropathy, not elsewhere classified with focal glomerulonephritis

N07.2 Hereditary nephropathy, not elsewhere classified with diffuse membranous glomerulonephritis

N07.3 Hereditary nephropathy, not elsewhere classified with diffuse mesangial proliferative glomerulonephritis

N07.4 Hereditary nephropathy, not elsewhere classified with diffuse endocapillary proliferative glomerulonephritis

N07.5 Hereditary nephropathy, not elsewhere classified with diffuse mesangiocapillary glomerulonephritis
Hereditary nephropathy, not elsewhere classified with membranoproliferative glomerulonephritis, types 1 and 3, or NOS

N07.6 Hereditary nephropathy, not elsewhere classified with dense deposit disease
Hereditary nephropathy, not elsewhere classified with membranoproliferative glomerulonephritis, type 2

N07.7 Hereditary nephropathy, not elsewhere classified with diffuse crescentic glomerulonephritis
Hereditary nephropathy, not elsewhere classified with extracapillary glomerulonephritis

N07.8 Hereditary nephropathy, not elsewhere classified with other morphologic lesions
Hereditary nephropathy, not elsewhere classified with proliferative glomerulonephritis NOS

N07.9 Hereditary nephropathy, not elsewhere classified with unspecified morphologic lesions

N08 Glomerular disorders in diseases classified elsewhere
Glomerulonephritis
Nephritis
Nephropathy
Code first underlying disease, such as:
amyloidosis (E85.-)
congenital syphilis (A50.5)
cryoglobulinemia (D89.1)
disseminated intravascular coagulation (D65)
gout (M1A.-, M10.-)
microscopic polyangiitis (M31.7)
multiple myeloma (C90.0-)
sepsis (A40.0-A41.9)
sickle-cell disease (D57.0-D57.8)
Excludes1 glomerulonephritis, nephritis and nephropathy (in):
antiglomerular basement membrane disease (M31.0)
diabetes (E08-E13 with .21)
gonococcal (A54.21)
Goodpasture's syndrome (M31.0)
hemolytic-uremic syndrome (D59.3)
lupus (M32.14)
mumps (B26.83)
syphilis (A52.75)
systemic lupus erythematosus (M32.14)
Wegener's granulomatosis (M31.31)
pyelonephritis in diseases classified elsewhere (N16)
renal tubulo-interstitial disorders classified elsewhere (N16)

RENAL TUBULO-INTERSTITIAL DISEASES (N10-N16)

Includes pyelonephritis
Excludes1 pyeloureteritis cystica (N28.85)

N10 Acute pyelonephritis ⬅
Acute infectious interstitial nephritis
Acute pyelitis
Acute tubulo-interstitial nephritis ⬅
Hemoglobin nephrosis
Myoglobin nephrosis
Use additional code (B95-B97), to identify infectious agent

● **N11 Chronic tubulo-interstitial nephritis**
Includes chronic infectious interstitial nephritis
chronic pyelitis
chronic pyelonephritis
Use additional code (B95-B97), to identify infectious agent

N11.0 Nonobstructive reflux-associated chronic pyelonephritis
Pyelonephritis (chronic) associated with (vesicoureteral) reflux
Excludes1 vesicoureteral reflux NOS (N13.70)

N11.1 Chronic obstructive pyelonephritis
Pyelonephritis (chronic) associated with anomaly of pelviureteric junction
Pyelonephritis (chronic) associated with anomaly of pyeloureteric junction
Pyelonephritis (chronic) associated with crossing of vessel
Pyelonephritis (chronic) associated with kinking of ureter
Pyelonephritis (chronic) associated with obstruction of ureter
Pyelonephritis (chronic) associated with stricture of pelviureteric junction
Pyelonephritis (chronic) associated with stricture of ureter
Excludes1 calculous pyelonephritis (N20.9)
obstructive uropathy (N13.-)

CHAPTER 14 (N00-N99)

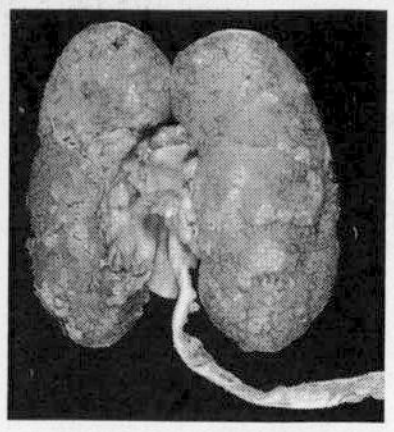

Figure 14-3 Acute pyelonephritis. Cortical surface exhibits grayish white areas of inflammation and abscess formation. (From Kumar: Robbins and Cotran: Pathologic Basis of Disease, ed 8, Saunders, An Imprint of Elsevier, 2009)

Item 14–5 Pyelonephritis is an infection of the kidneys and ureters and may be chronic or acute in one or both kidneys.

N11.8 Other chronic tubulo-interstitial nephritis
Nonobstructive chronic pyelonephritis NOS

N11.9 Chronic tubulo-interstitial nephritis, unspecified
Chronic interstitial nephritis NOS
Chronic pyelitis NOS
Chronic pyelonephritis NOS

N12 Tubulo-interstitial nephritis, not specified as acute or chronic
Interstitial nephritis NOS
Pyelitis NOS
Pyelonephritis NOS
Excludes1 calculous pyelonephritis (N2Ø.9)

● **N13 Obstructive and reflux uropathy**
Excludes2 calculus of kidney and ureter without hydronephrosis (N2Ø.-)
congenital obstructive defects of renal pelvis and ureter (Q62.Ø-Q62.3)
hydronephrosis with ureteropelvic junction obstruction (Q62.1)
obstructive pyelonephritis (N11.1)

N13.Ø Hydronephrosis with ureteropelvic junction obstruction ◀
Hydronephrosis due to acquired occlusion of ureteropelvic junction ◀
Excludes2 Hydronephrosis with ureteropelvic junction obstruction due to calculus (N13.2) ◀

N13.1 Hydronephrosis with ureteral stricture, not elsewhere classified
Excludes1 hydronephrosis with ureteral stricture with infection (N13.6)

N13.2 Hydronephrosis with renal and ureteral calculous obstruction
Excludes1 hydronephrosis with renal and ureteral calculous obstruction with infection (N13.6)

● **N13.3 Other and unspecified hydronephrosis**
Excludes1 hydronephrosis with infection (N13.6)
N13.3Ø Unspecified hydronephrosis
N13.39 Other hydronephrosis

N13.4 Hydroureter
Excludes1 congenital hydroureter (Q62.3-)
hydroureter with infection (N13.6)
vesicoureteral-reflux with hydroureter (N13.73-)

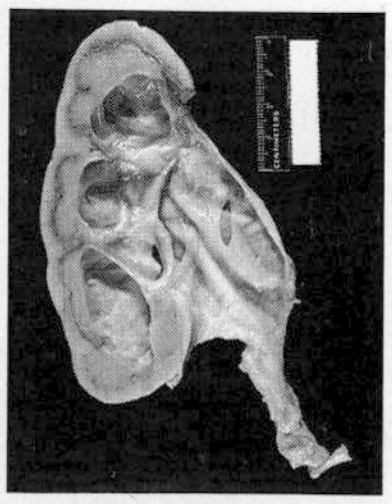

Figure 14-4 Hydronephrosis of the kidney, with marked dilatation of pelvis and calyces and thinning of renal parenchyma. (From Kumar: Robbins and Cotran: Pathologic Basis of Disease, ed 8, Saunders, An Imprint of Elsevier, 2009)

N13.5 Crossing vessel and stricture of ureter without hydronephrosis
Kinking and stricture of ureter without hydronephrosis
Excludes1 crossing vessel and stricture of ureter without hydronephrosis with infection (N13.6)

N13.6 Pyonephrosis
Conditions in N13.Ø-N13.5 with infection ⬅
Obstructive uropathy with infection
Use additional code (B95-B97), to identify infectious agent

● **N13.7 Vesicoureteral-reflux**
Excludes1 reflux-associated pyelonephritis (N11.Ø)
N13.7Ø Vesicoureteral-reflux, unspecified
Occurs when urine flows from bladder back into ureters
Vesicoureteral-reflux NOS
N13.71 Vesicoureteral-reflux without reflux nephropathy
● **N13.72 Vesicoureteral-reflux with reflux nephropathy without hydroureter**
N13.721 Vesicoureteral-reflux with reflux nephropathy without hydroureter, unilateral
N13.722 Vesicoureteral-reflux with reflux nephropathy without hydroureter, bilateral
N13.729 Vesicoureteral-reflux with reflux nephropathy without hydroureter, unspecified
● **N13.73 Vesicoureteral-reflux with reflux nephropathy with hydroureter**
N13.731 Vesicoureteral-reflux with reflux nephropathy with hydroureter, unilateral
N13.732 Vesicoureteral-reflux with reflux nephropathy with hydroureter, bilateral
N13.739 Vesicoureteral-reflux with reflux nephropathy with hydroureter, unspecified

N13.8 Other obstructive and reflux uropathy
Urinary tract obstruction due to specified cause
Code first, if applicable, any causal condition first, such as:
enlarged prostate (N4Ø.1)

N13.9 Obstructive and reflux uropathy, unspecified
Urinary tract obstruction NOS

● **N14 Drug- and heavy-metal-induced tubulo-interstitial and tubular conditions**
Code first poisoning due to drug or toxin, if applicable (T36-T65 with fifth or sixth character 1-4 or 6)
Use additional code for adverse effect, if applicable, to identify drug (T36-T5Ø with fifth or sixth character 5)
N14.Ø Analgesic nephropathy
N14.1 Nephropathy induced by other drugs, medicaments and biological substances
N14.2 Nephropathy induced by unspecified drug, medicament or biological substance
N14.3 Nephropathy induced by heavy metals
N14.4 Toxic nephropathy, not elsewhere classified

● **N15 Other renal tubulo-interstitial diseases**
N15.Ø Balkan nephropathy
Balkan endemic nephropathy
N15.1 Renal and perinephric abscess
N15.8 Other specified renal tubulo-interstitial diseases
N15.9 Renal tubulo-interstitial disease, unspecified
Infection of kidney NOS
Excludes1 urinary tract infection NOS (N39.Ø)

N16 Renal tubulo-interstitial disorders in diseases classified elsewhere
Pyelonephritis
Tubulo-interstitial nephritis
Code first *underlying disease, such as:*
brucellosis (A23.Ø-A23.9)
cryoglobulinemia (D89.1)
glycogen storage disease (E74.Ø)
leukemia (C91-C95)
lymphoma (C81.Ø-C85.9, C96.Ø-C96.9)
multiple myeloma (C9Ø.Ø-)
sepsis (A4Ø.Ø-A41.9)
Wilson's disease (E83.Ø)
Excludes1 diphtheritic pyelonephritis and tubulo-interstitial nephritis (A36.84)
pyelonephritis and tubulo-interstitial nephritis in candidiasis (B37.49)
pyelonephritis and tubulo-interstitial nephritis in cystinosis (E72.Ø4)
pyelonephritis and tubulo-interstitial nephritis in salmonella infection (AØ2.25)
pyelonephritis and tubulo-interstitial nephritis in sarcoidosis (D86.84)
pyelonephritis and tubulo-interstitial nephritis in sicca syndrome [Sjogren's] (M35.Ø4)
pyelonephritis and tubulo-interstitial nephritis in systemic lupus erythematosus (M32.15)
pyelonephritis and tubulo-interstitial nephritis in toxoplasmosis (B58.83)
renal tubular degeneration in diabetes (EØ8-E13 with .29)
syphilitic pyelonephritis and tubulo-interstitial nephritis (A52.75)

ACUTE KIDNEY FAILURE AND CHRONIC KIDNEY DISEASE (N17-N19)

Excludes2 congenital renal failure (P96.Ø)
drug- and heavy-metal-induced tubulo-interstitial and tubular conditions (N14.-)
extrarenal uremia (R39.2)
hemolytic-uremic syndrome (D59.3)
hepatorenal syndrome (K76.7)
postpartum hepatorenal syndrome (O9Ø.4)
posttraumatic renal failure (T79.5)
prerenal uremia (R39.2)
renal failure complicating abortion or ectopic or molar pregnancy (OØØ-OØ7, OØ8.4)
renal failure following labor and delivery (O9Ø.4)
renal failure postprocedural (N99.Ø)

● **N17 Acute kidney failure**
Code also associated underlying condition
Excludes1 posttraumatic renal failure (T79.5)
N17.Ø Acute kidney failure with tubular necrosis
Acute tubular necrosis
Renal tubular necrosis
Tubular necrosis NOS
N17.1 Acute kidney failure with acute cortical necrosis
Acute cortical necrosis
Cortical necrosis NOS
Renal cortical necrosis
N17.2 Acute kidney failure with medullary necrosis
Medullary [papillary] necrosis NOS
Acute medullary [papillary] necrosis
Renal medullary [papillary] necrosis
N17.8 Other acute kidney failure
N17.9 Acute kidney failure, unspecified
Acute kidney injury (nontraumatic)
Excludes2 traumatic kidney injury (S37.Ø-)

Item 14–6 Decreased blood flow is the usual cause of **acute renal failure** that offers a good prognosis for recovery.
Chronic renal failure is usually the result of long-standing kidney disease and is a very serious condition that generally results in death.

● **N18 Chronic kidney disease (CKD)**
Code first *any associated:*
diabetic chronic kidney disease (EØ8.22, EØ9.22, E1Ø.22, E11.22, E13.22)
hypertensive chronic kidney disease (I12.-, I13.-)
Use additional code to identify kidney transplant status, if applicable, (Z94.Ø)
N18.1 Chronic kidney disease, stage 1
N18.2 Chronic kidney disease, stage 2 (mild)
N18.3 Chronic kidney disease, stage 3 (moderate)
N18.4 Chronic kidney disease, stage 4 (severe)
N18.5 Chronic kidney disease, stage 5
Excludes1 chronic kidney disease, stage 5 requiring chronic dialysis (N18.6)
N18.6 End stage renal disease
Chronic kidney disease requiring chronic dialysis
Use additional code to identify dialysis status (Z99.2)
N18.9 Chronic kidney disease, unspecified
Chronic renal disease
Chronic renal failure NOS
Chronic renal insufficiency
Chronic uremia

N19 Unspecified kidney failure
Uremia NOS
Excludes1 acute kidney failure (N17.-)
chronic kidney disease (N18.-)
chronic uremia (N18.9)
extrarenal uremia (R39.2)
prerenal uremia (R39.2)
renal insufficiency (acute) (N28.9)
uremia of newborn (P96.Ø)

UROLITHIASIS (N2Ø-N23)

● **N2Ø Calculus of kidney and ureter**
Calculous pyelonephritis
Excludes1 nephrocalcinosis (E83.5)
that with hydronephrosis (N13.2)
N2Ø.Ø Calculus of kidney
Nephrolithiasis NOS
Renal calculus
Renal stone
Staghorn calculus
Stone in kidney
N2Ø.1 Calculus of ureter
Ureteric stone
N2Ø.2 Calculus of kidney with calculus of ureter
N2Ø.9 Urinary calculus, unspecified

● **N21 Calculus of lower urinary tract**
Includes calculus of lower urinary tract with cystitis and urethritis
N21.Ø Calculus in bladder
Calculus in diverticulum of bladder
Urinary bladder stone
Excludes2 staghorn calculus (N2Ø.Ø)
N21.1 Calculus in urethra
Excludes2 calculus of prostate (N42.Ø)
N21.8 Other lower urinary tract calculus
N21.9 Calculus of lower urinary tract, unspecified
Excludes1 calculus of urinary tract NOS (N2Ø.9)

CHAPTER 14 (NØØ-N99)

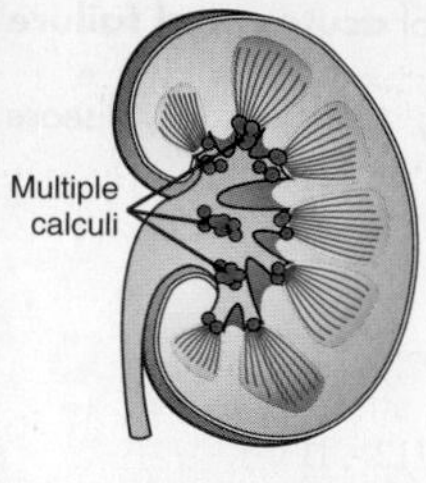

Figure 14-5 Multiple urinary calculi.

N22 Calculus of urinary tract in diseases classified elsewhere
Code first underlying disease, such as:
gout (M1A.-, M1Ø.-)
schistosomiasis (B65.Ø-B65.9)

N23 Unspecified renal colic

OTHER DISORDERS OF KIDNEY AND URETER (N25-N29)

Excludes2 disorders of kidney and ureter with urolithiasis (N2Ø-N23)

● **N25 Disorders resulting from impaired renal tubular function**
Excludes1 metabolic disorders classifiable to E7Ø-E88

N25.Ø Renal osteodystrophy
Azotemic osteodystrophy
Phosphate-losing tubular disorders
Renal rickets
Renal short stature

N25.1 Nephrogenic diabetes insipidus
Excludes1 diabetes insipidus NOS (E23.2)

● **N25.8 Other disorders resulting from impaired renal tubular function**

N25.81 Secondary hyperparathyroidism of renal origin
Excludes1 secondary hyperparathyroidism, non-renal (E21.1)

N25.89 Other disorders resulting from impaired renal tubular function
Hypokalemic nephropathy
Lightwood-Albright syndrome
Renal tubular acidosis NOS

N25.9 Disorder resulting from impaired renal tubular function, unspecified

● **N26 Unspecified contracted kidney**
Excludes1 contracted kidney due to hypertension (I12.-)
diffuse sclerosing glomerulonephritis (NØ5.8.-)
hypertensive nephrosclerosis (arteriolar) (arteriosclerotic) (I12.-)
small kidney of unknown cause (N27.-)

N26.1 Atrophy of kidney (terminal)
N26.2 Page kidney
N26.9 Renal sclerosis, unspecified

● **N27 Small kidney of unknown cause**
Includes oligonephronia

N27.Ø Small kidney, unilateral
N27.1 Small kidney, bilateral
N27.9 Small kidney, unspecified

● **N28 Other disorders of kidney and ureter, not elsewhere classified**

N28.Ø Ischemia and infarction of kidney
Renal artery embolism
Renal artery obstruction
Renal artery occlusion
Renal artery thrombosis
Renal infarct
Excludes1 atherosclerosis of renal artery (extrarenal part) (I7Ø.1)
congenital stenosis of renal artery (Q27.1)
Goldblatt's kidney (I7Ø.1)

N28.1 Cyst of kidney, acquired
Cyst (multiple)(solitary) of kidney, acquired
Excludes1 cystic kidney disease (congenital) (Q61.-)

● **N28.8 Other specified disorders of kidney and ureter**
Excludes1 hydroureter (N13.4)
ureteric stricture with hydronephrosis (N13.1)
ureteric stricture without hydronephrosis (N13.5)

N28.81 Hypertrophy of kidney
N28.82 Megaloureter
N28.83 Nephroptosis
N28.84 Pyelitis cystica
N28.85 Pyeloureteritis cystica
N28.86 Ureteritis cystica
N28.89 Other specified disorders of kidney and ureter

N28.9 Disorder of kidney and ureter, unspecified
Nephropathy NOS
Renal disease (acute) NOS
Renal insufficiency (acute)
Excludes1 chronic renal insufficiency (N18.9)
unspecified nephritic syndrome (NØ5.-)

N29 Other disorders of kidney and ureter in diseases classified elsewhere
Code first underlying disease, such as:
amyloidosis (E85.-)
nephrocalcinosis (E83.5)
schistosomiasis (B65.Ø-B65.9)
Excludes1 disorders of kidney and ureter in:
cystinosis (E72.Ø)
gonorrhea (A54.21)
syphilis (A52.75)
tuberculosis (A18.11)

OTHER DISEASES OF THE URINARY SYSTEM (N3Ø-N39)

Excludes1 urinary infection (complicating):
abortion or ectopic or molar pregnancy (OØØ-OØ7, OØ8.8)
pregnancy, childbirth and the puerperium (O23.-, O75.3, O86.2-)

● **N3Ø Cystitis**
Infection of bladder and irritation in lower urinary tract
Use additional code to identify infectious agent (B95-B97)
Excludes1 prostatocystitis (N41.3)

● **N3Ø.Ø Acute cystitis**
Excludes1 irradiation cystitis (N3Ø.4-)
trigonitis (N3Ø.3-)

N3Ø.ØØ Acute cystitis without hematuria
N3Ø.Ø1 Acute cystitis with hematuria

● **N3Ø.1 Interstitial cystitis (chronic)**
Ongoing infection of kidney glomeruli and tubules

N3Ø.1Ø Interstitial cystitis (chronic) without hematuria
N3Ø.11 Interstitial cystitis (chronic) with hematuria

● **N3Ø.2 Other chronic cystitis**

N3Ø.2Ø Other chronic cystitis without hematuria
N3Ø.21 Other chronic cystitis with hematuria

● **N3Ø.3 Trigonitis**
Inflammation of triangular area of bladder (where the ureters and urethra come together)
Urethrotrigonitis

N3Ø.3Ø Trigonitis without hematuria
N3Ø.31 Trigonitis with hematuria

● **N3Ø.4 Irradiation cystitis**

N3Ø.4Ø Irradiation cystitis without hematuria
N3Ø.41 Irradiation cystitis with hematuria

● **N30.8 Other cystitis**
Abscess of bladder
N30.80 Other cystitis without hematuria
N30.81 Other cystitis with hematuria

● **N30.9 Cystitis, unspecified**
N30.90 Cystitis, unspecified without hematuria
N30.91 Cystitis, unspecified with hematuria

● **N31 Neuromuscular dysfunction of bladder, not elsewhere classified**
Use additional code to identify any associated urinary incontinence (N39.3-N39.4-)
Excludes1 cord bladder NOS (G95.89)
neurogenic bladder due to cauda equina syndrome (G83.4)
neuromuscular dysfunction due to spinal cord lesion (G95.89)

N31.0 Uninhibited neuropathic bladder, not elsewhere classified
N31.1 Reflex neuropathic bladder, not elsewhere classified
N31.2 Flaccid neuropathic bladder, not elsewhere classified
Atonic (motor) (sensory) neuropathic bladder
Diminished tone of bladder muscle
Autonomous neuropathic bladder
Nonreflex neuropathic bladder
N31.8 Other neuromuscular dysfunction of bladder
N31.9 Neuromuscular dysfunction of bladder, unspecified
Neurogenic bladder dysfunction NOS

● **N32 Other disorders of bladder**
Excludes2 calculus of bladder (N21.0)
cystocele (N81.1-)
hernia or prolapse of bladder, female (N81.1-)

N32.0 Bladder-neck obstruction
Bladder-neck stenosis (acquired)
Excludes1 congenital bladder-neck obstruction (Q64.3-)
N32.1 Vesicointestinal fistula
Vesicorectal fistula
N32.2 Vesical fistula, not elsewhere classified
Excludes1 fistula between bladder and female genital tract (N82.0-N82.1)
N32.3 Diverticulum of bladder
Formation of sac from a herniation of wall of bladder
Excludes1 congenital diverticulum of bladder (Q64.6)
diverticulitis of bladder (N30.8-)

● **N32.8 Other specified disorders of bladder**
N32.81 Overactive bladder
Detrusor muscle hyperactivity
Excludes1 frequent urination due to specified bladder condition- code to condition
N32.89 Other specified disorders of bladder
Bladder hemorrhage
Bladder hypertrophy
Calcified bladder
Contracted bladder
N32.9 Bladder disorder, unspecified

N33 Bladder disorders in diseases classified elsewhere
Code first underlying disease, such as:
schistosomiasis (B65.0-B65.9)
Excludes1 bladder disorder in syphilis (A52.76)
bladder disorder in tuberculosis (A18.12)
candidal cystitis (B37.41)
chlamydial cystitis(A56.01)
cystitis in gonorrhea (A54.01)
cystitis in neurogenic bladder (N31.-)
diphtheritic cystitis (A36.85)
syphilitic cystitis (A52.76)
trichomonal cystitis (A59.03)

● **N34 Urethritis and urethral syndrome**
Use additional code (B95-B97), to identify infectious agent
Excludes2 Reiter's disease (M02.3-)
urethritis in diseases with a predominantly sexual mode of transmission (A50-A64)
urethrotrigonitis (N30.3-)

N34.0 Urethral abscess
Abscess (of) Cowper's gland
Abscess (of) Littré's gland
Abscess (of) urethral (gland)
Periurethral abscess
Excludes1 urethral caruncle (N36.2)
N34.1 Nonspecific urethritis
Nongonococcal urethritis
Nonvenereal urethritis
N34.2 Other urethritis
Inflammation of urethra
Meatitis, urethral
Postmenopausal urethritis
Ulcer of urethra (meatus)
Urethritis NOS
N34.3 Urethral syndrome, unspecified

● **N35 Urethral stricture**
Narrowing of lumen of urethra caused by scarring due to infection or injury
Excludes1 congenital urethral stricture (Q64.3-)
postprocedural urethral stricture (N99.1-)

● **N35.0 Post-traumatic urethral stricture**
Urethral stricture due to injury
Excludes1 postprocedural urethral stricture (N99.1-)
● **N35.01 Post-traumatic urethral stricture, male**
N35.010 Post-traumatic urethral stricture, male, meatal
N35.011 Post-traumatic bulbous urethral stricture
N35.012 Post-traumatic membranous urethral stricture
N35.013 Post-traumatic anterior urethral stricture
N35.014 Post-traumatic urethral stricture, male, unspecified
● **N35.02 Post-traumatic urethral stricture, female**
N35.021 Urethral stricture due to childbirth
N35.028 Other post-traumatic urethral stricture, female

● **N35.1 Postinfective urethral stricture, not elsewhere classified**
Excludes1 urethral stricture associated with schistosomiasis (B65.-, N29)
gonococcal urethral stricture (A54.01)
syphilitic urethral stricture (A52.76)
● **N35.11 Postinfective urethral stricture, not elsewhere classified, male**
N35.111 Postinfective urethral stricture, not elsewhere classified, male, meatal
N35.112 Postinfective bulbous urethral stricture, not elsewhere classified
N35.113 Postinfective membranous urethral stricture, not elsewhere classified
N35.114 Postinfective anterior urethral stricture, not elsewhere classified
N35.119 Postinfective urethral stricture, not elsewhere classified, male, unspecified
N35.12 Postinfective urethral stricture, not elsewhere classified, female
N35.8 Other urethral stricture
Excludes1 postprocedural urethral stricture (N99.1-)
N35.9 Urethral stricture, unspecified

● **N36 Other disorders of urethra**

N36.0 Urethral fistula

Urethroperineal fistula
Urethrorectal fistula
Urinary fistula NOS

Excludes1 urethroscrotal fistula (N50.89) ⬅ Revised
urethrovaginal fistula (N82.1)
urethrovesicovaginal fistula (N82.1)

N36.1 Urethral diverticulum

N36.2 Urethral caruncle

● **N36.4 Urethral functional and muscular disorders**

Use additional code to identify associated urinary stress incontinence (N39.3)

N36.41 Hypermobility of urethra

N36.42 Intrinsic sphincter deficiency (ISD)

N36.43 Combined hypermobility of urethra and intrinsic sphincter deficiency

N36.44 Muscular disorders of urethra

Bladder sphincter dyssynergy

N36.5 Urethral false passage

N36.8 Other specified disorders of urethra

Excludes1 congenital urethrocele (Q64.7) ◀
female urethrocele (N81.0) ◀

N36.9 Urethral disorder, unspecified

N37 Urethral disorders in diseases classified elsewhere

Code first underlying disease

Excludes1 urethritis (in):
candidal infection (B37.41)
chlamydial (A56.01)
gonorrhea (A54.01)
syphilis (A52.76)
trichomonal infection (A59.03)
tuberculosis (A18.13)

● **N39 Other disorders of urinary system**

Excludes2 hematuria NOS (R31.-)
recurrent or persistent hematuria (N02.-)
recurrent or persistent hematuria with specified morphological lesion (N02.-)
proteinuria NOS (R80.-)

N39.0 Urinary tract infection, site not specified

Use additional code (B95-B97), to identify infectious agent

Excludes1 candidiasis of urinary tract (B37.4-)
neonatal urinary tract infection (P39.3)
urinary tract infection of specified site, such as:
cystitis (N30.-)
urethritis (N34.-)

N39.3 Stress incontinence (female) (male)

Code also any associated overactive bladder (N32.81)

Excludes1 mixed incontinence (N39.46)

● **N39.4 Other specified urinary incontinence**

Code also any associated overactive bladder (N32.81)

Excludes1 enuresis NOS (R32)
functional urinary incontinence (R39.81)
urinary incontinence associated with cognitive impairment (R39.81)
urinary incontinence NOS (R32)
urinary incontinence of nonorganic origin (F98.0)

N39.41 Urge incontinence

Excludes1 mixed incontinence (N39.46)

N39.42 Incontinence without sensory awareness

Insensible (urinary) incontinence ◀

N39.43 Post-void dribbling

N39.44 Nocturnal enuresis

N39.45 Continuous leakage

N39.46 Mixed incontinence

Urge and stress incontinence

● **N39.49 Other specified urinary incontinence**

N39.490 Overflow incontinence

N39.491 Coital incontinence ◀

N39.492 Postural (urinary) incontinence ◀

N39.498 Other specified urinary incontinence

Reflex incontinence
Total incontinence

N39.8 Other specified disorders of urinary system

N39.9 Disorder of urinary system, unspecified

DISEASES OF MALE GENITAL ORGANS (N40-N53)

★(See Plate 387 on page NAP-5.)

● **N40 Benign prostatic hyperplasia** ⬅

Includes adenofibromatous hypertrophy of prostate
benign hypertrophy of the prostate
Enlargement of prostate gland usually occurring with age and causing obstructed urine flow
benign prostatic hypertrophy
BPH
enlarged prostate ◀
nodular prostate
polyp of prostate

Excludes1 benign neoplasms of prostate (adenoma, benign) (fibroadenoma) (fibroma) (myoma) (D29.1)
malignant neoplasm of prostate (C61)

N40.0 Benign prostatic hyperplasia without lower urinary tract symptoms ⬅

Enlarged prostate without LUTS
Enlarged prostate NOS

N40.1 Benign prostatic hyperplasia with lower urinary tract symptoms ⬅

Enlarged prostate with LUTS

Use additional code for associated symptoms, when specified:
incomplete bladder emptying (R39.14)
nocturia (R35.1)
straining on urination (R39.16)
urinary frequency (R35.0)
urinary hesitancy (R39.11)
urinary incontinence (N39.4-)
urinary obstruction (N13.8)
urinary retention (R33.8)
urinary urgency (R39.15)
weak urinary stream (R39.12)

N40.2 Nodular prostate without lower urinary tract symptoms

Nodular prostate without LUTS

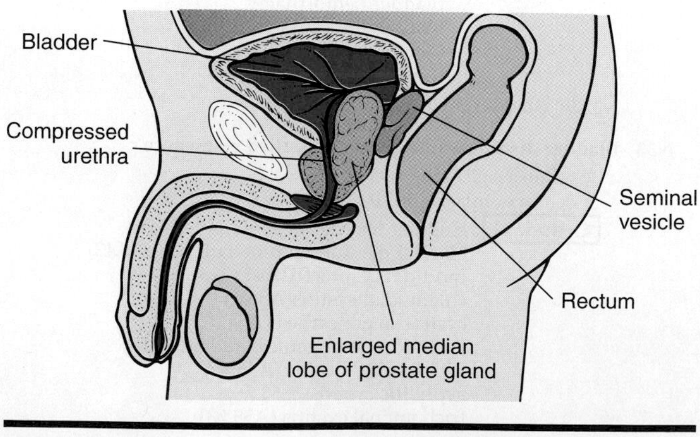

Figure 14-6 Benign prostatic hyperplasia. (From Shiland: Mastering Healthcare Terminology, ed 3, St. Louis, Mosby, 2010)

N40.3 **Nodular prostate with lower urinary tract symptoms**
Use additional code for associated symptoms, when specified:
incomplete bladder emptying (R39.14)
nocturia (R35.1)
straining on urination (R39.16)
urinary frequency (R35.0)
urinary hesitancy (R39.11)
urinary incontinence (N39.4-)
urinary obstruction (N13.8)
urinary retention (R33.8)
urinary urgency (R39.15)
weak urinary stream (R39.12)

● N41 **Inflammatory diseases of prostate**
Use additional code (B95-B97), to identify infectious agent
N41.0 **Acute prostatitis**
N41.1 **Chronic prostatitis**
N41.2 **Abscess of prostate**
N41.3 **Prostatocystitis**
N41.4 **Granulomatous prostatitis**
N41.8 **Other inflammatory diseases of prostate**
N41.9 **Inflammatory disease of prostate, unspecified**
Prostatitis NOS

● N42 **Other and unspecified disorders of prostate**
N42.0 **Calculus of prostate**
Prostatic stone
N42.1 **Congestion and hemorrhage of prostate**
Excludes1 enlarged prostate (N40.-)
hematuria (R31.-)
hyperplasia of prostate (N40.-)
inflammatory diseases of prostate (N41.-)
● N42.3 **Dysplasia of prostate**
N42.30 **Unspecified dysplasia of prostate** ◀
N42.31 **Prostatic intraepithelial neoplasia** ◀
PIN ◀
Prostatic intraepithelial neoplasia I (PIN I) ◀
Prostatic intraepithelial neoplasia II (PIN II) ◀
Excludes1 prostatic intraepithelial neoplasia III (PIN III) (D07.5) ◀
N42.32 **Atypical small acinar proliferation of prostate** ◀
N42.39 **Other dysplasia of prostate** ◀
● N42.8 **Other specified disorders of prostate**
N42.81 **Prostatodynia syndrome**
Painful prostate syndrome
N42.82 **Prostatosis syndrome**
N42.83 **Cyst of prostate**
N42.89 **Other specified disorders of prostate**
N42.9 **Disorder of prostate, unspecified**

● N43 **Hydrocele and spermatocele**
Includes hydrocele of spermatic cord, testis or tunica vaginalis
Excludes1 congenital hydrocele (P83.5)
N43.0 **Encysted hydrocele**
N43.1 **Infected hydrocele**
Use additional code (B95-B97), to identify infectious agent
N43.2 **Other hydrocele**
N43.3 **Hydrocele, unspecified**

Item 14-7 Hydrocele is a sac of fluid accumulating in the testes membrane.

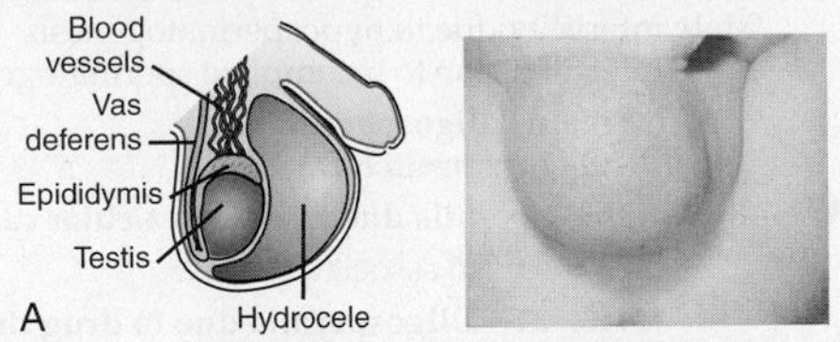

Figure 14-7 A. Hydrocele. **B.** Newborn with large right hydrocele. (**B** from Behrman: Nelson Textbook of Pediatrics, ed 18, Saunders, An Imprint of Elsevier, 2007)

● N43.4 **Spermatocele of epididymis**
Spermatic cyst
N43.40 **Spermatocele of epididymis, unspecified**
N43.41 **Spermatocele of epididymis, single**
N43.42 **Spermatocele of epididymis, multiple**

● N44 **Noninflammatory disorders of testis**
● N44.0 **Torsion of testis**
N44.00 **Torsion of testis, unspecified**
N44.01 **Extravaginal torsion of spermatic cord**
N44.02 **Intravaginal torsion of spermatic cord**
Torsion of spermatic cord NOS
N44.03 **Torsion of appendix testis**
N44.04 **Torsion of appendix epididymis**
N44.1 **Cyst of tunica albuginea testis**
N44.2 **Benign cyst of testis**
N44.8 **Other noninflammatory disorders of the testis**

● N45 **Orchitis and epididymitis**
Orchitis *is inflammation of one or both of the testes as a result of mumps or other infection, trauma, or metastasis.* ***Epididymitis*** *is inflammation of the tubular structure that connects the testicle with the vas deferens.*
Use additional code (B95-B97), to identify infectious agent
N45.1 **Epididymitis**
N45.2 **Orchitis**
N45.3 **Epididymo-orchitis**
N45.4 **Abscess of epididymis or testis**

● N46 **Male infertility**
Excludes1 vasectomy status (Z98.52)
● N46.0 **Azoospermia**
Absolute male infertility
Male infertility due to germinal (cell) aplasia
Male infertility due to spermatogenic arrest (complete)
N46.01 **Organic azoospermia**
Azoospermia NOS
● N46.02 **Azoospermia due to extratesticular causes**
Code also associated cause
N46.021 **Azoospermia due to drug therapy**
N46.022 **Azoospermia due to infection**
N46.023 **Azoospermia due to obstruction of efferent ducts**
N46.024 **Azoospermia due to radiation**
N46.025 **Azoospermia due to systemic disease**
N46.029 **Azoospermia due to other extratesticular causes**

Item 14-8 Male infertility is the inability of the female sex partner to conceive after one year of unprotected intercourse.

Azoospermia is no sperm ejaculated and **oligospermia** is few sperm ejaculated—both resulting in infertility. Extratesticular causes such as injury, infections, radiation, and chemotherapy may also cause male infertility.

● **N46.1 Oligospermia**
Male infertility due to germinal cell desquamation
Male infertility due to hypospermatogenesis
Male infertility due to incomplete spermatogenic arrest

N46.11 Organic oligospermia
Oligospermia NOS

● **N46.12 Oligospermia due to extratesticular causes**
Code also associated cause

N46.121 Oligospermia due to drug therapy
N46.122 Oligospermia due to infection
N46.123 Oligospermia due to obstruction of efferent ducts
N46.124 Oligospermia due to radiation
N46.125 Oligospermia due to systemic disease
N46.129 Oligospermia due to other extratesticular causes

N46.8 Other male infertility
N46.9 Male infertility, unspecified

● **N47 Disorders of prepuce**
N47.Ø Adherent prepuce, newborn
N47.1 Phimosis
N47.2 Paraphimosis
N47.3 Deficient foreskin
N47.4 Benign cyst of prepuce
N47.5 Adhesions of prepuce and glans penis
N47.6 Balanoposthitis
Use additional code (B95-B97), to identify infectious agent
Excludes1 balanitis (N48.1)
N47.7 Other inflammatory diseases of prepuce
Use additional code (B95-B97), to identify infectious agent
N47.8 Other disorders of prepuce

● **N48 Other disorders of penis**
N48.Ø Leukoplakia of penis
Balanitis xerotica obliterans
Kraurosis of penis
Lichen sclerosus of external male genital organs
Excludes1 carcinoma in situ of penis (DØ7.4)
N48.1 Balanitis
Use additional code (B95-B97), to identify infectious agent
Excludes1 amebic balanitis (AØ6.8)
balanitis xerotica obliterans (N48.Ø)
candidal balanitis (B37.42)
gonococcal balanitis (A54.23)
herpesviral [herpes simplex] balanitis (A6Ø.Ø1)

● **N48.2 Other inflammatory disorders of penis**
Use additional code (B95-B97), to identify infectious agent
Excludes1 balanitis (N48.1)
balanitis xerotica obliterans (N48.Ø)
balanoposthitis (N47.6)

N48.21 Abscess of corpus cavernosum and penis
N48.22 Cellulitis of corpus cavernosum and penis
N48.29 Other inflammatory disorders of penis

● **N48.3 Priapism**
Painful erection
Code first *underlying cause*

N48.3Ø Priapism, unspecified
N48.31 Priapism due to trauma
N48.32 Priapism due to disease classified elsewhere
N48.33 Priapism, drug-induced
N48.39 Other priapism

N48.5 Ulcer of penis
N48.6 Induration penis plastica
Peyronie's disease
Plastic induration of penis

● **N48.8 Other specified disorders of penis**
N48.81 Thrombosis of superficial vein of penis
N48.82 Acquired torsion of penis
Acquired torsion of penis NOS
Excludes1 congenital torsion of penis (Q55.63)
N48.83 Acquired buried penis
Excludes1 congenital hidden penis (Q55.64)
N48.89 Other specified disorders of penis

N48.9 Disorder of penis, unspecified

● **N49 Inflammatory disorders of male genital organs, not elsewhere classified**
Use additional code (B95-B97), to identify infectious agent
Excludes1 inflammation of penis (N48.1, N48.2-)
orchitis and epididymitis (N45.-)

N49.Ø Inflammatory disorders of seminal vesicle
Vesiculitis NOS
N49.1 Inflammatory disorders of spermatic cord, tunica vaginalis and vas deferens
Vasitis
N49.2 Inflammatory disorders of scrotum
N49.3 Fournier gangrene
N49.8 Inflammatory disorders of other specified male genital organs
Inflammation of multiple sites in male genital organs
N49.9 Inflammatory disorder of unspecified male genital organ
Abscess of unspecified male genital organ
Boil of unspecified male genital organ
Carbuncle of unspecified male genital organ
Cellulitis of unspecified male genital organ

● **N5Ø Other and unspecified disorders of male genital organs**
Excludes2 torsion of testis (N44.Ø-)

N5Ø.Ø Atrophy of testis
N5Ø.1 Vascular disorders of male genital organs
Hematocele, NOS, of male genital organs
Hemorrhage of male genital organs
Thrombosis of male genital organs
N5Ø.3 Cyst of epididymis

Item 14–9 Seminal vesiculitis is an inflammation of the seminal vesicle. Spermatocele is a benign cystic accumulation of sperm arising from the head of the epididymis. Torsion of the testis is a medical emergency occurring most commonly in boys 7 to 12 years of age and results from a congenital abnormality of the covering of the testis allowing the testis to twist within its sac and cutting off the blood supply to the testis.

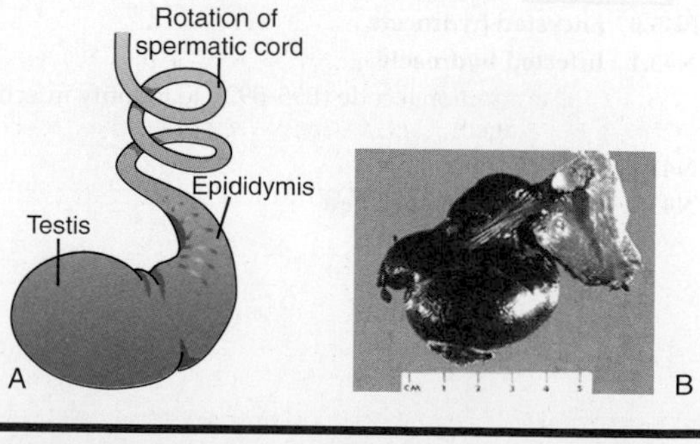

Figure 14-8 A. Torsion of testis. **B.** Torsion of the testis. (**B** from Kumar: Robbins and Cotran: Pathologic Basis of Disease, ed 8, Saunders, An Imprint of Elsevier, 2009)

● **N5Ø.8 Other specified disorders of male genital organs**
● **N5Ø.81 Testicular pain** ◀
N5Ø.811 Right testicular pain ◀
N5Ø.812 Left testicular pain ◀
N5Ø.819 Testicular pain, unspecified ◀
N5Ø.82 Scrotal pain ◀
N5Ø.89 Other specified disorders of the male genital organs ◀
Atrophy of scrotum, seminal vesicle, spermatic cord, tunica vaginalis and vas deferens ◀
Chylocele, tunica vaginalis (nonfilarial) NOS ◀
Edema of scrotum, seminal vesicle, spermatic cord, tunica vaginalis and vas deferens ◀
Hypertrophy of scrotum, seminal vesicle, spermatic cord, tunica vaginalis and vas deferens ◀
Stricture of spermatic cord, tunica vaginalis, and vas deferens ◀
Ulcer of scrotum, seminal vesicle, spermatic cord, testis, tunica vaginalis and vas deferens ◀
Urethroscrotal fistula ◀
N5Ø.9 Disorder of male genital organs, unspecified

N51 Disorders of male genital organs in diseases classified elsewhere
Code first underlying disease, such as:
filariasis (B74.Ø-B74.9)
Excludes1 amebic balanitis (AØ6.8)
candidal balanitis (B37.42)
gonococcal balanitis (A54.23)
gonococcal prostatitis (A54.22)
herpesviral [herpes simplex] balanitis (A6Ø.Ø1)
trichomonal prostatitis (A59.Ø2)
tuberculous prostatitis (A18.14)

● **N52 Male erectile dysfunction**
Excludes1 psychogenic impotence (F52.21)
● **N52.Ø Vasculogenic erectile dysfunction**
N52.Ø1 Erectile dysfunction due to arterial insufficiency
N52.Ø2 Corporo-venous occlusive erectile dysfunction
N52.Ø3 Combined arterial insufficiency and corporo-venous occlusive erectile dysfunction
N52.1 Erectile dysfunction due to diseases classified elsewhere
Code first underlying disease
N52.2 Drug-induced erectile dysfunction
● **N52.3 Postprocedural erectile dysfunction** ⬅
N52.31 Erectile dysfunction following radical prostatectomy
N52.32 Erectile dysfunction following radical cystectomy
N52.33 Erectile dysfunction following urethral surgery
N52.34 Erectile dysfunction following simple prostatectomy
N52.35 Erectile dysfunction following radiation therapy ◀
N52.36 Erectile dysfunction following interstitial seed therapy ◀
N52.37 Erectile dysfunction following prostate ablative therapy ◀
Erectile dysfunction following cryotherapy ◀
Erectile dysfunction following other prostate ablative therapies
Erectile dysfunction following ultrasound ablative therapies ◀
N52.39 Other and unspecified postprocedural erectile dysfunction ⬅
N52.8 Other male erectile dysfunction
N52.9 Male erectile dysfunction, unspecified
Impotence NOS

● **N53 Other male sexual dysfunction**
Excludes1 psychogenic sexual dysfunction (F52.-)
● **N53.1 Ejaculatory dysfunction**
Excludes1 premature ejaculation (F52.4)
N53.11 Retarded ejaculation
N53.12 Painful ejaculation
N53.13 Anejaculatory orgasm
N53.14 Retrograde ejaculation
N53.19 Other ejaculatory dysfunction
Ejaculatory dysfunction NOS
N53.8 Other male sexual dysfunction
N53.9 Unspecified male sexual dysfunction

DISORDERS OF BREAST (N6Ø-N65)

Excludes1 disorders of breast associated with childbirth (O91-O92)

● **N6Ø Benign mammary dysplasia**
Benign lumpiness of breast
Includes fibrocystic mastopathy
● **N6Ø.Ø Solitary cyst of breast**
Cyst of breast
N6Ø.Ø1 Solitary cyst of right breast
N6Ø.Ø2 Solitary cyst of left breast
N6Ø.Ø9 Solitary cyst of unspecified breast
● **N6Ø.1 Diffuse cystic mastopathy**
Cystic breast
Fibrocystic disease of breast
Excludes1 diffuse cystic mastopathy with epithelial proliferation (N6Ø.3-)
N6Ø.11 Diffuse cystic mastopathy of right breast
N6Ø.12 Diffuse cystic mastopathy of left breast
N6Ø.19 Diffuse cystic mastopathy of unspecified breast
● **N6Ø.2 Fibroadenosis of breast**
Adenofibrosis of breast
Excludes2 fibroadenoma of breast (D24.-)
N6Ø.21 Fibroadenosis of right breast
N6Ø.22 Fibroadenosis of left breast
N6Ø.29 Fibroadenosis of unspecified breast
● **N6Ø.3 Fibrosclerosis of breast**
Cystic mastopathy with epithelial proliferation
N6Ø.31 Fibrosclerosis of right breast
N6Ø.32 Fibrosclerosis of left breast
N6Ø.39 Fibrosclerosis of unspecified breast
● **N6Ø.4 Mammary duct ectasia**
N6Ø.41 Mammary duct ectasia of right breast
N6Ø.42 Mammary duct ectasia of left breast
N6Ø.49 Mammary duct ectasia of unspecified breast

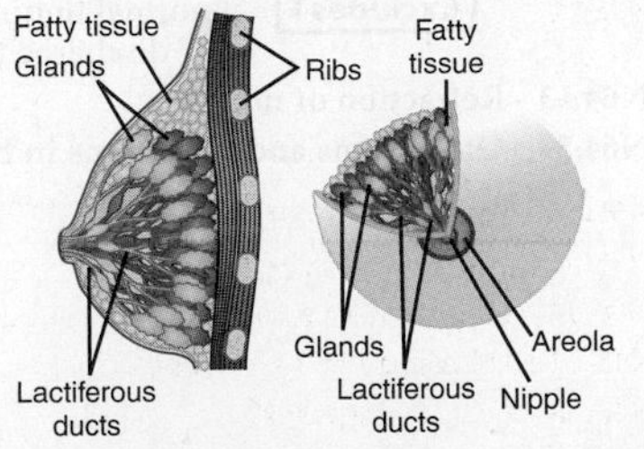

Figure 14-9 Breast.

● N60.8 **Other benign mammary dysplasias**
N60.81 **Other benign mammary dysplasias of right breast**
N60.82 **Other benign mammary dysplasias of left breast**
N60.89 **Other benign mammary dysplasias of unspecified breast**

● N60.9 **Unspecified benign mammary dysplasia**
N60.91 **Unspecified benign mammary dysplasia of right breast**
N60.92 **Unspecified benign mammary dysplasia of left breast**
N60.99 **Unspecified benign mammary dysplasia of unspecified breast**

● N61 **Inflammatory disorders of breast**
Excludes1 inflammatory carcinoma of breast (C50.9)
inflammatory disorder of breast associated with childbirth (O91.-)
neonatal infective mastitis (P39.0)
thrombophlebitis of breast [Mondor's disease] (I80.8)

N61.0 **Mastitis without abscess** ◀
Infective mastitis (acute) (nonpuerperal) (subacute) ◀
Mastitis (acute) (nonpuerperal) (subacute) NOS ◀
Cellulitis (acute) (nonpuerperal) (subacute) of breast NOS ◀
Cellulitis (acute) (nonpuerperal) (subacute) of nipple NOS ◀

N61.1 **Abscess of the breast and nipple** ◀
Abscess (acute) (chronic) (nonpuerperal) of areola ◀
Abscess (acute) (chronic) (nonpuerperal) of breast ◀
Carbuncle of breast ◀
Mastitis with abscess ◀

N62 **Hypertrophy of breast**
Gynecomastia
Hypertrophy of breast NOS
Massive pubertal hypertrophy of breast
Excludes1 breast engorgement of newborn (P83.4)
disproportion of reconstructed breast (N65.1)

N63 **Unspecified lump in breast**
Nodule(s) NOS in breast

● N64 **Other disorders of breast**
Excludes2 mechanical complication of breast prosthesis and implant (T85.4-)

N64.0 **Fissure and fistula of nipple**
N64.1 **Fat necrosis of breast**
Fat necrosis (segmental) of breast
Code first breast necrosis due to breast graft (T85.898) ⬅
N64.2 **Atrophy of breast**
N64.3 **Galactorrhea not associated with childbirth**
Excessive or spontaneous flow of milk
N64.4 **Mastodynia**

● N64.5 **Other signs and symptoms in breast**
Excludes2 abnormal findings on diagnostic imaging of breast (R92.-)
N64.51 **Induration of breast**
N64.52 **Nipple discharge**
Excludes1 abnormal findings in nipple discharge (R89.-)
N64.53 **Retraction of nipple**
N64.59 **Other signs and symptoms in breast**

● N64.8 **Other specified disorders of breast**
N64.81 **Ptosis of breast**
Excludes1 ptosis of native breast in relation to reconstructed breast (N65.1)
N64.82 **Hypoplasia of breast**
Micromastia
Excludes1 congenital absence of breast (Q83.0)
hypoplasia of native breast in relation to reconstructed breast (N65.1)
N64.89 **Other specified disorders of breast**
Galactocele
Subinvolution of breast (postlactational)

N64.9 **Disorder of breast, unspecified**

● N65 **Deformity and disproportion of reconstructed breast**
N65.0 **Deformity of reconstructed breast**
Contour irregularity in reconstructed breast
Excess tissue in reconstructed breast
Misshapen reconstructed breast
N65.1 **Disproportion of reconstructed breast**
Breast asymmetry between native breast and reconstructed breast
Disproportion between native breast and reconstructed breast

INFLAMMATORY DISEASES OF FEMALE PELVIC ORGANS (N70-N77)

Excludes1 inflammatory diseases of female pelvic organs complicating:
abortion or ectopic or molar pregnancy (O00-O07, O08.0)
pregnancy, childbirth and the puerperium (O23.-, O75.3, O85, O86.-)

★ **(See Plate 360 on page NAP-32.)**

● N70 **Salpingitis and oophoritis**
Oophoritis = inflammation of ovary
Salpingitis = inflammation of fallopian tube
Includes abscess (of) fallopian tube
abscess (of) ovary
pyosalpinx
salpingo-oophoritis
tubo-ovarian abscess
tubo-ovarian inflammatory disease
Use additional code (B95-B97), to identify infectious agent
Excludes1 gonococcal infection (A54.24)
tuberculous infection (A18.17)

● N70.0 **Acute salpingitis and oophoritis**
N70.01 **Acute salpingitis**
N70.02 **Acute oophoritis**
N70.03 **Acute salpingitis and oophoritis**

● N70.1 **Chronic salpingitis and oophoritis**
Hydrosalpinx
N70.11 **Chronic salpingitis**
N70.12 **Chronic oophoritis**
N70.13 **Chronic salpingitis and oophoritis**

● N70.9 **Salpingitis and oophoritis, unspecified**
N70.91 **Salpingitis, unspecified**
N70.92 **Oophoritis, unspecified**
N70.93 **Salpingitis and oophoritis, unspecified**

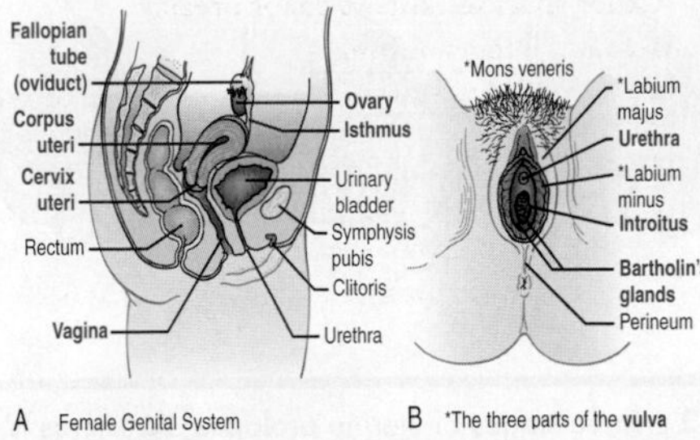

Figure 14-10 A. Female genital system. **B.** External female genital system. (From Buck CJ: Step-by-Step Medical Coding, ed 2016, St. Louis, Elsevier, 2016)

Item 14-10 Salpingitis is an infection of one or both fallopian tubes. **Oophoritis** is an infection of one or both ovaries.

● **N71 Inflammatory disease of uterus, except cervix**

Includes endo (myo) metritis
metritis
myometritis
pyometra
uterine abscess

Use additional code (B95-B97), to identify infectious agent

Excludes1 hyperplastic endometritis (N85.Ø-)
infection of uterus following delivery (O85, O86.-)

N71.Ø Acute inflammatory disease of uterus

N71.1 Chronic inflammatory disease of uterus

N71.9 Inflammatory disease of uterus, unspecified

N72 Inflammatory disease of cervix uteri

Includes cervicitis (with or without erosion or ectropion)
endocervicitis (with or without erosion or ectropion)
exocervicitis (with or without erosion or ectropion)

Use additional code (B95-B97), to identify infectious agent

Excludes1 erosion and ectropion of cervix without cervicitis (N86)

● **N73 Other female pelvic inflammatory diseases**

Use additional code (B95-B97), to identify infectious agent

N73.Ø Acute parametritis and pelvic cellulitis
Abscess of broad ligament
Abscess of parametrium
Pelvic cellulitis, female

N73.1 Chronic parametritis and pelvic cellulitis
Any condition in N73.Ø specified as chronic

Excludes1 tuberculous parametritis and pelvic cellutis (A18.17)

N73.2 Unspecified parametritis and pelvic cellulitis
Any condition in N73.Ø unspecified whether acute or chronic

N73.3 Female acute pelvic peritonitis

N73.4 Female chronic pelvic peritonitis

Excludes1 tuberculous pelvic (female) peritonitis (A18.17)

N73.5 Female pelvic peritonitis, unspecified

N73.6 Female pelvic peritoneal adhesions (postinfective)

Excludes2 postprocedural pelvic peritoneal adhesions (N99.4)

N73.8 Other specified female pelvic inflammatory diseases

N73.9 Female pelvic inflammatory disease, unspecified
Female pelvic infection or inflammation NOS

N74 Female pelvic inflammatory disorders in diseases classified elsewhere

Code first underlying disease

Excludes1 chlamydial cervicitis (A56.Ø2)
chlamydial pelvic inflammatory disease (A56.11)
gonococcal cervicitis (A54.Ø3)
gonococcal pelvic inflammatory disease (A54.24)
herpesviral [herpes simplex] cervicitis (A6Ø.Ø3)
herpesviral [herpes simplex] pelvic inflammatory disease (A6Ø.Ø9)
syphilitic cervicitis (A52.76)
syphilitic pelvic inflammatory disease (A52.76)
trichomonal cervicitis (A59.Ø9)
tuberculous cervicitis (A18.16)
tuberculous pelvic inflammatory disease (A18.17)

● **N75 Diseases of Bartholin's gland**

N75.Ø Cyst of Bartholin's gland
Cysts filled with liquid or semisolid material

N75.1 Abscess of Bartholin's gland
Localized collection of pus

N75.8 Other diseases of Bartholin's gland
Bartholinitis

N75.9 Disease of Bartholin's gland, unspecified

● **N76 Other inflammation of vagina and vulva**

Use additional code (B95-B97), to identify infectious agent

Excludes2 senile (atrophic) vaginitis (N95.2)
vulvar vestibulitis (N94.81Ø)

N76.Ø Acute vaginitis
Acute vulvovaginitis
Vaginitis NOS
Vulvovaginitis NOS

N76.1 Subacute and chronic vaginitis
Chronic vulvovaginitis
Subacute vulvovaginitis

N76.2 Acute vulvitis
Vulvitis NOS

N76.3 Subacute and chronic vulvitis

N76.4 Abscess of vulva
Furuncle of vulva

N76.5 Ulceration of vagina

N76.6 Ulceration of vulva

● **N76.8 Other specified inflammation of vagina and vulva**

N76.81 Mucositis (ulcerative) of vagina and vulva

Code also type of associated therapy, such as:
antineoplastic and immunosuppressive drugs (T45.1X-)
radiological procedure and radiotherapy (Y84.2)

Excludes2 gastrointestinal mucositis (ulcerative) (K92.81)
nasal mucositis (ulcerative) (J34.81)
oral mucositis (ulcerative) (K12.3-)

N76.89 Other specified inflammation of vagina and vulva

● **N77 Vulvovaginal ulceration and inflammation in diseases classified elsewhere**

N77.Ø Ulceration of vulva in diseases classified elsewhere

Code first underlying disease, such as:
Behçet's disease (M35.2)

Excludes1 ulceration of vulva in gonococcal infection (A54.Ø2)
ulceration of vulva in herpesviral [herpes simplex] infection (A6Ø.Ø4)
ulceration of vulva in syphilis (A51.Ø)
ulceration of vulva in tuberculosis (A18.18)

N77.1 Vaginitis, vulvitis and vulvovaginitis in diseases classified elsewhere
Code first underlying disease, such as:
pinworm (B8Ø)
Excludes1 candidial vulvovaginitis (B37.3)
chlamydial vulvovaginitis (A56.Ø2)
gonococcal vulvovaginitis (A54.Ø2)
herpesviral [herpes simplex] vulvovaginitis (A6Ø.Ø4)
trichomonal vulvovaginitis (A59.Ø1)
tuberculous vulvovaginitis (A18.18)
vulvovaginitis in early syphilis (A51.Ø)
vulvovaginitis in late syphilis (A52.76)

NONINFLAMMATORY DISORDERS OF FEMALE GENITAL TRACT (N8Ø-N98)

● **N8Ø Endometriosis**
N8Ø.Ø Endometriosis of uterus
Adenomyosis
Excludes1 stromal endometriosis (D39.Ø)
N8Ø.1 Endometriosis of ovary
N8Ø.2 Endometriosis of fallopian tube
N8Ø.3 Endometriosis of pelvic peritoneum
N8Ø.4 Endometriosis of rectovaginal septum and vagina
N8Ø.5 Endometriosis of intestine
N8Ø.6 Endometriosis in cutaneous scar
N8Ø.8 Other endometriosis
N8Ø.9 Endometriosis, unspecified

● **N81 Female genital prolapse**
Excludes1 genital prolapse complicating pregnancy, labor or delivery (O34.5-)
prolapse and hernia of ovary and fallopian tube (N83.4-) ◄
prolapse of vaginal vault after hysterectomy (N99.3)
N81.Ø Urethrocele
Excludes1 urethrocele with cystocele (N81.1-)
urethrocele with prolapse of uterus (N81.2-N81.4)
● **N81.1 Cystocele**
Cystocele with urethrocele
Cystourethrocele
Excludes1 cystocele with prolapse of uterus (N81.2-N81.4)
N81.1Ø Cystocele, unspecified
Prolapse of (anterior) vaginal wall NOS
N81.11 Cystocele, midline
N81.12 Cystocele, lateral
Paravaginal cystocele

Item 14–11 Endometriosis is a condition for which no clear cause has been identified. Endometrial tissue is expelled from the uterus into the abdominal cavity and can implant onto a variety of organs. Classification is based on the site of implant of the endometrial tissue.

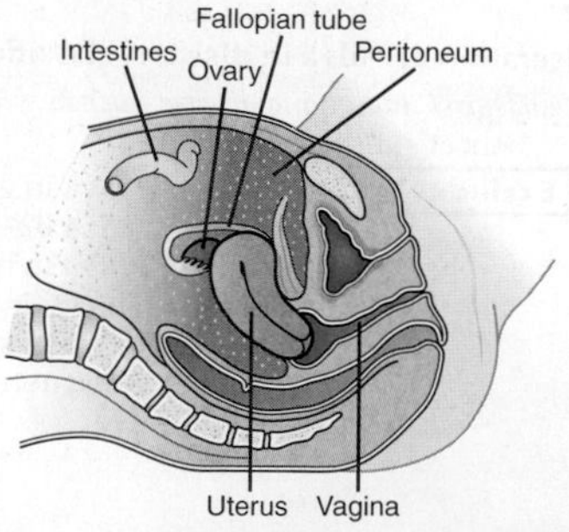

Figure 14-11 Sites of potential endometrial implants.

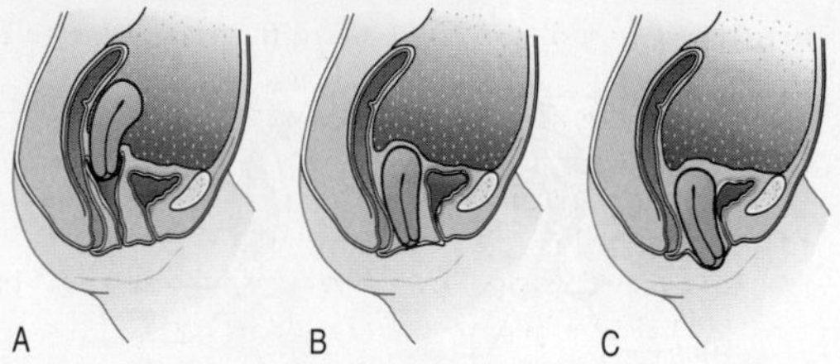

Figure 14-12 Three stages of uterine prolapse. **A.** Uterus is prolapsed. **B.** Vagina and uterus are prolapsed (incomplete uterovaginal prolapse). **C.** Vagina and uterus are completely prolapsed and are exposed through the external genitalia (complete uterovaginal prolapse).

N81.2 Incomplete uterovaginal prolapse
First degree uterine prolapse
Prolapse of cervix NOS
Second degree uterine prolapse
Excludes1 cervical stump prolaspe (N81.85)
N81.3 Complete uterovaginal prolapse
Procidentia (uteri) NOS
Third degree uterine prolapse
N81.4 Uterovaginal prolapse, unspecified
Prolapse of uterus NOS
N81.5 Vaginal enterocele
Excludes1 enterocele with prolapse of uterus (N81.2-N81.4)
N81.6 Rectocele
Prolapse of posterior vaginal wall
Use additional code for any associated fecal incontinence, if applicable (R15.-)
Excludes2 perineocele (N81.81)
rectal prolapse (K62.3)
rectocele with prolapse of uterus (N81.2-N81.4)
● **N81.8 Other female genital prolapse**
N81.81 Perineocele
N81.82 Incompetence or weakening of pubocervical tissue
N81.83 Incompetence or weakening of rectovaginal tissue
N81.84 Pelvic muscle wasting
Disuse atrophy of pelvic muscles and anal sphincter
N81.85 Cervical stump prolapse
N81.89 Other female genital prolapse
Deficient perineum
Old laceration of muscles of pelvic floor
N81.9 Female genital prolapse, unspecified

● **N82 Fistulae involving female genital tract**
Excludes1 vesicointestinal fistulae (N32.1)
N82.Ø Vesicovaginal fistula
N82.1 Other female urinary-genital tract fistulae
Cervicovesical fistula
Ureterovaginal fistula
Urethrovaginal fistula
Uteroureteric fistula
Uterovesical fistula
N82.2 Fistula of vagina to small intestine
N82.3 Fistula of vagina to large intestine
Rectovaginal fistula
N82.4 Other female intestinal-genital tract fistulae
Intestinouterine fistula
N82.5 Female genital tract-skin fistulae
Uterus to abdominal wall fistula
Vaginoperineal fistula
N82.8 Other female genital tract fistulae
N82.9 Female genital tract fistula, unspecified

CHAPTER 14 (NØØ-N99)

● N83 **Noninflammatory disorders of ovary, fallopian tube and broad ligament**
Excludes2 hydrosalpinx (N70.1-)

● N83.0 **Follicular cyst of ovary**
Cyst of graafian follicle
Hemorrhagic follicular cyst (of ovary)
N83.00 **Follicular cyst of ovary, unspecified side** ◀
N83.01 **Follicular cyst of right ovary** ◀
N83.02 **Follicular cyst of left ovary** ◀

● N83.1 **Corpus luteum cyst**
Hemorrhagic corpus luteum cyst
N83.10 **Corpus luteum cyst of ovary, unspecified side** ◀
N83.11 **Corpus luteum cyst of right ovary** ◀
N83.12 **Corpus luteum cyst of left ovary** ◀

● N83.2 **Other and unspecified ovarian cysts**
Excludes1 developmental ovarian cyst (Q50.1)
neoplastic ovarian cyst (D27.-)
polycystic ovarian syndrome (E28.2)
Stein-Leventhal syndrome (E28.2)

● N83.20 **Unspecified ovarian cysts**
N83.201 **Unspecified ovarian cyst, right side** ◀
N83.202 **Unspecified ovarian cyst, left side** ◀
N83.209 **Unspecified ovarian cyst, unspecified side** ◀
Ovarian cyst, NOS ◀

● N83.29 **Other ovarian cysts**
Retention cyst of ovary
Simple cyst of ovary
N83.291 **Other ovarian cyst, right side** ◀
N83.292 **Other ovarian cyst, left side** ◀
N83.299 **Other ovarian cyst, unspecified side** ◀

● N83.3 **Acquired atrophy of ovary and fallopian tube**

● N83.31 **Acquired atrophy of ovary**
N83.311 **Acquired atrophy of right ovary** ◀
N83.312 **Acquired atrophy of left ovary** ◀
N83.319 **Acquired atrophy of ovary, unspecified side** ◀
Acquired atrophy of ovary, NOS ◀

● N83.32 **Acquired atrophy of fallopian tube**
N83.321 **Acquired atrophy of right fallopian tube** ◀
N83.322 **Acquired atrophy of left fallopian tube** ◀
N83.329 **Acquired atrophy of fallopian tube, unspecified side** ◀
Acquired atrophy of fallopian tube, NOS ◀

● N83.33 **Acquired atrophy of ovary and fallopian tube**
N83.331 **Acquired atrophy of right ovary and fallopian tube** ◀
N83.332 **Acquired atrophy of left ovary and fallopian tube** ◀
N83.339 **Acquired atrophy of ovary and fallopian tube, unspecified side** ◀
Acquired atrophy of ovary and fallopian tube, NOS ◀

● N83.4 **Prolapse and hernia of ovary and fallopian tube**
N83.40 **Prolapse and hernia of ovary and fallopian tube, unspecified side** ◀
Prolapse and hernia of ovary and fallopian tube, NOS ◀
N83.41 **Prolapse and hernia of right ovary and fallopian tube** ◀
N83.42 **Prolapse and hernia of left ovary and fallopian tube** ◀

● N83.5 **Torsion of ovary, ovarian pedicle and fallopian tube**
Torsion of accessory tube

● N83.51 **Torsion of ovary and ovarian pedicle**
N83.511 **Torsion of right ovary and ovarian pedicle** ◀
N83.512 **Torsion of left ovary and ovarian pedicle** ◀
N83.519 **Torsion of ovary and ovarian pedicle, unspecified side** ◀
Torsion of ovary and ovarian pedicle, NOS ◀

● N83.52 **Torsion of fallopian tube**
Torsion of hydatid of Morgagni
N83.521 **Torsion of right fallopian tube** ◀
N83.522 **Torsion of left fallopian tube** ◀
N83.529 **Torsion of fallopian tube, unspecified side** ◀
Torsion of fallopian tube, NOS ◀

N83.53 **Torsion of ovary, ovarian pedicle and fallopian tube**

N83.6 **Hematosalpinx**
Excludes1 hematosalpinx (with) (in):
hematocolpos (N89.7)
hematometra (N85.7)
tubal pregnancy (O00.1-) ⟸

N83.7 **Hematoma of broad ligament**

N83.8 **Other noninflammatory disorders of ovary, fallopian tube and broad ligament**
Broad ligament laceration syndrome [Allen-Masters]

N83.9 **Noninflammatory disorder of ovary, fallopian tube and broad ligament, unspecified**

● N84 **Polyp of female genital tract**
Excludes1 adenomatous polyp (D28.-)
placental polyp (O90.89)

N84.0 **Polyp of corpus uteri**
Polyp of endometrium
Polyp of uterus NOS
Excludes1 polypoid endometrial hyperplasia (N85.0-)

N84.1 **Polyp of cervix uteri**
Mucous polyp of cervix

N84.2 **Polyp of vagina**

N84.3 **Polyp of vulva**
Polyp of labia

N84.8 **Polyp of other parts of female genital tract**

N84.9 **Polyp of female genital tract, unspecified**

● N85 **Other noninflammatory disorders of uterus, except cervix**
Excludes1 endometriosis (N80.-)
inflammatory diseases of uterus (N71.-)
noninflammatory disorders of cervix, except malposition (N86-N88)
polyp of corpus uteri (N84.0)
uterine prolapse (N81.-)

● N85.0 **Endometrial hyperplasia**
N85.00 **Endometrial hyperplasia, unspecified**
Hyperplasia (adenomatous) (cystic) (glandular) of endometrium
Hyperplastic endometritis
N85.01 **Benign endometrial hyperplasia**
Endometrial hyperplasia (complex) (simple) without atypia
N85.02 **Endometrial intraepithelial neoplasia [EIN]**
Endometrial hyperplasia with atypia
Excludes1 malignant neoplasm of endometrium (with endometrial intraepithelial neoplasia [EIN]) (C54.1)

CHAPTER 14 (N00-N99)

N85.2 Hypertrophy of uterus
Bulky or enlarged uterus
Excludes1 puerperal hypertrophy of uterus (O90.89)

N85.3 Subinvolution of uterus
Excludes1 puerperal subinvolution of uterus (O90.89)

N85.4 Malposition of uterus
Anteversion of uterus
Retroflexion of uterus
Retroversion of uterus
Excludes1 malposition of uterus complicating pregnancy, labor or delivery (O34.5-, O65.5)

N85.5 Inversion of uterus
Excludes1 current obstetric trauma (O71.2)
postpartum inversion of uterus (O71.2)

N85.6 Intrauterine synechiae

N85.7 Hematometra
Hematosalpinx with hematometra
Excludes1 hematometra with hematocolpos (N89.7)

N85.8 Other specified noninflammatory disorders of uterus
Atrophy of uterus, acquired
Fibrosis of uterus NOS

N85.9 Noninflammatory disorder of uterus, unspecified
Disorder of uterus NOS

N86 Erosion and ectropion of cervix uteri
Decubitus (trophic) ulcer of cervix
Eversion of cervix
Excludes1 erosion and ectropion of cervix with cervicitis (N72)

● **N87 Dysplasia of cervix uteri**
Excludes1 abnormal results from cervical cytologic examination without histologic confirmation (R87.61-)
carcinoma in situ of cervix uteri (D06.-)
cervical intraepithelial neoplasia III [CIN III] (D06.-)
HGSIL of cervix (R87.613)
severe dysplasia of cervix uteri (D06.-)

N87.0 Mild cervical dysplasia
Cervical intraepithelial neoplasia I [CIN I]

N87.1 Moderate cervical dysplasia
Cervical intraepithelial neoplasia II [CIN II]

N87.9 Dysplasia of cervix uteri, unspecified
Anaplasia of cervix
Cervical atypism
Cervical dysplasia NOS

● **N88 Other noninflammatory disorders of cervix uteri**
Excludes2 inflammatory disease of cervix (N72)
polyp of cervix (N84.1)

N88.0 Leukoplakia of cervix uteri

N88.1 Old laceration of cervix uteri
Adhesions of cervix
Excludes1 current obstetric trauma (O71.3)

N88.2 Stricture and stenosis of cervix uteri
Excludes1 stricture and stenosis of cervix uteri complicating labor (O65.5)

N88.3 Incompetence of cervix uteri
Investigation and management of (suspected) cervical incompetence in a nonpregnant woman
Excludes1 cervical incompetence complicating pregnancy (O34.3-)

N88.4 Hypertrophic elongation of cervix uteri

N88.8 Other specified noninflammatory disorders of cervix uteri
Excludes1 current obstetric trauma (O71.3)

N88.9 Noninflammatory disorder of cervix uteri, unspecified

● **N89 Other noninflammatory disorders of vagina**
Excludes1 abnormal results from vaginal cytologic examination without histologic confirmation (R87.62-)
carcinoma in situ of vagina (D07.2)
HGSIL of vagina (R87.623)
inflammation of vagina (N76.-)
senile (atrophic) vaginitis (N95.2)
severe dysplasia of vagina (D07.2)
trichomonal leukorrhea (A59.00)
vaginal intraepithelial neoplasia [VAIN], grade III (D07.2)

N89.0 Mild vaginal dysplasia
Vaginal intraepithelial neoplasia [VAIN], grade I

N89.1 Moderate vaginal dysplasia
Vaginal intraepithelial neoplasia [VAIN], grade II

N89.3 Dysplasia of vagina, unspecified

N89.4 Leukoplakia of vagina

N89.5 Stricture and atresia of vagina
Vaginal adhesions
Vaginal stenosis
Excludes1 congenital atresia or stricture (Q52.4)
postprocedural adhesions of vagina (N99.2)

N89.6 Tight hymenal ring
Rigid hymen
Tight introitus
Excludes1 imperforate hymen (Q52.3)

N89.7 Hematocolpos
Hematocolpos with hematometra or hematosalpinx

N89.8 Other specified noninflammatory disorders of vagina
Leukorrhea NOS
Old vaginal laceration
Pessary ulcer of vagina
Excludes1 current obstetric trauma (O70.-, O71.4, O71.7-O71.8)
old laceration involving muscles of pelvic floor (N81.8)

N89.9 Noninflammatory disorder of vagina, unspecified

● **N90 Other noninflammatory disorders of vulva and perineum**
Excludes1 anogenital (venereal) warts (A63.0)
carcinoma in situ of vulva (D07.1)
condyloma acuminatum (A63.0)
current obstetric trauma (O70.-, O71.7-O71.8)
inflammation of vulva (N76.-)
severe dysplasia of vulva (D07.1)
vulvar intraepithelial neoplasm III [VIN III] (D07.1)

N90.0 Mild vulvar dysplasia
Vulvar intraepithelial neoplasia [VIN], grade I

N90.1 Moderate vulvar dysplasia
Vulvar intraepithelial neoplasia [VIN], grade II

N90.3 Dysplasia of vulva, unspecified

N90.4 Leukoplakia of vulva
Dystrophy of vulva
Kraurosis of vulva
Lichen sclerosus of external female genital organs

N90.5 Atrophy of vulva
Stenosis of vulva

● **N90.6 Hypertrophy of vulva**

N90.60 Unspecified hypertrophy of vulva ◀
Unspecified hypertrophy of labia ◀

N90.61 Childhood asymmetric labium majus enlargement ◀
CALME ◀

N90.69 Other specified hypertrophy of vulva ◀
Other specified hypertrophy of labia ◀

N90.7 Vulvar cyst

● **N90.8 Other specified noninflammatory disorders of vulva and perineum**
● **N90.81 Female genital mutilation status**
Female genital cutting status
N90.810 Female genital mutilation status, unspecified
Female genital cutting status, unspecified
Female genital mutilation status NOS
N90.811 Female genital mutilation Type I status
Clitorectomy status
Female genital cutting Type I status
N90.812 Female genital mutilation Type II status
Clitorectomy with excision of labia minora status
Female genital cutting Type II status
N90.813 Female genital mutilation Type III status
Female genital cutting Type III status
Infibulation status
N90.818 Other female genital mutilation status
Female genital cutting Type IV status
Female genital mutilation Type IV status
Other female genital cutting status
N90.89 Other specified noninflammatory disorders of vulva and perineum
Adhesions of vulva
Hypertrophy of clitoris
N90.9 Noninflammatory disorder of vulva and perineum, unspecified

● **N91 Absent, scanty and rare menstruation**
Excludes1 ovarian dysfunction (E28.-)
N91.0 Primary amenorrhea
N91.1 Secondary amenorrhea
N91.2 Amenorrhea, unspecified
N91.3 Primary oligomenorrhea
N91.4 Secondary oligomenorrhea
N91.5 Oligomenorrhea, unspecified
Hypomenorrhea NOS

● **N92 Excessive, frequent and irregular menstruation**
Excludes1 postmenopausal bleeding (N95.0)
precocious puberty (menstruation) (E30.1)
N92.0 Excessive and frequent menstruation with regular cycle
Heavy periods NOS
Menorrhagia NOS
Polymenorrhea
N92.1 Excessive and frequent menstruation with irregular cycle
Irregular intermenstrual bleeding
Irregular, shortened intervals between menstrual bleeding
Menometrorrhagia
Metrorrhagia
N92.2 Excessive menstruation at puberty
Excessive bleeding associated with onset of menstrual periods
Pubertal menorrhagia
Puberty bleeding
N92.3 Ovulation bleeding
Regular intermenstrual bleeding
N92.4 Excessive bleeding in the premenopausal period
Climacteric menorrhagia or metrorrhagia
Menopausal menorrhagia or metrorrhagia
Preclimacteric menorrhagia or metrorrhagia
Premenopausal menorrhagia or metrorrhagia
N92.5 Other specified irregular menstruation
N92.6 Irregular menstruation, unspecified
Irregular bleeding NOS
Irregular periods NOS
Excludes1 irregular menstruation with:
lengthened intervals or scanty bleeding (N91.3-N91.5)
shortened intervals or excessive bleeding (N92.1)

● **N93 Other abnormal uterine and vaginal bleeding**
Excludes1 neonatal vaginal hemorrhage (P54.6)
precocious puberty (menstruation) (E30.1)
pseudomenses (P54.6)
N93.0 Postcoital and contact bleeding
N93.1 Pre-pubertal vaginal bleeding ◀
N93.8 Other specified abnormal uterine and vaginal bleeding
Dysfunctional or functional uterine or vaginal bleeding NOS
N93.9 Abnormal uterine and vaginal bleeding, unspecified

● **N94 Pain and other conditions associated with female genital organs and menstrual cycle**
N94.0 Mittelschmerz
Ovulation pain
● **N94.1 Dyspareunia**
Painful intercourse/coitus
Excludes1 psychogenic dyspareunia (F52.6)
N94.10 Unspecified dyspareunia ◀
N94.11 Superficial (introital) dyspareunia ◀
N94.12 Deep dyspareunia ◀
N94.19 Other specified dyspareunia ◀
N94.2 Vaginismus
Vagina tightness
Excludes1 psychogenic vaginismus (F52.5)
N94.3 Premenstrual tension syndrome
AKA: PMS
Premenstrual dysphoric disorder
Code also associated menstrual migraine (G43.82-, G43.83-)
Excludes1 Premenstrual dysphoric disorder (F32.81) ◀
N94.4 Primary dysmenorrhea
Lifelong painful menstruation
N94.5 Secondary dysmenorrhea
Later onset of painful menstruation
N94.6 Dysmenorrhea, unspecified
Excludes1 psychogenic dysmenorrhea (F45.8)
● **N94.8 Other specified conditions associated with female genital organs and menstrual cycle**
● **N94.81 Vulvodynia**
N94.810 Vulvar vestibulitis
N94.818 Other vulvodynia
N94.819 Vulvodynia, unspecified
Vulvodynia NOS
N94.89 Other specified conditions associated with female genital organs and menstrual cycle
N94.9 Unspecified condition associated with female genital organs and menstrual cycle

CHAPTER 14 (N00-N99)

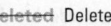

● N95 **Menopausal and other perimenopausal disorders**
Menopausal and other perimenopausal disorders due to naturally occurring (age-related) menopause and perimenopause
Excludes1 excessive bleeding in the premenopausal period (N92.4)
menopausal and perimenopausal disorders due to artificial or premature menopause (E89.4-, E28.31-)
premature menopause (E28.31-)
Excludes2 postmenopausal osteoporosis (M81.Ø-)
postmenopausal osteoporosis with current pathological fracture (M8Ø.Ø-)
postmenopausal urethritis (N34.2)

N95.Ø **Postmenopausal bleeding**

N95.1 **Menopausal and female climacteric states**
Symptoms such as flushing, sleeplessness, headache, lack of concentration, associated with natural (age-related) menopause
Use additional code for associated symptoms
Excludes1 asymptomatic menopausal state (Z78.Ø)
symptoms associated with artificial menopause (E89.41)
symptoms associated with premature menopause (E28.31Ø)

N95.2 **Postmenopausal atrophic vaginitis**
Senile (atrophic) vaginitis

N95.8 **Other specified menopausal and perimenopausal disorders**

N95.9 **Unspecified menopausal and perimenopausal disorder**

N96 **Recurrent pregnancy loss**
Investigation or care in a nonpregnant woman with history of recurrent pregnancy loss
Excludes1 recurrent pregnancy loss with current pregnancy (O26.2-)

● N97 **Female infertility**
Includes inability to achieve a pregnancy
sterility, female NOS
Excludes1 female infertility associated with:
hypopituitarism (E23.Ø)
Stein-Leventhal syndrome (E28.2)
Excludes2 incompetence of cervix uteri (N88.3)

N97.Ø **Female infertility associated with anovulation**

N97.1 **Female infertility of tubal origin**
Female infertility associated with congenital anomaly of tube
Female infertility due to tubal block
Female infertility due to tubal occlusion
Female infertility due to tubal stenosis

N97.2 **Female infertility of uterine origin**
Female infertility associated with congenital anomaly of uterus
Female infertility due to nonimplantation of ovum

N97.8 **Female infertility of other origin**

N97.9 **Female infertility, unspecified**

● N98 **Complications associated with artificial fertilization**

N98.Ø **Infection associated with artificial insemination**

N98.1 **Hyperstimulation of ovaries**
Hyperstimulation of ovaries NOS
Hyperstimulation of ovaries associated with induced ovulation

N98.2 **Complications of attempted introduction of fertilized ovum following in vitro fertilization**

N98.3 **Complications of attempted introduction of embryo in embryo transfer**

N98.8 **Other complications associated with artificial fertilization**

N98.9 **Complication associated with artificial fertilization, unspecified**

INTRAOPERATIVE AND POSTPROCEDURAL COMPLICATIONS AND DISORDERS OF GENITOURINARY SYSTEM, NOT ELSEWHERE CLASSIFIED (N99)

● N99 **Intraoperative and postprocedural complications and disorders of genitourinary system, not elsewhere classified**
Excludes2 irradiation cystitis (N3Ø.4-)
postoophorectomy osteoporosis with current pathological fracture (M8Ø.8-)
postoophorectomy osteoporosis without current pathological fracture (M81.8)

N99.Ø **Postprocedural (acute) (chronic) kidney failure**
Use additional code to type of kidney disease

● N99.1 **Postprocedural urethral stricture**
Postcatheterization urethral stricture

● N99.11 **Postprocedural urethral stricture, male**

N99.11Ø **Postprocedural urethral stricture, male, meatal**

N99.111 **Postprocedural bulbous urethral stricture**

N99.112 **Postprocedural membranous urethral stricture**

N99.113 **Postprocedural anterior bulbous urethral stricture** (Revised)

N99.114 **Postprocedural urethral stricture, male, unspecified**

N99.115 **Postprocedural fossa navicularis urethral stricture** ◄

N99.12 **Postprocedural urethral stricture, female**

N99.2 **Postprocedural adhesions of vagina**

N99.3 **Prolapse of vaginal vault after hysterectomy**

N99.4 **Postprocedural pelvic peritoneal adhesions**
Excludes2 pelvic peritoneal adhesions NOS (N73.6)
postinfective pelvic peritoneal adhesions (N73.6)

● N99.5 **Complications of stoma of urinary tract**
Excludes2 mechanical complication of urinary catheter (T83.Ø-) (Revised)

● N99.51 **Complication of cystostomy**

N99.51Ø **Cystostomy hemorrhage**

N99.511 **Cystostomy infection**

N99.512 **Cystostomy malfunction**

N99.518 **Other cystostomy complication**

● N99.52 **Complication of incontinent external stoma of urinary tract** (Revised)

N99.52Ø **Hemorrhage of incontinent external stoma of urinary tract** (Revised)

N99.521 **Infection of incontinent external stoma of urinary tract** (Revised)

N99.522 **Malfunction of incontinent external stoma of urinary tract** (Revised)

N99.523 **Herniation of incontinent stoma of urinary tract** ◄

N99.524 **Stenosis of incontinent stoma of urinary tract** ◄

N99.528 **Other complication of incontinent external stoma of urinary tract** (Revised)

● N99.53 Complication of continent stoma of urinary tract ⟸
N99.530 Hemorrhage of continent stoma of urinary tract ⟸
N99.531 Infection of continent stoma of urinary tract ⟸
N99.532 Malfunction of continent stoma of urinary tract ⟸
N99.533 Herniation of continent stoma of urinary tract ◀
N99.534 Stenosis of continent stoma of urinary tract ◀
N99.538 Other complication of continent stoma of urinary tract ⟸

● N99.6 Intraoperative hemorrhage and hematoma of a genitourinary system organ or structure complicating a procedure

Excludes1 intraoperative hemorrhage and hematoma of a genitourinary system organ or structure due to accidental puncture or laceration during a procedure (N99.7-)

N99.61 Intraoperative hemorrhage and hematoma of a genitourinary system organ or structure complicating a genitourinary system procedure
N99.62 Intraoperative hemorrhage and hematoma of a genitourinary system organ or structure complicating other procedure

● N99.7 Accidental puncture and laceration of a genitourinary system organ or structure during a procedure
N99.71 Accidental puncture and laceration of a genitourinary system organ or structure during a genitourinary system procedure
N99.72 Accidental puncture and laceration of a genitourinary system organ or structure during other procedure

● N99.8 Other intraoperative and postprocedural complications and disorders of genitourinary system
N99.81 Other intraoperative complications of genitourinary system
● N99.82 Postprocedural hemorrhage of a genitourinary system organ or structure following a procedure ⟸
N99.820 Postprocedural hemorrhage of a genitourinary system organ or structure following a genitourinary system procedure ⟸
N99.821 Postprocedural hemorrhage of a genitourinary system organ or structure following other procedure ⟸
N99.83 Residual ovary syndrome
● N99.84 Postprocedural hematoma and seroma of a genitourinary system organ or structure following a procedure ◀
N99.840 Postprocedural hematoma of a genitourinary system organ or structure following a genitourinary system procedure ◀
N99.841 Postprocedural hematoma of a genitourinary system organ or structure following other procedure ◀
N99.842 Postprocedural seroma of a genitourinary system organ or structure following a genitourinary system procedure ◀
N99.843 Postprocedural seroma of a genitourinary system organ or structure following other procedure ◀
N99.89 Other postprocedural complications and disorders of genitourinary system

CHAPTER 14 (N00-N99)

CHAPTER 15

PREGNANCY, CHILDBIRTH AND THE PUERPERIUM (O00-O9A)

OGCR Chapter-Specific Coding Guidelines

15. Chapter 15: Pregnancy, Childbirth, and the Puerperium (O00-O9A)

a. General Rules for Obstetric Cases

1) Codes from chapter 15 and sequencing priority

Obstetric cases require codes from chapter 15, codes in the range O00-O9A, Pregnancy, Childbirth, and the Puerperium. Chapter 15 codes have sequencing priority over codes from other chapters. Additional codes from other chapters may be used in conjunction with chapter 15 codes to further specify conditions. Should the provider document that the pregnancy is incidental to the encounter, then code Z33.1, Pregnant state, incidental, should be used in place of any chapter 15 codes. It is the provider's responsibility to state that the condition being treated is not affecting the pregnancy.

2) Chapter 15 codes used only on the maternal record

Chapter 15 codes are to be used only on the maternal record, never on the record of the newborn.

3) Final character for trimester

The majority of codes in Chapter 15 have a final character indicating the trimester of pregnancy. The timeframes for the trimesters are indicated at the beginning of the chapter. If trimester is not a component of a code it is because the condition always occurs in a specific trimester, or the concept of trimester of pregnancy is not applicable. Certain codes have characters for only certain trimesters because the condition does not occur in all trimesters, but it may occur in more than just one.

Assignment of the final character for trimester should be based on the provider's documentation of the trimester (or number of weeks) for the current admission/encounter. This applies to the assignment of trimester for pre-existing conditions as well as those that develop during or are due to the pregnancy. The provider's documentation of the number of weeks may be used to assign the appropriate code identifying the trimester.

Whenever delivery occurs during the current admission, and there is an "in childbirth" option for the obstetric complication being coded, the "in childbirth" code should be assigned.

4) Selection of trimester for inpatient admissions that encompass more than one trimester

In instances when a patient is admitted to a hospital for complications of pregnancy during one trimester and remains in the hospital into a subsequent trimester, the trimester character for the antepartum complication code should be assigned on the basis of the trimester when the complication developed, not the trimester of the discharge. If the condition developed prior to the current admission/encounter or represents a pre-existing condition, the trimester character for the trimester at the time of the admission/encounter should be assigned.

5) Unspecified trimester

Each category that includes codes for trimester has a code for "unspecified trimester." The "unspecified trimester" code should rarely be used, such as when the documentation in the record is insufficient to determine the trimester and it is not possible to obtain clarification.

6) 7th character for Fetus Identification

Where applicable, a 7th character is to be assigned for certain categories (O31, O32, O33.3 - O33.6, O35, O36, O40, O41, O60.1, O60.2, O64, and O69) to identify the fetus for which the complication code applies.

Assign 7th character "0":

- For single gestations
- When the documentation in the record is insufficient to determine the fetus affected and it is not possible to obtain clarification.
- When it is not possible to clinically determine which fetus is affected.

b. Selection of OB Principal or First-listed Diagnosis

1) Routine outpatient prenatal visits

For routine outpatient prenatal visits when no complications are present, a code from category Z34, Encounter for supervision of normal pregnancy, should be used as the first-listed diagnosis. These codes should not be used in conjunction with chapter 15 codes.

2) *Supervision of High-Risk Pregnancy*

Codes from category O09, Supervision of high-risk pregnancy, are intended for use only during the prenatal period. For complications during the labor or delivery episode as a result of a high-risk pregnancy, assign the applicable complication codes from Chapter 15. If there are no complications during the labor or delivery episode, assign code O80, Encounter for full-term uncomplicated delivery.

For routine prenatal outpatient visits for patients with high-risk pregnancies, a code from category O09, Supervision of high-risk pregnancy, should be used as the first-listed diagnosis. Secondary chapter 15 codes may be used in conjunction with these codes if appropriate.

3) Episodes when no delivery occurs

In episodes when no delivery occurs, the principal diagnosis should correspond to the principal complication of the pregnancy which necessitated the encounter. Should more than one complication exist, all of which are treated or monitored, any of the complications codes may be sequenced first.

4) When a delivery occurs

When an obstetric patient is admitted and delivers during that admission, the condition that prompted the admission should be sequenced as the principal diagnosis. If multiple conditions prompted the admission, sequence the one most related to the delivery as the principal diagnosis. A code for any complication of the delivery should be assigned as an additional diagnosis. In cases of cesarean delivery, if the patient was admitted with a condition that resulted in the performance of a cesarean procedure, that condition should be selected as the principal diagnosis. If the reason for the admission was unrelated to the condition resulting in the cesarean delivery, the condition related to the reason for the admission should be selected as the principal diagnosis.

5) Outcome of delivery

A code from category Z37, Outcome of delivery, should be included on every maternal record when a delivery has occurred. These codes are not to be used on subsequent records or on the newborn record.

c. Pre-existing conditions versus conditions due to the pregnancy

Certain categories in Chapter 15 distinguish between conditions of the mother that existed prior to pregnancy (pre-existing) and those that are a direct result of pregnancy. When assigning codes from Chapter 15, it is important to assess if a condition was pre-existing prior to pregnancy or developed during or due to the pregnancy in order to assign the correct code.

Categories that do not distinguish between pre-existing and pregnancy-related conditions may be used for either. It is acceptable to use codes specifically for the puerperium with codes complicating pregnancy and childbirth if a condition arises postpartum during the delivery encounter.

d. Pre-existing hypertension in pregnancy

Category O10, Pre-existing hypertension complicating pregnancy, childbirth and the puerperium, includes codes for hypertensive heart and hypertensive chronic kidney disease. When assigning one of the O10 codes that includes hypertensive heart disease or hypertensive chronic kidney disease, it is necessary to add a secondary code from the appropriate hypertension category to specify the type of heart failure or chronic kidney disease.

See Section I.C.9. Hypertension.

e. Fetal Conditions Affecting the Management of the Mother

1) Codes from categories O35 and O36

Codes from categories O35, Maternal care for known or suspected fetal abnormality and damage, and O36, Maternal care for other fetal problems, are assigned only when the fetal condition is actually responsible for modifying the management of the mother, i.e., by requiring diagnostic studies, additional observation, special care, or termination of pregnancy. The fact that the fetal condition exists does not justify assigning a code from this series to the mother's record.

2) In utero surgery

In cases when surgery is performed on the fetus, a diagnosis code from category O35, Maternal care for known or suspected fetal abnormality and damage, should be assigned identifying the fetal condition. Assign the appropriate procedure code for the procedure performed.

No code from Chapter 16, the perinatal codes, should be used on the mother's record to identify fetal conditions. Surgery performed in utero on a fetus is still to be coded as an obstetric encounter.

f. HIV Infection in Pregnancy, Childbirth and the Puerperium

During pregnancy, childbirth or the puerperium, a patient admitted because of an HIV-related illness should receive a principal diagnosis from subcategory O98.7-, Human immunodeficiency [HIV] disease complicating pregnancy, childbirth and the puerperium, followed by the code(s) for the HIV-related illness(es).

Patients with asymptomatic HIV infection status admitted during pregnancy, childbirth, or the puerperium should receive codes of O98.7- and Z21, Asymptomatic human immunodeficiency virus [HIV] infection status.

g. Diabetes mellitus in pregnancy

Diabetes mellitus is a significant complicating factor in pregnancy. Pregnant women who are diabetic should be assigned a code from category O24, Diabetes mellitus in pregnancy, childbirth, and the puerperium, first, followed by the appropriate diabetes code(s) (E08-E13) from Chapter 4.

h. Long term use of insulin and oral hypoglycemics
Code Z79.4, Long-term (current) use of insulin **or code Z79.84, Long-term (current) use of oral hypoglycemic drugs,** should also be assigned if the diabetes mellitus is being treated with insulin **or oral medications. If the patient is treated with both oral medications and insulin, only the code for insulin-controlled should be assigned.**

i. Gestational (pregnancy induced) diabetes
Gestational (pregnancy induced) diabetes can occur during the second and third trimester of pregnancy in women who were not diabetic prior to pregnancy. Gestational diabetes can cause complications in the pregnancy similar to those of pre-existing diabetes mellitus. It also puts the woman at greater risk of developing diabetes after the pregnancy. Codes for gestational diabetes are in subcategory O24.4, Gestational diabetes mellitus. No other code from category O24, Diabetes mellitus in pregnancy, childbirth, and the puerperium, should be used with a code from O24.4.

The codes under subcategory O24.4 include diet controlled, insulin controlled**, and controlled by oral hypoglycemic drugs.** If a patient with gestational diabetes is treated with both diet and insulin, only the code for insulin-controlled is required. **If a patient with gestational diabetes is treated with both diet and oral hypoglycemic medications, only the code for "controlled by oral hypoglycemic drugs" is required.** Code Z79.4, Long-term (current) use of insulin **or code Z79.84, Long-term (current) use of oral hypoglycemic drugs,** should not be assigned with codes from subcategory O24.4.

An abnormal glucose tolerance in pregnancy is assigned a code from subcategory O99.81, Abnormal glucose complicating pregnancy, childbirth, and the puerperium.

j. Sepsis and septic shock complicating abortion, pregnancy, childbirth and the puerperium
When assigning a chapter 15 code for sepsis complicating abortion, pregnancy, childbirth, and the puerperium, a code for the specific type of infection should be assigned as an additional diagnosis. If severe sepsis is present, a code from subcategory R65.2, Severe sepsis, and code(s) for associated organ dysfunction(s) should also be assigned as additional diagnoses.

k. Puerperal sepsis
Code O85, Puerperal sepsis, should be assigned with a secondary code to identify the causal organism (e.g., for a bacterial infection, assign a code from category B95-B96, Bacterial infections in conditions classified elsewhere). A code from category A4Ø, Streptococcal sepsis, or A41, Other sepsis, should not be used for puerperal sepsis. If applicable, use additional codes to identify severe sepsis (R65.2-) and any associated acute organ dysfunction.

l. Alcohol and tobacco use during pregnancy, childbirth and the puerperium

1) Alcohol use during pregnancy, childbirth and the puerperium
Codes under subcategory O99.31, Alcohol use complicating pregnancy, childbirth, and the puerperium, should be assigned for any pregnancy case when a mother uses alcohol during the pregnancy or postpartum. A secondary code from category F1Ø, Alcohol related disorders, should also be assigned to identify manifestations of the alcohol use.

2) Tobacco use during pregnancy, childbirth and the puerperium
Codes under subcategory O99.33, Smoking (tobacco) complicating pregnancy, childbirth, and the puerperium, should be assigned for any pregnancy case when a mother uses any type of tobacco product during the pregnancy or postpartum. A secondary code from category F17, Nicotine dependence, should also be assigned to identify the type of nicotine dependence.

m. Poisoning, toxic effects, adverse effects and underdosing in a pregnant patient
A code from subcategory O9A.2, Injury, poisoning and certain other consequences of external causes complicating pregnancy, childbirth, and the puerperium, should be sequenced first, followed by the appropriate injury, poisoning, toxic effect, adverse effect or underdosing code, and then the additional code(s) that specifies the condition caused by the poisoning, toxic effect, adverse effect or underdosing.

See Section I.C.19. Adverse effects, poisoning, underdosing and toxic effects.

n. Normal Delivery, Code O8Ø

1) Encounter for full term uncomplicated delivery
Code O8Ø should be assigned when a woman is admitted for a full-term normal delivery and delivers a single, healthy infant without any complications antepartum, during the delivery, or postpartum during the delivery episode. Code O8Ø is always a principal diagnosis. It is not to be used if any other code from chapter 15 is needed to describe a current complication of the antenatal, delivery, or perinatal period. Additional codes from other chapters may be used with code O8Ø if they are not related to or are in any way complicating the pregnancy.

2) Uncomplicated delivery with resolved antepartum complication
Code O8Ø may be used if the patient had a complication at some point during the pregnancy, but the complication is not present at the time of the admission for delivery.

3) Outcome of delivery for O8Ø
Z37.Ø, Single live birth, is the only outcome of delivery code appropriate for use with O8Ø.

o. The Peripartum and Postpartum Periods

1) Peripartum and Postpartum periods
The postpartum period begins immediately after delivery and continues for six weeks following delivery. The peripartum period is defined as the last month of pregnancy to five months postpartum.

2) Peripartum and postpartum complication
A postpartum complication is any complication occurring within the six-week period.

3) Pregnancy-related complications after 6 week period
Chapter 15 codes may also be used to describe pregnancy-related complications after the peripartum or postpartum period if the provider documents that a condition is pregnancy related.

4) Admission for routine postpartum care following delivery outside hospital
When the mother delivers outside the hospital prior to admission and is admitted for routine postpartum care and no complications are noted, code Z39.Ø, Encounter for care and examination of mother immediately after delivery, should be assigned as the principal diagnosis.

5) Pregnancy associated cardiomyopathy
Pregnancy associated cardiomyopathy, code O9Ø.3, is unique in that it may be diagnosed in the third trimester of pregnancy but may continue to progress months after delivery. For this reason, it is referred to as peripartum cardiomyopathy. Code O9Ø.3 is only for use when the cardiomyopathy develops as a result of pregnancy in a woman who did not have pre-existing heart disease.

p. Code O94, Sequelae of complication of pregnancy, childbirth, and the puerperium

1) Code O94
Code O94, Sequelae of complication of pregnancy, childbirth, and the puerperium, is for use in those cases when an initial complication of a pregnancy develops a sequelae requiring care or treatment at a future date.

2) After the initial postpartum period
This code may be used at any time after the initial postpartum period.

3) Sequencing of Code O94
This code, like all sequela codes, is to be sequenced following the code describing the sequelae of the complication.

q. *Termination of Pregnancy and Spontaneous abortions*

1) Abortion with Liveborn Fetus
When an attempted termination of pregnancy results in a liveborn fetus assign code Z33.2, Encounter for elective termination of pregnancy and a code from category Z37, Outcome of Delivery.

2) Retained Products of Conception following an abortion
Subsequent encounters for retained products of conception following a spontaneous abortion or elective termination of pregnancy are assigned the appropriate code from category OØ3, Spontaneous abortion, or codes OØ7.4, Failed attempted termination of pregnancy without complication and Z33.2, Encounter for elective termination of pregnancy. This advice is appropriate even when the patient was discharged previously with a discharge diagnosis of complete abortion.

3) Complications leading to abortion
Codes from Chapter 15 may be used as additional codes to identify any documented complications of the pregnancy in conjunction with codes in categories in OØ7 and OØ8.

r. Abuse in a pregnant patient
For suspected or confirmed cases of abuse of a pregnant patient, a code(s) from subcategories O9A.3, Physical abuse complicating pregnancy, childbirth, and the puerperium, O9A.4, Sexual abuse complicating pregnancy, childbirth, and the puerperium, and O9A.5, Psychological abuse complicating pregnancy, childbirth, and the puerperium, should be sequenced first, followed by the appropriate codes (if applicable) to identify any associated current injury due to physical abuse, sexual abuse, and the perpetrator of abuse.

See Section I.C.19. Adult and child abuse, neglect and other maltreatment.

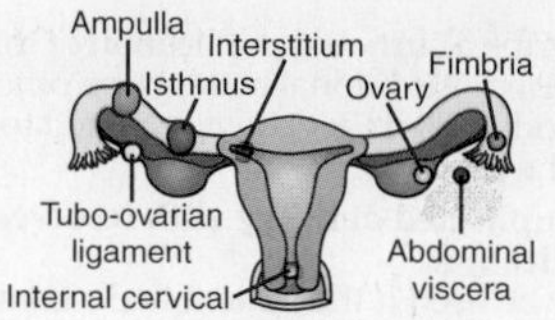

Figure 15-1 Implantation sites of ectopic pregnancy.

Item 15-1 **Ectopic** pregnancy most often occurs in the fallopian tube. Pregnancy outside the uterus may end in a lifethreatening rupture.

★**(See Plate 375 on page NAP-4.)**

CHAPTER 15

PREGNANCY, CHILDBIRTH AND THE PUERPERIUM (O00-O9A)

Note: CODES FROM THIS CHAPTER ARE FOR USE ONLY ON MATERNAL RECORDS, NEVER ON NEWBORN RECORDS

Codes from this chapter are for use for conditions related to or aggravated by the pregnancy, childbirth, or by the puerperium (maternal causes or obstetric causes)

Trimesters are counted from the first day of the last menstrual period. They are defined as follows:

1st trimester - less than 14 weeks 0 days

2nd trimester - 14 weeks 0 days to less than 28 weeks 0 days

3rd trimester - 28 weeks 0 days until delivery

Use additional code from category Z3A, Weeks of gestation, to identify the specific week of the pregnancy, if known. ⇦

Excludes1 supervision of normal pregnancy (Z34.-)

Excludes2 mental and behavioral disorders associated with the puerperium (F53)
obstetrical tetanus (A34)
postpartum necrosis of pituitary gland (E23.0)
puerperal osteomalacia (M83.0)

This chapter contains the following blocks:

O00-O08	Pregnancy with abortive outcome
O09	Supervision of high risk pregnancy
O10-O16	Edema, proteinuria and hypertensive disorders in pregnancy, childbirth and the puerperium
O20-O29	Other maternal disorders predominantly related to pregnancy
O30-O48	Maternal care related to the fetus and amniotic cavity and possible delivery problems
O60-O77	Complications of labor and delivery
O80, O82	Encounter for delivery
O85-O92	Complications predominantly related to the puerperium
O94-O9A	Other obstetric conditions, not elsewhere classified

PREGNANCY WITH ABORTIVE OUTCOME (O00-O08)

Excludes1 continuing pregnancy in multiple gestation after abortion of one fetus or more (O31.1-, O31.3-)

● **O00 Ectopic pregnancy**

Includes ruptured ectopic pregnancy

Use additional code from category O08 to identify any associated complication

● **O00.0 Abdominal pregnancy**

Excludes1 maternal care for viable fetus in abdominal pregnancy (O36.7-)

O00.00 Abdominal pregnancy without intrauterine pregnancy ◀
Abdominal pregnancy NOS ◀

O00.01 Abdominal pregnancy with intrauterine pregnancy ◀

Item 15-2 A **hydatidiform** mole is an overproduction of placental tissue. The tumor secretes a hormone, chorionic gonadotropic hormone (CGH), that indicates a positive pregnancy test. There is no viable fetus. More than 80% of hydatidiform moles are noncancerous.

● **O00.1 Tubal pregnancy**
Fallopian pregnancy
Rupture of (fallopian) tube due to pregnancy
Tubal abortion

O00.10 Tubal pregnancy without intrauterine pregnancy ◀
Tubal pregnancy NOS ◀

O00.11 Tubal pregnancy with intrauterine pregnancy ◀

● **O00.2 Ovarian pregnancy**

O00.20 Ovarian pregnancy without intrauterine pregnancy ◀
Ovarian pregnancy NOS ◀

O00.21 Ovarian pregnancy with intrauterine pregnancy ◀

● **O00.8 Other ectopic pregnancy**
Cervical pregnancy
Cornual pregnancy
Intraligamentous pregnancy
Mural pregnancy

O00.80 Other ectopic pregnancy without intrauterine pregnancy ◀
Other ectopic pregnancy NOS ◀

O00.81 Other ectopic pregnancy with intrauterine pregnancy ◀

● **O00.9 Ectopic pregnancy, unspecified**

O00.90 Unspecified ectopic pregnancy without intrauterine pregnancy ◀
Ectopic pregnancy NOS ◀

O00.91 Unspecified ectopic pregnancy with intrauterine pregnancy ◀

● **O01 Hydatidiform mole**

Use additional code from category O08 to identify any associated complication

Excludes1 chorioadenoma (destruens) (D39.2)
malignant hydatidiform mole (D39.2)

O01.0 Classical hydatidiform mole
Complete hydatidiform mole

O01.1 Incomplete and partial hydatidiform mole

O01.9 Hydatidiform mole, unspecified
Trophoblastic disease NOS
Vesicular mole NOS

● **O02 Other abnormal products of conception**

Use additional code from category O08 to identify any associated complication

Excludes1 papyraceous fetus (O31.0-)

O02.0 Blighted ovum and nonhydatidiform mole
Carneous mole
Fleshy mole
Intrauterine mole NOS
Molar pregnancy NEC
Pathological ovum

O02.1 Missed abortion
Early fetal death, before completion of 20 weeks of gestation, with retention of dead fetus

Excludes1 failed induced abortion (O07.-)
fetal death (intrauterine) (late) (O36.4)
missed abortion with blighted ovum (O02.0)
missed abortion with hydatidiform mole (O01.-)
missed abortion with nonhydatidiform (O02.0)
missed abortion with other abnormal products of conception (O02.8-)
missed delivery (O36.4)
stillbirth (P95)

● **O02.8 Other specified abnormal products of conception**

Excludes1 abnormal products of conception with blighted ovum (O02.0)
abnormal products of conception with hydatidiform mole (O01.-)
abnormal products of conception with nonhydatidiform mole (O02.0)

O02.81 Inappropriate change in quantitative human chorionic gonadotropin (hCG) in early pregnancy

Biochemical pregnancy
Chemical pregnancy
Inappropriate level of quantitative human chorionic gonadotropin (hCG) for gestational age in early pregnancy

O02.89 Other abnormal products of conception

O02.9 Abnormal product of conception, unspecified

● **O03 Spontaneous abortion**

Note: Incomplete abortion includes retained products of conception following spontaneous abortion.

Includes miscarriage

O03.0 Genital tract and pelvic infection following incomplete spontaneous abortion

Endometritis following incomplete spontaneous abortion
Oophoritis following incomplete spontaneous abortion
Parametritis following incomplete spontaneous abortion
Pelvic peritonitis following incomplete spontaneous abortion
Salpingitis following incomplete spontaneous abortion
Salpingo-oophoritis following incomplete spontaneous abortion

Excludes1 sepsis following incomplete spontaneous abortion (O03.37)
urinary tract infection following incomplete spontaneous abortion (O03.38)

O03.1 Delayed or excessive hemorrhage following incomplete spontaneous abortion

Afibrinogenemia following incomplete spontaneous abortion
Defibrination syndrome following incomplete spontaneous abortion
Hemolysis following incomplete spontaneous abortion
Intravascular coagulation following incomplete spontaneous abortion

O03.2 Embolism following incomplete spontaneous abortion

Air embolism following incomplete spontaneous abortion
Amniotic fluid embolism following incomplete spontaneous abortion
Blood-clot embolism following incomplete spontaneous abortion
Embolism NOS following incomplete spontaneous abortion
Fat embolism following incomplete spontaneous abortion
Pulmonary embolism following incomplete spontaneous abortion
Pyemic embolism following incomplete spontaneous abortion
Septic or septicopyemic embolism following incomplete spontaneous abortion
Soap embolism following incomplete spontaneous abortion

● **O03.3 Other and unspecified complications following incomplete spontaneous abortion**

O03.30 Unspecified complication following incomplete spontaneous abortion

O03.31 Shock following incomplete spontaneous abortion

Circulatory collapse following incomplete spontaneous abortion
Shock (postprocedural) following incomplete spontaneous abortion

Excludes1 shock due to infection following incomplete spontaneous abortion (O03.37)

O03.32 Renal failure following incomplete spontaneous abortion

Kidney failure (acute) following incomplete spontaneous abortion
Oliguria following incomplete spontaneous abortion
Renal shutdown following incomplete spontaneous abortion
Renal tubular necrosis following incomplete spontaneous abortion
Uremia following incomplete spontaneous abortion

O03.33 Metabolic disorder following incomplete spontaneous abortion

O03.34 Damage to pelvic organs following incomplete spontaneous abortion

Laceration, perforation, tear or chemical damage of bladder following incomplete spontaneous abortion
Laceration, perforation, tear or chemical damage of bowel following incomplete spontaneous abortion
Laceration, perforation, tear or chemical damage of broad ligament following incomplete spontaneous abortion
Laceration, perforation, tear or chemical damage of cervix following incomplete spontaneous abortion
Laceration, perforation, tear or chemical damage of periurethral tissue following incomplete spontaneous abortion
Laceration, perforation, tear or chemical damage of uterus following incomplete spontaneous abortion
Laceration, perforation, tear or chemical damage of vagina following incomplete spontaneous abortion

O03.35 Other venous complications following incomplete spontaneous abortion

O03.36 Cardiac arrest following incomplete spontaneous abortion

O03.37 Sepsis following incomplete spontaneous abortion

Use additional code to identify infectious agent (B95-B97)
Use additional code to identify severe sepsis, if applicable (R65.2-)

Excludes1 septic or septicopyemic embolism following incomplete spontaneous abortion (O03.2)

O03.38 Urinary tract infection following incomplete spontaneous abortion

Cystitis following incomplete spontaneous abortion

O03.39 Incomplete spontaneous abortion with other complications

CHAPTER 15 (O00-O9A)

O03.4 Incomplete spontaneous abortion without complication

O03.5 Genital tract and pelvic infection following complete or unspecified spontaneous abortion

Endometritis following complete or unspecified spontaneous abortion
Oophoritis following complete or unspecified spontaneous abortion
Parametritis following complete or unspecified spontaneous abortion
Pelvic peritonitis following complete or unspecified spontaneous abortion
Salpingitis following complete or unspecified spontaneous abortion
Salpingo-oophoritis following complete or unspecified spontaneous abortion

Excludes1 sepsis following complete or unspecified spontaneous abortion (O03.87)
urinary tract infection following complete or unspecified spontaneous abortion (O03.88)

O03.6 Delayed or excessive hemorrhage following complete or unspecified spontaneous abortion

Afibrinogenemia following complete or unspecified spontaneous abortion
Defibrination syndrome following complete or unspecified spontaneous abortion
Hemolysis following complete or unspecified spontaneous abortion
Intravascular coagulation following complete or unspecified spontaneous abortion

O03.7 Embolism following complete or unspecified spontaneous abortion

Air embolism following complete or unspecified spontaneous abortion
Amniotic fluid embolism following complete or unspecified spontaneous abortion
Blood-clot embolism following complete or unspecified spontaneous abortion
Embolism NOS following complete or unspecified spontaneous abortion
Fat embolism following complete or unspecified spontaneous abortion
Pulmonary embolism following complete or unspecified spontaneous abortion
Pyemic embolism following complete or unspecified spontaneous abortion
Septic or septicopyemic embolism following complete or unspecified spontaneous abortion
Soap embolism following complete or unspecified spontaneous abortion

● **O03.8 Other and unspecified complications following complete or unspecified spontaneous abortion**

O03.80 Unspecified complication following complete or unspecified spontaneous abortion

O03.81 Shock following complete or unspecified spontaneous abortion

Circulatory collapse following complete or unspecified spontaneous abortion
Shock (postprocedural) following complete or unspecified spontaneous abortion

Excludes1 shock due to infection following complete or unspecified spontaneous abortion (O03.87)

O03.82 Renal failure following complete or unspecified spontaneous abortion

Kidney failure (acute) following complete or unspecified spontaneous abortion
Oliguria following complete or unspecified spontaneous abortion
Renal shutdown following complete or unspecified spontaneous abortion
Renal tubular necrosis following complete or unspecified spontaneous abortion
Uremia following complete or unspecified spontaneous abortion

O03.83 Metabolic disorder following complete or unspecified spontaneous abortion

O03.84 Damage to pelvic organs following complete or unspecified spontaneous abortion

Laceration, perforation, tear or chemical damage of bladder following complete or unspecified spontaneous abortion
Laceration, perforation, tear or chemical damage of bowel following complete or unspecified spontaneous abortion
Laceration, perforation, tear or chemical damage of broad ligament following complete or unspecified spontaneous abortion
Laceration, perforation, tear or chemical damage of cervix following complete or unspecified spontaneous abortion
Laceration, perforation, tear or chemical damage of periurethral tissue following complete or unspecified spontaneous abortion
Laceration, perforation, tear or chemical damage of uterus following complete or unspecified spontaneous abortion
Laceration, perforation, tear or chemical damage of vagina following complete or unspecified spontaneous abortion

O03.85 Other venous complications following complete or unspecified spontaneous abortion

O03.86 Cardiac arrest following complete or unspecified spontaneous abortion

O03.87 Sepsis following complete or unspecified spontaneous abortion

Use additional code to identify infectious agent (B95-B97)
Use additional code to identify severe sepsis, if applicable (R65.2-)

Excludes1 septic or septicopyemic embolism following complete or unspecified spontaneous abortion (O03.7)

O03.88 Urinary tract infection following complete or unspecified spontaneous abortion

Cystitis following complete or unspecified spontaneous abortion

O03.89 Complete or unspecified spontaneous abortion with other complications

O03.9 Complete or unspecified spontaneous abortion without complication

Miscarriage NOS
Spontaneous abortion NOS

CHAPTER 15 (O00-O9A)

● **O04 Complications following (induced) termination of pregnancy**

Includes complications following (induced) termination of pregnancy

Excludes1 encounter for elective termination of pregnancy, uncomplicated (Z33.2)
failed attempted termination of pregnancy (O07.-)

O04.5 Genital tract and pelvic infection following (induced) termination of pregnancy

Endometritis following (induced) termination of pregnancy
Oophoritis following (induced) termination of pregnancy
Parametritis following (induced) termination of pregnancy
Pelvic peritonitis following (induced) termination of pregnancy
Salpingitis following (induced) termination of pregnancy
Salpingo-oophoritis following (induced) termination of pregnancy

Excludes1 sepsis following (induced) termination of pregnancy (O04.87)
urinary tract infection following (induced) termination of pregnancy (O04.88)

O04.6 Delayed or excessive hemorrhage following (induced) termination of pregnancy

Afibrinogenemia following (induced) termination of pregnancy
Defibrination syndrome following (induced) termination of pregnancy
Hemolysis following (induced) termination of pregnancy
Intravascular coagulation following (induced) termination of pregnancy

O04.7 Embolism following (induced) termination of pregnancy

Air embolism following (induced) termination of pregnancy
Amniotic fluid embolism following (induced) termination of pregnancy
Blood-clot embolism following (induced) termination of pregnancy
Embolism NOS following (induced) termination of pregnancy
Fat embolism following (induced) termination of pregnancy
Pulmonary embolism following (induced) termination of pregnancy
Pyemic embolism following (induced) termination of pregnancy
Septic or septicopyemic embolism following (induced) termination of pregnancy
Soap embolism following (induced) termination of pregnancy

● **O04.8 (Induced) termination of pregnancy with other and unspecified complications**

O04.80 (Induced) termination of pregnancy with unspecified complications

O04.81 Shock following (induced) termination of pregnancy

Circulatory collapse following (induced) termination of pregnancy
Shock (postprocedural) following (induced) termination of pregnancy

Excludes1 shock due to infection following (induced) termination of pregnancy (O04.87)

O04.82 Renal failure following (induced) termination of pregnancy

Kidney failure (acute) following (induced) termination of pregnancy
Oliguria following (induced) termination of pregnancy
Renal shutdown following (induced) termination of pregnancy
Renal tubular necrosis following (induced) termination of pregnancy
Uremia following (induced) termination of pregnancy

O04.83 Metabolic disorder following (induced) termination of pregnancy

O04.84 Damage to pelvic organs following (induced) termination of pregnancy

Laceration, perforation, tear or chemical damage of bladder following (induced) termination of pregnancy
Laceration, perforation, tear or chemical damage of bowel following (induced) termination of pregnancy
Laceration, perforation, tear or chemical damage of broad ligament following (induced) termination of pregnancy
Laceration, perforation, tear or chemical damage of cervix following (induced) termination of pregnancy
Laceration, perforation, tear or chemical damage of periurethral tissue following (induced) termination of pregnancy
Laceration, perforation, tear or chemical damage of uterus following (induced) termination of pregnancy
Laceration, perforation, tear or chemical damage of vagina following (induced) termination of pregnancy

O04.85 Other venous complications following (induced) termination of pregnancy

O04.86 Cardiac arrest following (induced) termination of pregnancy

O04.87 Sepsis following (induced) termination of pregnancy

Use additional code to identify infectious agent (B95-B97)
Use additional code to identify severe sepsis, if applicable (R65.2-)

Excludes1 septic or septicopyemic embolism following (induced) termination of pregnancy (O04.7)

O04.88 Urinary tract infection following (induced) termination of pregnancy

Cystitis following (induced) termination of pregnancy

O04.89 (Induced) termination of pregnancy with other complications

O07 Failed attempted termination of pregnancy

Includes failure of attempted induction of termination of pregnancy
incomplete elective abortion

Excludes1 incomplete spontaneous abortion (O03.0-)

O07.0 Genital tract and pelvic infection following failed attempted termination of pregnancy
Endometritis following failed attempted termination of pregnancy
Oophoritis following failed attempted termination of pregnancy
Parametritis following failed attempted termination of pregnancy
Pelvic peritonitis following failed attempted termination of pregnancy
Salpingitis following failed attempted termination of pregnancy
Salpingo-oophoritis following failed attempted termination of pregnancy

Excludes1 sepsis following failed attempted termination of pregnancy (O07.37)
urinary tract infection following failed attempted termination of pregnancy (O07.38)

O07.1 Delayed or excessive hemorrhage following failed attempted termination of pregnancy
Afibrinogenemia following failed attempted termination of pregnancy
Defibrination syndrome following failed attempted termination of pregnancy
Hemolysis following failed attempted termination of pregnancy
Intravascular coagulation following failed attempted termination of pregnancy

O07.2 Embolism following failed attempted termination of pregnancy
Air embolism following failed attempted termination of pregnancy
Amniotic fluid embolism following failed attempted termination of pregnancy
Blood-clot embolism following failed attempted termination of pregnancy
Embolism NOS following failed attempted termination of pregnancy
Fat embolism following failed attempted termination of pregnancy
Pulmonary embolism following failed attempted termination of pregnancy
Pyemic embolism following failed attempted termination of pregnancy
Septic or septicopyemic embolism following failed attempted termination of pregnancy
Soap embolism following failed attempted termination of pregnancy

O07.3 Failed attempted termination of pregnancy with other and unspecified complications

O07.30 Failed attempted termination of pregnancy with unspecified complications

O07.31 Shock following failed attempted termination of pregnancy
Circulatory collapse following failed attempted termination of pregnancy
Shock (postprocedural) following failed attempted termination of pregnancy

Excludes1 shock due to infection following failed attempted termination of pregnancy (O07.37)

O07.32 Renal failure following failed attempted termination of pregnancy
Kidney failure (acute) following failed attempted termination of pregnancy
Oliguria following failed attempted termination of pregnancy
Renal shutdown following failed attempted termination of pregnancy
Renal tubular necrosis following failed attempted termination of pregnancy
Uremia following failed attempted termination of pregnancy

O07.33 Metabolic disorder following failed attempted termination of pregnancy

O07.34 Damage to pelvic organs following failed attempted termination of pregnancy
Laceration, perforation, tear or chemical damage of bladder following failed attempted termination of pregnancy
Laceration, perforation, tear or chemical damage of bowel following failed attempted termination of pregnancy
Laceration, perforation, tear or chemical damage of broad ligament following failed attempted termination of pregnancy
Laceration, perforation, tear or chemical damage of cervix following failed attempted termination of pregnancy
Laceration, perforation, tear or chemical damage of periurethral tissue following failed attempted termination of pregnancy
Laceration, perforation, tear or chemical damage of uterus following failed attempted termination of pregnancy
Laceration, perforation, tear or chemical damage of vagina following failed attempted termination of pregnancy

O07.35 Other venous complications following failed attempted termination of pregnancy

O07.36 Cardiac arrest following failed attempted termination of pregnancy

O07.37 Sepsis following failed attempted termination of pregnancy
Use additional code (B95-B97), to identify infectious agent
Use additional code (R65.2-) to identify severe sepsis, if applicable

Excludes1 septic or septicopyemic embolism following failed attempted termination of pregnancy (O07.2)

O07.38 Urinary tract infection following failed attempted termination of pregnancy
Cystitis following failed attempted termination of pregnancy

O07.39 Failed attempted termination of pregnancy with other complications

O07.4 Failed attempted termination of pregnancy without complication

● **O08 Complications following ectopic and molar pregnancy**
This category is for use with categories O00-O02 to identify any associated complications.

O08.0 Genital tract and pelvic infection following ectopic and molar pregnancy
Endometritis following ectopic and molar pregnancy
Oophoritis following ectopic and molar pregnancy
Parametritis following ectopic and molar pregnancy
Pelvic peritonitis following ectopic and molar pregnancy
Salpingitis following ectopic and molar pregnancy
Salpingo-oophoritis following ectopic and molar pregnancy
Excludes1 sepsis following ectopic and molar pregnancy (O08.82)
urinary tract infection (O08.83)

O08.1 Delayed or excessive hemorrhage following ectopic and molar pregnancy
Afibrinogenemia following ectopic and molar pregnancy
Defibrination syndrome following ectopic and molar pregnancy
Hemolysis following ectopic and molar pregnancy
Intravascular coagulation following ectopic and molar pregnancy
Excludes1 delayed or excessive hemorrhage due to incomplete abortion (O03.1)

O08.2 Embolism following ectopic and molar pregnancy
Air embolism following ectopic and molar pregnancy
Amniotic fluid embolism following ectopic and molar pregnancy
Blood-clot embolism following ectopic and molar pregnancy
Embolism NOS following ectopic and molar pregnancy
Fat embolism following ectopic and molar pregnancy
Pulmonary embolism following ectopic and molar pregnancy
Pyemic embolism following ectopic and molar pregnancy
Septic or septicopyemic embolism following ectopic and molar pregnancy
Soap embolism following ectopic and molar pregnancy

O08.3 Shock following ectopic and molar pregnancy
Circulatory collapse following ectopic and molar pregnancy
Shock (postprocedural) following ectopic and molar pregnancy
Excludes1 shock due to infection following ectopic and molar pregnancy (O08.82)

O08.4 Renal failure following ectopic and molar pregnancy
Kidney failure (acute) following ectopic and molar pregnancy
Oliguria following ectopic and molar pregnancy
Renal shutdown following ectopic and molar pregnancy
Renal tubular necrosis following ectopic and molar pregnancy
Uremia following ectopic and molar pregnancy

O08.5 Metabolic disorders following an ectopic and molar pregnancy

O08.6 Damage to pelvic organs and tissues following an ectopic and molar pregnancy
Laceration, perforation, tear or chemical damage of bladder following an ectopic and molar pregnancy
Laceration, perforation, tear or chemical damage of bowel following an ectopic and molar pregnancy
Laceration, perforation, tear or chemical damage of broad ligament following an ectopic and molar pregnancy
Laceration, perforation, tear or chemical damage of cervix following an ectopic and molar pregnancy
Laceration, perforation, tear or chemical damage of periurethral tissue following an ectopic and molar pregnancy
Laceration, perforation, tear or chemical damage of uterus following an ectopic and molar pregnancy
Laceration, perforation, tear or chemical damage of vagina following an ectopic and molar pregnancy

O08.7 Other venous complications following an ectopic and molar pregnancy

● **O08.8 Other complications following an ectopic and molar pregnancy**

O08.81 Cardiac arrest following an ectopic and molar pregnancy

O08.82 Sepsis following ectopic and molar pregnancy
Use additional code (B95-B97), to identify infectious agent
Use additional code (R65.2-) to identify severe sepsis, if applicable
Excludes1 septic or septicopyemic embolism following ectopic and molar pregnancy (O08.2)

O08.83 Urinary tract infection following an ectopic and molar pregnancy
Cystitis following an ectopic and molar pregnancy

O08.89 Other complications following an ectopic and molar pregnancy

O08.9 Unspecified complication following an ectopic and molar pregnancy

SUPERVISION OF HIGH RISK PREGNANCY (O09)

● **O09 Supervision of high risk pregnancy**

● **O09.0 Supervision of pregnancy with history of infertility**

O09.00 Supervision of pregnancy with history of infertility, unspecified trimester

O09.01 Supervision of pregnancy with history of infertility, first trimester

O09.02 Supervision of pregnancy with history of infertility, second trimester

O09.03 Supervision of pregnancy with history of infertility, third trimester

● **O09.1 Supervision of pregnancy with history of ectopic pregnancy**

O09.10 Supervision of pregnancy with history of ectopic pregnancy, unspecified trimester

O09.11 Supervision of pregnancy with history of ectopic pregnancy, first trimester

O09.12 Supervision of pregnancy with history of ectopic pregnancy, second trimester

O09.13 Supervision of pregnancy with history of ectopic pregnancy, third trimester

● O09.A Supervision of pregnancy with history of molar pregnancy ◀
O09.A0 Supervision of pregnancy with history of molar pregnancy, unspecified trimester ◀
O09.A1 Supervision of pregnancy with history of molar pregnancy, first trimester ◀
O09.A2 Supervision of pregnancy with history of molar pregnancy, second trimester ◀
O09.A3 Supervision of pregnancy with history of molar pregnancy, third trimester ◀

● O09.2 Supervision of pregnancy with other poor reproductive or obstetric history
Excludes2 pregnancy care for patient with history of recurrent pregnancy loss (O26.2-)

● O09.21 Supervision of pregnancy with history of pre-term labor
O09.211 Supervision of pregnancy with history of pre-term labor, first trimester
O09.212 Supervision of pregnancy with history of pre-term labor, second trimester
O09.213 Supervision of pregnancy with history of pre-term labor, third trimester
O09.219 Supervision of pregnancy with history of pre-term labor, unspecified trimester

● O09.29 Supervision of pregnancy with other poor reproductive or obstetric history
Supervision of pregnancy with history of neonatal death
Supervision of pregnancy with history of stillbirth
O09.291 Supervision of pregnancy with other poor reproductive or obstetric history, first trimester
O09.292 Supervision of pregnancy with other poor reproductive or obstetric history, second trimester
O09.293 Supervision of pregnancy with other poor reproductive or obstetric history, third trimester
O09.299 Supervision of pregnancy with other poor reproductive or obstetric history, unspecified trimester

● O09.3 Supervision of pregnancy with insufficient antenatal care
Supervision of concealed pregnancy
Supervision of hidden pregnancy
O09.30 Supervision of pregnancy with insufficient antenatal care, unspecified trimester
O09.31 Supervision of pregnancy with insufficient antenatal care, first trimester
O09.32 Supervision of pregnancy with insufficient antenatal care, second trimester
O09.33 Supervision of pregnancy with insufficient antenatal care, third trimester

● O09.4 Supervision of pregnancy with grand multiparity
O09.40 Supervision of pregnancy with grand multiparity, unspecified trimester
O09.41 Supervision of pregnancy with grand multiparity, first trimester
O09.42 Supervision of pregnancy with grand multiparity, second trimester
O09.43 Supervision of pregnancy with grand multiparity, third trimester

● O09.5 Supervision of elderly primigravida and multigravida
Pregnancy for a female 35 years and older at expected date of delivery

● O09.51 Supervision of elderly primigravida
O09.511 Supervision of elderly primigravida, first trimester
O09.512 Supervision of elderly primigravida, second trimester
O09.513 Supervision of elderly primigravida, third trimester
O09.519 Supervision of elderly primigravida, unspecified trimester

● O09.52 Supervision of elderly multigravida
O09.521 Supervision of elderly multigravida, first trimester
O09.522 Supervision of elderly multigravida, second trimester
O09.523 Supervision of elderly multigravida, third trimester
O09.529 Supervision of elderly multigravida, unspecified trimester

● O09.6 Supervision of young primigravida and multigravida
Supervision of pregnancy for a female less than 16 years old at expected date of delivery

● O09.61 Supervision of young primigravida
O09.611 Supervision of young primigravida, first trimester
O09.612 Supervision of young primigravida, second trimester
O09.613 Supervision of young primigravida, third trimester
O09.619 Supervision of young primigravida, unspecified trimester

● O09.62 Supervision of young multigravida
O09.621 Supervision of young multigravida, first trimester
O09.622 Supervision of young multigravida, second trimester
O09.623 Supervision of young multigravida, third trimester
O09.629 Supervision of young multigravida, unspecified trimester

● O09.7 Supervision of high risk pregnancy due to social problems
O09.70 Supervision of high risk pregnancy due to social problems, unspecified trimester
O09.71 Supervision of high risk pregnancy due to social problems, first trimester
O09.72 Supervision of high risk pregnancy due to social problems, second trimester
O09.73 Supervision of high risk pregnancy due to social problems, third trimester

● O09.8 Supervision of other high risk pregnancies

● O09.81 Supervision of pregnancy resulting from assisted reproductive technology
Supervision of pregnancy resulting from in-vitro fertilization
Excludes2 gestational carrier status (Z33.3) ◀
O09.811 Supervision of pregnancy resulting from assisted reproductive technology, first trimester
O09.812 Supervision of pregnancy resulting from assisted reproductive technology, second trimester
O09.813 Supervision of pregnancy resulting from assisted reproductive technology, third trimester
O09.819 Supervision of pregnancy resulting from assisted reproductive technology, unspecified trimester

● **O09.82 Supervision of pregnancy with history of in utero procedure during previous pregnancy**

O09.821 Supervision of pregnancy with history of in utero procedure during previous pregnancy, first trimester

O09.822 Supervision of pregnancy with history of in utero procedure during previous pregnancy, second trimester

O09.823 Supervision of pregnancy with history of in utero procedure during previous pregnancy, third trimester

O09.829 Supervision of pregnancy with history of in utero procedure during previous pregnancy, unspecified trimester

Excludes1 supervision of pregnancy affected by in utero procedure during current pregnancy (O35.7)

● **O09.89 Supervision of other high risk pregnancies**

O09.891 Supervision of other high risk pregnancies, first trimester

O09.892 Supervision of other high risk pregnancies, second trimester

O09.893 Supervision of other high risk pregnancies, third trimester

O09.899 Supervision of other high risk pregnancies, unspecified trimester

● **O09.9 Supervision of high risk pregnancy, unspecified**

O09.90 Supervision of high risk pregnancy, unspecified, unspecified trimester

O09.91 Supervision of high risk pregnancy, unspecified, first trimester

O09.92 Supervision of high risk pregnancy, unspecified, second trimester

O09.93 Supervision of high risk pregnancy, unspecified, third trimester

EDEMA, PROTEINURIA AND HYPERTENSIVE DISORDERS IN PREGNANCY, CHILDBIRTH AND THE PUERPERIUM (O10-O16)

● **O10 Pre-existing hypertension complicating pregnancy, childbirth and the puerperium**

Includes pre-existing hypertension with pre-existing proteinuria complicating pregnancy, childbirth and the puerperium

Excludes2 pre-existing hypertension with superimposed pre-eclampsia complicating pregnancy, childbirth and the puerperium (O11.-)

● **O10.0 Pre-existing essential hypertension complicating pregnancy, childbirth and the puerperium**

Any condition in I10 specified as a reason for obstetric care during pregnancy, childbirth or the puerperium

● **O10.01 Pre-existing essential hypertension complicating pregnancy**

O10.011 Pre-existing essential hypertension complicating pregnancy, first trimester

O10.012 Pre-existing essential hypertension complicating pregnancy, second trimester

O10.013 Pre-existing essential hypertension complicating pregnancy, third trimester

O10.019 Pre-existing essential hypertension complicating pregnancy, unspecified trimester

O10.02 Pre-existing essential hypertension complicating childbirth

O10.03 Pre-existing essential hypertension complicating the puerperium

● **O10.1 Pre-existing hypertensive heart disease complicating pregnancy, childbirth and the puerperium**

Any condition in I11 specified as a reason for obstetric care during pregnancy, childbirth or the puerperium

Use additional code from I11 to identify the type of hypertensive heart disease

● **O10.11 Pre-existing hypertensive heart disease complicating pregnancy**

O10.111 Pre-existing hypertensive heart disease complicating pregnancy, first trimester

O10.112 Pre-existing hypertensive heart disease complicating pregnancy, second trimester

O10.113 Pre-existing hypertensive heart disease complicating pregnancy, third trimester

O10.119 Pre-existing hypertensive heart disease complicating pregnancy, unspecified trimester

O10.12 Pre-existing hypertensive heart disease complicating childbirth

O10.13 Pre-existing hypertensive heart disease complicating the puerperium

● **O10.2 Pre-existing hypertensive chronic kidney disease complicating pregnancy, childbirth and the puerperium**

Any condition in I12 specified as a reason for obstetric care during pregnancy, childbirth or the puerperium

Use additional code from I12 to identify the type of hypertensive chronic kidney disease

● **O10.21 Pre-existing hypertensive chronic kidney disease complicating pregnancy**

O10.211 Pre-existing hypertensive chronic kidney disease complicating pregnancy, first trimester

O10.212 Pre-existing hypertensive chronic kidney disease complicating pregnancy, second trimester

O10.213 Pre-existing hypertensive chronic kidney disease complicating pregnancy, third trimester

O10.219 Pre-existing hypertensive chronic kidney disease complicating pregnancy, unspecified trimester

O10.22 Pre-existing hypertensive chronic kidney disease complicating childbirth

O10.23 Pre-existing hypertensive chronic kidney disease complicating the puerperium

CHAPTER 15 (O00-O9A)

● O10.3 **Pre-existing hypertensive heart and chronic kidney disease complicating pregnancy, childbirth and the puerperium**
Any condition in I13 specified as a reason for obstetric care during pregnancy, childbirth or the puerperium
Use additional code from I13 to identify the type of hypertensive heart and chronic kidney disease

● O10.31 **Pre-existing hypertensive heart and chronic kidney disease complicating pregnancy**
O10.311 **Pre-existing hypertensive heart and chronic kidney disease complicating pregnancy, first trimester**
O10.312 **Pre-existing hypertensive heart and chronic kidney disease complicating pregnancy, second trimester**
O10.313 **Pre-existing hypertensive heart and chronic kidney disease complicating pregnancy, third trimester**
O10.319 **Pre-existing hypertensive heart and chronic kidney disease complicating pregnancy, unspecified trimester**

O10.32 **Pre-existing hypertensive heart and chronic kidney disease complicating childbirth**
O10.33 **Pre-existing hypertensive heart and chronic kidney disease complicating the puerperium**

● O10.4 **Pre-existing secondary hypertension complicating pregnancy, childbirth and the puerperium**
Any condition in I15 specified as a reason for obstetric care during pregnancy, childbirth or the puerperium
Use additional code from I15 to identify the type of secondary hypertension

● O10.41 **Pre-existing secondary hypertension complicating pregnancy**
O10.411 **Pre-existing secondary hypertension complicating pregnancy, first trimester**
O10.412 **Pre-existing secondary hypertension complicating pregnancy, second trimester**
O10.413 **Pre-existing secondary hypertension complicating pregnancy, third trimester**
O10.419 **Pre-existing secondary hypertension complicating pregnancy, unspecified trimester**

O10.42 **Pre-existing secondary hypertension complicating childbirth**
O10.43 **Pre-existing secondary hypertension complicating the puerperium**

● O10.9 **Unspecified pre-existing hypertension complicating pregnancy, childbirth and the puerperium**

● O10.91 **Unspecified pre-existing hypertension complicating pregnancy**
O10.911 **Unspecified pre-existing hypertension complicating pregnancy, first trimester**
O10.912 **Unspecified pre-existing hypertension complicating pregnancy, second trimester**
O10.913 **Unspecified pre-existing hypertension complicating pregnancy, third trimester**
O10.919 **Unspecified pre-existing hypertension complicating pregnancy, unspecified trimester**

O10.92 **Unspecified pre-existing hypertension complicating childbirth**
O10.93 **Unspecified pre-existing hypertension complicating the puerperium**

● O11 **Pre-existing hypertension with pre-eclampsia**
Includes conditions in O10 complicated by pre-eclampsia
pre-eclampsia superimposed pre-existing hypertension
Use additional code from O10 to identify the type of hypertension

O11.1 **Pre-existing hypertension with pre-eclampsia, first trimester**
O11.2 **Pre-existing hypertension with pre-eclampsia, second trimester**
O11.3 **Pre-existing hypertension with pre-eclampsia, third trimester**
O11.4 **Pre-existing hypertension with pre-eclampsia, complicating childbirth** ◀
O11.5 **Pre-existing hypertension with pre-eclampsia, complicating the puerperium** ◀
O11.9 **Pre-existing hypertension with pre-eclampsia, unspecified trimester**

● O12 **Gestational [pregnancy-induced] edema and proteinuria without hypertension**

● O12.0 **Gestational edema**
O12.00 **Gestational edema, unspecified trimester**
O12.01 **Gestational edema, first trimester**
O12.02 **Gestational edema, second trimester**
O12.03 **Gestational edema, third trimester**
O12.04 **Gestational edema, complicating childbirth** ◀
O12.05 **Gestational edema, complicating the puerperium** ◀

● O12.1 **Gestational proteinuria**
O12.10 **Gestational proteinuria, unspecified trimester**
O12.11 **Gestational proteinuria, first trimester**
O12.12 **Gestational proteinuria, second trimester**
O12.13 **Gestational proteinuria, third trimester**
O12.14 **Gestational proteinuria, complicating childbirth** ◀
O12.15 **Gestational proteinuria, complicating the puerperium** ◀

● O12.2 **Gestational edema with proteinuria**
O12.20 **Gestational edema with proteinuria, unspecified trimester**
O12.21 **Gestational edema with proteinuria, first trimester**
O12.22 **Gestational edema with proteinuria, second trimester**
O12.23 **Gestational edema with proteinuria, third trimester**
O12.24 **Gestational edema with proteinuria, complicating childbirth** ◀
O12.25 **Gestational edema with proteinuria, complicating the puerperium** ◀

● O13 **Gestational [pregnancy-induced] hypertension without significant proteinuria**
Includes gestational hypertension NOS
transient hypertension of pregnancy ◀

O13.1 **Gestational [pregnancy-induced] hypertension without significant proteinuria, first trimester**
O13.2 **Gestational [pregnancy-induced] hypertension without significant proteinuria, second trimester**
O13.3 **Gestational [pregnancy-induced] hypertension without significant proteinuria, third trimester**
O13.4 **Gestational [pregnancy-induced] hypertension without significant proteinuria, complicating childbirth** ◀
O13.5 **Gestational [pregnancy-induced] hypertension without significant proteinuria, complicating the puerperium** ◀
O13.9 **Gestational [pregnancy-induced] hypertension without significant proteinuria, unspecified trimester**

● O14 Pre-eclampsia
Excludes1 pre-existing hypertension with pre-eclampsia (O11)
● O14.0 Mild to moderate pre-eclampsia
O14.00 Mild to moderate pre-eclampsia, unspecified trimester
O14.02 Mild to moderate pre-eclampsia, second trimester
O14.03 Mild to moderate pre-eclampsia, third trimester
O14.04 Mild to moderate pre-eclampsia, complicating childbirth ◀
O14.05 Mild to moderate pre-eclampsia, complicating the puerperium ◀
● O14.1 Severe pre-eclampsia
Excludes1 HELLP syndrome (O14.2-)
H=hemolysis, EL=elevated liver enzymes, LP=low platelet count
O14.10 Severe pre-eclampsia, unspecified trimester
O14.12 Severe pre-eclampsia, second trimester
O14.13 Severe pre-eclampsia, third trimester
O14.14 Severe pre-eclampsia complicating childbirth ◀
O14.15 Severe pre-eclampsia, complicating the puerperium ◀
● O14.2 HELLP syndrome
Severe pre-eclampsia with hemolysis, elevated liver enzymes and low platelet count (HELLP)
O14.20 HELLP syndrome (HELLP), unspecified trimester
O14.22 HELLP syndrome (HELLP), second trimester
O14.23 HELLP syndrome (HELLP), third trimester
O14.24 HELLP syndrome, complicating childbirth ◀
O14.25 HELLP syndrome, complicating the puerperium ◀
● O14.9 Unspecified pre-eclampsia
O14.90 Unspecified pre-eclampsia, unspecified trimester
O14.92 Unspecified pre-eclampsia, second trimester
O14.93 Unspecified pre-eclampsia, third trimester
O14.94 Unspecified pre-eclampsia, complicating childbirth ◀
O14.95 Unspecified pre-eclampsia, complicating the puerperium ◀

● O15 Eclampsia
Includes convulsions following conditions in O10-O14 and O16
● O15.0 Eclampsia complicating pregnancy ⬅
O15.00 Eclampsia complicating pregnancy, unspecified trimester ⬅
O15.02 Eclampsia complicating pregnancy, second trimester ⬅
O15.03 Eclampsia complicating pregnancy, third trimester ⬅
O15.1 Eclampsia complicating labor ⬅
O15.2 Eclampsia complicating the puerperium ⬅
O15.9 Eclampsia, unspecified as to time period
Eclampsia NOS

● O16 Unspecified maternal hypertension
O16.1 Unspecified maternal hypertension, first trimester
O16.2 Unspecified maternal hypertension, second trimester
O16.3 Unspecified maternal hypertension, third trimester
O16.4 Unspecified maternal hypertension, complicating childbirth ◀
O16.5 Unspecified maternal hypertension, complicating the puerperium ◀
O16.9 Unspecified maternal hypertension, unspecified trimester

OTHER MATERNAL DISORDERS PREDOMINANTLY RELATED TO PREGNANCY (O20-O29)

Excludes2 maternal care related to the fetus and amniotic cavity and possible delivery problems (O30-O48)
maternal diseases classifiable elsewhere but complicating pregnancy, labor and delivery, and the puerperium (O98-O99)

● O20 Hemorrhage in early pregnancy
Includes hemorrhage before completion of 20 weeks gestation
Excludes1 pregnancy with abortive outcome (O00-O08)
O20.0 Threatened abortion
Hemorrhage specified as due to threatened abortion
O20.8 Other hemorrhage in early pregnancy
O20.9 Hemorrhage in early pregnancy, unspecified

● O21 Excessive vomiting in pregnancy
O21.0 Mild hyperemesis gravidarum
Hyperemesis gravidarum, mild or unspecified, starting before the end of the 20th week of gestation
O21.1 Hyperemesis gravidarum with metabolic disturbance
Hyperemesis gravidarum, starting before the end of the 20th week of gestation, with metabolic disturbance such as carbohydrate depletion
Hyperemesis gravidarum, starting before the end of the 20th week of gestation, with metabolic disturbance such as dehydration
Hyperemesis gravidarum, starting before the end of the 20th week of gestation, with metabolic disturbance such as electrolyte imbalance
O21.2 Late vomiting of pregnancy
Excessive vomiting starting after 20 completed weeks of gestation
O21.8 Other vomiting complicating pregnancy
Vomiting due to diseases classified elsewhere, complicating pregnancy
Use additional code, to identify cause
O21.9 Vomiting of pregnancy, unspecified

● O22 Venous complications and hemorrhoids in pregnancy
Excludes1 venous complications of:
abortion NOS (O03.9)
ectopic or molar pregnancy (O08.7)
failed attempted abortion (O07.35)
induced abortion (O04.85)
spontaneous abortion (O03.89)
Excludes2 obstetric pulmonary embolism (O88.-)
venous complications and hemorrhoids of childbirth and the puerperium (O87.-)
● O22.0 Varicose veins of lower extremity in pregnancy
Varicose veins NOS in pregnancy
O22.00 Varicose veins of lower extremity in pregnancy, unspecified trimester
O22.01 Varicose veins of lower extremity in pregnancy, first trimester
O22.02 Varicose veins of lower extremity in pregnancy, second trimester
O22.03 Varicose veins of lower extremity in pregnancy, third trimester
● O22.1 Genital varices in pregnancy
Perineal varices in pregnancy
Vaginal varices in pregnancy
Vulval varices in pregnancy
O22.10 Genital varices in pregnancy, unspecified trimester
O22.11 Genital varices in pregnancy, first trimester
O22.12 Genital varices in pregnancy, second trimester
O22.13 Genital varices in pregnancy, third trimester

CHAPTER 15 (O00-O9A)

● **O22.2 Superficial thrombophlebitis in pregnancy**
Phlebitis in pregnancy NOS
Thrombophlebitis of legs in pregnancy
Thrombosis in pregnancy NOS
Use additional code to identify the superficial thrombophlebitis (I80.0-)

O22.20 Superficial thrombophlebitis in pregnancy, unspecified trimester
O22.21 Superficial thrombophlebitis in pregnancy, first trimester
O22.22 Superficial thrombophlebitis in pregnancy, second trimester
O22.23 Superficial thrombophlebitis in pregnancy, third trimester

● **O22.3 Deep phlebothrombosis in pregnancy**
Deep vein thrombosis, antepartum
Use additional code to identify the deep vein thrombosis (I82.4-, I82.5-, I82.62-. I82.72-)
Use additional code, if applicable, for associated long-term (current) use of anticoagulants (Z79.01)

O22.30 Deep phlebothrombosis in pregnancy, unspecified trimester
O22.31 Deep phlebothrombosis in pregnancy, first trimester
O22.32 Deep phlebothrombosis in pregnancy, second trimester
O22.33 Deep phlebothrombosis in pregnancy, third trimester

● **O22.4 Hemorrhoids in pregnancy**

O22.40 Hemorrhoids in pregnancy, unspecified trimester
O22.41 Hemorrhoids in pregnancy, first trimester
O22.42 Hemorrhoids in pregnancy, second trimester
O22.43 Hemorrhoids in pregnancy, third trimester

● **O22.5 Cerebral venous thrombosis in pregnancy**
Cerebrovenous sinus thrombosis in pregnancy

O22.50 Cerebral venous thrombosis in pregnancy, unspecified trimester
O22.51 Cerebral venous thrombosis in pregnancy, first trimester
O22.52 Cerebral venous thrombosis in pregnancy, second trimester
O22.53 Cerebral venous thrombosis in pregnancy, third trimester

● **O22.8 Other venous complications in pregnancy**

● **O22.8X Other venous complications in pregnancy**

O22.8X1 Other venous complications in pregnancy, first trimester
O22.8X2 Other venous complications in pregnancy, second trimester
O22.8X3 Other venous complications in pregnancy, third trimester
O22.8X9 Other venous complications in pregnancy, unspecified trimester

● **O22.9 Venous complication in pregnancy, unspecified**
Gestational phlebitis NOS
Gestational phlebopathy NOS
Gestational thrombosis NOS

O22.90 Venous complication in pregnancy, unspecified, unspecified trimester
O22.91 Venous complication in pregnancy, unspecified, first trimester
O22.92 Venous complication in pregnancy, unspecified, second trimester
O22.93 Venous complication in pregnancy, unspecified, third trimester

● **O23 Infections of genitourinary tract in pregnancy**
Use additional code to identify organism (B95.-, B96.-)
Excludes2 gonococcal infections complicating pregnancy, childbirth and the puerperium (O98.2)
infections with a predominantly sexual mode of transmission NOS complicating pregnancy, childbirth and the puerperium (O98.3)
syphilis complicating pregnancy, childbirth and the puerperium (O98.1)
tuberculosis of genitourinary system complicating pregnancy, childbirth and the puerperium (O98.0)
venereal disease NOS complicating pregnancy, childbirth and the puerperium (O98.3)

● **O23.0 Infections of kidney in pregnancy**
Pyelonephritis in pregnancy

O23.00 Infections of kidney in pregnancy, unspecified trimester
O23.01 Infections of kidney in pregnancy, first trimester
O23.02 Infections of kidney in pregnancy, second trimester
O23.03 Infections of kidney in pregnancy, third trimester

● **O23.1 Infections of bladder in pregnancy**

O23.10 Infections of bladder in pregnancy, unspecified trimester
O23.11 Infections of bladder in pregnancy, first trimester
O23.12 Infections of bladder in pregnancy, second trimester
O23.13 Infections of bladder in pregnancy, third trimester

● **O23.2 Infections of urethra in pregnancy**

O23.20 Infections of urethra in pregnancy, unspecified trimester
O23.21 Infections of urethra in pregnancy, first trimester
O23.22 Infections of urethra in pregnancy, second trimester
O23.23 Infections of urethra in pregnancy, third trimester

● **O23.3 Infections of other parts of urinary tract in pregnancy**

O23.30 Infections of other parts of urinary tract in pregnancy, unspecified trimester
O23.31 Infections of other parts of urinary tract in pregnancy, first trimester
O23.32 Infections of other parts of urinary tract in pregnancy, second trimester
O23.33 Infections of other parts of urinary tract in pregnancy, third trimester

● **O23.4 Unspecified infection of urinary tract in pregnancy**

O23.40 Unspecified infection of urinary tract in pregnancy, unspecified trimester
O23.41 Unspecified infection of urinary tract in pregnancy, first trimester
O23.42 Unspecified infection of urinary tract in pregnancy, second trimester
O23.43 Unspecified infection of urinary tract in pregnancy, third trimester

● **O23.5 Infections of the genital tract in pregnancy**

● **O23.51 Infection of cervix in pregnancy**

O23.511 Infections of cervix in pregnancy, first trimester
O23.512 Infections of cervix in pregnancy, second trimester
O23.513 Infections of cervix in pregnancy, third trimester
O23.519 Infections of cervix in pregnancy, unspecified trimester

● **O23.52 Salpingo-oophoritis in pregnancy**
Oophoritis = inflammation of ovary
Salpingitis = inflammation of fallopian tube
Oophoritis in pregnancy
Salpingitis in pregnancy

O23.521 Salpingo-oophoritis in pregnancy, first trimester

O23.522 Salpingo-oophoritis in pregnancy, second trimester

O23.523 Salpingo-oophoritis in pregnancy, third trimester

O23.529 Salpingo-oophoritis in pregnancy, unspecified trimester

● **O23.59 Infection of other part of genital tract in pregnancy**

O23.591 Infection of other part of genital tract in pregnancy, first trimester

O23.592 Infection of other part of genital tract in pregnancy, second trimester

O23.593 Infection of other part of genital tract in pregnancy, third trimester

O23.599 Infection of other part of genital tract in pregnancy, unspecified trimester

● **O23.9 Unspecified genitourinary tract infection in pregnancy**
Genitourinary tract infection in pregnancy NOS

O23.90 Unspecified genitourinary tract infection in pregnancy, unspecified trimester

O23.91 Unspecified genitourinary tract infection in pregnancy, first trimester

O23.92 Unspecified genitourinary tract infection in pregnancy, second trimester

O23.93 Unspecified genitourinary tract infection in pregnancy, third trimester

OGCR Section I.C.15.g.

Diabetes mellitus in pregnancy

Diabetes mellitus is a significant complicating factor in pregnancy. Pregnant women who are diabetic should be assigned a code from category O24, Diabetes mellitus in pregnancy, childbirth, and the puerperium, first, followed by the appropriate diabetes code(s) (E08-E13) from Chapter 4.

● **O24 Diabetes mellitus in pregnancy, childbirth, and the puerperium**

● **O24.0 Pre-existing type 1 diabetes mellitus, in pregnancy, childbirth and the puerperium** ⬅
Juvenile onset diabetes mellitus, in pregnancy, childbirth and the puerperium
Ketosis-prone diabetes mellitus in pregnancy, childbirth and the puerperium
Use additional code from category E10 to further identify any manifestations

● **O24.01 Pre-existing type 1 diabetes mellitus, in pregnancy** ⬅

O24.011 Pre-existing type 1 diabetes mellitus, in pregnancy, first trimester ⬅

O24.012 Pre-existing type 1 diabetes mellitus, in pregnancy, second trimester ⬅

O24.013 Pre-existing type 1 diabetes mellitus, in pregnancy, third trimester ⬅

O24.019 Pre-existing type 1 diabetes mellitus, in pregnancy, unspecified trimester ⬅

O24.02 Pre-existing type 1 diabetes mellitus, in childbirth ⬅

O24.03 Pre-existing type 1 diabetes mellitus, in the puerperium ⬅

● **O24.1 Pre-existing type 2 diabetes mellitus, in pregnancy, childbirth and the puerperium** ⬅
Insulin-resistant diabetes mellitus in pregnancy, childbirth and the puerperium
Use additional code (for):
from category E11 to further identify any manifestations
long-term (current) use of insulin (Z79.4)

● **O24.11 Pre-existing type 2 diabetes mellitus, in pregnancy** ⬅

O24.111 Pre-existing type 2 diabetes mellitus, in pregnancy, first trimester ⬅

O24.112 Pre-existing type 2 diabetes mellitus, in pregnancy, second trimester ⬅

O24.113 Pre-existing type 2 diabetes mellitus, in pregnancy, third trimester ⬅

O24.119 Pre-existing type 2 diabetes mellitus, in pregnancy, unspecified trimester ⬅

O24.12 Pre-existing type 2 diabetes mellitus, in childbirth ⬅

O24.13 Pre-existing type 2 diabetes mellitus, in the puerperium ⬅

● **O24.3 Unspecified pre-existing diabetes mellitus in pregnancy, childbirth and the puerperium**
Use additional code (for):
from category E11 to further identify any manifestation
long-term (current) use of insulin (Z79.4)

● **O24.31 Unspecified pre-existing diabetes mellitus in pregnancy**

O24.311 Unspecified pre-existing diabetes mellitus in pregnancy, first trimester

O24.312 Unspecified pre-existing diabetes mellitus in pregnancy, second trimester

O24.313 Unspecified pre-existing diabetes mellitus in pregnancy, third trimester

O24.319 Unspecified pre-existing diabetes mellitus in pregnancy, unspecified trimester

O24.32 Unspecified pre-existing diabetes mellitus in childbirth

O24.33 Unspecified pre-existing diabetes mellitus in the puerperium

● **O24.4 Gestational diabetes mellitus**
Diabetes mellitus arising in pregnancy
Gestational diabetes mellitus NOS

● **O24.41 Gestational diabetes mellitus in pregnancy**

O24.410 Gestational diabetes mellitus in pregnancy, diet controlled

O24.414 Gestational diabetes mellitus in pregnancy, insulin controlled

O24.415 Gestational diabetes mellitus in pregnancy, controlled by oral hypoglycemic drugs ◀
Gestational diabetes mellitus in pregnancy, controlled by oral antidiabetic drugs ◀

O24.419 Gestational diabetes mellitus in pregnancy, unspecified control

CHAPTER 15 (O00-O9A)

● **O24.42 Gestational diabetes mellitus in childbirth**
O24.420 Gestational diabetes mellitus in childbirth, diet controlled
O24.424 Gestational diabetes mellitus in childbirth, insulin controlled
O24.425 Gestational diabetes mellitus in childbirth, controlled by oral hypoglycemic drugs ◀
Gestational diabetes mellitus in childbirth, controlled by oral antidiabetic drugs ◀
O24.429 Gestational diabetes mellitus in childbirth, unspecified control

OGCR Section I.C.15.i.

Gestational (pregnancy induced) diabetes

Gestational (pregnancy induced) diabetes can occur during the second and third trimester of pregnancy in women who were not diabetic prior to pregnancy. Gestational diabetes can cause complications in the pregnancy similar to those of pre-existing diabetes mellitus. It also puts the woman at greater risk of developing diabetes after the pregnancy. Codes for gestational diabetes are in subcategory O24.4, Gestational diabetes mellitus. No other code from category O24, Diabetes mellitus in pregnancy, childbirth, and the puerperium, should be used with a code from O24.4

The codes under subcategory O24.4 include diet controlled, insulin controlled, **and controlled by oral hypoglycemic drugs.** If a patient with gestational diabetes is treated with both diet and insulin, only the code for insulin-controlled is required. **If a patient with gestational diabetes is treated with both diet and oral hypoglycemic medications, only the code for "controlled by oral hypoglycemic drugs" is required.** Code Z79.4, Long-term (current) use of insulin **or code Z79.84, Long-term (current) use of oral hypoglycemic drugs,** should not be assigned with codes from subcategory O24.4.

An abnormal glucose tolerance in pregnancy is assigned a code from subcategory O99.81, Abnormal glucose complicating pregnancy, childbirth, and the puerperium.

● **O24.43 Gestational diabetes mellitus in the puerperium**
O24.430 Gestational diabetes mellitus in the puerperium, diet controlled
O24.434 Gestational diabetes mellitus in the puerperium, insulin controlled
O24.435 Gestational diabetes mellitus in puerperium, controlled by oral hypoglycemic drugs ◀
Gestational diabetes mellitus in puerperium, controlled by oral antidiabetic drugs ◀
O24.439 Gestational diabetes mellitus in the puerperium, unspecified control

● **O24.8 Other pre-existing diabetes mellitus in pregnancy, childbirth, and the puerperium**
Use additional code (for):
from categories E08, E09 and E13 to further identify any manifestation
long-term (current) use of insulin (Z79.4)

● **O24.81 Other pre-existing diabetes mellitus in pregnancy**
O24.811 Other pre-existing diabetes mellitus in pregnancy, first trimester
O24.812 Other pre-existing diabetes mellitus in pregnancy, second trimester
O24.813 Other pre-existing diabetes mellitus in pregnancy, third trimester
O24.819 Other pre-existing diabetes mellitus in pregnancy, unspecified trimester

O24.82 Other pre-existing diabetes mellitus in childbirth
O24.83 Other pre-existing diabetes mellitus in the puerperium

● **O24.9 Unspecified diabetes mellitus in pregnancy, childbirth and the puerperium**
Use additional code for long-term (current) use of insulin (Z79.4)
Unknown whether patient was diabetic before pregnancy occurred

● **O24.91 Unspecified diabetes mellitus in pregnancy**
O24.911 Unspecified diabetes mellitus in pregnancy, first trimester
O24.912 Unspecified diabetes mellitus in pregnancy, second trimester
O24.913 Unspecified diabetes mellitus in pregnancy, third trimester
O24.919 Unspecified diabetes mellitus in pregnancy, unspecified trimester

O24.92 Unspecified diabetes mellitus in childbirth
O24.93 Unspecified diabetes mellitus in the puerperium

● **O25 Malnutrition in pregnancy, childbirth and the puerperium**

● **O25.1 Malnutrition in pregnancy**
O25.10 Malnutrition in pregnancy, unspecified trimester
O25.11 Malnutrition in pregnancy, first trimester
O25.12 Malnutrition in pregnancy, second trimester
O25.13 Malnutrition in pregnancy, third trimester

O25.2 Malnutrition in childbirth
O25.3 Malnutrition in the puerperium

● **O26 Maternal care for other conditions predominantly related to pregnancy**

● **O26.0 Excessive weight gain in pregnancy**
Excludes2 gestational edema (O12.0, O12.2)
O26.00 Excessive weight gain in pregnancy, unspecified trimester
O26.01 Excessive weight gain in pregnancy, first trimester
O26.02 Excessive weight gain in pregnancy, second trimester
O26.03 Excessive weight gain in pregnancy, third trimester

● **O26.1 Low weight gain in pregnancy**
O26.10 Low weight gain in pregnancy, unspecified trimester
O26.11 Low weight gain in pregnancy, first trimester
O26.12 Low weight gain in pregnancy, second trimester
O26.13 Low weight gain in pregnancy, third trimester

● **O26.2 Pregnancy care for patient with recurrent pregnancy loss**
O26.20 Pregnancy care for patient with recurrent pregnancy loss, unspecified trimester
O26.21 Pregnancy care for patient with recurrent pregnancy loss, first trimester
O26.22 Pregnancy care for patient with recurrent pregnancy loss, second trimester
O26.23 Pregnancy care for patient with recurrent pregnancy loss, third trimester

● **O26.3 Retained intrauterine contraceptive device in pregnancy**
O26.30 Retained intrauterine contraceptive device in pregnancy, unspecified trimester
O26.31 Retained intrauterine contraceptive device in pregnancy, first trimester
O26.32 Retained intrauterine contraceptive device in pregnancy, second trimester
O26.33 Retained intrauterine contraceptive device in pregnancy, third trimester

● **O26.4 Herpes gestationis**
- **O26.40 Herpes gestationis, unspecified trimester**
- **O26.41 Herpes gestationis, first trimester**
- **O26.42 Herpes gestationis, second trimester**
- **O26.43 Herpes gestationis, third trimester**

● **O26.5 Maternal hypotension syndrome**
Supine hypotensive syndrome
- **O26.50 Maternal hypotension syndrome, unspecified trimester**
- **O26.51 Maternal hypotension syndrome, first trimester**
- **O26.52 Maternal hypotension syndrome, second trimester**
- **O26.53 Maternal hypotension syndrome, third trimester**

● **O26.6 Liver and biliary tract disorders in pregnancy, childbirth and the puerperium**
Use additional code to identify the specific disorder
Excludes2 hepatorenal syndrome following labor and delivery (O90.4)

● **O26.61 Liver and biliary tract disorders in pregnancy**
- **O26.611 Liver and biliary tract disorders in pregnancy, first trimester**
- **O26.612 Liver and biliary tract disorders in pregnancy, second trimester**
- **O26.613 Liver and biliary tract disorders in pregnancy, third trimester**
- **O26.619 Liver and biliary tract disorders in pregnancy, unspecified trimester**

O26.62 Liver and biliary tract disorders in childbirth
O26.63 Liver and biliary tract disorders in the puerperium

● **O26.7 Subluxation of symphysis (pubis) in pregnancy, childbirth and the puerperium**
Excludes1 traumatic separation of symphysis (pubis) during childbirth (O71.6)

● **O26.71 Subluxation of symphysis (pubis) in pregnancy**
- **O26.711 Subluxation of symphysis (pubis) in pregnancy, first trimester**
- **O26.712 Subluxation of symphysis (pubis) in pregnancy, second trimester**
- **O26.713 Subluxation of symphysis (pubis) in pregnancy, third trimester**
- **O26.719 Subluxation of symphysis (pubis) in pregnancy, unspecified trimester**

O26.72 Subluxation of symphysis (pubis) in childbirth
O26.73 Subluxation of symphysis (pubis) in the puerperium

● **O26.8 Other specified pregnancy related conditions**

● **O26.81 Pregnancy related exhaustion and fatigue**
- **O26.811 Pregnancy related exhaustion and fatigue, first trimester**
- **O26.812 Pregnancy related exhaustion and fatigue, second trimester**
- **O26.813 Pregnancy related exhaustion and fatigue, third trimester**
- **O26.819 Pregnancy related exhaustion and fatigue, unspecified trimester**

● **O26.82 Pregnancy related peripheral neuritis**
- **O26.821 Pregnancy related peripheral neuritis, first trimester**
- **O26.822 Pregnancy related peripheral neuritis, second trimester**
- **O26.823 Pregnancy related peripheral neuritis, third trimester**
- **O26.829 Pregnancy related peripheral neuritis, unspecified trimester**

● **O26.83 Pregnancy related renal disease**
Use additional code to identify the specific disorder
- **O26.831 Pregnancy related renal disease, first trimester**
- **O26.832 Pregnancy related renal disease, second trimester**
- **O26.833 Pregnancy related renal disease, third trimester**
- **O26.839 Pregnancy related renal disease, unspecified trimester**

● **O26.84 Uterine size-date discrepancy complicating pregnancy**
Excludes1 encounter for suspected problem with fetal growth ruled out (Z03.74)
- **O26.841 Uterine size-date discrepancy, first trimester**
- **O26.842 Uterine size-date discrepancy, second trimester**
- **O26.843 Uterine size-date discrepancy, third trimester**
- **O26.849 Uterine size-date discrepancy, unspecified trimester**

● **O26.85 Spotting complicating pregnancy**
- **O26.851 Spotting complicating pregnancy, first trimester**
- **O26.852 Spotting complicating pregnancy, second trimester**
- **O26.853 Spotting complicating pregnancy, third trimester**
- **O26.859 Spotting complicating pregnancy, unspecified trimester**

O26.86 Pruritic urticarial papules and plaques of pregnancy (PUPPP)
Polymorphic eruption of pregnancy

● **O26.87 Cervical shortening**
Excludes1 encounter for suspected cervical shortening ruled out (Z03.75)
- **O26.872 Cervical shortening, second trimester**
- **O26.873 Cervical shortening, third trimester**
- **O26.879 Cervical shortening, unspecified trimester**

● **O26.89 Other specified pregnancy related conditions**
- **O26.891 Other specified pregnancy related conditions, first trimester**
- **O26.892 Other specified pregnancy related conditions, second trimester**
- **O26.893 Other specified pregnancy related conditions, third trimester**
- **O26.899 Other specified pregnancy related conditions, unspecified trimester**

● **O26.9 Pregnancy related conditions, unspecified**
- **O26.90 Pregnancy related conditions, unspecified, unspecified trimester**
- **O26.91 Pregnancy related conditions, unspecified, first trimester**
- **O26.92 Pregnancy related conditions, unspecified, second trimester**
- **O26.93 Pregnancy related conditions, unspecified, third trimester**

- O28 **Abnormal findings on antenatal screening of mother**
  - **Excludes1** diagnostic findings classified elsewhere - see Alphabetical Index
  - O28.0 **Abnormal hematological finding on antenatal screening of mother**
  - O28.1 **Abnormal biochemical finding on antenatal screening of mother**
  - O28.2 **Abnormal cytological finding on antenatal screening of mother**
  - O28.3 **Abnormal ultrasonic finding on antenatal screening of mother**
  - O28.4 **Abnormal radiological finding on antenatal screening of mother**
  - O28.5 **Abnormal chromosomal and genetic finding on antenatal screening of mother**
  - O28.8 **Other abnormal findings on antenatal screening of mother**
  - O28.9 **Unspecified abnormal findings on antenatal screening of mother**

- O29 **Complications of anesthesia during pregnancy**
  - **Includes** maternal complications arising from the administration of a general, regional or local anesthetic, analgesic or other sedation during pregnancy
  - Use additional code, if necessary, to identify the complication
  - **Excludes2** complications of anesthesia during labor and delivery (O74.-)
    complications of anesthesia during the puerperium (O89.-)
  - O29.0 **Pulmonary complications of anesthesia during pregnancy**
    - O29.01 **Aspiration pneumonitis due to anesthesia during pregnancy**
      - Inhalation of stomach contents or secretions NOS due to anesthesia during pregnancy
      - Mendelson's syndrome due to anesthesia during pregnancy
      - O29.011 **Aspiration pneumonitis due to anesthesia during pregnancy, first trimester**
      - O29.012 **Aspiration pneumonitis due to anesthesia during pregnancy, second trimester**
      - O29.013 **Aspiration pneumonitis due to anesthesia during pregnancy, third trimester**
      - O29.019 **Aspiration pneumonitis due to anesthesia during pregnancy, unspecified trimester**
    - O29.02 **Pressure collapse of lung due to anesthesia during pregnancy**
      - O29.021 **Pressure collapse of lung due to anesthesia during pregnancy, first trimester**
      - O29.022 **Pressure collapse of lung due to anesthesia during pregnancy, second trimester**
      - O29.023 **Pressure collapse of lung due to anesthesia during pregnancy, third trimester**
      - O29.029 **Pressure collapse of lung due to anesthesia during pregnancy, unspecified trimester**
    - O29.09 **Other pulmonary complications of anesthesia during pregnancy**
      - O29.091 **Other pulmonary complications of anesthesia during pregnancy, first trimester**
      - O29.092 **Other pulmonary complications of anesthesia during pregnancy, second trimester**
      - O29.093 **Other pulmonary complications of anesthesia during pregnancy, third trimester**
      - O29.099 **Other pulmonary complications of anesthesia during pregnancy, unspecified trimester**
  - O29.1 **Cardiac complications of anesthesia during pregnancy**
    - O29.11 **Cardiac arrest due to anesthesia during pregnancy**
      - O29.111 **Cardiac arrest due to anesthesia during pregnancy, first trimester**
      - O29.112 **Cardiac arrest due to anesthesia during pregnancy, second trimester**
      - O29.113 **Cardiac arrest due to anesthesia during pregnancy, third trimester**
      - O29.119 **Cardiac arrest due to anesthesia during pregnancy, unspecified trimester**
    - O29.12 **Cardiac failure due to anesthesia during pregnancy**
      - O29.121 **Cardiac failure due to anesthesia during pregnancy, first trimester**
      - O29.122 **Cardiac failure due to anesthesia during pregnancy, second trimester**
      - O29.123 **Cardiac failure due to anesthesia during pregnancy, third trimester**
      - O29.129 **Cardiac failure due to anesthesia during pregnancy, unspecified trimester**
    - O29.19 **Other cardiac complications of anesthesia during pregnancy**
      - O29.191 **Other cardiac complications of anesthesia during pregnancy, first trimester**
      - O29.192 **Other cardiac complications of anesthesia during pregnancy, second trimester**
      - O29.193 **Other cardiac complications of anesthesia during pregnancy, third trimester**
      - O29.199 **Other cardiac complications of anesthesia during pregnancy, unspecified trimester**
  - O29.2 **Central nervous system complications of anesthesia during pregnancy**
    - O29.21 **Cerebral anoxia due to anesthesia during pregnancy**
      - O29.211 **Cerebral anoxia due to anesthesia during pregnancy, first trimester**
      - O29.212 **Cerebral anoxia due to anesthesia during pregnancy, second trimester**
      - O29.213 **Cerebral anoxia due to anesthesia during pregnancy, third trimester**
      - O29.219 **Cerebral anoxia due to anesthesia during pregnancy, unspecified trimester**

O29.29 Other central nervous system complications of anesthesia during pregnancy
O29.291 Other central nervous system complications of anesthesia during pregnancy, first trimester
O29.292 Other central nervous system complications of anesthesia during pregnancy, second trimester
O29.293 Other central nervous system complications of anesthesia during pregnancy, third trimester
O29.299 Other central nervous system complications of anesthesia during pregnancy, unspecified trimester

O29.3 Toxic reaction to local anesthesia during pregnancy
O29.3X Toxic reaction to local anesthesia during pregnancy
O29.3X1 Toxic reaction to local anesthesia during pregnancy, first trimester
O29.3X2 Toxic reaction to local anesthesia during pregnancy, second trimester
O29.3X3 Toxic reaction to local anesthesia during pregnancy, third trimester
O29.3X9 Toxic reaction to local anesthesia during pregnancy, unspecified trimester

O29.4 Spinal and epidural anesthesia induced headache during pregnancy
O29.40 Spinal and epidural anesthesia induced headache during pregnancy, unspecified trimester
O29.41 Spinal and epidural anesthesia induced headache during pregnancy, first trimester
O29.42 Spinal and epidural anesthesia induced headache during pregnancy, second trimester
O29.43 Spinal and epidural anesthesia induced headache during pregnancy, third trimester

O29.5 Other complications of spinal and epidural anesthesia during pregnancy
O29.5X Other complications of spinal and epidural anesthesia during pregnancy
O29.5X1 Other complications of spinal and epidural anesthesia during pregnancy, first trimester
O29.5X2 Other complications of spinal and epidural anesthesia during pregnancy, second trimester
O29.5X3 Other complications of spinal and epidural anesthesia during pregnancy, third trimester
O29.5X9 Other complications of spinal and epidural anesthesia during pregnancy, unspecified trimester

O29.6 Failed or difficult intubation for anesthesia during pregnancy
O29.60 Failed or difficult intubation for anesthesia during pregnancy, unspecified trimester
O29.61 Failed or difficult intubation for anesthesia during pregnancy, first trimester
O29.62 Failed or difficult intubation for anesthesia during pregnancy, second trimester
O29.63 Failed or difficult intubation for anesthesia during pregnancy, third trimester

O29.8 Other complications of anesthesia during pregnancy
O29.8X Other complications of anesthesia during pregnancy
O29.8X1 Other complications of anesthesia during pregnancy, first trimester
O29.8X2 Other complications of anesthesia during pregnancy, second trimester
O29.8X3 Other complications of anesthesia during pregnancy, third trimester
O29.8X9 Other complications of anesthesia during pregnancy, unspecified trimester

O29.9 Unspecified complication of anesthesia during pregnancy
O29.90 Unspecified complication of anesthesia during pregnancy, unspecified trimester
O29.91 Unspecified complication of anesthesia during pregnancy, first trimester
O29.92 Unspecified complication of anesthesia during pregnancy, second trimester
O29.93 Unspecified complication of anesthesia during pregnancy, third trimester

MATERNAL CARE RELATED TO THE FETUS AND AMNIOTIC CAVITY AND POSSIBLE DELIVERY PROBLEMS (O30-O48)

O30 Multiple gestation
Code also any complications specific to multiple gestation
O30.0 Twin pregnancy
O30.00 Twin pregnancy, unspecified number of placenta and unspecified number of amniotic sacs
O30.001 Twin pregnancy, unspecified number of placenta and unspecified number of amniotic sacs, first trimester
O30.002 Twin pregnancy, unspecified number of placenta and unspecified number of amniotic sacs, second trimester
O30.003 Twin pregnancy, unspecified number of placenta and unspecified number of amniotic sacs, third trimester
O30.009 Twin pregnancy, unspecified number of placenta and unspecified number of amniotic sacs, unspecified trimester
O30.01 Twin pregnancy, monochorionic/monoamniotic
Twin pregnancy, one placenta, one amniotic sac
Excludes1 conjoined twins (O30.02-)
O30.011 Twin pregnancy, monochorionic/monoamniotic, first trimester
O30.012 Twin pregnancy, monochorionic/monoamniotic, second trimester
O30.013 Twin pregnancy, monochorionic/monoamniotic, third trimester
O30.019 Twin pregnancy, monochorionic/monoamniotic, unspecified trimester
O30.02 Conjoined twin pregnancy
O30.021 Conjoined twin pregnancy, first trimester
O30.022 Conjoined twin pregnancy, second trimester
O30.023 Conjoined twin pregnancy, third trimester
O30.029 Conjoined twin pregnancy, unspecified trimester

● O30.03 Twin pregnancy, monochorionic/diamniotic
Twin pregnancy, one placenta, two amniotic sacs
- O30.031 Twin pregnancy, monochorionic/diamniotic, first trimester
- O30.032 Twin pregnancy, monochorionic/diamniotic, second trimester
- O30.033 Twin pregnancy, monochorionic/diamniotic, third trimester
- O30.039 Twin pregnancy, monochorionic/diamniotic, unspecified trimester

● O30.04 Twin pregnancy, dichorionic/diamniotic
Twin pregnancy, two placentae, two amniotic sacs
- O30.041 Twin pregnancy, dichorionic/diamniotic, first trimester
- O30.042 Twin pregnancy, dichorionic/diamniotic, second trimester
- O30.043 Twin pregnancy, dichorionic/diamniotic, third trimester
- O30.049 Twin pregnancy, dichorionic/diamniotic, unspecified trimester

● O30.09 Twin pregnancy, unable to determine number of placenta and number of amniotic sacs
- O30.091 Twin pregnancy, unable to determine number of placenta and number of amniotic sacs, first trimester
- O30.092 Twin pregnancy, unable to determine number of placenta and number of amniotic sacs, second trimester
- O30.093 Twin pregnancy, unable to determine number of placenta and number of amniotic sacs, third trimester
- O30.099 Twin pregnancy, unable to determine number of placenta and number of amniotic sacs, unspecified trimester

● O30.1 Triplet pregnancy

● O30.10 Triplet pregnancy, unspecified number of placenta and unspecified number of amniotic sacs
- O30.101 Triplet pregnancy, unspecified number of placenta and unspecified number of amniotic sacs, first trimester
- O30.102 Triplet pregnancy, unspecified number of placenta and unspecified number of amniotic sacs, second trimester
- O30.103 Triplet pregnancy, unspecified number of placenta and unspecified number of amniotic sacs, third trimester
- O30.109 Triplet pregnancy, unspecified number of placenta and unspecified number of amniotic sacs, unspecified trimester

● O30.11 Triplet pregnancy with two or more monochorionic fetuses
- O30.111 Triplet pregnancy with two or more monochorionic fetuses, first trimester
- O30.112 Triplet pregnancy with two or more monochorionic fetuses, second trimester
- O30.113 Triplet pregnancy with two or more monochorionic fetuses, third trimester
- O30.119 Triplet pregnancy with two or more monochorionic fetuses, unspecified trimester

● O30.12 Triplet pregnancy with two or more monoamniotic fetuses
- O30.121 Triplet pregnancy with two or more monoamniotic fetuses, first trimester
- O30.122 Triplet pregnancy with two or more monoamniotic fetuses, second trimester
- O30.123 Triplet pregnancy with two or more monoamniotic fetuses, third trimester
- O30.129 Triplet pregnancy with two or more monoamniotic fetuses, unspecified trimester

● O30.19 Triplet pregnancy, unable to determine number of placenta and number of amniotic sacs
- O30.191 Triplet pregnancy, unable to determine number of placenta and number of amniotic sacs, first trimester
- O30.192 Triplet pregnancy, unable to determine number of placenta and number of amniotic sacs, second trimester
- O30.193 Triplet pregnancy, unable to determine number of placenta and number of amniotic sacs, third trimester
- O30.199 Triplet pregnancy, unable to determine number of placenta and number of amniotic sacs, unspecified trimester

● O30.2 Quadruplet pregnancy

● O30.20 Quadruplet pregnancy, unspecified number of placenta and unspecified number of amniotic sacs
- O30.201 Quadruplet pregnancy, unspecified number of placenta and unspecified number of amniotic sacs, first trimester
- O30.202 Quadruplet pregnancy, unspecified number of placenta and unspecified number of amniotic sacs, second trimester
- O30.203 Quadruplet pregnancy, unspecified number of placenta and unspecified number of amniotic sacs, third trimester
- O30.209 Quadruplet pregnancy, unspecified number of placenta and unspecified number of amniotic sacs, unspecified trimester

● O30.21 Quadruplet pregnancy with two or more monochorionic fetuses
- O30.211 Quadruplet pregnancy with two or more monochorionic fetuses, first trimester
- O30.212 Quadruplet pregnancy with two or more monochorionic fetuses, second trimester
- O30.213 Quadruplet pregnancy with two or more monochorionic fetuses, third trimester
- O30.219 Quadruplet pregnancy with two or more monochorionic fetuses, unspecified trimester

● O30.22 Quadruplet pregnancy with two or more monoamniotic fetuses
- O30.221 Quadruplet pregnancy with two or more monoamniotic fetuses, first trimester
- O30.222 Quadruplet pregnancy with two or more monoamniotic fetuses, second trimester
- O30.223 Quadruplet pregnancy with two or more monoamniotic fetuses, third trimester
- O30.229 Quadruplet pregnancy with two or more monoamniotic fetuses, unspecified trimester

● O30.29 Quadruplet pregnancy, unable to determine number of placenta and number of amniotic sacs
- O30.291 Quadruplet pregnancy, unable to determine number of placenta and number of amniotic sacs, first trimester
- O30.292 Quadruplet pregnancy, unable to determine number of placenta and number of amniotic sacs, second trimester
- O30.293 Quadruplet pregnancy, unable to determine number of placenta and number of amniotic sacs, third trimester
- O30.299 Quadruplet pregnancy, unable to determine number of placenta and number of amniotic sacs, unspecified trimester

● O30.8 Other specified multiple gestation

Multiple gestation pregnancy greater then quadruplets

● O30.80 Other specified multiple gestation, unspecified number of placenta and unspecified number of amniotic sacs
- O30.801 Other specified multiple gestation, unspecified number of placenta and unspecified number of amniotic sacs, first trimester
- O30.802 Other specified multiple gestation, unspecified number of placenta and unspecified number of amniotic sacs, second trimester
- O30.803 Other specified multiple gestation, unspecified number of placenta and unspecified number of amniotic sacs, third trimester
- O30.809 Other specified multiple gestation, unspecified number of placenta and unspecified number of amniotic sacs, unspecified trimester

● O30.81 Other specified multiple gestation with two or more monochorionic fetuses
- O30.811 Other specified multiple gestation with two or more monochorionic fetuses, first trimester
- O30.812 Other specified multiple gestation with two or more monochorionic fetuses, second trimester
- O30.813 Other specified multiple gestation with two or more monochorionic fetuses, third trimester
- O30.819 Other specified multiple gestation with two or more monochorionic fetuses, unspecified trimester

● O30.82 Other specified multiple gestation with two or more monoamniotic fetuses
- O30.821 Other specified multiple gestation with two or more monoamniotic fetuses, first trimester
- O30.822 Other specified multiple gestation with two or more monoamniotic fetuses, second trimester
- O30.823 Other specified multiple gestation with two or more monoamniotic fetuses, third trimester
- O30.829 Other specified multiple gestation with two or more monoamniotic fetuses, unspecified trimester

● O30.89 Other specified multiple gestation, unable to determine number of placenta and number of amniotic sacs
- O30.891 Other specified multiple gestation, unable to determine number of placenta and number of amniotic sacs, first trimester
- O30.892 Other specified multiple gestation, unable to determine number of placenta and number of amniotic sacs, second trimester
- O30.893 Other specified multiple gestation, unable to determine number of placenta and number of amniotic sacs, third trimester
- O30.899 Other specified multiple gestation, unable to determine number of placenta and number of amniotic sacs, unspecified trimester

● O30.9 Multiple gestation, unspecified

Multiple pregnancy NOS

- O30.90 Multiple gestation, unspecified, unspecified trimester
- O30.91 Multiple gestation, unspecified, first trimester
- O30.92 Multiple gestation, unspecified, second trimester
- O30.93 Multiple gestation, unspecified, third trimester

CHAPTER 15 (O00-O9A)

● **O31   Complications specific to multiple gestation**

> **Excludes2**   delayed delivery of second twin, triplet, etc. (O63.2)
> malpresentation of one fetus or more (O32.9)
> placental transfusion syndromes (O43.0-)

One of the following 7th characters is to be assigned to each code under category O31. 7th character Ø is for single gestations and multiple gestations where the fetus is unspecified. 7th characters 1 through 9 are for cases of multiple gestations to identify the fetus for which the code applies. The appropriate code from category O30, Multiple gestation, must also be assigned when assigning a code from category O31 that has a 7th character of 1 through 9.

Ø	not applicable or unspecified
1	fetus 1
2	fetus 2
3	fetus 3
4	fetus 4
5	fetus 5
9	other fetus

● **O31.0   Papyraceous fetus**
> Fetus compressus

X● **O31.00   Papyraceous fetus, unspecified trimester**

X● **O31.01   Papyraceous fetus, first trimester**

X● **O31.02   Papyraceous fetus, second trimester**

X● **O31.03   Papyraceous fetus, third trimester**

● **O31.1   Continuing pregnancy after spontaneous abortion of one fetus or more**

X● **O31.10   Continuing pregnancy after spontaneous abortion of one fetus or more, unspecified trimester**

X● **O31.11   Continuing pregnancy after spontaneous abortion of one fetus or more, first trimester**

X● **O31.12   Continuing pregnancy after spontaneous abortion of one fetus or more, second trimester**

X● **O31.13   Continuing pregnancy after spontaneous abortion of one fetus or more, third trimester**

● **O31.2   Continuing pregnancy after intrauterine death of one fetus or more**

X● **O31.20   Continuing pregnancy after intrauterine death of one fetus or more, unspecified trimester**

X● **O31.21   Continuing pregnancy after intrauterine death of one fetus or more, first trimester**

X● **O31.22   Continuing pregnancy after intrauterine death of one fetus or more, second trimester**

X● **O31.23   Continuing pregnancy after intrauterine death of one fetus or more, third trimester**

● **O31.3   Continuing pregnancy after elective fetal reduction of one fetus or more**
> Continuing pregnancy after selective termination of one fetus or more

X● **O31.30   Continuing pregnancy after elective fetal reduction of one fetus or more, unspecified trimester**

X● **O31.31   Continuing pregnancy after elective fetal reduction of one fetus or more, first trimester**

X● **O31.32   Continuing pregnancy after elective fetal reduction of one fetus or more, second trimester**

X● **O31.33   Continuing pregnancy after elective fetal reduction of one fetus or more, third trimester**

● **O31.8   Other complications specific to multiple gestation**

● **O31.8X   Other complications specific to multiple gestation**

● **O31.8X1   Other complications specific to multiple gestation, first trimester**

● **O31.8X2   Other complications specific to multiple gestation, second trimester**

● **O31.8X3   Other complications specific to multiple gestation, third trimester**

● **O31.8X9   Other complications specific to multiple gestation, unspecified trimester**

● **O32   Maternal care for malpresentation of fetus**

> **Includes**   the listed conditions as a reason for observation, hospitalization or other obstetric care of the mother, or for cesarean delivery before onset of labor

> **Excludes1**   malpresentation of fetus with obstructed labor (O64.-)

One of the following 7th characters is to be assigned to each code under category O32. 7th character Ø is for single gestations and multiple gestations where the fetus is unspecified. 7th characters 1 through 9 are for cases of multiple gestations to identify the fetus for which the code applies. The appropriate code from category O30, Multiple gestation, must also be assigned when assigning a code from category O32 that has a 7th character of 1 through 9.

Ø	not applicable or unspecified
1	fetus 1
2	fetus 2
3	fetus 3
4	fetus 4
5	fetus 5
9	other fetus

X● **O32.0   Maternal care for unstable lie**

X● **O32.1   Maternal care for breech presentation**
> Maternal care for buttocks presentation
> Maternal care for complete breech
> Maternal care for frank breech
> **Excludes1**   footling presentation (O32.8)
> incomplete breech (O32.8)

X● **O32.2   Maternal care for transverse and oblique lie**
> Maternal care for oblique presentation
> Maternal care for transverse presentation

X● **O32.3   Maternal care for face, brow and chin presentation**

X● **O32.4   Maternal care for high head at term**
> Maternal care for failure of head to enter pelvic brim

X● **O32.6   Maternal care for compound presentation**

X● **O32.8   Maternal care for other malpresentation of fetus**
> Maternal care for footling presentation
> Maternal care for incomplete breech

X● **O32.9   Maternal care for malpresentation of fetus, unspecified**

● **O33   Maternal care for disproportion**

> **Includes**   the listed conditions as a reason for observation, hospitalization or other obstetric care of the mother, or for cesarean delivery before onset of labor

> **Excludes1**   disproportion with obstructed labor (O65-O66)

O33.0   Maternal care for disproportion due to deformity of maternal pelvic bones
> Maternal care for disproportion due to pelvic deformity causing disproportion NOS

O33.1   Maternal care for disproportion due to generally contracted pelvis
> Maternal care for disproportion due to contracted pelvis NOS causing disproportion

◀ New   ◀═ Revised   ~~deleted~~ Deleted   **OGCR** Official Guidelines   **X** Assign placeholder X   ● Use Additional Character(s)

Excludes 1	Excludes 2	Includes	Use additional	Code first	Code also	Unspecified

O33.2 Maternal care for disproportion due to inlet contraction of pelvis

Maternal care for disproportion due to inlet contraction (pelvis) causing disproportion

X● O33.3 Maternal care for disproportion due to outlet contraction of pelvis

Maternal care for disproportion due to mid-cavity contraction (pelvis)

Maternal care for disproportion due to outlet contraction (pelvis)

One of the following 7th characters is to be assigned to code O33.3. 7th character Ø is for single gestations and multiple gestations where the fetus is unspecified. 7th characters 1 through 9 are for cases of multiple gestations to identify the fetus for which the code applies. The appropriate code from category O3Ø, Multiple gestation, must also be assigned when assigning code O33.3 with a 7th character of 1 through 9.

Ø	not applicable or unspecified
1	fetus 1
2	fetus 2
3	fetus 3
4	fetus 4
5	fetus 5
9	other fetus

X● O33.4 Maternal care for disproportion of mixed maternal and fetal origin

One of the following 7th characters is to be assigned to code O33.4. 7th character Ø is for single gestations and multiple gestations where the fetus is unspecified. 7th characters 1 through 9 are for cases of multiple gestations to identify the fetus for which the code applies. The appropriate code from category O3Ø, Multiple gestation, must also be assigned when assigning code O33.4 with a 7th character of 1 through 9.

Ø	not applicable or unspecified
1	fetus 1
2	fetus 2
3	fetus 3
4	fetus 4
5	fetus 5
9	other fetus

X● O33.5 Maternal care for disproportion due to unusually large fetus

Maternal care for disproportion due to disproportion of fetal origin with normally formed fetus

Maternal care for disproportion due to fetal disproportion NOS

One of the following 7th characters is to be assigned to code O33.5. 7th character Ø is for single gestations and multiple gestations where the fetus is unspecified. 7th characters 1 through 9 are for cases of multiple gestations to identify the fetus for which the code applies. The appropriate code from category O3Ø, Multiple gestation, must also be assigned when assigning code O33.5 with a 7th character of 1 through 9.

Ø	not applicable or unspecified
1	fetus 1
2	fetus 2
3	fetus 3
4	fetus 4
5	fetus 5
9	other fetus

X● O33.6 Maternal care for disproportion due to hydrocephalic fetus

One of the following 7th characters is to be assigned to code O33.6. 7th character Ø is for single gestations and multiple gestations where the fetus is unspecified. 7th characters 1 through 9 are for cases of multiple gestations to identify the fetus for which the code applies. The appropriate code from category O3Ø, Multiple gestation, must also be assigned when assigning code O33.6 with a 7th character of 1 through 9.

Ø	not applicable or unspecified
1	fetus 1
2	fetus 2
3	fetus 3
4	fetus 4
5	fetus 5
9	other fetus

X● O33.7 Maternal care for disproportion due to other fetal deformities

Maternal care for disproportion due to fetal ascites

Maternal care for disproportion due to fetal hydrops

Maternal care for disproportion due to fetal meningomyelocele

Maternal care for disproportion due to fetal sacral teratoma

Maternal care for disproportion due to fetal tumor

Excludes1 obstructed labor due to other fetal deformities (O66.3)

One of the following 7th characters is to be assigned to code O33.7. 7th character Ø is for single gestations and multiple gestations where the fetus is unspecified. 7th characters 1 through 9 are for cases of multiple gestations to identify the fetus for which the code applies. The appropriate code from category O3Ø, Multiple gestation, must also be assigned when assigning code O33.7 with a 7th character of 1 through 9. ◀

Ø	not applicable or unspecified ◀
1	fetus 1 ◀
2	fetus 2 ◀
3	fetus 3 ◀
4	fetus 4 ◀
5	fetus 5 ◀
9	other fetus ◀

O33.8 Maternal care for disproportion of other origin

O33.9 Maternal care for disproportion, unspecified

Maternal care for disproportion due to cephalopelvic disproportion NOS

Maternal care for disproportion due to fetopelvic disproportion NOS

● O34 Maternal care for abnormality of pelvic organs

Includes the listed conditions as a reason for hospitalization or other obstetric care of the mother, or for cesarean delivery before onset of labor

Code first any associated obstructed labor (O65.5)

Use additional code for specific condition

● O34.Ø Maternal care for congenital malformation of uterus

Maternal care for double uterus ◀

Maternal care for uterus bicornis ◀

O34.ØØ Maternal care for unspecified congenital malformation of uterus, unspecified trimester

O34.Ø1 Maternal care for unspecified congenital malformation of uterus, first trimester

O34.Ø2 Maternal care for unspecified congenital malformation of uterus, second trimester

O34.Ø3 Maternal care for unspecified congenital malformation of uterus, third trimester

● O34.1 Maternal care for benign tumor of corpus uteri
Excludes2 maternal care for benign tumor of cervix (O34.4-)
maternal care for malignant neoplasm of uterus (O9A.1-)
O34.10 Maternal care for benign tumor of corpus uteri, unspecified trimester
O34.11 Maternal care for benign tumor of corpus uteri, first trimester
O34.12 Maternal care for benign tumor of corpus uteri, second trimester
O34.13 Maternal care for benign tumor of corpus uteri, third trimester
● O34.2 Maternal care due to uterine scar from previous surgery
● O34.21 Maternal care for scar from previous cesarean delivery
O34.211 Maternal care for low transverse scar from previous cesarean delivery ◀
O34.212 Maternal care for vertical scar from previous cesarean delivery ◀
Maternal care for classical scar from previous cesarean delivery ◀
O34.219 Maternal care for unspecified type scar from previous cesarean delivery ◀
O34.29 Maternal care due to uterine scar from other previous surgery
Maternal care due to uterine scar from other transmural uterine incision ◀
● O34.3 Maternal care for cervical incompetence
Maternal care for cerclage with or without cervical incompetence
Maternal care for Shirodkar suture with or without cervical incompetence
O34.30 Maternal care for cervical incompetence, unspecified trimester
O34.31 Maternal care for cervical incompetence, first trimester
O34.32 Maternal care for cervical incompetence, second trimester
O34.33 Maternal care for cervical incompetence, third trimester
● O34.4 Maternal care for other abnormalities of cervix
O34.40 Maternal care for other abnormalities of cervix, unspecified trimester
O34.41 Maternal care for other abnormalities of cervix, first trimester
O34.42 Maternal care for other abnormalities of cervix, second trimester
O34.43 Maternal care for other abnormalities of cervix, third trimester
● O34.5 Maternal care for other abnormalities of gravid uterus
● O34.51 Maternal care for incarceration of gravid uterus
O34.511 Maternal care for incarceration of gravid uterus, first trimester
O34.512 Maternal care for incarceration of gravid uterus, second trimester
O34.513 Maternal care for incarceration of gravid uterus, third trimester
O34.519 Maternal care for incarceration of gravid uterus, unspecified trimester
● O34.52 Maternal care for prolapse of gravid uterus
O34.521 Maternal care for prolapse of gravid uterus, first trimester
O34.522 Maternal care for prolapse of gravid uterus, second trimester
O34.523 Maternal care for prolapse of gravid uterus, third trimester
O34.529 Maternal care for prolapse of gravid uterus, unspecified trimester
● O34.53 Maternal care for retroversion of gravid uterus
O34.531 Maternal care for retroversion of gravid uterus, first trimester
O34.532 Maternal care for retroversion of gravid uterus, second trimester
O34.533 Maternal care for retroversion of gravid uterus, third trimester
O34.539 Maternal care for retroversion of gravid uterus, unspecified trimester
● O34.59 Maternal care for other abnormalities of gravid uterus
O34.591 Maternal care for other abnormalities of gravid uterus, first trimester
O34.592 Maternal care for other abnormalities of gravid uterus, second trimester
O34.593 Maternal care for other abnormalities of gravid uterus, third trimester
O34.599 Maternal care for other abnormalities of gravid uterus, unspecified trimester
● O34.6 Maternal care for abnormality of vagina
Excludes2 maternal care for vaginal varices in pregnancy (O22.1-)
O34.60 Maternal care for abnormality of vagina, unspecified trimester
O34.61 Maternal care for abnormality of vagina, first trimester
O34.62 Maternal care for abnormality of vagina, second trimester
O34.63 Maternal care for abnormality of vagina, third trimester
● O34.7 Maternal care for abnormality of vulva and perineum
Excludes2 maternal care for perineal and vulval varices in pregnancy (O22.1-)
O34.70 Maternal care for abnormality of vulva and perineum, unspecified trimester
O34.71 Maternal care for abnormality of vulva and perineum, first trimester
O34.72 Maternal care for abnormality of vulva and perineum, second trimester
O34.73 Maternal care for abnormality of vulva and perineum, third trimester
● O34.8 Maternal care for other abnormalities of pelvic organs
O34.80 Maternal care for other abnormalities of pelvic organs, unspecified trimester
O34.81 Maternal care for other abnormalities of pelvic organs, first trimester
O34.82 Maternal care for other abnormalities of pelvic organs, second trimester
O34.83 Maternal care for other abnormalities of pelvic organs, third trimester
● O34.9 Maternal care for abnormality of pelvic organ, unspecified
O34.90 Maternal care for abnormality of pelvic organ, unspecified, unspecified trimester
O34.91 Maternal care for abnormality of pelvic organ, unspecified, first trimester
O34.92 Maternal care for abnormality of pelvic organ, unspecified, second trimester
O34.93 Maternal care for abnormality of pelvic organ, unspecified, third trimester

● O35 **Maternal care for known or suspected fetal abnormality and damage**

Includes the listed conditions in the fetus as a reason for hospitalization or other obstetric care to the mother, or for termination of pregnancy

Code also any associated maternal condition

Excludes1 encounter for suspected maternal and fetal conditions ruled out (Z03.7-)

One of the following 7th characters is to be assigned to each code under category O35. 7th character 0 is for single gestations and multiple gestations where the fetus is unspecified. 7th characters 1 through 9 are for cases of multiple gestations to identify the fetus for which the code applies. The appropriate code from category O30, Multiple gestation, must also be assigned when assigning a code from category O35 that has a 7th character of 1 through 9.

0	not applicable or unspecified
1	fetus 1
2	fetus 2
3	fetus 3
4	fetus 4
5	fetus 5
9	other fetus

X● O35.0 **Maternal care for (suspected) central nervous system malformation in fetus**
Maternal care for fetal anencephaly
Maternal care for fetal hydrocephalus
Maternal care for fetal spina bifida
Excludes2 chromosomal abnormality in fetus (O35.1)

X● O35.1 **Maternal care for (suspected) chromosomal abnormality in fetus**

X● O35.2 **Maternal care for (suspected) hereditary disease in fetus**
Excludes2 chromosomal abnormality in fetus (O35.1)

OGCR Section I.C.15.e.l.

Fetal Conditions Affecting the Management of the Mother

1) Code from categories O35 and O36

Codes from categories O35, Maternal care for known or suspected fetal abnormality and damage, and O36, Maternal care for other fetal problems, are assigned only when the fetal condition is actually responsible for modifying the management of the mother, i.e., by requiring diagnostic studies, additional observation, special care, or termination of pregnancy. The fact that the fetal condition exists does not justify assigning a code from this series to the mother's record.

2) In utero surgery

In cases when surgery is performed on the fetus, a diagnosis code from category O35, Maternal care for known or suspected fetal abnormality and damage, should be assigned identifying the fetal condition. Assign the appropriate procedure code for the procedure performed.

No code from Chapter 16, the perinatal codes, should be used on the mother's record to identify fetal conditions. Surgery performed in utero on a fetus is still to be coded as an obstetric encounter.

X● O35.3 **Maternal care for (suspected) damage to fetus from viral disease in mother**
Maternal care for damage to fetus from maternal cytomegalovirus infection
Maternal care for damage to fetus from maternal rubella

X● O35.4 **Maternal care for (suspected) damage to fetus from alcohol**

X● O35.5 **Maternal care for (suspected) damage to fetus by drugs**
Maternal care for damage to fetus from drug addiction

X● O35.6 **Maternal care for (suspected) damage to fetus by radiation**

X● O35.7 **Maternal care for (suspected) damage to fetus by other medical procedures**
Maternal care for damage to fetus by amniocentesis
Maternal care for damage to fetus by biopsy procedures
Maternal care for damage to fetus by hematological investigation
Maternal care for damage to fetus by intrauterine contraceptive device
Maternal care for damage to fetus by intrauterine surgery

X● O35.8 **Maternal care for other (suspected) fetal abnormality and damage**
Maternal care for damage to fetus from maternal listeriosis
Maternal care for damage to fetus from maternal toxoplasmosis

X● O35.9 **Maternal care for (suspected) fetal abnormality and damage, unspecified**

● O36 **Maternal care for other fetal problems**

Includes the listed conditions in the fetus as a reason for hospitalization or other obstetric care of the mother, or for termination of pregnancy

Excludes1 encounter for suspected maternal and fetal conditions ruled out (Z03.7-)
placental transfusion syndromes (O43.0-)

Excludes2 labor and delivery complicated by fetal stress (O77.-)

One of the following 7th characters is to be assigned to each code under category O36. 7th character 0 is for single gestations and multiple gestations where the fetus is unspecified. 7th characters 1 through 9 are for cases of multiple gestations to identify the fetus for which the code applies. The appropriate code from category O30, Multiple gestation, must also be assigned when assigning a code from category O36 that has a 7th character of 1 through 9.

0	not applicable or unspecified
1	fetus 1
2	fetus 2
3	fetus 3
4	fetus 4
5	fetus 5
9	other fetus

● O36.0 **Maternal care for rhesus isoimmunization**
Maternal care for Rh incompatibility (with hydrops fetalis)

● O36.01 **Maternal care for anti-D [Rh] antibodies**

● O36.011 **Maternal care for anti-D [Rh] antibodies, first trimester**

● O36.012 **Maternal care for anti-D [Rh] antibodies, second trimester**

● O36.013 **Maternal care for anti-D [Rh] antibodies, third trimester**

● O36.019 **Maternal care for anti-D [Rh] antibodies, unspecified trimester**

● O36.09 **Maternal care for other rhesus isoimmunization**

● O36.091 **Maternal care for other rhesus isoimmunization, first trimester**

● O36.092 **Maternal care for other rhesus isoimmunization, second trimester**

● O36.093 **Maternal care for other rhesus isoimmunization, third trimester**

● O36.099 **Maternal care for other rhesus isoimmunization, unspecified trimester**

CHAPTER 15 (O00-O9A)

● O36.1 **Maternal care for other isoimmunization**
Maternal care for ABO isoimmunization

● O36.11 **Maternal care for Anti-A sensitization**
Maternal care for isoimmunization NOS (with hydrops fetalis)

● O36.111 **Maternal care for Anti-A sensitization, first trimester**

● O36.112 **Maternal care for Anti-A sensitization, second trimester**

● O36.113 **Maternal care for Anti-A sensitization, third trimester**

● O36.119 **Maternal care for Anti-A sensitization, unspecified trimester**

● O36.19 **Maternal care for other isoimmunization**
Maternal care for Anti-B sensitization

● O36.191 **Maternal care for other isoimmunization, first trimester**

● O36.192 **Maternal care for other isoimmunization, second trimester**

● O36.193 **Maternal care for other isoimmunization, third trimester**

● O36.199 **Maternal care for other isoimmunization, unspecified trimester**

● O36.2 **Maternal care for hydrops fetalis**
Maternal care for hydrops fetalis NOS
Maternal care for hydrops fetalis not associated with isoimmunization

Excludes1 hydrops fetalis associated with ABO isoimmunization (O36.1-)
hydrops fetalis associated with rhesus isoimmunization (O36.Ø-)

● O36.2Ø **Maternal care for hydrops fetalis, unspecified trimester**

● O36.21 **Maternal care for hydrops fetalis, first trimester**

● O36.22 **Maternal care for hydrops fetalis, second trimester**

● O36.23 **Maternal care for hydrops fetalis, third trimester**

● O36.4 **Maternal care for intrauterine death**
Maternal care for intrauterine fetal death NOS
Maternal care for intrauterine fetal death after completion of 2Ø weeks of gestation
Maternal care for late fetal death
Maternal care for missed delivery

Excludes1 missed abortion (OØ2.1)
stillbirth (P95)

● O36.5 **Maternal care for known or suspected poor fetal growth**

● O36.51 **Maternal care for known or suspected placental insufficiency**

● O36.511 **Maternal care for known or suspected placental insufficiency, first trimester**

● O36.512 **Maternal care for known or suspected placental insufficiency, second trimester**

● O36.513 **Maternal care for known or suspected placental insufficiency, third trimester**

● O36.519 **Maternal care for known or suspected placental insufficiency, unspecified trimester**

● O36.59 **Maternal care for other known or suspected poor fetal growth**
Maternal care for known or suspected light-for-dates NOS
Maternal care for known or suspected small-for-dates NOS

● O36.591 **Maternal care for other known or suspected poor fetal growth, first trimester**

● O36.592 **Maternal care for other known or suspected poor fetal growth, second trimester**

● O36.593 **Maternal care for other known or suspected poor fetal growth, third trimester**

● O36.599 **Maternal care for other known or suspected poor fetal growth, unspecified trimester**

● O36.6 **Maternal care for excessive fetal growth**
Maternal care for known or suspected large-for-dates

X● O36.6Ø **Maternal care for excessive fetal growth, unspecified trimester**

X● O36.61 **Maternal care for excessive fetal growth, first trimester**

X● O36.62 **Maternal care for excessive fetal growth, second trimester**

X● O36.63 **Maternal care for excessive fetal growth, third trimester**

● O36.7 **Maternal care for viable fetus in abdominal pregnancy**

X● O36.7Ø **Maternal care for viable fetus in abdominal pregnancy, unspecified trimester**

X● O36.71 **Maternal care for viable fetus in abdominal pregnancy, first trimester**

X● O36.72 **Maternal care for viable fetus in abdominal pregnancy, second trimester**

X● O36.73 **Maternal care for viable fetus in abdominal pregnancy, third trimester**

● O36.8 **Maternal care for other specified fetal problems**

X● O36.8Ø **Pregnancy with inconclusive fetal viability**
Encounter to determine fetal viability of pregnancy

● O36.81 **Decreased fetal movements**

● O36.812 **Decreased fetal movements, second trimester**

● O36.813 **Decreased fetal movements, third trimester**

● O36.819 **Decreased fetal movements, unspecified trimester**

● O36.82 **Fetal anemia and thrombocytopenia**

● O36.821 **Fetal anemia and thrombocytopenia, first trimester**

● O36.822 **Fetal anemia and thrombocytopenia, second trimester**

● O36.823 **Fetal anemia and thrombocytopenia, third trimester**

● O36.829 **Fetal anemia and thrombocytopenia, unspecified trimester**

● O36.89 **Maternal care for other specified fetal problems**

● O36.891 **Maternal care for other specified fetal problems, first trimester**

● O36.892 **Maternal care for other specified fetal problems, second trimester**

● O36.893 **Maternal care for other specified fetal problems, third trimester**

● O36.899 **Maternal care for other specified fetal problems, unspecified trimester**

● O36.9 Maternal care for fetal problem, unspecified

X● O36.90 Maternal care for fetal problem, unspecified, unspecified trimester

X● O36.91 Maternal care for fetal problem, unspecified, first trimester

X● O36.92 Maternal care for fetal problem, unspecified, second trimester

X● O36.93 Maternal care for fetal problem, unspecified, third trimester

● O40 Polyhydramnios

Overabundance of amniotic fluid

Includes hydramnios

Excludes1 encounter for suspected maternal and fetal conditions ruled out (Z03.7-)

One of the following 7th characters is to be assigned to each code under category O40. 7th character 0 is for single gestations and multiple gestations where the fetus is unspecified. 7th characters 1 through 9 are for cases of multiple gestations to identify the fetus for which the code applies. The appropriate code from category O30, Multiple gestation, must also be assigned when assigning a code from category O40 that has a 7th character of 1 through 9.

0	not applicable or unspecified
1	fetus 1
2	fetus 2
3	fetus 3
4	fetus 4
5	fetus 5
9	other fetus

X● O40.1 Polyhydramnios, first trimester

X● O40.2 Polyhydramnios, second trimester

X● O40.3 Polyhydramnios, third trimester

X● O40.9 Polyhydramnios, unspecified trimester

● O41 Other disorders of amniotic fluid and membranes

Excludes1 encounter for suspected maternal and fetal conditions ruled out (Z03.7-)

One of the following 7th characters is to be assigned to each code under category O41. 7th character 0 is for single gestations and multiple gestations where the fetus is unspecified. 7th characters 1 through 9 are for cases of multiple gestations to identify the fetus for which the code applies. The appropriate code from category O30, Multiple gestation, must also be assigned when assigning a code from category O41 that has a 7th character of 1 through 9.

0	not applicable or unspecified
1	fetus 1
2	fetus 2
3	fetus 3
4	fetus 4
5	fetus 5
9	other fetus

● O41.0 Oligohydramnios

Scant volume of amniotic fluid

Oligohydramnios without rupture of membranes

X● O41.00 Oligohydramnios, unspecified trimester

X● O41.01 Oligohydramnios, first trimester

X● O41.02 Oligohydramnios, second trimester

X● O41.03 Oligohydramnios, third trimester

● O41.1 Infection of amniotic sac and membranes

● O41.10 Infection of amniotic sac and membranes, unspecified

● O41.101 Infection of amniotic sac and membranes, unspecified, first trimester

● O41.102 Infection of amniotic sac and membranes, unspecified, second trimester

● O41.103 Infection of amniotic sac and membranes, unspecified, third trimester

● O41.109 Infection of amniotic sac and membranes, unspecified, unspecified trimester

● O41.12 Chorioamnionitis

● O41.121 Chorioamnionitis, first trimester

● O41.122 Chorioamnionitis, second trimester

● O41.123 Chorioamnionitis, third trimester

● O41.129 Chorioamnionitis, unspecified trimester

● O41.14 Placentitis

● O41.141 Placentitis, first trimester

● O41.142 Placentitis, second trimester

● O41.143 Placentitis, third trimester

● O41.149 Placentitis, unspecified trimester

● O41.8 Other specified disorders of amniotic fluid and membranes

● O41.8X Other specified disorders of amniotic fluid and membranes

● O41.8X1 Other specified disorders of amniotic fluid and membranes, first trimester

● O41.8X2 Other specified disorders of amniotic fluid and membranes, second trimester

● O41.8X3 Other specified disorders of amniotic fluid and membranes, third trimester

● O41.8X9 Other specified disorders of amniotic fluid and membranes, unspecified trimester

● O41.9 Disorder of amniotic fluid and membranes, unspecified

X● O41.90 Disorder of amniotic fluid and membranes, unspecified, unspecified trimester

X● O41.91 Disorder of amniotic fluid and membranes, unspecified, first trimester

X● O41.92 Disorder of amniotic fluid and membranes, unspecified, second trimester

X● O41.93 Disorder of amniotic fluid and membranes, unspecified, third trimester

● O42 Premature rupture of membranes

● O42.0 Premature rupture of membranes, onset of labor within 24 hours of rupture

O42.00 Premature rupture of membranes, onset of labor within 24 hours of rupture, unspecified weeks of gestation

● O42.01 Preterm premature rupture of membranes, onset of labor within 24 hours of rupture

Premature rupture of membranes before 37 completed weeks of gestation

O42.011 Preterm premature rupture of membranes, onset of labor within 24 hours of rupture, first trimester

O42.012 Preterm premature rupture of membranes, onset of labor within 24 hours of rupture, second trimester

O42.013 Preterm premature rupture of membranes, onset of labor within 24 hours of rupture, third trimester

O42.019 Preterm premature rupture of membranes, onset of labor within 24 hours of rupture, unspecified trimester

O42.02 Full-term premature rupture of membranes, onset of labor within 24 hours of rupture

Premature rupture of membranes at or after 37 completed weeks of gestation, onset of labor within 24 hours of rupture ⬅

CHAPTER 15 (O00-O9A)

● O42.1 **Premature rupture of membranes, onset of labor more than 24 hours following rupture**

O42.10 **Premature rupture of membranes, onset of labor more than 24 hours following rupture, unspecified weeks of gestation**

● O42.11 **Preterm premature rupture of membranes, onset of labor more than 24 hours following rupture**

Premature rupture of membranes before 37 completed weeks of gestation

O42.111 **Preterm premature rupture of membranes, onset of labor more than 24 hours following rupture, first trimester**

O42.112 **Preterm premature rupture of membranes, onset of labor more than 24 hours following rupture, second trimester**

O42.113 **Preterm premature rupture of membranes, onset of labor more than 24 hours following rupture, third trimester**

O42.119 **Preterm premature rupture of membranes, onset of labor more than 24 hours following rupture, unspecified trimester**

O42.12 **Full-term premature rupture of membranes, onset of labor more than 24 hours following rupture**

Premature rupture of membranes at or after 37 completed weeks of gestation, onset of labor more than 24 hours following rupture ◄

● O42.9 **Premature rupture of membranes, unspecified as to length of time between rupture and onset of labor**

O42.90 **Premature rupture of membranes, unspecified as to length of time between rupture and onset of labor, unspecified weeks of gestation**

● O42.91 **Preterm premature rupture of membranes, unspecified as to length of time between rupture and onset of labor**

Premature rupture of membranes before 37 completed weeks of gestation

O42.911 **Preterm premature rupture of membranes, unspecified as to length of time between rupture and onset of labor, first trimester**

O42.912 **Preterm premature rupture of membranes, unspecified as to length of time between rupture and onset of labor, second trimester**

O42.913 **Preterm premature rupture of membranes, unspecified as to length of time between rupture and onset of labor, third trimester**

O42.919 **Preterm premature rupture of membranes, unspecified as to length of time between rupture and onset of labor, unspecified trimester**

O42.92 **Full-term premature rupture of membranes, unspecified as to length of time between rupture and onset of labor**

Premature rupture of membranes at or after 37 completed weeks of gestation, unspecified as to length of time between rupture and onset of labor ◄

● O43 **Placental disorders**

Excludes2 maternal care for poor fetal growth due to placental insufficiency (O36.5-)
placenta previa (O44.-)
placental polyp (O90.89)
placentitis (O41.14-)
premature separation of placenta [abruptio placentae] (O45.-)

● O43.0 **Placental transfusion syndromes**

● O43.01 **Fetomaternal placental transfusion syndrome**

Maternofetal placental transfusion syndrome

O43.011 **Fetomaternal placental transfusion syndrome, first trimester**

O43.012 **Fetomaternal placental transfusion syndrome, second trimester**

O43.013 **Fetomaternal placental transfusion syndrome, third trimester**

O43.019 **Fetomaternal placental transfusion syndrome, unspecified trimester**

● O43.02 **Fetus-to-fetus placental transfusion syndrome**

O43.021 **Fetus-to-fetus placental transfusion syndrome, first trimester**

O43.022 **Fetus-to-fetus placental transfusion syndrome, second trimester**

O43.023 **Fetus-to-fetus placental transfusion syndrome, third trimester**

O43.029 **Fetus-to-fetus placental transfusion syndrome, unspecified trimester**

● O43.1 **Malformation of placenta**

● O43.10 **Malformation of placenta, unspecified**

Abnormal placenta NOS

O43.101 **Malformation of placenta, unspecified, first trimester**

O43.102 **Malformation of placenta, unspecified, second trimester**

O43.103 **Malformation of placenta, unspecified, third trimester**

O43.109 **Malformation of placenta, unspecified, unspecified trimester**

● O43.11 **Circumvallate placenta**

O43.111 **Circumvallate placenta, first trimester**

O43.112 **Circumvallate placenta, second trimester**

O43.113 **Circumvallate placenta, third trimester**

O43.119 **Circumvallate placenta, unspecified trimester**

● O43.12 **Velamentous insertion of umbilical cord**

O43.121 **Velamentous insertion of umbilical cord, first trimester**

O43.122 **Velamentous insertion of umbilical cord, second trimester**

O43.123 **Velamentous insertion of umbilical cord, third trimester**

O43.129 **Velamentous insertion of umbilical cord, unspecified trimester**

● O43.19 **Other malformation of placenta**

O43.191 **Other malformation of placenta, first trimester**

O43.192 **Other malformation of placenta, second trimester**

O43.193 **Other malformation of placenta, third trimester**

O43.199 **Other malformation of placenta, unspecified trimester**

● O43.2 Morbidly adherent placenta
Code also associated third stage postpartum hemorrhage, if applicable (O72.0)
Excludes1 retained placenta (O73.-)
● O43.21 Placenta accreta
O43.211 Placenta accreta, first trimester
O43.212 Placenta accreta, second trimester
O43.213 Placenta accreta, third trimester
O43.219 Placenta accreta, unspecified trimester
● O43.22 Placenta increta
O43.221 Placenta increta, first trimester
O43.222 Placenta increta, second trimester
O43.223 Placenta increta, third trimester
O43.229 Placenta increta, unspecified trimester
● O43.23 Placenta percreta
O43.231 Placenta percreta, first trimester
O43.232 Placenta percreta, second trimester
O43.233 Placenta percreta, third trimester
O43.239 Placenta percreta, unspecified trimester
● O43.8 Other placental disorders
● O43.81 Placental infarction
O43.811 Placental infarction, first trimester
O43.812 Placental infarction, second trimester
O43.813 Placental infarction, third trimester
O43.819 Placental infarction, unspecified trimester
● O43.89 Other placental disorders
Placental dysfunction
O43.891 Other placental disorders, first trimester
O43.892 Other placental disorders, second trimester
O43.893 Other placental disorders, third trimester
O43.899 Other placental disorders, unspecified trimester
● O43.9 Unspecified placental disorder
O43.90 Unspecified placental disorder, unspecified trimester
O43.91 Unspecified placental disorder, first trimester
O43.92 Unspecified placental disorder, second trimester
O43.93 Unspecified placental disorder, third trimester
● O44 Placenta previa
● O44.0 Complete placenta previa NOS or without hemorrhage ⬅
Placenta previa NOS ◀
O44.00 Complete placenta previa NOS or without hemorrhage, unspecified trimester ⬅
O44.01 Complete placenta previa NOS or without hemorrhage, first trimester ⬅
O44.02 Complete placenta previa NOS or without hemorrhage, second trimester ⬅
O44.03 Complete placenta previa NOS or without hemorrhage, third trimester ⬅

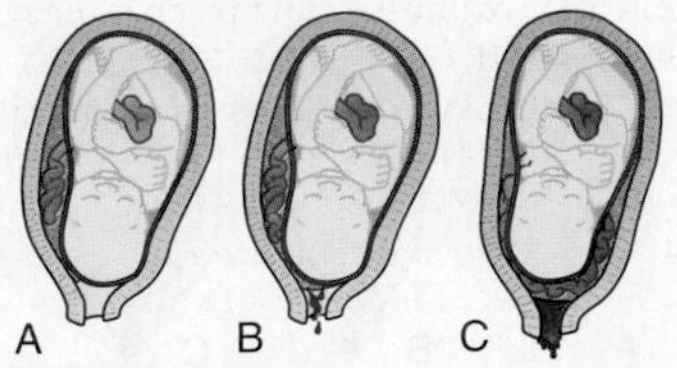

Figure 15-2 **A.** Marginal placento previa. **B.** Partial placenta previa. **C.** Total placento previa.

Item 15-3 Placenta previa is a condition in which the opening of the cervix is obstructed by the displaced placenta. The three types, marginal, partial, and total, are varying degrees of placenta displacement. Placenta abruption is the premature breaking away of the placenta from the site of the uterine implant before the delivery of the fetus.

● O44.1 Complete placenta previa with hemorrhage ⬅
Excludes1 labor and delivery complicated by hemorrhage from vasa previa (O69.4)
O44.10 Complete placenta previa with hemorrhage, unspecified trimester ⬅
O44.11 Complete placenta previa with hemorrhage, first trimester ⬅
O44.12 Complete placenta previa with hemorrhage, second trimester ⬅
O44.13 Complete placenta previa with hemorrhage, third trimester ⬅
● O44.2 Partial placenta previa without hemorrhage ◀
Marginal placenta previa, NOS or without hemorrhage ◀
O44.20 Partial placenta previa NOS or without hemorrhage, unspecified trimester ◀
O44.21 Partial placenta previa NOS or without hemorrhage, first trimester ◀
O44.22 Partial placenta previa NOS or without hemorrhage, second trimester ◀
O44.23 Partial placenta previa NOS or without hemorrhage, third trimester ◀
● O44.3 Partial placenta previa with hemorrhage ◀
Marginal placenta previa with hemorrhage ◀
O44.30 Partial placenta previa with hemorrhage, unspecified trimester ◀
O44.31 Partial placenta previa with hemorrhage, first trimester ◀
O44.32 Partial placenta previa with hemorrhage, second trimester ◀
O44.33 Partial placenta previa with hemorrhage, third trimester ◀
● O44.4 Low lying placenta NOS or without hemorrhage ◀
Low implantation of placenta NOS or without hemorrhage ◀
O44.40 Low lying placenta NOS or without hemorrhage, unspecified trimester ◀
O44.41 Low lying placenta NOS or without hemorrhage, first trimester ◀
O44.42 Low lying placenta NOS or without hemorrhage, second trimester ◀
O44.43 Low lying placenta NOS or without hemorrhage, third trimester ◀
● O44.5 Low lying placenta with hemorrhage ◀
Low implantation of placenta with hemorrhage ◀
O44.50 Low lying placenta with hemorrhage, unspecified trimester ◀
O44.51 Low lying placenta with hemorrhage, first trimester ◀
O44.52 Low lying placenta with hemorrhage, second trimester ◀
O44.53 Low lying placenta with hemorrhage, third trimester ◀

CHAPTER 15 (O00-O9A)

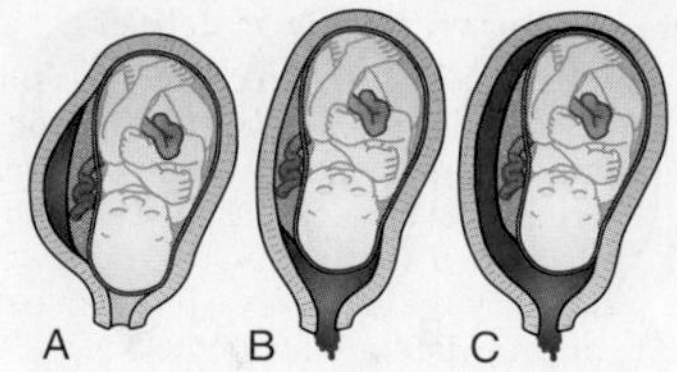

Figure 15-3 Abruptio placentae is classified according to the grade of separation of the placenta from the uterine wall. **A.** Mild separation in which hemorrhage is internal. **B.** Moderate separation in which there is external hemorrhage. **C.** Severe separation in which there is external hemorrhage and extreme separation.

● **O45 Premature separation of placenta [abruptio placentae]**

● **O45.Ø Premature separation of placenta with coagulation defect**

● **O45.ØØ Premature separation of placenta with coagulation defect, unspecified**

O45.ØØ1 Premature separation of placenta with coagulation defect, unspecified, first trimester

O45.ØØ2 Premature separation of placenta with coagulation defect, unspecified, second trimester

O45.ØØ3 Premature separation of placenta with coagulation defect, unspecified, third trimester

O45.ØØ9 Premature separation of placenta with coagulation defect, unspecified, unspecified trimester

● **O45.Ø1 Premature separation of placenta with afibrinogenemia**

Premature separation of placenta with hypofibrinogenemia

O45.Ø11 Premature separation of placenta with afibrinogenemia, first trimester

O45.Ø12 Premature separation of placenta with afibrinogenemia, second trimester

O45.Ø13 Premature separation of placenta with afibrinogenemia, third trimester

O45.Ø19 Premature separation of placenta with afibrinogenemia, unspecified trimester

● **O45.Ø2 Premature separation of placenta with disseminated intravascular coagulation**

O45.Ø21 Premature separation of placenta with disseminated intravascular coagulation, first trimester

O45.Ø22 Premature separation of placenta with disseminated intravascular coagulation, second trimester

O45.Ø23 Premature separation of placenta with disseminated intravascular coagulation, third trimester

O45.Ø29 Premature separation of placenta with disseminated intravascular coagulation, unspecified trimester

● **O45.Ø9 Premature separation of placenta with other coagulation defect**

O45.Ø91 Premature separation of placenta with other coagulation defect, first trimester

O45.Ø92 Premature separation of placenta with other coagulation defect, second trimester

O45.Ø93 Premature separation of placenta with other coagulation defect, third trimester

O45.Ø99 Premature separation of placenta with other coagulation defect, unspecified trimester

● **O45.8 Other premature separation of placenta**

● **O45.8X Other premature separation of placenta**

O45.8X1 Other premature separation of placenta, first trimester

O45.8X2 Other premature separation of placenta, second trimester

O45.8X3 Other premature separation of placenta, third trimester

O45.8X9 Other premature separation of placenta, unspecified trimester

● **O45.9 Premature separation of placenta, unspecified**

Abruptio placentae NOS

O45.9Ø Premature separation of placenta, unspecified, unspecified trimester

O45.91 Premature separation of placenta, unspecified, first trimester

O45.92 Premature separation of placenta, unspecified, second trimester

O45.93 Premature separation of placenta, unspecified, third trimester

● **O46 Antepartum hemorrhage, not elsewhere classified**

Excludes1 hemorrhage in early pregnancy (O2Ø.-)
intrapartum hemorrhage NEC (O67.-)
placenta previa (O44.-)
premature separation of placenta [abruptio placentae] (O45.-)

● **O46.Ø Antepartum hemorrhage with coagulation defect**

● **O46.ØØ Antepartum hemorrhage with coagulation defect, unspecified**

O46.ØØ1 Antepartum hemorrhage with coagulation defect, unspecified, first trimester

O46.ØØ2 Antepartum hemorrhage with coagulation defect, unspecified, second trimester

O46.ØØ3 Antepartum hemorrhage with coagulation defect, unspecified, third trimester

O46.ØØ9 Antepartum hemorrhage with coagulation defect, unspecified, unspecified trimester

● **O46.Ø1 Antepartum hemorrhage with afibrinogenemia**

Antepartum hemorrhage with hypofibrinogenemia

O46.Ø11 Antepartum hemorrhage with afibrinogenemia, first trimester

O46.Ø12 Antepartum hemorrhage with afibrinogenemia, second trimester

O46.Ø13 Antepartum hemorrhage with afibrinogenemia, third trimester

O46.Ø19 Antepartum hemorrhage with afibrinogenemia, unspecified trimester

● **O46.Ø2 Antepartum hemorrhage with disseminated intravascular coagulation**

O46.Ø21 Antepartum hemorrhage with disseminated intravascular coagulation, first trimester

O46.Ø22 Antepartum hemorrhage with disseminated intravascular coagulation, second trimester

O46.Ø23 Antepartum hemorrhage with disseminated intravascular coagulation, third trimester

O46.Ø29 Antepartum hemorrhage with disseminated intravascular coagulation, unspecified trimester

● **O46.09 Antepartum hemorrhage with other coagulation defect**

O46.091 Antepartum hemorrhage with other coagulation defect, first trimester

O46.092 Antepartum hemorrhage with other coagulation defect, second trimester

O46.093 Antepartum hemorrhage with other coagulation defect, third trimester

O46.099 Antepartum hemorrhage with other coagulation defect, unspecified trimester

● **O46.8 Other antepartum hemorrhage**

● **O46.8x Other antepartum hemorrhage**

O46.8x1 Other antepartum hemorrhage, first trimester

O46.8x2 Other antepartum hemorrhage, second trimester

O46.8x3 Other antepartum hemorrhage, third trimester

O46.8x9 Other antepartum hemorrhage, unspecified trimester

● **O46.9 Antepartum hemorrhage, unspecified**

O46.90 Antepartum hemorrhage, unspecified, unspecified trimester

O46.91 Antepartum hemorrhage, unspecified, first trimester

O46.92 Antepartum hemorrhage, unspecified, second trimester

O46.93 Antepartum hemorrhage, unspecified, third trimester

● **O47 False labor**

Includes Braxton Hicks contractions
threatened labor

Excludes1 preterm labor (O60.-)

● **O47.0 False labor before 37 completed weeks of gestation**

O47.00 False labor before 37 completed weeks of gestation, unspecified trimester

O47.02 False labor before 37 completed weeks of gestation, second trimester

O47.03 False labor before 37 completed weeks of gestation, third trimester

O47.1 False labor at or after 37 completed weeks of gestation

O47.9 False labor, unspecified

● **O48 Late pregnancy**

O48.0 Post-term pregnancy

Pregnancy over 40 completed weeks to 42 completed weeks gestation

O48.1 Prolonged pregnancy

Pregnancy which has advanced beyond 42 completed weeks gestation

COMPLICATIONS OF LABOR AND DELIVERY (O60-O77)

● **O60 Preterm labor**

Includes onset (spontaneous) of labor before 37 completed weeks of gestation

Excludes1 false labor (O47.0-)
threatened labor NOS (O47.0-)

● **O60.0 Preterm labor without delivery**

O60.00 Preterm labor without delivery, unspecified trimester

O60.02 Preterm labor without delivery, second trimester

O60.03 Preterm labor without delivery, third trimester

● **O60.1 Preterm labor with preterm delivery**

One of the following 7th characters is to be assigned to each code under subcategory O60.1. 7th character 0 is for single gestations and multiple gestations where the fetus is unspecified. 7th characters 1 through 9 are for cases of multiple gestations to identify the fetus for which the code applies. The appropriate code from category O30, Multiple gestation, must also be assigned when assigning a code from subcategory O60.1 that has a 7th character of 1 through 9.

0	not applicable or unspecified
1	fetus 1
2	fetus 2
3	fetus 3
4	fetus 4
5	fetus 5
9	other fetus

X● **O60.10 Preterm labor with preterm delivery, unspecified trimester**

Preterm labor with delivery NOS

X● **O60.12 Preterm labor second trimester with preterm delivery second trimester**

X● **O60.13 Preterm labor second trimester with preterm delivery third trimester**

X● **O60.14 Preterm labor third trimester with preterm delivery third trimester**

● **O60.2 Term delivery with preterm labor**

One of the following 7th characters is to be assigned to each code under subcategory O60.2. 7th character 0 is for single gestations and multiple gestations where the fetus is unspecified. 7th characters 1 through 9 are for cases of multiple gestations to identify the fetus for which the code applies. The appropriate code from category O30, Multiple gestation, must also be assigned when assigning a code from subcategory O60.2 that has a 7th character of 1 through 9.

0	not applicable or unspecified
1	fetus 1
2	fetus 2
3	fetus 3
4	fetus 4
5	fetus 5
9	other fetus

X● **O60.20 Term delivery with preterm labor, unspecified trimester**

X● **O60.22 Term delivery with preterm labor, second trimester**

X● **O60.23 Term delivery with preterm labor, third trimester**

● **O61 Failed induction of labor**

O61.0 Failed medical induction of labor

Failed induction (of labor) by oxytocin
Failed induction (of labor) by prostaglandins

O61.1 Failed instrumental induction of labor

Failed mechanical induction (of labor)
Failed surgical induction (of labor)

O61.8 Other failed induction of labor

O61.9 Failed induction of labor, unspecified

CHAPTER 15 (O00-O9A)

● O62 **Abnormalities of forces of labor**

O62.0 **Primary inadequate contractions**
Failure of cervical dilatation
Primary hypotonic uterine dysfunction
Uterine inertia during latent phase of labor

O62.1 **Secondary uterine inertia**
Arrested active phase of labor
Secondary hypotonic uterine dysfunction

O62.2 **Other uterine inertia**
Atony of uterus without hemorrhage
Atony of uterus NOS
Desultory labor
Hypotonic uterine dysfunction NOS
Irregular labor
Poor contractions
Slow slope active phase of labor
Uterine inertia NOS
Excludes1 atony of uterus with hemorrhage (postpartum) (O72.1)
postpartum atony of uterus without hemorrhage (O75.89)

O62.3 **Precipitate labor**

O62.4 **Hypertonic, incoordinate, and prolonged uterine contractions**
Cervical spasm
Contraction ring dystocia
Dyscoordinate labor
Hour-glass contraction of uterus
Hypertonic uterine dysfunction
Incoordinate uterine action
Tetanic contractions
Uterine dystocia NOS
Uterine spasm
Excludes1 dystocia (fetal) (maternal) NOS (O66.9)

O62.8 **Other abnormalities of forces of labor**

O62.9 **Abnormality of forces of labor, unspecified**

● O63 **Long labor**

O63.0 **Prolonged first stage (of labor)**

O63.1 **Prolonged second stage (of labor)**

O63.2 **Delayed delivery of second twin, triplet, etc.**

O63.9 **Long labor, unspecified**
Prolonged labor NOS

● O64 **Obstructed labor due to malposition and malpresentation of fetus**

One of the following 7th characters is to be assigned to each code under category O64. 7th character 0 is for single gestations and multiple gestations where the fetus is unspecified. 7th characters 1 through 9 are for cases of multiple gestations to identify the fetus for which the code applies. The appropriate code from category O30, Multiple gestation, must also be assigned when assigning a code from category O64 that has a 7th character of 1 through 9.

0	not applicable or unspecified
1	fetus 1
2	fetus 2
3	fetus 3
4	fetus 4
5	fetus 5
9	other fetus

X● O64.0 **Obstructed labor due to incomplete rotation of fetal head**
Deep transverse arrest
Obstructed labor due to persistent occipitoiliac (position)
Obstructed labor due to persistent occipitoposterior (position)
Obstructed labor due to persistent occipitosacral (position)
Obstructed labor due to persistent occipitotransverse (position)

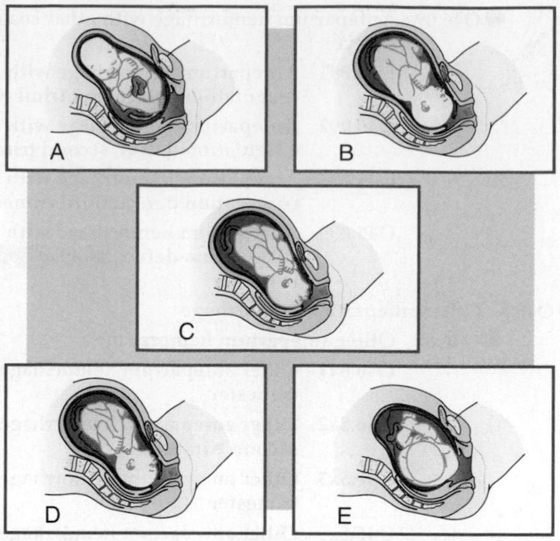

Figure 15-4 Five types of malposition and malpresentation of the fetus: **A.** Breech. **B.** Vertex. **C.** Face. **D.** Brow. **E.** Shoulder.

X● O64.1 **Obstructed labor due to breech presentation**
Obstructed labor due to buttocks presentation
Obstructed labor due to complete breech presentation
Obstructed labor due to frank breech presentation

X● O64.2 **Obstructed labor due to face presentation**
Obstructed labor due to chin presentation

X● O64.3 **Obstructed labor due to brow presentation**

X● O64.4 **Obstructed labor due to shoulder presentation**
Prolapsed arm
Excludes1 impacted shoulders (O66.0)
shoulder dystocia (O66.0)

X● O64.5 **Obstructed labor due to compound presentation**

X● O64.8 **Obstructed labor due to other malposition and malpresentation**
Obstructed labor due to footling presentation
Obstructed labor due to incomplete breech presentation

X● O64.9 **Obstructed labor due to malposition and malpresentation, unspecified**

● O65 **Obstructed labor due to maternal pelvic abnormality**

O65.0 **Obstructed labor due to deformed pelvis**

O65.1 **Obstructed labor due to generally contracted pelvis**

O65.2 **Obstructed labor due to pelvic inlet contraction**

O65.3 **Obstructed labor due to pelvic outlet and mid-cavity contraction**

O65.4 **Obstructed labor due to fetopelvic disproportion, unspecified**
Excludes1 dystocia due to abnormality of fetus (O66.2-O66.3)

O65.5 **Obstructed labor due to abnormality of maternal pelvic organs**
Obstructed labor due to conditions listed in O34.-
Use additional code to identify abnormality of pelvic organs O34.-

O65.8 **Obstructed labor due to other maternal pelvic abnormalities**

O65.9 **Obstructed labor due to maternal pelvic abnormality, unspecified**

CHAPTER 15 (O00-O9A)

◄ New ◄ Revised ~~deleted~~ Deleted OGCR Official Guidelines X Assign placeholder X ● Use Additional Character(s)
Excludes 1 | Excludes 2 | Includes | Use additional | Code first | Code also | Unspecified

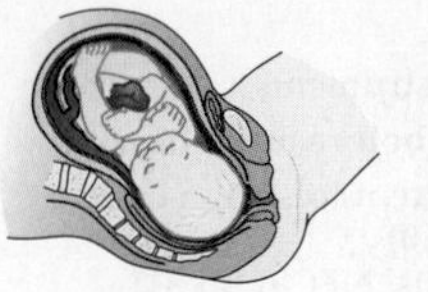

Figure 15-5 Hydrocephalic fetus causing disproportion.

● O66 Other obstructed labor

O66.0 Obstructed labor due to shoulder dystocia
Impacted shoulders

O66.1 Obstructed labor due to locked twins

O66.2 Obstructed labor due to unusually large fetus

O66.3 Obstructed labor due to other abnormalities of fetus
Dystocia due to fetal ascites
Dystocia due to fetal hydrops
Dystocia due to fetal meningomyelocele
Dystocia due to fetal sacral teratoma
Dystocia due to fetal tumor
Dystocia due to hydrocephalic fetus
Use additional code to identify cause of obstruction

● O66.4 Failed trial of labor

O66.40 Failed trial of labor, unspecified

O66.41 Failed attempted vaginal birth after previous cesarean delivery
Code first rupture of uterus, if applicable (O71.0-, O71.1)

O66.5 Attempted application of vacuum extractor and forceps
Attempted application of vacuum or forceps, with subsequent delivery by forceps or cesarean delivery

O66.6 Obstructed labor due to other multiple fetuses

O66.8 Other specified obstructed labor
Use additional code to identify cause of obstruction

O66.9 Obstructed labor, unspecified
Dystocia NOS
Fetal dystocia NOS
Maternal dystocia NOS

● O67 Labor and delivery complicated by intrapartum hemorrhage, not elsewhere classified

Excludes1 antepartum hemorrhage NEC (O46.-)
placenta previa (O44.-)
premature separation of placenta [abruptio placentae] (O45.-)

Excludes2 postpartum hemorrhage (O72.-)

O67.0 Intrapartum hemorrhage with coagulation defect
Intrapartum hemorrhage (excessive) associated with afibrinogenemia
Intrapartum hemorrhage (excessive) associated with disseminated intravascular coagulation
Intrapartum hemorrhage (excessive) associated with hyperfibrinolysis
Intrapartum hemorrhage (excessive) associated with hypofibrinogenemia

O67.8 Other intrapartum hemorrhage
Excessive intrapartum hemorrhage

O67.9 Intrapartum hemorrhage, unspecified

O68 Labor and delivery complicated by abnormality of fetal acid-base balance
Fetal acidemia complicating labor and delivery
Fetal acidosis complicating labor and delivery
Fetal alkalosis complicating labor and delivery
Fetal metabolic acidemia complicating labor and delivery

Excludes1 fetal stress NOS (O77.9)
labor and delivery complicated by electrocardiographic evidence of fetal stress (O77.8)
labor and delivery complicated by ultrasonic evidence of fetal stress (O77.8)

Excludes2 abnormality in fetal heart rate or rhythm (O76)
labor and delivery complicated by meconium in amniotic fluid (O77.0)

● O69 Labor and delivery complicated by umbilical cord complications

One of the following 7th characters is to be assigned to each code under category O69. 7th character 0 is for single gestations and multiple gestations where the fetus is unspecified. 7th characters 1 through 9 are for cases of multiple gestations to identify the fetus for which the code applies. The appropriate code from category O30, Multiple gestation, must also be assigned when assigning a code from category O69 that has a 7th character of 1 through 9.

0	not applicable or unspecified
1	fetus 1
2	fetus 2
3	fetus 3
4	fetus 4
5	fetus 5
9	other fetus

X● O69.0 Labor and delivery complicated by prolapse of cord

X● O69.1 Labor and delivery complicated by cord around neck, with compression

Excludes1 labor and delivery complicated by cord around neck, without compression (O69.81)

X● O69.2 Labor and delivery complicated by other cord entanglement, with compression
Labor and delivery complicated by compression of cord NOS
Labor and delivery complicated by entanglement of cords of twins in monoamniotic sac
Labor and delivery complicated by knot in cord

Excludes1 labor and delivery complicated by other cord entanglement, without compression (O69.82)

X● O69.3 Labor and delivery complicated by short cord

X● O69.4 Labor and delivery complicated by vasa previa
Labor and delivery complicated by hemorrhage from vasa previa

X● O69.5 Labor and delivery complicated by vascular lesion of cord
Labor and delivery complicated by cord bruising
Labor and delivery complicated by cord hematoma
Labor and delivery complicated by thrombosis of umbilical vessels

● O69.8 Labor and delivery complicated by other cord complications

X● O69.81 Labor and delivery complicated by cord around neck, without compression

X● O69.82 Labor and delivery complicated by other cord entanglement, without compression

X● O69.89 Labor and delivery complicated by other cord complications

X● O69.9 Labor and delivery complicated by cord complication, unspecified

● O70 Perineal laceration during delivery

Includes episiotomy extended by laceration

Excludes1 obstetric high vaginal laceration alone (O71.4)

O70.0 First degree perineal laceration during delivery
Perineal laceration, rupture or tear involving fourchette during delivery
Perineal laceration, rupture or tear involving labia during delivery
Perineal laceration, rupture or tear involving skin during delivery
Perineal laceration, rupture or tear involving vagina during delivery
Perineal laceration, rupture or tear involving vulva during delivery
Slight perineal laceration, rupture or tear during delivery

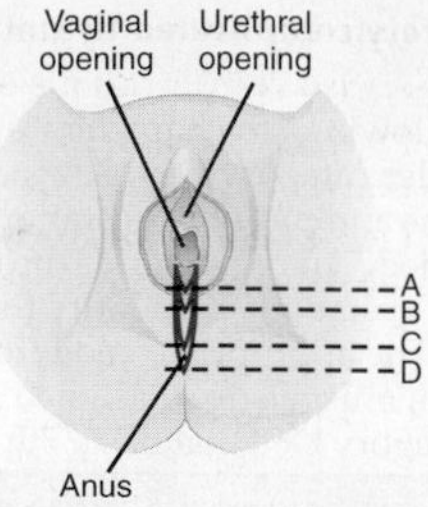

Figure 15-6 Perineal lacerations: **A.** First-degree is laceration of superficial tissues. **B.** Second-degree is limited to the pelvic floor and may involve the perineal or vaginal muscles. **C.** Third-degree involves the anal sphincter. **D.** Fourth-degree involves anal or rectal mucosa.

O7Ø.1 Second degree perineal laceration during delivery
Perineal laceration, rupture or tear during delivery as in O7Ø.Ø, also involving pelvic floor
Perineal laceration, rupture or tear during delivery as in O7Ø.Ø, also involving perineal muscles
Perineal laceration, rupture or tear during delivery as in O7Ø.Ø, also involving vaginal muscles
Excludes1 perineal laceration involving anal sphincter (O7Ø.2)

● **O7Ø.2 Third degree perineal laceration during delivery**
Perineal laceration, rupture or tear during delivery as in O7Ø.1, also involving anal sphincter
Perineal laceration, rupture or tear during delivery as in O7Ø.1, also involving rectovaginal septum
Perineal laceration, rupture or tear during delivery as in O7Ø.1, also involving sphincter NOS
Excludes1 anal sphincter tear during delivery without third degree perineal laceration (O7Ø.4)
perineal laceration involving anal or rectal mucosa (O7Ø.3)

O7Ø.2Ø Third degree perineal laceration during delivery, unspecified ◀

O7Ø.21 Third degree perineal laceration during delivery, IIIa ◀
Third degree perineal laceration during delivery with less than 5Ø% of external anal sphincter (EAS) thickness torn ◀

O7Ø.22 Third degree perineal laceration during delivery, IIIb ◀
Third degree perineal laceration during delivery with more than 5Ø% external anal sphincter (EAS) thickness torn ◀

O7Ø.23 Third degree perineal laceration during delivery, IIIc ◀
Third degree perineal laceration during delivery with both external anal sphincter (EAS) and internal anal sphincter (IAS) torn ◀

O7Ø.3 Fourth degree perineal laceration during delivery
Perineal laceration, rupture or tear during delivery as in O7Ø.2, also involving anal mucosa
Perineal laceration, rupture or tear during delivery as in O7Ø.2, also involving rectal mucosa

O7Ø.4 Anal sphincter tear complicating delivery, not associated with third degree laceration
Excludes1 anal sphincter tear with third degree perineal laceration (O7Ø.2)

O7Ø.9 Perineal laceration during delivery, unspecified

● **O71 Other obstetric trauma**
Includes obstetric damage from instruments

● **O71.Ø Rupture of uterus (spontaneous) before onset of labor**
Excludes1 disruption of (current) cesarean delivery wound (O9Ø.Ø)
laceration of uterus, NEC (O71.81)

O71.ØØ Rupture of uterus before onset of labor, unspecified trimester

O71.Ø2 Rupture of uterus before onset of labor, second trimester

O71.Ø3 Rupture of uterus before onset of labor, third trimester

O71.1 Rupture of uterus during labor
Rupture of uterus not stated as occurring before onset of labor
Excludes1 disruption of cesarean delivery wound (O9Ø.Ø)
laceration of uterus, NEC (O71.81)

O71.2 Postpartum inversion of uterus

O71.3 Obstetric laceration of cervix
Annular detachment of cervix

O71.4 Obstetric high vaginal laceration alone
Laceration of vaginal wall without perineal laceration
Excludes1 obstetric high vaginal laceration with perineal laceration (O7Ø.-)

O71.5 Other obstetric injury to pelvic organs
Obstetric injury to bladder
Obstetric injury to urethra
Excludes2 obstetric periurethral trauma (O71.82)

O71.6 Obstetric damage to pelvic joints and ligaments
Obstetric avulsion of inner symphyseal cartilage
Obstetric damage to coccyx
Obstetric traumatic separation of symphysis (pubis)

O71.7 Obstetric hematoma of pelvis
Obstetric hematoma of perineum
Obstetric hematoma of vagina
Obstetric hematoma of vulva

● **O71.8 Other specified obstetric trauma**

O71.81 Laceration of uterus, not elsewhere classified

O71.82 Other specified trauma to perineum and vulva
Obstetric periurethral trauma

O71.89 Other specified obstetric trauma

O71.9 Obstetric trauma, unspecified

● **O72 Postpartum hemorrhage**
Includes hemorrhage after delivery of fetus or infant

O72.Ø Third-stage hemorrhage
Hemorrhage associated with retained, trapped or adherent placenta
Retained placenta NOS
Code also type of adherent placenta (O43.2-)

O72.1 Other immediate postpartum hemorrhage
Hemorrhage following delivery of placenta
Postpartum hemorrhage (atonic) NOS
Uterine atony with hemorrhage
Excludes1 uterine atony NOS (O62.2)
uterine atony without hemorrhage (O62.2)
postpartum atony of uterus without hemorrhage (O75.89)

O72.2 Delayed and secondary postpartum hemorrhage
Hemorrhage associated with retained portions of placenta or membranes after the first 24 hours following delivery of placenta
Retained products of conception NOS, following delivery

O72.3 Postpartum coagulation defects
Postpartum afibrinogenemia
Postpartum fibrinolysis

● **O73 Retained placenta and membranes, without hemorrhage**
Excludes1 placenta accreta (O43.21-)
placenta increta (O43.22-)
placenta percreta (O43.23-)

O73.0 Retained placenta without hemorrhage
Adherent placenta, without hemorrhage
Trapped placenta without hemorrhage

O73.1 Retained portions of placenta and membranes, without hemorrhage
Retained products of conception following delivery, without hemorrhage

● **O74 Complications of anesthesia during labor and delivery**
Includes maternal complications arising from the administration of a general, regional or local anesthetic, analgesic or other sedation during labor and delivery
Use additional code, if applicable, to identify specific complication

O74.0 Aspiration pneumonitis due to anesthesia during labor and delivery
Inhalation of stomach contents or secretions NOS due to anesthesia during labor and delivery
Mendelson's syndrome due to anesthesia during labor and delivery

O74.1 Other pulmonary complications of anesthesia during labor and delivery

O74.2 Cardiac complications of anesthesia during labor and delivery

O74.3 Central nervous system complications of anesthesia during labor and delivery

O74.4 Toxic reaction to local anesthesia during labor and delivery

O74.5 Spinal and epidural anesthesia-induced headache during labor and delivery

O74.6 Other complications of spinal and epidural anesthesia during labor and delivery

O74.7 Failed or difficult intubation for anesthesia during labor and delivery

O74.8 Other complications of anesthesia during labor and delivery

O74.9 Complication of anesthesia during labor and delivery, unspecified

● **O75 Other complications of labor and delivery, not elsewhere classified**
Excludes2 puerperal (postpartum) infection (O86.-)
puerperal (postpartum) sepsis (O85)

O75.0 Maternal distress during labor and delivery

O75.1 Shock during or following labor and delivery
Obstetric shock following labor and delivery

O75.2 Pyrexia during labor, not elsewhere classified

O75.3 Other infection during labor
Sepsis during labor
Use additional code (B95-B97), to identify infectious agent

O75.4 Other complications of obstetric surgery and procedures
Cardiac arrest following obstetric surgery or procedures
Cardiac failure following obstetric surgery or procedures
Cerebral anoxia following obstetric surgery or procedures
Pulmonary edema following obstetric surgery or procedures
Use additional code to identify specific complication
Excludes2 complications of anesthesia during labor and delivery (O74.-)
disruption of obstetrical (surgical) wound (O90.0-O90.1)
hematoma of obstetrical (surgical) wound (O90.2)
infection of obstetrical (surgical) wound (O86.0)

O75.5 Delayed delivery after artificial rupture of membranes

● **O75.8 Other specified complications of labor and delivery**

O75.81 Maternal exhaustion complicating labor and delivery

O75.82 Onset (spontaneous) of labor after 37 completed weeks of gestation but before 39 completed weeks gestation, with delivery by (planned) cesarean section
Delivery by (planned) cesarean section occurring after 37 completed weeks of gestation but before 39 completed weeks gestation due to (spontaneous) onset of labor
Code first to specify reason for planned cesarean section such as:
cephalopelvic disproportion (normally formed fetus) (O33.9)
previous cesarean delivery (O34.21)

O75.89 Other specified complications of labor and delivery

O75.9 Complication of labor and delivery, unspecified

O76 Abnormality in fetal heart rate and rhythm complicating labor and delivery
Depressed fetal heart rate tones complicating labor and delivery
Fetal bradycardia complicating labor and delivery
Fetal heart rate decelerations complicating labor and delivery
Fetal heart rate irregularity complicating labor and delivery
Fetal heart rate abnormal variability complicating labor and delivery
Fetal tachycardia complicating labor and delivery
Non-reassuring fetal heart rate or rhythm complicating labor and delivery
Excludes1 fetal stress NOS (O77.9)
labor and delivery complicated by electrocardiographic evidence of fetal stress (O77.8)
labor and delivery complicated by ultrasonic evidence of fetal stress (O77.8)
Excludes2 fetal metabolic acidemia (O68)
other fetal stress (O77.0-O77.1)

● **O77 Other fetal stress complicating labor and delivery**

O77.0 Labor and delivery complicated by meconium in amniotic fluid

O77.1 Fetal stress in labor or delivery due to drug administration

O77.8 Labor and delivery complicated by other evidence of fetal stress
Labor and delivery complicated by electrocardiographic evidence of fetal stress
Labor and delivery complicated by ultrasonic evidence of fetal stress
Excludes1 abnormality of fetal acid-base balance (O68)
abnormality in fetal heart rate or rhythm (O76)
fetal metabolic acidemia (O68)

O77.9 Labor and delivery complicated by fetal stress, unspecified
Excludes1 abnormality of fetal acid-base balance (O68)
abnormality in fetal heart rate or rhythm (O76)
fetal metabolic acidemia (O68)

CHAPTER 15 (O00-O9A)

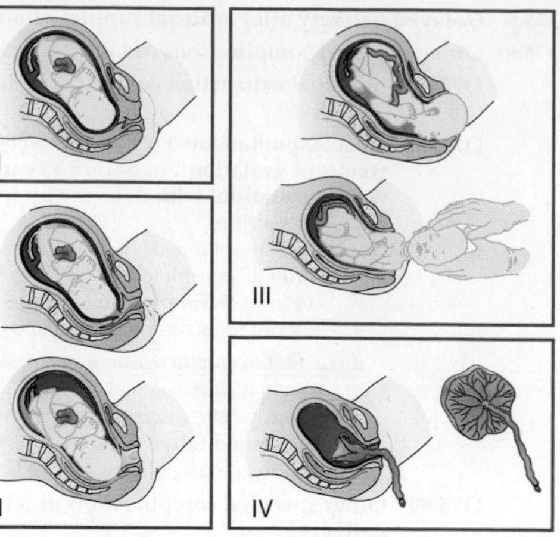

Figure 15-7 The four stages of normal delivery: **I.** Lightening, which occurs 2 to 4 weeks before birth, at which time the fetus turns with head toward the vagina. **II.** Regular contractions begin, the amniotic sac ruptures, and dilation is complete. **III.** Delivery of the head and rotation. **IV.** Expulsion of placenta.

OGCR Section I.C., Chapter 15.n.

Normal Delivery, Code O8Ø

1) Encounter for full term uncomplicated delivery

Code O8Ø should be assigned when a woman is admitted for a full-term normal delivery and delivers a single, healthy infant without any complications antepartum, during the delivery, or postpartum during the delivery episode. Code O8Ø is always a principal diagnosis. It is not to be used if any other code from chapter 15 is needed to describe a current complication of the antenatal, delivery, or perinatal period. Additional codes from other chapters may be used with code O8Ø if they are not related to or are in any way complicating the pregnancy.

2) Uncomplicated delivery with resolved antepartum complication

Code O8Ø may be used if the patient had a complication at some point during the pregnancy, but the complication is not present at the time of the admission for delivery.

3) Outcome of delivery for O8Ø

Z37.Ø, Single live brith, is the only outcome of delivery code appropriate for use with O8Ø.

ENCOUNTER FOR DELIVERY (O8Ø-O82)

O8Ø Encounter for full-term uncomplicated delivery
Delivery requiring minimal or no assistance, with or without episiotomy, without fetal manipulation [e.g., rotation version] or instrumentation [forceps] of a spontaneous, cephalic, vaginal, full-term, single, live-born infant. This code is for use as a single diagnosis code and is not to be used with any other code from chapter 15.
Use additional code to indicate outcome of delivery (Z37.Ø)

O82 Encounter for cesarean delivery without indication
Use additional code to indicate outcome of delivery (Z37.Ø)

COMPLICATIONS PREDOMINANTLY RELATED TO THE PUERPERIUM (O85-O92)

Excludes2 mental and behavioral disorders associated with the puerperium (F53)
obstetrical tetanus (A34)
puerperal osteomalacia (M83.Ø)

O85 Puerperal sepsis
Postpartum sepsis
Puerperal peritonitis
Puerperal pyemia
Use additional code (B95-B97), to identify infectious agent
Use additional code (R65.2-) to identify severe sepsis, if applicable
Excludes1 fever of unknown origin following delivery (O86.4)
genital tract infection following delivery (O86.1-)
obstetric pyemic and septic embolism (O88.3-)
puerperal septic thrombophlebitis (O86.81)
urinary tract infection following delivery (O86.2-)
Excludes2 sepsis during labor (O75.3)

● **O86 Other puerperal infections**
Use additional code (B95-B97), to identify infectious agent
Excludes2 infection during labor (O75.3)
obstetrical tetanus (A34)

O86.Ø Infection of obstetric surgical wound
Infected cesarean delivery wound following delivery
Infected perineal repair following delivery

● **O86.1 Other infection of genital tract following delivery**
O86.11 Cervicitis following delivery
O86.12 Endometritis following delivery
O86.13 Vaginitis following delivery
O86.19 Other infection of genital tract following delivery

● **O86.2 Urinary tract infection following delivery**
O86.2Ø Urinary tract infection following delivery, unspecified
Puerperal urinary tract infection NOS
O86.21 Infection of kidney following delivery
O86.22 Infection of bladder following delivery
Infection of urethra following delivery
O86.29 Other urinary tract infection following delivery

O86.4 Pyrexia of unknown origin following delivery
Puerperal infection NOS following delivery
Puerperal pyrexia NOS following delivery
Excludes2 pyrexia during labor (O75.2)

● **O86.8 Other specified puerperal infections**
O86.81 Puerperal septic thrombophlebitis
O86.89 Other specified puerperal infections

● **O87 Venous complications and hemorrhoids in the puerperium**
Includes venous complications in labor, delivery and the puerperium
Excludes2 obstetric embolism (O88.-)
puerperal septic thrombophlebitis (O86.81)
venous complications in pregnancy (O22.-)

O87.Ø Superficial thrombophlebitis in the puerperium
Puerperal phlebitis NOS
Puerperal thrombosis NOS

O87.1 Deep phlebothrombosis in the puerperium
Deep vein thrombosis, postpartum
Pelvic thrombophlebitis, postpartum
Use additional code to identify the deep vein thrombosis (I82.4-, I82.5-, I82.62-. I82.72-)
Use additional code, if applicable, for associated long-term (current) use of anticoagulants (Z79.Ø1)

◀ New ◀ Revised ~~deleted~~ Deleted **OGCR** Official Guidelines X Assign placeholder X ● Use Additional Character(s)
Excludes 1 Excludes 2 Includes Use additional Code first Code also Unspecified

O87.2 Hemorrhoids in the puerperium

O87.3 Cerebral venous thrombosis in the puerperium
Cerebrovenous sinus thrombosis in the puerperium

O87.4 Varicose veins of lower extremity in the puerperium

O87.8 Other venous complications in the puerperium
Genital varices in the puerperium

O87.9 Venous complication in the puerperium, unspecified
Puerperal phlebopathy NOS

O88 Obstetric embolism

Excludes1 embolism complicating abortion NOS (O03.2)
embolism complicating ectopic or molar pregnancy (O08.2)
embolism complicating failed attempted abortion (O07.2)
embolism complicating induced abortion (O04.7)
embolism complicating spontaneous abortion (O03.2, O03.7)

● **O88.0 Obstetric air embolism**

● **O88.01 Obstetric air embolism in pregnancy**

O88.011 Air embolism in pregnancy, first trimester

O88.012 Air embolism in pregnancy, second trimester

O88.013 Air embolism in pregnancy, third trimester

O88.019 Air embolism in pregnancy, unspecified trimester

O88.02 Air embolism in childbirth

O88.03 Air embolism in the puerperium

● **O88.1 Amniotic fluid embolism**
Anaphylactoid syndrome in pregnancy

● **O88.11 Amniotic fluid embolism in pregnancy**

O88.111 Amniotic fluid embolism in pregnancy, first trimester

O88.112 Amniotic fluid embolism in pregnancy, second trimester

O88.113 Amniotic fluid embolism in pregnancy, third trimester

O88.119 Amniotic fluid embolism in pregnancy, unspecified trimester

O88.12 Amniotic fluid embolism in childbirth

O88.13 Amniotic fluid embolism in the puerperium

● **O88.2 Obstetric thromboembolism**

● **O88.21 Thromboembolism in pregnancy**
Obstetric (pulmonary) embolism NOS

O88.211 Thromboembolism in pregnancy, first trimester

O88.212 Thromboembolism in pregnancy, second trimester

O88.213 Thromboembolism in pregnancy, third trimester

O88.219 Thromboembolism in pregnancy, unspecified trimester

O88.22 Thromboembolism in childbirth

O88.23 Thromboembolism in the puerperium
Puerperal (pulmonary) embolism NOS

● **O88.3 Obstetric pyemic and septic embolism**

● **O88.31 Pyemic and septic embolism in pregnancy**

O88.311 Pyemic and septic embolism in pregnancy, first trimester

O88.312 Pyemic and septic embolism in pregnancy, second trimester

O88.313 Pyemic and septic embolism in pregnancy, third trimester

O88.319 Pyemic and septic embolism in pregnancy, unspecified trimester

O88.32 Pyemic and septic embolism in childbirth

O88.33 Pyemic and septic embolism in the puerperium

● **O88.8 Other obstetric embolism**
Obstetric fat embolism

● **O88.81 Other embolism in pregnancy**

O88.811 Other embolism in pregnancy, first trimester

O88.812 Other embolism in pregnancy, second trimester

O88.813 Other embolism in pregnancy, third trimester

O88.819 Other embolism in pregnancy, unspecified trimester

O88.82 Other embolism in childbirth

O88.83 Other embolism in the puerperium

● **O89 Complications of anesthesia during the puerperium**

Includes maternal complications arising from the administration of a general, regional or local anesthetic, analgesic or other sedation during the puerperium

Use additional code, if applicable, to identify specific complication

● **O89.0 Pulmonary complications of anesthesia during the puerperium**

O89.01 Aspiration pneumonitis due to anesthesia during the puerperium
Inhalation of stomach contents or secretions NOS due to anesthesia during the puerperium
Mendelson's syndrome due to anesthesia during the puerperium

O89.09 Other pulmonary complications of anesthesia during the puerperium

O89.1 Cardiac complications of anesthesia during the puerperium

O89.2 Central nervous system complications of anesthesia during the puerperium

O89.3 Toxic reaction to local anesthesia during the puerperium

O89.4 Spinal and epidural anesthesia-induced headache during the puerperium

O89.5 Other complications of spinal and epidural anesthesia during the puerperium

O89.6 Failed or difficult intubation for anesthesia during the puerperium

O89.8 Other complications of anesthesia during the puerperium

O89.9 Complication of anesthesia during the puerperium, unspecified

CHAPTER 15 (O00-O9A)

● **O90 Complications of the puerperium, not elsewhere classified**

O90.0 Disruption of cesarean delivery wound
Dehiscence of cesarean delivery wound
Excludes1 rupture of uterus (spontaneous) before onset of labor (O71.0-)
rupture of uterus during labor (O71.1)

O90.1 Disruption of perineal obstetric wound
Disruption of wound of episiotomy
Disruption of wound of perineal laceration
Secondary perineal tear

O90.2 Hematoma of obstetric wound

O90.3 Peripartum cardiomyopathy
Conditions in I42.- arising during pregnancy and the puerperium
Excludes1 pre-existing heart disease complicating pregnancy and the puerperium (O99.4-)

O90.4 Postpartum acute kidney failure
Hepatorenal syndrome following labor and delivery

O90.5 Postpartum thyroiditis

O90.6 Postpartum mood disturbance
Postpartum blues
Postpartum sadness
Postpartum dysphoria
Excludes1 postpartum depression (F53)
puerperal psychosis (F53)

● **O90.8 Other complications of the puerperium, not elsewhere classified**

O90.81 Anemia of the puerperium
Postpartum anemia NOS
Excludes1 pre-existing anemia complicating the puerperium (O99.03)

O90.89 Other complications of the puerperium, not elsewhere classified
Placental polyp

O90.9 Complication of the puerperium, unspecified

● **O91 Infections of breast associated with pregnancy, the puerperium and lactation**
Use additional code to identify infection

● **O91.0 Infection of nipple associated with pregnancy, the puerperium and lactation**

● **O91.01 Infection of nipple associated with pregnancy**
Gestational abscess of nipple

O91.011 Infection of nipple associated with pregnancy, first trimester

O91.012 Infection of nipple associated with pregnancy, second trimester

O91.013 Infection of nipple associated with pregnancy, third trimester

O91.019 Infection of nipple associated with pregnancy, unspecified trimester

O91.02 Infection of nipple associated with the puerperium
Puerperal abscess of nipple

O91.03 Infection of nipple associated with lactation
Abscess of nipple associated with lactation

● **O91.1 Abscess of breast associated with pregnancy, the puerperium and lactation**

● **O91.11 Abscess of breast associated with pregnancy**
Gestational mammary abscess
Gestational purulent mastitis
Gestational subareolar abscess

O91.111 Abscess of breast associated with pregnancy, first trimester

O91.112 Abscess of breast associated with pregnancy, second trimester

O91.113 Abscess of breast associated with pregnancy, third trimester

O91.119 Abscess of breast associated with pregnancy, unspecified trimester

O91.12 Abscess of breast associated with the puerperium
Puerperal mammary abscess
Puerperal purulent mastitis
Puerperal subareolar abscess

O91.13 Abscess of breast associated with lactation
Mammary abscess associated with lactation
Purulent mastitis associated with lactation
Subareolar abscess associated with lactation

● **O91.2 Nonpurulent mastitis associated with pregnancy, the puerperium and lactation**

● **O91.21 Nonpurulent mastitis associated with pregnancy**
Gestational interstitial mastitis
Gestational lymphangitis of breast
Gestational mastitis NOS
Gestational parenchymatous mastitis

O91.211 Nonpurulent mastitis associated with pregnancy, first trimester

O91.212 Nonpurulent mastitis associated with pregnancy, second trimester

O91.213 Nonpurulent mastitis associated with pregnancy, third trimester

O91.219 Nonpurulent mastitis associated with pregnancy, unspecified trimester

O91.22 Nonpurulent mastitis associated with the puerperium
Puerperal interstitial mastitis
Puerperal lymphangitis of breast
Puerperal mastitis NOS
Puerperal parenchymatous mastitis

O91.23 Nonpurulent mastitis associated with lactation
Interstitial mastitis associated with lactation
Lymphangitis of breast associated with lactation
Mastitis NOS associated with lactation
Parenchymatous mastitis associated with lactation

● **O92 Other disorders of breast and disorders of lactation associated with pregnancy and the puerperium**

● **O92.0 Retracted nipple associated with pregnancy, the puerperium, and lactation**

● **O92.01 Retracted nipple associated with pregnancy**

O92.011 Retracted nipple associated with pregnancy, first trimester

O92.012 Retracted nipple associated with pregnancy, second trimester

O92.013 Retracted nipple associated with pregnancy, third trimester

O92.019 Retracted nipple associated with pregnancy, unspecified trimester

O92.02 Retracted nipple associated with the puerperium

O92.03 Retracted nipple associated with lactation

● **O92.1 Cracked nipple associated with pregnancy, the puerperium, and lactation**
Fissure of nipple, gestational or puerperal

● **O92.11 Cracked nipple associated with pregnancy**

O92.111 Cracked nipple associated with pregnancy, first trimester

O92.112 Cracked nipple associated with pregnancy, second trimester

O92.113 Cracked nipple associated with pregnancy, third trimester

O92.119 Cracked nipple associated with pregnancy, unspecified trimester

O92.12 Cracked nipple associated with the puerperium

O92.13 Cracked nipple associated with lactation

● **O92.2 Other and unspecified disorders of breast associated with pregnancy and the puerperium**
- **O92.20 Unspecified disorder of breast associated with pregnancy and the puerperium**
- **O92.29 Other disorders of breast associated with pregnancy and the puerperium**

O92.3 Agalactia
Primary agalactia
Excludes1 elective agalactia (O92.5)
secondary agalactia (O92.5)
therapeutic agalactia (O92.5)

O92.4 Hypogalactia

O92.5 Suppressed lactation
Elective agalactia
Secondary agalactia
Therapeutic agalactia
Excludes1 primary agalactia (O92.3)

O92.6 Galactorrhea

● **O92.7 Other and unspecified disorders of lactation**
- **O92.70 Unspecified disorders of lactation**
- **O92.79 Other disorders of lactation**
  Puerperal galactocele

OTHER OBSTETRIC CONDITIONS, NOT ELSEWHERE CLASSIFIED (O94-O9A)

O94 Sequelae of complication of pregnancy, childbirth, and the puerperium
Note: This category is to be used to indicate conditions in O00-O77.-, O85-O94 and O98-O9A.- as the cause of late effects. The 'sequelae' include conditions specified as such, or as late effects, which may occur at any time after the puerperium.
Code first condition resulting from (sequela) of complication of pregnancy, childbirth, and the puerperium

O98 Maternal infectious and parasitic diseases classifiable elsewhere but complicating pregnancy, childbirth and the puerperium
Includes the listed conditions when complicating the pregnant state, when aggravated by the pregnancy, or as a reason for obstetric care
Use additional code (Chapter 1), to identify specific infectious or parasitic disease
Excludes2 herpes gestationis (O26.4-)
infectious carrier state (O99.82-, O99.83-)
obstetrical tetanus (A34)
puerperal infection (O86.-)
puerperal sepsis (O85)
when the reason for maternal care is that the disease is known or suspected to have affected the fetus (O35-O36)

● **O98.0 Tuberculosis complicating pregnancy, childbirth and the puerperium**
Conditions in A15-A19
- ● **O98.01 Tuberculosis complicating pregnancy**
  - **O98.011 Tuberculosis complicating pregnancy, first trimester**
  - **O98.012 Tuberculosis complicating pregnancy, second trimester**
  - **O98.013 Tuberculosis complicating pregnancy, third trimester**
  - **O98.019 Tuberculosis complicating pregnancy, unspecified trimester**
- **O98.02 Tuberculosis complicating childbirth**
- **O98.03 Tuberculosis complicating the puerperium**

● **O98.1 Syphilis complicating pregnancy, childbirth and the puerperium**
Conditions in A50-A53
- ● **O98.11 Syphilis complicating pregnancy**
  - **O98.111 Syphilis complicating pregnancy, first trimester**
  - **O98.112 Syphilis complicating pregnancy, second trimester**
  - **O98.113 Syphilis complicating pregnancy, third trimester**
  - **O98.119 Syphilis complicating pregnancy, unspecified trimester**
- **O98.12 Syphilis complicating childbirth**
- **O98.13 Syphilis complicating the puerperium**

● **O98.2 Gonorrhea complicating pregnancy, childbirth and the puerperium**
Conditions in A54.-
- ● **O98.21 Gonorrhea complicating pregnancy**
  - **O98.211 Gonorrhea complicating pregnancy, first trimester**
  - **O98.212 Gonorrhea complicating pregnancy, second trimester**
  - **O98.213 Gonorrhea complicating pregnancy, third trimester**
  - **O98.219 Gonorrhea complicating pregnancy, unspecified trimester**
- **O98.22 Gonorrhea complicating childbirth**
- **O98.23 Gonorrhea complicating the puerperium**

● **O98.3 Other infections with a predominantly sexual mode of transmission complicating pregnancy, childbirth and the puerperium**
Conditions in A55-A64
- ● **O98.31 Other infections with a predominantly sexual mode of transmission complicating pregnancy**
  - **O98.311 Other infections with a predominantly sexual mode of transmission complicating pregnancy, first trimester**
  - **O98.312 Other infections with a predominantly sexual mode of transmission complicating pregnancy, second trimester**
  - **O98.313 Other infections with a predominantly sexual mode of transmission complicating pregnancy, third trimester**
  - **O98.319 Other infections with a predominantly sexual mode of transmission complicating pregnancy, unspecified trimester**
- **O98.32 Other infections with a predominantly sexual mode of transmission complicating childbirth**
- **O98.33 Other infections with a predominantly sexual mode of transmission complicating the puerperium**

● **O98.4 Viral hepatitis complicating pregnancy, childbirth and the puerperium**
Conditions in B15-B19
- ● **O98.41 Viral hepatitis complicating pregnancy**
  - **O98.411 Viral hepatitis complicating pregnancy, first trimester**
  - **O98.412 Viral hepatitis complicating pregnancy, second trimester**
  - **O98.413 Viral hepatitis complicating pregnancy, third trimester**
  - **O98.419 Viral hepatitis complicating pregnancy, unspecified trimester**
- **O98.42 Viral hepatitis complicating childbirth**
- **O98.43 Viral hepatitis complicating the puerperium**

● O98.5 **Other viral diseases complicating pregnancy, childbirth and the puerperium**
Conditions in A80-B09, B25-B34, R87.81-, R87.82-
Excludes1 human immunodeficiency virus [HIV] disease complicating pregnancy, childbirth and the puerperium (O98.7-)

● O98.51 **Other viral diseases complicating pregnancy**
O98.511 **Other viral diseases complicating pregnancy, first trimester**
O98.512 **Other viral diseases complicating pregnancy, second trimester**
O98.513 **Other viral diseases complicating pregnancy, third trimester**
O98.519 **Other viral diseases complicating pregnancy, unspecified trimester**

O98.52 **Other viral diseases complicating childbirth**
O98.53 **Other viral diseases complicating the puerperium**

● O98.6 **Protozoal diseases complicating pregnancy, childbirth and the puerperium**
Conditions in B50-B64

● O98.61 **Protozoal diseases complicating pregnancy**
O98.611 **Protozoal diseases complicating pregnancy, first trimester**
O98.612 **Protozoal diseases complicating pregnancy, second trimester**
O98.613 **Protozoal diseases complicating pregnancy, third trimester**
O98.619 **Protozoal diseases complicating pregnancy, unspecified trimester**

O98.62 **Protozoal diseases complicating childbirth**
O98.63 **Protozoal diseases complicating the puerperium**

● O98.7 **Human immunodeficiency virus [HIV] disease complicating pregnancy, childbirth and the puerperium**
Use additional code to identify the type of HIV disease:
Acquired immune deficiency syndrome (AIDS) (B20)
Asymptomatic HIV status (Z21)
HIV positive NOS (Z21)
Symptomatic HIV disease (B20)

OGCR Section I.C.15.f.

HIV Infection in Pregnancy, Childbirth and the Puerperium

During pregnancy, childbirth or the puerperium, a patient admitted because of an HIV-related illness should receive a principal diagnosis from subcategory O98.7-. Human immunodeficiency [HIV] disease complicating pregnancy, childbirth and the puerperium, followed by the code(s) for the HIV-related illness(es).

Patients with asymptomatic HIV infection status admitted during pregnancy, childbirth, or the puerperium should receive codes of O98.7- and Z21, Asymptomatic human immunodeficiency virus [HIV] infection status.

● O98.71 **Human immunodeficiency virus [HIV] disease complicating pregnancy**
O98.711 **Human immunodeficiency virus [HIV] disease complicating pregnancy, first trimester**
O98.712 **Human immunodeficiency virus [HIV] disease complicating pregnancy, second trimester**
O98.713 **Human immunodeficiency virus [HIV] disease complicating pregnancy, third trimester**
O98.719 **Human immunodeficiency virus [HIV] disease complicating pregnancy, unspecified trimester**

O98.72 **Human immunodeficiency virus [HIV] disease complicating childbirth**
O98.73 **Human immunodeficiency virus [HIV] disease complicating the puerperium**

● O98.8 **Other maternal infectious and parasitic diseases complicating pregnancy, childbirth and the puerperium**

● O98.81 **Other maternal infectious and parasitic diseases complicating pregnancy**
O98.811 **Other maternal infectious and parasitic diseases complicating pregnancy, first trimester**
O98.812 **Other maternal infectious and parasitic diseases complicating pregnancy, second trimester**
O98.813 **Other maternal infectious and parasitic diseases complicating pregnancy, third trimester**
O98.819 **Other maternal infectious and parasitic diseases complicating pregnancy, unspecified trimester**

O98.82 **Other maternal infectious and parasitic diseases complicating childbirth**
O98.83 **Other maternal infectious and parasitic diseases complicating the puerperium**

● O98.9 **Unspecified maternal infectious and parasitic disease complicating pregnancy, childbirth and the puerperium**

● O98.91 **Unspecified maternal infectious and parasitic disease complicating pregnancy**
O98.911 **Unspecified maternal infectious and parasitic disease complicating pregnancy, first trimester**
O98.912 **Unspecified maternal infectious and parasitic disease complicating pregnancy, second trimester**
O98.913 **Unspecified maternal infectious and parasitic disease complicating pregnancy, third trimester**
O98.919 **Unspecified maternal infectious and parasitic disease complicating pregnancy, unspecified trimester**

O98.92 **Unspecified maternal infectious and parasitic disease complicating childbirth**
O98.93 **Unspecified maternal infectious and parasitic disease complicating the puerperium**

● O99 **Other maternal diseases classifiable elsewhere but complicating pregnancy, childbirth and the puerperium**
Includes: conditions which complicate the pregnant state, are aggravated by the pregnancy or are a main reason for obstetric care
Use additional code to identify specific condition
Excludes2 when the reason for maternal care is that the condition is known or suspected to have affected the fetus (O35-O36)

● O99.0 **Anemia complicating pregnancy, childbirth and the puerperium**
Conditions in D50-D64
Excludes1 anemia arising in the puerperium (O90.81)
postpartum anemia NOS (O90.81)

● O99.01 **Anemia complicating pregnancy**
O99.011 **Anemia complicating pregnancy, first trimester**
O99.012 **Anemia complicating pregnancy, second trimester**
O99.013 **Anemia complicating pregnancy, third trimester**
O99.019 **Anemia complicating pregnancy, unspecified trimester**

O99.02 **Anemia complicating childbirth**
O99.03 **Anemia complicating the puerperium**
Excludes1 postpartum anemia not pre-existing prior to delivery (O90.81)

● **O99.1 Other diseases of the blood and blood-forming organs and certain disorders involving the immune mechanism complicating pregnancy, childbirth and the puerperium**
Conditions in D65-D89
Excludes2 hemorrhage with coagulation defects (O45.-, O46.Ø-, O67.Ø, O72.3)

● **O99.11 Other diseases of the blood and blood-forming organs and certain disorders involving the immune mechanism complicating pregnancy**

O99.111 Other diseases of the blood and blood-forming organs and certain disorders involving the immune mechanism complicating pregnancy, first trimester

O99.112 Other diseases of the blood and blood-forming organs and certain disorders involving the immune mechanism complicating pregnancy, second trimester

O99.113 Other diseases of the blood and blood-forming organs and certain disorders involving the immune mechanism complicating pregnancy, third trimester

O99.119 Other diseases of the blood and blood-forming organs and certain disorders involving the immune mechanism complicating pregnancy, unspecified trimester

O99.12 Other diseases of the blood and blood-forming organs and certain disorders involving the immune mechanism complicating childbirth

O99.13 Other diseases of the blood and blood-forming organs and certain disorders involving the immune mechanism complicating the puerperium

● **O99.2 Endocrine, nutritional and metabolic diseases complicating pregnancy, childbirth and the puerperium**
Conditions in EØØ-E88
Excludes2 diabetes mellitus (O24.-)
malnutrition (O25.-)
postpartum thyroiditis (O9Ø.5)

● **O99.21 Obesity complicating pregnancy, childbirth, and the puerperium**
Use additional code to identify the type of obesity (E66.-)

O99.21Ø Obesity complicating pregnancy, unspecified trimester

O99.211 Obesity complicating pregnancy, first trimester

O99.212 Obesity complicating pregnancy, second trimester

O99.213 Obesity complicating pregnancy, third trimester

O99.214 Obesity complicating childbirth

O99.215 Obesity complicating the puerperium

● **O99.28 Other endocrine, nutritional and metabolic diseases complicating pregnancy, childbirth and the puerperium**

O99.28Ø Endocrine, nutritional and metabolic diseases complicating pregnancy, unspecified trimester

O99.281 Endocrine, nutritional and metabolic diseases complicating pregnancy, first trimester

O99.282 Endocrine, nutritional and metabolic diseases complicating pregnancy, second trimester

O99.283 Endocrine, nutritional and metabolic diseases complicating pregnancy, third trimester

O99.284 Endocrine, nutritional and metabolic diseases complicating childbirth

O99.285 Endocrine, nutritional and metabolic diseases complicating the puerperium

● **O99.3 Mental disorders and diseases of the nervous system complicating pregnancy, childbirth and the puerperium**

● **O99.31 Alcohol use complicating pregnancy, childbirth, and the puerperium**
Use additional code(s) from F1Ø to identify manifestations of the alcohol use

O99.31Ø Alcohol use complicating pregnancy, unspecified trimester

O99.311 Alcohol use complicating pregnancy, first trimester

O99.312 Alcohol use complicating pregnancy, second trimester

O99.313 Alcohol use complicating pregnancy, third trimester

O99.314 Alcohol use complicating childbirth

O99.315 Alcohol use complicating the puerperium

● **O99.32 Drug use complicating pregnancy, childbirth, and the puerperium**
Use additional code(s) from F11-F16 and F18-F19 to identify manifestations of the drug use

O99.32Ø Drug use complicating pregnancy, unspecified trimester

O99.321 Drug use complicating pregnancy, first trimester

O99.322 Drug use complicating pregnancy, second trimester

O99.323 Drug use complicating pregnancy, third trimester

O99.324 Drug use complicating childbirth

O99.325 Drug use complicating the puerperium

● **O99.33 Tobacco use disorder complicating pregnancy, childbirth, and the puerperium** ⟸
Smoking complicating pregnancy, childbirth, and the puerperium ◀
Use additional code from category F17 to identify type of tobacco nicotine dependence ◀

O99.33Ø Smoking (tobacco) complicating pregnancy, unspecified trimester

O99.331 Smoking (tobacco) complicating pregnancy, first trimester

O99.332 Smoking (tobacco) complicating pregnancy, second trimester

O99.333 Smoking (tobacco) complicating pregnancy, third trimester

O99.334 Smoking (tobacco) complicating childbirth

O99.335 Smoking (tobacco) complicating the puerperium

● O99.34 **Other mental disorders complicating pregnancy, childbirth, and the puerperium**
Conditions in FØ1-FØ9 and F2Ø-F99
Excludes2 postpartum mood disturbance (O9Ø.6)
postnatal psychosis (F53)
puerperal psychosis (F53)

O99.34Ø **Other mental disorders complicating pregnancy, unspecified trimester**
O99.341 **Other mental disorders complicating pregnancy, first trimester**
O99.342 **Other mental disorders complicating pregnancy, second trimester**
O99.343 **Other mental disorders complicating pregnancy, third trimester**
O99.344 **Other mental disorders complicating childbirth**
O99.345 **Other mental disorders complicating the puerperium**

● O99.35 **Diseases of the nervous system complicating pregnancy, childbirth, and the puerperium**
Conditions in GØØ-G99
Excludes2 pregnancy related peripheral neuritis (O26.8-)

O99.35Ø **Diseases of the nervous system complicating pregnancy, unspecified trimester**
O99.351 **Diseases of the nervous system complicating pregnancy, first trimester**
O99.352 **Diseases of the nervous system complicating pregnancy, second trimester**
O99.353 **Diseases of the nervous system complicating pregnancy, third trimester**
O99.354 **Diseases of the nervous system complicating childbirth**
O99.355 **Diseases of the nervous system complicating the puerperium**

● O99.4 **Diseases of the circulatory system complicating pregnancy, childbirth and the puerperium**
Conditions in IØØ-I99
Excludes1 peripartum cardiomyopathy (O9Ø.3)
Excludes2 hypertensive disorders (O1Ø-O16)
obstetric embolism (O88.-)
venous complications and cerebrovenous sinus thrombosis in labor, childbirth and the puerperium (O87.-)
venous complications and cerebrovenous sinus thrombosis in pregnancy (O22.-)

● O99.41 **Diseases of the circulatory system complicating pregnancy**
O99.411 **Diseases of the circulatory system complicating pregnancy, first trimester**
O99.412 **Diseases of the circulatory system complicating pregnancy, second trimester**
O99.413 **Diseases of the circulatory system complicating pregnancy, third trimester**
O99.419 **Diseases of the circulatory system complicating pregnancy, unspecified trimester**

O99.42 **Diseases of the circulatory system complicating childbirth**
O99.43 **Diseases of the circulatory system complicating the puerperium**

● O99.5 **Diseases of the respiratory system complicating pregnancy, childbirth and the puerperium**
Conditions in JØØ-J99

● O99.51 **Diseases of the respiratory system complicating pregnancy**
O99.511 **Diseases of the respiratory system complicating pregnancy, first trimester**
O99.512 **Diseases of the respiratory system complicating pregnancy, second trimester**
O99.513 **Diseases of the respiratory system complicating pregnancy, third trimester**
O99.519 **Diseases of the respiratory system complicating pregnancy, unspecified trimester**

O99.52 **Diseases of the respiratory system complicating childbirth**
O99.53 **Diseases of the respiratory system complicating the puerperium**

● O99.6 **Diseases of the digestive system complicating pregnancy, childbirth and the puerperium**
Conditions in KØØ-K93
Excludes2 hemorrhoids in pregnancy (O22.4-) ◀
liver and biliary tract disorders in pregnancy, childbirth and the puerperium (O26.6-)

● O99.61 **Diseases of the digestive system complicating pregnancy**
O99.611 **Diseases of the digestive system complicating pregnancy, first trimester**
O99.612 **Diseases of the digestive system complicating pregnancy, second trimester**
O99.613 **Diseases of the digestive system complicating pregnancy, third trimester**
O99.619 **Diseases of the digestive system complicating pregnancy, unspecified trimester**

O99.62 **Diseases of the digestive system complicating childbirth**
O99.63 **Diseases of the digestive system complicating the puerperium**

● O99.7 **Diseases of the skin and subcutaneous tissue complicating pregnancy, childbirth and the puerperium**
Conditions in LØØ-L99
Excludes2 herpes gestationis (O26.4)
pruritic urticarial papules and plaques of pregnancy (PUPPP) (O26.86)

● O99.71 **Diseases of the skin and subcutaneous tissue complicating pregnancy**
O99.711 **Diseases of the skin and subcutaneous tissue complicating pregnancy, first trimester**
O99.712 **Diseases of the skin and subcutaneous tissue complicating pregnancy, second trimester**
O99.713 **Diseases of the skin and subcutaneous tissue complicating pregnancy, third trimester**
O99.719 **Diseases of the skin and subcutaneous tissue complicating pregnancy, unspecified trimester**

O99.72 **Diseases of the skin and subcutaneous tissue complicating childbirth**
O99.73 **Diseases of the skin and subcutaneous tissue complicating the puerperium**

● **O99.8 Other specified diseases and conditions complicating pregnancy, childbirth and the puerperium**
Conditions in D00-D48, H00-H95, M00-N99, and Q00-Q99
Use additional code to identify condition
Excludes2 genitourinary infections in pregnancy (O23.-)
infection of genitourinary tract following delivery (O86.1-O86.3)
malignant neoplasm complicating pregnancy, childbirth and the puerperium (O9A.1-)
maternal care for known or suspected abnormality of maternal pelvic organs (O34.-)
postpartum acute kidney failure (O90.4)
traumatic injuries in pregnancy (O9A.2-)

● **O99.81 Abnormal glucose complicating pregnancy, childbirth and the puerperium**
Excludes1 gestational diabetes (O24.4-)
O99.810 Abnormal glucose complicating pregnancy
O99.814 Abnormal glucose complicating childbirth
O99.815 Abnormal glucose complicating the puerperium

● **O99.82 Streptococcus B carrier state complicating pregnancy, childbirth and the puerperium**
Excludes1 Carrier of streptococcus group B (GBS) in a nonpregnant woman (Z22.330) ◀
O99.820 Streptococcus B carrier state complicating pregnancy
O99.824 Streptococcus B carrier state complicating childbirth
O99.825 Streptococcus B carrier state complicating the puerperium

● **O99.83 Other infection carrier state complicating pregnancy, childbirth and the puerperium**
Use additional code to identify the carrier state (Z22.-)
O99.830 Other infection carrier state complicating pregnancy
O99.834 Other infection carrier state complicating childbirth
O99.835 Other infection carrier state complicating the puerperium

● **O99.84 Bariatric surgery status complicating pregnancy, childbirth and the puerperium**
Gastric banding status complicating pregnancy, childbirth and the puerperium
Gastric bypass status for obesity complicating pregnancy, childbirth and the puerperium
Obesity surgery status complicating pregnancy, childbirth and the puerperium
O99.840 Bariatric surgery status complicating pregnancy, unspecified trimester
O99.841 Bariatric surgery status complicating pregnancy, first trimester
O99.842 Bariatric surgery status complicating pregnancy, second trimester
O99.843 Bariatric surgery status complicating pregnancy, third trimester
O99.844 Bariatric surgery status complicating childbirth
O99.845 Bariatric surgery status complicating the puerperium

O99.89 Other specified diseases and conditions complicating pregnancy, childbirth and the puerperium

OGCR Section I.C.2.l.3.

Malignant neoplasm in a pregnant patient

When a pregnant woman has a malignant neoplasm, a code from subcategory O9A.1-, Malignant neoplasm complicating pregnancy, childbirth, and the puerperium, should be sequenced first, followed by the appropriate code from Chapter 2 to indicate the type of neoplasm.

● **O9A Maternal malignant neoplasms, traumatic injuries and abuse classifiable elsewhere but complicating pregnancy, childbirth and the puerperium**

● **O9A.1 Malignant neoplasm complicating pregnancy, childbirth and the puerperium**
Conditions in C00-C96
Use additional code to identify neoplasm
Excludes2 maternal care for benign tumor of corpus uteri (O34.1-)
maternal care for benign tumor of cervix (O34.4-)

● **O9A.11 Malignant neoplasm complicating pregnancy**
O9A.111 Malignant neoplasm complicating pregnancy, first trimester
O9A.112 Malignant neoplasm complicating pregnancy, second trimester
O9A.113 Malignant neoplasm complicating pregnancy, third trimester
O9A.119 Malignant neoplasm complicating pregnancy, unspecified trimester

O9A.12 Malignant neoplasm complicating childbirth
O9A.13 Malignant neoplasm complicating the puerperium

● **O9A.2 Injury, poisoning and certain other consequences of external causes complicating pregnancy, childbirth and the puerperium**
Conditions in S00-T88, except T74 and T76
Use additional code(s) to identify the injury or poisoning
Excludes2 physical, sexual and psychological abuse complicating pregnancy, childbirth and the puerperium (O9A.3-, O9A.4-, O9A.5-)

● **O9A.21 Injury, poisoning and certain other consequences of external causes complicating pregnancy**
O9A.211 Injury, poisoning and certain other consequences of external causes complicating pregnancy, first trimester
O9A.212 Injury, poisoning and certain other consequences of external causes complicating pregnancy, second trimester
O9A.213 Injury, poisoning and certain other consequences of external causes complicating pregnancy, third trimester
O9A.219 Injury, poisoning and certain other consequences of external causes complicating pregnancy, unspecified trimester

O9A.22 Injury, poisoning and certain other consequences of external causes complicating childbirth
O9A.23 Injury, poisoning and certain other consequences of external causes complicating the puerperium

CHAPTER 15 (O00-O9A)

● **O9A.3 Physical abuse complicating pregnancy, childbirth and the puerperium**
Conditions in T74.11 or T76.11
Use additional code (if applicable):
to identify any associated current injury due to physical abuse
to identify the perpetrator of abuse (YØ7.-)
Excludes2 sexual abuse complicating pregnancy, childbirth and the puerperium (O9A.4)

● **O9A.31 Physical abuse complicating pregnancy**
O9A.311 Physical abuse complicating pregnancy, first trimester
O9A.312 Physical abuse complicating pregnancy, second trimester
O9A.313 Physical abuse complicating pregnancy, third trimester
O9A.319 Physical abuse complicating pregnancy, unspecified trimester

O9A.32 Physical abuse complicating childbirth
O9A.33 Physical abuse complicating the puerperium

● **O9A.4 Sexual abuse complicating pregnancy, childbirth and the puerperium**
Conditions in T74.21 or T76.21
Use additional code (if applicable):
to identify any associated current injury due to sexual abuse
to identify the perpetrator of abuse (YØ7.-)

● **O9A.41 Sexual abuse complicating pregnancy**
O9A.411 Sexual abuse complicating pregnancy, first trimester
O9A.412 Sexual abuse complicating pregnancy, second trimester
O9A.413 Sexual abuse complicating pregnancy, third trimester
O9A.419 Sexual abuse complicating pregnancy, unspecified trimester

O9A.42 Sexual abuse complicating childbirth
O9A.43 Sexual abuse complicating the puerperium

● **O9A.5 Psychological abuse complicating pregnancy, childbirth and the puerperium**
Conditions in T74.31 or T76.31
Use additional code to identify the perpetrator of abuse (YØ7.-)

● **O9A.51 Psychological abuse complicating pregnancy**
O9A.511 Psychological abuse complicating pregnancy, first trimester
O9A.512 Psychological abuse complicating pregnancy, second trimester
O9A.513 Psychological abuse complicating pregnancy, third trimester
O9A.519 Psychological abuse complicating pregnancy, unspecified trimester

O9A.52 Psychological abuse complicating childbirth
O9A.53 Psychological abuse complicating the puerperium

CHAPTER 16

CERTAIN CONDITIONS ORIGINATING IN THE PERINATAL PERIOD (PØØ-P96)

OGCR Chapter-Specific Coding Guidelines

16. Chapter 16: Certain Conditions Originating in the Perinatal Period (PØØ-P96)

For coding and reporting purposes the perinatal period is defined as before birth through the 28th day following birth. The following guidelines are provided for reporting purposes

a. General Perinatal Rules

1) Use of Chapter 16 Codes

Codes in this chapter are never for use on the maternal record. Codes from Chapter 15, the obstetric chapter, are never permitted on the newborn record. Chapter 16 codes may be used throughout the life of the patient if the condition is still present.

2) Principal Diagnosis for Birth Record

When coding the birth episode in a newborn record, assign a code from category Z38, Liveborn infants according to place of birth and type of delivery, as the principal diagnosis. A code from category Z38 is assigned only once, to a newborn at the time of birth. If a newborn is transferred to another institution, a code from category Z38 should not be used at the receiving hospital.

A code from category Z38 is used only on the newborn record, not on the mother's record.

3) Use of Codes from other Chapters with Codes from Chapter 16

Codes from other chapters may be used with codes from chapter 16 if the codes from the other chapters provide more specific detail. Codes for signs and symptoms may be assigned when a definitive diagnosis has not been established. If the reason for the encounter is a perinatal condition, the code from chapter 16 should be sequenced first.

4) Use of Chapter 16 Codes after the Perinatal Period

Should a condition originate in the perinatal period, and continue throughout the life of the patient, the perinatal code should continue to be used regardless of the patient's age.

5) Birth process or community acquired conditions

If a newborn has a condition that may be either due to the birth process or community acquired and the documentation does not indicate which it is, the default is due to the birth process and the code from Chapter 16 should be used. If the condition is community-acquired, a code from Chapter 16 should not be assigned.

6) Code all clinically significant conditions

All clinically significant conditions noted on routine newborn examination should be coded. A condition is clinically significant if it requires:

- clinical evaluation; or
- therapeutic treatment; or
- diagnostic procedures; or
- extended length of hospital stay; or
- increased nursing care and/or monitoring; or
- has implications for future health care needs

Note: The perinatal guidelines listed above are the same as the general coding guidelines for "additional diagnoses", except for the final point regarding implications for future health care needs. Codes should be assigned for conditions that have been specified by the provider as having implications for future health care needs.

b. Observation and Evaluation of Newborns for Suspected Conditions not Found

1) Assign a code from category Z05, Observation and evaluation of newborns and infants for suspected conditions ruled out, to identify those instances when a healthy newborn is evaluated for a suspected condition that is determined after study not to be present. Do not use a code from category Z05 when the patient has identified signs or symptoms of a suspected problem; in such cases code the sign or symptom.

2) A code from category Z05 may also be assigned as a principal or first-listed code for readmissions or encounters when the code from category Z38 code no longer applies. Codes from category Z05 are for use only for healthy newborns and infants for which no condition after study is found to be present.

3) Z05 on a birth record

A code from category Z05 is to be used as a secondary code after the code from category Z38, Liveborn infants according to place of birth and type of delivery.

c. Coding Additional Perinatal Diagnoses

1) Assigning codes for conditions that require treatment

Assign codes for conditions that require treatment or further investigation, prolong the length of stay, or require resource utilization.

2) Codes for conditions specified as having implications for future health care needs

Assign codes for conditions that have been specified by the provider as having implications for future health care needs.

Note: This guideline should not be used for adult patients.

d. Prematurity and Fetal Growth Retardation

Providers utilize different criteria in determining prematurity. A code for prematurity should not be assigned unless it is documented. Assignment of codes in categories PØ5, Disorders of newborn related to slow fetal growth and fetal malnutrition, and PØ7, Disorders of newborn related to short gestation and low birth weight, not elsewhere classified, should be based on the recorded birth weight and estimated gestational age. Codes from category PØ5 should not be assigned with codes from category PØ7.

When both birth weight and gestational age are available, two codes from category PØ7 should be assigned, with the code for birth weight sequenced before the code for gestational age.

e. Low birth weight and immaturity status

Codes from category PØ7, Disorders of newborn related to short gestation and low birth weight, not elsewhere classified, are for use for a child or adult who was premature or had a low birth weight as a newborn and this is affecting the patient's current health status.

See Section I.C.21. Factors influencing health status and contact with health services, Status.

f. Bacterial Sepsis of Newborn

Category P36, Bacterial sepsis of newborn, includes congenital sepsis. If a perinate is documented as having sepsis without documentation of congenital or community acquired, the default is congenital and a code from category P36 should be assigned. If the P36 code includes the causal organism, an additional code from category B95, Streptococcus, Staphylococcus, and Enterococcus as the cause of diseases classified elsewhere, or B96, Other bacterial agents as the cause of diseases classified elsewhere, should not be assigned. If the P36 code does not include the causal organism, assign an additional code from category B96. If applicable, use additional codes to identify severe sepsis (R65.2-) and any associated acute organ dysfunction.

g. Stillbirth

Code P95, Stillbirth, is only for use in institutions that maintain separate records for stillbirths. No other code should be used with P95. Code P95 should not be used on the mother's record.

CHAPTER 16 (PØØ-P96)

CHAPTER 16

CERTAIN CONDITIONS ORIGINATING IN THE PERINATAL PERIOD (P00-P96)

Note: Codes from this chapter are for use on newborn records only, never on maternal records.

Includes   conditions that have their origin in the fetal or perinatal period (before birth through the first 28 days after birth) even if morbidity occurs later

Excludes2   congenital malformations, deformations and chromosomal abnormalities (Q00-Q99)
endocrine, nutritional and metabolic diseases (E00-E88)
injury, poisoning and certain other consequences of external causes (S00-T88)
neoplasms (C00-D49)
tetanus neonatorum (A33)

This chapter contains the following blocks:

P00-P04	Newborn affected by maternal factors and by complications of pregnancy, labor, and delivery
P05-P08	Disorders of newborns related to length of gestation and fetal growth
P09	Abnormal findings on neonatal screening
P10-P15	Birth trauma
P19-P29	Respiratory and cardiovascular disorders specific to the perinatal period
P35-P39	Infections specific to the perinatal period
P50-P61	Hemorrhagic and hematological disorders of newborn
P70-P74	Transitory endocrine and metabolic disorders specific to newborn
P76-P78	Digestive system disorders of newborn
P80-P83	Conditions involving the integument and temperature regulation of newborn
P84	Other problems with newborn
P90-P96	Other disorders originating in the perinatal period

NEWBORN AFFECTED BY MATERNAL FACTORS AND BY COMPLICATIONS OF PREGNANCY, LABOR, AND DELIVERY (P00–P04)

Note: These codes are for use when the listed maternal conditions are specified as the cause of confirmed morbidity or potential morbidity which have their origin in the perinatal period (before birth through the first 28 days after birth). ◀▪▪

● **P00**   **Newborn affected by maternal conditions that may be unrelated to present pregnancy** ◀▪▪

Code first any current condition in newborn

Excludes2   encounter for observation of newborn for suspected diseases and conditions ruled out (Z05.-) ◀
newborn affected by maternal complications of pregnancy (P01.-) ◀
newborn affected by maternal endocrine and metabolic disorders (P70–P74)
newborn affected by noxious substances transmitted via placenta or breast milk (P04.-)

P00.0   **Newborn affected by maternal hypertensive disorders** ◀▪▪
Newborn affected by maternal conditions classifiable to O10-O11, O13-O16 ◀▪▪

P00.1   **Newborn affected by maternal renal and urinary tract diseases** ◀▪▪
Newborn affected by maternal conditions classifiable to N00-N39 ◀▪▪

P00.2   **Newborn affected by maternal infectious and parasitic diseases** ◀▪▪
Newborn affected by maternal infectious disease classifiable to A00-B99, J09 and J10 ◀▪▪

Excludes1   infections specific to the perinatal period (P35-P39)
maternal genital tract or other localized infections (P00.8)

P00.3   **Newborn affected by other maternal circulatory and respiratory diseases** ◀▪▪
Newborn affected by maternal conditions classifiable to I00-I99, J00-J99, Q20-Q34 and not included in P00.0, P00.2 ◀▪▪

P00.4   **Newborn affected by maternal nutritional disorders** ◀▪▪
Newborn affected by maternal disorders classifiable to E40-E64 ◀▪▪
Maternal malnutrition NOS

P00.5   **Newborn affected by maternal injury** ◀▪▪
Newborn affected by maternal conditions classifiable to O9A.2- ◀▪▪

P00.6   **Newborn affected by surgical procedure on mother** ◀▪▪
Newborn affected by amniocentesis ◀▪▪

Excludes1   Cesarean delivery for present delivery (P03.4)
damage to placenta from amniocentesis, cesarean delivery or surgical induction (P02.1)
previous surgery to uterus or pelvic organs (P03.89)

Excludes2   newborn affected by complication of (fetal) intrauterine procedure (P96.5)

P00.7   **Newborn affected by other medical procedures on mother, not elsewhere classified** ◀▪▪
Newborn affected by radiation to mother ◀▪▪

Excludes1   damage to placenta from amniocentesis, cesarean delivery or surgical induction (P02.1)
newborn affected by other complications of labor and delivery (P03.-)

● **P00.8**   **Newborn affected by other maternal conditions** ◀▪▪

P00.81   **Newborn affected by periodontal disease in mother** ◀▪▪

P00.89   **Newborn affected by other maternal conditions** ◀▪▪
Newborn affected by conditions classifiable to T80-T88 ◀▪▪
Newborn affected by maternal genital tract or other localized infections ◀▪▪
Newborn affected by maternal systemic lupus erythematosus ◀▪▪

P00.9   **Newborn affected by unspecified maternal condition** ◀▪▪

● **P01**   **Newborn affected by maternal complications of pregnancy** ◀▪▪

Code first any current condition in newborn

Excludes2   encounter for observation of newborn for suspected diseases and conditions ruled out (Z05.-) ◀

P01.0   **Newborn affected by incompetent cervix** ◀▪▪

P01.1   **Newborn affected by premature rupture of membranes** ◀▪▪

P01.2   **Newborn affected by oligohydramnios** ◀▪▪

Excludes1   oligohydramnios due to premature rupture of membranes (P01.1)

P01.3   **Newborn affected by polyhydramnios** ◀▪▪
Excess of amniotic fluid, usually > 2000 mL
Newborn affected by hydramnios ◀▪▪

P01.4   **Newborn affected by ectopic pregnancy** ◀▪▪
Newborn affected by abdominal pregnancy ◀▪▪

P01.5   **Newborn affected by multiple pregnancy** ◀▪▪
Newborn affected by triplet (pregnancy) ◀▪▪
Newborn affected by twin (pregnancy) ◀▪▪

P01.6   **Newborn affected by maternal death** ◀▪▪

P01.7   **Newborn affected by malpresentation before labor** ◀▪▪
Newborn affected by breech presentation before labor ◀▪▪
Newborn affected by external version before labor ◀▪▪
Newborn affected by face presentation before labor ◀▪▪
Newborn affected by transverse lie before labor ◀▪▪
Newborn affected by unstable lie before labor ◀▪▪

P01.8   **Newborn affected by other maternal complications of pregnancy** ◀▪▪

P01.9   **Newborn affected by maternal complication of pregnancy, unspecified** ◀▪▪

● P02 Newborn affected by complications of placenta, cord and membranes ⬅

Code first any current condition in newborn

Excludes2 encounter for observation of newborn for suspected diseases and conditions ruled out (Z05.-) ◀

P02.0 Newborn affected by placenta previa ⬅

P02.1 Newborn affected by other forms of placental separation and hemorrhage ⬅

Newborn affected by abruptio placenta ⬅
Newborn affected by accidental hemorrhage ⬅
Newborn affected by antepartum hemorrhage ⬅
Newborn affected by damage to placenta from amniocentesis, cesarean delivery or surgical induction ⬅
Newborn affected by maternal blood loss ⬅
Newborn affected by premature separation of placenta ⬅

● P02.2 Newborn affected by other and unspecified morphological and functional abnormalities of placenta ⬅

P02.20 Newborn affected by unspecified morphological and functional abnormalities of placenta ⬅

P02.29 Newborn affected by other morphological and functional abnormalities of placenta ⬅

Newborn affected by placental dysfunction ⬅
Newborn affected by placental infarction ⬅
Newborn affected by placental insufficiency ⬅

P02.3 Newborn affected by placental transfusion syndromes ⬅

Newborn affected by placental and cord abnormalities resulting in twin-to-twin or other transplacental transfusion ⬅

P02.4 Newborn affected by prolapsed cord ⬅

P02.5 Newborn affected by other compression of umbilical cord ⬅

Newborn affected by umbilical cord (tightly) around neck ⬅
Newborn affected by entanglement of umbilical cord ⬅
Newborn affected by knot in umbilical cord ⬅

● P02.6 Newborn affected by other and unspecified conditions of umbilical cord ⬅

P02.60 Newborn affected by unspecified conditions of umbilical cord ⬅

P02.69 Newborn affected by other conditions of umbilical cord ⬅

Newborn affected by short umbilical cord ⬅
Newborn affected by vasa previa ⬅

Excludes1 newborn affected by single umbilical artery (Q27.0)

P02.7 Newborn affected by chorioamnionitis ⬅

Inflammation of chorion and amnion
Newborn affected by amnionitis ⬅
Newborn affected by membranitis ⬅
Newborn affected by placentitis ⬅

P02.8 Newborn affected by other abnormalities of membranes ⬅

P02.9 Newborn affected by abnormality of membranes, unspecified ⬅

● P03 Newborn affected by other complications of labor and delivery ⬅

Code first any current condition in newborn

Excludes2 encounter for observation of newborn for suspected diseases and conditions ruled out (Z05.-) ◀

P03.0 Newborn affected by breech delivery and extraction ⬅

P03.1 Newborn affected by other malpresentation, malposition and disproportion during labor and delivery ⬅

Newborn affected by contracted pelvis ⬅
Newborn affected by conditions classifiable to O64-O66 ⬅
Newborn affected by persistent occipitoposterior ⬅
Newborn affected by transverse lie ⬅

P03.2 Newborn affected by forceps delivery ⬅

P03.3 Newborn affected by delivery by vacuum extractor [ventouse] ⬅

P03.4 Newborn affected by Cesarean delivery ⬅

P03.5 Newborn affected by precipitate delivery ⬅

Newborn affected by rapid second stage ⬅

P03.6 Newborn affected by abnormal uterine contractions ⬅

Newborn affected by conditions classifiable to O62.-, except O62.3 ⬅
Newborn affected by hypertonic labor ⬅
Newborn affected by uterine inertia ⬅

● P03.8 Newborn affected by other specified complications of labor and delivery ⬅

● P03.81 Newborn affected by abnormality in fetal (intrauterine) heart rate or rhythm ⬅

Excludes1 neonatal cardiac dysrhythmia (P29.1-)

P03.810 Newborn affected by abnormality in fetal (intrauterine) heart rate or rhythm before the onset of labor ⬅

P03.811 Newborn affected by abnormality in fetal (intrauterine) heart rate or rhythm during labor ⬅

P03.819 Newborn affected by abnormality in fetal (intrauterine) heart rate or rhythm, unspecified as to time of onset ⬅

P03.82 Meconium passage during delivery

Excludes1 meconium aspiration (P24.00, P24.01)
meconium staining (P96.83)

P03.89 Newborn affected by other specified complications of labor and delivery ⬅

Newborn affected by abnormality of maternal soft tissues ⬅
Newborn affected by conditions classifiable to O60-O75 and by procedures used in labor and delivery not included in P02.- and P03.0-P03.6 ⬅
Newborn affected by induction of labor ⬅

P03.9 Newborn affected by complication of labor and delivery, unspecified ⬅

● P04 Newborn affected by noxious substances transmitted via placenta or breast milk ⬅

Includes nonteratogenic effects of substances transmitted via placenta

Excludes2 congenital malformations (Q00-Q99)
encounter for observation of newborn for suspected diseases and conditions ruled out (Z05.-) ◀
neonatal jaundice from excessive hemolysis due to drugs or toxins transmitted from mother (P58.4)
newborn in contact with and (suspected) exposures hazardous to health not transmitted via placenta or breast milk (Z77.-)

P04.0 Newborn affected by maternal anesthesia and analgesia in pregnancy, labor and delivery ⬅

Newborn affected by reactions and intoxications from maternal opiates and tranquilizers administered during labor and delivery ⬅

P04.1 Newborn affected by other maternal medication ⬅

Newborn affected by cancer chemotherapy ⬅
Newborn affected by cytotoxic drugs ⬅

Excludes1 dysmorphism due to warfarin (Q86.2)
fetal hydantoin syndrome (Q86.1)
maternal use of drugs of addiction (P04.4-)

CHAPTER 16 (P00-P96)

P04.2 Newborn affected by maternal use of tobacco
Newborn affected by exposure in utero to tobacco smoke

Excludes2 newborn exposure to environmental tobacco smoke (P96.81)

P04.3 Newborn affected by maternal use of alcohol

Excludes1 fetal alcohol syndrome (Q86.0)

● P04.4 Newborn affected by maternal use of drugs of addiction

P04.41 Newborn affected by maternal use of cocaine
'Crack baby'

P04.49 Newborn affected by maternal use of other drugs of addiction

Excludes2 newborn affected by maternal anesthesia and analgesia (P04.0)
withdrawal symptoms from maternal use of drugs of addiction (P96.1)

P04.5 Newborn affected by maternal use of nutritional chemical substances

P04.6 Newborn affected by maternal exposure to environmental chemical substances

P04.8 Newborn affected by other maternal noxious substances

P04.9 Newborn affected by maternal noxious substance, unspecified

OGCR Section I.C.16.d.

Prematurity and Fetal Growth Retardation

Providers utilize different criteria in determining prematurity. A code for prematurity should not be assigned unless it is documented. Assignment of codes in categories P05, Disorders of newborn related to slow fetal growth and fetal malnutrition, and P07, Disorders of newborn related to short gestation and low birth weight, not elsewhere classified, should be based on the recorded birth weight and estimated gestational age. Codes from category P05 should not be assigned with codes from category P07.

When both birth weight and gestational age are available, two codes from category P07 should be assigned, with the code for birth weight sequenced before the code for gestational age.

A code from P05 and codes from P07.2 and P07.3 may be used to specify weeks of gestation as documented by the provider in the record.

DISORDERS OF NEWBORN RELATED TO LENGTH OF GESTATION AND FETAL GROWTH (P05-P08)

● P05 Disorders of newborn related to slow fetal growth and fetal malnutrition

● P05.0 Newborn light for gestational age
Newborn light-for-dates
Weight below but length above 10th percentile for gestational age

P05.00 Newborn light for gestational age, unspecified weight

P05.01 Newborn light for gestational age, less than 500 grams

P05.02 Newborn light for gestational age, 500-749 grams

P05.03 Newborn light for gestational age, 750-999 grams

P05.04 Newborn light for gestational age, 1000-1249 grams

P05.05 Newborn light for gestational age, 1250-1499 grams

P05.06 Newborn light for gestational age, 1500-1749 grams

P05.07 Newborn light for gestational age, 1750-1999 grams

P05.08 Newborn light for gestational age, 2000-2499 grams

P05.09 Newborn light for gestational age, 2500 grams and over
Newborn light for gestational age, other

● P05.1 Newborn small for gestational age
Newborn small-and-light-for-dates
Newborn small-for-dates
Weight and length below 10th percentile for gestational age

P05.10 Newborn small for gestational age, unspecified weight

P05.11 Newborn small for gestational age, less than 500 grams

P05.12 Newborn small for gestational age, 500-749 grams

P05.13 Newborn small for gestational age, 750-999 grams

P05.14 Newborn small for gestational age, 1000-1249 grams

P05.15 Newborn small for gestational age, 1250-1499 grams

P05.16 Newborn small for gestational age, 1500-1749 grams

P05.17 Newborn small for gestational age, 1750-1999 grams

P05.18 Newborn small for gestational age, 2000-2499 grams

P05.19 Newborn small for gestational age, other
Newborn small for gestational age, 2500 grams and over

P05.2 Newborn affected by fetal (intrauterine) malnutrition not light or small for gestational age
Infant, not light or small for gestational age, showing signs of fetal malnutrition, such as dry, peeling skin and loss of subcutaneous tissue

Excludes1 newborn affected by fetal malnutrition with light for gestational age (P05.0-)
newborn affected by fetal malnutrition with small for gestational age (P05.1-)

P05.9 Newborn affected by slow intrauterine growth, unspecified
Newborn affected by fetal growth retardation NOS

● P07 Disorders of newborn related to short gestation and low birth weight, not elsewhere classified

Note: When both birth weight and gestational age of the newborn are available, both should be coded with birth weight sequenced before gestational age.

Includes the listed conditions, without further specification, as the cause of morbidity or additional care, in newborn

● P07.0 Extremely low birth weight newborn
Newborn birth weight 999 g. or less

Excludes1 low birth weight due to slow fetal growth and fetal malnutrition (P05.-)

P07.00 Extremely low birth weight newborn, unspecified weight

P07.01 Extremely low birth weight newborn, less than 500 grams

P07.02 Extremely low birth weight newborn, 500-749 grams

P07.03 Extremely low birth weight newborn, 750-999 grams

CHAPTER 16 (P00-P96)

● **P07.1 Other low birth weight newborn**
Newborn birth weight 1000-2499 g.
Excludes1 low birth weight due to slow fetal growth and fetal malnutrition (P05.-) ◀

P07.10 Other low birth weight newborn, unspecified weight

P07.14 Other low birth weight newborn, 1000-1249 grams

P07.15 Other low birth weight newborn, 1250-1499 grams

P07.16 Other low birth weight newborn, 1500-1749 grams

P07.17 Other low birth weight newborn, 1750-1999 grams

P07.18 Other low birth weight newborn, 2000-2499 grams

● **P07.2 Extreme immaturity of newborn**
Less than 28 completed weeks (less than 196 completed days) of gestation

P07.20 Extreme immaturity of newborn, unspecified weeks of gestation
Gestational age less than 28 completed weeks NOS

P07.21 Extreme immaturity of newborn, gestational age less than 23 completed weeks
Extreme immaturity of newborn, gestational age less than 23 weeks, 0 days

P07.22 Extreme immaturity of newborn, gestational age 23 completed weeks
Extreme immaturity of newborn, gestational age 23 weeks, 0 days through 23 weeks, 6 days

P07.23 Extreme immaturity of newborn, gestational age 24 completed weeks
Extreme immaturity of newborn, gestational age 24 weeks, 0 days through 24 weeks, 6 days

P07.24 Extreme immaturity of newborn, gestational age 25 completed weeks
Extreme immaturity of newborn, gestational age 25 weeks, 0 days through 25 weeks, 6 days

P07.25 Extreme immaturity of newborn, gestational age 26 completed weeks
Extreme immaturity of newborn, gestational age 26 weeks, 0 days through 26 weeks, 6 days

P07.26 Extreme immaturity of newborn, gestational age 27 completed weeks
Extreme immaturity of newborn, gestational age 27 weeks, 0 days through 27 weeks, 6 days

● **P07.3 Preterm [premature] newborn [other]**
28 completed weeks or more but less than 37 completed weeks (196 completed days but less than 259 completed days) of gestation
Prematurity NOS

P07.30 Preterm newborn, unspecified weeks of gestation

P07.31 Preterm newborn, gestational age 28 completed weeks
Preterm newborn, gestational age 28 weeks, 0 days through 28 weeks, 6 days

P07.32 Preterm newborn, gestational age 29 completed weeks
Preterm newborn, gestational age 29 weeks, 0 days through 29 weeks, 6 days

P07.33 Preterm newborn, gestational age 30 completed weeks
Preterm newborn, gestational age 30 weeks, 0 days through 30 weeks, 6 days

P07.34 Preterm newborn, gestational age 31 completed weeks
Preterm newborn, gestational age 31 weeks, 0 days through 31 weeks, 6 days

P07.35 Preterm newborn, gestational age 32 completed weeks
Preterm newborn, gestational age 32 weeks, 0 days through 32 weeks, 6 days

P07.36 Preterm newborn, gestational age 33 completed weeks
Preterm newborn, gestational age 33 weeks, 0 days through 33 weeks, 6 days

P07.37 Preterm newborn, gestational age 34 completed weeks
Preterm newborn, gestational age 34 weeks, 0 days through 34 weeks, 6 days

P07.38 Preterm newborn, gestational age 35 completed weeks
Preterm newborn, gestational age 35 weeks, 0 days through 35 weeks, 6 days

P07.39 Preterm newborn, gestational age 36 completed weeks
Preterm newborn, gestational age 36 weeks, 0 days through 36 weeks, 6 days

● **P08 Disorders of newborn related to long gestation and high birth weight**
Note: When both birth weight and gestational age of the newborn are available, priority of assignment should be given to birth weight.
Includes the listed conditions, without further specification, as causes of morbidity or additional care, in newborn

P08.0 Exceptionally large newborn baby
Usually implies a birth weight of 4500 g. or more
Excludes1 syndrome of infant of diabetic mother (P70.1)
syndrome of infant of mother with gestational diabetes (P70.0)

P08.1 Other heavy for gestational age newborn
Other newborn heavy- or large-for-dates regardless of period of gestation
Usually implies a birth weight of 4000 g. to 4499 g.
Excludes1 newborn with a birth weight of 4500 or more (P08.0)
syndrome of infant of diabetic mother (P70.1)
syndrome of infant of mother with gestational diabetes (P70.0)

● **P08.2 Late newborn, not heavy for gestational age**

P08.21 Post-term newborn
Newborn with gestation period over 40 completed weeks to 42 completed weeks

P08.22 Prolonged gestation of newborn
Newborn with gestation period over 42 completed weeks (294 days or more), not heavy- or large-for-dates
Postmaturity NOS

ABNORMAL FINDINGS ON NEONATAL SCREENING (P09)

P09 Abnormal findings on neonatal screening
Use additional code to identify signs, symptoms and conditions associated with the screening
Excludes2 nonspecific serologic evidence of human immunodeficiency virus [HIV] (R75)

CHAPTER 16 (P00-P96)

BIRTH TRAUMA (P10-P15)

● **P10 Intracranial laceration and hemorrhage due to birth injury**
Excludes1 intracranial hemorrhage of newborn NOS (P52.9)
intracranial hemorrhage of newborn due to anoxia or hypoxia (P52.-)
nontraumatic intracranial hemorrhage of newborn (P52.-)

P10.0 Subdural hemorrhage due to birth injury
Subdural hematoma (localized) due to birth injury
Excludes1 subdural hemorrhage accompanying tentorial tear (P10.4)

P10.1 Cerebral hemorrhage due to birth injury

P10.2 Intraventricular hemorrhage due to birth injury

P10.3 Subarachnoid hemorrhage due to birth injury

P10.4 Tentorial tear due to birth injury
Pertaining to tentorium of cerebellum (extension of dura mater that separates cerebellum from inferior portion of occipital lobes)

P10.8 Other intracranial lacerations and hemorrhages due to birth injury

P10.9 Unspecified intracranial laceration and hemorrhage due to birth injury

Item 16-1 The **peripheral nervous system** consists of 31 pairs of spinal nerves, 12 pairs of cranial nerves, and the autonomic nerves, which are divided into the parasympathetic and sympathetic nerves. The cranial nerves are: olfactory (I), optic (II), oculomotor (III), trochlear (IV), trigeminal (V), abducens (VI), facial (VII), vestibulocochlear (VIII), glossopharyngeal (IX), vagus (X), accessory (XI), and hypoglossal (XII).

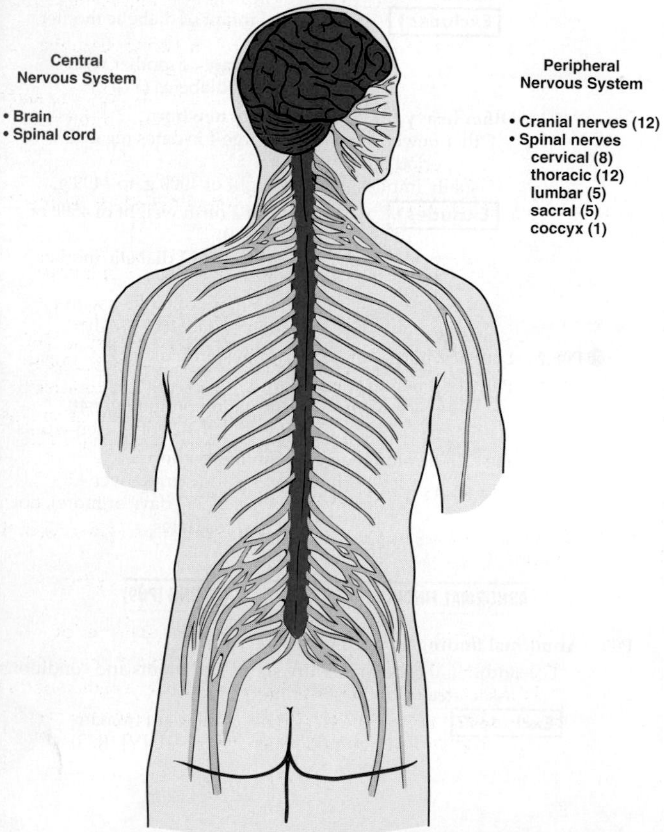

Figure 16-1 The central nervous system consists of the brain and spinal cord. The peripheral nervous system consists of nerves that lie outside the skull and spinal cord. (From Stoy: Mosby's EMT-Basic Textbook, ed 2, St. Louis, Mosby, 2007)

● **P11 Other birth injuries to central nervous system**

P11.0 Cerebral edema due to birth injury

P11.1 Other specified brain damage due to birth injury

P11.2 Unspecified brain damage due to birth injury

P11.3 Birth injury to facial nerve
Facial palsy due to birth injury

P11.4 Birth injury to other cranial nerves

P11.5 Birth injury to spine and spinal cord
Fracture of spine due to birth injury

P11.9 Birth injury to central nervous system, unspecified

● **P12 Birth injury to scalp**

P12.0 Cephalhematoma due to birth injury

P12.1 Chignon (from vacuum extraction) due to birth injury

P12.2 Epicranial subaponeurotic hemorrhage due to birth injury
Subgaleal hemorrhage

P12.3 Bruising of scalp due to birth injury

P12.4 Injury of scalp of newborn due to monitoring equipment
Sampling incision of scalp of newborn
Scalp clip (electrode) injury of newborn

● **P12.8 Other birth injuries to scalp**

P12.81 Caput succedaneum

P12.89 Other birth injuries to scalp

P12.9 Birth injury to scalp, unspecified

● **P13 Birth injury to skeleton**
Excludes2 birth injury to spine (P11.5)

P13.0 Fracture of skull due to birth injury

P13.1 Other birth injuries to skull
Excludes1 cephalhematoma (P12.0)

P13.2 Birth injury to femur

P13.3 Birth injury to other long bones

P13.4 Fracture of clavicle due to birth injury

P13.8 Birth injuries to other parts of skeleton

P13.9 Birth injury to skeleton, unspecified

● **P14 Birth injury to peripheral nervous system**

P14.0 Erb's paralysis due to birth injury

P14.1 Klumpke's paralysis due to birth injury

P14.2 Phrenic nerve paralysis due to birth injury

P14.3 Other brachial plexus birth injuries

P14.8 Birth injuries to other parts of peripheral nervous system

P14.9 Birth injury to peripheral nervous system, unspecified

● **P15 Other birth injuries**

P15.0 Birth injury to liver
Rupture of liver due to birth injury

P15.1 Birth injury to spleen
Rupture of spleen due to birth injury

P15.2 Sternomastoid injury due to birth injury

P15.3 Birth injury to eye
Subconjunctival hemorrhage due to birth injury
Traumatic glaucoma due to birth injury

P15.4 Birth injury to face
Facial congestion due to birth injury

P15.5 Birth injury to external genitalia

P15.6 Subcutaneous fat necrosis due to birth injury

P15.8 Other specified birth injuries

P15.9 Birth injury, unspecified

RESPIRATORY AND CARDIOVASCULAR DISORDERS SPECIFIC TO THE PERINATAL PERIOD (P19-P29)

● **P19 Metabolic acidemia in newborn**
Includes metabolic acidemia in newborn
P19.0 Metabolic acidemia in newborn first noted before onset of labor
P19.1 Metabolic acidemia in newborn first noted during labor
P19.2 Metabolic acidemia noted at birth
P19.9 Metabolic acidemia, unspecified

● **P22 Respiratory distress of newborn**
Excludes1 respiratory arrest of newborn (P28.81)
respiratory failure of newborn NOS (P28.5)
P22.0 Respiratory distress syndrome of newborn
Cardiorespiratory distress syndrome of newborn
Hyaline membrane disease
Idiopathic respiratory distress syndrome [IRDS or RDS] of newborn
Pulmonary hypoperfusion syndrome
Respiratory distress syndrome, type I
P22.1 Transient tachypnea of newborn
Idiopathic tachypnea of newborn
Respiratory distress syndrome, type II
Wet lung syndrome
P22.8 Other respiratory distress of newborn
P22.9 Respiratory distress of newborn, unspecified

● **P23 Congenital pneumonia**
Includes infective pneumonia acquired in utero or during birth
Excludes1 neonatal pneumonia resulting from aspiration (P24.-)
P23.0 Congenital pneumonia due to viral agent
Use additional code (B97) to identify organism
Excludes1 congenital rubella pneumonitis (P35.0)
P23.1 Congenital pneumonia due to Chlamydia
P23.2 Congenital pneumonia due to staphylococcus
P23.3 Congenital pneumonia due to streptococcus, group B
P23.4 Congenital pneumonia due to Escherichia coli
P23.5 Congenital pneumonia due to Pseudomonas
P23.6 Congenital pneumonia due to other bacterial agents
Congenital pneumonia due to Hemophilus influenzae
Congenital pneumonia due to Klebsiella pneumoniae
Congenital pneumonia due to Mycoplasma
Congenital pneumonia due to Streptococcus, except group B
Use additional code (B95-B96) to identify organism
P23.8 Congenital pneumonia due to other organisms
P23.9 Congenital pneumonia, unspecified

● **P24 Neonatal aspiration**
Includes aspiration in utero and during delivery
● **P24.0 Meconium aspiration**
Excludes1 meconium passage (without aspiration) during delivery (P03.82)
meconium staining (P96.83)
P24.00 Meconium aspiration without respiratory symptoms
Meconium aspiration NOS
P24.01 Meconium aspiration with respiratory symptoms
Meconium aspiration pneumonia
Meconium aspiration pneumonitis
Meconium aspiration syndrome NOS
Use additional code to identify any secondary pulmonary hypertension, if applicable (I27.2)
● **P24.1 Neonatal aspiration of (clear) amniotic fluid and mucus**
Neonatal aspiration of liquor (amnii)
P24.10 Neonatal aspiration of (clear) amniotic fluid and mucus without respiratory symptoms
Neonatal aspiration of amniotic fluid and mucus NOS
P24.11 Neonatal aspiration of (clear) amniotic fluid and mucus with respiratory symptoms
Neonatal aspiration of amniotic fluid and mucus with pneumonia
Neonatal aspiration of amniotic fluid and mucus with pneumonitis
Use additional code to identify any secondary pulmonary hypertension, if applicable (I27.2)
● **P24.2 Neonatal aspiration of blood**
P24.20 Neonatal aspiration of blood without respiratory symptoms
Neonatal aspiration of blood NOS
P24.21 Neonatal aspiration of blood with respiratory symptoms
Neonatal aspiration of blood with pneumonia
Neonatal aspiration of blood with pneumonitis
Use additional code to identify any secondary pulmonary hypertension, if applicable (I27.2)
● **P24.3 Neonatal aspiration of milk and regurgitated food**
Neonatal aspiration of stomach contents
P24.30 Neonatal aspiration of milk and regurgitated food without respiratory symptoms
Neonatal aspiration of milk and regurgitated food NOS
P24.31 Neonatal aspiration of milk and regurgitated food with respiratory symptoms
Neonatal aspiration of milk and regurgitated food with pneumonia
Neonatal aspiration of milk and regurgitated food with pneumonitis
Use additional code to identify any secondary pulmonary hypertension, if applicable (I27.2)
● **P24.8 Other neonatal aspiration**
P24.80 Other neonatal aspiration without respiratory symptoms
Neonatal aspiration NEC
P24.81 Other neonatal aspiration with respiratory symptoms
Neonatal aspiration pneumonia NEC
Neonatal aspiration with pneumonitis NEC
Neonatal aspiration with pneumonia NOS
Neonatal aspiration with pneumonitis NOS
Use additional code to identify any secondary pulmonary hypertension, if applicable (I27.2)
P24.9 Neonatal aspiration, unspecified

● **P25 Interstitial emphysema and related conditions originating in the perinatal period**
P25.0 Interstitial emphysema originating in the perinatal period
P25.1 Pneumothorax originating in the perinatal period
P25.2 Pneumomediastinum originating in the perinatal period
P25.3 Pneumopericardium originating in the perinatal period
P25.8 Other conditions related to interstitial emphysema originating in the perinatal period

● **P26 Pulmonary hemorrhage originating in the perinatal period**
Excludes1 acute idiopathic hemorrhage in infants over 28 days old (R04.81)
P26.0 Tracheobronchial hemorrhage originating in the perinatal period
P26.1 Massive pulmonary hemorrhage originating in the perinatal period
P26.8 Other pulmonary hemorrhages originating in the perinatal period
P26.9 Unspecified pulmonary hemorrhage originating in the perinatal period

● **P27 Chronic respiratory disease originating in the perinatal period**
Excludes1 respiratory distress of newborn (P22.0-P22.9)
P27.0 Wilson-Mikity syndrome
Pulmonary dysmaturity
P27.1 Bronchopulmonary dysplasia originating in the perinatal period
P27.8 Other chronic respiratory diseases originating in the perinatal period
Congenital pulmonary fibrosis
Ventilator lung in newborn
P27.9 Unspecified chronic respiratory disease originating in the perinatal period

● **P28 Other respiratory conditions originating in the perinatal period**
Excludes1 congenital malformations of the respiratory system (Q30-Q34)
P28.0 Primary atelectasis of newborn
Failure of lungs to expand properly at birth
Primary failure to expand terminal respiratory units
Pulmonary hypoplasia associated with short gestation
Pulmonary immaturity NOS
● **P28.1 Other and unspecified atelectasis of newborn**
P28.10 Unspecified atelectasis of newborn
Atelectasis of newborn NOS
P28.11 Resorption atelectasis without respiratory distress syndrome
Excludes1 resorption atelectasis with respiratory distress syndrome (P22.0)
P28.19 Other atelectasis of newborn
Partial atelectasis of newborn
Secondary atelectasis of newborn
P28.2 Cyanotic attacks of newborn
Excludes1 apnea of newborn (P28.3-P28.4)
P28.3 Primary sleep apnea of newborn
Central sleep apnea of newborn
Obstructive sleep apnea of newborn
Sleep apnea of newborn NOS
P28.4 Other apnea of newborn
Apnea of prematurity
Obstructive apnea of newborn
Excludes1 obstructive sleep apnea of newborn (P28.3)
P28.5 Respiratory failure of newborn
Excludes1 respiratory arrest of newborn (P28.81)
respiratory distress of newborn (P22.0-)
● **P28.8 Other specified respiratory conditions of newborn**
P28.81 Respiratory arrest of newborn
P28.89 Other specified respiratory conditions of newborn
Congenital laryngeal stridor
Sniffles in newborn
Snuffles in newborn
Excludes1 early congenital syphilitic rhinitis (A50.05)
P28.9 Respiratory condition of newborn, unspecified
Respiratory depression in newborn

● **P29 Cardiovascular disorders originating in the perinatal period**
Excludes1 congenital malformations of the circulatory system (Q20-Q28)
P29.0 Neonatal cardiac failure
● **P29.1 Neonatal cardiac dysrhythmia**
P29.11 Neonatal tachycardia
P29.12 Neonatal bradycardia
P29.2 Neonatal hypertension
P29.3 Persistent fetal circulation
Delayed closure of ductus arteriosus
(Persistent) pulmonary hypertension of newborn
P29.4 Transient myocardial ischemia in newborn
● **P29.8 Other cardiovascular disorders originating in the perinatal period**
P29.81 Cardiac arrest of newborn
P29.89 Other cardiovascular disorders originating in the perinatal period
P29.9 Cardiovascular disorder originating in the perinatal period, unspecified

INFECTIONS SPECIFIC TO THE PERINATAL PERIOD (P35-P39)

Infections acquired in utero, during birth via the umbilicus, or during the first 28 days after birth
Excludes2 asymptomatic human immunodeficiency virus [HIV] infection status (Z21)
congenital gonococcal infection (A54.-)
congenital pneumonia (P23.-)
congenital syphilis (A50.-)
human immunodeficiency virus [HIV] disease (B20)
infant botulism (A48.51)
infectious diseases not specific to the perinatal period (A00-B99, J09, J10.-)
intestinal infectious disease (A00-A09)
laboratory evidence of human immunodeficiency virus [HIV] (R75)
tetanus neonatorum (A33)

● **P35 Congenital viral diseases**
Includes infections acquired in utero or during birth
P35.0 Congenital rubella syndrome
Congenital rubella pneumonitis
P35.1 Congenital cytomegalovirus infection
Viruses transmitted by multiple routes that cause mild/subclinical infection
P35.2 Congenital herpesviral [herpes simplex] infection
P35.3 Congenital viral hepatitis
P35.8 Other congenital viral diseases
Congenital varicella [chickenpox]
P35.9 Congenital viral disease, unspecified

● **P36 Bacterial sepsis of newborn**
Includes congenital sepsis
Use additional code(s), if applicable, to identify severe sepsis (R65.2-) and associated acute organ dysfunction(s)
P36.0 Sepsis of newborn due to streptococcus, group B
● **P36.1 Sepsis of newborn due to other and unspecified streptococci**
P36.10 Sepsis of newborn due to unspecified streptococci
P36.19 Sepsis of newborn due to other streptococci
P36.2 Sepsis of newborn due to Staphylococcus aureus

● **P36.3 Sepsis of newborn due to other and unspecified staphylococci**
- **P36.30 Sepsis of newborn due to unspecified staphylococci**
- **P36.39 Sepsis of newborn due to other staphylococci**

P36.4 Sepsis of newborn due to Escherichia coli

P36.5 Sepsis of newborn due to anaerobes

P36.8 Other bacterial sepsis of newborn
Use additional code from category B96 to identify organism

P36.9 Bacterial sepsis of newborn, unspecified

● **P37 Other congenital infectious and parasitic diseases**
Excludes2 congenital syphilis (A5Ø.-)
infectious neonatal diarrhea (AØØ-AØ9)
necrotizing enterocolitis in newborn (P77.-)
noninfectious neonatal diarrhea (P78.3)
ophthalmia neonatorum due to gonococcus (A54.31)
tetanus neonatorum (A33)

P37.Ø Congenital tuberculosis

P37.1 Congenital toxoplasmosis
Parasitic infection, often causing mild flu-like illness
Hydrocephalus due to congenital toxoplasmosis

P37.2 Neonatal (disseminated) listeriosis
Acquired transplacentally or during/after parturition in which symptoms are those of sepsis

P37.3 Congenital falciparum malaria

P37.4 Other congenital malaria

P37.5 Neonatal candidiasis

P37.8 Other specified congenital infectious and parasitic diseases

P37.9 Congenital infectious or parasitic disease, unspecified

● **P38 Omphalitis of newborn**
Inflammation of umbilicus
Excludes1 omphalitis not of newborn (LØ8.82)
tetanus omphalitis (A33)
umbilical hemorrhage of newborn (P51.-)

P38.1 Omphalitis with mild hemorrhage

P38.9 Omphalitis without hemorrhage
Omphalitis of newborn NOS

● **P39 Other infections specific to the perinatal period**
Use additional code to identify organism or specific infection

P39.Ø Neonatal infective mastitis
Excludes1 breast engorgement of newborn (P83.4)
noninfective mastitis of newborn (P83.4)

P39.1 Neonatal conjunctivitis and dacryocystitis
Neonatal chlamydial conjunctivitis
Ophthalmia neonatorum NOS
Neonate = newborn
Excludes1 gonococcal conjunctivitis (A54.31)

P39.2 Intra-amniotic infection affecting newborn, not elsewhere classified

P39.3 Neonatal urinary tract infection

P39.4 Neonatal skin infection
Neonatal pyoderma
Excludes1 pemphigus neonatorum (LØØ)
staphylococcal scalded skin syndrome (LØØ)

P39.8 Other specified infections specific to the perinatal period

P39.9 Infection specific to the perinatal period, unspecified

HEMORRHAGIC AND HEMATOLOGICAL DISORDERS OF NEWBORN (P5Ø-P61)

Excludes1 congenital stenosis and stricture of bile ducts (Q44.3)
Crigler-Najjar syndrome (E8Ø.5)
Dubin-Johnson syndrome (E8Ø.6)
Gilbert syndrome (E8Ø.4)
hereditary hemolytic anemias (D55-D58)

● **P5Ø Newborn affected by intrauterine (fetal) blood loss**
Excludes1 congenital anemia from intrauterine (fetal) blood loss (P61.3)

P5Ø.Ø Newborn affected by intrauterine (fetal) blood loss from vasa previa

P5Ø.1 Newborn affected by intrauterine (fetal) blood loss from ruptured cord

P5Ø.2 Newborn affected by intrauterine (fetal) blood loss from placenta

P5Ø.3 Newborn affected by hemorrhage into co-twin

P5Ø.4 Newborn affected by hemorrhage into maternal circulation

P5Ø.5 Newborn affected by intrauterine (fetal) blood loss from cut end of co-twin's cord

P5Ø.8 Newborn affected by other intrauterine (fetal) blood loss

P5Ø.9 Newborn affected by intrauterine (fetal) blood loss, unspecified
Newborn affected by fetal hemorrhage NOS

● **P51 Umbilical hemorrhage of newborn**
Excludes1 omphalitis with mild hemorrhage (P38.1)
umbilical hemorrhage from cut end of co-twins cord (P5Ø.5)

P51.Ø Massive umbilical hemorrhage of newborn

P51.8 Other umbilical hemorrhages of newborn
Slipped umbilical ligature NOS

P51.9 Umbilical hemorrhage of newborn, unspecified

● **P52 Intracranial nontraumatic hemorrhage of newborn**
Includes intracranial hemorrhage due to anoxia or hypoxia
Excludes1 intracranial hemorrhage due to birth injury (P1Ø.-)
intracranial hemorrhage due to other injury (SØ6.-)

P52.Ø Intraventricular (nontraumatic) hemorrhage, grade 1, of newborn
Subependymal hemorrhage (without intraventricular extension)
Bleeding into germinal matrix

P52.1 Intraventricular (nontraumatic) hemorrhage, grade 2, of newborn
Subependymal hemorrhage with intraventricular extension
Bleeding into ventricle

● **P52.2 Intraventricular (nontraumatic) hemorrhage, grade 3 and grade 4, of newborn**
- **P52.21 Intraventricular (nontraumatic) hemorrhage, grade 3, of newborn**
  Subependymal hemorrhage with intraventricular extension with enlargement of ventricle
- **P52.22 Intraventricular (nontraumatic) hemorrhage, grade 4, of newborn**
  Bleeding into cerebral cortex
  Subependymal hemorrhage with intracerebral extension

P52.3 Unspecified intraventricular (nontraumatic) hemorrhage of newborn

CHAPTER 16 (PØØ-P96)

P52.4 **Intracerebral (nontraumatic) hemorrhage of newborn**
P52.5 **Subarachnoid (nontraumatic) hemorrhage of newborn**
P52.6 **Cerebellar (nontraumatic) and posterior fossa hemorrhage of newborn**
P52.8 **Other intracranial (nontraumatic) hemorrhages of newborn**
P52.9 **Intracranial (nontraumatic) hemorrhage of newborn, unspecified**

P53 **Hemorrhagic disease of newborn**
Vitamin K deficiency of newborn

● P54 **Other neonatal hemorrhages**
Excludes1 newborn affected by (intrauterine) blood loss (P5Ø.-)
pulmonary hemorrhage originating in the perinatal period (P26.-)
P54.Ø **Neonatal hematemesis**
Vomiting of blood
Excludes1 neonatal hematemesis due to swallowed maternal blood (P78.2)
P54.1 **Neonatal melena**
Dark-colored feces stained with blood pigments
Excludes1 neonatal melena due to swallowed maternal blood (P78.2)
P54.2 **Neonatal rectal hemorrhage**
P54.3 **Other neonatal gastrointestinal hemorrhage**
P54.4 **Neonatal adrenal hemorrhage**
P54.5 **Neonatal cutaneous hemorrhage**
Neonatal bruising
Neonatal ecchymoses
Neonatal petechiae
Neonatal superficial hematomata
Excludes2 bruising of scalp due to birth injury (P12.3)
cephalhematoma due to birth injury (P12.Ø)
P54.6 **Neonatal vaginal hemorrhage**
Neonatal pseudomenses
P54.8 **Other specified neonatal hemorrhages**
P54.9 **Neonatal hemorrhage, unspecified**

● P55 **Hemolytic disease of newborn**
AKA erythroblastosis fetalis and is due to Rh isoimmunization, result of Rh blood factor incompatibilities between mother (Rh negative) and fetus (Rh positive)
P55.Ø **Rh isoimmunization of newborn**
P55.1 **ABO isoimmunization of newborn**
P55.8 **Other hemolytic diseases of newborn**
P55.9 **Hemolytic disease of newborn, unspecified**

● P56 **Hydrops fetalis due to hemolytic disease**
Caused by maternal sensitization to fetal blood group antigen
Excludes1 hydrops fetalis NOS (P83.2)
P56.Ø **Hydrops fetalis due to isoimmunization**
● P56.9 **Hydrops fetalis due to other and unspecified hemolytic disease**
P56.9Ø **Hydrops fetalis due to unspecified hemolytic disease**
P56.99 **Hydrops fetalis due to other hemolytic disease**

● P57 **Kernicterus**
High levels of bilirubin in blood, with severe neural symptoms
P57.Ø **Kernicterus due to isoimmunization**
P57.8 **Other specified kernicterus**
Excludes1 Crigler-Najjar syndrome (E8Ø.5)
P57.9 **Kernicterus, unspecified**

● P58 **Neonatal jaundice due to other excessive hemolysis**
Excludes1 jaundice due to isoimmunization (P55-P57)
P58.Ø **Neonatal jaundice due to bruising**
P58.1 **Neonatal jaundice due to bleeding**
P58.2 **Neonatal jaundice due to infection**
P58.3 **Neonatal jaundice due to polycythemia**
● P58.4 **Neonatal jaundice due to drugs or toxins transmitted from mother or given to newborn**
Code first *poisoning due to drug or toxin, if applicable (T36-T65 with fifth or sixth character 1-4 or 6)*
Use additional code for adverse effect, if applicable, to identify drug (T36-T5Ø with fifth or sixth character 5)
P58.41 **Neonatal jaundice due to drugs or toxins transmitted from mother**
P58.42 **Neonatal jaundice due to drugs or toxins given to newborn**
P58.5 **Neonatal jaundice due to swallowed maternal blood**
P58.8 **Neonatal jaundice due to other specified excessive hemolysis**
P58.9 **Neonatal jaundice due to excessive hemolysis, unspecified**

● P59 **Neonatal jaundice from other and unspecified causes**
Excludes1 jaundice due to inborn errors of metabolism (E7Ø-E88)
kernicterus (P57.-)
P59.Ø **Neonatal jaundice associated with preterm delivery**
Hyperbilirubinemia of prematurity
Jaundice due to delayed conjugation associated with preterm delivery
P59.1 **Inspissated bile syndrome**
● P59.2 **Neonatal jaundice from other and unspecified hepatocellular damage**
Excludes1 congenital viral hepatitis (P35.3)
P59.2Ø **Neonatal jaundice from unspecified hepatocellular damage**
P59.29 **Neonatal jaundice from other hepatocellular damage**
Neonatal giant cell hepatitis
Neonatal (idiopathic) hepatitis
P59.3 **Neonatal jaundice from breast milk inhibitor**
P59.8 **Neonatal jaundice from other specified causes**
P59.9 **Neonatal jaundice, unspecified**
Neonatal physiological jaundice (intense)(prolonged) NOS

P6Ø **Disseminated intravascular coagulation of newborn**
Defibrination syndrome of newborn

● P61 **Other perinatal hematological disorders**
Excludes1 transient hypogammaglobulinemia of infancy (D8Ø.7)
P61.Ø **Transient neonatal thrombocytopenia**
Lack of sufficient numbers of circulating thrombocytes (platelets)
Neonatal thrombocytopenia due to exchange transfusion
Neonatal thrombocytopenia due to idiopathic maternal thrombocytopenia
Neonatal thrombocytopenia due to isoimmunization
P61.1 **Polycythemia neonatorum**
Neonate = newborn
P61.2 **Anemia of prematurity**
P61.3 **Congenital anemia from fetal blood loss**
P61.4 **Other congenital anemias, not elsewhere classified**
Congenital anemia NOS

CHAPTER 16 (PØØ-P96)

◀ New ◀ Revised ~~deleted~~ Deleted **OGCR** Official Guidelines X Assign placeholder X ● Use Additional Character(s)
Excludes 1 | Excludes 2 | Includes | Use additional | Code first | Code also | Unspecified

P61.5 Transient neonatal neutropenia
Low levels of granulocytic neutrophilic white blood cells
Excludes1 congenital neutropenia (nontransient) (D70.0)

P61.6 Other transient neonatal disorders of coagulation

P61.8 Other specified perinatal hematological disorders

P61.9 Perinatal hematological disorder, unspecified

TRANSITORY ENDOCRINE AND METABOLIC DISORDERS SPECIFIC TO NEWBORN (P70-P74)

Includes transitory endocrine and metabolic disturbances caused by the infant's response to maternal endocrine and metabolic factors, or its adjustment to extrauterine environment

● **P70 Transitory disorders of carbohydrate metabolism specific to newborn**

P70.0 Syndrome of infant of mother with gestational diabetes
Newborn (with hypoglycemia) affected by maternal gestational diabetes
Excludes1 newborn (with hypoglycemia) affected by maternal (pre-existing) diabetes mellitus (P70.1)
syndrome of infant of a diabetic mother (P70.1)

P70.1 Syndrome of infant of a diabetic mother
Newborn (with hypoglycemia) affected by maternal (pre-existing) diabetes mellitus
Excludes1 newborn (with hypoglycemia) affected by maternal gestational diabetes (P70.0)
syndrome of infant of mother with gestational diabetes (P70.0)

P70.2 Neonatal diabetes mellitus

P70.3 Iatrogenic neonatal hypoglycemia

P70.4 Other neonatal hypoglycemia
Transitory neonatal hypoglycemia

P70.8 Other transitory disorders of carbohydrate metabolism of newborn

P70.9 Transitory disorder of carbohydrate metabolism of newborn, unspecified

● **P71 Transitory neonatal disorders of calcium and magnesium metabolism**

P71.0 Cow's milk hypocalcemia in newborn

P71.1 Other neonatal hypocalcemia
Excludes1 neonatal hypoparathyroidism (P71.4)

P71.2 Neonatal hypomagnesemia

P71.3 Neonatal tetany without calcium or magnesium deficiency
Neonatal tetany NOS

P71.4 Transitory neonatal hypoparathyroidism

P71.8 Other transitory neonatal disorders of calcium and magnesium metabolism

P71.9 Transitory neonatal disorder of calcium and magnesium metabolism, unspecified

● **P72 Other transitory neonatal endocrine disorders**
Excludes1 congenital hypothyroidism with or without goiter (E03.0-E03.1)
dyshormogenetic goiter (E07.1)
Pendred's syndrome (E07.1)

P72.0 Neonatal goiter, not elsewhere classified
Transitory congenital goiter with normal functioning

P72.1 Transitory neonatal hyperthyroidism
Neonatal thyrotoxicosis

P72.2 Other transitory neonatal disorders of thyroid function, not elsewhere classified
Transitory neonatal hypothyroidism

P72.8 Other specified transitory neonatal endocrine disorders

P72.9 Transitory neonatal endocrine disorder, unspecified

● **P74 Other transitory neonatal electrolyte and metabolic disturbances**

P74.0 Late metabolic acidosis of newborn
Excludes1 (fetal) metabolic acidosis of newborn (P19)

P74.1 Dehydration of newborn

P74.2 Disturbances of sodium balance of newborn

P74.3 Disturbances of potassium balance of newborn

P74.4 Other transitory electrolyte disturbances of newborn

P74.5 Transitory tyrosinemia of newborn

P74.6 Transitory hyperammonemia of newborn

P74.8 Other transitory metabolic disturbances of newborn
Amino-acid metabolic disorders described as transitory

P74.9 Transitory metabolic disturbance of newborn, unspecified

DIGESTIVE SYSTEM DISORDERS OF NEWBORN (P76-P78)

● **P76 Other intestinal obstruction of newborn**

P76.0 Meconium plug syndrome
Fetal stool obstruction in large intestine, present at birth; may be symptom of organic disease.
Meconium ileus NOS
Excludes1 meconium ileus in cystic fibrosis (E84.11)

P76.1 Transitory ileus of newborn
Temporary obstruction of ileus (small intestine)
Excludes1 Hirschsprung's disease (Q43.1)

P76.2 Intestinal obstruction due to inspissated milk
Being thickened, dried, or made less fluid

P76.8 Other specified intestinal obstruction of newborn
Excludes1 intestinal obstruction classifiable to K56.-

P76.9 Intestinal obstruction of newborn, unspecified

● **P77 Necrotizing enterocolitis of newborn**

P77.1 Stage 1 necrotizing enterocolitis in newborn
Necrotizing enterocolitis without pneumatosis, without perforation

P77.2 Stage 2 necrotizing enterocolitis in newborn
Necrotizing enterocolitis with pneumatosis, without perforation

P77.3 Stage 3 necrotizing enterocolitis in newborn
Necrotizing enterocolitis with perforation
Necrotizing enterocolitis with pneumatosis and perforation

P77.9 Necrotizing enterocolitis in newborn, unspecified
Necrotizing enterocolitis in newborn, NOS

● **P78 Other perinatal digestive system disorders**
Excludes1 cystic fibrosis (E84.0-E84.9)
neonatal gastrointestinal hemorrhages (P54.0-P54.3)

P78.0 Perinatal intestinal perforation
Meconium peritonitis

P78.1 Other neonatal peritonitis
Neonatal peritonitis NOS

P78.2 Neonatal hematemesis and melena due to swallowed maternal blood

P78.3 Noninfective neonatal diarrhea
Neonatal diarrhea NOS

● **P78.8 Other specified perinatal digestive system disorders**

P78.81 Congenital cirrhosis (of liver)

P78.82 Peptic ulcer of newborn

P78.83 Newborn esophageal reflux
Neonatal esophageal reflux

P78.89 Other specified perinatal digestive system disorders

P78.9 Perinatal digestive system disorder, unspecified

CHAPTER 16 (P00-P96)

CONDITIONS INVOLVING THE INTEGUMENT AND TEMPERATURE REGULATION OF NEWBORN (P80-P83)

● **P80 Hypothermia of newborn**

P80.0 Cold injury syndrome
Severe and usually chronic hypothermia associated with a pink flushed appearance, edema and neurological and biochemical abnormalities.
Excludes1 mild hypothermia of newborn (P80.8)

P80.8 Other hypothermia of newborn
Mild hypothermia of newborn

P80.9 Hypothermia of newborn, unspecified

● **P81 Other disturbances of temperature regulation of newborn**

P81.0 Environmental hyperthermia of newborn

P81.8 Other specified disturbances of temperature regulation of newborn

P81.9 Disturbance of temperature regulation of newborn, unspecified
Fever of newborn NOS

● **P83 Other conditions of integument specific to newborn**
Excludes1 congenital malformations of skin and integument (Q80-Q84)
hydrops fetalis due to hemolytic disease (P56.-)
neonatal skin infection (P39.4)
staphylococcal scalded skin syndrome (L00)
Excludes2 cradle cap (L21.0)
diaper [napkin] dermatitis (L22)

P83.0 Sclerema neonatorum
Neonate = newborn

P83.1 Neonatal erythema toxicum
Benign, generalized, transient pustules that become firm vesicles

P83.2 Hydrops fetalis not due to hemolytic disease
Severe, life-threatening problem of severe edema (swelling) as result of too much fluid leaving blood and entering tissue
Hydrops fetalis NOS

● **P83.3 Other and unspecified edema specific to newborn**

P83.30 Unspecified edema specific to newborn

P83.39 Other edema specific to newborn

P83.4 Breast engorgement of newborn
Noninfective mastitis of newborn

P83.5 Congenital hydrocele

P83.6 Umbilical polyp of newborn

P83.8 Other specified conditions of integument specific to newborn
Bronze baby syndrome
Neonatal scleroderma
Urticaria neonatorum

P83.9 Condition of the integument specific to newborn, unspecified

OTHER PROBLEMS WITH NEWBORN (P84)

P84 Other problems with newborn
Acidemia of newborn
Acidosis of newborn
Anoxia of newborn NOS
Asphyxia of newborn NOS
Hypercapnia of newborn
Hypoxemia of newborn
Hypoxia of newborn NOS
Mixed metabolic and respiratory acidosis of newborn
Excludes1 intracranial hemorrhage due to anoxia or hypoxia (P52.-)
hypoxic ischemic encephalopathy [HIE] (P91.6-)
late metabolic acidosis of newborn (P74.0)

OTHER DISORDERS ORIGINATING IN THE PERINATAL PERIOD (P90-P96)

P90 Convulsions of newborn
Excludes1 benign myoclonic epilepsy in infancy (G40.3-)
benign neonatal convulsions (familial) (G40.3-)

● **P91 Other disturbances of cerebral status of newborn**

P91.0 Neonatal cerebral ischemia

P91.1 Acquired periventricular cysts of newborn

P91.2 Neonatal cerebral leukomalacia
Degeneration of white matter adjacent to cerebral ventricles following cerebral hypoxia or brain ischemia in neonates
Periventricular leukomalacia

P91.3 Neonatal cerebral irritability

P91.4 Neonatal cerebral depression

P91.5 Neonatal coma

● **P91.6 Hypoxic ischemic encephalopathy [HIE]**

P91.60 Hypoxic ischemic encephalopathy [HIE], unspecified

P91.61 Mild hypoxic ischemic encephalopathy [HIE]

P91.62 Moderate hypoxic ischemic encephalopathy [HIE]

P91.63 Severe hypoxic ischemic encephalopathy [HIE]

P91.8 Other specified disturbances of cerebral status of newborn

P91.9 Disturbance of cerebral status of newborn, unspecified

● **P92 Feeding problems of newborn**
Excludes1 feeding problems in child over 28 days old (R63.3)

● **P92.0 Vomiting of newborn**
Excludes1 vomiting of child over 28 days old (R11.-)

P92.01 Bilious vomiting of newborn
Excludes1 bilious vomiting in child over 28 days old (R11.14)

P92.09 Other vomiting of newborn
Excludes1 regurgitation of food in newborn (P92.1)

P92.1 Regurgitation and rumination of newborn

P92.2 Slow feeding of newborn

P92.3 Underfeeding of newborn

P92.4 Overfeeding of newborn

P92.5 Neonatal difficulty in feeding at breast

P92.6 Failure to thrive in newborn
Excludes1 failure to thrive in child over 28 days old (R62.51)

P92.8 Other feeding problems of newborn

P92.9 Feeding problem of newborn, unspecified

● **P93 Reactions and intoxications due to drugs administered to newborn**

Includes reactions and intoxications due to drugs administered to fetus affecting newborn

Excludes1 jaundice due to drugs or toxins transmitted from mother or given to newborn (P58.4-)
reactions and intoxications from maternal opiates, tranquilizers and other medication (P04.0-P04.1, P04.4)
withdrawal symptoms from maternal use of drugs of addiction (P96.1)
withdrawal symptoms from therapeutic use of drugs in newborn (P96.2)

P93.0 Grey baby syndrome
Grey syndrome from chloramphenicol administration in newborn

P93.8 Other reactions and intoxications due to drugs administered to newborn
Use additional code for adverse effect, if applicable, to identify drug (T36-T50 with fifth or sixth character 5)

● **P94 Disorders of muscle tone of newborn**

P94.0 Transient neonatal myasthenia gravis
Excludes1 myasthenia gravis (G70.0)

P94.1 Congenital hypertonia

P94.2 Congenital hypotonia
Floppy baby syndrome, unspecified

P94.8 Other disorders of muscle tone of newborn

P94.9 Disorder of muscle tone of newborn, unspecified

P95 Stillbirth
Deadborn fetus NOS
Fetal death of unspecified cause
Stillbirth NOS

Excludes1 maternal care for intrauterine death (O36.4)
missed abortion (O02.1)
outcome of delivery, stillbirth (Z37.1, Z37.3, Z37.4, Z37.7)

OGCR Section I.C.16.g.

Stillbirth

Code P95, Stillbirth, is only for use for institutions that maintain separate records for stillbirths. No other code should be used with P95. Code P95 should not be used on the mother's record.

● **P96 Other conditions originating in the perinatal period**

P96.0 Congenital renal failure
Uremia of newborn

P96.1 Neonatal withdrawal symptoms from maternal use of drugs of addiction
Drug withdrawal syndrome in infant of dependent mother
Neonatal abstinence syndrome

Excludes1 reactions and intoxications from maternal opiates and tranquilizers administered during labor and delivery (P04.0)

P96.2 Withdrawal symptoms from therapeutic use of drugs in newborn

P96.3 Wide cranial sutures of newborn
Neonatal craniotabes

P96.5 Complication to newborn due to (fetal) intrauterine procedure
Excludes2 newborn affected by amniocentesis (P00.6) ◄

● **P96.8 Other specified conditions originating in the perinatal period**

P96.81 Exposure to (parental) (environmental) tobacco smoke in the perinatal period
Excludes2 newborn affected by in utero exposure to tobacco (P04.2)
exposure to environmental tobacco smoke after the perinatal period (Z77.22)

P96.82 Delayed separation of umbilical cord

P96.83 Meconium staining
Excludes1 meconium aspiration (P24.00, P24.01)
meconium passage during delivery (P03.82)

P96.89 Other specified conditions originating in the perinatal period
Use additional code to specify condition

P96.9 Condition originating in the perinatal period, unspecified
Congenital debility NOS

CHAPTER 16 (P00-P96)

CHAPTER 17

CONGENITAL MALFORMATIONS, DEFORMATIONS AND CHROMOSOMAL ABNORMALITIES (Q00-Q99)

OGCR Chapter-Specific Coding Guidelines

17. Chapter 17: Congenital malformations, deformations, and chromosomal abnormalities (Q00-Q99)

Assign an appropriate code(s) from categories Q00-Q99, Congenital malformations, deformations, and chromosomal abnormalities when a malformation/deformation or chromosomal abnormality is documented. A malformation/deformation/ or chromosomal abnormality may be the principal/first-listed diagnosis on a record or a secondary diagnosis.

When a malformation/deformation/or chromosomal abnormality does not have a unique code assignment, assign additional code(s) for any manifestations that may be present.

When the code assignment specifically identifies the malformation/deformation/or chromosomal abnormality, manifestations that are an inherent component of the anomaly should not be coded separately. Additional codes should be assigned for manifestations that are not an inherent component.

Codes from Chapter 17 may be used throughout the life of the patient. If a congenital malformation or deformity has been corrected, a personal history code should be used to identify the history of the malformation or deformity. Although present at birth, malformation/deformation/or chromosomal abnormality may not be identified until later in life. Whenever the condition is diagnosed by the physician, it is appropriate to assign a code from codes Q00-Q99.

For the birth admission, the appropriate code from category Z38, Liveborn infants, according to place of birth and type of delivery, should be sequenced as the principal diagnosis, followed by any congenital anomaly codes, Q00-Q99.

CHAPTER 17

CONGENITAL MALFORMATIONS, DEFORMATIONS AND CHROMOSOMAL ABNORMALITIES (Q00-Q99)

Note: Codes from this chapter are not for use on maternal or fetal records

Excludes2 inborn errors of metabolism (E70-E88)

This chapter contains the following blocks:

Q00-Q07	Congenital malformations of the nervous system
Q10-Q18	Congenital malformations of eye, ear, face and neck
Q20-Q28	Congenital malformations of the circulatory system
Q30-Q34	Congenital malformations of the respiratory system
Q35-Q37	Cleft lip and cleft palate
Q38-Q45	Other congenital malformations of the digestive system
Q50-Q56	Congenital malformations of genital organs
Q60-Q64	Congenital malformations of the urinary system
Q65-Q79	Congenital malformations and deformations of the musculoskeletal system
Q80-Q89	Other congenital malformations
Q90-Q99	Chromosomal abnormalities, not elsewhere classified

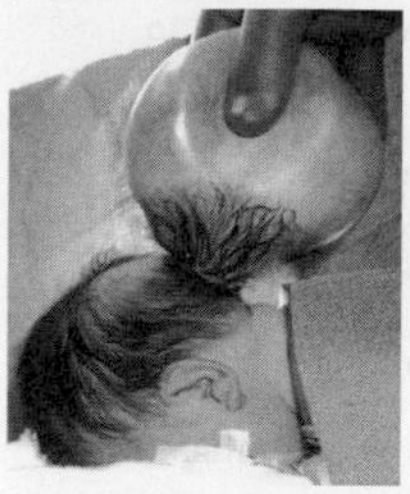

Figure 17-1 An infant with a large occipital encephalocele. The large skin-covered encephalocele is visible. (From Townsend: Sabiston Textbook of Surgery, ed 19, Saunders, An Imprint of Elsevier, 2012)

CONGENITAL MALFORMATIONS OF THE NERVOUS SYSTEM (Q00–Q07)

● **Q00 Anencephaly and similar malformations**

Q00.0 Anencephaly

Absence of skull with cerebral hemispheres missing or reduced to small masses attached to base of cranium

Acephaly
Acrania
Amyelencephaly
Hemianencephaly
Hemicephaly

Q00.1 Craniorachischisis

Developmental anomaly consisting of fissure of cranium and vertebral column

Q00.2 Iniencephaly

Developmental anomaly characterized by enlargement of foramen magnum and absence of laminae and spinous processes of cervical, dorsal

● **Q01 Encephalocele**

Sac-like protrusions of brain and membranes visible through an opening in skull

Includes Arnold-Chiari syndrome, type III
encephalocystocele
encephalomyelocele
hydroencephalocele
hydromeningocele, cranial
meningocele, cerebral
meningoencephalocele

Excludes1 Meckel-Gruber syndrome (Q61.9)

Q01.0 Frontal encephalocele
Q01.1 Nasofrontal encephalocele
Q01.2 Occipital encephalocele
Q01.8 Encephalocele of other sites
Q01.9 Encephalocele, unspecified

Q02 Microcephaly

Head size measures significantly below normal based on standardized charts

Includes hydromicrocephaly
micrencephalon

Excludes1 Meckel-Gruber syndrome (Q61.9)

● **Q03 Congenital hydrocephalus**

Accumulation of cerebrospinal fluid in ventricles resulting in swelling and enlargement

Includes hydrocephalus in newborn

Excludes1 Arnold-Chiari syndrome, type II (Q07.0-)
acquired hydrocephalus (G91.-)
hydrocephalus due to congenital toxoplasmosis (P37.1)
hydrocephalus with spina bifida (Q05.0-Q05.4)

Q03.0 Malformations of aqueduct of Sylvius

Anomaly of aqueduct of Sylvius
Obstruction of aqueduct of Sylvius, congenital
Stenosis of aqueduct of Sylvius

Q03.1 Atresia of foramina of Magendie and Luschka

Dandy-Walker syndrome

Q03.8 Other congenital hydrocephalus

Q03.9 Congenital hydrocephalus, unspecified

● **Q04 Other congenital malformations of brain**
Excludes1 cyclopia (Q87.0)
macrocephaly (Q75.3)

Q04.0 Congenital malformations of corpus callosum
Agenesis of corpus callosum

Q04.1 Arhinencephaly
Congenital absence of olfactory bulbs, tract, or nerves

Q04.2 Holoprosencephaly
Failure of cleavage of forebrain (prosencephalon) resulting in incomplete or absent cortical separation and deficits in midline facial development

Q04.3 Other reduction deformities of brain
Absence of part of brain
Agyria
Agenesis of part of brain
Cerebral cortex are not fully formed, brain surface is smooth
Aplasia of part of brain
Hydranencephaly
Hypoplasia of part of brain
Lissencephaly
Congenital malformation or absence of convolutions of cerebral cortex
Microgyria
Malformation of brain characterized by excessive number of small convolutions (gyri) on surface
Pachygyria
Reduction in number of sulci of cerebrum
Excludes1 congenital malformations of corpus callosum (Q04.0)

Q04.4 Septo-optic dysplasia of brain

Q04.5 Megalencephaly
Abnormally large brain

Q04.6 Congenital cerebral cysts
Porencephaly
Schizencephaly
Excludes1 acquired porencephalic cyst (G93.0)

Q04.8 Other specified congenital malformations of brain
Arnold-Chiari syndrome, type IV
Macrogyria

Q04.9 Congenital malformation of brain, unspecified
Congenital anomaly NOS of brain
Congenital deformity NOS of brain
Congenital disease or lesion NOS of brain
Multiple anomalies NOS of brain, congenital

● **Q05 Spina bifida**
Developmental anomaly characterized by defective closure of vertebral arch, through which spinal cord and meninges may protrude
Includes hydromeningocele (spinal)
meningocele (spinal)
meningomyelocele
myelocele
myelomeningocele
rachischisis
spina bifida (aperta)(cystica)
syringomyelocele

Use additional code for any associated paraplegia (paraparesis) (G82.2-)
Excludes1 Arnold-Chiari syndrome, type II (Q07.0-)
spina bifida occulta (Q76.0)

Q05.0 Cervical spina bifida with hydrocephalus

Q05.1 Thoracic spina bifida with hydrocephalus
Dorsal spina bifida with hydrocephalus
Thoracolumbar spina bifida with hydrocephalus

Q05.2 Lumbar spina bifida with hydrocephalus
Lumbosacral spina bifida with hydrocephalus

Q05.3 Sacral spina bifida with hydrocephalus

Q05.4 Unspecified spina bifida with hydrocephalus

Q05.5 Cervical spina bifida without hydrocephalus

Q05.6 Thoracic spina bifida without hydrocephalus
Dorsal spina bifida NOS
Thoracolumbar spina bifida NOS

Q05.7 Lumbar spina bifida without hydrocephalus
Lumbosacral spina bifida NOS

Q05.8 Sacral spina bifida without hydrocephalus

Q05.9 Spina bifida, unspecified

● **Q06 Other congenital malformations of spinal cord**

Q06.0 Amyelia
Congenital absence of spinal cord

Q06.1 Hypoplasia and dysplasia of spinal cord
Underdevelopment of spinal cord
Atelomyelia
Congenitally incomplete development of spinal cord
Myelatelia
Myelodysplasia of spinal cord
Defective development of spinal cord, especially lower segments

Q06.2 Diastematomyelia
Congenital anomaly, associated with spina bifida, in which spinal cord is split into halves and surrounded by dural sac

Q06.3 Other congenital cauda equina malformations

Q06.4 Hydromyelia
Dilation of central canal of spinal cord with increased fluid accumulation
Hydrorachis

Q06.8 Other specified congenital malformations of spinal cord

Q06.9 Congenital malformation of spinal cord, unspecified
Congenital anomaly NOS of spinal cord
Congenital deformity NOS of spinal cord
Congenital disease or lesion NOS of spinal cord

● **Q07 Other congenital malformations of nervous system**
Excludes2 congenital central alveolar hypoventilation syndrome (G47.35)
familial dysautonomia [Riley-Day] (G90.1)
neurofibromatosis (nonmalignant) (Q85.0-)

● **Q07.0 Arnold-Chiari syndrome**
Herniation of cerebellar tonsils and vermis through foramen magnum into spinal canal
Arnold-Chiari syndrome, type II
Excludes1 Arnold-Chiari syndrome, type III (Q01.-)
Arnold-Chiari syndrome, type IV (Q04.8)

Q07.00 Arnold-Chiari syndrome without spina bifida or hydrocephalus

Q07.01 Arnold-Chiari syndrome with spina bifida

Q07.02 Arnold-Chiari syndrome with hydrocephalus

Q07.03 Arnold-Chiari syndrome with spina bifida and hydrocephalus

Q07.8 Other specified congenital malformations of nervous system
Agenesis of nerve
Displacement of brachial plexus
Jaw-winking syndrome
Marcus Gunn's syndrome

Q07.9 Congenital malformation of nervous system, unspecified
Congenital anomaly NOS of nervous system
Congenital deformity NOS of nervous system
Congenital disease or lesion NOS of nervous system

CHAPTER 17 (Q00-Q99)

CONGENITAL MALFORMATIONS OF EYE, EAR, FACE AND NECK (Q10-Q18)

Excludes2 cleft lip and cleft palate (Q35-Q37)
congenital malformation of cervical spine (Q05.0, Q05.5, Q67.5, Q76.0-Q76.4)
congenital malformation of larynx (Q31.-)
congenital malformation of lip NEC (Q38.0)
congenital malformation of nose (Q30.-)
congenital malformation of parathyroid gland (Q89.2)
congenital malformation of thyroid gland (Q89.2)

● **Q10 Congenital malformations of eyelid, lacrimal apparatus and orbit**

Excludes1 cryptophthalmos NOS (Q11.2)
cryptophthalmos syndrome (Q87.0)

Q10.0 Congenital ptosis
Prolapse or drooping of upper eyelid from paralysis of third nerve or from sympathetic innervations

Q10.1 Congenital ectropion
Outward turning of eyelid

Q10.2 Congenital entropion
Inward turning of eyelid

Q10.3 Other congenital malformations of eyelid
Ablepharon
Blepharophimosis, congenital
Coloboma of eyelid
Congenital absence or agenesis of cilia
Congenital absence or agenesis of eyelid
Congenital accessory eyelid
Congenital accessory eye muscle
Congenital malformation of eyelid NOS

Q10.4 Absence and agenesis of lacrimal apparatus
Congenital absence of punctum lacrimale

Q10.5 Congenital stenosis and stricture of lacrimal duct

Q10.6 Other congenital malformations of lacrimal apparatus
Congenital malformation of lacrimal apparatus NOS

Q10.7 Congenital malformation of orbit

● **Q11 Anophthalmos, microphthalmos and macrophthalmos**
Absence of eye and optic pit

Q11.0 Cystic eyeball

Q11.1 Other anophthalmos
Anophthalmos NOS
Agenesis of eye
Absence of eye
Aplasia of eye

Q11.2 Microphthalmos
Partial absence of eye and optic pit
Cryptophthalmos NOS
Dysplasia of eye
Hypoplasia of eye
Rudimentary eye
Excludes1 cryptophthalmos syndrome (Q87.0)

Q11.3 Macrophthalmos
Congenital enlargement of eyes
Excludes1 macrophthalmos in congenital glaucoma (Q15.0)

● **Q12 Congenital lens malformations**

Q12.0 Congenital cataract

Q12.1 Congenital displaced lens

Q12.2 Coloboma of lens

Q12.3 Congenital aphakia

Q12.4 Spherophakia
Smaller, more spherical optic lens than normal

Q12.8 Other congenital lens malformations
Microphakia

Q12.9 Congenital lens malformation, unspecified

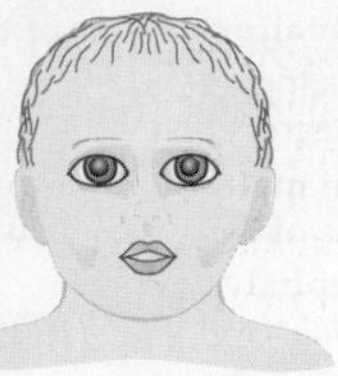

Figure 17-2 Bilateral congenital **hydrophthalmia,** in which the eyes are very large in comparison to the other facial features due to glaucoma.

● **Q13 Congenital malformations of anterior segment of eye**

Q13.0 Coloboma of iris
Coloboma NOS

Q13.1 Absence of iris
Aniridia
Use additional code for associated glaucoma (H42)

Q13.2 Other congenital malformations of iris
Anisocoria, congenital
Atresia of pupil
Congenital malformation of iris NOS
Corectopia

Q13.3 Congenital corneal opacity

Q13.4 Other congenital corneal malformations
Congenital malformation of cornea NOS
Microcornea
Peter's anomaly

Q13.5 Blue sclera
Condition of unusual blueness of sclera; not harmful

● **Q13.8 Other congenital malformations of anterior segment of eye**

Q13.81 Rieger's anomaly
Use additional code for associated glaucoma (H42)

Q13.89 Other congenital malformations of anterior segment of eye

Q13.9 Congenital malformation of anterior segment of eye, unspecified

● **Q14 Congenital malformations of posterior segment of eye**

Excludes2 optic nerve hypoplasia (H47.03-)

Q14.0 Congenital malformation of vitreous humor
Congenital vitreous opacity

Q14.1 Congenital malformation of retina
Congenital retinal aneurysm

Q14.2 Congenital malformation of optic disc
Coloboma of optic disc

Q14.3 Congenital malformation of choroid

Q14.8 Other congenital malformations of posterior segment of eye
Coloboma of the fundus

Q14.9 Congenital malformation of posterior segment of eye, unspecified

CHAPTER 17 (Q00-Q99)

● **Q15 Other congenital malformations of eye**

Excludes1 congenital nystagmus (H55.01)
ocular albinism (E70.31-)
optic nerve hypoplasia (H47.03-)
retinitis pigmentosa (H35.52)

Q15.0 Congenital glaucoma
Axenfeld's anomaly
Buphthalmos
Congenital syndrome characterized by port-wine nevus covering portions of face and cranium
Glaucoma of childhood
Glaucoma of newborn
Hydrophthalmos
Keratoglobus, congenital, with glaucoma
Macrocornea with glaucoma
Macrophthalmos in congenital glaucoma
Megalocornea with glaucoma

Q15.8 Other specified congenital malformations of eye

Q15.9 Congenital malformation of eye, unspecified
Congenital anomaly of eye
Congenital deformity of eye

● **Q16 Congenital malformations of ear causing impairment of hearing**

Excludes1 congenital deafness (H90.-)

Q16.0 Congenital absence of (ear) auricle

Q16.1 Congenital absence, atresia and stricture of auditory canal (external)
Congenital atresia or stricture of osseous meatus

Q16.2 Absence of eustachian tube

Q16.3 Congenital malformation of ear ossicles
Congenital fusion of ear ossicles

Q16.4 Other congenital malformations of middle ear
Congenital malformation of middle ear NOS

Q16.5 Congenital malformation of inner ear
Congenital anomaly of membranous labyrinth
Congenital anomaly of organ of Corti

Q16.9 Congenital malformation of ear causing impairment of hearing, unspecified
Congenital absence of ear NOS

● **Q17 Other congenital malformations of ear**

Excludes1 congenital malformations of ear with impairment of hearing (Q16.0-Q16.9)
preauricular sinus (Q18.1)

Q17.0 Accessory auricle
Accessory tragus
Polyotia
Preauricular appendage or tag
Supernumerary ear
Supernumerary lobule

Q17.1 Macrotia
Enlarged ears

Q17.2 Microtia
An abnormally small or underdeveloped external ear

Q17.3 Other misshapen ear
Pointed ear

Q17.4 Misplaced ear
Low-set ears

Excludes1 cervical auricle (Q18.2)

Q17.5 Prominent ear
Bat ear

Q17.8 Other specified congenital malformations of ear
Congenital absence of lobe of ear

Q17.9 Congenital malformation of ear, unspecified
Congenital anomaly of ear NOS

● **Q18 Other congenital malformations of face and neck**

Excludes1 cleft lip and cleft palate (Q35-Q37)
conditions classified to Q67.0-Q67.4
congenital malformations of skull and face bones (Q75.-)
cyclopia (Q87.0)
dentofacial anomalies [including malocclusion] (M26.-)
malformation syndromes affecting facial appearance (Q87.0)
persistent thyroglossal duct (Q89.2)

Q18.0 Sinus, fistula and cyst of branchial cleft
Branchial vestige
Brachial remnants (cysts, fistula, skin tags) that are developmental anomalies

Q18.1 Preauricular sinus and cyst
Fistula of auricle, congenital
Cervicoaural fistula
Abnormal passage in neck originating from first branchial cleft

Q18.2 Other branchial cleft malformations
Branchial cleft malformation NOS
Cervical auricle
Otocephaly

Q18.3 Webbing of neck
Pterygium colli
Thick fold of skin on side of neck

Q18.4 Macrostomia
Results from failure of union of maxillary and mandibular processes, results in abnormally large mouth

Q18.5 Microstomia

Q18.6 Macrocheilia
Excessive size of lips
Hypertrophy of lip, congenital

Q18.7 Microcheilia
Abnormal smallness of lips

Q18.8 Other specified congenital malformations of face and neck
Medial cyst of face and neck
Medial fistula of face and neck
Medial sinus of face and neck

Q18.9 Congenital malformation of face and neck, unspecified
Congenital anomaly NOS of face and neck

CONGENITAL MALFORMATIONS OF THE CIRCULATORY SYSTEM (Q20-Q28)

● **Q20 Congenital malformations of cardiac chambers and connections**

Excludes1 dextrocardia with situs inversus (Q89.3)
mirror-image atrial arrangement with situs inversus (Q89.3)

Q20.0 Common arterial trunk
Persistent truncus arteriosus

Excludes1 aortic septal defect (Q21.4)

Q20.1 Double outlet right ventricle
Taussig-Bing syndrome

Q20.2 Double outlet left ventricle

Q20.3 Discordant ventriculoarterial connection
Dextrotransposition of aorta
Transposition of great vessels (complete)

Q20.4 Double inlet ventricle
Common ventricle
Cor triloculare biatriatum
Single ventricle

Q20.5 Discordant atrioventricular connection
Corrected transposition
Levotransposition
Ventricular inversion

Q20.6 Isomerism of atrial appendages
Isomerism of atrial appendages with asplenia or polysplenia

Q20.8 Other congenital malformations of cardiac chambers and connections
Cor binoculare

Q20.9 Congenital malformation of cardiac chambers and connections, unspecified

CHAPTER 17 (Q00-Q99)

◀ New ◀ Revised ~~deleted~~ Deleted **OGCR** Official Guidelines **X** Assign placeholder X ● Use Additional Character(s)
Excludes1 Excludes2 Includes Use additional Code first Code also Unspecified

● **Q21 Congenital malformations of cardiac septa**
Excludes1 acquired cardiac septal defect (I51.0)

Q21.0 Ventricular septal defect
Roger's disease

Q21.1 Atrial septal defect
Coronary sinus defect
Patent or persistent foramen ovale
Patent or persistent ostium secundum defect (type II)
Patent or persistent sinus venosus defect

Q21.2 Atrioventricular septal defect
Common atrioventricular canal
Endocardial cushion defect
Ostium primum atrial septal defect (type I)

Q21.3 Tetralogy of Fallot
Ventricular septal defect with pulmonary stenosis or atresia, dextroposition of aorta and hypertrophy of right ventricle.

Q21.4 Aortopulmonary septal defect
Aortic septal defect
Aortopulmonary window

Q21.8 Other congenital malformations of cardiac septa
Eisenmenger's defect
Pentalogy of Fallot
Excludes1 Eisenmenger's complex (I27.8)
Eisenmenger's syndrome (I27.8)

Q21.9 Congenital malformation of cardiac septum, unspecified
Septal (heart) defect NOS

● **Q22 Congenital malformations of pulmonary and tricuspid valves**

Q22.0 Pulmonary valve atresia

Q22.1 Congenital pulmonary valve stenosis

Q22.2 Congenital pulmonary valve insufficiency
Congenital pulmonary valve regurgitation

Q22.3 Other congenital malformations of pulmonary valve
Congenital malformation of pulmonary valve NOS
Supernumerary cusps of pulmonary valve

Q22.4 Congenital tricuspid stenosis
Congenital tricuspid atresia

Q22.5 Ebstein's anomaly
Malformation of tricuspid valve

Q22.6 Hypoplastic right heart syndrome

Q22.8 Other congenital malformations of tricuspid valve

Q22.9 Congenital malformation of tricuspid valve, unspecified

● **Q23 Congenital malformations of aortic and mitral valves**

Q23.0 Congenital stenosis of aortic valve
Congenital aortic atresia
Congenital aortic stenosis NOS
Excludes1 congenital stenosis of aortic valve in hypoplastic left heart syndrome (Q23.4)
congenital subaortic stenosis (Q24.4)
supravalvular aortic stenosis (congenital) (Q25.3)

Q23.1 Congenital insufficiency of aortic valve
Bicuspid aortic valve
Congenital aortic insufficiency

Q23.2 Congenital mitral stenosis
Congenital mitral atresia

Q23.3 Congenital mitral insufficiency

Q23.4 Hypoplastic left heart syndrome

Q23.8 Other congenital malformations of aortic and mitral valves

Q23.9 Congenital malformation of aortic and mitral valves, unspecified

● **Q24 Other congenital malformations of heart**
Excludes1 endocardial fibroelastosis (I42.4)

Q24.0 Dextrocardia
Heart is located in right hemithorax
Excludes1 dextrocardia with situs inversus (Q89.3)
isomerism of atrial appendages (with asplenia or polysplenia) (Q20.6)
mirror-image atrial arrangement with situs inversus (Q89.3)

Q24.1 Levocardia
Normal position of heart but related structures on wrong side

Q24.2 Cor triatriatum
Congenital heart defect; left atrium is subdivided

Q24.3 Pulmonary infundibular stenosis
Subvalvular pulmonic stenosis

Q24.4 Congenital subaortic stenosis

Q24.5 Malformation of coronary vessels
Congenital coronary (artery) aneurysm

Q24.6 Congenital heart block

Q24.8 Other specified congenital malformations of heart
Congenital diverticulum of left ventricle
Congenital malformation of myocardium
Congenital malformation of pericardium
Malposition of heart
Uhl's disease

Q24.9 Congenital malformation of heart, unspecified
Congenital anomaly of heart
Congenital disease of heart

● **Q25 Congenital malformations of great arteries**

Q25.0 Patent ductus arteriosus
Fetal blood vessel connecting left pulmonary artery directly to descending aorta
Patent ductus Botallo
Persistent ductus arteriosus

Q25.1 Coarctation of aorta
Coarctation of aorta (preductal) (postductal)
Stenosis of aorta ◀

● **Q25.2 Atresia of aorta**

Q25.21 Interruption of aortic arch ◀
Atresia of aortic arch ◀

Q25.29 Other atresia of aorta ◀
Atresia of aorta ◀

Q25.3 Supravalvular aortic stenosis
Excludes1 congenital aortic stenosis NOS (Q23.0)
congenital stenosis of aortic valve (Q23.0)

● **Q25.4 Other congenital malformations of aorta**
Excludes1 hypoplasia of aorta in hypoplastic left heart syndrome (Q23.4)

Q25.40 Congenital malformation of aorta unspecified ◀

Q25.41 Absence and aplasia of aorta ◀

Q25.42 Hypoplasia of aorta ◀

Q25.43 Congenital aneurysm of aorta ◀
Congenital aneurysm of aortic root ◀
Congenital aneurysm of aortic sinus ◀

Q25.44 Congenital dilation of aorta ◀

Q25.45 Double aortic arch ◀
Vascular ring of aorta ◀

Q25.46 Tortuous aortic arch ◀
Persistent convolutions of aortic arch ◀

Q25.47 Right aortic arch ◀
Persistent right aortic arch ◀

Q25.48 Anomalous origin of subclavian artery ◀

Q25.49 Other congenital malformations of aorta ◀

Q25.5 Atresia of pulmonary artery

Q25.6 Stenosis of pulmonary artery
Supravalvular pulmonary stenosis

● **Q25.7 Other congenital malformations of pulmonary artery**

Q25.71 Coarctation of pulmonary artery

Q25.72 Congenital pulmonary arteriovenous malformation
Congenital pulmonary arteriovenous aneurysm

Q25.79 Other congenital malformations of pulmonary artery
Aberrant pulmonary artery
Agenesis of pulmonary artery
Congenital aneurysm of pulmonary artery
Congenital anomaly of pulmonary artery
Hypoplasia of pulmonary artery

Q25.8 Other congenital malformations of other great arteries

Q25.9 Congenital malformation of great arteries, unspecified

● **Q26 Congenital malformations of great veins**

Q26.Ø Congenital stenosis of vena cava
Congenital stenosis of vena cava (inferior)(superior)

Q26.1 Persistent left superior vena cava

Q26.2 Total anomalous pulmonary venous connection
Total anomalous pulmonary venous return [TAPVR], subdiaphragmatic
Total anomalous pulmonary venous return [TAPVR], supradiaphragmatic

Q26.3 Partial anomalous pulmonary venous connection
Partial anomalous pulmonary venous return

Q26.4 Anomalous pulmonary venous connection, unspecified

Q26.5 Anomalous portal venous connection

Q26.6 Portal vein-hepatic artery fistula

Q26.8 Other congenital malformations of great veins
Absence of vena cava (inferior) (superior)
Azygos continuation of inferior vena cava
Persistent left posterior cardinal vein
Scimitar syndrome

Q26.9 Congenital malformation of great vein, unspecified
Congenital anomaly of vena cava (inferior) (superior) NOS

● **Q27 Other congenital malformations of peripheral vascular system**

Excludes2 anomalies of cerebral and precerebral vessels (Q28.Ø-Q28.3)
anomalies of coronary vessels (Q24.5)
anomalies of pulmonary artery (Q25.5-Q25.7)
congenital retinal aneurysm (Q14.1)
hemangioma and lymphangioma (D18.-)

Q27.Ø Congenital absence and hypoplasia of umbilical artery
Single umbilical artery

Q27.1 Congenital renal artery stenosis

Q27.2 Other congenital malformations of renal artery
Congenital malformation of renal artery NOS
Multiple renal arteries

● **Q27.3 Arteriovenous malformation (peripheral)**
Arteriovenous aneurysm

Excludes1 acquired arteriovenous aneurysm (I77.Ø)

Excludes2 arteriovenous malformation of cerebral vessels (Q28.2)
arteriovenous malformation of precerebral vessels (Q28.Ø)

Q27.30 Arteriovenous malformation, site unspecified

Q27.31 Arteriovenous malformation of vessel of upper limb

Q27.32 Arteriovenous malformation of vessel of lower limb

Q27.33 Arteriovenous malformation of digestive system vessel

Q27.34 Arteriovenous malformation of renal vessel

Q27.39 Arteriovenous malformation, other site

Q27.4 Congenital phlebectasia

Q27.8 Other specified congenital malformations of peripheral vascular system
Absence of peripheral vascular system
Atresia of peripheral vascular system
Congenital aneurysm (peripheral)
Congenital stricture, artery
Congenital varix

Excludes1 arteriovenous malformation (Q27.3-)

Q27.9 Congenital malformation of peripheral vascular system, unspecified
Anomaly of artery or vein NOS

● **Q28 Other congenital malformations of circulatory system**

Excludes1 congenital aneurysm NOS (Q27.8)
congenital coronary aneurysm (Q24.5)
ruptured cerebral arteriovenous malformation (I6Ø.8)
ruptured malformation of precerebral vessels (I72.Ø)

Excludes2 congenital peripheral aneurysm (Q27.8)
congenital pulmonary aneurysm (Q25.79)
congenital retinal aneurysm (Q14.1)

Q28.Ø Arteriovenous malformation of precerebral vessels
Congenital arteriovenous precerebral aneurysm (nonruptured)

Q28.1 Other malformations of precerebral vessels
Congenital malformation of precerebral vessels NOS
Congenital precerebral aneurysm (nonruptured)

Q28.2 Arteriovenous malformation of cerebral vessels
Arteriovenous malformation of brain NOS
Congenital arteriovenous cerebral aneurysm (nonruptured)

Q28.3 Other malformations of cerebral vessels
Congenital cerebral aneurysm (nonruptured)
Congenital malformation of cerebral vessels NOS
Developmental venous anomaly

Q28.8 Other specified congenital malformations of circulatory system
Congenital aneurysm, specified site NEC
Spinal vessel anomaly

Q28.9 Congenital malformation of circulatory system, unspecified

CONGENITAL MALFORMATIONS OF THE RESPIRATORY SYSTEM (Q3Ø-Q34)

● **Q3Ø Congenital malformations of nose**

Excludes1 congenital deviation of nasal septum (Q67.4)

Q3Ø.Ø Choanal atresia
Atresia of nares (anterior) (posterior)
Congenital stenosis of nares (anterior) (posterior)

Q3Ø.1 Agenesis and underdevelopment of nose
Congenital absent of nose

Q3Ø.2 Fissured, notched and cleft nose

Q3Ø.3 Congenital perforated nasal septum

Q3Ø.8 Other congenital malformations of nose
Accessory nose
Congenital anomaly of nasal sinus wall

Q3Ø.9 Congenital malformation of nose, unspecified

● **Q31 Congenital malformations of larynx**

Excludes1 congenital laryngeal stridor NOS (P28.89)

Q31.Ø Web of larynx
Glottic web of larynx
Subglottic web of larynx
Web of larynx NOS

Q31.1 Congenital subglottic stenosis

Q31.2 Laryngeal hypoplasia

Q31.3 Laryngocele

Q31.5 Congenital laryngomalacia

Q31.8 Other congenital malformations of larynx
Absence of larynx
Agenesis of larynx
Atresia of larynx
Congenital cleft thyroid cartilage
Congenital fissure of epiglottis
Congenital stenosis of larynx NEC
Posterior cleft of cricoid cartilage

Q31.9 Congenital malformation of larynx, unspecified

● **Q32 Congenital malformations of trachea and bronchus**
Excludes1 congenital bronchiectasis (Q33.4)

Q32.0 Congenital tracheomalacia

Q32.1 Other congenital malformations of trachea
Atresia of trachea
Congenital anomaly of tracheal cartilage
Congenital dilatation of trachea
Congenital malformation of trachea
Congenital stenosis of trachea
Congenital tracheocele

Q32.2 Congenital bronchomalacia

Q32.3 Congenital stenosis of bronchus

Q32.4 Other congenital malformations of bronchus
Absence of bronchus
Agenesis of bronchus
Atresia of bronchus
Congenital diverticulum of bronchus
Congenital malformation of bronchus NOS

● **Q33 Congenital malformations of lung**

Q33.0 Congenital cystic lung
Congenital cystic lung disease
Congenital honeycomb lung
Congenital polycystic lung disease
Excludes1 cystic fibrosis (E84.0)
cystic lung disease, acquired or unspecified (J98.4)

Q33.1 Accessory lobe of lung
Azygos lobe (fissured), lung

Q33.2 Sequestration of lung

Q33.3 Agenesis of lung
Congenital absence of lung (lobe)

Q33.4 Congenital bronchiectasis

Q33.5 Ectopic tissue in lung

Q33.6 Congenital hypoplasia and dysplasia of lung
Excludes1 pulmonary hypoplasia associated with short gestation (P28.0)

Q33.8 Other congenital malformations of lung

Q33.9 Congenital malformation of lung, unspecified

● **Q34 Other congenital malformations of respiratory system**
Excludes2 congenital central alveolar hypoventilation syndrome (G47.35)

Q34.0 Anomaly of pleura

Q34.1 Congenital cyst of mediastinum

Q34.8 Other specified congenital malformations of respiratory system
Atresia of nasopharynx

Q34.9 Congenital malformation of respiratory system, unspecified
Congenital absence of respiratory system
Congenital anomaly of respiratory system NOS

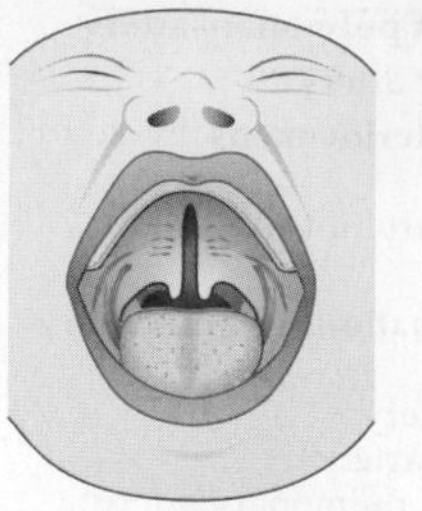

Figure 17-3 Cleft palate.

CLEFT LIP AND CLEFT PALATE (Q35-Q37)

Use additional code to identify associated malformation of the nose (Q30.2)
Excludes1 Robin's syndrome (Q87.0)

● **Q35 Cleft palate**
Includes fissure of palate
palatoschisis
Excludes1 cleft palate with cleft lip (Q37.-)

Q35.1 Cleft hard palate

Q35.3 Cleft soft palate

Q35.5 Cleft hard palate with cleft soft palate

Q35.7 Cleft uvula

Q35.9 Cleft palate, unspecified
Cleft palate NOS

● **Q36 Cleft lip**
Includes cheiloschisis
congenital fissure of lip
harelip
labium leporinum
Excludes1 cleft lip with cleft palate (Q37.-)

Q36.0 Cleft lip, bilateral

Q36.1 Cleft lip, median

Q36.9 Cleft lip, unilateral
Cleft lip NOS

● **Q37 Cleft palate with cleft lip**
Includes cheilopalatoschisis

Q37.0 Cleft hard palate with bilateral cleft lip

Q37.1 Cleft hard palate with unilateral cleft lip
Cleft hard palate with cleft lip NOS

Q37.2 Cleft soft palate with bilateral cleft lip

Q37.3 Cleft soft palate with unilateral cleft lip
Cleft soft palate with cleft lip NOS

Q37.4 Cleft hard and soft palate with bilateral cleft lip

Q37.5 Cleft hard and soft palate with unilateral cleft lip
Cleft hard and soft palate with cleft lip NOS

Q37.8 Unspecified cleft palate with bilateral cleft lip

Q37.9 Unspecified cleft palate with unilateral cleft lip
Cleft palate with cleft lip NOS

OTHER CONGENITAL MALFORMATIONS OF THE DIGESTIVE SYSTEM (Q38-Q45)

● **Q38 Other congenital malformations of tongue, mouth and pharynx**
Excludes1 dentofacial anomalies (M26.-)
macrostomia (Q18.4)
microstomia (Q18.5)

Q38.0 Congenital malformations of lips, not elsewhere classified
Congenital fistula of lip
Congenital malformation of lip NOS
Van der Woude's syndrome
Excludes1 cleft lip (Q36.-)
cleft lip with cleft palate (Q37.-)
macrocheilia (Q18.6)
microcheilia (Q18.7)

Q38.1 Ankyloglossia
Restricted movement of tongue resulting in speech difficulty
Tongue tie

Q38.2 Macroglossia
Excessive size of tongue
Congenital hypertrophy of tongue

Q38.3 Other congenital malformations of tongue
Aglossia
Bifid tongue
Congenital adhesion of tongue
Congenital fissure of tongue
Congenital malformation of tongue NOS
Double tongue
Hypoglossia
Hypoplasia of tongue
Microglossia

Q38.4 Congenital malformations of salivary glands and ducts
Atresia of salivary glands and ducts
Congenital absence of salivary glands and ducts
Congenital accessory salivary glands and ducts
Congenital fistula of salivary gland

Q38.5 Congenital malformations of palate, not elsewhere classified
Congenital absence of uvula
Congenital malformation of palate NOS
Congenital high arched palate
Excludes1 cleft palate (Q35.-)
cleft palate with cleft lip (Q37.-)

Q38.6 Other congenital malformations of mouth
Congenital malformation of mouth NOS

Q38.7 Congenital pharyngeal pouch
Congenital diverticulum of pharynx
Excludes1 pharyngeal pouch syndrome (D82.1)

Q38.8 Other congenital malformations of pharynx
Congenital malformation of pharynx NOS
Imperforate pharynx

● **Q39 Congenital malformations of esophagus**

Q39.0 Atresia of esophagus without fistula
Atresia of esophagus NOS

Q39.1 Atresia of esophagus with tracheo-esophageal fistula
Atresia of esophagus with broncho-esophageal fistula

Q39.2 Congenital tracheo-esophageal fistula without atresia
Congenital tracheo-esophageal fistula NOS

Q39.3 Congenital stenosis and stricture of esophagus

Q39.4 Esophageal web

Q39.5 Congenital dilatation of esophagus
Congenital cardiospasm

Q39.6 Congenital diverticulum of esophagus
Congenital esophageal pouch

Q39.8 Other congenital malformations of esophagus
Congenital absence of esophagus
Congenital displacement of esophagus
Congenital duplication of esophagus

Q39.9 Congenital malformation of esophagus, unspecified

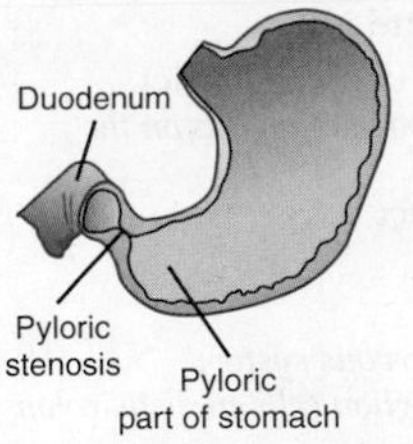

Figure 17-4 Pyloric stenosis.

● **Q40 Other congenital malformations of upper alimentary tract**

Q40.0 Congenital hypertrophic pyloric stenosis
Congenital or infantile constriction
Congenital or infantile hypertrophy
Congenital or infantile spasm
Congenital or infantile stenosis
Congenital or infantile stricture

Q40.1 Congenital hiatus hernia
Congenital displacement of cardia through esophageal hiatus
Excludes1 congenital diaphragmatic hernia (Q79.0)

Q40.2 Other specified congenital malformations of stomach
Congenital displacement of stomach
Congenital diverticulum of stomach
Congenital hourglass stomach
Congenital duplication of stomach
Megalogastria
Microgastria

Q40.3 Congenital malformation of stomach, unspecified

Q40.8 Other specified congenital malformations of upper alimentary tract

Q40.9 Congenital malformation of upper alimentary tract, unspecified
Congenital anomaly of upper alimentary tract
Congenital deformity of upper alimentary tract

● **Q41 Congenital absence, atresia and stenosis of small intestine**
Includes congenital obstruction, occlusion or stricture of small intestine or intestine NOS
Excludes1 cystic fibrosis with intestinal manifestation (E84.11)
meconium ileus NOS (without cystic fibrosis) (P76.0)

Q41.0 Congenital absence, atresia and stenosis of duodenum

Q41.1 Congenital absence, atresia and stenosis of jejunum
Apple peel syndrome
Imperforate jejunum

Q41.2 Congenital absence, atresia and stenosis of ileum

Q41.8 Congenital absence, atresia and stenosis of other specified parts of small intestine

Q41.9 Congenital absence, atresia and stenosis of small intestine, part unspecified
Congenital absence, atresia and stenosis of intestine NOS

● **Q42 Congenital absence, atresia and stenosis of large intestine**
Includes congenital obstruction, occlusion and stricture of large intestine

Q42.0 Congenital absence, atresia and stenosis of rectum with fistula

Q42.1 Congenital absence, atresia and stenosis of rectum without fistula
Imperforate rectum

Q42.2 Congenital absence, atresia and stenosis of anus with fistula

Q42.3 Congenital absence, atresia and stenosis of anus without fistula
Imperforate anus

Q42.8 Congenital absence, atresia and stenosis of other parts of large intestine

Q42.9 Congenital absence, atresia and stenosis of large intestine, part unspecified

CHAPTER 17 (Q00-Q99)

● Q43 Other congenital malformations of intestine

Q43.Ø Meckel's diverticulum (displaced) (hypertrophic)
Congenital abnormality in which a pouch remains on the lower end of the small intestine
Persistent omphalomesenteric duct
Persistent vitelline duct

Q43.1 Hirschsprung's disease
Developmental disorder of enteric nervous system characterized by absence of ganglion cells in distal colon resulting in functional obstruction
Aganglionosis
Congenital (aganglionic) megacolon

Q43.2 Other congenital functional disorders of colon
Congenital dilatation of colon

Q43.3 Congenital malformations of intestinal fixation
Congenital omental, anomalous adhesions [bands]
Congenital peritoneal adhesions [bands]
Incomplete rotation of cecum and colon
Insufficient rotation of cecum and colon
Jackson's membrane
Malrotation of colon
Rotation failure of cecum and colon
Universal mesentery

Q43.4 Duplication of intestine

Q43.5 Ectopic anus
Anal opening in abnormal location

Q43.6 Congenital fistula of rectum and anus
Excludes1 congenital fistula of anus with absence, atresia and stenosis (Q42.2)
congenital fistula of rectum with absence, atresia and stenosis (Q42.Ø)
congenital rectovaginal fistula (Q52.2)
congenital urethrorectal fistula (Q64.73)
pilonidal fistula or sinus (LØ5.-)

Q43.7 Persistent cloaca
Malformation in which rectum, vagina, and urinary tract form one channel AKA congenital cloaca
Cloaca NOS

Q43.8 Other specified congenital malformations of intestine
Congenital blind loop syndrome
Congenital diverticulitis, colon
Congenital diverticulum, intestine
Dolichocolon
Megaloappendix
Megaloduodenum
Microcolon
Transposition of appendix
Transposition of colon
Transposition of intestine

Q43.9 Congenital malformation of intestine, unspecified

● Q44 Congenital malformations of gallbladder, bile ducts and liver

Q44.Ø Agenesis, aplasia and hypoplasia of gallbladder
Congenital absence of gallbladder

Q44.1 Other congenital malformations of gallbladder
Congenital malformation of gallbladder NOS
Intrahepatic gallbladder

Q44.2 Atresia of bile ducts

Q44.3 Congenital stenosis and stricture of bile ducts

Q44.4 Choledochal cyst

Q44.5 Other congenital malformations of bile ducts
Accessory hepatic duct
Biliary duct duplication
Congenital malformation of bile duct NOS
Cystic duct duplication

Q44.6 Cystic disease of liver
Fibrocystic disease of liver

Q44.7 Other congenital malformations of liver
Accessory liver
Alagille's syndrome
Congenital absence of liver
Congenital hepatomegaly
Congenital malformation of liver NOS

● Q45 Other congenital malformations of digestive system
Excludes2 congenital diaphragmatic hernia (Q79.Ø)
congenital hiatus hernia (Q4Ø.1)

Q45.Ø Agenesis, aplasia and hypoplasia of pancreas
Congenital absence of pancreas

Q45.1 Annular pancreas

Q45.2 Congenital pancreatic cyst

Q45.3 Other congenital malformations of pancreas and pancreatic duct
Accessory pancreas
Congenital malformation of pancreas or pancreatic duct NOS
Excludes1 congenital diabetes mellitus (E1Ø.-)
cystic fibrosis (E84.Ø-E84.9)
fibrocystic disease of pancreas (E84.-)
neonatal diabetes mellitus (P7Ø.2)

Q45.8 Other specified congenital malformations of digestive system
Absence (complete) (partial) of alimentary tract NOS
Duplication of digestive system
Malposition, congenital of digestive system

Q45.9 Congenital malformation of digestive system, unspecified
Congenital anomaly of digestive system
Congenital deformity of digestive system

CONGENITAL MALFORMATIONS OF GENITAL ORGANS (Q5Ø-Q56)

Excludes1 androgen insensitivity syndrome (E34.5-)
syndromes associated with anomalies in the number and form of chromosomes (Q9Ø-Q99)

● Q5Ø Congenital malformations of ovaries, fallopian tubes and broad ligaments

● Q5Ø.Ø Congenital absence of ovary
Excludes1 Turner's syndrome (Q96.-)

Q5Ø.Ø1 Congenital absence of ovary, unilateral

Q5Ø.Ø2 Congenital absence of ovary, bilateral

Q5Ø.1 Developmental ovarian cyst

Q5Ø.2 Congenital torsion of ovary

● Q5Ø.3 Other congenital malformations of ovary

Q5Ø.31 Accessory ovary

Q5Ø.32 Ovarian streak
Inadequate ovaries with absent follicular and hormonal function
46, XX with streak gonads

Q5Ø.39 Other congenital malformation of ovary
Congenital malformation of ovary NOS

Q5Ø.4 Embryonic cyst of fallopian tube
Fimbrial cyst

Q5Ø.5 Embryonic cyst of broad ligament
Epoophoron cyst
Parovarian cyst

Q5Ø.6 Other congenital malformations of fallopian tube and broad ligament
Absence of fallopian tube and broad ligament
Accessory fallopian tube and broad ligament
Atresia of fallopian tube and broad ligament
Congenital malformation of fallopian tube or broad ligament NOS

● Q51 Congenital malformations of uterus and cervix

Q51.Ø Agenesis and aplasia of uterus
Congenital absence of uterus

● Q51.1 Doubling of uterus with doubling of cervix and vagina

Q51.1Ø Doubling of uterus with doubling of cervix and vagina without obstruction
Doubling of uterus with doubling of cervix and vagina NOS

Q51.11 Doubling of uterus with doubling of cervix and vagina with obstruction

Q51.2 Other doubling of uterus
Doubling of uterus NOS
Septate uterus, complete or partial

Q51.3 Bicornate uterus
Bicornate uterus, complete or partial
Birth defect in which uterus has two separate 'horns' that form top of uterus

Q51.4 Unicornate uterus
Unicornate uterus with or without a separate uterine horn
Uterus with only one functioning horn
Uterus with half being undeveloped

Q51.5 Agenesis and aplasia of cervix
Congenital absence of cervix

Q51.6 Embryonic cyst of cervix

Q51.7 Congenital fistulae between uterus and digestive and urinary tracts

● **Q51.8 Other congenital malformations of uterus and cervix**

● **Q51.81 Other congenital malformations of uterus**

Q51.810 Arcuate uterus
Arcuatus uterus

Q51.811 Hypoplasia of uterus

Q51.818 Other congenital malformations of uterus
Müllerian anomaly of uterus NEC

● **Q51.82 Other congenital malformations of cervix**

Q51.820 Cervical duplication

Q51.821 Hypoplasia of cervix

Q51.828 Other congenital malformations of cervix

Q51.9 Congenital malformation of uterus and cervix, unspecified

● **Q52 Other congenital malformations of female genitalia**

Q52.0 Congenital absence of vagina
Vaginal agenesis, total or partial

● **Q52.1 Doubling of vagina**
Excludes1 doubling of vagina with doubling of uterus and cervix (Q51.1-)

Q52.10 Doubling of vagina, unspecified
Septate vagina NOS

Q52.11 Transverse vaginal septum

● **Q52.12 Longitudinal vaginal septum**
~~Longitudinal vaginal septum with or without obstruction~~

Q52.120 Longitudinal vaginal septum, nonobstructing ◀

Q52.121 Longitudinal vaginal septum, obstructing, right side ◀

Q52.122 Longitudinal vaginal septum, obstructing, left side ◀

Q52.123 Longitudinal vaginal septum, microperforate, right side ◀

Q52.124 Longitudinal vaginal septum, microperforate, left side ◀

Q52.129 Other and unspecified longitudinal vaginal septum ◀

Q52.2 Congenital rectovaginal fistula
Excludes1 cloaca (Q43.7)

Q52.3 Imperforate hymen
Membrane (hymen) completely closes vaginal orifice

Q52.4 Other congenital malformations of vagina
Canal of Nuck cyst, congenital
Congenital malformation of vagina NOS
Embryonic vaginal cyst
Gartner's duct cyst

Q52.5 Fusion of labia

Q52.6 Congenital malformation of clitoris

● **Q52.7 Other and unspecified congenital malformations of vulva**

Q52.70 Unspecified congenital malformations of vulva
Congenital malformation of vulva NOS

Q52.71 Congenital absence of vulva

Q52.79 Other congenital malformations of vulva
Congenital cyst of vulva

Q52.8 Other specified congenital malformations of female genitalia

Q52.9 Congenital malformation of female genitalia, unspecified

● **Q53 Undescended and ectopic testicle**

● **Q53.0 Ectopic testis**

Q53.00 Ectopic testis, unspecified

Q53.01 Ectopic testis, unilateral

Q53.02 Ectopic testes, bilateral

● **Q53.1 Undescended testicle, unilateral**

Q53.10 Unspecified undescended testicle, unilateral

Q53.11 Abdominal testis, unilateral

Q53.12 Ectopic perineal testis, unilateral

● **Q53.2 Undescended testicle, bilateral**

Q53.20 Undescended testicle, unspecified, bilateral

Q53.21 Abdominal testis, bilateral

Q53.22 Ectopic perineal testis, bilateral

Q53.9 Undescended testicle, unspecified
Cryptorchism NOS

● **Q54 Hypospadias**
Birth defect of male; urethra opens in abnormal location on shaft
Excludes1 epispadias (Q64.0)

Q54.0 Hypospadias, balanic
Hypospadias, coronal
Hypospadias, glandular

Q54.1 Hypospadias, penile

Q54.2 Hypospadias, penoscrotal

Q54.3 Hypospadias, perineal

Q54.4 Congenital chordee
Chordee without hypospadias

Q54.8 Other hypospadias
Hypospadias with intersex state

Q54.9 Hypospadias, unspecified

Item 17–1 Testes form in the abdomen of the male and only descend into the scrotum during normal embryonic development. "Ectopic" testes are out of their normal place or "retained" (left behind) in the abdomen. Crypto (hidden) orchism (testicle) is a major risk factor for testicular cancer.

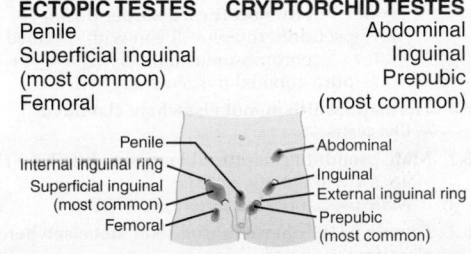

ECTOPIC TESTES	CRYPTORCHID TESTES
Penile	Abdominal
Superficial inguinal (most common)	Inguinal
Femoral	Prepubic (most common)

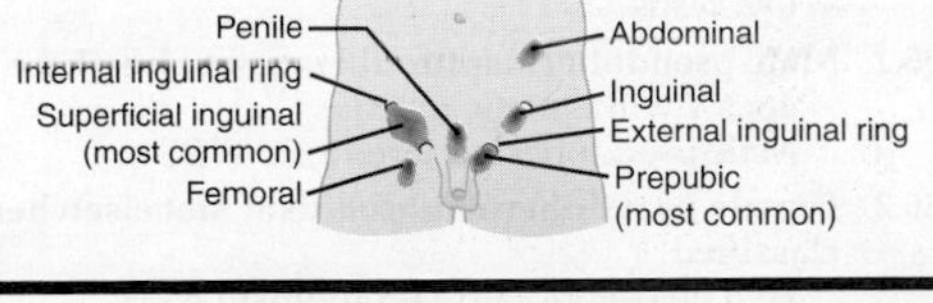

Figure 17-5 Undescended testes and the positions of the testes in various types of cryptorchidism or abnormal paths of descent.

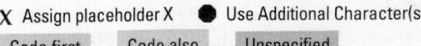

● **Q55 Other congenital malformations of male genital organs**
Excludes1 congenital hydrocele (P83.5)
hypospadias (Q54.-)
Q55.0 Absence and aplasia of testis
Monorchism
Q55.1 Hypoplasia of testis and scrotum
Fusion of testes
● **Q55.2 Other and unspecified congenital malformations of testis and scrotum**
Q55.20 Unspecified congenital malformations of testis and scrotum
Congenital malformation of testis or scrotum NOS
Q55.21 Polyorchism
Developmental anomaly characterized by presence of more than two testes
Q55.22 Retractile testis
Q55.23 Scrotal transposition
Q55.29 Other congenital malformations of testis and scrotum
Q55.3 Atresia of vas deferens
Code first any associated cystic fibrosis (E84.-)
Q55.4 Other congenital malformations of vas deferens, epididymis, seminal vesicles and prostate
Absence or aplasia of prostate
Absence or aplasia of spermatic cord
Congenital malformation of vas deferens, epididymis, seminal vesicles or prostate NOS
Q55.5 Congenital absence and aplasia of penis
● **Q55.6 Other congenital malformations of penis**
Q55.61 Curvature of penis (lateral)
Q55.62 Hypoplasia of penis
Underdevelopment penis
Micropenis
Q55.63 Congenital torsion of penis
Excludes1 acquired torsion of penis (N48.82)
Q55.64 Hidden penis
Buried penis
Concealed penis
Excludes1 acquired buried penis (N48.83)
Q55.69 Other congenital malformation of penis
Congenital malformation of penis NOS
Q55.7 Congenital vasocutaneous fistula
Abnormal opening between vas deferens and skin
Q55.8 Other specified congenital malformations of male genital organs
Q55.9 Congenital malformation of male genital organ, unspecified
Congenital anomaly of male genital organ
Congenital deformity of male genital organ

● **Q56 Indeterminate sex and pseudohermaphroditism**
Internal reproductive organs are opposite external physical characteristics.
Excludes1 46,XX true hermaphrodite (Q99.1)
androgen insensitivity syndrome (E34.5-)
chimera 46,XX/46,XY true hermaphrodite (Q99.0)
female pseudohermaphroditism with adrenocortical disorder (E25.-)
pseudohermaphroditism with specified chromosomal anomaly (Q96-Q99)
pure gonadal dysgenesis (Q99.1)
Q56.0 Hermaphroditism, not elsewhere classified
Ovotestis
Q56.1 Male pseudohermaphroditism, not elsewhere classified
46, XY with streak gonads
Male pseudohermaphroditism NOS
Q56.2 Female pseudohermaphroditism, not elsewhere classified
Female pseudohermaphroditism NOS
Q56.3 Pseudohermaphroditism, unspecified
Q56.4 Indeterminate sex, unspecified
Ambiguous genitalia

CONGENITAL MALFORMATIONS OF THE URINARY SYSTEM (Q60-Q64)

● **Q60 Renal agenesis and other reduction defects of kidney**
Includes congenital absence of kidney
congenital atrophy of kidney
infantile atrophy of kidney
Q60.0 Renal agenesis, unilateral
Q60.1 Renal agenesis, bilateral
Q60.2 Renal agenesis, unspecified
Q60.3 Renal hypoplasia, unilateral
Q60.4 Renal hypoplasia, bilateral
Q60.5 Renal hypoplasia, unspecified
Q60.6 Potter's syndrome

● **Q61 Cystic kidney disease**
Cysts that develop in failing kidney due to end-stage renal disease
Excludes1 acquired cyst of kidney (N28.1)
Potter's syndrome (Q60.6)
● **Q61.0 Congenital renal cyst**
Q61.00 Congenital renal cyst, unspecified
Cyst of kidney NOS (congenital)
Q61.01 Congenital single renal cyst
Q61.02 Congenital multiple renal cysts
● **Q61.1 Polycystic kidney, infantile type**
Polycystic kidney, autosomal recessive
Q61.11 Cystic dilatation of collecting ducts
Q61.19 Other polycystic kidney, infantile type
Q61.2 Polycystic kidney, adult type
Polycystic kidney, autosomal dominant
Q61.3 Polycystic kidney, unspecified
Q61.4 Renal dysplasia
Multicystic dysplastic kidney
Multicystic kidney (development)
Multicystic kidney disease
Multicystic renal dysplasia
Excludes1 polycystic kidney disease (Q61.11-Q61.3)
Q61.5 Medullary cystic kidney
Nephronopthisis
Sponge kidney NOS
Q61.8 Other cystic kidney diseases
Fibrocystic kidney
Fibrocystic renal degeneration or disease
Q61.9 Cystic kidney disease, unspecified
Meckel-Gruber syndrome

● **Q62 Congenital obstructive defects of renal pelvis and congenital malformations of ureter**
Q62.0 Congenital hydronephrosis
● **Q62.1 Congenital occlusion of ureter**
Atresia and stenosis of ureter
Q62.10 Congenital occlusion of ureter, unspecified
Q62.11 Congenital occlusion of ureteropelvic junction
Q62.12 Congenital occlusion of ureterovesical orifice
Q62.2 Congenital megaureter
Congenital dilatation of ureter
● **Q62.3 Other obstructive defects of renal pelvis and ureter**
Q62.31 Congenital ureterocele, orthotopic
Q62.32 Cecoureterocele
Ectopic ureterocele
Q62.39 Other obstructive defects of renal pelvis and ureter
Ureteropelvic junction obstruction NOS
Q62.4 Agenesis of ureter
Congenital absence ureter

Q62.5 Duplication of ureter
Accessory ureter
Double ureter

● **Q62.6 Malposition of ureter**
Q62.60 Malposition of ureter, unspecified
Q62.61 Deviation of ureter
Q62.62 Displacement of ureter
Q62.63 Anomalous implantation of ureter
Ectopia of ureter
Ectopic ureter
Q62.69 Other malposition of ureter

Q62.7 Congenital vesico-uretero-renal reflux
Q62.8 Other congenital malformations of ureter
Anomaly of ureter NOS

● **Q63 Other congenital malformations of kidney**
Excludes1 congenital nephrotic syndrome (N04.-)
Q63.0 Accessory kidney
Q63.1 Lobulated, fused and horseshoe kidney
Q63.2 Ectopic kidney
Congenital displaced kidney
Malrotation of kidney
Q63.3 Hyperplastic and giant kidney
Compensatory hypertrophy of kidney
Q63.8 Other specified congenital malformations of kidney
Congenital renal calculi
Q63.9 Congenital malformation of kidney, unspecified

● **Q64 Other congenital malformations of urinary system**
Q64.0 Epispadias
Urethral opening somewhere on dorsum of penis
Excludes1 hypospadias (Q54.-)

● **Q64.1 Exstrophy of urinary bladder**
Bladder is exposed, inside out, and protrudes through abdominal wall
Q64.10 Exstrophy of urinary bladder, unspecified
Ectopia vesicae
Q64.11 Supravesical fissure of urinary bladder
Q64.12 Cloacal extrophy of urinary bladder
Q64.19 Other exstrophy of urinary bladder
Extroversion of bladder

Q64.2 Congenital posterior urethral valves

● **Q64.3 Other atresia and stenosis of urethra and bladder neck**
Q64.31 Congenital bladder neck obstruction
Congenital obstruction of vesicourethral orifice
Q64.32 Congenital stricture of urethra
Q64.33 Congenital stricture of urinary meatus
Q64.39 Other atresia and stenosis of urethra and bladder neck
Atresia and stenosis of urethra and bladder neck NOS

Q64.4 Malformation of urachus
Cyst of urachus
Patent urachus
Prolapse of urachus
Q64.5 Congenital absence of bladder and urethra
Q64.6 Congenital diverticulum of bladder

● **Q64.7 Other and unspecified congenital malformations of bladder and urethra**
Excludes1 congenital prolapse of bladder (mucosa) (Q79.4)
Q64.70 Unspecified congenital malformation of bladder and urethra
Malformation of bladder or urethra NOS
Q64.71 Congenital prolapse of urethra
Q64.72 Congenital prolapse of urinary meatus
Q64.73 Congenital urethrorectal fistula
Q64.74 Double urethra
Q64.75 Double urinary meatus
Q64.79 Other congenital malformations of bladder and urethra

Q64.8 Other specified congenital malformations of urinary system
Q64.9 Congenital malformation of urinary system, unspecified
Congenital anomaly NOS of urinary system
Congenital deformity NOS of urinary system

CONGENITAL MALFORMATIONS AND DEFORMATIONS OF THE MUSCULOSKELETAL SYSTEM (Q65-Q79)

● **Q65 Congenital deformities of hip**
Excludes1 clicking hip (R29.4)

● **Q65.0 Congenital dislocation of hip, unilateral**
Q65.00 Congenital dislocation of unspecified hip, unilateral
Q65.01 Congenital dislocation of right hip, unilateral
Q65.02 Congenital dislocation of left hip, unilateral

Q65.1 Congenital dislocation of hip, bilateral
Q65.2 Congenital dislocation of hip, unspecified

● **Q65.3 Congenital partial dislocation of hip, unilateral**
Q65.30 Congenital partial dislocation of unspecified hip, unilateral
Q65.31 Congenital partial dislocation of right hip, unilateral
Q65.32 Congenital partial dislocation of left hip, unilateral

Q65.4 Congenital partial dislocation of hip, bilateral
Q65.5 Congenital partial dislocation of hip, unspecified
Q65.6 Congenital unstable hip
Congenital dislocatable hip

● **Q65.8 Other congenital deformities of hip**
Q65.81 Congenital coxa valga
Q65.82 Congenital coxa vara
Q65.89 Other specified congenital deformities of hip
Anteversion of femoral neck
Congenital acetabular dysplasia

Q65.9 Congenital deformity of hip, unspecified

● **Q66 Congenital deformities of feet**
Excludes1 reduction defects of feet (Q72.-)
valgus deformities (acquired) (M21.0-)
varus deformities (acquired) (M21.1-)

Q66.0 Congenital talipes equinovarus
Heel is turned inward from midline and foot is plantar flexed; AKA clubfoot
Q66.1 Congenital talipes calcaneovarus
Deformity of foot in which heel is turned toward midline of body and anterior of foot is elevated

● **Q66.2 Congenital metatarsus (primus) varus**
Angulation of first metatarsal bone toward midline of body
Q66.21 Congenital metatarsus primus varus ◀
Q66.22 Congenital metatarsus adductus ◀
Congenital metatarsus varus ◀

Q66.3 Other congenital varus deformities of feet
Hallux varus, congenital
Q66.4 Congenital talipes calcaneovalgus

● **Q66.5 Congenital pes planus**
Congenital flat foot
Congenital rigid flat foot
Congenital spastic (everted) flat foot
Excludes1 pes planus, acquired (M21.4)
Q66.50 Congenital pes planus, unspecified foot
Q66.51 Congenital pes planus, right foot
Q66.52 Congenital pes planus, left foot

Q66.6 Other congenital valgus deformities of feet
Inward angulation
Congenital metatarsus valgus
Q66.7 Congenital pes cavus

Item 17–2 Equinus foot is a term referring to the hoof of a horse. The deformity is usually congenital or spastic. Talipes equinovarus is referred to as clubfoot. The foot tends to be smaller than normal, with the heel pointing downward and the forefoot turning inward. The heel cord (Achilles tendon) is tight, causing the heel to be drawn up toward the leg.

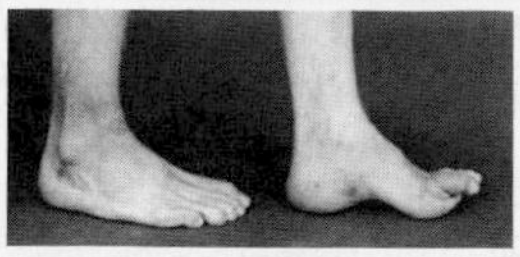

Figure 17-6 Supination and cavus deformity of forefoot. *(Courtesy Jay Cummings, MD.)* (From Canale: Campbell's Operative Orthopaedics, ed 11, Mosby, Inc., 2007)

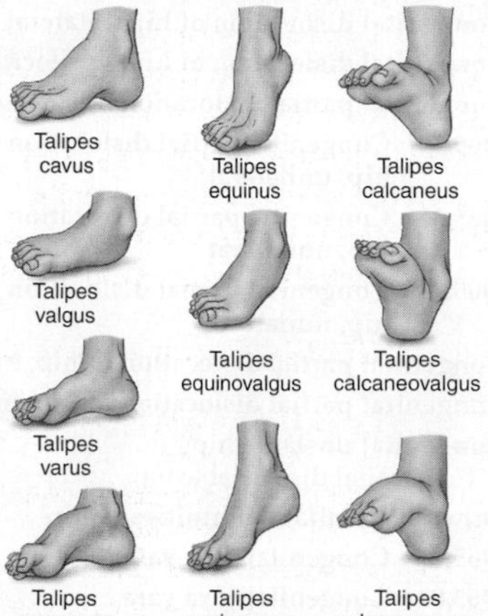

Figure 17-7 Talipes. (From Dorland: Dorland's Illustrated Medical Dictionary, ed 31, Saunders, 2007, p 1893)

● **Q66.8 Other congenital deformities of feet**
Q66.80 Congenital vertical talus deformity, unspecified foot
Q66.81 Congenital vertical talus deformity, right foot
Q66.82 Congenital vertical talus deformity, left foot
Q66.89 Other specified congenital deformities of feet
Congenital asymmetric talipes
Congenital clubfoot NOS
Congenital talipes NOS
Congenital tarsal coalition
Hammer toe, congenital

Q66.9 Congenital deformity of feet, unspecified

● **Q67 Congenital musculoskeletal deformities of head, face, spine and chest**
Excludes1 congenital malformation syndromes classified to Q87.-
Potter's syndrome (Q60.6)

Q67.0 Congenital facial asymmetry
Q67.1 Congenital compression facies
Q67.2 Dolichocephaly
Long head dimension
Q67.3 Plagiocephaly
Asymmetric shape of head resulting from irregular closure of cranial sutures
Q67.4 Other congenital deformities of skull, face and jaw
Congenital depressions in skull
Congenital hemifacial atrophy or hypertrophy
Deviation of nasal septum, congenital
Squashed or bent nose, congenital
Excludes1 dentofacial anomalies [including malocclusion] (M26.-)
syphilitic saddle nose (A50.5)

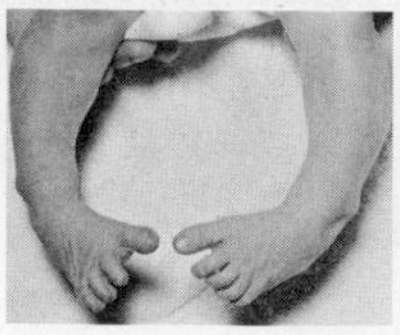

Figure 17-8 Mild to moderate inbowing of the lower leg. (From Jones KL: Smith's Recognizable Patterns of Human Malformation, ed 6, Philadelphia, Saunders, 2005)

Q67.5 Congenital deformity of spine
Congenital postural scoliosis
Congenital scoliosis NOS
Excludes1 infantile idiopathic scoliosis (M41.0)
scoliosis due to congenital bony malformation (Q76.3)

Q67.6 Pectus excavatum
Congenital funnel chest
Funnel-shaped chest depression
Q67.7 Pectus carinatum
Congenital pigeon chest
Q67.8 Other congenital deformities of chest
Congenital deformity of chest wall NOS

● **Q68 Other congenital musculoskeletal deformities**
Excludes1 reduction defects of limb(s) (Q71-Q73)
Excludes2 congenital myotonic chondrodystrophy (G71.13)

Q68.0 Congenital deformity of sternocleidomastoid muscle
Congenital contracture of sternocleidomastoid (muscle)
Congenital (sternomastoid) torticollis
Sternomastoid tumor (congenital)
Q68.1 Congenital deformity of finger(s) and hand
Congenital clubfinger
Spade-like hand (congenital)
Q68.2 Congenital deformity of knee
Congenital dislocation of knee
Congenital genu recurvatum
Hyperextension of knee resulting from hypermobility
Q68.3 Congenital bowing of femur
Excludes1 anteversion of femur (neck) (Q65.89)
Q68.4 Congenital bowing of tibia and fibula
Q68.5 Congenital bowing of long bones of leg, unspecified
Q68.6 Discoid meniscus
Q68.8 Other specified congenital musculoskeletal deformities
Congenital deformity of clavicle
Congenital deformity of elbow
Congenital deformity of forearm
Congenital deformity of scapula
Congenital deformity of wrist
Congenital dislocation of elbow
Congenital dislocation of shoulder
Congenital dislocation of wrist

● **Q69 Polydactyly**
AKA hyperdactyly, consists of supernumerary fingers or toes
Q69.0 Accessory finger(s)
Q69.1 Accessory thumb(s)
Q69.2 Accessory toe(s)
Accessory hallux
Q69.9 Polydactyly, unspecified
Supernumerary digit(s) NOS

● **Q70 Syndactyly**
Webbing between distal phalanges of adjacent digits
● **Q70.0 Fused fingers**
Complex syndactyly of fingers with synostosis
Q70.00 Fused fingers, unspecified hand
Q70.01 Fused fingers, right hand
Q70.02 Fused fingers, left hand
Q70.03 Fused fingers, bilateral

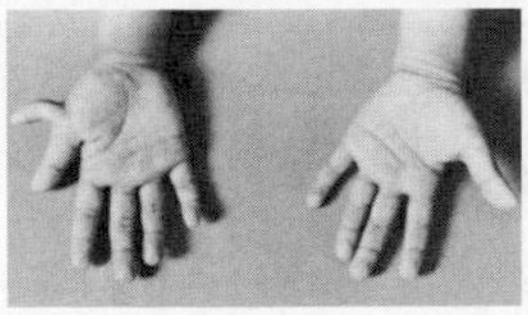

Figure 17-9 Polydactyly, congenital duplicated thumb. (From DeLee: DeLee and Drez's Orthopaedic Sports Medicine, ed 3, Saunders, An Imprint of Elsevier, 2009)

● Q70.1 Webbed fingers
Simple syndactyly of fingers without synostosis
Q70.10 Webbed fingers, unspecified hand
Q70.11 Webbed fingers, right hand
Q70.12 Webbed fingers, left hand
Q70.13 Webbed fingers, bilateral

● Q70.2 Fused toes
Complex syndactyly of toes with synostosis
Q70.20 Fused toes, unspecified foot
Q70.21 Fused toes, right foot
Q70.22 Fused toes, left foot
Q70.23 Fused toes, bilateral

● Q70.3 Webbed toes
Simple syndactyly of toes without synostosis
Q70.30 Webbed toes, unspecified foot
Q70.31 Webbed toes, right foot
Q70.32 Webbed toes, left foot
Q70.33 Webbed toes, bilateral

Q70.4 Polysyndactyly, unspecified
Excludes1 specified syndactyly of hand and feet - code to specified conditions (Q70.0- -Q70.3-)
Extra and webbed digits

Q70.9 Syndactyly, unspecified
Symphalangy NOS

● Q71 Reduction defects of upper limb

● Q71.0 Congenital complete absence of upper limb
Q71.00 Congenital complete absence of unspecified upper limb
Q71.01 Congenital complete absence of right upper limb
Q71.02 Congenital complete absence of left upper limb
Q71.03 Congenital complete absence of upper limb, bilateral

● Q71.1 Congenital absence of upper arm and forearm with hand present
Q71.10 Congenital absence of unspecified upper arm and forearm with hand present
Q71.11 Congenital absence of right upper arm and forearm with hand present
Q71.12 Congenital absence of left upper arm and forearm with hand present
Q71.13 Congenital absence of upper arm and forearm with hand present, bilateral

● Q71.2 Congenital absence of both forearm and hand
Q71.20 Congenital absence of both forearm and hand, unspecified upper limb
Q71.21 Congenital absence of both forearm and hand, right upper limb
Q71.22 Congenital absence of both forearm and hand, left upper limb
Q71.23 Congenital absence of both forearm and hand, bilateral

● Q71.3 Congenital absence of hand and finger
Q71.30 Congenital absence of unspecified hand and finger
Q71.31 Congenital absence of right hand and finger
Q71.32 Congenital absence of left hand and finger
Q71.33 Congenital absence of hand and finger, bilateral

● Q71.4 Longitudinal reduction defect of radius
Clubhand (congenital)
Radial clubhand
Q71.40 Longitudinal reduction defect of unspecified radius
Q71.41 Longitudinal reduction defect of right radius
Q71.42 Longitudinal reduction defect of left radius
Q71.43 Longitudinal reduction defect of radius, bilateral

● Q71.5 Longitudinal reduction defect of ulna
Q71.50 Longitudinal reduction defect of unspecified ulna
Q71.51 Longitudinal reduction defect of right ulna
Q71.52 Longitudinal reduction defect of left ulna
Q71.53 Longitudinal reduction defect of ulna, bilateral

● Q71.6 Lobster-claw hand
Q71.60 Lobster-claw hand, unspecified hand
Q71.61 Lobster-claw right hand
Q71.62 Lobster-claw left hand
Q71.63 Lobster-claw hand, bilateral

● Q71.8 Other reduction defects of upper limb
● Q71.81 Congenital shortening of upper limb
Q71.811 Congenital shortening of right upper limb
Q71.812 Congenital shortening of left upper limb
Q71.813 Congenital shortening of upper limb, bilateral
Q71.819 Congenital shortening of unspecified upper limb
● Q71.89 Other reduction defects of upper limb
Q71.891 Other reduction defects of right upper limb
Q71.892 Other reduction defects of left upper limb
Q71.893 Other reduction defects of upper limb, bilateral
Q71.899 Other reduction defects of unspecified upper limb

● Q71.9 Unspecified reduction defect of upper limb
Q71.90 Unspecified reduction defect of unspecified upper limb
Q71.91 Unspecified reduction defect of right upper limb
Q71.92 Unspecified reduction defect of left upper limb
Q71.93 Unspecified reduction defect of upper limb, bilateral

● Q72 Reduction defects of lower limb

● Q72.0 Congenital complete absence of lower limb
Q72.00 Congenital complete absence of unspecified lower limb
Q72.01 Congenital complete absence of right lower limb
Q72.02 Congenital complete absence of left lower limb
Q72.03 Congenital complete absence of lower limb, bilateral

● Q72.1 Congenital absence of thigh and lower leg with foot present
Q72.10 Congenital absence of unspecified thigh and lower leg with foot present
Q72.11 Congenital absence of right thigh and lower leg with foot present
Q72.12 Congenital absence of left thigh and lower leg with foot present
Q72.13 Congenital absence of thigh and lower leg with foot present, bilateral

CHAPTER 17 (Q00-Q99)

● Q72.2 Congenital absence of both lower leg and foot
Q72.20 Congenital absence of both lower leg and foot, unspecified lower limb
Q72.21 Congenital absence of both lower leg and foot, right lower limb
Q72.22 Congenital absence of both left lower leg and foot, left lower limb
Q72.23 Congenital absence of both lower leg and foot, bilateral

● Q72.3 Congenital absence of foot and toe(s)
Q72.30 Congenital absence of unspecified foot and toe(s)
Q72.31 Congenital absence of right foot and toe(s)
Q72.32 Congenital absence of left foot and toe(s)
Q72.33 Congenital absence of foot and toe(s), bilateral

● Q72.4 Longitudinal reduction defect of femur
Proximal femoral focal deficiency
Q72.40 Longitudinal reduction defect of unspecified femur
Q72.41 Longitudinal reduction defect of right femur
Q72.42 Longitudinal reduction defect of left femur
Q72.43 Longitudinal reduction defect of femur, bilateral

● Q72.5 Longitudinal reduction defect of tibia
Q72.50 Longitudinal reduction defect of unspecified tibia
Q72.51 Longitudinal reduction defect of right tibia
Q72.52 Longitudinal reduction defect of left tibia
Q72.53 Longitudinal reduction defect of tibia, bilateral

● Q72.6 Longitudinal reduction defect of fibula
Q72.60 Longitudinal reduction defect of unspecified fibula
Q72.61 Longitudinal reduction defect of right fibula
Q72.62 Longitudinal reduction defect of left fibula
Q72.63 Longitudinal reduction defect of fibula, bilateral

● Q72.7 Split foot
Q72.70 Split foot, unspecified lower limb
Q72.71 Split foot, right lower limb
Q72.72 Split foot, left lower limb
Q72.73 Split foot, bilateral

● Q72.8 Other reduction defects of lower limb
● Q72.81 Congenital shortening of lower limb
Q72.811 Congenital shortening of right lower limb
Q72.812 Congenital shortening of left lower limb
Q72.813 Congenital shortening of lower limb, bilateral
Q72.819 Congenital shortening of unspecified lower limb
● Q72.89 Other reduction defects of lower limb
Q72.891 Other reduction defects of right lower limb
Q72.892 Other reduction defects of left lower limb
Q72.893 Other reduction defects of lower limb, bilateral
Q72.899 Other reduction defects of unspecified lower limb

● Q72.9 Unspecified reduction defect of lower limb
Q72.90 Unspecified reduction defect of unspecified lower limb
Q72.91 Unspecified reduction defect of right lower limb
Q72.92 Unspecified reduction defect of left lower limb
Q72.93 Unspecified reduction defect of lower limb, bilateral

● Q73 Reduction defects of unspecified limb
Q73.0 Congenital absence of unspecified limb(s)
Amelia NOS
Q73.1 Phocomelia, unspecified limb(s)
Phocomelia NOS
Absence/shortening of long bones primarily as a result of thalidomide
Q73.8 Other reduction defects of unspecified limb(s)
Longitudinal reduction deformity of unspecified limb(s)
Ectromelia of limb NOS
Gross hypoplasia or aplasia of one or more long bones of limb(s)
Hemimelia of limb NOS
Absence of one-half of long bone
Reduction defect of limb NOS

● Q74 Other congenital malformations of limb(s)
Excludes1 polydactyly (Q69.-)
reduction defect of limb (Q71-Q73)
syndactyly (Q70.-)
Q74.0 Other congenital malformations of upper limb(s), including shoulder girdle
Accessory carpal bones
Cleidocranial dysostosis
Congenital pseudarthrosis of clavicle
Macrodactylia (fingers)
Madelung's deformity
Radioulnar synostosis
Sprengel's deformity
Triphalangeal thumb
Q74.1 Congenital malformation of knee
Congenital absence of patella
Congenital dislocation of patella
Congenital genu valgum
Congenital genu varum
Rudimentary patella
Excludes1 congenital dislocation of knee (Q68.2)
congenital genu recurvatum (Q68.2)
nail patella syndrome (Q87.2)
Q74.2 Other congenital malformations of lower limb(s), including pelvic girdle
Congenital fusion of sacroiliac joint
Congenital malformation of ankle joint
Congenital malformation of sacroiliac joint
Excludes1 anteversion of femur (neck) (Q65.89)
Q74.3 Arthrogryposis multiplex congenita
Q74.8 Other specified congenital malformations of limb(s)
Q74.9 Unspecified congenital malformation of limb(s)
Congenital anomaly of limb(s) NOS

● Q75 Other congenital malformations of skull and face bones
Excludes1 congenital malformation of face NOS (Q18.-)
congenital malformation syndromes classified to Q87.-
dentofacial anomalies [including malocclusion] (M26.-)
musculoskeletal deformities of head and face (Q67.0-Q67.4)
skull defects associated with congenital anomalies of brain such as:
anencephaly (Q00.0)
encephalocele (Q01.-)
hydrocephalus (Q03.-)
microcephaly (Q02)
Q75.0 Craniosynostosis
Premature closure of sutures of skull
Acrocephaly
Imperfect fusion of skull
Oxycephaly
Trigonocephaly
Q75.1 Craniofacial dysostosis
Congential deformity of head
Crouzon's disease

Item 17–3 Anencephalus is a congenital deformity of the cranial vault. **Craniosynostosis,** also known as craniostenosis and stenocephaly, signifies any form of congenital deformity of the skull that results from the premature closing of the sutures of the skull. **Iniencephaly** is a deformity in which the head and neck are flexed backward to a great extent and the head is very large in comparison to the shortened body.

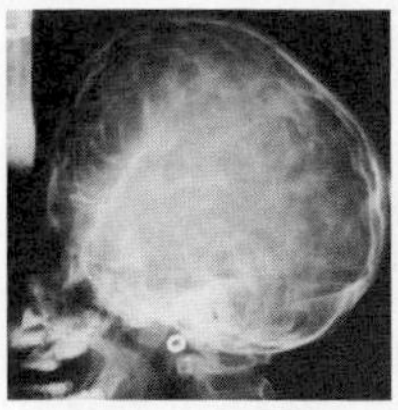

Figure 17-10 Generalized craniosynostosis in a 4-year-old girl without symptoms or signs of increased intracranial pressure. (From Bell WE, McCormick WF: Increased Intracranial Pressure in Children, ed 2, Philadelphia, WB Saunders, 1978, p 116)

Q75.2 Hypertelorism

Q75.3 Macrocephaly
Unusually large size of head; AKA megalocephaly

Q75.4 Mandibulofacial dysostosis
Franceschetti syndrome
Treacher Collins syndrome

Q75.5 Oculomandibular dysostosis
Ossification of occular and mandibular bones

Q75.8 Other specified congenital malformations of skull and face bones
Absence of skull bone, congenital
Congenital deformity of forehead
Platybasia

Q75.9 Congenital malformation of skull and face bones, unspecified
Congenital anomaly of face bones NOS
Congenital anomaly of skull NOS

● **Q76 Congenital malformations of spine and bony thorax**
Excludes1 congenital musculoskeletal deformities of spine and chest (Q67.5-Q67.8)

Q76.0 Spina bifida occulta
Excludes1 meningocele (spinal) (Q05.-)
spina bifida (aperta) (cystica) (Q05.-)

Q76.1 Klippel-Feil syndrome
Cervical fusion syndrome

Q76.2 Congenital spondylolisthesis
Congenital spondylolysis
Excludes1 spondylolisthesis (acquired) (M43.1-)
spondylolysis (acquired) (M43.0-)

Q76.3 Congenital scoliosis due to congenital bony malformation
Hemivertebra fusion or failure of segmentation with scoliosis

● **Q76.4 Other congenital malformations of spine, not associated with scoliosis**

● **Q76.41 Congenital kyphosis**
Abnormal increase in convexity curvature of thoracic spinal column; AKA humpback

Q76.411 Congenital kyphosis, occipito-atlanto-axial region
Q76.412 Congenital kyphosis, cervical region
Q76.413 Congenital kyphosis, cervicothoracic region
Q76.414 Congenital kyphosis, thoracic region
Q76.415 Congenital kyphosis, thoracolumbar region
Q76.419 Congenital kyphosis, unspecified region

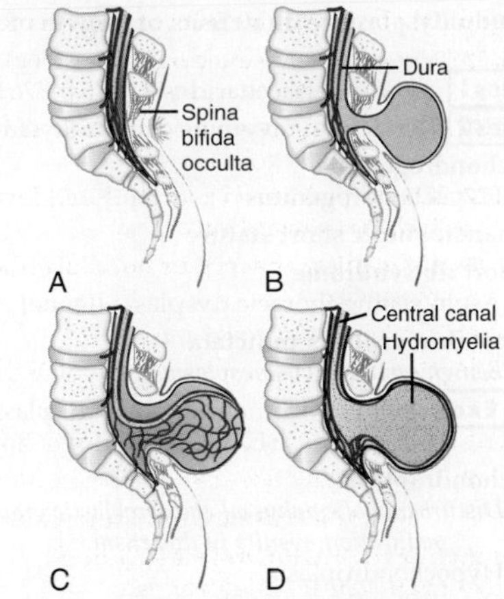

Figure 17-11 A. Spina bifida occulta. **B.** Meningocele. **C.** Myelomeningocele. **D.** Myelocystocele (syringomyelocele) or hydromyelia.

Item 17–4 Spina bifida is a midline spinal defect in which one or more vertebrae fail to fuse, leaving an opening in the vertebral canal. When the defect is not visible, it is called spina bifida occulta, and when it is visible, it is called spina bifida cystica.

● **Q76.42 Congenital lordosis**
An abnormal increase in curvature of lumbar spine (sway back)

Q76.425 Congenital lordosis, thoracolumbar region
Q76.426 Congenital lordosis, lumbar region
Q76.427 Congenital lordosis, lumbosacral region
Q76.428 Congenital lordosis, sacral and sacrococcygeal region
Q76.429 Congenital lordosis, unspecified region

Q76.49 Other congenital malformations of spine, not associated with scoliosis
Congenital absence of vertebra NOS
Congenital fusion of spine NOS
Congenital malformation of lumbosacral (joint) (region) NOS
Congenital malformation of spine NOS
Hemivertebra NOS
Malformation of spine NOS
Platyspondylisis NOS
Supernumerary vertebra NOS

Q76.5 Cervical rib
Supernumerary rib in cervical region

Q76.6 Other congenital malformations of ribs
Accessory rib
Congenital absence of rib
Congenital fusion of ribs
Congenital malformation of ribs NOS
Excludes1 short rib syndrome (Q77.2)

Q76.7 Congenital malformation of sternum
Congenital absence of sternum
Sternum bifidum

Q76.8 Other congenital malformations of bony thorax

Q76.9 Congenital malformation of bony thorax, unspecified

● Q77 Osteochondrodysplasia with defects of growth of tubular bones and spine
Excludes1 mucopolysaccharidosis (E76.Ø-E76.3)
Excludes2 congenital myotonic chondrodystrophy (G71.13)
Q77.Ø Achondrogenesis
Hypochondrogenesis
Q77.1 Thanatophoric short stature
Q77.2 Short rib syndrome
Asphyxiating thoracic dysplasia [Jeune]
Q77.3 Chondrodysplasia punctata
Benign cartilaginous neoplasms
Excludes1 rhizomelic chondrodysplasia punctata (E71.43)
Q77.4 Achondroplasia
Disturbance of epiphyseal chondroblastic growth and maturation, results in dwarfism
Hypochondroplasia
Osteosclerosis congenita
Q77.5 Diastrophic dysplasia
Q77.6 Chondroectodermal dysplasia
Defective development of skin, hair, teeth, with polydactyly and defect of cardiac septum
Ellis-van Creveld syndrome
Q77.7 Spondyloepiphyseal dysplasia
Q77.8 Other osteochondrodysplasia with defects of growth of tubular bones and spine
Q77.9 Osteochondrodysplasia with defects of growth of tubular bones and spine, unspecified

● Q78 Other osteochondrodysplasias
Disorder of development of bone and cartilage; common cause of dwarfism
Excludes2 congenital myotonic chondrodystrophy (G71.13)
Q78.Ø Osteogenesis imperfecta
Fragilitas ossium
Osteopsathyrosis
Q78.1 Polyostotic fibrous dysplasia
Albright(-McCune)(-Sternberg) syndrome
Q78.2 Osteopetrosis
Abnormally dense bone; AKA marble bones disease, ivory bones
Albers-Schönberg syndrome
Osteosclerosis NOS
Q78.3 Progressive diaphyseal dysplasia
Camurati-Engelmann syndrome
Q78.4 Enchondromatosis
Thinning of overlying cortex of bone and distorted length
Maffucci's syndrome
Ollier's disease
Q78.5 Metaphyseal dysplasia
Disturbance in enchondral bone growth, causing ends of shafts to remain larger than normal in circumference
Pyle's syndrome
Q78.6 Multiple congenital exostoses
Diaphyseal aclasis
Q78.8 Other specified osteochondrodysplasias
Osteopoikilosis
Q78.9 Osteochondrodysplasia, unspecified
Chondrodystrophy NOS
AKA skeletal dysplasia (dwarfism) caused by genetic mutations affecting hyaline cartilage capping long bones and vertebrae
Osteodystrophy NOS

● Q79 Congenital malformations of musculoskeletal system, not elsewhere classified
Excludes2 congenital (sternomastoid) torticollis (Q68.Ø)
Q79.Ø Congenital diaphragmatic hernia
Excludes1 congenital hiatus hernia (Q4Ø.1)
Q79.1 Other congenital malformations of diaphragm
Absence of diaphragm
Congenital malformation of diaphragm NOS
Eventration of diaphragm
Q79.2 Exomphalos
Abdominal hernia in which part of intestine protrudes at umbilicus; AKA exomphalos and exumbilication
Omphalocele
Excludes1 umbilical hernia (K42.-)
Q79.3 Gastroschisis
Congenital fissure of anterior abdominal wall often with protrusion of small/large intestine
Q79.4 Prune belly syndrome
Congenital prolapse of bladder mucosa
Eagle-Barrett syndrome
● Q79.5 Other congenital malformations of abdominal wall
Excludes1 umbilical hernia (K42.-)
Q79.51 Congenital hernia of bladder
Q79.59 Other congenital malformations of abdominal wall
Q79.6 Ehlers-Danlos syndrome
Group of inherited disorders of connective tissue; AKA cutis hyperelastica
Q79.8 Other congenital malformations of musculoskeletal system
Absence of muscle
Absence of tendon
Accessory muscle
Amyotrophia congenita
Congenital constricting bands
Congenital shortening of tendon
Poland syndrome
Q79.9 Congenital malformation of musculoskeletal system, unspecified
Congenital anomaly of musculoskeletal system NOS
Congenital deformity of musculoskeletal system NOS

OTHER CONGENITAL MALFORMATIONS (Q8Ø-Q89)

● Q8Ø Congenital ichthyosis
Characterized by increased keratinization, resulting in noninflammatory scaling of skin
Excludes1 Refsum's disease (G6Ø.1)
Q8Ø.Ø Ichthyosis vulgaris
Q8Ø.1 X-linked ichthyosis
Q8Ø.2 Lamellar ichthyosis
Collodion baby
Q8Ø.3 Congenital bullous ichthyosiform erythroderma
Q8Ø.4 Harlequin fetus
Q8Ø.8 Other congenital ichthyosis
Q8Ø.9 Congenital ichthyosis, unspecified

● Q81 Epidermolysis bullosa
Loosening of epidermis
Q81.Ø Epidermolysis bullosa simplex
Excludes1 Cockayne's syndrome (Q87.1)
Q81.1 Epidermolysis bullosa letalis
Herlitz' syndrome
Q81.2 Epidermolysis bullosa dystrophica
Q81.8 Other epidermolysis bullosa
Q81.9 Epidermolysis bullosa, unspecified

CHAPTER 17 (QØØ-Q99)

● **Q82 Other congenital malformations of skin**
Excludes1 acrodermatitis enteropathica (E83.2)
congenital erythropoietic porphyria (E80.0)
pilonidal cyst or sinus (L05.-)
Sturge-Weber (-Dimitri) syndrome (Q85.8)

Q82.0 Hereditary lymphedema
Characterized by swelling of subcutaneous tissue caused by obstruction of lymphatic vessels and resulting edema of lymph fluid

Q82.1 Xeroderma pigmentosum
Dry, rough, discolored state of skin, and formation of scaly desquamation

Q82.2 Mastocytosis
Characterized by infiltrates of mast cells in tissues/organs
Urticaria pigmentosa
Excludes1 malignant mastocytosis (C96.2)

Q82.3 Incontinentia pigmenti
Characterized by hyperpigmented cutaneous

Q82.4 Ectodermal dysplasia (anhidrotic)
Absence/deficiency of tissues/structures, including teeth, hair, nails, and certain glands
Excludes1 Ellis-van Creveld syndrome (Q77.6)

Q82.5 Congenital non-neoplastic nevus
Birthmark NOS
Flammeus Nevus
Portwine Nevus
Sanguineous Nevus
Strawberry Nevus
Vascular Nevus NOS
Verrucous Nevus
Excludes2 Café au lait spots (L81.3)
lentigo (L81.4)
nevus NOS (D22.-)
araneus nevus (I78.1)
melanocytic nevus (D22.-)
pigmented nevus (D22.-)
spider nevus (I78.1)
stellar nevus (I78.1)

Q82.6 Congenital sacral dimple ◀
Parasacral dimple ◀
Excludes2 pilonidal cyst with abscess (L05.01) ◀
pilonidal cyst without abscess (L05.91) ◀

Q82.8 Other specified congenital malformations of skin
Abnormal palmar creases
Accessory skin tags
Benign familial pemphigus [Hailey-Hailey]
Congenital poikiloderma
Cutis laxa (hyperelastica)
Dermatoglyphic anomalies
Inherited keratosis palmaris et plantaris
Keratosis follicularis [Darier-White]
Excludes1 Ehlers-Danlos syndrome (Q79.6)

Q82.9 Congenital malformation of skin, unspecified

● **Q83 Congenital malformations of breast**
Excludes2 absence of pectoral muscle (Q79.8)
hypoplasia of breast (N64.82)
micromastia (N64.82)

Q83.0 Congenital absence of breast with absent nipple

Q83.1 Accessory breast
Supernumerary breast

Q83.2 Absent nipple

Q83.3 Accessory nipple
Supernumerary nipple

Q83.8 Other congenital malformations of breast

Q83.9 Congenital malformation of breast, unspecified

● **Q84 Other congenital malformations of integument**

Q84.0 Congenital alopecia
Congenital atrichosis

Q84.1 Congenital morphological disturbances of hair, not elsewhere classified
Beaded hair
Monilethrix
Pili annulati
Excludes1 Menkes' kinky hair syndrome (E83.0)

Q84.2 Other congenital malformations of hair
Congenital hypertrichosis
Congenital malformation of hair NOS
Persistent lanugo

Q84.3 Anonychia
Absence of nail
Excludes1 nail patella syndrome (Q87.2)

Q84.4 Congenital leukonychia
Opaque, whitish discoloration of nails; AKA leukopathia unguium

Q84.5 Enlarged and hypertrophic nails
Congenital onychauxis
Pachyonychia

Q84.6 Other congenital malformations of nails
Congenital clubnail
Congenital koilonychia
Congenital malformation of nail NOS

Q84.8 Other specified congenital malformations of integument
Aplasia cutis congenita

Q84.9 Congenital malformation of integument, unspecified
Congenital anomaly of integument NOS
Congenital deformity of integument NOS

● **Q85 Phakomatoses, not elsewhere classified**
Excludes1 ataxia telangiectasia [Louis-Bar] (G11.3)
familial dysautonomia [Riley-Day] (G90.1)

● **Q85.0 Neurofibromatosis (nonmalignant)**
Developmental changes in nervous system and other structures, with formation of neurofibromas

Q85.00 Neurofibromatosis, unspecified

Q85.01 Neurofibromatosis, type 1
Von Recklinghausen disease

Q85.02 Neurofibromatosis, type 2
Acoustic neurofibromatosis

Q85.03 Schwannomatosis

Q85.09 Other neurofibromatosis

Q85.1 Tuberous sclerosis
Bourneville's disease
Epiloia

Q85.8 Other phakomatoses, not elsewhere classified
Peutz-Jeghers Syndrome
Sturge-Weber(-Dimitri) syndrome
von Hippel-Lindau syndrome
Excludes1 Meckel-Gruber syndrome (Q61.9)

Q85.9 Phakomatosis, unspecified
Hamartosis NOS

● **Q86 Congenital malformation syndromes due to known exogenous causes, not elsewhere classified**
Excludes2 iodine-deficiency-related hypothyroidism (E00-E02)
nonteratogenic effects of substances transmitted via placenta or breast milk (P04.-)

Q86.0 Fetal alcohol syndrome (dysmorphic)

Q86.1 Fetal hydantoin syndrome
Meadow's syndrome

Q86.2 Dysmorphism due to warfarln

Q86.8 Other congenital malformation syndromes due to known exogenous causes

● **Q87 Other specified congenital malformation syndromes affecting multiple systems**
Use additional code(s) to identify all associated manifestations

Q87.0 Congenital malformation syndromes predominantly affecting facial appearance
Acrocephalopolysyndactyly
Acrocephalosyndactyly [Apert]
Cryptophthalmos syndrome
Cyclopia
Goldenhar syndrome
Moebius syndrome
Oro-facial-digital syndrome
Robin syndrome
Whistling face

Q87.1 Congenital malformation syndromes predominantly associated with short stature
Aarskog syndrome
Cockayne syndrome
De Lange syndrome
Dubowitz syndrome
Noonan syndrome
Prader-Willi syndrome
Robinow-Silverman-Smith syndrome
Russell-Silver syndrome
Seckel syndrome
Excludes1 Ellis-van Creveld syndrome (Q77.6)
Smith-Lemli-Opitz syndrome (E78.72)

Q87.2 Congenital malformation syndromes predominantly involving limbs
Holt-Oram syndrome
Klippel-Trenaunay-Weber syndrome
Nail patella syndrome
Rubinstein-Taybi syndrome
Sirenomelia syndrome
Thrombocytopenia with absent radius [TAR] syndrome
VATER syndrome

Q87.3 Congenital malformation syndromes involving early overgrowth
Beckwith-Wiedemann syndrome
Sotos' syndrome
Weaver syndrome

● **Q87.4 Marfan's syndrome**
Q87.40 Marfan's syndrome, unspecified
● **Q87.41 Marfan's syndrome with cardiovascular manifestations**
Q87.410 Marfan's syndrome with aortic dilation
Q87.418 Marfan's syndrome with other cardiovascular manifestations
Q87.42 Marfan's syndrome with ocular manifestations
Q87.43 Marfan's syndrome with skeletal manifestation

Q87.5 Other congenital malformation syndromes with other skeletal changes

● **Q87.8 Other specified congenital malformation syndromes, not elsewhere classified**
Excludes1 Zellweger syndrome (E71.510)
Q87.81 Alport syndrome
Progressive sensorineural hearing loss, progressive pyelonephritis or glomerulonephritis, and ocular defects
Use additional code to identify stage of chronic kidney disease (N18.1-N18.6)
Q87.82 Arterial tortuosity syndrome ◄
Q87.89 Other specified congenital malformation syndromes, not elsewhere classified
Laurence-Moon (-Bardet)-Biedl syndrome

● **Q89 Other congenital malformations, not elsewhere classified**
● **Q89.0 Congenital absence and malformations of spleen**
Excludes1 isomerism of atrial appendages (with asplenia or polysplenia) (Q20.6)
Q89.01 Asplenia (congenital)
Q89.09 Congenital malformations of spleen
Congenital splenomegaly

Q89.1 Congenital malformations of adrenal gland
Excludes1 adrenogenital disorders (E25.-)
congenital adrenal hyperplasia (E25.0)

Q89.2 Congenital malformations of other endocrine glands
Congenital malformation of parathyroid or thyroid gland
Persistent thyroglossal duct
Thyroglossal cyst
Excludes1 congenital goiter (E03.0)
congenital hypothyroidism (E03.1)

Q89.3 Situs inversus
Lateral transposition of viscera of thorax and abdomen
Dextrocardia with situs inversus
Mirror-image atrial arrangement with situs inversus
Situs inversus or transversus abdominalis
Situs inversus or transversus thoracis
Transposition of abdominal viscera
Transposition of thoracic viscera
Excludes1 dextrocardia NOS (Q24.0)

Q89.4 Conjoined twins
Craniopagus
Dicephaly
Pygopagus
Thoracopagus

Q89.7 Multiple congenital malformations, not elsewhere classified
Multiple congenital anomalies NOS
Multiple congenital deformities NOS
Excludes1 congenital malformation syndromes affecting multiple systems (Q87.-)

Q89.8 Other specified congenital malformations
Use additional code(s) to identify all associated manifestations

Q89.9 Congenital malformation, unspecified
Congenital anomaly NOS
Congenital deformity NOS

CHROMOSOMAL ABNORMALITIES, NOT ELSEWHERE CLASSIFIED (Q90-Q99)

Excludes2 mitochondrial metabolic disorders (E88.4-)

● **Q90 Down syndrome**
Use additional code(s) to identify any associated physical conditions and degree of intellectual disabilities (F70-F79)
Q90.0 Trisomy 21, nonmosaicism (meiotic nondisjunction)
Trisomy 21, nondisjunction, accounts for 95% of Downs syndrome cases
Q90.1 Trisomy 21, mosaicism (mitotic nondisjunction)
Q90.2 Trisomy 21, translocation
Q90.9 Down syndrome, unspecified
Trisomy 21 NOS

● **Q91 Trisomy 18 and Trisomy 13**
Q91.0 Trisomy 18, nonmosaicism (meiotic nondisjunction)
Q91.1 Trisomy 18, mosaicism (mitotic nondisjunction)
Q91.2 Trisomy 18, translocation
Q91.3 Trisomy 18, unspecified
Q91.4 Trisomy 13, nonmosaicism (meiotic nondisjunction)
Q91.5 Trisomy 13, mosaicism (mitotic nondisjunction)
Q91.6 Trisomy 13, translocation
Q91.7 Trisomy 13, unspecified

● **Q92 Other trisomies and partial trisomies of the autosomes, not elsewhere classified**

Includes unbalanced translocations and insertions

Excludes1 trisomies of chromosomes 13, 18, 21 (Q90-Q91)

Q92.0 Whole chromosome trisomy, nonmosaicism (meiotic nondisjunction)

Q92.1 Whole chromosome trisomy, mosaicism (mitotic nondisjunction)

Q92.2 Partial trisomy

Less than whole arm duplicated

Whole arm or more duplicated

Excludes1 partial trisomy due to unbalanced translocation (Q92.5)

Q92.5 Duplications with other complex rearrangements

Partial trisomy due to unbalanced translocations

Code also any associated deletions due to unbalanced translocations, inversions and insertions (Q93.7)

● **Q92.6 Marker chromosomes**

Trisomies due to dicentrics

Trisomies due to extra rings

Trisomies due to isochromosomes

Individual with marker heterochromatin

Q92.61 Marker chromosomes in normal individual

Q92.62 Marker chromosomes in abnormal individual

Q92.7 Triploidy and polyploidy

Q92.8 Other specified trisomies and partial trisomies of autosomes

Duplications identified by fluorescence in situ hybridization (FISH)

Duplications identified by in situ hybridization (ISH)

Duplications seen only at prometaphase

Q92.9 Trisomy and partial trisomy of autosomes, unspecified

● **Q93 Monosomies and deletions from the autosomes, not elsewhere classified**

Q93.0 Whole chromosome monosomy, nonmosaicism (meiotic nondisjunction)

Q93.1 Whole chromosome monosomy, mosaicism (mitotic nondisjunction)

Q93.2 Chromosome replaced with ring, dicentric or isochromosome

Q93.3 Deletion of short arm of chromosome 4

Wolff-Hirschorn syndrome

Q93.4 Deletion of short arm of chromosome 5

Cri-du-chat syndrome

Q93.5 Other deletions of part of a chromosome

Angelman syndrome

Q93.7 Deletions with other complex rearrangements

Deletions due to unbalanced translocations, inversions and insertions

Code also any associated duplications due to unbalanced translocations, inversions and insertions (Q92.5)

● **Q93.8 Other deletions from the autosomes**

Q93.81 Velo-cardio-facial syndrome

Deletion 22q11.2

Q93.88 Other microdeletions Miller-Dieker syndrome

Smith-Magenis syndrome

Q93.89 Other deletions from the autosomes

Deletions identified by fluorescence in situ hybridization (FISH)

Deletions identified by in situ hybridization (ISH)

Deletions seen only at prometaphase

Q93.9 Deletion from autosomes, unspecified

● **Q95 Balanced rearrangements and structural markers, not elsewhere classified**

Includes Robertsonian and balanced reciprocal translocations and insertions

Q95.0 Balanced translocation and insertion in normal individual

Q95.1 Chromosome inversion in normal individual

Q95.2 Balanced autosomal rearrangement in abnormal individual

Q95.3 Balanced sex/autosomal rearrangement in abnormal individual

Q95.5 Individual with autosomal fragile site

Q95.8 Other balanced rearrangements and structural markers

Q95.9 Balanced rearrangement and structural marker, unspecified

● **Q96 Turner's syndrome**

Caused by missing or incomplete X chromosome affecting growth and sexual development

Excludes1 Noonan syndrome (Q87.1)

Q96.0 Karyotype 45, X

Q96.1 Karyotype 46, X iso (Xq)

Karyotype 46, isochromosome Xq

Q96.2 Karyotype 46, X with abnormal sex chromosome, except iso (Xq)

Karyotype 46, X with abnormal sex chromosome, except isochromosome Xq

Q96.3 Mosaicism, 45, X/46, XX or XY

Q96.4 Mosaicism, 45, X/other cell line(s) with abnormal sex chromosome

Q96.8 Other variants of Turner's syndrome

Q96.9 Turner's syndrome, unspecified

● **Q97 Other sex chromosome abnormalities, female phenotype, not elsewhere classified**

Excludes1 Turner's syndrome (Q96.-)

Q97.0 Karyotype 47, XXX

Q97.1 Female with more than three X chromosomes

Q97.2 Mosaicism, lines with various numbers of X chromosomes

Q97.3 Female with 46, XY karyotype

Q97.8 Other specified sex chromosome abnormalities, female phenotype

Q97.9 Sex chromosome abnormality, female phenotype, unspecified

● **Q98 Other sex chromosome abnormalities, male phenotype, not elsewhere classified**

Q98.0 Klinefelter syndrome karyotype 47, XXY

Q98.1 Klinefelter syndrome, male with more than two X chromosomes

Q98.3 Other male with 46, XX karyotype

Q98.4 Klinefelter syndrome, unspecified

Q98.5 Karyotype 47, XYY

Q98.6 Male with structurally abnormal sex chromosome

Q98.7 Male with sex chromosome mosaicism

Q98.8 Other specified sex chromosome abnormalities, male phenotype

Q98.9 Sex chromosome abnormality, male phenotype, unspecified

● **Q99 Other chromosome abnormalities, not elsewhere classified**

Q99.0 Chimera 46, XX/46, XY

Chimera 46, XX/46, XY true hermaphrodite

Q99.1 46, XX true hermaphrodite

46, XX with streak gonads

46, XY with streak gonads

Pure gonadal dysgenesis

Q99.2 Fragile X chromosome

Fragile X syndrome

Q99.8 Other specified chromosome abnormalities

Q99.9 Chromosomal abnormality, unspecified

CHAPTER 17 (Q00-Q99)

CHAPTER 18

SYMPTOMS, SIGNS AND ABNORMAL CLINICAL AND LABORATORY FINDINGS, NOT ELSEWHERE CLASSIFIED (RØØ-R99)

OGCR Chapter-Specific Coding Guidelines

18. Chapter 18: Symptoms, signs, and abnormal clinical and laboratory findings, not elsewhere classified (RØØ-R99)
Chapter 18 includes symptoms, signs, abnormal results of clinical or other investigative procedures, and ill-defined conditions regarding which no diagnosis classifiable elsewhere is recorded. Signs and symptoms that point to a specific diagnosis have been assigned to a category in other chapters of the classification.

a. Use of symptom codes
Codes that describe symptoms and signs are acceptable for reporting purposes when a related definitive diagnosis has not been established (confirmed) by the provider.

b. Use of a symptom code with a definitive diagnosis code
Codes for signs and symptoms may be reported in addition to a related definitive diagnosis when the sign or symptom is not routinely associated with that diagnosis, such as the various signs and symptoms associated with complex syndromes. The definitive diagnosis code should be sequenced before the symptom code.

Signs or symptoms that are associated routinely with a disease process should not be assigned as additional codes, unless otherwise instructed by the classification.

c. Combination codes that include symptoms
ICD-10-CM contains a number of combination codes that identify both the definitive diagnosis and common symptoms of that diagnosis. When using one of these combination codes, an additional code should not be assigned for the symptom.

d. Repeated falls
Code R29.6, Repeated falls, is for use for encounters when a patient has recently fallen and the reason for the fall is being investigated.

Code Z91.81, History of falling, is for use when a patient has fallen in the past and is at risk for future falls. When appropriate, both codes R29.6 and Z91.81 may be assigned together.

e. Coma scale
The coma scale codes (R4Ø.2-) can be used in conjunction with traumatic brain injury codes, acute cerebrovascular disease or sequelae of cerebrovascular disease codes. These codes are primarily for use by trauma registries, but they may be used in any setting where this information is collected. **The coma scale may also be used to assess the status of the central nervous system for other non-trauma conditions, such as monitoring patients in the intensive care unit regardless of medical condition.** The coma scale codes should be sequenced after the diagnosis code(s).

These codes, one from each subcategory, are needed to complete the scale. The 7th character indicates when the scale was recorded. The 7th character should match for all three codes.

At a minimum, report the initial score documented on presentation at your facility. This may be a score from the emergency medicine technician (EMT) or in the emergency department. If desired, a facility may choose to capture multiple coma scale scores.

Assign code R4Ø.24, Glasgow coma scale, total score, when only the total score is documented in the medical record and not the individual score(s).

f. Functional quadriplegia
Functional quadriplegia (code R53.2) is the lack of ability to use one's limbs or to ambulate due to extreme debility. It is not associated with neurologic deficit or injury, and code R53.2 should not be used for cases of neurologic quadriplegia. It should only be assigned if functional quadriplegia is specifically documented in the medical record.

g. SIRS due to Non-Infectious Process
The systemic inflammatory response syndrome (SIRS) can develop as a result of certain non-infectious disease processes, such as trauma, malignant neoplasm, or pancreatitis. When SIRS is documented with a noninfectious condition, and no subsequent infection is documented, the code for the underlying condition, such as an injury, should be assigned, followed by code R65.1Ø, Systemic inflammatory response syndrome (SIRS) of non-infectious origin without acute organ dysfunction, or code R65.11, Systemic inflammatory response syndrome (SIRS) of non-infectious origin with acute organ dysfunction. If an associated acute organ dysfunction is documented, the appropriate code(s) for the specific type of organ dysfunction(s) should be assigned in addition to code R65.11. If acute organ dysfunction is documented, but it cannot be determined if the acute organ dysfunction is associated with SIRS or due to another condition (e.g., directly due to the trauma), the provider should be queried.

h. Death NOS
Code R99, Ill-defined and unknown cause of mortality, is only for use in the very limited circumstance when a patient who has already died is brought into an emergency department or other healthcare facility and is pronounced dead upon arrival. It does not represent the discharge disposition of death.

i. NIHSS Stroke Scale
The NIH stroke scale (NIHSS) codes (R29.7- -) can be used in conjunction with acute stroke codes (I63) to identify the patient's neurological status and the severity of the stroke. The stroke scale codes should be sequenced after the acute stroke diagnosis code(s).

At a minimum, report the initial score documented. If desired, a facility may choose to capture multiple stroke scale scores.

See Section I.B.14. for information concerning the medical record documentation that may be used for assignment of the NIHSS codes.

OGCR Section I.B.4.

Signs and symptoms

Codes that describe symptoms and signs, as opposed to diagnoses, are acceptable for reporting purposes when a related definitive diagnosis has not been established (confirmed) by the provider. Chapter 18 of ICD-10-CM, Symptoms, Signs, and Abnormal Clinical and Laboratory Findings, Not Elsewhere Classified (codes RØØ.Ø-R99) contains many, but not all codes for symptoms.

CHAPTER 18

SYMPTOMS, SIGNS AND ABNORMAL CLINICAL AND LABORATORY FINDINGS, NOT ELSEWHERE CLASSIFIED (RØØ-R99)

Note: This chapter includes symptoms, signs, abnormal results of clinical or other investigative procedures, and ill-defined conditions regarding which no diagnosis classifiable elsewhere is recorded.

Signs and symptoms that point rather definitely to a given diagnosis have been assigned to a category in other chapters of the classification. In general, categories in this chapter include the less well-defined conditions and symptoms that, without the necessary study of the case to establish a final diagnosis, point perhaps equally to two or more diseases or to two or more systems of the body. Practically all categories in the chapter could be designated 'not otherwise specified', 'unknown etiology' or 'transient'. The Alphabetical Index should be consulted to determine which symptoms and signs are to be allocated here and which to other chapters. The residual subcategories, numbered .8, are generally provided for other relevant symptoms that cannot be allocated elsewhere in the classification.

The conditions and signs or symptoms included in categories RØØ-R94 consist of:

(a) cases for which no more specific diagnosis can be made even after all the facts bearing on the case have been investigated;
(b) signs or symptoms existing at the time of initial encounter that proved to be transient and whose causes could not be determined;
(c) provisional diagnosis in a patient who failed to return for further investigation or care;
(d) cases referred elsewhere for investigation or treatment before the diagnosis was made;
(e) cases in which a more precise diagnosis was not available for any other reason;
(f) certain symptoms, for which supplementary information is provided, that represent important problems in medical care in their own right.

Excludes2 abnormal findings on antenatal screening of mother (O28.-)
certain conditions originating in the perinatal period (PØ4-P96)
signs and symptoms classified in the body system chapters
signs and symptoms of breast (N63, N64.5)

This chapter contains the following blocks:

RØØ-RØ9	Symptoms and signs involving the circulatory and respiratory systems
R1Ø-R19	Symptoms and signs involving the digestive system and abdomen
R2Ø-R23	Symptoms and signs involving the skin and subcutaneous tissue
R25-R29	Symptoms and signs involving the nervous and musculoskeletal systems
R3Ø-R39	Symptoms and signs involving the genitourinary system
R4Ø-R46	Symptoms and signs involving cognition, perception, emotional state and behavior
R47-R49	Symptoms and signs involving speech and voice
R5Ø-R69	General symptoms and signs
R7Ø-R79	Abnormal findings on examination of blood, without diagnosis
R8Ø-R82	Abnormal findings on examination of urine, without diagnosis
R83-R89	Abnormal findings on examination of other body fluids, substances and tissues, without diagnosis
R9Ø-R94	Abnormal findings on diagnostic imaging and in function studies, without diagnosis
R97	Abnormal tumor markers
R99	Ill-defined and unknown cause of mortality

SYMPTOMS AND SIGNS INVOLVING THE CIRCULATORY AND RESPIRATORY SYSTEMS (RØØ-RØ9)

● **RØØ Abnormalities of heart beat**

Excludes1 abnormalities originating in the perinatal period (P29.1-)

Excludes2 specified arrhythmias (I47-I49) ◀

RØØ.Ø Tachycardia, unspecified
Rapid heart rate >1ØØ beats
Rapid heart beat
Sinoauricular tachycardia NOS
Sinus [sinusal] tachycardia NOS
Excludes1 neonatal tachycardia (P29.11)
paroxysmal tachycardia (I47.-)

RØØ.1 Bradycardia, unspecified
Slow heart rate, <6Ø
Sinoatrial bradycardia
Sinus bradycardia
Slow heart beat
Vagal bradycardia
Use additional code for adverse effect, if applicable, to identify drug (T36-T5Ø with fifth or sixth character 5)
Excludes1 neonatal bradycardia (P29.12)

RØØ.2 Palpitations
Awareness of heart beat

RØØ.8 Other abnormalities of heart beat

RØØ.9 Unspecified abnormalities of heart beat

● **R01 Cardiac murmurs and other cardiac sounds**
Excludes1 cardiac murmurs and sounds originating in the perinatal period (P29.8)

R01.0 Benign and innocent cardiac murmurs
Functional cardiac murmur

R01.1 Cardiac murmur, unspecified
Cardiac bruit NOS
Heart murmur NOS
Systolic murmur NOS ◀

R01.2 Other cardiac sounds
Cardiac dullness, increased or decreased
Precordial friction

OGCR Section I.C.9.a.7.

Hypertension, Transient
Assign code R03.0, Elevated blood pressure reading without diagnosis of hypertension, unless patient has an established diagnosis of hypertension. Assign code O13.-, Gestational [pregnancy-induced] hypertension with significant proteinuria, or O14.-, Pre-eclampsia, for transient hypertension of pregnancy.

● **R03 Abnormal blood-pressure reading, without diagnosis**

R03.0 Elevated blood-pressure reading, without diagnosis of hypertension
Note: This category is to be used to record an episode of elevated blood pressure in a patient in whom no formal diagnosis of hypertension has been made, or as an isolated incidental finding.

R03.1 Nonspecific low blood-pressure reading
Excludes1 hypotension (I95.-)
maternal hypotension syndrome (O26.5-)
neurogenic orthostatic hypotension (G90.3)

● **R04 Hemorrhage from respiratory passages**

R04.0 Epistaxis
Hemorrhage from nose
Nosebleed

R04.1 Hemorrhage from throat
Excludes2 hemoptysis (R04.2)

R04.2 Hemoptysis
Blood-stained sputum
Cough with hemorrhage

● **R04.8 Hemorrhage from other sites in respiratory passages**

R04.81 Acute idiopathic pulmonary hemorrhage in infants
AIPHI
Acute idiopathic hemorrhage in infants over 28 days old
Excludes1 perinatal pulmonary hemorrhage (P26.-)
von Willebrand's disease (D68.0)

R04.89 Hemorrhage from other sites in respiratory passages
Pulmonary hemorrhage NOS

R04.9 Hemorrhage from respiratory passages, unspecified

R05 Cough
Excludes1 cough with hemorrhage (R04.2)
smoker's cough (J41.0)

● **R06 Abnormalities of breathing**
Excludes1 acute respiratory distress syndrome (J80)
respiratory arrest (R09.2)
respiratory arrest of newborn (P28.81)
respiratory distress syndrome of newborn (P22.-)
respiratory failure (J96.-)
respiratory failure of newborn (P28.5)

● **R06.0 Dyspnea**
Excludes1 tachypnea NOS (R06.82)
transient tachypnea of newborn (P22.1)

R06.00 Dyspnea, unspecified

R06.01 Orthopnea

R06.02 Shortness of breath

R06.09 Other forms of dyspnea

R06.1 Stridor
Harsh, high-pitched breath sound
Excludes1 congenital laryngeal stridor (P28.89)
laryngismus (stridulus) (J38.5)

R06.2 Wheezing
Excludes1 Asthma (J45.-)

R06.3 Periodic breathing
Cheyne-Stokes breathing
An abnormal pattern of breathing with gradually increasing and decreasing tidal volume with some periods of apnea

R06.4 Hyperventilation
Excludes1 psychogenic hyperventilation (F45.8)

R06.5 Mouth breathing
Excludes2 dry mouth NOS (R68.2)

R06.6 Hiccough
Excludes1 psychogenic hiccough (F45.8)

R06.7 Sneezing

● **R06.8 Other abnormalities of breathing**

R06.81 Apnea, not elsewhere classified
Apnea NOS
Excludes1 apnea (of) newborn (P28.4)
sleep apnea (G47.3-)
sleep apnea of newborn (primary) (P28.3)

R06.82 Tachypnea, not elsewhere classified
Tachypnea NOS
Excludes1 transitory tachypnea of newborn (P22.1)

R06.83 Snoring

R06.89 Other abnormalities of breathing
Breath-holding (spells)
Sighing

R06.9 Unspecified abnormalities of breathing

● **R07 Pain in throat and chest**
Excludes1 epidemic myalgia (B33.0)
Excludes2 jaw pain R68.84
pain in breast (N64.4)

R07.0 Pain in throat
Excludes1 chronic sore throat (J31.2)
sore throat (acute) NOS (J02.9)
Excludes2 dysphagia (R13.1-)
pain in neck (M54.2)

R07.1 Chest pain on breathing
Painful respiration

R07.2 Precordial pain

● **R07.8 Other chest pain**
R07.81 Pleurodynia
Pleurodynia NOS
Excludes1 epidemic pleurodynia (B33.0)
R07.82 Intercostal pain
R07.89 Other chest pain
Anterior chest-wall pain NOS
R07.9 Chest pain, unspecified

● **R09 Other symptoms and signs involving the circulatory and respiratory system**
Excludes1 acute respiratory distress syndrome (J80)
respiratory arrest of newborn (P28.81)
respiratory distress syndrome of newborn (P22.0)
respiratory failure (J96.-)
respiratory failure of newborn (P28.5)

● **R09.0 Asphyxia and hypoxemia**
Excludes1 asphyxia due to carbon monoxide (T58.-)
asphyxia due to foreign body in respiratory tract (T17.-)
birth (intrauterine) asphyxia (P84)
hypercapnia (R06.4)
hyperventilation (R06.4)
traumatic asphyxia (T71.-)
R09.01 Asphyxia
R09.02 Hypoxemia

R09.1 Pleurisy
Occurs when double membrane (pleura) lining chest cavity and lung surface becomes inflamed causing sharp pain on inspiration/expiration
Excludes1 pleurisy with effusion (J90)

R09.2 Respiratory arrest
Cardiorespiratory failure
Excludes1 cardiac arrest (I46.-)
respiratory arrest of newborn (P28.81)
respiratory distress of newborn (P22.0)
respiratory failure (J96.-)
respiratory failure of newborn (P28.5)
respiratory insufficiency (R06.89)
respiratory insufficiency of newborn (P28.5)

R09.3 Abnormal sputum
Abnormal amount of sputum
Abnormal color of sputum
Abnormal odor of sputum
Excessive sputum
Excludes1 blood-stained sputum (R04.2)

● **R09.8 Other specified symptoms and signs involving the circulatory and respiratory systems**
R09.81 Nasal congestion
R09.82 Postnasal drip
R09.89 Other specified symptoms and signs involving the circulatory and respiratory systems
Bruit (arterial)
Abnormal chest percussion
Feeling of foreign body in throat
Friction sounds in chest
Chest tympany
Choking sensation
Rales
Wet rattling, clicking, crackling sounds on auscultation
Weak pulse
Excludes2 foreign body in throat (T17.2-)
wheezing (R06.2)

SYMPTOMS AND SIGNS INVOLVING THE DIGESTIVE SYSTEM AND ABDOMEN (R10-R19)

Excludes2 congenital or infantile pylorospasm (Q40.0) ◀
gastrointestinal hemorrhage (K92.0-K92.2) ◀
intestinal obstruction (K56.-) ◀
newborn gastrointestinal hemorrhage (P54.0-P54.3) ◀
newborn intestinal obstruction (P76.-) ◀
pylorospasm (K31.3) ◀
signs and symptoms involving the urinary system (R30-R39) ◀
symptoms referable to female genital organs (N94.-) ◀
symptoms referable to male genital organs (N48-N50) ◀

● **R10 Abdominal and pelvic pain**
Excludes1 renal colic (N23)
Excludes2 dorsalgia (M54.-)
flatulence and related conditions (R14.-)

R10.0 Acute abdomen
Severe abdominal pain (generalized) (with abdominal rigidity)
Excludes1 abdominal rigidity NOS (R19.3)
generalized abdominal pain NOS (R10.84)
localized abdominal pain (R10.1-R10.3-)

● **R10.1 Pain localized to upper abdomen**
R10.10 Upper abdominal pain, unspecified
R10.11 Right upper quadrant pain
R10.12 Left upper quadrant pain
R10.13 Epigastric pain
Dyspepsia
Excludes1 functional dyspepsia (K30)

R10.2 Pelvic and perineal pain
Excludes1 vulvodynia (N94.81)

● **R10.3 Pain localized to other parts of lower abdomen**
R10.30 Lower abdominal pain, unspecified
R10.31 Right lower quadrant pain
R10.32 Left lower quadrant pain
R10.33 Periumbilical pain

● **R10.8 Other abdominal pain**
● **R10.81 Abdominal tenderness**
Abdominal tenderness NOS
R10.811 Right upper quadrant abdominal tenderness
R10.812 Left upper quadrant abdominal tenderness
R10.813 Right lower quadrant abdominal tenderness
R10.814 Left lower quadrant abdominal tenderness
R10.815 Periumbilic abdominal tenderness
R10.816 Epigastric abdominal tenderness
R10.817 Generalized abdominal tenderness
R10.819 Abdominal tenderness, unspecified site

CHAPTER 18 (R00-R99)

- **R10.82 Rebound abdominal tenderness**
  - **R10.821 Right upper quadrant rebound abdominal tenderness**
  - **R10.822 Left upper quadrant rebound abdominal tenderness**
  - **R10.823 Right lower quadrant rebound abdominal tenderness**
  - **R10.824 Left lower quadrant rebound abdominal tenderness**
  - **R10.825 Periumbilic rebound abdominal tenderness**
  - **R10.826 Epigastric rebound abdominal tenderness**
  - **R10.827 Generalized rebound abdominal tenderness**
  - **R10.829 Rebound abdominal tenderness, unspecified site**

R10.83 Colic
Colic NOS
Infantile colic
Excludes1 colic in adult and child over 12 months old (R10.84)

R10.84 Generalized abdominal pain
Excludes1 generalized abdominal pain associated with acute abdomen (R10.0)

R10.9 Unspecified abdominal pain

R11 Nausea and vomiting
Excludes1 cyclical vomiting associated with migraine (G43.A-)
excessive vomiting in pregnancy (O21.-)
hematemesis (K92.0)
neonatal hematemesis (P54.0)
newborn vomiting (P92.0-)
psychogenic vomiting (F50.89)
vomiting associated with bulimia nervosa (F50.2)
vomiting following gastrointestinal surgery (K91.0)

R11.0 Nausea
Nausea NOS
Nausea without vomiting

R11.1 Vomiting

- **R11.10 Vomiting, unspecified**
  Vomiting NOS
- **R11.11 Vomiting without nausea**
- **R11.12 Projectile vomiting**
- **R11.13 Vomiting of fecal matter**
- **R11.14 Bilious vomiting**
  Bilious emesis

R11.2 Nausea with vomiting, unspecified
Persistent nausea with vomiting NOS

R12 Heartburn
Excludes1 dyspepsia NOS (R10.13)
functional dyspepsia (K30)

R13 Aphagia and dysphagia

R13.0 Aphagia
Inability to swallow
Excludes1 psychogenic aphagia (F50.9)

R13.1 Dysphagia
Difficulty swallowing
Code first, if applicable, dysphagia following cerebrovascular disease (I69. with final characters -91)
Excludes1 psychogenic dysphagia (F45.8)

- **R13.10 Dysphagia, unspecified**
  Difficulty in swallowing NOS
- **R13.11 Dysphagia, oral phase**
- **R13.12 Dysphagia, oropharyngeal phase**
- **R13.13 Dysphagia, pharyngeal phase**
- **R13.14 Dysphagia, pharyngoesophageal phase**
- **R13.19 Other dysphagia**
  Cervical dysphagia
  Neurogenic dysphagia

R14 Flatulence and related conditions
Excludes1 psychogenic aerophagy (F45.8)

R14.0 Abdominal distension (gaseous)
Bloating
Tympanites (abdominal) (intestinal)

R14.1 Gas pain

R14.2 Eructation
Belching air from stomach through mouth

R14.3 Flatulence

R15 Fecal incontinence
Includes encopresis NOS
Excludes1 fecal incontinence of nonorganic origin (F98.1)

R15.0 Incomplete defecation
Excludes1 constipation (K59.0-)
fecal impaction (K56.41)

R15.1 Fecal smearing
Fecal soiling

R15.2 Fecal urgency

R15.9 Full incontinence of feces
Fecal incontinence NOS

R16 Hepatomegaly and splenomegaly, not elsewhere classified
Enlargement of liver or spleen

R16.0 Hepatomegaly, not elsewhere classified
Hepatomegaly NOS

R16.1 Splenomegaly, not elsewhere classified
Splenomegaly NOS

R16.2 Hepatomegaly with splenomegaly, not elsewhere classified
Hepatosplenomegaly NOS

R17 Unspecified jaundice
Excludes1 neonatal jaundice (P55, P57-P59)

R18 Ascites
Includes fluid in peritoneal cavity
Excludes1 ascites in alcoholic cirrhosis (K70.31)
ascites in alcoholic hepatitis (K70.11)
ascites in toxic liver disease with chronic active hepatitis (K71.51)

R18.0 Malignant ascites
Code first malignancy, such as:
malignant neoplasm of ovary (C56.-)
secondary malignant neoplasm of retroperitoneum and peritoneum (C78.6)

R18.8 Other ascites
Ascites NOS
Peritoneal effusion (chronic)

● **R19 Other symptoms and signs involving the digestive system and abdomen**
Excludes1 acute abdomen (R10.0)

● **R19.0 Intra-abdominal and pelvic swelling, mass and lump**
Excludes1 abdominal distension (gaseous) (R14.-)
ascites (R18.-)

R19.00 Intra-abdominal and pelvic swelling, mass and lump, unspecified site
R19.01 Right upper quadrant abdominal swelling, mass and lump
R19.02 Left upper quadrant abdominal swelling, mass and lump
R19.03 Right lower quadrant abdominal swelling, mass and lump
R19.04 Left lower quadrant abdominal swelling, mass and lump
R19.05 Periumbilic swelling, mass or lump
Diffuse or generalized umbilical swelling or mass
R19.06 Epigastric swelling, mass or lump
R19.07 Generalized intra-abdominal and pelvic swelling, mass and lump
Diffuse or generalized intra-abdominal swelling or mass NOS
Diffuse or generalized pelvic swelling or mass NOS
R19.09 Other intra-abdominal and pelvic swelling, mass and lump

● **R19.1 Abnormal bowel sounds**
R19.11 Absent bowel sounds
R19.12 Hyperactive bowel sounds
R19.15 Other abnormal bowel sounds
Abnormal bowel sounds NOS

R19.2 Visible peristalsis
Hyperperistalsis

● **R19.3 Abdominal rigidity**
Excludes1 abdominal rigidity with severe abdominal pain (R10.0)

R19.30 Abdominal rigidity, unspecified site
R19.31 Right upper quadrant abdominal rigidity
R19.32 Left upper quadrant abdominal rigidity
R19.33 Right lower quadrant abdominal rigidity
R19.34 Left lower quadrant abdominal rigidity
R19.35 Periumbilic abdominal rigidity
R19.36 Epigastric abdominal rigidity
R19.37 Generalized abdominal rigidity

R19.4 Change in bowel habit
Excludes1 constipation (K59.0-)
functional diarrhea (K59.1)

R19.5 Other fecal abnormalities
Abnormal stool color
Bulky stools
Mucus in stools
Occult blood in feces
Occult blood in stools
Excludes1 melena (K92.1)
neonatal melena (P54.1)

R19.6 Halitosis

R19.7 Diarrhea, unspecified
Diarrhea NOS
Excludes1 functional diarrhea (K59.1)
neonatal diarrhea (P78.3)
psychogenic diarrhea (F45.8)

R19.8 Other specified symptoms and signs involving the digestive system and abdomen

SYMPTOMS AND SIGNS INVOLVING THE SKIN AND SUBCUTANEOUS TISSUE (R20-R23)

Excludes2 symptoms relating to breast (N64.4-N64.5)

● **R20 Disturbances of skin sensation**
Excludes1 dissociative anesthesia and sensory loss (F44.6)
psychogenic disturbances (F45.8)

R20.0 Anesthesia of skin
Loss of sensation
R20.1 Hypoesthesia of skin
Unpleasant abnormal sensation
R20.2 Paresthesia of skin
Abnormal touch sensation, including burning, prickling, often in absence of external stimulus
Formication
Pins and needles
Tingling skin
Excludes1 acroparesthesia (I73.8)
R20.3 Hyperesthesia
R20.8 Other disturbances of skin sensation
R20.9 Unspecified disturbances of skin sensation

R21 Rash and other nonspecific skin eruption
Includes rash NOS
Excludes1 specified type of rash- code to condition
vesicular eruption (R23.8)

● **R22 Localized swelling, mass and lump of skin and subcutaneous tissue**
Includes subcutaneous nodules (localized) (superficial)
Excludes1 abnormal findings on diagnostic imaging (R90-R93)
edema (R60.-)
enlarged lymph nodes (R59.-)
localized adiposity (E65)
swelling of joint (M25.4-)

R22.0 Localized swelling, mass and lump, head
R22.1 Localized swelling, mass and lump, neck
R22.2 Localized swelling, mass and lump, trunk
Excludes1 intra-abdominal or pelvic mass and lump (R19.0-)
intra-abdominal or pelvic swelling (R19.0-)
Excludes2 breast mass and lump (N63)

● **R22.3 Localized swelling, mass and lump, upper limb**
R22.30 Localized swelling, mass and lump, unspecified upper limb
R22.31 Localized swelling, mass and lump, right upper limb
R22.32 Localized swelling, mass and lump, left upper limb
R22.33 Localized swelling, mass and lump, upper limb, bilateral

● **R22.4 Localized swelling, mass and lump, lower limb**
R22.40 Localized swelling, mass and lump, unspecified lower limb
R22.41 Localized swelling, mass and lump, right lower limb
R22.42 Localized swelling, mass and lump, left lower limb
R22.43 Localized swelling, mass and lump, lower limb, bilateral

R22.9 Localized swelling, mass and lump, unspecified

CHAPTER 18 (R00-R99)

● **R23 Other skin changes**

R23.0 Cyanosis

Excludes1 acrocyanosis (I73.8)
cyanotic attacks of newborn (P28.2)

R23.1 Pallor

Clammy skin

R23.2 Flushing

Excessive blushing

Code first, if applicable, menopausal and female climacteric states (N95.1)

R23.3 Spontaneous ecchymoses

Small hemorrhagic spot of skin; AKA black and blue spot

Petechiae

Excludes1 ecchymoses of newborn (P54.5)
purpura (D69.-)

R23.4 Changes in skin texture

Desquamation of skin
Scaling of skin
Induration of skin

Excludes1 epidermal thickening NOS (L85.9)

R23.8 Other skin changes

R23.9 Unspecified skin changes

SYMPTOMS AND SIGNS INVOLVING THE NERVOUS AND MUSCULOSKELETAL SYSTEMS (R25-R29)

● **R25 Abnormal involuntary movements**

Excludes1 specific movement disorders (G20-G26)
stereotyped movement disorders (F98.4)
tic disorders (F95.-)

R25.0 Abnormal head movements

R25.1 Tremor, unspecified

Excludes1 chorea NOS (G25.5)
essential tremor (G25.0)
hysterical tremor (F44.4)
intention tremor (G25.2)

R25.2 Cramp and spasm

Excludes2 carpopedal spasm (R29.0)
charley-horse (M62.831)
infantile spasms (G40.4-)
muscle spasm of back (M62.830)
muscle spasm of calf (M62.831)

R25.3 Fasciculation

Twitching NOS

R25.8 Other abnormal involuntary movements

R25.9 Unspecified abnormal involuntary movements

● **R26 Abnormalities of gait and mobility**

Excludes1 ataxia NOS (R27.0)
hereditary ataxia (G11.-)
locomotor (syphilitic) ataxia (A52.11)
immobility syndrome (paraplegic) (M62.3)

R26.0 Ataxic gait

Staggering gait

R26.1 Paralytic gait

Spastic gait

R26.2 Difficulty in walking, not elsewhere classified

Excludes1 falling (R29.6)
unsteadiness on feet (R26.81)

● **R26.8 Other abnormalities of gait and mobility**

R26.81 Unsteadiness on feet

R26.89 Other abnormalities of gait and mobility

R26.9 Unspecified abnormalities of gait and mobility

● **R27 Other lack of coordination**

Excludes1 ataxic gait (R26.0)
hereditary ataxia (G11.-)
vertigo NOS (R42)

R27.0 Ataxia, unspecified

Excludes1 ataxia following cerebrovascular disease (I69. with final characters -93)

R27.8 Other lack of coordination

R27.9 Unspecified lack of coordination

● **R29 Other symptoms and signs involving the nervous and musculoskeletal systems**

R29.0 Tetany

Hyperexcitability of nerves and muscles characterized by spasm, twitching, and cramps

Carpopedal spasm

Excludes1 hysterical tetany (F44.5)
neonatal tetany (P71.3)
parathyroid tetany (E20.9)
post-thyroidectomy tetany (E89.2)

R29.1 Meningismus

R29.2 Abnormal reflex

Excludes2 abnormal pupillary reflex (H57.0)
hyperactive gag reflex (J39.2)
vasovagal reaction or syncope (R55)

R29.3 Abnormal posture

R29.4 Clicking hip

Excludes1 congenital deformities of hip (Q65.-)

R29.5 Transient paralysis

Code first any associated spinal cord injury (S14.0, S14.1-, S24.0, S24.1-, S34.0-, S34.1-)

Excludes1 transient ischemic attack (G45.9)

R29.6 Repeated falls

Falling
Tendency to fall

Excludes2 at risk for falling (Z91.81)
history of falling (Z91.81)

OGCR Section I.C.18.d.

> Repeated falls
>
> Code R29.6, Repeated falls, is for use for encounters when a patient has recently fallen and the reason for the fall is being investigated.
>
> Code Z91.81, History of falling, is for use when a patient has fallen in the past and is at risk for future falls.When appropriate, both codes R29.6 and Z91.81 may be assigned together.

● **R29.7 National Institutes of Health Stroke Scale (NIHSS) score** ◀

Code first the type of cerebral infarction (I63-) ◀

● **R29.70 NIHSS score 0-9** ◀

R29.700 NIHSS score 0 ◀
R29.701 NIHSS score 1 ◀
R29.702 NIHSS score 2 ◀
R29.703 NIHSS score 3 ◀
R29.704 NIHSS score 4 ◀
R29.705 NIHSS score 5 ◀
R29.706 NIHSS score 6 ◀
R29.707 NIHSS score 7 ◀
R29.708 NIHSS score 8 ◀
R29.709 NIHSS score 9 ◀

OGCR Section I.C.18.i.

NIHSS Stroke Scale

The NIH stroke scale (NIHSS) codes (R29.7- -) can be used in conjunction with acute stroke codes (I63) to identify the patient's neurological status and the severity of the stroke. The stroke scale codes should be sequenced after the acute stroke diagnosis code(s).

At a minimum, report the initial score documented. If desired, a facility may choose to capture multiple stroke scale scores.

● **R29.71 NIHSS score 10-19** ◀
- **R29.710 NIHSS score 10** ◀
- **R29.711 NIHSS score 11** ◀
- **R29.712 NIHSS score 12** ◀
- **R29.713 NIHSS score 13** ◀
- **R29.714 NIHSS score 14** ◀
- **R29.715 NIHSS score 15** ◀
- **R29.716 NIHSS score 16** ◀
- **R29.717 NIHSS score 17** ◀
- **R29.718 NIHSS score 18** ◀
- **R29.719 NIHSS score 19** ◀

● **R29.72 NIHSS score 20-29** ◀
- **R29.720 NIHSS score 20** ◀
- **R29.721 NIHSS score 21** ◀
- **R29.722 NIHSS score 22** ◀
- **R29.723 NIHSS score 23** ◀
- **R29.724 NIHSS score 24** ◀
- **R29.725 NIHSS score 25** ◀
- **R29.726 NIHSS score 26** ◀
- **R29.727 NIHSS score 27** ◀
- **R29.728 NIHSS score 28** ◀
- **R29.729 NIHSS score 29** ◀

● **R29.73 NIHSS score 30-39** ◀
- **R29.730 NIHSS score 30** ◀
- **R29.731 NIHSS score 31** ◀
- **R29.732 NIHSS score 32** ◀
- **R29.733 NIHSS score 33** ◀
- **R29.734 NIHSS score 34** ◀
- **R29.735 NIHSS score 35** ◀
- **R29.736 NIHSS score 36** ◀
- **R29.737 NIHSS score 37** ◀
- **R29.738 NIHSS score 38** ◀
- **R29.739 NIHSS score 39** ◀

● **R29.74 NIHSS score 40-42** ◀
- **R29.740 NIHSS score 40** ◀
- **R29.741 NIHSS score 41** ◀
- **R29.742 NIHSS score 42** ◀

● **R29.8 Other symptoms and signs involving the nervous and musculoskeletal systems**

● **R29.81 Other symptoms and signs involving the nervous system**

R29.810 Facial weakness
Facial droop
Excludes1 Bell's palsy (G51.0)
facial weakness following cerebrovascular disease (I69. with final characters -92)

R29.818 Other symptoms and signs involving the nervous system

● **R29.89 Other symptoms and signs involving the musculoskeletal system**
Excludes2 pain in limb (M79.6-)

R29.890 Loss of height
Excludes1 osteoporosis (M80-M81)

R29.891 Ocular torticollis
Excludes1 congenital (sterno-mastoid) torticollis Q68.0
psychogenic torticollis (F45.8)
spasmodic torticollis (G24.3)
torticollis due to birth injury (P15.8)
torticollis NOS M43.6

R29.898 Other symptoms and signs involving the musculoskeletal system

● **R29.9 Unspecified symptoms and signs involving the nervous and musculoskeletal systems**

R29.90 Unspecified symptoms and signs involving the nervous system

R29.91 Unspecified symptoms and signs involving the musculoskeletal system

SYMPTOMS AND SIGNS INVOLVING THE GENITOURINARY SYSTEM (R30-R39)

● **R30 Pain associated with micturition**
Excludes1 psychogenic pain associated with micturition (F45.8)

R30.0 Dysuria
Painful urination
Strangury

R30.1 Vesical tenesmus
Straining to urinate

R30.9 Painful micturition, unspecified
Painful urination NOS

● **R31 Hematuria**
Excludes1 hematuria included with underlying conditions, such as:
acute cystitis with hematuria (N30.01)
recurrent and persistent hematuria in glomerular diseases (N02.-)

R31.0 Gross hematuria

R31.1 Benign essential microscopic hematuria

● **R31.2 Other microscopic hematuria**

R31.21 Asymptomatic microscopic hematuria ◀
AMH ◀

R31.29 Other microscopic hematuria ◀

R31.9 Hematuria, unspecified

R32 Unspecified urinary incontinence
Enuresis NOS
Excludes1 functional urinary incontinence (R39.81)
nonorganic enuresis (F98.0)
stress incontinence and other specified urinary incontinence (N39.3-N39.4-)
urinary incontinence associated with cognitive impairment (R39.81)

● **R33 Retention of urine**
Excludes1 psychogenic retention of urine (F45.8)

R33.0 Drug induced retention of urine
Use additional code for adverse effect, if applicable, to identify drug (T36-T50 with fifth or sixth character 5)

R33.8 Other retention of urine
Code first, if applicable, any causal condition, such as:
enlarged prostate (N40.1)

R33.9 Retention of urine, unspecified

R34 Anuria and oliguria

Excludes1 anuria and oliguria complicating abortion or ectopic or molar pregnancy (O00-O07, O08.4)
anuria and oliguria complicating pregnancy (O26.83-)
anuria and oliguria complicating the puerperium (O90.4)

● **R35 Polyuria**
Passage of excessive volume of urine
Code first, if applicable, any causal condition, such as:
enlarged prostate (N40.1)
Excludes1 psychogenic polyuria (F45.8)

R35.0 Frequency of micturition
Discharge or passage of urine; AKA uresis

R35.1 Nocturia
Urinary frequency at night

R35.8 Other polyuria
Polyuria NOS

● **R36 Urethral discharge**

R36.0 Urethral discharge without blood

R36.1 Hematospermia
Presence of blood in semen

R36.9 Urethral discharge, unspecified
Penile discharge NOS
Urethrorrhea

R37 Sexual dysfunction, unspecified

● **R39 Other and unspecified symptoms and signs involving the genitourinary system**

R39.0 Extravasation of urine
Leakage, discharge

● **R39.1 Other difficulties with micturition**
Code first, if applicable, any causal condition, such as:
enlarged prostate (N40.1)

R39.11 Hesitancy of micturition

R39.12 Poor urinary stream
Weak urinary steam

R39.13 Splitting of urinary stream

R39.14 Feeling of incomplete bladder emptying

R39.15 Urgency of urination
Excludes1 urge incontinence (N39.41, N39.46)

R39.16 Straining to void

● **R39.19 Other difficulties with micturition**

R39.191 Need to immediately re-void ◀

R39.192 Position dependent micturition ◀

R39.198 Other difficulties with micturition ◀

R39.2 Extrarenal uremia
Prerenal uremia
Excludes1 uremia NOS (N19)

● **R39.8 Other symptoms and signs involving the genitourinary system**

R39.81 Functional urinary incontinence
Urinary incontinence due to cognitive impairment, or severe physical disability or immobility
Excludes1 stress incontinence and other specified urinary incontinence (N39.3-N39.4-)
urinary incontinence NOS (R32)

R39.82 Chronic bladder pain ◀

R39.89 Other symptoms and signs involving the genitourinary system

R39.9 Unspecified symptoms and signs involving the genitourinary system

SYMPTOMS AND SIGNS INVOLVING COGNITION, PERCEPTION, EMOTIONAL STATE AND BEHAVIOR (R40-R46)

Excludes2 symptoms and signs constituting part of a pattern of mental disorder (F01-F99) ◀

● **R40 Somnolence, stupor and coma**

Excludes1 neonatal coma (P91.5)
somnolence, stupor and coma in diabetes (E08-E13)
somnolence, stupor and coma in hepatic failure (K72.-)
somnolence, stupor and coma in hypoglycemia (nondiabetic) (E15)

R40.0 Somnolence
Drowsiness
Excludes1 coma (R40.2-)

R40.1 Stupor
Lowered level of consciousness
Catatonic stupor
Semicoma
Excludes1 catatonic schizophrenia (F20.2)
coma (R40.2-)
depressive stupor (F31-F33)
dissociative stupor (F44.2)
manic stupor (F30.2)

OGCR Section I.C.18.e.

Coma scale

The coma scale codes (R40.2-) can be used in conjunction with traumatic brain injury codes, acute cerebrovascular disease or sequelae of cerebrovascular disease codes. These codes are primarily for use by trauma registries, but they may be used in any setting where this information is collected. **The coma scale may also be used to assess the status of the central nervous system for other non-trauma conditions, such as monitoring patients in the intensive care unit regardless of medical condition.** The coma scale codes should be sequenced after the diagnosis code(s).

These codes, one from each subcategory, are needed to complete the scale. The 7th character indicates when the scale was recorded. The 7th character should match for all three codes.

At a minimum, report the initial score documented on presentation at your facility. This may be a score from the emergency medicine technician (EMT) or in the emergency department. If desired, a facility may choose to capture multiple coma scale scores.

Assign code R40.24, Glasgow coma scale, total score, when only the total score is documented in the medical record and not the individual score(s).

● **R40.2 Coma**
Code first any associated:
fracture of skull (S02.-)
intracranial injury (S06.-)

Note: One code from each subcategory R40.21-R40-23 is required to complete the coma scale ⬅

R40.20 Unspecified coma
Coma NOS
Unconsciousness NOS

● **R40.21 Coma scale, eyes open**
The following appropriate 7th character is to be added to subcategory R40.21-:

0	unspecified time
1	in the field [EMT or ambulance]
2	at arrival to emergency department
3	at hospital admission
4	24 hours or more after hospital admission

● **R40.211 Coma scale, eyes open, never**

● **R40.212 Coma scale, eyes open, to pain**

● **R40.213 Coma scale, eyes open, to sound**

● **R40.214 Coma scale, eyes open, spontaneous**

● R40.22 **Coma scale, best verbal response**

The following appropriate 7th character is to be added to subcategory R40.22-:

0	unspecified time
1	in the field [EMT or ambulance]
2	at arrival to emergency department
3	at hospital admission
4	24 hours or more after hospital admission

● R40.221 **Coma scale, best verbal response, none**

● R40.222 **Coma scale, best verbal response, incomprehensible words**

● R40.223 **Coma scale, best verbal response, inappropriate words**

● R40.224 **Coma scale, best verbal response, confused conversation**

● R40.225 **Coma scale, best verbal response, oriented**

● R40.23 **Coma scale, best motor response**

The following appropriate 7th character is to be added to subcategory R40.23-:

0	unspecified time
1	in the field [EMT or ambulance]
2	at arrival to emergency department
3	at hospital admission
4	24 hours or more after hospital admission

● R40.231 **Coma scale, best motor response, none**

● R40.232 **Coma scale, best motor response, extension**

Glasgow Coma Scale

Eye Opening Response • Spontaneous--open with blinking at baseline	4 points
• To verbal stimuli, command, speech	3 points
• To pain only (not applied to face)	2 points
• No response	1 point
Verbal Response • Oriented	5 points
• Confused conversation, but able to answer questions	4 points
• Inappropriate words	3 points
• Incomprehensible speech	2 points
• No response	1 point
Motor Response • Obeys commands for movement	6 points
• Purposeful movement to painful stimulus	5 points
• Withdraws in response to pain	4 points
• Flexion in response to pain (decorticate posturing)	3 points
• Extension response in response to pain (decerebrate posturing)	2 points
• No response	1 point
Categorization: Coma: No eye opening, no ability to follow commands, no word verbalizations (3-8)	
Head Injury Classification: Severe Head Injury--GCS score of 8 or less; Moderate Head Injury--GCS score of 9 to 12; Mild head injury--GCS score of 13 to 15	
(Adapted from: Advanced Trauma Life Support: Course for Physicians, American College of Surgeons, 1993). http://www.bt.cdc.gov/masscasulatires/gscale.asp	

Figure 18-1

● R40.233 **Coma scale, best motor response, abnormal**

● R40.234 **Coma scale, best motor response, flexion withdrawal**

● R40.235 **Coma scale, best motor response, localizes pain**

● R40.236 **Coma scale, best motor response, obeys commands**

● R40.24 **Glasgow coma scale, total score**

Note: Assign a code from subcategory R40.24, when only the total coma score is documented ◀

The following appropriate 7th character is to be added to subcategory R40.24-: ◀

0	unspecified time ◀
1	in the field [EMT or ambulance] ◀
2	at arrival to emergency department ◀
3	at hospital admission ◀
4	24 hours or more after hospital admission ◀

● R40.241 **Glasgow coma scale score 13-15**

● R40.242 **Glasgow coma scale score 9-12**

● R40.243 **Glasgow coma scale score 3-8**

● R40.244 **Other coma, without documented Glasgow coma scale score, or with partial score reported**

R40.3 **Persistent vegetative state**

R40.4 **Transient alteration of awareness**

● R41 **Other symptoms and signs involving cognitive functions and awareness**

Excludes1 dissociative [conversion] disorders (F44.-)
mild cognitive impairment, so stated (G31.84)

R41.0 **Disorientation, unspecified**
Confusion NOS
Delirium NOS

R41.1 **Anterograde amnesia**

R41.2 **Retrograde amnesia**

R41.3 **Other amnesia**
Amnesia NOS
Memory loss NOS

Excludes1 amnestic disorder due to known physiologic condition (F04)
amnestic syndrome due to psychoactive substance use (F10-F19 with 5th character .6)
mild memory disturbance due to known physiological condition (F06.8)
transient global amnesia (G45.4)

R41.4 **Neurologic neglect syndrome**
Asomatognosia
Hemi-akinesia
Hemi-inattention
Hemispatial neglect
Left-sided neglect
Sensory neglect
Visuospatial neglect

Excludes1 visuospatial deficit (R41.842)

● R41.8 **Other symptoms and signs involving cognitive functions and awareness**

R41.81 **Age-related cognitive decline**
Senility NOS

R41.82 **Altered mental status, unspecified**
Change in mental status NOS

Excludes1 altered level of consciousness (R40.-)
altered mental status due to known condition - code to condition
delirium NOS (R41.0)

R41.83 **Borderline intellectual functioning**
IQ level 71 to 84

Excludes1 intellectual disabilities (F70-F79)

CHAPTER 18 (R00-R99)

● R41.84 **Other specified cognitive deficit**
Excludes1 cognitive deficits as sequelae of cerebrovascular disease (I69.01-, I69.11-, I69.21-, I69.31-, I69.81-, I69.91-) ◀
R41.840 **Attention and concentration deficit**
Excludes1 attention-deficit hyperactivity disorders (F90.-)
R41.841 **Cognitive communication deficit**
R41.842 **Visuospatial deficit**
R41.843 **Psychomotor deficit**
R41.844 **Frontal lobe and executive function deficit**
R41.89 **Other symptoms and signs involving cognitive functions and awareness**
Anosognosia
R41.9 **Unspecified symptoms and signs involving cognitive functions and awareness**

R42 **Dizziness and giddiness**
Light-headedness
Vertigo NOS
Excludes1 vertiginous syndromes (H81.-)
vertigo from infrasound (T75.23)

● R43 **Disturbances of smell and taste**
R43.0 **Anosmia**
Absence of sense of smell; AKA anosphresia and olfactory anesthesia
R43.1 **Parosmia**
R43.2 **Parageusia**
Perversion of sense of taste or bad taste in mouth; AKA dysgeusia
R43.8 **Other disturbances of smell and taste**
Mixed disturbance of smell and taste
R43.9 **Unspecified disturbances of smell and taste**

● R44 **Other symptoms and signs involving general sensations and perceptions**
Excludes1 alcoholic hallucinations (F1.5)
hallucinations in drug psychosis (F11-F19 with .5)
hallucinations in mood disorders with psychotic symptoms (F30.2, F31.5, F32.3, F33.3)
hallucinations in schizophrenia, schizotypal and delusional disorders (F20-F29)
Excludes2 disturbances of skin sensation (R20.-)
R44.0 **Auditory hallucinations**
R44.1 **Visual hallucinations**
R44.2 **Other hallucinations**
R44.3 **Hallucinations, unspecified**
R44.8 **Other symptoms and signs involving general sensations and perceptions**
R44.9 **Unspecified symptoms and signs involving general sensations and perceptions**

● R45 **Symptoms and signs involving emotional state**
R45.0 **Nervousness**
Nervous tension
R45.1 **Restlessness and agitation**
R45.2 **Unhappiness**
R45.3 **Demoralization and apathy**
Excludes1 anhedonia (R45.84)
R45.4 **Irritability and anger**
R45.5 **Hostility**
R45.6 **Violent behavior**
R45.7 **State of emotional shock and stress, unspecified**
● R45.8 **Other symptoms and signs involving emotional state**
R45.81 **Low self-esteem**
R45.82 **Worries**
R45.83 **Excessive crying of child, adolescent or adult**
Excludes1 excessive crying of infant (baby) R68.11
R45.84 **Anhedonia**
Total loss of feeling of pleasure in pleasurable acts
● R45.85 **Homicidal and suicidal ideations**
Excludes1 suicide attempt (T14.91)
R45.850 **Homicidal ideations**
R45.851 **Suicidal ideations**
R45.86 **Emotional lability**
R45.87 **Impulsiveness**
R45.89 **Other symptoms and signs involving emotional state**

● R46 **Symptoms and signs involving appearance and behavior**
Excludes1 appearance and behavior in schizophrenia, schizotypal and delusional disorders (F20-F29)
mental and behavioral disorders (F01-F99)
R46.0 **Very low level of personal hygiene**
R46.1 **Bizarre personal appearance**
R46.2 **Strange and inexplicable behavior**
R46.3 **Overactivity**
R46.4 **Slowness and poor responsiveness**
Excludes1 stupor (R40.1)
R46.5 **Suspiciousness and marked evasiveness**
R46.6 **Undue concern and preoccupation with stressful events**
R46.7 **Verbosity and circumstantial detail obscuring reason for contact**
● R46.8 **Other symptoms and signs involving appearance and behavior**
R46.81 **Obsessive-compulsive behavior**
Excludes1 obsessive-compulsive disorder (F42-) ⬅
R46.89 **Other symptoms and signs involving appearance and behavior**

SYMPTOMS AND SIGNS INVOLVING SPEECH AND VOICE (R47-R49)

● R47 **Speech disturbances, not elsewhere classified**
Excludes1 autism (F84.0)
cluttering (F80.81)
specific developmental disorders of speech and language (F80.-)
stuttering (F80.81)
● R47.0 **Dysphasia and aphasia**
R47.01 **Aphasia**
Excludes1 aphasia following cerebrovascular disease (I69. with final characters -20)
progressive isolated aphasia (G31.01)
R47.02 **Dysphasia**
Impairment in comprehension of speech, caused by left-sided brain damage
Excludes1 dysphasia following cerebrovascular disease (I69. with final characters -21)

◀ New ⬅ Revised ~~deleted~~ Deleted OGCR Official Guidelines X Assign placeholder X ● Use Additional Character(s)
Excludes 1 Excludes 2 Includes Use additional Code first Code also Unspecified

R47.1 **Dysarthria and anarthria**
Motor speech disorder
Excludes1 dysarthria following cerebrovascular disease (I69. with final characters -22)

● R47.8 **Other speech disturbances**
Excludes1 dysarthria following cerebrovascular disease (I69. with final characters -28)

R47.81 **Slurred speech**

R47.82 **Fluency disorder in conditions classified elsewhere**
Stuttering in conditions classified elsewhere
Code first underlying disease or condition, such as:
Parkinson's disease (G2Ø)
Excludes1 adult onset fluency disorder (F98.5)
childhood onset fluency disorder (F8Ø.81)
fluency disorder (stuttering) following cerebrovascular disease (I69. with final characters -23)

R47.89 **Other speech disturbances**

R47.9 **Unspecified speech disturbances**

● R48 **Dyslexia and other symbolic dysfunctions, not elsewhere classified**
Excludes1 specific developmental disorders of scholastic skills (F81.-)

R48.Ø **Dyslexia and alexia**

R48.1 **Agnosia**
Loss of ability to recognize objects, persons, sounds, shapes, or smells
Astereognosia (astereognosis)
Autotopagnosia
Excludes1 visual object agnosia (R48.3)

R48.2 **Apraxia**
Loss of ability to execute or carry out learned purposeful movements
Excludes1 apraxia following cerebrovascular disease (I69. with final characters -9Ø)

R48.3 **Visual agnosia**
Prosopagnosia
Simultanagnosia (asimultagnosia)

R48.8 **Other symbolic dysfunctions**
Acalculia
Difficulty performing simple mathematical tasks resulting from neurological injury
Agraphia

R48.9 **Unspecified symbolic dysfunctions**

● R49 **Voice and resonance disorders**
Excludes1 psychogenic voice and resonance disorders (F44.4)

R49.Ø **Dysphonia**
Hoarseness

R49.1 **Aphonia**
Loss of voice

● R49.2 **Hypernasality and hyponasality**

R49.21 **Hypernasality**

R49.22 **Hyponasality**

R49.8 **Other voice and resonance disorders**

R49.9 **Unspecified voice and resonance disorder**
Change in voice NOS
Resonance disorder NOS

GENERAL SYMPTOMS AND SIGNS (R5Ø-R69)

● R5Ø **Fever of other and unknown origin**
Excludes1 chills without fever (R68.83)
febrile convulsions (R56.Ø-)
fever of unknown origin during labor (O75.2)
fever of unknown origin in newborn (P81.9)
hypothermia due to illness (R68.Ø)
malignant hyperthermia due to anesthesia (T88.3)
puerperal pyrexia NOS (O86.4)

R5Ø.2 **Drug induced fever**
Use additional code for adverse effect, if applicable, to identify drug (T36-T5Ø with fifth or sixth character 5)
Excludes1 postvaccination (postimmunization) fever (R5Ø.83)

● R5Ø.8 **Other specified fever**

R5Ø.81 **Fever presenting with conditions classified elsewhere**
Code first underlying condition when associated fever is present, such as with:
leukemia (C91-C95)
neutropenia (D7Ø.-)
sickle-cell disease (D57.-)

R5Ø.82 **Postprocedural fever**
Excludes1 postprocedural infection (T81.4-) ◄
posttransfusion fever (R5Ø.84)
postvaccination (postimmunization) fever (R5Ø.83)

R5Ø.83 **Postvaccination fever**
Postimmunization fever

R5Ø.84 **Febrile nonhemolytic transfusion reaction**
FNHTR
Posttransfusion fever

R5Ø.9 **Fever, unspecified**
Fever NOS
Fever of unknown origin [FUO]
Fever with chills
Fever with rigors
Hyperpyrexia NOS
Persistent fever
Pyrexia NOS

R51 **Headache**
Facial pain NOS
Excludes1 atypical face pain (G5Ø.1)
migraine and other headache syndromes (G43-G44)
trigeminal neuralgia (G5Ø.Ø)

R52 **Pain, unspecified**
Acute pain NOS
Generalized pain NOS
Pain NOS
Excludes1 acute and chronic pain, not elsewhere classified (G89.-)
localized pain, unspecified type - code to pain by site, such as:
abdomen pain (R1Ø.-)
back pain (M54.9)
breast pain (N64.4)
chest pain (RØ7.1-RØ7.9)
ear pain (H92.Ø-)
eye pain (H57.1)
headache (R51)
joint pain (M25.5-)
limb pain (M79.6-)
lumbar region pain (M54.5)
pelvic and perineal pain (R1Ø.2)
shoulder pain (M25.51-)
spine pain (M54.-)
throat pain (RØ7.Ø)
tongue pain (K14.6)
tooth pain (KØ8.8)
renal colic (N23)
pain disorders exclusively related to psychological factors (F45.41)

CHAPTER 18 (RØØ-R99)

● R53 Malaise and fatigue

R53.0 Neoplastic (malignant) related fatigue

Code first associated neoplasm

R53.1 Weakness

Asthenia NOS

Excludes1 age-related weakness (R54)
muscle weakness (M62.8-)
sarcopenia (M62.84) ◀
senile asthenia (R54)

R53.2 Functional quadriplegia

Complete immobility due to severe physical disability or frailty

Excludes1 frailty NOS (R54)
hysterical paralysis (F44.4)
immobility syndrome (M62.3)
neurologic quadriplegia (G82.5-)
quadriplegia (G82.50)

● R53.8 Other malaise and fatigue

Excludes1 combat exhaustion and fatigue (F43.0)
congenital debility (P96.9)
exhaustion and fatigue due to depressive episode (F32.-)
exhaustion and fatigue due to excessive exertion (T73.3)
exhaustion and fatigue due to exposure (T73.2)
exhaustion and fatigue due to heat (T67.-)
exhaustion and fatigue due to pregnancy (O26.8-)
exhaustion and fatigue due to recurrent depressive episode (F33)
exhaustion and fatigue due to senile debility (R54)

R53.81 Other malaise

Chronic debility
Debility NOS
General physical deterioration
Malaise NOS
Nervous debility

Excludes1 age-related physical debility (R54)

R53.82 Chronic fatigue, unspecified

Chronic fatigue syndrome NOS

Excludes1 postviral fatigue syndrome (G93.3)

R53.83 Other fatigue

Fatigue NOS
Lack of energy
Lethargy
Tiredness

R54 Age-related physical debility

Frailty
Old age
Senescence
Senile asthenia
Senile debility

Excludes1 age-related cognitive decline (R41.81)
sarcopenia (M62.84) ◀
senile psychosis (F03)
senility NOS (R41.81)

R55 Syncope and collapse

Blackout
Fainting
Vasovagal attack

Excludes1 cardiogenic shock (R57.0)
carotid sinus syncope (G90.01)
heat syncope (T67.1)
neurocirculatory asthenia (F45.8)
neurogenic orthostatic hypotension (G90.3)
orthostatic hypotension (I95.1)
postprocedural shock (T81.1-)
psychogenic syncope (F48.8)
shock NOS (R57.9)
shock complicating or following abortion or ectopic or molar pregnancy (O00-O07, O08.3)
shock complicating or following labor and delivery (O75.1)
Stokes-Adams attack (I45.9)
unconsciousness NOS (R40.2-)

● R56 Convulsions, not elsewhere classified

Excludes1 dissociative convulsions and seizures (F44.5)
epileptic convulsions and seizures (G40.-)
newborn convulsions and seizures (P90)

● R56.0 Febrile convulsions

R56.00 Simple febrile convulsions

Febrile convulsion NOS
Febrile seizure NOS

R56.01 Complex febrile convulsions

Atypical febrile seizure
Complex febrile seizure
Complicated febrile seizure

Excludes1 status epilepticus (G40.901)

R56.1 Post traumatic seizures

Excludes1 post traumatic epilepsy (G40.-)

R56.9 Unspecified convulsions

Convulsion disorder
Fit NOS
Recurrent convulsions
Seizure(s) (convulsive) NOS

● R57 Shock, not elsewhere classified

Excludes1 anaphylactic shock NOS (T78.2)
anaphylactic reaction or shock due to adverse food reaction (T78.0-)
anaphylactic shock due to adverse effect of correct drug or medicament properly administered (T88.6)
anaphylactic shock due to serum (T80.5-)
anesthetic shock (T88.3)
electric shock (T75.4)
obstetric shock (O75.1)
postprocedural shock (T81.1-)
psychic shock (F43.0)
septic shock (R65.21)
shock complicating or following ectopic or molar pregnancy (O00-O07, O08.3)
shock due to lightning (T75.01)
traumatic shock (T79.4)
toxic shock syndrome (A48.3)

R57.0 Cardiogenic shock

R57.1 Hypovolemic shock

Decreased blood volume (loss)

R57.8 Other shock

R57.9 Shock, unspecified

Failure of peripheral circulation NOS

Resulting in significant blood pressure drop

R58 Hemorrhage, not elsewhere classified
Hemorrhage NOS
Excludes1 hemorrhage included with underlying conditions, such as:
acute duodenal ulcer with hemorrhage (K26.Ø)
acute gastritis with bleeding (K29.Ø1)
ulcerative enterocolitis with rectal bleeding (K51.Ø1)

● **R59 Enlarged lymph nodes**
Includes swollen glands
Excludes1 lymphadenitis NOS (I88.9)
acute lymphadenitis (LØ4.-)
chronic lymphadenitis (I88.1)
mesenteric (acute) (chronic) lymphadenitis (I88.Ø)

R59.Ø Localized enlarged lymph nodes

R59.1 Generalized enlarged lymph nodes
Lymphadenopathy NOS

R59.9 Enlarged lymph nodes, unspecified

● **R6Ø Edema, not elsewhere classified**
Excludes1 angioneurotic edema (T78.3)
ascites (R18.-)
cerebral edema (G93.6)
cerebral edema due to birth injury (P11.Ø)
edema of larynx (J38.4)
edema of nasopharynx (J39.2)
edema of pharynx (J39.2)
gestational edema (O12.Ø-)
hereditary edema (Q82.Ø)
hydrops fetalis NOS (P83.2)
hydrothorax (J94.8)
nutritional edema (E4Ø-E46)
hydrops fetalis NOS (P83.2)
newborn edema (P83.3)
pulmonary edema (J81.-)

R6Ø.Ø Localized edema

R6Ø.1 Generalized edema

R6Ø.9 Edema, unspecified
Fluid retention NOS

R61 Generalized hyperhidrosis
Excessive sweating
Night sweats
Secondary hyperhidrosis
Code first, if applicable, menopausal and female climacteric states (N95.1)
Excludes1 focal (primary) (secondary) hyperhidrosis (L74.5-)
Frey's syndrome (L74.52)
localized (primary) (secondary) hyperhidrosis (L74.5-)

● **R62 Lack of expected normal physiological development in childhood and adults**
Excludes1 delayed puberty (E3Ø.Ø)
gonadal dysgenesis (Q99.1)
hypopituitarism (E23.Ø)

R62.Ø Delayed milestone in childhood
Delayed attainment of expected physiological developmental stage
Late talker
Late walker

● **R62.5 Other and unspecified lack of expected normal physiological development in childhood**
Excludes1 HIV disease resulting in failure to thrive (B2Ø)
physical retardation due to malnutrition (E45)

R62.5Ø Unspecified lack of expected normal physiological development in childhood
Infantilism NOS

R62.51 Failure to thrive (child)
Failure to gain weight
Excludes1 failure to thrive in child under 28 days old (P92.6)

R62.52 Short stature (child)
Lack of growth
Physical retardation
Short stature NOS
Excludes1 short stature due to endocrine disorder (E34.3)

R62.59 Other lack of expected normal physiological development in childhood

R62.7 Adult failure to thrive

● **R63 Symptoms and signs concerning food and fluid intake**
Excludes1 bulimia NOS (F5Ø.2)
eating disorders of nonorganic origin (F5Ø.-)
malnutrition (E4Ø-E46)

R63.Ø Anorexia
Loss of appetite
Excludes1 anorexia nervosa (F5Ø.Ø-)
loss of appetite of nonorganic origin (F5Ø.89) ◄

R63.1 Polydipsia
Excessive thirst

R63.2 Polyphagia
Excessive eating
Hyperalimentation NOS

R63.3 Feeding difficulties
Feeding problem (elderly) (infant) NOS
Excludes1 feeding problems of newborn (P92.-)
infant feeding disorder of nonorganic origin (F98.2-)

R63.4 Abnormal weight loss

R63.5 Abnormal weight gain
Excludes1 excessive weight gain in pregnancy (O26.Ø-)
obesity (E66.-)

R63.6 Underweight
Use additional code to identify body mass index (BMI), if known (Z68.-)
Excludes1 abnormal weight loss (R63.4)
anorexia nervosa (F5Ø.Ø-)
malnutrition (E4Ø-E46)

R63.8 Other symptoms and signs concerning food and fluid intake

R64 Cachexia
Wasting syndrome
Code first underlying condition, if known
Excludes1 abnormal weight loss (R63.4)
nutritional marasmus (E41)

OGCR Section I.C.18.g.

SIRS due to Non-Infectious Process

The systemic inflammatory response syndrome (SIRS) can develop as a result of certain non-infectious disease processes, such as trauma, malignant neoplasm, or pancreatitis. When SIRS is documented with a noninfectious condition, and no subsequent infection is documented, the code for the underlying condition, such as an injury, should be assigned, followed by code R65.10. Systemic inflammatory response syndrome (SIRS) of non-infectious origin without acute organ dysfunction, or code R65.11, Systemic inflammatory response syndrome (SIRS) of non-infectious origin with acute organ dysfunction. If an associated acute organ dysfunction is documented, the appropriate code(s) for the specific type of organ dysfunction(s) should be assigned in addition to code R65.11. If acute organ dysfunction is documented, but it cannot be determined if the acute organ dysfunction is associated with SIRS or due to another condition (e.g., directly due to the trauma), the provider should be queried.

● **R65 Symptoms and signs specifically associated with systemic inflammation and infection**

● **R65.1 Systemic inflammatory response syndrome (SIRS) of non-infectious origin**

Code first underlying condition, such as:
heatstroke (T67.0)
injury and trauma (S00-T88)

Excludes1 sepsis - code to infection
severe sepsis (R65.2)

R65.10 Systemic inflammatory response syndrome (SIRS) of non-infectious origin without acute organ dysfunction

Systemic inflammatory response syndrome (SIRS) NOS

R65.11 Systemic inflammatory response syndrome (SIRS) of non-infectious origin with acute organ dysfunction

Use additional code to identify specific acute organ dysfunction, such as:
acute kidney failure (N17.-)
acute respiratory failure (J96.0-)
critical illness myopathy (G72.81)
critical illness polyneuropathy (G62.81)
disseminated intravascular coagulopathy [DIC] (D65)
encephalopathy (metabolic) (septic) (G93.41)
hepatic failure (K72.0-)

● **R65.2 Severe sepsis**

Infection with associated acute organ dysfunction
Sepsis with acute organ dysfunction
Sepsis with multiple organ dysfunction
Systemic inflammatory response syndrome due to infectious process with acute organ dysfunction

Code first underlying infection, such as:
infection following a procedure (T81.4-) (Revised)
infections following infusion, transfusion and therapeutic injection (T80.2-)
puerperal sepsis (O85)
sepsis following complete or unspecified spontaneous abortion (O03.87)
sepsis following ectopic and molar pregnancy (O08.82)
sepsis following incomplete spontaneous abortion (O03.37)
sepsis following (induced) termination of pregnancy (O04.87)
sepsis NOS (A41.9)

Use additional code to identify specific acute organ dysfunction, such as:
acute kidney failure (N17.-)
acute respiratory failure (J96.0-)
critical illness myopathy (G72.81)
critical illness polyneuropathy (G62.81)
disseminated intravascular coagulopathy [DIC] (D65)
encephalopathy (metabolic) (septic) (G93.41)
hepatic failure (K72.0-)

R65.20 Severe sepsis without septic shock

Severe sepsis NOS

R65.21 Severe sepsis with septic shock

● **R68 Other general symptoms and signs**

R68.0 Hypothermia, not associated with low environmental temperature

Excludes1 hypothermia NOS (accidental) (T68)
hypothermia due to anesthesia (T88.51)
hypothermia due to low environmental temperature (T68)
newborn hypothermia (P80.-)

● **R68.1 Nonspecific symptoms peculiar to infancy**

Excludes1 colic, infantile (R10.83)
neonatal cerebral irritability (P91.3)
teething syndrome (K00.7)

R68.11 Excessive crying of infant (baby)

Excludes1 excessive crying of child, adolescent, or adult (R45.83)

R68.12 Fussy infant (baby)

Irritable infant

R68.13 Apparent life threatening event in infant (ALTE)

Apparent life threatening event in newborn

Code first confirmed diagnosis, if known

Use additional code(s) for associated signs and symptoms if no confirmed diagnosis established, or if signs and symptoms are not associated routinely with confirmed diagnosis, or provide additional information for cause of ALTE

R68.19 Other nonspecific symptoms peculiar to infancy

R68.2 Dry mouth, unspecified

Excludes1 dry mouth due to dehydration (E86.0)
dry mouth due to sicca syndrome [Sjögren] (M35.0-)
salivary gland hyposecretion (K11.7)

R68.3 Clubbing of fingers

Clubbing of nails

Excludes1 congenital clubfinger (Q68.1)

● **R68.8 Other general symptoms and signs**

R68.81 Early satiety

R68.82 Decreased libido

Decreased sexual desire

R68.83 Chills (without fever)

Chills NOS

Excludes1 chills with fever (R50.9)

R68.84 Jaw pain

Mandibular pain
Maxilla pain

Excludes1 temporomandibular joint arthralgia (M26.62-) (Revised)

R68.89 Other general symptoms and signs

R69 Illness, unspecified

Unknown and unspecified cases of morbidity

ABNORMAL FINDINGS ON EXAMINATION OF BLOOD, WITHOUT DIAGNOSIS (R70-R79)

Excludes2 abnormal findings on antenatal screening of mother (O28.-) ◀
abnormalities of lipids (E78.-) ◀
abnormalities of platelets and thrombocytes (D69.-) ◀
abnormalities of white blood cells classified elsewhere (D70-D72) ◀
coagulation hemorrhagic disorders (D65-D68) ◀
diagnostic abnormal findings classified elsewhere —*see* Alphabetical Index ◀
hemorrhagic and hematological disorders of newborn (P50-P61) ◀

● **R70 Elevated erythrocyte sedimentation rate and abnormality of plasma viscosity**

R70.0 Elevated erythrocyte sedimentation rate

R70.1 Abnormal plasma viscosity

CHAPTER 18 (R00-R99)

◀ New ⬅ Revised ~~deleted~~ Deleted **OGCR** Official Guidelines X Assign placeholder X ● Use Additional Character(s)
Excludes 1 | Excludes 2 | Includes | Use additional | Code first | Code also | Unspecified

● **R71 Abnormality of red blood cells**
Excludes1 anemias (D5Ø-D64)
anemia of premature infant (P61.2)
benign (familial) polycythemia (D75.Ø)
congenital anemias (P61.2-P61.4)
newborn anemia due to isoimmunization (P55.-)
polycythemia neonatorum (P61.1)
polycythemia NOS (D75.1)
polycythemia vera (D45)
secondary polycythemia (D75.1)

R71.Ø Precipitous drop in hematocrit
Drop (precipitous) in hemoglobin
Drop in hematocrit
Blood volume that is red blood cells

R71.8 Other abnormality of red blood cells
Abnormal red-cell morphology NOS
Abnormal red-cell volume NOS
Anisocytosis
Red blood cells of unequal size
Poikilocytosis
Red blood cells of abnormal shape

● **R73 Elevated blood glucose level**
Excludes1 diabetes mellitus (EØ8-E13)
diabetes mellitus in pregnancy, childbirth and the puerperium (O24.-)
neonatal disorders (P7Ø.Ø-P7Ø.2)
postsurgical hypoinsulinemia (E89.1)

● **R73.Ø Abnormal glucose**
Excludes1 abnormal glucose in pregnancy (O99.81-)
diabetes mellitus (EØ8-E13)
dysmetabolic syndrome X (E88.81)
gestational diabetes (O24.4-)
glycosuria (R81)
hypoglycemia (E16.2)

R73.Ø1 Impaired fasting glucose
Elevated fasting glucose

R73.Ø2 Impaired glucose tolerance (oral)
Elevated glucose tolerance

R73.Ø3 Prediabetes ◀
Latent diabetes ◀

R73.Ø9 Other abnormal glucose
Abnormal glucose NOS
Abnormal non-fasting glucose tolerance
~~Prediabetes~~

R73.9 Hyperglycemia, unspecified

● **R74 Abnormal serum enzyme levels**

R74.Ø Nonspecific elevation of levels of transaminase and lactic acid dehydrogenase [LDH]

R74.8 Abnormal levels of other serum enzymes
Abnormal level of acid phosphatase
Abnormal level of alkaline phosphatase
Abnormal level of amylase
Abnormal level of lipase [triacylglycerol lipase]

R74.9 Abnormal serum enzyme level, unspecified

OGCR Section I.C.1.2.e and f.

Patients with inconclusive HIV serology

e. Patients with inconclusive HIV serology, but no definitive diagnosis or manifestations of the illness, may be assigned code R75, Inconclusive laboratory evidence of human immunodeficiency virus [HIV].

f. Previously diagnosed HIV-related illness

Patients with any known prior diagnosis of an HIV-related illness should be coded to B2Ø. Once a patient has developed an HIV-related illness, the patient should always be assigned code B2Ø on every subsequent admission/encounter. Patients previously diagnosed with any HIV illness (B2Ø) should never be assigned to R75 or Z21, Asymptomatic human immunodeficiency virus [HIV] infection status.

R75 Inconclusive laboratory evidence of human immunodeficiency virus [HIV]
Nonconclusive HIV-test finding in infants
Excludes1 asymptomatic human immunodeficiency virus [HIV] infection status (Z21)
human immunodeficiency virus [HIV] disease (B2Ø)

● **R76 Other abnormal immunological findings in serum**

R76.Ø Raised antibody titer
Excludes1 isoimmunization in pregnancy (O36.Ø-O36.1)
isoimmunization affecting newborn (P55.-)

● **R76.1 Nonspecific reaction to test for tuberculosis**

R76.11 Nonspecific reaction to tuberculin skin test without active tuberculosis
Abnormal result of Mantoux test
PPD positive
Tuberculin (skin test) positive
Tuberculin (skin test) reactor
Excludes1 nonspecific reaction to cell mediated immunity measurement of gamma interferon antigen response without active tuberculosis (R76.12)

R76.12 Nonspecific reaction to cell mediated immunity measurement of gamma interferon antigen response without active tuberculosis
Nonspecific reaction to QuantiFERON-TB test (QFT) without active tuberculosis
Excludes1 nonspecific reaction to tuberculin skin test without active tuberculosis (R76.11)
positive tuberculin skin test (R76.11)

R76.8 Other specified abnormal immunological findings in serum
Raised level of immunoglobulins NOS

R76.9 Abnormal immunological finding in serum, unspecified

● **R77 Other abnormalities of plasma proteins**
Excludes1 disorders of plasma-protein metabolism (E88.Ø)

R77.Ø Abnormality of albumin

R77.1 Abnormality of globulin
Hyperglobulinemia NOS

R77.2 Abnormality of alphafetoprotein

R77.8 Other specified abnormalities of plasma proteins

R77.9 Abnormality of plasma protein, unspecified

CHAPTER 18 (RØØ-R99)

● **R78 Findings of drugs and other substances, not normally found in blood**

Use additional code to identify any retained foreign body, if applicable (Z18.-)

Excludes1 mental or behavioral disorders due to psychoactive substance use (F1Ø-F19)

R78.Ø Finding of alcohol in blood

Use additional external cause code (Y9Ø.-), for detail regarding alcohol level.

R78.1 Finding of opiate drug in blood

R78.2 Finding of cocaine in blood

R78.3 Finding of hallucinogen in blood

R78.4 Finding of other drugs of addictive potential in blood

R78.5 Finding of other psychotropic drug in blood

R78.6 Finding of steroid agent in blood

● **R78.7 Finding of abnormal level of heavy metals in blood**

R78.71 Abnormal lead level in blood

Excludes1 lead poisoning (T56.Ø-)

R78.79 Finding of abnormal level of heavy metals in blood

● **R78.8 Finding of other specified substances, not normally found in blood**

R78.81 Bacteremia

Blood poisoning/bacteremia

Excludes1 sepsis-code to specified infection ⇐

R78.89 Finding of other specified substances, not normally found in blood

Finding of abnormal level of lithium in blood

R78.9 Finding of unspecified substance, not normally found in blood

● **R79 Other abnormal findings of blood chemistry**

Use additional code to identify any retained foreign body, if applicable (Z18.-)

Excludes1 abnormality of fluid, electrolyte or acid-base balance (E86-E87)
asymptomatic hyperuricemia (E79.Ø)
hyperglycemia NOS (R73.9)
hypoglycemia NOS (E16.2)
neonatal hypoglycemia (P7Ø.3-P7Ø.4)
specific findings indicating disorder of amino-acid metabolism (E7Ø-E72)
specific findings indicating disorder of carbohydrate metabolism (E73-E74)
specific findings indicating disorder of lipid metabolism (E75.-)

R79.Ø Abnormal level of blood mineral

Abnormal blood level of cobalt
Abnormal blood level of copper
Abnormal blood level of iron
Abnormal blood level of magnesium
Abnormal blood level of mineral NEC
Abnormal blood level of zinc

Excludes1 abnormal level of lithium (R78.89)
disorders of mineral metabolism (E83.-)
neonatal hypomagnesemia (P71.2)
nutritional mineral deficiency (E58-E61)

R79.1 Abnormal coagulation profile

Abnormal or prolonged bleeding time
Abnormal or prolonged coagulation time
Abnormal or prolonged partial thromboplastin time [PTT]
Abnormal or prolonged prothrombin time [PT]

Excludes1 coagulation defects (D68.-)

● **R79.8 Other specified abnormal findings of blood chemistry**

R79.81 Abnormal blood-gas level

R79.82 Elevated C-reactive protein (CRP)

R79.89 Other specified abnormal findings of blood chemistry

R79.9 Abnormal finding of blood chemistry, unspecified

ABNORMAL FINDINGS ON EXAMINATION OF URINE, WITHOUT DIAGNOSIS (R8Ø-R82)

Excludes1 abnormal findings on antenatal screening of mother (O28.-)
diagnostic abnormal findings classified elsewhere - see Alphabetical Index
specific findings indicating disorder of amino-acid metabolism (E7Ø-E72)
specific findings indicating disorder of carbohydrate metabolism (E73-E74)

● **R8Ø Proteinuria**

Excludes1 gestational proteinuria (O12.1-)

R8Ø.Ø Isolated proteinuria

Idiopathic proteinuria

Excludes1 isolated proteinuria with specific morphological lesion (NØ6.-)

R8Ø.1 Persistent proteinuria, unspecified

R8Ø.2 Orthostatic proteinuria, unspecified

Postural proteinuria

R8Ø.3 Bence Jones proteinuria

R8Ø.8 Other proteinuria

R8Ø.9 Proteinuria, unspecified

Albuminuria NOS

R81 Glycosuria

Excludes1 renal glycosuria (E74.8)

● **R82 Other and unspecified abnormal findings in urine**

Includes chromoabnormalities in urine

Use additional code to identify any retained foreign body, if applicable (Z18.-)

Excludes2 hematuria (R31.-)

R82.Ø Chyluria

White milky urine

Excludes1 filarial chyluria (B74.-)

R82.1 Myoglobinuria

Presence of myoglobin (iron containing protein) in urine

R82.2 Biliuria

Presence of bile pigments/salts in urine

R82.3 Hemoglobinuria

Presence of hemoglobin in urine

Excludes1 hemoglobinuria due to hemolysis from external causes NEC (D59.6)
hemoglobinuria due to paroxysmal nocturnal [Marchiafava-Micheli] (D59.5)

R82.4 Acetonuria

Ketonuria

R82.5 Elevated urine levels of drugs, medicaments and biological substances

Elevated urine levels of catecholamines
Elevated urine levels of indoleacetic acid
Elevated urine levels of 17-ketosteroids
Elevated urine levels of steroids

R82.6 Abnormal urine levels of substances chiefly nonmedicinal as to source

Abnormal urine level of heavy metals

● **R82.7 Abnormal findings on microbiological examination of urine**

Excludes1 colonization status (Z22.-)

R82.71 Bacteriuria ◀

R82.79 Other abnormal findings on microbiological examination of urine ◀

Positive culture findings of urine ◀

R82.8 Abnormal findings on cytological and histological examination of urine

● R82.9 **Other and unspecified abnormal findings in urine**

R82.90 **Unspecified abnormal findings in urine**

R82.91 **Other chromoabnormalities of urine**
Chromoconversion (dipstick)
Idiopathic dipstick converts positive for blood with no cellular forms in sediment
Excludes1 hemoglobinuria (R82.3)
myoglobinuria (R82.1)

R82.99 **Other abnormal findings in urine**
Cells and casts in urine
Crystalluria
Melanuria

ABNORMAL FINDINGS ON EXAMINATION OF OTHER BODY FLUIDS, SUBSTANCES AND TISSUES, WITHOUT DIAGNOSIS (R83-R89)

Excludes1 abnormal findings on antenatal screening of mother (O28.-)
diagnostic abnormal findings classified elsewhere - see Alphabetical Index

Excludes2 abnormal findings on examination of blood, without diagnosis (R7Ø-R79)
abnormal findings on examination of urine, without diagnosis (R8Ø-R82)
abnormal tumor markers (R97.-)

● R83 **Abnormal findings in cerebrospinal fluid**

R83.Ø **Abnormal level of enzymes in cerebrospinal fluid**

R83.1 **Abnormal level of hormones in cerebrospinal fluid**

R83.2 **Abnormal level of other drugs, medicaments and biological substances in cerebrospinal fluid**

R83.3 **Abnormal level of substances chiefly nonmedicinal as to source in cerebrospinal fluid**

R83.4 **Abnormal immunological findings in cerebrospinal fluid**

R83.5 **Abnormal microbiological findings in cerebrospinal fluid**
Positive culture findings in cerebrospinal fluid
Excludes1 colonization status (Z22.-)

R83.6 **Abnormal cytological findings in cerebrospinal fluid**

R83.8 **Other abnormal findings in cerebrospinal fluid**
Abnormal chromosomal findings in cerebrospinal fluid

R83.9 **Unspecified abnormal finding in cerebrospinal fluid**

● R84 **Abnormal findings in specimens from respiratory organs and thorax**

Includes abnormal findings in bronchial washings
abnormal findings in nasal secretions
abnormal findings in pleural fluid
abnormal findings in sputum
abnormal findings in throat scrapings

Excludes1 blood-stained sputum (RØ4.2)

R84.Ø **Abnormal level of enzymes in specimens from respiratory organs and thorax**

R84.1 **Abnormal level of hormones in specimens from respiratory organs and thorax**

R84.2 **Abnormal level of other drugs, medicaments and biological substances in specimens from respiratory organs and thorax**

R84.3 **Abnormal level of substances chiefly nonmedicinal as to source in specimens from respiratory organs and thorax**

R84.4 **Abnormal immunological findings in specimens from respiratory organs and thorax**

R84.5 **Abnormal microbiological findings in specimens from respiratory organs and thorax**
Positive culture findings in specimens from respiratory organs and thorax
Excludes1 colonization status (Z22.-)

R84.6 **Abnormal cytological findings in specimens from respiratory organs and thorax**

R84.7 **Abnormal histological findings in specimens from respiratory organs and thorax**

R84.8 **Other abnormal findings in specimens from respiratory organs and thorax**
Abnormal chromosomal findings in specimens from respiratory organs and thorax

R84.9 **Unspecified abnormal finding in specimens from respiratory organs and thorax**

● R85 **Abnormal findings in specimens from digestive organs and abdominal cavity**

Includes abnormal findings in peritoneal fluid
abnormal findings in saliva

Excludes1 cloudy peritoneal dialysis effluent (R88.Ø)
fecal abnormalities (R19.5)

R85.Ø **Abnormal level of enzymes in specimens from digestive organs and abdominal cavity**

R85.1 **Abnormal level of hormones in specimens from digestive organs and abdominal cavity**

R85.2 **Abnormal level of other drugs, medicaments and biological substances in specimens from digestive organs and abdominal cavity**

R85.3 **Abnormal level of substances chiefly nonmedicinal as to source in specimens from digestive organs and abdominal cavity**

R85.4 **Abnormal immunological findings in specimens from digestive organs and abdominal cavity**

R85.5 **Abnormal microbiological findings in specimens from digestive organs and abdominal cavity**
Positive culture findings in specimens from digestive organs and abdominal cavity
Excludes1 colonization status (Z22.-)

● R85.6 **Abnormal cytological findings in specimens from digestive organs and abdominal cavity**

● R85.61 **Abnormal cytologic smear of anus**

Excludes1 abnormal cytological findings in specimens from other digestive organs and abdominal cavity (R85.69)
carcinoma in situ of anus (histologically confirmed) (DØ1.3)
anal intraepithelial neoplasia I [AIN I] (K62.82)
anal intraepithelial neoplasia II [AIN II] (K62.82)
anal intraepithelial neoplasia III [AIN III] (DØ1.3)
dysplasia (mild) (moderate) of anus (histologically confirmed) (K62.82)
severe dysplasia of anus (histologically confirmed) (DØ1.3)

Excludes2 anal high risk human papillomavirus (HPV) DNA test positive (R85.81)
anal low risk human papillomavirus (HPV) DNA test positive (R85.82)

R85.61Ø **Atypical squamous cells of undetermined significance on cytologic smear of anus (ASC-US)**

R85.611 **Atypical squamous cells cannot exclude high grade squamous intraepithelial lesion on cytologic smear of anus (ASC-H)**

R85.612 **Low grade squamous intraepithelial lesion on cytologic smear of anus (LGSIL)**

R85.613 **High grade squamous intraepithelial lesion on cytologic smear of anus (HGSIL)**

R85.614 **Cytologic evidence of malignancy on smear of anus**

CHAPTER 18 (RØØ-R99)

R85.615 **Unsatisfactory cytologic smear of anus**
Inadequate sample of cytologic smear of anus

R85.616 **Satisfactory anal smear but lacking transformation zone**

R85.618 **Other abnormal cytological findings on specimens from anus**

R85.619 **Unspecified abnormal cytological findings in specimens from anus**
Abnormal anal cytology NOS
Atypical glandular cells of anus NOS

R85.69 **Abnormal cytological findings in specimens from other digestive organs and abdominal cavity**

R85.7 **Abnormal histological findings in specimens from digestive organs and abdominal cavity**

● R85.8 **Other abnormal findings in specimens from digestive organs and abdominal cavity**

R85.81 **Anal high risk human papillomavirus (HPV) DNA test positive**
Excludes1 anogenital warts due to human papillomavirus (HPV) (A63.0)
condyloma acuminatum (A63.0)

R85.82 **Anal low risk human papillomavirus (HPV) DNA test positive**
Use additional code for associated human papillomavirus (B97.7)

R85.89 **Other abnormal findings in specimens from digestive organs and abdominal cavity**
Abnormal chromosomal findings in specimens from digestive organs and abdominal cavity

R85.9 **Unspecified abnormal finding in specimens from digestive organs and abdominal cavity**

● R86 **Abnormal findings in specimens from male genital organs**
Includes abnormal findings in prostatic secretions
abnormal findings in semen, seminal fluid
abnormal spermatozoa
Excludes1 azoospermia (N46.0-)
oligospermia (N46.1-)

R86.0 **Abnormal level of enzymes in specimens from male genital organs**

R86.1 **Abnormal level of hormones in specimens from male genital organs**

R86.2 **Abnormal level of other drugs, medicaments and biological substances in specimens from male genital organs**

R86.3 **Abnormal level of substances chiefly nonmedicinal as to source in specimens from male genital organs**

R86.4 **Abnormal immunological findings in specimens from male genital organs**

R86.5 **Abnormal microbiological findings in specimens from male genital organs**
Positive culture findings in specimens from male genital organs
Excludes1 colonization status (Z22.-)

R86.6 **Abnormal cytological findings in specimens from male genital organs**

R86.7 **Abnormal histological findings in specimens from male genital organs**

R86.8 **Other abnormal findings in specimens from male genital organs**
Abnormal chromosomal findings in specimens from male genital organs

R86.9 **Unspecified abnormal finding in specimens from male genital organs**

● R87 **Abnormal findings in specimens from female genital organs**
Includes abnormal findings in secretion and smears from cervix uteri
abnormal findings in secretion and smears from vagina
abnormal findings in secretion and smears from vulva

R87.0 **Abnormal level of enzymes in specimens from female genital organs**

R87.1 **Abnormal level of hormones in specimens from female genital organs**

R87.2 **Abnormal level of other drugs, medicaments and biological substances in specimens from female genital organs**

R87.3 **Abnormal level of substances chiefly nonmedicinal as to source in specimens from female genital organs**

R87.4 **Abnormal immunological findings in specimens from female genital organs**

R87.5 **Abnormal microbiological findings in specimens from female genital organs**
Positive culture findings in specimens from female genital organs
Excludes1 colonization status (Z22.-)

● R87.6 **Abnormal cytological findings in specimens from female genital organs**

● R87.61 **Abnormal cytological findings in specimens from cervix uteri**
Excludes1 abnormal cytological findings in specimens from other female genital organs (R87.69)
abnormal cytological findings in specimens from vagina (R87.62-)
carcinoma in situ of cervix uteri (histologically confirmed) (D06.-)
cervical intraepithelial neoplasia I [CIN I] (N87.0)
cervical intraepithelial neoplasia II [CIN II] (N87.1)
cervical intraepithelial neoplasia III [CIN III] (D06.-)
dysplasia (mild) (moderate) of cervix uteri (histologically confirmed) (N87.-)
severe dysplasia of cervix uteri (histologically confirmed) (D06.-)
Excludes2 cervical high risk human papillomavirus (HPV) DNA test positive (R87.810)
cervical low risk human papillomavirus (HPV) DNA test positive (R87.820)

R87.610 **Atypical squamous cells of undetermined significance on cytologic smear of cervix (ASC-US)**

R87.611 **Atypical squamous cells cannot exclude high grade squamous intraepithelial lesion on cytologic smear of cervix (ASC-H)**

R87.612 **Low grade squamous intraepithelial lesion on cytologic smear of cervix (LGSIL)**

R87.613 **High grade squamous intraepithelial lesion on cytologic smear of cervix (HGSIL)**

R87.614 **Cytologic evidence of malignancy on smear of cervix**

R87.615 **Unsatisfactory cytologic smear of cervix**
Inadequate sample of cytologic smear of cervix

R87.616 Satisfactory cervical smear but lacking transformation zone

R87.618 Other abnormal cytological findings on specimens from cervix uteri

R87.619 Unspecified abnormal cytological findings in specimens from cervix uteri
Abnormal cervical cytology NOS
Abnormal Papanicolaou smear of cervix NOS
Abnormal thin preparation smear of cervix NOS
Atypical endocervial cells of cervix NOS
Atypical endometrial cells of cervix NOS
Atypical glandular cells of cervix NOS

● **R87.62 Abnormal cytological findings in specimens from vagina**
Use additional code to identify acquired absence of uterus and cervix, if applicable (Z90.71-)
Excludes1 abnormal cytological findings in specimens from cervix uteri (R87.61-)
abnormal cytological findings in specimens from other female genital organs (R87.69)
carcinoma in situ of vagina (histologically confirmed) (D07.2)
vaginal intraepithelial neoplasia I [VAIN I] (N89.0)
vaginal intraepithelial neoplasia II [VAIN II] (N89.1)
vaginal intraepithelial neoplasia III [VAIN III] (D07.2)
dysplasia (mild) (moderate) of vagina (histologically confirmed) (N89.-)
severe dysplasia of vagina (histologically confirmed) (D07.2)
Excludes2 vaginal high risk human papillomavirus (HPV) DNA test positive (R87.811)
vaginal low risk human papillomavirus (HPV) DNA test positive (R87.821)

R87.620 Atypical squamous cells of undetermined significance on cytologic smear of vagina (ASC-US)

R87.621 Atypical squamous cells cannot exclude high grade squamous intraepithelial lesion on cytologic smear of vagina (ASC-H)

R87.622 Low grade squamous intraepithelial lesion on cytologic smear of vagina (LGSIL)

R87.623 High grade squamous intraepithelial lesion on cytologic smear of vagina (HGSIL)

R87.624 Cytologic evidence of malignancy on smear of vagina

R87.625 Unsatisfactory cytologic smear of vagina
Inadequate sample of cytologic smear of vagina

R87.628 Other abnormal cytological findings on specimens from vagina

R87.629 Unspecified abnormal cytological findings in specimens from vagina
Abnormal Papanicolaou smear of vagina NOS
Abnormal thin preparation smear of vagina NOS
Abnormal vaginal cytology NOS
Atypical endocervical cells of vagina NOS
Atypical endometrial cells of vagina NOS
Atypical glandular cells of vagina NOS

R87.69 Abnormal cytological findings in specimens from other female genital organs
Abnormal cytological findings in specimens from female genital organs NOS
Excludes1 dysplasia of vulva (histologically confirmed) (N90.0-N90.3)

R87.7 Abnormal histological findings in specimens from female genital organs
Excludes1 carcinoma in situ (histologically confirmed) of female genital organs (D06-D07.3)
cervical intraepithelial neoplasia I [CIN I] (N87.0)
cervical intraepithelial neoplasia II [CIN II] (N87.1)
cervical intraepithelial neoplasia III [CIN III] (D06.-)
dysplasia (mild) (moderate) of cervix uteri (histologically confirmed) (N87.-)
dysplasia (mild) (moderate) of vagina (histologically confirmed) (N89.-)
vaginal intraepithelial neoplasia I [VAIN I] (N89.0)
vaginal intraepithelial neoplasia II [VAIN II] (N89.1)
vaginal intraepithelial neoplasia III [VAIN III] (D07.2)
severe dysplasia of cervix uteri (histologically confirmed) (D06.-)
severe dysplasia of vagina (histologically confirmed) (D07.2)

● **R87.8 Other abnormal findings in specimens from female genital organs**

● **R87.81 High risk human papillomavirus (HPV) DNA test positive from female genital organs**
Excludes1 anogenital warts due to human papillomavirus (HPV) (A63.0)
condyloma acuminatum (A63.0)

R87.810 Cervical high risk human papillomavirus (HPV) DNA test positive

R87.811 Vaginal high risk human papillomavirus (HPV) DNA test positive

● **R87.82 Low risk human papillomavirus (HPV) DNA test positive from female genital organs**
Use additional code for associated human papillomavirus (B97.7)

R87.820 Cervical low risk human papillomavirus (HPV) DNA test positive

R87.821 Vaginal low risk human papillomavirus (HPV) DNA test positive

R87.89 Other abnormal findings in specimens from female genital organs
Abnormal chromosomal findings in specimens from female genital organs

R87.9 Unspecified abnormal finding in specimens from female genital organs

CHAPTER 18 (R00-R99)

● **R88 Abnormal findings in other body fluids and substances**
R88.Ø Cloudy (hemodialysis) (peritoneal) dialysis effluent
R88.8 Abnormal findings in other body fluids and substances

● **R89 Abnormal findings in specimens from other organs, systems and tissues**
Includes abnormal findings in nipple discharge
abnormal findings in synovial fluid
abnormal findings in wound secretions
R89.Ø Abnormal level of enzymes in specimens from other organs, systems and tissues
R89.1 Abnormal level of hormones in specimens from other organs, systems and tissues
R89.2 Abnormal level of other drugs, medicaments and biological substances in specimens from other organs, systems and tissues
R89.3 Abnormal level of substances chiefly nonmedicinal as to source in specimens from other organs, systems and tissues
R89.4 Abnormal immunological findings in specimens from other organs, systems and tissues
R89.5 Abnormal microbiological findings in specimens from other organs, systems and tissues
Positive culture findings in specimens from other organs, systems and tissues
Excludes1 colonization status (Z22.-)
R89.6 Abnormal cytological findings in specimens from other organs, systems and tissues
R89.7 Abnormal histological findings in specimens from other organs, systems and tissues
R89.8 Other abnormal findings in specimens from other organs, systems and tissues
Abnormal chromosomal findings in specimens from other organs, systems and tissues
R89.9 Unspecified abnormal finding in specimens from other organs, systems and tissues

ABNORMAL FINDINGS ON DIAGNOSTIC IMAGING AND IN FUNCTION STUDIES, WITHOUT DIAGNOSIS (R9Ø-R94)

Includes nonspecific abnormal findings on diagnostic imaging by computerized axial tomography [CAT scan]
nonspecific abnormal findings on diagnostic imaging by magnetic resonance imaging [MRI][NMR]
nonspecific abnormal findings on diagnostic imaging by positron emission tomography [PET scan]
nonspecific abnormal findings on diagnostic imaging by thermography
nonspecific abnormal findings on diagnostic imaging by ultrasound [echogram]
nonspecific abnormal findings on diagnostic imaging by X-ray examination
Excludes1 abnormal findings on antenatal screening of mother (O28.-)
diagnostic abnormal findings classified elsewhere - see Alphabetical Index

● **R9Ø Abnormal findings on diagnostic imaging of central nervous system**
R9Ø.Ø Intracranial space-occupying lesion found on diagnostic imaging of central nervous system
● **R9Ø.8 Other abnormal findings on diagnostic imaging of central nervous system**
R9Ø.81 Abnormal echoencephalogram
R9Ø.82 White matter disease, unspecified
R9Ø.89 Other abnormal findings on diagnostic imaging of central nervous system
Other cerebrovascular abnormality found on diagnostic imaging of central nervous system

● **R91 Abnormal findings on diagnostic imaging of lung**
R91.1 Solitary pulmonary nodule
Coin lesion lung
Solitary pulmonary nodule, subsegmental branch of the bronchial tree
R91.8 Other nonspecific abnormal finding of lung field
Lung mass NOS found on diagnostic imaging of lung
Pulmonary infiltrate NOS
Shadow, lung

● **R92 Abnormal and inconclusive findings on diagnostic imaging of breast**
R92.Ø Mammographic microcalcification found on diagnostic imaging of breast
Excludes2 mammographic calcification (calculus) found on diagnostic imaging of breast (R92.1)
R92.1 Mammographic calcification found on diagnostic imaging of breast
Mammographic calculus found on diagnostic imaging of breast
R92.2 Inconclusive mammogram
Dense breasts NOS
Inconclusive mammogram NEC
Inconclusive mammography due to dense breasts
Inconclusive mammography NEC
R92.8 Other abnormal and inconclusive findings on diagnostic imaging of breast

● **R93 Abnormal findings on diagnostic imaging of other body structures**
R93.Ø Abnormal findings on diagnostic imaging of skull and head, not elsewhere classified
Excludes1 intracranial space-occupying lesion found on diagnostic imaging (R9Ø.Ø)
R93.1 Abnormal findings on diagnostic imaging of heart and coronary circulation
Abnormal echocardiogram NOS
Abnormal heart shadow
R93.2 Abnormal findings on diagnostic imaging of liver and biliary tract
Nonvisualization of gallbladder
R93.3 Abnormal findings on diagnostic imaging of other parts of digestive tract
● **R93.4 Abnormal findings on diagnostic imaging of urinary organs**
Excludes2 hypertrophy of kidney (N28.81) ◀
R93.41 Abnormal radiologic findings on diagnostic imaging of renal pelvis, ureter, or bladder ◀
Filling defect of bladder found on diagnostic imaging ◀
Filling defect of renal pelvis found on diagnostic imaging ◀
Filling defect of ureter found on diagnostic imaging ◀
● **R93.42 Abnormal radiologic findings on diagnostic imaging of kidney** ◀
R93.421 Abnormal radiologic findings on diagnostic imaging of right kidney ◀
R93.422 Abnormal radiologic findings on diagnostic imaging of left kidney ◀
R93.429 Abnormal radiologic findings on diagnostic imaging of unspecified kidney ◀
R93.49 Abnormal radiologic findings on diagnostic imaging of other urinary organs ◀

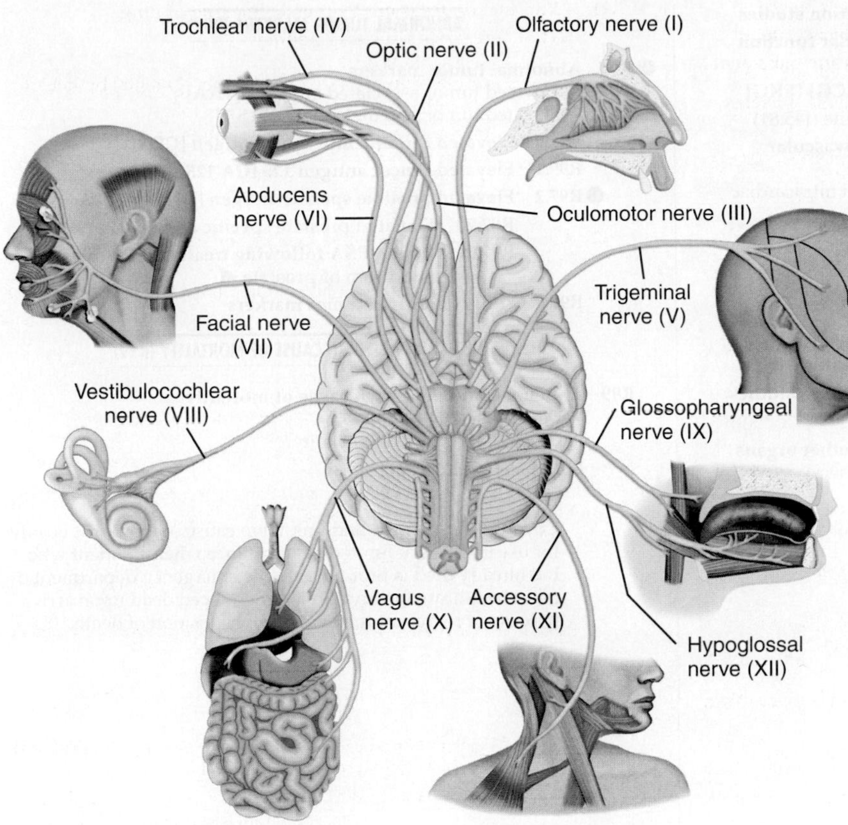

Figure 18-2 Cranial nerves. (From Patton and Thibodeau: Anatomy and physiology, ed 7, St. Louis, Mosby, 2009)

R93.5 Abnormal findings on diagnostic imaging of other abdominal regions, including retroperitoneum

R93.6 Abnormal findings on diagnostic imaging of limbs

Excludes2 abnormal finding in skin and subcutaneous tissue (R93.8)

R93.7 Abnormal findings on diagnostic imaging of other parts of musculoskeletal system

Excludes2 abnormal findings on diagnostic imaging of skull (R93.Ø)

R93.8 Abnormal findings on diagnostic imaging of other specified body structures

Abnormal finding by radioisotope localization of placenta

Abnormal radiological finding in skin and subcutaneous tissue

Mediastinal shift

R93.9 Diagnostic imaging inconclusive due to excess body fat of patient

● **R94 Abnormal results of function studies**

Includes abnormal results of radionuclide [radioisotope] uptake studies

abnormal results of scintigraphy

● **R94.Ø Abnormal results of function studies of central nervous system**

R94.Ø1 Abnormal electroencephalogram [EEG]

R94.Ø2 Abnormal brain scan

R94.Ø9 Abnormal results of other function studies of central nervous system

● **R94.1 Abnormal results of function studies of peripheral nervous system and special senses**

● **R94.11 Abnormal results of function studies of eye**

R94.11Ø Abnormal electro-oculogram [EOG]

R94.111 Abnormal electroretinogram [ERG]

Abnormal retinal function study

R94.112 Abnormal visually evoked potential [VEP]

R94.113 Abnormal oculomotor study

R94.118 Abnormal results of other function studies of eye

● **R94.12 Abnormal results of function studies of ear and other special senses**

R94.12Ø Abnormal auditory function study

R94.121 Abnormal vestibular function study

R94.128 Abnormal results of other function studies of ear and other special senses

● **R94.13 Abnormal results of function studies of peripheral nervous system**

R94.13Ø Abnormal response to nerve stimulation, unspecified

R94.131 Abnormal electromyogram [EMG]

Excludes1 electromyogram of eye (R94.113)

R94.138 Abnormal results of other function studies of peripheral nervous system

R94.2 Abnormal results of pulmonary function studies

Reduced ventilatory capacity

Reduced vital capacity

Item 18–1 The **peripheral nervous system** consists of 31 pairs of spinal nerves, 12 pairs of cranial nerves, and the autonomic nerves, which are divided into the parasympathetic and sympathetic nerves. The cranial nerves are: olfactory (I), optic (II), oculomotor (III), trochlear (IV), trigeminal (V), abducens (VI), facial (VII), vestibulocochlear (VIII), glossopharyngeal (IX), vagus (X), accessory (XI), and hypoglossal (XII).

● **R94.3 Abnormal results of cardiovascular function studies**

R94.30 Abnormal result of cardiovascular function study, unspecified

R94.31 Abnormal electrocardiogram [ECG] [EKG]

Excludes1 long QT syndrome (I45.81)

R94.39 Abnormal result of other cardiovascular function study

Abnormal electrophysiological intracardiac studies
Abnormal phonocardiogram
Abnormal vectorcardiogram

R94.4 Abnormal results of kidney function studies

Abnormal renal function test

R94.5 Abnormal results of liver function studies

R94.6 Abnormal results of thyroid function studies

R94.7 Abnormal results of other endocrine function studies

Excludes2 abnormal glucose (R73.0-)

R94.8 Abnormal results of function studies of other organs and systems

Abnormal basal metabolic rate [BMR]
Abnormal bladder function test
Abnormal splenic function test

ABNORMAL TUMOR MARKERS (R97)

● **R97 Abnormal tumor markers**

Elevated tumor associated antigens [TAA]
Elevated tumor specific antigens [TSA]

R97.0 Elevated carcinoembryonic antigen [CEA]

R97.1 Elevated cancer antigen 125 [CA 125]

● **R97.2 Elevated prostate specific antigen [PSA]**

R97.20 Elevated prostate specific antigen [PSA] ◀

R97.21 Rising PSA following treatment for malignant neoplasm of prostate ◀

R97.8 Other abnormal tumor markers

ILL-DEFINED AND UNKNOWN CAUSE OF MORTALITY (R99)

R99 Ill-defined and unknown cause of mortality

Death (unexplained) NOS
Unspecified cause of mortality

OGCR Section I.C.18.h.

Death NOS

Code R99, Ill-defined and unknown cause of mortality, is only for use in the very limited circumstance when a patient who has already died is brought into the emergency department or other healthcare facility and is pronounced dead upon arrival. It does not represent the discharge disposition of death.

CHAPTER 19

INJURY, POISONING AND CERTAIN OTHER CONSEQUENCES OF EXTERNAL CAUSES (SØØ-T88)

OGCR Chapter-Specific Coding Guidelines

19. Chapter 19: Injury, poisoning, and certain other consequences of external causes (SØØ-T88)

a. Application of 7th Characters in Chapter 19

Most categories in chapter 19 have a 7th character requirement for each applicable code. Most categories in this chapter have three 7th character values (with the exception of fractures): A, initial encounter, D, subsequent encounter and S, sequela. Categories for traumatic fractures have additional 7th character values. **While the patient may be seen by a new or different provider over the course of treatment for an injury, assignment of the 7th character is based on whether the patient is undergoing active treatment and not whether the provider is seeing the patient for the first time.**

For complication codes, active treatment refers to treatment for the condition described by the code, even though it may be related to an earlier precipitating problem. For example, code T84.5ØXA, Infection and inflammatory reaction due to unspecified internal joint prosthesis, initial encounter, is used when active treatment is provided for the infection, even though the condition relates to the prosthetic device, implant or graft that was placed at a previous encounter.

7th character "A", initial encounter is used **for each encounter where** the patient is receiving active treatment for the condition.

7th character "D" subsequent encounter is used for encounters after the patient has **completed** active treatment of the condition and is receiving routine care for the condition during the healing or recovery phase.

The aftercare Z codes should not be used for aftercare for conditions such as injuries or poisonings, where 7th characters are provided to identify subsequent care. For example, for aftercare of an injury, assign the acute injury code with the 7th character "D" (subsequent encounter).

7th character "S", sequela, is for use for complications or conditions that arise as a direct result of a condition, such as scar formation after a burn. The scars are sequelae of the burn. When using 7th character "S", it is necessary to use both the injury code that precipitated the sequela and the code for the sequela itself. The "S" is added only to the injury code, not the sequela code. The 7th character "S" identifies the injury responsible for the sequela. The specific type of sequela (e.g. scar) is sequenced first, followed by the injury code.

See Section I.B.1Ø. Sequelae, (Late Effects)

b. Coding of Injuries

When coding injuries, assign separate codes for each injury unless a combination code is provided, in which case the combination code is assigned. Code TØ7, Unspecified multiple injuries should not be assigned in the inpatient setting unless information for a more specific code is not available. Traumatic injury codes (SØØ-T14.9) are not to be used for normal, healing surgical wounds or to identify complications of surgical wounds.

The code for the most serious injury, as determined by the provider and the focus of treatment, is sequenced first.

1) Superficial injuries

Superficial injuries such as abrasions or contusions are not coded when associated with more severe injuries of the same site.

2) Primary injury with damage to nerves/blood vessels

When a primary injury results in minor damage to peripheral nerves or blood vessels, the primary injury is sequenced first with additional code(s) for injuries to nerves and spinal cord (such as category SØ4), and/or injury to blood vessels (such as category S15). When the primary injury is to the blood vessels or nerves, that injury should be sequenced first.

c. Coding of Traumatic Fractures

The principles of multiple coding of injuries should be followed in coding fractures. Fractures of specified sites are coded individually by site in accordance with both the provisions within categories SØ2, S12, S22, S32, S42, S49, S52, S59, S62, S72, S79, S82, S89, S92 and the level of detail furnished by medical record content.

A fracture not indicated as open or closed should be coded to closed. A fracture not indicated whether displaced or not displaced should be coded to displaced.

More specific guidelines are as follows:

1) Initial vs. Subsequent Encounter for Fractures

Traumatic fractures are coded using the appropriate 7th character for initial encounter (A, B, C) **for each encounter where** the patient is receiving active treatment for the fracture. The appropriate 7th character for initial encounter should also be assigned for a patient who delayed seeking treatment for the fracture or nonunion.

Fractures are coded using the appropriate 7th character for subsequent care for encounters after the patient has completed active treatment of the fracture and is receiving routine care for the fracture during the healing or recovery phase.

Care for complications of surgical treatment for fracture repairs during the healing or recovery phase should be coded with the appropriate complication codes.

Care of complications of fractures, such as malunion and nonunion, should be reported with the appropriate 7th character for subsequent care with nonunion (K, M, N,) or subsequent care with malunion (P, Q, R).

Malunion/nonunion: The appropriate 7th character for initial encounter should also be assigned for a patient who delayed seeking treatment for the fracture or nonunion.

The open fracture designations in the assignment of the 7th character for fractures of the forearm, femur and lower leg, including ankle are based on the Gustilo open fracture classification. When the Gustilo classification type is not specified for an open fracture, the 7th character for open fracture type I or II should be assigned (B, E, H, M, Q).

A code from category M8Ø, not a traumatic fracture code, should be used for any patient with known osteoporosis who suffers a fracture, even if the patient had a minor fall or trauma, if that fall or trauma would not usually break a normal, healthy bone.

See Section I.C.13. Osteoporosis.

The aftercare Z codes should not be used for aftercare for traumatic fractures. For aftercare of a traumatic fracture, assign the acute fracture code with the appropriate 7th character.

2) Multiple fractures sequencing

Multiple fractures are sequenced in accordance with the severity of the fracture.

d. Coding of Burns and Corrosions

The ICD-10-CM makes a distinction between burns and corrosions. The burn codes are for thermal burns, except sunburns, that come from a heat source, such as a fire or hot appliance. The burn codes are also for burns resulting from electricity and radiation. Corrosions are burns due to chemicals. The guidelines are the same for burns and corrosions.

Current burns (T2Ø-T25) are classified by depth, extent and by agent (X code). Burns are classified by depth as first degree (erythema), second degree (blistering), and third degree (full-thickness involvement). Burns of the eye and internal organs (T26-T28) are classified by site, but not by degree.

1) Sequencing of burn and related condition codes

Sequence first the code that reflects the highest degree of burn when more than one burn is present.

a. When the reason for the admission or encounter is for treatment of external multiple burns, sequence first the code that reflects the burn of the highest degree.

b. When a patient has both internal and external burns, the circumstances of admission govern the selection of the principal diagnosis or first-listed diagnosis.

c. When a patient is admitted for burn injuries and other related conditions such as smoke inhalation and/or respiratory failure, the circumstances of admission govern the selection of the principal or first-listed diagnosis.

2) Burns of the same local site
Classify burns of the same local site (three-character category level, T2Ø-T28) but of different degrees to the subcategory identifying the highest degree recorded in the diagnosis.

3) Non-healing burns
Non-healing burns are coded as acute burns.
Necrosis of burned skin should be coded as a non-healed burn.

4) Infected Burn
For any documented infected burn site, use an additional code for the infection.

5) Assign separate codes for each burn site
When coding burns, assign separate codes for each burn site. Category T3Ø, Burn and corrosion, body region unspecified is extremely vague and should rarely be used.

6) Burns and Corrosions Classified According to Extent of Body Surface Involved
Assign codes from category T31, Burns classified according to extent of body surface involved, or T32, Corrosions classified according to extent of body surface involved, when the site of the burn is not specified or when there is a need for additional data. It is advisable to use category T31 as additional coding when needed to provide data for evaluating burn mortality, such as that needed by burn units. It is also advisable to use category T31 as an additional code for reporting purposes when there is mention of a third-degree burn involving 2Ø percent or more of the body surface.

Categories T31 and T32 are based on the classic "rule of nines" in estimating body surface involved: head and neck are assigned nine percent, each arm nine percent, each leg 18 percent, the anterior trunk 18 percent, posterior trunk 18 percent, and genitalia one percent. Providers may change these percentage assignments where necessary to accommodate infants and children who have proportionately larger heads than adults, and patients who have large buttocks, thighs, or abdomen that involve burns.

7) Encounters for treatment of sequela of burns
Encounters for the treatment of the late effects of burns or corrosions (i.e., scars or joint contractures) should be coded with a burn or corrosion code with the 7th character "S" for sequela.

8) Sequelae with a late effect code and current burn
When appropriate, both a code for a current burn or corrosion with 7th character "A" or "D" and a burn or corrosion code with 7th character "S" may be assigned on the same record (when both a current burn and sequelae of an old burn exist). Burns and corrosions do not heal at the same rate and a current healing wound may still exist with sequela of a healed burn or corrosion.

See Section I.B.1Ø. Sequela, (Late Effects)

9) Use of an external cause code with burns and corrosions
An external cause code should be used with burns and corrosions to identify the source and intent of the burn, as well as the place where it occurred.

e. Adverse Effects, Poisoning , Underdosing and Toxic Effects
Codes in categories T36-T65 are combination codes that include the substance that was taken as well as the intent. No additional external cause code is required for poisonings, toxic effects, adverse effects and underdosing codes.

1) Do not code directly from the Table of Drugs
Do not code directly from the Table of Drugs and Chemicals. Always refer back to the Tabular List.

2) Use as many codes as necessary to describe
Use as many codes as necessary to describe completely all drugs, medicinal or biological substances.

3) If the same code would describe the causative agent
If the same code would describe the causative agent for more than one adverse reaction, poisoning, toxic effect or underdosing, assign the code only once.

4) If two or more drugs, medicinal or biological substances
If two or more drugs, medicinal or biological substances are reported, code each individually unless a combination code is listed in the Table of Drugs and Chemicals.

5) The occurrence of drug toxicity is classified in ICD-10-CM as follows:

(a) Adverse Effect
When coding an adverse effect of a drug that has been correctly prescribed and properly administered, assign the appropriate code for the nature of the adverse effect followed by the appropriate code for the adverse effect of the drug (T36-T5Ø). The code for the drug should have a 5th or 6th character "5" (for example T36.ØX5-) Examples of the nature of an adverse effect are tachycardia, delirium, gastrointestinal hemorrhaging, vomiting, hypokalemia, hepatitis, renal failure, or respiratory failure.

(b) Poisoning
When coding a poisoning or reaction to the improper use of a medication (e.g., overdose, wrong substance given or taken in error, wrong route of administration), first assign the appropriate code from categories T36-T5Ø. The poisoning codes have an associated intent as their 5th or 6th character (accidental, intentional self-harm, assault and undetermined). **If the intent of the poisoning is unknown or unspecified, code the intent as accidental intent. The undetermined intent is only for use if the documentation in the record specifies that the intent cannot be determined.** Use additional code(s) for all manifestations of poisonings.

If there is also a diagnosis of abuse or dependence of the substance, the abuse or dependence is assigned as an additional code.

Examples of poisoning include:

(i) Error was made in drug prescription
Errors made in drug prescription or in the administration of the drug by provider, nurse, patient, or other person.

(ii) Overdose of a drug intentionally taken If an overdose of a drug was intentionally taken or administered and resulted in drug toxicity, it would be coded as a poisoning.

(iii) Nonprescribed drug taken with correctly prescribed and properly administered drug.
If a nonprescribed drug or medicinal agent was taken in combination with a correctly prescribed and properly administered drug, any drug toxicity or other reaction resulting from the interaction of the two drugs would be classified as a poisoning.

(iv) Interaction of drug(s) and alcohol.
When a reaction results from the interaction of a drug(s) and alcohol, this would be classified as poisoning.

See Section I.C.4. if poisoning is the result of insulin pump malfunctions.

(c) Underdosing
Underdosing refers to taking less of a medication than is prescribed by a provider or a manufacturer's instruction. For

underdosing, assign the code from categories T36-T50 (fifth or sixth character "6").

Codes for underdosing should never be assigned as principal or first-listed codes. If a patient has a relapse or exacerbation of the medical condition for which the drug is prescribed because of the reduction in dose, then the medical condition itself should be coded.

Noncompliance (Z91.12-, Z91.13-) or complication of care (Y63.6-Y63.9) codes are to be used with an underdosing code to indicate intent, if known.

(d) Toxic Effects

When a harmful substance is ingested or comes in contact with a person, this is classified as a toxic effect. The toxic effect codes are in categories T51-T65.

Toxic effect codes have an associated intent: accidental, intentional self-harm, assault and undetermined.

f. Adult and child abuse, neglect and other maltreatment

Sequence first the appropriate code from categories T74.- (Adult and child abuse, neglect and other maltreatment, confirmed) or T76.- (Adult and child abuse, neglect and other maltreatment, suspected) for abuse, neglect and other maltreatment, followed by any accompanying mental health or injury code(s).

If the documentation in the medical record states abuse or neglect it is coded as confirmed (T74.-). It is coded as suspected if it is documented as suspected (T76.-).

For cases of confirmed abuse or neglect an external cause code from the assault section (X92-**Y09**) should be added to identify the cause of any physical injuries. A perpetrator code (Y07) should be added when the perpetrator of the abuse is known. For suspected cases of abuse or neglect, do not report external cause or perpetrator code.

If a suspected case of abuse, neglect or mistreatment is ruled out during an encounter code Z04.71, Encounter for examination and observation following alleged physical adult abuse, ruled out, or code Z04.72, Encounter for examination and observation following alleged child physical abuse, ruled out, should be used, not a code from T76.

If a suspected case of alleged rape or sexual abuse is ruled out during an encounter code Z04.41, Encounter for examination and observation following alleged **adult rape** or code Z04.42, Encounter for examination and observation following alleged **child** rape, should be used, not a code from T76.

See Section I.C.15. Abuse in a pregnant patient.

g. Complications of care

1) General guidelines for complications of care

(a) Documentation of complications of care

See Section I.B.16. for information on documentation of complications of care.

2) Pain due to medical devices

Pain associated with devices, implants or grafts left in a surgical site (for example painful hip prosthesis) is assigned to the appropriate code(s) found in Chapter 19, Injury, poisoning, and certain other consequences of external causes. Specific codes for pain due to medical devices are found in the T code section of the ICD-10-CM. Use additional code(s) from category G89 to identify acute or chronic pain due to presence of the device, implant or graft (G89.18 or G89.28).

3) Transplant complications

(a) Transplant complications other than kidney

Codes under category T86, Complications of transplanted organs and tissues, are for use for both complications and rejection of transplanted organs. A transplant complication code is only assigned if the complication affects the function of the transplanted organ. Two codes are required to fully describe a transplant complication: the appropriate code from category T86 and a secondary code that identifies the complication.

Pre-existing conditions or conditions that develop after the transplant are not coded as complications unless they affect the function of the transplanted organs.

See I.C.21. for transplant organ removal status

See I.C.2. for malignant neoplasm associated with transplanted organ.

(b) Kidney transplant complications

Patients who have undergone kidney transplant may still have some form of chronic kidney disease (CKD) because the kidney transplant may not fully restore kidney function. Code T86.1- should be assigned for documented complications of a kidney transplant, such as transplant failure or rejection or other transplant complication. Code T86.1- should not be assigned for post kidney transplant patients who have chronic kidney (CKD) unless a transplant complication such as transplant failure or rejection is documented. If the documentation is unclear as to whether the patient has a complication of the transplant, query the provider.

Conditions that affect the function of the transplanted kidney, other than CKD, should be assigned a code from subcategory T86.1, Complications of transplanted organ, Kidney, and a secondary code that identifies the complication.

For patients with CKD following a kidney transplant, but who do not have a complication such as failure or rejection, *see section I.C.14. Chronic kidney disease and kidney transplant status.*

4) Complication codes that include the external cause

As with certain other T codes, some of the complications of care codes have the external cause included in the code. The code includes the nature of the complication as well as the type of procedure that caused the complication. No external cause code indicating the type of procedure is necessary for these codes.

5) Complications of care codes within the body system chapters

Intraoperative and postprocedural complication codes are found within the body system chapters with codes specific to the organs and structures of that body system. These codes should be sequenced first, followed by a code(s) for the specific complication, if applicable.

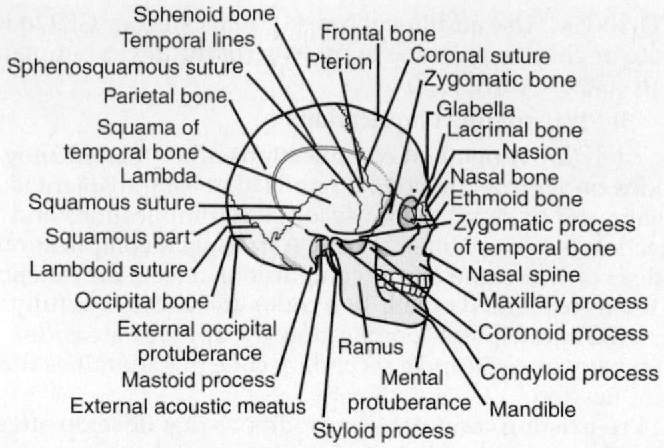

Figure 19-1 Lateral view of skull.

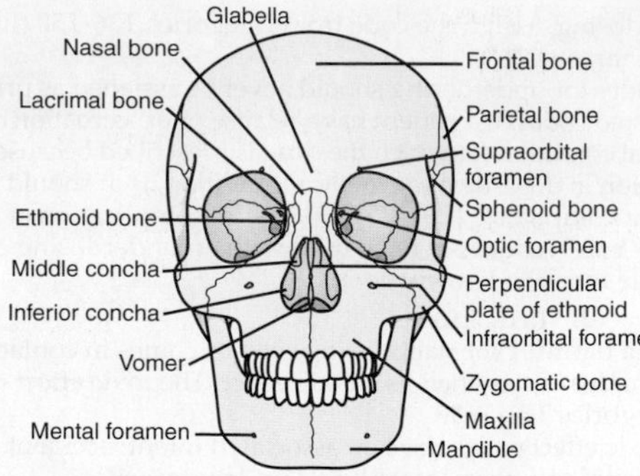

Figure 19-2 Frontal view of skull.

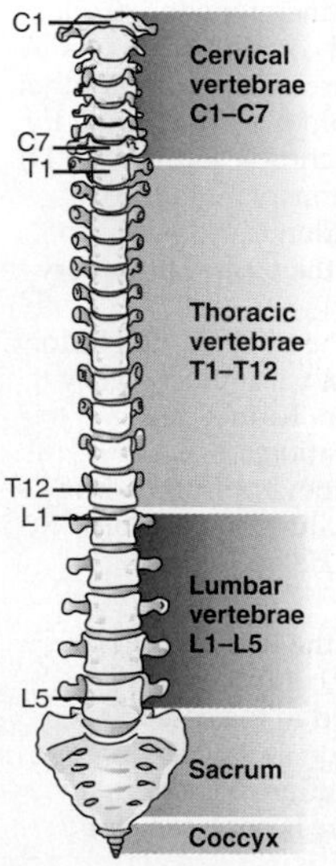

Figure 19-3 Anterior view of vertebral column.

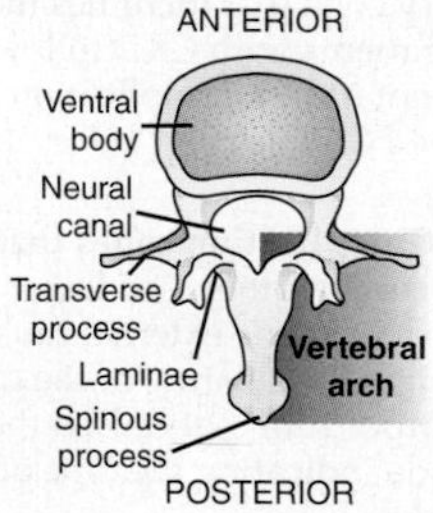

Figure 19-4 Vertebra viewed from above.

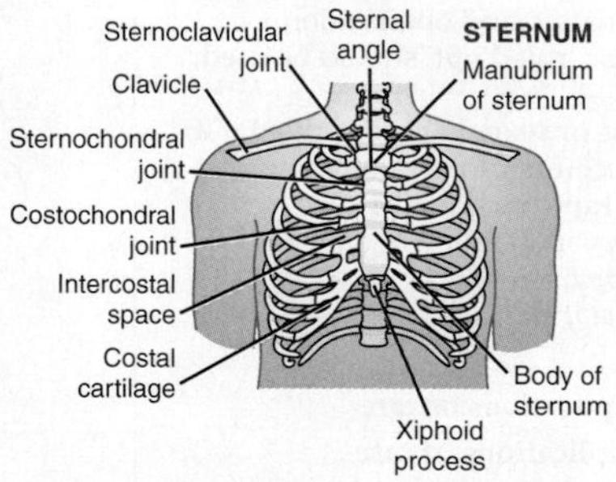

Figure 19-5 Anterior view of rib cage.

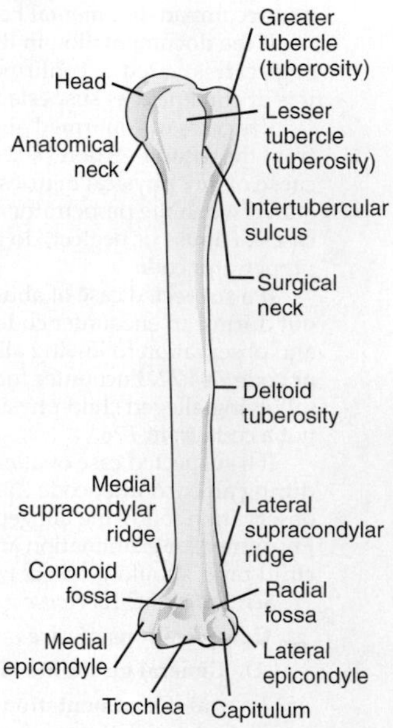

Figure 19-6 Anterior aspect of left humerus.

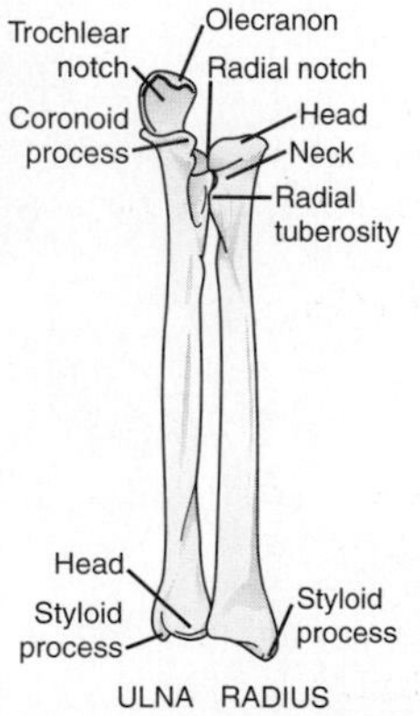

Figure 19-7 Anterior aspect of left radius and ulna.

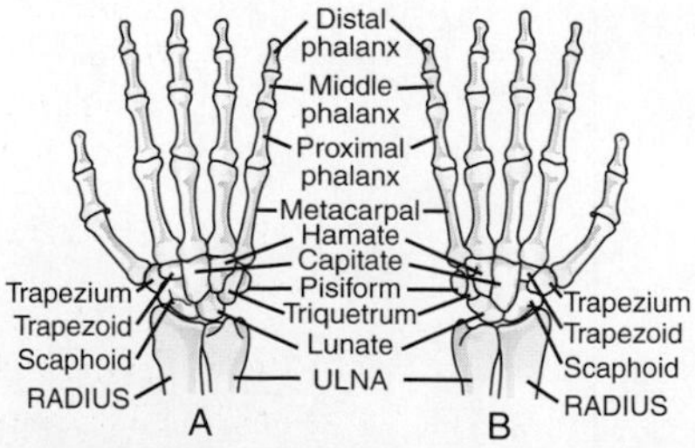

Figure 19-8 Right hand and wrist: **A.** Dorsal surface. **B.** Palmar surface.

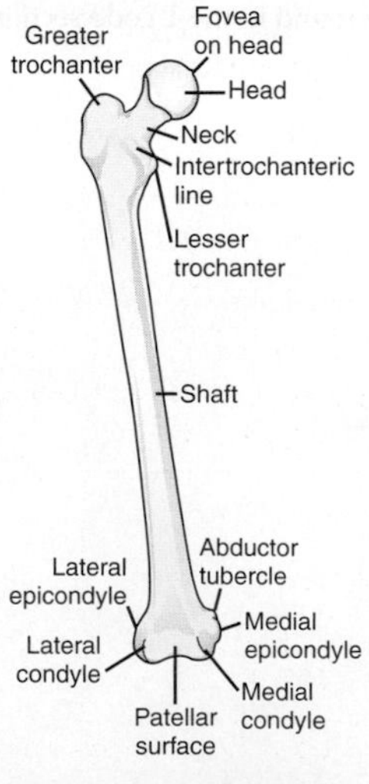

Figure 19-9 Anterior aspect of right femur.

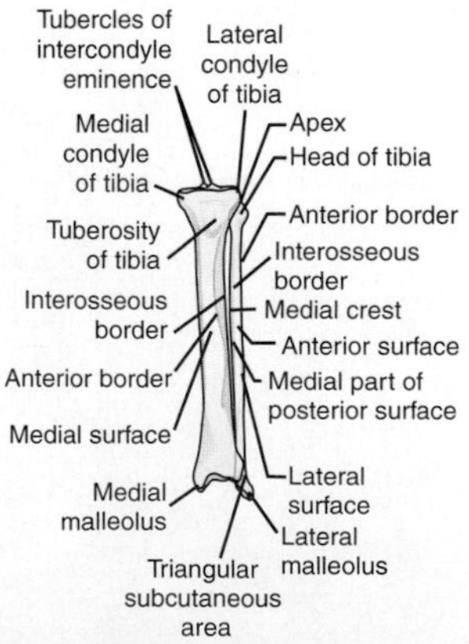

Figure 19-10 Anterior aspect of left tibia and fibula.

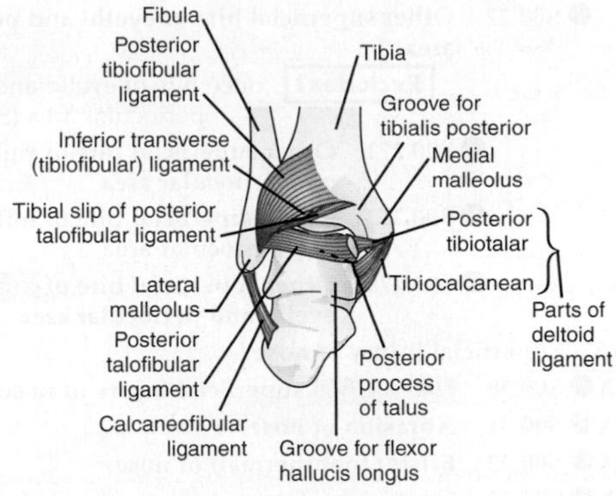

Figure 19-11 Posterior aspect of the left ankle joint.

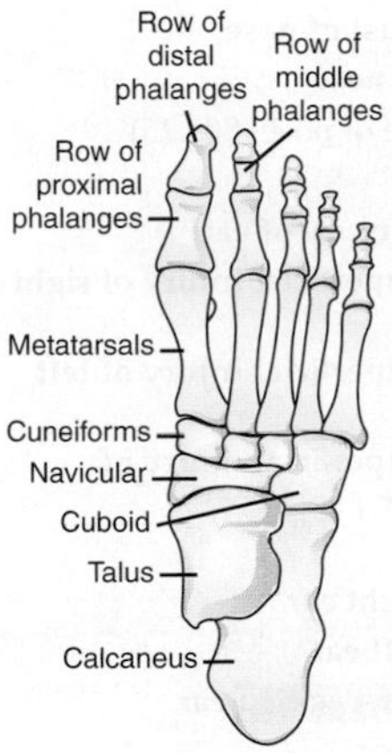

Figure 19-12 Right foot viewed from above.

CHAPTER 19

INJURY, POISONING AND CERTAIN OTHER CONSEQUENCES OF EXTERNAL CAUSES (SØØ-T88)

Note: Use secondary code(s) from Chapter 2Ø, External causes of morbidity, to indicate cause of injury. Codes within the T section that include the external cause do not require an additional external cause code.

Use additional code to identify any retained foreign body, if applicable (Z18.-)

Excludes1 birth trauma (P1Ø-P15)
obstetric trauma (O7Ø-O71)

Note: The chapter uses the S-section for coding different types of injuries related to single body regions and the T-section to cover injuries to unspecified body regions as well as poisoning and certain other consequences of external causes.

This chapter contains the following blocks:

SØØ-SØ9	Injuries to the head
S1Ø-S19	Injuries to the neck
S2Ø-S29	Injuries to the thorax
S3Ø-S39	Injuries to the abdomen, lower back, lumbar spine, pelvis and external genitals
S4Ø-S49	Injuries to the shoulder and upper arm
S5Ø-S59	Injuries to the elbow and forearm
S6Ø-S69	Injuries to the wrist, hand, and fingers
S7Ø-S79	Injuries to the hip and thigh
S8Ø-S89	Injuries to the knee and lower leg
S9Ø-S99	Injuries to the ankle and foot
TØ7	Injuries involving multiple body regions
T14	Injury of unspecified body region
T15-T19	Effects of foreign body entering through natural orifice
T2Ø-T32	Burns and corrosions
T2Ø-T25	Burns and corrosions of external body surface, specified by site
T26-T28	Burns and corrosions confined to eye and internal organs
T3Ø-T32	Burns and corrosions of multiple and unspecified body regions
T33-T34	Frostbite
T36-T5Ø	Poisoning by, adverse effect of and underdosing of drugs, medicaments and biological substances
T51-T65	Toxic effects of substances chiefly nonmedicinal as to source
T66-T78	Other and unspecified effects of external causes
T79	Certain early complications of trauma
T8Ø-T88	Complications of surgical and medical care, not elsewhere classified

INJURIES TO THE HEAD (SØØ-SØ9)

Includes injuries of ear
injuries of eye
injuries of face [any part]
injuries of gum
injuries of jaw
injuries of oral cavity
injuries of palate
injuries of periocular area
injuries of scalp
injuries of temporomandibular joint area
injuries of tongue
injuries of tooth

Code also for any associated infection

Excludes2 burns and corrosions (T2Ø-T32)
effects of foreign body in ear (T16)
effects of foreign body in larynx (T17.3)
effects of foreign body in mouth NOS (T18.Ø)
effects of foreign body in nose (T17.Ø-T17.1)
effects of foreign body in pharynx (T17.2)
effects of foreign body on external eye (T15.-)
frostbite (T33-T34)
insect bite or sting, venomous (T63.4)

● **SØØ Superficial injury of head**

Excludes1 diffuse cerebral contusion (SØ6.2-)
focal cerebral contusion (SØ6.3-)
injury of eye and orbit (SØ5.-)
open wound of head (SØ1.-)

The appropriate 7th character is to be added to each code from category SØØ

A	initial encounter *All encounters involving diagnosis and treatment*
D	subsequent encounter *Encounters during the healing phase*
S	sequela

● **SØØ.Ø Superficial injury of scalp**

X● **SØØ.ØØ Unspecified superficial injury of scalp**

X● **SØØ.Ø1 Abrasion of scalp**

X● **SØØ.Ø2 Blister (nonthermal) of scalp**

X● **SØØ.Ø3 Contusion of scalp**
Bruise of scalp
Hematoma of scalp

X● **SØØ.Ø4 External constriction of part of scalp**

X● **SØØ.Ø5 Superficial foreign body of scalp**
Splinter in the scalp

X● **SØØ.Ø6 Insect bite (nonvenomous) of scalp**

X● **SØØ.Ø7 Other superficial bite of scalp**
Excludes1 open bite of scalp (SØ1.Ø5)

CHAPTER 19 (SØØ-T88)

● S00.1 Contusion of eyelid and periocular area
Black eye
Excludes2 contusion of eyeball and orbital tissues (S05.1)
X● S00.10 Contusion of unspecified eyelid and periocular area
X● S00.11 Contusion of right eyelid and periocular area
X● S00.12 Contusion of left eyelid and periocular area
● S00.2 Other and unspecified superficial injuries of eyelid and periocular area
Excludes2 superficial injury of conjunctiva and cornea (S05.0-)
● S00.20 Unspecified superficial injury of eyelid and periocular area
● S00.201 Unspecified superficial injury of right eyelid and periocular area
● S00.202 Unspecified superficial injury of left eyelid and periocular area
● S00.209 Unspecified superficial injury of unspecified eyelid and periocular area
● S00.21 Abrasion of eyelid and periocular area
● S00.211 Abrasion of right eyelid and periocular area
● S00.212 Abrasion of left eyelid and periocular area
● S00.219 Abrasion of unspecified eyelid and periocular area
● S00.22 Blister (nonthermal) of eyelid and periocular area
● S00.221 Blister (nonthermal) of right eyelid and periocular area
● S00.222 Blister (nonthermal) of left eyelid and periocular area
● S00.229 Blister (nonthermal) of unspecified eyelid and periocular area
● S00.24 External constriction of eyelid and periocular area
● S00.241 External constriction of right eyelid and periocular area
● S00.242 External constriction of left eyelid and periocular area
● S00.249 External constriction of unspecified eyelid and periocular area
● S00.25 Superficial foreign body of eyelid and periocular area
Splinter of eyelid and periocular area
Excludes2 retained foreign body in eyelid (H02.81-)
● S00.251 Superficial foreign body of right eyelid and periocular area
● S00.252 Superficial foreign body of left eyelid and periocular area
● S00.259 Superficial foreign body of unspecified eyelid and periocular area
● S00.26 Insect bite (nonvenomous) of eyelid and periocular area
● S00.261 Insect bite (nonvenomous) of right eyelid and periocular area
● S00.262 Insect bite (nonvenomous) of left eyelid and periocular area
● S00.269 Insect bite (nonvenomous) of unspecified eyelid and periocular area
● S00.27 Other superficial bite of eyelid and periocular area
Excludes1 open bite of eyelid and periocular area (S01.15)
● S00.271 Other superficial bite of right eyelid and periocular area
● S00.272 Other superficial bite of left eyelid and periocular area
● S00.279 Other superficial bite of unspecified eyelid and periocular area
● S00.3 Superficial injury of nose
X● S00.30 Unspecified superficial injury of nose
X● S00.31 Abrasion of nose
X● S00.32 Blister (nonthermal) of nose
X● S00.33 Contusion of nose
Bruise of nose
Hematoma of nose
X● S00.34 External constriction of nose
X● S00.35 Superficial foreign body of nose
Splinter in the nose
X● S00.36 Insect bite (nonvenomous) of nose
X● S00.37 Other superficial bite of nose
Excludes1 open bite of nose (S01.25)
● S00.4 Superficial injury of ear
● S00.40 Unspecified superficial injury of ear
● S00.401 Unspecified superficial injury of right ear
● S00.402 Unspecified superficial injury of left ear
● S00.409 Unspecified superficial injury of unspecified ear
● S00.41 Abrasion of ear
● S00.411 Abrasion of right ear
● S00.412 Abrasion of left ear
● S00.419 Abrasion of unspecified ear
● S00.42 Blister (nonthermal) of ear
● S00.421 Blister (nonthermal) of right ear
● S00.422 Blister (nonthermal) of left ear
● S00.429 Blister (nonthermal) of unspecified ear
● S00.43 Contusion of ear
Bruise of ear
Hematoma of ear
● S00.431 Contusion of right ear
● S00.432 Contusion of left ear
● S00.439 Contusion of unspecified ear
● S00.44 External constriction of ear
● S00.441 External constriction of right ear
● S00.442 External constriction of left ear
● S00.449 External constriction of unspecified ear
● S00.45 Superficial foreign body of ear
Splinter in the ear
● S00.451 Superficial foreign body of right ear
● S00.452 Superficial foreign body of left ear
● S00.459 Superficial foreign body of unspecified ear
● S00.46 Insect bite (nonvenomous) of ear
● S00.461 Insect bite (nonvenomous) of right ear
● S00.462 Insect bite (nonvenomous) of left ear
● S00.469 Insect bite (nonvenomous) of unspecified ear

● S00.47 Other superficial bite of ear
Excludes1 open bite of ear (S01.35)
● S00.471 Other superficial bite of right ear
● S00.472 Other superficial bite of left ear
● S00.479 Other superficial bite of unspecified ear

● S00.5 Superficial injury of lip and oral cavity
● S00.50 Unspecified superficial injury of lip and oral cavity
● S00.501 Unspecified superficial injury of lip
● S00.502 Unspecified superficial injury of oral cavity
● S00.51 Abrasion of lip and oral cavity
● S00.511 Abrasion of lip
● S00.512 Abrasion of oral cavity
● S00.52 Blister (nonthermal) of lip and oral cavity
● S00.521 Blister (nonthermal) of lip
● S00.522 Blister (nonthermal) of oral cavity
● S00.53 Contusion of lip and oral cavity
● S00.531 Contusion of lip
Bruise of lip
Hematoma of oral cavity
● S00.532 Contusion of oral cavity
Bruise of lip
Hematoma of oral cavity
● S00.54 External constriction of lip and oral cavity
● S00.541 External constriction of lip
● S00.542 External constriction of oral cavity
● S00.55 Superficial foreign body of lip and oral cavity
● S00.551 Superficial foreign body of lip
Splinter of lip and oral cavity
● S00.552 Superficial foreign body of oral cavity
Splinter of lip and oral cavity
● S00.56 Insect bite (nonvenomous) of lip and oral cavity
● S00.561 Insect bite (nonvenomous) of lip
● S00.562 Insect bite (nonvenomous) of oral cavity
● S00.57 Other superficial bite of lip and oral cavity
● S00.571 Other superficial bite of lip
Excludes1 open bite of lip (S01.551)
● S00.572 Other superficial bite of oral cavity
Excludes1 open bite of oral cavity (S01.552)

● S00.8 Superficial injury of other parts of head
Superficial injuries of face [any part] ◀
X● S00.80 Unspecified superficial injury of other part of head
X● S00.81 Abrasion of other part of head
X● S00.82 Blister (nonthermal) of other part of head
X● S00.83 Contusion of other part of head
Bruise of other part of head
Hematoma of other part of head
X● S00.84 External constriction of other part of head
X● S00.85 Superficial foreign body of other part of head
Splinter in other part of head
X● S00.86 Insect bite (nonvenomous) of other part of head
X● S00.87 Other superficial bite of other part of head
Excludes1 open bite of other part of head (S01.85)

● S00.9 Superficial injury of unspecified part of head
X● S00.90 Unspecified superficial injury of unspecified part of head
X● S00.91 Abrasion of unspecified part of head
X● S00.92 Blister (nonthermal) of unspecified part of head
X● S00.93 Contusion of unspecified part of head
Bruise of head
Hematoma of head
X● S00.94 External constriction of unspecified part of head
X● S00.95 Superficial foreign body of unspecified part of head
Splinter of head
X● S00.96 Insect bite (nonvenomous) of unspecified part of head
X● S00.97 Other superficial bite of unspecified part of head
Excludes1 open bite of head (S01.95)

● S01 Open wound of head
Code also any associated:
injury of cranial nerve (S04.-)
injury of muscle and tendon of head (S09.1-)
intracranial injury (S06.-)
wound infection
Excludes1 open skull fracture (S02.- with 7th character B)
Excludes2 injury of eye and orbit (S05.-)
traumatic amputation of part of head (S08.-)

The appropriate 7th character is to be added to each code from category S01

A	initial encounter
D	subsequent encounter
S	sequela

● S01.0 Open wound of scalp
Excludes1 avulsion of scalp (S08.0)
X● S01.00 Unspecified open wound of scalp
X● S01.01 Laceration without foreign body of scalp
X● S01.02 Laceration with foreign body of scalp
X● S01.03 Puncture wound without foreign body of scalp
X● S01.04 Puncture wound with foreign body of scalp
X● S01.05 Open bite of scalp
Bite of scalp NOS
Excludes1 superficial bite of scalp (S00.06, S00.07-)

● S01.1 Open wound of eyelid and periocular area
Open wound of eyelid and periocular area with or without involvement of lacrimal passages
● S01.10 Unspecified open wound of eyelid and periocular area
● S01.101 Unspecified open wound of right eyelid and periocular area
● S01.102 Unspecified open wound of left eyelid and periocular area
● S01.109 Unspecified open wound of unspecified eyelid and periocular area
● S01.11 Laceration without foreign body of eyelid and periocular area
● S01.111 Laceration without foreign body of right eyelid and periocular area
● S01.112 Laceration without foreign body of left eyelid and periocular area
● S01.119 Laceration without foreign body of unspecified eyelid and periocular area
● S01.12 Laceration with foreign body of eyelid and periocular area
● S01.121 Laceration with foreign body of right eyelid and periocular area
● S01.122 Laceration with foreign body of left eyelid and periocular area
● S01.129 Laceration with foreign body of unspecified eyelid and periocular area

● S01.13 Puncture wound without foreign body of eyelid and periocular area
● S01.131 Puncture wound without foreign body of right eyelid and periocular area
● S01.132 Puncture wound without foreign body of left eyelid and periocular area
● S01.139 Puncture wound without foreign body of unspecified eyelid and periocular area
● S01.14 Puncture wound with foreign body of eyelid and periocular area
● S01.141 Puncture wound with foreign body of right eyelid and periocular area
● S01.142 Puncture wound with foreign body of left eyelid and periocular area
● S01.149 Puncture wound with foreign body of unspecified eyelid and periocular area
● S01.15 Open bite of eyelid and periocular area
Bite of eyelid and periocular area NOS
Excludes1 superficial bite of eyelid and periocular area (S00.26, S00.27)
● S01.151 Open bite of right eyelid and periocular area
● S01.152 Open bite of left eyelid and periocular area
● S01.159 Open bite of unspecified eyelid and periocular area
● S01.2 Open wound of nose
X● S01.20 Unspecified open wound of nose
X● S01.21 Laceration without foreign body of nose
X● S01.22 Laceration with foreign body of nose
X● S01.23 Puncture wound without foreign body of nose
X● S01.24 Puncture wound with foreign body of nose
X● S01.25 Open bite of nose
Bite of nose NOS
Excludes1 superficial bite of nose (S00.36, S00.37)
● S01.3 Open wound of ear
● S01.30 Unspecified open wound of ear
● S01.301 Unspecified open wound of right ear
● S01.302 Unspecified open wound of left ear
● S01.309 Unspecified open wound of unspecified ear
● S01.31 Laceration without foreign body of ear
● S01.311 Laceration without foreign body of right ear
● S01.312 Laceration without foreign body of left ear
● S01.319 Laceration without foreign body of unspecified ear
● S01.32 Laceration with foreign body of ear
● S01.321 Laceration with foreign body of right ear
● S01.322 Laceration with foreign body of left ear
● S01.329 Laceration with foreign body of unspecified ear
● S01.33 Puncture wound without foreign body of ear
● S01.331 Puncture wound without foreign body of right ear
● S01.332 Puncture wound without foreign body of left ear
● S01.339 Puncture wound without foreign body of unspecified ear
● S01.34 Puncture wound with foreign body of ear
● S01.341 Puncture wound with foreign body of right ear
● S01.342 Puncture wound with foreign body of left ear
● S01.349 Puncture wound with foreign body of unspecified ear
● S01.35 Open bite of ear
Bite of ear NOS
Excludes1 superficial bite of ear (S00.46, S00.47)
● S01.351 Open bite of right ear
● S01.352 Open bite of left ear
● S01.359 Open bite of unspecified ear
● S01.4 Open wound of cheek and temporomandibular area
● S01.40 Unspecified open wound of cheek and temporomandibular area
● S01.401 Unspecified open wound of right cheek and temporomandibular area
● S01.402 Unspecified open wound of left cheek and temporomandibular area
● S01.409 Unspecified open wound of unspecified cheek and temporomandibular area
● S01.41 Laceration without foreign body of cheek and temporomandibular area
● S01.411 Laceration without foreign body of right cheek and temporomandibular area
● S01.412 Laceration without foreign body of left cheek and temporomandibular area
● S01.419 Laceration without foreign body of unspecified cheek and temporomandibular area
● S01.42 Laceration with foreign body of cheek and temporomandibular area
● S01.421 Laceration with foreign body of right cheek and temporomandibular area
● S01.422 Laceration with foreign body of left cheek and temporomandibular area
● S01.429 Laceration with foreign body of unspecified cheek and temporomandibular area
● S01.43 Puncture wound without foreign body of cheek and temporomandibular area
● S01.431 Puncture wound without foreign body of right cheek and temporomandibular area
● S01.432 Puncture wound without foreign body of left cheek and temporomandibular area
● S01.439 Puncture wound without foreign body of unspecified cheek and temporomandibular area
● S01.44 Puncture wound with foreign body of cheek and temporomandibular area
● S01.441 Puncture wound with foreign body of right cheek and temporomandibular area
● S01.442 Puncture wound with foreign body of left cheek and temporomandibular area
● S01.449 Puncture wound with foreign body of unspecified cheek and temporomandibular area

◀ New ◀ Revised ~~deleted~~ Deleted OGCR Official Guidelines X Assign placeholder X ● Use Additional Character(s)
Excludes 1 | Excludes 2 | Includes | Use additional | Code first | Code also | Unspecified

● S01.45 Open bite of cheek and temporomandibular area
Bite of cheek and temporomandibular area NOS
Excludes2 superficial bite of cheek and temporomandibular area (S00.86, S00.87)
● **S01.451 Open bite of right cheek and temporomandibular area**
● **S01.452 Open bite of left cheek and temporomandibular area**
● **S01.459 Open bite of unspecified cheek and temporomandibular area**

● S01.5 Open wound of lip and oral cavity
Excludes2 tooth dislocation (S03.2)
tooth fracture (S02.5)
● S01.50 Unspecified open wound of lip and oral cavity
● **S01.501 Unspecified open wound of lip**
● **S01.502 Unspecified open wound of oral cavity**
● S01.51 Laceration of lip and oral cavity without foreign body
● **S01.511 Laceration without foreign body of lip**
● **S01.512 Laceration without foreign body of oral cavity**
● S01.52 Laceration of lip and oral cavity with foreign body
● **S01.521 Laceration with foreign body of lip**
● **S01.522 Laceration with foreign body of oral cavity**
● S01.53 Puncture wound of lip and oral cavity without foreign body
● **S01.531 Puncture wound without foreign body of lip**
● **S01.532 Puncture wound without foreign body of oral cavity**
● S01.54 Puncture wound of lip and oral cavity with foreign body
● **S01.541 Puncture wound with foreign body of lip**
● **S01.542 Puncture wound with foreign body of oral cavity**
● S01.55 Open bite of lip and oral cavity
● **S01.551 Open bite of lip**
Bite of lip NOS
Excludes1 superficial bite of lip (S00.571)
● **S01.552 Open bite of oral cavity**
Bite of oral cavity NOS
Excludes1 superficial bite of oral cavity (S00.572)

● S01.8 Open wound of other parts of head
X● **S01.80 Unspecified open wound of other part of head**
X● **S01.81 Laceration without foreign body of other part of head**
X● **S01.82 Laceration with foreign body of other part of head**
X● **S01.83 Puncture wound without foreign body of other part of head**
X● **S01.84 Puncture wound with foreign body of other part of head**
X● **S01.85 Open bite of other part of head**
Bite of other part of head NOS
Excludes1 superficial bite of other part of head (S00.85)

● S01.9 Open wound of unspecified part of head
X● **S01.90 Unspecified open wound of unspecified part of head**
X● **S01.91 Laceration without foreign body of unspecified part of head**
X● **S01.92 Laceration with foreign body of unspecified part of head**
X● **S01.93 Puncture wound without foreign body of unspecified part of head**
X● **S01.94 Puncture wound with foreign body of unspecified part of head**
X● **S01.95 Open bite of unspecified part of head**
Bite of head NOS
Excludes1 superficial bite of head NOS (S00.97)

● **S02 Fracture of skull and facial bones**
Note: A fracture not indicated as open or closed should be coded to closed
The appropriate 7th character is to be added to each code from category S02

A	initial encounter for closed fracture
B	initial encounter for open fracture
D	subsequent encounter for fracture with routine healing
G	subsequent encounter for fracture with delayed healing
K	subsequent encounter for fracture with nonunion
S	sequela

Code also any associated intracranial injury (S06.-)

X● S02.0 Fracture of vault of skull
Fracture of frontal bone
Fracture of parietal bone
● S02.1 Fracture of base of skull
Excludes1 orbit NOS (S02.8)
Excludes2 orbital floor (S02.3-)
● S02.10 Unspecified fracture of base of skull
● **S02.101 Fracture of base of skull, right side** ◀
● **S02.102 Fracture of base of skull, left side** ◀
● **S02.109 Fracture of base of skull, unspecified side** ◀
● S02.11 Fracture of occiput
● **S02.110 Type I occipital condyle fracture, unspecified side**
● **S02.111 Type II occipital condyle fracture, unspecified side**
● **S02.112 Type III occipital condyle fracture, unspecified side**
● **S02.113 Unspecified occipital condyle fracture**
● **S02.118 Other fracture of occiput, unspecified side**
● **S02.119 Unspecified fracture of occiput**
● **S02.11A Type I occipital condyle fracture, right side**
● **S02.11B Type I occipital condyle fracture, left side**
● **S02.11C Type II occipital condyle fracture, right side**
● **S02.11D Type II occipital condyle fracture, left side**
● **S02.11E Type III occipital condyle fracture, right side**
● **S02.11F Type III occipital condyle fracture, left side**
● **S02.11G Other fracture of occiput, right side**
● **S02.11H Other fracture of occiput, left side**

CHAPTER 19 (S00-T88)

X● S02.19 **Other fracture of base of skull**
Fracture of anterior fossa of base of skull
Fracture of ethmoid sinus
Fracture of frontal sinus
Fracture of middle fossa of base of skull
Fracture of orbital roof
Fracture of posterior fossa of base of skull
Fracture of sphenoid
Fracture of temporal bone

X● S02.2 **Fracture of nasal bones**

● S02.3 **Fracture of orbital floor**
Excludes1 orbit NOS (S02.8)
Excludes2 orbital roof (S02.1-)

X● S02.30 **Fracture of orbital floor, unspecified side**
X● S02.31 **Fracture of orbital floor, right side**
X● S02.32 **Fracture of orbital floor, left side**

● S02.4 **Fracture of malar, maxillary and zygoma bones**
Fracture of superior maxilla
Fracture of upper jaw (bone)
Fracture of zygomatic process of temporal bone

● S02.40 **Fracture of malar, maxillary and zygoma bones, unspecified**
● S02.400 **Malar fracture unspecified side**
● S02.401 **Maxillary fracture, unspecified side**
● S02.402 **Zygomatic fracture, unspecified side**
● S02.40A **Malar fracture, right side**
● S02.40B **Malar fracture, left side**
● S02.40C **Maxillary fracture, right side**
● S02.40D **Maxillary fracture, left side**
● S02.40E **Zygomatic fracture, right side**
● S02.40F **Zygomatic fracture, left side**

● S02.41 **LeFort fracture**
● S02.411 **LeFort I fracture**
● S02.412 **LeFort II fracture**
● S02.413 **LeFort III fracture**

X● S02.42 **Fracture of alveolus of maxilla**

X● S02.5 **Fracture of tooth (traumatic) Broken tooth**
Excludes1 cracked tooth (nontraumatic) (K03.81)

● S02.6 **Fracture of mandible**
Fracture of lower jaw (bone)

● S02.60 **Fracture of mandible of unspecified site**
● S02.600 **Fracture of unspecified part of body of mandible, unspecified side**
● S02.601 **Fracture of unspecified part of body of right mandible**
● S02.602 **Fracture of unspecified part of body of left mandible**
● S02.609 **Fracture of mandible, unspecified**

● S02.61 **Fracture of condylar process of mandible**
● S02.610 **Fracture of condylar process of mandible, unspecified side**
● S02.611 **Fracture of condylar process of right mandible**
● S02.612 **Fracture of condylar process of left mandible**

● S02.62 **Fracture of subcondylar process of mandible**
● S02.620 **Fracture of subcondylar process of mandible, unspecified side**
● S02.621 **Fracture of subcondylar process of right mandible**
● S02.622 **Fracture of subcondylar process of left mandible**

● S02.63 **Fracture of coronoid process of mandible**
● S02.630 **Fracture of coronoid process of mandible, unspecified side**
● S02.631 **Fracture of coronoid process of right mandible**
● S02.632 **Fracture of coronoid process of left mandible**

● S02.64 **Fracture of ramus of mandible**
● S02.640 **Fracture of ramus of mandible, unspecified side**
● S02.641 **Fracture of ramus of right mandible**
● S02.642 **Fracture of ramus of left mandible**

● S02.65 **Fracture of angle of mandible**
● S02.650 **Fracture of angle of mandible, unspecified side**
● S02.651 **Fracture of angle of right mandible**
● S02.652 **Fracture of angle of left mandible**

X● S02.66 **Fracture of symphysis of mandible**

● S02.67 **Fracture of alveolus of mandible**
● S02.670 **Fracture of alveolus of mandible, unspecified side**
● S02.671 **Fracture of alveolus of right mandible**
● S02.672 **Fracture of alveolus of left mandible**

X● S02.69 **Fracture of mandible of other specified site**

● S02.8 **Fractures of other specified skull and facial bones**
Fracture of orbit NOS
Fracture of palate
Excludes1 fracture of orbital floor (S02.3-)
fracture of orbital roof (S02.1-)

X● S02.80 **Fracture of other specified skull and facial bones, unspecified side**
X● S02.81 **Fracture of other specified skull and facial bones, right side**
X● S02.82 **Fracture of other specified skull and facial bones, left side**

● S02.9 **Fracture of unspecified skull and facial bones**
X● S02.91 **Unspecified fracture of skull**
X● S02.92 **Unspecified fracture of facial bones**

● S03 **Dislocation and sprain of joints and ligaments of head**
Includes avulsion of joint (capsule) or ligament of head
laceration of cartilage, joint (capsule) or ligament of head
sprain of cartilage, joint (capsule) or ligament of head
traumatic hemarthrosis of joint or ligament of head
traumatic rupture of joint or ligament of head
traumatic subluxation of joint or ligament of head
traumatic tear of joint or ligament of head
Code also any associated open wound
Excludes2 Strain of muscle or tendon of head (S09.1)
The appropriate 7th character is to be added to each code from category S03

A	initial encounter
D	subsequent encounter
S	sequela

● S03.0 **Dislocation of jaw**
Dislocation of jaw (cartilage) (meniscus)
Dislocation of mandible
Dislocation of temporomandibular (joint)

X● S03.00 **Dislocation of jaw, unspecified side**
X● S03.01 **Dislocation of jaw, right side**
X● S03.02 **Dislocation of jaw, left side**
X● S03.03 **Dislocation of jaw, bilateral side**

X● S03.1 **Dislocation of septal cartilage of nose**
X● S03.2 **Dislocation of tooth**

● S03.4 **Sprain of jaw**
Sprain of temporomandibular (joint) (ligament)

X● S03.40 **Sprain of jaw, unspecified side**
X● S03.41 **Sprain of jaw, right side**
X● S03.42 **Sprain of jaw, left side**
X● S03.43 **Sprain of jaw, bilateral side**

X● S03.8 **Sprain of joints and ligaments of other parts of head**
X● S03.9 **Sprain of joints and ligaments of unspecified parts of head**

● **S04 Injury of cranial nerve**
The selection of side should be based on the side of the body being affected
Code first any associated intracranial injury (S06.-)
Code also any associated:
open wound of head (S01.-)
skull fracture (S02.-)
The appropriate 7th character is to be added to each code from category S04

A	initial encounter
D	subsequent encounter
S	sequela

● **S04.0 Injury of optic nerve and pathways**
Use additional code to identify any visual field defect or blindness (H53.4-, H54)
● **S04.01 Injury of optic nerve**
Injury of 2nd cranial nerve
● **S04.011 Injury of optic nerve, right eye**
● **S04.012 Injury of optic nerve, left eye**
● **S04.019 Injury of optic nerve, unspecified eye**
Injury of optic nerve NOS
X● **S04.02 Injury of optic chiasm**
● **S04.03 Injury of optic tract and pathways**
Injury of optic radiation
● **S04.031 Injury of optic tract and pathways, right eye**
● **S04.032 Injury of optic tract and pathways, left eye**
● **S04.039 Injury of optic tract and pathways, unspecified eye**
Injury of optic tract and pathways NOS
● **S04.04 Injury of visual cortex**
● **S04.041 Injury of visual cortex, right eye**
● **S04.042 Injury of visual cortex, left eye**
● **S04.049 Injury of visual cortex, unspecified eye**
Injury of visual cortex NOS

● **S04.1 Injury of oculomotor nerve**
Injury of 3rd cranial nerve
X● **S04.10 Injury of oculomotor nerve, unspecified side**
X● **S04.11 Injury of oculomotor nerve, right side**
X● **S04.12 Injury of oculomotor nerve, left side**
● **S04.2 Injury of trochlear nerve**
Injury of 4th cranial nerve
X● **S04.20 Injury of trochlear nerve, unspecified side**
X● **S04.21 Injury of trochlear nerve, right side**
X● **S04.22 Injury of trochlear nerve, left side**
● **S04.3 Injury of trigeminal nerve**
Injury of 5th cranial nerve
X● **S04.30 Injury of trigeminal nerve, unspecified side**
X● **S04.31 Injury of trigeminal nerve, right side**
X● **S04.32 Injury of trigeminal nerve, left side**
● **S04.4 Injury of abducent nerve**
Injury of 6th cranial nerve
X● **S04.40 Injury of abducent nerve, unspecified side**
X● **S04.41 Injury of abducent nerve, right side**
X● **S04.42 Injury of abducent nerve, left side**
● **S04.5 Injury of facial nerve**
Injury of 7th cranial nerve
X● **S04.50 Injury of facial nerve, unspecified side**
X● **S04.51 Injury of facial nerve, right side**
X● **S04.52 Injury of facial nerve, left side**
● **S04.6 Injury of acoustic nerve**
Injury of auditory nerve
Injury of 8th cranial nerve
X● **S04.60 Injury of acoustic nerve, unspecified side**
X● **S04.61 Injury of acoustic nerve, right side**
X● **S04.62 Injury of acoustic nerve, left side**
● **S04.7 Injury of accessory nerve**
Injury of 11th cranial nerve
X● **S04.70 Injury of accessory nerve, unspecified side**
X● **S04.71 Injury of accessory nerve, right side**
X● **S04.72 Injury of accessory nerve, left side**

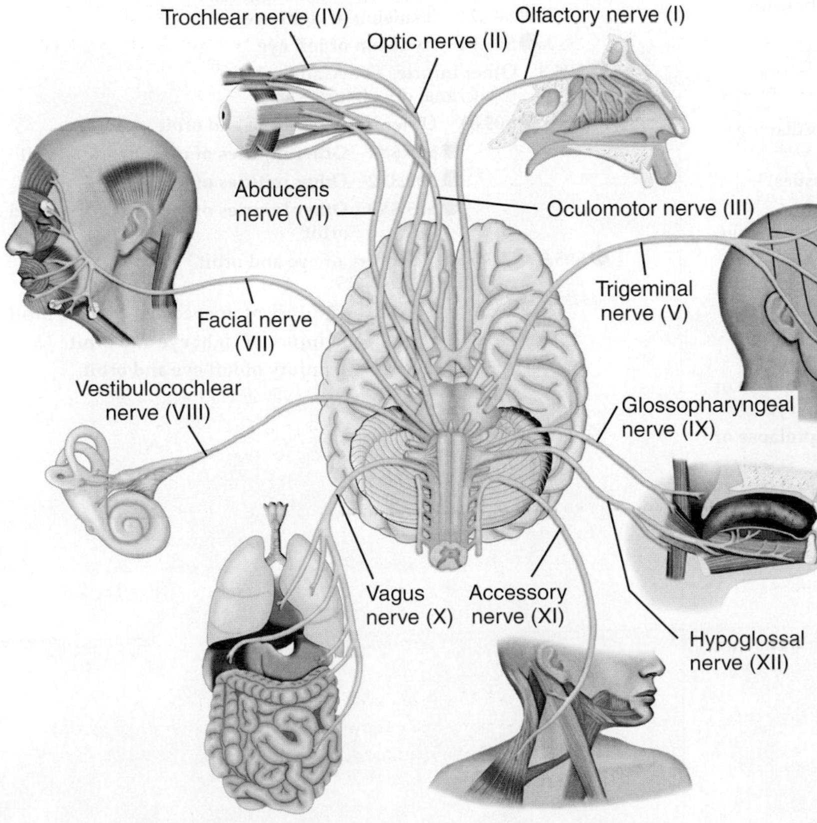

Figure 19-13 Cranial nerves. (From Patton and Thibodeau: Anatomy and physiology, ed 7, St. Louis, Mosby, 2009)

● S04.8 **Injury of other cranial nerves**

● S04.81 **Injury of olfactory [1st] nerve**

● S04.811 **Injury of olfactory [1st] nerve, right side**

● S04.812 **Injury of olfactory [1st] nerve, left side**

● S04.819 **Injury of olfactory [1st] nerve, unspecified side**

● S04.89 **Injury of other cranial nerves**

Injury of vagus [10th] nerve

● S04.891 **Injury of other cranial nerves, right side**

● S04.892 **Injury of other cranial nerves, left side**

● S04.899 **Injury of other cranial nerves, unspecified side**

X● S04.9 **Injury of unspecified cranial nerve**

● S05 **Injury of eye and orbit**

Includes open wound of eye and orbit

Excludes2 2nd cranial [optic] nerve injury (S04.0-)
3rd cranial [oculomotor] nerve injury (S04.1-)
open wound of eyelid and periocular area (S01.1-)
orbital bone fracture (S02.1-, S02.3-, S02.8-)
superficial injury of eyelid (S00.1-S00.2)

The appropriate 7th character is to be added to each code from category S05

A	initial encounter
D	subsequent encounter
S	sequela

● S05.0 **Injury of conjunctiva and corneal abrasion without foreign body**

Excludes1 foreign body in conjunctival sac (T15.1)
foreign body in cornea (T15.0)

X● S05.00 **Injury of conjunctiva and corneal abrasion without foreign body, unspecified eye**

X● S05.01 **Injury of conjunctiva and corneal abrasion without foreign body, right eye**

X● S05.02 **Injury of conjunctiva and corneal abrasion without foreign body, left eye**

● S05.1 **Contusion of eyeball and orbital tissues**

Traumatic hyphema

Excludes2 black eye NOS (S00.1)
contusion of eyelid and periocular area (S00.1)

X● S05.10 **Contusion of eyeball and orbital tissues, unspecified eye**

X● S05.11 **Contusion of eyeball and orbital tissues, right eye**

X● S05.12 **Contusion of eyeball and orbital tissues, left eye**

● S05.2 **Ocular laceration and rupture with prolapse or loss of intraocular tissue**

X● S05.20 **Ocular laceration and rupture with prolapse or loss of intraocular tissue, unspecified eye**

X● S05.21 **Ocular laceration and rupture with prolapse or loss of intraocular tissue, right eye**

X● S05.22 **Ocular laceration and rupture with prolapse or loss of intraocular tissue, left eye**

● S05.3 **Ocular laceration without prolapse or loss of intraocular tissue**

Laceration of eye NOS

X● S05.30 **Ocular laceration without prolapse or loss of intraocular tissue, unspecified eye**

X● S05.31 **Ocular laceration without prolapse or loss of intraocular tissue, right eye**

X● S05.32 **Ocular laceration without prolapse or loss of intraocular tissue, left eye**

● S05.4 **Penetrating wound of orbit with or without foreign body**

Excludes2 retained (old) foreign body following penetrating wound in orbit (H05.5-)

X● S05.40 **Penetrating wound of orbit with or without foreign body, unspecified eye**

X● S05.41 **Penetrating wound of orbit with or without foreign body, right eye**

X● S05.42 **Penetrating wound of orbit with or without foreign body, left eye**

● S05.5 **Penetrating wound with foreign body of eyeball**

Excludes2 retained (old) intraocular foreign body (H44.6-, H44.7)

X● S05.50 **Penetrating wound with foreign body of unspecified eyeball**

X● S05.51 **Penetrating wound with foreign body of right eyeball**

X● S05.52 **Penetrating wound with foreign body of left eyeball**

● S05.6 **Penetrating wound without foreign body of eyeball**

Ocular penetration NOS

X● S05.60 **Penetrating wound without foreign body of unspecified eyeball**

X● S05.61 **Penetrating wound without foreign body of right eyeball**

X● S05.62 **Penetrating wound without foreign body of left eyeball**

● S05.7 **Avulsion of eye**

Traumatic enucleation

X● S05.70 **Avulsion of unspecified eye**

X● S05.71 **Avulsion of right eye**

X● S05.72 **Avulsion of left eye**

● S05.8 **Other injuries of eye and orbit**

Lacrimal duct injury

● S05.8X **Other injuries of eye and orbit**

● S05.8X1 **Other injuries of right eye and orbit**

● S05.8X2 **Other injuries of left eye and orbit**

● S05.8X9 **Other injuries of unspecified eye and orbit**

● S05.9 **Unspecified injury of eye and orbit**

Injury of eye NOS

X● S05.90 **Unspecified injury of unspecified eye and orbit**

X● S05.91 **Unspecified injury of right eye and orbit**

X● S05.92 **Unspecified injury of left eye and orbit**

● **S06 Intracranial injury**
Includes traumatic brain injury
Code also any associated:
open wound of head (S01.-)
skull fracture (S02.-)
Excludes1 head injury NOS (S09.90)
The appropriate 7th character is to be added to each code from category S06

A	initial encounter
D	subsequent encounter
S	sequela

● **S06.0 Concussion**
Commotio cerebri
Excludes1 concussion with other intracranial injuries classified in subcategories S06.1- to S06.6- , S06.81- and S06.82- code to specified intracranial injury

● **S06.0X Concussion**
● **S06.0X0 Concussion without loss of consciousness**
● **S06.0X1 Concussion with loss of consciousness of 30 minutes or less**
~~S06.0X2 Concussion with loss of consciousness of 31 minutes to 59 minutes~~
~~S06.0X3 Concussion with loss of consciousness of 1 hour to 5 hours 59 minutes~~
~~S06.0X4 Concussion with loss of consciousness of 6 hours to 24 hours~~
~~S06.0X5 Concussion with loss of consciousness greater than 24 hours with return to pre-existing conscious level~~
~~S06.0X6 Concussion with loss of consciousness greater than 24 hours without return to pre-existing conscious level with patient surviving~~
~~S06.0X7 Concussion with loss of consciousness of any duration with death due to brain injury prior to regaining consciousness~~
~~S06.0X8 Concussion with loss of consciousness of any duration with death due to other cause prior to regaining consciousness~~
● **S06.0X9 Concussion with loss of consciousness of unspecified duration**
Concussion NOS

● **S06.1 Traumatic cerebral edema**
Diffuse traumatic cerebral edema
Focal traumatic cerebral edema

● **S06.1X Traumatic cerebral edema**
● **S06.1X0 Traumatic cerebral edema without loss of consciousness**
● **S06.1X1 Traumatic cerebral edema with loss of consciousness of 30 minutes or less**
● **S06.1X2 Traumatic cerebral edema with loss of consciousness of 31 minutes to 59 minutes**
● **S06.1X3 Traumatic cerebral edema with loss of consciousness of 1 hour to 5 hours 59 minutes**
● **S06.1X4 Traumatic cerebral edema with loss of consciousness of 6 hours to 24 hours**
● **S06.1X5 Traumatic cerebral edema with loss of consciousness greater than 24 hours with return to pre-existing conscious level**
● **S06.1X6 Traumatic cerebral edema with loss of consciousness greater than 24 hours without return to pre-existing conscious level with patient surviving**
● **S06.1X7 Traumatic cerebral edema with loss of consciousness of any duration with death due to brain injury prior to regaining consciousness**
● **S06.1X8 Traumatic cerebral edema with loss of consciousness of any duration with death due to other cause prior to regaining consciousness**
● **S06.1X9 Traumatic cerebral edema with loss of consciousness of unspecified duration**
Traumatic cerebral edema NOS

● **S06.2 Diffuse traumatic brain injury**
Diffuse axonal brain injury
Excludes1 traumatic diffuse cerebral edema (S06.1X-)

● **S06.2X Diffuse traumatic brain injury**
● **S06.2X0 Diffuse traumatic brain injury without loss of consciousness**
● **S06.2X1 Diffuse traumatic brain injury with loss of consciousness of 30 minutes or less**
● **S06.2X2 Diffuse traumatic brain injury with loss of consciousness of 31 minutes to 59 minutes**
● **S06.2X3 Diffuse traumatic brain injury with loss of consciousness of 1 hour to 5 hours 59 minutes**
● **S06.2X4 Diffuse traumatic brain injury with loss of consciousness of 6 hours to 24 hours**
● **S06.2X5 Diffuse traumatic brain injury with loss of consciousness greater than 24 hours with return to pre-existing conscious levels**
● **S06.2X6 Diffuse traumatic brain injury with loss of consciousness greater than 24 hours without return to pre-existing conscious level with patient surviving**
● **S06.2X7 Diffuse traumatic brain injury with loss of consciousness of any duration with death due to brain injury prior to regaining consciousness**
● **S06.2X8 Diffuse traumatic brain injury with loss of consciousness of any duration with death due to other cause prior to regaining consciousness**
● **S06.2X9 Diffuse traumatic brain injury with loss of consciousness of unspecified duration**
Diffuse traumatic brain injury NOS

● SØ6.3 Focal traumatic brain injury

Excludes1 any condition classifiable to SØ6.4-SØ6.6
focal cerebral edema (SØ6.1)

● SØ6.3Ø Unspecified focal traumatic brain injury

● SØ6.3ØØ Unspecified focal traumatic brain injury without loss of consciousness

● SØ6.3Ø1 Unspecified focal traumatic brain injury with loss of consciousness of 3Ø minutes or less

● SØ6.3Ø2 Unspecified focal traumatic brain injury with loss of consciousness of 31 minutes to 59 minutes

● SØ6.3Ø3 Unspecified focal traumatic brain injury with loss of consciousness of 1 hour to 5 hours 59 minutes

● SØ6.3Ø4 Unspecified focal traumatic brain injury with loss of consciousness of 6 hours to 24 hours

● SØ6.3Ø5 Unspecified focal traumatic brain injury with loss of consciousness greater than 24 hours with return to pre-existing conscious level

● SØ6.3Ø6 Unspecified focal traumatic brain injury with loss of consciousness greater than 24 hours without return to pre-existing conscious level with patient surviving

● SØ6.3Ø7 Unspecified focal traumatic brain injury with loss of consciousness of any duration with death due to brain injury prior to regaining consciousness

● SØ6.3Ø8 Unspecified focal traumatic brain injury with loss of consciousness of any duration with death due to other cause prior to regaining consciousness

● SØ6.3Ø9 Unspecified focal traumatic brain injury with loss of consciousness of unspecified duration
Unspecified focal traumatic brain injury NOS

● SØ6.31 Contusion and laceration of right cerebrum

● SØ6.31Ø Contusion and laceration of right cerebrum without loss of consciousness

● SØ6.311 Contusion and laceration of right cerebrum with loss of consciousness of 3Ø minutes or less

● SØ6.312 Contusion and laceration of right cerebrum with loss of consciousness of 31 minutes to 59 minutes

● SØ6.313 Contusion and laceration of right cerebrum with loss of consciousness of 1 hour to 5 hours 59 minutes

● SØ6.314 Contusion and laceration of right cerebrum with loss of consciousness of 6 hours to 24 hours

● SØ6.315 Contusion and laceration of right cerebrum with loss of consciousness greater than 24 hours with return to pre-existing conscious level

● SØ6.316 Contusion and laceration of right cerebrum with loss of consciousness greater than 24 hours without return to pre-existing conscious level with patient surviving

● SØ6.317 Contusion and laceration of right cerebrum with loss of consciousness of any duration with death due to brain injury prior to regaining consciousness

● SØ6.318 Contusion and laceration of right cerebrum with loss of consciousness of any duration with death due to other cause prior to regaining consciousness

● SØ6.319 Contusion and laceration of right cerebrum with loss of consciousness of unspecified duration
Contusion and laceration of right cerebrum NOS

● SØ6.32 Contusion and laceration of left cerebrum

● SØ6.32Ø Contusion and laceration of left cerebrum without loss of consciousness

● SØ6.321 Contusion and laceration of left cerebrum with loss of consciousness of 3Ø minutes or less

● SØ6.322 Contusion and laceration of left cerebrum with loss of consciousness of 31 minutes to 59 minutes

● SØ6.323 Contusion and laceration of left cerebrum with loss of consciousness of 1 hour to 5 hours 59 minutes

● SØ6.324 Contusion and laceration of left cerebrum with loss of consciousness of 6 hours to 24 hours

● SØ6.325 Contusion and laceration of left cerebrum with loss of consciousness greater than 24 hours with return to pre-existing conscious level

● SØ6.326 Contusion and laceration of left cerebrum with loss of consciousness greater than 24 hours without return to pre-existing conscious level with patient surviving

● SØ6.327 Contusion and laceration of left cerebrum with loss of consciousness of any duration with death due to brain injury prior to regaining consciousness

● SØ6.328 Contusion and laceration of left cerebrum with loss of consciousness of any duration with death due to other cause prior to regaining consciousness

● SØ6.329 Contusion and laceration of left cerebrum with loss of consciousness of unspecified duration
Contusion and laceration of left cerebrum NOS

● SØ6.33 Contusion and laceration of cerebrum, unspecified

● SØ6.33Ø Contusion and laceration of cerebrum, unspecified, without loss of consciousness

● SØ6.331 Contusion and laceration of cerebrum, unspecified, with loss of consciousness of 3Ø minutes or less

● SØ6.332 Contusion and laceration of cerebrum, unspecified, with loss of consciousness of 31 minutes to 59 minutes

● SØ6.333 Contusion and laceration of cerebrum, unspecified, with loss of consciousness of 1 hour to 5 hours 59 minutes

● SØ6.334 Contusion and laceration of cerebrum, unspecified, with loss of consciousness of 6 hours to 24 hours

● SØ6.335 Contusion and laceration of cerebrum, unspecified, with loss of consciousness greater than 24 hours with return to pre-existing conscious level

● S06.336 Contusion and laceration of cerebrum, unspecified, with loss of consciousness greater than 24 hours without return to pre-existing conscious level with patient surviving

● S06.337 Contusion and laceration of cerebrum, unspecified, with loss of consciousness of any duration with death due to brain injury prior to regaining consciousness

● S06.338 Contusion and laceration of cerebrum, unspecified, with loss of consciousness of any duration with death due to other cause prior to regaining consciousness

● S06.339 Contusion and laceration of cerebrum, unspecified, with loss of consciousness of unspecified duration
Contusion and laceration of cerebrum NOS

● S06.34 Traumatic hemorrhage of right cerebrum
Traumatic intracerebral hemorrhage and hematoma of right cerebrum

● S06.340 Traumatic hemorrhage of right cerebrum without loss of consciousness

● S06.341 Traumatic hemorrhage of right cerebrum with loss of consciousness of 30 minutes or less

● S06.342 Traumatic hemorrhage of right cerebrum with loss of consciousness of 31 minutes to 59 minutes

● S06.343 Traumatic hemorrhage of right cerebrum with loss of consciousness of 1 hours to 5 hours 59 minutes

● S06.344 Traumatic hemorrhage of right cerebrum with loss of consciousness of 6 hours to 24 hours

● S06.345 Traumatic hemorrhage of right cerebrum with loss of consciousness greater than 24 hours with return to pre-existing conscious level

● S06.346 Traumatic hemorrhage of right cerebrum with loss of consciousness greater than 24 hours without return to pre-existing conscious level with patient surviving

● S06.347 Traumatic hemorrhage of right cerebrum with loss of consciousness of any duration with death due to brain injury prior to regaining consciousness

● S06.348 Traumatic hemorrhage of right cerebrum with loss of consciousness of any duration with death due to other cause prior to regaining consciousness

● S06.349 Traumatic hemorrhage of right cerebrum with loss of consciousness of unspecified duration
Traumatic hemorrhage of right cerebrum NOS

● S06.35 Traumatic hemorrhage of left cerebrum
Traumatic intracerebral hemorrhage and hematoma of left cerebrum

● S06.350 Traumatic hemorrhage of left cerebrum without loss of consciousness

● S06.351 Traumatic hemorrhage of left cerebrum with loss of consciousness of 30 minutes or less

● S06.352 Traumatic hemorrhage of left cerebrum with loss of consciousness of 31 minutes to 59 minutes

● S06.353 Traumatic hemorrhage of left cerebrum with loss of consciousness of 1 hours to 5 hours 59 minutes

● S06.354 Traumatic hemorrhage of left cerebrum with loss of consciousness of 6 hours to 24 hours

● S06.355 Traumatic hemorrhage of left cerebrum with loss of consciousness greater than 24 hours with return to pre-existing conscious level

● S06.356 Traumatic hemorrhage of left cerebrum with loss of consciousness greater than 24 hours without return to pre-existing conscious level with patient surviving

● S06.357 Traumatic hemorrhage of left cerebrum with loss of consciousness of any duration with death due to brain injury prior to regaining consciousness

● S06.358 Traumatic hemorrhage of left cerebrum with loss of consciousness of any duration with death due to other cause prior to regaining consciousness

● S06.359 Traumatic hemorrhage of left cerebrum with loss of consciousness of unspecified duration
Traumatic hemorrhage of left cerebrum NOS

● S06.36 Traumatic hemorrhage of cerebrum, unspecified
Traumatic intracerebral hemorrhage and hematoma, unspecified

● S06.360 Traumatic hemorrhage of cerebrum, unspecified, without loss of consciousness

● S06.361 Traumatic hemorrhage of cerebrum, unspecified, with loss of consciousness of 30 minutes or less

● S06.362 Traumatic hemorrhage of cerebrum, unspecified, with loss of consciousness of 31 minutes to 59 minutes

● S06.363 Traumatic hemorrhage of cerebrum, unspecified, with loss of consciousness of 1 hours to 5 hours 59 minutes

● S06.364 Traumatic hemorrhage of cerebrum, unspecified, with loss of consciousness of 6 hours to 24 hours

● S06.365 Traumatic hemorrhage of cerebrum, unspecified, with loss of consciousness greater than 24 hours with return to pre-existing conscious level

● S06.366 Traumatic hemorrhage of cerebrum, unspecified, with loss of consciousness greater than 24 hours without return to pre-existing conscious level with patient surviving

● S06.367 Traumatic hemorrhage of cerebrum, unspecified, with loss of consciousness of any duration with death due to brain injury prior to regaining consciousness

● S06.368 Traumatic hemorrhage of cerebrum, unspecified, with loss of consciousness of any duration with death due to other cause prior to regaining consciousness

● S06.369 Traumatic hemorrhage of cerebrum, unspecified, with loss of consciousness of unspecified duration
Traumatic hemorrhage of cerebrum NOS

- S06.37 **Contusion, laceration, and hemorrhage of cerebellum**
  - S06.370 **Contusion, laceration, and hemorrhage of cerebellum without loss of consciousness**
  - S06.371 **Contusion, laceration, and hemorrhage of cerebellum with loss of consciousness of 30 minutes or less**
  - S06.372 **Contusion, laceration, and hemorrhage of cerebellum with loss of consciousness of 31 minutes to 59 minutes**
  - S06.373 **Contusion, laceration, and hemorrhage of cerebellum with loss of consciousness of 1 hour to 5 hours 59 minutes**
  - S06.374 **Contusion, laceration, and hemorrhage of cerebellum with loss of consciousness of 6 hours to 24 hours**
  - S06.375 **Contusion, laceration, and hemorrhage of cerebellum with loss of consciousness greater than 24 hours with return to pre-existing conscious level**
  - S06.376 **Contusion, laceration, and hemorrhage of cerebellum with loss of consciousness greater than 24 hours without return to pre-existing conscious level with patient surviving**
  - S06.377 **Contusion, laceration, and hemorrhage of cerebellum with loss of consciousness of any duration with death due to brain injury prior to regaining consciousness**
  - S06.378 **Contusion, laceration, and hemorrhage of cerebellum with loss of consciousness of any duration with death due to other cause prior to regaining consciousness**
  - S06.379 **Contusion, laceration, and hemorrhage of cerebellum with loss of consciousness of unspecified duration**
    Contusion, laceration, and hemorrhage of cerebellum NOS
- S06.38 **Contusion, laceration, and hemorrhage of brainstem**
  - S06.380 **Contusion, laceration, and hemorrhage of brainstem without loss of consciousness**
  - S06.381 **Contusion, laceration, and hemorrhage of brainstem with loss of consciousness of 30 minutes or less**
  - S06.382 **Contusion, laceration, and hemorrhage of brainstem with loss of consciousness of 31 minutes to 59 minutes**
  - S06.383 **Contusion, laceration, and hemorrhage of brainstem with loss of consciousness of 1 hour to 5 hours 59 minutes**
  - S06.384 **Contusion, laceration, and hemorrhage of brainstem with loss of consciousness of 6 hours to 24 hours**
  - S06.385 **Contusion, laceration, and hemorrhage of brainstem with loss of consciousness greater than 24 hours with return to pre-existing conscious level**
  - S06.386 **Contusion, laceration, and hemorrhage of brainstem with loss of consciousness greater than 24 hours without return to pre-existing conscious level with patient surviving**
  - S06.387 **Contusion, laceration, and hemorrhage of brainstem with loss of consciousness of any duration with death due to brain injury prior to regaining consciousness**
  - S06.388 **Contusion, laceration, and hemorrhage of brainstem with loss of consciousness of any duration with death due to other cause prior to regaining consciousness**
  - S06.389 **Contusion, laceration, and hemorrhage of brainstem with loss of consciousness of unspecified duration**
    Contusion, laceration, and hemorrhage of brainstem NOS

- S06.4 **Epidural hemorrhage**
  Situated outside dura mater
  Extradural hemorrhage NOS
  Intracranial hemorrhage due to trauma
  Extradural hemorrhage (traumatic)
  - S06.4X **Epidural hemorrhage**
    - S06.4X0 **Epidural hemorrhage without loss of consciousness**
    - S06.4X1 **Epidural hemorrhage with loss of consciousness of 30 minutes or less**
    - S06.4X2 **Epidural hemorrhage with loss of consciousness of 31 minutes to 59 minutes**
    - S06.4X3 **Epidural hemorrhage with loss of consciousness of 1 hour to 5 hours 59 minutes**
    - S06.4X4 **Epidural hemorrhage with loss of consciousness of 6 hours to 24 hours**
    - S06.4X5 **Epidural hemorrhage with loss of consciousness greater than 24 hours with return to pre-existing conscious level**
    - S06.4X6 **Epidural hemorrhage with loss of consciousness greater than 24 hours without return to pre-existing conscious level with patient surviving**
    - S06.4X7 **Epidural hemorrhage with loss of consciousness of any duration with death due to brain injury prior to regaining consciousness**
    - S06.4X8 **Epidural hemorrhage with loss of consciousness of any duration with death due to other causes prior to regaining consciousness**
    - S06.4X9 **Epidural hemorrhage with loss of consciousness of unspecified duration**
      Epidural hemorrhage NOS

- S06.5 **Traumatic subdural hemorrhage**
  - S06.5X **Traumatic subdural hemorrhage**
    - S06.5X0 **Traumatic subdural hemorrhage without loss of consciousness**
    - S06.5X1 **Traumatic subdural hemorrhage with loss of consciousness of 30 minutes or less**
    - S06.5X2 **Traumatic subdural hemorrhage with loss of consciousness of 31 minutes to 59 minutes**
    - S06.5X3 **Traumatic subdural hemorrhage with loss of consciousness of 1 hour to 5 hours 59 minutes**
    - S06.5X4 **Traumatic subdural hemorrhage with loss of consciousness of 6 hours to 24 hours**
    - S06.5X5 **Traumatic subdural hemorrhage with loss of consciousness greater than 24 hours with return to pre-existing conscious level**
    - S06.5X6 **Traumatic subdural hemorrhage with loss of consciousness greater than 24 hours without return to pre-existing conscious level with patient surviving**
    - S06.5X7 **Traumatic subdural hemorrhage with loss of consciousness of any duration with death due to brain injury before regaining consciousness**
    - S06.5X8 **Traumatic subdural hemorrhage with loss of consciousness of any duration with death due to other cause before regaining consciousness**
    - S06.5X9 **Traumatic subdural hemorrhage with loss of consciousness of unspecified duration**
      Traumatic subdural hemorrhage NOS
- S06.6 **Traumatic subarachnoid hemorrhage**
  Between arachnoid and pia mater
  - S06.6X **Traumatic subarachnoid hemorrhage**
    - S06.6X0 **Traumatic subarachnoid hemorrhage without loss of consciousness**
    - S06.6X1 **Traumatic subarachnoid hemorrhage with loss of consciousness of 30 minutes or less**
    - S06.6X2 **Traumatic subarachnoid hemorrhage with loss of consciousness of 31 minutes to 59 minutes**
    - S06.6X3 **Traumatic subarachnoid hemorrhage with loss of consciousness of 1 hour to 5 hours 59 minutes**
    - S06.6X4 **Traumatic subarachnoid hemorrhage with loss of consciousness of 6 hours to 24 hours**
    - S06.6X5 **Traumatic subarachnoid hemorrhage with loss of consciousness greater than 24 hours with return to pre-existing conscious level**
    - S06.6X6 **Traumatic subarachnoid hemorrhage with loss of consciousness greater than 24 hours without return to pre-existing conscious level with patient surviving**
    - S06.6X7 **Traumatic subarachnoid hemorrhage with loss of consciousness of any duration with death due to brain injury prior to regaining consciousness**
    - S06.6X8 **Traumatic subarachnoid hemorrhage with loss of consciousness of any duration with death due to other cause prior to regaining consciousness**
    - S06.6X9 **Traumatic subarachnoid hemorrhage with loss of consciousness of unspecified duration**
      Traumatic subarachnoid hemorrhage NOS
- S06.8 **Other specified intracranial injuries**
  - S06.81 **Injury of right internal carotid artery, intracranial portion, not elsewhere classified**
    - S06.810 **Injury of right internal carotid artery, intracranial portion, not elsewhere classified without loss of consciousness**
    - S06.811 **Injury of right internal carotid artery, intracranial portion, not elsewhere classified with loss of consciousness of 30 minutes or less**
    - S06.812 **Injury of right internal carotid artery, intracranial portion, not elsewhere classified with loss of consciousness of 31 minutes to 59 minutes**
    - S06.813 **Injury of right internal carotid artery, intracranial portion, not elsewhere classified with loss of consciousness of 1 hour to 5 hours 59 minutes**
    - S06.814 **Injury of right internal carotid artery, intracranial portion, not elsewhere classified with loss of consciousness of 6 hours to 24 hours**
    - S06.815 **Injury of right internal carotid artery, intracranial portion, not elsewhere classified with loss of consciousness greater than 24 hours with return to pre-existing conscious level**
    - S06.816 **Injury of right internal carotid artery, intracranial portion, not elsewhere classified with loss of consciousness greater than 24 hours without return to pre-existing conscious level with patient surviving**
    - S06.817 **Injury of right internal carotid artery, intracranial portion, not elsewhere classified with loss of consciousness of any duration with death due to brain injury prior to regaining consciousness**
    - S06.818 **Injury of right internal carotid artery, intracranial portion, not elsewhere classified with loss of consciousness of any duration with death due to other cause prior to regaining consciousness**
    - S06.819 **Injury of right internal carotid artery, intracranial portion, not elsewhere classified with loss of consciousness of unspecified duration**
      Injury of right internal carotid artery, intracranial portion, not elsewhere classified NOS

CHAPTER 19 (S00-T88)

● S06.82 **Injury of left internal carotid artery, intracranial portion, not elsewhere classified**

● S06.820 **Injury of left internal carotid artery, intracranial portion, not elsewhere classified without loss of consciousness**

● S06.821 **Injury of left internal carotid artery, intracranial portion, not elsewhere classified with loss of consciousness of 30 minutes or less**

● S06.822 **Injury of left internal carotid artery, intracranial portion, not elsewhere classified with loss of consciousness of 31 minutes to 59 minutes**

● S06.823 **Injury of left internal carotid artery, intracranial portion, not elsewhere classified with loss of consciousness of 1 hour to 5 hours 59 minutes**

● S06.824 **Injury of left internal carotid artery, intracranial portion, not elsewhere classified with loss of consciousness of 6 hours to 24 hours**

● S06.825 **Injury of left internal carotid artery, intracranial portion, not elsewhere classified with loss of consciousness greater than 24 hours with return to pre-existing conscious level**

● S06.826 **Injury of left internal carotid artery, intracranial portion, not elsewhere classified with loss of consciousness greater than 24 hours without return to pre-existing conscious level with patient surviving**

● S06.827 **Injury of left internal carotid artery, intracranial portion, not elsewhere classified with loss of consciousness of any duration with death due to brain injury prior to regaining consciousness**

● S06.828 **Injury of left internal carotid artery, intracranial portion, not elsewhere classified with loss of consciousness of any duration with death due to other cause prior to regaining consciousness**

● S06.829 **Injury of left internal carotid artery, intracranial portion, not elsewhere classified with loss of consciousness of unspecified duration**

Injury of left internal carotid artery, intracranial portion, not elsewhere classified NOS

● S06.89 **Other specified intracranial injury**

Excludes1 concussion (S06.0X-) ◀

● S06.890 **Other specified intracranial injury without loss of consciousness**

● S06.891 **Other specified intracranial injury with loss of consciousness of 30 minutes or less**

● S06.892 **Other specified intracranial injury with loss of consciousness of 31 minutes to 59 minutes**

● S06.893 **Other specified intracranial injury with loss of consciousness of 1 hour to 5 hours 59 minutes**

● S06.894 **Other specified intracranial injury with loss of consciousness of 6 hours to 24 hours**

● S06.895 **Other specified intracranial injury with loss of consciousness greater than 24 hours with return to pre-existing conscious level**

● S06.896 **Other specified intracranial injury with loss of consciousness greater than 24 hours without return to pre-existing conscious level with patient surviving**

● S06.897 **Other specified intracranial injury with loss of consciousness of any duration with death due to brain injury prior to regaining consciousness**

● S06.898 **Other specified intracranial injury with loss of consciousness of any duration with death due to other cause prior to regaining consciousness**

● S06.899 **Other specified intracranial injury with loss of consciousness of unspecified duration**

● S06.9 **Unspecified intracranial injury**

Brain injury NOS

Head injury NOS with loss of consciousness

Traumatic brain injury NOS ◀

Excludes1 conditions classifiable to S06.0- to S06.8-code to specified intracranial injury ◀

head injury NOS (S09.90)

● S06.9X **Unspecified intracranial injury**

● S06.9X0 **Unspecified intracranial injury without loss of consciousness**

● S06.9X1 **Unspecified intracranial injury with loss of consciousness of 30 minutes or less**

● S06.9X2 **Unspecified intracranial injury with loss of consciousness of 31 minutes to 59 minutes**

● S06.9X3 **Unspecified intracranial injury with loss of consciousness of 1 hour to 5 hours 59 minutes**

● S06.9X4 **Unspecified intracranial injury with loss of consciousness of 6 hours to 24 hours**

● S06.9X5 **Unspecified intracranial injury with loss of consciousness greater than 24 hours with return to pre-existing conscious level**

● S06.9X6 **Unspecified intracranial injury with loss of consciousness greater than 24 hours without return to pre-existing conscious level with patient surviving**

● S06.9X7 **Unspecified intracranial injury with loss of consciousness of any duration with death due to brain injury prior to regaining consciousness**

● S06.9X8 **Unspecified intracranial injury with loss of consciousness of any duration with death due to other cause prior to regaining consciousness**

● S06.9X9 **Unspecified intracranial injury with loss of consciousness of unspecified duration**

● **S07 Crushing injury of head**
Use additional code for all associated injuries, such as:
intracranial injuries (S06.-)
skull fractures (S02.-)
The appropriate 7th character is to be added to each code from category S07
A initial encounter
D subsequent encounter
S sequela

X● **S07.0 Crushing injury of face**
X● **S07.1 Crushing injury of skull**
X● **S07.8 Crushing injury of other parts of head**
X● **S07.9 Crushing injury of head, part unspecified**

● **S08 Avulsion and traumatic amputation of part of head**
An amputation not identified as partial or complete should be coded to complete
The appropriate 7th character is to be added to each code from category S08
A initial encounter
D subsequent encounter
S sequela

X● **S08.0 Avulsion of scalp**
● **S08.1 Traumatic amputation of ear**
● **S08.11 Complete traumatic amputation of ear**
● **S08.111 Complete traumatic amputation of right ear**
● **S08.112 Complete traumatic amputation of left ear**
● **S08.119 Complete traumatic amputation of unspecified ear**
● **S08.12 Partial traumatic amputation of ear**
● **S08.121 Partial traumatic amputation of right ear**
● **S08.122 Partial traumatic amputation of left ear**
● **S08.129 Partial traumatic amputation of unspecified ear**
● **S08.8 Traumatic amputation of other parts of head**
● **S08.81 Traumatic amputation of nose**
● **S08.811 Complete traumatic amputation of nose**
● **S08.812 Partial traumatic amputation of nose**
X● **S08.89 Traumatic amputation of other parts of head**

● **S09 Other and unspecified injuries of head**
The appropriate 7th character is to be added to each code from category S09
A initial encounter
D subsequent encounter
S sequela

X● **S09.0 Injury of blood vessels of head, not elsewhere classified**
Excludes1 injury of cerebral blood vessels (S06.-)
injury of precerebral blood vessels (S15.-)
● **S09.1 Injury of muscle and tendon of head**
Code also any associated open wound (S01.-)
Excludes2 sprain to joints and ligament of head (S03.9)
X● **S09.10 Unspecified injury of muscle and tendon of head**
Injury of muscle and tendon of head NOS
X● **S09.11 Strain of muscle and tendon of head**
X● **S09.12 Laceration of muscle and tendon of head**
X● **S09.19 Other specified injury of muscle and tendon of head**
● **S09.2 Traumatic rupture of ear drum**
Excludes1 traumatic rupture of ear drum due to blast injury (S09.31-)
X● **S09.20 Traumatic rupture of unspecified ear drum**
X● **S09.21 Traumatic rupture of right ear drum**
X● **S09.22 Traumatic rupture of left ear drum**
● **S09.3 Other specified and unspecified injury of middle and inner ear**
Excludes1 injury to ear NOS (S09.91-)
Excludes2 injury to external ear (S00.4-, S01.3-, S08.1-)
● **S09.30 Unspecified injury of middle and inner ear**
● **S09.301 Unspecified injury of right middle and inner ear**
● **S09.302 Unspecified injury of left middle and inner ear**
● **S09.309 Unspecified injury of unspecified middle and inner ear**
● **S09.31 Primary blast injury of ear**
Blast injury of ear NOS
● **S09.311 Primary blast injury of right ear**
● **S09.312 Primary blast injury of left ear**
● **S09.313 Primary blast injury of ear, bilateral**
● **S09.319 Primary blast injury of unspecified ear**
● **S09.39 Other specified injury of middle and inner ear**
Secondary blast injury to ear
● **S09.391 Other specified injury of right middle and inner ear**
● **S09.392 Other specified injury of left middle and inner ear**
● **S09.399 Other specified injury of unspecified middle and inner ear**
X● **S09.8 Other specified injuries of head**
● **S09.9 Unspecified injury of face and head**
X● **S09.90 Unspecified injury of head**
Head injury NOS
Excludes1 brain injury NOS (S06.9-)
head injury NOS with loss of consciousness (S06.9-)
intracranial injury NOS (S06.9-)
X● **S09.91 Unspecified injury of ear**
Injury of ear NOS
X● **S09.92 Unspecified injury of nose**
Injury of nose NOS
X● **S09.93 Unspecified injury of face**
Injury of face NOS

INJURIES TO THE NECK (S10-S19)

Includes injuries of nape
injuries of supraclavicular region
injuries of throat
Excludes2 burns and corrosions (T20-T32)
effects of foreign body in esophagus (T18.1)
effects of foreign body in larynx (T17.3)
effects of foreign body in pharynx (T17.2)
effects of foreign body in trachea (T17.4)
frostbite (T33-T34)
insect bite or sting, venomous (T63.4)

● **S10 Superficial injury of neck**
The appropriate 7th character is to be added to each code from category S10
A initial encounter
D subsequent encounter
S sequela

X● **S10.0 Contusion of throat**
Contusion of cervical esophagus
Contusion of larynx
Contusion of pharynx
Contusion of trachea

● S10.1 **Other and unspecified superficial injuries of throat**
- X● S10.10 **Unspecified superficial injuries of throat**
- X● S10.11 **Abrasion of throat**
- X● S10.12 **Blister (nonthermal) of throat**
- X● S10.14 **External constriction of part of throat**
- X● S10.15 **Superficial foreign body of throat**
  Splinter in the throat
- X● S10.16 **Insect bite (nonvenomous) of throat**
- X● S10.17 **Other superficial bite of throat**
  Excludes1 open bite of throat (S11.85)

● S10.8 **Superficial injury of other specified parts of neck**
- X● S10.80 **Unspecified superficial injury of other specified part of neck**
- X● S10.81 **Abrasion of other specified part of neck**
- X● S10.82 **Blister (nonthermal) of other specified part of neck**
- X● S10.83 **Contusion of other specified part of neck**
- X● S10.84 **External constriction of other specified part of neck**
- X● S10.85 **Superficial foreign body of other specified part of neck**
  Splinter in other part of neck
- X● S10.86 **Insect bite of other specified part of neck**
- X● S10.87 **Other superficial bite of other specified part of neck**
  Excludes1 open bite of other specified parts of neck (S11.85)

● S10.9 **Superficial injury of unspecified part of neck**
- X● S10.90 **Unspecified superficial injury of unspecified part of neck**
- X● S10.91 **Abrasion of unspecified part of neck**
- X● S10.92 **Blister (nonthermal) of unspecified part of neck**
- X● S10.93 **Contusion of unspecified part of neck**
- X● S10.94 **External constriction of unspecified part of neck**
- X● S10.95 **Superficial foreign body of unspecified part of neck**
- X● S10.96 **Insect bite of unspecified part of neck**
- X● S10.97 **Other superficial bite of unspecified part of neck**

● S11 **Open wound of neck**

Code also any associated:
spinal cord injury (S14.0, S14.1-)
wound infection

Excludes2 open fracture of vertebra (S12.- with 7th character B)

The appropriate 7th character is to be added to each code from category S11

A	initial encounter
D	subsequent encounter
S	sequela

● S11.0 **Open wound of larynx and trachea**

● S11.01 **Open wound of larynx**
Excludes2 open wound of vocal cord (S11.03)
- ● S11.011 **Laceration without foreign body of larynx**
- ● S11.012 **Laceration with foreign body of larynx**
- ● S11.013 **Puncture wound without foreign body of larynx**
- ● S11.014 **Puncture wound with foreign body of larynx**
- ● S11.015 **Open bite of larynx**
  Bite of larynx NOS
- ● S11.019 **Unspecified open wound of larynx**

● S11.02 **Open wound of trachea**
Open wound of cervical trachea
Open wound of trachea NOS
Excludes2 open wound of thoracic trachea (S27.5-)
- ● S11.021 **Laceration without foreign body of trachea**
- ● S11.022 **Laceration with foreign body of trachea**
- ● S11.023 **Puncture wound without foreign body of trachea**
- ● S11.024 **Puncture wound with foreign body of trachea**
- ● S11.025 **Open bite of trachea**
  Bite of trachea NOS
- ● S11.029 **Unspecified open wound of trachea**

● S11.03 **Open wound of vocal cord**
- ● S11.031 **Laceration without foreign body of vocal cord**
- ● S11.032 **Laceration with foreign body of vocal cord**
- ● S11.033 **Puncture wound without foreign body of vocal cord**
- ● S11.034 **Puncture wound with foreign body of vocal cord**
- ● S11.035 **Open bite of vocal cord**
  Bite of vocal cord NOS
- ● S11.039 **Unspecified open wound of vocal cord**

● S11.1 **Open wound of thyroid gland**
- X● S11.10 **Unspecified open wound of thyroid gland**
- X● S11.11 **Laceration without foreign body of thyroid gland**
- X● S11.12 **Laceration with foreign body of thyroid gland**
- X● S11.13 **Puncture wound without foreign body of thyroid gland**
- X● S11.14 **Puncture wound with foreign body of thyroid gland**
- X● S11.15 **Open bite of thyroid gland**
  Bite of thyroid gland NOS

● S11.2 **Open wound of pharynx and cervical esophagus**
Excludes1 open wound of esophagus NOS (S27.8-)
- X● S11.20 **Unspecified open wound of pharynx and cervical esophagus**
- X● S11.21 **Laceration without foreign body of pharynx and cervical esophagus**
- X● S11.22 **Laceration with foreign body of pharynx and cervical esophagus**
- X● S11.23 **Puncture wound without foreign body of pharynx and cervical esophagus**
- X● S11.24 **Puncture wound with foreign body of pharynx and cervical esophagus**
- X● S11.25 **Open bite of pharynx and cervical esophagus**
  Bite of pharynx and cervical esophagus NOS

● S11.8 **Open wound of other specified parts of neck**
- X● S11.80 **Unspecified open specified wound of other part of neck**
- X● S11.81 **Laceration without foreign body of other specified part of neck**
- X● S11.82 **Laceration with foreign body of other specified part of neck**
- X● S11.83 **Puncture wound without foreign body of other specified part of neck**
- X● S11.84 **Puncture wound with foreign body of other specified part of neck**
- X● S11.85 **Open bite of other specified part of neck**
  Bite of other part of neck NOS
  Excludes1 superficial bite of other specified part of neck (S10.87)
- X● S11.89 **Other open wound of other part of neck**

● **S11.9 Open wound of unspecified part of neck**
- X● **S11.90** Unspecified open wound of unspecified part of neck
- X● **S11.91** Laceration without foreign body of unspecified part of neck
- X● **S11.92** Laceration with foreign body of unspecified part of neck
- X● **S11.93** Puncture wound without foreign body of unspecified part of neck
- X● **S11.94** Puncture wound with foreign body of unspecified part of neck
- X● **S11.95** Open bite of unspecified part of neck
  Bite of neck NOS
  Excludes1 superficial bite of neck (S10.97)

● **S12 Fracture of cervical vertebra and other parts of neck**

Note: A fracture not indicated as displaced or nondisplaced should be coded to displaced

A fracture not indicated as open or closed should be coded to closed

Includes fracture of cervical neural arch
fracture of cervical spine
fracture of cervical spinous process
fracture of cervical transverse process
fracture of cervical vertebral arch
fracture of neck

Code first any associated cervical spinal cord injury (S14.0, S14.1-)

The appropriate 7th character is to be added to all codes from subcategories S12.0-S12.6

A	initial encounter for closed fracture
B	initial encounter for open fracture
D	subsequent encounter for fracture with routine healing
G	subsequent encounter for fracture with delayed healing
K	subsequent encounter for fracture with nonunion
S	sequela

● **S12.0 Fracture of first cervical vertebra**
Atlas
- ● **S12.00** Unspecified fracture of first cervical vertebra
  - ● **S12.000** Unspecified displaced fracture of first cervical vertebra
  - ● **S12.001** Unspecified nondisplaced fracture of first cervical vertebra
- X● **S12.01** Stable burst fracture of first cervical vertebra
- X● **S12.02** Unstable burst fracture of first cervical vertebra
- ● **S12.03** Posterior arch fracture of first cervical vertebra
  - ● **S12.030** Displaced posterior arch fracture of first cervical vertebra
  - ● **S12.031** Nondisplaced posterior arch fracture of first cervical vertebra
- ● **S12.04** Lateral mass fracture of first cervical vertebra
  - ● **S12.040** Displaced lateral mass fracture of first cervical vertebra
  - ● **S12.041** Nondisplaced lateral mass fracture of first cervical vertebra
- ● **S12.09** Other fracture of first cervical vertebra
  - ● **S12.090** Other displaced fracture of first cervical vertebra
  - ● **S12.091** Other nondisplaced fracture of first cervical vertebra

● **S12.1 Fracture of second cervical vertebra**
Axis
- ● **S12.10** Unspecified fracture of second cervical vertebra
  - ● **S12.100** Unspecified displaced fracture of second cervical vertebra
  - ● **S12.101** Unspecified nondisplaced fracture of second cervical vertebra
- ● **S12.11** Type II dens fracture
  - ● **S12.110** Anterior displaced Type II dens fracture
  - ● **S12.111** Posterior displaced Type II dens fracture
  - ● **S12.112** Nondisplaced Type II dens fracture
- ● **S12.12** Other dens fracture
  - ● **S12.120** Other displaced dens fracture
  - ● **S12.121** Other nondisplaced dens fracture
- ● **S12.13** Unspecified traumatic spondylolisthesis of second cervical vertebra
  - ● **S12.130** Unspecified traumatic displaced spondylolisthesis of second cervical vertebra
  - ● **S12.131** Unspecified traumatic nondisplaced spondylolisthesis of second cervical vertebra
- X● **S12.14** Type III traumatic spondylolisthesis of second cervical vertebra
- ● **S12.15** Other traumatic spondylolisthesis of second cervical vertebra
  - ● **S12.150** Other traumatic displaced spondylolisthesis of second cervical vertebra
  - ● **S12.151** Other traumatic nondisplaced spondylolisthesis of second cervical vertebra
- ● **S12.19** Other fracture of second cervical vertebra
  - ● **S12.190** Other displaced fracture of second cervical vertebra
  - ● **S12.191** Other nondisplaced fracture of second cervical vertebra

● **S12.2 Fracture of third cervical vertebra**
- ● **S12.20** Unspecified fracture of third cervical vertebra
  - ● **S12.200** Unspecified displaced fracture of third cervical vertebra
  - ● **S12.201** Unspecified nondisplaced fracture of third cervical vertebra
- ● **S12.23** Unspecified traumatic spondylolisthesis of third cervical vertebra
  - ● **S12.230** Unspecified traumatic displaced spondylolisthesis of third cervical vertebra
  - ● **S12.231** Unspecified traumatic nondisplaced spondylolisthesis of third cervical vertebra
- X● **S12.24** Type III traumatic spondylolisthesis of third cervical vertebra
- ● **S12.25** Other traumatic spondylolisthesis of third cervical vertebra
  - ● **S12.250** Other traumatic displaced spondylolisthesis of third cervical vertebra
  - ● **S12.251** Other traumatic nondisplaced spondylolisthesis of third cervical vertebra
- ● **S12.29** Other fracture of third cervical vertebra
  - ● **S12.290** Other displaced fracture of third cervical vertebra
  - ● **S12.291** Other nondisplaced fracture of third cervical vertebra

● **S12.3 Fracture of fourth cervical vertebra**
- ● **S12.30** Unspecified fracture of fourth cervical vertebra
  - ● **S12.300** Unspecified displaced fracture of fourth cervical vertebra
  - ● **S12.301** Unspecified nondisplaced fracture of fourth cervical vertebra

CHAPTER 19 (S00-T88)

● S12.33 Unspecified traumatic spondylolisthesis of fourth cervical vertebra
  ● S12.330 Unspecified traumatic displaced spondylolisthesis of fourth cervical vertebra
  ● S12.331 Unspecified traumatic nondisplaced spondylolisthesis of fourth cervical vertebra
X ● S12.34 Type III traumatic spondylolisthesis of fourth cervical vertebra
● S12.35 Other traumatic spondylolisthesis of fourth cervical vertebra
  ● S12.350 Other traumatic displaced spondylolisthesis of fourth cervical vertebra
  ● S12.351 Other traumatic nondisplaced spondylolisthesis of fourth cervical vertebra
● S12.39 Other fracture of fourth cervical vertebra
  ● S12.390 Other displaced fracture of fourth cervical vertebra
  ● S12.391 Other nondisplaced fracture of fourth cervical vertebra
● S12.4 Fracture of fifth cervical vertebra
  ● S12.40 Unspecified fracture of fifth cervical vertebra
    ● S12.400 Unspecified displaced fracture of fifth cervical vertebra
    ● S12.401 Unspecified nondisplaced fracture of fifth cervical vertebra
  ● S12.43 Unspecified traumatic spondylolisthesis of fifth cervical vertebra
    ● S12.430 Unspecified traumatic displaced spondylolisthesis of fifth cervical vertebra
    ● S12.431 Unspecified traumatic nondisplaced spondylolisthesis of fifth cervical vertebra
  X ● S12.44 Type III traumatic spondylolisthesis of fifth cervical vertebra
  ● S12.45 Other traumatic spondylolisthesis of fifth cervical vertebra
    ● S12.450 Other traumatic displaced spondylolisthesis of fifth cervical vertebra
    ● S12.451 Other traumatic nondisplaced spondylolisthesis of fifth cervical vertebra
  ● S12.49 Other fracture of fifth cervical vertebra
    ● S12.490 Other displaced fracture of fifth cervical vertebra
    ● S12.491 Other nondisplaced fracture of fifth cervical vertebra
● S12.5 Fracture of sixth cervical vertebra
  ● S12.50 Unspecified fracture of sixth cervical vertebra
    ● S12.500 Unspecified displaced fracture of sixth cervical vertebra
    ● S12.501 Unspecified nondisplaced fracture of sixth cervical vertebra
  ● S12.53 Unspecified traumatic spondylolisthesis of sixth cervical vertebra
    ● S12.530 Unspecified traumatic displaced spondylolisthesis of sixth cervical vertebra
    ● S12.531 Unspecified traumatic nondisplaced spondylolisthesis of sixth cervical vertebra

X ● S12.54 Type III traumatic spondylolisthesis of sixth cervical vertebra
● S12.55 Other traumatic spondylolisthesis of sixth cervical vertebra
  ● S12.550 Other traumatic displaced spondylolisthesis of sixth cervical vertebra
  ● S12.551 Other traumatic nondisplaced spondylolisthesis of sixth cervical vertebra
● S12.59 Other fracture of sixth cervical vertebra
  ● S12.590 Other displaced fracture of sixth cervical vertebra
  ● S12.591 Other nondisplaced fracture of sixth cervical vertebra
● S12.6 Fracture of seventh cervical vertebra
  S12.60 Unspecified fracture of seventh cervical vertebra
    ● S12.600 Unspecified displaced fracture of seventh cervical vertebra
    ● S12.601 Unspecified nondisplaced fracture of seventh cervical vertebra
  ● S12.63 Unspecified traumatic spondylolisthesis of seventh cervical vertebra
    ● S12.630 Unspecified traumatic displaced spondylolisthesis of seventh cervical vertebra
    ● S12.631 Unspecified traumatic nondisplaced spondylolisthesis of seventh cervical vertebra
  X ● S12.64 Type III traumatic spondylolisthesis of seventh cervical vertebra
  ● S12.65 Other traumatic spondylolisthesis of seventh cervical vertebra
    ● S12.650 Other traumatic displaced spondylolisthesis of seventh cervical vertebra
    ● S12.651 Other traumatic nondisplaced spondylolisthesis of seventh cervical vertebra
  ● S12.69 Other fracture of seventh cervical vertebra
    ● S12.690 Other displaced fracture of seventh cervical vertebra
    ● S12.691 Other nondisplaced fracture of seventh cervical vertebra
X ● S12.8 Fracture of other parts of neck
  Hyoid bone   Thyroid cartilage
  Larynx   Trachea
  The appropriate 7th character is to be added to code S12.8

A	initial encounter
D	subsequent encounter
S	sequela

X ● S12.9 Fracture of neck, unspecified
  Fracture of neck NOS
  Fracture of cervical spine NOS
  Fracture of cervical vertebra NOS
  The appropriate 7th character is to be added to code S12.9

A	initial encounter
D	subsequent encounter
S	sequela

● S13 **Dislocation and sprain of joints and ligaments at neck level**

Includes avulsion of joint or ligament at neck level
laceration of cartilage, joint or ligament at neck level
sprain of cartilage, joint or ligament at neck level
traumatic hemarthrosis of joint or ligament at neck level
traumatic rupture of joint or ligament at neck level
traumatic subluxation of joint or ligament at neck level
traumatic tear of joint or ligament at neck level

Code also any associated open wound

Excludes2 strain of muscle or tendon at neck level (S16.1)

The appropriate 7th character is to be added to each code from category S13

A	initial encounter
D	subsequent encounter
S	sequela

X● S13.Ø **Traumatic rupture of cervical intervertebral disc**

Excludes1 rupture or displacement (nontraumatic) of cervical intervertebral disc NOS (M5Ø.-)

● S13.1 **Subluxation and dislocation of cervical vertebra**

Code also any associated:
open wound of neck (S11.-)
spinal cord injury (S14.1-)

Excludes2 fracture of cervical vertebrae (S12.Ø-S12.3-)

● S13.1Ø **Subluxation and dislocation of unspecified cervical vertebrae**

● S13.1ØØ **Subluxation of unspecified cervical vertebrae**

● S13.1Ø1 **Dislocation of unspecified cervical vertebrae**

● S13.11 **Subluxation and dislocation of C_0/C_1 cervical vertebrae**
Subluxation and dislocation of atlantooccipital joint
Subluxation and dislocation of atloidooccipital joint
Subluxation and dislocation of occipitoatloid joint

● S13.11Ø **Subluxation of C_0/C_1 cervical vertebrae**

● S13.111 **Dislocation of C_0/C_1 cervical vertebrae**

● S13.12 **Subluxation and dislocation of C_1/C_2 cervical vertebrae**
Subluxation and dislocation of atlantoaxial joint

● S13.12Ø **Subluxation of C_1/C_2 cervical vertebrae**

● S13.121 **Dislocation of C_1/C_2 cervical vertebrae**

● S13.13 **Subluxation and dislocation of C_2/C_3 cervical vertebrae**

● S13.13Ø **Subluxation of C_2/C_3 cervical vertebrae**

● S13.131 **Dislocation of C_2/C_3 cervical vertebrae**

● S13.14 **Subluxation and dislocation of C_3/C_4 cervical vertebrae**

● S13.14Ø **Subluxation of C_3/C_4 cervical vertebrae**

● S13.141 **Dislocation of C_3/C_4 cervical vertebrae**

● S13.15 **Subluxation and dislocation of C_4/C_5 cervical vertebrae**

● S13.15Ø **Subluxation of C_4/C_5 cervical vertebrae**

● S13.151 **Dislocation of C_4/C_5 cervical vertebrae**

● S13.16 **Subluxation and dislocation of C_5/C_6 cervical vertebrae**

● S13.16Ø **Subluxation of C_5/C_6 cervical vertebrae**

● S13.161 **Dislocation of C_5/C_6 cervical vertebrae**

● S13.17 **Subluxation and dislocation of C_6/C_7 cervical vertebrae**

● S13.17Ø **Subluxation of C_6/C_7 cervical vertebrae**

● S13.171 **Dislocation of C_6/C_7 cervical vertebrae**

● S13.18 **Subluxation and dislocation of C_7/T_1 cervical vertebrae**

● S13.18Ø **Subluxation of C_7/T_1 cervical vertebrae**

● S13.181 **Dislocation of C_7/T_1 cervical vertebrae**

● S13.2 **Dislocation of other and unspecified parts of neck**

X● S13.2Ø **Dislocation of unspecified parts of neck**

X● S13.29 **Dislocation of other parts of neck**

X● S13.4 **Sprain of ligaments of cervical spine**
Sprain of anterior longitudinal (ligament), cervical
Sprain of atlanto-axial (joints)
Sprain of atlanto-occipital (joints)
Whiplash injury of cervical spine

X● S13.5 **Sprain of thyroid region**
Sprain of cricoarytenoid (joint) (ligament)
Sprain of cricothyroid (joint) (ligament)
Sprain of thyroid cartilage

X● S13.8 **Sprain of joints and ligaments of other parts of neck**

X● S13.9 **Sprain of joints and ligaments of unspecified parts of neck**

● S14 **Injury of nerves and spinal cord at neck level**

Note: Code to highest level of cervical cord injury

Code also any associated:
fracture of cervical vertebra (S12.Ø--S12.6.-)
open wound of neck (S11.-)
transient paralysis (R29.5)

The appropriate 7th character is to be added to each code from category S14

A	initial encounter
D	subsequent encounter
S	sequela

X● S14.Ø **Concussion and edema of cervical spinal cord**

● S14.1 **Other and unspecified injuries of cervical spinal cord**

● S14.1Ø **Unspecified injury of cervical spinal cord**

● S14.1Ø1 **Unspecified injury at C_1 level of cervical spinal cord**

● S14.1Ø2 **Unspecified injury at C_2 level of cervical spinal cord**

● S14.1Ø3 **Unspecified injury at C_3 level of cervical spinal cord**

● S14.1Ø4 **Unspecified injury at C_4 level of cervical spinal cord**

● S14.1Ø5 **Unspecified injury at C_5 level of cervical spinal cord**

● S14.1Ø6 **Unspecified injury at C_6 level of cervical spinal cord**

● S14.1Ø7 **Unspecified injury at C_7 level of cervical spinal cord**

● S14.1Ø8 **Unspecified injury at C_8 level of cervical spinal cord**

● S14.1Ø9 **Unspecified injury at unspecified level of cervical spinal cord**
Injury of cervical spinal cord NOS

● **S14.11**   Complete lesion of cervical spinal cord
- ● **S14.111**   Complete lesion at C_1 level of cervical spinal cord
- ● **S14.112**   Complete lesion at C_2 level of cervical spinal cord
- ● **S14.113**   Complete lesion at C_3 level of cervical spinal cord
- ● **S14.114**   Complete lesion at C_4 level of cervical spinal cord
- ● **S14.115**   Complete lesion at C_5 level of cervical spinal cord
- ● **S14.116**   Complete lesion at C_6 level of cervical spinal cord
- ● **S14.117**   Complete lesion at C_7 level of cervical spinal cord
- ● **S14.118**   Complete lesion at C_8 level of cervical spinal cord
- ● **S14.119**   Complete lesion at unspecified level of cervical spinal cord

● **S14.12**   Central cord syndrome of cervical spinal cord
- ● **S14.121**   Central cord syndrome at C_1 level of cervical spinal cord
- ● **S14.122**   Central cord syndrome at C_2 level of cervical spinal cord
- ● **S14.123**   Central cord syndrome at C_3 level of cervical spinal cord
- ● **S14.124**   Central cord syndrome at C_4 level of cervical spinal cord
- ● **S14.125**   Central cord syndrome at C_5 level of cervical spinal cord
- ● **S14.126**   Central cord syndrome at C_6 level of cervical spinal cord
- ● **S14.127**   Central cord syndrome at C_7 level of cervical spinal cord
- ● **S14.128**   Central cord syndrome at C_8 level of cervical spinal cord
- ● **S14.129**   Central cord syndrome at unspecified level of cervical spinal cord

● **S14.13**   Anterior cord syndrome of cervical spinal cord
- ● **S14.131**   Anterior cord syndrome at C_1 level of cervical spinal cord
- ● **S14.132**   Anterior cord syndrome at C_2 level of cervical spinal cord
- ● **S14.133**   Anterior cord syndrome at C_3 level of cervical spinal cord
- ● **S14.134**   Anterior cord syndrome at C_4 level of cervical spinal cord
- ● **S14.135**   Anterior cord syndrome at C_5 level of cervical spinal cord
- ● **S14.136**   Anterior cord syndrome at C_6 level of cervical spinal cord
- ● **S14.137**   Anterior cord syndrome at C_7 level of cervical spinal cord
- ● **S14.138**   Anterior cord syndrome at C_8 level of cervical spinal cord
- ● **S14.139**   Anterior cord syndrome at unspecified level of cervical spinal cord

● **S14.14**   Brown-Séquard syndrome of cervical spinal cord
- ● **S14.141**   Brown-Séquard syndrome at C_1 level of cervical spinal cord
- ● **S14.142**   Brown-Séquard syndrome at C_2 level of cervical spinal cord
- ● **S14.143**   Brown-Séquard syndrome at C_3 level of cervical spinal cord
- ● **S14.144**   Brown-Séquard syndrome at C_4 level of cervical spinal cord
- ● **S14.145**   Brown-Séquard syndrome at C_5 level of cervical spinal cord
- ● **S14.146**   Brown-Séquard syndrome at C_6 level of cervical spinal cord
- ● **S14.147**   Brown-Séquard syndrome at C_7 level of cervical spinal cord
- ● **S14.148**   Brown-Séquard syndrome at C_8 level of cervical spinal cord
- ● **S14.149**   Brown-Séquard syndrome at unspecified level of cervical spinal cord

● **S14.15**   Other incomplete lesions of cervical spinal cord
> Incomplete lesion of cervical spinal cord NOS
> Posterior cord syndrome of cervical spinal cord
- ● **S14.151**   Other incomplete lesion at C_1 level of cervical spinal cord
- ● **S14.152**   Other incomplete lesion at C_2 level of cervical spinal cord
- ● **S14.153**   Other incomplete lesion at C_3 level of cervical spinal cord
- ● **S14.154**   Other incomplete lesion at C_4 level of cervical spinal cord
- ● **S14.155**   Other incomplete lesion at C_5 level of cervical spinal cord
- ● **S14.156**   Other incomplete lesion at C_6 level of cervical spinal cord
- ● **S14.157**   Other incomplete lesion at C_7 level of cervical spinal cord
- ● **S14.158**   Other incomplete lesion at C_8 level of cervical spinal cord
- ● **S14.159**   Other incomplete lesion at unspecified level of cervical spinal cord

X ● **S14.2**   Injury of nerve root of cervical spine
X ● **S14.3**   Injury of brachial plexus
X ● **S14.4**   Injury of peripheral nerves of neck
X ● **S14.5**   Injury of cervical sympathetic nerves
X ● **S14.8**   Injury of other specified nerves of neck
X ● **S14.9**   Injury of unspecified nerves of neck

● **S15**   Injury of blood vessels at neck level
> Code also any associated open wound (S11.-)
>
> The appropriate 7th character is to be added to each code from category S15

A	initial encounter
D	subsequent encounter
S	sequela

● **S15.0**   Injury of carotid artery of neck
> Injury of carotid artery (common) (external) (internal, extracranial portion)
> Injury of carotid artery NOS
>
> **Excludes1**   injury of internal carotid artery, intracranial portion (S06.8)

- ● **S15.00**   Unspecified injury of carotid artery
  - ● **S15.001**   Unspecified injury of right carotid artery
  - ● **S15.002**   Unspecified injury of left carotid artery
  - ● **S15.009**   Unspecified injury of unspecified carotid artery
- ● **S15.01**   Minor laceration of carotid artery
  > Incomplete transection of carotid artery
  > Laceration of carotid artery NOS
  > Superficial laceration of carotid artery
  - ● **S15.011**   Minor laceration of right carotid artery
  - ● **S15.012**   Minor laceration of left carotid artery
  - ● **S15.019**   Minor laceration of unspecified carotid artery

---

◀ New   ⬅▥ Revised   ~~deleted~~ Deleted   **OGCR** Official Guidelines   **X** Assign placeholder X   ● Use Additional Character(s)

| Excludes 1 | Excludes 2 | Includes | Use additional | Code first | Code also | Unspecified |

● S15.02 Major laceration of carotid artery
Complete transection of carotid artery
Traumatic rupture of carotid artery
● S15.021 Major laceration of right carotid artery
● S15.022 Major laceration of left carotid artery
● S15.029 Major laceration of unspecified carotid artery
● S15.09 Other specified injury of carotid artery
● S15.091 Other specified injury of right carotid artery
● S15.092 Other specified injury of left carotid artery
● S15.099 Other specified injury of unspecified carotid artery
● S15.1 Injury of vertebral artery
● S15.10 Unspecified injury of vertebral artery
● S15.101 Unspecified injury of right vertebral artery
● S15.102 Unspecified injury of left vertebral artery
● S15.109 Unspecified injury of unspecified vertebral artery
● S15.11 Minor laceration of vertebral artery
Incomplete transection of vertebral artery
Laceration of vertebral artery NOS
Superficial laceration of vertebral artery
● S15.111 Minor laceration of right vertebral artery
● S15.112 Minor laceration of left vertebral artery
● S15.119 Minor laceration of unspecified vertebral artery
● S15.12 Major laceration of vertebral artery
Complete transection of vertebral artery
Traumatic rupture of vertebral artery
● S15.121 Major laceration of right vertebral artery
● S15.122 Major laceration of left vertebral artery
● S15.129 Major laceration of unspecified vertebral artery
● S15.19 Other specified injury of vertebral artery
● S15.191 Other specified injury of right vertebral artery
● S15.192 Other specified injury of left vertebral artery
● S15.199 Other specified injury of unspecified vertebral artery
● S15.2 Injury of external jugular vein
● S15.20 Unspecified injury of external jugular vein
● S15.201 Unspecified injury of right external jugular vein
● S15.202 Unspecified injury of left external jugular vein
● S15.209 Unspecified injury of unspecified external jugular vein
● S15.21 Minor laceration of external jugular vein
Incomplete transection of external jugular vein
Laceration of external jugular vein NOS
Superficial laceration of external jugular vein
● S15.211 Minor laceration of right external jugular vein
● S15.212 Minor laceration of left external jugular vein
● S15.219 Minor laceration of unspecified external jugular vein
● S15.22 Major laceration of external jugular vein
Complete transection of external jugular vein
Traumatic rupture of external jugular vein
● S15.221 Major laceration of right external jugular vein
● S15.222 Major laceration of left external jugular vein
● S15.229 Major laceration of unspecified external jugular vein
● S15.29 Other specified injury of external jugular vein
● S15.291 Other specified injury of right external jugular vein
● S15.292 Other specified injury of left external jugular vein
● S15.299 Other specified injury of unspecified external jugular vein
● S15.3 Injury of internal jugular vein
● S15.30 Unspecified injury of internal jugular vein
● S15.301 Unspecified injury of right internal jugular vein
● S15.302 Unspecified injury of left internal jugular vein
● S15.309 Unspecified injury of unspecified internal jugular vein
● S15.31 Minor laceration of internal jugular vein
Incomplete transection of internal jugular vein
Laceration of internal jugular vein NOS
Superficial laceration of internal jugular vein
● S15.311 Minor laceration of right internal jugular vein
● S15.312 Minor laceration of left internal jugular vein
● S15.319 Minor laceration of unspecified internal jugular vein
● S15.32 Major laceration of internal jugular vein
Complete transection of internal jugular vein
Traumatic rupture of internal jugular vein
● S15.321 Major laceration of right internal jugular vein
● S15.322 Major laceration of left internal jugular vein
● S15.329 Major laceration of unspecified internal jugular vein
● S15.39 Other specified injury of internal jugular vein
● S15.391 Other specified injury of right internal jugular vein
● S15.392 Other specified injury of left internal jugular vein
● S15.399 Other specified injury of unspecified internal jugular vein
X● S15.8 Injury of other specified blood vessels at neck level
X● S15.9 Injury of unspecified blood vessel at neck level
● S16 Injury of muscle, fascia and tendon at neck level
Code also any associated open wound (S11.-)
Excludes2 sprain of joint or ligament at neck level (S13.9)
The appropriate 7th character is to be added to each code from category S16

A	initial encounter
D	subsequent encounter
S	sequela

X● S16.1 Strain of muscle, fascia and tendon at neck level
X● S16.2 Laceration of muscle, fascia and tendon at neck level
X● S16.8 Other specified injury of muscle, fascia and tendon at neck level
X● S16.9 Unspecified injury of muscle, fascia and tendon at neck level

● S17 **Crushing injury of neck**
Use additional code for all associated injuries, such as:
injury of blood vessels (S15.-)
open wound of neck (S11.-)
spinal cord injury (S14.0, S14.1-)
vertebral fracture (S12.0--S12.3-)
The appropriate 7th character is to be added to each code from category S17

A	initial encounter
D	subsequent encounter
S	sequela

X● **S17.0 Crushing injury of larynx and trachea**
X● **S17.8 Crushing injury of other specified parts of neck**
X● **S17.9 Crushing injury of neck, part unspecified**

● S19 **Other and unspecified injuries of neck**
The appropriate 7th character is to be added to each code from category S19

A	initial encounter
D	subsequent encounter
S	sequela

● **S19.8 Other specified injuries of neck**
X● **S19.80 Other specified injuries of unspecified part of neck**
X● **S19.81 Other specified injuries of larynx**
X● **S19.82 Other specified injuries of cervical trachea**
Excludes2 other specified injury of thoracic trachea (S27.5-)
X● **S19.83 Other specified injuries of vocal cord**
X● **S19.84 Other specified injuries of thyroid gland**
X● **S19.85 Other specified injuries of pharynx and cervical esophagus**
X● **S19.89 Other specified injuries of other specified part of neck**
X● **S19.9 Unspecified injury of neck**

INJURIES TO THE THORAX (S20-S29)

Includes injuries of breast
injuries of chest (wall)
injuries of interscapular area

Excludes2 burns and corrosions (T20-T32)
effects of foreign body in bronchus (T17.5)
effects of foreign body in esophagus (T18.1)
effects of foreign body in lung (T17.8)
effects of foreign body in trachea (T17.4)
frostbite (T33-T34)
injuries of axilla
injuries of clavicle
injuries of scapular region
injuries of shoulder
insect bite or sting, venomous (T63.4)

● S20 **Superficial injury of thorax**
The appropriate 7th character is to be added to each code from category S20

A	initial encounter
D	subsequent encounter
S	sequela

● **S20.0 Contusion of breast**
X● **S20.00 Contusion of breast, unspecified breast**
X● **S20.01 Contusion of right breast**
X● **S20.02 Contusion of left breast**

● **S20.1 Other and unspecified superficial injuries of breast**
● **S20.10 Unspecified superficial injuries of breast**
● **S20.101 Unspecified superficial injuries of breast, right breast**
● **S20.102 Unspecified superficial injuries of breast, left breast**
● **S20.109 Unspecified superficial injuries of breast, unspecified breast**
● **S20.11 Abrasion of breast**
● **S20.111 Abrasion of breast, right breast**
● **S20.112 Abrasion of breast, left breast**
● **S20.119 Abrasion of breast, unspecified breast**
● **S20.12 Blister (nonthermal) of breast**
● **S20.121 Blister (nonthermal) of breast, right breast**
● **S20.122 Blister (nonthermal) of breast, left breast**
● **S20.129 Blister (nonthermal) of breast, unspecified breast**
● **S20.14 External constriction of part of breast**
● **S20.141 External constriction of part of breast, right breast**
● **S20.142 External constriction of part of breast, left breast**
● **S20.149 External constriction of part of breast, unspecified breast**
● **S20.15 Superficial foreign body of breast**
Splinter in the breast
● **S20.151 Superficial foreign body of breast, right breast**
● **S20.152 Superficial foreign body of breast, left breast**
● **S20.159 Superficial foreign body of breast, unspecified breast**
● **S20.16 Insect bite (nonvenomous) of breast**
● **S20.161 Insect bite (nonvenomous) of breast, right breast**
● **S20.162 Insect bite (nonvenomous) of breast, left breast**
● **S20.169 Insect bite (nonvenomous) of breast, unspecified breast**
● **S20.17 Other superficial bite of breast**
Excludes1 open bite of breast (S21.05-)
● **S20.171 Other superficial bite of breast, right breast**
● **S20.172 Other superficial bite of breast, left breast**
● **S20.179 Other superficial bite of breast, unspecified breast**
● **S20.2 Contusion of thorax**
X● **S20.20 Contusion of thorax, unspecified**
● **S20.21 Contusion of front wall of thorax**
● **S20.211 Contusion of right front wall of thorax**
● **S20.212 Contusion of left front wall of thorax**
● **S20.219 Contusion of unspecified front wall of thorax**
● **S20.22 Contusion of back wall of thorax**
● **S20.221 Contusion of right back wall of thorax**
● **S20.222 Contusion of left back wall of thorax**
● **S20.229 Contusion of unspecified back wall of thorax**

- S20.3 Other and unspecified superficial injuries of front wall of thorax
  - S20.30 Unspecified superficial injuries of front wall of thorax
    - S20.301 Unspecified superficial injuries of right front wall of thorax
    - S20.302 Unspecified superficial injuries of left front wall of thorax
    - S20.309 Unspecified superficial injuries of unspecified front wall of thorax
  - S20.31 Abrasion of front wall of thorax
    - S20.311 Abrasion of right front wall of thorax
    - S20.312 Abrasion of left front wall of thorax
    - S20.319 Abrasion of unspecified front wall of thorax
  - S20.32 Blister (nonthermal) of front wall of thorax
    - S20.321 Blister (nonthermal) of right front wall of thorax
    - S20.322 Blister (nonthermal) of left front wall of thorax
    - S20.329 Blister (nonthermal) of unspecified front wall of thorax
  - S20.34 External constriction of front wall of thorax
    - S20.341 External constriction of right front wall of thorax
    - S20.342 External constriction of left front wall of thorax
    - S20.349 External constriction of unspecified front wall of thorax
  - S20.35 Superficial foreign body of front wall of thorax
    Splinter in front wall of thorax
    - S20.351 Superficial foreign body of right front wall of thorax
    - S20.352 Superficial foreign body of left front wall of thorax
    - S20.359 Superficial foreign body of unspecified front wall of thorax
  - S20.36 Insect bite (nonvenomous) of front wall of thorax
    - S20.361 Insect bite (nonvenomous) of right front wall of thorax
    - S20.362 Insect bite (nonvenomous) of left front wall of thorax
    - S20.369 Insect bite (nonvenomous) of unspecified front wall of thorax
  - S20.37 Other superficial bite of front wall of thorax
    Excludes1 open bite of front wall of thorax (S21.14)
    - S20.371 Other superficial bite of right front wall of thorax
    - S20.372 Other superficial bite of left front wall of thorax
    - S20.379 Other superficial bite of unspecified front wall of thorax
- S20.4 Other and unspecified superficial injuries of back wall of thorax
  - S20.40 Unspecified superficial injuries of back wall of thorax
    - S20.401 Unspecified superficial injuries of right back wall of thorax
    - S20.402 Unspecified superficial injuries of left back wall of thorax
    - S20.409 Unspecified superficial injuries of unspecified back wall of thorax
  - S20.41 Abrasion of back wall of thorax
    - S20.411 Abrasion of right back wall of thorax
    - S20.412 Abrasion of left back wall of thorax
    - S20.419 Abrasion of unspecified back wall of thorax
  - S20.42 Blister (nonthermal) of back wall of thorax
    - S20.421 Blister (nonthermal) of right back wall of thorax
    - S20.422 Blister (nonthermal) of left back wall of thorax
    - S20.429 Blister (nonthermal) of unspecified back wall of thorax
  - S20.44 External constriction of back wall of thorax
    - S20.441 External constriction of right back wall of thorax
    - S20.442 External constriction of left back wall of thorax
    - S20.449 External constriction of unspecified back wall of thorax
  - S20.45 Superficial foreign body of back wall of thorax
    Splinter of back wall of thorax
    - S20.451 Superficial foreign body of right back wall of thorax
    - S20.452 Superficial foreign body of left back wall of thorax
    - S20.459 Superficial foreign body of unspecified back wall of thorax
  - S20.46 Insect bite (nonvenomous) of back wall of thorax
    - S20.461 Insect bite (nonvenomous) of right back wall of thorax
    - S20.462 Insect bite (nonvenomous) of left back wall of thorax
    - S20.469 Insect bite (nonvenomous) of unspecified back wall of thorax
  - S20.47 Other superficial bite of back wall of thorax
    Excludes1 open bite of back wall of thorax (S21.24)
    - S20.471 Other superficial bite of right back wall of thorax
    - S20.472 Other superficial bite of left back wall of thorax
    - S20.479 Other superficial bite of unspecified back wall of thorax
- S20.9 Superficial injury of unspecified parts of thorax
  Excludes1 contusion of thorax NOS (S20.20)
  - X S20.90 Unspecified superficial injury of unspecified parts of thorax
    Superficial injury of thoracic wall NOS
  - X S20.91 Abrasion of unspecified parts of thorax
  - X S20.92 Blister (nonthermal) of unspecified parts of thorax
  - X S20.94 External constriction of unspecified parts of thorax
  - X S20.95 Superficial foreign body of unspecified parts of thorax
    Splinter in thorax NOS
  - X S20.96 Insect bite (nonvenomous) of unspecified parts of thorax
  - X S20.97 Other superficial bite of unspecified parts of thorax
    Excludes1 open bite of thorax NOS (S21.95)

CHAPTER 19 (S00-T88)

Item 19–1 Pneumothorax is a collection of gas (positive air pressure) in the pleural space resulting in the lung collapsing. A tension pneumothorax is life-threatening and is a result of air in the pleural space causing a displacement in the mediastinal structures and cardiopulmonary function compromise. A traumatic pneumothorax results from blunt or penetrating injury that disrupts the parietal/visceral pleura. **Hemothorax** is blood or bloody fluid in the pleural cavity as a result of traumatic blood vessel rupture or inflammation of the lungs from pneumonia.

● S21 Open wound of thorax
Code also any associated injury such as:
injury of heart (S26.-)
injury of intrathoracic organs (S27.-)
rib fracture (S22.3-, S22.4-)
spinal cord injury (S24.0-, S24.1-)
traumatic hemothorax (S27.1)
traumatic hemopneumothorax (S27.3)
traumatic pneumothorax (S27.0)
wound infection
Excludes1 traumatic amputation (partial) of thorax (S28.1)
The appropriate 7th character is to be added to each code from category S21

A	initial encounter
D	subsequent encounter
S	sequela

● S21.0 Open wound of breast
● S21.00 Unspecified open wound of breast
● S21.001 Unspecified open wound of right breast
● S21.002 Unspecified open wound of left breast
● S21.009 Unspecified open wound of unspecified breast
● S21.01 Laceration without foreign body of breast
● S21.011 Laceration without foreign body of right breast
● S21.012 Laceration without foreign body of left breast
● S21.019 Laceration without foreign body of unspecified breast
● S21.02 Laceration with foreign body of breast
● S21.021 Laceration with foreign body of right breast
● S21.022 Laceration with foreign body of left breast
● S21.029 Laceration with foreign body of unspecified breast
● S21.03 Puncture wound without foreign body of breast
● S21.031 Puncture wound without foreign body of right breast
● S21.032 Puncture wound without foreign body of left breast
● S21.039 Puncture wound without foreign body of unspecified breast
● S21.04 Puncture wound with foreign body of breast
● S21.041 Puncture wound with foreign body of right breast
● S21.042 Puncture wound with foreign body of left breast
● S21.049 Puncture wound with foreign body of unspecified breast
● S21.05 Open bite of breast
Bite of breast NOS
Excludes1 superficial bite of breast (S20.17)
● S21.051 Open bite of right breast
● S21.052 Open bite of left breast
● S21.059 Open bite of unspecified breast

● S21.1 Open wound of front wall of thorax without penetration into thoracic cavity
Open wound of chest without penetration into thoracic cavity
● S21.10 Unspecified open wound of front wall of thorax without penetration into thoracic cavity
● S21.101 Unspecified open wound of right front wall of thorax without penetration into thoracic cavity
● S21.102 Unspecified open wound of left front wall of thorax without penetration into thoracic cavity
● S21.109 Unspecified open wound of unspecified front wall of thorax without penetration into thoracic cavity
● S21.11 Laceration without foreign body of front wall of thorax without penetration into thoracic cavity
● S21.111 Laceration without foreign body of right front wall of thorax without penetration into thoracic cavity
● S21.112 Laceration without foreign body of left front wall of thorax without penetration into thoracic cavity
● S21.119 Laceration without foreign body of unspecified front wall of thorax without penetration into thoracic cavity
● S21.12 Laceration with foreign body of front wall of thorax without penetration into thoracic cavity
● S21.121 Laceration with foreign body of right front wall of thorax without penetration into thoracic cavity
● S21.122 Laceration with foreign body of left front wall of thorax without penetration into thoracic cavity
● S21.129 Laceration with foreign body of unspecified front wall of thorax without penetration into thoracic cavity
● S21.13 Puncture wound without foreign body of front wall of thorax without penetration into thoracic cavity
● S21.131 Puncture wound without foreign body of right front wall of thorax without penetration into thoracic cavity
● S21.132 Puncture wound without foreign body of left front wall of thorax without penetration into thoracic cavity
● S21.139 Puncture wound without foreign body of unspecified front wall of thorax without penetration into thoracic cavity
● S21.14 Puncture wound with foreign body of front wall of thorax without penetration into thoracic cavity
● S21.141 Puncture wound with foreign body of right front wall of thorax without penetration into thoracic cavity
● S21.142 Puncture wound with foreign body of left front wall of thorax without penetration into thoracic cavity
● S21.149 Puncture wound with foreign body of unspecified front wall of thorax without penetration into thoracic cavity

● S21.15 Open bite of front wall of thorax without penetration into thoracic cavity
Bite of front wall of thorax NOS
Excludes1 superficial bite of front wall of thorax (S20.37)

● S21.151 Open bite of right front wall of thorax without penetration into thoracic cavity

● S21.152 Open bite of left front wall of thorax without penetration into thoracic cavity

● S21.159 Open bite of unspecified front wall of thorax without penetration into thoracic cavity

● S21.2 Open wound of back wall of thorax without penetration into thoracic cavity

● S21.20 Unspecified open wound of back wall of thorax without penetration into thoracic cavity

● S21.201 Unspecified open wound of right back wall of thorax without penetration into thoracic cavity

● S21.202 Unspecified open wound of left back wall of thorax without penetration into thoracic cavity

● S21.209 Unspecified open wound of unspecified back wall of thorax without penetration into thoracic cavity

● S21.21 Laceration without foreign body of back wall of thorax without penetration into thoracic cavity

● S21.211 Laceration without foreign body of right back wall of thorax without penetration into thoracic cavity

● S21.212 Laceration without foreign body of left back wall of thorax without penetration into thoracic cavity

● S21.219 Laceration without foreign body of unspecified back wall of thorax without penetration into thoracic cavity

● S21.22 Laceration with foreign body of back wall of thorax without penetration into thoracic cavity

● S21.221 Laceration with foreign body of right back wall of thorax without penetration into thoracic cavity

● S21.222 Laceration with foreign body of left back wall of thorax without penetration into thoracic cavity

● S21.229 Laceration with foreign body of unspecified back wall of thorax without penetration into thoracic cavity

● S21.23 Puncture wound without foreign body of back wall of thorax without penetration into thoracic cavity

● S21.231 Puncture wound without foreign body of right back wall of thorax without penetration into thoracic cavity

● S21.232 Puncture wound without foreign body of left back wall of thorax without penetration into thoracic cavity

● S21.239 Puncture wound without foreign body of unspecified back wall of thorax without penetration into thoracic cavity

● S21.24 Puncture wound with foreign body of back wall of thorax without penetration into thoracic cavity

● S21.241 Puncture wound with foreign body of right back wall of thorax without penetration into thoracic cavity

● S21.242 Puncture wound with foreign body of left back wall of thorax without penetration into thoracic cavity

● S21.249 Puncture wound with foreign body of unspecified back wall of thorax without penetration into thoracic cavity

● S21.25 Open bite of back wall of thorax without penetration into thoracic cavity
Bite of back wall of thorax NOS
Excludes1 superficial bite of back wall of thorax (S20.47)

● S21.251 Open bite of right back wall of thorax without penetration into thoracic cavity

● S21.252 Open bite of left back wall of thorax without penetration into thoracic cavity

● S21.259 Open bite of unspecified back wall of thorax without penetration into thoracic cavity

● S21.3 Open wound of front wall of thorax with penetration into thoracic cavity
Open wound of chest with penetration into thoracic cavity

● S21.30 Unspecified open wound of front wall of thorax with penetration into thoracic cavity

● S21.301 Unspecified open wound of right front wall of thorax with penetration into thoracic cavity

● S21.302 Unspecified open wound of left front wall of thorax with penetration into thoracic cavity

● S21.309 Unspecified open wound of unspecified front wall of thorax with penetration into thoracic cavity

● S21.31 Laceration without foreign body of front wall of thorax with penetration into thoracic cavity

● S21.311 Laceration without foreign body of right front wall of thorax with penetration into thoracic cavity

● S21.312 Laceration without foreign body of left front wall of thorax with penetration into thoracic cavity

● S21.319 Laceration without foreign body of unspecified front wall of thorax with penetration into thoracic cavity

● S21.32 Laceration with foreign body of front wall of thorax with penetration into thoracic cavity

● S21.321 Laceration with foreign body of right front wall of thorax with penetration into thoracic cavity

● S21.322 Laceration with foreign body of left front wall of thorax with penetration into thoracic cavity

● S21.329 Laceration with foreign body of unspecified front wall of thorax with penetration into thoracic cavity

● S21.33 Puncture wound without foreign body of front wall of thorax with penetration into thoracic cavity
● S21.331 Puncture wound without foreign body of right front wall of thorax with penetration into thoracic cavity
● S21.332 Puncture wound without foreign body of left front wall of thorax with penetration into thoracic cavity
● S21.339 Puncture wound without foreign body of unspecified front wall of thorax with penetration into thoracic cavity
● S21.34 Puncture wound with foreign body of front wall of thorax with penetration into thoracic cavity
● S21.341 Puncture wound with foreign body of right front wall of thorax with penetration into thoracic cavity
● S21.342 Puncture wound with foreign body of left front wall of thorax with penetration into thoracic cavity
● S21.349 Puncture wound with foreign body of unspecified front wall of thorax with penetration into thoracic cavity
● S21.35 Open bite of front wall of thorax with penetration into thoracic cavity
Excludes1 superficial bite of front wall of thorax (S20.37)
● S21.351 Open bite of right front wall of thorax with penetration into thoracic cavity
● S21.352 Open bite of left front wall of thorax with penetration into thoracic cavity
● S21.359 Open bite of unspecified front wall of thorax with penetration into thoracic cavity
● S21.4 Open wound of back wall of thorax with penetration into thoracic cavity
● S21.40 Unspecified open wound of back wall of thorax with penetration into thoracic cavity
● S21.401 Unspecified open wound of right back wall of thorax with penetration into thoracic cavity
● S21.402 Unspecified open wound of left back wall of thorax with penetration into thoracic cavity
● S21.409 Unspecified open wound of unspecified back wall of thorax with penetration into thoracic cavity
● S21.41 Laceration without foreign body of back wall of thorax with penetration into thoracic cavity
● S21.411 Laceration without foreign body of right back wall of thorax with penetration into thoracic cavity
● S21.412 Laceration without foreign body of left back wall of thorax with penetration into thoracic cavity
● S21.419 Laceration without foreign body of unspecified back wall of thorax with penetration into thoracic cavity
● S21.42 Laceration with foreign body of back wall of thorax with penetration into thoracic cavity
● S21.421 Laceration with foreign body of right back wall of thorax with penetration into thoracic cavity
● S21.422 Laceration with foreign body of left back wall of thorax with penetration into thoracic cavity
● S21.429 Laceration with foreign body of unspecified back wall of thorax with penetration into thoracic cavity
● S21.43 Puncture wound without foreign body of back wall of thorax with penetration into thoracic cavity
● S21.431 Puncture wound without foreign body of right back wall of thorax with penetration into thoracic cavity
● S21.432 Puncture wound without foreign body of left back wall of thorax with penetration into thoracic cavity
● S21.439 Puncture wound without foreign body of unspecified back wall of thorax with penetration into thoracic cavity
● S21.44 Puncture wound with foreign body of back wall of thorax with penetration into thoracic cavity
● S21.441 Puncture wound with foreign body of right back wall of thorax with penetration into thoracic cavity
● S21.442 Puncture wound with foreign body of left back wall of thorax with penetration into thoracic cavity
● S21.449 Puncture wound with foreign body of unspecified back wall of thorax with penetration into thoracic cavity
● S21.45 Open bite of back wall of thorax with penetration into thoracic cavity
Bite of back wall of thorax NOS
Excludes1 superficial bite of back wall of thorax (S20.47)
● S21.451 Open bite of right back wall of thorax with penetration into thoracic cavity
● S21.452 Open bite of left back wall of thorax with penetration into thoracic cavity
● S21.459 Open bite of unspecified back wall of thorax with penetration into thoracic cavity
● S21.9 Open wound of unspecified part of thorax
Open wound of thoracic wall NOS
X● S21.90 Unspecified open wound of unspecified part of thorax
X● S21.91 Laceration without foreign body of unspecified part of thorax
X● S21.92 Laceration with foreign body of unspecified part of thorax
X● S21.93 Puncture wound without foreign body of unspecified part of thorax
X● S21.94 Puncture wound with foreign body of unspecified part of thorax
X● S21.95 Open bite of unspecified part of thorax
Excludes1 superficial bite of thorax (S20.97)

● **S22   Fracture of rib(s), sternum and thoracic spine**

Note: A fracture not indicated as displaced or nondisplaced should be coded to displaced

A fracture not indicated as open or closed should be coded to closed

Includes   fracture of thoracic neural arch
fracture of thoracic spinous process
fracture of thoracic transverse process
fracture of thoracic vertebra
fracture of thoracic vertebral arch

Code first any associated:
injury of intrathoracic organ (S27.-)
spinal cord injury (S24.0-, S24.1-)

Excludes1   transection of thorax (S28.1)
Excludes2   fracture of clavicle (S42.0-)
fracture of scapula (S42.1-)

The appropriate 7th character is to be added to each code from category S22

A   initial encounter for closed fracture
B   initial encounter for open fracture
D   subsequent encounter for fracture with routine healing
G   subsequent encounter for fracture with delayed healing
K   subsequent encounter for fracture with nonunion
S   sequela

● **S22.0   Fracture of thoracic vertebra**

● **S22.00   Fracture of unspecified thoracic vertebra**

● S22.000   Wedge compression fracture of unspecified thoracic vertebra
● S22.001   Stable burst fracture of unspecified thoracic vertebra
● S22.002   Unstable burst fracture of unspecified thoracic vertebra
● S22.008   Other fracture of unspecified thoracic vertebra
● S22.009   Unspecified fracture of unspecified thoracic vertebra

● **S22.01   Fracture of first thoracic vertebra**

● S22.010   Wedge compression fracture of first thoracic vertebra
● S22.011   Stable burst fracture of first thoracic vertebra
● S22.012   Unstable burst fracture of first thoracic vertebra
● S22.018   Other fracture of first thoracic vertebra
● S22.019   Unspecified fracture of first thoracic vertebra

● **S22.02   Fracture of second thoracic vertebra**

● S22.020   Wedge compression fracture of second thoracic vertebra
● S22.021   Stable burst fracture of second thoracic vertebra
● S22.022   Unstable burst fracture of second thoracic vertebra
● S22.028   Other fracture of second thoracic vertebra
● S22.029   Unspecified fracture of second thoracic vertebra

● **S22.03   Fracture of third thoracic vertebra**

● S22.030   Wedge compression fracture of third thoracic vertebra
● S22.031   Stable burst fracture of third thoracic vertebra
● S22.032   Unstable burst fracture of third thoracic vertebra
● S22.038   Other fracture of third thoracic vertebra
● S22.039   Unspecified fracture of third thoracic vertebra

● **S22.04   Fracture of fourth thoracic vertebra**

● S22.040   Wedge compression fracture of fourth thoracic vertebra
● S22.041   Stable burst fracture of fourth thoracic vertebra
● S22.042   Unstable burst fracture of fourth thoracic vertebra
● S22.048   Other fracture of fourth thoracic vertebra
● S22.049   Unspecified fracture of fourth thoracic vertebra

● **S22.05   Fracture of T_5-T_6 vertebra**

● S22.050   Wedge compression fracture of T_5-T_6 vertebra
● S22.051   Stable burst fracture of T_5-T_6 vertebra
● S22.052   Unstable burst fracture of T_5-T_6 vertebra
● S22.058   Other fracture of T_5-T_6 vertebra
● S22.059   Unspecified fracture of T_5-T_6 vertebra

● **S22.06   Fracture of T_7-T_8 vertebra**

● S22.060   Wedge compression fracture of T_7-T_8 vertebra
● S22.061   Stable burst fracture of T_7-T_8 vertebra
● S22.062   Unstable burst fracture of T_7-T_8 vertebra
● S22.068   Other fracture of T_7-T_8 thoracic vertebra
● S22.069   Unspecified fracture of T_7-T_8 vertebra

● **S22.07   Fracture of T_9-T_{10} vertebra**

● S22.070   Wedge compression fracture of T_9-T_{10} vertebra
● S22.071   Stable burst fracture of T_9-T_{10} vertebra
● S22.072   Unstable burst fracture of T_9-T_{10} vertebra
● S22.078   Other fracture of T_9-T_{10} vertebra
● S22.079   Unspecified fracture of T_9-T_{10} vertebra

● **S22.08   Fracture of T_{11}-T_{12} vertebra**

● S22.080   Wedge compression fracture of T_{11}-T_{12} vertebra
● S22.081   Stable burst fracture of T_{11}-T_{12} vertebra
● S22.082   Unstable burst fracture of T_{11}-T_{12} vertebra
● S22.088   Other fracture of T_{11}-T_{12} vertebra
● S22.089   Unspecified fracture of T_{11}-T_{12} vertebra

● **S22.2   Fracture of sternum**

X● S22.20   Unspecified fracture of sternum
X● S22.21   Fracture of manubrium
X● S22.22   Fracture of body of sternum
X● S22.23   Sternal manubrial dissociation
X● S22.24   Fracture of xiphoid process

● **S22.3 Fracture of one rib**

X● S22.31   Fracture of one rib, right side
X● S22.32   Fracture of one rib, left side
X● S22.39   Fracture of one rib, unspecified side

● **S22.4   Multiple fractures of ribs**
Fractures of two or more ribs

Excludes1   flail chest (S22.5-)

X● S22.41   Multiple fractures of ribs, right side
X● S22.42   Multiple fractures of ribs, left side
X● S22.43   Multiple fractures of ribs, bilateral
X● S22.49   Multiple fractures of ribs, unspecified side

X● **S22.5   Flail chest**
Unstable chest due to sternum and/or rib fracture

X● **S22.9   Fracture of bony thorax, part unspecified**

● S23 Dislocation and sprain of joints and ligaments of thorax

Includes avulsion of joint or ligament of thorax
laceration of cartilage, joint or ligament of thorax
sprain of cartilage, joint or ligament of thorax
traumatic hemarthrosis of joint or ligament of thorax
traumatic rupture of joint or ligament of thorax
traumatic subluxation of joint or ligament of thorax
traumatic tear of joint or ligament of thorax

Code also any associated open wound

Excludes2 dislocation, sprain of sternoclavicular joint (S43.2, S43.6)
strain of muscle or tendon of thorax (S29.01-)

The appropriate 7th character is to be added to each code from category S23

A	initial encounter
D	subsequent encounter
S	sequela

X● S23.0 Traumatic rupture of thoracic intervertebral disc

Excludes1 rupture or displacement (nontraumatic) of thoracic intervertebral disc NOS (M51.- with fifth character 4)

● S23.1 Subluxation and dislocation of thoracic vertebra

Code also any associated
open wound of thorax (S21.-)
spinal cord injury (S24.0-, S24.1-)

Excludes2 fracture of thoracic vertebrae (S22.0-)

● S23.10 Subluxation and dislocation of unspecified thoracic vertebra
● S23.100 Subluxation of unspecified thoracic vertebra
● S23.101 Dislocation of unspecified thoracic vertebra
● S23.11 Subluxation and dislocation of T_1/T_2 thoracic vertebra
● S23.110 Subluxation of T_1/T_2 thoracic vertebra
● S23.111 Dislocation of T_1/T_2 thoracic vertebra
● S23.12 Subluxation and dislocation of T_2/T_3-T_3/T_4 thoracic vertebra
● S23.120 Subluxation of T_2/T_3 thoracic vertebra
● S23.121 Dislocation of T_2/T_3 thoracic vertebra
● S23.122 Subluxation of T_3/T_4 thoracic vertebra
● S23.123 Dislocation of T_3/T_4 thoracic vertebra
● S23.13 Subluxation and dislocation of T_4/T_5-T_5/T_6 thoracic vertebra
● S23.130 Subluxation of T_4/T_5 thoracic vertebra
● S23.131 Dislocation of T_4/T_5 thoracic vertebra
● S23.132 Subluxation of T_5/T_6 thoracic vertebra
● S23.133 Dislocation of T_5/T_6 thoracic vertebra
● S23.14 Subluxation and dislocation of T_6/T_7-T_7/T_8 thoracic vertebra
● S23.140 Subluxation of T_6/T_7 thoracic vertebra
● S23.141 Dislocation of T_6/T_7 thoracic vertebra
● S23.142 Subluxation of T_7/T_8 thoracic vertebra
● S23.143 Dislocation of T_7/T_8 thoracic vertebra
● S23.15 Subluxation and dislocation of T_8/T_9-T_9/T_{10} thoracic vertebra
● S23.150 Subluxation of T_8/T_9 thoracic vertebra
● S23.151 Dislocation of T_8/T_9 thoracic vertebra
● S23.152 Subluxation of T_9/T_{10} thoracic vertebra
● S23.153 Dislocation of T_9/T_{10} thoracic vertebra
● S23.16 Subluxation and dislocation of T_{10}/T_{11}-T_{11}/T_{12} thoracic vertebra
● S23.160 Subluxation of T_{10}/T_{11} thoracic vertebra
● S23.161 Dislocation of T_{10}/T_{11} thoracic vertebra
● S23.162 Subluxation of T_{11}/T_{12} thoracic vertebra
● S23.163 Dislocation of T_{11}/T_{12} thoracic vertebra
● S23.17 Subluxation and dislocation of T_{12}/L_1 thoracic vertebra
● S23.170 Subluxation of T_{12}/L_1 thoracic vertebra
● S23.171 Dislocation of T_{12}/L_1 thoracic vertebra

● S23.2 Dislocation of other and unspecified parts of thorax
X● S23.20 Dislocation of unspecified part of thorax
X● S23.29 Dislocation of other parts of thorax

X● S23.3 Sprain of ligaments of thoracic spine

● S23.4 Sprain of ribs and sternum
X● S23.41 Sprain of ribs
● S23.42 Sprain of sternum
● S23.420 Sprain of sternoclavicular (joint) (ligament)
● S23.421 Sprain of chondrosternal joint
● S23.428 Other sprain of sternum
● S23.429 Unspecified sprain of sternum

X● S23.8 Sprain of other specified parts of thorax

X● S23.9 Sprain of unspecified parts of thorax

● S24 Injury of nerves and spinal cord at thorax level

Note: Code to highest level of thoracic spinal cord injury.
Injuries to the spinal cord (S24.0 and S24.1) refer to the cord level and not bone level injury, and can affect nerve roots at and below the level given.

Code also any associated:
fracture of thoracic vertebra (S22.0-)
open wound of thorax (S21.-)
transient paralysis (R29.5)

Excludes2 injury of brachial plexus (S14.3)

The appropriate 7th character is to be added to each code from category S24

A	initial encounter
D	subsequent encounter
S	sequela

X● S24.0 Concussion and edema of thoracic spinal cord

● S24.1 Other and unspecified injuries of thoracic spinal cord
● S24.10 Unspecified injury of thoracic spinal cord
● S24.101 Unspecified injury at T_1 level of thoracic spinal cord
● S24.102 Unspecified injury at T_2-T_6 level of thoracic spinal cord
● S24.103 Unspecified injury at T_7-T_{10} level of thoracic spinal cord
● S24.104 Unspecified injury at T_{11}-T_{12} level of thoracic spinal cord
● S24.109 Unspecified injury at unspecified level of thoracic spinal cord
Injury of thoracic spinal cord NOS
● S24.11 Complete lesion of thoracic spinal cord
● S24.111 Complete lesion at T_1 level of thoracic spinal cord
● S24.112 Complete lesion at T_2-T_6 level of thoracic spinal cord
● S24.113 Complete lesion at T_7-T_{10} level of thoracic spinal cord
● S24.114 Complete lesion at T_{11}-T_{12} level of thoracic spinal cord
● S24.119 Complete lesion at unspecified level of thoracic spinal cord

CHAPTER 19 (S00-T88)

◀ New ◀ Revised ~~deleted~~ Deleted OGCR Official Guidelines X Assign placeholder X ● Use Additional Character(s)
Excludes 1 Excludes 2 Includes Use additional Code first Code also Unspecified

● **S24.13 Anterior cord syndrome of thoracic spinal cord**
- ● **S24.131 Anterior cord syndrome at T_1 level of thoracic spinal cord**
- ● **S24.132 Anterior cord syndrome at T_2-T_6 level of thoracic spinal cord**
- ● **S24.133 Anterior cord syndrome at T_7-T_{10} level of thoracic spinal cord**
- ● **S24.134 Anterior cord syndrome at T_{11}-T_{12} level of thoracic spinal cord**
- ● **S24.139 Anterior cord syndrome at unspecified level of thoracic spinal cord**

● **S24.14 Brown-Séquard syndrome of thoracic spinal cord**
- ● **S24.141 Brown-Séquard syndrome at T_1 level of thoracic spinal cord**
- ● **S24.142 Brown-Séquard syndrome at T_2-T_6 level of thoracic spinal cord**
- ● **S24.143 Brown-Séquard syndrome at T_7-T_{10} level of thoracic spinal cord**
- ● **S24.144 Brown-Séquard syndrome at T_{11}-T_{12} level of thoracic spinal cord**
- ● **S24.149 Brown-Séquard syndrome at unspecified level of thoracic spinal cord**

● **S24.15 Other incomplete lesions of thoracic spinal cord**
Incomplete lesion of thoracic spinal cord NOS
Posterior cord syndrome of thoracic spinal cord
- ● **S24.151 Other incomplete lesion at T_1 level of thoracic spinal cord**
- ● **S24.152 Other incomplete lesion at T_2-T_6 level of thoracic spinal cord**
- ● **S24.153 Other incomplete lesion at T_7-T_{10} level of thoracic spinal cord**
- ● **S24.154 Other incomplete lesion at T_{11}-T_{12} level of thoracic spinal cord**
- ● **S24.159 Other incomplete lesion at unspecified level of thoracic spinal cord**

X● **S24.2 Injury of nerve root of thoracic spine**
X● **S24.3 Injury of peripheral nerves of thorax**
X● **S24.4 Injury of thoracic sympathetic nervous system**
Injury of cardiac plexus
Injury of esophageal plexus
Injury of pulmonary plexus
Injury of stellate ganglion
Injury of thoracic sympathetic ganglion
X● **S24.8 Injury of other specified nerves of thorax**
X● **S24.9 Injury of unspecified nerve of thorax**

● **S25 Injury of blood vessels of thorax**
The appropriate 7th character is to be added to each code from category S25
A	initial encounter
D	subsequent encounter
S	sequela

Code also any associated open wound (S21.-)

● **S25.0 Injury of thoracic aorta**
Injury of aorta NOS
- X● **S25.00 Unspecified injury of thoracic aorta**
- X● **S25.01 Minor laceration of thoracic aorta**
Incomplete transection of thoracic aorta
Laceration of thoracic aorta NOS
Superficial laceration of thoracic aorta
- X● **S25.02 Major laceration of thoracic aorta**
Complete transection of thoracic aorta
Traumatic rupture of thoracic aorta
- X● **S25.09 Other specified injury of thoracic aorta**

● **S25.1 Injury of innominate or subclavian artery**
- ● **S25.10 Unspecified injury of innominate or subclavian artery**
  - ● **S25.101 Unspecified injury of right innominate or subclavian artery**
  - ● **S25.102 Unspecified injury of left innominate or subclavian artery**
  - ● **S25.109 Unspecified injury of unspecified innominate or subclavian artery**
- ● **S25.11 Minor laceration of innominate or subclavian artery**
Incomplete transection of innominate or subclavian artery
Laceration of innominate or subclavian artery NOS
Superficial laceration of innominate or subclavian artery
  - ● **S25.111 Minor laceration of right innominate or subclavian artery**
  - ● **S25.112 Minor laceration of left innominate or subclavian artery**
  - ● **S25.119 Minor laceration of unspecified innominate or subclavian artery**
- ● **S25.12 Major laceration of innominate or subclavian artery**
Complete transection of innominate or subclavian artery
Traumatic rupture of innominate or subclavian artery
  - ● **S25.121 Major laceration of right innominate or subclavian artery**
  - ● **S25.122 Major laceration of left innominate or subclavian artery**
  - ● **S25.129 Major laceration of unspecified innominate or subclavian artery**
- ● **S25.19 Other specified injury of innominate or subclavian artery**
  - ● **S25.191 Other specified injury of right innominate or subclavian artery**
  - ● **S25.192 Other specified injury of left innominate or subclavian artery**
  - ● **S25.199 Other specified injury of unspecified innominate or subclavian artery**

● **S25.2 Injury of superior vena cava**
Injury of vena cava NOS
- X● **S25.20 Unspecified injury of superior vena cava**
- X● **S25.21 Minor laceration of superior vena cava**
Incomplete transection of superior vena cava
Laceration of superior vena cava NOS
Superficial laceration of superior vena cava
- X● **S25.22 Major laceration of superior vena cava**
Complete transection of superior vena cava
Traumatic rupture of superior vena cava
- X● **S25.29 Other specified injury of superior vena cava**

● **S25.3 Injury of innominate or subclavian vein**
- ● **S25.30 Unspecified injury of innominate or subclavian vein**
  - ● **S25.301 Unspecified injury of right innominate or subclavian vein**
  - ● **S25.302 Unspecified injury of left innominate or subclavian vein**
  - ● **S25.309 Unspecified injury of unspecified innominate or subclavian vein**

● S25.31 Minor laceration of innominate or subclavian vein
Incomplete transection of innominate or subclavian vein
Laceration of innominate or subclavian vein NOS
Superficial laceration of innominate or subclavian vein
● S25.311 Minor laceration of right innominate or subclavian vein
● S25.312 Minor laceration of left innominate or subclavian vein
● S25.319 Minor laceration of unspecified innominate or subclavian vein
● S25.32 Major laceration of innominate or subclavian vein
Complete transection of innominate or subclavian vein
Traumatic rupture of innominate or subclavian vein
● S25.321 Major laceration of right innominate or subclavian vein
● S25.322 Major laceration of left innominate or subclavian vein
● S25.329 Major laceration of unspecified innominate or subclavian vein
● S25.39 Other specified injury of innominate or subclavian vein
● S25.391 Other specified injury of right innominate or subclavian vein
● S25.392 Other specified injury of left innominate or subclavian vein
● S25.399 Other specified injury of unspecified innominate or subclavian vein
● S25.4 Injury of pulmonary blood vessels
● S25.40 Unspecified injury of pulmonary blood vessels
● S25.401 Unspecified injury of right pulmonary blood vessels
● S25.402 Unspecified injury of left pulmonary blood vessels
● S25.409 Unspecified injury of unspecified pulmonary blood vessels
● S25.41 Minor laceration of pulmonary blood vessels
Incomplete transection of pulmonary blood vessels
Laceration of pulmonary blood vessels NOS
Superficial laceration of pulmonary blood vessels
● S25.411 Minor laceration of right pulmonary blood vessels
● S25.412 Minor laceration of left pulmonary blood vessels
● S25.419 Minor laceration of unspecified pulmonary blood vessels
● S25.42 Major laceration of pulmonary blood vessels
Complete transection of pulmonary blood vessels
Traumatic rupture of pulmonary blood vessels
● S25.421 Major laceration of right pulmonary blood vessels
● S25.422 Major laceration of left pulmonary blood vessels
● S25.429 Major laceration of unspecified pulmonary blood vessels
● S25.49 Other specified injury of pulmonary blood vessels
● S25.491 Other specified injury of right pulmonary blood vessels
● S25.492 Other specified injury of left pulmonary blood vessels
● S25.499 Other specified injury of unspecified pulmonary blood vessels
● S25.5 Injury of intercostal blood vessels
● S25.50 Unspecified injury of intercostal blood vessels
● S25.501 Unspecified injury of intercostal blood vessels, right side
● S25.502 Unspecified injury of intercostal blood vessels, left side
● S25.509 Unspecified injury of intercostal blood vessels, unspecified side
● S25.51 Laceration of intercostal blood vessels
● S25.511 Laceration of intercostal blood vessels, right side
● S25.512 Laceration of intercostal blood vessels, left side
● S25.519 Laceration of intercostal blood vessels, unspecified side
● S25.59 Other specified injury of intercostal blood vessels
● S25.591 Other specified injury of intercostal blood vessels, right side
● S25.592 Other specified injury of intercostal blood vessels, left side
● S25.599 Other specified injury of intercostal blood vessels, unspecified side
● S25.8 Injury of other blood vessels of thorax
Injury of azygos vein
Injury of mammary artery or vein
● S25.80 Unspecified injury of other blood vessels of thorax
● S25.801 Unspecified injury of other blood vessels of thorax, right side
● S25.802 Unspecified injury of other blood vessels of thorax, left side
● S25.809 Unspecified injury of other blood vessels of thorax, unspecified side
● S25.81 Laceration of other blood vessels of thorax
● S25.811 Laceration of other blood vessels of thorax, right side
● S25.812 Laceration of other blood vessels of thorax, left side
● S25.819 Laceration of other blood vessels of thorax, unspecified side
● S25.89 Other specified injury of other blood vessels of thorax
● S25.891 Other specified injury of other blood vessels of thorax, right side
● S25.892 Other specified injury of other blood vessels of thorax, left side
● S25.899 Other specified injury of other blood vessels of thorax, unspecified side
● S25.9 Injury of unspecified blood vessel of thorax
X● S25.90 Unspecified injury of unspecified blood vessel of thorax
X● S25.91 Laceration of unspecified blood vessel of thorax
X● S25.99 Other specified injury of unspecified blood vessel of thorax

Item 19–2 Pneumothorax is a collection of gas (positive air pressure) in the pleural space resulting in the lung collapsing. A tension pneumothorax is life-threatening and is a result of air in the pleural space causing a displacement in the mediastinal structures and cardiopulmonary function compromise. A traumatic pneumothorax results from blunt or penetrating injury that disrupts the parietal/visceral pleura. **Hemothorax** is blood or bloody fluid in the pleural cavity as a result of traumatic blood vessel rupture or inflammation of the lungs from pneumonia.

● **S26 Injury of heart**

The appropriate 7th character is to be added to each code from category S26

A initial encounter
D subsequent encounter
S sequela

Code also any associated:
open wound of thorax (S21.-)
traumatic hemopneumothorax (S27.2)
traumatic hemothorax (S27.1)
traumatic pneumothorax (S27.Ø)

● **S26.Ø Injury of heart with hemopericardium**
Hemopericardium: effusion of blood within pericardium
X● **S26.ØØ Unspecified injury of heart with hemopericardium**
X● **S26.Ø1 Contusion of heart with hemopericardium**
● **S26.Ø2 Laceration of heart with hemopericardium**
● **S26.Ø2Ø Mild laceration of heart with hemopericardium**
Laceration of heart without penetration of heart chamber
● **S26.Ø21 Moderate laceration of heart with hemopericardium**
Laceration of heart with penetration of heart chamber
● **S26.Ø22 Major laceration of heart with hemopericardium**
Laceration of heart with penetration of multiple heart chambers
X● **S26.Ø9 Other injury of heart with hemopericardium**

● **S26.1 Injury of heart without hemopericardium**
Hemopericardium: effusion of blood within pericardium
X● **S26.1Ø Unspecified injury of heart without hemopericardium**
X● **S26.11 Contusion of heart without hemopericardium**
X● **S26.12 Laceration of heart without hemopericardium**
X● **S26.19 Other injury of heart without hemopericardium**

● **S26.9 Injury of heart, unspecified with or without hemopericardium**
Hemopericardium: effusion of blood within pericardium
X● **S26.9Ø Unspecified injury of heart, unspecified with or without hemopericardium**
X● **S26.91 Contusion of heart, unspecified with or without hemopericardium**
X● **S26.92 Laceration of heart, unspecified with or without hemopericardium**
Laceration of heart NOS
X● **S26.99 Other injury of heart, unspecified with or without hemopericardium**

● **S27 Injury of other and unspecified intrathoracic organs**

Code also any associated open wound of thorax (S21.-)

Excludes2 injury of cervical esophagus (S1Ø-S19)
injury of trachea (cervical) (S1Ø-S19)

The appropriate 7th character is to be added to each code from category S27

A initial encounter
D subsequent encounter
S sequela

X● **S27.Ø Traumatic pneumothorax**
Excludes1 spontaneous pneumothorax (J93.-)
X● **S27.1 Traumatic hemothorax**
X● **S27.2 Traumatic hemopneumothorax**
● **S27.3 Other and unspecified injuries of lung**
● **S27.3Ø Unspecified injury of lung**
● **S27.3Ø1 Unspecified injury of lung, unilateral**
● **S27.3Ø2 Unspecified injury of lung, bilateral**
● **S27.3Ø9 Unspecified injury of lung, unspecified**
● **S27.31 Primary blast injury of lung**
Blast injury of lung NOS
● **S27.311 Primary blast injury of lung, unilateral**
● **S27.312 Primary blast injury of lung, bilateral**
● **S27.319 Primary blast injury of lung, unspecified**
● **S27.32 Contusion of lung**
● **S27.321 Contusion of lung, unilateral**
● **S27.322 Contusion of lung, bilateral**
● **S27.329 Contusion of lung, unspecified**
● **S27.33 Laceration of lung**
● **S27.331 Laceration of lung, unilateral**
● **S27.332 Laceration of lung, bilateral**
● **S27.339 Laceration of lung, unspecified**
● **S27.39 Other injuries of lung**
Secondary blast injury of lung
● **S27.391 Other injuries of lung, unilateral**
● **S27.392 Other injuries of lung, bilateral**
● **S27.399 Other injuries of lung, unspecified**
● **S27.4 Injury of bronchus**
● **S27.4Ø Unspecified injury of bronchus**
● **S27.4Ø1 Unspecified injury of bronchus, unilateral**
● **S27.4Ø2 Unspecified injury of bronchus, bilateral**
● **S27.4Ø9 Unspecified injury of bronchus, unspecified**
● **S27.41 Primary blast injury of bronchus**
Blast injury of bronchus NOS
● **S27.411 Primary blast injury of bronchus, unilateral**
● **S27.412 Primary blast injury of bronchus, bilateral**
● **S27.419 Primary blast injury of bronchus, unspecified**

CHAPTER 19 (SØØ-T88)

S27.42 Contusion of bronchus
S27.421 Contusion of bronchus, unilateral
S27.422 Contusion of bronchus, bilateral
S27.429 Contusion of bronchus, unspecified
S27.43 Laceration of bronchus
S27.431 Laceration of bronchus, unilateral
S27.432 Laceration of bronchus, bilateral
S27.439 Laceration of bronchus, unspecified
S27.49 Other injury of bronchus
Secondary blast injury of bronchus
S27.491 Other injury of bronchus, unilateral
S27.492 Other injury of bronchus, bilateral
S27.499 Other injury of bronchus, unspecified
S27.5 Injury of thoracic trachea
X S27.5Ø Unspecified injury of thoracic trachea
X S27.51 Primary blast injury of thoracic trachea
Blast injury of thoracic trachea NOS
X S27.52 Contusion of thoracic trachea
X S27.53 Laceration of thoracic trachea
X S27.59 Other injury of thoracic trachea
Secondary blast injury of thoracic trachea
S27.6 Injury of pleura
X S27.6Ø Unspecified injury of pleura
X S27.63 Laceration of pleura
X S27.69 Other injury of pleura
S27.8 Injury of other specified intrathoracic organs
S27.8Ø Injury of diaphragm
S27.8Ø2 Contusion of diaphragm
S27.8Ø3 Laceration of diaphragm
S27.8Ø8 Other injury of diaphragm
S27.8Ø9 Unspecified injury of diaphragm
S27.81 Injury of esophagus (thoracic part)
S27.812 Contusion of esophagus (thoracic part)
S27.813 Laceration of esophagus (thoracic part)
S27.818 Other injury of esophagus (thoracic part)
S27.819 Unspecified injury of esophagus (thoracic part)
S27.89 Injury of other specified intrathoracic organs
Injury of lymphatic thoracic duct
Injury of thymus gland
S27.892 Contusion of other specified intrathoracic organs
S27.893 Laceration of other specified intrathoracic organs
S27.898 Other injury of other specified intrathoracic organs
S27.899 Unspecified injury of other specified intrathoracic organs
X S27.9 Injury of unspecified intrathoracic organ
S28 Crushing injury of thorax, and traumatic amputation of part of thorax
The appropriate 7th character is to be added to each code from category S28

A	initial encounter
D	subsequent encounter
S	sequela

X S28.Ø Crushed chest
Use additional code for all associated injuries
Excludes1 flail chest (S22.5)
X S28.1 Traumatic amputation (partial) of part of thorax, except breast
S28.2 Traumatic amputation of breast
S28.21 Complete traumatic amputation of breast
Traumatic amputation of breast NOS
S28.211 Complete traumatic amputation of right breast
S28.212 Complete traumatic amputation of left breast
S28.219 Complete traumatic amputation of unspecified breast
S28.22 Partial traumatic amputation of breast
S28.221 Partial traumatic amputation of right breast
S28.222 Partial traumatic amputation of left breast
S28.229 Partial traumatic amputation of unspecified breast
S29 Other and unspecified injuries of thorax
Code also any associated open wound (S21.-)
The appropriate 7th character is to be added to each code from category S29

A	initial encounter
D	subsequent encounter
S	sequela

S29.Ø Injury of muscle and tendon at thorax level
S29.ØØ Unspecified injury of muscle and tendon of thorax
S29.ØØ1 Unspecified injury of muscle and tendon of front wall of thorax
S29.ØØ2 Unspecified injury of muscle and tendon of back wall of thorax
S29.ØØ9 Unspecified injury of muscle and tendon of unspecified wall of thorax
S29.Ø1 Strain of muscle and tendon of thorax
S29.Ø11 Strain of muscle and tendon of front wall of thorax
S29.Ø12 Strain of muscle and tendon of back wall of thorax
S29.Ø19 Strain of muscle and tendon of unspecified wall of thorax
S29.Ø2 Laceration of muscle and tendon of thorax
S29.Ø21 Laceration of muscle and tendon of front wall of thorax
S29.Ø22 Laceration of muscle and tendon of back wall of thorax
S29.Ø29 Laceration of muscle and tendon of unspecified wall of thorax
S29.Ø9 Other injury of muscle and tendon of thorax
S29.Ø91 Other injury of muscle and tendon of front wall of thorax
S29.Ø92 Other injury of muscle and tendon of back wall of thorax
S29.Ø99 Other injury of muscle and tendon of unspecified wall of thorax
X S29.8 Other specified injuries of thorax
X S29.9 Unspecified injury of thorax

CHAPTER 19 (SØØ-T88)

INJURIES TO THE ABDOMEN, LOWER BACK, LUMBAR SPINE PELVIS AND EXTERNAL GENITALS (S30-S39)

Includes injuries to the abdominal wall
injuries to the anus
injuries to the buttock
injuries to the external genitalia
injuries to the flank
injuries to the groin

Excludes2 burns and corrosions (T20-T32)
effects of foreign body in anus and rectum (T18.5)
effects of foreign body in genitourinary tract (T19.-)
effects of foreign body in stomach, small intestine and colon (T18.2-T18.4)
frostbite (T33-T34)
insect bite or sting, venomous (T63.4)

● **S30 Superficial injury of abdomen, lower back, pelvis and external genitals**
Excludes2 superficial injury of hip (S70.-)
The appropriate 7th character is to be added to each code from category S30

A	initial encounter
D	subsequent encounter
S	sequela

X● **S30.0 Contusion of lower back and pelvis**
Contusion of buttock
X● **S30.1 Contusion of abdominal wall**
Contusion of flank
Contusion of groin
● **S30.2 Contusion of external genital organs**
● **S30.20 Contusion of unspecified external genital organ**
● **S30.201 Contusion of unspecified external genital organ, male**
● **S30.202 Contusion of unspecified external genital organ, female**
X● **S30.21 Contusion of penis**
X● **S30.22 Contusion of scrotum and testes**
X● **S30.23 Contusion of vagina and vulva**
X● **S30.3 Contusion of anus**
● **S30.8 Other superficial injuries of abdomen, lower back, pelvis and external genitals**
● **S30.81 Abrasion of abdomen, lower back, pelvis and external genitals**
● **S30.810 Abrasion of lower back and pelvis**
● **S30.811 Abrasion of abdominal wall**
● **S30.812 Abrasion of penis**
● **S30.813 Abrasion of scrotum and testes**
● **S30.814 Abrasion of vagina and vulva**
● **S30.815 Abrasion of unspecified external genital organs, male**
● **S30.816 Abrasion of unspecified external genital organs, female**
● **S30.817 Abrasion of anus**
● **S30.82 Blister (nonthermal) of abdomen, lower back, pelvis and external genitals**
● **S30.820 Blister (nonthermal) of lower back and pelvis**
● **S30.821 Blister (nonthermal) of abdominal wall**
● **S30.822 Blister (nonthermal) of penis**
● **S30.823 Blister (nonthermal) of scrotum and testes**
● **S30.824 Blister (nonthermal) of vagina and vulva**
● **S30.825 Blister (nonthermal) of unspecified external genital organs, male**
● **S30.826 Blister (nonthermal) of unspecified external genital organs, female**
● **S30.827 Blister (nonthermal) of anus**
● **S30.84 External constriction of abdomen, lower back, pelvis and external genitals**
● **S30.840 External constriction of lower back and pelvis**
● **S30.841 External constriction of abdominal wall**
● **S30.842 External constriction of penis**
Hair tourniquet syndrome of penis
Use additional cause code to identify the constricting item (W49.0-)
● **S30.843 External constriction of scrotum and testes**
● **S30.844 External constriction of vagina and vulva**
● **S30.845 External constriction of unspecified external genital organs, male**
● **S30.846 External constriction of unspecified external genital organs, female**
● **S30.85 Superficial foreign body of abdomen, lower back, pelvis and external genitals**
Splinter in the abdomen, lower back, pelvis and external genitals
● **S30.850 Superficial foreign body of lower back and pelvis**
● **S30.851 Superficial foreign body of abdominal wall**
● **S30.852 Superficial foreign body of penis**
● **S30.853 Superficial foreign body of scrotum and testes**
● **S30.854 Superficial foreign body of vagina and vulva**
● **S30.855 Superficial foreign body of unspecified external genital organs, male**
● **S30.856 Superficial foreign body of unspecified external genital organs, female**
● **S30.857 Superficial foreign body of anus**
● **S30.86 Insect bite (nonvenomous) of abdomen, lower back, pelvis and external genitals**
● **S30.860 Insect bite (nonvenomous) of lower back and pelvis**
● **S30.861 Insect bite (nonvenomous) of abdominal wall**
● **S30.862 Insect bite (nonvenomous) of penis**
● **S30.863 Insect bite (nonvenomous) of scrotum and testes**
● **S30.864 Insect bite (nonvenomous) of vagina and vulva**
● **S30.865 Insect bite (nonvenomous) of unspecified external genital organs, male**
● **S30.866 Insect bite (nonvenomous) of unspecified external genital organs, female**
● **S30.867 Insect bite (nonvenomous) of anus**

CHAPTER 19 (S00-T88)

● S30.87 **Other superficial bite of abdomen, lower back, pelvis and external genitals**
Excludes1 open bite of abdomen, lower back, pelvis and external genitals (S31.05, S31.15, S31.25, S31.35, S31.45, S31.55)

● S30.870 **Other superficial bite of lower back and pelvis**
● S30.871 **Other superficial bite of abdominal wall**
● S30.872 **Other superficial bite of penis**
● S30.873 **Other superficial bite of scrotum and testes**
● S30.874 **Other superficial bite of vagina and vulva**
● S30.875 **Other superficial bite of unspecified external genital organs, male**
● S30.876 **Other superficial bite of unspecified external genital organs, female**
● S30.877 **Other superficial bite of anus**

● S30.9 **Unspecified superficial injury of abdomen, lower back, pelvis and external genitals**
X● S30.91 **Unspecified superficial injury of lower back and pelvis**
X● S30.92 **Unspecified superficial injury of abdominal wall**
X● S30.93 **Unspecified superficial injury of penis**
X● S30.94 **Unspecified superficial injury of scrotum and testes**
X● S30.95 **Unspecified superficial injury of vagina and vulva**
X● S30.96 **Unspecified superficial injury of unspecified external genital organs, male**
X● S30.97 **Unspecified superficial injury of unspecified external genital organs, female**
X● S30.98 **Unspecified superficial injury of anus**

● S31 **Open wound of abdomen, lower back, pelvis and external genitals**
Code also any associated:
spinal cord injury (S24.0, S24.1-, S34.0-, S34.1-)
wound infection
Excludes1 traumatic amputation of part of abdomen, lower back and pelvis (S38.2-, S38.3)
Excludes2 open wound of hip (S71.00-S71.02)
open fracture of pelvis (S32.1--S32.9 with 7th character B)

The appropriate 7th character is to be added to each code from category S31

A	initial encounter
D	subsequent encounter
S	sequela

● S31.0 **Open wound of lower back and pelvis**
● S31.00 **Unspecified open wound of lower back and pelvis**
● S31.000 **Unspecified open wound of lower back and pelvis without penetration into retroperitoneum**
Unspecified open wound of lower back and pelvis NOS
● S31.001 **Unspecified open wound of lower back and pelvis with penetration into retroperitoneum**

● S31.01 **Laceration without foreign body of lower back and pelvis**
● S31.010 **Laceration without foreign body of lower back and pelvis without penetration into retroperitoneum**
Laceration without foreign body of lower back and pelvis NOS
● S31.011 **Laceration without foreign body of lower back and pelvis with penetration into retroperitoneum**

● S31.02 **Laceration with foreign body of lower back and pelvis**
● S31.020 **Laceration with foreign body of lower back and pelvis without penetration into retroperitoneum**
Laceration with foreign body of lower back and pelvis NOS
● S31.021 **Laceration with foreign body of lower back and pelvis with penetration into retroperitoneum**

● S31.03 **Puncture wound without foreign body of lower back and pelvis**
● S31.030 **Puncture wound without foreign body of lower back and pelvis without penetration into retroperitoneum**
Puncture wound without foreign body of lower back and pelvis NOS
● S31.031 **Puncture wound without foreign body of lower back and pelvis with penetration into retroperitoneum**

● S31.04 **Puncture wound with foreign body of lower back and pelvis**
● S31.040 **Puncture wound with foreign body of lower back and pelvis without penetration into retroperitoneum**
Puncture wound with foreign body of lower back and pelvis NOS
● S31.041 **Puncture wound with foreign body of lower back and pelvis with penetration into retroperitoneum**

● S31.05 **Open bite of lower back and pelvis**
Bite of lower back and pelvis NOS
Excludes1 superficial bite of lower back and pelvis (S30.860, S30.870)
● S31.050 **Open bite of lower back and pelvis without penetration into retroperitoneum**
Open bite of lower back and pelvis NOS
● S31.051 **Open bite of lower back and pelvis with penetration into retroperitoneum**

● S31.1 **Open wound of abdominal wall without penetration into peritoneal cavity**
Open wound of abdominal wall NOS
Excludes2 open wound of abdominal wall with penetration into peritoneal cavity (S31.6-)
● S31.10 **Unspecified open wound of abdominal wall without penetration into peritoneal cavity**
● S31.100 **Unspecified open wound of abdominal wall, right upper quadrant without penetration into peritoneal cavity**
● S31.101 **Unspecified open wound of abdominal wall, left upper quadrant without penetration into peritoneal cavity**

CHAPTER 19 (S00-T88)

S31.1Ø2 Unspecified open wound of abdominal wall, epigastric region without penetration into peritoneal cavity

S31.1Ø3 Unspecified open wound of abdominal wall, right lower quadrant without penetration into peritoneal cavity

S31.1Ø4 Unspecified open wound of abdominal wall, left lower quadrant without penetration into peritoneal cavity

S31.1Ø5 Unspecified open wound of abdominal wall, periumbilic region without penetration into peritoneal cavity

S31.1Ø9 Unspecified open wound of abdominal wall, unspecified quadrant without penetration into peritoneal cavity

Unspecified open wound of abdominal wall NOS

S31.11 Laceration without foreign body of abdominal wall without penetration into peritoneal cavity

S31.11Ø Laceration without foreign body of abdominal wall, right upper quadrant without penetration into peritoneal cavity

S31.111 Laceration without foreign body of abdominal wall, left upper quadrant without penetration into peritoneal cavity

S31.112 Laceration without foreign body of abdominal wall, epigastric region without penetration into peritoneal cavity

S31.113 Laceration without foreign body of abdominal wall, right lower quadrant without penetration into peritoneal cavity

S31.114 Laceration without foreign body of abdominal wall, left lower quadrant without penetration into peritoneal cavity

S31.115 Laceration without foreign body of abdominal wall, periumbilic region without penetration into peritoneal cavity

S31.119 Laceration without foreign body of abdominal wall, unspecified quadrant without penetration into peritoneal cavity

S31.12 Laceration with foreign body of abdominal wall without penetration into peritoneal cavity

S31.12Ø Laceration of abdominal wall with foreign body, right upper quadrant without penetration into peritoneal cavity

S31.121 Laceration of abdominal wall with foreign body, left upper quadrant without penetration into peritoneal cavity

S31.122 Laceration of abdominal wall with foreign body, epigastric region without penetration into peritoneal cavity

S31.123 Laceration of abdominal wall with foreign body, right lower quadrant without penetration into peritoneal cavity

S31.124 Laceration of abdominal wall with foreign body, left lower quadrant without penetration into peritoneal cavity

S31.125 Laceration of abdominal wall with foreign body, periumbilic region without penetration into peritoneal cavity

S31.129 Laceration of abdominal wall with foreign body, unspecified quadrant without penetration into peritoneal cavity

S31.13 Puncture wound of abdominal wall without foreign body without penetration into peritoneal cavity

S31.13Ø Puncture wound of abdominal wall without foreign body, right upper quadrant without penetration into peritoneal cavity

S31.131 Puncture wound of abdominal wall without foreign body, left upper quadrant without penetration into peritoneal cavity

S31.132 Puncture wound of abdominal wall without foreign body, epigastric region without penetration into peritoneal cavity

S31.133 Puncture wound of abdominal wall without foreign body, right lower quadrant without penetration into peritoneal cavity

S31.134 Puncture wound of abdominal wall without foreign body, left lower quadrant without penetration into peritoneal cavity

S31.135 Puncture wound of abdominal wall without foreign body, periumbilic region without penetration into peritoneal cavity

S31.139 Puncture wound of abdominal wall without foreign body, unspecified quadrant without penetration into peritoneal cavity

S31.14 Puncture wound of abdominal wall with foreign body without penetration into peritoneal cavity

S31.14Ø Puncture wound of abdominal wall with foreign body, right upper quadrant without penetration into peritoneal cavity

S31.141 Puncture wound of abdominal wall with foreign body, left upper quadrant without penetration into peritoneal cavity

S31.142 Puncture wound of abdominal wall with foreign body, epigastric region without penetration into peritoneal cavity

S31.143 Puncture wound of abdominal wall with foreign body, right lower quadrant without penetration into peritoneal cavity

S31.144 Puncture wound of abdominal wall with foreign body, left lower quadrant without penetration into peritoneal cavity

S31.145 Puncture wound of abdominal wall with foreign body, periumbilic region without penetration into peritoneal cavity

S31.149 Puncture wound of abdominal wall with foreign body, unspecified quadrant without penetration into peritoneal cavity

● S31.15 Open bite of abdominal wall without penetration into peritoneal cavity
Bite of abdominal wall NOS
Excludes1 superficial bite of abdominal wall (S30.871)
● S31.150 Open bite of abdominal wall, right upper quadrant without penetration into peritoneal cavity
● S31.151 Open bite of abdominal wall, left upper quadrant without penetration into peritoneal cavity
● S31.152 Open bite of abdominal wall, epigastric region without penetration into peritoneal cavity
● S31.153 Open bite of abdominal wall, right lower quadrant without penetration into peritoneal cavity
● S31.154 Open bite of abdominal wall, left lower quadrant without penetration into peritoneal cavity
● S31.155 Open bite of abdominal wall, periumbilic region without penetration into peritoneal cavity
● S31.159 Open bite of abdominal wall, unspecified quadrant without penetration into peritoneal cavity

● S31.2 Open wound of penis
X● S31.20 Unspecified open wound of penis
X● S31.21 Laceration without foreign body of penis
X● S31.22 Laceration with foreign body of penis
X● S31.23 Puncture wound without foreign body of penis
X● S31.24 Puncture wound with foreign body of penis
X● S31.25 Open bite of penis
Bite of penis NOS
Excludes1 superficial bite of penis (S30.862, S30.872)

● S31.3 Open wound of scrotum and testes
X● S31.30 Unspecified open wound of scrotum and testes
X● S31.31 Laceration without foreign body of scrotum and testes
X● S31.32 Laceration with foreign body of scrotum and testes
X● S31.33 Puncture wound without foreign body of scrotum and testes
X● S31.34 Puncture wound with foreign body of scrotum and testes
X● S31.35 Open bite of scrotum and testes
Bite of scrotum and testes NOS
Excludes1 superficial bite of scrotum and testes (S30.863, S30.873)

● S31.4 Open wound of vagina and vulva
Excludes1 injury to vagina and vulva during delivery (O70.-, O71.4)
X● S31.40 Unspecified open wound of vagina and vulva
X● S31.41 Laceration without foreign body of vagina and vulva
X● S31.42 Laceration with foreign body of vagina and vulva
X● S31.43 Puncture wound without foreign body of vagina and vulva
X● S31.44 Puncture wound with foreign body of vagina and vulva
X● S31.45 Open bite of vagina and vulva
Bite of vagina and vulva NOS
Excludes1 superficial bite of vagina and vulva (S30.864, S30.874)

● S31.5 Open wound of unspecified external genital organs
Excludes1 traumatic amputation of external genital organs (S38.21, S38.22)
● S31.50 Unspecified open wound of unspecified external genital organs
● S31.501 Unspecified open wound of unspecified external genital organs, male
● S31.502 Unspecified open wound of unspecified external genital organs, female
● S31.51 Laceration without foreign body of unspecified external genital organs
● S31.511 Laceration without foreign body of unspecified external genital organs, male
● S31.512 Laceration without foreign body of unspecified external genital organs, female
● S31.52 Laceration with foreign body of unspecified external genital organs
● S31.521 Laceration with foreign body of unspecified external genital organs, male
● S31.522 Laceration with foreign body of unspecified external genital organs, female
● S31.53 Puncture wound without foreign body of unspecified external genital organs
● S31.531 Puncture wound without foreign body of unspecified external genital organs, male
● S31.532 Puncture wound without foreign body of unspecified external genital organs, female
● S31.54 Puncture wound with foreign body of unspecified external genital organs
● S31.541 Puncture wound with foreign body of unspecified external genital organs, male
● S31.542 Puncture wound with foreign body of unspecified external genital organs, female
● S31.55 Open bite of unspecified external genital organs
Bite of unspecified external genital organs NOS
Excludes1 superficial bite of unspecified external genital organs (S30.865, S30.866, S30.875, S30.876)
● S31.551 Open bite of unspecified external genital organs, male
● S31.552 Open bite of unspecified external genital organs, female

● S31.6 Open wound of abdominal wall with penetration into peritoneal cavity
● S31.60 Unspecified open wound of abdominal wall with penetration into peritoneal cavity
● S31.600 Unspecified open wound of abdominal wall, right upper quadrant with penetration into peritoneal cavity
● S31.601 Unspecified open wound of abdominal wall, left upper quadrant with penetration into peritoneal cavity
● S31.602 Unspecified open wound of abdominal wall, epigastric region with penetration into peritoneal cavity

● S31.603 Unspecified open wound of abdominal wall, right lower quadrant with penetration into peritoneal cavity

● S31.604 Unspecified open wound of abdominal wall, left lower quadrant with penetration into peritoneal cavity

● S31.605 Unspecified open wound of abdominal wall, periumbilic region with penetration into peritoneal cavity

● S31.609 Unspecified open wound of abdominal wall, unspecified quadrant with penetration into peritoneal cavity

● S31.61 Laceration without foreign body of abdominal wall with penetration into peritoneal cavity

● S31.610 Laceration without foreign body of abdominal wall, right upper quadrant with penetration into peritoneal cavity

● S31.611 Laceration without foreign body of abdominal wall, left upper quadrant with penetration into peritoneal cavity

● S31.612 Laceration without foreign body of abdominal wall, epigastric region with penetration into peritoneal cavity

● S31.613 Laceration without foreign body of abdominal wall, right lower quadrant with penetration into peritoneal cavity

● S31.614 Laceration without foreign body of abdominal wall, left lower quadrant with penetration into peritoneal cavity

● S31.615 Laceration without foreign body of abdominal wall, periumbilic region with penetration into peritoneal cavity

● S31.619 Laceration without foreign body of abdominal wall, unspecified quadrant with penetration into peritoneal cavity

● S31.62 Laceration with foreign body of abdominal wall with penetration into peritoneal cavity

● S31.620 Laceration with foreign body of abdominal wall, right upper quadrant with penetration into peritoneal cavity

● S31.621 Laceration with foreign body of abdominal wall, left upper quadrant with penetration into peritoneal cavity

● S31.622 Laceration with foreign body of abdominal wall, epigastric region with penetration into peritoneal cavity

● S31.623 Laceration with foreign body of abdominal wall, right lower quadrant with penetration into peritoneal cavity

● S31.624 Laceration with foreign body of abdominal wall, left lower quadrant with penetration into peritoneal cavity

● S31.625 Laceration with foreign body of abdominal wall, periumbilic region with penetration into peritoneal cavity

● S31.629 Laceration with foreign body of abdominal wall, unspecified quadrant with penetration into peritoneal cavity

● S31.63 Puncture wound without foreign body of abdominal wall with penetration into peritoneal cavity

● S31.630 Puncture wound without foreign body of abdominal wall, right upper quadrant with penetration into peritoneal cavity

● S31.631 Puncture wound without foreign body of abdominal wall, left upper quadrant with penetration into peritoneal cavity

● S31.632 Puncture wound without foreign body of abdominal wall, epigastric region with penetration into peritoneal cavity

● S31.633 Puncture wound without foreign body of abdominal wall, right lower quadrant with penetration into peritoneal cavity

● S31.634 Puncture wound without foreign body of abdominal wall, left lower quadrant with penetration into peritoneal cavity

● S31.635 Puncture wound without foreign body of abdominal wall, periumbilic region with penetration into peritoneal cavity

● S31.639 Puncture wound without foreign body of abdominal wall, unspecified quadrant with penetration into peritoneal cavity

● S31.64 Puncture wound with foreign body of abdominal wall with penetration into peritoneal cavity

● S31.640 Puncture wound with foreign body of abdominal wall, right upper quadrant with penetration into peritoneal cavity

● S31.641 Puncture wound with foreign body of abdominal wall, left upper quadrant with penetration into peritoneal cavity

● S31.642 Puncture wound with foreign body of abdominal wall, epigastric region with penetration into peritoneal cavity

● S31.643 Puncture wound with foreign body of abdominal wall, right lower quadrant with penetration into peritoneal cavity

● S31.644 Puncture wound with foreign body of abdominal wall, left lower quadrant with penetration into peritoneal cavity

● S31.645 Puncture wound with foreign body of abdominal wall, periumbilic region with penetration into peritoneal cavity

● S31.649 Puncture wound with foreign body of abdominal wall, unspecified quadrant with penetration into peritoneal cavity

● S31.65 **Open bite of abdominal wall with penetration into peritoneal cavity**
Excludes1 superficial bite of abdominal wall (S30.861, S30.871)
● S31.650 **Open bite of abdominal wall, right upper quadrant with penetration into peritoneal cavity**
● S31.651 **Open bite of abdominal wall, left upper quadrant with penetration into peritoneal cavity**
● S31.652 **Open bite of abdominal wall, epigastric region with penetration into peritoneal cavity**
● S31.653 **Open bite of abdominal wall, right lower quadrant with penetration into peritoneal cavity**
● S31.654 **Open bite of abdominal wall, left lower quadrant with penetration into peritoneal cavity**
● S31.655 **Open bite of abdominal wall, periumbilic region with penetration into peritoneal cavity**
● S31.659 **Open bite of abdominal wall, unspecified quadrant with penetration into peritoneal cavity**

● S31.8 **Open wound of other parts of abdomen, lower back and pelvis**
● S31.80 **Open wound of unspecified buttock**
● S31.801 **Laceration without foreign body of unspecified buttock**
● S31.802 **Laceration with foreign body of unspecified buttock**
● S31.803 **Puncture wound without foreign body of unspecified buttock**
● S31.804 **Puncture wound with foreign body of unspecified buttock**
● S31.805 **Open bite of unspecified buttock**
Bite of buttock NOS
Excludes1 superficial bite of buttock (S30.870)
● S31.809 **Unspecified open wound of unspecified buttock**
● S31.81 **Open wound of right buttock**
● S31.811 **Laceration without foreign body of right buttock**
● S31.812 **Laceration with foreign body of right buttock**
● S31.813 **Puncture wound without foreign body of right buttock**
● S31.814 **Puncture wound with foreign body of right buttock**
● S31.815 **Open bite of right buttock**
Bite of right buttock NOS
Excludes1 superficial bite of buttock (S30.870)
● S31.819 **Unspecified open wound of right buttock**
● S31.82 **Open wound of left buttock**
● S31.821 **Laceration without foreign body of left buttock**
● S31.822 **Laceration with foreign body of left buttock**
● S31.823 **Puncture wound without foreign body of left buttock**
● S31.824 **Puncture wound with foreign body of left buttock**
● S31.825 **Open bite of left buttock**
Bite of left buttock NOS
Excludes1 superficial bite of buttock (S30.870)
● S31.829 **Unspecified open wound of left buttock**
● S31.83 **Open wound of anus**
● S31.831 **Laceration without foreign body of anus**
● S31.832 **Laceration with foreign body of anus**
● S31.833 **Puncture wound without foreign body of anus**
● S31.834 **Puncture wound with foreign body of anus**
● S31.835 **Open bite of anus**
Bite of anus NOS
Excludes1 superficial bite of anus (S30.877)
● S31.839 **Unspecified open wound of anus**

● S32 **Fracture of lumbar spine and pelvis**

Note: A fracture not indicated as displaced or nondisplaced should be coded to displaced

A fracture not indicated as opened or closed should be coded to closed

Includes fracture of lumbosacral neural arch
fracture of lumbosacral spinous process
fracture of lumbosacral transverse process
fracture of lumbosacral vertebra
fracture of lumbosacral vertebral arch

Code first any associated spinal cord and spinal nerve injury (S34.-)

Excludes1 transection of abdomen (S38.3)
Excludes2 fracture of hip NOS (S72.0-)

The appropriate 7th character is to be added to each code from category S32

A	initial encounter for closed fracture
B	initial encounter for open fracture
D	subsequent encounter for fracture with routine healing
G	subsequent encounter for fracture with delayed healing
K	subsequent encounter for fracture with nonunion
S	sequela

● S32.0 **Fracture of lumbar vertebra**
Fracture of lumbar spine NOS
● S32.00 **Fracture of unspecified lumbar vertebra**
● S32.000 **Wedge compression fracture of unspecified lumbar vertebra**
● S32.001 **Stable burst fracture of unspecified lumbar vertebra**
● S32.002 **Unstable burst fracture of unspecified lumbar vertebra**
● S32.008 **Other fracture of unspecified lumbar vertebra**
● S32.009 **Unspecified fracture of unspecified lumbar vertebra**
● S32.01 **Fracture of first lumbar vertebra**
● S32.010 **Wedge compression fracture of first lumbar vertebra**
● S32.011 **Stable burst fracture of first lumbar vertebra**
● S32.012 **Unstable burst fracture of first lumbar vertebra**
● S32.018 **Other fracture of first lumbar vertebra**
● S32.019 **Unspecified fracture of first lumbar vertebra**

● S32.02 **Fracture of second lumbar vertebra**
● S32.020 **Wedge compression fracture of second lumbar vertebra**
● S32.021 **Stable burst fracture of second lumbar vertebra**
● S32.022 **Unstable burst fracture of second lumbar vertebra**
● S32.028 **Other fracture of second lumbar vertebra**
● S32.029 **Unspecified fracture of second lumbar vertebra**
● S32.03 **Fracture of third lumbar vertebra**
● S32.030 **Wedge compression fracture of third lumbar vertebra**
● S32.031 **Stable burst fracture of third lumbar vertebra**
● S32.032 **Unstable burst fracture of third lumbar vertebra**
● S32.038 **Other fracture of third lumbar vertebra**
● S32.039 **Unspecified fracture of third lumbar vertebra**
● S32.04 **Fracture of fourth lumbar vertebra**
● S32.040 **Wedge compression fracture of fourth lumbar vertebra**
● S32.041 **Stable burst fracture of fourth lumbar vertebra**
● S32.042 **Unstable burst fracture of fourth lumbar vertebra**
● S32.048 **Other fracture of fourth lumbar vertebra**
● S32.049 **Unspecified fracture of fourth lumbar vertebra**
● S32.05 **Fracture of fifth lumbar vertebra**
● S32.050 **Wedge compression fracture of fifth lumbar vertebra**
● S32.051 **Stable burst fracture of fifth lumbar vertebra**
● S32.052 **Unstable burst fracture of fifth lumbar vertebra**
● S32.058 **Other fracture of fifth lumbar vertebra**
● S32.059 **Unspecified fracture of fifth lumbar vertebra**
● S32.1 **Fracture of sacrum**
For vertical fractures, code to most medial fracture extension
Use two codes if both a vertical and transverse fracture are present
Code also any associated fracture of pelvic ring (S32.8-)
X● S32.10 **Unspecified fracture of sacrum**
● S32.11 **Zone I fracture of sacrum**
Vertical sacral ala fracture of sacrum
● S32.110 **Nondisplaced Zone I fracture of sacrum**
● S32.111 **Minimally displaced Zone I fracture of sacrum**
● S32.112 **Severely displaced Zone I fracture of sacrum**
● S32.119 **Unspecified Zone I fracture of sacrum**
● S32.12 **Zone II fracture of sacrum**
Vertical foraminal region fracture of sacrum
● S32.120 **Nondisplaced Zone II fracture of sacrum**
● S32.121 **Minimally displaced Zone II fracture of sacrum**
● S32.122 **Severely displaced Zone II fracture of sacrum**
● S32.129 **Unspecified Zone II fracture of sacrum**
● S32.13 **Zone III fracture of sacrum**
Vertical fracture into spinal canal region of sacrum
● S32.130 **Nondisplaced Zone III fracture of sacrum**
● S32.131 **Minimally displaced Zone III fracture of sacrum**
● S32.132 **Severely displaced Zone III fracture of sacrum**
● S32.139 **Unspecified Zone III fracture of sacrum**
X● S32.14 **Type 1 fracture of sacrum**
Transverse flexion fracture of sacrum without displacement
X● S32.15 **Type 2 fracture of sacrum**
Transverse flexion fracture of sacrum with posterior displacement
X● S32.16 **Type 3 fracture of sacrum**
Transverse extension fracture of sacrum with anterior displacement
X● S32.17 **Type 4 fracture of sacrum**
Transverse segmental comminution of upper sacrum
X● S32.19 **Other fracture of sacrum**
X● S32.2 **Fracture of coccyx**
● S32.3 **Fracture of ilium**
Excludes1 fracture of ilium with associated disruption of pelvic ring (S32.8-)
● S32.30 **Unspecified fracture of ilium**
● S32.301 **Unspecified fracture of right ilium**
● S32.302 **Unspecified fracture of left ilium**
● S32.309 **Unspecified fracture of unspecified ilium**
● S32.31 **Avulsion fracture of ilium**
● S32.311 **Displaced avulsion fracture of right ilium**
● S32.312 **Displaced avulsion fracture of left ilium**
● S32.313 **Displaced avulsion fracture of unspecified ilium**
● S32.314 **Nondisplaced avulsion fracture of right ilium**
● S32.315 **Nondisplaced avulsion fracture of left ilium**
● S32.316 **Nondisplaced avulsion fracture of unspecified ilium**
● S32.39 **Other fracture of ilium**
● S32.391 **Other fracture of right ilium**
● S32.392 **Other fracture of left ilium**
● S32.399 **Other fracture of unspecified ilium**

CHAPTER 19 (S00-T88)

S32.4 Fracture of acetabulum
Code also any associated fracture of pelvic ring (S32.8-)
S32.40 Unspecified fracture of acetabulum
S32.401 Unspecified fracture of right acetabulum
S32.402 Unspecified fracture of left acetabulum
S32.409 Unspecified fracture of unspecified acetabulum
S32.41 Fracture of anterior wall of acetabulum
S32.411 Displaced fracture of anterior wall of right acetabulum
S32.412 Displaced fracture of anterior wall of left acetabulum
S32.413 Displaced fracture of anterior wall of unspecified acetabulum
S32.414 Nondisplaced fracture of anterior wall of right acetabulum
S32.415 Nondisplaced fracture of anterior wall of left acetabulum
S32.416 Nondisplaced fracture of anterior wall of unspecified acetabulum
S32.42 Fracture of posterior wall of acetabulum
S32.421 Displaced fracture of posterior wall of right acetabulum
S32.422 Displaced fracture of posterior wall of left acetabulum
S32.423 Displaced fracture of posterior wall of unspecified acetabulum
S32.424 Nondisplaced fracture of posterior wall of right acetabulum
S32.425 Nondisplaced fracture of posterior wall of left acetabulum
S32.426 Nondisplaced fracture of posterior wall of unspecified acetabulum
S32.43 Fracture of anterior column [iliopubic] of acetabulum
S32.431 Displaced fracture of anterior column [iliopubic] of right acetabulum
S32.432 Displaced fracture of anterior column [iliopubic] of left acetabulum
S32.433 Displaced fracture of anterior column [iliopubic] of unspecified acetabulum
S32.434 Nondisplaced fracture of anterior column [iliopubic] of right acetabulum
S32.435 Nondisplaced fracture of anterior column [iliopubic] of left acetabulum
S32.436 Nondisplaced fracture of anterior column [iliopubic] of unspecified acetabulum
S32.44 Fracture of posterior column [ilioischial] of acetabulum
S32.441 Displaced fracture of posterior column [ilioischial] of right acetabulum
S32.442 Displaced fracture of posterior column [ilioischial] of left acetabulum
S32.443 Displaced fracture of posterior column [ilioischial] of unspecified acetabulum
S32.444 Nondisplaced fracture of posterior column [ilioischial] of right acetabulum
S32.445 Nondisplaced fracture of posterior column [ilioischial] of left acetabulum
S32.446 Nondisplaced fracture of posterior column [ilioischial] of unspecified acetabulum
S32.45 Transverse fracture of acetabulum
S32.451 Displaced transverse fracture of right acetabulum
S32.452 Displaced transverse fracture of left acetabulum
S32.453 Displaced transverse fracture of unspecified acetabulum
S32.454 Nondisplaced transverse fracture of right acetabulum
S32.455 Nondisplaced transverse fracture of left acetabulum
S32.456 Nondisplaced transverse fracture of unspecified acetabulum
S32.46 Associated transverse-posterior fracture of acetabulum
S32.461 Displaced associated transverse-posterior fracture of right acetabulum
S32.462 Displaced associated transverse-posterior fracture of left acetabulum
S32.463 Displaced associated transverse-posterior fracture of unspecified acetabulum
S32.464 Nondisplaced associated transverse-posterior fracture of right acetabulum
S32.465 Nondisplaced associated transverse-posterior fracture of left acetabulum
S32.466 Nondisplaced associated transverse-posterior fracture of unspecified acetabulum
S32.47 Fracture of medial wall of acetabulum
S32.471 Displaced fracture of medial wall of right acetabulum
S32.472 Displaced fracture of medial wall of left acetabulum
S32.473 Displaced fracture of medial wall of unspecified acetabulum
S32.474 Nondisplaced fracture of medial wall of right acetabulum
S32.475 Nondisplaced fracture of medial wall of left acetabulum
S32.476 Nondisplaced fracture of medial wall of unspecified acetabulum
S32.48 Dome fracture of acetabulum
S32.481 Displaced dome fracture of right acetabulum
S32.482 Displaced dome fracture of left acetabulum
S32.483 Displaced dome fracture of unspecified acetabulum
S32.484 Nondisplaced dome fracture of right acetabulum
S32.485 Nondisplaced dome fracture of left acetabulum
S32.486 Nondisplaced dome fracture of unspecified acetabulum
S32.49 Other fracture of acetabulum
S32.491 Other fracture of right acetabulum
S32.492 Other fracture of left acetabulum
S32.499 Other fracture of unspecified acetabulum

● S32.5 Fracture of pubis
Excludes1 fracture of pubis with associated disruption of pelvic ring (S32.8-)
● S32.50 Unspecified fracture of pubis
● S32.501 Unspecified fracture of right pubis
● S32.502 Unspecified fracture of left pubis
● S32.509 Unspecified fracture of unspecified pubis
● S32.51 Fracture of superior rim of pubis
● S32.511 Fracture of superior rim of right pubis
● S32.512 Fracture of superior rim of left pubis
● S32.519 Fracture of superior rim of unspecified pubis
● S32.59 Other specified fracture of pubis
● S32.591 Other specified fracture of right pubis
● S32.592 Other specified fracture of left pubis
● S32.599 Other specified fracture of unspecified pubis
● S32.6 Fracture of ischium
Excludes1 fracture of ischium with associated disruption of pelvic ring (S32.8-)
● S32.60 Unspecified fracture of ischium
● S32.601 Unspecified fracture of right ischium
● S32.602 Unspecified fracture of left ischium
● S32.609 Unspecified fracture of unspecified ischium
● S32.61 Avulsion fracture of ischium
● S32.611 Displaced avulsion fracture of right ischium
● S32.612 Displaced avulsion fracture of left ischium
● S32.613 Displaced avulsion fracture of unspecified ischium
● S32.614 Nondisplaced avulsion fracture of right ischium
● S32.615 Nondisplaced avulsion fracture of left ischium
● S32.616 Nondisplaced avulsion fracture of unspecified ischium
● S32.69 Other specified fracture of ischium
● S32.691 Other specified fracture of right ischium
● S32.692 Other specified fracture of left ischium
● S32.699 Other specified fracture of unspecified ischium
● S32.8 Fracture of other parts of pelvis
Code also any associated:
fracture of acetabulum (S32.4-)
sacral fracture (S32.1-)
● S32.81 Multiple fractures of pelvis with disruption of pelvic ring
Multiple pelvic fractures with disruption of pelvic circle
● S32.810 Multiple fractures of pelvis with stable disruption of pelvic ring
● S32.811 Multiple fractures of pelvis with unstable disruption of pelvic ring
X● S32.82 Multiple fractures of pelvis without disruption of pelvic ring
Multiple pelvic fractures without disruption of pelvic circle
X● S32.89 Fracture of other parts of pelvis
X● S32.9 Fracture of unspecified parts of lumbosacral spine and pelvis
Fracture of lumbosacral spine NOS
Fracture of pelvis NOS

● S33 Dislocation and sprain of joints and ligaments of lumbar spine and pelvis
Includes avulsion of joint or ligament of lumbar spine and pelvis
laceration of cartilage, joint or ligament of lumbar spine and pelvis
sprain of cartilage, joint or ligament of lumbar spine and pelvis
traumatic hemarthrosis of joint or ligament of lumbar spine and pelvis
traumatic rupture of joint or ligament of lumbar spine and pelvis
traumatic subluxation of joint or ligament of lumbar spine and pelvis
traumatic tear of joint or ligament of lumbar spine and pelvis
Code also any associated open wound
Excludes1 nontraumatic rupture or displacement of lumbar intervertebral disc NOS (M51.-)
obstetric damage to pelvic joints and ligaments (O71.6)
Excludes2 dislocation and sprain of joints and ligaments of hip (S73.-)
strain of muscle of lower back and pelvis (S39.01-)
The appropriate 7th character is to be added to each code from category S33

A	initial encounter
D	subsequent encounter
S	sequela

X● S33.0 Traumatic rupture of lumbar intervertebral disc
Excludes1 rupture or displacement (nontraumatic) of lumbar intervertebral disc NOS (M51.- with fifth character 6)
● S33.1 Subluxation and dislocation of lumbar vertebra
Code also any associated:
open wound of abdomen, lower back and pelvis (S31)
spinal cord injury (S24.0, S24.1-, S34.0-, S34.1-)
Excludes2 fracture of lumbar vertebrae (S32.0-)
● S33.10 Subluxation and dislocation of unspecified lumbar vertebra
● S33.100 Subluxation of unspecified lumbar vertebra
● S33.101 Dislocation of unspecified lumbar vertebra
● S33.11 Subluxation and dislocation of L_1/L_2 lumbar vertebra
● S33.110 Subluxation of L_1/L_2 lumbar vertebra
● S33.111 Dislocation of L_1/L_2 lumbar vertebra
● S33.12 Subluxation and dislocation of L_2/L_3 lumbar vertebra
● S33.120 Subluxation of L_2/L_3 lumbar vertebra
● S33.121 Dislocation of L_2/L_3 lumbar vertebra
● S33.13 Subluxation and dislocation of L_3/L_4 lumbar vertebra
● S33.130 Subluxation of L_3/L_4 lumbar vertebra
● S33.131 Dislocation of L_3/L_4 lumbar vertebra
● S33.14 Subluxation and dislocation of L_4/L_5 lumbar vertebra
● S33.140 Subluxation of L_4/L_5 lumbar vertebra
● S33.141 Dislocation of L_4/L_5 lumbar vertebra
X● S33.2 Dislocation of sacroiliac and sacrococcygeal joint
● S33.3 Dislocation of other and unspecified parts of lumbar spine and pelvis
X● S33.30 Dislocation of unspecified parts of lumbar spine and pelvis
X● S33.39 Dislocation of other parts of lumbar spine and pelvis
X● S33.4 Traumatic rupture of symphysis pubis
X● S33.5 Sprain of ligaments of lumbar spine

CHAPTER 19 (S00-T88)

X● S33.6 **Sprain of sacroiliac joint**

X● S33.8 **Sprain of other parts of lumbar spine and pelvis**

X● S33.9 **Sprain of unspecified parts of lumbar spine and pelvis**

● S34 **Injury of lumbar and sacral spinal cord and nerves at abdomen, lower back and pelvis level**

Note: Code to highest level of lumbar cord injury

Injuries to the spinal cord (S34.Ø and S34.1) refer to the cord level and not bone level injury, and can affect nerve roots at and below the level given.

The appropriate 7th character is to be added to each code from category S34

A	initial encounter
D	subsequent encounter
S	sequela

Code also any associated:
fracture of vertebra (S22.Ø-, S32.Ø-)
open wound of abdomen, lower back and pelvis (S31.-)
transient paralysis (R29.5)

● S34.Ø **Concussion and edema of lumbar and sacral spinal cord**

X● S34.Ø1 **Concussion and edema of lumbar spinal cord**

X● S34.Ø2 **Concussion and edema of sacral spinal cord**
Concussion and edema of conus medullaris

● S34.1 **Other and unspecified injury of lumbar and sacral spinal cord**

● S34.1Ø **Unspecified injury to lumbar spinal cord**

● S34.1Ø1 **Unspecified injury to L_1 level of lumbar spinal cord**
Unspecified injury to lumbar spinal cord level 1 ◀

● S34.1Ø2 **Unspecified injury to L_2 level of lumbar spinal cord**
Unspecified injury to lumbar spinal cord level 2 ◀

● S34.1Ø3 **Unspecified injury to L_3 level of lumbar spinal cord**
Unspecified injury to lumbar spinal cord level 3 ◀

● S34.1Ø4 **Unspecified injury to L_4 level of lumbar spinal cord**
Unspecified injury to lumbar spinal cord level 4 ◀

● S34.1Ø5 **Unspecified injury to L_5 level of lumbar spinal cord**
Unspecified injury to lumbar spinal cord level 5 ◀

● S34.1Ø9 **Unspecified injury to unspecified level of lumbar spinal cord**

● S34.11 **Complete lesion of lumbar spinal cord**

● S34.111 **Complete lesion of L_1 level of lumbar spinal cord**
Complete lesion of lumbar spinal cord level 1 ◀

● S34.112 **Complete lesion of L_2 level of lumbar spinal cord**
Complete lesion of lumbar spinal cord level 2 ◀

● S34.113 **Complete lesion of L_3 level of lumbar spinal cord**
Complete lesion of lumbar spinal cord level 3 ◀

● S34.114 **Complete lesion of L_4 level of lumbar spinal cord**
Complete lesion of lumbar spinal cord level 4 ◀

● S34.115 **Complete lesion of L_5 level of lumbar spinal cord**
Complete lesion of lumbar spinal cord level 5 ◀

● S34.119 **Complete lesion of unspecified level of lumbar spinal cord**

● S34.12 **Incomplete lesion of lumbar spinal cord**

● S34.121 **Incomplete lesion of L_1 level of lumbar spinal cord**
Incomplete lesion of lumbar spinal cord level 1 ◀

● S34.122 **Incomplete lesion of L_2 level of lumbar spinal cord**
Incomplete lesion of lumbar spinal cord level 2 ◀

● S34.123 **Incomplete lesion of L_3 level of lumbar spinal cord**
Incomplete lesion of lumbar spinal cord level 3 ◀

● S34.124 **Incomplete lesion of L_4 level of lumbar spinal cord**
Incomplete lesion of lumbar spinal cord level 4 ◀

● S34.125 **Incomplete lesion of L_5 level of lumbar spinal cord**
Incomplete lesion of lumbar spinal cord level 5 ◀

● S34.129 **Incomplete lesion of unspecified level of lumbar spinal cord**

● S34.13 **Other and unspecified injury to sacral spinal cord**
Other injury to conus medullaris

● S34.131 **Complete lesion of sacral spinal cord**
Complete lesion of conus medullaris

● S34.132 **Incomplete lesion of sacral spinal cord**
Incomplete lesion of conus medullaris

● S34.139 **Unspecified injury to sacral spinal cord**
Unspecified injury of conus medullaris

● S34.2 **Injury of nerve root of lumbar and sacral spine**

X● S34.21 **Injury of nerve root of lumbar spine**

X● S34.22 **Injury of nerve root of sacral spine**

X● S34.3 **Injury of cauda equina**

X● S34.4 **Injury of lumbosacral plexus**

X● S34.5 **Injury of lumbar, sacral and pelvic sympathetic nerves**
Injury of celiac ganglion or plexus
Injury of hypogastric plexus
Injury of mesenteric plexus (inferior) (superior)
Injury of splanchnic nerve

X● S34.6 **Injury of peripheral nerve(s) at abdomen, lower back and pelvis level**

X● S34.8 **Injury of other nerves at abdomen, lower back and pelvis level**

X● S34.9 **Injury of unspecified nerves at abdomen, lower back and pelvis level**

● S35 **Injury of blood vessels at abdomen, lower back and pelvis level**

The appropriate 7th character is to be added to each code from category S35

A	initial encounter
D	subsequent encounter
S	sequela

Code also any associated open wound (S31.-)

● S35.Ø **Injury of abdominal aorta**

Excludes1 injury of aorta NOS (S25.Ø)

X● S35.ØØ **Unspecified injury of abdominal aorta**

X● S35.Ø1 **Minor laceration of abdominal aorta**
Incomplete transection of abdominal aorta
Laceration of abdominal aorta NOS
Superficial laceration of abdominal aorta

X● S35.Ø2 **Major laceration of abdominal aorta**
Complete transection of abdominal aorta
Traumatic rupture of abdominal aorta

X● S35.Ø9 **Other injury of abdominal aorta**

◀ New ⟸ Revised ~~deleted~~ Deleted **OGCR** Official Guidelines X Assign placeholder X ● Use Additional Character(s)
Excludes 1 | Excludes 2 | Includes | Use additional | Code first | Code also | Unspecified

● S35.1 **Injury of inferior vena cava**
Injury of hepatic vein
Excludes1 injury of vena cava NOS (S25.2)
X● S35.10 **Unspecified injury of inferior vena cava**
X● S35.11 **Minor laceration of inferior vena cava**
Incomplete transection of inferior vena cava
Laceration of inferior vena cava NOS
Superficial laceration of inferior vena cava
X● S35.12 **Major laceration of inferior vena cava**
Complete transection of inferior vena cava
Traumatic rupture of inferior vena cava
X● S35.19 **Other injury of inferior vena cava**
● S35.2 **Injury of celiac or mesenteric artery and branches**
● S35.21 **Injury of celiac artery**
● S35.211 **Minor laceration of celiac artery**
Incomplete transection of celiac artery
Laceration of celiac artery NOS
Superficial laceration of celiac artery
● S35.212 **Major laceration of celiac artery**
Complete transection of celiac artery
Traumatic rupture of celiac artery
● S35.218 **Other injury of celiac artery**
● S35.219 **Unspecified injury of celiac artery**
● S35.22 **Injury of superior mesenteric artery**
● S35.221 **Minor laceration of superior mesenteric artery**
Incomplete transection of superior mesenteric artery
Laceration of superior mesenteric artery NOS
Superficial laceration of superior mesenteric artery
● S35.222 **Major laceration of superior mesenteric artery**
Complete transection of superior mesenteric artery
Traumatic rupture of superior mesenteric artery
● S35.228 **Other injury of superior mesenteric artery**
● S35.229 **Unspecified injury of superior mesenteric artery**
● S35.23 **Injury of inferior mesenteric artery**
● S35.231 **Minor laceration of inferior mesenteric artery**
Incomplete transection of inferior mesenteric artery
Laceration of inferior mesenteric artery NOS
Superficial laceration of inferior mesenteric artery
● S35.232 **Major laceration of inferior mesenteric artery**
Complete transection of inferior mesenteric artery
Traumatic rupture of inferior mesenteric artery
● S35.238 **Other injury of inferior mesenteric artery**
● S35.239 **Unspecified injury of inferior mesenteric artery**
● S35.29 **Injury of branches of celiac and mesenteric artery**
Injury of gastric artery
Injury of gastroduodenal artery
Injury of hepatic artery
Injury of splenic artery
● S35.291 **Minor laceration of branches of celiac and mesenteric artery**
Incomplete transection of branches of celiac and mesenteric artery
Laceration of branches of celiac and mesenteric artery NOS
Superficial laceration of branches of celiac and mesenteric artery
● S35.292 **Major laceration of branches of celiac and mesenteric artery**
Complete transection of branches of celiac and mesenteric artery
Traumatic rupture of branches of celiac and mesenteric artery
● S35.298 **Other injury of branches of celiac and mesenteric artery**
● S35.299 **Unspecified injury of branches of celiac and mesenteric artery**
● S35.3 **Injury of portal or splenic vein and branches**
● S35.31 **Injury of portal vein**
● S35.311 **Laceration of portal vein**
● S35.318 **Other specified injury of portal vein**
● S35.319 **Unspecified injury of portal vein**
● S35.32 **Injury of splenic vein**
● S35.321 **Laceration of splenic vein**
● S35.328 **Other specified injury of splenic vein**
● S35.329 **Unspecified injury of splenic vein**
● S35.33 **Injury of superior mesenteric vein**
● S35.331 **Laceration of superior mesenteric vein**
● S35.338 **Other specified injury of superior mesenteric vein**
● S35.339 **Unspecified injury of superior mesenteric vein**
● S35.34 **Injury of inferior mesenteric vein**
● S35.341 **Laceration of inferior mesenteric vein**
● S35.348 **Other specified injury of inferior mesenteric vein**
● S35.349 **Unspecified injury of inferior mesenteric vein**
● S35.4 **Injury of renal blood vessels**
● S35.40 **Unspecified injury of renal blood vessel**
● S35.401 **Unspecified injury of right renal artery**
● S35.402 **Unspecified injury of left renal artery**
● S35.403 **Unspecified injury of unspecified renal artery**
● S35.404 **Unspecified injury of right renal vein**
● S35.405 **Unspecified injury of left renal vein**
● S35.406 **Unspecified injury of unspecified renal vein**

CHAPTER 19 (S00-T88)

- ● S35.41 Laceration of renal blood vessel
  - ● S35.411 Laceration of right renal artery
  - ● S35.412 Laceration of left renal artery
  - ● S35.413 Laceration of unspecified renal artery
  - ● S35.414 Laceration of right renal vein
  - ● S35.415 Laceration of left renal vein
  - ● S35.416 Laceration of unspecified renal vein
- ● S35.49 Other specified injury of renal blood vessel
  - ● S35.491 Other specified injury of right renal artery
  - ● S35.492 Other specified injury of left renal artery
  - ● S35.493 Other specified injury of unspecified renal artery
  - ● S35.494 Other specified injury of right renal vein
  - ● S35.495 Other specified injury of left renal vein
  - ● S35.496 Other specified injury of unspecified renal vein

● S35.5 Injury of iliac blood vessels
- X● S35.50 Injury of unspecified iliac blood vessel(s)
- ● S35.51 Injury of iliac artery or vein
  Injury of hypogastric artery or vein
  - ● S35.511 Injury of right iliac artery
  - ● S35.512 Injury of left iliac artery
  - ● S35.513 Injury of unspecified iliac artery
  - ● S35.514 Injury of right iliac vein
  - ● S35.515 Injury of left iliac vein
  - ● S35.516 Injury of unspecified iliac vein
- ● S35.53 Injury of uterine artery or vein
  - ● S35.531 Injury of right uterine artery
  - ● S35.532 Injury of left uterine artery
  - ● S35.533 Injury of unspecified uterine artery
  - ● S35.534 Injury of right uterine vein
  - ● S35.535 Injury of left uterine vein
  - ● S35.536 Injury of unspecified uterine vein
- X● S35.59 Injury of other iliac blood vessels

● S35.8 Injury of other blood vessels at abdomen, lower back and pelvis level
Injury of ovarian artery or vein
- ● S35.8X Injury of other blood vessels at abdomen, lower back and pelvis level
  - ● S35.8X1 Laceration of other blood vessels at abdomen, lower back and pelvis level
  - ● S35.8X8 Other specified injury of other blood vessels at abdomen, lower back and pelvis level
  - ● S35.8X9 Unspecified injury of other blood vessels at abdomen, lower back and pelvis level

● S35.9 Injury of unspecified blood vessel at abdomen, lower back and pelvis level
- X● S35.90 Unspecified injury of unspecified blood vessel at abdomen, lower back and pelvis level
- X● S35.91 Laceration of unspecified blood vessel at abdomen, lower back and pelvis level
- X● S35.99 Other specified injury of unspecified blood vessel at abdomen, lower back and pelvis level

● S36 Injury of intra-abdominal organs

The appropriate 7th character is to be added to each code from category S36

A	initial encounter
D	subsequent encounter
S	sequela

Code also any associated open wound (S31.-)

● S36.0 Injury of spleen
- X● S36.00 Unspecified injury of spleen
- ● S36.02 Contusion of spleen
  - ● S36.020 Minor contusion of spleen
    Contusion of spleen less than 2 cm
  - ● S36.021 Major contusion of spleen
    Contusion of spleen greater than 2 cm
  - ● S36.029 Unspecified contusion of spleen
- ● S36.03 Laceration of spleen
  - ● S36.030 Superficial (capsular) laceration of spleen
    Laceration of spleen less than 1 cm
    Minor laceration of spleen
  - ● S36.031 Moderate laceration of spleen
    Laceration of spleen 1 to 3 cm
  - ● S36.032 Major laceration of spleen
    Avulsion of spleen
    Laceration of spleen greater than 3 cm
    Massive laceration of spleen
    Multiple moderate lacerations of spleen
    Stellate laceration of spleen
  - ● S36.039 Unspecified laceration of spleen
- X● S36.09 Other injury of spleen

● S36.1 Injury of liver and gallbladder and bile duct
- ● S36.11 Injury of liver
  - ● S36.112 Contusion of liver
  - ● S36.113 Laceration of liver, unspecified degree
  - ● S36.114 Minor laceration of liver
    Laceration involving capsule only, or, without significant involvement of hepatic parenchyma [i.e., less than 1 cm deep]
  - ● S36.115 Moderate laceration of liver
    Laceration involving parenchyma but without major disruption of parenchyma [i.e., less than 10 cm long and less than 3 cm deep]
  - ● S36.116 Major laceration of liver
    Laceration with significant disruption of hepatic parenchyma [i.e., greater than 10 cm long and 3 cm deep]
    Multiple moderate lacerations, with or without hematoma
    Stellate laceration of liver
  - ● S36.118 Other injury of liver
  - ● S36.119 Unspecified injury of liver
- ● S36.12 Injury of gallbladder
  - ● S36.122 Contusion of gallbladder
  - ● S36.123 Laceration of gallbladder
  - ● S36.128 Other injury of gallbladder
  - ● S36.129 Unspecified injury of gallbladder
- X● S36.13 Injury of bile duct

● **S36.2**   Injury of pancreas
   ● **S36.20**   Unspecified injury of pancreas
     ● **S36.200**   Unspecified injury of head of pancreas
     ● **S36.201**   Unspecified injury of body of pancreas
     ● **S36.202**   Unspecified injury of tail of pancreas
     ● **S36.209**   Unspecified injury of unspecified part of pancreas
   ● **S36.22**   Contusion of pancreas
     ● **S36.220**   Contusion of head of pancreas
     ● **S36.221**   Contusion of body of pancreas
     ● **S36.222**   Contusion of tail of pancreas
     ● **S36.229**   Contusion of unspecified part of pancreas
   ● **S36.23**   Laceration of pancreas, unspecified degree
     ● **S36.230**   Laceration of head of pancreas, unspecified degree
     ● **S36.231**   Laceration of body of pancreas, unspecified degree
     ● **S36.232**   Laceration of tail of pancreas, unspecified degree
     ● **S36.239**   Laceration of unspecified part of pancreas, unspecified degree
   ● **S36.24**   Minor laceration of pancreas
     ● **S36.240**   Minor laceration of head of pancreas
     ● **S36.241**   Minor laceration of body of pancreas
     ● **S36.242**   Minor laceration of tail of pancreas
     ● **S36.249**   Minor laceration of unspecified part of pancreas
   ● **S36.25**   Moderate laceration of pancreas
     ● **S36.250**   Moderate laceration of head of pancreas
     ● **S36.251**   Moderate laceration of body of pancreas
     ● **S36.252**   Moderate laceration of tail of pancreas
     ● **S36.259**   Moderate laceration of unspecified part of pancreas
   ● **S36.26**   Major laceration of pancreas
     ● **S36.260**   Major laceration of head of pancreas
     ● **S36.261**   Major laceration of body of pancreas
     ● **S36.262**   Major laceration of tail of pancreas
     ● **S36.269**   Major laceration of unspecified part of pancreas
   ● **S36.29**   Other injury of pancreas
     ● **S36.290**   Other injury of head of pancreas
     ● **S36.291**   Other injury of body of pancreas
     ● **S36.292**   Other injury of tail of pancreas
     ● **S36.299**   Other injury of unspecified part of pancreas
● **S36.3**   Injury of stomach
   X ● **S36.30**   Unspecified injury of stomach
   X ● **S36.32**   Contusion of stomach
   X ● **S36.33**   Laceration of stomach
   X ● **S36.39**   Other injury of stomach
● **S36.4**   Injury of small intestine
   ● **S36.40**   Unspecified injury of small intestine
     ● **S36.400**   Unspecified injury of duodenum
     ● **S36.408**   Unspecified injury of other part of small intestine
     ● **S36.409**   Unspecified injury of unspecified part of small intestine

● **S36.41**   Primary blast injury of small intestine
     Blast injury of small intestine NOS
     ● **S36.410**   Primary blast injury of duodenum
     ● **S36.418**   Primary blast injury of other part of small intestine
     ● **S36.419**   Primary blast injury of unspecified part of small intestine
   ● **S36.42**   Contusion of small intestine
     ● **S36.420**   Contusion of duodenum
     ● **S36.428**   Contusion of other part of small intestine
     ● **S36.429**   Contusion of unspecified part of small intestine
   ● **S36.43**   Laceration of small intestine
     ● **S36.430**   Laceration of duodenum
     ● **S36.438**   Laceration of other part of small intestine
     ● **S36.439**   Laceration of unspecified part of small intestine
   ● **S36.49**   Other injury of small intestine
     ● **S36.490**   Other injury of duodenum
     ● **S36.498**   Other injury of other part of small intestine
     ● **S36.499**   Other injury of unspecified part of small intestine
● **S36.5**   Injury of colon
   Excludes2   injury of rectum (S36.6-)
   ● **S36.50**   Unspecified injury of colon
     ● **S36.500**   Unspecified injury of ascending [right] colon
     ● **S36.501**   Unspecified injury of transverse colon
     ● **S36.502**   Unspecified injury of descending [left] colon
     ● **S36.503**   Unspecified injury of sigmoid colon
     ● **S36.508**   Unspecified injury of other part of colon
     ● **S36.509**   Unspecified injury of unspecified part of colon
   ● **S36.51**   Primary blast injury of colon
     Blast injury of colon NOS
     ● **S36.510**   Primary blast injury of ascending [right] colon
     ● **S36.511**   Primary blast injury of transverse colon
     ● **S36.512**   Primary blast injury of descending [left] colon
     ● **S36.513**   Primary blast injury of sigmoid colon
     ● **S36.518**   Primary blast injury of other part of colon
     ● **S36.519**   Primary blast injury of unspecified part of colon
   ● **S36.52**   Contusion of colon
     ● **S36.520**   Contusion of ascending [right] colon
     ● **S36.521**   Contusion of transverse colon
     ● **S36.522**   Contusion of descending [left] colon
     ● **S36.523**   Contusion of sigmoid colon
     ● **S36.528**   Contusion of other part of colon
     ● **S36.529**   Contusion of unspecified part of colon
   ● **S36.53**   Laceration of colon
     ● **S36.530**   Laceration of ascending [right] colon
     ● **S36.531**   Laceration of transverse colon
     ● **S36.532**   Laceration of descending [left] colon
     ● **S36.533**   Laceration of sigmoid colon
     ● **S36.538**   Laceration of other part of colon
        S36.539   Laceration of unspecified part of colon ·

◀ New   ◀▥ Revised   ~~deleted~~ Deleted   **OGCR** Official Guidelines   X Assign placeholder X   ● Use Additional Character(s)

Excludes 1   Excludes 2   Includes   Use additional   Code first   Code also   Unspecified

● S36.59 Other injury of colon
Secondary blast injury of colon
● S36.590 Other injury of ascending [right] colon
● S36.591 Other injury of transverse colon
● S36.592 Other injury of descending [left] colon
● S36.593 Other injury of sigmoid colon
● S36.598 Other injury of other part of colon
● S36.599 Other injury of unspecified part of colon
● S36.6 Injury of rectum
X● S36.60 Unspecified injury of rectum
X● S36.61 Primary blast injury of rectum
Blast injury of rectum NOS
X● S36.62 Contusion of rectum
X● S36.63 Laceration of rectum
X● S36.69 Other injury of rectum
Secondary blast injury of rectum
● S36.8 Injury of other intra-abdominal organs
X● S36.81 Injury of peritoneum
● S36.89 Injury of other intra-abdominal organs
Injury of retroperitoneum
● S36.892 Contusion of other intra-abdominal organs
● S36.893 Laceration of other intra-abdominal organs
● S36.898 Other injury of other intra-abdominal organs
S36.899 Unspecified injury of other intra-abdominal organs
● S36.9 Injury of unspecified intra-abdominal organ
X● S36.90 Unspecified injury of unspecified intra-abdominal organ
X● S36.92 Contusion of unspecified intra-abdominal organ
X● S36.93 Laceration of unspecified intra-abdominal organ
X● S36.99 Other injury of unspecified intra-abdominal organ
● S37 Injury of urinary and pelvic organs
Code also any associated open wound (S31.-)
Excludes1 obstetric trauma to pelvic organs (O71.-)
Excludes2 injury of peritoneum (S36.81)
injury of retroperitoneum (S36.89-)
The appropriate 7th character is to be added to each code from category S37

A	initial encounter
D	subsequent encounter
S	sequela

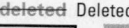

● S37.0 Injury of kidney
Excludes2 acute kidney injury (nontraumatic) (N17.9)
● S37.00 Unspecified injury of kidney
● S37.001 Unspecified injury of right kidney
● S37.002 Unspecified injury of left kidney
● S37.009 Unspecified injury of unspecified kidney
● S37.01 Minor contusion of kidney
Contusion of kidney less than 2 cm
Contusion of kidney NOS
● S37.011 Minor contusion of right kidney
● S37.012 Minor contusion of left kidney
● S37.019 Minor contusion of unspecified kidney
● S37.02 Major contusion of kidney
Contusion of kidney greater than 2 cm
● S37.021 Major contusion of right kidney
● S37.022 Major contusion of left kidney
● S37.029 Major contusion of unspecified kidney
● S37.03 Laceration of kidney, unspecified degree
● S37.031 Laceration of right kidney, unspecified degree
● S37.032 Laceration of left kidney, unspecified degree
● S37.039 Laceration of unspecified kidney, unspecified degree
● S37.04 Minor laceration of kidney
Laceration of kidney less than 1 cm
● S37.041 Minor laceration of right kidney
● S37.042 Minor laceration of left kidney
● S37.049 Minor laceration of unspecified kidney
● S37.05 Moderate laceration of kidney
Laceration of kidney 1 to 3 cm
● S37.051 Moderate laceration of right kidney
● S37.052 Moderate laceration of left kidney
● S37.059 Moderate laceration of unspecified kidney
● S37.06 Major laceration of kidney
Avulsion of kidney
Laceration of kidney greater than 3 cm
Massive laceration of kidney
Multiple moderate lacerations of kidney
Stellate laceration of kidney
● S37.061 Major laceration of right kidney
● S37.062 Major laceration of left kidney
● S37.069 Major laceration of unspecified kidney
● S37.09 Other injury of kidney
● S37.091 Other injury of right kidney
● S37.092 Other injury of left kidney
● S37.099 Other injury of unspecified kidney
● S37.1 Injury of ureter
X● S37.10 Unspecified injury of ureter
X● S37.12 Contusion of ureter
X● S37.13 Laceration of ureter
X● S37.19 Other injury of ureter
● S37.2 Injury of bladder
X● S37.20 Unspecified injury of bladder
X● S37.22 Contusion of bladder
X● S37.23 Laceration of bladder
X● S37.29 Other injury of bladder
● S37.3 Injury of urethra
X● S37.30 Unspecified injury of urethra
X● S37.32 Contusion of urethra
X● S37.33 Laceration of urethra
X● S37.39 Other injury of urethra
● S37.4 Injury of ovary
● S37.40 Unspecified injury of ovary
● S37.401 Unspecified injury of ovary, unilateral
● S37.402 Unspecified injury of ovary, bilateral
● S37.409 Unspecified injury of ovary, unspecified
● S37.42 Contusion of ovary
● S37.421 Contusion of ovary, unilateral
● S37.422 Contusion of ovary, bilateral
● S37.429 Contusion of ovary, unspecified

● S37.43 Laceration of ovary
● S37.431 Laceration of ovary, unilateral
● S37.432 Laceration of ovary, bilateral
● S37.439 Laceration of ovary, unspecified
● S37.49 Other injury of ovary
● S37.491 Other injury of ovary, unilateral
● S37.492 Other injury of ovary, bilateral
● S37.499 Other injury of ovary, unspecified
● S37.5 Injury of fallopian tube
● S37.50 Unspecified injury of fallopian tube
● S37.501 Unspecified injury of fallopian tube, unilateral
● S37.502 Unspecified injury of fallopian tube, bilateral
● S37.509 Unspecified injury of fallopian tube, unspecified
● S37.51 Primary blast injury of fallopian tube
Blast injury of fallopian tube NOS
● S37.511 Primary blast injury of fallopian tube, unilateral
● S37.512 Primary blast injury of fallopian tube, bilateral
● S37.519 Primary blast injury of fallopian tube, unspecified
● S37.52 Contusion of fallopian tube
● S37.521 Contusion of fallopian tube, unilateral
● S37.522 Contusion of fallopian tube, bilateral
● S37.529 Contusion of fallopian tube, unspecified
● S37.53 Laceration of fallopian tube
● S37.531 Laceration of fallopian tube, unilateral
● S37.532 Laceration of fallopian tube, bilateral
● S37.539 Laceration of fallopian tube, unspecified
● S37.59 Other injury of fallopian tube
Secondary blast injury of fallopian tube
● S37.591 Other injury of fallopian tube, unilateral
● S37.592 Other injury of fallopian tube, bilateral
● S37.599 Other injury of fallopian tube, unspecified
● S37.6 Injury of uterus
Excludes1 injury to gravid uterus (O9A.2-)
injury to uterus during delivery (O71.-)
X● S37.60 Unspecified injury of uterus
X● S37.62 Contusion of uterus
X● S37.63 Laceration of uterus
X● S37.69 Other injury of uterus
● S37.8 Injury of other urinary and pelvic organs
● S37.81 Injury of adrenal gland
● S37.812 Contusion of adrenal gland
● S37.813 Laceration of adrenal gland
● S37.818 Other injury of adrenal gland
● S37.819 Unspecified injury of adrenal gland
● S37.82 Injury of prostate
● S37.822 Contusion of prostate
● S37.823 Laceration of prostate
● S37.828 Other injury of prostate
● S37.829 Unspecified injury of prostate
● S37.89 Injury of other urinary and pelvic organ
● S37.892 Contusion of other urinary and pelvic organ
● S37.893 Laceration of other urinary and pelvic organ
● S37.898 Other injury of other urinary and pelvic organ
● S37.899 Unspecified injury of other urinary and pelvic organ
● S37.9 Injury of unspecified urinary and pelvic organ
X● S37.90 Unspecified injury of unspecified urinary and pelvic organ
X● S37.92 Contusion of unspecified urinary and pelvic organ
X● S37.93 Laceration of unspecified urinary and pelvic organ
X● S37.99 Other injury of unspecified urinary and pelvic organ

● **S38 Crushing injury and traumatic amputation of abdomen, lower back, pelvis and external genitals**
An amputation not identified as partial or complete should be coded to complete
The appropriate 7th character is to be added to each code from category S38

A	initial encounter
D	subsequent encounter
S	sequela

● S38.0 Crushing injury of external genital organs
Use additional code for any associated injuries
● S38.00 Crushing injury of unspecified external genital organs
● S38.001 Crushing injury of unspecified external genital organs, male
● S38.002 Crushing injury of unspecified external genital organs, female
X● S38.01 Crushing injury of penis
X● S38.02 Crushing injury of scrotum and testis
X● S38.03 Crushing injury of vulva
X● S38.1 Crushing injury of abdomen, lower back, and pelvis
Use additional code for all associated injuries, such as:
fracture of thoracic or lumbar spine and pelvis (S22.0-, S32.-)
injury to intra-abdominal organs (S36.-)
injury to urinary and pelvic organs (S37.-)
open wound of abdominal wall (S31.-)
spinal cord injury (S34.0, S34.1-)
Excludes2 crushing injury of external genital organs (S38.0-)
● S38.2 Traumatic amputation of external genital organs
● S38.21 Traumatic amputation of female external genital organs
Traumatic amputation of clitoris
Traumatic amputation of labium (majus) (minus)
Traumatic amputation of vulva
● S38.211 Complete traumatic amputation of female external genital organs
● S38.212 Partial traumatic amputation of female external genital organs
● S38.22 Traumatic amputation of penis
● S38.221 Complete traumatic amputation of penis
● S38.222 Partial traumatic amputation of penis
● S38.23 Traumatic amputation of scrotum and testis
● S38.231 Complete traumatic amputation of scrotum and testis
● S38.232 Partial traumatic amputation of scrotum and testis
X● S38.3 Transection (partial) of abdomen

● S39 Other and unspecified injuries of abdomen, lower back, pelvis and external genitals

Code also any associated open wound (S31.-)

Excludes2 sprain of joints and ligaments of lumbar spine and pelvis (S33.-)

The appropriate 7th character is to be added to each code from category S39

A	initial encounter
D	subsequent encounter
S	sequela

● S39.0 Injury of muscle, fascia and tendon of abdomen, lower back and pelvis

● S39.00 Unspecified injury of muscle, fascia and tendon of abdomen, lower back and pelvis

● S39.001 Unspecified injury of muscle, fascia and tendon of abdomen

● S39.002 Unspecified injury of muscle, fascia and tendon of lower back

● S39.003 Unspecified injury of muscle, fascia and tendon of pelvis

● S39.01 Strain of muscle, fascia and tendon of abdomen, lower back and pelvis

● S39.011 Strain of muscle, fascia and tendon of abdomen

● S39.012 Strain of muscle, fascia and tendon of lower back

● S39.013 Strain of muscle, fascia and tendon of pelvis

● S39.02 Laceration of muscle, fascia and tendon of abdomen, lower back and pelvis

● S39.021 Laceration of muscle, fascia and tendon of abdomen

● S39.022 Laceration of muscle, fascia and tendon of lower back

● S39.023 Laceration of muscle, fascia and tendon of pelvis

● S39.09 Other injury of muscle, fascia and tendon of abdomen, lower back and pelvis

● S39.091 Other injury of muscle, fascia and tendon of abdomen

● S39.092 Other injury of muscle, fascia and tendon of lower back

● S39.093 Other injury of muscle, fascia and tendon of pelvis

● S39.8 Other specified injuries of abdomen, lower back, pelvis and external genitals

X● S39.81 Other specified injuries of abdomen

X● S39.82 Other specified injuries of lower back

X● S39.83 Other specified injuries of pelvis

● S39.84 Other specified injuries of external genitals

● S39.840 Fracture of corpus cavernosum penis

● S39.848 Other specified injuries of external genitals

● S39.9 Unspecified injury of abdomen, lower back, pelvis and external genitals

X● S39.91 Unspecified injury of abdomen

X● S39.92 Unspecified injury of lower back

X● S39.93 Unspecified injury of pelvis

X● S39.94 Unspecified injury of external genitals

INJURIES TO THE SHOULDER AND UPPER ARM (S40-S49)

Includes injuries of axilla injuries of scapular region

Excludes2 burns and corrosions (T20-T32)
frostbite (T33-T34)
injuries of elbow (S50-S59)
insect bite or sting, venomous (T63.4)

● S40 Superficial injury of shoulder and upper arm

The appropriate 7th character is to be added to each code from category S40

A	initial encounter
D	subsequent encounter
S	sequela

● S40.0 Contusion of shoulder and upper arm

● S40.01 Contusion of shoulder

● S40.011 Contusion of right shoulder

● S40.012 Contusion of left shoulder

● S40.019 Contusion of unspecified shoulder

● S40.02 Contusion of upper arm

● S40.021 Contusion of right upper arm

● S40.022 Contusion of left upper arm

● S40.029 Contusion of unspecified upper arm

● S40.2 Other superficial injuries of shoulder

● S40.21 Abrasion of shoulder

● S40.211 Abrasion of right shoulder

● S40.212 Abrasion of left shoulder

● S40.219 Abrasion of unspecified shoulder

● S40.22 Blister (nonthermal) of shoulder

● S40.221 Blister (nonthermal) of right shoulder

● S40.222 Blister (nonthermal) of left shoulder

● S40.229 Blister (nonthermal) of unspecified shoulder

● S40.24 External constriction of shoulder

● S40.241 External constriction of right shoulder

● S40.242 External constriction of left shoulder

● S40.249 External constriction of unspecified shoulder

● S40.25 Superficial foreign body of shoulder

Splinter in the shoulder

● S40.251 Superficial foreign body of right shoulder

● S40.252 Superficial foreign body of left shoulder

● S40.259 Superficial foreign body of unspecified shoulder

● S40.26 Insect bite (nonvenomous) of shoulder

● S40.261 Insect bite (nonvenomous) of right shoulder

● S40.262 Insect bite (nonvenomous) of left shoulder

● S40.269 Insect bite (nonvenomous) of unspecified shoulder

● S40.27 Other superficial bite of shoulder

Excludes1 open bite of shoulder (S41.05)

● S40.271 Other superficial bite of right shoulder

● S40.272 Other superficial bite of left shoulder

● S40.279 Other superficial bite of unspecified shoulder

CHAPTER 19 (S00-T88)

● S40.8 Other superficial injuries of upper arm
● S40.81 Abrasion of upper arm
● S40.811 Abrasion of right upper arm
● S40.812 Abrasion of left upper arm
● S40.819 Abrasion of unspecified upper arm
● S40.82 Blister (nonthermal) of upper arm
● S40.821 Blister (nonthermal) of right upper arm
● S40.822 Blister (nonthermal) of left upper arm
● S40.829 Blister (nonthermal) of unspecified upper arm
● S40.84 External constriction of upper arm
● S40.841 External constriction of right upper arm
● S40.842 External constriction of left upper arm
● S40.849 External constriction of unspecified upper arm
● S40.85 Superficial foreign body of upper arm
Splinter in the upper arm
● S40.851 Superficial foreign body of right upper arm
● S40.852 Superficial foreign body of left upper arm
● S40.859 Superficial foreign body of unspecified upper arm
● S40.86 Insect bite (nonvenomous) of upper arm
● S40.861 Insect bite (nonvenomous) of right upper arm
● S40.862 Insect bite (nonvenomous) of left upper arm
● S40.869 Insect bite (nonvenomous) of unspecified upper arm
● S40.87 Other superficial bite of upper arm
Excludes1 open bite of upper arm (S41.14)
Excludes2 other superficial bite of shoulder (S40.27-)
● S40.871 Other superficial bite of right upper arm
● S40.872 Other superficial bite of left upper arm
● S40.879 Other superficial bite of unspecified upper arm
● S40.9 Unspecified superficial injury of shoulder and upper arm
● S40.91 Unspecified superficial injury of shoulder
● S40.911 Unspecified superficial injury of right shoulder
● S40.912 Unspecified superficial injury of left shoulder
● S40.919 Unspecified superficial injury of unspecified shoulder
● S40.92 Unspecified superficial injury of upper arm
● S40.921 Unspecified superficial injury of right upper arm
● S40.922 Unspecified superficial injury of left upper arm
● S40.929 Unspecified superficial injury of unspecified upper arm

● S41 Open wound of shoulder and upper arm
Code also any associated wound infection
Excludes1 traumatic amputation of shoulder and upper arm (S48.-)
Excludes2 open fracture of shoulder and upper arm (S42.- with 7th character B or C)

The appropriate 7th character is to be added to each code from category S41

A	initial encounter
D	subsequent encounter
S	sequela

● S41.0 Open wound of shoulder
● S41.00 Unspecified open wound of shoulder
● S41.001 Unspecified open wound of right shoulder
● S41.002 Unspecified open wound of left shoulder
● S41.009 Unspecified open wound of unspecified shoulder
● S41.01 Laceration without foreign body of shoulder
● S41.011 Laceration without foreign body of right shoulder
● S41.012 Laceration without foreign body of left shoulder
● S41.019 Laceration without foreign body of unspecified shoulder
● S41.02 Laceration with foreign body of shoulder
● S41.021 Laceration with foreign body of right shoulder
● S41.022 Laceration with foreign body of left shoulder
● S41.029 Laceration with foreign body of unspecified shoulder
● S41.03 Puncture wound without foreign body of shoulder
● S41.031 Puncture wound without foreign body of right shoulder
● S41.032 Puncture wound without foreign body of left shoulder
● S41.039 Puncture wound without foreign body of unspecified shoulder
● S41.04 Puncture wound with foreign body of shoulder
● S41.041 Puncture wound with foreign body of right shoulder
● S41.042 Puncture wound with foreign body of left shoulder
● S41.049 Puncture wound with foreign body of unspecified shoulder
● S41.05 Open bite of shoulder
Bite of shoulder NOS
Excludes1 superficial bite of shoulder (S40.27)
● S41.051 Open bite of right shoulder
● S41.052 Open bite of left shoulder
● S41.059 Open bite of unspecified shoulder
● S41.1 Open wound of upper arm
● S41.10 Unspecified open wound of upper arm
● S41.101 Unspecified open wound of right upper arm
● S41.102 Unspecified open wound of left upper arm
● S41.109 Unspecified open wound of unspecified upper arm

● S41.11 Laceration without foreign body of upper arm
● S41.111 Laceration without foreign body of right upper arm
● S41.112 Laceration without foreign body of left upper arm
● S41.119 Laceration without foreign body of unspecified upper arm
● S41.12 Laceration with foreign body of upper arm
● S41.121 Laceration with foreign body of right upper arm
● S41.122 Laceration with foreign body of left upper arm
● S41.129 Laceration with foreign body of unspecified upper arm
● S41.13 Puncture wound without foreign body of upper arm
● S41.131 Puncture wound without foreign body of right upper arm
● S41.132 Puncture wound without foreign body of left upper arm
● S41.139 Puncture wound without foreign body of unspecified upper arm
● S41.14 Puncture wound with foreign body of upper arm
● S41.141 Puncture wound with foreign body of right upper arm
● S41.142 Puncture wound with foreign body of left upper arm
● S41.149 Puncture wound with foreign body of unspecified upper arm
● S41.15 Open bite of upper arm
Bite of upper arm NOS
Excludes1 superficial bite of upper arm (S40.87)
● S41.151 Open bite of right upper arm
● S41.152 Open bite of left upper arm
● S41.159 Open bite of unspecified upper arm

● S42 Fracture of shoulder and upper arm
Note: A fracture not indicated as displaced or nondisplaced should be coded to displaced
A fracture not indicated as open or closed should be coded to closed
Excludes1 traumatic amputation of shoulder and upper arm (S48.-)
The appropriate 7th character is to be added to all codes from category S42

A	initial encounter for closed fracture
B	initial encounter for open fracture
D	subsequent encounter for fracture with routine healing
G	subsequent encounter for fracture with delayed healing
K	subsequent encounter for fracture with nonunion
P	subsequent encounter for fracture with malunion
S	sequela

● S42.0 Fracture of clavicle
● S42.00 Fracture of unspecified part of clavicle
● S42.001 Fracture of unspecified part of right clavicle
● S42.002 Fracture of unspecified part of left clavicle
● S42.009 Fracture of unspecified part of unspecified clavicle
● S42.01 Fracture of sternal end of clavicle
● S42.011 Anterior displaced fracture of sternal end of right clavicle
● S42.012 Anterior displaced fracture of sternal end of left clavicle
● S42.013 Anterior displaced fracture of sternal end of unspecified clavicle
Displaced fracture of sternal end of clavicle NOS
● S42.014 Posterior displaced fracture of sternal end of right clavicle
● S42.015 Posterior displaced fracture of sternal end of left clavicle
● S42.016 Posterior displaced fracture of sternal end of unspecified clavicle
● S42.017 Nondisplaced fracture of sternal end of right clavicle
● S42.018 Nondisplaced fracture of sternal end of left clavicle
● S42.019 Nondisplaced fracture of sternal end of unspecified clavicle
● S42.02 Fracture of shaft of clavicle
● S42.021 Displaced fracture of shaft of right clavicle
● S42.022 Displaced fracture of shaft of left clavicle
● S42.023 Displaced fracture of shaft of unspecified clavicle
● S42.024 Nondisplaced fracture of shaft of right clavicle
● S42.025 Nondisplaced fracture of shaft of left clavicle
● S42.026 Nondisplaced fracture of shaft of unspecified clavicle
● S42.03 Fracture of lateral end of clavicle
Fracture of acromial end of clavicle
● S42.031 Displaced fracture of lateral end of right clavicle
● S42.032 Displaced fracture of lateral end of left clavicle
● S42.033 Displaced fracture of lateral end of unspecified clavicle
● S42.034 Nondisplaced fracture of lateral end of right clavicle
● S42.035 Nondisplaced fracture of lateral end of left clavicle
● S42.036 Nondisplaced fracture of lateral end of unspecified clavicle
● S42.1 Fracture of scapula
● S42.10 Fracture of unspecified part of scapula
● S42.101 Fracture of unspecified part of scapula, right shoulder
● S42.102 Fracture of unspecified part of scapula, left shoulder
● S42.109 Fracture of unspecified part of scapula, unspecified shoulder
● S42.11 Fracture of body of scapula
● S42.111 Displaced fracture of body of scapula, right shoulder
● S42.112 Displaced fracture of body of scapula, left shoulder
● S42.113 Displaced fracture of body of scapula, unspecified shoulder
● S42.114 Nondisplaced fracture of body of scapula, right shoulder
● S42.115 Nondisplaced fracture of body of scapula, left shoulder
● S42.116 Nondisplaced fracture of body of scapula, unspecified shoulder

● S42.12 Fracture of acromial process
● S42.121 Displaced fracture of acromial process, right shoulder
● S42.122 Displaced fracture of acromial process, left shoulder
● S42.123 Displaced fracture of acromial process, unspecified shoulder
● S42.124 Nondisplaced fracture of acromial process, right shoulder
● S42.125 Nondisplaced fracture of acromial process, left shoulder
● S42.126 Nondisplaced fracture, of acromial process, unspecified shoulder
● S42.13 Fracture of coracoid process
● S42.131 Displaced fracture of coracoid process, right shoulder
● S42.132 Displaced fracture of coracoid process, left shoulder
● S42.133 Displaced fracture of coracoid process, unspecified shoulder
● S42.134 Nondisplaced fracture of coracoid process, right shoulder
● S42.135 Nondisplaced fracture of coracoid process, left shoulder
● S42.136 Nondisplaced fracture of coracoid process, unspecified shoulder
● S42.14 Fracture of glenoid cavity of scapula
● S42.141 Displaced fracture of glenoid cavity of scapula, right shoulder
● S42.142 Displaced fracture of glenoid cavity of scapula, left shoulder
● S42.143 Displaced fracture of glenoid cavity of scapula, unspecified shoulder
● S42.144 Nondisplaced fracture of glenoid cavity of scapula, right shoulder
● S42.145 Nondisplaced fracture of glenoid cavity of scapula, left shoulder
● S42.146 Nondisplaced fracture of glenoid cavity of scapula, unspecified shoulder
● S42.15 Fracture of neck of scapula
● S42.151 Displaced fracture of neck of scapula, right shoulder
● S42.152 Displaced fracture of neck of scapula, left shoulder
● S42.153 Displaced fracture of neck of scapula, unspecified shoulder
● S42.154 Nondisplaced fracture of neck of scapula, right shoulder
● S42.155 Nondisplaced fracture of neck of scapula, left shoulder
● S42.156 Nondisplaced fracture of neck of scapula, unspecified shoulder
● S42.19 Fracture of other part of scapula
● S42.191 Fracture of other part of scapula, right shoulder
● S42.192 Fracture of other part of scapula, left shoulder
● S42.199 Fracture of other part of scapula, unspecified shoulder

● S42.2 Fracture of upper end of humerus
Fracture of proximal end of humerus
Excludes2 fracture of shaft of humerus (S42.3-)
physeal fracture of upper end of humerus (S49.0-)
● S42.20 Unspecified fracture of upper end of humerus
● S42.201 Unspecified fracture of upper end of right humerus
● S42.202 Unspecified fracture of upper end of left humerus
● S42.209 Unspecified fracture of upper end of unspecified humerus
● S42.21 Unspecified fracture of surgical neck of humerus
Fracture of neck of humerus NOS
● S42.211 Unspecified displaced fracture of surgical neck of right humerus
● S42.212 Unspecified displaced fracture of surgical neck of left humerus
● S42.213 Unspecified displaced fracture of surgical neck of unspecified humerus
● S42.214 Unspecified nondisplaced fracture of surgical neck of right humerus
● S42.215 Unspecified nondisplaced fracture of surgical neck of left humerus
● S42.216 Unspecified nondisplaced fracture of surgical neck of unspecified humerus
● S42.22 2-part fracture of surgical neck of humerus
● S42.221 2-part displaced fracture of surgical neck of right humerus
● S42.222 2-part displaced fracture of surgical neck of left humerus
● S42.223 2-part displaced fracture of surgical neck of unspecified humerus
● S42.224 2-part nondisplaced fracture of surgical neck of right humerus
● S42.225 2-part nondisplaced fracture of surgical neck of left humerus
● S42.226 2-part nondisplaced fracture of surgical neck of unspecified humerus
● S42.23 3-part fracture of surgical neck of humerus
● S42.231 3-part fracture of surgical neck of right humerus
● S42.232 3-part fracture of surgical neck of left humerus
● S42.239 3-part fracture of surgical neck of unspecified humerus
● S42.24 4-part fracture of surgical neck of humerus
● S42.241 4-part fracture of surgical neck of right humerus
● S42.242 4-part fracture of surgical neck of left humerus
● S42.249 4-part fracture of surgical neck of unspecified humerus
● S42.25 Fracture of greater tuberosity of humerus
● S42.251 Displaced fracture of greater tuberosity of right humerus
● S42.252 Displaced fracture of greater tuberosity of left humerus
● S42.253 Displaced fracture of greater tuberosity of unspecified humerus
● S42.254 Nondisplaced fracture of greater tuberosity of right humerus
● S42.255 Nondisplaced fracture of greater tuberosity of left humerus
● S42.256 Nondisplaced fracture of greater tuberosity of unspecified humerus

● S42.26 **Fracture of lesser tuberosity of humerus**
- ● S42.261 **Displaced fracture of lesser tuberosity of right humerus**
- ● S42.262 **Displaced fracture of lesser tuberosity of left humerus**
- ● S42.263 **Displaced fracture of lesser tuberosity of unspecified humerus**
- ● S42.264 **Nondisplaced fracture of lesser tuberosity of right humerus**
- ● S42.265 **Nondisplaced fracture of lesser tuberosity of left humerus**
- ● S42.266 **Nondisplaced fracture of lesser tuberosity of unspecified humerus**

● S42.27 **Torus fracture of upper end of humerus**

The appropriate 7th character is to be added to all codes in subcategory S42.27

A	initial encounter for closed fracture
D	subsequent encounter for fracture with routine healing
G	subsequent encounter for fracture with delayed healing
K	subsequent encounter for fracture with nonunion
P	subsequent encounter for fracture with malunion
S	sequela

- ● S42.271 **Torus fracture of upper end of right humerus**
- ● S42.272 **Torus fracture of upper end of left humerus**
- ● S42.279 **Torus fracture of upper end of unspecified humerus**

● S42.29 **Other fracture of upper end of humerus**

Fracture of anatomical neck of humerus
Fracture of articular head of humerus

- ● S42.291 **Other displaced fracture of upper end of right humerus**
- ● S42.292 **Other displaced fracture of upper end of left humerus**
- ● S42.293 **Other displaced fracture of upper end of unspecified humerus**
- ● S42.294 **Other nondisplaced fracture of upper end of right humerus**
- ● S42.295 **Other nondisplaced fracture of upper end of left humerus**
- ● S42.296 **Other nondisplaced fracture of upper end of unspecified humerus**

● S42.3 **Fracture of shaft of humerus**

Fracture of humerus NOS
Fracture of upper arm NOS

Excludes2 physeal fractures of upper end of humerus (S49.Ø-)
physeal fractures of lower end of humerus (S49.1-)

● S42.3Ø **Unspecified fracture of shaft of humerus**
- ● S42.3Ø1 **Unspecified fracture of shaft of humerus, right arm**
- ● S42.3Ø2 **Unspecified fracture of shaft of humerus, left arm**
- ● S42.3Ø9 **Unspecified fracture of shaft of humerus, unspecified arm**

● S42.31 **Greenstick fracture of shaft of humerus**

The appropriate 7th character is to be added to all codes in subcategory S42.31

A	initial encounter for closed fracture
D	subsequent encounter for fracture with routine healing
G	subsequent encounter for fracture with delayed healing
K	subsequent encounter for fracture with nonunion
P	subsequent encounter for fracture with malunion
S	sequela

- ● S42.311 **Greenstick fracture of shaft of humerus, right arm**
- ● S42.312 **Greenstick fracture of shaft of humerus, left arm**
- ● S42.319 **Greenstick fracture of shaft of humerus, unspecified arm**

● S42.32 **Transverse fracture of shaft of humerus**
- ● S42.321 **Displaced transverse fracture of shaft of humerus, right arm**
- ● S42.322 **Displaced transverse fracture of shaft of humerus, left arm**
- ● S42.323 **Displaced transverse fracture of shaft of humerus, unspecified arm**
- ● S42.324 **Nondisplaced transverse fracture of shaft of humerus, right arm**
- ● S42.325 **Nondisplaced transverse fracture of shaft of humerus, left arm**
- ● S42.326 **Nondisplaced transverse fracture of shaft of humerus, unspecified arm**

● S42.33 **Oblique fracture of shaft of humerus**
- ● S42.331 **Displaced oblique fracture of shaft of humerus, right arm**
- ● S42.332 **Displaced oblique fracture of shaft of humerus, left arm**
- ● S42.333 **Displaced oblique fracture of shaft of humerus, unspecified arm**
- ● S42.334 **Nondisplaced oblique fracture of shaft of humerus, right arm**
- ● S42.335 **Nondisplaced oblique fracture of shaft of humerus, left arm**
- ● S42.336 **Nondisplaced oblique fracture of shaft of humerus, unspecified arm**

● S42.34 **Spiral fracture of shaft of humerus**
- ● S42.341 **Displaced spiral fracture of shaft of humerus, right arm**
- ● S42.342 **Displaced spiral fracture of shaft of humerus, left arm**
- ● S42.343 **Displaced spiral fracture of shaft of humerus, unspecified arm**
- ● S42.344 **Nondisplaced spiral fracture of shaft of humerus, right arm**
- ● S42.345 **Nondisplaced spiral fracture of shaft of humerus, left arm**
- ● S42.346 **Nondisplaced spiral fracture of shaft of humerus, unspecified arm**

● S42.35 **Comminuted fracture of shaft of humerus**
- ● S42.351 **Displaced comminuted fracture of shaft of humerus, right arm**
- ● S42.352 **Displaced comminuted fracture of shaft of humerus, left arm**
- ● S42.353 **Displaced comminuted fracture of shaft of humerus, unspecified arm**

● S42.354 Nondisplaced comminuted fracture of shaft of humerus, right arm
● S42.355 Nondisplaced comminuted fracture of shaft of humerus, left arm
● S42.356 Nondisplaced comminuted fracture of shaft of humerus, unspecified arm

● S42.36 Segmental fracture of shaft of humerus
● S42.361 Displaced segmental fracture of shaft of humerus, right arm
● S42.362 Displaced segmental fracture of shaft of humerus, left arm
● S42.363 Displaced segmental fracture of shaft of humerus, unspecified arm
● S42.364 Nondisplaced segmental fracture of shaft of humerus, right arm
● S42.365 Nondisplaced segmental fracture of shaft of humerus, left arm
● S42.366 Nondisplaced segmental fracture of shaft of humerus, unspecified arm

● S42.39 Other fracture of shaft of humerus
● S42.391 Other fracture of shaft of right humerus
● S42.392 Other fracture of shaft of left humerus
● S42.399 Other fracture of shaft of unspecified humerus

● S42.4 Fracture of lower end of humerus
Fracture of distal end of humerus
Excludes2 fracture of shaft of humerus (S42.3-)
physeal fracture of lower end of humerus (S49.1-)

● S42.40 Unspecified fracture of lower end of humerus
Fracture of elbow NOS
● S42.401 Unspecified fracture of lower end of right humerus
● S42.402 Unspecified fracture of lower end of left humerus
● S42.409 Unspecified fracture of lower end of unspecified humerus

● S42.41 Simple supracondylar fracture without intercondylar fracture of humerus
● S42.411 Displaced simple supracondylar fracture without intercondylar fracture of right humerus
● S42.412 Displaced simple supracondylar fracture without intercondylar fracture of left humerus
● S42.413 Displaced simple supracondylar fracture without intercondylar fracture of unspecified humerus
● S42.414 Nondisplaced simple supracondylar fracture without intercondylar fracture of right humerus
● S42.415 Nondisplaced simple supracondylar fracture without intercondylar fracture of left humerus
● S42.416 Nondisplaced simple supracondylar fracture without intercondylar fracture of unspecified humerus

● S42.42 Comminuted supracondylar fracture without intercondylar fracture of humerus
● S42.421 Displaced comminuted supracondylar fracture without intercondylar fracture of right humerus
● S42.422 Displaced comminuted supracondylar fracture without intercondylar fracture of left humerus
● S42.423 Displaced comminuted supracondylar fracture without intercondylar fracture of unspecified humerus
● S42.424 Nondisplaced comminuted supracondylar fracture without intercondylar fracture of right humerus
● S42.425 Nondisplaced comminuted supracondylar fracture without intercondylar fracture of left humerus
● S42.426 Nondisplaced comminuted supracondylar fracture without intercondylar fracture of unspecified humerus

● S42.43 Fracture (avulsion) of lateral epicondyle of humerus
● S42.431 Displaced fracture (avulsion) of lateral epicondyle of right humerus
● S42.432 Displaced fracture (avulsion) of lateral epicondyle of left humerus
● S42.433 Displaced fracture (avulsion) of lateral epicondyle of unspecified humerus
● S42.434 Nondisplaced fracture (avulsion) of lateral epicondyle of right humerus
● S42.435 Nondisplaced fracture (avulsion) of lateral epicondyle of left humerus
● S42.436 Nondisplaced fracture (avulsion) of lateral epicondyle of unspecified humerus

● S42.44 Fracture (avulsion) of medial epicondyle of humerus
● S42.441 Displaced fracture (avulsion) of medial epicondyle of right humerus
● S42.442 Displaced fracture (avulsion) of medial epicondyle of left humerus
● S42.443 Displaced fracture (avulsion) of medial epicondyle of unspecified humerus
● S42.444 Nondisplaced fracture (avulsion) of medial epicondyle of right humerus
● S42.445 Nondisplaced fracture (avulsion) of medial epicondyle of left humerus
● S42.446 Nondisplaced fracture (avulsion) of medial epicondyle of unspecified humerus
● S42.447 Incarcerated fracture (avulsion) of medial epicondyle of right humerus
● S42.448 Incarcerated fracture (avulsion) of medial epicondyle of left humerus
● S42.449 Incarcerated fracture (avulsion) of medial epicondyle of unspecified humerus

● S42.45 Fracture of lateral condyle of humerus
Fracture of capitellum of humerus
● S42.451 Displaced fracture of lateral condyle of right humerus
● S42.452 Displaced fracture of lateral condyle of left humerus
● S42.453 Displaced fracture of lateral condyle of unspecified humerus
● S42.454 Nondisplaced fracture of lateral condyle of right humerus
● S42.455 Nondisplaced fracture of lateral condyle of left humerus
● S42.456 Nondisplaced fracture of lateral condyle of unspecified humerus

CHAPTER 19 (S00-T88)

● S42.46 **Fracture of medial condyle of humerus**
Trochlea fracture of humerus
● S42.461 **Displaced fracture of medial condyle of right humerus**
● S42.462 **Displaced fracture of medial condyle of left humerus**
● S42.463 **Displaced fracture of medial condyle of unspecified humerus**
● S42.464 **Nondisplaced fracture of medial condyle of right humerus**
● S42.465 **Nondisplaced fracture of medial condyle of left humerus**
● S42.466 **Nondisplaced fracture of medial condyle of unspecified humerus**
● S42.47 **Transcondylar fracture of humerus**
● S42.471 **Displaced transcondylar fracture of right humerus**
● S42.472 **Displaced transcondylar fracture of left humerus**
● S42.473 **Displaced transcondylar fracture of unspecified humerus**
● S42.474 **Nondisplaced transcondylar fracture of right humerus**
● S42.475 **Nondisplaced transcondylar fracture of left humerus**
● S42.476 **Nondisplaced transcondylar fracture of unspecified humerus**
● S42.48 **Torus fracture of lower end of humerus**
The appropriate 7th character is to be added to all codes in subcategory S42.48

A	initial encounter for closed fracture
D	subsequent encounter for fracture with routine healing
G	subsequent encounter for fracture with delayed healing
K	subsequent encounter for fracture with nonunion
P	subsequent encounter for fracture with malunion
S	sequela

● S42.481 **Torus fracture of lower end of right humerus**
● S42.482 **Torus fracture of lower end of left humerus**
● S42.489 **Torus fracture of lower end of unspecified humerus**
● S42.49 **Other fracture of lower end of humerus**
● S42.491 **Other displaced fracture of lower end of right humerus**
● S42.492 **Other displaced fracture of lower end of left humerus**
● S42.493 **Other displaced fracture of lower end of unspecified humerus**
● S42.494 **Other nondisplaced fracture of lower end of right humerus**
● S42.495 **Other nondisplaced fracture of lower end of left humerus**
● S42.496 **Other nondisplaced fracture of lower end of unspecified humerus**
● S42.9 **Fracture of shoulder girdle, part unspecified**
Fracture of shoulder NOS
X● S42.90 **Fracture of unspecified shoulder girdle, part unspecified**
X● S42.91 **Fracture of right shoulder girdle, part unspecified**
X● S42.92 **Fracture of left shoulder girdle, part unspecified**

● S43 **Dislocation and sprain of joints and ligaments of shoulder girdle**
Includes avulsion of joint or ligament of shoulder girdle
laceration of cartilage, joint or ligament of shoulder girdle
sprain of cartilage, joint or ligament of shoulder girdle
traumatic hemarthrosis of joint or ligament of shoulder girdle
traumatic rupture of joint or ligament of shoulder girdle
traumatic subluxation of joint or ligament of shoulder girdle
traumatic tear of joint or ligament of shoulder girdle
Code also any associated open wound
Excludes2 strain of muscle, fascia and tendon of shoulder and upper arm (S46.-)
The appropriate 7th character is to be added to each code from category S43

A	initial encounter
D	subsequent encounter
S	sequela

● S43.0 **Subluxation and dislocation of shoulder joint**
Dislocation of glenohumeral joint
Subluxation of glenohumeral joint
● S43.00 **Unspecified subluxation and dislocation of shoulder joint**
Dislocation of humerus NOS
Subluxation of humerus NOS
● S43.001 **Unspecified subluxation of right shoulder joint**
● S43.002 **Unspecified subluxation of left shoulder joint**
● S43.003 **Unspecified subluxation of unspecified shoulder joint**
● S43.004 **Unspecified dislocation of right shoulder joint**
● S43.005 **Unspecified dislocation of left shoulder joint**
● S43.006 **Unspecified dislocation of unspecified shoulder joint**
● S43.01 **Anterior subluxation and dislocation of humerus**
● S43.011 **Anterior subluxation of right humerus**
● S43.012 **Anterior subluxation of left humerus**
● S43.013 **Anterior subluxation of unspecified humerus**
● S43.014 **Anterior dislocation of right humerus**
● S43.015 **Anterior dislocation of left humerus**
● S43.016 **Anterior dislocation of unspecified humerus**
● S43.02 **Posterior subluxation and dislocation of humerus**
● S43.021 **Posterior subluxation of right humerus**
● S43.022 **Posterior subluxation of left humerus**
● S43.023 **Posterior subluxation of unspecified humerus**
● S43.024 **Posterior dislocation of right humerus**
● S43.025 **Posterior dislocation of left humerus**
● S43.026 **Posterior dislocation of unspecified humerus**

CHAPTER 19 (S00-T88)

S43.03 Inferior subluxation and dislocation of humerus
S43.031 Inferior subluxation of right humerus
S43.032 Inferior subluxation of left humerus
S43.033 Inferior subluxation of unspecified humerus
S43.034 Inferior dislocation of right humerus
S43.035 Inferior dislocation of left humerus
S43.036 Inferior dislocation of unspecified humerus
S43.08 Other subluxation and dislocation of shoulder joint
S43.081 Other subluxation of right shoulder joint
S43.082 Other subluxation of left shoulder joint
S43.083 Other subluxation of unspecified shoulder joint
S43.084 Other dislocation of right shoulder joint
S43.085 Other dislocation of left shoulder joint
S43.086 Other dislocation of unspecified shoulder joint
S43.1 Subluxation and dislocation of acromioclavicular joint
S43.10 Unspecified dislocation of acromioclavicular joint
S43.101 Unspecified dislocation of right acromioclavicular joint
S43.102 Unspecified dislocation of left acromioclavicular joint
S43.109 Unspecified dislocation of unspecified acromioclavicular joint
S43.11 Subluxation of acromioclavicular joint
S43.111 Subluxation of right acromioclavicular joint
S43.112 Subluxation of left acromioclavicular joint
S43.119 Subluxation of unspecified acromioclavicular joint
S43.12 Dislocation of acromioclavicular joint, 100%-200% displacement
S43.121 Dislocation of right acromioclavicular joint, 100%-200% displacement
S43.122 Dislocation of left acromioclavicular joint, 100%-200% displacement
S43.129 Dislocation of unspecified acromioclavicular joint, 100%-200% displacement
S43.13 Dislocation of acromioclavicular joint, greater than 200% displacement
S43.131 Dislocation of right acromioclavicular joint, greater than 200% displacement
S43.132 Dislocation of left acromioclavicular joint, greater than 200% displacement
S43.139 Dislocation of unspecified acromioclavicular joint, greater than 200% displacement
S43.14 Inferior dislocation of acromioclavicular joint
S43.141 Inferior dislocation of right acromioclavicular joint
S43.142 Inferior dislocation of left acromioclavicular joint
S43.149 Inferior dislocation of unspecified acromioclavicular joint
S43.15 Posterior dislocation of acromioclavicular joint
S43.151 Posterior dislocation of right acromioclavicular joint
S43.152 Posterior dislocation of left acromioclavicular joint
S43.159 Posterior dislocation of unspecified acromioclavicular joint
S43.2 Subluxation and dislocation of sternoclavicular joint
S43.20 Unspecified subluxation and dislocation of sternoclavicular joint
S43.201 Unspecified subluxation of right sternoclavicular joint
S43.202 Unspecified subluxation of left sternoclavicular joint
S43.203 Unspecified subluxation of unspecified sternoclavicular joint
S43.204 Unspecified dislocation of right sternoclavicular joint
S43.205 Unspecified dislocation of left sternoclavicular joint
S43.206 Unspecified dislocation of unspecified sternoclavicular joint
S43.21 Anterior subluxation and dislocation of sternoclavicular joint
S43.211 Anterior subluxation of right sternoclavicular joint
S43.212 Anterior subluxation of left sternoclavicular joint
S43.213 Anterior subluxation of unspecified sternoclavicular joint
S43.214 Anterior dislocation of right sternoclavicular joint
S43.215 Anterior dislocation of left sternoclavicular joint
S43.216 Anterior dislocation of unspecified sternoclavicular joint
S43.22 Posterior subluxation and dislocation of sternoclavicular joint
S43.221 Posterior subluxation of right sternoclavicular joint
S43.222 Posterior subluxation of left sternoclavicular joint
S43.223 Posterior subluxation of unspecified sternoclavicular joint
S43.224 Posterior dislocation of right sternoclavicular joint
S43.225 Posterior dislocation of left sternoclavicular joint
S43.226 Posterior dislocation of unspecified sternoclavicular joint
S43.3 Subluxation and dislocation of other and unspecified parts of shoulder girdle
S43.30 Subluxation and dislocation of unspecified parts of shoulder girdle
Dislocation of shoulder girdle NOS
Subluxation of shoulder girdle NOS
S43.301 Subluxation of unspecified parts of right shoulder girdle
S43.302 Subluxation of unspecified parts of left shoulder girdle
S43.303 Subluxation of unspecified parts of unspecified shoulder girdle
S43.304 Dislocation of unspecified parts of right shoulder girdle
S43.305 Dislocation of unspecified parts of left shoulder girdle
S43.306 Dislocation of unspecified parts of unspecified shoulder girdle

● **S43.31 Subluxation and dislocation of scapula**
  ● S43.311 Subluxation of right scapula
  ● S43.312 Subluxation of left scapula
  ● S43.313 Subluxation of unspecified scapula
  ● S43.314 Dislocation of right scapula
  ● S43.315 Dislocation of left scapula
  ● S43.316 Dislocation of unspecified scapula
● **S43.39 Subluxation and dislocation of other parts of shoulder girdle**
  ● S43.391 Subluxation of other parts of right shoulder girdle
  ● S43.392 Subluxation of other parts of left shoulder girdle
  ● S43.393 Subluxation of other parts of unspecified shoulder girdle
  ● S43.394 Dislocation of other parts of right shoulder girdle
  ● S43.395 Dislocation of other parts of left shoulder girdle
  ● S43.396 Dislocation of other parts of unspecified shoulder girdle
● **S43.4 Sprain of shoulder joint**
  ● S43.40 Unspecified sprain of shoulder joint
    ● S43.401 Unspecified sprain of right shoulder joint
    ● S43.402 Unspecified sprain of left shoulder joint
    ● S43.409 Unspecified sprain of unspecified shoulder joint
  ● **S43.41 Sprain of coracohumeral (ligament)**
    ● S43.411 Sprain of right coracohumeral (ligament)
    ● S43.412 Sprain of left coracohumeral (ligament)
    ● S43.419 Sprain of unspecified coracohumeral (ligament)
  ● **S43.42 Sprain of rotator cuff capsule**
    Encounters during the healing phase
    | **Excludes1** | rotator cuff syndrome (complete) (incomplete), not specified as traumatic (M75.1-) |

    | **Excludes2** | injury of tendon of rotator cuff (S46.0-) |

    ● S43.421 Sprain of right rotator cuff capsule
    ● S43.422 Sprain of left rotator cuff capsule
    ● S43.429 Sprain of unspecified rotator cuff capsule
  ● **S43.43 Superior glenoid labrum lesion**
    SLAP lesion
    ● S43.431 Superior glenoid labrum lesion of right shoulder
    ● S43.432 Superior glenoid labrum lesion of left shoulder
    ● S43.439 Superior glenoid labrum lesion of unspecified shoulder
  ● **S43.49 Other sprain of shoulder joint**
    ● S43.491 Other sprain of right shoulder joint
    ● S43.492 Other sprain of left shoulder joint
    ● S43.499 Other sprain of unspecified shoulder joint
● **S43.5 Sprain of acromioclavicular joint**
    Sprain of acromioclavicular ligament
  X● S43.50 Sprain of unspecified acromioclavicular joint
  X● S43.51 Sprain of right acromioclavicular joint
  X● S43.52 Sprain of left acromioclavicular joint

● **S43.6 Sprain of sternoclavicular joint**
  X● S43.60 Sprain of unspecified sternoclavicular joint
  X● S43.61 Sprain of right sternoclavicular joint
  X● S43.62 Sprain of left sternoclavicular joint
● **S43.8 Sprain of other specified parts of shoulder girdle**
  X● S43.80 Sprain of other specified parts of unspecified shoulder girdle
  X● S43.81 Sprain of other specified parts of right shoulder girdle
  X● S43.82 Sprain of other specified parts of left shoulder girdle
● **S43.9 Sprain of unspecified parts of shoulder girdle**
  X● S43.90 Sprain of unspecified parts of unspecified shoulder girdle
    Sprain of shoulder girdle NOS
  X● S43.91 Sprain of unspecified parts of right shoulder girdle
  X● S43.92 Sprain of unspecified parts of left shoulder girdle

● **S44 Injury of nerves at shoulder and upper arm level**
    Code also any associated open wound (S41.-)
    | **Excludes2** | injury of brachial plexus (S14.3-) |

    The appropriate 7th character is to be added to each code from category S44

    | A | initial encounter |
    | D | subsequent encounter |
    | S | sequela |

  ● **S44.0 Injury of ulnar nerve at upper arm level**
    | **Excludes1** | ulnar nerve NOS (S54.0) |
    X● S44.00 Injury of ulnar nerve at upper arm level, unspecified arm
    X● S44.01 Injury of ulnar nerve at upper arm level, right arm
    X● S44.02 Injury of ulnar nerve at upper arm level, left arm
  ● **S44.1 Injury of median nerve at upper arm level**
    | **Excludes1** | median nerve NOS (S54.1) |
    X● S44.10 Injury of median nerve at upper arm level, unspecified arm
    X● S44.11 Injury of median nerve at upper arm level, right arm
    X● S44.12 Injury of median nerve at upper arm level, left arm
  ● **S44.2 Injury of radial nerve at upper arm level**
    | **Excludes1** | radial nerve NOS (S54.2) |
    X● S44.20 Injury of radial nerve at upper arm level, unspecified arm
    X● S44.21 Injury of radial nerve at upper arm level, right arm
    X● S44.22 Injury of radial nerve at upper arm level, left arm
  ● **S44.3 Injury of axillary nerve**
    X● S44.30 Injury of axillary nerve, unspecified arm
    X● S44.31 Injury of axillary nerve, right arm
    X● S44.32 Injury of axillary nerve, left arm
  ● **S44.4 Injury of musculocutaneous nerve**
    X● S44.40 Injury of musculocutaneous nerve, unspecified arm
    X● S44.41 Injury of musculocutaneous nerve, right arm
    X● S44.42 Injury of musculocutaneous nerve, left arm

● S44.5 Injury of cutaneous sensory nerve at shoulder and upper arm level
X● S44.50 Injury of cutaneous sensory nerve at shoulder and upper arm level, unspecified arm
X● S44.51 Injury of cutaneous sensory nerve at shoulder and upper arm level, right arm
X● S44.52 Injury of cutaneous sensory nerve at shoulder and upper arm level, left arm
● S44.8 Injury of other nerves at shoulder and upper arm level
● S44.8X Injury of other nerves at shoulder and upper arm level
● S44.8X1 Injury of other nerves at shoulder and upper arm level, right arm
● S44.8X2 Injury of other nerves at shoulder and upper arm level, left arm
● S44.8X9 Injury of other nerves at shoulder and upper arm level, unspecified arm
● S44.9 Injury of unspecified nerve at shoulder and upper arm level
X● S44.90 Injury of unspecified nerve at shoulder and upper arm level, unspecified arm
X● S44.91 Injury of unspecified nerve at shoulder and upper arm level, right arm
X● S44.92 Injury of unspecified nerve at shoulder and upper arm level, left arm

● S45 Injury of blood vessels at shoulder and upper arm level
Code also any associated open wound (S41.-)
Excludes2 injury of subclavian artery (S25.1)
injury of subclavian vein (S25.3)
The appropriate 7th character is to be added to each code from category S45

A	initial encounter
D	subsequent encounter
S	sequela

● S45.0 Injury of axillary artery
● S45.00 Unspecified injury of axillary artery
● S45.001 Unspecified injury of axillary artery, right side
● S45.002 Unspecified injury of axillary artery, left side
● S45.009 Unspecified injury of axillary artery, unspecified side
● S45.01 Laceration of axillary artery
● S45.011 Laceration of axillary artery, right side
● S45.012 Laceration of axillary artery, left side
● S45.019 Laceration of axillary artery, unspecified side
● S45.09 Other specified injury of axillary artery
● S45.091 Other specified injury of axillary artery, right side
● S45.092 Other specified injury of axillary artery, left side
● S45.099 Other specified injury of axillary artery, unspecified side
● S45.1 Injury of brachial artery
● S45.10 Unspecified injury of brachial artery
● S45.101 Unspecified injury of brachial artery, right side
● S45.102 Unspecified injury of brachial artery, left side
● S45.109 Unspecified injury of brachial artery, unspecified side
● S45.11 Laceration of brachial artery
● S45.111 Laceration of brachial artery, right side
● S45.112 Laceration of brachial artery, left side
● S45.119 Laceration of brachial artery, unspecified side
● S45.19 Other specified injury of brachial artery
● S45.191 Other specified injury of brachial artery, right side
● S45.192 Other specified injury of brachial artery, left side
● S45.199 Other specified injury of brachial artery, unspecified side
● S45.2 Injury of axillary or brachial vein
● S45.20 Unspecified injury of axillary or brachial vein
● S45.201 Unspecified injury of axillary or brachial vein, right side
● S45.202 Unspecified injury of axillary or brachial vein, left side
● S45.209 Unspecified injury of axillary or brachial vein, unspecified side
● S45.21 Laceration of axillary or brachial vein
● S45.211 Laceration of axillary or brachial vein, right side
● S45.212 Laceration of axillary or brachial vein, left side
● S45.219 Laceration of axillary or brachial vein, unspecified side
● S45.29 Other specified injury of axillary or brachial vein
● S45.291 Other specified injury of axillary or brachial vein, right side
● S45.292 Other specified injury of axillary or brachial vein, left side
● S45.299 Other specified injury of axillary or brachial vein, unspecified side
● S45.3 Injury of superficial vein at shoulder and upper arm level
● S45.30 Unspecified injury of superficial vein at shoulder and upper arm level
● S45.301 Unspecified injury of superficial vein at shoulder and upper arm level, right arm
● S45.302 Unspecified injury of superficial vein at shoulder and upper arm level, left arm
● S45.309 Unspecified injury of superficial vein at shoulder and upper arm level, unspecified arm
● S45.31 Laceration of superficial vein at shoulder and upper arm level
● S45.311 Laceration of superficial vein at shoulder and upper arm level, right arm
● S45.312 Laceration of superficial vein at shoulder and upper arm level, left arm
● S45.319 Laceration of superficial vein at shoulder and upper arm level, unspecified arm
● S45.39 Other specified injury of superficial vein at shoulder and upper arm level
● S45.391 Other specified injury of superficial vein at shoulder and upper arm level, right arm
● S45.392 Other specified injury of superficial vein at shoulder and upper arm level, left arm
● S45.399 Other specified injury of superficial vein at shoulder and upper arm level, unspecified arm

CHAPTER 19 (S00-T88)

S45.8 Injury of other specified blood vessels at shoulder and upper arm level

S45.80 Unspecified injury of other specified blood vessels at shoulder and upper arm level

S45.801 Unspecified injury of other specified blood vessels at shoulder and upper arm level, right arm

S45.802 Unspecified injury of other specified blood vessels at shoulder and upper arm level, left arm

S45.809 Unspecified injury of other specified blood vessels at shoulder and upper arm level, unspecified arm

S45.81 Laceration of other specified blood vessels at shoulder and upper arm level

S45.811 Laceration of other specified blood vessels at shoulder and upper arm level, right arm

S45.812 Laceration of other specified blood vessels at shoulder and upper arm level, left arm

S45.819 Laceration of other specified blood vessels at shoulder and upper arm level, unspecified arm

S45.89 Other specified injury of other specified blood vessels at shoulder and upper arm level

S45.891 Other specified injury of other specified blood vessels at shoulder and upper arm level, right arm

S45.892 Other specified injury of other specified blood vessels at shoulder and upper arm level, left arm

S45.899 Other specified injury of other specified blood vessels at shoulder and upper arm level, unspecified arm

S45.9 Injury of unspecified blood vessel at shoulder and upper arm level

S45.90 Unspecified injury of unspecified blood vessel at shoulder and upper arm level

S45.901 Unspecified injury of unspecified blood vessel at shoulder and upper arm level, right arm

S45.902 Unspecified injury of unspecified blood vessel at shoulder and upper arm level, left arm

S45.909 Unspecified injury of unspecified blood vessel at shoulder and upper arm level, unspecified arm

S45.91 Laceration of unspecified blood vessel at shoulder and upper arm level

S45.911 Laceration of unspecified blood vessel at shoulder and upper arm level, right arm

S45.912 Laceration of unspecified blood vessel at shoulder and upper arm level, left arm

S45.919 Laceration of unspecified blood vessel at shoulder and upper arm level, unspecified arm

S45.99 Other specified injury of unspecified blood vessel at shoulder and upper arm level

S45.991 Other specified injury of unspecified blood vessel at shoulder and upper arm level, right arm

S45.992 Other specified injury of unspecified blood vessel at shoulder and upper arm level, left arm

S45.999 Other specified injury of unspecified blood vessel at shoulder and upper arm level, unspecified arm

S46 Injury of muscle, fascia and tendon at shoulder and upper arm level

Code also any associated open wound (S41.-)

Excludes2 injury of muscle, fascia and tendon at elbow (S56.-)
sprain of joints and ligaments of shoulder girdle (S43.9)

The appropriate 7th character is to be added to each code from category S46

A	initial encounter
D	subsequent encounter
S	sequela

S46.0 Injury of muscle(s) and tendon(s) of the rotator cuff of shoulder

S46.00 Unspecified injury of muscle(s) and tendon(s) of the rotator cuff of shoulder

S46.001 Unspecified injury of muscle(s) and tendon(s) of the rotator cuff of right shoulder

S46.002 Unspecified injury of muscle(s) and tendon(s) of the rotator cuff of left shoulder

S46.009 Unspecified injury of muscle(s) and tendon(s) of the rotator cuff of unspecified shoulder

S46.01 Strain of muscle(s) and tendon(s) of the rotator cuff of shoulder

Acute onset due to trauma to rotator cuff muscle/tendon

S46.011 Strain of muscle(s) and tendon(s) of the rotator cuff of right shoulder

S46.012 Strain of muscle(s) and tendon(s) of the rotator cuff of left shoulder

S46.019 Strain of muscle(s) and tendon(s) of the rotator cuff of unspecified shoulder

S46.02 Laceration of muscle(s) and tendon(s) of the rotator cuff of shoulder

S46.021 Laceration of muscle(s) and tendon(s) of the rotator cuff of right shoulder

S46.022 Laceration of muscle(s) and tendon(s) of the rotator cuff of left shoulder

S46.029 Laceration of muscle(s) and tendon(s) of the rotator cuff of unspecified shoulder

S46.09 Other injury of muscle(s) and tendon(s) of the rotator cuff of shoulder

S46.091 Other injury of muscle(s) and tendon(s) of the rotator cuff of right shoulder

S46.092 Other injury of muscle(s) and tendon(s) of the rotator cuff of left shoulder

S46.099 Other injury of muscle(s) and tendon(s) of the rotator cuff of unspecified shoulder

S46.1 Injury of muscle, fascia and tendon of long head of biceps

S46.10 Unspecified injury of muscle, fascia and tendon of long head of biceps

S46.101 Unspecified injury of muscle, fascia and tendon of long head of biceps, right arm

S46.102 Unspecified injury of muscle, fascia and tendon of long head of biceps, left arm

S46.109 Unspecified injury of muscle, fascia and tendon of long head of biceps, unspecified arm

- S46.11 Strain of muscle, fascia and tendon of long head of biceps
  - S46.111 Strain of muscle, fascia and tendon of long head of biceps, right arm
  - S46.112 Strain of muscle, fascia and tendon of long head of biceps, left arm
  - S46.119 Strain of muscle, fascia and tendon of long head of biceps, unspecified arm
- S46.12 Laceration of muscle, fascia and tendon of long head of biceps
  - S46.121 Laceration of muscle, fascia and tendon of long head of biceps, right arm
  - S46.122 Laceration of muscle, fascia and tendon of long head of biceps, left arm
  - S46.129 Laceration of muscle, fascia and tendon of long head of biceps, unspecified arm
- S46.19 Other injury of muscle, fascia and tendon of long head of biceps
  - S46.191 Other injury of muscle, fascia and tendon of long head of biceps, right arm
  - S46.192 Other injury of muscle, fascia and tendon of long head of biceps, left arm
  - S46.199 Other injury of muscle, fascia and tendon of long head of biceps, unspecified arm

S46.2 Injury of muscle, fascia and tendon of other parts of biceps

- S46.20 Unspecified injury of muscle, fascia and tendon of other parts of biceps
  - S46.201 Unspecified injury of muscle, fascia and tendon of other parts of biceps, right arm
  - S46.202 Unspecified injury of muscle, fascia and tendon of other parts of biceps, left arm
  - S46.209 Unspecified injury of muscle, fascia and tendon of other parts of biceps, unspecified arm
- S46.21 Strain of muscle, fascia and tendon of other parts of biceps
  - S46.211 Strain of muscle, fascia and tendon of other parts of biceps, right arm
  - S46.212 Strain of muscle, fascia and tendon of other parts of biceps, left arm
  - S46.219 Strain of muscle, fascia and tendon of other parts of biceps, unspecified arm
- S46.22 Laceration of muscle, fascia and tendon of other parts of biceps
  - S46.221 Laceration of muscle, fascia and tendon of other parts of biceps, right arm
  - S46.222 Laceration of muscle, fascia and tendon of other parts of biceps, left arm
  - S46.229 Laceration of muscle, fascia and tendon of other parts of biceps, unspecified arm
- S46.29 Other injury of muscle, fascia and tendon of other parts of biceps
  - S46.291 Other injury of muscle, fascia and tendon of other parts of biceps, right arm
  - S46.292 Other injury of muscle, fascia and tendon of other parts of biceps, left arm
  - S46.299 Other injury of muscle, fascia and tendon of other parts of biceps, unspecified arm

S46.3 Injury of muscle, fascia and tendon of triceps

- S46.30 Unspecified injury of muscle, fascia and tendon of triceps
  - S46.301 Unspecified injury of muscle, fascia and tendon of triceps, right arm
  - S46.302 Unspecified injury of muscle, fascia and tendon of triceps, left arm
  - S46.309 Unspecified injury of muscle, fascia and tendon of triceps, unspecified arm
- S46.31 Strain of muscle, fascia and tendon of triceps
  - S46.311 Strain of muscle, fascia and tendon of triceps, right arm
  - S46.312 Strain of muscle, fascia and tendon of triceps, left arm
  - S46.319 Strain of muscle, fascia and tendon of triceps, unspecified arm
- S46.32 Laceration of muscle, fascia and tendon of triceps
  - S46.321 Laceration of muscle, fascia and tendon of triceps, right arm
  - S46.322 Laceration of muscle, fascia and tendon of triceps, left arm
  - S46.329 Laceration of muscle, fascia and tendon of triceps, unspecified arm
- S46.39 Other injury of muscle, fascia and tendon of triceps
  - S46.391 Other injury of muscle, fascia and tendon of triceps, right arm
  - S46.392 Other injury of muscle, fascia and tendon of triceps, left arm
  - S46.399 Other injury of muscle, fascia and tendon of triceps, unspecified arm

S46.8 Injury of other muscles, fascia and tendons at shoulder and upper arm level

- S46.80 Unspecified injury of other muscles, fascia and tendons at shoulder and upper arm level
  - S46.801 Unspecified injury of other muscles, fascia and tendons at shoulder and upper arm level, right arm
  - S46.802 Unspecified injury of other muscles, fascia and tendons at shoulder and upper arm level, left arm
  - S46.809 Unspecified injury of other muscles, fascia and tendons at shoulder and upper arm level, unspecified arm
- S46.81 Strain of other muscles, fascia and tendons at shoulder and upper arm level
  - S46.811 Strain of other muscles, fascia and tendons at shoulder and upper arm level, right arm
  - S46.812 Strain of other muscles, fascia and tendons at shoulder and upper arm level, left arm
  - S46.819 Strain of other muscles, fascia and tendons at shoulder and upper arm level, unspecified arm

CHAPTER 19 (S00-T88)

- S46.82 Laceration of other muscles, fascia and tendons at shoulder and upper arm level
  - S46.821 Laceration of other muscles, fascia and tendons at shoulder and upper arm level, right arm
  - S46.822 Laceration of other muscles, fascia and tendons at shoulder and upper arm level, left arm
  - S46.829 Laceration of other muscles, fascia and tendons at shoulder and upper arm level, unspecified arm
- S46.89 Other injury of other muscles, fascia and tendons at shoulder and upper arm level
  - S46.891 Other injury of other muscles, fascia and tendons at shoulder and upper arm level, right arm
  - S46.892 Other injury of other muscles, fascia and tendons at shoulder and upper arm level, left arm
  - S46.899 Other injury of other muscles, fascia and tendons at shoulder and upper arm level, unspecified arm

S46.9 Injury of unspecified muscle, fascia and tendon at shoulder and upper arm level

- S46.90 Unspecified injury of unspecified muscle, fascia and tendon at shoulder and upper arm level
  - S46.901 Unspecified injury of unspecified muscle, fascia and tendon at shoulder and upper arm level, right arm
  - S46.902 Unspecified injury of unspecified muscle, fascia and tendon at shoulder and upper arm level, left arm
  - S46.909 Unspecified injury of unspecified muscle, fascia and tendon at shoulder and upper arm level, unspecified arm
- S46.91 Strain of unspecified muscle, fascia and tendon at shoulder and upper arm level
  - S46.911 Strain of unspecified muscle, fascia and tendon at shoulder and upper arm level, right arm
  - S46.912 Strain of unspecified muscle, fascia and tendon at shoulder and upper arm level, left arm
  - S46.919 Strain of unspecified muscle, fascia and tendon at shoulder and upper arm level, unspecified arm
- S46.92 Laceration of unspecified muscle, fascia and tendon at shoulder and upper arm level
  - S46.921 Laceration of unspecified muscle, fascia and tendon at shoulder and upper arm level, right arm
  - S46.922 Laceration of unspecified muscle, fascia and tendon at shoulder and upper arm level, left arm
  - S46.929 Laceration of unspecified muscle, fascia and tendon at shoulder and upper arm level, unspecified arm
- S46.99 Other injury of unspecified muscle, fascia and tendon at shoulder and upper arm level
  - S46.991 Other injury of unspecified muscle, fascia and tendon at shoulder and upper arm level, right arm
  - S46.992 Other injury of unspecified muscle, fascia and tendon at shoulder and upper arm level, left arm
  - S46.999 Other injury of unspecified muscle, fascia and tendon at shoulder and upper arm level, unspecified arm

S47 Crushing injury of shoulder and upper arm

Use additional code for all associated injuries

Excludes2 crushing injury of elbow (S57.Ø-)

The appropriate 7th character is to be added to each code from category S47

A	initial encounter
D	subsequent encounter
S	sequela

- X S47.1 Crushing injury of right shoulder and upper arm
- X S47.2 Crushing injury of left shoulder and upper arm
- X S47.9 Crushing injury of shoulder and upper arm, unspecified arm

S48 Traumatic amputation of shoulder and upper arm

An amputation not identified as partial or complete should be coded to complete

Excludes1 traumatic amputation at elbow level (S58.Ø)

The appropriate 7th character is to be added to each code from category S48

A	initial encounter
D	subsequent encounter
S	sequela

S48.Ø Traumatic amputation at shoulder joint

- S48.Ø1 Complete traumatic amputation at shoulder joint
  - S48.Ø11 Complete traumatic amputation at right shoulder joint
  - S48.Ø12 Complete traumatic amputation at left shoulder joint
  - S48.Ø19 Complete traumatic amputation at unspecified shoulder joint
- S48.Ø2 Partial traumatic amputation at shoulder joint
  - S48.Ø21 Partial traumatic amputation at right shoulder joint
  - S48.Ø22 Partial traumatic amputation at left shoulder joint
  - S48.Ø29 Partial traumatic amputation at unspecified shoulder joint

S48.1 Traumatic amputation at level between shoulder and elbow

- S48.11 Complete traumatic amputation at level between shoulder and elbow
  - S48.111 Complete traumatic amputation at level between right shoulder and elbow
  - S48.112 Complete traumatic amputation at level between left shoulder and elbow
  - S48.119 Complete traumatic amputation at level between unspecified shoulder and elbow
- S48.12 Partial traumatic amputation at level between shoulder and elbow
  - S48.121 Partial traumatic amputation at level between right shoulder and elbow
  - S48.122 Partial traumatic amputation at level between left shoulder and elbow
  - S48.129 Partial traumatic amputation at level between unspecified shoulder and elbow

● S48.9 Traumatic amputation of shoulder and upper arm, level unspecified
● S48.91 Complete traumatic amputation of shoulder and upper arm, level unspecified
● S48.911 Complete traumatic amputation of right shoulder and upper arm, level unspecified
● S48.912 Complete traumatic amputation of left shoulder and upper arm, level unspecified
● S48.919 Complete traumatic amputation of unspecified shoulder and upper arm, level unspecified
● S48.92 Partial traumatic amputation of shoulder and upper arm, level unspecified
● S48.921 Partial traumatic amputation of right shoulder and upper arm, level unspecified
● S48.922 Partial traumatic amputation of left shoulder and upper arm, level unspecified
● S48.929 Partial traumatic amputation of unspecified shoulder and upper arm, level unspecified

● S49 Other and unspecified injuries of shoulder and upper arm

The appropriate 7th character is to be added to each code from subcategories S49.0 and S49.1

A	initial encounter for closed fracture
D	subsequent encounter for fracture with routine healing
G	subsequent encounter for fracture with delayed healing
K	subsequent encounter for fracture with nonunion
P	subsequent encounter for fracture with malunion
S	sequela

● S49.0 Physeal fracture of upper end of humerus
● S49.00 Unspecified physeal fracture of upper end of humerus
● S49.001 Unspecified physeal fracture of upper end of humerus, right arm
● S49.002 Unspecified physeal fracture of upper end of humerus, left arm
● S49.009 Unspecified physeal fracture of upper end of humerus, unspecified arm
● S49.01 Salter-Harris Type I physeal fracture of upper end of humerus
● S49.011 Salter-Harris Type I physeal fracture of upper end of humerus, right arm
● S49.012 Salter-Harris Type I physeal fracture of upper end of humerus, left arm
● S49.019 Salter-Harris Type I physeal fracture of upper end of humerus, unspecified arm
● S49.02 Salter-Harris Type II physeal fracture of upper end of humerus
● S49.021 Salter-Harris Type II physeal fracture of upper end of humerus, right arm
● S49.022 Salter-Harris Type II physeal fracture of upper end of humerus, left arm
● S49.029 Salter-Harris Type II physeal fracture of upper end of humerus, unspecified arm
● S49.03 Salter-Harris Type III physeal fracture of upper end of humerus
● S49.031 Salter-Harris Type III physeal fracture of upper end of humerus, right arm
● S49.032 Salter-Harris Type III physeal fracture of upper end of humerus, left arm
● S49.039 Salter-Harris Type III physeal fracture of upper end of humerus, unspecified arm

Item 19-3 SALTER-HARRIS TYPE 1: epiphysis is completely separated from end of bone, or metaphysic growth plate remains attached to epiphysis

SALTER-HARRIS TYPE 2: epiphysis and growth plate are partially separated from metaphysis, which is cracked—most common type

SALTER-HARRIS TYPE 3: fracture occurring through epiphysis and separates part of epiphysis and growth plate from metaphysis fracture, usually at distal end of tibia

SALTER-HARRIS TYPE 4: fracture runs through epiphysis, across growth plate, into metaphysic, surgery is required to restore joint surface to normal and align growth plate

● S49.04 Salter-Harris Type IV physeal fracture of upper end of humerus
● S49.041 Salter-Harris Type IV physeal fracture of upper end of humerus, right arm
● S49.042 Salter-Harris Type IV physeal fracture of upper end of humerus, left arm
● S49.049 Salter-Harris Type IV physeal fracture of upper end of humerus, unspecified arm
● S49.09 Other physeal fracture of upper end of humerus
● S49.091 Other physeal fracture of upper end of humerus, right arm
● S49.092 Other physeal fracture of upper end of humerus, left arm
● S49.099 Other physeal fracture of upper end of humerus, unspecified arm
● S49.1 Physeal fracture of lower end of humerus
● S49.10 Unspecified physeal fracture of lower end of humerus
● S49.101 Unspecified physeal fracture of lower end of humerus, right arm
● S49.102 Unspecified physeal fracture of lower end of humerus, left arm
● S49.109 Unspecified physeal fracture of lower end of humerus, unspecified arm
● S49.11 Salter-Harris Type I physeal fracture of lower end of humerus
● S49.111 Salter-Harris Type I physeal fracture of lower end of humerus, right arm
● S49.112 Salter-Harris Type I physeal fracture of lower end of humerus, left arm
● S49.119 Salter-Harris Type I physeal fracture of lower end of humerus, unspecified arm
● S49.12 Salter-Harris Type II physeal fracture of lower end of humerus
● S49.121 Salter-Harris Type II physeal fracture of lower end of humerus, right arm
● S49.122 Salter-Harris Type II physeal fracture of lower end of humerus, left arm
● S49.129 Salter-Harris Type II physeal fracture of lower end of humerus, unspecified arm
● S49.13 Salter-Harris Type III physeal fracture of lower end of humerus
● S49.131 Salter-Harris Type III physeal fracture of lower end of humerus, right arm
● S49.132 Salter-Harris Type III physeal fracture of lower end of humerus, left arm
● S49.139 Salter-Harris Type III physeal fracture of lower end of humerus, unspecified arm

CHAPTER 19 (S00-T88)

● S49.14 Salter-Harris Type IV physeal fracture of lower end of humerus
● S49.141 Salter-Harris Type IV physeal fracture of lower end of humerus, right arm
● S49.142 Salter-Harris Type IV physeal fracture of lower end of humerus, left arm
● S49.149 Salter-Harris Type IV physeal fracture of lower end of humerus, unspecified arm
● S49.19 Other physeal fracture of lower end of humerus
● S49.191 Other physeal fracture of lower end of humerus, right arm
● S49.192 Other physeal fracture of lower end of humerus, left arm
● S49.199 Other physeal fracture of lower end of humerus, unspecified arm
● S49.8 Other specified injuries of shoulder and upper arm

The appropriate 7th character is to be added to each code in subcategory S49.8

A initial encounter
D subsequent encounter
S sequela

X● S49.80 Other specified injuries of shoulder and upper arm, unspecified arm
X● S49.81 Other specified injuries of right shoulder and upper arm
X● S49.82 Other specified injuries of left shoulder and upper arm
● S49.9 Unspecified injury of shoulder and upper arm

The appropriate 7th character is to be added to each code in subcategory S49.9

A initial encounter
D subsequent encounter
S sequela

X● S49.90 Unspecified injury of shoulder and upper arm, unspecified arm
X● S49.91 Unspecified injury of right shoulder and upper arm
X● S49.92 Unspecified injury of left shoulder and upper arm

INJURIES TO THE ELBOW AND FOREARM (S50-S59)

Excludes2 burns and corrosions (T20-T32)
frostbite (T33-T34)
injuries of wrist and hand (S60-S69)
insect bite or sting, venomous (T63.4)

● S50 Superficial injury of elbow and forearm

Excludes2 superficial injury of wrist and hand (S60.-)

The appropriate 7th character is to be added to each code from category S50

A initial encounter
D subsequent encounter
S sequela

● S50.0 Contusion of elbow
X● S50.00 Contusion of unspecified elbow
X● S50.01 Contusion of right elbow
X● S50.02 Contusion of left elbow
● S50.1 Contusion of forearm
X● S50.10 Contusion of unspecified forearm
X● S50.11 Contusion of right forearm
X● S50.12 Contusion of left forearm
● S50.3 Other superficial injuries of elbow
● S50.31 Abrasion of elbow
● S50.311 Abrasion of right elbow
● S50.312 Abrasion of left elbow
● S50.319 Abrasion of unspecified elbow
● S50.32 Blister (nonthermal) of elbow
● S50.321 Blister (nonthermal) of right elbow
● S50.322 Blister (nonthermal) of left elbow
● S50.329 Blister (nonthermal) of unspecified elbow
● S50.34 External constriction of elbow
● S50.341 External constriction of right elbow
● S50.342 External constriction of left elbow
● S50.349 External constriction of unspecified elbow
● S50.35 Superficial foreign body of elbow
Splinter in the elbow
● S50.351 Superficial foreign body of right elbow
● S50.352 Superficial foreign body of left elbow
● S50.359 Superficial foreign body of unspecified elbow
● S50.36 Insect bite (nonvenomous) of elbow
● S50.361 Insect bite (nonvenomous) of right elbow
● S50.362 Insect bite (nonvenomous) of left elbow
● S50.369 Insect bite (nonvenomous) of unspecified elbow
● S50.37 Other superficial bite of elbow

Excludes1 open bite of elbow (S51.04)

● S50.371 Other superficial bite of right elbow
● S50.372 Other superficial bite of left elbow
● S50.379 Other superficial bite of unspecified elbow
● S50.8 Other superficial injuries of forearm
● S50.81 Abrasion of forearm
● S50.811 Abrasion of right forearm
● S50.812 Abrasion of left forearm
● S50.819 Abrasion of unspecified forearm
● S50.82 Blister (nonthermal) of forearm
● S50.821 Blister (nonthermal) of right forearm
● S50.822 Blister (nonthermal) of left forearm
● S50.829 Blister (nonthermal) of unspecified forearm
● S50.84 External constriction of forearm
● S50.841 External constriction of right forearm
● S50.842 External constriction of left forearm
● S50.849 External constriction of unspecified forearm
● S50.85 Superficial foreign body of forearm
Splinter in the forearm
● S50.851 Superficial foreign body of right forearm
● S50.852 Superficial foreign body of left forearm
● S50.859 Superficial foreign body of unspecified forearm
● S50.86 Insect bite (nonvenomous) of forearm
● S50.861 Insect bite (nonvenomous) of right forearm
● S50.862 Insect bite (nonvenomous) of left forearm
● S50.869 Insect bite (nonvenomous) of unspecified forearm

- S50.87 Other superficial bite of forearm
  - Excludes1 open bite of forearm (S51.84)
  - S50.871 Other superficial bite of right forearm
  - S50.872 Other superficial bite of left forearm
  - S50.879 Other superficial bite of unspecified forearm
- S50.9 Unspecified superficial injury of elbow and forearm
  - S50.90 Unspecified superficial injury of elbow
    - S50.901 Unspecified superficial injury of right elbow
    - S50.902 Unspecified superficial injury of left elbow
    - S50.909 Unspecified superficial injury of unspecified elbow
  - S50.91 Unspecified superficial injury of forearm
    - S50.911 Unspecified superficial injury of right forearm
    - S50.912 Unspecified superficial injury of left forearm
    - S50.919 Unspecified superficial injury of unspecified forearm

S51 Open wound of elbow and forearm

Code also any associated wound infection

Excludes1 open fracture of elbow and forearm (S52.- with open fracture 7th character)
traumatic amputation of elbow and forearm (S58.-)

Excludes2 open wound of wrist and hand (S61.-)

The appropriate 7th character is to be added to each code from category S51

A	initial encounter
D	subsequent encounter
S	sequela

- S51.0 Open wound of elbow
  - S51.00 Unspecified open wound of elbow
    - S51.001 Unspecified open wound of right elbow
    - S51.002 Unspecified open wound of left elbow
    - S51.009 Unspecified open wound of unspecified elbow
      Open wound of elbow NOS
  - S51.01 Laceration without foreign body of elbow
    - S51.011 Laceration without foreign body of right elbow
    - S51.012 Laceration without foreign body of left elbow
    - S51.019 Laceration without foreign body of unspecified elbow
  - S51.02 Laceration with foreign body of elbow
    - S51.021 Laceration with foreign body of right elbow
    - S51.022 Laceration with foreign body of left elbow
    - S51.029 Laceration with foreign body of unspecified elbow
  - S51.03 Puncture wound without foreign body of elbow
    - S51.031 Puncture wound without foreign body of right elbow
    - S51.032 Puncture wound without foreign body of left elbow
    - S51.039 Puncture wound without foreign body of unspecified elbow
  - S51.04 Puncture wound with foreign body of elbow
    - S51.041 Puncture wound with foreign body of right elbow
    - S51.042 Puncture wound with foreign body of left elbow
    - S51.049 Puncture wound with foreign body of unspecified elbow
  - S51.05 Open bite of elbow
    Bite of elbow NOS
    Excludes1 superficial bite of elbow (S50.36, S50.37)
    - S51.051 Open bite, right elbow
    - S51.052 Open bite, left elbow
    - S51.059 Open bite, unspecified elbow
- S51.8 Open wound of forearm
  Excludes2 open wound of elbow (S51.0-)
  - S51.80 Unspecified open wound of forearm
    - S51.801 Unspecified open wound of right forearm
    - S51.802 Unspecified open wound of left forearm
    - S51.809 Unspecified open wound of unspecified forearm
      Open wound of forearm NOS
  - S51.81 Laceration without foreign body of forearm
    - S51.811 Laceration without foreign body of right forearm
    - S51.812 Laceration without foreign body of left forearm
    - S51.819 Laceration without foreign body of unspecified forearm
  - S51.82 Laceration with foreign body of forearm
    - S51.821 Laceration with foreign body of right forearm
    - S51.822 Laceration with foreign body of left forearm
    - S51.829 Laceration with foreign body of unspecified forearm
  - S51.83 Puncture wound without foreign body of forearm
    - S51.831 Puncture wound without foreign body of right forearm
    - S51.832 Puncture wound without foreign body of left forearm
    - S51.839 Puncture wound without foreign body of unspecified forearm
  - S51.84 Puncture wound with foreign body of forearm
    - S51.841 Puncture wound with foreign body of right forearm
    - S51.842 Puncture wound with foreign body of left forearm
    - S51.849 Puncture wound with foreign body of unspecified forearm
  - S51.85 Open bite of forearm
    Bite of forearm NOS
    Excludes1 superficial bite of forearm (S50.86, S50.87)
    - S51.851 Open bite of right forearm
    - S51.852 Open bite of left forearm
    - S51.859 Open bite of unspecified forearm

CHAPTER 19 (S00-T88)

● S52 Fracture of forearm

Note: A fracture not identified as displaced or nondisplaced should be coded to displaced

A fracture not designated as open or closed should be coded to closed

The open fracture designations are based on the Gustilo open fracture classification

Excludes1 traumatic amputation of forearm (S58.-)

Excludes2 fracture at wrist and hand level (S62.-)

The appropriate 7th character is to be added to all codes from category S52

A	initial encounter for closed fracture
B	initial encounter for open fracture type I or II initial encounter for open fracture NOS
C	initial encounter for open fracture type IIIA, IIIB, or IIIC
D	subsequent encounter for closed fracture with routine healing
E	subsequent encounter for open fracture type I or II with routine healing
F	subsequent encounter for open fracture type IIIA, IIIB, or IIIC with routine healing
G	subsequent encounter for closed fracture with delayed healing
H	subsequent encounter for open fracture type I or II with delayed healing
J	subsequent encounter for open fracture type IIIA, IIIB, or IIIC with delayed healing
K	subsequent encounter for closed fracture with nonunion
M	subsequent encounter for open fracture type I or II with nonunion
N	subsequent encounter for open fracture type IIIA, IIIB, or IIIC with nonunion
P	subsequent encounter for closed fracture with malunion
Q	subsequent encounter for open fracture type I or II with malunion
R	subsequent encounter for open fracture type IIIA, IIIB, or IIIC with malunion
S	sequela

● S52.0 Fracture of upper end of ulna

Fracture of proximal end of ulna

Excludes2 fracture of elbow NOS (S42.40-)
fractures of shaft of ulna (S52.2-)

● S52.00 Unspecified fracture of upper end of ulna

● S52.001 Unspecified fracture of upper end of right ulna

● S52.002 Unspecified fracture of upper end of left ulna

● S52.009 Unspecified fracture of upper end of unspecified ulna

● S52.01 Torus fracture of upper end of ulna

The appropriate 7th character is to be added to all codes in subcategory S52.01

A	initial encounter for closed fracture
D	subsequent encounter for fracture with routine healing
G	subsequent encounter for fracture with delayed healing
K	subsequent encounter for fracture with nonunion
P	subsequent encounter for fracture with malunion
S	sequela

● S52.011 Torus fracture of upper end of right ulna

● S52.012 Torus fracture of upper end of left ulna

● S52.019 Torus fracture of upper end of unspecified ulna

● S52.02 Fracture of olecranon process without intraarticular extension of ulna

● S52.021 Displaced fracture of olecranon process without intraarticular extension of right ulna

● S52.022 Displaced fracture of olecranon process without intraarticular extension of left ulna

● S52.023 Displaced fracture of olecranon process without intraarticular extension of unspecified ulna

● S52.024 Nondisplaced fracture of olecranon process without intraarticular extension of right ulna

● S52.025 Nondisplaced fracture of olecranon process without intraarticular extension of left ulna

● S52.026 Nondisplaced fracture of olecranon process without intraarticular extension of unspecified ulna

● S52.03 Fracture of olecranon process with intraarticular extension of ulna

● S52.031 Displaced fracture of olecranon process with intraarticular extension of right ulna

● S52.032 Displaced fracture of olecranon process with intraarticular extension of left ulna

● S52.033 Displaced fracture of olecranon process with intraarticular extension of unspecified ulna

● S52.034 Nondisplaced fracture of olecranon process with intraarticular extension of right ulna

● S52.035 Nondisplaced fracture of olecranon process with intraarticular extension of left ulna

● S52.036 Nondisplaced fracture of olecranon process with intraarticular extension of unspecified ulna

● S52.04 Fracture of coronoid process of ulna

● S52.041 Displaced fracture of coronoid process of right ulna

● S52.042 Displaced fracture of coronoid process of left ulna

● S52.043 Displaced fracture of coronoid process of unspecified ulna

● S52.044 Nondisplaced fracture of coronoid process of right ulna

● S52.045 Nondisplaced fracture of coronoid process of left ulna

● S52.046 Nondisplaced fracture of coronoid process of unspecified ulna

● S52.09 Other fracture of upper end of ulna

● S52.091 Other fracture of upper end of right ulna

● S52.092 Other fracture of upper end of left ulna

● S52.099 Other fracture of upper end of unspecified ulna

● S52.1 Fracture of upper end of radius

Fracture of proximal end of radius

Excludes2 physeal fractures of upper end of radius (S59.2-)
fracture of shaft of radius (S52.3-)

● S52.10 Unspecified fracture of upper end of radius

● S52.101 Unspecified fracture of upper end of right radius

● S52.102 Unspecified fracture of upper end of left radius

● S52.109 Unspecified fracture of upper end of unspecified radius

● S52.11 Torus fracture of upper end of radius
The appropriate 7th character is to be added to all codes in subcategory S52.11

A	initial encounter for closed fracture
D	subsequent encounter for fracture with routine healing
G	subsequent encounter for fracture with delayed healing
K	subsequent encounter for fracture with nonunion
P	subsequent encounter for fracture with malunion
S	sequela

● S52.111 Torus fracture of upper end of right radius
● S52.112 Torus fracture of upper end of left radius
● S52.119 Torus fracture of upper end of unspecified radius
● S52.12 Fracture of head of radius
● S52.121 Displaced fracture of head of right radius
● S52.122 Displaced fracture of head of left radius
● S52.123 Displaced fracture of head of unspecified radius
● S52.124 Nondisplaced fracture of head of right radius
● S52.125 Nondisplaced fracture of head of left radius
● S52.126 Nondisplaced fracture of head of unspecified radius
● S52.13 Fracture of neck of radius
● S52.131 Displaced fracture of neck of right radius
● S52.132 Displaced fracture of neck of left radius
● S52.133 Displaced fracture of neck of unspecified radius
● S52.134 Nondisplaced fracture of neck of right radius
● S52.135 Nondisplaced fracture of neck of left radius
● S52.136 Nondisplaced fracture of neck of unspecified radius
● S52.18 Other fracture of upper end of radius
● S52.181 Other fracture of upper end of right radius
● S52.182 Other fracture of upper end of left radius
● S52.189 Other fracture of upper end of unspecified radius
● S52.2 Fracture of shaft of ulna
● S52.20 Unspecified fracture of shaft of ulna
Fracture of ulna NOS
● S52.201 Unspecified fracture of shaft of right ulna
● S52.202 Unspecified fracture of shaft of left ulna
● S52.209 Unspecified fracture of shaft of unspecified ulna

● S52.21 Greenstick fracture of shaft of ulna
The appropriate 7th character is to be added to all codes in subcategory S52.21

A	initial encounter for closed fracture
D	subsequent encounter for fracture with routine healing
G	subsequent encounter for fracture with delayed healing
K	subsequent encounter for fracture with nonunion
P	subsequent encounter for fracture with malunion
S	sequela

● S52.211 Greenstick fracture of shaft of right ulna
● S52.212 Greenstick fracture of shaft of left ulna
● S52.219 Greenstick fracture of shaft of unspecified ulna
● S52.22 Transverse fracture of shaft of ulna
● S52.221 Displaced transverse fracture of shaft of right ulna
● S52.222 Displaced transverse fracture of shaft of left ulna
● S52.223 Displaced transverse fracture of shaft of unspecified ulna
● S52.224 Nondisplaced transverse fracture of shaft of right ulna
● S52.225 Nondisplaced transverse fracture of shaft of left ulna
● S52.226 Nondisplaced transverse fracture of shaft of unspecified ulna
● S52.23 Oblique fracture of shaft of ulna
● S52.231 Displaced oblique fracture of shaft of right ulna
● S52.232 Displaced oblique fracture of shaft of left ulna
● S52.233 Displaced oblique fracture of shaft of unspecified ulna
● S52.234 Nondisplaced oblique fracture of shaft of right ulna
● S52.235 Nondisplaced oblique fracture of shaft of left ulna
● S52.236 Nondisplaced oblique fracture of shaft of unspecified ulna
● S52.24 Spiral fracture of shaft of ulna
● S52.241 Displaced spiral fracture of shaft of ulna, right arm
● S52.242 Displaced spiral fracture of shaft of ulna, left arm
● S52.243 Displaced spiral fracture of shaft of ulna, unspecified arm
● S52.244 Nondisplaced spiral fracture of shaft of ulna, right arm
● S52.245 Nondisplaced spiral fracture of shaft of ulna, left arm
● S52.246 Nondisplaced spiral fracture of shaft of ulna, unspecified arm

- S52.25 Comminuted fracture of shaft of ulna
  - S52.251 Displaced comminuted fracture of shaft of ulna, right arm
  - S52.252 Displaced comminuted fracture of shaft of ulna, left arm
  - S52.253 Displaced comminuted fracture of shaft of ulna, unspecified arm
  - S52.254 Nondisplaced comminuted fracture of shaft of ulna, right arm
  - S52.255 Nondisplaced comminuted fracture of shaft of ulna, left arm
  - S52.256 Nondisplaced comminuted fracture of shaft of ulna, unspecified arm
- S52.26 Segmental fracture of shaft of ulna
  - S52.261 Displaced segmental fracture of shaft of ulna, right arm
  - S52.262 Displaced segmental fracture of shaft of ulna, left arm
  - S52.263 Displaced segmental fracture of shaft of ulna, unspecified arm
  - S52.264 Nondisplaced segmental fracture of shaft of ulna, right arm
  - S52.265 Nondisplaced segmental fracture of shaft of ulna, left arm
  - S52.266 Nondisplaced segmental fracture of shaft of ulna, unspecified arm
- S52.27 Monteggia's fracture of ulna

  Fracture of upper shaft of ulna with dislocation of radial head
  - S52.271 Monteggia's fracture of right ulna
  - S52.272 Monteggia's fracture of left ulna
  - S52.279 Monteggia's fracture of unspecified ulna
- S52.28 Bent bone of ulna
  - S52.281 Bent bone of right ulna
  - S52.282 Bent bone of left ulna
  - S52.283 Bent bone of unspecified ulna
- S52.29 Other fracture of shaft of ulna
  - S52.291 Other fracture of shaft of right ulna
  - S52.292 Other fracture of shaft of left ulna
  - S52.299 Other fracture of shaft of unspecified ulna

- S52.3 Fracture of shaft of radius
  - S52.30 Unspecified fracture of shaft of radius
    - S52.301 Unspecified fracture of shaft of right radius
    - S52.302 Unspecified fracture of shaft of left radius
    - S52.309 Unspecified fracture of shaft of unspecified radius
  - S52.31 Greenstick fracture of shaft of radius

    The appropriate 7th character is to be added to all codes in subcategory S52.31

A	initial encounter for closed fracture
D	subsequent encounter for fracture with routine healing
G	subsequent encounter for fracture with delayed healing
K	subsequent encounter for fracture with nonunion
P	subsequent encounter for fracture with malunion
S	sequela

    - S52.311 Greenstick fracture of shaft of radius, right arm
    - S52.312 Greenstick fracture of shaft of radius, left arm
    - S52.319 Greenstick fracture of shaft of radius, unspecified arm
  - S52.32 Transverse fracture of shaft of radius
    - S52.321 Displaced transverse fracture of shaft of right radius
    - S52.322 Displaced transverse fracture of shaft of left radius
    - S52.323 Displaced transverse fracture of shaft of unspecified radius
    - S52.324 Nondisplaced transverse fracture of shaft of right radius
    - S52.325 Nondisplaced transverse fracture of shaft of left radius
    - S52.326 Nondisplaced transverse fracture of shaft of unspecified radius
  - S52.33 Oblique fracture of shaft of radius
    - S52.331 Displaced oblique fracture of shaft of right radius
    - S52.332 Displaced oblique fracture of shaft of left radius
    - S52.333 Displaced oblique fracture of shaft of unspecified radius
    - S52.334 Nondisplaced oblique fracture of shaft of right radius
    - S52.335 Nondisplaced oblique fracture of shaft of left radius
    - S52.336 Nondisplaced oblique fracture of shaft of unspecified radius
  - S52.34 Spiral fracture of shaft of radius
    - S52.341 Displaced spiral fracture of shaft of radius, right arm
    - S52.342 Displaced spiral fracture of shaft of radius, left arm
    - S52.343 Displaced spiral fracture of shaft of radius, unspecified arm
    - S52.344 Nondisplaced spiral fracture of shaft of radius, right arm
    - S52.345 Nondisplaced spiral fracture of shaft of radius, left arm
    - S52.346 Nondisplaced spiral fracture of shaft of radius, unspecified arm
  - S52.35 Comminuted fracture of shaft of radius
    - S52.351 Displaced comminuted fracture of shaft of radius, right arm
    - S52.352 Displaced comminuted fracture of shaft of radius, left arm
    - S52.353 Displaced comminuted fracture of shaft of radius, unspecified arm
    - S52.354 Nondisplaced comminuted fracture of shaft of radius, right arm
    - S52.355 Nondisplaced comminuted fracture of shaft of radius, left arm
    - S52.356 Nondisplaced comminuted fracture of shaft of radius, unspecified arm
  - S52.36 Segmental fracture of shaft of radius
    - S52.361 Displaced segmental fracture of shaft of radius, right arm
    - S52.362 Displaced segmental fracture of shaft of radius, left arm
    - S52.363 Displaced segmental fracture of shaft of radius, unspecified arm
    - S52.364 Nondisplaced segmental fracture of shaft of radius, right arm
    - S52.365 Nondisplaced segmental fracture of shaft of radius, left arm
    - S52.366 Nondisplaced segmental fracture of shaft of radius, unspecified arm

S52.37 Galeazzi's fracture
Fracture of lower shaft of radius with radioulnar joint dislocation
S52.371 Galeazzi's fracture of right radius
S52.372 Galeazzi's fracture of left radius
S52.379 Galeazzi's fracture of unspecified radius
S52.38 Bent bone of radius
S52.381 Bent bone of right radius
S52.382 Bent bone of left radius
S52.389 Bent bone of unspecified radius
S52.39 Other fracture of shaft of radius
S52.391 Other fracture of shaft of radius, right arm
S52.392 Other fracture of shaft of radius, left arm
S52.399 Other fracture of shaft of radius, unspecified arm
S52.5 Fracture of lower end of radius
Fracture of distal end of radius
Excludes2 physeal fractures of lower end of radius (S59.2-)
S52.50 Unspecified fracture of the lower end of radius
S52.501 Unspecified fracture of the lower end of right radius
S52.502 Unspecified fracture of the lower end of left radius
S52.509 Unspecified fracture of the lower end of unspecified radius
S52.51 Fracture of radial styloid process
S52.511 Displaced fracture of right radial styloid process
S52.512 Displaced fracture of left radial styloid process
S52.513 Displaced fracture of unspecified radial styloid process
S52.514 Nondisplaced fracture of right radial styloid process
S52.515 Nondisplaced fracture of left radial styloid process
S52.516 Nondisplaced fracture of unspecified radial styloid process
S52.52 Torus fracture of lower end of radius
The appropriate 7th character is to be added to all codes in subcategory S52.52

A	initial encounter for closed fracture
D	subsequent encounter for fracture with routine healing
G	subsequent encounter for fracture with delayed healing
K	subsequent encounter for fracture with nonunion
P	subsequent encounter for fracture with malunion
S	sequela

S52.521 Torus fracture of lower end of right radius
S52.522 Torus fracture of lower end of left radius
S52.529 Torus fracture of lower end of unspecified radius
S52.53 Colles' fracture
S52.531 Colles' fracture of right radius
S52.532 Colles' fracture of left radius
S52.539 Colles' fracture of unspecified radius
S52.54 Smith's fracture
S52.541 Smith's fracture of right radius
S52.542 Smith's fracture of left radius
S52.549 Smith's fracture of unspecified radius
S52.55 Other extraarticular fracture of lower end of radius
S52.551 Other extraarticular fracture of lower end of right radius
S52.552 Other extraarticular fracture of lower end of left radius
S52.559 Other extraarticular fracture of lower end of unspecified radius
S52.56 Barton's fracture
S52.561 Barton's fracture of right radius
S52.562 Barton's fracture of left radius
S52.569 Barton's fracture of unspecified radius
S52.57 Other intraarticular fracture of lower end of radius
S52.571 Other intraarticular fracture of lower end of right radius
S52.572 Other intraarticular fracture of lower end of left radius
S52.579 Other intraarticular fracture of lower end of unspecified radius
S52.59 Other fractures of lower end of radius
S52.591 Other fractures of lower end of right radius
S52.592 Other fractures of lower end of left radius
S52.599 Other fractures of lower end of unspecified radius
S52.6 Fracture of lower end of ulna
S52.60 Unspecified fracture of lower end of ulna
S52.601 Unspecified fracture of lower end of right ulna
S52.602 Unspecified fracture of lower end of left ulna
S52.609 Unspecified fracture of lower end of unspecified ulna
S52.61 Fracture of ulna styloid process
S52.611 Displaced fracture of right ulna styloid process
S52.612 Displaced fracture of left ulna styloid process
S52.613 Displaced fracture of unspecified ulna styloid process
S52.614 Nondisplaced fracture of right ulna styloid process
S52.615 Nondisplaced fracture of left ulna styloid process
S52.616 Nondisplaced fracture of unspecified ulna styloid process

● S52.62 **Torus fracture of lower end of ulna**
The appropriate 7th character is to be added to all codes in subcategory S52.62

A	initial encounter for closed fracture
D	subsequent encounter for fracture with routine healing
G	subsequent encounter for fracture with delayed healing
K	subsequent encounter for fracture with nonunion
P	subsequent encounter for fracture with malunion
S	sequela

● S52.621 **Torus fracture of lower end of right ulna**
● S52.622 **Torus fracture of lower end of left ulna**
● S52.629 **Torus fracture of lower end of unspecified ulna**
● S52.69 **Other fracture of lower end of ulna**
● S52.691 **Other fracture of lower end of right ulna**
● S52.692 **Other fracture of lower end of left ulna**
● S52.699 **Other fracture of lower end of unspecified ulna**
● S52.9 **Unspecified fracture of forearm**
X● S52.90 **Unspecified fracture of unspecified forearm**
X● S52.91 **Unspecified fracture of right forearm**
X● S52.92 **Unspecified fracture of left forearm**

● S53 **Dislocation and sprain of joints and ligaments of elbow**
Includes avulsion of joint or ligament of elbow
laceration of cartilage, joint or ligament of elbow
sprain of cartilage, joint or ligament of elbow
traumatic hemarthrosis of joint or ligament of elbow
traumatic rupture of joint or ligament of elbow
traumatic subluxation of joint or ligament of elbow
traumatic tear of joint or ligament of elbow
Code also any associated open wound
Excludes2 strain of muscle, fascia and tendon at forearm level (S56.-)
The appropriate 7th character is to be added to each code from category S53

A	initial encounter
D	subsequent encounter
S	sequela

● S53.0 **Subluxation and dislocation of radial head**
Dislocation of radiohumeral joint
Subluxation of radiohumeral joint
Excludes1 Monteggia's fracture-dislocation (S52.27-)
● S53.00 **Unspecified subluxation and dislocation of radial head**
● S53.001 **Unspecified subluxation of right radial head**
● S53.002 **Unspecified subluxation of left radial head**
● S53.003 **Unspecified subluxation of unspecified radial head**
● S53.004 **Unspecified dislocation of right radial head**
● S53.005 **Unspecified dislocation of left radial head**
● S53.006 **Unspecified dislocation of unspecified radial head**
● S53.01 **Anterior subluxation and dislocation of radial head**
Anteriomedial subluxation and dislocation of radial head
● S53.011 **Anterior subluxation of right radial head**
● S53.012 **Anterior subluxation of left radial head**
● S53.013 **Anterior subluxation of unspecified radial head**
● S53.014 **Anterior dislocation of right radial head**
● S53.015 **Anterior dislocation of left radial head**
● S53.016 **Anterior dislocation of unspecified radial head**
● S53.02 **Posterior subluxation and dislocation of radial head**
Posteriolateral subluxation and dislocation of radial head
● S53.021 **Posterior subluxation of right radial head**
● S53.022 **Posterior subluxation of left radial head**
● S53.023 **Posterior subluxation of unspecified radial head**
● S53.024 **Posterior dislocation of right radial head**
● S53.025 **Posterior dislocation of left radial head**
● S53.026 **Posterior dislocation of unspecified radial head**
● S53.03 **Nursemaid's elbow**
● S53.031 **Nursemaid's elbow, right elbow**
● S53.032 **Nursemaid's elbow, left elbow**
● S53.033 **Nursemaid's elbow, unspecified elbow**
● S53.09 **Other subluxation and dislocation of radial head**
● S53.091 **Other subluxation of right radial head**
● S53.092 **Other subluxation of left radial head**
● S53.093 **Other subluxation of unspecified radial head**
● S53.094 **Other dislocation of right radial head**
● S53.095 **Other dislocation of left radial head**
● S53.096 **Other dislocation of unspecified radial head**
● S53.1 **Subluxation and dislocation of ulnohumeral joint**
Subluxation and dislocation of elbow NOS
Excludes1 dislocation of radial head alone (S53.0-)
● S53.10 **Unspecified subluxation and dislocation of ulnohumeral joint**
● S53.101 **Unspecified subluxation of right ulnohumeral joint**
● S53.102 **Unspecified subluxation of left ulnohumeral joint**
● S53.103 **Unspecified subluxation of unspecified ulnohumeral joint**
● S53.104 **Unspecified dislocation of right ulnohumeral joint**
● S53.105 **Unspecified dislocation of left ulnohumeral joint**
● S53.106 **Unspecified dislocation of unspecified ulnohumeral joint**

● S53.11 Anterior subluxation and dislocation of ulnohumeral joint
● S53.111 Anterior subluxation of right ulnohumeral joint
● S53.112 Anterior subluxation of left ulnohumeral joint
● S53.113 Anterior subluxation of unspecified ulnohumeral joint
● S53.114 Anterior dislocation of right ulnohumeral joint
● S53.115 Anterior dislocation of left ulnohumeral joint
● S53.116 Anterior dislocation of unspecified ulnohumeral joint
● S53.12 Posterior subluxation and dislocation of ulnohumeral joint
● S53.121 Posterior subluxation of right ulnohumeral joint
● S53.122 Posterior subluxation of left ulnohumeral joint
● S53.123 Posterior subluxation of unspecified ulnohumeral joint
● S53.124 Posterior dislocation of right ulnohumeral joint
● S53.125 Posterior dislocation of left ulnohumeral joint
● S53.126 Posterior dislocation of unspecified ulnohumeral joint
● S53.13 Medial subluxation and dislocation of ulnohumeral joint
● S53.131 Medial subluxation of right ulnohumeral joint
● S53.132 Medial subluxation of left ulnohumeral joint
● S53.133 Medial subluxation of unspecified ulnohumeral joint
● S53.134 Medial dislocation of right ulnohumeral joint
● S53.135 Medial dislocation of left ulnohumeral joint
● S53.136 Medial dislocation of unspecified ulnohumeral joint
● S53.14 Lateral subluxation and dislocation of ulnohumeral joint
● S53.141 Lateral subluxation of right ulnohumeral joint
● S53.142 Lateral subluxation of left ulnohumeral joint
● S53.143 Lateral subluxation of unspecified ulnohumeral joint
● S53.144 Lateral dislocation of right ulnohumeral joint
● S53.145 Lateral dislocation of left ulnohumeral joint
● S53.146 Lateral dislocation of unspecified ulnohumeral joint
● S53.19 Other subluxation and dislocation of ulnohumeral joint
● S53.191 Other subluxation of right ulnohumeral joint
● S53.192 Other subluxation of left ulnohumeral joint
● S53.193 Other subluxation of unspecified ulnohumeral joint
● S53.194 Other dislocation of right ulnohumeral joint
● S53.195 Other dislocation of left ulnohumeral joint
● S53.196 Other dislocation of unspecified ulnohumeral joint

● S53.2 Traumatic rupture of radial collateral ligament
Excludes1 sprain of radial collateral ligament NOS (S53.43-)
X● S53.20 Traumatic rupture of unspecified radial collateral ligament
X● S53.21 Traumatic rupture of right radial collateral ligament
X● S53.22 Traumatic rupture of left radial collateral ligament

● S53.3 Traumatic rupture of ulnar collateral ligament
Excludes1 sprain of ulnar collateral ligament (S53.44-)
X● S53.30 Traumatic rupture of unspecified ulnar collateral ligament
X● S53.31 Traumatic rupture of right ulnar collateral ligament
X● S53.32 Traumatic rupture of left ulnar collateral ligament

● S53.4 Sprain of elbow
Excludes2 traumatic rupture of radial collateral ligament (S53.2-)
traumatic rupture of ulnar collateral ligament (S53.3-)
● S53.40 Unspecified sprain of elbow
● S53.401 Unspecified sprain of right elbow
● S53.402 Unspecified sprain of left elbow
● S53.409 Unspecified sprain of unspecified elbow
Sprain of elbow NOS
● S53.41 Radiohumeral (joint) sprain
● S53.411 Radiohumeral (joint) sprain of right elbow
● S53.412 Radiohumeral (joint) sprain of left elbow
● S53.419 Radiohumeral (joint) sprain of unspecified elbow
● S53.42 Ulnohumeral (joint) sprain
● S53.421 Ulnohumeral (joint) sprain of right elbow
● S53.422 Ulnohumeral (joint) sprain of left elbow
● S53.429 Ulnohumeral (joint) sprain of unspecified elbow

● S53.43 Radial collateral ligament sprain
● S53.431 Radial collateral ligament sprain of right elbow
● S53.432 Radial collateral ligament sprain of left elbow
● S53.439 Radial collateral ligament sprain of unspecified elbow
● S53.44 Ulnar collateral ligament sprain
● S53.441 Ulnar collateral ligament sprain of right elbow
● S53.442 Ulnar collateral ligament sprain of left elbow
● S53.449 Ulnar collateral ligament sprain of unspecified elbow
● S53.49 Other sprain of elbow
● S53.491 Other sprain of right elbow
● S53.492 Other sprain of left elbow
● S53.499 Other sprain of unspecified elbow

● S54 Injury of nerves at forearm level
Code also any associated open wound (S51.-)
Excludes2 injury of nerves at wrist and hand level (S64.-)
The appropriate 7th character is to be added to each code from category S54

A	initial encounter
D	subsequent encounter
S	sequela

● S54.0 Injury of ulnar nerve at forearm level
Injury of ulnar nerve NOS
X● S54.00 Injury of ulnar nerve at forearm level, unspecified arm
X● S54.01 Injury of ulnar nerve at forearm level, right arm
X● S54.02 Injury of ulnar nerve at forearm level, left arm
● S54.1 Injury of median nerve at forearm level
Injury of median nerve NOS
X● S54.10 Injury of median nerve at forearm level, unspecified arm
X● S54.11 Injury of median nerve at forearm level, right arm
X● S54.12 Injury of median nerve at forearm level, left arm
● S54.2 Injury of radial nerve at forearm level
Injury of radial nerve NOS
X● S54.20 Injury of radial nerve at forearm level, unspecified arm
X● S54.21 Injury of radial nerve at forearm level, right arm
X● S54.22 Injury of radial nerve at forearm level, left arm
● S54.3 Injury of cutaneous sensory nerve at forearm level
X● S54.30 Injury of cutaneous sensory nerve at forearm level, unspecified arm
X● S54.31 Injury of cutaneous sensory nerve at forearm level, right arm
X● S54.32 Injury of cutaneous sensory nerve at forearm level, left arm
● S54.8 Injury of other nerves at forearm level
● S54.8X Injury of other nerves at forearm level ⬅
● S54.8X1 Injury of other nerves at forearm level, right arm ⬅
● S54.8X2 Injury of other nerves at forearm level, left arm ⬅
● S54.8X9 Injury of other nerves at forearm level, unspecified arm ⬅
● S54.9 Injury of unspecified nerve at forearm level
X● S54.90 Injury of unspecified nerve at forearm level, unspecified arm
X● S54.91 Injury of unspecified nerve at forearm level, right arm
X● S54.92 Injury of unspecified nerve at forearm level, left arm

● S55 Injury of blood vessels at forearm level
Code also any associated open wound (S51.-)
Excludes2 injury of blood vessels at wrist and hand level (S65.-)
injury of brachial vessels (S45.1-S45.2)
The appropriate 7th character is to be added to each code from category S55

A	initial encounter
D	subsequent encounter
S	sequela

● S55.0 Injury of ulnar artery at forearm level
● S55.00 Unspecified injury of ulnar artery at forearm level
● S55.001 Unspecified injury of ulnar artery at forearm level, right arm
● S55.002 Unspecified injury of ulnar artery at forearm level, left arm
● S55.009 Unspecified injury of ulnar artery at forearm level, unspecified arm
● S55.01 Laceration of ulnar artery at forearm level
● S55.011 Laceration of ulnar artery at forearm level, right arm
● S55.012 Laceration of ulnar artery at forearm level, left arm
● S55.019 Laceration of ulnar artery at forearm level, unspecified arm
● S55.09 Other specified injury of ulnar artery at forearm level
● S55.091 Other specified injury of ulnar artery at forearm level, right arm
● S55.092 Other specified injury of ulnar artery at forearm level, left arm
● S55.099 Other specified injury of ulnar artery at forearm level, unspecified arm
● S55.1 Injury of radial artery at forearm level
● S55.10 Unspecified injury of radial artery at forearm level
● S55.101 Unspecified injury of radial artery at forearm level, right arm
● S55.102 Unspecified injury of radial artery at forearm level, left arm
● S55.109 Unspecified injury of radial artery at forearm level, unspecified arm
● S55.11 Laceration of radial artery at forearm level
● S55.111 Laceration of radial artery at forearm level, right arm
● S55.112 Laceration of radial artery at forearm level, left arm
● S55.119 Laceration of radial artery at forearm level, unspecified arm
● S55.19 Other specified injury of radial artery at forearm level
● S55.191 Other specified injury of radial artery at forearm level, right arm
● S55.192 Other specified injury of radial artery at forearm level, left arm
● S55.199 Other specified injury of radial artery at forearm level, unspecified arm

◀ New ⬅ Revised ~~deleted~~ Deleted **OGCR** Official Guidelines X Assign placeholder X ● Use Additional Character(s)
Excludes 1 Excludes 2 Includes Use additional Code first Code also Unspecified

● S55.2 Injury of vein at forearm level

● S55.20 Unspecified injury of vein at forearm level

● S55.201 Unspecified injury of vein at forearm level, right arm

● S55.202 Unspecified injury of vein at forearm level, left arm

● S55.209 Unspecified injury of vein at forearm level, unspecified arm

● S55.21 Laceration of vein at forearm level

● S55.211 Laceration of vein at forearm level, right arm

● S55.212 Laceration of vein at forearm level, left arm

● S55.219 Laceration of vein at forearm level, unspecified arm

● S55.29 Other specified injury of vein at forearm level

● S55.291 Other specified injury of vein at forearm level, right arm

● S55.292 Other specified injury of vein at forearm level, left arm

● S55.299 Other specified injury of vein at forearm level, unspecified arm

● S55.8 Injury of other blood vessels at forearm level

● S55.80 Unspecified injury of other blood vessels at forearm level

● S55.801 Unspecified injury of other blood vessels at forearm level, right arm

● S55.802 Unspecified injury of other blood vessels at forearm level, left arm

● S55.809 Unspecified injury of other blood vessels at forearm level, unspecified arm

● S55.81 Laceration of other blood vessels at forearm level

● S55.811 Laceration of other blood vessels at forearm level, right arm

● S55.812 Laceration of other blood vessels at forearm level, left arm

● S55.819 Laceration of other blood vessels at forearm level, unspecified arm

● S55.89 Other specified injury of other blood vessels at forearm level

● S55.891 Other specified injury of other blood vessels at forearm level, right arm

● S55.892 Other specified injury of other blood vessels at forearm level, left arm

● S55.899 Other specified injury of other blood vessels at forearm level, unspecified arm

● S55.9 Injury of unspecified blood vessel at forearm level

● S55.90 Unspecified injury of unspecified blood vessel at forearm level

● S55.901 Unspecified injury of unspecified blood vessel at forearm level, right arm

● S55.902 Unspecified injury of unspecified blood vessel at forearm level, left arm

● S55.909 Unspecified injury of unspecified blood vessel at forearm level, unspecified arm

● S55.91 Laceration of unspecified blood vessel at forearm level

● S55.911 Laceration of unspecified blood vessel at forearm level, right arm

● S55.912 Laceration of unspecified blood vessel at forearm level, left arm

● S55.919 Laceration of unspecified blood vessel at forearm level, unspecified arm

● S55.99 Other specified injury of unspecified blood vessel at forearm level

● S55.991 Other specified injury of unspecified blood vessel at forearm level, right arm

● S55.992 Other specified injury of unspecified blood vessel at forearm level, left arm

● S55.999 Other specified injury of unspecified blood vessel at forearm level, unspecified arm

● S56 Injury of muscle, fascia and tendon at forearm level

Code also any associated open wound (S51.-)

Excludes2 injury of muscle, fascia and tendon at or below wrist (S66.-)
sprain of joints and ligaments of elbow (S53.4-)

The appropriate 7th character is to be added to each code from category S56

A	initial encounter
D	subsequent encounter
S	sequela

● S56.0 Injury of flexor muscle, fascia and tendon of thumb at forearm level

● S56.00 Unspecified injury of flexor muscle, fascia and tendon of thumb at forearm level

● S56.001 Unspecified injury of flexor muscle, fascia and tendon of right thumb at forearm level

● S56.002 Unspecified injury of flexor muscle, fascia and tendon of left thumb at forearm level

● S56.009 Unspecified injury of flexor muscle, fascia and tendon of unspecified thumb at forearm level

● S56.01 Strain of flexor muscle, fascia and tendon of thumb at forearm level

● S56.011 Strain of flexor muscle, fascia and tendon of right thumb at forearm level

● S56.012 Strain of flexor muscle, fascia and tendon of left thumb at forearm level

● S56.019 Strain of flexor muscle, fascia and tendon of unspecified thumb at forearm level

● S56.02 Laceration of flexor muscle, fascia and tendon of thumb at forearm level

● S56.021 Laceration of flexor muscle, fascia and tendon of right thumb at forearm level

● S56.022 Laceration of flexor muscle, fascia and tendon of left thumb at forearm level

● S56.029 Laceration of flexor muscle, fascia and tendon of unspecified thumb at forearm level

● S56.09 Other injury of flexor muscle, fascia and tendon of thumb at forearm level

● S56.091 Other injury of flexor muscle, fascia and tendon of right thumb at forearm level

● S56.092 Other injury of flexor muscle, fascia and tendon of left thumb at forearm level

● S56.099 Other injury of flexor muscle, fascia and tendon of unspecified thumb at forearm level

CHAPTER 19 (S00-T88)

S56.1 Injury of flexor muscle, fascia and tendon of other and unspecified finger at forearm level

S56.10 Unspecified injury of flexor muscle, fascia and tendon of other and unspecified finger at forearm level

S56.101 Unspecified injury of flexor muscle, fascia and tendon of right index finger at forearm level

S56.102 Unspecified injury of flexor muscle, fascia and tendon of left index finger at forearm level

S56.103 Unspecified injury of flexor muscle, fascia and tendon of right middle finger at forearm level

S56.104 Unspecified injury of flexor muscle, fascia and tendon of left middle finger at forearm level

S56.105 Unspecified injury of flexor muscle, fascia and tendon of right ring finger at forearm level

S56.106 Unspecified injury of flexor muscle, fascia and tendon of left ring finger at forearm level

S56.107 Unspecified injury of flexor muscle, fascia and tendon of right little finger at forearm level

S56.108 Unspecified injury of flexor muscle, fascia and tendon of left little finger at forearm level

S56.109 Unspecified injury of flexor muscle, fascia and tendon of unspecified finger at forearm level

S56.11 Strain of flexor muscle, fascia and tendon of other and unspecified finger at forearm level

S56.111 Strain of flexor muscle, fascia and tendon of right index finger at forearm level

S56.112 Strain of flexor muscle, fascia and tendon of left index finger at forearm level

S56.113 Strain of flexor muscle, fascia and tendon of right middle finger at forearm level

S56.114 Strain of flexor muscle, fascia and tendon of left middle finger at forearm level

S56.115 Strain of flexor muscle, fascia and tendon of right ring finger at forearm level

S56.116 Strain of flexor muscle, fascia and tendon of left ring finger at forearm level

S56.117 Strain of flexor muscle, fascia and tendon of right little finger at forearm level

S56.118 Strain of flexor muscle, fascia and tendon of left little finger at forearm level

S56.119 Strain of flexor muscle, fascia and tendon of finger of unspecified finger at forearm level

S56.12 Laceration of flexor muscle, fascia and tendon of other and unspecified finger at forearm level

S56.121 Laceration of flexor muscle, fascia and tendon of right index finger at forearm level

S56.122 Laceration of flexor muscle, fascia and tendon of left index finger at forearm level

S56.123 Laceration of flexor muscle, fascia and tendon of right middle finger at forearm level

S56.124 Laceration of flexor muscle, fascia and tendon of left middle finger at forearm level

S56.125 Laceration of flexor muscle, fascia and tendon of right ring finger at forearm level

S56.126 Laceration of flexor muscle, fascia and tendon of left ring finger at forearm level

S56.127 Laceration of flexor muscle, fascia and tendon of right little finger at forearm level

S56.128 Laceration of flexor muscle, fascia and tendon of left little finger at forearm level

S56.129 Laceration of flexor muscle, fascia and tendon of unspecified finger at forearm level

S56.19 Other injury of flexor muscle, fascia and tendon of other and unspecified finger at forearm level

S56.191 Other injury of flexor muscle, fascia and tendon of right index finger at forearm level

S56.192 Other injury of flexor muscle, fascia and tendon of left index finger at forearm level

S56.193 Other injury of flexor muscle, fascia and tendon of right middle finger at forearm level

S56.194 Other injury of flexor muscle, fascia and tendon of left middle finger at forearm level

S56.195 Other injury of flexor muscle, fascia and tendon of right ring finger at forearm level

S56.196 Other injury of flexor muscle, fascia and tendon of left ring finger at forearm level

S56.197 Other injury of flexor muscle, fascia and tendon of right little finger at forearm level

S56.198 Other injury of flexor muscle, fascia and tendon of left little finger at forearm level

S56.199 Other injury of flexor muscle, fascia and tendon of unspecified finger at forearm level

S56.2 Injury of other flexor muscle, fascia and tendon at forearm level

S56.20 Unspecified injury of other flexor muscle, fascia and tendon at forearm level

S56.201 Unspecified injury of other flexor muscle, fascia and tendon at forearm level, right arm

S56.202 Unspecified injury of other flexor muscle, fascia and tendon at forearm level, left arm

S56.209 Unspecified injury of other flexor muscle, fascia and tendon at forearm level, unspecified arm

S56.21 Strain of other flexor muscle, fascia and tendon at forearm level

S56.211 Strain of other flexor muscle, fascia and tendon at forearm level, right arm

S56.212 Strain of other flexor muscle, fascia and tendon at forearm level, left arm

S56.219 Strain of other flexor muscle, fascia and tendon at forearm level, unspecified arm

- S56.22 Laceration of other flexor muscle, fascia and tendon at forearm level
  - S56.221 Laceration of other flexor muscle, fascia and tendon at forearm level, right arm
  - S56.222 Laceration of other flexor muscle, fascia and tendon at forearm level, left arm
  - S56.229 Laceration of other flexor muscle, fascia and tendon at forearm level, unspecified arm
- S56.29 Other injury of other flexor muscle, fascia and tendon at forearm level
  - S56.291 Other injury of other flexor muscle, fascia and tendon at forearm level, right arm
  - S56.292 Other injury of other flexor muscle, fascia and tendon at forearm level, left arm
  - S56.299 Other injury of other flexor muscle, fascia and tendon at forearm level, unspecified arm

S56.3 Injury of extensor or abductor muscles, fascia and tendons of thumb at forearm level

- S56.30 Unspecified injury of extensor or abductor muscles, fascia and tendons of thumb at forearm level
  - S56.301 Unspecified injury of extensor or abductor muscles, fascia and tendons of right thumb at forearm level
  - S56.302 Unspecified injury of extensor or abductor muscles, fascia and tendons of left thumb at forearm level
  - S56.309 Unspecified injury of extensor or abductor muscles, fascia and tendons of unspecified thumb at forearm level
- S56.31 Strain of extensor or abductor muscles, fascia and tendons of thumb at forearm level
  - S56.311 Strain of extensor or abductor muscles, fascia and tendons of right thumb at forearm level
  - S56.312 Strain of extensor or abductor muscles, fascia and tendons of left thumb at forearm level
  - S56.319 Strain of extensor or abductor muscles, fascia and tendons of unspecified thumb at forearm level
- S56.32 Laceration of extensor or abductor muscles, fascia and tendons of thumb at forearm level
  - S56.321 Laceration of extensor or abductor muscles, fascia and tendons of right thumb at forearm level
  - S56.322 Laceration of extensor or abductor muscles, fascia and tendons of left thumb at forearm level
  - S56.329 Laceration of extensor or abductor muscles, fascia and tendons of unspecified thumb at forearm level
- S56.39 Other injury of extensor or abductor muscles, fascia and tendons of thumb at forearm level
  - S56.391 Other injury of extensor or abductor muscles, fascia and tendons of right thumb at forearm level
  - S56.392 Other injury of extensor or abductor muscles, fascia and tendons of left thumb at forearm level
  - S56.399 Other injury of extensor or abductor muscles, fascia and tendons of unspecified thumb at forearm level

S56.4 Injury of extensor muscle, fascia and tendon of other and unspecified finger at forearm level

- S56.40 Unspecified injury of extensor muscle, fascia and tendon of other and unspecified finger at forearm level
  - S56.401 Unspecified injury of extensor muscle, fascia and tendon of right index finger at forearm level
  - S56.402 Unspecified injury of extensor muscle, fascia and tendon of left index finger at forearm level
  - S56.403 Unspecified injury of extensor muscle, fascia and tendon of right middle finger at forearm level
  - S56.404 Unspecified injury of extensor muscle, fascia and tendon of left middle finger at forearm level
  - S56.405 Unspecified injury of extensor muscle, fascia and tendon of right ring finger at forearm level
  - S56.406 Unspecified injury of extensor muscle, fascia and tendon of left ring finger at forearm level
  - S56.407 Unspecified injury of extensor muscle, fascia and tendon of right little finger at forearm level
  - S56.408 Unspecified injury of extensor muscle, fascia and tendon of left little finger at forearm level
  - S56.409 Unspecified injury of extensor muscle, fascia and tendon of unspecified finger at forearm level
- S56.41 Strain of extensor muscle, fascia and tendon of other and unspecified finger at forearm level
  - S56.411 Strain of extensor muscle, fascia and tendon of right index finger at forearm level
  - S56.412 Strain of extensor muscle, fascia and tendon of left index finger at forearm level
  - S56.413 Strain of extensor muscle, fascia and tendon of right middle finger at forearm level
  - S56.414 Strain of extensor muscle, fascia and tendon of left middle finger at forearm level
  - S56.415 Strain of extensor muscle, fascia and tendon of right ring finger at forearm level
  - S56.416 Strain of extensor muscle, fascia and tendon of left ring finger at forearm level
  - S56.417 Strain of extensor muscle, fascia and tendon of right little finger at forearm level
  - S56.418 Strain of extensor muscle, fascia and tendon of left little finger at forearm level
  - S56.419 Strain of extensor muscle, fascia and tendon of finger, unspecified finger at forearm level

CHAPTER 19 (S00-T88)

- S56.42 Laceration of extensor muscle, fascia and tendon of other and unspecified finger at forearm level
  - S56.421 Laceration of extensor muscle, fascia and tendon of right index finger at forearm level
  - S56.422 Laceration of extensor muscle, fascia and tendon of left index finger at forearm level
  - S56.423 Laceration of extensor muscle, fascia and tendon of right middle finger at forearm level
  - S56.424 Laceration of extensor muscle, fascia and tendon of left middle finger at forearm level
  - S56.425 Laceration of extensor muscle, fascia and tendon of right ring finger at forearm level
  - S56.426 Laceration of extensor muscle, fascia and tendon of left ring finger at forearm level
  - S56.427 Laceration of extensor muscle, fascia and tendon of right little finger at forearm level
  - S56.428 Laceration of extensor muscle, fascia and tendon of left little finger at forearm level
  - S56.429 Laceration of extensor muscle, fascia and tendon of unspecified finger at forearm level
- S56.49 Other injury of extensor muscle, fascia and tendon of other and unspecified finger at forearm level
  - S56.491 Other injury of extensor muscle, fascia and tendon of right index finger at forearm level
  - S56.492 Other injury of extensor muscle, fascia and tendon of left index finger at forearm level
  - S56.493 Other injury of extensor muscle, fascia and tendon of right middle finger at forearm level
  - S56.494 Other injury of extensor muscle, fascia and tendon of left middle finger at forearm level
  - S56.495 Other injury of extensor muscle, fascia and tendon of right ring finger at forearm level
  - S56.496 Other injury of extensor muscle, fascia and tendon of left ring finger at forearm level
  - S56.497 Other injury of extensor muscle, fascia and tendon of right little finger at forearm level
  - S56.498 Other injury of extensor muscle, fascia and tendon of left little finger at forearm level
  - S56.499 Other injury of extensor muscle, fascia and tendon of unspecified finger at forearm level

- S56.5 Injury of other extensor muscle, fascia and tendon at forearm level
  - S56.50 Unspecified injury of other extensor muscle, fascia and tendon at forearm level
    - S56.501 Unspecified injury of other extensor muscle, fascia and tendon at forearm level, right arm
    - S56.502 Unspecified injury of other extensor muscle, fascia and tendon at forearm level, left arm
    - S56.509 Unspecified injury of other extensor muscle, fascia and tendon at forearm level, unspecified arm
  - S56.51 Strain of other extensor muscle, fascia and tendon at forearm level
    - S56.511 Strain of other extensor muscle, fascia and tendon at forearm level, right arm
    - S56.512 Strain of other extensor muscle, fascia and tendon at forearm level, left arm
    - S56.519 Strain of other extensor muscle, fascia and tendon at forearm level, unspecified arm
  - S56.52 Laceration of other extensor muscle, fascia and tendon at forearm level
    - S56.521 Laceration of other extensor muscle, fascia and tendon at forearm level, right arm
    - S56.522 Laceration of other extensor muscle, fascia and tendon at forearm level, left arm
    - S56.529 Laceration of other extensor muscle, fascia and tendon at forearm level, unspecified arm
  - S56.59 Other injury of other extensor muscle, fascia and tendon at forearm level
    - S56.591 Other injury of other extensor muscle, fascia and tendon at forearm level, right arm
    - S56.592 Other injury of other extensor muscle, fascia and tendon at forearm level, left arm
    - S56.599 Other injury of other extensor muscle, fascia and tendon at forearm level, unspecified arm
- S56.8 Injury of other muscles, fascia and tendons at forearm level
  - S56.80 Unspecified injury of other muscles, fascia and tendons at forearm level
    - S56.801 Unspecified injury of other muscles, fascia and tendons at forearm level, right arm
    - S56.802 Unspecified injury of other muscles, fascia and tendons at forearm level, left arm
    - S56.809 Unspecified injury of other muscles, fascia and tendons at forearm level, unspecified arm
  - S56.81 Strain of other muscles, fascia and tendons at forearm level
    - S56.811 Strain of other muscles, fascia and tendons at forearm level, right arm
    - S56.812 Strain of other muscles, fascia and tendons at forearm level, left arm
    - S56.819 Strain of other muscles, fascia and tendons at forearm level, unspecified arm
  - S56.82 Laceration of other muscles, fascia and tendons at forearm level
    - S56.821 Laceration of other muscles, fascia and tendons at forearm level, right arm
    - S56.822 Laceration of other muscles, fascia and tendons at forearm level, left arm
    - S56.829 Laceration of other muscles, fascia and tendons at forearm level, unspecified arm

● S56.89   Other injury of other muscles, fascia and tendons at forearm level
    ● S56.891   Other injury of other muscles, fascia and tendons at forearm level, right arm
    ● S56.892   Other injury of other muscles, fascia and tendons at forearm level, left arm
    ● S56.899   Other injury of other muscles, fascia and tendons at forearm level, unspecified arm

● S56.9   Injury of unspecified muscles, fascia and tendons at forearm level
    ● S56.90   Unspecified injury of unspecified muscles, fascia and tendons at forearm level
        ● S56.901   Unspecified injury of unspecified muscles, fascia and tendons at forearm level, right arm
        ● S56.902   Unspecified injury of unspecified muscles, fascia and tendons at forearm level, left arm
        ● S56.909   Unspecified injury of unspecified muscles, fascia and tendons at forearm level, unspecified arm
    ● S56.91   Strain of unspecified muscles, fascia and tendons at forearm level
        ● S56.911   Strain of unspecified muscles, fascia and tendons at forearm level, right arm
        ● S56.912   Strain of unspecified muscles, fascia and tendons at forearm level, left arm
        ● S56.919   Strain of unspecified muscles, fascia and tendons at forearm level, unspecified arm
    ● S56.92   Laceration of unspecified muscles, fascia and tendons at forearm level
        ● S56.921   Laceration of unspecified muscles, fascia and tendons at forearm level, right arm
        ● S56.922   Laceration of unspecified muscles, fascia and tendons at forearm level, left arm
        ● S56.929   Laceration of unspecified muscles, fascia and tendons at forearm level, unspecified arm
    ● S56.99   Other injury of unspecified muscles, fascia and tendons at forearm level
        ● S56.991   Other injury of unspecified muscles, fascia and tendons at forearm level, right arm
        ● S56.992   Other injury of unspecified muscles, fascia and tendons at forearm level, left arm
        ● S56.999   Other injury of unspecified muscles, fascia and tendons at forearm level, unspecified arm

● S57   Crushing injury of elbow and forearm
    Use additional code(s) for all associated injuries
    Excludes2   crushing injury of wrist and hand (S67.-)
    The appropriate 7th character is to be added to each code from category S57

A	initial encounter
D	subsequent encounter
S	sequela

    ● S57.0   Crushing injury of elbow
        X ● S57.00   Crushing injury of unspecified elbow
        X ● S57.01   Crushing injury of right elbow
        X ● S57.02   Crushing injury of left elbow

● S57.8   Crushing injury of forearm
    X ● S57.80   Crushing injury of unspecified forearm
    X ● S57.81   Crushing injury of right forearm
    X ● S57.82   Crushing injury of left forearm

● S58   Traumatic amputation of elbow and forearm
    An amputation not identified as partial or complete should be coded to complete
    Excludes1   traumatic amputation of wrist and hand (S68.-)
    The appropriate 7th character is to be added to each code from category S58

A	initial encounter
D	subsequent encounter
S	sequela

    ● S58.0   Traumatic amputation at elbow level
        ● S58.01   Complete traumatic amputation at elbow level
            ● S58.011   Complete traumatic amputation at elbow level, right arm
            ● S58.012   Complete traumatic amputation at elbow level, left arm
            ● S58.019   Complete traumatic amputation at elbow level, unspecified arm
        ● S58.02   Partial traumatic amputation at elbow level
            ● S58.021   Partial traumatic amputation at elbow level, right arm
            ● S58.022   Partial traumatic amputation at elbow level, left arm
            ● S58.029   Partial traumatic amputation at elbow level, unspecified arm
    ● S58.1   Traumatic amputation at level between elbow and wrist
        ● S58.11   Complete traumatic amputation at level between elbow and wrist
            ● S58.111   Complete traumatic amputation at level between elbow and wrist, right arm
            ● S58.112   Complete traumatic amputation at level between elbow and wrist, left arm
            ● S58.119   Complete traumatic amputation at level between elbow and wrist, unspecified arm
        ● S58.12   Partial traumatic amputation at level between elbow and wrist
            ● S58.121   Partial traumatic amputation at level between elbow and wrist, right arm
            ● S58.122   Partial traumatic amputation at level between elbow and wrist, left arm
            ● S58.129   Partial traumatic amputation at level between elbow and wrist, unspecified arm
    ● S58.9   Traumatic amputation of forearm, level unspecified
        Excludes1   traumatic amputation of wrist (S68.-)
        ● S58.91   Complete traumatic amputation of forearm, level unspecified
            ● S58.911   Complete traumatic amputation of right forearm, level unspecified
            ● S58.912   Complete traumatic amputation of left forearm, level unspecified
            ● S58.919   Complete traumatic amputation of unspecified forearm, level unspecified
        ● S58.92   Partial traumatic amputation of forearm, level unspecified
            ● S58.921   Partial traumatic amputation of right forearm, level unspecified
            ● S58.922   Partial traumatic amputation of left forearm, level unspecified
            ● S58.929   Partial traumatic amputation of unspecified forearm, level unspecified

Item 19-4 SALTER-HARRIS TYPE 1: epiphysis is completely separated from end of bone, or metaphysic growth plate remains attached to epiphysis

SALTER-HARRIS TYPE 2: epiphysis and growth plate are partially separated from metaphysis, which is cracked—most common type

SALTER-HARRIS TYPE 3: fracture occurring through epiphysis and separates part of epiphysis and growth plate from metaphysis fracture, usually at distal end of tibia

SALTER-HARRIS TYPE 4: fracture runs through epiphysis, across growth plate, into metaphysic, surgery is required to restore joint surface to normal and align growth plate

● **S59 Other and unspecified injuries of elbow and forearm**

Excludes2 other and unspecified injuries of wrist and hand (S69.-)

The appropriate 7th character is to be added to each code from subcategories S59.0, S59.1, and S59.2

A	initial encounter for closed fracture
D	subsequent encounter for fracture with routine healing
G	subsequent encounter for fracture with delayed healing
K	subsequent encounter for fracture with nonunion
P	subsequent encounter for fracture with malunion
S	sequela

● **S59.0 Physeal fracture of lower end of ulna**
- ● **S59.00 Unspecified physeal fracture of lower end of ulna**
  - ● **S59.001 Unspecified physeal fracture of lower end of ulna, right arm**
  - ● **S59.002 Unspecified physeal fracture of lower end of ulna, left arm**
  - ● **S59.009 Unspecified physeal fracture of lower end of ulna, unspecified arm**
- ● **S59.01 Salter-Harris Type I physeal fracture of lower end of ulna**
  - ● **S59.011 Salter-Harris Type I physeal fracture of lower end of ulna, right arm**
  - ● **S59.012 Salter-Harris Type I physeal fracture of lower end of ulna, left arm**
  - ● **S59.019 Salter-Harris Type I physeal fracture of lower end of ulna, unspecified arm**
- ● **S59.02 Salter-Harris Type II physeal fracture of lower end of ulna**
  - ● **S59.021 Salter-Harris Type II physeal fracture of lower end of ulna, right arm**
  - ● **S59.022 Salter-Harris Type II physeal fracture of lower end of ulna, left arm**
  - ● **S59.029 Salter-Harris Type II physeal fracture of lower end of ulna, unspecified arm**
- ● **S59.03 Salter-Harris Type III physeal fracture of lower end of ulna**
  - ● **S59.031 Salter-Harris Type III physeal fracture of lower end of ulna, right arm**
  - ● **S59.032 Salter-Harris Type III physeal fracture of lower end of ulna, left arm**
  - ● **S59.039 Salter-Harris Type III physeal fracture of lower end of ulna, unspecified arm**
- ● **S59.04 Salter-Harris Type IV physeal fracture of lower end of ulna**
  - ● **S59.041 Salter-Harris Type IV physeal fracture of lower end of ulna, right arm**
  - ● **S59.042 Salter-Harris Type IV physeal fracture of lower end of ulna, left arm**
  - ● **S59.049 Salter-Harris Type IV physeal fracture of lower end of ulna, unspecified arm**
- ● **S59.09 Other physeal fracture of lower end of ulna**
  - ● **S59.091 Other physeal fracture of lower end of ulna, right arm**
  - ● **S59.092 Other physeal fracture of lower end of ulna, left arm**
  - ● **S59.099 Other physeal fracture of lower end of ulna, unspecified arm**

● **S59.1 Physeal fracture of upper end of radius**
- ● **S59.10 Unspecified physeal fracture of upper end of radius**
  - ● **S59.101 Unspecified physeal fracture of upper end of radius, right arm**
  - ● **S59.102 Unspecified physeal fracture of upper end of radius, left arm**
  - ● **S59.109 Unspecified physeal fracture of upper end of radius, unspecified arm**
- ● **S59.11 Salter-Harris Type I physeal fracture of upper end of radius**
  - ● **S59.111 Salter-Harris Type I physeal fracture of upper end of radius, right arm**
  - ● **S59.112 Salter-Harris Type I physeal fracture of upper end of radius, left arm**
  - ● **S59.119 Salter-Harris Type I physeal fracture of upper end of radius, unspecified arm**
- ● **S59.12 Salter-Harris Type II physeal fracture of upper end of radius**
  - ● **S59.121 Salter-Harris Type II physeal fracture of upper end of radius, right arm**
  - ● **S59.122 Salter-Harris Type II physeal fracture of upper end of radius, left arm**
  - ● **S59.129 Salter-Harris Type II physeal fracture of upper end of radius, unspecified arm**
- ● **S59.13 Salter-Harris Type III physeal fracture of upper end of radius**
  - ● **S59.131 Salter-Harris Type III physeal fracture of upper end of radius, right arm**
  - ● **S59.132 Salter-Harris Type III physeal fracture of upper end of radius, left arm**
  - ● **S59.139 Salter-Harris Type III physeal fracture of upper end of radius, unspecified arm**
- ● **S59.14 Salter-Harris Type IV physeal fracture of upper end of radius**
  - ● **S59.141 Salter-Harris Type IV physeal fracture of upper end of radius, right arm**
  - ● **S59.142 Salter-Harris Type IV physeal fracture of upper end of radius, left arm**
  - ● **S59.149 Salter-Harris Type IV physeal fracture of upper end of radius, unspecified arm**
- ● **S59.19 Other physeal fracture of upper end of radius**
  - ● **S59.191 Other physeal fracture of upper end of radius, right arm**
  - ● **S59.192 Other physeal fracture of upper end of radius, left arm**
  - ● **S59.199 Other physeal fracture of upper end of radius, unspecified arm**

● **S59.2 Physeal fracture of lower end of radius**
- ● **S59.20 Unspecified physeal fracture of lower end of radius**
  - ● **S59.201 Unspecified physeal fracture of lower end of radius, right arm**
  - ● **S59.202 Unspecified physeal fracture of lower end of radius, left arm**
  - ● **S59.209 Unspecified physeal fracture of lower end of radius, unspecified arm**

- S59.21 Salter-Harris Type I physeal fracture of lower end of radius
  - S59.211 Salter-Harris Type I physeal fracture of lower end of radius, right arm
  - S59.212 Salter-Harris Type I physeal fracture of lower end of radius, left arm
  - S59.219 Salter-Harris Type I physeal fracture of lower end of radius, unspecified arm
- S59.22 Salter-Harris Type II physeal fracture of lower end of radius
  - S59.221 Salter-Harris Type II physeal fracture of lower end of radius, right arm
  - S59.222 Salter-Harris Type II physeal fracture of lower end of radius, left arm
  - S59.229 Salter-Harris Type II physeal fracture of lower end of radius, unspecified arm
- S59.23 Salter-Harris Type III physeal fracture of lower end of radius
  - S59.231 Salter-Harris Type III physeal fracture of lower end of radius, right arm
  - S59.232 Salter-Harris Type III physeal fracture of lower end of radius, left arm
  - S59.239 Salter-Harris Type III physeal fracture of lower end of radius, unspecified arm
- S59.24 Salter-Harris Type IV physeal fracture of lower end of radius
  - S59.241 Salter-Harris Type IV physeal fracture of lower end of radius, right arm
  - S59.242 Salter-Harris Type IV physeal fracture of lower end of radius, left arm
  - S59.249 Salter-Harris Type IV physeal fracture of lower end of radius, unspecified arm
- S59.29 Other physeal fracture of lower end of radius
  - S59.291 Other physeal fracture of lower end of radius, right arm
  - S59.292 Other physeal fracture of lower end of radius, left arm
  - S59.299 Other physeal fracture of lower end of radius, unspecified arm

S59.8 Other specified injuries of elbow and forearm

The appropriate 7th character is to be added to each code in subcategory S59.8

A	initial encounter
D	subsequent encounter
S	sequela

- S59.80 Other specified injuries of elbow
  - S59.801 Other specified injuries of right elbow
  - S59.802 Other specified injuries of left elbow
  - S59.809 Other specified injuries of unspecified elbow
- S59.81 Other specified injuries of forearm
  - S59.811 Other specified injuries right forearm
  - S59.812 Other specified injuries left forearm
  - S59.819 Other specified injuries unspecified forearm

S59.9 Unspecified injury of elbow and forearm

The appropriate 7th character is to be added to each code in subcategory S59.9

A	initial encounter
D	subsequent encounter
S	sequela

- S59.90 Unspecified injury of elbow
  - S59.901 Unspecified injury of right elbow
  - S59.902 Unspecified injury of left elbow
  - S59.909 Unspecified injury of unspecified elbow
- S59.91 Unspecified injury of forearm
  - S59.911 Unspecified injury of right forearm
  - S59.912 Unspecified injury of left forearm
  - S59.919 Unspecified injury of unspecified forearm

INJURIES TO THE WRIST, HAND AND FINGERS (S60-S69)

Excludes2 burns and corrosions (T20-T32)
frostbite (T33-T34)
insect bite or sting, venomous (T63.4)

S60 Superficial injury of wrist, hand and fingers

The appropriate 7th character is to be added to each code from category S60

A	initial encounter
D	subsequent encounter
S	sequela

S60.0 Contusion of finger without damage to nail

Excludes1 contusion involving nail (matrix) (S60.1)

- X S60.00 Contusion of unspecified finger without damage to nail
  - Contusion of finger(s) NOS
- S60.01 Contusion of thumb without damage to nail
  - S60.011 Contusion of right thumb without damage to nail
  - S60.012 Contusion of left thumb without damage to nail
  - S60.019 Contusion of unspecified thumb without damage to nail
- S60.02 Contusion of index finger without damage to nail
  - S60.021 Contusion of right index finger without damage to nail
  - S60.022 Contusion of left index finger without damage to nail
  - S60.029 Contusion of unspecified index finger without damage to nail
- S60.03 Contusion of middle finger without damage to nail
  - S60.031 Contusion of right middle finger without damage to nail
  - S60.032 Contusion of left middle finger without damage to nail
  - S60.039 Contusion of unspecified middle finger without damage to nail
- S60.04 Contusion of ring finger without damage to nail
  - S60.041 Contusion of right ring finger without damage to nail
  - S60.042 Contusion of left ring finger without damage to nail
  - S60.049 Contusion of unspecified ring finger without damage to nail

CHAPTER 19 (S00-T88)

- S60.05 Contusion of little finger without damage to nail
  - S60.051 Contusion of right little finger without damage to nail
  - S60.052 Contusion of left little finger without damage to nail
  - S60.059 Contusion of unspecified little finger without damage to nail
- S60.1 Contusion of finger with damage to nail
  - X S60.10 Contusion of unspecified finger with damage to nail
  - S60.11 Contusion of thumb with damage to nail
    - S60.111 Contusion of right thumb with damage to nail
    - S60.112 Contusion of left thumb with damage to nail
    - S60.119 Contusion of unspecified thumb with damage to nail
  - S60.12 Contusion of index finger with damage to nail
    - S60.121 Contusion of right index finger with damage to nail
    - S60.122 Contusion of left index finger with damage to nail
    - S60.129 Contusion of unspecified index finger with damage to nail
  - S60.13 Contusion of middle finger with damage to nail
    - S60.131 Contusion of right middle finger with damage to nail
    - S60.132 Contusion of left middle finger with damage to nail
    - S60.139 Contusion of unspecified middle finger with damage to nail
  - S60.14 Contusion of ring finger with damage to nail
    - S60.141 Contusion of right ring finger with damage to nail
    - S60.142 Contusion of left ring finger with damage to nail
    - S60.149 Contusion of unspecified ring finger with damage to nail
  - S60.15 Contusion of little finger with damage to nail
    - S60.151 Contusion of right little finger with damage to nail
    - S60.152 Contusion of left little finger with damage to nail
    - S60.159 Contusion of unspecified little finger with damage to nail
- S60.2 Contusion of wrist and hand

  Excludes2 contusion of fingers (S60.0-, S60.1-)
  - S60.21 Contusion of wrist
    - S60.211 Contusion of right wrist
    - S60.212 Contusion of left wrist
    - S60.219 Contusion of unspecified wrist
  - S60.22 Contusion of hand
    - S60.221 Contusion of right hand
    - S60.222 Contusion of left hand
    - S60.229 Contusion of unspecified hand
- S60.3 Other superficial injuries of thumb
  - S60.31 Abrasion of thumb
    - S60.311 Abrasion of right thumb
    - S60.312 Abrasion of left thumb
    - S60.319 Abrasion of unspecified thumb
  - S60.32 Blister (nonthermal) of thumb
    - S60.321 Blister (nonthermal) of right thumb
    - S60.322 Blister (nonthermal) of left thumb
    - S60.329 Blister (nonthermal) of unspecified thumb
  - S60.34 External constriction of thumb

    Hair tourniquet syndrome of thumb

    Use additional cause code to identify the constricting item (W49.0-)
    - S60.341 External constriction of right thumb
    - S60.342 External constriction of left thumb
    - S60.349 External constriction of unspecified thumb
  - S60.35 Superficial foreign body of thumb

    Splinter in the thumb
    - S60.351 Superficial foreign body of right thumb
    - S60.352 Superficial foreign body of left thumb
    - S60.359 Superficial foreign body of unspecified thumb
  - S60.36 Insect bite (nonvenomous) of thumb
    - S60.361 Insect bite (nonvenomous) of right thumb
    - S60.362 Insect bite (nonvenomous) of left thumb
    - S60.369 Insect bite (nonvenomous) of unspecified thumb
  - S60.37 Other superficial bite of thumb

    Excludes1 open bite of thumb (S61.05-, S61.15-)
    - S60.371 Other superficial bite of right thumb
    - S60.372 Other superficial bite of left thumb
    - S60.379 Other superficial bite of unspecified thumb
  - S60.39 Other superficial injuries of thumb
    - S60.391 Other superficial injuries of right thumb
    - S60.392 Other superficial injuries of left thumb
    - S60.399 Other superficial injuries of unspecified thumb
- S60.4 Other superficial injuries of other fingers
  - S60.41 Abrasion of fingers
    - S60.410 Abrasion of right index finger
    - S60.411 Abrasion of left index finger
    - S60.412 Abrasion of right middle finger
    - S60.413 Abrasion of left middle finger
    - S60.414 Abrasion of right ring finger
    - S60.415 Abrasion of left ring finger
    - S60.416 Abrasion of right little finger
    - S60.417 Abrasion of left little finger
    - S60.418 Abrasion of other finger

      Abrasion of specified finger with unspecified laterality
    - S60.419 Abrasion of unspecified finger
  - S60.42 Blister (nonthermal) of fingers
    - S60.420 Blister (nonthermal) of right index finger
    - S60.421 Blister (nonthermal) of left index finger
    - S60.422 Blister (nonthermal) of right middle finger
    - S60.423 Blister (nonthermal) of left middle finger
    - S60.424 Blister (nonthermal) of right ring finger
    - S60.425 Blister (nonthermal) of left ring finger
    - S60.426 Blister (nonthermal) of right little finger
    - S60.427 Blister (nonthermal) of left little finger

- S60.428 **Blister (nonthermal) of other finger**
  Blister (nonthermal) of specified finger with unspecified laterality
- S60.429 **Blister (nonthermal) of unspecified finger**

S60.44 **External constriction of fingers**
Hair tourniquet syndrome of finger
Use additional cause code to identify the constricting item (W49.0-)

- S60.440 **External constriction of right index finger**
- S60.441 **External constriction of left index finger**
- S60.442 **External constriction of right middle finger**
- S60.443 **External constriction of left middle finger**
- S60.444 **External constriction of right ring finger**
- S60.445 **External constriction of left ring finger**
- S60.446 **External constriction of right little finger**
- S60.447 **External constriction of left little finger**
- S60.448 **External constriction of other finger**
  External constriction of specified finger with unspecified laterality
- S60.449 **External constriction of unspecified finger**

S60.45 **Superficial foreign body of fingers**
Splinter in the finger(s)

- S60.450 **Superficial foreign body of right index finger**
- S60.451 **Superficial foreign body of left index finger**
- S60.452 **Superficial foreign body of right middle finger**
- S60.453 **Superficial foreign body of left middle finger**
- S60.454 **Superficial foreign body of right ring finger**
- S60.455 **Superficial foreign body of left ring finger**
- S60.456 **Superficial foreign body of right little finger**
- S60.457 **Superficial foreign body of left little finger**
- S60.458 **Superficial foreign body of other finger**
  Superficial foreign body of specified finger with unspecified laterality
- S60.459 **Superficial foreign body of unspecified finger**

S60.46 **Insect bite (nonvenomous) of fingers**

- S60.460 **Insect bite (nonvenomous) of right index finger**
- S60.461 **Insect bite (nonvenomous) of left index finger**
- S60.462 **Insect bite (nonvenomous) of right middle finger**
- S60.463 **Insect bite (nonvenomous) of left middle finger**
- S60.464 **Insect bite (nonvenomous) of right ring finger**
- S60.465 **Insect bite (nonvenomous) of left ring finger**
- S60.466 **Insect bite (nonvenomous) of right little finger**
- S60.467 **Insect bite (nonvenomous) of left little finger**
- S60.468 **Insect bite (nonvenomous) of other finger**
  Insect bite (nonvenomous) of specified finger with unspecified laterality
- S60.469 **Insect bite (nonvenomous) of unspecified finger**

S60.47 **Other superficial bite of fingers**
Excludes1 open bite of fingers (S61.25-, S61.35-)

- S60.470 **Other superficial bite of right index finger**
- S60.471 **Other superficial bite of left index finger**
- S60.472 **Other superficial bite of right middle finger**
- S60.473 **Other superficial bite of left middle finger**
- S60.474 **Other superficial bite of right ring finger**
- S60.475 **Other superficial bite of left ring finger**
- S60.476 **Other superficial bite of right little finger**
- S60.477 **Other superficial bite of left little finger**
- S60.478 **Other superficial bite of other finger**
  Other superficial bite of specified finger with unspecified laterality
- S60.479 **Other superficial bite of unspecified finger**

S60.5 **Other superficial injuries of hand**
Excludes2 superficial injuries of fingers (S60.3-, S60.4-)

S60.51 **Abrasion of hand**
- S60.511 **Abrasion of right hand**
- S60.512 **Abrasion of left hand**
- S60.519 **Abrasion of unspecified hand**

S60.52 **Blister (nonthermal) of hand**
- S60.521 **Blister (nonthermal) of right hand**
- S60.522 **Blister (nonthermal) of left hand**
- S60.529 **Blister (nonthermal) of unspecified hand**

S60.54 **External constriction of hand**
- S60.541 **External constriction of right hand**
- S60.542 **External constriction of left hand**
- S60.549 **External constriction of unspecified hand**

S60.55 **Superficial foreign body of hand**
Splinter in the hand
- S60.551 **Superficial foreign body of right hand**
- S60.552 **Superficial foreign body of left hand**
- S60.559 **Superficial foreign body of unspecified hand**

S60.56 **Insect bite (nonvenomous) of hand**
- S60.561 **Insect bite (nonvenomous) of right hand**
- S60.562 **Insect bite (nonvenomous) of left hand**
- S60.569 **Insect bite (nonvenomous) of unspecified hand**

CHAPTER 19 (S00-T88)

● S60.57 Other superficial bite of hand
Excludes1 open bite of hand (S61.45-)
● S60.571 Other superficial bite of hand of right hand
● S60.572 Other superficial bite of hand of left hand
● S60.579 Other superficial bite of hand of unspecified hand
● S60.8 Other superficial injuries of wrist
● S60.81 Abrasion of wrist
● S60.811 Abrasion of right wrist
● S60.812 Abrasion of left wrist
● S60.819 Abrasion of unspecified wrist
● S60.82 Blister (nonthermal) of wrist
● S60.821 Blister (nonthermal) of right wrist
● S60.822 Blister (nonthermal) of left wrist
● S60.829 Blister (nonthermal) of unspecified wrist
● S60.84 External constriction of wrist
● S60.841 External constriction of right wrist
● S60.842 External constriction of left wrist
● S60.849 External constriction of unspecified wrist
● S60.85 Superficial foreign body of wrist
Splinter in the wrist
● S60.851 Superficial foreign body of right wrist
● S60.852 Superficial foreign body of left wrist
● S60.859 Superficial foreign body of unspecified wrist
● S60.86 Insect bite (nonvenomous) of wrist
● S60.861 Insect bite (nonvenomous) of right wrist
● S60.862 Insect bite (nonvenomous) of left wrist
● S60.869 Insect bite (nonvenomous) of unspecified wrist
● S60.87 Other superficial bite of wrist
Excludes1 open bite of wrist (S61.55)
● S60.871 Other superficial bite of right wrist
● S60.872 Other superficial bite of left wrist
● S60.879 Other superficial bite of unspecified wrist
● S60.9 Unspecified superficial injury of wrist, hand and fingers
● S60.91 Unspecified superficial injury of wrist
● S60.911 Unspecified superficial injury of right wrist
● S60.912 Unspecified superficial injury of left wrist
● S60.919 Unspecified superficial injury of unspecified wrist
● S60.92 Unspecified superficial injury of hand
● S60.921 Unspecified superficial injury of right hand
● S60.922 Unspecified superficial injury of left hand
● S60.929 Unspecified superficial injury of unspecified hand
● S60.93 Unspecified superficial injury of thumb
● S60.931 Unspecified superficial injury of right thumb
● S60.932 Unspecified superficial injury of left thumb
● S60.939 Unspecified superficial injury of unspecified thumb
● S60.94 Unspecified superficial injury of other fingers
● S60.940 Unspecified superficial injury of right index finger
● S60.941 Unspecified superficial injury of left index finger
● S60.942 Unspecified superficial injury of right middle finger
● S60.943 Unspecified superficial injury of left middle finger
● S60.944 Unspecified superficial injury of right ring finger
● S60.945 Unspecified superficial injury of left ring finger
● S60.946 Unspecified superficial injury of right little finger
● S60.947 Unspecified superficial injury of left little finger
● S60.948 Unspecified superficial injury of other finger
Unspecified superficial injury of specified finger with unspecified laterality
● S60.949 Unspecified superficial injury of unspecified finger

● S61 Open wound of wrist, hand and fingers
Code also any associated wound infection
Excludes1 open fracture of wrist, hand and finger (S62.- with 7th character B)
traumatic amputation of wrist and hand (S68.-)

The appropriate 7th character is to be added to each code from category S61

A	initial encounter
D	subsequent encounter
S	sequela

● S61.0 Open wound of thumb without damage to nail
Excludes1 open wound of thumb with damage to nail (S61.1-)
● S61.00 Unspecified open wound of thumb without damage to nail
● S61.001 Unspecified open wound of right thumb without damage to nail
● S61.002 Unspecified open wound of left thumb without damage to nail
● S61.009 Unspecified open wound of unspecified thumb without damage to nail
● S61.01 Laceration without foreign body of thumb without damage to nail
● S61.011 Laceration without foreign body of right thumb without damage to nail
● S61.012 Laceration without foreign body of left thumb without damage to nail
● S61.019 Laceration without foreign body of unspecified thumb without damage to nail
● S61.02 Laceration with foreign body of thumb without damage to nail
● S61.021 Laceration with foreign body of right thumb without damage to nail
● S61.022 Laceration with foreign body of left thumb without damage to nail
● S61.029 Laceration with foreign body of unspecified thumb without damage to nail

CHAPTER 19 (S00-T88)

● S61.03 Puncture wound without foreign body of thumb without damage to nail
● S61.031 Puncture wound without foreign body of right thumb without damage to nail
● S61.032 Puncture wound without foreign body of left thumb without damage to nail
● S61.039 Puncture wound without foreign body of unspecified thumb without damage to nail
● S61.04 Puncture wound with foreign body of thumb without damage to nail
● S61.041 Puncture wound with foreign body of right thumb without damage to nail
● S61.042 Puncture wound with foreign body of left thumb without damage to nail
● S61.049 Puncture wound with foreign body of unspecified thumb without damage to nail
● S61.05 Open bite of thumb without damage to nail
Bite of thumb NOS
Excludes1 superficial bite of thumb (S60.36-, S60.37-)
● S61.051 Open bite of right thumb without damage to nail
● S61.052 Open bite of left thumb without damage to nail
● S61.059 Open bite of unspecified thumb without damage to nail
● S61.1 Open wound of thumb with damage to nail
● S61.10 Unspecified open wound of thumb with damage to nail
● S61.101 Unspecified open wound of right thumb with damage to nail
● S61.102 Unspecified open wound of left thumb with damage to nail
● S61.109 Unspecified open wound of unspecified thumb with damage to nail
● S61.11 Laceration without foreign body of thumb with damage to nail
● S61.111 Laceration without foreign body of right thumb with damage to nail
● S61.112 Laceration without foreign body of left thumb with damage to nail
● S61.119 Laceration without foreign body of unspecified thumb with damage to nail
● S61.12 Laceration with foreign body of thumb with damage to nail
● S61.121 Laceration with foreign body of right thumb with damage to nail
● S61.122 Laceration with foreign body of left thumb with damage to nail
● S61.129 Laceration with foreign body of unspecified thumb with damage to nail
● S61.13 Puncture wound without foreign body of thumb with damage to nail
● S61.131 Puncture wound without foreign body of right thumb with damage to nail
● S61.132 Puncture wound without foreign body of left thumb with damage to nail
● S61.139 Puncture wound without foreign body of unspecified thumb with damage to nail
● S61.14 Puncture wound with foreign body of thumb with damage to nail
● S61.141 Puncture wound with foreign body of right thumb with damage to nail
● S61.142 Puncture wound with foreign body of left thumb with damage to nail
● S61.149 Puncture wound with foreign body of unspecified thumb with damage to nail
● S61.15 Open bite of thumb with damage to nail
Bite of thumb with damage to nail NOS
Excludes1 superficial bite of thumb (S60.36-, S60.37-)
● S61.151 Open bite of right thumb with damage to nail
● S61.152 Open bite of left thumb with damage to nail
● S61.159 Open bite of unspecified thumb with damage to nail
● S61.2 Open wound of other finger without damage to nail
Excludes1 open wound of finger involving nail (matrix) (S61.3-)
Excludes2 open wound of thumb without damage to nail (S61.0-)
● S61.20 Unspecified open wound of other finger without damage to nail
● S61.200 Unspecified open wound of right index finger without damage to nail
● S61.201 Unspecified open wound of left index finger without damage to nail
● S61.202 Unspecified open wound of right middle finger without damage to nail
● S61.203 Unspecified open wound of left middle finger without damage to nail
● S61.204 Unspecified open wound of right ring finger without damage to nail
● S61.205 Unspecified open wound of left ring finger without damage to nail
● S61.206 Unspecified open wound of right little finger without damage to nail
● S61.207 Unspecified open wound of left little finger without damage to nail
● S61.208 Unspecified open wound of other finger without damage to nail
Unspecified open wound of specified finger with unspecified laterality without damage to nail
● S61.209 Unspecified open wound of unspecified finger without damage to nail
● S61.21 Laceration without foreign body of finger without damage to nail
● S61.210 Laceration without foreign body of right index finger without damage to nail
● S61.211 Laceration without foreign body of left index finger without damage to nail
● S61.212 Laceration without foreign body of right middle finger without damage to nail
● S61.213 Laceration without foreign body of left middle finger without damage to nail

CHAPTER 19 (S00-T88)

● S61.214 **Laceration without foreign body of right ring finger without damage to nail**

● S61.215 **Laceration without foreign body of left ring finger without damage to nail**

● S61.216 **Laceration without foreign body of right little finger without damage to nail**

● S61.217 **Laceration without foreign body of left little finger without damage to nail**

● S61.218 **Laceration without foreign body of other finger without damage to nail**
Laceration without foreign body of specified finger with unspecified laterality without damage to nail

● S61.219 **Laceration without foreign body of unspecified finger without damage to nail**

● S61.22 **Laceration with foreign body of finger without damage to nail**

● S61.220 **Laceration with foreign body of right index finger without damage to nail**

● S61.221 **Laceration with foreign body of left index finger without damage to nail**

● S61.222 **Laceration with foreign body of right middle finger without damage to nail**

● S61.223 **Laceration with foreign body of left middle finger without damage to nail**

● S61.224 **Laceration with foreign body of right ring finger without damage to nail**

● S61.225 **Laceration with foreign body of left ring finger without damage to nail**

● S61.226 **Laceration with foreign body of right little finger without damage to nail**

● S61.227 **Laceration with foreign body of left little finger without damage to nail**

● S61.228 **Laceration with foreign body of other finger without damage to nail**
Laceration with foreign body of specified finger with unspecified laterality without damage to nail

● S61.229 **Laceration with foreign body of unspecified finger without damage to nail**

● S61.23 **Puncture wound without foreign body of finger without damage to nail**

● S61.230 **Puncture wound without foreign body of right index finger without damage to nail**

● S61.231 **Puncture wound without foreign body of left index finger without damage to nail**

● S61.232 **Puncture wound without foreign body of right middle finger without damage to nail**

● S61.233 **Puncture wound without foreign body of left middle finger without damage to nail**

● S61.234 **Puncture wound without foreign body of right ring finger without damage to nail**

● S61.235 **Puncture wound without foreign body of left ring finger without damage to nail**

● S61.236 **Puncture wound without foreign body of right little finger without damage to nail**

● S61.237 **Puncture wound without foreign body of left little finger without damage to nail**

● S61.238 **Puncture wound without foreign body of other finger without damage to nail**
Puncture wound without foreign body of specified finger with unspecified laterality without damage to nail

● S61.239 **Puncture wound without foreign body of unspecified finger without damage to nail**

● S61.24 **Puncture wound with foreign body of finger without damage to nail**

● S61.240 **Puncture wound with foreign body of right index finger without damage to nail**

● S61.241 **Puncture wound with foreign body of left index finger without damage to nail**

● S61.242 **Puncture wound with foreign body of right middle finger without damage to nail**

● S61.243 **Puncture wound with foreign body of left middle finger without damage to nail**

● S61.244 **Puncture wound with foreign body of right ring finger without damage to nail**

● S61.245 **Puncture wound with foreign body of left ring finger without damage to nail**

● S61.246 **Puncture wound with foreign body of right little finger without damage to nail**

● S61.247 **Puncture wound with foreign body of left little finger without damage to nail**

● S61.248 **Puncture wound with foreign body of other finger without damage to nail**
Puncture wound with foreign body of specified finger with unspecified laterality without damage to nail

● S61.249 **Puncture wound with foreign body of unspecified finger without damage to nail**

● S61.25 **Open bite of finger without damage to nail**
Bite of finger without damage to nail NOS
Excludes1 superficial bite of finger (S60.46-, S60.47-)

● S61.250 **Open bite of right index finger without damage to nail**

● S61.251 **Open bite of left index finger without damage to nail**

● S61.252 **Open bite of right middle finger without damage to nail**

● S61.253 **Open bite of left middle finger without damage to nail**

● S61.254 **Open bite of right ring finger without damage to nail**

● S61.255 **Open bite of left ring finger without damage to nail**

● S61.256 **Open bite of right little finger without damage to nail**

● S61.257 **Open bite of left little finger without damage to nail**

● S61.258 **Open bite of other finger without damage to nail**
Open bite of specified finger with unspecified laterality without damage to nail

● S61.259 **Open bite of unspecified finger without damage to nail**

◀ New ◀ Revised ~~deleted~~ Deleted **OGCR** Official Guidelines **X** Assign placeholder X ● Use Additional Character(s)
Excludes 1 | Excludes 2 | Includes | Use additional | Code first | Code also | Unspecified

● S61.3 Open wound of other finger with damage to nail
● S61.30 Unspecified open wound of finger with damage to nail
● S61.300 Unspecified open wound of right index finger with damage to nail
● S61.301 Unspecified open wound of left index finger with damage to nail
● S61.302 Unspecified open wound of right middle finger with damage to nail
● S61.303 Unspecified open wound of left middle finger with damage to nail
● S61.304 Unspecified open wound of right ring finger with damage to nail
● S61.305 Unspecified open wound of left ring finger with damage to nail
● S61.306 Unspecified open wound of right little finger with damage to nail
● S61.307 Unspecified open wound of left little finger with damage to nail
● S61.308 Unspecified open wound of other finger with damage to nail
Unspecified open wound of specified finger with unspecified laterality with damage to nail
● S61.309 Unspecified open wound of unspecified finger with damage to nail
● S61.31 Laceration without foreign body of finger with damage to nail
● S61.310 Laceration without foreign body of right index finger with damage to nail
● S61.311 Laceration without foreign body of left index finger with damage to nail
● S61.312 Laceration without foreign body of right middle finger with damage to nail
● S61.313 Laceration without foreign body of left middle finger with damage to nail
● S61.314 Laceration without foreign body of right ring finger with damage to nail
● S61.315 Laceration without foreign body of left ring finger with damage to nail
● S61.316 Laceration without foreign body of right little finger with damage to nail
● S61.317 Laceration without foreign body of left little finger with damage to nail
● S61.318 Laceration without foreign body of other finger with damage to nail
Laceration without foreign body of specified finger with unspecified laterality with damage to nail
● S61.319 Laceration without foreign body of unspecified finger with damage to nail
● S61.32 Laceration with foreign body of finger with damage to nail
● S61.320 Laceration with foreign body of right index finger with damage to nail
● S61.321 Laceration with foreign body of left index finger with damage to nail
● S61.322 Laceration with foreign body of right middle finger with damage to nail
● S61.323 Laceration with foreign body of left middle finger with damage to nail
● S61.324 Laceration with foreign body of right ring finger with damage to nail
● S61.325 Laceration with foreign body of left ring finger with damage to nail
● S61.326 Laceration with foreign body of right little finger with damage to nail
● S61.327 Laceration with foreign body of left little finger with damage to nail
● S61.328 Laceration with foreign body of other finger with damage to nail
Laceration with foreign body of specified finger with unspecified laterality with damage to nail
● S61.329 Laceration with foreign body of unspecified finger with damage to nail
● S61.33 Puncture wound without foreign body of finger with damage to nail
● S61.330 Puncture wound without foreign body of right index finger with damage to nail
● S61.331 Puncture wound without foreign body of left index finger with damage to nail
● S61.332 Puncture wound without foreign body of right middle finger with damage to nail
● S61.333 Puncture wound without foreign body of left middle finger with damage to nail
● S61.334 Puncture wound without foreign body of right ring finger with damage to nail
● S61.335 Puncture wound without foreign body of left ring finger with damage to nail
● S61.336 Puncture wound without foreign body of right little finger with damage to nail
● S61.337 Puncture wound without foreign body of left little finger with damage to nail
● S61.338 Puncture wound without foreign body of other finger with damage to nail
Puncture wound without foreign body of specified finger with unspecified laterality with damage to nail
● S61.339 Puncture wound without foreign body of unspecified finger with damage to nail
● S61.34 Puncture wound with foreign body of finger with damage to nail
● S61.340 Puncture wound with foreign body of right index finger with damage to nail
● S61.341 Puncture wound with foreign body of left index finger with damage to nail
● S61.342 Puncture wound with foreign body of right middle finger with damage to nail
● S61.343 Puncture wound with foreign body of left middle finger with damage to nail
● S61.344 Puncture wound with foreign body of right ring finger with damage to nail
● S61.345 Puncture wound with foreign body of left ring finger with damage to nail
● S61.346 Puncture wound with foreign body of right little finger with damage to nail
● S61.347 Puncture wound with foreign body of left little finger with damage to nail
● S61.348 Puncture wound with foreign body of other finger with damage to nail
Puncture wound with foreign body of specified finger with unspecified laterality with damage to nail
● S61.349 Puncture wound with foreign body of unspecified finger with damage to nail

CHAPTER 19 (S00-T88)

● S61.35 Open bite of finger with damage to nail
Bite of finger with damage to nail NOS
Excludes1 superficial bite of finger (S60.46-, S60.47-)
● S61.350 Open bite of right index finger with damage to nail
● S61.351 Open bite of left index finger with damage to nail
● S61.352 Open bite of right middle finger with damage to nail
● S61.353 Open bite of left middle finger with damage to nail
● S61.354 Open bite of right ring finger with damage to nail
● S61.355 Open bite of left ring finger with damage to nail
● S61.356 Open bite of right little finger with damage to nail
● S61.357 Open bite of left little finger with damage to nail
● S61.358 Open bite of other finger with damage to nail
Open bite of specified finger with unspecified laterality with damage to nail
● S61.359 Open bite of unspecified finger with damage to nail

● S61.4 Open wound of hand
● S61.40 Unspecified open wound of hand
● S61.401 Unspecified open wound of right hand
● S61.402 Unspecified open wound of left hand
● S61.409 Unspecified open wound of unspecified hand
● S61.41 Laceration without foreign body of hand
● S61.411 Laceration without foreign body of right hand
● S61.412 Laceration without foreign body of left hand
● S61.419 Laceration without foreign body of unspecified hand
● S61.42 Laceration with foreign body of hand
● S61.421 Laceration with foreign body of right hand
● S61.422 Laceration with foreign body of left hand
● S61.429 Laceration with foreign body of unspecified hand
● S61.43 Puncture wound without foreign body of hand
● S61.431 Puncture wound without foreign body of right hand
● S61.432 Puncture wound without foreign body of left hand
● S61.439 Puncture wound without foreign body of unspecified hand
● S61.44 Puncture wound with foreign body of hand
● S61.441 Puncture wound with foreign body of right hand
● S61.442 Puncture wound with foreign body of left hand
● S61.449 Puncture wound with foreign body of unspecified hand
● S61.45 Open bite of hand
Bite of hand NOS
Excludes1 superficial bite of hand (S60.56-, S60.57-)
● S61.451 Open bite of right hand
● S61.452 Open bite of left hand
● S61.459 Open bite of unspecified hand

● S61.5 Open wound of wrist
● S61.50 Unspecified open wound of wrist
● S61.501 Unspecified open wound of right wrist
● S61.502 Unspecified open wound of left wrist
● S61.509 Unspecified open wound of unspecified wrist
● S61.51 Laceration without foreign body of wrist
● S61.511 Laceration without foreign body of right wrist
● S61.512 Laceration without foreign body of left wrist
● S61.519 Laceration without foreign body of unspecified wrist
● S61.52 Laceration with foreign body of wrist
● S61.521 Laceration with foreign body of right wrist
● S61.522 Laceration with foreign body of left wrist
● S61.529 Laceration with foreign body of unspecified wrist
● S61.53 Puncture wound without foreign body of wrist
● S61.531 Puncture wound without foreign body of right wrist
● S61.532 Puncture wound without foreign body of left wrist
● S61.539 Puncture wound without foreign body of unspecified wrist
● S61.54 Puncture wound with foreign body of wrist
● S61.541 Puncture wound with foreign body of right wrist
● S61.542 Puncture wound with foreign body of left wrist
● S61.549 Puncture wound with foreign body of unspecified wrist
● S61.55 Open bite of wrist
Bite of wrist NOS
Excludes1 superficial bite of wrist (S60.86-, S60.87-)
● S61.551 Open bite of right wrist
● S61.552 Open bite of left wrist
● S61.559 Open bite of unspecified wrist

● **S62 Fracture at wrist and hand level**
Note: A fracture not indicated as displaced or nondisplaced should be coded to displaced
A fracture not indicated as open or closed should be coded to closed
Excludes1 traumatic amputation of wrist and hand (S68.-)
Excludes2 fracture of distal parts of ulna and radius (S52.-)
The appropriate 7th character is to be added to each code from category S62

A	initial encounter for closed fracture
B	initial encounter for open fracture
D	subsequent encounter for fracture with routine healing
G	subsequent encounter for fracture with delayed healing
K	subsequent encounter for fracture with nonunion
P	subsequent encounter for fracture with malunion
S	sequela

● S62.0 Fracture of navicular [scaphoid] bone of wrist
● S62.00 Unspecified fracture of navicular [scaphoid] bone of wrist
● S62.001 Unspecified fracture of navicular [scaphoid] bone of right wrist
● S62.002 Unspecified fracture of navicular [scaphoid] bone of left wrist
● S62.009 Unspecified fracture of navicular [scaphoid] bone of unspecified wrist

CHAPTER 19 (S00-T88)

● S62.01 Fracture of distal pole of navicular [scaphoid] bone of wrist
Fracture of volar tuberosity of navicular [scaphoid] bone of wrist
● S62.011 Displaced fracture of distal pole of navicular [scaphoid] bone of right wrist
● S62.012 Displaced fracture of distal pole of navicular [scaphoid] bone of left wrist
● S62.013 Displaced fracture of distal pole of navicular [scaphoid] bone of unspecified wrist
● S62.014 Nondisplaced fracture of distal pole of navicular [scaphoid] bone of right wrist
● S62.015 Nondisplaced fracture of distal pole of navicular [scaphoid] bone of left wrist
● S62.016 Nondisplaced fracture of distal pole of navicular [scaphoid] bone of unspecified wrist
● S62.02 Fracture of middle third of navicular [scaphoid] bone of wrist
● S62.021 Displaced fracture of middle third of navicular [scaphoid] bone of right wrist
● S62.022 Displaced fracture of middle third of navicular [scaphoid] bone of left wrist
● S62.023 Displaced fracture of middle third of navicular [scaphoid] bone of unspecified wrist
● S62.024 Nondisplaced fracture of middle third of navicular [scaphoid] bone of right wrist
● S62.025 Nondisplaced fracture of middle third of navicular [scaphoid] bone of left wrist
● S62.026 Nondisplaced fracture of middle third of navicular [scaphoid] bone of unspecified wrist
● S62.03 Fracture of proximal third of navicular [scaphoid] bone of wrist
● S62.031 Displaced fracture of proximal third of navicular [scaphoid] bone of right wrist
● S62.032 Displaced fracture of proximal third of navicular [scaphoid] bone of left wrist
● S62.033 Displaced fracture of proximal third of navicular [scaphoid] bone of unspecified wrist
● S62.034 Nondisplaced fracture of proximal third of navicular [scaphoid] bone of right wrist
● S62.035 Nondisplaced fracture of proximal third of navicular [scaphoid] bone of left wrist
● S62.036 Nondisplaced fracture of proximal third of navicular [scaphoid] bone of unspecified wrist
● S62.1 Fracture of other and unspecified carpal bone(s)
Excludes2 fracture of scaphoid of wrist (S62.0-)
● S62.10 Fracture of unspecified carpal bone
Fracture of wrist NOS
● S62.101 Fracture of unspecified carpal bone, right wrist
● S62.102 Fracture of unspecified carpal bone, left wrist
● S62.109 Fracture of unspecified carpal bone, unspecified wrist
● S62.11 Fracture of triquetrum [cuneiform] bone of wrist
● S62.111 Displaced fracture of triquetrum [cuneiform] bone, right wrist
● S62.112 Displaced fracture of triquetrum [cuneiform] bone, left wrist
● S62.113 Displaced fracture of triquetrum [cuneiform] bone, unspecified wrist
● S62.114 Nondisplaced fracture of triquetrum [cuneiform] bone, right wrist
● S62.115 Nondisplaced fracture of triquetrum [cuneiform] bone, left wrist
● S62.116 Nondisplaced fracture of triquetrum [cuneiform] bone, unspecified wrist
● S62.12 Fracture of lunate [semilunar]
● S62.121 Displaced fracture of lunate [semilunar], right wrist
● S62.122 Displaced fracture of lunate [semilunar], left wrist
● S62.123 Displaced fracture of lunate [semilunar], unspecified wrist
● S62.124 Nondisplaced fracture of lunate [semilunar], right wrist
● S62.125 Nondisplaced fracture of lunate [semilunar], left wrist
● S62.126 Nondisplaced fracture of lunate [semilunar], unspecified wrist
● S62.13 Fracture of capitate [os magnum] bone
● S62.131 Displaced fracture of capitate [os magnum] bone, right wrist
● S62.132 Displaced fracture of capitate [os magnum] bone, left wrist
● S62.133 Displaced fracture of capitate [os magnum] bone, unspecified wrist
● S62.134 Nondisplaced fracture of capitate [os magnum] bone, right wrist
● S62.135 Nondisplaced fracture of capitate [os magnum] bone, left wrist
● S62.136 Nondisplaced fracture of capitate [os magnum] bone, unspecified wrist
● S62.14 Fracture of body of hamate [unciform] bone
Fracture of hamate [unciform] bone NOS
● S62.141 Displaced fracture of body of hamate [unciform] bone, right wrist
● S62.142 Displaced fracture of body of hamate [unciform] bone, left wrist
● S62.143 Displaced fracture of body of hamate [unciform] bone, unspecified wrist
● S62.144 Nondisplaced fracture of body of hamate [unciform] bone, right wrist
● S62.145 Nondisplaced fracture of body of hamate [unciform] bone, left wrist
● S62.146 Nondisplaced fracture of body of hamate [unciform] bone, unspecified wrist
● S62.15 Fracture of hook process of hamate [unciform] bone
Fracture of unciform process of hamate [unciform] bone
● S62.151 Displaced fracture of hook process of hamate [unciform] bone, right wrist
● S62.152 Displaced fracture of hook process of hamate [unciform] bone, left wrist
● S62.153 Displaced fracture of hook process of hamate [unciform] bone, unspecified wrist
● S62.154 Nondisplaced fracture of hook process of hamate [unciform] bone, right wrist
● S62.155 Nondisplaced fracture of hook process of hamate [unciform] bone, left wrist
● S62.156 Nondisplaced fracture of hook process of hamate [unciform] bone, unspecified wrist

CHAPTER 19 (S00-T88)

- ● S62.16   Fracture of pisiform
  - ● S62.161   Displaced fracture of pisiform, right wrist
  - ● S62.162   Displaced fracture of pisiform, left wrist
  - ● S62.163   Displaced fracture of pisiform, unspecified wrist
  - ● S62.164   Nondisplaced fracture of pisiform, right wrist
  - ● S62.165   Nondisplaced fracture of pisiform, left wrist
  - ● S62.166   Nondisplaced fracture of pisiform, unspecified wrist
- ● S62.17   Fracture of trapezium [larger multangular]
  - ● S62.171   Displaced fracture of trapezium [larger multangular], right wrist
  - ● S62.172   Displaced fracture of trapezium [larger multangular], left wrist
  - ● S62.173   Displaced fracture of trapezium [larger multangular], unspecified wrist
  - ● S62.174   Nondisplaced fracture of trapezium [larger multangular], right wrist
  - ● S62.175   Nondisplaced fracture of trapezium [larger multangular], left wrist
  - ● S62.176   Nondisplaced fracture of trapezium [larger multangular], unspecified wrist
- ● S62.18   Fracture of trapezoid [smaller multangular]
  - ● S62.181   Displaced fracture of trapezoid [smaller multangular], right wrist
  - ● S62.182   Displaced fracture of trapezoid [smaller multangular], left wrist
  - ● S62.183   Displaced fracture of trapezoid [smaller multangular], unspecified wrist
  - ● S62.184   Nondisplaced fracture of trapezoid [smaller multangular], right wrist
  - ● S62.185   Nondisplaced fracture of trapezoid [smaller multangular], left wrist
  - ● S62.186   Nondisplaced fracture of trapezoid [smaller multangular], unspecified wrist
- ● S62.2   Fracture of first metacarpal bone
  - ● S62.20   Unspecified fracture of first metacarpal bone
    - ● S62.201   Unspecified fracture of first metacarpal bone, right hand
    - ● S62.202   Unspecified fracture of first metacarpal bone, left hand
    - ● S62.209   Unspecified fracture of first metacarpal bone, unspecified hand
  - ● S62.21   Bennett's fracture
    - ● S62.211   Bennett's fracture, right hand
    - ● S62.212   Bennett's fracture, left hand
    - ● S62.213   Bennett's fracture, unspecified hand
  - ● S62.22   Rolando's fracture
    - ● S62.221   Displaced Rolando's fracture, right hand
    - ● S62.222   Displaced Rolando's fracture, left hand
    - ● S62.223   Displaced Rolando's fracture, unspecified hand
    - ● S62.224   Nondisplaced Rolando's fracture, right hand
    - ● S62.225   Nondisplaced Rolando's fracture, left hand
    - ● S62.226   Nondisplaced Rolando's fracture, unspecified hand

- ● S62.23   Other fracture of base of first metacarpal bone
  - ● S62.231   Other displaced fracture of base of first metacarpal bone, right hand
  - ● S62.232   Other displaced fracture of base of first metacarpal bone, left hand
  - ● S62.233   Other displaced fracture of base of first metacarpal bone, unspecified hand
  - ● S62.234   Other nondisplaced fracture of base of first metacarpal bone, right hand
  - ● S62.235   Other nondisplaced fracture of base of first metacarpal bone, left hand
  - ● S62.236   Other nondisplaced fracture of base of first metacarpal bone, unspecified hand
- ● S62.24   Fracture of shaft of first metacarpal bone
  - ● S62.241   Displaced fracture of shaft of first metacarpal bone, right hand
  - ● S62.242   Displaced fracture of shaft of first metacarpal bone, left hand
  - ● S62.243   Displaced fracture of shaft of first metacarpal bone, unspecified hand
  - ● S62.244   Nondisplaced fracture of shaft of first metacarpal bone, right hand
  - ● S62.245   Nondisplaced fracture of shaft of first metacarpal bone, left hand
  - ● S62.246   Nondisplaced fracture of shaft of first metacarpal bone, unspecified hand
- ● S62.25   Fracture of neck of first metacarpal bone
  - ● S62.251   Displaced fracture of neck of first metacarpal bone, right hand
  - ● S62.252   Displaced fracture of neck of first metacarpal bone, left hand
  - ● S62.253   Displaced fracture of neck of first metacarpal bone, unspecified hand
  - ● S62.254   Nondisplaced fracture of neck of first metacarpal bone, right hand
  - ● S62.255   Nondisplaced fracture of neck of first metacarpal bone, left hand
  - ● S62.256   Nondisplaced fracture of neck of first metacarpal bone, unspecified hand
- ● S62.29   Other fracture of first metacarpal bone
  - ● S62.291   Other fracture of first metacarpal bone, right hand
  - ● S62.292   Other fracture of first metacarpal bone, left hand
  - ● S62.299   Other fracture of first metacarpal bone, unspecified hand
- ● S62.3   Fracture of other and unspecified metacarpal bone
  - **Excludes2**   fracture of first metacarpal bone (S62.2-)
  - ● S62.30   Unspecified fracture of other metacarpal bone
    - ● S62.300   Unspecified fracture of second metacarpal bone, right hand
    - ● S62.301   Unspecified fracture of second metacarpal bone, left hand
    - ● S62.302   Unspecified fracture of third metacarpal bone, right hand
    - ● S62.303   Unspecified fracture of third metacarpal bone, left hand
    - ● S62.304   Unspecified fracture of fourth metacarpal bone, right hand
    - ● S62.305   Unspecified fracture of fourth metacarpal bone, left hand
    - ● S62.306   Unspecified fracture of fifth metacarpal bone, right hand
    - ● S62.307   Unspecified fracture of fifth metacarpal bone, left hand

S62.308 Unspecified fracture of other metacarpal bone
Unspecified fracture of specified metacarpal bone with unspecified laterality
S62.309 Unspecified fracture of unspecified metacarpal bone
S62.31 Displaced fracture of base of other metacarpal bone
S62.310 Displaced fracture of base of second metacarpal bone, right hand
S62.311 Displaced fracture of base of second metacarpal bone, left hand
S62.312 Displaced fracture of base of third metacarpal bone, right hand
S62.313 Displaced fracture of base of third metacarpal bone, left hand
S62.314 Displaced fracture of base of fourth metacarpal bone, right hand
S62.315 Displaced fracture of base of fourth metacarpal bone, left hand
S62.316 Displaced fracture of base of fifth metacarpal bone, right hand
S62.317 Displaced fracture of base of fifth metacarpal bone, left hand
S62.318 Displaced fracture of base of other metacarpal bone
Displaced fracture of base of specified metacarpal bone with unspecified laterality
S62.319 Displaced fracture of base of unspecified metacarpal bone
S62.32 Displaced fracture of shaft of other metacarpal bone
S62.320 Displaced fracture of shaft of second metacarpal bone, right hand
S62.321 Displaced fracture of shaft of second metacarpal bone, left hand
S62.322 Displaced fracture of shaft of third metacarpal bone, right hand
S62.323 Displaced fracture of shaft of third metacarpal bone, left hand
S62.324 Displaced fracture of shaft of fourth metacarpal bone, right hand
S62.325 Displaced fracture of shaft of fourth metacarpal bone, left hand
S62.326 Displaced fracture of shaft of fifth metacarpal bone, right hand
S62.327 Displaced fracture of shaft of fifth metacarpal bone, left hand
S62.328 Displaced fracture of shaft of other metacarpal bone
Displaced fracture of shaft of specified metacarpal bone with unspecified laterality
S62.329 Displaced fracture of shaft of unspecified metacarpal bone
S62.33 Displaced fracture of neck of other metacarpal bone
S62.330 Displaced fracture of neck of second metacarpal bone, right hand
S62.331 Displaced fracture of neck of second metacarpal bone, left hand
S62.332 Displaced fracture of neck of third metacarpal bone, right hand
S62.333 Displaced fracture of neck of third metacarpal bone, left hand
S62.334 Displaced fracture of neck of fourth metacarpal bone, right hand
S62.335 Displaced fracture of neck of fourth metacarpal bone, left hand
S62.336 Displaced fracture of neck of fifth metacarpal bone, right hand
S62.337 Displaced fracture of neck of fifth metacarpal bone, left hand
S62.338 Displaced fracture of neck of other metacarpal bone
Displaced fracture of neck of specified metacarpal bone with unspecified laterality
S62.339 Displaced fracture of neck of unspecified metacarpal bone
S62.34 Nondisplaced fracture of base of other metacarpal bone
S62.340 Nondisplaced fracture of base of second metacarpal bone, right hand
S62.341 Nondisplaced fracture of base of second metacarpal bone, left hand
S62.342 Nondisplaced fracture of base of third metacarpal bone, right hand
S62.343 Nondisplaced fracture of base of third metacarpal bone, left hand
S62.344 Nondisplaced fracture of base of fourth metacarpal bone, right hand
S62.345 Nondisplaced fracture of base of fourth metacarpal bone, left hand
S62.346 Nondisplaced fracture of base of fifth metacarpal bone, right hand
S62.347 Nondisplaced fracture of base of fifth metacarpal bone, left hand
S62.348 Nondisplaced fracture of base of other metacarpal bone
Nondisplaced fracture of base of specified metacarpal bone with unspecified laterality
S62.349 Nondisplaced fracture of base of unspecified metacarpal bone
S62.35 Nondisplaced fracture of shaft of other metacarpal bone
S62.350 Nondisplaced fracture of shaft of second metacarpal bone, right hand
S62.351 Nondisplaced fracture of shaft of second metacarpal bone, left hand
S62.352 Nondisplaced fracture of shaft of third metacarpal bone, right hand
S62.353 Nondisplaced fracture of shaft of third metacarpal bone, left hand
S62.354 Nondisplaced fracture of shaft of fourth metacarpal bone, right hand
S62.355 Nondisplaced fracture of shaft of fourth metacarpal bone, left hand
S62.356 Nondisplaced fracture of shaft of fifth metacarpal bone, right hand
S62.357 Nondisplaced fracture of shaft of fifth metacarpal bone, left hand
S62.358 Nondisplaced fracture of shaft of other metacarpal bone
Nondisplaced fracture of shaft of specified metacarpal bone with unspecified laterality
S62.359 Nondisplaced fracture of shaft of unspecified metacarpal bone

- S62.36 Nondisplaced fracture of neck of other metacarpal bone
  - S62.360 Nondisplaced fracture of neck of second metacarpal bone, right hand
  - S62.361 Nondisplaced fracture of neck of second metacarpal bone, left hand
  - S62.362 Nondisplaced fracture of neck of third metacarpal bone, right hand
  - S62.363 Nondisplaced fracture of neck of third metacarpal bone, left hand
  - S62.364 Nondisplaced fracture of neck of fourth metacarpal bone, right hand
  - S62.365 Nondisplaced fracture of neck of fourth metacarpal bone, left hand
  - S62.366 Nondisplaced fracture of neck of fifth metacarpal bone, right hand
  - S62.367 Nondisplaced fracture of neck of fifth metacarpal bone, left hand
  - S62.368 Nondisplaced fracture of neck of other metacarpal bone
    Nondisplaced fracture of neck of specified metacarpal bone with unspecified laterality
  - S62.369 Nondisplaced fracture of neck of unspecified metacarpal bone
- S62.39 Other fracture of other metacarpal bone
  - S62.390 Other fracture of second metacarpal bone, right hand
  - S62.391 Other fracture of second metacarpal bone, left hand
  - S62.392 Other fracture of third metacarpal bone, right hand
  - S62.393 Other fracture of third metacarpal bone, left hand
  - S62.394 Other fracture of fourth metacarpal bone, right hand
  - S62.395 Other fracture of fourth metacarpal bone, left hand
  - S62.396 Other fracture of fifth metacarpal bone, right hand
  - S62.397 Other fracture of fifth metacarpal bone, left hand
  - S62.398 Other fracture of other metacarpal bone
    Other fracture of specified metacarpal bone with unspecified laterality
  - S62.399 Other fracture of unspecified metacarpal bone

- S62.5 Fracture of thumb
  - S62.50 Fracture of unspecified phalanx of thumb
    - S62.501 Fracture of unspecified phalanx of right thumb
    - S62.502 Fracture of unspecified phalanx of left thumb
    - S62.509 Fracture of unspecified phalanx of unspecified thumb
  - S62.51 Fracture of proximal phalanx of thumb
    - S62.511 Displaced fracture of proximal phalanx of right thumb
    - S62.512 Displaced fracture of proximal phalanx of left thumb
    - S62.513 Displaced fracture of proximal phalanx of unspecified thumb
    - S62.514 Nondisplaced fracture of proximal phalanx of right thumb
    - S62.515 Nondisplaced fracture of proximal phalanx of left thumb
    - S62.516 Nondisplaced fracture of proximal phalanx of unspecified thumb
  - S62.52 Fracture of distal phalanx of thumb
    - S62.521 Displaced fracture of distal phalanx of right thumb
    - S62.522 Displaced fracture of distal phalanx of left thumb
    - S62.523 Displaced fracture of distal phalanx of unspecified thumb
    - S62.524 Nondisplaced fracture of distal phalanx of right thumb
    - S62.525 Nondisplaced fracture of distal phalanx of left thumb
    - S62.526 Nondisplaced fracture of distal phalanx of unspecified thumb

- S62.6 Fracture of other and unspecified finger(s)
  Excludes2 fracture of thumb (S62.5-)
  - S62.60 Fracture of unspecified phalanx of finger
    - S62.600 Fracture of unspecified phalanx of right index finger
    - S62.601 Fracture of unspecified phalanx of left index finger
    - S62.602 Fracture of unspecified phalanx of right middle finger
    - S62.603 Fracture of unspecified phalanx of left middle finger
    - S62.604 Fracture of unspecified phalanx of right ring finger
    - S62.605 Fracture of unspecified phalanx of left ring finger
    - S62.606 Fracture of unspecified phalanx of right little finger
    - S62.607 Fracture of unspecified phalanx of left little finger
    - S62.608 Fracture of unspecified phalanx of other finger
      Fracture of unspecified phalanx of specified finger with unspecified laterality
    - S62.609 Fracture of unspecified phalanx of unspecified finger
  - S62.61 Displaced fracture of proximal phalanx of finger
    - S62.610 Displaced fracture of proximal phalanx of right index finger
    - S62.611 Displaced fracture of proximal phalanx of left index finger
    - S62.612 Displaced fracture of proximal phalanx of right middle finger
    - S62.613 Displaced fracture of proximal phalanx of left middle finger
    - S62.614 Displaced fracture of proximal phalanx of right ring finger
    - S62.615 Displaced fracture of proximal phalanx of left ring finger
    - S62.616 Displaced fracture of proximal phalanx of right little finger
    - S62.617 Displaced fracture of proximal phalanx of left little finger
    - S62.618 Displaced fracture of proximal phalanx of other finger
      Displaced fracture of proximal phalanx of specified finger with unspecified laterality
    - S62.619 Displaced fracture of proximal phalanx of unspecified finger

- S62.62 Displaced fracture of medial phalanx of finger
  - S62.620 Displaced fracture of medial phalanx of right index finger
  - S62.621 Displaced fracture of medial phalanx of left index finger
  - S62.622 Displaced fracture of medial phalanx of right middle finger
  - S62.623 Displaced fracture of medial phalanx of left middle finger
  - S62.624 Displaced fracture of medial phalanx of right ring finger
  - S62.625 Displaced fracture of medial phalanx of left ring finger
  - S62.626 Displaced fracture of medial phalanx of right little finger
  - S62.627 Displaced fracture of medial phalanx of left little finger
  - S62.628 Displaced fracture of medial phalanx of other finger
    Displaced fracture of medial phalanx of specified finger with unspecified laterality
  - S62.629 Displaced fracture of medial phalanx of unspecified finger
- S62.63 Displaced fracture of distal phalanx of finger
  - S62.630 Displaced fracture of distal phalanx of right index finger
  - S62.631 Displaced fracture of distal phalanx of left index finger
  - S62.632 Displaced fracture of distal phalanx of right middle finger
  - S62.633 Displaced fracture of distal phalanx of left middle finger
  - S62.634 Displaced fracture of distal phalanx of right ring finger
  - S62.635 Displaced fracture of distal phalanx of left ring finger
  - S62.636 Displaced fracture of distal phalanx of right little finger
  - S62.637 Displaced fracture of distal phalanx of left little finger
  - S62.638 Displaced fracture of distal phalanx of other finger
    Displaced fracture of distal phalanx of specified finger with unspecified laterality
  - S62.639 Displaced fracture of distal phalanx of unspecified finger
- S62.64 Nondisplaced fracture of proximal phalanx of finger
  - S62.640 Nondisplaced fracture of proximal phalanx of right index finger
  - S62.641 Nondisplaced fracture of proximal phalanx of left index finger
  - S62.642 Nondisplaced fracture of proximal phalanx of right middle finger
  - S62.643 Nondisplaced fracture of proximal phalanx of left middle finger
  - S62.644 Nondisplaced fracture of proximal phalanx of right ring finger
  - S62.645 Nondisplaced fracture of proximal phalanx of left ring finger
  - S62.646 Nondisplaced fracture of proximal phalanx of right little finger
  - S62.647 Nondisplaced fracture of proximal phalanx of left little finger
  - S62.648 Nondisplaced fracture of proximal phalanx of other finger
    Nondisplaced fracture of proximal phalanx of specified finger with unspecified laterality
  - S62.649 Nondisplaced fracture of proximal phalanx of unspecified finger
- S62.65 Nondisplaced fracture of medial phalanx of finger
  - S62.650 Nondisplaced fracture of medial phalanx of right index finger
  - S62.651 Nondisplaced fracture of medial phalanx of left index finger
  - S62.652 Nondisplaced fracture of medial phalanx of right middle finger
  - S62.653 Nondisplaced fracture of medial phalanx of left middle finger
  - S62.654 Nondisplaced fracture of medial phalanx of right ring finger
  - S62.655 Nondisplaced fracture of medial phalanx of left ring finger
  - S62.656 Nondisplaced fracture of medial phalanx of right little finger
  - S62.657 Nondisplaced fracture of medial phalanx of left little finger
  - S62.658 Nondisplaced fracture of medial phalanx of other finger
    Nondisplaced fracture of medial phalanx of specified finger with unspecified laterality
  - S62.659 Nondisplaced fracture of medial phalanx of unspecified finger
- S62.66 Nondisplaced fracture of distal phalanx of finger
  - S62.660 Nondisplaced fracture of distal phalanx of right index finger
  - S62.661 Nondisplaced fracture of distal phalanx of left index finger
  - S62.662 Nondisplaced fracture of distal phalanx of right middle finger
  - S62.663 Nondisplaced fracture of distal phalanx of left middle finger
  - S62.664 Nondisplaced fracture of distal phalanx of right ring finger
  - S62.665 Nondisplaced fracture of distal phalanx of left ring finger
  - S62.666 Nondisplaced fracture of distal phalanx of right little finger
  - S62.667 Nondisplaced fracture of distal phalanx of left little finger
  - S62.668 Nondisplaced fracture of distal phalanx of other finger
    Nondisplaced fracture of distal phalanx of specified finger with unspecified laterality
  - S62.669 Nondisplaced fracture of distal phalanx of unspecified finger
- S62.9 Unspecified fracture of wrist and hand
  - X S62.90 Unspecified fracture of unspecified wrist and hand
  - X S62.91 Unspecified fracture of right wrist and hand
  - X S62.92 Unspecified fracture of left wrist and hand

CHAPTER 19 (S00-T88)

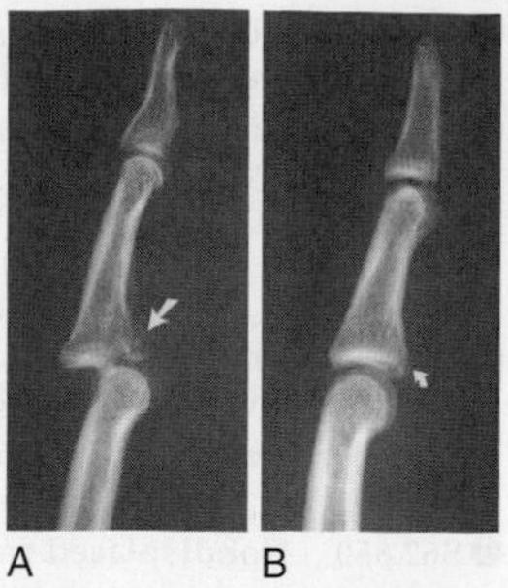

Figure 19-14 Dislocation including displacement and subluxation. (From Grainger & Allison's Diagnostic Radiology: A Textbook of Medical Imaging, ed 4, Churchill Livingstone, 2001)

● **S63 Dislocation and sprain of joints and ligaments at wrist and hand level**

Includes avulsion of joint or ligament at wrist and hand level
laceration of cartilage, joint or ligament at wrist and hand level
sprain of cartilage, joint or ligament at wrist and hand level
traumatic hemarthrosis of joint or ligament at wrist and hand level
traumatic rupture of joint or ligament at wrist and hand level
traumatic subluxation of joint or ligament at wrist and hand level
traumatic tear of joint or ligament at wrist and hand level

Code also any associated open wound

Excludes2 strain of muscle, fascia and tendon of wrist and hand (S66.-)

The appropriate 7th character is to be added to each code from category S63

A initial encounter
D subsequent encounter
S sequela

● **S63.Ø Subluxation and dislocation of wrist and hand joints**

● **S63.ØØ Unspecified subluxation and dislocation of wrist and hand**
Dislocation of carpal bone NOS
Dislocation of distal end of radius NOS
Subluxation of carpal bone NOS
Subluxation of distal end of radius NOS

● **S63.ØØ1 Unspecified subluxation of right wrist and hand**

● **S63.ØØ2 Unspecified subluxation of left wrist and hand**

● **S63.ØØ3 Unspecified subluxation of unspecified wrist and hand**

● **S63.ØØ4 Unspecified dislocation of right wrist and hand**

● **S63.ØØ5 Unspecified dislocation of left wrist and hand**

● **S63.ØØ6 Unspecified dislocation of unspecified wrist and hand**

● **S63.Ø1 Subluxation and dislocation of distal radioulnar joint**

● **S63.Ø11 Subluxation of distal radioulnar joint of right wrist**

● **S63.Ø12 Subluxation of distal radioulnar joint of left wrist**

● **S63.Ø13 Subluxation of distal radioulnar joint of unspecified wrist**

● **S63.Ø14 Dislocation of distal radioulnar joint of right wrist**

● **S63.Ø15 Dislocation of distal radioulnar joint of left wrist**

● **S63.Ø16 Dislocation of distal radioulnar joint of unspecified wrist**

● **S63.Ø2 Subluxation and dislocation of radiocarpal joint**

● **S63.Ø21 Subluxation of radiocarpal joint of right wrist**

● **S63.Ø22 Subluxation of radiocarpal joint of left wrist**

● **S63.Ø23 Subluxation of radiocarpal joint of unspecified wrist**

● **S63.Ø24 Dislocation of radiocarpal joint of right wrist**

● **S63.Ø25 Dislocation of radiocarpal joint of left wrist**

● **S63.Ø26 Dislocation of radiocarpal joint of unspecified wrist**

● **S63.Ø3 Subluxation and dislocation of midcarpal joint**

● **S63.Ø31 Subluxation of midcarpal joint of right wrist**

● **S63.Ø32 Subluxation of midcarpal joint of left wrist**

● **S63.Ø33 Subluxation of midcarpal joint of unspecified wrist**

● **S63.Ø34 Dislocation of midcarpal joint of right wrist**

● **S63.Ø35 Dislocation of midcarpal joint of left wrist**

● **S63.Ø36 Dislocation of midcarpal joint of unspecified wrist**

● **S63.Ø4 Subluxation and dislocation of carpometacarpal joint of thumb**

Excludes2 interphalangeal subluxation and dislocation of thumb (S63.1-)

● **S63.Ø41 Subluxation of carpometacarpal joint of right thumb**

● **S63.Ø42 Subluxation of carpometacarpal joint of left thumb**

● **S63.Ø43 Subluxation of carpometacarpal joint of unspecified thumb**

● **S63.Ø44 Dislocation of carpometacarpal joint of right thumb**

● **S63.Ø45 Dislocation of carpometacarpal joint of left thumb**

● **S63.Ø46 Dislocation of carpometacarpal joint of unspecified thumb**

● **S63.Ø5 Subluxation and dislocation of other carpometacarpal joint**

Excludes2 subluxation and dislocation of carpometacarpal joint of thumb (S63.Ø4-)

● **S63.Ø51 Subluxation of other carpometacarpal joint of right hand**

● **S63.Ø52 Subluxation of other carpometacarpal joint of left hand**

● **S63.Ø53 Subluxation of other carpometacarpal joint of unspecified hand**

● **S63.Ø54 Dislocation of other carpometacarpal joint of right hand**

● **S63.Ø55 Dislocation of other carpometacarpal joint of left hand**

● **S63.Ø56 Dislocation of other carpometacarpal joint of unspecified hand**

- S63.06 Subluxation and dislocation of metacarpal (bone), proximal end
  - S63.061 Subluxation of metacarpal (bone), proximal end of right hand
  - S63.062 Subluxation of metacarpal (bone), proximal end of left hand
  - S63.063 Subluxation of metacarpal (bone), proximal end of unspecified hand
  - S63.064 Dislocation of metacarpal (bone), proximal end of right hand
  - S63.065 Dislocation of metacarpal (bone), proximal end of left hand
  - S63.066 Dislocation of metacarpal (bone), proximal end of unspecified hand
- S63.07 Subluxation and dislocation of distal end of ulna
  - S63.071 Subluxation of distal end of right ulna
  - S63.072 Subluxation of distal end of left ulna
  - S63.073 Subluxation of distal end of unspecified ulna
  - S63.074 Dislocation of distal end of right ulna
  - S63.075 Dislocation of distal end of left ulna
  - S63.076 Dislocation of distal end of unspecified ulna
- S63.09 Other subluxation and dislocation of wrist and hand
  - S63.091 Other subluxation of right wrist and hand
  - S63.092 Other subluxation of left wrist and hand
  - S63.093 Other subluxation of unspecified wrist and hand
  - S63.094 Other dislocation of right wrist and hand
  - S63.095 Other dislocation of left wrist and hand
  - S63.096 Other dislocation of unspecified wrist and hand

- S63.1 Subluxation and dislocation of thumb
  - S63.10 Unspecified subluxation and dislocation of thumb
    - S63.101 Unspecified subluxation of right thumb
    - S63.102 Unspecified subluxation of left thumb
    - S63.103 Unspecified subluxation of unspecified thumb
    - S63.104 Unspecified dislocation of right thumb
    - S63.105 Unspecified dislocation of left thumb
    - S63.106 Unspecified dislocation of unspecified thumb
  - S63.11 Subluxation and dislocation of metacarpophalangeal joint of thumb
    - S63.111 Subluxation of metacarpophalangeal joint of right thumb
    - S63.112 Subluxation of metacarpophalangeal joint of left thumb
    - S63.113 Subluxation of metacarpophalangeal joint of unspecified thumb
    - S63.114 Dislocation of metacarpophalangeal joint of right thumb
    - S63.115 Dislocation of metacarpophalangeal joint of left thumb
    - S63.116 Dislocation of metacarpophalangeal joint of unspecified thumb
  - S63.12 Subluxation and dislocation of unspecified interphalangeal joint of thumb
    - S63.121 Subluxation of unspecified interphalangeal joint of right thumb
    - S63.122 Subluxation of unspecified interphalangeal joint of left thumb
    - S63.123 Subluxation of unspecified interphalangeal joint of unspecified thumb
    - S63.124 Dislocation of unspecified interphalangeal joint of right thumb
    - S63.125 Dislocation of unspecified interphalangeal joint of left thumb
    - S63.126 Dislocation of unspecified interphalangeal joint of unspecified thumb
  - S63.13 Subluxation and dislocation of proximal interphalangeal joint of thumb
    - S63.131 Subluxation of proximal interphalangeal joint of right thumb
    - S63.132 Subluxation of proximal interphalangeal joint of left thumb
    - S63.133 Subluxation of proximal interphalangeal joint of unspecified thumb
    - S63.134 Dislocation of proximal interphalangeal joint of right thumb
    - S63.135 Dislocation of proximal interphalangeal joint of left thumb
    - S63.136 Dislocation of proximal interphalangeal joint of unspecified thumb
  - S63.14 Subluxation and dislocation of distal interphalangeal joint of thumb
    - S63.141 Subluxation of distal interphalangeal joint of right thumb
    - S63.142 Subluxation of distal interphalangeal joint of left thumb
    - S63.143 Subluxation of distal interphalangeal joint of unspecified thumb
    - S63.144 Dislocation of distal interphalangeal joint of right thumb
    - S63.145 Dislocation of distal interphalangeal joint of left thumb
    - S63.146 Dislocation of distal interphalangeal joint of unspecified thumb

- S63.2 Subluxation and dislocation of other finger(s)

  Excludes2 subluxation and dislocation of thumb (S63.1-)

  - S63.20 Unspecified subluxation of other finger
    - S63.200 Unspecified subluxation of right index finger
    - S63.201 Unspecified subluxation of left index finger
    - S63.202 Unspecified subluxation of right middle finger
    - S63.203 Unspecified subluxation of left middle finger
    - S63.204 Unspecified subluxation of right ring finger
    - S63.205 Unspecified subluxation of left ring finger
    - S63.206 Unspecified subluxation of right little finger
    - S63.207 Unspecified subluxation of left little finger
    - S63.208 Unspecified subluxation of other finger

      Unspecified subluxation of specified finger with unspecified laterality
    - S63.209 Unspecified subluxation of unspecified finger

● S63.21 Subluxation of metacarpophalangeal joint of finger
● S63.210 Subluxation of metacarpophalangeal joint of right index finger
● S63.211 Subluxation of metacarpophalangeal joint of left index finger
● S63.212 Subluxation of metacarpophalangeal joint of right middle finger
● S63.213 Subluxation of metacarpophalangeal joint of left middle finger
● S63.214 Subluxation of metacarpophalangeal joint of right ring finger
● S63.215 Subluxation of metacarpophalangeal joint of left ring finger
● S63.216 Subluxation of metacarpophalangeal joint of right little finger
● S63.217 Subluxation of metacarpophalangeal joint of left little finger
● S63.218 Subluxation of metacarpophalangeal joint of other finger
Subluxation of metacarpophalangeal joint of specified finger with unspecified laterality
● S63.219 Subluxation of metacarpophalangeal joint of unspecified finger
● S63.22 Subluxation of unspecified interphalangeal joint of finger
● S63.220 Subluxation of unspecified interphalangeal joint of right index finger
● S63.221 Subluxation of unspecified interphalangeal joint of left index finger
● S63.222 Subluxation of unspecified interphalangeal joint of right middle finger
● S63.223 Subluxation of unspecified interphalangeal joint of left middle finger
● S63.224 Subluxation of unspecified interphalangeal joint of right ring finger
● S63.225 Subluxation of unspecified interphalangeal joint of left ring finger
● S63.226 Subluxation of unspecified interphalangeal joint of right little finger
● S63.227 Subluxation of unspecified interphalangeal joint of left little finger
● S63.228 Subluxation of unspecified interphalangeal joint of other finger
Subluxation of unspecified interphalangeal joint of specified finger with unspecified laterality
● S63.229 Subluxation of unspecified interphalangeal joint of unspecified finger
● S63.23 Subluxation of proximal interphalangeal joint of finger
● S63.230 Subluxation of proximal interphalangeal joint of right index finger
● S63.231 Subluxation of proximal interphalangeal joint of left index finger
● S63.232 Subluxation of proximal interphalangeal joint of right middle finger
● S63.233 Subluxation of proximal interphalangeal joint of left middle finger
● S63.234 Subluxation of proximal interphalangeal joint of right ring finger
● S63.235 Subluxation of proximal interphalangeal joint of left ring finger
● S63.236 Subluxation of proximal interphalangeal joint of right little finger
● S63.237 Subluxation of proximal interphalangeal joint of left little finger
● S63.238 Subluxation of proximal interphalangeal joint of other finger
Subluxation of proximal interphalangeal joint of specified finger with unspecified laterality
● S63.239 Subluxation of proximal interphalangeal joint of unspecified finger
● S63.24 Subluxation of distal interphalangeal joint of finger
● S63.240 Subluxation of distal interphalangeal joint of right index finger
● S63.241 Subluxation of distal interphalangeal joint of left index finger
● S63.242 Subluxation of distal interphalangeal joint of right middle finger
● S63.243 Subluxation of distal interphalangeal joint of left middle finger
● S63.244 Subluxation of distal interphalangeal joint of right ring finger
● S63.245 Subluxation of distal interphalangeal joint of left ring finger
● S63.246 Subluxation of distal interphalangeal joint of right little finger
● S63.247 Subluxation of distal interphalangeal joint of left little finger
● S63.248 Subluxation of distal interphalangeal joint of other finger
Subluxation of distal interphalangeal joint of specified finger with unspecified laterality
● S63.249 Subluxation of distal interphalangeal joint of unspecified finger
● S63.25 Unspecified dislocation of other finger
● S63.250 Unspecified dislocation of right index finger
● S63.251 Unspecified dislocation of left index finger
● S63.252 Unspecified dislocation of right middle finger
● S63.253 Unspecified dislocation of left middle finger
● S63.254 Unspecified dislocation of right ring finger
● S63.255 Unspecified dislocation of left ring finger
● S63.256 Unspecified dislocation of right little finger
● S63.257 Unspecified dislocation of left little finger

CHAPTER 19 (SØØ-T88)

● S63.258 Unspecified dislocation of other finger
Unspecified dislocation of specified finger with unspecified laterality
● S63.259 Unspecified dislocation of unspecified finger
Unspecified dislocation of specified finger with unspecified laterality
● S63.26 Dislocation of metacarpophalangeal joint of finger
● S63.260 Dislocation of metacarpophalangeal joint of right index finger
● S63.261 Dislocation of metacarpophalangeal joint of left index finger
● S63.262 Dislocation of metacarpophalangeal joint of right middle finger
● S63.263 Dislocation of metacarpophalangeal joint of left middle finger
● S63.264 Dislocation of metacarpophalangeal joint of right ring finger
● S63.265 Dislocation of metacarpophalangeal joint of left ring finger
● S63.266 Dislocation of metacarpophalangeal joint of right little finger
● S63.267 Dislocation of metacarpophalangeal joint of left little finger
● S63.268 Dislocation of metacarpophalangeal joint of other finger
Dislocation of metacarpophalangeal joint of specified finger with unspecified laterality
● S63.269 Dislocation of metacarpophalangeal joint of unspecified finger
● S63.27 Dislocation of unspecified interphalangeal joint of finger
● S63.270 Dislocation of unspecified interphalangeal joint of right index finger
● S63.271 Dislocation of unspecified interphalangeal joint of left index finger
● S63.272 Dislocation of unspecified interphalangeal joint of right middle finger
● S63.273 Dislocation of unspecified interphalangeal joint of left middle finger
● S63.274 Dislocation of unspecified interphalangeal joint of right ring finger
● S63.275 Dislocation of unspecified interphalangeal joint of left ring finger
● S63.276 Dislocation of unspecified interphalangeal joint of right little finger
● S63.277 Dislocation of unspecified interphalangeal joint of left little finger
● S63.278 Dislocation of unspecified interphalangeal joint of other finger
Dislocation of unspecified interphalangeal joint of specified finger with unspecified laterality
● S63.279 Dislocation of unspecified interphalangeal joint of unspecified finger
Dislocation of unspecified interphalangeal joint of specified finger without specified laterality

● S63.28 Dislocation of proximal interphalangeal joint of finger
● S63.280 Dislocation of proximal interphalangeal joint of right index finger
● S63.281 Dislocation of proximal interphalangeal joint of left index finger
● S63.282 Dislocation of proximal interphalangeal joint of right middle finger
● S63.283 Dislocation of proximal interphalangeal joint of left middle finger
● S63.284 Dislocation of proximal interphalangeal joint of right ring finger
● S63.285 Dislocation of proximal interphalangeal joint of left ring finger
● S63.286 Dislocation of proximal interphalangeal joint of right little finger
● S63.287 Dislocation of proximal interphalangeal joint of left little finger
● S63.288 Dislocation of proximal interphalangeal joint of other finger
Dislocation of proximal interphalangeal joint of specified finger with unspecified laterality
● S63.289 Dislocation of proximal interphalangeal joint of unspecified finger
● S63.29 Dislocation of distal interphalangeal joint of finger
● S63.290 Dislocation of distal interphalangeal joint of right index finger
● S63.291 Dislocation of distal interphalangeal joint of left index finger
● S63.292 Dislocation of distal interphalangeal joint of right middle finger
● S63.293 Dislocation of distal interphalangeal joint of left middle finger
● S63.294 Dislocation of distal interphalangeal joint of right ring finger
● S63.295 Dislocation of distal interphalangeal joint of left ring finger
● S63.296 Dislocation of distal interphalangeal joint of right little finger
● S63.297 Dislocation of distal interphalangeal joint of left little finger
● S63.298 Dislocation of distal interphalangeal joint of other finger
Dislocation of distal interphalangeal joint of specified finger with unspecified laterality
● S63.299 Dislocation of distal interphalangeal joint of unspecified finger
● S63.3 Traumatic rupture of ligament of wrist
● S63.30 Traumatic rupture of unspecified ligament of wrist
● S63.301 Traumatic rupture of unspecified ligament of right wrist
● S63.302 Traumatic rupture of unspecified ligament of left wrist
● S63.309 Traumatic rupture of unspecified ligament of unspecified wrist

● S63.31 Traumatic rupture of collateral ligament of wrist
- ● S63.311 Traumatic rupture of collateral ligament of right wrist
- ● S63.312 Traumatic rupture of collateral ligament of left wrist
- ● S63.319 Traumatic rupture of collateral ligament of unspecified wrist

● S63.32 Traumatic rupture of radiocarpal ligament
- ● S63.321 Traumatic rupture of right radiocarpal ligament
- ● S63.322 Traumatic rupture of left radiocarpal ligament
- ● S63.329 Traumatic rupture of unspecified radiocarpal ligament

● S63.33 Traumatic rupture of ulnocarpal (palmar) ligament
- ● S63.331 Traumatic rupture of right ulnocarpal (palmar) ligament
- ● S63.332 Traumatic rupture of left ulnocarpal (palmar) ligament
- ● S63.339 Traumatic rupture of unspecified ulnocarpal (palmar) ligament

● S63.39 Traumatic rupture of other ligament of wrist
- ● S63.391 Traumatic rupture of other ligament of right wrist
- ● S63.392 Traumatic rupture of other ligament of left wrist
- ● S63.399 Traumatic rupture of other ligament of unspecified wrist

● S63.4 Traumatic rupture of ligament of finger at metacarpophalangeal and interphalangeal joint(s)

● S63.40 Traumatic rupture of unspecified ligament of finger at metacarpophalangeal and interphalangeal joint
- ● S63.400 Traumatic rupture of unspecified ligament of right index finger at metacarpophalangeal and interphalangeal joint
- ● S63.401 Traumatic rupture of unspecified ligament of left index finger at metacarpophalangeal and interphalangeal joint
- ● S63.402 Traumatic rupture of unspecified ligament of right middle finger at metacarpophalangeal and interphalangeal joint
- ● S63.403 Traumatic rupture of unspecified ligament of left middle finger at metacarpophalangeal and interphalangeal joint
- ● S63.404 Traumatic rupture of unspecified ligament of right ring finger at metacarpophalangeal and interphalangeal joint
- ● S63.405 Traumatic rupture of unspecified ligament of left ring finger at metacarpophalangeal and interphalangeal joint
- ● S63.406 Traumatic rupture of unspecified ligament of right little finger at metacarpophalangeal and interphalangeal joint
- ● S63.407 Traumatic rupture of unspecified ligament of left little finger at metacarpophalangeal and interphalangeal joint
- ● S63.408 Traumatic rupture of unspecified ligament of other finger at metacarpophalangeal and interphalangeal joint
  - Traumatic rupture of unspecified ligament of specified finger with unspecified laterality at metacarpophalangeal and interphalangeal joint
- ● S63.409 Traumatic rupture of unspecified ligament of unspecified finger at metacarpophalangeal and interphalangeal joint

● S63.41 Traumatic rupture of collateral ligament of finger at metacarpophalangeal and interphalangeal joint
- ● S63.410 Traumatic rupture of collateral ligament of right index finger at metacarpophalangeal and interphalangeal joint
- ● S63.411 Traumatic rupture of collateral ligament of left index finger at metacarpophalangeal and interphalangeal joint
- ● S63.412 Traumatic rupture of collateral ligament of right middle finger at metacarpophalangeal and interphalangeal joint
- ● S63.413 Traumatic rupture of collateral ligament of left middle finger at metacarpophalangeal and interphalangeal joint
- ● S63.414 Traumatic rupture of collateral ligament of right ring finger at metacarpophalangeal and interphalangeal joint
- ● S63.415 Traumatic rupture of collateral ligament of left ring finger at metacarpophalangeal and interphalangeal joint
- ● S63.416 Traumatic rupture of collateral ligament of right little finger at metacarpophalangeal and interphalangeal joint
- ● S63.417 Traumatic rupture of collateral ligament of left little finger at metacarpophalangeal and interphalangeal joint
- ● S63.418 Traumatic rupture of collateral ligament of other finger at metacarpophalangeal and interphalangeal joint
  - Traumatic rupture of collateral ligament of specified finger with unspecified laterality at metacarpophalangeal and interphalangeal joint
- ● S63.419 Traumatic rupture of collateral ligament of unspecified finger at metacarpophalangeal and interphalangeal joint

● S63.42 Traumatic rupture of palmar ligament of finger at metacarpophalangeal and interphalangeal joint
- ● S63.420 Traumatic rupture of palmar ligament of right index finger at metacarpophalangeal and interphalangeal joint
- ● S63.421 Traumatic rupture of palmar ligament of left index finger at metacarpophalangeal and interphalangeal joint

● S63.422 **Traumatic rupture of palmar ligament of right middle finger at metacarpophalangeal and interphalangeal joint**

● S63.423 **Traumatic rupture of palmar ligament of left middle finger at metacarpophalangeal and interphalangeal joint**

● S63.424 **Traumatic rupture of palmar ligament of right ring finger at metacarpophalangeal and interphalangeal joint**

● S63.425 **Traumatic rupture of palmar ligament of left ring finger at metacarpophalangeal and interphalangeal joint**

● S63.426 **Traumatic rupture of palmar ligament of right little finger at metacarpophalangeal and interphalangeal joint**

● S63.427 **Traumatic rupture of palmar ligament of left little finger at metacarpophalangeal and interphalangeal joint**

● S63.428 **Traumatic rupture of palmar ligament of other finger at metacarpophalangeal and interphalangeal joint**
Traumatic rupture of palmar ligament of specified finger with unspecified laterality at metacarpophalangeal and interphalangeal joint

● S63.429 **Traumatic rupture of palmar ligament of unspecified finger at metacarpophalangeal and interphalangeal joint**

● S63.43 **Traumatic rupture of volar plate of finger at metacarpophalangeal and interphalangeal joint**

● S63.430 **Traumatic rupture of volar plate of right index finger at metacarpophalangeal and interphalangeal joint**

● S63.431 **Traumatic rupture of volar plate of left index finger at metacarpophalangeal and interphalangeal joint**

● S63.432 **Traumatic rupture of volar plate of right middle finger at metacarpophalangeal and interphalangeal joint**

● S63.433 **Traumatic rupture of volar plate of left middle finger at metacarpophalangeal and interphalangeal joint**

● S63.434 **Traumatic rupture of volar plate of right ring finger at metacarpophalangeal and interphalangeal joint**

● S63.435 **Traumatic rupture of volar plate of left ring finger at metacarpophalangeal and interphalangeal joint**

● S63.436 **Traumatic rupture of volar plate of right little finger at metacarpophalangeal and interphalangeal joint**

● S63.437 **Traumatic rupture of volar plate of left little finger at metacarpophalangeal and interphalangeal joint**

● S63.438 **Traumatic rupture of volar plate of other finger at metacarpophalangeal and interphalangeal joint**
Traumatic rupture of volar plate of specified finger with unspecified laterality at metacarpophalangeal and interphalangeal joint

● S63.439 **Traumatic rupture of volar plate of unspecified finger at metacarpophalangeal and interphalangeal joint**

● S63.49 **Traumatic rupture of other ligament of finger at metacarpophalangeal and interphalangeal joint**

● S63.490 **Traumatic rupture of other ligament of right index finger at metacarpophalangeal and interphalangeal joint**

● S63.491 **Traumatic rupture of other ligament of left index finger at metacarpophalangeal and interphalangeal joint**

● S63.492 **Traumatic rupture of other ligament of right middle finger at metacarpophalangeal and interphalangeal joint**

● S63.493 **Traumatic rupture of other ligament of left middle finger at metacarpophalangeal and interphalangeal joint**

● S63.494 **Traumatic rupture of other ligament of right ring finger at metacarpophalangeal and interphalangeal joint**

● S63.495 **Traumatic rupture of other ligament of left ring finger at metacarpophalangeal and interphalangeal joint**

● S63.496 **Traumatic rupture of other ligament of right little finger at metacarpophalangeal and interphalangeal joint**

● S63.497 **Traumatic rupture of other ligament of left little finger at metacarpophalangeal and interphalangeal joint**

● S63.498 **Traumatic rupture of other ligament of other finger at metacarpophalangeal and interphalangeal joint**
Traumatic rupture of ligament of specified finger with unspecified laterality at metacarpophalangeal and interphalangeal joint

● S63.499 **Traumatic rupture of other ligament of unspecified finger at metacarpophalangeal and interphalangeal joint**

● S63.5 **Other and unspecified sprain of wrist**

● S63.50 **Unspecified sprain of wrist**

● S63.501 **Unspecified sprain of right wrist**

● S63.502 **Unspecified sprain of left wrist**

● S63.509 **Unspecified sprain of unspecified wrist**

● S63.51 **Sprain of carpal (joint)**

● S63.511 **Sprain of carpal joint of right wrist**

● S63.512 **Sprain of carpal joint of left wrist**

● S63.519 **Sprain of carpal joint of unspecified wrist**

CHAPTER 19 (SØØ-T88)

● S63.52   Sprain of radiocarpal joint
> **Excludes1**   traumatic rupture of radiocarpal ligament (S63.32-)

    ● S63.521   Sprain of radiocarpal joint of right wrist
    ● S63.522   Sprain of radiocarpal joint of left wrist
    ● S63.529   Sprain of radiocarpal joint of unspecified wrist

● S63.59   Other specified sprain of wrist
    ● S63.591   Other specified sprain of right wrist
    ● S63.592   Other specified sprain of left wrist
    ● S63.599   Other specified sprain of unspecified wrist

● S63.6   Other and unspecified sprain of finger(s)
> **Excludes1**   traumatic rupture of ligament of finger at metacarpophalangeal and interphalangeal joint(s) (S63.4-)

 ● S63.60   Unspecified sprain of thumb
    ● S63.601   Unspecified sprain of right thumb
    ● S63.602   Unspecified sprain of left thumb
    ● S63.609   Unspecified sprain of unspecified thumb

 ● S63.61   Unspecified sprain of other and unspecified finger(s)
    ● S63.610   Unspecified sprain of right index finger
    ● S63.611   Unspecified sprain of left index finger
    ● S63.612   Unspecified sprain of right middle finger
    ● S63.613   Unspecified sprain of left middle finger
    ● S63.614   Unspecified sprain of right ring finger
    ● S63.615   Unspecified sprain of left ring finger
    ● S63.616   Unspecified sprain of right little finger
    ● S63.617   Unspecified sprain of left little finger
    ● S63.618   Unspecified sprain of other finger
> Unspecified sprain of specified finger with unspecified laterality

    ● S63.619   Unspecified sprain of unspecified finger

 ● S63.62   Sprain of interphalangeal joint of thumb
    ● S63.621   Sprain of interphalangeal joint of right thumb
    ● S63.622   Sprain of interphalangeal joint of left thumb
    ● S63.629   Sprain of interphalangeal joint of unspecified thumb

 ● S63.63   Sprain of interphalangeal joint of other and unspecified finger(s)
    ● S63.630   Sprain of interphalangeal joint of right index finger
    ● S63.631   Sprain of interphalangeal joint of left index finger
    ● S63.632   Sprain of interphalangeal joint of right middle finger
    ● S63.633   Sprain of interphalangeal joint of left middle finger
    ● S63.634   Sprain of interphalangeal joint of right ring finger
    ● S63.635   Sprain of interphalangeal joint of left ring finger
    ● S63.636   Sprain of interphalangeal joint of right little finger
    ● S63.637   Sprain of interphalangeal joint of left little finger

    ● S63.638   Sprain of interphalangeal joint of other finger
    ● S63.639   Sprain of interphalangeal joint of unspecified finger

 ● S63.64   Sprain of metacarpophalangeal joint of thumb
    ● S63.641   Sprain of metacarpophalangeal joint of right thumb
    ● S63.642   Sprain of metacarpophalangeal joint of left thumb
    ● S63.649   Sprain of metacarpophalangeal joint of unspecified thumb

 ● S63.65   Sprain of metacarpophalangeal joint of other and unspecified finger(s)
    ● S63.650   Sprain of metacarpophalangeal joint of right index finger
    ● S63.651   Sprain of metacarpophalangeal joint of left index finger
    ● S63.652   Sprain of metacarpophalangeal joint of right middle finger
    ● S63.653   Sprain of metacarpophalangeal joint of left middle finger
    ● S63.654   Sprain of metacarpophalangeal joint of right ring finger
    ● S63.655   Sprain of metacarpophalangeal joint of left ring finger
    ● S63.656   Sprain of metacarpophalangeal joint of right little finger
    ● S63.657   Sprain of metacarpophalangeal joint of left little finger
    ● S63.658   Sprain of metacarpophalangeal joint of other finger
> Sprain of metacarpophalangeal joint of specified finger with unspecified laterality

    ● S63.659   Sprain of metacarpophalangeal joint of unspecified finger

 ● S63.68   Other sprain of thumb
    ● S63.681   Other sprain of right thumb
    ● S63.682   Other sprain of left thumb
    ● S63.689   Other sprain of unspecified thumb

 ● S63.69   Other sprain of other and unspecified finger(s)
    ● S63.690   Other sprain of right index finger
    ● S63.691   Other sprain of left index finger
    ● S63.692   Other sprain of right middle finger
    ● S63.693   Other sprain of left middle finger
    ● S63.694   Other sprain of right ring finger
    ● S63.695   Other sprain of left ring finger
    ● S63.696   Other sprain of right little finger
    ● S63.697   Other sprain of left little finger
    ● S63.698   Other sprain of other finger
> Other sprain of specified finger with unspecified laterality

    ● S63.699   Other sprain of unspecified finger

● S63.8   Sprain of other part of wrist and hand
 ● S63.8X   Sprain of other part of wrist and hand
    ● S63.8X1   Sprain of other part of right wrist and hand
    ● S63.8X2   Sprain of other part of left wrist and hand
    ● S63.8X9   Sprain of other part of unspecified wrist and hand

● S63.9   Sprain of unspecified part of wrist and hand
 X ● S63.90   Sprain of unspecified part of unspecified wrist and hand
 X ● S63.91   Sprain of unspecified part of right wrist and hand
 X ● S63.92   Sprain of unspecified part of left wrist and hand

---

● **S64 Injury of nerves at wrist and hand level**

The appropriate 7th character is to be added to each code from category S64

A	initial encounter
D	subsequent encounter
S	sequela

Code also any associated open wound (S61.-)

● **S64.0 Injury of ulnar nerve at wrist and hand level**

X● **S64.00 Injury of ulnar nerve at wrist and hand level of unspecified arm**

X● **S64.01 Injury of ulnar nerve at wrist and hand level of right arm**

X● **S64.02 Injury of ulnar nerve at wrist and hand level of left arm**

● **S64.1 Injury of median nerve at wrist and hand level**

X● **S64.10 Injury of median nerve at wrist and hand level of unspecified arm**

X● **S64.11 Injury of median nerve at wrist and hand level of right arm**

X● **S64.12 Injury of median nerve at wrist and hand level of left arm**

● **S64.2 Injury of radial nerve at wrist and hand level**

X● **S64.20 Injury of radial nerve at wrist and hand level of unspecified arm**

X● **S64.21 Injury of radial nerve at wrist and hand level of right arm**

X● **S64.22 Injury of radial nerve at wrist and hand level of left arm**

● **S64.3 Injury of digital nerve of thumb**

X● **S64.30 Injury of digital nerve of unspecified thumb**

X● **S64.31 Injury of digital nerve of right thumb**

X● **S64.32 Injury of digital nerve of left thumb**

● **S64.4 Injury of digital nerve of other and unspecified finger**

X● **S64.40 Injury of digital nerve of unspecified finger**

● **S64.49 Injury of digital nerve of other finger**

● **S64.490 Injury of digital nerve of right index finger**

● **S64.491 Injury of digital nerve of left index finger**

● **S64.492 Injury of digital nerve of right middle finger**

● **S64.493 Injury of digital nerve of left middle finger**

● **S64.494 Injury of digital nerve of right ring finger**

● **S64.495 Injury of digital nerve of left ring finger**

● **S64.496 Injury of digital nerve of right little finger**

● **S64.497 Injury of digital nerve of left little finger**

● **S64.498 Injury of digital nerve of other finger**

Injury of digital nerve of specified finger with unspecified laterality

● **S64.8 Injury of other nerves at wrist and hand level**

● **S64.8X Injury of other nerves at wrist and hand level**

● **S64.8X1 Injury of other nerves at wrist and hand level of right arm**

● **S64.8X2 Injury of other nerves at wrist and hand level of left arm**

● **S64.8X9 Injury of other nerves at wrist and hand level of unspecified arm**

● **S64.9 Injury of unspecified nerve at wrist and hand level**

X● **S64.90 Injury of unspecified nerve at wrist and hand level of unspecified arm**

X● **S64.91 Injury of unspecified nerve at wrist and hand level of right arm**

X● **S64.92 Injury of unspecified nerve at wrist and hand level of left arm**

● **S65 Injury of blood vessels at wrist and hand level**

The appropriate 7th character is to be added to each code from category S65

A	initial encounter
D	subsequent encounter
S	sequela

Code also any associated open wound (S61.-)

● **S65.0 Injury of ulnar artery at wrist and hand level**

● **S65.00 Unspecified injury of ulnar artery at wrist and hand level**

● **S65.001 Unspecified injury of ulnar artery at wrist and hand level of right arm**

● **S65.002 Unspecified injury of ulnar artery at wrist and hand level of left arm**

● **S65.009 Unspecified injury of ulnar artery at wrist and hand level of unspecified arm**

● **S65.01 Laceration of ulnar artery at wrist and hand level**

● **S65.011 Laceration of ulnar artery at wrist and hand level of right arm**

● **S65.012 Laceration of ulnar artery at wrist and hand level of left arm**

● **S65.019 Laceration of ulnar artery at wrist and hand level of unspecified arm**

● **S65.09 Other specified injury of ulnar artery at wrist and hand level**

● **S65.091 Other specified injury of ulnar artery at wrist and hand level of right arm**

● **S65.092 Other specified injury of ulnar artery at wrist and hand level of left arm**

● **S65.099 Other specified injury of ulnar artery at wrist and hand level of unspecified arm**

● **S65.1 Injury of radial artery at wrist and hand level**

● **S65.10 Unspecified injury of radial artery at wrist and hand level**

● **S65.101 Unspecified injury of radial artery at wrist and hand level of right arm**

● **S65.102 Unspecified injury of radial artery at wrist and hand level of left arm**

● **S65.109 Unspecified injury of radial artery at wrist and hand level of unspecified arm**

● **S65.11 Laceration of radial artery at wrist and hand level**

● **S65.111 Laceration of radial artery at wrist and hand level of right arm**

● **S65.112 Laceration of radial artery at wrist and hand level of left arm**

● **S65.119 Laceration of radial artery at wrist and hand level of unspecified arm**

● **S65.19 Other specified injury of radial artery at wrist and hand level**

● **S65.191 Other specified injury of radial artery at wrist and hand level of right arm**

● **S65.192 Other specified injury of radial artery at wrist and hand level of left arm**

● **S65.199 Other specified injury of radial artery at wrist and hand level of unspecified arm**

CHAPTER 19 (SØØ-T88)

- S65.2 Injury of superficial palmar arch
  - S65.20 Unspecified injury of superficial palmar arch
    - S65.201 Unspecified injury of superficial palmar arch of right hand
    - S65.202 Unspecified injury of superficial palmar arch of left hand
    - S65.209 Unspecified injury of superficial palmar arch of unspecified hand
  - S65.21 Laceration of superficial palmar arch
    - S65.211 Laceration of superficial palmar arch of right hand
    - S65.212 Laceration of superficial palmar arch of left hand
    - S65.219 Laceration of superficial palmar arch of unspecified hand
  - S65.29 Other specified injury of superficial palmar arch
    - S65.291 Other specified injury of superficial palmar arch of right hand
    - S65.292 Other specified injury of superficial palmar arch of left hand
    - S65.299 Other specified injury of superficial palmar arch of unspecified hand
- S65.3 Injury of deep palmar arch
  - S65.30 Unspecified injury of deep palmar arch
    - S65.301 Unspecified injury of deep palmar arch of right hand
    - S65.302 Unspecified injury of deep palmar arch of left hand
    - S65.309 Unspecified injury of deep palmar arch of unspecified hand
  - S65.31 Laceration of deep palmar arch
    - S65.311 Laceration of deep palmar arch of right hand
    - S65.312 Laceration of deep palmar arch of left hand
    - S65.319 Laceration of deep palmar arch of unspecified hand
  - S65.39 Other specified injury of deep palmar arch
    - S65.391 Other specified injury of deep palmar arch of right hand
    - S65.392 Other specified injury of deep palmar arch of left hand
    - S65.399 Other specified injury of deep palmar arch of unspecified hand
- S65.4 Injury of blood vessel of thumb
  - S65.40 Unspecified injury of blood vessel of thumb
    - S65.401 Unspecified injury of blood vessel of right thumb
    - S65.402 Unspecified injury of blood vessel of left thumb
    - S65.409 Unspecified injury of blood vessel of unspecified thumb
  - S65.41 Laceration of blood vessel of thumb
    - S65.411 Laceration of blood vessel of right thumb
    - S65.412 Laceration of blood vessel of left thumb
    - S65.419 Laceration of blood vessel of unspecified thumb
  - S65.49 Other specified injury of blood vessel of thumb
    - S65.491 Other specified injury of blood vessel of right thumb
    - S65.492 Other specified injury of blood vessel of left thumb
    - S65.499 Other specified injury of blood vessel of unspecified thumb
- S65.5 Injury of blood vessel of other and unspecified finger
  - S65.50 Unspecified injury of blood vessel of other and unspecified finger
    - S65.500 Unspecified injury of blood vessel of right index finger
    - S65.501 Unspecified injury of blood vessel of left index finger
    - S65.502 Unspecified injury of blood vessel of right middle finger
    - S65.503 Unspecified injury of blood vessel of left middle finger
    - S65.504 Unspecified injury of blood vessel of right ring finger
    - S65.505 Unspecified injury of blood vessel of left ring finger
    - S65.506 Unspecified injury of blood vessel of right little finger
    - S65.507 Unspecified injury of blood vessel of left little finger
    - S65.508 Unspecified injury of blood vessel of other finger
      Unspecified injury of blood vessel of specified finger with unspecified laterality
    - S65.509 Unspecified injury of blood vessel of unspecified finger
  - S65.51 Laceration of blood vessel of other and unspecified finger
    - S65.510 Laceration of blood vessel of right index finger
    - S65.511 Laceration of blood vessel of left index finger
    - S65.512 Laceration of blood vessel of right middle finger
    - S65.513 Laceration of blood vessel of left middle finger
    - S65.514 Laceration of blood vessel of right ring finger
    - S65.515 Laceration of blood vessel of left ring finger
    - S65.516 Laceration of blood vessel of right little finger
    - S65.517 Laceration of blood vessel of left little finger
    - S65.518 Laceration of blood vessel of other finger
      Laceration of blood vessel of specified finger with unspecified laterality
    - S65.519 Laceration of blood vessel of unspecified finger
  - S65.59 Other specified injury of blood vessel of other and unspecified finger
    - S65.590 Other specified injury of blood vessel of right index finger
    - S65.591 Other specified injury of blood vessel of left index finger
    - S65.592 Other specified injury of blood vessel of right middle finger
    - S65.593 Other specified injury of blood vessel of left middle finger
    - S65.594 Other specified injury of blood vessel of right ring finger
    - S65.595 Other specified injury of blood vessel of left ring finger

● S65.596 **Other specified injury of blood vessel of right little finger**

● S65.597 **Other specified injury of blood vessel of left little finger**

● S65.598 **Other specified injury of blood vessel of other finger**
Other specified injury of blood vessel of specified finger with unspecified laterality

● S65.599 **Other specified injury of blood vessel of unspecified finger**

● S65.8 **Injury of other blood vessels at wrist and hand level**

● S65.80 **Unspecified injury of other blood vessels at wrist and hand level**

● S65.801 **Unspecified injury of other blood vessels at wrist and hand level of right arm**

● S65.802 **Unspecified injury of other blood vessels at wrist and hand level of left arm**

● S65.809 **Unspecified injury of other blood vessels at wrist and hand level of unspecified arm**

● S65.81 **Laceration of other blood vessels at wrist and hand level**

● S65.811 **Laceration of other blood vessels at wrist and hand level of right arm**

● S65.812 **Laceration of other blood vessels at wrist and hand level of left arm**

● S65.819 **Laceration of other blood vessels at wrist and hand level of unspecified arm**

● S65.89 **Other specified injury of other blood vessels at wrist and hand level**

● S65.891 **Other specified injury of other blood vessels at wrist and hand level of right arm**

● S65.892 **Other specified injury of other blood vessels at wrist and hand level of left arm**

● S65.899 **Other specified injury of other blood vessels at wrist and hand level of unspecified arm**

● S65.9 **Injury of unspecified blood vessel at wrist and hand level**

● S65.90 **Unspecified injury of unspecified blood vessel at wrist and hand level**

● S65.901 **Unspecified injury of unspecified blood vessel at wrist and hand level of right arm**

● S65.902 **Unspecified injury of unspecified blood vessel at wrist and hand level of left arm**

● S65.909 **Unspecified injury of unspecified blood vessel at wrist and hand level of unspecified arm**

● S65.91 **Laceration of unspecified blood vessel at wrist and hand level**

● S65.911 **Laceration of unspecified blood vessel at wrist and hand level of right arm**

● S65.912 **Laceration of unspecified blood vessel at wrist and hand level of left arm**

● S65.919 **Laceration of unspecified blood vessel at wrist and hand level of unspecified arm**

● S65.99 **Other specified injury of unspecified blood vessel at wrist and hand level**

● S65.991 **Other specified injury of unspecified blood vessel at wrist and hand of right arm**

● S65.992 **Other specified injury of unspecified blood vessel at wrist and hand of left arm**

● S65.999 **Other specified injury of unspecified blood vessel at wrist and hand of unspecified arm**

● S66 **Injury of muscle, fascia and tendon at wrist and hand level**

Code also any associated open wound (S61.-)

Excludes2 sprain of joints and ligaments of wrist and hand (S63.-)

The appropriate 7th character is to be added to each code from category S66

A	initial encounter
D	subsequent encounter
S	sequela

● S66.0 **Injury of long flexor muscle, fascia and tendon of thumb at wrist and hand level**

● S66.00 **Unspecified injury of long flexor muscle, fascia and tendon of thumb at wrist and hand level**

● S66.001 **Unspecified injury of long flexor muscle, fascia and tendon of right thumb at wrist and hand level**

● S66.002 **Unspecified injury of long flexor muscle, fascia and tendon of left thumb at wrist and hand level**

● S66.009 **Unspecified injury of long flexor muscle, fascia and tendon of unspecified thumb at wrist and hand level**

● S66.01 **Strain of long flexor muscle, fascia and tendon of thumb at wrist and hand level**

● S66.011 **Strain of long flexor muscle, fascia and tendon of right thumb at wrist and hand level**

● S66.012 **Strain of long flexor muscle, fascia and tendon of left thumb at wrist and hand level**

● S66.019 **Strain of long flexor muscle, fascia and tendon of unspecified thumb at wrist and hand level**

● S66.02 **Laceration of long flexor muscle, fascia and tendon of thumb at wrist and hand level**

● S66.021 **Laceration of long flexor muscle, fascia and tendon of right thumb at wrist and hand level**

● S66.022 **Laceration of long flexor muscle, fascia and tendon of left thumb at wrist and hand level**

● S66.029 **Laceration of long flexor muscle, fascia and tendon of unspecified thumb at wrist and hand level**

● S66.09 **Other specified injury of long flexor muscle, fascia and tendon of thumb at wrist and hand level**

● S66.091 **Other specified injury of long flexor muscle, fascia and tendon of right thumb at wrist and hand level**

● S66.092 **Other specified injury of long flexor muscle, fascia and tendon of left thumb at wrist and hand level**

● S66.099 **Other specified injury of long flexor muscle, fascia and tendon of unspecified thumb at wrist and hand level**

CHAPTER 19 (S00-T88)

● S66.1 **Injury of flexor muscle, fascia and tendon of other and unspecified finger at wrist and hand level**

Excludes2 injury of long flexor muscle, fascia and tendon of thumb at wrist and hand level (S66.0-)

● S66.10 **Unspecified injury of flexor muscle, fascia and tendon of other and unspecified finger at wrist and hand level**

● S66.100 **Unspecified injury of flexor muscle, fascia and tendon of right index finger at wrist and hand level**

● S66.101 **Unspecified injury of flexor muscle, fascia and tendon of left index finger at wrist and hand level**

● S66.102 **Unspecified injury of flexor muscle, fascia and tendon of right middle finger at wrist and hand level**

● S66.103 **Unspecified injury of flexor muscle, fascia and tendon of left middle finger at wrist and hand level**

● S66.104 **Unspecified injury of flexor muscle, fascia and tendon of right ring finger at wrist and hand level**

● S66.105 **Unspecified injury of flexor muscle, fascia and tendon of left ring finger at wrist and hand level**

● S66.106 **Unspecified injury of flexor muscle, fascia and tendon of right little finger at wrist and hand level**

● S66.107 **Unspecified injury of flexor muscle, fascia and tendon of left little finger at wrist and hand level**

● S66.108 **Unspecified injury of flexor muscle, fascia and tendon of other finger at wrist and hand level**

Unspecified injury of flexor muscle, fascia and tendon of specified finger with unspecified laterality at wrist and hand level

● S66.109 **Unspecified injury of flexor muscle, fascia and tendon of unspecified finger at wrist and hand level**

● S66.11 **Strain of flexor muscle, fascia and tendon of other and unspecified finger at wrist and hand level**

● S66.110 **Strain of flexor muscle, fascia and tendon of right index finger at wrist and hand level**

● S66.111 **Strain of flexor muscle, fascia and tendon of left index finger at wrist and hand level**

● S66.112 **Strain of flexor muscle, fascia and tendon of right middle finger at wrist and hand level**

● S66.113 **Strain of flexor muscle, fascia and tendon of left middle finger at wrist and hand level**

● S66.114 **Strain of flexor muscle, fascia and tendon of right ring finger at wrist and hand level**

● S66.115 **Strain of flexor muscle, fascia and tendon of left ring finger at wrist and hand level**

● S66.116 **Strain of flexor muscle, fascia and tendon of right little finger at wrist and hand level**

● S66.117 **Strain of flexor muscle, fascia and tendon of left little finger at wrist and hand level**

● S66.118 **Strain of flexor muscle, fascia and tendon of other finger at wrist and hand level**

Strain of flexor muscle, fascia and tendon of specified finger with unspecified laterality at wrist and hand level

● S66.119 **Strain of flexor muscle, fascia and tendon of unspecified finger at wrist and hand level**

● S66.12 **Laceration of flexor muscle, fascia and tendon of other and unspecified finger at wrist and hand level**

● S66.120 **Laceration of flexor muscle, fascia and tendon of right index finger at wrist and hand level**

● S66.121 **Laceration of flexor muscle, fascia and tendon of left index finger at wrist and hand level**

● S66.122 **Laceration of flexor muscle, fascia and tendon of right middle finger at wrist and hand level**

● S66.123 **Laceration of flexor muscle, fascia and tendon of left middle finger at wrist and hand level**

● S66.124 **Laceration of flexor muscle, fascia and tendon of right ring finger at wrist and hand level**

● S66.125 **Laceration of flexor muscle, fascia and tendon of left ring finger at wrist and hand level**

● S66.126 **Laceration of flexor muscle, fascia and tendon of right little finger at wrist and hand level**

● S66.127 **Laceration of flexor muscle, fascia and tendon of left little finger at wrist and hand level**

● S66.128 **Laceration of flexor muscle, fascia and tendon of other finger at wrist and hand level**

Laceration of flexor muscle, fascia and tendon of specified finger with unspecified laterality at wrist and hand level

● S66.129 **Laceration of flexor muscle, fascia and tendon of unspecified finger at wrist and hand level**

● S66.19 **Other injury of flexor muscle, fascia and tendon of other and unspecified finger at wrist and hand level**

● S66.190 **Other injury of flexor muscle, fascia and tendon of right index finger at wrist and hand level**

● S66.191 **Other injury of flexor muscle, fascia and tendon of left index finger at wrist and hand level**

● S66.192 **Other injury of flexor muscle, fascia and tendon of right middle finger at wrist and hand level**

● S66.193 **Other injury of flexor muscle, fascia and tendon of left middle finger at wrist and hand level**

● S66.194 **Other injury of flexor muscle, fascia and tendon of right ring finger at wrist and hand level**

● S66.195 **Other injury of flexor muscle, fascia and tendon of left ring finger at wrist and hand level**

● S66.196 **Other injury of flexor muscle, fascia and tendon of right little finger at wrist and hand level**

● S66.197 **Other injury of flexor muscle, fascia and tendon of left little finger at wrist and hand level**

● S66.198 Other injury of flexor muscle, fascia and tendon of other finger at wrist and hand level
Other injury of flexor muscle, fascia and tendon of specified finger with unspecified laterality at wrist and hand level

● S66.199 Other injury of flexor muscle, fascia and tendon of unspecified finger at wrist and hand level

● S66.2 Injury of extensor muscle, fascia and tendon of thumb at wrist and hand level

● S66.20 Unspecified injury of extensor muscle, fascia and tendon of thumb at wrist and hand level

● S66.201 Unspecified injury of extensor muscle, fascia and tendon of right thumb at wrist and hand level

● S66.202 Unspecified injury of extensor muscle, fascia and tendon of left thumb at wrist and hand level

● S66.209 Unspecified injury of extensor muscle, fascia and tendon of unspecified thumb at wrist and hand level

● S66.21 Strain of extensor muscle, fascia and tendon of thumb at wrist and hand level

● S66.211 Strain of extensor muscle, fascia and tendon of right thumb at wrist and hand level

● S66.212 Strain of extensor muscle, fascia and tendon of left thumb at wrist and hand level

● S66.219 Strain of extensor muscle, fascia and tendon of unspecified thumb at wrist and hand level

● S66.22 Laceration of extensor muscle, fascia and tendon of thumb at wrist and hand level

● S66.221 Laceration of extensor muscle, fascia and tendon of right thumb at wrist and hand level

● S66.222 Laceration of extensor muscle, fascia and tendon of left thumb at wrist and hand level

● S66.229 Laceration of extensor muscle, fascia and tendon of unspecified thumb at wrist and hand level

● S66.29 Other specified injury of extensor muscle, fascia and tendon of thumb at wrist and hand level

● S66.291 Other specified injury of extensor muscle, fascia and tendon of right thumb at wrist and hand level

● S66.292 Other specified injury of extensor muscle, fascia and tendon of left thumb at wrist and hand level

● S66.299 Other specified injury of extensor muscle, fascia and tendon of unspecified thumb at wrist and hand level

● S66.3 Injury of extensor muscle, fascia and tendon of other and unspecified finger at wrist and hand level

Excludes2 injury of extensor muscle, fascia and tendon of thumb at wrist and hand level (S66.2-)

● S66.30 Unspecified injury of extensor muscle, fascia and tendon of other and unspecified finger at wrist and hand level

● S66.300 Unspecified injury of extensor muscle, fascia and tendon of right index finger at wrist and hand level

● S66.301 Unspecified injury of extensor muscle, fascia and tendon of left index finger at wrist and hand level

● S66.302 Unspecified injury of extensor muscle, fascia and tendon of right middle finger at wrist and hand level

● S66.303 Unspecified injury of extensor muscle, fascia and tendon of left middle finger at wrist and hand level

● S66.304 Unspecified injury of extensor muscle, fascia and tendon of right ring finger at wrist and hand level

● S66.305 Unspecified injury of extensor muscle, fascia and tendon of left ring finger at wrist and hand level

● S66.306 Unspecified injury of extensor muscle, fascia and tendon of right little finger at wrist and hand level

● S66.307 Unspecified injury of extensor muscle, fascia and tendon of left little finger at wrist and hand level

● S66.308 Unspecified injury of extensor muscle, fascia and tendon of other finger at wrist and hand level
Unspecified injury of extensor muscle, fascia and tendon of specified finger with unspecified laterality at wrist and hand level

● S66.309 Unspecified injury of extensor muscle, fascia and tendon of unspecified finger at wrist and hand level

● S66.31 Strain of extensor muscle, fascia and tendon of other and unspecified finger at wrist and hand level

● S66.310 Strain of extensor muscle, fascia and tendon of right index finger at wrist and hand level

● S66.311 Strain of extensor muscle, fascia and tendon of left index finger at wrist and hand level

● S66.312 Strain of extensor muscle, fascia and tendon of right middle finger at wrist and hand level

● S66.313 Strain of extensor muscle, fascia and tendon of left middle finger at wrist and hand level

● S66.314 Strain of extensor muscle, fascia and tendon of right ring finger at wrist and hand level

● S66.315 Strain of extensor muscle, fascia and tendon of left ring finger at wrist and hand level

● S66.316 Strain of extensor muscle, fascia and tendon of right little finger at wrist and hand level

● S66.317 Strain of extensor muscle, fascia and tendon of left little finger at wrist and hand level

● S66.318 Strain of extensor muscle, fascia and tendon of other finger at wrist and hand level
Strain of extensor muscle, fascia and tendon of specified finger with unspecified laterality at wrist and hand level

● S66.319 Strain of extensor muscle, fascia and tendon of unspecified finger at wrist and hand level

CHAPTER 19 (S00-T88)

● S66.32 **Laceration of extensor muscle, fascia and tendon of other and unspecified finger at wrist and hand level**

● S66.320 **Laceration of extensor muscle, fascia and tendon of right index finger at wrist and hand level**

● S66.321 **Laceration of extensor muscle, fascia and tendon of left index finger at wrist and hand level**

● S66.322 **Laceration of extensor muscle, fascia and tendon of right middle finger at wrist and hand level**

● S66.323 **Laceration of extensor muscle, fascia and tendon of left middle finger at wrist and hand level**

● S66.324 **Laceration of extensor muscle, fascia and tendon of right ring finger at wrist and hand level**

● S66.325 **Laceration of extensor muscle, fascia and tendon of left ring finger at wrist and hand level**

● S66.326 **Laceration of extensor muscle, fascia and tendon of right little finger at wrist and hand level**

● S66.327 **Laceration of extensor muscle, fascia and tendon of left little finger at wrist and hand level**

● S66.328 **Laceration of extensor muscle, fascia and tendon of other finger at wrist and hand level**

Laceration of extensor muscle, fascia and tendon of specified finger with unspecified laterality at wrist and hand level

● S66.329 **Laceration of extensor muscle, fascia and tendon of unspecified finger at wrist and hand level**

● S66.39 **Other injury of extensor muscle, fascia and tendon of other and unspecified finger at wrist and hand level**

● S66.390 **Other injury of extensor muscle, fascia and tendon of right index finger at wrist and hand level**

● S66.391 **Other injury of extensor muscle, fascia and tendon of left index finger at wrist and hand level**

● S66.392 **Other injury of extensor muscle, fascia and tendon of right middle finger at wrist and hand level**

● S66.393 **Other injury of extensor muscle, fascia and tendon of left middle finger at wrist and hand level**

● S66.394 **Other injury of extensor muscle, fascia and tendon of right ring finger at wrist and hand level**

● S66.395 **Other injury of extensor muscle, fascia and tendon of left ring finger at wrist and hand level**

● S66.396 **Other injury of extensor muscle, fascia and tendon of right little finger at wrist and hand level**

● S66.397 **Other injury of extensor muscle, fascia and tendon of left little finger at wrist and hand level**

● S66.398 **Other injury of extensor muscle, fascia and tendon of other finger at wrist and hand level**

Other injury of extensor muscle, fascia and tendon of specified finger with unspecified laterality at wrist and hand level

● S66.399 **Other injury of extensor muscle, fascia and tendon of unspecified finger at wrist and hand level**

● S66.4 **Injury of intrinsic muscle, fascia and tendon of thumb at wrist and hand level**

● S66.40 **Unspecified injury of intrinsic muscle, fascia and tendon of thumb at wrist and hand level**

● S66.401 **Unspecified injury of intrinsic muscle, fascia and tendon of right thumb at wrist and hand level**

● S66.402 **Unspecified injury of intrinsic muscle, fascia and tendon of left thumb at wrist and hand level**

● S66.409 **Unspecified injury of intrinsic muscle, fascia and tendon of unspecified thumb at wrist and hand level**

● S66.41 **Strain of intrinsic muscle, fascia and tendon of thumb at wrist and hand level**

● S66.411 **Strain of intrinsic muscle, fascia and tendon of right thumb at wrist and hand level**

● S66.412 **Strain of intrinsic muscle, fascia and tendon of left thumb at wrist and hand level**

● S66.419 **Strain of intrinsic muscle, fascia and tendon of unspecified thumb at wrist and hand level**

● S66.42 **Laceration of intrinsic muscle, fascia and tendon of thumb at wrist and hand level**

● S66.421 **Laceration of intrinsic muscle, fascia and tendon of right thumb at wrist and hand level**

● S66.422 **Laceration of intrinsic muscle, fascia and tendon of left thumb at wrist and hand level**

● S66.429 **Laceration of intrinsic muscle, fascia and tendon of unspecified thumb at wrist and hand level**

● S66.49 **Other specified injury of intrinsic muscle, fascia and tendon of thumb at wrist and hand level**

● S66.491 **Other specified injury of intrinsic muscle, fascia and tendon of right thumb at wrist and hand level**

● S66.492 **Other specified injury of intrinsic muscle, fascia and tendon of left thumb at wrist and hand level**

● S66.499 **Other specified injury of intrinsic muscle, fascia and tendon of unspecified thumb at wrist and hand level**

● S66.5 **Injury of intrinsic muscle, fascia and tendon of other and unspecified finger at wrist and hand level**

Excludes2 injury of intrinsic muscle, fascia and tendon of thumb at wrist and hand level (S66.4-)

● S66.50 **Unspecified injury of intrinsic muscle, fascia and tendon of other and unspecified finger at wrist and hand level**

● S66.500 **Unspecified injury of intrinsic muscle, fascia and tendon of right index finger at wrist and hand level**

● S66.501 **Unspecified injury of intrinsic muscle, fascia and tendon of left index finger at wrist and hand level**

● S66.502 **Unspecified injury of intrinsic muscle, fascia and tendon of right middle finger at wrist and hand level**

● S66.503 **Unspecified injury of intrinsic muscle, fascia and tendon of left middle finger at wrist and hand level**

● S66.504 **Unspecified injury of intrinsic muscle, fascia and tendon of right ring finger at wrist and hand level**

● S66.505 Unspecified injury of intrinsic muscle, fascia and tendon of left ring finger at wrist and hand level

● S66.506 Unspecified injury of intrinsic muscle, fascia and tendon of right little finger at wrist and hand level

● S66.507 Unspecified injury of intrinsic muscle, fascia and tendon of left little finger at wrist and hand level

● S66.508 Unspecified injury of intrinsic muscle, fascia and tendon of other finger at wrist and hand level

Unspecified injury of intrinsic muscle, fascia and tendon of specified finger with unspecified laterality at wrist and hand level

● S66.509 Unspecified injury of intrinsic muscle, fascia and tendon of unspecified finger at wrist and hand level

● S66.51 Strain of intrinsic muscle, fascia and tendon of other and unspecified finger at wrist and hand level

● S66.510 Strain of intrinsic muscle, fascia and tendon of right index finger at wrist and hand level

● S66.511 Strain of intrinsic muscle, fascia and tendon of left index finger at wrist and hand level

● S66.512 Strain of intrinsic muscle, fascia and tendon of right middle finger at wrist and hand level

● S66.513 Strain of intrinsic muscle, fascia and tendon of left middle finger at wrist and hand level

● S66.514 Strain of intrinsic muscle, fascia and tendon of right ring finger at wrist and hand level

● S66.515 Strain of intrinsic muscle, fascia and tendon of left ring finger at wrist and hand level

● S66.516 Strain of intrinsic muscle, fascia and tendon of right little finger at wrist and hand level

● S66.517 Strain of intrinsic muscle, fascia and tendon of left little finger at wrist and hand level

● S66.518 Strain of intrinsic muscle, fascia and tendon of other finger at wrist and hand level

Strain of intrinsic muscle, fascia and tendon of specified finger with unspecified laterality at wrist and hand level

● S66.519 Strain of intrinsic muscle, fascia and tendon of unspecified finger at wrist and hand level

● S66.52 Laceration of intrinsic muscle, fascia and tendon of other and unspecified finger at wrist and hand level

● S66.520 Laceration of intrinsic muscle, fascia and tendon of right index finger at wrist and hand level

● S66.521 Laceration of intrinsic muscle, fascia and tendon of left index finger at wrist and hand level

● S66.522 Laceration of intrinsic muscle, fascia and tendon of right middle finger at wrist and hand level

● S66.523 Laceration of intrinsic muscle, fascia and tendon of left middle finger at wrist and hand level

● S66.524 Laceration of intrinsic muscle, fascia and tendon of right ring finger at wrist and hand level

● S66.525 Laceration of intrinsic muscle, fascia and tendon of left ring finger at wrist and hand level

● S66.526 Laceration of intrinsic muscle, fascia and tendon of right little finger at wrist and hand level

● S66.527 Laceration of intrinsic muscle, fascia and tendon of left little finger at wrist and hand level

● S66.528 Laceration of intrinsic muscle, fascia and tendon of other finger at wrist and hand level

Laceration of intrinsic muscle, fascia and tendon of specified finger with unspecified laterality at wrist and hand level

● S66.529 Laceration of intrinsic muscle, fascia and tendon of unspecified finger at wrist and hand level

● S66.59 Other injury of intrinsic muscle, fascia and tendon of other and unspecified finger at wrist and hand level

● S66.590 Other injury of intrinsic muscle, fascia and tendon of right index finger at wrist and hand level

● S66.591 Other injury of intrinsic muscle, fascia and tendon of left index finger at wrist and hand level

● S66.592 Other injury of intrinsic muscle, fascia and tendon of right middle finger at wrist and hand level

● S66.593 Other injury of intrinsic muscle, fascia and tendon of left middle finger at wrist and hand level

● S66.594 Other injury of intrinsic muscle, fascia and tendon of right ring finger at wrist and hand level

● S66.595 Other injury of intrinsic muscle, fascia and tendon of left ring finger at wrist and hand level

● S66.596 Other injury of intrinsic muscle, fascia and tendon of right little finger at wrist and hand level

● S66.597 Other injury of intrinsic muscle, fascia and tendon of left little finger at wrist and hand level

● S66.598 Other injury of intrinsic muscle, fascia and tendon of other finger at wrist and hand level

Other injury of intrinsic muscle, fascia and tendon of specified finger with unspecified laterality at wrist and hand level

● S66.599 Other injury of intrinsic muscle, fascia and tendon of unspecified finger at wrist and hand level

CHAPTER 19 (S00-T88)

● S66.8 Injury of other specified muscles, fascia and tendons at wrist and hand level

● S66.80 Unspecified injury of other specified muscles, fascia and tendons at wrist and hand level

● S66.801 Unspecified injury of other specified muscles, fascia and tendons at wrist and hand level, right hand

● S66.802 Unspecified injury of other specified muscles, fascia and tendons at wrist and hand level, left hand

● S66.809 Unspecified injury of other specified muscles, fascia and tendons at wrist and hand level, unspecified hand

● S66.81 Strain of other specified muscles, fascia and tendons at wrist and hand level

● S66.811 Strain of other specified muscles, fascia and tendons at wrist and hand level, right hand

● S66.812 Strain of other specified muscles, fascia and tendons at wrist and hand level, left hand

● S66.819 Strain of other specified muscles, fascia and tendons at wrist and hand level, unspecified hand

● S66.82 Laceration of other specified muscles, fascia and tendons at wrist and hand level

● S66.821 Laceration of other specified muscles, fascia and tendons at wrist and hand level, right hand

● S66.822 Laceration of other specified muscles, fascia and tendons at wrist and hand level, left hand

● S66.829 Laceration of other specified muscles, fascia and tendons at wrist and hand level, unspecified hand

● S66.89 Other injury of other specified muscles, fascia and tendons at wrist and hand level

● S66.891 Other injury of other specified muscles, fascia and tendons at wrist and hand level, right hand

● S66.892 Other injury of other specified muscles, fascia and tendons at wrist and hand level, left hand

● S66.899 Other injury of other specified muscles, fascia and tendons at wrist and hand level, unspecified hand

● S66.9 Injury of unspecified muscle, fascia and tendon at wrist and hand level

● S66.90 Unspecified injury of unspecified muscle, fascia and tendon at wrist and hand level

● S66.901 Unspecified injury of unspecified muscle, fascia and tendon at wrist and hand level, right hand

● S66.902 Unspecified injury of unspecified muscle, fascia and tendon at wrist and hand level, left hand

● S66.909 Unspecified injury of unspecified muscle, fascia and tendon at wrist and hand level, unspecified hand

● S66.91 Strain of unspecified muscle, fascia and tendon at wrist and hand level

● S66.911 Strain of unspecified muscle, fascia and tendon at wrist and hand level, right hand

● S66.912 Strain of unspecified muscle, fascia and tendon at wrist and hand level, left hand

● S66.919 Strain of unspecified muscle, fascia and tendon at wrist and hand level, unspecified hand

● S66.92 Laceration of unspecified muscle, fascia and tendon at wrist and hand level

● S66.921 Laceration of unspecified muscle, fascia and tendon at wrist and hand level, right hand

● S66.922 Laceration of unspecified muscle, fascia and tendon at wrist and hand level, left hand

● S66.929 Laceration of unspecified muscle, fascia and tendon at wrist and hand level, unspecified hand

● S66.99 Other injury of unspecified muscle, fascia and tendon at wrist and hand level

● S66.991 Other injury of unspecified muscle, fascia and tendon at wrist and hand level, right hand

● S66.992 Other injury of unspecified muscle, fascia and tendon at wrist and hand level, left hand

● S66.999 Other injury of unspecified muscle, fascia and tendon at wrist and hand level, unspecified hand

● S67 Crushing injury of wrist, hand and fingers

Use additional code for all associated injuries, such as:
fracture of wrist and hand (S62.-)
open wound of wrist and hand (S61.-)

The appropriate 7th character is to be added to each code from category S67

A	initial encounter
D	subsequent encounter
S	sequela

● S67.Ø Crushing injury of thumb

X● S67.ØØ Crushing injury of unspecified thumb

X● S67.Ø1 Crushing injury of right thumb

X● S67.Ø2 Crushing injury of left thumb

● S67.1 Crushing injury of other and unspecified finger(s)

Excludes2 crushing injury of thumb (S67.Ø-)

X● S67.1Ø Crushing injury of unspecified finger(s)

● S67.19 Crushing injury of other finger(s)

● S67.19Ø Crushing injury of right index finger

● S67.191 Crushing injury of left index finger

● S67.192 Crushing injury of right middle finger

● S67.193 Crushing injury of left middle finger

● S67.194 Crushing injury of right ring finger

● S67.195 Crushing injury of left ring finger

● S67.196 Crushing injury of right little finger

● S67.197 Crushing injury of left little finger

● S67.198 Crushing injury of other finger
Crushing injury of specified finger with unspecified laterality

● S67.2 Crushing injury of hand

Excludes2 crushing injury of fingers (S67.1-)
crushing injury of thumb (S67.Ø-)

X● S67.2Ø Crushing injury of unspecified hand

X● S67.21 Crushing injury of right hand

X● S67.22 Crushing injury of left hand

● S67.3 Crushing injury of wrist

X● S67.3Ø Crushing injury of unspecified wrist

X● S67.31 Crushing injury of right wrist

X● S67.32 Crushing injury of left wrist

● S67.4 Crushing injury of wrist and hand
Excludes1 crushing injury of hand alone (S67.2-)
crushing injury of wrist alone (S67.3-)
Excludes2 crushing injury of fingers (S67.1-)
crushing injury of thumb (S67.Ø-)
X● S67.4Ø Crushing injury of unspecified wrist and hand
X● S67.41 Crushing injury of right wrist and hand
X● S67.42 Crushing injury of left wrist and hand
● S67.9 Crushing injury of unspecified part(s) of wrist, hand and fingers
X● S67.9Ø Crushing injury of unspecified part(s) of unspecified wrist, hand and fingers
X● S67.91 Crushing injury of unspecified part(s) of right wrist, hand and fingers
X● S67.92 Crushing injury of unspecified part(s) of left wrist, hand and fingers

● S68 Traumatic amputation of wrist, hand and fingers
An amputation not identified as partial or complete should be coded to complete
The appropriate 7th character is to be added to each code from category S68

A	initial encounter
D	subsequent encounter
S	sequela

● S68.Ø Traumatic metacarpophalangeal amputation of thumb
Traumatic amputation of thumb NOS
● S68.Ø1 Complete traumatic metacarpophalangeal amputation of thumb
● S68.Ø11 Complete traumatic metacarpophalangeal amputation of right thumb
● S68.Ø12 Complete traumatic metacarpophalangeal amputation of left thumb
● S68.Ø19 Complete traumatic metacarpophalangeal amputation of unspecified thumb
● S68.Ø2 Partial traumatic metacarpophalangeal amputation of thumb
● S68.Ø21 Partial traumatic metacarpophalangeal amputation of right thumb
● S68.Ø22 Partial traumatic metacarpophalangeal amputation of left thumb
● S68.Ø29 Partial traumatic metacarpophalangeal amputation of unspecified thumb
● S68.1 Traumatic metacarpophalangeal amputation of other and unspecified finger
Traumatic amputation of finger NOS
Excludes2 traumatic metacarpophalangeal amputation of thumb (S68.Ø-)
● S68.11 Complete traumatic metacarpophalangeal amputation of other and unspecified finger
● S68.11Ø Complete traumatic metacarpophalangeal amputation of right index finger
● S68.111 Complete traumatic metacarpophalangeal amputation of left index finger
● S68.112 Complete traumatic metacarpophalangeal amputation of right middle finger
● S68.113 Complete traumatic metacarpophalangeal amputation of left middle finger
● S68.114 Complete traumatic metacarpophalangeal amputation of right ring finger
● S68.115 Complete traumatic metacarpophalangeal amputation of left ring finger
● S68.116 Complete traumatic metacarpophalangeal amputation of right little finger
● S68.117 Complete traumatic metacarpophalangeal amputation of left little finger
● S68.118 Complete traumatic metacarpophalangeal amputation of other finger
Complete traumatic metacarpophalangeal amputation of specified finger with unspecified laterality
● S68.119 Complete traumatic metacarpophalangeal amputation of unspecified finger
● S68.12 Partial traumatic metacarpophalangeal amputation of other and unspecified finger
● S68.12Ø Partial traumatic metacarpophalangeal amputation of right index finger
● S68.121 Partial traumatic metacarpophalangeal amputation of left index finger
● S68.122 Partial traumatic metacarpophalangeal amputation of right middle finger
● S68.123 Partial traumatic metacarpophalangeal amputation of left middle finger
● S68.124 Partial traumatic metacarpophalangeal amputation of right ring finger
● S68.125 Partial traumatic metacarpophalangeal amputation of left ring finger
● S68.126 Partial traumatic metacarpophalangeal amputation of right little finger
● S68.127 Partial traumatic metacarpophalangeal amputation of left little finger
● S68.128 Partial traumatic metacarpophalangeal amputation of other finger
Partial traumatic metacarpophalangeal amputation of specified finger with unspecified laterality
● S68.129 Partial traumatic metacarpophalangeal amputation of unspecified finger
● S68.4 Traumatic amputation of hand at wrist level
Traumatic amputation of hand NOS
Traumatic amputation of wrist
● S68.41 Complete traumatic amputation of hand at wrist level
● S68.411 Complete traumatic amputation of right hand at wrist level
● S68.412 Complete traumatic amputation of left hand at wrist level
● S68.419 Complete traumatic amputation of unspecified hand at wrist level

● S68.42 Partial traumatic amputation of hand at wrist level
- ● S68.421 Partial traumatic amputation of right hand at wrist level
- ● S68.422 Partial traumatic amputation of left hand at wrist level
- ● S68.429 Partial traumatic amputation of unspecified hand at wrist level

● S68.5 Traumatic transphalangeal amputation of thumb
Traumatic interphalangeal joint amputation of thumb

● S68.51 Complete traumatic transphalangeal amputation of thumb
- ● S68.511 Complete traumatic transphalangeal amputation of right thumb
- ● S68.512 Complete traumatic transphalangeal amputation of left thumb
- ● S68.519 Complete traumatic transphalangeal amputation of unspecified thumb

● S68.52 Partial traumatic transphalangeal amputation of thumb
- ● S68.521 Partial traumatic transphalangeal amputation of right thumb
- ● S68.522 Partial traumatic transphalangeal amputation of left thumb
- ● S68.529 Partial traumatic transphalangeal amputation of unspecified thumb

● S68.6 Traumatic transphalangeal amputation of other and unspecified finger

● S68.61 Complete traumatic transphalangeal amputation of other and unspecified finger(s)
- ● S68.610 Complete traumatic transphalangeal amputation of right index finger
- ● S68.611 Complete traumatic transphalangeal amputation of left index finger
- ● S68.612 Complete traumatic transphalangeal amputation of right middle finger
- ● S68.613 Complete traumatic transphalangeal amputation of left middle finger
- ● S68.614 Complete traumatic transphalangeal amputation of right ring finger
- ● S68.615 Complete traumatic transphalangeal amputation of left ring finger
- ● S68.616 Complete traumatic transphalangeal amputation of right little finger
- ● S68.617 Complete traumatic transphalangeal amputation of left little finger
- ● S68.618 Complete traumatic transphalangeal amputation of other finger
  Complete traumatic transphalangeal amputation of specified finger with unspecified laterality
- ● S68.619 Complete traumatic transphalangeal amputation of unspecified finger

● S68.62 Partial traumatic transphalangeal amputation of other and unspecified finger
- ● S68.620 Partial traumatic transphalangeal amputation of right index finger
- ● S68.621 Partial traumatic transphalangeal amputation of left index finger
- ● S68.622 Partial traumatic transphalangeal amputation of right middle finger
- ● S68.623 Partial traumatic transphalangeal amputation of left middle finger
- ● S68.624 Partial traumatic transphalangeal amputation of right ring finger
- ● S68.625 Partial traumatic transphalangeal amputation of left ring finger
- ● S68.626 Partial traumatic transphalangeal amputation of right little finger
- ● S68.627 Partial traumatic transphalangeal amputation of left little finger
- ● S68.628 Partial traumatic transphalangeal amputation of other finger
  Partial traumatic transphalangeal amputation of specified finger with unspecified laterality
- ● S68.629 Partial traumatic transphalangeal amputation of unspecified finger

● S68.7 Traumatic transmetacarpal amputation of hand

● S68.71 Complete traumatic transmetacarpal amputation of hand
- ● S68.711 Complete traumatic transmetacarpal amputation of right hand
- ● S68.712 Complete traumatic transmetacarpal amputation of left hand
- ● S68.719 Complete traumatic transmetacarpal amputation of unspecified hand

● S68.72 Partial traumatic transmetacarpal amputation of hand
- ● S68.721 Partial traumatic transmetacarpal amputation of right hand
- ● S68.722 Partial traumatic transmetacarpal amputation of left hand
- ● S68.729 Partial traumatic transmetacarpal amputation of unspecified hand

● S69 Other and unspecified injuries of wrist, hand and finger(s)
The appropriate 7th character is to be added to each code from category S69

A	initial encounter
D	subsequent encounter
S	sequela

● S69.8 Other specified injuries of wrist, hand and finger(s)
- X● S69.80 Other specified injuries of unspecified wrist, hand and finger(s)
- X● S69.81 Other specified injuries of right wrist, hand and finger(s)
- X● S69.82 Other specified injuries of left wrist, hand and finger(s)

● S69.9 Unspecified injury of wrist, hand and finger(s)
- X● S69.90 Unspecified injury of unspecified wrist, hand and finger(s)
- X● S69.91 Unspecified injury of right wrist, hand and finger(s)
- X● S69.92 Unspecified injury of left wrist, hand and finger(s)

INJURIES TO THE HIP AND THIGH (S70-S79)

Excludes2 burns and corrosions (T20-T32)
frostbite (T33-T34)
snake bite (T63.0-)
venomous insect bite or sting (T63.4-)

● **S70 Superficial injury of hip and thigh**
The appropriate 7th character is to be added to each code from category S70

A initial encounter
D subsequent encounter
S sequela

● **S70.0 Contusion of hip**
X● **S70.00 Contusion of unspecified hip**
X● **S70.01 Contusion of right hip**
X● **S70.02 Contusion of left hip**

● **S70.1 Contusion of thigh**
X● **S70.10 Contusion of unspecified thigh**
X● **S70.11 Contusion of right thigh**
X● **S70.12 Contusion of left thigh**

● **S70.2 Other superficial injuries of hip**
● **S70.21 Abrasion of hip**
● **S70.211 Abrasion, right hip**
● **S70.212 Abrasion, left hip**
● **S70.219 Abrasion, unspecified hip**
● **S70.22 Blister (nonthermal) of hip**
● **S70.221 Blister (nonthermal), right hip**
● **S70.222 Blister (nonthermal), left hip**
● **S70.229 Blister (nonthermal), unspecified hip**
● **S70.24 External constriction of hip**
● **S70.241 External constriction, right hip**
● **S70.242 External constriction, left hip**
● **S70.249 External constriction, unspecified hip**
● **S70.25 Superficial foreign body of hip**
Splinter in the hip
● **S70.251 Superficial foreign body, right hip**
● **S70.252 Superficial foreign body, left hip**
● **S70.259 Superficial foreign body, unspecified hip**
● **S70.26 Insect bite (nonvenomous) of hip**
● **S70.261 Insect bite (nonvenomous), right hip**
● **S70.262 Insect bite (nonvenomous), left hip**
● **S70.269 Insect bite (nonvenomous), unspecified hip**
● **S70.27 Other superficial bite of hip**
Excludes1 open bite of hip (S71.05-)
● **S70.271 Other superficial bite of hip, right hip**
● **S70.272 Other superficial bite of hip, left hip**
● **S70.279 Other superficial bite of hip, unspecified hip**

● **S70.3 Other superficial injuries of thigh**
● **S70.31 Abrasion of thigh**
● **S70.311 Abrasion, right thigh**
● **S70.312 Abrasion, left thigh**
● **S70.319 Abrasion, unspecified thigh**
● **S70.32 Blister (nonthermal) of thigh**
● **S70.321 Blister (nonthermal), right thigh**
● **S70.322 Blister (nonthermal), left thigh**
● **S70.329 Blister (nonthermal), unspecified thigh**
● **S70.34 External constriction of thigh**
● **S70.341 External constriction, right thigh**
● **S70.342 External constriction, left thigh**
● **S70.349 External constriction, unspecified thigh**
● **S70.35 Superficial foreign body of thigh**
Splinter in the thigh
● **S70.351 Superficial foreign body, right thigh**
● **S70.352 Superficial foreign body, left thigh**
● **S70.359 Superficial foreign body, unspecified thigh**
● **S70.36 Insect bite (nonvenomous) of thigh**
● **S70.361 Insect bite (nonvenomous), right thigh**
● **S70.362 Insect bite (nonvenomous), left thigh**
● **S70.369 Insect bite (nonvenomous), unspecified thigh**
● **S70.37 Other superficial bite of thigh**
Excludes1 open bite of thigh (S71.15)
● **S70.371 Other superficial bite of right thigh**
● **S70.372 Other superficial bite of left thigh**
● **S70.379 Other superficial bite of unspecified thigh**

● **S70.9 Unspecified superficial injury of hip and thigh**
● **S70.91 Unspecified superficial injury of hip**
● **S70.911 Unspecified superficial injury of right hip**
● **S70.912 Unspecified superficial injury of left hip**
● **S70.919 Unspecified superficial injury of unspecified hip**
● **S70.92 Unspecified superficial injury of thigh**
● **S70.921 Unspecified superficial injury of right thigh**
● **S70.922 Unspecified superficial injury of left thigh**
● **S70.929 Unspecified superficial injury of unspecified thigh**

● **S71 Open wound of hip and thigh**
Code also any associated wound infection
Excludes1 open fracture of hip and thigh (S72.-)
traumatic amputation of hip and thigh (S78.-)
Excludes2 bite of venomous animal (T63.-)
open wound of ankle, foot and toes (S91.-)
open wound of knee and lower leg (S81.-)
The appropriate 7th character is to be added to each code from category S71

A initial encounter
D subsequent encounter
S sequela

● **S71.0 Open wound of hip**
● **S71.00 Unspecified open wound of hip**
● **S71.001 Unspecified open wound, right hip**
● **S71.002 Unspecified open wound, left hip**
● **S71.009 Unspecified open wound, unspecified hip**
● **S71.01 Laceration without foreign body of hip**
● **S71.011 Laceration without foreign body, right hip**
● **S71.012 Laceration without foreign body, left hip**
● **S71.019 Laceration without foreign body, unspecified hip**

- S71.02 Laceration with foreign body of hip
  - S71.021 Laceration with foreign body, right hip
  - S71.022 Laceration with foreign body, left hip
  - S71.029 Laceration with foreign body, unspecified hip
- S71.03 Puncture wound without foreign body of hip
  - S71.031 Puncture wound without foreign body, right hip
  - S71.032 Puncture wound without foreign body, left hip
  - S71.039 Puncture wound without foreign body, unspecified hip
- S71.04 Puncture wound with foreign body of hip
  - S71.041 Puncture wound with foreign body, right hip
  - S71.042 Puncture wound with foreign body, left hip
  - S71.049 Puncture wound with foreign body, unspecified hip
- S71.05 Open bite of hip
  Bite of hip NOS
  Excludes1 superficial bite of hip (S70.26, S70.27)
  - S71.051 Open bite, right hip
  - S71.052 Open bite, left hip
  - S71.059 Open bite, unspecified hip

S71.1 Open wound of thigh

- S71.10 Unspecified open wound of thigh
  - S71.101 Unspecified open wound, right thigh
  - S71.102 Unspecified open wound, left thigh
  - S71.109 Unspecified open wound, unspecified thigh
- S71.11 Laceration without foreign body of thigh
  - S71.111 Laceration without foreign body, right thigh
  - S71.112 Laceration without foreign body, left thigh
  - S71.119 Laceration without foreign body, unspecified thigh
- S71.12 Laceration with foreign body of thigh
  - S71.121 Laceration with foreign body, right thigh
  - S71.122 Laceration with foreign body, left thigh
  - S71.129 Laceration with foreign body, unspecified thigh
- S71.13 Puncture wound without foreign body of thigh
  - S71.131 Puncture wound without foreign body, right thigh
  - S71.132 Puncture wound without foreign body, left thigh
  - S71.139 Puncture wound without foreign body, unspecified thigh
- S71.14 Puncture wound with foreign body of thigh
  - S71.141 Puncture wound with foreign body, right thigh
  - S71.142 Puncture wound with foreign body, left thigh
  - S71.149 Puncture wound with foreign body, unspecified thigh
- S71.15 Open bite of thigh
  Bite of thigh NOS
  Excludes1 superficial bite of thigh (S70.37-)
  - S71.151 Open bite, right thigh
  - S71.152 Open bite, left thigh
  - S71.159 Open bite, unspecified thigh

S72 Fracture of femur

Note: A fracture not indicated as displaced or nondisplaced should be coded to displaced

A fracture not indicated as open or closed should be coded to closed

The open fracture designations are based on the Gustilo open fracture classification

Excludes1 traumatic amputation of hip and thigh (S78.-)

Excludes2 fracture of lower leg and ankle (S82.-)
fracture of foot (S92.-)
periprosthetic fracture of prosthetic implant of hip (T84.040, T84.041)

The appropriate 7th character is to be added to all codes from category S72

A	initial encounter for closed fracture
B	initial encounter for open fracture type I or II initial encounter for open fracture NOS
C	initial encounter for open fracture type IIIA, IIIB, or IIIC
D	subsequent encounter for closed fracture with routine healing
E	subsequent encounter for open fracture type I or II with routine healing
F	subsequent encounter for open fracture type IIIA, IIIB, or IIIC with routine healing
G	subsequent encounter for closed fracture with delayed healing
H	subsequent encounter for open fracture type I or II with delayed healing
J	subsequent encounter for open fracture type IIIA, IIIB, or IIIC with delayed healing
K	subsequent encounter for closed fracture with nonunion
M	subsequent encounter for open fracture type I or II with nonunion
N	subsequent encounter for open fracture type IIIA, IIIB, or IIIC with nonunion
P	subsequent encounter for closed fracture with malunion
Q	subsequent encounter for open fracture type I or II with malunion
R	subsequent encounter for open fracture type IIIA, IIIB, or IIIC with malunion
S	sequela

S72.0 Fracture of head and neck of femur

Excludes2 physeal fracture of upper end of femur (S79.0-)

- S72.00 Fracture of unspecified part of neck of femur
  Fracture of hip NOS
  Fracture of neck of femur NOS
  - S72.001 Fracture of unspecified part of neck of right femur
  - S72.002 Fracture of unspecified part of neck of left femur
  - S72.009 Fracture of unspecified part of neck of unspecified femur
- S72.01 Unspecified intracapsular fracture of femur
  Subcapital fracture of femur
  - S72.011 Unspecified intracapsular fracture of right femur
  - S72.012 Unspecified intracapsular fracture of left femur
  - S72.019 Unspecified intracapsular fracture of unspecified femur

CHAPTER 19 (S00-T88)

● S72.02 **Fracture of epiphysis (separation) (upper) of femur**
Transepiphyseal fracture of femur
Fracture and separation across growth plate
Excludes1 capital femoral epiphyseal fracture (pediatric) of femur (S79.01-)
Salter-Harris Type I physeal fracture of upper end of femur (S79.01-)
● S72.021 **Displaced fracture of epiphysis (separation) (upper) of right femur**
● S72.022 **Displaced fracture of epiphysis (separation) (upper) of left femur**
● S72.023 **Displaced fracture of epiphysis (separation) (upper) of unspecified femur**
● S72.024 **Nondisplaced fracture of epiphysis (separation) (upper) of right femur**
● S72.025 **Nondisplaced fracture of epiphysis (separation) (upper) of left femur**
● S72.026 **Nondisplaced fracture of epiphysis (separation) (upper) of unspecified femur**

● S72.03 **Midcervical fracture of femur**
Transcervical fracture of femur NOS
● S72.031 **Displaced midcervical fracture of right femur**
● S72.032 **Displaced midcervical fracture of left femur**
● S72.033 **Displaced midcervical fracture of unspecified femur**
● S72.034 **Nondisplaced midcervical fracture of right femur**
● S72.035 **Nondisplaced midcervical fracture of left femur**
● S72.036 **Nondisplaced midcervical fracture of unspecified femur**

● S72.04 **Fracture of base of neck of femur**
Cervicotrochanteric fracture of femur
● S72.041 **Displaced fracture of base of neck of right femur**
● S72.042 **Displaced fracture of base of neck of left femur**
● S72.043 **Displaced fracture of base of neck of unspecified femur**
● S72.044 **Nondisplaced fracture of base of neck of right femur**
● S72.045 **Nondisplaced fracture of base of neck of left femur**
● S72.046 **Nondisplaced fracture of base of neck of unspecified femur**

● S72.05 **Unspecified fracture of head of femur**
Fracture of head of femur NOS
● S72.051 **Unspecified fracture of head of right femur**
● S72.052 **Unspecified fracture of head of left femur**
● S72.059 **Unspecified fracture of head of unspecified femur**

● S72.06 **Articular fracture of head of femur**
● S72.061 **Displaced articular fracture of head of right femur**
● S72.062 **Displaced articular fracture of head of left femur**
● S72.063 **Displaced articular fracture of head of unspecified femur**
● S72.064 **Nondisplaced articular fracture of head of right femur**
● S72.065 **Nondisplaced articular fracture of head of left femur**
● S72.066 **Nondisplaced articular fracture of head of unspecified femur**

● S72.09 **Other fracture of head and neck of femur**
● S72.091 **Other fracture of head and neck of right femur**
● S72.092 **Other fracture of head and neck of left femur**
● S72.099 **Other fracture of head and neck of unspecified femur**

● S72.1 **Pertrochanteric fracture**
Fracture extending close to, but not into, joint
● S72.10 **Unspecified trochanteric fracture of femur**
Fracture of trochanter NOS
● S72.101 **Unspecified trochanteric fracture of right femur**
● S72.102 **Unspecified trochanteric fracture of left femur**
● S72.109 **Unspecified trochanteric fracture of unspecified femur**

● S72.11 **Fracture of greater trochanter of femur**
● S72.111 **Displaced fracture of greater trochanter of right femur**
● S72.112 **Displaced fracture of greater trochanter of left femur**
● S72.113 **Displaced fracture of greater trochanter of unspecified femur**
● S72.114 **Nondisplaced fracture of greater trochanter of right femur**
● S72.115 **Nondisplaced fracture of greater trochanter of left femur**
● S72.116 **Nondisplaced fracture of greater trochanter of unspecified femur**

● S72.12 **Fracture of lesser trochanter of femur**
● S72.121 **Displaced fracture of lesser trochanter of right femur**
● S72.122 **Displaced fracture of lesser trochanter of left femur**
● S72.123 **Displaced fracture of lesser trochanter of unspecified femur**
● S72.124 **Nondisplaced fracture of lesser trochanter of right femur**
● S72.125 **Nondisplaced fracture of lesser trochanter of left femur**
● S72.126 **Nondisplaced fracture of lesser trochanter of unspecified femur**

● S72.13 **Apophyseal fracture of femur**
Pertaining to articulations between articular facets of adjacent vertebrae
Excludes1 chronic (nontraumatic) slipped upper femoral epiphysis (M93.0-)
● S72.131 **Displaced apophyseal fracture of right femur**
● S72.132 **Displaced apophyseal fracture of left femur**
● S72.133 **Displaced apophyseal fracture of unspecified femur**
● S72.134 **Nondisplaced apophyseal fracture of right femur**
● S72.135 **Nondisplaced apophyseal fracture of left femur**
● S72.136 **Nondisplaced apophyseal fracture of unspecified femur**

- ● S72.14 Intertrochanteric fracture of femur
  - ● S72.141 Displaced intertrochanteric fracture of right femur
  - ● S72.142 Displaced intertrochanteric fracture of left femur
  - ● S72.143 Displaced intertrochanteric fracture of unspecified femur
  - ● S72.144 Nondisplaced intertrochanteric fracture of right femur
  - ● S72.145 Nondisplaced intertrochanteric fracture of left femur
  - ● S72.146 Nondisplaced intertrochanteric fracture of unspecified femur
- ● S72.2 Subtrochanteric fracture of femur

  Subtrochanteric: inferior to trochanter
  - X● S72.21 Displaced subtrochanteric fracture of right femur
  - X● S72.22 Displaced subtrochanteric fracture of left femur
  - X● S72.23 Displaced subtrochanteric fracture of unspecified femur
  - X● S72.24 Nondisplaced subtrochanteric fracture of right femur
  - X● S72.25 Nondisplaced subtrochanteric fracture of left femur
  - X● S72.26 Nondisplaced subtrochanteric fracture of unspecified femur
- ● S72.3 Fracture of shaft of femur
  - ● S72.30 Unspecified fracture of shaft of femur
    - ● S72.301 Unspecified fracture of shaft of right femur
    - ● S72.302 Unspecified fracture of shaft of left femur
    - ● S72.309 Unspecified fracture of shaft of unspecified femur
  - ● S72.32 Transverse fracture of shaft of femur
    - ● S72.321 Displaced transverse fracture of shaft of right femur
    - ● S72.322 Displaced transverse fracture of shaft of left femur
    - ● S72.323 Displaced transverse fracture of shaft of unspecified femur
    - ● S72.324 Nondisplaced transverse fracture of shaft of right femur
    - ● S72.325 Nondisplaced transverse fracture of shaft of left femur
    - ● S72.326 Nondisplaced transverse fracture of shaft of unspecified femur
  - ● S72.33 Oblique fracture of shaft of femur
    - ● S72.331 Displaced oblique fracture of shaft of right femur
    - ● S72.332 Displaced oblique fracture of shaft of left femur
    - ● S72.333 Displaced oblique fracture of shaft of unspecified femur
    - ● S72.334 Nondisplaced oblique fracture of shaft of right femur
    - ● S72.335 Nondisplaced oblique fracture of shaft of left femur
    - ● S72.336 Nondisplaced oblique fracture of shaft of unspecified femur
  - ● S72.34 Spiral fracture of shaft of femur
    - ● S72.341 Displaced spiral fracture of shaft of right femur
    - ● S72.342 Displaced spiral fracture of shaft of left femur
    - ● S72.343 Displaced spiral fracture of shaft of unspecified femur
    - ● S72.344 Nondisplaced spiral fracture of shaft of right femur
    - ● S72.345 Nondisplaced spiral fracture of shaft of left femur
    - ● S72.346 Nondisplaced spiral fracture of shaft of unspecified femur
  - ● S72.35 Comminuted fracture of shaft of femur
    - ● S72.351 Displaced comminuted fracture of shaft of right femur
    - ● S72.352 Displaced comminuted fracture of shaft of left femur
    - ● S72.353 Displaced comminuted fracture of shaft of unspecified femur
    - ● S72.354 Nondisplaced comminuted fracture of shaft of right femur
    - ● S72.355 Nondisplaced comminuted fracture of shaft of left femur
    - ● S72.356 Nondisplaced comminuted fracture of shaft of unspecified femur
  - ● S72.36 Segmental fracture of shaft of femur
    - ● S72.361 Displaced segmental fracture of shaft of right femur
    - ● S72.362 Displaced segmental fracture of shaft of left femur
    - ● S72.363 Displaced segmental fracture of shaft of unspecified femur
    - ● S72.364 Nondisplaced segmental fracture of shaft of right femur
    - ● S72.365 Nondisplaced segmental fracture of shaft of left femur
    - ● S72.366 Nondisplaced segmental fracture of shaft of unspecified femur
  - ● S72.39 Other fracture of shaft of femur
    - ● S72.391 Other fracture of shaft of right femur
    - ● S72.392 Other fracture of shaft of left femur
    - ● S72.399 Other fracture of shaft of unspecified femur
- ● S72.4 Fracture of lower end of femur

  Fracture of distal end of femur

  Excludes2 fracture of shaft of femur (S72.3-)
  physeal fracture of lower end of femur (S79.1-)
  - ● S72.40 Unspecified fracture of lower end of femur
    - ● S72.401 Unspecified fracture of lower end of right femur
    - ● S72.402 Unspecified fracture of lower end of left femur
    - ● S72.409 Unspecified fracture of lower end of unspecified femur
  - ● S72.41 Unspecified condyle fracture of lower end of femur

    Condyle fracture of femur NOS
    - ● S72.411 Displaced unspecified condyle fracture of lower end of right femur
    - ● S72.412 Displaced unspecified condyle fracture of lower end of left femur
    - ● S72.413 Displaced unspecified condyle fracture of lower end of unspecified femur
    - ● S72.414 Nondisplaced unspecified condyle fracture of lower end of right femur
    - ● S72.415 Nondisplaced unspecified condyle fracture of lower end of left femur
    - ● S72.416 Nondisplaced unspecified condyle fracture of lower end of unspecified femur

CHAPTER 19 (SØØ-T88)

- S72.42 Fracture of lateral condyle of femur
  - S72.421 Displaced fracture of lateral condyle of right femur
  - S72.422 Displaced fracture of lateral condyle of left femur
  - S72.423 Displaced fracture of lateral condyle of unspecified femur
  - S72.424 Nondisplaced fracture of lateral condyle of right femur
  - S72.425 Nondisplaced fracture of lateral condyle of left femur
  - S72.426 Nondisplaced fracture of lateral condyle of unspecified femur
- S72.43 Fracture of medial condyle of femur
  - S72.431 Displaced fracture of medial condyle of right femur
  - S72.432 Displaced fracture of medial condyle of left femur
  - S72.433 Displaced fracture of medial condyle of unspecified femur
  - S72.434 Nondisplaced fracture of medial condyle of right femur
  - S72.435 Nondisplaced fracture of medial condyle of left femur
  - S72.436 Nondisplaced fracture of medial condyle of unspecified femur
- S72.44 Fracture of lower epiphysis (separation) of femur

  Excludes1 Salter-Harris Type I physeal fracture of lower end of femur (S79.11-)
  - S72.441 Displaced fracture of lower epiphysis (separation) of right femur
  - S72.442 Displaced fracture of lower epiphysis (separation) of left femur
  - S72.443 Displaced fracture of lower epiphysis (separation) of unspecified femur
  - S72.444 Nondisplaced fracture of lower epiphysis (separation) of right femur
  - S72.445 Nondisplaced fracture of lower epiphysis (separation) of left femur
  - S72.446 Nondisplaced fracture of lower epiphysis (separation) of unspecified femur
- S72.45 Supracondylar fracture without intracondylar extension of lower end of femur

  Supracondylar fracture of lower end of femur NOS

  Excludes1 supracondylar fracture with intracondylar extension of lower end of femur (S72.46-)
  - S72.451 Displaced supracondylar fracture without intracondylar extension of lower end of right femur
  - S72.452 Displaced supracondylar fracture without intracondylar extension of lower end of left femur
  - S72.453 Displaced supracondylar fracture without intracondylar extension of lower end of unspecified femur
  - S72.454 Nondisplaced supracondylar fracture without intracondylar extension of lower end of right femur
  - S72.455 Nondisplaced supracondylar fracture without intracondylar extension of lower end of left femur
  - S72.456 Nondisplaced supracondylar fracture without intracondylar extension of lower end of unspecified femur
- S72.46 Supracondylar fracture with intracondylar extension of lower end of femur

  Excludes1 supracondylar fracture without intracondylar extension of lower end of femur (S72.45-)
  - S72.461 Displaced supracondylar fracture with intracondylar extension of lower end of right femur
  - S72.462 Displaced supracondylar fracture with intracondylar extension of lower end of left femur
  - S72.463 Displaced supracondylar fracture with intracondylar extension of lower end of unspecified femur
  - S72.464 Nondisplaced supracondylar fracture with intracondylar extension of lower end of right femur
  - S72.465 Nondisplaced supracondylar fracture with intracondylar extension of lower end of left femur
  - S72.466 Nondisplaced supracondylar fracture with intracondylar extension of lower end of unspecified femur
- S72.47 Torus fracture of lower end of femur

  The appropriate 7th character is to be added to all codes in subcategory S72.47

A	initial encounter for closed fracture
D	subsequent encounter for fracture with routine healing
G	subsequent encounter for fracture with delayed healing
K	subsequent encounter for fracture with nonunion
P	subsequent encounter for fracture with malunion
S	sequela

  - S72.471 Torus fracture of lower end of right femur
  - S72.472 Torus fracture of lower end of left femur
  - S72.479 Torus fracture of lower end of unspecified femur
- S72.49 Other fracture of lower end of femur
  - S72.491 Other fracture of lower end of right femur
  - S72.492 Other fracture of lower end of left femur
  - S72.499 Other fracture of lower end of unspecified femur
- S72.8 Other fracture of femur
  - S72.8X Other fracture of femur
    - S72.8X1 Other fracture of right femur
    - S72.8X2 Other fracture of left femur
    - S72.8X9 Other fracture of unspecified femur
- S72.9 Unspecified fracture of femur

  Fracture of thigh NOS

  Fracture of upper leg NOS

  Excludes1 fracture of hip NOS (S72.00-, S72.01-)
  - X S72.90 Unspecified fracture of unspecified femur
  - X S72.91 Unspecified fracture of right femur
  - X S72.92 Unspecified fracture of left femur

CHAPTER 19 (S00-T88)

● S73 Dislocation and sprain of joint and ligaments of hip

Includes avulsion of joint or ligament of hip
laceration of cartilage, joint or ligament of hip
sprain of cartilage, joint or ligament of hip
traumatic hemarthrosis of joint or ligament of hip
traumatic rupture of joint or ligament of hip
traumatic subluxation of joint or ligament of hip
traumatic tear of joint or ligament of hip

Code also any associated open wound

Excludes2 strain of muscle, fascia and tendon of hip and thigh (S76.-)

The appropriate 7th character is to be added to each code from category S73

A initial encounter
D subsequent encounter
S sequela

● S73.0 Subluxation and dislocation of hip
Out of position
Excludes2 dislocation and subluxation of hip prosthesis (T84.020, T84.021)

● S73.00 Unspecified subluxation and dislocation of hip
Dislocation of hip NOS
Subluxation of hip NOS

● S73.001 Unspecified subluxation of right hip
● S73.002 Unspecified subluxation of left hip
● S73.003 Unspecified subluxation of unspecified hip
● S73.004 Unspecified dislocation of right hip
● S73.005 Unspecified dislocation of left hip
● S73.006 Unspecified dislocation of unspecified hip

● S73.01 Posterior subluxation and dislocation of hip
● S73.011 Posterior subluxation of right hip
● S73.012 Posterior subluxation of left hip
● S73.013 Posterior subluxation of unspecified hip
● S73.014 Posterior dislocation of right hip
● S73.015 Posterior dislocation of left hip
● S73.016 Posterior dislocation of unspecified hip

● S73.02 Obturator subluxation and dislocation of hip
● S73.021 Obturator subluxation of right hip
● S73.022 Obturator subluxation of left hip
● S73.023 Obturator subluxation of unspecified hip
● S73.024 Obturator dislocation of right hip
● S73.025 Obturator dislocation of left hip
● S73.026 Obturator dislocation of unspecified hip

● S73.03 Other anterior dislocation of hip
● S73.031 Other anterior subluxation of right hip
● S73.032 Other anterior subluxation of left hip
● S73.033 Other anterior subluxation of unspecified hip
● S73.034 Other anterior dislocation of right hip
● S73.035 Other anterior dislocation of left hip
● S73.036 Other anterior dislocation of unspecified hip

● S73.04 Central dislocation of hip
● S73.041 Central subluxation of right hip
● S73.042 Central subluxation of left hip
● S73.043 Central subluxation of unspecified hip
● S73.044 Central dislocation of right hip
● S73.045 Central dislocation of left hip
● S73.046 Central dislocation of unspecified hip

● S73.1 Sprain of hip
● S73.10 Unspecified sprain of hip
● S73.101 Unspecified sprain of right hip
● S73.102 Unspecified sprain of left hip
● S73.109 Unspecified sprain of unspecified hip

● S73.11 Iliofemoral ligament sprain of hip
● S73.111 Iliofemoral ligament sprain of right hip
● S73.112 Iliofemoral ligament sprain of left hip
● S73.119 Iliofemoral ligament sprain of unspecified hip

● S73.12 Ischiocapsular (ligament) sprain of hip
● S73.121 Ischiocapsular ligament sprain of right hip
● S73.122 Ischiocapsular ligament sprain of left hip
● S73.129 Ischiocapsular ligament sprain of unspecified hip

● S73.19 Other sprain of hip
● S73.191 Other sprain of right hip
● S73.192 Other sprain of left hip
● S73.199 Other sprain of unspecified hip

● S74 Injury of nerves at hip and thigh level

Code also any associated open wound (S71.-)

Excludes2 injury of nerves at ankle and foot level (S94.-)
injury of nerves at lower leg level (S84.-)

The appropriate 7th character is to be added to each code from category S74

A initial encounter
D subsequent encounter
S sequela

● S74.0 Injury of sciatic nerve at hip and thigh level
X● S74.00 Injury of sciatic nerve at hip and thigh level, unspecified leg
X● S74.01 Injury of sciatic nerve at hip and thigh level, right leg
X● S74.02 Injury of sciatic nerve at hip and thigh level, left leg

● S74.1 Injury of femoral nerve at hip and thigh level
X● S74.10 Injury of femoral nerve at hip and thigh level, unspecified leg
X● S74.11 Injury of femoral nerve at hip and thigh level, right leg
X● S74.12 Injury of femoral nerve at hip and thigh level, left leg

● S74.2 Injury of cutaneous sensory nerve at hip and thigh level
X● S74.20 Injury of cutaneous sensory nerve at hip and thigh level, unspecified leg
X● S74.21 Injury of cutaneous sensory nerve at hip and high level, right leg
X● S74.22 Injury of cutaneous sensory nerve at hip and thigh level, left leg

● S74.8 Injury of other nerves at hip and thigh level
● S74.8X Injury of other nerves at hip and thigh level
● S74.8X1 Injury of other nerves at hip and thigh level, right leg
● S74.8X2 Injury of other nerves at hip and thigh level, left leg
● S74.8X9 Injury of other nerves at hip and thigh level, unspecified leg

● S74.9 Injury of unspecified nerve at hip and thigh level
X● S74.90 Injury of unspecified nerve at hip and thigh level, unspecified leg
X● S74.91 Injury of unspecified nerve at hip and thigh level, right leg
X● S74.92 Injury of unspecified nerve at hip and thigh level, left leg

● S75 Injury of blood vessels at hip and thigh level
Code also any associated open wound (S71.-)
Excludes2 injury of blood vessels at lower leg level (S85.-)
injury of popliteal artery (S85.0)
The appropriate 7th character is to be added to each code from category S75
A initial encounter
D subsequent encounter
S sequela

● S75.0 Injury of femoral artery
● S75.00 Unspecified injury of femoral artery
● S75.001 Unspecified injury of femoral artery, right leg
● S75.002 Unspecified injury of femoral artery, left leg
● S75.009 Unspecified injury of femoral artery, unspecified leg
● S75.01 Minor laceration of femoral artery
Incomplete transection of femoral artery
Laceration of femoral artery NOS
Superficial laceration of femoral artery
● S75.011 Minor laceration of femoral artery, right leg
● S75.012 Minor laceration of femoral artery, left leg
● S75.019 Minor laceration of femoral artery, unspecified leg
● S75.02 Major laceration of femoral artery
Complete transection of femoral artery
Traumatic rupture of femoral artery
● S75.021 Major laceration of femoral artery, right leg
● S75.022 Major laceration of femoral artery, left leg
● S75.029 Major laceration of femoral artery, unspecified leg
● S75.09 Other specified injury of femoral artery
● S75.091 Other specified injury of femoral artery, right leg
● S75.092 Other specified injury of femoral artery, left leg
● S75.099 Other specified injury of femoral artery, unspecified leg
● S75.1 Injury of femoral vein at hip and thigh level
● S75.10 Unspecified injury of femoral vein at hip and thigh level
● S75.101 Unspecified injury of femoral vein at hip and thigh level, right leg
● S75.102 Unspecified injury of femoral vein at hip and thigh level, left leg
● S75.109 Unspecified injury of femoral vein at hip and thigh level, unspecified leg
● S75.11 Minor laceration of femoral vein at hip and thigh level
Incomplete transection of femoral vein at hip and thigh level
Laceration of femoral vein at hip and thigh level NOS
Superficial laceration of femoral vein at hip and thigh level
● S75.111 Minor laceration of femoral vein at hip and thigh level, right leg
● S75.112 Minor laceration of femoral vein at hip and thigh level, left leg
● S75.119 Minor laceration of femoral vein at hip and thigh level, unspecified leg
● S75.12 Major laceration of femoral vein at hip and thigh level
Complete transection of femoral vein at hip and thigh level
Traumatic rupture of femoral vein at hip and thigh level
● S75.121 Major laceration of femoral vein at hip and thigh level, right leg
● S75.122 Major laceration of femoral vein at hip and thigh level, left leg
● S75.129 Major laceration of femoral vein at hip and thigh level, unspecified leg
● S75.19 Other specified injury of femoral vein at hip and thigh level
● S75.191 Other specified injury of femoral vein at hip and thigh level, right leg
● S75.192 Other specified injury of femoral vein at hip and thigh level, left leg
● S75.199 Other specified injury of femoral vein at hip and thigh level, unspecified leg
● S75.2 Injury of greater saphenous vein at hip and thigh level
Excludes1 greater saphenous vein NOS (S85.3)
● S75.20 Unspecified injury of greater saphenous vein at hip and thigh level
● S75.201 Unspecified injury of greater saphenous vein at hip and thigh level, right leg
● S75.202 Unspecified injury of greater saphenous vein at hip and thigh level, left leg
● S75.209 Unspecified injury of greater saphenous vein at hip and thigh level, unspecified leg
● S75.21 Minor laceration of greater saphenous vein at hip and thigh level
Incomplete transection of greater saphenous vein at hip and thigh level
Laceration of greater saphenous vein at hip and thigh level NOS
Superficial laceration of greater saphenous vein at hip and thigh level
● S75.211 Minor laceration of greater saphenous vein at hip and thigh level, right leg
● S75.212 Minor laceration of greater saphenous vein at hip and thigh level, left leg
● S75.219 Minor laceration of greater saphenous vein at hip and thigh level, unspecified leg
● S75.22 Major laceration of greater saphenous vein at hip and thigh level
Complete transection of greater saphenous vein at hip and thigh level
Traumatic rupture of greater saphenous vein at hip and thigh level
● S75.221 Major laceration of greater saphenous vein at hip and thigh level, right leg
● S75.222 Major laceration of greater saphenous vein at hip and thigh level, left leg
● S75.229 Major laceration of greater saphenous vein at hip and thigh level, unspecified leg

CHAPTER 19 (S00-T88)

- S75.29 Other specified injury of greater saphenous vein at hip and thigh level
  - S75.291 Other specified injury of greater saphenous vein at hip and thigh level, right leg
  - S75.292 Other specified injury of greater saphenous vein at hip and thigh level, left leg
  - S75.299 Other specified injury of greater saphenous vein at hip and thigh level, unspecified leg
- S75.8 Injury of other blood vessels at hip and thigh level
  - S75.80 Unspecified injury of other blood vessels at hip and thigh level
    - S75.801 Unspecified injury of other blood vessels at hip and thigh level, right leg
    - S75.802 Unspecified injury of other blood vessels at hip and thigh level, left leg
    - S75.809 Unspecified injury of other blood vessels at hip and thigh level, unspecified leg
  - S75.81 Laceration of other blood vessels at hip and thigh level
    - S75.811 Laceration of other blood vessels at hip and thigh level, right leg
    - S75.812 Laceration of other blood vessels at hip and thigh level, left leg
    - S75.819 Laceration of other blood vessels at hip and thigh level, unspecified leg
  - S75.89 Other specified injury of other blood vessels at hip and thigh level
    - S75.891 Other specified injury of other blood vessels at hip and thigh level, right leg
    - S75.892 Other specified injury of other blood vessels at hip and thigh level, left leg
    - S75.899 Other specified injury of other blood vessels at hip and thigh level, unspecified leg
- S75.9 Injury of unspecified blood vessel at hip and thigh level
  - S75.90 Unspecified injury of unspecified blood vessel at hip and thigh level
    - S75.901 Unspecified injury of unspecified blood vessel at hip and thigh level, right leg
    - S75.902 Unspecified injury of unspecified blood vessel at hip and thigh level, left leg
    - S75.909 Unspecified injury of unspecified blood vessel at hip and thigh level, unspecified leg
  - S75.91 Laceration of unspecified blood vessel at hip and thigh level
    - S75.911 Laceration of unspecified blood vessel at hip and thigh level, right leg
    - S75.912 Laceration of unspecified blood vessel at hip and thigh level, left leg
    - S75.919 Laceration of unspecified blood vessel at hip and thigh level, unspecified leg
  - S75.99 Other specified injury of unspecified blood vessel at hip and thigh level
    - S75.991 Other specified injury of unspecified blood vessel at hip and thigh level, right leg
    - S75.992 Other specified injury of unspecified blood vessel at hip and thigh level, left leg
    - S75.999 Other specified injury of unspecified blood vessel at hip and thigh level, unspecified leg

S76 Injury of muscle, fascia and tendon at hip and thigh level

Code also any associated open wound (S71.-)

Excludes2 injury of muscle, fascia and tendon at lower leg level (S86)
sprain of joint and ligament of hip (S73.1)

The appropriate 7th character is to be added to each code from category S76

A	initial encounter
D	subsequent encounter
S	sequela

- S76.0 Injury of muscle, fascia and tendon of hip
  - S76.00 Unspecified injury of muscle, fascia and tendon of hip
    - S76.001 Unspecified injury of muscle, fascia and tendon of right hip
    - S76.002 Unspecified injury of muscle, fascia and tendon of left hip
    - S76.009 Unspecified injury of muscle, fascia and tendon of unspecified hip
  - S76.01 Strain of muscle, fascia and tendon of hip
    - S76.011 Strain of muscle, fascia and tendon of right hip
    - S76.012 Strain of muscle, fascia and tendon of left hip
    - S76.019 Strain of muscle, fascia and tendon of unspecified hip
  - S76.02 Laceration of muscle, fascia and tendon of hip
    - S76.021 Laceration of muscle, fascia and tendon of right hip
    - S76.022 Laceration of muscle, fascia and tendon of left hip
    - S76.029 Laceration of muscle, fascia and tendon of unspecified hip
  - S76.09 Other specified injury of muscle, fascia and tendon of hip
    - S76.091 Other specified injury of muscle, fascia and tendon of right hip
    - S76.092 Other specified injury of muscle, fascia and tendon of left hip
    - S76.099 Other specified injury of muscle, fascia and tendon of unspecified hip
- S76.1 Injury of quadriceps muscle, fascia and tendon
  Injury of patellar ligament (tendon)
  - S76.10 Unspecified injury of quadriceps muscle, fascia and tendon
    - S76.101 Unspecified injury of right quadriceps muscle, fascia and tendon
    - S76.102 Unspecified injury of left quadriceps muscle, fascia and tendon
    - S76.109 Unspecified injury of unspecified quadriceps muscle, fascia and tendon
  - S76.11 Strain of quadriceps muscle, fascia and tendon
    - S76.111 Strain of right quadriceps muscle, fascia and tendon
    - S76.112 Strain of left quadriceps muscle, fascia and tendon
    - S76.119 Strain of unspecified quadriceps muscle, fascia and tendon
  - S76.12 Laceration of quadriceps muscle, fascia and tendon
    - S76.121 Laceration of right quadriceps muscle, fascia and tendon
    - S76.122 Laceration of left quadriceps muscle, fascia and tendon
    - S76.129 Laceration of unspecified quadriceps muscle, fascia and tendon

● S76.19 Other specified injury of quadriceps muscle, fascia and tendon
● S76.191 Other specified injury of right quadriceps muscle, fascia and tendon
● S76.192 Other specified injury of left quadriceps muscle, fascia and tendon
● S76.199 Other specified injury of unspecified quadriceps muscle, fascia and tendon
● S76.2 Injury of adductor muscle, fascia and tendon of thigh
● S76.20 Unspecified injury of adductor muscle, fascia and tendon of thigh
● S76.201 Unspecified injury of adductor muscle, fascia and tendon of right thigh
● S76.202 Unspecified injury of adductor muscle, fascia and tendon of left thigh
● S76.209 Unspecified injury of adductor muscle, fascia and tendon of unspecified thigh
● S76.21 Strain of adductor muscle, fascia and tendon of thigh
● S76.211 Strain of adductor muscle, fascia and tendon of right thigh
● S76.212 Strain of adductor muscle, fascia and tendon of left thigh
● S76.219 Strain of adductor muscle, fascia and tendon of unspecified thigh
● S76.22 Laceration of adductor muscle, fascia and tendon of thigh
● S76.221 Laceration of adductor muscle, fascia and tendon of right thigh
● S76.222 Laceration of adductor muscle, fascia and tendon of left thigh
● S76.229 Laceration of adductor muscle, fascia and tendon of unspecified thigh
● S76.29 Other injury of adductor muscle, fascia and tendon of thigh
● S76.291 Other injury of adductor muscle, fascia and tendon of right thigh
● S76.292 Other injury of adductor muscle, fascia and tendon of left thigh
● S76.299 Other injury of adductor muscle, fascia and tendon of unspecified thigh
● S76.3 Injury of muscle, fascia and tendon of the posterior muscle group at thigh level
● S76.30 Unspecified injury of muscle, fascia and tendon of the posterior muscle group at thigh level
● S76.301 Unspecified injury of muscle, fascia and tendon of the posterior muscle group at thigh level, right thigh
● S76.302 Unspecified injury of muscle, fascia and tendon of the posterior muscle group at thigh level, left thigh
● S76.309 Unspecified injury of muscle, fascia and tendon of the posterior muscle group at thigh level, unspecified thigh
● S76.31 Strain of muscle, fascia and tendon of the posterior muscle group at thigh level
● S76.311 Strain of muscle, fascia and tendon of the posterior muscle group at thigh level, right thigh
● S76.312 Strain of muscle, fascia and tendon of the posterior muscle group at thigh level, left thigh
● S76.319 Strain of muscle, fascia and tendon of the posterior muscle group at thigh level, unspecified thigh
● S76.32 Laceration of muscle, fascia and tendon of the posterior muscle group at thigh level
● S76.321 Laceration of muscle, fascia and tendon of the posterior muscle group at thigh level, right thigh
● S76.322 Laceration of muscle, fascia and tendon of the posterior muscle group at thigh level, left thigh
● S76.329 Laceration of muscle, fascia and tendon of the posterior muscle group at thigh level, unspecified thigh
● S76.39 Other specified injury of muscle, fascia and tendon of the posterior muscle group at thigh level
● S76.391 Other specified injury of muscle, fascia and tendon of the posterior muscle group at thigh level, right thigh
● S76.392 Other specified injury of muscle, fascia and tendon of the posterior muscle group at thigh level, left thigh
● S76.399 Other specified injury of muscle, fascia and tendon of the posterior muscle group at thigh level, unspecified thigh
● S76.8 Injury of other specified muscles, fascia and tendons at thigh level
● S76.80 Unspecified injury of other specified muscles, fascia and tendons at thigh level
● S76.801 Unspecified injury of other specified muscles, fascia and tendons at thigh level, right thigh
● S76.802 Unspecified injury of other specified muscles, fascia and tendons at thigh level, left thigh
● S76.809 Unspecified injury of other specified muscles, fascia and tendons at thigh level, unspecified thigh
● S76.81 Strain of other specified specified muscles, fascia and tendons at thigh level
● S76.811 Strain of other specified muscles, fascia and tendons at thigh level, right thigh
● S76.812 Strain of other specified muscles, fascia and tendons at thigh level, left thigh
● S76.819 Strain of other specified muscles, fascia and tendons at thigh level, unspecified thigh
● S76.82 Laceration of other specified muscles, fascia and tendons at thigh level
● S76.821 Laceration of other specified muscles, fascia and tendons at thigh level, right thigh
● S76.822 Laceration of other specified muscles, fascia and tendons at thigh level, left thigh
● S76.829 Laceration of other specified muscles, fascia and tendons at thigh level, unspecified thigh
● S76.89 Other injury of other specified muscles, fascia and tendons at thigh level
● S76.891 Other injury of other specified muscles, fascia and tendons at thigh level, right thigh
● S76.892 Other injury of other specified muscles, fascia and tendons at thigh level, left thigh
● S76.899 Other injury of other specified muscles, fascia and tendons at thigh level, unspecified thigh

CHAPTER 19 (S00-T88)

● **S76.9** **Injury of unspecified muscles, fascia and tendons at thigh level**

  ● **S76.90** Unspecified injury of unspecified muscles, fascia and tendons at thigh level

    ● **S76.901** Unspecified injury of unspecified muscles, fascia and tendons at thigh level, right thigh

    ● **S76.902** Unspecified injury of unspecified muscles, fascia and tendons at thigh level, left thigh

    ● **S76.909** Unspecified injury of unspecified muscles, fascia and tendons at thigh level, unspecified thigh

  ● **S76.91** Strain of unspecified muscles, fascia and tendons at thigh level

    ● **S76.911** Strain of unspecified muscles, fascia and tendons at thigh level, right thigh

    ● **S76.912** Strain of unspecified muscles, fascia and tendons at thigh level, left thigh

    ● **S76.919** Strain of unspecified muscles fascia and tendons at thigh level, unspecified thigh

  ● **S76.92** Laceration of unspecified muscles, fascia and tendons at thigh level

    ● **S76.921** Laceration of unspecified muscles, fascia and tendons at thigh level, right thigh

    ● **S76.922** Laceration of unspecified muscles, fascia and tendons at thigh level, left thigh

    ● **S76.929** Laceration of unspecified muscles, fascia and tendons at thigh level, unspecified thigh

  ● **S76.99** Other specified injury of unspecified muscles, fascia and tendons at thigh level

    ● **S76.991** Other specified injury of unspecified muscles, fascia and tendons at thigh level, right thigh

    ● **S76.992** Other specified injury of unspecified muscles, fascia and tendons at thigh level, left thigh

    ● **S76.999** Other specified injury of unspecified muscles, fascia and tendons at thigh level, unspecified thigh

● **S77** **Crushing injury of hip and thigh**

  Use additional code(s) for all associated injuries

  Excludes2 crushing injury of ankle and foot (S97.-)

            crushing injury of lower leg (S87.-)

  The appropriate 7th character is to be added to each code from category S77

A	initial encounter
D	subsequent encounter
S	sequela

  ● **S77.0** Crushing injury of hip

    X● **S77.00** Crushing injury of unspecified hip

    X● **S77.01** Crushing injury of right hip

    X● **S77.02** Crushing injury of left hip

  ● **S77.1** Crushing injury of thigh

    X● **S77.10** Crushing injury of unspecified thigh

    X● **S77.11** Crushing injury of right thigh

    X● **S77.12** Crushing injury of left thigh

  ● **S77.2** Crushing injury of hip with thigh

    X● **S77.20** Crushing injury of unspecified hip with thigh

    X● **S77.21** Crushing injury of right hip with thigh

    X● **S77.22** Crushing injury of left hip with thigh

● **S78** **Traumatic amputation of hip and thigh**

  An amputation not identified as partial or complete should be coded to complete

  Excludes1 traumatic amputation of knee (S88.0-)

  The appropriate 7th character is to be added to each code from category S78

A	initial encounter
D	subsequent encounter
S	sequela

  ● **S78.0** Traumatic amputation at hip joint

    ● **S78.01** Complete traumatic amputation at hip joint

      ● **S78.011** Complete traumatic amputation at right hip joint

      ● **S78.012** Complete traumatic amputation at left hip joint

      ● **S78.019** Complete traumatic amputation at unspecified hip joint

    ● **S78.02** Partial traumatic amputation at hip joint

      ● **S78.021** Partial traumatic amputation at right hip joint

      ● **S78.022** Partial traumatic amputation at left hip joint

      ● **S78.029** Partial traumatic amputation at unspecified hip joint

  ● **S78.1** Traumatic amputation at level between hip and knee

    Excludes1 traumatic amputation of knee (S88.0-)

    ● **S78.11** Complete traumatic amputation at level between hip and knee

      ● **S78.111** Complete traumatic amputation at level between right hip and knee

      ● **S78.112** Complete traumatic amputation at level between left hip and knee

      ● **S78.119** Complete traumatic amputation at level between unspecified hip and knee

    ● **S78.12** Partial traumatic amputation at level between hip and knee

      ● **S78.121** Partial traumatic amputation at level between right hip and knee

      ● **S78.122** Partial traumatic amputation at level between left hip and knee

      ● **S78.129** Partial traumatic amputation at level between unspecified hip and knee

  ● **S78.9** Traumatic amputation of hip and thigh, level unspecified

    ● **S78.91** Complete traumatic amputation of hip and thigh, level unspecified

      ● **S78.911** Complete traumatic amputation of right hip and thigh, level unspecified

      ● **S78.912** Complete traumatic amputation of left hip and thigh, level unspecified

      ● **S78.919** Complete traumatic amputation of unspecified hip and thigh, level unspecified

    ● **S78.92** Partial traumatic amputation of hip and thigh, level unspecified

      ● **S78.921** Partial traumatic amputation of right hip and thigh, level unspecified

      ● **S78.922** Partial traumatic amputation of left hip and thigh, level unspecified

      ● **S78.929** Partial traumatic amputation of unspecified hip and thigh, level unspecified

◀ New   ⬅ Revised   ~~deleted~~ Deleted   **OGCR** Official Guidelines   **X** Assign placeholder X   ● Use Additional Character(s)

Excludes 1   Excludes 2   Includes   Use additional   Code first   Code also   Unspecified

CHAPTER 19 (S00-T88)

Item 19–5 SALTER-HARRIS TYPE 1: epiphysis is completely separated from end of bone, or metaphysic growth plate remains attached to epiphysis

SALTER-HARRIS TYPE 2: epiphysis and growth plate are partially separated from metaphysis, which is cracked—most common type

SALTER-HARRIS TYPE 3: fracture occurring through epiphysis and separates part of epiphysis and growth plate from metaphysis fracture, usually at distal end of tibia

SALTER-HARRIS TYPE 4: fracture runs through epiphysis, across growth plate, into metaphysic, surgery is required to restore joint surface to normal and align growth plate

● **S79 Other and unspecified injuries of hip and thigh**

Note: A fracture not indicated as open or closed should be coded to closed

The appropriate 7th character is to be added to each code from subcategories S79.Ø and S79.1

A	initial encounter for closed fracture
D	subsequent encounter for fracture with routine healing
G	subsequent encounter for fracture with delayed healing
K	subsequent encounter for fracture with nonunion
P	subsequent encounter for fracture with malunion
S	sequela

● **S79.Ø Physeal fracture of upper end of femur**

Excludes1 apophyseal fracture of upper end of femur (S72.13-)
nontraumatic slipped upper femoral epiphysis (M93.Ø-)

● **S79.ØØ Unspecified physeal fracture of upper end of femur**

● **S79.ØØ1 Unspecified physeal fracture of upper end of right femur**

● **S79.ØØ2 Unspecified physeal fracture of upper end of left femur**

● **S79.ØØ9 Unspecified physeal fracture of upper end of unspecified femur**

● **S79.Ø1 Salter-Harris Type I physeal fracture of upper end of femur**

Acute on chronic slipped capital femoral epiphysis (traumatic)
Acute slipped capital femoral epiphysis (traumatic)
Capital femoral epiphyseal fracture

Excludes1 chronic slipped upper femoral epiphysis (nontraumatic) (M93.Ø2-)

● **S79.Ø11 Salter-Harris Type I physeal fracture of upper end of right femur**

● **S79.Ø12 Salter-Harris Type I physeal fracture of upper end of left femur**

● **S79.Ø19 Salter-Harris Type I physeal fracture of upper end of unspecified femur**

● **S79.Ø9 Other physeal fracture of upper end of femur**

● **S79.Ø91 Other physeal fracture of upper end of right femur**

● **S79.Ø92 Other physeal fracture of upper end of left femur**

● **S79.Ø99 Other physeal fracture of upper end of unspecified femur**

● **S79.1 Physeal fracture of lower end of femur**

● **S79.1Ø Unspecified physeal fracture of lower end of femur**

● **S79.1Ø1 Unspecified physeal fracture of lower end of right femur**

● **S79.1Ø2 Unspecified physeal fracture of lower end of left femur**

● **S79.1Ø9 Unspecified physeal fracture of lower end of unspecified femur**

● **S79.11 Salter-Harris Type I physeal fracture of lower end of femur**

● **S79.111 Salter-Harris Type I physeal fracture of lower end of right femur**

● **S79.112 Salter-Harris Type I physeal fracture of lower end of left femur**

● **S79.119 Salter-Harris Type I physeal fracture of lower end of unspecified femur**

● **S79.12 Salter-Harris Type II physeal fracture of lower end of femur**

● **S79.121 Salter-Harris Type II physeal fracture of lower end of right femur**

● **S79.122 Salter-Harris Type II physeal fracture of lower end of left femur**

● **S79.129 Salter-Harris Type II physeal fracture of lower end of unspecified femur**

● **S79.13 Salter-Harris Type III physeal fracture of lower end of femur**

● **S79.131 Salter-Harris Type III physeal fracture of lower end of right femur**

● **S79.132 Salter-Harris Type III physeal fracture of lower end of left femur**

● **S79.139 Salter-Harris Type III physeal fracture of lower end of unspecified femur**

● **S79.14 Salter-Harris Type IV physeal fracture of lower end of femur**

● **S79.141 Salter-Harris Type IV physeal fracture of lower end of right femur**

● **S79.142 Salter-Harris Type IV physeal fracture of lower end of left femur**

● **S79.149 Salter-Harris Type IV physeal fracture of lower end of unspecified femur**

● **S79.19 Other physeal fracture of lower end of femur**

● **S79.191 Other physeal fracture of lower end of right femur**

● **S79.192 Other physeal fracture of lower end of left femur**

● **S79.199 Other physeal fracture of lower end of unspecified femur**

● **S79.8 Other specified injuries of hip and thigh**

The appropriate 7th character is to be added to each code in subcategory S79.8

A	initial encounter
D	subsequent encounter
S	sequela

● **S79.81 Other specified injuries of hip**

● **S79.811 Other specified injuries of right hip**

● **S79.812 Other specified injuries of left hip**

● **S79.819 Other specified injuries of unspecified hip**

● **S79.82 Other specified injuries of thigh**

● **S79.821 Other specified injuries of right thigh**

● **S79.822 Other specified injuries of left thigh**

● **S79.829 Other specified injuries of unspecified thigh**

● **S79.9 Unspecified injury of hip and thigh**

The appropriate 7th character is to be added to each code in subcategory S79.9

A	initial encounter
D	subsequent encounter
S	sequela

● **S79.91 Unspecified injury of hip**

● **S79.911 Unspecified injury of right hip**

● **S79.912 Unspecified injury of left hip**

● **S79.919 Unspecified injury of unspecified hip**

CHAPTER 19 (SØØ-T88)

● S79.92   Unspecified injury of thigh
  ● S79.921   Unspecified injury of right thigh
  ● S79.922   Unspecified injury of left thigh
  ● S79.929   Unspecified injury of unspecified thigh

INJURIES TO THE KNEE AND LOWER LEG (S80-S89)

Excludes2   burns and corrosions (T20-T32)
     frostbite (T33-T34)
     injuries of ankle and foot, except fracture of ankle and malleolus (S90-S99)
     insect bite or sting, venomous (T63.4)

● S80   Superficial injury of knee and lower leg
   Excludes2   superficial injury of ankle and foot (S90.-)
   The appropriate 7th character is to be added to each code from category S80

> A   initial encounter
> D   subsequent encounter
> S   sequela

 ● S80.0   Contusion of knee
  X ● S80.00   Contusion of unspecified knee
  X ● S80.01   Contusion of right knee
  X ● S80.02   Contusion of left knee
 ● S80.1   Contusion of lower leg
  X ● S80.10   Contusion of unspecified lower leg
  X ● S80.11   Contusion of right lower leg
  X ● S80.12   Contusion of left lower leg
 ● S80.2   Other superficial injuries of knee
  ● S80.21   Abrasion of knee
   ● S80.211   Abrasion, right knee
   ● S80.212   Abrasion, left knee
   ● S80.219   Abrasion, unspecified knee
  ● S80.22   Blister (nonthermal) of knee
   ● S80.221   Blister (nonthermal), right knee
   ● S80.222   Blister (nonthermal), left knee
   ● S80.229   Blister (nonthermal), unspecified knee
  ● S80.24   External constriction of knee
   ● S80.241   External constriction, right knee
   ● S80.242   External constriction, left knee
   ● S80.249   External constriction, unspecified knee
  ● S80.25   Superficial foreign body of knee
     Splinter in the knee
   ● S80.251   Superficial foreign body, right knee
   ● S80.252   Superficial foreign body, left knee
   ● S80.259   Superficial foreign body, unspecified knee
  ● S80.26   Insect bite (nonvenomous) of knee
   ● S80.261   Insect bite (nonvenomous), right knee
   ● S80.262   Insect bite (nonvenomous), left knee
   ● S80.269   Insect bite (nonvenomous), unspecified knee
  ● S80.27   Other superficial bite of knee
     Excludes1   open bite of knee (S81.05-)
   ● S80.271   Other superficial bite of right knee
   ● S80.272   Other superficial bite of left knee
   ● S80.279   Other superficial bite of unspecified knee
 ● S80.8   Other superficial injuries of lower leg
  ● S80.81   Abrasion of lower leg
   ● S80.811   Abrasion, right lower leg
   ● S80.812   Abrasion, left lower leg
   ● S80.819   Abrasion, unspecified lower leg

  ● S80.82   Blister (nonthermal) of lower leg
   ● S80.821   Blister (nonthermal), right lower leg
   ● S80.822   Blister (nonthermal), left lower leg
   ● S80.829   Blister (nonthermal), unspecified lower leg
  ● S80.84   External constriction of lower leg
   ● S80.841   External constriction, right lower leg
   ● S80.842   External constriction, left lower leg
   ● S80.849   External constriction, unspecified lower leg
  ● S80.85   Superficial foreign body of lower leg
     Splinter in the lower leg
   ● S80.851   Superficial foreign body, right lower leg
   ● S80.852   Superficial foreign body, left lower leg
   ● S80.859   Superficial foreign body, unspecified lower leg
  ● S80.86   Insect bite (nonvenomous) of lower leg
   ● S80.861   Insect bite (nonvenomous), right lower leg
   ● S80.862   Insect bite (nonvenomous), left lower leg
   ● S80.869   Insect bite (nonvenomous), unspecified lower leg
  ● S80.87   Other superficial bite of lower leg
     Excludes1   open bite of lower leg (S81.85-)
   ● S80.871   Other superficial bite, right lower leg
   ● S80.872   Other superficial bite, left lower leg
   ● S80.879   Other superficial bite, unspecified lower leg
 ● S80.9   Unspecified superficial injury of knee and lower leg
  ● S80.91   Unspecified superficial injury of knee
   ● S80.911   Unspecified superficial injury of right knee
   ● S80.912   Unspecified superficial injury of left knee
   ● S80.919   Unspecified superficial injury of unspecified knee
  ● S80.92   Unspecified superficial injury of lower leg
   ● S80.921   Unspecified superficial injury of right lower leg
   ● S80.922   Unspecified superficial injury of left lower leg
   ● S80.929   Unspecified superficial injury of unspecified lower leg

● S81   Open wound of knee and lower leg
   Code also any associated wound infection
   Excludes1   open fracture of knee and lower leg (S82.-)
     traumatic amputation of lower leg (S88.-)
   Excludes2   open wound of ankle and foot (S91.-)
   The appropriate 7th character is to be added to each code from category S81

> A   initial encounter
> D   subsequent encounter
> S   sequela

 ● S81.0   Open wound of knee
  ● S81.00   Unspecified open wound of knee
   ● S81.001   Unspecified open wound, right knee
   ● S81.002   Unspecified open wound, left knee
   ● S81.009   Unspecified open wound, unspecified knee

CHAPTER 19 (S00-T88)

● S81.01 Laceration without foreign body of knee
● S81.011 Laceration without foreign body, right knee
● S81.012 Laceration without foreign body, left knee
● S81.019 Laceration without foreign body, unspecified knee
● S81.02 Laceration with foreign body of knee
● S81.021 Laceration with foreign body, right knee
● S81.022 Laceration with foreign body, left knee
● S81.029 Laceration with foreign body, unspecified knee
● S81.03 Puncture wound without foreign body of knee
● S81.031 Puncture wound without foreign body, right knee
● S81.032 Puncture wound without foreign body, left knee
● S81.039 Puncture wound without foreign body, unspecified knee
● S81.04 Puncture wound with foreign body of knee
● S81.041 Puncture wound with foreign body, right knee
● S81.042 Puncture wound with foreign body, left knee
● S81.049 Puncture wound with foreign body, unspecified knee
● S81.05 Open bite of knee
Bite of knee NOS
Excludes1 superficial bite of knee (S8Ø.27-)
● S81.051 Open bite, right knee
● S81.052 Open bite, left knee
● S81.059 Open bite, unspecified knee
● S81.8 Open wound of lower leg
● S81.80 Unspecified open wound of lower leg
● S81.801 Unspecified open wound, right lower leg
● S81.802 Unspecified open wound, left lower leg
● S81.809 Unspecified open wound, unspecified lower leg
● S81.81 Laceration without foreign body of lower leg
● S81.811 Laceration without foreign body, right lower leg
● S81.812 Laceration without foreign body, left lower leg
● S81.819 Laceration without foreign body, unspecified lower leg
● S81.82 Laceration with foreign body of lower leg
● S81.821 Laceration with foreign body, right lower leg
● S81.822 Laceration with foreign body, left lower leg
● S81.829 Laceration with foreign body, unspecified lower leg
● S81.83 Puncture wound without foreign body of lower leg
● S81.831 Puncture wound without foreign body, right lower leg
● S81.832 Puncture wound without foreign body, left lower leg
● S81.839 Puncture wound without foreign body, unspecified lower leg
● S81.84 Puncture wound with foreign body of lower leg
● S81.841 Puncture wound with foreign body, right lower leg
● S81.842 Puncture wound with foreign body, left lower leg
● S81.849 Puncture wound with foreign body, unspecified lower leg
● S81.85 Open bite of lower leg
Bite of lower leg NOS
Excludes1 superficial bite of lower leg (S8Ø.86-, S8Ø.87-)
● S81.851 Open bite, right lower leg
● S81.852 Open bite, left lower leg
● S81.859 Open bite, unspecified lower leg

● S82 Fracture of lower leg, including ankle

Note: A fracture not indicated as displaced or nondisplaced should be coded to displaced

A fracture not indicated as open or closed should be coded to closed

The open fracture designations are based on the Gustilo open fracture classification

Includes fracture of malleolus
Excludes1 traumatic amputation of lower leg (S88.-)
Excludes2 fracture of foot, except ankle (S92.-)
periprosthetic fracture of prosthetic implant of knee (T84.Ø42, T84.Ø43)

The appropriate 7th character is to be added to all codes from category S82

A	initial encounter for closed fracture
B	initial encounter for open fracture type I or II initial encounter for open fracture NOS
C	initial encounter for open fracture type IIIA, IIIB, or IIIC
D	subsequent encounter for closed fracture with routine healing
E	subsequent encounter for open fracture type I or II with routine healing
F	subsequent encounter for open fracture type IIIA, IIIB, or IIIC with routine healing
G	subsequent encounter for closed fracture with delayed healing
H	subsequent encounter for open fracture type I or II with delayed healing
J	subsequent encounter for open fracture type IIIA, IIIB, or IIIC with delayed healing
K	subsequent encounter for closed fracture with nonunion
M	subsequent encounter for open fracture type I or II with nonunion
N	subsequent encounter for open fracture type IIIA, IIIB, or IIIC with nonunion
P	subsequent encounter for closed fracture with malunion
Q	subsequent encounter for open fracture type I or II with malunion
R	subsequent encounter for open fracture type IIIA, IIIB, or IIIC with malunion
S	sequela

● S82.Ø Fracture of patella
Knee cap
● S82.ØØ Unspecified fracture of patella
● S82.ØØ1 Unspecified fracture of right patella
● S82.ØØ2 Unspecified fracture of left patella
● S82.ØØ9 Unspecified fracture of unspecified patella

CHAPTER 19 (SØØ-T88)

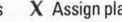

● S82.01 Osteochondral fracture of patella
● S82.011 Displaced osteochondral fracture of right patella
● S82.012 Displaced osteochondral fracture of left patella
● S82.013 Displaced osteochondral fracture of unspecified patella
● S82.014 Nondisplaced osteochondral fracture of right patella
● S82.015 Nondisplaced osteochondral fracture of left patella
● S82.016 Nondisplaced osteochondral fracture of unspecified patella
● S82.02 Longitudinal fracture of patella
● S82.021 Displaced longitudinal fracture of right patella
● S82.022 Displaced longitudinal fracture of left patella
● S82.023 Displaced longitudinal fracture of unspecified patella
● S82.024 Nondisplaced longitudinal fracture of right patella
● S82.025 Nondisplaced longitudinal fracture of left patella
● S82.026 Nondisplaced longitudinal fracture of unspecified patella
● S82.03 Transverse fracture of patella
● S82.031 Displaced transverse fracture of right patella
● S82.032 Displaced transverse fracture of left patella
● S82.033 Displaced transverse fracture of unspecified patella
● S82.034 Nondisplaced transverse fracture of right patella
● S82.035 Nondisplaced transverse fracture of left patella
● S82.036 Nondisplaced transverse fracture of unspecified patella
● S82.04 Comminuted fracture of patella
● S82.041 Displaced comminuted fracture of right patella
● S82.042 Displaced comminuted fracture of left patella
● S82.043 Displaced comminuted fracture of unspecified patella
● S82.044 Nondisplaced comminuted fracture of right patella
● S82.045 Nondisplaced comminuted fracture of left patella
● S82.046 Nondisplaced comminuted fracture of unspecified patella
● S82.09 Other fracture of patella
● S82.091 Other fracture of right patella
● S82.092 Other fracture of left patella
● S82.099 Other fracture of unspecified patella
● S82.1 Fracture of upper end of tibia
Fracture of proximal end of tibia
Excludes2 fracture of shaft of tibia (S82.2-)
physeal fracture of upper end of tibia (S89.0-)
● S82.10 Unspecified fracture of upper end of tibia
● S82.101 Unspecified fracture of upper end of right tibia
● S82.102 Unspecified fracture of upper end of left tibia
● S82.109 Unspecified fracture of upper end of unspecified tibia

● S82.11 Fracture of tibial spine
● S82.111 Displaced fracture of right tibial spine
● S82.112 Displaced fracture of left tibial spine
● S82.113 Displaced fracture of unspecified tibial spine
● S82.114 Nondisplaced fracture of right tibial spine
● S82.115 Nondisplaced fracture of left tibial spine
● S82.116 Nondisplaced fracture of unspecified tibial spine
● S82.12 Fracture of lateral condyle of tibia
● S82.121 Displaced fracture of lateral condyle of right tibia
● S82.122 Displaced fracture of lateral condyle of left tibia
● S82.123 Displaced fracture of lateral condyle of unspecified tibia
● S82.124 Nondisplaced fracture of lateral condyle of right tibia
● S82.125 Nondisplaced fracture of lateral condyle of left tibia
● S82.126 Nondisplaced fracture of lateral condyle of unspecified tibia
● S82.13 Fracture of medial condyle of tibia
● S82.131 Displaced fracture of medial condyle of right tibia
● S82.132 Displaced fracture of medial condyle of left tibia
● S82.133 Displaced fracture of medial condyle of unspecified tibia
● S82.134 Nondisplaced fracture of medial condyle of right tibia
● S82.135 Nondisplaced fracture of medial condyle of left tibia
● S82.136 Nondisplaced fracture of medial condyle of unspecified tibia
● S82.14 Bicondylar fracture of tibia
Fracture of tibial plateau NOS
● S82.141 Displaced bicondylar fracture of right tibia
● S82.142 Displaced bicondylar fracture of left tibia
● S82.143 Displaced bicondylar fracture of unspecified tibia
● S82.144 Nondisplaced bicondylar fracture of right tibia
● S82.145 Nondisplaced bicondylar fracture of left tibia
● S82.146 Nondisplaced bicondylar fracture of unspecified tibia
● S82.15 Fracture of tibial tuberosity
● S82.151 Displaced fracture of right tibial tuberosity
● S82.152 Displaced fracture of left tibial tuberosity
● S82.153 Displaced fracture of unspecified tibial tuberosity
● S82.154 Nondisplaced fracture of right tibial tuberosity
● S82.155 Nondisplaced fracture of left tibial tuberosity
● S82.156 Nondisplaced fracture of unspecified tibial tuberosity

● S82.16 Torus fracture of upper end of tibia

The appropriate 7th character is to be added to all codes in subcategory S82.16

A	initial encounter for closed fracture
D	subsequent encounter for fracture with routine healing
G	subsequent encounter for fracture with delayed healing
K	subsequent encounter for fracture with nonunion
P	subsequent encounter for fracture with malunion
S	sequela

● S82.161 Torus fracture of upper end of right tibia

● S82.162 Torus fracture of upper end of left tibia

● S82.169 Torus fracture of upper end of unspecified tibia

● S82.19 Other fracture of upper end of tibia

● S82.191 Other fracture of upper end of right tibia

● S82.192 Other fracture of upper end of left tibia

● S82.199 Other fracture of upper end of unspecified tibia

● S82.2 Fracture of shaft of tibia

● S82.20 Unspecified fracture of shaft of tibia

Fracture of tibia NOS

● S82.201 Unspecified fracture of shaft of right tibia

● S82.202 Unspecified fracture of shaft of left tibia

● S82.209 Unspecified fracture of shaft of unspecified tibia

● S82.22 Transverse fracture of shaft of tibia

● S82.221 Displaced transverse fracture of shaft of right tibia

● S82.222 Displaced transverse fracture of shaft of left tibia

● S82.223 Displaced transverse fracture of shaft of unspecified tibia

● S82.224 Nondisplaced transverse fracture of shaft of right tibia

● S82.225 Nondisplaced transverse fracture of shaft of left tibia

● S82.226 Nondisplaced transverse fracture of shaft of unspecified tibia

● S82.23 Oblique fracture of shaft of tibia

● S82.231 Displaced oblique fracture of shaft of right tibia

● S82.232 Displaced oblique fracture of shaft of left tibia

● S82.233 Displaced oblique fracture of shaft of unspecified tibia

● S82.234 Nondisplaced oblique fracture of shaft of right tibia

● S82.235 Nondisplaced oblique fracture of shaft of left tibia

● S82.236 Nondisplaced oblique fracture of shaft of unspecified tibia

● S82.24 Spiral fracture of shaft of tibia

Toddler fracture

● S82.241 Displaced spiral fracture of shaft of right tibia

● S82.242 Displaced spiral fracture of shaft of left tibia

● S82.243 Displaced spiral fracture of shaft of unspecified tibia

● S82.244 Nondisplaced spiral fracture of shaft of right tibia

● S82.245 Nondisplaced spiral fracture of shaft of left tibia

● S82.246 Nondisplaced spiral fracture of shaft of unspecified tibia

● S82.25 Comminuted fracture of shaft of tibia

● S82.251 Displaced comminuted fracture of shaft of right tibia

● S82.252 Displaced comminuted fracture of shaft of left tibia

● S82.253 Displaced comminuted fracture of shaft of unspecified tibia

● S82.254 Nondisplaced comminuted fracture of shaft of right tibia

● S82.255 Nondisplaced comminuted fracture of shaft of left tibia

● S82.256 Nondisplaced comminuted fracture of shaft of unspecified tibia

● S82.26 Segmental fracture of shaft of tibia

● S82.261 Displaced segmental fracture of shaft of right tibia

● S82.262 Displaced segmental fracture of shaft of left tibia

● S82.263 Displaced segmental fracture of shaft of unspecified tibia

● S82.264 Nondisplaced segmental fracture of shaft of right tibia

● S82.265 Nondisplaced segmental fracture of shaft of left tibia

● S82.266 Nondisplaced segmental fracture of shaft of unspecified tibia

● S82.29 Other fracture of shaft of tibia

● S82.291 Other fracture of shaft of right tibia

● S82.292 Other fracture of shaft of left tibia

● S82.299 Other fracture of shaft of unspecified tibia

● S82.3 Fracture of lower end of tibia

Excludes1 bimalleolar fracture of lower leg (S82.84-)
fracture of medial malleolus alone (S82.5-)
Maisonneuve's fracture (S82.86-)
pilon fracture of distal tibia (S82.87-)
trimalleolar fractures of lower leg (S82.85-)

● S82.30 Unspecified fracture of lower end of tibia

● S82.301 Unspecified fracture of lower end of right tibia

● S82.302 Unspecified fracture of lower end of left tibia

● S82.309 Unspecified fracture of lower end of unspecified tibia

CHAPTER 19 (S00-T88)

● S82.31 Torus fracture of lower end of tibia

The appropriate 7th character is to be added to all codes in subcategory S82.31

A	initial encounter for closed fracture
D	subsequent encounter for fracture with routine healing
G	subsequent encounter for fracture with delayed healing
K	subsequent encounter for fracture with nonunion
P	subsequent encounter for fracture with malunion
S	sequela

● S82.311 Torus fracture of lower end of right tibia

● S82.312 Torus fracture of lower end of left tibia

● S82.319 Torus fracture of lower end of unspecified tibia

● S82.39 Other fracture of lower end of tibia

● S82.391 Other fracture of lower end of right tibia

● S82.392 Other fracture of lower end of left tibia

● S82.399 Other fracture of lower end of unspecified tibia

● S82.4 Fracture of shaft of fibula

Excludes2 fracture of lateral malleolus alone (S82.6-)

● S82.40 Unspecified fracture of shaft of fibula

● S82.401 Unspecified fracture of shaft of right fibula

● S82.402 Unspecified fracture of shaft of left fibula

● S82.409 Unspecified fracture of shaft of unspecified fibula

● S82.42 Transverse fracture of shaft of fibula

● S82.421 Displaced transverse fracture of shaft of right fibula

● S82.422 Displaced transverse fracture of shaft of left fibula

● S82.423 Displaced transverse fracture of shaft of unspecified fibula

● S82.424 Nondisplaced transverse fracture of shaft of right fibula

● S82.425 Nondisplaced transverse fracture of shaft of left fibula

● S82.426 Nondisplaced transverse fracture of shaft of unspecified fibula

● S82.43 Oblique fracture of shaft of fibula

● S82.431 Displaced oblique fracture of shaft of right fibula

● S82.432 Displaced oblique fracture of shaft of left fibula

● S82.433 Displaced oblique fracture of shaft of unspecified fibula

● S82.434 Nondisplaced oblique fracture of shaft of right fibula

● S82.435 Nondisplaced oblique fracture of shaft of left fibula

● S82.436 Nondisplaced oblique fracture of shaft of unspecified fibula

● S82.44 Spiral fracture of shaft of fibula

● S82.441 Displaced spiral fracture of shaft of right fibula

● S82.442 Displaced spiral fracture of shaft of left fibula

● S82.443 Displaced spiral fracture of shaft of unspecified fibula

● S82.444 Nondisplaced spiral fracture of shaft of right fibula

● S82.445 Nondisplaced spiral fracture of shaft of left fibula

● S82.446 Nondisplaced spiral fracture of shaft of unspecified fibula

● S82.45 Comminuted fracture of shaft of fibula

● S82.451 Displaced comminuted fracture of shaft of right fibula

● S82.452 Displaced comminuted fracture of shaft of left fibula

● S82.453 Displaced comminuted fracture of shaft of unspecified fibula

● S82.454 Nondisplaced comminuted fracture of shaft of right fibula

● S82.455 Nondisplaced comminuted fracture of shaft of left fibula

● S82.456 Nondisplaced comminuted fracture of shaft of unspecified fibula

● S82.46 Segmental fracture of shaft of fibula

● S82.461 Displaced segmental fracture of shaft of right fibula

● S82.462 Displaced segmental fracture of shaft of left fibula

● S82.463 Displaced segmental fracture of shaft of unspecified fibula

● S82.464 Nondisplaced segmental fracture of shaft of right fibula

● S82.465 Nondisplaced segmental fracture of shaft of left fibula

● S82.466 Nondisplaced segmental fracture of shaft of unspecified fibula

● S82.49 Other fracture of shaft of fibula

● S82.491 Other fracture of shaft of right fibula

● S82.492 Other fracture of shaft of left fibula

● S82.499 Other fracture of shaft of unspecified fibula

● S82.5 Fracture of medial malleolus

Excludes1 pilon fracture of distal tibia (S82.87-)
Salter-Harris type III of lower end of tibia (S89.13-)
Salter-Harris type IV of lower end of tibia (S89.14-)

X● S82.51 Displaced fracture of medial malleolus of right tibia

X● S82.52 Displaced fracture of medial malleolus of left tibia

X● S82.53 Displaced fracture of medial malleolus of unspecified tibia

X● S82.54 Nondisplaced fracture of medial malleolus of right tibia

X● S82.55 Nondisplaced fracture of medial malleolus of left tibia

X● S82.56 Nondisplaced fracture of medial malleolus of unspecified tibia

● S82.6 Fracture of lateral malleolus
Excludes1 pilon fracture of distal tibia (S82.87-)
X● S82.61 Displaced fracture of lateral malleolus of right fibula
X● S82.62 Displaced fracture of lateral malleolus of left fibula
X● S82.63 Displaced fracture of lateral malleolus of unspecified fibula
X● S82.64 Nondisplaced fracture of lateral malleolus of right fibula
X● S82.65 Nondisplaced fracture of lateral malleolus of left fibula
X● S82.66 Nondisplaced fracture of lateral malleolus of unspecified fibula
● S82.8 Other fractures of lower leg
● S82.81 Torus fracture of upper end of fibula
The appropriate 7th character is to be added to all codes in subcategory S82.81

A	initial encounter for closed fracture
D	subsequent encounter for fracture with routine healing
G	subsequent encounter for fracture with delayed healing
K	subsequent encounter for fracture with nonunion
P	subsequent encounter for fracture with malunion
S	sequela

● S82.811 Torus fracture of upper end of right fibula
● S82.812 Torus fracture of upper end of left fibula
● S82.819 Torus fracture of upper end of unspecified fibula
● S82.82 Torus fracture of lower end of fibula
The appropriate 7th character is to be added to all codes in subcategory S82.82

A	initial encounter for closed fracture
D	subsequent encounter for fracture with routine healing
G	subsequent encounter for fracture with delayed healing
K	subsequent encounter for fracture with nonunion
P	subsequent encounter for fracture with malunion
S	sequela

● S82.821 Torus fracture of lower end of right fibula
● S82.822 Torus fracture of lower end of left fibula
● S82.829 Torus fracture of lower end of unspecified fibula
● S82.83 Other fracture of upper and lower end of fibula
● S82.831 Other fracture of upper and lower end of right fibula
● S82.832 Other fracture of upper and lower end of left fibula
● S82.839 Other fracture of upper and lower end of unspecified fibula
● S82.84 Bimalleolar fracture of lower leg
● S82.841 Displaced bimalleolar fracture of right lower leg
● S82.842 Displaced bimalleolar fracture of left lower leg
● S82.843 Displaced bimalleolar fracture of unspecified lower leg
● S82.844 Nondisplaced bimalleolar fracture of right lower leg
● S82.845 Nondisplaced bimalleolar fracture of left lower leg
● S82.846 Nondisplaced bimalleolar fracture of unspecified lower leg
● S82.85 Trimalleolar fracture of lower leg
● S82.851 Displaced trimalleolar fracture of right lower leg
● S82.852 Displaced trimalleolar fracture of left lower leg
● S82.853 Displaced trimalleolar fracture of unspecified lower leg
● S82.854 Nondisplaced trimalleolar fracture of right lower leg
● S82.855 Nondisplaced trimalleolar fracture of left lower leg
● S82.856 Nondisplaced trimalleolar fracture of unspecified lower leg
● S82.86 Maisonneuve's fracture
● S82.861 Displaced Maisonneuve's fracture of right leg
● S82.862 Displaced Maisonneuve's fracture of left leg
● S82.863 Displaced Maisonneuve's fracture of unspecified leg
● S82.864 Nondisplaced Maisonneuve's fracture of right leg
● S82.865 Nondisplaced Maisonneuve's fracture of left leg
● S82.866 Nondisplaced Maisonneuve's fracture of unspecified leg
● S82.87 Pilon fracture of tibia
● S82.871 Displaced pilon fracture of right tibia
● S82.872 Displaced pilon fracture of left tibia
● S82.873 Displaced pilon fracture of unspecified tibia
● S82.874 Nondisplaced pilon fracture of right tibia
● S82.875 Nondisplaced pilon fracture of left tibia
● S82.876 Nondisplaced pilon fracture of unspecified tibia
● S82.89 Other fractures of lower leg
Fracture of ankle NOS
● S82.891 Other fracture of right lower leg
● S82.892 Other fracture of left lower leg
● S82.899 Other fracture of unspecified lower leg
● S82.9 Unspecified fracture of lower leg
X● S82.90 Unspecified fracture of unspecified lower leg
X● S82.91 Unspecified fracture of right lower leg
X● S82.92 Unspecified fracture of left lower leg

CHAPTER 19 (S00-T88)

● S83 **Dislocation and sprain of joints and ligaments of knee**

Includes avulsion of joint or ligament of knee
laceration of cartilage, joint or ligament of knee
sprain of cartilage, joint or ligament of knee
traumatic hemarthrosis of joint or ligament of knee
traumatic rupture of joint or ligament of knee
traumatic subluxation of joint or ligament of knee
traumatic tear of joint or ligament of knee

Code also any associated open wound

Excludes1 derangement of patella (M22.Ø-M22.3)
injury of patellar ligament (tendon) (S76.1-)
internal derangement of knee (M23.-)
old dislocation of knee (M24.36)
pathological dislocation of knee (M24.36)
recurrent dislocation of knee (M22.Ø)

Excludes2 strain of muscle, fascia and tendon of lower leg (S86.-)

The appropriate 7th character is to be added to each code from category S83

A	initial encounter
D	subsequent encounter
S	sequela

● S83.Ø **Subluxation and dislocation of patella**
● S83.ØØ **Unspecified subluxation and dislocation of patella**
● S83.ØØ1 Unspecified subluxation of right patella
● S83.ØØ2 Unspecified subluxation of left patella
● S83.ØØ3 Unspecified subluxation of unspecified patella
● S83.ØØ4 Unspecified dislocation of right patella
● S83.ØØ5 Unspecified dislocation of left patella
● S83.ØØ6 Unspecified dislocation of unspecified patella
● S83.Ø1 **Lateral subluxation and dislocation of patella**
● S83.Ø11 Lateral subluxation of right patella
● S83.Ø12 Lateral subluxation of left patella
● S83.Ø13 Lateral subluxation of unspecified patella
● S83.Ø14 Lateral dislocation of right patella
● S83.Ø15 Lateral dislocation of left patella
● S83.Ø16 Lateral dislocation of unspecified patella
● S83.Ø9 **Other subluxation and dislocation of patella**
● S83.Ø91 Other subluxation of right patella
● S83.Ø92 Other subluxation of left patella
● S83.Ø93 Other subluxation of unspecified patella
● S83.Ø94 Other dislocation of right patella
● S83.Ø95 Other dislocation of left patella
● S83.Ø96 Other dislocation of unspecified patella
● S83.1 **Subluxation and dislocation of knee**
Excludes2 instability of knee prosthesis (T84.Ø22, T84.Ø23)
● S83.1Ø **Unspecified subluxation and dislocation of knee**
● S83.1Ø1 Unspecified subluxation of right knee
● S83.1Ø2 Unspecified subluxation of left knee
● S83.1Ø3 Unspecified subluxation of unspecified knee
● S83.1Ø4 Unspecified dislocation of right knee
● S83.1Ø5 Unspecified dislocation of left knee
● S83.1Ø6 Unspecified dislocation of unspecified knee
● S83.11 **Anterior subluxation and dislocation of proximal end of tibia**
Posterior subluxation and dislocation of distal end of femur
● S83.111 Anterior subluxation of proximal end of tibia, right knee
● S83.112 Anterior subluxation of proximal end of tibia, left knee
● S83.113 Anterior subluxation of proximal end of tibia, unspecified knee
● S83.114 Anterior dislocation of proximal end of tibia, right knee
● S83.115 Anterior dislocation of proximal end of tibia, left knee
● S83.116 Anterior dislocation of proximal end of tibia, unspecified knee
● S83.12 **Posterior subluxation and dislocation of proximal end of tibia**
Anterior dislocation of distal end of femur
● S83.121 Posterior subluxation of proximal end of tibia, right knee
● S83.122 Posterior subluxation of proximal end of tibia, left knee
● S83.123 Posterior subluxation of proximal end of tibia, unspecified knee
● S83.124 Posterior dislocation of proximal end of tibia, right knee
● S83.125 Posterior dislocation of proximal end of tibia, left knee
● S83.126 Posterior dislocation of proximal end of tibia, unspecified knee
● S83.13 **Medial subluxation and dislocation of proximal end of tibia**
● S83.131 Medial subluxation of proximal end of tibia, right knee
● S83.132 Medial subluxation of proximal end of tibia, left knee
● S83.133 Medial subluxation of proximal end of tibia, unspecified knee
● S83.134 Medial dislocation of proximal end of tibia, right knee
● S83.135 Medial dislocation of proximal end of tibia, left knee
● S83.136 Medial dislocation of proximal end of tibia, unspecified knee
● S83.14 **Lateral subluxation and dislocation of proximal end of tibia**
● S83.141 Lateral subluxation of proximal end of tibia, right knee
● S83.142 Lateral subluxation of proximal end of tibia, left knee
● S83.143 Lateral subluxation of proximal end of tibia, unspecified knee
● S83.144 Lateral dislocation of proximal end of tibia, right knee
● S83.145 Lateral dislocation of proximal end of tibia, left knee
● S83.146 Lateral dislocation of proximal end of tibia, unspecified knee
● S83.19 **Other subluxation and dislocation of knee**
● S83.191 Other subluxation of right knee
● S83.192 Other subluxation of left knee
● S83.193 Other subluxation of unspecified knee
● S83.194 Other dislocation of right knee
● S83.195 Other dislocation of left knee
● S83.196 Other dislocation of unspecified knee

● **S83.2**　**Tear of meniscus, current injury**
　　Excludes1　old bucket-handle tear (M23.2)
　● **S83.20**　Tear of unspecified meniscus, current injury
　　　　Tear of meniscus of knee NOS
　　● **S83.200**　Bucket-handle tear of unspecified meniscus, current injury, right knee
　　● **S83.201**　Bucket-handle tear of unspecified meniscus, current injury, left knee
　　● **S83.202**　Bucket-handle tear of unspecified meniscus, current injury, unspecified knee
　　● **S83.203**　Other tear of unspecified meniscus, current injury, right knee
　　● **S83.204**　Other tear of unspecified meniscus, current injury, left knee
　　● **S83.205**　Other tear of unspecified meniscus, current injury, unspecified knee
　　● **S83.206**　Unspecified tear of unspecified meniscus, current injury, right knee
　　● **S83.207**　Unspecified tear of unspecified meniscus, current injury, left knee
　　● **S83.209**　Unspecified tear of unspecified meniscus, current injury, unspecified knee
　● **S83.21**　Bucket-handle tear of medial meniscus, current injury
　　● **S83.211**　Bucket-handle tear of medial meniscus, current injury, right knee
　　● **S83.212**　Bucket-handle tear of medial meniscus, current injury, left knee
　　● **S83.219**　Bucket-handle tear of medial meniscus, current injury, unspecified knee
　● **S83.22**　Peripheral tear of medial meniscus, current injury
　　● **S83.221**　Peripheral tear of medial meniscus, current injury, right knee
　　● **S83.222**　Peripheral tear of medial meniscus, current injury, left knee
　　● **S83.229**　Peripheral tear of medial meniscus, current injury, unspecified knee
　● **S83.23**　Complex tear of medial meniscus, current injury
　　● **S83.231**　Complex tear of medial meniscus, current injury, right knee
　　● **S83.232**　Complex tear of medial meniscus, current injury, left knee
　　● **S83.239**　Complex tear of medial meniscus, current injury, unspecified knee
　● **S83.24**　Other tear of medial meniscus, current injury
　　● **S83.241**　Other tear of medial meniscus, current injury, right knee
　　● **S83.242**　Other tear of medial meniscus, current injury, left knee
　　● **S83.249**　Other tear of medial meniscus, current injury, unspecified knee
　● **S83.25**　Bucket-handle tear of lateral meniscus, current injury
　　● **S83.251**　Bucket-handle tear of lateral meniscus, current injury, right knee
　　● **S83.252**　Bucket-handle tear of lateral meniscus, current injury, left knee
　　● **S83.259**　Bucket-handle tear of lateral meniscus, current injury, unspecified knee

● **S83.26**　Peripheral tear of lateral meniscus, current injury
　● **S83.261**　Peripheral tear of lateral meniscus, current injury, right knee
　● **S83.262**　Peripheral tear of lateral meniscus, current injury, left knee
　● **S83.269**　Peripheral tear of lateral meniscus, current injury, unspecified knee
● **S83.27**　Complex tear of lateral meniscus, current injury
　● **S83.271**　Complex tear of lateral meniscus, current injury, right knee
　● **S83.272**　Complex tear of lateral meniscus, current injury, left knee
　● **S83.279**　Complex tear of lateral meniscus, current injury, unspecified knee
● **S83.28**　Other tear of lateral meniscus, current injury
　● **S83.281**　Other tear of lateral meniscus, current injury, right knee
　● **S83.282**　Other tear of lateral meniscus, current injury, left knee
　● **S83.289**　Other tear of lateral meniscus, current injury, unspecified knee
● **S83.3**　Tear of articular cartilage of knee, current
　X● **S83.30**　Tear of articular cartilage of unspecified knee, current
　X● **S83.31**　Tear of articular cartilage of right knee, current
　X● **S83.32**　Tear of articular cartilage of left knee, current
● **S83.4**　Sprain of collateral ligament of knee
　● **S83.40**　Sprain of unspecified collateral ligament of knee
　　● **S83.401**　Sprain of unspecified collateral ligament of right knee
　　● **S83.402**　Sprain of unspecified collateral ligament of left knee
　　● **S83.409**　Sprain of unspecified collateral ligament of unspecified knee
　● **S83.41**　Sprain of medial collateral ligament of knee
　　　Sprain of tibial collateral ligament
　　● **S83.411**　Sprain of medial collateral ligament of right knee
　　● **S83.412**　Sprain of medial collateral ligament of left knee
　　● **S83.419**　Sprain of medial collateral ligament of unspecified knee
　● **S83.42**　Sprain of lateral collateral ligament of knee
　　　Sprain of fibular collateral ligament
　　● **S83.421**　Sprain of lateral collateral ligament of right knee
　　● **S83.422**　Sprain of lateral collateral ligament of left knee
　　● **S83.429**　Sprain of lateral collateral ligament of unspecified knee
● **S83.5**　Sprain of cruciate ligament of knee
　● **S83.50**　Sprain of unspecified cruciate ligament of knee
　　● **S83.501**　Sprain of unspecified cruciate ligament of right knee
　　● **S83.502**　Sprain of unspecified cruciate ligament of left knee
　　● **S83.509**　Sprain of unspecified cruciate ligament of unspecified knee
　● **S83.51**　Sprain of anterior cruciate ligament of knee
　　● **S83.511**　Sprain of anterior cruciate ligament of right knee
　　● **S83.512**　Sprain of anterior cruciate ligament of left knee
　　● **S83.519**　Sprain of anterior cruciate ligament of unspecified knee

CHAPTER 19 (S00-T88)

- S83.52 Sprain of posterior cruciate ligament of knee
  - S83.521 Sprain of posterior cruciate ligament of right knee
  - S83.522 Sprain of posterior cruciate ligament of left knee
  - S83.529 Sprain of posterior cruciate ligament of unspecified knee
- S83.6 Sprain of the superior tibiofibular joint and ligament
  - X S83.60 Sprain of the superior tibiofibular joint and ligament, unspecified knee
  - X S83.61 Sprain of the superior tibiofibular joint and ligament, right knee
  - X S83.62 Sprain of the superior tibiofibular joint and ligament, left knee
- S83.8 Sprain of other specified parts of knee
  - S83.8X Sprain of other specified parts of knee
    - S83.8X1 Sprain of other specified parts of right knee
    - S83.8X2 Sprain of other specified parts of left knee
    - S83.8X9 Sprain of other specified parts of unspecified knee
- S83.9 Sprain of unspecified site of knee
  - X S83.90 Sprain of unspecified site of unspecified knee
  - X S83.91 Sprain of unspecified site of right knee
  - X S83.92 Sprain of unspecified site of left knee

S84 Injury of nerves at lower leg level

Code also any associated open wound (S81.-)

Excludes2 injury of nerves at ankle and foot level (S94.-)

The appropriate 7th character is to be added to each code from category S84

A	initial encounter
D	subsequent encounter
S	sequela

- S84.0 Injury of tibial nerve at lower leg level
  - X S84.00 Injury of tibial nerve at lower leg level, unspecified leg
  - X S84.01 Injury of tibial nerve at lower leg level, right leg
  - X S84.02 Injury of tibial nerve at lower leg level, left leg
- S84.1 Injury of peroneal nerve at lower leg level
  - X S84.10 Injury of peroneal nerve at lower leg level, unspecified leg
  - X S84.11 Injury of peroneal nerve at lower leg level, right leg
  - X S84.12 Injury of peroneal nerve at lower leg level, left leg
- S84.2 Injury of cutaneous sensory nerve at lower leg level
  - X S84.20 Injury of cutaneous sensory nerve at lower leg level, unspecified leg
  - X S84.21 Injury of cutaneous sensory nerve at lower leg level, right leg
  - X S84.22 Injury of cutaneous sensory nerve at lower leg level, left leg
- S84.8 Injury of other nerves at lower leg level
  - S84.80 Injury of other nerves at lower leg level
    - S84.801 Injury of other nerves at lower leg level, right leg
    - S84.802 Injury of other nerves at lower leg level, left leg
    - S84.809 Injury of other nerves at lower leg level, unspecified leg
- S84.9 Injury of unspecified nerve at lower leg level
  - X S84.90 Injury of unspecified nerve at lower leg level, unspecified leg
  - X S84.91 Injury of unspecified nerve at lower leg level, right leg
  - X S84.92 Injury of unspecified nerve at lower leg level, left leg

S85 Injury of blood vessels at lower leg level

Code also any associated open wound (S81.-)

Excludes2 injury of blood vessels at ankle and foot level (S95.-)

The appropriate 7th character is to be added to each code from category S85

A	initial encounter
D	subsequent encounter
S	sequela

- S85.0 Injury of popliteal artery
  - S85.00 Unspecified injury of popliteal artery
    - S85.001 Unspecified injury of popliteal artery, right leg
    - S85.002 Unspecified injury of popliteal artery, left leg
    - S85.009 Unspecified injury of popliteal artery, unspecified leg
  - S85.01 Laceration of popliteal artery
    - S85.011 Laceration of popliteal artery, right leg
    - S85.012 Laceration of popliteal artery, left leg
    - S85.019 Laceration of popliteal artery, unspecified leg
  - S85.09 Other specified injury of popliteal artery
    - S85.091 Other specified injury of popliteal artery, right leg
    - S85.092 Other specified injury of popliteal artery, left leg
    - S85.099 Other specified injury of popliteal artery, unspecified leg
- S85.1 Injury of tibial artery
  - S85.10 Unspecified injury of unspecified tibial artery
    Injury of tibial artery NOS
    - S85.101 Unspecified injury of unspecified tibial artery, right leg
    - S85.102 Unspecified injury of unspecified tibial artery, left leg
    - S85.109 Unspecified injury of unspecified tibial artery, unspecified leg
  - S85.11 Laceration of unspecified tibial artery
    - S85.111 Laceration of unspecified tibial artery, right leg
    - S85.112 Laceration of unspecified tibial artery, left leg
    - S85.119 Laceration of unspecified tibial artery, unspecified leg
  - S85.12 Other specified injury of unspecified tibial artery
    - S85.121 Other specified injury of unspecified tibial artery, right leg
    - S85.122 Other specified injury of unspecified tibial artery, left leg
    - S85.129 Other specified injury of unspecified tibial artery, unspecified leg
  - S85.13 Unspecified injury of anterior tibial artery
    - S85.131 Unspecified injury of anterior tibial artery, right leg
    - S85.132 Unspecified injury of anterior tibial artery, left leg
    - S85.139 Unspecified injury of anterior tibial artery, unspecified leg
  - S85.14 Laceration of anterior tibial artery
    - S85.141 Laceration of anterior tibial artery, right leg
    - S85.142 Laceration of anterior tibial artery, left leg
    - S85.149 Laceration of anterior tibial artery, unspecified leg

- S85.15 Other specified injury of anterior tibial artery
  - S85.151 Other specified injury of anterior tibial artery, right leg
  - S85.152 Other specified injury of anterior tibial artery, left leg
  - S85.159 Other specified injury of anterior tibial artery, unspecified leg
- S85.16 Unspecified injury of posterior tibial artery
  - S85.161 Unspecified injury of posterior tibial artery, right leg
  - S85.162 Unspecified injury of posterior tibial artery, left leg
  - S85.169 Unspecified injury of posterior tibial artery, unspecified leg
- S85.17 Laceration of posterior tibial artery
  - S85.171 Laceration of posterior tibial artery, right leg
  - S85.172 Laceration of posterior tibial artery, left leg
  - S85.179 Laceration of posterior tibial artery, unspecified leg
- S85.18 Other specified injury of posterior tibial artery
  - S85.181 Other specified injury of posterior tibial artery, right leg
  - S85.182 Other specified injury of posterior tibial artery, left leg
  - S85.189 Other specified injury of posterior tibial artery, unspecified leg

S85.2 Injury of peroneal artery
- S85.20 Unspecified injury of peroneal artery
  - S85.201 Unspecified injury of peroneal artery, right leg
  - S85.202 Unspecified injury of peroneal artery, left leg
  - S85.209 Unspecified injury of peroneal artery, unspecified leg
- S85.21 Laceration of peroneal artery
  - S85.211 Laceration of peroneal artery, right leg
  - S85.212 Laceration of peroneal artery, left leg
  - S85.219 Laceration of peroneal artery, unspecified leg
- S85.29 Other specified injury of peroneal artery
  - S85.291 Other specified injury of peroneal artery, right leg
  - S85.292 Other specified injury of peroneal artery, left leg
  - S85.299 Other specified injury of peroneal artery, unspecified leg

S85.3 Injury of greater saphenous vein at lower leg level
Injury of greater saphenous vein NOS
Injury of saphenous vein NOS
- S85.30 Unspecified injury of greater saphenous vein at lower leg level
  - S85.301 Unspecified injury of greater saphenous vein at lower leg level, right leg
  - S85.302 Unspecified injury of greater saphenous vein at lower leg level, left leg
  - S85.309 Unspecified injury of greater saphenous vein at lower leg level, unspecified leg
- S85.31 Laceration of greater saphenous vein at lower leg level
  - S85.311 Laceration of greater saphenous vein at lower leg level, right leg
  - S85.312 Laceration of greater saphenous vein at lower leg level, left leg
  - S85.319 Laceration of greater saphenous vein at lower leg level, unspecified leg
- S85.39 Other specified injury of greater saphenous vein at lower leg level
  - S85.391 Other specified injury of greater saphenous vein at lower leg level, right leg
  - S85.392 Other specified injury of greater saphenous vein at lower leg level, left leg
  - S85.399 Other specified injury of greater saphenous vein at lower leg level, unspecified leg

S85.4 Injury of lesser saphenous vein at lower leg level
- S85.40 Unspecified injury of lesser saphenous vein at lower leg level
  - S85.401 Unspecified injury of lesser saphenous vein at lower leg level, right leg
  - S85.402 Unspecified injury of lesser saphenous vein at lower leg level, left leg
  - S85.409 Unspecified injury of lesser saphenous vein at lower leg level, unspecified leg
- S85.41 Laceration of lesser saphenous vein at lower leg level
  - S85.411 Laceration of lesser saphenous vein at lower leg level, right leg
  - S85.412 Laceration of lesser saphenous vein at lower leg level, left leg
  - S85.419 Laceration of lesser saphenous vein at lower leg level, unspecified leg
- S85.49 Other specified injury of lesser saphenous vein at lower leg level
  - S85.491 Other specified injury of lesser saphenous vein at lower leg level, right leg
  - S85.492 Other specified injury of lesser saphenous vein at lower leg level, left leg
  - S85.499 Other specified injury of lesser saphenous vein at lower leg level, unspecified leg

S85.5 Injury of popliteal vein
- S85.50 Unspecified injury of popliteal vein
  - S85.501 Unspecified injury of popliteal vein, right leg
  - S85.502 Unspecified injury of popliteal vein, left leg
  - S85.509 Unspecified injury of popliteal vein, unspecified leg
- S85.51 Laceration of popliteal vein
  - S85.511 Laceration of popliteal vein, right leg
  - S85.512 Laceration of popliteal vein, left leg
  - S85.519 Laceration of popliteal vein, unspecified leg

- S85.59 Other specified injury of popliteal vein
  - S85.591 Other specified injury of popliteal vein, right leg
  - S85.592 Other specified injury of popliteal vein, left leg
  - S85.599 Other specified injury of popliteal vein, unspecified leg
- S85.8 Injury of other blood vessels at lower leg level
  - S85.80 Unspecified injury of other blood vessels at lower leg level
    - S85.801 Unspecified injury of other blood vessels at lower leg level, right leg
    - S85.802 Unspecified injury of other blood vessels at lower leg level, left leg
    - S85.809 Unspecified injury of other blood vessels at lower leg level, unspecified leg
  - S85.81 Laceration of other blood vessels at lower leg level
    - S85.811 Laceration of other blood vessels at lower leg level, right leg
    - S85.812 Laceration of other blood vessels at lower leg level, left leg
    - S85.819 Laceration of other blood vessels at lower leg level, unspecified leg
  - S85.89 Other specified injury of other blood vessels at lower leg level
    - S85.891 Other specified injury of other blood vessels at lower leg level, right leg
    - S85.892 Other specified injury of other blood vessels at lower leg level, left leg
    - S85.899 Other specified injury of other blood vessels at lower leg level, unspecified leg
- S85.9 Injury of unspecified blood vessel at lower leg level
  - S85.90 Unspecified injury of unspecified blood vessel at lower leg level
    - S85.901 Unspecified injury of unspecified blood vessel at lower leg level, right leg
    - S85.902 Unspecified injury of unspecified blood vessel at lower leg level, left leg
    - S85.909 Unspecified injury of unspecified blood vessel at lower leg level, unspecified leg
  - S85.91 Laceration of unspecified blood vessel at lower leg level
    - S85.911 Laceration of unspecified blood vessel at lower leg level, right leg
    - S85.912 Laceration of unspecified blood vessel at lower leg level, left leg
    - S85.919 Laceration of unspecified blood vessel at lower leg level, unspecified leg
  - S85.99 Other specified injury of unspecified blood vessel at lower leg level
    - S85.991 Other specified injury of unspecified blood vessel at lower leg level, right leg
    - S85.992 Other specified injury of unspecified blood vessel at lower leg level, left leg
    - S85.999 Other specified injury of unspecified blood vessel at lower leg level, unspecified leg

S86 Injury of muscle, fascia and tendon at lower leg level

Code also any associated open wound (S81.-)

Excludes2 injury of muscle, fascia and tendon at ankle (S96.-)
injury of patellar ligament (tendon) (S76.1-)
sprain of joints and ligaments of knee (S83.-)

The appropriate 7th character is to be added to each code from category S86

A	initial encounter
D	subsequent encounter
S	sequela

- S86.0 Injury of Achilles tendon
  - S86.00 Unspecified injury of Achilles tendon
    - S86.001 Unspecified injury of right Achilles tendon
    - S86.002 Unspecified injury of left Achilles tendon
    - S86.009 Unspecified injury of unspecified Achilles tendon
  - S86.01 Strain of Achilles tendon
    - S86.011 Strain of right Achilles tendon
    - S86.012 Strain of left Achilles tendon
    - S86.019 Strain of unspecified Achilles tendon
  - S86.02 Laceration of Achilles tendon
    - S86.021 Laceration of right Achilles tendon
    - S86.022 Laceration of left Achilles tendon
    - S86.029 Laceration of unspecified Achilles tendon
  - S86.09 Other specified injury of Achilles tendon
    - S86.091 Other specified injury of right Achilles tendon
    - S86.092 Other specified injury of left Achilles tendon
    - S86.099 Other specified injury of unspecified Achilles tendon
- S86.1 Injury of other muscle(s) and tendon(s) of posterior muscle group at lower leg level
  - S86.10 Unspecified injury of other muscle(s) and tendon(s) of posterior muscle group at lower leg level
    - S86.101 Unspecified injury of other muscle(s) and tendon(s) of posterior muscle group at lower leg level, right leg
    - S86.102 Unspecified injury of other muscle(s) and tendon(s) of posterior muscle group at lower leg level, left leg
    - S86.109 Unspecified injury of other muscle(s) and tendon(s) of posterior muscle group at lower leg level, unspecified leg
  - S86.11 Strain of other muscle(s) and tendon(s) of posterior muscle group at lower leg level
    - S86.111 Strain of other muscle(s) and tendon(s) of posterior muscle group at lower leg level, right leg
    - S86.112 Strain of other muscle(s) and tendon(s) of posterior muscle group at lower leg level, left leg
    - S86.119 Strain of other muscle(s) and tendon(s) of posterior muscle group at lower leg level, unspecified leg

CHAPTER 19 (S00-T88)

◄ New ⟸ Revised ~~deleted~~ Deleted OGCR Official Guidelines X Assign placeholder X ● Use Additional Character(s)
Excludes 1 Excludes 2 Includes Use additional Code first Code also Unspecified

● S86.12 Laceration of other muscle(s) and tendon(s) of posterior muscle group at lower leg level
● S86.121 Laceration of other muscle(s) and tendon(s) of posterior muscle group at lower leg level, right leg
● S86.122 Laceration of other muscle(s) and tendon(s) of posterior muscle group at lower leg level, left leg
● S86.129 Laceration of other muscle(s) and tendon(s) of posterior muscle group at lower leg level, unspecified leg
● S86.19 Other injury of other muscle(s) and tendon(s) of posterior muscle group at lower leg level
● S86.191 Other injury of other muscle(s) and tendon(s) of posterior muscle group at lower leg level, right leg
● S86.192 Other injury of other muscle(s) and tendon(s) of posterior muscle group at lower leg level, left leg
● S86.199 Other injury of other muscle(s) and tendon(s) of posterior muscle group at lower leg level, unspecified leg
● S86.2 Injury of muscle(s) and tendon(s) of anterior muscle group at lower leg level
● S86.20 Unspecified injury of muscle(s) and tendon(s) of anterior muscle group at lower leg level
● S86.201 Unspecified injury of muscle(s) and tendon(s) of anterior muscle group at lower leg level, right leg
● S86.202 Unspecified injury of muscle(s) and tendon(s) of anterior muscle group at lower leg level, left leg
● S86.209 Unspecified injury of muscle(s) and tendon(s) of anterior muscle group at lower leg level, unspecified leg
● S86.21 Strain of muscle(s) and tendon(s) of anterior muscle group at lower leg level
● S86.211 Strain of muscle(s) and tendon(s) of anterior muscle group at lower leg level, right leg
● S86.212 Strain of muscle(s) and tendon(s) of anterior muscle group at lower leg level, left leg
● S86.219 Strain of muscle(s) and tendon(s) of anterior muscle group at lower leg level, unspecified leg
● S86.22 Laceration of muscle(s) and tendon(s) of anterior muscle group at lower leg level
● S86.221 Laceration of muscle(s) and tendon(s) of anterior muscle group at lower leg level, right leg
● S86.222 Laceration of muscle(s) and tendon(s) of anterior muscle group at lower leg level, left leg
● S86.229 Laceration of muscle(s) and tendon(s) of anterior muscle group at lower leg level, unspecified leg
● S86.29 Other injury of muscle(s) and tendon(s) of anterior muscle group at lower leg level
● S86.291 Other injury of muscle(s) and tendon(s) of anterior muscle group at lower leg level, right leg
● S86.292 Other injury of muscle(s) and tendon(s) of anterior muscle group at lower leg level, left leg
● S86.299 Other injury of muscle(s) and tendon(s) of anterior muscle group at lower leg level, unspecified leg
● S86.3 Injury of muscle(s) and tendon(s) of peroneal muscle group at lower leg level
● S86.30 Unspecified injury of muscle(s) and tendon(s) of peroneal muscle group at lower leg level
● S86.301 Unspecified injury of muscle(s) and tendon(s) of peroneal muscle group at lower leg level, right leg
● S86.302 Unspecified injury of muscle(s) and tendon(s) of peroneal muscle group at lower leg level, left leg
● S86.309 Unspecified injury of muscle(s) and tendon(s) of peroneal muscle group at lower leg level, unspecified leg
● S86.31 Strain of muscle(s) and tendon(s) of peroneal muscle group at lower leg level
● S86.311 Strain of muscle(s) and tendon(s) of peroneal muscle group at lower leg level, right leg
● S86.312 Strain of muscle(s) and tendon(s) of peroneal muscle group at lower leg level, left leg
● S86.319 Strain of muscle(s) and tendon(s) of peroneal muscle group at lower leg level, unspecified leg
● S86.32 Laceration of muscle(s) and tendon(s) of peroneal muscle group at lower leg level
● S86.321 Laceration of muscle(s) and tendon(s) of peroneal muscle group at lower leg level, right leg
● S86.322 Laceration of muscle(s) and tendon(s) of peroneal muscle group at lower leg level, left leg
● S86.329 Laceration of muscle(s) and tendon(s) of peroneal muscle group at lower leg level, unspecified leg
● S86.39 Other injury of muscle(s) and tendon(s) of peroneal muscle group at lower leg level
● S86.391 Other injury of muscle(s) and tendon(s) of peroneal muscle group at lower leg level, right leg
● S86.392 Other injury of muscle(s) and tendon(s) of peroneal muscle group at lower leg level, left leg
● S86.399 Other injury of muscle(s) and tendon(s) of peroneal muscle group at lower leg level, unspecified leg
● S86.8 Injury of other muscles and tendons at lower leg level
● S86.80 Unspecified injury of other muscles and tendons at lower leg level
● S86.801 Unspecified injury of other muscle(s) and tendon(s) at lower leg level, right leg
● S86.802 Unspecified injury of other muscle(s) and tendon(s) at lower leg level, left leg
● S86.809 Unspecified injury of other muscle(s) and tendon(s) at lower leg level, unspecified leg
● S86.81 Strain of other muscles and tendons at lower leg level
● S86.811 Strain of other muscle(s) and tendon(s) at lower leg level, right leg
● S86.812 Strain of other muscle(s) and tendon(s) at lower leg level, left leg
● S86.819 Strain of other muscle(s) and tendon(s) at lower leg level, unspecified leg

● S86.82 Laceration of other muscles and tendons at lower leg level
● S86.821 Laceration of other muscle(s) and tendon(s) at lower leg level, right leg
● S86.822 Laceration of other muscle(s) and tendon(s) at lower leg level, left leg
● S86.829 Laceration of other muscle(s) and tendon(s) at lower leg level, unspecified leg
● S86.89 Other injury of other muscles and tendons at lower leg level
● S86.891 Other injury of other muscle(s) and tendon(s) at lower leg level, right leg
● S86.892 Other injury of other muscle(s) and tendon(s) at lower leg level, left leg
● S86.899 Other injury of other muscle(s) and tendon(s) at lower leg level, unspecified leg
● S86.9 Injury of unspecified muscle and tendon at lower leg level
● S86.90 Unspecified injury of unspecified muscle and tendon at lower leg level
● S86.901 Unspecified injury of unspecified muscle(s) and tendon(s) at lower leg level, right leg
● S86.902 Unspecified injury of unspecified muscle(s) and tendon(s) at lower leg level, left leg
● S86.909 Unspecified injury of unspecified muscle(s) and tendon(s) at lower leg level, unspecified leg
● S86.91 Strain of unspecified muscle and tendon at lower leg level
● S86.911 Strain of unspecified muscle(s) and tendon(s) at lower leg level, right leg
● S86.912 Strain of unspecified muscle(s) and tendon(s) at lower leg level, left leg
● S86.919 Strain of unspecified muscle(s) and tendon(s) at lower leg level, unspecified leg
● S86.92 Laceration of unspecified muscle and tendon at lower leg level
● S86.921 Laceration of unspecified muscle(s) and tendon(s) at lower leg level, right leg
● S86.922 Laceration of unspecified muscle(s) and tendon(s) at lower leg level, left leg
● S86.929 Laceration of unspecified muscle(s) and tendon(s) at lower leg level, unspecified leg
● S86.99 Other injury of unspecified muscle and tendon at lower leg level
● S86.991 Other injury of unspecified muscle(s) and tendon(s) at lower leg level, right leg
● S86.992 Other injury of unspecified muscle(s) and tendon(s) at lower leg level, left leg
● S86.999 Other injury of unspecified muscle(s) and tendon(s) at lower leg level, unspecified leg

● S87 Crushing injury of lower leg

Use additional code(s) for all associated injuries

Excludes2 crushing injury of ankle and foot (S97.-)

The appropriate 7th character is to be added to each code from category S87

A	initial encounter
D	subsequent encounter
S	sequela

● S87.0 Crushing injury of knee
X● S87.00 Crushing injury of unspecified knee
X● S87.01 Crushing injury of right knee
X● S87.02 Crushing injury of left knee
● S87.8 Crushing injury of lower leg
X● S87.80 Crushing injury of unspecified lower leg
X● S87.81 Crushing injury of right lower leg
X● S87.82 Crushing injury of left lower leg

● S88 Traumatic amputation of lower leg

An amputation not identified as partial or complete should be coded to complete

Excludes1 traumatic amputation of ankle and foot (S98.-)

The appropriate 7th character is to be added to each code from category S88

A	initial encounter
D	subsequent encounter
S	sequela

● S88.0 Traumatic amputation at knee level
● S88.01 Complete traumatic amputation at knee level
● S88.011 Complete traumatic amputation at knee level, right lower leg
● S88.012 Complete traumatic amputation at knee level, left lower leg
● S88.019 Complete traumatic amputation at knee level, unspecified lower leg
● S88.02 Partial traumatic amputation at knee level
● S88.021 Partial traumatic amputation at knee level, right lower leg
● S88.022 Partial traumatic amputation at knee level, left lower leg
● S88.029 Partial traumatic amputation at knee level, unspecified lower leg
● S88.1 Traumatic amputation at level between knee and ankle
● S88.11 Complete traumatic amputation at level between knee and ankle
● S88.111 Complete traumatic amputation at level between knee and ankle, right lower leg
● S88.112 Complete traumatic amputation at level between knee and ankle, left lower leg
● S88.119 Complete traumatic amputation at level between knee and ankle, unspecified lower leg
● S88.12 Partial traumatic amputation at level between knee and ankle
● S88.121 Partial traumatic amputation at level between knee and ankle, right lower leg
● S88.122 Partial traumatic amputation at level between knee and ankle, left lower leg
● S88.129 Partial traumatic amputation at level between knee and ankle, unspecified lower leg

S88.9 Traumatic amputation of lower leg, level unspecified

S88.91 Complete traumatic amputation of lower leg, level unspecified

S88.911 Complete traumatic amputation of right lower leg, level unspecified

S88.912 Complete traumatic amputation of left lower leg, level unspecified

S88.919 Complete traumatic amputation of unspecified lower leg, level unspecified

S88.92 Partial traumatic amputation of lower leg, level unspecified

S88.921 Partial traumatic amputation of right lower leg, level unspecified

S88.922 Partial traumatic amputation of left lower leg, level unspecified

S88.929 Partial traumatic amputation of unspecified lower leg, level unspecified

S89 Other and unspecified injuries of lower leg

Note: A fracture not indicated as open or closed should be coded to closed

Excludes2 other and unspecified injuries of ankle and foot (S99.-)

The appropriate 7th character is to be added to each code from subcategories S89.0, S89.1, S89.2, and S89.3

A	initial encounter for closed fracture
D	subsequent encounter for fracture with routine healing
G	subsequent encounter for fracture with delayed healing
K	subsequent encounter for fracture with nonunion
P	subsequent encounter for fracture with malunion
S	sequela

S89.0 Physeal fracture of upper end of tibia

S89.00 Unspecified physeal fracture of upper end of tibia

S89.001 Unspecified physeal fracture of upper end of right tibia

S89.002 Unspecified physeal fracture of upper end of left tibia

S89.009 Unspecified physeal fracture of upper end of unspecified tibia

S89.01 Salter-Harris Type I physeal fracture of upper end of tibia

S89.011 Salter-Harris Type I physeal fracture of upper end of right tibia

S89.012 Salter-Harris Type I physeal fracture of upper end of left tibia

S89.019 Salter-Harris Type I physeal fracture of upper end of unspecified tibia

S89.02 Salter-Harris Type II physeal fracture of upper end of tibia

S89.021 Salter-Harris Type II physeal fracture of upper end of right tibia

S89.022 Salter-Harris Type II physeal fracture of upper end of left tibia

S89.029 Salter-Harris Type II physeal fracture of upper end of unspecified tibia

S89.03 Salter-Harris Type III physeal fracture of upper end of tibia

S89.031 Salter-Harris Type III physeal fracture of upper end of right tibia

S89.032 Salter-Harris Type III physeal fracture of upper end of left tibia

S89.039 Salter-Harris Type III physeal fracture of upper end of unspecified tibia

S89.04 Salter-Harris Type IV physeal fracture of upper end of tibia

S89.041 Salter-Harris Type IV physeal fracture of upper end of right tibia

S89.042 Salter-Harris Type IV physeal fracture of upper end of left tibia

S89.049 Salter-Harris Type IV physeal fracture of upper end of unspecified tibia

S89.09 Other physeal fracture of upper end of tibia

S89.091 Other physeal fracture of upper end of right tibia

S89.092 Other physeal fracture of upper end of left tibia

S89.099 Other physeal fracture of upper end of unspecified tibia

S89.1 Physeal fracture of lower end of tibia

S89.10 Unspecified physeal fracture of lower end of tibia

S89.101 Unspecified physeal fracture of lower end of right tibia

S89.102 Unspecified physeal fracture of lower end of left tibia

S89.109 Unspecified physeal fracture of lower end of unspecified tibia

S89.11 Salter-Harris Type I physeal fracture of lower end of tibia

S89.111 Salter-Harris Type I physeal fracture of lower end of right tibia

S89.112 Salter-Harris Type I physeal fracture of lower end of left tibia

S89.119 Salter-Harris Type I physeal fracture of lower end of unspecified tibia

S89.12 Salter-Harris Type II physeal fracture of lower end of tibia

S89.121 Salter-Harris Type II physeal fracture of lower end of right tibia

S89.122 Salter-Harris Type II physeal fracture of lower end of left tibia

S89.129 Salter-Harris Type II physeal fracture of lower end of unspecified tibia

S89.13 Salter-Harris Type III physeal fracture of lower end of tibia

Excludes1 fracture of medial malleolus (adult) (S82.5-)

S89.131 Salter-Harris Type III physeal fracture of lower end of right tibia

S89.132 Salter-Harris Type III physeal fracture of lower end of left tibia

S89.139 Salter-Harris Type III physeal fracture of lower end of unspecified tibia

S89.14 Salter-Harris Type IV physeal fracture of lower end of tibia

Excludes1 fracture of medial malleolus (adult) (S82.5-)

S89.141 Salter-Harris Type IV physeal fracture of lower end of right tibia

S89.142 Salter-Harris Type IV physeal fracture of lower end of left tibia

S89.149 Salter-Harris Type IV physeal fracture of lower end of unspecified tibia

S89.19 Other physeal fracture of lower end of tibia

S89.191 Other physeal fracture of lower end of right tibia

S89.192 Other physeal fracture of lower end of left tibia

S89.199 Other physeal fracture of lower end of unspecified tibia

● S89.2 Physeal fracture of upper end of fibula
● S89.20 Unspecified physeal fracture of upper end of fibula
● S89.201 Unspecified physeal fracture of upper end of right fibula
● S89.202 Unspecified physeal fracture of upper end of left fibula
● S89.209 Unspecified physeal fracture of upper end of unspecified fibula
● S89.21 Salter-Harris Type I physeal fracture of upper end of fibula
● S89.211 Salter-Harris Type I physeal fracture of upper end of right fibula
● S89.212 Salter-Harris Type I physeal fracture of upper end of left fibula
● S89.219 Salter-Harris Type I physeal fracture of upper end of unspecified fibula
● S89.22 Salter-Harris Type II physeal fracture of upper end of fibula
● S89.221 Salter-Harris Type II physeal fracture of upper end of right fibula
● S89.222 Salter-Harris Type II physeal fracture of upper end of left fibula
● S89.229 Salter-Harris Type II physeal fracture of upper end of unspecified fibula
● S89.29 Other physeal fracture of upper end of fibula
● S89.291 Other physeal fracture of upper end of right fibula
● S89.292 Other physeal fracture of upper end of left fibula
● S89.299 Other physeal fracture of upper end of unspecified fibula
● S89.3 Physeal fracture of lower end of fibula
● S89.30 Unspecified physeal fracture of lower end of fibula
● S89.301 Unspecified physeal fracture of lower end of right fibula
● S89.302 Unspecified physeal fracture of lower end of left fibula
● S89.309 Unspecified physeal fracture of lower end of unspecified fibula
● S89.31 Salter-Harris Type I physeal fracture of lower end of fibula
● S89.311 Salter-Harris Type I physeal fracture of lower end of right fibula
● S89.312 Salter-Harris Type I physeal fracture of lower end of left fibula
● S89.319 Salter-Harris Type I physeal fracture of lower end of unspecified fibula
● S89.32 Salter-Harris Type II physeal fracture of lower end of fibula
● S89.321 Salter-Harris Type II physeal fracture of lower end of right fibula
● S89.322 Salter-Harris Type II physeal fracture of lower end of left fibula
● S89.329 Salter-Harris Type II physeal fracture of lower end of unspecified fibula
● S89.39 Other physeal fracture of lower end of fibula
● S89.391 Other physeal fracture of lower end of right fibula
● S89.392 Other physeal fracture of lower end of left fibula
● S89.399 Other physeal fracture of lower end of unspecified fibula
● S89.8 Other specified injuries of lower leg

The appropriate 7th character is to be added to each code in subcategory S89.8

A initial encounter
D subsequent encounter
S sequela

X● S89.80 Other specified injuries of unspecified lower leg
X● S89.81 Other specified injuries of right lower leg
X● S89.82 Other specified injuries of left lower leg
● S89.9 Unspecified injury of lower leg

The appropriate 7th character is to be added to each code in subcategory S89.9

A initial encounter
D subsequent encounter
S sequela

X● S89.90 Unspecified injury of unspecified lower leg
X● S89.91 Unspecified injury of right lower leg
X● S89.92 Unspecified injury of left lower leg

INJURIES TO THE ANKLE AND FOOT (S90-S99)

Excludes2 burns and corrosions (T20-T32)
fracture of ankle and malleolus (S82.-)
frostbite (T33-T34)
insect bite or sting, venomous (T63.4)

● S90 Superficial injury of ankle, foot and toes

The appropriate 7th character is to be added to each code from category S90

A initial encounter
D subsequent encounter
S sequela

● S90.0 Contusion of ankle
X● S90.00 Contusion of unspecified ankle
X● S90.01 Contusion of right ankle
X● S90.02 Contusion of left ankle
● S90.1 Contusion of toe without damage to nail
● S90.11 Contusion of great toe without damage to nail
● S90.111 Contusion of right great toe without damage to nail
● S90.112 Contusion of left great toe without damage to nail
● S90.119 Contusion of unspecified great toe without damage to nail
● S90.12 Contusion of lesser toe without damage to nail
● S90.121 Contusion of right lesser toe(s) without damage to nail
● S90.122 Contusion of left lesser toe(s) without damage to nail
● S90.129 Contusion of unspecified lesser toe(s) without damage to nail
Contusion of toe NOS
● S90.2 Contusion of toe with damage to nail
● S90.21 Contusion of great toe with damage to nail
● S90.211 Contusion of right great toe with damage to nail
● S90.212 Contusion of left great toe with damage to nail
● S90.219 Contusion of unspecified great toe with damage to nail

● S90.22   Contusion of lesser toe with damage to nail
    ● S90.221   Contusion of right lesser toe(s) with damage to nail
    ● S90.222   Contusion of left lesser toe(s) with damage to nail
    ● S90.229   Contusion of unspecified lesser toe(s) with damage to nail
● S90.3   Contusion of foot
    Excludes2   contusion of toes (S90.1-, S90.2-)
X ● S90.30   Contusion of unspecified foot
         Contusion of foot NOS
X ● S90.31   Contusion of right foot
X ● S90.32   Contusion of left foot
● S90.4   Other superficial injuries of toe
    ● S90.41   Abrasion of toe
       ● S90.411   Abrasion, right great toe
       ● S90.412   Abrasion, left great toe
       ● S90.413   Abrasion, unspecified great toe
       ● S90.414   Abrasion, right lesser toe(s)
       ● S90.415   Abrasion, left lesser toe(s)
       ● S90.416   Abrasion, unspecified lesser toe(s)
    ● S90.42   Blister (nonthermal) of toe
       ● S90.421   Blister (nonthermal), right great toe
       ● S90.422   Blister (nonthermal), left great toe
       ● S90.423   Blister (nonthermal), unspecified great toe
       ● S90.424   Blister (nonthermal), right lesser toe(s)
       ● S90.425   Blister (nonthermal), left lesser toe(s)
       ● S90.426   Blister (nonthermal), unspecified lesser toe(s)
    ● S90.44   External constriction of toe
        Hair tourniquet syndrome of toe
       ● S90.441   External constriction, right great toe
       ● S90.442   External constriction, left great toe
       ● S90.443   External constriction, unspecified great toe
       ● S90.444   External constriction, right lesser toe(s)
       ● S90.445   External constriction, left lesser toe(s)
       ● S90.446   External constriction, unspecified lesser toe(s)
    ● S90.45   Superficial foreign body of toe
        Splinter in the toe
       ● S90.451   Superficial foreign body, right great toe
       ● S90.452   Superficial foreign body, left great toe
       ● S90.453   Superficial foreign body, unspecified great toe
       ● S90.454   Superficial foreign body, right lesser toe(s)
       ● S90.455   Superficial foreign body, left lesser toe(s)
       ● S90.456   Superficial foreign body, unspecified lesser toe(s)
    ● S90.46   Insect bite (nonvenomous) of toe
       ● S90.461   Insect bite (nonvenomous), right great toe
       ● S90.462   Insect bite (nonvenomous), left great toe
       ● S90.463   Insect bite (nonvenomous), unspecified great toe
       ● S90.464   Insect bite (nonvenomous), right lesser toe(s)
       ● S90.465   Insect bite (nonvenomous), left lesser toe(s)
       ● S90.466   Insect bite (nonvenomous), unspecified lesser toe(s)

● S90.47   Other superficial bite of toe
    Excludes1   open bite of toe (S91.15-, S91.25-)
    ● S90.471   Other superficial bite of right great toe
    ● S90.472   Other superficial bite of left great toe
    ● S90.473   Other superficial bite of unspecified great toe
    ● S90.474   Other superficial bite of right lesser toe(s)
    ● S90.475   Other superficial bite of left lesser toe(s)
    ● S90.476   Other superficial bite of unspecified lesser toe(s)
● S90.5   Other superficial injuries of ankle
    ● S90.51   Abrasion of ankle
       ● S90.511   Abrasion, right ankle
       ● S90.512   Abrasion, left ankle
       ● S90.519   Abrasion, unspecified ankle
    ● S90.52   Blister (nonthermal) of ankle
       ● S90.521   Blister (nonthermal), right ankle
       ● S90.522   Blister (nonthermal), left ankle
       ● S90.529   Blister (nonthermal), unspecified ankle
    ● S90.54   External constriction of ankle
       ● S90.541   External constriction, right ankle
       ● S90.542   External constriction, left ankle
       ● S90.549   External constriction, unspecified ankle
    ● S90.55   Superficial foreign body of ankle
        Splinter in the ankle
       ● S90.551   Superficial foreign body, right ankle
       ● S90.552   Superficial foreign body, left ankle
       ● S90.559   Superficial foreign body, unspecified ankle
    ● S90.56   Insect bite (nonvenomous) of ankle
       ● S90.561   Insect bite (nonvenomous), right ankle
       ● S90.562   Insect bite (nonvenomous), left ankle
       ● S90.569   Insect bite (nonvenomous), unspecified ankle
    ● S90.57   Other superficial bite of ankle
       Excludes1   open bite of ankle (S91.05-)
       ● S90.571   Other superficial bite of ankle, right ankle
       ● S90.572   Other superficial bite of ankle, left ankle
       ● S90.579   Other superficial bite of ankle, unspecified ankle
● S90.8   Other superficial injuries of foot
    ● S90.81   Abrasion of foot
       ● S90.811   Abrasion, right foot
       ● S90.812   Abrasion, left foot
       ● S90.819   Abrasion, unspecified foot
    ● S90.82   Blister (nonthermal) of foot
       ● S90.821   Blister (nonthermal), right foot
       ● S90.822   Blister (nonthermal), left foot
       ● S90.829   Blister (nonthermal), unspecified foot
    ● S90.84   External constriction of foot
       ● S90.841   External constriction, right foot
       ● S90.842   External constriction, left foot
       ● S90.849   External constriction, unspecified foot
    ● S90.85   Superficial foreign body of foot
        Splinter in the foot
       ● S90.851   Superficial foreign body, right foot
       ● S90.852   Superficial foreign body, left foot
       ● S90.859   Superficial foreign body, unspecified foot

● S90.86 Insect bite (nonvenomous) of foot
● S90.861 Insect bite (nonvenomous), right foot
● S90.862 Insect bite (nonvenomous), left foot
● S90.869 Insect bite (nonvenomous), unspecified foot
● S90.87 Other superficial bite of foot
Excludes1 open bite of foot (S91.35-)
● S90.871 Other superficial bite of right foot
● S90.872 Other superficial bite of left foot
● S90.879 Other superficial bite of unspecified foot
● S90.9 Unspecified superficial injury of ankle, foot and toe
● S90.91 Unspecified superficial injury of ankle
● S90.911 Unspecified superficial injury of right ankle
● S90.912 Unspecified superficial injury of left ankle
● S90.919 Unspecified superficial injury of unspecified ankle
● S90.92 Unspecified superficial injury of foot
● S90.921 Unspecified superficial injury of right foot
● S90.922 Unspecified superficial injury of left foot
● S90.929 Unspecified superficial injury of unspecified foot
S90.93 Unspecified superficial injury of toes
● S90.931 Unspecified superficial injury of right great toe
● S90.932 Unspecified superficial injury of left great toe
● S90.933 Unspecified superficial injury of unspecified great toe
● S90.934 Unspecified superficial injury of right lesser toe(s)
● S90.935 Unspecified superficial injury of left lesser toe(s)
● S90.936 Unspecified superficial injury of unspecified lesser toe(s)

● **S91 Open wound of ankle, foot and toes**
Code also any associated wound infection
Excludes1 open fracture of ankle, foot and toes (S92.-with 7th character B)
traumatic amputation of ankle and foot (S98.-)
The appropriate 7th character is to be added to each code from category S91

A	initial encounter
D	subsequent encounter
S	sequela

● S91.0 Open wound of ankle
● S91.00 Unspecified open wound of ankle
● S91.001 Unspecified open wound, right ankle
● S91.002 Unspecified open wound, left ankle
● S91.009 Unspecified open wound, unspecified ankle
● S91.01 Laceration without foreign body of ankle
● S91.011 Laceration without foreign body, right ankle
● S91.012 Laceration without foreign body, left ankle
● S91.019 Laceration without foreign body, unspecified ankle
● S91.02 Laceration with foreign body of ankle
● S91.021 Laceration with foreign body, right ankle
● S91.022 Laceration with foreign body, left ankle
● S91.029 Laceration with foreign body, unspecified ankle
● S91.03 Puncture wound without foreign body of ankle
● S91.031 Puncture wound without foreign body, right ankle
● S91.032 Puncture wound without foreign body, left ankle
● S91.039 Puncture wound without foreign body, unspecified ankle
● S91.04 Puncture wound with foreign body of ankle
● S91.041 Puncture wound with foreign body, right ankle
● S91.042 Puncture wound with foreign body, left ankle
● S91.049 Puncture wound with foreign body, unspecified ankle
● S91.05 Open bite of ankle
Excludes1 superficial bite of ankle (S90.56-, S90.57-)
● S91.051 Open bite, right ankle
● S91.052 Open bite, left ankle
● S91.059 Open bite, unspecified ankle
● S91.1 Open wound of toe without damage to nail
● S91.10 Unspecified open wound of toe without damage to nail
● S91.101 Unspecified open wound of right great toe without damage to nail
● S91.102 Unspecified open wound of left great toe without damage to nail
● S91.103 Unspecified open wound of unspecified great toe without damage to nail
● S91.104 Unspecified open wound of right lesser toe(s) without damage to nail
● S91.105 Unspecified open wound of left lesser toe(s) without damage to nail
● S91.106 Unspecified open wound of unspecified lesser toe(s) without damage to nail
● S91.109 Unspecified open wound of unspecified toe(s) without damage to nail
● S91.11 Laceration without foreign body of toe without damage to nail
● S91.111 Laceration without foreign body of right great toe without damage to nail
● S91.112 Laceration without foreign body of left great toe without damage to nail
● S91.113 Laceration without foreign body of unspecified great toe without damage to nail
● S91.114 Laceration without foreign body of right lesser toe(s) without damage to nail
● S91.115 Laceration without foreign body of left lesser toe(s) without damage to nail
● S91.116 Laceration without foreign body of unspecified lesser toe(s) without damage to nail
● S91.119 Laceration without foreign body of unspecified toe without damage to nail

- S91.12 Laceration with foreign body of toe without damage to nail
  - S91.121 Laceration with foreign body of right great toe without damage to nail
  - S91.122 Laceration with foreign body of left great toe without damage to nail
  - S91.123 Laceration with foreign body of unspecified great toe without damage to nail
  - S91.124 Laceration with foreign body of right lesser toe(s) without damage to nail
  - S91.125 Laceration with foreign body of left lesser toe(s) without damage to nail
  - S91.126 Laceration with foreign body of unspecified lesser toe(s) without damage to nail
  - S91.129 Laceration with foreign body of unspecified toe(s) without damage to nail
- S91.13 Puncture wound without foreign body of toe without damage to nail
  - S91.131 Puncture wound without foreign body of right great toe without damage to nail
  - S91.132 Puncture wound without foreign body of left great toe without damage to nail
  - S91.133 Puncture wound without foreign body of unspecified great toe without damage to nail
  - S91.134 Puncture wound without foreign body of right lesser toe(s) without damage to nail
  - S91.135 Puncture wound without foreign body of left lesser toe(s) without damage to nail
  - S91.136 Puncture wound without foreign body of unspecified lesser toe(s) without damage to nail
  - S91.139 Puncture wound without foreign body of unspecified toe(s) without damage to nail
- S91.14 Puncture wound with foreign body of toe without damage to nail
  - S91.141 Puncture wound with foreign body of right great toe without damage to nail
  - S91.142 Puncture wound with foreign body of left great toe without damage to nail
  - S91.143 Puncture wound with foreign body of unspecified great toe without damage to nail
  - S91.144 Puncture wound with foreign body of right lesser toe(s) without damage to nail
  - S91.145 Puncture wound with foreign body of left lesser toe(s) without damage to nail
  - S91.146 Puncture wound with foreign body of unspecified lesser toe(s) without damage to nail
  - S91.149 Puncture wound with foreign body of unspecified toe(s) without damage to nail
- S91.15 Open bite of toe without damage to nail

  Bite of toe NOS

  Excludes1 superficial bite of toe (S90.46-, S90.47-)
  - S91.151 Open bite of right great toe without damage to nail
  - S91.152 Open bite of left great toe without damage to nail
  - S91.153 Open bite of unspecified great toe without damage to nail
  - S91.154 Open bite of right lesser toe(s) without damage to nail
  - S91.155 Open bite of left lesser toe(s) without damage to nail
  - S91.156 Open bite of unspecified lesser toe(s) without damage to nail
  - S91.159 Open bite of unspecified toe(s) without damage to nail
- S91.2 Open wound of toe with damage to nail
  - S91.20 Unspecified open wound of toe with damage to nail
    - S91.201 Unspecified open wound of right great toe with damage to nail
    - S91.202 Unspecified open wound of left great toe with damage to nail
    - S91.203 Unspecified open wound of unspecified great toe with damage to nail
    - S91.204 Unspecified open wound of right lesser toe(s) with damage to nail
    - S91.205 Unspecified open wound of left lesser toe(s) with damage to nail
    - S91.206 Unspecified open wound of unspecified lesser toe(s) with damage to nail
    - S91.209 Unspecified open wound of unspecified toe(s) with damage to nail
  - S91.21 Laceration without foreign body of toe with damage to nail
    - S91.211 Laceration without foreign body of right great toe with damage to nail
    - S91.212 Laceration without foreign body of left great toe with damage to nail
    - S91.213 Laceration without foreign body of unspecified great toe with damage to nail
    - S91.214 Laceration without foreign body of right lesser toe(s) with damage to nail
    - S91.215 Laceration without foreign body of left lesser toe(s) with damage to nail
    - S91.216 Laceration without foreign body of unspecified lesser toe(s) with damage to nail
    - S91.219 Laceration without foreign body of unspecified toe(s) with damage to nail
  - S91.22 Laceration with foreign body of toe with damage to nail
    - S91.221 Laceration with foreign body of right great toe with damage to nail
    - S91.222 Laceration with foreign body of left great toe with damage to nail
    - S91.223 Laceration with foreign body of unspecified great toe with damage to nail
    - S91.224 Laceration with foreign body of right lesser toe(s) with damage to nail
    - S91.225 Laceration with foreign body of left lesser toe(s) with damage to nail
    - S91.226 Laceration with foreign body of unspecified lesser toe(s) with damage to nail
    - S91.229 Laceration with foreign body of unspecified toe(s) with damage to nail

CHAPTER 19 (S00-T88)

- S91.23 Puncture wound without foreign body of toe with damage to nail
  - S91.231 Puncture wound without foreign body of right great toe with damage to nail
  - S91.232 Puncture wound without foreign body of left great toe with damage to nail
  - S91.233 Puncture wound without foreign body of unspecified great toe with damage to nail
  - S91.234 Puncture wound without foreign body of right lesser toe(s) with damage to nail
  - S91.235 Puncture wound without foreign body of left lesser toe(s) with damage to nail
  - S91.236 Puncture wound without foreign body of unspecified lesser toe(s) with damage to nail
  - S91.239 Puncture wound without foreign body of unspecified toe(s) with damage to nail
- S91.24 Puncture wound with foreign body of toe with damage to nail
  - S91.241 Puncture wound with foreign body of right great toe with damage to nail
  - S91.242 Puncture wound with foreign body of left great toe with damage to nail
  - S91.243 Puncture wound with foreign body of unspecified great toe with damage to nail
  - S91.244 Puncture wound with foreign body of right lesser toe(s) with damage to nail
  - S91.245 Puncture wound with foreign body of left lesser toe(s) with damage to nail
  - S91.246 Puncture wound with foreign body of unspecified lesser toe(s) with damage to nail
  - S91.249 Puncture wound with foreign body of unspecified toe(s) with damage to nail
- S91.25 Open bite of toe with damage to nail
  Bite of toe with damage to nail NOS
  Excludes1 superficial bite of toe (S90.46-, S90.47-)
  - S91.251 Open bite of right great toe with damage to nail
  - S91.252 Open bite of left great toe with damage to nail
  - S91.253 Open bite of unspecified great toe with damage to nail
  - S91.254 Open bite of right lesser toe(s) with damage to nail
  - S91.255 Open bite of left lesser toe(s) with damage to nail
  - S91.256 Open bite of unspecified lesser toe(s) with damage to nail
  - S91.259 Open bite of unspecified toe(s) with damage to nail
- S91.3 Open wound of foot
  - S91.30 Unspecified open wound of foot
    - S91.301 Unspecified open wound, right foot
    - S91.302 Unspecified open wound, left foot
    - S91.309 Unspecified open wound, unspecified foot
  - S91.31 Laceration without foreign body of foot
    - S91.311 Laceration without foreign body, right foot
    - S91.312 Laceration without foreign body, left foot
    - S91.319 Laceration without foreign body, unspecified foot
  - S91.32 Laceration with foreign body of foot
    - S91.321 Laceration with foreign body, right foot
    - S91.322 Laceration with foreign body, left foot
    - S91.329 Laceration with foreign body, unspecified foot
  - S91.33 Puncture wound without foreign body of foot
    - S91.331 Puncture wound without foreign body, right foot
    - S91.332 Puncture wound without foreign body, left foot
    - S91.339 Puncture wound without foreign body, unspecified foot
  - S91.34 Puncture wound with foreign body of foot
    - S91.341 Puncture wound with foreign body, right foot
    - S91.342 Puncture wound with foreign body, left foot
    - S91.349 Puncture wound with foreign body, unspecified foot
  - S91.35 Open bite of foot
    Excludes1 superficial bite of foot (S90.86-, S90.87-)
    - S91.351 Open bite, right foot
    - S91.352 Open bite, left foot
    - S91.359 Open bite, unspecified foot

S92 Fracture of foot and toe, except ankle

Note: A fracture not indicated as displaced or nondisplaced should be coded to displaced

A fracture not indicated as open or closed should be coded to closed

Excludes1 traumatic amputation of ankle and foot (S98.-)

Excludes2 fracture of ankle (S82.-)
fracture of malleolus (S82.-)

The appropriate 7th character is to be added to each code from category S92

A	initial encounter for closed fracture
B	initial encounter for open fracture
D	subsequent encounter for fracture with routine healing
G	subsequent encounter for fracture with delayed healing
K	subsequent encounter for fracture with nonunion
P	subsequent encounter for fracture with malunion
S	sequela

- S92.0 Fracture of calcaneus
  Heel bone Os calcis
  Excludes2 Physeal fracture of calcaneus (S99.0-) ◄
  - S92.00 Unspecified fracture of calcaneus
    - S92.001 Unspecified fracture of right calcaneus
    - S92.002 Unspecified fracture of left calcaneus
    - S92.009 Unspecified fracture of unspecified calcaneus
  - S92.01 Fracture of body of calcaneus
    - S92.011 Displaced fracture of body of right calcaneus
    - S92.012 Displaced fracture of body of left calcaneus

◄ New ⟵ Revised ~~deleted~~ Deleted OGCR Official Guidelines X Assign placeholder X ● Use Additional Character(s)
Excludes 1 | Excludes 2 | Includes | Use additional | Code first | Code also | Unspecified

- S92.013 Displaced fracture of body of unspecified calcaneus
- S92.014 Nondisplaced fracture of body of right calcaneus
- S92.015 Nondisplaced fracture of body of left calcaneus
- S92.016 Nondisplaced fracture of body of unspecified calcaneus

S92.02 Fracture of anterior process of calcaneus

- S92.021 Displaced fracture of anterior process of right calcaneus
- S92.022 Displaced fracture of anterior process of left calcaneus
- S92.023 Displaced fracture of anterior process of unspecified calcaneus
- S92.024 Nondisplaced fracture of anterior process of right calcaneus
- S92.025 Nondisplaced fracture of anterior process of left calcaneus
- S92.026 Nondisplaced fracture of anterior process of unspecified calcaneus

S92.03 Avulsion fracture of tuberosity of calcaneus

- S92.031 Displaced avulsion fracture of tuberosity of right calcaneus
- S92.032 Displaced avulsion fracture of tuberosity of left calcaneus
- S92.033 Displaced avulsion fracture of tuberosity of unspecified calcaneus
- S92.034 Nondisplaced avulsion fracture of tuberosity of right calcaneus
- S92.035 Nondisplaced avulsion fracture of tuberosity of left calcaneus
- S92.036 Nondisplaced avulsion fracture of tuberosity of unspecified calcaneus

S92.04 Other fracture of tuberosity of calcaneus

- S92.041 Displaced other fracture of tuberosity of right calcaneus
- S92.042 Displaced other fracture of tuberosity of left calcaneus
- S92.043 Displaced other fracture of tuberosity of unspecified calcaneus
- S92.044 Nondisplaced other fracture of tuberosity of right calcaneus
- S92.045 Nondisplaced other fracture of tuberosity of left calcaneus
- S92.046 Nondisplaced other fracture of tuberosity of unspecified calcaneus

S92.05 Other extraarticular fracture of calcaneus

- S92.051 Displaced other extraarticular fracture of right calcaneus
- S92.052 Displaced other extraarticular fracture of left calcaneus
- S92.053 Displaced other extraarticular fracture of unspecified calcaneus
- S92.054 Nondisplaced other extraarticular fracture of right calcaneus
- S92.055 Nondisplaced other extraarticular fracture of left calcaneus
- S92.056 Nondisplaced other extraarticular fracture of unspecified calcaneus

S92.06 Intraarticular fracture of calcaneus

- S92.061 Displaced intraarticular fracture of right calcaneus
- S92.062 Displaced intraarticular fracture of left calcaneus
- S92.063 Displaced intraarticular fracture of unspecified calcaneus
- S92.064 Nondisplaced intraarticular fracture of right calcaneus
- S92.065 Nondisplaced intraarticular fracture of left calcaneus
- S92.066 Nondisplaced intraarticular fracture of unspecified calcaneus

S92.1 Fracture of talus

Astragalus

S92.10 Unspecified fracture of talus

- S92.101 Unspecified fracture of right talus
- S92.102 Unspecified fracture of left talus
- S92.109 Unspecified fracture of unspecified talus

S92.11 Fracture of neck of talus

- S92.111 Displaced fracture of neck of right talus
- S92.112 Displaced fracture of neck of left talus
- S92.113 Displaced fracture of neck of unspecified talus
- S92.114 Nondisplaced fracture of neck of right talus
- S92.115 Nondisplaced fracture of neck of left talus
- S92.116 Nondisplaced fracture of neck of unspecified talus

S92.12 Fracture of body of talus

- S92.121 Displaced fracture of body of right talus
- S92.122 Displaced fracture of body of left talus
- S92.123 Displaced fracture of body of unspecified talus
- S92.124 Nondisplaced fracture of body of right talus
- S92.125 Nondisplaced fracture of body of left talus
- S92.126 Nondisplaced fracture of body of unspecified talus

S92.13 Fracture of posterior process of talus

- S92.131 Displaced fracture of posterior process of right talus
- S92.132 Displaced fracture of posterior process of left talus
- S92.133 Displaced fracture of posterior process of unspecified talus
- S92.134 Nondisplaced fracture of posterior process of right talus
- S92.135 Nondisplaced fracture of posterior process of left talus
- S92.136 Nondisplaced fracture of posterior process of unspecified talus

S92.14 Dome fracture of talus

Excludes1 osteochondritis dissecans (M93.2)

- S92.141 Displaced dome fracture of right talus
- S92.142 Displaced dome fracture of left talus
- S92.143 Displaced dome fracture of unspecified talus
- S92.144 Nondisplaced dome fracture of right talus
- S92.145 Nondisplaced dome fracture of left talus
- S92.146 Nondisplaced dome fracture of unspecified talus

- S92.15 Avulsion fracture (chip fracture) of talus
  - S92.151 Displaced avulsion fracture (chip fracture) of right talus
  - S92.152 Displaced avulsion fracture (chip fracture) of left talus
  - S92.153 Displaced avulsion fracture (chip fracture) of unspecified talus
  - S92.154 Nondisplaced avulsion fracture (chip fracture) of right talus
  - S92.155 Nondisplaced avulsion fracture (chip fracture) of left talus
  - S92.156 Nondisplaced avulsion fracture (chip fracture) of unspecified talus
- S92.19 Other fracture of talus
  - S92.191 Other fracture of right talus
  - S92.192 Other fracture of left talus
  - S92.199 Other fracture of unspecified talus
- S92.2 Fracture of other and unspecified tarsal bone(s)
  - S92.20 Fracture of unspecified tarsal bone(s)
    - S92.201 Fracture of unspecified tarsal bone(s) of right foot
    - S92.202 Fracture of unspecified tarsal bone(s) of left foot
    - S92.209 Fracture of unspecified tarsal bone(s) of unspecified foot
  - S92.21 Fracture of cuboid bone
    - S92.211 Displaced fracture of cuboid bone of right foot
    - S92.212 Displaced fracture of cuboid bone of left foot
    - S92.213 Displaced fracture of cuboid bone of unspecified foot
    - S92.214 Nondisplaced fracture of cuboid bone of right foot
    - S92.215 Nondisplaced fracture of cuboid bone of left foot
    - S92.216 Nondisplaced fracture of cuboid bone of unspecified foot
  - S92.22 Fracture of lateral cuneiform
    - S92.221 Displaced fracture of lateral cuneiform of right foot
    - S92.222 Displaced fracture of lateral cuneiform of left foot
    - S92.223 Displaced fracture of lateral cuneiform of unspecified foot
    - S92.224 Nondisplaced fracture of lateral cuneiform of right foot
    - S92.225 Nondisplaced fracture of lateral cuneiform of left foot
    - S92.226 Nondisplaced fracture of lateral cuneiform of unspecified foot
  - S92.23 Fracture of intermediate cuneiform
    - S92.231 Displaced fracture of intermediate cuneiform of right foot
    - S92.232 Displaced fracture of intermediate cuneiform of left foot
    - S92.233 Displaced fracture of intermediate cuneiform of unspecified foot
    - S92.234 Nondisplaced fracture of intermediate cuneiform of right foot
    - S92.235 Nondisplaced fracture of intermediate cuneiform of left foot
    - S92.236 Nondisplaced fracture of intermediate cuneiform of unspecified foot
  - S92.24 Fracture of medial cuneiform
    - S92.241 Displaced fracture of medial cuneiform of right foot
    - S92.242 Displaced fracture of medial cuneiform of left foot
    - S92.243 Displaced fracture of medial cuneiform of unspecified foot
    - S92.244 Nondisplaced fracture of medial cuneiform of right foot
    - S92.245 Nondisplaced fracture of medial cuneiform of left foot
    - S92.246 Nondisplaced fracture of medial cuneiform of unspecified foot
  - S92.25 Fracture of navicular [scaphoid] of foot
    - S92.251 Displaced fracture of navicular [scaphoid] of right foot
    - S92.252 Displaced fracture of navicular [scaphoid] of left foot
    - S92.253 Displaced fracture of navicular [scaphoid] of unspecified foot
    - S92.254 Nondisplaced fracture of navicular [scaphoid] of right foot
    - S92.255 Nondisplaced fracture of navicular [scaphoid] of left foot
    - S92.256 Nondisplaced fracture of navicular [scaphoid] of unspecified foot
- S92.3 Fracture of metatarsal bone(s)

  Excludes2 Physeal fracture of metatarsal (S99.1-) ◀

  - S92.30 Fracture of unspecified metatarsal bone(s)
    - S92.301 Fracture of unspecified metatarsal bone(s), right foot
    - S92.302 Fracture of unspecified metatarsal bone(s), left foot
    - S92.309 Fracture of unspecified metatarsal bone(s), unspecified foot
  - S92.31 Fracture of first metatarsal bone
    - S92.311 Displaced fracture of first metatarsal bone, right foot
    - S92.312 Displaced fracture of first metatarsal bone, left foot
    - S92.313 Displaced fracture of first metatarsal bone, unspecified foot
    - S92.314 Nondisplaced fracture of first metatarsal bone, right foot
    - S92.315 Nondisplaced fracture of first metatarsal bone, left foot
    - S92.316 Nondisplaced fracture of first metatarsal bone, unspecified foot
  - S92.32 Fracture of second metatarsal bone
    - S92.321 Displaced fracture of second metatarsal bone, right foot
    - S92.322 Displaced fracture of second metatarsal bone, left foot
    - S92.323 Displaced fracture of second metatarsal bone, unspecified foot
    - S92.324 Nondisplaced fracture of second metatarsal bone, right foot
    - S92.325 Nondisplaced fracture of second metatarsal bone, left foot
    - S92.326 Nondisplaced fracture of second metatarsal bone, unspecified foot
  - S92.33 Fracture of third metatarsal bone
    - S92.331 Displaced fracture of third metatarsal bone, right foot
    - S92.332 Displaced fracture of third metatarsal bone, left foot
    - S92.333 Displaced fracture of third metatarsal bone, unspecified foot

S92.334 Nondisplaced fracture of third metatarsal bone, right foot
S92.335 Nondisplaced fracture of third metatarsal bone, left foot
S92.336 Nondisplaced fracture of third metatarsal bone, unspecified foot
S92.34 Fracture of fourth metatarsal bone
S92.341 Displaced fracture of fourth metatarsal bone, right foot
S92.342 Displaced fracture of fourth metatarsal bone, left foot
S92.343 Displaced fracture of fourth metatarsal bone, unspecified foot
S92.344 Nondisplaced fracture of fourth metatarsal bone, right foot
S92.345 Nondisplaced fracture of fourth metatarsal bone, left foot
S92.346 Nondisplaced fracture of fourth metatarsal bone, unspecified foot
S92.35 Fracture of fifth metatarsal bone
S92.351 Displaced fracture of fifth metatarsal bone, right foot
S92.352 Displaced fracture of fifth metatarsal bone, left foot
S92.353 Displaced fracture of fifth metatarsal bone, unspecified foot
S92.354 Nondisplaced fracture of fifth metatarsal bone, right foot
S92.355 Nondisplaced fracture of fifth metatarsal bone, left foot
S92.356 Nondisplaced fracture of fifth metatarsal bone, unspecified foot
S92.4 Fracture of great toe
Excludes2 Physeal fracture of phalanx of toe (S99.2-) ◀
S92.40 Unspecified fracture of great toe
S92.401 Displaced unspecified fracture of right great toe
S92.402 Displaced unspecified fracture of left great toe
S92.403 Displaced unspecified fracture of unspecified great toe
S92.404 Nondisplaced unspecified fracture of right great toe
S92.405 Nondisplaced unspecified fracture of left great toe
S92.406 Nondisplaced unspecified fracture of unspecified great toe
S92.41 Fracture of proximal phalanx of great toe
S92.411 Displaced fracture of proximal phalanx of right great toe
S92.412 Displaced fracture of proximal phalanx of left great toe
S92.413 Displaced fracture of proximal phalanx of unspecified great toe
S92.414 Nondisplaced fracture of proximal phalanx of right great toe
S92.415 Nondisplaced fracture of proximal phalanx of left great toe
S92.416 Nondisplaced fracture of proximal phalanx of unspecified great toe
S92.42 Fracture of distal phalanx of great toe
S92.421 Displaced fracture of distal phalanx of right great toe
S92.422 Displaced fracture of distal phalanx of left great toe
S92.423 Displaced fracture of distal phalanx of unspecified great toe
S92.424 Nondisplaced fracture of distal phalanx of right great toe
S92.425 Nondisplaced fracture of distal phalanx of left great toe
S92.426 Nondisplaced fracture of distal phalanx of unspecified great toe
S92.49 Other fracture of great toe
S92.491 Other fracture of right great toe
S92.492 Other fracture of left great toe
S92.499 Other fracture of unspecified great toe
S92.5 Fracture of lesser toe(s)
Excludes2 Physeal fracture of phalanx of toe (S99.2-) ◀
S92.50 Unspecified fracture of lesser toe(s)
S92.501 Displaced unspecified fracture of right lesser toe(s)
S92.502 Displaced unspecified fracture of left lesser toe(s)
S92.503 Displaced unspecified fracture of unspecified lesser toe(s)
S92.504 Nondisplaced unspecified fracture of right lesser toe(s)
S92.505 Nondisplaced unspecified fracture of left lesser toe(s)
S92.506 Nondisplaced unspecified fracture of unspecified lesser toe(s)
S92.51 Fracture of proximal phalanx of lesser toe(s)
S92.511 Displaced fracture of proximal phalanx of right lesser toe(s)
S92.512 Displaced fracture of proximal phalanx of left lesser toe(s)
S92.513 Displaced fracture of proximal phalanx of unspecified lesser toe(s)
S92.514 Nondisplaced fracture of proximal phalanx of right lesser toe(s)
S92.515 Nondisplaced fracture of proximal phalanx of left lesser toe(s)
S92.516 Nondisplaced fracture of proximal phalanx of unspecified lesser toe(s)
S92.52 Fracture of medial phalanx of lesser toe(s)
S92.521 Displaced fracture of medial phalanx of right lesser toe(s)
S92.522 Displaced fracture of medial phalanx of left lesser toe(s)
S92.523 Displaced fracture of medial phalanx of unspecified lesser toe(s)
S92.524 Nondisplaced fracture of medial phalanx of right lesser toe(s)
S92.525 Nondisplaced fracture of medial phalanx of left lesser toe(s)
S92.526 Nondisplaced fracture of medial phalanx of unspecified lesser toe(s)
S92.53 Fracture of distal phalanx of lesser toe(s)
S92.531 Displaced fracture of distal phalanx of right lesser toe(s)
S92.532 Displaced fracture of distal phalanx of left lesser toe(s)
S92.533 Displaced fracture of distal phalanx of unspecified lesser toe(s)
S92.534 Nondisplaced fracture of distal phalanx of right lesser toe(s)
S92.535 Nondisplaced fracture of distal phalanx of left lesser toe(s)
S92.536 Nondisplaced fracture of distal phalanx of unspecified lesser toe(s)

● S92.59 Other fracture of lesser toe(s)
● S92.591 Other fracture of right lesser toe(s)
● S92.592 Other fracture of left lesser toe(s)
● S92.599 Other fracture of unspecified lesser toe(s)
● S92.8 Other fracture of foot, except ankle ◀
● S92.81 Other fracture of foot ◀
Sesamoid fracture of foot
● S92.811 Other fracture of right foot
● S92.812 Other fracture of left foot
● S92.819 Other fracture of unspecified foot
● S92.9 Unspecified fracture of foot and toe
● S92.90 Unspecified fracture of foot
● S92.901 Unspecified fracture of right foot
● S92.902 Unspecified fracture of left foot
● S92.909 Unspecified fracture of unspecified foot
● S92.91 Unspecified fracture of toe
● S92.911 Unspecified fracture of right toe(s)
● S92.912 Unspecified fracture of left toe(s)
● S92.919 Unspecified fracture of unspecified toe(s)

● S93 Dislocation and sprain of joints and ligaments at ankle, foot and toe level

Includes avulsion of joint or ligament of ankle, foot and toe
laceration of cartilage, joint or ligament of ankle, foot and toe
sprain of cartilage, joint or ligament of ankle, foot and toe
traumatic hemarthrosis of joint or ligament of ankle, foot and toe
traumatic rupture of joint or ligament of ankle, foot and toe
traumatic subluxation of joint or ligament of ankle, foot and toe
traumatic tear of joint or ligament of ankle, foot and toe

Code also any associated open wound

Excludes2 strain of muscle and tendon of ankle and foot (S96.-)

The appropriate 7th character is to be added to each code from category S93

A initial encounter
D subsequent encounter
S sequela

● S93.0 Subluxation and dislocation of ankle joint
Subluxation and dislocation of astragalus
Subluxation and dislocation of fibula, lower end
Subluxation and dislocation of talus
Subluxation and dislocation of tibia, lower end
X● S93.01 Subluxation of right ankle joint
X● S93.02 Subluxation of left ankle joint
X● S93.03 Subluxation of unspecified ankle joint
X● S93.04 Dislocation of right ankle joint
X● S93.05 Dislocation of left ankle joint
X● S93.06 Dislocation of unspecified ankle joint
● S93.1 Subluxation and dislocation of toe
● S93.10 Unspecified subluxation and dislocation of toe
Dislocation of toe NOS
Subluxation of toe NOS
● S93.101 Unspecified subluxation of right toe(s)
● S93.102 Unspecified subluxation of left toe(s)
● S93.103 Unspecified subluxation of unspecified toe(s)
● S93.104 Unspecified dislocation of right toe(s)
● S93.105 Unspecified dislocation of left toe(s)
● S93.106 Unspecified dislocation of unspecified toe(s)
● S93.11 Dislocation of interphalangeal joint
● S93.111 Dislocation of interphalangeal joint of right great toe
● S93.112 Dislocation of interphalangeal joint of left great toe
● S93.113 Dislocation of interphalangeal joint of unspecified great toe
● S93.114 Dislocation of interphalangeal joint of right lesser toe(s)
● S93.115 Dislocation of interphalangeal joint of left lesser toe(s)
● S93.116 Dislocation of interphalangeal joint of unspecified lesser toe(s)
● S93.119 Dislocation of interphalangeal joint of unspecified toe(s)
● S93.12 Dislocation of metatarsophalangeal joint
● S93.121 Dislocation of metatarsophalangeal joint of right great toe
● S93.122 Dislocation of metatarsophalangeal joint of left great toe
● S93.123 Dislocation of metatarsophalangeal joint of unspecified great toe
● S93.124 Dislocation of metatarsophalangeal joint of right lesser toe(s)
● S93.125 Dislocation of metatarsophalangeal joint of left lesser toe(s)
● S93.126 Dislocation of metatarsophalangeal joint of unspecified lesser toe(s)
● S93.129 Dislocation of metatarsophalangeal joint of unspecified toe(s)
● S93.13 Subluxation of interphalangeal joint
● S93.131 Subluxation of interphalangeal joint of right great toe
● S93.132 Subluxation of interphalangeal joint of left great toe
● S93.133 Subluxation of interphalangeal joint of unspecified great toe
● S93.134 Subluxation of interphalangeal joint of right lesser toe(s)
● S93.135 Subluxation of interphalangeal joint of left lesser toe(s)
● S93.136 Subluxation of interphalangeal joint of unspecified lesser toe(s)
● S93.139 Subluxation of interphalangeal joint of unspecified toe(s)
● S93.14 Subluxation of metatarsophalangeal joint
● S93.141 Subluxation of metatarsophalangeal joint of right great toe
● S93.142 Subluxation of metatarsophalangeal joint of left great toe
● S93.143 Subluxation of metatarsophalangeal joint of unspecified great toe
● S93.144 Subluxation of metatarsophalangeal joint of right lesser toe(s)
● S93.145 Subluxation of metatarsophalangeal joint of left lesser toe(s)
● S93.146 Subluxation of metatarsophalangeal joint of unspecified lesser toe(s)
● S93.149 Subluxation of metatarsophalangeal joint of unspecified toe(s)

● S93.3 Subluxation and dislocation of foot
Excludes2 dislocation of toe (S93.1-)
● S93.30 Unspecified subluxation and dislocation of foot
Dislocation of foot NOS
Subluxation of foot NOS
● S93.301 Unspecified subluxation of right foot
● S93.302 Unspecified subluxation of left foot
● S93.303 Unspecified subluxation of unspecified foot
● S93.304 Unspecified dislocation of right foot
● S93.305 Unspecified dislocation of left foot
● S93.306 Unspecified dislocation of unspecified foot
● S93.31 Subluxation and dislocation of tarsal joint
● S93.311 Subluxation of tarsal joint of right foot
● S93.312 Subluxation of tarsal joint of left foot
● S93.313 Subluxation of tarsal joint of unspecified foot
● S93.314 Dislocation of tarsal joint of right foot
● S93.315 Dislocation of tarsal joint of left foot
● S93.316 Dislocation of tarsal joint of unspecified foot
● S93.32 Subluxation and dislocation of tarsometatarsal joint
● S93.321 Subluxation of tarsometatarsal joint of right foot
● S93.322 Subluxation of tarsometatarsal joint of left foot
● S93.323 Subluxation of tarsometatarsal joint of unspecified foot
● S93.324 Dislocation of tarsometatarsal joint of right foot
● S93.325 Dislocation of tarsometatarsal joint of left foot
● S93.326 Dislocation of tarsometatarsal joint of unspecified foot
● S93.33 Other subluxation and dislocation of foot
● S93.331 Other subluxation of right foot
● S93.332 Other subluxation of left foot
● S93.333 Other subluxation of unspecified foot
● S93.334 Other dislocation of right foot
● S93.335 Other dislocation of left foot
● S93.336 Other dislocation of unspecified foot
● S93.4 Sprain of ankle
Injury to ligaments when one or more is stretched/torn
Excludes2 injury of Achilles tendon (S86.0-)
● S93.40 Sprain of unspecified ligament of ankle
Sprain of ankle NOS
Sprained ankle NOS
● S93.401 Sprain of unspecified ligament of right ankle
● S93.402 Sprain of unspecified ligament of left ankle
● S93.409 Sprain of unspecified ligament of unspecified ankle
● S93.41 Sprain of calcaneofibular ligament
● S93.411 Sprain of calcaneofibular ligament of right ankle
● S93.412 Sprain of calcaneofibular ligament of left ankle
● S93.419 Sprain of calcaneofibular ligament of unspecified ankle
● S93.42 Sprain of deltoid ligament
● S93.421 Sprain of deltoid ligament of right ankle
● S93.422 Sprain of deltoid ligament of left ankle
● S93.429 Sprain of deltoid ligament of unspecified ankle
● S93.43 Sprain of tibiofibular ligament
● S93.431 Sprain of tibiofibular ligament of right ankle
● S93.432 Sprain of tibiofibular ligament of left ankle
● S93.439 Sprain of tibiofibular ligament of unspecified ankle
● S93.49 Sprain of other ligament of ankle
Sprain of internal collateral ligament
Sprain of talofibular ligament
● S93.491 Sprain of other ligament of right ankle
● S93.492 Sprain of other ligament of left ankle
● S93.499 Sprain of other ligament of unspecified ankle
● S93.5 Sprain of toe
● S93.50 Unspecified sprain of toe
● S93.501 Unspecified sprain of right great toe
● S93.502 Unspecified sprain of left great toe
● S93.503 Unspecified sprain of unspecified great toe
● S93.504 Unspecified sprain of right lesser toe(s)
● S93.505 Unspecified sprain of left lesser toe(s)
● S93.506 Unspecified sprain of unspecified lesser toe(s)
● S93.509 Unspecified sprain of unspecified toe(s)
● S93.51 Sprain of interphalangeal joint of toe
● S93.511 Sprain of interphalangeal joint of right great toe
● S93.512 Sprain of interphalangeal joint of left great toe
● S93.513 Sprain of interphalangeal joint of unspecified great toe
● S93.514 Sprain of interphalangeal joint of right lesser toe(s)
● S93.515 Sprain of interphalangeal joint of left lesser toe(s)
● S93.516 Sprain of interphalangeal joint of unspecified lesser toe(s)
● S93.519 Sprain of interphalangeal joint of unspecified toe(s)
● S93.52 Sprain of metatarsophalangeal joint of toe
● S93.521 Sprain of metatarsophalangeal joint of right great toe
● S93.522 Sprain of metatarsophalangeal joint of left great toe
● S93.523 Sprain of metatarsophalangeal joint of unspecified great toe
● S93.524 Sprain of metatarsophalangeal joint of right lesser toe(s)
● S93.525 Sprain of metatarsophalangeal joint of left lesser toe(s)
● S93.526 Sprain of metatarsophalangeal joint of unspecified lesser toe(s)
● S93.529 Sprain of metatarsophalangeal joint of unspecified toe(s)

● S93.6 Sprain of foot
Excludes2 sprain of metatarsophalangeal joint of toe (S93.52-)
sprain of toe (S93.5-)
● S93.60 Unspecified sprain of foot
● S93.601 Unspecified sprain of right foot
● S93.602 Unspecified sprain of left foot
● S93.609 Unspecified sprain of unspecified foot
● S93.61 Sprain of tarsal ligament of foot
● S93.611 Sprain of tarsal ligament of right foot
● S93.612 Sprain of tarsal ligament of left foot
● S93.619 Sprain of tarsal ligament of unspecified foot
● S93.62 Sprain of tarsometatarsal ligament of foot
● S93.621 Sprain of tarsometatarsal ligament of right foot
● S93.622 Sprain of tarsometatarsal ligament of left foot
● S93.629 Sprain of tarsometatarsal ligament of unspecified foot
● S93.69 Other sprain of foot
● S93.691 Other sprain of right foot
● S93.692 Other sprain of left foot
● S93.699 Other sprain of unspecified foot

● S94 Injury of nerves at ankle and foot level
The appropriate 7th character is to be added to each code from category S94

A	initial encounter
D	subsequent encounter
S	sequela

Code also any associated open wound (S91.-)
● S94.0 Injury of lateral plantar nerve
X● S94.00 Injury of lateral plantar nerve, unspecified leg
X● S94.01 Injury of lateral plantar nerve, right leg
X● S94.02 Injury of lateral plantar nerve, left leg
● S94.1 Injury of medial plantar nerve
X● S94.10 Injury of medial plantar nerve, unspecified leg
X● S94.11 Injury of medial plantar nerve, right leg
X● S94.12 Injury of medial plantar nerve, left leg
● S94.2 Injury of deep peroneal nerve at ankle and foot level
Injury of terminal, lateral branch of deep peroneal nerve
X● S94.20 Injury of deep peroneal nerve at ankle and foot level, unspecified leg
X● S94.21 Injury of deep peroneal nerve at ankle and foot level, right leg
X● S94.22 Injury of deep peroneal nerve at ankle and foot level, left leg
● S94.3 Injury of cutaneous sensory nerve at ankle and foot level
X● S94.30 Injury of cutaneous sensory nerve at ankle and foot level, unspecified leg
X● S94.31 Injury of cutaneous sensory nerve at ankle and foot level, right leg
X● S94.32 Injury of cutaneous sensory nerve at ankle and foot level, left leg
● S94.8 Injury of other nerves at ankle and foot level
● S94.8X Injury of other nerves at ankle and foot level
● S94.8X1 Injury of other nerves at ankle and foot level, right leg
● S94.8X2 Injury of other nerves at ankle and foot level, left leg
● S94.8X9 Injury of other nerves at ankle and foot level, unspecified leg
● S94.9 Injury of unspecified nerve at ankle and foot level
X● S94.90 Injury of unspecified nerve at ankle and foot level, unspecified leg
X● S94.91 Injury of unspecified nerve at ankle and foot level, right leg
X● S94.92 Injury of unspecified nerve at ankle and foot level, left leg

● S95 Injury of blood vessels at ankle and foot level
Code also any associated open wound (S91.-)
Excludes2 injury of posterior tibial artery and vein (S85.1-, S85.8-)
The appropriate 7th character is to be added to each code from category S95

A	initial encounter
D	subsequent encounter
S	sequela

● S95.0 Injury of dorsal artery of foot
● S95.00 Unspecified injury of dorsal artery of foot
● S95.001 Unspecified injury of dorsal artery of right foot
● S95.002 Unspecified injury of dorsal artery of left foot
● S95.009 Unspecified injury of dorsal artery of unspecified foot
● S95.01 Laceration of dorsal artery of foot
● S95.011 Laceration of dorsal artery of right foot
● S95.012 Laceration of dorsal artery of left foot
● S95.019 Laceration of dorsal artery of unspecified foot
● S95.09 Other specified injury of dorsal artery of foot
● S95.091 Other specified injury of dorsal artery of right foot
● S95.092 Other specified injury of dorsal artery of left foot
● S95.099 Other specified injury of dorsal artery of unspecified foot
● S95.1 Injury of plantar artery of foot
● S95.10 Unspecified injury of plantar artery of foot
● S95.101 Unspecified injury of plantar artery of right foot
● S95.102 Unspecified injury of plantar artery of left foot
● S95.109 Unspecified injury of plantar artery of unspecified foot
● S95.11 Laceration of plantar artery of foot
● S95.111 Laceration of plantar artery of right foot
● S95.112 Laceration of plantar artery of left foot
● S95.119 Laceration of plantar artery of unspecified foot
● S95.19 Other specified injury of plantar artery of foot
● S95.191 Other specified injury of plantar artery of right foot
● S95.192 Other specified injury of plantar artery of left foot
● S95.199 Other specified injury of plantar artery of unspecified foot

● S95.2 Injury of dorsal vein of foot
● S95.20 Unspecified injury of dorsal vein of foot
● S95.201 Unspecified injury of dorsal vein of right foot
● S95.202 Unspecified injury of dorsal vein of left foot
● S95.209 Unspecified injury of dorsal vein of unspecified foot
● S95.21 Laceration of dorsal vein of foot
● S95.211 Laceration of dorsal vein of right foot
● S95.212 Laceration of dorsal vein of left foot
● S95.219 Laceration of dorsal vein of unspecified foot
● S95.29 Other specified injury of dorsal vein of foot
● S95.291 Other specified injury of dorsal vein of right foot
● S95.292 Other specified injury of dorsal vein of left foot
● S95.299 Other specified injury of dorsal vein of unspecified foot
● S95.8 Injury of other blood vessels at ankle and foot level
● S95.80 Unspecified injury of other blood vessels at ankle and foot level
● S95.801 Unspecified injury of other blood vessels at ankle and foot level, right leg
● S95.802 Unspecified injury of other blood vessels at ankle and foot level, left leg
● S95.809 Unspecified injury of other blood vessels at ankle and foot level, unspecified leg
● S95.81 Laceration of other blood vessels at ankle and foot level
● S95.811 Laceration of other blood vessels at ankle and foot level, right leg
● S95.812 Laceration of other blood vessels at ankle and foot level, left leg
● S95.819 Laceration of other blood vessels at ankle and foot level, unspecified leg
● S95.89 Other specified injury of other blood vessels at ankle and foot level
● S95.891 Other specified injury of other blood vessels at ankle and foot level, right leg
● S95.892 Other specified injury of other blood vessels at ankle and foot level, left leg
● S95.899 Other specified injury of other blood vessels at ankle and foot level, unspecified leg
● S95.9 Injury of unspecified blood vessel at ankle and foot level
● S95.90 Unspecified injury of unspecified blood vessel at ankle and foot level
● S95.901 Unspecified injury of unspecified blood vessel at ankle and foot level, right leg
● S95.902 Unspecified injury of unspecified blood vessel at ankle and foot level, left leg
● S95.909 Unspecified injury of unspecified blood vessel at ankle and foot level, unspecified leg
● S95.91 Laceration of unspecified blood vessel at ankle and foot level
● S95.911 Laceration of unspecified blood vessel at ankle and foot level, right leg
● S95.912 Laceration of unspecified blood vessel at ankle and foot level, left leg
● S95.919 Laceration of unspecified blood vessel at ankle and foot level, unspecified leg
● S95.99 Other specified injury of unspecified blood vessel at ankle and foot level
● S95.991 Other specified injury of unspecified blood vessel at ankle and foot level, right leg
● S95.992 Other specified injury of unspecified blood vessel at ankle and foot level, left leg
● S95.999 Other specified injury of unspecified blood vessel at ankle and foot level, unspecified leg

● S96 Injury of muscle and tendon at ankle and foot level

Code also any associated open wound (S91.-)

Excludes2 injury of Achilles tendon (S86.0-)
sprain of joints and ligaments of ankle and foot (S93.-)

The appropriate 7th character is to be added to each code from category S96

A	initial encounter
D	subsequent encounter
S	sequela

● S96.0 Injury of muscle and tendon of long flexor muscle of toe at ankle and foot level
● S96.00 Unspecified injury of muscle and tendon of long flexor muscle of toe at ankle and foot level
● S96.001 Unspecified injury of muscle and tendon of long flexor muscle of toe at ankle and foot level, right foot
● S96.002 Unspecified injury of muscle and tendon of long flexor muscle of toe at ankle and foot level, left foot
● S96.009 Unspecified injury of muscle and tendon of long flexor muscle of toe at ankle and foot level, unspecified foot
● S96.01 Strain of muscle and tendon of long flexor muscle of toe at ankle and foot level
● S96.011 Strain of muscle and tendon of long flexor muscle of toe at ankle and foot level, right foot
● S96.012 Strain of muscle and tendon of long flexor muscle of toe at ankle and foot level, left foot
● S96.019 Strain of muscle and tendon of long flexor muscle of toe at ankle and foot level, unspecified foot
● S96.02 Laceration of muscle and tendon of long flexor muscle of toe at ankle and foot level
● S96.021 Laceration of muscle and tendon of long flexor muscle of toe at ankle and foot level, right foot
● S96.022 Laceration of muscle and tendon of long flexor muscle of toe at ankle and foot level, left foot
● S96.029 Laceration of muscle and tendon of long flexor muscle of toe at ankle and foot level, unspecified foot
● S96.09 Other injury of muscle and tendon of long flexor muscle of toe at ankle and foot level
● S96.091 Other injury of muscle and tendon of long flexor muscle of toe at ankle and foot level, right foot
● S96.092 Other injury of muscle and tendon of long flexor muscle of toe at ankle and foot level, left foot
● S96.099 Other injury of muscle and tendon of long flexor muscle of toe at ankle and foot level, unspecified foot

CHAPTER 19 (S00-T88)

● S96.1 Injury of muscle and tendon of long extensor muscle of toe at ankle and foot level

● S96.10 Unspecified injury of muscle and tendon of long extensor muscle of toe at ankle and foot level

● S96.101 Unspecified injury of muscle and tendon of long extensor muscle of toe at ankle and foot level, right foot

● S96.102 Unspecified injury of muscle and tendon of long extensor muscle of toe at ankle and foot level, left foot

● S96.109 Unspecified injury of muscle and tendon of long extensor muscle of toe at ankle and foot level, unspecified foot

● S96.11 Strain of muscle and tendon of long extensor muscle of toe at ankle and foot level

● S96.111 Strain of muscle and tendon of long extensor muscle of toe at ankle and foot level, right foot

● S96.112 Strain of muscle and tendon of long extensor muscle of toe at ankle and foot level, left foot

● S96.119 Strain of muscle and tendon of long extensor muscle of toe at ankle and foot level, unspecified foot

● S96.12 Laceration of muscle and tendon of long extensor muscle of toe at ankle and foot level

● S96.121 Laceration of muscle and tendon of long extensor muscle of toe at ankle and foot level, right foot

● S96.122 Laceration of muscle and tendon of long extensor muscle of toe at ankle and foot level, left foot

● S96.129 Laceration of muscle and tendon of long extensor muscle of toe at ankle and foot level, unspecified foot

● S96.19 Other specified injury of muscle and tendon of long extensor muscle of toe at ankle and foot level

● S96.191 Other specified injury of muscle and tendon of long extensor muscle of toe at ankle and foot level, right foot

● S96.192 Other specified injury of muscle and tendon of long extensor muscle of toe at ankle and foot level, left foot

● S96.199 Other specified injury of muscle and tendon of long extensor muscle of toe at ankle and foot level, unspecified foot

● S96.2 Injury of intrinsic muscle and tendon at ankle and foot level

● S96.20 Unspecified injury of intrinsic muscle and tendon at ankle and foot level

● S96.201 Unspecified injury of intrinsic muscle and tendon at ankle and foot level, right foot

● S96.202 Unspecified injury of intrinsic muscle and tendon at ankle and foot level, left foot

● S96.209 Unspecified injury of intrinsic muscle and tendon at ankle and foot level, unspecified foot

● S96.21 Strain of intrinsic muscle and tendon at ankle and foot level

● S96.211 Strain of intrinsic muscle and tendon at ankle and foot level, right foot

● S96.212 Strain of intrinsic muscle and tendon at ankle and foot level, left foot

● S96.219 Strain of intrinsic muscle and tendon at ankle and foot level, unspecified foot

● S96.22 Laceration of intrinsic muscle and tendon at ankle and foot level

● S96.221 Laceration of intrinsic muscle and tendon at ankle and foot level, right foot

● S96.222 Laceration of intrinsic muscle and tendon at left ankle and foot level, left foot

● S96.229 Laceration of intrinsic muscle and tendon at ankle and foot level, unspecified foot

● S96.29 Other specified injury of intrinsic muscle and tendon at ankle and foot level

● S96.291 Other specified injury of intrinsic muscle and tendon at ankle and foot level, right foot

● S96.292 Other specified injury of intrinsic muscle and tendon at ankle and foot level, left foot

● S96.299 Other specified injury of intrinsic muscle and tendon at ankle and foot level, unspecified foot

● S96.8 Injury of other specified muscles and tendons at ankle and foot level

● S96.80 Unspecified injury of other specified muscles and tendons at ankle and foot level

● S96.801 Unspecified injury of other specified muscles and tendons at ankle and foot level, right foot

● S96.802 Unspecified injury of other specified muscles and tendons at ankle and foot level, left foot

● S96.809 Unspecified injury of other specified muscles and tendons at ankle and foot level, unspecified foot

● S96.81 Strain of other specified muscles and tendons at ankle and foot level

● S96.811 Strain of other specified muscles and tendons at ankle and foot level, right foot

● S96.812 Strain of other specified muscles and tendons at ankle and foot level, left foot

● S96.819 Strain of other specified muscles and tendons at ankle and foot level, unspecified foot

● S96.82 Laceration of other specified muscles and tendons at ankle and foot level

● S96.821 Laceration of other specified muscles and tendons at ankle and foot level, right foot

● S96.822 Laceration of other specified muscles and tendons at ankle and foot level, left foot

● S96.829 Laceration of other specified muscles and tendons at ankle and foot level, unspecified foot

● S96.89 Other specified injury of other specified muscles and tendons at ankle and foot level

● S96.891 Other specified injury of other specified muscles and tendons at ankle and foot level, right foot

● S96.892 Other specified injury of other specified muscles and tendons at ankle and foot level, left foot

● S96.899 Other specified injury of other specified muscles and tendons at ankle and foot level, unspecified foot

● S96.9 Injury of unspecified muscle and tendon at ankle and foot level
● S96.90 Unspecified injury of unspecified muscle and tendon at ankle and foot level
● S96.901 Unspecified injury of unspecified muscle and tendon at ankle and foot level, right foot
● S96.902 Unspecified injury of unspecified muscle and tendon at ankle and foot level, left foot
● S96.909 Unspecified injury of unspecified muscle and tendon at ankle and foot level, unspecified foot
● S96.91 Strain of unspecified muscle and tendon at ankle and foot level
● S96.911 Strain of unspecified muscle and tendon at ankle and foot level, right foot
● S96.912 Strain of unspecified muscle and tendon at ankle and foot level, left foot
● S96.919 Strain of unspecified muscle and tendon at ankle and foot level, unspecified foot
● S96.92 Laceration of unspecified muscle and tendon at ankle and foot level
● S96.921 Laceration of unspecified muscle and tendon at ankle and foot level, right foot
● S96.922 Laceration of unspecified muscle and tendon at ankle and foot level, left foot
● S96.929 Laceration of unspecified muscle and tendon at ankle and foot level, unspecified foot
● S96.99 Other specified injury of unspecified muscle and tendon at ankle and foot level
● S96.991 Other specified injury of unspecified muscle and tendon at ankle and foot level, right foot
● S96.992 Other specified injury of unspecified muscle and tendon at ankle and foot level, left foot
● S96.999 Other specified injury of unspecified muscle and tendon at ankle and foot level, unspecified foot

● S97 Crushing injury of ankle and foot

Use additional code(s) for all associated injuries

The appropriate 7th character is to be added to each code from category S97

A	initial encounter
D	subsequent encounter
S	sequela

● S97.0 Crushing injury of ankle
X● S97.00 Crushing injury of unspecified ankle
X● S97.01 Crushing injury of right ankle
X● S97.02 Crushing injury of left ankle
● S97.1 Crushing injury of toe
● S97.10 Crushing injury of unspecified toe(s)
● S97.101 Crushing injury of unspecified right toe(s)
● S97.102 Crushing injury of unspecified left toe(s)
● S97.109 Crushing injury of unspecified toe(s)
Crushing injury of toe NOS
● S97.11 Crushing injury of great toe
● S97.111 Crushing injury of right great toe
● S97.112 Crushing injury of left great toe
● S97.119 Crushing injury of unspecified great toe
● S97.12 Crushing injury of lesser toe(s)
● S97.121 Crushing injury of right lesser toe(s)
● S97.122 Crushing injury of left lesser toe(s)
● S97.129 Crushing injury of lesser toe(s), unspecified toe(s)
● S97.8 Crushing injury of foot
X● S97.80 Crushing injury of foot, unspecified side
Crushing injury of foot NOS
X● S97.81 Crushing injury of right foot
X● S97.82 Crushing injury of left foot

● S98 Traumatic amputation of ankle and foot

An amputation not identified as partial or complete should be coded to complete

The appropriate 7th character is to be added to each code from category S98

A	initial encounter
D	subsequent encounter
S	sequela

● S98.0 Traumatic amputation of foot at ankle level
● S98.01 Complete traumatic amputation of foot at ankle level
● S98.011 Complete traumatic amputation of right foot at ankle level
● S98.012 Complete traumatic amputation of left foot at ankle level
● S98.019 Complete traumatic amputation of unspecified foot at ankle level
● S98.02 Partial traumatic amputation of foot at ankle level
● S98.021 Partial traumatic amputation of right foot at ankle level
● S98.022 Partial traumatic amputation of left foot at ankle level
● S98.029 Partial traumatic amputation of unspecified foot at ankle level
● S98.1 Traumatic amputation of one toe
● S98.11 Complete traumatic amputation of great toe
● S98.111 Complete traumatic amputation of right great toe
● S98.112 Complete traumatic amputation of left great toe
● S98.119 Complete traumatic amputation of unspecified great toe
● S98.12 Partial traumatic amputation of great toe
● S98.121 Partial traumatic amputation of right great toe
● S98.122 Partial traumatic amputation of left great toe
● S98.129 Partial traumatic amputation of unspecified great toe
● S98.13 Complete traumatic amputation of one lesser toe
Traumatic amputation of toe NOS
● S98.131 Complete traumatic amputation of one right lesser toe
● S98.132 Complete traumatic amputation of one left lesser toe
● S98.139 Complete traumatic amputation of one unspecified lesser toe

● S98.14 Partial traumatic amputation of one lesser toe
● S98.141 Partial traumatic amputation of one right lesser toe
● S98.142 Partial traumatic amputation of one left lesser toe
● S98.149 Partial traumatic amputation of one unspecified lesser toe
● S98.2 Traumatic amputation of two or more lesser toes
● S98.21 Complete traumatic amputation of two or more lesser toes
● S98.211 Complete traumatic amputation of two or more right lesser toes
● S98.212 Complete traumatic amputation of two or more left lesser toes
● S98.219 Complete traumatic amputation of two or more unspecified lesser toes
● S98.22 Partial traumatic amputation of two or more lesser toes
● S98.221 Partial traumatic amputation of two or more right lesser toes
● S98.222 Partial traumatic amputation of two or more left lesser toes
● S98.229 Partial traumatic amputation of two or more unspecified lesser toes
● S98.3 Traumatic amputation of midfoot
● S98.31 Complete traumatic amputation of midfoot
● S98.311 Complete traumatic amputation of right midfoot
● S98.312 Complete traumatic amputation of left midfoot
● S98.319 Complete traumatic amputation of unspecified midfoot
● S98.32 Partial traumatic amputation of midfoot
● S98.321 Partial traumatic amputation of right midfoot
● S98.322 Partial traumatic amputation of left midfoot
● S98.329 Partial traumatic amputation of unspecified midfoot
● S98.9 Traumatic amputation of foot, level unspecified
● S98.91 Complete traumatic amputation of foot, level unspecified
● S98.911 Complete traumatic amputation of right foot, level unspecified
● S98.912 Complete traumatic amputation of left foot, level unspecified
● S98.919 Complete traumatic amputation of unspecified foot, level unspecified
● S98.92 Partial traumatic amputation of foot, level unspecified
● S98.921 Partial traumatic amputation of right foot, level unspecified
● S98.922 Partial traumatic amputation of left foot, level unspecified
● S98.929 Partial traumatic amputation of unspecified foot, level unspecified

● S99 Other and unspecified injuries of ankle and foot
● S99.0 Physeal fracture of calcaneus ◀

The appropriate 7th character is to be added to each code from subcategories S99.0 ◀

A	initial encounter for closed fracture ◀
B	initial encounter for open fracture ◀
D	subsequent encounter for fracture with routine healing ◀
G	subsequent encounter for fracture with delayed healing ◀
K	subsequent encounter for fracture with nonunion ◀
P	subsequent encounter for fracture with malunion ◀
S	sequela ◀

● S99.00 Unspecified physeal fracture of calcaneus ◀
● S99.001 Unspecified physeal fracture of right calcaneus ◀
● S99.002 Unspecified physeal fracture of left calcaneus ◀
● S99.009 Unspecified physeal fracture of unspecified calcaneus ◀
● S99.01 Salter-Harris Type I physeal fracture of calcaneus ◀
● S99.011 Salter-Harris Type I physeal fracture of right calcaneus ◀
● S99.012 Salter-Harris Type I physeal fracture of left calcaneus ◀
● S99.019 Salter-Harris Type I physeal fracture of unspecified calcaneus ◀
● S99.02 Salter-Harris Type II physeal fracture of calcaneus ◀
● S99.021 Salter-Harris Type II physeal fracture of right calcaneus ◀
● S99.022 Salter-Harris Type II physeal fracture of left calcaneus ◀
● S99.029 Salter-Harris Type II physeal fracture of unspecified calcaneus ◀
● S99.03 Salter-Harris Type III physeal fracture of calcaneus ◀
● S99.031 Salter-Harris Type III physeal fracture of right calcaneus ◀
● S99.032 Salter-Harris Type III physeal fracture of left calcaneus ◀
● S99.039 Salter-Harris Type III physeal fracture of unspecified calcaneus ◀
● S99.04 Salter-Harris Type IV physeal fracture of calcaneus ◀
● S99.041 Salter-Harris Type IV physeal fracture of right calcaneus ◀
● S99.042 Salter-Harris Type IV physeal fracture of left calcaneus ◀
● S99.049 Salter-Harris Type IV physeal fracture of unspecified calcaneus ◀
● S99.09 Other physeal fracture of calcaneus ◀
● S99.091 Other physeal fracture of right calcaneus ◀
● S99.092 Other physeal fracture of left calcaneus ◀
● S99.099 Other physeal fracture of unspecified calcaneus ◀

CHAPTER 19 (S00-T88)

● **S99.1 Physeal fracture of metatarsal** ◀

The appropriate 7th character is to be added to each code from subcategories S99.1 ◀

A	initial encounter for closed fracture ◀
B	initial encounter for open fracture ◀
D	subsequent encounter for fracture with routine healing ◀
G	subsequent encounter for fracture with delayed healing ◀
K	subsequent encounter for fracture with nonunion ◀
P	subsequent encounter for fracture with malunion ◀
S	sequela ◀

● **S99.10 Unspecified physeal fracture of metatarsal** ◀

● **S99.101 Unspecified physeal fracture of right metatarsal** ◀

● **S99.102 Unspecified physeal fracture of left metatarsal** ◀

● **S99.109 Unspecified physeal fracture of unspecified metatarsal** ◀

● **S99.11 Salter-Harris Type I physeal fracture of metatarsal** ◀

● **S99.111 Salter-Harris Type I physeal fracture of right metatarsal** ◀

● **S99.112 Salter-Harris Type I physeal fracture of left metatarsal** ◀

● **S99.119 Salter-Harris Type I physeal fracture of unspecified metatarsal** ◀

● **S99.12 Salter-Harris Type II physeal fracture of metatarsal** ◀

● **S99.121 Salter-Harris Type II physeal fracture of right metatarsal** ◀

● **S99.122 Salter-Harris Type II physeal fracture of left metatarsal** ◀

● **S99.129 Salter-Harris Type II physeal fracture of unspecified metatarsal** ◀

● **S99.13 Salter-Harris Type III physeal fracture of metatarsal** ◀

● **S99.131 Salter-Harris Type III physeal fracture of right metatarsal** ◀

● **S99.132 Salter-Harris Type III physeal fracture of left metatarsal** ◀

● **S99.139 Salter-Harris Type III physeal fracture of unspecified metatarsal** ◀

● **S99.14 Salter-Harris Type IV physeal fracture of metatarsal** ◀

● **S99.141 Salter-Harris Type IV physeal fracture of right metatarsal** ◀

● **S99.142 Salter-Harris Type IV physeal fracture of left metatarsal** ◀

● **S99.149 Salter-Harris Type IV physeal fracture of unspecified metatarsal** ◀

● **S99.19 Other physeal fracture of metatarsal** ◀

● **S99.191 Other physeal fracture of right metatarsal** ◀

● **S99.192 Other physeal fracture of left metatarsal** ◀

● **S99.199 Other physeal fracture of unspecified metatarsal** ◀

● **S99.2 Physeal fracture of phalanx of toe** ◀

The appropriate 7th character is to be added to each code from subcategories S99.2 ◀

A	initial encounter for closed fracture ◀
B	initial encounter for open fracture ◀
D	subsequent encounter for fracture with routine healing ◀
G	subsequent encounter for fracture with delayed healing ◀
K	subsequent encounter for fracture with nonunion ◀
P	subsequent encounter for fracture with malunion ◀
S	sequela ◀

● **S99.20 Unspecified physeal fracture of phalanx of toe** ◀

● **S99.201 Unspecified physeal fracture of phalanx of right toe** ◀

● **S99.202 Unspecified physeal fracture of phalanx of right toe** ◀

● **S99.209 Unspecified physeal fracture of phalanx of unspecified toe** ◀

● **S99.21 Salter-Harris Type I physeal fracture of phalanx of toe** ◀

● **S99.211 Salter-Harris Type I physeal fracture of phalanx of right toe** ◀

● **S99.212 Salter-Harris Type I physeal fracture of phalanx of left toe** ◀

● **S99.219 Salter-Harris Type I physeal fracture of phalanx of unspecified toe** ◀

● **S99.22 Salter-Harris Type II physeal fracture of phalanx of toe** ◀

● **S99.221 Salter-Harris Type II physeal fracture of phalanx of right toe** ◀

● **S99.222 Salter-Harris Type II physeal fracture of phalanx of left toe** ◀

● **S99.229 Salter-Harris Type II physeal fracture of phalanx of unspecified toe** ◀

● **S99.23 Salter-Harris Type III physeal fracture of phalanx of toe** ◀

● **S99.231 Salter-Harris Type III physeal fracture of phalanx of right toe** ◀

● **S99.232 Salter-Harris Type III physeal fracture of phalanx of left toe** ◀

● **S99.239 Salter-Harris Type III physeal fracture of phalanx of unspecified toe** ◀

● **S99.24 Salter-Harris Type IV physeal fracture of phalanx of toe** ◀

● **S99.241 Salter-Harris Type IV physeal fracture of phalanx of right toe** ◀

● **S99.242 Salter-Harris Type IV physeal fracture of phalanx of left toe** ◀

● **S99.249 Salter-Harris Type IV physeal fracture of phalanx of unspecified toe** ◀

● **S99.29 Other physeal fracture of phalanx of toe** ◀

● **S99.291 Other physeal fracture of phalanx of right toe** ◀

● **S99.292 Other physeal fracture of phalanx of left toe** ◀

● **S99.299 Other physeal fracture of phalanx of unspecified toe** ◀

● **S99.8   Other specified injuries of ankle and foot**
The appropriate 7th character is to be added to each
code from subcategory S99.8 ◄

A	initial encounter ◄
D	subsequent encounter ◄
S	sequela ◄

● **S99.81   Other specified injuries of ankle**
  ● S99.811   Other specified injuries of right ankle
  ● S99.812   Other specified injuries of left ankle
  ● S99.819   Other specified injuries of unspecified ankle

● **S99.82   Other specified injuries of foot**
  ● S99.821   Other specified injuries of right foot
  ● S99.822   Other specified injuries of left foot
  ● S99.829   Other specified injuries of unspecified foot

● **S99.9   Unspecified injury of ankle and foot**
The appropriate 7th character is to be added to each
code from subcategory S99.9 ◄

A	initial encounter ◄
D	subsequent encounter ◄
S	sequela ◄

● **S99.91   Unspecified injury of ankle**
  ● S99.911   Unspecified injury of right ankle
  ● S99.912   Unspecified injury of left ankle
  ● S99.919   Unspecified injury of unspecified ankle

● **S99.92   Unspecified injury of foot**
  ● S99.921   Unspecified injury of right foot
  ● S99.922   Unspecified injury of left foot
  ● S99.929   Unspecified injury of unspecified foot

INJURY, POISONING AND CERTAIN OTHER CONSEQUENCES OF EXTERNAL CAUSES (T07-T88)

INJURIES INVOLVING MULTIPLE BODY REGIONS (T07)

Excludes1	burns and corrosions (T20-T32)
	frostbite (T33-T34)
	insect bite or sting, venomous (T63.4)
	sunburn (L55.-)

T07   Unspecified multiple injuries

Excludes1	injury NOS (T14)

INJURY OF UNSPECIFIED BODY REGION (T14)

● **T14   Injury of unspecified body region**

Excludes1	multiple unspecified injuries (T07)

T14.8   Other injury of unspecified body region
Abrasion NOS   Fracture NOS
Contusion NOS   Skin injury NOS
Crush injury NOS   Vascular injury NOS

● **T14.9   Unspecified injury**
T14.90   Injury, unspecified
Injury NOS
T14.91   Suicide attempt
Attempted suicide NOS

EFFECTS OF FOREIGN BODY ENTERING THROUGH NATURAL ORIFICE (T15-T19)

Excludes2	foreign body accidentally left in operation wound (T81.5-)
	foreign body in penetrating wound - see open wound by body region
	residual foreign body in soft tissue (M79.5)
	splinter, without open wound - see superficial injury by body region

● **T15   Foreign body on external eye**

Excludes2	foreign body in penetrating wound of orbit and eye ball (S05.4-, S05.5-)
	open wound of eyelid and periocular area (S01.1-)
	retained foreign body in eyelid (H02.8-)
	retained (old) foreign body in penetrating wound of orbit and eye ball (H05.5-, H44.6-, H44.7-)
	superficial foreign body of eyelid and periocular area (S00.25-)

The appropriate 7th character is to be added to each code from
category T15

A	initial encounter
D	subsequent encounter
S	sequela

● **T15.0   Foreign body in cornea**
  X ● T15.00   Foreign body in cornea, unspecified eye
  X ● T15.01   Foreign body in cornea, right eye
  X ● T15.02   Foreign body in cornea, left eye
● **T15.1   Foreign body in conjunctival sac**
  X ● T15.10   Foreign body in conjunctival sac, unspecified eye
  X ● T15.11   Foreign body in conjunctival sac, right eye
  X ● T15.12   Foreign body in conjunctival sac, left eye
● **T15.8   Foreign body in other and multiple parts of external eye**
  Foreign body in lacrimal punctum
  X ● T15.80   Foreign body in other and multiple parts of external eye, unspecified eye
  X ● T15.81   Foreign body in other and multiple parts of external eye, right eye
  X ● T15.82   Foreign body in other and multiple parts of external eye, left eye
● **T15.9   Foreign body on external eye, part unspecified**
  X ● T15.90   Foreign body on external eye, part unspecified, unspecified eye
  X ● T15.91   Foreign body on external eye, part unspecified, right eye
  X ● T15.92   Foreign body on external eye, part unspecified, left eye

● **T16   Foreign body in ear**

Includes	foreign body in auditory canal

The appropriate 7th character is to be added to each code from
category T16

A	initial encounter
D	subsequent encounter
S	sequela

  X ● T16.1   Foreign body in right ear
  X ● T16.2   Foreign body in left ear
  X ● T16.9   Foreign body in ear, unspecified ear

● **T17   Foreign body in respiratory tract**
The appropriate 7th character is to be added to each code from
category T17

A	initial encounter
D	subsequent encounter
S	sequela

  X ● T17.0   Foreign body in nasal sinus
  X ● T17.1   Foreign body in nostril
  Foreign body in nose NOS

◄ New   ◄▥ Revised   ~~deleted~~ Deleted   **OGCR** Official Guidelines   X Assign placeholder X   ● Use Additional Character(s)

Excludes 1	Excludes 2	Includes	Use additional	Code first	Code also	Unspecified

- **T17.2 Foreign body in pharynx**
  Foreign body in nasopharynx
  Foreign body in throat NOS
  - **T17.20 Unspecified foreign body in pharynx**
    - **T17.200 Unspecified foreign body in pharynx causing asphyxiation**
    - **T17.208 Unspecified foreign body in pharynx causing other injury**
  - **T17.21 Gastric contents in pharynx**
    Aspiration of gastric contents into pharynx
    Vomitus in pharynx
    - **T17.210 Gastric contents in pharynx causing asphyxiation**
    - **T17.218 Gastric contents in pharynx causing other injury**
  - **T17.22 Food in pharynx**
    Bones in pharynx
    Seeds in pharynx
    - **T17.220 Food in pharynx causing asphyxiation**
    - **T17.228 Food in pharynx causing other injury**
  - **T17.29 Other foreign object in pharynx**
    - **T17.290 Other foreign object in pharynx causing asphyxiation**
    - **T17.298 Other foreign object in pharynx causing other injury**
- **T17.3 Foreign body in larynx**
  - **T17.30 Unspecified foreign body in larynx**
    - **T17.300 Unspecified foreign body in larynx causing asphyxiation**
    - **T17.308 Unspecified foreign body in larynx causing other injury**
  - **T17.31 Gastric contents in larynx**
    Aspiration of gastric contents into larynx
    Vomitus in larynx
    - **T17.310 Gastric contents in larynx causing asphyxiation**
    - **T17.318 Gastric contents in larynx causing other injury**
  - **T17.32 Food in larynx**
    Bones in larynx (Revised)
    Seeds in larynx
    - **T17.320 Food in larynx causing asphyxiation**
    - **T17.328 Food in larynx causing other injury**
  - **T17.39 Other foreign object in larynx**
    - **T17.390 Other foreign object in larynx causing asphyxiation**
    - **T17.398 Other foreign object in larynx causing other injury**
- **T17.4 Foreign body in trachea**
  - **T17.40 Unspecified foreign body in trachea**
    - **T17.400 Unspecified foreign body in trachea causing asphyxiation**
    - **T17.408 Unspecified foreign body in trachea causing other injury**
  - **T17.41 Gastric contents in trachea**
    Aspiration of gastric contents into trachea
    Vomitus in trachea
    - **T17.410 Gastric contents in trachea causing asphyxiation**
    - **T17.418 Gastric contents in trachea causing other injury**
  - **T17.42 Food in trachea**
    Bones in trachea
    Seeds in trachea
    - **T17.420 Food in trachea causing asphyxiation**
    - **T17.428 Food in trachea causing other injury**
  - **T17.49 Other foreign object in trachea**
    - **T17.490 Other foreign object in trachea causing asphyxiation**
    - **T17.498 Other foreign object in trachea causing other injury**
- **T17.5 Foreign body in bronchus**
  - **T17.50 Unspecified foreign body in bronchus**
    - **T17.500 Unspecified foreign body in bronchus causing asphyxiation**
    - **T17.508 Unspecified foreign body in bronchus causing other injury**
  - **T17.51 Gastric contents in bronchus**
    Aspiration of gastric contents into bronchus
    Vomitus in bronchus
    - **T17.510 Gastric contents in bronchus causing asphyxiation**
    - **T17.518 Gastric contents in bronchus causing other injury**
  - **T17.52 Food in bronchus**
    Bones in bronchus
    Seeds in bronchus
    - **T17.520 Food in bronchus causing asphyxiation**
    - **T17.528 Food in bronchus causing other injury**
  - **T17.59 Other foreign object in bronchus**
    - **T17.590 Other foreign object in bronchus causing asphyxiation**
    - **T17.598 Other foreign object in bronchus causing other injury**
- **T17.8 Foreign body in other parts of respiratory tract**
  Foreign body in bronchioles
  Foreign body in lung
  - **T17.80 Unspecified foreign body in other parts of respiratory tract**
    - **T17.800 Unspecified foreign body in other parts of respiratory tract causing asphyxiation**
    - **T17.808 Unspecified foreign body in other parts of respiratory tract causing other injury**
  - **T17.81 Gastric contents in other parts of respiratory tract**
    Aspiration of gastric contents into other parts of respiratory tract
    Vomitus in other parts of respiratory tract
    - **T17.810 Gastric contents in other parts of respiratory tract causing asphyxiation**
    - **T17.818 Gastric contents in other parts of respiratory tract causing other injury**
  - **T17.82 Food in other parts of respiratory tract**
    Bones in other parts of respiratory tract
    Seeds in other parts of respiratory tract
    - **T17.820 Food in other parts of respiratory tract causing asphyxiation**
    - **T17.828 Food in other parts of respiratory tract causing other injury**
  - **T17.89 Other foreign object in other parts of respiratory tract**
    - **T17.890 Other foreign object in other parts of respiratory tract causing asphyxiation**
    - **T17.898 Other foreign object in other parts of respiratory tract causing other injury**
- **T17.9 Foreign body in respiratory tract, part unspecified**
  - **T17.90 Unspecified foreign body in respiratory tract, part unspecified**
    - **T17.900 Unspecified foreign body in respiratory tract, part unspecified causing asphyxiation**
    - **T17.908 Unspecified foreign body in respiratory tract, part unspecified causing other injury**

● **T17.91 Gastric contents in respiratory tract, part unspecified**
Aspiration of gastric contents into respiratory tract, part unspecified
Vomitus in trachea respiratory tract, part unspecified

● **T17.910 Gastric contents in respiratory tract, part unspecified causing asphyxiation**

● **T17.918 Gastric contents in respiratory tract, part unspecified causing other injury**

● **T17.92 Food in respiratory tract, part unspecified**
Bones in respiratory tract, part unspecified
Seeds in respiratory tract, part unspecified

● **T17.920 Food in respiratory tract, part unspecified causing asphyxiation**

● **T17.928 Food in respiratory tract, part unspecified causing other injury**

● **T17.99 Other foreign object in respiratory tract, part unspecified**

● **T17.990 Other foreign object in respiratory tract, part unspecified in causing asphyxiation**

● **T17.998 Other foreign object in respiratory tract, part unspecified causing other injury**

● **T18 Foreign body in alimentary tract**
Excludes2 foreign body in pharynx (T17.2-)
The appropriate 7th character is to be added to each code from category T18

A	initial encounter
D	subsequent encounter
S	sequela

X● **T18.0 Foreign body in mouth**

X● **T18.1 Foreign body in esophagus**
Excludes2 foreign body in respiratory tract (T17.-)

● **T18.10 Unspecified foreign body in esophagus**

● **T18.100 Unspecified foreign body in esophagus causing compression of trachea**
Unspecified foreign body in esophagus causing obstruction of respiration

● **T18.108 Unspecified foreign body in esophagus causing other injury**

● **T18.11 Gastric contents in esophagus**
Vomitus in esophagus

● **T18.110 Gastric contents in esophagus causing compression of trachea**
Gastric contents in esophagus causing obstruction of respiration

● **T18.118 Gastric contents in esophagus causing other injury**

● **T18.12 Food in esophagus**
Bones in esophagus
Seeds in esophagus

● **T18.120 Food in esophagus causing compression of trachea**
Food in esophagus causing obstruction of respiration

● **T18.128 Food in esophagus causing other injury**

● **T18.19 Other foreign object in esophagus**

● **T18.190 Other foreign object in esophagus causing compression of trachea**
Other foreign body in esophagus causing obstruction of respiration

● **T18.198 Other foreign object in esophagus causing other injury**

X● **T18.2 Foreign body in stomach**

X● **T18.3 Foreign body in small intestine**

X● **T18.4 Foreign body in colon**

X● **T18.5 Foreign body in anus and rectum**
Foreign body in rectosigmoid (junction)

X● **T18.8 Foreign body in other parts of alimentary tract**

X● **T18.9 Foreign body of alimentary tract, part unspecified**
Foreign body in digestive system NOS
Swallowed foreign body NOS

● **T19 Foreign body in genitourinary tract**
Excludes2 complications due to implanted mesh (T83.7-)
mechanical complications of contraceptive device (intrauterine) (vaginal) (T83.3-)
presence of contraceptive device (intrauterine) (vaginal) (Z97.5)
The appropriate 7th character is to be added to each code from category T19

A	initial encounter
D	subsequent encounter
S	sequela

X● **T19.0 Foreign body in urethra**

X● **T19.1 Foreign body in bladder**

X● **T19.2 Foreign body in vulva and vagina**

X● **T19.3 Foreign body in uterus**

X● **T19.4 Foreign body in penis**

X● **T19.8 Foreign body in other parts of genitourinary tract**

X● **T19.9 Foreign body in genitourinary tract, part unspecified**

BURNS AND CORROSIONS (T20-T32)

Includes burns (thermal) from electrical heating appliances
burns (thermal) from electricity
burns (thermal) from flame
burns (thermal) from friction
burns (thermal) from hot air and hot gases
burns (thermal) from hot objects
burns (thermal) from lightning
burns (thermal) from radiation chemical
burn [corrosion] (external) (internal) scalds

Excludes2 erythema [dermatitis] ab igne (L59.0)
radiation-related disorders of the skin and subcutaneous tissue (L55-L59)
sunburn (L55.-)

OGCR Section I.C.19.d.

Burns and Corrosions

The ICD-10-CM makes a distinction between burn and corrosions. The burn codes are for thermal burns, except sunburns, that come from a heat source, such as a fire or hot appliance. The burn codes are also for burns resulting from electricity and radiation. Corrosions are burns due to chemicals. The guidelines for burns and corrosions are the same.

Current burns (T20-T25) are classified by depth, extent and by agent (X code). Burns are classified by depth as first degree (erythema), second degree (blistering), and third degree (full-thickness involvement). Burns of the eye and internal organs (T26-T28) are classified by site, but not by degree.

1) Sequencing of burn and related condition codes

Sequence first the code that reflects the highest degree of burn when more than one burn is present.

a. When the reason for the admission or encounter is for treatment of external multiple burns, sequence first the code that reflects the burn of the highest degree.

b. When a patient has both internal and external burns, the circumstances of admission govern the selection of the principal diagnosis or first-listed diagnosis.

c. When a patient is admitted for burn injuries and other related conditions such as smoke inhalation and/or respiratory failure, the circumstances of admission govern the selection of the principal or first-listed diagnosis.

2) Burns of the same local site

Classify burns of the same local site (three-character category level, T20-T28) but of different degrees to the subcategory identifying the highest degree recorded in the diagnosis.

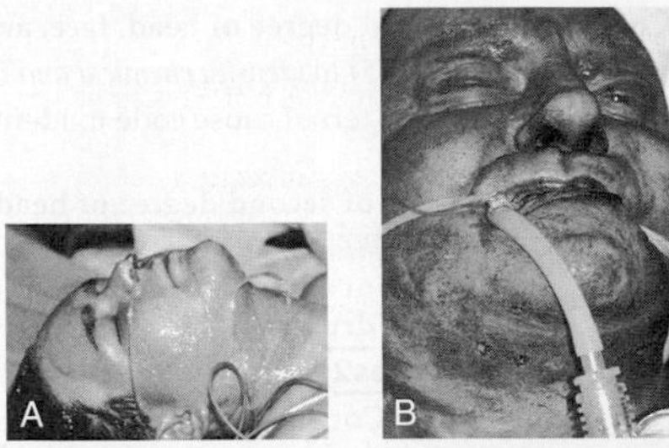

Figure 19-15 **A.** Second-degree burn. **B.** Third-degree burn. (From Cummings: Otolaryngology: Head & Neck Surgery, ed 4, Mosby, 2005)

BURNS AND CORROSIONS OF EXTERNAL BODY SURFACE, SPECIFIED BY SITE (T20-T25)

Includes burns and corrosions of first degree [erythema]
burns and corrosions of second degree [blisters] [epidermal loss]
burns and corrosions of third degree [deep necrosis of underlying tissue] [full-thickness skin loss]

Use additional code from category T31 or T32 to identify extent of body surface involved

● **T20 Burn and corrosion of head, face, and neck**

Excludes2 burn and corrosion of ear drum (T28.41, T28.91)
burn and corrosion of eye and adnexa (T26.-)
burn and corrosion of mouth and pharynx (T28.0)

The appropriate 7th character is to be added to each code from category T20

A	initial encounter
D	subsequent encounter
S	sequela

● **T20.0 Burn of unspecified degree of head, face, and neck**
Use additional external cause code to identify the source, place and intent of the burn (X00-X19, X75-X77, X96-X98, Y92)

X● **T20.00** **Burn of unspecified degree of head, face, and neck, unspecified site**
● **T20.01** **Burn of unspecified degree of ear [any part, except ear drum]**
Excludes2 burn of ear drum (T28.41-)
● **T20.011** **Burn of unspecified degree of right ear [any part, except ear drum]**
● **T20.012** **Burn of unspecified degree of left ear [any part, except ear drum]**
● **T20.019** **Burn of unspecified degree of unspecified ear [any part, except ear drum]**
X● **T20.02** **Burn of unspecified degree of lip(s)**
X● **T20.03** **Burn of unspecified degree of chin**
X● **T20.04** **Burn of unspecified degree of nose (septum)**
X● **T20.05** **Burn of unspecified degree of scalp [any part]**
X● **T20.06** **Burn of unspecified degree of forehead and cheek**
X● **T20.07** **Burn of unspecified degree of neck**
X● **T20.09** **Burn of unspecified degree of multiple sites of head, face, and neck**

● **T20.1 Burn of first degree of head, face, and neck**
Use additional external cause code to identify the source, place and intent of the burn (X00-X19, X75-X77, X96-X98, Y92)

X● **T20.10** **Burn of first degree of head, face, and neck, unspecified site**
● **T20.11** **Burn of first degree of ear [any part, except ear drum]**
Excludes2 burn of ear drum (T28.41-)
● **T20.111** **Burn of first degree of right ear [any part, except ear drum]**
● **T20.112** **Burn of first degree of left ear [any part, except ear drum]**
● **T20.119** **Burn of first degree of unspecified ear [any part, except ear drum]**
X● **T20.12** **Burn of first degree of lip(s)**
X● **T20.13** **Burn of first degree of chin**
X● **T20.14** **Burn of first degree of nose (septum)**
X● **T20.15** **Burn of first degree of scalp [any part]**
X● **T20.16** **Burn of first degree of forehead and cheek**
X● **T20.17** **Burn of first degree of neck**
X● **T20.19** **Burn of first degree of multiple sites of head, face, and neck**

● **T20.2 Burn of second degree of head, face, and neck**
Use additional external cause code to identify the source, place and intent of the burn (X00-X19, X75-X77, X96-X98, Y92)

X● **T20.20** **Burn of second degree of head, face, and neck, unspecified site**
● **T20.21** **Burn of second degree of ear [any part, except ear drum]**
Excludes2 burn of ear drum (T28.41-)
● **T20.211** **Burn of second degree of right ear [any part, except ear drum]**
● **T20.212** **Burn of second degree of left ear [any part, except ear drum]**
● **T20.219** **Burn of second degree of unspecified ear [any part, except ear drum]**
X● **T20.22** **Burn of second degree of lip(s)**
X● **T20.23** **Burn of second degree of chin**
X● **T20.24** **Burn of second degree of nose (septum)**
X● **T20.25** **Burn of second degree of scalp [any part]**
X● **T20.26** **Burn of second degree of forehead and cheek**
X● **T20.27** **Burn of second degree of neck**
X● **T20.29** **Burn of second degree of multiple sites of head, face, and neck**

● **T20.3 Burn of third degree of head, face, and neck**
Use additional external cause code to identify the source, place and intent of the burn (X00-X19, X75-X77, X96-X98, Y92)

X● **T20.30** **Burn of third degree of head, face, and neck, unspecified site**
● **T20.31** **Burn of third degree of ear [any part, except ear drum]**
Excludes2 burn of ear drum (T28.41-)
● **T20.311** **Burn of third degree of right ear [any part, except ear drum]**
● **T20.312** **Burn of third degree of left ear [any part, except ear drum]**
● **T20.319** **Burn of third degree of unspecified ear [any part, except ear drum]**

X● T20.32 Burn of third degree of lip(s)
X● T20.33 Burn of third degree of chin
X● T20.34 Burn of third degree of nose (septum)
X● T20.35 Burn of third degree of scalp [any part]
X● T20.36 Burn of third degree of forehead and cheek
X● T20.37 Burn of third degree of neck
X● T20.39 Burn of third degree of multiple sites of head, face, and neck

● **T20.4 Corrosion of unspecified degree of head, face, and neck**
Code first (T51-T65) to identify chemical and intent
Use additional external cause code to identify place (Y92)

X● T20.40 Corrosion of unspecified degree of head, face, and neck, unspecified site
● T20.41 Corrosion of unspecified degree of ear [any part, except ear drum]
Excludes2 corrosion of ear drum (T28.91-)
● T20.411 Corrosion of unspecified degree of right ear [any part, except ear drum]
● T20.412 Corrosion of unspecified degree of left ear [any part, except ear drum]
● T20.419 Corrosion of unspecified degree of unspecified ear [any part, except ear drum]
X● T20.42 Corrosion of unspecified degree of lip(s)
X● T20.43 Corrosion of unspecified degree of chin
X● T20.44 Corrosion of unspecified degree of nose (septum)
X● T20.45 Corrosion of unspecified degree of scalp [any part]
X● T20.46 Corrosion of unspecified degree of forehead and cheek
X● T20.47 Corrosion of unspecified degree of neck
X● T20.49 Corrosion of unspecified degree of multiple sites of head, face, and neck

● **T20.5 Corrosion of first degree of head, face, and neck**
Code first (T51-T65) to identify chemical and intent
Use additional external cause code to identify place (Y92)

X● T20.50 Corrosion of first degree of head, face, and neck, unspecified site
● T20.51 Corrosion of first degree of ear [any part, except ear drum]
Excludes2 corrosion of ear drum (T28.91-)
● T20.511 Corrosion of first degree of right ear [any part, except ear drum]
● T20.512 Corrosion of first degree of left ear [any part, except ear drum]
● T20.519 Corrosion of first degree of unspecified ear [any part, except ear drum]
X● T20.52 Corrosion of first degree of lip(s)
X● T20.53 Corrosion of first degree of chin
X● T20.54 Corrosion of first degree of nose (septum)
X● T20.55 Corrosion of first degree of scalp [any part]
X● T20.56 Corrosion of first degree of forehead and cheek
X● T20.57 Corrosion of first degree of neck
X● T20.59 Corrosion of first degree of multiple sites of head, face, and neck

● **T20.6 Corrosion of second degree of head, face, and neck**
Code first (T51-T65) to identify chemical and intent
Use additional external cause code to identify place (Y92)

X● T20.60 Corrosion of second degree of head, face, and neck, unspecified site
● T20.61 Corrosion of second degree of ear [any part, except ear drum]
Excludes2 corrosion of ear drum (T28.91-)
● T20.611 Corrosion of second degree of right ear [any part, except ear drum]
● T20.612 Corrosion of second degree of left ear [any part, except ear drum]
● T20.619 Corrosion of second degree of unspecified ear [any part, except ear drum]
X● T20.62 Corrosion of second degree of lip(s)
X● T20.63 Corrosion of second degree of chin
X● T20.64 Corrosion of second degree of nose (septum)
X● T20.65 Corrosion of second degree of scalp [any part]
X● T20.66 Corrosion of second degree of forehead and cheek
X● T20.67 Corrosion of second degree of neck
X● T20.69 Corrosion of second degree of multiple sites of head, face, and neck

● **T20.7 Corrosion of third degree of head, face, and neck**
Code first (T51-T65) to identify chemical and intent
Use additional external cause code to identify place (Y92)

X● T20.70 Corrosion of third degree of head, face, and neck, unspecified site
● T20.71 Corrosion of third degree of ear [any part, except ear drum]
Excludes2 corrosion of ear drum (T28.91-)
● T20.711 Corrosion of third degree of right ear [any part, except ear drum]
● T20.712 Corrosion of third degree of left ear [any part, except ear drum]
● T20.719 Corrosion of third degree of unspecified ear [any part, except ear drum]
X● T20.72 Corrosion of third degree of lip(s)
X● T20.73 Corrosion of third degree of chin
X● T20.74 Corrosion of third degree of nose (septum)
X● T20.75 Corrosion of third degree of scalp [any part]
X● T20.76 Corrosion of third degree of forehead and cheek
X● T20.77 Corrosion of third degree of neck
X● T20.79 Corrosion of third degree of multiple sites of head, face, and neck

● T21 Burn and corrosion of trunk

Includes burns and corrosion of hip region

Excludes2 burns and corrosion of axilla (T22.- with fifth character 4)
burns and corrosion of scapular region (T22.- with fifth character 6)
burns and corrosion of shoulder (T22.- with fifth character 5)

The appropriate 7th character is to be added to each code from category T21

A initial encounter
D subsequent encounter
S sequela

● T21.0 Burn of unspecified degree of trunk
Use additional external cause code to identify the source, place and intent of the burn (X00-X19, X75-X77, X96-X98, Y92)

X● T21.00 Burn of unspecified degree of trunk, unspecified site

X● T21.01 Burn of unspecified degree of chest wall
Burn of of unspecified degree of breast

X● T21.02 Burn of unspecified degree of abdominal wall
Burn of unspecified degree of flank
Burn of unspecified degree of groin

X● T21.03 Burn of unspecified degree of upper back
Burn of unspecified degree of interscapular region

X● T21.04 Burn of unspecified degree of lower back

X● T21.05 Burn of unspecified degree of buttock
Burn of unspecified degree of anus

X● T21.06 Burn of unspecified degree of male genital region
Burn of unspecified degree of penis
Burn of unspecified degree of scrotum
Burn of unspecified degree of testis

X● T21.07 Burn of unspecified degree of female genital region
Burn of unspecified degree of labium (majus) (minus)
Burn of unspecified degree of perineum
Burn of unspecified degree of vulva
Excludes2 burn of vagina (T28.3)

X● T21.09 Burn of unspecified degree of other site of trunk

● T21.1 Burn of first degree of trunk
Use additional external cause code to identify the source, place and intent of the burn (X00-X19, X75-X77, X96-X98, Y92)

X● T21.10 Burn of first degree of trunk, unspecified site

X● T21.11 Burn of first degree of chest wall
Burn of first degree of breast

X● T21.12 Burn of first degree of abdominal wall
Burn of first degree of flank
Burn of first degree of groin

X● T21.13 Burn of first degree of upper back
Burn of first degree of interscapular region

X● T21.14 Burn of first degree of lower back

X● T21.15 Burn of first degree of buttock
Burn of first degree of anus

X● T21.16 Burn of first degree of male genital region
Burn of first degree of penis
Burn of first degree of scrotum
Burn of first degree of testis

X● T21.17 Burn of first degree of female genital region
Burn of first degree of labium (majus) (minus)
Burn of first degree of perineum
Burn of first degree of vulva
Excludes2 burn of vagina (T28.3)

X● T21.19 Burn of first degree of other site of trunk

● T21.2 Burn of second degree of trunk
Use additional external cause code to identify the source, place and intent of the burn (X00-X19, X75-X77, X96-X98, Y92)

X● T21.20 Burn of second degree of trunk, unspecified site

X● T21.21 Burn of second degree of chest wall
Burn of second degree of breast

X● T21.22 Burn of second degree of abdominal wall
Burn of second degree of flank
Burn of second degree of groin

X● T21.23 Burn of second degree of upper back
Burn of second degree of interscapular region

X● T21.24 Burn of second degree of lower back

X● T21.25 Burn of second degree of buttock
Burn of second degree of anus

X● T21.26 Burn of second degree of male genital region
Burn of second degree of penis
Burn of second degree of scrotum
Burn of second degree of testis

X● T21.27 Burn of second degree of female genital region
Burn of second degree of labium (majus) (minus)
Burn of second degree of perineum
Burn of second degree of vulva
Excludes2 burn of vagina (T28.3)

X● T21.29 Burn of second degree of other site of trunk

● T21.3 Burn of third degree of trunk
Use additional external cause code to identify the source, place and intent of the burn (X00-X19, X75-X77, X96-X98, Y92)

X● T21.30 Burn of third degree of trunk, unspecified site

X● T21.31 Burn of third degree of chest wall
Burn of third degree of breast

X● T21.32 Burn of third degree of abdominal wall
Burn of third degree of flank
Burn of third degree of groin

X● T21.33 Burn of third degree of upper back
Burn of third degree of interscapular region

X● T21.34 Burn of third degree of lower back

X● T21.35 Burn of third degree of buttock
Burn of third degree of anus

X● T21.36 Burn of third degree of male genital region
Burn of third degree of penis
Burn of third degree of scrotum
Burn of third degree of testis

X● T21.37 Burn of third degree of female genital region
Burn of third degree of labium (majus) (minus)
Burn of third degree of perineum
Burn of third degree of vulva
Excludes2 burn of vagina (T28.3)

X● T21.39 Burn of third degree of other site of trunk

CHAPTER 19 (S00-T88)

● T21.4 **Corrosion of unspecified degree of trunk**
Code first (T51-T65) to identify chemical and intent
Use additional external cause code to identify place (Y92)

X● T21.40 **Corrosion of unspecified degree of trunk, unspecified site**

X● T21.41 **Corrosion of unspecified degree of chest wall**
Corrosion of unspecified degree of breast

X● T21.42 **Corrosion of unspecified degree of abdominal wall**
Corrosion of unspecified degree of flank
Corrosion of unspecified degree of groin

X● T21.43 **Corrosion of unspecified degree of upper back**
Corrosion of unspecified degree of interscapular region

X● T21.44 **Corrosion of unspecified degree of lower back**

X● T21.45 **Corrosion of unspecified degree of buttock**
Corrosion of unspecified degree of anus

X● T21.46 **Corrosion of unspecified degree of male genital region**
Corrosion of unspecified degree of penis
Corrosion of unspecified degree of scrotum
Corrosion of unspecified degree of testis

X● T21.47 **Corrosion of unspecified degree of female genital region**
Corrosion of unspecified degree of labium (majus) (minus)
Corrosion of unspecified degree of perineum
Corrosion of unspecified degree of vulva
Excludes2 corrosion of vagina (T28.8)

X● T21.49 **Corrosion of unspecified degree of other site of trunk**

● T21.5 **Corrosion of first degree of trunk**
Code first (T51-T65) to identify chemical and intent
Use additional external cause code to identify place (Y92)

X● T21.50 **Corrosion of first degree of trunk, unspecified site**

X● T21.51 **Corrosion of first degree of chest wall**
Corrosion of first degree of breast

X● T21.52 **Corrosion of first degree of abdominal wall**
Corrosion of first degree of flank
Corrosion of first degree of groin

X● T21.53 **Corrosion of first degree of upper back**
Corrosion of first degree of interscapular region

X● T21.54 **Corrosion of first degree of lower back**

X● T21.55 **Corrosion of first degree of buttock**
Corrosion of first degree of anus

X● T21.56 **Corrosion of first degree of male genital region**
Corrosion of first degree of penis
Corrosion of first degree of scrotum
Corrosion of first degree of testis

X● T21.57 **Corrosion of first degree of female genital region**
Corrosion of first degree of labium (majus) (minus)
Corrosion of first degree of perineum
Corrosion of first degree of vulva
Excludes2 corrosion of vagina (T28.8)

X● T21.59 **Corrosion of first degree of other site of trunk**

● T21.6 **Corrosion of second degree of trunk**
Code first (T51-T65) to identify chemical and intent
Use additional external cause code to identify place (Y92)

X● T21.60 **Corrosion of second degree of trunk, unspecified site**

X● T21.61 **Corrosion of second degree of chest wall**
Corrosion of second degree of breast

X● T21.62 **Corrosion of second degree of abdominal wall**
Corrosion of second degree of flank
Corrosion of second degree of groin

X● T21.63 **Corrosion of second degree of upper back**
Corrosion of second degree of interscapular region

X● T21.64 **Corrosion of second degree of lower back**

X● T21.65 **Corrosion of second degree of buttock**
Corrosion of second degree of anus

X● T21.66 **Corrosion of second degree of male genital region**
Corrosion of second degree of penis
Corrosion of second degree of scrotum
Corrosion of second degree of testis

X● T21.67 **Corrosion of second degree of female genital region**
Corrosion of second degree of labium (majus) (minus)
Corrosion of second degree of perineum
Corrosion of second degree of vulva
Excludes2 corrosion of vagina (T28.8)

X● T21.69 **Corrosion of second degree of other site of trunk**

● T21.7 **Corrosion of third degree of trunk**
Code first (T51-T65) to identify chemical and intent
Use additional external cause code to identify place (Y92)

X● T21.70 **Corrosion of third degree of trunk, unspecified site**

X● T21.71 **Corrosion of third degree of chest wall**
Corrosion of third degree of breast

X● T21.72 **Corrosion of third degree of abdominal wall**
Corrosion of third degree of flank
Corrosion of third degree of groin

X● T21.73 **Corrosion of third degree of upper back**
Corrosion of third degree of interscapular region

X● T21.74 **Corrosion of third degree of lower back**

X● T21.75 **Corrosion of third degree of buttock**
Corrosion of third degree of anus

X● T21.76 **Corrosion of third degree of male genital region**
Corrosion of third degree of penis
Corrosion of third degree of scrotum
Corrosion of third degree of testis

X● T21.77 **Corrosion of third degree of female genital region**
Corrosion of third degree of labium (majus) (minus)
Corrosion of third degree of perineum
Corrosion of third degree of vulva
Excludes2 corrosion of vagina (T28.8)

X● T21.79 **Corrosion of third degree of other site of trunk**

● **T22 Burn and corrosion of shoulder and upper limb, except wrist and hand**

Excludes2 burn and corrosion of interscapular region (T21.-)
burn and corrosion of wrist and hand (T23.-)

The appropriate 7th character is to be added to each code from category T22

A	initial encounter
D	subsequent encounter
S	sequela

● **T22.0 Burn of unspecified degree of shoulder and upper limb, except wrist and hand**
Use additional external cause code to identify the source, place and intent of the burn (X00-X19, X75-X77, X96-X98, Y92)

X● **T22.00** Burn of unspecified degree of shoulder and upper limb, except wrist and hand, unspecified site

● **T22.01** Burn of unspecified degree of forearm
● **T22.011** Burn of unspecified degree of right forearm
● **T22.012** Burn of unspecified degree of left forearm
● **T22.019** Burn of unspecified degree of unspecified forearm

● **T22.02** Burn of unspecified degree of elbow
● **T22.021** Burn of unspecified degree of right elbow
● **T22.022** Burn of unspecified degree of left elbow
● **T22.029** Burn of unspecified degree of unspecified elbow

● **T22.03** Burn of unspecified degree of upper arm
● **T22.031** Burn of unspecified degree of right upper arm
● **T22.032** Burn of unspecified degree of left upper arm
● **T22.039** Burn of unspecified degree of unspecified upper arm

● **T22.04** Burn of unspecified degree of axilla
● **T22.041** Burn of unspecified degree of right axilla
● **T22.042** Burn of unspecified degree of left axilla
● **T22.049** Burn of unspecified degree of unspecified axilla

● **T22.05** Burn of unspecified degree of shoulder
● **T22.051** Burn of unspecified degree of right shoulder
● **T22.052** Burn of unspecified degree of left shoulder
● **T22.059** Burn of unspecified degree of unspecified shoulder

● **T22.06** Burn of unspecified degree of scapular region
● **T22.061** Burn of unspecified degree of right scapular region
● **T22.062** Burn of unspecified degree of left scapular region
● **T22.069** Burn of unspecified degree of unspecified scapular region

● **T22.09** Burn of unspecified degree of multiple sites of shoulder and upper limb, except wrist and hand
● **T22.091** Burn of unspecified degree of multiple sites of right shoulder and upper limb, except wrist and hand
● **T22.092** Burn of unspecified degree of multiple sites of left shoulder and upper limb, except wrist and hand
● **T22.099** Burn of unspecified degree of multiple sites of unspecified shoulder and upper limb, except wrist and hand

● **T22.1 Burn of first degree of shoulder and upper limb, except wrist and hand**
Use additional external cause code to identify the source, place and intent of the burn (X00-X19, X75-X77, X96-X98, Y92)

X● **T22.10** Burn of first degree of shoulder and upper limb, except wrist and hand, unspecified site

● **T22.11** Burn of first degree of forearm
● **T22.111** Burn of first degree of right forearm
● **T22.112** Burn of first degree of left forearm
● **T22.119** Burn of first degree of unspecified forearm

● **T22.12** Burn of first degree of elbow
● **T22.121** Burn of first degree of right elbow
● **T22.122** Burn of first degree of left elbow
● **T22.129** Burn of first degree of unspecified elbow

● **T22.13** Burn of first degree of upper arm
● **T22.131** Burn of first degree of right upper arm
● **T22.132** Burn of first degree of left upper arm
● **T22.139** Burn of first degree of unspecified upper arm

● **T22.14** Burn of first degree of axilla
● **T22.141** Burn of first degree of right axilla
● **T22.142** Burn of first degree of left axilla
● **T22.149** Burn of first degree of unspecified axilla

● **T22.15** Burn of first degree of shoulder
● **T22.151** Burn of first degree of right shoulder
● **T22.152** Burn of first degree of left shoulder
● **T22.159** Burn of first degree of unspecified shoulder

● **T22.16** Burn of first degree of scapular region
● **T22.161** Burn of first degree of right scapular region
● **T22.162** Burn of first degree of left scapular region
● **T22.169** Burn of first degree of unspecified scapular region

● **T22.19** Burn of first degree of multiple sites of shoulder and upper limb, except wrist and hand
● **T22.191** Burn of first degree of multiple sites of right shoulder and upper limb, except wrist and hand
● **T22.192** Burn of first degree of multiple sites of left shoulder and upper limb, except wrist and hand
● **T22.199** Burn of first degree of multiple sites of unspecified shoulder and upper limb, except wrist and hand

CHAPTER 19 (S00-T88)

● T22.2 Burn of second degree of shoulder and upper limb, except wrist and hand
Use additional external cause code to identify the source, place and intent of the burn (XØØ-X19, X75-X77, X96-X98, Y92)
X● T22.2Ø Burn of second degree of shoulder and upper limb, except wrist and hand, unspecified site
● T22.21 Burn of second degree of forearm
● T22.211 Burn of second degree of right forearm
● T22.212 Burn of second degree of left forearm
● T22.219 Burn of second degree of unspecified forearm
● T22.22 Burn of second degree of elbow
● T22.221 Burn of second degree of right elbow
● T22.222 Burn of second degree of left elbow
● T22.229 Burn of second degree of unspecified elbow
● T22.23 Burn of second degree of upper arm
● T22.231 Burn of second degree of right upper arm
● T22.232 Burn of second degree of left upper arm
● T22.239 Burn of second degree of unspecified upper arm
● T22.24 Burn of second degree of axilla
● T22.241 Burn of second degree of right axilla
● T22.242 Burn of second degree of left axilla
● T22.249 Burn of second degree of unspecified axilla
● T22.25 Burn of second degree of shoulder
● T22.251 Burn of second degree of right shoulder
● T22.252 Burn of second degree of left shoulder
● T22.259 Burn of second degree of unspecified shoulder
● T22.26 Burn of second degree of scapular region
● T22.261 Burn of second degree of right scapular region
● T22.262 Burn of second degree of left scapular region
● T22.269 Burn of second degree of unspecified scapular region
● T22.29 Burn of second degree of multiple sites of shoulder and upper limb, except wrist and hand
● T22.291 Burn of second degree of multiple sites of right shoulder and upper limb, except wrist and hand
● T22.292 Burn of second degree of multiple sites of left shoulder and upper limb, except wrist and hand
● T22.299 Burn of second degree of multiple sites of unspecified shoulder and upper limb, except wrist and hand
● T22.3 Burn of third degree of shoulder and upper limb, except wrist and hand
Use additional external cause code to identify the source, place and intent of the burn (XØØ-X19, X75-X77, X96-X98, Y92)
X● T22.3Ø Burn of third degree of shoulder and upper limb, except wrist and hand, unspecified site
● T22.31 Burn of third degree of forearm
● T22.311 Burn of third degree of right forearm
● T22.312 Burn of third degree of left forearm
● T22.319 Burn of third degree of unspecified forearm
● T22.32 Burn of third degree of elbow
● T22.321 Burn of third degree of right elbow
● T22.322 Burn of third degree of left elbow
● T22.329 Burn of third degree of unspecified elbow
● T22.33 Burn of third degree of upper arm
● T22.331 Burn of third degree of right upper arm
● T22.332 Burn of third degree of left upper arm
● T22.339 Burn of third degree of unspecified upper arm
● T22.34 Burn of third degree of axilla
● T22.341 Burn of third degree of right axilla
● T22.342 Burn of third degree of left axilla
● T22.349 Burn of third degree of unspecified axilla
● T22.35 Burn of third degree of shoulder
● T22.351 Burn of third degree of right shoulder
● T22.352 Burn of third degree of left shoulder
● T22.359 Burn of third degree of unspecified shoulder
● T22.36 Burn of third degree of scapular region
● T22.361 Burn of third degree of right scapular region
● T22.362 Burn of third degree of left scapular region
● T22.369 Burn of third degree of unspecified scapular region
● T22.39 Burn of third degree of multiple sites of shoulder and upper limb, except wrist and hand
● T22.391 Burn of third degree of multiple sites of right shoulder and upper limb, except wrist and hand
● T22.392 Burn of third degree of multiple sites of left shoulder and upper limb, except wrist and hand
● T22.399 Burn of third degree of multiple sites of unspecified shoulder and upper limb, except wrist and hand
● T22.4 Corrosion of unspecified degree of shoulder and upper limb, except wrist and hand
Code first (T51-T65) to identify chemical and intent
Use additional external cause code to identify place (Y92)
X● T22.4Ø Corrosion of unspecified degree of shoulder and upper limb, except wrist and hand, unspecified site
● T22.41 Corrosion of unspecified degree of forearm
● T22.411 Corrosion of unspecified degree of right forearm
● T22.412 Corrosion of unspecified degree of left forearm
● T22.419 Corrosion of unspecified degree of unspecified forearm
● T22.42 Corrosion of unspecified degree of elbow
● T22.421 Corrosion of unspecified degree of right elbow
● T22.422 Corrosion of unspecified degree of left elbow
● T22.429 Corrosion of unspecified degree of unspecified elbow
● T22.43 Corrosion of unspecified degree of upper arm
● T22.431 Corrosion of unspecified degree of right upper arm
● T22.432 Corrosion of unspecified degree of left upper arm
● T22.439 Corrosion of unspecified degree of unspecified upper arm

● **T22.44** Corrosion of unspecified degree of axilla
● **T22.441** Corrosion of unspecified degree of right axilla
● **T22.442** Corrosion of unspecified degree of left axilla
● **T22.449** Corrosion of unspecified degree of unspecified axilla
● **T22.45** Corrosion of unspecified degree of shoulder
● **T22.451** Corrosion of unspecified degree of right shoulder
● **T22.452** Corrosion of unspecified degree of left shoulder
● **T22.459** Corrosion of unspecified degree of unspecified shoulder
● **T22.46** Corrosion of unspecified degree of scapular region
● **T22.461** Corrosion of unspecified degree of right scapular region
● **T22.462** Corrosion of unspecified degree of left scapular region
● **T22.469** Corrosion of unspecified degree of unspecified scapular region
● **T22.49** Corrosion of unspecified degree of multiple sites of shoulder and upper limb, except wrist and hand
● **T22.491** Corrosion of unspecified degree of multiple sites of right shoulder and upper limb, except wrist and hand
● **T22.492** Corrosion of unspecified degree of multiple sites of left shoulder and upper limb, except wrist and hand
● **T22.499** Corrosion of unspecified degree of multiple sites of unspecified shoulder and upper limb, except wrist and hand

● **T22.5** **Corrosion of first degree of shoulder and upper limb, except wrist and hand**
Code first (T51-T65) to identify chemical and intent
Use additional external cause code to identify place (Y92)

X● **T22.50** Corrosion of first degree of shoulder and upper limb, except wrist and hand unspecified site
● **T22.51** Corrosion of first degree of forearm
● **T22.511** Corrosion of first degree of right forearm
● **T22.512** Corrosion of first degree of left forearm
● **T22.519** Corrosion of first degree of unspecified forearm
● **T22.52** Corrosion of first degree of elbow
● **T22.521** Corrosion of first degree of right elbow
● **T22.522** Corrosion of first degree of left elbow
● **T22.529** Corrosion of first degree of unspecified elbow
● **T22.53** Corrosion of first degree of upper arm
● **T22.531** Corrosion of first degree of right upper arm
● **T22.532** Corrosion of first degree of left upper arm
● **T22.539** Corrosion of first degree of unspecified upper arm
● **T22.54** Corrosion of first degree of axilla
● **T22.541** Corrosion of first degree of right axilla
● **T22.542** Corrosion of first degree of left axilla
● **T22.549** Corrosion of first degree of unspecified axilla
● **T22.55** Corrosion of first degree of shoulder
● **T22.551** Corrosion of first degree of right shoulder
● **T22.552** Corrosion of first degree of left shoulder
● **T22.559** Corrosion of first degree of unspecified shoulder
● **T22.56** Corrosion of first degree of scapular region
● **T22.561** Corrosion of first degree of right scapular region
● **T22.562** Corrosion of first degree of left scapular region
● **T22.569** Corrosion of first degree of unspecified scapular region
● **T22.59** Corrosion of first degree of multiple sites of shoulder and upper limb, except wrist and hand
● **T22.591** Corrosion of first degree of multiple sites of right shoulder and upper limb, except wrist and hand
● **T22.592** Corrosion of first degree of multiple sites of left shoulder and upper limb, except wrist and hand
● **T22.599** Corrosion of first degree of multiple sites of unspecified shoulder and upper limb, except wrist and hand

● **T22.6** **Corrosion of second degree of shoulder and upper limb, except wrist and hand**
Code first (T51-T65) to identify chemical and intent
Use additional external cause code to identify place (Y92)

X● **T22.60** Corrosion of second degree of shoulder and upper limb, except wrist and hand, unspecified site
● **T22.61** Corrosion of second degree of forearm
● **T22.611** Corrosion of second degree of right forearm
● **T22.612** Corrosion of second degree of left forearm
● **T22.619** Corrosion of second degree of unspecified forearm
● **T22.62** Corrosion of second degree of elbow
● **T22.621** Corrosion of second degree of right elbow
● **T22.622** Corrosion of second degree of left elbow
● **T22.629** Corrosion of second degree of unspecified elbow
● **T22.63** Corrosion of second degree of upper arm
● **T22.631** Corrosion of second degree of right upper arm
● **T22.632** Corrosion of second degree of left upper arm
● **T22.639** Corrosion of second degree of unspecified upper arm
● **T22.64** Corrosion of second degree of axilla
● **T22.641** Corrosion of second degree of right axilla
● **T22.642** Corrosion of second degree of left axilla
● **T22.649** Corrosion of second degree of unspecified axilla
● **T22.65** Corrosion of second degree of shoulder
● **T22.651** Corrosion of second degree of right shoulder
● **T22.652** Corrosion of second degree of left shoulder
● **T22.659** Corrosion of second degree of unspecified shoulder

CHAPTER 19 (SØ-T88)

● T22.66 Corrosion of second degree of scapular region
● T22.661 Corrosion of second degree of right scapular region
● T22.662 Corrosion of second degree of left scapular region
● T22.669 Corrosion of second degree of unspecified scapular region
● T22.69 Corrosion of second degree of multiple sites of shoulder and upper limb, except wrist and hand
● T22.691 Corrosion of second degree of multiple sites of right shoulder and upper limb, except wrist and hand
● T22.692 Corrosion of second degree of multiple sites of left shoulder and upper limb, except wrist and hand
● T22.699 Corrosion of second degree of multiple sites of unspecified shoulder and upper limb, except wrist and hand
● T22.7 Corrosion of third degree of shoulder and upper limb, except wrist and hand
Code first (T51-T65) to identify chemical and intent
Use additional external cause code to identify place (Y92)
X● T22.70 Corrosion of third degree of shoulder and upper limb, except wrist and hand, unspecified site
● T22.71 Corrosion of third degree of forearm
● T22.711 Corrosion of third degree of right forearm
● T22.712 Corrosion of third degree of left forearm
● T22.719 Corrosion of third degree of unspecified forearm
● T22.72 Corrosion of third degree of elbow
● T22.721 Corrosion of third degree of right elbow
● T22.722 Corrosion of third degree of left elbow
● T22.729 Corrosion of third degree of unspecified elbow
● T22.73 Corrosion of third degree of upper arm
● T22.731 Corrosion of third degree of right upper arm
● T22.732 Corrosion of third degree of left upper arm
● T22.739 Corrosion of third degree of unspecified upper arm
● T22.74 Corrosion of third degree of axilla
● T22.741 Corrosion of third degree of right axilla
● T22.742 Corrosion of third degree of left axilla
● T22.749 Corrosion of third degree of unspecified axilla
● T22.75 Corrosion of third degree of shoulder
● T22.751 Corrosion of third degree of right shoulder
● T22.752 Corrosion of third degree of left shoulder
● T22.759 Corrosion of third degree of unspecified shoulder
● T22.76 Corrosion of third degree of scapular region
● T22.761 Corrosion of third degree of right scapular region
● T22.762 Corrosion of third degree of left scapular region
● T22.769 Corrosion of third degree of unspecified scapular region
● T22.79 Corrosion of third degree of multiple sites of shoulder and upper limb, except wrist and hand
● T22.791 Corrosion of third degree of multiple sites of right shoulder and upper limb, except wrist and hand
● T22.792 Corrosion of third degree of multiple sites of left shoulder and upper limb, except wrist and hand
● T22.799 Corrosion of third degree of multiple sites of unspecified shoulder and upper limb, except wrist and hand

● **T23 Burn and corrosion of wrist and hand**

The appropriate 7th character is to be added to each code from category T23

A	initial encounter
D	subsequent encounter
S	sequela

● T23.0 Burn of unspecified degree of wrist and hand
Use additional external cause code to identify the source, place and intent of the burn (X00-X19, X75-X77, X96-X98, Y92)
● T23.00 Burn of unspecified degree of hand, unspecified site
● T23.001 Burn of unspecified degree of right hand, unspecified site
● T23.002 Burn of unspecified degree of left hand, unspecified site
● T23.009 Burn of unspecified degree of unspecified hand, unspecified site
● T23.01 Burn of unspecified degree of thumb (nail)
● T23.011 Burn of unspecified degree of right thumb (nail)
● T23.012 Burn of unspecified degree of left thumb (nail)
● T23.019 Burn of unspecified degree of unspecified thumb (nail)
● T23.02 Burn of unspecified degree of single finger (nail) except thumb
● T23.021 Burn of unspecified degree of single right finger (nail) except thumb
● T23.022 Burn of unspecified degree of single left finger (nail) except thumb
● T23.029 Burn of unspecified degree of unspecified single finger (nail) except thumb
● T23.03 Burn of unspecified degree of multiple fingers (nail), not including thumb
● T23.031 Burn of unspecified degree of multiple right fingers (nail), not including thumb
● T23.032 Burn of unspecified degree of multiple left fingers (nail), not including thumb
● T23.039 Burn of unspecified degree of unspecified multiple fingers (nail), not including thumb
● T23.04 Burn of unspecified degree of multiple fingers (nail), including thumb
● T23.041 Burn of unspecified degree of multiple right fingers (nail), including thumb
● T23.042 Burn of unspecified degree of multiple left fingers (nail), including thumb
● T23.049 Burn of unspecified degree of unspecified multiple fingers (nail), including thumb

● T23.05 Burn of unspecified degree of palm
● T23.051 Burn of unspecified degree of right palm
● T23.052 Burn of unspecified degree of left palm
● T23.059 Burn of unspecified degree of unspecified palm
● T23.06 Burn of unspecified degree of back of hand
● T23.061 Burn of unspecified degree of back of right hand
● T23.062 Burn of unspecified degree of back of left hand
● T23.069 Burn of unspecified degree of back of unspecified hand
● T23.07 Burn of unspecified degree of wrist
● T23.071 Burn of unspecified degree of right wrist
● T23.072 Burn of unspecified degree of left wrist
● T23.079 Burn of unspecified degree of unspecified wrist
● T23.09 Burn of unspecified degree of multiple sites of wrist and hand
● T23.091 Burn of unspecified degree of multiple sites of right wrist and hand
● T23.092 Burn of unspecified degree of multiple sites of left wrist and hand
● T23.099 Burn of unspecified degree of multiple sites of unspecified wrist and hand

● T23.1 Burn of first degree of wrist and hand

Use additional external cause code to identify the source, place and intent of the burn (X00-X19, X75-X77, X96-X98, Y92)

● T23.10 Burn of first degree of hand, unspecified site
● T23.101 Burn of first degree of right hand, unspecified site
● T23.102 Burn of first degree of left hand, unspecified site
● T23.109 Burn of first degree of unspecified hand, unspecified site
● T23.11 Burn of first degree of thumb (nail)
● T23.111 Burn of first degree of right thumb (nail)
● T23.112 Burn of first degree of left thumb (nail)
● T23.119 Burn of first degree of unspecified thumb (nail)
● T23.12 Burn of first degree of single finger (nail) except thumb
● T23.121 Burn of first degree of single right finger (nail) except thumb
● T23.122 Burn of first degree of single left finger (nail) except thumb
● T23.129 Burn of first degree of unspecified single finger (nail) except thumb
● T23.13 Burn of first degree of multiple fingers (nail), not including thumb
● T23.131 Burn of first degree of multiple right fingers (nail), not including thumb
● T23.132 Burn of first degree of multiple left fingers (nail), not including thumb
● T23.139 Burn of first degree of unspecified multiple fingers (nail), not including thumb
● T23.14 Burn of first degree of multiple fingers (nail), including thumb
● T23.141 Burn of first degree of multiple right fingers (nail), including thumb
● T23.142 Burn of first degree of multiple left fingers (nail), including thumb
● T23.149 Burn of first degree of unspecified multiple fingers (nail), including thumb
● T23.15 Burn of first degree of palm
● T23.151 Burn of first degree of right palm
● T23.152 Burn of first degree of left palm
● T23.159 Burn of first degree of unspecified palm
● T23.16 Burn of first degree of back of hand
● T23.161 Burn of first degree of back of right hand
● T23.162 Burn of first degree of back of left hand
● T23.169 Burn of first degree of back of unspecified hand
● T23.17 Burn of first degree of wrist
● T23.171 Burn of first degree of right wrist
● T23.172 Burn of first degree of left wrist
● T23.179 Burn of first degree of unspecified wrist
● T23.19 Burn of first degree of multiple sites of wrist and hand
● T23.191 Burn of first degree of multiple sites of right wrist and hand
● T23.192 Burn of first degree of multiple sites of left wrist and hand
● T23.199 Burn of first degree of multiple sites of unspecified wrist and hand

● T23.2 Burn of second degree of wrist and hand

Use additional external cause code to identify the source, place and intent of the burn (X00-X19, X75-X77, X96-X98, Y92)

● T23.20 Burn of second degree of hand, unspecified site
● T23.201 Burn of second degree of right hand, unspecified site
● T23.202 Burn of second degree of left hand, unspecified site
● T23.209 Burn of second degree of unspecified hand, unspecified site
● T23.21 Burn of second degree of thumb (nail)
● T23.211 Burn of second degree of right thumb (nail)
● T23.212 Burn of second degree of left thumb (nail)
● T23.219 Burn of second degree of unspecified thumb (nail)
● T23.22 Burn of second degree of single finger (nail) except thumb
● T23.221 Burn of second degree of single right finger (nail) except thumb
● T23.222 Burn of second degree of single left finger (nail) except thumb
● T23.229 Burn of second degree of unspecified single finger (nail) except thumb
● T23.23 Burn of second degree of multiple fingers (nail), not including thumb
● T23.231 Burn of second degree of multiple right fingers (nail), not including thumb
● T23.232 Burn of second degree of multiple left fingers (nail), not including thumb
● T23.239 Burn of second degree of unspecified multiple fingers (nail), not including thumb

CHAPTER 19 (S00-T88)

- ● T23.24 Burn of second degree of multiple fingers (nail), including thumb
  - ● T23.241 Burn of second degree of multiple right fingers (nail), including thumb
  - ● T23.242 Burn of second degree of multiple left fingers (nail), including thumb
  - ● T23.249 Burn of second degree of unspecified multiple fingers (nail), including thumb
- ● T23.25 Burn of second degree of palm
  - ● T23.251 Burn of second degree of right palm
  - ● T23.252 Burn of second degree of left palm
  - ● T23.259 Burn of second degree of unspecified palm
- ● T23.26 Burn of second degree of back of hand
  - ● T23.261 Burn of second degree of back of right hand
  - ● T23.262 Burn of second degree of back of left hand
  - ● T23.269 Burn of second degree of back of unspecified hand
- ● T23.27 Burn of second degree of wrist
  - ● T23.271 Burn of second degree of right wrist
  - ● T23.272 Burn of second degree of left wrist
  - ● T23.279 Burn of second degree of unspecified wrist
- ● T23.29 Burn of second degree of multiple sites of wrist and hand
  - ● T23.291 Burn of second degree of multiple sites of right wrist and hand
  - ● T23.292 Burn of second degree of multiple sites of left wrist and hand
  - ● T23.299 Burn of second degree of multiple sites of unspecified wrist and hand

● T23.3 Burn of third degree of wrist and hand

Use additional external cause code to identify the source, place and intent of the burn (X00-X19, X75-X77, X96-X98, Y92)

- ● T23.30 Burn of third degree of hand, unspecified site
  - ● T23.301 Burn of third degree of right hand, unspecified site
  - ● T23.302 Burn of third degree of left hand, unspecified site
  - ● T23.309 Burn of third degree of unspecified hand, unspecified site
- ● T23.31 Burn of third degree of thumb (nail)
  - ● T23.311 Burn of third degree of right thumb (nail)
  - ● T23.312 Burn of third degree of left thumb (nail)
  - ● T23.319 Burn of third degree of unspecified thumb (nail)
- ● T23.32 Burn of third degree of single finger (nail) except thumb
  - ● T23.321 Burn of third degree of single right finger (nail) except thumb
  - ● T23.322 Burn of third degree of single left finger (nail) except thumb
  - ● T23.329 Burn of third degree of unspecified single finger (nail) except thumb
- ● T23.33 Burn of third degree of multiple fingers (nail), not including thumb
  - ● T23.331 Burn of third degree of multiple right fingers (nail), not including thumb
  - ● T23.332 Burn of third degree of multiple left fingers (nail), not including thumb
  - ● T23.339 Burn of third degree of unspecified multiple fingers (nail), not including thumb
- ● T23.34 Burn of third degree of multiple fingers (nail), including thumb
  - ● T23.341 Burn of third degree of multiple right fingers (nail), including thumb
  - ● T23.342 Burn of third degree of multiple left fingers (nail), including thumb
  - ● T23.349 Burn of third degree of unspecified multiple fingers (nail), including thumb
- ● T23.35 Burn of third degree of palm
  - ● T23.351 Burn of third degree of right palm
  - ● T23.352 Burn of third degree of left palm
  - ● T23.359 Burn of third degree of unspecified palm
- ● T23.36 Burn of third degree of back of hand
  - ● T23.361 Burn of third degree of back of right hand
  - ● T23.362 Burn of third degree of back of left hand
  - ● T23.369 Burn of third degree of back of unspecified hand
- ● T23.37 Burn of third degree of wrist
  - ● T23.371 Burn of third degree of right wrist
  - ● T23.372 Burn of third degree of left wrist
  - ● T23.379 Burn of third degree of unspecified wrist
- ● T23.39 Burn of third degree of multiple sites of wrist and hand
  - ● T23.391 Burn of third degree of multiple sites of right wrist and hand
  - ● T23.392 Burn of third degree of multiple sites of left wrist and hand
  - ● T23.399 Burn of third degree of multiple sites of unspecified wrist and hand

● T23.4 Corrosion of unspecified degree of wrist and hand

Code first (T51-T65) to identify chemical and intent

Use additional external cause code to identify place (Y92)

- ● T23.40 Corrosion of unspecified degree of hand, unspecified site
  - ● T23.401 Corrosion of unspecified degree of right hand, unspecified site
  - ● T23.402 Corrosion of unspecified degree of left hand, unspecified site
  - ● T23.409 Corrosion of unspecified degree of unspecified hand, unspecified site
- ● T23.41 Corrosion of unspecified degree of thumb (nail)
  - ● T23.411 Corrosion of unspecified degree of right thumb (nail)
  - ● T23.412 Corrosion of unspecified degree of left thumb (nail)
  - ● T23.419 Corrosion of unspecified degree of unspecified thumb (nail)

CHAPTER 19 (S00-T88)

T23.42 Corrosion of unspecified degree of single finger (nail) except thumb
T23.421 Corrosion of unspecified degree of single right finger (nail) except thumb
T23.422 Corrosion of unspecified degree of single left finger (nail) except thumb
T23.429 Corrosion of unspecified degree of unspecified single finger (nail) except thumb
T23.43 Corrosion of unspecified degree of multiple fingers (nail), not including thumb
T23.431 Corrosion of unspecified degree of multiple right fingers (nail), not including thumb
T23.432 Corrosion of unspecified degree of multiple left fingers (nail), not including thumb
T23.439 Corrosion of unspecified degree of unspecified multiple fingers (nail), not including thumb
T23.44 Corrosion of unspecified degree of multiple fingers (nail), including thumb
T23.441 Corrosion of unspecified degree of multiple right fingers (nail), including thumb
T23.442 Corrosion of unspecified degree of multiple left fingers (nail), including thumb
T23.449 Corrosion of unspecified degree of unspecified multiple fingers (nail), including thumb
T23.45 Corrosion of unspecified degree of palm
T23.451 Corrosion of unspecified degree of right palm
T23.452 Corrosion of unspecified degree of left palm
T23.459 Corrosion of unspecified degree of unspecified palm
T23.46 Corrosion of unspecified degree of back of hand
T23.461 Corrosion of unspecified degree of back of right hand
T23.462 Corrosion of unspecified degree of back of left hand
T23.469 Corrosion of unspecified degree of back of unspecified hand
T23.47 Corrosion of unspecified degree of wrist
T23.471 Corrosion of unspecified degree of right wrist
T23.472 Corrosion of unspecified degree of left wrist
T23.479 Corrosion of unspecified degree of unspecified wrist
T23.49 Corrosion of unspecified degree of multiple sites of wrist and hand
T23.491 Corrosion of unspecified degree of multiple sites of right wrist and hand
T23.492 Corrosion of unspecified degree of multiple sites of left wrist and hand
T23.499 Corrosion of unspecified degree of multiple sites of unspecified wrist and hand

T23.5 Corrosion of first degree of wrist and hand
Code first (*T51-T65*) *to identify chemical and intent*
Use additional external cause code to identify place (Y92)
T23.50 Corrosion of first degree of hand, unspecified site
T23.501 Corrosion of first degree of right hand, unspecified site
T23.502 Corrosion of first degree of left hand, unspecified site
T23.509 Corrosion of first degree of unspecified hand, unspecified site
T23.51 Corrosion of first degree of thumb (nail)
T23.511 Corrosion of first degree of right thumb (nail)
T23.512 Corrosion of first degree of left thumb (nail)
T23.519 Corrosion of first degree of unspecified thumb (nail)
T23.52 Corrosion of first degree of single finger (nail) except thumb
T23.521 Corrosion of first degree of single right finger (nail) except thumb
T23.522 Corrosion of first degree of single left finger (nail) except thumb
T23.529 Corrosion of first degree of unspecified single finger (nail) except thumb
T23.53 Corrosion of first degree of multiple fingers (nail), not including thumb
T23.531 Corrosion of first degree of multiple right fingers (nail), not including thumb
T23.532 Corrosion of first degree of multiple left fingers (nail), not including thumb
T23.539 Corrosion of first degree of unspecified multiple fingers (nail), not including thumb
T23.54 Corrosion of first degree of multiple fingers (nail), including thumb
T23.541 Corrosion of first degree of multiple right fingers (nail), including thumb
T23.542 Corrosion of first degree of multiple left fingers (nail), including thumb
T23.549 Corrosion of first degree of unspecified multiple fingers (nail), including thumb
T23.55 Corrosion of first degree of palm
T23.551 Corrosion of first degree of right palm
T23.552 Corrosion of first degree of left palm
T23.559 Corrosion of first degree of unspecified palm
T23.56 Corrosion of first degree of back of hand
T23.561 Corrosion of first degree of back of right hand
T23.562 Corrosion of first degree of back of left hand
T23.569 Corrosion of first degree of back of unspecified hand
T23.57 Corrosion of first degree of wrist
T23.571 Corrosion of first degree of right wrist
T23.572 Corrosion of first degree of left wrist
T23.579 Corrosion of first degree of unspecified wrist

● T23.59 Corrosion of first degree of multiple sites of wrist and hand
- ● T23.591 Corrosion of first degree of multiple sites of right wrist and hand
- ● T23.592 Corrosion of first degree of multiple sites of left wrist and hand
- ● T23.599 Corrosion of first degree of multiple sites of unspecified wrist and hand

● T23.6 Corrosion of second degree of wrist and hand
Code first (T51-T65) to identify chemical and intent
Use additional external cause code to identify place (Y92)

● T23.60 Corrosion of second degree of hand, unspecified site
- ● T23.601 Corrosion of second degree of right hand, unspecified site
- ● T23.602 Corrosion of second degree of left hand, unspecified site
- ● T23.609 Corrosion of second degree of unspecified hand, unspecified site

● T23.61 Corrosion of second degree of thumb (nail)
- ● T23.611 Corrosion of second degree of right thumb (nail)
- ● T23.612 Corrosion of second degree of left thumb (nail)
- ● T23.619 Corrosion of second degree of unspecified thumb (nail)

● T23.62 Corrosion of second degree of single finger (nail) except thumb
- ● T23.621 Corrosion of second degree of single right finger (nail) except thumb
- ● T23.622 Corrosion of second degree of single left finger (nail) except thumb
- ● T23.629 Corrosion of second degree of unspecified single finger (nail) except thumb

● T23.63 Corrosion of second degree of multiple fingers (nail), not including thumb
- ● T23.631 Corrosion of second degree of multiple right fingers (nail), not including thumb
- ● T23.632 Corrosion of second degree of multiple left fingers (nail), not including thumb
- ● T23.639 Corrosion of second degree of unspecified multiple fingers (nail), not including thumb

● T23.64 Corrosion of second degree of multiple fingers (nail), including thumb
- ● T23.641 Corrosion of second degree of multiple right fingers (nail), including thumb
- ● T23.642 Corrosion of second degree of multiple left fingers (nail), including thumb
- ● T23.649 Corrosion of second degree of unspecified multiple fingers (nail), including thumb

● T23.65 Corrosion of second degree of palm
- ● T23.651 Corrosion of second degree of right palm
- ● T23.652 Corrosion of second degree of left palm
- ● T23.659 Corrosion of second degree of unspecified palm

● T23.66 Corrosion of second degree of back of hand
- ● T23.661 Corrosion of second degree back of right hand
- ● T23.662 Corrosion of second degree back of left hand
- ● T23.669 Corrosion of second degree back of unspecified hand

● T23.67 Corrosion of second degree of wrist
- ● T23.671 Corrosion of second degree of right wrist
- ● T23.672 Corrosion of second degree of left wrist
- ● T23.679 Corrosion of second degree of unspecified wrist

● T23.69 Corrosion of second degree of multiple sites of wrist and hand
- ● T23.691 Corrosion of second degree of multiple sites of right wrist and hand
- ● T23.692 Corrosion of second degree of multiple sites of left wrist and hand
- ● T23.699 Corrosion of second degree of multiple sites of unspecified wrist and hand

● T23.7 Corrosion of third degree of wrist and hand
Code first (T51-T65) to identify chemical and intent
Use additional external cause code to identify place (Y92)

● T23.70 Corrosion of third degree of hand, unspecified site
- ● T23.701 Corrosion of third degree of right hand, unspecified site
- ● T23.702 Corrosion of third degree of left hand, unspecified site
- ● T23.709 Corrosion of third degree of unspecified hand, unspecified site

● T23.71 Corrosion of third degree of thumb (nail)
- ● T23.711 Corrosion of third degree of right thumb (nail)
- ● T23.712 Corrosion of third degree of left thumb (nail)
- ● T23.719 Corrosion of third degree of unspecified thumb (nail)

● T23.72 Corrosion of third degree of single finger (nail) except thumb
- ● T23.721 Corrosion of third degree of single right finger (nail) except thumb
- ● T23.722 Corrosion of third degree of single left finger (nail) except thumb
- ● T23.729 Corrosion of third degree of unspecified single finger (nail) except thumb

● T23.73 Corrosion of third degree of multiple fingers (nail), not including thumb
- ● T23.731 Corrosion of third degree of multiple right fingers (nail), not including thumb
- ● T23.732 Corrosion of third degree of multiple left fingers (nail), not including thumb
- ● T23.739 Corrosion of third degree of unspecified multiple fingers (nail), not including thumb

T23.74 Corrosion of third degree of multiple fingers (nail), including thumb
- T23.741 Corrosion of third degree of multiple right fingers (nail), including thumb
- T23.742 Corrosion of third degree of multiple left fingers (nail), including thumb
- T23.749 Corrosion of third degree of unspecified multiple fingers (nail), including thumb

T23.75 Corrosion of third degree of palm
- T23.751 Corrosion of third degree of right palm
- T23.752 Corrosion of third degree of left palm
- T23.759 Corrosion of third degree of unspecified palm

T23.76 Corrosion of third degree of back of hand
- T23.761 Corrosion of third degree of back of right hand
- T23.762 Corrosion of third degree of back of left hand
- T23.769 Corrosion of third degree of back of unspecified hand

T23.77 Corrosion of third degree of wrist
- T23.771 Corrosion of third degree of right wrist
- T23.772 Corrosion of third degree of left wrist
- T23.779 Corrosion of third degree of unspecified wrist

T23.79 Corrosion of third degree of multiple sites of wrist and hand
- T23.791 Corrosion of third degree of multiple sites of right wrist and hand
- T23.792 Corrosion of third degree of multiple sites of left wrist and hand
- T23.799 Corrosion of third degree of multiple sites of unspecified wrist and hand

T24 Burn and corrosion of lower limb, except ankle and foot

Excludes2 burn and corrosion of ankle and foot (T25.-)
burn and corrosion of hip region (T21.-)

The appropriate 7th character is to be added to each code from category T24

A	initial encounter
D	subsequent encounter
S	sequela

T24.0 Burn of unspecified degree of lower limb, except ankle and foot

Use additional external cause code to identify the source, place and intent of the burn (X00-X19, X75-X77, X96-X98, Y92)

T24.00 Burn of unspecified degree of unspecified site of lower limb, except ankle and foot
- T24.001 Burn of unspecified degree of unspecified site of right lower limb, except ankle and foot
- T24.002 Burn of unspecified degree of unspecified site of left lower limb, except ankle and foot
- T24.009 Burn of unspecified degree of unspecified site of unspecified lower limb, except ankle and foot

T24.01 Burn of unspecified degree of thigh
- T24.011 Burn of unspecified degree of right thigh
- T24.012 Burn of unspecified degree of left thigh
- T24.019 Burn of unspecified degree of unspecified thigh

T24.02 Burn of unspecified degree of knee
- T24.021 Burn of unspecified degree of right knee
- T24.022 Burn of unspecified degree of left knee
- T24.029 Burn of unspecified degree of unspecified knee

T24.03 Burn of unspecified degree of lower leg
- T24.031 Burn of unspecified degree of right lower leg
- T24.032 Burn of unspecified degree of left lower leg
- T24.039 Burn of unspecified degree of unspecified lower leg

T24.09 Burn of unspecified degree of multiple sites of lower limb, except ankle and foot
- T24.091 Burn of unspecified degree of multiple sites of right lower limb, except ankle and foot
- T24.092 Burn of unspecified degree of multiple sites of left lower limb, except ankle and foot
- T24.099 Burn of unspecified degree of multiple sites of unspecified lower limb, except ankle and foot

T24.1 Burn of first degree of lower limb, except ankle and foot

Use additional external cause code to identify the source, place and intent of the burn (X00-X19, X75-X77, X96-X98, Y92)

T24.10 Burn of first degree of unspecified site of lower limb, except ankle and foot
- T24.101 Burn of first degree of unspecified site of right lower limb, except ankle and foot
- T24.102 Burn of first degree of unspecified site of left lower limb, except ankle and foot
- T24.109 Burn of first degree of unspecified site of unspecified lower limb, except ankle and foot

T24.11 Burn of first degree of thigh
- T24.111 Burn of first degree of right thigh
- T24.112 Burn of first degree of left thigh
- T24.119 Burn of first degree of unspecified thigh

T24.12 Burn of first degree of knee
- T24.121 Burn of first degree of right knee
- T24.122 Burn of first degree of left knee
- T24.129 Burn of first degree of unspecified knee

T24.13 Burn of first degree of lower leg
- T24.131 Burn of first degree of right lower leg
- T24.132 Burn of first degree of left lower leg
- T24.139 Burn of first degree of unspecified lower leg

T24.19 Burn of first degree of multiple sites of lower limb, except ankle and foot
- T24.191 Burn of first degree of multiple sites of right lower limb, except ankle and foot
- T24.192 Burn of first degree of multiple sites of left lower limb, except ankle and foot
- T24.199 Burn of first degree of multiple sites of unspecified lower limb, except ankle and foot

- T24.2 **Burn of second degree of lower limb, except ankle and foot**
  Use additional external cause code to identify the source, place and intent of the burn (X00-X19, X75-X77, X96-X98, Y92)
  - T24.20 **Burn of second degree of unspecified site of lower limb, except ankle and foot**
    - T24.201 **Burn of second degree of unspecified site of right lower limb, except ankle and foot**
    - T24.202 **Burn of second degree of unspecified site of left lower limb, except ankle and foot**
    - T24.209 **Burn of second degree of unspecified site of unspecified lower limb, except ankle and foot**
  - T24.21 **Burn of second degree of thigh**
    - T24.211 **Burn of second degree of right thigh**
    - T24.212 **Burn of second degree of left thigh**
    - T24.219 **Burn of second degree of unspecified thigh**
  - T24.22 **Burn of second degree of knee**
    - T24.221 **Burn of second degree of right knee**
    - T24.222 **Burn of second degree of left knee**
    - T24.229 **Burn of second degree of unspecified knee**
  - T24.23 **Burn of second degree of lower leg**
    - T24.231 **Burn of second degree of right lower leg**
    - T24.232 **Burn of second degree of left lower leg**
    - T24.239 **Burn of second degree of unspecified lower leg**
  - T24.29 **Burn of second degree of multiple sites of lower limb, except ankle and foot**
    - T24.291 **Burn of second degree of multiple sites of right lower limb, except ankle and foot**
    - T24.292 **Burn of second degree of multiple sites of left lower limb, except ankle and foot**
    - T24.299 **Burn of second degree of multiple sites of unspecified lower limb, except ankle and foot**
- T24.3 **Burn of third degree of lower limb, except ankle and foot**
  Use additional external cause code to identify the source, place and intent of the burn (X00-X19, X75-X77, X96-X98, Y92)
  - T24.30 **Burn of third degree of unspecified site of lower limb, except ankle and foot**
    - T24.301 **Burn of third degree of unspecified site of right lower limb, except ankle and foot**
    - T24.302 **Burn of third degree of unspecified site of left lower limb, except ankle and foot**
    - T24.309 **Burn of third degree of unspecified site of unspecified lower limb, except ankle and foot**
  - T24.31 **Burn of third degree of thigh**
    - T24.311 **Burn of third degree of right thigh**
    - T24.312 **Burn of third degree of left thigh**
    - T24.319 **Burn of third degree of unspecified thigh**
  - T24.32 **Burn of third degree of knee**
    - T24.321 **Burn of third degree of right knee**
    - T24.322 **Burn of third degree of left knee**
    - T24.329 **Burn of third degree of unspecified knee**
  - T24.33 **Burn of third degree of lower leg**
    - T24.331 **Burn of third degree of right lower leg**
    - T24.332 **Burn of third degree of left lower leg**
    - T24.339 **Burn of third degree of unspecified lower leg**
  - T24.39 **Burn of third degree of multiple sites of lower limb, except ankle and foot**
    - T24.391 **Burn of third degree of multiple sites of right lower limb, except ankle and foot**
    - T24.392 **Burn of third degree of multiple sites of left lower limb, except ankle and foot**
    - T24.399 **Burn of third degree of multiple sites of unspecified lower limb, except ankle and foot**
- T24.4 **Corrosion of unspecified degree of lower limb, except ankle and foot**
  Code first (T51-T65) to identify chemical and intent
  Use additional external cause code to identify place (Y92)
  - T24.40 **Corrosion of unspecified degree of unspecified site of lower limb, except ankle and foot**
    - T24.401 **Corrosion of unspecified degree of unspecified site of right lower limb, except ankle and foot**
    - T24.402 **Corrosion of unspecified degree of unspecified site of left lower limb, except ankle and foot**
    - T24.409 **Corrosion of unspecified degree of unspecified site of unspecified lower limb, except ankle and foot**
  - T24.41 **Corrosion of unspecified degree of thigh**
    - T24.411 **Corrosion of unspecified degree of right thigh**
    - T24.412 **Corrosion of unspecified degree of left thigh**
    - T24.419 **Corrosion of unspecified degree of unspecified thigh**
  - T24.42 **Corrosion of unspecified degree of knee**
    - T24.421 **Corrosion of unspecified degree of right knee**
    - T24.422 **Corrosion of unspecified degree of left knee**
    - T24.429 **Corrosion of unspecified degree of unspecified knee**
  - T24.43 **Corrosion of unspecified degree of lower leg**
    - T24.431 **Corrosion of unspecified degree of right lower leg**
    - T24.432 **Corrosion of unspecified degree of left lower leg**
    - T24.439 **Corrosion of unspecified degree of unspecified lower leg**
  - T24.49 **Corrosion of unspecified degree of multiple sites of lower limb, except ankle and foot**
    - T24.491 **Corrosion of unspecified degree of multiple sites of right lower limb, except ankle and foot**
    - T24.492 **Corrosion of unspecified degree of multiple sites of left lower limb, except ankle and foot**
    - T24.499 **Corrosion of unspecified degree of multiple sites of unspecified lower limb, except ankle and foot**

● T24.5 Corrosion of first degree of lower limb, except ankle and foot
Code first (T51-T65) to identify chemical and intent
Use additional external cause code to identify place (Y92)
● T24.50 Corrosion of first degree of unspecified site of lower limb, except ankle and foot
● T24.501 Corrosion of first degree of unspecified site of right lower limb, except ankle and foot
● T24.502 Corrosion of first degree of unspecified site of left lower limb, except ankle and foot
● T24.509 Corrosion of first degree of unspecified site of unspecified lower limb, except ankle and foot
● T24.51 Corrosion of first degree of thigh
● T24.511 Corrosion of first degree of right thigh
● T24.512 Corrosion of first degree of left thigh
● T24.519 Corrosion of first degree of unspecified thigh
● T24.52 Corrosion of first degree of knee
● T24.521 Corrosion of first degree of right knee
● T24.522 Corrosion of first degree of left knee
● T24.529 Corrosion of first degree of unspecified knee
● T24.53 Corrosion of first degree of lower leg
● T24.531 Corrosion of first degree of right lower leg
● T24.532 Corrosion of first degree of left lower leg
● T24.539 Corrosion of first degree of unspecified lower leg
● T24.59 Corrosion of first degree of multiple sites of lower limb, except ankle and foot
● T24.591 Corrosion of first degree of multiple sites of right lower limb, except ankle and foot
● T24.592 Corrosion of first degree of multiple sites of left lower limb, except ankle and foot
● T24.599 Corrosion of first degree of multiple sites of unspecified lower limb, except ankle and foot
● T24.6 Corrosion of second degree of lower limb, except ankle and foot
Code first (T51-T65) to identify chemical and intent
Use additional external cause code to identify place (Y92)
● T24.60 Corrosion of second degree of unspecified site of lower limb, except ankle and foot
● T24.601 Corrosion of second degree of unspecified site of right lower limb, except ankle and foot
● T24.602 Corrosion of second degree of unspecified site of left lower limb, except ankle and foot
● T24.609 Corrosion of second degree of unspecified site of unspecified lower limb, except ankle and foot
● T24.61 Corrosion of second degree of thigh
● T24.611 Corrosion of second degree of right thigh
● T24.612 Corrosion of second degree of left thigh
● T24.619 Corrosion of second degree of unspecified thigh
● T24.62 Corrosion of second degree of knee
● T24.621 Corrosion of second degree of right knee
● T24.622 Corrosion of second degree of left knee
● T24.629 Corrosion of second degree of unspecified knee
● T24.63 Corrosion of second degree of lower leg
● T24.631 Corrosion of second degree of right lower leg
● T24.632 Corrosion of second degree of left lower leg
● T24.639 Corrosion of second degree of unspecified lower leg
● T24.69 Corrosion of second degree of multiple sites of lower limb, except ankle and foot
● T24.691 Corrosion of second degree of multiple sites of right lower limb, except ankle and foot
● T24.692 Corrosion of second degree of multiple sites of left lower limb, except ankle and foot
● T24.699 Corrosion of second degree of multiple sites of unspecified lower limb, except ankle and foot
● T24.7 Corrosion of third degree of lower limb, except ankle and foot
Code first (T51-T65) to identify chemical and intent
Use additional external cause code to identify place (Y92)
● T24.70 Corrosion of third degree of unspecified site of lower limb, except ankle and foot
● T24.701 Corrosion of third degree of unspecified site of right lower limb, except ankle and foot
● T24.702 Corrosion of third degree of unspecified site of left lower limb, except ankle and foot
● T24.709 Corrosion of third degree of unspecified site of unspecified lower limb, except ankle and foot
● T24.71 Corrosion of third degree of thigh
● T24.711 Corrosion of third degree of right thigh
● T24.712 Corrosion of third degree of left thigh
● T24.719 Corrosion of third degree of unspecified thigh
● T24.72 Corrosion of third degree of knee
● T24.721 Corrosion of third degree of right knee
● T24.722 Corrosion of third degree of left knee
● T24.729 Corrosion of third degree of unspecified knee
● T24.73 Corrosion of third degree of lower leg
● T24.731 Corrosion of third degree of right lower leg
● T24.732 Corrosion of third degree of left lower leg
● T24.739 Corrosion of third degree of unspecified lower leg
● T24.79 Corrosion of third degree of multiple sites of lower limb, except ankle and foot
● T24.791 Corrosion of third degree of multiple sites of right lower limb, except ankle and foot
● T24.792 Corrosion of third degree of multiple sites of left lower limb, except ankle and foot
● T24.799 Corrosion of third degree of multiple sites of unspecified lower limb, except ankle and foot

CHAPTER 19 (S00-T88)

● T25 Burn and corrosion of ankle and foot
The appropriate 7th character is to be added to each code from category T25

A	initial encounter
D	subsequent encounter
S	sequela

● T25.0 Burn of unspecified degree of ankle and foot
Use additional external cause code to identify the source, place and intent of the burn (X00-X19, X75-X77, X96-X98, Y92)
● T25.01 Burn of unspecified degree of ankle
● T25.011 Burn of unspecified degree of right ankle
● T25.012 Burn of unspecified degree of left ankle
● T25.019 Burn of unspecified degree of unspecified ankle
● T25.02 Burn of unspecified degree of foot
Excludes2 burn of unspecified degree of toe(s) (nail) (T25.03-)
● T25.021 Burn of unspecified degree of right foot
● T25.022 Burn of unspecified degree of left foot
● T25.029 Burn of unspecified degree of unspecified foot
● T25.03 Burn of unspecified degree of toe(s) (nail)
● T25.031 Burn of unspecified degree of right toe(s) (nail)
● T25.032 Burn of unspecified degree of left toe(s) (nail)
● T25.039 Burn of unspecified degree of unspecified toe(s) (nail)
● T25.09 Burn of unspecified degree of multiple sites of ankle and foot
● T25.091 Burn of unspecified degree of multiple sites of right ankle and foot
● T25.092 Burn of unspecified degree of multiple sites of left ankle and foot
● T25.099 Burn of unspecified degree of multiple sites of unspecified ankle and foot
● T25.1 Burn of first degree of ankle and foot
Use additional external cause code to identify the source, place and intent of the burn (X00-X19, X75-X77, X96-X98, Y92)
● T25.11 Burn of first degree of ankle
● T25.111 Burn of first degree of right ankle
● T25.112 Burn of first degree of left ankle
● T25.119 Burn of first degree of unspecified ankle
● T25.12 Burn of first degree of foot
Excludes2 burn of first degree of toe(s) (nail) (T25.13-)
● T25.121 Burn of first degree of right foot
● T25.122 Burn of first degree of left foot
● T25.129 Burn of first degree of unspecified foot
● T25.13 Burn of first degree of toe(s) (nail)
● T25.131 Burn of first degree of right toe(s) (nail)
● T25.132 Burn of first degree of left toe(s) (nail)
● T25.139 Burn of first degree of unspecified toe(s) (nail)
● T25.19 Burn of first degree of multiple sites of ankle and foot
● T25.191 Burn of first degree of multiple sites of right ankle and foot
● T25.192 Burn of first degree of multiple sites of left ankle and foot
● T25.199 Burn of first degree of multiple sites of unspecified ankle and foot
● T25.2 Burn of second degree of ankle and foot
Use additional external cause code to identify the source, place and intent of the burn (X00-X19, X75-X77, X96-X98, Y92)
● T25.21 Burn of second degree of ankle
● T25.211 Burn of second degree of right ankle
● T25.212 Burn of second degree of left ankle
● T25.219 Burn of second degree of unspecified ankle
● T25.22 Burn of second degree of foot
Excludes2 burn of second degree of toe(s) (nail) (T25.23-)
● T25.221 Burn of second degree of right foot
● T25.222 Burn of second degree of left foot
● T25.229 Burn of second degree of unspecified foot
● T25.23 Burn of second degree of toe(s) (nail)
● T25.231 Burn of second degree of right toe(s) (nail)
● T25.232 Burn of second degree of left toe(s) (nail)
● T25.239 Burn of second degree of unspecified toe(s) (nail)
● T25.29 Burn of second degree of multiple sites of ankle and foot
● T25.291 Burn of second degree of multiple sites of right ankle and foot
● T25.292 Burn of second degree of multiple sites of left ankle and foot
● T25.299 Burn of second degree of multiple sites of unspecified ankle and foot
● T25.3 Burn of third degree of ankle and foot
Use additional external cause code to identify the source, place and intent of the burn (X00-X19, X75-X77, X96-X98, Y92)
● T25.31 Burn of third degree of ankle
● T25.311 Burn of third degree of right ankle
● T25.312 Burn of third degree of left ankle
● T25.319 Burn of third degree of unspecified ankle
● T25.32 Burn of third degree of foot
Excludes2 burn of third degree of toe(s) (nail) (T25.33-)
● T25.321 Burn of third degree of right foot
● T25.322 Burn of third degree of left foot
● T25.329 Burn of third degree of unspecified foot
● T25.33 Burn of third degree of toe(s) (nail)
● T25.331 Burn of third degree of right toe(s) (nail)
● T25.332 Burn of third degree of left toe(s) (nail)
● T25.339 Burn of third degree of unspecified toe(s) (nail)
● T25.39 Burn of third degree of multiple sites of ankle and foot
● T25.391 Burn of third degree of multiple sites of right ankle and foot
● T25.392 Burn of third degree of multiple sites of left ankle and foot
● T25.399 Burn of third degree of multiple sites of unspecified ankle and foot

● **T25.4 Corrosion of unspecified degree of ankle and foot**
Code first (T51-T65) to identify chemical and intent
Use additional external cause code to identify place (Y92)
● **T25.41 Corrosion of unspecified degree of ankle**
● **T25.411 Corrosion of unspecified degree of right ankle**
● **T25.412 Corrosion of unspecified degree of left ankle**
● **T25.419 Corrosion of unspecified degree of unspecified ankle**
● **T25.42 Corrosion of unspecified degree of foot**
Excludes2 corrosion of unspecified degree of toe(s) (nail) (T25.43-)
● **T25.421 Corrosion of unspecified degree of right foot**
● **T25.422 Corrosion of unspecified degree of left foot**
● **T25.429 Corrosion of unspecified degree of unspecified foot**
● **T25.43 Corrosion of unspecified degree of toe(s) (nail)**
● **T25.431 Corrosion of unspecified degree of right toe(s) (nail)**
● **T25.432 Corrosion of unspecified degree of left toe(s) (nail)**
● **T25.439 Corrosion of unspecified degree of unspecified toe(s) (nail)**
● **T25.49 Corrosion of unspecified degree of multiple sites of ankle and foot**
● **T25.491 Corrosion of unspecified degree of multiple sites of right ankle and foot**
● **T25.492 Corrosion of unspecified degree of multiple sites of left ankle and foot**
● **T25.499 Corrosion of unspecified degree of multiple sites of unspecified ankle and foot**

● **T25.5 Corrosion of first degree of ankle and foot**
Code first (T51-T65) to identify chemical and intent
Use additional external cause code to identify place (Y92)
● **T25.51 Corrosion of first degree of ankle**
● **T25.511 Corrosion of first degree of right ankle**
● **T25.512 Corrosion of first degree of left ankle**
● **T25.519 Corrosion of first degree of unspecified ankle**
● **T25.52 Corrosion of first degree of foot**
Excludes2 corrosion of first degree of toe(s) (nail) (T25.53-)
● **T25.521 Corrosion of first degree of right foot**
● **T25.522 Corrosion of first degree of left foot**
● **T25.529 Corrosion of first degree of unspecified foot**
● **T25.53 Corrosion of first degree of toe(s) (nail)**
● **T25.531 Corrosion of first degree of right toe(s) (nail)**
● **T25.532 Corrosion of first degree of left toe(s) (nail)**
● **T25.539 Corrosion of first degree of unspecified toe(s) (nail)**
● **T25.59 Corrosion of first degree of multiple sites of ankle and foot**
● **T25.591 Corrosion of first degree of multiple sites of right ankle and foot**
● **T25.592 Corrosion of first degree of multiple sites of left ankle and foot**
● **T25.599 Corrosion of first degree of multiple sites of unspecified ankle and foot**

● **T25.6 Corrosion of second degree of ankle and foot**
Code first (T51-T65) to identify chemical and intent
Use additional external cause code to identify place (Y92)
● **T25.61 Corrosion of second degree of ankle**
● **T25.611 Corrosion of second degree of right ankle**
● **T25.612 Corrosion of second degree of left ankle**
● **T25.619 Corrosion of second degree of unspecified ankle**
● **T25.62 Corrosion of second degree of foot**
Excludes2 corrosion of second degree of toe(s) (nail) (T25.63-)
● **T25.621 Corrosion of second degree of right foot**
● **T25.622 Corrosion of second degree of left foot**
● **T25.629 Corrosion of second degree of unspecified foot**
● **T25.63 Corrosion of second degree of toe(s) (nail)**
● **T25.631 Corrosion of second degree of right toe(s) (nail)**
● **T25.632 Corrosion of second degree of left toe(s) (nail)**
● **T25.639 Corrosion of second degree of unspecified toe(s) (nail)**
● **T25.69 Corrosion of second degree of multiple sites of ankle and foot**
● **T25.691 Corrosion of second degree of right ankle and foot**
● **T25.692 Corrosion of second degree of left ankle and foot**
● **T25.699 Corrosion of second degree of unspecified ankle and foot**

● **T25.7 Corrosion of third degree of ankle and foot**
Code first (T51-T65) to identify chemical and intent
Use additional external cause code to identify place (Y92)
● **T25.71 Corrosion of third degree of ankle**
● **T25.711 Corrosion of third degree of right ankle**
● **T25.712 Corrosion of third degree of left ankle**
● **T25.719 Corrosion of third degree of unspecified ankle**
● **T25.72 Corrosion of third degree of foot**
Excludes2 corrosion of third degree of toe(s) (nail) (T25.73-)
● **T25.721 Corrosion of third degree of right foot**
● **T25.722 Corrosion of third degree of left foot**
● **T25.729 Corrosion of third degree of unspecified foot**
● **T25.73 Corrosion of third degree of toe(s) (nail)**
● **T25.731 Corrosion of third degree of right toe(s) (nail)**
● **T25.732 Corrosion of third degree of left toe(s) (nail)**
● **T25.739 Corrosion of third degree of unspecified toe(s) (nail)**
● **T25.79 Corrosion of third degree of multiple sites of ankle and foot**
● **T25.791 Corrosion of third degree of multiple sites of right ankle and foot**
● **T25.792 Corrosion of third degree of multiple sites of left ankle and foot**
● **T25.799 Corrosion of third degree of multiple sites of unspecified ankle and foot**

BURNS AND CORROSIONS CONFINED TO EYE AND INTERNAL ORGANS (T26-T28)

● **T26 Burn and corrosion confined to eye and adnexa**

The appropriate 7th character is to be added to each code from category T26

A	initial encounter
D	subsequent encounter
S	sequela

● **T26.0 Burn of eyelid and periocular area**

Use additional external cause code to identify the source, place and intent of the burn (X00-X19, X75-X77, X96-X98, Y92)

X● **T26.00 Burn of unspecified eyelid and periocular area**

X● **T26.01 Burn of right eyelid and periocular area**

X● **T26.02 Burn of left eyelid and periocular area**

● **T26.1 Burn of cornea and conjunctival sac**

Use additional external cause code to identify the source, place and intent of the burn (X00-X19, X75-X77, X96-X98, Y92)

X● **T26.10 Burn of cornea and conjunctival sac, unspecified eye**

X● **T26.11 Burn of cornea and conjunctival sac, right eye**

X● **T26.12 Burn of cornea and conjunctival sac, left eye**

● **T26.2 Burn with resulting rupture and destruction of eyeball**

Use additional external cause code to identify the source, place and intent of the burn (X00-X19, X75-X77, X96-X98, Y92)

X● **T26.20 Burn with resulting rupture and destruction of unspecified eyeball**

X● **T26.21 Burn with resulting rupture and destruction of right eyeball**

X● **T26.22 Burn with resulting rupture and destruction of left eyeball**

● **T26.3 Burns of other specified parts of eye and adnexa**

Use additional external cause code to identify the source, place and intent of the burn (X00-X19, X75-X77, X96-X98, Y92)

X● **T26.30 Burns of other specified parts of unspecified eye and adnexa**

X● **T26.31 Burns of other specified parts of right eye and adnexa**

X● **T26.32 Burns of other specified parts of left eye and adnexa**

● **T26.4 Burn of eye and adnexa, part unspecified**

Use additional external cause code to identify the source, place and intent of the burn (X00-X19, X75-X77, X96-X98, Y92)

X● **T26.40 Burn of unspecified eye and adnexa, part unspecified**

X● **T26.41 Burn of right eye and adnexa, part unspecified**

X● **T26.42 Burn of left eye and adnexa, part unspecified**

● **T26.5 Corrosion of eyelid and periocular area**

Code first (T51-T65) to identify chemical and intent

Use additional external cause code to identify place (Y92)

X● **T26.50 Corrosion of unspecified eyelid and periocular area**

X● **T26.51 Corrosion of right eyelid and periocular area**

X● **T26.52 Corrosion of left eyelid and periocular area**

● **T26.6 Corrosion of cornea and conjunctival sac**

Code first (T51-T65) to identify chemical and intent

Use additional external cause code to identify place (Y92)

X● **T26.60 Corrosion of cornea and conjunctival sac, unspecified eye**

X● **T26.61 Corrosion of cornea and conjunctival sac, right eye**

X● **T26.62 Corrosion of cornea and conjunctival sac, left eye**

● **T26.7 Corrosion with resulting rupture and destruction of eyeball**

Code first (T51-T65) to identify chemical and intent

Use additional external cause code to identify place (Y92)

X● **T26.70 Corrosion with resulting rupture and destruction of unspecified eyeball**

X● **T26.71 Corrosion with resulting rupture and destruction of right eyeball**

X● **T26.72 Corrosion with resulting rupture and destruction of left eyeball**

● **T26.8 Corrosions of other specified parts of eye and adnexa**

Code first (T51-T65) to identify chemical and intent

Use additional external cause code to identify place (Y92)

X● **T26.80 Corrosions of other specified parts of unspecified eye and adnexa**

X● **T26.81 Corrosions of other specified parts of right eye and adnexa**

X● **T26.82 Corrosions of other specified parts of left eye and adnexa**

● **T26.9 Corrosion of eye and adnexa, part unspecified**

Code first (T51-T65) to identify chemical and intent

Use additional external cause code to identify place (Y92)

X● **T26.90 Corrosion of unspecified eye and adnexa, part unspecified**

X● **T26.91 Corrosion of right eye and adnexa, part unspecified**

X● **T26.92 Corrosion of left eye and adnexa, part unspecified**

● **T27 Burn and corrosion of respiratory tract**

Use additional external cause code to identify the source and intent of the burn (X00-X19, X75-X77, X96-X98)

Use additional external cause code to identify place (Y92)

The appropriate 7th character is to be added to each code from category T27

A	initial encounter
D	subsequent encounter
S	sequela

X● **T27.0 Burn of larynx and trachea**

X● **T27.1 Burn involving larynx and trachea with lung**

X● **T27.2 Burn of other parts of respiratory tract**

Burn of thoracic cavity

X● **T27.3 Burn of respiratory tract, part unspecified**

Code first (T51-T65) to identify chemical and intent for codes T27.4-T27.7

X● **T27.4 Corrosion of larynx and trachea**

X● **T27.5 Corrosion involving larynx and trachea with lung**

X● **T27.6 Corrosion of other parts of respiratory tract**

X● **T27.7 Corrosion of respiratory tract, part unspecified**

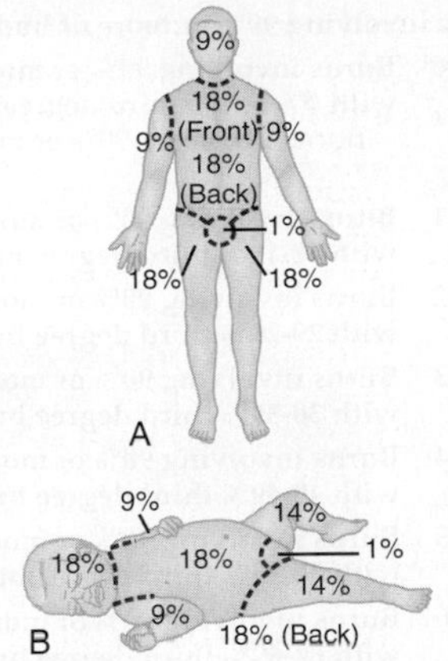

Figure 19-16 Rule of nines: percentages of total body area. (From Marx: Rosen's Emergency Medicine: Concepts and Clinical Practice, ed 6, Mosby, 2006)

● **T28 Burn and corrosion of other internal organs**

Use additional external cause code to identify the source and intent of the burn (X00-X19, X75-X77, X96-X98)

Use additional external cause code to identify place (Y92)

The appropriate 7th character is to be added to each code from category T28

A	initial encounter
D	subsequent encounter
S	sequela

X● **T28.0** Burn of mouth and pharynx
X● **T28.1** Burn of esophagus
X● **T28.2** Burn of other parts of alimentary tract
X● **T28.3** Burn of internal genitourinary organs
X● **T28.4** Burns of other and unspecified internal organs
X● **T28.40** Burn of unspecified internal organ
● **T28.41** Burn of ear drum
● **T28.411** Burn of right ear drum
● **T28.412** Burn of left ear drum
● **T28.419** Burn of unspecified ear drum
X● **T28.49** Burn of other internal organ
Code first (T51-T65) to identify chemical and intent for T28.5-T28.9-
X● **T28.5** Corrosion of mouth and pharynx
X● **T28.6** Corrosion of esophagus
X● **T28.7** Corrosion of other parts of alimentary tract
X● **T28.8** Corrosion of internal genitourinary organs
● **T28.9** Corrosions of other and unspecified internal organs
X● **T28.90** Corrosions of unspecified internal organs
● **T28.91** Corrosions of ear drum
● **T28.911** Corrosions of right ear drum
● **T28.912** Corrosions of left ear drum
● **T28.919** Corrosions of unspecified ear drum
X● **T28.99** Corrosions of other internal organs

OGCR Section I.C.19.d.5.

Assign separate code for each burn site
When coding burns, assign separate codes for each burn site. Category T30, Burn and corrosion, body region unspecified is extremely vague and should rarely be used.

BURNS AND CORROSIONS OF MULTIPLE AND UNSPECIFIED BODY REGIONS (T30-T32)

● **T30 Burn and corrosion, body region unspecified**
T30.0 Burn of unspecified body region, unspecified degree
This code is not for inpatient use. Code to specified site and degree of burns
Burn NOS
Multiple burns NOS
T30.4 Corrosion of unspecified body region, unspecified degree
This code is not for inpatient use. Code to specified site and degree of corrosion
Corrosion NOS
Multiple corrosion NOS

● **T31 Burns classified according to extent of body surface involved**
Note: This category is to be used as the primary code only when the site of the burn is unspecified. It should be used as a supplementary code with categories T20-T25 when the site is specified.
T31.0 Burns involving less than 10% of body surface
● **T31.1** Burns involving 10-19% of body surface
T31.10 Burns involving 10-19% of body surface with 0% to 9% third degree burns
Burns involving 10-19% of body surface NOS
T31.11 Burns involving 10-19% of body surface with 10-19% third degree burns
● **T31.2** Burns involving 20-29% of body surface
T31.20 Burns involving 20-29% of body surface with 0% to 9% third degree burns
Burns involving 20-29% of body surface NOS
T31.21 Burns involving 20-29% of body surface with 10-19% third degree burns
T31.22 Burns involving 20-29% of body surface with 20-29% third degree burns
● **T31.3** Burns involving 30-39% of body surface
T31.30 Burns involving 30-39% of body surface with 0% to 9% third degree burns
Burns involving 30-39% of body surface NOS
T31.31 Burns involving 30-39% of body surface with 10-19% third degree burns
T31.32 Burns involving 30-39% of body surface with 20-29% third degree burns
T31.33 Burns involving 30-39% of body surface with 30-39% third degree burns
● **T31.4** Burns involving 40-49% of body surface
T31.40 Burns involving 40-49% of body surface with 0% to 9% third degree burns
Burns involving 40-49% of body surface NOS
T31.41 Burns involving 40-49% of body surface with 10-19% third degree burns
T31.42 Burns involving 40-49% of body surface with 20-29% third degree burns
T31.43 Burns involving 40-49% of body surface with 30-39% third degree burns
T31.44 Burns involving 40-49% of body surface with 40-49% third degree burns

CHAPTER 19 (S00-T88)

● T31.5 Burns involving 50-59% of body surface
- T31.50 Burns involving 50-59% of body surface with 0% to 9% third degree burns
  - Burns involving 50-59% of body surface NOS
- T31.51 Burns involving 50-59% of body surface with 10-19% third degree burns
- T31.52 Burns involving 50-59% of body surface with 20-29% third degree burns
- T31.53 Burns involving 50-59% of body surface with 30-39% third degree burns
- T31.54 Burns involving 50-59% of body surface with 40-49% third degree burns
- T31.55 Burns involving 50-59% of body surface with 50-59% third degree burns

● T31.6 Burns involving 60-69% of body surface
- T31.60 Burns involving 60-69% of body surface with 0% to 9% third degree burns
  - Burns involving 60-69% of body surface NOS
- T31.61 Burns involving 60-69% of body surface with 10-19% third degree burns
- T31.62 Burns involving 60-69% of body surface with 20-29% third degree burns
- T31.63 Burns involving 60-69% of body surface with 30-39% third degree burns
- T31.64 Burns involving 60-69% of body surface with 40-49% third degree burns
- T31.65 Burns involving 60-69% of body surface with 50-59% third degree burns
- T31.66 Burns involving 60-69% of body surface with 60-69% third degree burns

● T31.7 Burns involving 70-79% of body surface
- T31.70 Burns involving 70-79% of body surface with 0% to 9% third degree burns
  - Burns involving 70-79% of body surface NOS
- T31.71 Burns involving 70-79% of body surface with 10-19% third degree burns
- T31.72 Burns involving 70-79% of body surface with 20-29% third degree burns
- T31.73 Burns involving 70-79% of body surface with 30-39% third degree burns
- T31.74 Burns involving 70-79% of body surface with 40-49% third degree burns
- T31.75 Burns involving 70-79% of body surface with 50-59% third degree burns
- T31.76 Burns involving 70-79% of body surface with 60-69% third degree burns
- T31.77 Burns involving 70-79% of body surface with 70-79% third degree burns

● T31.8 Burns involving 80-89% of body surface
- T31.80 Burns involving 80-89% of body surface with 0% to 9% third degree burns
  - Burns involving 80-89% of body surface NOS
- T31.81 Burns involving 80-89% of body surface with 10-19% third degree burns
- T31.82 Burns involving 80-89% of body surface with 20-29% third degree burns
- T31.83 Burns involving 80-89% of body surface with 30-39% third degree burns
- T31.84 Burns involving 80-89% of body surface with 40-49% third degree burns
- T31.85 Burns involving 80-89% of body surface with 50-59% third degree burns
- T31.86 Burns involving 80-89% of body surface with 60-69% third degree burns
- T31.87 Burns involving 80-89% of body surface with 70-79% third degree burns
- T31.88 Burns involving 80-89% of body surface with 80-89% third degree burns

● T31.9 Burns involving 90% or more of body surface
- T31.90 Burns involving 90% or more of body surface with 0% to 9% third degree burns
  - Burns involving 90% or more of body surface NOS
- T31.91 Burns involving 90% or more of body surface with 10-19% third degree burns
- T31.92 Burns involving 90% or more of body surface with 20-29% third degree burns
- T31.93 Burns involving 90% or more of body surface with 30-39% third degree burns
- T31.94 Burns involving 90% or more of body surface with 40-49% third degree burns
- T31.95 Burns involving 90% or more of body surface with 50-59% third degree burns
- T31.96 Burns involving 90% or more of body surface with 60-69% third degree burns
- T31.97 Burns involving 90% or more of body surface with 70-79% third degree burns
- T31.98 Burns involving 90% or more of body surface with 80-89% third degree burns
- T31.99 Burns involving 90% or more of body surface with 90% or more third degree burns

● **T32 Corrosions classified according to extent of body surface involved**

Note: This category is to be used as the primary code only when the site of the corrosion is unspecified. It may be used as a supplementary code with categories T20-T25 when the site is specified.

- T32.0 Corrosions involving less than 10% of body surface

● T32.1 Corrosions involving 10-19% of body surface
- T32.10 Corrosions involving 10-19% of body surface with 0% to 9% third degree corrosion
  - Corrosions involving 10-19% of body surface NOS
- T32.11 Corrosions involving 10-19% of body surface with 10-19% third degree corrosion

● T32.2 Corrosions involving 20-29% of body surface
- T32.20 Corrosions involving 20-29% of body surface with 0% to 9% third degree corrosion
- T32.21 Corrosions involving 20-29% of body surface with 10-19% third degree corrosion
- T32.22 Corrosions involving 20-29% of body surface with 20-29% third degree corrosion

● T32.3 Corrosions involving 30-39% of body surface
- T32.30 Corrosions involving 30-39% of body surface with 0% to 9% third degree corrosion
- T32.31 Corrosions involving 30-39% of body surface with 10-19% third degree corrosion
- T32.32 Corrosions involving 30-39% of body surface with 20-29% third degree corrosion
- T32.33 Corrosions involving 30-39% of body surface with 30-39% third degree corrosion

● T32.4 Corrosions involving 40-49% of body surface
- T32.40 Corrosions involving 40-49% of body surface with 0% to 9% third degree corrosion
- T32.41 Corrosions involving 40-49% of body surface with 10-19% third degree corrosion
- T32.42 Corrosions involving 40-49% of body surface with 20-29% third degree corrosion
- T32.43 Corrosions involving 40-49% of body surface with 30-39% third degree corrosion
- T32.44 Corrosions involving 40-49% of body surface with 40-49% third degree corrosion

● **T32.5**   Corrosions involving 50-59% of body surface

     T32.50   Corrosions involving 50-59% of body surface with 0% to 9% third degree corrosion

     T32.51   Corrosions involving 50-59% of body surface with 10-19% third degree corrosion

     T32.52   Corrosions involving 50-59% of body surface with 20-29% third degree corrosion

     T32.53   Corrosions involving 50-59% of body surface with 30-39% third degree corrosion

     T32.54   Corrosions involving 50-59% of body surface with 40-49% third degree corrosion

     T32.55   Corrosions involving 50-59% of body surface with 50-59% third degree corrosion

● **T32.6**   Corrosions involving 60-69% of body surface

     T32.60   Corrosions involving 60-69% of body surface with 0% to 9% third degree corrosion

     T32.61   Corrosions involving 60-69% of body surface with 10-19% third degree corrosion

     T32.62   Corrosions involving 60-69% of body surface with 20-29% third degree corrosion

     T32.63   Corrosions involving 60-69% of body surface with 30-39% third degree corrosion

     T32.64   Corrosions involving 60-69% of body surface with 40-49% third degree corrosion

     T32.65   Corrosions involving 60-69% of body surface with 50-59% third degree corrosion

     T32.66   Corrosions involving 60-69% of body surface with 60-69% third degree corrosion

● **T32.7**   Corrosions involving 70-79% of body surface

     T32.70   Corrosions involving 70-79% of body surface with 0% to 9% third degree corrosion

     T32.71   Corrosions involving 70-79% of body surface with 10-19% third degree corrosion

     T32.72   Corrosions involving 70-79% of body surface with 20-29% third degree corrosion

     T32.73   Corrosions involving 70-79% of body surface with 30-39% third degree corrosion

     T32.74   Corrosions involving 70-79% of body surface with 40-49% third degree corrosion

     T32.75   Corrosions involving 70-79% of body surface with 50-59% third degree corrosion

     T32.76   Corrosions involving 70-79% of body surface with 60-69% third degree corrosion

     T32.77   Corrosions involving 70-79% of body surface with 70-79% third degree corrosion

● **T32.8**   Corrosions involving 80-89% of body surface

     T32.80   Corrosions involving 80-89% of body surface with 0% to 9% third degree corrosion

     T32.81   Corrosions involving 80-89% of body surface with 10-19% third degree corrosion

     T32.82   Corrosions involving 80-89% of body surface with 20-29% third degree corrosion

     T32.83   Corrosions involving 80-89% of body surface with 30-39% third degree corrosion

     T32.84   Corrosions involving 80-89% of body surface with 40-49% third degree corrosion

     T32.85   Corrosions involving 80-89% of body surface with 50-59% third degree corrosion

     T32.86   Corrosions involving 80-89% of body surface with 60-69% third degree corrosion

     T32.87   Corrosions involving 80-89% of body surface with 70-79% third degree corrosion

     T32.88   Corrosions involving 80-89% of body surface with 80-89% third degree corrosion

● **T32.9**   Corrosions involving 90% or more of body surface

     T32.90   Corrosions involving 90% or more of body surface with 0% to 9% third degree corrosion

     T32.91   Corrosions involving 90% or more of body surface with 10-19% third degree corrosion

     T32.92   Corrosions involving 90% or more of body surface with 20-29% third degree corrosion

     T32.93   Corrosions involving 90% or more of body surface with 30-39% third degree corrosion

     T32.94   Corrosions involving 90% or more of body surface with 40-49% third degree corrosion

     T32.95   Corrosions involving 90% or more of body surface with 50-59% third degree corrosion

     T32.96   Corrosions involving 90% or more of body surface with 60-69% third degree corrosion

     T32.97   Corrosions involving 90% or more of body surface with 70-79% third degree corrosion

     T32.98   Corrosions involving 90% or more of body surface with 80-89% third degree corrosion

     T32.99   Corrosions involving 90% or more of body surface with 90% or more third degree corrosion

FROSTBITE (T33-T34)

| **Excludes2** | hypothermia and other effects of reduced temperature (T68, T69.-) |

● **T33**   **Superficial frostbite**

     Includes   frostbite with partial thickness skin loss

     The appropriate 7th character is to be added to each code from category T33

A	initial encounter
D	subsequent encounter
S	sequela

   ● **T33.0**   **Superficial frostbite of head**

      ● **T33.01**   Superficial frostbite of ear

        ● **T33.011**   Superficial frostbite of right ear

        ● **T33.012**   Superficial frostbite of left ear

        ● **T33.019**   Superficial frostbite of unspecified ear

     X ● **T33.02**   Superficial frostbite of nose

     X ● **T33.09**   Superficial frostbite of other part of head

   X ● **T33.1**   Superficial frostbite of neck

   X ● **T33.2**   Superficial frostbite of thorax

   X ● **T33.3**   Superficial frostbite of abdominal wall, lower back and pelvis

   ● **T33.4**   Superficial frostbite of arm

      | **Excludes2** | superficial frostbite of wrist and hand (T33.5-) |

     X ● **T33.40**   Superficial frostbite of unspecified arm

     X ● **T33.41**   Superficial frostbite of right arm

     X ● **T33.42**   Superficial frostbite of left arm

   ● **T33.5**   **Superficial frostbite of wrist, hand, and fingers**

      ● **T33.51**   Superficial frostbite of wrist

        ● **T33.511**   Superficial frostbite of right wrist

        ● **T33.512**   Superficial frostbite of left wrist

        ● **T33.519**   Superficial frostbite of unspecified wrist

      ● **T33.52**   Superficial frostbite of hand

        | **Excludes2** | superficial frostbite of fingers (T33.53-) |

        ● **T33.521**   Superficial frostbite of right hand

        ● **T33.522**   Superficial frostbite of left hand

        ● **T33.529**   Superficial frostbite of unspecified hand

● T33.53 Superficial frostbite of finger(s)
● T33.531 Superficial frostbite of right finger(s)
● T33.532 Superficial frostbite of left finger(s)
● T33.539 Superficial frostbite of unspecified finger(s)
● T33.6 Superficial frostbite of hip and thigh
X● T33.60 Superficial frostbite of unspecified hip and thigh
X● T33.61 Superficial frostbite of right hip and thigh
X● T33.62 Superficial frostbite of left hip and thigh
● T33.7 Superficial frostbite of knee and lower leg
Excludes2 superficial frostbite of ankle and foot (T33.8-)
X● T33.70 Superficial frostbite of unspecified knee and lower leg
X● T33.71 Superficial frostbite of right knee and lower leg
X● T33.72 Superficial frostbite of left knee and lower leg
● T33.8 Superficial frostbite of ankle, foot, and toe(s)
● T33.81 Superficial frostbite of ankle
● T33.811 Superficial frostbite of right ankle
● T33.812 Superficial frostbite of left ankle
● T33.819 Superficial frostbite of unspecified ankle
● T33.82 Superficial frostbite of foot
● T33.821 Superficial frostbite of right foot
● T33.822 Superficial frostbite of left foot
● T33.829 Superficial frostbite of unspecified foot
● T33.83 Superficial frostbite of toe(s)
● T33.831 Superficial frostbite of right toe(s)
● T33.832 Superficial frostbite of left toe(s)
● T33.839 Superficial frostbite of unspecified toe(s)
● T33.9 Superficial frostbite of other and unspecified sites
X● T33.90 Superficial frostbite of unspecified sites
Superficial frostbite NOS
X● T33.99 Superficial frostbite of other sites
Superficial frostbite of leg NOS
Superficial frostbite of trunk NOS
● T34 Frostbite with tissue necrosis
The appropriate 7th character is to be added to each code from category T34

A	initial encounter
D	subsequent encounter
S	sequela

● T34.0 Frostbite with tissue necrosis of head
● T34.01 Frostbite with tissue necrosis of ear
● T34.011 Frostbite with tissue necrosis of right ear
● T34.012 Frostbite with tissue necrosis of left ear
● T34.019 Frostbite with tissue necrosis of unspecified ear
X● T34.02 Frostbite with tissue necrosis of nose
X● T34.09 Frostbite with tissue necrosis of other part of head
X● T34.1 Frostbite with tissue necrosis of neck
X● T34.2 Frostbite with tissue necrosis of thorax
X● T34.3 Frostbite with tissue necrosis of abdominal wall, lower back and pelvis
● T34.4 Frostbite with tissue necrosis of arm
Excludes2 frostbite with tissue necrosis of wrist and hand (T34.5-)
X● T34.40 Frostbite with tissue necrosis of unspecified arm
X● T34.41 Frostbite with tissue necrosis of right arm
X● T34.42 Frostbite with tissue necrosis of left arm
● T34.5 Frostbite with tissue necrosis of wrist, hand, and finger(s)
● T34.51 Frostbite with tissue necrosis of wrist
● T34.511 Frostbite with tissue necrosis of right wrist
● T34.512 Frostbite with tissue necrosis of left wrist
● T34.519 Frostbite with tissue necrosis of unspecified wrist
● T34.52 Frostbite with tissue necrosis of hand
Excludes2 frostbite with tissue necrosis of finger(s) (T34.53-)
● T34.521 Frostbite with tissue necrosis of right hand
● T34.522 Frostbite with tissue necrosis of left hand
● T34.529 Frostbite with tissue necrosis of unspecified hand
● T34.53 Frostbite with tissue necrosis of finger(s)
● T34.531 Frostbite with tissue necrosis of right finger(s)
● T34.532 Frostbite with tissue necrosis of left finger(s)
● T34.539 Frostbite with tissue necrosis of unspecified finger(s)
● T34.6 Frostbite with tissue necrosis of hip and thigh
X● T34.60 Frostbite with tissue necrosis of unspecified hip and thigh
X● T34.61 Frostbite with tissue necrosis of right hip and thigh
X● T34.62 Frostbite with tissue necrosis of left hip and thigh
● T34.7 Frostbite with tissue necrosis of knee and lower leg
Excludes2 frostbite with tissue necrosis of ankle and foot (T34.8-)
X● T34.70 Frostbite with tissue necrosis of unspecified knee and lower leg
X● T34.71 Frostbite with tissue necrosis of right knee and lower leg
X● T34.72 Frostbite with tissue necrosis of left knee and lower leg
● T34.8 Frostbite with tissue necrosis of ankle, foot, and toe(s)
● T34.81 Frostbite with tissue necrosis of ankle
● T34.811 Frostbite with tissue necrosis of right ankle
● T34.812 Frostbite with tissue necrosis of left ankle
● T34.819 Frostbite with tissue necrosis of unspecified ankle

● **T34.82 Frostbite with tissue necrosis of foot**
● **T34.821 Frostbite with tissue necrosis of right foot**
● **T34.822 Frostbite with tissue necrosis of left foot**
● **T34.829 Frostbite with tissue necrosis of unspecified foot**
● **T34.83 Frostbite with tissue necrosis of toe(s)**
● **T34.831 Frostbite with tissue necrosis of right toe(s)**
● **T34.832 Frostbite with tissue necrosis of left toe(s)**
● **T34.839 Frostbite with tissue necrosis of unspecified toe(s)**
● **T34.9 Frostbite with tissue necrosis of other and unspecified sites**
X● **T34.90 Frostbite with tissue necrosis of unspecified sites**
Frostbite with tissue necrosis NOS
X● **T34.99 Frostbite with tissue necrosis of other sites**
Frostbite with tissue necrosis of leg NOS
Frostbite with tissue necrosis of trunk NOS

OGCR See Section I.C.19.e.

Adverse Effects, Poisoning , Underdosing and Toxic Effects
Codes in categories T36-T65 are combination codes that include the substance that was taken as well as the intent. No additional external cause code is required for poisonings, toxic effects, adverse effects and underdosing codes.

POISONING BY, ADVERSE EFFECTS OF AND UNDERDOSING OF DRUGS MEDICAMENTS AND BIOLOGICAL SUBSTANCES (T36-T50)

Includes adverse effect of correct substance properly administered
poisoning by overdose of substance
poisoning by wrong substance given or taken in error
underdosing by (inadvertently) (deliberately) taking less substance than prescribed or instructed

Code first, for adverse effects, the nature of the adverse effect, such as:
adverse effect NOS (T88.7)
aspirin gastritis (K29.-)
blood disorders (D56-D76)
contact dermatitis (L23-L25)
dermatitis due to substances taken internally (L27.-)
nephropathy (N14.0-N14.2)

Note: The drug giving rise to the adverse effect should be identified by use of codes from categories T36-T50 with fifth or sixth character 5.

Use additional code(s) to specify:
manifestations of poisoning
underdosing or failure in dosage during medical and surgical care (Y63.6, Y63.8-Y63.9)
underdosing of medication regimen (Z91.12-, Z91.13-)

Excludes1 toxic reaction to local anesthesia in pregnancy (O29.3-)

Excludes2 abuse and dependence of psychoactive substances (F10-F19)
abuse of non-dependence-producing substances (F55.-)
drug reaction and poisoning affecting newborn (P00-P96)
pathological drug intoxication (inebriation) (F10-F19)

● **T36 Poisoning by, adverse effect of and underdosing of systemic antibiotics**

Excludes1 antineoplastic antibiotics (T45.1-)
locally applied antibiotic NEC (T49.0)
topically used antibiotic for ear, nose and throat (T49.6)
topically used antibiotic for eye (T49.5)

The appropriate 7th character is to be added to each code from category T36

A	initial encounter
D	subsequent encounter
S	sequela

● **T36.0 Poisoning by, adverse effect of and underdosing of penicillins**
● **T36.0X Poisoning by, adverse effect of and underdosing of penicillins**
● **T36.0X1 Poisoning by penicillins, accidental (unintentional)**
Poisoning by penicillins NOS
● **T36.0X2 Poisoning by penicillins, intentional self-harm**
● **T36.0X3 Poisoning by penicillins, assault**
● **T36.0X4 Poisoning by penicillins, undetermined**
● **T36.0X5 Adverse effect of penicillins**
● **T36.0X6 Underdosing of penicillins**
● **T36.1 Poisoning by, adverse effect of and underdosing of cephalosporins and other betalactam antibiotics**
● **T36.1X Poisoning by, adverse effect of and underdosing of cephalosporins and other beta-lactam antibiotics**
● **T36.1X1 Poisoning by cephalosporins and other beta-lactam antibiotics, accidental (unintentional)**
Poisoning by cephalosporins and other beta-lactam antibiotics NOS
● **T36.1X2 Poisoning by cephalosporins and other beta-lactam antibiotics, intentional self-harm**
● **T36.1X3 Poisoning by cephalosporins and other beta-lactam antibiotics, assault**
● **T36.1X4 Poisoning by cephalosporins and other beta-lactam antibiotics, undetermined**
● **T36.1X5 Adverse effect of cephalosporins and other beta-lactam antibiotics**
● **T36.1X6 Underdosing of cephalosporins and other beta-lactam antibiotics**
● **T36.2 Poisoning by, adverse effect of and underdosing of chloramphenicol group**
● **T36.2X Poisoning by, adverse effect of and underdosing of chloramphenicol group**
● **T36.2X1 Poisoning by chloramphenicol group, accidental (unintentional)**
Poisoning by chloramphenicol group NOS
● **T36.2X2 Poisoning by chloramphenicol group, intentional self-harm**
● **T36.2X3 Poisoning by chloramphenicol group, assault**
● **T36.2X4 Poisoning by chloramphenicol group, undetermined**
● **T36.2X5 Adverse effect of chloramphenicol group**
● **T36.2X6 Underdosing of chloramphenicol group**

● **T36.3 Poisoning by, adverse effect of and underdosing of macrolides**

● **T36.3X Poisoning by, adverse effect of and underdosing of macrolides**

● **T36.3X1 Poisoning by macrolides, accidental (unintentional)**

Poisoning by macrolides NOS

● **T36.3X2 Poisoning by macrolides, intentional self-harm**

● **T36.3X3 Poisoning by macrolides, assault**

● **T36.3X4 Poisoning by macrolides, undetermined**

● **T36.3X5 Adverse effect of macrolides**

● **T36.3X6 Underdosing of macrolides**

● **T36.4 Poisoning by, adverse effect of and underdosing of tetracyclines**

● **T36.4X Poisoning by, adverse effect of and underdosing of tetracyclines**

● **T36.4X1 Poisoning by tetracyclines, accidental (unintentional)**

Poisoning by tetracyclines NOS

● **T36.4X2 Poisoning by tetracyclines, intentional self-harm**

● **T36.4X3 Poisoning by tetracyclines, assault**

● **T36.4X4 Poisoning by tetracyclines, undetermined**

● **T36.4X5 Adverse effect of tetracyclines**

● **T36.4X6 Underdosing of tetracyclines**

● **T36.5 Poisoning by, adverse effect of and underdosing of aminoglycosides**

Poisoning by, adverse effect of and underdosing of streptomycin

● **T36.5X Poisoning by, adverse effect of and underdosing of aminoglycosides**

● **T36.5X1 Poisoning by aminoglycosides, accidental (unintentional)**

Poisoning by aminoglycosides NOS

● **T36.5X2 Poisoning by aminoglycosides, intentional self-harm**

● **T36.5X3 Poisoning by aminoglycosides, assault**

● **T36.5X4 Poisoning by aminoglycosides, undetermined**

● **T36.5X5 Adverse effect of aminoglycosides**

● **T36.5X6 Underdosing of aminoglycosides**

● **T36.6 Poisoning by, adverse effect of and underdosing of rifampicins**

● **T36.6X Poisoning by, adverse effect of and underdosing of rifampicins**

● **T36.6X1 Poisoning by rifampicins, accidental (unintentional)**

Poisoning by rifampicins NOS

● **T36.6X2 Poisoning by rifampicins, intentional self-harm**

● **T36.6X3 Poisoning by rifampicins, assault**

● **T36.6X4 Poisoning by rifampicins, undetermined**

● **T36.6X5 Adverse effect of rifampicins**

● **T36.6X6 Underdosing of rifampicins**

● **T36.7 Poisoning by, adverse effect of and underdosing of antifungal antibiotics, systemically used**

● **T36.7X Poisoning by, adverse effect of and underdosing of antifungal antibiotics, systemically used**

● **T36.7X1 Poisoning by antifungal antibiotics, systemically used, accidental (unintentional)**

Poisoning by antifungal antibiotics, systemically used NOS

● **T36.7X2 Poisoning by antifungal antibiotics, systemically used, intentional self-harm**

● **T36.7X3 Poisoning by antifungal antibiotics, systemically used, assault**

● **T36.7X4 Poisoning by antifungal antibiotics, systemically used, undetermined**

● **T36.7X5 Adverse effect of antifungal antibiotics, systemically used**

● **T36.7X6 Underdosing of antifungal antibiotics, systemically used**

● **T36.8 Poisoning by, adverse effect of and underdosing of other systemic antibiotics**

● **T36.8X Poisoning by, adverse effect of and underdosing of other systemic antibiotics**

● **T36.8X1 Poisoning by other systemic antibiotics, accidental (unintentional)**

Poisoning by other systemic antibiotics NOS

● **T36.8X2 Poisoning by other systemic antibiotics, intentional self-harm**

● **T36.8X3 Poisoning by other systemic antibiotics, assault**

● **T36.8X4 Poisoning by other systemic antibiotics, undetermined**

● **T36.8X5 Adverse effect of other systemic antibiotics**

● **T36.8X6 Underdosing of other systemic antibiotics**

● **T36.9 Poisoning by, adverse effect of and underdosing of unspecified systemic antibiotic**

X● **T36.91 Poisoning by unspecified systemic antibiotic, accidental (unintentional)**

Poisoning by systemic antibiotic NOS

X● **T36.92 Poisoning by unspecified systemic antibiotic, intentional self-harm**

X● **T36.93 Poisoning by unspecified systemic antibiotic, assault**

X● **T36.94 Poisoning by unspecified systemic antibiotic, undetermined**

X● **T36.95 Adverse effect of unspecified systemic antibiotic**

X● **T36.96 Underdosing of unspecified systemic antibiotic**

● **T37 Poisoning by, adverse effect of and underdosing of other systemic anti-infectives and antiparasitics**

Excludes1 anti-infectives topically used for ear, nose and throat (T49.6-)
anti-infectives topically used for eye (T49.5-)
locally applied anti-infectives NEC (T49.Ø-)

The appropriate 7th character is to be added to each code from category T37

A initial encounter
D subsequent encounter
S sequela

● **T37.Ø Poisoning by, adverse effect of and underdosing of sulfonamides**

● **T37.ØX Poisoning by, adverse effect of and underdosing of sulfonamides**

● **T37.ØX1 Poisoning by sulfonamides, accidental (unintentional)**

Poisoning by sulfonamides NOS

● **T37.ØX2 Poisoning by sulfonamides, intentional self-harm**

● **T37.ØX3 Poisoning by sulfonamides, assault**

● **T37.ØX4 Poisoning by sulfonamides, undetermined**

● **T37.ØX5 Adverse effect of sulfonamides**

● **T37.ØX6 Underdosing of sulfonamides**

● T37.1 **Poisoning by, adverse effect of and underdosing of antimycobacterial drugs**
Excludes1 rifampicins (T36.6-) streptomycin (T36.5-)
● T37.1X **Poisoning by, adverse effect of and underdosing of antimycobacterial drugs**
● T37.1X1 **Poisoning by antimycobacterial drugs, accidental (unintentional)**
Poisoning by antimycobacterial drugs NOS
● T37.1X2 **Poisoning by antimycobacterial drugs, intentional self-harm**
● T37.1X3 **Poisoning by antimycobacterial drugs, assault**
● T37.1X4 **Poisoning by antimycobacterial drugs, undetermined**
● T37.1X5 **Adverse effect of antimycobacterial drugs**
● T37.1X6 **Underdosing of antimycobacterial drugs**
● T37.2 **Poisoning by, adverse effect of and underdosing of antimalarials and drugs acting on other blood protozoa**
Excludes1 hydroxyquinoline derivatives (T37.8-)
● T37.2X **Poisoning by, adverse effect of and underdosing of antimalarials and drugs acting on other blood protozoa**
● T37.2X1 **Poisoning by antimalarials and drugs acting on other blood protozoa, accidental (unintentional)**
Poisoning by antimalarials and drugs acting on other blood protozoa NOS
● T37.2X2 **Poisoning by antimalarials and drugs acting on other blood protozoa, intentional self-harm**
● T37.2X3 **Poisoning by antimalarials and drugs acting on other blood protozoa, assault**
● T37.2X4 **Poisoning by antimalarials and drugs acting on other blood protozoa, undetermined**
● T37.2X5 **Adverse effect of antimalarials and drugs acting on other blood protozoa**
● T37.2X6 **Underdosing of antimalarials and drugs acting on other blood protozoa**
● T37.3 **Poisoning by, adverse effect of and underdosing of other antiprotozoal drugs**
● T37.3X **Poisoning by, adverse effect of and underdosing of other antiprotozoal drugs**
● T37.3X1 **Poisoning by other antiprotozoal drugs, accidental (unintentional)**
Poisoning by other antiprotozoal drugs NOS
● T37.3X2 **Poisoning by other antiprotozoal drugs, intentional self-harm**
● T37.3X3 **Poisoning by other antiprotozoal drugs, assault**
● T37.3X4 **Poisoning by other antiprotozoal drugs, undetermined**
● T37.3X5 **Adverse effect of other antiprotozoal drugs**
● T37.3X6 **Underdosing of other antiprotozoal drugs**
● T37.4 **Poisoning by, adverse effect of and underdosing of anthelminthics**
● T37.4X **Poisoning by, adverse effect of and underdosing of anthelminthics**
● T37.4X1 **Poisoning by anthelminthics, accidental (unintentional)**
Poisoning by anthelminthics NOS
● T37.4X2 **Poisoning by anthelminthics, intentional self-harm**
● T37.4X3 **Poisoning by anthelminthics, assault**
● T37.4X4 **Poisoning by anthelminthics, undetermined**
● T37.4X5 **Adverse effect of anthelminthics**
● T37.4X6 **Underdosing of anthelminthics**
● T37.5 **Poisoning by, adverse effect of and underdosing of antiviral drugs**
Excludes1 amantadine (T42.8-)
cytarabine (T45.1-)
● T37.5X **Poisoning by, adverse effect of and underdosing of antiviral drugs**
● T37.5X1 **Poisoning by antiviral drugs, accidental (unintentional)**
Poisoning by antiviral drugs NOS
● T37.5X2 **Poisoning by antiviral drugs, intentional self-harm**
● T37.5X3 **Poisoning by antiviral drugs, assault**
● T37.5X4 **Poisoning by antiviral drugs, undetermined**
● T37.5X5 **Adverse effect of antiviral drugs**
● T37.5X6 **Underdosing of antiviral drugs**
● T37.8 **Poisoning by, adverse effect of and underdosing of other specified systemic anti-infectives and antiparasitics**
Poisoning by, adverse effect of and underdosing of hydroxyquinoline derivatives
Excludes1 antimalarial drugs (T37.2-)
● T37.8X **Poisoning by, adverse effect of and underdosing of other specified systemic anti-infectives and antiparasitics**
● T37.8X1 **Poisoning by other specified systemic anti-infectives and antiparasitics, accidental (unintentional)**
Poisoning by other specified systemic anti-infectives and antiparasitics NOS
● T37.8X2 **Poisoning by other specified systemic anti-infectives and antiparasitics, intentional self-harm**
● T37.8X3 **Poisoning by other specified systemic anti-infectives and antiparasitics, assault**
● T37.8X4 **Poisoning by other specified systemic anti-infectives and antiparasitics, undetermined**
● T37.8X5 **Adverse effect of other specified systemic anti-infectives and antiparasitics**
● T37.8X6 **Underdosing of other specified systemic anti-infectives and antiparasitics**
● T37.9 **Poisoning by, adverse effect of and underdosing of unspecified systemic anti-infective and antiparasitics**
X● T37.91 **Poisoning by unspecified systemic anti-infective and antiparasitics, accidental (unintentional)**
Poisoning by, adverse effect of and underdosing of systemic anti-infective and antiparasitics NOS
X● T37.92 **Poisoning by unspecified systemic anti-infective and antiparasitics, intentional self-harm**
X● T37.93 **Poisoning by unspecified systemic anti-infective and antiparasitics, assault**
X● T37.94 **Poisoning by unspecified systemic anti-infective and antiparasitics, undetermined**
X● T37.95 **Adverse effect of unspecified systemic anti-infective and antiparasitic**
X● T37.96 **Underdosing of unspecified systemic anti-infectives and antiparasitics**

CHAPTER 19 (S00-T88)

● T38 Poisoning by, adverse effect of and underdosing of hormones and their synthetic substitutes and antagonists, not elsewhere classified

Excludes1 mineralocorticoids and their antagonists (T50.0-)
oxytocic hormones (T48.0-)
parathyroid hormones and derivatives (T50.9-)

The appropriate 7th character is to be added to each code from category T38

A	initial encounter
D	subsequent encounter
S	sequela

● T38.0 Poisoning by, adverse effect of and underdosing of glucocorticoids and synthetic analogues

Excludes1 glucocorticoids, topically used (T49.-)

● T38.0X Poisoning by, adverse effect of and underdosing of glucocorticoids and synthetic analogues

● T38.0X1 Poisoning by glucocorticoids and synthetic analogues, accidental (unintentional)
Poisoning by glucocorticoids and synthetic analogues NOS

● T38.0X2 Poisoning by glucocorticoids and synthetic analogues, intentional self-harm

● T38.0X3 Poisoning by glucocorticoids and synthetic analogues, assault

● T38.0X4 Poisoning by glucocorticoids and synthetic analogues, undetermined

● T38.0X5 Adverse effect of glucocorticoids and synthetic analogues

● T38.0X6 Underdosing of glucocorticoids and synthetic analogues

● T38.1 Poisoning by, adverse effect of and underdosing of thyroid hormones and substitutes

● T38.1X Poisoning by, adverse effect of and underdosing of thyroid hormones and substitutes

● T38.1X1 Poisoning by thyroid hormones and substitutes, accidental (unintentional)
Poisoning by thyroid hormones and substitutes NOS

● T38.1X2 Poisoning by thyroid hormones and substitutes, intentional self-harm

● T38.1X3 Poisoning by thyroid hormones and substitutes, assault

● T38.1X4 Poisoning by thyroid hormones and substitutes, undetermined

● T38.1X5 Adverse effect of thyroid hormones and substitutes

● T38.1X6 Underdosing of thyroid hormones and substitutes

● T38.2 Poisoning by, adverse effect of and underdosing of antithyroid drugs

● T38.2X Poisoning by, adverse effect of and underdosing of antithyroid drugs

● T38.2X1 Poisoning by antithyroid drugs, accidental (unintentional)
Poisoning by antithyroid drugs NOS

● T38.2X2 Poisoning by antithyroid drugs, intentional self-harm

● T38.2X3 Poisoning by antithyroid drugs, assault

● T38.2X4 Poisoning by antithyroid drugs, undetermined

● T38.2X5 Adverse effect of antithyroid drugs

● T38.2X6 Underdosing of antithyroid drugs

● T38.3 Poisoning by, adverse effect of and underdosing of insulin and oral hypoglycemic [antidiabetic] drugs

● T38.3X Poisoning by, adverse effect of and underdosing of insulin and oral hypoglycemic [antidiabetic] drugs

● T38.3X1 Poisoning by insulin and oral hypoglycemic [antidiabetic] drugs, accidental (unintentional)
Poisoning by insulin and oral hypoglycemic [antidiabetic] drugs NOS

● T38.3X2 Poisoning by insulin and oral hypoglycemic [antidiabetic] drugs, intentional self-harm

● T38.3X3 Poisoning by insulin and oral hypoglycemic [antidiabetic] drugs, assault

● T38.3X4 Poisoning by insulin and oral hypoglycemic [antidiabetic] drugs, undetermined

● T38.3X5 Adverse effect of insulin and oral hypoglycemic [antidiabetic] drugs

● T38.3X6 Underdosing of insulin and oral hypoglycemic [antidiabetic] drugs

● T38.4 Poisoning by, adverse effect of and underdosing of oral contraceptives
Poisoning by, adverse effect of and underdosing of multiple- and single-ingredient oral contraceptive preparations

● T38.4X Poisoning by, adverse effect of and underdosing of oral contraceptives

● T38.4X1 Poisoning by oral contraceptives, accidental (unintentional)
Poisoning by oral contraceptives NOS

● T38.4X2 Poisoning by oral contraceptives, intentional self-harm

● T38.4X3 Poisoning by oral contraceptives, assault

● T38.4X4 Poisoning by oral contraceptives, undetermined

● T38.4X5 Adverse effect of oral contraceptives

● T38.4X6 Underdosing of oral contraceptives

● T38.5 Poisoning by, adverse effect of and underdosing of other estrogens and progestogens
Poisoning by, adverse effect of and underdosing of estrogens and progestogens mixtures and substitutes

● T38.5X Poisoning by, adverse effect of and underdosing of other estrogens and progestogens

● T38.5X1 Poisoning by other estrogens and progestogens, accidental (unintentional)
Poisoning by other estrogens and progestogens NOS

● T38.5X2 Poisoning by other estrogens and progestogens, intentional self-harm

● T38.5X3 Poisoning by other estrogens and progestogens, assault

● T38.5X4 Poisoning by other estrogens and progestogens, undetermined

● T38.5X5 Adverse effect of other estrogens and progestogens

● T38.5X6 Underdosing of other estrogens and progestogens

- T38.6 **Poisoning by, adverse effect of and underdosing of antigonadotrophins, antiestrogens, antiandrogens, not elsewhere classified**
  Poisoning by, adverse effect of and underdosing of tamoxifen
  - T38.6X **Poisoning by, adverse effect of and underdosing of antigonadotrophins, antiestrogens, antiandrogens, not elsewhere classified**
    - T38.6X1 **Poisoning by antigonadotrophins, antiestrogens, antiandrogens, not elsewhere classified, accidental (unintentional)**
      Poisoning by antigonadotrophins, antiestrogens, antiandrogens, not elsewhere classified NOS
    - T38.6X2 **Poisoning by antigonadotrophins, antiestrogens, antiandrogens, not elsewhere classified, intentional self-harm**
    - T38.6X3 **Poisoning by antigonadotrophins, antiestrogens, antiandrogens, not elsewhere classified, assault**
    - T38.6X4 **Poisoning by antigonadotrophins, antiestrogens, antiandrogens, not elsewhere classified, undetermined**
    - T38.6X5 **Adverse effect of antigonadotrophins, antiestrogens, antiandrogens, not elsewhere classified**
    - T38.6X6 **Underdosing of antigonadotrophins, antiestrogens, antiandrogens, not elsewhere classified**
- T38.7 **Poisoning by, adverse effect of and underdosing of androgens and anabolic congeners**
  - T38.7X **Poisoning by, adverse effect of and underdosing of androgens and anabolic congeners**
    - T38.7X1 **Poisoning by androgens and anabolic congeners, accidental (unintentional)**
      Poisoning by androgens and anabolic congeners NOS
    - T38.7X2 **Poisoning by androgens and anabolic congeners, intentional self-harm**
    - T38.7X3 **Poisoning by androgens and anabolic congeners, assault**
    - T38.7X4 **Poisoning by androgens and anabolic congeners, undetermined**
    - T38.7X5 **Adverse effect of androgens and anabolic congeners**
    - T38.7X6 **Underdosing of androgens and anabolic congeners**
- T38.8 **Poisoning by, adverse effect of and underdosing of other and unspecified hormones and synthetic substitutes**
  - T38.80 **Poisoning by, adverse effect of and underdosing of unspecified hormones and synthetic substitutes**
    - T38.801 **Poisoning by unspecified hormones and synthetic substitutes, accidental (unintentional)**
      Poisoning by unspecified hormones and synthetic substitutes NOS
    - T38.802 **Poisoning by unspecified hormones and synthetic substitutes, intentional self-harm**
    - T38.803 **Poisoning by unspecified hormones and synthetic substitutes, assault**
    - T38.804 **Poisoning by unspecified hormones and synthetic substitutes, undetermined**
    - T38.805 **Adverse effect of unspecified hormones and synthetic substitutes**
    - T38.806 **Underdosing of unspecified hormones and synthetic substitutes**
  - T38.81 **Poisoning by, adverse effect of and underdosing of anterior pituitary [adenohypophyseal] hormones**
    - T38.811 **Poisoning by anterior pituitary [adenohypophyseal] hormones, accidental (unintentional)**
      Poisoning by anterior pituitary [adenohypophyseal] hormones NOS
    - T38.812 **Poisoning by anterior pituitary [adenohypophyseal] hormones, intentional self-harm**
    - T38.813 **Poisoning by anterior pituitary [adenohypophyseal] hormones, assault**
    - T38.814 **Poisoning by anterior pituitary [adenohypophyseal] hormones, undetermined**
    - T38.815 **Adverse effect of anterior pituitary [adenohypophyseal] hormones**
    - T38.816 **Underdosing of anterior pituitary [adenohypophyseal] hormones**
  - T38.89 **Poisoning by, adverse effect of and underdosing of other hormones and synthetic substitutes**
    - T38.891 **Poisoning by other hormones and synthetic substitutes, accidental (unintentional)**
      Poisoning by other hormones and synthetic substitutes NOS
    - T38.892 **Poisoning by other hormones and synthetic substitutes, intentional self-harm**
    - T38.893 **Poisoning by other hormones and synthetic substitutes, assault**
    - T38.894 **Poisoning by other hormones and synthetic substitutes, undetermined**
    - T38.895 **Adverse effect of other hormones and synthetic substitutes**
    - T38.896 **Underdosing of other hormones and synthetic substitutes**
- T38.9 **Poisoning by, adverse effect of and underdosing of other and unspecified hormone antagonists**
  - T38.90 **Poisoning by, adverse effect of and underdosing of unspecified hormone antagonists**
    - T38.901 **Poisoning by unspecified hormone antagonists, accidental (unintentional)**
      Poisoning by unspecified hormone antagonists NOS
    - T38.902 **Poisoning by unspecified hormone antagonists, intentional self-harm**
    - T38.903 **Poisoning by unspecified hormone antagonists, assault**
    - T38.904 **Poisoning by unspecified hormone antagonists, undetermined**
    - T38.905 **Adverse effect of unspecified hormone antagonists**
    - T38.906 **Underdosing of unspecified hormone antagonists**

T38.99 **Poisoning by, adverse effect of and underdosing of other hormone antagonists**

T38.991 **Poisoning by other hormone antagonists, accidental (unintentional)**
Poisoning by other hormone antagonists NOS

T38.992 **Poisoning by other hormone antagonists, intentional self-harm**

T38.993 **Poisoning by other hormone antagonists, assault**

T38.994 **Poisoning by other hormone antagonists, undetermined**

T38.995 **Adverse effect of other hormone antagonists**

T38.996 **Underdosing of other hormone antagonists**

T39 **Poisoning by, adverse effect of and underdosing of nonopioid analgesics, antipyretics and antirheumatics**

The appropriate 7th character is to be added to each code from category T39

A	initial encounter
D	subsequent encounter
S	sequela

T39.0 **Poisoning by, adverse effect of and underdosing of salicylates**

T39.01 **Poisoning by, adverse effect of and underdosing of aspirin**
Poisoning by, adverse effect of and underdosing of acetylsalicylic acid

T39.011 **Poisoning by aspirin, accidental (unintentional)**

T39.012 **Poisoning by aspirin, intentional self-harm**

T39.013 **Poisoning by aspirin, assault**

T39.014 **Poisoning by aspirin, undetermined**

T39.015 **Adverse effect of aspirin**

T39.016 **Underdosing of aspirin**

T39.09 **Poisoning by, adverse effect of and underdosing of other salicylates**

T39.091 **Poisoning by salicylates, accidental (unintentional)**
Poisoning by salicylates NOS

T39.092 **Poisoning by salicylates, intentional self-harm**

T39.093 **Poisoning by salicylates, assault**

T39.094 **Poisoning by salicylates, undetermined**

T39.095 **Adverse effect of salicylates**

T39.096 **Underdosing of salicylates**

T39.1 **Poisoning by, adverse effect of and underdosing of 4-Aminophenol derivatives**

T39.1X **Poisoning by, adverse effect of and underdosing of 4-Aminophenol derivatives**

T39.1X1 **Poisoning by 4-Aminophenol derivatives, accidental (unintentional)**
Poisoning by 4-Aminophenol derivatives NOS

T39.1X2 **Poisoning by 4-Aminophenol derivatives, intentional self-harm**

T39.1X3 **Poisoning by 4-Aminophenol derivatives, assault**

T39.1X4 **Poisoning by 4-Aminophenol derivatives, undetermined**

T39.1X5 **Adverse effect of 4-Aminophenol derivatives**

T39.1X6 **Underdosing of 4-Aminophenol derivatives**

T39.2 **Poisoning by, adverse effect of and underdosing of pyrazolone derivatives**

T39.2X **Poisoning by, adverse effect of and underdosing of pyrazolone derivatives**

T39.2X1 **Poisoning by pyrazolone derivatives, accidental (unintentional)**
Poisoning by pyrazolone derivatives NOS

T39.2X2 **Poisoning by pyrazolone derivatives, intentional self-harm**

T39.2X3 **Poisoning by pyrazolone derivatives, assault**

T39.2X4 **Poisoning by pyrazolone derivatives, undetermined**

T39.2X5 **Adverse effect of pyrazolone derivatives**

T39.2X6 **Underdosing of pyrazolone derivatives**

T39.3 **Poisoning by, adverse effect of and underdosing of other nonsteroidal anti-inflammatory drugs [NSAID]**

T39.31 **Poisoning by, adverse effect of and underdosing of propionic acid derivatives**
Poisoning by, adverse effect of and underdosing of fenoprofen
Poisoning by, adverse effect of and underdosing of flurbiprofen
Poisoning by, adverse effect of and underdosing of ibuprofen
Poisoning by, adverse effect of and underdosing of ketoprofen
Poisoning by, adverse effect of and underdosing of naproxen
Poisoning by, adverse effect of and underdosing of oxaprozin

T39.311 **Poisoning by propionic acid derivatives, accidental (unintentional)**

T39.312 **Poisoning by propionic acid derivatives, intentional self-harm**

T39.313 **Poisoning by propionic acid derivatives, assault**

T39.314 **Poisoning by propionic acid derivatives, undetermined**

T39.315 **Adverse effect of propionic acid derivatives**

T39.316 **Underdosing of propionic acid derivatives**

T39.39 **Poisoning by, adverse effect of and underdosing of other nonsteroidal anti-inflammatory drugs [NSAID]**

T39.391 **Poisoning by other nonsteroidal anti-inflammatory drugs [NSAID], accidental (unintentional)**
Poisoning by other nonsteroidal anti-inflammatory drugs NOS

T39.392 **Poisoning by other nonsteroidal anti-inflammatory drugs [NSAID], intentional self-harm**

T39.393 **Poisoning by other nonsteroidal anti-inflammatory drugs [NSAID], assault**

T39.394 **Poisoning by other nonsteroidal anti-inflammatory drugs [NSAID], undetermined**

T39.395 **Adverse effect of other nonsteroidal anti-inflammatory drugs [NSAID]**

T39.396 **Underdosing of other nonsteroidal anti-inflammatory drugs [NSAID]**

● T39.4 **Poisoning by, adverse effect of and underdosing of antirheumatics, not elsewhere classified**

Excludes1 poisoning by, adverse effect of and underdosing of glucocorticoids (T38.0-)
poisoning by, adverse effect of and underdosing of salicylates (T39.0-)

● T39.4X **Poisoning by, adverse effect of and underdosing of antirheumatics, not elsewhere classified**

● T39.4X1 **Poisoning by antirheumatics, not elsewhere classified, accidental (unintentional)**
Poisoning by antirheumatics, not elsewhere classified NOS

● T39.4X2 **Poisoning by antirheumatics, not elsewhere classified, intentional self-harm**

● T39.4X3 **Poisoning by antirheumatics, not elsewhere classified, assault**

● T39.4X4 **Poisoning by antirheumatics, not elsewhere classified, undetermined**

● T39.4X5 **Adverse effect of antirheumatics, not elsewhere classified**

● T39.4X6 **Underdosing of antirheumatics, not elsewhere classified**

● T39.8 **Poisoning by, adverse effect of and underdosing of other nonopioid analgesics and antipyretics, not elsewhere classified**

● T39.8X **Poisoning by, adverse effect of and underdosing of other nonopioid analgesics and antipyretics, not elsewhere classified**

● T39.8X1 **Poisoning by other nonopioid analgesics and antipyretics, not elsewhere classified, accidental (unintentional)**
Poisoning by other nonopioid analgesics and antipyretics, not elsewhere classified NOS

● T39.8X2 **Poisoning by other nonopioid analgesics and antipyretics, not elsewhere classified, intentional self-harm**

● T39.8X3 **Poisoning by other nonopioid analgesics and antipyretics, not elsewhere classified, assault**

● T39.8X4 **Poisoning by other nonopioid analgesics and antipyretics, not elsewhere classified, undetermined**

● T39.8X5 **Adverse effect of other nonopioid analgesics and antipyretics, not elsewhere classified**

● T39.8X6 **Underdosing of other nonopioid analgesics and antipyretics, not elsewhere classified**

● T39.9 **Poisoning by, adverse effect of and underdosing of unspecified nonopioid analgesic, antipyretic and antirheumatic**

X● T39.91 **Poisoning by unspecified nonopioid analgesic, antipyretic and antirheumatic, accidental (unintentional)**
Poisoning by nonopioid analgesic, antipyretic and antirheumatic NOS

X● T39.92 **Poisoning by unspecified nonopioid analgesic, antipyretic and antirheumatic, intentional self-harm**

X● T39.93 **Poisoning by unspecified nonopioid analgesic, antipyretic and antirheumatic, assault**

X● T39.94 **Poisoning by unspecified nonopioid analgesic, antipyretic and antirheumatic, undetermined**

X● T39.95 **Adverse effect of unspecified nonopioid analgesic, antipyretic and antirheumatic**

X● T39.96 **Underdosing of unspecified nonopioid analgesic, antipyretic and antirheumatic**

● T40 **Poisoning by, adverse effect of and underdosing of narcotics and psychodysleptics [hallucinogens]**

Excludes2 drug dependence and related mental and behavioral disorders due to psychoactive substance use (F10.-F19.-)

The appropriate 7th character is to be added to each code from category T40

A	initial encounter
D	subsequent encounter
S	sequela

● T40.0 **Poisoning by, adverse effect of and underdosing of opium**

● T40.0X **Poisoning by, adverse effect of and underdosing of opium**

● T40.0X1 **Poisoning by opium, accidental (unintentional)**
Poisoning by opium NOS

● T40.0X2 **Poisoning by opium, intentional self-harm**

● T40.0X3 **Poisoning by opium, assault**

● T40.0X4 **Poisoning by opium, undetermined**

● T40.0X5 **Adverse effect of opium**

● T40.0X6 **Underdosing of opium**

● T40.1 **Poisoning by and adverse effect of heroin**

● T40.1X **Poisoning by and adverse effect of heroin**

● T40.1X1 **Poisoning by heroin, accidental (unintentional)**
Poisoning by heroin NOS

● T40.1X2 **Poisoning by heroin, intentional self-harm**

● T40.1X3 **Poisoning by heroin, assault**

● T40.1X4 **Poisoning by heroin, undetermined**

● T40.2 **Poisoning by, adverse effect of and underdosing of other opioids**

● T40.2X **Poisoning by, adverse effect of and underdosing of other opioids**

● T40.2X1 **Poisoning by other opioids, accidental (unintentional)**
Poisoning by other opioids NOS

● T40.2X2 **Poisoning by other opioids, intentional self-harm**

● T40.2X3 **Poisoning by other opioids, assault**

● T40.2X4 **Poisoning by other opioids, undetermined**

● T40.2X5 **Adverse effect of other opioids**

● T40.2X6 **Underdosing of other opioids**

● T40.3 **Poisoning by, adverse effect of and underdosing of methadone**

● T40.3X **Poisoning by, adverse effect of and underdosing of methadone**

● T40.3X1 **Poisoning by methadone, accidental (unintentional)**
Poisoning by methadone NOS

● T40.3X2 **Poisoning by methadone, intentional self-harm**

● T40.3X3 **Poisoning by methadone, assault**

● T40.3X4 **Poisoning by methadone, undetermined**

● T40.3X5 **Adverse effect of methadone**

● T40.3X6 **Underdosing of methadone**

CHAPTER 19 (S00-T88)

- T40.4 **Poisoning by, adverse effect of and underdosing of other synthetic narcotics**
  - T40.4X **Poisoning by, adverse effect of and underdosing of other synthetic narcotics**
    - T40.4X1 **Poisoning by other synthetic narcotics, accidental (unintentional)**
      Poisoning by other synthetic narcotics NOS
    - T40.4X2 **Poisoning by other synthetic narcotics, intentional self-harm**
    - T40.4X3 **Poisoning by other synthetic narcotics, assault**
    - T40.4X4 **Poisoning by other synthetic narcotics, undetermined**
    - T40.4X5 **Adverse effect of other synthetic narcotics**
    - T40.4X6 **Underdosing of other synthetic narcotics**
- T40.5 **Poisoning by, adverse effect of and underdosing of cocaine**
  - T40.5X **Poisoning by, adverse effect of and underdosing of cocaine**
    - T40.5X1 **Poisoning by cocaine, accidental (unintentional)**
      Poisoning by cocaine NOS
    - T40.5X2 **Poisoning by cocaine, intentional self-harm**
    - T40.5X3 **Poisoning by cocaine, assault**
    - T40.5X4 **Poisoning by cocaine, undetermined**
    - T40.5X5 **Adverse effect of cocaine**
    - T40.5X6 **Underdosing of cocaine**
- T40.6 **Poisoning by, adverse effect of and underdosing of other and unspecified narcotics**
  - T40.60 **Poisoning by, adverse effect of and underdosing of unspecified narcotics**
    - T40.601 **Poisoning by unspecified narcotics, accidental (unintentional)**
      Poisoning by narcotics NOS
    - T40.602 **Poisoning by unspecified narcotics, intentional self-harm**
    - T40.603 **Poisoning by unspecified narcotics, assault**
    - T40.604 **Poisoning by unspecified narcotics, undetermined**
    - T40.605 **Adverse effect of unspecified narcotics**
    - T40.606 **Underdosing of unspecified narcotics**
  - T40.69 **Poisoning by, adverse effect of and underdosing of other narcotics**
    - T40.691 **Poisoning by other narcotics, accidental (unintentional)**
      Poisoning by other narcotics NOS
    - T40.692 **Poisoning by other narcotics, intentional self-harm**
    - T40.693 **Poisoning by other narcotics, assault**
    - T40.694 **Poisoning by other narcotics, undetermined**
    - T40.695 **Adverse effect of other narcotics**
    - T40.696 **Underdosing of other narcotics**
- T40.7 **Poisoning by, adverse effect of and underdosing of cannabis (derivatives)**
  - T40.7X **Poisoning by, adverse effect of and underdosing of cannabis (derivatives)**
    - T40.7X1 **Poisoning by cannabis (derivatives), accidental (unintentional)**
      Poisoning by cannabis NOS
    - T40.7X2 **Poisoning by cannabis (derivatives), intentional self-harm**
    - T40.7X3 **Poisoning by cannabis (derivatives), assault**
    - T40.7X4 **Poisoning by cannabis (derivatives), undetermined**
    - T40.7X5 **Adverse effect of cannabis (derivatives)**
    - T40.7X6 **Underdosing of cannabis (derivatives)**
- T40.8 **Poisoning by and adverse effect of lysergide [LSD]**
  - T40.8X **Poisoning by and adverse effect of lysergide [LSD]**
    - T40.8X1 **Poisoning by lysergide [LSD], accidental (unintentional)**
      Poisoning by lysergide [LSD] NOS
    - T40.8X2 **Poisoning by lysergide [LSD], intentional self-harm**
    - T40.8X3 **Poisoning by lysergide [LSD], assault**
    - T40.8X4 **Poisoning by lysergide [LSD], undetermined**
- T40.9 **Poisoning by, adverse effect of and underdosing of other and unspecified psychodysleptics [hallucinogens]**
  - T40.90 **Poisoning by, adverse effect of and underdosing of unspecified psychodysleptics [hallucinogens]**
    - T40.901 **Poisoning by unspecified psychodysleptics [hallucinogens], accidental (unintentional)**
    - T40.902 **Poisoning by unspecified psychodysleptics [hallucinogens], intentional self-harm**
    - T40.903 **Poisoning by unspecified psychodysleptics [hallucinogens], assault**
    - T40.904 **Poisoning by unspecified psychodysleptics [hallucinogens], undetermined**
    - T40.905 **Adverse effect of unspecified psychodysleptics [hallucinogens]**
    - T40.906 **Underdosing of unspecified psychodysleptics**
  - T40.99 **Poisoning by, adverse effect of and underdosing of other psychodysleptics [hallucinogens]**
    - T40.991 **Poisoning by other psychodysleptics [hallucinogens], accidental (unintentional)**
      Poisoning by other psychodysleptics [hallucinogens] NOS
    - T40.992 **Poisoning by other psychodysleptics [hallucinogens], intentional self-harm**
    - T40.993 **Poisoning by other psychodysleptics [hallucinogens], assault**
    - T40.994 **Poisoning by other psychodysleptics [hallucinogens], undetermined**
    - T40.995 **Adverse effect of other psychodysleptics [hallucinogens]**
    - T40.996 **Underdosing of other psychodysleptics**

● **T41 Poisoning by, adverse effect of and underdosing of anesthetics and therapeutic gases**

Excludes1 benzodiazepines (T42.4-)
cocaine (T40.5-)
complications of anesthesia during pregnancy (O29.-)
complications of anesthesia during labor and delivery (O74.-)
complications of anesthesia during the puerperium (O89.-) opioids (T40.0-T40.2-)

The appropriate 7th character is to be added to each code from category T41

A initial encounter
D subsequent encounter
S sequela

● **T41.0 Poisoning by, adverse effect of and underdosing of inhaled anesthetics**

Excludes1 oxygen (T41.5-)

● **T41.0X Poisoning by, adverse effect of and underdosing of inhaled anesthetics**

● **T41.0X1 Poisoning by inhaled anesthetics, accidental (unintentional)**
Poisoning by inhaled anesthetics NOS

● **T41.0X2 Poisoning by inhaled anesthetics, intentional self-harm**

● **T41.0X3 Poisoning by inhaled anesthetics, assault**

● **T41.0X4 Poisoning by inhaled anesthetics, undetermined**

● **T41.0X5 Adverse effect of inhaled anesthetics**

● **T41.0X6 Underdosing of inhaled anesthetics**

● **T41.1 Poisoning by, adverse effect of and underdosing of intravenous anesthetics**
Poisoning by, adverse effect of and underdosing of thiobarbiturates

● **T41.1X Poisoning by, adverse effect of and underdosing of intravenous anesthetics**

● **T41.1X1 Poisoning by intravenous anesthetics, accidental (unintentional)**
Poisoning by intravenous anesthetics NOS

● **T41.1X2 Poisoning by intravenous anesthetics, intentional self-harm**

● **T41.1X3 Poisoning by intravenous anesthetics, assault**

● **T41.1X4 Poisoning by intravenous anesthetics, undetermined**

● **T41.1X5 Adverse effect of intravenous anesthetics**

● **T41.1X6 Underdosing of intravenous anesthetics**

● **T41.2 Poisoning by, adverse effect of and underdosing of other and unspecified general anesthetics**

● **T41.20 Poisoning by, adverse effect of and underdosing of unspecified general anesthetics**

● **T41.201 Poisoning by unspecified general anesthetics, accidental (unintentional)**
Poisoning by general anesthetics NOS

● **T41.202 Poisoning by unspecified general anesthetics, intentional self-harm**

● **T41.203 Poisoning by unspecified general anesthetics, assault**

● **T41.204 Poisoning by unspecified general anesthetics, undetermined**

● **T41.205 Adverse effect of unspecified general anesthetics**

● **T41.206 Underdosing of unspecified general anesthetics**

● **T41.29 Poisoning by, adverse effect of and underdosing of other general anesthetics**

● **T41.291 Poisoning by other general anesthetics, accidental (unintentional)**
Poisoning by other general anesthetics NOS

● **T41.292 Poisoning by other general anesthetics, intentional self-harm**

● **T41.293 Poisoning by other general anesthetics, assault**

● **T41.294 Poisoning by other general anesthetics, undetermined**

● **T41.295 Adverse effect of other general anesthetics**

● **T41.296 Underdosing of other general anesthetics**

● **T41.3 Poisoning by, adverse effect of and underdosing of local anesthetics**
Cocaine (topical)

Excludes2 poisoning by cocaine used as a central nervous system stimulant (T40.5X1-T40.5X4)

● **T41.3X Poisoning by, adverse effect of and underdosing of local anesthetics**

● **T41.3X1 Poisoning by local anesthetics, accidental (unintentional)**
Poisoning by local anesthetics NOS

● **T41.3X2 Poisoning by local anesthetics, intentional self-harm**

● **T41.3X3 Poisoning by local anesthetics, assault**

● **T41.3X4 Poisoning by local anesthetics, undetermined**

● **T41.3X5 Adverse effect of local anesthetics**

● **T41.3X6 Underdosing of local anesthetics**

● **T41.4 Poisoning by, adverse effect of and underdosing of unspecified anesthetic**

X● **T41.41 Poisoning by unspecified anesthetic, accidental (unintentional)**
Poisoning by anesthetic NOS

X● **T41.42 Poisoning by unspecified anesthetic, intentional self-harm**

X● **T41.43 Poisoning by unspecified anesthetic, assault**

X● **T41.44 Poisoning by unspecified anesthetic, undetermined**

X● **T41.45 Adverse effect of unspecified anesthetic**

X● **T41.46 Underdosing of unspecified anesthetics**

● **T41.5 Poisoning by, adverse effect of and underdosing of therapeutic gases**

● **T41.5X Poisoning by, adverse effect of and underdosing of therapeutic gases**

● **T41.5X1 Poisoning by therapeutic gases, accidental (unintentional)**
Poisoning by therapeutic gases NOS

● **T41.5X2 Poisoning by therapeutic gases, intentional self-harm**

● **T41.5X3 Poisoning by therapeutic gases, assault**

● **T41.5X4 Poisoning by therapeutic gases, undetermined**

● **T41.5X5 Adverse effect of therapeutic gases**

● **T41.5X6 Underdosing of therapeutic gases**

CHAPTER 19 (S00-T88)

● T42 **Poisoning by, adverse effect of and underdosing of antiepileptic, sedative-hypnotic and antiparkinsonism drugs**

Excludes2 drug dependence and related mental and behavioral disorders due to psychoactive substance use (F1Ø.--F19.-)

The appropriate 7th character is to be added to each code from category T42

A	initial encounter
D	subsequent encounter
S	sequela

● T42.Ø **Poisoning by, adverse effect of and underdosing of hydantoin derivatives**

● T42.ØX **Poisoning by, adverse effect of and underdosing of hydantoin derivatives**

● T42.ØX1 **Poisoning by hydantoin derivatives, accidental (unintentional)**
Poisoning by hydantoin derivatives NOS

● T42.ØX2 **Poisoning by hydantoin derivatives, intentional self-harm**

● T42.ØX3 **Poisoning by hydantoin derivatives, assault**

● T42.ØX4 **Poisoning by hydantoin derivatives, undetermined**

● T42.ØX5 **Adverse effect of hydantoin derivatives**

● T42.ØX6 **Underdosing of hydantoin derivatives**

● T42.1 **Poisoning by, adverse effect of and underdosing of iminostilbenes**
Poisoning by, adverse effect of and underdosing of carbamazepine

● T42.1X **Poisoning by, adverse effect of and underdosing of iminostilbenes**

● T42.1X1 **Poisoning by iminostilbenes, accidental (unintentional)**
Poisoning by iminostilbenes NOS

● T42.1X2 **Poisoning by iminostilbenes, intentional self-harm**

● T42.1X3 **Poisoning by iminostilbenes, assault**

● T42.1X4 **Poisoning by iminostilbenes, undetermined**

● T42.1X5 **Adverse effect of iminostilbenes**

● T42.1X6 **Underdosing of iminostilbenes**

● T42.2 **Poisoning by, adverse effect of and underdosing of succinimides and oxazolidinediones**

● T42.2X **Poisoning by, adverse effect of and underdosing of succinimides and oxazolidinediones**

● T42.2X1 **Poisoning by succinimides and oxazolidinediones, accidental (unintentional)**
Poisoning by succinimides and oxazolidinediones NOS

● T42.2X2 **Poisoning by succinimides and oxazolidinediones, intentional self-harm**

● T42.2X3 **Poisoning by succinimides and oxazolidinediones, assault**

● T42.2X4 **Poisoning by succinimides and oxazolidinediones, undetermined**

● T42.2X5 **Adverse effect of succinimides and oxazolidinediones**

● T42.2X6 **Underdosing of succinimides and oxazolidinediones**

● T42.3 **Poisoning by, adverse effect of and underdosing of barbiturates**

Excludes1 poisoning by, adverse effect of and underdosing of thiobarbiturates (T41.1-)

● T42.3X **Poisoning by, adverse effect of and underdosing of barbiturates**

● T42.3X1 **Poisoning by barbiturates, accidental (unintentional)**
Poisoning by barbiturates NOS

● T42.3X2 **Poisoning by barbiturates, intentional self-harm**

● T42.3X3 **Poisoning by barbiturates, assault**

● T42.3X4 **Poisoning by barbiturates, undetermined**

● T42.3X5 **Adverse effect of barbiturates**

● T42.3X6 **Underdosing of barbiturates**

● T42.4 **Poisoning by, adverse effect of and underdosing of benzodiazepines**

● T42.4X **Poisoning by, adverse effect of and underdosing of benzodiazepines**

● T42.4X1 **Poisoning by benzodiazepines, accidental (unintentional)**
Poisoning by benzodiazepines NOS

● T42.4X2 **Poisoning by benzodiazepines, intentional self-harm**

● T42.4X3 **Poisoning by benzodiazepines, assault**

● T42.4X4 **Poisoning by benzodiazepines, undetermined**

● T42.4X5 **Adverse effect of benzodiazepines**

● T42.4X6 **Underdosing of benzodiazepines**

● T42.5 **Poisoning by, adverse effect of and underdosing of mixed antiepileptics**

● T42.5X **Poisoning by, adverse effect of and underdosing of antiepileptics**

● T42.5X1 **Poisoning by mixed antiepileptics, accidental (unintentional)**
Poisoning by mixed antiepileptics NOS

● T42.5X2 **Poisoning by mixed antiepileptics, intentional self-harm**

● T42.5X3 **Poisoning by mixed antiepileptics, assault**

● T42.5X4 **Poisoning by mixed antiepileptics, undetermined**

● T42.5X5 **Adverse effect of mixed antiepileptics**

● T42.5X6 **Underdosing of mixed antiepileptics**

● T42.6 **Poisoning by, adverse effect of and underdosing of other antiepileptic and sedative-hypnotic drugs**
Poisoning by, adverse effect of and underdosing of methaqualone
Poisoning by, adverse effect of and underdosing of valproic acid

Excludes1 poisoning by, adverse effect of and underdosing of carbamazepine (T42.1-)

● T42.6X **Poisoning by, adverse effect of and underdosing of other antiepileptic and sedative-hypnotic drugs**

● T42.6X1 **Poisoning by other antiepileptic and sedative-hypnotic drugs, accidental (unintentional)**
Poisoning by other antiepileptic and sedative-hypnotic drugs NOS

● T42.6X2 **Poisoning by other antiepileptic and sedative-hypnotic drugs, intentional self-harm**

● **T42.6X3 Poisoning by other antiepileptic and sedative-hypnotic drugs, assault**

● **T42.6X4 Poisoning by other antiepileptic and sedative-hypnotic drugs, undetermined**

● **T42.6X5 Adverse effect of other antiepileptic and sedative-hypnotic drugs**

● **T42.6X6 Underdosing of other antiepileptic and sedative-hypnotic drugs**

● **T42.7 Poisoning by, adverse effect of and underdosing of unspecified antiepileptic and sedative-hypnotic drugs**

X● **T42.71 Poisoning by unspecified antiepileptic and sedative-hypnotic drugs, accidental (unintentional)**

Poisoning by antiepileptic and sedative-hypnotic drugs NOS

X● **T42.72 Poisoning by unspecified antiepileptic and sedative-hypnotic drugs, intentional self-harm**

X● **T42.73 Poisoning by unspecified antiepileptic and sedative-hypnotic drugs, assault**

X● **T42.74 Poisoning by unspecified antiepileptic and sedative-hypnotic drugs, undetermined**

X● **T42.75 Adverse effect of unspecified antiepileptic and sedative-hypnotic drugs**

X● **T42.76 Underdosing of unspecified antiepileptic and sedative-hypnotic drugs**

● **T42.8 Poisoning by, adverse effect of and underdosing of antiparkinsonism drugs and other central muscle-tone depressants**

Poisoning by, adverse effect of and underdosing of amantadine

● **T42.8X Poisoning by, adverse effect of and underdosing of antiparkinsonism drugs and other central muscle-tone depressants**

● **T42.8X1 Poisoning by antiparkinsonism drugs and other central muscle-tone depressants, accidental (unintentional)**

Poisoning by antiparkinsonism drugs and other central muscle-tone depressants NOS

● **T42.8X2 Poisoning by antiparkinsonism drugs and other central muscle-tone depressants, intentional self-harm**

● **T42.8X3 Poisoning by antiparkinsonism drugs and other central muscle-tone depressants, assault**

● **T42.8X4 Poisoning by antiparkinsonism drugs and other central muscle-tone depressants, undetermined**

● **T42.8X5 Adverse effect of antiparkinsonism drugs and other central muscle-tone depressants**

● **T42.8X6 Underdosing of antiparkinsonism drugs and other central muscle-tone depressants**

● **T43 Poisoning by, adverse effect of and underdosing of psychotropic drugs, not elsewhere classified**

Excludes1 appetite depressants (T50.5-)
barbiturates (T42.3-)
benzodiazepines (T42.4-)
methaqualone (T42.6-)
psychodysleptics [hallucinogens] (T40.7-T40.9-)

Excludes2 drug dependence and related mental and behavioral disorders due to psychoactive substance use (F10.--F19.-)

The appropriate 7th character is to be added to each code from category T43

A	initial encounter
D	subsequent encounter
S	sequela

● **T43.0 Poisoning by, adverse effect of and underdosing of tricyclic and tetracyclic antidepressants**

● **T43.01 Poisoning by, adverse effect of and underdosing of tricyclic antidepressants**

● **T43.011 Poisoning by tricyclic antidepressants, accidental (unintentional)**

Poisoning by tricyclic antidepressants NOS

● **T43.012 Poisoning by tricyclic antidepressants, intentional self-harm**

● **T43.013 Poisoning by tricyclic antidepressants, assault**

● **T43.014 Poisoning by tricyclic antidepressants, undetermined**

● **T43.015 Adverse effect of tricyclic antidepressants**

● **T43.016 Underdosing of tricyclic antidepressants**

● **T43.02 Poisoning by, adverse effect of and underdosing of tetracyclic antidepressants**

● **T43.021 Poisoning by tetracyclic antidepressants, accidental (unintentional)**

Poisoning by tetracyclic antidepressants NOS

● **T43.022 Poisoning by tetracyclic antidepressants, intentional self-harm**

● **T43.023 Poisoning by tetracyclic antidepressants, assault**

● **T43.024 Poisoning by tetracyclic antidepressants, undetermined**

● **T43.025 Adverse effect of tetracyclic antidepressants**

● **T43.026 Underdosing of tetracyclic antidepressants**

● T43.1 Poisoning by, adverse effect of and underdosing of monoamine-oxidase-inhibitor antidepressants

● T43.1X Poisoning by, adverse effect of and underdosing of monoamine-oxidase-inhibitor antidepressants

● T43.1X1 Poisoning by monoamine-oxidase-inhibitor antidepressants, accidental (unintentional)
Poisoning by monoamine-oxidase-inhibitor antidepressants NOS

● T43.1X2 Poisoning by monoamine-oxidase-inhibitor antidepressants, intentional self-harm

● T43.1X3 Poisoning by monoamine-oxidase-inhibitor antidepressants, assault

● T43.1X4 Poisoning by monoamine-oxidase-inhibitor antidepressants, undetermined

● T43.1X5 Adverse effect of monoamine-oxidase-inhibitor antidepressants

● T43.1X6 Underdosing of monoamine-oxidase-inhibitor antidepressants

● T43.2 Poisoning by, adverse effect of and underdosing of other and unspecified antidepressants

● T43.20 Poisoning by, adverse effect of and underdosing of unspecified antidepressants

● T43.201 Poisoning by unspecified antidepressants, accidental (unintentional)
Poisoning by antidepressants NOS

● T43.202 Poisoning by unspecified antidepressants, intentional self-harm

● T43.203 Poisoning by unspecified antidepressants, assault

● T43.204 Poisoning by unspecified antidepressants, undetermined

● T43.205 Adverse effect of unspecified antidepressants

● T43.206 Underdosing of unspecified antidepressants

● T43.21 Poisoning by, adverse effect of and underdosing of selective serotonin and norepinephrine reuptake inhibitors
Poisoning by, adverse effect of and underdosing of SSNRI antidepressants

● T43.211 Poisoning by selective serotonin and norepinephrine reuptake inhibitors, accidental (unintentional)

● T43.212 Poisoning by selective serotonin and norepinephrine reuptake inhibitors, intentional self-harm

● T43.213 Poisoning by selective serotonin and norepinephrine reuptake inhibitors, assault

● T43.214 Poisoning by selective serotonin and norepinephrine reuptake inhibitors, undetermined

● T43.215 Adverse effect of selective serotonin and norepinephrine reuptake inhibitors

● T43.216 Underdosing of selective serotonin and norepinephrine reuptake inhibitors

● T43.22 Poisoning by, adverse effect of and underdosing of selective serotonin reuptake inhibitors
Poisoning by, adverse effect of and underdosing of SSRI antidepressants

● T43.221 Poisoning by selective serotonin reuptake inhibitors, accidental (unintentional)

● T43.222 Poisoning by selective serotonin reuptake inhibitors, intentional self-harm

● T43.223 Poisoning by selective serotonin reuptake inhibitors, assault

● T43.224 Poisoning by selective serotonin reuptake inhibitors, undetermined

● T43.225 Adverse effect of selective serotonin reuptake inhibitors

● T43.226 Underdosing of selective serotonin reuptake inhibitors

● T43.29 Poisoning by, adverse effect of and underdosing of other antidepressants

● T43.291 Poisoning by other antidepressants, accidental (unintentional)
Poisoning by other antidepressants NOS

● T43.292 Poisoning by other antidepressants, intentional self-harm

● T43.293 Poisoning by other antidepressants, assault

● T43.294 Poisoning by other antidepressants, undetermined

● T43.295 Adverse effect of other antidepressants

● T43.296 Underdosing of other antidepressants

● T43.3 Poisoning by, adverse effect of and underdosing of phenothiazine antipsychotics and neuroleptics

● T43.3X Poisoning by, adverse effect of and underdosing of phenothiazine antipsychotics and neuroleptics

● T43.3X1 Poisoning by phenothiazine antipsychotics and neuroleptics, accidental (unintentional)
Poisoning by phenothiazine antipsychotics and neuroleptics NOS

● T43.3X2 Poisoning by phenothiazine antipsychotics and neuroleptics, intentional self-harm

● T43.3X3 Poisoning by phenothiazine antipsychotics and neuroleptics, assault

● T43.3X4 Poisoning by phenothiazine antipsychotics and neuroleptics, undetermined

● T43.3X5 Adverse effect of phenothiazine antipsychotics and neuroleptics

● T43.3X6 Underdosing of phenothiazine antipsychotics and neuroleptics

● T43.4 Poisoning by, adverse effect of and underdosing of butyrophenone and thiothixene neuroleptics

● T43.4X Poisoning by, adverse effect of and underdosing of butyrophenone and thiothixene neuroleptics

● T43.4X1 Poisoning by butyrophenone and thiothixene neuroleptics, accidental (unintentional)
Poisoning by butyrophenone and thiothixene neuroleptics NOS

● T43.4X2 Poisoning by butyrophenone and thiothixene neuroleptics, intentional self-harm

● T43.4X3 Poisoning by butyrophenone and thiothixene neuroleptics, assault

● T43.4X4 Poisoning by butyrophenone and thiothixene neuroleptics, undetermined

● T43.4X5 Adverse effect of butyrophenone and thiothixene neuroleptics

● T43.4X6 Underdosing of butyrophenone and thiothixene neuroleptics

T43.5 Poisoning by, adverse effect of and underdosing of other and unspecified antipsychotics and neuroleptics
Excludes1 poisoning by, adverse effect of and underdosing of rauwolfia (T46.5-)

T43.50 Poisoning by, adverse effect of and underdosing of unspecified antipsychotics and neuroleptics

T43.501 Poisoning by unspecified antipsychotics and neuroleptics, accidental (unintentional)
Poisoning by antipsychotics and neuroleptics NOS

T43.502 Poisoning by unspecified antipsychotics and neuroleptics, intentional self-harm

T43.503 Poisoning by unspecified antipsychotics and neuroleptics, assault

T43.504 Poisoning by unspecified antipsychotics and neuroleptics, undetermined

T43.505 Adverse effect of unspecified antipsychotics and neuroleptics

T43.506 Underdosing of unspecified antipsychotics and neuroleptics

T43.59 Poisoning by, adverse effect of and underdosing of other antipsychotics and neuroleptics

T43.591 Poisoning by other antipsychotics and neuroleptics, accidental (unintentional)
Poisoning by other antipsychotics and neuroleptics NOS

T43.592 Poisoning by other antipsychotics and neuroleptics, intentional self-harm

T43.593 Poisoning by other antipsychotics and neuroleptics, assault

T43.594 Poisoning by other antipsychotics and neuroleptics, undetermined

T43.595 Adverse effect of other antipsychotics and neuroleptics

T43.596 Underdosing of other antipsychotics and neuroleptics

T43.6 Poisoning by, adverse effect of and underdosing of psychostimulants
Excludes1 poisoning by, adverse effect of and underdosing of cocaine (T40.5-)

T43.60 Poisoning by, adverse effect of and underdosing of unspecified psychostimulant

T43.601 Poisoning by unspecified psychostimulants, accidental (unintentional)
Poisoning by psychostimulants NOS

T43.602 Poisoning by unspecified psychostimulants, intentional self-harm

T43.603 Poisoning by unspecified psychostimulants, assault

T43.604 Poisoning by unspecified psychostimulants, undetermined

T43.605 Adverse effect of unspecified psychostimulants

T43.606 Underdosing of unspecified psychostimulants

T43.61 Poisoning by, adverse effect of and underdosing of caffeine

T43.611 Poisoning by caffeine, accidental (unintentional)
Poisoning by caffeine NOS

T43.612 Poisoning by caffeine, intentional self-harm

T43.613 Poisoning by caffeine, assault

T43.614 Poisoning by caffeine, undetermined

T43.615 Adverse effect of caffeine

T43.616 Underdosing of caffeine

T43.62 Poisoning by, adverse effect of and underdosing of amphetamines
Poisoning by, adverse effect of and underdosing of methamphetamines

T43.621 Poisoning by amphetamines, accidental (unintentional)
Poisoning by amphetamines NOS

T43.622 Poisoning by amphetamines, intentional self-harm

T43.623 Poisoning by amphetamines, assault

T43.624 Poisoning by amphetamines, undetermined

T43.625 Adverse effect of amphetamines

T43.626 Underdosing of amphetamines

T43.63 Poisoning by, adverse effect of and underdosing of methylphenidate

T43.631 Poisoning by methylphenidate, accidental (unintentional)
Poisoning by methylphenidate NOS

T43.632 Poisoning by methylphenidate, intentional self-harm

T43.633 Poisoning by methylphenidate, assault

T43.634 Poisoning by methylphenidate, undetermined

T43.635 Adverse effect of methylphenidate

T43.636 Underdosing of methylphenidate

T43.69 Poisoning by, adverse effect of and underdosing of other psychostimulants

T43.691 Poisoning by other psychostimulants, accidental (unintentional)
Poisoning by other psychostimulants NOS

T43.692 Poisoning by other psychostimulants, intentional self-harm

T43.693 Poisoning by other psychostimulants, assault

T43.694 Poisoning by other psychostimulants, undetermined

T43.695 Adverse effect of other psychostimulants

T43.696 Underdosing of other psychostimulants

T43.8 Poisoning by, adverse effect of and underdosing of other psychotropic drugs

T43.8X Poisoning by, adverse effect of and underdosing of other psychotropic drugs

T43.8X1 Poisoning by other psychotropic drugs, accidental (unintentional)
Poisoning by other psychotropic drugs NOS

T43.8X2 Poisoning by other psychotropic drugs, intentional self-harm

T43.8X3 Poisoning by other psychotropic drugs, assault

T43.8X4 Poisoning by other psychotropic drugs, undetermined

T43.8X5 Adverse effect of other psychotropic drugs

T43.8X6 Underdosing of other psychotropic drugs

CHAPTER 19 (S00-T88)

● T43.9 **Poisoning by, adverse effect of and underdosing of unspecified psychotropic drug**

X● T43.91 **Poisoning by unspecified psychotropic drug, accidental (unintentional)**
Poisoning by psychotropic drug NOS

X● T43.92 **Poisoning by unspecified psychotropic drug, intentional self-harm**

X● T43.93 **Poisoning by unspecified psychotropic drug, assault**

X● T43.94 **Poisoning by unspecified psychotropic drug, undetermined**

X● T43.95 **Adverse effect of unspecified psychotropic drug**

X● T43.96 **Underdosing of unspecified psychotropic drug**

● T44 **Poisoning by, adverse effect of and underdosing of drugs primarily affecting the autonomic nervous system**

The appropriate 7th character is to be added to each code from category T44

A	initial encounter
D	subsequent encounter
S	sequela

● T44.0 **Poisoning by, adverse effect of and underdosing of anticholinesterase agents**

● T44.0X **Poisoning by, adverse effect of and underdosing of anticholinesterase agents**

● T44.0X1 **Poisoning by anticholinesterase agents, accidental (unintentional)**
Poisoning by anticholinesterase agents NOS

● T44.0X2 **Poisoning by anticholinesterase agents, intentional self-harm**

● T44.0X3 **Poisoning by anticholinesterase agents, assault**

● T44.0X4 **Poisoning by anticholinesterase agents, undetermined**

● T44.0X5 **Adverse effect of anticholinesterase agents**

● T44.0X6 **Underdosing of anticholinesterase agents**

● T44.1 **Poisoning by, adverse effect of and underdosing of other parasympathomimetics [cholinergics]**

● T44.1X **Poisoning by, adverse effect of and underdosing of other parasympathomimetics [cholinergics]**

● T44.1X1 **Poisoning by other parasympathomimetics [cholinergics], accidental (unintentional)**
Poisoning by other parasympathomimetics [cholinergics] NOS

● T44.1X2 **Poisoning by other parasympathomimetics [cholinergics], intentional self-harm**

● T44.1X3 **Poisoning by other parasympathomimetics [cholinergics], assault**

● T44.1X4 **Poisoning by other parasympathomimetics [cholinergics], undetermined**

● T44.1X5 **Adverse effect of other parasympathomimetics [cholinergics]**

● T44.1X6 **Underdosing of other parasympathomimetics**

● T44.2 **Poisoning by, adverse effect of and underdosing of ganglionic blocking drugs**

● T44.2X **Poisoning by, adverse effect of and underdosing of ganglionic blocking drugs**

● T44.2X1 **Poisoning by ganglionic blocking drugs, accidental (unintentional)**
Poisoning by ganglionic blocking drugs NOS

● T44.2X2 **Poisoning by ganglionic blocking drugs, intentional self-harm**

● T44.2X3 **Poisoning by ganglionic blocking drugs, assault**

● T44.2X4 **Poisoning by ganglionic blocking drugs, undetermined**

● T44.2X5 **Adverse effect of ganglionic blocking drugs**

● T44.2X6 **Underdosing of ganglionic blocking drugs**

● T44.3 **Poisoning by, adverse effect of and underdosing of other parasympatholytics [anticholinergics and antimuscarinics] and spasmolytics**
Poisoning by, adverse effect of and underdosing of papaverine

● T44.3X **Poisoning by, adverse effect of and underdosing of other parasympatholytics [anticholinergics and antimuscarinics] and spasmolytics**

● T44.3X1 **Poisoning by other parasympatholytics [anticholinergics and antimuscarinics] and spasmolytics, accidental (unintentional)**
Poisoning by other parasympatholytics [anticholinergics and antimuscarinics] and spasmolytics NOS

● T44.3X2 **Poisoning by other parasympatholytics [anticholinergics and antimuscarinics] and spasmolytics, intentional self-harm**

● T44.3X3 **Poisoning by other parasympatholytics [anticholinergics and antimuscarinics] and spasmolytics, assault**

● T44.3X4 **Poisoning by other parasympatholytics [anticholinergics and antimuscarinics] and spasmolytics, undetermined**

● T44.3X5 **Adverse effect of other parasympatholytics [anticholinergics and antimuscarinics] and spasmolytics**

● T44.3X6 **Underdosing of other parasympatholytics [anticholinergics and antimuscarinics] and spasmolytics**

● T44.4 **Poisoning by, adverse effect of and underdosing of predominantly alpha-adrenoreceptor agonists**
Poisoning by, adverse effect of and underdosing of metaraminol

● T44.4X **Poisoning by, adverse effect of and underdosing of predominantly alpha-adrenoreceptor agonists**

● T44.4X1 **Poisoning by predominantly alpha-adrenoreceptor agonists, accidental (unintentional)**
Poisoning by predominantly alpha-adrenoreceptor agonists NOS

● T44.4X2 **Poisoning by predominantly alpha-adrenoreceptor agonists, intentional self-harm**

● T44.4X3 **Poisoning by predominantly alpha-adrenoreceptor agonists, assault**

● T44.4X4 **Poisoning by predominantly alpha-adrenoreceptor agonists, undetermined**

● T44.4X5 **Adverse effect of predominantly alpha-adrenoreceptor agonists**

● T44.4X6 **Underdosing of predominantly alpha-adrenoreceptor agonists**

● **T44.5 Poisoning by, adverse effect of and underdosing of predominantly beta-adrenoreceptor agonists**
Excludes1 poisoning by, adverse effect of and underdosing of beta-adrenoreceptor agonists used in asthma therapy (T48.6-)

● **T44.5X Poisoning by, adverse effect of and underdosing of predominantly beta-adrenoreceptor agonists**

● **T44.5X1 Poisoning by predominantly beta-adrenoreceptor agonists, accidental (unintentional)**
Poisoning by predominantly beta-adrenoreceptor agonists NOS

● **T44.5X2 Poisoning by predominantly beta-adrenoreceptor agonists, intentional self-harm**

● **T44.5X3 Poisoning by predominantly beta-adrenoreceptor agonists, assault**

● **T44.5X4 Poisoning by predominantly beta-adrenoreceptor agonists, undetermined**

● **T44.5X5 Adverse effect of predominantly beta-adrenoreceptor agonists**

● **T44.5X6 Underdosing of predominantly beta-adrenoreceptor agonists**

● **T44.6 Poisoning by, adverse effect of and underdosing of alpha-adrenoreceptor antagonists**
Excludes1 poisoning by, adverse effect of and underdosing of ergot alkaloids (T48.0)

● **T44.6X Poisoning by, adverse effect of and underdosing of alpha-adrenoreceptor antagonists**

● **T44.6X1 Poisoning by alpha-adrenoreceptor antagonists, accidental (unintentional)**
Poisoning by alpha-adrenoreceptor antagonists NOS

● **T44.6X2 Poisoning by alpha-adrenoreceptor antagonists, intentional self-harm**

● **T44.6X3 Poisoning by alpha-adrenoreceptor antagonists, assault**

● **T44.6X4 Poisoning by alpha-adrenoreceptor antagonists, undetermined**

● **T44.6X5 Adverse effect of alpha-adrenoreceptor antagonists**

● **T44.6X6 Underdosing of alpha-adrenoreceptor antagonists**

● **T44.7 Poisoning by, adverse effect of and underdosing of beta-adrenoreceptor antagonists**

● **T44.7X Poisoning by, adverse effect of and underdosing of beta-adrenoreceptor antagonists**

● **T44.7X1 Poisoning by beta-adrenoreceptor antagonists, accidental (unintentional)**
Poisoning by beta-adrenoreceptor antagonists NOS

● **T44.7X2 Poisoning by beta-adrenoreceptor antagonists, intentional self-harm**

● **T44.7X3 Poisoning by beta-adrenoreceptor antagonists, assault**

● **T44.7X4 Poisoning by beta-adrenoreceptor antagonists, undetermined**

● **T44.7X5 Adverse effect of beta-adrenoreceptor antagonists**

● **T44.7X6 Underdosing of beta-adrenoreceptor antagonists**

● **T44.8 Poisoning by, adverse effect of and underdosing of centrally-acting and adrenergic-neuron-blocking agents**
Excludes1 poisoning by, adverse effect of and underdosing of clonidine (T46.5)
poisoning by, adverse effect of and underdosing of guanethidine (T46.5)

● **T44.8X Poisoning by, adverse effect of and underdosing of centrally-acting and adrenergic-neuron-blocking agents**

● **T44.8X1 Poisoning by centrally-acting and adrenergic-neuron-blocking agents, accidental (unintentional)**
Poisoning by centrally-acting and adrenergic-neuron-blocking agents NOS

● **T44.8X2 Poisoning by centrally-acting and adrenergic-neuron-blocking agents, intentional self-harm**

● **T44.8X3 Poisoning by centrally-acting and adrenergic-neuron-blocking agents, assault**

● **T44.8X4 Poisoning by centrally-acting and adrenergic-neuron-blocking agents, undetermined**

● **T44.8X5 Adverse effect of centrally-acting and adrenergic-neuron-blocking agents**

● **T44.8X6 Underdosing of centrally-acting and adrenergic-neuron-blocking agents**

● **T44.9 Poisoning by, adverse effect of and underdosing of other and unspecified drugs primarily affecting the autonomic nervous system**
Poisoning by, adverse effect of and underdosing of drug stimulating both alpha and beta-adrenoreceptors

● **T44.90 Poisoning by, adverse effect of and underdosing of unspecified drugs primarily affecting the autonomic nervous system**

● **T44.901 Poisoning by unspecified drugs primarily affecting the autonomic nervous system, accidental (unintentional)**
Poisoning by unspecified drugs primarily affecting the autonomic nervous system NOS

● **T44.902 Poisoning by unspecified drugs primarily affecting the autonomic nervous system, intentional self-harm**

● **T44.903 Poisoning by unspecified drugs primarily affecting the autonomic nervous system, assault**

● **T44.904 Poisoning by unspecified drugs primarily affecting the autonomic nervous system, undetermined**

● **T44.905 Adverse effect of unspecified drugs primarily affecting the autonomic nervous system**

● **T44.906 Underdosing of unspecified drugs primarily affecting the autonomic nervous system**

CHAPTER 19 (S00-T88)

T44.99 **Poisoning by, adverse effect of and underdosing of other drugs primarily affecting the autonomic nervous system**

T44.991 **Poisoning by other drug primarily affecting the autonomic nervous system, accidental (unintentional)**
Poisoning by other drugs primarily affecting the autonomic nervous system NOS

T44.992 **Poisoning by other drug primarily affecting the autonomic nervous system, intentional self-harm**

T44.993 **Poisoning by other drug primarily affecting the autonomic nervous system, assault**

T44.994 **Poisoning by other drug primarily affecting the autonomic nervous system, undetermined**

T44.995 **Adverse effect of other drug primarily affecting the autonomic nervous system**

T44.996 **Underdosing of other drug primarily affecting the autonomic nervous system**

T45 **Poisoning by, adverse effect of and underdosing of primarily systemic and hematological agents, not elsewhere classified**

The appropriate 7th character is to be added to each code from category T45

A	initial encounter
D	subsequent encounter
S	sequela

T45.Ø **Poisoning by, adverse effect of and underdosing of antiallergic and antiemetic drugs**

Excludes1 poisoning by, adverse effect of and underdosing of phenothiazine-based neuroleptics (T43.3)

T45.ØX **Poisoning by, adverse effect of and underdosing of antiallergic and antiemetic drugs**

T45.ØX1 **Poisoning by antiallergic and antiemetic drugs, accidental (unintentional)**
Poisoning by antiallergic and antiemetic drugs NOS

T45.ØX2 **Poisoning by antiallergic and antiemetic drugs, intentional self-harm**

T45.ØX3 **Poisoning by antiallergic and antiemetic drugs, assault**

T45.ØX4 **Poisoning by antiallergic and antiemetic drugs, undetermined**

T45.ØX5 **Adverse effect of antiallergic and antiemetic drugs**

T45.ØX6 **Underdosing of antiallergic and antiemetic drugs**

T45.1 **Poisoning by, adverse effect of and underdosing of antineoplastic and immunosuppressive drugs**

Excludes1 poisoning by, adverse effect of and underdosing of tamoxifen (T38.6)

T45.1X **Poisoning by, adverse effect of and underdosing of antineoplastic and immunosuppressive drugs**

T45.1X1 **Poisoning by antineoplastic and immunosuppressive drugs, accidental (unintentional)**
Poisoning by antineoplastic and immunosuppressive drugs NOS

T45.1X2 **Poisoning by antineoplastic and immunosuppressive drugs, intentional self-harm**

T45.1X3 **Poisoning by antineoplastic and immunosuppressive drugs, assault**

T45.1X4 **Poisoning by antineoplastic and immunosuppressive drugs, undetermined**

T45.1X5 **Adverse effect of antineoplastic and immunosuppressive drugs**

T45.1X6 **Underdosing of antineoplastic and immunosuppressive drugs**

T45.2 **Poisoning by, adverse effect of and underdosing of vitamins**

Excludes2 poisoning by, adverse effect of and underdosing of nicotinic acid (derivatives) (T46.7)
poisoning by, adverse effect of and underdosing of iron (T45.4)
poisoning by, adverse effect of and underdosing of vitamin K (T45.7)

T45.2X **Poisoning by, adverse effect of and underdosing of vitamins**

T45.2X1 **Poisoning by vitamins, accidental (unintentional)**
Poisoning by vitamins NOS

T45.2X2 **Poisoning by vitamins, intentional self-harm**

T45.2X3 **Poisoning by vitamins, assault**

T45.2X4 **Poisoning by vitamins, undetermined**

T45.2X5 **Adverse effect of vitamins**

T45.2X6 **Underdosing of vitamins**

Excludes1 vitamin deficiencies (E50-E56)

T45.3 **Poisoning by, adverse effect of and underdosing of enzymes**

T45.3X **Poisoning by, adverse effect of and underdosing of enzymes**

T45.3X1 **Poisoning by enzymes, accidental (unintentional)**
Poisoning by enzymes NOS

T45.3X2 **Poisoning by enzymes, intentional self-harm**

T45.3X3 **Poisoning by enzymes, assault**

T45.3X4 **Poisoning by enzymes, undetermined**

T45.3X5 **Adverse effect of enzymes**

T45.3X6 **Underdosing of enzymes**

T45.4 **Poisoning by, adverse effect of and underdosing of iron and its compounds**

T45.4X **Poisoning by, adverse effect of and underdosing of iron and its compounds**

T45.4X1 **Poisoning by iron and its compounds, accidental (unintentional)**
Poisoning by iron and its compounds NOS

T45.4X2 **Poisoning by iron and its compounds, intentional self-harm**

T45.4X3 **Poisoning by iron and its compounds, assault**

T45.4X4 **Poisoning by iron and its compounds, undetermined**

T45.4X5 **Adverse effect of iron and its compounds**

T45.4X6 **Underdosing of iron and its compounds**

Excludes1 iron deficiency (E61.1)

T45.5 Poisoning by, adverse effect of and underdosing of anticoagulants and antithrombotic drugs

T45.51 Poisoning by, adverse effect of and underdosing of anticoagulants

T45.511 Poisoning by anticoagulants, accidental (unintentional)
Poisoning by anticoagulants NOS

T45.512 Poisoning by anticoagulants, intentional self-harm

T45.513 Poisoning by anticoagulants, assault

T45.514 Poisoning by anticoagulants, undetermined

T45.515 Adverse effect of anticoagulants

T45.516 Underdosing of anticoagulants

T45.52 Poisoning by, adverse effect of and underdosing of antithrombotic drugs
Poisoning by, adverse effect of and underdosing of antiplatelet drugs
Excludes2 poisoning by, adverse effect of and underdosing of aspirin (T39.Ø1-)
poisoning by, adverse effect of and underdosing of acetylsalicylic acid (T39.Ø1-)

T45.521 Poisoning by antithrombotic drugs, accidental (unintentional)
Poisoning by antithrombotic drug NOS

T45.522 Poisoning by antithrombotic drugs, intentional self-harm

T45.523 Poisoning by antithrombotic drugs, assault

T45.524 Poisoning by antithrombotic drugs, undetermined

T45.525 Adverse effect of antithrombotic drugs

T45.526 Underdosing of antithrombotic drugs

T45.6 Poisoning by, adverse effect of and underdosing of fibrinolysis-affecting drugs

T45.6Ø Poisoning by, adverse effect of and underdosing of unspecified fibrinolysis-affecting drugs

T45.6Ø1 Poisoning by unspecified fibrinolysis-affecting drugs, accidental (unintentional)
Poisoning by fibrinolysis-affecting drug NOS

T45.6Ø2 Poisoning by unspecified fibrinolysis-affecting drugs, intentional self-harm

T45.6Ø3 Poisoning by unspecified fibrinolysis-affecting drugs, assault

T45.6Ø4 Poisoning by unspecified fibrinolysis-affecting drugs, undetermined

T45.6Ø5 Adverse effect of unspecified fibrinolysis-affecting drugs

T45.6Ø6 Underdosing of unspecified fibrinolysis-affecting drugs

T45.61 Poisoning by, adverse effect of and underdosing of thrombolytic drugs

T45.611 Poisoning by thrombolytic drug, accidental (unintentional)
Poisoning by thrombolytic drug NOS

T45.612 Poisoning by thrombolytic drug, intentional self-harm

T45.613 Poisoning by thrombolytic drug, assault

T45.614 Poisoning by thrombolytic drug, undetermined

T45.615 Adverse effect of thrombolytic drugs

T45.616 Underdosing of thrombolytic drugs

T45.62 Poisoning by, adverse effect of and underdosing of hemostatic drugs

T45.621 Poisoning by hemostatic drug, accidental (unintentional)
Poisoning by hemostatic drug NOS

T45.622 Poisoning by hemostatic drug, intentional self-harm

T45.623 Poisoning by hemostatic drug, assault

T45.624 Poisoning by hemostatic drug, undetermined

T45.625 Adverse effect of hemostatic drug

T45.626 Underdosing of hemostatic drugs

T45.69 Poisoning by, adverse effect of and underdosing of other fibrinolysis-affecting drugs

T45.691 Poisoning by other fibrinolysis-affecting drugs, accidental (unintentional)
Poisoning by other fibrinolysis-affecting drug NOS

T45.692 Poisoning by other fibrinolysis-affecting drugs, intentional self-harm

T45.693 Poisoning by other fibrinolysis-affecting drugs, assault

T45.694 Poisoning by other fibrinolysis-affecting drugs, undetermined

T45.695 Adverse effect of other fibrinolysis-affecting drugs

T45.696 Underdosing of other fibrinolysis-affecting drugs

T45.7 Poisoning by, adverse effect of and underdosing of anticoagulant antagonists, vitamin K and other coagulants

T45.7X Poisoning by, adverse effect of and underdosing of anticoagulant antagonists, vitamin K and other coagulants

T45.7X1 Poisoning by anticoagulant antagonists, vitamin K and other coagulants, accidental (unintentional)
Poisoning by anticoagulant antagonists, vitamin K and other coagulants NOS

T45.7X2 Poisoning by anticoagulant antagonists, vitamin K and other coagulants, intentional self-harm

T45.7X3 Poisoning by anticoagulant antagonists, vitamin K and other coagulants, assault

T45.7X4 Poisoning by anticoagulant antagonists, vitamin K and other coagulants, undetermined

T45.7X5 Adverse effect of anticoagulant antagonists, vitamin K and other coagulants

T45.7X6 Underdosing of anticoagulant antagonist, vitamin K and other coagulants
Excludes1 vitamin K deficiency (E56.1)

● T45.8 **Poisoning by, adverse effect of and underdosing of other primarily systemic and hematological agents**
Poisoning by, adverse effect of and underdosing of liver preparations and other antianemic agents
Poisoning by, adverse effect of and underdosing of natural blood and blood products
Poisoning by, adverse effect of and underdosing of plasma substitute
Excludes2 poisoning by, adverse effect of and underdosing of immunoglobulin (T5Ø.Z1)
poisoning by, adverse effect of and underdosing of iron (T45.4)
transfusion reactions (T8Ø.-)

● T45.8X **Poisoning by, adverse effect of and underdosing of other primarily systemic and hematological agents**

● T45.8X1 **Poisoning by other primarily systemic and hematological agents, accidental (unintentional)**
Poisoning by other primarily systemic and hematological agents NOS

● T45.8X2 **Poisoning by other primarily systemic and hematological agents, intentional self-harm**

● T45.8X3 **Poisoning by other primarily systemic and hematological agents, assault**

● T45.8X4 **Poisoning by other primarily systemic and hematological agents, undetermined**

● T45.8X5 **Adverse effect of other primarily systemic and hematological agents**

● T45.8X6 **Underdosing of other primarily systemic and hematological agents**

● T45.9 **Poisoning by, adverse effect of and underdosing of unspecified primarily systemic and hematological agent**

X● T45.91 **Poisoning by unspecified primarily systemic and hematological agent, accidental (unintentional)**
Poisoning by primarily systemic and hematological agent NOS

X● T45.92 **Poisoning by unspecified primarily systemic and hematological agent, intentional self-harm**

X● T45.93 **Poisoning by unspecified primarily systemic and hematological agent, assault**

X● T45.94 **Poisoning by unspecified primarily systemic and hematological agent, undetermined**

X● T45.95 **Adverse effect of unspecified primarily systemic and hematological agent**

X● T45.96 **Underdosing of unspecified primarily systemic and hematological agent**

● T46 **Poisoning by, adverse effect of and underdosing of agents primarily affecting the cardiovascular system**
Excludes1 poisoning by, adverse effect of and underdosing of metaraminol (T44.4)

The appropriate 7th character is to be added to each code from category T46

A	initial encounter
D	subsequent encounter
S	sequela

● T46.Ø **Poisoning by, adverse effect of and underdosing of cardiac-stimulant glycosides and drugs of similar action**

● T46.ØX **Poisoning by, adverse effect of and underdosing of cardiac-stimulant glycosides and drugs of similar action**

● T46.ØX1 **Poisoning by cardiac-stimulant glycosides and drugs of similar action, accidental (unintentional)**
Poisoning by cardiac-stimulant glycosides and drugs of similar action NOS

● T46.ØX2 **Poisoning by cardiac-stimulant glycosides and drugs of similar action, intentional self-harm**

● T46.ØX3 **Poisoning by cardiac-stimulant glycosides and drugs of similar action, assault**

● T46.ØX4 **Poisoning by cardiac-stimulant glycosides and drugs of similar action, undetermined**

● T46.ØX5 **Adverse effect of cardiac-stimulant glycosides and drugs of similar action**

● T46.ØX6 **Underdosing of cardiac-stimulant glycosides and drugs of similar action**

● T46.1 **Poisoning by, adverse effect of and underdosing of calcium-channel blockers**

● T46.1X **Poisoning by, adverse effect of and underdosing of calcium-channel blockers**

● T46.1X1 **Poisoning by calcium-channel blockers, accidental (unintentional)**
Poisoning by calcium-channel blockers NOS

● T46.1X2 **Poisoning by calcium-channel blockers, intentional self-harm**

● T46.1X3 **Poisoning by calcium-channel blockers, assault**

● T46.1X4 **Poisoning by calcium-channel blockers, undetermined**

● T46.1X5 **Adverse effect of calcium-channel blockers**

● T46.1X6 **Underdosing of calcium-channel blockers**

● T46.2 **Poisoning by, adverse effect of and underdosing of other antidysrhythmic drugs, not elsewhere classified**
Excludes1 poisoning by, adverse effect of and underdosing of beta-adrenoreceptor antagonists (T44.7-)

● T46.2X **Poisoning by, adverse effect of and underdosing of other antidysrhythmic drugs**

● T46.2X1 **Poisoning by other antidysrhythmic drugs, accidental (unintentional)**
Poisoning by other antidysrhythmic drugs NOS

● T46.2X2 **Poisoning by other antidysrhythmic drugs, intentional self-harm**

● T46.2X3 **Poisoning by other antidysrhythmic drugs, assault**

● T46.2X4 **Poisoning by other antidysrhythmic drugs, undetermined**

● T46.2X5 **Adverse effect of other antidysrhythmic drugs**

● T46.2X6 **Underdosing of other antidysrhythmic drugs**

● T46.3 **Poisoning by, adverse effect of and underdosing of coronary vasodilators**
Poisoning by, adverse effect of and underdosing of dipyridamole
Excludes1 poisoning by, adverse effect of and underdosing of calcium-channel blockers (T46.1)

● T46.3X **Poisoning by, adverse effect of and underdosing of coronary vasodilators**

● T46.3X1 **Poisoning by coronary vasodilators, accidental (unintentional)**
Poisoning by coronary vasodilators NOS

● T46.3X2 **Poisoning by coronary vasodilators, intentional self-harm**

● T46.3X3 **Poisoning by coronary vasodilators, assault**

● T46.3X4 **Poisoning by coronary vasodilators, undetermined**

● T46.3X5　Adverse effect of coronary
　　　　　　vasodilators
● T46.3X6　Underdosing of coronary vasodilators

● T46.4　Poisoning by, adverse effect of and underdosing of
　　　　　angiotensin-converting-enzyme inhibitors

　● T46.4X　Poisoning by, adverse effect of and
　　　　　　underdosing of angiotensin-converting-enzyme
　　　　　　inhibitors

　　● T46.4X1　Poisoning by angiotensin-converting-
　　　　　　　　enzyme inhibitors, accidental
　　　　　　　　(unintentional)
　　　　　　　　　Poisoning by angiotensin-
　　　　　　　　　　converting-enzyme inhibitors
　　　　　　　　　　NOS

　　● T46.4X2　Poisoning by angiotensin-converting-
　　　　　　　　enzyme inhibitors, intentional
　　　　　　　　self-harm

　　● T46.4X3　Poisoning by angiotensin-converting-
　　　　　　　　enzyme inhibitors, assault

　　● T46.4X4　Poisoning by angiotensin-converting-
　　　　　　　　enzyme inhibitors, undetermined

　　● T46.4X5　Adverse effect of angiotensin-
　　　　　　　　converting-enzyme inhibitors

　　● T46.4X6　Underdosing of angiotensin-
　　　　　　　　converting-enzyme inhibitors

● T46.5　Poisoning by, adverse effect of and underdosing of other
　　　　　antihypertensive drugs

　　Excludes2　poisoning by, adverse effect of and
　　　　　　　　underdosing of beta-adrenoreceptor
　　　　　　　　antagonists (T44.7)
　　　　　　　poisoning by, adverse effect of and
　　　　　　　　underdosing of calcium-channel
　　　　　　　　blockers (T46.1)
　　　　　　　poisoning by, adverse effect of
　　　　　　　　and underdosing of diuretics
　　　　　　　　(T50.0-T50.2)

　● T46.5X　Poisoning by, adverse effect of and
　　　　　　underdosing of other antihypertensive drugs

　　● T46.5X1　Poisoning by other antihypertensive
　　　　　　　　drugs, accidental (unintentional)
　　　　　　　　　Poisoning by other antihypertensive
　　　　　　　　　　drugs NOS

　　● T46.5X2　Poisoning by other antihypertensive
　　　　　　　　drugs, intentional self-harm

　　● T46.5X3　Poisoning by other antihypertensive
　　　　　　　　drugs, assault

　　● T46.5X4　Poisoning by other antihypertensive
　　　　　　　　drugs, undetermined

　　● T46.5X5　Adverse effect of other
　　　　　　　　antihypertensive drugs

　　● T46.5X6　Underdosing of other
　　　　　　　　antihypertensive drugs

● T46.6　Poisoning by, adverse effect of and underdosing of
　　　　　antihyperlipidemic and antiarteriosclerotic drugs

　● T46.6X　Poisoning by, adverse effect of and
　　　　　　underdosing of antihyperlipidemic and
　　　　　　antiarteriosclerotic drugs

　　● T46.6X1　Poisoning by antihyperlipidemic and
　　　　　　　　antiarteriosclerotic drugs, accidental
　　　　　　　　(unintentional)
　　　　　　　　　Poisoning by antihyperlipidemic and
　　　　　　　　　　antiarteriosclerotic drugs NOS

　　● T46.6X2　Poisoning by antihyperlipidemic and
　　　　　　　　antiarteriosclerotic drugs, intentional
　　　　　　　　self-harm

　　● T46.6X3　Poisoning by antihyperlipidemic and
　　　　　　　　antiarteriosclerotic drugs, assault

　　● T46.6X4　Poisoning by antihyperlipidemic
　　　　　　　　and antiarteriosclerotic drugs,
　　　　　　　　undetermined

● T46.6X5　Adverse effect of antihyperlipidemic
　　　　　　and antiarteriosclerotic drugs
● T46.6X6　Underdosing of antihyperlipidemic
　　　　　　and antiarteriosclerotic drugs

● T46.7　Poisoning by, adverse effect of and underdosing of
　　　　　peripheral vasodilators
　　　　　Poisoning by, adverse effect of and underdosing of
　　　　　　nicotinic acid (derivatives)

　　Excludes1　poisoning by, adverse effect of and
　　　　　　　　underdosing of papaverine (T44.3)

　● T46.7X　Poisoning by, adverse effect of and
　　　　　　underdosing of peripheral vasodilators

　　● T46.7X1　Poisoning by peripheral vasodilators,
　　　　　　　　accidental (unintentional)
　　　　　　　　　Poisoning by peripheral vasodilators
　　　　　　　　　　NOS

　　● T46.7X2　Poisoning by peripheral vasodilators,
　　　　　　　　intentional self-harm

　　● T46.7X3　Poisoning by peripheral vasodilators,
　　　　　　　　assault

　　● T46.7X4　Poisoning by peripheral vasodilators,
　　　　　　　　undetermined

　　● T46.7X5　Adverse effect of peripheral
　　　　　　　　vasodilators

　　● T46.7X6　Underdosing of peripheral
　　　　　　　　vasodilators

● T46.8　Poisoning by, adverse effect of and underdosing of
　　　　　antivaricose drugs, including sclerosing agents

　● T46.8X　Poisoning by, adverse effect of and
　　　　　　underdosing of antivaricose drugs, including
　　　　　　sclerosing agents

　　● T46.8X1　Poisoning by antivaricose drugs,
　　　　　　　　including sclerosing agents,
　　　　　　　　accidental (unintentional)
　　　　　　　　　Poisoning by antivaricose drugs,
　　　　　　　　　　including sclerosing agents
　　　　　　　　　　NOS

　　● T46.8X2　Poisoning by antivaricose drugs,
　　　　　　　　including sclerosing agents,
　　　　　　　　intentional self-harm

　　● T46.8X3　Poisoning by antivaricose drugs,
　　　　　　　　including sclerosing agents, assault

　　● T46.8X4　Poisoning by antivaricose drugs,
　　　　　　　　including sclerosing agents,
　　　　　　　　undetermined

　　● T46.8X5　Adverse effect of antivaricose drugs,
　　　　　　　　including sclerosing agents

　　● T46.8X6　Underdosing of antivaricose drugs,
　　　　　　　　including sclerosing agents

● T46.9　Poisoning by, adverse effect of and underdosing of
　　　　　other and unspecified agents primarily affecting the
　　　　　cardiovascular system

　● T46.90　Poisoning by, adverse effect of and
　　　　　　underdosing of unspecified agents primarily
　　　　　　affecting the cardiovascular system

　　● T46.901　Poisoning by unspecified agents
　　　　　　　　primarily affecting the cardiovascular
　　　　　　　　system, accidental (unintentional)

　　● T46.902　Poisoning by unspecified agents
　　　　　　　　primarily affecting the cardiovascular
　　　　　　　　system, intentional self-harm

　　● T46.903　Poisoning by unspecified agents
　　　　　　　　primarily affecting the cardiovascular
　　　　　　　　system, assault

　　● T46.904　Poisoning by unspecified agents
　　　　　　　　primarily affecting the cardiovascular
　　　　　　　　system, undetermined

　　● T46.905　Adverse effect of unspecified agents
　　　　　　　　primarily affecting the cardiovascular
　　　　　　　　system

　　● T46.906　Underdosing of unspecified agents
　　　　　　　　primarily affecting the cardiovascular
　　　　　　　　system

CHAPTER 19 (S00-T88)

- T46.99 **Poisoning by, adverse effect of and underdosing of other agents primarily affecting the cardiovascular system**
  - T46.991 **Poisoning by other agents primarily affecting the cardiovascular system, accidental (unintentional)**
  - T46.992 **Poisoning by other agents primarily affecting the cardiovascular system, intentional self-harm**
  - T46.993 **Poisoning by other agents primarily affecting the cardiovascular system, assault**
  - T46.994 **Poisoning by other agents primarily affecting the cardiovascular system, undetermined**
  - T46.995 **Adverse effect of other agents primarily affecting the cardiovascular system**
  - T46.996 **Underdosing of other agents primarily affecting the cardiovascular system**

T47 Poisoning by, adverse effect of and underdosing of agents primarily affecting the gastrointestinal system

The appropriate 7th character is to be added to each code from category T47

A	initial encounter
D	subsequent encounter
S	sequela

- T47.Ø **Poisoning by, adverse effect of and underdosing of histamine H2-receptor blockers**
  - T47.ØX **Poisoning by, adverse effect of and underdosing of histamine H2-receptor blockers**
    - T47.ØX1 **Poisoning by histamine H2-receptor blockers, accidental (unintentional)**
      Poisoning by histamine H2-receptor blockers NOS
    - T47.ØX2 **Poisoning by histamine H2-receptor blockers, intentional self-harm**
    - T47.ØX3 **Poisoning by histamine H2-receptor blockers, assault**
    - T47.ØX4 **Poisoning by histamine H2-receptor blockers, undetermined**
    - T47.ØX5 **Adverse effect of histamine H2-receptor blockers**
    - T47.ØX6 **Underdosing of histamine H2-receptor blockers**
- T47.1 **Poisoning by, adverse effect of and underdosing of other antacids and anti-gastric-secretion drugs**
  - T47.1X **Poisoning by, adverse effect of and underdosing of other antacids and anti-gastric-secretion drugs**
    - T47.1X1 **Poisoning by other antacids and anti-gastric-secretion drugs, accidental (unintentional)**
      Poisoning by other antacids and anti-gastric-secretion drugs NOS
    - T47.1X2 **Poisoning by other antacids and anti-gastric-secretion drugs, intentional self-harm**
    - T47.1X3 **Poisoning by other antacids and anti-gastric-secretion drugs, assault**
    - T47.1X4 **Poisoning by other antacids and anti-gastric-secretion drugs, undetermined**
    - T47.1X5 **Adverse effect of other antacids and anti-gastric-secretion drugs**
    - T47.1X6 **Underdosing of other antacids and anti-gastric-secretion drugs**
- T47.2 **Poisoning by, adverse effect of and underdosing of stimulant laxatives**
  - T47.2X **Poisoning by, adverse effect of and underdosing of stimulant laxatives**
    - T47.2X1 **Poisoning by stimulant laxatives, accidental (unintentional)**
      Poisoning by stimulant laxatives NOS
    - T47.2X2 **Poisoning by stimulant laxatives, intentional self-harm**
    - T47.2X3 **Poisoning by stimulant laxatives, assault**
    - T47.2X4 **Poisoning by stimulant laxatives, undetermined**
    - T47.2X5 **Adverse effect of stimulant laxatives**
    - T47.2X6 **Underdosing of stimulant laxatives**
- T47.3 **Poisoning by, adverse effect of and underdosing of saline and osmotic laxatives**
  - T47.3X **Poisoning by and adverse effect of saline and osmotic laxatives**
    - T47.3X1 **Poisoning by saline and osmotic laxatives, accidental (unintentional)**
      Poisoning by saline and osmotic laxatives NOS
    - T47.3X2 **Poisoning by saline and osmotic laxatives, intentional self-harm**
    - T47.3X3 **Poisoning by saline and osmotic laxatives, assault**
    - T47.3X4 **Poisoning by saline and osmotic laxatives, undetermined**
    - T47.3X5 **Adverse effect of saline and osmotic laxatives**
    - T47.3X6 **Underdosing of saline and osmotic laxatives**
- T47.4 **Poisoning by, adverse effect of and underdosing of other laxatives**
  - T47.4X **Poisoning by, adverse effect of and underdosing of other laxatives**
    - T47.4X1 **Poisoning by other laxatives, accidental (unintentional)**
      Poisoning by other laxatives NOS
    - T47.4X2 **Poisoning by other laxatives, intentional self-harm**
    - T47.4X3 **Poisoning by other laxatives, assault**
    - T47.4X4 **Poisoning by other laxatives, undetermined**
    - T47.4X5 **Adverse effect of other laxatives**
    - T47.4X6 **Underdosing of other laxatives**
- T47.5 **Poisoning by, adverse effect of and underdosing of digestants**
  - T47.5X **Poisoning by, adverse effect of and underdosing of digestants**
    - T47.5X1 **Poisoning by digestants, accidental (unintentional)**
      Poisoning by digestants NOS
    - T47.5X2 **Poisoning by digestants, intentional self-harm**
    - T47.5X3 **Poisoning by digestants, assault**
    - T47.5X4 **Poisoning by digestants, undetermined**
    - T47.5X5 **Adverse effect of digestants**
    - T47.5X6 **Underdosing of digestants**

● T47.6   Poisoning by, adverse effect of and underdosing of antidiarrheal drugs

> Excludes2   poisoning by, adverse effect of and underdosing of systemic antibiotics and other anti-infectives (T36-T37)

  ● T47.6X   Poisoning by, adverse effect of and underdosing of antidiarrheal drugs

    ● T47.6X1   Poisoning by antidiarrheal drugs, accidental (unintentional)
         Poisoning by antidiarrheal drugs NOS

    ● T47.6X2   Poisoning by antidiarrheal drugs, intentional self-harm

    ● T47.6X3   Poisoning by antidiarrheal drugs, assault

    ● T47.6X4   Poisoning by antidiarrheal drugs, undetermined

    ● T47.6X5   Adverse effect of antidiarrheal drugs

    ● T47.6X6   Underdosing of antidiarrheal drugs

● T47.7   Poisoning by, adverse effect of and underdosing of emetics

  ● T47.7X   Poisoning by, adverse effect of and underdosing of emetics

    ● T47.7X1   Poisoning by emetics, accidental (unintentional)
         Poisoning by emetics NOS

    ● T47.7X2   Poisoning by emetics, intentional self-harm

    ● T47.7X3   Poisoning by emetics, assault

    ● T47.7X4   Poisoning by emetics, undetermined

    ● T47.7X5   Adverse effect of emetics

    ● T47.7X6   Underdosing of emetics

● T47.8   Poisoning by, adverse effect of and underdosing of other agents primarily affecting gastrointestinal system

  ● T47.8X   Poisoning by, adverse effect of and underdosing of other agents primarily affecting gastrointestinal system

    ● T47.8X1   Poisoning by other agents primarily affecting gastrointestinal system, accidental (unintentional)
         Poisoning by other agents primarily affecting gastrointestinal system NOS

    ● T47.8X2   Poisoning by other agents primarily affecting gastrointestinal system, intentional self-harm

    ● T47.8X3   Poisoning by other agents primarily affecting gastrointestinal system, assault

    ● T47.8X4   Poisoning by other agents primarily affecting gastrointestinal system, undetermined

    ● T47.8X5   Adverse effect of other agents primarily affecting gastrointestinal system

    ● T47.8X6   Underdosing of other agents primarily affecting gastrointestinal system

● T47.9   Poisoning by, adverse effect of and underdosing of unspecified agents primarily affecting the gastrointestinal system

  X ● T47.91   Poisoning by unspecified agents primarily affecting the gastrointestinal system, accidental (unintentional)
         Poisoning by agents primarily affecting the gastrointestinal system NOS

  X ● T47.92   Poisoning by unspecified agents primarily affecting the gastrointestinal system, intentional self-harm

  X ● T47.93   Poisoning by unspecified agents primarily affecting the gastrointestinal system, assault

  X ● T47.94   Poisoning by unspecified agents primarily affecting the gastrointestinal system, undetermined

  X ● T47.95   Adverse effect of unspecified agents primarily affecting the gastrointestinal system

  X ● T47.96   Underdosing of unspecified agents primarily affecting the gastrointestinal system

● T48   Poisoning by, adverse effect of and underdosing of agents primarily acting on smooth and skeletal muscles and the respiratory system

> The appropriate 7th character is to be added to each code from category T48

> | A | initial encounter |
> | D | subsequent encounter |
> | S | sequela |

  ● T48.0   Poisoning by, adverse effect of and underdosing of oxytocic drugs

> Excludes1   poisoning by, adverse effect of and underdosing of estrogens, progestogens and antagonists (T38.4-T38.6)

  ● T48.0X   Poisoning by, adverse effect of and underdosing of oxytocic drugs

    ● T48.0X1   Poisoning by oxytocic drugs, accidental (unintentional)
         Poisoning by oxytocic drugs NOS

    ● T48.0X2   Poisoning by oxytocic drugs, intentional self-harm

    ● T48.0X3   Poisoning by oxytocic drugs, assault

    ● T48.0X4   Poisoning by oxytocic drugs, undetermined

    ● T48.0X5   Adverse effect of oxytocic drugs

    ● T48.0X6   Underdosing of oxytocic drugs

● T48.1   Poisoning by, adverse effect of and underdosing of skeletal muscle relaxants [neuromuscular blocking agents]

  ● T48.1X   Poisoning by, adverse effect of and underdosing of skeletal muscle relaxants [neuromuscular blocking agents]

    ● T48.1X1   Poisoning by skeletal muscle relaxants [neuromuscular blocking agents], accidental (unintentional)
         Poisoning by skeletal muscle relaxants [neuromuscular blocking agents] NOS

    ● T48.1X2   Poisoning by skeletal muscle relaxants [neuromuscular blocking agents], intentional self-harm

    ● T48.1X3   Poisoning by skeletal muscle relaxants [neuromuscular blocking agents], assault

    ● T48.1X4   Poisoning by skeletal muscle relaxants [neuromuscular blocking agents], undetermined

    ● T48.1X5   Adverse effect of skeletal muscle relaxants [neuromuscular blocking agents]

    ● T48.1X6   Underdosing of skeletal muscle relaxants [neuromuscular blocking agents]

- T48.2 **Poisoning by, adverse effect of and underdosing of other and unspecified drugs acting on muscles**
  - T48.20 **Poisoning by, adverse effect of and underdosing of unspecified drugs acting on muscles**
    - T48.201 **Poisoning by unspecified drugs acting on muscles, accidental (unintentional)**
      Poisoning by unspecified drugs acting on muscles NOS
    - T48.202 **Poisoning by unspecified drugs acting on muscles, intentional self-harm**
    - T48.203 **Poisoning by unspecified drugs acting on muscles, assault**
    - T48.204 **Poisoning by unspecified drugs acting on muscles, undetermined**
    - T48.205 **Adverse effect of unspecified drugs acting on muscles**
    - T48.206 **Underdosing of unspecified drugs acting on muscles**
  - T48.29 **Poisoning by, adverse effect of and underdosing of other drugs acting on muscles**
    - T48.291 **Poisoning by other drugs acting on muscles, accidental (unintentional)**
      Poisoning by other drugs acting on muscles NOS
    - T48.292 **Poisoning by other drugs acting on muscles, intentional self-harm**
    - T48.293 **Poisoning by other drugs acting on muscles, assault**
    - T48.294 **Poisoning by other drugs acting on muscles, undetermined**
    - T48.295 **Adverse effect of other drugs acting on muscles**
    - T48.296 **Underdosing of other drugs acting on muscles**
- T48.3 **Poisoning by, adverse effect of and underdosing of antitussives**
  - T48.3X **Poisoning by, adverse effect of and underdosing of antitussives**
    - T48.3X1 **Poisoning by antitussives, accidental (unintentional)**
      Poisoning by antitussives NOS
    - T48.3X2 **Poisoning by antitussives, intentional self-harm**
    - T48.3X3 **Poisoning by antitussives, assault**
    - T48.3X4 **Poisoning by antitussives, undetermined**
    - T48.3X5 **Adverse effect of antitussives**
    - T48.3X6 **Underdosing of antitussives**
- T48.4 **Poisoning by, adverse effect of and underdosing of expectorants**
  - T48.4X **Poisoning by, adverse effect of and underdosing of expectorants**
    - T48.4X1 **Poisoning by expectorants, accidental (unintentional)**
      Poisoning by expectorants NOS
    - T48.4X2 **Poisoning by expectorants, intentional self-harm**
    - T48.4X3 **Poisoning by expectorants, assault**
    - T48.4X4 **Poisoning by expectorants, undetermined**
    - T48.4X5 **Adverse effect of expectorants**
    - T48.4X6 **Underdosing of expectorants**
- T48.5 **Poisoning by, adverse effect of and underdosing of other anti-common-cold drugs**
  Poisoning by, adverse effect of and underdosing of decongestants
  Excludes2 poisoning by, adverse effect of and underdosing of antipyretics, NEC (T39.9-)
  poisoning by, adverse effect of and underdosing of non-steroidal antiinflammatory drugs (T39.3-)
  poisoning by, adverse effect of and underdosing of salicylates (T39.0-)
  - T48.5X **Poisoning by, adverse effect of and underdosing of other anti-common-cold drugs**
    - T48.5X1 **Poisoning by other anti-common-cold drugs, accidental (unintentional)**
      Poisoning by other anti-common-cold drugs NOS
    - T48.5X2 **Poisoning by other anti-common-cold drugs, intentional self-harm**
    - T48.5X3 **Poisoning by other anti-common-cold drugs, assault**
    - T48.5X4 **Poisoning by other anti-common-cold drugs, undetermined**
    - T48.5X5 **Adverse effect of other anti-common-cold drugs**
    - T48.5X6 **Underdosing of other anti-common-cold drugs**
- T48.6 **Poisoning by, adverse effect of and underdosing of antiasthmatics, not elsewhere classified**
  Poisoning by, adverse effect of and underdosing of beta-adrenoreceptor agonists used in asthma therapy
  Excludes1 poisoning by, adverse effect of and underdosing of beta-adrenoreceptor agonists not used in asthma therapy (T44.5)
  poisoning by, adverse effect of and underdosing of anterior pituitary [adenohypophyseal] hormones (T38.8)
  - T48.6X **Poisoning by, adverse effect of and underdosing of antiasthmatics**
    - T48.6X1 **Poisoning by antiasthmatics, accidental (unintentional)**
      Poisoning by antiasthmatics NOS
    - T48.6X2 **Poisoning by antiasthmatics, intentional self-harm**
    - T48.6X3 **Poisoning by antiasthmatics, assault**
    - T48.6X4 **Poisoning by antiasthmatics, undetermined**
    - T48.6X5 **Adverse effect of antiasthmatics**
    - T48.6X6 **Underdosing of antiasthmatics**
- T48.9 **Poisoning by, adverse effect of and underdosing of other and unspecified agents primarily acting on the respiratory system**
  - T48.90 **Poisoning by, adverse effect of and underdosing of unspecified agents primarily acting on the respiratory system**
    - T48.901 **Poisoning by unspecified agents primarily acting on the respiratory system, accidental (unintentional)**
    - T48.902 **Poisoning by unspecified agents primarily acting on the respiratory system, intentional self-harm**
    - T48.903 **Poisoning by unspecified agents primarily acting on the respiratory system, assault**
    - T48.904 **Poisoning by unspecified agents primarily acting on the respiratory system, undetermined**

CHAPTER 19 (S00-T88)

T48.905 Adverse effect of unspecified agents primarily acting on the respiratory system

T48.906 Underdosing of unspecified agents primarily acting on the respiratory system

T48.99 Poisoning by, adverse effect of and underdosing of other agents primarily acting on the respiratory system

T48.991 Poisoning by other agents primarily acting on the respiratory system, accidental (unintentional)

T48.992 Poisoning by other agents primarily acting on the respiratory system, intentional self-harm

T48.993 Poisoning by other agents primarily acting on the respiratory system, assault

T48.994 Poisoning by other agents primarily acting on the respiratory system, undetermined

T48.995 Adverse effect of other agents primarily acting on the respiratory system

T48.996 Underdosing of other agents primarily acting on the respiratory system

T49 Poisoning by, adverse effect of and underdosing of topical agents primarily affecting skin and mucous membrane and by ophthalmological, otorhinorlaryngological and dental drugs

Includes poisoning by, adverse effect of and underdosing of glucocorticoids, topically used

The appropriate 7th character is to be added to each code from category T49

A	initial encounter
D	subsequent encounter
S	sequela

T49.0 Poisoning by, adverse effect of and underdosing of local antifungal, anti-infective and anti-inflammatory drugs

T49.0X Poisoning by, adverse effect of and underdosing of local antifungal, anti-infective and anti-inflammatory drugs

T49.0X1 Poisoning by local antifungal, anti-infective and anti-inflammatory drugs, accidental (unintentional)
Poisoning by local antifungal, anti-infective and anti-inflammatory drugs NOS

T49.0X2 Poisoning by local antifungal, anti-infective and anti-inflammatory drugs, intentional self-harm

T49.0X3 Poisoning by local antifungal, anti-infective and anti-inflammatory drugs, assault

T49.0X4 Poisoning by local antifungal, anti-infective and anti-inflammatory drugs, undetermined

T49.0X5 Adverse effect of local antifungal, anti-infective and anti-inflammatory drugs

T49.0X6 Underdosing of local antifungal, anti-infective and anti-inflammatory drugs

T49.1 Poisoning by, adverse effect of and underdosing of antipruritics

T49.1X Poisoning by, adverse effect of and underdosing of antipruritics

T49.1X1 Poisoning by antipruritics, accidental (unintentional)
Poisoning by antipruritics NOS

T49.1X2 Poisoning by antipruritics, intentional self-harm

T49.1X3 Poisoning by antipruritics, assault

T49.1X4 Poisoning by antipruritics, undetermined

T49.1X5 Adverse effect of antipruritics

T49.1X6 Underdosing of antipruritics

T49.2 Poisoning by, adverse effect of and underdosing of local astringents and local detergents

T49.2X Poisoning by, adverse effect of and underdosing of local astringents and local detergents

T49.2X1 Poisoning by local astringents and local detergents, accidental (unintentional)
Poisoning by local astringents and local detergents NOS

T49.2X2 Poisoning by local astringents and local detergents, intentional self-harm

T49.2X3 Poisoning by local astringents and local detergents, assault

T49.2X4 Poisoning by local astringents and local detergents, undetermined

T49.2X5 Adverse effect of local astringents and local detergents

T49.2X6 Underdosing of local astringents and local detergents

T49.3 Poisoning by, adverse effect of and underdosing of emollients, demulcents and protectants

T49.3X Poisoning by, adverse effect of and underdosing of emollients, demulcents and protectants

T49.3X1 Poisoning by emollients, demulcents and protectants, accidental (unintentional)
Poisoning by emollients, demulcents and protectants NOS

T49.3X2 Poisoning by emollients, demulcents and protectants, intentional self-harm

T49.3X3 Poisoning by emollients, demulcents and protectants, assault

T49.3X4 Poisoning by emollients, demulcents and protectants, undetermined

T49.3X5 Adverse effect of emollients, demulcents and protectants

T49.3X6 Underdosing of emollients, demulcents and protectants

T49.4 Poisoning by, adverse effect of and underdosing of keratolytics, keratoplastics, and other hair treatment drugs and preparations

T49.4X Poisoning by, adverse effect of and underdosing of keratolytics, keratoplastics, and other hair treatment drugs and preparations

T49.4X1 Poisoning by keratolytics, keratoplastics, and other hair treatment drugs and preparations, accidental (unintentional)
Poisoning by keratolytics, keratoplastics, and other hair treatment drugs and preparations NOS

T49.4X2 Poisoning by keratolytics, keratoplastics, and other hair treatment drugs and preparations, intentional self-harm

T49.4X3 Poisoning by keratolytics, keratoplastics, and other hair treatment drugs and preparations, assault

T49.4X4 Poisoning by keratolytics, keratoplastics, and other hair treatment drugs and preparations, undetermined

T49.4X5 Adverse effect of keratolytics, keratoplastics, and other hair treatment drugs and preparations

T49.4X6 Underdosing of keratolytics, keratoplastics, and other hair treatment drugs and preparations

CHAPTER 19 (S00-T88)

● **T49.5 Poisoning by, adverse effect of and underdosing of ophthalmological drugs and preparations**

● **T49.5X Poisoning by, adverse effect of and underdosing of ophthalmological drugs and preparations**

● **T49.5X1 Poisoning by ophthalmological drugs and preparations, accidental (unintentional)**

Poisoning by ophthalmological drugs and preparations NOS

● **T49.5X2 Poisoning by ophthalmological drugs and preparations, intentional self-harm**

● **T49.5X3 Poisoning by ophthalmological drugs and preparations, assault**

● **T49.5X4 Poisoning by ophthalmological drugs and preparations, undetermined**

● **T49.5X5 Adverse effect of ophthalmological drugs and preparations**

● **T49.5X6 Underdosing of ophthalmological drugs and preparations**

● **T49.6 Poisoning by, adverse effect of and underdosing of otorhinolaryngological drugs and preparations**

● **T49.6X Poisoning by, adverse effect of and underdosing of otorhinolaryngological drugs and preparations**

● **T49.6X1 Poisoning by otorhinolaryngological drugs and preparations, accidental (unintentional)**

Poisoning by otorhinolaryngological drugs and preparations NOS

● **T49.6X2 Poisoning by otorhinolaryngological drugs and preparations, intentional self-harm**

● **T49.6X3 Poisoning by otorhinolaryngological drugs and preparations, assault**

● **T49.6X4 Poisoning by otorhinolaryngological drugs and preparations, undetermined**

● **T49.6X5 Adverse effect of otorhinolaryngological drugs and preparations**

● **T49.6X6 Underdosing of otorhinolaryngological drugs and preparations**

● **T49.7 Poisoning by, adverse effect of and underdosing of dental drugs, topically applied**

● **T49.7X Poisoning by, adverse effect of and underdosing of dental drugs, topically applied**

● **T49.7X1 Poisoning by dental drugs, topically applied, accidental (unintentional)**

Poisoning by dental drugs, topically applied NOS

● **T49.7X2 Poisoning by dental drugs, topically applied, intentional self-harm**

● **T49.7X3 Poisoning by dental drugs, topically applied, assault**

● **T49.7X4 Poisoning by dental drugs, topically applied, undetermined**

● **T49.7X5 Adverse effect of dental drugs, topically applied**

● **T49.7X6 Underdosing of dental drugs, topically applied**

● **T49.8 Poisoning by, adverse effect of and underdosing of other topical agents**

Poisoning by, adverse effect of and underdosing of spermicides

● **T49.8X Poisoning by, adverse effect of and underdosing of other topical agents**

● **T49.8X1 Poisoning by other topical agents, accidental (unintentional)**

Poisoning by other topical agents NOS

● **T49.8X2 Poisoning by other topical agents, intentional self-harm**

● **T49.8X3 Poisoning by other topical agents, assault**

● **T49.8X4 Poisoning by other topical agents, undetermined**

● **T49.8X5 Adverse effect of other topical agents**

● **T49.8X6 Underdosing of other topical agents**

● **T49.9 Poisoning by, adverse effect of and underdosing of unspecified topical agent**

X● **T49.91 Poisoning by unspecified topical agent, accidental (unintentional)**

X● **T49.92 Poisoning by unspecified topical agent, intentional self-harm**

X● **T49.93 Poisoning by unspecified topical agent, assault**

X● **T49.94 Poisoning by unspecified topical agent, undetermined**

X● **T49.95 Adverse effect of unspecified topical agent**

X● **T49.96 Underdosing of unspecified topical agent**

● **T50 Poisoning by, adverse effect of and underdosing of diuretics and other and unspecified drugs, medicaments and biological substances**

The appropriate 7th character is to be added to each code from category T5Ø

A	initial encounter
D	subsequent encounter
S	sequela

● **T5Ø.Ø Poisoning by, adverse effect of and underdosing of mineralocorticoids and their antagonists**

● **T5Ø.ØX Poisoning by, adverse effect of and underdosing of mineralocorticoids and their antagonists**

● **T5Ø.ØX1 Poisoning by mineralocorticoids and their antagonists, accidental (unintentional)**

Poisoning by mineralocorticoids and their antagonists NOS

● **T5Ø.ØX2 Poisoning by mineralocorticoids and their antagonists, intentional self-harm**

● **T5Ø.ØX3 Poisoning by mineralocorticoids and their antagonists, assault**

● **T5Ø.ØX4 Poisoning by mineralocorticoids and their antagonists, undetermined**

● **T5Ø.ØX5 Adverse effect of mineralocorticoids and their antagonists**

● **T5Ø.ØX6 Underdosing of mineralocorticoids and their antagonists**

● **T5Ø.1 Poisoning by, adverse effect of and underdosing of loop [high-ceiling] diuretics**

● **T5Ø.1X Poisoning by, adverse effect of and underdosing of loop [high-ceiling] diuretics**

● **T5Ø.1X1 Poisoning by loop [high-ceiling] diuretics, accidental (unintentional)**

Poisoning by loop [high-ceiling] diuretics NOS

● **T5Ø.1X2 Poisoning by loop [high-ceiling] diuretics, intentional self-harm**

● **T5Ø.1X3 Poisoning by loop [high-ceiling] diuretics, assault**

T50.1X4 **Poisoning by loop [high-ceiling] diuretics, undetermined**
T50.1X5 **Adverse effect of loop [high-ceiling] diuretics**
T50.1X6 **Underdosing of loop [high-ceiling] diuretics**

T50.2 **Poisoning by, adverse effect of and underdosing of carbonic-anhydrase inhibitors, benzothiadiazides and other diuretics**
Poisoning by, adverse effect of and underdosing of acetazolamide

T50.2X **Poisoning by, adverse effect of and underdosing of carbonic-anhydrase inhibitors, benzothiadiazides and other diuretics**
T50.2X1 **Poisoning by carbonic-anhydrase inhibitors, benzothiadiazides and other diuretics, accidental (unintentional)**
Poisoning by carbonic-anhydrase inhibitors, benzothiadiazides and other diuretics NOS
T50.2X2 **Poisoning by carbonic-anhydrase inhibitors, benzothiadiazides and other diuretics, intentional self-harm**
T50.2X3 **Poisoning by carbonic-anhydrase inhibitors, benzothiadiazides and other diuretics, assault**
T50.2X4 **Poisoning by carbonic-anhydrase inhibitors, benzothiadiazides and other diuretics, undetermined**
T50.2X5 **Adverse effect of carbonic-anhydrase inhibitors, benzothiadiazides and other diuretics**
T50.2X6 **Underdosing of carbonic-anhydrase inhibitors, benzothiadiazides and other diuretics**

T50.3 **Poisoning by, adverse effect of and underdosing of electrolytic, caloric and water-balance agents**
Poisoning by, adverse effect of and underdosing of oral rehydration salts

T50.3X **Poisoning by, adverse effect of and underdosing of electrolytic, caloric and water-balance agents**
T50.3X1 **Poisoning by electrolytic, caloric and water-balance agents, accidental (unintentional)**
Poisoning by electrolytic, caloric and water-balance agents NOS
T50.3X2 **Poisoning by electrolytic, caloric and water-balance agents, intentional self-harm**
T50.3X3 **Poisoning by electrolytic, caloric and water-balance agents, assault**
T50.3X4 **Poisoning by electrolytic, caloric and water-balance agents, undetermined**
T50.3X5 **Adverse effect of electrolytic, caloric and water-balance agents**
T50.3X6 **Underdosing of electrolytic, caloric and water-balance agents**

T50.4 **Poisoning by, adverse effect of and underdosing of drugs affecting uric acid metabolism**

T50.4X **Poisoning by, adverse effect of and underdosing of drugs affecting uric acid metabolism**
T50.4X1 **Poisoning by drugs affecting uric acid metabolism, accidental (unintentional)**
Poisoning by drugs affecting uric acid metabolism NOS
T50.4X2 **Poisoning by drugs affecting uric acid metabolism, intentional self-harm**
T50.4X3 **Poisoning by drugs affecting uric acid metabolism, assault**
T50.4X4 **Poisoning by drugs affecting uric acid metabolism, undetermined**
T50.4X5 **Adverse effect of drugs affecting uric acid metabolism**
T50.4X6 **Underdosing of drugs affecting uric acid metabolism**

T50.5 **Poisoning by, adverse effect of and underdosing of appetite depressants**

T50.5X **Poisoning by, adverse effect of and underdosing of appetite depressants**
T50.5X1 **Poisoning by appetite depressants, accidental (unintentional)**
Poisoning by appetite depressants NOS
T50.5X2 **Poisoning by appetite depressants, intentional self-harm**
T50.5X3 **Poisoning by appetite depressants, assault**
T50.5X4 **Poisoning by appetite depressants, undetermined**
T50.5X5 **Adverse effect of appetite depressants**
T50.5X6 **Underdosing of appetite depressants**

T50.6 **Poisoning by, adverse effect of and underdosing of antidotes and chelating agents**
Poisoning by, adverse effect of and underdosing of alcohol deterrents

T50.6X **Poisoning by, adverse effect of and underdosing of antidotes and chelating agents**
T50.6X1 **Poisoning by antidotes and chelating agents, accidental (unintentional)**
Poisoning by antidotes and chelating agents NOS
T50.6X2 **Poisoning by antidotes and chelating agents, intentional self-harm**
T50.6X3 **Poisoning by antidotes and chelating agents, assault**
T50.6X4 **Poisoning by antidotes and chelating agents, undetermined**
T50.6X5 **Adverse effect of antidotes and chelating agents**
T50.6X6 **Underdosing of antidotes and chelating agents**

T50.7 **Poisoning by, adverse effect of and underdosing of analeptics and opioid receptor antagonists**

T50.7X **Poisoning by, adverse effect of and underdosing of analeptics and opioid receptor antagonists**
T50.7X1 **Poisoning by analeptics and opioid receptor antagonists, accidental (unintentional)**
Poisoning by analeptics and opioid receptor antagonists NOS
T50.7X2 **Poisoning by analeptics and opioid receptor antagonists, intentional self-harm**
T50.7X3 **Poisoning by analeptics and opioid receptor antagonists, assault**
T50.7X4 **Poisoning by analeptics and opioid receptor antagonists, undetermined**
T50.7X5 **Adverse effect of analeptics and opioid receptor antagonists**
T50.7X6 **Underdosing of analeptics and opioid receptor antagonists**

- ● T50.8 Poisoning by, adverse effect of and underdosing of diagnostic agents
  - ● T50.8X Poisoning by, adverse effect of and underdosing of diagnostic agents
    - ● T50.8X1 Poisoning by diagnostic agents, accidental (unintentional)
      Poisoning by diagnostic agents NOS
    - ● T50.8X2 Poisoning by diagnostic agents, intentional self-harm
    - ● T50.8X3 Poisoning by diagnostic agents, assault
    - ● T50.8X4 Poisoning by diagnostic agents, undetermined
    - ● T50.8X5 Adverse effect of diagnostic agents
    - ● T50.8X6 Underdosing of diagnostic agents
- ● T50.A Poisoning by, adverse effect of and underdosing of bacterial vaccines
  - ● T50.A1 Poisoning by, adverse effect of and underdosing of pertussis vaccine, including combinations with a pertussis component
    - ● T50.A11 Poisoning by pertussis vaccine, including combinations with a pertussis component, accidental (unintentional)
    - ● T50.A12 Poisoning by pertussis vaccine, including combinations with a pertussis component, intentional self-harm
    - ● T50.A13 Poisoning by pertussis vaccine, including combinations with a pertussis component, assault
    - ● T50.A14 Poisoning by pertussis vaccine, including combinations with a pertussis component, undetermined
    - ● T50.A15 Adverse effect of pertussis vaccine, including combinations with a pertussis component
    - ● T50.A16 Underdosing of pertussis vaccine, including combinations with a pertussis component
  - ● T50.A2 Poisoning by, adverse effect of and underdosing of mixed bacterial vaccines without a pertussis component
    - ● T50.A21 Poisoning by mixed bacterial vaccines without a pertussis component, accidental (unintentional)
    - ● T50.A22 Poisoning by mixed bacterial vaccines without a pertussis component, intentional self-harm
    - ● T50.A23 Poisoning by mixed bacterial vaccines without a pertussis component, assault
    - ● T50.A24 Poisoning by mixed bacterial vaccines without a pertussis component, undetermined
    - ● T50.A25 Adverse effect of mixed bacterial vaccines without a pertussis component
    - ● T50.A26 Underdosing of mixed bacterial vaccines without a pertussis component
  - ● T50.A9 Poisoning by, adverse effect of and underdosing of other bacterial vaccines
    - ● T50.A91 Poisoning by other bacterial vaccines, accidental (unintentional)
    - ● T50.A92 Poisoning by other bacterial vaccines, intentional self-harm
    - ● T50.A93 Poisoning by other bacterial vaccines, assault
    - ● T50.A94 Poisoning by other bacterial vaccines, undetermined
    - ● T50.A95 Adverse effect of other bacterial vaccines
    - ● T50.A96 Underdosing of other bacterial vaccines
- ● T50.B Poisoning by, adverse effect of and underdosing of viral vaccines
  - ● T50.B1 Poisoning by, adverse effect of and underdosing of smallpox vaccines
    - ● T50.B11 Poisoning by smallpox vaccines, accidental (unintentional)
    - ● T50.B12 Poisoning by smallpox vaccines, intentional self-harm
    - ● T50.B13 Poisoning by smallpox vaccines, assault
    - ● T50.B14 Poisoning by smallpox vaccines, undetermined
    - ● T50.B15 Adverse effect of smallpox vaccines
    - ● T50.B16 Underdosing of smallpox vaccines
  - ● T50.B9 Poisoning by, adverse effect of and underdosing of other viral vaccines
    - ● T50.B91 Poisoning by other viral vaccines, accidental (unintentional)
    - ● T50.B92 Poisoning by other viral vaccines, intentional self-harm
    - ● T50.B93 Poisoning by other viral vaccines, assault
    - ● T50.B94 Poisoning by other viral vaccines, undetermined
    - ● T50.B95 Adverse effect of other viral vaccines
    - ● T50.B96 Underdosing of other viral vaccines
- ● T50.Z Poisoning by, adverse effect of and underdosing of other vaccines and biological substances
  - ● T50.Z1 Poisoning by, adverse effect of and underdosing of immunoglobulin
    - ● T50.Z11 Poisoning by immunoglobulin, accidental (unintentional)
    - ● T50.Z12 Poisoning by immunoglobulin, intentional self-harm
    - ● T50.Z13 Poisoning by immunoglobulin, assault
    - ● T50.Z14 Poisoning by immunoglobulin, undetermined
    - ● T50.Z15 Adverse effect of immunoglobulin
    - ● T50.Z16 Underdosing of immunoglobulin

- T50.Z9 **Poisoning by, adverse effect of and underdosing of other vaccines and biological substances**
  - T50.Z91 **Poisoning by other vaccines and biological substances, accidental (unintentional)**
  - T50.Z92 **Poisoning by other vaccines and biological substances, intentional self-harm**
  - T50.Z93 **Poisoning by other vaccines and biological substances, assault**
  - T50.Z94 **Poisoning by other vaccines and biological substances, undetermined**
  - T50.Z95 **Adverse effect of other vaccines and biological substances**
  - T50.Z96 **Underdosing of other vaccines and biological substances**

T50.9 **Poisoning by, adverse effect of and underdosing of other and unspecified drugs, medicaments and biological substances**

- T50.90 **Poisoning by, adverse effect of and underdosing of unspecified drugs, medicaments and biological substances**
  - T50.901 **Poisoning by unspecified drugs, medicaments and biological substances, accidental (unintentional)**
  - T50.902 **Poisoning by unspecified drugs, medicaments and biological substances, intentional self-harm**
  - T50.903 **Poisoning by unspecified drugs, medicaments and biological substances, assault**
  - T50.904 **Poisoning by unspecified drugs, medicaments and biological substances, undetermined**
  - T50.905 **Adverse effect of unspecified drugs, medicaments and biological substances**
  - T50.906 **Underdosing of unspecified drugs, medicaments and biological substances**
- T50.99 **Poisoning by, adverse effect of and underdosing of other drugs, medicaments and biological substances**
  - T50.991 **Poisoning by other drugs, medicaments and biological substances, accidental (unintentional)**
  - T50.992 **Poisoning by other drugs, medicaments and biological substances, intentional self-harm**
  - T50.993 **Poisoning by other drugs, medicaments and biological substances, assault**
  - T50.994 **Poisoning by other drugs, medicaments and biological substances, undetermined**
  - T50.995 **Adverse effect of other drugs, medicaments and biological substances**
  - T50.996 **Underdosing of other drugs, medicaments and biological substances**

TOXIC EFFECTS OF SUBSTANCES CHIEFLY NONMEDICINAL AS TO SOURCE (T51-T65)

Note: When no intent is indicated code to accidental. Undetermined intent is only for use when there is specific documentation in the record that the intent of the toxic effect cannot be determined.

Use additional code(s): for all associated manifestations of toxic effect, such as:
respiratory conditions due to external agents (J60-J70)
personal history of foreign body fully removed (Z87.821)
to identify any retained foreign body, if applicable (Z18.-)

Excludes1 contact with and (suspected) exposure to toxic substances (Z77.-)

T51 **Toxic effect of alcohol**

The appropriate 7th character is to be added to each code from category T51

A	initial encounter
D	subsequent encounter
S	sequela

T51.0 **Toxic effect of ethanol**
Toxic effect of ethyl alcohol

Excludes2 acute alcohol intoxication or 'hangover' effects (F10.129, F10.229, F10.929)
drunkenness (F10.129, F10.229, F10.929)
pathological alcohol intoxication (F10.129, F10.229, F10.929)

- T51.0X **Toxic effect of ethanol**
  - T51.0X1 **Toxic effect of ethanol, accidental (unintentional)**
    Toxic effect of ethanol NOS
  - T51.0X2 **Toxic effect of ethanol, intentional self-harm**
  - T51.0X3 **Toxic effect of ethanol, assault**
  - T51.0X4 **Toxic effect of ethanol, undetermined**

T51.1 **Toxic effect of methanol**
Toxic effect of methyl alcohol

- T51.1X **Toxic effect of methanol**
  - T51.1X1 **Toxic effect of methanol, accidental (unintentional)**
    Toxic effect of methanol NOS
  - T51.1X2 **Toxic effect of methanol, intentional self-harm**
  - T51.1X3 **Toxic effect of methanol, assault**
  - T51.1X4 **Toxic effect of methanol, undetermined**

T51.2 **Toxic effect of 2-Propanol**
Toxic effect of isopropyl alcohol

- T51.2X **Toxic effect of 2-Propanol**
  - T51.2X1 **Toxic effect of 2-Propanol, accidental (unintentional)**
    Toxic effect of 2-Propanol NOS
  - T51.2X2 **Toxic effect of 2-Propanol, intentional self-harm**
  - T51.2X3 **Toxic effect of 2-Propanol, assault**
  - T51.2X4 **Toxic effect of 2-Propanol, undetermined**

T51.3 **Toxic effect of fusel oil**
Toxic effect of amyl alcohol
Toxic effect of butyl [1-butanol] alcohol
Toxic effect of propyl [1-propanol] alcohol

- T51.3X **Toxic effect of fusel oil**
  - T51.3X1 **Toxic effect of fusel oil, accidental (unintentional)**
    Toxic effect of fusel oil NOS
  - T51.3X2 **Toxic effect of fusel oil, intentional self-harm**
  - T51.3X3 **Toxic effect of fusel oil, assault**
  - T51.3X4 **Toxic effect of fusel oil, undetermined**

● T51.8 Toxic effect of other alcohols
● T51.8X Toxic effect of other alcohols
● T51.8X1 Toxic effect of other alcohols, accidental (unintentional)
Toxic effect of other alcohols NOS
● T51.8X2 Toxic effect of other alcohols, intentional self-harm
● T51.8X3 Toxic effect of other alcohols, assault
● T51.8X4 Toxic effect of other alcohols, undetermined
● T51.9 Toxic effect of unspecified alcohol
X● T51.91 Toxic effect of unspecified alcohol, accidental (unintentional)
X● T51.92 Toxic effect of unspecified alcohol, intentional self-harm
X● T51.93 Toxic effect of unspecified alcohol, assault
X● T51.94 Toxic effect of unspecified alcohol, undetermined

● T52 Toxic effect of organic solvents
Excludes1 halogen derivatives of aliphatic and aromatic hydrocarbons (T53.-)
The appropriate 7th character is to be added to each code from category T52

A	initial encounter
D	subsequent encounter
S	sequela

● T52.Ø Toxic effects of petroleum products
Toxic effects of gasoline [petrol]
Toxic effects of kerosene [paraffin oil]
Toxic effects of paraffin wax
Toxic effects of ether petroleum
Toxic effects of naphtha petroleum
Toxic effects of spirit petroleum
● T52.ØX Toxic effects of petroleum products
● T52.ØX1 Toxic effect of petroleum products, accidental (unintentional)
Toxic effects of petroleum products NOS
● T52.ØX2 Toxic effect of petroleum products, intentional self-harm
● T52.ØX3 Toxic effect of petroleum products, assault
● T52.ØX4 Toxic effect of petroleum products, undetermined
● T52.1 Toxic effects of benzene
Excludes1 homologues of benzene (T52.2)
nitroderivatives and aminoderivatives of benzene and its homologues (T65.3)
● T52.1X Toxic effects of benzene
● T52.1X1 Toxic effect of benzene, accidental (unintentional)
Toxic effects of benzene NOS
● T52.1X2 Toxic effect of benzene, intentional self-harm
● T52.1X3 Toxic effect of benzene, assault
● T52.1X4 Toxic effect of benzene, undetermined
● T52.2 Toxic effects of homologues of benzene
Toxic effects of toluene [methylbenzene]
Toxic effects of xylene [dimethylbenzene]
● T52.2X Toxic effects of homologues of benzene
● T52.2X1 Toxic effect of homologues of benzene, accidental (unintentional)
Toxic effects of homologues of benzene NOS
● T52.2X2 Toxic effect of homologues of benzene, intentional self-harm
● T52.2X3 Toxic effect of homologues of benzene, assault
● T52.2X4 Toxic effect of homologues of benzene, undetermined
● T52.3 Toxic effects of glycols
● T52.3X Toxic effects of glycols
● T52.3X1 Toxic effect of glycols, accidental (unintentional)
Toxic effects of glycols NOS
● T52.3X2 Toxic effect of glycols, intentional self-harm
● T52.3X3 Toxic effect of glycols, assault
● T52.3X4 Toxic effect of glycols, undetermined
● T52.4 Toxic effects of ketones
● T52.4X Toxic effects of ketones
● T52.4X1 Toxic effect of ketones, accidental (unintentional)
Toxic effects of ketones NOS
● T52.4X2 Toxic effect of ketones, intentional self-harm
● T52.4X3 Toxic effect of ketones, assault
● T52.4X4 Toxic effect of ketones, undetermined
● T52.8 Toxic effects of other organic solvents
● T52.8X Toxic effects of other organic solvents
● T52.8X1 Toxic effect of other organic solvents, accidental (unintentional)
Toxic effects of other organic solvents NOS
● T52.8X2 Toxic effect of other organic solvents, intentional self-harm
● T52.8X3 Toxic effect of other organic solvents, assault
● T52.8X4 Toxic effect of other organic solvents, undetermined
● T52.9 Toxic effects of unspecified organic solvent
X● T52.91 Toxic effect of unspecified organic solvent, accidental (unintentional)
X● T52.92 Toxic effect of unspecified organic solvent, intentional self-harm
X● T52.93 Toxic effect of unspecified organic solvent, assault
X● T52.94 Toxic effect of unspecified organic solvent, undetermined

● T53 Toxic effect of halogen derivatives of aliphatic and aromatic hydrocarbons
The appropriate 7th character is to be added to each code from category T53

A	initial encounter
D	subsequent encounter
S	sequela

● T53.Ø Toxic effects of carbon tetrachloride
Toxic effects of tetrachloromethane
● T53.ØX Toxic effects of carbon tetrachloride
● T53.ØX1 Toxic effect of carbon tetrachloride, accidental (unintentional)
Toxic effects of carbon tetrachloride NOS
● T53.ØX2 Toxic effect of carbon tetrachloride, intentional self-harm
● T53.ØX3 Toxic effect of carbon tetrachloride, assault
● T53.ØX4 Toxic effect of carbon tetrachloride, undetermined

● T53.1 Toxic effects of chloroform
Toxic effects of trichloromethane
● T53.1X Toxic effects of chloroform
● T53.1X1 Toxic effect of chloroform, accidental (unintentional)
Toxic effects of chloroform NOS
● T53.1X2 Toxic effect of chloroform, intentional self-harm
● T53.1X3 Toxic effect of chloroform, assault
● T53.1X4 Toxic effect of chloroform, undetermined
● T53.2 Toxic effects of trichloroethylene
Toxic effects of trichloroethene
● T53.2X Toxic effects of trichloroethylene
● T53.2X1 Toxic effect of trichloroethylene, accidental (unintentional)
Toxic effects of trichloroethylene NOS
● T53.2X2 Toxic effect of trichloroethylene, intentional self-harm
● T53.2X3 Toxic effect of trichloroethylene, assault
● T53.2X4 Toxic effect of trichloroethylene, undetermined
● T53.3 Toxic effects of tetrachloroethylene
Toxic effects of perchloroethylene
Toxic effect of tetrachloroethene
● T53.3X Toxic effects of tetrachloroethylene
● T53.3X1 Toxic effect of tetrachloroethylene, accidental (unintentional)
Toxic effects of tetrachloroethylene NOS
● T53.3X2 Toxic effect of tetrachloroethylene, intentional self-harm
● T53.3X3 Toxic effect of tetrachloroethylene, assault
● T53.3X4 Toxic effect of tetrachloroethylene, undetermined
● T53.4 Toxic effects of dichloromethane
Toxic effects of methylene chloride
● T53.4X Toxic effects of dichloromethane
● T53.4X1 Toxic effect of dichloromethane, accidental (unintentional)
Toxic effects of dichloromethane NOS
● T53.4X2 Toxic effect of dichloromethane, intentional self-harm
● T53.4X3 Toxic effect of dichloromethane, assault
● T53.4X4 Toxic effect of dichloromethane, undetermined
● T53.5 Toxic effects of chlorofluorocarbons
● T53.5X Toxic effects of chlorofluorocarbons
● T53.5X1 Toxic effect of chlorofluorocarbons, accidental (unintentional)
Toxic effects of chlorofluorocarbons NOS
● T53.5X2 Toxic effect of chlorofluorocarbons, intentional self-harm
● T53.5X3 Toxic effect of chlorofluorocarbons, assault
● T53.5X4 Toxic effect of chlorofluorocarbons, undetermined

● T53.6 Toxic effects of other halogen derivatives of aliphatic hydrocarbons
● T53.6X Toxic effects of other halogen derivatives of aliphatic hydrocarbons
● T53.6X1 Toxic effect of other halogen derivatives of aliphatic hydrocarbons, accidental (unintentional)
Toxic effects of other halogen derivatives of aliphatic hydrocarbons NOS
● T53.6X2 Toxic effect of other halogen derivatives of aliphatic hydrocarbons, intentional self-harm
● T53.6X3 Toxic effect of other halogen derivatives of aliphatic hydrocarbons, assault
● T53.6X4 Toxic effect of other halogen derivatives of aliphatic hydrocarbons, undetermined
● T53.7 Toxic effects of other halogen derivatives of aromatic hydrocarbons
● T53.7X Toxic effects of other halogen derivatives of aromatic hydrocarbons
● T53.7X1 Toxic effect of other halogen derivatives of aromatic hydrocarbons, accidental (unintentional)
Toxic effects of other halogen derivatives of aromatic hydrocarbons NOS
● T53.7X2 Toxic effect of other halogen derivatives of aromatic hydrocarbons, intentional self-harm
● T53.7X3 Toxic effect of other halogen derivatives of aromatic hydrocarbons, assault
● T53.7X4 Toxic effect of other halogen derivatives of aromatic hydrocarbons, undetermined
● T53.9 Toxic effects of unspecified halogen derivatives of aliphatic and aromatic hydrocarbons
X● T53.91 Toxic effect of unspecified halogen derivatives of aliphatic and aromatic hydrocarbons, accidental (unintentional)
X● T53.92 Toxic effect of unspecified halogen derivatives of aliphatic and aromatic hydrocarbons, intentional self-harm
X● T53.93 Toxic effect of unspecified halogen derivatives of aliphatic and aromatic hydrocarbons, assault
X● T53.94 Toxic effect of unspecified halogen derivatives of aliphatic and aromatic hydrocarbons, undetermined

● T54 Toxic effect of corrosive substances
The appropriate 7th character is to be added to each code from category T54

A	initial encounter
D	subsequent encounter
S	sequela

● T54.0 Toxic effects of phenol and phenol homologues
● T54.0X Toxic effects of phenol and phenol homologues
● T54.0X1 Toxic effect of phenol and phenol homologues, accidental (unintentional)
Toxic effects of phenol and phenol homologues NOS
● T54.0X2 Toxic effect of phenol and phenol homologues, intentional self-harm
● T54.0X3 Toxic effect of phenol and phenol homologues, assault
● T54.0X4 Toxic effect of phenol and phenol homologues, undetermined

CHAPTER 19 (S00-T88)

● **T54.1**   **Toxic effects of other corrosive organic compounds**
- ● **T54.1X**   **Toxic effects of other corrosive organic compounds**
  - ● **T54.1X1**   **Toxic effect of other corrosive organic compounds, accidental (unintentional)**
    Toxic effects of other corrosive organic compounds NOS
  - ● **T54.1X2**   **Toxic effect of other corrosive organic compounds, intentional self-harm**
  - ● **T54.1X3**   **Toxic effect of other corrosive organic compounds, assault**
  - ● **T54.1X4**   **Toxic effect of other corrosive organic compounds, undetermined**

● **T54.2**   **Toxic effects of corrosive acids and acid-like substances**
  Toxic effects of hydrochloric acid
  Toxic effects of sulfuric acid
- ● **T54.2X**   **Toxic effects of corrosive acids and acid-like substances**
  - ● **T54.2X1**   **Toxic effect of corrosive acids and acid-like substances, accidental (unintentional)**
    Toxic effects of corrosive acids and acid-like substances NOS
  - ● **T54.2X2**   **Toxic effect of corrosive acids and acid-like substances, intentional self-harm**
  - ● **T54.2X3**   **Toxic effect of corrosive acids and acid-like substances, assault**
  - ● **T54.2X4**   **Toxic effect of corrosive acids and acid-like substances, undetermined**

● **T54.3**   **Toxic effects of corrosive alkalis and alkali-like substances**
  Toxic effects of potassium hydroxide
  Toxic effects of sodium hydroxide
- ● **T54.3X**   **Toxic effects of corrosive alkalis and alkali-like substances**
  - ● **T54.3X1**   **Toxic effect of corrosive alkalis and alkali-like substances, accidental (unintentional)**
    Toxic effects of corrosive alkalis and alkali-like substances NOS
  - ● **T54.3X2**   **Toxic effect of corrosive alkalis and alkali-like substances, intentional self-harm**
  - ● **T54.3X3**   **Toxic effect of corrosive alkalis and alkali-like substances, assault**
  - ● **T54.3X4**   **Toxic effect of corrosive alkalis and alkali-like substances, undetermined**

● **T54.9**   **Toxic effects of unspecified corrosive substance**
- X ● **T54.91**   **Toxic effect of unspecified corrosive substance, accidental (unintentional)**
- X ● **T54.92**   **Toxic effect of unspecified corrosive substance, intentional self-harm**
- X ● **T54.93**   **Toxic effect of unspecified corrosive substance, assault**
- X ● **T54.94**   **Toxic effect of unspecified corrosive substance, undetermined**

● **T55**   **Toxic effect of soaps and detergents**
  The appropriate 7th character is to be added to each code from category T55

A	initial encounter
D	subsequent encounter
S	sequela

- ● **T55.0**   **Toxic effect of soaps**
  - ● **T55.0X**   **Toxic effect of soaps**
    - ● **T55.0X1**   **Toxic effect of soaps, accidental (unintentional)**
      Toxic effect of soaps NOS
    - ● **T55.0X2**   **Toxic effect of soaps, intentional self-harm**
    - ● **T55.0X3**   **Toxic effect of soaps, assault**
    - ● **T55.0X4**   **Toxic effect of soaps, undetermined**
- ● **T55.1**   **Toxic effect of detergents**
  - ● **T55.1X**   **Toxic effect of detergents**
    - ● **T55.1X1**   **Toxic effect of detergents, accidental (unintentional)**
      Toxic effect of detergents NOS
    - ● **T55.1X2**   **Toxic effect of detergents, intentional self-harm**
    - ● **T55.1X3**   **Toxic effect of detergents, assault**
    - ● **T55.1X4**   **Toxic effect of detergents, undetermined**

● **T56**   **Toxic effect of metals**

Includes   toxic effects of fumes and vapors of metals
toxic effects of metals from all sources, except medicinal substances

Use additional code to identify any retained metal foreign body, if applicable (Z18.0-, T18.1-)

Excludes1   arsenic and its compounds (T57.0)
manganese and its compounds (T57.2)

The appropriate 7th character is to be added to each code from category T56

A	initial encounter
D	subsequent encounter
S	sequela

- ● **T56.0**   **Toxic effects of lead and its compounds**
  - ● **T56.0X**   **Toxic effects of lead and its compounds**
    - ● **T56.0X1**   **Toxic effect of lead and its compounds, accidental (unintentional)**
      Toxic effects of lead and its compounds NOS
    - ● **T56.0X2**   **Toxic effect of lead and its compounds, intentional self-harm**
    - ● **T56.0X3**   **Toxic effect of lead and its compounds, assault**
    - ● **T56.0X4**   **Toxic effect of lead and its compounds, undetermined**
- ● **T56.1**   **Toxic effects of mercury and its compounds**
  - ● **T56.1X**   **Toxic effects of mercury and its compounds**
    - ● **T56.1X1**   **Toxic effect of mercury and its compounds, accidental (unintentional)**
      Toxic effects of mercury and its compounds NOS
    - ● **T56.1X2**   **Toxic effect of mercury and its compounds, intentional self-harm**
    - ● **T56.1X3**   **Toxic effect of mercury and its compounds, assault**
    - ● **T56.1X4**   **Toxic effect of mercury and its compounds, undetermined**

● T56.2   Toxic effects of chromium and its compounds
  ● T56.2X   Toxic effects of chromium and its compounds
    ● T56.2X1   Toxic effect of chromium and its compounds, accidental (unintentional)
      Toxic effects of chromium and its compounds NOS
    ● T56.2X2   Toxic effect of chromium and its compounds, intentional self-harm
    ● T56.2X3   Toxic effect of chromium and its compounds, assault
    ● T56.2X4   Toxic effect of chromium and its compounds, undetermined
● T56.3   Toxic effects of cadmium and its compounds
  ● T56.3X   Toxic effects of cadmium and its compounds
    ● T56.3X1   Toxic effect of cadmium and its compounds, accidental (unintentional)
      Toxic effects of cadmium and its compounds NOS
    ● T56.3X2   Toxic effect of cadmium and its compounds, intentional self-harm
    ● T56.3X3   Toxic effect of cadmium and its compounds, assault
    ● T56.3X4   Toxic effect of cadmium and its compounds, undetermined
● T56.4   Toxic effects of copper and its compounds
  ● T56.4X   Toxic effects of copper and its compounds
    ● T56.4X1   Toxic effect of copper and its compounds, accidental (unintentional)
      Toxic effects of copper and its compounds NOS
    ● T56.4X2   Toxic effect of copper and its compounds, intentional self-harm
    ● T56.4X3   Toxic effect of copper and its compounds, assault
    ● T56.4X4   Toxic effect of copper and its compounds, undetermined
● T56.5   Toxic effects of zinc and its compounds
  ● T56.5X   Toxic effects of zinc and its compounds
    ● T56.5X1   Toxic effect of zinc and its compounds, accidental (unintentional)
      Toxic effects of zinc and its compounds NOS
    ● T56.5X2   Toxic effect of zinc and its compounds, intentional self-harm
    ● T56.5X3   Toxic effect of zinc and its compounds, assault
    ● T56.5X4   Toxic effect of zinc and its compounds, undetermined
● T56.6   Toxic effects of tin and its compounds
  ● T56.6X   Toxic effects of tin and its compounds
    ● T56.6X1   Toxic effect of tin and its compounds, accidental (unintentional)
      Toxic effects of tin and its compounds NOS
    ● T56.6X2   Toxic effect of tin and its compounds, intentional self-harm
    ● T56.6X3   Toxic effect of tin and its compounds, assault
    ● T56.6X4   Toxic effect of tin and its compounds, undetermined

● T56.7   Toxic effects of beryllium and its compounds
  ● T56.7X   Toxic effects of beryllium and its compounds
    ● T56.7X1   Toxic effect of beryllium and its compounds, accidental (unintentional)
      Toxic effects of beryllium and its compounds NOS
    ● T56.7X2   Toxic effect of beryllium and its compounds, intentional self-harm
    ● T56.7X3   Toxic effect of beryllium and its compounds, assault
    ● T56.7X4   Toxic effect of beryllium and its compounds, undetermined
● T56.8   Toxic effects of other metals
  ● T56.81   Toxic effect of thallium
    ● T56.811   Toxic effect of thallium, accidental (unintentional)
      Toxic effect of thallium NOS
    ● T56.812   Toxic effect of thallium, intentional self-harm
    ● T56.813   Toxic effect of thallium, assault
    ● T56.814   Toxic effect of thallium, undetermined
  ● T56.89   Toxic effects of other metals
    ● T56.891   Toxic effect of other metals, accidental (unintentional)
      Toxic effects of other metals NOS
    ● T56.892   Toxic effect of other metals, intentional self-harm
    ● T56.893   Toxic effect of other metals, assault
    ● T56.894   Toxic effect of other metals, undetermined
● T56.9   Toxic effects of unspecified metal
  X ● T56.91   Toxic effect of unspecified metal, accidental (unintentional)
  X ● T56.92   Toxic effect of unspecified metal, intentional self-harm
  X ● T56.93   Toxic effect of unspecified metal, assault
  X ● T56.94   Toxic effect of unspecified metal, undetermined

● T57   Toxic effect of other inorganic substances
  The appropriate 7th character is to be added to each code from category T57

> | A | initial encounter |
> | D | subsequent encounter |
> | S | sequela |

● T57.0   Toxic effect of arsenic and its compounds
  ● T57.0X   Toxic effect of arsenic and its compounds
    ● T57.0X1   Toxic effect of arsenic and its compounds, accidental (unintentional)
      Toxic effect of arsenic and its compounds NOS
    ● T57.0X2   Toxic effect of arsenic and its compounds, intentional self-harm
    ● T57.0X3   Toxic effect of arsenic and its compounds, assault
    ● T57.0X4   Toxic effect of arsenic and its compounds, undetermined

CHAPTER 19 (S00–T88)

● T57.1 **Toxic effect of phosphorus and its compounds**
Excludes1 organophosphate insecticides (T60.0)
● T57.1X **Toxic effect of phosphorus and its compounds**
● T57.1X1 **Toxic effect of phosphorus and its compounds, accidental (unintentional)**
Toxic effect of phosphorus and its compounds NOS
● T57.1X2 **Toxic effect of phosphorus and its compounds, intentional self-harm**
● T57.1X3 **Toxic effect of phosphorus and its compounds, assault**
● T57.1X4 **Toxic effect of phosphorus and its compounds, undetermined**
● T57.2 **Toxic effect of manganese and its compounds**
● T57.2X **Toxic effect of manganese and its compounds**
● T57.2X1 **Toxic effect of manganese and its compounds, accidental (unintentional)**
Toxic effect of manganese and its compounds NOS
● T57.2X2 **Toxic effect of manganese and its compounds, intentional self-harm**
● T57.2X3 **Toxic effect of manganese and its compounds, assault**
● T57.2X4 **Toxic effect of manganese and its compounds, undetermined**
● T57.3 **Toxic effect of hydrogen cyanide**
● T57.3X **Toxic effect of hydrogen cyanide**
● T57.3X1 **Toxic effect of hydrogen cyanide, accidental (unintentional)**
Toxic effect of hydrogen cyanide NOS
● T57.3X2 **Toxic effect of hydrogen cyanide, intentional self-harm**
● T57.3X3 **Toxic effect of hydrogen cyanide, assault**
● T57.3X4 **Toxic effect of hydrogen cyanide, undetermined**
● T57.8 **Toxic effect of other specified inorganic substances**
● T57.8X **Toxic effect of other specified inorganic substances**
● T57.8X1 **Toxic effect of other specified inorganic substances, accidental (unintentional)**
Toxic effect of other specified inorganic substances NOS
● T57.8X2 **Toxic effect of other specified inorganic substances, intentional self-harm**
● T57.8X3 **Toxic effect of other specified inorganic substances, assault**
● T57.8X4 **Toxic effect of other specified inorganic substances, undetermined**
● T57.9 **Toxic effect of unspecified inorganic substance**
X● T57.91 **Toxic effect of unspecified inorganic substance, accidental (unintentional)**
X● T57.92 **Toxic effect of unspecified inorganic substance, intentional self-harm**
X● T57.93 **Toxic effect of unspecified inorganic substance, assault**
X● T57.94 **Toxic effect of unspecified inorganic substance, undetermined**

● T58 **Toxic effect of carbon monoxide**
Includes asphyxiation from carbon monoxide
toxic effect of carbon monoxide from all sources
The appropriate 7th character is to be added to each code from category T58

A	initial encounter
D	subsequent encounter
S	sequela

● T58.0 **Toxic effect of carbon monoxide from motor vehicle exhaust**
Toxic effect of exhaust gas from gas engine
Toxic effect of exhaust gas from motor pump
X● T58.01 **Toxic effect of carbon monoxide from motor vehicle exhaust, accidental (unintentional)**
X● T58.02 **Toxic effect of carbon monoxide from motor vehicle exhaust, intentional self-harm**
X● T58.03 **Toxic effect of carbon monoxide from motor vehicle exhaust, assault**
X● T58.04 **Toxic effect of carbon monoxide from motor vehicle exhaust, undetermined**
● T58.1 **Toxic effect of carbon monoxide from utility gas**
Toxic effect of acetylene
Toxic effect of gas NOS used for lighting, heating, cooking
Toxic effect of water gas
X● T58.11 **Toxic effect of carbon monoxide from utility gas, accidental (unintentional)**
X● T58.12 **Toxic effect of carbon monoxide from utility gas, intentional self-harm**
X● T58.13 **Toxic effect of carbon monoxide from utility gas, assault**
X● T58.14 **Toxic effect of carbon monoxide from utility gas, undetermined**
● T58.2 **Toxic effect of carbon monoxide from incomplete combustion of other domestic fuels**
Toxic effect of carbon monoxide from incomplete combustion of coal, coke, kerosene, wood
● T58.2X **Toxic effect of carbon monoxide from incomplete combustion of other domestic fuels**
● T58.2X1 **Toxic effect of carbon monoxide from incomplete combustion of other domestic fuels, accidental (unintentional)**
● T58.2X2 **Toxic effect of carbon monoxide from incomplete combustion of other domestic fuels, intentional self-harm**
● T58.2X3 **Toxic effect of carbon monoxide from incomplete combustion of other domestic fuels, assault**
● T58.2X4 **Toxic effect of carbon monoxide from incomplete combustion of other domestic fuels, undetermined**
● T58.8 **Toxic effect of carbon monoxide from other source**
Toxic effect of carbon monoxide from blast furnace gas
Toxic effect of carbon monoxide from fuels in industrial use
Toxic effect of carbon monoxide from kiln vapor
● T58.8X **Toxic effect of carbon monoxide from other source**
● T58.8X1 **Toxic effect of carbon monoxide from other source, accidental (unintentional)**
● T58.8X2 **Toxic effect of carbon monoxide from other source, intentional self-harm**
● T58.8X3 **Toxic effect of carbon monoxide from other source, assault**
● T58.8X4 **Toxic effect of carbon monoxide from other source, undetermined**

CHAPTER 19 (S00-T88)

◀ New ⟸ Revised ~~deleted~~ Deleted OCGR Official Guidelines X Assign placeholder X ● Use Additional Character(s)
Excludes 1 Excludes 2 Includes Use additional Code first Code also Unspecified

- ● T58.9 Toxic effect of carbon monoxide from unspecified source
  - X● T58.91 Toxic effect of carbon monoxide from unspecified source, accidental (unintentional)
  - X● T58.92 Toxic effect of carbon monoxide from unspecified source, intentional self-harm
  - X● T58.93 Toxic effect of carbon monoxide from unspecified source, assault
  - X● T58.94 Toxic effect of carbon monoxide from unspecified source, undetermined

● T59 Toxic effect of other gases, fumes and vapors

Includes aerosol propellants

Excludes1 chlorofluorocarbons (T53.5)

The appropriate 7th character is to be added to each code from category T59

A	initial encounter
D	subsequent encounter
S	sequela

- ● T59.0 Toxic effect of nitrogen oxides
  - ● T59.0X Toxic effect of nitrogen oxides
    - ● T59.0X1 Toxic effect of nitrogen oxides, accidental (unintentional)
      Toxic effect of nitrogen oxides NOS
    - ● T59.0X2 Toxic effect of nitrogen oxides, intentional self-harm
    - ● T59.0X3 Toxic effect of nitrogen oxides, assault
    - ● T59.0X4 Toxic effect of nitrogen oxides, undetermined
- ● T59.1 Toxic effect of sulfur dioxide
  - ● T59.1X Toxic effect of sulfur dioxide
    - ● T59.1X1 Toxic effect of sulfur dioxide, accidental (unintentional)
      Toxic effect of sulfur dioxide NOS
    - ● T59.1X2 Toxic effect of sulfur dioxide, intentional self-harm
    - ● T59.1X3 Toxic effect of sulfur dioxide, assault
    - ● T59.1X4 Toxic effect of sulfur dioxide, undetermined
- ● T59.2 Toxic effect of formaldehyde
  - ● T59.2X Toxic effect of formaldehyde
    - ● T59.2X1 Toxic effect of formaldehyde, accidental (unintentional)
      Toxic effect of formaldehyde NOS
    - ● T59.2X2 Toxic effect of formaldehyde, intentional self-harm
    - ● T59.2X3 Toxic effect of formaldehyde, assault
    - ● T59.2X4 Toxic effect of formaldehyde, undetermined
- ● T59.3 Toxic effect of lacrimogenic gas
  Toxic effect of tear gas
  - ● T59.3X Toxic effect of lacrimogenic gas
    - ● T59.3X1 Toxic effect of lacrimogenic gas, accidental (unintentional)
      Toxic effect of lacrimogenic gas NOS
    - ● T59.3X2 Toxic effect of lacrimogenic gas, intentional self-harm
    - ● T59.3X3 Toxic effect of lacrimogenic gas, assault
    - ● T59.3X4 Toxic effect of lacrimogenic gas, undetermined
- ● T59.4 Toxic effect of chlorine gas
  - ● T59.4X Toxic effect of chlorine gas
    - ● T59.4X1 Toxic effect of chlorine gas, accidental (unintentional)
      Toxic effect of chlorine gas NOS
    - ● T59.4X2 Toxic effect of chlorine gas, intentional self-harm
    - ● T59.4X3 Toxic effect of chlorine gas, assault
    - ● T59.4X4 Toxic effect of chlorine gas, undetermined
- ● T59.5 Toxic effect of fluorine gas and hydrogen fluoride
  - ● T59.5X Toxic effect of fluorine gas and hydrogen fluoride
    - ● T59.5X1 Toxic effect of fluorine gas and hydrogen fluoride, accidental (unintentional)
      Toxic effect of fluorine gas and hydrogen fluoride NOS
    - ● T59.5X2 Toxic effect of fluorine gas and hydrogen fluoride, intentional self-harm
    - ● T59.5X3 Toxic effect of fluorine gas and hydrogen fluoride, assault
    - ● T59.5X4 Toxic effect of fluorine gas and hydrogen fluoride, undetermined
- ● T59.6 Toxic effect of hydrogen sulfide
  - ● T59.6X Toxic effect of hydrogen sulfide
    - ● T59.6X1 Toxic effect of hydrogen sulfide, accidental (unintentional)
      Toxic effect of hydrogen sulfide NOS
    - ● T59.6X2 Toxic effect of hydrogen sulfide, intentional self-harm
    - ● T59.6X3 Toxic effect of hydrogen sulfide, assault
    - ● T59.6X4 Toxic effect of hydrogen sulfide, undetermined
- ● T59.7 Toxic effect of carbon dioxide
  - ● T59.7X Toxic effect of carbon dioxide
    - ● T59.7X1 Toxic effect of carbon dioxide, accidental (unintentional)
      Toxic effect of carbon dioxide NOS
    - ● T59.7X2 Toxic effect of carbon dioxide, intentional self-harm
    - ● T59.7X3 Toxic effect of carbon dioxide, assault
    - ● T59.7X4 Toxic effect of carbon dioxide, undetermined
- ● T59.8 Toxic effect of other specified gases, fumes and vapors
  - ● T59.81 Toxic effect of smoke
    Smoke inhalation
    Excludes2 toxic effect of cigarette (tobacco) smoke (T65.22-)
    - ● T59.811 Toxic effect of smoke, accidental (unintentional)
      Toxic effect of smoke NOS
    - ● T59.812 Toxic effect of smoke, intentional self-harm
    - ● T59.813 Toxic effect of smoke, assault
    - ● T59.814 Toxic effect of smoke, undetermined
  - ● T59.89 Toxic effect of other specified gases, fumes and vapors
    - ● T59.891 Toxic effect of other specified gases, fumes and vapors, accidental (unintentional)
    - ● T59.892 Toxic effect of other specified gases, fumes and vapors, intentional self-harm
    - ● T59.893 Toxic effect of other specified gases, fumes and vapors, assault
    - ● T59.894 Toxic effect of other specified gases, fumes and vapors, undetermined

● T59.9 **Toxic effect of unspecified gases, fumes and vapors**
X● T59.91 **Toxic effect of unspecified gases, fumes and vapors, accidental (unintentional)**
X● T59.92 **Toxic effect of unspecified gases, fumes and vapors, intentional self-harm**
X● T59.93 **Toxic effect of unspecified gases, fumes and vapors, assault**
X● T59.94 **Toxic effect of unspecified gases, fumes and vapors, undetermined**

● T60 **Toxic effect of pesticides**
Includes toxic effect of wood preservatives
The appropriate 7th character is to be added to each code from category T60

A initial encounter
D subsequent encounter
S sequela

● T60.0 **Toxic effect of organophosphate and carbamate insecticides**
● T60.0X **Toxic effect of organophosphate and carbamate insecticides**
● T60.0X1 **Toxic effect of organophosphate and carbamate insecticides, accidental (unintentional)**
Toxic effect of organophosphate and carbamate insecticides NOS
● T60.0X2 **Toxic effect of organophosphate and carbamate insecticides, intentional self-harm**
● T60.0X3 **Toxic effect of organophosphate and carbamate insecticides, assault**
● T60.0X4 **Toxic effect of organophosphate and carbamate insecticides, undetermined**
● T60.1 **Toxic effect of halogenated insecticides**
Excludes1 chlorinated hydrocarbon (T53.-)
● T60.1X **Toxic effect of halogenated insecticides**
● T60.1X1 **Toxic effect of halogenated insecticides, accidental (unintentional)**
Toxic effect of halogenated insecticides NOS
● T60.1X2 **Toxic effect of halogenated insecticides, intentional self-harm**
● T60.1X3 **Toxic effect of halogenated insecticides, assault**
● T60.1X4 **Toxic effect of halogenated insecticides, undetermined**
● T60.2 **Toxic effect of other insecticides**
● T60.2X **Toxic effect of other insecticides**
● T60.2X1 **Toxic effect of other insecticides, accidental (unintentional)**
Toxic effect of other insecticides NOS
● T60.2X2 **Toxic effect of other insecticides, intentional self-harm**
● T60.2X3 **Toxic effect of other insecticides, assault**
● T60.2X4 **Toxic effect of other insecticides, undetermined**
● T60.3 **Toxic effect of herbicides and fungicides**
● T60.3X **Toxic effect of herbicides and fungicides**
● T60.3X1 **Toxic effect of herbicides and fungicides, accidental (unintentional)**
Toxic effect of herbicides and fungicides NOS
● T60.3X2 **Toxic effect of herbicides and fungicides, intentional self-harm**
● T60.3X3 **Toxic effect of herbicides and fungicides, assault**
● T60.3X4 **Toxic effect of herbicides and fungicides, undetermined**
● T60.4 **Toxic effect of rodenticides**
Excludes1 strychnine and its salts (T65.1)
thallium (T56.81-)
● T60.4X **Toxic effect of rodenticides**
● T60.4X1 **Toxic effect of rodenticides, accidental (unintentional)**
Toxic effect of rodenticides NOS
● T60.4X2 **Toxic effect of rodenticides, intentional self-harm**
● T60.4X3 **Toxic effect of rodenticides, assault**
● T60.4X4 **Toxic effect of rodenticides, undetermined**
● T60.8 **Toxic effect of other pesticides**
● T60.8X **Toxic effect of other pesticides**
● T60.8X1 **Toxic effect of other pesticides, accidental (unintentional)**
Toxic effect of other pesticides NOS
● T60.8X2 **Toxic effect of other pesticides, intentional self-harm**
● T60.8X3 **Toxic effect of other pesticides, assault**
● T60.8X4 **Toxic effect of other pesticides, undetermined**
● T60.9 **Toxic effect of unspecified pesticide**
X● T60.91 **Toxic effect of unspecified pesticide, accidental (unintentional)**
X● T60.92 **Toxic effect of unspecified pesticide, intentional self-harm**
X● T60.93 **Toxic effect of unspecified pesticide, assault**
X● T60.94 **Toxic effect of unspecified pesticide, undetermined**

● T61 **Toxic effect of noxious substances eaten as seafood**
Excludes1 allergic reaction to food, such as:
anaphylactic reaction or shock due to adverse food reaction (T78.0-)
bacterial foodborne intoxications (A05.-)
dermatitis (L23.6, L25.4, L27.2)
food protein-induced enterocolitis syndrome (K52.21) ◀
food protein-induced enteropathy (K52.22) ◀
gastroenteritis (noninfective) (K52.29) ◀
toxic effect of aflatoxin and other mycotoxins (T64)
toxic effect of cyanides (T65.0-)
toxic effect of harmful algae bloom (T65.82-)
toxic effect of hydrogen cyanide (T57.3-)
toxic effect of mercury (T56.1-)
toxic effect of red tide (T65.82-)
The appropriate 7th character is to be added to each code from category T61

A initial encounter
D subsequent encounter
S sequela

● T61.0 **Ciguatera fish poisoning**
X● T61.01 **Ciguatera fish poisoning, accidental (unintentional)**
X● T61.02 **Ciguatera fish poisoning, intentional self-harm**
X● T61.03 **Ciguatera fish poisoning, assault**
X● T61.04 **Ciguatera fish poisoning, undetermined**
● T61.1 **Scombroid fish poisoning**
Histamine-like syndrome
X● T61.11 **Scombroid fish poisoning, accidental (unintentional)**
X● T61.12 **Scombroid fish poisoning, intentional self-harm**
X● T61.13 **Scombroid fish poisoning, assault**
X● T61.14 **Scombroid fish poisoning, undetermined**

● T61.7 Other fish and shellfish poisoning
● T61.77 Other fish poisoning
● T61.771 Other fish poisoning, accidental (unintentional)
● T61.772 Other fish poisoning, intentional self-harm
● T61.773 Other fish poisoning, assault
● T61.774 Other fish poisoning, undetermined
● T61.78 Other shellfish poisoning
● T61.781 Other shellfish poisoning, accidental (unintentional)
● T61.782 Other shellfish poisoning, intentional self-harm
● T61.783 Other shellfish poisoning, assault
● T61.784 Other shellfish poisoning, undetermined
● T61.8 Toxic effect of other seafood
● T61.8X Toxic effect of other seafood
● T61.8X1 Toxic effect of other seafood, accidental (unintentional)
● T61.8X2 Toxic effect of other seafood, intentional self-harm
● T61.8X3 Toxic effect of other seafood, assault
● T61.8X4 Toxic effect of other seafood, undetermined
● T61.9 Toxic effect of unspecified seafood
X● T61.91 Toxic effect of unspecified seafood, accidental (unintentional)
X● T61.92 Toxic effect of unspecified seafood, intentional self-harm
X● T61.93 Toxic effect of unspecified seafood, assault
X● T61.94 Toxic effect of unspecified seafood, undetermined

● T62 Toxic effect of other noxious substances eaten as food

Excludes1 allergic reaction to food, such as:
anaphylactic shock (reaction) due to adverse food reaction (T78.0-)
dermatitis (L23.6, L25.4, L27.2)
food protein-induced enterocolitis syndrome (K52.21) ◀
food protein-induced enteropathy (K52.22) ◀
gastroenteritis (noninfective) (K52.29) ◀
bacterial food borne intoxications (A05.-)
toxic effect of aflatoxin and other mycotoxins (T64)
toxic effect of cyanides (T65.0-)
toxic effect of hydrogen cyanide (T57.3-)
toxic effect of mercury (T56.1-)

The appropriate 7th character is to be added to each code from category T62

A initial encounter
D subsequent encounter
S sequela

● T62.0 Toxic effect of ingested mushrooms
● T62.0X Toxic effect of ingested mushrooms
● T62.0X1 Toxic effect of ingested mushrooms, accidental (unintentional)
Toxic effect of ingested mushrooms NOS
● T62.0X2 Toxic effect of ingested mushrooms, intentional self-harm
● T62.0X3 Toxic effect of ingested mushrooms, assault
● T62.0X4 Toxic effect of ingested mushrooms, undetermined
● T62.1 Toxic effect of ingested berries
● T62.1X Toxic effect of ingested berries
● T62.1X1 Toxic effect of ingested berries, accidental (unintentional)
Toxic effect of ingested berries NOS
● T62.1X2 Toxic effect of ingested berries, intentional self-harm
● T62.1X3 Toxic effect of ingested berries, assault
● T62.1X4 Toxic effect of ingested berries, undetermined
● T62.2 Toxic effect of other ingested (parts of) plant(s)
● T62.2X Toxic effect of other ingested (parts of) plant(s)
● T62.2X1 Toxic effect of other ingested (parts of) plant(s), accidental (unintentional)
Toxic effect of other ingested (parts of) plant(s) NOS
● T62.2X2 Toxic effect of other ingested (parts of) plant(s), intentional self-harm
● T62.2X3 Toxic effect of other ingested (parts of) plant(s), assault
● T62.2X4 Toxic effect of other ingested (parts of) plant(s), undetermined
● T62.8 Toxic effect of other specified noxious substances eaten as food
● T62.8X Toxic effect of other specified noxious substances eaten as food
● T62.8X1 Toxic effect of other specified noxious substances eaten as food, accidental (unintentional)
Toxic effect of other specified noxious substances eaten as food NOS
● T62.8X2 Toxic effect of other specified noxious substances eaten as food, intentional self-harm
● T62.8X3 Toxic effect of other specified noxious substances eaten as food, assault
● T62.8X4 Toxic effect of other specified noxious substances eaten as food, undetermined
● T62.9 Toxic effect of unspecified noxious substance eaten as food
X● T62.91 Toxic effect of unspecified noxious substance eaten as food, accidental (unintentional)
Toxic effect of unspecified noxious substance eaten as food NOS
X● T62.92 Toxic effect of unspecified noxious substance eaten as food, intentional self-harm
X● T62.93 Toxic effect of unspecified noxious substance eaten as food, assault
X● T62.94 Toxic effect of unspecified noxious substance eaten as food, undetermined

● T63 Toxic effect of contact with venomous animals and plants

Includes bite or touch of venomous animal
pricked or stuck by thorn or leaf

Excludes2 ingestion of toxic animal or plant (T61.-, T62.-)

The appropriate 7th character is to be added to each code from category T63

A initial encounter
D subsequent encounter
S sequela

● T63.0 Toxic effect of snake venom
● T63.00 Toxic effect of unspecified snake venom
● T63.001 Toxic effect of unspecified snake venom, accidental (unintentional)
Toxic effect of unspecified snake venom NOS
● T63.002 Toxic effect of unspecified snake venom, intentional self-harm
● T63.003 Toxic effect of unspecified snake venom, assault
● T63.004 Toxic effect of unspecified snake venom, undetermined

CHAPTER 19 (S00-T88)

● T63.01 Toxic effect of rattlesnake venom
● T63.011 Toxic effect of rattlesnake venom, accidental (unintentional)
Toxic effect of rattlesnake venom NOS
● T63.012 Toxic effect of rattlesnake venom, intentional self-harm
● T63.013 Toxic effect of rattlesnake venom, assault
● T63.014 Toxic effect of rattlesnake venom, undetermined
● T63.02 Toxic effect of coral snake venom
● T63.021 Toxic effect of coral snake venom, accidental (unintentional)
Toxic effect of coral snake venom NOS
● T63.022 Toxic effect of coral snake venom, intentional self-harm
● T63.023 Toxic effect of coral snake venom, assault
● T63.024 Toxic effect of coral snake venom, undetermined
● T63.03 Toxic effect of taipan venom
● T63.031 Toxic effect of taipan venom, accidental (unintentional)
Toxic effect of taipan venom NOS
● T63.032 Toxic effect of taipan venom, intentional self-harm
● T63.033 Toxic effect of taipan venom, assault
● T63.034 Toxic effect of taipan venom, undetermined
● T63.04 Toxic effect of cobra venom
● T63.041 Toxic effect of cobra venom, accidental (unintentional)
Toxic effect of cobra venom NOS
● T63.042 Toxic effect of cobra venom, intentional self-harm
● T63.043 Toxic effect of cobra venom, assault
● T63.044 Toxic effect of cobra venom, undetermined
● T63.06 Toxic effect of venom of other North and South American snake
● T63.061 Toxic effect of venom of other North and South American snake, accidental (unintentional)
Toxic effect of venom of other North and South American snake NOS
● T63.062 Toxic effect of venom of other North and South American snake, intentional self-harm
● T63.063 Toxic effect of venom of other North and South American snake, assault
● T63.064 Toxic effect of venom of other North and South American snake, undetermined
● T63.07 Toxic effect of venom of other Australian snake
● T63.071 Toxic effect of venom of other Australian snake, accidental (unintentional)
Toxic effect of venom of other Australian snake NOS
● T63.072 Toxic effect of venom of other Australian snake, intentional self-harm
● T63.073 Toxic effect of venom of other Australian snake, assault
● T63.074 Toxic effect of venom of other Australian snake, undetermined
● T63.08 Toxic effect of venom of other African and Asian snake
● T63.081 Toxic effect of venom of other African and Asian snake, accidental (unintentional)
Toxic effect of venom of other African and Asian snake NOS
● T63.082 Toxic effect of venom of other African and Asian snake, intentional self-harm
● T63.083 Toxic effect of venom of other African and Asian snake, assault
● T63.084 Toxic effect of venom of other African and Asian snake, undetermined
● T63.09 Toxic effect of venom of other snake
● T63.091 Toxic effect of venom of other snake, accidental (unintentional)
Toxic effect of venom of other snake NOS
● T63.092 Toxic effect of venom of other snake, intentional self-harm
● T63.093 Toxic effect of venom of other snake, assault
● T63.094 Toxic effect of venom of other snake, undetermined
● T63.1 Toxic effect of venom of other reptiles
● T63.11 Toxic effect of venom of gila monster
● T63.111 Toxic effect of venom of gila monster, accidental (unintentional)
Toxic effect of venom of gila monster NOS
● T63.112 Toxic effect of venom of gila monster, intentional self-harm
● T63.113 Toxic effect of venom of gila monster, assault
● T63.114 Toxic effect of venom of gila monster, undetermined
● T63.12 Toxic effect of venom of other venomous lizard
● T63.121 Toxic effect of venom of other venomous lizard, accidental (unintentional)
Toxic effect of venom of other venomous lizard NOS
● T63.122 Toxic effect of venom of other venomous lizard, intentional self-harm
● T63.123 Toxic effect of venom of other venomous lizard, assault
● T63.124 Toxic effect of venom of other venomous lizard, undetermined
● T63.19 Toxic effect of venom of other reptiles
● T63.191 Toxic effect of venom of other reptiles, accidental (unintentional)
Toxic effect of venom of other reptiles NOS
● T63.192 Toxic effect of venom of other reptiles, intentional self-harm
● T63.193 Toxic effect of venom of other reptiles, assault
● T63.194 Toxic effect of venom of other reptiles, undetermined
● T63.2 Toxic effect of venom of scorpion
● T63.2X Toxic effect of venom of scorpion
● T63.2X1 Toxic effect of venom of scorpion, accidental (unintentional)
Toxic effect of venom of scorpion NOS
● T63.2X2 Toxic effect of venom of scorpion, intentional self-harm

● T63.2X3　Toxic effect of venom of scorpion, assault
● T63.2X4　Toxic effect of venom of scorpion, undetermined
● T63.3　**Toxic effect of venom of spider**
　● T63.30　Toxic effect of unspecified spider venom
　　● T63.301　Toxic effect of unspecified spider venom, accidental (unintentional)
　　● T63.302　Toxic effect of unspecified spider venom, intentional self-harm
　　● T63.303　Toxic effect of unspecified spider venom, assault
　　● T63.304　Toxic effect of unspecified spider venom, undetermined
　● T63.31　Toxic effect of venom of black widow spider
　　● T63.311　Toxic effect of venom of black widow spider, accidental (unintentional)
　　● T63.312　Toxic effect of venom of black widow spider, intentional self-harm
　　● T63.313　Toxic effect of venom of black widow spider, assault
　　● T63.314　Toxic effect of venom of black widow spider, undetermined
　● T63.32　Toxic effect of venom of tarantula
　　● T63.321　Toxic effect of venom of tarantula, accidental (unintentional)
　　● T63.322　Toxic effect of venom of tarantula, intentional self-harm
　　● T63.323　Toxic effect of venom of tarantula, assault
　　● T63.324　Toxic effect of venom of tarantula, undetermined
　● T63.33　Toxic effect of venom of brown recluse spider
　　● T63.331　Toxic effect of venom of brown recluse spider, accidental (unintentional)
　　● T63.332　Toxic effect of venom of brown recluse spider, intentional self-harm
　　● T63.333　Toxic effect of venom of brown recluse spider, assault
　　● T63.334　Toxic effect of venom of brown recluse spider, undetermined
　● T63.39　Toxic effect of venom of other spider
　　● T63.391　Toxic effect of venom of other spider, accidental (unintentional)
　　● T63.392　Toxic effect of venom of other spider, intentional self-harm
　　● T63.393　Toxic effect of venom of other spider, assault
　　● T63.394　Toxic effect of venom of other spider, undetermined
● T63.4　**Toxic effect of venom of other arthropods**
　● T63.41　Toxic effect of venom of centipedes and venomous millipedes
　　● T63.411　Toxic effect of venom of centipedes and venomous millipedes, accidental (unintentional)
　　● T63.412　Toxic effect of venom of centipedes and venomous millipedes, intentional self-harm
　　● T63.413　Toxic effect of venom of centipedes and venomous millipedes, assault
　　● T63.414　Toxic effect of venom of centipedes and venomous millipedes, undetermined

● T63.42　Toxic effect of venom of ants
　● T63.421　Toxic effect of venom of ants, accidental (unintentional)
　● T63.422　Toxic effect of venom of ants, intentional self-harm
　● T63.423　Toxic effect of venom of ants, assault
　● T63.424　Toxic effect of venom of ants, undetermined
● T63.43　Toxic effect of venom of caterpillars
　● T63.431　Toxic effect of venom of caterpillars, accidental (unintentional)
　● T63.432　Toxic effect of venom of caterpillars, intentional self-harm
　● T63.433　Toxic effect of venom of caterpillars, assault
　● T63.434　Toxic effect of venom of caterpillars, undetermined
● T63.44　Toxic effect of venom of bees
　● T63.441　Toxic effect of venom of bees, accidental (unintentional)
　● T63.442　Toxic effect of venom of bees, intentional self-harm
　● T63.443　Toxic effect of venom of bees, assault
　● T63.444　Toxic effect of venom of bees, undetermined
● T63.45　Toxic effect of venom of hornets
　● T63.451　Toxic effect of venom of hornets, accidental (unintentional)
　● T63.452　Toxic effect of venom of hornets, intentional self-harm
　● T63.453　Toxic effect of venom of hornets, assault
　● T63.454　Toxic effect of venom of hornets, undetermined
● T63.46　Toxic effect of venom of wasps
　　Toxic effect of yellow jacket
　● T63.461　Toxic effect of venom of wasps, accidental (unintentional)
　● T63.462　Toxic effect of venom of wasps, intentional self-harm
　● T63.463　Toxic effect of venom of wasps, assault
　● T63.464　Toxic effect of venom of wasps, undetermined
● T63.48　Toxic effect of venom of other arthropod
　● T63.481　Toxic effect of venom of other arthropod, accidental (unintentional)
　● T63.482　Toxic effect of venom of other arthropod, intentional self-harm
　● T63.483　Toxic effect of venom of other arthropod, assault
　● T63.484　Toxic effect of venom of other arthropod, undetermined
● T63.5　**Toxic effect of contact with venomous fish**
　Excludes2　poisoning by ingestion of fish (T61.-)
　● T63.51　Toxic effect of contact with stingray
　　● T63.511　Toxic effect of contact with stingray, accidental (unintentional)
　　● T63.512　Toxic effect of contact with stingray, intentional self-harm
　　● T63.513　Toxic effect of contact with stingray, assault
　　● T63.514　Toxic effect of contact with stingray, undetermined

◀ New　◀▥ Revised　~~deleted~~ Deleted　**OGCR** Official Guidelines　X Assign placeholder X　● Use Additional Character(s)
Excludes 1　Excludes 2　Includes　Use additional　Code first　Code also　Unspecified

● **T63.59**   Toxic effect of contact with other venomous fish
- ● **T63.591**   Toxic effect of contact with other venomous fish, accidental (unintentional)
- ● **T63.592**   Toxic effect of contact with other venomous fish, intentional self-harm
- ● **T63.593**   Toxic effect of contact with other venomous fish, assault
- ● **T63.594**   Toxic effect of contact with other venomous fish, undetermined

● **T63.6**   Toxic effect of contact with other venomous marine animals

> **Excludes1**   sea-snake venom (T63.09)
> **Excludes2**   poisoning by ingestion of shellfish (T61.78-)

- ● **T63.61**   Toxic effect of contact with Portugese Man-o-war
  - Toxic effect of contact with bluebottle
  - ● **T63.611**   Toxic effect of contact with Portugese Man-o-war, accidental (unintentional)
  - ● **T63.612**   Toxic effect of contact with Portugese Man-o-war, intentional self-harm
  - ● **T63.613**   Toxic effect of contact with Portugese Man-o-war, assault
  - ● **T63.614**   Toxic effect of contact with Portugese Man-o-war, undetermined
- ● **T63.62**   Toxic effect of contact with other jellyfish
  - ● **T63.621**   Toxic effect of contact with other jellyfish, accidental (unintentional)
  - ● **T63.622**   Toxic effect of contact with other jellyfish, intentional self-harm
  - ● **T63.623**   Toxic effect of contact with other jellyfish, assault
  - ● **T63.624**   Toxic effect of contact with other jellyfish, undetermined
- ● **T63.63**   Toxic effect of contact with sea anemone
  - ● **T63.631**   Toxic effect of contact with sea anemone, accidental (unintentional)
  - ● **T63.632**   Toxic effect of contact with sea anemone, intentional self-harm
  - ● **T63.633**   Toxic effect of contact with sea anemone, assault
  - ● **T63.634**   Toxic effect of contact with sea anemone, undetermined
- ● **T63.69**   Toxic effect of contact with other venomous marine animals
  - ● **T63.691**   Toxic effect of contact with other venomous marine animals, accidental (unintentional)
  - ● **T63.692**   Toxic effect of contact with other venomous marine animals, intentional self-harm
  - ● **T63.693**   Toxic effect of contact with other venomous marine animals, assault
  - ● **T63.694**   Toxic effect of contact with other venomous marine animals, undetermined

● **T63.7**   Toxic effect of contact with venomous plant
- ● **T63.71**   Toxic effect of contact with venomous marine plant
  - ● **T63.711**   Toxic effect of contact with venomous marine plant, accidental (unintentional)
  - ● **T63.712**   Toxic effect of contact with venomous marine plant, intentional self-harm
  - ● **T63.713**   Toxic effect of contact with venomous marine plant, assault
  - ● **T63.714**   Toxic effect of contact with venomous marine plant, undetermined

- ● **T63.79**   Toxic effect of contact with other venomous plant
  - ● **T63.791**   Toxic effect of contact with other venomous plant, accidental (unintentional)
  - ● **T63.792**   Toxic effect of contact with other venomous plant, intentional self-harm
  - ● **T63.793**   Toxic effect of contact with other venomous plant, assault
  - ● **T63.794**   Toxic effect of contact with other venomous plant, undetermined

● **T63.8**   Toxic effect of contact with other venomous animals
- ● **T63.81**   Toxic effect of contact with venomous frog

  > **Excludes1**   contact with nonvenomous frog (W62.0)

  - ● **T63.811**   Toxic effect of contact with venomous frog, accidental (unintentional)
  - ● **T63.812**   Toxic effect of contact with venomous frog, intentional self-harm
  - ● **T63.813**   Toxic effect of contact with venomous frog, assault
  - ● **T63.814**   Toxic effect of contact with venomous frog, undetermined
- ● **T63.82**   Toxic effect of contact with venomous toad

  > **Excludes1**   contact with nonvenomous toad (W62.1)

  - ● **T63.821**   Toxic effect of contact with venomous toad, accidental (unintentional)
  - ● **T63.822**   Toxic effect of contact with venomous toad, intentional self-harm
  - ● **T63.823**   Toxic effect of contact with venomous toad, assault
  - ● **T63.824**   Toxic effect of contact with venomous toad, undetermined
- ● **T63.83**   Toxic effect of contact with other venomous amphibian

  > **Excludes1**   contact with nonvenomous amphibian (W62.9)

  - ● **T63.831**   Toxic effect of contact with other venomous amphibian, accidental (unintentional)
  - ● **T63.832**   Toxic effect of contact with other venomous amphibian, intentional self-harm
  - ● **T63.833**   Toxic effect of contact with other venomous amphibian, assault
  - ● **T63.834**   Toxic effect of contact with other venomous amphibian, undetermined
- ● **T63.89**   Toxic effect of contact with other venomous animals
  - ● **T63.891**   Toxic effect of contact with other venomous animals, accidental (unintentional)
  - ● **T63.892**   Toxic effect of contact with other venomous animals, intentional self-harm
  - ● **T63.893**   Toxic effect of contact with other venomous animals, assault
  - ● **T63.894**   Toxic effect of contact with other venomous animals, undetermined

● **T63.9**   Toxic effect of contact with unspecified venomous animal
- X ● **T63.91**   Toxic effect of contact with unspecified venomous animal, accidental (unintentional)
- X ● **T63.92**   Toxic effect of contact with unspecified venomous animal, intentional self-harm
- X ● **T63.93**   Toxic effect of contact with unspecified venomous animal, assault
- X ● **T63.94**   Toxic effect of contact with unspecified venomous animal, undetermined

● T64 Toxic effect of aflatoxin and other mycotoxin food contaminants
The appropriate 7th character is to be added to each code from category T64

A	initial encounter
D	subsequent encounter
S	sequela

● T64.0 Toxic effect of aflatoxin
X● T64.01 Toxic effect of aflatoxin, accidental (unintentional)
X● T64.02 Toxic effect of aflatoxin, intentional self-harm
X● T64.03 Toxic effect of aflatoxin, assault
X● T64.04 Toxic effect of aflatoxin, undetermined
● T64.8 Toxic effect of other mycotoxin food contaminants
X● T64.81 Toxic effect of other mycotoxin food contaminants, accidental (unintentional)
X● T64.82 Toxic effect of other mycotoxin food contaminants, intentional self-harm
X● T64.83 Toxic effect of other mycotoxin food contaminants, assault
X● T64.84 Toxic effect of other mycotoxin food contaminants, undetermined

● T65 Toxic effect of other and unspecified substances
The appropriate 7th character is to be added to each code from category T65

A	initial encounter
D	subsequent encounter
S	sequela

● T65.0 Toxic effect of cyanides
Excludes1 hydrogen cyanide (T57.3-)
● T65.0X Toxic effect of cyanides
● T65.0X1 Toxic effect of cyanides, accidental (unintentional)
Toxic effect of cyanides NOS
● T65.0X2 Toxic effect of cyanides, intentional self-harm
● T65.0X3 Toxic effect of cyanides, assault
● T65.0X4 Toxic effect of cyanides, undetermined
● T65.1 Toxic effect of strychnine and its salts
● T65.1X Toxic effect of strychnine and its salts
● T65.1X1 Toxic effect of strychnine and its salts, accidental (unintentional)
Toxic effect of strychnine and its salts NOS
● T65.1X2 Toxic effect of strychnine and its salts, intentional self-harm
● T65.1X3 Toxic effect of strychnine and its salts, assault
● T65.1X4 Toxic effect of strychnine and its salts, undetermined
● T65.2 Toxic effect of tobacco and nicotine
Excludes2 nicotine dependence (F17.-)
● T65.21 Toxic effect of chewing tobacco
● T65.211 Toxic effect of chewing tobacco, accidental (unintentional)
Toxic effect of chewing tobacco NOS
● T65.212 Toxic effect of chewing tobacco, intentional self-harm
● T65.213 Toxic effect of chewing tobacco, assault
● T65.214 Toxic effect of chewing tobacco, undetermined
● T65.22 Toxic effect of tobacco cigarettes
Toxic effect of tobacco smoke
Use additional code for exposure to second hand tobacco smoke (Z57.31, Z77.22)
● T65.221 Toxic effect of tobacco cigarettes, accidental (unintentional)
Toxic effect of tobacco cigarettes NOS
● T65.222 Toxic effect of tobacco cigarettes, intentional self-harm
● T65.223 Toxic effect of tobacco cigarettes, assault
● T65.224 Toxic effect of tobacco cigarettes, undetermined
● T65.29 Toxic effect of other tobacco and nicotine
● T65.291 Toxic effect of other tobacco and nicotine, accidental (unintentional)
Toxic effect of other tobacco and nicotine NOS
● T65.292 Toxic effect of other tobacco and nicotine, intentional self-harm
● T65.293 Toxic effect of other tobacco and nicotine, assault
● T65.294 Toxic effect of other tobacco and nicotine, undetermined
● T65.3 Toxic effect of nitroderivatives and aminoderivatives of benzene and its homologues
Toxic effect of anilin [benzenamine]
Toxic effect of nitrobenzene
Toxic effect of trinitrotoluene
● T65.3X Toxic effect of nitroderivatives and aminoderivatives of benzene and its homologues
● T65.3X1 Toxic effect of nitroderivatives and aminoderivatives of benzene and its homologues, accidental (unintentional)
Toxic effect of nitroderivatives and aminoderivatives of benzene and its homologues NOS
● T65.3X2 Toxic effect of nitroderivatives and aminoderivatives of benzene and its homologues, intentional self-harm
● T65.3X3 Toxic effect of nitroderivatives and aminoderivatives of benzene and its homologues, assault
● T65.3X4 Toxic effect of nitroderivatives and aminoderivatives of benzene and its homologues, undetermined
● T65.4 Toxic effect of carbon disulfide
● T65.4X Toxic effect of carbon disulfide
● T65.4X1 Toxic effect of carbon disulfide, accidental (unintentional)
Toxic effect of carbon disulfide NOS
● T65.4X2 Toxic effect of carbon disulfide, intentional self-harm
● T65.4X3 Toxic effect of carbon disulfide, assault
● T65.4X4 Toxic effect of carbon disulfide, undetermined

CHAPTER 19 (S00-T88)

● T65.5 **Toxic effect of nitroglycerin and other nitric acids and esters**
Toxic effect of 1,2,3-Propanetriol trinitrate
● T65.5X **Toxic effect of nitroglycerin and other nitric acids and esters**
● T65.5X1 **Toxic effect of nitroglycerin and other nitric acids and esters, accidental (unintentional)**
Toxic effect of nitroglycerin and other nitric acids and esters NOS
● T65.5X2 **Toxic effect of nitroglycerin and other nitric acids and esters, intentional self-harm**
● T65.5X3 **Toxic effect of nitroglycerin and other nitric acids and esters, assault**
● T65.5X4 **Toxic effect of nitroglycerin and other nitric acids and esters, undetermined**
● T65.6 **Toxic effect of paints and dyes, not elsewhere classified**
● T65.6X **Toxic effect of paints and dyes, not elsewhere classified**
● T65.6X1 **Toxic effect of paints and dyes, not elsewhere classified, accidental (unintentional)**
Toxic effect of paints and dyes NOS
● T65.6X2 **Toxic effect of paints and dyes, not elsewhere classified, intentional self-harm**
● T65.6X3 **Toxic effect of paints and dyes, not elsewhere classified, assault**
● T65.6X4 **Toxic effect of paints and dyes, not elsewhere classified, undetermined**
● T65.8 **Toxic effect of other specified substances**
● T65.81 **Toxic effect of latex**
● T65.811 **Toxic effect of latex, accidental (unintentional)**
Toxic effect of latex NOS
● T65.812 **Toxic effect of latex, intentional self-harm**
● T65.813 **Toxic effect of latex, assault**
● T65.814 **Toxic effect of latex, undetermined**
● T65.82 **Toxic effect of harmful algae and algae toxins**
Toxic effect of (harmful) algae bloom NOS
Toxic effect of blue-green algae bloom
Toxic effect of brown tide
Toxic effect of cyanobacteria bloom
Toxic effect of Florida red tide
Toxic effect of pfiesteria piscicida
Toxic effect of red tide
● T65.821 **Toxic effect of harmful algae and algae toxins, accidental (unintentional)**
Toxic effect of harmful algae and algae toxins NOS
● T65.822 **Toxic effect of harmful algae and algae toxins, intentional self-harm**
● T65.823 **Toxic effect of harmful algae and algae toxins, assault**
● T65.824 **Toxic effect of harmful algae and algae toxins, undetermined**
● T65.83 **Toxic effect of fiberglass**
● T65.831 **Toxic effect of fiberglass, accidental (unintentional)**
Toxic effect of fiberglass NOS
● T65.832 **Toxic effect of fiberglass, intentional self-harm**
● T65.833 **Toxic effect of fiberglass, assault**
● T65.834 **Toxic effect of fiberglass, undetermined**
● T65.89 **Toxic effect of other specified substances**
● T65.891 **Toxic effect of other specified substances, accidental (unintentional)**
Toxic effect of other specified substances NOS
● T65.892 **Toxic effect of other specified substances, intentional self-harm**
● T65.893 **Toxic effect of other specified substances, assault**
● T65.894 **Toxic effect of other specified substances, undetermined**
● T65.9 **Toxic effect of unspecified substance**
X● T65.91 **Toxic effect of unspecified substance, accidental (unintentional)**
Poisoning NOS
X● T65.92 **Toxic effect of unspecified substance, intentional self-harm**
X● T65.93 **Toxic effect of unspecified substance, assault**
X● T65.94 **Toxic effect of unspecified substance, undetermined**

OTHER AND UNSPECIFIED EFFECTS OF EXTERNAL CAUSES (T66-T78)

● T66 **Radiation sickness, unspecified**
Excludes1 specified adverse effects of radiation, such as:
burns (T2Ø-T31)
leukemia (C91-C95)
radiation gastroenteritis and colitis (K52.Ø)
radiation pneumonitis (J7Ø.Ø)
radiation related disorders of the skin and subcutaneous tissue (L55-L59)
sunburn (L55.-)

The appropriate 7th character is to be added to code T66

A	initial encounter
D	subsequent encounter
S	sequela

● T67 **Effects of heat and light**
Excludes1 erythema [dermatitis] ab igne (L59.Ø)
malignant hyperpyrexia due to anesthesia (T88.3)
radiation-related disorders of the skin and subcutaneous tissue (L55-L59)
Excludes2 burns (T2Ø-T31)
sunburn (L55.-)
sweat disorder due to heat (L74-L75)

The appropriate 7th character is to be added to each code from category T67

A	initial encounter
D	subsequent encounter
S	sequela

X● T67.Ø **Heatstroke and sunstroke**
Heat apoplexy
Heat pyrexia
Siriasis
Thermoplegia
Use additional code(s) to identify any associated complications of heatstroke, such as:
coma and stupor (R4Ø.-)
systemic inflammatory response syndrome (R65.1-)
X● T67.1 **Heat syncope**
Heat collapse
X● T67.2 **Heat cramp**
X● T67.3 **Heat exhaustion, anhydrotic**
Heat prostration due to water depletion
Excludes1 heat exhaustion due to salt depletion (T67.4)

X● T67.4 **Heat exhaustion due to salt depletion**
Heat prostration due to salt (and water) depletion

X● T67.5 **Heat exhaustion, unspecified**
Heat prostration NOS

X● T67.6 **Heat fatigue, transient**

X● T67.7 **Heat edema**

X● T67.8 **Other effects of heat and light**

X● T67.9 **Effect of heat and light, unspecified**

X● T68 **Hypothermia**
Accidental hypothermia
Hypothermia NOS
Use additional code to identify source of exposure:
Exposure to excessive cold of man-made origin (W93)
Exposure to excessive cold of natural origin (X31)
Excludes1 hypothermia following anesthesia (T88.51)
hypothermia not associated with low environmental temperature (R68.Ø)
hypothermia of newborn (P8Ø.-)
Excludes2 frostbite (T33-T34)
The appropriate 7th character is to be added to code T68

A	initial encounter
D	subsequent encounter
S	sequela

● T69 **Other effects of reduced temperature**
Use additional code to identify source of exposure:
Exposure to excessive cold of man-made origin (W93)
Exposure to excessive cold of natural origin (X31)
Excludes2 frostbite (T33-T34)
The appropriate 7th character is to be added to each code from category T69

A	initial encounter
D	subsequent encounter
S	sequela

● T69.Ø **Immersion hand and foot**

● T69.Ø1 **Immersion hand**

● T69.Ø11 **Immersion hand, right hand**

● T69.Ø12 **Immersion hand, left hand**

● T69.Ø19 **Immersion hand, unspecified hand**

● T69.Ø2 **Immersion foot**
Trench foot

● T69.Ø21 **Immersion foot, right foot**

● T69.Ø22 **Immersion foot, left foot**

● T69.Ø29 **Immersion foot, unspecified foot**

X● T69.1 **Chilblains**

X● T69.8 **Other specified effects of reduced temperature**

X● T69.9 **Effect of reduced temperature, unspecified**

● T7Ø **Effects of air pressure and water pressure**
The appropriate 7th character is to be added to each code from category T7Ø

A	initial encounter
D	subsequent encounter
S	sequela

X● T7Ø.Ø **Otitic barotrauma**
Aero-otitis media
Effects of change in ambient atmospheric pressure or water pressure on ears

X● T7Ø.1 **Sinus barotrauma**
Aerosinusitis
Effects of change in ambient atmospheric pressure on sinuses

● T7Ø.2 **Other and unspecified effects of high altitude**
Excludes2 polycythemia due to high altitude (D75.1)

X● T7Ø.2Ø **Unspecified effects of high altitude**

X● T7Ø.29 **Other effects of high altitude**
Alpine sickness
Anoxia due to high altitude
Barotrauma NOS
Hypobaropathy
Mountain sickness

X● T7Ø.3 **Caisson disease [decompression sickness]**
Compressed-air disease
Diver's palsy or paralysis

X● T7Ø.4 **Effects of high-pressure fluids**
Hydraulic jet injection (industrial)
Pneumatic jet injection (industrial)
Traumatic jet injection (industrial)

X● T7Ø.8 **Other effects of air pressure and water pressure**

X● T7Ø.9 **Effect of air pressure and water pressure, unspecified**

● T71 **Asphyxiation**
Mechanical suffocation
Traumatic suffocation
Excludes1 acute respiratory distress (syndrome) (J8Ø)
anoxia due to high altitude (T7Ø.2)
asphyxia NOS (RØ9.Ø1)
asphyxia from carbon monoxide (T58.-)
asphyxia from inhalation of food or foreign body (T17.-)
asphyxia from other gases, fumes and vapors (T59.-)
respiratory distress (syndrome) in newborn (P22.-)
The appropriate 7th character is to be added to each code from category T71

A	initial encounter
D	subsequent encounter
S	sequela

● T71.1 **Asphyxiation due to mechanical threat to breathing**
Suffocation due to mechanical threat to breathing

● T71.11 **Asphyxiation due to smothering under pillow**

● T71.111 **Asphyxiation due to smothering under pillow, accidental**
Asphyxiation due to smothering under pillow NOS

● T71.112 **Asphyxiation due to smothering under pillow, intentional self-harm**

● T71.113 **Asphyxiation due to smothering under pillow, assault**

● T71.114 **Asphyxiation due to smothering under pillow, undetermined**

● T71.12 **Asphyxiation due to plastic bag**

● T71.121 **Asphyxiation due to plastic bag, accidental**
Asphyxiation due to plastic bag NOS

● T71.122 **Asphyxiation due to plastic bag, intentional self-harm**

● T71.123 **Asphyxiation due to plastic bag, assault**

● T71.124 **Asphyxiation due to plastic bag, undetermined**

CHAPTER 19 (SØØ-T88)

● T71.13 **Asphyxiation due to being trapped in bed linens**

● T71.131 **Asphyxiation due to being trapped in bed linens, accidental**
Asphyxiation due to being trapped in bed linens NOS

● T71.132 **Asphyxiation due to being trapped in bed linens, intentional self-harm**

● T71.133 **Asphyxiation due to being trapped in bed linens, assault**

● T71.134 **Asphyxiation due to being trapped in bed linens, undetermined**

● T71.14 **Asphyxiation due to smothering under another person's body (in bed)**

● T71.141 **Asphyxiation due to smothering under another person's body (in bed), accidental**
Asphyxiation due to smothering under another person's body (in bed) NOS

● T71.143 **Asphyxiation due to smothering under another person's body (in bed), assault**

● T71.144 **Asphyxiation due to smothering under another person's body (in bed), undetermined**

● T71.15 **Asphyxiation due to smothering in furniture**

● T71.151 **Asphyxiation due to smothering in furniture, accidental**
Asphyxiation due to smothering in furniture NOS

● T71.152 **Asphyxiation due to smothering in furniture, intentional self-harm**

● T71.153 **Asphyxiation due to smothering in furniture, assault**

● T71.154 **Asphyxiation due to smothering in furniture, undetermined**

● T71.16 **Asphyxiation due to hanging**
Hanging by window shade cord
Use additional code for any associated injuries, such as:
crushing injury of neck (S17.-)
fracture of cervical vertebrae (S12.Ø-S12.2-)
open wound of neck (S11.-)

● T71.161 **Asphyxiation due to hanging, accidental**
Asphyxiation due to hanging NOS
Hanging NOS

● T71.162 **Asphyxiation due to hanging, intentional self-harm**

● T71.163 **Asphyxiation due to hanging, assault**

● T71.164 **Asphyxiation due to hanging, undetermined**

● T71.19 **Asphyxiation due to mechanical**
Threat to breathing due to other causes

● T71.191 **Asphyxiation due to mechanical threat to breathing due to other causes, accidental**
Asphyxiation due to other causes NOS

● T71.192 **Asphyxiation due to mechanical threat to breathing due to other causes, intentional self-harm**

● T71.193 **Asphyxiation due to mechanical threat to breathing due to other causes, assault**

● T71.194 **Asphyxiation due to mechanical threat to breathing due to other causes, undetermined**

● T71.2 **Asphyxiation due to systemic oxygen deficiency due to low oxygen content in ambient air**
Suffocation due to systemic oxygen deficiency due to low oxygen content in ambient air

X● T71.2Ø **Asphyxiation due to systemic oxygen deficiency due to low oxygen content in ambient air due to unspecified cause**

X● T71.21 **Asphyxiation due to cave-in or falling earth**
Use additional code for any associated cataclysm (X34-X38)

● T71.22 **Asphyxiation due to being trapped in a car trunk**

● T71.221 **Asphyxiation due to being trapped in a car trunk, accidental**

● T71.222 **Asphyxiation due to being trapped in a car trunk, intentional self-harm**

● T71.223 **Asphyxiation due to being trapped in a car trunk, assault**

● T71.224 **Asphyxiation due to being trapped in a car trunk, undetermined**

● T71.23 **Asphyxiation due to being trapped in a (discarded) refrigerator**

● T71.231 **Asphyxiation due to being trapped in a (discarded) refrigerator, accidental**

● T71.232 **Asphyxiation due to being trapped in a (discarded) refrigerator, intentional self-harm**

● T71.233 **Asphyxiation due to being trapped in a (discarded) refrigerator, assault**

● T71.234 **Asphyxiation due to being trapped in a (discarded) refrigerator, undetermined**

X● T71.29 **Asphyxiation due to being trapped in other low oxygen environment**

X● T71.9 **Asphyxiation due to unspecified cause**
Suffocation (by strangulation) due to unspecified cause
Suffocation NOS
Systemic oxygen deficiency due to low oxygen content in ambient air due to unspecified cause
Systemic oxygen deficiency due to mechanical threat to breathing due to unspecified cause
Traumatic asphyxia NOS

● T73 **Effects of other deprivation**
The appropriate 7th character is to be added to each code from category T73

A	initial encounter
D	subsequent encounter
S	sequela

X● T73.Ø **Starvation**
Deprivation of food

X● T73.1 **Deprivation of water**

X● T73.2 **Exhaustion due to exposure**

X● T73.3 **Exhaustion due to excessive exertion**
Exhaustion due to overexertion

X● T73.8 **Other effects of deprivation**

X● T73.9 **Effect of deprivation, unspecified**

●T74 **Adult and child abuse, neglect and other maltreatment, confirmed**

Use additional code, if applicable, to identify any associated current injury

Use additional external cause code to identify perpetrator, if known (Y07.-)

Excludes1 abuse and maltreatment in pregnancy (O9A.3-, O9A.4-, O9A.5-)
adult and child maltreatment, suspected (T76.-)

The appropriate 7th character is to be added to each code from category T74

A	initial encounter
D	subsequent encounter
S	sequela

●T74.0 **Neglect or abandonment, confirmed**

X●T74.01 **Adult neglect or abandonment, confirmed**

X●T74.02 **Child neglect or abandonment, confirmed**

●T74.1 **Physical abuse, confirmed**

Excludes2 sexual abuse (T74.2-)

X●T74.11 **Adult physical abuse, confirmed**

X●T74.12 **Child physical abuse, confirmed**

Excludes2 shaken infant syndrome (T74.4)

●T74.2 **Sexual abuse, confirmed**

Rape, confirmed
Sexual assault, confirmed

X●T74.21 **Adult sexual abuse, confirmed**

X●T74.22 **Child sexual abuse, confirmed**

●T74.3 **Psychological abuse, confirmed**

X●T74.31 **Adult psychological abuse, confirmed**

X●T74.32 **Child psychological abuse, confirmed**

X●T74.4 **Shaken infant syndrome**

●T74.9 **Unspecified maltreatment, confirmed**

X●T74.91 **Unspecified adult maltreatment, confirmed**

X●T74.92 **Unspecified child maltreatment, confirmed**

●T75 **Other and unspecified effects of other external causes**

Excludes1 adverse effects NEC (T78.-)

Excludes2 burns (electric) (T20-T31)

The appropriate 7th character is to be added to each code from category T75

A	initial encounter
D	subsequent encounter
S	sequela

●T75.0 **Effects of lightning**

Struck by lightning

X●T75.00 **Unspecified effects of lightning**

Struck by lightning NOS

X●T75.01 **Shock due to being struck by lightning**

X●T75.09 **Other effects of lightning**

Use additional code for other effects of lightning

X●T75.1 **Unspecified effects of drowning and nonfatal submersion**

Immersion

Excludes1 specified effects of drowning code to effects

●T75.2 **Effects of vibration**

X●T75.20 **Unspecified effects of vibration**

X●T75.21 **Pneumatic hammer syndrome**

X●T75.22 **Traumatic vasospastic syndrome**

X●T75.23 **Vertigo from infrasound**

Excludes1 vertigo NOS (R42)

X●T75.29 **Other effects of vibration**

X●T75.3 **Motion sickness**

Airsickness
Seasickness
Travel sickness

Use additional external cause code to identify vehicle or type of motion (Y92.81-, Y93.5-)

X●T75.4 **Electrocution**

Shock from electric current
Shock from electroshock gun (taser)

●T75.8 **Other specified effects of external causes**

X●T75.81 **Effects of abnormal gravitation [G] forces**

X●T75.82 **Effects of weightlessness**

X●T75.89 **Other specified effects of external causes**

●T76 **Adult and child abuse, neglect and other maltreatment, suspected**

Use additional code, if applicable, to identify any associated current injury

Excludes1 adult and child maltreatment, confirmed (T74.-)
suspected abuse and maltreatment in pregnancy (O9A.3-, O9A.4-, O9A.5-)
suspected adult physical abuse, ruled out (Z04.71)
suspected adult sexual abuse, ruled out (Z04.41)
suspected child physical abuse, ruled out (Z04.72)
suspected child sexual abuse, ruled out (Z04.42)

The appropriate 7th character is to be added to each code from category T76

A	initial encounter
D	subsequent encounter
S	sequela

●T76.0 **Neglect or abandonment, suspected**

X●T76.01 **Adult neglect or abandonment, suspected**

X●T76.02 **Child neglect or abandonment, suspected**

●T76.1 **Physical abuse, suspected**

X●T76.11 **Adult physical abuse, suspected**

X●T76.12 **Child physical abuse, suspected**

●T76.2 **Sexual abuse, suspected**

Rape, suspected
Sexual abuse, suspected

Excludes1 alleged abuse, ruled out (Z04.7)

X●T76.21 **Adult sexual abuse, suspected**

X●T76.22 **Child sexual abuse, suspected**

●T76.3 **Psychological abuse, suspected**

X●T76.31 **Adult psychological abuse, suspected**

X●T76.32 **Child psychological abuse, suspected**

●T76.9 **Unspecified maltreatment, suspected**

X●T76.91 **Unspecified adult maltreatment, suspected**

X●T76.92 **Unspecified child maltreatment, suspected**

● T78 **Adverse effects, not elsewhere classified**

Excludes2 complications of surgical and medical care NEC (T80-T88)

The appropriate 7th character is to be added to each code from category T78

A	initial encounter
D	subsequent encounter
S	sequela

● T78.0 **Anaphylactic reaction due to food**

Anaphylactic reaction due to adverse food reaction
Anaphylactic shock or reaction due to nonpoisonous foods
Anaphylactoid reaction due to food

X● T78.00 **Anaphylactic reaction due to unspecified food**

X● T78.01 **Anaphylactic reaction due to peanuts**

X● T78.02 **Anaphylactic reaction due to shellfish (crustaceans)**

X● T78.03 **Anaphylactic reaction due to other fish**

X● T78.04 **Anaphylactic reaction due to fruits and vegetables**

X● T78.05 **Anaphylactic reaction due to tree nuts and seeds**

Excludes2 anaphylactic reaction due to peanuts (T78.01) ◀

X● T78.06 **Anaphylactic reaction due to food additives**

X● T78.07 **Anaphylactic reaction due to milk and dairy products**

X● T78.08 **Anaphylactic reaction due to eggs**

X● T78.09 **Anaphylactic reaction due to other food products**

X● T78.1 **Other adverse food reactions, not elsewhere classified**

Use additional code to identify the type of reaction, if applicable ⬅

Excludes1 anaphylactic reaction or shock due to adverse food reaction (T78.0-)
anaphylactic reaction due to food (T78.0-)
bacterial food borne intoxications (A05.-)

Excludes2 allergic and dietetic gastroenteritis and colitis (K52.29) ⬅
allergic rhinitis due to food (J30.5)
dermatitis due to food in contact with skin (L23.6, L24.6, L25.4)
dermatitis due to ingested food (L27.2)
food protein-induced enterocolitis syndrome (K52.21) ◀
food protein-induced enteropathy (K52.22) ◀

X● T78.2 **Anaphylactic shock, unspecified**

Occurs when allergic response triggers large quantities of histamines, prostaglandins, leukotrienes resulting in systemic vasodilation

Allergic shock
Anaphylactic reaction
Anaphylaxis

Excludes1 anaphylactic reaction or shock due to adverse effect of correct medicinal substance properly administered (T88.6)
anaphylactic reaction or shock due to adverse food reaction (T78.0-)
anaphylactic reaction or shock due to serum (T80.5-)

X● T78.3 **Angioneurotic edema**

Allergic angioedema
Giant urticaria
Vascular disorder resulting from abnormalities of autonomic nervous system fibers supplying blood vessels
Quincke's edema

Excludes1 serum urticaria (T80.6-)
urticaria (L50.-)

● T78.4 **Other and unspecified allergy**

Excludes1 specified types of allergic reaction such as:
allergic diarrhea (K52.29) ⬅
allergic gastroenteritis and colitis (K52.29 ⬅)
dermatitis (L23-L25, L27.-)
food protein-induced enterocolitis syndrome (K52.21) ◀
food protein-induced enteropathy (K52.22) ◀
hay fever (J30.1)

X● T78.40 **Allergy, unspecified**

Allergic reaction NOS
Hypersensitivity NOS

X● T78.41 **Arthus phenomenon**

Arthus reaction

X● T78.49 **Other allergy**

X● T78.8 **Other adverse effects, not elsewhere classified**

CERTAIN EARLY COMPLICATIONS OF TRAUMA (T79)

● T79 **Certain early complications of trauma, not elsewhere classified**

Excludes2 acute respiratory distress syndrome (J80)
complications occurring during or following medical procedures (T80-T88)
complications of surgical and medical care NEC (T80-T88)
newborn respiratory distress syndrome (P22.0)

The appropriate 7th character is to be added to each code from category T79

A	initial encounter
D	subsequent encounter
S	sequela

X● T79.0 **Air embolism (traumatic)**

Excludes1 air embolism complicating abortion or ectopic or molar pregnancy (O00-O07, O08.2)
air embolism complicating pregnancy, childbirth and the puerperium (O88.0)
air embolism following infusion, transfusion, and therapeutic injection (T80.0)
air embolism following procedure NEC (T81.7-)

X● T79.1 **Fat embolism (traumatic)**

Excludes1 fat embolism complicating:
abortion or ectopic or molar pregnancy (O00-O07, O08.2)
pregnancy, childbirth and the puerperium (O88.8)

X● T79.2 **Traumatic secondary and recurrent hemorrhage and seroma**

X● **T79.4 Traumatic shock**
Shock (immediate) (delayed) following injury
Excludes1 anaphylactic shock due to adverse food reaction (T78.0-)
anaphylactic shock due to correct medicinal substance properly administered (T88.6)
anaphylactic shock due to serum (T80.5-)
anaphylactic shock NOS (T78.2)
anesthetic shock (T88.2)
electric shock (T75.4)
nontraumatic shock NEC (R57.-)
obstetric shock (O75.1)
postprocedural shock (T81.1-)
septic shock (R65.21)
shock complicating abortion or ectopic or molar pregnancy (O00-O07, O08.3)
shock due to lightning (T75.01)
shock NOS (R57.9)

X● **T79.5 Traumatic anuria**
Crush syndrome
Renal failure following crushing

X● **T79.6 Traumatic ischemia of muscle**
Traumatic rhabdomyolysis
Volkmann's ischemic contracture
Excludes2 anterior tibial syndrome (M76.8)
compartment syndrome (traumatic) (T79.A-)
nontraumatic ischemia of muscle (M62.2-)

X● **T79.7 Traumatic subcutaneous emphysema**
Excludes1 emphysema NOS (J43)
emphysema (subcutaneous) resulting from a procedure (T81.82)

● **T79.A Traumatic compartment syndrome**
Excludes1 fibromyalgia (M79.7)
nontraumatic compartment syndrome (M79.A-)
traumatic ischemic infarction of muscle (T79.6)

X● **T79.A0 Compartment syndrome, unspecified**
Compartment syndrome NOS

● **T79.A1 Traumatic compartment syndrome of upper extremity**
Traumatic compartment syndrome of shoulder, arm, forearm, wrist, hand, and fingers

● **T79.A11 Traumatic compartment syndrome of right upper extremity**

● **T79.A12 Traumatic compartment syndrome of left upper extremity**

● **T79.A19 Traumatic compartment syndrome of unspecified upper extremity**

● **T79.A2 Traumatic compartment syndrome of lower extremity**
Traumatic compartment syndrome of hip, buttock, thigh, leg, foot, and toes

● **T79.A21 Traumatic compartment syndrome of right lower extremity**

● **T79.A22 Traumatic compartment syndrome of left lower extremity**

● **T79.A29 Traumatic compartment syndrome of unspecified lower extremity**

X● **T79.A3 Traumatic compartment syndrome of abdomen**

X● **T79.A9 Traumatic compartment syndrome of other sites**

X● **T79.8 Other early complications of trauma**

X● **T79.9 Unspecified early complication of trauma**

COMPLICATIONS OF SURGICAL AND MEDICAL CARE NOT ELSEWHERE CLASSIFIED (T80-T88)

Use additional code for adverse effect, if applicable, to identify drug (T36-T50 with fifth or sixth character 5)

Use additional code(s) to identify the specified condition resulting from the complication.

Use additional code to identify devices involved and details of circumstances (Y62-Y82)

Excludes2 any encounters with medical care for postprocedural conditions in which no complications are present, such as:
artificial opening status (Z93.-)
closure of external stoma (Z43.-)
fitting and adjustment of external prosthetic device (Z44.-)
burns and corrosions from local applications and irradiation (T20-T32)
complications of surgical procedures during pregnancy, childbirth and the puerperium (O00-O9A)
mechanical complication of respirator [ventilator] (J95.850)
poisoning and toxic effects of drugs and chemicals (T36-T65 with fifth or sixth character 1-4 or 6)
postprocedural fever (R50.82)
specified complications classified elsewhere, such as:
cerebrospinal fluid leak from spinal puncture (G97.0)
colostomy malfunction (K94.0-)
disorders of fluid and electrolyte imbalance (E86-E87)
functional disturbances following cardiac surgery (I97.0-I97.1)
intraoperative and postprocedural complications of specified body systems (D78.-, E36.-, E89.-, G97.3-, G97.4, H59.3-, H59.-, H95.2-, H95.3, I97.4-, I97.5, J95.6-, J95.7, K91.6-, L76.-, M96.-, N99.-)
ostomy complications (J95.0-, K94.-, N99.5-)
postgastric surgery syndromes (K91.1)
postlaminectomy syndrome NEC (M96.1)
postmastectomy lymphedema syndrome (I97.2)
postsurgical blind-loop syndrome (K91.2)
ventilator associated pneumonia (J95.851)

● **T80 Complications following infusion, transfusion and therapeutic injection**
Includes complications following perfusion
Excludes2 bone marrow transplant rejection (T86.01)
febrile nonhemolytic transfusion reaction (R50.84)
fluid overload due to transfusion (E87.71)
posttransfusion purpura (D69.51)
transfusion associated circulatory overload (TACO) (E87.71)
transfusion (red blood cell) associated hemochromatosis (E83.111)
transfusion related acute lung injury (TRALI) (J95.84)

The appropriate 7th character is to be added to each code from category T80

A	initial encounter
D	subsequent encounter
S	sequela

X● **T80.0 Air embolism following infusion, transfusion and therapeutic injection**

CHAPTER 19 (S00-T88)

X● **T80.1 Vascular complications following infusion, transfusion and therapeutic injection**

Use additional code to identify the vascular complication

Excludes2 extravasation of vesicant agent (T80.81-)
infiltration of vesicant agent (T80.81-)
vascular complications specified as due to prosthetic devices, implants and grafts (T82.8- T83.8-, T84.8-, T85.8-) ⬅
postprocedural vascular complications (T81.7-)

● **T80.2 Infections following infusion, transfusion and therapeutic injection**

Use additional code to identify the specific infection, such as:
sepsis (A41.9)

Use additional code (R65.2-) to identify severe sepsis, if applicable

Excludes2 infections specified as due to prosthetic devices, implants and grafts (T82.6-T82.7, T83.5-T83.6, T84.5-T84.7, T85.7)
postprocedural infections (T81.4-) ⬅

● **T80.21 Infection due to central venous catheter**

Infection due to pulmonary artery catheter (Swan-Ganz catheter) ◀

● **T80.211 Bloodstream infection due to central venous catheter**

Catheter-related bloodstream infection (CRBSI) NOS
Central line-associated bloodstream infection (CLABSI)
Bloodstream infection due to Hickman catheter
Bloodstream infection due to peripherally inserted central catheter (PICC)
Bloodstream infection due to portacath (port-a-cath)
Bloodstream infection due to pulmonary artery catheter ◀
Bloodstream infection due to triple lumen catheter
Bloodstream infection due to umbilical venous catheter

● **T80.212 Local infection due to central venous catheter**

Exit or insertion site infection
Local infection due to Hickman catheter
Local infection due to peripherally inserted central catheter (PICC)
Local infection due to portacath (port-a-cath)
Local infection due to pulmonary artery catheter ◀
Local infection due to triple lumen catheter
Local infection due to umbilical venous catheter
Port or reservoir infection
Tunnel infection

● **T80.218 Other infection due to central venous catheter**

Other central line-associated infection
Other infection due to Hickman catheter
Other infection due to peripherally inserted central catheter (PICC)
Other infection due to portacath (port-a-cath)
Other infection due to pulmonary artery catheter ◀
Other infection due to triple lumen catheter
Other infection due to umbilical venous catheter

● **T80.219 Unspecified infection due to central venous catheter**

Central line-associated infection NOS
Unspecified infection due to Hickman catheter
Unspecified infection due to peripherally inserted central catheter (PICC)
Unspecified infection due to portacath (port-a-cath)
Unspecified infection due to pulmonary artery catheter ◀
Unspecified infection due to triple lumen catheter
Unspecified infection due to umbilical venous catheter

X● **T80.22 Acute infection following transfusion, infusion, or injection of blood and blood products**

X● **T80.29 Infection following other infusion, transfusion and therapeutic injection**

● **T80.3 ABO incompatibility reaction due to transfusion of blood or blood products**

Excludes1 minor blood group antigens reactions (Duffy) (E) (K(ell)) (Kidd) (Lewis) (M) (N) (P) (S) (T80.A)

X● **T80.30 ABO incompatibility reaction due to transfusion of blood or blood products, unspecified**

ABO incompatibility blood transfusion NOS
Reaction to ABO incompatibility from transfusion NOS

● **T80.31 ABO incompatibility with hemolytic transfusion reaction**

● **T80.310 ABO incompatibility with acute hemolytic transfusion reaction**

ABO incompatibility with hemolytic transfusion reaction less than 24 hours after transfusion
Acute hemolytic transfusion reaction (AHTR) due to ABO incompatibility

● **T80.311 ABO incompatibility with delayed hemolytic transfusion reaction**

ABO incompatibility with hemolytic transfusion reaction 24 hours or more after transfusion
Delayed hemolytic transfusion reaction (DHTR) due to ABO incompatibility

● T80.319 **ABO incompatibility with hemolytic transfusion reaction, unspecified**
ABO incompatibility with hemolytic transfusion reaction at unspecified time after transfusion
Hemolytic transfusion reaction (HTR) due to ABO incompatibility NOS

X● T80.39 **Other ABO incompatibility reaction due to transfusion of blood or blood products**
Delayed serologic transfusion reaction (DSTR) from ABO incompatibility
Other ABO incompatible blood transfusion
Other reaction to ABO incompatible blood transfusion

● T80.4 **Rh incompatibility reaction due to transfusion of blood or blood products**
Reaction due to incompatibility of Rh antigens (C) (c) (D) (E) (e)

X● T80.40 **Rh incompatibility reaction due to transfusion of blood or blood products, unspecified**
Reaction due to Rh factor in transfusion NOS
Rh incompatible blood transfusion NOS

● T80.41 **Rh incompatibility with hemolytic transfusion reaction**

● T80.410 **Rh incompatibility with acute hemolytic transfusion reaction**
Acute hemolytic transfusion reaction (AHTR) due to Rh incompatibility
Rh incompatibility with hemolytic transfusion reaction less than 24 hours after transfusion

● T80.411 **Rh incompatibility with delayed hemolytic transfusion reaction**
Delayed hemolytic transfusion reaction (DHTR) due to Rh incompatibility
Rh incompatibility with hemolytic transfusion reaction 24 hours or more after transfusion

● T80.419 **Rh incompatibility with hemolytic transfusion reaction, unspecified**
Rh incompatibility with hemolytic transfusion reaction at unspecified time after transfusion
Hemolytic transfusion reaction (HTR) due to Rh incompatibility NOS

X● T80.49 **Other Rh incompatibility reaction due to transfusion of blood or blood products**
Delayed serologic transfusion reaction (DSTR) from Rh incompatibility
Other reaction to Rh incompatible blood transfusion

● T80.A **Non-ABO incompatibility reaction due to transfusion of blood or blood products**
Reaction due to incompatibility of minor antigens (Duffy) (Kell) (Kidd) (Lewis) (M) (N) (P) (S)

X● T80.A0 **Non-ABO incompatibility reaction due to transfusion of blood or blood products, unspecified**
Non-ABO antigen incompatibility reaction from transfusion NOS

● T80.A1 **Non-ABO incompatibility with hemolytic transfusion reaction**

● T80.A10 **Non-ABO incompatibility with acute hemolytic transfusion reaction**
Acute hemolytic transfusion reaction (AHTR) due to non-ABO incompatibility
Non-ABO incompatibility with hemolytic transfusion reaction less than 24 hours after transfusion

● T80.A11 **Non-ABO incompatibility with delayed hemolytic transfusion reaction**
Delayed hemolytic transfusion reaction (DHTR) due to non-ABO incompatibility
Non-ABO incompatibility with hemolytic transfusion reaction 24 or more hours after transfusion

● T80.A19 **Non-ABO incompatibility with hemolytic transfusion reaction, unspecified**
Hemolytic transfusion reaction (HTR) due to non-ABO incompatibility NOS
Non-ABO incompatibility with hemolytic transfusion reaction at unspecified time after transfusion

X● T80.A9 **Other non-ABO incompatibility reaction due to transfusion of blood or blood products**
Delayed serologic transfusion reaction (DSTR) from non-ABO incompatibility
Other reaction to non-ABO incompatible blood transfusion

● T80.5 **Anaphylactic reaction due to serum**
Allergic reaction due to serum
Anaphylactic shock due to serum
Anaphylactoid reaction due to serum
Anaphylaxis due to serum
Excludes1 ABO incompatibility reaction due to transfusion of blood or blood products (T80.3-)
allergic reaction or shock NOS (T78.2)
anaphylactic reaction or shock NOS (T78.2)
anaphylactic reaction or shock due to adverse effect of correct medicinal substance properly administered (T88.6)
other serum reaction (T80.6-)

X● T80.51 **Anaphylactic reaction due to administration of blood and blood products**

X● T80.52 **Anaphylactic reaction due to vaccination**

X● T80.59 **Anaphylactic reaction due to other serum**

● T80.6 **Other serum reactions**
Intoxication by serum
Protein sickness
Serum rash
Serum sickness
Serum urticaria
Excludes2 serum hepatitis (B16-B19)

X● T80.61 **Other serum reaction due to administration of blood and blood products**

X● T80.62 **Other serum reaction due to vaccination**

X● T80.69 **Other serum reaction due to other serum**

● T80.8 **Other complications following infusion, transfusion and therapeutic injection**

● T80.81 **Extravasation of vesicant agent**
Infiltration of vesicant agent

● T80.810 **Extravasation of vesicant antineoplastic chemotherapy**
Infiltration of vesicant antineoplastic chemotherapy

● T80.818 **Extravasation of other vesicant agent**
Infiltration of other vesicant agent

X● T80.89 **Other complications following infusion, transfusion and therapeutic injection**
Delayed serologic transfusion reaction (DSTR), unspecified incompatibility
Use additional code to identify graft-versus-host reaction, if applicable, (D89.81-)

● T80.9 **Unspecified complication following infusion, transfusion and therapeutic injection**

X● T80.90 **Unspecified complication following infusion and therapeutic injection**

● T80.91 **Hemolytic transfusion reaction, unspecified incompatibility**
Excludes1 ABO incompatibility with hemolytic transfusion reaction (T80.31-)
Non-ABO incompatibility with hemolytic transfusion reaction (T80.A1-)
Rh incompatibility with hemolytic transfusion reaction (T80.41-)

● T80.910 **Acute hemolytic transfusion reaction, unspecified incompatibility**

● T80.911 **Delayed hemolytic transfusion reaction, unspecified incompatibility**

● T80.919 **Hemolytic transfusion reaction, unspecified incompatibility, unspecified as acute or delayed**
Hemolytic transfusion reaction NOS

X● T80.92 **Unspecified transfusion reaction**
Transfusion reaction NOS

● T81 **Complications of procedures, not elsewhere classified**
Use additional code for adverse effect, if applicable, to identify drug (T36-T50 with fifth or sixth character 5)
Excludes2 complications following immunization (T88.0-T88.1)
complications following infusion, transfusion and therapeutic injection (T80.-)
complications of transplanted organs and tissue (T86.-)
poisoning and toxic effects of drugs and chemicals (T36-T65 with fifth or sixth character 1-4 or 6)
specified complications classified elsewhere, such as:
complication of prosthetic devices, implants and grafts (T82-T85)
dermatitis due to drugs and medicaments (L23.3, L24.4, L25.1, L27.0-L27.1)
endosseous dental implant failure (M27.6-)
floppy iris syndrome (IFIS) (intraoperative) H21.81
intraoperative and postprocedural complications of specific body system (D78.-, E36.-, E89.-, G97.3-, G97.4, H59.3-, H59.-, H95.2-, H95.3, I97.4-, I97.5, J95, K91.-, L76.-, M96.-, N99.-)
ostomy complications (J95.0-, K94.-, N99.5-)
plateau iris syndrome (post-iridectomy) (postprocedural) H21.82

The appropriate 7th character is to be added to each code from category T81

A	initial encounter
D	subsequent encounter
S	sequela

● T81.1 **Postprocedural shock**
Shock during or resulting from a procedure, not elsewhere classified
Excludes1 anaphylactic shock NOS (T78.2)
anaphylactic shock due to correct substance properly administered (T88.6)
anaphylactic shock due to serum (T80.5-)
anesthetic shock (T88.2)
electric shock (T75.4)
obstetric shock (O75.1)
septic shock (R65.21)
shock following abortion or ectopic or molar pregnancy (O00-O07, O08.3)
traumatic shock (T79.4)

X● T81.10 **Postprocedural shock unspecified**
Collapse NOS during or resulting from a procedure, not elsewhere classified
Postprocedural failure of peripheral circulation
Postprocedural shock NOS

X● T81.11 **Postprocedural cardiogenic shock**

X● T81.12 **Postprocedural septic shock**
Postprocedural endotoxic shock resulting from a procedure, not elsewhere classified
Postprocedural gram-negative shock resulting from a procedure, not elsewhere classified
Code first underlying infection
Use additional code, to identify any associated acute organ dysfunction, if applicable

X● T81.19 **Other postprocedural shock**
Postprocedural hypovolemic shock

CHAPTER 19 (S00-T88)

● T81.3 **Disruption of wound, not elsewhere classified**
Disruption of any suture materials or other closure methods
Excludes1 breakdown (mechanical) of permanent sutures (T85.612)
displacement of permanent sutures (T85.622)
disruption of cesarean delivery wound (O90.0)
disruption of perineal obstetric wound (O90.1)
mechanical complication of permanent sutures NEC (T85.692)

X● T81.30 **Disruption of wound, unspecified**
Disruption of wound NOS

X● T81.31 **Disruption of external operation (surgical) wound, not elsewhere classified**
Excludes1 dehiscence of amputation stump (T87.81)
Dehiscence of operation wound NOS
Disruption of operation wound NOS
Disruption or dehiscence of closure of cornea
Disruption or dehiscence of closure of mucosa
Disruption or dehiscence of closure of skin and subcutaneous tissue
Full-thickness skin disruption or dehiscence
Superficial disruption or dehiscence of operation wound

X● T81.32 **Disruption of internal operation (surgical) wound, not elsewhere classified**
Deep disruption or dehiscence of operation wound NOS
Disruption or dehiscence of closure of internal organ or other internal tissue
Disruption or dehiscence of closure of muscle or muscle flap
Disruption or dehiscence of closure of ribs or rib cage
Disruption or dehiscence of closure of skull or craniotomy
Disruption or dehiscence of closure of sternum or sternotomy
Disruption or dehiscence of closure of tendon or ligament
Disruption or dehiscence of closure of superficial or muscular fascia

X● T81.33 **Disruption of traumatic injury wound repair**
Disruption or dehiscence of closure of traumatic laceration (external) (internal)

X● T81.4 **Infection following a procedure**
Intra-abdominal abscess following a procedure
Postprocedural infection, not elsewhere classified
Sepsis following a procedure
Stitch abscess following a procedure
Subphrenic abscess following a procedure
Wound abscess following a procedure
Use additional code to identify infection
Use additional code (R65.2-) to identify severe sepsis, if applicable
Excludes1 obstetric surgical wound infection (O86.0)
postprocedural fever NOS (R50.82)
postprocedural retroperitoneal abscess (K68.11)
Excludes2 bleb associated endophthalmitis (H59.4-)
infection due to infusion, transfusion and therapeutic injection (T80.2-)
infection due to prosthetic devices, implants and grafts (T82.6-T82.7, T83.5-T83.6, T84.5-T84.7, T85.7)

● T81.5 **Complications of foreign body accidentally left in body following procedure**

● T81.50 **Unspecified complication of foreign body accidentally left in body following procedure**

● T81.500 **Unspecified complication of foreign body accidentally left in body following surgical operation**

● T81.501 **Unspecified complication of foreign body accidentally left in body following infusion or transfusion**

● T81.502 **Unspecified complication of foreign body accidentally left in body following kidney dialysis**

● T81.503 **Unspecified complication of foreign body accidentally left in body following injection or immunization**

● T81.504 **Unspecified complication of foreign body accidentally left in body following endoscopic examination**

● T81.505 **Unspecified complication of foreign body accidentally left in body following heart catheterization**

● T81.506 **Unspecified complication of foreign body accidentally left in body following aspiration, puncture or other catheterization**

● T81.507 **Unspecified complication of foreign body accidentally left in body following removal of catheter or packing**

● T81.508 **Unspecified complication of foreign body accidentally left in body following other procedure**

● T81.509 **Unspecified complication of foreign body accidentally left in body following unspecified procedure**

● T81.51 **Adhesions due to foreign body accidentally left in body following procedure**

● T81.510 **Adhesions due to foreign body accidentally left in body following surgical operation**

● T81.511 **Adhesions due to foreign body accidentally left in body following infusion or transfusion**

● T81.512 **Adhesions due to foreign body accidentally left in body following kidney dialysis**

● T81.513 **Adhesions due to foreign body accidentally left in body following injection or immunization**

● T81.514 **Adhesions due to foreign body accidentally left in body following endoscopic examination**

● T81.515 **Adhesions due to foreign body accidentally left in body following heart catheterization**

● T81.516 **Adhesions due to foreign body accidentally left in body following aspiration, puncture or other catheterization**

● T81.517 **Adhesions due to foreign body accidentally left in body following removal of catheter or packing**

● T81.518 **Adhesions due to foreign body accidentally left in body following other procedure**

● T81.519 **Adhesions due to foreign body accidentally left in body following unspecified procedure**

CHAPTER 19 (S00-T88)

● T81.52 Obstruction due to foreign body accidentally left in body following procedure

● T81.520 Obstruction due to foreign body accidentally left in body following surgical operation

● T81.521 Obstruction due to foreign body accidentally left in body following infusion or transfusion

● T81.522 Obstruction due to foreign body accidentally left in body following kidney dialysis

● T81.523 Obstruction due to foreign body accidentally left in body following injection or immunization

● T81.524 Obstruction due to foreign body accidentally left in body following endoscopic examination

● T81.525 Obstruction due to foreign body accidentally left in body following heart catheterization

● T81.526 Obstruction due to foreign body accidentally left in body following aspiration, puncture or other catheterization

● T81.527 Obstruction due to foreign body accidentally left in body following removal of catheter or packing

● T81.528 Obstruction due to foreign body accidentally left in body following other procedure

● T81.529 Obstruction due to foreign body accidentally left in body following unspecified procedure

● T81.53 Perforation due to foreign body accidentally left in body following procedure

● T81.530 Perforation due to foreign body accidentally left in body following surgical operation

● T81.531 Perforation due to foreign body accidentally left in body following infusion or transfusion

● T81.532 Perforation due to foreign body accidentally left in body following kidney dialysis

● T81.533 Perforation due to foreign body accidentally left in body following injection or immunization

● T81.534 Perforation due to foreign body accidentally left in body following endoscopic examination

● T81.535 Perforation due to foreign body accidentally left in body following heart catheterization

● T81.536 Perforation due to foreign body accidentally left in body following aspiration, puncture or other catheterization

● T81.537 Perforation due to foreign body accidentally left in body following removal of catheter or packing

● T81.538 Perforation due to foreign body accidentally left in body following other procedure

● T81.539 Perforation due to foreign body accidentally left in body following unspecified procedure

● T81.59 Other complications of foreign body accidentally left in body following procedure

Excludes2 obstruction or perforation due to prosthetic devices and implants intentionally left in body (T82.Ø-T82.5, T83.Ø-T83.4, T83.7, T84.Ø-T84.4, T85.Ø-T85.6)

● T81.590 Other complications of foreign body accidentally left in body following surgical operation

● T81.591 Other complications of foreign body accidentally left in body following infusion or transfusion

● T81.592 Other complications of foreign body accidentally left in body following kidney dialysis

● T81.593 Other complications of foreign body accidentally left in body following injection or immunization

● T81.594 Other complications of foreign body accidentally left in body following endoscopic examination

● T81.595 Other complications of foreign body accidentally left in body following heart catheterization

● T81.596 Other complications of foreign body accidentally left in body following aspiration, puncture or other catheterization

● T81.597 Other complications of foreign body accidentally left in body following removal of catheter or packing

● T81.598 Other complications of foreign body accidentally left in body following other procedure

● T81.599 Other complications of foreign body accidentally left in body following unspecified procedure

● T81.6 Acute reaction to foreign substance accidentally left during a procedure

Excludes2 complications of foreign body accidentally left in body cavity or operation wound following procedure (T81.5-)

X● T81.60 Unspecified acute reaction to foreign substance accidentally left during a procedure

X● T81.61 Aseptic peritonitis due to foreign substance accidentally left during a procedure

Chemical peritonitis

X● T81.69 Other acute reaction to foreign substance accidentally left during a procedure

● **T81.7 Vascular complications following a procedure, not elsewhere classified**
Air embolism following procedure NEC
Phlebitis or thrombophlebitis resulting from a procedure
Excludes1 embolism complicating abortion or ectopic or molar pregnancy (O00-O07, O08.2)
embolism complicating pregnancy, childbirth and the puerperium (O88.-)
traumatic embolism (T79.0)
Excludes2 embolism due to prosthetic devices, implants and grafts (T82.8, T83.81, T84.8-, T85.1-) ◄
embolism following infusion, transfusion and therapeutic injection (T80.0)

● **T81.71 Complication of artery following a procedure, not elsewhere classified**
● **T81.710 Complication of mesenteric artery following a procedure, not elsewhere classified**
● **T81.711 Complication of renal artery following a procedure, not elsewhere classified**
● **T81.718 Complication of other artery following a procedure, not elsewhere classified**
● **T81.719 Complication of unspecified artery following a procedure, not elsewhere classified**

X● **T81.72 Complication of vein following a procedure, not elsewhere classified**

● **T81.8 Other complications of procedures, not elsewhere classified**
Excludes2 hypothermia following anesthesia (T88.51)
malignant hyperpyrexia due to anesthesia (T88.3)

X● **T81.81 Complication of inhalation therapy**
X● **T81.82 Emphysema (subcutaneous) resulting from a procedure**
X● **T81.83 Persistent postprocedural fistula**
X● **T81.89 Other complications of procedures, not elsewhere classified**
Use additional code to specify complication, such as:
postprocedural delirium (F05)

X● **T81.9 Unspecified complication of procedure**

● **T82 Complications of cardiac and vascular prosthetic devices, implants and grafts**
Excludes2 failure and rejection of transplanted organs and tissue (T86.-)

The appropriate 7th character is to be added to each code from category T82

A	initial encounter
D	subsequent encounter
S	sequela

● **T82.0 Mechanical complication of heart valve prosthesis**
Mechanical complication of artificial heart valve
Excludes1 mechanical complication of biological heart valve graft (T82.22-)

X● **T82.01 Breakdown (mechanical) of heart valve prosthesis**
X● **T82.02 Displacement of heart valve prosthesis**
Malposition of heart valve prosthesis
X● **T82.03 Leakage of heart valve prosthesis**
X● **T82.09 Other mechanical complication of heart valve prosthesis**
Obstruction (mechanical) of heart valve prosthesis
Perforation of heart valve prosthesis
Protrusion of heart valve prosthesis

● **T82.1 Mechanical complication of cardiac electronic device**

● **T82.11 Breakdown (mechanical) of cardiac electronic device**
● **T82.110 Breakdown (mechanical) of cardiac electrode**
● **T82.111 Breakdown (mechanical) of cardiac pulse generator (battery)**
● **T82.118 Breakdown (mechanical) of other cardiac electronic device**
● **T82.119 Breakdown (mechanical) of unspecified cardiac electronic device**

● **T82.12 Displacement of cardiac electronic device**
Malposition of cardiac electronic device
● **T82.120 Displacement of cardiac electrode**
● **T82.121 Displacement of cardiac pulse generator (battery)**
● **T82.128 Displacement of other cardiac electronic device**
● **T82.129 Displacement of unspecified cardiac electronic device**

● **T82.19 Other mechanical complication of cardiac electronic device**
Leakage of cardiac electronic device
Obstruction of cardiac electronic device
Perforation of cardiac electronic device
Protrusion of cardiac electronic device
● **T82.190 Other mechanical complication of cardiac electrode**
● **T82.191 Other mechanical complication of cardiac pulse generator (battery)**
● **T82.198 Other mechanical complication of other cardiac electronic device**
● **T82.199 Other mechanical complication of unspecified cardiac device**

● **T82.2 Mechanical complication of coronary artery bypass graft and biological heart valve graft**
Excludes1 mechanical complication of artificial heart valve prosthesis (T82.0-)

● **T82.21 Mechanical complication of coronary artery bypass graft**
● **T82.211 Breakdown (mechanical) of coronary artery bypass graft**
● **T82.212 Displacement of coronary artery bypass graft**
Malposition of coronary artery bypass graft
● **T82.213 Leakage of coronary artery bypass graft**
● **T82.218 Other mechanical complication of coronary artery bypass graft**
Obstruction, mechanical of coronary artery bypass graft
Perforation of coronary artery bypass graft
Protrusion of coronary artery bypass graft

CHAPTER 19 (S00-T88)

● T82.22 **Mechanical complication of biological heart valve graft**

● T82.221 **Breakdown (mechanical) of biological heart valve graft**

● T82.222 **Displacement of biological heart valve graft**
Malposition of biological heart valve graft

● T82.223 **Leakage of biological heart valve graft**

● T82.228 **Other mechanical complication of biological heart valve graft**
Obstruction of biological heart valve graft
Perforation of biological heart valve graft
Protrusion of biological heart valve graft

● T82.3 **Mechanical complication of other vascular grafts**

● T82.31 **Breakdown (mechanical) of other vascular grafts**

● T82.310 **Breakdown (mechanical) of aortic (bifurcation) graft (replacement)**

● T82.311 **Breakdown (mechanical) of carotid arterial graft (bypass)**

● T82.312 **Breakdown (mechanical) of femoral arterial graft (bypass)**

● T82.318 **Breakdown (mechanical) of other vascular grafts**

● T82.319 **Breakdown (mechanical) of unspecified vascular grafts**

● T82.32 **Displacement of other vascular grafts**
Malposition of other vascular grafts

● T82.320 **Displacement of aortic (bifurcation) graft (replacement)**

● T82.321 **Displacement of carotid arterial graft (bypass)**

● T82.322 **Displacement of femoral arterial graft (bypass)**

● T82.328 **Displacement of other vascular grafts**

● T82.329 **Displacement of unspecified vascular grafts**

● T82.33 **Leakage of other vascular grafts**

● T82.330 **Leakage of aortic (bifurcation) graft (replacement)**

● T82.331 **Leakage of carotid arterial graft (bypass)**

● T82.332 **Leakage of femoral arterial graft (bypass)**

● T82.338 **Leakage of other vascular grafts**

● T82.339 **Leakage of unspecified vascular graft**

● T82.39 **Other mechanical complication of other vascular grafts**
Obstruction (mechanical) of other vascular grafts
Perforation of other vascular grafts
Protrusion of other vascular grafts

● T82.390 **Other mechanical complication of aortic (bifurcation) graft (replacement)**

● T82.391 **Other mechanical complication of carotid arterial graft (bypass)**

● T82.392 **Other mechanical complication of femoral arterial graft (bypass)**

● T82.398 **Other mechanical complication of other vascular grafts**

● T82.399 **Other mechanical complication of unspecified vascular grafts**

● T82.4 **Mechanical complication of vascular dialysis catheter**
Mechanical complication of hemodialysis catheter
Excludes1 mechanical complication of intraperitoneal dialysis catheter (T85.62)

X● T82.41 **Breakdown (mechanical) of vascular dialysis catheter**

X● T82.42 **Displacement of vascular dialysis catheter**
Malposition of vascular dialysis catheter

X● T82.43 **Leakage of vascular dialysis catheter**

X● T82.49 **Other complication of vascular dialysis catheter**
Obstruction (mechanical) of vascular dialysis catheter
Perforation of vascular dialysis catheter
Protrusion of vascular dialysis catheter

● T82.5 **Mechanical complication of other cardiac and vascular devices and implants**
Excludes2 mechanical complication of epidural and subdural infusion catheter (T85.61)

● T82.51 **Breakdown (mechanical) of other cardiac and vascular devices and implants**

● T82.510 **Breakdown (mechanical) of surgically created arteriovenous fistula**

● T82.511 **Breakdown (mechanical) of surgically created arteriovenous shunt**

● T82.512 **Breakdown (mechanical) of artificial heart**

● T82.513 **Breakdown (mechanical) of balloon (counterpulsation) device**

● T82.514 **Breakdown (mechanical) of infusion catheter**

● T82.515 **Breakdown (mechanical) of umbrella device**

● T82.518 **Breakdown (mechanical) of other cardiac and vascular devices and implants**

● T82.519 **Breakdown (mechanical) of unspecified cardiac and vascular devices and implants**

● T82.52 **Displacement of other cardiac and vascular devices and implants**
Malposition of other cardiac and vascular devices and implants

● T82.520 **Displacement of surgically created arteriovenous fistula**

● T82.521 **Displacement of surgically created arteriovenous shunt**

● T82.522 **Displacement of artificial heart**

● T82.523 **Displacement of balloon (counterpulsation) device**

● T82.524 **Displacement of infusion catheter**

● T82.525 **Displacement of umbrella device**

● T82.528 **Displacement of other cardiac and vascular devices and implants**

● T82.529 **Displacement of unspecified cardiac and vascular devices and implants**

● T82.53 **Leakage of other cardiac and vascular devices and implants**

● T82.530 **Leakage of surgically created arteriovenous fistula**

● T82.531 **Leakage of surgically created arteriovenous shunt**

● T82.532 **Leakage of artificial heart**

● T82.533 **Leakage of balloon (counterpulsation) device**

● T82.534 **Leakage of infusion catheter**

● T82.535 **Leakage of umbrella device**

● T82.538 **Leakage of other cardiac and vascular devices and implants**

● T82.539 **Leakage of unspecified cardiac and vascular devices and implants**

CHAPTER 19 (SØ-T88)

● **T82.59**   **Other mechanical complication of other cardiac and vascular devices and implants**
     Obstruction (mechanical) of other cardiac and vascular devices and implants
     Perforation of other cardiac and vascular devices and implants
     Protrusion of other cardiac and vascular devices and implants

    ● **T82.590**   **Other mechanical complication of surgically created arteriovenous fistula**

    ● **T82.591**   **Other mechanical complication of surgically created arteriovenous shunt**

    ● **T82.592**   **Other mechanical complication of artificial heart**

    ● **T82.593**   **Other mechanical complication of balloon (counterpulsation) device**

    ● **T82.594**   **Other mechanical complication of infusion catheter**

    ● **T82.595**   **Other mechanical complication of umbrella device**

    ● **T82.598**   **Other mechanical complication of other cardiac and vascular devices and implants**

    ● **T82.599**   **Other mechanical complication of unspecified cardiac and vascular devices and implants**

X ● **T82.6**   **Infection and inflammatory reaction due to cardiac valve prosthesis**
     Use additional code to identify infection

X ● **T82.7**   **Infection and inflammatory reaction due to other cardiac and vascular devices, implants and grafts**
     Use additional code to identify infection

● **T82.8**   **Other specified complications of cardiac and vascular prosthetic devices, implants and grafts**

   ● **T82.81**   **Embolism due to cardiac and vascular prosthetic devices, implants and grafts** ◀▪▬

    ● **T82.817**   **Embolism due to cardiac prosthetic devices, implants and grafts**

    ● **T82.818**   **Embolism due to vascular prosthetic devices, implants and grafts**

   ● **T82.82**   **Fibrosis due to cardiac and vascular prosthetic devices, implants and grafts** ◀▪▬

    ● **T82.827**   **Fibrosis due to cardiac prosthetic devices, implants and grafts**

    ● **T82.828**   **Fibrosis due to vascular prosthetic devices, implants and grafts**

   ● **T82.83**   **Hemorrhage due to cardiac and vascular prosthetic devices, implants and grafts** ◀▪▬

    ● **T82.837**   **Hemorrhage due to cardiac prosthetic devices, implants and grafts**

    ● **T82.838**   **Hemorrhage due to vascular prosthetic devices, implants and grafts**

   ● **T82.84**   **Pain due to cardiac and vascular prosthetic devices, implants and grafts** ◀▪▬

    ● **T82.847**   **Pain due to cardiac prosthetic devices, implants and grafts**

    ● **T82.848**   **Pain due to vascular prosthetic devices, implants and grafts**

● **T82.85**   **Stenosis due to cardiac and vascular prosthetic devices, implants and grafts** ◀▪▬

   ● **T82.855**   **Stenosis of coronary artery stent** ◀
     In-stent stenosis (restenosis) of coronary artery stent ◀
     Restenosis of coronary artery stent ◀

   ● **T82.856**   **Stenosis of peripheral vascular stent** ◀
     In-stent stenosis (restenosis) of peripheral vascular stent ◀
     Restenosis of peripheral vascular stent ◀

   ● **T82.857**   **Stenosis of other cardiac prosthetic devices, implants and grafts**

   ● **T82.858**   **Stenosis of other vascular prosthetic devices, implants and grafts**

● **T82.86**   **Thrombosis of cardiac and vascular prosthetic devices, implants and grafts**

   ● **T82.867**   **Thrombosis due to cardiac prosthetic devices, implants and grafts**

   ● **T82.868**   **Thrombosis due to vascular prosthetic devices, implants and grafts**

● **T82.89**   **Other specified complication of cardiac and vascular prosthetic devices, implants and grafts**

   ● **T82.897**   **Other specified complication of cardiac prosthetic devices, implants and grafts**

   ● **T82.898**   **Other specified complication of vascular prosthetic devices, implants and grafts**

X ● **T82.9**   **Unspecified complication of cardiac and vascular prosthetic device, implant and graft**

● **T83**   **Complications of genitourinary prosthetic devices, implants and grafts**
   Excludes2   failure and rejection of transplanted organs and tissue (T86.-)

   The appropriate 7th character is to be added to each code from category T83

    A   initial encounter
    D   subsequent encounter
    S   sequela

● **T83.0**   **Mechanical complication of urinary catheter** ◀▪▬
   Excludes2   complications of stoma of urinary tract (N99.5-)

   ● **T83.01**   **Breakdown (mechanical) of urinary catheter** ◀▪▬

    ● **T83.010**   **Breakdown (mechanical) of cystostomy catheter**

    ● **T83.011**   **Breakdown (mechanical) of indwelling urethral catheter**

    ● **T83.012**   **Breakdown (mechanical) of nephrostomy catheter**

    ● **T83.018**   **Breakdown (mechanical) of other urinary catheter** ◀▪▬
     Breakdown (mechanical) of Hopkins catheter
     Breakdown (mechanical) of ileostomy catheter
     Breakdown (mechanical) urostomy catheter

CHAPTER 19 (S00-T88)

● T83.02 **Displacement of urinary catheter** ⬅
Malposition of urinary catheter ⬅
● T83.020 **Displacement of cystostomy catheter**
● T83.021 **Displacement of indwelling urethral catheter**
● T83.022 **Displacement of nephrostomy catheter**
● T83.028 **Displacement of other urinary catheter** ⬅
Displacement of Hopkins catheter ◀
Displacement of ileostomy catheter ◀
Displacement of urostomy catheter ◀
● T83.03 **Leakage of urinary catheter** ⬅
● T83.030 **Leakage of cystostomy catheter**
● T83.031 **Leakage of indwelling urethral catheter**
● T83.032 **Leakage of nephrostomy catheter**
● T83.038 **Leakage of other urinary catheter** ⬅
Leakage of Hopkins catheter ◀
Leakage of ileostomy catheter ◀
Leakage of urostomy catheter ◀
● T83.09 **Other mechanical complication of urinary catheter** ⬅
Obstruction (mechanical) of urinary catheter ⬅
Perforation of urinary catheter ⬅
Protrusion of urinary catheter ⬅
● T83.090 **Other mechanical complication of cystostomy catheter**
● T83.091 **Other mechanical complication of indwelling urethral catheter**
● T83.092 **Other mechanical complication of nephrostomy catheter**
● T83.098 **Other mechanical complication of other urinary catheter** ⬅
Other mechanical complication of Hopkins catheter ◀
Other mechanical complication of ileostomy catheter ◀
Other mechanical complication of urostomy catheter ◀
● T83.1 **Mechanical complication of other urinary devices and implants**
● T83.11 **Breakdown (mechanical) of other urinary devices and implants**
● T83.110 **Breakdown (mechanical) of urinary electronic stimulator device**
Excludes2 Breakdown (mechanical) of electrode (lead) for sacral nerve neurostimulator (T85.111) ◀
Breakdown (mechanical) of implanted electronic sacral neurostimulator, pulse generator or receiver (T85.113) ◀
● T83.111 **Breakdown (mechanical) of implanted urinary sphincter**
● T83.112 **Breakdown (mechanical) of indwelling ureteral stent**
● T83.113 **Breakdown (mechanical) of other urinary stents**
Breakdown (mechanical) of ileal conduit stent ◀
Breakdown (mechanical) of nephroureteral stent ◀
● T83.118 **Breakdown (mechanical) of other urinary devices and implants**
● T83.12 **Displacement of other urinary devices and implants**
Malposition of other urinary devices and implants
● T83.120 **Displacement of urinary electronic stimulator device**
Excludes2 Displacement of electrode (lead) for sacral nerve neurostimulator (T85.121) ◀
Displacement of implanted electronic sacral neurostimulator, pulse generator or receiver (T85.123) ◀
● T83.121 **Displacement of implanted urinary sphincter**
● T83.122 **Displacement of indwelling ureteral stent**
● T83.123 **Displacement of other urinary stents**
Displacement of ileal conduit stent ◀
Displacement of nephroureteral stent ◀
● T83.128 **Displacement of other urinary devices and implants**
● T83.19 **Other mechanical complication of other urinary devices and implants**
Leakage of other urinary devices and implants
Obstruction (mechanical) of other urinary devices and implants
Perforation of other urinary devices and implants
Protrusion of other urinary devices and implants
● T83.190 **Other mechanical complication of urinary electronic stimulator device**
Excludes2 Other mechanical complication of electrode (lead) for sacral nerve neurostimulator (T85.191) ◀
Other mechanical complication of implanted electronic sacral neurostimulator, pulse generator or receiver (T85.193) ◀
● T83.191 **Other mechanical complication of implanted urinary sphincter**
● T83.192 **Other mechanical complication of indwelling ureteral stent**
● T83.193 **Other mechanical complication of other urinary stent**
Other mechanical complication of ileal conduit stent ◀
Other mechanical complication of nephroureteral stent ◀
● T83.198 **Other mechanical complication of other urinary devices and implants**
● T83.2 **Mechanical complication of graft of urinary organ**
X● T83.21 **Breakdown (mechanical) of graft of urinary organ**
X● T83.22 **Displacement of graft of urinary organ**
Malposition of graft of urinary organ
X● T83.23 **Leakage of graft of urinary organ**
X● T83.24 **Erosion of graft of urinary organ**

X● **T83.25 Exposure of graft of urinary organ**

X● **T83.29 Other mechanical complication of graft of urinary organ**
Obstruction (mechanical) of graft of urinary organ
Perforation of graft of urinary organ
Protrusion of graft of urinary organ

● **T83.3 Mechanical complication of intrauterine contraceptive device**

X● **T83.31 Breakdown (mechanical) of intrauterine contraceptive device**

X● **T83.32 Displacement of intrauterine contraceptive device**
Malposition of intrauterine contraceptive device
Missing string of intrauterine contraceptive device ◀

X● **T83.39 Other mechanical complication of intrauterine contraceptive device**
Leakage of intrauterine contraceptive device
Obstruction (mechanical) of intrauterine contraceptive device
Perforation of intrauterine contraceptive device
Protrusion of intrauterine contraceptive device

● **T83.4 Mechanical complication of other prosthetic devices, implants and grafts of genital tract**

● **T83.41 Breakdown (mechanical) of other prosthetic devices, implants and grafts of genital tract**

● **T83.410 Breakdown (mechanical) of implanted penile prosthesis**
Breakdown (mechanical) of penile prosthesis cylinder ◀
Breakdown (mechanical) of penile prosthesis pump ◀
Breakdown (mechanical) of penile prosthesis reservoir ◀

● **T83.411 Breakdown (mechanical) of implanted testicular prosthesis** ◀

● **T83.418 Breakdown (mechanical) of other prosthetic devices, implants and grafts of genital tract**

● **T83.42 Displacement of other prosthetic devices, implants and grafts of genital tract**
Malposition of other prosthetic devices, implants and grafts of genital tract

● **T83.420 Displacement of implanted penile prosthesis**
Displacement of penile prosthesis cylinder ◀
Displacement of penile prosthesis pump ◀
Displacement of penile prosthesis reservoir ◀

● **T83.421 Displacement of implanted testicular prosthesis** ◀

● **T83.428 Displacement of other prosthetic devices, implants and grafts of genital tract**

● **T83.49 Other mechanical complication of other prosthetic devices, implants and grafts of genital tract**
Leakage of other prosthetic devices, implants and grafts of genital tract
Obstruction, mechanical of other prosthetic devices, implants and grafts of genital tract
Perforation of other prosthetic devices, implants and grafts of genital tract
Protrusion of other prosthetic devices, implants and grafts of genital tract

● **T83.490 Other mechanical complication of implanted penile prosthesis**
Other mechanical complication of penile prosthesis cylinder ◀
Other mechanical complication of penile prosthesis pump ◀
Other mechanical complication of penile prosthesis reservoir ◀

● **T83.491 Other mechanical complication of implanted testicular prosthesis**

● **T83.498 Other mechanical complication of other prosthetic devices, implants and grafts of genital tract**

● **T83.5 Infection and inflammatory reaction due to prosthetic device, implant and graft in urinary system**
Use additional code to identify infection

● **T83.51 Infection and inflammatory reaction due to urinary catheter**
Excludes2 complications of stoma of urinary tract (N99.5-)

● **T83.510 Infection and inflammatory reaction due to cystostomy catheter**

● **T83.511 Infection and inflammatory reaction due to indwelling urethral catheter**

● **T83.512 Infection and inflammatory reaction due to nephrostomy catheter**

● **T83.518 Infection and inflammatory reaction due to other urinary catheter**
Infection and inflammatory reaction due to Hopkins catheter ◀
Infection and inflammatory reaction due to ileostomy catheter ◀
Infection and inflammatory reaction due to urostomy catheter ◀

● **T83.59 Infection and inflammatory reaction due to prosthetic device, implant and graft in urinary system**

● **T83.590 Infection and inflammatory reaction due to implanted urinary neurostimulation device**
Excludes2 Infection and inflammatory reaction due to electrode lead of sacral nerve neurostimulator (T85.732) ◀
Infection and inflammatory reaction due to pulse generator or receiver of sacral nerve neurostimulator (T85.734) ◀

● **T83.591 Infection and inflammatory reaction due to implanted urinary sphincter**

● **T83.592 Infection and inflammatory reaction due to indwelling ureteral stent**

● **T83.593 Infection and inflammatory reaction due to other urinary stents**
Infection and inflammatory reaction due to ileal conduit stents ◀
Infection and inflammatory reaction due to nephroureteral stent ◀

● **T83.598 Infection and inflammatory reaction due to other prosthetic device, implant and graft in urinary system**

● T83.6 **Infection and inflammatory reaction due to prosthetic device, implant and graft in genital tract**
Use additional code to identify infection

● T83.61 **Infection and inflammatory reaction due to implanted penile prosthesis**
Infection and inflammatory reaction due to penile prosthesis cylinder ◀
Infection and inflammatory reaction due to penile prosthesis pump ◀
Infection and inflammatory reaction due to penile prosthesis reservoir ◀

● T83.62 **Infection and inflammatory reaction due to implanted testicular prosthesis**

● T83.69 **Infection and inflammatory reaction due to other prosthetic device, implant and graft in genital tract**

● T83.7 **Complications due to implanted mesh and other prosthetic materials**

● T83.71 **Erosion of implanted mesh and other prosthetic materials to surrounding organ or tissue**

● T83.711 **Erosion of implanted vaginal mesh to surrounding organ or tissue** ⬅
Erosion of implanted vaginal mesh into pelvic floor muscles ⬅

● T83.712 **Erosion of implanted urethral mesh to surrounding organ or tissue**
Erosion of implanted female urethral sling ◀
Erosion of implanted male urethral sling ◀
Erosion of implanted urethral mesh into pelvic floor muscles ◀

● T83.713 **Erosion of implanted urethral bulking agent to surrounding organ or tissue**

● T83.714 **Erosion of implanted ureteral bulking agent to surrounding organ or tissue**

● T83.718 **Erosion of other implanted mesh to organ or tissue**

● T83.719 **Erosion of other prosthetic materials to surrounding organ or tissue**

● T83.72 **Exposure of implanted mesh and other prosthetic materials into surrounding organ or tissue**
Extrusion of implanted mesh ◀

● T83.721 **Exposure of implanted vaginal mesh into vagina** ⬅
Exposure of implanted vaginal mesh through vaginal wall ⬅

● T83.722 **Exposure of implanted urethral mesh into urethra**
Exposure of implanted female urethral sling ◀
Exposure of implanted male urethral sling ◀
Exposure of implanted urethral mesh through urethral wall ◀

● T83.723 **Exposure of implanted urethral bulking agent into urethra**

● T83.724 **Exposure of implanted ureteral bulking agent into ureter**

● T83.728 **Exposure of other implanted mesh into organ or tissue**

● T83.729 **Exposure of other prosthetic materials into organ or tissue**

X● T83.79 **Other specified complications due to other genitourinary prosthetic materials**

● T83.8 **Other specified complications of genitourinary prosthetic devices, implants and grafts**

X● T83.81 **Embolism due to genitourinary prosthetic devices, implants and grafts**

X● T83.82 **Fibrosis due to genitourinary prosthetic devices, implants and grafts**

X● T83.83 **Hemorrhage due to genitourinary prosthetic devices, implants and grafts**

X● T83.84 **Pain due to genitourinary prosthetic devices, implants and grafts**

X● T83.85 **Stenosis due to genitourinary prosthetic devices, implants and grafts**

X● T83.86 **Thrombosis due to genitourinary prosthetic devices, implants and grafts**

X● T83.89 **Other specified complication of genitourinary prosthetic devices, implants and grafts**

X● T83.9 **Unspecified complication of genitourinary prosthetic device, implant and graft**

● T84 **Complications of internal orthopedic prosthetic devices, implants and grafts**
Excludes2 failure and rejection of transplanted organs and tissues (T86.-)
fracture of bone following insertion of orthopedic implant, joint prosthesis or bone plate (M96.6)

The appropriate 7th character is to be added to each code from category T84

A	initial encounter
D	subsequent encounter
S	sequela

● T84.0 **Mechanical complication of internal joint prosthesis**

● T84.01 **Broken internal joint prosthesis**
Breakage (fracture) of prosthetic joint
Broken prosthetic joint implant
Excludes1 periprosthetic joint implant fracture (T84.04)

● T84.010 **Broken internal right hip prosthesis**

● T84.011 **Broken internal left hip prosthesis**

● T84.012 **Broken internal right knee prosthesis**

● T84.013 **Broken internal left knee prosthesis**

● T84.018 **Broken internal joint prosthesis, other site**
Use additional code to identify the joint (Z96.6-)

● T84.019 **Broken internal joint prosthesis, unspecified site**

● T84.02 **Dislocation of internal joint prosthesis**
Instability of internal joint prosthesis
Subluxation of internal joint prosthesis

● T84.020 **Dislocation of internal right hip prosthesis**

● T84.021 **Dislocation of internal left hip prosthesis**

● T84.022 **Instability of internal right knee prosthesis**

● T84.023 **Instability of internal left knee prosthesis**

● T84.028 **Dislocation of other internal joint prosthesis**
Use additional code to identify the joint (Z96.6-)

● T84.029 **Dislocation of unspecified internal joint prosthesis**

- T84.03 **Mechanical loosening of internal prosthetic joint**
  Aseptic loosening of prosthetic joint
  - T84.030 **Mechanical loosening of internal right hip prosthetic joint**
  - T84.031 **Mechanical loosening of internal left hip prosthetic joint**
  - T84.032 **Mechanical loosening of internal right knee prosthetic joint**
  - T84.033 **Mechanical loosening of internal left knee prosthetic joint**
  - T84.038 **Mechanical loosening of other internal prosthetic joint**
    Use additional code to identify the joint (Z96.6-)
  - T84.039 **Mechanical loosening of unspecified internal prosthetic joint**
- ~~T84.04 Periprosthetic fracture around internal prosthetic joint~~
  - ~~T84.040 Periprosthetic fracture around internal prosthetic right hip joint~~
  - ~~T84.041 Periprosthetic fracture around internal prosthetic left hip joint~~
  - ~~T84.042 Periprosthetic fracture around internal prosthetic right knee joint~~
  - ~~T84.043 Periprosthetic fracture around internal prosthetic left knee joint~~
  - ~~T84.048 Periprosthetic fracture around other internal prosthetic joint~~
  - ~~T84.049 Periprosthetic fracture around unspecified internal prosthetic joint~~
- T84.05 **Periprosthetic osteolysis of internal prosthetic joint**
  Use additional code to identify major osseous defect, if applicable (M89.7-)
  - T84.050 **Periprosthetic osteolysis of internal prosthetic right hip joint**
  - T84.051 **Periprosthetic osteolysis of internal prosthetic left hip joint**
  - T84.052 **Periprosthetic osteolysis of internal prosthetic right knee joint**
  - T84.053 **Periprosthetic osteolysis of internal prosthetic left knee joint**
  - T84.058 **Periprosthetic osteolysis of other internal prosthetic joint**
    Use additional code to identify the joint (Z96.6-)
  - T84.059 **Periprosthetic osteolysis of unspecified internal prosthetic joint**
- T84.06 **Wear of articular bearing surface of internal prosthetic joint**
  - T84.060 **Wear of articular bearing surface of internal prosthetic right hip joint**
  - T84.061 **Wear of articular bearing surface of internal prosthetic left hip joint**
  - T84.062 **Wear of articular bearing surface of internal prosthetic right knee joint**
  - T84.063 **Wear of articular bearing surface of internal prosthetic left knee joint**
  - T84.068 **Wear of articular bearing surface of other internal prosthetic joint**
    Use additional code to identify the joint (Z96.6-)
  - T84.069 **Wear of articular bearing surface of unspecified internal prosthetic joint**
- T84.09 **Other mechanical complication of internal joint prosthesis**
  Prosthetic joint implant failure NOS
  - T84.090 **Other mechanical complication of internal right hip prosthesis**
  - T84.091 **Other mechanical complication of internal left hip prosthesis**
  - T84.092 **Other mechanical complication of internal right knee prosthesis**
  - T84.093 **Other mechanical complication of internal left knee prosthesis**
  - T84.098 **Other mechanical complication of other internal joint prosthesis**
    Use additional code to identify the joint (Z96.6-)
  - T84.099 **Other mechanical complication of unspecified internal joint prosthesis**

- T84.1 **Mechanical complication of internal fixation device of bones of limb**
  Excludes2 mechanical complication of internal fixation device of bones of feet (T84.2-)
  mechanical complication of internal fixation device of bones of fingers (T84.2-)
  mechanical complication of internal fixation device of bones of hands (T84.2-)
  mechanical complication of internal fixation device of bones of toes (T84.2-)
- T84.11 **Breakdown (mechanical) of internal fixation device of bones of limb**
  - T84.110 **Breakdown (mechanical) of internal fixation device of right humerus**
  - T84.111 **Breakdown (mechanical) of internal fixation device of left humerus**
  - T84.112 **Breakdown (mechanical) of internal fixation device of bone of right forearm**
  - T84.113 **Breakdown (mechanical) of internal fixation device of bone of left forearm**
  - T84.114 **Breakdown (mechanical) of internal fixation device of right femur**
  - T84.115 **Breakdown (mechanical) of internal fixation device of left femur**
  - T84.116 **Breakdown (mechanical) of internal fixation device of bone of right lower leg**
  - T84.117 **Breakdown (mechanical) of internal fixation device of bone of left lower leg**
  - T84.119 **Breakdown (mechanical) of internal fixation device of unspecified bone of limb**
- T84.12 **Displacement of internal fixation device of bones of limb**
  Malposition of internal fixation device of bones of limb
  - T84.120 **Displacement of internal fixation device of right humerus**
  - T84.121 **Displacement of internal fixation device of left humerus**
  - T84.122 **Displacement of internal fixation device of bone of right forearm**
  - T84.123 **Displacement of internal fixation device of bone of left forearm**
  - T84.124 **Displacement of internal fixation device of right femur**
  - T84.125 **Displacement of internal fixation device of left femur**
  - T84.126 **Displacement of internal fixation device of bone of right lower leg**
  - T84.127 **Displacement of internal fixation device of bone of left lower leg**
  - T84.129 **Displacement of internal fixation device of unspecified bone of limb**

CHAPTER 19 (S00-T88)

● T84.19 **Other mechanical complication of internal fixation device of bones of limb**
Obstruction (mechanical) of internal fixation device of bones of limb
Perforation of internal fixation device of bones of limb
Protrusion of internal fixation device of bones of limb

● T84.190 **Other mechanical complication of internal fixation device of right humerus**

● T84.191 **Other mechanical complication of internal fixation device of left humerus**

● T84.192 **Other mechanical complication of internal fixation device of bone of right forearm**

● T84.193 **Other mechanical complication of internal fixation device of bone of left forearm**

● T84.194 **Other mechanical complication of internal fixation device of right femur**

● T84.195 **Other mechanical complication of internal fixation device of left femur**

● T84.196 **Other mechanical complication of internal fixation device of bone of right lower leg**

● T84.197 **Other mechanical complication of internal fixation device of bone of left lower leg**

● T84.199 **Other mechanical complication of internal fixation device of unspecified bone of limb**

● T84.2 **Mechanical complication of internal fixation device of other bones**

● T84.21 **Breakdown (mechanical) of internal fixation device of other bones**

● T84.210 **Breakdown (mechanical) of internal fixation device of bones of hand and fingers**

● T84.213 **Breakdown (mechanical) of internal fixation device of bones of foot and toes**

● T84.216 **Breakdown (mechanical) of internal fixation device of vertebrae**

● T84.218 **Breakdown (mechanical) of internal fixation device of other bones**

● T84.22 **Displacement of internal fixation device of other bones**
Malposition of internal fixation device of other bones

● T84.220 **Displacement of internal fixation device of bones of hand and fingers**

● T84.223 **Displacement of internal fixation device of bones of foot and toes**

● T84.226 **Displacement of internal fixation device of vertebrae**

● T84.228 **Displacement of internal fixation device of other bones**

● T84.29 **Other mechanical complication of internal fixation device of other bones**
Obstruction (mechanical) of internal fixation device of other bones
Perforation of internal fixation device of other bones
Protrusion of internal fixation device of other bones

● T84.290 **Other mechanical complication of internal fixation device of bones of hand and fingers**

● T84.293 **Other mechanical complication of internal fixation device of bones of foot and toes**

● T84.296 **Other mechanical complication of internal fixation device of vertebrae**

● T84.298 **Other mechanical complication of internal fixation device of other bones**

● T84.3 **Mechanical complication of other bone devices, implants and grafts**
Excludes2 other complications of bone graft (T86.83-)

● T84.31 **Breakdown (mechanical) of other bone devices, implants and grafts**

● T84.310 **Breakdown (mechanical) of electronic bone stimulator**

● T84.318 **Breakdown (mechanical) of other bone devices, implants and grafts**

● T84.32 **Displacement of other bone devices, implants and grafts**
Malposition of other bone devices, implants and grafts

● T84.320 **Displacement of electronic bone stimulator**

● T84.328 **Displacement of other bone devices, implants and grafts**

● T84.39 **Other mechanical complication of other bone devices, implants and grafts**
Obstruction (mechanical) of other bone devices, implants and grafts
Perforation of other bone devices, implants and grafts
Protrusion of other bone devices, implants and grafts

● T84.390 **Other mechanical complication of electronic bone stimulator**

● T84.398 **Other mechanical complication of other bone devices, implants and grafts**

● T84.4 **Mechanical complication of other internal orthopedic devices, implants and grafts**

● T84.41 **Breakdown (mechanical) of other internal orthopedic devices, implants and grafts**

● T84.410 **Breakdown (mechanical) of muscle and tendon graft**

● T84.418 **Breakdown (mechanical) of other internal orthopedic devices, implants and grafts**

● T84.42 **Displacement of other internal orthopedic devices, implants and grafts**
Malposition of other internal orthopedic devices, implants and grafts

● T84.420 **Displacement of muscle and tendon graft**

● T84.428 **Displacement of other internal orthopedic devices, implants and grafts**

New · Revised · ~~deleted~~ Deleted · OGCR Official Guidelines · X Assign placeholder X · ● Use Additional Character(s)
Excludes1 · Excludes2 · Includes · Use additional · Code first · Code also · Unspecified

● **T84.49 Other mechanical complication of other internal orthopedic devices, implants and grafts**
Mechanical complication of other internal orthopedic devices, implants and grafts NOS
Obstruction (mechanical) of other internal orthopedic devices, implants and grafts
Perforation of other internal orthopedic devices, implants and grafts
Protrusion of other internal orthopedic devices, implants and grafts

● **T84.490 Other mechanical complication of muscle and tendon graft**

● **T84.498 Other mechanical complication of other internal orthopedic devices, implants and grafts**

● **T84.5 Infection and inflammatory reaction due to internal joint prosthesis**
Use additional code to identify infection

X● **T84.50 Infection and inflammatory reaction due to unspecified internal joint prosthesis**

X● **T84.51 Infection and inflammatory reaction due to internal right hip prosthesis**

X● **T84.52 Infection and inflammatory reaction due to internal left hip prosthesis**

X● **T84.53 Infection and inflammatory reaction due to internal right knee prosthesis**

X● **T84.54 Infection and inflammatory reaction due to internal left knee prosthesis**

X● **T84.59 Infection and inflammatory reaction due to other internal joint prosthesis**

● **T84.6 Infection and inflammatory reaction due to internal fixation device**
Use additional code to identify infection

X● **T84.60 Infection and inflammatory reaction due to internal fixation device of unspecified site**

● **T84.61 Infection and inflammatory reaction due to internal fixation device of arm**

● **T84.610 Infection and inflammatory reaction due to internal fixation device of right humerus**

● **T84.611 Infection and inflammatory reaction due to internal fixation device of left humerus**

● **T84.612 Infection and inflammatory reaction due to internal fixation device of right radius**

● **T84.613 Infection and inflammatory reaction due to internal fixation device of left radius**

● **T84.614 Infection and inflammatory reaction due to internal fixation device of right ulna**

● **T84.615 Infection and inflammatory reaction due to internal fixation device of left ulna**

● **T84.619 Infection and inflammatory reaction due to internal fixation device of unspecified bone of arm**

● **T84.62 Infection and inflammatory reaction due to internal fixation device of leg**

● **T84.620 Infection and inflammatory reaction due to internal fixation device of right femur**

● **T84.621 Infection and inflammatory reaction due to internal fixation device of left femur**

● **T84.622 Infection and inflammatory reaction due to internal fixation device of right tibia**

● **T84.623 Infection and inflammatory reaction due to internal fixation device of left tibia**

● **T84.624 Infection and inflammatory reaction due to internal fixation device of right fibula**

● **T84.625 Infection and inflammatory reaction due to internal fixation device of left fibula**

● **T84.629 Infection and inflammatory reaction due to internal fixation device of unspecified bone of leg**

X● **T84.63 Infection and inflammatory reaction due to internal fixation device of spine**

X● **T84.69 Infection and inflammatory reaction due to internal fixation device of other site**

● **T84.7 Infection and inflammatory reaction due to other internal orthopedic prosthetic devices, implants and grafts**
Use additional code to identify infection

● **T84.8 Other specified complications of internal orthopedic prosthetic devices, implants and grafts**

X● **T84.81 Embolism due to internal orthopedic prosthetic devices, implants and grafts**

X● **T84.82 Fibrosis due to internal orthopedic prosthetic devices, implants and grafts**

X● **T84.83 Hemorrhage due to internal orthopedic prosthetic devices, implants and grafts**

X● **T84.84 Pain due to internal orthopedic prosthetic devices, implants and grafts**

X● **T84.85 Stenosis due to internal orthopedic prosthetic devices, implants and grafts**

X● **T84.86 Thrombosis due to internal orthopedic prosthetic devices, implants and grafts**

X● **T84.89 Other specified complication of internal orthopedic prosthetic devices, implants and grafts**

X● **T84.9 Unspecified complication of internal orthopedic prosthetic device, implant and graft**

● **T85 Complications of other internal prosthetic devices, implants and grafts**
Excludes2 failure and rejection of transplanted organs and tissue (T86.-)
The appropriate 7th character is to be added to each code from category T85

A	initial encounter
D	subsequent encounter
S	sequela

● **T85.0 Mechanical complication of ventricular intracranial (communicating) shunt**

X● **T85.01 Breakdown (mechanical) of ventricular intracranial (communicating) shunt**

X● **T85.02 Displacement of ventricular intracranial (communicating) shunt**
Malposition of ventricular intracranial (communicating) shunt

X● **T85.03 Leakage of ventricular intracranial (communicating) shunt**

X● **T85.09 Other mechanical complication of ventricular intracranial (communicating) shunt**
Obstruction (mechanical) of ventricular intracranial (communicating) shunt
Perforation of ventricular intracranial (communicating) shunt
Protrusion of ventricular intracranial (communicating) shunt

CHAPTER 19 (S00-T88)

● **T85.1 Mechanical complication of implanted electronic stimulator of nervous system**

● **T85.11 Breakdown (mechanical) of implanted electronic stimulator of nervous system**

● **T85.11Ø Breakdown (mechanical) of implanted electronic neurostimulator of brain electrode (lead)**

● **T85.111 Breakdown (mechanical) of implanted electronic neurostimulator of peripheral nerve electrode (lead)**
Breakdown of electrode (lead) for cranial nerve neurostimulators ◀
Breakdown of electrode (lead) for gastric neurostimulator ◀
Breakdown of electrode (lead) for sacral nerve neurostimulator ◀
Breakdown of electrode (lead) for vagal nerve neurostimulators ◀

● **T85.112 Breakdown (mechanical) of implanted electronic neurostimulator of spinal cord electrode (lead)**

● **T85.113 Breakdown (mechanical) of implanted electronic neurostimulator, generator**
Breakdown (mechanical) of implanted electronic neurostimuator generator, brain, peripheral, gastric, spinal ◀
Breakdown (mechanical) of implanted electronic sacral neurostimulator, pulse generator or receiver ◀

● **T85.118 Breakdown (mechanical) of other implanted electronic stimulator of nervous system**

● **T85.12 Displacement of implanted electronic stimulator of nervous system**
Malposition of implanted electronic stimulator of nervous system

● **T85.12Ø Displacement of implanted electronic neurostimulator of brain electrode (lead)**

● **T85.121 Displacement of implanted electronic neurostimulator of peripheral nerve electrode (lead)**
Displacement of electrode (lead) for cranial nerve neurostimulators ◀
Displacement of electrode (lead) for gastric neurostimulator ◀
Displacement of electrode (lead) for sacral nerve neurostimulator ◀
Displacement of electrode (lead) for vagal nerve neurostimulators ◀

● **T85.122 Displacement of implanted electronic neurostimulator of spinal cord electrode (lead)**

● **T85.123 Displacement of implanted electronic neurostimulator, generator**
Displacement of implanted electronic neurostimulator generator, brain, peripheral, gastric, spinal ◀
Displacement of implanted electronic sacral neurostimulator, pulse generator or receiver ◀

● **T85.128 Displacement of other implanted electronic stimulator of nervous system**

● **T85.19 Other mechanical complication of implanted electronic stimulator of nervous system**
Leakage of implanted electronic stimulator of nervous system
Obstruction (mechanical) of implanted electronic stimulator of nervous system
Perforation of implanted electronic stimulator of nervous system
Protrusion of implanted electronic stimulator of nervous system

● **T85.19Ø Other mechanical complication of implanted electronic neurostimulator of brain electrode (lead)**

● **T85.191 Other mechanical complication of implanted electronic neurostimulator of peripheral nerve electrode (lead)**
Other mechanical complication of electrode (lead) for cranial nerve neurostimulators ◀
Other mechanical complication of electrode (lead) for gastric neurostimulator ◀
Other mechanical complication of electrode (lead) for sacral nerve neurostimulator ◀
Other mechanical complication of electrode (lead) for vagal nerve neurostimulators ◀

● **T85.192 Other mechanical complication of implanted electronic neurostimulator of spinal cord electrode (lead)**

● **T85.193 Other mechanical complication of implanted electronic neurostimulator, generator**
Other mechanical complication of implanted electronic neurostimulator generator, brain, peripheral, gastric, spinal ◀
Other mechanical complication of implanted electronic sacral neurostimulator, pulse generator or receiver ◀

● **T85.199 Other mechanical complication of other implanted electronic stimulator of nervous system**

● **T85.2 Mechanical complication of intraocular lens**

X● **T85.21 Breakdown (mechanical) of intraocular lens**

X● **T85.22 Displacement of intraocular lens**
Malposition of intraocular lens

X● **T85.29 Other mechanical complication of intraocular lens**
Obstruction (mechanical) of intraocular lens
Perforation of intraocular lens
Protrusion of intraocular lens

● **T85.3 Mechanical complication of other ocular prosthetic devices, implants and grafts**
Excludes2 other complications of corneal graft (T86.84-)

● **T85.31 Breakdown (mechanical) of other ocular prosthetic devices, implants and grafts**

● **T85.31Ø Breakdown (mechanical) of prosthetic orbit of right eye**

● **T85.311 Breakdown (mechanical) of prosthetic orbit of left eye**

● **T85.318 Breakdown (mechanical) of other ocular prosthetic devices, implants and grafts**

● **T85.32 Displacement of other ocular prosthetic devices, implants and grafts**
Malposition of other ocular prosthetic devices, implants and grafts
● **T85.320 Displacement of prosthetic orbit of right eye**
● **T85.321 Displacement of prosthetic orbit of left eye**
● **T85.328 Displacement of other ocular prosthetic devices, implants and grafts**
● **T85.39 Other mechanical complication of other ocular prosthetic devices, implants and grafts**
Obstruction (mechanical) of other ocular prosthetic devices, implants and grafts
Perforation of other ocular prosthetic devices, implants and grafts
Protrusion of other ocular prosthetic devices, implants and grafts
● **T85.390 Other mechanical complication of prosthetic orbit of right eye**
● **T85.391 Other mechanical complication of prosthetic orbit of left eye**
● **T85.398 Other mechanical complication of other ocular prosthetic devices, implants and grafts**
● **T85.4 Mechanical complication of breast prosthesis and implant**
X● **T85.41 Breakdown (mechanical) of breast prosthesis and implant**
X● **T85.42 Displacement of breast prosthesis and implant**
Malposition of breast prosthesis and implant
X● **T85.43 Leakage of breast prosthesis and implant**
X● **T85.44 Capsular contracture of breast implant**
X● **T85.49 Other mechanical complication of breast prosthesis and implant**
Obstruction (mechanical) of breast prosthesis and implant
Perforation of breast prosthesis and implant
Protrusion of breast prosthesis and implant
● **T85.5 Mechanical complication of gastrointestinal prosthetic devices, implants and grafts**
● **T85.51 Breakdown (mechanical) of gastrointestinal prosthetic devices, implants and grafts**
● **T85.510 Breakdown (mechanical) of bile duct prosthesis**
● **T85.511 Breakdown (mechanical) of esophageal anti-reflux device**
● **T85.518 Breakdown (mechanical) of other gastrointestinal prosthetic devices, implants and grafts**
● **T85.52 Displacement of gastrointestinal prosthetic devices, implants and grafts**
Malposition of gastrointestinal prosthetic devices, implants and grafts
● **T85.520 Displacement of bile duct prosthesis**
● **T85.521 Displacement of esophageal anti-reflux device**
● **T85.528 Displacement of other gastrointestinal prosthetic devices, implants and grafts**
● **T85.59 Other mechanical complication of gastrointestinal prosthetic devices, implants and**
Obstruction, mechanical of gastrointestinal prosthetic devices, implants and grafts
Perforation of gastrointestinal prosthetic devices, implants and grafts
Protrusion of gastrointestinal prosthetic devices, implants and grafts
● **T85.590 Other mechanical complication of bile duct prosthesis**
● **T85.591 Other mechanical complication of esophageal anti-reflux device**
● **T85.598 Other mechanical complication of other gastrointestinal prosthetic devices, implants and grafts**
● **T85.6 Mechanical complication of other specified internal and external prosthetic devices, implants and grafts**
● **T85.61 Breakdown (mechanical) of other specified internal prosthetic devices, implants and grafts**
● **T85.610 Breakdown (mechanical) of cranial or spinal infusion catheter**
Breakdown (mechanical) of epidural infusion catheter ◀
Breakdown (mechanical) of intrathecal infusion catheter ◀
Breakdown (mechanical) of subarachnoid infusion catheter ◀
Breakdown (mechanical) of subdural infusion catheter ◀
● **T85.611 Breakdown (mechanical) of intraperitoneal dialysis catheter**
Excludes1 mechanical complication of vascular dialysis catheter (T82.4-)
● **T85.612 Breakdown (mechanical) of permanent sutures**
Excludes1 mechanical complication of permanent (wire) suture used in bone repair (T84.1-T84.2)
● **T85.613 Breakdown (mechanical) of artificial skin graft and decellularized allodermis**
Failure of artificial skin graft and decellularized allodermis
Non-adherence of artificial skin graft and decellularized allodermis
Poor incorporation of artificial skin graft and decellularized allodermis
Shearing of artificial skin graft and decellularized allodermis
● **T85.614 Breakdown (mechanical) of insulin pump**
● **T85.615 Breakdown (mechanical) of other nervous system device, implant or graft**
Breakdown (mechanical) of intrathecal infusion pump ◀
● **T85.618 Breakdown (mechanical) of other specified internal prosthetic devices, implants and grafts**

CHAPTER 19 (S00-T88)

● T85.62 **Displacement of other specified internal prosthetic devices, implants and grafts**
Malposition of other specified internal prosthetic devices, implants and grafts

● T85.620 **Displacement of cranial or spinal infusion catheter**
Displacement of epidural infusion catheter ◀
Displacement of intrathecal infusion catheter ◀
Displacement of subarachnoid infusion catheter ◀
Displacement of subdural infusion catheter ◀

● T85.621 **Displacement of intraperitoneal dialysis catheter**
Excludes1 mechanical complication of vascular dialysis catheter (T82.4-)

● T85.622 **Displacement of permanent sutures**
Excludes1 mechanical complication of permanent (wire) suture used in bone repair (T84.1-T84.2)

● T85.623 **Displacement of artificial skin graft and decellularized allodermis**
Dislodgement of artificial skin graft and decellularized allodermis
Displacement of artificial skin graft and decellularized allodermis

● T85.624 **Displacement of insulin pump**

● T85.625 **Displacement of other nervous system device, implant or graft**
Displacement of intrathecal infusion pump ◀

● T85.628 **Displacement of other specified internal prosthetic devices, implants and grafts**

● T85.63 **Leakage of other specified internal prosthetic devices, implants and grafts**

● T85.630 **Leakage of cranial or spinal infusion catheter**
Leakage of epidural infusion catheter ◀
Leakage of intrathecal infusion catheter ◀
Leakage of subdural infusion catheter ◀
Leakage of subarachnoid infusion catheter ◀

● T85.631 **Leakage of intraperitoneal dialysis catheter**
Excludes1 mechanical complication of vascular dialysis catheter (T82.4)

● T85.633 **Leakage of insulin pump**

● T85.635 **Leakage of other nervous system device, implant or graft**
Leakage of intrathecal infusion pump ◀

● T85.638 **Leakage of other specified internal prosthetic devices, implants and grafts**

● T85.69 **Other mechanical complication of other specified internal prosthetic devices, implants and grafts**
Obstruction, mechanical of other specified internal prosthetic devices, implants and grafts
Perforation of other specified internal prosthetic devices, implants and grafts
Protrusion of other specified internal prosthetic devices, implants and grafts

● T85.690 **Other mechanical complication of cranial or spinal infusion catheter**
Other mechanical complication of epidural infusion catheter ◀
Other mechanical complication of intrathecal infusion catheter ◀
Other mechanical complication of subarachnoid infusion catheter ◀
Other mechanical complication of subdural infusion catheter ◀

● T85.691 **Other mechanical complication of intraperitoneal dialysis catheter**
Excludes1 mechanical complication of vascular dialysis catheter (T82.4)

● T85.692 **Other mechanical complication of permanent sutures**
Excludes1 mechanical complication of permanent (wire) suture used in bone repair (T84.1-T84.2)

● T85.693 **Other mechanical complication of artificial skin graft and decellularized allodermis**

● T85.694 **Other mechanical complication of insulin pump**

● T85.695 **Other mechanical complication of other nervous system device, implant or graft**
Other mechanical complication of intrathecal infusion pump ◀

● T85.698 **Other mechanical complication of other specified internal prosthetic devices, implants and grafts**
Mechanical complication of nonabsorbable surgical material NOS

● T85.7 **Infection and inflammatory reaction due to other internal prosthetic devices, implants and grafts**
Use additional code to identify infection

X● T85.71 **Infection and inflammatory reaction due to peritoneal dialysis catheter**

X● T85.72 **Infection and inflammatory reaction due to insulin pump**

● T85.73 **Infection and inflammatory reaction due to nervous system devices, implants and graft**

● T85.730 **Infection and inflammatory reaction due to ventricular intracranial (communicating) shunt**

● T85.731 **Infection and inflammatory reaction due to implanted electronic neurostimulator of brain, electrode (lead)**

●T85.732 **Infection and inflammatory reaction due to implanted electronic neurostimulator of peripheral nerve, electrode (lead)**
Infection and inflammatory reaction due to electrode (lead) for cranial nerve neurostimulators
Infection and inflammatory reaction due to electrode (lead) for gastric neurostimulator ◄
Infection and inflammatory reaction due to electrode (lead) for sacral nerve neurostimulator ◄
Infection and inflammatory reaction due to electrode (lead) for vagal nerve neurostimulators ◄

●T85.733 **Infection and inflammatory reaction due to implanted electronic neurostimulator of spinal cord, electrode (lead)** ◄

●T85.734 **Infection and inflammatory reaction due to implanted electronic neurostimulator, generator** ◄
Generator pocket infection ◄

●T85.735 **Infection and inflammatory reaction due to cranial or spinal infusion catheter** ◄
Infection and inflammatory reaction due to epidural catheter ◄
Infection and inflammatory reaction due to intrathecal infusion catheter ◄
Infection and inflammatory reaction due to subarachnoid catheter ◄
Infection and inflammatory reaction due to subdural catheter ◄

●T85.738 **Infection and inflammatory reaction due to other nervous system device, implant or graft** ◄
Infection and inflammatory reaction due to intrathecal infusion pump ◄

X●T85.79 **Infection and inflammatory reaction due to other internal prosthetic devices, implants and grafts**

●T85.8 **Other specified complications of internal prosthetic devices, implants and grafts, not elsewhere classified**

●T85.81 **Embolism due to internal prosthetic devices, implants and grafts, not elsewhere classified**

●T85.810 **Embolism due to nervous system prosthetic devices, implants and grafts**

●T85.818 **Embolism due to other internal prosthetic devices, implants and grafts**

●T85.82 **Fibrosis due to internal prosthetic devices, implants and grafts, not elsewhere classified**

●T85.820 **Fibrosis due to nervous system prosthetic devices, implants and grafts**

●T85.828 **Fibrosis due to other internal prosthetic devices, implants and grafts**

●T85.83 **Hemorrhage due to internal prosthetic devices, implants and grafts, not elsewhere classified**

●T85.830 **Hemorrhage due to nervous system prosthetic devices, implants and grafts**

●T85.838 **Hemorrhage due to other internal prosthetic devices, implants and grafts**

●T85.84 **Pain due to internal prosthetic devices, implants and grafts, not elsewhere classified**

●T85.840 **Pain due to nervous system prosthetic devices, implants and grafts**

●T85.848 **Pain due to other internal prosthetic devices, implants and grafts**

●T85.85 **Stenosis due to internal prosthetic devices, implants and grafts, not elsewhere classified**

●T85.850 **Stenosis due to nervous system prosthetic devices, implants and grafts**

●T85.858 **Stenosis due to other internal prosthetic devices, implants and grafts**

●T85.86 **Thrombosis due to internal prosthetic devices, implants and grafts, not elsewhere classified**

●T85.860 **Thrombosis due to nervous system prosthetic devices, implants and grafts**

●T85.868 **Thrombosis due to other internal prosthetic devices, implants and grafts**

●T85.89 **Other specified complication of internal prosthetic devices, implants and grafts, not elsewhere classified**

●T85.890 **Other specified complication of nervous system prosthetic devices, implants and grafts**

●T85.898 **Other specified complication of other internal prosthetic devices, implants and grafts**

X●T85.9 **Unspecified complication of internal prosthetic device, implant and graft**
Complication of internal prosthetic device, implant and graft NOS

●T86 **Complications of transplanted organs and tissue**
Use additional code to identify other transplant complications, such as:
graft-versus-host disease (D89.81-)
malignancy associated with organ transplant (C80.2)
post-transplant lymphoproliferative disorders (PTLD) (D47.Z1)

●T86.0 **Complications of bone marrow transplant**
T86.00 **Unspecified complication of bone marrow transplant**
T86.01 **Bone marrow transplant rejection**
T86.02 **Bone marrow transplant failure**
T86.03 **Bone marrow transplant infection**
T86.09 **Other complications of bone marrow transplant**

●T86.1 **Complications of kidney transplant**
T86.10 **Unspecified complication of kidney transplant**
T86.11 **Kidney transplant rejection**
T86.12 **Kidney transplant failure**
T86.13 **Kidney transplant infection**
Use additional code to specify infection
T86.19 **Other complication of kidney transplant**

CHAPTER 19 (S00-T88)

OGCR Section I.C.19.g.3.

Organ Transplant Complications

Transplant Complications

(a) Transplant complications other than kidney

Codes under category T86, Complications of transplanted organs and tissues, are for use for both complications and rejection of transplanted organs. A transplant complication code is only assigned if the complication affects the function of the transplanted organ. Two codes are required to fully describe a transplant complication: the appropriate code from category T86 and a secondary code that identifies the complication.

Pre-existing conditions or conditions that develop after the transplant are not coded as complications unless they affect the function of the transplanted organs.

See I.C.21 for transplant organ removal status

See I.C.2 for malignant neoplasm associated with transplanted organ.

● **T86.2 Complications of heart transplant**

Excludes1 complication of:
artificial heart device (T82.5)
heart-lung transplant (T86.3)

T86.20 Unspecified **complication of heart transplant**

T86.21 Heart transplant rejection

T86.22 Heart transplant failure

T86.23 Heart transplant infection

Use additional code to specify infection

● **T86.29 Other complications of heart transplant**

T86.290 Cardiac allograft vasculopathy

Excludes1 atherosclerosis of coronary arteries (I25.75-, I25.76-, I25.81-)

T86.298 Other complications of heart transplant

● **T86.3 Complications of heart-lung transplant**

T86.30 Unspecified **complication of heart-lung transplant**

T86.31 Heart-lung transplant rejection

T86.32 Heart-lung transplant failure

T86.33 Heart-lung transplant infection

Use additional code to specify infection

T86.39 Other complications of heart-lung transplant

● **T86.4 Complications of liver transplant**

T86.40 Unspecified **complication of liver transplant**

T86.41 Liver transplant rejection

T86.42 Liver transplant failure

T86.43 Liver transplant infection

Use additional code to identify infection, such as:
Cytomegalovirus (CMV) infection (B25.-)

T86.49 Other complications of liver transplant

● **T86.5 Complications of stem cell transplant**

Complications from stem cells from peripheral blood
Complications from stem cells from umbilical cord

● **T86.8 Complications of other transplanted organs and tissues**

● **T86.81 Complications of lung transplant**

Excludes1 complication of heart-lung transplant (T86.3-)

T86.810 Lung transplant rejection

T86.811 Lung transplant failure

T86.812 Lung transplant infection

Use additional code to specify infection

T86.818 Other complications of lung transplant

T86.819 Unspecified **complication of lung transplant**

● **T86.82 Complications of skin graft (allograft) (autograft)**

Excludes2 complication of artificial skin graft (T85.693)

T86.820 Skin graft (allograft) rejection

T86.821 Skin graft (allograft) (autograft) failure

T86.822 Skin graft (allograft) (autograft) infection

Use additional code to specify infection

T86.828 Other complications of skin graft (allograft) (autograft)

T86.829 Unspecified **complication of skin graft (allograft) (autograft)**

● **T86.83 Complications of bone graft**

Excludes2 mechanical complications of bone graft (T84.3-)

T86.830 Bone graft rejection

T86.831 Bone graft failure

T86.832 Bone graft infection

Use additional code to specify infection

T86.838 Other complications of bone graft

T86.839 Unspecified **complication of bone graft**

● **T86.84 Complications of corneal transplant**

Excludes2 mechanical complications of corneal graft (T85.3-)

T86.840 Corneal transplant rejection

T86.841 Corneal transplant failure

T86.842 Corneal transplant infection

Use additional code to specify infection

T86.848 Other complications of corneal transplant

T86.849 Unspecified **complication of corneal transplant**

● **T86.85 Complication of intestine transplant**

T86.850 Intestine transplant rejection

T86.851 Intestine transplant failure

T86.852 Intestine transplant infection

Use additional code to specify infection

T86.858 Other complications of intestine transplant

T86.859 Unspecified **complication of intestine transplant**

● T86.89 **Complications of other transplanted tissue**
Transplant failure or rejection of pancreas
T86.890 **Other transplanted tissue rejection**
T86.891 **Other transplanted tissue failure**
T86.892 **Other transplanted tissue infection**
Use additional code to specify infection
T86.898 **Other complications of other transplanted tissue**
T86.899 **Unspecified complication of other transplanted tissue**

● T86.9 **Complication of unspecified transplanted organ and tissue**
T86.90 **Unspecified complication of unspecified transplanted organ and tissue**
T86.91 **Unspecified transplanted organ and tissue rejection**
T86.92 **Unspecified transplanted organ and tissue failure**
T86.93 **Unspecified transplanted organ and tissue infection**
Use additional code to specify infection
T86.99 **Other complications of unspecified transplanted organ and tissue**

● T87 **Complications peculiar to reattachment and amputation**
● T87.Ø **Complications of reattached (part of) upper extremity**
● T87.ØX **Complications of reattached (part of) upper extremity**
T87.ØX1 **Complications of reattached (part of) right upper extremity**
T87.ØX2 **Complications of reattached (part of) left upper extremity**
T87.ØX9 **Complications of reattached (part of) unspecified upper extremity**
● T87.1 **Complications of reattached (part of) lower extremity**
● T87.1X **Complications of reattached (part of) lower extremity**
T87.1X1 **Complications of reattached (part of) right lower extremity**
T87.1X2 **Complications of reattached (part of) left lower extremity**
T87.1X9 **Complications of reattached (part of) unspecified lower extremity**
T87.2 **Complications of other reattached body part**
● T87.3 **Neuroma of amputation stump**
T87.3Ø **Neuroma of amputation stump, unspecified extremity**
T87.31 **Neuroma of amputation stump, right upper extremity**
T87.32 **Neuroma of amputation stump, left upper extremity**
T87.33 **Neuroma of amputation stump, right lower extremity**
T87.34 **Neuroma of amputation stump, left lower extremity**
● T87.4 **Infection of amputation stump**
T87.4Ø **Infection of amputation stump, unspecified extremity**
T87.41 **Infection of amputation stump, right upper extremity**
T87.42 **Infection of amputation stump, left upper extremity**
T87.43 **Infection of amputation stump, right lower extremity**
T87.44 **Infection of amputation stump, left lower extremity**
● T87.5 **Necrosis of amputation stump**
T87.5Ø **Necrosis of amputation stump, unspecified extremity**
T87.51 **Necrosis of amputation stump, right upper extremity**
T87.52 **Necrosis of amputation stump, left upper extremity**
T87.53 **Necrosis of amputation stump, right lower extremity**
T87.54 **Necrosis of amputation stump, left lower extremity**
● T87.8 **Other complications of amputation stump**
T87.81 **Dehiscence of amputation stump**
T87.89 **Other complications of amputation stump**
Amputation stump contracture
Amputation stump contracture of next proximal joint
Amputation stump flexion
Amputation stump edema
Amputation stump hematoma
Excludes2 phantom limb syndrome (G54.6-G54.7)
T87.9 **Unspecified complications of amputation stump**

● T88 **Other complications of surgical and medical care, not elsewhere classified**
Excludes2 complication following infusion, transfusion and therapeutic injection (T8Ø.-)
complication following procedure NEC (T81.-)
complications of anesthesia in labor and delivery (O74.-)
complications of anesthesia in pregnancy (O29.-)
complications of anesthesia in puerperium (O89.-)
complications of devices, implants and grafts (T82-T85)
complications of obstetric surgery and procedure (O75.4)
dermatitis due to drugs and medicaments (L23.3, L24.4, L25.1, L27.Ø-L27.1)
poisoning and toxic effects of drugs and chemicals (T36-T65 with fifth or sixth character 1-4 or 6)
specified complications classified elsewhere

The appropriate 7th character is to be added to each code from category T88

A	initial encounter
D	subsequent encounter
S	sequela

X● T88.Ø **Infection following immunization**
Sepsis following immunization
X● T88.1 **Other complications following immunization, not elsewhere classified**
Generalized vaccinia
Rash following immunization
Excludes1 vaccinia not from vaccine (BØ8.Ø11)
Excludes2 anaphylactic shock due to serum (T8Ø.5-)
other serum reactions (T8Ø.6-)
postimmunization arthropathy (MØ2.2)
postimmunization encephalitis (GØ4.Ø2)
postimmunization fever (R5Ø.83)

CHAPTER 19 (SØØ-T88)

X● T88.2 **Shock due to anesthesia**
Use additional code for adverse effect, if applicable, to identify drug (T41.- with fifth or sixth character 5)
Excludes1 complications of anesthesia (in):
labor and delivery (O74.-)
pregnancy (O29.-)
puerperium (O89.-)
postprocedural shock NOS (T81.1-)

X● T88.3 **Malignant hyperthermia due to anesthesia**
Use additional code for adverse effect, if applicable, to identify drug (T41.- with fifth or sixth character 5)

X● T88.4 **Failed or difficult intubation**

● T88.5 **Other complications of anesthesia**
Use additional code for adverse effect, if applicable, to identify drug (T41.- with fifth or sixth character 5)

X● T88.51 **Hypothermia following anesthesia**

X● T88.52 **Failed moderate sedation during procedure**
Failed conscious sedation during procedure
Excludes2 personal history of failed moderate sedation (Z92.83)

X● T88.53 **Unintended awareness under general anesthesia during procedure** ◀
Excludes2 personal history of unintended awareness under general anesthesia (Z92.84) ◀

X● T88.59 **Other complications of anesthesia**

X● T88.6 **Anaphylactic reaction due to adverse effect of correct drug or medicament properly administered**
Anaphylactic shock due to adverse effect of correct drug or medicament properly administered
Anaphylactoid reaction NOS
Use additional code for adverse effect, if applicable, to identify drug (T36-T5Ø with fifth or sixth character 5)
Excludes1 anaphylactic reaction due to serum (T8Ø.5-)
anaphylactic shock or reaction due to adverse food reaction (T78.Ø-)

X● T88.7 **Unspecified adverse effect of drug or medicament**
Drug hypersensitivity NOS
Drug reaction NOS
Use additional code for adverse effect, if applicable, to identify drug (T36-T5Ø with fifth or sixth character 5)
Excludes1 specified adverse effects of drugs and medicaments (AØØ-R94 and T8Ø-T88.6, T88.8)

X● T88.8 **Other specified complications of surgical and medical care, not elsewhere classified**
Use additional code to identify the complication

X● T88.9 **Complication of surgical and medical care, unspecified**

CHAPTER 20

EXTERNAL CAUSES OF MORBIDITY (V00-Y99)

OGCR Chapter-Specific Coding Guidelines

20. Chapter 20: External Causes of Morbidity (V00-Y99)

The external causes of morbidity codes should never be sequenced as the first-listed or principal diagnosis.

External cause codes are intended to provide data for injury research and evaluation of injury prevention strategies. These codes capture how the injury or health condition happened (cause), the intent (unintentional or accidental; or intentional, such as suicide or assault), the place where the event occurred the activity of the patient at the time of the event, and the person's status (e.g., civilian, military).

There is no national requirement for mandatory ICD-10-CM external cause code reporting. Unless a provider is subject to a state-based external cause code reporting mandate or these codes are required by a particular payer, reporting of ICD-10-CM codes in Chapter 20, External Causes of Morbidity, is not required. In the absence of a mandatory reporting requirement, providers are encouraged to voluntarily report external cause codes, as they provide valuable data for injury research and evaluation of injury prevention strategies.

a. General External Cause Coding Guidelines

1) Used with any code in the range of A00.0-T88.9, Z00-Z99

An external cause code may be used with any code in the range of A00.0-T88.9, Z00-Z99, classification that is a health condition due to an external cause. Though they are most applicable to injuries, they are also valid for use with such things as infections or diseases due to an external source, and other health conditions, such as a heart attack that occurs during strenuous physical activity.

2) External cause code used for length of treatment

Assign the external cause code, with the appropriate 7th character (initial encounter, subsequent encounter or sequela) for each encounter for which the injury or condition is being treated.

Most categories in chapter 20 have a 7th character requirement for each applicable code. Most categories in this chapter have three 7th character values: A, initial encounter, D, subsequent encounter and S, sequela. While the patient may be seen by a new or different provider over the course of treatment for an injury or condition, assignment of the 7th character for external cause should match the 7th character of the code assigned for the associated injury or condition for the encounter.

3) Use the full range of external cause codes

Use the full range of external cause codes to completely describe the cause, the intent, the place of occurrence and if applicable, the activity of the patient at the time of the event, and the patient's status, for all injuries, and other health conditions due to an external cause.

4) Assign as many external cause codes as necessary

Assign as many external cause codes as necessary to fully explain each cause. If only one external code can be recorded, assign the code most related to the principal diagnosis.

5) The selection of the appropriate external cause code

The selection of the appropriate external cause code is guided by the Alphabetic Index of External Causes and by Inclusion and Exclusion notes in the Tabular List.

6) External cause code can never be a principal diagnosis

An external cause code can never be a principal (first-listed) diagnosis.

7) Combination external cause codes

Certain of the external cause codes are combination codes that identify sequential events that result in an injury, such as a fall which results in striking against an object. The injury may be due to either event or both. The combination external cause code used should correspond to the sequence of events regardless of which caused the most serious injury.

8) No external cause code needed in certain circumstances

No external cause code from Chapter 20 is needed if the external cause and intent are included in a code from another chapter (e.g. T36.0X1- Poisoning by penicillins, accidental (unintentional)).

b. Place of Occurrence Guideline

Codes from category Y92, Place of occurrence of the external cause, are secondary codes for use after other external cause codes to identify the location of the patient at the time of injury or other condition.

Generally, a place of occurrence code is **assigned** only once, at the initial encounter for treatment. **However, in the rare instance that a new injury occurs during hospitalization, an additional place of occurrence code may be assigned.** No 7th characters are used for Y92. Only one code from Y92 should be recorded on a medical record.

Do not use place of occurrence code Y92.9 if the place is not stated or is not applicable.

c. Activity Code

Assign a code from category Y93, Activity code, to describe the activity of the patient at the time the injury or other health condition occurred.

An activity code is used only once, at the initial encounter for treatment. Only one code from Y93 should be recorded on a medical record.

The activity codes are not applicable to poisonings, adverse effects, misadventures or sequela.

Do not assign Y93.9, Unspecified activity, if the activity is not stated.

A code from category Y93 is appropriate for use with external cause and intent codes if identifying the activity provides additional information about the event.

d. Place of Occurrence, Activity, and Status Codes Used with other External Cause Code

When applicable, place of occurrence, activity, and external cause status codes are sequenced after the main external cause code(s). Regardless of the number of external cause codes assigned, there should be only one place of occurrence code, one activity code, and one external cause status code assigned to an encounter.

e. If the Reporting Format Limits the Number of External Cause Codes

If the reporting format limits the number of external cause codes that can be used in reporting clinical data, report the code for the cause/intent most related to the principal diagnosis. If the format permits capture of additional external cause codes, the cause/intent, including medical misadventures, of the additional events should be reported rather than the codes for place, activity, or external status.

f. Multiple External Cause Coding Guidelines

More than one external cause code is required to fully describe the external cause of an illness or injury. The assignment of external cause codes should be sequenced in the following priority:

If two or more events cause separate injuries, an external cause code should be assigned for each cause. The first-listed external cause code will be selected in the following order:

External codes for child and adult abuse take priority over all other external cause codes.

See Section I.C.19., Child and Adult abuse guidelines.

External codes for terrorism events take priority over all other external cause codes except child and adult abuse.

External cause codes for cataclysmic events take priority over all other external cause codes except child and adult abuse and terrorism.

External cause codes for transport accidents take priority over all other external cause codes except cataclysmic events, child and adult abuse and terrorism.

Activity and external cause status codes are assigned following all causal (intent) external cause codes.

The first-listed external cause code should correspond to the cause of the most serious diagnosis due to an assault, accident, or self-harm, following the order of hierarchy listed above.

g. Child and Adult Abuse Guideline

Adult and child abuse, neglect and maltreatment are classified as assault. Any of the assault codes may be used to indicate the external cause of any injury resulting from the confirmed abuse.

For confirmed cases of abuse, neglect and maltreatment, when the perpetrator is known, a code from YØ7, Perpetrator of maltreatment and neglect, should accompany any other assault codes.

See Section I.C.19. Adult and child abuse, neglect and other maltreatment

h. Unknown or Undetermined Intent Guideline

If the intent (accident, self-harm, assault) of the cause of an injury or other condition is unknown or unspecified, code the intent as accidental intent. All transport accident categories assume accidental intent.

1) Use of undetermined intent

External cause codes for events of undetermined intent are only for use if the documentation in the record specifies that the intent cannot be determined.

i. Sequelae (Late Effects) of External Cause Guidelines

1) Sequelae external cause codes

Sequela are reported using the external cause code with the 7th character "S" for sequela. These codes should be used with any report of a late effect or sequela resulting from a previous injury.

See Section I.B.1Ø. Sequela, (Late Effects)

2) Sequela external cause code with a related current injury

A sequela external cause code should never be used with a related current nature of injury code.

3) Use of sequela external cause codes for subsequent visits

Use a late effect external cause code for subsequent visits when a late effect of the initial injury is being treated. Do not use a late effect external cause code for subsequent visits for follow-up care (e.g., to assess healing, to receive rehabilitative therapy) of the injury when no late effect of the injury has been documented.

j. Terrorism Guidelines

1) Cause of injury identified by the Federal Government (FBI) as terrorism

When the cause of an injury is identified by the Federal Government (FBI) as terrorism, the first-listed external cause code should be a code from category Y38, Terrorism. The definition of terrorism employed by the FBI is found at the inclusion note at the beginning of category Y38. Use additional code for place of occurrence (Y92.-). More than one Y38 code may be assigned if the injury is the result of more than one mechanism of terrorism.

2) Cause of an injury is suspected to be the result of terrorism

When the cause of an injury is suspected to be the result of terrorism a code from category Y38 should not be assigned. Suspected cases should be classified as assault.

3) Code Y38.9, Terrorism, secondary effects

Assign code Y38.9, Terrorism, secondary effects, for conditions occurring subsequent to the terrorist event. This code should not be assigned for conditions that are due to the initial terrorist act.

It is acceptable to assign code Y38.9 with another code from Y38 if there is an injury due to the initial terrorist event and an injury that is a subsequent result of the terrorist event.

k. External cause status

A code from category Y99, External cause status, should be assigned whenever any other external cause code is assigned for an encounter, including an Activity code, except for the events noted below. Assign a code from category Y99, External cause status, to indicate the work status of the person at the time the event occurred. The status code indicates whether the event occurred during military activity, whether a non-military person was at work, whether an individual including a student or volunteer was involved in a non-work activity at the time of the causal event.

A code from Y99, External cause status, should be assigned, when applicable, with other external cause codes, such as transport accidents and falls. The external cause status codes are not applicable to poisonings, adverse effects, misadventures or late effects.

Do not assign a code from category Y99 if no other external cause codes (cause, activity) are applicable for the encounter.

An external cause status code is used only once, at the initial encounter for treatment. Only one code from Y99 should be recorded on a medical record.

Do not assign code Y99.9, Unspecified external cause status, if the status is not stated.

CHAPTER 20

EXTERNAL CAUSES OF MORBIDITY (VØØ-Y99)

Note: This chapter permits the classification of environmental events and circumstances as the cause of injury, and other adverse effects. Where a code from this section is applicable, it is intended that it shall be used secondary to a code from another chapter of the Classification indicating the nature of the condition. Most often, the condition will be classifiable to Chapter 19, Injury, poisoning and certain other consequences of external causes (SØØ-T88). Other conditions that may be stated to be due to external causes are classified in Chapters I to XVIII. For these conditions, codes from Chapter 2Ø should be used to provide additional information as to the cause of the condition.

This chapter contains the following blocks:

VØØ-X58	Accidents
VØØ-V99	Transport accidents
VØØ-VØ9	Pedestrian injured in transport accident
V1Ø-V19	Pedal cycle rider injured in transport accident
V2Ø-V29	Motorcycle rider injured in transport accident
V3Ø-V39	Occupant of three-wheeled motor vehicle injured in transport accident
V4Ø-V49	Car occupant injured in transport accident
V5Ø-V59	Occupant of pick-up truck or van injured in transport accident
V6Ø-V69	Occupant of heavy transport vehicle injured in transport accident
V7Ø-V79	Bus occupant injured in transport accident
V8Ø-V89	Other land transport accidents
V9Ø-V94	Water transport accidents
V95-V97	Air and space transport accidents
V98-V99	Other and unspecified transport accidents
WØØ-X58	Other external causes of accidental injury
WØØ-W19	Slipping, tripping, stumbling and falls
W2Ø-W49	Exposure to inanimate mechanical forces
W5Ø-W64	Exposure to animate mechanical forces
W65-W74	Accidental non-transport drowning and submersion
W85-W99	Exposure to electric current, radiation and extreme ambient air temperature and pressure
XØØ-XØ8	Exposure to smoke, fire and flames
X1Ø-X19	Contact with heat and hot substances
X3Ø-X39	Exposure to forces of nature
X5Ø	Overexertion and strenuous or repetitive movements ◀
X52, X58	Accidental exposure to other specified factors
X71-X83	Intentional self-harm
X92-YØ9 ⬅	Assault
Y21-Y33	Event of undetermined intent
Y35-Y38	Legal intervention, operations of war, military operations, and terrorism
Y62-Y84	Complications of medical and surgical care
Y62-Y69	Misadventures to patients during surgical and medical care
Y7Ø-Y82	Medical devices associated with adverse incidents in diagnostic and therapeutic use
Y83-Y84	Surgical and other medical procedures as the cause of abnormal reaction of the patient, or of later complication, without mention of misadventure at the time of the procedure
Y9Ø-Y99	Supplementary factors related to causes of morbidity classified elsewhere

ACCIDENTS (VØØ-X58)

TRANSPORT ACCIDENTS (VØØ-V99)

Note: This section is structured in 12 groups. Those relating to land transport accidents (VØØ-V89) reflect the victim's mode of transport and are subdivided to identify the victim's 'counterpart' or the type of event. The vehicle of which the injured person is an occupant is identified in the first two characters since it is seen as the most important factor to identify for prevention purposes. A transport accident is one in which the vehicle involved must be moving or running or in use for transport purposes at the time of the accident. ◀

Use additional code to identify:
Airbag injury (W22.1)
Type of street or road (Y92.4-)
Use of cellular telephone and other electronic equipment at the time of the transport accident (Y93.C-)

Excludes1 agricultural vehicles in stationary use or maintenance (W31.-)
assault by crashing of motor vehicle (YØ3.-)
automobile or motor cycle in stationary use or maintenance - code to type of accident
crashing of motor vehicle, undetermined intent (Y32)
intentional self-harm by crashing of motor vehicle (X82)

Excludes2 transport accidents due to cataclysm (X34-X38)

Note: Definitions related to transport accidents: ⬅

(a) A transport accident (VØØ-V99) is any accident involving a device designed primarily for, or used at the time primarily for, conveying persons or good from one place to another. ⬅

(b) A public highway [trafficway] or street is the entire width between property lines (or other boundary lines) of land open to the public as a matter of right or custom for purposes of moving persons or property from one place to another. A roadway is that part of the public highway designed, improved and customarily used for vehicular traffic.

(c) A traffic accident is any vehicle accident occurring on the public highway [i.e., originating on, terminating on, or involving a vehicle partially on the highway]. A vehicle accident is assumed to have occurred on the public highway unless another place is specified, except in the case of accidents involving only off-road motor vehicles, which are classified as nontraffic accidents unless the contrary is stated.

(d) A nontraffic accident is any vehicle accident that occurs entirely in any place other than a public highway.

(e) A pedestrian is any person involved in an accident who was not at the time of the accident riding in or on a motor vehicle, railway train, streetcar or animal-drawn or other vehicle, or on a pedal cycle or animal. This includes, a person changing a tire, working on a parked car, or a person on foot. It also includes the user of a pedestrian conveyance such as a baby-stroller, ice-skates, skis, sled, roller skates, a skateboard, nonmotorized or motorized wheelchair, motorized mobility scooter, or nonmotorized scooter. ⬅

(f) A driver is an occupant of a transport vehicle who is operating or intending to operate it.

(g) A passenger is any occupant of a transport vehicle other than the driver, except a person traveling on the outside of the vehicle.

(h) A person on the outside of a vehicle is any person being transported by a vehicle but not occupying the space normally reserved for the driver or passengers, or the space intended for the transport of property. This includes a person travelling on the bodywork, bumper, fender, roof, running board or step of a vehicle, as well as, hanging on the outside of the vehicle. ⬅

(i) A pedal cycle is any land transport vehicle operated solely by nonmotorized pedals including a bicycle or tricycle.

(j) A pedal cyclist is any person riding a pedal cycle or in a sidecar or trailer attached to a pedal cycle.

CHAPTER 2Ø (VØ1-Y99)

(k) A motorcycle is a two-wheeled motor vehicle with one or two riding saddles and sometimes with a third wheel for the support of a sidecar. The sidecar is considered part of the motorcycle. This includes a moped, motor scooter, or motorized bicycle.
(l) A motorcycle rider is any person riding a motorcycle or in a sidecar or trailer attached to the motorcycle.
(m) A three-wheeled motor vehicle is a motorized tricycle designed primarily for on-road use. This includes a motor-driven tricycle, a motorized rickshaw, or a three-wheeled motor car.
(n) A car [automobile] is a four-wheeled motor vehicle designed primarily for carrying up to 7 persons. A trailer being towed by the car is considered part of the car. It does not include a van or minivan—see definition (o)
(o) A pick-up truck or van is a four or six-wheeled motor vehicle designed for carrying passengers as well as property or cargo weighing less than the local limit for classification as a heavy goods vehicle, and not requiring a special driver's license. This includes a minivan and a sport-utility vehicle (SUV).
(p) A heavy transport vehicle is a motor vehicle designed primarily for carrying property, meeting local criteria for classification as a heavy goods vehicle in terms of weight and requiring a special driver's license.
(q) A bus (coach) is a motor vehicle designed or adapted primarily for carrying more than 1Ø passengers, and requiring a special driver's license.
(r) A railway train or railway vehicle is any device, with or without freight or passenger cars coupled to it, designed for traffic on a railway track. This includes subterranean (subways) or elevated trains.
(s) A streetcar is a device designed and used primarily for transporting passengers within a municipality, running on rails, usually subject to normal traffic control signals, and operated principally on a right-of-way that forms part of the roadway. This includes a tram or trolley that runs on rails. A trailer being towed by a streetcar is considered part of the streetcar.
(t) A special vehicle mainly used on industrial premises is a motor vehicle designed primarily for use within the buildings and premises of industrial or commercial establishments. This includes battery-powered airport passenger vehicles or baggage/mail trucks, forklifts, coal-cars in a coal mine, logging cars and trucks used in mines or quarries.
(u) A special vehicle mainly used in agriculture is a motor vehicle designed specifically for use in farming and agriculture (horticulture), to work the land, tend and harvest crops and transport materials on the farm. This includes harvesters, farm machinery and tractor and trailers.
(v) A special construction vehicle is a motor vehicle designed specifically for use on construction and demolition sites. This includes bulldozers, diggers, earth levellers, dump trucks, backhoes, front-end loaders, pavers, and mechanical shovels.
(w) A special all-terrain vehicle is a motor vehicle of special design to enable it to negotiate over rough or soft terrain, snow or sand. Examples of special design are high construction, special wheels and tires, tracks, and support on a cushion of air. This includes snow mobiles, all-terrain vehicles (ATV), and dune buggies. It does not include passenger vehicle designated as sport utility vehicles (SUV).
(x) A watercraft is any device designed for transporting passengers or goods on water. This includes motor or sail boats, ships, and hovercraft.
(y) An aircraft is any device for transporting passengers or goods in the air. This includes hot-air balloons, gliders, helicopters and airplanes.
(z) A military vehicle is any motorized vehicle operating on a public roadway owned by the military and being operated by a member of the military.

PEDESTRIAN INJURED IN TRANSPORT ACCIDENT (VØØ-VØ9)

Includes person changing tire on transport vehicle
person examining engine of vehicle broken down in (on side of) road

Excludes1 fall due to non-transport collision with other person (WØ3)
pedestrian on foot falling (slipping) on ice and snow (WØØ.-)
struck or bumped by another person (W51)

● **VØØ Pedestrian conveyance accident**

Use additional place of occurrence and activity external cause codes, if known (Y92.-, Y93.-)

Excludes1 collision with another person without fall (W51)
fall due to person on foot colliding with another person on foot (WØ3)
fall from non-moving wheelchair, nonmotorized scooter and motorized mobility scooter without collision (WØ5.-)
pedestrian (conveyance) collision with other land transport vehicle (VØ1-VØ9)
pedestrian on foot falling (slipping) on ice and snow (WØØ.-)

The appropriate 7th character is to be added to each code from category VØØ

A	initial encounter
D	subsequent encounter
S	sequela

● **VØØ.Ø Pedestrian on foot injured in collision with pedestrian conveyance**

X● **VØØ.Ø1 Pedestrian on foot injured in collision with roller-skater**

X● **VØØ.Ø2 Pedestrian on foot injured in collision with skateboarder**

X● **VØØ.Ø9 Pedestrian on foot injured in collision with other pedestrian conveyance**

● **VØØ.1 Rolling-type pedestrian conveyance accident**

Excludes1 accident with babystroller (VØØ.82-)
accident with wheelchair (powered) (VØØ.81-)
accident with motorized mobility scooter (VØØ.83-)

● **VØØ.11 In-line roller-skate accident**

● **VØØ.111 Fall from in-line roller-skates**

● **VØØ.112 In-line roller-skater colliding with stationary object**

● **VØØ.118 Other in-line roller-skate accident**

Excludes1 roller-skater collision with other land transport vehicle (VØ1-VØ9 with 5th character 1)

● **VØØ.12 Non-in-line roller-skate accident**

● **VØØ.121 Fall from non-in-line roller-skates**

● **VØØ.122 Non-in-line roller-skater colliding with stationary object**

● **VØØ.128 Other non-in-line roller-skating accident**

Excludes1 roller-skater collision with other land transport vehicle (VØ1-VØ9 with 5th character 1)

● V00.13 Skateboard accident
● V00.131 Fall from skateboard
● V00.132 Skateboarder colliding with stationary object
● V00.138 Other skateboard accident
Excludes1 skateboarder collision with other land transport vehicle (V01-V09 with 5th character 2)

● V00.14 Scooter (nonmotorized) accident
Excludes1 motorscooter accident (V20-V29)
● V00.141 Fall from scooter (nonmotorized)
● V00.142 Scooter (nonmotorized) colliding with stationary object
● V00.148 Other scooter (nonmotorized) accident
Excludes1 scooter (non-motorized) collision with other land transport vehicle (V01-V09 with fifth character 9)

● V00.15 Heelies accident
Rolling shoe
Wheeled shoe
Wheelies accident
● V00.151 Fall from heelies
● V00.152 Heelies colliding with stationary object
● V00.158 Other heelies accident

● V00.18 Accident on other rolling-type pedestrian conveyance
● V00.181 Fall from other rolling-type pedestrian conveyance
● V00.182 Pedestrian on other rolling-type pedestrian conveyance colliding with stationary object
● V00.188 Other accident on other rolling-type pedestrian conveyance

● V00.2 Gliding-type pedestrian conveyance accident
● V00.21 Ice-skates accident
● V00.211 Fall from ice-skates
● V00.212 Ice-skater colliding with stationary object
● V00.218 Other ice-skates accident
Excludes1 ice-skater collision with other land transport vehicle (V01-V09 with 5th digit 9)

● V00.22 Sled accident
● V00.221 Fall from sled
● V00.222 Sledder colliding with stationary object
● V00.228 Other sled accident
Excludes1 sled collision with other land transport vehicle (V01-V09 with 5th digit 9)

● V00.28 Other gliding-type pedestrian conveyance accident
● V00.281 Fall from other gliding-type pedestrian conveyance
● V00.282 Pedestrian on other gliding-type pedestrian conveyance colliding with stationary object
● V00.288 Other accident on other gliding-type pedestrian conveyance
Excludes1 gliding-type pedestrian conveyance collision with other land transport vehicle (V01-V09 with 5th digit 9)

● V00.3 Flat-bottomed pedestrian conveyance accident
● V00.31 Snowboard accident
● V00.311 Fall from snowboard
● V00.312 Snowboarder colliding with stationary object
● V00.318 Other snowboard accident
Excludes1 snowboarder collision with other land transport vehicle (V01-V09 with 5th digit 9)

● V00.32 Snow-ski accident
● V00.321 Fall from snow-skis
● V00.322 Snow-skier colliding with stationary object
● V00.328 Other snow-ski accident
Excludes1 snow-skier collision with other land transport vehicle (V01-V09 with 5th digit 9)

● V00.38 Other flat-bottomed pedestrian conveyance accident
● V00.381 Fall from other flat-bottomed pedestrian conveyance
● V00.382 Pedestrian on other flat-bottomed pedestrian conveyance colliding with stationary object
● V00.388 Other accident on other flat-bottomed pedestrian conveyance

● V00.8 Accident on other pedestrian conveyance
● V00.81 Accident with wheelchair (powered)
● V00.811 Fall from moving wheelchair (powered)
Excludes1 fall from non-moving wheelchair (W05.0)
● V00.812 Wheelchair (powered) colliding with stationary object
● V00.818 Other accident with wheelchair (powered)

● V00.82 Accident with babystroller
● V00.821 Fall from babystroller
● V00.822 Babystroller colliding with stationary object
● V00.828 Other accident with babystroller

CHAPTER 20 (V01-Y99)

● V00.83 **Accident with motorized mobility scooter**

● V00.831 **Fall from motorized mobility scooter**

Excludes1 fall from non-moving motorized mobility scooter (W05.2)

● V00.832 **Motorized mobility scooter colliding with stationary object**

● V00.838 **Other accident with motorized mobility scooter**

● V00.89 **Accident on other pedestrian conveyance**

● V00.891 **Fall from other pedestrian conveyance**

● V00.892 **Pedestrian on other pedestrian conveyance colliding with stationary object**

● V00.898 **Other accident on other pedestrian conveyance**

Excludes1 other pedestrian (conveyance) collision with other land transport vehicle (V01-V09 with 5th digit 9)

● V01 **Pedestrian injured in collision with pedal cycle**

The appropriate 7th character is to be added to each code from category V01

A	initial encounter
D	subsequent encounter
S	sequela

● V01.0 **Pedestrian injured in collision with pedal cycle in nontraffic accident**

X● V01.00 **Pedestrian on foot injured in collision with pedal cycle in nontraffic accident**

Pedestrian NOS injured in collision with pedal cycle in nontraffic accident

X● V01.01 **Pedestrian on roller-skates injured in collision with pedal cycle in nontraffic accident**

X● V01.02 **Pedestrian on skateboard injured in collision with pedal cycle in nontraffic accident**

X● V01.09 **Pedestrian with other conveyance injured in collision with pedal cycle in nontraffic accident**

Pedestrian with babystroller injured in collision with pedal cycle in nontraffic accident
Pedestrian in wheelchair (powered) injured in collision with pedal cycle in nontraffic accident
Pedestrian in motorized mobility scooter injured in collision with pedal cycle in nontraffic accident
Pedestrian on ice-skates injured in collision with pedal cycle in nontraffic accident
Pedestrian on nonmotorized scooter injured in collision with pedal cycle in nontraffic accident
Pedestrian on sled injured in collision with pedal cycle in nontraffic accident
Pedestrian on snowboard injured in collision with pedal cycle in nontraffic accident
Pedestrian on snow-skis injured in collision with pedal cycle in nontraffic accident

● V01.1 **Pedestrian injured in collision with pedal cycle in traffic accident**

X● V01.10 **Pedestrian on foot injured in collision with pedal cycle in traffic accident**

Pedestrian NOS injured in collision with pedal cycle in traffic accident

X● V01.11 **Pedestrian on roller-skates injured in collision with pedal cycle in traffic accident**

X● V01.12 **Pedestrian on skateboard injured in collision with pedal cycle in traffic accident**

X● V01.19 **Pedestrian with other conveyance injured in collision with pedal cycle in traffic accident**

Pedestrian with babystroller injured in collision with pedal cycle in traffic accident
Pedestrian in wheelchair (powered) injured in collision with pedal cycle in traffic accident
Pedestrian in motorized mobility scooter injured in collision with pedal cycle in traffic accident
Pedestrian on ice-skates injured in collision with pedal cycle in traffic accident
Pedestrian on nonmotorized scooter injured in collision with pedal cycle in traffic accident
Pedestrian on sled injured in collision with pedal cycle in traffic accident
Pedestrian on snowboard injured in collision with pedal cycle in traffic accident
Pedestrian on snow-skis injured in collision with pedal cycle in traffic accident

● V01.9 **Pedestrian injured in collision with pedal cycle, unspecified whether traffic or nontraffic accident**

X● V01.90 **Pedestrian on foot injured in collision with pedal cycle, unspecified whether traffic or nontraffic accident**

Pedestrian NOS injured in collision with pedal cycle, unspecified whether traffic or nontraffic accident

X● V01.91 **Pedestrian on roller-skates injured in collision with pedal cycle, unspecified whether traffic or nontraffic accident**

X● V01.92 **Pedestrian on skateboard injured in collision with pedal cycle, unspecified whether traffic or nontraffic accident**

X● V01.99 **Pedestrian with other conveyance injured in collision with pedal cycle, unspecified whether traffic or nontraffic accident**

Pedestrian with babystroller injured in collision with pedal cycle, unspecified whether traffic or nontraffic accident
Pedestrian in wheelchair (powered) injured in collision with pedal cycle, unspecified whether traffic or nontraffic accident
Pedestrian in motorized mobility scooter injured in collision with pedal cycle, unspecified whether traffic or nontraffic accident
Pedestrian on ice-skates injured in collision with pedal cycle unspecified, whether traffic or nontraffic accident
Pedestrian on nonmotorized scooter injured in collision with pedal cycle, unspecified whether traffic or nontraffic accident
Pedestrian on sled injured in collision with pedal cycle unspecified, whether traffic or nontraffic accident
Pedestrian on snowboard injured in collision with pedal cycle, unspecified whether traffic or nontraffic accident
Pedestrian on snow-skis injured in collision with pedal cycle, unspecified whether traffic or nontraffic accident

● **VØ2 Pedestrian injured in collision with two- or three-wheeled motor vehicle**

The appropriate 7th character is to be added to each code from category VØ2

A	initial encounter
D	subsequent encounter
S	sequela

● **VØ2.Ø Pedestrian injured in collision with two- or three-wheeled motor vehicle in nontraffic accident**

X● **VØ2.ØØ Pedestrian on foot injured in collision with two- or three-wheeled motor vehicle in nontraffic accident**

Pedestrian NOS injured in collision with two- or three-wheeled motor vehicle in nontraffic accident

X● **VØ2.Ø1 Pedestrian on roller-skates injured in collision with two- or three-wheeled motor vehicle in nontraffic accident**

X● **VØ2.Ø2 Pedestrian on skateboard injured in collision with two- or three-wheeled motor vehicle in nontraffic accident**

X● **VØ2.Ø9 Pedestrian with other conveyance injured in collision with two- or three-wheeled motor vehicle in nontraffic accident**

Pedestrian with babystroller injured in collision with two- or three-wheeled motor vehicle in nontraffic accident

Pedestrian on ice-skates injured in collision with two- or three-wheeled motor vehicle in nontraffic accident

Pedestrian in wheelchair (powered) injured in collision with two- or three-wheeled motor vehicle in nontraffic accident

Pedestrian in motorized mobility scooter injured in collision with two- or three-wheeled motor vehicle in nontraffic accident

Pedestrian on nonmotorized scooter injured in collision with two- or three-wheeled motor vehicle in nontraffic accident

Pedestrian on sled injured in collision with two- or three-wheeled motor vehicle in nontraffic accident

Pedestrian on snowboard injured in collision with two- or three-wheeled motor vehicle in nontraffic accident

Pedestrian on snow-skis injured in collision with two- or three-wheeled motor vehicle in nontraffic accident

● **VØ2.1 Pedestrian injured in collision with two- or three-wheeled motor vehicle in traffic accident**

X● **VØ2.1Ø Pedestrian on foot injured in collision with two- or three-wheeled motor vehicle in traffic accident**

Pedestrian NOS injured in collision with two- or three-wheeled motor vehicle in traffic accident

X● **VØ2.11 Pedestrian on roller-skates injured in collision with two- or three-wheeled motor vehicle in traffic accident**

X● **VØ2.12 Pedestrian on skateboard injured in collision with two- or three-wheeled motor vehicle in traffic accident**

X● **VØ2.19 Pedestrian with other conveyance injured in collision with two- or three-wheeled motor vehicle in traffic accident**

Pedestrian with babystroller injured in collision with two- or three-wheeled motor vehicle in traffic accident

Pedestrian in wheelchair (powered) injured in collision with two- or three-wheeled motor vehicle in traffic accident

Pedestrian in motorized mobility scooter injured in collision with two- or three-wheeled motor vehicle in traffic accident

Pedestrian on ice-skates injured in collision with two- or three-wheeled motor vehicle in traffic accident

Pedestrian on nonmotorized scooter injured in collision with two- or three-wheeled motor vehicle in traffic accident

Pedestrian on sled injured in collision with two- or three-wheeled motor vehicle in traffic accident

Pedestrian on snowboard injured in collision with two- or three-wheeled motor vehicle in traffic accident

Pedestrian on snow-skis injured in collision with two- or three-wheeled motor vehicle in traffic accident

● **VØ2.9 Pedestrian injured in collision with two- or three-wheeled motor vehicle, unspecified whether traffic or nontraffic accident**

X● **VØ2.9Ø Pedestrian on foot injured in collision with two- or three-wheeled motor vehicle, unspecified whether traffic or nontraffic accident**

Pedestrian NOS injured in collision with two- or three-wheeled motor vehicle, unspecified whether traffic or nontraffic accident

X● **VØ2.91 Pedestrian on roller-skates injured in collision with two- or three-wheeled motor vehicle, unspecified whether traffic or nontraffic accident**

X● **VØ2.92 Pedestrian on skateboard injured in collision with two- or three-wheeled motor vehicle, unspecified whether traffic or nontraffic accident**

X● **V02.99 Pedestrian with other conveyance injured in collision with two- or three-wheeled motor vehicle, unspecified whether traffic or nontraffic accident**

Pedestrian with babystroller injured in collision with two- or three-wheeled motor vehicle, unspecified whether traffic or nontraffic accident

Pedestrian in wheelchair (powered) injured in collision with two- or three-wheeled motor vehicle, unspecified whether traffic or nontraffic accident

Pedestrian in motorized mobility scooter injured in collision with two- or three-wheeled motor vehicle, unspecified whether traffic or nontraffic accident

Pedestrian on ice-skates injured in collision with two- or three-wheeled motor vehicle, unspecified whether traffic or nontraffic accident

Pedestrian on nonmotorized scooter injured in collision with two- or three-wheeled motor vehicle, unspecified whether traffic or nontraffic accident

Pedestrian on sled injured in collision with two- or three-wheeled motor vehicle, unspecified whether traffic or nontraffic accident

Pedestrian on snowboard injured in collision with two- or three-wheeled motor vehicle, unspecified whether traffic or nontraffic accident

Pedestrian on snow-skis injured in collision with two- or three-wheeled motor vehicle, unspecified whether traffic or nontraffic accident

● **V03 Pedestrian injured in collision with car, pick-up truck or van**

The appropriate 7th character is to be added to each code from category V03

A	initial encounter
D	subsequent encounter
S	sequela

● **V03.0 Pedestrian injured in collision with car, pick-up truck or van in nontraffic accident**

X● **V03.00 Pedestrian on foot injured in collision with car, pick-up truck or van in nontraffic accident**

Pedestrian NOS injured in collision with car, pick-up truck or van in nontraffic accident

X● **V03.01 Pedestrian on roller-skates injured in collision with car, pick-up truck or van in nontraffic accident**

X● **V03.02 Pedestrian on skateboard injured in collision with car, pick-up truck or van in nontraffic accident**

X● **V03.09 Pedestrian with other conveyance injured in collision with car, pick-up truck or van in nontraffic accident**

Pedestrian with babystroller injured in collision with car, pick-up truck or van in nontraffic accident

Pedestrian in wheelchair (powered) injured in collision with car, pick-up truck or van in nontraffic accident

Pedestrian in motorized mobility scooter injured in collision with car, pick-up truck or van in nontraffic accident

Pedestrian on ice-skates injured in collision with car, pick-up truck or van in nontraffic accident

Pedestrian on nonmotorized scooter injured in collision with car, pick-up truck or van in nontraffic accident

Pedestrian on sled injured in collision with car, pick-up truck or van in nontraffic accident

Pedestrian on snowboard injured in collision with car, pick-up truck or van in nontraffic accident

Pedestrian on snow-skis injured in collision with car, pick-up truck or van in nontraffic accident

● **V03.1 Pedestrian injured in collision with car, pick-up truck or van in traffic accident**

X● **V03.10 Pedestrian on foot injured in collision with car, pick-up truck or van in traffic accident**

Pedestrian NOS injured in collision with car, pick-up truck or van in traffic accident

X● **V03.11 Pedestrian on roller-skates injured in collision with car, pick-up truck or van in traffic accident**

X● **V03.12 Pedestrian on skateboard injured in collision with car, pick-up truck or van in traffic accident**

X● **V03.19 Pedestrian with other conveyance injured in collision with car, pick-up truck or van in traffic accident**

Pedestrian with babystroller injured in collision with car, pick-up truck or van in traffic accident

Pedestrian in wheelchair (powered) injured in collision with car, pick-up truck or van in traffic accident

Pedestrian in motorized mobility scooter injured in collision with car, pick-up truck or van in traffic accident

Pedestrian on ice-skates injured in collision with car, pick-up truck or van in traffic accident

Pedestrian on nonmotorized scooter injured in collision with car, pick-up truck or van in traffic accident

Pedestrian on sled injured in collision with car, pick-up truck or van in traffic accident

Pedestrian on snowboard injured in collision with car, pick-up truck or van in traffic accident

Pedestrian on snow-skis injured in collision with car, pick-up truck or van in traffic accident

● **VØ3.9 Pedestrian injured in collision with car, pick-up truck or van, unspecified whether traffic or nontraffic accident**

X● **VØ3.90 Pedestrian on foot injured in collision with car, pick-up truck or van, unspecified whether traffic or nontraffic accident**
Pedestrian NOS injured in collision with car, pick-up truck or van, unspecified whether traffic or nontraffic accident

X● **VØ3.91 Pedestrian on roller-skates injured in collision with car, pick-up truck or van, unspecified whether traffic or nontraffic accident**

X● **VØ3.92 Pedestrian on skateboard injured in collision with car, pick-up truck or van, unspecified whether traffic or nontraffic accident**

X● **VØ3.99 Pedestrian with other conveyance injured in collision with car, pick-up truck or van, unspecified whether traffic or nontraffic accident**
Pedestrian with babystroller injured in collision with car, pick-up truck or van, unspecified whether traffic or nontraffic accident
Pedestrian in wheelchair (powered) injured in collision with car, pick-up truck or van, unspecified whether traffic or nontraffic accident
Pedestrian in motorized mobility scooter injured in collision with car, pick-up truck or van, unspecified whether traffic or nontraffic accident
Pedestrian on ice-skates injured in collision with car, pick-up truck or van, unspecified whether traffic or nontraffic accident
Pedestrian on nonmotorized scooter injured in collision with car, pick-up truck or van, unspecified whether traffic or nontraffic accident
Pedestrian on sled injured in collision with car, pick-up truck or van in nontraffic accident
Pedestrian on snowboard injured in collision with car, pick-up truck or van, unspecified whether traffic or nontraffic accident
Pedestrian on snow-skis injured in collision with car, pick-up truck or van, unspecified whether traffic or nontraffic accident

● **VØ4 Pedestrian injured in collision with heavy transport vehicle or bus**

Excludes1 pedestrian injured in collision with military vehicle (VØ9.Ø1, VØ9.21)

The appropriate 7th character is to be added to each code from category VØ4

A	initial encounter
D	subsequent encounter
S	sequela

● **VØ4.Ø Pedestrian injured in collision with heavy transport vehicle or bus in nontraffic accident**

X● **VØ4.ØØ Pedestrian on foot injured in collision with heavy transport vehicle or bus in nontraffic accident**
Pedestrian NOS injured in collision with heavy transport vehicle or bus in nontraffic accident

X● **VØ4.Ø1 Pedestrian on roller-skates injured in collision with heavy transport vehicle or bus in nontraffic accident**

X● **VØ4.Ø2 Pedestrian on skateboard injured in collision with heavy transport vehicle or bus in nontraffic accident**

X● **VØ4.Ø9 Pedestrian with other conveyance injured in collision with heavy transport vehicle or bus in nontraffic accident**
Pedestrian with babystroller injured in collision with heavy transport vehicle or bus in nontraffic accident
Pedestrian in wheelchair (powered) injured in collision with heavy transport vehicle or bus in nontraffic accident
Pedestrian in motorized mobility scooter injured in collision with heavy transport vehicle or bus in nontraffic accident
Pedestrian on ice-skates injured in collision with heavy transport vehicle or bus in nontraffic accident
Pedestrian on nonmotorized scooter injured in collision with heavy transport vehicle or bus in nontraffic accident
Pedestrian on sled injured in collision with heavy transport vehicle or bus in nontraffic accident
Pedestrian on snowboard injured in collision with heavy transport vehicle or bus in nontraffic accident
Pedestrian on snow-skis injured in collision with heavy transport vehicle or bus in nontraffic accident

● **VØ4.1 Pedestrian injured in collision with heavy transport vehicle or bus in traffic accident**

X● **VØ4.1Ø Pedestrian on foot injured in collision with heavy transport vehicle or bus in traffic accident**
Pedestrian NOS injured in collision with heavy transport vehicle or bus in traffic accident

X● **VØ4.11 Pedestrian on roller-skates injured in collision with heavy transport vehicle or bus in traffic accident**

X● **VØ4.12 Pedestrian on skateboard injured in collision with heavy transport vehicle or bus in traffic accident**

X● **VØ4.19 Pedestrian with other conveyance injured in collision with heavy transport vehicle or bus in traffic accident**
Pedestrian with babystroller injured in collision with heavy transport vehicle or bus in traffic accident
Pedestrian in wheelchair (powered) injured in collision with heavy transport vehicle or bus in traffic accident
Pedestrian in motorized mobility scooter injured in collision with heavy transport vehicle or bus in traffic accident
Pedestrian on ice-skates injured in collision with heavy transport vehicle or bus in traffic accident
Pedestrian on nonmotorized scooter injured in collision with heavy transport vehicle or bus in traffic accident
Pedestrian on sled injured in collision with heavy transport vehicle or bus in traffic accident
Pedestrian on snowboard injured in collision with heavy transport vehicle or bus in traffic accident
Pedestrian on snow-skis injured in collision with heavy transport vehicle or bus in traffic accident

● V04.9 **Pedestrian injured in collision with heavy transport vehicle or bus, unspecified whether traffic or nontraffic accident**

X● V04.90 **Pedestrian on foot injured in collision with heavy transport vehicle or bus, unspecified whether traffic or nontraffic accident**

Pedestrian NOS injured in collision with heavy transport vehicle or bus, unspecified whether traffic or nontraffic accident

X● V04.91 **Pedestrian on roller-skates injured in collision with heavy transport vehicle or bus, unspecified whether traffic or nontraffic accident**

X● V04.92 **Pedestrian on skateboard injured in collision with heavy transport vehicle or bus, unspecified whether traffic or nontraffic accident**

X● V04.99 **Pedestrian with other conveyance injured in collision with heavy transport vehicle or bus, unspecified whether traffic or nontraffic accident**

Pedestrian with babystroller injured in collision with heavy transport vehicle or bus, unspecified whether traffic or nontraffic accident

Pedestrian in wheelchair (powered) injured in collision with heavy transport vehicle or bus, unspecified whether traffic or nontraffic accident

Pedestrian in motorized mobility scooter injured in collision with heavy transport vehicle or bus, unspecified whether traffic or nontraffic accident

Pedestrian on ice-skates injured in collision with heavy transport vehicle or bus, unspecified whether traffic or nontraffic accident

Pedestrian on nonmotorized scooter injured in collision with heavy transport vehicle or bus, unspecified whether traffic or nontraffic accident

Pedestrian on sled injured in collision with heavy transport vehicle or bus, unspecified whether traffic or nontraffic accident

Pedestrian on snowboard injured in collision with heavy transport vehicle or bus, unspecified whether traffic or nontraffic accident

Pedestrian on snow-skis injured in collision with heavy transport vehicle or bus, unspecified whether traffic or nontraffic accident

● V05 **Pedestrian injured in collision with railway train or railway vehicle**

The appropriate 7th character is to be added to each code from category V05

A	initial encounter
D	subsequent encounter
S	sequela

● V05.0 **Pedestrian injured in collision with railway train or railway vehicle in nontraffic accident**

X● V05.00 **Pedestrian on foot injured in collision with railway train or railway vehicle in nontraffic accident**

Pedestrian NOS injured in collision with railway train or railway vehicle in nontraffic accident

X● V05.01 **Pedestrian on roller-skates injured in collision with railway train or railway vehicle in nontraffic accident**

X● V05.02 **Pedestrian on skateboard injured in collision with railway train or railway vehicle in nontraffic accident**

X● V05.09 **Pedestrian with other conveyance injured in collision with railway train or railway vehicle in nontraffic accident**

Pedestrian with babystroller injured in collision with railway train or railway vehicle in nontraffic accident

Pedestrian in wheelchair (powered) injured in collision with railway train or railway vehicle in nontraffic accident

Pedestrian in motorized mobility scooter injured in collision with railway train or railway vehicle in nontraffic accident

Pedestrian on ice-skates injured in collision with railway train or railway vehicle in nontraffic accident

Pedestrian on nonmotorized scooter injured in collision with railway train or railway vehicle in nontraffic accident

Pedestrian on sled injured in collision with railway train or railway vehicle in nontraffic accident

Pedestrian on snowboard injured in collision with railway train or railway vehicle in nontraffic accident

Pedestrian on snow-skis injured in collision with railway train or railway vehicle in nontraffic accident

● V05.1 **Pedestrian injured in collision with railway train or railway vehicle in traffic accident**

X● V05.10 **Pedestrian on foot injured in collision with railway train or railway vehicle in traffic accident**

Pedestrian NOS injured in collision with railway train or railway vehicle in traffic accident

X● V05.11 **Pedestrian on roller-skates injured in collision with railway train or railway vehicle in traffic accident**

X● V05.12 **Pedestrian on skateboard injured in collision with railway train or railway vehicle in traffic accident**

X● V05.19 **Pedestrian with other conveyance injured in collision with railway train or railway vehicle in traffic accident**

Pedestrian with babystroller injured in collision with railway train or railway vehicle in traffic accident

Pedestrian in wheelchair (powered) injured in collision with railway train or railway vehicle in traffic accident

Pedestrian in motorized mobility scooter injured in collision with railway train or railway vehicle in traffic accident

Pedestrian on ice-skates injured in collision with railway train or railway vehicle in traffic accident

Pedestrian on nonmotorized scooter injured in collision with railway train or railway vehicle in traffic accident

Pedestrian on sled injured in collision with railway train or railway vehicle in traffic accident

Pedestrian on snowboard injured in collision with railway train or railway vehicle in traffic accident

Pedestrian on snow-skis injured in collision with railway train or railway vehicle in traffic accident

● **V05.9 Pedestrian injured in collision with railway train or railway vehicle, unspecified whether traffic or nontraffic accident**

X● **V05.90 Pedestrian on foot injured in collision with railway train or railway vehicle, unspecified whether traffic or nontraffic accident**

Pedestrian NOS injured in collision with railway train or railway vehicle, unspecified whether traffic or nontraffic accident

X● **V05.91 Pedestrian on roller-skates injured in collision with railway train or railway vehicle, unspecified whether traffic or nontraffic accident**

X● **V05.92 Pedestrian on skateboard injured in collision with railway train or railway vehicle, unspecified whether traffic or nontraffic accident**

X● **V05.99 Pedestrian with other conveyance injured in collision with railway train or railway vehicle, unspecified whether traffic or nontraffic accident**

Pedestrian with babystroller injured in collision with railway train or railway vehicle, unspecified whether traffic or nontraffic

Pedestrian in wheelchair (powered) injured in collision with railway train or railway vehicle, unspecified whether traffic or nontraffic

Pedestrian in motorized mobility scooter injured in collision with railway train or railway vehicle, unspecified whether traffic or nontraffic

Pedestrian on ice-skates injured in collision with railway train or railway vehicle, unspecified whether traffic or nontraffic

Pedestrian on nonmotorized scooter injured in collision with railway train or railway vehicle, unspecified whether traffic or nontraffic

Pedestrian on sled injured in collision with railway train or railway vehicle, unspecified whether traffic or nontraffic

Pedestrian on snowboard injured in collision with railway train or railway vehicle, unspecified whether traffic or nontraffic

Pedestrian on snow-skis injured in collision with railway train or railway vehicle, unspecified whether traffic or nontraffic

● **V06 Pedestrian injured in collision with other nonmotor vehicle**

Includes collision with animal-drawn vehicle, animal being ridden, nonpowered streetcar

Excludes1 pedestrian injured in collision with pedestrian conveyance (V00.0-)

The appropriate 7th character is to be added to each code from category V06

A initial encounter
D subsequent encounter
S sequela

● **V06.0 Pedestrian injured in collision with other nonmotor vehicle in nontraffic accident**

X● **V06.00 Pedestrian on foot injured in collision with other nonmotor vehicle in nontraffic accident**

Pedestrian NOS injured in collision with other nonmotor vehicle in nontraffic accident

X● **V06.01 Pedestrian on roller-skates injured in collision with other nonmotor vehicle in nontraffic accident**

X● **V06.02 Pedestrian on skateboard injured in collision with other nonmotor vehicle in nontraffic accident**

X● **V06.09 Pedestrian with other conveyance injured in collision with other nonmotor vehicle in nontraffic accident**

Pedestrian with babystroller injured in collision with other nonmotor vehicle in nontraffic accident

Pedestrian in wheelchair (powered) injured in collision with other nonmotor vehicle in nontraffic accident

Pedestrian in motorized mobility scooter injured in collision with other nonmotor vehicle in nontraffic accident

Pedestrian on ice-skates injured in collision with other nonmotor vehicle in nontraffic accident

Pedestrian on nonmotorized scooter injured in collision with other nonmotor vehicle in nontraffic accident

Pedestrian on sled injured in collision with other nonmotor vehicle in nontraffic accident

Pedestrian on snowboard injured in collision with other nonmotor vehicle in nontraffic accident

Pedestrian on snow-skis injured in collision with other nonmotor vehicle in nontraffic accident

● **V06.1 Pedestrian injured in collision with other nonmotor vehicle in traffic accident**

X● **V06.10 Pedestrian on foot injured in collision with other nonmotor vehicle in traffic accident**

Pedestrian NOS injured in collision with other nonmotor vehicle in traffic accident

X● **V06.11 Pedestrian on roller-skates injured in collision with other nonmotor vehicle in traffic accident**

X● **V06.12 Pedestrian on skateboard injured in collision with other nonmotor vehicle in traffic accident**

X● **V06.19 Pedestrian with other conveyance injured in collision with other nonmotor vehicle in traffic accident**

Pedestrian with babystroller injured in collision with other nonmotor vehicle in nontraffic accident

Pedestrian in wheelchair (powered) injured in collision with other nonmotor vehicle in traffic accident

Pedestrian in motorized mobility scooter injured in collision with other nonmotor vehicle in traffic accident

Pedestrian on ice-skates injured in collision with other nonmotor vehicle in traffic accident

Pedestrian on nonmotorized scooter injured in collision with other nonmotor vehicle in traffic accident

Pedestrian on sled injured in collision with other nonmotor vehicle in traffic accident

Pedestrian on snowboard injured in collision with other nonmotor vehicle in traffic accident

Pedestrian on snow-skis injured in collision with other nonmotor vehicle in traffic accident

CHAPTER 20 (V01-Y99)

● V06.9 **Pedestrian injured in collision with other nonmotor vehicle, unspecified whether traffic or nontraffic accident**

X● V06.90 **Pedestrian on foot injured in collision with other nonmotor vehicle, unspecified whether traffic or nontraffic accident**
Pedestrian NOS injured in collision with other nonmotor vehicle, unspecified whether traffic or nontraffic accident

X● V06.91 **Pedestrian on roller-skates injured in collision with other nonmotor vehicle, unspecified whether traffic or nontraffic accident**

X● V06.92 **Pedestrian on skateboard injured in collision with other nonmotor vehicle, unspecified whether traffic or nontraffic accident**

X● V06.99 **Pedestrian with other conveyance injured in collision with other nonmotor vehicle, unspecified whether traffic or nontraffic accident**
Pedestrian with babystroller injured in collision with other nonmotor vehicle, unspecified whether traffic or nontraffic accident
Pedestrian in wheelchair (powered) injured in collision with other nonmotor vehicle, unspecified whether traffic or nontraffic accident
Pedestrian in motorized mobility scooter injured in collision with other nonmotor vehicle, unspecified whether traffic or nontraffic accident
Pedestrian on ice-skates injured in collision with other nonmotor vehicle, unspecified whether traffic or nontraffic accident
Pedestrian on nonmotorized scooter injured in collision with other nonmotor vehicle, unspecified whether traffic or nontraffic accident
Pedestrian on sled injured in collision with other nonmotor vehicle, unspecified whether traffic or nontraffic accident
Pedestrian on snowboard injured in collision with other nonmotor vehicle, unspecified whether traffic or nontraffic accident
Pedestrian on snow-skis injured in collision with other nonmotor vehicle, unspecified whether traffic or nontraffic accident

● V09 **Pedestrian injured in other and unspecified transport accidents**

The appropriate 7th character is to be added to each code from category V09

A initial encounter
D subsequent encounter
S sequela

● V09.0 **Pedestrian injured in nontraffic accident involving other and unspecified motor vehicles**

X● V09.00 **Pedestrian injured in nontraffic accident involving unspecified motor vehicles**

X● V09.01 **Pedestrian injured in nontraffic accident involving military vehicle**

X● V09.09 **Pedestrian injured in nontraffic accident involving other motor vehicles**
Pedestrian injured in nontraffic accident by special vehicle

X● V09.1 **Pedestrian injured in unspecified nontraffic accident**

● V09.2 **Pedestrian injured in traffic accident involving other and unspecified motor vehicles**

X● V09.20 **Pedestrian injured in traffic accident involving unspecified motor vehicles**

X● V09.21 **Pedestrian injured in traffic accident involving military vehicle**

X● V09.29 **Pedestrian injured in traffic accident involving other motor vehicles**

X● V09.3 **Pedestrian injured in unspecified traffic accident**

X● V09.9 **Pedestrian injured in unspecified transport accident**

PEDAL CYCLE RIDER INJURED IN TRANSPORT ACCIDENT (V10-V19)

Includes any non-motorized vehicle, excluding an animal-drawn vehicle, or a sidecar or trailer attached to the pedal cycle

Excludes2 rupture of pedal cycle tire (W37.0)

● V10 **Pedal cycle rider injured in collision with pedestrian or animal**

Excludes1 pedal cycle rider collision with animal-drawn vehicle or animal being ridden (V16.-)

The appropriate 7th character is to be added to each code from category V10

A initial encounter
D subsequent encounter
S sequela

X● V10.0 **Pedal cycle driver injured in collision with pedestrian or animal in nontraffic accident**

X● V10.1 **Pedal cycle passenger injured in collision with pedestrian or animal in nontraffic accident**

X● V10.2 **Unspecified pedal cyclist injured in collision with pedestrian or animal in nontraffic accident**

X● V10.3 **Person boarding or alighting a pedal cycle injured in collision with pedestrian or animal**

X● V10.4 **Pedal cycle driver injured in collision with pedestrian or animal in traffic accident**

X● V10.5 **Pedal cycle passenger injured in collision with pedestrian or animal in traffic accident**

X● V10.9 **Unspecified pedal cyclist injured in collision with pedestrian or animal in traffic accident**

● V11 **Pedal cycle rider injured in collision with other pedal cycle**

The appropriate 7th character is to be added to each code from category V11

A initial encounter
D subsequent encounter
S sequela

X● V11.0 **Pedal cycle driver injured in collision with other pedal cycle in nontraffic accident**

X● V11.1 **Pedal cycle passenger injured in collision with other pedal cycle in nontraffic accident**

X● V11.2 **Unspecified pedal cyclist injured in collision with other pedal cycle in nontraffic accident**

X● V11.3 **Person boarding or alighting a pedal cycle injured in collision with other pedal cycle**

X● V11.4 **Pedal cycle driver injured in collision with other pedal cycle in traffic accident**

X● V11.5 **Pedal cycle passenger injured in collision with other pedal cycle in traffic accident**

X● V11.9 **Unspecified pedal cyclist injured in collision with other pedal cycle in traffic accident**

● **V12 Pedal cycle rider injured in collision with two- or three-wheeled motor vehicle**

The appropriate 7th character is to be added to each code from category V12

A	initial encounter
D	subsequent encounter
S	sequela

X● **V12.0 Pedal cycle driver injured in collision with two- or three-wheeled motor vehicle in nontraffic accident**

X● **V12.1 Pedal cycle passenger injured in collision with two- or three-wheeled motor vehicle in nontraffic accident**

X● **V12.2 Unspecified pedal cyclist injured in collision with two- or three-wheeled motor vehicle in nontraffic accident**

X● **V12.3 Person boarding or alighting a pedal cycle injured in collision with two- or three-wheeled motor vehicle**

X● **V12.4 Pedal cycle driver injured in collision with two- or three-wheeled motor vehicle in traffic accident**

X● **V12.5 Pedal cycle passenger injured in collision with two- or three-wheeled motor vehicle in traffic accident**

X● **V12.9 Unspecified pedal cyclist injured in collision with two- or three-wheeled motor vehicle in traffic accident**

● **V13 Pedal cycle rider injured in collision with car, pick-up truck or van**

The appropriate 7th character is to be added to each code from category V13

A	initial encounter
D	subsequent encounter
S	sequela

X● **V13.0 Pedal cycle driver injured in collision with car, pick-up truck or van in nontraffic accident**

X● **V13.1 Pedal cycle passenger injured in collision with car, pick-up truck or van in nontraffic accident**

X● **V13.2 Unspecified pedal cyclist injured in collision with car, pick-up truck or van in nontraffic accident**

X● **V13.3 Person boarding or alighting a pedal cycle injured in collision with car, pick-up truck or van**

X● **V13.4 Pedal cycle driver injured in collision with car, pick-up truck or van in traffic accident**

X● **V13.5 Pedal cycle passenger injured in collision with car, pick-up truck or van in traffic accident**

X● **V13.9 Unspecified pedal cyclist injured in collision with car, pick-up truck or van in traffic accident**

● **V14 Pedal cycle rider injured in collision with heavy transport vehicle or bus**

Excludes1 pedal cycle rider injured in collision with military vehicle (V19.81)

The appropriate 7th character is to be added to each code from category V14

A	initial encounter
D	subsequent encounter
S	sequela

X● **V14.0 Pedal cycle driver injured in collision with heavy transport vehicle or bus in nontraffic accident**

X● **V14.1 Pedal cycle passenger injured in collision with heavy transport vehicle or bus in nontraffic accident**

X● **V14.2 Unspecified pedal cyclist injured in collision with heavy transport vehicle or bus in nontraffic accident**

X● **V14.3 Person boarding or alighting a pedal cycle injured in collision with heavy transport vehicle or bus**

X● **V14.4 Pedal cycle driver injured in collision with heavy transport vehicle or bus in traffic accident**

X● **V14.5 Pedal cycle passenger injured in collision with heavy transport vehicle or bus in traffic accident**

X● **V14.9 Unspecified pedal cyclist injured in collision with heavy transport vehicle or bus in traffic accident**

● **V15 Pedal cycle rider injured in collision with railway train or railway vehicle**

The appropriate 7th character is to be added to each code from category V15

A	initial encounter
D	subsequent encounter
S	sequela

X● **V15.0 Pedal cycle driver injured in collision with railway train or railway vehicle in nontraffic accident**

X● **V15.1 Pedal cycle passenger injured in collision with railway train or railway vehicle in nontraffic accident**

X● **V15.2 Unspecified pedal cyclist injured in collision with railway train or railway vehicle in nontraffic accident**

X● **V15.3 Person boarding or alighting a pedal cycle injured in collision with railway train or railway vehicle**

X● **V15.4 Pedal cycle driver injured in collision with railway train or railway vehicle in traffic accident**

X● **V15.5 Pedal cycle passenger injured in collision with railway train or railway vehicle in traffic accident**

X● **V15.9 Unspecified pedal cyclist injured in collision with railway train or railway vehicle in traffic accident**

● **V16 Pedal cycle rider injured in collision with other nonmotor vehicle**

Includes collision with animal-drawn vehicle, animal being ridden, streetcar

The appropriate 7th character is to be added to each code from category V16

A	initial encounter
D	subsequent encounter
S	sequela

X● **V16.0 Pedal cycle driver injured in collision with other nonmotor vehicle in nontraffic accident**

X● **V16.1 Pedal cycle passenger injured in collision with other nonmotor vehicle in nontraffic accident**

X● **V16.2 Unspecified pedal cyclist injured in collision with other nonmotor vehicle in nontraffic accident**

X● **V16.3 Person boarding or alighting a pedal cycle injured in collision with other nonmotor vehicle in nontraffic accident**

X● **V16.4 Pedal cycle driver injured in collision with other nonmotor vehicle in traffic accident**

X● **V16.5 Pedal cycle passenger injured in collision with other nonmotor vehicle in traffic accident**

X● **V16.9 Unspecified pedal cyclist injured in collision with other nonmotor vehicle in traffic accident**

● **V17 Pedal cycle rider injured in collision with fixed or stationary object**

The appropriate 7th character is to be added to each code from category V17

A	initial encounter
D	subsequent encounter
S	sequela

X● **V17.0 Pedal cycle driver injured in collision with fixed or stationary object in nontraffic accident**

X● **V17.1 Pedal cycle passenger injured in collision with fixed or stationary object in nontraffic accident**

X● **V17.2 Unspecified pedal cyclist injured in collision with fixed or stationary object in nontraffic accident**

X● **V17.3 Person boarding or alighting a pedal cycle injured in collision with fixed or stationary object**

X● **V17.4 Pedal cycle driver injured in collision with fixed or stationary object in traffic accident**

X● **V17.5 Pedal cycle passenger injured in collision with fixed or stationary object in traffic accident**

X● **V17.9 Unspecified pedal cyclist injured in collision with fixed or stationary object in traffic accident**

● **V18 Pedal cycle rider injured in noncollision transport accident**

Includes fall or thrown from pedal cycle (without antecedent collision)
overturning pedal cycle NOS
overturning pedal cycle without collision

The appropriate 7th character is to be added to each code from category V18

A	initial encounter
D	subsequent encounter
S	sequela

X● **V18.Ø Pedal cycle driver injured in noncollision transport accident in nontraffic accident**

X● **V18.1 Pedal cycle passenger injured in noncollision transport accident in nontraffic accident**

X● **V18.2 Unspecified pedal cyclist injured in noncollision transport accident in nontraffic accident**

X● **V18.3 Person boarding or alighting a pedal cycle injured in noncollision transport accident**

X● **V18.4 Pedal cycle driver injured in noncollision transport accident in traffic accident**

X● **V18.5 Pedal cycle passenger injured in noncollision transport accident in traffic accident**

X● **V18.9 Unspecified pedal cyclist injured in noncollision transport accident in traffic accident**

● **V19 Pedal cycle rider injured in other and unspecified transport accidents**

The appropriate 7th character is to be added to each code from category V19

A	initial encounter
D	subsequent encounter
S	sequela

● **V19.Ø Pedal cycle driver injured in collision with other and unspecified motor vehicles in nontraffic accident**

X● **V19.ØØ Pedal cycle driver injured in collision with unspecified motor vehicles in nontraffic accident**

X● **V19.Ø9 Pedal cycle driver injured in collision with other motor vehicles in nontraffic accident**

● **V19.1 Pedal cycle passenger injured in collision with other and unspecified motor vehicles in nontraffic accident**

X● **V19.1Ø Pedal cycle passenger injured in collision with unspecified motor vehicles in nontraffic accident**

X● **V19.19 Pedal cycle passenger injured in collision with other motor vehicles in nontraffic accident**

● **V19.2 Unspecified pedal cyclist injured in collision with other and unspecified motor vehicles in nontraffic accident**

X● **V19.2Ø Unspecified pedal cyclist injured in collision with unspecified motor vehicles in nontraffic accident**

Pedal cycle collision NOS, nontraffic

X● **V19.29 Unspecified pedal cyclist injured in collision with other motor vehicles in nontraffic accident**

X● **V19.3 Pedal cyclist (driver) (passenger) injured in unspecified nontraffic accident**

Pedal cycle accident NOS, nontraffic
Pedal cyclist injured in nontraffic accident NOS

● **V19.4 Pedal cycle driver injured in collision with other and unspecified motor vehicles in traffic accident**

X● **V19.4Ø Pedal cycle driver injured in collision with unspecified motor vehicles in traffic accident**

X● **V19.49 Pedal cycle driver injured in collision with other motor vehicles in traffic accident**

● **V19.5 Pedal cycle passenger injured in collision with other and unspecified motor vehicles in traffic accident**

X● **V19.5Ø Pedal cycle passenger injured in collision with unspecified motor vehicles in traffic accident**

X● **V19.59 Pedal cycle passenger injured in collision with other motor vehicles in traffic accident**

● **V19.6 Unspecified pedal cyclist injured in collision with other and unspecified motor vehicles in traffic accident**

X● **V19.6Ø Unspecified pedal cyclist injured in collision with unspecified motor vehicles in traffic accident**

Pedal cycle collision NOS (traffic)

X● **V19.69 Unspecified pedal cyclist injured in collision with other motor vehicles in traffic accident**

● **V19.8 Pedal cyclist (driver) (passenger) injured in other specified transport accidents**

X● **V19.81 Pedal cyclist (driver) (passenger) injured in transport accident with military vehicle**

X● **V19.88 Pedal cyclist (driver) (passenger) injured in other specified transport accidents**

X● **V19.9 Pedal cyclist (driver) (passenger) injured in unspecified traffic accident**

Pedal cycle accident NOS

MOTORCYCLE RIDER INJURED IN TRANSPORT ACCIDENT (V2Ø-V29)

Includes moped motorcycle with sidecar motorized bicycle motor scooter

Excludes1 three-wheeled motor vehicle (V3Ø-V39)

● **V2Ø Motorcycle rider injured in collision with pedestrian or animal**

Excludes1 motorcycle rider collision with animal-drawn vehicle or animal being ridden (V26.-)

The appropriate 7th character is to be added to each code from category V2Ø

A	initial encounter
D	subsequent encounter
S	sequela

X● **V2Ø.Ø Motorcycle driver injured in collision with pedestrian or animal in nontraffic accident**

X● **V2Ø.1 Motorcycle passenger injured in collision with pedestrian or animal in nontraffic accident**

X● **V2Ø.2 Unspecified motorcycle rider injured in collision with pedestrian or animal in nontraffic accident**

X● **V2Ø.3 Person boarding or alighting a motorcycle injured in collision with pedestrian or animal**

X● **V2Ø.4 Motorcycle driver injured in collision with pedestrian or animal in traffic accident**

X● **V2Ø.5 Motorcycle passenger injured in collision with pedestrian or animal in traffic accident**

X● **V2Ø.9 Unspecified motorcycle rider injured in collision with pedestrian or animal in traffic accident**

● **V21 Motorcycle rider injured in collision with pedal cycle**

The appropriate 7th character is to be added to each code from category V21

A	initial encounter
D	subsequent encounter
S	sequela

X● **V21.Ø Motorcycle driver injured in collision with pedal cycle in nontraffic accident**

X● **V21.1 Motorcycle passenger injured in collision with pedal cycle in nontraffic accident**

X● **V21.2 Unspecified motorcycle rider injured in collision with pedal cycle in nontraffic accident**

X● **V21.3 Person boarding or alighting a motorcycle injured in collision with pedal cycle**

X● **V21.4 Motorcycle driver injured in collision with pedal cycle in traffic accident**

X● **V21.5 Motorcycle passenger injured in collision with pedal cycle in traffic accident**

X● **V21.9 Unspecified motorcycle rider injured in collision with pedal cycle in traffic accident**

● **V22 Motorcycle rider injured in collision with two- or three-wheeled motor vehicle**

The appropriate 7th character is to be added to each code from category V22

A	initial encounter
D	subsequent encounter
S	sequela

X● **V22.0 Motorcycle driver injured in collision with two- or three-wheeled motor vehicle in nontraffic accident**

X● **V22.1 Motorcycle passenger injured in collision with two- or three-wheeled motor vehicle in nontraffic accident**

X● **V22.2 Unspecified motorcycle rider injured in collision with two- or three-wheeled motor vehicle in nontraffic accident**

X● **V22.3 Person boarding or alighting a motorcycle injured in collision with two- or three-wheeled motor vehicle**

X● **V22.4 Motorcycle driver injured in collision with two- or three-wheeled motor vehicle in traffic accident**

X● **V22.5 Motorcycle passenger injured in collision with two- or three-wheeled motor vehicle in traffic accident**

X● **V22.9 Unspecified motorcycle rider injured in collision with two- or three-wheeled motor vehicle in traffic accident**

● **V23 Motorcycle rider injured in collision with car, pick-up truck or van**

The appropriate 7th character is to be added to each code from category V23

A	initial encounter
D	subsequent encounter
S	sequela

X● **V23.0 Motorcycle driver injured in collision with car, pick-up truck or van in nontraffic accident**

X● **V23.1 Motorcycle passenger injured in collision with car, pick-up truck or van in nontraffic accident**

X● **V23.2 Unspecified motorcycle rider injured in collision with car, pick-up truck or van in nontraffic accident**

X● **V23.3 Person boarding or alighting a motorcycle injured in collision with car, pick-up truck or van**

X● **V23.4 Motorcycle driver injured in collision with car, pick-up truck or van in traffic accident**

X● **V23.5 Motorcycle passenger injured in collision with car, pick-up truck or van in traffic accident**

X● **V23.9 Unspecified motorcycle rider injured in collision with car, pick-up truck or van in traffic accident**

● **V24 Motorcycle rider injured in collision with heavy transport vehicle or bus**

Excludes1 motorcycle rider injured in collision with military vehicle (V29.81)

The appropriate 7th character is to be added to each code from category V24

A	initial encounter
D	subsequent encounter
S	sequela

X● **V24.0 Motorcycle driver injured in collision with heavy transport vehicle or bus in nontraffic accident**

X● **V24.1 Motorcycle passenger injured in collision with heavy transport vehicle or bus in nontraffic accident**

X● **V24.2 Unspecified motorcycle rider injured in collision with heavy transport vehicle or bus in nontraffic accident**

X● **V24.3 Person boarding or alighting a motorcycle injured in collision with heavy transport vehicle or bus**

X● **V24.4 Motorcycle driver injured in collision with heavy transport vehicle or bus in traffic accident**

X● **V24.5 Motorcycle passenger injured in collision with heavy transport vehicle or bus in traffic accident**

X● **V24.9 Unspecified motorcycle rider injured in collision with heavy transport vehicle or bus in traffic accident**

● **V25 Motorcycle rider injured in collision with railway train or railway vehicle**

The appropriate 7th character is to be added to each code from category V25

A	initial encounter
D	subsequent encounter
S	sequela

X● **V25.0 Motorcycle driver injured in collision with railway train or railway vehicle in nontraffic accident**

X● **V25.1 Motorcycle passenger injured in collision with railway train or railway vehicle in nontraffic accident**

X● **V25.2 Unspecified motorcycle rider injured in collision with railway train or railway vehicle in nontraffic accident**

X● **V25.3 Person boarding or alighting a motorcycle injured in collision with railway train or railway vehicle**

X● **V25.4 Motorcycle driver injured in collision with railway train or railway vehicle in traffic accident**

X● **V25.5 Motorcycle passenger injured in collision with railway train or railway vehicle in traffic accident**

X● **V25.9 Unspecified motorcycle rider injured in collision with railway train or railway vehicle in traffic accident**

● **V26 Motorcycle rider injured in collision with other nonmotor vehicle**

Includes collision with animal-drawn vehicle, animal being ridden, streetcar

The appropriate 7th character is to be added to each code from category V26

A	initial encounter
D	subsequent encounter
S	sequela

X● **V26.0 Motorcycle driver injured in collision with other nonmotor vehicle in nontraffic accident**

X● **V26.1 Motorcycle passenger injured in collision with other nonmotor vehicle in nontraffic accident**

X● **V26.2 Unspecified motorcycle rider injured in collision with other nonmotor vehicle in nontraffic accident**

X● **V26.3 Person boarding or alighting a motorcycle injured in collision with other nonmotor vehicle**

X● **V26.4 Motorcycle driver injured in collision with other nonmotor vehicle in traffic accident**

X● **V26.5 Motorcycle passenger injured in collision with other nonmotor vehicle in traffic accident**

X● **V26.9 Unspecified motorcycle rider injured in collision with other nonmotor vehicle in traffic accident**

● **V27 Motorcycle rider injured in collision with fixed or stationary object**

The appropriate 7th character is to be added to each code from category V27

A	initial encounter
D	subsequent encounter
S	sequela

X● **V27.0 Motorcycle driver injured in collision with fixed or stationary object in nontraffic accident**

X● **V27.1 Motorcycle passenger injured in collision with fixed or stationary object in nontraffic accident**

X● **V27.2 Unspecified motorcycle rider injured in collision with fixed or stationary object in nontraffic accident**

X● **V27.3 Person boarding or alighting a motorcycle injured in collision with fixed or stationary object**

X● **V27.4 Motorcycle driver injured in collision with fixed or stationary object in traffic accident**

X● **V27.5 Motorcycle passenger injured in collision with fixed or stationary object in traffic accident**

X● **V27.9 Unspecified motorcycle rider injured in collision with fixed or stationary object in traffic accident**

● V28 Motorcycle rider injured in noncollision transport accident

Includes fall or thrown from motorcycle (without antecedent collision)
overturning motorcycle NOS
overturning motorcycle without collision

The appropriate 7th character is to be added to each code from category V28

A	initial encounter
D	subsequent encounter
S	sequela

X● V28.0 Motorcycle driver injured in noncollision transport accident in nontraffic accident

X● V28.1 Motorcycle passenger injured in noncollision transport accident in nontraffic accident

X● V28.2 Unspecified motorcycle rider injured in noncollision transport accident in nontraffic accident

X● V28.3 Person boarding or alighting a motorcycle injured in noncollision transport accident

X● V28.4 Motorcycle driver injured in noncollision transport accident in traffic accident

X● V28.5 Motorcycle passenger injured in noncollision transport accident in traffic accident

X● V28.9 Unspecified motorcycle rider injured in noncollision transport accident in traffic accident

● V29 Motorcycle rider injured in other and unspecified transport accidents

The appropriate 7th character is to be added to each code from category V29

A	initial encounter
D	subsequent encounter
S	sequela

● V29.0 Motorcycle driver injured in collision with other and unspecified motor vehicles in nontraffic accident

X● V29.00 Motorcycle driver injured in collision with unspecified motor vehicles in nontraffic accident

X● V29.09 Motorcycle driver injured in collision with other motor vehicles in nontraffic accident

● V29.1 Motorcycle passenger injured in collision with other and unspecified motor vehicles in nontraffic accident

X● V29.10 Motorcycle passenger injured in collision with unspecified motor vehicles in nontraffic accident

X● V29.19 Motorcycle passenger injured in collision with other motor vehicles in nontraffic accident

● V29.2 Unspecified motorcycle rider injured in collision with other and unspecified motor vehicles in nontraffic accident

X● V29.20 Unspecified motorcycle rider injured in collision with unspecified motor vehicles in nontraffic accident
Motorcycle collision NOS, nontraffic

X● V29.29 Unspecified motorcycle rider injured in collision with other motor vehicles in nontraffic accident

X● V29.3 Motorcycle rider (driver) (passenger) injured in unspecified nontraffic accident
Motorcycle accident NOS, nontraffic
Motorcycle rider injured in nontraffic accident NOS

● V29.4 Motorcycle driver injured in collision with other and unspecified motor vehicles in traffic accident

X● V29.40 Motorcycle driver injured in collision with unspecified motor vehicles in traffic accident

X● V29.49 Motorcycle driver injured in collision with other motor vehicles in traffic accident

● V29.5 Motorcycle passenger injured in collision with other and unspecified motor vehicles in traffic accident

X● V29.50 Motorcycle passenger injured in collision with unspecified motor vehicles in traffic accident

X● V29.59 Motorcycle passenger injured in collision with other motor vehicles in traffic accident

● V29.6 Unspecified motorcycle rider injured in collision with other and unspecified motor vehicles in traffic accident

X● V29.60 Unspecified motorcycle rider injured in collision with unspecified motor vehicles in traffic accident
Motorcycle collision NOS (traffic)

X● V29.69 Unspecified motorcycle rider injured in collision with other motor vehicles in traffic accident

● V29.8 Motorcycle rider (driver) (passenger) injured in other specified transport accidents

X● V29.81 Motorcycle rider (driver) (passenger) injured in transport accident with military vehicle

X● V29.88 Motorcycle rider (driver) (passenger) injured in other specified transport accidents

X● V29.9 Motorcycle rider (driver) (passenger) injured in unspecified traffic accident
Motorcycle accident NOS

OCCUPANT OF THREE-WHEELED MOTOR VEHICLE INJURED IN TRANSPORT ACCIDENT (V30-V39)

Includes motorized tricycle
motorized rickshaw
three-wheeled motor car

Excludes1 all-terrain vehicles (V86.-)
motorcycle with sidecar (V20-V29)
vehicle designed primarily for off-road use (V86.-)

● V30 Occupant of three-wheeled motor vehicle injured in collision with pedestrian or animal

Excludes1 three-wheeled motor vehicle collision with animal-drawn vehicle or animal being ridden (V36.-)

The appropriate 7th character is to be added to each code from category V30

A	initial encounter
D	subsequent encounter
S	sequela

X● V30.0 Driver of three-wheeled motor vehicle injured in collision with pedestrian or animal in nontraffic accident

X● V30.1 Passenger in three-wheeled motor vehicle injured in collision with pedestrian or animal in nontraffic accident

X● V30.2 Person on outside of three-wheeled motor vehicle injured in collision with pedestrian or animal in nontraffic accident

X● V30.3 Unspecified occupant of three-wheeled motor vehicle injured in collision with pedestrian or animal in nontraffic accident

X● V30.4 Person boarding or alighting a three-wheeled motor vehicle injured in collision with pedestrian or animal

X● V30.5 Driver of three-wheeled motor vehicle injured in collision with pedestrian or animal in traffic accident

X● V30.6 Passenger in three-wheeled motor vehicle injured in collision with pedestrian or animal in traffic accident

X● V30.7 Person on outside of three-wheeled motor vehicle injured in collision with pedestrian or animal in traffic accident

X● V30.9 Unspecified occupant of three-wheeled motor vehicle injured in collision with pedestrian or animal in traffic accident

● **V31 Occupant of three-wheeled motor vehicle injured in collision with pedal cycle**

The appropriate 7th character is to be added to each code from category V31

A	initial encounter
D	subsequent encounter
S	sequela

X● **V31.0 Driver of three-wheeled motor vehicle injured in collision with pedal cycle in nontraffic accident**

X● **V31.1 Passenger in three-wheeled motor vehicle injured in collision with pedal cycle in nontraffic accident**

X● **V31.2 Person on outside of three-wheeled motor vehicle injured in collision with pedal cycle in nontraffic accident**

X● **V31.3 Unspecified occupant of three-wheeled motor vehicle injured in collision with pedal cycle in nontraffic accident**

X● **V31.4 Person boarding or alighting a three-wheeled motor vehicle injured in collision with pedal cycle**

X● **V31.5 Driver of three-wheeled motor vehicle injured in collision with pedal cycle in traffic accident**

X● **V31.6 Passenger in three-wheeled motor vehicle injured in collision with pedal cycle in traffic accident**

X● **V31.7 Person on outside of three-wheeled motor vehicle injured in collision with pedal cycle in traffic accident**

X● **V31.9 Unspecified occupant of three-wheeled motor vehicle injured in collision with pedal cycle in traffic accident**

● **V32 Occupant of three-wheeled motor vehicle injured in collision with two- or three-wheeled motor vehicle**

The appropriate 7th character is to be added to each code from category V32

A	initial encounter
D	subsequent encounter
S	sequela

X● **V32.0 Driver of three-wheeled motor vehicle injured in collision with two- or three-wheeled motor vehicle in nontraffic accident**

X● **V32.1 Passenger in three-wheeled motor vehicle injured in collision with two- or three-wheeled motor vehicle in nontraffic accident**

X● **V32.2 Person on outside of three-wheeled motor vehicle injured in collision with two- or three-wheeled motor vehicle in nontraffic accident**

X● **V32.3 Unspecified occupant of three-wheeled motor vehicle injured in collision with two- or three-wheeled motor vehicle in nontraffic accident**

X● **V32.4 Person boarding or alighting a three-wheeled motor vehicle injured in collision with two- or three-wheeled motor vehicle**

X● **V32.5 Driver of three-wheeled motor vehicle injured in collision with two- or three-wheeled motor vehicle in traffic accident**

X● **V32.6 Passenger in three-wheeled motor vehicle injured in collision with two- or three-wheeled motor vehicle in traffic accident**

X● **V32.7 Person on outside of three-wheeled motor vehicle injured in collision with two- or three-wheeled motor vehicle in traffic accident**

X● **V32.9 Unspecified occupant of three-wheeled motor vehicle injured in collision with two- or three-wheeled motor vehicle in traffic accident**

● **V33 Occupant of three-wheeled motor vehicle injured in collision with car, pick-up truck or van**

The appropriate 7th character is to be added to each code from category V33

A	initial encounter
D	subsequent encounter
S	sequela

X● **V33.0 Driver of three-wheeled motor vehicle injured in collision with car, pick-up truck or van in nontraffic accident**

X● **V33.1 Passenger in three-wheeled motor vehicle injured in collision with car, pick-up truck or van in nontraffic accident**

X● **V33.2 Person on outside of three-wheeled motor vehicle injured in collision with car, pick-up truck or van in nontraffic accident**

X● **V33.3 Unspecified occupant of three-wheeled motor vehicle injured in collision with car, pick-up truck or van in nontraffic accident**

X● **V33.4 Person boarding or alighting a three-wheeled motor vehicle injured in collision with car, pick-up truck or van**

X● **V33.5 Driver of three-wheeled motor vehicle injured in collision with car, pick-up truck or van in traffic accident**

X● **V33.6 Passenger in three-wheeled motor vehicle injured in collision with car, pick-up truck or van in traffic accident**

X● **V33.7 Person on outside of three-wheeled motor vehicle injured in collision with car, pick-up truck or van in traffic accident**

X● **V33.9 Unspecified occupant of three-wheeled motor vehicle injured in collision with car, pick-up truck or van in traffic accident**

● **V34 Occupant of three-wheeled motor vehicle injured in collision with heavy transport vehicle or bus**

Excludes1 occupant of three-wheeled motor vehicle injured in collision with military vehicle (V39.81)

The appropriate 7th character is to be added to each code from category V34

A	initial encounter
D	subsequent encounter
S	sequela

X● **V34.0 Driver of three-wheeled motor vehicle injured in collision with heavy transport vehicle or bus in nontraffic accident**

X● **V34.1 Passenger in three-wheeled motor vehicle injured in collision with heavy transport vehicle or bus in nontraffic accident**

X● **V34.2 Person on outside of three-wheeled motor vehicle injured in collision with heavy transport vehicle or bus in nontraffic accident**

X● **V34.3 Unspecified occupant of three-wheeled motor vehicle injured in collision with heavy transport vehicle or bus in nontraffic accident**

X● **V34.4 Person boarding or alighting a three-wheeled motor vehicle injured in collision with heavy transport vehicle or bus**

X● **V34.5 Driver of three-wheeled motor vehicle injured in collision with heavy transport vehicle or bus in traffic accident**

X● **V34.6 Passenger in three-wheeled motor vehicle injured in collision with heavy transport vehicle or bus in traffic accident**

X● **V34.7 Person on outside of three-wheeled motor vehicle injured in collision with heavy transport vehicle or bus in traffic accident**

X● **V34.9 Unspecified occupant of three-wheeled motor vehicle injured in collision with heavy transport vehicle or bus in traffic accident**

● **V35 Occupant of three-wheeled motor vehicle injured in collision with railway train or railway vehicle**

The appropriate 7th character is to be added to each code from category V35

A	initial encounter
D	subsequent encounter
S	sequela

X● **V35.0 Driver of three-wheeled motor vehicle injured in collision with railway train or railway vehicle in nontraffic accident**

X● **V35.1 Passenger in three-wheeled motor vehicle injured in collision with railway train or railway vehicle in nontraffic accident**

X● **V35.2 Person on outside of three-wheeled motor vehicle injured in collision with railway train or railway vehicle in nontraffic accident**

X● **V35.3 Unspecified occupant of three-wheeled motor vehicle injured in collision with railway train or railway vehicle in nontraffic accident**

X● **V35.4 Person boarding or alighting a three-wheeled motor vehicle injured in collision with railway train or railway vehicle**

X● **V35.5 Driver of three-wheeled motor vehicle injured in collision with railway train or railway vehicle in traffic accident**

X● **V35.6 Passenger in three-wheeled motor vehicle injured in collision with railway train or railway vehicle in traffic accident**

X● **V35.7 Person on outside of three-wheeled motor vehicle injured in collision with railway train or railway vehicle in traffic accident**

X● **V35.9 Unspecified occupant of three-wheeled motor vehicle injured in collision with railway train or railway vehicle in traffic accident**

● **V36 Occupant of three-wheeled motor vehicle injured in collision with other nonmotor vehicle**

Includes collision with animal-drawn vehicle, animal being ridden, streetcar

The appropriate 7th character is to be added to each code from category V36

A	initial encounter
D	subsequent encounter
S	sequela

X● **V36.0 Driver of three-wheeled motor vehicle injured in collision with other nonmotor vehicle in nontraffic accident**

X● **V36.1 Passenger in three-wheeled motor vehicle injured in collision with other nonmotor vehicle in nontraffic accident**

X● **V36.2 Person on outside of three-wheeled motor vehicle injured in collision with other nonmotor vehicle in nontraffic accident**

X● **V36.3 Unspecified occupant of three-wheeled motor vehicle injured in collision with other nonmotor vehicle in nontraffic accident**

X● **V36.4 Person boarding or alighting a three-wheeled motor vehicle injured in collision with other nonmotor vehicle**

X● **V36.5 Driver of three-wheeled motor vehicle injured in collision with other nonmotor vehicle in traffic accident**

X● **V36.6 Passenger in three-wheeled motor vehicle injured in collision with other nonmotor vehicle in traffic accident**

X● **V36.7 Person on outside of three-wheeled motor vehicle injured in collision with other nonmotor vehicle in traffic accident**

X● **V36.9 Unspecified occupant of three-wheeled motor vehicle injured in collision with other nonmotor vehicle in traffic accident**

● **V37 Occupant of three-wheeled motor vehicle injured in collision with fixed or stationary object**

The appropriate 7th character is to be added to each code from category V37

A	initial encounter
D	subsequent encounter
S	sequela

X● **V37.0 Driver of three-wheeled motor vehicle injured in collision with fixed or stationary object in nontraffic accident**

X● **V37.1 Passenger in three-wheeled motor vehicle injured in collision with fixed or stationary object in nontraffic accident**

X● **V37.2 Person on outside of three-wheeled motor vehicle injured in collision with fixed or stationary object in nontraffic accident**

X● **V37.3 Unspecified occupant of three-wheeled motor vehicle injured in collision with fixed or stationary object in nontraffic accident**

X● **V37.4 Person boarding or alighting a three-wheeled motor vehicle injured in collision with fixed or stationary object**

X● **V37.5 Driver of three-wheeled motor vehicle injured in collision with fixed or stationary object in traffic accident**

X● **V37.6 Passenger in three-wheeled motor vehicle injured in collision with fixed or stationary object in traffic accident**

X● **V37.7 Person on outside of three-wheeled motor vehicle injured in collision with fixed or stationary object in traffic accident**

X● **V37.9 Unspecified occupant of three-wheeled motor vehicle injured in collision with fixed or stationary object in traffic accident**

● **V38 Occupant of three-wheeled motor vehicle injured in noncollision transport accident**

Includes fall or thrown from three-wheeled motor vehicle
overturning of three-wheeled motor vehicle NOS
overturning of three-wheeled motor vehicle without collision

The appropriate 7th character is to be added to each code from category V38

A	initial encounter
D	subsequent encounter
S	sequela

X● **V38.0 Driver of three-wheeled motor vehicle injured in noncollision transport accident in nontraffic accident**

X● **V38.1 Passenger in three-wheeled motor vehicle injured in noncollision transport accident in nontraffic accident**

X● **V38.2 Person on outside of three-wheeled motor vehicle injured in noncollision transport accident in nontraffic accident**

X● **V38.3 Unspecified occupant of three-wheeled motor vehicle injured in noncollision transport accident in nontraffic accident**

X● **V38.4 Person boarding or alighting a three-wheeled motor vehicle injured in noncollision transport accident**

X● **V38.5 Driver of three-wheeled motor vehicle injured in noncollision transport accident in traffic accident**

X● **V38.6 Passenger in three-wheeled motor vehicle injured in noncollision transport accident in traffic accident**

X● **V38.7 Person on outside of three-wheeled motor vehicle injured in noncollision transport accident in traffic accident**

X● **V38.9 Unspecified occupant of three-wheeled motor vehicle injured in noncollision transport accident in traffic accident**

● V39 **Occupant of three-wheeled motor vehicle injured in other and unspecified transport accidents**

The appropriate 7th character is to be added to each code from category V39

A	initial encounter
D	subsequent encounter
S	sequela

● V39.0 **Driver of three-wheeled motor vehicle injured in collision with other and unspecified motor vehicles in nontraffic accident**

X● V39.00 **Driver of three-wheeled motor vehicle injured in collision with unspecified motor vehicles in nontraffic accident**

X● V39.09 **Driver of three-wheeled motor vehicle injured in collision with other motor vehicles in nontraffic accident**

● V39.1 **Passenger in three-wheeled motor vehicle injured in collision with other and unspecified motor vehicles in nontraffic accident**

X● V39.10 **Passenger in three-wheeled motor vehicle injured in collision with unspecified motor vehicles in nontraffic accident**

X● V39.19 **Passenger in three-wheeled motor vehicle injured in collision with other motor vehicles in nontraffic accident**

● V39.2 **Unspecified occupant of three-wheeled motor vehicle injured in collision with other and unspecified motor vehicles in nontraffic accident**

X● V39.20 **Unspecified occupant of three-wheeled motor vehicle injured in collision with unspecified motor vehicles in nontraffic accident**

Collision NOS involving three-wheeled motor vehicle, nontraffic

X● V39.29 **Unspecified occupant of three-wheeled motor vehicle injured in collision with other motor vehicles in nontraffic accident**

X● V39.3 **Occupant (driver) (passenger) of three-wheeled motor vehicle injured in unspecified nontraffic accident**

Accident NOS involving three-wheeled motor vehicle, nontraffic

Occupant of three-wheeled motor vehicle injured in nontraffic accident NOS

● V39.4 **Driver of three-wheeled motor vehicle injured in collision with other and unspecified motor vehicles in traffic accident**

X● V39.40 **Driver of three-wheeled motor vehicle injured in collision with unspecified motor vehicles in traffic accident**

X● V39.49 **Driver of three-wheeled motor vehicle injured in collision with other motor vehicles in traffic accident**

● V39.5 **Passenger in three-wheeled motor vehicle injured in collision with other and unspecified motor vehicles in traffic accident**

X● V39.50 **Passenger in three-wheeled motor vehicle injured in collision with unspecified motor vehicles in traffic accident**

X● V39.59 **Passenger in three-wheeled motor vehicle injured in collision with other motor vehicles in traffic accident**

● V39.6 **Unspecified occupant of three-wheeled motor vehicle injured in collision with other and unspecified motor vehicles in traffic accident**

X● V39.60 **Unspecified occupant of three-wheeled motor vehicle injured in collision with unspecified motor vehicles in traffic accident**

Collision NOS involving three-wheeled motor vehicle (traffic)

X● V39.69 **Unspecified occupant of three-wheeled motor vehicle injured in collision with other motor vehicles in traffic accident**

● V39.8 **Occupant (driver) (passenger) of three-wheeled motor vehicle injured in other specified transport accidents**

X● V39.81 **Occupant (driver) (passenger) of three-wheeled motor vehicle injured in transport accident with military vehicle**

X● V39.89 **Occupant (driver) (passenger) of three-wheeled motor vehicle injured in other specified transport accidents**

X● V39.9 **Occupant (driver) (passenger) of three-wheeled motor vehicle injured in unspecified traffic accident**

Accident NOS involving three-wheeled motor vehicle

CAR OCCUPANT INJURED IN TRANSPORT ACCIDENT (V40-V49)

Includes a four-wheeled motor vehicle designed primarily for carrying passengers

automobile (pulling a trailer or camper)

Excludes1 bus (V50-V59)

minibus (V50-V59)

minivan (V50-V59)

motorcoach (V70-V79)

pick-up truck (V50-V59)

sport utility vehicle (SUV) (V50-V59)

● V40 **Car occupant injured in collision with pedestrian or animal**

Excludes1 car collision with animal-drawn vehicle or animal being ridden (V46.-)

The appropriate 7th character is to be added to each code from category V40

A	initial encounter
D	subsequent encounter
S	sequela

X● V40.0 **Car driver injured in collision with pedestrian or animal in nontraffic accident**

X● V40.1 **Car passenger injured in collision with pedestrian or animal in nontraffic accident**

X● V40.2 **Person on outside of car injured in collision with pedestrian or animal in nontraffic accident**

X● V40.3 **Unspecified car occupant injured in collision with pedestrian or animal in nontraffic accident**

X● V40.4 **Person boarding or alighting a car injured in collision with pedestrian or animal**

X● V40.5 **Car driver injured in collision with pedestrian or animal in traffic accident**

X● V40.6 **Car passenger injured in collision with pedestrian or animal in traffic accident**

X● V40.7 **Person on outside of car injured in collision with pedestrian or animal in traffic accident**

X● V40.9 **Unspecified car occupant injured in collision with pedestrian or animal in traffic accident**

● V41 **Car occupant injured in collision with pedal cycle**

The appropriate 7th character is to be added to each code from category V41

A	initial encounter
D	subsequent encounter
S	sequela

X● V41.0 **Car driver injured in collision with pedal cycle in nontraffic accident**

X● V41.1 **Car passenger injured in collision with pedal cycle in nontraffic accident**

X● V41.2 **Person on outside of car injured in collision with pedal cycle in nontraffic accident**

X● V41.3 **Unspecified car occupant injured in collision with pedal cycle in nontraffic accident**

X● V41.4 **Person boarding or alighting a car injured in collision with pedal cycle**

X● V41.5 **Car driver injured in collision with pedal cycle in traffic accident**

X● V41.6 **Car passenger injured in collision with pedal cycle in traffic accident**

X● V41.7 Person on outside of car injured in collision with pedal cycle in traffic accident

X● V41.9 Unspecified car occupant injured in collision with pedal cycle in traffic accident

● V42 Car occupant injured in collision with two- or three-wheeled motor vehicle

The appropriate 7th character is to be added to each code from category V42

A	initial encounter
D	subsequent encounter
S	sequela

X● V42.0 Car driver injured in collision with two- or three-wheeled motor vehicle in nontraffic accident

X● V42.1 Car passenger injured in collision with two- or three-wheeled motor vehicle in nontraffic accident

X● V42.2 Person on outside of car injured in collision with two- or three-wheeled motor vehicle in nontraffic accident

X● V42.3 Unspecified car occupant injured in collision with two- or three-wheeled motor vehicle in nontraffic accident

X● V42.4 Person boarding or alighting a car injured in collision with two- or three-wheeled motor vehicle

X● V42.5 Car driver injured in collision with two- or three-wheeled motor vehicle in traffic accident

X● V42.6 Car passenger injured in collision with two- or three-wheeled motor vehicle in traffic accident

X● V42.7 Person on outside of car injured in collision with two- or three-wheeled motor vehicle in traffic accident

X● V42.9 Unspecified car occupant injured in collision with two- or three-wheeled motor vehicle in traffic accident

● V43 Car occupant injured in collision with car, pick-up truck or van

The appropriate 7th character is to be added to each code from category V43

A	initial encounter
D	subsequent encounter
S	sequela

● V43.0 Car driver injured in collision with car, pick-up truck or van in nontraffic accident

X● V43.01 Car driver injured in collision with sport utility vehicle in nontraffic accident

X● V43.02 Car driver injured in collision with other type car in nontraffic accident

X● V43.03 Car driver injured in collision with pick-up truck in nontraffic accident

X● V43.04 Car driver injured in collision with van in nontraffic accident

● V43.1 Car passenger injured in collision with car, pick-up truck or van in nontraffic accident

X● V43.11 Car passenger injured in collision with sport utility vehicle in nontraffic accident

X● V43.12 Car passenger injured in collision with other type car in nontraffic accident

X● V43.13 Car passenger injured in collision with pick-up in nontraffic accident

X● V43.14 Car passenger injured in collision with van in nontraffic accident

● V43.2 Person on outside of car injured in collision with car, pick-up truck or van in nontraffic accident

X● V43.21 Person on outside of car injured in collision with sport utility vehicle in nontraffic accident

X● V43.22 Person on outside of car injured in collision with other type car in nontraffic accident

X● V43.23 Person on outside of car injured in collision with pick-up truck in nontraffic accident

X● V43.24 Person on outside of car injured in collision with van in nontraffic accident

● V43.3 Unspecified car occupant injured in collision with car, pick-up truck or van in nontraffic accident

X● V43.31 Unspecified car occupant injured in collision with sport utility vehicle in nontraffic accident

X● V43.32 Unspecified car occupant injured in collision with other type car in nontraffic accident

X● V43.33 Unspecified car occupant injured in collision with pick-up truck in nontraffic accident

X● V43.34 Unspecified car occupant injured in collision with van in nontraffic accident

● V43.4 Person boarding or alighting a car injured in collision with car, pick-up truck or van

X● V43.41 Person boarding or alighting a car injured in collision with sport utility vehicle

X● V43.42 Person boarding or alighting a car injured in collision with other type car

X● V43.43 Person boarding or alighting a car injured in collision with pick-up truck

X● V43.44 Person boarding or alighting a car injured in collision with van

● V43.5 Car driver injured in collision with car, pick-up truck or van in traffic accident

X● V43.51 Car driver injured in collision with sport utility vehicle in traffic accident

X● V43.52 Car driver injured in collision with other type car in traffic accident

X● V43.53 Car driver injured in collision with pick-up truck in traffic accident

X● V43.54 Car driver injured in collision with van in traffic accident

● V43.6 Car passenger injured in collision with car, pick-up truck or van in traffic accident

X● V43.61 Car passenger injured in collision with sport utility vehicle in traffic accident

X● V43.62 Car passenger injured in collision with other type car in traffic accident

X● V43.63 Car passenger injured in collision with pick-up truck in traffic accident

X● V43.64 Car passenger injured in collision with van in traffic accident

● V43.7 Person on outside of car injured in collision with car, pick-up truck or van in traffic accident

X● V43.71 Person on outside of car injured in collision with sport utility vehicle in traffic accident

X● V43.72 Person on outside of car injured in collision with other type car in traffic accident

X● V43.73 Person on outside of car injured in collision with pick-up truck in traffic accident

X● V43.74 Person on outside of car injured in collision with van in traffic accident

● V43.9 Unspecified car occupant injured in collision with car, pick-up truck or van in traffic accident

X● V43.91 Unspecified car occupant injured in collision with sport utility vehicle in traffic accident

X● V43.92 Unspecified car occupant injured in collision with other type car in traffic accident

X● V43.93 Unspecified car occupant injured in collision with pick-up truck in traffic accident

X● V43.94 Unspecified car occupant injured in collision with van in traffic accident

● V44 Car occupant injured in collision with heavy transport vehicle or bus

Excludes1 car occupant injured in collision with military vehicle (V49.81)

The appropriate 7th character is to be added to each code from category V44

A initial encounter
D subsequent encounter
S sequela

X● V44.0 Car driver injured in collision with heavy transport vehicle or bus in nontraffic accident

X● V44.1 Car passenger injured in collision with heavy transport vehicle or bus in nontraffic accident

X● V44.2 Person on outside of car injured in collision with heavy transport vehicle or bus in nontraffic accident

X● V44.3 Unspecified car occupant injured in collision with heavy transport vehicle or bus in nontraffic accident

X● V44.4 Person boarding or alighting a car injured in collision with heavy transport vehicle or bus

X● V44.5 Car driver injured in collision with heavy transport vehicle or bus in traffic accident

X● V44.6 Car passenger injured in collision with heavy transport vehicle or bus in traffic accident

X● V44.7 Person on outside of car injured in collision with heavy transport vehicle or bus in traffic accident

X● V44.9 Unspecified car occupant injured in collision with heavy transport vehicle or bus in traffic accident

● V45 Car occupant injured in collision with railway train or railway vehicle

The appropriate 7th character is to be added to each code from category V45

A initial encounter
D subsequent encounter
S sequela

X● V45.0 Car driver injured in collision with railway train or railway vehicle in nontraffic accident

X● V45.1 Car passenger injured in collision with railway train or railway vehicle in nontraffic accident

X● V45.2 Person on outside of car injured in collision with railway train or railway vehicle in nontraffic accident

X● V45.3 Unspecified car occupant injured in collision with railway train or railway vehicle in nontraffic accident

X● V45.4 Person boarding or alighting a car injured in collision with railway train or railway vehicle

X● V45.5 Car driver injured in collision with railway train or railway vehicle in traffic accident

X● V45.6 Car passenger injured in collision with railway train or railway vehicle in traffic accident

X● V45.7 Person on outside of car injured in collision with railway train or railway vehicle in traffic accident

X● V45.9 Unspecified car occupant injured in collision with railway train or railway vehicle in traffic accident

● V46 Car occupant injured in collision with other nonmotor vehicle

Includes collision with animal-drawn vehicle, animal being ridden, streetcar

The appropriate 7th character is to be added to each code from category V46

A initial encounter
D subsequent encounter
S sequela

X● V46.0 Car driver injured in collision with other nonmotor vehicle in nontraffic accident

X● V46.1 Car passenger injured in collision with other nonmotor vehicle in nontraffic accident

X● V46.2 Person on outside of car injured in collision with other nonmotor vehicle in nontraffic accident

X● V46.3 Unspecified car occupant injured in collision with other nonmotor vehicle in nontraffic accident

X● V46.4 Person boarding or alighting a car injured in collision with other nonmotor vehicle

X● V46.5 Car driver injured in collision with other nonmotor vehicle in traffic accident

X● V46.6 Car passenger injured in collision with other nonmotor vehicle in traffic accident

X● V46.7 Person on outside of car injured in collision with other nonmotor vehicle in traffic accident

X● V46.9 Unspecified car occupant injured in collision with other nonmotor vehicle in traffic accident

● V47 Car occupant injured in collision with fixed or stationary object

The appropriate 7th character is to be added to each code from category V47

A initial encounter
D subsequent encounter
S sequela

X● V47.0 Car driver injured in collision with fixed or stationary object in nontraffic accident

~~V47.01 Driver of sport utility vehicle injured in collision with fixed or stationary object in nontraffic accident~~

~~V47.02 Driver of other type car injured in collision with fixed or stationary object in nontraffic accident~~

X● V47.1 Car passenger injured in collision with fixed or stationary object in nontraffic accident

~~V47.11 Passenger of sport utility vehicle injured in collision with fixed or stationary object in nontraffic accident~~

~~V47.12 Passenger of other type car injured in collision with fixed or stationary object in nontraffic accident~~

X● V47.2 Person on outside of car injured in collision with fixed or stationary object in nontraffic accident

X● V47.3 Unspecified car occupant injured in collision with fixed or stationary object in nontraffic accident

~~V47.31 Unspecified occupant of sport utility vehicle injured in collision with fixed or stationary object in nontraffic accident~~

~~V47.32 Unspecified occupant of other type car injured in collision with fixed or stationary object in nontraffic accident~~

X● V47.4 Person boarding or alighting a car injured in collision with fixed or stationary object

X● V47.5 Car driver injured in collision with fixed or stationary object in traffic accident

~~V47.51 Driver of sport utility vehicle injured in collision with fixed or stationary object in traffic accident~~

~~V47.52 Driver of other type car injured in collision with fixed or stationary object in traffic accident~~

X● V47.6 Car passenger injured in collision with fixed or stationary object in traffic accident

~~V47.61 Passenger of sport utility vehicle injured in collision with fixed or stationary object in traffic accident~~

~~V47.62 Passenger of other type car injured in collision with fixed or stationary object in traffic accident~~

X● V47.7 Person on outside of car injured in collision with fixed or stationary object in traffic accident

X● V47.9 Unspecified car occupant injured in collision with fixed or stationary object in traffic accident

~~V47.91 Unspecified occupant of sport utility vehicle injured in collision with fixed or stationary object in traffic accident~~

~~V47.92 Unspecified occupant of other type car injured in collision with fixed or stationary object in traffic accident~~

CHAPTER 20 (V01-Y99)

● **V48 Car occupant injured in noncollision transport accident**

Includes overturning car NOS
overturning car without collision

The appropriate 7th character is to be added to each code from category V48

A	initial encounter
D	subsequent encounter
S	sequela

X● **V48.Ø Car driver injured in noncollision transport accident in nontraffic accident**

X● **V48.1 Car passenger injured in noncollision transport accident in nontraffic accident**

X● **V48.2 Person on outside of car injured in noncollision transport accident in nontraffic accident**

X● **V48.3 Unspecified car occupant injured in noncollision transport accident in nontraffic accident**

X● **V48.4 Person boarding or alighting a car injured in noncollision transport accident**

X● **V48.5 Car driver injured in noncollision transport accident in traffic accident**

X● **V48.6 Car passenger injured in noncollision transport accident in traffic accident**

X● **V48.7 Person on outside of car injured in noncollision transport accident in traffic accident**

X● **V48.9 Unspecified car occupant injured in noncollision transport accident in traffic accident**

● **V49 Car occupant injured in other and unspecified transport accidents**

The appropriate 7th character is to be added to each code from category V49

A	initial encounter
D	subsequent encounter
S	sequela

● **V49.Ø Driver injured in collision with other and unspecified motor vehicles in nontraffic accident**

X● **V49.ØØ Driver injured in collision with unspecified motor vehicles in nontraffic accident**

X● **V49.Ø9 Driver injured in collision with other motor vehicles in nontraffic accident**

● **V49.1 Passenger injured in collision with other and unspecified motor vehicles in nontraffic accident**

X● **V49.1Ø Passenger injured in collision with unspecified motor vehicles in nontraffic accident**

X● **V49.19 Passenger injured in collision with other motor vehicles in nontraffic accident**

● **V49.2 Unspecified car occupant injured in collision with other and unspecified motor vehicles in nontraffic accident**

X● **V49.2Ø Unspecified car occupant injured in collision with unspecified motor vehicles in nontraffic accident**
Car collision NOS, nontraffic

X● **V49.29 Unspecified car occupant injured in collision with other motor vehicles in nontraffic accident**

X● **V49.3 Car occupant (driver) (passenger) injured in unspecified nontraffic accident**
Car accident NOS, nontraffic
Car occupant injured in nontraffic accident NOS

● **V49.4 Driver injured in collision with other and unspecified motor vehicles in traffic accident**

X● **V49.4Ø Driver injured in collision with unspecified motor vehicles in traffic accident**

X● **V49.49 Driver injured in collision with other motor vehicles in traffic accident**

● **V49.5 Passenger injured in collision with other and unspecified motor vehicles in traffic accident**

X● **V49.5Ø Passenger injured in collision with unspecified motor vehicles in traffic accident**

X● **V49.59 Passenger injured in collision with other motor vehicles in traffic accident**

● **V49.6 Unspecified car occupant injured in collision with other and unspecified motor vehicles in traffic accident**

X● **V49.6Ø Unspecified car occupant injured in collision with unspecified motor vehicles in traffic accident**
Car collision NOS (traffic)

X● **V49.69 Unspecified car occupant injured in collision with other motor vehicles in traffic accident**

● **V49.8 Car occupant (driver) (passenger) injured in other specified transport accidents**

X● **V49.81 Car occupant (driver) (passenger) injured in transport accident with military vehicle**

X● **V49.88 Car occupant (driver) (passenger) injured in other specified transport accidents**

X● **V49.9 Car occupant (driver) (passenger) injured in unspecified traffic accident**
Car accident NOS

OCCUPANT OF PICK-UP TRUCK OR VAN INJURED IN TRANSPORT ACCIDENT (V5Ø-V59)

Includes a four- or six-wheel motor vehicle designed primarily for carrying passengers and property but weighing less than the local limit for classification as a heavy goods vehicle
minibus
minivan
sport utility vehicle (SUV)
truck
van

Excludes1 heavy transport vehicle (V6Ø-V69)

● **V5Ø Occupant of pick-up truck or van injured in collision with pedestrian or animal**

Excludes1 pick-up truck or van collision with animal-drawn vehicle or animal being ridden (V56.-)

The appropriate 7th character is to be added to each code from category V5Ø

A	initial encounter
D	subsequent encounter
S	sequela

X● **V5Ø.Ø Driver of pick-up truck or van injured in collision with pedestrian or animal in nontraffic accident**

X● **V5Ø.1 Passenger in pick-up truck or van injured in collision with pedestrian or animal in nontraffic accident**

X● **V5Ø.2 Person on outside of pick-up truck or van injured in collision with pedestrian or animal in nontraffic accident**

X● **V5Ø.3 Unspecified occupant of pick-up truck or van injured in collision with pedestrian or animal in nontraffic accident**

X● **V5Ø.4 Person boarding or alighting a pick-up truck or van injured in collision with pedestrian or animal**

X● **V5Ø.5 Driver of pick-up truck or van injured in collision with pedestrian or animal in traffic accident**

X● **V5Ø.6 Passenger in pick-up truck or van injured in collision with pedestrian or animal in traffic accident**

X● **V5Ø.7 Person on outside of pick-up truck or van injured in collision with pedestrian or animal in traffic accident**

X● **V5Ø.9 Unspecified occupant of pick-up truck or van injured in collision with pedestrian or animal in traffic accident**

CHAPTER 2Ø (VØ1-Y99)

● V51 Occupant of pick-up truck or van injured in collision with pedal cycle

The appropriate 7th character is to be added to each code from category V51

A	initial encounter
D	subsequent encounter
S	sequela

X● V51.0 Driver of pick-up truck or van injured in collision with pedal cycle in nontraffic accident

X● V51.1 Passenger in pick-up truck or van injured in collision with pedal cycle in nontraffic accident

X● V51.2 Person on outside of pick-up truck or van injured in collision with pedal cycle in nontraffic accident

X● V51.3 Unspecified occupant of pick-up truck or van injured in collision with pedal cycle in nontraffic accident

X● V51.4 Person boarding or alighting a pick-up truck or van injured in collision with pedal cycle

X● V51.5 Driver of pick-up truck or van injured in collision with pedal cycle in traffic accident

X● V51.6 Passenger in pick-up truck or van injured in collision with pedal cycle in traffic accident

X● V51.7 Person on outside of pick-up truck or van injured in collision with pedal cycle in traffic accident

X● V51.9 Unspecified occupant of pick-up truck or van injured in collision with pedal cycle in traffic accident

● V52 Occupant of pick-up truck or van injured in collision with two- or three-wheeled motor vehicle

The appropriate 7th character is to be added to each code from category V52

A	initial encounter
D	subsequent encounter
S	sequela

X● V52.0 Driver of pick-up truck or van injured in collision with two- or three-wheeled motor vehicle in nontraffic accident

X● V52.1 Passenger in pick-up truck or van injured in collision with two- or three-wheeled motor vehicle in nontraffic accident

X● V52.2 Person on outside of pick-up truck or van injured in collision with two- or three-wheeled motor vehicle in nontraffic accident

X● V52.3 Unspecified occupant of pick-up truck or van injured in collision with two- or three-wheeled motor vehicle in nontraffic accident

X● V52.4 Person boarding or alighting a pick-up truck or van injured in collision with two- or three-wheeled motor vehicle

X● V52.5 Driver of pick-up truck or van injured in collision with two- or three-wheeled motor vehicle in traffic accident

X● V52.6 Passenger in pick-up truck or van injured in collision with two- or three-wheeled motor vehicle in traffic accident

X● V52.7 Person on outside of pick-up truck or van injured in collision with two- or three-wheeled motor vehicle in traffic accident

X● V52.9 Unspecified occupant of pick-up truck or van injured in collision with two- or three-wheeled motor vehicle in traffic accident

● V53 Occupant of pick-up truck or van injured in collision with car, pick-up truck or van

The appropriate 7th character is to be added to each code from category V53

A	initial encounter
D	subsequent encounter
S	sequela

X● V53.0 Driver of pick-up truck or van injured in collision with car, pick-up truck or van in nontraffic accident

X● V53.1 Passenger in pick-up truck or van injured in collision with car, pick-up truck or van in nontraffic accident

X● V53.2 Person on outside of pick-up truck or van injured in collision with car, pick-up truck or van in nontraffic accident

X● V53.3 Unspecified occupant of pick-up truck or van injured in collision with car, pick-up truck or van in nontraffic accident

X● V53.4 Person boarding or alighting a pick-up truck or van injured in collision with car, pick-up truck or van

X● V53.5 Driver of pick-up truck or van injured in collision with car, pick-up truck or van in traffic accident

X● V53.6 Passenger in pick-up truck or van injured in collision with car, pick-up truck or van in traffic accident

X● V53.7 Person on outside of pick-up truck or van injured in collision with car, pick-up truck or van in traffic accident

X● V53.9 Unspecified occupant of pick-up truck or van injured in collision with car, pick-up truck or van in traffic accident

● V54 Occupant of pick-up truck or van injured in collision with heavy transport vehicle or bus

Excludes1 occupant of pick-up truck or van injured in collision with military vehicle (V59.81)

The appropriate 7th character is to be added to each code from category V54

A	initial encounter
D	subsequent encounter
S	sequela

X● V54.0 Driver of pick-up truck or van injured in collision with heavy transport vehicle or bus in nontraffic accident

X● V54.1 Passenger in pick-up truck or van injured in collision with heavy transport vehicle or bus in nontraffic accident

X● V54.2 Person on outside of pick-up truck or van injured in collision with heavy transport vehicle or bus in nontraffic accident

X● V54.3 Unspecified occupant of pick-up truck or van injured in collision with heavy transport vehicle or bus in nontraffic accident

X● V54.4 Person boarding or alighting a pick-up truck or van injured in collision with heavy transport vehicle or bus

X● V54.5 Driver of pick-up truck or van injured in collision with heavy transport vehicle or bus in traffic accident

X● V54.6 Passenger in pick-up truck or van injured in collision with heavy transport vehicle or bus in traffic accident

X● V54.7 Person on outside of pick-up truck or van injured in collision with heavy transport vehicle or bus in traffic accident

X● V54.9 Unspecified occupant of pick-up truck or van injured in collision with heavy transport vehicle or bus in traffic accident

● V55 Occupant of pick-up truck or van injured in collision with railway train or railway vehicle

The appropriate 7th character is to be added to each code from category V55

A	initial encounter
D	subsequent encounter
S	sequela

X● **V55.0** **Driver of pick-up truck or van injured in collision with railway train or railway vehicle in nontraffic accident**

X● **V55.1** **Passenger in pick-up truck or van injured in collision with railway train or railway vehicle in nontraffic accident**

X● **V55.2** **Person on outside of pick-up truck or van injured in collision with railway train or railway vehicle in nontraffic accident**

X● **V55.3** **Unspecified occupant of pick-up truck or van injured in collision with railway train or railway vehicle in nontraffic accident**

X● **V55.4** **Person boarding or alighting a pick-up truck or van injured in collision with railway train or railway vehicle**

X● **V55.5** **Driver of pick-up truck or van injured in collision with railway train or railway vehicle in traffic accident**

X● **V55.6** **Passenger in pick-up truck or van injured in collision with railway train or railway vehicle in traffic accident**

X● **V55.7** **Person on outside of pick-up truck or van injured in collision with railway train or railway vehicle in traffic accident**

X● **V55.9** **Unspecified occupant of pick-up truck or van injured in collision with railway train or railway vehicle in traffic accident**

● V56 Occupant of pick-up truck or van injured in collision with other nonmotor vehicle

Includes collision with animal-drawn vehicle, animal being ridden, streetcar

The appropriate 7th character is to be added to each code from category V56

A	initial encounter
D	subsequent encounter
S	sequela

X● **V56.0** **Driver of pick-up truck or van injured in collision with other nonmotor vehicle in nontraffic accident**

X● **V56.1** **Passenger in pick-up truck or van injured in collision with other nonmotor vehicle in nontraffic accident**

X● **V56.2** **Person on outside of pick-up truck or van injured in collision with other nonmotor vehicle in nontraffic accident**

X● **V56.3** **Unspecified occupant of pick-up truck or van injured in collision with other nonmotor vehicle in nontraffic accident**

X● **V56.4** **Person boarding or alighting a pick-up truck or van injured in collision with other nonmotor vehicle**

X● **V56.5** **Driver of pick-up truck or van injured in collision with other nonmotor vehicle in traffic accident**

X● **V56.6** **Passenger in pick-up truck or van injured in collision with other nonmotor vehicle in traffic accident**

X● **V56.7** **Person on outside of pick-up truck or van injured in collision with other nonmotor vehicle in traffic accident**

X● **V56.9** **Unspecified occupant of pick-up truck or van injured in collision with other nonmotor vehicle in traffic accident**

● V57 Occupant of pick-up truck or van injured in collision with fixed or stationary object

The appropriate 7th character is to be added to each code from category V57

A	initial encounter
D	subsequent encounter
S	sequela

X● **V57.0** **Driver of pick-up truck or van injured in collision with fixed or stationary object in nontraffic accident**

X● **V57.1** **Passenger in pick-up truck or van injured in collision with fixed or stationary object in nontraffic accident**

X● **V57.2** **Person on outside of pick-up truck or van injured in collision with fixed or stationary object in nontraffic accident**

X● **V57.3** **Unspecified occupant of pick-up truck or van injured in collision with fixed or stationary object in nontraffic accident**

X● **V57.4** **Person boarding or alighting a pick-up truck or van injured in collision with fixed or stationary object**

X● **V57.5** **Driver of pick-up truck or van injured in collision with fixed or stationary object in traffic accident**

X● **V57.6** **Passenger in pick-up truck or van injured in collision with fixed or stationary object in traffic accident**

X● **V57.7** **Person on outside of pick-up truck or van injured in collision with fixed or stationary object in traffic accident**

X● **V57.9** **Unspecified occupant of pick-up truck or van injured in collision with fixed or stationary object in traffic accident**

● V58 Occupant of pick-up truck or van injured in noncollision transport accident

Includes overturning pick-up truck or van NOS
overturning pick-up truck or van without collision

The appropriate 7th character is to be added to each code from category V58

A	initial encounter
D	subsequent encounter
S	sequela

X● **V58.0** **Driver of pick-up truck or van injured in noncollision transport accident in nontraffic accident**

X● **V58.1** **Passenger in pick-up truck or van injured in noncollision transport accident in nontraffic accident**

X● **V58.2** **Person on outside of pick-up truck or van injured in noncollision transport accident in nontraffic accident**

X● **V58.3** **Unspecified occupant of pick-up truck or van injured in noncollision transport accident in nontraffic accident**

X● **V58.4** **Person boarding or alighting a pick-up truck or van injured in noncollision transport accident**

X● **V58.5** **Driver of pick-up truck or van injured in noncollision transport accident in traffic accident**

X● **V58.6** **Passenger in pick-up truck or van injured in noncollision transport accident in traffic accident**

X● **V58.7** **Person on outside of pick-up truck or van injured in noncollision transport accident in traffic accident**

X● **V58.9** **Unspecified occupant of pick-up truck or van injured in noncollision transport accident in traffic accident**

● **V59 Occupant of pick-up truck or van injured in other and unspecified transport accidents**

The appropriate 7th character is to be added to each code from category V59

A	initial encounter
D	subsequent encounter
S	sequela

● **V59.0 Driver of pick-up truck or van injured in collision with other and unspecified motor vehicles in nontraffic accident**

X● **V59.00 Driver of pick-up truck or van injured in collision with unspecified motor vehicles in nontraffic accident**

X● **V59.09 Driver of pick-up truck or van injured in collision with other motor vehicles in nontraffic accident**

● **V59.1 Passenger in pick-up truck or van injured in collision with other and unspecified motor vehicles in nontraffic accident**

X● **V59.10 Passenger in pick-up truck or van injured in collision with unspecified motor vehicles in nontraffic accident**

X● **V59.19 Passenger in pick-up truck or van injured in collision with other motor vehicles in nontraffic accident**

● **V59.2 Unspecified occupant of pick-up truck or van injured in collision with other and unspecified motor vehicles in nontraffic accident**

X● **V59.20 Unspecified occupant of pick-up truck or van injured in collision with unspecified motor vehicles in nontraffic accident**

Collision NOS involving pick-up truck or van, nontraffic

X● **V59.29 Unspecified occupant of pick-up truck or van injured in collision with other motor vehicles in nontraffic accident**

X● **V59.3 Occupant (driver) (passenger) of pick-up truck or van injured in unspecified nontraffic accident**

Accident NOS involving pick-up truck or van, nontraffic

Occupant of pick-up truck or van injured in nontraffic accident NOS

● **V59.4 Driver of pick-up truck or van injured in collision with other and unspecified motor vehicles in traffic accident**

X● **V59.40 Driver of pick-up truck or van injured in collision with unspecified motor vehicles in traffic accident**

X● **V59.49 Driver of pick-up truck or van injured in collision with other motor vehicles in traffic accident**

● **V59.5 Passenger in pick-up truck or van injured in collision with other and unspecified motor vehicles in traffic accident**

X● **V59.50 Passenger in pick-up truck or van injured in collision with unspecified motor vehicles in traffic accident**

X● **V59.59 Passenger in pick-up truck or van injured in collision with other motor vehicles in traffic accident**

● **V59.6 Unspecified occupant of pick-up truck or van injured in collision with other and unspecified motor vehicles in traffic accident**

X● **V59.60 Unspecified occupant of pick-up truck or van injured in collision with unspecified motor vehicles in traffic accident**

Collision NOS involving pick-up truck or van (traffic)

X● **V59.69 Unspecified occupant of pick-up truck or van injured in collision with other motor vehicles in traffic accident**

● **V59.8 Occupant (driver) (passenger) of pick-up truck or van injured in other specified transport accidents**

X● **V59.81 Occupant (driver) (passenger) of pick-up truck or van injured in transport accident with military vehicle**

X● **V59.88 Occupant (driver) (passenger) of pick-up truck or van injured in other specified transport accidents**

X● **V59.9 Occupant (driver) (passenger) of pick-up truck or van injured in unspecified traffic accident**

Accident NOS involving pick-up truck or van

OCCUPANT OF HEAVY TRANSPORT VEHICLE INJURED IN TRANSPORT ACCIDENT (V60-V69)

Includes 18 wheeler
armored car
panel truck

Excludes1 bus
motorcoach

● **V60 Occupant of heavy transport vehicle injured in collision with pedestrian or animal**

Excludes1 heavy transport vehicle collision with animal-drawn vehicle or animal being ridden (V66.-)

The appropriate 7th character is to be added to each code from category V60

A	initial encounter
D	subsequent encounter
S	sequela

X● **V60.0 Driver of heavy transport vehicle injured in collision with pedestrian or animal in nontraffic accident**

X● **V60.1 Passenger in heavy transport vehicle injured in collision with pedestrian or animal in nontraffic accident**

X● **V60.2 Person on outside of heavy transport vehicle injured in collision with pedestrian or animal in nontraffic accident**

X● **V60.3 Unspecified occupant of heavy transport vehicle injured in collision with pedestrian or animal in nontraffic accident**

X● **V60.4 Person boarding or alighting a heavy transport vehicle injured in collision with pedestrian or animal**

X● **V60.5 Driver of heavy transport vehicle injured in collision with pedestrian or animal in traffic accident**

X● **V60.6 Passenger in heavy transport vehicle injured in collision with pedestrian or animal in traffic accident**

X● **V60.7 Person on outside of heavy transport vehicle injured in collision with pedestrian or animal in traffic accident**

X● **V60.9 Unspecified occupant of heavy transport vehicle injured in collision with pedestrian or animal in traffic accident**

● **V61 Occupant of heavy transport vehicle injured in collision with pedal cycle**

The appropriate 7th character is to be added to each code from category V61

A	initial encounter
D	subsequent encounter
S	sequela

X● **V61.0 Driver of heavy transport vehicle injured in collision with pedal cycle in nontraffic accident**

X● **V61.1 Passenger in heavy transport vehicle injured in collision with pedal cycle in nontraffic accident**

X● **V61.2 Person on outside of heavy transport vehicle injured in collision with pedal cycle in nontraffic accident**

X● **V61.3 Unspecified occupant of heavy transport vehicle injured in collision with pedal cycle in nontraffic accident**

X● **V61.4 Person boarding or alighting a heavy transport vehicle injured in collision with pedal cycle while boarding or alighting**

X● **V61.5 Driver of heavy transport vehicle injured in collision with pedal cycle in traffic accident**

X● V61.6 **Passenger in heavy transport vehicle injured in collision with pedal cycle in traffic accident**

X● V61.7 **Person on outside of heavy transport vehicle injured in collision with pedal cycle in traffic accident**

X● V61.9 **Unspecified occupant of heavy transport vehicle injured in collision with pedal cycle in traffic accident**

● **V62 Occupant of heavy transport vehicle injured in collision with two- or three-wheeled motor vehicle**

The appropriate 7th character is to be added to each code from category V62

A	initial encounter
D	subsequent encounter
S	sequela

X● V62.0 **Driver of heavy transport vehicle injured in collision with two- or three-wheeled motor vehicle in nontraffic accident**

X● V62.1 **Passenger in heavy transport vehicle injured in collision with two- or three-wheeled motor vehicle in nontraffic accident**

X● V62.2 **Person on outside of heavy transport vehicle injured in collision with two- or three-wheeled motor vehicle in nontraffic accident**

X● V62.3 **Unspecified occupant of heavy transport vehicle injured in collision with two- or three-wheeled motor vehicle in nontraffic accident**

X● V62.4 **Person boarding or alighting a heavy transport vehicle injured in collision with two- or three-wheeled motor vehicle**

X● V62.5 **Driver of heavy transport vehicle injured in collision with two- or three-wheeled motor vehicle in traffic accident**

X● V62.6 **Passenger in heavy transport vehicle injured in collision with two- or three-wheeled motor vehicle in traffic accident**

X● V62.7 **Person on outside of heavy transport vehicle injured in collision with two- or three-wheeled motor vehicle in traffic accident**

X● V62.9 **Unspecified occupant of heavy transport vehicle injured in collision with two- or three-wheeled motor vehicle in traffic accident**

● **V63 Occupant of heavy transport vehicle injured in collision with car, pick-up truck or van**

The appropriate 7th character is to be added to each code from category V63

A	initial encounter
D	subsequent encounter
S	sequela

X● V63.0 **Driver of heavy transport vehicle injured in collision with car, pick-up truck or van in nontraffic accident**

X● V63.1 **Passenger in heavy transport vehicle injured in collision with car, pick-up truck or van in nontraffic accident**

X● V63.2 **Person on outside of heavy transport vehicle injured in collision with car, pick-up truck or van in nontraffic accident**

X● V63.3 **Unspecified occupant of heavy transport vehicle injured in collision with car, pick-up truck or van in nontraffic accident**

X● V63.4 **Person boarding or alighting a heavy transport vehicle injured in collision with car, pick-up truck or van**

X● V63.5 **Driver of heavy transport vehicle injured in collision with car, pick-up truck or van in traffic accident**

X● V63.6 **Passenger in heavy transport vehicle injured in collision with car, pick-up truck or van in traffic accident**

X● V63.7 **Person on outside of heavy transport vehicle injured in collision with car, pick-up truck or van in traffic accident**

X● V63.9 **Unspecified occupant of heavy transport vehicle injured in collision with car, pick-up truck or van in traffic accident**

● **V64 Occupant of heavy transport vehicle injured in collision with heavy transport vehicle or bus**

Excludes1 occupant of heavy transport vehicle injured in collision with military vehicle (V69.81)

The appropriate 7th character is to be added to each code from category V64

A	initial encounter
D	subsequent encounter
S	sequela

X● V64.0 **Driver of heavy transport vehicle injured in collision with heavy transport vehicle or bus in nontraffic accident**

X● V64.1 **Passenger in heavy transport vehicle injured in collision with heavy transport vehicle or bus in nontraffic accident**

X● V64.2 **Person on outside of heavy transport vehicle injured in collision with heavy transport vehicle or bus in nontraffic accident**

X● V64.3 **Unspecified occupant of heavy transport vehicle injured in collision with heavy transport vehicle or bus in nontraffic accident**

X● V64.4 **Person boarding or alighting a heavy transport vehicle injured in collision with heavy transport vehicle or bus while boarding or alighting**

X● V64.5 **Driver of heavy transport vehicle injured in collision with heavy transport vehicle or bus in traffic accident**

X● V64.6 **Passenger in heavy transport vehicle injured in collision with heavy transport vehicle or bus in traffic accident**

X● V64.7 **Person on outside of heavy transport vehicle injured in collision with heavy transport vehicle or bus in traffic accident**

X● V64.9 **Unspecified occupant of heavy transport vehicle injured in collision with heavy transport vehicle or bus in traffic accident**

● **V65 Occupant of heavy transport vehicle injured in collision with railway train or railway vehicle**

The appropriate 7th character is to be added to each code from category V65

A	initial encounter
D	subsequent encounter
S	sequela

X● V65.0 **Driver of heavy transport vehicle injured in collision with railway train or railway vehicle in nontraffic accident**

X● V65.1 **Passenger in heavy transport vehicle injured in collision with railway train or railway vehicle in nontraffic accident**

X● V65.2 **Person on outside of heavy transport vehicle injured in collision with railway train or railway vehicle in nontraffic accident**

X● V65.3 **Unspecified occupant of heavy transport vehicle injured in collision with railway train or railway vehicle in nontraffic accident**

X● V65.4 **Person boarding or alighting a heavy transport vehicle injured in collision with railway train or railway vehicle**

X● V65.5 **Driver of heavy transport vehicle injured in collision with railway train or railway vehicle in traffic accident**

X● V65.6 **Passenger in heavy transport vehicle injured in collision with railway train or railway vehicle in traffic accident**

X● V65.7 **Person on outside of heavy transport vehicle injured in collision with railway train or railway vehicle in traffic accident**

X● V65.9 **Unspecified occupant of heavy transport vehicle injured in collision with railway train or railway vehicle in traffic accident**

● **V66 Occupant of heavy transport vehicle injured in collision with other nonmotor vehicle**

Includes collision with animal-drawn vehicle, animal being ridden, streetcar

The appropriate 7th character is to be added to each code from category V66

A	initial encounter
D	subsequent encounter
S	sequela

X● **V66.0 Driver of heavy transport vehicle injured in collision with other nonmotor vehicle in nontraffic accident**

X● **V66.1 Passenger in heavy transport vehicle injured in collision with other nonmotor vehicle in nontraffic accident**

X● **V66.2 Person on outside of heavy transport vehicle injured in collision with other nonmotor vehicle in nontraffic accident**

X● **V66.3 Unspecified occupant of heavy transport vehicle injured in collision with other nonmotor vehicle in nontraffic accident**

X● **V66.4 Person boarding or alighting a heavy transport vehicle injured in collision with other nonmotor vehicle**

X● **V66.5 Driver of heavy transport vehicle injured in collision with other nonmotor vehicle in traffic accident**

X● **V66.6 Passenger in heavy transport vehicle injured in collision with other nonmotor vehicle in traffic accident**

X● **V66.7 Person on outside of heavy transport vehicle injured in collision with other nonmotor vehicle in traffic accident**

X● **V66.9 Unspecified occupant of heavy transport vehicle injured in collision with other nonmotor vehicle in traffic accident**

● **V67 Occupant of heavy transport vehicle injured in collision with fixed or stationary object**

The appropriate 7th character is to be added to each code from category V67

A	initial encounter
D	subsequent encounter
S	sequela

X● **V67.0 Driver of heavy transport vehicle injured in collision with fixed or stationary object in nontraffic accident**

X● **V67.1 Passenger in heavy transport vehicle injured in collision with fixed or stationary object in nontraffic accident**

X● **V67.2 Person on outside of heavy transport vehicle injured in collision with fixed or stationary object in nontraffic accident**

X● **V67.3 Unspecified occupant of heavy transport vehicle injured in collision with fixed or stationary object in nontraffic accident**

X● **V67.4 Person boarding or alighting a heavy transport vehicle injured in collision with fixed or stationary object**

X● **V67.5 Driver of heavy transport vehicle injured in collision with fixed or stationary object in traffic accident**

X● **V67.6 Passenger in heavy transport vehicle injured in collision with fixed or stationary object in traffic accident**

X● **V67.7 Person on outside of heavy transport vehicle injured in collision with fixed or stationary object in traffic accident**

X● **V67.9 Unspecified occupant of heavy transport vehicle injured in collision with fixed or stationary object in traffic accident**

● **V68 Occupant of heavy transport vehicle injured in noncollision transport accident**

Includes overturning heavy transport vehicle NOS
overturning heavy transport vehicle without collision

The appropriate 7th character is to be added to each code from category V68

A	initial encounter
D	subsequent encounter
S	sequela

X● **V68.0 Driver of heavy transport vehicle injured in noncollision transport accident in nontraffic accident**

X● **V68.1 Passenger in heavy transport vehicle injured in noncollision transport accident in nontraffic accident**

X● **V68.2 Person on outside of heavy transport vehicle injured in noncollision transport accident in nontraffic accident**

X● **V68.3 Unspecified occupant of heavy transport vehicle injured in noncollision transport accident in nontraffic accident**

X● **V68.4 Person boarding or alighting a heavy transport vehicle injured in noncollision transport accident**

X● **V68.5 Driver of heavy transport vehicle injured in noncollision transport accident in traffic accident**

X● **V68.6 Passenger in heavy transport vehicle injured in noncollision transport accident in traffic accident**

X● **V68.7 Person on outside of heavy transport vehicle injured in noncollision transport accident in traffic accident**

X● **V68.9 Unspecified occupant of heavy transport vehicle injured in noncollision transport accident in traffic accident**

● **V69 Occupant of heavy transport vehicle injured in other and unspecified transport accidents**

The appropriate 7th character is to be added to each code from category V69

A	initial encounter
D	subsequent encounter
S	sequela

● **V69.0 Driver of heavy transport vehicle injured in collision with other and unspecified motor vehicles in nontraffic accident**

X● **V69.00 Driver of heavy transport vehicle injured in collision with unspecified motor vehicles in nontraffic accident**

X● **V69.09 Driver of heavy transport vehicle injured in collision with other motor vehicles in nontraffic accident**

● **V69.1 Passenger in heavy transport vehicle injured in collision with other and unspecified motor vehicles in nontraffic accident**

X● **V69.10 Passenger in heavy transport vehicle injured in collision with unspecified motor vehicles in nontraffic accident**

X● **V69.19 Passenger in heavy transport vehicle injured in collision with other motor vehicles in nontraffic accident**

● **V69.2 Unspecified occupant of heavy transport vehicle injured in collision with other and unspecified motor vehicles in nontraffic accident**

X● **V69.20 Unspecified occupant of heavy transport vehicle injured in collision with unspecified motor vehicles in nontraffic accident**

Collision NOS involving heavy transport vehicle, nontraffic

X● **V69.29 Unspecified occupant of heavy transport vehicle injured in collision with other motor vehicles in nontraffic accident**

CHAPTER 20 (V01-Y99)

X● V69.3 **Occupant (driver) (passenger) of heavy transport vehicle injured in unspecified nontraffic accident**
Accident NOS involving heavy transport vehicle, nontraffic
Occupant of heavy transport vehicle injured in nontraffic accident NOS

● V69.4 **Driver of heavy transport vehicle injured in collision with other and unspecified motor vehicles in traffic accident**

X● V69.40 **Driver of heavy transport vehicle injured in collision with unspecified motor vehicles in traffic accident**

X● V69.49 **Driver of heavy transport vehicle injured in collision with other motor vehicles in traffic accident**

● V69.5 **Passenger in heavy transport vehicle injured in collision with other and unspecified motor vehicles in traffic accident**

X● V69.50 **Passenger in heavy transport vehicle injured in collision with unspecified motor vehicles in traffic accident**

X● V69.59 **Passenger in heavy transport vehicle injured in collision with other motor vehicles in traffic accident**

● V69.6 **Unspecified occupant of heavy transport vehicle injured in collision with other and unspecified motor vehicles in traffic accident**

X● V69.60 **Unspecified occupant of heavy transport vehicle injured in collision with unspecified motor vehicles in traffic accident**
Collision NOS involving heavy transport vehicle (traffic)

X● V69.69 **Unspecified occupant of heavy transport vehicle injured in collision with other motor vehicles in traffic accident**

● V69.8 **Occupant (driver) (passenger) of heavy transport vehicle injured in other specified transport accidents**

X● V69.81 **Occupant (driver) (passenger) of heavy transport vehicle injured in transport accidents with military vehicle**

X● V69.88 **Occupant (driver) (passenger) of heavy transport vehicle injured in other specified transport accidents**

X● V69.9 **Occupant (driver) (passenger) of heavy transport vehicle injured in unspecified traffic accident**
Accident NOS involving heavy transport vehicle

BUS OCCUPANT INJURED IN TRANSPORT ACCIDENT (V70-V79)

Includes motorcoach
Excludes1 minibus (V50-V59)

● V70 **Bus occupant injured in collision with pedestrian or animal**
Excludes1 bus collision with animal-drawn vehicle or animal being ridden (V76.-)

The appropriate 7th character is to be added to each code from category V70

A	initial encounter
D	subsequent encounter
S	sequela

X● V70.0 **Driver of bus injured in collision with pedestrian or animal in nontraffic accident**

X● V70.1 **Passenger on bus injured in collision with pedestrian or animal in nontraffic accident**

X● V70.2 **Person on outside of bus injured in collision with pedestrian or animal in nontraffic accident**

X● V70.3 **Unspecified occupant of bus injured in collision with pedestrian or animal in nontraffic accident**

X● V70.4 **Person boarding or alighting from bus injured in collision with pedestrian or animal**

X● V70.5 **Driver of bus injured in collision with pedestrian or animal in traffic accident**

X● V70.6 **Passenger on bus injured in collision with pedestrian or animal in traffic accident**

X● V70.7 **Person on outside of bus injured in collision with pedestrian or animal in traffic accident**

X● V70.9 **Unspecified occupant of bus injured in collision with pedestrian or animal in traffic accident**

● V71 **Bus occupant injured in collision with pedal cycle**

The appropriate 7th character is to be added to each code from category V71

A	initial encounter
D	subsequent encounter
S	sequela

X● V71.0 **Driver of bus injured in collision with pedal cycle in nontraffic accident**

X● V71.1 **Passenger on bus injured in collision with pedal cycle in nontraffic accident**

X● V71.2 **Person on outside of bus injured in collision with pedal cycle in nontraffic accident**

X● V71.3 **Unspecified occupant of bus injured in collision with pedal cycle in nontraffic accident**

X● V71.4 **Person boarding or alighting from bus injured in collision with pedal cycle**

X● V71.5 **Driver of bus injured in collision with pedal cycle in traffic accident**

X● V71.6 **Passenger on bus injured in collision with pedal cycle in traffic accident**

X● V71.7 **Person on outside of bus injured in collision with pedal cycle in traffic accident**

X● V71.9 **Unspecified occupant of bus injured in collision with pedal cycle in traffic accident**

● V72 **Bus occupant injured in collision with two- or three-wheeled motor vehicle**

The appropriate 7th character is to be added to each code from category V72

A	initial encounter
D	subsequent encounter
S	sequela

X● V72.0 **Driver of bus injured in collision with two- or three-wheeled motor vehicle in nontraffic accident**

X● V72.1 **Passenger on bus injured in collision with two- or three-wheeled motor vehicle in nontraffic accident**

X● V72.2 **Person on outside of bus injured in collision with two- or three-wheeled motor vehicle in nontraffic accident**

X● V72.3 **Unspecified occupant of bus injured in collision with two- or three-wheeled motor vehicle in nontraffic accident**

X● V72.4 **Person boarding or alighting from bus injured in collision with two- or three-wheeled motor vehicle**

X● V72.5 **Driver of bus injured in collision with two- or three-wheeled motor vehicle in traffic accident**

X● V72.6 **Passenger on bus injured in collision with two- or three-wheeled motor vehicle in traffic accident**

X● V72.7 **Person on outside of bus injured in collision with two- or three-wheeled motor vehicle in traffic accident**

X● V72.9 **Unspecified occupant of bus injured in collision with two- or three-wheeled motor vehicle in traffic accident**

● **V73 Bus occupant injured in collision with car, pick-up truck or van**

The appropriate 7th character is to be added to each code from category V73

A initial encounter
D subsequent encounter
S sequela

X● **V73.0** Driver of bus injured in collision with car, pick-up truck or van in nontraffic accident

X● **V73.1** Passenger on bus injured in collision with car, pick-up truck or van in nontraffic accident

X● **V73.2** Person on outside of bus injured in collision with car, pick-up truck or van in nontraffic accident

X● **V73.3** Unspecified occupant of bus injured in collision with car, pick-up truck or van in nontraffic accident

X● **V73.4** Person boarding or alighting from bus injured in collision with car, pick-up truck or van

X● **V73.5** Driver of bus injured in collision with car, pick-up truck or van in traffic accident

X● **V73.6** Passenger on bus injured in collision with car, pick-up truck or van in traffic accident

X● **V73.7** Person on outside of bus injured in collision with car, pick-up truck or van in traffic accident

X● **V73.9** Unspecified occupant of bus injured in collision with car, pick-up truck or van in traffic accident

● **V74 Bus occupant injured in collision with heavy transport vehicle or bus**

Excludes1 bus occupant injured in collision with military vehicle (V79.81)

The appropriate 7th character is to be added to each code from category V74

A initial encounter
D subsequent encounter
S sequela

X● **V74.0** Driver of bus injured in collision with heavy transport vehicle or bus in nontraffic accident

X● **V74.1** Passenger on bus injured in collision with heavy transport vehicle or bus in nontraffic accident

X● **V74.2** Person on outside of bus injured in collision with heavy transport vehicle or bus in nontraffic accident

X● **V74.3** Unspecified occupant of bus injured in collision with heavy transport vehicle or bus in nontraffic accident

X● **V74.4** Person boarding or alighting from bus injured in collision with heavy transport vehicle or bus

X● **V74.5** Driver of bus injured in collision with heavy transport vehicle or bus in traffic accident

X● **V74.6** Passenger on bus injured in collision with heavy transport vehicle or bus in traffic accident

X● **V74.7** Person on outside of bus injured in collision with heavy transport vehicle or bus in traffic accident

X● **V74.9** Unspecified occupant of bus injured in collision with heavy transport vehicle or bus in traffic accident

● **V75 Bus occupant injured in collision with railway train or railway vehicle**

The appropriate 7th character is to be added to each code from category V75

A initial encounter
D subsequent encounter
S sequela

X● **V75.0** Driver of bus injured in collision with railway train or railway vehicle in nontraffic accident

X● **V75.1** Passenger on bus injured in collision with railway train or railway vehicle in nontraffic accident

X● **V75.2** Person on outside of bus injured in collision with railway train or railway vehicle in nontraffic accident

X● **V75.3** Unspecified occupant of bus injured in collision with railway train or railway vehicle in nontraffic accident

X● **V75.4** Person boarding or alighting from bus injured in collision with railway train or railway vehicle

X● **V75.5** Driver of bus injured in collision with railway train or railway vehicle in traffic accident

X● **V75.6** Passenger on bus injured in collision with railway train or railway vehicle in traffic accident

X● **V75.7** Person on outside of bus injured in collision with railway train or railway vehicle in traffic accident

X● **V75.9** Unspecified occupant of bus injured in collision with railway train or railway vehicle in traffic accident

● **V76 Bus occupant injured in collision with other nonmotor vehicle**

Includes collision with animal-drawn vehicle, animal being ridden, streetcar

The appropriate 7th character is to be added to each code from category V76

A initial encounter
D subsequent encounter
S sequela

X● **V76.0** Driver of bus injured in collision with other nonmotor vehicle in nontraffic accident

X● **V76.1** Passenger on bus injured in collision with other nonmotor vehicle in nontraffic accident

X● **V76.2** Person on outside of bus injured in collision with other nonmotor vehicle in nontraffic accident

X● **V76.3** Unspecified occupant of bus injured in collision with other nonmotor vehicle in nontraffic accident

X● **V76.4** Person boarding or alighting from bus injured in collision with other nonmotor vehicle

X● **V76.5** Driver of bus injured in collision with other nonmotor vehicle in traffic accident

X● **V76.6** Passenger on bus injured in collision with other nonmotor vehicle in traffic accident

X● **V76.7** Person on outside of bus injured in collision with other nonmotor vehicle in traffic accident

X● **V76.9** Unspecified occupant of bus injured in collision with other nonmotor vehicle in traffic accident

● **V77 Bus occupant injured in collision with fixed or stationary object**

The appropriate 7th character is to be added to each code from category V77

A initial encounter
D subsequent encounter
S sequela

X● **V77.0** Driver of bus injured in collision with fixed or stationary object in nontraffic accident

X● **V77.1** Passenger on bus injured in collision with fixed or stationary object in nontraffic accident

X● **V77.2** Person on outside of bus injured in collision with fixed or stationary object in nontraffic accident

X● **V77.3** Unspecified occupant of bus injured in collision with fixed or stationary object in nontraffic accident

X● **V77.4** Person boarding or alighting from bus injured in collision with fixed or stationary object

X● **V77.5** Driver of bus injured in collision with fixed or stationary object in traffic accident

X● **V77.6** Passenger on bus injured in collision with fixed or stationary object in traffic accident

X● **V77.7** Person on outside of bus injured in collision with fixed or stationary object in traffic accident

X● **V77.9** Unspecified occupant of bus injured in collision with fixed or stationary object in traffic accident

● V78 **Bus occupant injured in noncollision transport accident**
Includes overturning bus NOS
overturning bus without collision
The appropriate 7th character is to be added to each code from category V78
A initial encounter
D subsequent encounter
S sequela

X● V78.0 **Driver of bus injured in noncollision transport accident in nontraffic accident**
X● V78.1 **Passenger on bus injured in noncollision transport accident in nontraffic accident**
X● V78.2 **Person on outside of bus injured in noncollision transport accident in nontraffic accident**
X● V78.3 **Unspecified occupant of bus injured in noncollision transport accident in nontraffic accident**
X● V78.4 **Person boarding or alighting from bus injured in noncollision transport accident**
X● V78.5 **Driver of bus injured in noncollision transport accident in traffic accident**
X● V78.6 **Passenger on bus injured in noncollision transport accident in traffic accident**
X● V78.7 **Person on outside of bus injured in noncollision transport accident in traffic accident**
X● V78.9 **Unspecified occupant of bus injured in noncollision transport accident in traffic accident**

● V79 **Bus occupant injured in other and unspecified transport accidents**
The appropriate 7th character is to be added to each code from category V79
A initial encounter
D subsequent encounter
S sequela

● V79.0 **Driver of bus injured in collision with other and unspecified motor vehicles in nontraffic accident**
X● V79.00 **Driver of bus injured in collision with unspecified motor vehicles in nontraffic accident**
X● V79.09 **Driver of bus injured in collision with other motor vehicles in nontraffic accident**
● V79.1 **Passenger on bus injured in collision with other and unspecified motor vehicles in nontraffic accident**
X● V79.10 **Passenger on bus injured in collision with unspecified motor vehicles in nontraffic accident**
X● V79.19 **Passenger on bus injured in collision with other motor vehicles in nontraffic accident**
● V79.2 **Unspecified bus occupant injured in collision with other and unspecified motor vehicles in nontraffic accident**
X● V79.20 **Unspecified bus occupant injured in collision with unspecified motor vehicles in nontraffic accident**
Bus collision NOS, nontraffic
X● V79.29 **Unspecified bus occupant injured in collision with other motor vehicles in nontraffic accident**
X● V79.3 **Bus occupant (driver) (passenger) injured in unspecified nontraffic accident**
Bus accident NOS, nontraffic
Bus occupant injured in nontraffic accident NOS
● V79.4 **Driver of bus injured in collision with other and unspecified motor vehicles in traffic accident**
X● V79.40 **Driver of bus injured in collision with unspecified motor vehicles in traffic accident**
X● V79.49 **Driver of bus injured in collision with other motor vehicles in traffic accident**
● V79.5 **Passenger on bus injured in collision with other and unspecified motor vehicles in traffic accident**
X● V79.50 **Passenger on bus injured in collision with unspecified motor vehicles in traffic accident**
X● V79.59 **Passenger on bus injured in collision with other motor vehicles in traffic accident**
● V79.6 **Unspecified bus occupant injured in collision with other and unspecified motor vehicles in traffic accident**
X● V79.60 **Unspecified bus occupant injured in collision with unspecified motor vehicles in traffic accident**
Bus collision NOS (traffic)
X● V79.69 **Unspecified bus occupant injured in collision with other motor vehicles in traffic accident**
● V79.8 **Bus occupant (driver) (passenger) injured in other specified transport accidents**
X● V79.81 **Bus occupant (driver) (passenger) injured in transport accidents with military vehicle**
X● V79.88 **Bus occupant (driver) (passenger) injured in other specified transport accidents**
X● V79.9 **Bus occupant (driver) (passenger) injured in unspecified traffic accident**
Bus accident NOS

OTHER LAND TRANSPORT ACCIDENTS (V80-V89)

● V80 **Animal-rider or occupant of animal-drawn vehicle injured in transport accident**
The appropriate 7th character is to be added to each code from category V80
A initial encounter
D subsequent encounter
S sequela

● V80.0 **Animal-rider or occupant of animal drawn vehicle injured by fall from or being thrown from animal or animal-drawn vehicle in noncollision accident**
● V80.01 **Animal-rider injured by fall from or being thrown from animal in noncollision accident**
● V80.010 **Animal-rider injured by fall from or being thrown from horse in noncollision accident**
● V80.018 **Animal-rider injured by fall from or being thrown from other animal in noncollision accident**
X● V80.02 **Occupant of animal-drawn vehicle injured by fall from or being thrown from animal-drawn vehicle in noncollision accident**
Overturning animal-drawn vehicle NOS
Overturning animal-drawn vehicle without collision
● V80.1 **Animal-rider or occupant of animal-drawn vehicle injured in collision with pedestrian or animal**
Excludes1 animal-rider or animal-drawn vehicle collision with animal-drawn vehicle or animal being ridden (V80.7)
X● V80.11 **Animal-rider injured in collision with pedestrian or animal**
X● V80.12 **Occupant of animal-drawn vehicle injured in collision with pedestrian or animal**
● V80.2 **Animal-rider or occupant of animal-drawn vehicle injured in collision with pedal cycle**
X● V80.21 **Animal-rider injured in collision with pedal cycle**
X● V80.22 **Occupant of animal-drawn vehicle injured in collision with pedal cycle**

● V80.3 **Animal-rider or occupant of animal-drawn vehicle injured in collision with two- or three-wheeled motor vehicle**

X● V80.31 **Animal-rider injured in collision with two- or three-wheeled motor vehicle**

X● V80.32 **Occupant of animal-drawn vehicle injured in collision with two- or three-wheeled motor vehicle**

● V80.4 **Animal-rider or occupant of animal-drawn vehicle injured in collision with car, pick-up truck, van, heavy transport vehicle or bus**

Excludes1 animal-rider injured in collision with military vehicle (V80.910)
occupant of animal-drawn vehicle injured in collision with military vehicle (V80.920)

X● V80.41 **Animal-rider injured in collision with car, pick-up truck, van, heavy transport vehicle or bus**

X● V80.42 **Occupant of animal-drawn vehicle injured in collision with car, pick-up truck, van, heavy transport vehicle or bus**

● V80.5 **Animal-rider or occupant of animal-drawn vehicle injured in collision with other specified motor vehicle**

X● V80.51 **Animal-rider injured in collision with other specified motor vehicle**

X● V80.52 **Occupant of animal-drawn vehicle injured in collision with other specified motor vehicle**

● V80.6 **Animal-rider or occupant of animal-drawn vehicle injured in collision with railway train or railway vehicle**

X● V80.61 **Animal-rider injured in collision with railway train or railway vehicle**

X● V80.62 **Occupant of animal-drawn vehicle injured in collision with railway train or railway vehicle**

● V80.7 **Animal-rider or occupant of animal-drawn vehicle injured in collision with other nonmotor vehicles**

● V80.71 **Animal-rider or occupant of animal-drawn vehicle injured in collision with animal being ridden**

● V80.710 **Animal-rider injured in collision with other animal being ridden**

● V80.711 **Occupant of animal-drawn vehicle injured in collision with animal being ridden**

● V80.72 **Animal-rider or occupant of animal-drawn vehicle injured in collision with other animal-drawn vehicle**

● V80.720 **Animal-rider injured in collision with animal-drawn vehicle**

● V80.721 **Occupant of animal-drawn vehicle injured in collision with other animal-drawn vehicle**

● V80.73 **Animal-rider or occupant of animal-drawn vehicle injured in collision with streetcar**

● V80.730 **Animal-rider injured in collision with streetcar**

● V80.731 **Occupant of animal-drawn vehicle injured in collision with streetcar**

● V80.79 **Animal-rider or occupant of animal-drawn vehicle injured in collision with other nonmotor vehicles**

● V80.790 **Animal-rider injured in collision with other nonmotor vehicles**

● V80.791 **Occupant of animal-drawn vehicle injured in collision with other nonmotor vehicles**

● V80.8 **Animal-rider or occupant of animal-drawn vehicle injured in collision with fixed or stationary object**

X● V80.81 **Animal-rider injured in collision with fixed or stationary object**

X● V80.82 **Occupant of animal-drawn vehicle injured in collision with fixed or stationary object**

● V80.9 **Animal-rider or occupant of animal-drawn vehicle injured in other and unspecified transport accidents**

● V80.91 **Animal-rider injured in other and unspecified transport accidents**

● V80.910 **Animal-rider injured in transport accident with military vehicle**

● V80.918 **Animal-rider injured in other transport accident**

● V80.919 **Animal-rider injured in unspecified transport accident**
Animal rider accident NOS

● V80.92 **Occupant of animal-drawn vehicle injured in other and unspecified transport accidents**

● V80.920 **Occupant of animal-drawn vehicle injured in transport accident with military vehicle**

● V80.928 **Occupant of animal-drawn vehicle injured in other transport accident**

● V80.929 **Occupant of animal-drawn vehicle injured in unspecified transport accident**
Animal-drawn vehicle accident NOS

● V81 **Occupant of railway train or railway vehicle injured in transport accident**

Includes derailment of railway train or railway vehicle
person on outside of train

Excludes1 streetcar (V82.-)

The appropriate 7th character is to be added to each code from category V81

A initial encounter
D subsequent encounter
S sequela

X● V81.0 **Occupant of railway train or railway vehicle injured in collision with motor vehicle in nontraffic accident**

Excludes1 occupant of railway train or railway vehicle injured due to collision with military vehicle (V81.83)

X● V81.1 **Occupant of railway train or railway vehicle injured in collision with motor vehicle in traffic accident**

Excludes1 occupant of railway train or railway vehicle injured due to collision with military vehicle (V81.83)

X● V81.2 **Occupant of railway train or railway vehicle injured in collision with or hit by rolling stock**

X● V81.3 **Occupant of railway train or railway vehicle injured in collision with other object**
Railway collision NOS

X● V81.4 **Person injured while boarding or alighting from railway train or railway vehicle**

X● V81.5 **Occupant of railway train or railway vehicle injured by fall in railway train or railway vehicle**

X● V81.6 **Occupant of railway train or railway vehicle injured by fall from railway train or railway vehicle**

X● V81.7 **Occupant of railway train or railway vehicle injured in derailment without antecedent collision**

CHAPTER 20 (V01-Y99)

●V81.8 **Occupant of railway train or railway vehicle injured in other specified railway accidents**

X●V81.81 **Occupant of railway train or railway vehicle injured due to explosion or fire on train**

X●V81.82 **Occupant of railway train or railway vehicle injured due to object falling onto train**
Occupant of railway train or railway vehicle injured due to falling earth onto train
Occupant of railway train or railway vehicle injured due to falling rocks onto train
Occupant of railway train or railway vehicle injured due to falling snow onto train
Occupant of railway train or railway vehicle injured due to falling trees onto train

X●V81.83 **Occupant of railway train or railway vehicle injured due to collision with military vehicle**

X●V81.89 **Occupant of railway train or railway vehicle injured due to other specified railway accident**

X●V81.9 **Occupant of railway train or railway vehicle injured in unspecified railway accident**
Railway accident NOS

●V82 **Occupant of powered streetcar injured in transport accident**

Includes interurban electric car
person on outside of streetcar
tram (car)
trolley (car)

Excludes1 bus (V70-V79)
motorcoach (V70-V79)
nonpowered streetcar (V76.-)
train (V81.-)

The appropriate 7th character is to be added to each code from category V82

A	initial encounter
D	subsequent encounter
S	sequela

X●V82.0 **Occupant of streetcar injured in collision with motor vehicle in nontraffic accident**

X●V82.1 **Occupant of streetcar injured in collision with motor vehicle in traffic accident**

X●V82.2 **Occupant of streetcar injured in collision with or hit by rolling stock**

X●V82.3 **Occupant of streetcar injured in collision with other object**

Excludes1 collision with animal-drawn vehicle or animal being ridden (V82.8)

X●V82.4 **Person injured while boarding or alighting from streetcar**

X●V82.5 **Occupant of streetcar injured by fall in streetcar**

Excludes1 fall in streetcar:
while boarding or alighting (V82.4)
with antecedent collision (V82.0-V82.3)

X●V82.6 **Occupant of streetcar injured by fall from streetcar**

Excludes1 fall from streetcar:
while boarding or alighting (V82.4)
with antecedent collision (V82.0-V82.3)

X●V82.7 **Occupant of streetcar injured in derailment without antecedent collision**

Excludes1 occupant of streetcar injured in derailment with antecedent collision (V82.0-V82.3)

X●V82.8 **Occupant of streetcar injured in other specified transport accidents**
Streetcar collision with military vehicle
Streetcar collision with train or nonmotor vehicles

X●V82.9 **Occupant of streetcar injured in unspecified traffic accident**
Streetcar accident NOS

●V83 **Occupant of special vehicle mainly used on industrial premises injured in transport accident**

Includes battery-powered airport passenger vehicle
battery-powered truck (baggage) (mail)
coal-car in mine
forklift (truck)
logging car
self-propelled industrial truck
station baggage truck (powered)
tram, truck, or tub (powered) in mine or quarry

Excludes1 special construction vehicles (V85.-)
special industrial vehicle in stationary use or maintenance (W31.-)

The appropriate 7th character is to be added to each code from category V83

A	initial encounter
D	subsequent encounter
S	sequela

X●V83.0 **Driver of special industrial vehicle injured in traffic accident**

X●V83.1 **Passenger of special industrial vehicle injured in traffic accident**

X●V83.2 **Person on outside of special industrial vehicle injured in traffic accident**

X●V83.3 **Unspecified occupant of special industrial vehicle injured in traffic accident**

X●V83.4 **Person injured while boarding or alighting from special industrial vehicle**

X●V83.5 **Driver of special industrial vehicle injured in nontraffic accident**

X●V83.6 **Passenger of special industrial vehicle injured in nontraffic accident**

X●V83.7 **Person on outside of special industrial vehicle injured in nontraffic accident**

X●V83.9 **Unspecified occupant of special industrial vehicle injured in nontraffic accident**
Special-industrial-vehicle accident NOS

●V84 **Occupant of special vehicle mainly used in agriculture injured in transport accident**

Includes self-propelled farm machinery
tractor (and trailer)

Excludes1 animal-powered farm machinery accident (W30.8-)
contact with combine harvester (W30.0)
special agricultural vehicle in stationary use or maintenance (W30.-)

The appropriate 7th character is to be added to each code from category V84

A	initial encounter
D	subsequent encounter
S	sequela

X●V84.0 **Driver of special agricultural vehicle injured in traffic accident**

X●V84.1 **Passenger of special agricultural vehicle injured in traffic accident**

X●V84.2 **Person on outside of special agricultural vehicle injured in traffic accident**

X●V84.3 **Unspecified occupant of special agricultural vehicle injured in traffic accident**

X●V84.4 **Person injured while boarding or alighting from special agricultural vehicle**

X●V84.5 **Driver of special agricultural vehicle injured in nontraffic accident**

X●V84.6 **Passenger of special agricultural vehicle injured in nontraffic accident**

X●V84.7 **Person on outside of special agricultural vehicle injured in nontraffic accident**

X●V84.9 **Unspecified occupant of special agricultural vehicle injured in nontraffic accident**
Special-agricultural vehicle accident NOS

● V85 Occupant of special construction vehicle injured in transport accident

Includes bulldozer
digger
dump truck
earth-leveller
mechanical shovel
road-roller

Excludes1 special industrial vehicle (V83.-)
special construction vehicle in stationary use or maintenance (W31.-)

The appropriate 7th character is to be added to each code from category V85

A	initial encounter
D	subsequent encounter
S	sequela

X● V85.0 Driver of special construction vehicle injured in traffic accident

X● V85.1 Passenger of special construction vehicle injured in traffic accident

X● V85.2 Person on outside of special construction vehicle injured in traffic accident

X● V85.3 Unspecified occupant of special construction vehicle injured in traffic accident

X● V85.4 Person injured while boarding or alighting from special construction vehicle

X● V85.5 Driver of special construction vehicle injured in nontraffic accident

X● V85.6 Passenger of special construction vehicle injured in nontraffic accident

X● V85.7 Person on outside of special construction vehicle injured in nontraffic accident

X● V85.9 Unspecified occupant of special construction vehicle injured in nontraffic accident
Special-construction-vehicle accident NOS

● V86 Occupant of special all-terrain or other off-road motor vehicle, injured in transport accident

Excludes1 special all-terrain vehicle in stationary use or maintenance (W31.-)
sport-utility vehicle (V50-V59)
three-wheeled motor vehicle designed for on-road use (V30-V39)

The appropriate 7th character is to be added to each code from category V86

A	initial encounter
D	subsequent encounter
S	sequela

● V86.0 Driver of special all-terrain or other off-road motor vehicle injured in traffic accident

X● V86.01 Driver of ambulance or fire engine injured in traffic accident

X● V86.02 Driver of snowmobile injured in traffic accident

X● V86.03 Driver of dune buggy injured in traffic accident

X● V86.04 Driver of military vehicle injured in traffic accident

X● V86.09 Driver of other off-road special all-terrain or other off-road vehicle injured in traffic accident
Driver of dirt bike injured in traffic accident
Driver of go cart injured in traffic accident
Driver of golf cart injured in traffic accident

● V86.1 Passenger of special all-terrain or other off-road motor vehicle injured in traffic accident

X● V86.11 Passenger of ambulance or fire engine injured in traffic accident

X● V86.12 Passenger of snowmobile injured in traffic accident

X● V86.13 Passenger of dune buggy injured in traffic accident

X● V86.14 Passenger of military vehicle injured in traffic accident

X● V86.19 Passenger of other off-road special all-terrain or other off-road off-road motor vehicle injured in traffic accident
Passenger of dirt bike injured in traffic accident
Passenger of go cart injured in traffic accident
Passenger of golf cart injured in traffic accident

● V86.2 Person on outside of special all-terrain or other off-road motor vehicle injured in traffic accident

X● V86.21 Person on outside of ambulance or fire engine injured in traffic accident

X● V86.22 Person on outside of snowmobile injured in traffic accident

X● V86.23 Person on outside of dune buggy injured in traffic accident

X● V86.24 Person on outside of military vehicle injured in traffic accident

X● V86.29 Person on outside of other special all-terrain or other off-road motor vehicle injured in traffic accident
Person on outside of dirt bike injured in traffic accident
Person on outside of go cart in traffic accident
Person on outside of golf cart injured in traffic accident

● V86.3 Unspecified occupant of special all-terrain or other off-road motor vehicle injured in traffic accident

X● V86.31 Unspecified occupant of ambulance or fire engine injured in traffic accident

X● V86.32 Unspecified occupant of snowmobile injured in traffic accident

X● V86.33 Unspecified occupant of dune buggy injured in traffic accident

X● V86.34 Unspecified occupant of military vehicle injured in traffic accident

X● V86.39 Unspecified occupant of other special all-terrain or other off-road motor vehicle injured in traffic accident
Unspecified occupant of dirt bike injured in traffic accident
Unspecified occupant of go cart injured in traffic accident
Unspecified occupant of golf cart injured in traffic accident

● V86.4 Person injured while boarding or alighting from special all-terrain or other off-road motor vehicle

X● V86.41 Person injured while boarding or alighting from ambulance or fire engine

X● V86.42 Person injured while boarding or alighting from snowmobile

X● V86.43 Person injured while boarding or alighting from dune buggy

X● V86.44 Person injured while boarding or alighting from military vehicle

X● V86.49 Person injured while boarding or alighting from other special all-terrain or other off-road motor vehicle
Person injured while boarding or alighting from dirt bike
Person injured while boarding or alighting from go cart
Person injured while boarding or alighting from golf cart

● V86.5 **Driver of special all-terrain or other off-road motor vehicle injured in nontraffic accident**

X● V86.51 **Driver of ambulance or fire engine injured in nontraffic accident**

X● V86.52 **Driver of snowmobile injured in nontraffic accident**

X● V86.53 **Driver of dune buggy injured in nontraffic accident**

X● V86.54 **Driver of military vehicle injured in nontraffic accident**

X● V86.59 **Driver of other off-road special all-terrain or other off-road motor vehicle injured in nontraffic accident**
Driver of dirt bike injured in nontraffic accident
Driver of go cart injured in nontraffic accident
Driver of golf cart injured in nontraffic accident

● V86.6 **Passenger of special all-terrain or other off-road motor vehicle injured in nontraffic accident**

X● V86.61 **Passenger of ambulance or fire engine injured in nontraffic accident**

X● V86.62 **Passenger of snowmobile injured in nontraffic accident**

X● V86.63 **Passenger of dune buggy injured in nontraffic accident**

X● V86.64 **Passenger of military vehicle injured in nontraffic accident**

X● V86.69 **Passenger of other special all-terrain or other off-road vehicle injured in nontraffic accident**
Passenger of dirt bike injured in nontraffic accident
Passenger of go cart injured in nontraffic accident
Passenger of golf cart injured in nontraffic accident

● V86.7 **Person on outside of special all-terrain or other off-road motor vehicle injured in nontraffic accident**

X● V86.71 **Person on outside of ambulance or fire engine injured in nontraffic accident**

X● V86.72 **Person on outside of snowmobile injured in nontraffic accident**

X● V86.73 **Person on outside of dune buggy injured in nontraffic accident**

X● V86.74 **Person on outside of military vehicle injured in nontraffic accident**

X● V86.79 **Person on outside of other special all-terrain or other off-road motor vehicles injured in nontraffic accident**
Person on outside of dirt bike injured in nontraffic accident
Person on outside of go cart injured in nontraffic accident
Person on outside of golf cart injured in nontraffic accident

● V86.9 **Unspecified occupant of special all-terrain or other off-road motor vehicle injured in nontraffic accident**

X● V86.91 **Unspecified occupant of ambulance or fire engine injured in nontraffic accident**

X● V86.92 **Unspecified occupant of snowmobile injured in nontraffic accident**

X● V86.93 **Unspecified occupant of dune buggy injured in nontraffic accident**

X● V86.94 **Unspecified occupant of military vehicle injured in nontraffic accident**

X● V86.99 **Unspecified occupant of other off-road special all-terrain or other off-road motor vehicle injured in nontraffic accident**
All-terrain motor-vehicle accident NOS
Off-road motor-vehicle accident NOS
Other motor-vehicle accident NOS
Unspecified occupant of dirt bike injured in nontraffic accident
Unspecified occupant of go cart injured in nontraffic accident
Unspecified occupant of golf cart injured in nontraffic accident
Unspecified occupant of race car injured in nontraffic accident

● V87 **Traffic accident of specified type but victim's mode of transport unknown**

Excludes1 collision involving:
pedal cycle (V10-V19)
pedestrian (V01-V09)

The appropriate 7th character is to be added to each code from category V87

A	initial encounter
D	subsequent encounter
S	sequela

X● V87.0 **Person injured in collision between car and two- or three-wheeled powered vehicle (traffic)**

X● V87.1 **Person injured in collision between other motor vehicle and two- or three-wheeled motor vehicle (traffic)**

X● V87.2 **Person injured in collision between car and pick-up truck or van (traffic)**

X● V87.3 **Person injured in collision between car and bus (traffic)**

X● V87.4 **Person injured in collision between car and heavy transport vehicle (traffic)**

X● V87.5 **Person injured in collision between heavy transport vehicle and bus (traffic)**

X● V87.6 **Person injured in collision between railway train or railway vehicle and car (traffic)**

X● V87.7 **Person injured in collision between other specified motor vehicles (traffic)**

X● V87.8 **Person injured in other specified noncollision transport accidents involving motor vehicle (traffic)**

X● V87.9 **Person injured in other specified (collision) (noncollision) transport accidents involving nonmotor vehicle (traffic)**

● V88 **Nontraffic accident of specified type but victim's mode of transport unknown**

Excludes1 collision involving:
pedal cycle (V10-V19)
pedestrian (V01-V09)

The appropriate 7th character is to be added to each code from category V88

A	initial encounter
D	subsequent encounter
S	sequela

X● V88.0 **Person injured in collision between car and two- or three-wheeled motor vehicle, nontraffic**

X● V88.1 **Person injured in collision between other motor vehicle and two- or three-wheeled motor vehicle, nontraffic**

X● V88.2 **Person injured in collision between car and pick-up truck or van, nontraffic**

X● **V88.3** **Person injured in collision between car and bus, nontraffic**

X● **V88.4** **Person injured in collision between car and heavy transport vehicle, nontraffic**

X● **V88.5** **Person injured in collision between heavy transport vehicle and bus, nontraffic**

X● **V88.6** **Person injured in collision between railway train or railway vehicle and car, nontraffic**

X● **V88.7** **Person injured in collision between other specified motor vehicle, nontraffic**

X● **V88.8** **Person injured in other specified noncollision transport accidents involving motor vehicle, nontraffic**

X● **V88.9** **Person injured in other specified (collision) (noncollision) transport accidents involving nonmotor vehicle, nontraffic**

● **V89** **Motor- or nonmotor-vehicle accident, type of vehicle unspecified**

The appropriate 7th character is to be added to each code from category V89

A	initial encounter
D	subsequent encounter
S	sequela

X● **V89.0** **Person injured in unspecified motor-vehicle accident, nontraffic**
Motor-vehicle accident NOS, nontraffic

X● **V89.1** **Person injured in unspecified nonmotor-vehicle accident, nontraffic**
Nonmotor-vehicle accident NOS (nontraffic)

X● **V89.2** **Person injured in unspecified motor-vehicle accident, traffic**
Motor-vehicle accident [MVA] NOS
Road (traffic) accident [RTA] NOS

X● **V89.3** **Person injured in unspecified nonmotor-vehicle accident, traffic**
Nonmotor-vehicle traffic accident NOS

X● **V89.9** **Person injured in unspecified vehicle accident**
Collision NOS

WATER TRANSPORT ACCIDENTS (V90-V94)

● **V90** **Drowning and submersion due to accident to watercraft**

Excludes1 civilian water transport accident involving military watercraft (V94.81-)
fall into water not from watercraft (W16.-)
military watercraft accident in military or war operations (Y36.0-, Y37.0-)
water-transport–related drowning or submersion without accident to watercraft (V92.-)

The appropriate 7th character is to be added to each code from category V90

A	initial encounter
D	subsequent encounter
S	sequela

● **V90.0** **Drowning and submersion due to watercraft overturning**

X● **V90.00** **Drowning and submersion due to merchant ship overturning**

X● **V90.01** **Drowning and submersion due to passenger ship overturning**
Drowning and submersion due to ferry-boat overturning
Drowning and submersion due to liner overturning

X● **V90.02** **Drowning and submersion due to fishing boat overturning**

X● **V90.03** **Drowning and submersion due to other powered watercraft overturning**
Drowning and submersion due to hovercraft (on open water) overturning
Drowning and submersion due to jet ski overturning

X● **V90.04** **Drowning and submersion due to sailboat overturning**

X● **V90.05** **Drowning and submersion due to canoe or kayak overturning**

X● **V90.06** **Drowning and submersion due to (nonpowered) inflatable craft overturning**

X● **V90.08** **Drowning and submersion due to other unpowered watercraft overturning**
Drowning and submersion due to windsurfer overturning

X● **V90.09** **Drowning and submersion due to unspecified watercraft overturning**
Drowning and submersion due to boat NOS overturning
Drowning and submersion due to ship NOS overturning
Drowning and submersion due to watercraft NOS overturning

● **V90.1** **Drowning and submersion due to watercraft sinking**

X● **V90.10** **Drowning and submersion due to merchant ship sinking**

X● **V90.11** **Drowning and submersion due to passenger ship sinking**
Drowning and submersion due to ferry-boat sinking
Drowning and submersion due to liner sinking

X● **V90.12** **Drowning and submersion due to fishing boat sinking**

X● **V90.13** **Drowning and submersion due to other powered watercraft sinking**
Drowning and submersion due to hovercraft (on open water) sinking
Drowning and submersion due to jet ski sinking

X● **V90.14** **Drowning and submersion due to sailboat sinking**

X● **V90.15** **Drowning and submersion due to canoe or kayak sinking**

X● **V90.16** **Drowning and submersion due to (nonpowered) inflatable craft sinking**

X● **V90.18** **Drowning and submersion due to other unpowered watercraft sinking**

X● **V90.19** **Drowning and submersion due to unspecified watercraft sinking**
Drowning and submersion due to boat NOS sinking
Drowning and submersion due to ship NOS sinking
Drowning and submersion due to watercraft NOS sinking

● **V90.2** **Drowning and submersion due to falling or jumping from burning watercraft**

X● **V90.20** **Drowning and submersion due to falling or jumping from burning merchant ship**

X● **V90.21** **Drowning and submersion due to falling or jumping from burning passenger ship**
Drowning and submersion due to falling or jumping from burning ferry-boat
Drowning and submersion due to falling or jumping from burning liner

X● **V90.22** **Drowning and submersion due to falling or jumping from burning fishing boat**

X● **V90.23** **Drowning and submersion due to falling or jumping from other burning powered watercraft**
Drowning and submersion due to falling and jumping from burning hovercraft (on open water)
Drowning and submersion due to falling and jumping from burning jet ski

X● **V90.24** **Drowning and submersion due to falling or jumping from burning sailboat**

X● **V90.25** **Drowning and submersion due to falling or jumping from burning canoe or kayak**

CHAPTER 20 (V01-Y99)

X● V90.26 **Drowning and submersion due to falling or jumping from burning (nonpowered) inflatable craft**

X● V90.27 **Drowning and submersion due to falling or jumping from burning water-skis**

X● V90.28 **Drowning and submersion due to falling or jumping from other burning unpowered watercraft**
Drowning and submersion due to falling and jumping from burning surf-board
Drowning and submersion due to falling and jumping from burning windsurfer

X● V90.29 **Drowning and submersion due to falling or jumping from unspecified burning watercraft**
Drowning and submersion due to falling or jumping from burning boat NOS
Drowning and submersion due to falling or jumping from burning ship NOS
Drowning and submersion due to falling or jumping from burning watercraft NOS

● V90.3 **Drowning and submersion due to falling or jumping from crushed watercraft**

X● V90.30 **Drowning and submersion due to falling or jumping from crushed merchant ship**

X● V90.31 **Drowning and submersion due to falling or jumping from crushed passenger ship**
Drowning and submersion due to falling and jumping from crushed ferry-boat
Drowning and submersion due to falling and jumping from crushed liner

X● V90.32 **Drowning and submersion due to falling or jumping from crushed fishing boat**

X● V90.33 **Drowning and submersion due to falling or jumping from other crushed powered watercraft**
Drowning and submersion due to falling and jumping from crushed hovercraft
Drowning and submersion due to falling and jumping from crushed jet ski

X● V90.34 **Drowning and submersion due to falling or jumping from crushed sailboat**

X● V90.35 **Drowning and submersion due to falling or jumping from crushed canoe or kayak**

X● V90.36 **Drowning and submersion due to falling or jumping from crushed (nonpowered) inflatable craft**

X● V90.37 **Drowning and submersion due to falling or jumping from crushed water-skis**

X● V90.38 **Drowning and submersion due to falling or jumping from other crushed unpowered watercraft**
Drowning and submersion due to falling and jumping from crushed surf-board
Drowning and submersion due to falling and jumping from crushed windsurfer

X● V90.39 **Drowning and submersion due to falling or jumping from crushed unspecified watercraft**
Drowning and submersion due to falling and jumping from crushed boat NOS
Drowning and submersion due to falling and jumping from crushed ship NOS
Drowning and submersion due to falling and jumping from crushed watercraft NOS

● V90.8 **Drowning and submersion due to other accident to watercraft**

X● V90.80 **Drowning and submersion due to other accident to merchant ship**

X● V90.81 **Drowning and submersion due to other accident to passenger ship**
Drowning and submersion due to other accident to ferry-boat
Drowning and submersion due to other accident to liner

X● V90.82 **Drowning and submersion due to other accident to fishing boat**

X● V90.83 **Drowning and submersion due to other accident to other powered watercraft**
Drowning and submersion due to other accident to hovercraft (on open water)
Drowning and submersion due to other accident to jet ski

X● V90.84 **Drowning and submersion due to other accident to sailboat**

X● V90.85 **Drowning and submersion due to other accident to canoe or kayak**

X● V90.86 **Drowning and submersion due to other accident to (nonpowered) inflatable craft**

X● V90.87 **Drowning and submersion due to other accident to water-skis**

X● V90.88 **Drowning and submersion due to other accident to other unpowered watercraft**
Drowning and submersion due to other accident to surf-board
Drowning and submersion due to other accident to windsurfer

X● V90.89 **Drowning and submersion due to other accident to unspecified watercraft**
Drowning and submersion due to other accident to boat NOS
Drowning and submersion due to other accident to ship NOS
Drowning and submersion due to other accident to watercraft NOS

● V91 **Other injury due to accident to watercraft**

Includes any injury except drowning and submersion as a result of an accident to watercraft

Excludes1 civilian water transport accident involving military watercraft (V94.81-)
military watercraft accident in military or war operations (Y36, Y37.-)

Excludes2 drowning and submersion due to accident to watercraft (V90.-)

The appropriate 7th character is to be added to each code from category V91

A	initial encounter
D	subsequent encounter
S	sequela

● V91.0 **Burn due to watercraft on fire**

Excludes1 burn from localized fire or explosion on board ship without accident to watercraft (V93.-)

X● V91.00 **Burn due to merchant ship on fire**

X● V91.01 **Burn due to passenger ship on fire**
Burn due to ferry-boat on fire
Burn due to liner on fire

X● V91.02 **Burn due to fishing boat on fire**

X● V91.03 **Burn due to other powered watercraft on fire**
Burn due to hovercraft (on open water) on fire
Burn due to jet ski on fire

X● V91.04 **Burn due to sailboat on fire**

X● V91.05 **Burn due to canoe or kayak on fire**

X● V91.06 **Burn due to (nonpowered) inflatable craft on fire**

X● V91.07 **Burn due to water-skis on fire**

X● V91.08 **Burn due to other unpowered watercraft on fire**

X● V91.09 **Burn due to unspecified watercraft on fire**
Burn due to boat NOS on fire
Burn due to ship NOS on fire
Burn due to watercraft NOS on fire

CHAPTER 20 (V01-Y99)

● V91.1 **Crushed between watercraft and other watercraft or other object due to collision**
Crushed by lifeboat after abandoning ship in a collision
Note: Select the specified type of watercraft that the victim was on at the time of the collision.

X● V91.10 **Crushed between merchant ship and other watercraft or other object due to collision**

X● V91.11 **Crushed between passenger ship and other watercraft or other object due to collision**
Crushed between ferry-boat and other watercraft or other object due to collision
Crushed between liner and other watercraft or other object due to collision

X● V91.12 **Crushed between fishing boat and other watercraft or other object due to collision**

X● V91.13 **Crushed between other powered watercraft and other watercraft or other object due to collision**
Crushed between hovercraft (on open water) and other watercraft or other object due to collision
Crushed between jet ski and other watercraft or other object due to collision

X● V91.14 **Crushed between sailboat and other watercraft or other object due to collision**

X● V91.15 **Crushed between canoe or kayak and other watercraft or other object due to collision**

X● V91.16 **Crushed between (nonpowered) inflatable craft and other watercraft or other object due to collision**

X● V91.18 **Crushed between other unpowered watercraft and other watercraft or other object due to collision**
Crushed between surfboard and other watercraft or other object due to collision
Crushed between windsurfer and other watercraft or other object due to collision

X● V91.19 **Crushed between unspecified watercraft and other watercraft or other object due to collision**
Crushed between boat NOS and other watercraft or other object due to collision
Crushed between ship NOS and other watercraft or other object due to collision
Crushed between watercraft NOS and other watercraft or other object due to collision

● V91.2 **Fall due to collision between watercraft and other watercraft or other object**
Fall while remaining on watercraft after collision
Note: Select the specified type of watercraft that the victim was on at the time of the collision.
Excludes1 crushed between watercraft and other watercraft and other object due to collision (V91.1-)
drowning and submersion due to falling from crushed watercraft (V90.3-)

X● V91.20 **Fall due to collision between merchant ship and other watercraft or other object**

X● V91.21 **Fall due to collision between passenger ship and other watercraft or other object**
Fall due to collision between ferry-boat and other watercraft or other object
Fall due to collision between liner and other watercraft or other object

X● V91.22 **Fall due to collision between fishing boat and other watercraft or other object**

X● V91.23 **Fall due to collision between other powered watercraft and other watercraft or other object**
Fall due to collision between hovercraft (on open water) and other watercraft or other object
Fall due to collision between jet ski and other watercraft or other object

X● V91.24 **Fall due to collision between sailboat and other watercraft or other object**

X● V91.25 **Fall due to collision between canoe or kayak and other watercraft or other object**

X● V91.26 **Fall due to collision between (nonpowered) inflatable craft and other watercraft or other object**

X● V91.29 **Fall due to collision between unspecified watercraft and other watercraft or other object**
Fall due to collision between boat NOS and other watercraft or other object
Fall due to collision between ship NOS and other watercraft or other object
Fall due to collision between watercraft NOS and other watercraft or other object

● V91.3 **Hit or struck by falling object due to accident to watercraft**
Hit or struck by falling object (part of damaged watercraft or other object) after falling or jumping from damaged watercraft
Excludes2 drowning or submersion due to fall or jumping from damaged watercraft (V90.2-, V90.3-)

X● V91.30 **Hit or struck by falling object due to accident to merchant ship**

X● V91.31 **Hit or struck by falling object due to accident to passenger ship**
Hit or struck by falling object due to accident to ferry-boat
Hit or struck by falling object due to accident to liner

X● V91.32 **Hit or struck by falling object due to accident to fishing boat**

X● V91.33 **Hit or struck by falling object due to accident to other powered watercraft**
Hit or struck by falling object due to accident to hovercraft (on open water)
Hit or struck by falling object due to accident to jet ski

X● V91.34 **Hit or struck by falling object due to accident to sailboat**

X● V91.35 **Hit or struck by falling object due to accident to canoe or kayak**

X● V91.36 **Hit or struck by falling object due to accident to (nonpowered) inflatable craft**

X● V91.37 **Hit or struck by falling object due to accident to water-skis**
Hit by water-skis after jumping off of waterskis

X● V91.38 **Hit or struck by falling object due to accident to other unpowered watercraft**
Hit or struck by surf-board after falling off damaged surf-board
Hit or struck by object after falling off damaged windsurfer

X● V91.39 **Hit or struck by falling object due to accident to unspecified watercraft**
Hit or struck by falling object due to accident to boat NOS
Hit or struck by falling object due to accident to ship NOS
Hit or struck by falling object due to accident to watercraft NOS

● V91.8 **Other injury due to other accident to watercraft**

X● V91.80 **Other injury due to other accident to merchant ship**

X● V91.81 **Other injury due to other accident to passenger ship**
Other injury due to other accident to ferry-boat
Other injury due to other accident to liner

X● V91.82 **Other injury due to other accident to fishing boat**

X● V91.83 **Other injury due to other accident to other powered watercraft**
Other injury due to other accident to hovercraft (on open water)
Other injury due to other accident to jet ski

X● V91.84 **Other injury due to other accident to sailboat**

X● V91.85 **Other injury due to other accident to canoe or kayak**

X● V91.86 **Other injury due to other accident to (nonpowered) inflatable craft**

X● V91.87 **Other injury due to other accident to water-skis**

X● V91.88 **Other injury due to other accident to other unpowered watercraft**
Other injury due to other accident to surf-board
Other injury due to other accident to windsurfer

X● V91.89 **Other injury due to other accident to unspecified watercraft**
Other injury due to other accident to boat NOS
Other injury due to other accident to ship NOS
Other injury due to other accident to watercraft NOS

● V92 **Drowning and submersion due to accident on board watercraft, without accident to watercraft**

Excludes1 civilian water transport accident involving military watercraft (V94.81-)
drowning or submersion due to accident to watercraft (V90-V91)
drowning or submersion of diver who voluntarily jumps from boat not involved in an accident (W16.711, W16.721)
fall into water without watercraft (W16.-)
military watercraft accident in military or war operations (Y36, Y37)

The appropriate 7th character is to be added to each code from category V92

A	initial encounter
D	subsequent encounter
S	sequela

● V92.0 **Drowning and submersion due to fall off watercraft**
Drowning and submersion due to fall from gangplank of watercraft
Drowning and submersion due to fall overboard watercraft

Excludes2 hitting head on object or bottom of body of water due to fall from watercraft (V94.0-)

X● V92.00 **Drowning and submersion due to fall off merchant ship**

X● V92.01 **Drowning and submersion due to fall off passenger ship**
Drowning and submersion due to fall off ferry-boat
Drowning and submersion due to fall off liner

X● V92.02 **Drowning and submersion due to fall off fishing boat**

X● V92.03 **Drowning and submersion due to fall off other powered watercraft**
Drowning and submersion due to fall off hovercraft (on open water)
Drowning and submersion due to fall off jet ski

X● V92.04 **Drowning and submersion due to fall off sailboat**

X● V92.05 **Drowning and submersion due to fall off canoe or kayak**

X● V92.06 **Drowning and submersion due to fall off (nonpowered) inflatable craft**

X● V92.07 **Drowning and submersion due to fall off water-skis**

Excludes1 drowning and submersion due to falling off burning water-skis (V90.27)
drowning and submersion due to falling off crushed water-skis (V90.37)
hit by boat while water-skiing NOS (V94.X)

X● V92.08 **Drowning and submersion due to fall off other unpowered watercraft**
Drowning and submersion due to fall off surf-board
Drowning and submersion due to fall off windsurfer

Excludes1 drowning and submersion due to fall off burning unpowered watercraft (V90.28)
drowning and submersion due to fall off crushed unpowered watercraft (V90.38)
drowning and submersion due to fall off damaged unpowered watercraft (V90.88)
drowning and submersion due to rider of nonpowered watercraft being hit by other watercraft (V94.-)
other injury due to rider of nonpowered watercraft being hit by other watercraft (V94.-)

X● V92.09 **Drowning and submersion due to fall off unspecified watercraft**
Drowning and submersion due to fall off boat NOS
Drowning and submersion due to fall off ship NOS
Drowning and submersion due to fall off watercraft NOS

● V92.1 **Drowning and submersion due to being thrown overboard by motion of watercraft**

Excludes1 drowning and submersion due to fall off surf-board (V92.08)
drowning and submersion due to fall off water-skis (V92.07)
drowning and submersion due to fall off windsurfer (V92.08)

X● V92.10 **Drowning and submersion due to being thrown overboard by motion of merchant ship**

X● V92.11 **Drowning and submersion due to being thrown overboard by motion of passenger ship**
Drowning and submersion due to being thrown overboard by motion of ferry-boat
Drowning and submersion due to being thrown overboard by motion of liner

CHAPTER 20 (V01-Y99)

X● V92.12 **Drowning and submersion due to being thrown overboard by motion of fishing boat**

X● V92.13 **Drowning and submersion due to being thrown overboard by motion of other powered watercraft**
Drowning and submersion due to being thrown overboard by motion of hovercraft

X● V92.14 **Drowning and submersion due to being thrown overboard by motion of sailboat**

X● V92.15 **Drowning and submersion due to being thrown overboard by motion of canoe or kayak**

X● V92.16 **Drowning and submersion due to being thrown overboard by motion of (nonpowered) inflatable craft**

X● V92.19 **Drowning and submersion due to being thrown overboard by motion of unspecified watercraft**
Drowning and submersion due to being thrown overboard by motion of boat NOS
Drowning and submersion due to being thrown overboard by motion of ship NOS
Drowning and submersion due to being thrown overboard by motion of watercraft NOS

● V92.2 **Drowning and submersion due to being washed overboard from watercraft**
Code first any associated cataclysm (X37.Ø-)

X● V92.2Ø **Drowning and submersion due to being washed overboard from merchant ship**

X● V92.21 **Drowning and submersion due to being washed overboard from passenger ship**
Drowning and submersion due to being washed overboard from ferry-boat
Drowning and submersion due to being washed overboard from liner

X● V92.22 **Drowning and submersion due to being washed overboard from fishing boat**

X● V92.23 **Drowning and submersion due to being washed overboard from other powered watercraft**
Drowning and submersion due to being washed overboard from hovercraft (on open water)
Drowning and submersion due to being washed overboard from jet ski

X● V92.24 **Drowning and submersion due to being washed overboard from sailboat**

X● V92.25 **Drowning and submersion due to being washed overboard from canoe or kayak**

X● V92.26 **Drowning and submersion due to being washed overboard from (nonpowered) inflatable craft**

X● V92.27 **Drowning and submersion due to being washed overboard from water-skis**
Excludes1 drowning and submersion due to fall off water-skis (V92.Ø7)

X● V92.28 **Drowning and submersion due to being washed overboard from other unpowered watercraft**
Drowning and submersion due to being washed overboard from surf-board
Drowning and submersion due to being washed overboard from windsurfer

X● V92.29 **Drowning and submersion due to being washed overboard from unspecified watercraft**
Drowning and submersion due to being washed overboard from boat NOS
Drowning and submersion due to being washed overboard from ship NOS
Drowning and submersion due to being washed overboard from watercraft NOS

● V93 **Other injury due to accident on board watercraft, without accident to watercraft**
Excludes1 civilian water transport accident involving military watercraft (V94.81-)
other injury due to accident to watercraft (V91.-)
military watercraft accident in military or war operations (Y36, Y37.-)
Excludes2 drowning and submersion due to accident on board watercraft, without accident to watercraft (V92.-)

The appropriate 7th character is to be added to each code from category V93

A	initial encounter
D	subsequent encounter
S	sequela

● V93.Ø **Burn due to localized fire on board watercraft**
Excludes1 burn due to watercraft on fire (V91.Ø-)

X● V93.ØØ **Burn due to localized fire on board merchant vessel**

X● V93.Ø1 **Burn due to localized fire on board passenger vessel**
Burn due to localized fire on board ferry-boat
Burn due to localized fire on board liner

X● V93.Ø2 **Burn due to localized fire on board fishing boat**

X● V93.Ø3 **Burn due to localized fire on board other powered watercraft**
Burn due to localized fire on board hovercraft
Burn due to localized fire on board jet ski

X● V93.Ø4 **Burn due to localized fire on board sailboat**

X● V93.Ø9 **Burn due to localized fire on board unspecified watercraft**
Burn due to localized fire on board boat NOS
Burn due to localized fire on board ship NOS
Burn due to localized fire on board watercraft NOS

● V93.1 **Other burn on board watercraft**
Burn due to source other than fire on board watercraft
Excludes1 burn due to watercraft on fire (V91.Ø-)

X● V93.1Ø **Other burn on board merchant vessel**

X● V93.11 **Other burn on board passenger vessel**
Other burn on board ferry-boat
Other burn on board liner

X● V93.12 **Other burn on board fishing boat**

X● V93.13 **Other burn on board other powered watercraft**
Other burn on board hovercraft
Other burn on board jet ski

X● V93.14 **Other burn on board sailboat**

X● V93.19 **Other burn on board unspecified watercraft**
Other burn on board boat NOS
Other burn on board ship NOS
Other burn on board watercraft NOS

● V93.2 **Heat exposure on board watercraft**
Excludes1 exposure to man-made heat not aboard watercraft (W92)
exposure to natural heat while on board watercraft (X3Ø)
exposure to sunlight while on board watercraft (X32)
Excludes2 burn due to fire on board watercraft (V93.Ø-)

X● V93.2Ø **Heat exposure on board merchant ship**

X● V93.21 **Heat exposure on board passenger ship**
Heat exposure on board ferry-boat
Heat exposure on board liner

X● V93.22 **Heat exposure on board fishing boat**

X● V93.23 **Heat exposure on board other powered watercraft**
Heat exposure on board hovercraft

X● V93.24 **Heat exposure on board sailboat**
X● V93.29 **Heat exposure on board unspecified watercraft**
Heat exposure on board boat NOS
Heat exposure on board ship NOS
Heat exposure on board watercraft NOS

● V93.3 **Fall on board watercraft**
Excludes1 fall due to collision of watercraft (V91.2-)
X● V93.30 **Fall on board merchant ship**
X● V93.31 **Fall on board passenger ship**
Fall on board ferry-boat
Fall on board liner
X● V93.32 **Fall on board fishing boat**
X● V93.33 **Fall on board other powered watercraft**
Fall on board hovercraft (on open water)
Fall on board jet ski
X● V93.34 **Fall on board sailboat**
X● V93.35 **Fall on board canoe or kayak**
X● V93.36 **Fall on board (nonpowered) inflatable craft**
X● V93.38 **Fall on board other unpowered watercraft**
X● V93.39 **Fall on board unspecified watercraft**
Fall on board boat NOS
Fall on board ship NOS
Fall on board watercraft NOS

● V93.4 **Struck by falling object on board watercraft**
Hit by falling object on board watercraft
Excludes1 struck by falling object due to accident to watercraft (V91.3)
X● V93.40 **Struck by falling object on merchant ship**
X● V93.41 **Struck by falling object on passenger ship**
Struck by falling object on ferry-boat
Struck by falling object on liner
X● V93.42 **Struck by falling object on fishing boat**
X● V93.43 **Struck by falling object on other powered watercraft**
Struck by falling object on hovercraft
X● V93.44 **Struck by falling object on sailboat**
X● V93.48 **Struck by falling object on other unpowered watercraft**
X● V93.49 **Struck by falling object on unspecified watercraft**

● V93.5 **Explosion on board watercraft**
Boiler explosion on steamship
Excludes2 fire on board watercraft (V93.0-)
X● V93.50 **Explosion on board merchant ship**
X● V93.51 **Explosion on board passenger ship**
Explosion on board ferry-boat
Explosion on board liner
X● V93.52 **Explosion on board fishing boat**
X● V93.53 **Explosion on board other powered watercraft**
Explosion on board hovercraft
Explosion on board jet ski
X● V93.54 **Explosion on board sailboat**
X● V93.59 **Explosion on board unspecified watercraft**
Explosion on board boat NOS
Explosion on board ship NOS
Explosion on board watercraft NOS

● V93.6 **Machinery accident on board watercraft**
Excludes1 machinery explosion on board watercraft (V93.4-)
machinery fire on board watercraft (V93.0-)
X● V93.60 **Machinery accident on board merchant ship**
X● V93.61 **Machinery accident on board passenger ship**
Machinery accident on board ferry-boat
Machinery accident on board liner
X● V93.62 **Machinery accident on board fishing boat**
X● V93.63 **Machinery accident on board other powered watercraft**
Machinery accident on board hovercraft
X● V93.64 **Machinery accident on board sailboat**
X● V93.69 **Machinery accident on board unspecified watercraft**
Machinery accident on board boat NOS
Machinery accident on board ship NOS
Machinery accident on board watercraft NOS

● V93.8 **Other injury due to other accident on board watercraft**
Accidental poisoning by gases or fumes on watercraft
X● V93.80 **Other injury due to other accident on board merchant ship**
X● V93.81 **Other injury due to other accident on board passenger ship**
Other injury due to other accident on board ferry-boat
Other injury due to other accident on board liner
X● V93.82 **Other injury due to other accident on board fishing boat**
X● V93.83 **Other injury due to other accident on board other powered watercraft**
Other injury due to other accident on board hovercraft
Other injury due to other accident on board jet ski
X● V93.84 **Other injury due to other accident on board sailboat**
X● V93.85 **Other injury due to other accident on board canoe or kayak**
X● V93.86 **Other injury due to other accident on board (nonpowered) inflatable craft**
X● V93.87 **Other injury due to other accident on board water-skis**
Hit or struck by object while waterskiing
X● V93.88 **Other injury due to other accident on board other unpowered watercraft**
Hit or struck by object while surfing
Hit or struck by object while on board windsurfer
X● V93.89 **Other injury due to other accident on board unspecified watercraft**
Other injury due to other accident on board boat NOS
Other injury due to other accident on board ship NOS
Other injury due to other accident on board watercraft NOS

● V94 **Other and unspecified water transport accidents**
Excludes1 military watercraft accidents in military or war operations (Y36, Y37)

The appropriate 7th character is to be added to each code from category V94

A	initial encounter
D	subsequent encounter
S	sequela

X● V94.0 **Hitting object or bottom of body of water due to fall from watercraft**
Excludes2 drowning and submersion due to fall from watercraft (V92.0-)
● V94.1 **Bather struck by watercraft**
Swimmer hit by watercraft
X● V94.11 **Bather struck by powered watercraft**
X● V94.12 **Bather struck by nonpowered watercraft**

CHAPTER 20 (V01-Y99)

● V94.2 **Rider of nonpowered watercraft struck by other watercraft**

X● V94.21 **Rider of nonpowered watercraft struck by other nonpowered watercraft**
Canoer hit by other nonpowered watercraft
Surfer hit by other nonpowered watercraft
Windsurfer hit by other nonpowered watercraft

X● V94.22 **Rider of nonpowered watercraft struck by powered watercraft**
Canoer hit by motorboat
Surfer hit by motorboat
Windsurfer hit by motorboat

● V94.3 **Injury to rider of (inflatable) watercraft being pulled behind other watercraft**

X● V94.31 **Injury to rider of (inflatable) recreational watercraft being pulled behind other watercraft**
Injury to rider of inner-tube pulled behind motor boat

X● V94.32 **Injury to rider of non-recreational watercraft being pulled behind other watercraft**
Injury to occupant of dingy being pulled behind boat or ship
Injury to occupant of life-raft being pulled behind boat or ship

X● V94.4 **Injury to barefoot water-skier**
Injury to person being pulled behind boat or ship

● V94.8 **Other water transport accident**

● V94.81 **Water transport accident involving military watercraft**

● V94.810 **Civilian watercraft involved in water transport accident with military watercraft**
Passenger on civilian watercraft injured due to accident with military watercraft

● V94.811 **Civilian in water injured by military watercraft**

● V94.818 **Other water transport accident involving military watercraft**

X● V94.89 **Other water transport accident**

X● V94.9 **Unspecified water transport accident**
Water transport accident NOS

AIR AND SPACE TRANSPORT ACCIDENTS (V95-V97)

Excludes1 military aircraft accidents in military or war operations (Y36, Y37)

● V95 **Accident to powered aircraft causing injury to occupant**

The appropriate 7th character is to be added to each code from category V95

A initial encounter
D subsequent encounter
S sequela

● V95.0 **Helicopter accident injuring occupant**

X● V95.00 **Unspecified helicopter accident injuring occupant**

X● V95.01 **Helicopter crash injuring occupant**

X● V95.02 **Forced landing of helicopter injuring occupant**

X● V95.03 **Helicopter collision injuring occupant**
Helicopter collision with any object, fixed, movable or moving

X● V95.04 **Helicopter fire injuring occupant**

X● V95.05 **Helicopter explosion injuring occupant**

X● V95.09 **Other helicopter accident injuring occupant**

● V95.1 **Ultralight, microlight or powered-glider accident injuring occupant**

X● V95.10 **Unspecified ultralight, microlight or powered-glider accident injuring occupant**

X● V95.11 **Ultralight, microlight or powered-glider crash injuring occupant**

X● V95.12 **Forced landing of ultralight, microlight or powered-glider injuring occupant**

X● V95.13 **Ultralight, microlight or powered-glider collision injuring occupant**
Ultralight, microlight or powered-glider collision with any object, fixed, movable or moving

X● V95.14 **Ultralight, microlight or powered-glider fire injuring occupant**

X● V95.15 **Ultralight, microlight or powered-glider explosion injuring occupant**

X● V95.19 **Other ultralight, microlight or powered-glider accident injuring occupant**

● V95.2 **Other private fixed-wing aircraft accident injuring occupant**

X● V95.20 **Unspecified accident to other private fixed-wing aircraft, injuring occupant**

X● V95.21 **Other private fixed-wing aircraft crash injuring occupant**

X● V95.22 **Forced landing of other private fixed-wing aircraft injuring occupant**

X● V95.23 **Other private fixed-wing aircraft collision injuring occupant**
Other private fixed-wing aircraft collision with any object, fixed, movable or moving

X● V95.24 **Other private fixed-wing aircraft fire injuring occupant**

X● V95.25 **Other private fixed-wing aircraft explosion injuring occupant**

X● V95.29 **Other accident to other private fixed-wing aircraft injuring occupant**

● V95.3 **Commercial fixed-wing aircraft accident injuring occupant**

X● V95.30 **Unspecified accident to commercial fixed-wing aircraft injuring occupant**

X● V95.31 **Commercial fixed-wing aircraft crash injuring occupant**

X● V95.32 **Forced landing of commercial fixed-wing aircraft injuring occupant**

X● V95.33 **Commercial fixed-wing aircraft collision injuring occupant**
Commercial fixed-wing aircraft collision with any object, fixed, movable or moving

X● V95.34 **Commercial fixed-wing aircraft fire injuring occupant**

X● V95.35 **Commercial fixed-wing aircraft explosion injuring occupant**

X● V95.39 **Other accident to commercial fixed-wing aircraft injuring occupant**

● V95.4 **Spacecraft accident injuring occupant**

X● V95.40 **Unspecified spacecraft accident injuring occupant**

X● V95.41 **Spacecraft crash injuring occupant**

X● V95.42 **Forced landing of spacecraft injuring occupant**

X● V95.43 **Spacecraft collision injuring occupant**
Spacecraft collision with any object, fixed, moveable or moving

X● V95.44 **Spacecraft fire injuring occupant**

X● V95.45 **Spacecraft explosion injuring occupant**

X● V95.49 **Other spacecraft accident injuring occupant**

X● V95.8 **Other powered aircraft accidents injuring occupant**

X● V95.9 **Unspecified aircraft accident injuring occupant**
Aircraft accident NOS
Air transport accident NOS

● V96 **Accident to nonpowered aircraft causing injury to occupant**
The appropriate 7th character is to be added to each code from category V96
A initial encounter
D subsequent encounter
S sequela

● V96.Ø **Balloon accident injuring occupant**
X● V96.ØØ **Unspecified balloon accident injuring occupant**
X● V96.Ø1 **Balloon crash injuring occupant**
X● V96.Ø2 **Forced landing of balloon injuring occupant**
X● V96.Ø3 **Balloon collision injuring occupant**
Balloon collision with any object, fixed, moveable or moving
X● V96.Ø4 **Balloon fire injuring occupant**
X● V96.Ø5 **Balloon explosion injuring occupant**
X● V96.Ø9 **Other balloon accident injuring occupant**
● V96.1 **Hang-glider accident injuring occupant**
X● V96.1Ø **Unspecified hang-glider accident injuring occupant**
X● V96.11 **Hang-glider crash injuring occupant**
X● V96.12 **Forced landing of hang-glider injuring occupant**
X● V96.13 **Hang-glider collision injuring occupant**
Hang-glider collision with any object, fixed, moveable or moving
X● V96.14 **Hang-glider fire injuring occupant**
X● V96.15 **Hang-glider explosion injuring occupant**
X● V96.19 **Other hang-glider accident injuring occupant**
● V96.2 **Glider (nonpowered) accident injuring occupant**
X● V96.2Ø **Unspecified glider (nonpowered) accident injuring occupant**
X● V96.21 **Glider (nonpowered) crash injuring occupant**
X● V96.22 **Forced landing of glider (nonpowered) injuring occupant**
X● V96.23 **Glider (nonpowered) collision injuring occupant**
Glider (nonpowered) collision with any object, fixed, moveable or moving
X● V96.24 **Glider (nonpowered) fire injuring occupant**
X● V96.25 **Glider (nonpowered) explosion injuring occupant**
X● V96.29 **Other glider (nonpowered) accident injuring occupant**
X● V96.8 **Other nonpowered-aircraft accidents injuring occupant**
Kite carrying a person accident injuring occupant
X● V96.9 **Unspecified nonpowered-aircraft accident injuring occupant**
Nonpowered-aircraft accident NOS

● V97 **Other specified air transport accidents**
The appropriate 7th character is to be added to each code from category V97
A initial encounter
D subsequent encounter
S sequela

X● V97.Ø **Occupant of aircraft injured in other specified air transport accidents**
Fall in, on or from aircraft in air transport accident
Excludes1 accident while boarding or alighting aircraft (V97.1)
X● V97.1 **Person injured while boarding or alighting from aircraft**
● V97.2 **Parachutist accident**
X● V97.21 **Parachutist entangled in object**
Parachutist landing in tree
X● V97.22 **Parachutist injured on landing**
X● V97.29 **Other parachutist accident**
● V97.3 **Person on ground injured in air transport accident**
X● V97.31 **Hit by object falling from aircraft**
Hit by crashing aircraft
Injured by aircraft hitting house
Injured by aircraft hitting car
X● V97.32 **Injured by rotating propeller**
X● V97.33 **Sucked into jet engine**
X● V97.39 **Other injury to person on ground due to air transport accident**
● V97.8 **Other air transport accidents, not elsewhere classified**
Excludes1 aircraft accident NOS (V95.9)
exposure to changes in air pressure during ascent or descent (W94.-)
● V97.81 **Air transport accident involving military aircraft**
● V97.81Ø **Civilian aircraft involved in air transport accident with military aircraft**
Passenger in civilian aircraft injured due to accident with military aircraft
● V97.811 **Civilian injured by military aircraft**
● V97.818 **Other air transport accident involving military aircraft**
X● V97.89 **Other air transport accidents, not elsewhere classified**
Injury from machinery on aircraft

OTHER AND UNSPECIFIED TRANSPORT ACCIDENTS (V98-V99)

Excludes1 vehicle accident, type of vehicle unspecified (V89.-)

● V98 **Other specified transport accidents**
The appropriate 7th character is to be added to each code from category V98
A initial encounter
D subsequent encounter
S sequela

X● V98.Ø **Accident to, on or involving cable-car, not on rails**
Caught or dragged by cable-car, not on rails
Fall or jump from cable-car, not on rails
Object thrown from or in cable-car, not on rails
X● V98.1 **Accident to, on or involving land-yacht**
X● V98.2 **Accident to, on or involving ice yacht**
X● V98.3 **Accident to, on or involving ski lift**
Accident to, on or involving ski chair-lift
Accident to, on or involving ski-lift with gondola
X● V98.8 **Other specified transport accidents**
X● V99 **Unspecified transport accident**
The appropriate 7th character is to be added to code V99
A initial encounter
D subsequent encounter
S sequela

OTHER EXTERNAL CAUSES OF ACCIDENTAL INJURY (W00-X58)

SLIPPING, TRIPPING, STUMBLING AND FALLS (W00-W19)

Excludes1 assault involving a fall (Y01-Y02)
fall from animal (V80.-)
fall (in) (from) machinery (in operation) (W28-W31)
fall (in) (from) transport vehicle (V01-V99)
intentional self-harm involving a fall (X80-X81)

Excludes2 at risk for fall (history of fall) Z91.81
fall (in) (from) burning building (X00.-)
fall into fire (X00-X04, X08-X09)

● **W00 Fall due to ice and snow**

Includes pedestrian on foot falling (slipping) on ice and snow

Excludes1 fall on (from) ice and snow involving pedestrian conveyance (V00.-)
fall from stairs and steps not due to ice and snow (W10.-)

The appropriate 7th character is to be added to each code from category W00

A	initial encounter
D	subsequent encounter
S	sequela

X● **W00.0 Fall on same level due to ice and snow**
X● **W00.1 Fall from stairs and steps due to ice and snow**
X● **W00.2 Other fall from one level to another due to ice and snow**
X● **W00.9 Unspecified fall due to ice and snow**

● **W01 Fall on same level from slipping, tripping and stumbling**

Includes fall on moving sidewalk

Excludes1 fall due to bumping (striking) against object (W18.0-)
fall in shower or bathtub (W18.2-)
fall on same level NOS (W18.30)
fall on same level from slipping, tripping and stumbling due to ice or snow (W00.0)
fall off or from toilet (W18.1-)
slipping, tripping and stumbling NOS (W18.40)
slipping, tripping and stumbling without falling (W18.4-)

The appropriate 7th character is to be added to each code from category W01

A	initial encounter
D	subsequent encounter
S	sequela

X● **W01.0 Fall on same level from slipping, tripping and stumbling without subsequent striking against object**
Falling over animal

● **W01.1 Fall on same level from slipping, tripping and stumbling with subsequent striking against object**

X● **W01.10 Fall on same level from slipping, tripping and stumbling with subsequent striking against unspecified object**

● **W01.11 Fall on same level from slipping, tripping and stumbling with subsequent striking against sharp object**

● **W01.110 Fall on same level from slipping, tripping and stumbling with subsequent striking against sharp glass**

● **W01.111 Fall on same level from slipping, tripping and stumbling with subsequent striking against power tool or machine**

● **W01.118 Fall on same level from slipping, tripping and stumbling with subsequent striking against other sharp object**

● **W01.119 Fall on same level from slipping, tripping and stumbling with subsequent striking against unspecified sharp object**

● **W01.19 Fall on same level from slipping, tripping and stumbling with subsequent striking against other object**

● **W01.190 Fall on same level from slipping, tripping and stumbling with subsequent striking against furniture**

● **W01.198 Fall on same level from slipping, tripping and stumbling with subsequent striking against other object**

X● **W03 Other fall on same level due to collision with another person**
Fall due to non-transport collision with other person

Excludes1 collision with another person without fall (W51)
crushed or pushed by a crowd or human stampede (W52)
fall involving pedestrian conveyance (V00-V09)
fall due to ice or snow (W00)
fall on same level NOS (W18.30)

The appropriate 7th character is to be added to code W03

A	initial encounter
D	subsequent encounter
S	sequela

X● **W04 Fall while being carried or supported by other persons**
Accidentally dropped while being carried

The appropriate 7th character is to be added to code W04

A	initial encounter
D	subsequent encounter
S	sequel

● **W05 Fall from non-moving wheelchair, nonmotorized scooter and motorized mobility scooter**

Excludes1 fall from moving wheelchair (powered) (V00.811)
fall from moving motorized mobility scooter (V00.831)
fall from nonmotorized scooter (V00.141)

The appropriate 7th character is to be added to each code from category W05

A	initial encounter
D	subsequent encounter
S	sequela

X● **W05.0 Fall from non-moving wheelchair**
X● **W05.1 Fall from non-moving nonmotorized scooter**
X● **W05.2 Fall from non-moving motorized mobility scooter**

CHAPTER 20 (V01-Y99)

X● **W06 Fall from bed**

The appropriate 7th character is to be added to code W06

A	initial encounter
D	subsequent encounter
S	sequela

X● **W07 Fall from chair**

The appropriate 7th character is to be added to code W07

A	initial encounter
D	subsequent encounter
S	sequela

X● **W08 Fall from other furniture**

The appropriate 7th character is to be added to code W08

A	initial encounter
D	subsequent encounter
S	sequela

● **W09 Fall on and from playground equipment**

Excludes1 fall involving recreational machinery (W31)

The appropriate 7th character is to be added to each code from category W09

A	initial encounter
D	subsequent encounter
S	sequela

X● **W09.0 Fall on or from playground slide**

X● **W09.1 Fall from playground swing**

X● **W09.2 Fall on or from jungle gym**

X● **W09.8 Fall on or from other playground equipment**

● **W10 Fall on and from stairs and steps**

Excludes1 fall from stairs and steps due to ice and snow (W00.1)

The appropriate 7th character is to be added to each code from category W10

A	initial encounter
D	subsequent encounter
S	sequela

X● **W10.0 Fall (on) (from) escalator**

X● **W10.1 Fall (on) (from) sidewalk curb**

X● **W10.2 Fall (on) (from) incline**

Fall (on) (from) ramp

X● **W10.8 Fall (on) (from) other stairs and steps**

X● **W10.9 Fall (on) (from) unspecified stairs and steps**

X● **W11 Fall on and from ladder**

The appropriate 7th character is to be added to code W11

A	initial encounter
D	subsequent encounter
S	sequela

X● **W12 Fall on and from scaffolding**

The appropriate 7th character is to be added to code W12

A	initial encounter
D	subsequent encounter
S	sequela

● **W13 Fall from, out of or through building or structure**

The appropriate 7th character is to be added to each code from category W13

A	initial encounter
D	subsequent encounter
S	sequela

X● **W13.0 Fall from, out of or through balcony**

Fall from, out of or through railing

X● **W13.1 Fall from, out of or through bridge**

X● **W13.2 Fall from, out of or through roof**

X● **W13.3 Fall through floor**

X● **W13.4 Fall from, out of or through window**

Excludes2 fall with subsequent striking against sharp glass (W01.110)

X● **W13.8 Fall from, out of or through other building or structure**

Fall from, out of or through viaduct
Fall from, out of or through wall
Fall from, out of or through flag-pole

X● **W13.9 Fall from, out of or through building, not otherwise specified**

Excludes1 collapse of a building or structure (W20.-)
fall or jump from burning building or structure (X00.-)

X● **W14 Fall from tree**

The appropriate 7th character is to be added to code W14

A	initial encounter
D	subsequent encounter
S	sequela

X● **W15 Fall from cliff**

The appropriate 7th character is to be added to code W15

A	initial encounter
D	subsequent encounter
S	sequela

● **W16 Fall, jump or diving into water**

Excludes1 accidental non-watercraft drowning and submersion not involving fall (W65-W74)
effects of air pressure from diving (W94.-)
fall into water from watercraft (V90-V94)
hitting an object or against bottom when falling from watercraft (V94.0)

Excludes2 striking or hitting diving board (W21.4)

The appropriate 7th character is to be added to each code from category W16

A	initial encounter
D	subsequent encounter
S	sequela

● **W16.0 Fall into swimming pool**

Fall into swimming pool NOS

Excludes1 fall into empty swimming pool (W17.3)

● **W16.01 Fall into swimming pool striking water surface**

● **W16.011 Fall into swimming pool striking water surface causing drowning and submersion**

Excludes1 drowning and submersion while in swimming pool without fall (W67)

● **W16.012 Fall into swimming pool striking water surface causing other injury**

● W16.02 Fall into swimming pool striking bottom
● W16.021 Fall into swimming pool striking bottom causing drowning and submersion
Excludes1 drowning and submersion while in swimming pool without fall (W67)
● W16.022 Fall into swimming pool striking bottom causing other injury
● W16.03 Fall into swimming pool striking wall
● W16.031 Fall into swimming pool striking wall causing drowning and submersion
Excludes1 drowning and submersion while in swimming pool without fall (W67)
● W16.032 Fall into swimming pool striking wall causing other injury
● W16.1 Fall into natural body of water
Fall into lake
Fall into open sea
Fall into river
Fall into stream
● W16.11 Fall into natural body of water striking water surface
● W16.111 Fall into natural body of water striking water surface causing drowning and submersion
Excludes1 drowning and submersion while in natural body of water without fall (W69)
● W16.112 Fall into natural body of water striking water surface causing other injury
● W16.12 Fall into natural body of water striking bottom
● W16.121 Fall into natural body of water striking bottom causing drowning and submersion
Excludes1 drowning and submersion while in natural body of water without fall (W69)
● W16.122 Fall into natural body of water striking bottom causing other injury
● W16.13 Fall into natural body of water striking side
● W16.131 Fall into natural body of water striking side causing drowning and submersion
Excludes1 drowning and submersion while in natural body of water without fall (W69)
● W16.132 Fall into natural body of water striking side causing other injury
● W16.2 Fall in (into) filled bathtub or bucket of water
● W16.21 Fall in (into) filled bathtub
Excludes1 fall into empty bathtub (W18.2)
● W16.211 Fall in (into) filled bathtub causing drowning and submersion
Excludes1 drowning and submersion while in filled bathtub without fall (W65)
● W16.212 Fall in (into) filled bathtub causing other injury
● W16.22 Fall in (into) bucket of water
● W16.221 Fall in (into) bucket of water causing drowning and submersion
● W16.222 Fall in (into) bucket of water causing other injury
● W16.3 Fall into other water
Fall into fountain
Fall into reservoir
● W16.31 Fall into other water striking water surface
● W16.311 Fall into other water striking water surface causing drowning and submersion
Excludes1 drowning and submersion while in other water without fall (W73)
● W16.312 Fall into other water striking water surface causing other injury
● W16.32 Fall into other water striking bottom
● W16.321 Fall into other water striking bottom causing drowning and submersion
Excludes1 drowning and submersion while in other water without fall (W73)
● W16.322 Fall into other water striking bottom causing other injury
● W16.33 Fall into other water striking wall
● W16.331 Fall into other water striking wall causing drowning and submersion
Excludes1 drowning and submersion while in other water without fall (W73)
● W16.332 Fall into other water striking wall causing other injury
● W16.4 Fall into unspecified water
X● W16.41 Fall into unspecified water causing drowning and submersion
X● W16.42 Fall into unspecified water causing other injury
● W16.5 Jumping or diving into swimming pool
● W16.51 Jumping or diving into swimming pool striking water surface
● W16.511 Jumping or diving into swimming pool striking water surface causing drowning and submersion
Excludes1 drowning and submersion while in swimming pool without jumping or diving (W67)
● W16.512 Jumping or diving into swimming pool striking water surface causing other injury
● W16.52 Jumping or diving into swimming pool striking bottom
● W16.521 Jumping or diving into swimming pool striking bottom causing drowning and submersion
Excludes1 drowning and submersion while in swimming pool without jumping or diving (W67)
● W16.522 Jumping or diving into swimming pool striking bottom causing other injury

● W16.53 **Jumping or diving into swimming pool striking wall**

● W16.531 **Jumping or diving into swimming pool striking wall causing drowning and submersion**

Excludes1 drowning and submersion while in swimming pool without jumping or diving (W67)

● W16.532 **Jumping or diving into swimming pool striking wall causing other injury**

● W16.6 **Jumping or diving into natural body of water**

Jumping or diving into lake
Jumping or diving into open sea
Jumping or diving into river
Jumping or diving into stream

● W16.61 **Jumping or diving into natural body of water striking water surface**

● W16.611 **Jumping or diving into natural body of water striking water surface causing drowning and submersion**

Excludes1 drowning and submersion while in natural body of water without jumping or diving (W69)

● W16.612 **Jumping or diving into natural body of water striking water surface causing other injury**

● W16.62 **Jumping or diving into natural body of water striking bottom**

● W16.621 **Jumping or diving into natural body of water striking bottom causing drowning and submersion**

Excludes1 drowning and submersion while in natural body of water without jumping or diving (W69)

● W16.622 **Jumping or diving into natural body of water striking bottom causing other injury**

● W16.7 **Jumping or diving from boat**

Excludes1 fall from boat into water - see watercraft accident (V9Ø-V94)

● W16.71 **Jumping or diving from boat striking water surface**

● W16.711 **Jumping or diving from boat striking water surface causing drowning and submersion**

● W16.712 **Jumping or diving from boat striking water surface causing other injury**

● W16.72 **Jumping or diving from boat striking bottom**

● W16.721 **Jumping or diving from boat striking bottom causing drowning and submersion**

● W16.722 **Jumping or diving from boat striking bottom causing other injury**

● W16.8 **Jumping or diving into other water**

Jumping or diving into fountain
Jumping or diving into reservoir

● W16.81 **Jumping or diving into other water striking water surface**

● W16.811 **Jumping or diving into other water striking water surface causing drowning and submersion**

Excludes1 drowning and submersion while in other water without jumping or diving (W73)

● W16.812 **Jumping or diving into other water striking water surface causing other injury**

● W16.82 **Jumping or diving into other water striking bottom**

● W16.821 **Jumping or diving into other water striking bottom causing drowning and submersion**

Excludes1 drowning and submersion while in other water without jumping or diving (W73)

● W16.822 **Jumping or diving into other water striking bottom causing other injury**

● W16.83 **Jumping or diving into other water striking wall**

● W16.831 **Jumping or diving into other water striking wall causing drowning and submersion**

Excludes1 drowning and submersion while in other water without jumping or diving (W73)

● W16.832 **Jumping or diving into other water striking wall causing other injury**

● W16.9 **Jumping or diving into unspecified water**

X● W16.91 **Jumping or diving into unspecified water causing drowning and submersion**

X● W16.92 **Jumping or diving into unspecified water causing other injury**

● W17 **Other fall from one level to another**

The appropriate 7th character is to be added to each code from category W17

A	initial encounter
D	subsequent encounter
S	sequela

X● W17.Ø **Fall into well**

X● W17.1 **Fall into storm drain or manhole**

X● W17.2 **Fall into hole**

Fall into pit

X● W17.3 **Fall into empty swimming pool**

Excludes1 fall into filled swimming pool (W16.Ø-)

X● W17.4 **Fall from dock**

● W17.8 **Other fall from one level to another**

X● W17.81 **Fall down embankment (hill)**

X● W17.82 **Fall from (out of) grocery cart**

Fall due to grocery cart tipping over

X● W17.89 **Other fall from one level to another**

Fall from cherry picker
Fall from lifting device
Fall from mobile elevated work platform [MEWP]
Fall from sky lift

CHAPTER 2Ø (VØ1-Y99)

◄ New ◄ Revised ~~deleted~~ Deleted OGCR Official Guidelines X Assign placeholder X ● Use Additional Character(s) Excludes 1 Excludes 2 Includes Use additional Code first Code also Unspecified

● W18 Other slipping, tripping and stumbling and falls

The appropriate 7th character is to be added to each code from category W18

A	initial encounter
D	subsequent encounter
S	sequela

● W18.0 Fall due to bumping against object

Striking against object with subsequent fall

Excludes1 fall on same level due to slipping, tripping, or stumbling with subsequent striking against object (W01.1-)

X● W18.00 Striking against unspecified object with subsequent fall

X● W18.01 Striking against sports equipment with subsequent fall

X● W18.02 Striking against glass with subsequent fall

X● W18.09 Striking against other object with subsequent fall

● W18.1 Fall from or off toilet

X● W18.11 Fall from or off toilet without subsequent striking against object

Fall from (off) toilet NOS

X● W18.12 Fall from or off toilet with subsequent striking against object

X● W18.2 Fall in (into) shower or empty bathtub

Excludes1 fall in full bathtub causing drowning or submersion (W16.21-)

● W18.3 Other and unspecified fall on same level

X● W18.30 Fall on same level, unspecified

X● W18.31 Fall on same level due to stepping on an object

Fall on same level due to stepping on an animal

Excludes1 slipping, tripping and stumbling without fall due to stepping on animal (W18.41)

X● W18.39 Other fall on same level

● W18.4 Slipping, tripping and stumbling without falling

Excludes1 collision with another person without fall (W51)

X● W18.40 Slipping, tripping and stumbling without falling, unspecified

X● W18.41 Slipping, tripping and stumbling without falling due to stepping on object

Slipping, tripping and stumbling without falling due to stepping on animal

Excludes1 slipping, tripping and stumbling with fall due to stepping on animal (W18.31)

X● W18.42 Slipping, tripping and stumbling without falling due to stepping into hole or opening

X● W18.43 Slipping, tripping and stumbling without falling due to stepping from one level to another

X● W18.49 Other slipping, tripping and stumbling without falling

X● W19 Unspecified fall

Accidental fall NOS

The appropriate 7th character is to be added to code W19

A	initial encounter
D	subsequent encounter
S	sequela

EXPOSURE TO INANIMATE MECHANICAL FORCES (W20-W49)

Excludes1 assault (X92-Y09) ◄
contact or collision with animals or persons (W50-W64)
exposure to inanimate mechanical forces involving military or war operations (Y36.-, Y37.-)
intentional self-harm (X71-X83)

● W20 Struck by thrown, projected or falling object

Code first any associated:
cataclysm (X34-X39)
lightning strike (T75.00)

Excludes1 falling object in machinery accident (W24, W28-W31)
falling object in transport accident (V01-V99)
object set in motion by explosion (W35-W40)
object set in motion by firearm (W32-W34)
struck by thrown sports equipment (W21.-)

The appropriate 7th character is to be added to each code from category W20

A	initial encounter
D	subsequent encounter
S	sequela

X● W20.0 Struck by falling object in cave-in

Excludes2 asphyxiation due to cave-in (T71.21)

X● W20.1 Struck by object due to collapse of building

Excludes1 struck by object due to collapse of burning building (X00.2, X02.2)

X● W20.8 Other cause of strike by thrown, projected or falling object

Excludes1 struck by thrown sports equipment (W21.-)

● W21 Striking against or struck by sports equipment

Excludes1 assault with sports equipment (Y08.0-)
striking against or struck by sports equipment with subsequent fall (W18.01)

The appropriate 7th character is to be added to each code from category W21

A	initial encounter
D	subsequent encounter
S	sequela

● W21.0 Struck by hit or thrown ball

X● W21.00 Struck by hit or thrown ball, unspecified type

X● W21.01 Struck by football

X● W21.02 Struck by soccer ball

X● W21.03 Struck by baseball

X● W21.04 Struck by golf ball

X● W21.05 Struck by basketball

X● W21.06 Struck by volleyball

X● W21.07 Struck by softball

X● W21.09 Struck by other hit or thrown ball

● W21.1 Struck by bat, racquet or club

X● W21.11 Struck by baseball bat

X● W21.12 Struck by tennis racquet

X● W21.13 Struck by golf club

X● W21.19 Struck by other bat, racquet or club

CHAPTER 20 (V01-Y99)

● W21.2 **Struck by hockey stick or puck**
● W21.21 **Struck by hockey stick**
● W21.210 **Struck by ice hockey stick**
● W21.211 **Struck by field hockey stick**
● W21.22 **Struck by hockey puck**
● W21.220 **Struck by ice hockey puck**
● W21.221 **Struck by field hockey puck**
● W21.3 **Struck by sports foot wear**
X● W21.31 **Struck by shoe cleats**
Stepped on by shoe cleats
X● W21.32 **Struck by skate blades**
Skated over by skate blades
X● W21.39 **Struck by other sports foot wear**
X● W21.4 **Striking against diving board**
Use additional code for subsequent falling into water, if applicable (W16.-)
● W21.8 **Striking against or struck by other sports equipment**
X● W21.81 **Striking against or struck by football helmet**
X● W21.89 **Striking against or struck by other sports equipment**
X● W21.9 **Striking against or struck by unspecified sports equipment**

● W22 **Striking against or struck by other objects**
Excludes1 striking against or struck by object with subsequent fall (W18.09)
The appropriate 7th character is to be added to each code from category W22

A	initial encounter
D	subsequent encounter
S	sequela

● W22.0 **Striking against stationary object**
Excludes1 striking against stationary sports equipment (W21.8)
X● W22.01 **Walked into wall**
X● W22.02 **Walked into lamppost**
X● W22.03 **Walked into furniture**
● W22.04 **Striking against wall of swimming pool**
● W22.041 **Striking against wall of swimming pool causing drowning and submersion**
Excludes1 drowning and submersion while swimming without striking against wall (W67)
● W22.042 **Striking against wall of swimming pool causing other injury**
X● W22.09 **Striking against other stationary object**
● W22.1 **Striking against or struck by automobile airbag**
X● W22.10 **Striking against or struck by unspecified automobile airbag**
X● W22.11 **Striking against or struck by driver side automobile airbag**
X● W22.12 **Striking against or struck by front passenger side automobile airbag**
X● W22.19 **Striking against or struck by other automobile airbag**
X● W22.8 **Striking against or struck by other objects**
Striking against or struck by object NOS
Excludes1 struck by thrown, projected or falling object (W20.-)

● W23 **Caught, crushed, jammed or pinched in or between objects**
Excludes1 injury caused by cutting or piercing instruments (W25-W27)
injury caused by firearms malfunction (W32.1, W33.1-, W34.1-)
injury caused by lifting and transmission devices (W24.-)
injury caused by machinery (W28-W31)
injury caused by nonpowered hand tools (W27.-)
injury caused by transport vehicle being used as a means of transportation (V01-V99)
injury caused by struck by thrown, projected or falling object (W20.-)
The appropriate 7th character is to be added to each code from category W23

A	initial encounter
D	subsequent encounter
S	sequela

X● W23.0 **Caught, crushed, jammed, or pinched between moving objects**
X● W23.1 **Caught, crushed, jammed, or pinched between stationary objects**

● W24 **Contact with lifting and transmission devices, not elsewhere classified**
Excludes1 transport accidents (V01-V99)
The appropriate 7th character is to be added to each code from category W24

A	initial encounter
D	subsequent encounter
S	sequela

X● W24.0 **Contact with lifting devices, not elsewhere classified**
Contact with chain hoist
Contact with drive belt
Contact with pulley (block)
X● W24.1 **Contact with transmission devices, not elsewhere classified**
Contact with transmission belt or cable

X● W25 **Contact with sharp glass**
Code first any associated:
injury due to flying glass from explosion or firearm discharge (W32-W40)
transport accident (V00-V99)
Excludes1 fall on same level due to slipping, tripping and stumbling with subsequent striking against sharp glass (W01.10)
striking against sharp glass with subsequent fall (W18.02)
Excludes2 glass embedded in skin (W45) ◀
The appropriate 7th character is to be added to code W25

A	initial encounter
D	subsequent encounter
S	sequela

● W26 **Contact with other sharp objects** ◀
Excludes2 sharp object(s) embedded in skin (W45) ◀
The appropriate 7th character is to be added to each code from category W26

A	initial encounter
D	subsequent encounter
S	sequela

X● W26.0 **Contact with knife**
Excludes1 contact with electric knife (W29.1)
X● W26.1 **Contact with sword or dagger**
X● W26.2 **Contact with edge of stiff paper** ◀
Paper cut ◀
X● W26.8 **Contact with other sharp object(s), not elsewhere classified** ◀
Contact with tin can lid ◀
X● W26.9 **Contact with unspecified sharp object(s)** ◀

CHAPTER 20 (V01-Y99)

◀ New ◀ Revised deleted Deleted OGCR Official Guidelines X Assign placeholder X ● Use Additional Character(s)
Excludes1 Excludes2 Includes Use additional Code first Code also Unspecified

●**W27 Contact with nonpowered hand tool**
The appropriate 7th character is to be added to each code from category W27
A initial encounter
D subsequent encounter
S sequela

X● **W27.0 Contact with workbench tool**
Contact with auger
Contact with axe
Contact with chisel
Contact with handsaw
Contact with screwdriver

X● **W27.1 Contact with garden tool**
Contact with hoe
Contact with nonpowered lawn mower
Contact with pitchfork
Contact with rake

X● **W27.2 Contact with scissors**

X● **W27.3 Contact with needle (sewing)**
Excludes1 contact with hypodermic needle (W46.-)

X● **W27.4 Contact with kitchen utensil**
Contact with fork
Contact with ice-pick
Contact with can-opener NOS

X● **W27.5 Contact with paper-cutter**

X● **W27.8 Contact with other nonpowered hand tool**
Contact with nonpowered sewing machine
Contact with shovel

X●**W28 Contact with powered lawn mower**
Powered lawn mower (commercial) (residential)
Excludes1 contact with nonpowered lawn mower (W27.1)
Excludes2 exposure to electric current (W86.-)
The appropriate 7th character is to be added to code W28
A initial encounter
D subsequent encounter
S sequela

●**W29 Contact with other powered hand tools and household machinery**
Excludes1 contact with commercial machinery (W31.82)
contact with hot household appliance (X15)
contact with nonpowered hand tool (W27.-)
exposure to electric current (W86)
The appropriate 7th character is to be added to each code from category W29
A initial encounter
D subsequent encounter
S sequela

X● **W29.0 Contact with powered kitchen appliance**
Contact with blender
Contact with can-opener
Contact with garbage disposal
Contact with mixer

X● **W29.1 Contact with electric knife**

X● **W29.2 Contact with other powered household machinery**
Contact with electric fan
Contact with powered dryer (clothes) (powered) (spin)
Contact with washing-machine
Contact with sewing machine

X● **W29.3 Contact with powered garden and outdoor hand tools and machinery**
Contact with chainsaw
Contact with edger
Contact with garden cultivator (tiller)
Contact with hedge trimmer
Contact with other powered garden tool
Excludes1 contact with powered lawn mower (W28)

X● **W29.4 Contact with nail gun**

X● **W29.8 Contact with other powered powered hand tools and household machinery**
Contact with do-it-yourself tool NOS

●**W30 Contact with agricultural machinery**
Includes animal-powered farm machine
Excludes1 agricultural transport vehicle accident (V01-V99)
explosion of grain store (W40.8)
exposure to electric current (W86.-)
The appropriate 7th character is to be added to each code from category W30
A initial encounter
D subsequent encounter
S sequela

X● **W30.0 Contact with combine harvester**
Contact with reaper
Contact with thresher

X● **W30.1 Contact with power take-off devices (PTO)**

X● **W30.2 Contact with hay derrick**

X● **W30.3 Contact with grain storage elevator**
Excludes1 explosion of grain store (W40.8)

● **W30.8 Contact with other specified agricultural machinery**

X● **W30.81 Contact with agricultural transport vehicle in stationary use**
Contact with agricultural transport vehicle under repair, not on public roadway
Excludes1 agricultural transport vehicle accident (V01-V99)

X● **W30.89 Contact with other specified agricultural machinery**

X● **W30.9 Contact with unspecified agricultural machinery**
Contact with farm machinery NOS

●**W31 Contact with other and unspecified machinery**
Excludes1 contact with agricultural machinery (W30.-)
contact with machinery in transport under own power or being towed by a vehicle (V01-V99)
exposure to electric current (W86)
The appropriate 7th character is to be added to each code from category W31
A initial encounter
D subsequent encounter
S sequela

X● **W31.0 Contact with mining and earth-drilling machinery**
Contact with bore or drill (land) (seabed)
Contact with shaft hoist
Contact with shaft lift
Contact with undercutter

X● **W31.1 Contact with metalworking machines**
Contact with abrasive wheel
Contact with forging machine
Contact with lathe
Contact with mechanical shears
Contact with metal drilling machine
Contact with milling machine
Contact with power press
Contact with rolling-mill
Contact with metal sawing machine

X● **W31.2 Contact with powered woodworking and forming machines**
Contact with band saw
Contact with bench saw
Contact with circular saw
Contact with molding machine
Contact with overhead plane
Contact with powered saw
Contact with radial saw
Contact with sander
Excludes1 nonpowered woodworking tools (W27.0)

CHAPTER 20 (V01-Y99)

X● **W31.3 Contact with prime movers**
Contact with gas turbine
Contact with internal combustion engine
Contact with steam engine
Contact with water driven turbine

● **W31.8 Contact with other specified machinery**

X● **W31.81 Contact with recreational machinery**
Contact with roller-coaster

X● **W31.82 Contact with other commercial machinery**
Contact with commercial electric fan
Contact with commercial kitchen appliances
Contact with commercial powered dryer (clothes) (powered) (spin)
Contact with commercial washing-machine
Contact with commercial sewing machine

Excludes1 contact with household machinery (W29.-)
contact with powered lawn mower (W28)

X● **W31.83 Contact with special construction vehicle in stationary use**
Contact with special construction vehicle under repair, not on public roadway

Excludes1 special construction vehicle accident (V01-V99)

X● **W31.89 Contact with other specified machinery**

X● **W31.9 Contact with unspecified machinery**
Contact with machinery NOS

● **W32 Accidental handgun discharge and malfunction**

Includes accidental discharge and malfunction of gun for single hand use
accidental discharge and malfunction of pistol
accidental discharge and malfunction of revolver
handgun discharge and malfunction NOS

Excludes1 accidental airgun discharge and malfunction (W34.010, W34.110)
accidental BB gun discharge and malfunction (W34.010, W34.110)
accidental pellet gun discharge and malfunction (W34.010, W34.110)
accidental shotgun discharge and malfunction (W33.01, W33.11)
assault by handgun discharge (X93)
handgun discharge involving legal intervention (Y35.0-)
handgun discharge involving military or war operations (Y36.4-)
intentional self-harm by handgun discharge (X72)
Very pistol discharge and malfunction (W34.09, W34.19)

The appropriate 7th character is to be added to each code from category W32

A	initial encounter
D	subsequent encounter
S	sequela

X● **W32.0 Accidental handgun discharge**

X● **W32.1 Accidental handgun malfunction**
Injury due to explosion of handgun (parts)
Injury due to malfunction of mechanism or component of handgun
Injury due to recoil of handgun
Powder burn from handgun

● **W33 Accidental rifle, shotgun and larger firearm discharge and malfunction**

Includes rifle, shotgun and larger firearm discharge and malfunction NOS

Excludes1 accidental airgun discharge and malfunction (W34.010, W34.110)
accidental BB gun discharge and malfunction (W34.010, W34.110)
accidental handgun discharge and malfunction (W32.-)
accidental pellet gun discharge and malfunction (W34.010, W34.110)
assault by rifle, shotgun and larger firearm discharge (X94)
firearm discharge involving legal intervention (Y35.0-)
firearm discharge involving military or war operations (Y36.4-)
intentional self-harm by rifle, shotgun and larger firearm discharge (X73)

The appropriate 7th character is to be added to each code from category W33

A	initial encounter
D	subsequent encounter
S	sequela

● **W33.0 Accidental rifle, shotgun and larger firearm discharge**

X● **W33.00 Accidental discharge of unspecified larger firearm**
Discharge of unspecified larger firearm NOS

X● **W33.01 Accidental discharge of shotgun**
Discharge of shotgun NOS

X● **W33.02 Accidental discharge of hunting rifle**
Discharge of hunting rifle NOS

X● **W33.03 Accidental discharge of machine gun**
Discharge of machine gun NOS

X● **W33.09 Accidental discharge of other larger firearm**
Discharge of other larger firearm NOS

● **W33.1 Accidental rifle, shotgun and larger firearm malfunction**
Injury due to explosion of rifle, shotgun and larger firearm (parts)
Injury due to malfunction of mechanism or component of rifle, shotgun and larger firearm
Injury due to piercing, cutting, crushing or pinching due to (by) slide trigger mechanism, scope or other gun part
Injury due to recoil of rifle, shotgun and larger firearm
Powder burn from rifle, shotgun and larger firearm

X● **W33.10 Accidental malfunction of unspecified larger firearm**
Malfunction of unspecified larger firearm NOS

X● **W33.11 Accidental malfunction of shotgun**
Malfunction of shotgun NOS

X● **W33.12 Accidental malfunction of hunting rifle**
Malfunction of hunting rifle NOS

X● **W33.13 Accidental malfunction of machine gun**
Malfunction of machine gun NOS

X● **W33.19 Accidental malfunction of other larger firearm**
Malfunction of other larger firearm NOS

● W34 Accidental discharge and malfunction from other and unspecified firearms and guns

The appropriate 7th character is to be added to each code from category W34

A initial encounter
D subsequent encounter
S sequela

● W34.0 Accidental discharge from other and unspecified firearms and guns

X● W34.00 Accidental discharge from unspecified firearms or gun

Discharge from firearm NOS
Gunshot wound NOS
Shot NOS

● W34.01 Accidental discharge of gas, air or spring-operated guns

● W34.010 Accidental discharge of airgun

Accidental discharge of BB gun
Accidental discharge of pellet gun

● W34.011 Accidental discharge of paintball gun

Accidental injury due to paintball discharge

● W34.018 Accidental discharge of other gas, air or spring-operated gun

X● W34.09 Accidental discharge from other specified firearms

Accidental discharge from Very pistol [flare]

● W34.1 Accidental malfunction from other and unspecified firearms and guns

X● W34.10 Accidental malfunction from unspecified firearms or gun

Firearm malfunction NOS

● W34.11 Accidental malfunction of gas, air or spring-operated guns

● W34.110 Accidental malfunction of airgun

Accidental malfunction of BB gun
Accidental malfunction of pellet gun

● W34.111 Accidental malfunction of paintball gun

Accidental injury due to paintball gun malfunction

● W34.118 Accidental malfunction of other gas, air or spring-operated gun

X● W34.19 Accidental malfunction from other specified firearms

Accidental malfunction from Very pistol [flare]

X● W35 Explosion and rupture of boiler

Excludes1 explosion and rupture of boiler on watercraft (V93.4)

The appropriate 7th character is to be added to code W35

A initial encounter
D subsequent encounter
S sequela

● W36 Explosion and rupture of gas cylinder

The appropriate 7th character is to be added to each code from category W36

A initial encounter
D subsequent encounter
S sequela

X● W36.1 Explosion and rupture of aerosol can

X● W36.2 Explosion and rupture of air tank

X● W36.3 Explosion and rupture of pressurized-gas tank

X● W36.8 Explosion and rupture of other gas cylinder

X● W36.9 Explosion and rupture of unspecified gas cylinder

● W37 Explosion and rupture of pressurized tire, pipe or hose

The appropriate 7th character is to be added to each code from category W37

A initial encounter
D subsequent encounter
S sequela

X● W37.0 Explosion of bicycle tire

X● W37.8 Explosion and rupture of other pressurized tire, pipe or hose

X● W38 Explosion and rupture of other specified pressurized devices

The appropriate 7th character is to be added to code W38

A initial encounter
D subsequent encounter
S sequela

X● W39 Discharge of firework

The appropriate 7th character is to be added to code W39

A initial encounter
D subsequent encounter
S sequela

● W40 Explosion of other materials

Excludes1 assault by explosive material (X96)
explosion involving legal intervention (Y35.1-)
explosion involving military or war operations (Y36.0-, Y36.2-)
intentional self-harm by explosive material (X75)

The appropriate 7th character is to be added to each code from category W40

A initial encounter
D subsequent encounter
S sequela

X● W40.0 Explosion of blasting material

Explosion of blasting cap
Explosion of detonator
Explosion of dynamite
Explosion of explosive (any) used in blasting operations

X● W40.1 Explosion of explosive gases

Explosion of acetylene
Explosion of butane
Explosion of coal gas
Explosion in mine NOS
Explosion of explosive gas
Explosion of fire damp
Explosion of gasoline fumes
Explosion of methane
Explosion of propane

X● W40.8 Explosion of other specified explosive materials

Explosion in dump NOS
Explosion in factory NOS
Explosion in grain store
Explosion in munitions

Excludes1 explosion involving legal intervention (Y35.1-)
explosion involving military or war operations (Y36.0-, Y36.2-)

X● W40.9 Explosion of unspecified explosive materials

Explosion NOS

● W42 Exposure to noise

The appropriate 7th character is to be added to each code from category W42

A initial encounter
D subsequent encounter
S sequela

X● W42.0 Exposure to supersonic waves

X● W42.9 Exposure to other noise

Exposure to sound waves NOS

CHAPTER 20 (V01-Y99)

● **W45 Foreign body or object entering through skin**

Includes foreign body or object embedded in skin ◀
nail embedded in skin ◀

Excludes2 contact with hand tools (nonpowered) (powered) (W27-W29)
contact with other sharp object(s) (W26.-)
contact with sharp glass (W25.-)
struck by objects (W20-W22)

The appropriate 7th character is to be added to each code from category W45

A initial encounter
D subsequent encounter
S sequela

X● **W45.0 Nail entering through skin**

~~W45.1 Paper entering through skin~~
~~Paper cut~~

~~W45.2 Lid of can entering through skin~~

X● **W45.8 Other foreign body or object entering through skin**
Splinter in skin NOS

● **W46 Contact with hypodermic needle**

The appropriate 7th character is to be added to each code from category W46

A initial encounter
D subsequent encounter
S sequela

X● **W46.0 Contact with hypodermic needle**
Hypodermic needle stick NOS

X● **W46.1 Contact with contaminated hypodermic needle**

● **W49 Exposure to other inanimate mechanical forces**

Includes exposure to abnormal gravitational [G] forces
exposure to inanimate mechanical forces NEC

Excludes1 exposure to inanimate mechanical forces involving military or war operations (Y36.-, Y37.-)

The appropriate 7th character is to be added to each code from category W49

A initial encounter
D subsequent encounter
S sequela

● **W49.0 Item causing external constriction**

X● **W49.01 Hair causing external constriction**

X● **W49.02 String or thread causing external constriction**

X● **W49.03 Rubber band causing external constriction**

X● **W49.04 Ring or other jewelry causing external constriction**

X● **W49.09 Other item causing external constriction**

X● **W49.9 Exposure to other inanimate mechanical forces**

EXPOSURE TO ANIMATE MECHANICAL FORCES (W50-W64)

Excludes1 toxic effect of contact with venomous animals and plants (T63.-)

● **W50 Accidental hit, strike, kick, twist, bite or scratch by another person**

Includes hit, strike, kick, twist, bite, or scratch by another person NOS

Excludes1 assault by bodily force (Y04)
struck by objects (W20-W22)

The appropriate 7th character is to be added to each code from category W50

A initial encounter
D subsequent encounter
S sequela

X● **W50.0 Accidental hit or strike by another person**
Hit or strike by another person NOS

X● **W50.1 Accidental kick by another person**
Kick by another person NOS

X● **W50.2 Accidental twist by another person**
Twist by another person NOS

X● **W50.3 Accidental bite by another person**
Human bite
Bite by another person NOS

X● **W50.4 Accidental scratch by another person**
Scratch by another person NOS

X● **W51 Accidental striking against or bumped into by another person**

Excludes1 assault by striking against or bumping into by another person (Y04.2)
fall due to collision with another person (W03)

The appropriate 7th character is to be added to code W51

A initial encounter
D subsequent encounter
S sequela

X● **W52 Crushed, pushed or stepped on by crowd or human stampede**
Crushed, pushed or stepped on by crowd or human stampede with or without fall

The appropriate 7th character is to be added to code W52

A initial encounter
D subsequent encounter
S sequela

● **W53 Contact with rodent**

Includes contact with saliva, feces or urine of rodent

The appropriate 7th character is to be added to each code from category W53

A initial encounter
D subsequent encounter
S sequela

● **W53.0 Contact with mouse**

X● **W53.01 Bitten by mouse**

X● **W53.09 Other contact with mouse**

● **W53.1 Contact with rat**

X● **W53.11 Bitten by rat**

X● **W53.19 Other contact with rat**

● **W53.2 Contact with squirrel**

X● **W53.21 Bitten by squirrel**

X● **W53.29 Other contact with squirrel**

● **W53.8 Contact with other rodent**

X● **W53.81 Bitten by other rodent**

X● **W53.89 Other contact with other rodent**

● **W54 Contact with dog**

Includes contact with saliva, feces or urine of dog

The appropriate 7th character is to be added to each code from category W54

A initial encounter
D subsequent encounter
S sequela

X● **W54.0 Bitten by dog**

X● **W54.1 Struck by dog**
Knocked over by dog

X● **W54.8 Other contact with dog**

CHAPTER 20 (V01-Y99)

● **W55 Contact with other mammals**

Includes contact with saliva, feces or urine of mammal

Excludes1 animal being ridden - see transport accidents
bitten or struck by dog (W54)
bitten or struck by rodent (W53.-)
contact with marine mammals (W56.X-)

The appropriate 7th character is to be added to each code from category W55

A	initial encounter
D	subsequent encounter
S	sequela

● **W55.Ø Contact with cat**
X● **W55.Ø1 Bitten by cat**
X● **W55.Ø3 Scratched by cat**
X● **W55.Ø9 Other contact with cat**

● **W55.1 Contact with horse**
X● **W55.11 Bitten by horse**
X● **W55.12 Struck by horse**
X● **W55.19 Other contact with horse**

● **W55.2 Contact with cow**
Contact with bull
X● **W55.21 Bitten by cow**
X● **W55.22 Struck by cow**
Gored by bull
X● **W55.29 Other contact with cow**

● **W55.3 Contact with other hoof stock**
Contact with goats
Contact with sheep
X● **W55.31 Bitten by other hoof stock**
X● **W55.32 Struck by other hoof stock**
Gored by goat
Gored by ram
X● **W55.39 Other contact with other hoof stock**

● **W55.4 Contact with pig**
X● **W55.41 Bitten by pig**
X● **W55.42 Struck by pig**
X● **W55.49 Other contact with pig**

● **W55.5 Contact with raccoon**
X● **W55.51 Bitten by raccoon**
X● **W55.52 Struck by raccoon**
X● **W55.59 Other contact with raccoon**

● **W55.8 Contact with other mammals**
X● **W55.81 Bitten by other mammals**
X● **W55.82 Struck by other mammals**
X● **W55.89 Other contact with other mammals**

● **W56 Contact with nonvenomous marine animal**

Excludes1 contact with venomous marine animal (T63.-)

The appropriate 7th character is to be added to each code from category W56

A	initial encounter
D	subsequent encounter
S	sequela

● **W56.Ø Contact with dolphin**
X● **W56.Ø1 Bitten by dolphin**
X● **W56.Ø2 Struck by dolphin**
X● **W56.Ø9 Other contact with dolphin**

● **W56.1 Contact with sea lion**
X● **W56.11 Bitten by sea lion**
X● **W56.12 Struck by sea lion**
X● **W56.19 Other contact with sea lion**

● **W56.2 Contact with orca**
Contact with killer whale
X● **W56.21 Bitten by orca**
X● **W56.22 Struck by orca**
X● **W56.29 Other contact with orca**

● **W56.3 Contact with other marine mammals**
X● **W56.31 Bitten by other marine mammals**
X● **W56.32 Struck by other marine mammals**
X● **W56.39 Other contact with other marine mammals**

● **W56.4 Contact with shark**
X● **W56.41 Bitten by shark**
X● **W56.42 Struck by shark**
X● **W56.49 Other contact with shark**

● **W56.5 Contact with other fish**
X● **W56.51 Bitten by other fish**
X● **W56.52 Struck by other fish**
X● **W56.59 Other contact with other fish**

● **W56.8 Contact with other nonvenomous marine animals**
X● **W56.81 Bitten by other nonvenomous marine animals**
X● **W56.82 Struck by other nonvenomous marine animals**
X● **W56.89 Other contact with other nonvenomous marine animals**

X● **W57 Bitten or stung by nonvenomous insect and other nonvenomous arthropods**

Excludes1 contact with venomous insects and arthropods (T63.2-, T63.3-, T63.4-)

The appropriate 7th character is to be added to code W57

A	initial encounter
D	subsequent encounter
S	sequela

● **W58 Contact with crocodile or alligator**

The appropriate 7th character is to be added to each code from category W58

A	initial encounter
D	subsequent encounter
S	sequela

● **W58.Ø Contact with alligator**
X● **W58.Ø1 Bitten by alligator**
X● **W58.Ø2 Struck by alligator**
X● **W58.Ø3 Crushed by alligator**
X● **W58.Ø9 Other contact with alligator**

● **W58.1 Contact with crocodile**
X● **W58.11 Bitten by crocodile**
X● **W58.12 Struck by crocodile**
X● **W58.13 Crushed by crocodile**
X● **W58.19 Other contact with crocodile**

● **W59 Contact with other nonvenomous reptiles**

Excludes1 contact with venomous reptile (T63.Ø-, T63.1-)

The appropriate 7th character is to be added to each code from category W59

A	initial encounter
D	subsequent encounter
S	sequela

● **W59.Ø Contact with nonvenomous lizards**
X● **W59.Ø1 Bitten by nonvenomous lizards**
X● **W59.Ø2 Struck by nonvenomous lizards**
X● **W59.Ø9 Other contact with nonvenomous lizards**
Exposure to nonvenomous lizards

CHAPTER 2Ø (VØ1-Y99)

●W59.1 Contact with nonvenomous snakes
X●W59.11 Bitten by nonvenomous snake
X●W59.12 Struck by nonvenomous snake
X●W59.13 Crushed by nonvenomous snake
X●W59.19 Other contact with nonvenomous snake
●W59.2 Contact with turtles
Excludes1 contact with tortoises (W59.8-)
X●W59.21 Bitten by turtle
X●W59.22 Struck by turtle
X●W59.29 Other contact with turtle
Exposure to turtles
●W59.8 Contact with other nonvenomous reptiles
X●W59.81 Bitten by other nonvenomous reptiles
X●W59.82 Struck by other nonvenomous reptiles
X●W59.83 Crushed by other nonvenomous reptiles
X●W59.89 Other contact with other nonvenomous reptiles

X●W6Ø Contact with nonvenomous plant thorns and spines and sharp leaves
Excludes1 contact with venomous plants (T63.X7-)
The appropriate 7th character is to be added to code W6Ø
A initial encounter
D subsequent encounter
S sequela

●W61 Contact with birds (domestic) (wild)
Includes contact with excreta of birds
The appropriate 7th character is to be added to each code from category W61
A initial encounter
D subsequent encounter
S sequela
●W61.Ø Contact with parrot
X●W61.Ø1 Bitten by parrot
X●W61.Ø2 Struck by parrot
X●W61.Ø9 Other contact with parrot
Exposure to parrots
●W61.1 Contact with macaw
X●W61.11 Bitten by macaw
X●W61.12 Struck by macaw
X●W61.19 Other contact with macaw
Exposure to macaws
●W61.2 Contact with other psittacines
X●W61.21 Bitten by other psittacines
X●W61.22 Struck by other psittacines
X●W61.29 Other contact with other psittacines
Exposure to other psittacines
●W61.3 Contact with chicken
X●W61.32 Struck by chicken
X●W61.33 Pecked by chicken
X●W61.39 Other contact with chicken
Exposure to chickens
●W61.4 Contact with turkey
X●W61.42 Struck by turkey
X●W61.43 Pecked by turkey
X●W61.49 Other contact with turkey
●W61.5 Contact with goose
X●W61.51 Bitten by goose
X●W61.52 Struck by goose
X●W61.59 Other contact with goose
●W61.6 Contact with duck
X●W61.61 Bitten by duck
X●W61.62 Struck by duck
X●W61.69 Other contact with duck
●W61.9 Contact with other birds
X●W61.91 Bitten by other birds
X●W61.92 Struck by other birds
X●W61.99 Other contact with other birds
Contact with bird NOS

●W62 Contact with nonvenomous amphibians
Excludes1 contact with venomous amphibians (T63.81-R63.83)
The appropriate 7th character is to be added to each code from category W62
A initial encounter
D subsequent encounter
S sequela
X●W62.Ø Contact with nonvenomous frogs
X●W62.1 Contact with nonvenomous toads
X●W62.9 Contact with other nonvenomous amphibians

X●W64 Exposure to other animate mechanical forces
Includes exposure to nonvenomous animal NOS
Excludes1 contact with venomous animal (T63.-)
The appropriate 7th character is to be added to code W64
A initial encounter
D subsequent encounter
S sequela

ACCIDENTAL NON-TRANSPORT DROWNING AND SUBMERSION (W65-W74)

Excludes1 accidental drowning and submersion due to fall into water (W16.-)
accidental drowning and submersion due to water transport accident (V9Ø.-, V92.-)
Excludes2 accidental drowning and submersion due to cataclysm (X34-X39)

X●W65 Accidental drowning and submersion while in bathtub
Excludes1 accidental drowning and submersion due to fall in (into) bathtub (W16.211)
The appropriate 7th character is to be added to code W65
A initial encounter
D subsequent encounter
S sequela

X●W67 Accidental drowning and submersion while in swimming pool
Excludes1 accidental drowning and submersion due to fall into swimming pool (W16.Ø11, W16.Ø21, W16.Ø31)
accidental drowning and submersion due to striking into wall of swimming pool (W22.Ø41)
The appropriate 7th character is to be added to code W67
A initial encounter
D subsequent encounter
S sequela

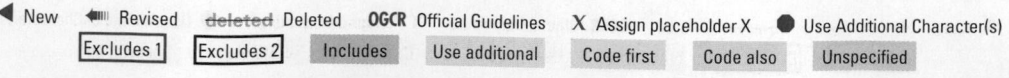

X●W69 Accidental drowning and submersion while in natural water
Accidental drowning and submersion while in lake
Accidental drowning and submersion while in open sea
Accidental drowning and submersion while in river
Accidental drowning and submersion while in stream
Excludes1 accidental drowning and submersion due to fall into natural body of water (W16.111, W16.121, W16.131)
The appropriate 7th character is to be added to code W69
A initial encounter
D subsequent encounter
S sequela

X● W73 Other specified cause of accidental non-transport drowning and submersion
Accidental drowning and submersion while in quenching tank
Accidental drowning and submersion while in reservoir
Excludes1 accidental drowning and submersion due to fall into other water (W16.311, W16.321, W16.331)
The appropriate 7th character is to be added to code W73
A initial encounter
D subsequent encounter
S sequela

X● W74 Unspecified cause of accidental drowning and submersion
Drowning NOS
The appropriate 7th character is to be added to code W74
A initial encounter
D subsequent encounter
S sequela

EXPOSURE TO ELECTRIC CURRENT, RADIATION AND EXTREME AMBIENT AIR TEMPERATURE AND PRESSURE (W85-W99)

Excludes1 exposure to:
failure in dosage of radiation or temperature during surgical and medical care (Y63.2-Y63.5)
lightning (T75.0-)
natural cold (X31)
natural heat (X30)
natural radiation NOS (X39)
radiological procedure and radiotherapy (Y84.2)
sunlight (X32)

X● W85 Exposure to electric transmission lines
Broken power line
The appropriate 7th character is to be added to code W85
A initial encounter
D subsequent encounter
S sequela

● W86 Exposure to other specified electric current
The appropriate 7th character is to be added to each code from category W86
A initial encounter
D subsequent encounter
S sequela

X● W86.0 Exposure to domestic wiring and appliances

X● W86.1 Exposure to industrial wiring, appliances and electrical machinery
Exposure to conductors
Exposure to control apparatus
Exposure to electrical equipment and machinery
Exposure to transformers

X● W86.8 Exposure to other electric current
Exposure to wiring and appliances in or on farm (not farmhouse)
Exposure to wiring and appliances outdoors
Exposure to wiring and appliances in or on public building
Exposure to wiring and appliances in or on residential institutions
Exposure to wiring and appliances in or on schools

● W88 Exposure to ionizing radiation
Excludes1 exposure to sunlight (X32)
The appropriate 7th character is to be added to each code from category W88
A initial encounter
D subsequent encounter
S sequela

X● W88.0 Exposure to X-rays

X● W88.1 Exposure to radioactive isotopes

X● W88.8 Exposure to other ionizing radiation

● W89 Exposure to man-made visible and ultraviolet light
Includes exposure to welding light (arc)
Excludes1 exposure to sunlight (X32) ◀
The appropriate 7th character is to be added to each code from category W89
A initial encounter
D subsequent encounter
S sequela

X● W89.0 Exposure to welding light (arc)

X● W89.1 Exposure to tanning bed

X● W89.8 Exposure to other man-made visible and ultraviolet light

X● W89.9 Exposure to unspecified man-made visible and ultraviolet light

● W90 Exposure to other nonionizing radiation
Excludes1 exposure to sunlight (X32)
The appropriate 7th character is to be added to each code from category W90
A initial encounter
D subsequent encounter
S sequela

X● W90.0 Exposure to radiofrequency

X● W90.1 Exposure to infrared radiation

X● W90.2 Exposure to laser radiation

X● W90.8 Exposure to other nonionizing radiation

X● W92 Exposure to excessive heat of man-made origin
The appropriate 7th character is to be added to code W92
A initial encounter
D subsequent encounter
S sequela

● W93 Exposure to excessive cold of man-made origin
The appropriate 7th character is to be added to each code from category W93
A initial encounter
D subsequent encounter
S sequela

● W93.0 Contact with or inhalation of dry ice

X● W93.01 Contact with dry ice

X● W93.02 Inhalation of dry ice

● W93.1 Contact with or inhalation of liquid air

X● W93.11 Contact with liquid air
Contact with liquid hydrogen
Contact with liquid nitrogen

X● W93.12 Inhalation of liquid air
Inhalation of liquid hydrogen
Inhalation of liquid nitrogen

X● W93.2 Prolonged exposure in deep freeze unit or refrigerator

X● W93.8 Exposure to other excessive cold of man-made origin

● **W94 Exposure to high and low air pressure and changes in air pressure**

The appropriate 7th character is to be added to each code from category W94

A	initial encounter
D	subsequent encounter
S	sequela

X● **W94.0 Exposure to prolonged high air pressure**

● **W94.1 Exposure to prolonged low air pressure**

X● **W94.11 Exposure to residence or prolonged visit at high altitude**

X● **W94.12 Exposure to other prolonged low air pressure**

● **W94.2 Exposure to rapid changes in air pressure during ascent**

X● **W94.21 Exposure to reduction in atmospheric pressure while surfacing from deep-water diving**

X● **W94.22 Exposure to reduction in atmospheric pressure while surfacing from underground**

X● **W94.23 Exposure to sudden change in air pressure in aircraft during ascent**

X● **W94.29 Exposure to other rapid changes in air pressure during ascent**

● **W94.3 Exposure to rapid changes in air pressure during descent**

X● **W94.31 Exposure to sudden change in air pressure in aircraft during descent**

X● **W94.32 Exposure to high air pressure from rapid descent in water**

X● **W94.39 Exposure to other rapid changes in air pressure during descent**

X● **W99 Exposure to other man-made environmental factors**

The appropriate 7th character is to be added to code W99

A	initial encounter
D	subsequent encounter
S	sequela

EXPOSURE TO SMOKE, FIRE AND FLAMES (X00-X08)

Excludes1 arson (X97)

Excludes2 explosions (W35-W40)
lightning (T75.0-)
transport accident (V01-V99)

● **X00 Exposure to uncontrolled fire in building or structure**

Includes conflagration in building or structure

Code first any associated cataclysm

Excludes2 exposure to ignition or melting of nightwear (X05)
exposure to ignition or melting of other clothing and apparel (X06.-)
exposure to other specified smoke, fire and flames (X08.-)

The appropriate 7th character is to be added to each code from category X00

A	initial encounter
D	subsequent encounter
S	sequela

X● **X00.0 Exposure to flames in uncontrolled fire in building or structure**

X● **X00.1 Exposure to smoke in uncontrolled fire in building or structure**

X● **X00.2 Injury due to collapse of burning building or structure in uncontrolled fire**

Excludes1 injury due to collapse of building not on fire (W20.1)

X● **X00.3 Fall from burning building or structure in uncontrolled fire**

X● **X00.4 Hit by object from burning building or structure in uncontrolled fire**

X● **X00.5 Jump from burning building or structure in uncontrolled fire**

X● **X00.8 Other exposure to uncontrolled fire in building or structure**

● **X01 Exposure to uncontrolled fire, not in building or structure**

Includes exposure to forest fire

The appropriate 7th character is to be added to each code from category X01

A	initial encounter
D	subsequent encounter
S	sequela

X● **X01.0 Exposure to flames in uncontrolled fire, not in building or structure**

X● **X01.1 Exposure to smoke in uncontrolled fire, not in building or structure**

X● **X01.3 Fall due to uncontrolled fire, not in building or structure**

X● **X01.4 Hit by object due to uncontrolled fire, not in building or structure**

X● **X01.8 Other exposure to uncontrolled fire, not in building or structure**

● **X02 Exposure to controlled fire in building or structure**

Includes exposure to fire in fireplace exposure to fire in stove

The appropriate 7th character is to be added to each code from category X02

A	initial encounter
D	subsequent encounter
S	sequela

X● **X02.0 Exposure to flames in controlled fire in building or structure**

X● **X02.1 Exposure to smoke in controlled fire in building or structure**

X● **X02.2 Injury due to collapse of burning building or structure in controlled fire**

Excludes1 injury due to collapse of building not on fire (W20.1)

X● **X02.3 Fall from burning building or structure in controlled fire**

X● **X02.4 Hit by object from burning building or structure in controlled fire**

X● **X02.5 Jump from burning building or structure in controlled fire**

X● **X02.8 Other exposure to controlled fire in building or structure**

● **X03 Exposure to controlled fire, not in building or structure**

Includes exposure to bon fire exposure to camp fire exposure to trash fire

The appropriate 7th character is to be added to each code from category X03

A	initial encounter
D	subsequent encounter
S	sequela

X● **X03.0 Exposure to flames in controlled fire, not in building or structure**

X● **X03.1 Exposure to smoke in controlled fire, not in building or structure**

X● **X03.3 Fall due to controlled fire, not in building or structure**

X● **X03.4 Hit by object due to controlled fire, not in building or structure**

X● **X03.8 Other exposure to controlled fire, not in building or structure**

X● XØ4 Exposure to ignition of highly flammable material
Exposure to ignition of gasoline
Exposure to ignition of kerosene
Exposure to ignition of petrol
Excludes2 exposure to ignition or melting of nightwear (XØ5)
exposure to ignition or melting of other clothing and apparel (XØ6)
The appropriate 7th character is to be added to code XØ4

A	initial encounter
D	subsequent encounter
S	sequela

X● XØ5 Exposure to ignition or melting of nightwear
Excludes2 exposure to uncontrolled fire in building or structure (XØØ.-)
exposure to uncontrolled fire, not in building or structure (XØ1.-)
exposure to controlled fire in building or structure (XØ2.-)
exposure to controlled fire, not in building or structure (XØ3.-)
exposure to ignition of highly flammable materials (XØ4.-)
The appropriate 7th character is to be added to code XØ5

A	initial encounter
D	subsequent encounter
S	sequela

● XØ6 Exposure to ignition or melting of other clothing and apparel
Excludes2 exposure to uncontrolled fire in building or structure (XØØ.-)
exposure to uncontrolled fire, not in building or structure (XØ1.-)
exposure to controlled fire in building or structure (XØ2.-)
exposure to controlled fire, not in building or structure (XØ3.-)
exposure to ignition of highly flammable materials (XØ4.-)
The appropriate 7th character is to be added to each code from category XØ6

A	initial encounter
D	subsequent encounter
S	sequela

X● XØ6.Ø Exposure to ignition of plastic jewelry
X● XØ6.1 Exposure to melting of plastic jewelry
X● XØ6.2 Exposure to ignition of other clothing and apparel
X● XØ6.3 Exposure to melting of other clothing and apparel

● XØ8 Exposure to other specified smoke, fire and flames
The appropriate 7th character is to be added to each code from category XØ8

A	initial encounter
D	subsequent encounter
S	sequela

● XØ8.Ø Exposure to bed fire
Exposure to mattress fire
X● XØ8.ØØ Exposure to bed fire due to unspecified burning material
X● XØ8.Ø1 Exposure to bed fire due to burning cigarette
X● XØ8.Ø9 Exposure to bed fire due to other burning material

● XØ8.1 Exposure to sofa fire
X● XØ8.1Ø Exposure to sofa fire due to unspecified burning material
X● XØ8.11 Exposure to sofa fire due to burning cigarette
X● XØ8.19 Exposure to sofa fire due to other burning material

● XØ8.2 Exposure to other furniture fire
X● XØ8.2Ø Exposure to other furniture fire due to unspecified burning material
X● XØ8.21 Exposure to other furniture fire due to burning cigarette
X● XØ8.29 Exposure to other furniture fire due to other burning material

X● XØ8.8 Exposure to other specified smoke, fire and flames

CONTACT WITH HEAT AND HOT SUBSTANCES (X1Ø-X19)

Excludes1 exposure to excessive natural heat (X3Ø)
exposure to fire and flames (XØØ-XØ9)

● X1Ø Contact with hot drinks, food, fats and cooking oils
The appropriate 7th character is to be added to each code from category X1Ø

A	initial encounter
D	subsequent encounter
S	sequela

X● X1Ø.Ø Contact with hot drinks
X● X1Ø.1 Contact with hot food
X● X1Ø.2 Contact with fats and cooking oils

● X11 Contact with hot tap-water
Includes contact with boiling tap-water
contact with boiling water NOS
Excludes1 contact with water heated on stove (X12)
The appropriate 7th character is to be added to each code from category X11

A	initial encounter
D	subsequent encounter
S	sequela

X● X11.Ø Contact with hot water in bath or tub
Excludes1 contact with running hot water in bath or tub (X11.1)
X● X11.1 Contact with running hot water
Contact with hot water running out of hose
Contact with hot water running out of tap
X● X11.8 Contact with other hot tap-water
Contact with hot water in bucket
Contact with hot tap-water NOS

X● X12 Contact with other hot fluids
Contact with water heated on stove
Excludes1 hot (liquid) metals (X18)
The appropriate 7th character is to be added to code X12

A	initial encounter
D	subsequent encounter
S	sequela

● X13 Contact with steam and other hot vapors
The appropriate 7th character is to be added to each code from category X13

A	initial encounter
D	subsequent encounter
S	sequela

X● X13.Ø Inhalation of steam and other hot vapors
X● X13.1 Other contact with steam and other hot vapors

●X14 Contact with hot air and other hot gases

The appropriate 7th character is to be added to each code from category X14

A	initial encounter
D	subsequent encounter
S	sequela

X●X14.0 Inhalation of hot air and gases

X●X14.1 Other contact with hot air and other hot gases

●X15 Contact with hot household appliances

Excludes1 contact with heating appliances (X16)
contact with powered household appliances (W29.-)
exposure to controlled fire in building or structure due to household appliance (X02.8)
exposure to household appliances electrical current (W86.0)

The appropriate 7th character is to be added to each code from category X15

A	initial encounter
D	subsequent encounter
S	sequela

X●X15.0 Contact with hot stove (kitchen)

X●X15.1 Contact with hot toaster

X●X15.2 Contact with hotplate

X●X15.3 Contact with hot saucepan or skillet

X●X15.8 Contact with other hot household appliances

Contact with cooker
Contact with kettle
Contact with light bulbs

X●X16 Contact with hot heating appliances, radiators and pipes

Excludes1 contact with powered appliances (W29.-)
exposure to controlled fire in building or structure due to appliance (X02.8)
exposure to industrial appliances electrical current (W86.1)

The appropriate 7th character is to be added to code X16

A	initial encounter
D	subsequent encounter
S	sequela

X●X17 Contact with hot engines, machinery and tools

Excludes1 contact with hot heating appliances, radiators and pipes (X16)
contact with hot household appliances (X15)

The appropriate 7th character is to be added to code X17

A	initial encounter
D	subsequent encounter
S	sequela

X●X18 Contact with other hot metals

Contact with liquid metal

The appropriate 7th character is to be added to code X18

A	initial encounter
D	subsequent encounter
S	sequela

X●X19 Contact with other heat and hot substances

Excludes1 objects that are not normally hot, e.g., an object made hot by a house fire (X00-X09)

The appropriate 7th character is to be added to code X19

A	initial encounter
D	subsequent encounter
S	sequela

EXPOSURE TO FORCES OF NATURE (X30-X39)

X●X30 Exposure to excessive natural heat

Exposure to excessive heat as the cause of sunstroke
Exposure to heat NOS

Excludes1 excessive heat of man-made origin (W92)
exposure to man-made radiation (W89)
exposure to sunlight (X32)
exposure to tanning bed (W89)

The appropriate 7th character is to be added to code X30

A	initial encounter
D	subsequent encounter
S	sequela

X●X31 Exposure to excessive natural cold

Excessive cold as the cause of chilblains NOS
Excessive cold as the cause of immersion foot or hand
Exposure to cold NOS
Exposure to weather conditions

Excludes1 cold of man-made origin (W93.-)
contact with or inhalation of dry ice (W93.-)
contact with or inhalation of liquefied gas (W93.-)

The appropriate 7th character is to be added to code X31

A	initial encounter
D	subsequent encounter
S	sequela

X●X32 Exposure to sunlight

Excludes1 ~~radiation-related disorders of the skin and subcutaneous tissue (L55-L59)~~
man-made radiation (tanning bed) (W89)

The appropriate 7th character is to be added to code X32

A	initial encounter
D	subsequent encounter
S	sequela

X●X34 Earthquake

Excludes2 tidal wave (tsunami) due to earthquake (X37.41)

The appropriate 7th character is to be added to code X34

A	initial encounter
D	subsequent encounter
S	sequela

X●X35 Volcanic eruption

Excludes2 tidal wave (tsunami) due to volcanic eruption (X37.41)

The appropriate 7th character is to be added to code X35

A	initial encounter
D	subsequent encounter
S	sequela

●X36 Avalanche, landslide and other earth movements

Includes victim of mudslide of cataclysmic nature

Excludes1 earthquake (X34)

Excludes2 transport accident involving collision with avalanche or landslide not in motion (V01-V99)

The appropriate 7th character is to be added to each code from category X36

A	initial encounter
D	subsequent encounter
S	sequela

X●X36.0 Collapse of dam or man-made structure causing earth movement

X●X36.1 Avalanche, landslide, or mudslide

X37 Cataclysmic storm
The appropriate 7th character is to be added to each code from category X37

A	initial encounter
D	subsequent encounter
S	sequela

X37.0 Hurricane
Storm surge
Typhoon
X37.1 Tornado
Cyclone
Twister
X37.2 Blizzard (snow) (ice)
X37.3 Dust storm
X37.4 Tidalwave
X37.41 Tidal wave due to earthquake or volcanic eruption
Tidal wave NOS
Tsunami
X37.42 Tidal wave due to storm
X37.43 Tidal wave due to landslide
X37.8 Other cataclysmic storms
Cloudburst
Torrential rain
Excludes2 flood (X38)
X37.9 Unspecified cataclysmic storm
Storm NOS
Excludes1 collapse of dam or man-made structure causing earth movement (X39.0)

X38 Flood
Flood arising from remote storm
Flood of cataclysmic nature arising from melting snow
Flood resulting directly from storm
Excludes1 collapse of dam or man-made structure causing earth movement (X39.0)
tidal wave NOS (X37.41)
tidal wave caused by storm (X37.2)
The appropriate 7th character is to be added to code X38

A	initial encounter
D	subsequent encounter
S	sequela

X39 Exposure to other forces of nature
The appropriate 7th character is to be added to each code from category X39

A	initial encounter
D	subsequent encounter
S	sequela

X39.0 Exposure to natural radiation
Excludes1 contact with and (suspected) exposure to radon and other naturally occuring radiation (Z77.123)
exposure to man-made radiation (W88-W90)
exposure to sunlight (X32)
X39.01 Exposure to radon
X39.08 Exposure to other natural radiation
X39.8 Other exposure to forces of nature

OVEREXERTION AND STRENUOUS OR REPETITIVE MOVEMENTS (X50)

X50 Overexertion and strenuous or repetitive movements
The appropriate 7th character is to be added to each code from category X50

A	initial encounter
D	subsequent encounter
S	sequela

X50.0 Overexertion from strenuous movement or load
Lifting heavy objects
Lifting weights
X50.1 Overexertion from prolonged static or awkward postures
Prolonged bending
Prolonged kneeling
Prolonged reaching
Prolonged sitting
Prolonged standing
Prolonged twisting
Static bending
Static kneeling
Static reaching
Static sitting
Static standing
Static twisting
X50.3 Overexertion from repetitive movements
Use of hand as hammer
Excludes2 Overuse from prolonged static or awkward postures (X50.1)
X50.9 Other and unspecified overexertion or strenuous movements or postures
Contact pressure
Contact stress

ACCIDENTAL EXPOSURE TO OTHER SPECIFIED FACTORS (X52, X58)

X52 Prolonged stay in weightless environment
Weightlessness in spacecraft (simulator)
The appropriate 7th character is to be added to code X52

A	initial encounter
D	subsequent encounter
S	sequela

X58 Exposure to other specified factors
Accident NOS
Exposure NOS
The appropriate 7th character is to be added to code X58

A	initial encounter
D	subsequent encounter
S	sequela

INTENTIONAL SELF-HARM (X71-X83)

Purposely self-inflicted injury
Suicide (attempted)

X71 Intentional self-harm by drowning and submersion
The appropriate 7th character is to be added to each code from category X71

A	initial encounter
D	subsequent encounter
S	sequela

X71.0 Intentional self-harm by drowning and submersion while in bathtub
X71.1 Intentional self-harm by drowning and submersion while in swimming pool
X71.2 Intentional self-harm by drowning and submersion after jump into swimming pool

X● X71.3 Intentional self-harm by drowning and submersion in natural water

X● X71.8 Other intentional self-harm by drowning and submersion

X● X71.9 Intentional self-harm by drowning and submersion, unspecified

X● X72 Intentional self-harm by handgun discharge

Intentional self-harm by gun for single hand use

Intentional self-harm by pistol

Intentional self-harm by revolver

Excludes1 Very pistol (X74.8)

The appropriate 7th character is to be added to code X72

A	initial encounter
D	subsequent encounter
S	sequela

● X73 Intentional self-harm by rifle, shotgun and larger firearm discharge

Excludes1 airgun (X74.Ø1)

The appropriate 7th character is to be added to each code from category X73

A	initial encounter
D	subsequent encounter
S	sequela

X● X73.Ø Intentional self-harm by shotgun discharge

X● X73.1 Intentional self-harm by hunting rifle discharge

X● X73.2 Intentional self-harm by machine gun discharge

X● X73.8 Intentional self-harm by other larger firearm discharge

X● X73.9 Intentional self-harm by unspecified larger firearm discharge

● X74 Intentional self-harm by other and unspecified firearm and gun discharge

The appropriate 7th character is to be added to each code from category X74

A	initial encounter
D	subsequent encounter
S	sequela

● X74.Ø Intentional self-harm by gas, air or spring-operated guns

X● X74.Ø1 Intentional self-harm by airgun

Intentional self-harm by BB gun discharge

Intentional self-harm by pellet gun discharge

X● X74.Ø2 Intentional self-harm by paintball gun

X● X74.Ø9 Intentional self-harm by other gas, air or spring-operated gun

X● X74.8 Intentional self-harm by other firearm discharge

Intentional self-harm by Very pistol [flare] discharge

X● X74.9 Intentional self-harm by unspecified firearm discharge

X● X75 Intentional self-harm by explosive material

The appropriate 7th character is to be added to code X75

A	initial encounter
D	subsequent encounter
S	sequela

X● X76 Intentional self-harm by smoke, fire and flames

The appropriate 7th character is to be added to code X76

A	initial encounter
D	subsequent encounter
S	sequela

● X77 Intentional self-harm by steam, hot vapors and hot objects

The appropriate 7th character is to be added to each code from category X77

A	initial encounter
D	subsequent encounter
S	sequela

X● X77.Ø Intentional self-harm by steam or hot vapors

X● X77.1 Intentional self-harm by hot tap water

X● X77.2 Intentional self-harm by other hot fluids

X● X77.3 Intentional self-harm by hot household appliances

X● X77.8 Intentional self-harm by other hot objects

X● X77.9 Intentional self-harm by unspecified hot objects

● X78 Intentional self-harm by sharp object

The appropriate 7th character is to be added to each code from category X78

A	initial encounter
D	subsequent encounter
S	sequela

X● X78.Ø Intentional self-harm by sharp glass

X● X78.1 Intentional self-harm by knife

X● X78.2 Intentional self-harm by sword or dagger

X● X78.8 Intentional self-harm by other sharp object

X● X78.9 Intentional self-harm by unspecified sharp object

X● X79 Intentional self-harm by blunt object

The appropriate 7th character is to be added to code X79

A	initial encounter
D	subsequent encounter
S	sequela

X● X8Ø Intentional self-harm by jumping from a high place

Intentional fall from one level to another

The appropriate 7th character is to be added to code X8Ø

A	initial encounter
D	subsequent encounter
S	sequela

● X81 Intentional self-harm by jumping or lying in front of moving object

The appropriate 7th character is to be added to each code from category X81

A	initial encounter
D	subsequent encounter
S	sequela

X● X81.Ø Intentional self-harm by jumping or lying in front of motor vehicle

X● X81.1 Intentional self-harm by jumping or lying in front of (subway) train

X● X81.8 Intentional self-harm by jumping or lying in front of other moving object

● X82 Intentional self-harm by crashing of motor vehicle

The appropriate 7th character is to be added to each code from category X82

A	initial encounter
D	subsequent encounter
S	sequela

X● X82.Ø Intentional collision of motor vehicle with other motor vehicle

X● X82.1 Intentional collision of motor vehicle with train

X● X82.2 Intentional collision of motor vehicle with tree

X● X82.8 Other intentional self-harm by crashing of motor vehicle

●X83 **Intentional self-harm by other specified means**

Excludes1 intentional self-harm by poisoning or contact with toxic substance - see Table of Drugs and Chemicals

The appropriate 7th character is to be added to each code from category X83

A initial encounter
D subsequent encounter
S sequela

X●X83.0 **Intentional self-harm by crashing of aircraft**

X●X83.1 **Intentional self-harm by electrocution**

X●X83.2 **Intentional self-harm by exposure to extremes of cold**

X●X83.8 **Intentional self-harm by other specified means**

ASSAULT (X92-Y09)

Includes homicide injuries inflicted by another person with intent to injure or kill, by any means

Excludes1 injuries due to legal intervention (Y35.-)
injuries due to operations of war (Y36.-)
injuries due to terrorism (Y38.-)

●X92 **Assault by drowning and submersion**

The appropriate 7th character is to be added to each code from category X92

A initial encounter
D subsequent encounter
S sequela

X●X92.0 **Assault by drowning and submersion while in bathtub**

X●X92.1 **Assault by drowning and submersion while in swimming pool**

X●X92.2 **Assault by drowning and submersion after push into swimming pool**

X●X92.3 **Assault by drowning and submersion in natural water**

X●X92.8 **Other assault by drowning and submersion**

X●X92.9 **Assault by drowning and submersion, unspecified**

X●X93 **Assault by handgun discharge**

Assault by discharge of gun for single hand use
Assault by discharge of pistol
Assault by discharge of revolver

Excludes1 Very pistol (X95.8)

The appropriate 7th character is to be added to code X93

A initial encounter
D subsequent encounter
S sequela

●X94 **Assault by rifle, shotgun and larger firearm discharge**

Excludes1 airgun (X95.01)

The appropriate 7th character is to be added to each code from category X94

A initial encounter
D subsequent encounter
S sequela

X●X94.0 **Assault by shotgun**

X●X94.1 **Assault by hunting rifle**

X●X94.2 **Assault by machine gun**

X●X94.8 **Assault by other larger firearm discharge**

X●X94.9 **Assault by unspecified larger firearm discharge**

●X95 **Assault by other and unspecified firearm and gun discharge**

The appropriate 7th character is to be added to each code from category X95

A initial encounter
D subsequent encounter
S sequela

●X95.0 **Assault by gas, air or spring-operated guns**

X●X95.01 **Assault by airgun discharge**
Assault by BB gun discharge
Assault by pellet gun discharge

X●X95.02 **Assault by paintball gun discharge**

X●X95.09 **Assault by other gas, air or spring-operated gun**

X●X95.8 **Assault by other firearm discharge**
Assault by very pistol [flare] discharge

X●X95.9 **Assault by unspecified firearm discharge**

●X96 **Assault by explosive material**

Excludes1 incendiary device (X97)
terrorism involving explosive material (Y38.2-)

The appropriate 7th character is to be added to each code from category X96

A initial encounter
D subsequent encounter
S sequela

X●X96.0 **Assault by antipersonnel bomb**

Excludes1 antipersonnel bomb use in military or war (Y36.2-)

X●X96.1 **Assault by gasoline bomb**

X●X96.2 **Assault by letter bomb**

X●X96.3 **Assault by fertilizer bomb**

X●X96.4 **Assault by pipe bomb**

X●X96.8 **Assault by other specified explosive**

X●X96.9 **Assault by unspecified explosive**

X●X97 **Assault by smoke, fire and flames**

Assault by arson
Assault by cigarettes
Assault by incendiary device

The appropriate 7th character is to be added to code X97

A initial encounter
D subsequent encounter
S sequela

●X98 **Assault by steam, hot vapors and hot objects**

The appropriate 7th character is to be added to each code from category X98

A initial encounter
D subsequent encounter
S sequela

X●X98.0 **Assault by steam or hot vapors**

X●X98.1 **Assault by hot tap water**

X●X98.2 **Assault by hot fluids**

X●X98.3 **Assault by hot household appliances**

X●X98.8 **Assault by other hot objects**

X●X98.9 **Assault by unspecified hot objects**

CHAPTER 20 (V01-Y99)

● X99 **Assault by sharp object**

Excludes1 assault by strike by sports equipment (Y08.0-)

The appropriate 7th character is to be added to each code from category X99

A	initial encounter
D	subsequent encounter
S	sequela

X● X99.0 **Assault by sharp glass**

X● X99.1 **Assault by knife**

X● X99.2 **Assault by sword or dagger**

X● X99.8 **Assault by other sharp object**

X● X99.9 **Assault by unspecified sharp object**
Assault by stabbing NOS

X● Y00 **Assault by blunt object**

Excludes1 assault by strike by sports equipment (Y08.0)

The appropriate 7th character is to be added to code Y00

A	initial encounter
D	subsequent encounter
S	sequela

X● Y01 **Assault by pushing from high place**

The appropriate 7th character is to be added to code Y01

A	initial encounter
D	subsequent encounter
S	sequela

● Y02 **Assault by pushing or placing victim in front of moving object**

The appropriate 7th character is to be added to each code from category Y02

A	initial encounter
D	subsequent encounter
S	sequela

X● Y02.0 **Assault by pushing or placing victim in front of motor vehicle**

X● Y02.1 **Assault by pushing or placing victim in front of (subway) train**

X● Y02.8 **Assault by pushing or placing victim in front of other moving object**

● Y03 **Assault by crashing of motor vehicle**

The appropriate 7th character is to be added to each code from category Y03

A	initial encounter
D	subsequent encounter
S	sequela

X● Y03.0 **Assault by being hit or run over by motor vehicle**

X● Y03.8 **Other assault by crashing of motor vehicle**

● Y04 **Assault by bodily force**

Excludes1 assault by:
submersion (X92.-)
use of weapon (X93-X95, X99, Y00)

The appropriate 7th character is to be added to each code from category Y04

A	initial encounter
D	subsequent encounter
S	sequela

X● Y04.0 **Assault by unarmed brawl or fight**

X● Y04.1 **Assault by human bite**

X● Y04.2 **Assault by strike against or bumped into by another person**

X● Y04.8 **Assault by other bodily force**
Assault by bodily force NOS

OGCR Section I.C.19.f.

Adult and child abuse, neglect and other maltreatment

Sequence first the appropriate code from categories T74.- or T76.- for abuse, neglect and other maltreatment, followed by any accompanying mental health or injury code(s).

If the documentation in the medical record states abuse or neglect it is coded as confirmed. It is coded as suspected if it is documented as suspected.

For cases of confirmed abuse or neglect an external cause code from the assault section (X92-Y08) should be added to identify the cause of any physical injuries. A perpetrator code (Y07) should be added when the perpetrator of the abuse is known. For suspected cases of abuse or neglect, do not report external cause or perpetrator code.

If a suspected case of abuse, neglect or mistreatment is ruled out during an encounter code Z04.71, Encounter for examination and observation following alleged physical adult abuse, ruled out, or code Z04.72, Encounter for examination and observation following alleged child physical abuse, ruled out, should be used, not a code from T76.

If a suspected case of alleged rape or sexual abuse is ruled out during an encounter code Z04.41, Encounter for examination and observation following alleged physical adult abuse, ruled out, or code Z04.42, Encounter for examination and observation following alleged rape or sexual abuse, ruled out, should be used, not a code from T76.

● Y07 **Perpetrator of assault, maltreatment and neglect**

Note: Codes from this category are for use only in cases of confirmed abuse (T74.-)

Selection of the correct perpetrator code is based on the relationship between the perpetrator and the victim

Includes perpetrator of abandonment
perpetrator of emotional neglect
perpetrator of mental cruelty
perpetrator of physical abuse
perpetrator of physical neglect
perpetrator of sexual abuse
perpetrator of torture

● Y07.0 **Spouse or partner, perpetrator of maltreatment and neglect**
Spouse or partner, perpetrator of maltreatment and neglect against spouse or partner

Y07.01 **Husband, perpetrator of maltreatment and neglect**

Y07.02 **Wife, perpetrator of maltreatment and neglect**

Y07.03 **Male partner, perpetrator of maltreatment and neglect**

Y07.04 **Female partner, perpetrator of maltreatment and neglect**

● Y07.1 **Parent (adoptive) (biological), perpetrator of maltreatment and neglect**

Y07.11 **Biological father, perpetrator of maltreatment and neglect**

Y07.12 **Biological mother, perpetrator of maltreatment and neglect**

Y07.13 **Adoptive father, perpetrator of maltreatment and neglect**

Y07.14 **Adoptive mother, perpetrator of maltreatment and neglect**

● Y07.4 **Other family member, perpetrator of maltreatment and neglect**

● Y07.41 **Sibling, perpetrator of maltreatment and neglect**

Excludes1 stepsibling, perpetrator of maltreatment and neglect (Y07.435, Y07.436)

Y07.410 **Brother, perpetrator of maltreatment and neglect**

Y07.411 **Sister, perpetrator of maltreatment and neglect**

CHAPTER 20 (V01-Y99)

● Y07.42 Foster parent, perpetrator of maltreatment and neglect
Y07.420 Foster father, perpetrator of maltreatment and neglect
Y07.421 Foster mother, perpetrator of maltreatment and neglect
● Y07.43 Stepparent or stepsibling, perpetrator of maltreatment and neglect
Y07.430 Stepfather, perpetrator of maltreatment and neglect
Y07.432 Male friend of parent (co-residing in household), perpetrator of maltreatment and neglect
Y07.433 Stepmother, perpetrator of maltreatment and neglect
Y07.434 Female friend of parent (co-residing in household), perpetrator of maltreatment and neglect
Y07.435 Stepbrother, perpetrator or maltreatment and neglect
Y07.436 Stepsister, perpetrator of maltreatment and neglect
● Y07.49 Other family member, perpetrator of maltreatment and neglect
Y07.490 Male cousin, perpetrator of maltreatment and neglect
Y07.491 Female cousin, perpetrator of maltreatment and neglect
Y07.499 Other family member, perpetrator of maltreatment and neglect
● Y07.5 Non-family member, perpetrator of maltreatment and neglect
Y07.50 Unspecified non-family member, perpetrator of maltreatment and neglect
● Y07.51 Daycare provider, perpetrator of maltreatment and neglect
Y07.510 At-home childcare provider, perpetrator of maltreatment and neglect
Y07.511 Daycare center childcare provider, perpetrator of maltreatment and neglect
Y07.512 At-home adultcare provider, perpetrator of maltreatment and neglect
Y07.513 Adultcare center provider, perpetrator of maltreatment and neglect
Y07.519 Unspecified daycare provider, perpetrator of maltreatment and neglect
● Y07.52 Healthcare provider, perpetrator of maltreatment and neglect
Y07.521 Mental health provider, perpetrator of maltreatment and neglect
Y07.528 Other therapist or healthcare provider, perpetrator of maltreatment and neglect
Nurse perpetrator of maltreatment and neglect
Occupational therapist perpetrator of maltreatment and neglect
Physical therapist perpetrator of maltreatment and neglect
Speech therapist perpetrator of maltreatment and neglect
Y07.529 Unspecified healthcare provider, perpetrator of maltreatment and neglect
Y07.53 Teacher or instructor, perpetrator of maltreatment and neglect
Coach, perpetrator of maltreatment and neglect
Y07.59 Other non-family member, perpetrator of maltreatment and neglect
Y07.9 Unspecified perpetrator of maltreatment and neglect

● Y08 Assault by other specified means
The appropriate 7th character is to be added to each code from category Y08

A	initial encounter
D	subsequent encounter
S	sequela

● Y08.0 Assault by strike by sport equipment
X● Y08.01 Assault by strike by hockey stick
X● Y08.02 Assault by strike by baseball bat
X● Y08.09 Assault by strike by other specified type of sport equipment
● Y08.8 Assault by other specified means
X● Y08.81 Assault by crashing of aircraft
X● Y08.89 Assault by other specified means

● Y09 Assault by unspecified means
Assassination (attempted) NOS
Homicide (attempted) NOS
Manslaughter (attempted) NOS
Murder (attempted) NOS

EVENT OF UNDETERMINED INTENT (Y21-Y33)

Undetermined intent is only for use when there is specific documentation in the record that the intent of the injury cannot be determined. If no such documentation is present, code to accidental (unintentional)

● Y21 Drowning and submersion, undetermined intent
The appropriate 7th character is to be added to each code from category Y21

A	initial encounter
D	subsequent encounter
S	sequela

X● Y21.0 Drowning and submersion while in bathtub, undetermined intent
X● Y21.1 Drowning and submersion after fall into bathtub, undetermined intent
X● Y21.2 Drowning and submersion while in swimming pool, undetermined intent
X● Y21.3 Drowning and submersion after fall into swimming pool, undetermined intent
X● Y21.4 Drowning and submersion in natural water, undetermined intent
X● Y21.8 Other drowning and submersion, undetermined intent
X● Y21.9 Unspecified drowning and submersion, undetermined intent

X● Y22 Handgun discharge, undetermined intent
Discharge of gun for single hand use, undetermined intent
Discharge of pistol, undetermined intent
Discharge of revolver, undetermined intent
Excludes2 very pistol (Y24.8)
The appropriate 7th character is to be added to code Y22

A	initial encounter
D	subsequent encounter
S	sequela

CHAPTER 20 (V01-Y99)

●Y23 Rifle, shotgun and larger firearm discharge, undetermined intent

Excludes2 airgun (Y24.0)

The appropriate 7th character is to be added to each code from category Y23

A	initial encounter
D	subsequent encounter
S	sequela

X●Y23.0 Shotgun discharge, undetermined intent

X●Y23.1 Hunting rifle discharge, undetermined intent

X●Y23.2 Military firearm discharge, undetermined intent

X●Y23.3 Machine gun discharge, undetermined intent

X●Y23.8 Other larger firearm discharge, undetermined intent

X●Y23.9 Unspecified larger firearm discharge, undetermined intent

●Y24 Other and unspecified firearm discharge, undetermined intent

The appropriate 7th character is to be added to each code from category Y24

A	initial encounter
D	subsequent encounter
S	sequela

X●Y24.0 Airgun discharge, undetermined intent

BB gun discharge, undetermined intent

Pellet gun discharge, undetermined intent

X●Y24.8 Other firearm discharge, undetermined intent

Paintball gun discharge, undetermined intent

Very pistol [flare] discharge, undetermined intent

X●Y24.9 Unspecified firearm discharge, undetermined intent

X●Y25 Contact with explosive material, undetermined intent

The appropriate 7th character is to be added to code Y25

A	initial encounter
D	subsequent encounter
S	sequela

X●Y26 Exposure to smoke, fire and flames, undetermined intent

The appropriate 7th character is to be added to code Y26

A	initial encounter
D	subsequent encounter
S	sequela

●Y27 Contact with steam, hot vapors and hot objects, undetermined intent

The appropriate 7th character is to be added to each code from category Y27

A	initial encounter
D	subsequent encounter
S	sequela

X●Y27.0 Contact with steam and hot vapors, undetermined intent

X●Y27.1 Contact with hot tap water, undetermined intent

X●Y27.2 Contact with hot fluids, undetermined intent

X●Y27.3 Contact with hot household appliance, undetermined intent

X●Y27.8 Contact with other hot objects, undetermined intent

X●Y27.9 Contact with unspecified hot objects, undetermined intent

●Y28 Contact with sharp object, undetermined intent

The appropriate 7th character is to be added to each code from category Y28

A	initial encounter
D	subsequent encounter
S	sequela

X●Y28.0 Contact with sharp glass, undetermined intent

X●Y28.1 Contact with knife, undetermined intent

X●Y28.2 Contact with sword or dagger, undetermined intent

X●Y28.8 Contact with other sharp object, undetermined intent

X●Y28.9 Contact with unspecified sharp object, undetermined intent

X●Y29 Contact with blunt object, undetermined intent

The appropriate 7th character is to be added to code Y29

A	initial encounter
D	subsequent encounter
S	sequela

X●Y30 Falling, jumping or pushed from a high place, undetermined intent

Victim falling from one level to another, undetermined intent

The appropriate 7th character is to be added to code Y30

A	initial encounter
D	subsequent encounter
S	sequela

X●Y31 Falling, lying or running before or into moving object, undetermined intent

The appropriate 7th character is to be added to code Y31

A	initial encounter
D	subsequent encounter
S	sequela

X●Y32 Crashing of motor vehicle, undetermined intent

The appropriate 7th character is to be added to code Y32

A	initial encounter
D	subsequent encounter
S	sequela

X●Y33 Other specified events, undetermined intent

The appropriate 7th character is to be added to code Y33

A	initial encounter
D	subsequent encounter
S	sequela

LEGAL INTERVENTION, OPERATIONS OF WAR, MILITARY OPERATIONS, AND TERRORISM (Y35-Y38)

Y35 Legal intervention

Includes any injury sustained as a result of an encounter with any law enforcement official, serving in any capacity at the time of the encounter, whether on-duty or off-duty. Includes: injury to law enforcement official, suspect and bystander

The appropriate 7th character is to be added to each code from category Y35

A	initial encounter
D	subsequent encounter
S	sequela

Y35.0 Legal intervention involving firearm discharge

Y35.00 Legal intervention involving unspecified firearm discharge
Legal intervention involving gunshot wound
Legal intervention involving shot NOS

Y35.001 Legal intervention involving unspecified firearm discharge, law enforcement official injured

Y35.002 Legal intervention involving unspecified firearm discharge, bystander injured

Y35.003 Legal intervention involving unspecified firearm discharge, suspect injured

Y35.01 Legal intervention involving injury by machine gun

Y35.011 Legal intervention involving injury by machine gun, law enforcement official injured

Y35.012 Legal intervention involving injury by machine gun, bystander injured

Y35.013 Legal intervention involving injury by machine gun, suspect injured

Y35.02 Legal intervention involving injury by handgun

Y35.021 Legal intervention involving injury by handgun, law enforcement official injured

Y35.022 Legal intervention involving injury by handgun, bystander injured

Y35.023 Legal intervention involving injury by handgun, suspect injured

Y35.03 Legal intervention involving injury by rifle pellet

Y35.031 Legal intervention involving injury by rifle pellet, law enforcement official injured

Y35.032 Legal intervention involving injury by rifle pellet, bystander injured

Y35.033 Legal intervention involving injury by rifle pellet, suspect injured

Y35.04 Legal intervention involving injury by rubber bullet

Y35.041 Legal intervention involving injury by rubber bullet, law enforcement official injured

Y35.042 Legal intervention involving injury by rubber bullet, bystander injured

Y35.043 Legal intervention involving injury by rubber bullet, suspect injured

Y35.09 Legal intervention involving other firearm discharge

Y35.091 Legal intervention involving other firearm discharge, law enforcement official injured

Y35.092 Legal intervention involving other firearm discharge, bystander injured

Y35.093 Legal intervention involving other firearm discharge, suspect injured

Y35.1 Legal intervention involving explosives

Y35.10 Legal intervention involving unspecified explosives

Y35.101 Legal intervention involving unspecified explosives, law enforcement official injured

Y35.102 Legal intervention involving unspecified explosives, bystander injured

Y35.103 Legal intervention involving unspecified explosives, suspect injured

Y35.11 Legal intervention involving injury by dynamite

Y35.111 Legal intervention involving injury by dynamite, law enforcement official injured

Y35.112 Legal intervention involving injury by dynamite, bystander injured

Y35.113 Legal intervention involving injury by dynamite, suspect injured

Y35.12 Legal intervention involving injury by explosive shell

Y35.121 Legal intervention involving injury by explosive shell, law enforcement official injured

Y35.122 Legal intervention involving injury by explosive shell, bystander injured

Y35.123 Legal intervention involving injury by explosive shell, suspect injured

Y35.19 Legal intervention involving other explosives
Legal intervention involving injury by grenade
Legal intervention involving injury by mortar bomb

Y35.191 Legal intervention involving other explosives, law enforcement official injured

Y35.192 Legal intervention involving other explosives, bystander injured

Y35.193 Legal intervention involving other explosives, suspect injured

Y35.2 Legal intervention involving gas
Legal intervention involving asphyxiation by gas
Legal intervention involving poisoning by gas

Y35.20 Legal intervention involving unspecified gas

Y35.201 Legal intervention involving unspecified gas, law enforcement official injured

Y35.202 Legal intervention involving unspecified gas, bystander injured

Y35.203 Legal intervention involving unspecified gas, suspect injured

CHAPTER 20 (V01-Y99)

● Y35.21 Legal intervention involving injury by tear gas
● Y35.211 Legal intervention involving injury by tear gas, law enforcement official injured
● Y35.212 Legal intervention involving injury by tear gas, bystander injured
● Y35.213 Legal intervention involving injury by tear gas, suspect injured
● Y35.29 Legal intervention involving other gas
● Y35.291 Legal intervention involving other gas, law enforcement official injured
● Y35.292 Legal intervention involving other gas, bystander injured
● Y35.293 Legal intervention involving other gas, suspect injured
● Y35.3 Legal intervention involving blunt objects
Legal intervention involving being hit or struck by blunt object
● Y35.30 Legal intervention involving unspecified blunt objects
● Y35.301 Legal intervention involving unspecified blunt objects, law enforcement official injured
● Y35.302 Legal intervention involving unspecified blunt objects, bystander injured
● Y35.303 Legal intervention involving unspecified blunt objects, suspect injured
● Y35.31 Legal intervention involving baton
● Y35.311 Legal intervention involving baton, law enforcement official injured
● Y35.312 Legal intervention involving baton, bystander injured
● Y35.313 Legal intervention involving baton, suspect injured
● Y35.39 Legal intervention involving other blunt objects
● Y35.391 Legal intervention involving other blunt objects, law enforcement official injured
● Y35.392 Legal intervention involving other blunt objects, bystander injured
● Y35.393 Legal intervention involving other blunt objects, suspect injured
● Y35.4 Legal intervention involving sharp objects
Legal intervention involving being cut by sharp objects
Legal intervention involving being stabbed by sharp objects
● Y35.40 Legal intervention involving unspecified sharp objects
● Y35.401 Legal intervention involving unspecified sharp objects, law enforcement official injured
● Y35.402 Legal intervention involving unspecified sharp objects, bystander injured
● Y35.403 Legal intervention involving unspecified sharp objects, suspect injured
● Y35.41 Legal intervention involving bayonet
● Y35.411 Legal intervention involving bayonet, law enforcement official injured
● Y35.412 Legal intervention involving bayonet, bystander injured
● Y35.413 Legal intervention involving bayonet, suspect injured
● Y35.49 Legal intervention involving other sharp objects
● Y35.491 Legal intervention involving other sharp objects, law enforcement official injured
● Y35.492 Legal intervention involving other sharp objects, bystander injured
● Y35.493 Legal intervention involving other sharp objects, suspect injured
● Y35.8 Legal intervention involving other specified means
● Y35.81 Legal intervention involving manhandling
● Y35.811 Legal intervention involving manhandling, law enforcement official injured
● Y35.812 Legal intervention involving manhandling, bystander injured
● Y35.813 Legal intervention involving manhandling, suspect injured
● Y35.89 Legal intervention involving other specified means
● Y35.891 Legal intervention involving other specified means, law enforcement official injured
● Y35.892 Legal intervention involving other specified means, bystander injured
● Y35.893 Legal intervention involving other specified means, suspect injured
● Y35.9 Legal intervention, means unspecified
X● Y35.91 Legal intervention, means unspecified, law enforcement official injured
X● Y35.92 Legal intervention, means unspecified, bystander injured
X● Y35.93 Legal intervention, means unspecified, suspect injured

● Y36 Operations of war
Includes injuries to military personnel and civilians caused by war, civil insurrection, and peacekeeping missions
Excludes1 injury to military personnel occurring during peacetime military operations (Y37.-)
military vehicles involved in transport accidents with non-military vehicle during peacetime (V09.01, V09.21, V19.81, V29.81, V39.81, V49.81, V59.81, V69.81, V79.81)

The appropriate 7th character is to be added to each code from category Y36

A	initial encounter
D	subsequent encounter
S	sequela

● Y36.0 War operations involving explosion of marine weapons
Weapons and military watercraft
● Y36.00 War operations involving explosion of unspecified marine weapon
War operations involving underwater blast NOS
● Y36.000 War operations involving explosion of unspecified marine weapon, military personnel
● Y36.001 War operations involving explosion of unspecified marine weapon, civilian
● Y36.01 War operations involving explosion of depth-charge
● Y36.010 War operations involving explosion of depth-charge, military personnel
● Y36.011 War operations involving explosion of depth-charge, civilian

Y36.02 War operations involving explosion of marine mine
War operations involving explosion of marine mine, at sea or in harbor
Y36.020 War operations involving explosion of marine mine, military personnel
Y36.021 War operations involving explosion of marine mine, civilian
Y36.03 War operations involving explosion of sea-based artillery shell
Y36.030 War operations involving explosion of sea-based artillery shell, military personnel
Y36.031 War operations involving explosion of sea-based artillery shell, civilian
Y36.04 War operations involving explosion of torpedo
Y36.040 War operations involving explosion of torpedo, military personnel
Y36.041 War operations involving explosion of torpedo, civilian
Y36.05 War operations involving accidental detonation of onboard marine weapons
Y36.050 War operations involving accidental detonation of onboard marine weapons, military personnel
Y36.051 War operations involving accidental detonation of onboard marine weapons, civilian
Y36.09 War operations involving explosion of other marine weapons
Y36.090 War operations involving explosion of other marine weapons, military personnel
Y36.091 War operations involving explosion of other marine weapons, civilian
Y36.1 War operations involving destruction of aircraft
Y36.10 War operations involving unspecified destruction of aircraft
Y36.100 War operations involving unspecified destruction of aircraft, military personnel
Y36.101 War operations involving unspecified destruction of aircraft, civilian
Y36.11 War operations involving destruction of aircraft due to enemy fire or explosives
War operations involving destruction of aircraft due to air to air missile
War operations involving destruction of aircraft due to explosive placed on aircraft
War operations involving destruction of aircraft due to rocket propelled grenade [RPG]
War operations involving destruction of aircraft due to small arms fire
War operations involving destruction of aircraft due to surface to air missile
Y36.110 War operations involving destruction of aircraft due to enemy fire or explosives, military personnel
Y36.111 War operations involving destruction of aircraft due to enemy fire or explosives, civilian
Y36.12 War operations involving destruction of aircraft due to collision with other aircraft
Y36.120 War operations involving destruction of aircraft due to collision with other aircraft, military personnel
Y36.121 War operations involving destruction of aircraft due to collision with other aircraft, civilian
Y36.13 War operations involving destruction of aircraft due to onboard fire
Y36.130 War operations involving destruction of aircraft due to onboard fire, military personnel
Y36.131 War operations involving destruction of aircraft due to onboard fire, civilian
Y36.14 War operations involving destruction of aircraft due to accidental detonation of onboard munitions and explosives
Y36.140 War operations involving destruction of aircraft due to accidental detonation of onboard munitions and explosives, military personnel
Y36.141 War operations involving destruction of aircraft due to accidental detonation of onboard munitions and explosives, civilian
Y36.19 War operations involving other destruction of aircraft
Y36.190 War operations involving other destruction of aircraft, military personnel
Y36.191 War operations involving other destruction of aircraft, civilian
Y36.2 War operations involving other explosions and fragments
Excludes1 war operations involving explosion of aircraft (Y36.1-)
war operations involving explosion of marine weapons (Y36.0-)
war operations involving explosion of nuclear weapons (Y36.5-)
war operations involving explosion occurring after cessation of hostilities (Y36.8-)
Y36.20 War operations involving unspecified explosion and fragments
War operations involving air blast NOS
War operations involving blast NOS
War operations involving blast fragments NOS
War operations involving blast wave NOS
War operations involving blast wind NOS
War operations involving explosion NOS
War operations involving explosion of bomb NOS
Y36.200 War operations involving unspecified explosion and fragments, military personnel
Y36.201 War operations involving unspecified explosion and fragments, civilian
Y36.21 War operations involving explosion of aerial bomb
Y36.210 War operations involving explosion of aerial bomb, military personnel
Y36.211 War operations involving explosion of aerial bomb, civilian
Y36.22 War operations involving explosion of guided missile
Y36.220 War operations involving explosion of guided missile, military personnel
Y36.221 War operations involving explosion of guided missile, civilian

Y36.23 War operations involving explosion of improvised explosive device [IED]
War operations involving explosion of person-borne improvised explosive device [IED]
War operations involving explosion of vehicle-borne improvised explosive device [IED]
War operations involving explosion of roadside improvised explosive device [IED]

Y36.230 War operations involving explosion of improvised explosive device [IED], military personnel

Y36.231 War operations involving explosion of improvised explosive device [IED], civilian

Y36.24 War operations involving explosion due to accidental detonation and discharge of own munitions or munitions launch device

Y36.240 War operations involving explosion due to accidental detonation and discharge of own munitions or munitions launch device, military personnel

Y36.241 War operations involving explosion due to accidental detonation and discharge of own munitions or munitions launch device, civilian

Y36.25 War operations involving fragments from munitions

Y36.250 War operations involving fragments from munitions, military personnel

Y36.251 War operations involving fragments from munitions, civilian

Y36.26 War operations involving fragments of improvised explosive device [IED]
War operations involving fragments of person-borne improvised explosive device [IED]
War operations involving fragments of vehicle-borne improvised explosive device [IED]
War operations involving fragments of roadside improvised explosive device [IED]

Y36.260 War operations involving fragments of improvised explosive device [IED], military personnel

Y36.261 War operations involving fragments of improvised explosive device [IED], civilian

Y36.27 War operations involving fragments from weapons

Y36.270 War operations involving fragments from weapons, military personnel

Y36.271 War operations involving fragments from weapons, civilian

Y36.29 War operations involving other explosions and fragments
War operations involving explosion of grenade
War operations involving explosions of land mine
War operations involving shrapnel NOS

Y36.290 War operations involving other explosions and fragments, military personnel

Y36.291 War operations involving other explosions and fragments, civilian

Y36.3 War operations involving fires, conflagrations and hot substances
War operations involving smoke, fumes, and heat from fires, conflagrations and hot substances

Excludes1 war operations involving fires and conflagrations aboard military aircraft (Y36.1-)
war operations involving fires and conflagrations aboard military watercraft (Y36.Ø-)
war operations involving fires and conflagrations caused indirectly by conventional weapons (Y36.2-)
war operations involving fires and thermal effects of nuclear weapons (Y36.53-)

Y36.3Ø War operations involving unspecified fire, conflagration and hot substance

Y36.3ØØ War operations involving unspecified fire, conflagration and hot substance, military personnel

Y36.3Ø1 War operations involving unspecified fire, conflagration and hot substance, civilian

Y36.31 War operations involving gasoline bomb
War operations involving incendiary bomb
War operations involving petrol bomb

Y36.31Ø War operations involving gasoline bomb, military personnel

Y36.311 War operations involving gasoline bomb, civilian

Y36.32 War operations involving incendiary bullet

Y36.32Ø War operations involving incendiary bullet, military personnel

Y36.321 War operations involving incendiary bullet, civilian

Y36.33 War operations involving flamethrower

Y36.33Ø War operations involving flamethrower, military personnel

Y36.331 War operations involving flamethrower, civilian

Y36.39 War operations involving other fires, conflagrations and hot substances

Y36.39Ø War operations involving other fires, conflagrations and hot substances, military personnel

Y36.391 War operations involving other fires, conflagrations and hot substances, civilian

Y36.4 War operations involving firearm discharge and other forms of conventional warfare

Y36.41 War operations involving rubber bullets

Y36.41Ø War operations involving rubber bullets, military personnel

Y36.411 War operations involving rubber bullets, civilian

Y36.42 War operations involving firearms pellets

Y36.42Ø War operations involving firearms pellets, military personnel

Y36.421 War operations involving firearms pellets, civilian

● **Y36.43 War operations involving other firearms discharge**
War operations involving bullets NOS
Excludes1 war operations involving munitions fragments (Y36.25-)
war operations involving incendiary bullets (Y36.32-)

● **Y36.430 War operations involving other firearms discharge, military personnel**

● **Y36.431 War operations involving other firearms discharge, civilian**

● **Y36.44 War operations involving unarmed hand to hand combat**
Excludes1 war operations involving combat using blunt or piercing object (Y36.45-)
war operations involving intentional restriction of air and airway (Y36.46-)
war operations involving unintentional restriction of air and airway (Y36.47-)

● **Y36.440 War operations involving unarmed hand to hand combat, military personnel**

● **Y36.441 War operations involving unarmed hand to hand combat, civilian**

● **Y36.45 War operations involving combat using blunt or piercing object**

● **Y36.450 War operations involving combat using blunt or piercing object, military personnel**

● **Y36.451 War operations involving combat using blunt or piercing object, civilian**

● **Y36.46 War operations involving intentional restriction of air and airway**

● **Y36.460 War operations involving intentional restriction of air and airway, military personnel**

● **Y36.461 War operations involving intentional restriction of air and airway, civilian**

● **Y36.47 War operations involving unintentional restriction of air and airway**

● **Y36.470 War operations involving unintentional restriction of air and airway, military personnel**

● **Y36.471 War operations involving unintentional restriction of air and airway, civilian**

● **Y36.49 War operations involving other forms of conventional warfare**

● **Y36.490 War operations involving other forms of conventional warfare, military personnel**

● **Y36.491 War operations involving other forms of conventional warfare, civilian**

● **Y36.5 War operations involving nuclear weapons**
War operations involving dirty bomb NOS

● **Y36.50 War operations involving unspecified effect of nuclear weapon**

● **Y36.500 War operations involving unspecified effect of nuclear weapon, military personnel**

● **Y36.501 War operations involving unspecified effect of nuclear weapon, civilian**

● **Y36.51 War operations involving direct blast effect of nuclear weapon**
War operations involving blast pressure of nuclear weapon

● **Y36.510 War operations involving direct blast effect of nuclear weapon, military personnel**

● **Y36.511 War operations involving direct blast effect of nuclear weapon, civilian**

● **Y36.52 War operations involving indirect blast effect of nuclear weapon**
War operations involving being thrown by blast of nuclear weapon
War operations involving being struck or crushed by blast debris of nuclear weapon

● **Y36.520 War operations involving indirect blast effect of nuclear weapon, military personnel**

● **Y36.521 War operations involving indirect blast effect of nuclear weapon, civilian**

● **Y36.53 War operations involving thermal radiation effect of nuclear weapon**
War operations involving direct heat from nuclear weapon
War operation involving fireball effects from nuclear weapon

● **Y36.530 War operations involving thermal radiation effect of nuclear weapon, military personnel**

● **Y36.531 War operations involving thermal radiation effect of nuclear weapon, civilian**

● **Y36.54 War operation involving nuclear radiation effects of nuclear weapon**
War operation involving acute radiation exposure from nuclear weapon
War operation involving exposure to immediate ionizing radiation from nuclear weapon
War operation involving fallout exposure from nuclear weapon
War operation involving secondary effects of nuclear weapons

● **Y36.540 War operation involving nuclear radiation effects of nuclear weapon, military personnel**

● **Y36.541 War operation involving nuclear radiation effects of nuclear weapon, civilian**

● **Y36.59 War operation involving other effects of nuclear weapons**

● **Y36.590 War operation involving other effects of nuclear weapons, military personnel**

● **Y36.591 War operation involving other effects of nuclear weapons, civilian**

● **Y36.6 War operations involving biological weapons**

● **Y36.6X War operations involving biological weapons**

● **Y36.6X0 War operations involving biological weapons, military personnel**

● **Y36.6X1 War operations involving biological weapons, civilian**

CHAPTER 20 (V01-Y99)

● Y36.7 **War operations involving chemical weapons and other forms of unconventional warfare**

Excludes1 war operations involving incendiary devices (Y36.3-, Y36.5-)

● Y36.7X **War operations involving chemical weapons and other forms of unconventional warfare**

● Y36.7X0 **War operations involving chemical weapons and other forms of unconventional warfare, military personnel**

● Y36.7X1 **War operations involving chemical weapons and other forms of unconventional warfare, civilian**

● Y36.8 **War operations occurring after cessation of hostilities**

War operations classifiable to categories Y36.0-Y36.8 but occurring after cessation of hostilities

● Y36.81 **Explosion of mine placed during war operations but exploding after cessation of hostilities**

● Y36.810 **Explosion of mine placed during war operations but exploding after cessation of hostilities, military personnel**

● Y36.811 **Explosion of mine placed during war operations but exploding after cessation of hostilities, civilian**

● Y36.82 **Explosion of bomb placed during war operations but exploding after cessation of hostilities**

● Y36.820 **Explosion of bomb placed during war operations but exploding after cessation of hostilities, military personnel**

● Y36.821 **Explosion of bomb placed during war operations but exploding after cessation of hostilities, civilian**

● Y36.88 **Other war operations occurring after cessation of hostilities**

● Y36.880 **Other war operations occurring after cessation of hostilities, military personnel**

● Y36.881 **Other war operations occurring after cessation of hostilities, civilian**

● Y36.89 **Unspecified war operations occurring after cessation of hostilities**

● Y36.890 **Unspecified war operations occurring after cessation of hostilities, military personnel**

● Y36.891 **Unspecified war operations occurring after cessation of hostilities, civilian**

● Y36.9 **Other and unspecified war operations**

X● Y36.90 **War operations, unspecified**

X● Y36.91 **War operations involving unspecified weapon of mass destruction [WMD]**

X● Y36.92 **War operations involving friendly fire**

● Y37 **Military operations**

Includes Injuries to military personnel and civilians occurring during peacetime on military property and during routine military exercises and operations

Excludes1 military aircraft involved in aircraft accident with civilian aircraft (V97.81-)
military vehicles involved in transport accident with civilian vehicle (V09.01, V09.21, V19.81, V29.81, V39.81, V49.81, V59.81, V69.81, V79.81)
military watercraft involved in water transport accident with civilian watercraft (V94.81-)
war operations (Y36.-)

The appropriate 7th character is to be added to each code from category Y37

A	initial encounter
D	subsequent encounter
S	sequela

● Y37.0 **Military operations involving explosion of marine weapons**

● Y37.00 **Military operations involving explosion of unspecified marine weapon**

Military operations involving underwater blast NOS

● Y37.000 **Military operations involving explosion of unspecified marine weapon, military personnel**

● Y37.001 **Military operations involving explosion of unspecified marine weapon, civilian**

● Y37.01 **Military operations involving explosion of depth-charge**

● Y37.010 **Military operations involving explosion of depth-charge, military personnel**

● Y37.011 **Military operations involving explosion of depth-charge, civilian**

● Y37.02 **Military operations involving explosion of marine mine**

Military operations involving explosion of marine mine, at sea or in harbor

● Y37.020 **Military operations involving explosion of marine mine, military personnel**

● Y37.021 **Military operations involving explosion of marine mine, civilian**

● Y37.03 **Military operations involving explosion of sea-based artillery shell**

● Y37.030 **Military operations involving explosion of sea-based artillery shell, military personnel**

● Y37.031 **Military operations involving explosion of sea-based artillery shell, civilian**

● Y37.04 **Military operations involving explosion of torpedo**

● Y37.040 **Military operations involving explosion of torpedo, military personnel**

● Y37.041 **Military operations involving explosion of torpedo, civilian**

● Y37.05 **Military operations involving accidental detonation of onboard marine weapons**

● Y37.050 **Military operations involving accidental detonation of onboard marine weapons, military personnel**

● Y37.051 **Military operations involving accidental detonation of onboard marine weapons, civilian**

◄ New ◄ Revised ~~deleted~~ Deleted OGCR Official Guidelines X Assign placeholder X ● Use Additional Character(s)
Excludes 1 | Excludes 2 | Includes | Use additional | Code first | Code also | Unspecified

● Y37.09 **Military operations involving explosion of other marine weapons**

● Y37.090 **Military operations involving explosion of other marine weapons, military personnel**

● Y37.091 **Military operations involving explosion of other marine weapons, civilian**

● Y37.1 **Military operations involving destruction of aircraft**

● Y37.10 **Military operations involving unspecified destruction of aircraft**

● Y37.100 **Military operations involving unspecified destruction of aircraft, military personnel**

● Y37.101 **Military operations involving unspecified destruction of aircraft, civilian**

● Y37.11 **Military operations involving destruction of aircraft due to enemy fire or explosives**

Military operations involving destruction of aircraft due to air to air missile

Military operations involving destruction of aircraft due to explosive placed on aircraft

Military operations involving destruction of aircraft due to rocket propelled grenade [RPG]

Military operations involving destruction of aircraft due to small arms fire

Military operations involving destruction of aircraft due to surface to air missile

● Y37.110 **Military operations involving destruction of aircraft due to enemy fire or explosives, military personnel**

● Y37.111 **Military operations involving destruction of aircraft due to enemy fire or explosives, civilian**

● Y37.12 **Military operations involving destruction of aircraft due to collision with other aircraft**

● Y37.120 **Military operations involving destruction of aircraft due to collision with other aircraft, military personnel**

● Y37.121 **Military operations involving destruction of aircraft due to collision with other aircraft, civilian**

● Y37.13 **Military operations involving destruction of aircraft due to onboard fire**

● Y37.130 **Military operations involving destruction of aircraft due to onboard fire, military personnel**

● Y37.131 **Military operations involving destruction of aircraft due to onboard fire, civilian**

● Y37.14 **Military operations involving destruction of aircraft due to accidental detonation of onboard munitions and explosives**

● Y37.140 **Military operations involving destruction of aircraft due to accidental detonation of onboard munitions and explosives, military personnel**

● Y37.141 **Military operations involving destruction of aircraft due to accidental detonation of onboard munitions and explosives, civilian**

● Y37.19 **Military operations involving other destruction of aircraft**

● Y37.190 **Military operations involving other destruction of aircraft, military personnel**

● Y37.191 **Military operations involving other destruction of aircraft, civilian**

● Y37.2 **Military operations involving other explosions and fragments**

Excludes1 military operations involving explosion of aircraft (Y37.1-)
military operations involving explosion of marine weapons (Y37.0-)
military operations involving explosion of nuclear weapons (Y37.5-)

● Y37.20 **Military operations involving unspecified explosion and fragments**

Military operations involving air blast NOS
Military operations involving blast NOS
Military operations involving blast fragments NOS
Military operations involving blast wave NOS
Military operations involving blast wind NOS
Military operations involving explosion NOS
Military operations involving explosion of bomb NOS

● Y37.200 **Military operations involving unspecified explosion and fragments, military personnel**

● Y37.201 **Military operations involving unspecified explosion and fragments, civilian**

● Y37.21 **Military operations involving explosion of aerial bomb**

● Y37.210 **Military operations involving explosion of aerial bomb, military personnel**

● Y37.211 **Military operations involving explosion of aerial bomb, civilian**

● Y37.22 **Military operations involving explosion of guided missile**

● Y37.220 **Military operations involving explosion of guided missile, military personnel**

● Y37.221 **Military operations involving explosion of guided missile, civilian**

● Y37.23 **Military operations involving explosion of improvised explosive device [IED]**

Military operations involving explosion of person-borne improvised explosive device [IED]

Military operations involving explosion of vehicle-borne improvised explosive device [IED]

Military operations involving explosion of roadside improvised explosive device [IED]

● Y37.230 **Military operations involving explosion of improvised explosive device [IED], military personnel**

● Y37.231 **Military operations involving explosion of improvised explosive device [IED], civilian**

● Y37.24 **Military operations involving explosion due to accidental detonation and discharge of own munitions or munitions launch device**

● Y37.240 **Military operations involving explosion due to accidental detonation and discharge of own munitions or munitions launch device, military personnel**

● Y37.241 **Military operations involving explosion due to accidental detonation and discharge of own munitions or munitions launch device, civilian**

CHAPTER 20 (V01-Y99)

● Y37.25 **Military operations involving fragments from munitions**

● Y37.250 **Military operations involving fragments from munitions, military personnel**

● Y37.251 **Military operations involving fragments from munitions, civilian**

● Y37.26 **Military operations involving fragments of improvised explosive device [IED]**

Military operations involving fragments of person-borne improvised explosive device [IED]

Military operations involving fragments of vehicle-borne improvised explosive device [IED]

Military operations involving fragments of roadside improvised explosive device [IED]

● Y37.260 **Military operations involving fragments of improvised explosive device [IED], military personnel**

● Y37.261 **Military operations involving fragments of improvised explosive device [IED], civilian**

● Y37.27 **Military operations involving fragments from weapons**

● Y37.270 **Military operations involving fragments from weapons, military personnel**

● Y37.271 **Military operations involving fragments from weapons, civilian**

● Y37.29 **Military operations involving other explosions and fragments**

Military operations involving explosion of grenade

Military operations involving explosions of land mine

Military operations involving shrapnel NOS

● Y37.290 **Military operations involving other explosions and fragments, military personnel**

● Y37.291 **Military operations involving other explosions and fragments, civilian**

● Y37.3 **Military operations involving fires, conflagrations and hot substances**

Military operations involving smoke, fumes, and heat from fires, conflagrations and hot substances

Excludes1 military operations involving fires and conflagrations aboard military aircraft (Y37.1-)

military operations involving fires and conflagrations aboard military watercraft (Y37.0-)

military operations involving fires and conflagrations caused indirectly by conventional weapons (Y37.2-)

military operations involving fires and thermal effects of nuclear weapons (Y36.53-)

● Y37.30 **Military operations involving unspecified fire, conflagration and hot substance**

● Y37.300 **Military operations involving unspecified fire, conflagration and hot substance, military personnel**

● Y37.301 **Military operations involving unspecified fire, conflagration and hot substance, civilian**

● Y37.31 **Military operations involving gasoline bomb**

Military operations involving incendiary bomb

Military operations involving petrol bomb

● Y37.310 **Military operations involving gasoline bomb, military personnel**

● Y37.311 **Military operations involving gasoline bomb, civilian**

● Y37.32 **Military operations involving incendiary bullet**

● Y37.320 **Military operations involving incendiary bullet, military personnel**

● Y37.321 **Military operations involving incendiary bullet, civilian**

● Y37.33 **Military operations involving flamethrower**

● Y37.330 **Military operations involving flamethrower, military personnel**

● Y37.331 **Military operations involving flamethrower, civilian**

● Y37.39 **Military operations involving other fires, conflagrations and hot substances**

● Y37.390 **Military operations involving other fires, conflagrations and hot substances, military personnel**

● Y37.391 **Military operations involving other fires, conflagrations and hot substances, civilian**

● Y37.4 **Military operations involving firearm discharge and other forms of conventional warfare**

● Y37.41 **Military operations involving rubber bullets**

● Y37.410 **Military operations involving rubber bullets, military personnel**

● Y37.411 **Military operations involving rubber bullets, civilian**

● Y37.42 **Military operations involving firearms pellets**

● Y37.420 **Military operations involving firearms pellets, military personnel**

● Y37.421 **Military operations involving firearms pellets, civilian**

● Y37.43 **Military operations involving other firearms discharge**

Military operations involving bullets NOS

Excludes1 military operations involving munitions fragments (Y37.25-)

military operations involving incendiary bullets (Y37.32-)

● Y37.430 **Military operations involving other firearms discharge, military personnel**

● Y37.431 **Military operations involving other firearms discharge, civilian**

● Y37.44 **Military operations involving unarmed hand to hand combat**

Excludes1 military operations involving combat using blunt or piercing object (Y37.45-)

military operations involving intentional restriction of air and airway (Y37.46-)

military operations involving unintentional restriction of air and airway (Y37.47-)

● Y37.440 **Military operations involving unarmed hand to hand combat, military personnel**

● Y37.441 **Military operations involving unarmed hand to hand combat, civilian**

● Y37.45 Military operations involving combat using blunt or piercing object
● Y37.450 Military operations involving combat using blunt or piercing object, military personnel
● Y37.451 Military operations involving combat using blunt or piercing object, civilian
● Y37.46 Military operations involving intentional restriction of air and airway
● Y37.460 Military operations involving intentional restriction of air and airway, military personnel
● Y37.461 Military operations involving intentional restriction of air and airway, civilian
● Y37.47 Military operations involving unintentional restriction of air and airway
● Y37.470 Military operations involving unintentional restriction of air and airway, military personnel
● Y37.471 Military operations involving unintentional restriction of air and airway, civilian
● Y37.49 Military operations involving other forms of conventional warfare
● Y37.490 Military operations involving other forms of conventional warfare, military personnel
● Y37.491 Military operations involving other forms of conventional warfare, civilian
● Y37.5 Military operations involving nuclear weapons
Military operation involving dirty bomb NOS
● Y37.50 Military operations involving unspecified effect of nuclear weapon
● Y37.500 Military operations involving unspecified effect of nuclear weapon, military personnel
● Y37.501 Military operations involving unspecified effect of nuclear weapon, civilian
● Y37.51 Military operations involving direct blast effect of nuclear weapon
Military operations involving blast pressure of nuclear weapon
● Y37.510 Military operations involving direct blast effect of nuclear weapon, military personnel
● Y37.511 Military operations involving direct blast effect of nuclear weapon, civilian
● Y37.52 Military operations involving indirect blast effect of nuclear weapon
Military operations involving being thrown by blast of nuclear weapon
Military operations involving being struck or crushed by blast debris of nuclear weapon
● Y37.520 Military operations involving indirect blast effect of nuclear weapon, military personnel
● Y37.521 Military operations involving indirect blast effect of nuclear weapon, civilian
● Y37.53 Military operations involving thermal radiation effect of nuclear weapon
Military operations involving direct heat from nuclear weapon
Military operation involving fireball effects from nuclear weapon
● Y37.530 Military operations involving thermal radiation effect of nuclear weapon, military personnel
● Y37.531 Military operations involving thermal radiation effect of nuclear weapon, civilian
● Y37.54 Military operation involving nuclear radiation effects of nuclear weapon
Military operation involving acute radiation exposure from nuclear weapon
Military operation involving exposure to immediate ionizing radiation from nuclear weapon
Military operation involving fallout exposure from nuclear weapon
Military operation involving secondary effects of nuclear weapons
● Y37.540 Military operation involving nuclear radiation effects of nuclear weapon, military personnel
● Y37.541 Military operation involving nuclear radiation effects of nuclear weapon, civilian
● Y37.59 Military operation involving other effects of nuclear weapons
● Y37.590 Military operation involving other effects of nuclear weapons, military personnel
● Y37.591 Military operation involving other effects of nuclear weapons, civilian
● Y37.6 Military operations involving biological weapons
● Y37.6X Military operations involving biological weapons
● Y37.6X0 Military operations involving biological weapons, military personnel
● Y37.6X1 Military operations involving biological weapons, civilian
● Y37.7 Military operations involving chemical weapons and other forms of unconventional warfare
Excludes1 military operations involving incendiary devices (Y36.3-, Y36.5-)
● Y37.7X Military operations involving chemical weapons and other forms of unconventional warfare
● Y37.7X0 Military operations involving chemical weapons and other forms of unconventional warfare, military personnel
● Y37.7X1 Military operations involving chemical weapons and other forms of unconventional warfare, civilian
● Y37.9 Other and unspecified military operations
X● Y37.90 Military operations, unspecified
X● Y37.91 Military operations involving unspecified weapon of mass destruction [WMD]
X● Y37.92 Military operations involving friendly fire

● Y38 **Terrorism**

These codes are for use to identify injuries resulting from the unlawful use of force or violence against persons or property to intimidate or coerce a government, the civilian population, or any segment thereof, in furtherance of political or social objective

Use additional code for place of occurrence (Y92.-)

The appropriate 7th character is to be added to each code from category Y38

A	initial encounter
D	subsequent encounter
S	sequela

● Y38.Ø **Terrorism involving explosion of marine weapons**
Terrorism involving depth-charge
Terrorism involving marine mine
Terrorism involving mine NOS, at sea or in harbor
Terrorism involving sea-based artillery shell
Terrorism involving torpedo
Terrorism involving underwater blast

● Y38.ØX **Terrorism involving explosion of marine weapons**

● Y38.ØX1 **Terrorism involving explosion of marine weapons, public safety official injured**

● Y38.ØX2 **Terrorism involving explosion of marine weapons, civilian injured**

● Y38.ØX3 **Terrorism involving explosion of marine weapons, terrorist injured**

● Y38.1 **Terrorism involving destruction of aircraft**
Terrorism involving aircraft burned
Terrorism involving aircraft exploded
Terrorism involving aircraft being shot down
Terrorism involving aircraft used as a weapon

● Y38.1X **Terrorism involving destruction of aircraft**

● Y38.1X1 **Terrorism involving destruction of aircraft, public safety official injured**

● Y38.1X2 **Terrorism involving destruction of aircraft, civilian injured**

● Y38.1X3 **Terrorism involving destruction of aircraft, terrorist injured**

● Y38.2 **Terrorism involving other explosions and fragments**
Terrorism involving antipersonnel (fragments) bomb
Terrorism involving blast NOS
Terrorism involving explosion NOS
Terrorism involving explosion of breech block
Terrorism involving explosion of cannon block
Terrorism involving explosion (fragments) of artillery shell
Terrorism involving explosion (fragments) of bomb
Terrorism involving explosion (fragments) of grenade
Terrorism involving explosion (fragments) of guided missile
Terrorism involving explosion (fragments) of land mine
Terrorism involving explosion of mortar bomb
Terrorism involving explosion of munitions
Terrorism involving explosion (fragments) of rocket
Terrorism involving explosion (fragments) of shell
Terrorism involving shrapnel
Terrorism involving mine NOS, on land

Excludes1 terrorism involving explosion of nuclear weapon (Y38.5)
terrorism involving suicide bomber (Y38.81)

● Y38.2X **Terrorism involving other explosions and fragments**

● Y38.2X1 **Terrorism involving other explosions and fragments, public safety official injured**

● Y38.2X2 **Terrorism involving other explosions and fragments, civilian injured**

● Y38.2X3 **Terrorism involving other explosions and fragments, terrorist injured**

● Y38.3 **Terrorism involving fires, conflagration and hot substances**
Terrorism involving conflagration NOS
Terrorism involving fire NOS
Terrorism involving petrol bomb

Excludes1 terrorism involving fire or heat of nuclear weapon (Y38.5)

● Y38.3X **Terrorism involving fires, conflagration and hot substances**

● Y38.3X1 **Terrorism involving fires, conflagration and hot substances, public safety official injured**

● Y38.3X2 **Terrorism involving fires, conflagration and hot substances, civilian injured**

● Y38.3X3 **Terrorism involving fires, conflagration and hot substances, terrorist injured**

● Y38.4 **Terrorism involving firearms**
Terrorism involving carbine bullet
Terrorism involving machine gun bullet
Terrorism involving pellets (shotgun)
Terrorism involving pistol bullet
Terrorism involving rifle bullet
Terrorism involving rubber (rifle) bullet

● Y38.4X **Terrorism involving firearms**

● Y38.4X1 **Terrorism involving firearms, public safety official injured**

● Y38.4X2 **Terrorism involving firearms, civilian injured**

● Y38.4X3 **Terrorism involving firearms, terrorist injured**

● Y38.5 **Terrorism involving nuclear weapons**
Terrorism involving blast effects of nuclear weapon
Terrorism involving exposure to ionizing radiation from nuclear weapon
Terrorism involving fireball effect of nuclear weapon
Terrorism involving heat from nuclear weapon

● Y38.5X **Terrorism involving nuclear weapons**

● Y38.5X1 **Terrorism involving nuclear weapons, public safety official injured**

● Y38.5X2 **Terrorism involving nuclear weapons, civilian injured**

● Y38.5X3 **Terrorism involving nuclear weapons, terrorist injured**

● Y38.6 **Terrorism involving biological weapons**
Terrorism involving anthrax
Terrorism involving cholera
A serious, often deadly, infectious disease of small intestine
Terrorism involving smallpox

● Y38.6X **Terrorism involving biological weapons**

● Y38.6X1 **Terrorism involving biological weapons, public safety official injured**

● Y38.6X2 **Terrorism involving biological weapons, civilian injured**

● Y38.6X3 **Terrorism involving biological weapons, terrorist injured**

● Y38.7 **Terrorism involving chemical weapons**
Terrorism involving gases, fumes, chemicals
Terrorism involving hydrogen cyanide
Terrorism involving phosgene
Terrorism involving sarin

● Y38.7X **Terrorism involving chemical weapons**

● Y38.7X1 **Terrorism involving chemical weapons, public safety official injured**

● Y38.7X2 **Terrorism involving chemical weapons, civilian injured**

● Y38.7X3 **Terrorism involving chemical weapons, terrorist injured**

Y38.8 Terrorism involving other and unspecified means

Y38.80 Terrorism involving unspecified means
Terrorism NOS

Y38.81 Terrorism involving suicide bomber

Y38.811 Terrorism involving suicide bomber, public safety official injured

Y38.812 Terrorism involving suicide bomber, civilian injured

Y38.89 Terrorism involving other means
Terrorism involving drowning and submersion
Terrorism involving lasers
Terrorism involving piercing or stabbing instruments

Y38.891 Terrorism involving other means, public safety official injured

Y38.892 Terrorism involving other means, civilian injured

Y38.893 Terrorism involving other means, terrorist injured

Y38.9 Terrorism, secondary effects

Note: This code is for use to identify conditions occurring subsequent to a terrorist attack not those that are due to the initial terrorist attack.

Y38.9X Terrorism, secondary effects

Y38.9X1 Terrorism, secondary effects, public safety official injured

Y38.9X2 Terrorism, secondary effects, civilian injured categories

COMPLICATIONS OF MEDICAL AND SURGICAL CARE (Y62-Y84)

Includes complications of medical devices surgical and medical procedures as the cause of abnormal reaction of the patient, or of later complication, without mention of misadventure at the time of the procedure

MISADVENTURES TO PATIENTS DURING SURGICAL AND MEDICAL CARE (Y62-Y69)

Excludes1 surgical and medical procedures as the cause of abnormal reaction of the patient, without mention of misadventure at the time of the procedure (Y83-Y84) ◀

Excludes2 breakdown or malfunctioning of medical device (during procedure) (after implantation) (ongoing use) (Y70-Y82)

Y62 Failure of sterile precautions during surgical and medical care

Y62.0 Failure of sterile precautions during surgical operation

Y62.1 Failure of sterile precautions during infusion or transfusion

Y62.2 Failure of sterile precautions during kidney dialysis and other perfusion

Y62.3 Failure of sterile precautions during injection or immunization

Y62.4 Failure of sterile precautions during endoscopic examination

Y62.5 Failure of sterile precautions during heart catheterization

Y62.6 Failure of sterile precautions during aspiration, puncture and other catheterization

Y62.8 Failure of sterile precautions during other surgical and medical care

Y62.9 Failure of sterile precautions during unspecified surgical and medical care

Y63 Failure in dosage during surgical and medical care

Excludes2 accidental overdose of drug or wrong drug given in error (T36-T50)

Y63.0 Excessive amount of blood or other fluid given during transfusion or infusion

Y63.1 Incorrect dilution of fluid used during infusion

Y63.2 Overdose of radiation given during therapy

Y63.3 Inadvertent exposure of patient to radiation during medical care

Y63.4 Failure in dosage in electroshock or insulin-shock therapy

Y63.5 Inappropriate temperature in local application and packing

Y63.6 Underdosing and nonadministration of necessary drug, medicament or biological substance

Y63.8 Failure in dosage during other surgical and medical care

Y63.9 Failure in dosage during unspecified surgical and medical care

Y64 Contaminated medical or biological substances

Y64.0 Contaminated medical or biological substance, transfused or infused

Y64.1 Contaminated medical or biological substance, injected or used for immunization

Y64.8 Contaminated medical or biological substance administered by other means

Y64.9 Contaminated medical or biological substance administered by unspecified means
Administered contaminated medical or biological substance NOS

Y65 Other misadventures during surgical and medical care

Y65.0 Mismatched blood in transfusion

Y65.1 Wrong fluid used in infusion

Y65.2 Failure in suture or ligature during surgical operation

Y65.3 Endotracheal tube wrongly placed during anesthetic procedure

Y65.4 Failure to introduce or to remove other tube or instrument

Y65.5 Performance of wrong procedure (operation)

Y65.51 Performance of wrong procedure (operation) on correct patient
Wrong device implanted into correct surgical site

Excludes1 performance of correct procedure (operation) on wrong side or body part (Y65.53)

Y65.52 Performance of procedure (operation) on patient not scheduled for surgery
Performance of procedure (operation) intended for another patient
Performance of procedure (operation) on wrong patient

Y65.53 Performance of correct procedure (operation) on wrong side or body part
Performance of correct procedure (operation) on wrong side
Performance of correct procedure (operation) on wrong site

Y65.8 Other specified misadventures during surgical and medical care

Y66 Nonadministration of surgical and medical care
Premature cessation of surgical and medical care

Excludes1 DNR status (Z66)
palliative care (Z51.5)

Y69 Unspecified misadventure during surgical and medical care

MEDICAL DEVICES ASSOCIATED WITH ADVERSE INCIDENTS IN DIAGNOSTIC AND THERAPEUTIC USE (Y70-Y82)

Includes breakdown or malfunction of medical devices (during use) (after implantation) (ongoing use)

Excludes2 breakdown or malfunctioning of medical device (after implantation) (during procedure) (ongoing use) (Y70-Y82) ◀
later complications following use of medical devices without breakdown or malfunctioning of device (Y83-Y84) ◀
misadventure to patients during surgical and medical care, classifiable to (Y62-Y69) ◀
surgical and other medical procedures as the cause of abnormal reaction of the patient, or of later complication, without mention of misadventure at the time of the procedure (Y83-Y84) ◀

● **Y70** **Anesthesiology devices associated with adverse incidents**
- Y70.0 **Diagnostic and monitoring anesthesiology devices associated with adverse incidents**
- Y70.1 **Therapeutic (nonsurgical) and rehabilitative anesthesiology devices associated with adverse incidents**
- Y70.2 **Prosthetic and other implants, materials and accessory anesthesiology devices associated with adverse incidents**
- Y70.3 **Surgical instruments, materials and anesthesiology devices (including sutures) associated with adverse incidents**
- Y70.8 **Miscellaneous anesthesiology devices associated with adverse incidents, not elsewhere classified**

● **Y71** **Cardiovascular devices associated with adverse incidents**
- Y71.0 **Diagnostic and monitoring cardiovascular devices associated with adverse incidents**
- Y71.1 **Therapeutic (nonsurgical) and rehabilitative cardiovascular devices associated with adverse incidents**
- Y71.2 **Prosthetic and other implants, materials and accessory cardiovascular devices associated with adverse incidents**
- Y71.3 **Surgical instruments, materials and cardiovascular devices (including sutures) associated with adverse incidents**
- Y71.8 **Miscellaneous cardiovascular devices associated with adverse incidents, not elsewhere classified**

● **Y72** **Otorhinolaryngological devices associated with adverse incidents**
- Y72.0 **Diagnostic and monitoring otorhinolaryngological devices associated with adverse incidents**
- Y72.1 **Therapeutic (nonsurgical) and rehabilitative otorhinolaryngological devices associated with adverse incidents**
- Y72.2 **Prosthetic and other implants, materials and accessory otorhinolaryngological devices associated with adverse incidents**
- Y72.3 **Surgical instruments, materials and otorhinolaryngological devices (including sutures) associated with adverse incidents**
- Y72.8 **Miscellaneous otorhinolaryngological devices associated with adverse incidents, not elsewhere classified**

● **Y73** **Gastroenterology and urology devices associated with adverse incidents**
- Y73.0 **Diagnostic and monitoring gastroenterology and urology devices associated with adverse incidents**
- Y73.1 **Therapeutic (nonsurgical) and rehabilitative gastroenterology and urology devices associated with adverse incidents**
- Y73.2 **Prosthetic and other implants, materials and accessory gastroenterology and urology devices associated with adverse incidents**
- Y73.3 **Surgical instruments, materials and gastroenterology and urology devices (including sutures) associated with adverse incidents**
- Y73.8 **Miscellaneous gastroenterology and urology devices associated with adverse incidents, not elsewhere classified**

● **Y74** **General hospital and personal-use devices associated with adverse incidents**
- Y74.0 **Diagnostic and monitoring general hospital and personal-use devices associated with adverse incidents**
- Y74.1 **Therapeutic (nonsurgical) and rehabilitative general hospital and personal-use devices associated with adverse incidents**
- Y74.2 **Prosthetic and other implants, materials and accessory general hospital and personal-use devices associated with adverse incidents**
- Y74.3 **Surgical instruments, materials and general hospital and personal-use devices (including sutures) associated with adverse incidents**
- Y74.8 **Miscellaneous general hospital and personal-use devices associated with adverse incidents, not elsewhere classified**

● **Y75** **Neurological devices associated with adverse incidents**
- Y75.0 **Diagnostic and monitoring neurological devices associated with adverse incidents**
- Y75.1 **Therapeutic (nonsurgical) and rehabilitative neurological devices associated with adverse incidents**
- Y75.2 **Prosthetic and other implants, materials and neurological devices associated with adverse incidents**
- Y75.3 **Surgical instruments, materials and neurological devices (including sutures) associated with adverse incidents**
- Y75.8 **Miscellaneous neurological devices associated with adverse incidents, not elsewhere classified**

● **Y76** **Obstetric and gynecological devices associated with adverse incidents**
- Y76.0 **Diagnostic and monitoring obstetric and gynecological devices associated with adverse incidents**
- Y76.1 **Therapeutic (nonsurgical) and rehabilitative obstetric and gynecological devices associated with adverse incidents**
- Y76.2 **Prosthetic and other implants, materials and accessory obstetric and gynecological devices associated with adverse incidents**
- Y76.3 **Surgical instruments, materials and obstetric and gynecological devices (including sutures) associated with adverse incidents**
- Y76.8 **Miscellaneous obstetric and gynecological devices associated with adverse incidents, not elsewhere classified**

● Y77 Ophthalmic devices associated with adverse incidents
- Y77.Ø Diagnostic and monitoring ophthalmic devices associated with adverse incidents
- Y77.1 Therapeutic (nonsurgical) and rehabilitative ophthalmic devices associated with adverse incidents
- Y77.2 Prosthetic and other implants, materials and accessory ophthalmic devices associated with adverse incidents
- Y77.3 Surgical instruments, materials and ophthalmic devices (including sutures) associated with adverse incidents
- Y77.8 Miscellaneous ophthalmic devices associated with adverse incidents, not elsewhere classified

● Y78 Radiological devices associated with adverse incidents
- Y78.Ø Diagnostic and monitoring radiological devices associated with adverse incidents
- Y78.1 Therapeutic (nonsurgical) and rehabilitative radiological devices associated with adverse incidents
- Y78.2 Prosthetic and other implants, materials and accessory radiological devices associated with adverse incidents
- Y78.3 Surgical instruments, materials and radiological devices (including sutures) associated with adverse incidents
- Y78.8 Miscellaneous radiological devices associated with adverse incidents, not elsewhere classified

● Y79 Orthopedic devices associated with adverse incidents
- Y79.Ø Diagnostic and monitoring orthopedic devices associated with adverse incidents
- Y79.1 Therapeutic (nonsurgical) and rehabilitative orthopedic devices associated with adverse incidents
- Y79.2 Prosthetic and other implants, materials and accessory orthopedic devices associated with adverse incidents
- Y79.3 Surgical instruments, materials and orthopedic devices (including sutures) associated with adverse incidents
- Y79.8 Miscellaneous orthopedic devices associated with adverse incidents, not elsewhere classified

● Y8Ø Physical medicine devices associated with adverse incidents
- Y8Ø.Ø Diagnostic and monitoring physical medicine devices associated with adverse incidents
- Y8Ø.1 Therapeutic (nonsurgical) and rehabilitative physical medicine devices associated with adverse incidents
- Y8Ø.2 Prosthetic and other implants, materials and accessory physical medicine devices associated with adverse incidents
- Y8Ø.3 Surgical instruments, materials and physical medicine devices (including sutures) associated with adverse incidents
- Y8Ø.8 Miscellaneous physical medicine devices associated with adverse incidents, not elsewhere classified

● Y81 General- and plastic-surgery devices associated with adverse incidents
- Y81.Ø Diagnostic and monitoring general- and plastic-surgery devices associated with adverse incidents
- Y81.1 Therapeutic (nonsurgical) and rehabilitative general- and plastic-surgery devices associated with adverse incidents
- Y81.2 Prosthetic and other implants, materials and accessory general- and plastic-surgery devices associated with adverse incidents
- Y81.3 Surgical instruments, materials and general- and plastic-surgery devices (including sutures) associated with adverse incidents
- Y81.8 Miscellaneous general- and plastic-surgery devices associated with adverse incidents, not elsewhere classified

● Y82 Other and unspecified medical devices associated with adverse incidents
- Y82.8 Other medical devices associated with adverse incidents
- Y82.9 Unspecified medical devices associated with adverse incidents

SURGICAL AND OTHER MEDICAL PROCEDURES AS THE CAUSE OF ABNORMAL REACTION OF THE PATIENT, OR OF LATER COMPLICATION, WITHOUT MENTION OF MISADVENTURE AT THE TIME OF THE PROCEDURE (Y83-Y84)

Excludes1 misadventures to patients during surgical and medical care, classifiable to (Y62-Y69)

Excludes2 breakdown or malfunctioning of medical device (after implantation) (during procedure) (ongoing use) (Y7Ø-Y82) ◀

● Y83 Surgical operation and other surgical procedures as the cause of abnormal reaction of the patient, or of later complication, without mention of misadventure at the time of the procedure
- Y83.Ø Surgical operation with transplant of whole organ as the cause of abnormal reaction of the patient, or of later complication, without mention of misadventure at the time of the procedure
- Y83.1 Surgical operation with implant of artificial internal device as the cause of abnormal reaction of the patient, or of later complication, without mention of misadventure at the time of the procedure
- Y83.2 Surgical operation with anastomosis, bypass or graft as the cause of abnormal reaction of the patient, or of later complication, without mention of misadventure at the time of the procedure
- Y83.3 Surgical operation with formation of external stoma as the cause of abnormal reaction of the patient, or of later complication, without mention of misadventure at the time of the procedure
- Y83.4 Other reconstructive surgery as the cause of abnormal reaction of the patient, or of later complication, without mention of misadventure at the time of the procedure
- Y83.5 Amputation of limb(s) as the cause of abnormal reaction of the patient, or of later complication, without mention of misadventure at the time of the procedure
- Y83.6 Removal of other organ (partial) (total) as the cause of abnormal reaction of the patient, or of later complication, without mention of misadventure at the time of the procedure
- Y83.8 Other surgical procedures as the cause of abnormal reaction of the patient, or of later complication, without mention of misadventure at the time of the procedure
- Y83.9 Surgical procedure, unspecified as the cause of abnormal reaction of the patient, or of later complication, without mention of misadventure at the time of the procedure

● Y84 Other medical procedures as the cause of abnormal reaction of the patient, or of later complication, without mention of misadventure at the time of the procedure
- Y84.Ø Cardiac catheterization as the cause of abnormal reaction of the patient, or of later complication, without mention of misadventure at the time of the procedure
- Y84.1 Kidney dialysis as the cause of abnormal reaction of the patient, or of later complication, without mention of misadventure at the time of the procedure
- Y84.2 Radiological procedure and radiotherapy as the cause of abnormal reaction of the patient, or of later complication, without mention of misadventure at the time of the procedure
- Y84.3 Shock therapy as the cause of abnormal reaction of the patient, or of later complication, without mention of misadventure at the time of the procedure
- Y84.4 Aspiration of fluid as the cause of abnormal reaction of the patient, or of later complication, without mention of misadventure at the time of the procedure
- Y84.5 Insertion of gastric or duodenal sound as the cause of abnormal reaction of the patient, or of later complication, without mention of misadventure at the time of the procedure
- Y84.6 Urinary catheterization as the cause of abnormal reaction of the patient, or of later complication, without mention of misadventure at the time of the procedure
- Y84.7 Blood-sampling as the cause of abnormal reaction of the patient, or of later complication, without mention of misadventure at the time of the procedure

Y84.8 **Other medical procedures as the cause of abnormal reaction of the patient, or of later complication, without mention of misadventure at the time of the procedure**

Y84.9 **Medical procedure, unspecified as the cause of abnormal reaction of the patient, or of later complication, without mention of misadventure at the time of the procedure**

SUPPLEMENTARY FACTORS RELATED TO CAUSES OF MORBIDITY CLASSIFIED ELSEWHERE (Y90-Y99)

Note: These categories may be used to provide supplementary information concerning causes of morbidity. They are not to be used for single-condition coding.

● Y90 **Evidence of alcohol involvement determined by blood alcohol level**

Code first any associated alcohol related disorders (F10)

Y90.0 **Blood alcohol level of less than 20 mg/100 ml**

Y90.1 **Blood alcohol level of 20-39 mg/100 ml**

Y90.2 **Blood alcohol level of 40-59 mg/100 ml**

Y90.3 **Blood alcohol level of 60-79 mg/100 ml**

Y90.4 **Blood alcohol level of 80-99 mg/100 ml**

Y90.5 **Blood alcohol level of 100-119 mg/100 ml**

Y90.6 **Blood alcohol level of 120-199 mg/100 ml**

Y90.7 **Blood alcohol level of 200-239 mg/100 ml**

Y90.8 **Blood alcohol level of 240 mg/100 ml or more**

Y90.9 **Presence of alcohol in blood, level not specified**

OGCR Section I.C.20.b.

Place of Occurrence Guideline

Codes from category Y92, Place of occurrence of the external cause, are secondary codes for use after other external cause codes to identify the location of the patient at the time of injury or other condition.

Generally, a place of occurrence code is assigned only once, at the initial encounter for treatment. However, in the rare instance that a new injury occurs during hospitalization, an additional place of occurrence code may be assigned. No 7th characters are used for Y92.

Only one code from Y92 should be recorded on a medical record.

A place of occurrence code should be used in conjunction with an activity code, Y93.

Do not use place of occurrence code Y92.9 if the place is not stated or is not applicable.

● Y92 **Place of occurrence of the external cause**

The following category is for use, when relevant, to identify the place of occurrence of the external cause. Use in conjunction with an activity code.

Place of occurrence should be recorded only at the initial encounter for treatment

● Y92.0 **Non-institutional (private) residence as the place of occurrence of the external cause**

Excludes1 abandoned or derelict house (Y92.89)
home under construction but not yet occupied (Y92.6-)
institutional place of residence (Y92.1-)

● Y92.00 **Unspecified non-institutional (private) residence as the place of occurrence of the external cause**

Y92.000 **Kitchen of unspecified non-institutional (private) residence as the place of occurrence of the external cause**

Y92.001 **Dining room of unspecified non-institutional (private) residence as the place of occurrence of the external cause**

Y92.002 **Bathroom of unspecified non-institutional (private) residence single-family (private) house as the place of occurrence of the external cause**

Y92.003 **Bedroom of unspecified non-institutional (private) residence as the place of occurrence of the external cause**

Y92.007 **Garden or yard of unspecified non-institutional (private) residence as the place of occurrence of the external cause**

Y92.008 **Other place in unspecified non-institutional (private) residence as the place of occurrence of the external cause**

Y92.009 **Unspecified place in unspecified non-institutional (private) residence as the place of occurrence of the external cause**

Home (NOS) as the place of occurrence of the external cause

● Y92.01 **Single-family non-institutional (private) house as the place of occurrence of the external cause**

Farmhouse as the place of occurrence of the external cause

Excludes1 barn (Y92.71)
chicken coop or hen house (Y92.72)
farm field (Y92.73)
orchard (Y92.74)
single family mobile home or trailer (Y92.02-)
slaughter house (Y92.86)

Y92.010 **Kitchen of single-family (private) house as the place of occurrence of the external cause**

Y92.011 **Dining room of single-family (private) house as the place of occurrence of the external cause**

Y92.012 **Bathroom of single-family (private) house as the place of occurrence of the external cause**

Y92.013 **Bedroom of single-family (private) house as the place of occurrence of the external cause**

Y92.014 **Private driveway to single-family (private) house as the place of occurrence of the external cause**

Y92.015 **Private garage of single-family (private) house as the place of occurrence of the external cause**

Y92.016 **Swimming pool in single-family (private) house or garden as the place of occurrence of the external cause**

Y92.017 **Garden or yard in single-family (private) house as the place of occurrence of the external cause**

Y92.018 **Other place in single-family (private) house as the place of occurrence of the external cause**

Y92.019 **Unspecified place in single-family (private) house as the place of occurrence of the external cause**

● **Y92.02** **Mobile home as the place of occurrence of the external cause**

Y92.020 **Kitchen in mobile home as the place of occurrence of the external cause**

Y92.021 **Dining room in mobile home as the place of occurrence of the external cause**

Y92.022 **Bathroom in mobile home as the place of occurrence of the external cause**

Y92.023 **Bedroom in mobile home as the place of occurrence of the external cause**

Y92.024 **Driveway of mobile home as the place of occurrence of the external cause**

Y92.025 **Garage of mobile home as the place of occurrence of the external cause**

Y92.026 **Swimming pool of mobile home as the place of occurrence of the external cause**

Y92.027 **Garden or yard of mobile home as the place of occurrence of the external cause**

Y92.028 **Other place in mobile home as the place of occurrence of the external cause**

Y92.029 **Unspecified place in mobile home as the place of occurrence of the external cause**

● **Y92.03** **Apartment as the place of occurrence of the external cause**

Condominium as the place of occurrence of the external cause

Co-op apartment as the place of occurrence of the external cause

Y92.030 **Kitchen in apartment as the place of occurrence of the external cause**

Y92.031 **Bathroom in apartment as the place of occurrence of the external cause**

Y92.032 **Bedroom in apartment as the place of occurrence of the external cause**

Y92.038 **Other place in apartment as the place of occurrence of the external cause**

Y92.039 **Unspecified place in apartment as the place of occurrence of the external cause**

● **Y92.04** **Boarding-house as the place of occurrence of the external cause**

Y92.040 **Kitchen in boarding-house as the place of occurrence of the external cause**

Y92.041 **Bathroom in boarding-house as the place of occurrence of the external cause**

Y92.042 **Bedroom in boarding-house as the place of occurrence of the external cause**

Y92.043 **Driveway of boarding-house as the place of occurrence of the external cause**

Y92.044 **Garage of boarding-house as the place of occurrence of the external cause**

Y92.045 **Swimming pool of boarding-house as the place of occurrence of the external cause**

Y92.046 **Garden or yard of boarding-house as the place of occurrence of the external cause**

Y92.048 **Other place in boarding-house as the place of occurrence of the external cause**

Y92.049 **Unspecified place in boarding-house as the place of occurrence of the external cause**

● **Y92.09** **Other non-institutional residence as the place of occurrence of the external cause**

Y92.090 **Kitchen in other non-institutional residence as the place of occurrence of the external cause**

Y92.091 **Bathroom in other non-institutional residence as the place of occurrence of the external cause**

Y92.092 **Bedroom in other non-institutional residence as the place of occurrence of the external cause**

Y92.093 **Driveway of other non-institutional residence as the place of occurrence of the external cause**

Y92.094 **Garage of other non-institutional residence as the place of occurrence of the external cause**

Y92.095 **Swimming pool of other non-institutional residence as the place of occurrence of the external cause**

Y92.096 **Garden or yard of other non-institutional residence as the place of occurrence of the external cause**

Y92.098 **Other place in other non-institutional residence as the place of occurrence of the external cause**

Y92.099 **Unspecified place in other non-institutional residence as the place of occurrence of the external cause**

● **Y92.1** **Institutional (nonprivate) residence as the place of occurrence of the external cause**

Y92.10 **Unspecified residential institution as the place of occurrence of the external cause**

● **Y92.11** **Children's home and orphanage as the place of occurrence of the external cause**

Y92.110 **Kitchen in children's home and orphanage as the place of occurrence of the external cause**

Y92.111 **Bathroom in children's home and orphanage as the place of occurrence of the external cause**

Y92.112 **Bedroom in children's home and orphanage as the place of occurrence of the external cause**

Y92.113 **Driveway of children's home and orphanage as the place of occurrence of the external cause**

Y92.114 **Garage of children's home and orphanage as the place of occurrence of the external cause**

Y92.115 **Swimming pool of children's home and orphanage as the place of occurrence of the external cause**

Y92.116 **Garden or yard of children's home and orphanage as the place of occurrence of the external cause**

Y92.118 **Other place in children's home and orphanage as the place of occurrence of the external cause**

Y92.119 **Unspecified place in children's home and orphanage as the place of occurrence of the external cause**

● Y92.12 Nursing home as the place of occurrence of the external cause
Home for the sick as the place of occurrence of the external cause
Hospice as the place of occurrence of the external cause
Y92.120 Kitchen in nursing home as the place of occurrence of the external cause
Y92.121 Bathroom in nursing home as the place of occurrence of the external cause
Y92.122 Bedroom in nursing home as the place of occurrence of the external cause
Y92.123 Driveway of nursing home as the place of occurrence of the external cause
Y92.124 Garage of nursing home as the place of occurrence of the external cause
Y92.125 Swimming pool of nursing home as the place of occurrence of the external cause
Y92.126 Garden or yard of nursing home as the place of occurrence of the external cause
Y92.128 Other place in nursing home as the place of occurrence of the external cause
Y92.129 Unspecified place in nursing home as the place of occurrence of the external cause

● Y92.13 Military base as the place of occurrence of the external cause
Excludes1 military training grounds (Y92.83)
Y92.130 Kitchen on military base as the place of occurrence of the external cause
Y92.131 Mess hall on military base as the place of occurrence of the external cause
Y92.133 Barracks on military base as the place of occurrence of the external cause
Y92.135 Garage on military base as the place of occurrence of the external cause
Y92.136 Swimming pool on military base as the place of occurrence of the external cause
Y92.137 Garden or yard on military base as the place of occurrence of the external cause
Y92.138 Other place on military base as the place of occurrence of the external cause
Y92.139 Unspecified place military base as the place of occurrence of the external cause

● Y92.14 Prison as the place of occurrence of the external cause
Y92.140 Kitchen in prison as the place of occurrence of the external cause
Y92.141 Dining room in prison as the place of occurrence of the external cause
Y92.142 Bathroom in prison as the place of occurrence of the external cause
Y92.143 Cell of prison as the place of occurrence of the external cause
Y92.146 Swimming pool of prison as the place of occurrence of the external cause
Y92.147 Courtyard of prison as the place of occurrence of the external cause
Y92.148 Other place in prison as the place of occurrence of the external cause
Y92.149 Unspecified place in prison as the place of occurrence of the external cause

● Y92.15 Reform school as the place of occurrence of the external cause
Y92.150 Kitchen in reform school as the place of occurrence of the external cause
Y92.151 Dining room in reform school as the place of occurrence of the external cause
Y92.152 Bathroom in reform school as the place of occurrence of the external cause
Y92.153 Bedroom in reform school as the place of occurrence of the external cause
Y92.154 Driveway of reform school as the place of occurrence of the external cause
Y92.155 Garage of reform school as the place of occurrence of the external cause
Y92.156 Swimming pool of reform school as the place of occurrence of the external cause
Y92.157 Garden or yard of reform school as the place of occurrence of the external cause
Y92.158 Other place in reform school as the place of occurrence of the external cause
Y92.159 Unspecified place in reform school as the place of occurrence of the external cause

● Y92.16 School dormitory as the place of occurrence of the external cause
Excludes1 reform school as the place of occurrence of the external cause (Y92.15-)
school buildings and grounds as the place of occurrence of the external cause (Y92.2-)
school sports and athletic areas as the place of occurrence of the external cause (Y92.3-)
Y92.160 Kitchen in school dormitory as the place of occurrence of the external cause
Y92.161 Dining room in school dormitory as the place of occurrence of the external cause
Y92.162 Bathroom in school dormitory as the place of occurrence of the external cause
Y92.163 Bedroom in school dormitory as the place of occurrence of the external cause
Y92.168 Other place in school dormitory as the place of occurrence of the external cause
Y92.169 Unspecified place in school dormitory as the place of occurrence of the external cause

● **Y92.19 Other specified residential institution as the place of occurrence of the external cause**

Y92.190 Kitchen in other specified residential institution as the place of occurrence of the external cause

Y92.191 Dining room in other specified residential institution as the place of occurrence of the external cause

Y92.192 Bathroom in other specified residential institution as the place of occurrence of the external cause

Y92.193 Bedroom in other specified residential institution as the place of occurrence of the external cause

Y92.194 Driveway of other specified residential institution as the place of occurrence of the external cause

Y92.195 Garage of other specified residential institution as the place of occurrence of the external cause

Y92.196 Pool of other specified residential institution as the place of occurrence of the external cause

Y92.197 Garden or yard of other specified residential institution as the place of occurrence of the external cause

Y92.198 Other place in other specified residential institution as the place of occurrence of the external cause

Y92.199 Unspecified place in other specified residential institution as the place of occurrence of the external cause

● **Y92.2 School, other institution and public administrative area as the place of occurrence of the external cause**

Building and adjacent grounds used by the general public or by a particular group of the public

Excludes1 building under construction as the place of occurrence of the external cause (Y92.6)
residential institution as the place of occurrence of the external cause (Y92.1)
school dormitory as the place of occurrence of the external cause (Y92.16-)
sports and athletics area of schools as the place of occurrence of the external cause (Y92.3-)

● **Y92.21 School (private) (public) (state) as the place of occurrence of the external cause**

Y92.210 Daycare center as the place of occurrence of the external cause

Y92.211 Elementary school as the place of occurrence of the external cause

Kindergarten as the place of occurrence of the external cause

Y92.212 Middle school as the place of occurrence of the external cause

Y92.213 High school as the place of occurrence of the external cause

Y92.214 College as the place of occurrence of the external cause

University as the place of occurrence of the external cause

Y92.215 Trade school as the place of occurrence of the external cause

Y92.218 Other school as the place of occurrence of the external cause

Y92.219 Unspecified school as the place of occurrence of the external cause

Y92.22 Religious institution as the place of occurrence of the external cause

Church as the place of occurrence of the external cause
Mosque as the place of occurrence of the external cause
Synagogue as the place of occurrence of the external cause

● **Y92.23 Hospital as the place of occurrence of the external cause**

Excludes1 ambulatory (outpatient) health services establishments (Y92.53-)
home for the sick as the place of occurrence of the external cause (Y92.12-)
hospice as the place of occurrence of the external cause (Y92.12-)
nursing home as the place of occurrence of the external cause (Y92.12-)

Y92.230 Patient room in hospital as the place of occurrence of the external cause

Y92.231 Patient bathroom in hospital as the place of occurrence of the external cause

Y92.232 Corridor of hospital as the place of occurrence of the external cause

Y92.233 Cafeteria of hospital as the place of occurrence of the external cause

Y92.234 Operating room of hospital as the place of occurrence of the external cause

Y92.238 Other place in hospital as the place of occurrence of the external cause

Y92.239 Unspecified place in hospital as the place of occurrence of the external cause

● **Y92.24 Public administrative building as the place of occurrence of the external cause**

Y92.240 Courthouse as the place of occurrence of the external cause

Y92.241 Library as the place of occurrence of the external cause

Y92.242 Post office as the place of occurrence of the external cause

Y92.243 City hall as the place of occurrence of the external cause

Y92.248 Other public administrative building as the place of occurrence of the external cause

● **Y92.25 Cultural building as the place of occurrence of the external cause**

Y92.250 Art gallery as the place of occurrence of the external cause

Y92.251 Museum as the place of occurrence of the external cause

Y92.252 Music hall as the place of occurrence of the external cause

Y92.253 Opera house as the place of occurrence of the external cause

Y92.254 Theater (live) as the place of occurrence of the external cause

Y92.258 Other cultural public building as the place of occurrence of the external cause

Y92.26 Movie house or cinema as the place of occurrence of the external cause

Y92.29 Other specified public building as the place of occurrence of the external cause

Assembly hall as the place of occurrence of the external cause
Clubhouse as the place of occurrence of the external cause

● Y92.3 **Sports and athletics area as the place of occurrence of the external cause**

● Y92.31 **Athletic court as the place of occurrence of the external cause**

Excludes1 tennis court in private home or garden (Y92.Ø9)

Y92.31Ø **Basketball court as the place of occurrence of the external cause**

Y92.311 **Squash court as the place of occurrence of the external cause**

Y92.312 **Tennis court as the place of occurrence of the external cause**

Y92.318 **Other athletic court as the place of occurrence of the external cause**

● Y92.32 **Athletic field as the place of occurrence of the external cause**

Y92.32Ø **Baseball field as the place of occurrence of the external cause**

Y92.321 **Football field as the place of occurrence of the external cause**

Y92.322 **Soccer field as the place of occurrence of the external cause**

Y92.328 **Other athletic field as the place of occurrence of the external cause**

Cricket field as the place of occurrence of the external cause

Hockey field as the place of occurrence of the external cause

● Y92.33 **Skating rink as the place of occurrence of the external cause**

Y92.33Ø **Ice skating rink (indoor) (outdoor) as the place of occurrence of the external cause**

Y92.331 **Roller skating rink as the place of occurrence of the external cause**

Y92.34 **Swimming pool (public) as the place of occurrence of the external cause**

Excludes1 swimming pool in private home or garden (Y92.Ø16)

Y92.39 **Other specified sports and athletic area as the place of occurrence of the external cause**

Golf-course as the place of occurrence of the external cause

Gymnasium as the place of occurrence of the external cause

Riding-school as the place of occurrence of the external cause

Stadium as the place of occurrence of the external cause

● Y92.4 **Street, highway and other paved roadways as the place of occurrence of the external cause** ◀

Excludes1 private driveway of residence (Y92.Ø14, Y92.Ø24, Y92.Ø43, Y92.Ø93, Y92.113, Y92.123, Y92.154, Y92.194)

● Y92.41 **Street and highway as the place of occurrence of the external cause**

Y92.41Ø **Unspecified street and highway as the place of occurrence of the external cause**

Road NOS as the place of occurrence of the external cause

Y92.411 **Interstate highway as the place of occurrence of the external cause**

Freeway as the place of occurrence of the external cause

Motorway as the place of occurrence of the external cause

Y92.412 **Parkway as the place of occurrence of the external cause**

Y92.413 **State road as the place of occurrence of the external cause**

Y92.414 **Local residential or business street as the place of occurrence of the external cause**

Y92.415 **Exit ramp or entrance ramp of street or highway as the place of occurrence of the external cause**

● Y92.48 **Other paved roadways as the place of occurrence of the external cause**

Y92.48Ø **Sidewalk as the place of occurrence of the external cause**

Y92.481 **Parking lot as the place of occurrence of the external cause**

Y92.482 **Bike path as the place of occurrence of the external cause**

Y92.488 **Other paved roadways as the place of occurrence of the external cause**

● Y92.5 **Trade and service area as the place of occurrence of the external cause**

Excludes1 garage in private home (Y92.Ø15)
schools and other public administration buildings (Y92.2-)

● Y92.51 **Private commercial establishments as the place of occurrence of the external cause**

Y92.51Ø **Bank as the place of occurrence of the external cause**

Y92.511 **Restaurant or café as the place of occurrence of the external cause**

Y92.512 **Supermarket, store or market as the place of occurrence of the external cause**

Y92.513 **Shop (commercial) as the place of occurrence of the external cause**

● Y92.52 **Service areas as the place of occurrence of the external cause**

Y92.52Ø **Airport as the place of occurrence of the external cause**

Y92.521 **Bus station as the place of occurrence of the external cause**

Y92.522 **Railway station as the place of occurrence of the external cause**

Y92.523 **Highway rest stop as the place of occurrence of the external cause**

Y92.524 **Gas station as the place of occurrence of the external cause**

Petroleum station as the place of occurrence of the external cause

Service station as the place of occurrence of the external cause

● Y92.53 **Ambulatory health services establishments as the place of occurrence of the external cause**

Y92.53Ø **Ambulatory surgery center as the place of occurrence of the external cause**

Outpatient surgery center, including that connected with a hospital as the place of occurrence of the external cause

Same day surgery center, including that connected with a hospital as the place of occurrence of the external cause

Y92.531 **Health care provider office as the place of occurrence of the external cause**

Physician office as the place of occurrence of the external cause

Y92.532 **Urgent care center as the place of occurrence of the external cause**

Y92.538 **Other ambulatory health services establishments as the place of occurrence of the external cause**

Y92.59 Other trade areas as the place of occurrence of the external cause
Office building as the place of occurrence of the external cause
Casino as the place of occurrence of the external cause
Garage (commercial) as the place of occurrence of the external cause
Hotel as the place of occurrence of the external cause
Radio or television station as the place of occurrence of the external cause
Shopping mall as the place of occurrence of the external cause
Warehouse as the place of occurrence of the external cause

● **Y92.6 Industrial and construction area as the place of occurrence of the external cause**

Y92.61 Building [any] under construction as the place of occurrence of the external cause

Y92.62 Dock or shipyard as the place of occurrence of the external cause
Dockyard as the place of occurrence of the external cause
Dry dock as the place of occurrence of the external cause
Shipyard as the place of occurrence of the external cause

Y92.63 Factory as the place of occurrence of the external cause
Factory building as the place of occurrence of the external cause
Factory premises as the place of occurrence of the external cause
Industrial yard as the place of occurrence of the external cause

Y92.64 Mine or pit as the place of occurrence of the external cause
Mine as the place of occurrence of the external cause

Y92.65 Oil rig as the place of occurrence of the external cause
Pit (coal) (gravel) (sand) as the place of occurrence of the external cause

Y92.69 Other specified industrial and construction area as the place of occurrence of the external cause
Gasworks as the place of occurrence of the external cause
Power-station (coal) (nuclear) (oil) as the place of occurrence of the external cause
Tunnel under construction as the place of occurrence of the external cause
Workshop as the place of occurrence of the external cause

● **Y92.7 Farm as the place of occurrence of the external cause**
Ranch as the place of occurrence of the external cause
Excludes1 farmhouse and home premises of farm (Y92.01-)

Y92.71 Barn as the place of occurrence of the external cause

Y92.72 Chicken coop as the place of occurrence of the external cause
Hen house as the place of occurrence of the external cause

Y92.73 Farm field as the place of occurrence of the external cause

Y92.74 Orchard as the place of occurrence of the external cause

Y92.79 Other farm location as the place of occurrence of the external cause

● **Y92.8 Other places as the place of occurrence of the external cause**

● **Y92.81 Transport vehicle as the place of occurrence of the external cause**
Excludes1 transport accidents (V00-V99)

Y92.810 Car as the place of occurrence of the external cause

Y92.811 Bus as the place of occurrence of the external cause

Y92.812 Truck as the place of occurrence of the external cause

Y92.813 Airplane as the place of occurrence of the external cause

Y92.814 Boat as the place of occurrence of the external cause

Y92.815 Train as the place of occurrence of the external cause

Y92.816 Subway car as the place of occurrence of the external cause

Y92.818 Other transport vehicle as the place of occurrence of the external cause

● **Y92.82 Wilderness area**

Y92.820 Desert as the place of occurrence of the external cause

Y92.821 Forest as the place of occurrence of the external cause

Y92.828 Other wilderness area as the place of occurrence of the external cause
Swamp as the place of occurrence of the external cause
Mountain as the place of occurrence of the external cause
Marsh as the place of occurrence of the external cause
Prairie as the place of occurrence of the external cause

● **Y92.83 Recreation area as the place of occurrence of the external cause**

Y92.830 Public park as the place of occurrence of the external cause

Y92.831 Amusement park as the place of occurrence of the external cause

Y92.832 Beach as the place of occurrence of the external cause
Seashore as the place of occurrence of the external cause

Y92.833 Campsite as the place of occurrence of the external cause

Y92.834 Zoological garden (zoo) as the place of occurrence of the external cause

Y92.838 Other recreation area as the place of occurrence of the external cause

Y92.84 Military training ground as the place of occurrence of the external cause

Y92.85 Railroad track as the place of occurrence of the external cause

Y92.86 Slaughter house as the place of occurrence of the external cause

Y92.89 Other specified places as the place of occurrence of the external cause
Derelict house as the place of occurrence of the external cause

OGCR Section I.C.20.b.

Do not use place of occurrence code Y92.9 if the place is not stated or is not applicable.

Y92.9 **Unspecified place or not applicable**

OGCR See Section I.C.20.c.

Activity Code

Assign a code from category Y93, Activity code, to describe the activity of the patient at the time the injury or other health condition occurred.

An activity code is used only once, at the initial encounter for treatment. Only one code from Y93 should be recorded on a medical record.

The activity codes are not applicable to poisonings, adverse effects, misadventures or sequela.

Do not assign Y93.9, Unspecified activity, if the activity is not stated.

A code from category Y93 is appropriate for use with external cause and intent codes if identifying the activity provides additional information about the event.

● **Y93 Activity codes**

Note: Category Y93 is provided for use to indicate the activity of the person seeking healthcare for an injury or health condition, such as a heart attack while shoveling snow, which resulted from, or was contributed to, by the activity. These codes are appropriate for use for both acute injuries, such as those from chapter 19, and conditions that are due to the long-term, cumulative effects of an activity, such as those from chapter 13. They are also appropriate for use with external cause codes for cause and intent if identifying the activity provides additional information on the event. These codes should be used in conjunction with codes for external cause status (Y99) and place of occurrence (Y92).

This section contains the following broad activity categories:

Y93.0 Activities involving walking and running
Y93.1 Activities involving water and water craft
Y93.2 Activities involving ice and snow
Y93.3 Activities involving climbing, rappelling, and jumping off
Y93.4 Activities involving dancing and other rhythmic movement
Y93.5 Activities involving other sports and athletics played individually
Y93.6 Activities involving other sports and athletics played as a team or group
Y93.7 Activities involving other specified sports and athletics
Y93.A Activities involving other cardiorespiratory exercise
Y93.B Activities involving other muscle strengthening exercises
Y93.C Activities involving computer technology and electronic devices
Y93.D Activities involving arts and handcrafts
Y93.E Activities involving personal hygiene and interior property and clothing maintenance
Y93.F Activities involving caregiving
Y93.G Activities involving food preparation, cooking and grilling
Y93.H Activities involving exterior property and land maintenance, building and construction
Y93.I Activities involving roller coasters and other types of external motion
Y93.J Activities involving playing musical instrument
Y93.K Activities involving animal care
Y93.8 Activities, other specified
Y93.9 Activity, unspecified

● **Y93.0 Activities involving walking and running**

Excludes1 Activity, walking an animal (Y93.K1)
Activity, walking or running on a treadmill (Y93.A1)

Y93.01 Activity, walking, marching and hiking
Activity, walking, marching and hiking on level or elevated terrain
Excludes1 activity, mountain climbing (Y93.31)

Y93.02 Activity, running

● **Y93.1 Activities involving water and water craft**

Excludes1 activities involving ice (Y93.2-)

Y93.11 Activity, swimming
Y93.12 Activity, springboard and platform diving
Y93.13 Activity, water polo
Y93.14 Activity, water aerobics and water exercise
Y93.15 Activity, underwater diving and snorkeling
Activity, SCUBA diving
Y93.16 Activity, rowing, canoeing, kayaking, rafting and tubing
Activity, canoeing, kayaking, rafting and tubing in calm and turbulent water
Y93.17 Activity, water skiing and wake boarding
Y93.18 Activity, surfing, windsurfing and boogie boarding
Activity, water sliding
Y93.19 Activity, other involving water and watercraft
Activity involving water NOS
Activity, parasailing
Activity, water survival training and testing

● **Y93.2 Activities involving ice and snow**

Excludes1 activity, shoveling ice and snow (Y93.H1)

Y93.21 Activity, ice skating
Activity, figure skating (singles) (pairs)
Activity, ice dancing
Excludes1 activity, ice hockey (Y93.22)
Y93.22 Activity, ice hockey
Y93.23 Activity, snow (alpine) (downhill) skiing, snow boarding, sledding, tobogganing and snow tubing
Excludes1 activity, cross country skiing (Y93.24)
Y93.24 Activity, cross country skiing
Activity, nordic skiing
Y93.29 Activity, other activity involving ice and snow
Activity, activity involving ice and snow NOS

● **Y93.3 Activities involving climbing, rappelling and jumping off**

Excludes1 activity, hiking on level or elevated terrain (Y93.01)
activity, jumping rope (Y93.56)
activity, trampoline jumping (Y93.44)

Y93.31 Activity, mountain climbing, rock climbing and wall climbing
Y93.32 Activity, rappelling
Y93.33 Activity, BASE jumping
Activity, building, Antenna, Span, Earth jumping
Y93.34 Activity, bungee jumping
Y93.35 Activity, hang gliding
Y93.39 Activity, other activity involving climbing, rappelling and jumping off

● **Y93.4 Activities involving dancing and other rhythmic movement**

Excludes1 activity, martial arts (Y93.75)

Y93.41 Activity, dancing
Y93.42 Activity, yoga
Y93.43 Activity, gymnastics
Activity, rhythmic gymnastics
Excludes1 activity, trampolining (Y93.44)
Y93.44 Activity, trampolining
Y93.45 Activity, cheerleading
Y93.49 Activity, other involving dancing and other rhythmic movements

CHAPTER 20 (V01-Y99)

● **Y93.5 Activities involving other sports and athletics played individually**
Excludes1 activity, dancing (Y93.41)
activity, gymnastic (Y93.43)
activity, trampolining (Y93.44)
activity, yoga (Y93.42)

Y93.51 Activity, roller skating (inline) and skateboarding

Y93.52 Activity, horseback riding

Y93.53 Activity, golf

Y93.54 Activity, bowling

Y93.55 Activity, bike riding

Y93.56 Activity, jumping rope

Y93.57 Activity, non-running track and field events
Excludes1 activity, running (any form) (Y93.Ø2)

Y93.59 Activity, other involving other sports and athletics played individually
Excludes1 activities involving climbing, rappelling, and jumping (Y93.3-)
activities involving ice and snow (Y93.2-)
activities involving walking and running (Y93.Ø-)
activities involving water and watercraft (Y93.1-)

● **Y93.6 Activities involving other sports and athletics played as a team or group**
Excludes1 activity, ice hockey (Y93.22)
activity, water polo (Y93.13)

Y93.61 Activity, American tackle football
Activity, football NOS

Y93.62 Activity, American flag or touch football

Y93.63 Activity, rugby

Y93.64 Activity, baseball
Activity, softball

Y93.65 Activity, lacrosse and field hockey

Y93.66 Activity, soccer

Y93.67 Activity, basketball

Y93.68 Activity, volleyball (beach) (court)

Y93.6A Activity, physical games generally associated with school recess, summer camp and children
Activity, capture the flag
Activity, dodge ball
Activity, four square
Activity, kickball

Y93.69 Activity, other involving other sports and athletics played as a team or group
Cricket

● **Y93.7 Activities involving other specified sports and athletics**

Y93.71 Activity, boxing

Y93.72 Activity, wrestling

Y93.73 Activity, racquet and hand sports
Activity, handball
Activity, racquetball
Activity, squash
Activity, tennis

Y93.74 Activity, frisbee
Activity, ultimate frisbee

Y93.75 Activity, martial arts
Activity, combatives

Y93.79 Activity, other specified sports and athletics
Excludes1 sports and athletics activities specified in categories Y93.Ø-Y93.6

● **Y93.A Activities involving other cardiorespiratory exercise**
Activities involving physical training

Y93.A1 Activity, exercise machines primarily for cardiorespiratory conditioning
Activity, elliptical and stepper machines
Activity, stationary bike
Activity, treadmill

Y93.A2 Activity, calisthenics
Activity, jumping jacks
Activity, warm up and cool down

Y93.A3 Activity, aerobic and step exercise

Y93.A4 Activity, circuit training

Y93.A5 Activity, obstacle course
Activity, challenge course
Activity, confidence course

Y93.A6 Activity, grass drills
Activity, guerilla drills

Y93.A9 Activity, other involving other cardiorespiratory exercise
Excludes1 activities involving cardiorespiratory exercise specified in categories Y93.Ø-Y93.7

● **Y93.B Activity involving other muscle strengthening exercises**

Y93.B1 Activity, exercise machines primarily for muscle strengthening

Y93.B2 Activity, push-ups, pull-ups, sit-ups

Y93.B3 Activity, free weights
Activity, barbells
Activity, dumbbells

Y93.B4 Activity, pilates

Y93.B9 Activity, other involving other muscle strengthening exercises
Excludes1 activities involving muscle strengthening specified in categories Y93.Ø-Y93.A

● **Y93.C Activities involving computer technology and electronic devices**
Excludes1 activity, electronic musical keyboard or instruments (Y93.J-)

Y93.C1 Activity, computer keyboarding
Activity, electronic game playing using keyboard or other stationary device

Y93.C2 Activity, hand held interactive electronic device
Activity, cellular telephone and communication device
Activity, electronic game playing using interactive device
Excludes1 activity, electronic game playing using keyboard or other stationary device (Y93.C1)

Y93.C9 Activity, other involving computer technology and electronic devices

● **Y93.D Activities involving arts and handcrafts**
Excludes1 activities involving playing musical instrument (Y93.J-)

Y93.D1 Knitting and crocheting

Y93.D2 Sewing

Y93.D3 Furniture building and finishing
Furniture repair

Y93.D9 Activity, other involving arts and handcrafts

● **Y93.E Activities involving personal hygiene and interior property and clothing maintenance**

Excludes1 activities involving cooking and grilling (Y93.G-)
activities involving exterior property and land maintenance, building and construction (Y93.H-)
activity involving caregiving (Y93.F-)
activity, dishwashing (Y93.G1)
activity, food preparation (Y93.G1)
activity, gardening (Y93.H2)

Y93.E1 Activity, personal bathing and showering

Y93.E2 Activity, laundry

Y93.E3 Activity, vacuuming

Y93.E4 Activity, ironing

Y93.E5 Activity, floor mopping and cleaning

Y93.E6 Activity, residential relocation
Activity, packing up and unpacking involved in moving to a new residence

Y93.E8 Activity, other personal hygiene activity

Y93.E9 Activity, other household maintenance

● **Y93.F Activities involving person providing caregiving**
Activity involving the provider of caregiving

Y93.F1 Activity, caregiving involving bathing

Y93.F2 Activity, caregiving involving lifting

Y93.F9 Activity, other caregiving

● **Y93.G Activities involving food preparation, cooking and grilling**

Y93.G1 Activity, food preparation and clean up
Activity, dishwashing

Y93.G2 Activity, grilling and smoking food

Y93.G3 Activity, cooking and baking
Activity, use of stove, oven and microwave oven

Y93.G9 Activity, other activity involving cooking and grilling

● **Y93.H Activities involving property and land maintenance, building and construction**

Y93.H1 Activity, digging, shoveling and raking
Activity, dirt digging
Activity, raking leaves
Activity, snow shoveling

Y93.H2 Activity, gardening and landscaping
Activity, pruning, trimming shrubs, weeding

Y93.H3 Activity, building and construction

Y93.H9 Activity, other activity involving property and land maintenance, building and construction

● **Y93.I Activities involving roller coasters and other types of external motion**

Y93.I1 Activity, rollercoaster riding

Y93.I9 Activity, other involving external motion

● **Y93.J Activities involving playing musical instrument**
Activity involving playing electric musical instrument

Y93.J1 Activity, piano playing
Activity, musical keyboard (electronic) playing

Y93.J2 Activity, drum and other percussion instrument playing

Y93.J3 Activity, string instrument playing

Y93.J4 Activity, winds and brass instrument playing

● **Y93.K Activities involving animal care**

Excludes1 activity, horseback riding (Y93.52)

Y93.K1 Activity, walking an animal

Y93.K2 Activity, milking an animal

Y93.K3 Activity, grooming and shearing an animal

Y93.K9 Activity, other activity involving animal care

● **Y93.8 Other activity**

Y93.81 Activity, refereeing a sports activity

Y93.82 Activity, spectator at an event

Y93.83 Activity, rough housing and horseplay

Y93.84 Activity, sleeping

Y93.85 Activity, choking game ◀
Activity, blackout game ◀
Activity, fainting game ◀
Activity, pass out game ◀

Y93.89 Activity, other specified

OGCR See Section I.C.20.c.

Do not assign Y93.9, Unspecified activity, if the activity is not stated.

● **Y93.9 Activity, unspecified**

Y95 Nosocomial condition

● **Y99 External cause status**

Note: A single code from category Y99 should be used in conjunction with the external cause code(s) assigned to a record to indicate the status of the person at the time the event occurred.

Y99.Ø Civilian activity done for income or pay
Civilian activity done for financial or other compensation

Excludes1 military activity (Y99.1)
volunteer activity (Y99.2)

Y99.1 Military activity

Excludes1 activity of off duty military personnel (Y99.8)

Y99.2 Volunteer activity

Excludes1 activity of child or other family member assisting in compensated work of other family member (Y99.8)

Y99.8 Other external cause status
Activity NEC
Activity of child or other family member assisting in compensated work of other family member
Hobby not done for income
Leisure activity
Off-duty activity of military personnel
Recreation or sport not for income or while a student
Student activity

Excludes1 civilian activity done for income or compensation (Y99.Ø)
military activity (Y99.1)

Y99.9 Unspecified external cause status

CHAPTER 21

FACTORS INFLUENCING HEALTH STATUS AND CONTACT WITH HEALTH SERVICES (Z00-Z99)

OGCR Chapter-Specific Coding Guidelines

21. **Chapter 21: Factors influencing health status and contact with health services (Z00-Z99)**

Note: The chapter specific guidelines provide additional information about the use of Z codes for specified encounters.

a. **Use of Z codes in any healthcare setting**

Z codes are for use in any healthcare setting. Z codes may be used as either a first-listed (principal diagnosis code in the inpatient setting) or secondary code, depending on the circumstances of the encounter. Certain Z codes may only be used as first-listed or principal diagnosis.

b. **Z Codes indicate a reason for an encounter**

Z codes are not procedure codes. A corresponding procedure code must accompany a Z code to describe any procedure performed.

c. **Categories of Z Codes**

1) **Contact/Exposure**

Category Z20 indicates contact with, and suspected exposure to, communicable diseases. These codes are for patients who do not show any sign or symptom of a disease but are suspected to have been exposed to it by close personal contact with an infected individual or are in an area where a disease is epidemic.

Category Z77, **Other contact with and (suspected) exposures hazardous to health,** indicates contact with and suspected exposures hazardous to health.

Contact/exposure codes may be used as a first-listed code to explain an encounter for testing, or, more commonly, as a secondary code to identify a potential risk.

2) **Inoculations and vaccinations**

Code Z23 is for encounters for inoculations and vaccinations. It indicates that a patient is being seen to receive a prophylactic inoculation against a disease. Procedure codes are required to identify the actual administration of the injection and the type(s) of immunizations given. Code Z23 may be used as a secondary code if the inoculation is given as a routine part of preventive health care, such as a well-baby visit.

3) **Status**

Status codes indicate that a patient is either a carrier of a disease or has the sequelae or residual of a past disease or condition. This includes such things as the presence of prosthetic or mechanical devices resulting from past treatment. A status code is informative, because the status may affect the course of treatment and its outcome. A status code is distinct from a history code. The history code indicates that the patient no longer has the condition.

A status code should not be used with a diagnosis code from one of the body system chapters, if the diagnosis code includes the information provided by the status code. For example, code Z94.1, Heart transplant status, should not be used with a code from subcategory T86.2, Complications of heart transplant. The status code does not provide additional information. The complication code indicates that the patient is a heart transplant patient.

For encounters for weaning from a mechanical ventilator, assign a code from subcategory J96.1, Chronic respiratory failure, followed by code Z99.11, Dependence on respirator [ventilator] status.

The status Z codes/categories are:

Z14 Genetic carrier
Genetic carrier status indicates that a person carries a gene, associated with a particular disease, which may be passed to offspring who may develop that disease. The person does not have the disease and is not at risk of developing the disease.

Z15 Genetic susceptibility to disease Genetic susceptibility indicates that a person has a gene that increases the risk of that person developing the disease.

Codes from category Z15 should not be used as principal or first-listed codes. If the patient has the condition to which he/she is susceptible, and that condition is the reason for the encounter, the code for the current condition should be sequenced first. If the patient is being seen for follow-up after completed treatment for this condition, and the condition no longer exists, a follow-up code should be sequenced first, followed by the appropriate personal history and genetic susceptibility codes. If the purpose of the encounter is genetic counseling associated with procreative management, code Z31.5, Encounter for genetic counseling, should be assigned as the first-listed code, followed by a code from category Z15. Additional codes should be assigned for any applicable family or personal history.

Z16 Resistance to antimicrobial drugs
This code indicates that a patient has a condition that is resistant to antimicrobial drug treatment. Sequence the infection code first.

Z17 Estrogen receptor status

Z18 Retained foreign body fragments

Z19 Hormone sensitivity malignancy status

Z21 Asymptomatic HIV infection status This code indicates that a patient has tested positive for HIV but has manifested no signs or symptoms of the disease.

Z22 Carrier of infectious disease Carrier status indicates that a person harbors the specific organisms of a disease without manifest symptoms and is capable of transmitting the infection.

Z28.3 Underimmunization status

Z33.1 Pregnant state, incidental This code is a secondary code only for use when the pregnancy is in no way complicating the reason for visit. Otherwise, a code from the obstetric chapter is required.

Z66 Do not resuscitate

This code may be used when it is documented by the provider that a patient is on do not resuscitate status at any time during the stay.

Z67 Blood type

Z68 Body mass index (BMI)
As with all other secondary diagnosis codes, the BMI codes should only be assigned when they meet the definition of a reportable diagnosis (see Section III, Reporting Additional Diagnoses).

Z74.01 Bed confinement status

Z76.82 Awaiting organ transplant status

Z78 Other specified health status

Code Z78.1, Physical restraint status, may be used when it is documented by the provider that a patient has been put in restraints during the current encounter. Please note that this code should not be reported when it is documented by the provider that a patient is temporarily restrained during a procedure.

Z79 Long-term (current) drug therapy

Codes from this category indicate a patient's continuous use of a prescribed drug (including such things as aspirin therapy) for the long-term treatment of a condition or for prophylactic use. It is not for use for patients who have addictions to drugs. This subcategory is not for use of medications for detoxification or maintenance programs to prevent withdrawal symptoms in patients with drug dependence (e.g., methadone maintenance for opiate dependence). Assign the appropriate code for the drug dependence instead.

Assign a code from Z79 if the patient is receiving a medication for an extended period as a prophylactic measure (such as for the prevention of deep vein thrombosis) or as treatment of a chronic condition (such as arthritis) or a disease requiring a lengthy course of treatment (such as cancer). Do not assign a code from category Z79 for medication being administered for a brief period of time to treat an acute illness or injury (such as a course of antibiotics to treat acute bronchitis).

Z88 Allergy status to drugs, medicaments and biological substances Except: Z88.9, Allergy status to unspecified drugs, medicaments and biological substances status

Z89 Acquired absence of limb

Z90 Acquired absence of organs, not elsewhere classified

Z91.0- Allergy status, other than to drugs and biological substances

Z92.82 Status post administration of tPA (rtPA) in a different facility within the last 24 hours prior to admission to a current facility Assign code Z92.82, Status post administration of tPA (rtPA) in a different facility within the last 24 hours prior to admission to current facility, as a secondary diagnosis when a patient is received by transfer into a facility and documentation indicates they were administered tissue plasminogen activator (tPA) within the last 24 hours prior to admission to the current facility. This guideline applies even if the patient is still receiving the tPA at the time they are received into the current facility. The appropriate code for the condition for which the tPA was administered (such as cerebrovascular disease or myocardial infarction) should be assigned first. Code Z92.82 is only applicable to the receiving facility record and not to the transferring facility record.

Z93	Artificial opening status
Z94	Transplanted organ and tissue status
Z95	Presence of cardiac and vascular implants and grafts
Z96	Presence of other functional implants
Z97	Presence of other devices
Z98	Other postprocedural states

Assign code Z98.85, Transplanted organ removal status, to indicate that a transplanted organ has been previously removed. This code should not be assigned for the encounter in which the transplanted organ is removed. The complication necessitating removal of the transplant organ should be assigned for that encounter.

See section I.C.19. for information on the coding of organ transplant complications.

Z99	Dependence on enabling machines and devices, not elsewhere classified

Note: Categories Z89-Z90 and Z93-Z99 are for use only if there are no complications or malfunctions of the organ or tissue replaced, the amputation site or the equipment on which the patient is dependent.

4) History (of)

There are two types of history Z codes, personal and family. Personal history codes explain a patient's past medical condition that no longer exists and is not receiving any treatment, but that has the potential for recurrence, and therefore may require continued monitoring.

Family history codes are for use when a patient has a family member(s) who has had a particular disease that causes the patient to be at higher risk of also contracting the disease.

Personal history codes may be used in conjunction with follow-up codes and family history codes may be used in conjunction with screening codes to explain the need for a test or procedure. History codes are also acceptable on any medical record regardless of the reason for visit. A history of an illness, even if no longer present, is important information that may alter the type of treatment ordered.

The history Z code categories are:

Z8Ø	Family history of primary malignant neoplasm
Z81	Family history of mental and behavioral disorders
Z82	Family history of certain disabilities and chronic diseases (leading to disablement)
Z83	Family history of other specific disorders
Z84	Family history of other conditions
Z85	Personal history of malignant neoplasm
Z86	Personal history of certain other diseases
Z87	Personal history of other diseases and conditions
Z91.4-	Personal history of psychological trauma, not elsewhere classified
Z91.5	Personal history of self-harm
Z91.8-	Other specified personal risk factors, not elsewhere classified Exception: Z91.83, Wandering in diseases classified elsewhere
Z92	Personal history of medical treatment Except: Z92.Ø, Personal history of contraception Except: Z92.82, Status post administration of tPA (rtPA) in a different facility within the last 24 hours prior to admission to a current facility

5) Screening

Screening is the testing for disease or disease precursors in seemingly well individuals so that early detection and treatment can be provided for those who test positive for the disease (e.g., screening mammogram).

The testing of a person to rule out or confirm a suspected diagnosis because the patient has some sign or symptom is a diagnostic examination, not a screening. In these cases, the sign or symptom is used to explain the reason for the test.

A screening code may be a first-listed code if the reason for the visit is specifically the screening exam. It may also be used as an additional code if the screening is done during an office visit for other health problems. A screening code is not necessary if the screening is inherent to a routine examination, such as a pap smear done during a routine pelvic examination.

Should a condition be discovered during the screening then the code for the condition may be assigned as an additional diagnosis.

The Z code indicates that a screening exam is planned. A procedure code is required to confirm that the screening was performed.

The screening Z codes/categories:

Z11	Encounter for screening for infectious and parasitic diseases
Z12	Encounter for screening for malignant neoplasms
Z13	Encounter for screening for other diseases and disorders Except: Z13.9, Encounter for screening, unspecified
Z36	Encounter for antenatal screening for mother

6) Observation

There are **three** observation Z code categories. They are for use in very limited circumstances when a person is being observed for a suspected condition that is ruled out. The observation codes are not for use if an injury or illness or any signs or symptoms related to the suspected condition are present. In such cases the diagnosis/symptom code is used with the corresponding external cause code.

The observation codes are to be used as principal diagnosis only. **The only exception to this is when the principal diagnosis is required to be a code from category Z38, Liveborn infants according to place of birth and type of delivery. Then a code from category Z05, Encounter for observation and evaluation of newborn for suspected diseases and conditions ruled out, is sequenced after the Z38 code.** Additional codes may be used in addition to the observation code but only if they are unrelated to the suspected condition being observed.

Codes from subcategory Z03.7 Encounter for suspected maternal and fetal conditions ruled out, may either be used as a first-listed or as an additional code assignment depending on the case. They are for use in very limited circumstances on a maternal record when an encounter is for a suspected maternal or fetal condition that is ruled out during that encounter (for example, a maternal or fetal condition may be suspected due to an abnormal test result). These codes should not be used when the condition is confirmed. In those cases, the confirmed condition should be coded. In addition, these codes are not for use if an illness or any signs or symptoms related to the suspected condition or problem are present. In such cases the diagnosis/symptom code is used.

Additional codes may be used in addition to the code from subcategory Z03.7, but only if they are unrelated to the suspected condition being evaluated.

Codes from subcategory Z03.7 may not be used for encounters for antenatal screening of mother. *See Section I.C.21. Screening.*

For encounters for suspected fetal condition that are inconclusive following testing and evaluation, assign the appropriate code from category O35, O36, O4Ø or O41.

The observation Z code categories:

ZØ3	Encounter for medical observation for suspected diseases and conditions ruled out
ZØ4	Encounter for examination and observation for other reasons Except: ZØ4.9, Encounter for examination and observation for unspecified reason
ZØ5	**Encounter for observation and evaluation of newborn for suspected diseases and conditions ruled out**

7) Aftercare

Aftercare visit codes cover situations when the initial treatment of a disease has been performed and the patient requires continued care during the healing or recovery phase, or for the long-term consequences of the disease. The aftercare Z code should not be used if treatment is directed at a current, acute disease. The diagnosis code is to be used in these cases.

Exceptions to this rule are codes Z51.Ø, Encounter for antineoplastic radiation therapy, and codes from subcategory Z51.1, Encounter for antineoplastic chemotherapy and immunotherapy. These codes are to be first-listed, followed by the diagnosis code when a patient's encounter is solely to receive radiation therapy, chemotherapy, or immunotherapy for the treatment of a neoplasm. If the reason for the encounter is more than one type of antineoplastic therapy, code Z51.Ø and a code from subcategory Z51.1 may be assigned together, in which case one of these codes would be reported as a secondary diagnosis.

The aftercare Z codes should also not be used for aftercare for injuries. For aftercare of an injury, assign the acute injury code with the appropriate 7th character (for subsequent encounter).

The aftercare codes are generally first-listed to explain the specific reason for the encounter. An aftercare code may be used as an additional code when some type of aftercare is provided in addition to the reason for admission and no diagnosis code is applicable. An example of this would be the closure of a colostomy during an encounter for treatment of another condition.

Aftercare codes should be used in conjunction with other aftercare codes or diagnosis codes to provide better detail on the specifics of an aftercare encounter visit, unless otherwise directed by the classification. Should a patient receive multiple types of antineoplastic therapy during the same encounter, code Z51.Ø, Encounter for antineoplastic radiation therapy, and codes from subcategory Z51.1, Encounter for antineoplastic chemotherapy and immunotherapy, may be used together on a record. The sequencing of multiple aftercare codes depends on the circumstances of the encounter.

Certain aftercare Z code categories need a secondary diagnosis code to describe the resolving condition or sequelae. For others, the condition is included in the code title.

Additional Z code aftercare category terms include fitting and adjustment, and attention to artificial openings.

Status Z codes may be used with aftercare Z codes to indicate the nature of the aftercare. For example code Z95.1, Presence of aortocoronary bypass graft, may be used with code Z48.812, Encounter for surgical aftercare following surgery on the circulatory system, to indicate the surgery for which the aftercare is being performed. A status code should not be used when the aftercare code indicates the type of status, such as using Z43.Ø, Encounter for attention to tracheostomy, with Z93.Ø, Tracheostomy status.

The aftercare Z category/codes:

Z42	Encounter for plastic and reconstructive surgery following medical procedure or healed injury
Z43	Encounter for attention to artificial openings
Z44	Encounter for fitting and adjustment of external prosthetic device
Z45	Encounter for adjustment and management of implanted device
Z46	Encounter for fitting and adjustment of other devices
Z47	Orthopedic aftercare
Z48	Encounter for other postprocedural aftercare
Z49	Encounter for care involving renal dialysis
Z51	Encounter for other aftercare **and medical care**

8) Follow-up

The follow-up codes are used to explain continuing surveillance following completed treatment of a disease, condition, or injury. They imply that the condition has been fully treated and no longer exists. They should not be confused with aftercare codes, or injury codes with a 7th character for subsequent encounter, that explain ongoing care of a healing condition or its sequelae. Follow-up codes may be used in conjunction with history codes to provide the full picture of the healed condition and its treatment. The follow-up code is sequenced first, followed by the history code.

A follow-up code may be used to explain multiple visits. Should a condition be found to have recurred on the follow-up visit, then the diagnosis code for the condition should be assigned in place of the follow-up code.

The follow-up Z code categories:

ZØ8	Encounter for follow-up examination after completed treatment for malignant neoplasm
ZØ9	Encounter for follow-up examination after completed treatment for conditions other than malignant neoplasm
Z39	Encounter for maternal postpartum care and examination

9) Donor

Codes in category Z52, Donors of organs and tissues, are used for living individuals who are donating blood or other body tissue. These codes are only for individuals donating for others, not for self-donations. They are not used to identify cadaveric donations.

1Ø) Counseling

Counseling Z codes are used when a patient or family member receives assistance in the aftermath of an illness or injury, or when support is required in coping with family or social problems. They are not used in conjunction with a diagnosis code when the counseling component of care is considered integral to standard treatment.

The counseling Z codes/categories:

Z3Ø.Ø-	Encounter for general counseling and advice on contraception
Z31.5	Encounter for genetic counseling
Z31.6-	Encounter for general counseling and advice on procreation
Z32.2	Encounter for childbirth instruction
Z32.3	Encounter for childcare instruction
Z69	Encounter for mental health services for victim and perpetrator of abuse
Z7Ø	Counseling related to sexual attitude, behavior and orientation
Z71	Persons encountering health services for other counseling and medical advice, not elsewhere classified
Z76.81	Expectant mother prebirth pediatrician visit

11) Encounters for Obstetrical and Reproductive Services

See Section I.C.15. Pregnancy, Childbirth, and the Puerperium, for further instruction on the use of these codes.

Z codes for pregnancy are for use in those circumstances when none of the problems or complications included in the codes from the Obstetrics chapter exist (a routine prenatal visit or postpartum care). Codes in category Z34, Encounter for supervision of normal pregnancy, are always first listed and are not to be used with any other code from the OB chapter.

Codes in category Z3A, Weeks of gestation, may be assigned to provide additional information about the pregnancy. **Category Z3A codes should not be assigned for pregnancies with abortive outcomes (categories OØØ-OØ8), elective termination of pregnancy (code Z33.32), nor for postpartum conditions, as category Z3A is not applicable to these conditions.** The date of the admission should be used to determine weeks of gestation for inpatient admissions that encompass more than one gestational week.

The outcome of delivery, category Z37, should be included on all maternal delivery records. It is always a secondary code. Codes in category Z37 should not be used on the newborn record.

Z codes for family planning (contraceptive) or procreative management and counseling should be included on an obstetric record either during the pregnancy or the postpartum stage, if applicable.

Z codes/categories for obstetrical and reproductive services:

Z3Ø	Encounter for contraceptive management
Z31	Encounter for procreative management
Z32.2	Encounter for childbirth instruction
Z32.3	Encounter for childcare instruction
Z33	Pregnant state
Z34	Encounter for supervision of normal pregnancy
Z36	Encounter for antenatal screening of mother
Z3A	Weeks of gestation
Z37	Outcome of delivery
Z39	Encounter for maternal postpartum care and examination
Z76.81	Expectant mother prebirth pediatrician visit

12) Newborns and Infants

See Section I.C.16. Newborn (Perinatal) Guidelines, for further instruction on the use of these codes.

Newborn Z codes/categories:

Z76.1	Encounter for health supervision and care of foundling
ZØØ.1-	Encounter for routine child health examination
Z38	Liveborn infants according to place of birth and type of delivery

13) Routine and administrative examinations

The Z codes allow for the description of encounters for routine examinations, such as, a general check-up, or, examinations for administrative purposes, such as, a pre-employment physical. The

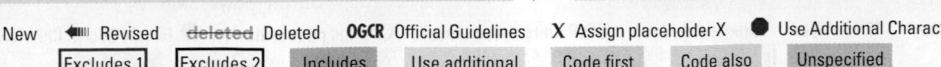

CHAPTER 21 (ZØØ-Z99)

codes are not to be used if the examination is for diagnosis of a suspected condition or for treatment purposes. In such cases the diagnosis code is used. During a routine exam, should a diagnosis or condition be discovered, it should be coded as an additional code. Pre-existing and chronic conditions and history codes may also be included as additional codes as long as the examination is for administrative purposes and not focused on any particular condition.

Some of the codes for routine health examinations distinguish between "with" and "without" abnormal findings. Code assignment depends on the information that is known at the time the encounter is being coded. For example, if no abnormal findings were found during the examination, but the encounter is being coded before test results are back, it is acceptable to assign the code for "without abnormal findings." When assigning a code for "with abnormal findings," additional code(s) should be assigned to identify the specific abnormal finding(s).

Pre-operative examination and pre-procedural laboratory examination Z codes are for use only in those situations when a patient is being cleared for a procedure or surgery and no treatment is given.

The Z codes/categories for routine and administrative examinations:

Z00	Encounter for general examination without complaint, suspected or reported diagnosis
Z01	Encounter for other special examination without complaint, suspected or reported diagnosis
Z02	Encounter for administrative examination Except: Z02.9, Encounter for administrative examinations, unspecified
Z32.0-	Encounter for pregnancy test

14) Miscellaneous Z codes

The miscellaneous Z codes capture a number of other health care encounters that do not fall into one of the other categories. Certain of these codes identify the reason for the encounter; others are for use as additional codes that provide useful information on circumstances that may affect a patient's care and treatment.

Prophylactic Organ Removal

For encounters specifically for prophylactic removal of an organ (such as prophylactic removal of breasts due to a genetic susceptibility to cancer or a family history of cancer), the principal or first-listed code should be a code from category Z40, Encounter for prophylactic surgery, followed by the appropriate codes to identify the associated risk factor (such as genetic susceptibility or family history).

If the patient has a malignancy of one site and is having prophylactic removal at another site to prevent either a new primary malignancy or metastatic disease, a code for the malignancy should also be assigned in addition to a code from subcategory Z40.0, Encounter for prophylactic surgery for risk factors related to malignant neoplasms. A Z40.0 code should not be assigned if the patient is having organ removal for treatment of a malignancy, such as the removal of the testes for the treatment of prostate cancer.

Miscellaneous Z codes/categories:

Z28	Immunization not carried out Except: Z28.3, Underimmunization status
Z29	**Encounter for other prophylactic measures**
Z40	Encounter for prophylactic surgery
Z41	Encounter for procedures for purposes other than remedying health state Except: Z41.9, Encounter for procedure for purposes other than remedying health state, unspecified
Z53	Persons encountering health services for specific procedures and treatment, not carried out
Z55	Problems related to education and literacy
Z56	Problems related to employment and unemployment
Z57	Occupational exposure to risk factors
Z58	Problems related to physical environment
Z59	Problems related to housing and economic circumstances
Z60	Problems related to social environment
Z62	Problems related to upbringing
Z63	Other problems related to primary support group, including family circumstances
Z64	Problems related to certain psychosocial circumstances
Z65	Problems related to other psychosocial circumstances
Z72	Problems related to lifestyle **Note: These codes should be assigned only when the documentation specifies that the patient has an associated problem**
Z73	Problems related to life management difficulty
Z74	Problems related to care provider dependency Except: Z74.01, Bed confinement status
Z75	Problems related to medical facilities and other health care
Z76.0	Encounter for issue of repeat prescription
Z76.3	Healthy person accompanying sick person
Z76.4	Other boarder to healthcare facility
Z76.5	Malingerer [conscious simulation]
Z91.1-	Patient's noncompliance with medical treatment and regimen
Z91.83	Wandering in diseases classified elsewhere
Z91.89	Other specified personal risk factors, not elsewhere classified

15) Nonspecific Z codes

Certain Z codes are so non-specific, or potentially redundant with other codes in the classification, that there can be little justification for their use in the inpatient setting. Their use in the outpatient setting should be limited to those instances when there is no further documentation to permit more precise coding. Otherwise, any sign or symptom or any other reason for visit that is captured in another code should be used.

Nonspecific Z codes/categories:

Z02.9	Encounter for administrative examinations, unspecified
Z04.9	Encounter for examination and observation for unspecified reason
Z13.9	Encounter for screening, unspecified
Z41.9	Encounter for procedure for purposes other than remedying health state, unspecified
Z52.9	Donor of unspecified organ or tissue
Z86.59	Personal history of other mental and behavioral disorders
Z88.9	Allergy status to unspecified drugs, medicaments and biological substances status
Z92.0	Personal history of contraception

16) Z Codes That May Only be Principal/First-Listed Diagnosis

The following Z codes/categories may only be reported as the principal/first-listed diagnosis, except when there are multiple encounters on the same day and the medical records for the encounters are combined:

Z00	Encounter for general examination without complaint, suspected or reported diagnosis Except: Z00.6
Z01	Encounter for other special examination without complaint, suspected or reported diagnosis
Z02	Encounter for administrative examination
Z03	Encounter for medical observation for suspected diseases and conditions ruled out
Z04	Encounter for examination and observation for other reasons
Z33.2	Encounter for elective termination of pregnancy
Z31.81	Encounter for male factor infertility in female patient
Z31.83	Encounter for assisted reproductive fertility procedure cycle
Z31.84	Encounter for fertility preservation procedure
Z34	Encounter for supervision of normal pregnancy
Z39	Encounter for maternal postpartum care and examination
Z38	Liveborn infants according to place of birth and type of delivery
Z42	Encounter for plastic and reconstructive surgery following medical procedure or healed injury
Z51.0	Encounter for antineoplastic radiation therapy
Z51.1-	Encounter for antineoplastic chemotherapy and immunotherapy
Z52	Donors of organs and tissues Except: Z52.9, Donor of unspecified organ or tissue
Z76.1	Encounter for health supervision and care of foundling
Z76.2	Encounter for health supervision and care of other healthy infant and child
Z99.12	Encounter for respirator [ventilator] dependence during power failure

CHAPTER 21

FACTORS INFLUENCING HEALTH STATUS AND CONTACT WITH HEALTH SERVICES (Z00-Z99)

Note: Z codes represent reasons for encounters. A corresponding procedure code must accompany a Z code if a procedure is performed. Categories Z00-Z99 are provided for occasions when circumstances other than a disease, injury or external cause classifiable to categories A00-Y89 are recorded as 'diagnoses' or 'problems.' This can arise in two main ways:

(a) When a person who may or may not be sick encounters the health services for some specific purpose, such as to receive limited care or service for a current condition, to donate an organ or tissue, to receive prophylactic vaccination (immunization), or to discuss a problem which is in itself not a disease or injury.

(b) When some circumstance or problem is present which influences the person's health status but is not in itself a current illness or injury.

This chapter contains the following blocks:

Z00-Z13	Persons encountering health services for examination
Z14-Z15	Genetic carrier and genetic susceptibility to disease
Z16	Resistance to antimicrobial drugs
Z17	Estrogen receptor status
Z18	Retained foreign body fragments
Z19	Hormone sensitivity malignancy status ◀
Z20-Z29	Persons with potential health hazards related to communicable diseases ◀
Z30-Z39	Persons encountering health services in circumstances related to reproduction
Z40-Z53	Encounters for other specific health care
Z55-Z65	Persons with potential health hazards related to socioeconomic and psychosocial circumstances
Z66	Do not resuscitate status
Z67	Blood type
Z68	Body mass index (BMI)
Z69-Z76	Persons encountering health services in other circumstances
Z77-Z99	Persons with potential health hazards related to family and personal history and certain conditions influencing health status

PERSONS ENCOUNTERING HEALTH SERVICES FOR EXAMINATIONS (Z00-Z13)

Note: Nonspecific abnormal findings disclosed at the time of these examinations are classified to categories R70-R94.

Excludes1 examinations related to pregnancy and reproduction (Z30-Z36, Z39.-)

● **Z00 Encounter for general examination without complaint, suspected or reported diagnosis**

Excludes1 encounter for examination for administrative purposes (Z02.-)

Excludes2 encounter for pre-procedural examinations (Z01.81-)
special screening examinations (Z11-Z13)

● **Z00.0 Encounter for general adult medical examination**

Encounter for adult periodic examination (annual) (physical) and any associated laboratory and radiologic examinations

Excludes1 encounter for examination of sign or symptom - code to sign or symptom
general health check-up of infant or child (Z00.12.-)

Z00.00 Encounter for general adult medical examination without abnormal findings

Encounter for adult health check-up NOS

Z00.01 Encounter for general adult medical examination with abnormal findings

Use additional code to identify abnormal findings

● **Z00.1 Encounter for newborn, infant and child health examinations**

● **Z00.11 Newborn health examination**

Health check for child under 29 days old

Use additional code to identify any abnormal findings

Excludes1 health check for child over 28 days old (Z00.12-)

Z00.110 Health examination for newborn under 8 days old

Health check for newborn under 8 days old

Z00.111 Health examination for newborn 8 to 28 days old

Health check for newborn 8 to 28 days old

Newborn weight check

● **Z00.12 Encounter for routine child health examination**

Encounter for development testing of infant or child

Health check (routine) for child over 28 days old

Excludes1 health check for child under 29 days old (Z00.11-)
health supervision of foundling or other healthy infant or child (Z76.1-Z76.2)
newborn health examination (Z00.11-)

Z00.121 Encounter for routine child health examination with abnormal findings

Use additional code to identify abnormal findings

Z00.129 Encounter for routine child health examination without abnormal findings

Encounter for routine child health examination NOS

Z00.2 Encounter for examination for period of rapid growth in childhood

Z00.3 Encounter for examination for adolescent development state

Encounter for puberty development state

Z00.5 Encounter for examination of potential donor of organ and tissue

Z00.6 Encounter for examination for normal comparison and control in clinical research program

Examination of participant or control in clinical research program

● **Z00.7 Encounter for examination for period of delayed growth in childhood**

Z00.70 Encounter for examination for period of delayed growth in childhood without abnormal findings

Z00.71 Encounter for examination for period of delayed growth in childhood with abnormal findings

Use additional code to identify abnormal findings

Z00.8 Encounter for other general examination

Encounter for health examination in population surveys

● **Z01 Encounter for other special examination without complaint, suspected or reported diagnosis**

Includes routine examination of specific system

Note: Codes from category Z01 represent the reason for the encounter. A separate procedure code is required to identify any examinations or procedures performed.

Excludes1 encounter for examination for administrative purposes (Z02.-)
encounter for examination for suspected conditions, proven not to exist (Z03.-)
encounter for laboratory and radiologic examinations as a component of general medical examinations (Z00.0-)
encounter for laboratory, radiologic and imaging examinations for sign(s) and symptom(s) - code to the sign(s) or symptom(s)

Excludes2 screening examinations (Z11-Z13)

● **Z01.0 Encounter for examination of eyes and vision**

Excludes1 examination for driving license (Z02.4)

Z01.00 Encounter for examination of eyes and vision without abnormal findings

Encounter for examination of eyes and vision NOS

Z01.01 Encounter for examination of eyes and vision with abnormal findings

Use additional code to identify abnormal findings

● **Z01.1 Encounter for examination of ears and hearing**

Z01.10 Encounter for examination of ears and hearing without abnormal findings

Encounter for examination of ears and hearing NOS

● **Z01.11 Encounter for examination of ears and hearing with abnormal findings**

Z01.110 Encounter for hearing examination following failed hearing screening

Z01.118 Encounter for examination of ears and hearing with other abnormal findings

Use additional code to identify abnormal findings

Z01.12 Encounter for hearing conservation and treatment

● **Z01.2 Encounter for dental examination and cleaning**

Z01.20 Encounter for dental examination and cleaning without abnormal findings

Encounter for dental examination and cleaning NOS

Z01.21 Encounter for dental examination and cleaning with abnormal findings

Use additional code to identify abnormal findings

● **Z01.3 Encounter for examination of blood pressure**

Z01.30 Encounter for examination of blood pressure without abnormal findings

Encounter for examination of blood pressure NOS

Z01.31 Encounter for examination of blood pressure with abnormal findings

Use additional code to identify abnormal findings

● **Z01.4 Encounter for gynecological examination**

Excludes2 pregnancy examination or test (Z32.0-)
routine examination for contraceptive maintenance (Z30.4-)

● **Z01.41 Encounter for routine gynecological examination**

Encounter for general gynecological examination with or without cervical smear
Encounter for gynecological examination (general) (routine) NOS
Encounter for pelvic examination (annual) (periodic)

Use additional code:
for screening for human papillomavirus, if applicable (Z11.51)
for screening vaginal pap smear, if applicable (Z12.72)
to identify acquired absence of uterus, if applicable (Z90.71-)

Excludes1 gynecologic examination status-post hysterectomy for malignant condition (Z08)
screening cervical pap smear not a part of a routine gynecological examination (Z12.4)

Z01.411 Encounter for gynecological examination (general) (routine) with abnormal findings

Use additional code to identify any abnormal findings ◀

Z01.419 Encounter for gynecological examination (general) (routine) without abnormal findings

Z01.42 Encounter for cervical smear to confirm findings of recent normal smear following initial abnormal smear

● **Z01.8 Encounter for other specified special examinations**

● **Z01.81 Encounter for preprocedural examinations**

Encounter for preoperative examinations
Encounter for radiological and imaging examinations as part of preprocedural examination

Z01.810 Encounter for preprocedural cardiovascular examination

Z01.811 Encounter for preprocedural respiratory examination

Z01.812 Encounter for preprocedural laboratory examination

Blood and urine tests prior to treatment or procedure

Z01.818 Encounter for other preprocedural examination

Encounter for preprocedural examination NOS
Encounter for examinations prior to antineoplastic chemotherapy

Z01.82 Encounter for allergy testing

Excludes1 encounter for antibody response examination (Z01.84)

Z01.83 Encounter for blood typing

Encounter for Rh typing

Z01.84 Encounter for antibody response examination

Encounter for immunity status testing

Excludes1 encounter for allergy testing (Z01.82)

Z01.89 Encounter for other specified special examinations

● **Z02 Encounter for administrative examination**

Z02.0 Encounter for examination for admission to educational institution
Encounter for examination for admission to preschool (education)
Encounter for examination for re-admission to school following illness or medical treatment

Z02.1 Encounter for pre-employment examination

Z02.2 Encounter for examination for admission to residential institution
Excludes1 examination for admission to prison (Z02.89)

Z02.3 Encounter for examination for recruitment to armed forces

Z02.4 Encounter for examination for driving license

Z02.5 Encounter for examination for participation in sport
Excludes1 blood-alcohol and blood-drug test (Z02.83)

Z02.6 Encounter for examination for insurance purposes

● **Z02.7 Encounter for issue of medical certificate**
Excludes1 encounter for general medical examination (Z00-Z01, Z02.0-Z02.6, Z02.8-Z02.9)

Z02.71 Encounter for disability determination
Encounter for issue of medical certificate of incapacity
Encounter for issue of medical certificate of invalidity

Z02.79 Encounter for issue of other medical certificate

● **Z02.8 Encounter for other administrative examinations**

Z02.81 Encounter for paternity testing

Z02.82 Encounter for adoption services

Z02.83 Encounter for blood-alcohol and blood-drug test
Use additional code for findings of alcohol or drugs in blood (R78.-)

Z02.89 Encounter for other administrative examinations
Encounter for examination for admission to prison
Encounter for examination for admission to summer camp
Encounter for immigration examination
Encounter for naturalization examination
Encounter for premarital examination
Excludes1 health supervision of foundling or other healthy infant or child (Z76.1-Z76.2)

Z02.9 Encounter for administrative examinations, unspecified

OGCR Section II.C.21.c.6.

Observation

There are **three** observation Z code categories. They are for use in very limited circumstances when a person is being observed for a suspected condition that is ruled out. The observation codes are not for use if an injury or illnesses or any signs or symptoms related to the suspected condition are present. In such cases the diagnosis/symptom code is used with the corresponding external cause code.

The observation codes are to be used as principal diagnosis only. **The only exception to this is when the principal diagnosis is required to be a code from category Z38, Liveborn infants according to place of birth and type of delivery. Then a code from category Z05, Encounter for observation and evaluation of newborn for suspected diseases and conditions ruled out, is sequenced after the Z38 code.** Additional codes may be used in addition to the observation code but only if they are unrelated to the suspected condition being observed.

Codes from subcategory Z03.7 Encounter for suspected maternal and fetal conditions ruled out, may either be used as a first listed or as an additional code assignment depending on the case. They are for use in very limited circumstances on a maternal record when an encounter is for a suspected maternal or fetal condition that is ruled out during that encounter (for example, a maternal or fetal condition may be suspected due to an abnormal test result). These codes should not be used when the condition is confirmed. In those cases, the confirmed condition should be coded. In addition, these codes are not for use if an illness or any signs or symptoms related to the suspected condition or problem are present. In such cases the diagnosis/symptom code is used.

Additional codes may be used in addition to the code from subcategory Z03.7, but only if they are unrelated to the suspected condition being evaluated.

Codes from subcategory Z03.7 may not be used for encounters for antenatal screening of mother. *See Section I.C.21. Screening.*

For encounters for suspected fetal condition that are inconclusive following testing and evaluation, assign the appropriate code from category O35, O36, O40 or O41.

The observation Z code categories:

Z03 Encounter for medical observation for suspected diseases and conditions ruled out

Z04 Encounter for examination and observation for other reasons
Except: Z04.9, Encounter for examination and observation for unspecified reason

Z05 Encounter for observation and evaluation of newborn for suspected diseases and conditions ruled out

● **Z03 Encounter for medical observation for suspected diseases and conditions ruled out**
This category is to be used when a person without a diagnosis is suspected of having an abnormal condition, without signs or symptoms, which requires study, but after examination and observation, is ruled out. This category is also for use for administrative and legal observation status.
Excludes1 contact with and (suspected) exposures hazardous to health (Z77.-)
newborn observation for suspected condition, ruled out (P00-P04)
person with feared complaint in whom no diagnosis is made (Z71.1)
signs or symptoms under study - code to signs or symptoms

Z03.6 Encounter for observation for suspected toxic effect from ingested substance ruled out
Encounter for observation for suspected adverse effect from drug
Encounter for observation for suspected poisoning

CHAPTER 21 (Z00-Z99)

● **Z03.7 Encounter for suspected maternal and fetal conditions ruled out**
Encounter for suspected maternal and fetal conditions not found
Excludes1 known or suspected fetal anomalies affecting management of mother, not ruled out (O26.-, O35.-, O36.-, O40.-, O41.-)

Z03.71 Encounter for suspected problem with amniotic cavity and membrane ruled out
Encounter for suspected oligohydramnios ruled out
Encounter for suspected polyhydramnios ruled out

Z03.72 Encounter for suspected placental problem ruled out

Z03.73 Encounter for suspected fetal anomaly ruled out

Z03.74 Encounter for suspected problem with fetal growth ruled out

Z03.75 Encounter for suspected cervical shortening ruled out

Z03.79 Encounter for other suspected maternal and fetal conditions ruled out

● **Z03.8 Encounter for observation for other suspected diseases and conditions ruled out**

● **Z03.81 Encounter for observation for suspected exposure to biological agents ruled out**

Z03.810 Encounter for observation for suspected exposure to anthrax ruled out

Z03.818 Encounter for observation for suspected exposure to other biological agents ruled out

Z03.89 Encounter for observation for other suspected diseases and conditions ruled out

● **Z04 Encounter for examination and observation for other reasons**
Includes encounter for examination for medicolegal reasons
This category is to be used when a person without a diagnosis is suspected of having an abnormal condition, without signs or symptoms, which requires study, but after examination and observation, is ruled-out. This category is also for use for administrative and legal observation status.

Z04.1 Encounter for examination and observation following transport accident
Excludes1 encounter for examination and observation following work accident (Z04.2)

Z04.2 Encounter for examination and observation following work accident

Z04.3 Encounter for examination and observation following other accident

● **Z04.4 Encounter for examination and observation following alleged rape**
Encounter for examination and observation of victim following alleged rape
Encounter for examination and observation of victim following alleged sexual abuse

Z04.41 Encounter for examination and observation following alleged adult rape
Suspected adult rape, ruled out
Suspected adult sexual abuse, ruled out

Z04.42 Encounter for examination and observation following alleged child rape
Suspected child rape, ruled out
Suspected child sexual abuse, ruled out

Z04.6 Encounter for general psychiatric examination, requested by authority

● **Z04.7 Encounter for examination and observation following alleged physical abuse**

Z04.71 Encounter for examination and observation following alleged adult physical abuse
Suspected adult physical abuse, ruled out
Excludes1 confirmed case of adult physical abuse (T74.-)
encounter for examination and observation following alleged adult sexual abuse (Z04.41)
suspected case of adult physical abuse, not ruled out (T76.-)

Z04.72 Encounter for examination and observation following alleged child physical abuse
Suspected child physical abuse, ruled out
Excludes1 confirmed case of child physical abuse (T74.-)
encounter for examination and observation following alleged child sexual abuse (Z04.42)
suspected case of child physical abuse, not ruled out (T76.-)

Z04.8 Encounter for examination and observation for other specified reasons
Encounter for examination and observation for request for expert evidence

Z04.9 Encounter for examination and observation for unspecified reason
Encounter for observation NOS

● **Z05 Encounter for observation and evaluation of newborn for suspected diseases and conditions ruled out** ◀
This category is to be used for newborns, within the neonatal period (the first 28 days of life), who are suspected of having an abnormal condition unrelated to exposure from the mother or the birth process, but without signs or symptoms, and which, after examination and observation, is ruled out. ◀
Excludes2 newborn observation for suspected condition, related to exposure from the mother or birth process (P00-P04) ◀

Z05.0 Observation and evaluation of newborn for suspected cardiac condition ruled out ◀

Z05.1 Observation and evaluation of newborn for suspected infectious condition ruled out ◀

Z05.2 Observation and evaluation of newborn for suspected neurological condition ruled out ◀

Z05.3 Observation and evaluation of newborn for suspected respiratory condition ruled out ◀

● **Z05.4 Observation and evaluation of newborn for suspected genetic, metabolic or immunologic condition ruled out** ◀

Z05.41 Observation and evaluation of newborn for suspected genetic condition ruled out ◀

Z05.42 Observation and evaluation of newborn for suspected metabolic condition ruled out ◀

Z05.43 Observation and evaluation of newborn for suspected immunologic condition ruled out ◀

Z05.5 Observation and evaluation of newborn for suspected gastrointestinal condition ruled out ◀

Z05.6 Observation and evaluation of newborn for suspected genitourinary condition ruled out ◀

● **Z05.7 Observation and evaluation of newborn for suspected skin, subcutaneous, musculoskeletal and connective tissue condition ruled out** ◀

Z05.71 Observation and evaluation of newborn for suspected skin and subcutaneous tissue condition ruled out ◀

Z05.72 Observation and evaluation of newborn for suspected musculoskeletal condition ruled out ◀

Z05.73 Observation and evaluation of newborn for suspected connective tissue condition ruled out ◀

Z05.8 **Observation and evaluation of newborn for other specified suspected condition ruled out** ◀

Z05.9 **Observation and evaluation of newborn for unspecified suspected condition ruled out** ◀

OGCR See Section II.C.21.c.8.

The follow-up codes are used to explain continuing surveillance following completed treatment of a disease, condition, or injury. They imply that the condition has been fully treated and no longer exists. They should not be confused with aftercare codes, or injury codes with 7th character "D," that explain ongoing care of a healing condition or its sequelae. Follow-up codes may be used in conjunction with history codes to provide the full picture of the healed condition and its treatment. The follow-up code is sequenced first, followed by the history code.

A follow-up code may be used to explain multiple visits. Should a condition be found to have recurred on the follow-up visit, then the diagnosis code for the condition should be assigned in place of the follow-up code.

The follow-up Z code categories:

Z08 Encounter for follow-up examination after completed treatment for malignant neoplasm

Z09 Encounter for follow-up examination after completed treatment for conditions other than malignant neoplasm

Z39 Encounter for maternal postpartum care and examination

Z08 Encounter for follow-up examination after completed treatment for malignant neoplasm

Medical surveillance following completed treatment

Use additional code to identify any acquired absence of organs (Z90.-)

Use additional code to identify the personal history of malignant neoplasm (Z85.-)

Excludes1 aftercare following medical care (Z43-Z49, Z51)

Z09 Encounter for follow-up examination after completed treatment for conditions other than malignant neoplasm

Medical surveillance following completed treatment

Use additional code to identify any applicable history of disease code (Z86.-, Z87.-)

Excludes1 aftercare following medical care (Z43-Z49, Z51)
surveillance of contraception (Z30.4-)
surveillance of prosthetic and other medical devices (Z44-Z46)

OGCR Section II.C.21.c.5.

Screening

Screening is the testing for disease or disease precursors in seemingly well individuals so that early detection and treatment can be provided for those who test positive for the disease (e.g., screening mammogram).

The testing of a person to rule out or confirm a suspected diagnosis because the patient has some sign or symptom is a diagnostic examination, not a screening. In these cases, the sign or symptom is used to explain the reason for the test.

A screening code may be a first listed code if the reason for the visit is specifically the screening exam. It may also be used as an additional code if the screening is done during an office visit for other health problems. A screening code is not necessary if the screening is inherent to a routine examination, such as a pap smear done during a routine pelvic examination.

Should a condition be discovered during the screening then the code for the condition may be assigned as an additional diagnosis.

The Z code indicates that a screening exam is planned. A procedure code is required to confirm that the screening was performed.

The screening Z codes /categories:

Z11 Encounter for screening for infectious and parasitic diseases

Z12 Encounter for screening for malignant neoplasms

Z13 Encounter for screening for other diseases and disorders
Except: Z13.9, Encounter for screening, unspecified

Z36 Encounter for antenatal screening for mother

● **Z11 Encounter for screening for infectious and parasitic diseases**

Screening is the testing for disease or disease precursors in asymptomatic individuals so that early detection and treatment can be provided for those who test positive for the disease.

Excludes1 encounter for diagnostic examination - code to sign or symptom

Z11.0 **Encounter for screening for intestinal infectious diseases**

Z11.1 **Encounter for screening for respiratory tuberculosis**

Z11.2 **Encounter for screening for other bacterial diseases**

Z11.3 **Encounter for screening for infections with a predominantly sexual mode of transmission**

Excludes2 encounter for screening for human immunodeficiency virus [HIV] (Z11.4)
encounter for screening for human papillomavirus (Z11.51)

Z11.4 **Encounter for screening for human immunodeficiency virus [HIV]**

● Z11.5 **Encounter for screening for other viral diseases**

Excludes2 encounter for screening for viral intestinal disease (Z11.0)

Z11.51 **Encounter for screening for human papillomavirus (HPV)**

Z11.59 **Encounter for screening for other viral diseases**

Z11.6 **Encounter for screening for other protozoal diseases and helminthiases**

Diseases or infestations caused by parasitic worms

Excludes2 encounter for screening for protozoal intestinal disease (Z11.0)

Z11.8 **Encounter for screening for other infectious and parasitic diseases**

Encounter for screening for chlamydia
Encounter for screening for rickettsial
Encounter for screening for spirochetal
Encounter for screening for mycoses

Z11.9 **Encounter for screening for infectious and parasitic diseases, unspecified**

● **Z12 Encounter for screening for malignant neoplasms**

Screening is the testing for disease or disease precursors in asymptomatic individuals so that early detection and treatment can be provided for those who test positive for the disease.

Use additional code to identify any family history of malignant neoplasm (Z80.-)

Excludes1 encounter for diagnostic examination - code to sign or symptom

Z12.0 **Encounter for screening for malignant neoplasm of stomach**

● Z12.1 **Encounter for screening for malignant neoplasm of intestinal tract**

Z12.10 **Encounter for screening for malignant neoplasm of intestinal tract, unspecified**

Z12.11 **Encounter for screening for malignant neoplasm of colon**

Encounter for screening colonoscopy NOS

Z12.12 **Encounter for screening for malignant neoplasm of rectum**

Z12.13 **Encounter for screening for malignant neoplasm of small intestine**

Z12.2 **Encounter for screening for malignant neoplasm of respiratory organs**

● Z12.3 **Encounter for screening for malignant neoplasm of breast**

Z12.31 **Encounter for screening mammogram for malignant neoplasm of breast**

Excludes1 inconclusive mammogram (R92.2)

Z12.39 **Encounter for other screening for malignant neoplasm of breast**

CHAPTER 21 (Z00-Z99)

Z12.4 Encounter for screening for malignant neoplasm of cervix
Encounter for screening pap smear for malignant neoplasm of cervix
Excludes1 when screening is part of general gynecological examination (Z01.4-)
Excludes2 encounter for screening for human papillomavirus (Z11.51) ◀

Z12.5 Encounter for screening for malignant neoplasm of prostate

Z12.6 Encounter for screening for malignant neoplasm of bladder

● **Z12.7 Encounter for screening for malignant neoplasm of other genitourinary organs**

Z12.71 Encounter for screening for malignant neoplasm of testis

Z12.72 Encounter for screening for malignant neoplasm of vagina
Vaginal pap smear status - post hysterectomy for non-malignant condition
Use additional code to identify acquired absence of uterus (Z90.71-)
Excludes1 vaginal pap smear status - post hysterectomy for malignant conditions (Z08)

Z12.73 Encounter for screening for malignant neoplasm of ovary

Z12.79 Encounter for screening for malignant neoplasm of other genitourinary organs

● **Z12.8 Encounter for screening for malignant neoplasm of other sites**

Z12.81 Encounter for screening for malignant neoplasm of oral cavity

Z12.82 Encounter for screening for malignant neoplasm of nervous system

Z12.83 Encounter for screening for malignant neoplasm of skin

Z12.89 Encounter for screening for malignant neoplasm of other sites

Z12.9 Encounter for screening for malignant neoplasm, site unspecified

● **Z13 Encounter for screening for other diseases and disorders**
Screening is the testing for disease or disease precursors in asymptomatic individuals so that early detection and treatment can be provided for those who test positive for the disease.
Excludes1 encounter for diagnostic examination - code to sign or symptom

Z13.0 Encounter for screening for diseases of the blood and blood-forming organs and certain disorders involving the immune mechanism

Z13.1 Encounter for screening for diabetes mellitus

● **Z13.2 Encounter for screening for nutritional, metabolic and other endocrine disorders**

Z13.21 Encounter for screening for nutritional disorder

● **Z13.22 Encounter for screening for metabolic disorder**

Z13.220 Encounter for screening for lipoid disorders
Encounter for screening for cholesterol level
Encounter for screening for hypercholesterolemia
Encounter for screening for hyperlipidemia

Z13.228 Encounter for screening for other metabolic disorders

Z13.29 Encounter for screening for other suspected endocrine disorder
Excludes1 encounter for screening for diabetes mellitus (Z13.1)

Z13.4 Encounter for screening for certain developmental disorders in childhood
Encounter for screening for developmental handicaps in early childhood
Excludes1 routine development testing of infant or child (Z00.1-)

Z13.5 Encounter for screening for eye and ear disorders
Excludes2 encounter for general hearing examination (Z01.1-)
encounter for general vision examination (Z01.0-)

Z13.6 Encounter for screening for cardiovascular disorders

● **Z13.7 Encounter for screening for genetic and chromosomal anomalies**
Excludes1 genetic testing for procreative management (Z31.4-)

Z13.71 Encounter for nonprocreative screening for genetic disease carrier status

Z13.79 Encounter for other screening for genetic and chromosomal anomalies

● **Z13.8 Encounter for screening for other specified diseases and disorders**
Excludes2 screening for malignant neoplasms (Z12.-)

● **Z13.81 Encounter for screening for digestive system disorders**

Z13.810 Encounter for screening for upper gastrointestinal disorder

Z13.811 Encounter for screening for lower gastrointestinal disorder
Excludes1 encounter for screening for intestinal infectious disease (Z11.0)

Z13.818 Encounter for screening for other digestive system disorders

● **Z13.82 Encounter for screening for musculoskeletal disorder**

Z13.820 Encounter for screening for osteoporosis

Z13.828 Encounter for screening for other musculoskeletal disorder

Z13.83 Encounter for screening for respiratory disorder NEC
Excludes1 encounter for screening for respiratory tuberculosis (Z11.1)

Z13.84 Encounter for screening for dental disorders

● **Z13.85 Encounter for screening for nervous system disorders**

Z13.850 Encounter for screening for traumatic brain injury

Z13.858 Encounter for screening for other nervous system disorders

Z13.88 Encounter for screening for disorder due to exposure to contaminants
Excludes1 those exposed to contaminants without suspected disorders (Z57-Z77.-)

Z13.89 Encounter for screening for other disorder
Encounter for screening for genitourinary disorders

Z13.9 Encounter for screening, unspecified

GENETIC CARRIER AND GENETIC SUSCEPTIBILITY TO DISEASE (Z14-Z15)

● **Z14 Genetic carrier**

● **Z14.0 Hemophilia A carrier**

Z14.01 Asymptomatic hemophilia A carrier

Z14.02 Symptomatic hemophilia A carrier

Z14.1 Cystic fibrosis carrier

Z14.8 Genetic carrier of other disease

● **Z15 Genetic susceptibility to disease**

Excludes1 chromosomal anomalies (Q90-Q99)

Includes confirmed abnormal gene

Use additional code, if applicable, for any associated family history of the disease (Z80-Z84)

● **Z15.0 Genetic susceptibility to malignant neoplasm**

Code first if applicable, any current malignant neoplasm (C00-C75, C81-C96)

Use additional code, if applicable, for any personal history of malignant neoplasm (Z85.-)

Z15.01 Genetic susceptibility to malignant neoplasm of breast

Z15.02 Genetic susceptibility to malignant neoplasm of ovary

Z15.03 Genetic susceptibility to malignant neoplasm of prostate

Z15.04 Genetic susceptibility to malignant neoplasm of endometrium

Z15.09 Genetic susceptibility to other malignant neoplasm

● **Z15.8 Genetic susceptibility to other disease**

Z15.81 Genetic susceptibility to multiple endocrine neoplasia [MEN]

Excludes1 multiple endocrine neoplasia [MEN] syndromes (E31.2-)

Z15.89 Genetic susceptibility to other disease

RESISTANCE TO ANTIMICROBIAL DRUGS (Z16)

● **Z16 Resistance to antimicrobial drugs**

Note: The codes in this category are provided for use as additional codes to identify the resistance and non-responsiveness of a condition to antimicrobial drugs.

Code first the infection

Excludes1 Methicillin resistant Staphylococcus aureus infection (A49.02)
Methicillin resistant Staphylococcus aureus infection in diseases classified elsewhere (B95.62)
Methicillin resistant Staphylococcus aureus pneumonia (J15.212)
Sepsis due to Methicillin resistant Staphylococcus aureus (A41.02)

● **Z16.1 Resistance to beta lactam antibiotics**

Z16.10 Resistance to unspecified beta lactam antibiotics

Z16.11 Resistance to penicillins
Resistance to amoxicillin
Resistance to ampicillin

Z16.12 Extended spectrum beta lactamase (ESBL) resistance

Z16.19 Resistance to other specified beta lactam antibiotics
Resistance to cephalosporins

● **Z16.2 Resistance to other antibiotics**

Z16.20 Resistance to unspecified antibiotic
Resistance to antibiotics NOS

Z16.21 Resistance to vancomycin

Z16.22 Resistance to vancomycin related antibiotics

Z16.23 Resistance to quinolones and fluoroquinolones

Z16.24 Resistance to multiple antibiotics

Z16.29 Resistance to other single specified antibiotic
Resistance to aminoglycosides
Resistance to macrolides
Resistance to sulfonamides
Resistance to tetracyclines

● **Z16.3 Resistance to other antimicrobial drugs**

Excludes1 resistance to antibiotics (Z16.1-, Z16.2-)

Z16.30 Resistance to unspecified antimicrobial drugs
Drug resistance NOS

Z16.31 Resistance to antiparasitic drug(s)
Resistance to quinine and related compounds

Z16.32 Resistance to antifungal drug(s)

Z16.33 Resistance to antiviral drug(s)

● **Z16.34 Resistance to antimycobacterial drug(s)**
Resistance to tuberculostatics

Z16.341 Resistance to single antimycobacterial drug
Resistance to antimycobacterial drug NOS

Z16.342 Resistance to multiple antimycobacterial drugs

Z16.35 Resistance to multiple antimicrobial drugs

Excludes1 Resistance to multiple antibiotics only (Z16.24)

Z16.39 Resistance to other specified antimicrobial drug

ESTROGEN RECEPTOR STATUS (Z17)

● **Z17 Estrogen receptor status**

Code first malignant neoplasm of breast (C50.-)

Z17.0 Estrogen receptor positive status [ER+]

Z17.1 Estrogen receptor negative status [ER-]

RETAINED FOREIGN BODY FRAGMENTS (Z18)

● **Z18 Retained foreign body fragments**

Includes embedded fragment (status)
embedded splinter (status)
retained foreign body status

Excludes1 artificial joint prosthesis status (Z96.6-)
foreign body accidentally left during a procedure (T81.5-)
foreign body entering through orifice (T15-T19)
in situ cardiac device (Z95.-)
organ or tissue replaced by means other than transplant (Z96.-, Z97.-)
organ or tissue replaced by transplant (Z94.-)
personal history of retained foreign body fully removed Z87.821
superficial foreign body (non-embedded splinter) - code to superficial foreign body, by site

● **Z18.0 Retained radioactive fragments**

Z18.01 Retained depleted uranium fragments

Z18.09 Other retained radioactive fragments
Other retained depleted isotope fragments
Retained nontherapeutic radioactive fragments

● **Z18.1 Retained metal fragments**

Excludes1 retained radioactive metal fragments (Z18.01-Z18.09)

Z18.10 Retained metal fragments, unspecified
Retained metal fragment NOS

Z18.11 Retained magnetic metal fragments

Z18.12 Retained nonmagnetic metal fragments

Z18.2 Retained plastic fragments
Acrylics fragments
Diethylhexylphthalates fragments
Isocyanate fragments

● **Z18.3 Retained organic fragments**

Z18.31 Retained animal quills or spines

Z18.32 Retained tooth

Z18.33 Retained wood fragments

Z18.39 Other retained organic fragments

● Z18.8 Other specified retained foreign body
Z18.81 Retained glass fragments
Z18.83 Retained stone or crystalline fragments
Retained concrete or cement fragments
Z18.89 Other specified retained foreign body fragments
Z18.9 Retained foreign body fragments, unspecified material

HORMONE SENSITIVITY MALIGNANCY STATUS (Z19) ◀

● Z19 Hormone sensitivity malignancy status ◀
Code first malignant neoplasm —*see* Table of Neoplasms, by site, malignant ◀
Z19.1 Hormone sensitive malignancy status ◀
Z19.2 Hormone resistant malignancy status ◀
Castrate resistant prostate malignancy status ◀

PERSONS WITH POTENTIAL HEALTH HAZARDS RELATED TO COMMUNICABLE DISEASES (Z20-Z29)

● Z20 Contact with and (suspected) exposure to communicable diseases
Excludes1 carrier of infectious disease (Z22.-)
diagnosed current infectious or parasitic disease - see Alphabetic Index
Excludes2 personal history of infectious and parasitic diseases (Z86.1-)
● Z20.0 Contact with and (suspected) exposure to intestinal infectious diseases
Z20.01 Contact with and (suspected) exposure to intestinal infectious diseases due to Escherichia coli (E. coli)
Z20.09 Contact with and (suspected) exposure to other intestinal infectious diseases
Z20.1 Contact with and (suspected) exposure to tuberculosis
Z20.2 Contact with and (suspected) exposure to infections with a predominantly sexual mode of transmission
Z20.3 Contact with and (suspected) exposure to rabies
Z20.4 Contact with and (suspected) exposure to rubella
Z20.5 Contact with and (suspected) exposure to viral hepatitis
Z20.6 Contact with and (suspected) exposure to human immunodeficiency virus [HIV]
Excludes1 asymptomatic human immunodeficiency virus [HIV]
HIV infection status (Z21)
Z20.7 Contact with and (suspected) exposure to pediculosis, acariasis and other infestations
● Z20.8 Contact with and (suspected) exposure to other communicable diseases
● Z20.81 Contact with and (suspected) exposure to other bacterial communicable diseases
Z20.810 Contact with and (suspected) exposure to anthrax
Z20.811 Contact with and (suspected) exposure to meningococcus
Z20.818 Contact with and (suspected) exposure to other bacterial communicable diseases
● Z20.82 Contact with and (suspected) exposure to other viral communicable diseases
Z20.820 Contact with and (suspected) exposure to varicella
Z20.828 Contact with and (suspected) exposure to other viral communicable diseases
Z20.89 Contact with and (suspected) exposure to other communicable diseases
Z20.9 Contact with and (suspected) exposure to unspecified communicable disease

Z21 Asymptomatic human immunodeficiency virus [HIV] infection status
HIV positive NOS
Code first Human immunodeficiency virus [HIV] disease complicating pregnancy, childbirth and the puerperium, if applicable (O98.7-)
Excludes1 acquired immunodeficiency syndrome (B20)
contact with human immunodeficiency virus [HIV] (Z20.6)
exposure to human immunodeficiency virus [HIV] (Z20.6)
human immunodeficiency virus [HIV] disease (B20)
inconclusive laboratory evidence of human immunodeficiency virus [HIV] (R75)

● Z22 Carrier of infectious disease
Includes colonization status
suspected carrier
Excludes2 carrier of viral hepatitis (B18.-) ◀
Z22.0 Carrier of typhoid
Z22.1 Carrier of other intestinal infectious diseases
Z22.2 Carrier of diphtheria
● Z22.3 Carrier of other specified bacterial diseases
Z22.31 Carrier of bacterial disease due to meningococci
● Z22.32 Carrier of bacterial disease due to staphylococci
Z22.321 Carrier or suspected carrier of Methicillin susceptible Staphylococcus aureus
MSSA colonization
Z22.322 Carrier or suspected carrier of Methicillin resistant Staphylococcus aureus
MRSA colonization
● Z22.33 Carrier of bacterial disease due to streptococci
Z22.330 Carrier of Group B streptococcus
Excludes1 Carrier of streptococcus group B (GBS) complicating pregnancy, childbirth and the puerperium (O99.82-) ◀
Z22.338 Carrier of other streptococcus
Z22.39 Carrier of other specified bacterial diseases
Z22.4 Carrier of infections with a predominantly sexual mode of transmission
~~Z22.5 Carrier of viral hepatitis~~
~~Z22.50 Carrier of unspecified viral hepatitis~~
~~Z22.51 Carrier of viral hepatitis B~~
~~Hepatitis B surface antigen [HBsAg] carrier~~
~~Z22.52 Carrier of viral hepatitis C~~
~~Z22.59 Carrier of other viral hepatitis~~
Z22.6 Carrier of human T-lymphotropic virus type-1 [HTLV-1] infection
Z22.8 Carrier of other infectious diseases
Z22.9 Carrier of infectious disease, unspecified

Z23 Encounter for immunization
Code first *any routine childhood examination*
Note: Procedure codes are required to identify the types of immunizations given.

● Z28 **Immunization not carried out and underimmunization status**
Includes vaccination not carried out
● Z28.0 **Immunization not carried out because of contraindication**
Z28.01 **Immunization not carried out because of acute illness of patient**
Z28.02 **Immunization not carried out because of chronic illness or condition of patient**
Z28.03 **Immunization not carried out because of immune compromised state of patient**
Z28.04 **Immunization not carried out because of patient allergy to vaccine or component**
Z28.09 **Immunization not carried out because of other contraindication**
Z28.1 **Immunization not carried out because of patient decision for reasons of belief or group pressure**
Immunization not carried out because of religious belief
● Z28.2 **Immunization not carried out because of patient decision for other and unspecified reason**
Z28.20 **Immunization not carried out because of patient decision for unspecified reason**
Z28.21 **Immunization not carried out because of patient refusal**
Z28.29 **Immunization not carried out because of patient decision for other reason**
Z28.3 **Underimmunization status**
Delinquent immunization status
Lapsed immunization schedule status
● Z28.8 **Immunization not carried out for other reason**
Z28.81 **Immunization not carried out due to patient having had the disease**
Z28.82 **Immunization not carried out because of caregiver refusal**
Immunization not carried out because of guardian refusal
Immunization not carried out because of parent refusal
Excludes1 immunization not carried out because of caregiver refusal because of religious belief (Z28.1)
Z28.89 **Immunization not carried out for other reason**
Z28.9 **Immunization not carried out for unspecified reason**

● Z29 **Encounter for other prophylactic measures** ◀
Excludes1 desensitization to allergens (Z51.6) ◀
prophylactic surgery (Z40.-) ◀
● Z29.1 **Encounter for prophylactic immunotherapy** ◀
Encounter for administration of immunoglobulin ◀
Z29.11 **Encounter for prophylactic immunotherapy for respiratory syncytial virus (RSV)** ◀
Z29.12 **Encounter for prophylactic antivenin** ◀
Z29.13 **Encounter for prophylactic Rho(D) immune globulin** ◀
Z29.14 **Encounter for prophylactic rabies immune globin** ◀
Z29.3 **Encounter for prophylactic fluoride administration** ◀
Z29.8 **Encounter for other specified prophylactic measures** ◀
Z29.9 **Encounter for prophylactic measures, unspecified** ◀

PERSONS ENCOUNTERING HEALTH SERVICES IN CIRCUMSTANCES RELATED TO REPRODUCTION (Z30-Z39)

● Z30 **Encounter for contraceptive management**
● Z30.0 **Encounter for general counseling and advice on contraception**
● Z30.01 **Encounter for initial prescription of contraceptives**
Excludes1 encounter for surveillance of contraceptives (Z30.4-)
Z30.011 **Encounter for initial prescription of contraceptive pills**
Z30.012 **Encounter for prescription of emergency contraception**
Encounter for postcoital contraception
Z30.013 **Encounter for initial prescription of injectable contraceptive**
Z30.014 **Encounter for initial prescription of intrauterine contraceptive device**
Excludes1 encounter for insertion of intrauterine contraceptive device (Z30.430, Z30.432)
Z30.015 **Encounter for initial prescription of vaginal ring hormonal contraceptive** ◀
Z30.016 **Encounter for initial prescription of transdermal patch hormonal contraceptive device** ◀
Z30.017 **Encounter for initial prescription of implantable subdermal contraceptive** ◀
Z30.018 **Encounter for initial prescription of other contraceptives**
Encounter for initial prescription of barrier contraception ◀
Encounter for initial prescription of diaphragm ◀
Z30.019 **Encounter for initial prescription of contraceptives, unspecified**
Z30.02 **Counseling and instruction in natural family planning to avoid pregnancy**
Z30.09 **Encounter for other general counseling and advice on contraception**
Encounter for family planning advice NOS
Z30.2 **Encounter for sterilization**
● Z30.4 **Encounter for surveillance of contraceptives**
Z30.40 **Encounter for surveillance of contraceptives, unspecified**
Z30.41 **Encounter for surveillance of contraceptive pills**
Encounter for repeat prescription for contraceptive pill
Z30.42 **Encounter for surveillance of injectable contraceptive**
● Z30.43 **Encounter for surveillance of intrauterine contraceptive device**
Z30.430 **Encounter for insertion of intrauterine contraceptive device**
Z30.431 **Encounter for routine checking of intrauterine contraceptive device**
Z30.432 **Encounter for removal of intrauterine contraceptive device**
Z30.433 **Encounter for removal and reinsertion of intrauterine contraceptive device**
Encounter for replacement of intrauterine contraceptive device

Z30.44 **Encounter for surveillance of vaginal ring hormonal contraceptive device** ◀

Z30.45 **Encounter for surveillance of transdermal patch hormonal contraceptive device** ◀

Z30.46 **Encounter for surveillance of implantable subdermal contraceptive** ◀
Encounter for checking, reinsertion or removal of implantable subdermal contraceptive ◀

Z30.49 **Encounter for surveillance of other contraceptives**
Encounter for surveillance of barrier contraception ◀
Encounter for surveillance of diaphragm ◀

Z30.8 **Encounter for other contraceptive management**
Encounter for postvasectomy sperm count
Encounter for routine examination for contraceptive maintenance
Excludes1 sperm count following sterilization reversal (Z31.42)
sperm count for fertility testing (Z31.41)

Z30.9 **Encounter for contraceptive management, unspecified**

● Z31 **Encounter for procreative management**
Excludes1 complications associated with artificial fertilization (N98.-)
female infertility (N97.-)
male infertility (N46.-)

Z31.0 **Encounter for reversal of previous sterilization**

● Z31.4 **Encounter for procreative investigation and testing**
Excludes1 postvasectomy sperm count (Z30.8)

Z31.41 **Encounter for fertility testing**
Encounter for fallopian tube patency testing
Encounter for sperm count for fertility testing

Z31.42 **Aftercare following sterilization reversal**
Sperm count following sterilization reversal

● Z31.43 **Encounter for genetic testing of female for procreative management**
Use additional code for recurrent pregnancy loss, if applicable (N96, O26.2-)
Excludes1 nonprocreative genetic testing (Z13.7-)

Z31.430 **Encounter of female for testing for genetic disease carrier status for procreative management**

Z31.438 **Encounter for other genetic testing of female for procreative management**

● Z31.44 **Encounter for genetic testing of male for procreative management**
Excludes1 nonprocreative genetic testing (Z13.7-)

Z31.440 **Encounter of male for testing for genetic disease carrier status for procreative management**

Z31.441 **Encounter for testing of male partner of patient with recurrent pregnancy loss**

Z31.448 **Encounter for other genetic testing of male for procreative management**

Z31.49 **Encounter for other procreative investigation and testing**

Z31.5 **Encounter for genetic counseling**

● Z31.6 **Encounter for general counseling and advice on procreation**

Z31.61 **Procreative counseling and advice using natural family planning**

Z31.62 **Encounter for fertility preservation counseling**
Encounter for fertility preservation counseling prior to cancer therapy
Encounter for fertility preservation counseling prior to surgical removal of gonads

Z31.69 **Encounter for other general counseling and advice on procreation**

Z31.7 **Encounter for procreative management and counseling for gestational carrier** ◀
Excludes1 pregnant state, gestational carrier (Z33.3) ◀

● Z31.8 **Encounter for other procreative management**

Z31.81 **Encounter for male factor infertility in female patient**

Z31.82 **Encounter for Rh incompatibility status**

Z31.83 **Encounter for assisted reproductive fertility procedure cycle**
Patient undergoing in vitro fertilization cycle
Use additional code to identify the type of infertility
Excludes1 pre-cycle diagnosis and testing - code to reason for encounter

Z31.84 **Encounter for fertility preservation procedure**
Encounter for fertility preservation procedure prior to cancer therapy
Encounter for fertility preservation procedure prior to surgical removal of gonads

Z31.89 **Encounter for other procreative management**

Z31.9 **Encounter for procreative management, unspecified**

● Z32 **Encounter for pregnancy test and childbirth and childcare instruction**

● Z32.0 **Encounter for pregnancy test**

Z32.00 **Encounter for pregnancy test, result unknown**
Encounter for pregnancy test NOS

Z32.01 **Encounter for pregnancy test, result positive**

Z32.02 **Encounter for pregnancy test, result negative**

Z32.2 **Encounter for childbirth instruction**

Z32.3 **Encounter for childcare instruction**
Encounter for prenatal or postpartum childcare instruction

● Z33 **Pregnant state**

Z33.1 **Pregnant state, incidental**
Pregnant state NOS
Excludes1 complications of pregnancy (O00-O9A)
pregnant state, gestational carrier (Z33.3) ◀

Z33.2 **Encounter for elective termination of pregnancy**
Excludes1 early fetal death with retention of dead fetus (O02.1)
late fetal death (O36.4)
spontaneous abortion (O03)

Z33.3 **Pregnant state, gestational carrier** ◀
Excludes1 encounter for procreative management and counseling for gestational carrier (Z31.7) ◀

● Z34 **Encounter for supervision of normal pregnancy**
Excludes1 any complication of pregnancy (O00-O9A)
encounter for pregnancy test (Z32.0-)
encounter for supervision of high risk pregnancy (O09.-)

● Z34.0 **Encounter for supervision of normal first pregnancy**

Z34.00 **Encounter for supervision of normal first pregnancy, unspecified trimester**

Z34.01 **Encounter for supervision of normal first pregnancy, first trimester**

Z34.02 **Encounter for supervision of normal first pregnancy, second trimester**

Z34.03 **Encounter for supervision of normal first pregnancy, third trimester**

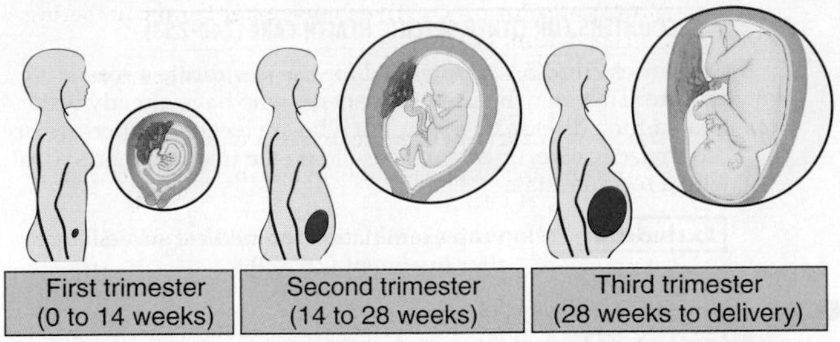

Figure 21-1 Trimesters. (From Shiland, Betsy J. Medical Terminology & Anatomy for ICD-10 Coding, ed 2, Mosby, 2015)

● **Z34.8 Encounter for supervision of other normal pregnancy**
- **Z34.80 Encounter for supervision of other normal pregnancy, unspecified trimester**
- **Z34.81 Encounter for supervision of other normal pregnancy, first trimester**
- **Z34.82 Encounter for supervision of other normal pregnancy, second trimester**
- **Z34.83 Encounter for supervision of other normal pregnancy, third trimester**

● **Z34.9 Encounter for supervision of normal pregnancy, unspecified**
- **Z34.90 Encounter for supervision of normal pregnancy, unspecified, unspecified trimester**
- **Z34.91 Encounter for supervision of normal pregnancy, unspecified, first trimester**
- **Z34.92 Encounter for supervision of normal pregnancy, unspecified, second trimester**
- **Z34.93 Encounter for supervision of normal pregnancy, unspecified, third trimester**

Z36 Encounter for antenatal screening of mother

Excludes1 abnormal findings on antenatal screening of mother (O28.-)
diagnostic examination - code to sign or symptom
encounter for suspected maternal and fetal conditions ruled out (Z03.7-)
suspected fetal condition affecting management of pregnancy - code to condition in Chapter 15

Excludes2 genetic counseling and testing (Z31.43-, Z31.5)
routine prenatal care (Z34)

● **Z3A Weeks of gestation**

Note: Codes from category Z3A are for use, only on the maternal record, to indicate the weeks of gestation of the pregnancy, if known. ⬅

Code first complications of pregnancy, childbirth and the puerperium (O00-O9A)

● **Z3A.0 Weeks of gestation of pregnancy, unspecified or less than 10 weeks**
- **Z3A.00 Weeks of gestation of pregnancy not specified**
- **Z3A.01 Less than 8 weeks gestation of pregnancy**
- **Z3A.08 8 weeks gestation of pregnancy**
- **Z3A.09 9 weeks gestation of pregnancy**

● **Z3A.1 Weeks of gestation of pregnancy, weeks 10-19**
- **Z3A.10 10 weeks gestation of pregnancy**
- **Z3A.11 11 weeks gestation of pregnancy**
- **Z3A.12 12 weeks gestation of pregnancy**
- **Z3A.13 13 weeks gestation of pregnancy**
- **Z3A.14 14 weeks gestation of pregnancy**
- **Z3A.15 15 weeks gestation of pregnancy**
- **Z3A.16 16 weeks gestation of pregnancy**
- **Z3A.17 17 weeks gestation of pregnancy**
- **Z3A.18 18 weeks gestation of pregnancy**
- **Z3A.19 19 weeks gestation of pregnancy**

● **Z3A.2 Weeks of gestation of pregnancy, weeks 20-29**
- **Z3A.20 20 weeks gestation of pregnancy**
- **Z3A.21 21 weeks gestation of pregnancy**
- **Z3A.22 22 weeks gestation of pregnancy**
- **Z3A.23 23 weeks gestation of pregnancy**
- **Z3A.24 24 weeks gestation of pregnancy**
- **Z3A.25 25 weeks gestation of pregnancy**
- **Z3A.26 26 weeks gestation of pregnancy**
- **Z3A.27 27 weeks gestation of pregnancy**
- **Z3A.28 28 weeks gestation of pregnancy**
- **Z3A.29 29 weeks gestation of pregnancy**

● **Z3A.3 Weeks of gestation of pregnancy, weeks 30-39**
- **Z3A.30 30 weeks gestation of pregnancy**
- **Z3A.31 31 weeks gestation of pregnancy**
- **Z3A.32 32 weeks gestation of pregnancy**
- **Z3A.33 33 weeks gestation of pregnancy**
- **Z3A.34 34 weeks gestation of pregnancy**
- **Z3A.35 35 weeks gestation of pregnancy**
- **Z3A.36 36 weeks gestation of pregnancy**
- **Z3A.37 37 weeks gestation of pregnancy**
- **Z3A.38 38 weeks gestation of pregnancy**
- **Z3A.39 39 weeks gestation of pregnancy**

● **Z3A.4 Weeks of gestation of pregnancy, weeks 40 or greater**
- **Z3A.40 40 weeks gestation of pregnancy**
- **Z3A.41 41 weeks gestation of pregnancy**
- **Z3A.42 42 weeks gestation of pregnancy**
- **Z3A.49 Greater than 42 weeks gestation of pregnancy**

● **Z37 Outcome of delivery**

This category is intended for use as an additional code to identify the outcome of delivery on the mother's record. It is not for use on the newborn record.

Excludes1 stillbirth (P95)

- **Z37.0 Single live birth**
- **Z37.1 Single stillbirth**
- **Z37.2 Twins, both liveborn**
- **Z37.3 Twins, one liveborn and one stillborn**
- **Z37.4 Twins, both stillborn**

● **Z37.5 Other multiple births, all liveborn**
- **Z37.50 Multiple births, unspecified, all liveborn**
- **Z37.51 Triplets, all liveborn**
- **Z37.52 Quadruplets, all liveborn**
- **Z37.53 Quintuplets, all liveborn**
- **Z37.54 Sextuplets, all liveborn**
- **Z37.59 Other multiple births, all liveborn**

CHAPTER 21 (Z00-Z99)

● Z37.6 **Other multiple births, some liveborn**
Z37.60 **Multiple births, unspecified, some liveborn**
Z37.61 **Triplets, some liveborn**
Z37.62 **Quadruplets, some liveborn**
Z37.63 **Quintuplets, some liveborn**
Z37.64 **Sextuplets, some liveborn**
Z37.69 **Other multiple births, some liveborn**
Z37.7 **Other multiple births, all stillborn**
Z37.9 **Outcome of delivery, unspecified**
Multiple birth NOS
Single birth NOS

● Z38 **Liveborn infants according to place of birth and type of delivery**
This category is for use as the principal code on the initial record of a newborn baby. It is to be used for the initial birth record only. It is not to be used on the mother's record.

● Z38.0 **Single liveborn infant, born in hospital**
Single liveborn infant, born in birthing center or other health care facility
Z38.00 **Single liveborn infant, delivered vaginally**
Z38.01 **Single liveborn infant, delivered by cesarean**
Z38.1 **Single liveborn infant, born outside hospital**
Z38.2 **Single liveborn infant, unspecified as to place of birth**
Single liveborn infant NOS
● Z38.3 **Twin liveborn infant, born in hospital**
Z38.30 **Twin liveborn infant, delivered vaginally**
Z38.31 **Twin liveborn infant, delivered by cesarean**
Z38.4 **Twin liveborn infant, born outside hospital**
Z38.5 **Twin liveborn infant, unspecified as to place of birth**
● Z38.6 **Other multiple liveborn infant, born in hospital**
Z38.61 **Triplet liveborn infant, delivered vaginally**
Z38.62 **Triplet liveborn infant, delivered by cesarean**
Z38.63 **Quadruplet liveborn infant, delivered vaginally**
Z38.64 **Quadruplet liveborn infant, delivered by cesarean**
Z38.65 **Quintuplet liveborn infant, delivered vaginally**
Z38.66 **Quintuplet liveborn infant, delivered by cesarean**
Z38.68 **Other multiple liveborn infant, delivered vaginally**
Z38.69 **Other multiple liveborn infant, delivered by cesarean**
Z38.7 **Other multiple liveborn infant, born outside hospital**
Z38.8 **Other multiple liveborn infant, unspecified as to place of birth**

● Z39 **Encounter for maternal postpartum care and examination**
Z39.0 **Encounter for care and examination of mother immediately after delivery**
Care and observation in uncomplicated cases when the delivery occurs outside a healthcare facility
Excludes1 care for postpartum complication - see Alphabetic index
Z39.1 **Encounter for care and examination of lactating mother**
Encounter for supervision of lactation
Excludes1 disorders of lactation (O92.-)
Z39.2 **Encounter for routine postpartum follow-up**

ENCOUNTERS FOR OTHER SPECIFIC HEALTH CARE (Z40-Z53)

Categories Z40-Z53 are intended for use to indicate a reason for care. They may be used for patients who have already been treated for a disease or injury, but who are receiving aftercare or prophylactic care, or care to consolidate the treatment, or to deal with a residual state

Excludes2 follow-up examination for medical surveillance after treatment (Z08-Z09)

● Z40 **Encounter for prophylactic surgery**
Excludes1 organ donations (Z52.-)
therapeutic organ removal - code to condition
● Z40.0 **Encounter for prophylactic surgery for risk factors related to malignant neoplasms**
Admission for prophylactic organ removal
Use additional code to identify risk factor
Z40.00 **Encounter for prophylactic removal of unspecified organ**
Z40.01 **Encounter for prophylactic removal of breast**
Z40.02 **Encounter for prophylactic removal of ovary**
Z40.09 **Encounter for prophylactic removal of other organ**
Z40.8 **Encounter for other prophylactic surgery**
Z40.9 **Encounter for prophylactic surgery, unspecified**

● Z41 **Encounter for procedures for purposes other than remedying health state**
Z41.1 **Encounter for cosmetic surgery**
Encounter for cosmetic breast implant
Encounter for cosmetic procedure
Excludes1 encounter for plastic and reconstructive surgery following medical procedure or healed injury (Z42.-)
encounter for post-mastectomy breast implantation (Z42.1)
Z41.2 **Encounter for routine and ritual male circumcision**
Z41.3 **Encounter for ear piercing**
Z41.8 **Encounter for other procedures for purposes other than remedying health state**
Z41.9 **Encounter for procedure for purposes other than remedying health state, unspecified**

● Z42 **Encounter for plastic and reconstructive surgery following medical procedure or healed injury**
Excludes1 encounter for cosmetic plastic surgery (Z41.1)
encounter for plastic surgery for treatment of current injury - code to relevent injury
Z42.1 **Encounter for breast reconstruction following mastectomy**
Excludes1 deformity and disproportion of reconstructed breast (N65.1-)
Z42.8 **Encounter for other plastic and reconstructive surgery following medical procedure or healed injury**

Z43 Encounter for attention to artificial openings

Includes closure of artificial openings
passage of sounds or bougies through artificial openings
reforming artificial openings
removal of catheter from artificial openings
toilet or cleansing of artificial openings

Excludes1 artificial opening status only, without need for care (Z93.-)
complications of external stoma (J95.0-, K94.-, N99.5-)

Excludes2 fitting and adjustment of prosthetic and other devices (Z44-Z46)

Z43.0 Encounter for attention to tracheostomy

Z43.1 Encounter for attention to gastrostomy

Z43.2 Encounter for attention to ileostomy

Z43.3 Encounter for attention to colostomy

Z43.4 Encounter for attention to other artificial openings of digestive tract

Z43.5 Encounter for attention to cystostomy

Z43.6 Encounter for attention to other artificial openings of urinary tract

Encounter for attention to nephrostomy
Encounter for attention to ureterostomy
Encounter for attention to urethrostomy

Z43.7 Encounter for attention to artificial vagina

Z43.8 Encounter for attention to other artificial openings

Z43.9 Encounter for attention to unspecified artificial opening

Z44 Encounter for fitting and adjustment of external prosthetic device

Includes removal or replacement of external prosthetic device

Excludes1 malfunction or other complications of device - see Alphabetical Index presence of prosthetic device (Z97.-)

Z44.0 Encounter for fitting and adjustment of artificial arm

Z44.00 Encounter for fitting and adjustment of unspecified artificial arm

Z44.001 Encounter for fitting and adjustment of unspecified right artificial arm

Z44.002 Encounter for fitting and adjustment of unspecified left artificial arm

Z44.009 Encounter for fitting and adjustment of unspecified artificial arm, unspecified arm

Z44.01 Encounter for fitting and adjustment of complete artificial arm

Z44.011 Encounter for fitting and adjustment of complete right artificial arm

Z44.012 Encounter for fitting and adjustment of complete left artificial arm

Z44.019 Encounter for fitting and adjustment of complete artificial arm, unspecified arm

Z44.02 Encounter for fitting and adjustment of partial artificial arm

Z44.021 Encounter for fitting and adjustment of partial artificial right arm

Z44.022 Encounter for fitting and adjustment of partial artificial left arm

Z44.029 Encounter for fitting and adjustment of partial artificial arm, unspecified arm

Z44.1 Encounter for fitting and adjustment of artificial leg

Z44.10 Encounter for fitting and adjustment of unspecified artificial leg

Z44.101 Encounter for fitting and adjustment of unspecified right artificial leg

Z44.102 Encounter for fitting and adjustment of unspecified left artificial leg

Z44.109 Encounter for fitting and adjustment of unspecified artificial leg, unspecified leg

Z44.11 Encounter for fitting and adjustment of complete artificial leg

Z44.111 Encounter for fitting and adjustment of complete right artificial leg

Z44.112 Encounter for fitting and adjustment of complete left artificial leg

Z44.119 Encounter for fitting and adjustment of complete artificial leg, unspecified leg

Z44.12 Encounter for fitting and adjustment of partial artificial leg

Z44.121 Encounter for fitting and adjustment of partial artificial right leg

Z44.122 Encounter for fitting and adjustment of partial artificial left leg

Z44.129 Encounter for fitting and adjustment of partial artificial leg, unspecified leg

Z44.2 Encounter for fitting and adjustment of artificial eye

Excludes1 mechanical complication of ocular prosthesis (T85.3)

Z44.20 Encounter for fitting and adjustment of artificial eye, unspecified

Z44.21 Encounter for fitting and adjustment of artificial right eye

Z44.22 Encounter for fitting and adjustment of artificial left eye

Z44.3 Encounter for fitting and adjustment of external breast prosthesis

Excludes1 complications of breast implant (T85.4-)
encounter for adjustment or removal of breast implant (Z45.81-)
encounter for initial breast implant insertion for cosmetic breast augmentation (Z41.1)
encounter for breast reconstruction following mastectomy (Z42.1)

Z44.30 Encounter for fitting and adjustment of external breast prosthesis, unspecified breast

Z44.31 Encounter for fitting and adjustment of external right breast prosthesis

Z44.32 Encounter for fitting and adjustment of external left breast prosthesis

Z44.8 Encounter for fitting and adjustment of other external prosthetic devices

Z44.9 Encounter for fitting and adjustment of unspecified external prosthetic device

CHAPTER 21 (Z00-Z99)

● **Z45 Encounter for adjustment and management of implanted device**

Includes removal or replacement of implanted device

Excludes1 malfunction or other complications of device - see Alphabetical Index

presence of prosthetic and other devices (Z95-Z97)

Excludes2 encounter for fitting and adjustment of non-implanted device (Z46.-)

● **Z45.0 Encounter for adjustment and management of cardiac device**

● **Z45.01 Encounter for adjustment and management of cardiac pacemaker**

Encounter for adjustment and management of cardiac resynchronization therapy pacemaker (CRT-P) ◀

Excludes1 encounter for adjustment and management of automatic implantable cardiac defibrillator with synchronous cardiac pacemaker (Z45.02)

Z45.010 Encounter for checking and testing of cardiac pacemaker pulse generator [battery]

Encounter for replacing cardiac pacemaker pulse generator [battery]

Z45.018 Encounter for adjustment and management of other part of cardiac pacemaker

Z45.02 Encounter for adjustment and management of automatic implantable cardiac defibrillator

Encounter for adjustment and management of automatic implantable cardiac defibrillator with synchronous cardiac pacemaker

Encounter for adjustment and management of cardiac resynchronization therapy defibrillator (CRT-D) ◀

Z45.09 Encounter for adjustment and management of other cardiac device

Z45.1 Encounter for adjustment and management of infusion pump

Z45.2 Encounter for adjustment and management of vascular access device

Encounter for adjustment and management of vascular catheters

Excludes1 encounter for adjustment and management of renal dialysis catheter (Z49.01)

● **Z45.3 Encounter for adjustment and management of implanted devices of the special senses**

Z45.31 Encounter for adjustment and management of implanted visual substitution device

● **Z45.32 Encounter for adjustment and management of implanted hearing device**

Excludes1 encounter for fitting and adjustment of hearing aide (Z46.1)

Z45.320 Encounter for adjustment and management of bone conduction device

Z45.321 Encounter for adjustment and management of cochlear device

Z45.328 Encounter for adjustment and management of other implanted hearing device

● **Z45.4 Encounter for adjustment and management of implanted nervous system device**

Z45.41 Encounter for adjustment and management of cerebrospinal fluid drainage device

Encounter for adjustment and management of cerebral ventricular (communicating) shunt

Z45.42 Encounter for adjustment and management of neuropacemaker (brain) (peripheral nerve) (spinal cord)

Z45.49 Encounter for adjustment and management of other implanted nervous system device

● **Z45.8 Encounter for adjustment and management of other implanted devices**

● **Z45.81 Encounter for adjustment or removal of breast implant**

Encounter for elective implant exchange (different material) (different size)

Encounter removal of tissue expander without synchronous insertion of permanent implant

Excludes1 complications of breast implant (T85.4-)

encounter for initial breast implant insertion for cosmetic breast augmentation (Z41.1)

encounter for breast reconstruction following mastectomy (Z42.1)

Z45.811 Encounter for adjustment or removal of right breast implant

Z45.812 Encounter for adjustment or removal of left breast implant

Z45.819 Encounter for adjustment or removal of unspecified breast implant

Z45.82 Encounter for adjustment or removal of myringotomy device (stent) (tube)

Z45.89 Encounter for adjustment and management of other implanted devices

Z45.9 Encounter for adjustment and management of unspecified implanted device

● **Z46 Encounter for fitting and adjustment of other devices**

Includes removal or replacement of other device

Excludes1 malfunction or other complications of device - see Alphabetical Index

Excludes2 encounter for fitting and management of implanted devices (Z45.-)

issue of repeat prescription only (Z76.0)

presence of prosthetic and other devices (Z95-Z97)

Z46.0 Encounter for fitting and adjustment of spectacles and contact lenses

Z46.1 Encounter for fitting and adjustment of hearing aid

Excludes1 encounter for adjustment and management of implanted hearing device (Z45.32-)

Z46.2 Encounter for fitting and adjustment of other devices related to nervous system and special senses

Excludes2 encounter for adjustment and management of implanted nervous system device (Z45.4-)

encounter for adjustment and management of implanted visual substitution device (Z45.31)

Z46.3 Encounter for fitting and adjustment of dental prosthetic device

Encounter for fitting and adjustment of dentures

Z46.4 Encounter for fitting and adjustment of orthodontic device

● **Z46.5 Encounter for fitting and adjustment of other gastrointestinal appliance and device**
Excludes1 encounter for attention to artificial openings of digestive tract (Z43.1-Z43.4)
Z46.51 Encounter for fitting and adjustment of gastric lap band
Z46.59 Encounter for fitting and adjustment of other gastrointestinal appliance and device
Z46.6 Encounter for fitting and adjustment of urinary device
Excludes2 attention to artificial openings of urinary tract (Z43.5, Z43.6)
● **Z46.8 Encounter for fitting and adjustment of other specified devices**
Z46.81 Encounter for fitting and adjustment of insulin pump
Encounter for insulin pump instruction and training
Encounter for insulin pump titration
Z46.82 Encounter for fitting and adjustment of non-vascular catheter
Z46.89 Encounter for fitting and adjustment of other specified devices
Encounter for fitting and adjustment of wheelchair
Z46.9 Encounter for fitting and adjustment of unspecified device

● **Z47 Orthopedic aftercare**
Excludes1 aftercare for healing fracture - code to fracture with 7th character D
Z47.1 Aftercare following joint replacement surgery
Use additional code to identify the joint (Z96.6-)
Z47.2 Encounter for removal of internal fixation device
Excludes1 encounter for adjustment of internal fixation device for fracture treatment - code to fracture with appropriate 7th character
encounter for removal of external fixation device - code to fracture with 7th character D
infection or inflammatory reaction to internal fixation device (T84.6-)
mechanical complication of internal fixation device (T84.1-)
● **Z47.3 Aftercare following explantation of joint prosthesis**
Aftercare following explantation of joint prosthesis, staged procedure
Encounter for joint prosthesis insertion following prior explantation of joint prosthesis
Z47.31 Aftercare following explantation of shoulder joint prosthesis
Excludes1 acquired absence of shoulder joint following prior explantation of shoulder joint prosthesis (Z89.23-)
shoulder joint prosthesis explantation status (Z89.23-)
Z47.32 Aftercare following explantation of hip joint prosthesis
Excludes1 acquired absence of hip joint following prior explantation of hip joint prosthesis (Z89.62-)
hip joint prosthesis explantation status (Z89.62-)
Z47.33 Aftercare following explantation of knee joint prosthesis
Excludes1 acquired absence of knee joint following prior explantation of knee prosthesis (Z89.52-)
knee joint prosthesis explantation status (Z89.52-)
● **Z47.8 Encounter for other orthopedic aftercare**
Z47.81 Encounter for orthopedic aftercare following surgical amputation
Use additional code to identify the limb amputated (Z89.-)
Z47.82 Encounter for orthopedic aftercare following scoliosis surgery
Z47.89 Encounter for other orthopedic aftercare

● **Z48 Encounter for other postprocedural aftercare**
Excludes1 encounter for follow-up examination after completed treatment (Z08-Z09)
Excludes2 encounter for attention to artificial openings (Z43.-)
encounter for fitting and adjustment of prosthetic and other devices (Z44-Z46)
● **Z48.0 Encounter for attention to dressings, sutures and drains**
Excludes1 encounter for planned postprocedural wound closure (Z48.1)
Z48.00 Encounter for change or removal of nonsurgical wound dressing
Encounter for change or removal of wound dressing NOS
Z48.01 Encounter for change or removal of surgical wound dressing
Z48.02 Encounter for removal of sutures
Encounter for removal of staples
Z48.03 Encounter for change or removal of drains
Z48.1 Encounter for planned postprocedural wound closure
Excludes1 encounter for attention to dressings and sutures (Z48.0-)
● **Z48.2 Encounter for aftercare following organ transplant**
Z48.21 Encounter for aftercare following heart transplant
Z48.22 Encounter for aftercare following kidney transplant
Z48.23 Encounter for aftercare following liver transplant
Z48.24 Encounter for aftercare following lung transplant
● **Z48.28 Encounter for aftercare following multiple organ transplant**
Z48.280 Encounter for aftercare following heart-lung transplant
Z48.288 Encounter for aftercare following multiple organ transplant
● **Z48.29 Encounter for aftercare following other organ transplant**
Z48.290 Encounter for aftercare following bone marrow transplant
Z48.298 Encounter for aftercare following other organ transplant
Z48.3 Aftercare following surgery for neoplasm
Use additional code to identify the neoplasm

CHAPTER 21 (Z00-Z99)

● **Z48.8 Encounter for other specified postprocedural aftercare**

● **Z48.81 Encounter for surgical aftercare following surgery on specified body systems**

These codes identify the body system requiring aftercare. They are for use in conjunction with other aftercare codes to fully explain the aftercare encounter. The condition treated should also be coded if still present.

Excludes1 aftercare for injury - code the injury with 7th character D
aftercare following surgery for neoplasm (Z48.3)

Excludes2 aftercare following organ transplant (Z48.2-)
orthopedic aftercare (Z47.-)

Z48.810 Encounter for surgical aftercare following surgery on the sense organs

Z48.811 Encounter for surgical aftercare following surgery on the nervous system

Excludes2 encounter for surgical aftercare following surgery on the sense organs (Z48.810)

Z48.812 Encounter for surgical aftercare following surgery on the circulatory system

Z48.813 Encounter for surgical aftercare following surgery on the respiratory system

Z48.814 Encounter for surgical aftercare following surgery on the teeth or oral cavity

Z48.815 Encounter for surgical aftercare following surgery on the digestive system

Z48.816 Encounter for surgical aftercare following surgery on the genitourinary system

Excludes1 encounter for aftercare following sterilization reversal (Z31.42)

Z48.817 Encounter for surgical aftercare following surgery on the skin and subcutaneous tissue

Z48.89 Encounter for other specified surgical aftercare

● **Z49 Encounter for care involving renal dialysis**

Code also associated end stage renal disease (N18.6)

● **Z49.0 Preparatory care for renal dialysis**

Encounter for dialysis instruction and training

Z49.01 Encounter for fitting and adjustment of extracorporeal dialysis catheter

Removal or replacement of renal dialysis catheter

Toilet or cleansing of renal dialysis catheter

Z49.02 Encounter for fitting and adjustment of peritoneal dialysis catheter

● **Z49.3 Encounter for adequacy testing for dialysis**

Z49.31 Encounter for adequacy testing for hemodialysis

Z49.32 Encounter for adequacy testing for peritoneal dialysis

Encounter for peritoneal equilibration test

● **Z51 Encounter for other aftercare and medical care** ⬅

Code also condition requiring care

Excludes1 follow-up examination after treatment (Z08-Z09)

Z51.0 Encounter for antineoplastic radiation therapy

● **Z51.1 Encounter for antineoplastic chemotherapy and immunotherapy**

Excludes2 encounter for chemotherapy and immunotherapy for nonneoplastic condition-code to condition

Z51.11 Encounter for antineoplastic chemotherapy

Z51.12 Encounter for antineoplastic immunotherapy

Z51.5 Encounter for palliative care

Z51.6 Encounter for desensitization to allergens ◀

● **Z51.8 Encounter for other specified aftercare**

Excludes1 holiday relief care (Z75.5)

Z51.81 Encounter for therapeutic drug level monitoring

Code also any long-term (current) drug therapy (Z79.-)

Excludes1 encounter for blood-drug test for administrative or medicolegal reasons (Z02.83)

Z51.89 Encounter for other specified aftercare

● **Z52 Donors of organs and tissues**

Includes autologous and other living donors

Excludes1 cadaveric donor - omit code
examination of potential donor (Z00.5)

● **Z52.0 Blood donor**

● **Z52.00 Unspecified blood donor**

Z52.000 Unspecified donor, whole blood

Z52.001 Unspecified donor, stem cells

Z52.008 Unspecified donor, other blood

● **Z52.01 Autologous blood donor**

Z52.010 Autologous donor, whole blood

Z52.011 Autologous donor, stem cells

Z52.018 Autologous donor, other blood

● **Z52.09 Other blood donor**

Volunteer donor

Z52.090 Other blood donor, whole blood

Z52.091 Other blood donor, stem cells

Z52.098 Other blood donor, other blood

● **Z52.1 Skin donor**

Z52.10 Skin donor, unspecified

Z52.11 Skin donor, autologous

Z52.19 Skin donor, other

● **Z52.2 Bone donor**

Z52.20 Bone donor, unspecified

Z52.21 Bone donor, autologous

Z52.29 Bone donor, other

Z52.3 Bone marrow donor

Z52.4 Kidney donor

Z52.5 Cornea donor

Z52.6 Liver donor

● Z52.8 **Donor of other specified organs or tissues**
● Z52.81 **Egg (Oocyte) donor**
Z52.810 **Egg (Oocyte) donor under age 35, anonymous recipient**
Egg donor under age 35 NOS
Z52.811 **Egg (Oocyte) donor under age 35, designated recipient**
Z52.812 **Egg (Oocyte) donor age 35 and over, anonymous recipient**
Egg donor age 35 and over NOS
Z52.813 **Egg (Oocyte) donor age 35 and over, designated recipient**
Z52.819 **Egg (Oocyte) donor, unspecified**
Z52.89 **Donor of other specified organs or tissues**
Z52.9 **Donor of unspecified organ or tissue**
Donor NOS

● Z53 **Persons encountering health services for specific procedures and treatment, not carried out**
● Z53.0 **Procedure and treatment not carried out because of contraindication**
Z53.01 **Procedure and treatment not carried out due to patient smoking**
Z53.09 **Procedure and treatment not carried out because of other contraindication**
Z53.1 **Procedure and treatment not carried out because of patient's decision for reasons of belief and group pressure**
● Z53.2 **Procedure and treatment not carried out because of patient's decision for other and unspecified reasons**
Z53.20 **Procedure and treatment not carried out because of patient's decision for unspecified reasons**
Z53.21 **Procedure and treatment not carried out due to patient leaving prior to being seen by health care provider**
Z53.29 **Procedure and treatment not carried out because of patient's decision for other reasons**
● Z53.3 **Procedure converted to open procedure** ◀
Z53.31 **Laparoscopic surgical procedure converted to open procedure** ◀
Z53.32 **Thoracoscopic surgical procedure converted to open procedure** ◀
Z53.33 **Arthroscopic surgical procedure converted to open procedure** ◀
Z53.39 **Other specified procedure converted to open procedure** ◀
Z53.8 **Procedure and treatment not carried out for other reasons**
Z53.9 **Procedure and treatment not carried out, unspecified reason**

PERSONS WITH POTENTIAL HEALTH HAZARDS RELATED TO SOCIOECONOMIC AND PSYCHOSOCIAL CIRCUMSTANCES (Z55-Z65)

● Z55 **Problems related to education and literacy**
Excludes1 disorders of psychological development (F80-F89)
Z55.0 **Illiteracy and low-level literacy**
Z55.1 **Schooling unavailable and unattainable**
Z55.2 **Failed school examinations**
Z55.3 **Underachievement in school**
Z55.4 **Educational maladjustment and discord with teachers and classmates**
Z55.8 **Other problems related to education and literacy**
Problems related to inadequate teaching
Z55.9 **Problems related to education and literacy, unspecified**
Academic problems NOS

● Z56 **Problems related to employment and unemployment**
Excludes2 occupational exposure to risk factors (Z57.-)
problems related to housing and economic circumstances (Z59.-)
Z56.0 **Unemployment, unspecified**
Z56.1 **Change of job**
Z56.2 **Threat of job loss**
Z56.3 **Stressful work schedule**
Z56.4 **Discord with boss and workmates**
Z56.5 **Uncongenial work environment**
Difficult conditions at work
Z56.6 **Other physical and mental strain related to work**
● Z56.8 **Other problems related to employment**
Z56.81 **Sexual harassment on the job**
Z56.82 **Military deployment status**
Individual (civilian or military) currently deployed in theater or in support of military war, peacekeeping and humanitarian operations
Z56.89 **Other problems related to employment**
Z56.9 **Unspecified problems related to employment**
Occupational problems NOS

● Z57 **Occupational exposure to risk factors**
Z57.0 **Occupational exposure to noise**
Z57.1 **Occupational exposure to radiation**
Z57.2 **Occupational exposure to dust**
● Z57.3 **Occupational exposure to other air contaminants**
Z57.31 **Occupational exposure to environmental tobacco smoke**
Excludes2 exposure to environmental tobacco smoke (Z77.22)
Z57.39 **Occupational exposure to other air contaminants**
Z57.4 **Occupational exposure to toxic agents in agriculture**
Occupational exposure to solids, liquids, gases or vapors in agriculture
Z57.5 **Occupational exposure to toxic agents in other industries**
Occupational exposure to solids, liquids, gases or vapors in other industries
Z57.6 **Occupational exposure to extreme temperature**
Z57.7 **Occupational exposure to vibration**
Z57.8 **Occupational exposure to other risk factors**
Z57.9 **Occupational exposure to unspecified risk factor**

● Z59 **Problems related to housing and economic circumstances**
Excludes2 problems related to upbringing (Z62.-)
Z59.0 **Homelessness**
Z59.1 **Inadequate housing**
Lack of heating
Restriction of space
Technical defects in home preventing adequate care
Unsatisfactory surroundings
Excludes1 problems related to the natural and physical environment (Z77.1-)
Z59.2 **Discord with neighbors, lodgers and landlord**
Z59.3 **Problems related to living in residential institution**
Boarding-school resident
Excludes1 institutional upbringing (Z62.2)
Z59.4 **Lack of adequate food and safe drinking water**
Inadequate drinking water supply
Excludes1 effects of hunger (T73.0)
inappropriate diet or eating habits (Z72.4)
malnutrition (E40-E46)
Z59.5 **Extreme poverty**
Z59.6 **Low income**
Z59.7 **Insufficient social insurance and welfare support**

Z59.8 **Other problems related to housing and economic circumstances**
Foreclosure on loan
Isolated dwelling
Problems with creditors

Z59.9 **Problem related to housing and economic circumstances, unspecified**

● Z60 **Problems related to social environment**

Z60.0 **Problems of adjustment to life-cycle transitions**
Empty nest syndrome
Phase of life problem
Problem with adjustment to retirement [pension]

Z60.2 **Problems related to living alone**

Z60.3 **Acculturation difficulty**
Problem with migration
Problem with social transplantation

Z60.4 **Social exclusion and rejection**
Exclusion and rejection on the basis of personal characteristics, such as unusual physical appearance, illness or behavior.
Excludes1 target of adverse discrimination such as for racial or religious reasons (Z60.5)

Z60.5 **Target of (perceived) adverse discrimination and persecution**
Excludes1 social exclusion and rejection (Z60.4)

Z60.8 **Other problems related to social environment**

Z60.9 **Problem related to social environment, unspecified**

● Z62 **Problems related to upbringing**
Includes current and past negative life events in childhood
current and past problems of a child related to upbringing
Excludes2 maltreatment syndrome (T74.-)
problems related to housing and economic circumstances (Z59.-)

Z62.0 **Inadequate parental supervision and control**

Z62.1 **Parental overprotection**

● Z62.2 **Upbringing away from parents**
Excludes1 problems with boarding school (Z59.3)

Z62.21 **Child in welfare custody**
Child in care of non-parental family member
Child in foster care
Excludes2 problem for parent due to child in welfare custody (Z63.5)

Z62.22 **Institutional upbringing**
Child living in orphanage or group home

Z62.29 **Other upbringing away from parents**

Z62.3 **Hostility towards and scapegoating of child**

Z62.6 **Inappropriate (excessive) parental pressure**

● Z62.8 **Other specified problems related to upbringing**

● Z62.81 **Personal history of abuse in childhood**

Z62.810 **Personal history of physical and sexual abuse in childhood**
Excludes1 current child physical abuse (T74.12, T76.12)
current child sexual abuse (T74.22, T76.22)

Z62.811 **Personal history of psychological abuse in childhood**
Excludes1 current child psychological abuse (T74.32, T76.32)

Z62.812 **Personal history of neglect in childhood**
Excludes1 current child neglect (T74.02, T76.02)

Z62.819 **Personal history of unspecified abuse in childhood**
Excludes1 current child abuse NOS (T74.92, T76.92)

● Z62.82 **Parent-child conflict**

Z62.820 **Parent-biological child conflict**
Parent-child problem NOS

Z62.821 **Parent-adopted child conflict**

Z62.822 **Parent-foster child conflict**

● Z62.89 **Other specified problems related to upbringing**

Z62.890 **Parent-child estrangement NEC**

Z62.891 **Sibling rivalry**

Z62.898 **Other specified problems related to upbringing**

Z62.9 **Problem related to upbringing, unspecified**

● Z63 **Other problems related to primary support group, including family circumstances**
Excludes2 maltreatment syndrome (T74.-, T76)
parent-child problems (Z62.-)
problems related to negative life events in childhood (Z62.-)
problems related to upbringing (Z62.-)

Z63.0 **Problems in relationship with spouse or partner**
Excludes1 counseling for spousal or partner abuse problems (Z69.1)
counseling related to sexual attitude, behavior, and orientation (Z70.-)

Z63.1 **Problems in relationship with in-laws**

● Z63.3 **Absence of family member**
Excludes1 absence of family member due to disappearance and death (Z63.4)
absence of family member due to separation and divorce (Z63.5)

Z63.31 **Absence of family member due to military deployment**
Individual or family affected by other family member being on military deployment
Excludes1 family disruption due to return of family member from military deployment (Z63.71)

Z63.32 **Other absence of family member**

Z63.4 **Disappearance and death of family member**
Assumed death of family member
Bereavement

Z63.5 **Disruption of family by separation and divorce**
Marital estrangement

Z63.6 **Dependent relative needing care at home**

● Z63.7 **Other stressful life events affecting family and household**

Z63.71 **Stress on family due to return of family member from military deployment**
Individual or family affected by family member having returned from military deployment (current or past conflict)

Z63.72 **Alcoholism and drug addiction in family**

Z63.79 **Other stressful life events affecting family and household**
Anxiety (normal) about sick person in family
Health problems within family
Ill or disturbed family member
Isolated family

◀ New ◀ Revised ~~deleted~~ Deleted **OCGR** Official Guidelines **X** Assign placeholder X ● Use Additional Character(s)
Excludes 1 Excludes 2 Includes Use additional Code first Code also Unspecified

Z63.8 Other specified problems related to primary support group
Family discord NOS
Family estrangement NOS
High expressed emotional level within family
Inadequate family support NOS
Inadequate or distorted communication within family

Z63.9 Problem related to primary support group, unspecified
Relationship disorder NOS

● **Z64 Problems related to certain psychosocial circumstances**

Z64.0 Problems related to unwanted pregnancy

Z64.1 Problems related to multiparity

Z64.4 Discord with counselors
Discord with probation officer
Discord with social worker

● **Z65 Problems related to other psychosocial circumstances**

Z65.0 Conviction in civil and criminal proceedings without imprisonment

Z65.1 Imprisonment and other incarceration

Z65.2 Problems related to release from prison

Z65.3 Problems related to other legal circumstances
Arrest
Child custody or support proceedings
Litigation
Prosecution

Z65.4 Victim of crime and terrorism
Victim of torture

Z65.5 Exposure to disaster, war and other hostilities
Excludes1 target of perceived discrimination or persecution (Z60.5)

Z65.8 Other specified problems related to psychosocial circumstances

Z65.9 Problem related to unspecified psychosocial circumstances

DO NOT RESUSCITATE STATUS (Z66)

Z66 Do not resuscitate
DNR status

BLOOD TYPE (Z67)

● **Z67 Blood type**

● **Z67.1 Type A blood**
Z67.10 Type A blood, Rh positive
Z67.11 Type A blood, Rh negative

● **Z67.2 Type B blood**
Z67.20 Type B blood, Rh positive
Z67.21 Type B blood, Rh negative

● **Z67.3 Type AB blood**
Z67.30 Type AB blood, Rh positive
Z67.31 Type AB blood, Rh negative

● **Z67.4 Type O blood**
Z67.40 Type O blood, Rh positive
Z67.41 Type O blood, Rh negative

● **Z67.9 Unspecified blood type**
Z67.90 Unspecified blood type, Rh positive
Z67.91 Unspecified blood type, Rh negative

BODY MASS INDEX [BMI] (Z68)

OGCR Section I.B.14.

General Coding Guidelines

14. Documentation for BMI, ***Depth of*** Non-pressure ulcers, Pressure Ulcer Stages, **Coma Scale, *and NIH Stroke Scale***

For the Body Mass Index (BMI), depth of non-pressure chronic ulcers, pressure ulcer stage, **coma scale, and NIH stroke scale (NIHSS) codes,** code assignment may be based on medical record documentation from clinicians who are not the patient's provider (i.e., physician or other qualified healthcare practitioner legally accountable for establishing the patient's diagnosis), since this information is typically documented by other clinicians involved in the care of the patient (e.g., a dietitian often documents the BMI, a nurse often documents the pressure ulcer stages, **and an emergency medical technician often documents the coma scale**). However, the associated diagnosis (such as overweight, obesity, **acute stroke,** or pressure ulcer) must be documented by the patient's provider. If there is conflicting medical record documentation, either from the same clinician or different clinicians, the patient's attending provider should be queried for clarification.

The BMI, **coma scale, and NIHSS** codes should only be reported as secondary diagnoses.

● **Z68 Body mass index [BMI]**
Kilograms per meters squared
Note: BMI adult codes are for use for persons 21 years of age or older.
BMI pediatric codes are for use for persons 2-20 years of age. These percentiles are based on the growth charts published by the Centers for Disease Control and Prevention (CDC)

Z68.1 Body mass index (BMI) 19 or less, adult

● **Z68.2 Body mass index (BMI) 20-29, adult**
Z68.20 Body mass index (BMI) 20.0-20.9, adult
Z68.21 Body mass index (BMI) 21.0-21.9, adult
Z68.22 Body mass index (BMI) 22.0-22.9, adult
Z68.23 Body mass index (BMI) 23.0-23.9, adult
Z68.24 Body mass index (BMI) 24.0-24.9, adult
Z68.25 Body mass index (BMI) 25.0-25.9, adult
Z68.26 Body mass index (BMI) 26.0-26.9, adult
Z68.27 Body mass index (BMI) 27.0-27.9, adult
Z68.28 Body mass index (BMI) 28.0-28.9, adult
Z68.29 Body mass index (BMI) 29.0-29.9, adult

● **Z68.3 Body mass index (BMI) 30-39, adult**
Z68.30 Body mass index (BMI) 30.0-30.9, adult
Z68.31 Body mass index (BMI) 31.0-31.9, adult
Z68.32 Body mass index (BMI) 32.0-32.9, adult
Z68.33 Body mass index (BMI) 33.0-33.9, adult
Z68.34 Body mass index (BMI) 34.0-34.9, adult
Z68.35 Body mass index (BMI) 35.0-35.9, adult
Z68.36 Body mass index (BMI) 36.0-36.9, adult
Z68.37 Body mass index (BMI) 37.0-37.9, adult
Z68.38 Body mass index (BMI) 38.0-38.9, adult
Z68.39 Body mass index (BMI) 39.0-39.9, adult

● **Z68.4 Body mass index (BMI) 40 or greater, adult**
Z68.41 Body mass index (BMI) 40.0-44.9, adult
Z68.42 Body mass index (BMI) 45.0-49.9, adult
Z68.43 Body mass index (BMI) 50-59.9, adult
Z68.44 Body mass index (BMI) 60.0-69.9, adult
Z68.45 Body mass index (BMI) 70 or greater, adult

CHAPTER 21 (Z00-Z99)

● Z68.5 **Body mass index (BMI) pediatric**
  Z68.51 **Body mass index (BMI) pediatric, less than 5th percentile for age**
  Z68.52 **Body mass index (BMI) pediatric, 5th percentile to less than 85th percentile for age**
  Z68.53 **Body mass index (BMI) pediatric, 85th percentile to less than 95th percentile for age**
  Z68.54 **Body mass index (BMI) pediatric, greater than or equal to 95th percentile for age**

PERSONS ENCOUNTERING HEALTH SERVICES IN OTHER CIRCUMSTANCES (Z69-Z76)

● Z69 **Encounter for mental health services for victim and perpetrator of abuse**
  Includes counseling for victims and perpetrators of abuse
● Z69.Ø **Encounter for mental health services for child abuse problems**
● Z69.Ø1 **Encounter for mental health services for parental child abuse**
  Z69.Ø1Ø **Encounter for mental health services for victim of parental child abuse**
  Z69.Ø11 **Encounter for mental health services for perpetrator of parental child abuse**
  Excludes1 encounter for mental health services for non-parental child abuse (Z69.Ø2-)
● Z69.Ø2 **Encounter for mental health services for non-parental child abuse**
  Z69.Ø2Ø **Encounter for mental health services for victim of non-parental child abuse**
  Z69.Ø21 **Encounter for mental health services for perpetrator of non- parental child abuse**
● Z69.1 **Encounter for mental health services for spousal or partner abuse problems**
  Z69.11 **Encounter for mental health services for victim of spousal or partner abuse**
  Z69.12 **Encounter for mental health services for perpetrator of spousal or partner abuse**
● Z69.8 **Encounter for mental health services for victim or perpetrator of other abuse**
  Z69.81 **Encounter for mental health services for victim of other abuse**
  Encounter for rape victim counseling
  Z69.82 **Encounter for mental health services for perpetrator of other abuse**

● Z7Ø **Counseling related to sexual attitude, behavior and orientation**
  Includes encounter for mental health services for sexual attitude, behavior and orientation
  Excludes2 contraceptive or procreative counseling (Z3Ø-Z31)
  Z7Ø.Ø **Counseling related to sexual attitude**
  Z7Ø.1 **Counseling related to patient's sexual behavior and orientation**
  Patient concerned regarding impotence
  Patient concerned regarding non-responsiveness
  Patient concerned regarding promiscuity
  Patient concerned regarding sexual orientation
  Z7Ø.2 **Counseling related to sexual behavior and orientation of third party**
  Advice sought regarding sexual behavior and orientation of child
  Advice sought regarding sexual behavior and orientation of partner
  Advice sought regarding sexual behavior and orientation of spouse
  Z7Ø.3 **Counseling related to combined concerns regarding sexual attitude, behavior and orientation**
  Z7Ø.8 **Other sex counseling**
  Encounter for sex education
  Z7Ø.9 **Sex counseling, unspecified**

● Z71 **Persons encountering health services for other counseling and medical advice, not elsewhere classified**
  Excludes2 contraceptive or procreation counseling (Z3Ø-Z31)
  sex counseling (Z7Ø.-)
  Z71.Ø **Person encountering health services to consult on behalf of another person**
  Person encountering health services to seek advice or treatment for non-attending third party
  Excludes2 anxiety (normal) about sick person in family (Z63.7)
  expectant (adoptive) parent(s) pre-birth pediatrician visit (Z76.81)
  Z71.1 **Person with feared health complaint in whom no diagnosis is made**
  Person encountering health services with feared condition which was not demonstrated
  Person encountering health services in which problem was normal state
  'Worried well'
  Excludes1 medical observation for suspected diseases and conditions proven not to exist (ZØ3.-)
  Z71.2 **Person consulting for explanation of examination or test findings**
  Z71.3 **Dietary counseling and surveillance**
  Use additional code for any associated underlying medical condition
  Use additional code to identify body mass index (BMI), if known (Z68.-)
● Z71.4 **Alcohol abuse counseling and surveillance**
  Use additional code for alcohol abuse or dependence (F1Ø.-)
  Z71.41 **Alcohol abuse counseling and surveillance of alcoholic**
  Z71.42 **Counseling for family member of alcoholic**
  Counseling for significant other, partner, or friend of alcoholic
● Z71.5 **Drug abuse counseling and surveillance**
  Use additional code for drug abuse or dependence (F11-F16, F18-F19)
  Z71.51 **Drug abuse counseling and surveillance of drug abuser**
  Z71.52 **Counseling for family member of drug abuser**
  Counseling for significant other, partner, or friend of drug abuser
  Z71.6 **Tobacco abuse counseling**
  Use additional code for nicotine dependence (F17.-)
  Z71.7 **Human immunodeficiency virus [HIV] counseling**
● Z71.8 **Other specified counseling**
  Excludes2 counseling for contraception (Z3Ø.Ø-)
  counseling for genetics (Z31.5)
  counseling for procreative management (Z31.6-)
  Z71.81 **Spiritual or religious counseling**
  Z71.89 **Other specified counseling**
  Z71.9 **Counseling, unspecified**
  Encounter for medical advice NOS

CHAPTER 21 (ZØØ-Z99)

● **Z72 Problems related to lifestyle**
Excludes2 problems related to life-management difficulty (Z73.-)
problems related to socioeconomic and psychosocial circumstances (Z55-Z65)

Z72.0 Tobacco use
Tobacco use NOS
Excludes1 history of tobacco dependence (Z87.891)
nicotine dependence (F17.2-)
tobacco dependence (F17.2-)
tobacco use during pregnancy (O99.33-)

Z72.3 Lack of physical exercise

Z72.4 Inappropriate diet and eating habits
Excludes1 behavioral eating disorders of infancy or childhood (F98.2.-F98.3)
eating disorders (F50.-)
lack of adequate food (Z59.4)
malnutrition and other nutritional deficiencies (E40-E64)

● **Z72.5 High risk sexual behavior**
Promiscuity
Excludes1 paraphilias (F65)

Z72.51 High risk heterosexual behavior

Z72.52 High risk homosexual behavior

Z72.53 High risk bisexual behavior

Z72.6 Gambling and betting
Excludes1 compulsive or pathological gambling (F63.0)

● **Z72.8 Other problems related to lifestyle**

● **Z72.81 Antisocial behavior**
Excludes1 conduct disorders (F91.-)

Z72.810 Child and adolescent antisocial behavior
Antisocial behavior (child) (adolescent) without manifest psychiatric disorder
Delinquency NOS
Group delinquency
Offenses in the context of gang membership
Stealing in company with others
Truancy from school

Z72.811 Adult antisocial behavior
Adult antisocial behavior without manifest psychiatric disorder

● **Z72.82 Problems related to sleep**

Z72.820 Sleep deprivation
Lack of adequate sleep
Excludes1 insomnia (G47.0-)

Z72.821 Inadequate sleep hygiene
Bad sleep habits
Irregular sleep habits
Unhealthy sleep wake schedule
Excludes1 insomnia (F51.0-, G47.0-)

Z72.89 Other problems related to lifestyle
Self-damaging behavior

Z72.9 Problem related to lifestyle, unspecified

● **Z73 Problems related to life management difficulty**
Excludes2 problems related to socioeconomic and psychosocial circumstances (Z55-Z65)

Z73.0 Burn-out

Z73.1 Type A behavior pattern

Z73.2 Lack of relaxation and leisure

Z73.3 Stress, not elsewhere classified
Physical and mental strain NOS
Excludes1 stress related to employment or unemployment (Z56.-)

Z73.4 Inadequate social skills, not elsewhere classified

Z73.5 Social role conflict, not elsewhere classified

Z73.6 Limitation of activities due to disability
Excludes1 care-provider dependency (Z74.-)

● **Z73.8 Other problems related to life management difficulty**

● **Z73.81 Behavioral insomnia of childhood**

Z73.810 Behavioral insomnia of childhood, sleep-onset association type

Z73.811 Behavioral insomnia of childhood, limit setting type

Z73.812 Behavioral insomnia of childhood, combined type

Z73.819 Behavioral insomnia of childhood, unspecified type

Z73.82 Dual sensory impairment

Z73.89 Other problems related to life management difficulty

Z73.9 Problem related to life management difficulty, unspecified

● **Z74 Problems related to care provider dependency**
Excludes2 dependence on enabling machines or devices NEC (Z99.-)

● **Z74.0 Reduced mobility**

Z74.01 Bed confinement status
Bedridden

Z74.09 Other reduced mobility
Chairridden
Reduced mobility NOS
Excludes2 wheelchair dependence (Z99.3)

Z74.1 Need for assistance with personal care

Z74.2 Need for assistance at home and no other household member able to render care

Z74.3 Need for continuous supervision

Z74.8 Other problems related to care provider dependency

Z74.9 Problem related to care provider dependency, unspecified

● **Z75 Problems related to medical facilities and other health care**

Z75.0 Medical services not available in home
Excludes1 no other household member able to render care (Z74.2)

Z75.1 Person awaiting admission to adequate facility elsewhere

Z75.2 Other waiting period for investigation and treatment

Z75.3 Unavailability and inaccessibility of health care facilities
Excludes1 bed unavailable (Z75.1)

Z75.4 Unavailability and inaccessibility of other helping agencies

Z75.5 Holiday relief care

Z75.8 Other problems related to medical facilities and other health care

Z75.9 Unspecified problem related to medical facilities and other health care

CHAPTER 21 (Z00-Z99)

● Z76 **Persons encountering health services in other circumstances**

Z76.0 **Encounter for issue of repeat prescription**
Encounter for issue of repeat prescription for appliance
Encounter for issue of repeat prescription for medicaments
Encounter for issue of repeat prescription for spectacles
Excludes2 issue of medical certificate (Z02.7)
repeat prescription for contraceptive (Z30.4-)

Z76.1 **Encounter for health supervision and care of foundling**

Z76.2 **Encounter for health supervision and care of other healthy infant and child**
Encounter for medical or nursing care or supervision of healthy infant under circumstances such as adverse socioeconomic conditions at home
Encounter for medical or nursing care or supervision of healthy infant under circumstances such as awaiting foster or adoptive placement
Encounter for medical or nursing care or supervision of healthy infant under circumstances such as maternal illness
Encounter for medical or nursing care or supervision of healthy infant under circumstances such as number of children at home preventing or interfering with normal care

Z76.3 **Healthy person accompanying sick person**

Z76.4 **Other boarder to healthcare facility**
Excludes1 homelessness (Z59.0)

Z76.5 **Malingerer [conscious simulation]**
Person feigning illness (with obvious motivation)
Excludes1 factitious disorder (F68.1-)
peregrinating patient (F68.1-)

● Z76.8 **Persons encountering health services in other specified circumstances**

Z76.81 **Expectant parent(s) prebirth pediatrician visit**
Pre-adoption pediatrician visit for adoptive parent(s)

Z76.82 **Awaiting organ transplant status**
Patient waiting for organ availability

Z76.89 **Persons encountering health services in other specified circumstances**
Persons encountering health services NOS

PERSONS WITH POTENTIAL HEALTH HAZARDS RELATED TO FAMILY AND PERSONAL HISTORY AND CERTAIN CONDITIONS INFLUENCING HEALTH STATUS (Z77-Z99)

Code also any follow-up examination (Z08-Z09)

● Z77 **Other contact with and (suspected) exposures hazardous to health**
Includes contact with and (suspected) exposures to potential hazards to health
Excludes2 contact with and (suspected) exposure to communicable diseases (Z20.-)
exposure to (parental) (environmental) tobacco smoke in the perinatal period (P96.81)
newborn affected by noxious substances transmitted via placenta or breast milk (P04.-) ◄
occupational exposure to risk factors (Z57.-)
retained foreign body (Z18.-)
retained foreign body fully removed (Z87.821)
toxic effects of substances chiefly nonmedicinal as to source (T51-T65)

● Z77.0 **Contact with and (suspected) exposure to hazardous, chiefly nonmedicinal, chemicals**

● Z77.01 **Contact with and (suspected) exposure to hazardous metals**

Z77.010 **Contact with and (suspected) exposure to arsenic**

Z77.011 **Contact with and (suspected) exposure to lead**

Z77.012 **Contact with and (suspected) exposure to uranium**
Excludes1 retained depleted uranium fragments (Z18.01)

Z77.018 **Contact with and (suspected) exposure to other hazardous metals**
Contact with and (suspected) exposure to chromium compounds
Contact with and (suspected) exposure to nickel dust

● Z77.02 **Contact with and (suspected) exposure to hazardous aromatic compounds**

Z77.020 **Contact with and (suspected) exposure to aromatic amines**

Z77.021 **Contact with and (suspected) exposure to benzene**

Z77.028 **Contact with and (suspected) exposure to other hazardous aromatic compounds**
Aromatic dyes NOS
Polycyclic aromatic hydrocarbons

● Z77.09 **Contact with and (suspected) exposure to other hazardous, chiefly nonmedicinal, chemicals**

Z77.090 **Contact with and (suspected) exposure to asbestos**

Z77.098 **Contact with and (suspected) exposure to other hazardous, chiefly nonmedicinal, chemicals**
Dyes NOS

● Z77.1 **Contact with and (suspected) exposure to environmental pollution and hazards in the physical environment**

● Z77.11 **Contact with and (suspected) exposure to environmental pollution**

Z77.110 **Contact with and (suspected) exposure to air pollution**

Z77.111 **Contact with and (suspected) exposure to water pollution**

Z77.112 **Contact with and (suspected) exposure to soil pollution**

Z77.118 **Contact with and (suspected) exposure to other environmental pollution**

● Z77.12 **Contact with and (suspected) exposure to hazards in the physical environment**

Z77.120 **Contact with and (suspected) exposure to mold (toxic)**

Z77.121 **Contact with and (suspected) exposure to harmful algae and algae toxins**
Contact with and (suspected) exposure to (harmful) algae bloom NOS
Contact with and (suspected) exposure to blue-green algae bloom
Contact with and (suspected) exposure to brown tide
Contact with and (suspected) exposure to cyanobacteria bloom
Contact with and (suspected) exposure to Florida red tide
Contact with and (suspected) exposure to pfiesteria piscicida
Contact with and (suspected) exposure to red tide

Z77.122 **Contact with and (suspected) exposure to noise**

Z77.123 **Contact with and (suspected) exposure to radon and other naturally occuring radiation**
Excludes2 radiation exposure as the cause of a confirmed condition (W88-W90, X39.0-)
radiation sickness NOS (T66)

Z77.128 **Contact with and (suspected) exposure to other hazards in the physical environment**

● Z77.2 **Contact with and (suspected) exposure to other hazardous substances**

Z77.21 **Contact with and (suspected) exposure to potentially hazardous body fluids**

Z77.22 **Contact with and (suspected) exposure to environmental tobacco smoke (acute) (chronic)**
Exposure to second hand tobacco smoke (acute) (chronic)
Passive smoking (acute) (chronic)
Excludes1 nicotine dependence (F17.-)
tobacco use (Z72.0)
Excludes2 occupational exposure to environmental tobacco smoke (Z57.31)

Z77.29 **Contact with and (suspected) exposure to other hazardous substances**

Z77.9 **Other contact with and (suspected) exposures hazardous to health**

● Z78 **Other specified health status**
Excludes2 asymptomatic human immunodeficiency virus [HIV] infection status (Z21)
postprocedural status (Z93-Z99)
sex reassignment status (Z87.890)

Z78.0 **Asymptomatic menopausal state**
Menopausal state NOS
Postmenopausal status NOS
Excludes2 symptomatic menopausal state (N95.1)

Z78.1 **Physical restraint status**
Excludes1 physical restraint due to a procedure - omit code

Z78.9 **Other specified health status**

● Z79 **Long term (current) drug therapy**
Includes long term (current) drug use for prophylactic purposes
Code also any therapeutic drug level monitoring (Z51.81)
Excludes2 drug abuse and dependence (F11-F19)
drug use complicating pregnancy, childbirth, and the puerperium (O99.32-)
long term (current) use of oral antidiabetic drugs (Z79.84) ◀
long term (current) use of oral hypoglycemic drugs (Z79.84) ◀

● Z79.0 **Long term (current) use of anticoagulants and antithrombotics/antiplatelets**
Excludes2 long term (current) use of aspirin (Z79.82)

Z79.01 **Long term (current) use of anticoagulants**

Z79.02 **Long term (current) use of antithrombotics/ antiplatelets**

Z79.1 **Long term (current) use of non-steroidal anti-inflammatories (NSAID)**
Excludes2 long term (current) use of aspirin (Z79.82)

Z79.2 **Long term (current) use of antibiotics**

Z79.3 **Long term (current) use of hormonal contraceptives**
Long term (current) use of birth control pill or patch

Z79.4 **Long term (current) use of insulin**

● Z79.5 **Long term (current) use of steroids**

Z79.51 **Long term (current) use of inhaled steroids**

Z79.52 **Long term (current) use of systemic steroids**

● Z79.8 **Other long term (current) drug therapy**

● Z79.81 **Long term (current) use of agents affecting estrogen receptors and estrogen levels**
Code first, *if applicable:*
malignant neoplasm of breast (C50.-)
malignant neoplasm of prostate (C61)
Use additional code, if applicable, to identify:
estrogen receptor positive status (Z17.0)
family history of breast cancer (Z80.3)
genetic susceptibility to malignant neoplasm (cancer) (Z15.0-)
personal history of breast cancer (Z85.3)
personal history of prostate cancer (Z85.46)
postmenopausal status (Z78.0)
Excludes1 hormone replacement therapy (postmenopausal) (Z79.890)

Z79.810 **Long term (current) use of selective estrogen receptor modulators (SERMs)**
Long term (current) use of raloxifene (Evista)
Long term (current) use of tamoxifen (Nolvadex)
Long term (current) use of toremifene (Fareston)

Z79.811 **Long term (current) use of aromatase inhibitors**
Long term (current) use of anastrozole (Arimidex)
Long term (current) use of exemestane (Aromasin)
Long term (current) use of letrozole (Femara)

Z79.818 **Long term (current) use of other agents affecting estrogen receptors and estrogen levels**
Long term (current) use of estrogen receptor downregulators
Long term (current) use of fulvestrant (Faslodex)
Long term (current) use of gonadotropin-releasing hormone (GnRH) agonist
Long term (current) use of goserelin acetate (Zoladex)
Long term (current) use of leuprolide acetate (leuprorelin) (Lupron)
Long term (current) use of megestrol acetate (Megace)

Z79.82 **Long term (current) use of aspirin**

Z79.83 **Long term (current) use of bisphosphonates**

Z79.84 **Long term (current) use of oral hypoglycemic drugs** ◀
Long term (current) use of oral antidiabetic drugs ◀
Excludes2 long term (current) use of insulin (Z79.4) ◀

● Z79.89 **Other long term (current) drug therapy**

Z79.890 **Hormone replacement therapy (postmenopausal)**

Z79.891 **Long term (current) use of opiate analgesic**
Long term (current) use of methadone for pain management
Excludes1 methodone use NOS (F11.9-) ◀
use of methodone for treatment of heroin addiction (F11.2-)

Z79.899 **Other long term (current) drug therapy**

CHAPTER 21 (Z00-Z99)

● Z80 **Family history of primary malignant neoplasm**

Z80.0 **Family history of malignant neoplasm of digestive organs**
Conditions classifiable to C15-C26

Z80.1 **Family history of malignant neoplasm of trachea, bronchus and lung**
Conditions classifiable to C33-C34

Z80.2 **Family history of malignant neoplasm of other respiratory and intrathoracic organs**
Conditions classifiable to C30-C32, C37-C39

Z80.3 **Family history of malignant neoplasm of breast**
Conditions classifiable to C50.-

● Z80.4 **Family history of malignant neoplasm of genital organs**
Conditions classifiable to C51-C63

Z80.41 **Family history of malignant neoplasm of ovary**

Z80.42 **Family history of malignant neoplasm of prostate**

Z80.43 **Family history of malignant neoplasm of testis**

Z80.49 **Family history of malignant neoplasm of other genital organs**

● Z80.5 **Family history of malignant neoplasm of urinary tract**
Conditions classifiable to C64-C68

Z80.51 **Family history of malignant neoplasm of kidney**

Z80.52 **Family history of malignant neoplasm of bladder**

Z80.59 **Family history of malignant neoplasm of other urinary tract organ**

Z80.6 **Family history of leukemia**
Conditions classifiable to C91-C95

Z80.7 **Family history of other malignant neoplasms of lymphoid, hematopoietic and related tissues**
Conditions classifiable to C81-C90, C96.-

Z80.8 **Family history of malignant neoplasm of other organs or systems**
Conditions classifiable to C00-C14, C40-C49, C69-C79

Z80.9 **Family history of malignant neoplasm, unspecified**
Conditions classifiable to C80.1

● Z81 **Family history of mental and behavioral disorders**

Z81.0 **Family history of intellectual disabilities**
Conditions classifiable to F70-F79

Z81.1 **Family history of alcohol abuse and dependence**
Conditions classifiable to F10.-

Z81.2 **Family history of tobacco abuse and dependence**
Conditions classifiable to F17.-

Z81.3 **Family history of other psychoactive substance abuse and dependence**
Conditions classifiable to F11-F16, F18-F19

Z81.4 **Family history of other substance abuse and dependence**
Conditions classifiable to F55

Z81.8 **Family history of other mental and behavioral disorders**
Conditions classifiable elsewhere in F01-F99

● Z82 **Family history of certain disabilities and chronic diseases (leading to disablement)**

Z82.0 **Family history of epilepsy and other diseases of the nervous system**
Conditions classifiable to G00-G99

Z82.1 **Family history of blindness and visual loss**
Conditions classifiable to H54.-

Z82.2 **Family history of deafness and hearing loss**
Conditions classifiable to H90-H91

Z82.3 **Family history of stroke**
Conditions classifiable to I60-I64

● Z82.4 **Family history of ischemic heart disease and other diseases of the circulatory system**
Conditions classifiable to I00-I52, I65-I99

Z82.41 **Family history of sudden cardiac death**

Z82.49 **Family history of ischemic heart disease and other diseases of the circulatory system**

Z82.5 **Family history of asthma and other chronic lower respiratory diseases**
Conditions classifiable to J40-J47
Excludes2 family history of other diseases of the respiratory system (Z83.6)

● Z82.6 **Family history of arthritis and other diseases of the musculoskeletal system and connective tissue**
Conditions classifiable to M00-M99

Z82.61 **Family history of arthritis**

Z82.62 **Family history of osteoporosis**

Z82.69 **Family history of other diseases of the musculoskeletal system and connective tissue**

● Z82.7 **Family history of congenital malformations, deformations and chromosomal abnormalities**
Conditions classifiable to Q00-Q99

Z82.71 **Family history of polycystic kidney**

Z82.79 **Family history of other congenital malformations, deformations and chromosomal abnormalities**

Z82.8 **Family history of other disabilities and chronic diseases leading to disablement, not elsewhere classified**

● Z83 **Family history of other specific disorders**
Excludes2 contact with and (suspected) exposure to communicable disease in the family (Z20.-)

Z83.0 **Family history of human immunodeficiency virus [HIV] disease**
Conditions classifiable to B20

Z83.1 **Family history of other infectious and parasitic diseases**
Conditions classifiable to A00-B19, B25-B94, B99

Z83.2 **Family history of diseases of the blood and blood-forming organs and certain disorders involving the immune mechanism**
Conditions classifiable to D50-D89

Z83.3 **Family history of diabetes mellitus**
Conditions classifiable to E08-E13

● Z83.4 **Family history of other endocrine, nutritional and metabolic diseases**
Conditions classifiable to E00-E07, E15-E88

Z83.41 **Family history of multiple endocrine neoplasia [MEN] syndrome**

Z83.42 **Family history of familial hypercholesterolemia** ◀

Z83.49 **Family history of other endocrine, nutritional and metabolic diseases**

● Z83.5 **Family history of eye and ear disorders**

● Z83.51 **Family history of eye disorders**
Conditions classifiable to H00-H53, H55-H59
Excludes2 family history of blindness and visual loss (Z82.1)

Z83.511 **Family history of glaucoma**

Z83.518 **Family history of other specified eye disorder**

Z83.52 **Family history of ear disorders**
Conditions classifiable to H60-H83, H92-H95
Excludes2 family history of deafness and hearing loss (Z82.2)

Z83.6 **Family history of other diseases of the respiratory system**
Conditions classifiable to J00-J39, J60-J99
Excludes2 family history of asthma and other chronic lower respiratory diseases (Z82.5)

● Z83.7 **Family history of diseases of the digestive system**
Conditions classifiable to K00-K93

Z83.71 **Family history of colonic polyps**
Excludes1 family history of malignant neoplasm of digestive organs (Z80.0)

Z83.79 **Family history of other diseases of the digestive system**

● Z84 **Family history of other conditions**

Z84.0 **Family history of diseases of the skin and subcutaneous tissue**
Conditions classifiable to L00-L99

Z84.1 **Family history of disorders of kidney and ureter**
Conditions classifiable to N00-N29

Z84.2 **Family history of other diseases of the genitourinary system**
Conditions classifiable to N30-N99

Z84.3 **Family history of consanguinity**

● Z84.8 **Family history of other specified conditions**

Z84.81 **Family history of carrier of genetic disease**

Z84.82 **Family history of sudden infant death syndrome** ◀
Family history of SIDS ◀

Z84.89 **Family history of other specified conditions**

● Z85 **Personal history of malignant neoplasm**

Code first any follow-up examination after treatment of malignant neoplasm (Z08)

Use additional code to identify:
- alcohol use and dependence (F10.-)
- exposure to environmental tobacco smoke (Z77.22)
- history of tobacco dependence (Z87.891) ⟸
- occupational exposure to environmental tobacco smoke (Z57.31)
- tobacco dependence (F17.-)
- tobacco use (Z72.0)

Excludes2 personal history of benign neoplasm (Z86.01-)
personal history of carcinoma-in-situ (Z86.00-)

● Z85.0 **Personal history of malignant neoplasm of digestive organs**

Z85.00 **Personal history of malignant neoplasm of unspecified digestive organ**

Z85.01 **Personal history of malignant neoplasm of esophagus**
Conditions classifiable to C15

● Z85.02 **Personal history of malignant neoplasm of stomach**

Z85.020 **Personal history of malignant carcinoid tumor of stomach**
Conditions classifiable to C7A.092

Z85.028 **Personal history of other malignant neoplasm of stomach**
Conditions classifiable to C16

● Z85.03 **Personal history of malignant neoplasm of large intestine**

Z85.030 **Personal history of malignant carcinoid tumor of large intestine**
Conditions classifiable to C7A.022-C7A.025, C7A.029

Z85.038 **Personal history of other malignant neoplasm of large intestine**
Conditions classifiable to C18

● Z85.04 **Personal history of malignant neoplasm of rectum, rectosigmoid junction, and anus**

Z85.040 **Personal history of malignant carcinoid tumor of rectum**
Conditions classifiable to C7A.026

Z85.048 **Personal history of other malignant neoplasm of rectum, rectosigmoid junction, and anus**
Conditions classifiable to C19-C21

Z85.05 **Personal history of malignant neoplasm of liver**
Conditions classifiable to C22

● Z85.06 **Personal history of malignant neoplasm of small intestine**

Z85.060 **Personal history of malignant carcinoid tumor of small intestine**
Conditions classifiable to C7A.01-

Z85.068 **Personal history of other malignant neoplasm of small intestine**
Conditions classifiable to C17

Z85.07 **Personal history of malignant neoplasm of pancreas**
Conditions classifiable to C25

Z85.09 **Personal history of malignant neoplasm of other digestive organs**

● Z85.1 **Personal history of malignant neoplasm of trachea, bronchus and lung**

● Z85.11 **Personal history of malignant neoplasm of bronchus and lung**

Z85.110 **Personal history of malignant carcinoid tumor of bronchus and lung**
Conditions classifiable to C7A.090

Z85.118 **Personal history of other malignant neoplasm of bronchus and lung**
Conditions classifiable to C34

Z85.12 **Personal history of malignant neoplasm of trachea**
Conditions classifiable to C33

● Z85.2 **Personal history of malignant neoplasm of other respiratory and intrathoracic organs**

Z85.20 **Personal history of malignant neoplasm of unspecified respiratory organ**

Z85.21 **Personal history of malignant neoplasm of larynx**
Conditions classifiable to C32

Z85.22 **Personal history of malignant neoplasm of nasal cavities, middle ear, and accessory sinuses**
Conditions classifiable to C30-C31

● Z85.23 **Personal history of malignant neoplasm of thymus**

Z85.230 **Personal history of malignant carcinoid tumor of thymus**
Conditions classifiable to C7A.091

Z85.238 **Personal history of other malignant neoplasm of thymus**
Conditions classifiable to C37

Z85.29 **Personal history of malignant neoplasm of other respiratory and intrathoracic organs**

Z85.3 **Personal history of malignant neoplasm of breast**
Conditions classifiable to C50.-

● Z85.4 **Personal history of malignant neoplasm of genital organs**
Conditions classifiable to C51-C63

Z85.40 **Personal history of malignant neoplasm of unspecified female genital organ**

Z85.41 **Personal history of malignant neoplasm of cervix uteri**

Z85.42 **Personal history of malignant neoplasm of other parts of uterus**

Z85.43 **Personal history of malignant neoplasm of ovary**

Z85.44 **Personal history of malignant neoplasm of other female genital organs**

Z85.45 **Personal history of malignant neoplasm of unspecified male genital organ**

Z85.46 **Personal history of malignant neoplasm of prostate**

Z85.47 **Personal history of malignant neoplasm of testis**

CHAPTER 21 (Z00-Z99)

Z85.48 **Personal history of malignant neoplasm of epididymis**

Z85.49 **Personal history of malignant neoplasm of other male genital organs**

● Z85.5 **Personal history of malignant neoplasm of urinary tract**
Conditions classifiable to C64-C68

Z85.50 **Personal history of malignant neoplasm of unspecified urinary tract organ**

Z85.51 **Personal history of malignant neoplasm of bladder**

● Z85.52 **Personal history of malignant neoplasm of kidney**
Excludes1 personal history of malignant neoplasm of renal pelvis (Z85.53)

Z85.520 **Personal history of malignant carcinoid tumor of kidney**
Conditions classifiable to C7A.093

Z85.528 **Personal history of other malignant neoplasm of kidney**
Conditions classifiable to C64

Z85.53 **Personal history of malignant neoplasm of renal pelvis**

Z85.54 **Personal history of malignant neoplasm of ureter**

Z85.59 **Personal history of malignant neoplasm of other urinary tract organ**

Z85.6 **Personal history of leukemia**
Conditions classifiable to C91-C95
Excludes1 leukemia in remission C91.0-C95.9 with 5th character 1

● Z85.7 **Personal history of other malignant neoplasms of lymphoid, hematopoietic and related tissues**

Z85.71 **Personal history of Hodgkin lymphoma**
Conditions classifiable to C81

Z85.72 **Personal history of non-Hodgkin lymphomas**
Conditions classifiable to C82-C85

Z85.79 **Personal history of other malignant neoplasms of lymphoid, hematopoietic and related tissues**
Conditions classifiable to C88-C90, C96
Excludes1 multiple myeloma in remission (C90.01)
plasma cell leukemia in remission (C90.11)
plasmacytoma in remission (C90.21)

● Z85.8 **Personal history of malignant neoplasms of other organs and systems**
Conditions classifiable to C00-C14, C40-C49, C69-C75, C7A.098, C76-C79 ⬅

● Z85.81 **Personal history of malignant neoplasm of lip, oral cavity, and pharynx**

Z85.810 **Personal history of malignant neoplasm of tongue**

Z85.818 **Personal history of malignant neoplasm of other sites of lip, oral cavity, and pharynx**

Z85.819 **Personal history of malignant neoplasm of unspecified site of lip, oral cavity, and pharynx**

● Z85.82 **Personal history of malignant neoplasm of skin**

Z85.820 **Personal history of malignant melanoma of skin**
Conditions classifiable to C43

Z85.821 **Personal history of Merkel cell carcinoma**
Conditions classifiable to C4A

Z85.828 **Personal history of other malignant neoplasm of skin**
Conditions classifiable to C44

● Z85.83 **Personal history of malignant neoplasm of bone and soft tissue**

Z85.830 **Personal history of malignant neoplasm of bone**

Z85.831 **Personal history of malignant neoplasm of soft tissue**
Excludes2 personal history of malignant neoplasm of skin (Z85.82-)

● Z85.84 **Personal history of malignant neoplasm of eye and nervous tissue**

Z85.840 **Personal history of malignant neoplasm of eye**

Z85.841 **Personal history of malignant neoplasm of brain**

Z85.848 **Personal history of malignant neoplasm of other parts of nervous tissue**

● Z85.85 **Personal history of malignant neoplasm of endocrine glands**

Z85.850 **Personal history of malignant neoplasm of thyroid**

Z85.858 **Personal history of malignant neoplasm of other endocrine glands**

Z85.89 **Personal history of malignant neoplasm of other organs and systems**

Z85.9 **Personal history of malignant neoplasm, unspecified**
Conditions classifiable to C7A.00, C80.1

● Z86 **Personal history of certain other diseases**
Code first any follow-up examination after treatment (Z09)

● Z86.0 **Personal history of in-situ and benign neoplasms and neoplasms of uncertain behavior**
Excludes2 personal history of malignant neoplasms (Z85.-)

● Z86.00 **Personal history of in-situ neoplasm**
Conditions classifiable to D00-D09 ◀

Z86.000 **Personal history of in-situ neoplasm of breast**

Z86.001 **Personal history of in-situ neoplasm of cervix uteri**
Personal history of cervical intraepithelial neoplasia III [CIN III] ◀

Z86.008 **Personal history of in-situ neoplasm of other site**
Personal history of vaginal intraepithelial neoplasia III [VAIN III] ◀
Personal history of vulvar intraepithelial neoplasia III [VIN III] ◀

● Z86.01 **Personal history of benign neoplasm**

Z86.010 **Personal history of colonic polyps**

Z86.011 **Personal history of benign neoplasm of the brain**

Z86.012 **Personal history of benign carcinoid tumor**

Z86.018 **Personal history of other benign neoplasm**

Z86.03 **Personal history of neoplasm of uncertain behavior**

● **Z86.1 Personal history of infectious and parasitic diseases**
Conditions classifiable to A00-B89, B99
Excludes1 personal history of infectious diseases specific to a body system sequelae of infectious and parasitic diseases (B90-B94)

Z86.11 Personal history of tuberculosis

Z86.12 Personal history of poliomyelitis

Z86.13 Personal history of malaria

Z86.14 Personal history of Methicillin resistant Staphylococcus aureus infection
Personal history of MRSA infection

Z86.19 Personal history of other infectious and parasitic diseases

Z86.2 Personal history of diseases of the blood and blood-forming organs and certain disorders involving the immune mechanism
Conditions classifiable to D50-D89

● **Z86.3 Personal history of endocrine, nutritional and metabolic diseases**
Conditions classifiable to E00-E88

Z86.31 Personal history of diabetic foot ulcer
Excludes2 current diabetic foot ulcer (E08.621, E09.621, E10.621, E11.621, E13.621)

Z86.32 Personal history of gestational diabetes
Personal history of conditions classifiable to O24.4-
Excludes1 gestational diabetes mellitus in current pregnancy (O24.4-)

Z86.39 Personal history of other endocrine, nutritional and metabolic disease

● **Z86.5 Personal history of mental and behavioral disorders**
Conditions classifiable to F40-F59

Z86.51 Personal history of combat and operational stress reaction

Z86.59 Personal history of other mental and behavioral disorders

● **Z86.6 Personal history of diseases of the nervous system and sense organs**
Conditions classifiable to G00-G99, H00-H95

Z86.61 Personal history of infections of the central nervous system
Personal history of encephalitis
Personal history of meningitis

Z86.69 Personal history of other diseases of the nervous system and sense organs

● **Z86.7 Personal history of diseases of the circulatory system**
Conditions classifiable to I00-I99
Excludes2 old myocardial infarction (I25.2)
personal history of anaphylactic shock (Z87.892)
postmyocardial infarction syndrome (I24.1)

● **Z86.71 Personal history of venous thrombosis and embolism**

Z86.711 Personal history of pulmonary embolism

Z86.718 Personal history of other venous thrombosis and embolism

Z86.72 Personal history of thrombophlebitis

Z86.73 Personal history of transient ischemic attack (TIA), and cerebral infarction without residual deficits
Personal history of prolonged reversible ischemic neurological deficit (PRIND)
Personal history of stroke NOS without residual deficits
Excludes1 personal history of traumatic brain injury (Z87.820)
sequelae of cerebrovascular disease (I69.-)

Z86.74 Personal history of sudden cardiac arrest
Personal history of sudden cardiac death successfully resuscitated

Z86.79 Personal history of other diseases of the circulatory system

● **Z87 Personal history of other diseases and conditions**
Code first *any follow-up examination after treatment (Z09)*

● **Z87.0 Personal history of diseases of the respiratory system**
Conditions classifiable to J00-J99

Z87.01 Personal history of pneumonia (recurrent)

Z87.09 Personal history of other diseases of the respiratory system

● **Z87.1 Personal history of diseases of the digestive system**
Conditions classifiable to K00-K93

Z87.11 Personal history of peptic ulcer disease

Z87.19 Personal history of other diseases of the digestive system

Z87.2 Personal history of diseases of the skin and subcutaneous tissue
Conditions classifiable to L00-L99
Excludes2 personal history of diabetic foot ulcer (Z86.31)

● **Z87.3 Personal history of diseases of the musculoskeletal system and connective tissue**
Conditions classifiable to M00-M99
Excludes2 personal history of (healed) traumatic fracture (Z87.81)

● **Z87.31 Personal history of (healed) nontraumatic fracture**

Z87.310 Personal history of (healed) osteoporosis fracture
Personal history of (healed) fragility fracture
Personal history of (healed) collapsed vertebra due to osteoporosis

Z87.311 Personal history of (healed) other pathological fracture
Personal history of (healed) collapsed vertebra NOS
Excludes2 personal history of osteoporosis fracture (Z87.310)

Z87.312 Personal history of (healed) stress fracture
Personal history of (healed) fatigue fracture

Z87.39 Personal history of other diseases of the musculoskeletal system and connective tissue

CHAPTER 21 (Z00-Z99)

● Z87.4 **Personal history of diseases of genitourinary system**
Conditions classifiable to N00-N99

● Z87.41 **Personal history of dysplasia of the female genital tract**
Excludes1 personal history of intraepithelial neoplasia III of female genital tract (Z87.001, Z87.008) ◀
personal history of malignant neoplasm of female genital tract (Z85.40-Z85.44)

Z87.410 **Personal history of cervical dysplasia**

Z87.411 **Personal history of vaginal dysplasia**

Z87.412 **Personal history of vulvar dysplasia**

Z87.42 **Personal history of other diseases of the female genital tract**

● Z87.43 **Personal history of diseases of male genital organs**

Z87.430 **Personal history of prostatic dysplasia**
Excludes1 personal history of malignant neoplasm of prostate (Z85.46)

Z87.438 **Personal history of other diseases of male genital organs**

● Z87.44 **Personal history of diseases of urinary system**
Excludes1 personal history of malignant neoplasm of cervix uteri (Z85.41)

Z87.440 **Personal history of urinary (tract) infections**

Z87.441 **Personal history of nephrotic syndrome**

Z87.442 **Personal history of urinary calculi**
Personal history of kidney stones

Z87.448 **Personal history of other diseases of urinary system**

● Z87.5 **Personal history of complications of pregnancy, childbirth and the puerperium**
Conditions classifiable to O00-O9A
Excludes2 recurrent pregnancy loss (N96)

Z87.51 **Personal history of pre-term labor**
Excludes1 current pregnancy with history of pre-term labor (O09.21-)

Z87.59 **Personal history of other complications of pregnancy, childbirth and the puerperium**
Personal history of trophoblastic disease

● Z87.7 **Personal history of (corrected) congenital malformations**
Conditions classifiable to Q00-Q89 that have been repaired or corrected
Excludes1 congenital malformations that have been partially corrected or repair but which still require medical treatment - code to condition
Excludes2 other postprocedural states (Z98.-)
personal history of medical treatment (Z92.-)
presence of cardiac and vascular implants and grafts (Z95.-)
presence of other devices (Z97.-)
presence of other functional implants (Z96.-)
transplanted organ and tissue status (Z94.-)

● Z87.71 **Personal history of (corrected) congenital malformations of genitourinary system**

Z87.710 **Personal history of (corrected) hypospadias**

Z87.718 **Personal history of other specified (corrected) congenital malformations of genitourinary system**

● Z87.72 **Personal history of (corrected) congenital malformations of nervous system and sense organs**

Z87.720 **Personal history of (corrected) congenital malformations of eye**

Z87.721 **Personal history of (corrected) congenital malformations of ear**

Z87.728 **Personal history of other specified (corrected) congenital malformations of nervous system and sense organs**

● Z87.73 **Personal history of (corrected) congenital malformations of digestive system**

Z87.730 **Personal history of (corrected) cleft lip and palate**

Z87.738 **Personal history of other specified (corrected) congenital malformations of digestive system**

Z87.74 **Personal history of (corrected) congenital malformations of heart and circulatory system**

Z87.75 **Personal history of (corrected) congenital malformations of respiratory system**

Z87.76 **Personal history of (corrected) congenital malformations of integument, limbs and musculoskeletal system**

● Z87.79 **Personal history of other (corrected) congenital malformations**

Z87.790 **Personal history of (corrected) congenital malformations of face and neck**

Z87.798 **Personal history of other (corrected) congenital malformations**

● Z87.8 **Personal history of other specified conditions**
Excludes2 personal history of self harm (Z91.5)

Z87.81 **Personal history of (healed) traumatic fracture**
Excludes2 personal history of (healed) nontraumatic fracture (Z87.31-)

● Z87.82 **Personal history of other (healed) physical injury and trauma**
Conditions classifiable to S00-T88, except traumatic fractures

Z87.820 **Personal history of traumatic brain injury**
Excludes1 personal history of transient ischemic attack (TIA), and cerebral infarction without residual deficits (Z86.73)

Z87.821 **Personal history of retained foreign body fully removed**

Z87.828 **Personal history of other (healed) physical injury and trauma**

● Z87.89 **Personal history of other specified conditions**

Z87.890 **Personal history of sex reassignment**

Z87.891 **Personal history of nicotine dependence**
Excludes1 current nicotine dependence (F17.2-)

Z87.892 **Personal history of anaphylaxis**
Code also allergy status such as:
allergy status to drugs, medicaments and biological substances (Z88.-)
allergy status, other than to drugs and biological substances (Z91.0-)

Z87.898 **Personal history of other specified conditions**

Z88 Allergy status to drugs, medicaments and biological substances
Excludes2 allergy status, other than to drugs and biological substances (Z91.0-)
- Z88.0 **Allergy status to penicillin**
- Z88.1 **Allergy status to other antibiotic agents status**
- Z88.2 **Allergy status to sulfonamides status**
- Z88.3 **Allergy status to other anti-infective agents status**
- Z88.4 **Allergy status to anesthetic agent status**
- Z88.5 **Allergy status to narcotic agent status**
- Z88.6 **Allergy status to analgesic agent status**
- Z88.7 **Allergy status to serum and vaccine status**
- Z88.8 **Allergy status to other drugs, medicaments and biological substances status**
- Z88.9 **Allergy status to unspecified drugs, medicaments and biological substances status**

Z89 Acquired absence of limb
Includes amputation status
postprocedural loss of limb
post-traumatic loss of limb
Excludes1 acquired deformities of limbs (M20-M21)
congenital absence of limbs (Q71-Q73)

Z89.0 Acquired absence of thumb and other finger(s)

Z89.01 Acquired absence of thumb
- Z89.011 **Acquired absence of right thumb**
- Z89.012 **Acquired absence of left thumb**
- Z89.019 **Acquired absence of unspecified thumb**

Z89.02 Acquired absence of other finger(s)
Excludes2 acquired absence of thumb (Z89.01-)
- Z89.021 **Acquired absence of right finger(s)**
- Z89.022 **Acquired absence of left finger(s)**
- Z89.029 **Acquired absence of unspecified finger(s)**

Z89.1 Acquired absence of hand and wrist

Z89.11 Acquired absence of hand
- Z89.111 **Acquired absence of right hand**
- Z89.112 **Acquired absence of left hand**
- Z89.119 **Acquired absence of unspecified hand**

Z89.12 Acquired absence of wrist
Disarticulation at wrist
- Z89.121 **Acquired absence of right wrist**
- Z89.122 **Acquired absence of left wrist**
- Z89.129 **Acquired absence of unspecified wrist**

Z89.2 Acquired absence of upper limb above wrist

Z89.20 Acquired absence of upper limb, unspecified level
- Z89.201 **Acquired absence of right upper limb, unspecified level**
- Z89.202 **Acquired absence of left upper limb, unspecified level**
- Z89.209 **Acquired absence of unspecified upper limb, unspecified level**
  Acquired absence of arm NOS

Z89.21 Acquired absence of upper limb below elbow
- Z89.211 **Acquired absence of right upper limb below elbow**
- Z89.212 **Acquired absence of left upper limb below elbow**
- Z89.219 **Acquired absence of unspecified upper limb below elbow**

Z89.22 Acquired absence of upper limb above elbow
Disarticulation at elbow
- Z89.221 **Acquired absence of right upper limb above elbow**
- Z89.222 **Acquired absence of left upper limb above elbow**
- Z89.229 **Acquired absence of unspecified upper limb above elbow**

Z89.23 Acquired absence of shoulder
Acquired absence of shoulder joint following explantation of shoulder joint prosthesis, with or without presence of antibiotic-impregnated cement spacer
- Z89.231 **Acquired absence of right shoulder**
- Z89.232 **Acquired absence of left shoulder**
- Z89.239 **Acquired absence of unspecified shoulder**

Z89.4 Acquired absence of toe(s), foot, and ankle

Z89.41 Acquired absence of great toe
- Z89.411 **Acquired absence of right great toe**
- Z89.412 **Acquired absence of left great toe**
- Z89.419 **Acquired absence of unspecified great toe**

Z89.42 Acquired absence of other toe(s)
Excludes2 acquired absence of great toe (Z89.41-)
- Z89.421 **Acquired absence of other right toe(s)**
- Z89.422 **Acquired absence of other left toe(s)**
- Z89.429 **Acquired absence of other toe(s), unspecified side**

Z89.43 Acquired absence of foot
- Z89.431 **Acquired absence of right foot**
- Z89.432 **Acquired absence of left foot**
- Z89.439 **Acquired absence of unspecified foot**

Z89.44 Acquired absence of ankle
Disarticulation of ankle
- Z89.441 **Acquired absence of right ankle**
- Z89.442 **Acquired absence of left ankle**
- Z89.449 **Acquired absence of unspecified ankle**

Z89.5 Acquired absence of leg below knee

Z89.51 Acquired absence of leg below knee
- Z89.511 **Acquired absence of right leg below knee**
- Z89.512 **Acquired absence of left leg below knee**
- Z89.519 **Acquired absence of unspecified leg below knee**

Z89.52 Acquired absence of knee
Acquired absence of knee joint following explantation of knee joint prosthesis, with or without presence of antibiotic-impregnated cement spacer
- Z89.521 **Acquired absence of right knee**
- Z89.522 **Acquired absence of left knee**
- Z89.529 **Acquired absence of unspecified knee**

CHAPTER 21 (Z00-Z99)

● Z89.6 **Acquired absence of leg above knee**

● Z89.61 **Acquired absence of leg above knee**
Acquired absence of leg NOS
Disarticulation at knee

Z89.611 **Acquired absence of right leg above knee**

Z89.612 **Acquired absence of left leg above knee**

Z89.619 **Acquired absence of unspecified leg above knee**

● Z89.62 **Acquired absence of hip**
Acquired absence of hip joint following explantation of hip joint prosthesis, with or without presence of antibiotic-impregnated cement spacer
Disarticulation at hip

Z89.621 **Acquired absence of right hip joint**

Z89.622 **Acquired absence of left hip joint**

Z89.629 **Acquired absence of unspecified hip joint**

Z89.9 **Acquired absence of limb, unspecified**

● Z90 **Acquired absence of organs, not elsewhere classified**

Includes postprocedural or post-traumatic loss of body part NEC

Excludes1 congenital absence - see Alphabetical Index

Excludes2 postprocedural absence of endocrine glands (E89.-)

● Z90.0 **Acquired absence of part of head and neck**

Z90.01 **Acquired absence of eye**

Z90.02 **Acquired absence of larynx**

Z90.09 **Acquired absence of other part of head and neck**
Acquired absence of nose
Excludes2 teeth (K08.1)

● Z90.1 **Acquired absence of breast and nipple**

Z90.10 **Acquired absence of unspecified breast and nipple**

Z90.11 **Acquired absence of right breast and nipple**

Z90.12 **Acquired absence of left breast and nipple**

Z90.13 **Acquired absence of bilateral breasts and nipples**

Z90.2 **Acquired absence of lung [part of]**

Z90.3 **Acquired absence of stomach [part of]**

● Z90.4 **Acquired absence of other specified parts of digestive tract**

● Z90.41 **Acquired absence of pancreas**
Code also exocrine pancreatic insufficiency (K86.81) ◀
Use additional code to identify any associated:
insulin use (Z79.4)
diabetes mellitus, postpancreatectomy (E13.-)

Z90.410 **Acquired total absence of pancreas**
Acquired absence of pancreas NOS

Z90.411 **Acquired partial absence of pancreas**

Z90.49 **Acquired absence of other specified parts of digestive tract**

Z90.5 **Acquired absence of kidney**

Z90.6 **Acquired absence of other parts of urinary tract**
Acquired absence of bladder

● Z90.7 **Acquired absence of genital organ(s)**
Excludes1 personal history of sex reassignment (Z87.890)
Excludes2 female genital mutilation status (N90.81-)

● Z90.71 **Acquired absence of cervix and uterus**

Z90.710 **Acquired absence of both cervix and uterus**
Acquired absence of uterus NOS
Status post total hysterectomy

Z90.711 **Acquired absence of uterus with remaining cervical stump**
Status post partial hysterectomy with remaining cervical stump

Z90.712 **Acquired absence of cervix with remaining uterus**

● Z90.72 **Acquired absence of ovaries**

Z90.721 **Acquired absence of ovaries, unilateral**

Z90.722 **Acquired absence of ovaries, bilateral**

Z90.79 **Acquired absence of other genital organ(s)**

● Z90.8 **Acquired absence of other organs**

Z90.81 **Acquired absence of spleen**

Z90.89 **Acquired absence of other organs**

● Z91 **Personal risk factors, not elsewhere classified**

Excludes2 contact with and (suspected) exposures hazardous to health (Z77.-)
exposure to pollution and other problems related to physical environment (Z77.1-)
occupational exposure to risk factors (Z57.-)
personal history of physical injury and trauma (Z87.81, Z87.82-)

● Z91.0 **Allergy status, other than to drugs and biological substances**
Excludes2 allergy status to drugs, medicaments, and biological substances (Z88.-)

● Z91.01 **Food allergy status**
Excludes2 food additives allergy status (Z91.02)

Z91.010 **Allergy to peanuts**

Z91.011 **Allergy to milk products**
Excludes1 lactose intolerance (E73.-)

Z91.012 **Allergy to eggs**

Z91.013 **Allergy to seafood**
Allergy to shellfish
Allergy to octopus or squid ink

Z91.018 **Allergy to other foods**
Allergy to nuts other than peanuts

Z91.02 **Food additives allergy status**

● Z91.03 **Insect allergy status**

Z91.030 **Bee allergy status**

Z91.038 **Other insect allergy status**

● Z91.04 **Nonmedicinal substance allergy status**

Z91.040 **Latex allergy status**
Latex sensitivity status

Z91.041 **Radiographic dye allergy status**
Allergy status to contrast media used for diagnostic X-ray procedure

Z91.048 **Other nonmedicinal substance allergy status**

Z91.09 **Other allergy status, other than to drugs and biological substances**

Z91.1 Patient's noncompliance with medical treatment and regimen

Z91.11 Patient's noncompliance with dietary regimen

Z91.12 Patient's intentional underdosing of medication regimen

Code first underdosing of medication (T36-T50) with fifth or sixth character 6

Excludes1 adverse effect of prescribed drug taken as directed - code to adverse effect
poisoning (overdose) - code to poisoning

Z91.120 Patient's intentional underdosing of medication regimen due to financial hardship

Z91.128 Patient's intentional underdosing of medication regimen for other reason

Z91.13 Patient's unintentional underdosing of medication regimen

Code first underdosing of medication (T36-T50) with fifth or sixth character 6

Excludes1 adverse effect of prescribed drug taken as directed - code to adverse effect
poisoning (overdose) - code to poisoning

Z91.130 Patient's unintentional underdosing of medication regimen due to age-related debility

Z91.138 Patient's unintentional underdosing of medication regimen for other reason

Z91.14 Patient's other noncompliance with medication regimen

Patient's underdosing of medication NOS

Z91.15 Patient's noncompliance with renal dialysis

Z91.19 Patient's noncompliance with other medical treatment and regimen

Z91.4 Personal history of psychological trauma, not elsewhere classified

Z91.41 Personal history of adult abuse

Excludes2 personal history of abuse in childhood (Z62.81-)

Z91.410 Personal history of adult physical and sexual abuse

Excludes1 current adult physical abuse (T74.11, T76.11)
current adult sexual abuse (T74.21, T76.11)

Z91.411 Personal history of adult psychological abuse

Z91.412 Personal history of adult neglect

Excludes1 current adult neglect (T74.01, T76.01)

Z91.419 Personal history of unspecified adult abuse

Z91.49 Other personal history of psychological trauma, not elsewhere classified

Z91.5 Personal history of self-harm

Personal history of parasuicide
Personal history of self-poisoning
Personal history of suicide attempt

Z91.8 Other specified personal risk factors, not elsewhere classified

Z91.81 History of falling

At risk for falling

Z91.82 Personal history of military deployment

Individual (civilian or military) with past history of military war, peacekeeping and humanitarian deployment (current or past conflict)
Returned from military deployment

Z91.83 Wandering in diseases classified elsewhere

Code first underlying disorder such as:
Alzheimer's disease (G30.-)
autism or pervasive developmental disorder (F84.-)
intellectual disabilities (F70-F79)
unspecified dementia with behavioral disturbance (F03.9-)

Z91.89 Other specified personal risk factors, not elsewhere classified

Z92 Personal history of medical treatment

Excludes2 postprocedural states (Z98.-)

Z92.0 Personal history of contraception

Excludes1 counseling or management of current contraceptive practices (Z30.-)
long term (current) use of contraception (Z79.3)
presence of (intrauterine) contraceptive device (Z97.5)

Z92.2 Personal history of drug therapy

Excludes2 long term (current) drug therapy (Z79.-)

Z92.21 Personal history of antineoplastic chemotherapy

Z92.22 Personal history of monoclonal drug therapy

Z92.23 Personal history of estrogen therapy

Z92.24 Personal history of steroid therapy

Z92.240 Personal history of inhaled steroid therapy

Z92.241 Personal history of systemic steroid therapy

Personal history of steroid therapy NOS

Z92.25 Personal history of immunosupression therapy

Excludes2 personal history of steroid therapy (Z92.24)

Z92.29 Personal history of other drug therapy

Z92.3 Personal history of irradiation

Personal history of exposure to therapeutic radiation

Excludes1 exposure to radiation in the physical environment (Z77.12)
occupational exposure to radiation (Z57.1)

CHAPTER 21 (Z00-Z99)

◄ New ◄ Revised ~~deleted~~ Deleted OGCR Official Guidelines X Assign placeholder X ● Use Additional Character(s)
Excludes1 Excludes2 Includes Use additional Code first Code also Unspecified

●Z92.8 **Personal history of other medical treatment**

Z92.81 **Personal history of extracorporeal membrane oxygenation (ECMO)**

Z92.82 **Status post administration of tPA (rtPA) in a different facility within the last 24 hours prior to admission to current facility**

Code first condition requiring tPA administration, such as:
acute cerebral infarction (I63.-)
acute myocardial infarction (I21.-, I22.-)

Z92.83 **Personal history of failed moderate sedation**
Personal history of failed conscious sedation
Excludes2 failed moderate sedation during procedure (T88.52)

Z92.84 **Personal history of unintended awareness under general anesthesia** ◀
Excludes2 unintended awareness under general anesthesia during procedure (T88.53) ◀

Z92.89 **Personal history of other medical treatment**

●Z93 **Artificial opening status**
Excludes1 artificial openings requiring attention or management (Z43.-)
complications of external stoma (J95.0-, K94.-, N99.5-)

Z93.0 **Tracheostomy status**

Z93.1 **Gastrostomy status**

Z93.2 **Ileostomy status**

Z93.3 **Colostomy status**

Z93.4 **Other artificial openings of gastrointestinal tract status**

●Z93.5 **Cystostomy status**

Z93.50 **Unspecified cystostomy status**

Z93.51 **Cutaneous-vesicostomy status**

Z93.52 **Appendico-vesicostomy status**

Z93.59 **Other cystostomy status**

Z93.6 **Other artificial openings of urinary tract status**
Nephrostomy status
Ureterostomy status
Urethrostomy status

Z93.8 **Other artificial opening status**

Z93.9 **Artificial opening status, unspecified**

●Z94 **Transplanted organ and tissue status**
Includes organ or tissue replaced by heterogenous or homogenous transplant
Excludes1 complications of transplanted organ or tissue - see Alphabetical Index
Excludes2 presence of vascular grafts (Z95.-)

Z94.0 **Kidney transplant status**

Z94.1 **Heart transplant status**
Excludes1 artificial heart status (Z95.812)
heart-valve replacement status (Z95.2-Z95.4)

Z94.2 **Lung transplant status**

Z94.3 **Heart and lungs transplant status**

Z94.4 **Liver transplant status**

Z94.5 **Skin transplant status**
Autogenous skin transplant status

Z94.6 **Bone transplant status**

Z94.7 **Corneal transplant status**

●Z94.8 **Other transplanted organ and tissue status**

Z94.81 **Bone marrow transplant status**

Z94.82 **Intestine transplant status**

Z94.83 **Pancreas transplant status**

Z94.84 **Stem cells transplant status**

Z94.89 **Other transplanted organ and tissue status**

Z94.9 **Transplanted organ and tissue status, unspecified**

●Z95 **Presence of cardiac and vascular implants and grafts**
Excludes1 complications of cardiac and vascular devices, implants and grafts (T82.-)

Z95.0 **Presence of cardiac pacemaker**
Presence of cardiac resynchronization therapy (CRT-P) pacemaker ◀
Excludes1 adjustment or management of cardiac device (Z45.0-) ◀
adjustment or management of cardiac pacemaker (Z45.0)
presence of automatic (implantable) cardiac defibrillator with synchronous cardiac pacemaker (Z95.810)

Z95.1 **Presence of aortocoronary bypass graft**
Presence of coronary artery bypass graft ◀

Z95.2 **Presence of prosthetic heart valve**
Presence of heart valve NOS

Z95.3 **Presence of xenogenic heart valve**

Z95.4 **Presence of other heart-valve replacement**

Z95.5 **Presence of coronary angioplasty implant and graft**
Excludes1 coronary angioplasty status without implant and graft (Z98.61)

●Z95.8 **Presence of other cardiac and vascular implants and grafts**

●Z95.81 **Presence of other cardiac implants and grafts**

Z95.810 **Presence of automatic (implantable) cardiac defibrillator**
Presence of automatic (implantable) cardiac defibrillator with synchronous cardiac pacemaker
Presence of cardiac resynchronization therapy defibrillator (CRT-D) ◀
Presence of cardioverter-defibrillator (ICD) ◀

Z95.811 **Presence of heart assist device**

Z95.812 **Presence of fully implantable artificial heart**

Z95.818 **Presence of other cardiac implants and grafts**

●Z95.82 **Presence of other vascular implants and grafts**

Z95.820 **Peripheral vascular angioplasty status with implants and grafts**
Excludes1 peripheral vascular angioplasty without implant and graft (Z98.62)

Z95.828 **Presence of other vascular implants and grafts**
Presence of intravascular prosthesis NEC

Z95.9 **Presence of cardiac and vascular implant and graft, unspecified**

●Z96 **Presence of other functional implants**
Excludes2 complications of internal prosthetic devices, implants and grafts (T82-T85)
fitting and adjustment of prosthetic and other devices (Z44-Z46)

Z96.0 **Presence of urogenital implants**

Z96.1 **Presence of intraocular lens**
Presence of pseudophakia

CHAPTER 21 (Z00-Z99)

● Z96.2 **Presence of otological and audiological implants**
- Z96.20 **Presence of otological and audiological implant, unspecified**
- Z96.21 **Cochlear implant status**
- Z96.22 **Myringotomy tube(s) status**
- Z96.29 **Presence of other otological and audiological implants**
  - Presence of bone-conduction hearing device
  - Presence of eustachian tube stent
  - Stapes replacement

Z96.3 **Presence of artificial larynx**

● Z96.4 **Presence of endocrine implants**
- Z96.41 **Presence of insulin pump (external) (internal)**
- Z96.49 **Presence of other endocrine implants**

Z96.5 **Presence of tooth-root and mandibular implants**

● Z96.6 **Presence of orthopedic joint implants**
- Z96.60 **Presence of unspecified orthopedic joint implant**
- ● Z96.61 **Presence of artificial shoulder joint**
  - Z96.611 **Presence of right artificial shoulder joint**
  - Z96.612 **Presence of left artificial shoulder joint**
  - Z96.619 **Presence of unspecified artificial shoulder joint**
- ● Z96.62 **Presence of artificial elbow joint**
  - Z96.621 **Presence of right artificial elbow joint**
  - Z96.622 **Presence of left artificial elbow joint**
  - Z96.629 **Presence of unspecified artificial elbow joint**
- ● Z96.63 **Presence of artificial wrist joint**
  - Z96.631 **Presence of right artificial wrist joint**
  - Z96.632 **Presence of left artificial wrist joint**
  - Z96.639 **Presence of unspecified artificial wrist joint**
- ● Z96.64 **Presence of artificial hip joint**
  - Hip-joint replacement (partial) (total)
  - Z96.641 **Presence of right artificial hip joint**
  - Z96.642 **Presence of left artificial hip joint**
  - Z96.643 **Presence of artificial hip joint, bilateral**
  - Z96.649 **Presence of unspecified artificial hip joint**
- ● Z96.65 **Presence of artificial knee joint**
  - Z96.651 **Presence of right artificial knee joint**
  - Z96.652 **Presence of left artificial knee joint**
  - Z96.653 **Presence of artificial knee joint, bilateral**
  - Z96.659 **Presence of unspecified artificial knee joint**
- ● Z96.66 **Presence of artificial ankle joint**
  - Z96.661 **Presence of right artificial ankle joint**
  - Z96.662 **Presence of left artificial ankle joint**
  - Z96.669 **Presence of unspecified artificial ankle joint**
- ● Z96.69 **Presence of other orthopedic joint implants**
  - Z96.691 **Finger-joint replacement of right hand**
  - Z96.692 **Finger-joint replacement of left hand**
  - Z96.693 **Finger-joint replacement, bilateral**
  - Z96.698 **Presence of other orthopedic joint implants**

Z96.7 **Presence of other bone and tendon implants**
- Presence of skull plate

● Z96.8 **Presence of other specified functional implants**
- Z96.81 **Presence of artificial skin**
- Z96.89 **Presence of other specified functional implants**

Z96.9 **Presence of functional implant, unspecified**

● Z97 **Presence of other devices**

Excludes1 complications of internal prosthetic devices, implants and grafts (T82-T85)
fitting and adjustment of prosthetic and other devices (Z44-Z46)

Excludes2 presence of cerebrospinal fluid drainage device (Z98.2)

Z97.0 **Presence of artificial eye**

● Z97.1 **Presence of artificial limb (complete) (partial)**
- Z97.10 **Presence of artificial limb (complete) (partial), unspecified**
- Z97.11 **Presence of artificial right arm (complete) (partial)**
- Z97.12 **Presence of artificial left arm (complete) (partial)**
- Z97.13 **Presence of artificial right leg (complete) (partial)**
- Z97.14 **Presence of artificial left leg (complete) (partial)**
- Z97.15 **Presence of artificial arms, bilateral (complete) (partial)**
- Z97.16 **Presence of artificial legs, bilateral (complete) (partial)**

Z97.2 **Presence of dental prosthetic device (complete) (partial)**
- Presence of dentures (complete) (partial)

Z97.3 **Presence of spectacles and contact lenses**

Z97.4 **Presence of external hearing-aid**

Z97.5 **Presence of (intrauterine) contraceptive device**

Excludes1 checking, reinsertion or removal of implantable subdermal contraceptive (Z30.46) ◀▮
checking, reinsertion or removal of intrauterine contraceptive device (Z30.43-) ◀

Z97.8 **Presence of other specified devices**

● **Z98 Other postprocedural states**
Excludes2 aftercare (Z43-Z49, Z51)
follow-up medical care (Z08-Z09)
postprocedural complication - see Alphabetical Index

Z98.0 Intestinal bypass and anastomosis status
Excludes2 bariatric surgery status (Z98.84)
gastric bypass status (Z98.84)
obesity surgery status (Z98.84)

Z98.1 Arthrodesis status

Z98.2 Presence of cerebrospinal fluid drainage device
Presence of CSF shunt

Z98.3 Post therapeutic collapse of lung status
Code first underlying disease

● **Z98.4 Cataract extraction status**
Use additional code to identify intraocular lens implant status (Z96.1)
Excludes1 aphakia (H27.0)

Z98.41 Cataract extraction status, right eye

Z98.42 Cataract extraction status, left eye

Z98.49 Cataract extraction status, unspecified eye

● **Z98.5 Sterilization status**
Excludes1 female infertility (N97.-)
male infertility (N46.-)

Z98.51 Tubal ligation status

Z98.52 Vasectomy status

● **Z98.6 Angioplasty status**

Z98.61 Coronary angioplasty status
Excludes1 coronary angioplasty status with implant and graft (Z95.5)

Z98.62 Peripheral vascular angioplasty status
Excludes1 peripheral vascular angioplasty status with implant and graft (Z95.820)

● **Z98.8 Other specified postprocedural states**

● **Z98.81 Dental procedure status**

Z98.810 Dental sealant status

Z98.811 Dental restoration status
Dental crown status
Dental fillings status

Z98.818 Other dental procedure status

Z98.82 Breast implant status
Excludes1 breast implant removal status (Z98.86)

Z98.83 Filtering (vitreous) bleb after glaucoma surgery status
Excludes1 inflammation (infection) of postprocedural bleb (H59.4-)

Z98.84 Bariatric surgery status
Gastric banding status
Gastric bypass status for obesity
Obesity surgery status
Excludes1 bariatric surgery status complicating pregnancy, childbirth, or the puerperium (O99.84)
Excludes2 intestinal bypass and anastomosis status (Z98.0)

Z98.85 Transplanted organ removal status
Transplanted organ previously removed due to complication, failure, rejection or infection
Excludes1 encounter for removal of transplanted organ -code to complication of transplanted organ (T86.-)

Z98.86 Personal history of breast implant removal

● **Z98.87 Personal history of in utero procedure**

Z98.870 Personal history of in utero procedure during pregnancy
Excludes2 complications from in utero procedure for current pregnancy (O35.7)
supervision of current pregnancy with history of in utero procedure during previous pregnancy (O09.82-)

Z98.871 Personal history of in utero procedure while a fetus

● **Z98.89 Other specified postprocedural states**

Z98.890 Other specified postprocedural states ◀
Personal history of surgery, not elsewhere classified ◀

Z98.891 History of uterine scar from previous surgery ◀
Excludes1 Maternal care due to uterine scar from previous surgery (O34.2-) ◀

● **Z99 Dependence on enabling machines and devices, not elsewhere classified**
Excludes1 cardiac pacemaker status (Z95.0)

Z99.0 Dependence on aspirator

● **Z99.1 Dependence on respirator**
Dependence on ventilator

Z99.11 Dependence on respirator [ventilator] status

Z99.12 Encounter for respirator [ventilator] dependence during power failure
Excludes1 mechanical complication of respirator [ventilator] (J95.850)

Z99.2 Dependence on renal dialysis
Hemodialysis status
Peritoneal dialysis status
Presence of arteriovenous shunt for dialysis
Renal dialysis status NOS
Excludes1 encounter for fitting and adjustment of dialysis catheter (Z49.0-)
Excludes2 noncompliance with renal dialysis (Z91.15) ◀

Z99.3 Dependence on wheelchair
Wheelchair confinement status
Code first cause of dependence, such as:
muscular dystrophy (G71.0)
obesity (E66.-)

● **Z99.8 Dependence on other enabling machines and devices**

Z99.81 Dependence on supplemental oxygen
Dependence on long-term oxygen

Z99.89 Dependence on other enabling machines and devices
Dependence on machine or device NOS

CHAPTER 21 (Z00-Z99)

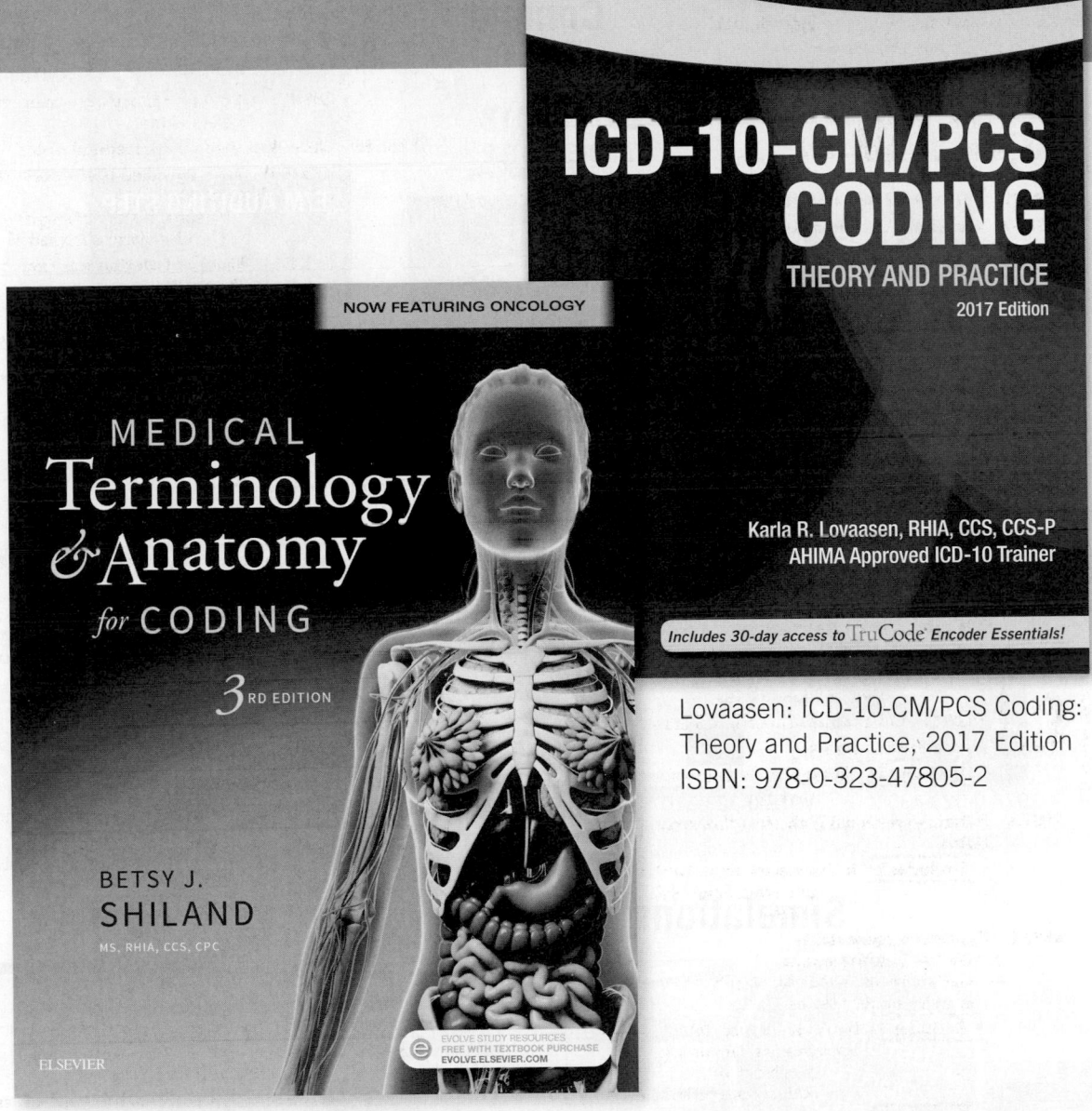

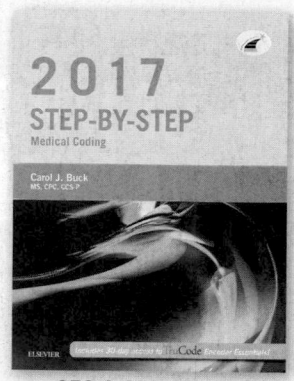

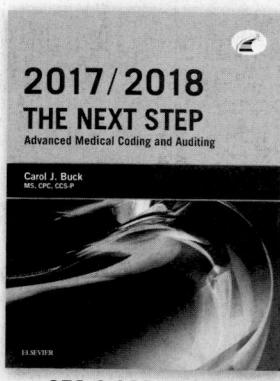

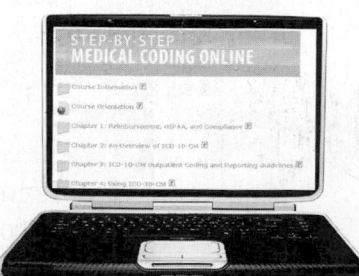